ATLAS OF ORAL AND MAXILLOFACIAL SURGERY

EDITION 2 VOLUME ONE

ATLAS OF ORAL AND MAXILLOFACIAL SURGERY

PAUL S. TIWANA, DDS, MD, MS, FACS, FACD
Francis J. Reichmann Professor and Chair
Division of Oral & Maxillofacial Surgery
College of Dentistry;
Professor
Department of Surgery
College of Medicine
The University of Oklahoma Health Sciences Center
Oklahoma City, Oklahoma
United States

DEEPAK KADEMANI, DMD, MD, FACS
President and Medical Director
Minnesota Oral & Facial Surgery
Fellowship Director
Oral/Head & Neck Oncologic and Reconstructive Surgery
Minneapolis, Minnesota
United States

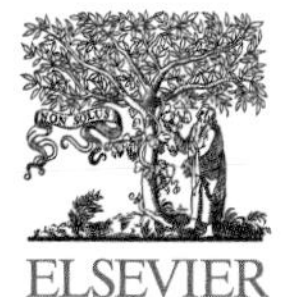
ELSEVIER

Elsevier
1600 John F. Kennedy Blvd.
Ste 1800
Philadelphia, PA 19103-2899

ATLAS OF ORAL AND MAXILLOFACIAL SURGERY, SECOND EDITION ISBN: 978-0-323-78963-9

Previous edition copyrighted 2016.

Senior Content Strategist: Lauren Boyle
Content Development Specialist: Deborah Poulson
Publishing Services Manager: Shereen Jameel
Senior Project Manager: Manikandan Chandrasekaran
Book Designer: Brian Salisbury

Printed in India

Last digit is the print number: 9 8 7 6 5 4 3 2 1

This book is dedicated to the following individuals:

To my family for all your love and support.

To my patients who have given me the privilege to care for them.

To students of our specialty in their quest for knowledge.

Deepak Kademani

This book is dedicated to the following individuals:

To my family; especially my wife Karen, and my daughters Jespreet (17), and Simran (15).

To my former residents and fellows.

Paul S. Tiwana

Section Editors

Richard Allen Finn, DDS
Professor
Oral and Maxillofacial Surgery Division
UT Southwestern Medical Center;
Chief
Oral and Maxillofacial Surgery
Veteran's Administration North Texas
Dallas, Texas
United States

Part I: Surgical Anatomy of the Head and Neck

Deepak G. Krishnan, DDS, FACS
Associate Professor—Surgery
Division of Oral Maxillofacial Surgery,
Department of Surgery
University of Cincinnati;
Oral Maxillofacial Surgeon
Cincinnati Children's Hospital and Medical Center
Cincinnati, Ohio
United States

Part II: Oral Surgery

Martin B. Steed, DDS, FACS
Professor and James B. Edwards Chair
Department of Oral and Maxillofacial Surgery
Medical University of South Carolina
James B. Edwards College of Dental Medicine
Charleston, South Carolina
United States

Part III: Implant Surgery

Steven M. Sullivan, DDS, FACS, FACD
Professor and Chair
Department of Surgical Sciences/Oral and Maxillofacial Surgery
University of Oklahoma College of Dentistry
Oklahoma City, Oklahoma
United States

Part IV: Orthognathic Surgery

Paul S. Tiwana, DDS, MD, MS, FACS, FACD
Francis J. Reichmann Professor and Chair
Division of Oral & Maxillofacial Surgery
College of Dentistry;
Professor
Department of Surgery
College of Medicine
The University of Oklahoma Health Sciences Center
Oklahoma City, Oklahoma
United States

Part V: Craniofacial Surgery

Ghali E. Ghali, DDS, MD, FACS, FRCS(Ed)
Director
Oral and Maxillofacial Surgery
Willis Knighton Health System
Shreveport, Louisiana
United States

Part VI: Cleft Lip and Palate

Alan S. Herford, DDS, MD
Chairman and Professor
Oral and Maxillofacial Surgery
Loma Linda University
Loma Linda, California
United States

Part VII: Craniomaxillofacial Trauma

Eric R. Carlson, DMD, MD, EdM, FACS
Professor and Kelly L. Krahwinkel Chairman
Department of Oral and Maxillofacial Surgery
University of Tennessee Graduate School of Medicine;
Director
Oral/Head and Neck Oncologic Surgery Fellowship
University of Tennessee Cancer Institute
Knoxville, Tennessee
United States

Part VIII: Benign Pathology

Deepak Kademani, DMD, MD, FACS
President and Medical Director
Minnesota Oral & Facial Surgery
Fellowship Director
Oral/Head & Neck Oncologic and Reconstructive Surgery
Minneapolis, Minnesota
United States

Part IX: Malignant Pathology

Brent B. Ward, DDS, MD, FACS, FACD
Professor, Chair and Fellowship Program Director
Oral and Maxillofacial Surgery
University of Michigan
Ann Arbor, Michigan
United States

Part X: Reconstructive Surgery

Gary F. Bouloux, MD, DDS, MDSc, FRACDS, FRACDS(OMS), FRCS (Eng), FACS
J. David Allen Family Professor
Division Chief
Oral and Maxillofacial Surgery
Department of Surgery
Emory University School of Medicine
Atlanta, Georgia
United States

Part XI: TMJ Surgery

Faisal A. Quereshy, MD, DDS, FACS
Professor/Program Director
Oral & Maxillofacial Surgery
Case Western Reserve University, Cleveland
Ohio
United States;
Medical Director
Facial Cosmetic Surgery
Visage Surgical Institute/V-Spa
Medina, Ohio
United States

Part XII: Facial Cosmetic Surgery

Joseph E. Cillo Jr., DMD, MPH, PhD, FACS
Division Chief and Program Director
Oral and Maxillofacial Surgery
Allegheny General Hospital;
Associate Professor
Oral and Maxillofacial Surgery
Allegheny General Hospital
Pittsburgh, Pennsylvania
United States

Part XIII: Obstructive Sleep Apnea

Contributors

A. Omar Abubaker, DMD, PhD
Professor and Chairman
Oral and Maxillofacial Surgery
VCU Medical Center
Richmond, Virginia
United States

Julio Acero, MD, DMD, PhD, FDSRCS, FEBOMFS
Full Professor Surgery
Alcala University;
Department Head
Oral and Maxillofacial Surgery
Ramon y Cajal University Hospital
Madrid, Spain

Ravi Agarwal, DDS
Program Director
Oral & Maxillofacial Surgery
Medstar Washington Hospital Center, Washington
District of Columbia
United States;
Chairman
Oral & Maxillofacial Surgery
Medstar Washington Hospital Center
Washington, District of Columbia
United States

Tara Aghaloo, DDS, MD, PhD
Professor
Oral and Maxillofacial Surgery
UCLA School of Dentistry
Los Angeles, California
United States

Maryam Akbari, DMD, MD, MPH
Oral and Maxillofacial Surgery
Mount Sinai
New York, New York
United States

Kyle P. Allen, MD, MPH
Tampa Bay Hearing and Balance Center;
Assistant Clinical Professor
Otolaryngology—Head and Neck Surgery
University of South Florida
Tampa, Florida
United States

Dror M. Allon, DMD
Director
Orthognathic and TMJ Surgery Unit;
Senior Lecturer
Oral and Maxillofacial Surgery
Tel Aviv University
Tel Aviv, Israel

Fernando Almeida, MD, PhD, DDS, FEBOMFS
Clinical Professor
Department of Surgery
Alcalá University (UAH);
Oral & Maxillofacial Surgeon
Department of Oral and Maxillofacial Surgery
University Hospital Ramón y Cajal
Madrid, Spain

Brian Alpert, DDS, FACS (Deceased)
Professor of Oral and Maxillofacial Surgery
University of Louisville School of Dentistry
Louisville, Kentucky
United States

Mehmet Ali Altay, DDS, PhD
Associate Professor
Oral and Maxillofacial Surgery
Akdeniz University, School of Dentistry
Antalya, Turkey

Felix Jose Amarista, DDS
Assistant Professor
Department of Oral and Maxillofacial Surgery
UT Health San Antonio
San Antonio, Texas
United States

Hatem Amer, MD
Associate Professor of Medicine
Division of Nephrology and Hypertension and
The William J von Liebig Center for Transplantation and
Clinical Regeneration
Mayo Clinic
Rochester, Minnesota
United States

Suganya Appugounder DMD, MS, FACS, MAJ, USAR, DC
Cleft and Craniofacial Surgery
Charleston Area Medical Center
Charleston, West Virginia
United States

Shyam Prasad Aravindaksha, BDS, MDS
Private Practice
Oral Maxillofacial Surgery
Greater Michigan Oral Surgeons
Flint, Michigan
United States

Sharon Aronovich, DMD
Clinical Associate Professor
Oral and Maxillofacial Surgery
University of Michigan
Ann Arbor, Michigan
United States

Leon Assael, BA, DMD, CMM
Professor Emeritus
Oral and Maxillofacial Surgery
Oregon Health & Science University
Portland, Oregon;
Affiliate Associate Professor
Public Health
University of California San Francisco
San Francisco, California
United States

Michael Awadallah, DDS, MD
Assistant Professor of Surgery
Weill Cornell Medicine
New York, New York
United States

Shahid R. Aziz, DMD, MD, FACS, FRCS (Ed)
Division Director
Oral & Maxillofacial Surgery
Hackensack University Medical Center;
Clinical Professor
Oral and Maxillofacial Surgery
Rutgers School of Dental Medicine
Newark, New Jersey;
Clinical Professor
Otolaryngology
Hackensack Meridian School of Medicine
Nutley, New Jersey
United States;
Visiting Professor
Oral and Maxillofacial Surgery
Update Dental College
Dhaka, Bangladesh

Shahrokh C. Bagheri, DMD, MD, FACS
Oral and Maxillofacial Surgeon
Georgia Oral and Facial Surgery
Atlanta, Georgia
United States

Jonathan Bailey, DMD, MD, FACS
Clinical Professor
Department of Surgery
Carle Illinois College of Medicine;
Associate Medical Director of Specialty Surgery
Division of Oral and Maxillofacial Surgery and Division of Head and Neck Cancer
Carle Foundation Hospital
Urbana, Illinois
United States

Andrew M. Baker, MD, DDS
Oral and Maxillofacial Surgery
Providence Cancer Institute
Portland, Oregon
United States

Karim Bakri, MBBS
Consultant
Division of Plastic Surgery
Mayo Clinic
Rochester, Minnesota
United States

Suzanne Barnes, DMD
Assistant Professor
Oral and Maxillofacial Surgery
University of Louisville
Louisville, Kentucky
United States

Brian Bast, DMD, MD
Professor and Chair
Oral and Maxillofacial Surgery
University of California, School of Dentistry
San Francisco, California
United States

Hussam Batal, DMD
Clinical Professor
Oral and Maxillofacial Surgery
Boston University Henry M. Goldman School of Dental Medicine
Boston, Massachusetts
United States

Dale A. Baur, DDS, MD
Professor and Chair, Vice Dean
Oral and Maxillofacial Surgery
Case Western Reserve University School of Dental Medicine;
Division Chief,
Oral and Maxillofacial Surgery
University Hospitals/Cleveland Medical Center
Cleveland, Ohio
United States

Edmond Bedrossian, DDS, FACD, FACOMS, FAO, FITI
Professor
Oral and Maxillofacial Surgery
University of the Pacific
San Francisco, California
United States

Edmond Armand Bedrossian, DDS
Private Practice
San Francisco, California
United States

R. Bryan Bell, MD, DDS, FACS, FRCS (Ed)
Physician Executive and Director
Division of Surgical Oncology, Radiation Oncology and Clinical Programs
Providence Cancer Institute;
Medical Director
Providence Head and Neck Cancer Program
Providence Cancer Institute;
Associate Member
Earle A. Chiles Research Institute
Providence Cancer Institute
Portland, Oregon
United States

David A. Bitonti, DMD
Clinical Associate Professor
Department of Surgery
F. Edward Hébert School of Medicine, Uniformed Services University of the Health Sciences
Bethesda, Maryland;
Dental Service Chief
Oral and Maxillofacial Surgeon
Hampton Veterans Affairs Medical Center
Hampton, Virginia
United States

Behnam Bohluli, DMD, FRCD(C)
Clinical Instructor
Oral and Maxillofacial Surgery
University of Toronto
Toronto, Ontario
Canada

Genevieve C. Bonin, BSc, MASc, DMD, FRCD(c), Dipl. ABOMS
Oral and Maxillofacial surgeon
Department of Oral and Maxillofacial Surgery
Verdun Hospital, University of Montreal
Montreal, Quebec
Canada

Gary F. Bouloux, MD, DDS, MDSc, FRACDS, FRACDS(OMS), FRCS (Eng), FACS
J. David Allen Family Professor
Division Chief
Oral and Maxillofacial Surgery
Department of Surgery
Emory University School of Medicine
Atlanta, Georgia
United States

Meaghan Bradley, DMD
Oral and Maxillofacial Surgery
Boston University
Boston, Massachusetts
United States

Omar Breik, BDSc (Hons) MBBS, MClinSc, FRACDS (OMS)
Consultant Maxillofacial/Head and Neck Surgeon
Department of Oral and Maxillofacial Surgery
Royal Brisbane and Women's Hospital;
Senior Lecturer
School of Dentistry/School of Medicine
University of Queensland
Brisbane, Queensland
Australia

Hans C. Brockhoff II, DDS, MD, FACS
Chief, Oral/Head and Neck Oncology and Microvascular Reconstructive Surgery
Oral and Maxillofacial Surgery
El Paso Children's Hospital, University Medical Center of El Paso;
Assistant Professor
Department of Surgery
Texas Tech University Health Sciences Center;
Program Director
El Paso Head & Neck and Microvascular Surgery Fellowship;
High Desert Oral & Facial Surgery
El Paso, Texas
United States

Daniel Buchbinder, DMD, MD
Professor and System Chief, Division of Maxillofacial Surgery
Department of Otolaryngology, Head and Neck Surgery
Icahn School of Medicine at Mount Sinai
New York, New York
United States

Tuan G. Bui, MD, DMD
Affiliate Assistant Professor
Oral and Maxillofacial Surgery
Oregon Health and Sciences University;
Head and Neck Surgical Associates
Portland, Oregon
United States

Patrick Byrne, MD, MBA
Chairman
The Head and Neck Institute
Cleveland Clinic
Cleveland, Ohio
United States

John Francis Caccamese Jr., MD, DMD, FACS
Professor and Vice Chairman
Oral-Maxillofacial Surgery
University of Maryland Dental School;
Clinical Professor
Pediatrics and Otorhinolaryngology
University of Maryland School of Medicine;
Co-Director
Randolph B. Capone Cleft Program at GBMC;
Adjunct Professor
Bioengineering
University of Maryland;
Baltimore, Maryland
United States

Ron Caloss, DDS, MD
Private Practice
Aligned Oral and Facial Surgery
Baptist Medical Center;
Professor
Oral and Maxillofacial Surgery
University of Mississippi Medical Center
Jackson, Mississippi
United States

Courtney Caplin, MD, DMD
Cosmetic Surgery Affiliates;
Clinical Assistant Professor
Oral and Maxillofacial Surgery
University of Oklahoma
Oklahoma City, Oklahoma
United States

Eric R. Carlson, DMD, MD, EdM, FACS
Professor and Kelly L. Krahwinkel Chairman
Department of Oral and Maxillofacial Surgery
University of Tennessee Graduate School of Medicine;
Director
Oral/Head and Neck Oncologic Surgery Fellowship
University of Tennessee Cancer Institute
Knoxville, Tennessee
United States

Nardy Casap, DMD, MD
Professor
Oral and Maxillofacial Surgery
Hebrew University-Hadassah Medical Center
Jerusalem, Israel

Carrie E. Cera Hill, MD, MBA
Pure Dermatology PLLC
Denver, Colorado
United States

Swagnik Chakrabarti, MBBS, MS, MCh
Chairperson
Chandan Cancer Institute
Lucknow, Uttar Pradesh
India

Ravi Chandran, DMD, PhD, FACS
Chairman and Residency Director
Oral and Maxillofacial Surgery/Pathology
University of Mississippi Medical Center
Jackson, Mississippi
United States

Blake Chaney, DDS, MD
Oral and Maxillofacial Surgery
University of Pittsburgh
Pittsburgh, Pennsylvania
United States

Allen C. Cheng, MD, DDS, FACS
Medical Director
Head and Neck Surgical Associates
Head and Neck Surgery;
Attending Surgeon
Providence Oral, Head and Neck
Providence Health;
Assistant Professor
Oral and Maxillofacial Surgery
Oregon Health Sciences University;
Medical Director
Oral/Head and Neck Oncology
Legacy Good Samaritan
Portland, Oregon
United States

Radhika Chigurupati, DMD, MS
Associate Professor
Oral and Maxillofacial Surgery
Boston University
Boston, Massachusetts
United States

Nam Cho, DDS, MD
Assistant Clinical Professor
Oral & Maxillofacial Surgery
Ostrow School of Dentistry
Los Angeles, California
United States

Joli Chou, DMD, MD
Associate Professor
Department of Oral and Maxillofacial Surgery
Sidney Kimmel Medical College
Thomas Jefferson University
Philadelphia, Pennsylvania
United States

Louis J. Christensen, DDS
Oral & Maxillofacial Surgery
HealthPartners;
Department of Oral & Maxillofacial Surgery
Regions Hospital
Saint Paul, Minnesota;
Assistant Clinical Professor
Division of Oral & Maxillofacial Surgery
University of Minnesota School of Dentistry
Minneapolis, Minnesota
United States

Joseph E. Cillo Jr., DMD, MPH, PhD, FACS
Division Chief and Program Director
Oral and Maxillofacial Surgery
Allegheny General Hospital;
Associate Professor
Oral and Maxillofacial Surgery
Allegheny General Hospital
Pittsburgh, Pennsylvania
United States

Scott T. Claiborne, DDS, MD
Minnesota Oral and Facial Surgery
Co-Fellowship Director
Oral/Head and Neck Oncologic and Reconstructive Surgery
Minneapolis, Minnesota
United States

David Collette, DMD, MD
Medical Director
The Oral Surgery Center Of Albuquerque
Albuquerque, New Mexico
United States

Gisela Contasti-Bocco, DDS
Assistant Professor
Orthodontics Department
Nova Southern University
Fort Lauderdale, Florida
United States

Bernard J. Costello, DMD, MD, FACS
Associate Dean for Faculty Affairs
Professor and Fellowship Program Director
Department of Oral and Maxillofacial Surgery
University of Pittsburgh, School of Dental Medicine;
Chief
Pediatric Oral and Maxillofacial Surgery Children's Hospital of Pittsburgh;
Professor and Fellowship Program Director
Department of Oral and Maxillofacial Surgery
University of Pittsburgh Medical Center Eye and Ear Institute UPMC
Pittsburgh, Pennsylvania
United States

Sebastian Cotofana, MD, PhD
Associate Professor of Anatomy
Department of Clinical Anatomy
Mayo Clinic
Rochester, Minnesota
United States

Marcus A. Couey, DDS, MD
Assistant Professor
Department of Oral and Maxillofacial Surgery
Boston University
Boston, Massachusetts
United States

Larry Cunningham Jr., MD, DDS
Professor and Chair
Oral and Maxillofacial Surgery
University of Pittsburgh School of Dental Medicine
Pittsburgh, Pennsylvania
United States

William J. Curtis, DMD, MD
Oral and Maxillofacial Surgery
Northern Nevada Oral & Maxillofacial Surgery
Reno, Nevada
United States

Angelo L. Cuzalina, MD, DDS
Cosmetic Surgery
Private Practice
Tulsa Surgical Arts;
Adjunctive Faculty
OSU Medical School
Otolaryngology Department
Tulsa, Oklahoma
United States

Rushil R. Dang, BDS, DMD
Maxillofacial Oncology and Reconstructive Surgery Fellow
Oral and Maxillofacial Surgery
Boston Medical Center and Boston University
Boston, Massachusetts
United States

Renie Daniel, MD, DMD, FACS
Assistant Professor
Department of Oral & Maxillofacial Surgery
The University of North Carolina
Chapel Hill, North Carolina
United States

David J. Dattilo, DDS
Director of Oral and Maxillofacial Surgery (Retired)
Allegheny Health System
Allegheny General
Hospital
Pittsburgh, Pennsylvania
United States;
Associate Professor of Surgery
Drexel University School of Medicine
Philadelphia, Pennsylvania
United States

Jeffrey S. Dean, DDS, MD, FACS
Oral and Maxillofacial Surgery
Dakota Dunes, South Dakota
United States

Shaun C. Desai, MD
Associate Professor
Facial Plastic and Reconstructive Surgery
Johns Hopkins University School of Medicine
Baltimore, Maryland
United States

Jasjit K. Dillon, MBBS, DDS, FDSRCS, FACS
Professor, Chief & Program Director
Oral & Maxillofacial Surgery
University of Washington
Seattle, Washington
United States

Jean-Charles Doucet, DMD, MD, MSc, FRCDC
Assistant Professor and Division Head of Oral and Maxillofacial Surgery
Oral and Maxillofacial Sciences
Dalhousie University;
Staff Surgeon
IWK Cleft Palate and Craniofacial Team
IWK Health Centre;
Staff Surgeon
Oral and Maxillofacial Surgery
QEII Health Science Centre
Halifax, Nova Scotia
Canada

Stephanie Joy Drew, DMD
Associate Professor
Emory School of Medicine
Atlanta, Georgia
United States

Donita Dyalram, DDS, MD, FACS
Associate Professor; Program Director/Associate Fellowship Director
Oral and Maxillofacial Surgery
University of Maryland Medical Center
Baltimore, Maryland
United States

Sean P. Edwards, DDS, MD
Clinical Associate Professor;
Director, Residency Program;
Chief, Pediatric Oral, and Maxillofacial Surgery
Oral and Maxillofacial Surgery/Hospital Dentistry
University of Michigan Health System
Ann Arbor, Michigan
United States

Hany Emam, BDS, MS, FACS
Associate Professor and Interim Chair
Oral and Maxillofacial Surgery
The Ohio State University College of Dentistry
Columbus, Ohio
United States

Max R. Emmerling, MD, DDS
Division of Oral and Maxillofacial Surgery
Cook County Health
Chicago, Illinois
United States

Mark Engelstad, DDS, MD, MHI
Associate Professor
Oral & Maxillofacial Surgery
Oregon Health & Science University
Portland, Oregon
United States

Helaman Erickson, DDS, MD, FACS
Oral and Maxillofacial Surgery
Permian Basin Oral Surgery and Dental Implant Center
Midland, Texas
United States

Maria Evasovich, MD
Associate Professor
Department of Surgery
University of Minnesota
Minneapolis, Minnesota
United States

Adam P. Fagin, DMD, MD
Private Practice
Peninsula Oral and Facial Surgery
San Mateo, California
United States

Christopher A. Fanelli, DDS, FRCD(C)
Private Practice
Interface—Centre for OMFS
London, Ontario
Canada;
Attending Surgeon—Consultant
Surgery—Oral Maxillofacial Surgery
London Health Sciences Centre, St Thomas Elgin General Hospital
St. Thomas, Ontario
Canada

Joseph J. Fantuzzo, MD, DDS, FACS
Clinical Associate Professor
Oral & Maxillofacial Surgery
University of Rochester Medical Center
Rochester, New York
United States

Tirbod Fattahi, DDS, MD, FACS
Professor and Chair
Department of Oral and Maxillofacial Surgery
University of Florida, College of Medicine
Jacksonville, Florida
United States

Rui P. Fernandes, MD, DMD, FACS, FRCS (Ed)
Professor
OMS, Neurosurgery, Orthopedic, Surgery
University of Florida College of Medicine
Jacksonville, Florida
United States

Richard Allen Finn, DDS
Professor
Surgery—Div OMFS
UTSWMC;
Chief
OMFS
Veteran's Administration North Texas
Dallas, Texas
United States

Peter B. Franco, DMD, FACS
Carolinas Center for Oral and Facial Surgery
Charlotte, North Carolina
United States

David Gailey, DDS, FACS
Surgical Cleft Director
Pediatric Surgery
Providence Children's Hospital;
President
Inland Oral Surgery
Spokane, Washington
United States

Pooja Gangwani, DDS, MPH
Assistant Professor
Oral and Maxillofacial Surgery
University of Rochester Medical Center
Rochester, New York
United States

Ghali E. Ghali, DDS, MD, FACS, FRCS(Ed)
Director
Oral and Maxillofacial Surgery
Willis Knighton Health System
Shreveport, Louisiana
United States

Waleed Gibreel, MBBS
Assistant Professor
Craniofacial Surgery
Division of Plastic Surgery
Mayo Clinic
Rochester, Minnesota
United States

Sabine C. Girod, MD, DDS, PhD, FACS
Professor Emeritus
Department of Surgery
School of Medicine, Stanford University
Stanford, California
United States

Brent Golden, DDS, MD, FACS
Fellowship Program Director
Pediatric Craniomaxillofacial Surgery
Orlando Health Arnold Palmer Medical Center
Orlando, Florida
United States

Jorge Gonzalez, DDS
Private Practice
Advanced Dental Implant Solutions
Fort Worth, Texas
United States

Marianela Gonzalez, DDS, MS
Clinical Associate Professor and Director
Oral and Maxillofacial Surgery
Texas A&M Health Science Center, College of Dentistry
Baylor University Dallas, Texas
United States

Eric J. Granquist, DMD, MD
Assistant Professor
Oral and Maxillofacial Surgery
University of Pennsylvania;
Director
UPenn Center For Temporomandibular Joint Disorders
Hospital of the University of Pennsylvania
Philadelphia, Pennsylvania
United States

Jaime Grant, MBChB, BDS (Hons), MRCS (Ed), FRCS (Ed) (OMFS)
Consultant Craniofacial/Maxillofacial Surgeon
Craniofacial/Maxillofacial Surgery
Birmingham Children's Hospital/Queen Elizabeth University Hospital
Birmingham, United Kingdom

Mingyang Liu Gray, MD, MPH
Resident Physician
Otolaryngology—Head and Neck Surgery
Icahn School of Medicine at Mount Sinai
New York, New York
United States

Cesar A. Guerrero, DDS
Private Practice
ClearChoice Houston
The Heights Hospital
Houston, Texas
United States

Danny Hadaya, DDS, PhD
Resident
Oral and Maxillofacial Surgery
UCLA School of Dentistry
Los Angeles, California
United States

David Hamlar, MD, DDS
Assistant Professor
Otolaryngology/Head and Neck Surgery
University of Minnesota Medical Center
Minneapolis, Minnesota
United States

Daniel A. Hammer, DDS, FACD, FACS
Vice Chair and Director of Research
Department of Oral and Maxillofacial Surgery and Dentistry
Naval Medical Center San Diego
San Diego, California;
Associate Professor of Surgery
Department of Surgery
Uniformed Services University
Bethesda, Maryland;
Voluntary Clinical Assistant Professor of Surgery
Department of Otolaryngology
UC San Diego School of Medicine,
San Diego, California
United States

Curtis Hanba, MD
Otolaryngology—Head and Neck Surgery
The University of Minnesota
Minneapolis, Minnesota
United States

Andrew Alistair Heggie, AM, MBBS, MDSc, BDSc, FRACDS (OMS), FFDRSC(I), FRCS (Ed)
Clinical Professor, Oral and Maxillofacial Surgery
Department of Plastic and Maxillofacial Surgery
Royal Children's Hospital of Melbourne
Parkville, Victoria
Australia

Mariana Henriquez, DDS
Santa Rosa Maxillofacial Surgery Center
Central University of Venezuela
Caracas, Venezuela

Andrew Henry, DMD, MD
Assistant Professor
Associate Director of Residency Training
Department of Oral and Maxillofacial Surgery
Boston University Goldman School of Dental Medicine
Boston, Massachusetts
United States

Alan S. Herford, DDS, MD
Chairman and Professor
Oral and Maxillofacial Surgery
Loma Linda University
Loma Linda, California
United States

Brandyn Herman, DMD
Assistant Professor
Oral and Maxillofacial Surgery
University of Kentucky College of Dentistry
Lexington, Kentucky
United States

David Hinkl, DMD
Oral and Maxillofacial Surgery
University of Oklahoma
Oklahoma City, Oklahoma
United States

Anthony David Holmes, AO, MB.BS, FRACS
Diplomate, American Board of Plastic Surgery
Clinical Professor, University of Melbourne
Dept. of Plastic and Maxillofacial Surgery
Royal Children's Hospital
Melbourne, Victoria
Australia

James B. Holton, DDS, MSD
Staff
Oral and Maxillofacial Surgery
UT Health Tyler
Tyler, Texas
United States

Mehran Hossaini-Zadeh, DMD
Professor and Chair
Oral and Maxillofacial Surgery
Temple University School of Dentistry
Philadelphia, Pennsylvania
United States

Reem H. Hossameldin, BDS, MSc, PhD
Associate Professor
Oral and Maxillofacial Surgery
Faculty of Dentistry, Cairo University
Cairo, Egypt

Tsung-yen Hsieh, MD
Assistant Professor
Department of Otolaryngology—Head & Neck Surgery, Division of Facial Plastic & Reconstructive Surgery
University of Cincinnati College of Medicine
Cincinnati, Ohio
United States

Allen Huang, DDS, MD
Assistant Professor
Oral and Maxillofacial Surgery
University of Southern California
Los Angeles, California
United States

Pamela J. Hughes, DDS
Oral and Maxillofacial Surgery
Kaiser Permanente
Portland, Oregon
United States

Tanisha Hutchinson, MD
Facial Plastic Surgery
Glasgold Group
Princeton, New Jersey
United States

Matthew R. Idle, BDS (Hons), MFDS, MBChB, FRCS (OMFS)
Consultant
Oral and Maxillofacial/Head and Neck Surgery
University Hospitals Birmingham
Birmingham, United Kingdom

Shyam Sunder Indrakanti, DDS, MD
Private Practice
Department of Oral and Maxillofacial Surgery
Parkland Memorial Hospital
Dallas, Texas
United States

Michael Jaskolka, DDS, MD, FACS
Director, Maxillofacial Surgery
Director, Cleft and Craniofacial Program
Physician Executive, Novant Health, Children's Institute, Coastal Region
Novant Health, New Hanover Regional Medical Center
Wilmington, North Carolina
United States

Jonathan James Jelmini, DDS, MD
Department of Oral and Maxillofacial Surgery
Oregon Health & Sciences University;
Resident
Trauma and Oral and Maxillofacial Surgery Service
Legacy Emanuel Medical Center
Portland, Oregon
United States

Ole T. Jensen, DDS, MS
Adjunct Professor
Department of Oral and Maxillofacial Surgery
School of Dentistry, University of Utah
Salt Lake City, Utah
United States

Ashok R. Jethwa, MD
Head and Neck Surgical Oncology/Microvascular Reconstruction
Otolaryngology
University of Minnesota
Minneapolis, Minnesota
United States

Baxter Jones, DDS
Resident
Department of Oral and Maxillofacial Surgery
Carle Foundation Hospital
Urbana, Illinois
United States

Deepak Kademani, DMD, MD, FACS
President and Medical Director
Minnesota Oral & Facial Surgery
Fellowship Director
Oral/Head & Neck Oncologic and Reconstructive Surgery
Minneapolis, Minnesota
United States

David R. Kang, MD, DDS
Medical Director
Surgery, Head & Neck Surgery
Methodist Dallas Medical Center
Dallas, Texas
United States

Herman Kao, DDS, MD
Vice Chairman
Oral and Maxillofacial Surgery
John Peter Smith Health Network;
Associate Professor
Surgery
TCU and UNTHSC Medical School
Fort Worth, Texas
United States

Vasiliki Karlis, DMD, MD, FACS
Associate Professor
Director OMS Training Program
Department of Oral and Maxillofacial Surgery
College of Dentistry
New York University
Bellevue Hospital Center
New York, New York
United States

Beomjune Kim, DMD, MD, FACS
Head and Neck/Microvascular Surgeon
Cancer Treatment Centers of America – Part of City of Hope
Newnan, Georgia
United States

D. David Kim, DMD, MD, FACS
Jack W. Gamble Endowed Chairman
Oral and Maxillofacial/Head and Neck Surgery
Louisiana State University Health Sciences Center Shreveport;
Edward and Freda Green Endowed Professor
Oral and Maxillofacial/Head and Neck Surgery
LSU Health Science Center Shreveport;
Fellowship Director, Head and Neck Oncology and Microvascular Reconstruction
Oral and Maxillofacial Surgery
LSU Health Science Center Shreveport
Shreveport, Louisiana
United States

Roderick Y. Kim, DDS, MD, MBA, FACS
Director of Research, Co-Fellowship Director, Vice Division Director
Oral and Maxillofacial Surgery
John Peter Smith Health Network;
Assistant Professor
Surgery
Texas Christian University
Fort Worth, Texas
United States

Paul Kloostra, DDS, MD
Fellowship Director
Cleft & Craniofacial Surgery
Charleston Area Medical Center
Charleston, West Virginia
United States

Antonia Kolokythas, DDS, MSc, MSed, FACS
Professor and Chair
Department of Oral and Maxillofacial Surgery
Augusta Univerity
Dental College of Georgia
Augusta, Georgia
United States

David A. Koppel, MB, BS, BDS, FDS, FRCS
Associate Professor
Faculty of Medicine/Faculty of Dental Medicine & Oral Health Sciences
McGill University
Montreal, Quebec
Canada

Deepak G. Krishnan, DDS, FACS
Associate Professor—Surgery
Division of Oral Maxillofacial Surgery, Department of Surgery
University of Cincinnati;
Oral Maxillofacial Surgeon
Division of Oral Maxillofacial Surgery
Department of Surgery
Cincinnati Children's Hospital and Medical Center
Cincinnati, Ohio
United States

Moni A. Kuriakose, MD, FRCS
Professor and Director
Surgical Oncology Chief Head and Neck Oncology
Mazumdar Shaw Cancer Center;
Director
Mazumdar Shaw Centre for Translational Research
Narayana Health Center
Bangalore, Karnataka
India

Li Han Lai, DDS
Oral and Maxillofacial Surgery
University of Washington
Seattle, Washington
United States

Zvi Laster, DMD
Maxillofacial Surgery Department
Poriya Governmental Hospital
Tiberias, Israel

Amir Laviv, DMD, MPH
Senior Lecturer
Department of Oral & Maxillofacial Surgery
Tel-Aviv University
Tel Aviv, Israel

Andrew W. C. Lee, MSc, DDS, MD, FRCD(C), FACS
Argyle Associates Oral & Maxillofacial Surgery
Department of Surgery
The Ottawa Hospital;
Lecturer
Faculty of Medicine
University of Ottawa
Ottawa, Canada

James B. Lewallen, DDS, MD, MSc
Private Practice
Southern Oral and Facial Surgery
Franklin, Tennessee
United States;
Affiliate Staff
Oral and Maxillofacial Surgery
Vanderbilt University Medical Center
Nashville, Tennessee
United States

Stanley Yung-Chuan Liu, MD, DDS, FACS
Associate Professor of Otolaryngology
And by Courtesy, of Plastic & Reconstructive Surgery
Director, Sleep Surgery Fellowship
Service Chief, Maxillofacial Surgery
Stanford University School of Medicine
Stanford, California
United States

Christian A. Loetscher, DDS, MS
Private Practice
Oral & Maxillofacial Surgery
Atlanta Oral & Maxillofacial Surgery, PC
Alpharetta, Georgia
United States

Patrick J. Louis, DDS, MD
Professor
Oral & Maxillofacial Surgery
University of Alabama at Birmingham;
Chairman
Oral & Maxillofacial Surgery
University of Alabama at Birmingham
Birmingham, Alabama
United States

Joshua E. Lubek, MD, DDS, FACS
Professor & Fellowship Director
Oral-Head & Neck Surgery/Microvascular Surgery
Marlene & Stewart Greenebaum Comprehensive Cancer Center &
Department of Oral & Maxillofacial Surgery
University of Maryland
Baltimore, Maryland
United States

Ricardo Lugo, DDS, MD
Assistant Clinical Professor
Department of Oral & Maxillofacial Surgery
University of California, San Francisco & Alameda Health System
Oakland, California
United States

Sofia Lyford-Pike, MD
Associate Professor
Otolaryngology Head and Neck Surgery
University of Minnesota
Minneapolis, Minnesota
United States

George M. Kushner, DMD, MD, FACS
Professor and Chairman
Oral and Maxillofacial Surgery
University of Louisville School of Dentistry
Louisville, Kentucky
United States

Colin MacIver, MBChB, FRCS, BDS, FDS, FRCS (Ed), FRCS (OMFS)
Consultant Maxillofacial/Head and Neck Surgeon
Maxillofacial Surgery
SSMC/Mayo Clinic Abu Dhabi;
Adjunct Professor
Department of Surgery
Khalifa University
Abu Dhabi
United Arab Emirates.

Stephen P. R. MacLeod, BDS, MB ChB, FDSRCS (ED&ENG), FRCS (ED), FFSTRCS (ED), FACS
Joseph R and Louise Ada Jarabak Professor of Surgery
Oral and Maxillofacial Surgery
Loyola University Medical Center
Maywood, Illinois
United States

Caitlin B. L. Magraw, MD, DDS, FACS
The Head and Neck Institute
Head and Neck Surgical Associates;
Associate Clinical Professor
Oral and Maxillofacial Surgery
Oregon Health and Sciences University
Portland, Oregon
United States

Nicholas M. Makhoul, BSc, DMD, MD, FRCD(C), FACS Dip ABOMS
Chair, Associate Dean
Oral and Maxillofacial Surgery
McGill University;
Associate Professor
Faculty of Dentistry
McGill University
Montreal, Quebec
Canada

Ashley E. Manlove, DMD, MD, FACS
Residency Program Director
Oral and Maxillofacial Surgery
Carle Foundation Hospital;
Director Cleft Lip and Palate Team
Oral and Maxillofacial Surgery
Carle Foundation Hospital
Urbana, Illinois
United States

Samir Mardini, MD
Professor and Chair
Plastic Surgery
Mayo Clinic
Rochester, Minnesota
United States

Michael R. Markiewicz, DDS, MD, MPH, FAAP, FACS, FRCD(c)
Professor and Chair
School of Dental Medicine
Oral and Maxillofacial Surgery
Clinical Professor
Department of Neurosurgery and Department of Surgery
Jacobs School of Medicine and Biomedical Sciences
University at Buffalo
Co-Director
Craniofacial Center of Western New York
John R. Oishei Children's Hospital
Attending Surgeon
Department of Head & Neck and Plastic & Reconstructive Surgery
Roswell Park Comprehensive Cancer Center
Buffalo, New York
United States

Jeffrey S. Marschall, DMD, MD, MS
Pediatric Craniomaxillofacial Surgery
Arnold Palmer Hospital for Children
Orlando, Florida
United States

Nigel Shaun Matthews, BDS, FDS, MBBS, FRCS, FRCS (OMFS)
Clinical Professor and Chairman
Associate Dean for Hospital Affairs
Director, TMJ Institute
Department of Oral and Maxillofacial Surgery
Indiana University School of Dentistry
Indianapolis, Indiana
United States

Joseph P. McCain, DMD, FACS
Oral & Maxillofacial Surgery
Massachusetts General Hospital—Harvard
Boston, Massachusetts
United States

J. Michael McCoy, DDS, FACS
Professor
Oral and Maxillofacial Surgery;
Professor
Pathology;
Professor
Radiology;
Medical Director
In-Patient Hyperbaric Oxygen Therapy
University of Tennessee Graduate School of Medicine
Knoxville, Tennessee
United States

Samuel J. McKenna, DDS, MD, FACS
Professor and Chairman
Oral and Maxillofacial Surgery
Vanderbilt University Medical Center
Nashville, Tennessee
United States

Daniel J. Meara, MS, MD, DMD, MHCDS, FACS
Chair
Oral and Maxillofacial Surgery & Hospital Dentistry
Christiana Care Health System;
Director of Research
Oral and Maxillofacial Surgery
Christiana Care Health System
Wilmington, Delaware;
Affiliate Faculty
Physical Therapy
University of Delaware
Newark, Delaware
United States

Paulo Jose Medeiros, DDS, MS, PhD
Professor and Chairman
Oral and Maxillofacial Surgery
Rio De Janiero State University
Rio De Janiero, Brazil

Pushkar Mehra, BDS, DMD, MS, FACS
Professor and Chair
Oral and Maxillofacial Surgery
Boston University Medical Center
Boston, Massachusetts
United States

Louis G. Mercuri, DDS, MS
Visiting Professor
Orthopaedic Surgery
Rush University Medical Center
Chicago Illinois
United States;
Consultant
Clinical Affairs
TMJ Concepts
Ventura, California
United States

Brett A. Miles, DDS, MD, FACS
Professor and Chair
Otolaryngology/Head and Neck Surgery
Northwell Health/Lenox Hill/Manhattan Eye Ear Hospital
New York, New York
United States

Meagan Miller, DDS
Oral and Maxillofacial Surgery
Loma Linda University
Loma Linda, California
United States

Justine Moe, MD, DDS, FRCDC, FACS
Clinical Assistant Professor and Residency Program Director
Oral and Maxillofacial Surgery
University of Michigan
Ann Arbor, Michigan
United States

Hwi Sean Moon, MD, DDS
Cleft and Craniofacial Surgery
El Paso Children's Hospital
El Paso, Texas
United States

Marina Morante Silva, MD, FEBOMFS
Department of Oral and Maxillofacial Surgery
University of Florida, College of Medicine
Jacksonville, Florida
United States

Christopher Morris, DDS, MD, FACS
Private Practice
Katy Center for Oral and Facial Surgery
Katy, Texas
United States

Dean Morton, BDS, MS
Professor
Department of Prosthodontics
Director
Center for Implant, Esthetic and Innovative Dentistry
Indiana University School of Dentistry
Indianapolis, Indiana
United States

Reza Movahed, DMD, FACS
Clinical Assistant Professor
Department of Orthodontics
Saint Louis University
Saint Louis, Missouri
United States

Elena Mujica, DDS
Private Practice
Santa Rosa Maxillofacial Surgery
Caracas, Venezuela

Robert Nadeau, DDS, MD, FACS
Interim Division Director and Program Director for Oral and Maxillofacial Surgery
Department of Developmental and Surgical Sciences
University of Minnesota;
Surgical Service Lead, OMS
M Health Fairview Hospitals and Clinics
Minneapolis, Minnesota
United States

John M. Nathan, MD, DDS
Division of Oral and Maxillofacial Surgery
Mayo Clinic
Rochester, Minnesota
United States

Gregory M. Ness, DDS, FACS
Professor Emeritus—Clinical
Oral and Maxillofacial Surgery and Anesthesiology
The Ohio State University College of Dentistry
Columbus, Ohio
United States

Craig Norbutt, DMD, MD
Assistant Clinical Professor
Oral & Maxillofacial Surgery
Carle Foundation Hospital
Champaign, Illinois
United States

Erik Jon Nuveen, MD, DMD, FAACS
Director of Fellowship
Cosmetic Surgery Affiliates
Oklahoma City, Oklahoma and Jacksonville Beach, Florida;
Voluntary Assistant Professor
Oral and Maxillofacial Surgery
The University of Oklahoma College of Dentistry
Oklahoma City, Oklahoma
United States

George Obeid, DDS
Senior Attending
Oral and Maxillofacial Surgery
Medstar Washington Hospital Center
Washington, District of Columbia
United States

Devin Joseph Okay, DDS
Attending Faculty
Department of Otolaryngology Head and Neck Surgery
Mount Sinai Health System;
Director
Division of Prosthodontics and Maxillofacial Prosthetics
Mount Sinai Health System
New York, New York
United States

Petra Olivieri, DMD, MD
Clinical Assistant Professor
Case Western Reserve University
MetroHealth Hospital
Department of Oral and Maxillofacial Surgery
Cleveland, Ohio
United States

Robert Ord, MB, BCh (Hons), BDS, FRCS, FACS, MS, MBA
Professor and Chairman
Oral and Maxillofacial Surgery
University of Maryland;
Professor
Oncology Program
Greenbaum Cancer Center
Baltimore, Maryland
United States

Daniel Oreadi, DMD
Associate Professor
Oral and Maxillofacial Surgery
Tufts University School of Dental Medicine
Boston, Massachusetts
United States

Neeraj Panchal, DDS, MD, MA
Assistant Professor
Oral and Maxillofacial Surgery
University of Pennsylvania;
Section Chief
Oral and Maxillofacial Surgery
Penn Presbyterian Medical Center;
Section Chief
Oral and Maxillofacial Surgery
Philadelphia Veterans Affairs Medical Center
Philadelphia, Pennsylvania
United States

Sat Parmar, BChD, BMBS, BMedSci, FDSRCS, FRCS Mr
Oral and Maxillofacial Surgery
University Hospitals Birmingham
Birmingham, United Kingdom

Ashish A. Patel, MD, DDS, FACS
Fellowship Director
Head and Neck Surgical Oncology and Microvascular Surgery
Providence Cancer Institute;
Director of Reconstructive Microsurgery
Head and Neck Institute
Head and Neck Surgical Associates;
Medical Director
Cranio-Oral and Maxillofacial and Neck Trauma
Legacy Emanuel Medical Center
Portland, Oregon
United States

Zachary S. Peacock, DMD, MD, FACS
Associate Professor of Oral and Maxillofacial Surgery
Massachusetts General Hospital
Harvard School of Dental Medicine
Boston, Massachusetts
United States

Karl Pennau, DDS
Oral & Maxillofacial Surgery
Oral Surgery Associates of Colorado Springs
Colorado Springs, Colorado
United States

Vincent J. Perciaccante, DDS, FACS
Adjunct Associate Professor
Department of Surgery, Division of Oral & Maxillofacial Surgery
Emory University School of Medicine
Atlanta, Georgia
United States;
Private Practice
South Oral and Maxillofacial Surgery
Peachtree City, Georgia
United States

Jon D. Perenack, MD, DDS
Adjunct Associate Clinical Professor and Director of Fellowship in Facial Cosmetic Surgery
Oral and Maxillofacial Surgery
Louisiana State University;
Medical and Surgical Director
Williamson Cosmetic Center and Perenack Esthetic Surgery
Baton Rouge, Louisiana
United States

Yuliya Petukhova, DDS
Oral and Maxillofacial Surgery Resident
Oral and Maxillofacial Surgery
Mayo Clinic
Rochester, Minnesota
United States

Laurence D. Pfeiffer, MD, DDS
Oral and Maxillofacial Surgeon
Department of Dentistry
Bassett Medical Center
Cooperstown, New York
United States

Matthew H. Pham, DMD, MD
Private Practice
Carolina's Center for Oral & Facial Surgery
Columbia, South Carolina
United States

John N. Phelan, PhD
Associate Professor (Retired)
Cell Biology
UT Southwestern Medical School
Dallas, Texas
United States

Joan Pi-Anfruns, DMD
Assistant Clinical Professor
Oral and Maxillofacial Surgery/Restorative Dentistry
UCLA School of Dentistry
Los Angeles, California
United States

Brendan H. G. Pierce, MD
Otolaryngology
Palo Alto Medical Foundation
Palo Alto, California
United States

Daniel Joseph Pinkston, DDS
ClearChoice Dental Implant Centers
St. Louis, Missouri
United States

Waldemar D. Polido, DDS, MS, PhD
Clinical Professor
Oral and Maxillofacial Surgery
Co-Director
Center for Implant, Esthetic and Innovative Dentistry
Indiana University School of Dentistry
Indianapolis, Indiana
United States

Jeffrey C. Posnick, DMD, MD, FRCS(C), FACS
Adjunct Professor
Plastic and Reconstructive Surgery
Johns Hopkins School of Medicine
Baltimore, Maryland
United States;
Professor Emeritus
Plastic and Reconstructive Surgery and Pediatrics
Georgetown University;
Professor
Oral and Maxillofacial Surgery
Howard University College of Dentistry
Washington DC, Washington
United States;
Professor of Orthodontics
University of Maryland
Baltimore College of Dental Surgery
Baltimore, Maryland
United States

David B. Powers, MD, DMD, FACS, FRCS (Ed)
Professor of Surgery
Director, Duke Craniomaxillofacial Trauma Program
Fellowship Director, Craniomaxillofacial Trauma and Reconstructive Surgery Fellowship
Vice Chair, Division of Plastic, Maxillofacial and Oral Surgery
Department of Surgery
Duke University Medical Center
Durham, North Carolina
United States

Janine Prange-Kiel, PhD
Associate Professor and Chief of Section of Anatomy
Department of Surgery
University of Texas Southwestern Medical Center
Dallas, Texas
United States

Prav Praveen, FRCS, MRCS, MBchBFDSRCS, FFDRCSI
Consultant Oral and Maxillofacial Surgeon
Oral and Maxillofacial Surgery
University Hospitals Birmingham NHS Trust
Birmingham, West Midlands
United Kingdom

David S. Precious, CM, DDS, MSc, FRCDC, FRCS, Dhc
Dean Emeritus and Professor
Oral and Maxillofacial Surgery
Dalhousie University
Halifax, Nova Scotia
Canada

Faisal A. Quereshy, MD, DDS, FACS
Professor/Program Director
Oral & Maxillofacial Surgery
Case Western Reserve University
Cleveland Ohio
United States;
Medical Director
Facial Cosmetic Surgery
Visage Surgical Institute/V-Spa
Medina, Ohio
United States

Peter D. Quinn, DMD, MD
Chief Executive Physician
University of Pennsylvania Health System
University of Pennsylvania;
Schoenleber Professor of Oral & Maxillofacial Surgery
University of Pennsylvania
School of Dental Medicine
Philadelphia, Pennsylvania
United States

Matthew Radant, MD, DDS
Assistant Clinical Professor
Department of Oral and Maxillofacial Surgery
The University of Oklahoma
Oklahoma City, Oklahoma
United States

Christopher K. Ray, DDS
Eastern Oklahoma Oral and Maxillofacial Surgeons;
Clinical Assistant Professor Department of Oral and Maxillofacial Surgery
The University of Oklahoma
Oklahoma City, Oklahoma
United States

Andrew Read-Fuller, DDS, MD, FACS, FACD
Clinical Assistant Professor and Graduate Program Director
Oral & Maxillofacial Surgery
Texas A&M University School of Dentistry
Dallas, Texas
United States

Likith Reddy, MD, DDS, FACS
Professor, Department Head
Oral and Maxillofacial Surgery
Texas A&M University School of Dentistry;
Section Chief
Oral & Maxillofacial Surgery
Baylor University Medical Center;
Clinical Professor
Texas A&M University School of Medicine
Dallas, Texas
United States

Shravan Renapurkar, BDS, DMD, FACS
Associate Professor
Oral and Maxillofacial Surgery
Virginia Commonwealth University
Richmond, Virginia
United States;
Program Director
Oral and Maxillofacial Surgery
Virginia Commonwealth University
Richmond, Virginia
United States

Johan P. Reyneke, B ChD, M ChD, FCMFOS (SA), PhD
Director
Centre for Orthognathic Surgery
Cape Town Mediclinic;
Extraordinary Professor
Maxillofacial and Oral Surgery
University of the Western Cape
Cape Town, South Africa;
Clinical Professor
Oral and Maxillofacial Surgery
University of Oklahoma
Oklahoma City, Oklahoma;
Clinical Professor
Oral and Maxillofacial Surgery
Florida University
Gainesville, Florida
United States

Fabio G. Ritto, DDS, MD, MS, PhD
Professor and Program Director
Oral and Maxillofacial Surgery
The University of Oklahoma Health Science Center
Oklahoma City, Oklahoma
United States

Carrie E. Robertson, MD
Associate Professor of Neurology
College of Medicine
Mayo Clinic
Rochester, Minnesota
United States

Jason Rogers, DDS
Oral and Maxillofacial Surgeon
Private Practice
Santa Rosa and Rohnert Park Oral Surgery
Santa Rosa, California
United States

Brian Louis Ruggiero, MD, DMD
Oral and Maxillofacial Surgery
University of Michigan
Ann Arbor, Michigan
United States

Ramon L. Ruiz, DMD, MD
Director
Pediatric Craniomaxillofacial Surgery
Arnold Palmer Hospital for Children;
Associate Professor
Department of Surgery
University of Central Florida College of Medicine
Orlando, Florida
United States

Mary Ann C. Sabino, DDS, PhD
Oral and Maxillofacial Surgery
Hennepin County Medical Center;
Adjunct Clinical Professor
Oral and Maxillofacial Surgery
University of Minnesota
Minneapolis, Minnesota
United States

Sepideh Sabooree, MD, DMD
Georgia Oral and Facial Reconstructive Surgery
Atlanta, Georgia
United States

Andrew Salama, MD, DDS, FACS
Chief
Oral and Maxillofacial Surgery
Northwell Health—Long Island Jewish Medical Center
New Hyde Park, New York
United States

Thomas J. Salinas, DDS
Professor
Dental Specialties
Mayo Clinic;
Professor
Department of Dental Specialties
Mayo Clinic
Rochester, Minnesota
United States

Nabil Samman, FRCS, FDSRCS
Formerly Professor of Oral and Maxillofacial Surgery
University of Hong Kong, Hong Kong
China

Sebastian Sauerbier, PhD, MD, DDS
Associate Professor
Department of Craniomaxillofacial Surgery
University Medical Center Freiburg
Freiburg, Germany

Thomas Schlieve, DDS, MD, FACS
Associate Professor
Residency Program Director
Department of Surgery, Division of Oral and Maxillofacial Surgery
UT Southwestern Medical Center
Parkland Memorial Hospital
Dallas, Texas
United States

Edward R. Schlissel, DDS, MS
Emeritus Professor
General Dentistry
School of Dental Medicine, Stony Brook University
Stony Brook, New York
United States

Rainer Schmelzeisen, MD, DDS, PhD, FRCS (London)
Medical Director Center of Dental Medicine
Department of Oral and Maxillofacial Surgery
University Medical Center Freiburg
Freiburg, Germany

Jocelyn M. Shand, MBBS (Melb), MDSc (Melb), BDS (Otago), FRACDS (OMS), FRCS (Edin), FDSRCS (Eng)
Head, Oral & Maxillofacial Surgery Program
Department of Plastic & Maxillofacial Surgery
The Royal Children's Hospital of Melbourne
Melbourne, Victoria
Australia

Kaushik H. Sharma, BDS, DMD, MPA
Adjunct Clinical Assistant Professor
Department of Oral & Maxillofacial Pathology, Medicine and Surgery
Temple University Kornberg School of Dentistry, Philadelphia
Pennsylvania
United States;
Oral/Head & Neck Oncologic and Microvascular Reconstructive Surgeon
Department of Oral and Maxillofacial Surgery
St Luke's University Hospital
Bethlehem, Pennsylvania
United States

Brett Shirley, DDS, MD, FACS
Oral and Maxillofacial Surgery
Ochsner LSU Health Science Center
Shreveport Louisiana
United States;
Maxillofacial Oncology and Reconstructive Surgery
John Peter Smith Hospital
Fort Worth, Texas
United States;
Oral and Maxillofacial Surgery
Piney Woods Oral and Maxillofacial Surgery
Nacogdoches, Texas
United States

Paul Shivers, MD, DMD
Clinical Instructor
Oral and Maxillofacial Surgery
University of Michigan
Ann Arbor, Michigan
United States

Raymond P. Shupak, MD, DMD, MBE
Assistant Professor
Geisinger Commonwealth School of Medicine
Department of Oral Medicine and Maxillofacial Surgery
Geisinger Health System
Danville, Pennsylvania
United States

Joseph E. Van Sickels, DDS, FACD, FICD, FACS
Professor and Program Director
Oral and Maxillofacial Surgery
University of Kentucky
Lexington, Kentucky
United States;
Robert D. Marciani Professor for Oral and Maxillofacial Surgery

Douglas P. Sinn, DDS
Clinical Professor
Department of Surgery, Division of Oral and Maxillofacial Surgery
UT Southwestern Medical Center
Dallas, Texas
United States

Kevin Smith, DDS, FACS, FACD
Professor and Residency Program Director
Oral and Maxillofacial Surgery
The University of Oklahoma;
Co-Director
JW Keys Cleft and Craniofacial Clinic
The University of Oklahoma, Oklahoma
City Oklahoma
United States;
Co-Director
MK Chapman Cleft and Craniofacial Clinic
The University of Tulsa
Tulsa, Oklahoma
United States

Miller H. Smith, DDS, MD, FRCD(C), FACS, FRCS (Edin)
Clinical Assistant Professor
Department of Surgery, Division of Oral Maxillofacial Surgery
Cumming School of Medicine—University of Calgary;
Private Practice
South Calgary Oral Maxillofacial Surgery
Calgary Alberta
Canada;
Clinical Assistant Professor
Faculty of Medicine & Dentistry
University of Alberta
Edmonton, Alberta
Canada

Luke C. Soletic, DDS, MD
Oral and Maxillofacial Surgery
NYU-Langone/Bellevue Hospital Center
New York University
Bellevue Hospital Center
New York, New York
United States

Joel Stanek, MD
Staff Physician
Otolaryngology - Head and Neck Surgery
Hennepin County Medical Center
Minneapolis, Minnesota
United States

David Stanton, MD, DMD (Deceased)
Associate Professor
Oral & Maxillofacial Surgery
University of Pennsylvania Health System;
Attending Surgeon
Oral & Maxillofacial Surgery
Children's Hospital of Philadelphia
Philadelphia, Pennsylvania
United States

Martin B. Steed, DDS, FACS
Professor and James B. Edwards Chair
Department of Oral and Maxillofacial Surgery
Medical University of South Carolina
James B. Edwards College of Dental Medicine
Charleston, South Carolina
United States

Mark Stevens, DDS
Professor Emeritus (Retired)
Department of Oral and Maxillofacial Surgery
Augusta University
Augusta, Georgia
United States

Marissa Suchyta, PhD
Research Fellow
Division of Plastic Surgery
Mayo Clinic
Rochester, Minnesota
United States

Steven M. Sullivan, DDS, FACS, FACD
Professor and Chair
Department of Surgical Sciences/Oral and Maxillofacial Surgery
University of Oklahoma College of Dentistry
Oklahoma City, Oklahoma
United States

Omotara Sulyman, MD
Otolaryngology
University of Minnesota
Minneapolis, Minnesota
United States

Srinivas M. Susarla, DMD, MD, FACS, FAAP
Associate Professor
Oral and Maxillofacial Surgery
University of Washington School of Dentistry;
Associate Professor
Surgery (Plastic)
University of Washington School of Medicine
Seattle, Washington
United States

David Knight Sylvester II, DDS
Assistant Clinical Professor
Oral & Maxillofacial Surgery
OU Health Sciences Center, Oklahoma
City Oklahoma
United States;
Private Practice Oral & Maxillofacial Surgeon
ClearChoice Dental Implant Centers
St. Louis, Missouri
United States

Jean-Claude Talmant, MD
Plastic Surgeon Head
Cleft Palate Team
Clinique Jules Verne
Nantes, France

Rahul Tandon, DMD, MD
Oral and Maxillofacial Surgeon
Private Practice
Hinsdale Oral & Maxillofacial Surgery
Hinsdale, Illinois
United States

Jayini Thakker, DDS, MD, FACS
Associate Professor, Program Director
Oral and Maxillofacial Surgery
Loma Linda University
Loma Linda, California
United States

Stone Thayer, MD, DMD, FACS
Assistant Professor
Plastic Surgery
Univ of California San Diego, San Diego
United States

Paul S. Tiwana, DDS, MD, MS, FACS, FACD
Francis J. Reichmann Professor and Chair
Division of Oral & Maxillofacial Surgery
College of Dentistry;
Professor
Department of Surgery
College of Medicine
The University of Oklahoma Health Sciences Center
Oklahoma City, Oklahoma
United States

Pasquale G. Tolomeo, MD, DDS
Cosmetic Surgery
Private Practice
Advanced Body Sculpting
Fall River, Massachusetts;
Cosmetic Surgery
Private Practice
Tulsa Surgical Arts
Tulsa, Oklahoma;
Adjunctive Faculty
Bellevue Oral & Maxillofacial Surgery
New York University
New York, New York
United States

Dan Q. Tran, DDS
Assistant Professor of Surgery
Oral and Maxillofacial Surgery
VCU Medical Center
Richmond, Virginia
United States

Trevor E. Treasure, DDS, MD, MBA, FRCD(C)
Assistant Professor
Oral and Maxillofacial Surgery
University of Texas-School of Dentistry
Houston, Texas
United States

David C. Trent, DDS, MD
Clinical Assistant Professor
Department of Oral and Maxillofacial Surgery
University of California—San Francisco
San Francisco California
United States;
Private Practice
Sacramento, California
United States

R. Gilbert Triplett, DDS, PhD
Regents Professor
Oral & Maxillofacial Surgery
Texas A&M University College of Dentistry
Dallas, Texas
United States

Greg Tull, DMD (Deceased)
Assistant Professor and Associate Program Director
Oral and Maxillofacial Surgery
University of Oklahoma
Oklahoma City, Oklahoma
United States

Michael D. Turner, DDS, MD, MSc, FACS
Associate Professor
Division of Oral and Maxillofacial Surgery
Icahn School of Medical School at Mount Sinai;
Chief of Oral and Maxillofacial Surgery
Division of Oral and Maxillofacial Surgery
Mount Sinai Hospital
New York, New York
United States

Timothy A. Turvey, DDS, FACS
Professor
Oral and Maxillofacial Surgery
University of North Carolina
Chapel Hill, North Carolina
United States

Rachel Uppgaard, DDS
Associate Professor
Developmental and Surgical Sciences
University of Minnesota
Minneapolis, Minnesota
United States

Craig E. Vigliante, DMD, MD
Oral and Maxillofacial Surgeon/Cosmetic Facial Surgeon
Private Practice
Potomac Surgical Arts, PC
Leesburg, Virginia;
Reston Advanced Oral & Cosmetic Facial Surgery, PLLC
Reston, Virginia
United States

Christopher F. Viozzi, MD, DDS, FACS
Consultant and Assistant Professor
Oral and Maxillofacial Surgery and Pediatric Adolescent Medicine
Mayo Clinic
Rochester, Minnesota
United States

John Vorrasi, DDS
Associate Professor, Program Director
Oral and Maxillofacial Surgery and Hospital Dentistry
University of Rochester
Rochester, New York
United States

Peter D. Waite, MPH, DDS, MD, FACS
Professor Emeritus
Oral and Maxillofacial Surgery
University of Alabama
Birmingham, Alabama
United States

Kenneth Wan, MBBS (1st Hons), BDSc (Hons), FRACDS (OMS)
Consultant in Oral & Maxillofacial Surgery
Fiona Stanley Hospital
Murdoch Western Australia
Australia;
Consultant
Oral and Maxillofacial Surgery
West Perth Oral & Maxillofacial Surgery
West Perth, Western Australia
Australia

Brent B. Ward, DDS, MD, FACS, FACD
Professor, Chair and Fellowship Program Director
Oral and Maxillofacial Surgery
University of Michigan
Ann Arbor, Michigan
United States

Todd R. Wentland, DDS, MD
Oral and Maxillofacial Surgery
John Peter Smith Hospital
Forth Worth, Texas;
Piney Woods Oral and Maxillofacial Surgery
Nacogdoches, Texas
United States

Fayette C. Williams, DDS, MD, FACS
Director, Division of Maxillofacial Oncology & Reconstructive Surgery
Oral & Maxillofacial Surgery
John Peter Smith Hospital
Fort Worth, Texas
United States

Jennifer E. Woerner, DMD, MD
Associate Professor
Department of Oral and Maxillofacial Surgery
Louisiana State University Health Sciences Center;
Fellowship Director of Craniofacial and Cleft Surgery
Department of Oral and Maxillofacial Surgery
Louisiana State University Health Sciences Center;
Associate Dean of Academic Affairs
School of Medicine
Louisiana State University Health Sciences Center
Shreveport, Louisiana
United States

Larry M. Wolford, DMD
Clinical Professor
Department of Oral and Maxillofacial Surgery
Texas A&M University College of Dentistry;
Clinical Professor
Department of Orthodontics
Texas A&M University College of Dentistry
Dallas, Texas
United States

Patrick Wong, DDS, MD
Oral and Maxillofacial Surgery
Texas A&M College of Dentistry
Dallas, Texas
United States

Brian M. Woo, DDS, MD, FACS
UCSF-Fresno/Community Medical Centers
Department of Oral and Maxillofacial Surgery
Program Director
Director Head and Neck Oncologic Surgery, Microvascular Reconstruction
Assistant Director Cleft Craniofacial Surgery
Fresno, California
United States

Mariusz K. Wrzosek, DMD, MD, FACS
Associate Professor
Oral & Maxillofacial Surgery
Loyola University Medical Center
Maywood, Illinois
United States

Duke Yamashita, DDS
Attending Staff
Plastic and Maxillofacial Surgery
Children Hospital Los Angeles
Los Angeles, California
United States;
Attending Staff
Dentistry, OMS
Rancho Los Amigos National Rehabilitation Center
Downey, California
United States

David M. Yates, DMD, MD, FACS
Division Chief of Cleft & Craniofacial Surgery
El Paso Children's Hospital
El Paso, Texas
United States

Melvyn Yeoh, DMD, MD
Associate Professor
Oral and Maxillofacial Surgery
University of Kentucky
Lexington, Kentucky
United States

Yedeh Ying, MD, DMD, FACS
Associate Professor
Oral and Maxillofacial Surgery
University of Alabama at Birmingham
Birmingham, Alabama
United States

George Zakhary, DDS, MD, FACS
Assistant Clinical Professor
Oral & Maxillofacial Surgery
University of California San Francisco
Fresno, California
United States

John R. Zuniga, DMD, MS, PhD
Robert V. Walker DDS Chair in Oral and Maxillofacial Surgery
Professor, Departments of Surgery and Neurology
University of Texas Southwestern
Dallas, Texas
United States

Foreword

2016 marked the introduction of the first edition of this comprehensive atlas of Oral and Maxillofacial Surgery and it quickly became the authoritative atlas for this discipline. Six years later (2022), the second edition of this treatise goes to press. Like all other surgical specialties, oral and maxillofacial surgery continues to rapidly evolve, and the new edition reflects the changing nature of surgery, the technological advances and the therapeutic modalities that have developed over this short timeframe. Why this atlas is titled Oral and Maxillofacial Surgery and not Craniomaxillofacial Surgery is bewildering. The title does not reflect the encompassing scope of surgery included in this book. This authoritative atlas will have appeal to multiple specialties from the traditional fields interested in facial, head, neck and oral surgery.

Having edited several textbooks involving multiple authors, I have experienced the complexities involved with the ambitious undertaking of this atlas. Deepak and Paul are very well organized and disciplined and have achieved success with this challenging task. They have recruited almost 300 contributors to provide 116 chapters for the new edition of this atlas. The work is divided into 13 sections which provides a comprehensive overview of the topics of: head and neck anatomy, oral surgery, implants, orthognathic surgery, craniofacial surgery, cleft lip and palate surgery, craniomaxillofacial trauma surgery, benign facial pathology surgery, malignant pathology involving the skull base, face and neck including the thyroid and parathyroid glands, reconstructive surgery including soft tissue, bone, cartilage, nerve, and facial transplantation, facial cosmetic surgery, TMJ surgery and obstructive sleep apnea surgery. This inclusive scope of practice is beyond most but embodies the multiple pathways available to contemporary surgeons wanting to pursue craniomaxillofacial surgery. The latest edition includes a separate section on obstructive sleep apnea surgery, which adds to the comprehensiveness of this edition. As with the first edition, the chapters are well illustrated and are encyclopedic.

Most of the authors are representative of the contemporary training of oral and maxillofacial surgeons including both dental and medical degrees, general surgery experience, as well as fellowship training. The commonality of most of the authors is their dental and medical background and surgical expertise dedicated exclusively to the head, face, oral cavity, and neck. Most of the chapters are co-authored by well known and experienced clinicians teamed with more nascent surgeons who are the future leaders of the specialty. Deepak and Paul are known internationally and have networked with many current and future leaders of the specialty. The international representation of the contributors (numerous countries on 6 continents) has an appealing draw and reflects the global practice of craniomaxillofacial surgery.

Deepak and Paul have similar educational backgrounds, credentials, and career pathways as well as being fellowship trained providers of surgical care. They are both very experienced clinicians and educators. Both have research experience, and both are active administratively with their respective institutions and with service commitments to multiple national and international organizations. Fellowship training pursued by Deepak was oncology and microvascular reconstruction, while Paul pursued fellowship in cleft and craniofacial surgery. The 2 editors have a dynamic synergism which is reflected in this high-quality comprehensive work. Their energy and enthusiasm for what they do is apparent. This atlas mirrors their love and dedication to their work, their patients, their residents and fellows, and to the future of craniomaxillofacial surgery.

by, Timothy A. Turvey, DDS, FACS

Foreword

I am honored to provide comment on the second edition of what I consider to be the most complete, and masterfully illustrated, atlas of oral and maxillofacial surgery ever published. This encyclopedic overview will enable our trainees, and practicing surgeons, to make evidence-based surgical decisions and afford our patients better outcomes. It is a stunning display in text, photographs, and illustration of the breadth and complexity of contemporary oral and maxillofacial surgery. A fledgling discipline that began formally in 1918 as "oral surgery," was propelled, in the first fifty years, by advances in office-based surgery, anesthesia, pharmacology, surgical instrumentation, sterile technique, and experiential wisdom gained from trauma surgery in two World Wars. Starting in the late '60s, and early '70s, our training programs were formalized and broadened to include more exposure to general surgery and surgical subspecialties. An explosion of knowledge in surgical instrumentation, reconstructive and craniofacial techniques, microsurgery, biomaterials, implants, and imaging in the last fifty years has brought us to the current state of our specialty. This remarkable tome is not only the quintessential reference in oral and maxillofacial surgery, but a testimonial to that century of progress.

Dr. Ira Rutkow in *American Surgery: An Illustrated History* stated that "there is no way to separate present day surgery, and one's own practice routines, from the experiences of all the surgeons and all the years that have gone before." This exceptional text brings an organized, consistent, visual pedagogic methodology covering office-based minor procedures to the most complicated head and neck reconstructive surgeries. In the late 19th century, the English novelist Samuel Butler once said, "Diseases come of their own accord, but cures come difficult and hard." Drs. Kademani and Tiwana have created an exceptional single-source reference for our most current understanding of maxillofacial surgical procedures. Contemporary therapeutic decisions must be based on fact, evidence, and experience. Only scientific evidence can adjudicate those difficult decisions we all make daily as surgeons. I personally am indebted to Deepak and Paul for this Herculean effort to synthesize the past, present, and future of our specialty.

—Peter D. Quinn, DMD, MD
Chief Physician Executive [emeritus]
University of Pennsylvania Health System
Schoenleber Professor-Oral & Maxillofacial Surgery
University of Pennsylvania School of Dental Medicine

Preface

The first edition of *Atlas of Oral and Maxillofacial Surgery* was received positively. While many operations do not change significantly with the passage of time, the incorporation of refinements to technique and new technology begins the process of reshaping old into new. These modifications in technique, and the ever-broadening depth of our specialty, provided us the impetus to write this updated edition.

Although our foundations are based in dentistry, the specialty of Oral and Maxillofacial Surgery has evolved to include both a medical and a dental basis of training. While variations in the scope of practice still occur in the specialty across regions of the world, we have observed that these gaps have perceptibly narrowed with time. This change has been driven through the globalization of educational experiences, research, and clinical fellowships. The latter is the most important in this process of driving the specialty forward into a *Pangaea*. This Atlas was written to take advantage of the unifying strengths of our specialty as the premier surgical specialty caring for oral, craniomaxillofacial, and head & neck conditions that require operative intervention. It provides a navigational aid that can guide both experienced surgeons and surgeons in training through new operations and provide a basis for refinements of already established operations in their repertoire. Each chapter is organized in a similar fashion, guiding surgeons through the complex anatomy, instrumentation, technical operative surgery, and modifications. Besides updating chapters from the first edition, many new chapters and a new section on Obstructive Sleep Apnea have been added. Our aim is that this Atlas will define and capture the current global perspective of Oral and Maxillofacial Surgery.

This book is written to provide practicing surgeons, residents, and students the most up-to-date reference for the technical performance and reasoning behind the many types of operations used in our specialty. From the basic to the most complex, readers will find that each chapter is sequentially organized to provide a comprehensive, concise, and practical description of the operative details needed for the contemporary surgical delivery of oral and maxillofacial surgical care. A formal section on relevant surgical anatomy has been incorporated to further assist the reader. Each chapter has been written by an expert surgeon and author who has a specific area of expertise. We would like to express our gratitude to all the section editors and authors for lending their time and expertise to the development of this Atlas.

It is our hope that the information presented here will continue to define the scope of practice of Oral and Maxillofacial Surgery and will provide a basis for education and training for surgeons in the future, with the goal of improving the quality of patient care across the world.

Acknowledgments

We are deeply grateful to our many friends and colleagues who have supported us and contributed to this Atlas. We wish to thank our section editors, Gary F. Bouloux, Eric R. Carlson, Joseph E. Cillo Jr., Richard Allen Finn, Ghali Ghali, Alan S. Herford, Deepak G. Krishnan, Faisal A. Quereshy, Martin Steed, Steven M. Sullivan, and Brent B. Ward, who worked tirelessly to complete their editorial efforts. We thank them immensely for sharing their expertise and for their confidence and support in bringing this project to fruition.

We are also indebted to the many authors who gave their time and expertise in contributing to this book to make it a reality. We owe a particular debt of gratitude to our artist on this project, Joe Chovan. His artistic interpretation of anatomy and surgical procedures has set a new standard for the specialty and was simply breathtaking.

Contents

PART V
Craniofacial Surgery

PART VI
Cleft Lip and Palate

PART VII
Craniomaxillofacial Trauma

VOLUME TWO

PART VIII
Benign Pathology

Video Contents

CHAPTER 1

The Neurocranium

Laurence D. Pfeiffer and John N. Phelan

The Neurocranium[1]

The oft-heard maxim "anatomy is destiny" was coined by Sigmund Freud in summary of his assertion that gender is the primary determinant of personality traits. For surgeons, the same quote can be applied to the importance of mastering the intricate construction of the portion of the human body for which they are responsible. Thorough comprehension of anatomy allows the surgeon to work safely and precisely, thereby optimizing restoration of health and minimizing morbidity. In this chapter, the structure of the neurocranium and how it relates to oral and maxillofacial surgery are examined.

The skull consists of the cranium (Fig. 1.1) and the mandible (Fig. 1.2). The cranium is divided into the neurocranium and the viscerocranium (see Fig. 1.1). The neurocranium encases the brain and is found above the orbits. Below the orbits, the viscerocranium, alternately called the *splanchnocranium* or midface, supports the nasal passages and the oral cavity and makes up the face.

The neurocranium may be considered in two parts: the roof, or cranial vault (also called by its Latin name, the *calvaria*), and the floor, or cranial base. The space within the neurocranium occupied by the brain is the cranial cavity. The calvaria is formed anteriorly by the frontal bone, posteriorly by part of the occipital bone, and laterally by the paired parietal bones and squamous portions of the temporal bones (Fig. 1.3). Although most bones develop by endochondral ossification, which involves the formation of a cartilaginous template that is gradually replaced by bone, the bones of the calvaria develop through intramembranous ossification, whereby mesenchymal cells forming a membrane over the brain condense into a collection of nodes and differentiate directly into osteoblasts. The osteoblasts secrete a matrix that becomes calcified, resulting in the formation of flattened bone within the membrane. The nodes or islands of bone enlarge radially, but at birth the bones of the calvaria are still separated from each other by the mesenchymal membrane.[2–4] The largest areas of noncalcified membrane, called *fontanelles*, are found where the frontal and occipital bones meet the parietal bones on the superior aspect of the calvaria (see Fig. 1.3). The failure of the calvarial bones to fuse prior to infancy allows the cranium to deform during passage through the birth canal and allows the volume of the neurocranium to continue to expand after birth to accommodate enlargement of the brain. Intramembranous ossification continues through infancy until the bones of the calvaria meet and form fibrous suture joints, which usually fuse during adulthood.

One or more of the sutures between the bones of the calvaria may prematurely fuse during fetal development. Virchow's law states that this event, called *craniosynostosis*, results in imbalanced development of the skull; enlargement perpendicular to the fused suture is limited, and enlargement of the area where the sutures remain open is correspondingly increased. The resulting malformation has the potential to cause compression of a portion of the brain, which may result in neurologic abnormalities.[5]

After fusion, the sutures remain visible on the external and internal surfaces of the calvaria (see Fig. 1.3). Along the midline, the sagittal suture is located between the left and right parietal bones. The vertex, a conceptual point indicating the apex of the skull, would be located on the sagittal suture on a perfect skull. On the internal surface of the calvaria, an indentation is normally visible along the midline that corresponds to the superior sagittal sinus, a venous sinus within the dura mater (this is discussed in more detail with the cranial base). The coronal suture runs between the frontal bone and parietal bones, and the lambdoid suture is found between the occipital bone and the parietal bones. The sagittal suture intersects the coronal suture at the bregma and the lambdoid suture at the lambda (Fig. 1.4).

Bilaterally on the calvaria, the squamosal suture is visible between the parietal bone and the squamous portion of the temporal bone. The area where the parietal, temporal, and occipital bones meet is called the *asterion*, which serves as a neurosurgical landmark. More anteriorly, the frontal, parietal, and temporal bones intersect with a bone involved in the formation of the cranial base, the sphenoid bone, to form an H-shaped suture called the *pterion* (Fig. 1.5). The middle meningeal artery, which arises from a branch of the external carotid artery called the *maxillary artery*, runs along the inside of the neurocranium and crosses the pterion. Trauma to the skull at the pterion can rupture the underlying middle meningeal artery, leading to a potentially fatal epidural hematoma.

The floor of the neurocranium is formed by the occipital, temporal, sphenoid, ethmoid, and frontal bones. The internal surface of the floor of the neurocranium, upon which the brain rests, is divided into the anterior, middle, and posterior cranial fossae (Fig. 1.6).

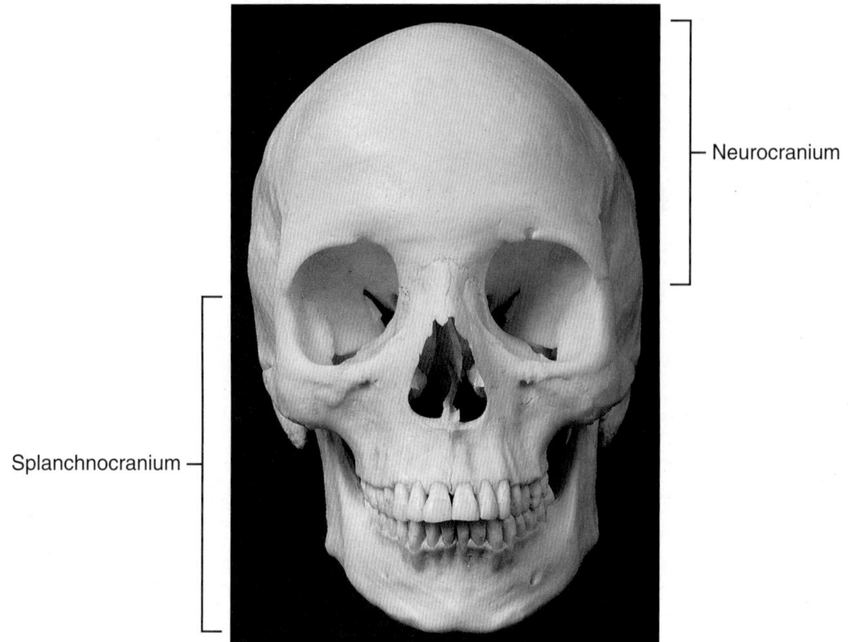

Figure 1.1 The cranium and its divisions. (From Abrahams PH, Spratt JD, Loukas M, van Schoor AN. *McMinn and Abrahams' Clinical Atlas of Human Anatomy*. 7th ed. St Louis, MO; Mosby; 2013.)

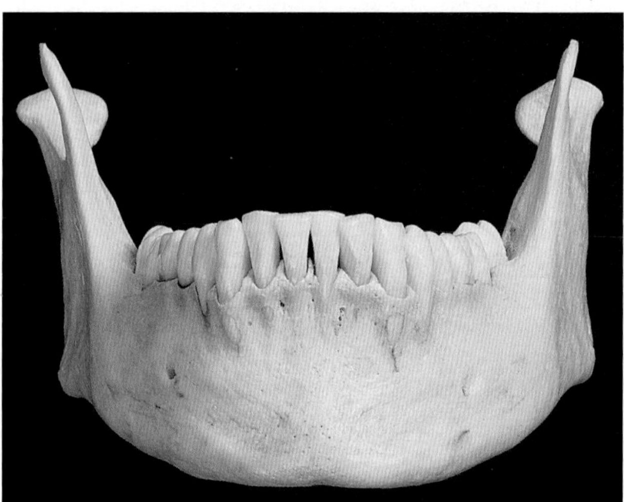

Figure 1.2 The mandible. (From Abrahams PH, Spratt JD, Loukas M, van Schoor AN. *McMinn and Abrahams' Clinical Atlas of Human Anatomy*. 7th ed. St Louis, MO; Mosby; 2013.)

The majority of the anterior cranial fossa consists of the orbital plates of the frontal bone, which form the roofs of the orbits. The orbital roofs bear impressions that mirror the undulating sulci and gyri of the overlying cerebrum. An explanation of how the gelatinous brain might influence the structure of rigid bone is found in Melvin Moss's functional matrix hypothesis, which states that the development of bone sequentially follows, and is thus dependent on, structural changes in the collections of developing soft tissues called *functional matrices*. The cerebrum would thus be a component of the functional matrix for which the associated bone is the frontal bone, or more specifically, the orbital plates of the frontal bone. Likewise, the superior sagittal sinus is a component of the functional matrix associated with the parietal bones, hence, the impression along the internal surface of the sagittal suture described earlier.

Part of the ethmoid bone is found between the orbital plates of the frontal bone (Fig. 1.7). The vertical ridge at the midline is the crista galli, named for its resemblance to a rooster's crest. The cerebral falx, a vertical sheet of dura mater separating the cerebral hemispheres, attaches to the crista galli. On either side of the crista galli are the cribriform plates, which have numerous perforations. Branches of the first cranial nerve, the olfactory nerve, pass through these perforations to reach the nasal cavity.

Posterior to the frontal and ethmoid bones are the lesser wings of the sphenoid bone, which form the posterior edge of the anterior cranial fossa. Extending posteriorly from the medial ends of the lesser wings are the anterior clinoid processes, to which attaches the cerebellar tentorium, a horizontal sheet of dura mater that separates the cerebrum from the cerebellum. The jugum, which is the flattened area between the anterior clinoid processes, supports the olfactory tracts.

The middle cranial fossa is formed by the greater wings and body of the sphenoid bone anteriorly and by the temporal bone posteriorly. The temporal lobes of the brain rest in the lateral recesses of this fossa. At the center of the middle cranial fossa is a portion of the body of the sphenoid bone called the *sella turcica,* which is named for its resemblance to a Turkish saddle. The pituitary gland hangs down from the brain and "sits" in this saddle. The depression for the gland in the center of the sella turcica is the hypophyseal fossa. On either side of the hypophyseal fossa is a concavity occupied by

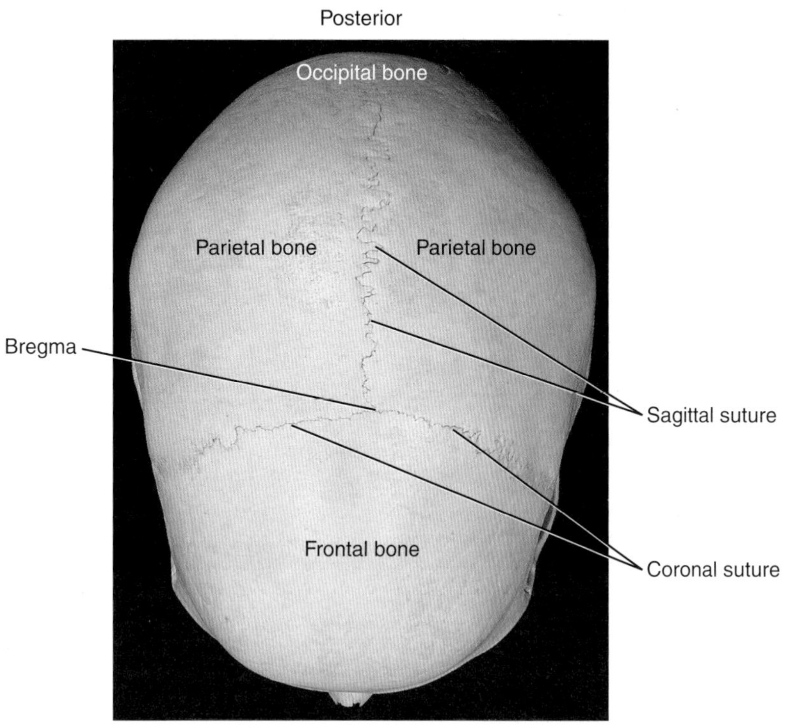

Figure 1.3 Superior view of the skull. (From Abrahams PH, Spratt JD, Loukas M, van Schoor AN. *McMinn and Abrahams' Clinical Atlas of Human Anatomy*. 7th ed. St Louis, MO; Mosby; 2013.)

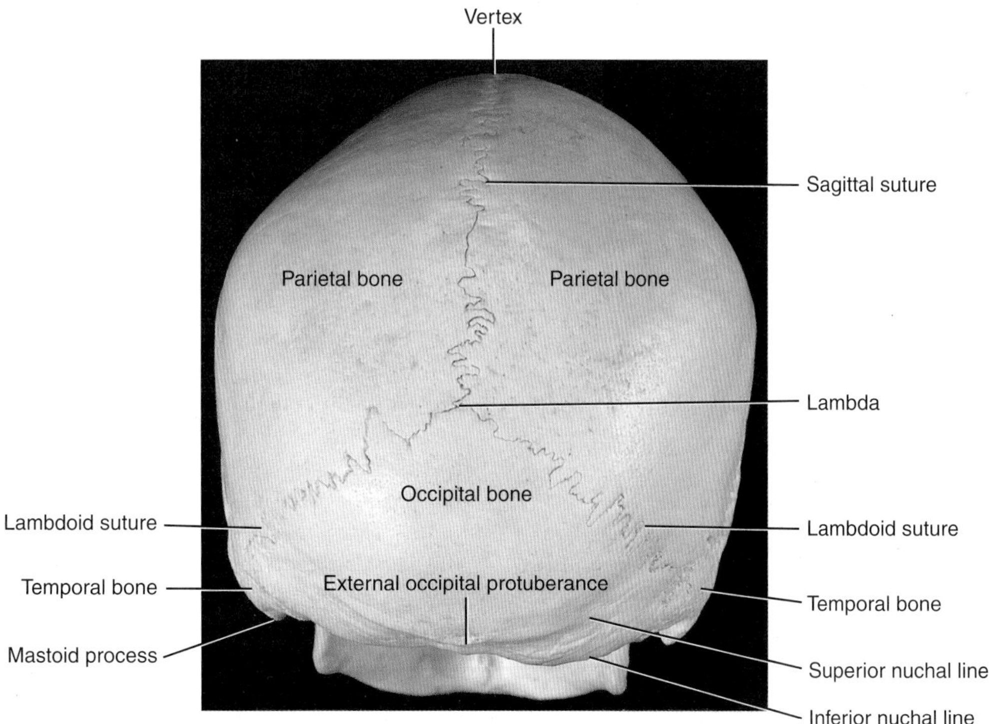

Figure 1.4 Posterior view of the skull. (From Abrahams PH, Spratt JD, Loukas M, van Schoor AN. *McMinn and Abrahams' Clinical Atlas of Human Anatomy*. 7th ed. St Louis, MO; Mosby; 2013.)

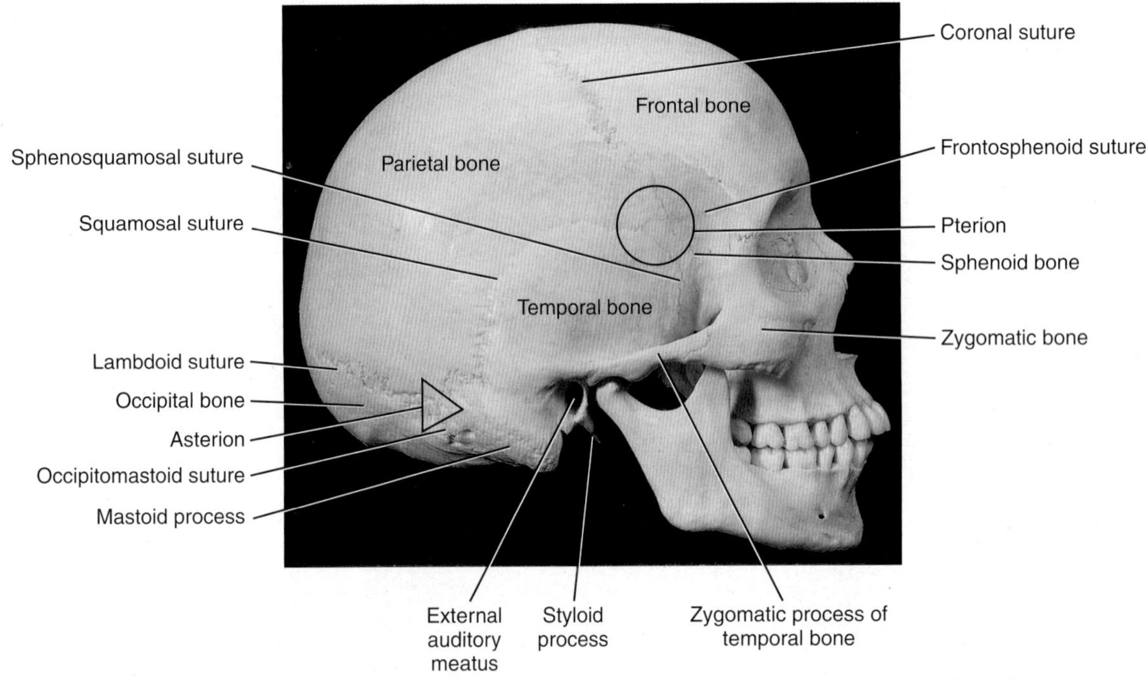

Figure 1.5 Lateral view of the skull. (From Abrahams PH, Spratt JD, Loukas M, van Schoor AN. *McMinn and Abrahams' Clinical Atlas of Human Anatomy*. 7th ed. St Louis, MO; Mosby; 2013.)

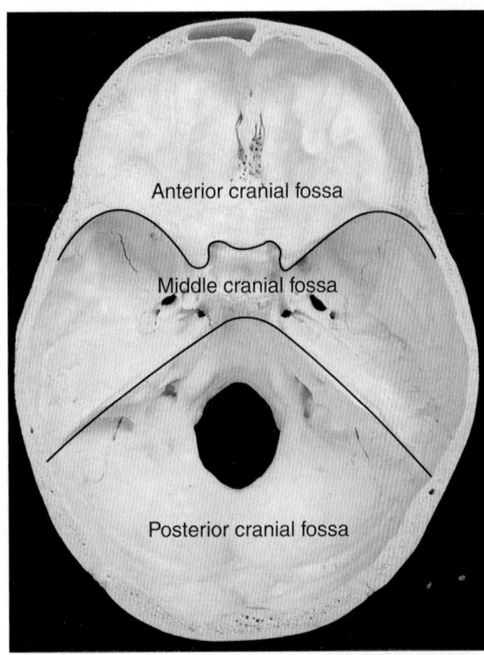

Figure 1.6 Divisions of the neurocranium. (From Abrahams PH, Spratt JD, Loukas M, van Schoor AN. *McMinn and Abrahams' Clinical Atlas of Human Anatomy*. 7th ed. St Louis, MO; Mosby; 2013.)

the cavernous sinus, another venous sinus in the dura mater. The internal carotid artery and the abducens nerve (cranial nerve VI) pass through this sinus, and the oculomotor nerve (cranial nerve III), the trochlear nerve (cranial nerve IV), and the first and second divisions of the trigeminal nerve (cranial nerve V) are embedded in the dura mater, forming the lateral wall of this sinus. The posterior portion of the sella turcica is the dorsum sellae, from which extend the posterior clinoid processes. These processes are another site of attachment for the cerebellar tentorium (Fig. 1.8).

There are several paired openings in the middle cranial fossa that allow passage of structures into and out of the cranial cavity. Just inferior to the overhanging portion of the lesser wing of the sphenoid are the optic canal and the superior orbital fissure. The optic canal passes through the lesser wing of the sphenoid bone and allows passage of the optic nerve (cranial nerve II), which is responsible for vision, and the ophthalmic artery, a branch of the internal carotid artery. The superior orbital fissure is a gap between the greater and lesser wings of the sphenoid. Three nerves supplying motor innervation to the extraocular muscles, the oculomotor nerve (cranial nerve III), the trochlear nerve (cranial nerve IV), and the abducens nerve (cranial nerve VI), and one sensory nerve, the ophthalmic division of the trigeminal nerve (cranial nerve V), pass through the superior orbital fissure to reach the orbit. The superior ophthalmic vein also passes through this fissure to drain blood from the orbit into the cavernous sinus.

Three pairs of foramina in the middle cranial fossa pass through the greater wing of the sphenoid bone. From anterior to posterior, they are the foramen rotundum, foramen ovale, and foramen spinosum. The second division, or maxillary division, of the trigeminal nerve passes through the foramen rotundum to reach the pterygopalatine fossa. The foramen ovale serves as the passageway that the third division, or mandibular division, of the trigeminal nerve, and often the lesser petrosal nerve, a branch of the glossopharyngeal nerve (cranial nerve IX), use to reach the infratemporal fossa. The middle meningeal artery travels from the infratemporal fossa

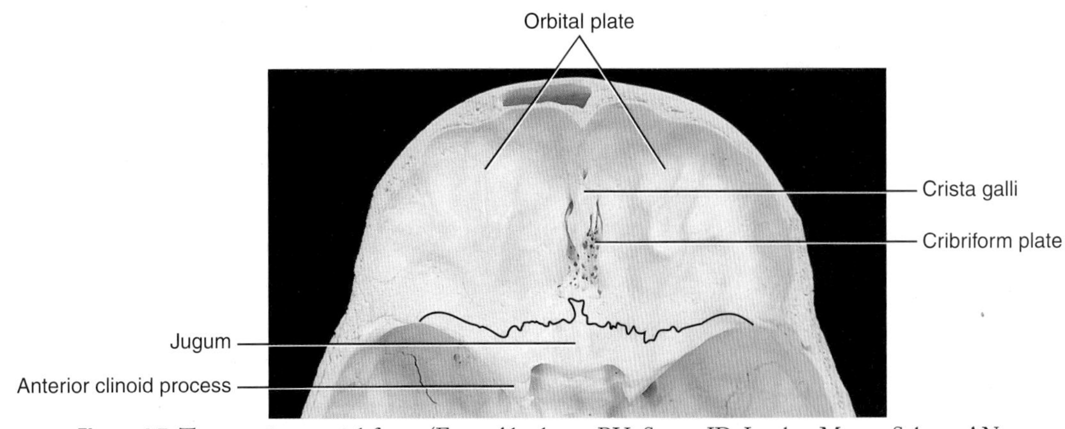

Figure 1.7 The anterior cranial fossa. (From Abrahams PH, Spratt JD, Loukas M, van Schoor AN. *McMinn and Abrahams' Clinical Atlas of Human Anatomy*. 7th ed. St Louis, MO; Mosby; 2013.)

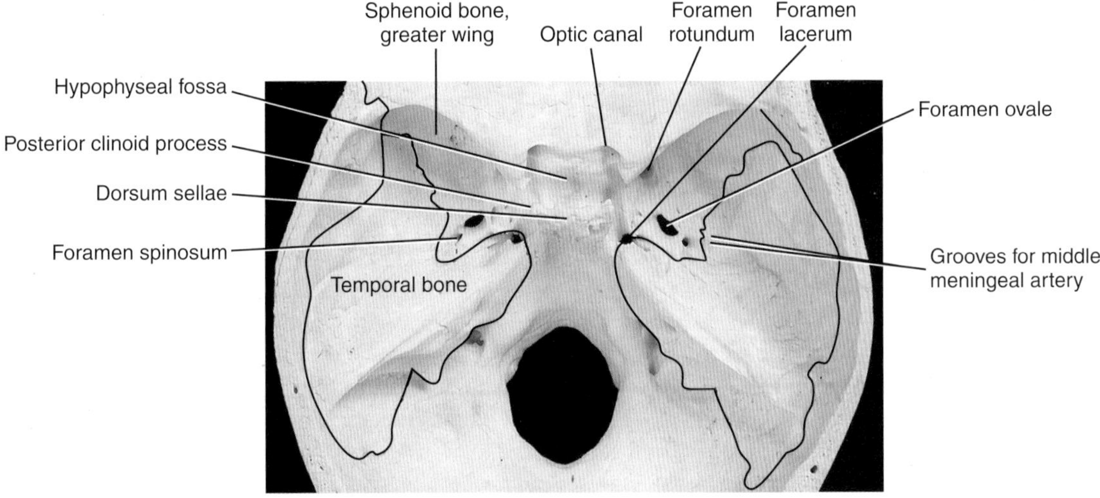

Not shown: Superior orbital fissure

Figure 1.8 The middle cranial fossa. (From Abrahams PH, Spratt JD, Loukas M, van Schoor AN. *McMinn and Abrahams' Clinical Atlas of Human Anatomy*. 7th ed. St Louis, MO; Mosby; 2013.)

to the middle cranial fossa by passing through the foramen spinosum. A series of grooves representing the paths of the branches of the middle meningeal artery, which supply the bone and dura mater between which they run, radiate laterally from the foramen spinosum across the middle cranial fossa and superiorly along the lateral aspect of the calvaria. The foramen spinosum also transmits one or more of the meningeal branches of the trigeminal nerve, which provide sensory innervation to the dura mater lining the middle cranial fossa.

Medial to the foramen ovale and foramen spinosum lies the foramen lacerum, which is a gap between the temporal and sphenoid bones that may be thought of as a very short vertical tunnel. The inferior end of this tunnel is completely blocked off by cartilage, and the only structures traversing the entire length of the foramen lacerum from its inferior to its superior opening are a few small blood vessels. Two structures of note travel part of the way through the foramen lacerum, however. The internal carotid artery enters the foramen lacerum from an opening in its wall that connects it to the carotid canal, which is described below. The artery then turns to access the cavernous sinus. A branch of the facial nerve (cranial nerve VII), the greater petrosal nerve, passes through the superior opening of the foramen lacerum, joins with the deep petrosal nerve, and leaves the foramen lacerum through an opening in its wall that leads to the pterygoid canal.

The occipital, sphenoid, and paired temporal and parietal bones contribute to the posterior cranial fossa, where the cerebellum and part of the brainstem are located. The foramen magnum is the large opening in the occipital bone that transmits the spinal cord and the vertebral arteries. The flat surface of the occipital and sphenoid bones anterior to the foramen magnum and posterior to the dorsum sellae is the clivus. The clivus is adjacent to the anterior surface of the pons, the middle portion of the brain stem. Superior to the foramen magnum and lateral to the clivus are the jugular tubercles, inferior to which are found the hypoglossal canals. In addition to the hypoglossal nerve (cranial nerve XII), the hypoglossal canal

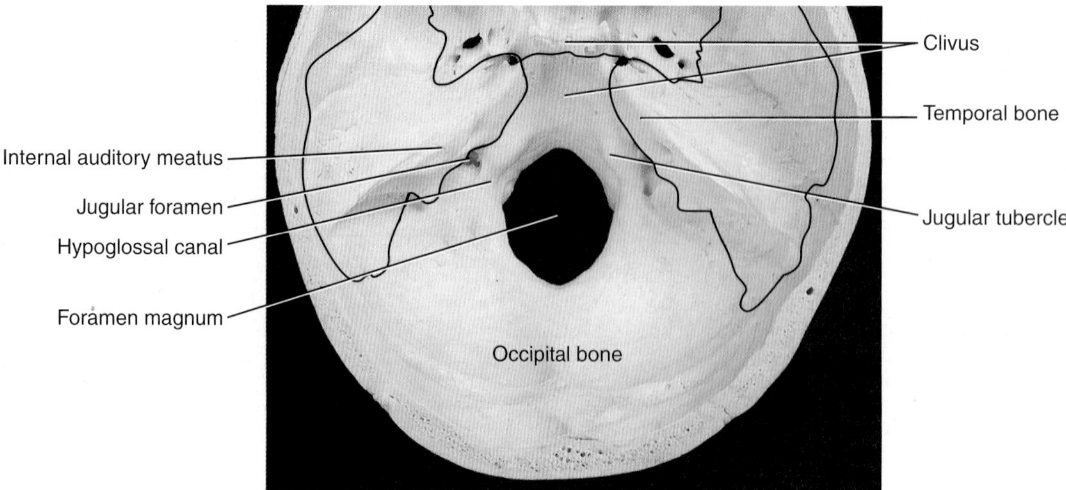

Figure 1.9 The posterior cranial fossa. (From Abrahams PH, Spratt JD, Loukas M, van Schoor AN. *McMinn and Abrahams' Clinical Atlas of Human Anatomy*. 7th ed. St Louis, MO; Mosby; 2013.)

transmits branches of the upper cervical spinal nerves that provide part of the sensory innervation to the dura mater lining the posterior cranial fossa (Fig. 1.9).

The hypoglossal nerve supplies motor innervation to the muscles of the tongue. Damage to the hypoglossal nerve may result in unilateral paralysis of the tongue. To test for hypoglossal nerve damage, the patient is asked to protrude (i.e., stick out) the tongue. Normally the tongue protrudes along the midline without deviating to either side; if motor innervation is lost to one side of the tongue, it deviates to the affected side.

Located superolateral to the jugular tubercle is a large gap between the temporal and occipital bones; this is the jugular foramen, which is named for the large vein it transmits, the internal jugular vein. The glossopharyngeal nerve (cranial nerve IX), the vagus nerve (cranial nerve X), and the accessory nerve (cranial nerve XI) pass through the jugular foramen. The glossopharyngeal nerve provides sensory and motor innervation to the pharynx and the tongue. The vagus nerve, in addition to carrying the majority of the body's parasympathetic innervation, sends motor and sensory branches to the pharynx and a branch to the posterior cranial fossa that is responsible for the remainder of the sensation to the dura mater in this area. The accessory nerve provides motor innervation to the sternocleidomastoid muscle of the neck and the trapezius muscle of the posterior neck and upper back.

Superior to the jugular foramen and inferior to the peak of the petrous portion of the temporal bone is the internal acoustic meatus, which is also called the *internal auditory meatus* or *canal.* The facial nerve (cranial nerve VII) and the vestibulocochlear nerve (cranial nerve VIII) enter this foramen. The facial nerve provides motor innervation to muscles used in facial expression; parasympathetic innervation to the lacrimal gland, glands of the nasal and oral mucosa, and two salivary glands; and the sensation of taste to the front of the tongue. The vestibulocochlear nerve is responsible for the sensations of hearing and balance.

Impressions for two of the dural venous sinuses, the superior sagittal and cavernous sinuses, have already been noted. The posterior cranial fossa also bears impressions corresponding to some of the dural sinuses, notably the bilateral sigmoid and transverse sinuses, and the centrally located confluence of sinuses. The dura mater is a bilaminar membrane; it has an external periosteal layer adherent to the internal surface of the cranial cavity and an internal meningeal layer continuous with the dura mater of the spinal cord. The periosteal and meningeal layers of the dura mater are fused except at the dural infoldings and at the dural venous sinuses. The infoldings are extensions of the meningeal layer of the dura that pass between parts of the brain to lend it structural support. Examples of the dural infoldings are the cerebral falx and the cerebellar tentorium mentioned earlier. The dural sinuses are channels between the two dural layers through which venous blood flows. The veins of the brain drain into the dural sinuses, which in turn drain into the internal jugular vein via the jugular foramen in the posterior cranial fossa.

Most of the dural venous sinuses lie within the margins of the dural infoldings. Running through the superior and inferior margins of the cerebral falx are the superior and inferior sagittal sinuses. The superior sagittal sinus begins anteriorly near the crista galli at the foramen cecum, an opening in the anterior cranial fossa where the frontal bone and the ethmoid bone meet. A vein from the nasal cavity enters the sinus through this foramen. The superior sagittal sinus runs posteriorly along the midline of the calvaria to the confluence of sinuses, a dilation that leaves an impression in the midline of the occipital bone.

Blood in the confluence of sinuses may drain laterally through the horizontally oriented left and right transverse sinuses, which run along the posterior and lateral margins of the cerebellar tentorium. At the base of the petrous portion of the temporal bones, the transverse sinuses are continuous with the sigmoid sinuses. These S-shaped sinuses continue inferiorly as the internal jugular veins at the level of the jugular foramina.

Blood from the orbit may pass through the superior orbital fissure via the superior ophthalmic vein and drain into the cavernous sinus. The cavernous sinus also receives blood from the brain via the superficial middle cerebral vein. Blood in the cavernous sinus may then pass posteriorly through the superior and inferior petrosal sinuses. The superior petrosal sinus runs along the margin of the cerebellar tentorium across the crest of the petrous portion of the temporal bone and empties into the junction of the transverse and sigmoid sinuses. The inferior petrosal sinus runs posteriorly in a very subtle groove between the petrous portion of the temporal bone and the occipital bone and drains directly into the origin of the internal jugular vein at the jugular foramen (Figs. 1.10 and 1.11).

Some of the foramina in the interior of the neurocranium lead directly to the viscerocranium and are not visible on the underside of an intact skull (Fig. 1.12). These include the openings in the cribriform plate, which lead to the nasal cavity; the optic canal and orbital fissures, which lead to the orbit; and the foramen rotundum, which leads to the pterygopalatine fossa. All but one of the remaining openings in the internal surface of the floor of the neurocranium are visible on its external surface. The foramen ovale and foramen spinosum open into the infratemporal fossa, which is a space

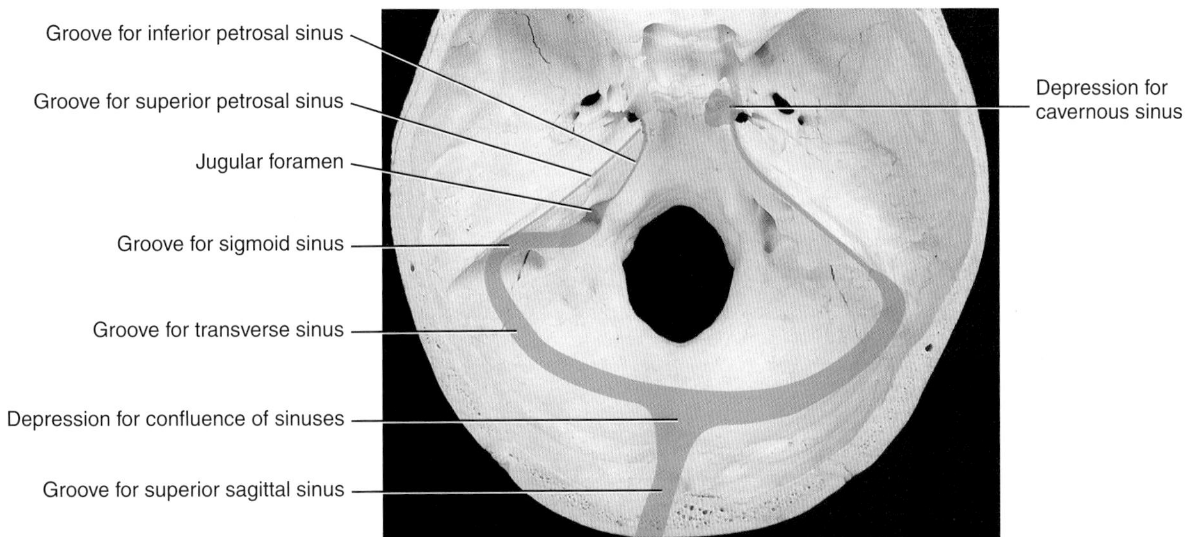

Figure 1.10 Grooves for the dural sinuses. (From Abrahams PH, Spratt JD, Loukas M, van Schoor AN. *McMinn and Abrahams' Clinical Atlas of Human Anatomy*. 7th ed. St Louis, MO; Mosby; 2013.)

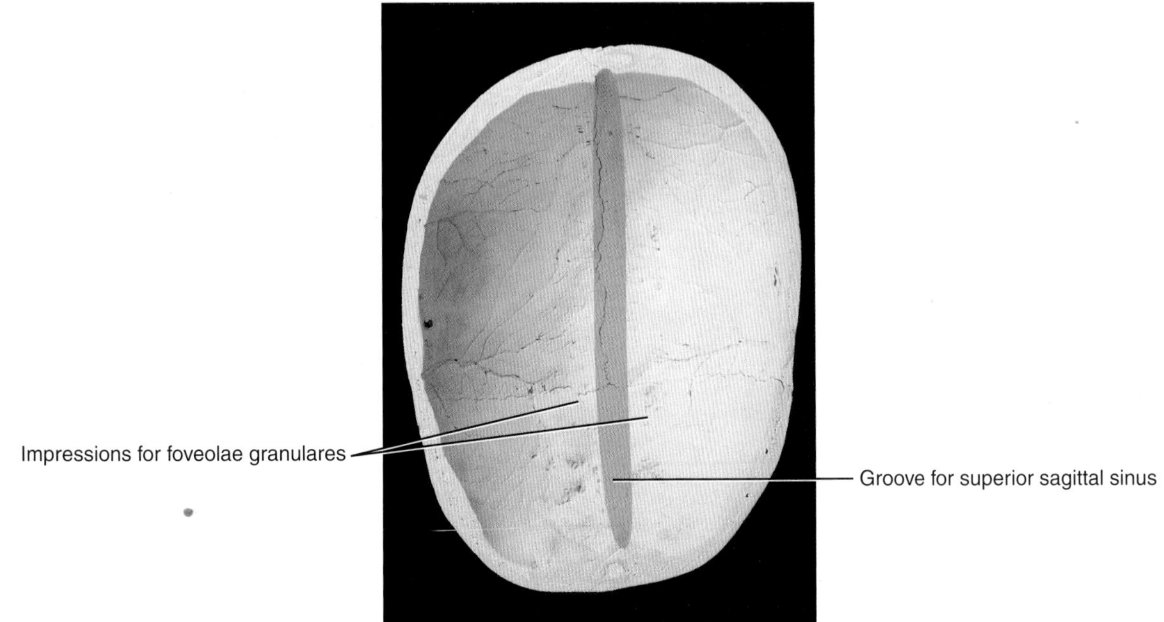

Figure 1.11 Underside of the calvaria. (From Abrahams PH, Spratt JD, Loukas M, van Schoor AN. *McMinn and Abrahams' Clinical Atlas of Human Anatomy*. 7th ed. St Louis, MO; Mosby; 2013.)

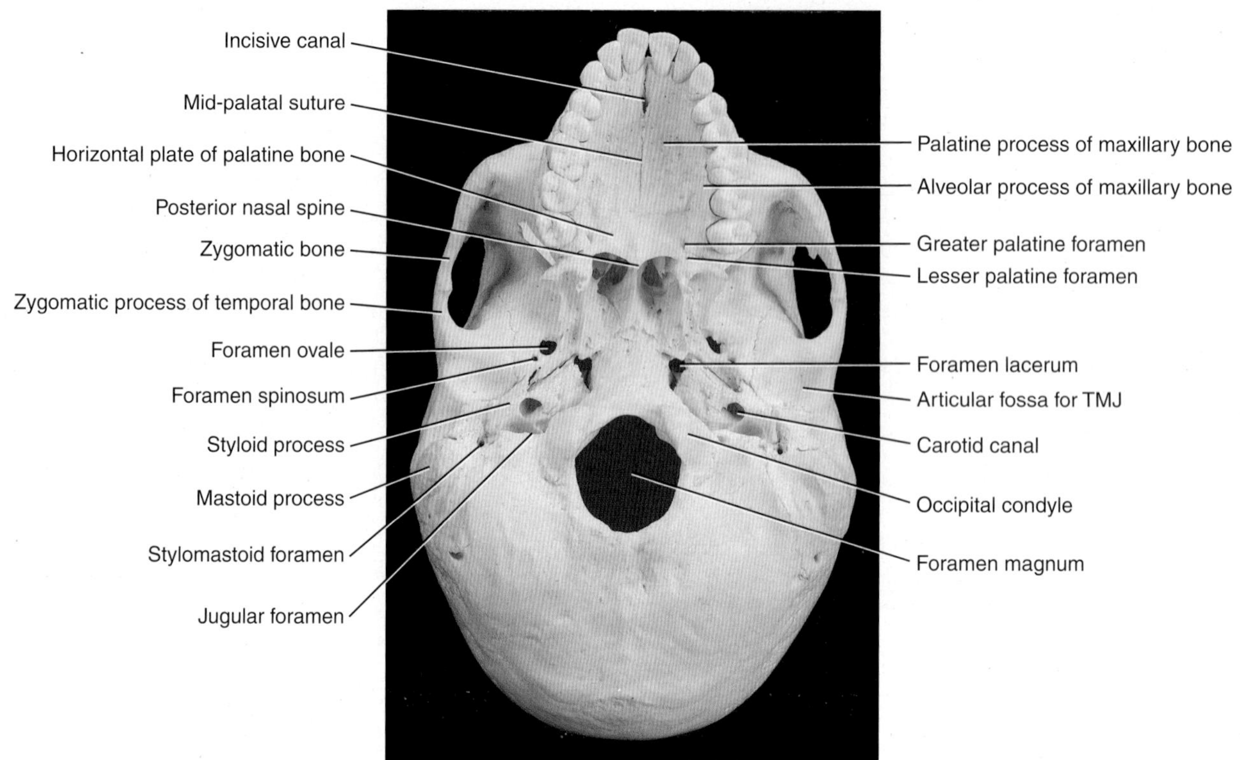

Figure 1.12 Underside of the cranium. *TMJ,* Temporomandibular joint. (From Abrahams PH, Spratt JD, Loukas M, van Schoor AN. *McMinn and Abrahams' Clinical Atlas of Human Anatomy*. 7th ed. St Louis, MO; Mosby; 2013.)

between the neurocranium and the viscerocranium. The foramen lacerum is located medial to the ovale and the spinosum; the jugular foramen, which transmits the internal jugular vein into the neck, is posterior to the spinosum. Between the lacerum and the spinosum is the carotid canal, which allows the internal carotid artery to enter the skull from the neck. The carotid canal is not visible on the internal surface of the floor of the neurocranium because it opens into the wall of the foramen lacerum.

The internal acoustic meatus is not visible externally on the neurocranium. After passing through the meatus from the posterior cranial fossa, the vestibulocochlear nerve ends in the sensory apparatus of the inner ear within the temporal bone. The facial nerve proceeds through the facial canal in the temporal bone and ultimately exits the skull through the stylomastoid foramen, located between the styloid and mastoid processes of the temporal bone at the base of the neurocranium.

The external surface of the occipital bone bears several notable structures. Lateral to the foramen magnum are two prominences, the occipital condyles, superior to which are the openings of the hypoglossal canals. The occipital condyles articulate with the first cervical vertebra to form the atlanto-occipital joint. The foramen magnum opens into the vertebral foramen of this vertebra; the sum of all of the vertebral foramina is the vertebral canal, which houses the spinal cord. The level of the foramen magnum is where the brain stem ends and the spinal cord begins.

Just anterior to the foramen magnum is the pharyngeal tubercle. The superior constrictor muscle, one of the muscles of the pharynx, attaches here.

The superior and inferior nuchal lines, two horizontal ridges that run parallel to each other, are found posterior to the foramen magnum. At the center of the superior nuchal line is the external occipital protuberance, or the inion. Muscles of the upper back and neck attach to these elevations.

Table 1.1 lists the structures passing through the foramina at the base of the neurocranium, and Table 1.2 presents the cranial nerves and their associated functions.

Table 1.1 Structures Passing Through the Foramina at the Base of the Neurocranium

Foramen	Structure
Cribriform plate	Cranial nerve (CN) I
Optic canal	CN II, ophthalmic artery, postganglionic sympathetic fibers
Superior orbital fissure	CN III, CN IV, CN V division 1, CN VI, ophthalmic veins, postganglionic sympathetic fibers
Foramen rotundum	CN V division 2
Foramen ovale	CN V division 3, lesser petrosal nerve
Foramen spinosum	Middle meningeal artery
Foramen lacerum	Greater petrosal nerve
Internal auditory meatus	CN VII, VIII
Jugular foramen	CN IX, X, XI, internal jugular vein
Hypoglossal canal	CN XII
Foramen magnum	Spinal cord, vertebral arteries, spinal component of CN XI, anterior and posterior spinal arteries

Table 1.2 Cranial Nerves and Function[6]

Nerve	Cranial Nerve	Somatic Motor	Branchial Motor	Visceral Motor	Visceral Sensory	General Sensory	Special Sensory	Function
Olfactory	I						✓	Smell
Optic	II						✓	Sight
Oculomotor	III	✓		✓				Moves pupil up (elevation) via superior rectus muscle, down (depression) via inferior rectus muscle, and in (adduction) via medial rectus muscle. Constricts pupil via constrictor pupillae muscle. Allows accommodation via medial rectus and constrictor pupillae muscles and ciliary body. Raises eyelid via levator palpebrae superioris muscle.
Trochlear	IV	✓						Moves pupil down (depression) and out (abduction) via superior oblique muscle.
Trigeminal	V		✓			✓		Motor to eight muscles, including muscles of mastication. Sensory to skin of face, oral mucosa, mandibular teeth, and dura mater.
Abducens	VI	✓						Moves pupil out (abduction) via lateral rectus muscle.
Facial	VII		✓	✓		✓	✓	Closes eye via orbicularis oculi muscle, motor to all other muscles of facial expression plus stapedius muscle, stylohyoid muscle, and posterior belly of digastric muscle. Parasympathetic influence on production of saliva (submandibular and sublingual glands) and tears (lacrimal gland). Provides taste to anterior two-thirds of tongue.

Continued

Table 1.2 Cranial Nerves and Function[6]—cont'd

Nerve	Cranial Nerve	Somatic Motor	Branchial Motor	Visceral Motor	Visceral Sensory	General Sensory	Special Sensory	Function
Vestibulocochlear	VIII						✓	Hearing, balance
Glossopharyngeal	IX		✓	✓	✓	✓	✓	Motor to stylopharyngeus muscle and other pharyngeal muscles. Sensory to middle ear. Parasympathetic influence on production of saliva (parotid gland). Provides taste to posterior one-third of tongue. Innervates carotid body and carotid sinus.
Vagus	X		✓	✓	✓	✓		Motor involvement in swallowing (pharyngeal muscles), elevation of palate (levator veli palatini muscle), and talking (laryngeal muscles). Sensory to skin around external ear. Parasympathetic innervation to viscera in thorax and abdomen. Provides taste to area of epiglottis.
Accessory	XI		✓					Elevates and rotates scapula via trapezius muscle. Turns head and flexes neck via sternocleidomastoid muscle.
Hypoglossal	XII	✓						Motor to all tongue muscles except palatoglossus (IX and X).

References

1. Garlick JA, Pfeiffer LD. *The Clinical Skull Manual.* Bloomington, IN: AuthorHouse Publishing; 2009.
2. Sonick M, Hwang D, Saadoun AP. *Implant Site Development.* Chichester, West Sussex, UK: Wiley-Blackwell; 2012.
3. Ranly DM. Craniofacial growth. *Dent Clin North Am.* 2000;44(3):457–470.
4. Rice DP. *Craniofacial Sutures: Development, Disease and Treatment.* Basel, Switzerland: Karger; 2008.
5. Pattisapu JV, Gegg CA, Olavarria G, et al. Craniosynostosis: diagnosis and surgical management. *Atlas Oral Maxillofac Surg Clin.* 2010;18(2):77–91.
6. Wilson-Pauwels L, Akesson EJ, Stewart PA. *Cranial Nerves.* PMPH-USA; 2008.

CHAPTER 2

The Orbit and Eye

Alan S. Herford, Trevor E. Treasure, and Rahul Tandon

Orbital surgery can be indicated for a variety of traumatic or pathologic conditions and for esthetic concerns in the contemporary practice of oral and maxillofacial surgery (OMS). OMS surgeons must be familiar with the complex anatomy of the orbital region, both for proper diagnosis and for subsequent treatment of these conditions. This chapter reviews the pertinent orbital anatomy for surgeons who perform orbital surgery. Unfamiliarity with orbital anatomy can have devastating consequences for the patient and the surgeon. Blindness, the most feared iatrogenic complication after internal orbital reconstruction, is fortunately rare. Frequently, deep orbital exploration is required to properly treat the patient's condition. Deep orbital exploration is safe provided that the anatomy and physiology of the orbit are considered before treatment. Clinically, this includes good visualization with proper lighting, gentle retraction of the globe/muscle cone, and careful subperiosteal dissection.

The Hard Tissue Anatomy

Bony Orbit

The bony orbit is not the straight, four-walled pyramid that is depicted in many textbooks (Fig. 2.1A). This simplistic view of the anatomy leads directly to inadequate orbital fracture repair and secondary deformities. Three of the four orbital walls have both concave and/or convex portions that should be reproduced when reconstruction is performed. Only the thick lateral wall of the orbit should be considered straight from anterior to posterior. More conical in shape, the orbit consists of a proximal apex and a distal base, both of which have thicker bone than any of the walls. The base of the cone is rotated laterally such that the visual axis diverges from the orbital axis by 23 degrees.[1]

The orbital entrance measures approximately 4 cm wide by 3.5 cm high.[1,2] The orbital rim is an important landmark for the structural dimension of the orbit: the orbit's maximum area is approximately 1 cm behind the rim; the apex is approximately 44 to 55 mm from the medial rim.[2] The lateral walls are approximately 90 degrees to each other; the medial walls are roughly parallel to each other and have a slight convexity proximal to distal. The total volume of the orbit is approximately 30 mL, with the globe comprising approximately 7 mL of the total (see Fig. 2.1B).[1,2] Seven bones form the internal orbit: the frontal, ethmoid, zygomatic, maxillary, lacrimal, palatine, and sphenoid bones (see Fig. 2.1A). Some of the bony walls are thick and resist fracture, whereas others are quite thin and fracture with regularity. Thin walls also allow easy transmission of infection and invasion by tumors from the paranasal sinuses.[1–3]

The surgeon should also be aware of asymmetry between the right and left orbits. One study demonstrated an average volume difference of 0.8 mL between the right and left orbits, and a 14% chance of 1.5 mL or greater difference between orbits. Orbital reconstruction has begun to employ virtual surgical planning using the contralateral, unaffected orbit to treat the traumatized orbit. The surgeon should be aware of possible differences and anticipate that custom plates may not fit correctly or will need adjustment based on this inherent asymmetry.[4]

Orbital Floor

Three bones form the floor of the orbit: the orbital process of the maxilla, the zygomatic bone, and the orbital plate of the palatine bone.[1–3] The orbital plate of the palatine bone is a crucial consideration in the treatment of deep fractures of the orbital floor. In most low-energy injuries of the orbital floor, this bone does not fracture and can be used as a sound ledge for orbital plates or mesh. It should be identified as a small, triangular-shaped bone posterior to the orbital plate of the maxilla and medial to the infraorbital/maxillary nerve.[5,6] Immediately behind the inferior rim, a concavity in the floor of about 15 mm extends past the inferior orbital fissure. This concavity becomes convex proximally as it approaches the orbital apex. Knowledge of this post-bulbar convexity aids in the reconstruction of the normal floor anatomy and helps to prevent late secondary enophthalmos.[5,7,8] Some surgeons routinely obliterate the inferior orbital fissure during fracture repair to prevent extraconal fat from herniating into the infratemporal fossa and thus contributing to secondary enophthalmos (Fig. 2.2).

The floor is also the roof of the maxillary sinus. The maxillary division of the trigeminal nerve (cranial nerve [CN] V2) leaves the foramen rotundum in the middle cranial fossa and enters the orbit in a confluence between the superior and inferior orbital fissures (see Fig. 2.1A). It continues anteriorly to enter the infraorbital canal in the orbital plate of the maxilla. The canal contains the infraorbital nerve, infraorbital branch of the maxillary artery, infraorbital veins, and postganglionic autonomic fibers from the pterygopalatine ganglion.[2,3]

The orbital floor and the medial wall are the most commonly fractured areas in orbital trauma. This high incidence can be attributed to the thinness of the orbital floor, which may measure only 0.5 mm thick. Inadequately treated posterior floor fractures can play a significant role in the etiology of posttraumatic enophthalmos.[5,7–10]

Orbital Roof

The orbital roof is composed of three bones. The frontal bone forms the major portion, and a small anterolateral portion of the zygoma and part of the lesser wing of the sphenoid bone posteriorly constitute the remainder.[1,3] The orbital roof has a concavity immediately behind the superior rim. Once past the concavity, the roof is mainly straight back to the orbital apex. Two important landmarks are found within the anterior roof: the lacrimal fossa anterolaterally and the trochlear fossa medially. Other important landmarks, situated at the junction with the lateral wall, are the superior orbital fissure (SOF) and the frontosphenoidal suture. The superior rim contains the supraorbital notch/foramen, found at the junction of the medial one-third and the lateral two-thirds. Injury through trauma or iatrogenic damage to the supraorbital neurovascular bundle may produce altered sensation of the forehead and brow.[1–3,11] The supratrochlear vessels are located medial to the supraorbital bundle. The supratrochlear artery is a branch of the ophthalmic artery, and the supratrochlear nerve is a terminal branch of the frontal nerve (CN V1).[1–3]

Lateral Wall

The lateral wall of the orbit is fairly straight from rim to apex and owes its strength to the two bones that form it: the greater wing of the sphenoid (GWS) and the zygomatic bone. Posteriorly, the lateral wall begins at the SOF and is composed primarily of the straight, thick GWS. Anteriorly, the GWS articulates with the orbital surface of the zygoma at the zygomaticosphenoidal suture. The zygoma contains two foramina and accompanying neurovascular bundles. The zygomaticofacial nerve is a purely sensory supply to the skin

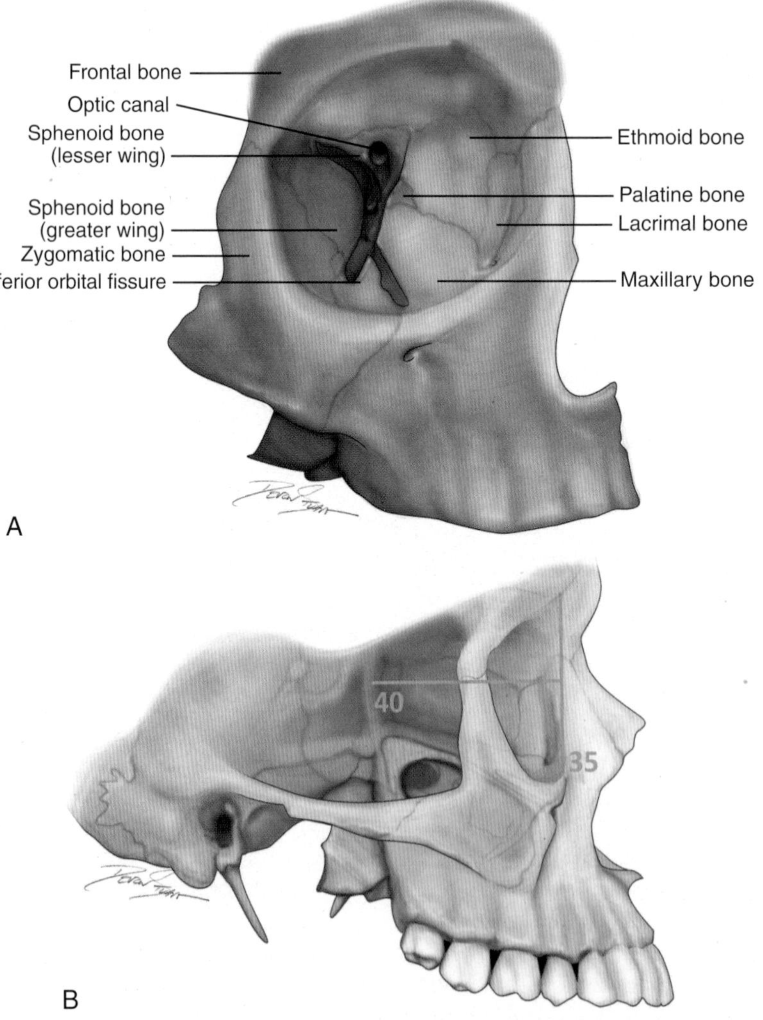

Figure 2.1 **A,** Bony orbit depicting the seven bones that form it: frontal, ethmoid, zygomatic, maxillary, lacrimal, palatine, and sphenoid. Also depicted are the associated fissures and canals. **B,** Sagittal view of the orbit demonstrating the volume, which is approximately 30 mL, with the globe comprising 7 mL of it.

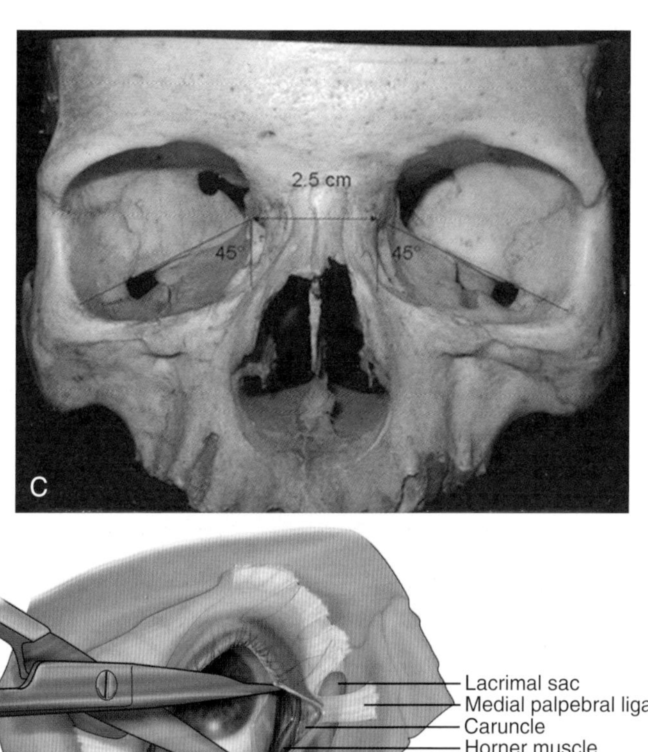

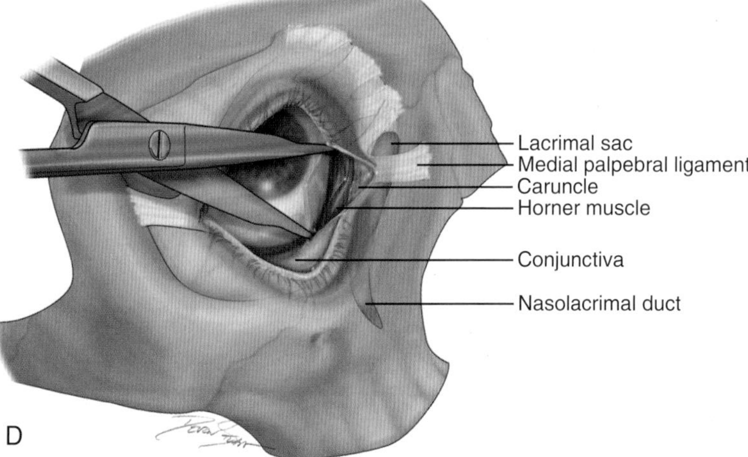

Figure 2.1 cont'd C, Frontal view of both orbits in which the angle formed by each lateral wall with its corresponding medial wall is approximately 45 degrees. The lateral walls themselves are nearly perpendicular to each other. **D,** Using Wescott scissors, the clinician can isolate the posterior lacrimal crest with careful dissection.

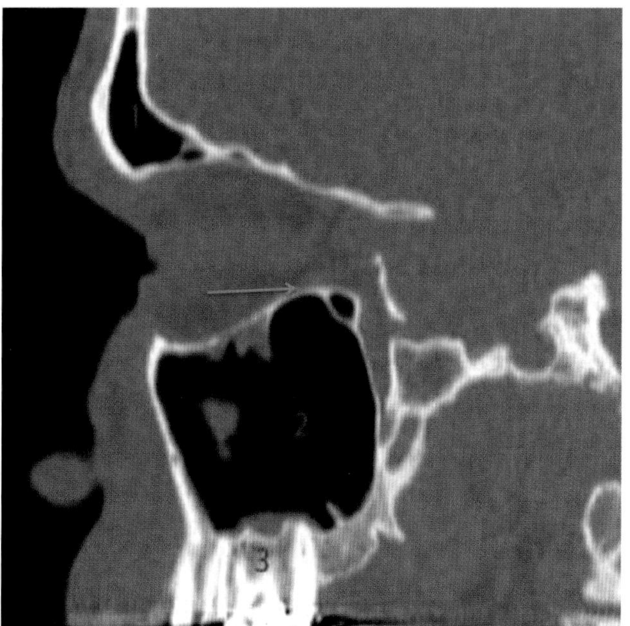

Figure 2.2 Sagittal computed tomography scan of the orbital floor showing the postbulbar bulge/convexity, which must be reproduced during reconstruction to prevent enophthalmos.

over the body of the zygoma. The zygomaticotemporal nerve carries sensory axons to the temporal fossa and postganglionic parasympathetic fibers of the pterygopalatine ganglion to the lacrimal gland by way of an anastomotic branch that connects V2 with the lacrimal nerve (a branch of CN V-1).[1,2] The Whitnall tubercle is a small, bony promontory inside the lateral orbital rim of the zygoma that serves as an attachment for several soft tissue structures.

The lateral walls should form a 45-degree angle at the orbital apex with the medial orbital walls and a 90-degree angle with each other in the axial plane (see Fig. 2.1C).[1] The recurrent meningeal branch of the ophthalmic artery exits the orbit near the posterior aspect of the frontosphenoidal suture at the meningeal foramen, which lies between the roof and lateral wall within the GWS. This artery then anastomoses with the middle meningeal artery, a branch off the first part of the maxillary artery, to supply the dura inside the skull.[2,11,12]

Medial Wall

The medial wall is bounded from anterior to posterior by four bones: the maxillary, lacrimal, and ethmoid bones and the lesser wing of the sphenoid. The lamina papyracea of the ethmoid bone is the thinnest bone in the medial wall, often fracturing in blowout fractures. The medial wall contains two foramina: the anterior ethmoidal foramen and the posterior ethmoidal foramen. The posterior ethmoidal neurovascular bundle is an important landmark for deep orbital dissection. As the surgeon dissects posteriorly, the posterior ethmoidal foramen is located 5 to 10 mm anterior to the optic canal.[1–3]

These foramina are located at the junction between the medial wall and the orbital roof at the frontoethmoidal suture,[13] which denotes the level of the cribriform plate. Both ethmoidal neurovascular bundles leave the orbit at the level of this suture to enter the roof of the nasal cavity.

The lacrimal sac fossa lies anteriorly between the anterior and posterior lacrimal crests (see Fig. 2.1D). The anterior lacrimal crest is within the frontal process of the maxilla, blending with the inferior orbital rim. The posterior lacrimal crest lies within the lacrimal bone. The medial wall displays a slight convexity in the axial plane from front to back, and this should be reproduced in a medial wall plate or mesh during fracture treatment.[1–3,6,7,14,15]

Orbital Apex

The orbital apex is a complex anatomic region that the surgeon must completely understand. All of the important nerves and blood vessels traverse this area. A complete review of the sphenoid bone anatomy is required to understand the orbital apex.[1] The two most important features of the orbital apex are the SOF and the optic canal (see Fig. 2.1A). The optic canal lies between the roof and the end of the medial wall at the orbital apex in the vertical dimension. The optic canal is entirely within the lesser wing of the sphenoid and is oriented laterally in the axial plane. The SOF is between the lesser and greater wings of the sphenoid and houses several important cranial nerves: the oculomotor nerve (CN III), the trochlear nerve (CN IV), the ophthalmic division of the trigeminal nerve (CN V1), and the abducens nerve (CN VI). CN III and VI enter the orbit inside the annulus of Zinn to run within the muscle cone (Fig. 2.3). The tendinous origin of the lateral rectus muscle divides the SOF into two compartments, one superior and one inferior. The area of the SOF encircled by the annulus of Zinn is called the *oculomotor foramen.* The ophthalmic nerve (CN V1) enters the orbit outside the annulus/muscle cone in the superior compartment to proceed forward as the frontal and lacrimal nerves. The trochlear nerve (CN IV) lies in the superior compartment, just outside the annulus of Zinn, in close proximity to the superior ophthalmic veins.[1,3,5,8,12,16,17]

The ophthalmic artery is the first branch off the internal carotid artery (ICA) after it enters the skull (Fig. 2.4). The artery lies below the optic nerve and runs forward in the dural-arachnoid sheath, eventually piercing and then emerging outside the sheath as it exits the optic canal lateral and inferior to the optic nerve. The central retinal artery (CRA) branches off the ophthalmic artery near the lateral rectus muscle origin and reenters the optic nerve sheath on the way to the retina. Because the CRA is an "end artery," the retina has no collateral arterial supply. The ophthalmic artery supplies the muscle cone, globe, and all superior orbital structures. The external carotid artery (ECA) contributes to the lower orbit through the maxillary, infraorbital, zygomaticofacial, and zygomaticotemporal arteries. Thus, the orbit has a dual blood supply from the ICA superiorly and the ECA inferiorly.[1,3,18–20]

The superior ophthalmic veins pass through the SOF outside the muscle cone in the superior compartment and drain to the cavernous sinus. The inferior ophthalmic veins pass through the inferior orbital fissure to communicate with the pterygoid plexus and anastomose with the superior ophthalmic veins posteriorly to drain to the cavernous sinus.[1,3,18,20–24]

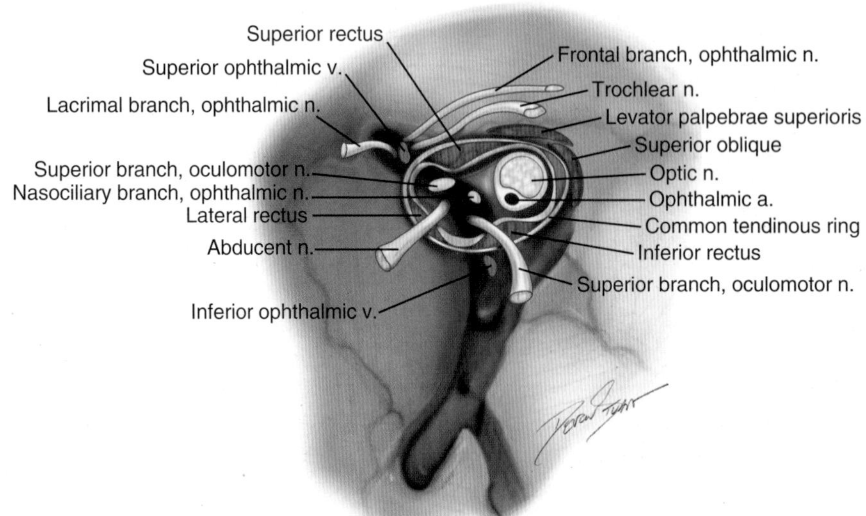

Figure 2.3 The annulus of Zinn encircles the superior orbital fissure, housing the oculomotor and abducens nerves within it. Note the trochlear nerve's position superior to the annulus.

Anteriorly, the superior and inferior ophthalmic veins can communicate with the angular vein on the face, creating the so-called danger triangle. The supposed lack of valves within the angular and ophthalmic veins would allow easy passage of bacterial emboli to the cavernous sinus.[1,3] In 2010, Zhang and Stringer[24] reported finding valves in cadavers using stereomicroscopy. The angular vein was found to drain into the facial vein or the superior ophthalmic vein in this study.

The Soft Tissue Anatomy

Eyelid Anatomy

The eyelids represent composite structures that cover the anterior globe and form the palpebral fissure (Fig. 2.5). The three layers of the lids are called *lamellae* (a single layer is a *lamella*).

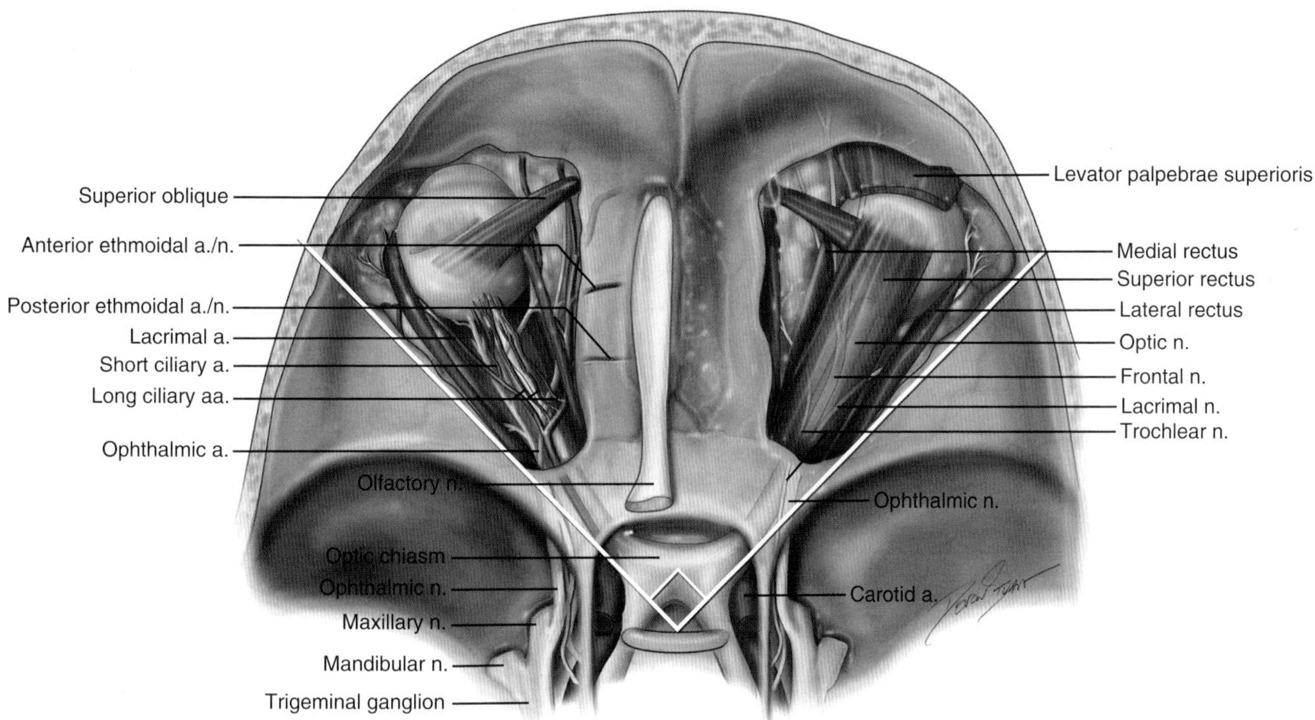

Figure 2.4 Horizontal section through the orbits shows branches of the ophthalmic artery *(left)* and the ophthalmic nerve *(right)*.

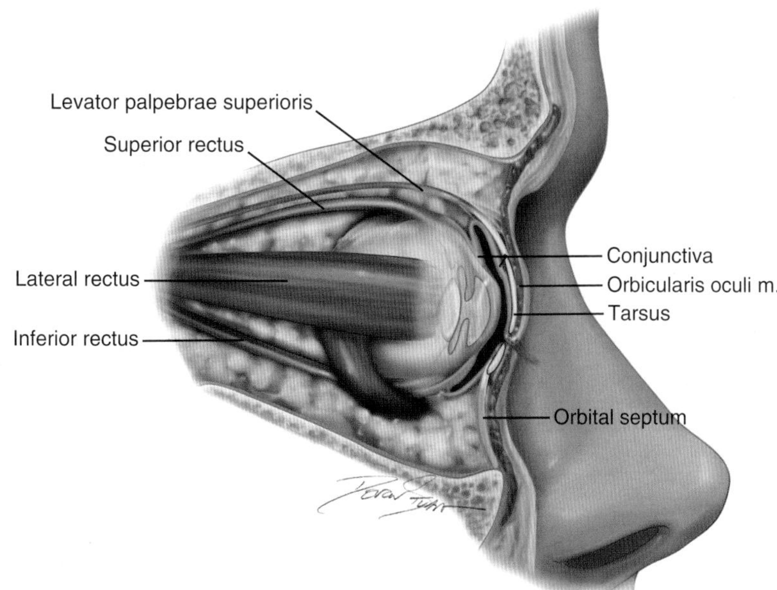

Figure 2.5 The upper and lower eyelids, which are both composed of three distinct layers: the external, middle, and internal layers.

There are three lamellae of the upper lids and three lamellae of the lower lids. In the upper lid, the anterior lamella consists of the skin and orbicularis oculi muscle; the middle lamella is composed of the orbital septum and levator aponeurosis; and the posterior lamella consists of the tarsal plate, Müller muscle, and palpebral conjunctivae. In the lower lid, the anterior lamella is composed of the skin and orbicularis oculi muscle; the middle layer consists of the orbital septum; and the posterior lamella consists of the palpebral conjunctiva, capsulopalpebral fascia (i.e., lower lid retractor), and tarsal plate. The medial and lateral locations where the two eyelids meet are referred to as the *canthi* (singular, *canthus*).[1,3,15,25]

Clinically the orbital septum is an important multilaminated structure. The septum of the upper lid is continuous with the lower, thereby surrounding the orbit 360 degrees.[1] The orbital septum restricts the extraconal fat within the internal orbit. With age, thinning of the orbital septum can occur, leading to anterior herniation of extraconal orbital fat, which may be corrected in cosmetic blepharoplasty. The septum meets the facial periosteum at the arcus marginalis, which closely follows the orbital rim except at the inferolateral region (see Fig. 2.5). On the zygoma, the arcus marginalis dips down onto the face below the orbital rim at the Eisler recess. This variation is important when performing preseptal approaches to the orbital floor. The periosteal incision must dip down laterally on the zygoma below the arcus marginalis in this area.[1] Violation of the orbital septum in this location may result in vertical scar contracture, producing lateral scleral show. Medially, the orbital septum runs in front of the trochlea and inserts into the posterior lacrimal crest.[1,15,26–31]

The dense, fibroelastic connective tissue known as the *tarsal plate* helps stabilize and support the lids. The upper and lower tarsal plates are different sizes in the vertical plane. The upper tarsal plate varies between 9 and 11 mm in height, and the lower tarsal plate is usually 4 to 5 mm in height. The superior tarsal fold in the upper lid is an important landmark for blepharoplasty and trauma approaches. This fold is normally at the junction of the superior border of the upper tarsal plate and the confluence of the orbital septum and levator aponeurosis. Oriented vertically, within the tarsal plates, there are usually 20 meibomian glands, which secrete an oil/sebaceous secretion onto the cornea. This lipid secretion stabilizes the tear film and prevents evaporation of the underlying aqueous layer.[1]

Medial and Lateral Canthal Tendons

In the medial and lateral canthal regions, thin skin overlies the anterior limbs of the tendons. The medial attachment of the upper and lower lids inserts at the anterior and posterior lacrimal crests, resulting in the medial canthus. The anterior limb of the medial canthal tendon (MCT) is more pronounced than its posterior counterpart. The anterior limb inserts into the anterior lacrimal crest of the frontal process of the maxilla. This thick anterior limb protects the common canaliculus and lacrimal sac, which lie below. The thinner posterior limb inserts into the posterior lacrimal crest, which is part of the lacrimal bone. A third vertical limb may be observed where the fascia thickens above the horizontal canthal tendons.[1] Between the anterior and posterior lacrimal crests lies the lacrimal sac fossa; this houses the lacrimal sac, which drains to the nose through the nasolacrimal duct. The vertical limb of the MCT protects the upper portion of the lacrimal sac. A deep head of pretarsal orbicularis oculi inserts onto the posterior lacrimal crest and is called the *Horner muscle* (Fig. 2.6). Identification of the anterior limb of the MCT is crucial when performing canthopexy.[1,7]

The lateral canthus anatomy is less complex than its medial counterpart. The lateral canthal tendon (LCT) has two limbs: the thicker posterior limb and the thinner anterior limb. The posterior limb inserts 4 to 5 mm inside the lateral rim of the zygoma at the Whitnall tubercle, which is 10 mm inferior to the frontozygomatic suture. The majority of the anterior limb is posterior to the orbital septum as it leaves the tarsal plate. Laterally, the anterior limb, periosteum, and orbital septum all blend together at the rim. Between the orbital septum and the anterior limb is a small collection of fat called the *Eisler fat pocket.* The posterior limb of the LCT is part of the structure known as the *lateral retinaculum.* This is a composite structure, and the components are known as the four Ls: the LCT, the lateral horn of the levator aponeurosis, the inferior suspensory ligament of Lockwood, and the check ligament of the lateral rectus muscle.[1,32] The lateral retinaculum inserts directly into the Whitnall tubercle of the zygoma.[1,7,15,25,32] In

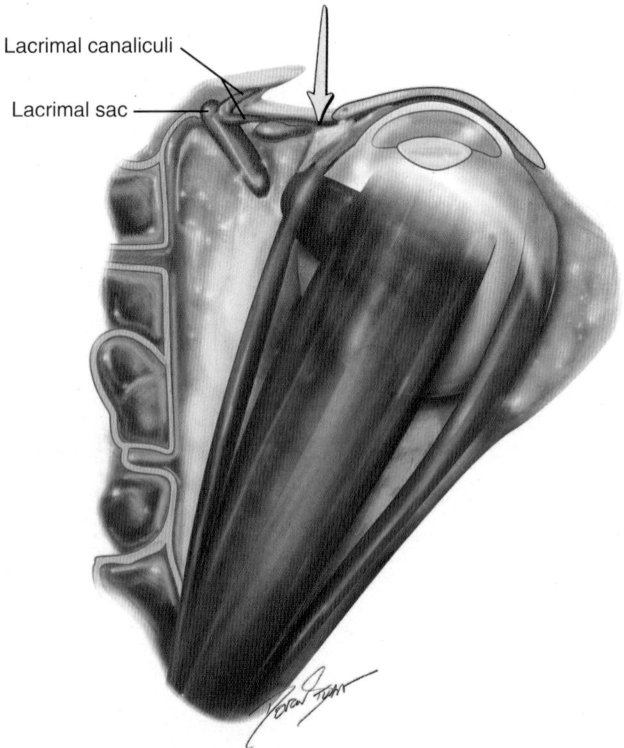

Figure 2.6 Sagittal section through the eyelids; note the attachment of the orbicularis oculi to the posterior lacrimal crest (Horner muscle).

northern European Caucasians, the lateral canthus is approximately 2 mm higher than the medial canthus. In Asians, the lateral canthus is 3 mm or more higher than the medial canthus.[33–36]

Nasolacrimal System and Lacrimal Glands

The paired almond-shaped lacrimal glands help to lubricate the eyes by producing reflex-induced tears. These exocrine glands are housed within the lacrimal fossa of the frontal bone in the lateral orbital roof. The blood supply is primarily from the lacrimal artery, a branch of the ophthalmic artery. Venous drainage from the gland is by the superior ophthalmic vein. Tears are produced by the main gland and accessory lacrimal glands.[1] The lacrimal gland secretes reflex-stimulated tears through postganglionic parasympathetic fibers that arise in the pterygopalatine ganglion. The movement of the eyelids distributes tears over the surface of the eye from lateral to medial.[1] Nonreflex tear secretion (i.e., basic secretion) comes from three sets of small mucin-secreting, goblet-type glands. The main lacrimal gland has an orbital lobe and a palpebral lobe. This division of the gland is produced by the lateral horn of the levator palpebrae muscle. Tear ducts (usually 6 to 12) empty into the superolateral fornix.[1,7,13,15,32]

Movement of tears to the nose occurs through a pump mechanism; the different heads of the orbicularis oculi milk tears to the lacrimal lake and puncta in the medial canthal region. The closing movements of the orbicularis oculi can produce a negative pressure within the lacrimal sac, thereby collecting tears at the puncta. The two puncta drain to the superior and inferior canaliculi, which either join together as a common canaliculus or empty directly into the lacrimal sac. Opening of the lids creates a positive pressure within the lacrimal sac, propelling tears into the nasolacrimal duct. The mucosal folds in the nasolacrimal duct form superior and inferior valvelike structures. The superior fold is known as the valve of Rosenmuller; the inferior fold is called the valve of Hasner.[1,3] Damage to the lacrimal drainage system, as can occur with nasoorbitoethmoid fractures and lacerations, interferes with tear drainage and can produce epiphora. The nasolacrimal duct is continuous above with the lacrimal sac fossa, which houses the lacrimal sac, and below with the inferior meatus of the lateral nasal wall.

Intraconal and Extraconal Orbital Fat

The orbital fat can be divided into two compartments by the muscle cone. Extraconal fat surrounds the muscle cone and is present within the bony orbit confined by the periorbita and orbital septum. In fractures of the orbit walls, this fat may herniate into the paranasal sinuses, infratemporal fossa, and possibly the anterior cranial fossa with blowout fractures of the orbital roof. During fracture treatment, this fat should be reduced into the bony orbit before reconstruction of the walls.[7,32]

The intraconal fat surrounds the optic nerve, blood vessels, and other sensory and motor nerves within the muscle cone. The intraconal fat is maintained by an intermuscular fascial system (i.e., intermuscular septa) that envelops the four rectus muscles, producing the cone shape.[1,28,29]

Orbital and Periorbital Muscles

The orbital muscles may be classified as intrinsic or extrinsic. There are seven skeletal muscles internally (intrinsic) within the bony orbit, six extraocular muscles, and the lone levator palpebrae muscle of the upper lid. All of the extraocular muscles originate at or near the annulus of Zinn, except the inferior oblique muscle (IOM). Thus, the four rectus, superior oblique, and levator palpebrae muscles all originate proximally and insert distally onto the globe or in the upper lid. The levator palpebrae muscle inserts into the tarsal plate of the upper lid through an aponeurosis that begins at the vertical equator of the globe.[1,3,32] The IOM originates in the anteromedial orbit, immediately lateral to the nasolacrimal duct behind the orbital rim. It travels obliquely below the inferior rectus and is encircled by the Lockwood ligament to insert on the globe. This places the muscle origin in jeopardy during orbital floor dissections. Subperiosteal dissection must be performed in the anteromedial orbit to avoid damage to this orbital muscle.[1,3,32]

The levator palpebrae muscle works in concert with a small, smooth muscle (i.e., the superior tarsal muscle, or the Müller muscle) to elevate the upper eyelid.[1,3] The levator palpebrae muscle is a voluntary skeletal muscle, innervated by the superior division of the oculomotor nerve (CN III). Damage from trauma or iatrogenic injury produces a severe ptosis of the upper lid. In the lower lid, the capsulopalpebral fascia is considered to be the retractor of the lid. This fascial extension from the inferior rectus travels forward to split and envelop the IOM. When the two limbs reunite, the resulting component is considered the transverse-oriented Lockwood ligament. The capsulopalpebral fascia then inserts into the inferior border of the lower tarsus. Some fibers may also travel forward to insert into the subcutaneous tissue below the tarsus to create a lower eyelid crease.[1]

The Müller muscle is an involuntary smooth muscle that originates from the levator palpebrae muscle and inserts into the superior edge of the tarsus. It is innervated by the sympathetic nervous system. The postganglionic sympathetic fibers travel from the superior cervical ganglion of the cervical trunk to the orbit by the ICA plexus and finally to the smooth muscle through the oculomotor nerve (CN III) and branches of the ophthalmic nerve (CN V1).[32] Interruption of these fibers produces Horner syndrome, with the characteristic ipsilateral mild ptosis, facial anhidrosis, miosis of the pupil, and pseudoexophthalmos. The inferior tarsal muscle of the lower eyelid arises from the capsulopalpebral fascia to insert into the lower tarsus.[1] However, in certain patients (or cadavers), it cannot be identified as easily as the superior Müller muscle.

The extrinsic muscles that constitute the majority of the eyelids are the fibers of the orbicularis oculi. The orbicularis oculi is innervated by the temporal and zygomatic branches of the facial nerve. The orbicularis oculi constitutes part of the anterior lamellae of the upper and lower lids and forms a sphincter around the palpebral fissure. The orbicularis oculi is divided into an orbital portion and a palpebral portion. The palpebral portion is further divided into pretarsal and preseptal portions.[1] Blinking or voluntary winking occurs through contraction of the palpebral portions, whereas forced closure occurs through contraction of the orbital portion.

The blood supply to the eyelids is through terminal vessels (arcades) of the ICA and ECA. The orbicularis oculi is an antagonist to the levator palpebrae and lower lid retractors and acts to close the eyelids/palpebral fissure. In the upper lid, the orbital portion of the orbicularis covers the corrugator and supercilii muscles. In the lower lid, the orbital portion of the orbicularis oculi covers the zygomaticus major, zygomaticus minor, levator anguli oris, levator labii superioris, and levator of the nasal alae muscles. The orbicularis oculi has its origins medially along the superomedial orbital rim and MCT and inferiorly along the inferomedial rim and frontal process of the maxilla. As with other muscles of facial expression, it is enveloped by the superficial musculoaponeurotic system (SMAS). The SMAS then inserts into the dermis of the facial skin.[1,3,15,32]

Summary

Familiarity with the orbital anatomy is of paramount importance for the surgeon performing orbital surgery. This knowledge reduces the possibility of complications, which can be devastating.

References

1. Zide BM, Jelks GW. *Surgical Anatomy of the Orbit*. New York: Raven Press; 1985.
2. Rene C. Update on orbital anatomy. *Eye (Lond)*. 2006;20(10):1119–1129.
3. Hollinshead W. *Anatomy for Surgeons*. 3rd ed. Philadelphia, Pennsylvania: Harper & Row; 1982.
4. Tandon R, Aljadeff L, Ji S, Finn RA. Anatomic variability of the human orbit. *J Oral Maxillofac Surg*. 2020;78(5):782–796.
5. Evans BT, Webb AAC. Post-traumatic orbital reconstruction: anatomical landmarks and the concept of the deep orbit. *Br J Oral Maxillofac Surg*. 2007;45(3):183–189.
6. Abed S, Shams P, Shen S, et al. Surgical anatomy of the Caucasian orbit: a cadaveric study of the cranio-orbital foramen. *Br J Oral Maxillofac Surg*. 2010;48(suppl 1):S6.
7. Hammer B. *Orbital Fractures: Diagnosis, Operative Treatment and Secondary Corrections*. Seattle, Washington: Hogrefe & Huber; 1995.
8. Kerans G, Evans BT, Webb AAC. Surgical anatomy of the deep orbit: assessment of individual variation to aid safe orbital dissection. *Br J Oral Maxillofac Surg*. 2011;49(suppl 1):S18.
9. Manson PN, Clifford CM, Su CT, et al. Mechanisms of global support and posttraumatic enophthalmos. I. The anatomy of the ligament sling and its relation to intramuscular cone orbital fat. *Plast Reconstr Surg*. 1986;77(2):193–202.
10. Worthington JP. Isolated posterior orbital floor fractures, diplopia and oculocardiac reflexes: a 10-year review. *Br J Oral Maxillofac Surg*. 2010;48(2):127–330.
11. Beden U, Edizer M, Elmali M, et al. Surgical anatomy of the deep lateral orbital wall. *Eur J Ophthalmol*. 2007;17(3):281–286.
12. Willems PWA, Farb RI, Agid R. Endovascular treatment of epistaxis. *Am J Neuroradiol*. 2009;30(9):1637–1645.
13. Gotwald TF, Menzler A, Beauchamp NJ, et al. Paranasal and orbital anatomy revisited: identification of the ethmoid arteries on coronal CT scans. *Crit Rev Comput Tomogr*. 2003;44(5):263–278.
14. Aviv RI, Casselman J. Orbital imaging. Part 1. Normal anatomy. *Clin Radiol*. 2005;60(3):279–287.
15. Bilyk JR. Periocular and orbital anatomy. *Curr Opin Ophthalmol*. 1995;6(5):53–58.
16. Daniels DL, Mark LP, Mafee MF, et al. Osseous anatomy of the orbital apex. *Am J Neuroradiol*. 1995;16(9):1929–1935.
17. Ettl A, Zwrtek K, Daxer A, Salomonowitz E. Anatomy of the orbital apex and cavernous sinus on high-resolution magnetic resonance images. *Surv Ophthalmol*. 2000;44(4):303–323.
18. Hayreh SS. Orbital vascular anatomy. *Eye (Lond)*. 2006;20(10):1130–1144.
19. McNab A. Orbital vascular anatomy and vascular lesions. *Orbit*. 2003;22(2):77–79.
20. Vignaud J, Hasso AN, Lasjaunias P, Clay C. Orbital vascular anatomy and embryology. *Radiology*. 1974;111(3):617–626.
21. Brismar J. Orbital phlebography. II. Anatomy of superior ophthalmic vein and its tributaries. *Acta Radiol Diagn (Stockh)*. 1974;15(5):481–496.
22. Bruna J. Orbital venography: examination methods, anatomy of the venous orbital system, normal orbital venogram. *Cesk Radiol*. 1972;26(5):299–303.
23. Dayton GO. Orbital venography: anatomy, technique, and diagnostic use. *Trans Am Ophthalmol Soc*. 1977;75:459–504.
24. Zhang J, Stringer MD. Ophthalmic and facial veins are not valveless. *Clin Exp Ophthalmol*. 2010;38(5):502–510.
25. Jelks GW, Jelks EB. The influence of orbital and eyelid anatomy on the palpebral aperture. *Clin Plast Surg*. 1991;18(1):183–195.
26. Hoffmann KT, Hosten N, Lemke AJ, et al. Septum orbitale: high-resolution MR in orbital anatomy. *Am J Neuroradiol*. 1998;19(1):91–94.
27. Jordan DR. Anatomy of the orbital septum. *Ophthal Plast Reconstr Surg*. 1993;9(2):150–151.
28. Koornneef L. Orbital septa: anatomy and function. *Ophthalmology*. 1979;86(4):876–880.
29. Koornneef L, Zonneveld FW. Orbital anatomy: the direct scanning of the orbit in three planes and their bearings on the treatment of motility disturbances of the eye after orbital "blow-out" fractures. *Acta Morphol Neerl-Scand*. 1985;23(3):229–246.
30. Meyer DR, Linberg JV, Wobig JL, McCormick SA. Anatomy of the orbital septum and associated eyelid connective tissues: implications for ptosis surgery. *Ophthal Plast Reconstr Surg*. 1991;7(2):104–113.
31. Putterman AM, Urist MJ. Surgical anatomy of the orbital septum. *Ann Ophthalmol*. 1974;6(3):290–294.
32. Turvey TA, Golden BA. Orbital anatomy for the surgeon. *Oral Maxillofac Surg Clin North Am*. 2012;24(4):525–536.
33. Rosenstein T, Talebzadeh N, Pogrel MA. Anatomy of the lateral canthal tendon. *Oral Surg Oral Med Oral Pathol Oral Radiol Endod*. 2000;89(1):24–28.
34. Gioia VM, Linberg JV, McCormick SA. The anatomy of the lateral canthal tendon. *Arch Ophthalmol*. 1987;105(4):529–532.
35. Ousterhout DK, Weil RB. The role of the lateral canthal tendon in lower eyelid laxity. *Plast Reconstr Surg*. 1982;69(4):620–623.
36. Parent AD, Das SK, Mallette RA, Haines DE. Significance of the lateral canthal tendon in craniofacial surgery. *Pediatr Neurosurg*. 1993;19(2):73–77.

CHAPTER 3

The Paranasal Sinuses

Shyam Prasad Aravindaksha

The literature on the anatomy and physiology of the paranasal sinuses goes back to the time of Galen (AD 130–201), who referred to the "porosity" of the bones of the head.[1] Leonardo da Vinci (1452–1519), whose classical sections of the head illustrate the maxillary antrum and the frontal sinus, apparently recognized the existence of these cavities as separate functional entities.[1] He also referred to the maxillary sinus as "the cavity of the bone which supports the cheek." In 1651 Highmore[2] was the first to give a detailed description of the maxillary antrum (antrum of Highmore). However, it was only in the late 19th century that the first detailed and systematic anatomic and pathologic descriptions of the paranasal sinuses were published by Zuckerkandl. These descriptions became even more valuable because they could be applied directly to patients and their problems.

The invention of the X-ray technique did not add much to the anatomic knowledge of the sinuses. However, computed tomography (CT), available since the mid-1970s, made the relationship between the largest sinuses and the ethmoids very clear, applying the knowledge that had been developed more than 100 years earlier. Comparisons of CT images with the drawings of Onodi, Grunwald, and Zuckerkandl demonstrate the incredible accuracy of the knowledge of these pioneers.[3]

The paranasal sinuses form a complex unit of four paired air-filled cavities at the entrance of the upper airway: the ethmoidal, sphenoidal, maxillary, and frontal sinuses (Fig. 3.1). Each of the sinuses is named according to the bone in which it is found. The paranasal sinuses develop as outgrowths from the nasal cavities and erode into the surrounding bones. All these cavities are lined by respiratory mucosa, which is ciliated and secretes mucus. All the paranasal sinuses open into the nasal cavity (Fig. 3.2). These sinuses are innervated by the branches of the trigeminal nerve (Fig. 3.3).

The paranasal sinuses start developing from ridges and furrows in the lateral nasal wall as early as the eighth week of embryogenesis, and they continue pneumatization until early adulthood.[4] As mentioned, each one is named after the skull bone in which it is located.[5,6] However, during the development of a sinus, pneumatization may involve adjacent bones; for example, the ethmoid sinus develops into the frontal, maxillary, or sphenoid bone, and the maxillary sinus extends into the zygomatic bone.

All sinuses are lined by a respiratory pseudostratified epithelium composed of four major types of cells: ciliated columnar cells, nonciliated columnar cells, goblet-type mucous cells, and basal cells.

This mucosa is directly attached to bone and is referred to as the *mucoperiosteum.* Although it is somewhat thinner, the mucoperiosteum of the sinuses is continuous with that of the nasal cavity through the various ostia of the sinuses.[7] The ostium is a natural opening through which the sinus cavity drains into the airway, either directly into the nasal cavity (sphenoid ostium) or indirectly by means of more complex anatomic structures (frontal recess).

Ethmoid Sinus

The ethmoid sinus begins forming in the third to fourth month of fetal life as evaginations of the lateral nasal wall. At birth the anterior ethmoid cells are aerated, whereas the posterior ethmoid cells are fluid filled. The posterior ethmoid air cells pneumatize with advancing age, and air replaces the fluid in these cells. The last air cells to finish forming are the anterior-most agger nasi and bulla cells.[8] When pneumatization is complete, the average size of the anterior ethmoid cells is 20–24 mm × 20–24 mm × 10–12 mm, and the average size of the posterior ethmoid cells is 20–21 mm × 20–22 mm × 10–12 mm.[3]

Ethmoid Air Cells

Within the labyrinth lie the ethmoid air cells, which are lined by pseudostratified ciliated columnar epithelium. The ethmoid air cells are bordered medially by the nasal cavity, laterally by the lamina papyracea, and superiorly by the fovea ethmoidalis. The basal lamina of the middle turbinate divides the ethmoid cells into anterior and posterior divisions.[9] The anterior cells empty into the middle meatus, and the posterior cells drain into the superior meatus.

Hajek[10] presented a simplified scheme to describe the location of the ethmoid air cells. Hajek's scheme depicted the air cells as existing in three sets of grooves, which form valleys between four lamellar projections of bone. Anteriorly the unciform groove (hiatus semilunaris) is formed by the unciform process anteriorly and the ethmoid bulla posteriorly; the hiatus semilunaris is the site of orifices to the frontal sinus, maxillary sinus, and anterior ethmoidal cells. The second groove is the middle meatus, which lies between the ethmoid bulla anteriorly and the middle turbinate posteriorly; the ethmoid bulla located in this lamella is often involved in nasofrontal duct obstruction. The third groove is the superior meatus, which is formed between the middle and superior

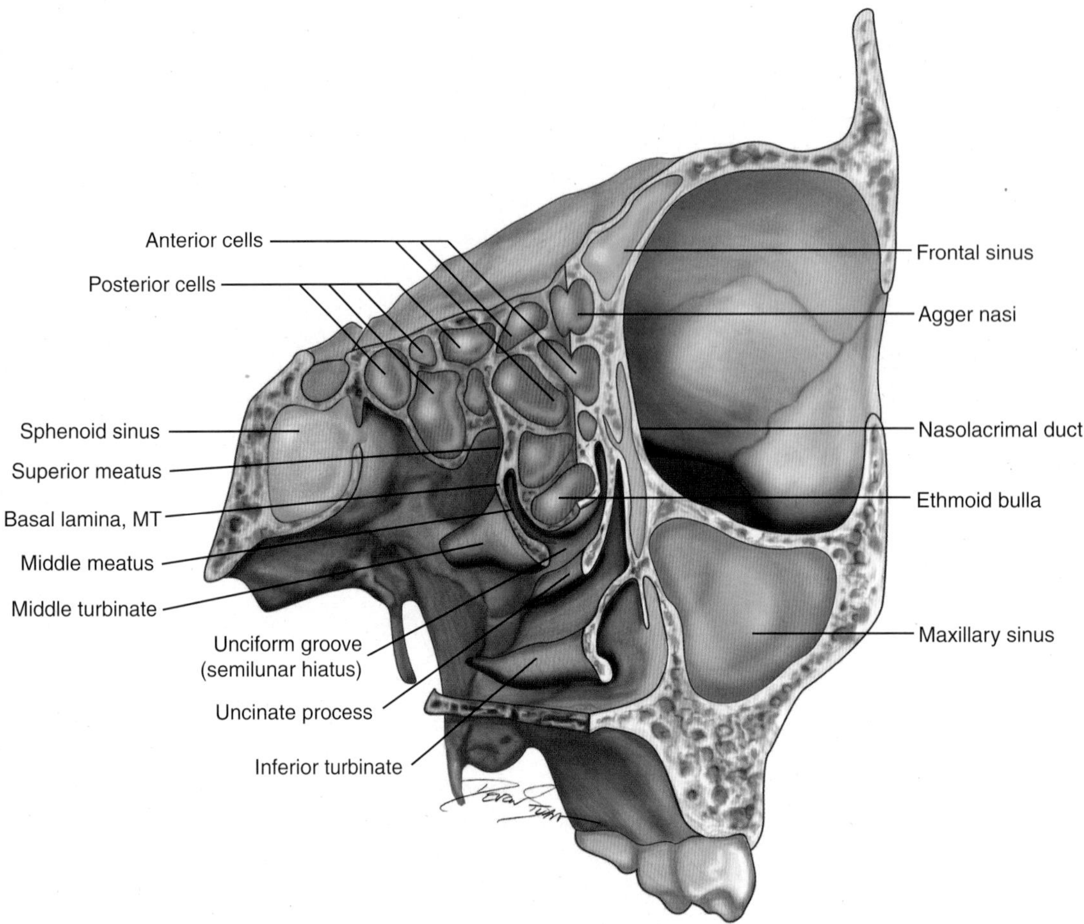

Figure 3.1 Paramedian view of the right nasal cavity, with coronal section through the maxillary sinus.

turbinates (Fig. 3.4).[5] The number of ethmoid cells varies by individual; however, seven smaller anterior cells and four larger posterior cells are typically present. The posterior air cells occasionally present as two very large air cells.[8] The uncinate groove is the most anterior and has three to four air cells at its superior border. At the middle meatus are one to two agger nasi cells, and posterior to the agger nasi is the ethmoid bulla that contains a superior and inferior cell.[11] The posterior ethmoid air cells drain via the superior meatus. The anterior ethmoid air cells drain via the middle meatus. Arterial supply to the ethmoid air cells is via the ethmoidal arteries that are branches from the ophthalmic artery. The anterior ethmoidal artery enters the anterior ethmoid foramen 24 mm posterior to the anterior lacrimal crest and supplies the anterior ethmoid air cells. The posterior ethmoidal artery enters the posterior ethmoid foramen 36 mm posterior to the anterior lacrimal crest and supplies the posterior ethmoidal air cells.[12] Venous drainage is via the named veins accompanying the arteries to the superior ophthalmic vein or pterygopalatine plexus. Lymphatic drainage from the anterior ethmoid cells is via the submandibular nodes, and the posterior ethmoid cells drain via the retropharyngeal nodes. Innervation is via anterior and posterior ethmoid nerves of the ophthalmic nerve (V1) and the posterior nasal branch of the maxillary nerve (V2).[3]

Maxillary Sinus

The maxillary sinus begins developing in the third week of gestation. In the twelfth week of gestation, the maxillary sinus forms as an ectodermal invagination from the middle meatal groove and grows internally to a size that at birth is approximately 7 mm × 4 mm × 4 mm and has a volume of 6 to 8 mL.[13] In utero the maxillary sinus is fluid filled; however, after birth the maxillary sinus pneumatizes in relation with biphasic rapid growth: during the first 3 years of life and then again from ages 7 to 12 years. By 12 years of age, the sinus is level with the floor of the nasal cavity[12]; however, as further pneumatization occurs into adulthood, with the eruption of the adult molars, the floor of the sinus descends to approximately 1 cm below the floor of the nasal cavity.[14]

The maxillary sinuses are paired paranasal sinuses that develop around the adult dentition to a volume of 15 mL, although the volume is smaller in children and enlarges with the sinus pneumatization that occurs with advancing age. These sinuses span from the region of the third molar posteriorly to the premolar teeth anteriorly. The dimensions of the sinus vary and range from 25 to 35 mm mesiodistal width, 36 to 45 mm vertical height, and 38 to 45 mm deep anteroposteriorly.[15] Mesiodistal width differences are usually attributed

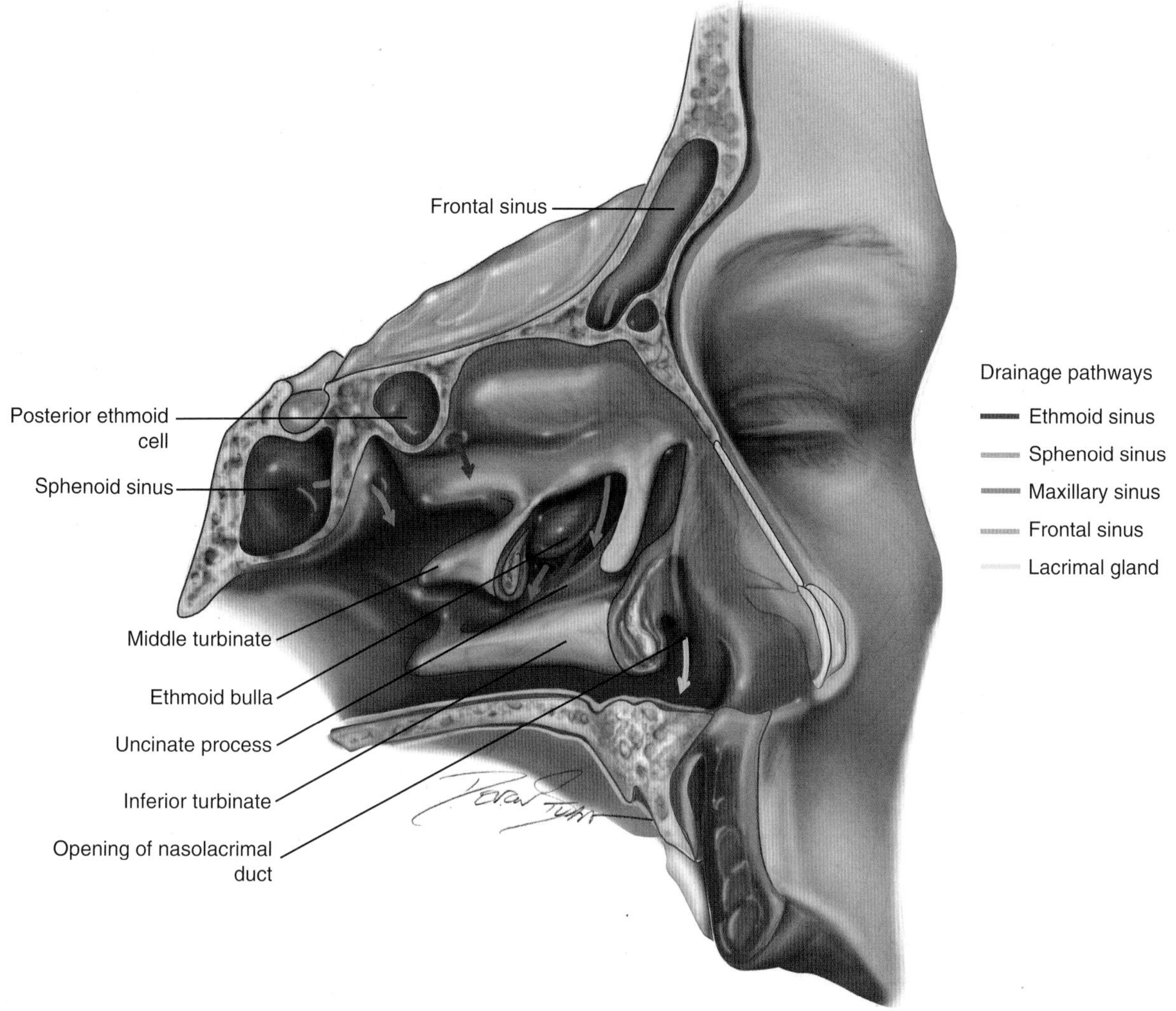

Frontal sinus
Posterior ethmoid cell
Sphenoid sinus
Middle turbinate
Ethmoid bulla
Uncinate process
Inferior turbinate
Opening of nasolacrimal duct
Drainage pathways
Ethmoid sinus
Sphenoid sinus
Maxillary sinus
Frontal sinus
Lacrimal gland

Figure 3.2 Lateral wall of the nasal cavity, illustrating the communication of the paranasal sinuses with the nasal cavity.

Anterior ethmoid n.
Septal branch of anterior ethmoid n.
Olfactory n.
Nasopalatine n.
Posterior superior lateral nasal nn.
Posterior inferior lateral nasal nn.

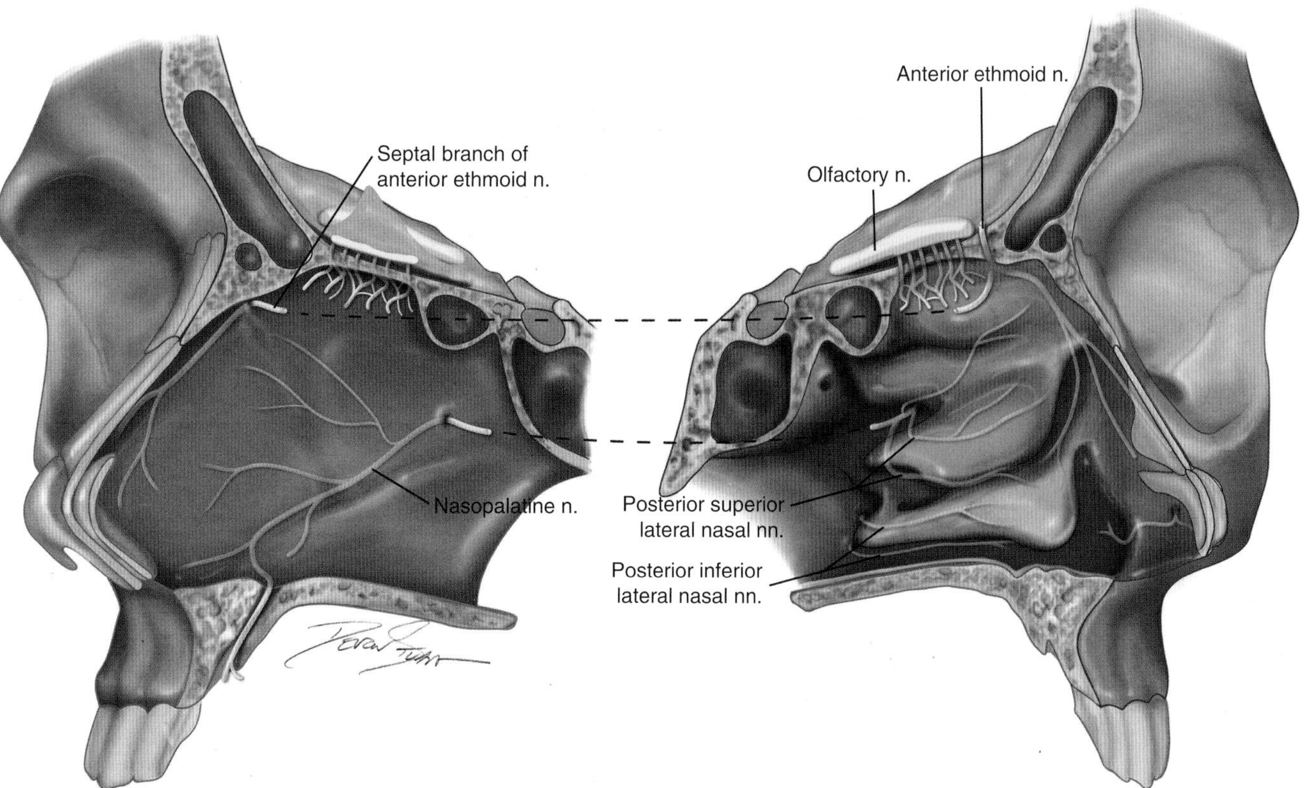

Figure 3.3 Nerve supply of the paranasal sinuses.

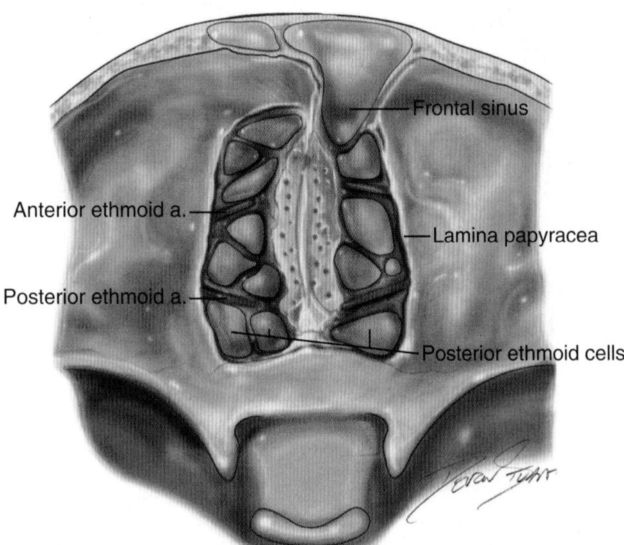

Figure 3.4 Diagram of the anatomy of an ethmoid air cell.

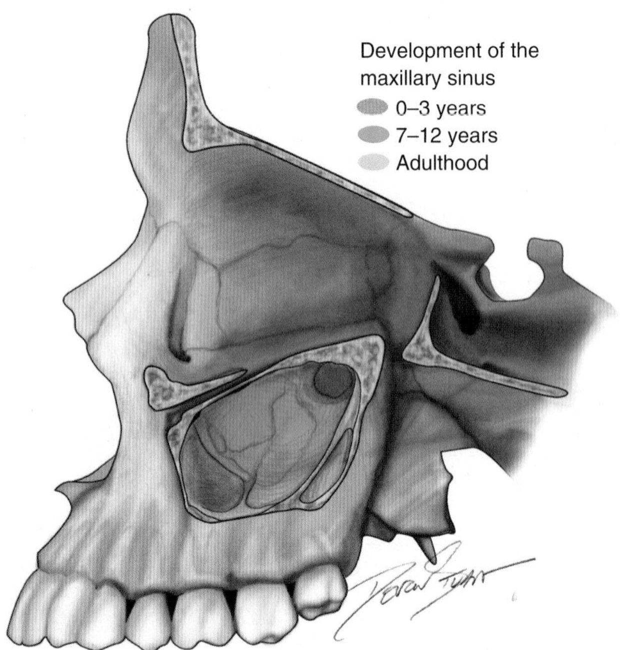

Figure 3.5 Sagittal view of the maxillary sinus anatomy.

to growth toward the zygomatic arch posteriorly rather than toward the canine teeth anteriorly.[8]

The maxillary sinus is shaped like a quadrangular pyramid, with the base facing the lateral nasal wall and the apex oriented at the zygomatic arch. The roof of the sinus contributes to the floor of the orbit, the floor faces the alveolar process, and the sinus proceeds deep and adjacent to the palate. The Schneiderian membrane lines the maxillary sinus and is composed of pseudostratified ciliated columnar epithelium. The concentration of cilia increases with proximity to the sinus ostium. The thickness of this membrane is 0.8 mm. Compared with the nasal mucosa, the antral mucosa is thinner and less vascular.[16] At birth, the maxillary sinus begins medial to the orbit, and its dimensions are largest anteroposteriorly. At 2 years of age, the sinus continues inferiorly below the medial orbit and continues to pneumatize laterally. By 4 years of age, the sinus reaches the infraorbital canal and continues laterally. By 9 years of age, inferior growth reaches the region of the hard palate. Pneumatization continues as the permanent teeth erupt.[17]

The roof of the maxillary sinus contributes to the floor of the orbit. The roof contains the infraorbital neurovascular bundle. The infraorbital foramen opens approximately 1 cm below the infraorbital rim.[18] The floor of the maxillary sinus abuts the alveolar process of the maxilla, frequently approximating the apices of the molar teeth (see the next section). The inferior extent of the sinus floor is 1 cm inferior to the floor of the nasal cavity. The medial wall of the maxillary sinus houses the sinus ostium at its superomedial aspect and the nasolacrimal duct, through which drainage of the lacrimal apparatus occurs. The maxillary sinus ostium empties into the posterior aspect of the semilunar hiatus. The nasolacrimal duct runs 4 to 9 mm anterior to the sinus ostium and empties at the anterior portion of the inferior meatus.[15]

Sinus development follows a three-compartment model described by Underwood[19] in which these compartments, frequently separated by septa, are associated with three different dental milestones. The anterior compartment forms around the primary molars between 8 and 24 months of age. The middle compartment forms around the adult first and second molars from 5 to 12 years of age. The posterior compartment forms around the third molars from 16 to 30 years of age.[19,20] The most inferior portion of the maxillary sinus is in the region of the first molar.[8] The distance from the sinus floor to the root tips of the teeth is longest for the first premolar and shortest for the second molar distobuccal root tip.[21] The roots of the maxillary first and second molars communicate with the floor of the maxillary sinus with an incidence of 40%.[22] The palatine roots of these teeth are 50% closer to the antral floor than to the palate, and in 20% of cases apical communication is present between the palatal roots of the maxillary first and second molars with the maxillary sinus (Fig. 3.5 and Table 3.1).[23]

Maxillary Septum

A *septum* is defined as a strut of bone that is at least 2.5 mm in height. Septa within the maxillary sinus are of two varieties. The primary septa are formed as part of the three-compartment model of sinus development and act as dividers of the anterior, middle, and posterior components; they are found between the roots of the second premolar and the first molar and the roots of the first and second molars, and distal to the roots of the third molar. Septa extrinsic to those of maxillary development are called *secondary septa* and occur as a result of pneumatization after dental extraction. The overall prevalence of septa present in any given maxillary sinus is 35%.[19] Septa in edentulous regions tend to be larger than those in partially edentulous regions, which are larger still than the dentate regions of the alveolus.[8] The presence of septae is pertinent for sinus lift procedures because they complicate the process of luxating the bony window to expose the sinus and increase the likelihood of sinus membrane perforation.

The size and number of maxillary sinus ostia are variable. Simon[23] found that the sinus ostium existed as a canal greater than 3 mm in mesiodistal width from the infundibulum to the antral opening in 82.7% of individuals, in contrast to the 13.7% in whom the ostium existed as just an opening. The average length of the sinus ostium is 5.55 mm, and it is oriented inferolaterally from the infundibulum to the antrum to drain the maxillary sinus into the hiatus semilunaris. Approximately 16% of individuals have an accessory ostium (i.e., an ostium opening outside the infundibulum and semilunar hiatus). The accessory ostium typically exists only as an opening and not as a canal, with an average length of 1.5 mm. The clinical significance of the ostium existing as a canal is an appreciation for how readily a canal obstruction can occur (Fig. 3.6).

Table 3.1 Distance From the Roots of the Maxillary Teeth to the Maxillary Sinus Floor

Root	Distance (mm)	SD
Buccal first premolar	6.18	1.60
Lingual first premolar	7.05	1.92
Second premolar	2.86	0.60
Mesiobuccal first molar	2.82	0.59
Palatal first molar	1.56	0.77
Distobuccal first molar	2.79	1.13
Mesiobuccal second molar	0.83	0.49
Palatal second molar	2.04	1.19
Distobuccal second molar	1.97	1.21

Data from Eberhardt JA, Torabinejad M, Christiansen EL. A computed tomographic study of the distances between the maxillary sinus floor and the apices of the maxillary posterior teeth. *Oral Surg Oral Med Oral Pathol.* 1992;73:345.

Harrison[24] presented the anatomic location of the superior alveolar nerves described in this section. The superior alveolar nerves are in intimate relationship to the maxillary sinus. The anterior superior alveolar (ASA) nerve arises 15 mm behind the infraorbital foramen and runs inferiorly in the anterior wall of the maxilla. Occasionally the ASA forms an elevation at the anterior part of the sinus cavity approximately 6 mm inferior to the infraorbital foramen on its way to supply the lateral nasal wall and septum and the anterior maxillary teeth. The middle superior alveolar (MSA) nerve often arises off the infraorbital nerve and courses along the posterolateral or anterior wall of the sinus to supply the premolar teeth. The posterior superior alveolar (PSA) nerve is a branch of the infraorbital nerve that branches off at the posterior end of the infraorbital canal. Two branches of this nerve are usually present: a smaller superior branch and the larger inferior branch. The superior branch of the PSA passes through the antrum and runs posteriorly along the maxillary tuberosity. The inferior branch supplies the molar teeth and joins the MSA and ASA to form the alveolar plexus. The significance of this presentation of the superior alveolar nerves is to point out an area at the anterior region of the maxilla where bone can be safely removed (e.g., Caldwell-Luc procedure), with minimal risk of damage to the superior alveolar nerves.

The maxillary sinus has many anastomoses and receives its arterial supply from the infraorbital, sphenopalatine, posterior lateral nasal, facial, pterygopalatine, greater palatine,

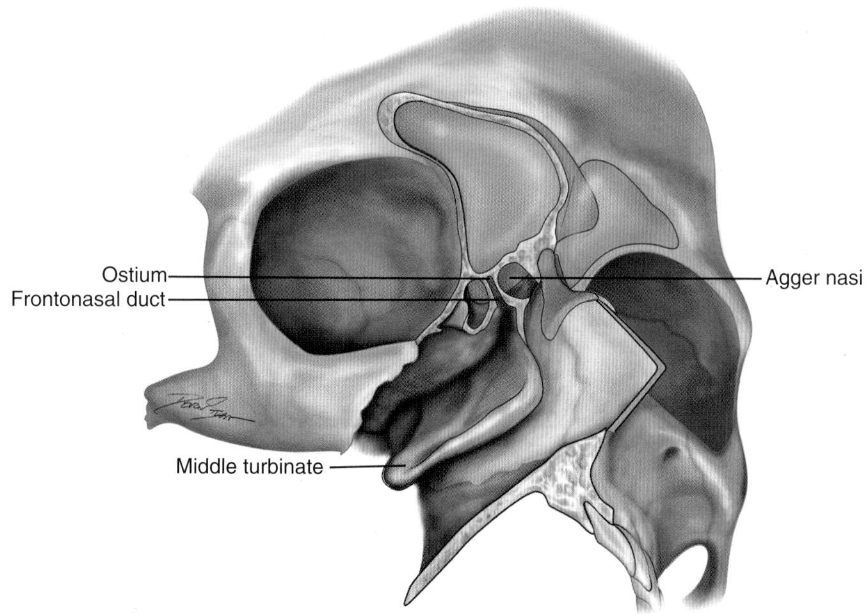

Figure 3.6 Coronal view of the osteomeatal complex.

and PSA arteries. Venous return from the maxillary sinus occurs anteriorly via the cavernous plexus that drains into the facial vein and posteriorly via the pterygoid plexus and to the internal jugular vein. Innervation of the maxillary sinus is via the anterior superior, middle superior, and PSA nerves. Lymphatic drainage occurs through the infraorbital foramen via the ostium to the submandibular lymphatic system.[14]

Frontal Sinus

The frontal sinuses are the most superior of the anterior sinuses. They are situated in the frontal bone between inner and outer plates. The inner plate, or posterior wall (separates the frontal sinus from the anterior cranial fossa), is much thinner than the outer wall and may be penetrated accidentally during surgery.[24] The septum between right and left sides is almost always asymmetrically placed and divides the frontal sinuses into two unequal sinuses. The larger sinus may pass across the midline and overlap the other. The sinuses often have incompletely separated recesses, which make the anatomy highly variable. Superficial surgical landmarks for the frontal sinus were described by Tubbs et al.[25] from adult cadaveric frontal sinus dissections. In their study of 70 adult cadavers, these investigators reported that the lateral wall of the frontal sinus never extended more than 5 mm lateral to a midpupillary line. At this same line and at a plane drawn through the supraorbital ridges, the roof of the frontal sinus was never higher than 12 mm, and in the midline, the roof of the frontal sinus never reached more than 4 cm above the nasion. The frontal sinus is separated from the orbit by a thin triangular plate.

Regarding the lateral extension of the frontal sinuses, the authors have observed several cases in which the lateral extension of the frontal sinuses extended more lateral than described by Tubbs et al.[25] Further, Maves[26] states that the degree of pneumatization of the frontal sinuses varies and that it may extend laterally as far as the sphenoid wing.

The ostium of the frontal sinus lies in the posteromedial aspect of the sinus floor. The front nasal duct opens into the anterior part of the middle meatus and the frontal recess or directly into the anterior end of the infundibulum (Fig. 3.7).

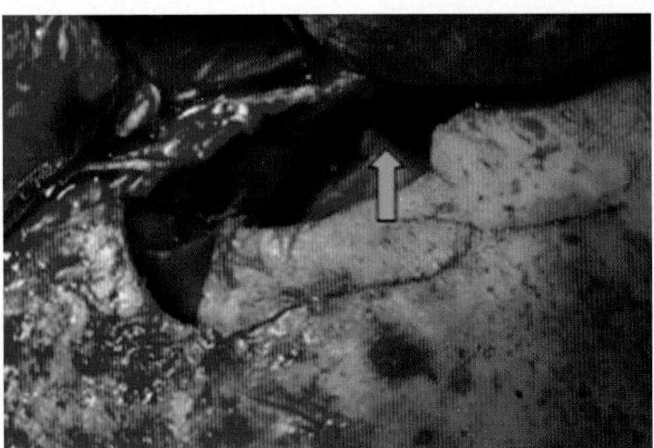

Figure 3.7 Frontonasal duct in situ *(arrow).*

This relationship to the infundibulum and middle meatus serves to protect the frontal sinus from the spread of disease in the osteomeatal complex. The agger nasi is intimately involved, in that the posterior wall of the agger nasi forms the anterior border of the frontal recess, which then passes posteromedially to the agger nasi and supraorbital cells. This recess is present in 77% of patients. In the other 23%, drainage occurs via a frontal sinus ostium.[27] There are also two patterns to the frontal sinus outflow tract: those that drain medial to the uncinate process and those that drain lateral to the uncinate process. Those that drain medially are more common and are significantly related to the presence of frontal sinusitis. The borders of the frontonasal duct are (1) the anterior border, which is the superior portion of the uncinate process; (2) the posterior border, which is the superior portion of the bulla ethmoidalis; (3) the medial border, which is formed by the conchal plate; and (4) the lateral border, which is the suprainfundibular plate.[18] The nasofrontal duct can safely be widened by removing the upper portion of the ground lamella of the ethmoid bulla at the posterior boundary of the nasofrontal duct with cutting forceps.[28]

Besides the different anterior ethmoid cell groups that could be related to the frontal infundibulum, other cells can originate from the frontal recess and, when present, are called the *frontal infundibular cells.* Bent and Kuhn[29] classified the frontal cells into four types:

- Type 1 is a single air cell above the agger nasi
- Type 2 is a group of small cells above the agger nasi but below the orbital roof
- Type 3 is a single cell extending from the agger nasi into the frontal sinus
- Type 4 is an isolated cell within the frontal sinus not contiguous with the agger nasi

The supraorbital and supratrochlear arteries, which branch off the ophthalmic artery, form the arterial supply of the frontal sinus. The superior ophthalmic vein provides venous drainage. Actual venous drainage for the inner table, however, is through the dura mater and the cranial periosteum for the outer table. These veins are in addition to the diploic veins and all venous structures that communicate in the venous plexuses of the inner table, periorbita, and cranial periosteum.

Sphenoid Sinus

The sphenoid sinuses are located at the skull base at the junction of the anterior and middle cerebral fossae. Their growth starts between the third and fourth months of fetal development, as an invagination of the nasal mucosa into the posterior portion of the cartilaginous nasal capsule.

Between birth and 3 years of age, the sphenoid is primarily a pit in the sphenoethmoid recess. Pneumatization of the sphenoid bone starts at age 3, extends toward the sella turcica by age 7, and reaches its final form in adolescence.[2] The two sinuses generally develop asymmetrically, separated by the intersinus bony septum. In some cases, because of this asymmetry, the intersinus septum goes off the midline and can have a posterior insertion on the bony carotid canal, in the lateral wall of the sphenoid.[30] For this reason, caution must be used when removing the septum in these cases because a brisk avulsion may result in carotid rupture.

Pneumatization of the sphenoid can invade the anterior and posterior clinoid processes, the posterior part of the nasal septum, and the vomer. The sphenoid sinus drains through a single ostium into the sphenoethmoid recess. This ostium is classically situated 7 cm from the base of the columella at an angle of 30 degrees to the floor of the nose in a parasagittal plane; this usually corresponds to a location halfway up the anterior wall of the sinus. The superior wall of the sphenoid sinus usually represents the floor of the sella turcica.

Depending on the extent of pneumatization, the sphenoid sinus can be classified into three types[2]:

1. Conchal: The area below the sella is a solid block of bone without pneumatization.
2. Presellar: The sphenoid is pneumatized to the level of the frontal plane of the sella and not beyond.
3. Sellar: The most common type, in which pneumatization extends into the body of the sphenoid beyond the floor of the sella, sometimes reaching the clivus.

The lateral wall of the sphenoid sinus can show various prominences, the most important being the carotid canal and the optic canal. The internal carotid artery, the most medial structure in the cavernous sinus, rests against the lateral surface of the sphenoid bone. Its prominence within the sphenoid varies from a focal bulge to a serpiginous elevation marking the full course of the intracavernous portion of the carotid artery from posteroinferior to posterosuperior (Fig. 3.8).[2] In some cases, even without advanced sinus disease, dehiscence in the bony margin can be present, and this should be particularly looked for on the CT scan.[30]

The optic canal is found in the posterosuperior angle between the lateral, posterior, and superior walls of the sinus, horizontally crossing the carotid canal from lateral to medial (see Fig. 3.8). Pneumatization of the sphenoid above and below the optic canal can result in a supraoptic recess and an infraoptic recess (the opticocarotid recess), respectively. The infraoptic recess lies between the optic nerve superiorly and the carotid canal inferiorly and can sometimes pneumatize the anterior clinoid process.[2]

The canals of two other nerves may be encountered in the lateral wall of the sphenoid sinus, below the level of the carotid canal: the second branch of the trigeminal nerve superiorly through the foramen rotundum and the vidian nerve in the pterygoid canal inferiorly (see Fig. 3.8).[2]

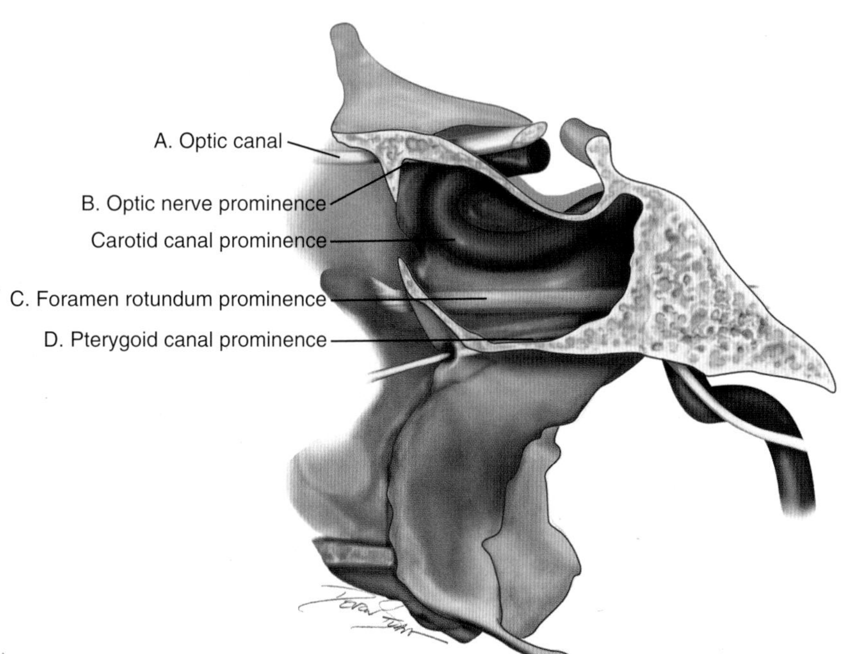

Figure 3.8 Simplified drawing of a lateral wall of the left sphenoid sinus. The optic canal (A) runs from anterolateral to posteromedial in the most superior aspect of the lateral wall. The carotid prominence (B) is usually seen at the junction of the posterior and lateral walls. Note the supraoptic recess (above A) and the infraoptic or opticocarotid recess (between A and B). The canals for the second branch of the trigeminal nerve (C) and the vidian nerve (D) can sometimes be endoscopically identified and define the superior and inferior boundaries of the lateral recess (between C and D) in a very pneumatized sphenoid.

References

1. Surgical anatomy of the paranasal sinuses. In: Kountakis SE, Onerci TM, eds. *Rhinologic and Sleep Apnea Surgical Techniques*. Berlin Heidelberg, Germany: Springer; 2007.
2. Surgical anatomy of the paranasal sinuses. In: Zoukaa B, Sargi RR, eds. *Rhinologic and Sleep Apnea Surgical Techniques*. Berlin Heidelberg, Germany: Springer; 2007.
3. Snow Jr JB, Ballenger JJ. Anatomy and physiology of the nose and paranasal sinuses. In: Snow JR JB, Ballenger JJ, eds. *Ballenger's Otorhinolaryngology Head and Neck Surgery*. 16th ed. Hamilton, Ontario: Decker; 2003.
4. Bolger WE. Anatomy of the paranasal sinuses. In: Kennedy DW, Bolger WE, Zinreich J, eds. *Diseases of the Sinuses: Diagnosis and Management*. New York: Decker; 2001.
5. Graney DO, Rice DH. Paranasal sinuses anatomy. In: Cummings CW, Fredrickson JM, Harker LA, et al., eds. *Otolaryngology Head and Neck Surgery*. 3rd ed. St Louis, Missouri: Mosby; 1998.
6. Van Cauwenberge P, Sys L, De Belder T, et al. Anatomy and physiology of the nose and the paranasal sinuses. *Immunol Allergy Clin North Am*. 2004;24:1–17.
7. Mosher HP. The applied anatomy and the intranasal surgery of the ethmoidal labyrinth. *Laryngoscope*. 1913;23:881.
8. Orrett E, Ogle RJ, Weinstock EF. Surgical anatomy of the nasal cavity and paranasal sinuses. *Oral Maxillofac Surg Clin North Am*. 2012;24(2):155–166.
9. Stammberger HR, Kennedy DW. Paranasal sinuses: anatomic terminology and nomenclature—the Anatomic Terminology Group. *Ann Otol Rhinol Laryngol Suppl*. 1995;167:7–16.
10. Ogle OE, Dym H. Surgery of the nose and paranasal sinuses. *Oral Maxillofac Surg Clin North Am*. 2012;24(2):13–14.
11. Ellis III E, Zide MF. Coronal approach. In: Ellis III E, Zide MF, eds. *Surgical Approaches to the Facial Skeleton*. 2nd ed. Philadelphia, Pennsylvania: Lippincott Williams & Wilkins; 2006.
12. Lawson W, Patel ZM, Lin FY. The development and pathologic processes that influence maxillary sinus pneumatization. *Anat Rec*. 2008;291(11):1554–1563.
13. Som P, Curtin H. *Head and Neck Imaging*. 5th ed. St. Louis, Missouri: Elsevier; 2011.
14. Smiler DG, Soltan M, Shostine MS, et al. *Oral and Maxillofacial Surgery*. 2nd ed. St Louis, Missouri: Mosby; 2009.
15. Van den Bergh JP, ten Bruggenkate CM, Disch FJ, et al. Anatomical aspects of sinus floor elevations. *Clin Oral Implants Res*. 2000;11(3):256–265.
16. Woo I, Le BT. Maxillary sinus floor elevation: review of anatomy and two techniques. *Implant Dent*. 2004;13(1):28–32.
17. Scuderi AJ, Harnsberger HR, Boyer RS. Pneumatization of the paranasal sinuses: normal features of importance to the accurate interpretation of CT scans and MR images. *Am J Roentgenol*. 1993;160(5):1101–1104.
18. Hitotsumatsu T, Matsushima T, Rhoton AL. Surgical anatomy of the midface and the midline skull base. *Operat Tech Neurosurg*. 1999;2:160.
19. Underwood AS. An inquiry into the anatomy and pathology of the maxillary sinus. *J Anat Physiol*. 1910;44(Pt 4):354–369.
20. Maestre-Ferrı́n L, Galán-Gil S, Rubio-Serrano M, et al. Maxillary sinus septa: a systematic review. *Med Oral Patol Oral Cir Bucal*. 2010;15(2):e383–e386.
21. Cenk K, Kivanc K, Selcen PY, et al. An assessment of the relationship between the maxillary sinus floor and the maxillary posterior teeth root tips using dental cone-beam computerized tomography. *Eur J Dent*. 2010;4(4):462–467.
22. Wallace JA. Transantral endodontic surgery. *Oral Surg Oral Med Oral Pathol*. 1996;82(1):80–83.
23. Simon E. Anatomy of the opening of the maxillary sinus. *Arch Otolaryngol*. 1939;29:640.
24. Harrison D. Surgical anatomy of maxillary and ethmoid sinuses. *Laryngoscope*. 1971;81(10):1658–1664.
25. Tubbs RS, Elton S, Salter G, et al. Superficial surgical landmarks for the frontal sinus. *J Neurosurg*. 2002;96(2):320–322.
26. Maves MD. Surgical anatomy of the head and neck. In: Bailey BJ, Johnson JT, Newlands SD, eds. *Head and Neck Surgery: Otolaryngology*. Vol 1. Philadelphia, Pennsylvania: Lippincott Williams & Wilkins; 2006.
27. Metson R. Endoscopic treatment of frontal sinusitis. *Laryngoscope*. 1992;102:712.
28. Kim KS, Kim HU, Chung IH, et al. Surgical anatomy of the nasofrontal duct: anatomical and computed tomographic analysis. *Laryngoscope*. 2001;111(4):603–608.
29. Bent J, Kuhn FA, Cuilty C. The frontal cell in frontal recess obstruction. *Am J Rhinol*. 1994;8:185–191.
30. Sethi DS, Stanley RE, Pillay PK. Endoscopic anatomy of the sphenoid sinus and sella turcica. *J Laryngol Otol*. 1995;109(5):951–955.

The Auditory System

Kyle P. Allen

Given the intimate association of the external auditory canal and middle ear space with the temporomandibular joint, it is necessary for oral and maxillofacial surgeons (OMS) to understand the auditory system. Disorders of the temporomandibular joint may sometimes present with primarily aural symptoms such as otalgia or aural fullness. This chapter describes the anatomy of the auditory system with an emphasis on information of interest to OMS.

The peripheral components of the auditory system are housed within or attached to the temporal bone. The auditory system can generally be broken down into several smaller components, including the external ear, the middle ear and mastoid, the inner ear, and the central auditory system. The course of the facial nerve within the fallopian canal of the temporal bone is also important. OMS will also be interested in the adjacent sphenoid bone, the mandibular nerve as it enters the skull base at the foramen ovale, and the middle meningeal artery passing through the foramen spinosum.

Temporal Bone

The temporal bones, which compose a portion of the lateral skull and skull base, have several components: the squamosa, petrous, mastoid, and tympanic portions, and the styloid process. These components are discussed briefly, with a focus on landmarks identified during surgical procedures.

The squamosa (Fig. 4.1) is the lateral, parasagittally oriented flat bone that composes a portion of the lateral skull. The temporalis muscle attaches on its lateral surface, and the middle meningeal artery runs in a groove on its medial surface. On the anterior, inferior surface of the lateral squama, the zygomatic process extends laterally and anteriorly to make up the posterior portion of the zygomatic arch. The zygomatic process is contiguous with a horizontally oriented structure known as the suprameatal crest or temporal line, which runs superior to the external auditory canal. The temporal line is a surgical landmark roughly approximating the level of the floor of the middle cranial fossa. The squamosa forms the superior and anterior aspects of the mandibular or glenoid fossa of the temporomandibular joint. The inferior articular tubercle forms the superior boundary of the mandibular fossa and is lined with a thin layer of cartilage.

The mastoid comprises the posterior temporal bone and is the site of attachment of the sternocleidomastoid, splenius capitis, longissimus capitis, and digastric muscles. The mastoid process is typically aerated with numerous bony air cells. These air cells communicate anteriorly with the mastoid antrum. A groove in the medial mastoid houses the dural sigmoid sinus. The superior border of the mastoid is the bony plate that separates the mastoid from the middle cranial fossa, known as the tegmen mastoideum. During a mastoidectomy (Fig. 4.2), the bone overlying the sigmoid sinus and the tegmen are used as landmarks to indicate the posterior and superior limits of dissection. Medially, dissection can be continued until the lateral semicircular canal is visualized through the mastoid antrum.

The petrous portion is a pyramidal-shaped bone with its apex pointing medially toward the clivus. During procedures within the middle cranial fossa, working on the superior surface, important structures can be identified as surgical landmarks. The arcuate eminence indicates the position of the underlying superior semicircular canal. Medial and anterior to the superior canal is the facial hiatus, where the greater superficial petrosal nerve (GSPN) exits the temporal bone to travel on the superior surface of the petrous bone.[1] The posterior, medial (Fig. 4.3) surface of the petrous portion of the temporal bone forms the anterior boundary of the posterior cranial fossa. The internal auditory canal is located in this region and contains the seventh and eight cranial nerves as they travel laterally. The complicated inferior surface of the petrous bone (see Fig. 4.1) includes the carotid canal and jugular bulb. The petrous apex is the most medial portion of the petrous bone, lying medial to the labyrinth. It is pneumatized in a minority of patients (30%) and otherwise composed of bone and marrow.

The styloid process is an elongated, narrow bony process arising from the undersurface of the temporal bone and extending inferiorly. It emanates just anterior to the stylomastoid foramen, where the facial nerve exits the fallopian canal.

The tympanic bone composes the bone of the external auditory canal, the structure of which is discussed in more detail later in the chapter. The anterior tympanic bone forms the posterior boundary of the glenoid fossa.

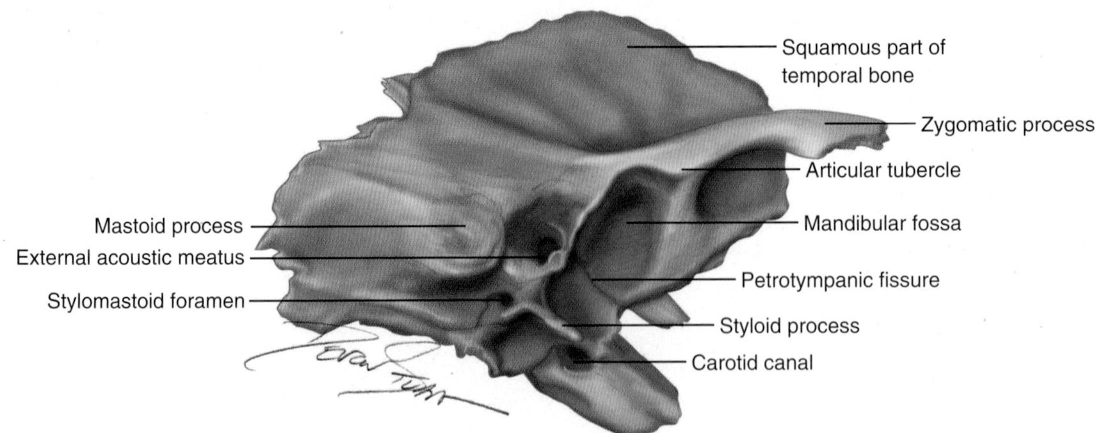

Figure 4.1 Inferolateral view of temporal bone.

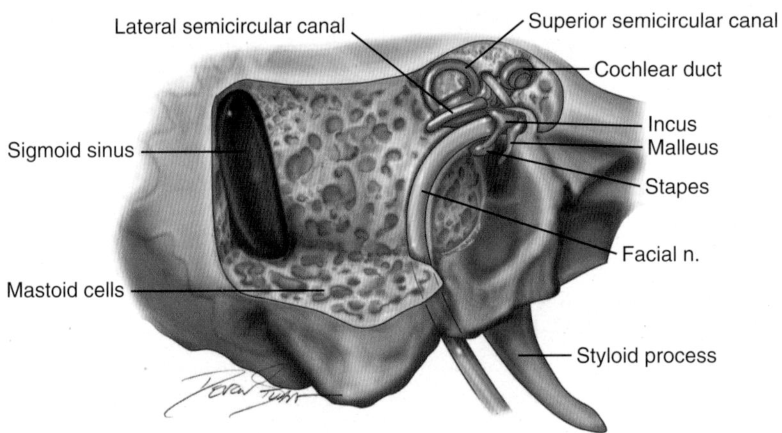

Figure 4.2 Lateral view of temporal bone, portion of mastoid cortex removed.

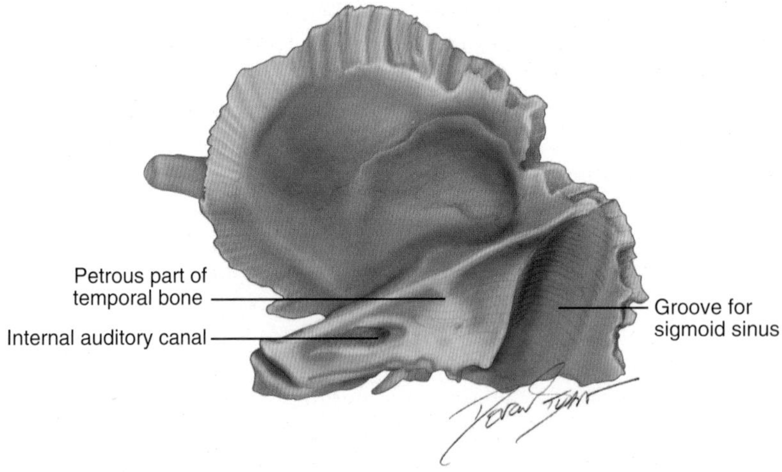

Figure 4.3 Medial view of temporal bone.

External Ear

Auricle

The auricle, or pinna, is the visible portion of the auditory system and is made up of a cartilaginous framework. This complex, three-dimensional structure collects sound energy and directs it to the conducting system of the middle ear.

The auricle begins to form during the sixth week of development, derived from the first and second branchial arch. Condensations of mesoderm form the six hillocks of His, which develop into identifiable portions of the auricle. The first through third hillocks form the tragus, crus helicis, and

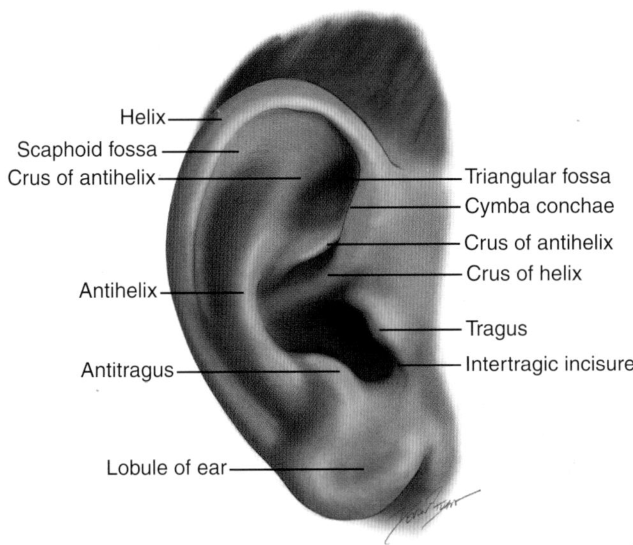

Figure 4.4 Auricle.

helix; the fourth through sixth form the antihelix, antitragus, and lobule.[2]

The adult auricle (Fig. 4.4) has a vertical height of 5 to 6 cm, and the helix sits 15 to 20 mm from the skin overlying the mastoid process.[3] The helix comprises the smooth superior and posterior margin of the auricle and terminates anteriorly in the crus helicis or root of the helix. The crus helicis divides the conchal bowl into the superiorly located concha cymba and the more inferiorly located concha cavum. The antihelix is a vertically oriented structure that separates the helix from the conchal bowl. Superiorly, the antihelix divides to form the superior and inferior crura. The depression found between the superior and inferior crura is known as the fossa triangularis. The tragus is a triangular structure anterior to the meatus of the external auditory canal. Positioned opposite the conchal bowl, posterior and inferior to the tragus, sits the antitragus. The lobule is the inferior-most portion of the auricle and is devoid of cartilage.

A number of rudimentary muscles attach to the auricle, which are of little clinical significance in humans. The extrinsic muscles reposition the auricle in relationship to the head and include the anterior and posterior auricular muscles. The posterior auricular muscles are routinely encountered while making a postauricular incision, and their disruption leads to no significant clinical deficit. The intrinsic muscles include the transverse, oblique auricular, tragal, antitragal, and minor and major helical muscles.

Arterial supply to the auricle is via branches from the external carotid system and includes contributions from the superficial temporal, posterior auricular, and occipital arteries. The venous drainage corresponds with the feeding arterial supply.

Sensory innervation of the auricle involves multiple cranial and cervical nerves. Sensation is provided by the auriculotemporal nerve (CN V), sensory components of the facial nerve, Arnold nerve (CN X), and the greater auricular nerve (C2–C3).

The auricle is a valuable source of cartilaginous grafting materials for procedures in which semirigid grafting material is desired. A large, flat graft can be harvested from the tragus without cosmetic deformity if the lateral tragal framework is preserved. The entirety of the concha cavum and cymba can be harvested if the crus helicis, antihelix, and antitragus are preserved to maintain the structural framework of the auricle.

External Auditory Canal

The external auditory canal (Fig. 4.5) is a structure made up of osseous and cartilaginous portions, extending from the conchal bowl to the tympanic membrane. From the concha, the external auditory canal is 2.5 cm in length, one-third of which is cartilaginous and two-thirds of which is osseous. The medial external auditory canal forms a groove known as the tympanic notch, which houses the tympanic annulus of the tympanic membrane. The anterior wall of the osseous canal makes up the posterior wall of the glenoid fossa of the temporomandibular joint.

The external auditory canal begins to form during the ninth week of embryogenesis and arises from the first branchial groove. The meatal plate, a solid core of ectoderm, extends toward the tympanic cavity. An intervening layer of mesoderm between the meatal plate and tympanic cavity persists at the fibrous layer of the tympanic membrane. The tympanic ring is ossified by the 15th week, leaving a superior defect in the ring known as the notch of Rivinus. Canalization of the ectoderm of the meatal plate begins at 21st week with canalization of the external auditory canal, a process that terminates at the 28th week of gestation. Developmental defects in this process can lead to canal stenosis or atresia.[4]

The external auditory canal reaches adult morphology at approximately 9 years of age. The neonatal external auditory canal is a short and relatively straight structure with a nearly horizontal positioned tympanic membrane. During growth, the canal lengthens and becomes more tortuous to protect the tympanic membrane, and the tympanic membrane assumes an oblique, anteromedial orientation with the posterior tympanic membrane situated lateral to the anterior portion. The skin overlying the lateral, cartilaginous canal is thicker than the skin of the osseous canal. This thicker skin contains the adnexal structures such as hair, sebaceous glands, and modified apocrine sweat glands, sometimes known as ceruminous glands.[5] The transition from hair-bearing to nonhair-bearing skin within the external auditory canal is a good surgical landmark for the transition from the cartilaginous to osseous canal. The skin of the osseous canal is thin and firmly adherent to the bone of the canal. Two suture lines are readily identified during surgery involving the external auditory canal. The tympanosquamous suture is located along the anterosuperior canal, and the tympanomastoid suture is located posteroinferiorly. The skin is more adherent at these sutures and can be difficult to elevate due to fibrous attachments.

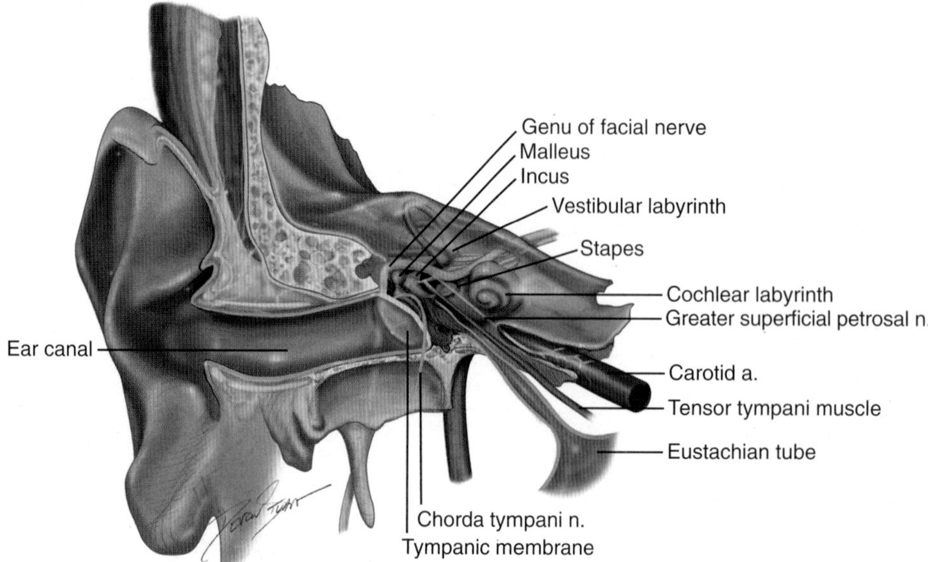

Figure 4.5 Anterior view of the auditory system with coronal section through the level of the external auditory canal.

Two commonly described natural dehiscences of the external auditory canal allow infection or neoplasm to spread from within the canal. The fissures of Santorini are defects of the cartilaginous canal due to natural cleavage planes within the cartilage of the anterior canal. This dehiscence allows neoplastic and infectious processes to spread to the anteriorly located parotid gland. The foramen of Huschke is an anteriorly located dehiscence formed due to incomplete ossification of the tympanic ring. This structure can also facilitate the spread of neoplasm or infection, and it is a source of spontaneous sialorrhea.[6] Furthermore, this bone defect allows for inadvertent entry into the external auditory canal, tympanic membrane perforation, and even ossicular injury during temporomandibular joint arthroscopy.[7]

Multiple cranial nerves provide sensory innervation of the external auditory canal, which can explain pain referred to the ear canal. The auriculotemporal branch of the mandibular nerve innervates the anterior aspect of the canal, whereas the auricular branch of the vagus nerve innervates the posterior canal. Branches of the facial and glossopharyngeal nerves also mediate sensory input. The contribution of the facial nerve, which also innervates a portion of the auricular concha, explains the vesicular eruption seen with facial paralysis due to viral reactivation in Ramsay Hunt syndrome.

Tympanic Membrane

The tympanic membrane is a three-layered structure separating the external auditory canal from the tympanic cavity of the middle ear. It measures roughly 1 cm in diameter. The tympanic membrane conveys sound energy to the ossicles within the middle ear and thereby to the inner ear at the oval window. The tympanic membrane firmly adheres to the malleus at the lateral process and the umbo. The membrane has a slight conical shape and is most depressed at the inferior tip of the malleus at the umbo (Fig. 4.6).

Most of the tympanic membrane is composed of three layers: an external layer of keratinizing squamous epithelium, a middle fibrous layer, and the mucosal medial layer within the tympanic cavity. This three-layered portion of the tympanic membrane is known as the pars tensa. The portion of the tympanic membrane between the lateral process of the malleus and the notch of Rivinus lacks a central fibrous layer and is known as the pars flaccida. Due to the lack of a fibrous layer, the pars flaccida is more compliant and is more susceptible to retraction due to the negative middle ear pressure created due to eustachian tube dysfunction.[8]

The auriculotemporal branch of the mandibular nerve provides predominant sensation to the tympanic membrane. The auricular branch of the vagus nerve and the tympanic branch of the glossopharyngeal nerve also provide sensory contributions.

Middle Ear and Mastoid

The middle ear is an air-filled space medial to the tympanic membrane (Fig. 4.7). It houses the ossicles, which convey the vibratory motion of the tympanic membrane to the oval window of the inner ear, thereby transmitting sound energy. The middle ear is lined with a modified respiratory epithelium containing ciliated and secreting cells. The volume of the tympanic cavity of the middle ear ranges from 0.5 to 1 cm^3.[9] The tympanic cavity communicates posterosuperiorly with the mastoid antrum via the aditus ad antrum, and thereby to the mastoid air cells. The total air volume of the middle ear and mastoid ranges from 1 to 21 cm^3.[10]

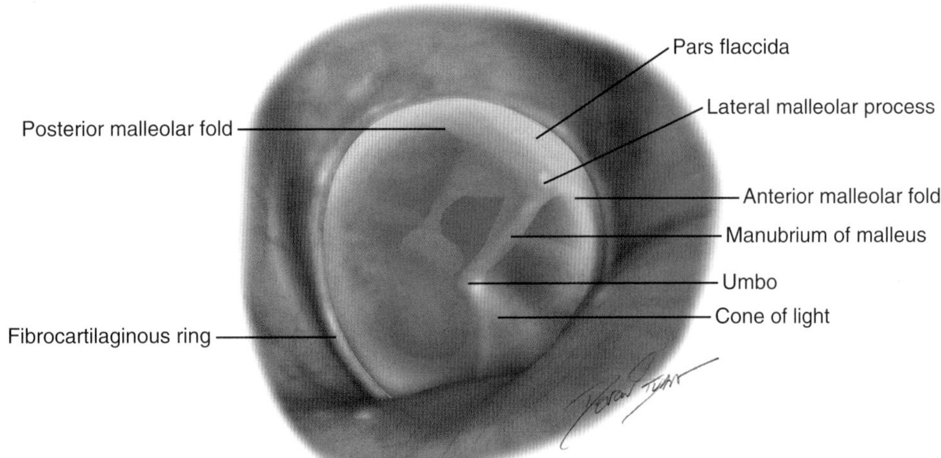

Figure 4.6 Right tympanic membrane.

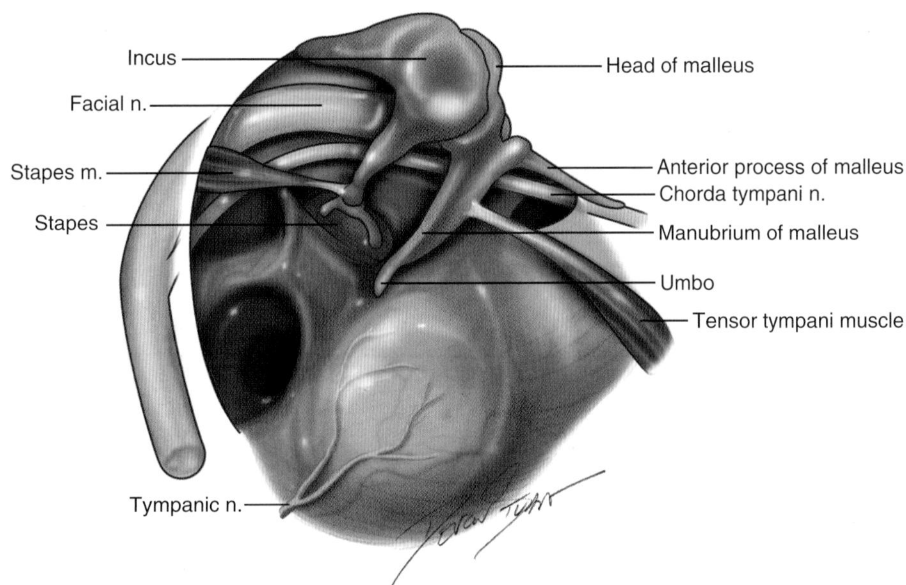

Figure 4.7 Middle ear, ossicles, and facial nerve.

Eustachian Tube

The middle ear communicates with the nasopharynx via the eustachian tube (see Fig. 4.5). With occasional opening, the eustachian tube allows the middle ear air pressure to equalize with that of the environment. The eustachian tube is 3.5 cm long and is composed of an osseous and cartilaginous portion. The eustachian tube orifice within the middle ear is located in the anterior tympanic cavity, originating inferior to the semicanal of the tensor tympani muscle and superior to the internal carotid artery. The proximal one-third of the eustachian tube is osseous, while the distal two-thirds, in continuity with the nasopharynx, is composed of cartilage. The orifice of the eustachian tube is seen in the nasopharynx as a raised structure named the torus tubarius. The four muscles associated with the eustachian tube are the tensor veli palatini, tensor tympani, levator veli palatini, and salpingopharyngeus. The primary muscle associated with opening of the eustachian tube is the levator veli palatini.

Ossicles and Middle Ear Musculature

The three ossicles of the middle ear include the malleus, incus, and stapes (see Fig. 4.7). The malleus is composed of the head, neck, lateral process, and manubrium. The head articulates with the body of the incus at the incudomalleolar joint, thereby transmitting vibrations from the tympanic membrane to the incus. The tensor tympani muscle attaches to the medial surface of the neck of the malleus. The incus is composed of the body, short process, long process, and lenticular process. The body articulates with the malleus head, and the lenticular process meets the stapes at the incudostapedial joint. The stapes is the smaller, stirrup-shaped ossicle that transmits mechanical energy to the inner ear fluids. The stapes superstructure is composed of the anterior and posterior crura, neck, and capitulum, which articulate with the lenticular process of the incus. The stapedius muscle tension attaches to the neck of the stapes. The crura of the stapes are fused to the footplate, which sits in the oval window of the vestibule. The footplate is supported within the oval window by the surrounding annular ligament.

Two skeletal muscles, described previously, are present within the middle ear. The stapedius muscle body runs vertically, medial to the mastoid segment of the facial nerve. The tendon is transmitted to the middle ear space through the pyramidal eminence. The stapedius muscle is innervated by the adjacent facial nerve. The stapedius muscle is activated by the stapedial reflex. Loud sound from either the contralateral or ipsilateral ear triggers muscle contraction, dampening mechanical vibration at the level of the stapes. The stapedial reflex requires intact facial and cochlear nerves and can be used for site-of-lesion testing. The tensor tympani muscle body runs adjacent to the eustachian tube, anterior to the middle ear space. The tendon enters the middle ear at the cochleariform process and attaches to the medial neck of the malleus. Activation of this nerve decreases the movement of the malleus and, thereby, the tympanic membrane. The muscle is innervated by a branch from the mandibular division of the trigeminal nerve.

Chorda Tympani Nerve

The chorda tympani nerve travels through the middle ear space. The nerve is unique in that it does not travel in a bony canal and is not surrounded by soft tissue. After branching from the mastoid segment of the facial nerve, the chorda tympani nerve enters the tympanic cavity at the posterior iter. The nerve travels anterosuperiorly, passing lateral to the long process of the incus and medial to the handle of the malleus. The nerve then exits the tympanic cavity at the anterior iter and travels to join the lingual nerve.

Inner Ear

The inner ear is a sensory organ that is responsible for sound perception and the sensation of acceleration. The anatomy and physiology of the inner ear are extremely complex.

The osseous labyrinth is composed of three main components: the vestibule, semicircular canals, and cochlea. The osseous labyrinth is lined with endosteum and filled with perilymph. The membranous labyrinth is housed within the perilymph of the osseous labyrinth. The membranous labyrinth contains endolymph and the sensory epithelium critical to its function.

Vestibule

The vestibule is an ovoid structure centrally located within the labyrinth. It is located medial to the middle ear, posterior to the cochlea, and anterior to the semicircular canals. The lateral wall of the vestibule contains the oval window, which abuts the middle ear space and is filled by the stapes footplate and annular ligament. The vestibule contains the two otolithic organs: the utricle and saccule. These otolithic organs sense gravitational and translational acceleration.

Semicircular Canals

The three semicircular canals sense rotational acceleration and communicate with the vestibule via five orifices. The lateral semicircular canal has two isolated openings into the vestibule, whereas the posterior and superior canals join to form the crus communis and join the vestibule as a unit at their posterior ends. The endolymphatic duct enters the labyrinth in the crus communi and communicates with the endolymphatic sac in the dura of the posterior cranial fossa. Each semicircular canal has an ampullated end that contains its sensory apparatus. The lateral and superior canals have ampullated ends in close proximity at their anterior ends and join the vestibule at its anterior and superior aspects. The ampullated end of the posterior canal is located on its inferior end and enters the vestibule inferiorly.

Cochlea

The cochlea is a snail-shaped structure with 2½ turns that is responsible for sound perception. The turns of the cochlea are coiled around the modiolus through which filaments of the cochlear nerve travel to innervate the cochlea (Fig. 4.8). Cross-sectional analysis of the lumen of the cochlea demonstrates three fluid spaces: the scala tympani, scala media, and scala vestibuli. On the inner wall of the cochlea, the osseous spiral lamina extends laterally to separate the scala vestibuli from scala tympani. At the cochlear apex, the osseous spiral lamina is deficient at the helicotrema, where the scala tympani and vestibuli join. The scala media is separated from the inferiorly located scala tympani by the basal membrane, and from the superiorly located scala vestibuli by the Reissner membrane. The scala tympani and vestibuli are filled with perilymph, whereas the centrally located scala media is filled with endolymph. The scala media also contains the organ of Corti and the auditory hair cells, which are responsible for audition. The scala tympani, in the basal turn of the cochlea, has an osseous deficiency known as the round window, in which the round window membrane is situated. The round window membrane sits 2 mm inferior to the oval window of the vestibule and separates the scala tympani from the tympanic cavity. By joining the basal turn of the cochlea near the round window in the scala tympani, the cochlear aqueduct allows communication with the subarachnoid space.

Internal Auditory Canal

The internal auditory canal transmits the facial and vestibulocochlear nerves from the brain stem to the periphery. The labyrinthine artery, a branch of the anterior inferior cerebellar artery, also courses through the internal auditory canal. The canal is, on average, 12 mm in length. The orifice of the

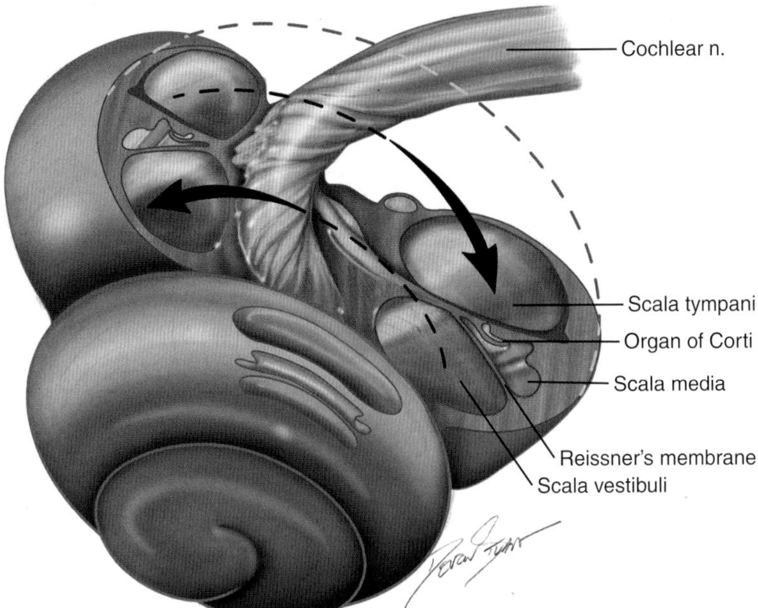

Figure 4.8 Cochlea and cochlear nerve.

canal communicating with the posterior fossa is known as the porus acusticus, and the most lateral aspect of the canal is the fundus. A cross section through the canal near the fundus demonstrates four distinct nerves within the lumen. The facial nerve is anterior and superior, the cochlear nerve is anterior and inferior, and the superior and inferior vestibular nerves are posteriorly situated within the canal. At the fundus, two osseous crests are present. The vertical crest, or Bill's bar, separates the anterior from posterior contents, and the transverse crest separates the superior from inferior contents.

Facial Nerve and Fallopian Canal

Although not a part of the auditory system, the facial nerve has a close association with the nerves and peripheral components of the organs of hearing and balance. The facial nerve runs within the fallopian canal, which is the longest osseous channel for any nerve in the body. The facial nerve can be subdivided into multiple segments: cisternal, intracanalicular, labyrinthine, tympanic, vertical, and extratemporal. When undertaking surgery of the temporal bone and lateral skull base, surgeons must have a detailed understanding of the facial nerve's course to avoid the devastating complication of facial nerve paralysis.

The facial nerve has motor and sensory components, and the sensory component is derived from the nervus intermedius at the brain stem. The nerve provides motor innervation to the mimetic musculature of the face, posterior belly of the digastric muscle, stylohyoid muscle, stapedius muscle, and auricular muscles. The nerve provides sensory input including taste sensation to the anterior two-thirds of the tongue and somatic sensation in the periauricular region. The nerve also carries preganglionic parasympathetic fibers destined for the lacrimal, submandibular, and sublingual glands.

The facial nerve leaves the brain stem at the pontomedullary junction, where it exits just anterior to the vestibulocochlear nerve. The cisternal segment of the nerve is 15 mm in length and travels within the cerebellopontine cistern to the internal auditory canal. The nerve enters the internal auditory canal at the porus acusticus, and the intracanalicular segment of the facial nerve is 12 mm in length. The nerve travels within the anterior superior portion of the internal auditory canal and is separated from the superior vestibular nerve by Bill's bar (vertical crest). The nerve exits the internal auditory canal at the meatal foramen and becomes the labyrinthine facial nerve. The meatal foramen is the narrowest portion of the fallopian canal with an average diameter of 0.7 mm.[11] The labyrinthine facial nerve is 3 to 4 mm in length and joins the geniculate ganglion. At the geniculate ganglion, the nerve makes its first turn, or genu, and becomes the tympanic facial nerve. With this first genu, the nerve makes a sharp turn from the anterosuperiorly directed labyrinthine segment to the posteroinferiorly oriented tympanic segment. The 8- to 11-mm tympanic segment of the facial nerve travels within the tympanic cavity of the middle ear and passes posterior superior to the oval window. The nerve courses superior to the cochleariform process along the inferior surface of the lateral semicircular canal. At the inferior margin of the lateral semicircular canal, it makes another turn (the second genu) and becomes the inferiorly directed vertical segment. The vertical segment travels 10 to 14 mm, as the longest segment of the intratemporal facial nerve, and exits the temporal bone at the stylomastoid foramen.

Within the temporal bone, there are three branches of the facial nerve. The first is the GSPN. The GSPN arises from the geniculate ganglion and travels anteriorly to the exit the temporal bone at the facial hiatus. The nerve then travels on the superior surface of the temporal bone, passes under V3, and enters the foramen lacerum. There, the GSPN joins the deep petrosal nerve and becomes the vidian nerve. The GSPN carries preganglionic parasympathetic fibers to the sphenopalatine ganglion and ultimately provides parasympathetic innervation to the lacrimal gland and mucous membranes of the nose and palate. The next intratemporal branch of the facial nerve is the nerve to the stapedius muscle within the vertical segment. The last intratemporal branch is the chorda tympani nerve. This nerve arises from the distal portion of the vertical facial nerve, courses superiorly and anteriorly, and enters the middle ear space. The nerve provides taste sensation to the lateral two-thirds of the tongue and provides preganglionic parasympathetic fibers, ultimately providing parasympathetic innervation to the submandibular and sublingual glands.

Summary

The auditory system has a complex anatomic and physiologic anatomic makeup. Though discussed with brevity in this chapter, there is a vast wealth of knowledge worth additional study for those interested. When operating in the vicinity of the temporal bone, detailed anatomic knowledge is required to avoid potentially devastating complications such as facial paralysis, hearing loss, and vertigo. This knowledge is gained via the study of anatomic treatises as well as cadaveric dissection prior to tackling surgical procedures in this region.

References

1. Shelton C, Brackmann DE, House WF. Middle fossa approach. In: Brackmann DE, Shelton C, Arriaga MA, eds. *Otologic Surgery*. Philadelphia, Pennsylvania: Saunders Elsevier; 2010.
2. Beahm EK, Walton RL. Auricular reconstruction for microtia: part I: anatomy, embryology, and clinical evaluation. *Plast Reconstr Surg*. 2002;109(7):2473–2482.
3. Becker DG, Lai SS, Wise JB, Steiger JD. Analysis in otoplasty. *Facial Plast Surg Clin North Am*. 2006;14(2):63–71.
4. Anson BJ, Donaldson JA. *Surgical Anatomy of the Temporal Bone and Ear*. Philadelphia, Pennsylvania: WB Saunders; 1981.
5. Marple BF, Roland PS. External auditory canal. In: Roland PS, Meyerhoff WL, Marple BF, eds. *Hearing Loss*. New York, New York: Thieme; 1997.
6. Sharma PD, Dawkins RS. Patent foramen of Huschke and spontaneous salivary fistula. *J Laryngol Otol*. 1984;98(1):83–85.
7. Herzog S, Fiese R. Persistent foramen of Huschke: possible risk factor for otologic complications after arthroscopy of the temporomandibular joint. *Oral Surg Oral Med Oral Pathol*. 1989;68(3):267–270.
8. Lim DJ. Tympanic membrane. Part II: pars flaccida. *Acta Otolaryngol*. 1968;66(6):515–532.
9. Gyo K, Goode RL, Miller CL. Effect of middle ear modification on umbo vibration: human temporal bone experiments with a new vibration measuring system. *Arch Otolaryngol Head Neck Surg*. 1986;112(12):1262–1268.
10. Molvaer OI, Vallersnes FM, Kringlebotn M. The size of the middle ear and the mastoid air cell. *Acta Otolaryngol*. 1978;85(1–2):24–32.
11. Gantz BJ, Gubbels SP, Samy RN. Surgery of the facial nerve. In: Gulya AJ, Minor LB, Poe DS, eds. *Glasscock-Shambaugh Surgery of the Ear*. Shelton, Connecticut: PMPH-USA; 2010.

CHAPTER 5

The Anatomy of the Face, Mouth, and Jaws

Christopher Morris

The oral and maxillofacial surgeon must have a firm grasp of facial anatomy and the surgical implications of the location and orientation of anatomic structures. This knowledge guides the surgeon in the planning of surgical approaches and in the reconstruction of traumatic or surgical defects.

The visceral cranium is the lower portion of the head that facilitates the visceral functions, including breathing, smelling, speaking, tasting, and swallowing. In this chapter, the anatomy of the region is addressed in a manner similar to a surgical approach, from superficial to deep, with the assessment of clinical points of interest as they relate to surgical access to the face.

The Skin

The skin is a complex organ, composed of superficial epidermis and underlying dermis, that provides sensation and protection. The anatomic and physiologic properties of the skin play an important role in the final esthetics of any facial surgical procedure (Fig. 5.1).

Gonzalez-Ulloa et al.[1] first described 14 distinct facial esthetic units where the skin has a uniform color, texture, thickness, and mobility throughout. Burget and Menick[2,3] expounded upon this concept. The relaxed skin tension lines (RSTLs) of the face generally provide excellent camouflage of incisions placed within or parallel to them. The lines of maximum extensibility are generally perpendicular to the RSTLs. Surgical approaches to the face should attempt to place incisions at the borders of facial subunits and parallel to RSTLs to minimize the effect of the final scar (Fig. 5.2).

The thickness and character of facial skin are also important when considering skin matches for reconstruction. For example, the skin of the nasal dorsum is nearly 3.3 times the thickness of the upper eyelid skin.[4] The skin of the face is also densely populated with pilosebaceous units, particularly in the forehead, nose, and chin (an area sometimes referred to as the T-zone), with a progressive decrease toward the lateral edges of the face.[5] This should be taken into consideration when planning skin resurfacing procedures that rely on the pilosebaceous units for reepithelialization.

The Fat Pads of the Face

The malar fat pad is a triangular structure superficial to the superficial musculoaponeurotic system (SMAS) and mimetic muscles. It is oriented with its base along the nasolabial fold and its apex at the zygomatic prominence. This structure descends and loses volume with age, resulting in the descent of the facial soft tissues associated with aging.[6]

The buccal fat pad is an important structure within the cheek. It has a central body and four processes: the buccal, pterygoid, pterygopalatine, and temporal (superficial and deep) processes.[7] The zygomatic and buccal branches of the facial nerve lie superficial to the buccal process, with the parotid duct running within it. Care should be taken when excising a portion of the buccal fat pad for cosmetic purposes or when using a pedicled buccal fat flap for oral-antral fistula closure.

Multiple other distinct fat pads have been described and should be taken into account, particularly when fat is injected as an adjunct to cosmetic surgery.[8]

The Superficial Musculoaponeurotic System

An understanding of the SMAS is fundamental to the facial surgeon because of the orientation of the SMAS and the neurovascular structures of the face.[9] The territorial distribution and details of the SMAS continue to be controversial; however, an understanding of the general principles and anatomic descriptions allows surgeons to draw their own conclusions.

The SMAS is a fanlike fibromuscular layer that encases the muscles of facial expression, similar to the superficial cervical fascia of the neck that encases the platysma in the neck. The SMAS connects the dermis to the underlying facial muscles via a three-dimensional architecture of collagen, elastic fibers, fat cells, and muscle fibers (Fig. 5.3).

The SMAS is continuous with the superficial temporal (temporoparietal) fascia superiorly and with the superficial cervical fascia of the platysma inferiorly. It lies superficial to the parotidomasseteric fascia. Anteriorly, the SMAS can

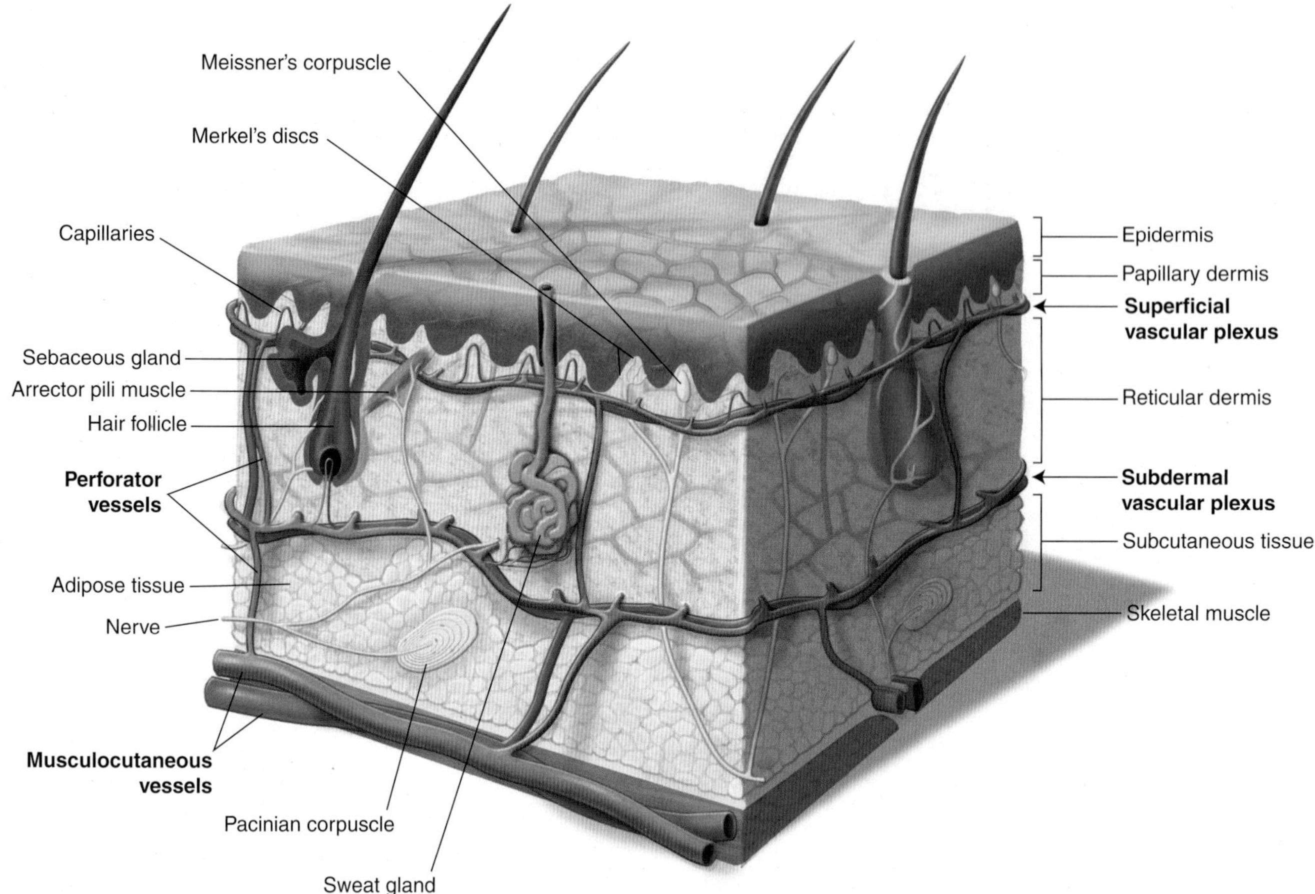

Figure 5.1 Schematic cross section of the skin containing the layers of the epidermis, dermis, and subcutaneous connective tissue. The position of the vascular supply is emphasized for reconstructive purposes. The superficial vascular plexus lies between the papillary and reticular dermal layers. The subdermal plexus lies between the reticular dermis and the subcutaneous layer. The musculocutaneous arteries provide blood supply deep to the subcutaneous tissue.

be extended to the approximate point of the facial artery and vein; however, it is of primary surgical relevance in the region overlying the parotid.[9] Anterior to the nasolabial fold, the innervation of the perioral musculature becomes more susceptible to injury as the SMAS becomes more fibrous and divides to form an investing fascia of the zygomaticus muscles.[10]

The Facial Layers of the Face: Regional Considerations

In the upper face, when elevating a coronal or forehead flap, dissection in the avascular plane between the periosteum and temporoparietal fascia protects the temporal branch of the facial nerve. During this dissection, it is important to note that the vessels and sensory nerves exit the bone via their various foramina and penetrate the layer being elevated; therefore, care must be taken in these areas.

In the temporal region, dissection should proceed deep to the superficial layer of the deep temporal fascia, within the temporal fat pad, to ensure that the temporal branch is sufficiently protected and elevated within the superficial temporal (temporoparietal) fascia.

The Facial Musculature

Six major muscle groups in the head assist with visceral functions: orbital muscles, masticatory muscles, muscles of facial expression, tongue muscles, pharynx muscles, and larynx muscles. This chapter focuses on the masticatory muscles, mimetic muscles (muscles of facial expression), and tongue muscles.

Masticatory Muscles

The muscles of mastication are derived from the first branchial arch and are innervated by the mandibular division of cranial nerve (CN) V (Fig. 5.4 and Table 5.1).

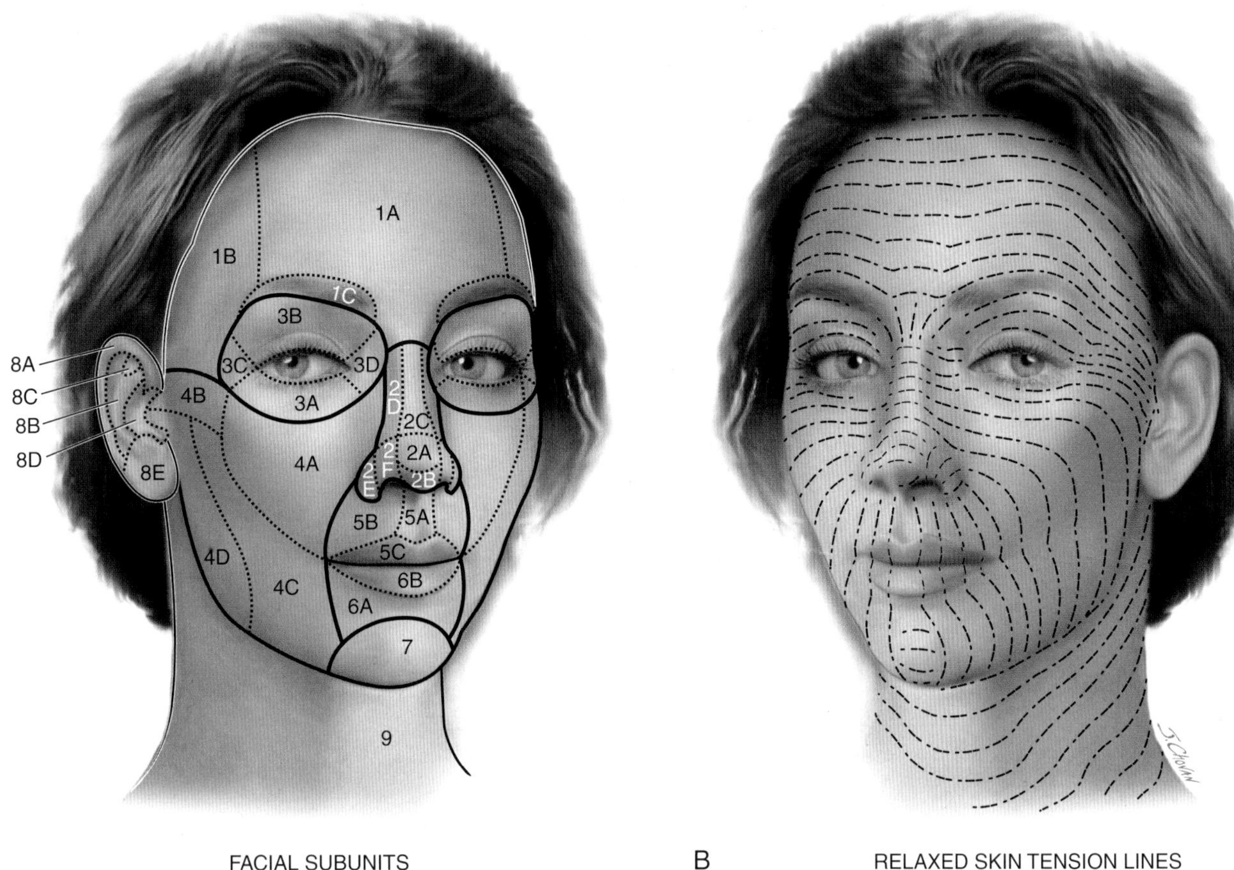

Figure 5.2 **A,** Facial esthetic subunits. Forehead subunits: *1A,* Central; *1B,* Lateral; *1C,* Eyebrow. Nasal subunits: *2A,* Tip; *2B,* Columellar; *2C,* Dorsal; *2D,* Right and left dorsal side wall; *2E,* Right and left alar base; *2F,* Right and left alar side wall. Periorbital subunits: *3A,* Lower eyelid; *3B,* Upper eyelid; *3C,* Lateral canthal; *3D,* Medial canthal. Cheek subunits: *4A,* Medial; *4B,* Zygomatic; *4C,* Lateral; *4D,* Buccal. Upper lip subunits: *5A,* Central; *5B,* Mucosal. Lower lip subunits: *6A,* Central; *6B,* Mucosal. *7,* Mental. Auricular subunits: *8A,* Helical; *8B,* Antihelical; *8C,* Triangular fossa; *8D,* Conchal; *8E,* Lobe. *9,* Neck. **B,** Relaxed skin tension lines.

Superficial Facial Musculature

The muscles of facial expression are superficial muscles that are innervated by branches of the facial nerve (CN VII); they are composed of the orbicularis oris and 23 paired muscles. Some have suggested that there are four layers of facial muscles; layer 4 is unique because these muscles are innervated from their superficial surface, whereas the muscles in layers 1 through 3 receive innervation from their deep surfaces (Table 5.2).[11]

Table 5.3 lists the muscles of facial expression with their general actions. An understanding of the general and more specific actions of the facial musculature can be helpful in the diagnosis of facial nerve deficits and in selective chemical denervation for esthetic purposes.

The buccinator muscle plays an important role in bolus formation and bolus control by pressing the cheek against the teeth during mastication.

Musculature of the Tongue

The musculature of the tongue is composed of four intrinsic and four extrinsic muscles (Fig. 5.5).

The intrinsic muscles of the tongue are the superior and inferior longitudinal muscles, the transverse muscles, and the vertical muscles. These muscles and the buccinators, innervated by CN VII, are responsible for bolus control during chewing. The extrinsic muscles are the genioglossus, hyoglossus, styloglossus, and palatoglossus muscles. All are innervated by the hypoglossal nerve (CN XII) with the exception of the palatoglossus muscles, which are innervated by the vagus nerve via the pharyngeal plexus. These muscles function to close the oropharyngeal opening via contraction of the palatoglossal arch during swallowing.

Deficit of the hypoglossal nerve results in a protruded tongue pointing toward the injury or lesion, which is due to

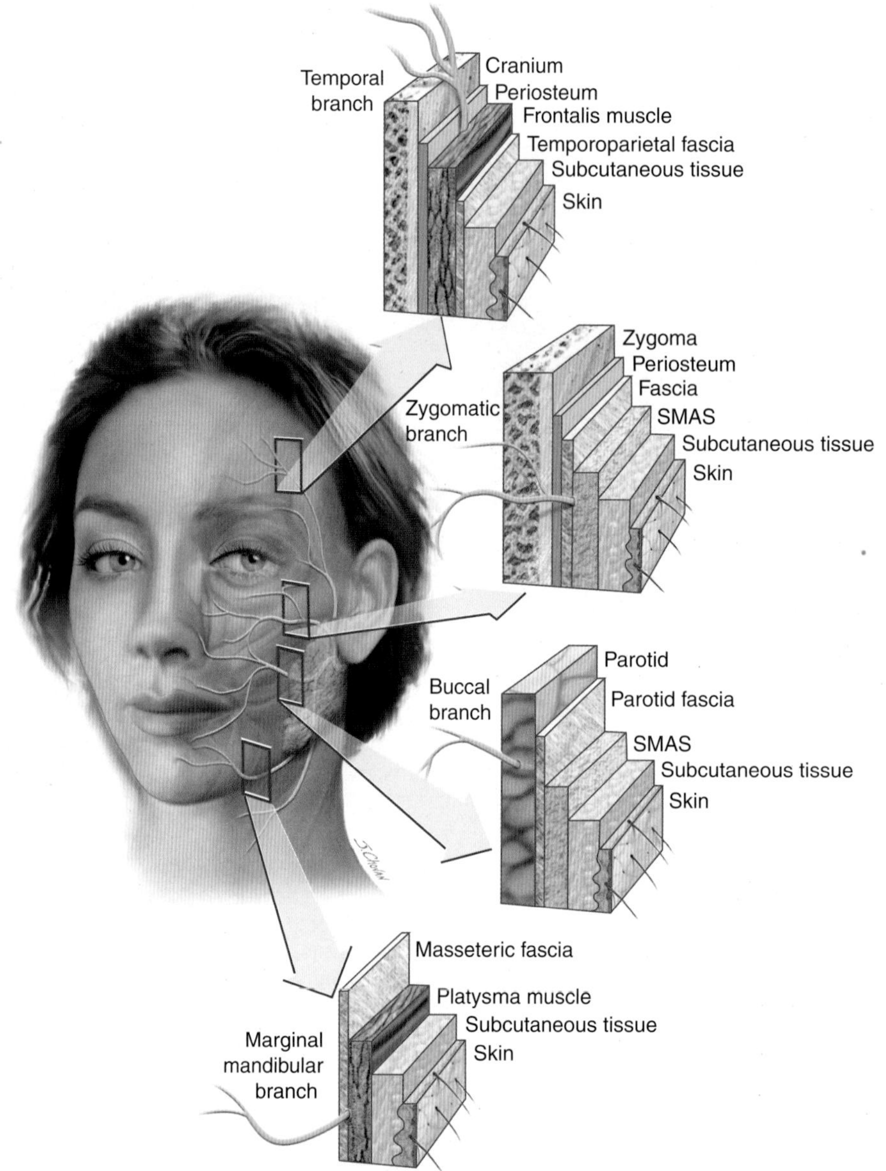

Figure 5.3 Fascial layers and superficial musculoaponeurotic system (SMAS). The regional position of the facial nerve is shown in relation to surgically important anatomic layers.

the fan-shaped insertion of the bilateral genioglossus muscles that cross the midline anteriorly.

The Facial Nerve

The trajectory of the facial nerve (CN VII) within the human face varies markedly from person to person. This makes the understanding of the anatomic literature and recognition of landmarks critical for a surgical approach to the face for any purpose. The trunk of the facial nerve leaves the stylomastoid foramen between 6 and 8 mm medial to the tympanomastoid suture and just lateral to the styloid process.[12] The trunk then enters the body of the parotid gland; at this point, the distribution and branching pattern of the facial nerve become quite variable.

The variability of the facial nerve has been well documented. Davis et al.[13] and Bąker and Conley[14] described the six most common nerve branching patterns. The following is a description of the most commonly accepted pattern, representing around 24% of individuals.

A general concept of facial nerve distribution is a division of the trunk into a superior temporofacial and an inferior cervicofacial division, separated into five rami. The five branches, or rami, of the facial nerve are the temporal (or frontal), zygomatic, buccal, marginal mandibular, and cervical

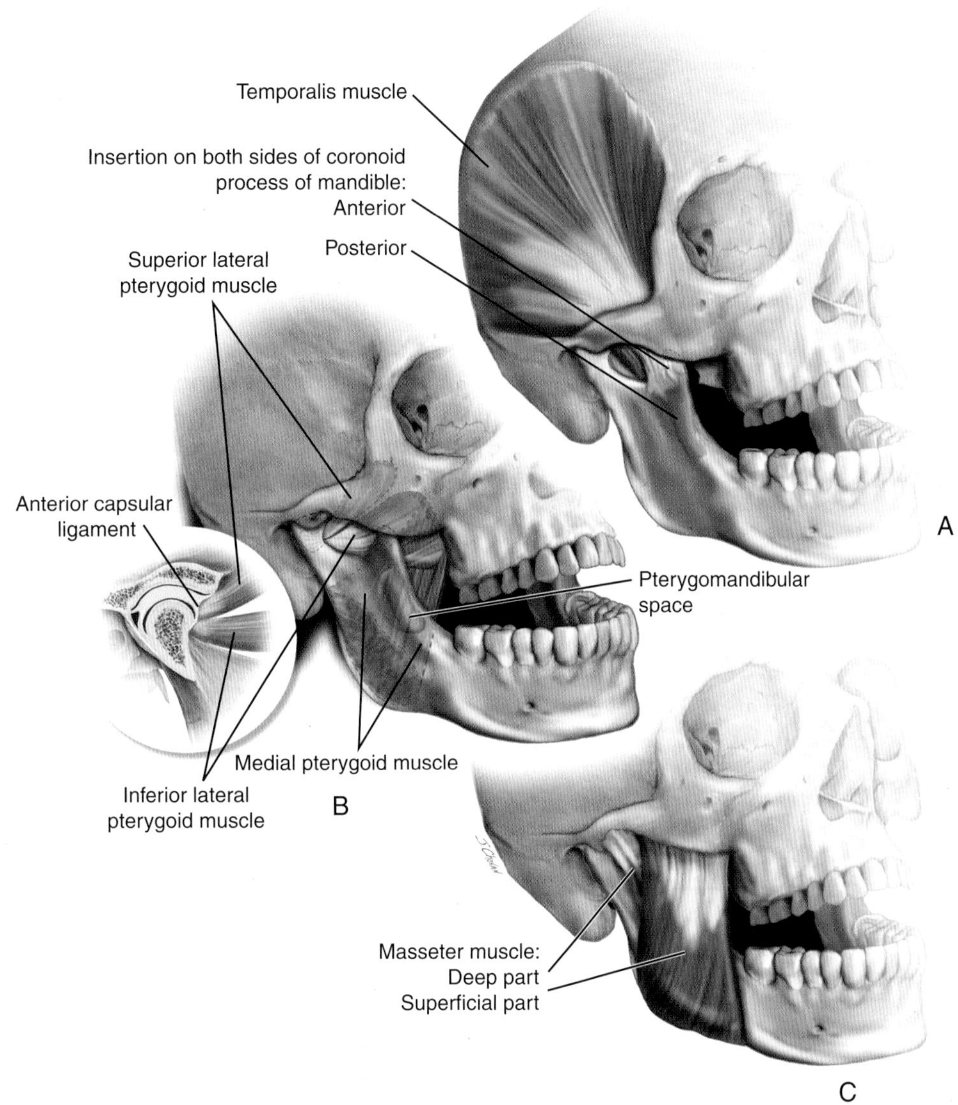

Figure 5.4 Muscles of mastication. **A,** Temporalis. **B,** Medial and lateral pterygoid. The pterygomandibular space between the mandible and the medial pterygoid is where local anesthetic is injected for a block of the inferior alveolar nerve. **C,** Masseter muscles.

Table 5.1 Muscles of Mastication

Muscle	Action	Innervation: CN V3
Masseter	Bilateral: Elevates and protrudes the mandible	Masseteric nerve
Temporalis	Bilateral: Elevates the mandible (vertical fibers)	Deep temporal nerves
	Bilateral: Retracts protruded mandible (horizontal fibers)	
Medial pterygoid	Bilateral: Elevates the mandible	Medial pterygoid nerve
Lateral pterygoid	Bilateral: Initiates mouth opening, protrudes mandible, and moves articular disk forward	Lateral pterygoid nerve
	Unilateral: Lateral movement while chewing	

CN, Cranial nerve.

rami. Typically, there are anastomoses between the buccal and zygomatic branches, but the temporal and mandibular branches are typically terminal branches without anastomoses and are therefore more affected by insult or injury. Because of the degree of morbidity associated with damage to these branches, this chapter focuses on characterizing the location of the facial nerve and its branches.

The temporal branch of the facial nerve requires additional consideration due to its complex anatomy. The temporal branch leaves the parotid and runs within the superficial

Table 5.2 Layers of Facial Musculature

Layer 1	Depressor anguli oris, zygomaticus minor, orbicularis oculi
Layer 2	Depressor labii inferioris, risorius, platysma, zygomaticus major, levator labii superioris alaeque nasi
Layer 3	Orbicularis oris, levator labii superioris
Layer 4	Mentalis, levator anguli oris, buccinator

temporal fascia (temporoparietal fascia/continuous with the SMAS) over the zygomatic arch to innervate the frontalis from its undersurface. The nerve passes over the arch between 8 and 35 cm anterior to the external auditory canal.[15]

More specifically, the temporal branch has between three and five rami; the most posterior ramus may be anterior or posterior to the superficial temporal vessels.[16] The most anterior branch is 2 cm posterior to the anterior extent of the zygomatic arch.[17] The plane of dissection in this area should be very superficial in relation to the superficial temporal fascia (temporoparietal fascia/SMAS), deep to the SMAS on the temporalis fascia, or within the temporal fat pad between the superficial and deep divisions of the temporalis fascia.

Several landmarks are available in the temporal region. Estimation of the temporal branch distribution can be made by drawing a triangle from the earlobe to the lateral brow and lateral extent of the highest forehead crease[18] or from a point 0.5 cm below the tragus to the lateral brow and 1.5 cm above the lateral brow.[19,20]

When approaching this area using a preauricular approach, it is prudent to incise through the superficial layer of the temporalis fascia and periosteum posterior to a point 8 mm anterior to the external auditory canal; if an anterior extension is required, it should be made superiorly, within the temporal hairline (Fig. 5.6).

In the lower face, the branches of the facial nerve are deep to the SMAS and become superficial anterior to the masseter muscle. The distribution of the marginal mandibular nerve must be discussed with regard to surgical approaches to the lower face because injury to this nerve results in paralysis of the lip and chin, producing a notable deformity; in addition, anastomoses with other branches are relatively rare (only 15% in one study[14]). The marginal mandibular nerve exits the parotid and travels anteriorly. Dingman and Grabb,[21] in their classic dissection study, identified the majority of marginal mandibular branches above the mandibular border; 19% exhibited a nerve up to 1 cm below the mandibular border posterior to the facial vessels. Anterior to the facial vessels, the nerve is above the mandibular border 100% of the time. The number of branches varies from one to four, but two branches are most common (67%).

The marginal mandibular nerve is protected throughout the majority of its course by the platysma muscle. About 2 cm lateral to the corner of the mouth, the nerve becomes more superficial. This is particularly important in relation to the deep muscles of facial expression (e.g., the mentalis and levator anguli oris), which are superficially innervated.[22]

In general, it is considered safe to make a submandibular incision a minimum of 1.5 cm below the inferior border of the mandible, ideally in a natural neck crease.[23] The marginal mandibular nerve can be protected by making an incision through the platysma and the superficial layer of the deep cervical fascia investing the submandibular gland, ligating the facial vessels, and superolaterally reflecting the nerve. Another approach, although somewhat more technique-sensitive, is

Table 5.3 Muscles of Facial Expression

Muscle	Innervation	General Action
Occipitofrontalis	Temporal	Elevates eyebrows, wrinkles forehead
Corrugator supercilii	Temporal	Eyebrows medial and down, squint
Procerus	Temporal/zygomatic	Eyebrows medial and down, frown
Orbicularis oculi	Temporal/zygomatic	Closes eyelid, contracts skin around eye
Zygomaticus major	Zygomatic/buccal	Elevates corner of mouth
Zygomaticus minor	Zygomatic/buccal	Elevates upper lip
Levator labii superioris	Zygomatic/buccal	Elevates upper lip and nasolabial fold
Levator labii superioris alaeque nasi	Zygomatic/buccal	Elevates upper lip, flares nostril
Risorius	Buccal	Pulls corner of mouth laterally, smile
Buccinator	Buccal	Pulls cheek against teeth, pulls cheeks from side to side
Levator anguli oris	Buccal	Pulls angle of mouth up and medially, deepens nasolabial fold
Orbicularis oris	Buccal	Closes and compresses lips
Nasalis	Buccal	Transverse: Compresses nostril Alar: Flares nostril
Depressor anguli oris	Buccal/marginal mandibular	Pulls corner of mouth down
Depressor labii inferioris	Marginal mandibular	Pulls down lower lip
Mentalis	Marginal mandibular	Elevates and protrudes lower lip, drinking
Platysma	Cervical	Depresses and wrinkles skin of lower face, mouth, and neck

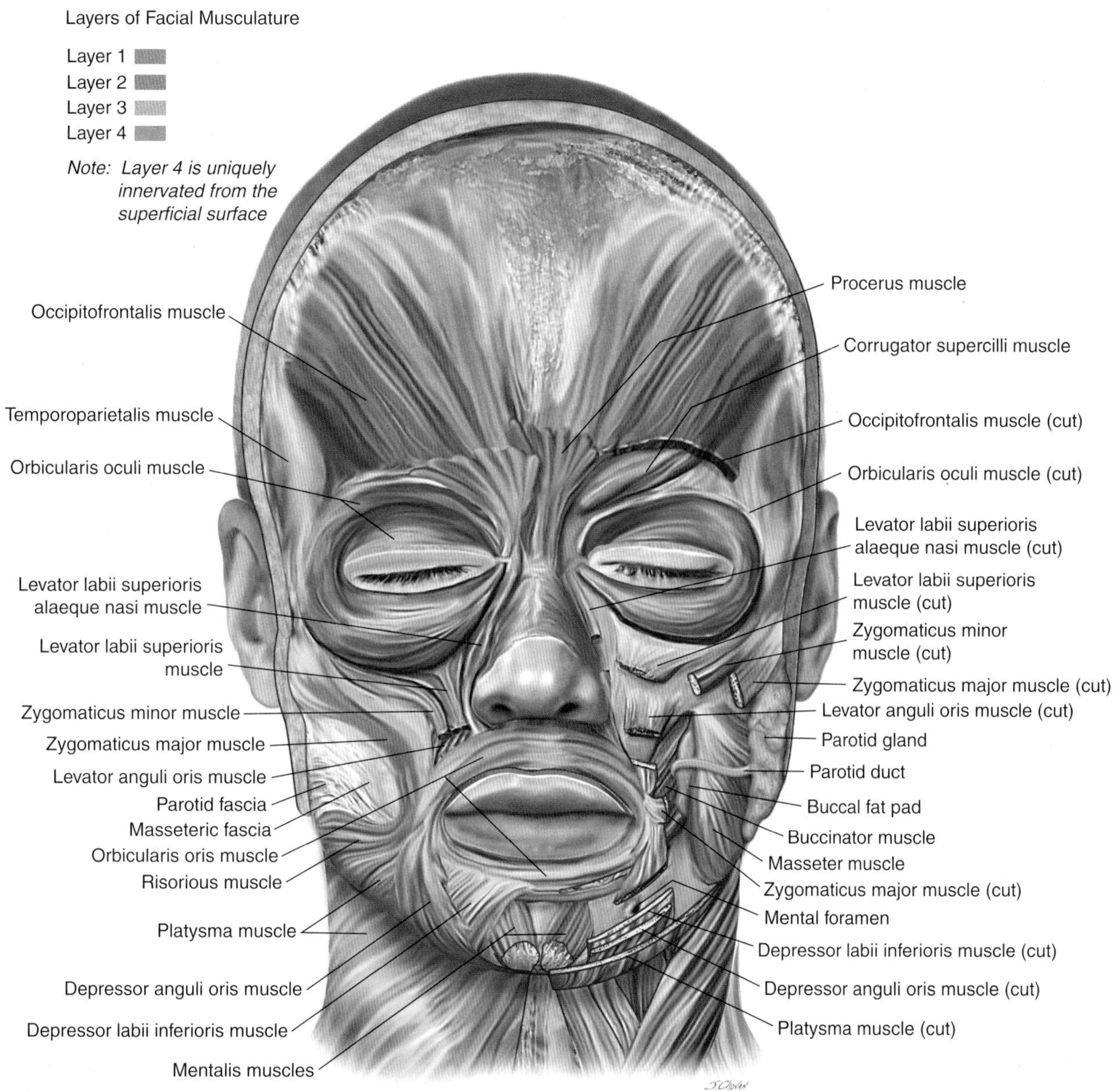

Figure 5.5 The muscles of facial expression.

to reflect the platysma superiorly and visually identify and protect the marginal branch of the facial nerve (Fig. 5.7).

The Ligaments and Adhesions of the Face

The retaining ligaments of the face are responsible for anchoring the overlying dermis to the facial skeleton and for maintenance of facial shape. The ligaments have been described as fasciocutaneous or osteocutaneous. The fasciocutaneous ligaments sequentially attach the dermis to the underlying fascia. These attachments are particularly strong in the central face, around the eyes, nose, lips, and chin. They are of intermediate strength over the lateral cheek and neck and looser over the temple and midcheek. Osteocutaneous ligaments are much stronger attachments that extend directly from the periosteum to the dermis. These are present as the zygomatic osteocutaneous ligaments, also referred to as the McGregor patch, and the mandibular cutaneous ligaments extending from the parasymphyseal region.[24]

These ligaments are functionally significant because weakening of these ligamentous systems results in the general pattern of descent in the aging face.

The Trigeminal Nerve: Cranial Nerve V

Sensation of the face is supplied by the trigeminal nerve, otherwise known as CN V. The technical aspects of local anesthesia are a fundamental prerequisite to facial surgery and are

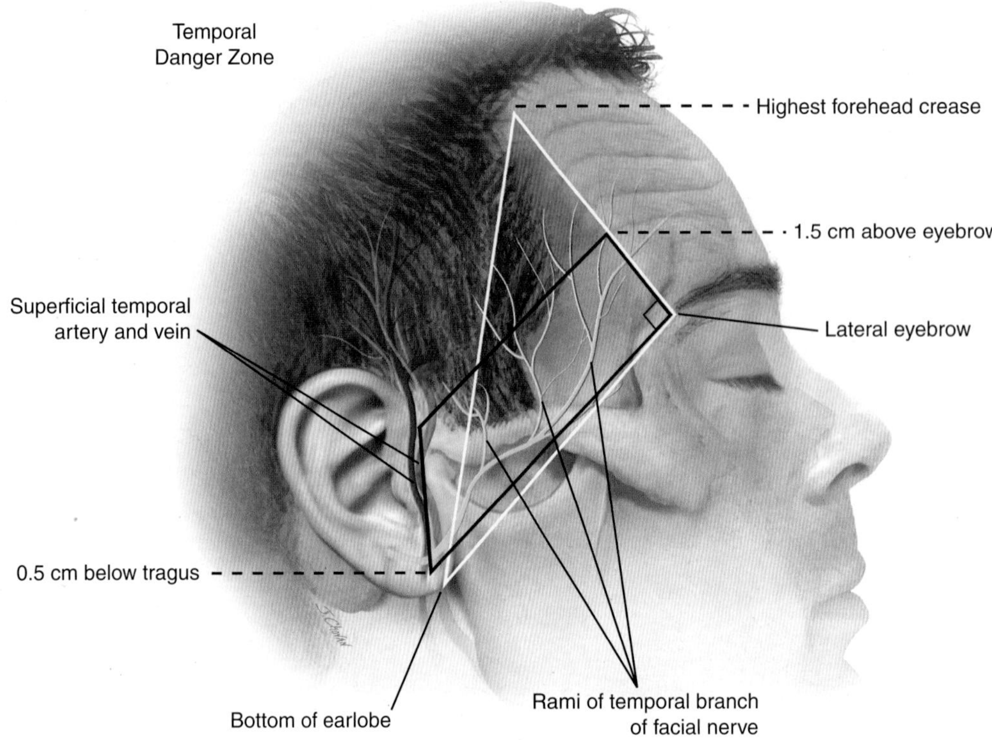

Figure 5.6 Temporal danger zone.

beyond the scope of this chapter.[25] In general, the three main branches of CN V provide sensation to the following.

1. **CN V1:** Cutaneous sensation to the eye, upper eyelid, forehead, nasal dorsum, anterior scalp to the vertex superiorly and the dura mater of the anterior cranial fossa. The ophthalmic and ciliary nerves provide sensation to the skin and conjunctiva of the upper eyelid and cornea, respectively. CN V1 also provides sensation to the upper nasal mucosa, the septal mucosa, and the mucosa of the frontal, ethmoidal, and sphenoidal sinuses.
2. **CN V2:** Cutaneous sensation to the cheek, side of the face, lower eyelid, side of the nose, and upper lip. Sensation to the maxillary dentition and mucosal sensation of the maxillary sinus are via the anterior, middle, and posterior superior alveolar nerves.
3. **CN V3:** Sensation to the lower lip, cheek, temple, anterior two-thirds of the tongue, floor of mouth, and mandibular dentition. The trunk of CN V3 has a large area of dural innervation in both the middle and posterior cranial fossa. The symptomology of temporomandibular joint dysfunction headache is directly related to this sensory distribution.

Knowledge of the location of the foramina of sensory nerves can limit the possibility of inadvertent neurosensory damage during dissection.

Other nerves that provide sensory innervation of the face include the great auricular nerve (C2–C3) and the lesser occipital nerve, which provide sensation to the skin of the ear (Fig. 5.8).

The Vascular Supply of the Face

The arterial supply of the face arises primarily from the external carotid systems. The central face, including the periorbital region, upper two-thirds of the nose, and central forehead, receives some anastomotic arterial supply via the ophthalmic division of the internal carotid artery.

The anterior face is densely populated with musculocutaneous perforating arteries, such as the facial and infraorbital arteries. Laterally, the face is supplied by larger, more anatomically consistent fasciocutaneous perforators, including the transverse facial, submental, and zygomatico-orbital arteries.[26] An understanding of the vascular supply of a given region is important when treatment planning involves the use of facial flaps for various facial defects, such as when the blood supply for a facelift depends on medially based musculocutaneous perforators.

The cutaneous angiosome concept provides some opportunity for surgical treatment planning, particularly when designing facial cutaneous flaps. Generally, the concept is that regional segments of bone, muscle, nerve, and overlying skin are supplied by a common vessel.[27]

Venous drainage of the face is primarily through the internal jugular vein. The facial vein and anterior division of the retromandibular vein join to become the facial vein that empties into the internal jugular vein. The internal jugular vein additionally receives venous return from the lingual, superior

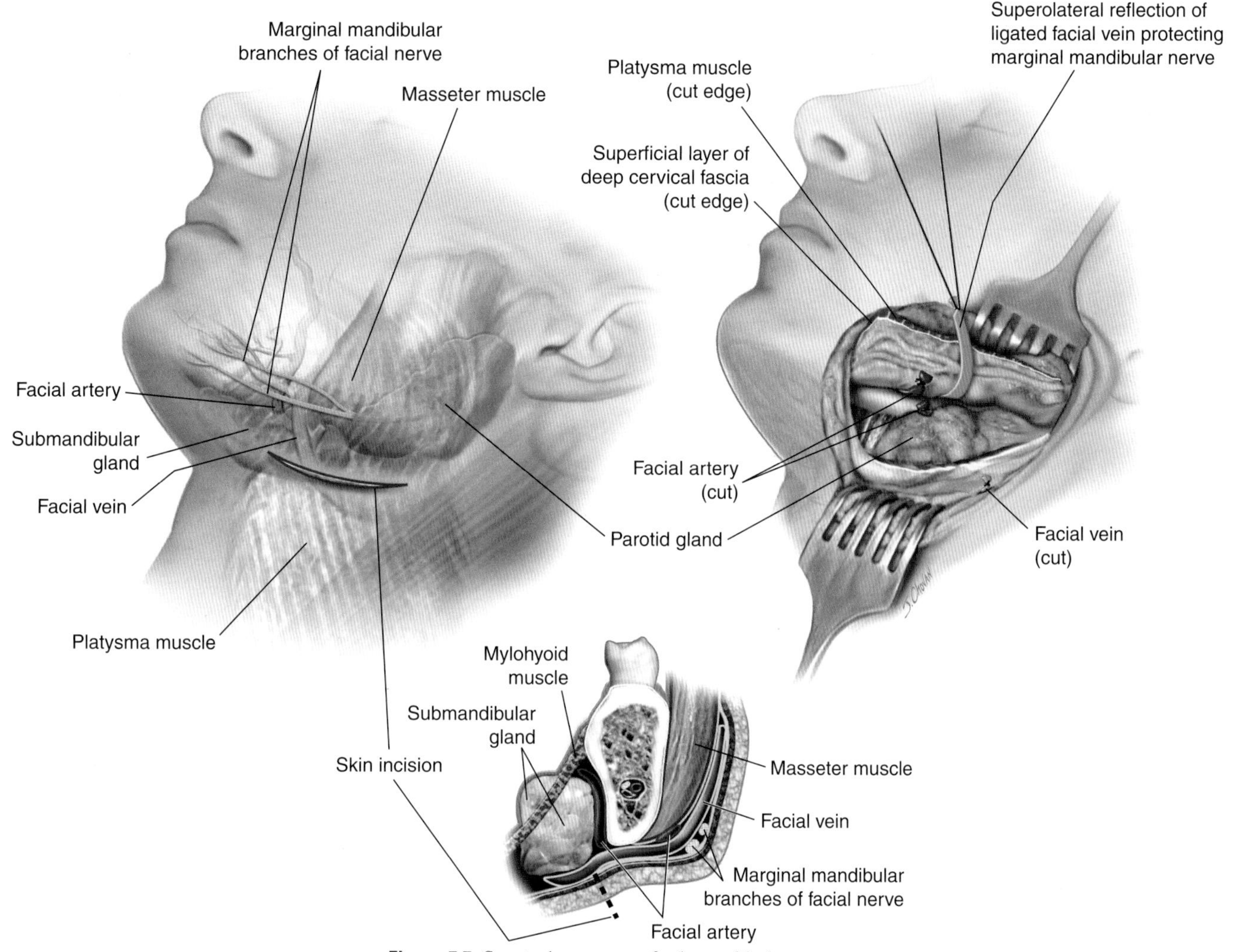

Figure 5.7 Surgical anatomy of submandibular access.

thyroid, and middle thyroid veins. The external jugular vein receives blood from the posterior division of the retromandibular vein and the posterior auricular vein.

Of clinical importance is the complex and extensive communication between extracranial veins and intracerebral veins. Many of these venous anastomoses may allow retrograde bacterial contamination and result in thrombosis of the cavernous sinus or devastating infections. The dangerous area of the face is a triangle formed by the corners of the mouth to the bridge of the nose; this area contains the angular vein that connects with the superior ophthalmic vein and cavernous sinus. The veins of the palatine tonsil also may be a conduit for infection because they connect with the pterygoid plexus and inferior ophthalmic vein and the cavernous sinus. Historically, this process was thought to be due to an anatomic deficiency of the valves in these veins; however, it is more likely due to relative proximity and the possibility of retrograde flow that allows for passage of bacteria into these vital areas (Figs. 5.9 and 5.10).[28,29]

Special Considerations

Maxilla and Mandible

The vascular supply to the maxilla and mandible is of particular importance to the facial surgeon in orthognathic and trauma surgery. Blood supply to the mandible after fracture or osteotomy is through a combination of centripetal blood flow from the periosteum and centrifugal flow from the inferior alveolar arteries. In an intact mandible, the blood supply is almost exclusively from the inferior alveolar artery; however, after traumatic or surgical insult, centripetal flow from the periosteum provides a sustaining arterial supply.[30,31]

In the maxilla, the vascular supply is somewhat more complex. Arterial anastomosis of the nasopalatine, descending palatine, and palatal vascular supply from the ascending pharyngeal artery and the ascending palatine branch of the facial artery supplies the intact maxilla. After down-fracture of the maxilla for orthognathic surgery, the blood supply of the ascending pharyngeal artery and the ascending

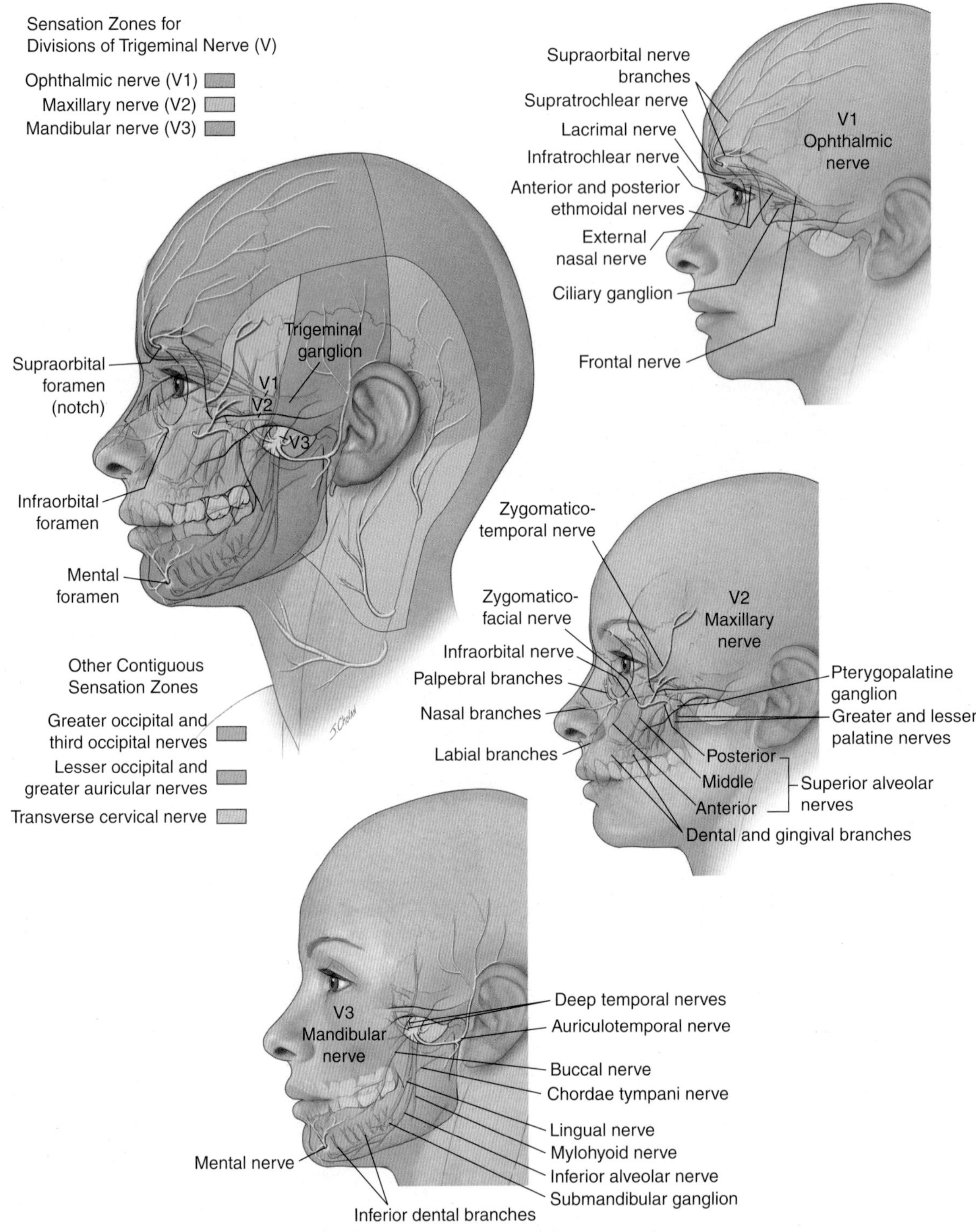

Figure 5.8 Sensory distribution of the trigeminal nerve.

palatine branch of the facial artery provide sustaining arterial supply.[32]

Temporomandibular Joint

The arterial supply to the temporomandibular joint (TMJ) is from the superficial temporal artery and from the maxillary artery posteriorly and the masseteric, posterior deep temporal, and lateral pterygoid arteries anteriorly. Venous drainage is via a plexus around the capsule and venous channels in the retrodiscal tissue.

Blood Supply to the Nose

The proximal vascular supply to the nose is from the ophthalmic artery via the anterior ethmoidal artery and the dorsal nasal and external nasal arteries. The facial artery

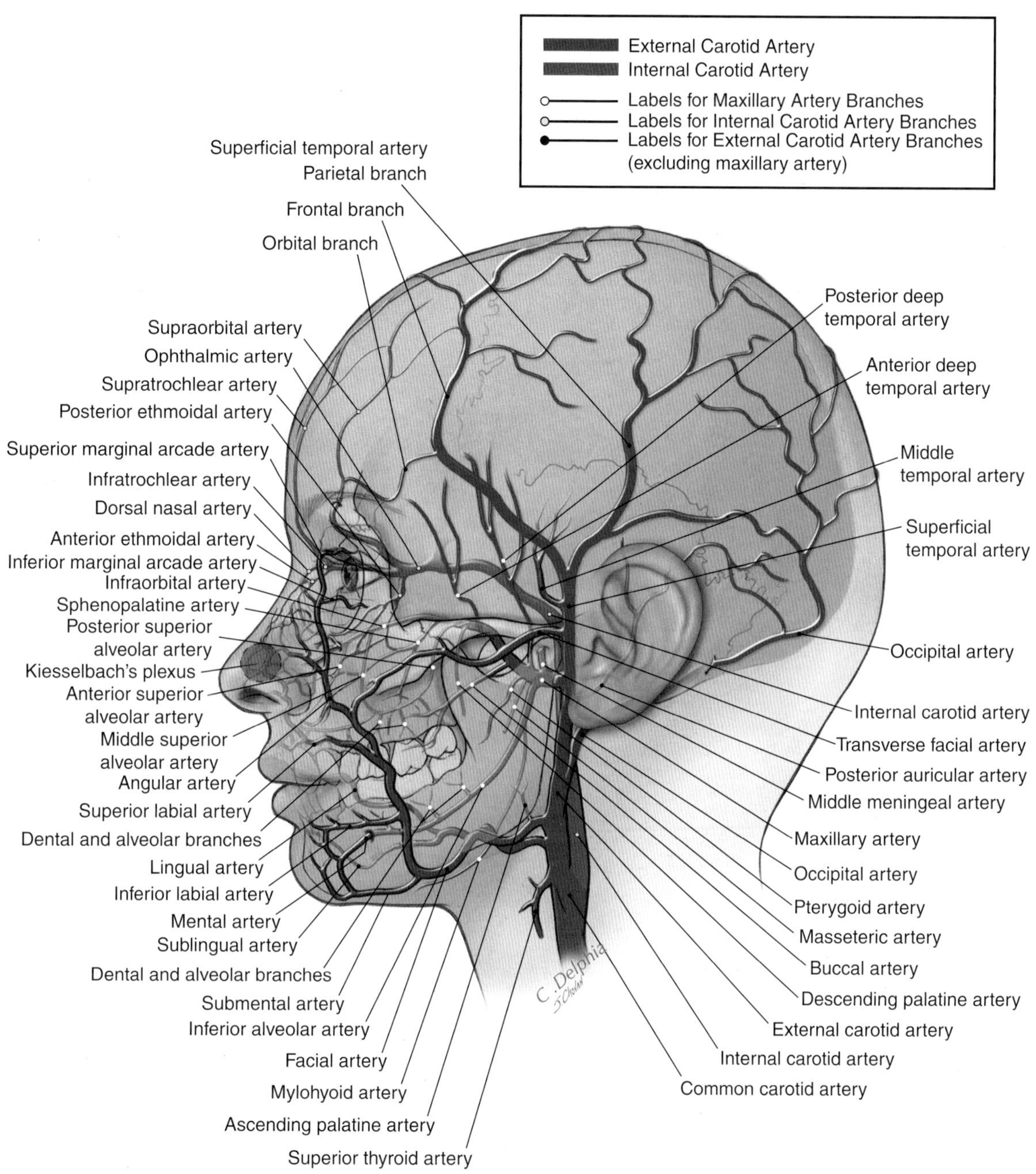

Figure 5.9 Arteries of the head and neck.

supplies the nasal tip via the superior labial and angular arteries. Disruption of the lateral nasal branch of the facial artery off the angular artery may result in loss of vascular supply to the nasal tip; this has implications in revision rhinoplasty.[33]

Kesselbach plexus is the rich vascular network of the nasal septum and is responsible for 90% of nosebleeds. Four arteries anastomose at this site: the nasopalatine branch of the descending palatine artery anastomoses with the septal branches of the sphenopalatine artery, the anterior ethmoidal artery, and the superior lateral branches of the superior labial branch of the facial artery (see Fig. 5.10).

The Oral Cavity

The oral cavity extends from the oral aperture to the palatoglossal fold. It contains the tongue and 20 deciduous (then 32 permanent) teeth. The musculature of the tongue was discussed earlier in this chapter.

The parotid duct (Stensen duct) is approximately 7 cm long; it exits the parotid gland and passes superficial to the masseter, then turns medially and passes through the buccinator to exit into the oral cavity at the level of the maxillary second molar. The approximate position of the duct can be

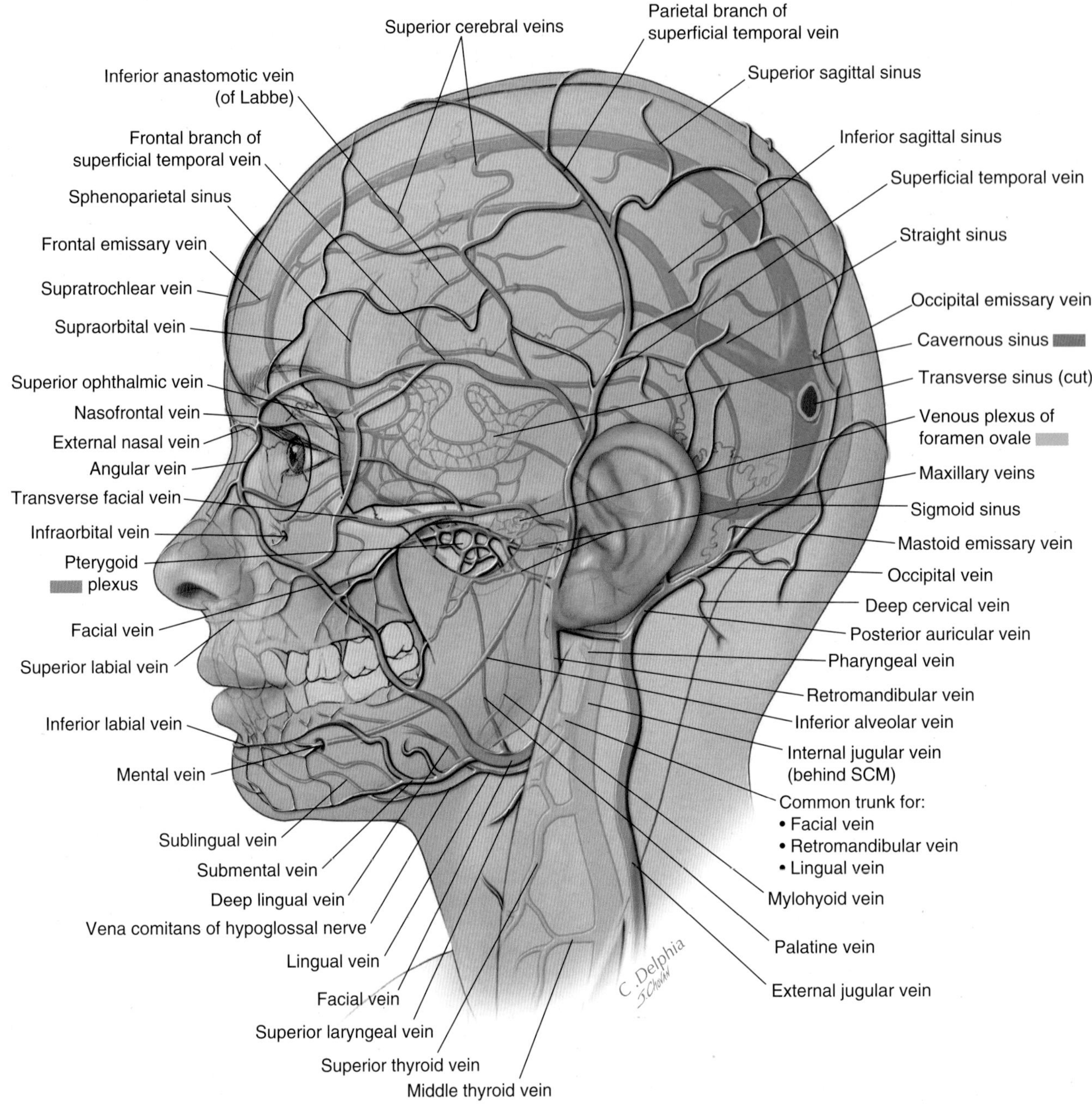

Figure 5.10 Veins of the head and neck.

estimated by drawing an imaginary line from the tragus to a midpoint between the upper lip and columella.[34]

In the floor of the mouth, the bilateral submandibular ducts empty on either side of the lingual frenum. The Wharton duct, which is approximately 5 cm in length, runs medial to the mylohyoid and lateral to the hyoglossus and genioglossus muscles. The lingual nerve descends laterally and, between the second and third molars, loops inferiorly to the duct, traveling superiorly and medially to innervate the muscles of the tongue; this makes almost a complete loop around the submandibular duct.

The sublingual glands drain inconspicuously into the floor of the mouth (Fig. 5.11).

The Temporomandibular Joint

The TMJ has been described as a ginglymoarthrodial joint because functionally it is composed of four articulating surfaces and two compartments (Fig. 5.12). The sliding, or arthrodial, upper compartment comprises the glenoid fossa, articular eminence of the temporal bone, and superior articular disk surface. The rotational, or ginglymoid, lower compartment is made up of the inferior articular disk surface and the condyle. The joint is surrounded by a fibrous capsule and has a synovial lining.

The articular disk is made up of dense, fibrous connective tissue, or fibrocartilage, and anatomically has three zones: the

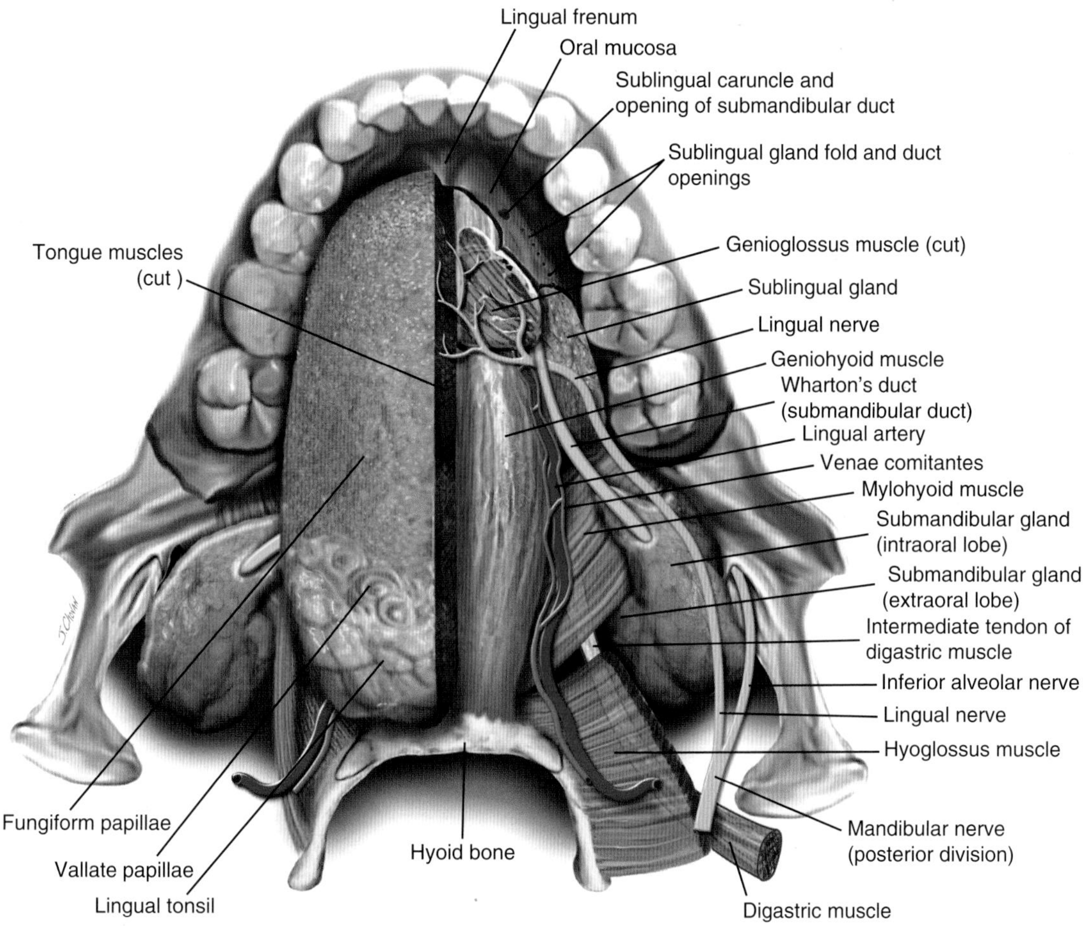

Figure 5.11 Anatomy of the floor of the mouth. The lingual nerve passes from lateral to medial inferior to the submandibular duct.

thick anterior zone, the thicker posterior zone, and the thin (avascular/aneural) intermediate zone.[35]

The disk is attached anteriorly to the articular eminence, condylar head, and joint capsule. The disk is attached posteriorly to the highly vascularized retrodiscal tissue. Medial and laterally the disk is attached to the capsule and neck of the condyle with attachment of the superior division of the lateral pterygoid muscle. There are three functional supporting ligaments of the TMJ: the collateral ligaments, the capsular ligaments, and the temporomandibular ligaments. The mandibular condyle is 15 to 20 mm wide (mediolaterally) and 8 to 10 mm long (anteroposteriorly). The vascular supply to the TMJ is discussed elsewhere in this chapter.

The Maxilla and Mandible

The osteology of the maxilla and mandible has been well described. However, understanding the anatomic positions of key structures aids in surgical treatment planning.

Design of a maxillary osteotomy should take into account the position of the infraorbital nerves bilaterally and the nasolacrimal canal. The infraorbital nerves are visualized during a standard dissection. The nasolacrimal canal orifice lies 10 to 21 mm from a horizontal line at the level of the piriform.[36]

In the mandible, the inferior alveolar nerve travels within the mandibular canal. This canal begins on the medial surface of the mandible posterior and behind the lingula. The neurovascular bundle descends inferiorly to its most inferior position at the first molar and then again ascends. Lateromedially, the canal is closest to the cortical plate in the third molar, with the greatest distance buccal to the first molar. Anteriorly, the nerve exits the mental foramen on the external surface of the mandible near the apex of the first and second premolar.[37]

The Nose

The surface anatomy of the nose is generally broken up into thirds. The upper third, also referred to as the *nasion* or *bony vault,* is made up of the paired nasal bones and the frontal process of the maxilla. Inferiorly, the nasal bones overlap with the upper lateral cartilages caudally for 6 to 8 mm; this is known as the keystone area and is the widest aspect of the nasal dorsum. This portion makes up the middle third, also referred to as the *upper cartilaginous vault.* The junction of the upper and lower lateral cartilages forms the scroll area. The lower one-third, also referred to as the *lobule* or *lower cartilaginous vault,* contains the lower lateral cartilages and their three subdivisions, the medial, middle, and lateral crura.

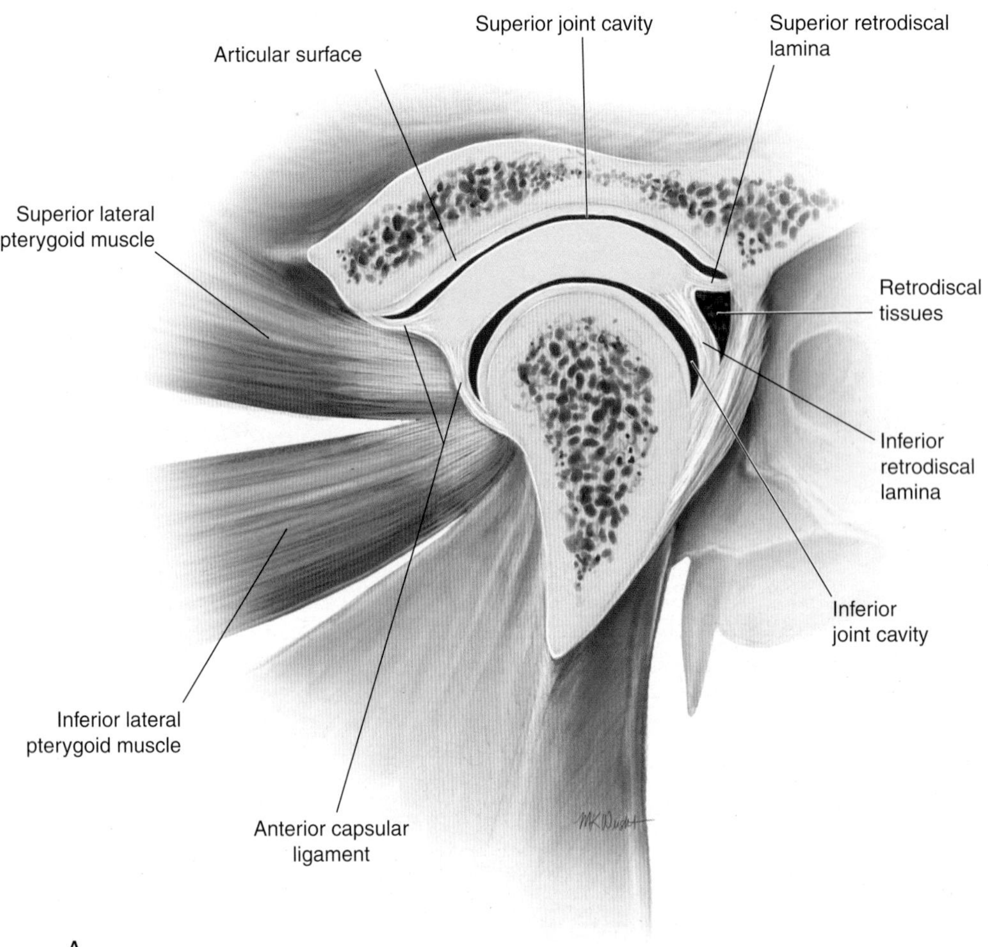

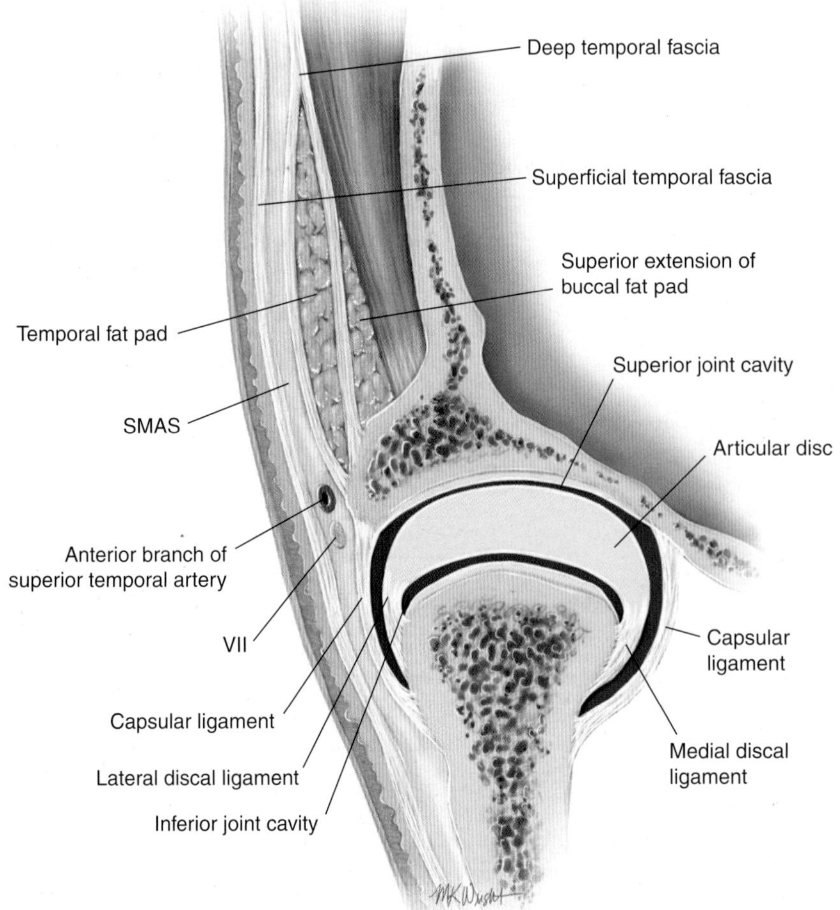

Figure 5.12 **A,** Lateral view of the temporomandibular joint. **B,** Anteroposterior view of the temporomandibular joint. Expanded view also shows the position of the facial nerve when in the temporal danger zone. Note that superior to the zygomatic arch, the temporalis fascia splits into superficial and deep with an intervening temporal fat pad. *SMAS*, Superficial musculoaponeurotic system.

The nasal septum is composed of the septal cartilage, the perpendicular plate of the ethmoid, and the vomer. The junction of the nasal septum and upper lateral cartilages forms the internal nasal valve; a normal angle is 10 to 15 degrees.[38] The external nasal valve is formed by the membranous septum, the caudal edge of the lateral crus of the lower lateral cartilage, and the soft tissue ala.[39]

Skin thickness is variable over the surface of the nose, and the thinnest skin is at the rhinion (0.6 mm). The skin is generally more mobile in the upper two-thirds of the nose and thicker and more adherent inferiorly.

Tip support mechanisms will be discussed more specifically in other parts of this text. The basic underlying anatomy as well as understanding the anatomic major and minor tip support mechanisms should guide the approach to the nasal skeleton. Vascular supply of the nose is discussed elsewhere in this chapter.

Summary

A comprehensive understanding of the anatomy of the face, mouth, and jaws is fundamental to facial surgery. Review of the anatomic features of a particular region before surgical access allows the surgeon to optimize cosmetic and functional results and limit iatrogenic injury.

References

1. Gonzalez-Ulloa M, Castillo A, Stevens E, et al. Preliminary study of the total restoration of the facial skin. *Plast Reconstr Surg.* 1946;13(3):151–161.
2. Burget GC, Menick FJ. The subunit principle in nasal reconstruction. *Plast Reconstr Surg.* 1985;76(2):239–247.
3. Burget GC, Menick FJ. Nasal reconstruction: seeking a fourth dimension. *Plast Reconstr Surg.* 1986;78(2):145–157.
4. Ha RY, Nojima K, Adams WP Jr, Brown SA. Analysis of facial skin thickness: defining the relative thickness index. *Plast Reconstr Surg.* 2005;115(6):1769–1773.
5. Pagnoni A, Kligman AM, el Gammal S, Stoudemayer T. Determination of density of follicles on various regions of the face by cyanoacrylate biopsy: correlation with sebum output. *Br J Dermatol.* 1994;131(6):862–865.
6. Gassner HG, Rafii A, Young A, Murakami C, Moe KS, Larrabee WF Jr. Surgical anatomy of the face: implications for modern face-lift techniques. *Arch Facial Plast Surg.* 2008;10(1):9–19.
7. Arce K. Buccal fat pad in maxillary reconstruction. *Atlas Oral Maxillofac Surg Clin North Am.* 2007;15(1):23–32.
8. Rohrich RJ, Pessa JE. The fat compartments of the face: anatomy and clinical implications for cosmetic surgery. *Plast Reconstr Surg.* 2007;119(7):2219–2227.
9. Mitz V, Peyronie M. The superficial musculo-aponeurotic system (SMAS) in the parotid and cheek area. *Plast Reconstr Surg.* 1976;58(1):80–88.
10. Barton FE Jr. The SMAS and the nasolabial fold. *Plast Reconstr Surg.* 1992;89(6):1054–1057.
11. Freilinger G, Gruber H, Happak W, Pechmann U. Surgical anatomy of the mimic muscle system and the facial nerve: importance for reconstructive and aesthetic surgery. *Plast Reconstr Surg.* 1987;80(5):686–690.
12. Tabb HG, Tannehill JF. The tympanomastoid fissure: a reliable approach to the facial nerve in parotid surgery. *South Med J.* 1973;66(11):1273–1276.
13. Davis RA, Anson BJ, Budinger JM, Kurth LR. Surgical anatomy of the facial nerve and parotid gland based upon a study of 350 cervicofacial halves. *Surg Gynecol Obstet.* 1956;102(4):385–412.
14. Baker DC, Conley J. Avoiding facial nerve injuries in rhytidectomy. Anatomical variations and pitfalls. *Plast Reconstr Surg.* 1979;64(6):781–795.
15. Al-Kayat A, Bramley P. A modified pre-auricular approach to the temporomandibular joint and malar arch. *Br J Oral Surg.* 1979;17(2):91–103.
16. Gosain AK, Sewall SR, Yousif NJ. The temporal branch of the facial nerve: how reliably can we predict its path? *Plast Reconstr Surg.* 1997;99(5):1224–1233.
17. Bernstein L, Nelson RH. Surgical anatomy of the extraparotid distribution of the facial nerve. *Arch Otolaryngol.* 1984;110(3):177–183.
18. Correia PdeC, Zani R. Surgical anatomy of the facial nerve, as related to ancillary operations in rhytidoplasty. *Plast Reconstr Surg.* 1973;52(5):549–552.
19. Pitanguy I. Facial cosmetic surgery: a 30-year perspective. *Plast Reconstr Surg.* 2000;105(4):1517–1526.
20. Pitanguy I, Ramos AS. The frontal branch of the facial nerve: the importance of its variations in face lifting. *Plast Reconstr Surg.* 1966;38(4):352–356.
21. Dingman RO, Grabb WC. Surgical anatomy of the mandibular ramus of the facial nerve based on the dissection of 100 facial halves. *Plast Reconstr Surg Transplant Bull.* 1962;29:266–272.
22. Liebman EP, Webster RC, Gaul JR, Griffin T. The marginal mandibular nerve in rhytidectomy and liposuction surgery. *Arch Otolaryngol Head Neck Surg.* 1988;114(2):179–181.
23. Ziarah HA, Atkinson ME. The surgical anatomy of the mandibular distribution of the facial nerve. *Br J Oral Surg.* 1981;19(3):159–170.
24. Furnas DW. The retaining ligaments of the cheek. *Plast Reconstr Surg.* 1989;83(1):11–16.
25. Zide BM, Swift R. How to block and tackle the face. *Plast Reconstr Surg.* 1998;101(3):840–851.
26. Whetzel TP, Mathes SJ. Arterial anatomy of the face: an analysis of vascular territories and perforating cutaneous vessels. *Plast Reconstr Surg.* 1992;89(4):591–603.
27. Taylor GI, Palmer JH. The vascular territories (angiosomes) of the body: experimental study and clinical applications. *Br J Plast Surg.* 1987;40(2):113–141.
28. Martin W. *Staphylococcus* infections of the face and lips. *Ann Surg.* 1922;76(1):13–27.
29. Zhang J, Stringer MD. Ophthalmic and facial veins are not valveless. *Clin Exp Ophthalmol.* 2010;38(5):502–510.
30. Bell WH, Levy BM. Revascularization and bone healing after anterior mandibular osteotomy. *J Oral Surg.* 1970;28(3):196–203.
31. Hellem S, Ostrup LT. Normal and retrograde blood supply to the body of the mandible in the dog. II. The role played by periosteomedullary and symphyseal anastomoses. *Int J Oral Surg.* 1981;10(1):31–42.
32. Bell WH. Revascularization and bone healing after anterior maxillary osteotomy: a study using adult rhesus monkeys. *J Oral Surg.* 1969;27(4):249–255.
33. Rohrich RJ, Gunter JP, Friedman RM. Nasal tip blood supply: an anatomic study validating the safety of the transcolumellar incision in rhinoplasty. *Plast Reconstr Surg.* 1995;95(5):795–799.
34. Cummings CW. *Cummings Otolaryngology Head and Neck Surgery.* 4th ed. Philadelphia: Mosby; 2005.
35. Poswillo D. Experimental reconstruction of the mandibular joint. *Int J Oral Surg.* 1974;3(6):400–411.
36. You ZH, Bell WH, Finn RA. Location of the nasolacrimal canal in relation to the high Le Fort I osteotomy. *J Oral Maxillofac Surg.* 1992;50(10):1075–1080.
37. Rajchel J, Ellis E III, Fonseca RJ. The anatomical location of the mandibular canal: its relationship to the sagittal ramus osteotomy. *Int J Adult Orthodon Orthognath Surg.* 1986;1(1):37–47.
38. Haight JS, Cole P. The site and function of the nasal valve. *Laryngoscope.* 1983;93(1):49–55.
39. Drumheller GW. Topology of the lateral nasal cartilages: the anatomical relationship of the lateral nasal to the greater alar cartilage, lateral crus. *Anat Rec.* 1973;176(3):321–327.

CHAPTER 6

The Salivary Glands

Brandyn Herman and Melvyn Yeoh

The human salivary gland system is composed of glands that are found in and around the mouth and throat. They can be divided into two distinct exocrine groups, the major salivary glands and the minor salivary glands. Collectively, the paired parotid, submandibular, and sublingual glands are referred to as the *major salivary glands* (Fig. 6.1). They all secrete saliva into the mouth through tubes called *salivary ducts.* The parotid duct, or Stensen duct, is located in the buccal mucosa adjacent to the upper molars; the submandibular duct, or Wharton duct, is found under the tongue in the anterior floor of the mouth; and the sublingual glands open through multiple small ducts in the floor of the mouth. In addition to these glands, many tiny glands, called minor salivary glands, are located in the lips, inner cheek area (buccal mucosa), and extensively in other linings of the mouth and throat. As a whole, salivary glands produce the saliva used to moisten the mouth, initiate digestion, and help protect teeth from decay.

General Anatomic Considerations

Histologically, the glands are all divided into lobules.[1] Specific blood vessels and nerves supplying the glands enter at the hilum and subsequently branch out into the lobules. The ducts follow the same general anatomic considerations applicable to all exocrine glands (Fig. 6.2). The acinus is the secretory end piece of the salivary gland. Acini produce and secrete the saliva into lumina formed by intercalated ducts.[1] The intercalated ducts then join each other to form striated ducts, finally draining into ducts located between the lobes of the gland. Cuboidal epithelial cells form the ductal epithelium and are partially covered by myoepithelial cells. The acinus unit is composed of excretory/secretory cells and surrounding myoepithelial cells. Human salivary gland acinar secretory cells can be broken down into two major types, serous and mucous; these are differentiated from one another by the chemical composition and morphologic profiles of the secretory granules within them.[2] Mucous secretory granules contain appreciable amounts of mucin and glycoconjugates. The distal ends of the mucous acinar units are surrounded by serous demilunes in the submandibular and sublingual glands. These serous demilunes secrete small amounts of serous saliva that mixes with the mucous saliva secreted by the majority of mucous cells in the mucous acinus.[3] In general, serous secretory granules contain a small amount of glycoconjugates and a large amount of water and ions, but some serous granules contain acidic glycoconjugates (these are termed *seromucous*).[4]

Parotid Gland

Anatomy

The parotid gland is the largest of the paired major salivary glands. The average gland weighs between 14 and 28 g. In men the gland averages 5.8 cm in the craniocaudal dimension and 3.4 cm in the ventrodorsal axis (it tends to be slightly smaller in women).[5–8] The intercalated ducts are long and thin.[6] The parotid gland has an abundance of fatty tissue in its parenchyma, with a ratio of adipose to acinar tissue of approximately 1:1.[1]

Although commonly mentioned as having distinct superficial and deep lobes, the parotid gland itself is actually not divided in this way anatomically. This nomenclature is based on using the facial nerve and its associated interstitial structures as a reference plane within the gland. The superficial portion is the region that overlies the lateral surface of the ramus of the mandible and masseter muscle, lateral to the facial nerve.[5] The deep portion refers to the smaller region behind and deep to the mandibular ramus, medial to the facial nerve, located between the mastoid process of the temporal bone and the ramus of the mandible.[5] Nearly 80% of the gland lies on the outer surface of the masseter muscle and the ascending ramus and angle of the mandible, lying caudal to and ventral to the external auditory canal and mastoid tip.[6] The remaining approximately 20% of the gland extends medially through an area known as the *stylomandibular tunnel.* This area is bounded ventrally by the posterior edge of the mandibular ramus, dorsally by the anterior borders of the sternocleidomastoid muscle and posterior belly of the digastric muscle, and more deeply and dorsally by the stylomandibular ligament, which extends from the tip of the styloid process to the angle and posterior edge of the mandible.[6] With these anatomic relationships in mind, it can be noted that the deep portion of the gland lies anterior to the styloid process, its musculature, and the carotid sheath, thereby placing this portion in the prestyloid compartment of the parapharyngeal space.[7,8]

The deep lobe portion of the parotid gland is located behind the lower jaw and base of the cranium and cannot be palpated

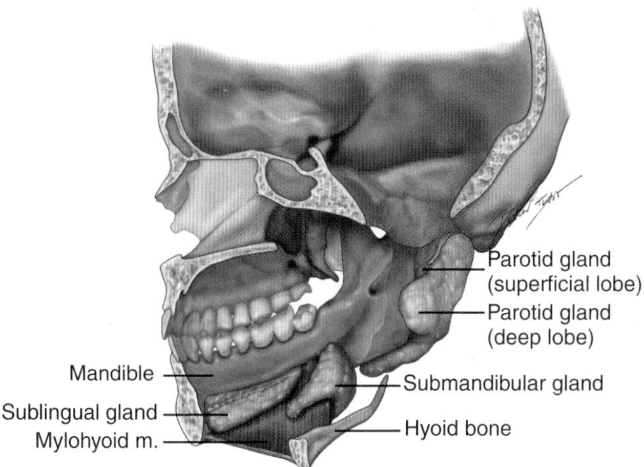

Figure 6.1 Sagittal illustration of the head showing the three major salivary glands: the parotid gland, the submandibular gland, and the sublingual gland.

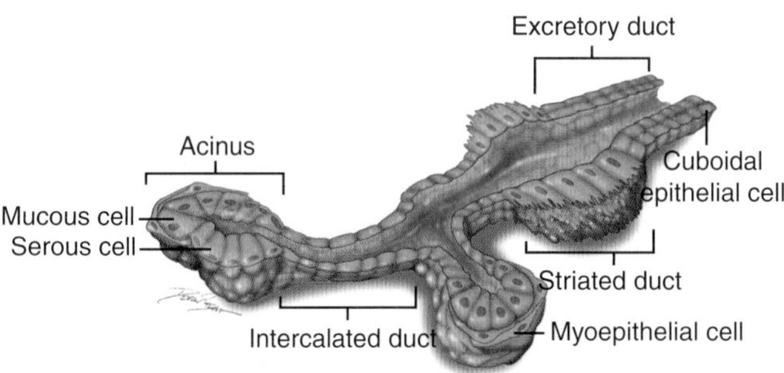

Figure 6.2 Histologic picture of a salivon.

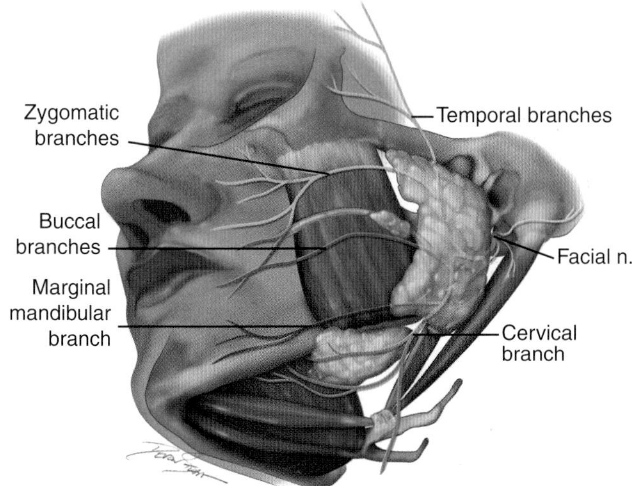

Figure 6.3 Lateral oblique illustration of the parotid gland and submandibular gland. The intimate relationship of the branches of the facial nerve and the parotid gland is illustrated.

under normal conditions. However, the superficial portion can be palpated as it overlies the ramus of the mandible. The parotid gland is irregular in shape, resembling a wedge that envelops the posterior border of the ascending ramus of the mandible (Fig. 6.3).[5] If viewed from its superficial surface, it extends medially to cover a portion of the masseter muscle. The body of the gland fills the space between the mandible and the surface bounded by the external auditory meatus and mastoid process. Deep to the ascending ramus, the gland extends forward variably to lie in contact with the medial pterygoid muscle.[5] Just below the condylar neck, above the medial pterygoid attachment, the gland extends between the two. Near the condyle, the gland lies between the capsule of the temporomandibular joint and external acoustic meatus. Laterally, at the junction of the mastoid process and sternocleidomastoid muscle, the gland lies directly on the posterior belly of the digastric muscle, styloid process, and stylohyoid muscle. These structures separate the gland from the internal carotid artery, internal jugular vein, and cranial nerves (CN) IX to CN XII.[5] A histologically distinct accessory parotid gland with both mucinous and serous acinar cells may also be seen lying anteriorly over the masseter muscle between the parotid duct and zygoma; its ducts empty directly into the parotid duct through one tributary.[9]

Fascia

The parotid gland is fixed by fibrous attachments at several important anatomic landmarks, including the external acoustic meatus, mastoid process, and fibrous sheath of the sternocleidomastoid.[10] The parotid fascia proper is an extension of the deep cervical fascia as it continues superiorly. This fascia splits into superficial and deep layers that completely enclose the gland, forming a dense, inelastic capsule that also covers the masseter muscle on the deep aspect of the parotid gland; this capsule often is referred to as the *parotid masseteric fascia.*[10] The superficial fascia is thicker, extending from the masseter and sternocleidomastoid muscles superiorly to the zygomatic arch. The thinner deep layer extends to the stylomandibular ligament, which separates the superficial and deep lobes of the parotid gland. Important as a surgical landmark, the stylomandibular ligament passes deep to the gland from the styloid process to the posterior border of the ascending ramus just above the angle, thereby also separating the parotid and submandibular glands.[10] The stylomandibular ligament and the mandibular ramus combine to form a tunnel through which a process of the gland can extend into the parapharyngeal space.

Stensen Duct

The parotid duct (Stensen duct) is 4 to 6 cm in length, 5 mm in diameter, and runs 13 mm inferior and parallel to the zygomatic arch.[10] Following a line from the floor of the external auditory meatus to just above the commissure of the lips, the duct exits the gland from its anteromedial surface and courses superficially over the masseter muscle and buccal fat pad.[5] It then turns medially at the anterior border of the muscle, at a near right angle, to pierce the buccinator muscle to empty into the oral cavity. The orifice into the oral cavity, known as the *parotid papilla,* typically can be found buccal to the upper second molars. In 20% of people, as the duct passes over the masseter, it may receive the duct of an accessory parotid gland that is usually slightly cranial to the Stensen duct.[11]

Neural Anatomy

The facial nerve is intimately associated with the parotid gland and has often been used to divide it into a larger superficial lobe and a smaller deep lobe (see Fig. 6.3). The main trunk is always located in the triangle formed by the mastoid, angle of the mandible, and cartilaginous ear canal. Within this triangle the main trunk can be found medial to the mastoid, almost at a point between the mandible and the cartilaginous ear canal.[10] The facial nerve is a mixed nerve carrying motor, sensory, and parasympathetic fibers; it has five intracranial segments and one extracranial segment.

The motor fibers originate from the facial nucleus of the pons. These fibers are joined by the nervus intermedius before entering the temporal bone through the internal acoustic meatus.[5] The nerve takes a tortuous course anteriorly toward the geniculate ganglion and then travels posteriorly along the medial wall of the tympanic cavity toward the second genu at the oval window.[5] The chorda tympani branches off the facial nerve just prior to entering the middle ear at a level 3 to 4 mm inferior to the oval window. The chorda tympani can be seen on otoscopy as it passes behind the tympanic membrane and between the handle of the malleus prior to exiting the skull via the petrotympanic fissure.[12] The facial nerve gives rise to three small branches just before it exits the skull: (1) the posterior auricular, (2) the posterior digastric, and (3) the stylohyoid nerves. As it exits the skull through the stylomastoid foramen, the facial nerve provides motor innervations for the muscles of facial expression.[13] After exiting the skull through the stylomastoid foramen, it courses anterolaterally around the styloid process, following the lateral surface of the posterior belly of the digastric muscle approximately 1 cm before piercing the posterior capsule of the parotid gland, where it splits into two main branches. This area of the facial nerve before it splits is an important surgical and anatomic landmark known as the *pes anserinus* (Latin for "goose's foot").[10] The upper temporofacial branch takes a vertical course, and the lower cervicofacial branch takes an anterior course. The two main branches continue within the gland, lateral to the posterior facial vein and external carotid artery. These two main branches eventually divide into five smaller branches: the temporal, zygomatic, buccal, marginal mandibular, and cervical branches.[14]

Six different branching anatomic patterns have been described, with rami often communicating between the branches, sometimes within the parotid gland but more often anterior to it.[15] The upper temporal and zygomatic branches are branches of the upper division, sharing the motor supply of the orbicularis oculi; the temporal branch alone supplies the forehead musculature. The marginal mandibular and cervical branches are branches of the lower division; the cervical branch supplies the platysma, and the remaining buccal and mandibular branches share the supply of the remaining facial muscles. The buccal branch demonstrates the most anatomic variability and cross-innervation, with the highest number of cross-innervations occurring between the zygomatic and buccal branches.[16] All muscles of facial expression receive motor innervations from the facial nerve on their deep surface except for the mentalis, buccinator, and levator anguli oris muscles.

Autonomic Nerve Innervation

The parotid gland is innervated by sympathetic and parasympathetic fibers (Fig. 6.4). The function of the sympathetic fibers is most likely vasoconstriction, whereas the function of the parasympathetic fibers (CN IX) is most likely secretory. The secretory parasympathetic innervation originates from the inferior salivatory nucleus in the medulla carrying preganglionic parasympathetic fibers through the jugular foramen.[5] The efferent fibers travel through the glossopharyngeal nerve. The Jacobsen nerve, a branch of the glossopharyngeal nerve found distal to the inferior ganglion, reenters the skull through the inferior tympanic canaliculus and proceeds into the middle ear, forming the tympanic plexus.[5] These fibers then continue into the middle cranial fossa as the lesser petrosal nerve, exiting through the foramen ovale to synapse in the otic ganglion.[10] The postganglionic parasympathetic fibers leave the otic ganglion at a level below the mandibular nerve and join the auriculotemporal nerve in the infratemporal fossa. These fibers are responsible for parotid gland salivary secretion. The superior cervical ganglion supplies the sympathetic innervation via postganglionic fibers that innervate the salivary and sweat glands and cutaneous blood vessels. Acetylcholine is the neurotransmitter for both postganglionic sympathetic and parasympathetic fibers.[17]

Arterial Supply

The transverse facial artery, a terminal branch of the external carotid artery, provides the gland's main arterial blood supply.[5] The external carotid artery enters the inferior surface of the gland and divides into two branches, the maxillary and superficial temporal arteries, at the junction between the middle and upper thirds of the gland. The superficial temporal artery gives off the transverse facial artery, which courses anteriorly between the zygoma and parotid duct to supply the parotid gland, parotid duct, and masseter muscle.[18] The maxillary artery courses in a forward and upward direction behind the condylar neck in the part of the parotid gland lying deep to it initially and subsequently emerges coursing into the infratemporal fossa.

Venous Drainage

The venous return is via the retromandibular vein, which is formed by the union of the maxillary and superficial temporal veins.[5] This vein courses through the gland to drain into both the external and internal jugular veins. The facial nerve lies superficial to the vessels, the artery is deeper, and the veins lie between them. The anatomy of the retromandibular vein varies, often bifurcating into anterior and posterior branches.[18]

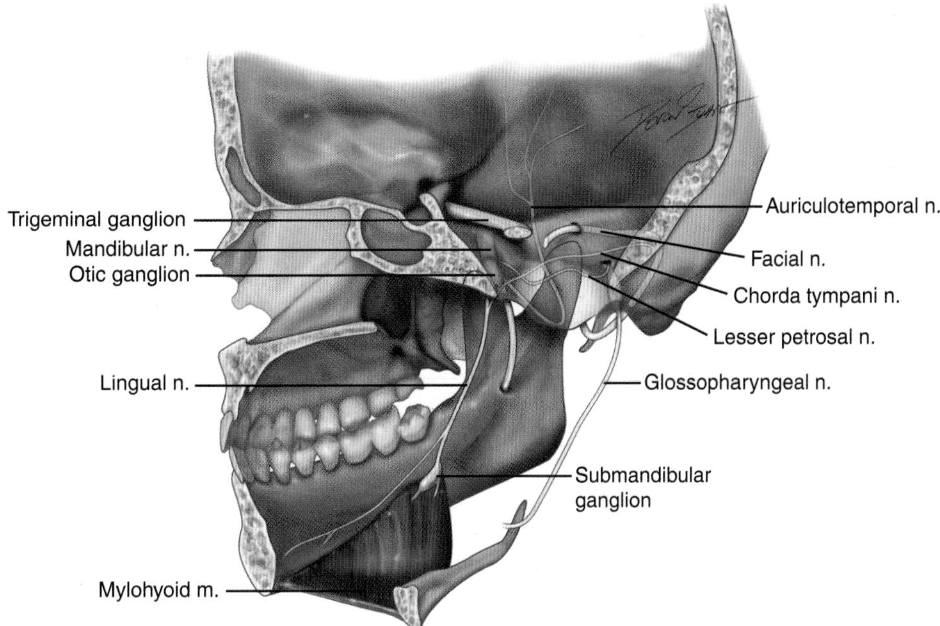

Figure 6.4 Illustration of the parasympathetic supply of the major salivary glands.

The superficial temporal vein typically enters the superior surface of the parotid gland and receives the internal maxillary vein to become the retromandibular vein, lying immediately deep to the marginal mandibular branch of the facial nerve.[18] Within the gland, it divides into anterior and posterior branches. The posterior branch joins the posterior auricular vein above the sternocleidomastoid muscle to form the external jugular vein. The anterior branch emerges from the gland to join the posterior facial vein to form the common facial vein.

Lymphatic Drainage

The lymphatic drainage of the parotid glands is rich and complex. The parotid is the only salivary gland with two nodal layers. Intraparenchymal lymph nodes, located within the parotid substance, receive drainage from the gland itself, external auditory canal, middle ear, soft palate, and posterior nasopharynx.[19] Periparotid lymph nodes, located in the superficial fascia between the glandular tissue and its capsule, serve as lymphatic basins for the scalp, auricle, eyelids, lacrimal glands, and temporal region.[5] Approximately 90% of the nodes are located in this superficial layer of nodes. Both of these systems drain into the superficial and deep cervical lymphatic chains.[11]

Submandibular Gland

Anatomy

The submandibular gland is the second largest salivary gland, about half the weight of the parotid gland, approximately 7 to 16 g.[5]

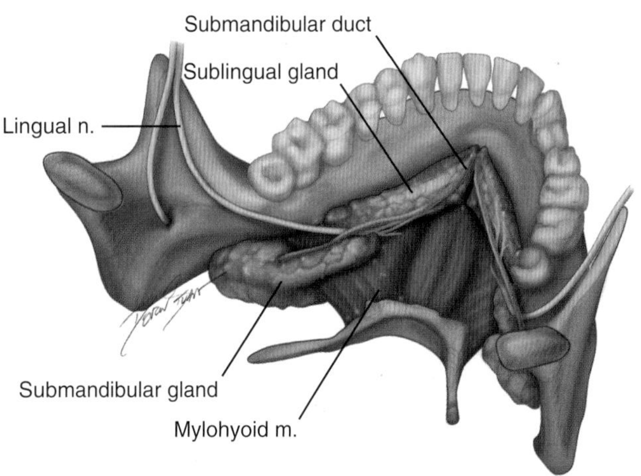

Figure 6.5 Posterior anterior view of the sublingual and submandibular glands.

It occupies most of the submandibular triangle of the neck, formed by the mandible and the anterior and posterior bellies of the digastric muscle (Fig. 6.5). The gland is often referred to as being folded around the dorsal free edge of the mylohyoid muscle.[5] Despite there being no separate lobes to the gland, it is often referred to as being divided by the mylohyoid muscle into a smaller anterior part and larger posterior part connected at the posterior free edge of the muscle. The larger posterior superficial lobe lies superficial and caudal to the mylohyoid muscle, whereas the smaller anterior deep portion lies above the mylohyoid muscle. It is a mixed serous and mucous gland, with about 10% of the acini being mucinous. In contrast to the parotid gland, the intercalated ducts are shorter and wider, and adipose tissue is not a significant component of the glandular parenchyma.[6] Often the gland sends a continuation of tissue with the submandibular duct under the mylohyoid muscle.[20]

Fascia

The submandibular gland is enclosed by the middle layer of the deep cervical fascia.[5]

Wharton Duct

The submandibular duct, also known as the Wharton duct, originates from the anterior surface of the deep portion of the gland, found between the hyoglossus and mylohyoid muscles on the genioglossus muscle. The duct travels 5 cm anteriorly toward the anterior floor of the mouth running superior to the hypoglossal nerve, deep to the lingual nerve and medial to the sublingual gland. It makes an almost 45-degree angle in both the sagittal and axial planes and exits in a papilla lateral to the lingual frenum in the anterior floor of the mouth.[6]

Neural Anatomy

Lying superficial to the submandibular gland are the lingual nerve and the submandibular ganglion, whereas deep to the gland is the hypoglossal nerve. The lingual nerve carries sensory innervations to the anterior two-thirds of the tongue and parasympathetic fibers to the gland itself from the superior salivatory nucleus in the pons, by way of the chorda tympani nerve.[5] The lingual nerve is found under the border of the mandible on the hyoglossus muscle above the hypoglossal nerve. It is attached to the submandibular gland by the submandibular ganglion and courses deep to the mylohyoid muscle to reach the tongue. The lingual nerve crosses the Wharton duct twice, being first lateral then inferior and then medial as it enters the tongue to provide sensation to the anterior two-thirds.

The motor function of the tongue is controlled by the hypoglossal nerve, which is inferior and medial to the posterior third of the gland just below the posterior belly of the digastric muscle.[21] It descends between the internal jugular vein and internal carotid artery, giving off branches of C1 that innervate the thyrohyoid and geniohyoid muscles while supplying the superior limb of the ansa cervicalis.[5] The hypoglossal nerve lies on the surface of the hyoglossus muscle and courses deep to the mylohyoid muscle to supply the tongue.

The marginal branch of the facial nerve runs in a subplatysmal plane within the superficial layer of the deep cervical fascia, continuous with the submandibular gland capsule.[22] The course of the nerve varies, and it commonly has multiple branches. Some studies have reported the nerve as being located above the mandibular border and outside of the submandibular triangle about 50% of the time.[23–25] It courses over the facial vessels as it travels upward to supply the depressor anguli oris and the depressor labii inferioris muscles.

Arterial Supply

The gland is supplied by the submental and sublingual arteries, branches of the lingual and facial arteries, with the facial artery serving as its main arterial blood supply.[22] The facial artery enters the triangle under the posterior belly of the digastric and stylohyoid muscles, running medially, and then hooks over to course superiorly deep to the gland.[22] It ascends to emerge above or through the upper border of the gland, running superiorly and adjacent to the inferior branches of the facial nerve into the face. The lingual artery runs deep to the digastric muscle along the lateral surface of the middle constrictor muscle, coursing anterior and medial to the hyoglossus muscle.[22]

Venous Drainage

The submandibular gland is drained mostly by the anterior facial vein as it courses inferiorly and posteriorly from the face to the inferior aspect of the mandible.[22] Superficial to the gland, the facial vein crosses the submandibular triangle to reach the anterior border of the mandible. It forms extensive anastomoses with the infraorbital and superior ophthalmic veins. Over the middle aspect of the gland, the anterior and posterior facial veins combine to form the common facial vein, which then courses lateral to the gland, exiting the submandibular triangle as it joins the internal jugular vein.[22]

Lymphatic Drainage

The submandibular gland's lymphatic drainage is into the submandibular nodes. These nodes can be classified into five subgroups: (1) preglandular, (2) postglandular, (3) prevascular, (4) postvascular, and (5) intracapsular.[26] Located between the gland and its fascia, but not within the glandular tissue itself, are the prevascular and postvascular lymph nodes, which drain the submandibular gland. They are closely approximated to the facial artery and vein at the gland's superior aspect and ultimately drain into the deep cervical and jugular chains.[27,28]

Sublingual Gland

Anatomy

The sublingual glands are the smallest pair of the major salivary glands, weighing only about 2 g.[5] They are almond-shaped and located above the mylohyoid muscle in the space between the mandible and genioglossus muscles, just below the oral mucosa deep to the sublingual folds opposite the lingual frenum.[29] The sublingual gland's medial contour is separated from the genioglossus muscle by the lingual nerve and the Wharton duct (Fig. 6.6). Unlike the other major salivary glands, it lacks a true fascial capsule and instead is covered by oral mucosa superiorly. It drains into the oral cavity through

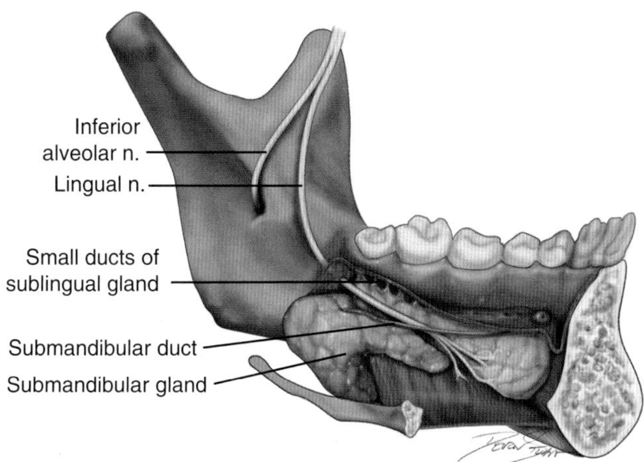

Figure 6.6 The positioning of the submandibular gland in relation to the mylohyoid muscle is illustrated in this sagittal view.

approximately 10 ducts, known as the *ducts of Rivinus,* from the gland's superior aspect.[6] Occasionally, some of the anterior ducts may collect into a larger common duct, known as the Bartholin duct, which empties into the Wharton duct.[7,27]

Neural Anatomy

The sublingual gland is supplied by both the sympathetic and parasympathetic nervous systems. The sympathetic innervation to the gland is derived from paravascular nerves from the cervical ganglion along the facial artery.[5] The presynaptic parasympathetic fibers of the facial nerve are carried by the chorda tympani to synapse in the submandibular ganglion, which then exits as postganglionic fibers to join the lingual nerve to supply the gland.[15]

Arterial Supply

The sublingual gland is supplied arterially via the sublingual and submental arteries, which are branches of the lingual and facial arteries, respectively.[6]

Venous Drainage

The venous drainage reflects the corresponding arterial supply.[6]

Lymphatic Drainage

The lymphatic drainage of the sublingual gland is through the submental and submandibular lymph nodes, the majority being through the submandibular nodes.[5]

Minor Salivary Glands

The minor salivary glands are situated beneath the mucosa of the oral cavity, palate, paranasal sinuses, pharynx, larynx, trachea, and bronchi. They are most numerous in the buccal, labial, palatal, and lingual regions.[5] Relatively few minor salivary glands are found in the gingiva, the anterior aspect of the hard palate, and the true vocal cords. They have the same basic structure as the major salivary glands but are either entirely mucous glands (on the hard palate) or mixed seromucous glands (sinonasal and oral cavities). It has been estimated that there are more than 750 minor salivary glands, ranging in size from 1 to 5 mm.[6] The majority of postganglionic parasympathetic innervation arises from the lingual nerve. The superior palatal glands, however, are innervated by the palatine nerves as they exit the sphenopalatine ganglion.[6] The blood supply and venous and lymphatic drainage of the minor salivary glands follow the supply of the oral cavity region in which they are located.[29]

Embryology

Salivary glands develop from solid epithelial buds that arise from the ectoderm of the primitive mouth. These buds invaginate into the surrounding mesenchyme. This invagination becomes an epithelial cord with a terminal bulb which later develops into the main duct, and through arborization, the body of the gland. Through development there are two distinct cell populations: an outer layer of columnar cells that form secreting acini and an inner layer of cells that produce the ductal system via repetitive bifurcation. Contractile myoepithelial cells arise from neural crest cells that surround the acini. Autonomic innervation stimulates acinar differentiation through sympathetic stimulation, and gland growth is influenced by the parasympathetic system.[30]

Imaging

With the advent of high-resolution 3D imaging via magnetic resonance imaging (MRI), computed tomography (CT), and ultrasound, the conventional sialogram no longer holds preference on being the imaging modality of choice for the salivary glands. Radiologists recommend obtaining CT for evaluation of inflammatory processes and MRI for imaging of tumors. CT has the advantage of demonstrating salivary gland disease and also assists in the identification of sialoliths. MRI offers superior visualization of mass/tumor borders, and in conjunction with contrast, it has the ability to differentiate solid mass versus cystic lesion and evaluate perineural invasion.[6]

High-quality clinical assessment coupled with gland morphology visualized on MRI and CT can have up to a 80% to 90% sensitivity in distinguishing benign and malignant lesions.[31] Clinicians must still be alert to low-grade tumors, such as mucoepidermoid carcinoma and acinic cell carcinoma, that may appear benign due to their smooth appearance, secondary to formation of a pseudocapsule. Benign lesions typically demonstrate low T1 signal intensity and high T2 signal intensity secondary to increased regions of serous and mucinous secretions. In contrast, low signal intensities in both T1 and T2 can have a more ominous prognosis and should alert the surgeon of a higher likelihood of metastatic disease.[6]

References

1. Amano O, Mizobe K, Bando Y, Sakiyama K. Anatomy and histology of rodent and human major salivary glands: overview of the Japan salivary gland society-sponsored workshop. *Acta Histochem Cytochem*. 2012;45(5):241–250.
2. Philips CJ, Tandler B, Nagato T. Evolution and divergence of salivary gland acinar cells: a format for understanding molecular evolution. In: Dobrosielski-Vergona K, ed. *Biology of the Salivary Glands*. Boca Raton, Florida: CRC Press; 1993.
3. Yamashina S, Tamaki H, Katsumata O. The serous demilune of rat sublingual gland is an artificial structure produced by conventional fixation. *Arch Histol Cytol*. 1999;62(4):347–354.
4. Munger BL. Mun[i]ger BL. Histochemical studies on seromucous- and mucous-secreting cells of human salivary glands. *Am J Anat*. 1964;115:411-429.
5. Holsinger FC, Bui DT. Anatomy, function, and evaluation of the salivary glands. In: Myers EN, Ferris RL, eds. *Salivary Gland Disorders*. Berlin, Germany: Springer; 2007.
6. Silvers AR, Som PM. Salivary glands. *Radiol Clin North Am*. 1998;36(5):941–966 (vi).
7. Mason DK, Chisolm DM. *Salivary Glands in Health and Disease*. London, United Kingdom: Saunders; 1975.
8. Batsakis JG. *Tumors of the Head and Neck: Clinical and Pathological Considerations*. 2nd ed. Baltimore, Maryland: Lippincott Williams & Wilkins; 1979.
9. Frommer J. The human accessory parotid gland: its incidence, nature, and significance. *Oral Surg Oral Med Oral Pathol*. 1977;43(5):671–676.
10. Nadershah M, Salama A. Removal of parotid, submandibular, and sublingual glands. *Oral Maxillofac Surg Clin North Am*. 2012;24(2):295–305 (x).
11. Hsu AK, Kutler DI. Indications, techniques, and complications of major salivary gland extirpation. *Oral Maxillofac Surg Clin North Am*. 2009;21(3):313–321.
12. Brennan PA. Chorda tympani. In: *Gray's Surgical Anatomy*. Amsterdam: Elsevier; 2020:91–96.
13. Greywoode JD, Ho HH, Artz GJ, Heffelfinger RN. Management of traumatic facial nerve injuries. *Facial Plast Surg*. 2010;26(6):511–518.
14. McKinney P, Katrana DJ. Prevention of injury to the great auricular nerve during rhytidectomy. *Plast Reconstr Surg*. 1980;66(5):675–679.
15. Davis RA, Anson BJ, Budinger JM, Kurth LR. Surgical anatomy of the facial nerve and parotid gland based upon a study of 350 cervicofacial halves. *Surg Gynecol Obstet*. 1956;102(4):385–412.
16. Gosain AK. Surgical anatomy of the facial nerve. *Clin Plast Surg*. 1995;22(2):241–251.
17. Agur AM, Dalley AF. *Grant's Atlas of Anatomy*. 12th ed. Baltimore, Maryland: Lippincott Williams & Wilkins; 2008.
18. Bhattacharyya N, Varvares MA. Anomalous relationship of the facial nerve and the retromandibular vein: a case report. *J Oral Maxillofac Surg*. 1999;57(1):75–76.
19. Garatea-Crelgo J, Gay-Escoda C, Bermejo B, Buenechea-Imaz R. Morphological study of the parotid lymph nodes. *J Cranio-Maxillo-Fac Surg*. 1993;21(5):207–209.
20. Woodburne RT, Burkel WE. *Essentials of Human Anatomy*. 8th ed. New York, New York: Oxford University Press; 1994.
21. Guerrissi JO, Taborda G. Endoscopic excision of the submandibular gland by an intraoral approach. *J Craniofac Surg*. 2001;12(3):299–303.
22. Carlson GW. The salivary glands. Embryology, anatomy, and surgical applications. *Surg Clin North Am*. 2000;80(1):261–273 (xii).
23. Dingman RO, Grabb WC. Surgical anatomy of the mandibular ramus of the facial nerve based on the dissection of 100 facial halves. *Plast Reconstr Surg Transplant Bull*. 1962;29:266–272.
24. Skandalakis JE, Gray SW, Rowe JS Jr. Surgical anatomy of the submandibular triangle. *Am Surg*. 1979;45(9):590–596.
25. Skandalakis JE, Gray SW, Rowe JS. The neck. In: Skandalakis JE, ed. *Anatomical Complications in General Surgery*. New York, New York: McGraw-Hill; 1983.
26. Portugal LG, Padhya TA, Gluckman JL. The neck: anatomy and physiology. In: Tami TA, Seiden AM, Cotton RT, et al., eds. *Otolaryngology: The Essentials*. New York, New York: Thieme; 2001.
27. Gray H. *Anatomy of the Human Body*. 30th ed. Philadelphia, Pennsylvania: Lea & Febiger; 1985.
28. Pownell PH, Brown OE, Pransky SM, Manning SC. Congenital abnormalities of the submandibular duct. *Int J Pediatr Otorhinolaryngol*. 1992;24(2):161–169.
29. Hollinshead WH. The neck: lymph nodes and lymphatics. In: Hollinshead WH, ed. *Anatomy for Surgeons, Volume 1: The Head and Neck*. 3rd ed. Philadelphia, Pennsylvania: Lippincott Williams & Wilkins; 1982.
30. Sperber GH, Sperber SM. *Craniofacial Embryogenetics and Development*. Raleigh, NC: PMPH USA; 2018:187–189.
31. Liu Y, Li J, Tan YR, Xiong P, Zhong LP. Accuracy of diagnosis of salivary gland tumors with the use of ultrasonography, computed tomography, and magnetic resonance imaging: a meta-analysis. *Oral Surg Oral Med Oral Pathol Oral Radiol*. 2015;119(2):238–245.e2.

CHAPTER 7

The Neck

Jeffrey S. Dean and Rahul Tandon

Although most oral and maxillofacial surgeons spend a great deal of time in the oral cavity and the associated maxillofacial region, the importance of understanding complete head and neck anatomy cannot be ignored. Trauma, superficial pathologic lesions, and infection are just a few of the reasons a maxillofacial surgeon requires a sound understanding of the anatomy of the neck. Malignant tumors in the maxillofacial region can spread through the lymphatic system to adjacent lymph nodes; therefore, a neck dissection is used to remove any suspicious lymph nodes. There are currently four classifications of neck dissection: radical, modified radical, selective, and extended.[1] This chapter focuses on the surgical anatomy of the neck and its relevance for the practicing oral and maxillofacial surgeon. Although many of the key anatomic sites have been identified and established, room remains for growth in both our knowledge of and approaches to this complex area.

Lymphatics (Fig. 7.1)

Before the importance of lymphatics in the organization of the neck is discussed, a brief overview of the main lymphatic duct, the thoracic duct, is imperative. The thoracic duct conveys lymph from the entire body back to the blood; however, the right side of the head and neck, right upper extremity, right lung, right side of the heart, and a portion of the liver all follow a different path. The path originates at the cisterna chili and enters the posterior mediastinum between the azygous vein and thoracic aorta. From there it courses to the left into the neck, anterior to the vertebral artery and vein, eventually entering the junction of the left subclavian and internal jugular veins.

Over the past three decades, advances have been made in our understanding of cervical fascial planes, lymphatic drainage patterns, preoperative staging, and extracapsular spread. Maximizing control and minimizing morbidity are concerns that have prompted modifications to the classic neck dissection. One modification in particular is the preservation of one or more nonlymphatic structures (e.g., spinal accessory nerve, internal jugular vein, and sternocleidomastoid muscle).[2] Further observations have indicated that the pattern of nodal disease depends on the primary site. These findings led to another neck dissection modification, the selective preservation of one or several lymph node groups.

Memorial Sloan-Kettering Cancer Center developed the lymph node regional definitions that are most widely used today. There are approximately 600 lymph nodes in the body, 200 of which are located in the neck. It is important to note that lymphatic flow is well organized and moves in a predictable path in the cervical region.[2] The neck is divided into six areas, or levels, ranging from submental and submandibular triangles toward the chest. These levels are identified by the Roman numerals I through VI. Oral cavity tumors have been found to metastasize to levels I through III,[3] whereas tumors of the lower neck (e.g., laryngeal cancer) tend to spread to lower levels (e.g., level III or IV). Level VII, which represented the lymph node groups in the superior mediastinum, is no longer used. Lymph nodes in nonneck regions are referred to by the name of their specific nodal groups.

Level I

Level I includes the submental and submandibular triangles. This level is itself subdivided. Level Ia is the submental triangle, bounded by the anterior bellies of the digastric and mylohyoid muscles. Level Ib is the triangle formed by the anterior and posterior bellies of the digastric muscle and body of the mandible.

Levels II, III, and IV

Levels II, III, and IV include nodes associated with the internal jugular vein, in addition to fibroadipose tissue located medial to the posterior border of the sternocleidomastoid and lateral to the border of the sternohyoid.

Level II

Level II refers to the upper third nodes, including the upper jugular, jugulodigastric, and upper posterior cervical nodes. It is bounded by the digastric muscle superiorly and the hyoid bone (clinical landmark) or the carotid bifurcation (surgical landmark) inferiorly. Level IIa contains nodes in the region anterior to the spinal accessory nerve, whereas level IIb contains those posterior to the nerve.

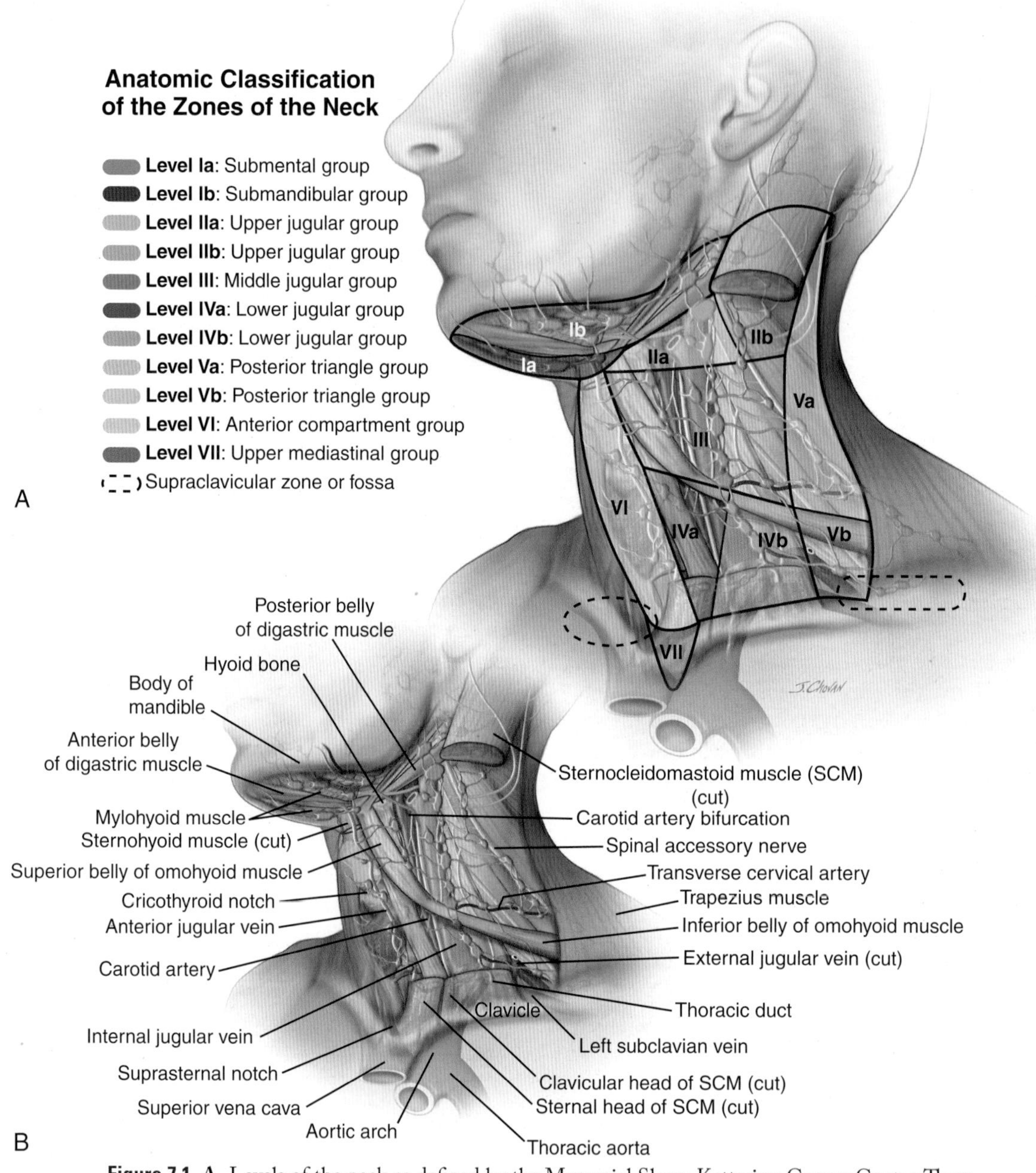

Figure 7.1 **A,** Levels of the neck as defined by the Memorial Sloan-Kettering Cancer Center. These six levels span the submental and submandibular triangles toward the chest and are important in organizing the neck anatomy for surgical procedures. **B,** Lymph nodes of the neck.

Level III

Level III includes the middle third jugular nodes, extending from the carotid bifurcation superiorly to the cricothyroid notch (clinical landmark), the inferior edge of the cricoid cartilage (radiologic landmark), or the omohyoid muscle (surgical landmark).

Level IV

Level IV contains the lower jugular nodes, extending from the omohyoid muscle superiorly to the clavicle inferiorly.

Level V

Level V refers to the posterior triangle group of lymph nodes located along the lower half of the spinal accessory nerve and the transverse cervical artery. The supraclavicular nodes are also included in this group. The posterior boundary is the anterior border of the trapezius muscle, the anterior boundary is the posterior border of the sternocleidomastoid muscle, and the inferior border is the clavicle.

Level VI

Level VI comprises the anterior compartment lymph nodes surrounding the midline visceral structures of the neck, extending from the level of the hyoid bone superiorly to the suprasternal notch inferiorly. On each side the lateral boundary is the medial border of the carotid sheath. Within this compartment are the perithyroidal lymph nodes, paratracheal lymph nodes, precricoid lymph nodes, and the lymph nodes along the recurrent laryngeal nerves.

If all the nodes are removed (levels I through V) and three structures are also removed (internal jugular vein, accessory nerve, and sternocleidomastoid muscle), a *radical* neck dissection has been performed. (The term *radical* is misleading; it simply refers to the fact that a complete neck dissection has been performed.) This procedure is indicated only if tumor spread to the neck is rather extensive. If the nodes from levels I through V are removed and one of the three structures is preserved, the procedure is called a *modified radical* neck dissection. If the operation does not involve all five levels, it is called a *selective* neck dissection.

Anatomic Triangles of the Neck (Fig. 7.2)

The triangles of the neck are bounded by the neck muscles with the sternocleidomastoid muscle dividing the neck into two major triangles, namely the anterior and posterior triangles, each with its own subdivisions. The sternocleidomastoid muscle passes obliquely across the neck, from the sternum and clavicle below to the mastoid process and occipital bone above. The side of the neck presents a somewhat quadrilateral outline limited by the lower border of the body of the mandible from above, an imaginary line extending from the angle of the mandible to the mastoid process and the anterior margin of the trapezius posteriorly, by the upper border of the clavicle from below, and by the midline of the neck anteriorly.

Anterior Triangle

The anterior triangle is bounded in front by the midline of the neck and behind by the anterior margin of the sternocleidomastoid. Its base, which is directed upward, is formed by the inferior border of the body of the mandible and a line extending from the angle of the mandible to the mastoid process; its apex is below, at the sternum. This space is subdivided into four smaller triangles by the digastric muscle above and the superior belly of the omohyoid muscle below. These smaller triangles are named the muscular (inferior carotid, omotracheal) triangle, the superior carotid (carotid) triangle, the submandibular (digastric) triangle, and the suprahyoid (submental) triangle. The anterior triangle is covered by integument, superficial fascia, the platysma, and deep fascia (Table 7.1).

Muscular (Omotracheal) Triangle

The muscular triangle is limited anteriorly by the median line of the neck from the hyoid bone superior to the sternum and behind by the anterior margin of the sternocleidomastoid (shares one margin with the anterior triangle), and the border is the superior belly of the omohyoid. The deep fascia contains branches of the supraclavicular nerves. Beneath these superficial structures are the sternohyoid and sternothyroid muscles, which together with the sternocleidomastoid conceal the lower part of the common carotid artery. This vessel, along with the internal jugular vein and vagus nerve, is enclosed within its sheath. The vein lies lateral to the artery on the right side of the neck but overlaps it below on the left side; the nerve lies between the artery and vein on a plane posterior to both. In front of the sheath are a few descending filaments from the ansa hypoglossi, and behind the sheath are the inferior thyroid artery, the recurrent nerve, and the sympathetic trunk. The medial side of this triangle contains the esophagus, trachea, thyroid gland and parathyroid glands, and lower part of the larynx. By cutting into the upper part of this space and slightly displacing the sternocleidomastoid, the surgeon may tie the common carotid artery below the omohyoid (Table 7.2).

Carotid Triangle

The superior carotid, or carotid, triangle is bounded from behind by the sternocleidomastoid, below by the superior belly of the omohyoid, and above by the stylohyoid and the posterior belly of the digastric. Within the deep fascia are branches of the facial and cutaneous cervical nerves. The floor of the superior carotid triangle is formed by parts of the thyrohyoid muscle, hyoglossus muscle, and the inferior and medial pharyngeal constrictor muscles. When dissected, this area contains the upper part of the common carotid artery, which bifurcates opposite the upper border of the thyroid cartilage into the external and internal carotid. These vessels are somewhat concealed from view by the anterior margin of the sternocleidomastoid, which overlaps them. The external and internal carotids lie side by side, and the external carotid is the more anterior of the two. The following branches of the external carotid are also met within this space: the superior thyroid, running forward and downward; the lingual, directly forward; the external maxillary, forward and upward; the occipital, backward; and the ascending pharyngeal, directly upward on the medial side of the internal carotid. The associated veins are the internal jugular, which lies on the lateral side of the common and internal carotid arteries, and veins corresponding to the above-mentioned branches of the external carotid (the superior thyroid and the lingual, common facial, ascending pharyngeal, and sometimes the occipital), all of which end in the internal jugular.

The nerves in this space should also be taken into consideration by the surgeon. In front of the sheath of the common carotid is the ramus descendens hypoglossi. The hypoglossal nerve crosses both the internal and external carotids above, curving around the origin of the occipital artery. Within the sheath, between the artery and vein and behind both, is the vagus nerve; behind the sheath is the sympathetic trunk. On the lateral sides of the vessels, the accessory nerve runs for a short distance before it pierces the sternocleidomastoid; on the medial side of the external carotid, just below the hyoid

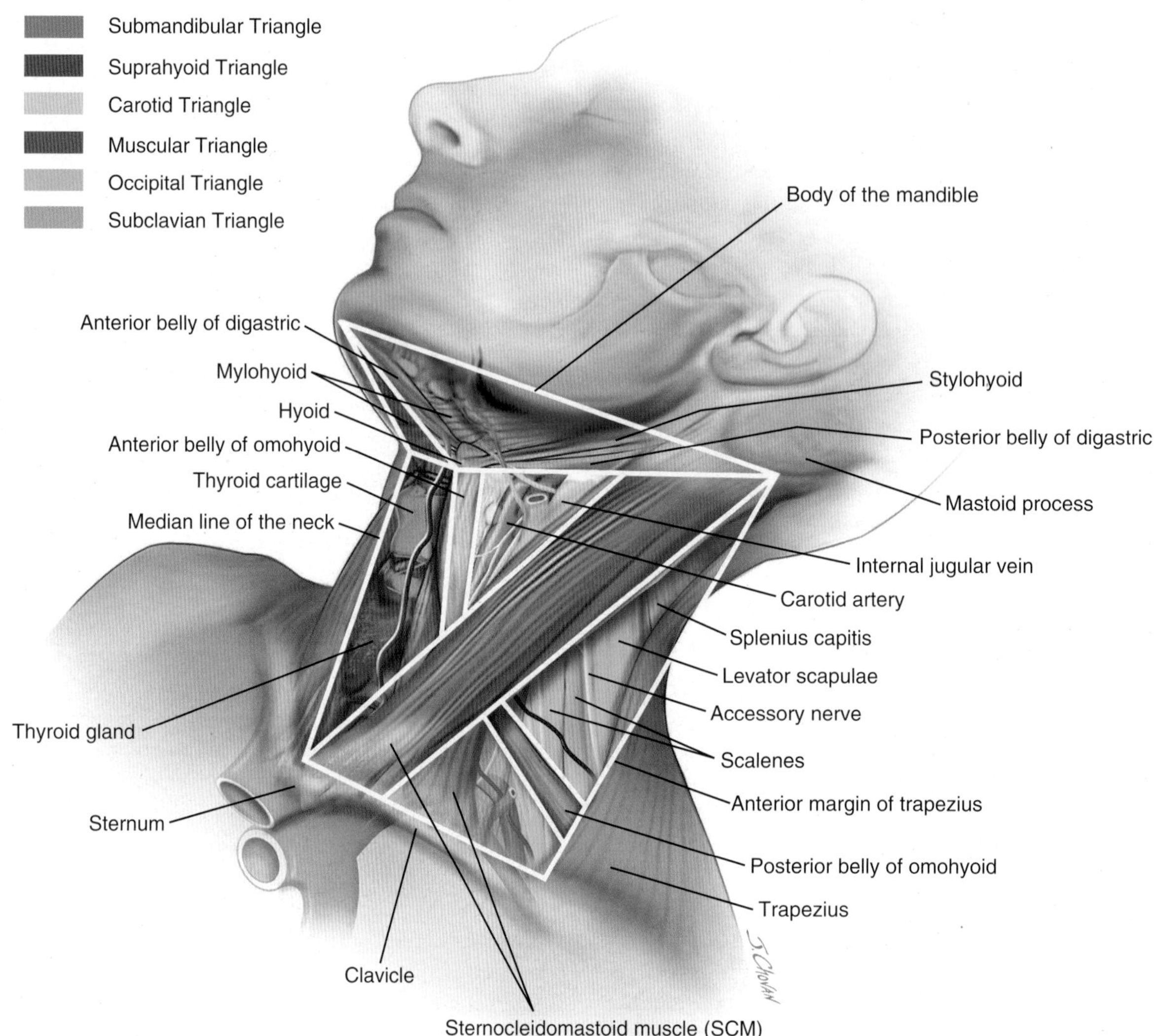

Figure 7.2 Anatomic triangles of the neck and their muscular borders. Also shown are both the arterial and venous supplies of the triangles.

bone, is the internal branch of the superior laryngeal nerve. More inferior is the external branch of the same nerve. The upper portion of the larynx and lower portion of the pharynx are also found in the front part of this space (Table 7.3).

Submaxillary (Digastric) Triangle

The submaxillary, or digastric, triangle corresponds to the region of the neck immediately beneath the body of the mandible. It is bounded above by the lower border of the body of the mandible and a line drawn from its angle to the mastoid process, and below by the posterior belly of the digastric and the stylohyoid. It is bordered in front by the anterior belly of the digastric. Within the deep fascia are branches of the facial nerve and ascending filaments of the cutaneous cervical nerve. The floor consists of the following muscles: mylohyoid, hyoglossus, and superior constrictor pharyngeal. The triangle is divided into an anterior and a posterior part by the stylomandibular ligament. The anterior part contains the submaxillary gland, superficial to which is the anterior facial vein; embedded in the gland is the external maxillary artery and its glandular branches. Beneath the gland, on the surface of the mylohyoid, are the submental artery and the mylohyoid artery and nerve. The posterior part of this triangle contains the external carotid artery, ascending deeply in the substance of the parotid gland; this vessel lies in front of and superficial to the internal carotid; it is crossed by the facial nerve and, during its course, gives off the posterior auricular, superficial temporal, and internal maxillary branches. More deeply are the internal carotid, the internal jugular vein, and the vagus nerve. These structures are separated from the external carotid by the styloglossus and stylopharyngeus muscles and the glossopharyngeal nerve (Table 7.4).

Suprahyoid Triangle

The suprahyoid triangle is limited from behind by the anterior belly of the digastric, in front of the midline of the neck between the mandible and the hyoid bone, and below by the

Table 7.1 The Anterior Triangle

The borders of the anterior triangle	Inferior border of the mandible—superior Midline of the neck—medial Anterior border sternocleidomastoid—lateral
Smaller triangles in the anterior triangle	Muscular (omotracheal) triangle Carotid triangle Submandibular triangle Submental triangle
Structures in the anterior triangle	Thyrohyoid, sternothyroid, sternohyoid muscles Thyroid gland, parathyroid glands, trachea, esophagus, larynx, submandibular gland, inferior portion of the parotid gland Common carotid artery, external carotid artery, internal carotid artery, superior and inferior thyroid artery, facial artery, lingual artery Internal jugular veins, common facial veins, lingual veins, superior and middle thyroid veins Vagus nerves, hypoglossal nerves, mylohyoid nerves, lingual nerves

Table 7.2 The Muscular (Omotracheal) Triangle

The borders of the muscular (omotracheal) triangle	Hyoid bone—superior Midline of the neck—medial Superior belly of the omohyoid and anterior sternocleidomastoid muscles—lateral
Structures in the muscular triangles	Thyroid gland, parathyroid glands, larynx, trachea, esophagus; thyrohyoid, sternothyroid and sternohyoid muscles; superior and inferior thyroid arteries, and anterior jugular veins

Table 7.3 The Carotid Triangle

The borders of the carotid triangle	Superior belly of the omohyoid muscle—anterior Posterior belly of the digastric muscle and stylohyoid muscle—superior Anterior border of the sternocleidomastoid muscle—posterior
Structures in the carotid triangle	Common and external carotid arteries and branches (excluding superficial temporal and posterior auricular artery). Internal jugular vein and corresponding branches to the arteries. Vagus nerve, hypoglossal nerve and sympathetic trunk, part of the accessory nerve, part of the superior laryngeal nerve

Table 7.4 The Submaxillary (Digastric Triangle)

The borders of the submaxillary (digastric) triangle	Inferior border of the mandible—superior Anterior belly of the digastric muscle—lateral Posterior belly of the digastric muscle—medial
Structures found in the submaxillary (digastric) triangle	Submaxillary gland, lymph nodes, inferior portion of the parotid gland. Facial artery and vein, submental artery and vein, lingual artery and vein. Mylohyoid nerve, hypoglossal nerve

body of the hyoid bone. The mylohyoid muscle helps to form the floor. It contains one or two lymph glands and some small veins, which unite to form the anterior jugular vein.

Posterior Triangle (Occipital and Supraclavicular Triangles)

The posterior triangle is bounded in front by the sternocleidomastoid and from behind by the anterior margin of the trapezius. Its base is formed by the middle third of the clavicle, and its apex is formed by the occipital bone. The space is crossed 2.5 cm above the clavicle by the inferior belly of the omohyoid, which divides it into two triangles, an upper (or occipital) triangle and a lower (or subclavian) triangle. Covering this triangle are the overlying skin, superficial and deep fascia, and platysma (Table 7.5).

Occipital Triangle

The larger division of the posterior triangle is bounded in front by the sternocleidomastoid and from behind, by the trapezius; it is limited inferiorly by the omohyoid. The floor is formed from above and downward by the splenius capitis, levator scapulae, and the medial and posterior scalenes. The accessory nerve is directed obliquely across the space from the sternocleidomastoid, which it pierces, to the inferior surface of the trapezius; below, the supraclavicular nerves and the transverse cervical vessels and the upper part of the brachial plexus cross the space. A chain of lymph glands is also found running along the posterior border of the sternocleidomastoid, from the mastoid process to the root of the neck (Table 7.6).

Supraclavicular Triangle

The smaller division of the posterior triangle is bounded above by the inferior belly of the omohyoid and below by the clavicle; its base is formed by the posterior border of the sternocleidomastoid. The floor consists of the first rib with the first digitation of the serratus anterior. The size of the supraclavicular triangle varies with the extent of attachment of the clavicular portions of the sternocleidomastoid and trapezius and also with the height at which the omohyoid crosses the neck. Its height also varies according to the position of the arm; it is diminished when the arm is raised because of the ascent of the clavicle, and it is increased when the arm is drawn downward, when the bone is depressed. Just above the level of the clavicle, the third portion of the subclavian artery curves laterally and downward from the lateral margin of the anterior scalene, across the first rib, to the axilla; this is the portion most commonly chosen for ligature of the vessel. Sometimes this vessel rises as high as 4 cm above the clavicle; occasionally, it passes in front of the anterior scalene or pierces the fibers of that muscle. The subclavian vein lies behind the clavicle and is not usually seen in this space; in some cases it rises as high as the artery, and it has even been seen to pass with that vessel behind the anterior scalene. The brachial plexus of nerves lies above the artery, in close contact with it. Passing transversely behind the clavicle are the transverse scapular vessels, and traversing its upper angle in the same direction are the transverse cervical artery and vein. The external jugular vein runs vertically downward behind the posterior border of the sternocleidomastoid, terminating in the subclavian vein; it receives the transverse cervical and transverse scapular veins, which form a plexus in front of the artery; occasionally a small vein crosses the clavicle from the cephalic. The small nerve to the subclavius crosses this triangle in the middle, and lymph glands are also found in this space (Table 7.7).

Fascial Layers of the Neck (Fig. 7.3)

The superficial cervical fascia is a subcutaneous layer containing varying amounts of fat, superficial lymph nodes, and other

Table 7.5 The Posterior Triangle

The borders of the posterior triangle	Posterior margin of the sternocleidomastoid muscle—anterior Anterior trapezius muscle—posterior Part of the clavicle—inferior
Structures found in the posterior triangle	Part of the subclavian artery, suprascapular artery, transverse cervical vessels of the thyrocervical trunk, external jugular vein, lymph nodes, spinal accessory nerve, trunks of the brachial plexus and fibers of the cervical plexus
Smaller triangles in the posterior triangle	Occipital triangle and supraclavicular triangle

Table 7.6 The Occipital Triangle

The borders of the occipital triangle	Posterior margin of the sternocleidomastoid muscle—anterior Anterior margin of the trapezius muscle—posterior Inferior belly of the omohyoid muscle—inferior
Structures found in the occipital triangle	Spinal accessory nerve, branches of the cervical plexus, upper part of the brachial plexus and supraclavicular nerve

Table 7.7 The Subclavian Triangle

The borders of the subclavian triangle	Inferior belly of the omohyoid muscle—superior Posterior margin of the sternocleidomastoid muscle—anterior Anterior margin of the trapezius muscle—posterior
Structures found in the supraclavicular triangle	Part of the subclavian artery, trunk of the brachial plexus, subclavius nerve, lymph nodes

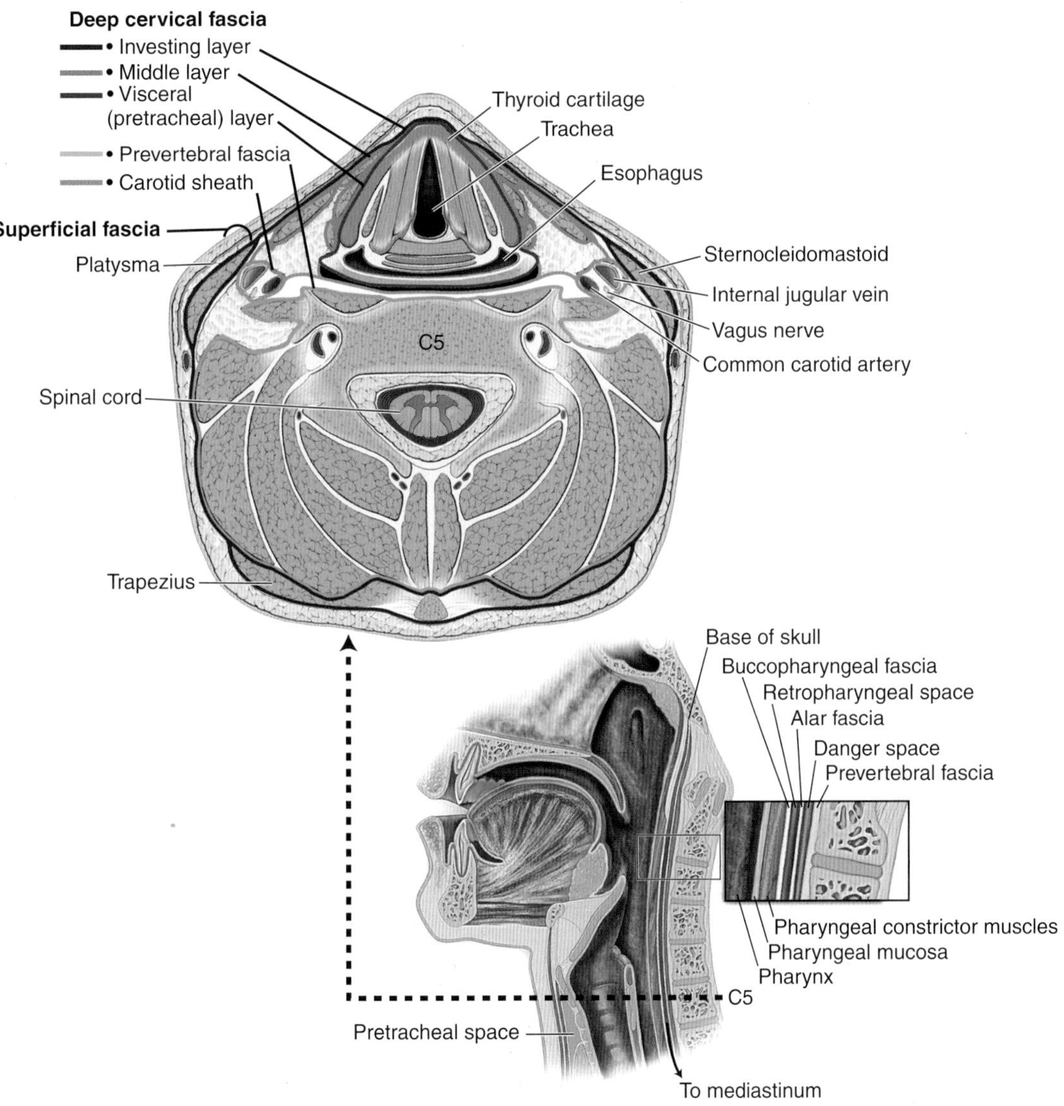

Figure 7.3 Fascial layers of the neck. These layers are important because they help compartmentalize the various anatomic structures of the neck.

vessels, which supply the surrounding cutaneous and muscular layers. Just deep to this layer is an intricate layer of deep cervical fascia, which wraps around the neck in a collar-like fashion. The fascia helps to organize and compartmentalize the anatomic structures of the neck. Between these compartments are spaces containing loose areolar tissue, through which potential routes exist for infections to spread from one site to another.

The platysma, discussed shortly, lies within the superficial fascia, and the sternocleidomastoid and trapezius are encircled and split by the deep investing fascia. The visceral (pretracheal) fascia lies deep to the deep investing fascia and forms a sheath around several structures within the neck (i.e., the pharynx, esophagus, trachea, and thyroid gland). The prevertebral fascia, which forms a fascial aspect over the floor of the posterior triangle, surrounds the cervical vertebral unit, which includes the cervical vertebrae, cervical portion of the spinal cord, anterior and posterior vertebral muscles, and the eight pairs of spinal nerves (including the phrenic nerve). The prevertebral fascia extends laterally on both sides to surround the brachial plexus and subclavian vessels, forming the axillary sheath.

The retropharyngeal space is located between the visceral fascia and the prevertebral fascia, extending from the base of the skull to the superior mediastinum. The loose connective tissue found within it allows a certain amount of up and down movement during swallowing. One subdivision of this space, called the *alar space,* is termed the "danger space" due to its potential to carry infective material or air from one compartment to another.

Muscles (Fig. 7.4)

Platysma

The platysma originates from the fascia overlying the pectoralis major and deltoid muscles and inserts into the

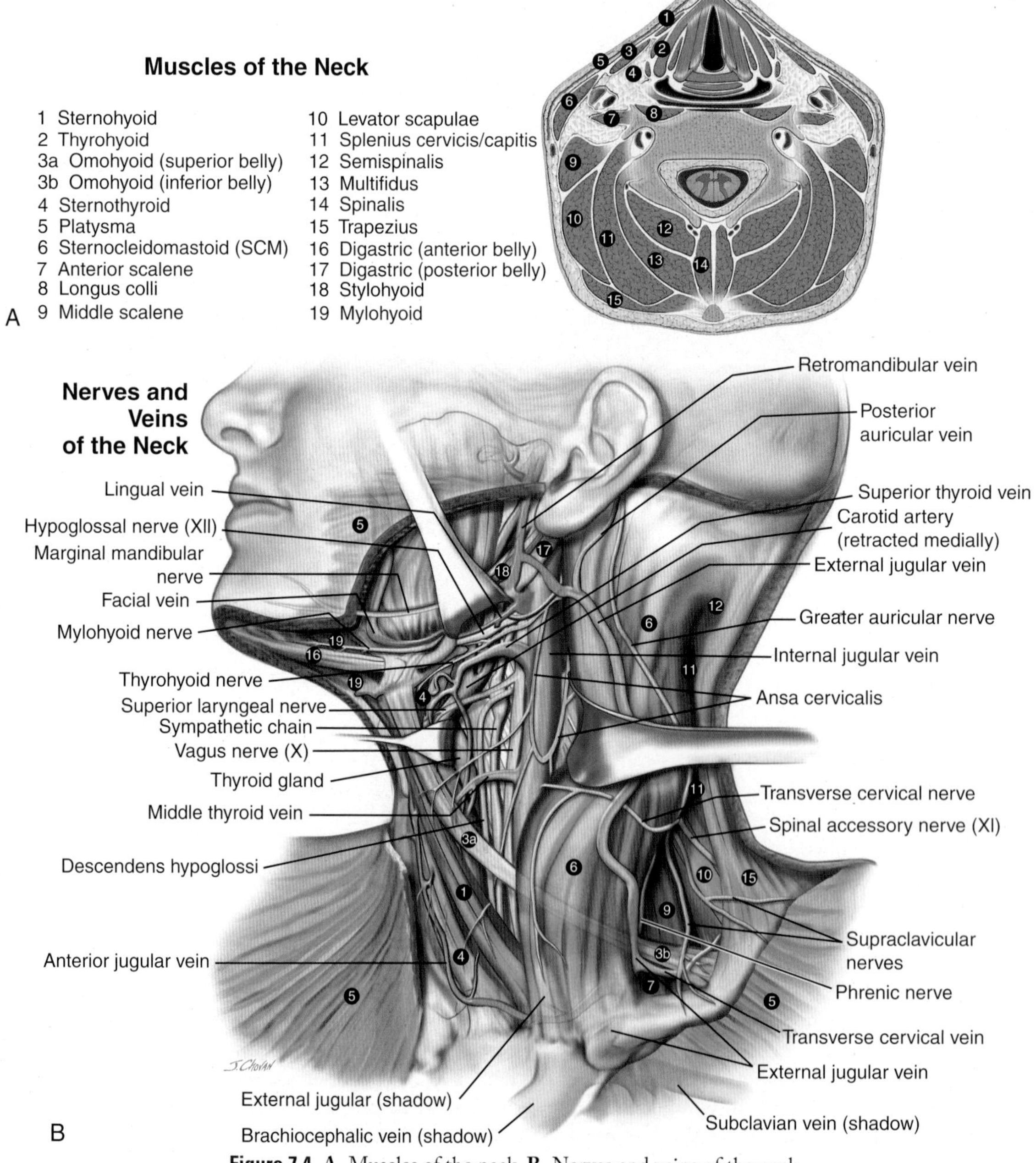

Figure 7.4 **A,** Muscles of the neck. **B,** Nerves and veins of the neck.

depression muscles of the corner of the mouth, the mandible, and the superficial muscular aponeurotic system layer of the face. It is innervated by the facial nerve (CN VII), more specifically its cervical branch. Its blood supply is from the branches of the submental and suprascapular arteries. The main function of the platysma is to wrinkle the neck, depress the corner of the mouth, increase the diameter of the neck, and assist in venous return. The surgeon must keep in mind several important considerations when operating on or near the platysma: the muscle increases blood supply to skin flaps, and it is absent in the midline. Additionally, the fibers of this muscle run in the opposite direction to that of the sternocleidomastoid.

Sternocleidomastoid

The sternocleidomastoid originates from the medial third of the clavicle (clavicular head) and the manubrium (sternal head). It inserts into the mastoid process and is innervated by the spinal accessory nerve (CN XI). It receives its blood supply from the occipital artery or directly from the external carotid artery (ECA) and from the superior thyroid and transverse cervical arteries. Its primary function is to turn the head toward the opposite side and tilt the head toward the ipsilateral shoulder. During surgery, it is important to leave the overlying fascia (superficial layer of deep cervical fascia); lateral retraction also exposes the submuscular recess.

Omohyoid

The omohyoid muscle is divided into two parts (superior and inferior bellies); nevertheless, the whole muscle originates at the upper border of the scapula and inserts into the intermediate tendon onto the clavicle and first rib and hyoid bone lateral to the sternohyoid muscle. It is innervated by the ansa cervicalis (anterior primary rami [APR] of C1, C2, and C3), and its vascular supply is from the inferior thyroid artery. It functions to depress the hyoid and tense the deep cervical fibers. It should be noted that it is absent in 10% of individuals. When present, though, it can act as a landmark, demarcating level III from level IV. The inferior belly lies superficial to the brachial plexus, phrenic nerve, and transverse cervical vessels. The superior belly lies superficial to the internal jugular vein.

Trapezius

The trapezius originates from the medial one-third of the superior nuchal line, external occipital protuberance, ligamentum nuchae, and the spinous process of C7 and T1–T12 (see Fig. 7.4B). It inserts into the lateral one-third of the clavicle, acromion process, and spine of the scapula and is innervated by the spinal accessory nerve (CN XI), in addition to the APR of C3 and C4. Its blood supply is from the transverse cervical artery or superficial cervical artery. It functions to elevate and rotate the scapula and stabilize the shoulder. Surgically, it delineates the posterior limit of level V neck dissections. Denervation of this muscle may result in shoulder drop and a winged scapula.

Digastric

The digastric muscle, much like the omohyoid, consists of two muscles, an anterior belly and a posterior belly. They originate at the digastric fossa of the mandible at the symphyseal border and insert at the hyoid bone via the intermediate tendon and mastoid process. The posterior belly is innervated by the facial nerve, and the anterior belly is innervated by the nerve to the mylohyoid. The posterior belly receives its blood supply from the occipital artery, whereas the anterior belly receives its blood supply from the submental branch of the facial artery. This muscle elevates the hyoid bone and depresses the mandible (assisting the lateral pterygoid). The posterior belly is superficial to the following structures: ECA, hypoglossal nerve, internal carotid artery, and internal jugular vein. The anterior belly is the landmark for identification of the mylohyoid for dissection of the submandibular triangle.

Blood Vessels (Fig. 7.5)

Blood supply to the neck can be divided according to the regional supply: anterior triangle, posterior triangle, and root of the neck.

The arteries of the anterior triangle are all derived from the common carotid artery, which ascends through the neck within the carotid sheath (see Fig. 7.5). It does not give off any branches until it reaches the level of the hyoid bone, at which point it divides into the internal carotid and external carotid arteries. The internal carotid artery gives off no branches as it moves upward to the base of the skull. The external carotid, however, extends upward toward the parotid region, giving off six collateral branches: the superior thyroid, lingual, facial, ascending pharyngeal, occipital, and posterior auricular arteries (see Fig. 7.4). The external artery ultimately terminates within the parotid region as two terminal branches: the superficial temporal artery and the maxillary artery. All veins of the anterior triangle, except the anterior jugular vein, drain to the internal jugular vein (see Fig. 7.4). The internal jugular vein travels within the carotid sheath, picking up the following tributaries as it descends: veins of the pharyngeal plexus, facial vein, lingual vein, superior thyroid vein, and the middle thyroid vein. After picking up these tributaries, the internal jugular vein passes under the sternocleidomastoid muscle, exiting the anterior triangle, and entering the root of the neck. Here it meets with the subclavian vein to form the brachiocephalic vein.

Within the posterior triangle of the neck, the subclavian artery supplies the majority of the arterial blood. Two cervical branches, the transverse cervical and suprascapular, pass anteriorly to the anterior scalene muscle and pin down the phrenic nerve to the

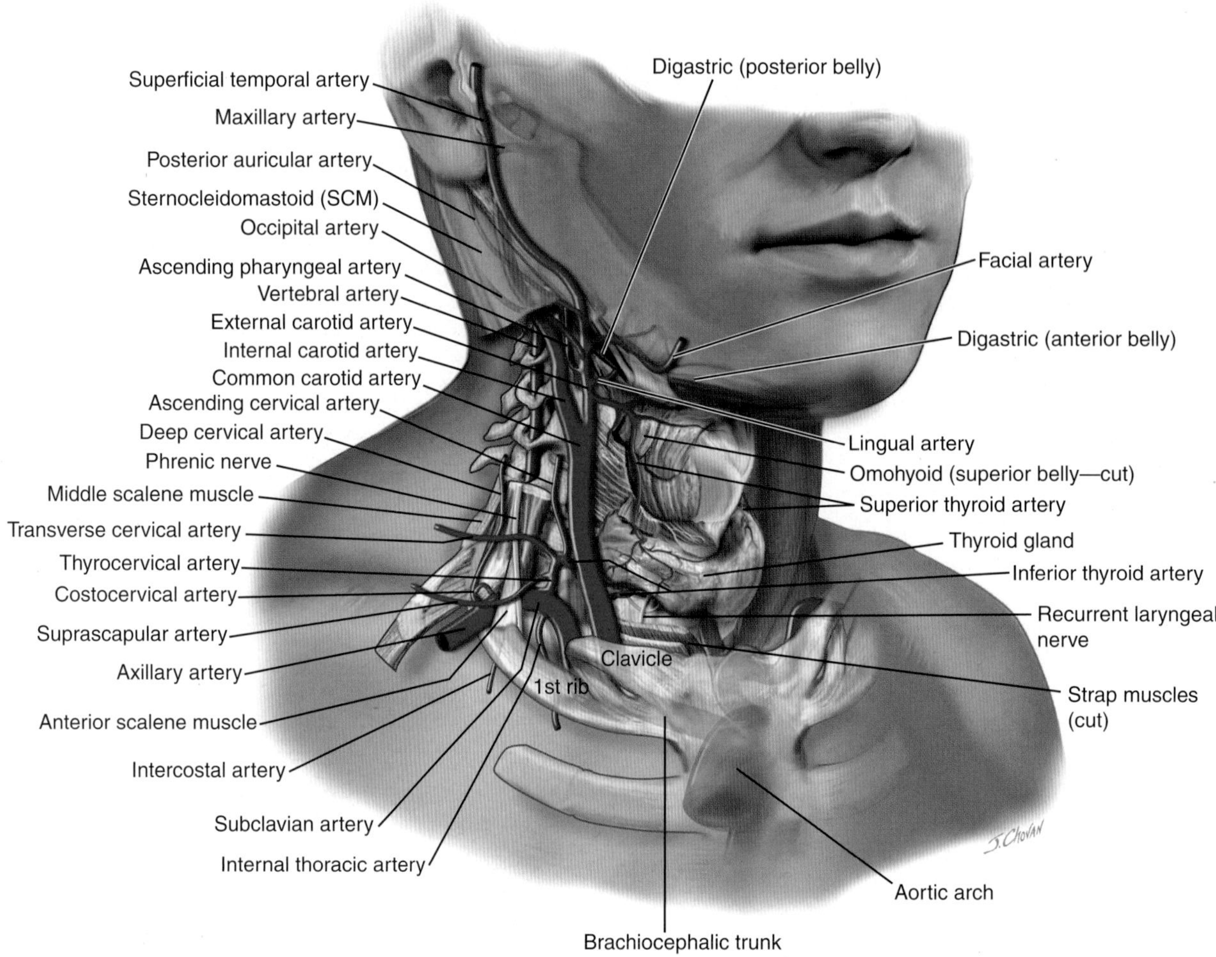

Figure 7.5 Arteries of the neck.

muscle (see Fig. 7.4). The external jugular vein moves obliquely and inferiorly over the sternocleidomastoid to enter the posterior triangle, where it picks up venous blood from three sources: the transverse cervical vein, suprascapular vein, and anterior jugular vein. The external jugular vein then joins with the subclavian vein and internal jugular vein to form the brachiocephalic vein.

The root of the neck also contains the source of many of the vessels that eventually supply the majority of the vascular supply of the neck. The subclavian artery arches superiorly over the first rib, becoming the axillary artery and giving off several branches such as the vertebral artery, which ascends in the root of the neck to the transverse foramen of the vertebrae C6 and enters the foramen magnum, internal thoracic artery, thyrocervical trunk, and costocervical trunk.

Nerves

Marginal Mandibular Nerve (see Fig. 7.2)

The marginal mandibular nerve is an important landmark, and care should be taken to ensure its preservation during neck dissections. It is most often injured during dissections at level Ib. It is located 1 cm anterior and inferior to the angle of the mandible at the mandibular notch, deep to the fascia of the submandibular gland (superficial layer of the deep cervical fascia) and superficial to the adventitia of the facial vein. It is important to note that more than one branch is often present, and during surgical procedures, the sensory branches associated with it are often sacrificed.

Spinal Accessory Nerve (see Fig. 7.2)

The spinal accessory nerve originates in the spinal nucleus and may extend to the fifth cervical segment. The motor neurons of this branch pass through two foramina, the foramen magnum and jugular foramen. From the foramen magnum it enters the skull posterior to the vertebral artery, and from the jugular foramen it exits the skull with CN IX and CN X, along with the internal jugular vein, which it subsequently crosses.

Phrenic Nerve (see Fig. 7.2)

The phrenic nerve (C3, C4, and C5) is the sole nerve supply to the diaphragm. It runs obliquely toward the midline on the anterior surface of the anterior scalene and is covered by prevertebral fascia. It also lies posterior and lateral to the carotid sheath. Both the suprascapular and transverse cervical arteries also pass anteriorly to the anterior scalene, clamping the phrenic nerve to that muscle.

Hypoglossal Nerve

The hypoglossal nucleus originates from the medulla oblongata, and the hypoglossal nerve arises from the cell bodies of the hypoglossal nucleus. The hypoglossal nerve exits the hypoglossal canal, lying deep to several important structures: the internal jugular vein, internal carotid artery, and CN IX, CN X, and CN XI. The path of this nerve is also important because it curves 90 degrees and passes between the internal jugular vein and the internal carotid artery. During its course, it is surrounded by a venous plexus called the *ranine veins*. It ends as it extends upward along the hyoglossus muscle and into the genioglossus, finally reaching the tip of the tongue.

Although metastatic neck disease is one of the most important factors in the spread of head and neck squamous cell carcinoma from primary sites, it is not encountered as frequently as some of the other potential pathologies associated with the neck. Trauma and infection are much more common in the typical maxillofacial practice, and, as such, it is important to understand the key anatomic landmarks in the neck. Control of the neck is one of the most important aspects of the successful management of these particular pathologies. In addition, communication with surgical colleagues regarding treatment and patient management mandates an understanding of important anatomic sites.

References

1. Nauman HH, Panje WR, Herbehold C, eds. *Head and Neck Surgery*. Vol. 3. Stuttgart, Germany: Thieme; 1997.
2. Suarez C, Rodrigo JP, Robbins KT, et al. Superselective neck dissection: rationale, indications, and results. *Eur Arch Oto-Rhino-Laryngol*. 2013;270(11):2815–2821.
3. Shah JP. Patterns of cervical lymph node metastasis from squamous carcinoma of the upper aerodigestive tract. *Am J Surg*. 1990;160(4):405–409.

CHAPTER 8

Fascial Spaces of the Head and Neck

Joseph E. Cillo Jr.

The fascia of the head and neck is composed of loose fibrous connective tissue envelopes and may be divided into the superficial and deep fascia. Between the fibers of the matrix are interstices that are filled with tissue fluid or ground substance that can readily break down when invaded by infection. The loose fibrous connective tissue that makes up the fascia of the head and neck is found in varying degrees of density with a tensile strength somewhat less than dense fibrous connective tissue located elsewhere in the body. There are 16 fascial spaces of the head and neck region, which are divided into four subtypes. These four subtypes are the fascial spaces of the face, suprahyoid fascial spaces, infrahyoid fascial spaces, and the fascial spaces of the neck (Table 8.1).

Superficial Fascia

The superficial fascia of the head and neck lies just under the skin, as it does throughout the entire body. It invests the superficially situated mimetic muscles (platysma, orbicularis oculi, and zygomaticus major and minor) and is located in distinct anatomic areas. It is composed of two layers, an outer fatty (*areolar cleavage plane*) layer and a thin inner membrane with a large number of elastic fibers (*superficial musculoaponeurotic system [SMAS]*).[1] The superficial fascia attaches the skin to the deep fascia, which covers and invests the structures lying deep to the skin while maintaining the movability of the skin, with the two layers allowing for separation during blunt dissection. The areolar cleavage plane overlies the lower masseter, is rhomboidal in shape, and is important in cosmetic surgery (such as in lower [cervicofacial] facelifts). Dissection is bloodless and provides safety for all facial nerve branches, as they are located outside of this plane.[2]

The SMAS is a fibromuscular fan like fascial extension of the platysma muscle that arises superiorly from the fascia over the zygomatic arch. The facial nerve lies deep to the SMAS and innervates the mimetic muscles of the forehead and midface from the ventral aspect of the muscles. The SMAS is continuous with the platysma muscle inferiorly and the superficial temporal fascia superiorly and is superficial to the parotideomasseteric fascia. It connects to the fascial musculature in the nasolabial, perioral, and periorbital regions. Location and anatomic identification of this layer are important in surgical manipulation for both reconstructive[3] and cosmetic[4] procedures.

Table 8.1 Fascial Space Subtypes

Fascial Space Subtype	Fascial Space Subtype Components
Fascial spaces of the face	Canine, buccal, parotid, infratemporal, masticatory spaces Masseteric Pterygomandibular Temporal
Suprahyoid fascial spaces	Sublingual, submental, submandibular, lateral pharyngeal, peritonsillar
Infrahyoid fascial spaces	Pretracheal
Fascial spaces of the neck	Retropharyngeal, danger, carotid sheath

Deep Fascia

The deep fascia begins at the anterior border of the masseter muscle and attaches to the superior temporal and nuchal lines. Posterior and inferior to these margins, it continues cranially as the pericranium. The deep facial fascia represents a continuation of the deep cervical fascia cephalad into the face and, more posterior, invests the muscles of mastication, the surgical importance of which is that the facial nerve branches within the cheek lie deep to this fascial layer.[1]

Fascial Spaces of the Face

The fascial spaces of the face are subdivided into five spaces: the canine space, the buccal space, the masticatory space (further divided into the masseteric, pterygomandibular, and temporal spaces), the parotid space, and the infratemporal space (Fig. 8.1A).

Canine Space

The canine space is located between the levator anguli oris and the levator labii superioris muscles. Infection spreads to this space through the root apices of the maxillary teeth, usually the canines. Direct surgical access is achieved through

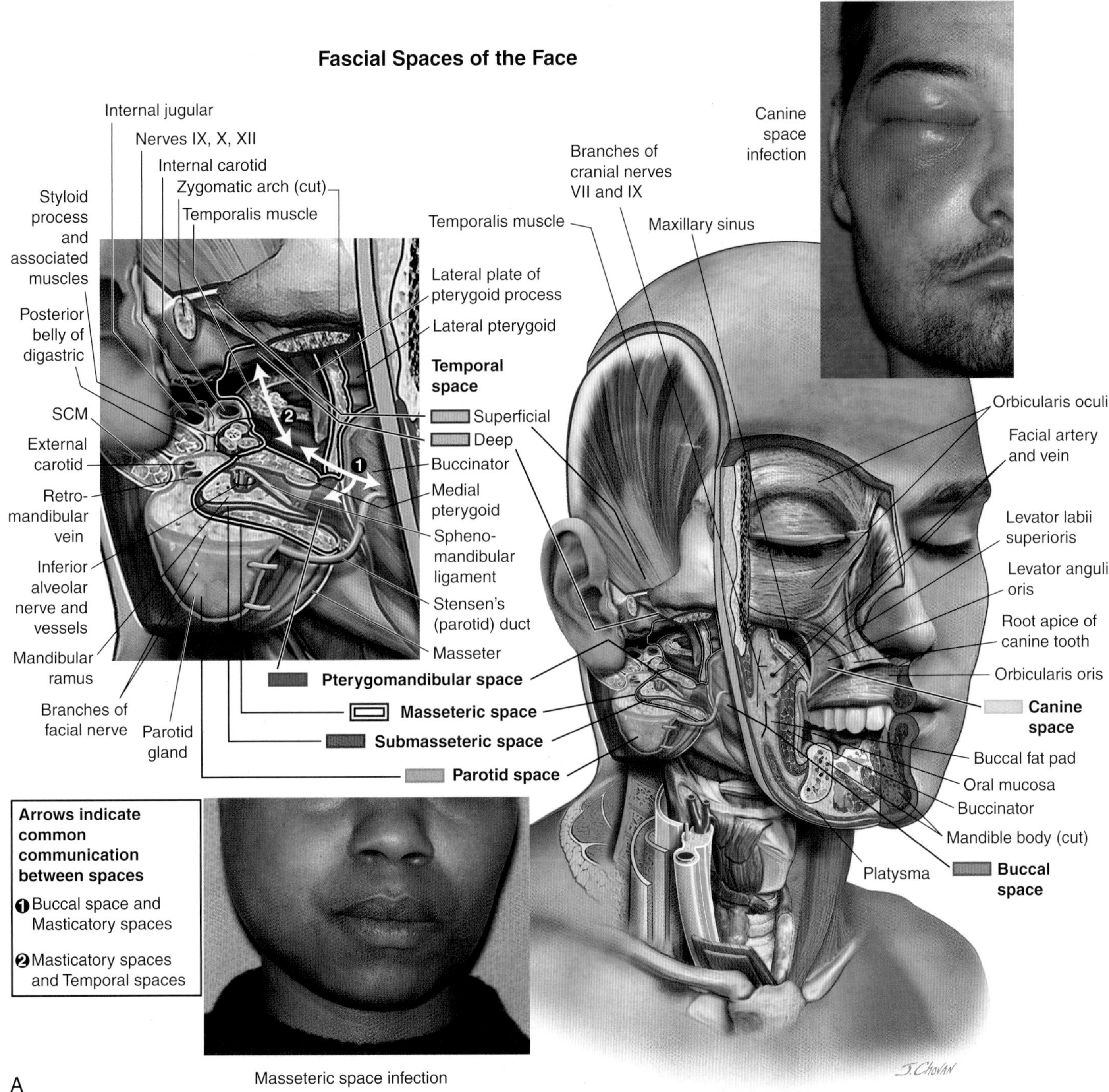

Figure 8.1 A, Fascial space anatomy of the face.

incision through the maxillary vestibular mucosa above the mucogingival junction (Fig. 8.1B).

Buccal Space

The buccal space is bounded anterior to the masticatory space and lateral to the buccinator muscle, with no true superior or inferior boundary, and consists of adipose tissue (the buccal fat pad that fills the greater part of the space), the Stensen duct, the facial artery and vein, lymphatic vessels, minor salivary glands, and branches of cranial nerves (CN) VII and IX. The buccal space frequently communicates posteriorly with the masticatory space because the parotideomasseteric fascia is sometimes incomplete along its medial course where it joins the buccopharyngeal fascia.[5] The parotid duct separates the buccal space into two equal-sized anterior and posterior compartments, with the facial vein located along the lateral margin of the buccinator muscle just anterior to transversely coursing the Stensen duct.[5]

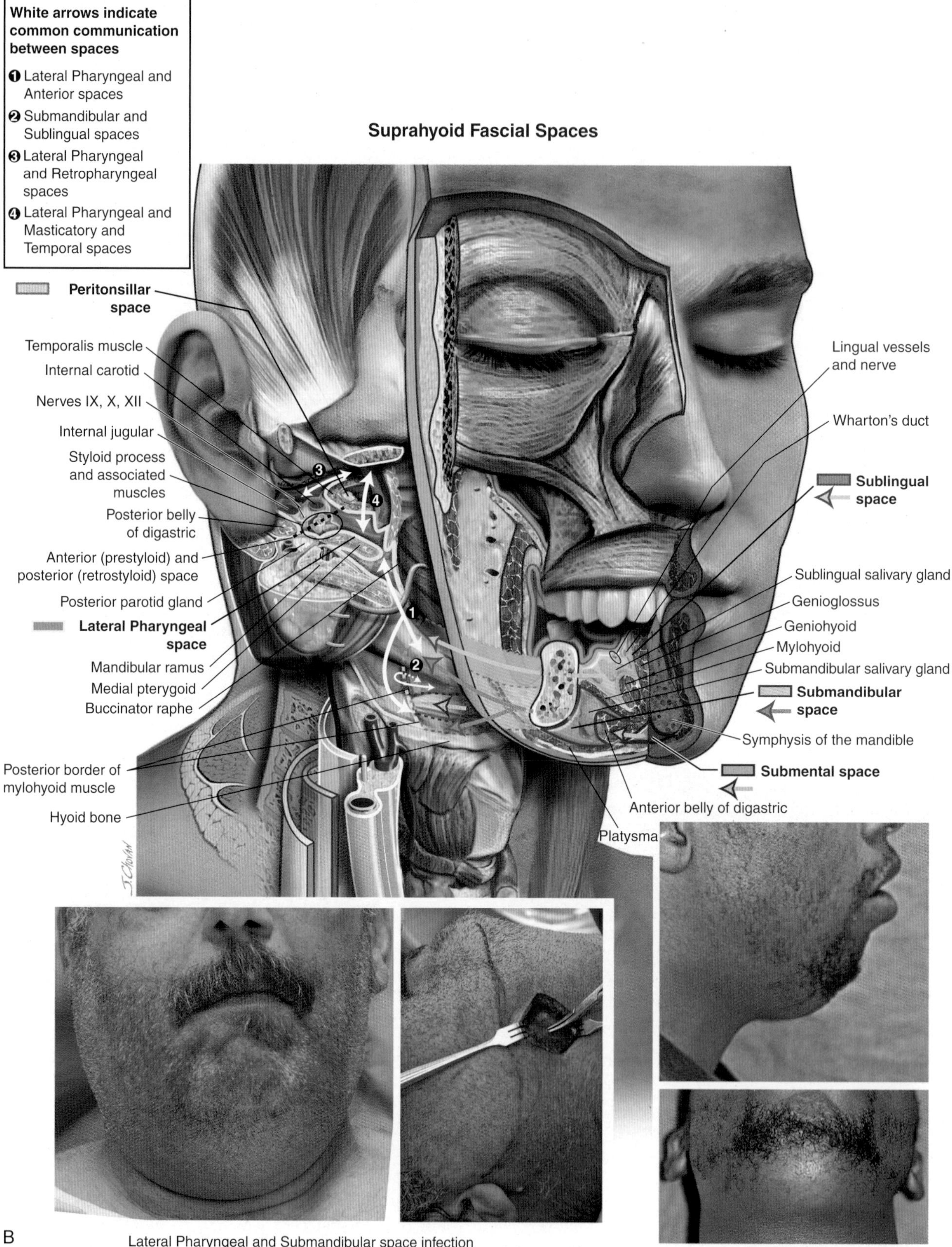
White arrows indicate common communication between spaces
1 Lateral Pharyngeal and Anterior spaces
2 Submandibular and Sublingual spaces
3 Lateral Pharyngeal and Retropharyngeal spaces
4 Lateral Pharyngeal and Masticatory and Temporal spaces
Suprahyoid Fascial Spaces
Peritonsillar space
Temporalis muscle
Internal carotid
Nerves IX, X, XII
Internal jugular
Styloid process and associated muscles
Posterior belly of digastric
Anterior (prestyloid) and posterior (retrostyloid) space
Posterior parotid gland
Lateral Pharyngeal space
Mandibular ramus
Medial pterygoid
Buccinator raphe
Posterior border of mylohyoid muscle
Hyoid bone
Lingual vessels and nerve
Wharton's duct
Sublingual space
Sublingual salivary gland
Genioglossus
Geniohyoid
Mylohyoid
Submandibular salivary gland
Submandibular space
Symphysis of the mandible
Submental space
Anterior belly of digastric
Platysma
B
Lateral Pharyngeal and Submandibular space infection
Submental space infection

Figure 8.1, cont'd B, Suprahyoid fascial spaces.

Continued

The buccal space may serve as a conduit as there is a lack of fascial compartmentalization in the superior, inferior, and posterior directions, which permits the spread of pathology both to and from the buccal space.[6] Surgical access to buccal space infections may be easily accomplished via the intraoral approach. However, more complicated infections or masses, directed by location within the buccal space and suspicion of malignancy, may require a preauricular or submandibular approach.

Parotid Space

The parotid space is formed by splitting the fascia of the investing layer of the deep cervical fascia and contains the parotid gland with the associated extraglandular and intraglandular lymph glands, the parotid portion of CN VII; the external carotid, internal maxillary, and superficial temporal arteries; and the retromandibular vein. Infection in this space may spread to the lateral pharyngeal spaces, as they communicate posteriorly and the fascia of the deep parotid space is thin and easily breached. However, primary infection in this compartment is rare and is generally blood-borne or retrograde through the parotid duct.

Masticatory Spaces

Masseteric Space (and Submasseteric Space)

The fascia that forms the borders of the masseteric space is a well-defined fibrous tissue that surrounds the muscles of mastication and contains the internal maxillary artery and the inferior alveolar nerve. It is bounded anteriorly by the mandible, posteriorly by the parotid gland, medially by the lateral pharyngeal space, and superiorly by the temporal space.

Most masseteric space infections are of odontogenic origin (e.g., molar teeth),[7] with trismus being the most pronounced clinical feature, and often preclude intraoral examination. Computed tomography (CT) or magnetic resonance imaging (MRI) may be an invaluable resource in the assessment of masseteric space infections, as it can often influence the surgical approach and distinguish abscess from cellulitis.[7] The submasseteric space is bounded laterally by the masseter muscle, medially by the mandible ramus, and posteriorly by the parotid gland. Infections are mostly of odontogenic origin (usually a mandibular third molar) and are often misdiagnosed as a parotid abscess or parotitis.[8] Intraoral surgical access to this space for simple, isolated abscesses is generally adequate to allow for drainage, but with extension into adjacent spaces, an extraoral submandibular approach may be required (Fig. 8.1C).

Pterygomandibular Space

The pterygomandibular space is bounded by the mandible laterally and medially and inferiorly by the medial pterygoid muscle. The posterior border is formed by the parotid gland as it curves medially around the posterior mandibular ramus and anteriorly by the pterygomandibular raphe, the fibrous junction of the buccinator and superior constrictor muscles. The inferior alveolar and lingual nerves, other structures in this space, are of particular importance in the administration of local anesthesia, including the inferior alveolar vessels, the sphenomandibular ligament, and the interpterygoid fascia.[9] Surgical access to this space may be achieved intraorally in the case of simple infections, but may require extraoral access when multiple adjacent spaces are involved.[10]

Temporal Space

The temporal fascia surrounds the temporalis muscle in a strong fibrous sheet that is divided into clearly distinguishable superficial and deep layers that originate from the same region with the muscle fibers of the two layers intermingled in the superior part of the muscle.[11] It attaches to the superior temporal line and passes inferiorly to the zygomatic arch. Superiorly, the temporal fascia and fibers of origin of the temporalis muscle blend into a firm aponeurosis, a flat fan of extremely dense and firm fibrous connective tissue. Communicating facial-zygomaticotemporal nerve branches piercing the fascial and muscular planes of the intermingled superficial and deep layers of the temporal fascia in the superior part of the muscle are important from a surgical perspective to prevent temporal hollowing that may occur due to surgical access procedures.[12]

Suprahyoid Fascial Spaces

Sublingual Space

The sublingual space is bounded between the mylohyoid muscle and the geniohyoid and genioglossus muscles. This space contains the lingual artery and nerve, the hypoglossal nerve, the glossopharyngeal nerve, the Wharton duct, and the sublingual salivary gland, which drains into the oral cavity through several small excretory ducts in the floor of the mouth and a major duct known as the Bartholin duct. Periapical molar infections may perforate the lingual mandible cortex above the mylohyoid line and spread to this space. Surgical access is easily achieved through an intraoral approach, but when other spaces are involved, extraoral access may be utilized, usually through a submandibular approach.

Submental Space

The submental space is bounded anteriorly by the symphysis of the mandible, laterally by the anterior bellies of the digastric muscles, superiorly by the mylohyoid muscle, and inferiorly by the superficial fascia of the platysma muscle. No vital structures traverse the submental space. This space is usually involved in odontogenic infections from the anterior mandibular teeth, as benign or malignant lesions in this area are rare.[13]

To drain these infections, the surgeon generally gains access through an extraoral incision below the chin. When infection has spread to this space, it represents one of the components (along with bilateral submandibular and sublingual space involvement) of Ludwig angina.

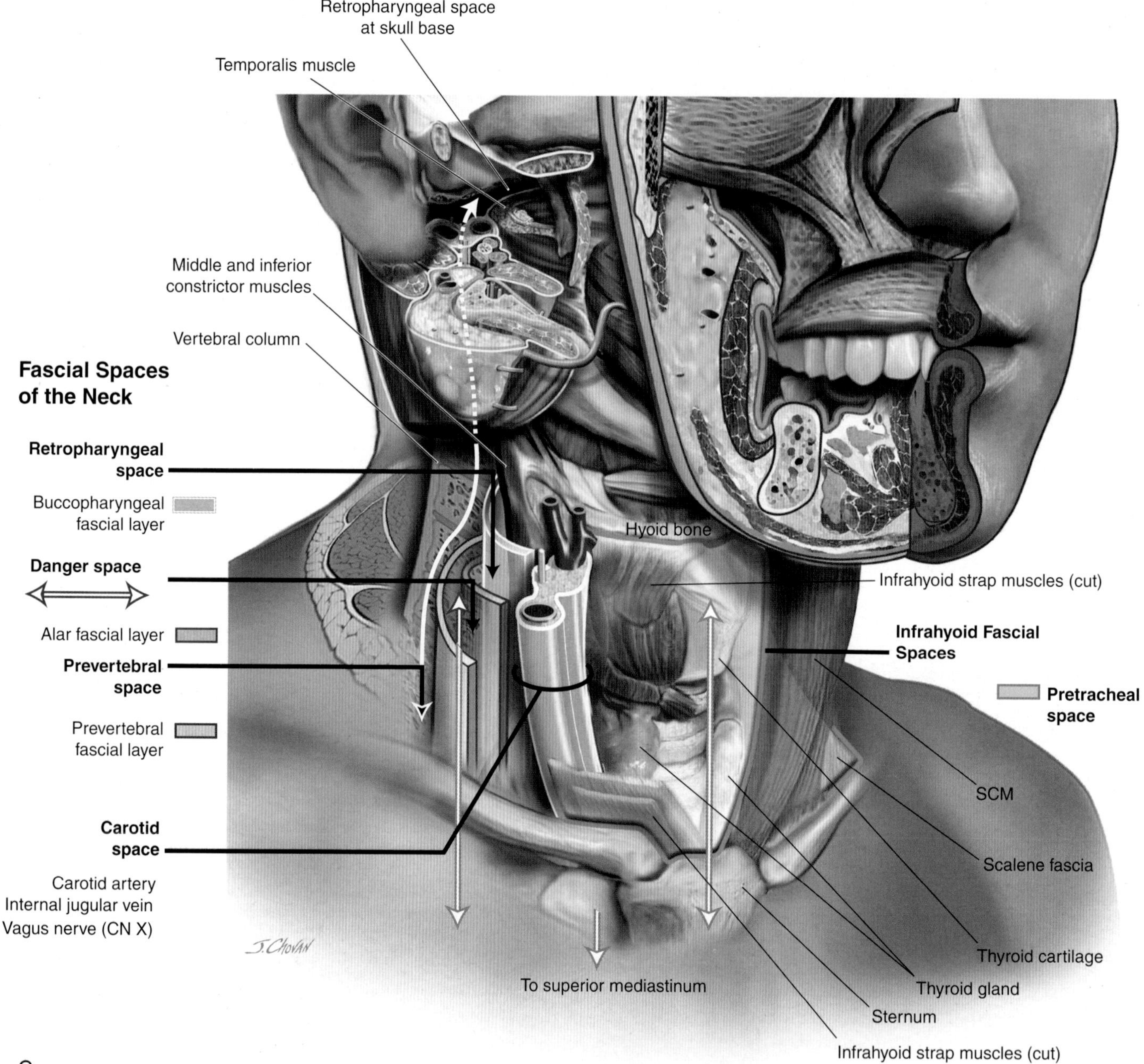

Figure 8.1, cont'd C, Fascial spaces of the neck. *SCM*, Sternocleidomastoid.

Submandibular Space

The submandibular space extends from the hyoid bone to the mucosa of the floor of the mouth and is bound anteriorly and laterally by the mandible and inferiorly by the superficial layer of the deep cervical fascia. The mylohyoid muscle separates it superiorly from the sublingual space, which communicates with it freely around the posterior border of the mylohyoid. The mylohyoid muscle also plays a key role in determining the direction of the spread of dental infections. It attaches to the mandible at an angle, leaving the apices of the second and third molars below the mylohyoid line and the apex of the first molar above. Periapical molar infections may perforate the lingual mandible cortex below the mylohyoid line and spread to the submandibular space.

The buccopharyngeal gap is a potentially dangerous connection between the submandibular and lateral pharyngeal spaces that is created by the styloglossus muscle as it passes between the middle and superior constrictors, which may allow infection to spread directly to the lateral pharyngeal space. Surgical access for drainage may be either intraoral or extraoral. When infection has spread to the bilateral submandibular spaces, it represents one of the components (along with submental and bilateral sublingual space involvement) of Ludwig angina. Surgical drainage in these situations is almost always through multiple extraoral incisions.

Lateral Pharyngeal Space

The lateral pharyngeal space (also called the parapharyngeal space) is an inverted cone with its base at the base of skull and its apex at the hyoid bone, and it is bounded posteriorly by the prevertebral fascia, anteriorly by the raphe of the buccinator and superior constrictors muscles, and laterally by the mandible and parotid fascia. The lateral pharyngeal space can be divided into anterior (prestyloid) and posterior (retrostyloid) compartments by the styloid process. The anterior compartment contains only fat, lymph nodes, and muscle, whereas the posterior compartment contains the carotid artery, the internal jugular vein, and CN IX through XII.

Odontogenic infections of the anterior space may present with pain, fever, neck swelling below the angle of the mandible, and trismus. Rotation of the neck away from the side of swelling causes severe pain from tension on the ipsilateral sternocleidomastoid muscle. As this space communicates with the other fascia spaces, spread of infection may also arise from numerous sources, including the tonsils, parotid, and submandibular, peritonsillar, masticator, or retropharyngeal spaces. Posterior space involvement may have more ominous signs. Lemierre syndrome may result from pharyngitis or tonsillitis with bacterial spread to the lateral pharyngeal space that may involve internal jugular vein thrombosis with septic emboli and metastatic infections that most frequently involve the lungs.[14] Warning signs of posterior involvement may include Horner syndrome or CN IX through XII palsies and may lead to complications that include septic jugular thrombophlebitis and carotid artery erosion or thrombosis.[15] Airway impingement due to medial bulging of the pharyngeal wall and supraglottic edema may occasionally occur, which may require the procurement of a stable airway by either tracheotomy or intubation.[16] The treatment of lateral pharyngeal space infections requires surgical drainage through either a transoral or an extraoral approach.[17] The intraoral approach may reach the anterior compartment but may be inadequate to completely access the posterior compartment. Extraoral access through a submandibular approach allows for adequate access to both compartments.

Peritonsillar Space

The peritonsillar space is a potential space of loose areolar tissue that surrounds the tonsil and is bounded laterally by the superior constrictors. Most abscesses occur in younger patients who present with fever, sore throat, and dysphagia. Local transoral incision and drainage is generally the method of choice for treatment, but treatment may include serial aspiration or surgical drainage with tonsillectomy. Peritonsillar abscess is a complication of acute tonsillitis that is rarely life threatening in itself but may spread to involve the lateral pharyngeal space. Lemierre syndrome may result from tonsillitis with bacterial spread to the lateral pharyngeal space that may involve internal jugular vein thrombosis with septic emboli.[14]

Infrahyoid Fascial Spaces

Pretracheal Space

The pretracheal space is bounded anteriorly by the investing cervical fascia, posteriorly by the visceral cervical fascia, superiorly by the attachments of the infrahyoid muscles and their fascia to the thyroid cartilage and to the hyoid bone, and continues into the anterior portion of the superior mediastinum bounded inferiorly by the sternum and scalene fascia. This space contains the infrahyoid strap muscles. Spread of infection to this space may occur directly by anterior perforations or rupture of the esophagus or indirectly by spread from the retrovisceral portion, around the sides of the esophagus and thyroid gland between the levels of the inferior thyroid artery and the oblique line of the thyroid cartilage. This space may allow infection to spread into the superior mediastinum, as these spaces communicate.

Fascial Spaces of the Neck

The fascial spaces of the neck all lie between the deep cervical fascia surrounding the pharynx anteriorly and the spine posteriorly. The retrovisceral space is divided into the retropharyngeal and danger spaces by the alar fascia and serves as the main route that oropharyngeal infections may use to descend into the mediastinum. The other fascial spaces of the neck include the prevertebral and carotid sheath spaces.

Retropharyngeal Space

The retropharyngeal space is bounded anteriorly by the constrictor muscles, posteriorly by the alar layer of the deep cervical fascia, and connects posteriorly to the danger space. Due to its deep location within the neck, pathologic lesions involving this space may be difficult or impossible to evaluate clinically, warranting the use of CT or MRI scans.[18] Patients with infections in this space may present with symptoms of fever, stiff neck, drooling, dysphagia, and bulging of the posterior pharyngeal wall. They may be complicated by the development of supraglottic edema with airway obstruction, aspiration pneumonia due to rupture of the abscess, and acute mediastinitis that may lead to empyema or pericardial effusions. Proximity to the danger space may allow infection to spread to the mediastinum to the level of the diaphragm and possibly posteriorly to the prevertebral space. Surgical drainage should be performed in the operating room via a transoral approach with the head down to prevent rupture during intubation and septic aspiration.

Danger Space

The danger space is bounded superiorly by the skull base, anteriorly by the alar fascia, posteriorly by the prevertebral fascia, and ends at the level of the diaphragm. Danger space infections may track from the anteriorly located retropharyngeal space between the buccopharyngeal fascia and alar fascia and pass inferiorly to the mediastinum and the pericardium, and they may result in conditions such as purulent pericarditis.[19]

Prevertebral Space

The prevertebral space is bounded by the anterior part of the cervical spine and the deep layer of the deep cervical fascia running between the transverse processes of the spine. It extends from the base of the skull into the mediastinum and ends at the level of the fourth thoracic vertebra. The prevertebral space contains the prevertebral muscles (longus colli and longus capitis), vertebral artery, vertebral vein, scalene muscles, phrenic nerve, and the proximal portion of the brachial plexus. When viewed on a lateral cephalometric radiograph, the normal dimensions of the prevertebral space in an adult are 4 mm at the C3 level, with a greater than 7 mm value indicating an abnormality such as pathology or infection.

Carotid Sheath Space

The carotid sheath space is composed of the conjoining of three cervical fasciae—the investing layer deep to the sternocleidomastoid muscle, the pretracheal layers, and the prevertebral layer of cervical fascia—and extends from the base of the skull to the root of the neck. It lies posterior to the parapharyngeal space, lateral to the retropharyngeal space, anterolateral to the prevertebral spaces, and medial to the parotid space and styloid process. It contains the common and internal carotid arteries, internal jugular vein, vagus nerve (CN X), deep cervical lymph nodes, carotid sinus nerve, and sympathetic fibers. Infections that usually arise from thrombosis of the internal jugular vein or from infected deep cervical lymph nodes that lie within the sheath tend to be localized within the cervical region between the hyoid and root of the neck, as the sheath closely adheres to the major vessels in this space.[20] Thrombosis of the jugular vein from a deep infection of the neck is not likely caused by direct infection of the carotid sheath but rather by the infectious material that follows tributaries of the internal jugular vein to reach the sheath.[21]

References

1. Stuzin JM, Baker TJ, Gordon HL. The relationship of the superficial and deep facial fascias: relevance to rhytidectomy and aging. *Plast Reconstr Surg*. 1992;89(3):441–449.
2. Mendelson BC, Freeman ME, Wu W, Huggins RJ. Surgical anatomy of the lower face: the premasseter space, the jowl, and the labiomandibular fold. *Aesthetic Plast Surg*. 2008;32(2):185–195.
3. Ambro BT, Goodstein LA, Morales RE, Taylor RJ. Evaluation of superficial musculoaponeurotic system flap and fat graft outcomes for benign and malignant parotid disease. *Otolaryngol Head Neck Surg*. 2013;148(6):949–954.
4. Trussler AP, Stephan P, Hatef D, Schaverien M, Meade R, Barton FE. The frontal branch of the facial nerve across the zygomatic arch: anatomical relevance of the high-SMAS technique. *Plast Reconstr Surg*. 2010;125(4):1221–1229.
5. Tart RP, Kotzur IM, Mancuso AA, Glantz MS, Mukherji SK. CT and MR imaging of the buccal space and buccal space masses. *Radiographics*. 1995;15(3):531–550.
6. Smoker WRK. Oral cavity. In: Som PM, Curtin HD, eds. *Head and Neck Imaging*. 3rd ed. St. Louis, Missouri: Mosby; 1996.
7. Schuknecht B, Stergiou G, Graetz K. Masticator space abscess derived from odontogenic infection: imaging manifestation and pathways of extension depicted by CT and MR in 30 patients. *Eur Radiol*. 2008;18(9):1972–1979.
8. Rai A, Rajput R, Khatua RK, Singh M. Submasseteric abscess: a rare head and neck abscess. *Indian J Dent Res*. 2011;22(1):166–168.
9. Khoury JN, Mihailidis S, Ghabriel M, Townsend G. Applied anatomy of the pterygomandibular space: improving the success of inferior alveolar nerve blocks. *Aust Dent J*. 2011;56(2):112–121.
10. Bratton TA, Jackson DC, Nkungula-Howlett T, Williams CW, Bennett CR. Management of complex multi-space odontogenic infections. *J Tenn Dent Assoc*. 2002;82(3):39–47.
11. Lee JY, Kim JN, Kim SH, et al. Anatomical verification and designation of the superficial layer of the temporalis muscle. *Clin Anat*. 2012;25(2):176–181.
12. Odobescu A, Williams HB, Gilardino MS. Description of a communication between the facial and zygomaticotemporal nerves. *J Plast Reconstr Aesthet Surg*. 2012;65(9):1188–1192.
13. Ural A, Imamoğlu M, Umit IA, et al. Neck masses confined to the submental space: our experience with 24 cases. *Ear Nose Throat J*. 2011;90(11):538–540.
14. Gupta S, Merchant SS. Lemierre's syndrome: rare, but life threatening: a case report with *Streptococcus intermedius*. *Case Rep Med*. 2012;2012:624065.
15. Reynolds SC, Chow AW. Severe soft tissue infections of the head and neck: a primer for critical care physicians. *Lung*. 2009;187(5):271–279.
16. Potter JK, Herford AS, Ellis E III. Tracheotomy versus endotracheal intubation for airway management in deep neck space infections. *J Oral Maxillofac Surg*. 2002;60(4):349–354.
17. Dzyak WR, Zide MF. Diagnosis and treatment of lateral pharyngeal space infections. *J Oral Maxillofac Surg*. 1984;42(4):243–249.
18. Debnam JM, Guha-Thakurta N. Retropharyngeal and prevertebral spaces: anatomic imaging and diagnosis. *Otolaryngol Clin North Am*. 2012;45(6):1293–1310.
19. Goodman LJ. Purulent pericarditis. *Curr Treat Options Cardiovasc Med*. 2000;2(4):343–350.
20. Anithakumari AM, Girish RB. Carotid space infection: a case report. *Indian J Otolaryngol Head Neck Surg*. 2006;58(1):95–97.
21. Dalley RW, Robertson WD, Oliverrio PJ. Overview of diagnostic imaging of the head and neck. In: Cummings CW, Fredrickson JM, Harker LA, et al., eds. *Otolaryngology, Head and Neck Surgery*. 3rd ed. St. Louis, Missouri: Mosby; 2006.

CHAPTER 9

Embryology of the Head and Neck

Janine Prange-Kiel

In the human embryo, all organs—including the structures of the head and neck—develop from three germ layers: ectoderm, mesoderm, and endoderm. These germ layers form during gastrulation, a differentiation process occurring at the beginning of week 3. (Note: All given time specifications refer to the gestational age of the embryo. Gestational age is determined by fertilization, which marks day 0.) Shortly after gastrulation has been completed, the formation of primordia, the earliest recognizable organ stages, starts in a process called organogenesis. By the end of week 8, organogenesis is completed, and during the remaining time of pregnancy, the fetal period, the organs continue to grow and mature.

Time Line of Head and Neck Development

In week 4, the brain develops at the cranial pole of the embryo by neurulation (discussed later). By the end of week 4, optic vesicles, which will substantially contribute to the formation of the eyes, have protruded from the developing brain. Together with the stomodeum, the primordium of the mouth, the optic vesicles are among the first discernible facial structures in the future head region. Starting on day 22, five pharyngeal arches begin to form and, in weeks 5 and 6, further differentiate into important structures in the head and neck region. At the same time, mesenchymal tissue around the developing brain starts to form the skull. In weeks 7 and 8, many facial structures, such as the jaw, nose, eyes, and ears, become more defined. During this late phase of organogenesis and in the following fetal period, the face takes on its characteristic human contours mostly by differential growth of its various structures. For example, early in organogenesis, the eyes are located at the lateral aspect of the developing head. During development, they appear to move closer to the midline because the portions of the face lateral to the eyes grow faster than the portion between the eyes.[1]

The proportions of facial structures change during prenatal development, in addition to the head-to-body ratio. In the early fetus (week 12), the head constitutes about one-third of the body length; this relation decreases to about one-quarter of the body length at the time of birth and continues to decrease during postnatal development.

Neurulation and Formation of Neural Crest Cells as a Prerequisite for Head and Neck Development (Fig. 9.1)

The formation of the head and neck strongly depends on the successful completion of neurulation (i.e., the formation of the central nervous system [CNS]). Early in week 4, parts of the most dorsal germ layer, the ectoderm, transform into the neural plate. The thickened epithelial cells, which form the neural plate, are located along the embryo's craniocaudal axis. The neuronal plate invaginates along this axis, and the resulting neuronal folds separate from the ectoderm and fuse to form the neural tube, which in turn will develop into the CNS. The free edges of the remaining surface ectoderm fuse over the neural tube and thereby build a continuous layer, which later will differentiate into epidermis. In humans, the fusion of the neural folds starts at two discrete points along the craniocaudal axis and proceeds in the cranial and caudal directions. The cranial portion of the neural tube, the future brain, closes completely on day 25.[2] Failure of this fusion results in anencephaly and is incompatible with postnatal life. In the US, anencephaly occurs with a prevalence of 2.46 per 10,000 live births[3] and is always accompanied by acrania, the partial or complete absence of the cranial vault (Fig. 9.2).

During the fusion of the neural folds into the neural tube, cells at the edge of the neural fold separate and form streaks of neural crest cells (NCCs) along the entire neural tube. NCCs undergo the epithelial-mesenchymal transition as they detach from the neural tube and migrate to various locations in the body. They form a vast array of structures, such as the ganglia of the autonomic nervous system, the enteric nervous system, and the adrenal medulla. In the head and neck region, NCCs give rise to much of the connective tissue in the craniofacial complex (skull, face, pharyngeal arches).[4–7] Therefore, neurocristopathies (i.e., the abnormal development of NCCs) often cause developmental defects that involve the craniofacial system (e.g., DiGeorge syndrome, Treacher Collins syndrome, and cleft formation).[8]

Skull Development

Neurocranium and Viscerocranium (Fig. 9.3)

Functionally, the cranium (skull) is composed of two parts: the neurocranium and the viscerocranium. The neurocranium surrounds and protects the brain and can be subdivided into the cranial base and the cranial vault. The viscerocranium comprises the facial skeleton and facilitates respiration and ingestion. The mesenchyme that forms the bones of the viscerocranium solely originates from NCCs, which migrate into the pharyngeal arches, whereas the material for bone formation in the neurocranium derives from both indigenous, cephalic mesoderm and NCCs.

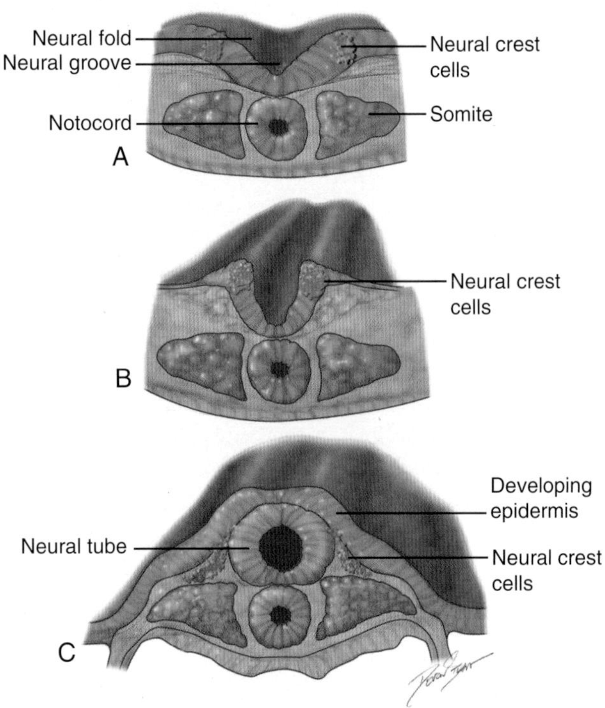

Figure 9.1 Neurulation (transverse section through embryonic disk). **A** and **B,** Neural folds and neural groove form from ectodermal tissue along the craniocaudal axis of the embryo. **C,** Merging of the neural folds results in the neural tube; the ectodermal tissue re-fuses over the neural tube. NCCs separate from the neural fold, undergo epithelial-mesenchymal transition, and migrate into various regions of the embryo.

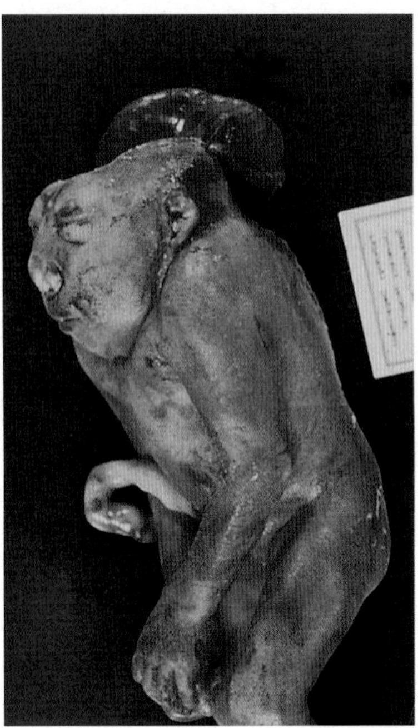

Figure 9.2 Newborn infant with acrania and meroencephaly. Failure of fusion of the cranial portion of the neural tube results in severe brain anomalies accompanied by faulty development of the cranial vault. (Courtesy of A.E. Chudley, M.D., Section of Genetics and Metabolism, Department of Pediatrics and Child Health, University of Manitoba, Children's Hospital, Winnipeg, Manitoba, Canada. As seen in Moore KL, Persaud PVR, Torchia NG. *The Developing Human*. 11th ed. Philadelphia, Pennsylvania: Saunders; 2020, Fig. 14.11B, p. 327.)

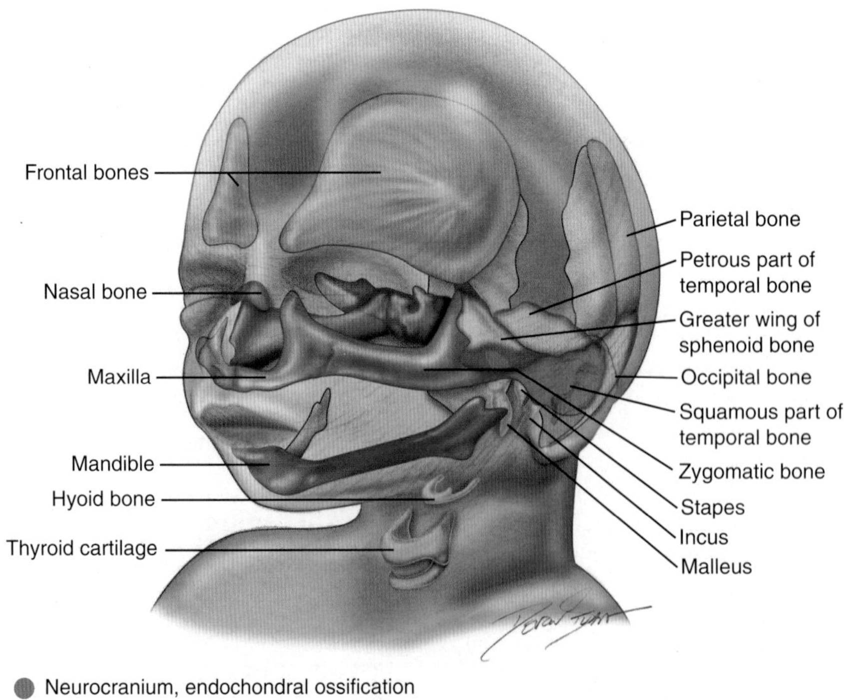

Figure 9.3 Skull development. Bones of the neurocranium and viscerocranium develop by endochondral and intramembranous ossification.

Intramembranous and Endochondral Ossification

In general, two types of bone formation can be distinguished, both of which are found in skull development. In intramembranous ossification, mesenchymal tissue condenses and forms a highly vascularized membranous sheath. Osteoblasts differentiate from mesenchymal precursor cells and deposit osteoid (unmineralized bone matrix), which is subsequently calcified. In endochondral ossification, chondrocytes, which also differentiate from mesenchyme, initially form a cartilaginous model of the future bone. Starting at primary centers of ossification, osteoblasts then gradually replace the cartilage with bone tissue.

The bones that constitute the cranial base (i.e., the base of the occipital bone, the body of the sphenoid bone, petrous and mastoid parts of the temporal bone, and the ethmoid bone) are formed by endochondral ossification. This also holds true for several bones of the viscerocranium, such as the bones of the middle ear, the styloid process of the temporal bone, and the hyoid bone. The remaining bones of the viscerocranium, such as the mandible, the maxillary and zygomatic bones, and the squamous part of the temporal bone, are formed by intramembranous ossification. Similarly, the bones that shape the cranial vault (frontal and parietal bones, parts of the occipital bone) are formed by intramembranous ossification.

The development of the temporomandibular joint starts at week 9 with the formation of the condylar process of the mandible, which is followed by the formation of the temporal portion of the joint (week 10). By week 14, the interarticular disk and the joint spaces have been formed.

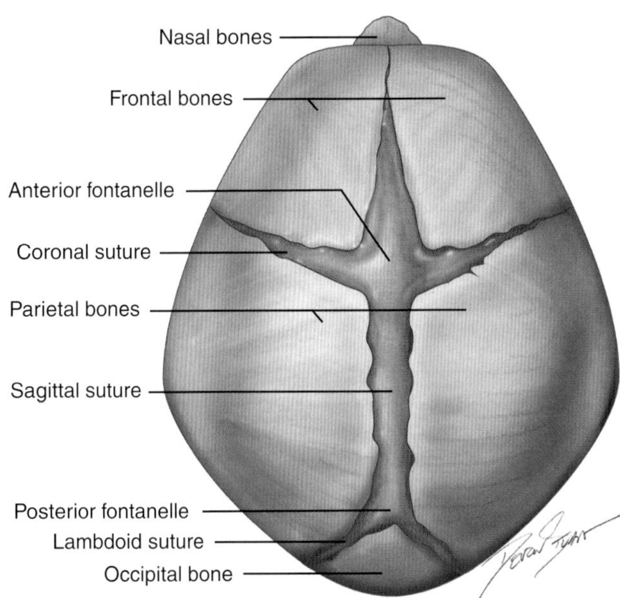

Figure 9.4 Development of the cranial vault. Sutures and fontanelles between the developing bones of the skull permit shifting of these bones during birth and provide space for additional growth of the bones.

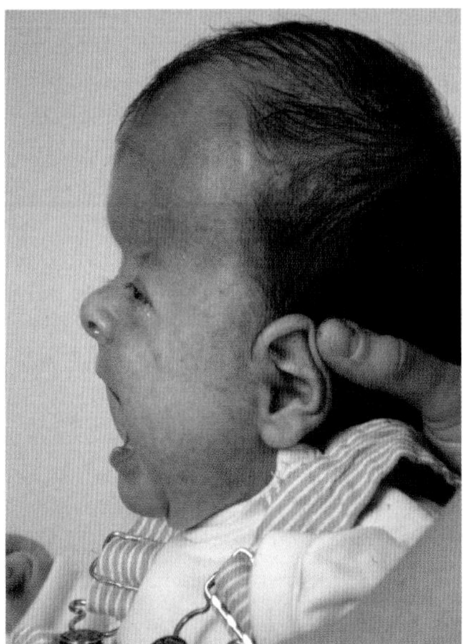

Figure 9.5 Craniosynostosis in an infant with Apert syndrome. Brachycephaly (skull shortened in anteroposterior direction) is caused by premature fusion of the coronary sutures. (From Cote C, Lerman J, Anderson B. *A Practice of Anesthesia for Infants and Children*. 6th ed. Philadelphia, Pennsylvania: Saunders; 2018.)

Sutures and Fontanelles (Fig. 9.4)

The bones of the cranial vault are joined by fibrous joints (syndesmoses), which are referred to as sutures. These sutures widen into larger fibrous areas, the fontanelles, in locations where more than two bones meet. Sutures and fontanelles allow for molding of the head while passing through the birth canal. Moreover, the sutures are the sides of pre- and postnatal growth of the cranial bones, and whereas the fontanelles usually close within the first 2 years of prenatal life, most of the sutures only close completely in adulthood. Coordinated growth of the CNS and its surrounding tissues (meninges, bones, and connective tissue) is essential for normal head development.[9,10]

Craniosynostosis (Fig. 9.5), the premature fusion of one or more cranial sutures, results in restriction of the growing brain and craniofacial deformities due to compensatory growth in areas that do not show premature fusion. The prevalence of this malformation ranges from 3.1 to 6.4 in 10,000 live births,[11] and the defect can occur as an isolated event or as a component of various syndromes. Depending on which of the sutures fuse prematurely, the shape of the skull is altered. For example, scaphocephaly, a long and narrow skull, is the result of early fusion of the sagittal suture, whereas brachycephaly, a skull shortened in the anteroposterior direction, is caused by premature fusion of both coronary sutures. Crouzon and Apert syndromes are two examples of syndromes associated with craniosynostosis of the coronary sutures. Mutations in a gene encoding for a fibroblast growth factor receptor cause both syndromes, which also feature deformation of other craniofacial structures, such as shallow orbits, hypertelorism, a hypoplastic midface region and maxilla, and mandibular prognathism.[12]

Special Sense Organs

A detailed description of the development of the special sense organs goes well beyond the scope of this text. In general, focal thickenings of the cranial surface ectoderm of the embryo, ectodermal placodes, appear around week 4 and form parts of the sense organs. The lens (or optic) placodes develop into the lens of the eye, the nasal (or olfactory) placodes produce the olfactory neurons, and the otic (or auditory) placodes form the otic vesicles, which develop into the membranous labyrinths of the inner ear, including the sensory cells for hearing and movement. The relationship between the placodes and the surrounding tissue is complex. On one hand, the surrounding tissue induces the development and further differentiation of the placodes; on the other hand, the placodes are essential for the development of the surrounding structures.[13]

Pharyngeal Arches

Overview (Fig. 9.6)

In phylogenetic terms, the pharyngeal arches derive from the gills of jawless fish. In humans, five pairs of pharyngeal arches (numbered 1 to 4 and 6) are located at the lateroventral aspects of the primitive oral cavity and the pharyngeal portion of the foregut. The first pair of pharyngeal arches forms in week 4 and is located just caudal to the primitive oral cavity. Subsequently, arches 2 through 4 and 6 develop in a craniocaudal sequence. The mesenchymal core of each arch is covered with ectoderm on the outside and with endoderm on the inside. The arches are separated from each other by pharyngeal membranes, which are double layers of endodermal and ectodermal tissue. The resulting indentations are called pharyngeal pouches and pharyngeal grooves (or clefts) on the inside and outside of the embryo, respectively. While the pouches and their endoderm develop into various important organs of the head and neck region, most of the grooves obliterate; only the first groove persists as the external acoustic meatus. Pharyngeal cysts and fistulas occur when the grooves do not completely obliterate.[14] Fistulas of the second pharyngeal groove are the most common type of pharyngeal fistulas; they usually open near the anterior border of the sternocleidomastoid muscle.

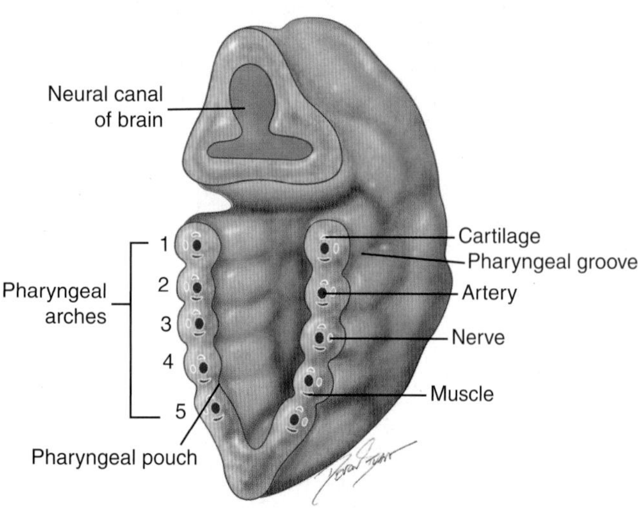

Figure 9.6 Pharyngeal arches. Five pharyngeal arches develop in a craniocaudal sequence. Each arch contains tissue that will differentiate into muscle, cartilage, blood vessels, and nerves.

Components of Each Arch: Muscle, Cartilage, Blood Vessel, and Nerve

The mesenchymal core of each arch, which receives contributions from the indigenous mesoderm as well as from NCCs, differentiates into connective tissue, musculature, and skeletal elements. Each pharyngeal arch also develops an aortic arch artery; these arteries are connected to each other and eventually differentiate into the definite aortic arch and its branches, which provide blood supply to the head and neck region. Furthermore, each pharyngeal arch contains a cranial nerve, which originates from the primitive brain. Each of these cranial nerves innervates muscles (motor innervation) and mucosa (sensory innervation) derived from the corresponding arch. Table 9.1 provides an overview of the skeletal elements, muscles, arteries, and nerves that are associated with each of the pharyngeal arches.

Pharyngeal Pouches

The inside of the pharyngeal pouches is lined with endodermal epithelium, which gives rise to various organs of the head and neck.

The first pharyngeal pouch extends to become the tympanic cavity and the pharyngotympanic tube. The first pharyngeal membrane differentiates into the tympanic membrane, and the first pharyngeal groove, which opposes the pouch, develops into the external acoustic meatus.

The second pharyngeal pouch develops into the palatine tonsil; its endoderm invaginates into the surrounding mesenchyme and forms tonsillar crypts. Subsequently, the tissue is infiltrated by lymphocytes, which derive from hematopoietic stem cells and form the lymphatic nodules of the tonsil.

Starting at week 6, the caudal portion of the third pharyngeal pouch extends ventrally. The pouches from both sides merge in the ventral midline and form the bilobed thymus. The endoderm of the pouches becomes the epithelial tissue of the thymus. Later, lymphocytes, infiltrate the space between the epithelial cells. The cranial part of the third pouch extends caudoventrally toward the thyroid gland and develops into the inferior parathyroid gland.

Parts of the fourth pouch also extend in the direction of the developing thyroid gland and form the superior parathyroid gland. The caudal portion of the fourth pouch develops into the ultimobranchial body, which fuses with the thyroid gland and gives rise to calcitonin-producing parafollicular cells (C cells).

Table 9.1 Structures Derived From the Pharyngeal Arches

Pharyngeal Arch	Arch Artery	Skeletal Elements	Muscles	Cranial Nerve
1	Terminal branch of maxillary artery	Endochondral ossification: incus, malleus, part of the sphenoid Intramembranous ossification: maxillary and zygomatic bone, squamous portion of temporal bone, mandible	Muscles of mastication, mylohyoid, anterior belly of digastric, tensor tympani, tensor veli palatini	Maxillary and mandibular divisions of trigeminal nerve (V_2 and V_3)
2	Stapedial artery (in the embryo), corticotympanic artery (in the adult)	Endochondral ossification: stapes, styloid process, parts of the hyoid	Muscles of facial expression, posterior belly of digastric, stylohyoid, stapedius	Facial nerve (VII)
3	Common carotid artery, root of internal carotid artery	Endochondral ossification: parts of the hyoid	Stylopharyngeus	Glossopharyngeal nerve (IX)
4	Arch of aorta (left), right subclavian artery (right), original sprouts of pulmonary artery	Laryngeal cartilages	Constrictors of pharynx, levator veli palatini, cricothyroid	Superior laryngeal branch of vagus nerve (X)
6	Ductus arteriosus, roots of definitive pulmonary arteries	Laryngeal cartilages	Intrinsic muscles of larynx	Recurrent laryngeal branch of vagus nerve (X)

Thyroid Gland

Approximately 24 days after fertilization, an endodermal thickening, the thyroid diverticulum, appears medially on the floor of the pharynx. The thyroid diverticulum migrates caudally into the mesenchyme of the neck through an opening in the dorsum of the developing tongue (foramen cecum). During its descent ventral to the hyoid bone and laryngeal structures, the developing thyroid remains connected to the pharynx via the thyroglossal duct. By week 7, the formation of the thyroid gland is completed, and the thyroglossal duct degenerates, leaving only the foramen cecum as a visible pit at the dorsum of the tongue. The endoderm of the thyroid diverticulum forms epithelial cords, which intermingle with mesenchyme to form the thyroid follicles. The pyramidal lobe, which can be seen in about 50% of all people, is a remnant of the descending thyroid tissue.

Failure of normal descent of the thymus, thyroid, or parathyroid tissue during embryonic development results in ectopic glandular tissue, which should not be mistaken for pathologic masses.[15,16] Ectopic thyroid tissue is the most common cause of congenital neck masses encountered in children. Although the masses often present asymptomatically, surgical removal is usually the treatment of choice to prevent infections.

Tongue

The tongue develops at the floor of the pharynx from material provided by pharyngeal arches 1 to 4. By the end of week 4, a median tongue bud is formed by the first pharyngeal arch. Very soon thereafter, distal tongue buds appear on each side of the median bud, overgrow the median tongue bud, and fuse to form the anterior two-thirds of the tongue. The line of fusion between the two distal tongue buds forms the median sulcus of the tongue. The posterior one-third of the tongue is formed from swellings of the pharyngeal arches 2 to 4. The terminal sulcus marks the line of fusion between the anterior two-thirds and the posterior one-third of the tongue. The foramen cecum, through which the thyroid gland descends, is located at the junction of the median and terminal sulci.

The mesenchyme of the pharyngeal arches provides the connective tissue and the vasculature of the tongue. Based on its origin from the first pharyngeal arch, the anterior two-thirds of the tongue receives its sensory innervation from the mandibular division of the trigeminal nerve. The posterior one-third of the tongue mostly derives from the third pharyngeal arch, and its sensory innervation is therefore provided by the glossopharyngeal nerve. Most extrinsic and intrinsic muscles of the tongue derive from myoblasts that migrate from the occipital mesenchyme into the tongue. These muscles are innervated by the hypoglossal nerve, which, like the myoblasts, migrates toward the tongue.

A branch of the facial nerve, namely the chorda tympani, and fibers from the glossopharyngeal and vagus nerves migrate into the tongue and innervate taste buds, which are formed by epithelial cells.

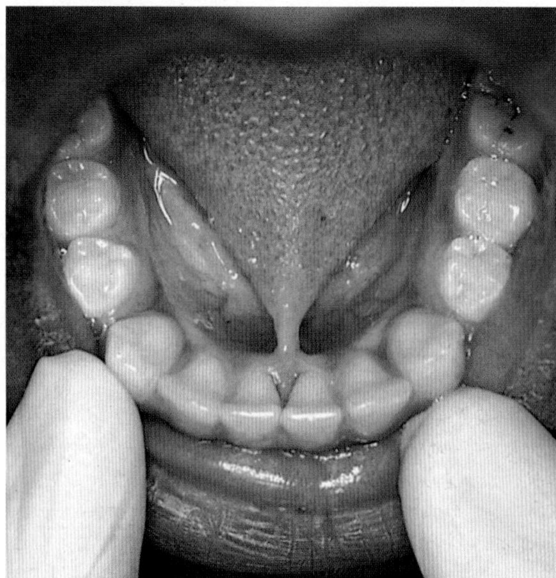

Figure 9.7 Ankyloglossia. A short frenulum ties the tongue to the floor of the mouth. (From Zitelli BJ, McIntire S, Nowalk A. *Atlas of Pediatric Physical Diagnosis*. 7th ed. Elsevier; 2017.)

In general, congenital anomalies of the tongue are rare, and most of the time they are part of a syndrome or sequence (e.g., macroglossia in Down syndrome, glossoptosis in Pierre Robin sequence). Ankyloglossia (Fig. 9.7), however, is a fairly frequent birth defect (prevalence ranges from less than 1% to 10%[17]) that may require surgical correction if it impedes feeding and speech development.[18]

Major Salivary Glands

Each salivary gland develops from a single epithelial bud through repetitive branching, eventually resulting in a secretory organ that stays connected with the oral cavity via its proximal duct.[19] The parotid salivary glands develop from oral ectoderm near the stomodeum and extend toward the ears, whereas the submandibular and sublingual salivary glands derive from invaginations of pharyngeal endoderm.

Facial Development

In week 4, the stomodeum is delineated by five prominences, which constitute the facial primordia. A single frontonasal prominence surrounds the ventrolateral portion of the forebrain above the stomodeum, paired maxillary prominences frame the lateral parts of the stomodeum, and paired mandibular prominences delineate the lower border of the stomodeum. The maxillary and mandibular prominences are parts of the first pharyngeal arch.

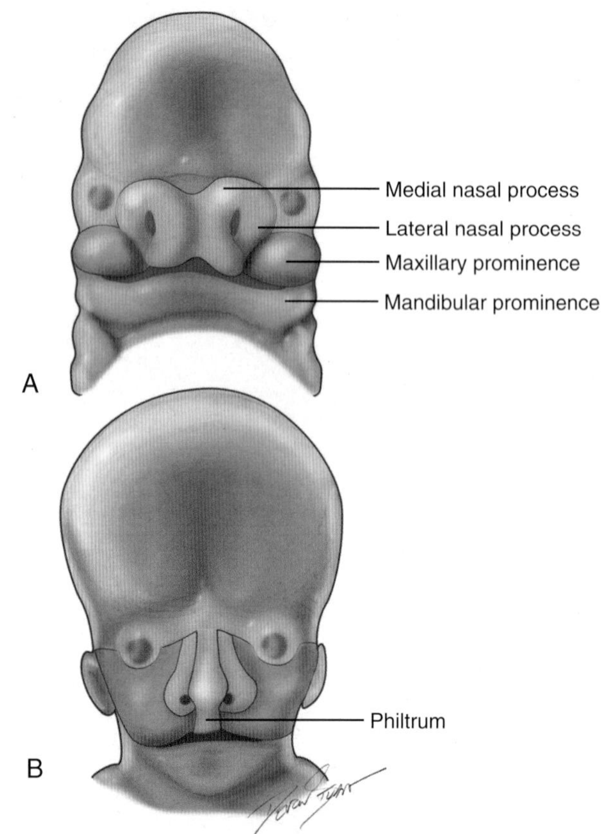

Figure 9.8 Facial development. **A,** A total of five prominences surround the stomodeum: a frontonasal prominence, from which the medial and lateral nasal processes derive, two maxillary prominences, and two mandibular prominences. **B,** Differential growth of these prominences results in the formation of the face.

Surface Structures (Fig. 9.8)

At the end of week 4, the nasal placodes develop on the inferolateral part of the frontolateral prominences. The mesenchymal tissue around the placodes starts to proliferate and forms medial and lateral nasal processes, while the placodes sink deeper into the tissue, causing the nasal pits to form. The lateral nasal processes later develop into the alae of the nose; the medial nasal processes merge to form not only the nasal septum, but also parts of the ethmoid bone, the cribriform plate, and the intermaxillary segment. The latter will form the philtrum and the premaxilla, which develops into the primary palate and becomes a part of the alveolar process of the maxilla. The frontonasal prominence also develops into the dorsum and apex of the nose and into the forehead.

The lateral nasal prominences on both sides are separated from the maxillary prominences by nasolacrimal grooves. Thickened ectoderm at the bottom of these grooves will descend into the underlying mesoderm and become hollow, thereby forming the nasolacrimal ducts and the lacrimal sacs of the eye, which become functional during the fetal period.

Starting in week 5, all prominences begin to fuse and shape the borders of the mouth and the nares. The maxillary prominences of both sides fuse with the premaxilla and with the caudal parts of the lateral nasal processes, thus closing the floor of the nasal pits and forming the maxilla and the upper lip. Laterally, the maxillary prominences merge with the mandibular prominences to form the cheeks. The lower lips and the mandible are formed entirely by the mandibular prominences.

Mesenchymal cells from the second pharyngeal arch migrate into the facial region and develop into the musculature of facial expression; the muscles of mastication derive from the first pharyngeal arch.

By week 6, a linear thickening of ectoderm appears on the surfaces of the mandibular and maxillary prominences, and through invagination, labiogingival grooves are formed between the lips and the anterior gums. A small area of ectoderm persists in the midline as a frenulum, which attaches the lips to the gingiva.

The auricle of the external ear develops from six auricular hillocks, which are formed from mesenchymal tissue of the first and second pharyngeal arch and are arranged on both sides of the first pharyngeal groove. The hillocks grow and coalesce to form the auricle. Due to its origin, the external ear is initially positioned at the base of the neck; it reaches its definite position only during the course of normal development of the derivatives of the pharyngeal arches. Therefore, many congenital syndromes associated with abnormal development of the pharyngeal arches, such as DiGeorge and Treacher Collins syndrome, also feature low-set ears.

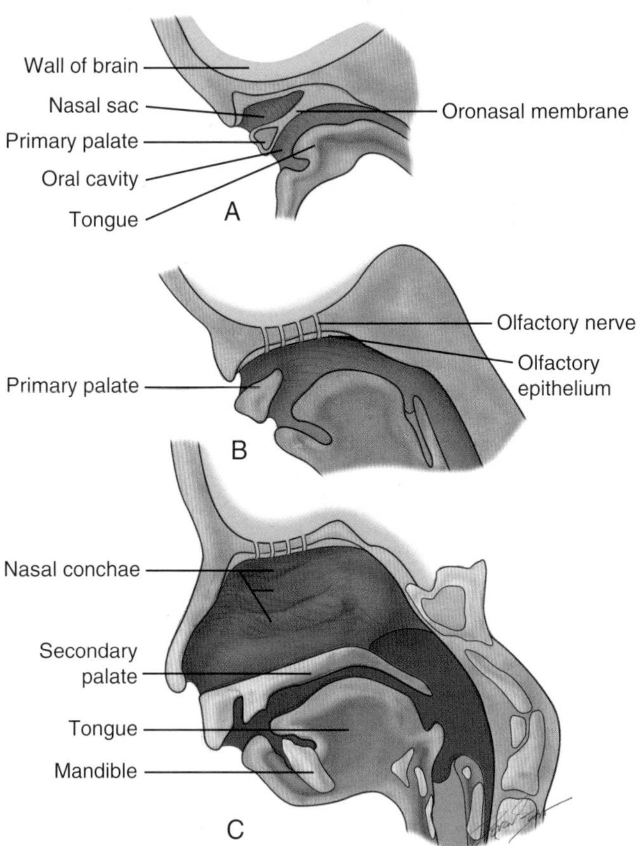

Figure 9.9 Development of the nasal cavity. **A**, The oronasal membrane separates the nasal sac and the oral cavity early in development. **B**, After rupture of the oronasal membrane, both cavities are connected. **C**, Formation of the secondary palate results in the re-separation of the nasal cavity and the oral cavity. The nasal conchae develop on the lateral wall late during organogenesis.

Development of the Nasal Cavities (Fig. 9.9)

The nasal pits deepen and form primordial nasal sacs, which are separated from the oral portion of the pharynx by an oronasal (nasobuccal) membrane. This membrane dissipates and thereby establishes a connection, the primitive choana, between the primary nasal cavities and the oral cavity. The nasal placodes become situated at the roof of the nasal cavity and differentiate into the olfactory epithelium, which becomes connected to the olfactory bulbs via olfactory nerves.

The superior, middle, and inferior conchae develop from elevations on the lateral walls of the nasal cavity late during organogenesis, whereas the paranasal sinuses only start to develop at the end of the fetal period. The extensions of the nasal cavities into the maxillary, frontal, sphenoid, and ethmoid bones start as diverticula of the lateral wall of the nasal cavities. The development of the paranasal sinuses continues into adolescence.[20]

The secondary nasal cavity becomes separated from the oral cavity again during the formation of the palate, when the palatal shelves fuse with each other, with the premaxilla, and with the nasal septum.

Development of the Palate (Fig. 9.10)

The palate separates the oral and nasal cavities and can be subdivided into the anterior hard palate and the posterior soft palate. Palate development is a two-step process. First, the primary palate derives from the frontonasal prominence. Later, the fusion of the palatal shelves, which derive from the maxillary prominences, forms the secondary palate.

The primary palate is formed early in week 6 by fusion of the medial nasal processes. It persists as a part of the maxilla and comprises the small portion of the adult hard palate anterior to the incisive foramen. Starting late in week 6, the secondary palate forms from the lateral palatine processes (palatal shelves), which extend medially from the internal walls of the maxillary prominences and project downward on either side of the tongue. During weeks 7 and 8, the palatal shelves first grow further vertically, then—within a few hours—ascend into a horizontal position above the tongue. Eventually, the two shelves meet in the midline, where they first form an epithelial seam. Upon degeneration of the epithelial tissue, the mesenchyme from both sides becomes continuous and the formation of the secondary palate is completed. Subsequently, the secondary palate fuses with the primary palate; together, they compose the definite palate. During weeks 9 to 12, the nasal septum, which is formed by the fused medial nasal processes (as discussed previously), fuses with the definite palate

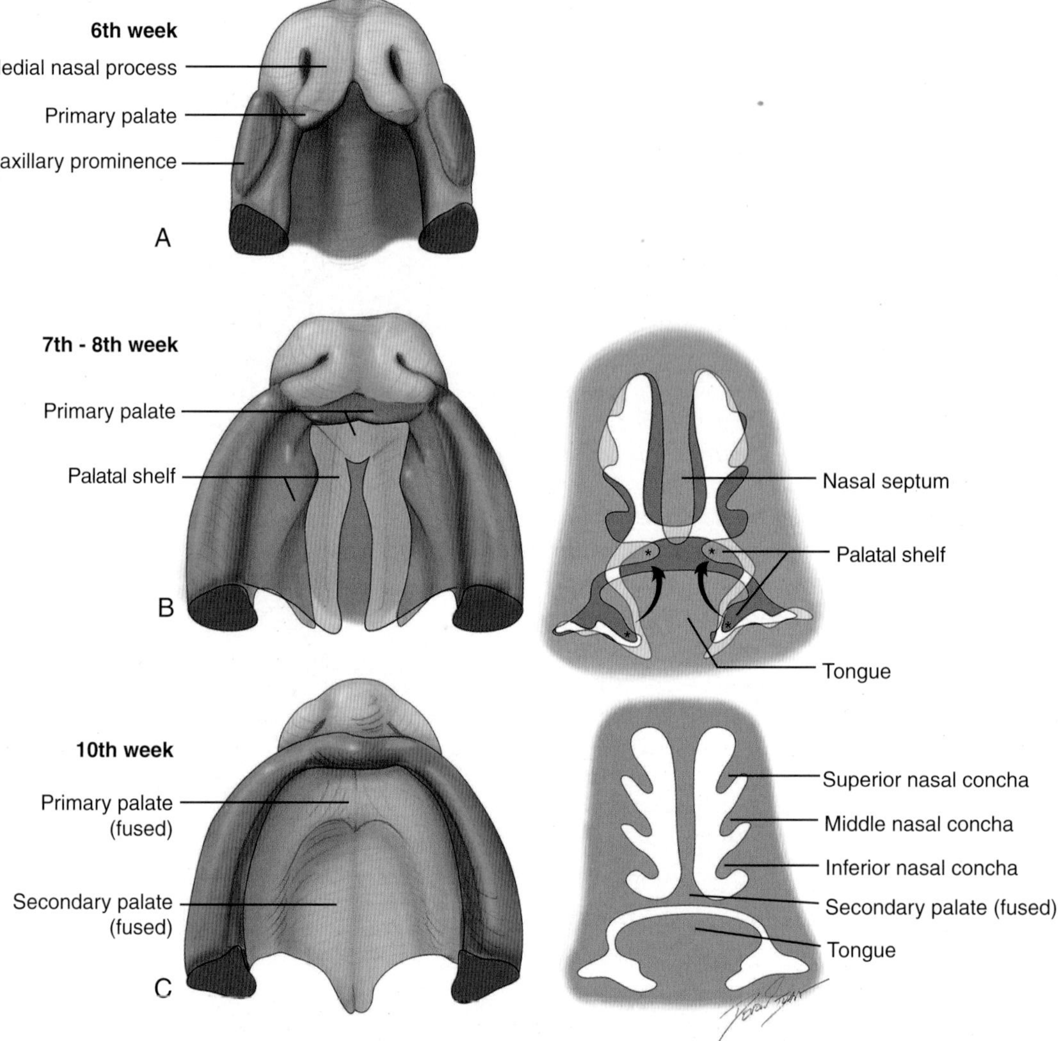

Figure 9.10 Development of the palate. **A,** Early in week 6, the medial nasal processes begin to fuse to form the primary palate. **B,** Palatal shelves extend from the lateral walls of the maxillary prominences and grow vertically during weeks 7 and 8 (shown in *purple*). Within a few hours the palatine shelves ascend into a horizontal position (shown in *light pink*, motion of the shelves indicated by the *arrows*). **C,** The palatine shelves fuse with each other and with the nasal septum to form the secondary palate. The secondary and primary palate are also fused.

and thereby completely separates the two nasal cavities from each other.

Bone tissue builds in the primary palate and the anterior portions of the palatal shelves to form the hard palate. The posterior portions of the shelves do not ossify but form the soft palate and the uvula. The palatal muscles (as well as the faucial muscles) are formed by the myogenic mesenchymal tissue of pharyngeal arches 1, 2, and 4 at the end of organogenesis and during early fetal life.

Cleft Lip and Palate (Fig. 9.11)

The formation of the upper lip and the palate is a complex series of events, during which the migration, growth, differentiation, and apoptosis of cells of various origins need to be coordinated.[21,22] Clefts of the lip or palate result from disruption of these events and can affect feeding, speech, hearing, appearance, and socialization. Cleft lip and palate are among the most common birth defects, occurring in approximately 1 in 700 live births.[22]

As the upper lip and primary palate differ in their origin from the secondary palate, two forms of cleft formations can be distinguished: anterior and posterior anomalies, with *anterior* and *posterior* referring to the position of the cleft relative to the incisive foramen.

Anterior cleft anomalies are often referred to as cleft lip with or without cleft palate. As mentioned earlier, the primary palate and the philtrum of the upper lip originate from fusion of the medial nasal processes. Fusion of these two structures with the maxillary prominences on both sides completes the formation of the upper lip and the alveolar portion of the maxilla. A partial or complete failure of the merged nasal

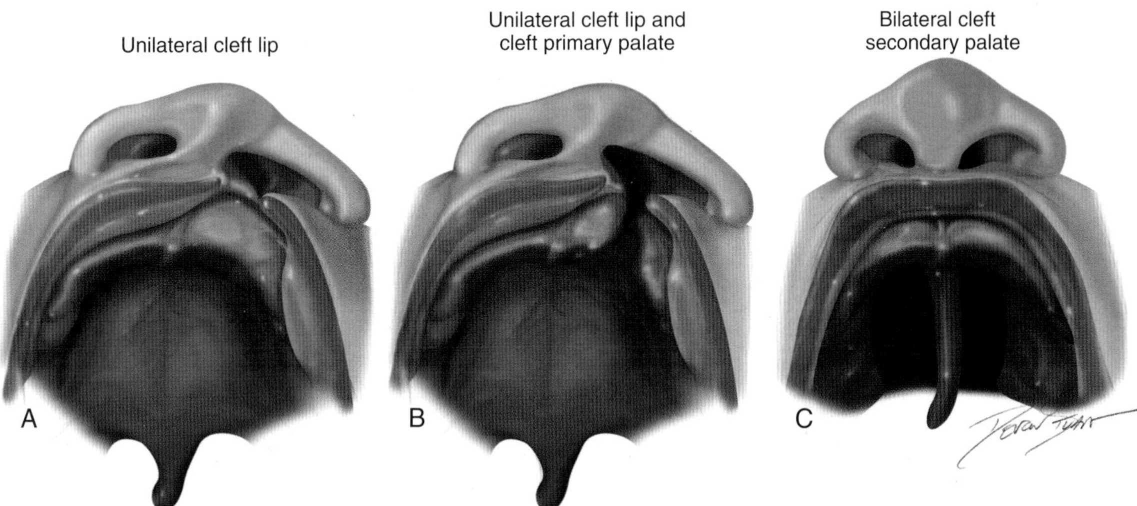

Figure 9.11 Cleft lip and palate. **A,** Anterior cleft without cleft palate. **B,** Anterior cleft with cleft anterior palate. **C,** Isolated posterior cleft (bilateral).

processes to unite with the maxillary prominences results in an anterior cleft anomaly, which affects the lip or the lip and the alveolar portion of the maxilla. Depending on whether only one or both maxillary prominences fail to fuse with the merged medial nasal processes, the cleft is unilateral or bilateral. Median cleft lip, which results from the failure of the medial nasal processes to fuse, is rare and usually associated with abnormal brain development.[23]

Posterior cleft anomalies are often referred to as isolated cleft palate. The posterior portions of the hard palate and the soft palate derive from the palatal shelves, which fuse in midline. Partial or complete failure of this fusion results in clefts of the secondary palate posterior to the incisive foramen, which can affect either the soft palate only or both the soft and the hard palate.

Although anterior and posterior cleft anomalies often occur together, they differ in their etiology as well as in their distribution with respect to sex, familial association, race, and geography.[24] For example, anterior cleft anomalies are observed more frequently in males, whereas posterior cleft anomalies are more prevalent in female newborns.[25] In a large portion (70%) of cases, the cleft lip and palate anomaly is an isolated occurrence (i.e., it is not associated with any other craniofacial anomaly). However, many syndromes, such as Stickler, Van der Woude, Crouzon, and Apert, feature cleft lip and palate. The etiology of cleft lip and palate is extremely complex, with contributions from both genetic and environmental factors.[21] A large number of genes have been identified to play a role in both syndromic and isolated forms of cleft lip and palate.[25] Maternal smoking and alcohol consumption as well as malnutrition are a few of the environmental influences associated with the induction of cleft anomalies.[22,25]

Anomalies Associated With the Development of the Pharyngeal Arches

Many complex craniofacial birth defects are associated with the development of the pharyngeal arches, of which only a small selection will be mentioned here.

Treacher Collins syndrome (Fig. 9.12) is a genetic disorder, in which migration of NCCs into the first pharyngeal arch is inhibited. Clinical features of the syndrome include hypoplasia of the mandible, maxilla, and zygomatic bones; cleft palate; abnormalities of the middle and external ear (including hearing loss due to atresia of the external ear canal); and lower eyelid abnormalities.[8]

22q11.2 deletion syndrome (also known as DiGeorge syndrome) is caused by deletions in the long arm of chromosome 22 and is associated with numerous phenotypes, including failure of pharyngeal pouches 3 and 4 to differentiate. This developmental deficit causes, among other symptoms, hypoparathyroidism with hypocalcemia, absence of the thymus with immune defects, and an interrupted aortic arch (narrowing of the aorta at the level of the ductus arteriosus).[26,27]

Pierre Robin sequence is characterized by micrognathia, which hinders normal tongue development and results in glossoptosis and consequential airway obstruction. Abnormal tongue development most likely also interferes with palate development, often causing cleft palate. No causal relationship between Pierre Robin sequence and a single genetic mutation is known, but it is often observed in conjunction with craniofacial syndromes, such as Stickler syndrome and 22q11.2 deletion syndrome.[28,29]

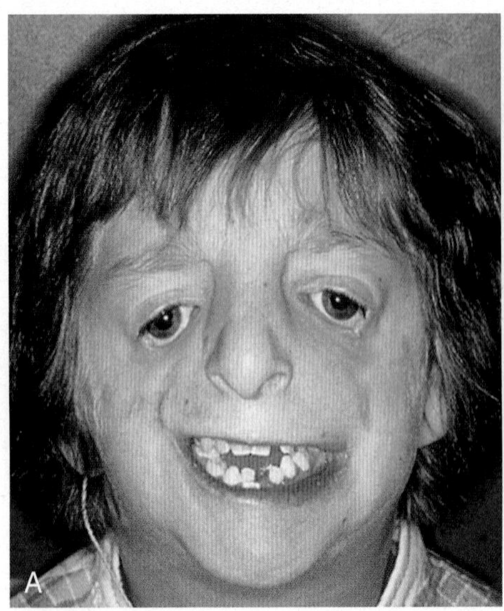
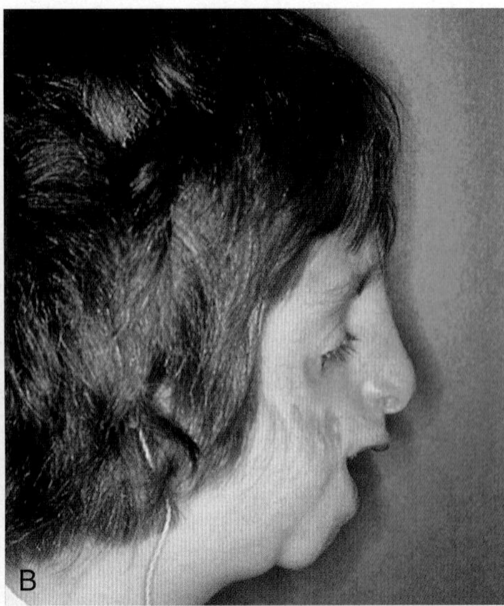

Figure 9.12 Child with Treacher Collins syndrome. Inhibited migration of neural crest cells (NCCs) into the first pharyngeal arch results in hypoplasia of the mandible, maxilla, and zygomatic bones, and in abnormalities of the lower eyelids. (From Kaban LB, Troulis MJ. *Pediatric Oral and Maxillofacial Surgery*. St. Louis, Missouri: Saunders; 2004.)

References

1. Chun-Hui Tsai A, Stool SE, Post JC. Phylogenetic aspects and embryology. In: Bluestone CD, Stool SE, Alper CM, et al., eds. *Pediatric Otolaryngology*. St. Louis, Missouri: Saunders; 2003.
2. Greene ND, Copp AJ. Development of the vertebrate central nervous system: formation of the neural tube. *Prenat Diagn*. 2009;29(4):303–311.
3. Mai CT, Isenburg JL, Canfield MA, et al. National Birth Defects Prevention Network. National population-based estimates for major birth defects, 2010-2014. *Birth Defects Res*. 2019;111(18):1420–1435.
4. Gong S-G. Cranial neural crest: migratory cell behavior and regulatory networks. *Exp Cell Res*. 2014;325(2):90–95.
5. Minoux M, Rijli FM. Molecular mechanisms of cranial neural crest cell migration and patterning in craniofacial development. *Development*. 2010;137(16):2605–2621.
6. Jiang X, Iseki S, Maxson RE, Sucov HM, Morriss-Kay GM. Tissue origins and interactions in the mammalian skull vault. *Dev Biol*. 2002;241(1):106–116.
7. Noden DM, Trainor PA. Relations and interactions between cranial mesoderm and neural crest populations. *J Anat*. 2005;207(5):575–601.
8. Trainor PA. Craniofacial birth defects: the role of neural crest cells in the etiology and pathogenesis of Treacher Collins syndrome and the potential for prevention. *Am J Med Genet*. 2010;152A(12):2984–2994.
9. Levi B, Wan DC, Wong VW, Nelson E, Hyun J, Longaker MT. Cranial suture biology: from pathways to patient care. *J Craniofac Surg*. 2012;23(1):13–19.
10. Tubbs RS, Bosmia AN, Cohen-Gadol AA. The human calvaria: a review of embryology, anatomy, pathology, and molecular development. *Childs Nerv Syst*. 2012;28(1):23–31.
11. Cornelissen M, Ottelander B, Rizopoulos D, et al. Increase of prevalence of craniosynostosis. *J Cranio-Maxillo-Fac Surg*. 2016;44(9):1273–1279.
12. Carinci F, Pezzetti F, Locci P, et al. Apert and Crouzon syndromes: clinical findings, genes and extracellular matrix. *J Craniofac Surg*. 2005;16(3):361–368.
13. Francis-West PH, Ladher RK, Schoenwolf GC. Development of the sensory organs. *Sci Prog*. 2002;85(Pt 2):151–173.
14. Acierno SP, Waldhausen JHT. Congenital cervical cysts, sinuses and fistulae. *Otolaryngol Clin North Am*. 2007;40(1):161–176 (vii-viii).
15. LaRiviere CA, Waldhausen JHT. Congenital cervical cysts, sinuses, and fistulae in pediatric surgery. *Surg Clin North Am*. 2012;92(3):583–597 (viii).
16. Nasseri F, Eftekhari F. Clinical and radiologic review of the normal and abnormal thymus: pearls and pitfalls. *Radiographics*. 2010;30(2):413–428.
17. Becker S, Mendez MD. *Ankyloglossia. In: StatPearls*. Treasure Island, FL: StatPearls Publishing; 2021. https://www.ncbi.nlm.nih.gov/books/NBK482295/.
18. Suter VGA, Bornstein MM. Ankyloglossia: facts and myths in diagnosis and treatment. *J Periodontol*. 2009;80(8):1204–1219.
19. de Paula F, Teshima THN, Hsieh R, Souza MM, Nico MMS, Lourenco SV. Overview of human salivary glands: highlights of morphology and developing processes. *Anat Rec*. 2017;300(7):1180–1188.
20. Jankowski R. Revisiting human nose anatomy: phylogenic and ontogenic perspectives. *Laryngoscope*. 2011;121(11):2461–2467.
21. Arosarena OA. Cleft lip and palate. *Otolaryngol Clin North Am*. 2007;40(1):27–60 (vi).
22. Mossey PA, Little J, Munger RG, Dixon MJ, Shaw WC. Cleft lip and palate. *Lancet*. 2009;374(9703):1773–1785.
23. de Boutray M, Beziat J-L, Yachouh J, Bigorre M, Gleizal A, Captier G. Median cleft of the upper lip: a new classification to guide treatment decisions. *J Cranio-Maxillo-Fac Surg*. 2016;44(6):664–671.
24. Schoenwolf GC, Bleyl SB, Brauer PR, Francis-West PH. In: *Larsen's Human Embryology*. 5th ed. Churchill Livingstone; 2015.
25. Dixon MJ, Marazita ML, Beaty TH, Murray JC. Cleft lip and palate: understanding genetic and environmental influences. *Nat Rev Genet*. 2011;12(3):167–178.
26. Cárdenas-Nieto D, Forero-Castro M, Esteban-Pérez C, et al. The 22q11.2 microdeletion in pediatric patients with cleft lip, palate, or both and congenital heart disease: a systematic review. *J Pediatr Genet*. 2020;9(1):1–8.
27. Marom T, Roth Y, Goldfarb A, et al. Head and neck manifestations of 22q11.2 deletion syndromes. *Eur Arch Oto-Rhino-Laryngol*. 2012;269(2):381–387.
28. Hsieh ST, Woo AS. Pierre Robin sequence. *Clin Plast Surg*. 2019;46(2):249–259.
29. Evans KN, Sie KC, Hopper RA, et al. Robin sequence: from diagnosis to development of an effective management plan. *Pediatrics*. 2011;127(5):936–948.

CHAPTER 10

Routine Extraction of Teeth

Rachel Uppgaard

Armamentarium

#1 Woodson elevator
#15 Blade/handle
#150 Maxillary universal forceps
#151 Mandibular universal forceps
#23 Cowhorn mandibular forceps
#301 Elevator
#40 Elevator
#74 Ash mandibular forceps
#77R Back action elevator
#9 Periosteal elevator
#99C or #1 Maxillary forceps
4 × 4 Gauze
Bite block/mouth prop
Bone rasp
Cryer/east-west elevator
Double-ended curette
EH01 Howard Elevator
Hemostat
Local anesthetic with vasoconstrictor
Minnesota retractor
Pharyngeal curtain (4 × 4 gauze)
Rongeurs
Saline irrigation
Suction

History of the Procedure

Simple extractions are a mainstay of oral and maxillofacial surgery. The first mention of tooth extraction was found in the writings of Hippocrates, and the procedure was described by the Roman Celsus in the first century AD. Tooth extractions were performed by tooth-drawers and lower barber-surgeons. In the 18th century, the first description of extraction instruments was published.[1] In modern times, advanced dental techniques permit the maintenance and restoration of teeth. Preventive dentistry provides dental patients with the knowledge and tools to better care for their teeth and maintain them long term. Yet, many patients require routine extractions and may be interested in the preservation of bone for future dental implants. Basic exodontia includes the use of instruments to reflect the marginal gingiva, perform simple luxation techniques and bone expansion, and to deliver the tooth. This chapter presents the basic instruments used for simple extractions, modifications for extracting teeth in different areas of the mouth, and tips to aid in the preservation of bone.

Indications for the Use of the Procedure

Prior to the procedure, it is imperative that the surgeon ascertain the status of the patient's systemic health via an interview at the initial consult appointment. The surgeon must identify not only the medical comorbidities of the patient but also the specific management of pathology that may be present with the tooth and recognize psychological considerations that may impact the patient's ability to tolerate the procedure. No aspect of simple tooth extraction is more important than the careful preoperative assessment of the patient and the management of various medical comorbidities. The preoperative examination must include an updated medical history, any indicated laboratory tests, physical exam including examination for associated pathology, oral exam, and dental radiographs. Consideration of the patient's ability to tolerate the procedure psychologically should be taken. Box 10.1 presents conditions that warrant extraction. It may be important to attempt to save the tooth through restorative, endodontic, and periodontic treatment.[2] Only if the initial therapy fails should the tooth be extracted.[3,4]

BOX 10.1 Indications for Tooth Extraction

- Carious and nonrestorable teeth
- Failed endodontic treatment
- Poor periodontal prognosis
- Impacted teeth and periapical pathology
- Necrotic teeth
- Supernumerary teeth
- Crowding/nonfunctional teeth
- Orthodontic considerations
- Deciduous teeth interfering with eruption of permanent teeth
- Root fracture
- Dental pain and unwillingness to undergo necessary treatment
- Interference with prosthodontic needs
- Pathology associated with the tooth

Data from McCaul LK, Jenkins WM, Kay EJ. The reasons for the extraction of various tooth types in Scotland: a 15-year follow up. *J Dent.* 2001;29(6):401–407.

Limitations and Contraindications

After a complete history and review of systems, the surgeon should further investigate comorbidities that may challenge patient safety during a routine dental extraction. Some examples include bleeding dyscrasias, liver disease, immunocompromise (secondary to metabolic derangements such as diabetes, cancer, or immunosuppressant medication), cardiac disease, and coronary artery disease. A thorough history of radiation and antiresorptive therapy should be explored and appropriate measures taken to maximize the healing potential of the patient.[5]

During the clinical and radiographic assessments, certain key findings should alert the surgeon that a routine dental extraction might need to be converted to a surgical approach. Such findings include teeth with gross amounts of decay through the furcation or below the level of the alveolus, bony pathology, tooth impaction, root dilacerations, and a previous history of endodontic therapy. Certain anatomic barriers may require additional skill and expertise, such as for the extraction of a maxillary molar in the presence of a pneumatized maxillary sinus or extraction of a mandibular molar with roots that approximate the inferior alveolar nerve canal.

TECHNIQUE: Instrumentation for Routine Extractions

A wide variety of forceps have been developed for specific surgical applications and surgeon preferences for specific teeth. Situations take precedence in daily practice, but the basic principle remains constant. The majority of dental extractions can be performed using a limited number of instruments.[6]

Instrumentation for Reflecting the Marginal Gingiva

Care should be taken prior to elevating the tooth and removing it with forceps to reflect the marginal gingiva. This may be done directly using the sharp end of the periosteal elevator to reflect the marginal gingiva from the bone, starting at one papilla and working the periosteal elevator across the buccal gingiva to the other papilla. The reflection of the tissue prevents maceration of the tissue via pressure from the elevators and forceps. It also may allow further reflection to visualize the bone and the furcation, if one is present. In some cases, a #15 blade may be used to make a sulcular incision prior to reflecting the marginal gingiva. It is important to make sure that the blade contacts the bone. Failure to incise through the periosteum will lead to challenges with reflecting the marginal gingiva and creating a flap when necessary.

Elevators

Many different types of elevators have specific applications for the extraction of teeth and tooth roots. The most common elevator is the straight elevator. The straight elevator is a single-bladed instrument that is placed between the tooth and the alveolar bone and used to put pressure between the tooth and the bone to expand the bone and to mobilize teeth and roots. The concave blade of the elevator is placed against the tooth or root to be extracted; the convex side is in contact with the alveolar bone. Care must be taken not to place the convex side of the elevator against an adjacent tooth. Because the elevator acts as a lever, the fulcrum must be against bone so as not to dislodge an adjacent tooth or restoration. The instrument is held in the palm of the hand with the index finger extended along the shaft of the elevator to control the forces applied to the tooth. Without the use of this technique, the elevator may slip and damage other oral tissues including the palate or floor of mouth. Rotation around the long axis of the instrument can achieve subluxation and mobilization of teeth and roots for extraction. As the tooth or root begins to mobilize, applying a more apical and interproximal position can optimize further mobilization (Fig. 10.1A). Start with a small elevator, and work up to a larger elevator or luxator (an elevator with a more flat blade). Once the tooth or root is mobile, delivery is feasible.

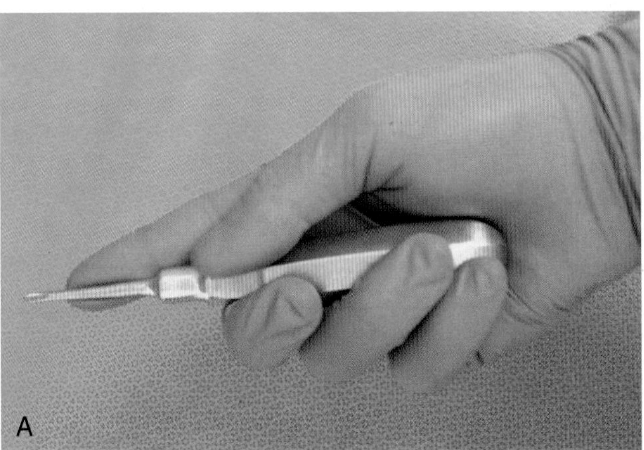

Figure 10.1 **A,** Correct way to hold a straight elevator; the index finger is placed near the blade.

Continued

TECHNIQUE: Instrumentation for Routine Extractions—cont'd

Specialized elevators are available for delivering fractured roots and root tips. One such elevator is the Cryer elevator. This is particularly useful when a single retained root from an extraction of a mandibular molar remains in the alveolar bone. A Cryer elevator is placed apically into the empty root socket, and the point of the blade is rotated toward the residual root. This action removes the interradicular bone and allows for engagement of the remaining root, and the remaining root can be lifted vertically out of the socket.

The above-mentioned techniques are important for surgeons performing basic exodontia, but it must be emphasized that elevators should not be used in all situations. For instance, caution must be exercised in the use of elevators when working with a fractured maxillary molar. Apical force applied with an elevator may push the root into the maxillary sinus. Instead, the root should be retrieved surgically, with removal of intraarticular bone for better access while limiting apical pressure.

Dental Extraction Forceps

Dental extraction forceps are principally used to grasp a tooth and apply a force that gives the surgeon leverage to expand the surrounding bone and deliver the tooth. Forceps are designed with two blades and handles joined by a hinge. The blades of extraction forceps are designed to grasp the buccal and lingual surfaces of the tooth. The concave shape of the blades allows the surgeon to apply the maximum surface area of the blades on the tooth, distributing the forces evenly and thus giving a greater degree of control. When holding the forceps, the further the distance from the hinge, the more force between the beaks. This results in better control of the tooth, and the forceps is less likely to slip. The beaks of the forceps are aimed in an apical direction toward the long axis of the tooth. It is important to visualize the placement of the beaks of the forceps to ensure that the soft tissue is not crushed via the beaks. Ensure that the beaks are seated as apically as possible to try and prevent the tooth from fracturing. If the beaks are more coronal and caries extend to the furcation, the crown could fracture making orientation and root removal more challenging. An assortment of forceps with blades and handles has been designed for specific teeth in the dental arch to enable the surgeon to achieve the most appropriate adaptation and to facilitate control of the forces applied to the tooth.

Maxillary Forceps

Extraction forceps for the six anterior maxillary teeth include maxillary universal forceps (#150) and maxillary straight forceps (#99C) in the American pattern forceps numbering system. The beaks of the forceps are applied labially and palatally and directed in an apical direction parallel to the roots of the anterior maxillary teeth. The maxillary straight forceps offers an advantage for maxillary anterior teeth, allowing easy forces applied apically, palatally, labially, and especially rotationally. The further posterior the extraction, the more difficult it is to use the straight forceps due to obstruction of the lower lip and mandibular teeth; in addition, the contour of the posterior maxillary teeth makes it difficult to adapt the beaks to the tooth surface. The maxillary universal forceps can be used in a similar fashion, but it has a curved beak and handle, which keeps them above the lip while still directing the beaks in an apical direction parallel to the roots of the teeth, avoiding iatrogenic injury. Additionally, these forceps can be used to extract maxillary posterior teeth (Fig. 10.1B and C).

Extraction forceps for the maxillary posterior teeth include the maxillary universal forceps and forceps with beaks specifically designed to fit more complex root forms, such as #89 and #90 forceps. These forceps have a concave palatal beak that can adapt to the palatal root surface and a pointed buccal beak that adapts to the buccal root bifurcation. The #53R and #53L are similar but with a more pointed palatal beak and a straight handle. These forceps can apply an excessive amount of force and fracture the maxillary tuberosity if used improperly.[7]

Mandibular Forceps

As with maxillary extraction forceps, multiple types of forceps have been designed specifically for the extraction of anterior and posterior mandibular teeth. These allow adaptation to root forms and tooth location in the dental arch. The forceps most often used for extraction of anterior mandibular teeth include the mandibular universal (#151) forceps and the Ash (#77) forceps. The Ash forceps have beaks angled at 90 degrees so that the handles extend directly out of the mouth parallel to the plane of occlusion. This allows for labial and lingual adaptation of the beaks without the handles interfering with the maxillary teeth, upper lip, and nose. These forceps can be used for the majority of mandibular teeth from second premolar to second premolar. Some providers use the Ash forceps for maxillary teeth as well. The mandibular universal forceps have angulated beaks and handles that allow for adaptation for all mandibular teeth. Additionally, the cowhorn (#23) forceps can be used efficiently for extraction of mandibular molars. The cowhorn forceps have pointed buccal and lingual beaks that can be placed in the furcation of the mandibular molars, allowing for vertical luxation as the handles are squeezed. Similar types of mandibular molar forceps have sharp beaks to fracture multirooted teeth so that the roots may be removed separately (Fig. 10.1D and E).

Continued

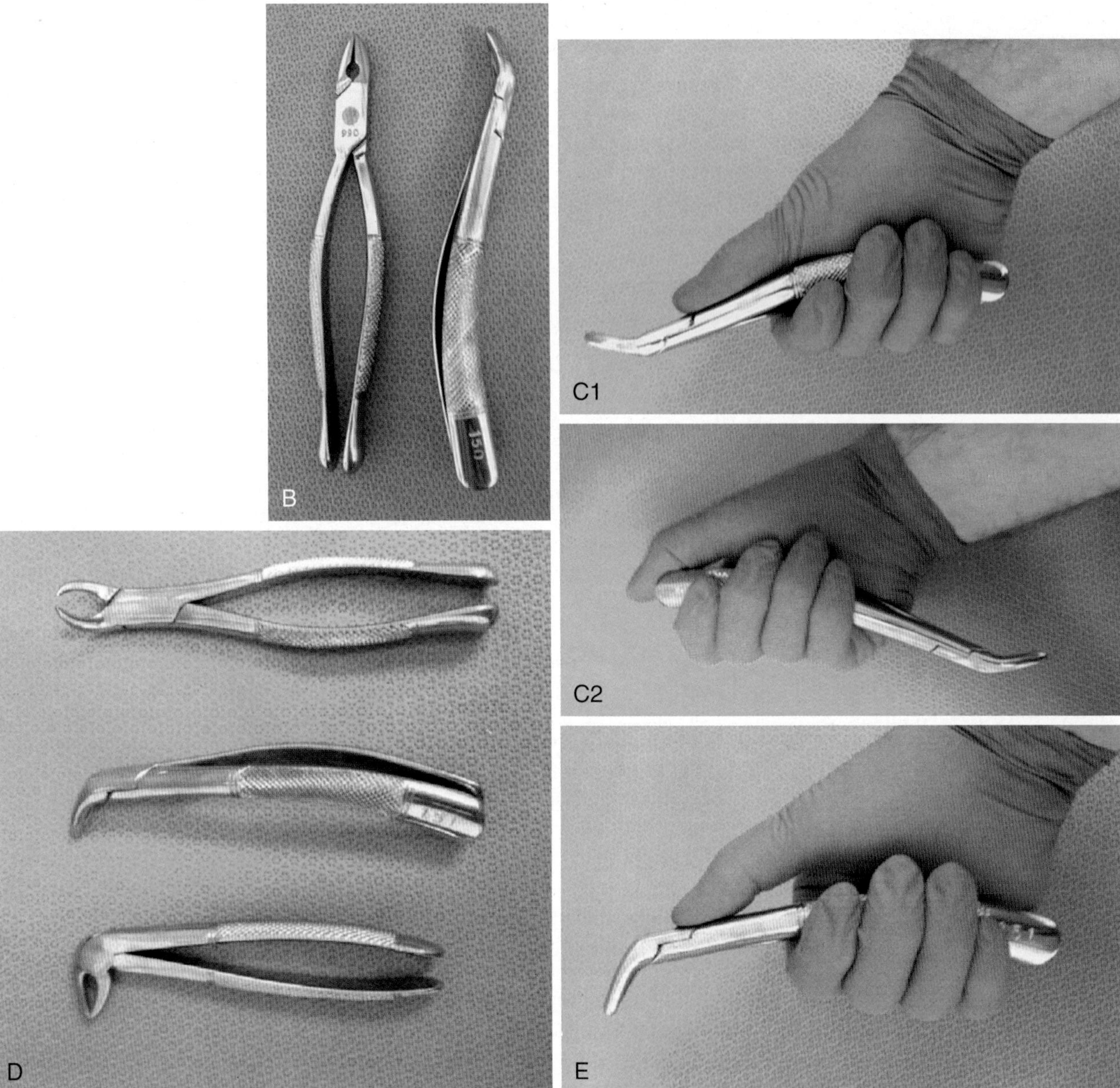

Figure 10.1 cont'd **B,** *Left,* Maxillary straight (#99C) extraction forceps; *right,* maxillary universal (#150) extraction forceps. **C1,** Traditional way to hold maxillary universal (#150) extraction forceps when approaching extractions from the front of the patient. **C2,** Backhanded technique for holding the maxillary universal (#150) forceps when approaching extractions from behind the patient. **D,** Mandibular extraction forceps: *top,* cowhorn (#23) forceps; *middle,* mandibular universal (#151) forceps; *bottom,* Ash (#77) forceps. **E,** Correct way to hold mandibular universal (#151) extraction forceps.

TECHNIQUE: Basic Principles for Simple Extractions

The surgeon must exercise skill and surgical technique to perform simple exodontia. The process involves the use of controlled force to expand the alveolus, separate the periodontal ligament, and deliver the tooth. Some factors attributing to the success of a simple tooth extraction include a sound knowledge of oral and dental anatomy, an understanding of the surgical techniques applied, and above all, surgical experience.

Surgeon-Patient Positioning

For optimal control of the procedure, the surgeon and patient must be in a proper chair position. This allows for ideal visibility, lighting, and access. For best visibility and access for mandibular extractions, the patient's mandible should be parallel the floor and should be at the level of the surgeon's elbow. For working on the patient's maxillary teeth, the patient's maxillary occlusal plane should be at 60 to 90 degrees with the floor. If the surgeon is left-handed, he or she should work in the 1 to 5 o'clock position. If the surgeon is right-handed, he or she should work in the 7 to 11 o'clock position. Some surgeons adapt these positions well, including sitting down for the procedure.

TECHNIQUE: Perioperative Management

Simple Dental Extraction

After a local anesthetic has been administered and takes effect, the surgeon usually begins by separating the superior portion of the attached gingiva from the tooth, typically with a #9 periosteal elevator or a #15 blade. At this point, a cotton gauze oral pharyngeal drape is placed to prevent displacement of the tooth into the oral pharynx and potential aspiration. As described above, the elevator is then used to mobilize or luxate the tooth. Place the elevator between the alveolus and the tooth and direct it apically, like a wedge, facilitating the coronal movement of the tooth or tooth root.[8] Effective elevation prevents injury to the adjacent teeth, maintains the integrity of the alveolar bony structure, and makes the forceps delivery simple.[9] Over time, the surgeon may develop the skill to deliver the tooth with the elevators in certain situations, avoiding the use of the extraction forceps.

The techniques for extracting teeth using dental extraction forceps differ, depending on the location in the dental arch. When extracting teeth, the right-handed surgeon is positioned in front and to the right of the patient; a left-handed surgeon is positioned in front and to the left. The index finger of the nondominant hand is placed labially, and the thumb palatally/lingually, firmly holding the alveolar process next to the tooth to be extracted. The beaks of the forceps are adapted to the buccal and lingual surfaces of the tooth with the beaks pointed apically, parallel to the long axis of the tooth.

Extraction of Maxillary Anterior Teeth

Extraction movements consist of applying gentle, controlled force apically. The alveolus is then expanded with repeated labial and then palatal movements, gradually increasing the force applied to the tooth (Fig. 10.2A and B). Because the

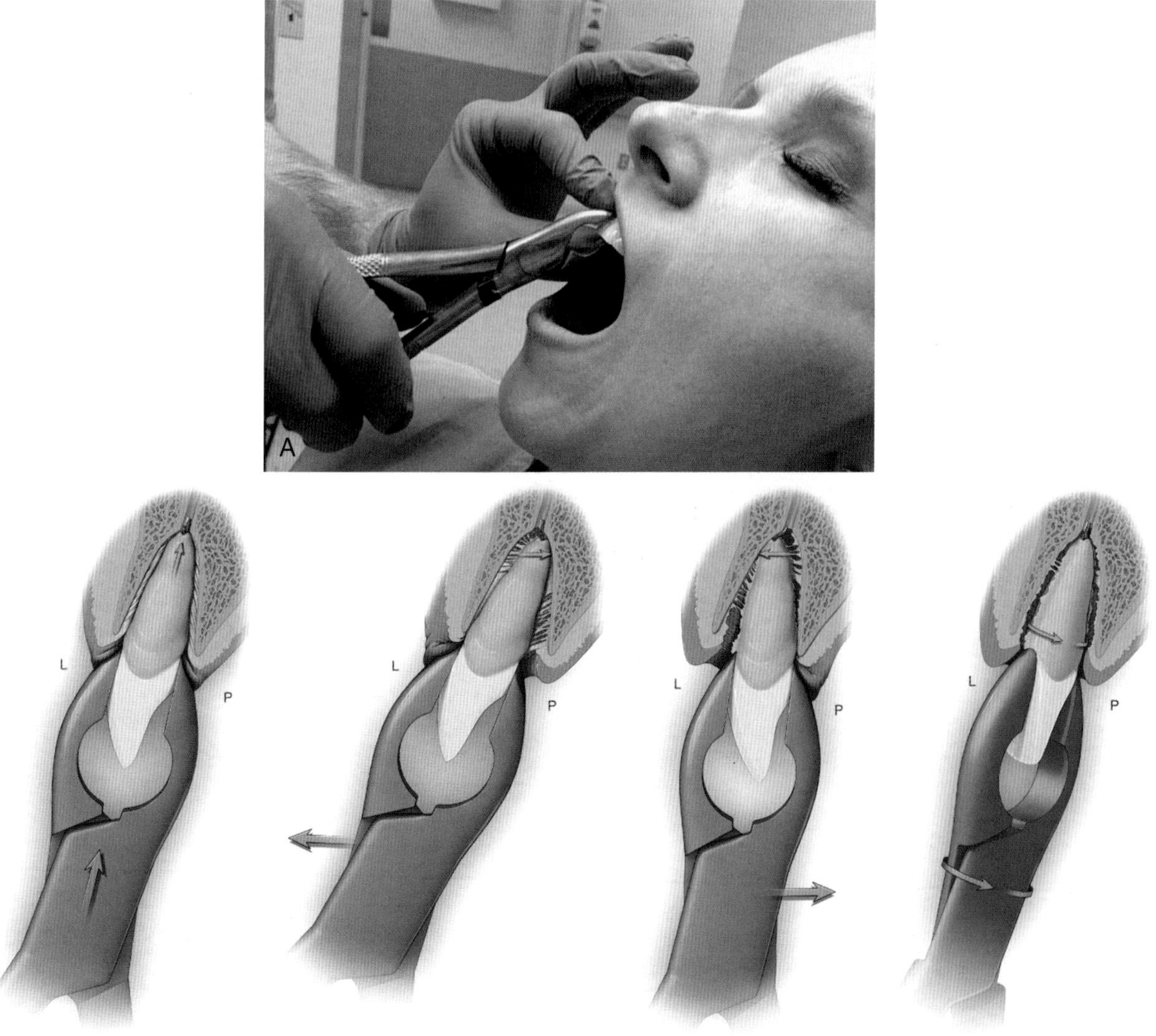

Figure 10.2 **A,** Extraction of a maxillary anterior tooth (central incisor). Forceps grasp the tooth, and fingers of the nondominant hand support the alveolar process. **B,** Extraction movements for maxillary anterior extractions: apply apical pressure, labial pressure, palatal pressure, and rotational movements to sever the periodontal ligament; delivery of the tooth is usually labial.

Continued

TECHNIQUE: Perioperative Management—cont'd

roots of the anterior maxillary teeth are somewhat conical, rotational movements with the dental extractions forceps can be applied, further severing the periodontal ligament and facilitating the delivery of the tooth. The tooth is then delivered with gentle traction, with care taken not to apply excessive force, because an abrupt delivery can result in the forceps injuring teeth in the opposing arch. The maxillary anterior teeth tend to be delivered buccally because the relative density of the buccal alveolar bone is less than that of the palatal alveolar bone, which results in a greater expansion of the buccal alveolus. Use caution not to place too much pressure on the buccal alveolar bone and risk fracturing the buccal plate.

Extraction of Mandibular Anterior Teeth and Premolars

The mandibular anterior teeth and premolars are extracted in a fashion similar to the use of the Ash extraction forceps. Continuous apical pressure is applied with the Ash forceps while buccal and lingual movements are gradually increased. Rotational movements may also be used, considering that the roots of these teeth are usually single and conical in shape (Fig. 10.2C and D).[10]

Extraction of Maxillary Premolars

Maxillary premolars are extracted with continuous apical pressure while buccolingual movements are applied. Approximately half of maxillary first premolars have two thin roots, so rotational movements should be avoided to prevent the fracture of the apical portion of the root. Occasionally, maxillary second premolars have two roots and are readily removed in a fashion similar to that of maxillary first molars (Fig. 10.2E and F).

Extraction of Maxillary First and Second Molars

The anatomy of maxillary molars differs from that of other teeth because they have three roots (two buccal roots and one large palatal root). The buccal and palatal roots are typically divergent, making what may look like a simple extraction more complex, with an increased likelihood of root

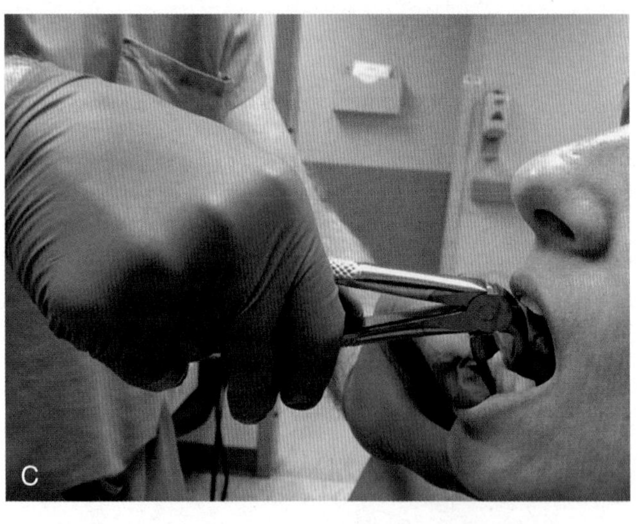

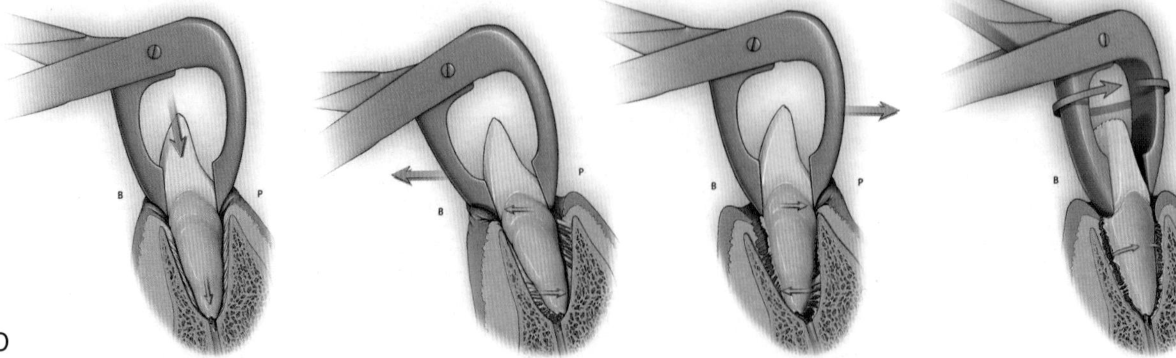

Figure 10.2, cont'd **C,** Correct way to hold mandibular Ash (#74) extraction forceps. **D,** Extraction movements for mandibular anterior and premolar extractions: apply apical pressure, buccal pressure, lingual pressure, and rotational movements to sever the periodontal ligament; delivery of the tooth is to the buccal side.

TECHNIQUE: Perioperative Management—cont'd

fractures.[11] Additionally, these teeth are in close proximity to the maxillary sinus, and careful radiographic interpretation can prevent possible antral involvement.[12] Because of these potential complications, in addition to the potential to fracture the buccal plate or the maxillary tuberosity, large initial forces should be avoided. Apical forces should be applied first; then slow, deliberate forces should be applied in the buccal and palatal directions, allowing the initial expansion of the surrounding alveolar bone. The buccal and lingual movements should slowly increase, facilitating the buccal delivery of the maxillary molars (Fig. 10.2G).

Continued

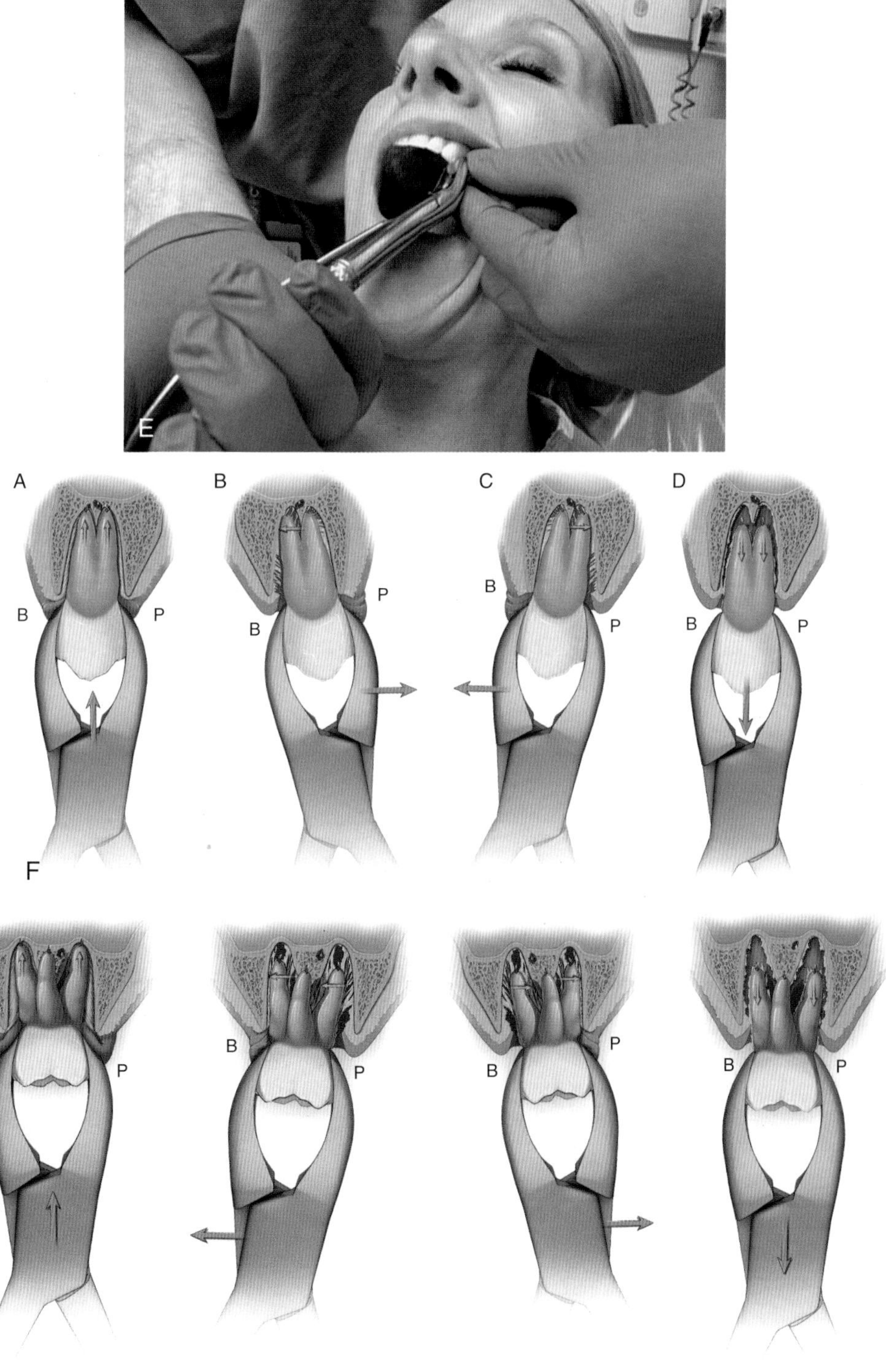

Figure 10.2, cont'd **E,** Extraction of maxillary left first premolar using the backhanded technique from the 11 o'clock position. **F,** Extraction movements. **G,** Universal (#150) extraction forceps engaging the bifurcation of the two buccal roots and palatal root of a maxillary molar. *A,* Apical; *B,* palatal; *C,* buccal; *D,* final extraction movement. *B,* Buccal; *P,* palatal.

TECHNIQUE: Perioperative Management—cont'd

Extraction of Mandibular First and Second Molars

Extraction of mandibular molars is often considered the most difficult due to the increased density of the posterior mandibular bone, the root form, and the proximity to the inferior alveolar nerve.[13] The extraction can be carried out with the use of a mandibular universal extraction forceps (#151) or cowhorn (#23) extraction forceps. The initial step involves seating the beak as apically as possible while applying heavy apical pressure to expand the alveolar bone. Because of the unique root anatomy and bifurcation of the mandibular molars, cowhorn (#23) extraction forceps are often utilized to facilitate the extraction of these teeth. The pointed beaks are placed into the buccal and lingual furcation, and a pumping motion is used while squeezing the forceps to displace the tooth coronally. Buccal and lingual rocking movements, in addition to figure-eight movements, can facilitate the expansion of the dense alveolar bone for delivery of the mandibular molar (Fig. 10.2H–I).

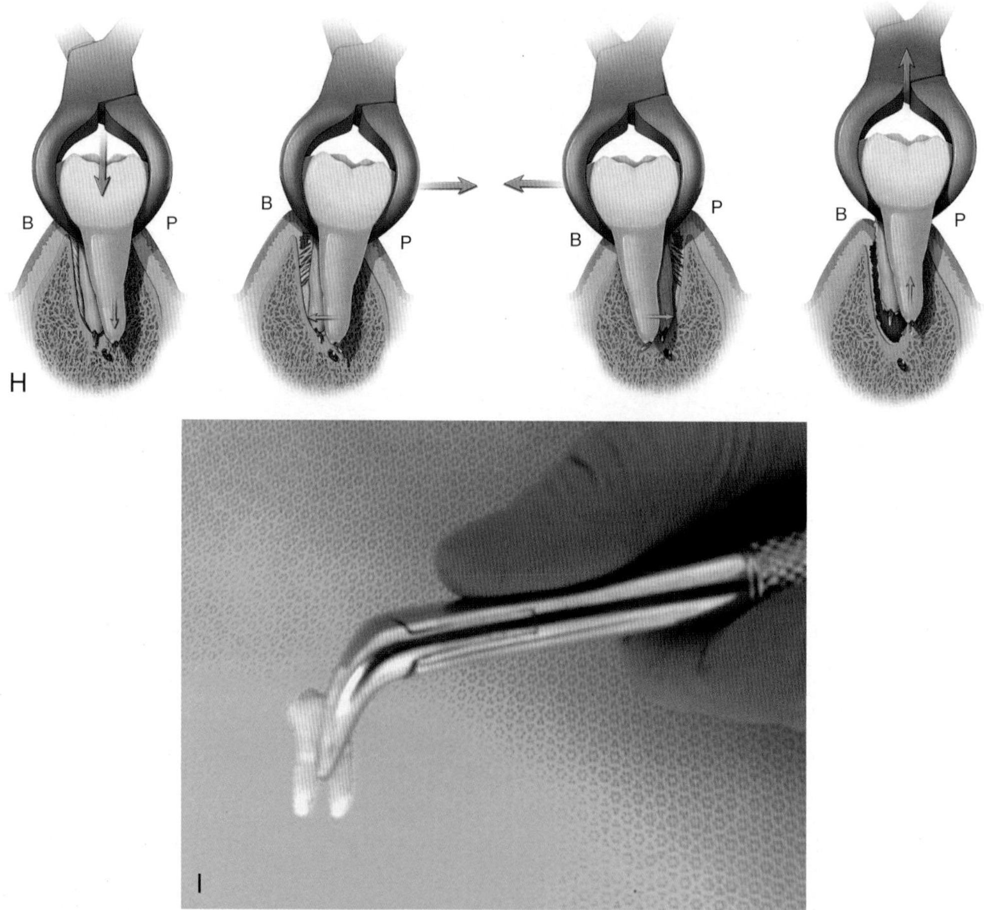

Figure 10.2, cont'd **H,** Extraction movement for mandibular molars: cowhorn seated into furcation, buccal-lingual movement, and pumping motion displacing coronally. **I,** Cowhorn (#23) extraction forceps engaging the bifurcation of a mandibular molar.

ALTERNATIVE TECHNIQUE: Atraumatic Extraction

Preservation of alveolar bone is the key to success in future restoration of the missing tooth with either a pontic of a bridge or endosseous implant.[14,15] The tooth extraction should be atraumatic, accomplished with the use of periotomes and small periosteal elevators, along with the techniques discussed earlier in the chapter.[16] The instruments mentioned at the beginning of the chapter are often adequate to extract the majority of teeth atraumatically. However, a root fractured off below the alveolar crest may prove very difficult to remove from the socket with elevators.[17] An interesting technique involves using the "root extractor" or an endodontic broach or file.

First, the canal of the fractured tooth is widened with a bur. Then the canal is engaged by the endodontic file. Finally, the root fragment is luxated coronally with the "root extractor" without excessive enlargement of the socket. Using an innovative method in which an endodontic file is used to engage the canal wall, the tooth fragment is slowly luxated and pulled out of the socket with practically no trauma to the alveolar bone or surrounding tissues.

Avoidance and Management of Intraoperative Complications

After extraction of the tooth has been completed, attention must be given to clearing the extraction site of any debris, loose or sharp pieces of bone, granulation tissue, or other pathology. Postoperative infections, bleeding, and edema are rare but possible.[18] A common cause of postoperative infection is the foreign body reaction to bone fragments or debris left in the extraction site or displaced underneath the gingival tissue.[19] It has been shown that a perioperative dose of antibiotics may reduce postoperative infection, pain, and dry socket after third molar extraction (although this has not been proven for routine dental extractions).[20] Chlorhexidine mouth rinse also has decreased the incidence of postoperative dry socket.[21] Residual granulation tissue is another reason for minor postoperative bleeding.[22] Curetting and irrigating of the extraction socket are performed to eliminate such potential complications. Appropriate use of bite blocks and mandibular support can limit jaw dislocations. As stated previously, the use of an oropharyngeal curtain can prevent aspiration of a tooth. If aspiration is suspected, a prompt chest radiograph should be ordered. If an oral-antral communication is encountered at the time of a maxillary molar extraction, an attempt should be made to primarily approximate the soft tissue of the dental extraction site and put the patient on antibiotics and sinus precautions. Nerve injuries and their management are discussed elsewhere in this text in detail.

Postoperative Considerations

Postoperative considerations should be discussed with all patients (Box 10.2). The patient's quality of life can be disrupted with regard to diet modification, opening of the mouth, and speech, even with nonsurgical extractions.[23] Most providers recommend a softer consistency diet after these procedures. Head elevation can reduce discomfort associated with swelling. The application of ice initially postoperatively has not been proven effective at reducing swelling.[24] Most patients require some form of prescribed medication for pain. The possibility of nausea, along with these medications, should be discussed. Hemostasis should be obtained before dismissal of the patient; additional information about hemostatic measures is routinely provided to the patient in written discharge instructions. A further medical workup should be initiated in patients with persistent bleeding.

BOX 10.2 Postoperative Considerations

Bleeding	Pain
Swelling	Bruising
Infection	Nausea
Hygiene	Diet

References

1. Hoffmann-Axthelm W. *History of Dentistry.* Chicago, Illinois: Quintessence; 1981.
2. Simon JF. Retain or extract: the decision process. *Quintessence Int.* 1999;30(12):851–854.
3. Hull PS, Worthington HV, Clerehugh V, Tsirba R, Davies RM, Clarkson JE. The reasons for tooth extractions in adults and their validation. *J Dent.* 1997;25(3–4):233–237.
4. McCaul LK, Jenkins WM, Kay EJ. The reasons for the extraction of various tooth types in Scotland: a 15-year follow up. *J Dent.* 2001;29(6): 401–407.
5. Ruggiero SL, Dodson TB, Assael LA, et al. American Association of Oral and Maxillofacial Surgeons position paper on bisphosphonate-related osteonecrosis of the jaw—2009 update. *J Oral Maxillofac Surg.* 2009;67(suppl 5):2–12.
6. Zambito RF, Zambito ML. Exodonture. Technique and art. *NY State Dent J.* 1992;58(3):33–37.
7. Dym H, Weiss A. Exodontia: tips and techniques for better outcomes. *Dent Clin North Am.* 2012;56(1):245–266 (x).
8. Sullivan SM. The principles of uncomplicated exodontia: simple steps for safe extractions. *Compend Contin Educ Dent.* 1999;20(1):48–52. 54, 56 passim.
9. Fonseca RJ, Turvey TA, Marciani RD. *Oral and Maxillofacial Surgery.* 2nd ed. St Louis, Missouri: Saunders; 2008.
10. Pedlar J, Frame JW. *Oral and Maxillofacial Surgery: An Objective Based Textbook.* 2nd ed. Philadelphia, Pennsylvania: Churchill Livingstone; 2007.
11. Lehtinen R, Ojala T. Rocking and twisting moments in extraction of teeth in the upper jaw. *Int J Oral Surg.* 1980;9(5):377–382.
12. Meijer GJ, Springer GJ, Koole R. [Complications during and after dentoalveolar surgery]. *Ned Tijdschr Tandheelkd.* 2004;111(5): 190–194.
13. Weinberg S. Oral surgery complications in general practice. *Dent J.* 1975;41(5):288–294. 299.
14. Chandra Sekar A, Praveen M, Saxena A, Gautam A. Immediate implant placement: a case report. *J Indian Prosthodont Soc.* 2012;12(2): 120–122.
15. Horowitz R, Holtzclaw D, Rosen PS. A review on alveolar ridge preservation following tooth extraction. *J Evid Based Dent Pract.* 2012;12(3):149–160.
16. Saund D, Dietrich T. Minimally-invasive tooth extraction: doorknobs and strings revisited. *Dent Update.* 2013;40(4):328–330. 325-6.
17. Simon JH. Root extrusion. Rationale and techniques. *Dent Clin North Am.* 1984;28(4): 909–921.
18. Venkateshwar GP, Padhye MN, Khosla AR, Kakkar ST. Complications of exodontia: a retrospective study. *Indian J Dent Res.* 2011;22(5): 633–638.
19. Adeyemo WL, Ladeinde AL, Ogunlewe MO. Influence of trans-operative complications on socket healing following dental extractions. *J Contemp Dent Pract.* 2007;8(1):52–59.
20. Lodi G, Figini L, Sardella A, Carrassi A, Del Fabbro M, Furness S. Antibiotics to prevent complications following tooth extractions. *Cochrane Database Syst Rev.* 2012;11:CD003811.
21. Dodson T. Prevention and treatment of dry socket. *Evid Based Dent.* 2013;14(1):13–14.
22. Dennis MJ. Exodontia for the general dentist: complications. *Todays FDA.* 2009;21(10):14–19.
23. Adeyemo WL, Taiwo OA, Oderinu OH, Adeyemi MF, Ladeinde AL, Ogunlewe MO. Oral health-related quality of life following non-surgical (routine) tooth extraction: a pilot study. *Contemp Clin Dent.* 2012;3(4): 427–432.
24. van der Westhuijzen AJ, Becker PJ, Morkel J, Roelse JA. A randomized observer blind comparison of bilateral facial ice pack therapy with no ice therapy following third molar surgery. *Int J Oral Maxillofac Surg.* 2005;34(3): 281–286.

CHAPTER 11

Surgical Extraction of Erupted Teeth

Greg Tull, David Hinkl, and Paul S. Tiwana

Armamentarium

#1 Periosteal elevator
4 × 4 Gauze
#9 Periosteal elevator
#15 Scalpel blade
#150/151 Forceps
#190/191 Elevators
Appropriate sutures
Bone file
Cryer elevator
Dental curette
Fissure #702/#703
Round bur #6, #8
Hemostat
Irrigation syringe/sterile saline
Local anesthetic with vasoconstrictor
Minnesota retractor
Molt curettes
Needle holder
Rongeurs
Small and large luxators
Small and large straight elevators
Surgical handpiece
Suture scissors
Suction
Bite block/mouth prop
Pharyngeal curtain

History of the Procedure

Oral hygiene via brushing and flossing was not a common practice in society until after World War II when soldiers returning from battle informed and educated America. Dentistry, specifically tooth removal, is one of the oldest medical forms of treatment, dating back to 7000 BC. Barbers and blacksmiths were actually the first specialists in dentistry during the Middle Ages.[1] They routinely removed infected teeth to alleviate pain without any forms of anesthesia. Most would say that dentistry was truly born in the 17th century. Pierre Fauchard was able to describe the decay process of teeth with details regarding acids and focused on preventative measures. In the 18th century, dentistry became its own discipline. During this time, dentures made of gold, silver, and ivory were introduced.[1] In the 19th century, the Baltimore College of Dentistry became the first dental school to give out DDS degrees and solidify North America as a world leader in dental education.[2]

One of the most consistent challenges that the oral and maxillofacial surgeon will encounter during their career is the surgical removal of erupted teeth. There is nothing more humbling than the surgical removal of a difficult tooth. Due to extensive caries, limited access to the oral field, patient anxiety, complex dental anatomy, and the density of surrounding alveolar bone are all contributing factors to difficult exodontia. Now more than ever, the surgical extraction of erupted teeth requires proper planning and execution through various techniques within our armamentarium.[3] The focus of tooth removal has shifted from simply alleviating pain and disease to preservation of alveolar bone for definitive reconstruction of the oral cavity.

The reputation of an oral and maxillofacial surgeon can often be determined by their ability to perform surgical exodontia.[2] As specialists, we are rarely referred simple extractions. Therefore, the development and proper training of exodontia techniques is the foundation of all things surgical within our field.[2]

The primary goal in the surgical removal of erupted teeth should be to deliver the tooth as atraumatically as possible, typically with a closed extraction technique. This is not always possible. Therefore, open techniques that provide improved access and safety must be mastered by the oral and maxillofacial surgeon. This chapter focuses on the surgical extraction techniques for treatment of erupted teeth.

Indications for the Use of the Procedure

The indications for proceeding with a surgical extraction are shown in Box 11.1. In some cases, surgical extractions are performed preventatively to avoid potential complications that may arise from using a simple closed technique, such as root and or alveolar bone fracture.[4] Assessment of the tooth anatomy, location, and adjacent structures is vital in determining if surgical technique is indicated as the immediate extraction approach. Bulbous or dilacerated root tips, fused teeth, abnormal tooth anomalies (i.e., dens in dente), or ankylosed teeth should be recognized in the radiographic examination, and therefore surgical technique should be used as the primary method to deliver these teeth from the socket.[4] Other

BOX 11.1 Indications

Unusual Root Morphology

Hypercementosis
Dilaceration of roots
Ankylosed or roots with abnormalities
Fusion/germination of teeth
Root fragments remaining in alveolar bone
Maxillary posterior teeth with roots in the maxillary sinus
Roots of teeth found below the gumline
Roots with large periapical lesions
Anticipated bone recontouring

indications for surgical extraction may be based on preventing damage to adjacent structures (i.e., dislodgement of a root tip into the maxillary sinus), recontouring of the bone surrounding the extracted tooth (i.e., supraerupted teeth), or removal of a large periapical lesion that cannot be fully removed through the socket with curettage alone.[5]

Limitations and Contraindications for Surgical Extractions

Review of the patient's medical history is imperative in determining any contraindications for proceeding with surgical dental extraction under local anesthetic. Conditions such as liver disease, bleeding dyscrasias, immunocompromised conditions, cardiac and coronary artery disease, history of radiation, and bisphosphonate therapy should be discussed and reviewed prior to extraction so that appropriate treatment measures can be taken.[6] Following the review of health history and systems, the clinician should proceed with radiographic and clinical examination to determine if the immediate extraction approach should be surgical.

Findings from radiographic and clinical assessment should be evaluated, and the risk to benefit ratio should be in the patient's favor prior to proceeding with surgical extraction. For instance, an asymptomatic root tip measuring less than 3 mm without periapical pathology enclosed in the alveolar bone, with elevated risk of local complications, such as dislodgement into the maxillary sinus or injury to the inferior alveolar, lingual, or mental nerves, should be left in place.[7] As a general rule, whenever the risks and surgical trauma necessary to remove the tooth outweigh the benefits to the patient, the root should be left in place. This should be recorded in the patient's chart and the patient informed of your decision.[7]

Various Techniques

When the determination has been made to proceed with a surgical extraction (Box 11.2), visualization of the area is paramount to achieve a desirable result. The primary goal of visualization requires reflection of tissue in a safe manner to protect nerves, vasculature, and oral tissues. Reflection of an adequate mucoperiosteal flap will provide adequate visualization, protect adjacent structures, and facilitate postoperative healing as compared with unintentionally traumatized soft tissue. When designing the flap, it is imperative that the base of the flap be wider than the coronal aspect to ensure adequate blood supply.[8] Most commonly, an envelope flap will provide the previously mentioned characteristics for surgical extractions. Begin by using a #15 blade, holding with firm pressure in the gingival sulcus against the bone at a 45-degree angle.[9] To make an envelope flap, extend the incision two teeth anterior and one tooth posterior to the tooth being removed.[8] If more access is necessary, a releasing incision may be performed anterior to the extraction site preserving the papilla, and with attention not to harm adjacent structures such as the mental nerve. Use the pointed end of the periosteal elevator to release the tissue from the bone, starting from the papilla, and advancing toward the keratinized mucosa, in a rotational motion, with care not to tear the thin alveolar mucosa.[9] After the flap is adequately elevated, a Minnesota retractor, or the spoon end of the periosteal elevator can be used to retract and protect the flap.[8]

BOX 11.2 Four Steps

1. Reflection of a mucoperiosteal flap
2. Removal of bone and exposure of the root surface
3. Extraction of the tooth with elevators or forceps
4. Curettage, irrigation, and suturing

Once the tissue has been reflected using a mucoperiosteal flap and adequate visualization has been achieved, a surgical bur with irrigation should be used to remove bone.

Bone removal around the tooth or teeth to be extracted should be evaluated based on the location of the tooth, remaining coronal tooth structure, and tooth position in the arch.

Single-Rooted Teeth

The first step is to obtain visualization and access by reflecting a full-thickness mucoperiosteal flap. Once visualization has been achieved there are four options for removing the tooth.[8]

1. Attempt to reseat the extraction forceps under direct visualization and remove the tooth with no surgical bone removal. This approach should be attempted, but a large amount of time should not be spent utilizing this technique.[8]
2. Grasp a small amount of buccal bone under the buccal beak of the forceps to obtain a better mechanical advantage and grasp the tooth root. A small amount of buccal bone is removed with the tooth. This technique has a disadvantage of loss of buccal alveolar structure.[8]

3. Use a periotome or straight elevator in the periodontal ligament space and advance it toward the apex. The periodontal ligament will be expanded as the elevator advances, acting as a wedge to displace the root occlusally. The small elevator is then followed with a large straight elevator and the tooth is luxated out of the socket.[8]
4. Proceed with surgical bone removal. Remove the buccal bone along the width of the tooth and approximately one-half to two-thirds the vertical depth of the tooth to be extracted until solid root structure is visible. This should be done using a surgical bur and irrigation. After removal of buccal bone that is of adequate width and vertical depth, use an elevator or straight forceps to deliver the tooth out of the socket. If there is difficulty in removing the tooth following bone removal and elevation, use the surgical bur and irrigation to make a purchase point large enough to insert an instrument to elevate the tooth out of the socket.[8]

Following removal of the tooth, use a bone file to smooth sharp bone edges, curette the socket, and irrigate the site using sterile saline. Attention should be directed to the base of the flap where it joins the bone, which is a common place for derby to settle. This may delay healing or even facilitate the development of subperiosteal abscess, and this site should be thoroughly irrigated before closure. Place the flap back into its original position and close using chromic or silk sutures.[9]

Multirooted Teeth

The process to reflect a flap and evaluate the area for bone removal should also be applied to surgical extractions for multirooted teeth. While holding the flap with the retractor, use the surgical bur with irrigation to removal buccal bone along the width of the tooth to be extracted and vertically to expose the cemento-enamel junction and furcation. Try to preserve 2 mm of bone margins at the mesial and distal alveolar margins.[8] Once the furcation is visible, two options are available depending on the surgeon's experience. If the crown of the tooth is still intact, the crown may be cut off with the surgical bur and irrigation to have better visualization of the roots for sectioning.[9] The crown may also be kept intact if the surgeon feels comfortable sectioning the roots of the tooth without direct visualization of the roots themselves. When sectioning teeth, a smaller #701 fissure bur and incomplete transection are recommended, keeping the lingual surface intact to avoid damage to lingual tissues.[8] Mandibular molars should be sectioned into mesial and distal roots. Maxillary molars should be sectioned into palatal, mesial, and distal roots. When sectioning mandibular molars, it is important to recall the close proximity of the lingual nerve to the crown; therefore, sectioning two-thirds to three-fourths through the crown and using an instrument to complete the fracture through the remaining tooth structure can be helpful in preventing injury to the lingual nerve.[9] Once the roots are sectioned, use an elevator to deliver each root out of the socket individually. Caution should be taken to not apply forces in an apical direction, which could dislodge the root into an undesirable location such as the submandibular space or maxillary sinus. After all of the roots have been removed from the socket, smooth sharp edges using a bone file, curette the socket, and irrigate with sterile saline. Return the flap to its original position and close using chromic or silk sutures[8] (Fig. 11.1).

Removal of Root Fragments and Tips

In the circumstance that a tooth breaks and a root tip or fragment remains in the socket, it is imperative to place the patient in a position that allows for excellent light, irrigation, and suction. If a nonsurgical extraction is being performed and the tooth has broken during the procedure, leaving the apical third of the tooth in the socket, attempt removal using a Cryer or elevator for larger fragments and a root tip pick for small fragments. Use caution and do not apply apical forces to the fragment to prevent dislodgement into adjacent spaces.[8]

If delivery of the fragment out of the socket is unsuccessful, immediately proceed with surgical technique. Reflect a flap and retract the tissue with a periosteal elevator. For larger fragments, remove buccal bone to expose the residual root and elevate the root tip out of the socket.

Once the residual fragment or root tip is delivered out of the socket, smooth bone with a bone file, curette, and irrigate with sterile saline. Replace the flap into its original position and close with resorbable or nonresorbable sutures of choice. The recommendation is to reapproximate the papilla utilizing a tension-free closure technique.[9]

Multiple Extractions

For sequencing of multiple extractions or full mouth extractions, maxillary teeth should be extracted first for the following reasons. Infiltration anesthetic has a more rapid onset and shorter effective time.[10] This allows the surgeon to begin the procedure sooner and prevent the delay of the surgery if profound anesthesia is lost in the maxilla.[8] During the extraction process, debris such as filling material, tooth segments, or bone chips may fall into the empty sockets of the lower teeth if the mandibular teeth are removed first. A potential disadvantage of extracting maxillary teeth first is that bleeding may interfere with visualization during the mandibular surgery. Extractions should begin with the most posterior tooth first. This allows the most efficiency in using dental elevators. The canine should be extracted last because removal of teeth on either side will weaken the bony socket and the extraction will likely be easier.[8]

The surgical approach to removing multiple teeth is similar to the removal of individual teeth with some slight modifications. A small envelope flap should be reflected, exposing the crestal bone around all teeth in a quadrant.[11] If removal of a tooth in a quadrant cannot be accomplished without significant force, buccal bone can easily be removed at this time. Luxation of all the teeth in a quadrant should be performed before extracting any teeth. The elevator may be place in the interproximal space, using adjacent teeth to fulcrum

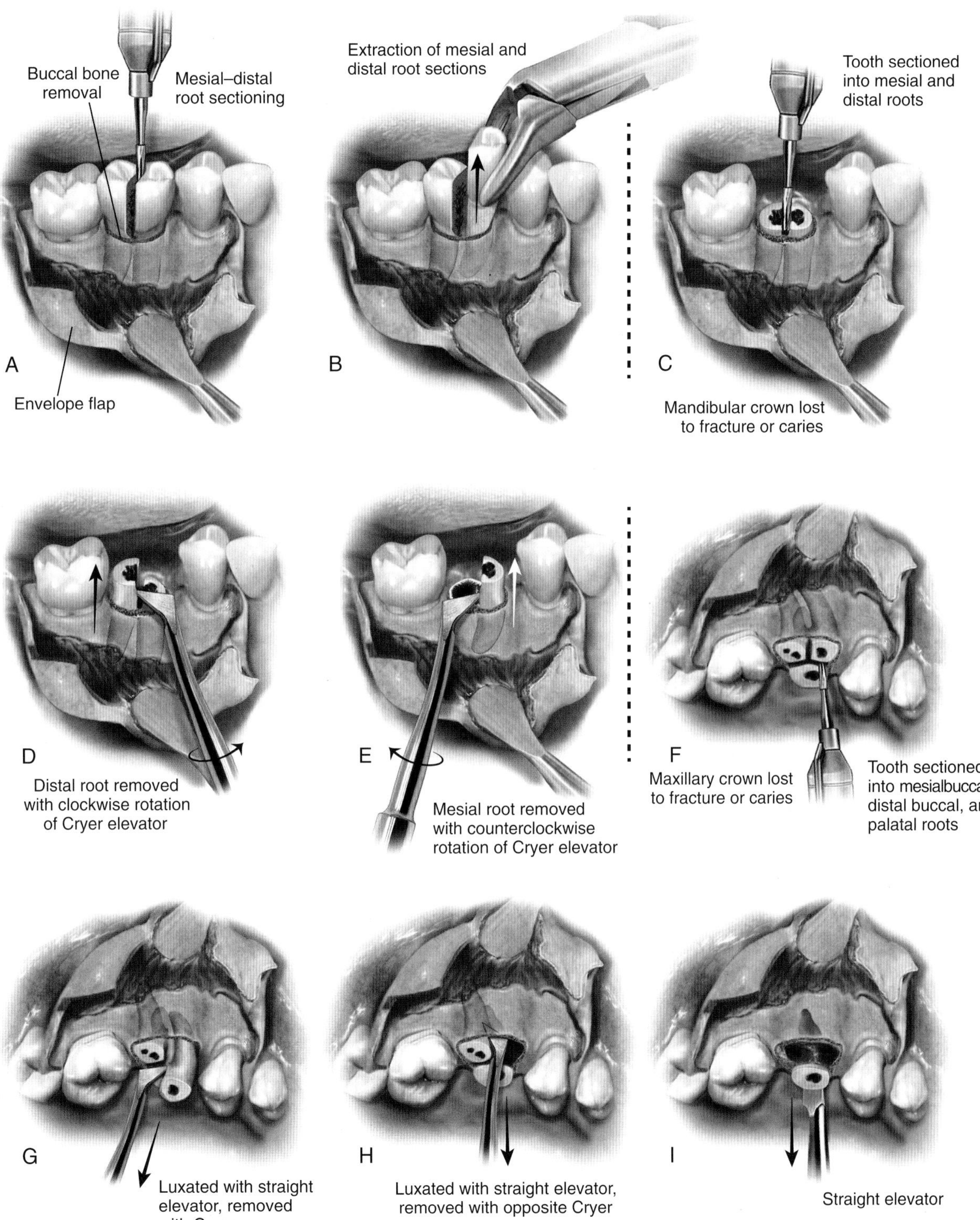

Figure 11.1 Sectioning of maxillary and mandibular molars. **A,** Visualization is achieved by reflecting an envelope flap, and buccal bone is removed to expose the furcation. The tooth is then sectioned in to mesial and distal roots. **B,** #151 Lower universal forceps are used to extract the mesial and distal roots separately. **C,** The crown of the lower first molar is lost from fracture of caries and is sectioned into mesial and distal roots. **D,** The distal root is extracted using a Cryer elevator. **E,** The mesial root is extracted with the opposite Cryer elevator. **F,** The crown of a maxillary molar has been lost to fracture or caries, and the roots are sectioned into mesial buccal, distal buccal, and palatal roots. **G,** The mesial buccal root is luxated with a small straight elevator and is then extracted with a Cryer elevator. **H,** The distal buccal root is luxated with a small straight elevator and is then extracted with the opposite Cryer elevator. **I,** The remaining palatal root is extracted with a small straight elevator.

luxation, since all teeth will be extracted. After extractions are completed, the buccal and lingual plates are preferably not compressed to maintain adequate alveolar width, especially if implants are part of the restorative plan. Any bone recontouring should be performed at this time, the soft tissue repositioned and the area palpated for any sharp areas or spicules.[11] Rongeurs and bone files are used to recontour any irregularities. The area is irrigated thoroughly with sterile saline. Any redundant tissue can be removed. All granulation tissue should be removed to avoid with postoperative bleeding. The surgeon should not attempt to gain primary closure over the extraction sites, as this will decrease the depth of the vestibule.[8] Interproximation of papilla can be performed, but this should not be attempted at the expense of a tension-free closure, loss of vestibular depth, and attached tissue. Interrupted or continuous sutures may be used, and the area should be sutured tension-free.[12]

ALTERNATIVE AND MODIFIED TECHNIQUES

An open window approach is indicated when a root tip remains in the socket and the buccocrestal bone must be maintained.[7] A #15 blade should be used to make an incision above the mucogingival junction in a vertical fashion extending to the papilla one tooth anterior to the retained root tip.[11] Once a soft tissue flap is reflected to expose to the bone overlying the root tip, a dental bur is used to remove this bone overlying the root tip and a root tip pick or elevator is inserted into the window and used to guide the root tip out of the socket[11] (Fig. 11.2).

Complications and Avoidance

Complications and avoidance of routine dental extractions are discussed in Chapter 10 of this textbook. Complications of surgical dental extractions include surgical damage to adjacent structures, root displacement into the maxillary sinus, the inferior alveolar canal or fascial spaces, sinus exposure, infections, bleeding, alveolar osteitis, paresthesia/anesthesia, and mandible fracture.[12] Displacement of a root tip is a rare but possible complication of surgical extractions. Mandibular molar roots can be dislodged into the submandibular space or the inferior alveolar canal. Maxillary molar root tips can be displaced into the maxillary sinus, buccal space, or infratemporal fossa.[13] Uninfected root tips can remain in place without postoperative complications.[12] The risk to benefit ratio should be in the patient's favor. When small root tips are adjacent to the max sinus or the inferior alveolar canal, it is not wise to remove them if attempted removal may force them into those structures.[7] If an oral-antral communication occurs, an attempt should be made to close the site primarily, and the patient should be prescribed antibiotics and sinus precautions.[12] Alveolar fracture is rare complication of surgical extractions and is more commonly encountered with routine dental extractions. Elderly patients are at a higher risk of alveolar fracture due to loss of bone density, elasticity, and strength. Patients with atrophic mandibles or mandibles with large intrabony defects are at an elevated risk for alveolar fracture.[13]

Postoperative Considerations

Postoperative considerations should be discussed with the patient prior to the procedure (Box 11.3). Pain, edema, trismus, and minor bleeding should be discussed with the patient prior to the procedure and addressed appropriately.[14] Bleeding is minimized by avoiding aggressive force, tearing of flaps, and excessive trauma to soft tissue.[14] Intraoperative and postoperative bleeding should be addressed with moist gauze and pressure. Use of additional sutures, gel foam, or local hemostatic agents such as tranexamic acid. Healthy patients should have minimal bleeding with clot formation from 6 to 12 hours.[15] Active bleeding after 12 hours is concerning, and the patient should be immediately reevaluated. Oozing from extraction sites should resolve 36 to 72 hours postextraction and should stop with pressure.[15] Active bleeding is determined if the mouth fills with blood immediately after removing gauze.[15] An incomplete (liver) clot is a mobile clot that disrupts the surgical site.[14] The surgeon should remove this defective clot to promote new

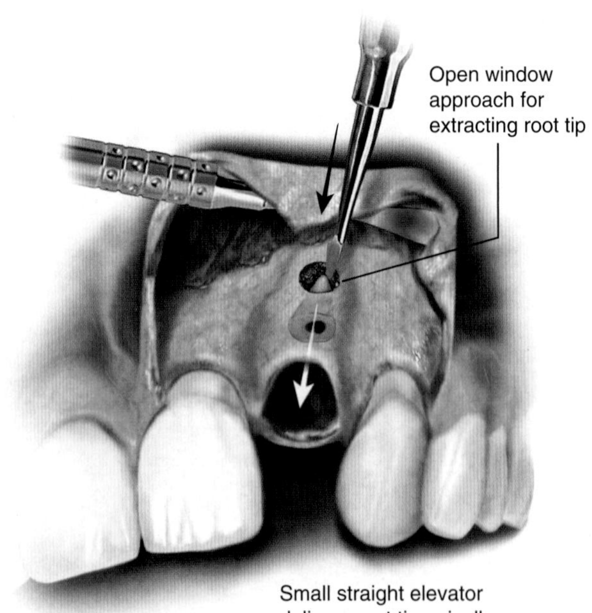

Figure 11.2 Open window approach for extracting a root tip. A three corned flap is reflected exposing the bone overlying the root tip. A surgical bur and irrigation are used to remove bone and gain access to the root tip. A small straight elevator is used to displace the root tip apically.

BOX 11.3 Postoperative Considerations

Bleeding

Swelling
Infection
Hygiene
Pain
Bruising
Nausea
Diet

healthy clot formation. Edema will occur 12 to 24 hours postoperatively, with a peak at 48 to 72 hours. Edema should begin to subside after 4 days with complete resolution at 5 to 7 days postoperatively. Edema should be managed with cold compress (minimize edema and reduce throbbing pain) and sleeping with the head in an elevated position to prevent additional swelling. Infection after surgical extractions is likely from debris remaining under the flap, and the adequate treatment typically includes debridement of the site and drainage.[15] Good tissue management will decrease infection rates, and curettage of infected tissue and irrigation of the site with saline or chlorohexidine will reduce bacterial load and lower the chance of infection.[15] Patients commonly presenting with a postoperative infection have a chief complaint of persistent pain, trismus, swelling that is not improving, foul taste, and/or drainage. Early recognition of infection is important to prevent cellulitis; the patient should be treated with an appropriate antibiotic. If an infection develops, incision and drainage should be performed to prevent further progression and involvement of the fascial planes which can lead to increased morbidity and potentially mortality.[15]

References

1. Ramos E, Santamaría J, Santamaría G, Barbier L, Arteagoitia I. Do systemic antibiotics prevent dry socket and infection after third molar extraction? A systematic review and meta-analysis. *Oral Surg Oral Med Oral Pathol Oral Radiol*. 2016;122(4):403–425.
2. Laskin D. Oral and maxillofacial surgery: the mystery behind the history. *J Oral Maxillofac Surg Med Pathol*. 2016;28(2):101–104.
3. Mitchell L, McCaul L, Mitchell D. *Oxford Handbook of Clinical Dentistry*. 5th ed. Oxford University Press; 2009.
4. Hull PS, Worthington HV, Clerehugh V, Tsirba R, Davies RM, Clarkson JE. The reasons for tooth extractions in adults and their validation. *J Dent*. 1997;25(3–4):233–237.
5. Fragiskos FD. *Oral Surgery*. 6th ed. Berlin: Springer; 2007.
6. Ruggiero SL, Dodson TB, Assael LA, et al. AAOMS position paper on bisphosphonate-related osteonecrosis of the Jaw 2009 update. *J Oral Maxillofac Surg*. 2009;67(5 Suppl):2–12.
7. Hooley J, Whitacre R. *A Self-Instructional Guide: The Removal of Teeth*. 3rd ed. Seattle: Stoma Press; 1983.
8. Hupp J, Ellis E, Tucker M. *Contemporary Oral and Maxillofacial Surgery*. 6th ed. St Louis, Missouri: Elsevier; 2014.
9. Pedlar J, Frame J. *Oral and Maxillofacial Surgery*. 2nd ed. Elsevier; 2007.
10. Dym H, Weiss A. Exodontia: tips and techniques for better outcomes. *Dent Clin North Am*. 2012;56(1):245–266, x.
11. Peterson L, Hupp J, Ellis E, Tucker M. *Contemporary Oral and Maxillofacial Surgery*. 4th ed. 4. St Louis, Missouri: Elsevier; 2003.
12. Brennan P, Ghali GE, Schliephake H, Cascarini L. *Maxillofacial Surgery*. 3rd ed. St Louis, Missouri: Elsevier; 2017.
13. Shigeishi H, Ohta K, Takechi M. Risk factors for postoperative complications following oral surgery. *J Appl Oral Sci*. 2015;23(4):419–423.
14. Pierse JE, Dym H, Clarkson E. Diagnosis and management of common postextraction complications. *Dent Clin North Am*. 2012;56(1):75–93, viii.
15. Fonseca RJ, Turvey TA, Marciani RD. *Oral and Maxillofacial Surgery*. 2nd ed. St Louis, Missouri: Saunders; 2008.

CHAPTER 12

Impacted Teeth

Louis J. Christensen and Mary Ann C. Sabino

Armamentarium

Each surgeon establishes an armamentarium for their individual surgical technique. However, most extractions of impacted teeth include instruments from the following list.[1] Alternative techniques that require specialized equipment are discussed in those sections in the chapter text.

#1 Periosteal elevator
#9 Periosteal elevator
#15 Scalpel blade
#150/151 Forceps
#190/191 Elevators
Appropriate sutures
Bone file
Cryer elevators
Dental curette
Fissure/round bur
Gilmore probe
Hemostat
Irrigation syringe/sterile saline
Local anesthetic with vasoconstrictor
Minnesota cheek retractor
Molt curettes
Needle holder
Rongeurs
Small and large luxators
Small and large straight elevators
Surgical handpiece
Suture scissors

Indications for Removal of Impacted Third Molars

The parameters of care published by the American Association of Oral and Maxillofacial Surgeons have established criteria for the extraction of impacted third molars. The indications for removal of impacted third molars include the following:

- Pain
- Pathology associated with tooth follicle (e.g., cysts, tumors)
- Abnormalities of tooth size or shape that preclude normal function
- Facilitation of the management or limitation of progression of periodontal disease[2]
- Resorption of third molar or adjacent tooth
- Facilitation of orthodontic tooth movement and promotion of stability of the dental occlusion
- Facilitation of prosthetic rehabilitation
- Tooth impeding the normal eruption of an adjacent tooth
- Tooth in the line of fracture
- Tooth involved in tumor resection
- Tooth interfering with orthognathic and/or reconstructive jaw surgery
- Preventive or prophylactic tooth removal, when indicated, for patients with medical or surgical conditions or treatments (e.g., organ transplants, alloplastic implants, antiresorptive therapy, chemotherapy, radiation therapy)
- Clinical findings of fractured tooth or teeth
- Facilitation of harvesting of autologous graft
- Impacted tooth (as defined previously)
- Anatomic position causing potential damage to adjacent teeth
- Patient's informed refusal of nonsurgical treatment options

Diagnostic Imaging

A panoramic radiograph is recommended for management of third molars, although periapical, maxillary, and/or mandibular radiographs and computed tomography may also be used. The goals of impacted tooth removal are to:

- Prevent pathology
- Preserve the periodontal health of adjacent teeth
- Optimize prosthetic rehabilitation
- Optimize management and/or healing of jaw fractures
- Optimize orthodontic results
- Aid in tumor resection
- Provide a healthy oral and maxillofacial environment for patients undergoing radiation therapy, chemotherapy, organ transplantation, or placement of alloplastic implants
- Prevent complications in orthognathic surgery

Cone beam computed tomography (CBCT) may be considered to better understand the relationship of impacted tooth roots and the inferior alveolar nerve.

Contraindications to Removal of Impacted Third Molars

The surgeon should consider three important clinical factors in deciding whether to extract an impacted third molar[3,4]:

- Patient of older age

- Compromised medical status
- Increased risk of damage to anatomic structures

Many classification systems correlate descriptive features of the tooth to the degree of difficulty in surgical extraction. The most common system, the Pell and Gregory classification (Fig. 12.1), incorporates two features:

1. The relationship of the impacted tooth to the anterior border of the ramus and the second molar
2. The depth of the impaction and the type of tissue overlying the impacted tooth

Other classification systems include one based on depth of impaction: soft tissue, partial bony impaction, and complete bony impaction. Another commonly used description is the Winter classification, which is based on the angulation of the impacted tooth (horizontal, vertical, mesioangular, or distoangular).

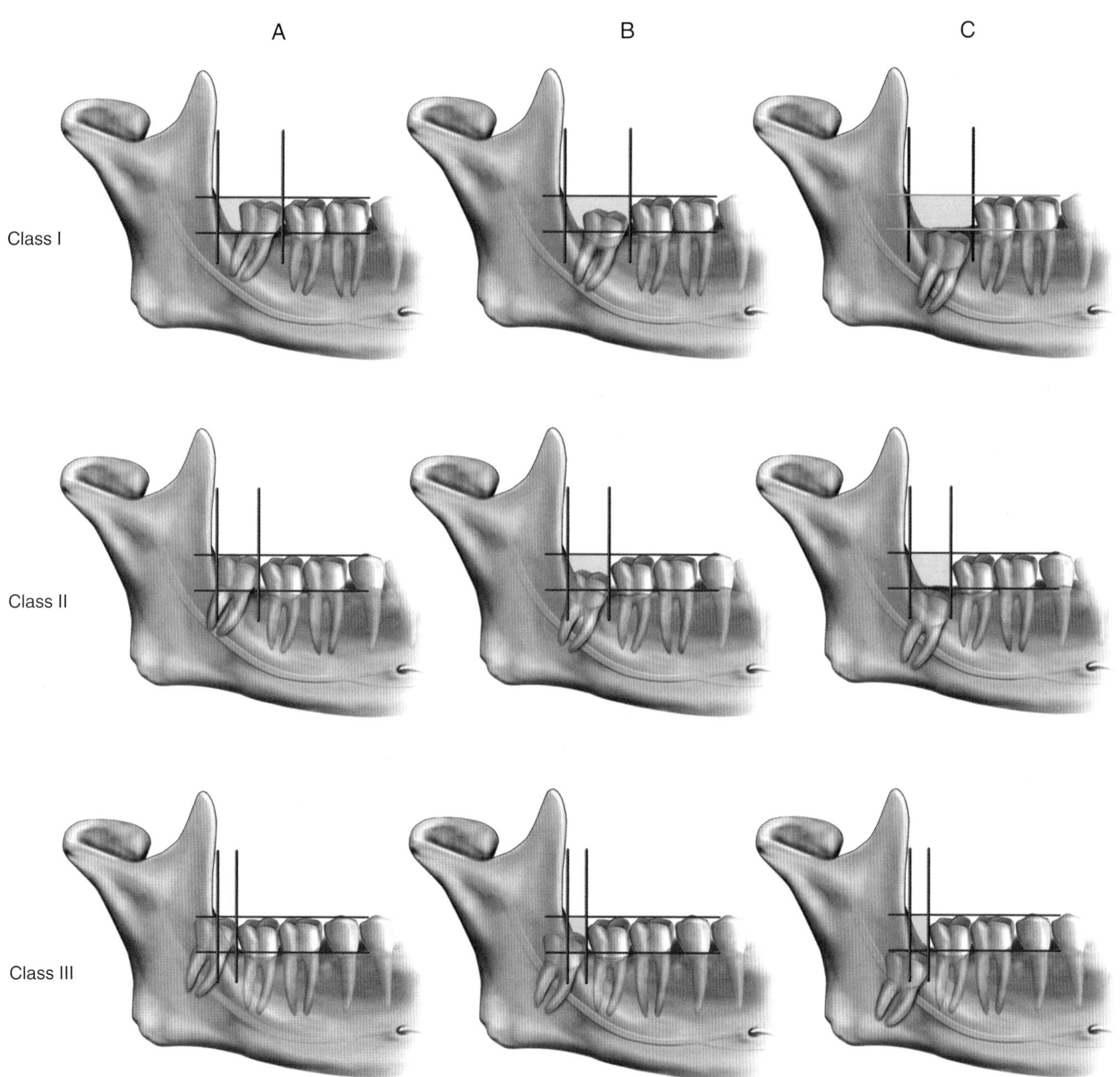

Figure 12.1 Pell and Gregory classification of impacted teeth. Class I/II/III describe the horizontal or anteroposterior (AP) position of the impacted third molar relative to the anterior border of the ascending ramus *(blue lines)*. Class A/B/C describe the vertical position of the impacted third molar relative to the mandibular occlusal plane *(red lines)*.

TECHNIQUE: Surgical Removal of Impacted Third Molars

Addressing the surgical removal of impacted teeth begins with access. Before a tooth can be extracted, clinically visualizing the surgical site is crucial. An envelope flap is most commonly used by surgeons in both the maxilla and mandible. The following considerations should be addressed when designing a surgical flap:

- Allow for complete visualization of the operative field.
- Prevent unnecessary trauma to the adjacent soft tissue when removing bone or teeth.
- Provide an adequate working area that allows for full removal of intrabony pathologic conditions when present.
- Place incisions over bone not planned for removal.
- Make sure the incision is long enough to allow for a flap that gives clear and adequate hard tissue visualization and permits easy retraction without tearing.
- Make sure the base of the flap is wider than the reflected free margin to ensure a proper blood supply to the reflected soft tissue.[4]

STEP 1A: Mandibular Incision

A sulcular incision is made from the distal end of the first molar posteriorly with a distobuccal release in the mandible, with an option to include a possible mesial vertical release for increased access (Fig. 12.2A). Multiple other variations have been discussed in the literature, such as a triangular flap, but they are not reviewed here.

Continued

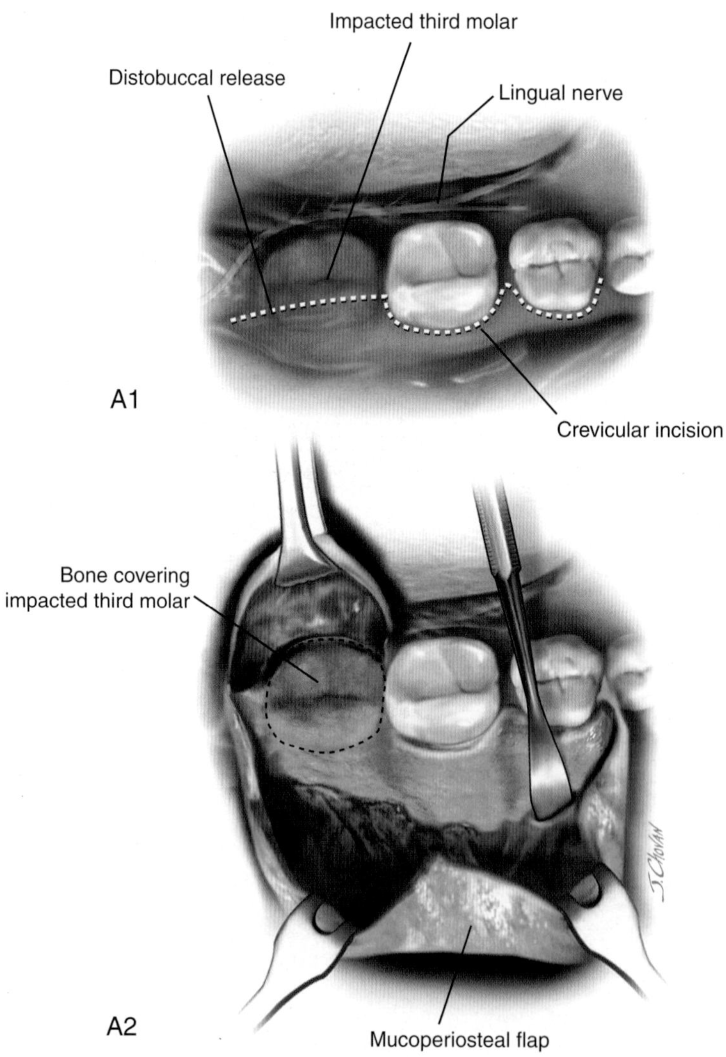

Figure 12.2 **A,** Incision design for surgical removal of impacted mandibular third molars. A mucoperiosteal flap using a crevicular incision with distobuccal release *(dashed line)* is created (A1), and the flap is elevated with a periosteal elevator (A2). An alternative design is an anterior vertical release with elevation of the flap.

TECHNIQUE: Surgical Removal of Impacted Third Molars—cont'd

STEP 1B: Maxillary Incision

In the maxilla, the same sulcular incision is created with a sharp #15 blade with a distobuccal release and an option of including a mesial vertical releasing incision for improved access (Fig. 12.2B). Multiple other variations, including the utilization of vertical releasing incisions, have been discussed in the literature but are not reviewed here.

Once the site has been visualized, the surgical plan can commence by following the subsequent routine steps, adjusted to the individual tooth and location.

STEP 2: Uncovering the Clinical Crown

After elevation of the mucoperiosteal flap, the bone covering the tooth is removed using a surgical handpiece and bur so that the impacted tooth can be visualized.

After the uncovering, a buccal trough is created to fully visualize the clinical crown. In some instances, as with horizontally impacted teeth, complete uncovering of the clinical crown is not possible (see Fig. 12.2B). Alternatively, for superficially impacted teeth and teeth in the maxilla, buccal bone may be removed with a Molt curette to expose the crown to the level of the cementoenamel junction (Fig. 12.2C).

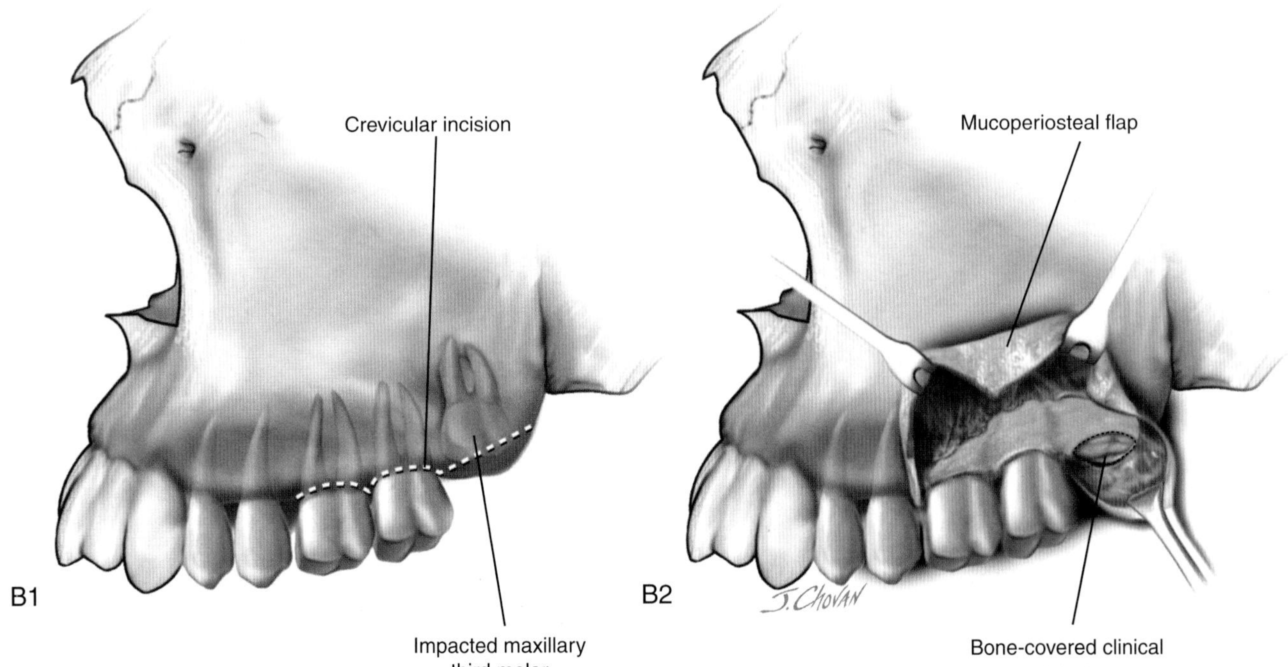

Figure 12.2, cont'd B, Incision design for surgical removal of impacted maxillary third molars. A mucoperiosteal flap using a crevicular incision with distobuccal release is created using a sharp #15 blade (B1). The flap is then elevated to uncover the clinical crown (B2). An alternative technique is raising a mesial vertical releasing incision and elevation with a periosteal elevator.

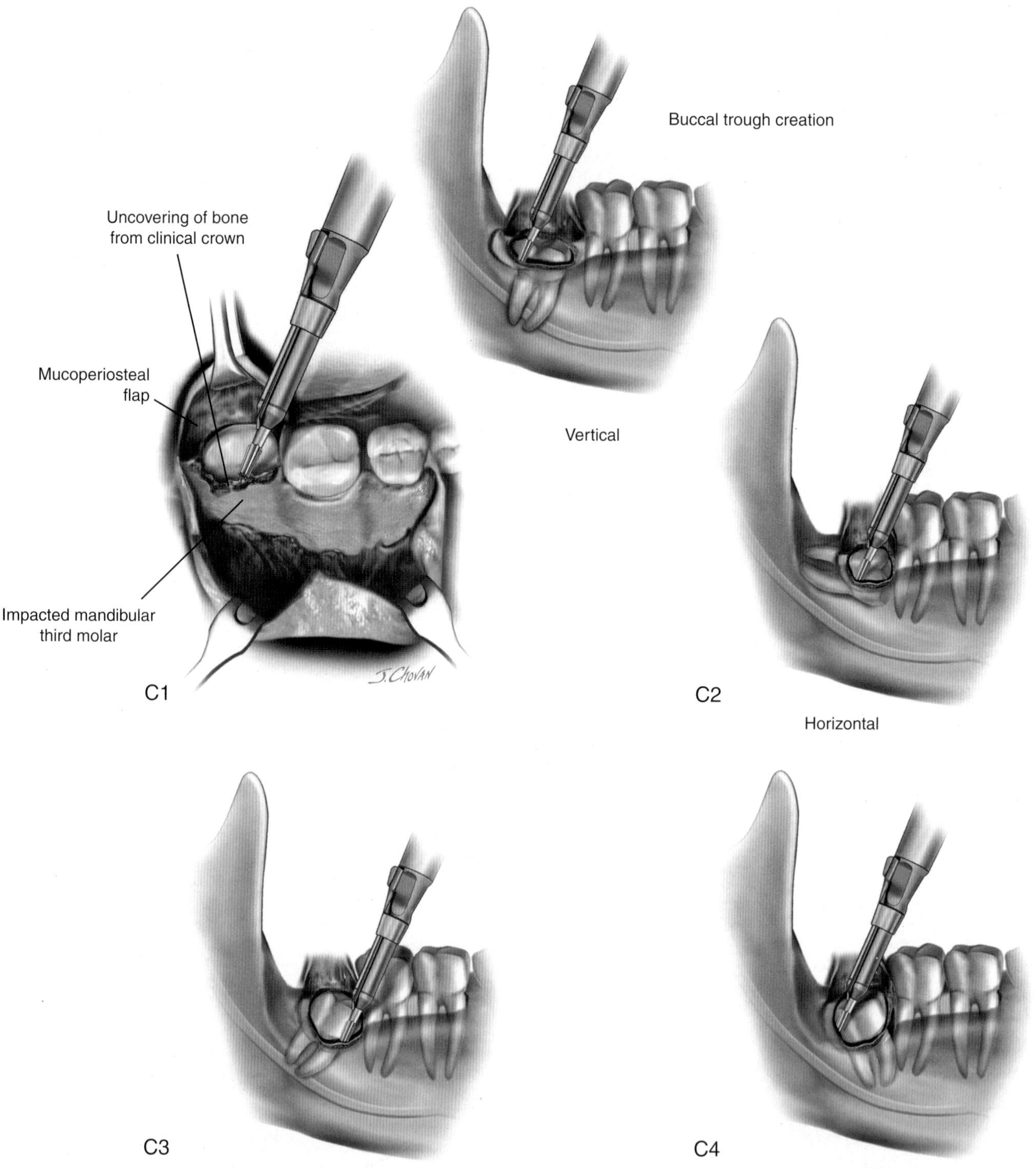

Figure 12.2, cont'd C, Uncovering a clinical crown. A fissure bur is used to uncover the clinical crown and create a buccal trough in vertical (C1), horizontal (C2), mesioangular (C3), and distoangular (C4) impactions using copious irrigation. In horizontal impactions, it may be difficult to uncover the crown in its entirety.

Continued

TECHNIQUE: Surgical Removal of Impacted Third Molars—cont'd

STEP 3: Sectioning the Clinical Crown and/or Roots

Once the crown has been uncovered, attempt elevation. If unable to elevate, consider sectioning the tooth. The surgical sectioning of impacted teeth varies, depending on the tooth's angulation, the number of roots, and the direction of root growth. Fig. 12.2D1–D4 represents the most common techniques, which are modified for each type of impaction. When possible, align the surgical bur parallel to the buccal groove but along the mesiobuccal cusp. This helps reduce the potential for a distal coronectomy. Section the clinical crown up to three-fourths of its buccal-lingual distance. Do not section the crown completely because of the potential for lingual cortical perforation and lingual nerve injury (Fig. 12.3).

After the clinical crown and roots have been sectioned, a small or large elevator is used to complete the section (Fig. 12.2D).

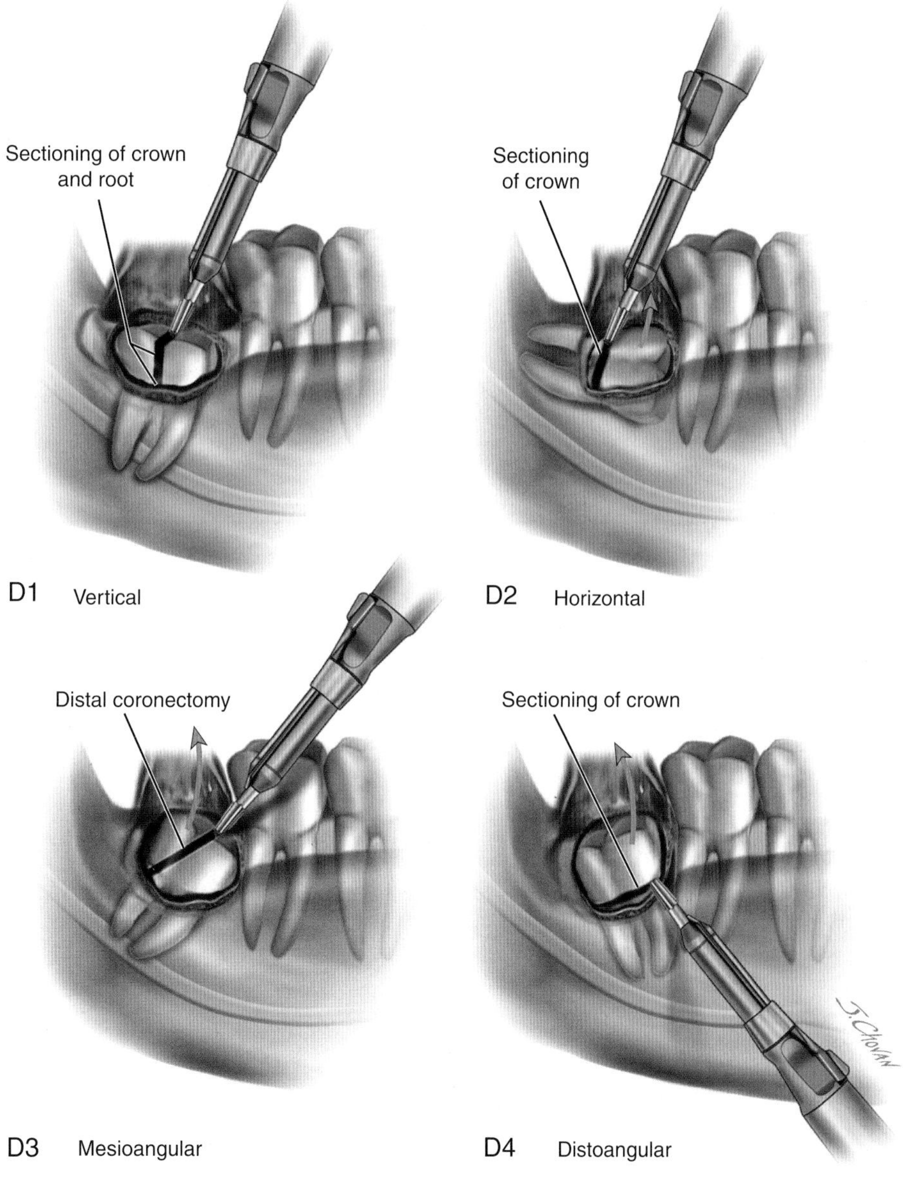

Figure 12.2, cont'd **D,** Sectioning of an impacted clinical crown and/or roots. In vertical impactions (D1), a fissure bur is used to section the clinical crown and roots into mesial and distal halves. The crown is sectioned separately from the roots in horizontal impactions (D2). Mesial and distal roots may require sectioning before retrieval. A distal coronectomy is performed in mesioangular impactions to allow elevation of roots in a distal/posterior direction (D3). In distoangular impactions (D4), the clinical crown must be sectioned to allow for the retrieval of roots. In some cases, roots may need to be sectioned before retrieval.

TECHNIQUE: Surgical Removal of Impacted Third Molars—cont'd

STEP 4: Elevation and Retrieval of Tooth Roots

A small/large elevator, small/large luxator, or Cryer elevators may be used to elevate retained roots. The root direction and number of roots dictate the degree of difficulty in removing tooth roots. Fig. 12.2E–F demonstrates common techniques and instruments used to elevate impacted retained roots. Remove any residual follicle with a dental curette and hemostat. If pathology is suspected, place the specimen in an appropriate container for transport and histopathologic analysis. Do not use excessive force during elevation or luxation of roots, especially in retrieving root tips, because this may force root tips apically and into potential spaces, such as the inferior alveolar nerve (IAN) canal and maxillary sinus (see Displacement of Root Tips later in the chapter).

If no mobility of the roots is noted, troughing of alveolar bone may be necessary to create a purchase point for the elevator.

STEP 5: Closure

After retrieval of all root tips, the area is copiously irrigated (including subperiosteal irrigation) and inspected for cortical perforation, damage to adjacent dentition, and encroachment of the IAN canal. Ensure adequate hemostasis and place hemostatic agents if necessary.

If necessary, place sutures to reapproximate flap margins.

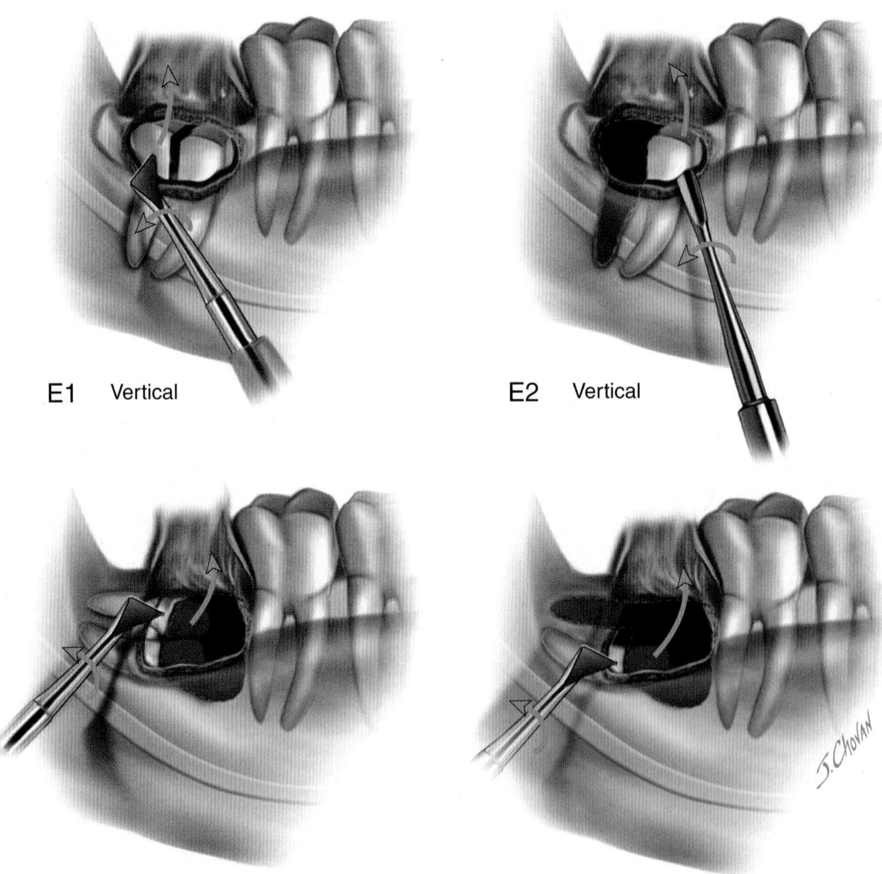

Figure 12.2, cont'd **E,** Delivery of impacted roots: vertical and horizontal impactions. After sectioning, a small perforation is created on the distal crown, and a Cryer elevator may be used to retrieve the distal half superiorly (E1), followed by elevation of the mesial root (E2). For horizontal impactions, a Cryer elevator may be used to elevate distal (E3) and mesial (E4) roots separately. Alternatively, a small luxator may be used to elevate roots.

Continued

Delivery of impacted roots
(mesioangular and distoangular)

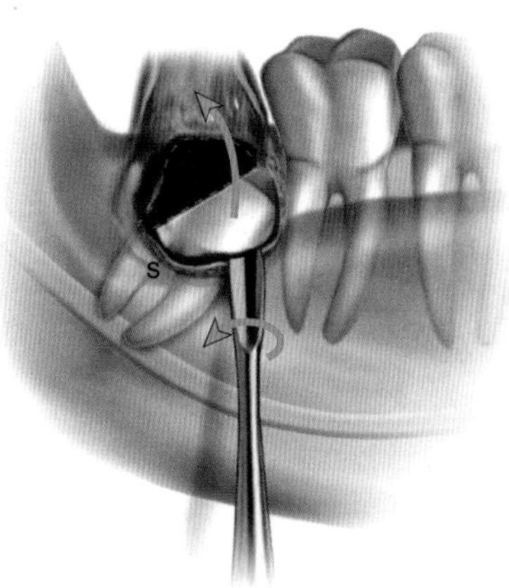

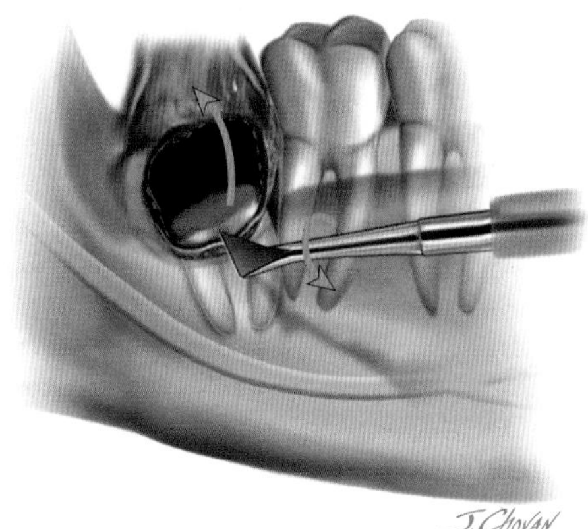

F1 Mesioangular F2 Distoangular

Figure 12.2, cont'd **F,** Delivery of roots: mesioangular and distoangular impactions. After a distal coronectomy, a small elevator or luxator may be used to elevate the mesioangular impaction in a posterior direction (F1). If the clinical crown is lodged under the distal cusp of the adjacent molar, the crown may be sectioned and the root elevated separately. In distoangular impactions, a Cryer elevator may be used to elevate both roots together (F2). Alternatively, the roots may be sectioned and delivered separately using a Cryer elevator or small luxator.

ALTERNATIVE TECHNIQUE 1: Elevation of a Lingual Flap

Elevation of a lingual flap has been described in the literature. This technique is more commonly used in the UK than in the US.[5,7–14] It is commonly used to increase exposure of the clinical crown for sectioning and to protect the lingual nerve during sectioning and possible perforation of the lingual cortex. The lingual nerve has been shown to vary greatly in its position relative to the alveolar crest and lingual plate in the third molar site, based on anatomic and radiologic studies.[7,8] Therefore, it is at great risk for damage during third molar surgery.

Elevation of a lingual flap has been shown to cause nerve injury, albeit transient. It is controversial whether the type of retractor used influences the onset of nerve paresthesias.[9,10] What is agreed upon is that most retractor-induced injuries are neurapraxic in nature and are transient. Permanent nerve damage is more commonly seen in direct injury to the lingual nerve due to cortical perforation, but it is also relatively uncommon.[10-14] This technique is discouraged because of the increased risk of damage to the lingual nerve in the region of the mandibular third molar. If lingual tissue must be elevated, it is important to use an appropriate retractor, insert it carefully in subperiosteal fashion, and contact the lingual plate (see Fig. 12.3).

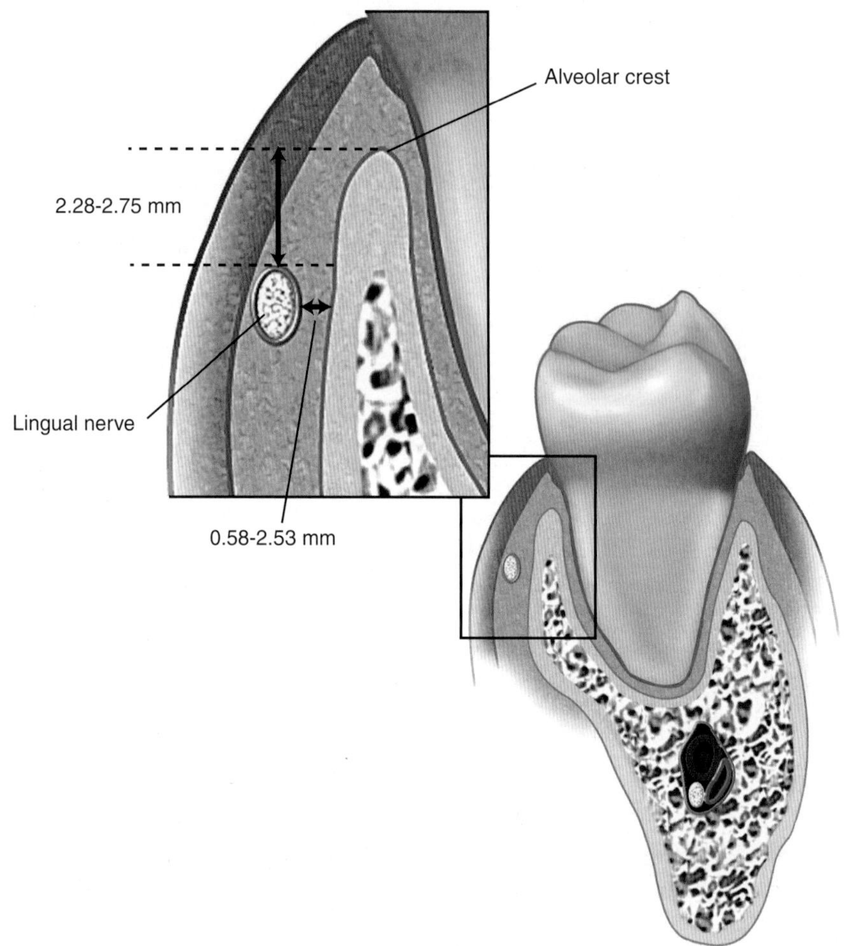

Figure 12.3 Position of lingual nerve. Mean distances of the lingual nerve from alveolar crest and lingual cortex based on cadaveric studies.

ALTERNATIVE TECHNIQUE 2: Partial Odontectomy/Coronectomy

The coronectomy technique was developed for cases in which roots of the mandibular third molar closely approximate the IAN canal and the risk of nerve damage exists.[15,16] This risk is commonly assessed by panoramic radiograph evaluation. The advent of CBCT technology has improved the ability to assess for the risk of nerve damage and allows the clinician to determine the exact position of the IAN canal in all three dimensions. This information has allowed the clinician and patient to have greater understanding of the risks associated with extraction of the impacted tooth. However, in the vast majority of cases, the treatment decision from panoramic evaluation was not altered by CBCT results.[17-20]

The most common technique has been described by Pogrel et al.[15] Surgical principles include the following:

- The tooth should not be mobile.
- There should be no infection involving the roots.
- The tooth should be vital without evidence of disease.
- The crown and coronal portion of roots should be removed until they are 2 to 3 mm below the level of the alveolar crest (Fig. 12.4).
- Retained root should not be mobilized.
- Endodontic therapy is not required and has been associated with an increased risk of infection.[21]

Long-term follow-up from coronectomy procedures has demonstrated that this procedure has minimal long-term complications.[22-24] The most common complications from this procedure, besides acute prolonged pain, are postoperative infection and migration of the roots. The highest reported rate of postoperative infection was 11%, with all being managed by PO antibiotics.[24] Migration of the roots typically occurred within the first 3 years of the procedure, and up to 5% of coronectomies had this complication.[22,23]

ALTERNATIVE TECHNIQUE 2: Partial Odontectomy/Coronectomy—cont'd

Surgical Technique

Preoperative prophylactic antibiotics and preoperative chlorhexidine or povidone-iodine rinse is used.

- A conventional buccal flap is raised and lingual tissues are retracted with a Walter lingual retractor to protect the lingual nerve.
- A 701 fissure bur is directed at a 45-degree angle to transect the clinical crown in its entirety such that it could be removed with a tissue forceps to minimize mobilization of retained root.
- Use of a lingual retractor is important due to the potential for cortical perforation and lingual nerve damage.
- A fissure bur is used to reduce remaining roots so that the roots are 2 to 3 mm inferior to the crest of the buccal and lingual plates. This allows for soft tissue healing over the coronectomy site.
- Do not attempt root canal treatment.
- Primary closure must be performed with one or more vertical mattress sutures.
- Radiographs should be taken immediately postoperatively, because in 30% of cases, retained roots have been shown to migrate superiorly (see Fig. 12.4).

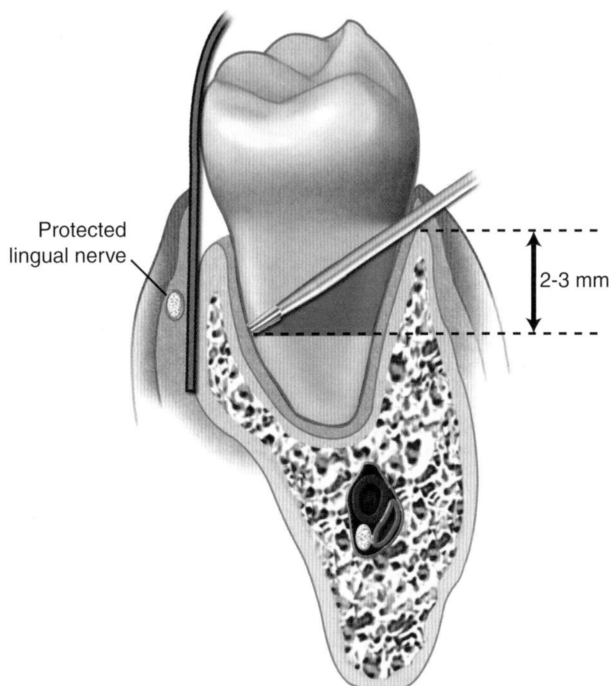

Figure 12.4 Coronectomy. Description of surgical technique. Note the protection of the lingual nerve using a retractor. The bur is angled at 45 degrees, and the remaining root surface has been removed such that it is 2 to 3 mm inferior to the alveolar crest *(shaded areas).*

Management of Intraoperative Complications

Bleeding

A thorough consultation that addresses a patient's past medical history, medications, and any history of bleeding problems can prepare the surgeon for potential bleeding complications intra- and postoperatively. If appropriate, coordinating with the patient's primary physician may be required before safe dentoalveolar surgery is performed in an anticoagulated/coagulopathic patient. Proper surgical technique should be exercised to avoid tearing flaps or excessive soft tissue injury.[4] Most intraoperative bleeding can be controlled with local measures, which may include oversuturing, application of topical thrombin, or use of a packing medium such as Gelfoam or oxidized cellulose or Surgicel.[25,26]

Nerve Damage

The two nerves most commonly at risk during impacted mandibular third molar surgery are the lingual nerve and the IAN. Retraction of a lingual flap has been previously discussed. IAN injury is most likely to occur in specific situations. The first and most commonly reported predisposing factor is complete bony impaction of mandibular third molars. The angulation classifications most commonly involved are mesioangular and vertical impaction. In some cases, nerve proximity to the root is indicated by an apparent narrowing of the IAN canal as it crosses the root or severe root dilaceration adjacent to the canal. Other well-documented radiographic signs are diversion of the path of the canal by the tooth; darkening of the apical end of the root, indicating that it is included within the canal; and interruption of the radiopaque white line of the canal.[4] Direct injuries include those that occur from anesthetic injections, crush injuries, injuries sustained during the extraction process or soft tissue management, and damage caused by the use of instruments. Indirect injuries to nerves can be the result of physiologic phenomena, including root infections, pressure from hematomas, and postsurgical edema.[26] When an injury to the lingual or IAN is diagnosed in the postoperative period, the surgeon should begin long-term planning for its management, including consideration of referral to a neurologist and/or microneurosurgeon.[4]

Retained Roots

Fracture of root tips is a common occurrence during extractions. Roots can be dilacerated or divergent. If the root tip is small (less than a few millimeters) and near vital structures, or if the removal of bone to retrieve the root tip would be excessive, the risks and benefits must be considered. Usually a small root remnant is of no consequence if it is not grossly infected. If the decision is made to leave it, the patient should be informed, radiographs taken, and complete documentation of the circumstances placed in the patient's record. The patient should be followed periodically to ensure uneventful healing.[1]

Displacement of Root Tips

Displacement of root tips is a rare occurrence. The most common areas of displacement are those that correspond to related anatomy; that is, the thin bone bordering the maxillary sinus and a thin lingual plate in the posterior aspect of the mandible. The third circumstance that must be considered is displacement of the maxillary third molar into the infratemporal fossa.[1] Immediate local retrieval should be attempted in all circumstances with the use of palpation, manipulation, and suction. Three-dimensional localization of the displaced tooth or root should be used for appropriate planning. For details on further surgical techniques and treatment, the reader is referred to the literature.

Sinus Perforation

Exposure of the maxillary sinus can occur during extraction of maxillary molars. Proper radiographic evaluation usually alerts the clinician to the possibility of this occurrence. Widely divergent roots and superiorly impacted roots increase the chance that the sinus floor may be removed or violated along with removal of the tooth. If the tooth roots are in close proximity to the sinus floor, less force should be used, and sectioning of the roots should be considered. The size of the communication determines the treatment:

- Small perforations (less than 2 mm) can often be treated with medical management and careful observation alone.
- Perforations 2 to 6 mm may require a collagen plug that is kept in place with figure-eight sutures.
- Perforations larger than 6 mm require a buccal or palatal advancement flap in addition to placement of a collagen plug.

All these treatments should be accompanied by antibiotics directed toward sinus microorganisms (*Streptococcus pneumoniae, Haemophilus influenzae,* and *Moraxella catarrhalis*) and sinus precautions (i.e., the patient should be advised to avoid nose blowing, sucking through straws, smoking, and forceful sneezing). Sequelae associated with infection include maxillary sinusitis and formation of a chronic oroantral fistula.[1,26]

Postoperative Complications Related to Removal of Impacted Third Molars

During the informed consent process, common complications related to the surgical removal of impacted teeth should be discussed. The prevention and management of complications shall only be briefly discussed in this chapter; readers are directed elsewhere[26,27] for excellent in-depth reviews. Common complications may include the following:

- Pain
- Bleeding
- Swelling
- Infection
- Damage to adjacent teeth or structures
- Nerve damage with resultant paresthesia
- Fracture
- Alveolar osteitis
- Oroantral communication

References

1. Saker M, Ogle OE, Dym H. Basic and complex exodontia and surgical management of impacted teeth. In: Fonseca RJ, Barber HD, Matheson JD, eds. *Oral and Maxillofacial Surgery* 2nd ed. Vol I. St Louis, Missouri: Saunders; 2009.
2. White RP Jr, Fisher EL, Phillips C, Tucker M, Moss KL, Offenbacher S. Visible third molars as risk indicator for increased periodontal probing depth. *J Oral Maxillofac Surg.* 2011;69(1):92–103.
3. Lieblich SE, Kleiman MA, Zak MJ. Dentoalveolar surgery: AAOMS parameters of care 2012. *J Oral Maxillofac Surg.* 2012;70(11 suppl 3):e1.
4. Peterson LJ, Ness GM. Impacted teeth. In: Miloro M, ed. *Peterson's Principles of Oral and Maxillofacial Surgery.* 2nd ed. Hamilton, Ontario: Decker; 2004.
5. Behnia H, Kheradvar A, Shahrokhi M. An anatomic study of the lingual nerve in the third molar region. *J Oral Maxillofac Surg.* 2000;58(6):649–651.
6. Assael LA. Indications for elective therapeutic third molar removal: the evidence is in. *J Oral Maxillofac Surg.* 2005;63(12):1691–1692.
7. Kiesselbach JE, Chamberlain JG. Clinical and anatomic observations on the relationship of the lingual nerve to the mandibular third molar region. *J Oral Maxillofac Surg.* 1984;42(9):565–567.
8. Miloro M, Halkias LE, Slone HW, Chakeres DW. Assessment of the lingual nerve in the third molar region using magnetic

resonance imaging. *J Oral Maxillofac Surg.* 1997;55(2):134–137.

9. Pogrel MA, Goldman KE. Lingual flap retraction for third molar removal. *J Oral Maxillofac Surg.* 2004;62(9):1125–1130.
10. Greenwood M, Langton SG, Rood JP. A comparison of broad and narrow retractors for lingual nerve protection during lower third molar surgery. *Br J Oral Maxillofac Surg.* 1994;32(2):114–117.
11. Rood JP. Permanent damage to inferior alveolar and lingual nerves during the removal of impacted mandibular third molars. Comparison of two methods of bone removal. *Br Dent J.* 1992;172(3):108–110.
12. Gomes AC, Vasconcelos BC, de Oliveira e Silva ED, da Silva LC. Lingual nerve damage after mandibular third molar surgery: a randomized clinical trial. *J Oral Maxillofac Surg.* 2005;63(10):1443–1446.
13. Pichler JW, Beirne OR. Lingual flap retraction and prevention of lingual nerve damage associated with third molar surgery: a systematic review of the literature. *Oral Surg Oral Med Oral Pathol Oral Radiol Endod.* 2001;91(4):395–401.
14. Gargallo-Albiol J, Buenechea-Imaz R, Gay-Escoda C. Lingual nerve protection during surgical removal of lower third molars. A prospective randomised study. *Int J Oral Maxillofac Surg.* 2000;29(4):268–271.
15. Pogrel MA, Lee JS, Muff DF. Coronectomy: a technique to protect the inferior alveolar nerve. *J Oral Maxillofac Surg.* 2004;62(12):1447–1452.
16. Renton T, Hankins M, Sproate C, McGurk M. A randomised controlled clinical trial to compare the incidence of injury to the inferior alveolar nerve as a result of coronectomy and removal of mandibular third molars. *Br J Oral Maxillofac Surg.* 2005;43(1):7–12.
17. Matzen LH, Christensen J, Hintze H, Schou S, Wenzel A. Influence of cone beam CT on treatment plan before surgical intervention of mandibular third molars and impact of radiographic factors on deciding on coronectomy vs surgical removal. *Dentomaxillofac Radiol.* 2013;42(1):98870341.
18. Manor Y, Abir R, Manor A, Kaffe I. Are different imaging methods affecting the treatment decision of extractions of mandibular third molars? *Dentomaxillofac Radiol.* 2017;46(1):20160233.
19. Szalma J, Vajta L, Lovász BV, Kiss C, Soós B, Lempel E. Identification of specific panoramic high-risk signs in impacted third molar cases in which cone beam computed tomography changes the treatment decision. *J Oral Maxillofac Surg.* 2020;78(7):1061–1070.
20. Baqain ZH, AlHadidi A, AbuKaraky A, Khader Y. Does the use of cone-beam computed tomography before mandibular third molar surgery impact treatment planning? *J Oral Maxillofac Surg.* 2020;78(7):1071–1077.
21. Sencimen M, Ortakoglu K, Aydin C, et al. Is endodontic treatment necessary during coronectomy procedure? *J Oral Maxillofac Surg.* 2010;68(10):2385–2390.
22. Leung YY, Cheung LK. Long-term morbidities of coronectomy on lower third molar. *Oral Surg Oral Med Oral Pathol Oral Radiol.* 2016;121(1):5–11.
23. Monaco G, D'Ambrosio M, De Santis G, Vignudelli E, Gatto MRA, Corinaldesi G. Coronectomy: a surgical option for impacted third molars in close proximity to the inferior alveolar nerve—a 5 year follow up study. *J Oral Maxillofac Surg.* 2019;77(6):1116–1124.
24. Pedersen MH, Bak J, Matzen LH, et al. Coronectomy of mandibular third molars: a clinical and radiological study of 231 cases with a mean follow-up period of 5.7 years. *Int J Oral Maxillofac Implants.* 2018;47(12):1596–1603.
25. Tolstunov L, Javid B, Keyes L, Nattestad A. Pericoronal ostectomy: an alternative surgical technique for management of mandibular third molars in close proximity to the inferior alveolar nerve. *J Oral Maxillofac Surg.* 2011;69(7):1858–1866.
26. Susarla SM, Blaeser BF, Magalnick D. Third molar surgery and associated complications. *Oral Maxillofac Surg Clin North Am.* 2003;15(2):177–186.
27. Bui CH, Seldin EB, Dodson TB. Types, frequencies, and risk factors for complications after third molar extraction. *J Oral Maxillofac Surg.* 2003;61(12):1379–1389.

CHAPTER 13

Canine Exposure

Shravan Renapurkar, Pamela J. Hughes, and Christopher K. Ray

Armamentarium

#15 Blade
#9 Periosteal elevator
3-0 Chromic gut suture
3-0 Silk suture
3-mm round bur/piezoelectric blade
Acid etch agent
Bonding agent
Composite resin
Cotton pledgets
Electrocautery
Handpiece
Local anesthetic syringe and cartridge
Minnesota retractor
Molt's curette
Needle holder
Orthodontic bracket with chain
Suture scissor

History of the Procedure

The canine is a critical tooth in determining facial esthetics and dental occlusion, and it affects the course of orthodontic treatment when there is a disturbance in its alignment or eruption.[1] The maxillary canine usually erupts before 13.9 years in females and before 14.6 years in males.[2] The maxillary canine is second only to the third molar in the rate of impaction and is significantly more frequently impacted than the mandibular canines.[3,4] Hence, this chapter specifies techniques related to maxillary canine, but they can possibly be applied to mandibular canines and other impacted teeth as well. When impacted, the maxillary canine necessitates multidisciplinary management among general/pediatric dentists, orthodontists, and surgeons to avoid adverse sequelae.[5]

The propensity toward the impaction of the maxillary canine has been attributed to various factors, including the tortuous eruption path by the canine between the sinus and orbit in route to the occlusal plane, local pathology, adjacent tooth dysmorphology, genetic predisposition, etc.[4,6–8] Critical to the management of canine impaction is its timely diagnosis, which is made by the correlation of characteristic clinical and radiographic findings.[9]

Once identified and diagnosed, options for the management of impacted canines include interceptive treatment by removal of deciduous teeth with judicious space maintenance, surgical exposure with orthodontic alignment, extraction, or observation.[10,11] Contemporary surgical exposure takes the form of both open and closed approaches, with consideration given to the location and degree of impaction.[12]

Indications for the Use of the Procedure

Canine impaction can lead to various potential sequelae, including cyst formation, infection, malposition, and migration of adjacent teeth; adjacent teeth root resorption; pain; and loss of arch length.[13,14] The most common complication is external root resorption of the incisors, which is often underdiagnosed and consequently improperly managed.[15] Timely diagnosis ascertained through vigilant clinical and radiographic examination also helps guide the treatment.

Clinical Exam

Initial clinical examination should include visual inspection and digital palpation of the palate and vestibule. However, according to Ericson and Kurol,[16] a canine bulge is seen in only 29% of children at 10 years of age. For this reason, lack of a bulge should not be considered pathognomonic for impaction, and additional clinical factors must be considered.

Signs of impaction of maxillary canine according to Bishara[9] include the following:

1. Delayed eruption of the permanent canine
2. Overretained deciduous canine (after age of 14 to 15 years)
3. Absence of a normal labial canine bulge along the alveolar ridge
4. Presence of a bulge on the palatal side of the alveolus
5. Distal tipping of the lateral incisor

It is possible that none of these clinical signs are present. Discovery of impacted canine based on clinical examination is relatively limited and should always be supplemented by radiographic exam.

Radiographic Exam

Radiographic imaging is an essential component in the management of canine impaction, especially when clinical signs are not evident. Radiographic evaluation of impacted teeth, including canines has experienced tremendous change in recent times, evolving from two-dimensional plain films to three-dimensional cone beam computed tomography (CBCT).

Two-Dimensional Radiography

Intraoral periapical films represented the initial application of radiography in canine impaction. The SLOB (same side lingual opposite buccal) rule (also known as Clark's rule and buccal object rule) has been traditionally utilized to derive canine location based on correlation of canine movement and change in X-ray beam angulation on successive periapical films. Ericson and Kurol cited a 90% success rate in the identification of palatal versus buccal location of an impacted canine with use of this principle.[17] Occlusal films/cephalometric films were often combined with periapical films and have traditionally served as adjuncts to further aid in localization.[14]

Each of the two-dimensional imaging modalities discussed thus far has been associated with significant limitations in accuracy, reliability, and detail.[14,17] Notwithstanding the historical prevalence of two-dimensional radiography, contemporary times have ushered in the much more widespread use of three-dimensional radiography.

Three-Dimensional Radiography

In the past, the use of computed tomography imaging was limited by cost, time, radiation exposure, and medicolegal concerns.[1,18] However, use of CBCT has only become more prevalent with contemporary decreases in radiation, cost, and other factors that once limited its application.[7] This modality is associated with much higher confidence, greater accuracy, and exact positioning[4] (Fig. 13.1A–D).

CBCT is not only better for location but also for identification of preexisting concomitant conditions such as resorption of lateral and central incisors.[15] Greater accuracy in the identification of root resorption can significantly alter comprehensive treatment planning, as excessive resorption indicates extraction and revision of treatment goals.[19] This accuracy in identification of root resorption has become increasingly prevalent over time. In 2000, Ericson estimated lateral incisor root resorption to be around 12% with the use of two-dimensional imaging, but with CBCT imaging, he found 38% of lateral incisors and 9% of central incisors had some form of resorption.[4,20,21] More recent studies have identified resorption rates as high as 74% of lateral incisors and 18% of central incisors adjacent to palatally impacted canines.[15]

Despite the improved localization and image detail of CBCT radiography, they do not warrant its application as a routine screening tool; rather, its tremendous advantages merit its use for detailed analysis and treatment planning, once impaction is suspected on clinical or routine (e.g., panoramic) screening radiographic exam.[10,22]

Selection of Procedure

Orthodontic considerations: The presence of adequate arch space for eruption of the impacted canine is a prerequisite for the procedure. The angulation and depth of impaction are important orthodontic considerations prior to choosing the treatment option as unfavorably impacted teeth would end up being difficult to reposition. To avoid periodontal defects after the eruption of the canine, the availability of adequate keratinized gingival soft tissue should be ascertained.

Following localization of the impacted canine and verification of its candidacy for exposure and orthodontic traction, various factors must be considered in determining the surgical approach for exposure.

Type of procedure: The choice of technique for surgical exposure of impacted teeth is usually based upon several criteria including:

1. Labio-palatal location of the canine
2. Coronal-apical position in relation to the mucogingival junction (MGJ)
3. Availability of attached gingiva

The basic techniques for performing the surgical exposure for further orthodontic eruption of impacted maxillary canine are gingivectomy, the apically positioned flap (APF) technique, and the closed flap technique.

Limitations and Contraindications

Although a great option to obtain desirable occlusal and esthetic results, surgical exposure of impacted canine and orthodontic eruption has some contraindications that could jeopardize the success and indicate extraction of the impacted canine. These include the following[9]:

1. Ankylosis of tooth
2. Severe root dilaceration
3. Severe retention or lack of arch space (lodged between lateral and incisor roots, horizontal placement), in which surgical uncovering and orthodontic extrusion will hold risks
4. First premolar is in the position of the canine; there is good occlusion and well aligned teeth
5. Pathological changes around the tooth (cysts, etc.)
6. Patient not willing to undergo orthodontic therapy

TECHNIQUE: Surgical Exposure of Impacted Maxillary Canine

The choice of the basic techniques for performing the surgical exposure for further orthodontic eruption of impacted maxillary canine as stated earlier can be by gingivectomy, via APF technique, or a closed flap technique (Fig. 13.2). The most appropriate technique is chosen based on clinical scenarios.

1. Gingivectomy technique can be utilized in both labial/buccal and palatal impactions when the canine cusp is coronal to MGJ with an adequate amount of keratinized gingiva and when the canine is not covered by significant amounts of bone.
2. The APF technique is most desirable in labially impacted canines and indicated when the canine crown is apical to MGJ but not too far apical where the flap cannot be sutured around the crown of the canine; the amount of attached gingiva is inadequate.

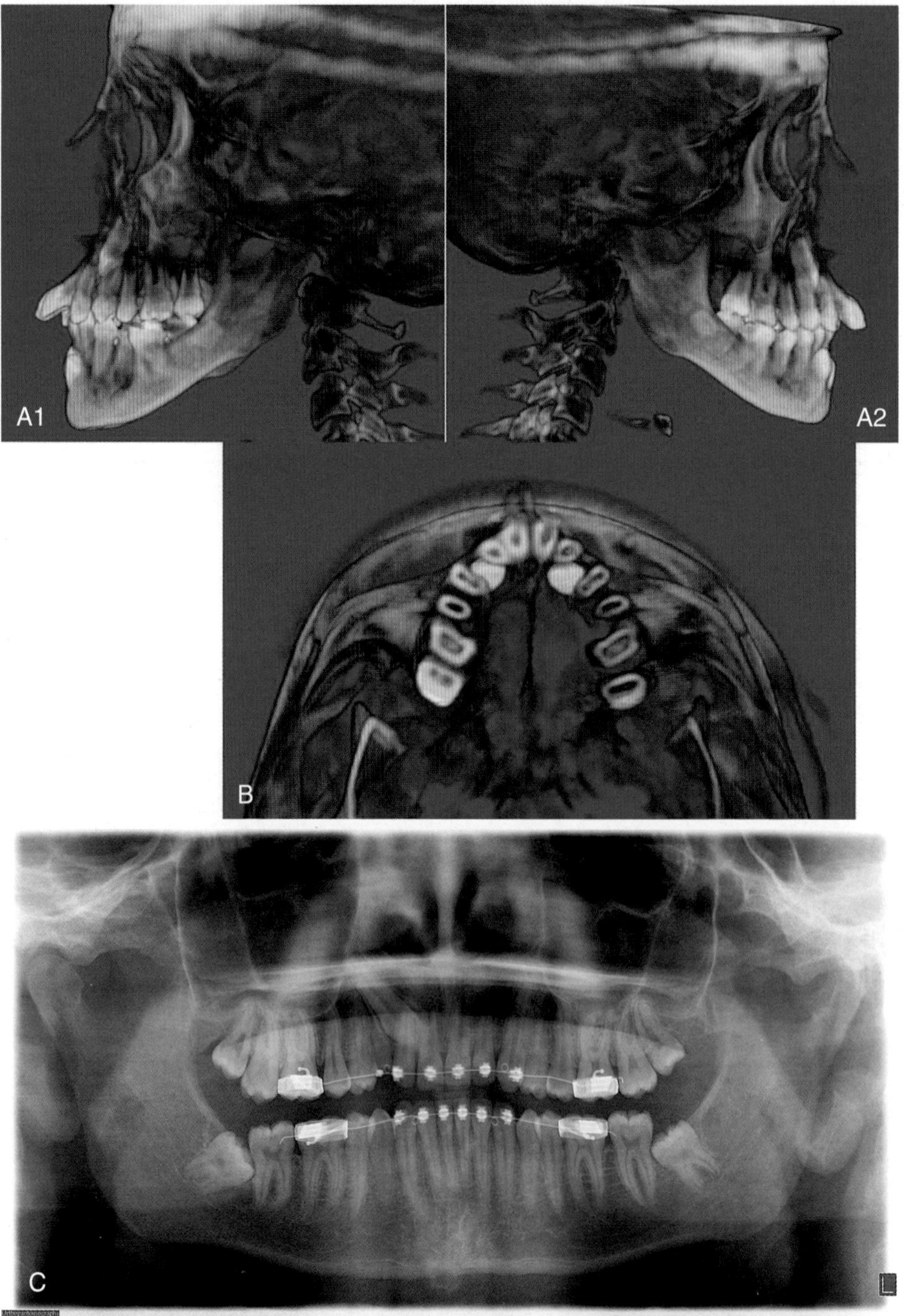

Figure 13.1 Three-dimensional reconstructions from a cone beam computed tomography (CBCT) scan showing bilateral palatally impacted canines. **A1–A2,** Right and left sagittal views. **B,** An axial cut makes localization easier. **C,** Panoramic radiographs can be utilized to localize impacted canines more successfully when combined with occlusal radiographs.

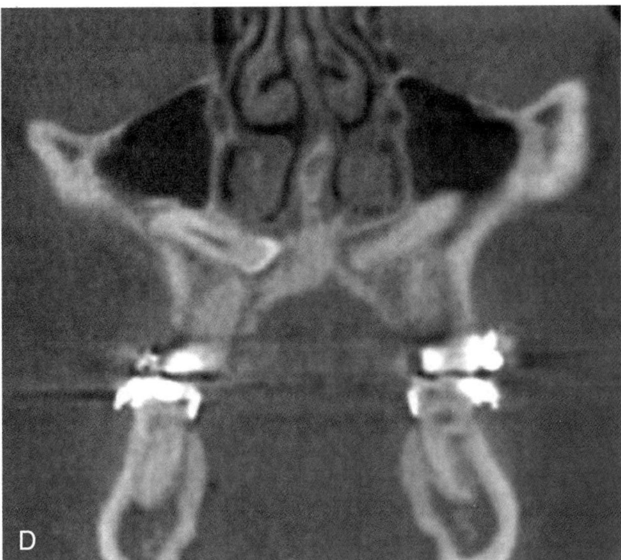

Figure 13.1, cont'd **D,** Coronal cut of CBCT showing the impacted canine with significant overlying bone and proximity with the floor of the nose. Surgical exposure would have high morbidity and low likelihood of successful orthodontic outcome. Risks and benefits must be weighed in deciding on extraction versus observation while collaborating with the orthodontist in formulating treatment decisions.

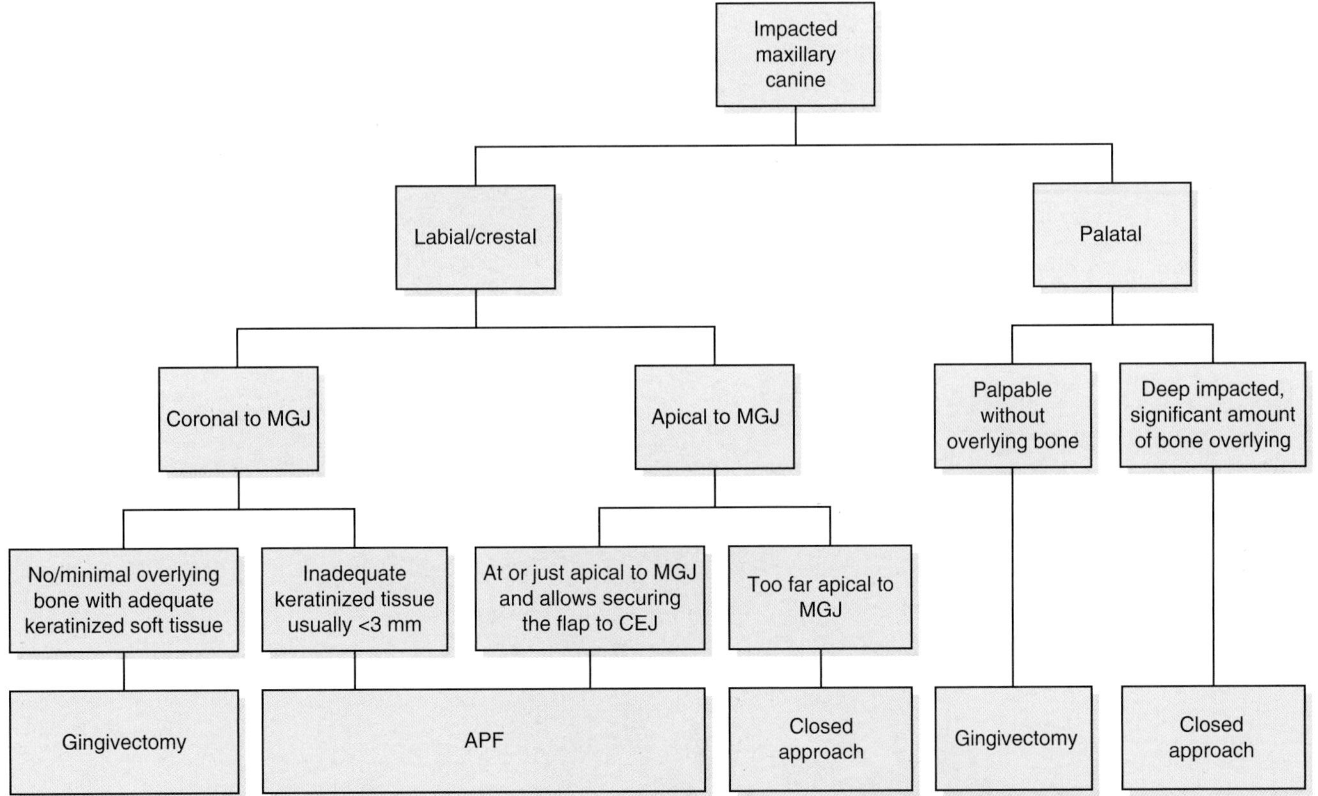

Figure 13.2 Treatment selection algorithm. Treatment selection is based on location, depth of impaction, and the amount of keratinized tissue available. *APF,* Apically positioned flap; *MGJ,* mucogingival junction.

TECHNIQUE: Surgical Exposure of Impacted Maxillary Canine—*cont'd*

3. The closed flap technique is performed in both labial and palatal impaction when the canine is high up in the alveolus and away from the MGJ.[2] In general, this technique can be performed virtually on any impacted canine or other teeth.

APF technique: (Fig 13.3A–D)

STEP 1: Incision

Examination of the area of impaction with attention to surface morphology, such as bulging, aids the surgeon in marking the extent of the incision and flap. A #15 blade is used to incise over the alveolar crest, extending to the line angle of adjacent teeth. Vertical release incisions are made beyond the MGJ to release the flap. Avoid incisions over a bony defect or the tooth crown itself, which could lead to breakdown or dehiscence with a subsequent undesirable periodontal defect.

STEP 2: Flap Elevation

A #9 periosteal elevator is used to reflect a full-thickness mucoperiosteal flap, extending from the crest to the unattached gingiva.

Continued

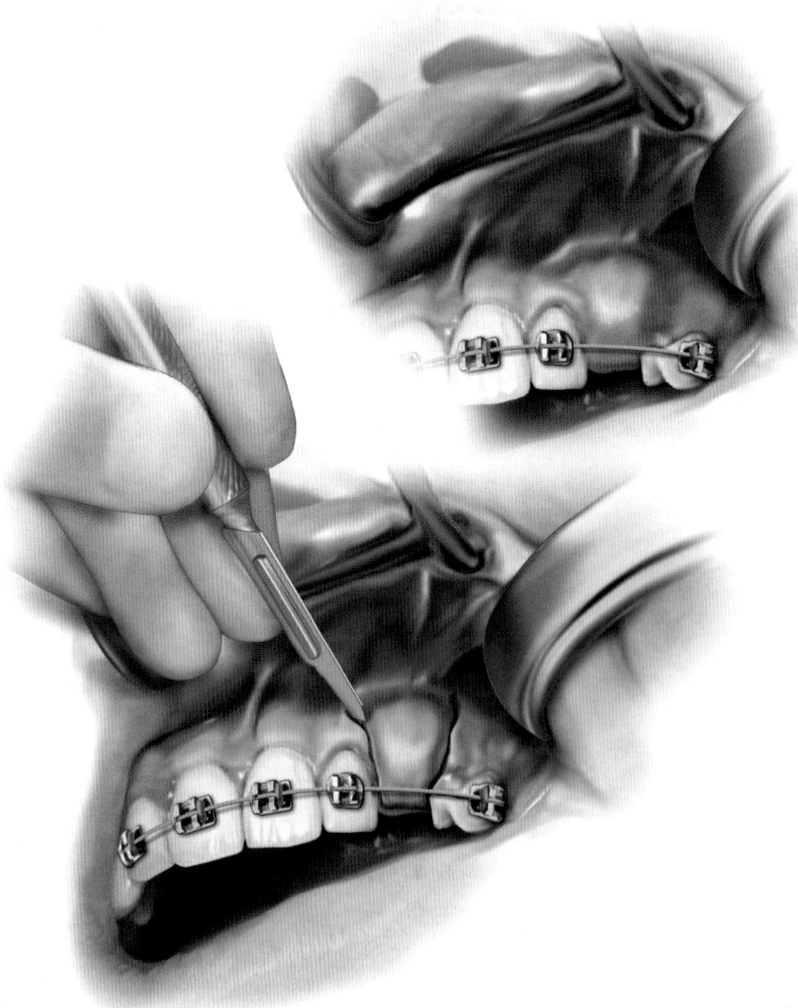

Figure 13.3 A, Incision.

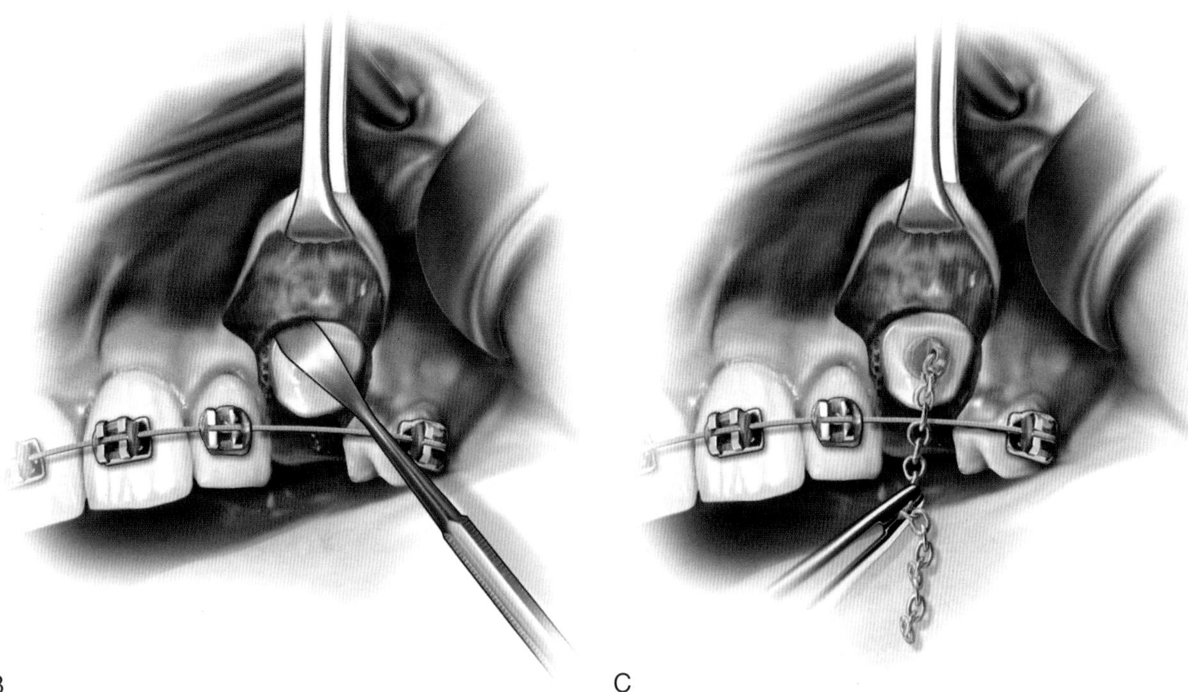

Figure 13.3, cont'd **B,** Flap elevation. **C,** Exposing the crown.

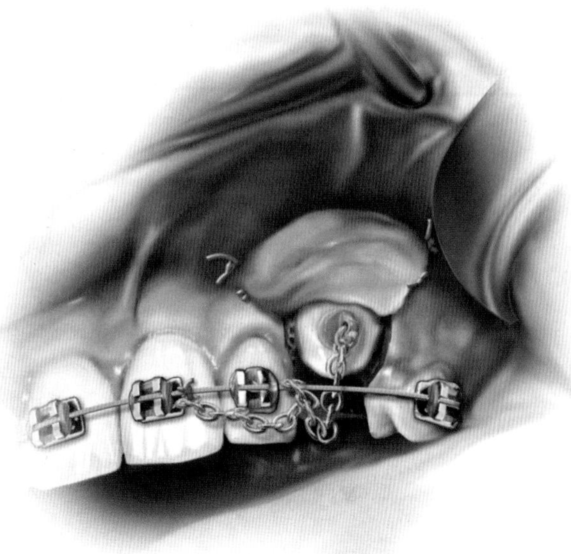

Figure 13.3, cont'd **D,** Bracket attachment and apical repositioning of the flap.

TECHNIQUE: Surgical Exposure of Impacted Maxillary Canine—*cont'd*

STEP 3: Exposing the Crown

Based on the clinical and radiographic findings, an adequate amount of coronal structure must be exposed both to bond the bracket and to allow optimal eruption of the tooth. Removal of bone around the crown can be performed with a Molt curette, rongeur, or drill. Care is taken to avoid damaging the coronal part of the tooth and to avoid exposure to or beyond the cementoenamel junction (CEJ). Bone in the path of eruption must also be removed.

STEP 4: Bracket Attachment

Once the crown has been exposed, hemostasis and isolation are performed to bond an orthodontic bracket with composite resin. Hemostasis is achieved by packing the pericoronal space with cotton pledgets soaked in local anesthetic containing epinephrine, electrocautery, radiosurgery, laser, or a combination of these modalities. Once the site is hemostatic, the bracket is bonded to the buccal side of the crown utilizing an adhesive bonding system. Bonding of the bracket is confirmed with a tug on the chain attached to the bracket.

STEP 5: Closure

The flap margin with attached gingiva is positioned at the CEJ of the impacted tooth and secured with sutures.

ALTERNATIVE TECHNIQUE 1 (WITH ONE ILLUSTRATION): Closed Technique: Buccal Impaction

STEP 1: Incision

A sulcular or crestal incision is made over the alveolar crest, extending to the line angle of adjacent teeth, with or without vertical releasing incisions.

STEP 2: Flap Elevation

A #9 periosteal elevator is used to reflect a full-thickness mucoperiosteal flap exposing the impacted tooth or associated bulge in the alveolus.

STEPS 3 AND 4: Exposure and Bonding

The crown should be exposed as previously described, and the orthodontic bracket and its associated chain are attached to the coronal tooth structure.

STEP 5: Closure

The flap is repositioned, and the incision is closed primarily with the chain extending through the flap margin.

CLOSED TECHNIQUE: Palatal Impaction (Fig 13.4A and B)

The APF is not applicable to a palatal impaction; however, there are two relevant flap-based variations when the impaction is associated with thick overlying bone or is not readily palpable. In these situations, a sulcular incision is made and a full-thickness mucoperiosteal flap is elevated on the palate. The impaction is localized by clinical and radiographic correlation. Bone overlying the impaction is removed, and the bracket is applied in the manner described previously, with the notable exception that the bracket is attached to the lingual aspect of the cusp. At this point, a window gingivectomy can be completed overlying the impaction so that the chain can be fed through the flap directly over the location of the impaction. Alternatively, the flap may be repositioned primarily and the chain may be fed through the line of closure. Passing of the chain through a window within the palatal flap has been favored by orthodontists, as it gives better control of tooth's eruptive forces. As with any form of closed flap without a window, the closed flap on the palate also has the disadvantage of having to perform reexposure in case the bracket debonds.

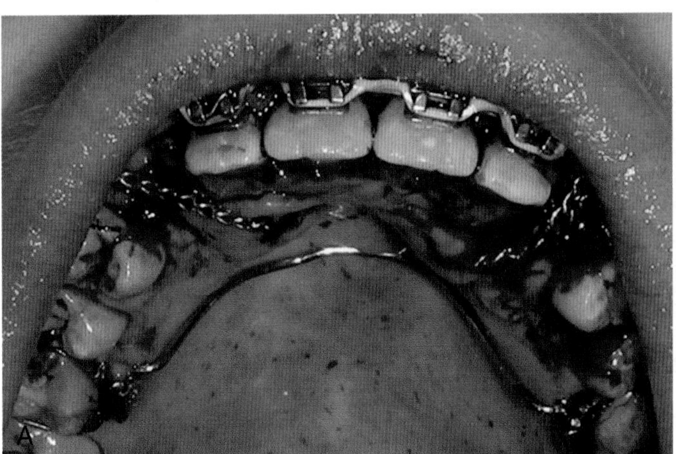

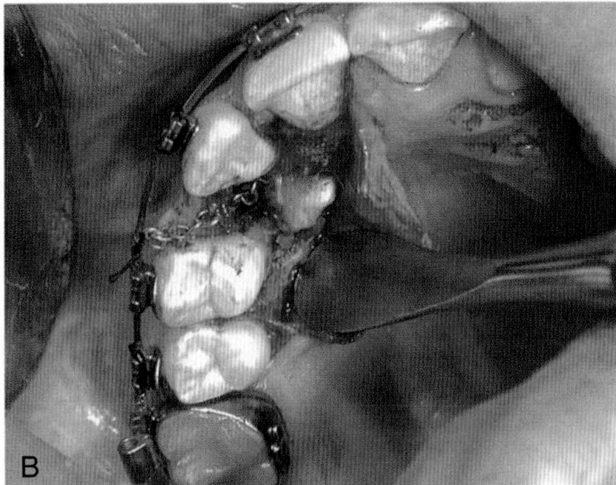

Figure 13.4 **A,** Closed technique chain fed through palatal mucosa. **B,** Closed technique with chain through incision line.

ALTERNATIVE TECHNIQUE 2: Gingivectomy Technique

In both buccal and palatal impactions, gingivectomy involves surgical exposure of the crown of an impacted tooth by removal of overlying buccal and palatal gingiva and bone. The prerequisite for success is the availability of attached gingiva, which is readily available palatally but requires scrutiny buccally. Buccally impacted canines may have a paucity of keratinized gingiva or keratinized gingiva of poor quality. In either case, an APF would result in more desirable outcome with regard to esthetics and overall periodontal support. However, if it is possible to expose the coronal portion of the tooth via gingivectomy in a manner that maintains a 2 to 3-mm band of thick, keratinized gingiva between the exposed tooth and the MGJ, the gingivectomy approach can be completed quickly and with little associated morbidity.

Avoidance and Management of Intraoperative Complications

Apart from choosing the right surgical exposure technique, the surgeon must consider several intraoperative details to obtain the best possible outcome.

1. Flap design: Inappropriate flap design can not only limit access intraoperatively but can also give rise to periodontal defects, including loss of keratinized gingiva. In both buccal and palatal impactions, crestal or sulcular incisions are recommended to stay within keratinized tissue. Placement of the incision in unattached mucosa can lead to clefting or a total lack of attached gingiva around the canine once it is pulled into position.
2. Proper hemostasis and isolation: Most bonding materials require adequate moisture control in the field while the bracket is being bonded. The absence of moisture control weakens the initial bond strength and predisposes the bracket to eventual debonding. In a closed technique setting, debonding would require further surgery to reexpose the tooth.
3. Tooth exposure: Approximately two-thirds of the crown must be exposed to obtain stable bracketing and application of orthodontic forces. Care should be taken to avoid damage to the coronal structure during bone removal and also to avoid exposure beyond the CEJ, which may cause external root resorption.

Postoperative Considerations

The postoperative considerations can be divided into two types:

1. Immediate operative considerations
   a. Oral hygiene maintenance
   b. Soft diet
   c. Postoperative pain
   d. Failure of the orthodontic bracket to bond to the tooth
   e. Surgical site infection
2. Long-term considerations
   a. Damage to the roots of adjacent teeth
   b. Failure to erupt
   c. Periodontal considerations:
      Dehiscence of the flap
      Lack of attached gingiva
   d. Devitalization of the pulp

References

1. Bedoya MM, Park JH. A review of the diagnosis and management of impacted maxillary canines. *J Am Dent Assoc.* 2009;140(12):1485–1493.
2. Felsenfeld AL, Aghaloo T. Surgical exposure of impacted teeth. *Oral Maxillofac Surg Clin North Am.* 2002;14(2):187–199.
3. Cooke J, Wang HL. Canine impactions: incidence and management. *Int J Periodontics Restorative Dent.* 2006;26(5):483–491.
4. Hamada Y, Timothius C, Shin D, John V. Canine impaction—a review of the prevalence, etiology, diagnosis and treatment. *Semin Orthod.* 2019;25:117.
5. Becker A, Chaushu S. Surgical treatment of impacted canines—what the orthodontist would like the surgeon to know. *Oral Maxillofac Surg Clin North Am.* 2015;27(3):449–458.
6. Alberto PL. Management of the impacted canine and second molar. *Oral Maxillofac Surg Clin North Am.* 2007;19(1):59–68, vi.
7. Chapokas AR, Almas K, Schincaglia GP. The impacted maxillary canine: a proposed classification for surgical exposure. *Oral Surg Oral Med Oral Pathol Oral Radiol.* 2012;113(2):222–228.
8. Peck S, Peck L, Kataja M. The palatally displaced canine as a dental anomaly of genetic origin. *Angle Orthod.* 1994;64(4):249–256.
9. Bishara SE. Clinical management of impacted maxillary canines. *Semin Orthod.* 1998;4(2):87–98.
10. Alqerban A, Jacobs R, Fieuws S, Willems G. Radiographic predictors for maxillary canine impaction. *Am J Orthod Dentofacial Orthop.* 2015;147(3):345–354.
11. Husain J, Burden D, McSherry P, Morris D, Allen M. Clinical Standards Committee of the Faculty of dental surgery, Royal College of surgeons of England. National clinical guidelines for management of the palatally ectopic maxillary canine. *Br Dent J.* 2012;213(4):171–176.
12. Sampaziotis D, Tsolakis IA, Bitsanis E, Tsolakis AI. Open versus closed surgical exposure of palatally impacted maxillary canines: comparison of the different treatment outcomes—a systematic review. *Eur J Orthod.* 2018;40(1):11–22.
13. Bishara SE. Impacted maxillary canines: a review. *Am J Orthod Dentofacial Orthop.* 1992;101(2):159–171.
14. Manne R, Gandikota C, Juvvadi SR, Rama HR, Anche S. Impacted canines: etiology, diagnosis, and orthodontic management. *J Pharm BioAllied Sci.* 2012;4(suppl 2):S234–S238.
15. Alemam AA, Abu Alhaija ES, Mortaja K, Al-Tawachi A. Incisor root resorption associated with palatally displaced maxillary canines: analysis and prediction using discriminant function analysis. *Am J Orthod Dentofacial Orthop.* 2020;157(1):80–90.
16. Ericson S, Kurol J. Longitudinal study and analysis of clinical supervision of maxillary canine eruption. *Community Dent Oral Epidemiol.* 1986;14(3):172–176.
17. Ericson S, Kurol J. Radiographic examination of ectopically erupting maxillary canines. *Am J Orthod Dentofacial Orthop.* 1987;91(6):483–492.
18. Elefteriadis JN, Athanasiou AE. Evaluation of impacted canines by means of computerized tomography. *Int J Adult Orthodon Orthognath Surg.* 1996;11(3):257–264.
19. Alqerban A, Jacobs R, Lambrechts P, Loozen G, Willems G. Root resorption of the maxillary lateral incisor caused by impacted canine: a literature review. *Clin Oral Investig.* 2009;13(3):247–255.
20. Ericson S, Kurol J. Incisor root resorptions due to ectopic maxillary canines imaged by computerized tomography: a comparative study in extracted teeth. *Angle Orthod.* 2000;70(4):276–283.
21. Ericson S, Kurol PJ. Resorption of incisors after ectopic eruption of maxillary canines: a CT study. *Angle Orthod.* 2000;70(6):415–423.
22. Alqerban A, Jacobs R, Fieuws S, Willems G. Predictors of root resorption associated with maxillary canine impaction in panoramic images. *Eur J Orthod.* 2016;38(3):292–299.

CHAPTER 14

Alveoloplasty

Stephanie Joy Drew

Armamentarium

Appropriate sutures
Bone files/rasp
Bone grafting materials/membranes
Drill with diamond burs or carbide (round and fissure)
Local anesthetic with vasoconstrictor
Osteotomes (thin curved and straight)
Piezo knife
Reciprocating saw
Rongeurs
Standard extraction setup with added instruments to aid in bone contouring

History of the Procedure

The historical use for alveoplasty was to create a smooth and wide denture base. This shape provides optimal stability for the removable prosthesis. In 1853 Willard[1] described contouring of the alveolar bone and contouring of the alveolar mucosa to obtain primary closure in preparation for denture placement. He stated that this should allow the patient to be restored sooner because the bone and tissue healed faster. In 1876 Beers[2] described radical alveolectomy with cutting forceps. This was aggressive treatment, and clinicians reverted to being more conservative over the next 50 years. The procedure was not looked on favorably because the bone underwent a tremendous amount of bone loss after the surgery. The bone loss was thought to be due to the periosteal stripping and large flaps developed to provide access for the bone contouring surgery. In 1923 Molt[3] recommended using models to plan the reshaping of the bone. His idea was to preserve bone and to maintain an appropriate vestibule.

In 1936 Dean[4] described his technique to preserve the labial cortex and contoured intraradicular bone. This allowed him to compress the labial plate. Not performing a mucoperiosteal dissection leads to less pain, swelling, and bone resorption.

In 1976 Michael and Barsoum[5] studied patients who had immediate denture placement and the amount of resorption associated with different surgical techniques, such as extraction without alveoplasty, extraction with labial alveolectomy, and extraction with intraseptal alveoplasty as described by Dean. The extractions alone had the least amount of bone loss; the labial alveoplasty had the most, even after 12 months.

The advent of implant dentistry has revolutionized the field. Now, contemporary therapy focuses on maintaining as much bone as possible to facilitate implant placement. Moreover, augmenting the alveolus for rehabilitation purposes is fairly standard procedure.

Indications for the Use of the Procedure

Reshaping of the alveolar bone has multiple indications in maxillofacial surgery. All techniques used provide resurfacing or restructuring of the alveolar bone to provide a functional skeletal relationship. The indications for alveoplasty range from debulking procedures for pathologic conditions of the bone to recontouring the bone in preparation for prosthetic rehabilitation.

Simple plasty of the alveolar bone is defined as the reshaping of the alveolar bone during dental extraction surgery. If the alveolus has a sharp edge, the bone must be smoothed down to help with the healing process and prevent sequestra formation and pain.

The contouring of the alveolus after extractions also aids in prosthetic rehabilitation, whether with dental implants or dentures. Any sharp bone projections or edges under dentures create pain when the prosthesis compresses and rubs against them. The shape of the ridges for denture fabrication should maintain as much width and adequate height as possible to distribute forces properly. Undercuts must be addressed to allow for smooth placement of the prosthesis. The goals are to lose as little bone as possible after extraction, to maintain a wide alveolar ridge with the ideal U shape, and to get rid of undercuts that prevent smooth use and placement of a removable prosthesis.

With respect to dental implant rehabilitation, the reshaping of the alveolus is done to provide a stable base for placement of the dental implants and to create enough room for the prosthetic components necessary to restore the dentition. This may require removing some of the bone, which may be counterintuitive to the protocols for creating dentures.

Limitations and Contraindications

Alveoplasty is limited by the local architecture and volume of bone in the surgical site. It is contraindicated if removing the bone would harm vital structures. It also is contraindicated if the patient does not need bone removed or recontoured.

Compression of the Alveolar Ridges

Compression is performed after extractions when the labial, buccal, and lingual or palatal plates are expanded and create undercuts. These undercuts may interfere with denture comfort. Compression is easily performed by applying finger pressure on the labial and palatal or buccal and lingual cortices to compress them together as tolerated by the tissues.

TECHNIQUE: Simple Alveoloplasty

Simple alveoloplasty can be done in conjunction with or after extraction of teeth. It is typically intended to remove sharp edges, bony prominences, or undercuts in preparation for prosthetic rehabilitation. This is a surgical technique that should be as conservative as possible (Fig. 14.1A and B).

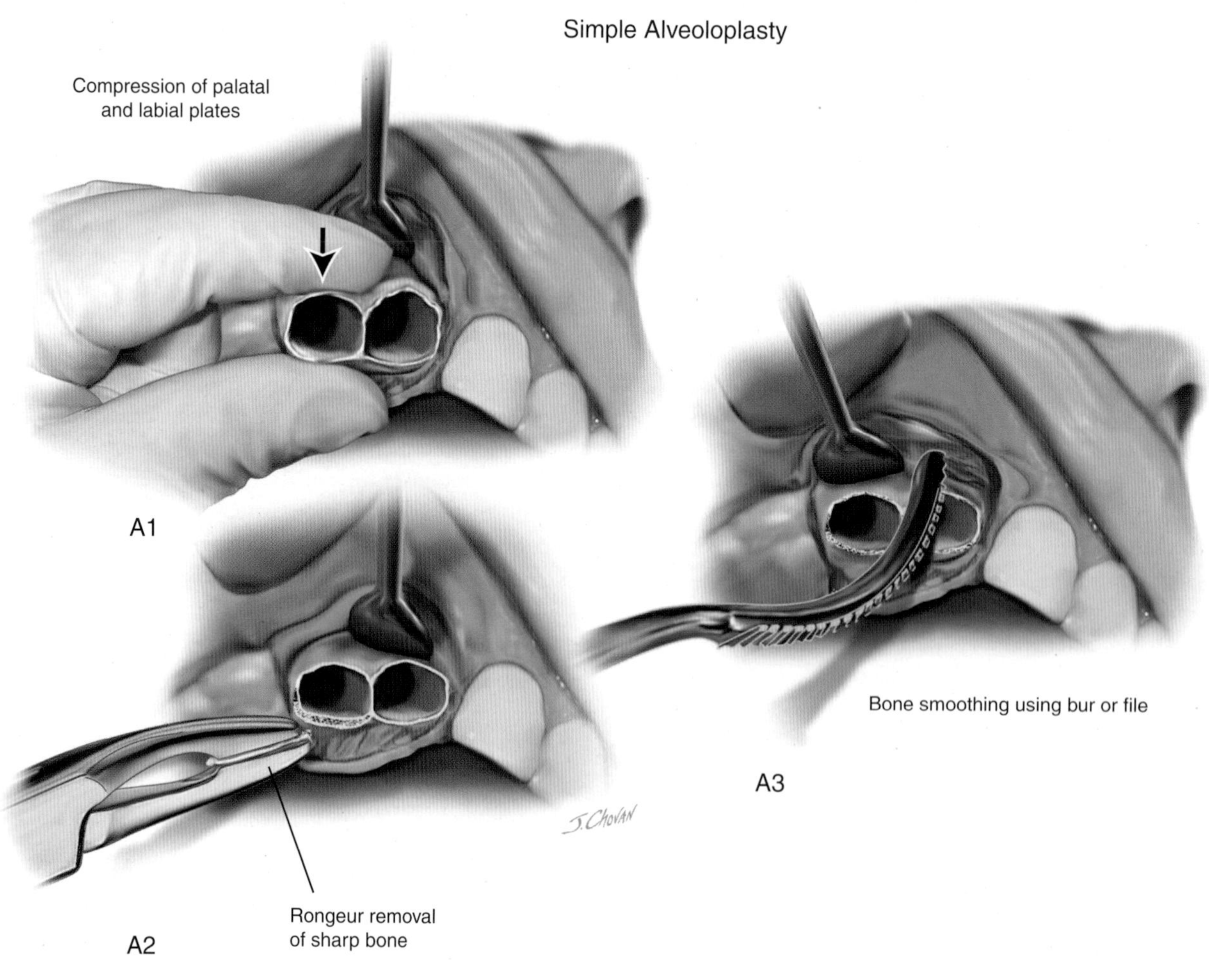

Figure 14.1 A1–A3, Simple alveoloplasty technique.

TECHNIQUE: Simple Alveoloplasty—cont'd

STEP 1: Incision

A full-thickness envelope flap is raised. The incision is made on the crest of the alveolus or in the gingival sulcus of the remaining teeth. The amount of reflection depends on how much bone needs to be exposed to complete the ostectomy. Minimal reflection may lessen postoperative edema, pain, and hematoma formation.

STEP 2: Bone Recontouring

Once the flap has been raised and bone exposed, a rongeurs, bone file, or rotary instrumentation is used to smooth or recontour the irregularity or undercut. Keep in mind that the more aggressive the removal of bone, the more resorption occurs (Fig. 14.1C and D).

STEP 3: Closure

Once the alveoloplasty has been performed, the area is irrigated thoroughly with sterile saline and then closed with sutures of choice.

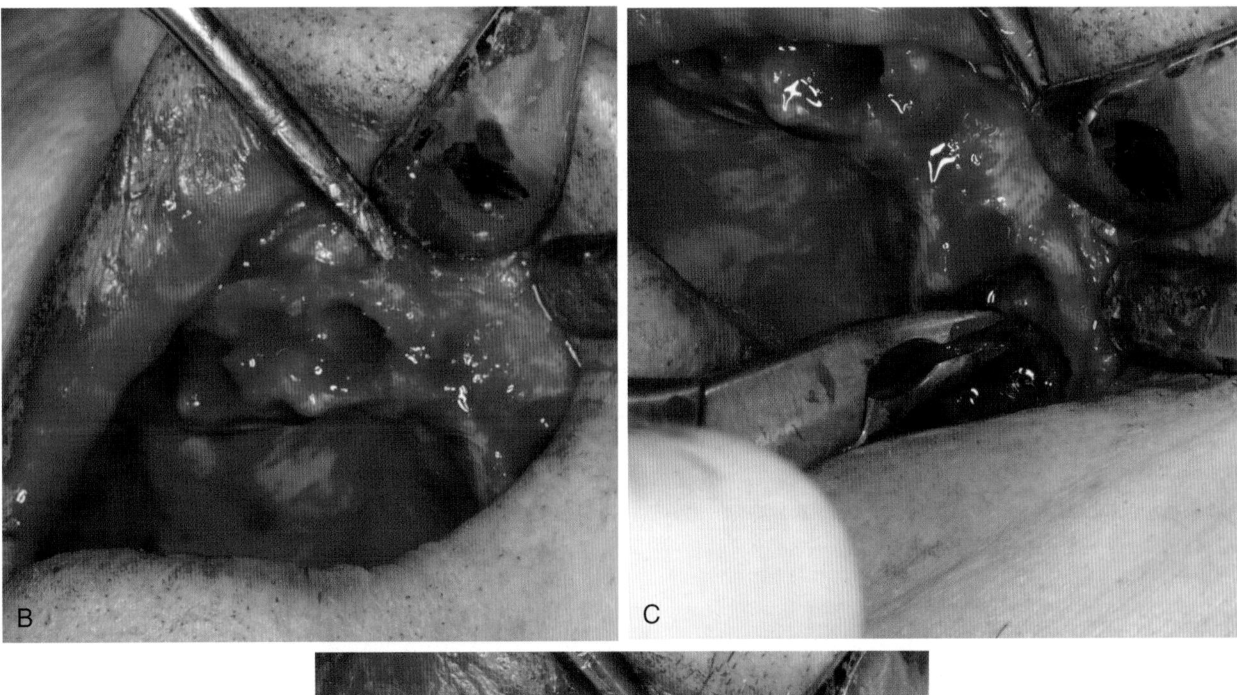

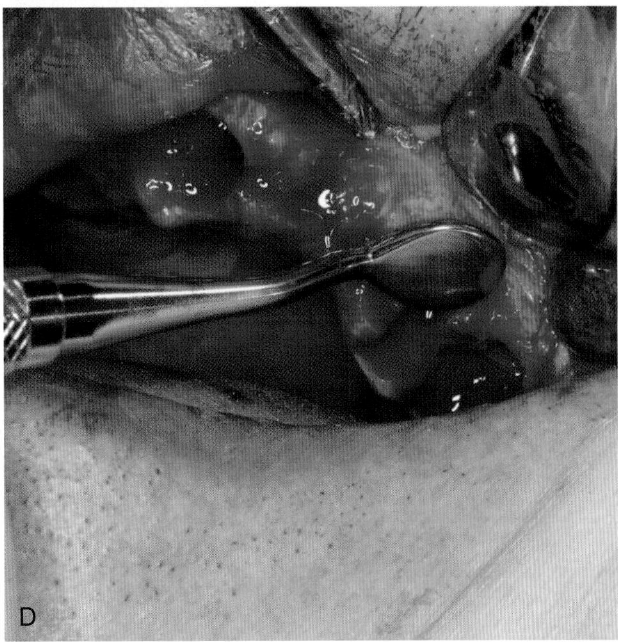

Figure 14.1, cont'd **B,** Sharp edges. **C,** Use of rongeurs. **D,** Bone file.

TECHNIQUE: Complex Maxillary Alveoloplasty/Alveolectomy

Anatomic considerations in the maxilla for reshaping of the alveolar bone include the maxillary sinus, nasal cavity/nasal floor, prominence of the canine eminences, palatal tori, and tuberosity anatomy. The incisive foramen and incisive nerve may be an issue when reshaping the anterior maxilla. The palatine vessels are also of concern in the posterior region. (Maxillary torus removal is reviewed in another chapter of the dentoalveolar section.)

Maxillary Tuberosity Reduction

Maxillary tuberosity reduction is usually soft tissue in nature due to the thick alveolar mucosa in the region. However, there are times when the issue is truly bone related. Perhaps supereruption of the dentition occurred and then the teeth were lost. Pneumatization of the sinus into the posterior maxillary alveolus may create a very thin layer of remaining bone between the oral cavity and the sinus cavity. If the tuberosity is vertically hypertrophic and needs to be removed to create interarch space for either dentures or dental implants, a panoramic film or computed tomography (CT) scan can demonstrate how much bone is left inferior to the sinus floor. This information helps guide the surgeon in making informed decisions about which technique to use to get a good result and to reduce the complication of oral antral communication.

TECHNIQUE: Soft Tissue Tuberosity Reduction

STEP 1: Incision
An elliptical incision is made on the occlusal aspect of the tuberosity, and the tissue inside the incision is removed.

STEP 2: Tissue Contouring
The tissue that surrounds the resultant defect is undermined, removing the fibrous submucosal tissue.

STEP 3: Closure
The edges of the wound are reapproximated.

TECHNIQUE: Bony Tuberosity Reduction

STEP 1: Incision
A crestal incision is made on the occlusal aspect of the tuberosity. The amount of extension of the incision depends on how much exposure is required for adequate bone removal.

STEP 2: Bone Recontouring
The desired amount of bone is removed. The amount of bone removal may be dictated by a surgical guide that was created from study models. Rotary instrumentation, a rongeurs, and a bone file may be used to remove bone.

STEP 3: Tissue Contouring
Redundant soft tissue is then trimmed, with care taken to avoid excessive removal of keratinized mucosa.

STEP 4: Closure
The area is irrigated thoroughly and closed primarily with sutures of choice.

ALTERNATIVE TECHNIQUE 1: Osteotomy With or Without Repositioning

Osteotomy with or without repositioning can be used to reposition sections of the alveolus to create better position for prosthetic rehabilitation. Alveolar vertical excess from unopposed teeth that have supraerupted and that create difficult surface topography for restoration in the maxillary posterior region can have an entire segment of the alveolus in this area repositioned superiorly with an osteotomy and rigid fixation. In this way, bone is not removed that may be needed for dental implant rehabilitation. This also creates interocclusal space needed for prosthetic components, and it can be used to reposition a segment of otherwise healthy super erupted teeth to the correct vertical position (Fig. 14.2A and B).

Incisions are created to maintain the periosteal blood supply to the segment, typically just above the mucogingival junction with a superior vertical release. Subperiosteal dissection is achieved superiorly to expose the lateral wall of the maxillary bone in the area of the planned osteotomy.

The lateral osteotomy is done with either a fine fissure bur or a piezo knife and the cuts are extended palatally from the buccal side. Care must be taken not to damage the palatal mucosa and blood supply to segments. Sometimes a small straight or curved chisel may be used.

The segment is positioned and stabilized in the correct orientation either with a surgical splint, if possible, or by hand manipulation and stabilized with rigid fixation.

Maxillary Posterior Segment

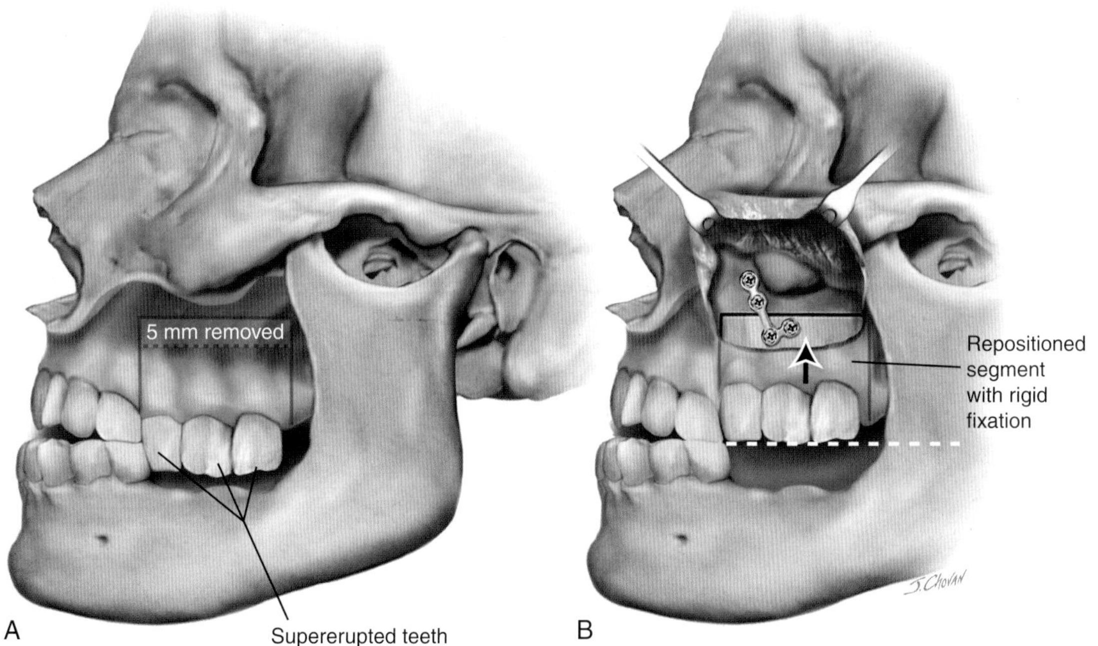

Figure 14.2 Maxillary posterior segment.

ALTERNATIVE TECHNIQUE 2: Mandibular Techniques

Most tori of the mandible are on the lingual surface by the premolar and canine region. The mucosa overlying these tori can be easily injured with function and often can be painful. The mucosa is very thin, and if a removable prosthesis is to be placed on this type of ridge, consideration should be given to smoothing down these tori before fabrication of the prosthesis. As with the maxillary torus, mandibular tori removal is discussed in another chapter of the dentoalveolar section.

Anterior Mandibular Knife Edge Ridge

Loss of the anterior mandibular teeth and eventual resorption of the alveolar bone may lead to severe thinning of the facial cortical bone to meet the lingual bone in the shape of a sharp knife edge ridge. Compression of the delicate overlying tissues creates point pressure from underneath and eventually the sharp edge cuts through the tissues, leading to ulceration and pain. Removal of this thin bone is indicated if this painful situation arises and a full or partial denture needs to be placed. If dental implants are to be considered as the prosthetic rehabilitation, this bone may be used as a wall to graft against to maintain bone height. Depending on the implant prosthesis to be made, it may also need to be removed to gain adequate interarch space for implant components. It is typically removed to the correct width needed for implant placement as measured on radiographic examination.

A crestal incision is made that preserves attached, keratinized gingiva. The tissues must be reflected in a subperiosteal fashion on the facial and lingual.

The sharp ridge is then removed with rongeurs, bur, or piezo knife. Careful planning so as not to take too much bone away is possible on newer imaging modalities, such as three-dimensional imaging or a surgical guide fabricated from study models. This information can also identify vital structures such as the mental foramen. This guides the surgeon and protects the soft tissues.

The area is irrigated, and the tissue flaps are primarily closed. Some redundant tissue may need to be removed. Care is taken to preserve as much keratinized mucosa as possible.

Ridge Splitting

Ridge splitting can be used to increase the width of the ridges for prosthetic rehabilitation. This can be done in the maxilla or mandible. Special customized distracters have also been created to gain significant width if necessary.

The incision for this technique is crestal, with minimal lateral dissection of the lateral and medial plates of bone. There has to be enough bone between the plates to split without creating lack of blood supply and further loss of bone.

Creating the Osteotomies

The least traumatic method of cutting the bone (osteotomes and/or a piezo knife) should be considered. An osteotomy is made along the crest of the ridge. At the most proximal and distal ends of the length of the superior cut, vertical cuts are made via tunneling of the soft tissues for access to the bone (Fig. 14.3A and B).

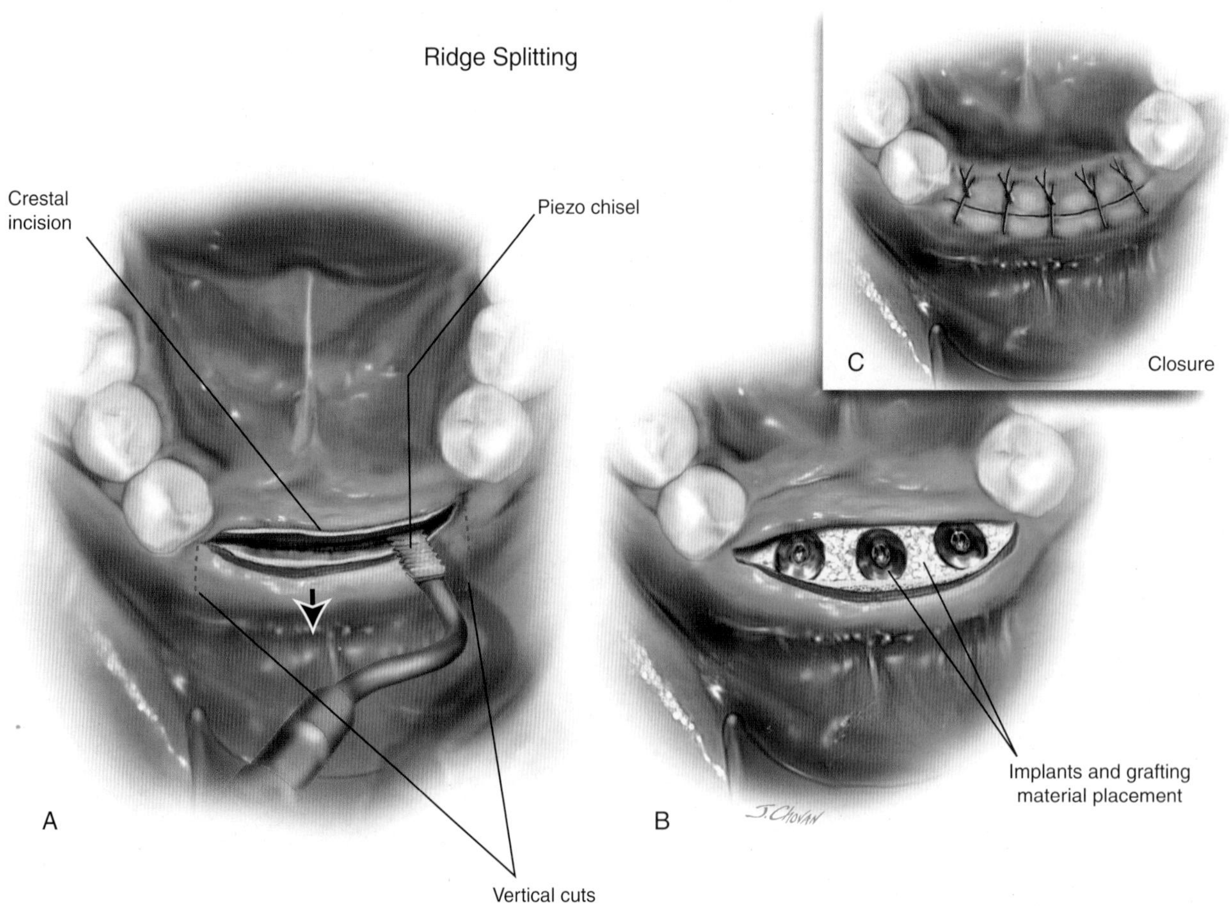

Figure 14.3 Ridge splitting.

A small osteotome is wedged and sequentially increased in size to start the separation of the plates. Once the plates have been widened, they need to be maintained; this can be done by placing a grafting material that does not absorb quickly or, if the plates are thick enough, dental implants may be placed immediately.

If a significant amount of width is needed, special distracters are available to slowly widen the plates of bone. The technique is as described; however, the distracters are placed and a latency period is observed before activation to follow the principles of alveolar distraction surgery.

Avoidance and Management of Intraoperative Complications

Intraoperative complications occur for several reasons with alveoplasty surgery. Expert command of normal surgical anatomy is essential to avoid damage to vital structures. This knowledge is also important in the evaluation of the malformed ridges of the patient in need of plasty surgery.

The position of the inferior alveolar nerve as it courses through the mandible directs the majority of decisions about recontouring the posterior portions of the mandible. Another concern is the position of the lingual nerve on the medial surface of the mandible against the alveolus, typically in the second molar region. This lingual region of bone may be sharp and thin and may need to be smoothed for denture fabrication.

In the mandible, the mental foramen is usually in a more relative superior position as the alveolus resorbs from pressure of a removable prosthesis, periodontal disease, and loss of teeth. The genial tubercles are also seen in a more superior position, as are the soft tissues of the floor of the mouth. Care must be taken to avoid Wharton's ducts of the submandibular glands and the lingual/floor of the mouth vasculature.

Muscle attachments become more superiorly positioned on the ridges in the patient who has loss in alveolar height. These may need to be repositioned with soft tissue surgery as part of the alveoloplasty procedure for preprosthetic treatment. This would be regarded as vestibuloplasty soft tissue surgery.

The maxilla has several key structures to take into account when planning surgery and avoiding complications. The nasal floor may be in close proximity with severe bone loss. If the nasal floor is perforated, this usually results in bleeding from the vascularized nasal mucosa. Simple nasal packing may be needed if it does not stop. In the midline of the palate in the anterior region, the incisive canal may be damaged if not protected during plasty surgery. If the incisive nerve must be sacrificed to help create a more stable base, the patient must be informed that the area supplied by this sensory branch will be anesthetic.

The maxillary sinuses are also potential barriers to obtaining good contour. As the bone is reshaped, the sinus may become exposed to the oral cavity. The surgeon must be prepared to handle this complication and must have the surgical skills to use adjunctive procedures, such as the buccal fat pad transfer, especially if primary closure is compromised.

Hemorrhage secondary to laceration of the greater palatine vessels or nasopalatine vessels may be possible if incisions and dissection are not carried out with care. These typically can be managed locally with injection of a local anesthetic with vasoconstrictor and compression and, if necessary, the use of cautery.

Overpreparation of the bone bed cannot be reversed easily. Careful planning with three-dimensional CT scanning and/or stone models help the surgeon plan how much bone to contour and ways to avoid vital structures. If too much bone is removed, consideration should be given to grafting with bone at the time of surgery, as long as the soft tissues are managed well and a good vascular supply remains to ensure the success of the grafting.

Postoperative Considerations

Pain, swelling, infection, and bleeding are all potential postoperative considerations with any surgery. In addition to these issues, nerve injury may occur and must be assessed if the injury is known or not evident at the time of surgery, in terms of management. Sequestra may form as a result of bone work that leaves spicules too thin to remain vascularized or pieces that come loose during surgery and get caught under the flap. These can lead to wound breakdown and infection and pain.

The timing of prosthetic rehabilitation is also important. If an immediate denture is to be delivered, the restorative dentist and/or surgeon may have to be involved to reline the prosthesis to allow for proper soft tissue healing. If dental implants are in the plan, the dentist may also have to recontour the temporary prosthesis and allow for soft tissue healing.

References

1. Willard AT. Preparing the mouth for full sets of artificial teeth. *Dent News Lett*. 1853;6:238.
2. Beers WG. Notes from practice. *Mo Dent J*. 1876;8:294.
3. Molt FF. The anesthetic and surgical problems in alveolectomy. *Dent Summ*. 1923;45:854.
4. Dean OT. Surgery for the denture patient. *J Am Dent Assoc*. 1936;23:2124.
5. Michael CG, Barsoum WM. Comparing ridge resorption with various surgical techniques in immediate dentures. *J Prosthet Dent*. 1976;35:142.

CHAPTER 15

Palatal and Lingual Torus Removal

Gregory M. Ness

Armamentarium

#1 Woodson elevator
#9 Molt periosteal elevator
#11 Scalpel blade and handle
Silk and gut sutures
Bone file
End-cutting rongeurs
Irrigation syringe and suction
Local anesthetic with vasoconstrictor
Needle holder and Dean scissors
Round or fissure burs, large acrylic bur
Straight and curved osteotomes and mallet
Straight or contraangle surgical handpiece

History of the Procedure

Palatal and mandibular lingual tori are relatively common bony outgrowths recognized since the 19th century as benign, typically incidental, findings. One of the first English-language papers describing tori was published in 1909 in the Proceedings of the Royal Society of Medicine (Surgical Section) by Rickman Godlee, who describes maxillary tori encountered by himself and dentist collaborators.[1] He refers to an earlier, detailed description in a German Festschrift commemorating Virchow's 70th birthday in 1891, and agreed with that paper by advising against torus removal in most cases. By the mid-20th century, numerous authors described the prevalence of both palatal and lingual (mandibular) tori in a variety of ethnic populations, nicely summarized by Garcia-Garcia.[2] Larger, more recent studies find tori in 10% to 50% of the population, with maxillary more common in women, and mandibular tori generally less frequent but, in most studies, more common in men.[3–6] Tori of the upper and lower jaws appear to occur together in the same patient infrequently.[6,7] Techniques for removing tori have been described in standard oral surgery textbooks since the mid-20th century and are largely unchanged, although some papers have proposed innovations such as guided surgery to address highly unusual circumstances.[8,9]

Indications for the Use of the Procedure

In most cases, palatal and lingual tori are benign, asymptomatic, and do not require removal. When a dental prosthesis will cover the palate, a large palatal torus will interfere with the prosthesis and may compromise its success. Similarly, the major connector or flange of a mandibular partial or complete denture cannot be adapted successfully to the alveolar ridge if mandibular tori are present. In these cases, tori should be removed.

In some patients, unusually large palatal tori are prone to traumatic injury to their thin mucosal covering, causing recurrent, painful ulcerations. Similarly, very large mandibular tori may either be subject to traumatic injury or, in extreme cases, interfere with tongue movement. In these situations tori are mechanical impediments to healthy oral function and should be removed.

Several authors have described techniques for the successful use of either maxillary or mandibular tori as donor sources of autogenous bone for intraoral grafting procedures.[10–13] In cases where the quantity of donor bone required matches the size of available tori, this is an attractive means to obtain the required bone from a site where bone removal may actually be advantageous to the patient.

Limitations and Contraindications

Because torus removal is almost always a routine, elective procedure, patients should be counseled in advance regarding the expected perioperative course and potential risks or complications. A clear indication should exist to justify the planned procedure. Any medical comorbidities that might complicate minor dentoalveolar surgery or its outcome should be managed to an optimized state, particularly those that might lead to excessive bleeding, reduced resistance to infection, or poor soft tissue healing. Any adjacent dentition should be healthy and demonstrate good oral hygiene before torus removal. As with all elective dentoalveolar surgery, the expected benefit of the operation should be weighed carefully against the potential risks. This is especially true in patients with serious health problems, and often it is elderly and potentially frail patients who seek torus removal as a step toward better dental prostheses.

TECHNIQUE: Palatal Torus Removal

STEP 1: Incision

Palatal tori are found in the posterior midline of the hard palate and vary widely in their size and morphology. Some are narrow in lateral dimension and elongated anteroposteriorly, and others are dome shaped. Large tori tend to be shaped in multiple lobes with varying symmetry, sometimes with deep clefts between the lobules. Often larger tori have relatively small bases and are thus somewhat pedicled at their connection to the hard palate. In all cases, the entire torus must be exposed to allow its removal. The morphology of a given torus dictates the incisions required to expose it.

The most commonly used incision design is a double-Y. A midline incision is made anteroposteriorly from a point several millimeters anterior to the margin of the torus. This full-thickness incision is carried to bone posteriorly until it reaches the most posterior visible point on the torus, or a point approximately a centimeter anterior to the hard-soft palate junction. Care should be taken to leave room for posterior releasing incisions to extend obliquely in a lateral and posterior direction from the posterior end of the midline incision without violating the soft palate. Completing these posterior releases is sometimes easier after the bulk of a large torus has been exposed or even removed. At the anterior end of the midline incision, oblique releasing incisions are extended laterally and anteriorly to end lateral to the lateral margins of the torus (Fig. 15.1A).

STEP 2: Soft Tissue Reflection

A #9 Molt periosteal elevator is used to reflect the thin overlying soft tissue from the torus. In tori with deep groves between lobes, a finer instrument such as a #1 Woodson elevator may help loosen the attachments without tearing the delicate mucosal layer. Usually the soft tissue is adherent in the surrounding clefts and grooves but covers the smooth surface of the torus loosely, allowing easy reflection of the full-thickness mucoperiosteal flap from the surface of the torus itself (Fig. 15.1B).

STEP 3: Ensure Full Exposure of the Torus

If the torus is large, it may be difficult to see and access its posterior margin. In such cases, subperiosteal dissection is carried along both lateral aspects of the torus working posteriorly, exposing a narrow margin of adjacent palatal bone. As the posterior margin of the torus is approached, the posterior releasing incisions, if not already made, may be created or extended as necessary to allow tension-free dissection around the posterolateral corners of the torus. A Seldin or similar retractor may be used to hold the laterally based soft tissue flaps away from the torus, or, if desired, the flaps may be sutured open by securing them to the alveolar mucosa with silk sutures (Fig. 15.1C).

STEP 4: Section the Torus

For larger or multilobar tori, a narrow fissure bur is used under irrigation to cut grooves into the torus, separating it into discrete segments. It is convenient to follow the clefts between lobes with the bur when these exist, although it may be necessary to further subdivide a large lobe by bisecting it. Anteroposterior osteotomies are easier to make than transverse ones, unless a contraangle surgical handpiece is used. A transverse osteotomy will be angled obliquely toward the posterior rather than perpendicular to the palate if made with a straight handpiece. The angle will depend on the access afforded by the patient's mouth opening and anterior dentition. In all cases, care must be taken to avoid cutting too deeply and scoring or cutting through the hard palate itself (Fig. 15.1D).

STEP 5: Create a Cleavage Plane

A fissure bur is used to create a horizontal osteotomy at the base of the anterior sections of the torus, typically to a depth of several millimeters. The osteotomy forms the beginning of a cleavage plane along which the section will be separated from the underlying palatal bone. Care must be taken to complete the osteotomy laterally through any cortical bone attaching the torus to the palate and to ensure that the deep part of the osteotomy remains superficial to the plane of the palatal bone. This is critical to avoid inadvertent removal of a full-thickness section of the hard palate with the torus segment, thus creating a communication into the nasal cavity.

The risk of cutting into the palate increases as the osteotomy is deepened because the straight handpiece must approach the palate from the anterior at an oblique angle. Thus, the surgeon's inclination to deepen the osteotomy with the handpiece in order to further reduce the segment's bony attachment to the palate must be tempered by awareness of the superior depth of the tip of the bur within the osteotomy (Fig. 15.1E).

STEP 6: Remove the Sections

An osteotome and mallet are used to cleave the segments from the hard palate, starting from the anterior and working posteriorly. When possible, an osteotome that is slightly wider than the segment can help avoid perforation of the palate as its corners can "ride" along the margin of cortical bone adjacent to the segment's base.

As each row of segments is removed, the newly exposed base of the next posterior segment is grooved as described in step 5. In central portions of a large torus that lack cortical walls, it may be possible to omit this step and proceed to removing the segment with the osteotome alone or by using a rongeur. If the rongeur is used, care must be taken to avoid excessive twisting force that may break the palatal bone and leave a perforation. In other cases where the palatal shelf bone is thin, fractured, or already partially perforated, the surgeon may elect to complete segment removal by reducing unstable segments with a bur, thereby avoiding stress on the palatal bone and further perforation (Fig. 15.1F).

TECHNIQUE: Palatal Torus Removal—cont'd

STEP 7: Smooth the Palatal Surface and Close

An acrylic bur under irrigation, a rongeur, or a bone file is used to smooth the residual bony surface once all segments of the torus have been removed. The wound is then thoroughly irrigated and the palatal soft tissue is replaced. Large tori may leave redundant soft tissue that is very thin along the flap margins, and this may be judiciously trimmed. If the flaps are reduced, the thinner margins should be sacrificed but the surgeon must avoid overreduction and consequent tension in the closure (Fig. 15.1G).

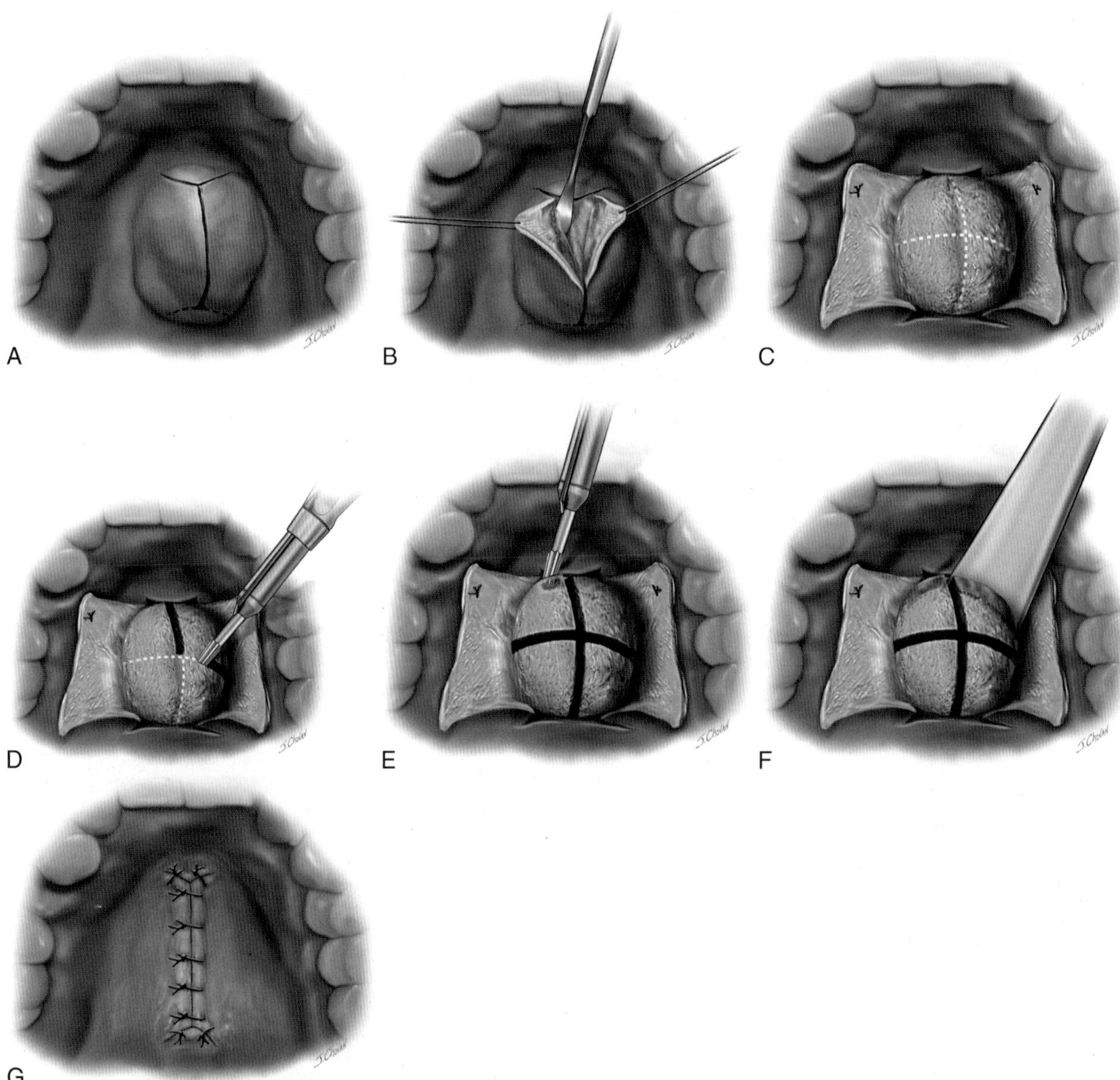

Figure 15.1 **A,** A Y-shaped incision is made as indicated to expose the torus. Dashed lines indicate posterior releasing incisions, which, for large tori, may be deferred until the torus is exposed or even removed. **B,** A periosteal elevator is used to create full-thickness flaps exposing the torus. **C,** The torus is exposed and, if helpful, the flaps secured laterally with sutures. **D,** The torus is sectioned using a surgical drill. **E,** The drill is then used to create a cleavage plane at the base of the torus, unless the torus is strongly pedunculated. **F,** A curved osteotome is used to separate the segments of torus from the bony palate. **G,** After smoothing the palatal bone and irrigation, the wound is closed with resorbable suture.

ALTERNATIVE TECHNIQUE 1: Reduction of Small Palatal Tori

If a palatal torus is dome shaped but formed in a single small lobule, it may be cleaved off in one single segment as described in steps 5 and 6. However, small, flat tori do not require sectioning or cleavage with an osteotome. Instead, they may be reduced as necessary with an acrylic bur under copious irrigation (Fig. 15.2).

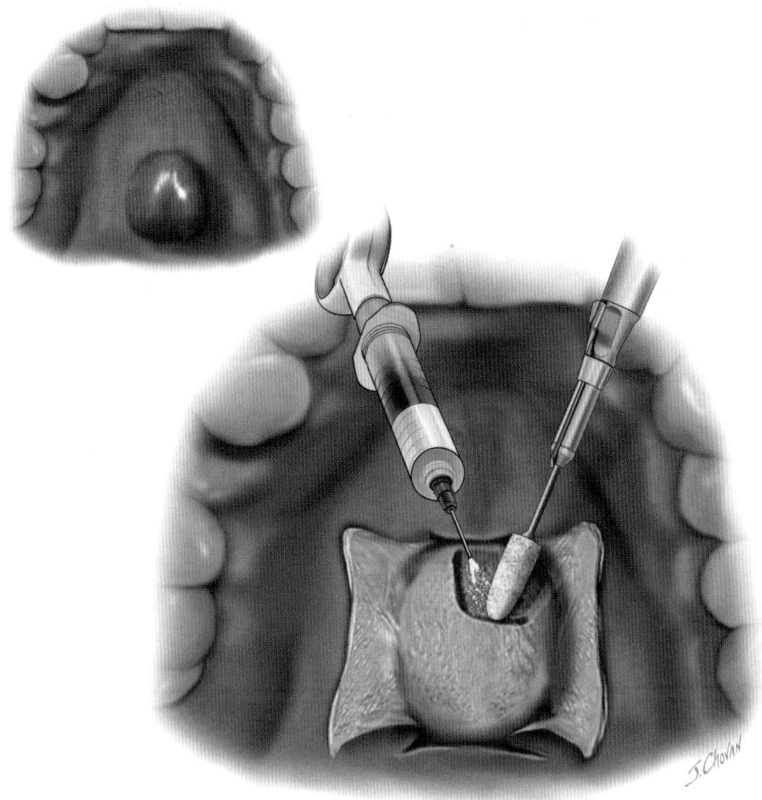

Figure 15.2 A small palatal torus may be removed with a large round or pear-shaped bur.

ALTERNATIVE TECHNIQUE 2: Palatal Splint for Postoperative Care

Many surgeons use a custom acrylic splint to cover the palate during the early postoperative period. The most common means of fabrication is to make a preoperative model of the patient's maxilla, then grind away the torus to the anticipated postoperative contour. It is better to under-reduce the model. A thick material vacuform or processed acrylic baseplate is then fabricated. After wound closure, the baseplate is lined with a self-curing soft tissue conditioning material, inserted into place, and trimmed of excess once it has set. The liner allows close adaptation to the surgical site, holding the flaps in place securely. It also usually makes the plate retentive during the short period of its use (1 to 2 weeks). Advocates claim reduced pain and fewer wound dehiscences using this technique.

TECHNIQUE: Lingual Torus Removal

STEP 1: Incision

Lingual tori are found on the alveolar ridge lingual to the mandibular canine and premolar area and vary dramatically in size and morphology. Some are flat and broad-based, and others are lobular and pedicled. Large lingual tori tend to be multilobular and occur in a strand, sometimes appearing to be stacked on one another, creating a horizontal shelf projecting medially from the alveolus. Other tori have small, pedicled bases except at their sides, where they have grown into congruence with adjacent lobules. For effective removal, the entire torus complex must be exposed.

An intrasulcular incision without release is created from near the lingual mandibular midline and extended to a point approximately 1 cm beyond the posterior extent of the tori. In edentulous patients, the incision is made on the crest of the alveolar ridge. If bilateral tori are to be removed in the same operation, the incision will extend around the dental arch to expose the opposite side in the same way. Although it is desirable to leave the midline soft tissue attached, this may be impractical in bilateral cases. A full-thickness mucoperiosteal flap is usually easily elevated with a Molt or Woodson elevator once the dissection is carried a few millimeters from the teeth to the crest of the ridge. To simplify this dissection further, especially when soft tissue forms a tightly bound collar around small, pedicled tori, local anesthetic may be injected directly under the periosteum at the torus base to balloon the tissue slightly (Fig. 15.3A).

STEP 2: Ensure Full Exposure of the Torus

If the tori are large, it may be difficult to see and access the inferior margin of the torus. A thin and somewhat friable layer of periosteum may remain attached inferiorly, but not easily seen or felt with an elevator. The lingual surface of the mandible curves outward and may be awkward to reach with an elevator, especially with large tori or when near the midline. Careful dissection at the initial exposure will reduce the risk of trauma to the mucosa or floor of the mouth later. In some cases it may be difficult to reach this inferior soft tissue attachment until the torus segment is mobile and it can be gently rotated and lifted superiorly to better access its inferior lingual surface.

A Seldin or similar retractor may be used to hold the soft tissue flaps and tongue medially, away from the tori. A Minnesota retractor may be more effective if the wound is larger (Fig. 15.3B).

STEP 3: Create a Cleavage Plane

Small, pedicled tori may be removed with an acrylic bur placed at their bases. Small but wide-based tori are easily reduced with a bur under irrigation. For larger tori, a fissure bur is used to create a vertical osteotomy at the junction of the tori and the alveolar bone, typically to a depth of several millimeters or more. The osteotomy forms the beginning of a cleavage plane along which the tori will be separated from the underlying mandible. When tori are pedicled, this osteotomy will follow the cleft already present, but for broader-based tori the surgeon must determine a plane that achieves the necessary exostosis reduction but leaves sufficient thickness of lingual cortex, especially when adjacent teeth are present. Care must also be taken to complete the osteotomy anteriorly and posteriorly through any cortical bone attaching a torus to the mandible. Furthermore, the osteotomy must be angled so that it parallels the native surface of the alveolus and lingual mandible. Often the best place to judge this angle is at the anterior margin of the tori, where the underlying alveolar contour may be visible. However, this can be difficult to judge in patients with larger or more anterior tori (Fig. 15.3C).

STEP 4: Remove the Tori

An osteotome and mallet are used to split the tori from the mandible by placing the osteotome in the groove just created and striking it with a mallet while an assistant supports the mandible from below. The osteotome should be directed along the plane of the intended split. Either a curved or a straight osteotome may be appropriate, depending on access to the site in individual patients.

When the cleavage plane has been established properly and the osteotome is directed along the correct angle, a bony fragment will split from the mandible which often includes the tori and a thin, tapering partial layer of cortical bone extending farther inferiorly. When this happens it usually creates an ideal lingual contour requiring little additional reduction of bone. Care must be taken when the fragment initially splits because it may still be tethered to the floor of the mouth by a periosteal attachment to this bone, as noted previously. If the fragment does not easily lift out of the wound without resistance, this periosteal attachment must be carefully dissected free to avoid unnecessary soft tissue trauma and swelling (Fig. 15.3D).

STEP 5: Smooth the Lingual Surface and Close

A bone file is often all that is necessary to smooth the residual bony surface once all segments of the torus have been removed. If larger bony prominences remain, an acrylic bur under irrigation is usually the best instrument for their removal, as rongeurs are often inadequate for reducing very dense, broad-based bony surfaces. It is not always necessary to remove every remnant of bony prominence if the prosthetic needs of the operation have been achieved, nor is it a goal to eliminate all undercuts from the lingual surface of the mandible. The wound is thoroughly irrigated, taking care to flush and suction clean the deepest part, and the soft tissue is repositioned and sutured. Edentulous areas may be closed with a running 3-0 plain or chromic gut suture, and circumdental sutures are effective in areas adjacent to teeth. Although not common, perforations in the flap may require closure separately. Generally, it is not necessary or advisable to attempt reduction of the redundant tissue that covered the tori (Fig. 15.3E).

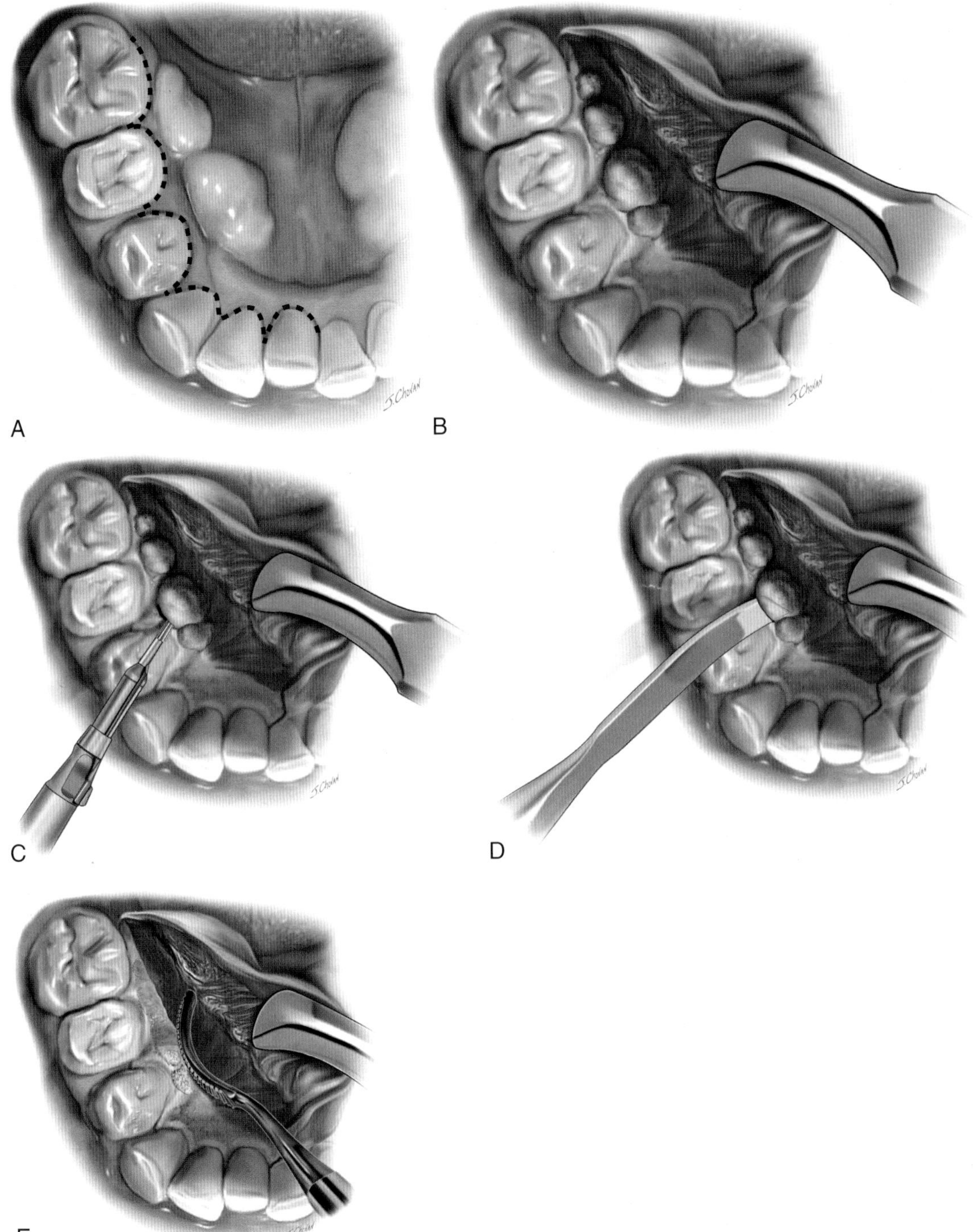

Figure 15.3 **A,** A sulcular incision is made as shown. **B,** The thin, soft tissue flap is carefully reflected to expose the tori. **C,** If necessary, a cleavage plane is established by cutting a groove along the superior border of the tori. **D,** An osteotome and mallet are used to separate the tori from the lingual alveolar bone. **E,** A pear-shaped bur is used as necessary to further reduce any sharp bony edges or prominent "plateaus" of tori remnants.

Avoidance and Management of Intraoperative Complications

Intraoperative complications from torus removal are uncommon. In the palate, inadvertent perforation of the palatal bone may occur. This will heal without difficulty provided that the overlying mucosa remains intact. If it does not, it may lead to a persistent oronasal fistula requiring delayed surgical repair. When the bone is perforated, care should be taken to make a secure, tension-free closure of soft tissue over the bony defect, even at the expense of rotating tissue to cover it and leaving a denuded patch elsewhere to heal by secondary intent.

In the mandible, the bleeding from within the surgical wound is generally minimal, but inadvertent perforation into the tissues of the floor of the mouth may generate bleeding in that tissue. Patients with bleeding tendencies who have lingual tori removed should be observed for floor of mouth swelling, potentially indicating an expanding hematoma, before they are discharged.

Postoperative Considerations

Postoperative complications arising from torus removal tend to parallel those seen with other forms of dentoalveolar surgery. Infection and serious bleeding are rare. Both lingual and palatal tori are often covered with very thin mucosa, which is friable and prone to dehiscence in the early postoperative period, if not during the procedure. Attempts to close a breakdown in this tissue are usually not warranted and may actually increase the size of the new wound. The patient may cleanse the area gently once or twice a day with a cotton swab moistened with half-strength peroxide or chlorhexidine mouth rinse.

References

1. Godlee RJ. The torus palatinus. *Proc R Soc Med (Surg Sect)*. 1909;2:175.
2. García-García AS, Martínez-González JM, Gómez-Font R, Soto-Rivadeneira A, Oviedo-Roldán L. Current status of the torus palatinus and torus mandibularis. *Med Oral Patol Oral Cir Bucal*. 2010;15(2):e353–e360.
3. Chohayeb AA, Volpe AR. Occurrence of torus palatinus and mandibularis among women of different ethnic groups. *Am J Dent*. 2001;14(5):278–280.
4. Shah DS, Sanghavi SJ, Chawda JD, Shah RM. Prevalence of torus palatinus and torus mandibularis in 1000 patients. *Indian J Dent Res*. 1992;3(4):107–110.
5. Haugen LK. Palatine and mandibular tori. A morphologic study in the current Norwegian population. *Acta Odontol Scand*. 1992;50(2):65–77.
6. Jainkittivong A, Langlais RP. Buccal and palatal exostoses: prevalence and concurrence with tori. *Oral Surg Oral Med Oral Pathol Oral Radiol Endod*. 2000;90(1):48–53.
7. Eggen S, Natvig B. Concurrence of torus mandibularis and torus palatinus. *Scand J Dent Res*. 1994;102(1):60–63.
8. Rocca JP, Raybaud H, Merigo E, et al. Er:YAG laser: a new technical approach to remove torus palatinus and torus mandibularis. *Case Rep Dent*. 2012;2012:487802..
9. de Carvalho RW, de Carvalho Bezerra Falcão PG, Antunes AA, de Luna Campos GJ, do Egito Vasconcelos BC. Guided surgery in unusual palatal torus. *J Craniofac Surg*. 2012;23(2):609–611.
10. Hassan KS, Alagl AS, Abdel-Hady A. Torus mandibularis bone chips combined with platelet rich plasma gel for treatment of intrabony osseous defects: clinical and radiographic evaluation. *Int J Oral Maxillofac Implants*. 2012;41(12):1519–1526.
11. Moraes Junior EF, Damante CA, Araujo SR. Torus palatinus: a graft option for alveolar ridge reconstruction. *Int J Periodontics Restorative Dent*. 2010;30(3):283–289.
12. Proussaefs P. Clinical and histologic evaluation of the use of mandibular tori as donor site for mandibular block autografts: report of three cases. *Int J Periodontics Restorative Dent*. 2006;26(1):43–51.
13. Ganz SD. Mandibular tori as a source for onlay bone graft augmentation: a surgical procedure. *Pract Periodontics Aesthet Dent*. 1997;9(9):973–982.

CHAPTER 16

Apicoectomy

Peter B. Franco, Luke C. Soletic, and Vasiliki Karlis

Armamentarium

#9 Molt periosteal elevator
#15 Scalpel blade
Amalgam applicator
Amalgam condenser
Appropriate sutures
Dental explorer
Gauze/cotton rolls/cotton pellets
Laser (optional)
Local anesthetic with vasoconstrictor
Needle holder
Periapical dental curette
Periodontal probe with 1-mm markings
Retractors
Retrograde filling material of choice
Saline and syringe for irrigation purposes
Scalpel handle
Scissors
Small, curved hemostat
Surgical burs: fissure and round
Surgical handpiece
Ultrasonic device with retrotips (optional)

History of the Procedure

Attempts have been made since the 1880s to remove the infected section of the root of a tooth and leave the remaining portion in the oral cavity.[1,2] Complete bone regeneration within previously infected periapical areas was demonstrated histologically in 1930.[3] Techniques referred to as "retrograde filling," "retrofill," or "retroseal" began to appear in the literature in the mid-20th century.[4,5] These terms can be defined as the resection and preparation of the root tip and insertion of a root-end filling in the prepared cavity while leaving the main portion of the tooth intact. Surgical endodontic success rates have dramatically improved over the years due to the development of new retrofilling materials and the increased use of ultrasonic preparation of the retrograde site. Periradicular surgery success rates had previously been documented at 60% to 70%, but these modern developments have since facilitated success rates over 90%.[6,7,8]

Indications for the Procedure

There are two main indications for apicoectomy in selected teeth.[9,10] The first category comprises teeth with active periapical pathology following adequate endodontic therapy. These are teeth with unresolved periapical lesions or that continue to be symptomatic following clinically sound conventional orthograde endodontic therapy (Figs. 16.1 and 16.2). As a common example in this situation, true periapical cysts generally do not resolve despite adequate orthograde endodontic therapy; therefore, they also require apicoectomy for resolution.[8]

The second category of teeth indicated for apicoectomy consists of those with active periapical pathology following inadequate endodontic therapy that cannot be retreated because of one or more of the following factors:

- Severely curved root(s)
- Presence of a post and core restoration
- Silver point filling
- Broken instrument in canal (i.e., file)
- Fracture at the apical third of the root
- Perforation of the apex
- Calcified canals

Prognostically, teeth without preoperative pain or acute inflammatory signs, with dense root canal obturations, and periapical lesions of 5 mm or less are associated with significantly higher postapicoectomy healing rates. Anterior teeth, both maxillary and mandibular, have demonstrated significantly higher healing rates than posterior teeth. Evidence has shown mandibular molars to have the lowest healing rates.[11]

Limitations and Contraindications

There are several contraindications to periradicular surgery. One such contraindication is teeth with short roots—the apicoectomy procedure reduces root length, potentially leading to an inadequate crown-to-root ratio and ultimately to early failure.

Another contraindication to apicoectomy is a tooth with a root that is inaccessible secondary to adjacent anatomic structures, such as the maxillary sinus, inferior alveolar nerve, mental nerve, greater palatine foramen, and incisive foramen. Teeth that are periodontally or restoratively hopeless are also not suitable for periradicular surgery. Appropriate caution should be given to medical comorbidities, as well as a history of antiresorptive medications.

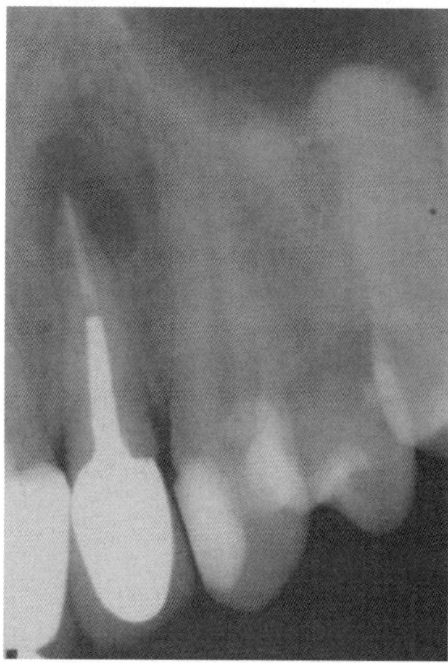

Figure 16.1 Periapical radiograph of tooth #10 showing sound endodontic therapy and well-fabricated restorative work. However, the presence of active periapical pathology is an indication for retrograde apicoectomy.

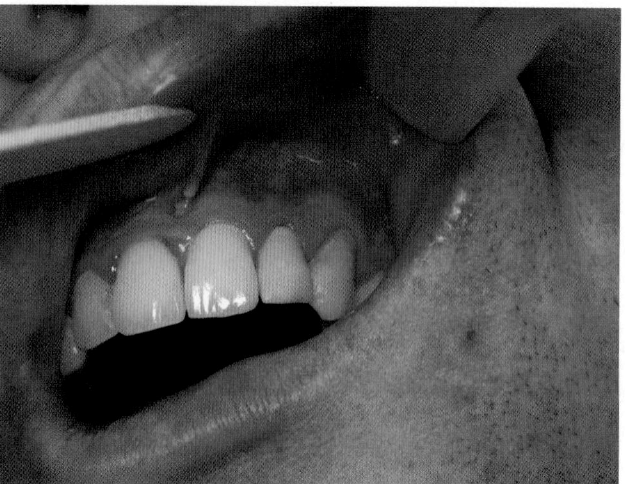

Figure 16.2 Clinical photograph of the patient from Figure 16.1, ready for the start of the surgical procedure.

TECHNIQUE: Apicoectomy

INCISION DESIGN

A surgical plan should be prepared before the initial incision is made. The design of the incision depends on several factors, including the tooth's position in the arch, the presence of fixed prosthodontic restorations, the extent of the periapical lesion, and gingival recession.

Several incision designs are commonly used to perform an apicoectomy. The first is the semilunar flap (Fig. 16.3A), which is traditionally used in the anterior maxilla. It is a crescent-shaped flap with the concave portion of the incision oriented cervically. As a caveat, accurate location of the root apex must be known for this incision to be successful. Wound-healing problems have been reported as a drawback of this incision; therefore, the incision must be made such that the closure is over intact bone.[12]

Another incision design is the sulcular flap (Fig. 16.3B). The incision is made in the gingival sulcus one tooth anterior to the tooth undergoing apicoectomy and is carried to one tooth posteriorly. After creation of the sulcular incision, one (or two) releasing incision is made at a slightly oblique angle so that the base of the flap is wider than the apex. These releasing incisions are made at the distal line angles of the two teeth immediately adjacent to the tooth in question to preserve the adjacent dental papilla. This is the incision design of choice if the surgeon is unsure of the exact location of the tooth apex, if there is a large periapical lesion, or if the patient requires bone grafting in the area. A disadvantage of the sulcular flap is gingival recession, which can be particularly unaesthetic in the region of the anterior maxilla, especially in dentition with fixed prostheses.[12]

The goal of minimizing postoperative recession has had increasing influence on incision design in the past two decades, particularly in the aesthetic zone. One such technique is the submarginal flap (Fig. 16.3C), which avoids reflection of the papilla and coronal portion of the gingiva. A horizontal incision is made no less than 2 mm from the sulcus of the included teeth, and a releasing incision is made mesially and distally. The submarginal flap is suitable for use in areas of gingival recession, as it can help minimize further recession.[13] Care must be taken not to place the incision within the free gingiva, which can worsen postoperative recession and cause interproximal papilla necrosis. The papilla base incision is a similar technique that can also be utilized in the aesthetic zone, which also avoids reflection of the papillae.[14]

After completion of any of the incisions just described, a full-thickness mucoperiosteal flap is raised (Fig. 16.3D), exposing the alveolar bone overlying the tooth's apex.

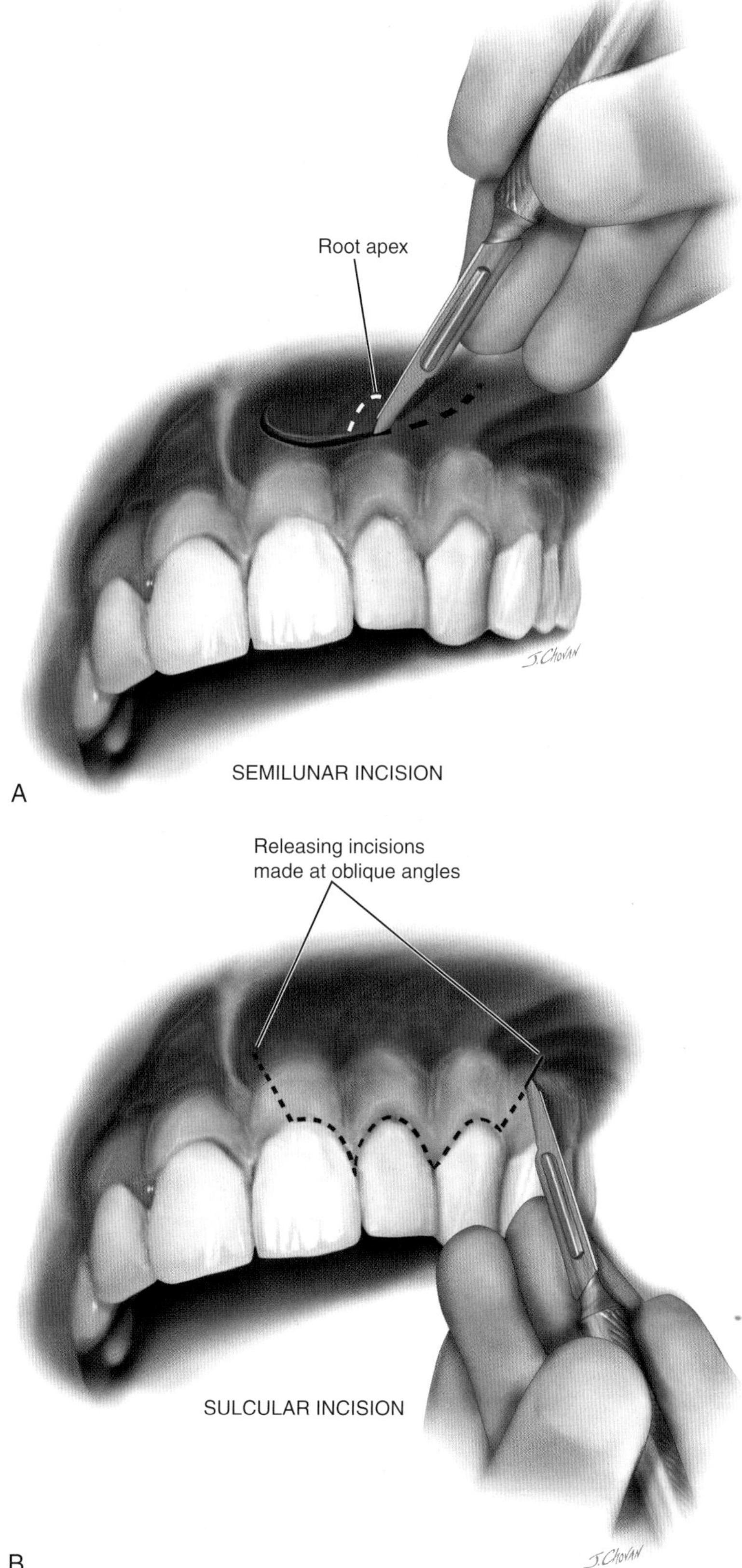

Figure 16.3 **A,** Illustration of a semilunar flap. Note that the complete incision is localized to the alveolar mucosa. **B,** Illustration of a sulcular flap. This incision can be performed with an anterior releasing incision, a posterior releasing incision, or both.

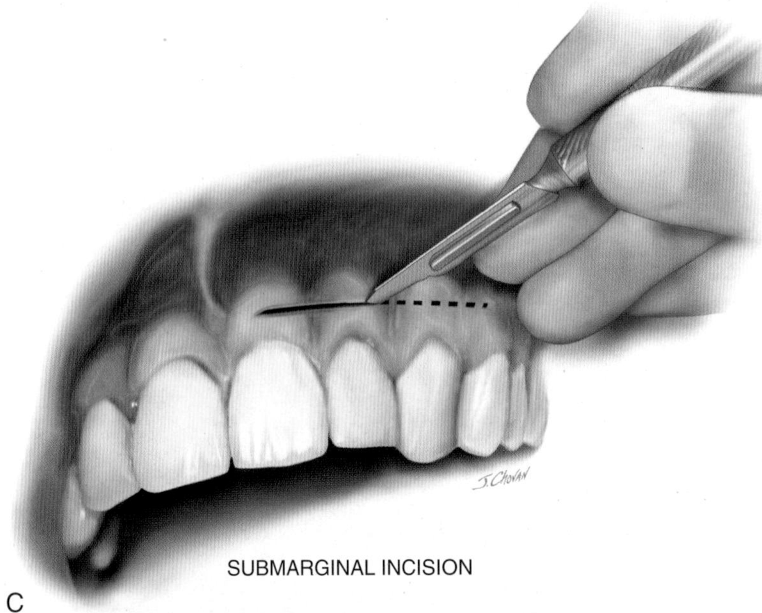

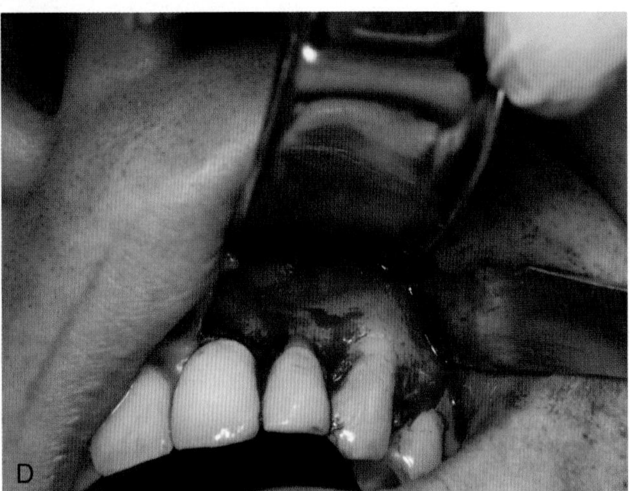

Figure 16.3, cont'd **C,** Illustration of a submarginal flap. This flap is essentially a combination of the sulcular flap and the semilunar flap. **D,** Clinical photograph of the patient from Figure 16.1 after elevation of the sulcular flap and full-thickness periosteal flap.

TECHNIQUE: Apicoectomy—*cont'd*

Visualization of the Root Apex

After flap elevation, the next step is to localize the lesion and visualize the apex. If the buccal bone has been perforated, this part of the surgery is simplified; simply debride the periapical tissue with a dental curette. If a thin shell of bone covers the root tip, use a dental curette to carefully lift the thinned cortical bone and then remove the periapical tissue (Fig. 16.4A).

If the buccal bone is found fully intact, the tooth's apex can be located on a periapical radiograph. This is accomplished by measuring the distance from the crest of the alveolar bone to the root apex. After determination of the root apex location, a surgical rotary handpiece with a small round bur or an ultrasonic device is used to create a bony window at the radiographically predetermined location, the root apex is visualized, and the periapical pathology is removed (Fig. 16.4B). After removal of the periapical pathology, obturation material (i.e., gutta-percha) may be visualized in the canal (Fig. 16.4C).

It is our recommendation that after removal of the periapical soft tissue pathology, the specimen be sent for histopathology. The American Academy of Oral and Maxillofacial Pathology has established clear guidelines regarding which tissues should be sent for histopathology. The academy's "Policy on Excised Tissue" can be found on the organization's website (www.aaomp.org).

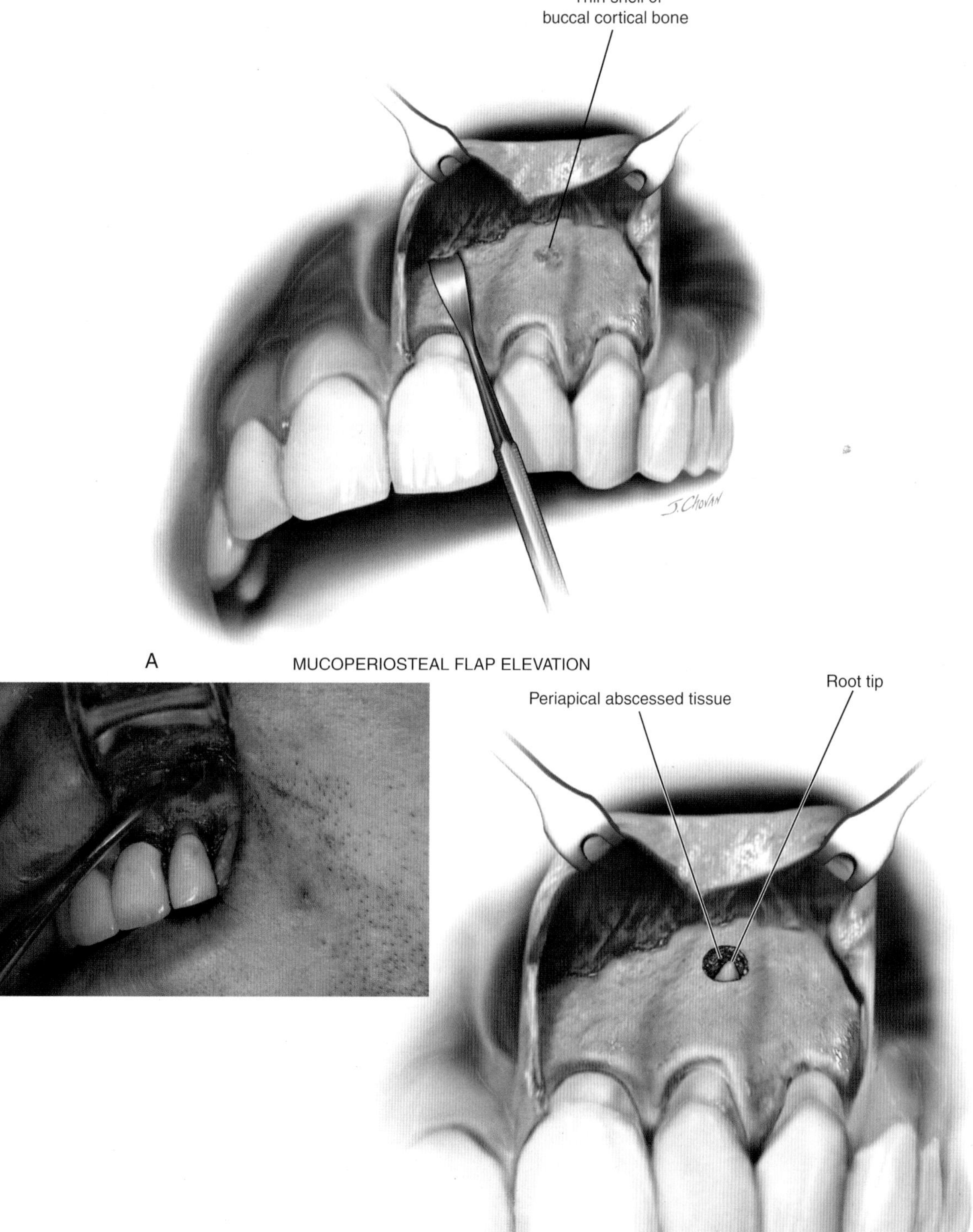

Figure 16.4 **A,** Illustration of elevation of the full-thickness flap root apex, identified with a thin shell of buccal cortical bone. This bone is removed with a dental curette, and the abscessed tissue is removed. **B1,** Clinical photograph of the creation of a buccal cortical window; the periosteal elevator points to the abscessed tissue. **B2,** Illustration after creation of the buccal cortical window.

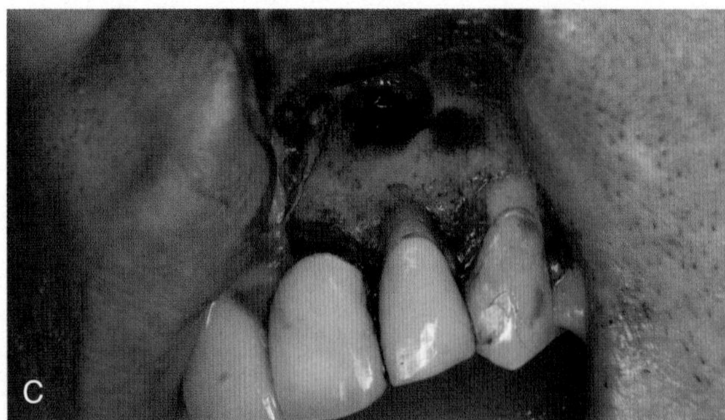

Figure 16.4, cont'd **C,** Clinical photograph after the removal of abscessed tissue; note the presence of gutta-percha.

TECHNIQUE: Apicoectomy—*cont'd*

Optic magnification is recommended with high-power surgical loupes at a minimum, while a surgical microscope provides the best visualization.

Apical Root Resection

Now that the root tip has been exposed, the terminal 2 to 3 mm of root length is resected with a fissure bur at a 45-degree angle to the long axis of the tooth (Fig. 16.5). This removes the portion of the root canal system that is most poorly sealed.[15] Furthermore, it has been demonstrated that a resection of the terminal 2 to 3 mm eliminates up to 93% of lateral canals.[8]

Root Preparation

After root resection, hemostasis must be obtained. A cotton roll soaked in a hemostatic agent or bone wax can be used to achieve adequate hemostasis. The root-end preparation within the root tip will be 2 to 3 mm in depth from the bevel in a longitudinal axis.

Successful root preparation is dependent on adequate retention form with buccolingual extension. This preparation can be performed using a surgical rotary handpiece or an ultrasonic device. Ultrasonic devices have been shown to reduce bacterial leakage, the frequency of perforation, and the amount of bevel required. Older literature reported an increased frequency of root fracture with ultrasonics.[16] On a lower intensity setting and with adequate irrigation, however, these devices do not directly damage the root.[17] Newer literature points to increased success rates with the use of ultrasonic versus traditional rotary handpieces.[18]

Lasers have also been used for root preparation during apicoectomy. Lasers can seal dentinal tubules by melting dentin, sterilize the affected area, and reduce postoperative pain. Furthermore, retrocavities prepared with the erbium: yttrium-aluminum-garnet (Er:YAG) laser have significantly lower microleakage.[19]

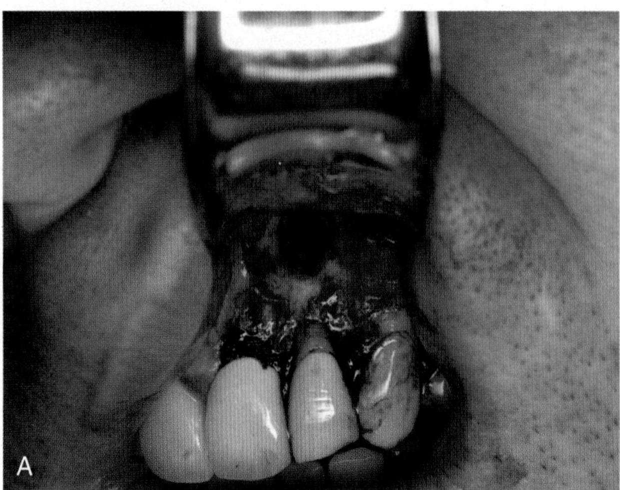

Figure 16.5 **A,** Clinical photograph of an apical root resection performed at a 45-degree angle.

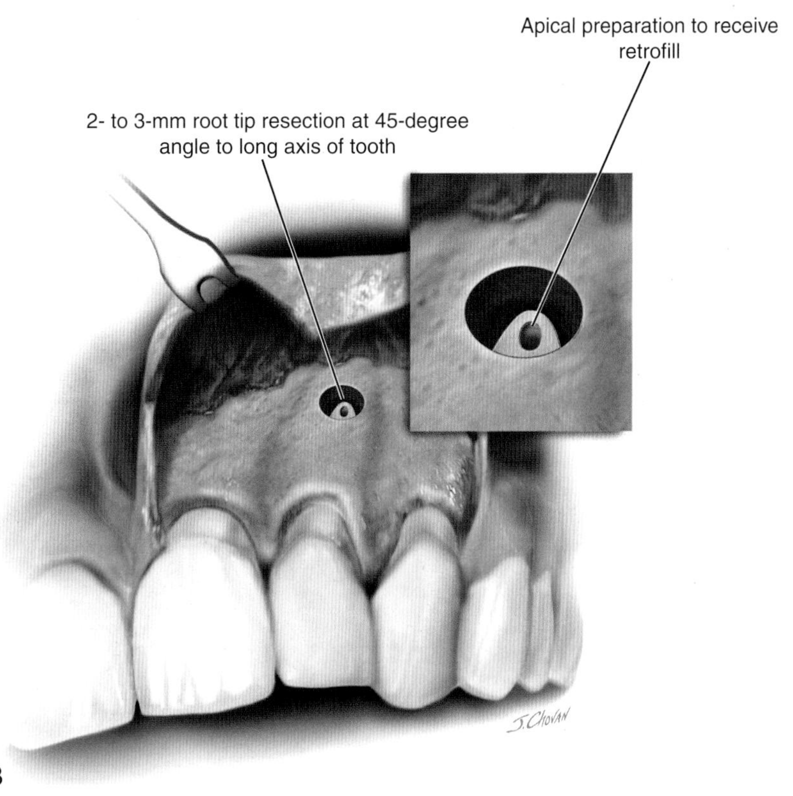

Figure 16.5, cont'd **B,** Illustration of an apical root resection with a close-up image of the apical root-end preparation; this involves removal of 2 to 3 mm of gutta-percha to allow for retrograde filling with the surgeon's material of choice.

TECHNIQUE: Apicoectomy—*cont'd*

Retrograde Fill

Once the terminal 2 to 3 mm of root tip has been resected and the site has been prepared, retrograde fill can be placed. This section discusses the different types of retrofilling materials currently available.

Dental amalgam has been the archetypal retrofilling material for many years due to several factors such as its ease of use, radiopacity, and low cost. However, amalgam has several drawbacks, including staining of tissues and sensitivity to moisture.[20] Fig. 16.6 depicts a completed retrofill with amalgam.

Mineral trioxide aggregate (MTA) was introduced as a retrofilling material in the mid-1990s. MTA has been shown to have excellent biocompatibility, which results in less of an inflammatory reaction than occurs with other materials. In addition, a cementum-like material has been shown to grow over the material, appearing as cellular cementum.[21] Studies also have linked MTA to the smallest amount of microleakage of the materials discussed in the literature, in addition to less marginal gap formation and better adaptation, which are important risk factors for failure of the apicoectomy.[22,23] Less-experienced practitioners often cite difficulty with handling as the major drawback to this material. MTA has generally shown high healing rates in the literature, notably 91% in a recent meta-analysis.[11]

Two commonly used reinforced zinc oxide–eugenol materials are Super-EBA and intermediate restorative material (IRM). They have been shown to have a better seal and therefore less microleakage than amalgam, but studies on their long-term performance are needed.[22] Recent reports have demonstrated that success rates for IRM and Super-EBA at 1 year postoperative are similar, at 91% for IRM and 82% for Super-EBA.[24]

Interest in the use of a dentin-bonded resin as a retrofill material has recently increased. Studies have shown that compared with resin-bonded retrofilling material, the dentin-bonded material shows adequate setting time, compressive strength, pH, and biocompatibility.[25]

Continued

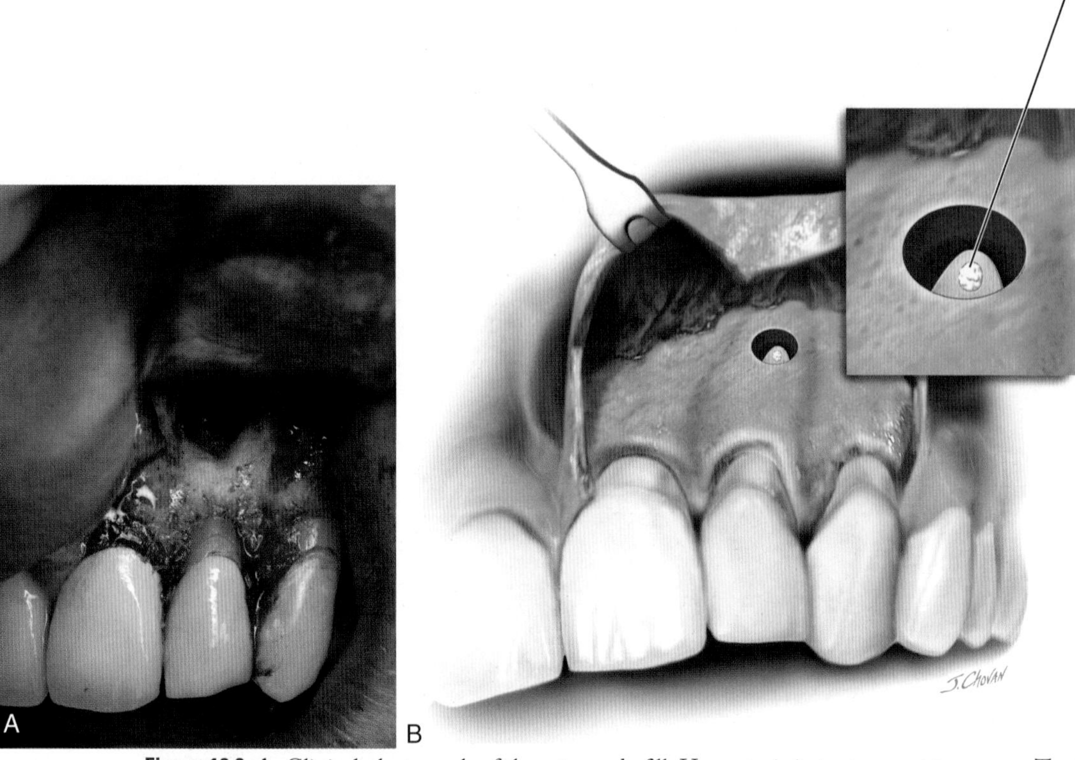

Figure 16.6 **A,** Clinical photograph of the retrograde fill. Hemostasis is tantamount to success. The authors recommend using lidocaine with vasoconstrictor-soaked cotton rolls before application of the retrofill. **B,** Illustration of the retrofill. The authors recommend mineral trioxide aggregate (MTA) as the retrofill material of choice.

TECHNIQUE: Apicoectomy—*cont'd*

Irrigation and Closure

After placement of the retrograde fill, a postoperative periapical radiograph is recommended to ensure adequate obturation. Following this radiographic verification, the surgical site is then carefully irrigated with copious normal saline. Finally, the flap is closed with interrupted sutures of the surgeon's choice, usually 3-0 or 4-0 chromic gut (Fig. 16.7).

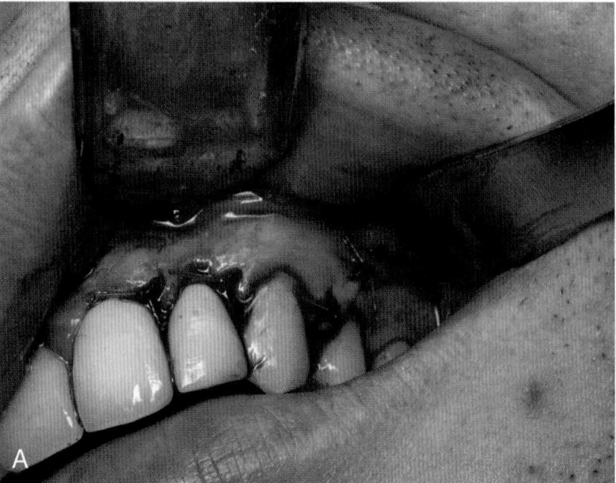

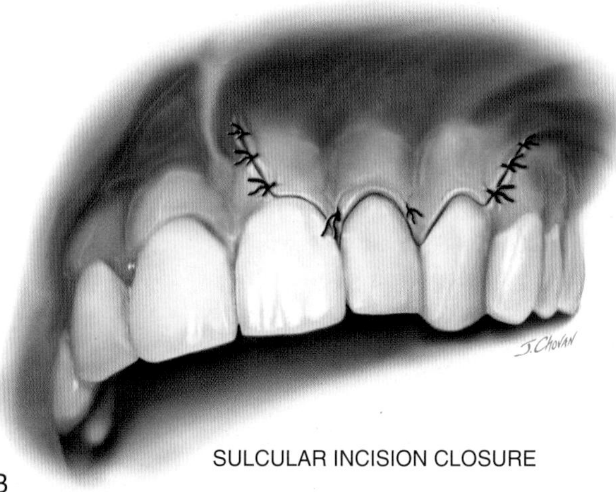

Figure 16.7 **A,** Clinical photograph of closure of the sulcular flap. The suture material used depends on the surgeon's preference; in this case, it was 3-0 chromic gut. **B,** Illustration of closure of the sulcular flap. Vertical mattress sutures typically are used to close the papilla in an interdental fashion.

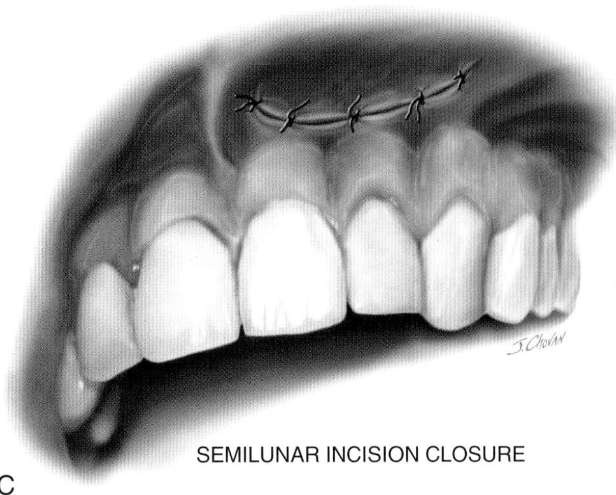

Figure 16.7,cont'd C, Illustration of closure of the semilunar flap. The sutures in this case are restricted to the alveolar mucosa; attached gingiva should not be included in the closure to avoid shortening lip length or vestibule height.

Avoidance and Management of Intraoperative Complications

Complete resection of the root terminus is imperative to a successful apicoectomy. Incomplete resection usually leads to one or both of two intraoperative complications: improper placement of the retrograde filling material and/or failure to completely remove excess material. Fig. 16.8 shows a postoperative periapical radiograph with adequate retrofill and a slight excess of amalgam particles that were imperceptible clinically.

An improperly placed retrofill results in an ineffective seal and increased microleakage. Excess material within the flap increases the likelihood of postoperative edema and infection. These two complications can potentially be avoided by taking a postoperative periapical radiograph. We recommend a postoperative radiograph after irrigation and cleansing of the surgical site. If one of the previously discussed complications is encountered, simply complete the root resection, remove any retrofill that was not placed correctly, replace the backfill, remove any excess material within the flap, irrigate carefully, and take a new radiograph.

A subset of complications relates to damage to anatomic structures. If apicoectomy is planned for a posterior maxillary tooth, attention must be paid to the bounds of the overlying maxillary sinus. If a perforation of the maxillary sinus occurs, several steps should be taken after completion of the procedure to prevent complications. Antibiotics should be considered, and routine sinus precautions are followed (e.g., sneezing with the mouth open, avoiding nose blowing, and using over-the-counter decongestants as needed). Small perforations will usually spontaneously resolve, but larger or persistent perforations will require surgical intervention.[26,27]

If a mandibular apicoectomy is planned, it is wise to consider several local anatomic factors. Mandibular incisor roots are in close proximity to one another, and it is quite possible to damage an adjacent root or to treat the wrong tooth in this region. In the canine/premolar region, the location of the mental foramen should be noted on a periapical or panoramic radiograph. In the molar region of the mandible, it is important to note the thickness of the buccal bone and the location of the inferior alveolar canal. Damage to the inferior alveolar and mental nerves is a risk. A recent study has demonstrated the incidence of altered sensation following mandibular apicoectomy treatment to be 14%, with higher incidence in premolar than molar regions.[28] As put forth in a joint 2016 position statement by the American Academy of Endodontists and the American Academy of Oral and

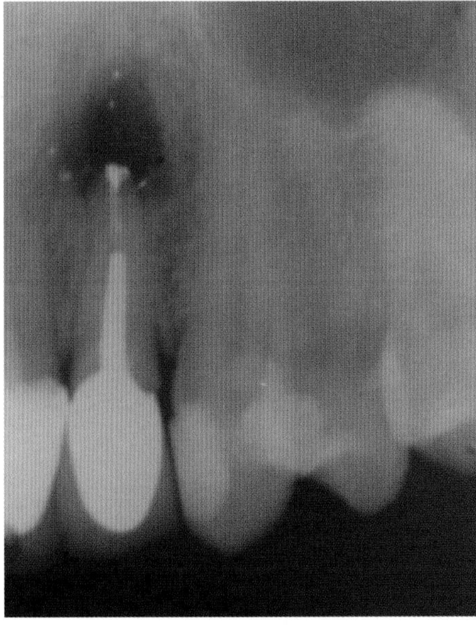

Figure 16.8 Postoperative periapical radiograph of the patient in Fig. 16.1 showing adequate retrofill of tooth #10. Some amalgam scatter can be seen.

Maxillofacial Radiology, limited field of view cone-beam computed tomography is the imaging modality of choice for presurgical treatment planning.[29]

Postoperative Considerations

Even if all excess material is removed, it is still possible for the oral mucosa to become discolored if amalgam is used for the retrofilling material. Thus, if the apicoectomy is planned for an anterior maxillary tooth in a patient with a high smile line, it is wise to avoid amalgam.

Wound dehiscence with the use of a semilunar flap has been well documented in the literature. An incorrectly designed flap can have insufficient vascular supply and possibly succumb to avascular necrosis. Additionally, although a flap may be clinically successful, its associated scar may compromise aesthetics.[26] Adherence to basic incision design principles, such as creating the base of the flap wider than the crest, placing incisions over healthy bone, and minding aesthetic areas help to minimize the incidence of postoperative complications.

References

1. Farrar JN. Radical and heroic treatment of alveolar abscess by amputation of roots of teeth. *Dent Cosm*. 1884;26:79.
2. Rhein ML. Amputation of the root as a radical cure in chronic alveolar abscess. *Dent Cosm*. 1890;32:904.
3. Coolidge ED. Root resection as a cure for chronic periapical infection: a histologic report of a case showing complete repair. *J Am Dent Assoc*. 1930;17:239.
4. Luks S. Root end amalgam technic in the practice of endodontics. *J Am Dent Assoc*. 1956;53(4):424–428.
5. Nicholls E. Retrograde filling of the root canal. *Oral Surg Oral Med Oral Pathol*. 1962;15:463–473.
6. Lieblich SE. Periapical surgery: clinical decision making. *Oral Maxillofac Surg Clin North Am*. 2002;14(2):179–186.
7. Lieblich SE. Endodontic surgery. *Dent Clin North Am*. 2012;56(1):121–132. viii-ix.
8. Kim S, Kratchman S. Modern endodontic surgery concepts and practice: a review. *J Endod*. 2006;32(7):601–623.
9. Fragiskos FD. *Oral Surgery, Apicoectomy*. Athens, Greece: Springer-Verlag; 2007.
10. von Arx T. Failed root canals: the case for apicoectomy (periradicular surgery). *J Oral Maxillofac Surg*. 2005;63(6):832–837.
11. von Arx T, Peñarrocha M, Jensen S. Prognostic factors in apical surgery with root-end filling: a meta-analysis. *J Endod*. 2010;36(6):957–973.
12. Velvart P, Peters CI. Soft tissue management in endodontic surgery. *J Endod*. 2005;31(1):4–16.
13. Kreisler M, Gockel R, Schmidt I, Kühl S, d'Hoedt B. Clinical evaluation of a modified marginal sulcular incision technique in endodontic surgery. *Oral Surg Oral Med Oral Pathol Oral Radiol Endod*. 2009;108(6):e22–e28.
14. von Arx A, Salvi GE. Incision techniques and flap designs for apical surgery in the anterior maxilla. *Eur J Esthet Dent*. 2008;3(2):110–126.
15. Lieblich SE, McGiverin B. Ultrasonic retrograde preparation. *Oral Maxillofac Surg Clin North Am*. 2002;14(2):167–172.
16. Abedi HR, Van Mierlo BL, Wilder-Smith P, Torabinejad M. Effects of ultrasonic root-end cavity preparation on the root apex. *Oral Surg Oral Med Oral Pathol Oral Radiol Endod*. 1995;80(2):207–213.
17. Gray GJ, Hatton JF, Holtzmann DJ, Jenkins DB, Nielsen CJ. Quality of root-end preparations using ultrasonic and rotary instrumentation in cadavers. *J Endod*. 2000;26(5):281–283.
18. Testori T, Capelli M, Milani S, Weinstein RL. Success and failure in periradicular surgery: a longitudinal retrospective analysis. *Oral Surg Oral Med Oral Pathol Oral Radiol Endod*. 1999;87(4):493–498.
19. Mohammadi Z. Laser applications in endodontics: an update review. *Int Dent J*. 2009;59(1):35–46.
20. Safavi K. Root end filling. *Oral Maxillofac Surg Clin North Am*. 2002;14(2):173–177.
21. Baek SH, Plenk H Jr, Kim S. Periapical tissue responses and cementum regeneration with amalgam, SuperEBA, and MTA as root-end filling materials. *J Endod*. 2005;31(6):444–449.
22. Fogel HM, Peikoff MD. Microleakage of root-end filling materials. *J Endod*. 2001;27(7):456–458.
23. Gatewood RS. Endodontic materials. *Dent Clin North Am*. 2007;51(3):695–712. vii.
24. Wälivaara DÅ, Abrahamsson P, Fogelin M, Isaksson S. Super-EBA and IRM as root-end fillings in periapical surgery with ultrasonic preparation: a prospective randomized clinical study of 206 consecutive teeth. *Oral Surg Oral Med Oral Pathol Oral Radiol Endod*. 2011;112(2):258–263.
25. Kim M, Ko H, Yang W, Lee Y, Kim S, Mante FK. A new resin-bonded retrograde filling material. *Oral Surg Oral Med Oral Pathol Oral Radiol Endod*. 2009;108(5):e111–e116.
26. Fink JB. Predicting the success and failure of surgical endodontic treatment. *Oral Maxillofac Surg Clin North Am*. 2002;14(2):153–165.
27. Freedman A, Horowitz I. Complications after apicoectomy in maxillary premolar and molar teeth. *Int J Oral Maxillofac Surg*. 1999;28(3):192–194.
28. Mainkar A, Zhu Q, Safavi K. Incidence of altered sensation after mandibular premolar and molar periapical surgery. *J Endod*. 2020;46(1):29–33.
29. Fayad M, et al. *Use of Cone Beam Computed Tomography in Endodontics—2015/2016 Update*. American Association of Endodontists; 2015. www.aae.org.

CHAPTER 17

Inferior Alveolar Nerve and Lingual Nerve Repair

Leon Assael

Armamentarium

#1 Periosteal elevator
#9 Periosteal elevator
#15 Scalpel blade
#150/#151 Forceps
#190/#191 Elevators
Appropriate sutures
Bone file
Binocular surgical microscope with video
Cryer elevators
Dental curette
Fissure/round bur
Gilmore probe
Hemostat
Irrigation syringe/sterile saline
Local anesthetic with vasoconstrictor
Microneurosurgical set
Minnesota cheek retractor
Molt curettes
Needle holder
Rongeurs
Seldin retractor
Small and large luxator
Small and large straight elevator
Surgical handpiece
Suture scissors

History of the Procedure

The great golden age anatomist Galen was uncertain of the role of peripheral nerves and initially did not distinguish them from tendons. Subsequently, he sectioned the recurring laryngeal nerve in pigs to demonstrate peripheral nerve action.[1] Injuries to peripheral nerves were poorly understood due to the nondiscrete nature of these injuries. However, in his 1795 treatise, John Haighton[2] reported that "an animate machine differs from an inanimate one in nothing more conspicuously than in its power of repairing its injuries." He identified the need for peripheral nerve continuity to preserve diaphragmatic function. His experiments on dogs, apparently after division of the vagus nerve in the neck (although he called it the VIII nerve), demonstrate the apparent ability of peripheral cranial nerves to undergo repair. He sectioned one side, both sides, and both sides in sequence over weeks to demonstrate not only the action of the peripheral nerve, but also its ability to undergo repair. His drawings of dissections completed in functionally restored animals demonstrate the spontaneous repair of peripheral nerves.

The first description of technique for reanastomosis of peripheral nerve neurotmesis is likely that of Gabriel Ferrara of Venice in 1608.[3] The first successful modern peripheral nerve repairs were performed during hand surgery for traumatic neurotmesis. In 1973 Millesi[4] emphasized the importance of fascicular alignment and perineural suturing to achieve favorable results in hand surgery. The results of hand surgery demonstrated the proof of motor and sensory recovery after neurotmesis could be obtained in humans.

Modern peripheral trigeminal nerve surgery was hampered by the development of access techniques and the irregular nature of referral for these sensory injuries which, compared with motor injuries of the hand, did not create as much disability for most. However, the presence of anesthesia dolorosa ineffectively treated with nerve ablation and the vexing issue of lingual nerve anesthesia and dysesthesia prompted surgeons in the 1970s to develop techniques for repair. Hausamen et al.[5] demonstrated a technique for the inferior alveolar nerve with interpositional grafting. Phillip Worthington, Ralph Merrill, Bruce Donoff, Michael (Tony) Pogrel, and John Gregg, among others, pioneered the advancement of these techniques in contemporary surgical practice. Today, large outcome studies demonstrating functional sensory recovery have established the utility of direct repair and interpositional grafting of peripheral trigeminal nerve injuries.

Indications for the Use of the Procedure

Peripheral trigeminal nerve injury can result from mechanical injury to the affected nerve after facial trauma or surgical intervention (Fig. 17.1). Mandible and zygomatico-orbital fractures commonly injure afferent V3 and V2, respectively. Frontal sinus and orbital fractures can produce neurosensory deficits of V1. However, the great majority of treated trigeminal neurosensory injuries result from elective oral surgical procedures. Removal of impacted mandibular third molars, mandibular fracture, mandibular tumors, and placement of dental implants commonly affect V3. In addition to

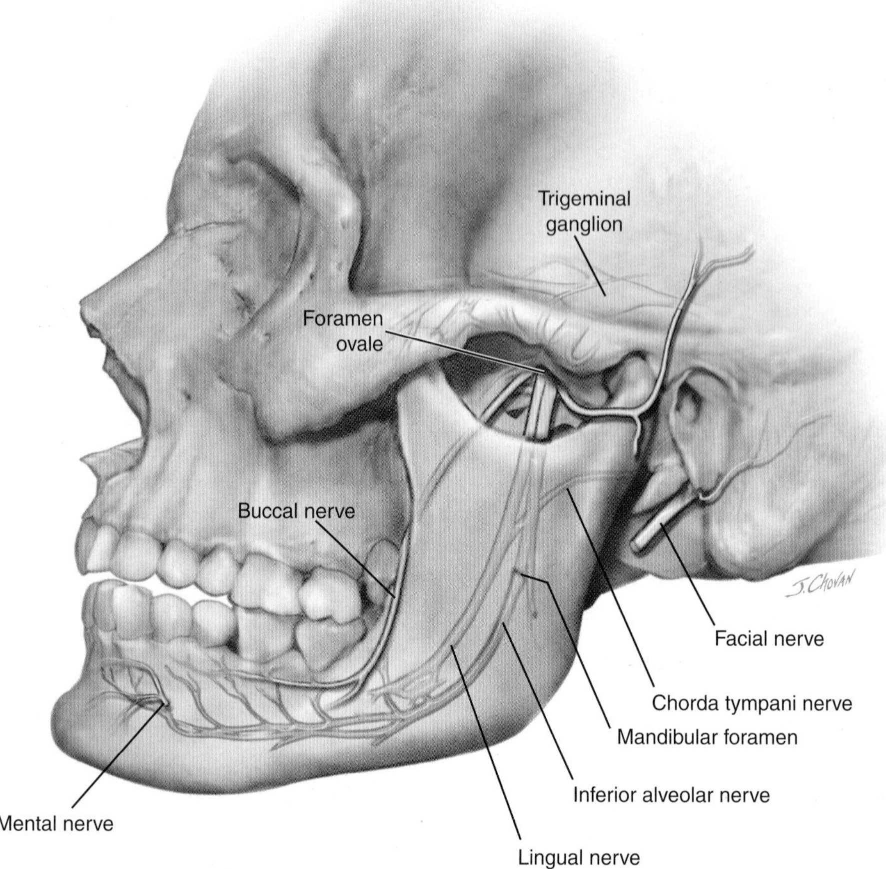

Fig. 17.1 Location of the lingual and inferior alveolar nerves.

mechanical injuries, chemical nerve injury of the trigeminal nerve results from endodontic medicaments, amide local anesthetics, and antiseptics such as alcohol. Thermal injury to the trigeminal nerve can occur from electrocautery, heat from rotary instruments, or heated dental surgical materials such as gutta-percha or methylmethacrylate (Fig. 17.2). Ischemic injury may occur due to endoneural or intravascular injection of epinephrine, radiation therapy, or infarction of the peripheral nerve vas neurosum.

Injuries to the sensory branches of the trigeminal nerve result in afferent defects characterized by alterations or absence of sensation. The alterations in sensation can be noxious or painful, or they may be innocuous, with mild tingling or just dullness. These findings can be briefly associated with touch stimulation or they can be continuous or exacerbated by stimulation.

Neuropathic pain and afferent somatosensory deficits can be spontaneous (due to no known cause) or anamnestically associated with procedures or trauma producing peripheral nerve injuries of branches of the trigeminal nerve. Spontaneous loss of sensation and spontaneous trigeminal neuropathic pain (including trigeminal neuralgia), while idiopathic, are variously postulated to be a result of viral illness, infarction of vas neurosum, vascular impingement, and neurodegenerative disorders among others. Surgical management of hypoesthesia or anesthesia is an established method, whereas procedures for dysesthesia and those resulting from spontaneous loss of sensation are less well defined, and recommendations for surgical management have been less well characterized in those cases.

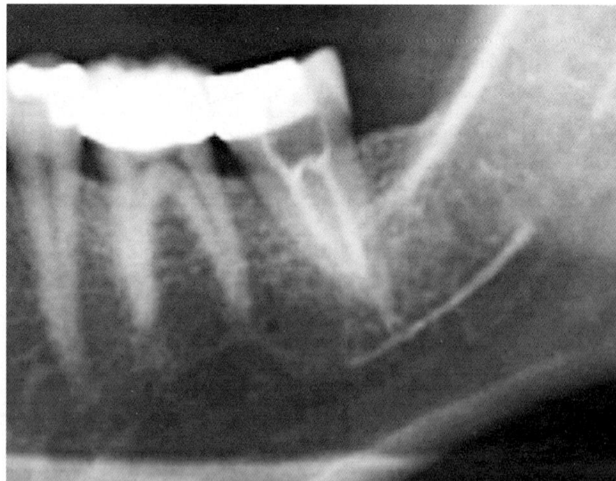

Fig. 17.2 Extrusion of root canal filling material past apex of second molar.

Over the course of surgical and nonsurgical treatment, the improvement of patients to the point of complete elimination of pain, paresthesia, and dysesthesia can be achieved in only a minority of patients. Despite these shortcomings, treatment is capable of reducing the impact of pain from an unbearable burden on the patient's well-being to a tolerable condition with substantial improvements in quality of life, as well as the achievement of functional sensory recovery, which is an afferent function to provide nonnoxious sensation to afford protection of structures, nociception, and proprioception. For patients with well-defined injuries and those with nociceptive inflammatory components, the prognosis is better yet with surgical intervention.

A variety of definitions of these conditions are used and are consistent with the characterization of neuropathic pain in a patient with a trigeminal nerve injury. The following definitions and clinical presentations are noted.

Hypoesthesia: A diminution of sensation, compared with a control stimulus, with the absence of pain. In such patients, sharp may feel dull. The patient produces errors in two-point and directional stimuli. No areas of anesthesia are present, and the findings are due either to decreased neural density (e.g., incomplete repair) without neurotmesis or to neuropraxia, and thus are transient.

Anesthesia: The absence of sensation with the absence of pain to any stimulus. These patients often treat the anesthetic part as a foreign body (e.g., a bolus). Hypersalivation, dysarthria, dysphagia, and speech articulation issues, among others, are noted when the perception of an absent body part is noted. This typically is due to neurotmesis, which may be physical separation, neuroma in continuity, lateral adhesive neuroma, kinking of the nerve, or some other impingement or infarction of the nerve.

Elicited neuropathic pain: With the absence of stimulus there is an absence of pain, but upon stimulus with what would normally produce no pain, a painful response is elicited. In such cases the patient withdraws from normally nonpainful activities, such as shaving, using lipstick, kissing, or chewing. This may be due to reafferentation without somatosensory modulation of pain fibers.

Spontaneous neuropathic pain: Prolonged neuropathic pain occurs and is persistent after the stimulus has been removed. This may be modulated by central nervous system mediation of pain.

Dysesthesia: A noxious response occurs to a stimulus; it may be elicited or spontaneous.

Hyperalgesia: An increased response occurs to a minimally noxious stimulus, for example, a pin produces a greater than expected and more prolonged pain response or a response not typical of the stimulus (e.g., burning).

Allodynia: A painful response occurs to an innocuous stimulus.

Hyperpathia: A prolonged and explosive pain response occurs to an innocuous stimulus; it may be continuous.

Anesthesia dolorosa: The persistence of pain after neurectomies or amputation of a body part. Although there is no afferent function (e.g., anesthesia is seen on examination), pain is perceived in the body part previously supplied by the nerve.

Diagnosis of the patient with an afferent sensation defect or neuropathic pain due to peripheral nerve injury includes an anamnestic assessment to determine the likely cause of injury, the time since injury, the evolution of the injury and sensation over time, and the effect on activities of daily living. It is important to determine whether nociceptive components to the pain remain (due to inflammation, infection, a persistent lesion, local inflammatory aspects, or mechanical impingement) that would explain afferent defects. Palpation of the site for redness, swelling, and pain, in addition to imaging with computed tomography (CT) to assess for pathologic defects, can be helpful. Limited areas of cherry-like redness in the tissue may be due to a neuroma, which in the case of inferior alveolar and lingual nerve injuries can fill third molar extraction sites and replace normal mucosal tissue. Magnetic resonance imaging (MRI), as noted below, of trigeminal peripheral nerve injuries may be useful in the assessment of neuroma and inflammation, which can produce a high signal and used in evaluation of deafferentation.

Afferent sensory defects should be carefully mapped. This can provide assistance in understanding the expected findings at surgery if intervention is carried out. The characteristics of any pain, whether constant or due to stimulation, are important in proportion to the stimulus or if sustained beyond the stimulus.

The diagnostic nerve block is a useful indicator of whether the injury is generating pain in the peripheral nerve and where in the nerve it is located. In general, the absence of both pain and sensation after peripheral nerve block indicates a peripheral mediation and source of that pain, generally due to a neuroma at the site of injury. However, the risk of false positives should be noted with regard to the potential that centrally mediated pain will result in an absence of pain after peripheral nerve block, but that pain is still dependent on a central nervous system (CNS) modulation. Thus, in many cases, the patient with centrally mediated pain has an alteration in that pain experience after peripheral nerve block. That alteration is usually toward mitigating the level of pain. For the patient with a peripheral source of pain, beginning the block with lidocaine anesthesia at the most peripheral site may determine whether a neuroma or perineural inflammation is a factor. For example, if the intent is to determine whether the injury is due to mechanical disturbance of a nerve at the time of surgery or whether it is in the location of the nerve block, it would be best for the patient to have a diagnostic block first at the site of possible mechanical injury (e.g., at the lingual crest for a third molar removal). If painful dysesthesia is persistent after this block, a Gow-Gates block (e.g., proximal to the site of nerve block) can be done to determine whether the location of injury is due to injection rather than surgery.

Diagnostic radiology for the patient with trigeminal nerve injury includes a panoramic radiograph, other local views of the injured site if needed, and a maxillofacial CT scan. MRI is sometimes helpful in locating sites of injury, inflammation, impingement, or masses. Imaging for neuropathic pain differs somewhat from that used for other patients with trigeminal nerve injury. An attempt to define the inflammatory aspects of the injury can be made with MRI of the region, including mapping of the site of nerve injury with three-dimensional reconstruction (Fig. 17.3).

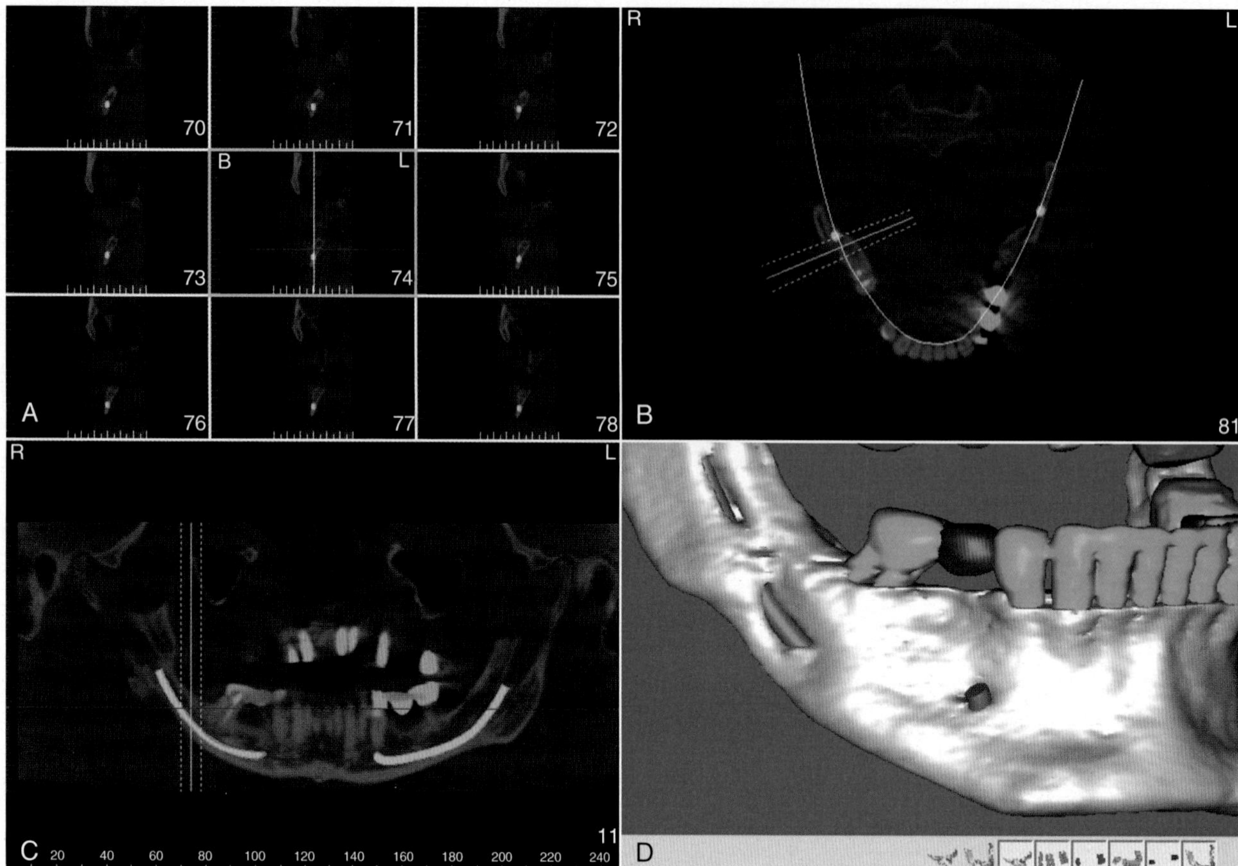

Fig. 17.3 A–D, Preoperative planning. Cone beam CT scan-generated views of inferior alveolar nerve position.

Neuromas can be identified, in addition to inflammation in the perineural tissues, bone, or associated soft tissues. The extent of perineural inflammation is particularly important in chemical nerve injury because this may not be completely apparent under the operating microscope. The need to resect associated bone or soft tissue also can be assessed with MRI. MRI neurography can be used to determine whether an inflammatory reaction or neural tissue turgor is apparent proximal to the injury. Deafferentation distal to the nerve can also sometimes be indicated on MRI neurography. CT or MRI of the brain is indicated to rule out a CNS lesion associated with the presence of neuropathic pain or to assess neurodegenerative findings, such as demyelinating diseases.

Limitations and Contraindications

All patients should be counseled regarding the lack of improvement of symptoms from peripheral nerve surgery. The most important prognostic factor in improvement is the length of time from injury to surgical intervention. In addition, the medical status of the patient must be considered. Medical management with neuroleptic medications also should be considered as a nonsurgical treatment option.

TECHNIQUE: Inferior Alveolar Nerve Repair

STEP 1: Patient Preparation

The patient is immobilized with a head rest, towels and tape, sandbags, or similar methods. Adjustments of patient position may be required after the microscope is in place following surgical access.

STEP 2: Incision

The ability to access the injured site transorally is usually possible and desirable, with full access to the inferior alveolar nerve from the lip to high in the infratemporal fossae via the transoral route, to the lingual nerve from the oral tongue to the chorda tympani insertion, and for the infraorbital nerve from the cheek to the internal orbit via a transoral/transantral approach. All repairs should be done under a two-headed, binocular operating microscope with the ability to visualize the operative site on a camera monitor; the ability to record is recommended. This allows both the surgeon and the assistant to visualize exactly the same site and from the same angle. It also allows the surgical team to operate via the microscope objectives or by observation on the monitor. This enables the surgical team to change hand position and gain access across a far greater range of variables than when operating with loupes (Fig. 17.4A).

STEP 3: Exposure and Osteotomy

Inferior alveolar nerve access can be performed via a crestal or buccal osteotomy. Using a saw or rotary instrument, the lateral and/or superior cortex is removed with attention towards retaining mechanical stability of the mandible; generally, the osteotomy cut is 3 to 5 mm deep to allow removal of the cortical bone. Of note is that the inferior alveolar nerve courses to the buccal side as it proceeds to the mental foramen. It often takes a buccal loop in the third molar area before returning toward the lingual side in the body. In addition, it may be tethered to the lingual side in the mental foramen as it releases the incisive nerve to the anterior mandible. Nearly one in five inferior alveolar nerves are bifid in the angle and posterior body of the mandible. Once the bone has been removed from the lateral cortex, nerve probes can enter the canal, and microcurettes can be used to relieve the bony canal laterally (Fig. 17.4B).

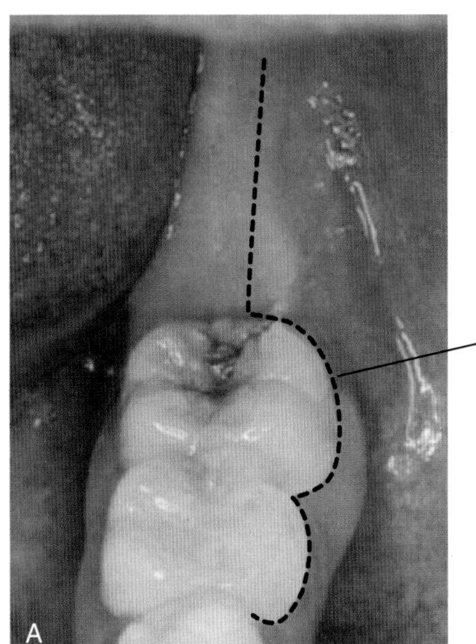

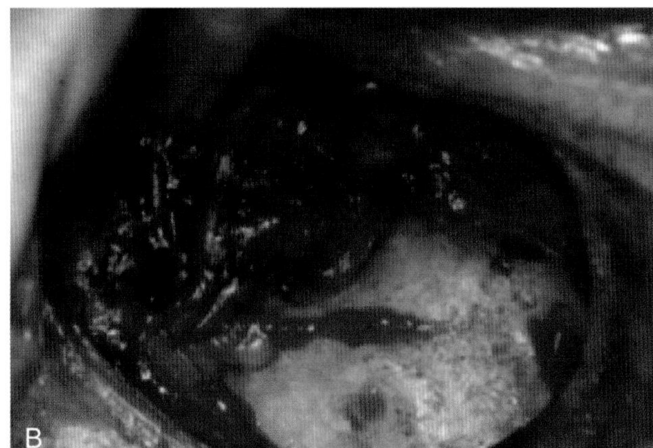

Fig. 17.4 **A,** Access incision and osteotomy to inferior alveolar nerve. **B,** Exposure of injured site on inferior alveolar nerve.

Continued

Technique: Inferior Alveolar Nerve Repair—cont'd

STEP 4: Lateralization of the Inferior Alveolar Nerve

The inferior alveolar nerve should be removed from its canal and lateralized at least 1 cm on each side of the injury. Attention to preservation of the vas neurosum and even small feeder vessels penetrating the vas neurosum can be made. Small branches to the pulps of teeth are neurovascular in nature; they sometimes can be preserved and should be, if possible. Although the main nutrient artery to a pulp may be severed, anastomotic blood supply from the periodontal ligament is likely to maintain vitality if the apices are not disturbed. Such proximity is especially an issue for lower second molar teeth. If held by the mental foramen distally, separating the incisive nerve or lateralizing it as well may be needed. The osteotomy for inferior alveolar nerve access should ensure that any entrapments have been eliminated and that any inflamed bone or granulation tissue has been removed.

ACCESS TECHNIQUE: Lingual Nerve Repair

STEP 1: Incision

Lingual nerve access can be obtained by repeating or creating a third molar or sagittal osteotomy incision from the temporal crest lateral/superiorly to the distal of the second molar and with an anterior buccal vestibular release. No releasing incisions are desirable on the lingual mucosa because these often tear into the parenchyma of the tongue. Once the buccal flap has been released, the lingual flap is elevated from the temporal crest to the premolar area, including the gingival papillae.

STEP 2: Retraction

With a peanut hemostat or sponge, the sublingual gland can be exposed with the lingual flap, revealing the distal lingual nerve and the conjunction with the Wharton duct lingual to the second molar. The proximal lingual nerve will be coursing in the infratemporal fossa anterior medially to the superior pharyngeal constrictor on the lingual crest of the mandible and lingual to the temporalis tendon. Leaving the temporalis tendon intact during the dissection is helpful in not confusing it with the proximal lingual nerve once released. Neuromas will often distort this anatomy and are often adherent to the lingual crest of the mandible making separation of the lingual nerve from the temporalis tendon, a necessary step.

STEP 3: Nerve Skeletonization

The proximal end of the lingual nerve must be distinguished from the temporalis tendon; careful preservation of this tendon when the flap is raised to its lingual aspect makes this distinction easier. Of note in the proximal dissection is that the chorda tympani joins the lingual nerve about 2 cm above the occlusal plane from the posterior and anterior branches to the pterygoid muscle; it should be preserved if noted. This dissection should reveal about 2.5 to 3 cm of lingual nerve, making the whole injury, in addition to tension-free repair or grafting, easier to understand (Fig. 17.5A–B).

STEP 4: Nerve Anastomoses Common to Both the Lingual and Inferior Alveolar Nerves

The goal in surgical repair is to have a contiguous nerve free of pathologic components. Amputation neuroma, lateral adhesive neuromas, and other neuromas in continuity should be removed. External pressure or kinking should be relieved. If the nerve is intact and a compressive neuropathy is the underlying cause of symptoms, external or internal neurolysis can play a role in improving sensation and reducing pain. For nerves with neurotmesis or resected neuromas, tension-free epineural repair is indicated. This typically is performed with sutures in the epineurium (e.g., proline 7-0 to 9-0, at least three to orient the nerve). Insufficient suturing may result in loss of coaptation during healing. Sealing of the epineurium with fibrin glue or Avitene BD can be performed as a way to promote early adaptation. Animal studies of nerve repair demonstrate partial restoration of tensile strength of the nerve in as little as 1 week after surgery (Fig. 17.5C–E).

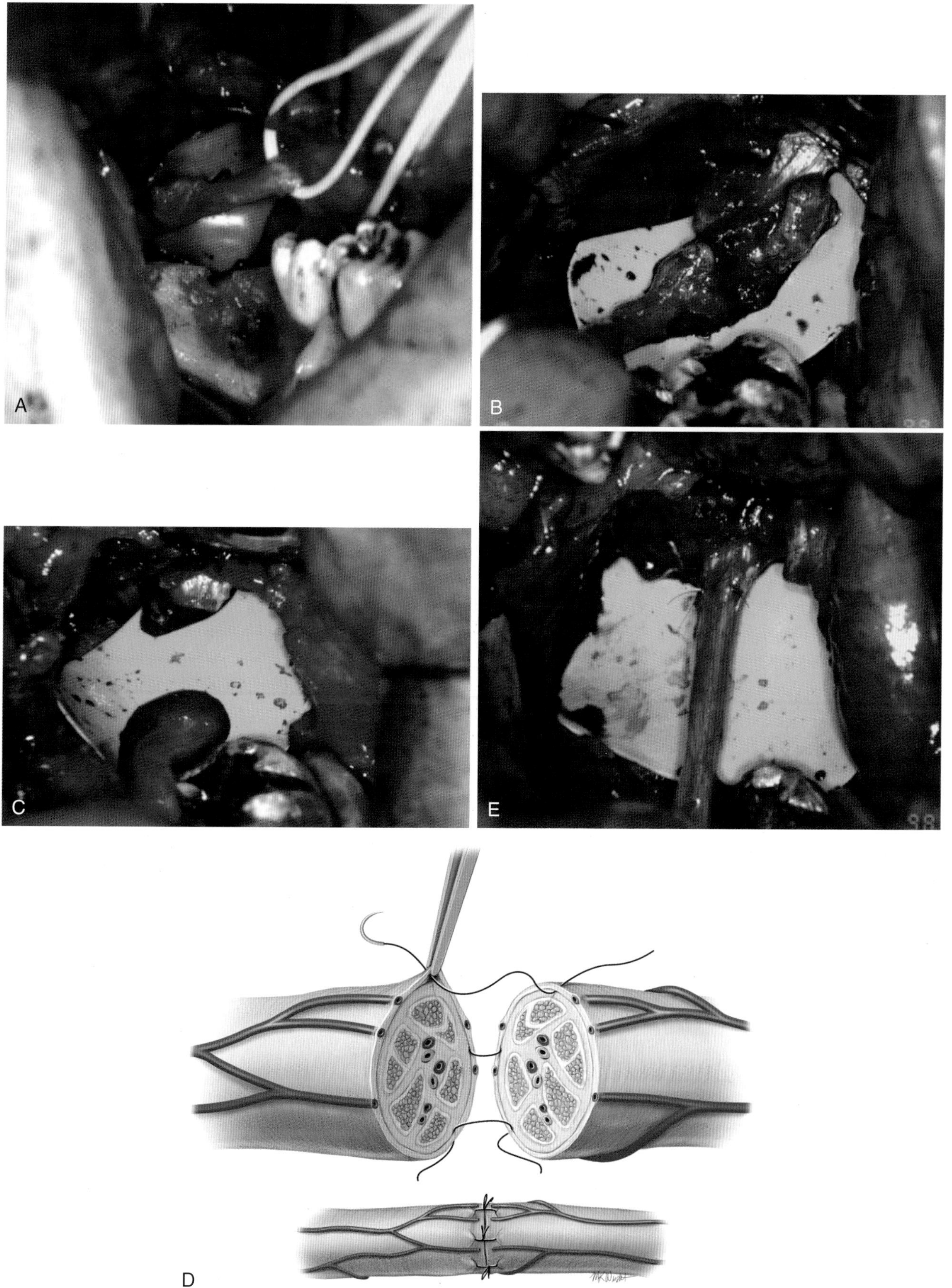

Fig. 17.5 **A,** Exposure of injured site on lingual nerve. **B,** Removal of neuromas, lateral or in continuity. **C,** Identified proximal distal nerve stumps. **D,** Epineural repair. **E,** Intraoperative view of completed epineural nerve repair.

ALTERNATIVE TECHNIQUES AND MODIFICATIONS

The surgical procedures for the patient with neuropathic pain associated with trigeminal nerve injury are not the same as for patients with simple sensory nerve injury. Consideration for greater resection of the injured portion of the nerve and replacement with a nerve graft is more likely because the persistence of pain may be due to continued perineural inflammation across any portion of the injured nerve. For example, chemical nerve injury due to endodontic procedures often leaves a leathery-appearing perineurium across up to centimeters of the inferior alveolar nerve. Identification of all the portions of the nerve demonstrating visual or MRI injury is needed to determine the amount of resection and nerve reanastomosis with cable graft. Experience in the past several years has been with Avance grafts (AxoGen) for this purpose. Vein grafts or autogenous great auricular or sural grafts also may be performed.

Neuropathic pain due to osteoradionecrosis or osteonecrosis often is also associated with ischemia. Relieving ischemia, such as with hyperbaric oxygen therapy or free flap surgery, often can reduce pain. It is unknown whether this pain reduction is due to increased tissue oxygen tension or to some other etiology.

Neurectomy, cryotherapy, and chemical denervation remain infrequent options for neuropathic pain. The time-honored technique of peripheral neurectomy remains in use, despite continued concerns about recidivism. In one recent study,[6] the rate of pain return after neurectomy was just 2 of 30 patients after 3 years of follow-up.

Avoidance and Management of Intraoperative Complications

Prevention of associated tissue trauma is especially important during dissection of the floor of the mouth. The sublingual plexus of veins as well as the sublingual artery and perforators on the lingual aspect of the mandible should be addressed carefully to ensure hemostasis. Muscles such as the superior pharyngeal constrictor should be released judiciously from their aponeurotic attachments if needed to avoid muscle bleeding and edema. Dissection within the mandible during inferior alveolar nerve repair should be performed to avoid damage to the teeth and perforation through the lingual aspect of the mandible where possible. The use of bone curettes can be helpful to avoid further injury to the inferior alveolar nerve during dissection of the mandible.

Postoperative Considerations

Peripheral nerve stimulators have been used to mitigate posttraumatic trigeminal neuropathic pain after repair.[7] Large case series and extensive follow-up are available to assess peripheral stimulators for the treatment of trigeminal postherpetic neuralgia. Johnson uses implanted subcutaneous pulse generators. Although these have provided 50% pain relief in 70% of patients, they may have less practical utility in V3-located injuries.[8]

Patients are advised not to smoke after nerve repair. Vitamin B complex can be useful in the treatment of neuropathic pain. In a blinded study,[9] the combination of B_1, B_6, and B_{12}, when used in an animal model, diminished pain behaviors associated with trigeminal induced traumatic neuropathic pain.

Neurosensory retraining exercises, with the assistance of occupational therapists, have been shown to mitigate symptoms and facilitate functional sensory recovery.

References

1. Gregg J. Historical perspectives on trigeminal nerve injuries. In: Miloro M, ed. *Trigeminal Nerve Injuries.* Berlin, Germany: Springer-Verlag; 2013.
2. Haighton J. An experimental inquiry concerning the reproduction of nerves. *Philos Trans R Soc Lond.* 1795;85:190.
3. Ferrara G. Nuova selva di cirugia, divisa in tre parti. Nella prima sono gli avvertimenti del manual, & artificioso modo di curare molte, e gravi infirmità del corpo humano. Nella seconda sono molti medicamenti esquisiti, con le figure de' ferri, ò instrumenti necessarii per essercitar l'arte della cirugia. Nella terza parimente si contengono molti rari medicamenti per distillationi, con le figure in ultimo de' vasi, e fornelli appartenenti all'arte distillatoriao. Venice: Sebastian Combi; 1608. [Translated in Little K, Zomorodi A, Selznick L, Friedman A: An eclectic history of peripheral nerve surgery, Neurosurg Clin North Am 15:109, 2004.]
4. Millesi H. Microsurgery of peripheral nerves. *Hand.* 1973;5(2):157–160.
5. Hausamen JE, Samii M, Schmidseder R. Restoring sensation to the cut inferior alveolar nerve by direct anastomosis or by free autologous nerve grafting. Experimental study in rabbits. *Plast Reconstr Surg.* 1974;54(1):83–87.
6. Agrawal SM, Kambalimath DH. Peripheral neurectomy: a minimally invasive treatment for trigeminal neuralgia. A retrospective study. *J Maxillofac Oral Surg.* 2011;10(3):195–198.
7. Lenchig S, Cohen J, Patin D. A minimally invasive surgical technique for the treatment of posttraumatic trigeminal neuropathic pain with peripheral nerve stimulation. *Pain Physician.* 2012;15(5):E725–E732.
8. Johnson MD, Burchiel KJ. Peripheral stimulation for treatment of trigeminal postherpetic neuralgia and trigeminal posttraumatic neuropathic pain: a pilot study. *Neurosurgery.* 2004;55(1):135–141.
9. Kopruszinski CM, Reis RC, Chichorro JG. B vitamins relieve neuropathic pain behaviors induced by infraorbital nerve constriction in rats. *Life Sci.* 2012;91(23–24):1187–1195.

CHAPTER 18

Odontogenic Infection

Dan Q. Tran and A. Omar Abubaker

Armamentarium

#15 Scalpel blade
¼ Penrose drains
3-0 Chromic gut
10-cc Syringe with 18-g needle
Appropriate sutures
Cricothyrotomy/tracheostomy kit
Culture swabs/tubes
Dental extraction kit:
  #9 Periosteal elevator
  Extraction forceps
  Straight elevator
Kelly clamp
Local anesthetic with vasoconstrictor
Mosquito curve hemostat
Needle electrocautery
Schnidt tonsil forceps

History of the Procedure

A court physician to the king of Württemberg, Wilhelm Friedrich von Ludwig, described the well-known condition of Ludwig's angina in 1836, but not until the early 20th century was the relationship between dental abscess and severe life-threatening neck swelling established.[1] Incision and drainage (I&D) of odontogenic abscess, in addition to dental extraction, has been a time-honored procedure performed by oral and maxillofacial surgeons. This operation relies on a thorough understanding of the fascial layers and the potential anatomic spaces through which infection can spread in the head and neck, as published in the classic anatomic studies done by Grodinsky and Holyoke from 1938 to 1939.[2–4] Prior to that, head and neck infection was common and often lethal. Osteomyelitis of the jaws was also a common and serious problem. At that time, erysipelas carried a 60% mortality rate. A discussion of the history of odontogenic infections is not complete without acknowledging the work in the modern and classic *Oral and Maxillofacial Infections* textbook by Topazian et al.[5]

Indications for the Use of the Procedure

Odontogenic infection with clinical or radiologic evidence of abscess collection warrants I&D via either a transcutaneous or a transoral approach, depending on the space involved, in addition to dental extraction. Modern protocols typically supplement the physical examination with a computed tomography (CT) scan with intravenous contrast dye to delineate the presence of a fluid collection and to localize the fascial spaces involved. Fascial space infection associated with an odontogenic source may include one or a combination of the spaces represented in Box 18.1.

BOX 18.1 Deep Fascial Space Involved in Odontogenic Infection

Deep fascial space infection associated with any tooth:
- Vestibular
- Buccal
- Subcutaneous

Deep fascial space infections associated with maxillary teeth:
- Canine
- Palatal
- Buccal
- Infratemporal
- Maxillary and other paranasal sinuses
- Cavernous sinus thrombosis

Deep fascial space infection associated with mandibular teeth:
- Space of the body of the mandible
- Submandibular
- Sublingual
- Submental
- Masticator (submasseteric, pterygomandibular, superficial temporal, deep temporal)

Deep fascial space infection of the neck and chest:
- Lateral pharyngeal (anterior and posterior compartments)
- Retropharyngeal
- Pretracheal
- Prevertebral
- Danger space
- Mediastinum

Limitations and Contraindications

The practice of I&D, along with eradication of the source of infection, is considered an urgent procedure and is rarely contraindicated in most circumstances. Trismus can make extractions and transoral approaches to drain the abscess challenging under local anesthesia, and many times general anesthesia is required. Medical comorbidities may require perioperative modification to optimize the patient for surgery and also may contribute to a poor or prolonged postoperative resolution of the infection.

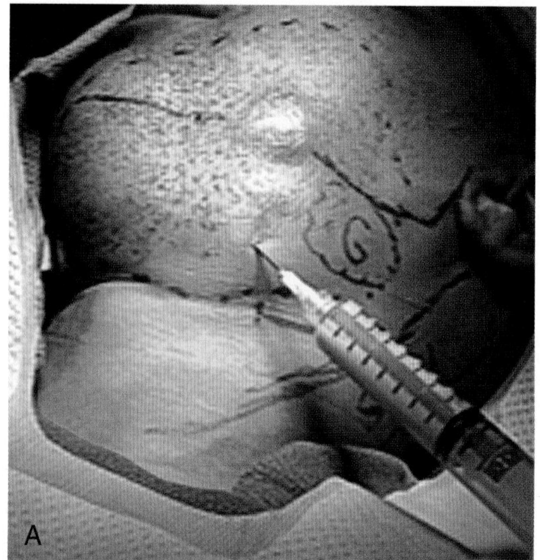

Figure 18.1 A, Aspiration of abscess with 10-cc syringe/18-gauge needle.

TECHNIQUE: Incision and Drainage of Fascial Space Infection of Odontogenic Origin

STEP 1: Securing Airway

Establishing a secure airway is paramount in cases of severe deep neck infection. Awake or sedated fiberoptic intubation might be necessary in cases of severe trismus or other airway compromise. Nasal intubation is relatively contraindicated in cases of retropharyngeal abscess due to potential iatrogenic disruption of posterior pharyngeal wall mucosa, increasing the risk of aspiration of infected material.[5] The surgeon should be prepared to perform surgical airway placement if a "cannot intubate, cannot ventilate" situation is encountered.

STEP 2: Aspiration of Abscess

After application of a topical cutaneous cleansing agent, abscess material is aspirated transcutaneously with a 10-cc syringe connected to an 18-gauge needle in a sterile fashion. If transmucosal aspiration is planned, a chlorhexidine oral rinse should be applied to minimize oral flora contamination. Aspirate should be sent as a microbiologic culture specimen (Fig. 18.1A). Care should be taken to not aspirate the entire abscess as it may make it difficult to find the fluid collection for definitive I&D.

STEP 3: Incision

Local anesthetic infiltration can be administered prior to incision. Various incision designs have been described depending on the fascial space involved. The skin incision should be long enough for the surgeon to easily introduce and manipulate the instrument of choice. The location and pattern of the skin and mucosal incision vary depending on the fascial space being drained (Fig. 18.1B and C).

STEP 4: Drainage and Culture

For submandibular abscess, the neck incision is approximately 2 to 4 cm just through skin below the angle of the mandible following a natural neck crease, inferior to the most inferior extent of swelling.[6] A mosquito hemostat or a Schnidt tonsil forceps is introduced through the skin, subcutaneous tissue, platysma muscle, and superficial layer of the deep cervical fascia until the inferior border of the mandible is encountered (Fig. 18.1D). Subperiosteal instrumentation of the lateral and medial aspect of the mandibular ramus is then performed if masticator space is also involved. Digital manipulation within the abscess cavity may help to disrupt the loculations. Purulent drainage can be cultured via the incision site, if aspirate was not previously obtained.

STEP 5: Irrigation and Drain Placement

All drainage sites should be irrigated with normal saline solution. Penrose drains (1/4") are then placed via incision sites and subsequently secured with 2-0 nylon sutures. An attempt should be made to place the tip of the drain in the center of the space being drained. The number of drains placed depends on the total number of fascial spaces involved (Fig. 18.1E).

Continued

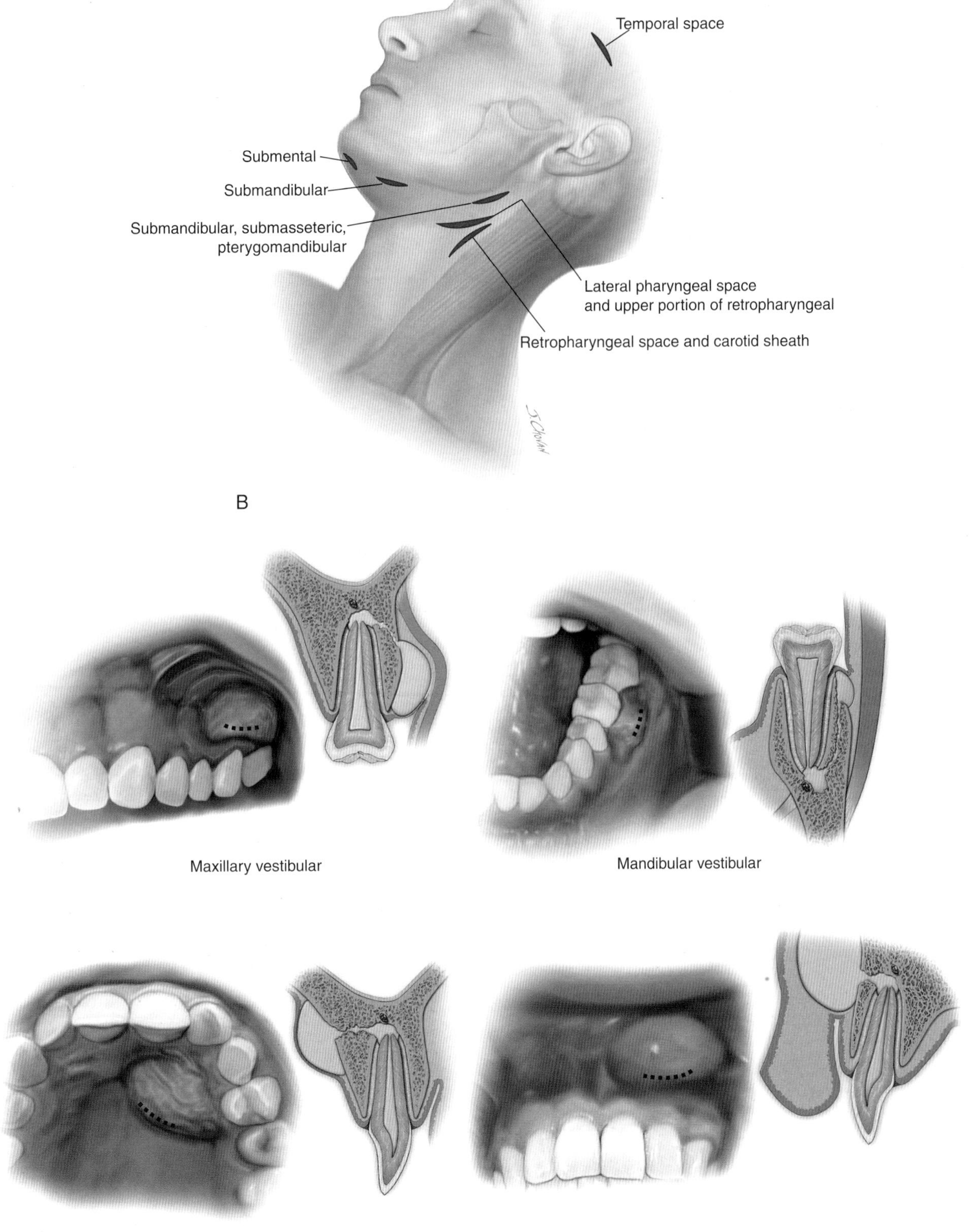

Figure 18.1, cont'd B, Various skin incision designs for incision and drainage (I&D) of deep fascial space infection. **C,** Various mucosal incision designs for I&D of vestibular and palatal abscess. Top left: Maxillary vestibular space I&D design. Top right: Mandibular vestibular space I&D design. Bottom left: Palatal space I&D design. Bottom right: Canine space I&D design.

TECHNIQUE: Incision and Drainage of Fascial Space Infection of Odontogenic Origin—*cont'd*

STEP 6: Removal of the Source of Infection by Dental Extraction

All infected teeth should be extracted to avoid possible reaccumulation of the abscess that may warrant a second trip to operating room. If extractions are performed in the same quadrant, gingival tissue should be loosely approximated with 3-0 chromic gut sutures to allow additional drainage postoperatively.

STEP 7: Decision on Extubation

Extubation in the operating room at the conclusion of the procedure should be discussed with the anesthesiologist. If the initial intubation is difficult, or if bilateral submandibular space infection is present, the surgeon should consider keeping the patient intubated in the intensive care unit (ICU) postoperatively for airway protection until neck involvement subsides. If airway assessment determines that reintubation is less difficult, if needed, one may attempt extubation in a controlled setting such as the ICU or the operating room.

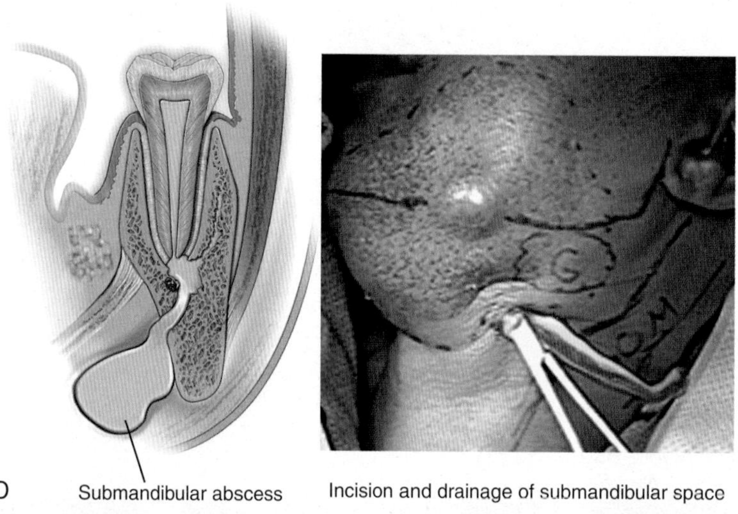

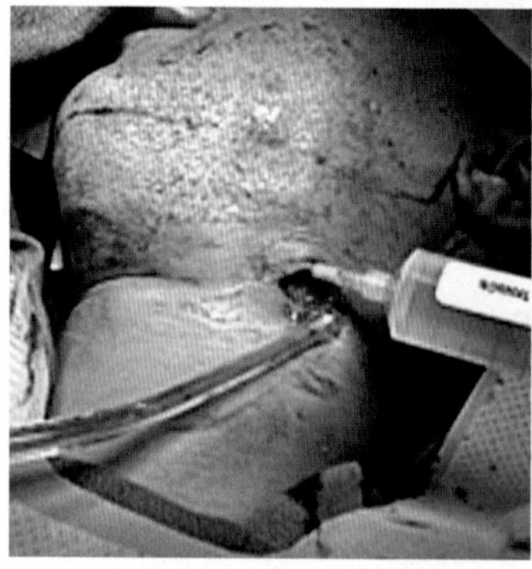

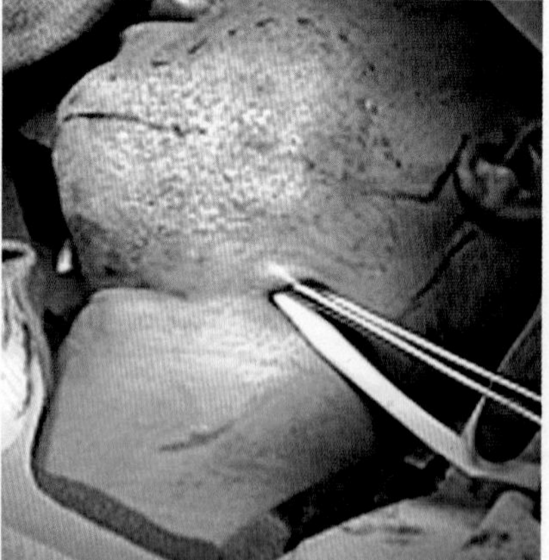

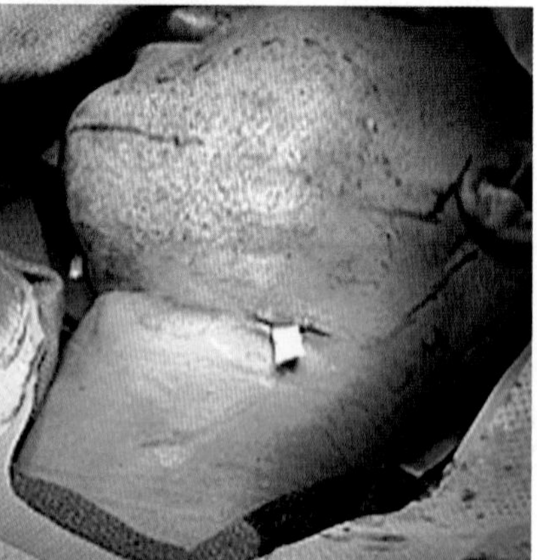

Figure 18.1, cont'd **D,** I&D of submandibular space. **E,** Irrigation and drain placement.

ALTERNATIVE TECHNIQUE 1: Incision and Drainage of Vestibular, Canine, and Palatal Space Abscess

For a vestibular or canine space abscess, a mosquito hemostat or a periosteal elevator is introduced via the vestibular incision into the involved space until the maxillary or mandibular buccal cortex is reached. For a palatal abscess, a palatal approach should be employed. Subperiosteal dissection may help to disrupt the loculations (Fig. 18.2).

ALTERNATIVE TECHNIQUE 2: Incision and Drainage of Lateral Pharyngeal and Retropharyngeal Space Abscess[6,7]

For lateral pharyngeal abscess, the submandibular approach as described earlier in this chapter will allow the surgeon to explore the lateral pharyngeal space by blunt finger dissection in the superomedial direction between the posterior belly of digastric and the sternocleidomastoid (SCM) muscles (Fig. 18.3A). However, the incision should be long enough to allow digital manipulation. Finger dissection of the lateral pharyngeal space is complete when the surgeon can palpate the endotracheal tube medially, the ipsilateral transverse processes of the vertebrae posteromedially, and the carotid sheath posterolaterally.

If the carotid sheath within the posterior compartment of the lateral pharyngeal space is involved, an anterior SCM approach may provide better access to the carotid artery or internal jugular vein. The incision is vertically oriented along the anterior border of the SCM beginning 3 cm inferior to the earlobe. A mosquito hemostat or a Schnidt tonsil forceps is introduced through the skin, subcutaneous tissue, platysma muscle, and superficial layer of the deep cervical fascia. The SCM is retracted posterolaterally to expose the carotid sheath. If it is involved, the sheath is then opened with subsequent proximal and distal vascular control in cases of vascular compromise.

For retropharyngeal abscess, the submandibular approach allows the surgeon to explore the suprahyoid component. If the infrahyoid portion was also involved, an anterior SCM approach should be selected. Finger dissection of the retropharyngeal space is a continuation of the complete dissection of the lateral pharyngeal space. The dissection is not complete until the surgeon can palpate the contralateral transverse processes of the vertebrae, the endotracheal tube from its posterior aspect, and, if necessary, the contralateral carotid sheath. The danger space, if involved, is entered by finger dissection through the alar fascia, which can be safely explored inferiorly as far as the T4 level (Fig. 18.3B and C).

In cases of descending mediastinal involvement, thoracic surgical consultation is necessary, and its management is not within the scope of this chapter.

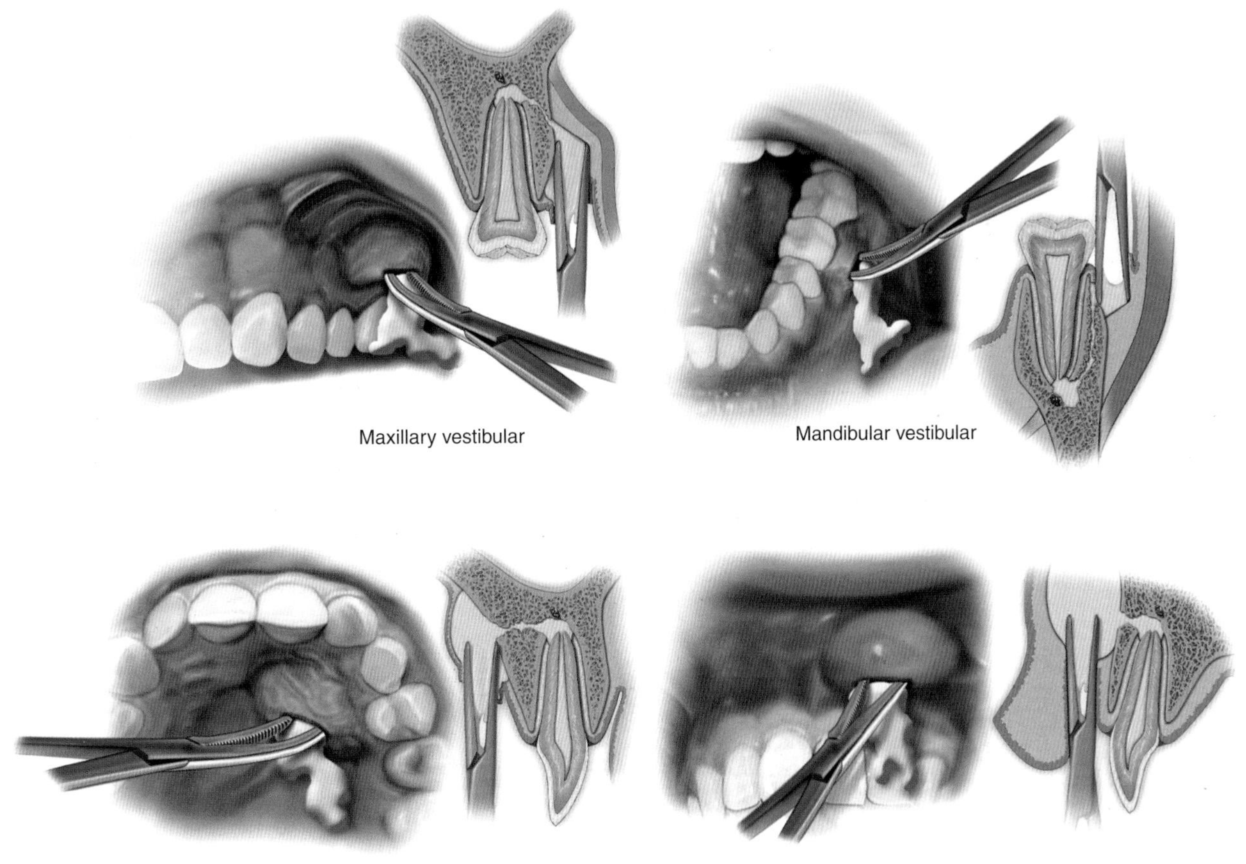

Figure 18.2 Incision and drainage (I&D) of vestibular, canine, and palatal space abscess. Top left: Maxillary vestibular space I&D. Top right: Mandibular vestibular space I&D. Bottom left: Palatal space I&D. Bottom right: Canine space I&D.

Avoidance and Management of Intraoperative Complications

Table 18.1 depicts the most commonly known intraoperative complications specific to the I&D of odontogenic infection. The most serious involve airway compromise.

Postoperative Considerations

If the patient is extubated at the end of the procedure with significant swelling, postoperative airway monitoring may include continuous pulse oximetry or admission to an observation bed setting such as a step-down unit. If a decision is made to keep the patient intubated in the ICU postoperatively, a cuff leak test should be performed to investigate airway patency prior to extubation. Alternatively, a Cook airway exchange catheter may be inserted below the tip of the endotracheal tube just above the carina before incompletely removing the endotracheal tube up to the level of the pharynx to access airway patency. If the airway is not patent, the existing endotracheal tube can be easily inserted using the Cook catheter as a guide. This tube exchanger is generally removed within 1 hour after extubation but can be left in place for up to 72 hours in cases of possible reintubation.[8,9]

Selection of empirical antibiotics is often institutionally driven; however, a combination of ampicillin/sulbactam and metronidazole is commonly used to provide broad-spectrum coverage. A bactericidal dosage of clindamycin (900 mg) is an alternative for the patient with a penicillin allergy. The antibiotic choice should be adjusted based on culture results. The use of a perioperative steroid to decrease airway edema is controversial. Its use may be beneficial but is contraindicated in diabetic or immunocompromised patients.

Subjective clinical improvement, especially pain reduction, is a good clinical indicator of infection resolution. The postoperative white blood cell count may be used, especially if there is a lack of resolution clinically. If this is the case, a repeat CT scan is necessary to determine if a recollection of the abscess is present. At that time a decision should be made to determine further treatment, such as performing additional I&D. Similarly, delayed infection resolution warrants a reevaluation of the effectiveness of the antibiotic.

There is no good evidence to show the benefits of drain irrigation or advancement. Typically, drains can be removed when they demonstrate a lack of purulent discharge.

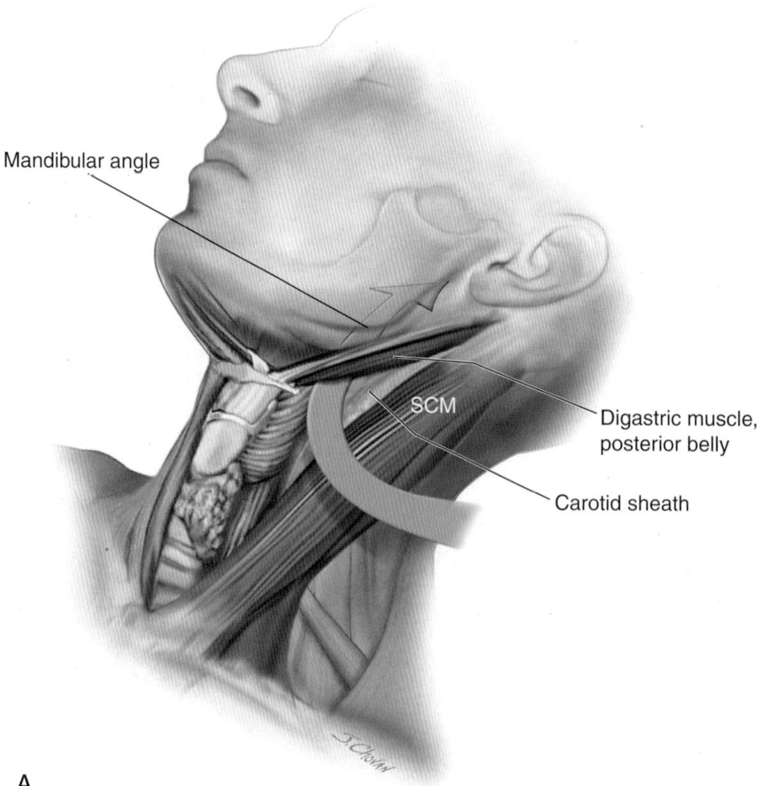

Figure 18.3 **A,** Incision and drainage (I&D) of lateral pharyngeal space abscess.

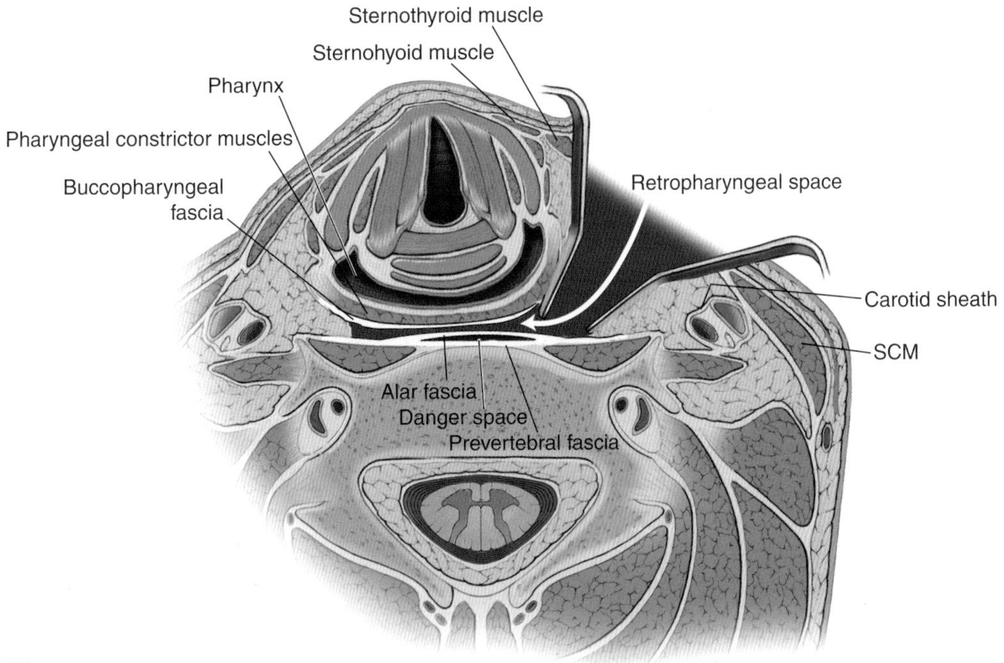

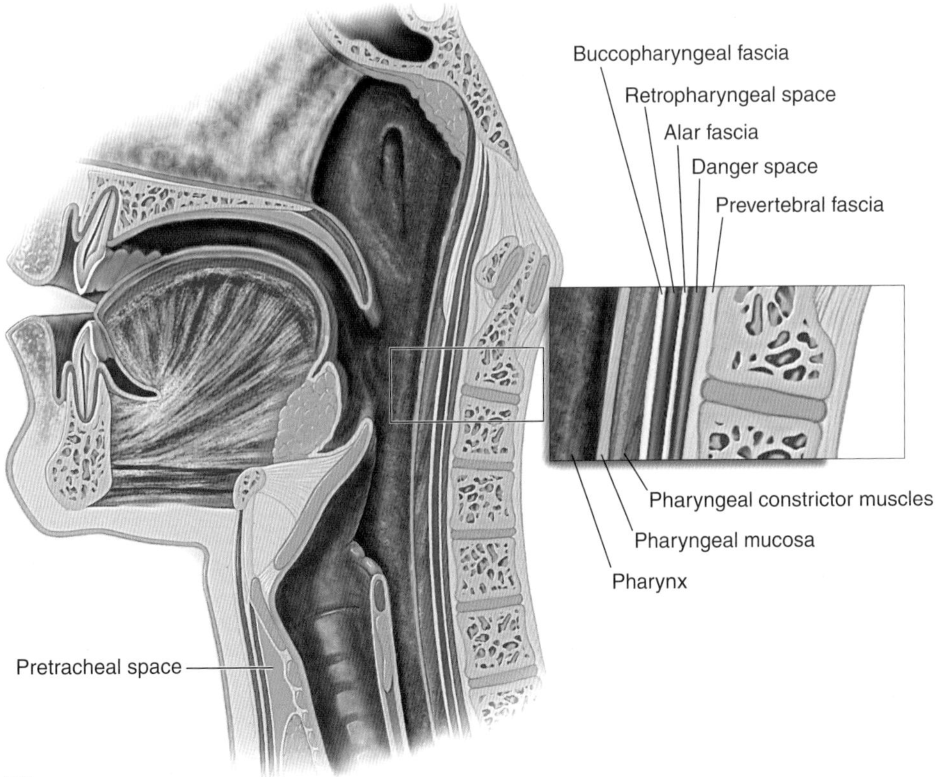

Figure 18.3, cont'd B1 and **B2,** Coronal and sagittal anatomic illustration for I&D of retropharyngeal space abscess.

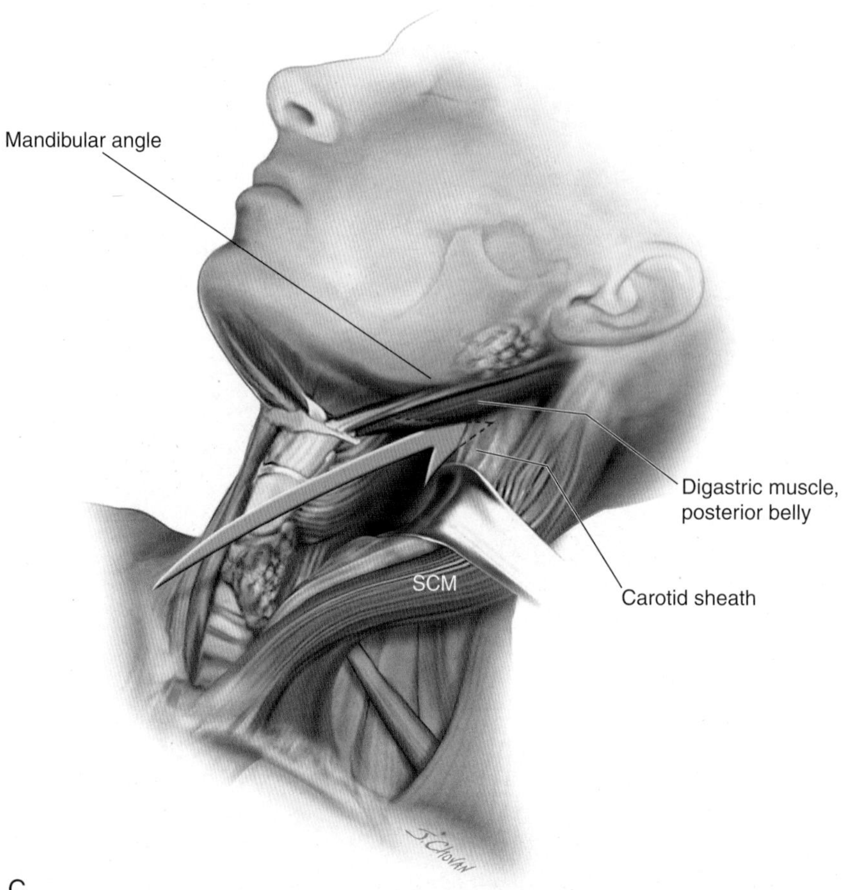

Figure 18.3, cont'd **C,** Surgical access for I&D of retropharyngeal abscess. *SCM*, Sternocleidomastoid.

Table 18.1 Most Common Perioperative Complications Associated with Incision and Drainage of Odontogenic Infection

Complication	Timing	Management
Airway obstruction	Preop Intraop	1. Anticipate surgical airway placement 2. Provide simultaneous supplemental oxygen with or without ventilator support via nasopharyngeal airway connected to anesthesia circuit
Aspiration of infected material	Intraop	1. Suction the airway prior to intubation 2. Cautious instrumentation of airway to avoid iatrogenic mucosal laceration during intubation
Incomplete drainage of abscess	Intraop Postop	1. Obtain preoperative CT scan with intravenous contrast dye to review all potential fascial spaces 2. Repeat CT scan in cases of reaccumulation of abscess and possible further incision and drainage

CT, Computed tomography.

References

1. Ludwig WF. Medicinishe correspondenz. *Blatt Des Würtembergischen Arztlichen Vercins.* 1836;6:26.
2. Grodinsky M, Holyoke EA. The fasciae and fascial spaces of the head, neck, and adjacent regions. *Am J Anat.* 1938;63:367.
3. Grodinsky M. Retropharyngeal and lateral pharyngeal abscesses. *Ann Surg.* 1939;110(2):177–199.
4. Grodinsky M. Ludwig's angina: an anatomical and clinical study with review of the literature. *Surgery.* 1939;5:678.
5. Topazian RG, Goldberg MH, Hupp JR. Odontogenic infections and deep fascial space infections of dental origin. In: Topazian RG, ed. *Oral and Maxillofacial Infections.* 4th ed. Philadelphia, Pennsylvania: WB Saunders; 2002.
6. Flynn TR. Surgical management of orofacial infections. *Atlas Oral Maxillofac Surg Clin North Am.* 2000;8(1):77–100.
7. Osborn TM, Assael LA, Bell RB. Deep space neck infection: principles of surgical management. *Oral Maxillofac Surg Clin North Am.* 2008;20(3):353–365.
8. Caplan RA, Benumof JL, Berry FA, et al. Practice guidelines for management of the difficult airway: a report by the American Society of Anesthesiologist Task Force on management of the difficult airway. *Anesthesiology.* 1993;78(3):597–602.
9. Schaeuble JC, Heidegger T. Strategies and algorithms for the management of the difficult airway: an update. *Trends Anaesth Crit Care.* 2012;2:208.

CHAPTER 19

Vestibuloplasty

Vincent J. Perciaccante and Deepak G. Krishnan

Armamentarium

#15 Scalpel handle and blades
#9 Periosteal elevator
#9 Periosteal elevator
1.1-mm Drill (9-mm, 11-mm long)
1.5-mm Screws (7-mm, 9-mm, and 1-mm long)
12 × 12-inch gauze to store graft
25-Gauge stainless steel wire
Adson tissue forceps
Appropriate sutures
Cotton tipped applicators
DeBakey tissue forceps
DeBakey tissue forceps
Dermatome
Impression compound
Iris scissors
Local anesthetic with vasoconstrictor
Metzenbaum scissors
Moist 4 × 4-inch gauze opened to single layer
Mosquito hemostats
Mosquito hemostats
Mosquito hemostats
Needle electrocautery
Obwegeser mandibular awl, 17.5 cm.
Obwegeser retractors, curved up, curved down (toe-in, toe-out)
Oral tissue conditioner
Peanut or Kitner sponges
Saline or sterile water, heated (water bath heater)
Seldin
Single and double skin hooks
Skin glue
Skin graft board
Skin Graft Preparation/Application
Skin Graft Procurement
Small osteotome and mallet
Stainless steel ruler
Stainless steel washers compatible with screws planned for use in attachment of stent
Sterile mineral oil
Sterile wooden tongue blades
Straight scissors
Surgical stent/denture
Tape
Vestibuloplasty Procedure
Waterproof surgical dressing
Weider retractor

History of the Procedure

The use of skin grafts to create a buccal vestibule in patients who present with inadequate soft tissue drape to support a denture base dates back to 1915 when Thiersch grafts were placed over the mandible via percutaneous pockets that were later opened to expose the underlying skin graft, providing a new sulcus.[1] Weiser[2] was likely the first to apply skin pouches perorally to the buccal vestibule. Pickrell,[3] Kilner and Jackson,[4] and Kazangian[5] all contributed publications to the literature on the evolving vestibuloplasty technique. A publication by Pichler and Trauner[6] in 1930 delineated many of the principles of this procedure (need for dissection close to the periosteum, hip skin donor site, allowing donor site to crust) that hold true to the present day. The lowering of the genioglossus muscles,[7] the mylohyoid muscles from the cuspid region posteriorly,[8] and of the mental foramen[9,10] added more versatility to the vestibuloplasty. Schuchardt reported on the skin grafting of the labiobuccal surface of the mandible in 1952.[11] In 1959 the technique of submucous vestibuloplasty in the maxilla was described by Obwegeser to extend fixed tissue on the alveolar ridge.[12,13] This procedure was found to be particularly useful in patients who showed alveolar resorption with resulting encroachment of the muscle attachments on the crest of the ridge. In 1963 Obwegeser presented total floor of the mouth lowering (LFM) by sectioning the mylohyoid as far forward as possible and sectioning parts of the genioglossus, which greatly enhanced the popularity of the vestibuloplasty.[9] Although the evolution of implants has made the vestibuloplasty procedure uncommon for increasing denture surface area, other pertinent indications remain for the technique, and it should continue to be part of the training of oral and maxillofacial surgeons. The typical atrophic mandibular ridge has a small line of attached mucosa at the crest of the ridge, whereas all of the remaining mucosa of the denture-bearing area can be elevated by the movement of the lips, cheeks, and tongue displacing a denture (Fig. 19.1). Split-thickness skin graft vestibuloplasty with grafting (VSG) and LFM procedures

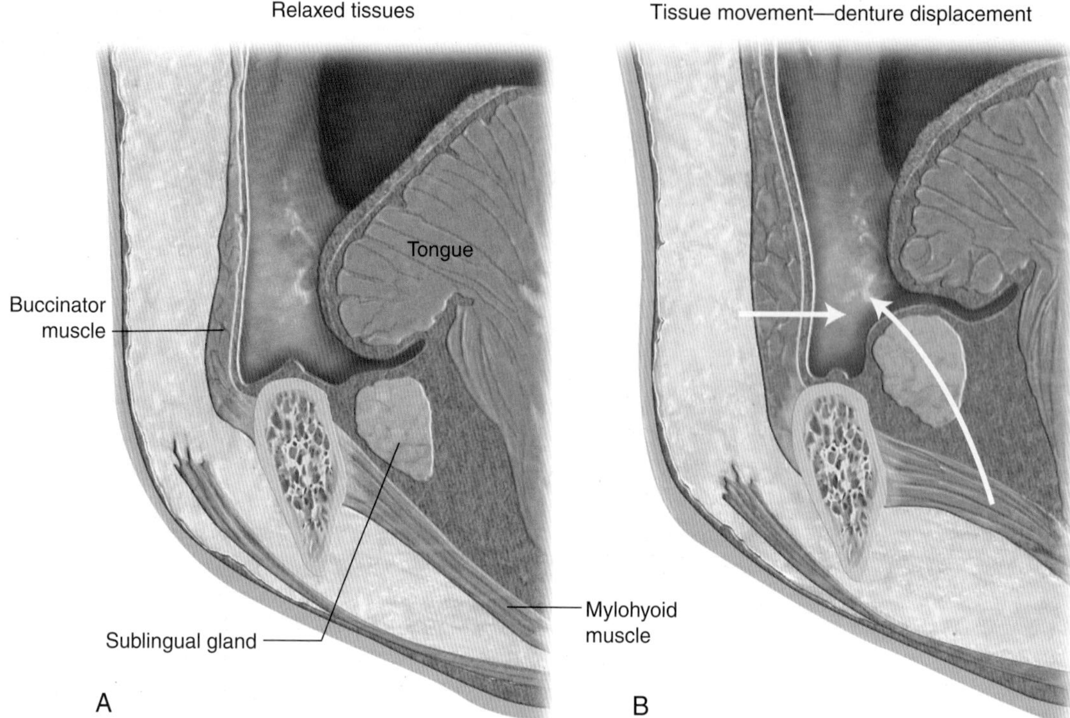

Figure 19.1 **A,** Buccal attachments and mylohyoid muscle relaxed. **B,** Elevation of buccal tissues and floor of mouth by contraction results in denture displacement.

result in a nondisplaceable tissue over the entire denture base. The graft's firm attachment to the periosteum ridge allows for denture stability even in cases where no significant ridge height can be created by the procedures.[1] An additional advantage offered by VSG and LFM surgery is that skin utilized in the grafts tends to react to pressure with a hyperkeratotic response, whereas mucosa tends to ulcerate under similar stress. Skin seems to be a more comfortable surface to the patient than mucosa. There are indications from the literature, such as a study by Landesman and colleagues,[14] that not only do VSG and LFM procedures not cause increased mandibular bone resorption, but they may also diminish the rate of resorption.

Indications for the Use of the Procedure

The main current indications for vestibuloplasty can be divided into four categories for the present discussion:

1. Ridge extension and lowering or otherwise altering the prosthesis and displacing submucous attachments to allow for better denture fit is the original indication for vestibuloplasty procedures in their many manifestations in the maxilla and mandible.
2. Procedures that attempt to reconstruct edentulous bone loss by various means frequently require vestibuloplasty procedures to complement and complete the osseous reconstruction. The compromised soft tissue drape resulting after such osseous augmentations can be markedly improved with soft tissue vestibuloplasties.
3. Inadequate or inappropriate soft tissue drape in cases where resection with or without grafting has been previously performed and prosthetic restoration demands improvement of the soft tissue drape.
4. Occasionally implants are placed so that they emerge in nonattached mucosa, and there are those who feel that the success of restorations based on these implants can be markedly improved with the creation of an attached mucosa/implant interface. The stability of the periimplant mucosa is important for the overall stability of the dental implant and the maintenance of bone health around an implant. Whether the stability is secured by nonkeratinized mucosa or keratinized attached mucosa is a point of discussion.[15] Some investigators report no difference in the maintenance of periimplant bone levels,[16] whereas others report an increased risk for periimplant bone loss when the implant is surrounded by alveolar mucosa.[17] Insufficient keratinized mucosa in the vicinity of implants does not necessarily mediate adverse effects on hygiene management.[16]

Limitations and Contraindications

The general health of the patient must be considered as a limiting factor in vestibuloplasty, as these procedures frequently require 2 to 3 hours of general anesthesia for completion. Patients who have been irradiated in the head and neck require extra precaution in all surgical procedures in the field of treatment. In mandibular vestibuloplasties, temporary or permanent mental nerve paresthesias are common, and the patient must understand this possibility prior to surgery and be able to tolerate these deficits. Donor and operative site pain can be significant, and those who feel they would do poorly with such a degree of postoperative pain should be excluded from these surgeries. Donor site color and texture will be altered, and this may dissuade some from the VSG procedure for cosmetic considerations. Mandibular ridges of less than 15 mm of body height are less likely to result in adequate vestibular depth after VSG and LFM; however, a broader immobile graft area after such procedures may improve denture-wearing ability even in the face of decreased mandibular bone height. Maxillary myotomies and grafts can be performed by open or closed techniques, and although 10 to 15 mm of ridge height and some palatal depth allow for more successful augmentations, the facial aspect of the maxilla allows for relocation of the muscle attachments more extensively without fear of muscle detachment complications than is possible in the mandible. Around the midline of the mandible, dissection in the supraperiosteal plane should end about 1 cm above the inferior border of the mandible to prevent mentalis detachment and resultant drooping of the chin.[1] Sharp mylohyoid ridge undercuts may be removed if excessive, but atrophy will occur after detachment of the mylohyoid in the LFM procedure. Sharpness of the genial tubercles will also atrophy after the genioglossus attachments are removed superiorly, but recontouring may be required if genial tubercles are large. Any recontouring procedures required should be done prior to VSG and LFM because it requires subperiosteal dissection. Healing of 2 to 3 months should be allowed prior to skin grafting over the area of excised bone.[1] Although skin grafts can be sutured in place, surgical stents allow for accurate adaptation to the labial-buccal and lingual areas. Most consider the surgical stent to be an important component of VSG and LFM procedures, and laboratory capabilities must exist for those who contemplate such preprosthetic surgeries.[1]

Technique: Graft Donor Sites

Because several vestibuloplasty techniques require a skin or mucosal graft, the technique for both of these procedures will be outlined prior to a discussion of techniques for vestibuloplasty. For obtaining a split-thickness skin graft, please refer to the reconstruction chapter of this text. If the determination is made to utilize a mucosal graft, it can be obtained from the palate or buccal mucosa. In the case of the palate, the graft is excised in a horseshoe shape in a supraperiosteal plane, whereas in the buccal mucosa a spindle-shaped graft is excised without muscle and as superficial to the lamina propria as possible. The palatal site is left to granulate in and may or may not be covered with a protective stent. The buccal mucosa graft site is closed with resorbable sutures in a superficial plane to prevent entrapment of muscle tissues in the scar, thereby minimizing the chance of trismus after healing. A study by Hashemi and colleagues[18] suggested that AlloDerm (Lifecell Corporation, Bridgewater, NJ) is a suitable alternative to mucosal and skin grafts in vestibuloplasty procedures. AlloDerm is donated human skin that is aseptically processed to remove all cells, maintaining only a skin matrix framework. Collagen and elastic fiber make up this US Food and Drug Administration-approved human tissue allograft, which has been in use since the early 1990s in burn injury treatment as well as in plastic and periodontal surgery.[19] Although AlloDerm overcomes many of the problems associated with mucosal and skin grafts, including donor site morbidity, it is associated with increased financial considerations.[19] Another allograft product is Mucograft (Geistlich Pharma North America, Inc., Princeton, NJ; Geistlich Pharma AG, Wolhusen, Switzerland).

Technique: Stents

All grafts are sutured inferiorly and superiorly to the vestibuloplasty site and held in place with a previously prepared surgical splint. Alternatively, grafts can be adapted closely to the undersurface of the stent and secured to it with Dermabond (Ethicon, Somerville, NJ). The stent is designed on a study model, and the borders of the stent are perforated so the green modeling compound can be heated and applied for border molding after the myotomy is completed. The molded stent is attached to the mandible or maxilla with circummandibular wires or screws.

TECHNIQUE: Vestibular Skin Grafting and Lowering of Floor of Mouth

STEP 1: Initial Incision and Dissection

A crestal incision is made with a #15 blade running from retromolar pad to retromolar pad at the junction of the free and attached gingiva in a supraperiosteal plane. As the supraperiosteal dissection proceeds, it is important to remove all of the soft tissue from the periosteum and displace it inferiorly. Failure to remove any soft tissue will result in graft mobility where it remains. Small periosteal perforations may occur but will not be as unfavorable as leaving soft tissue attached as long as they are less than 1 sq cm in size.[1] When a margin of mucosa is identified, double-ended skin hooks are applied and light tension is utilized to assist in the dissection from the periosteum with the front or back of the #15 blade, a periosteal elevator, or a peanut sponge. As the mental neurovascular bundle is approached, it is easily identified and left in the subperiosteal plane, and shallow dissection here avoids damage to this structure. Patient education should always include the possibility of mental nerve paresthesia/anesthesia. The posterior limit of the dissection should be at the external oblique line, whereas the anterior limit in the midline should not exceed 1 cm from the inferior border of the mandible to prevent sagging of the chin (Fig. 19.2A).

Continued

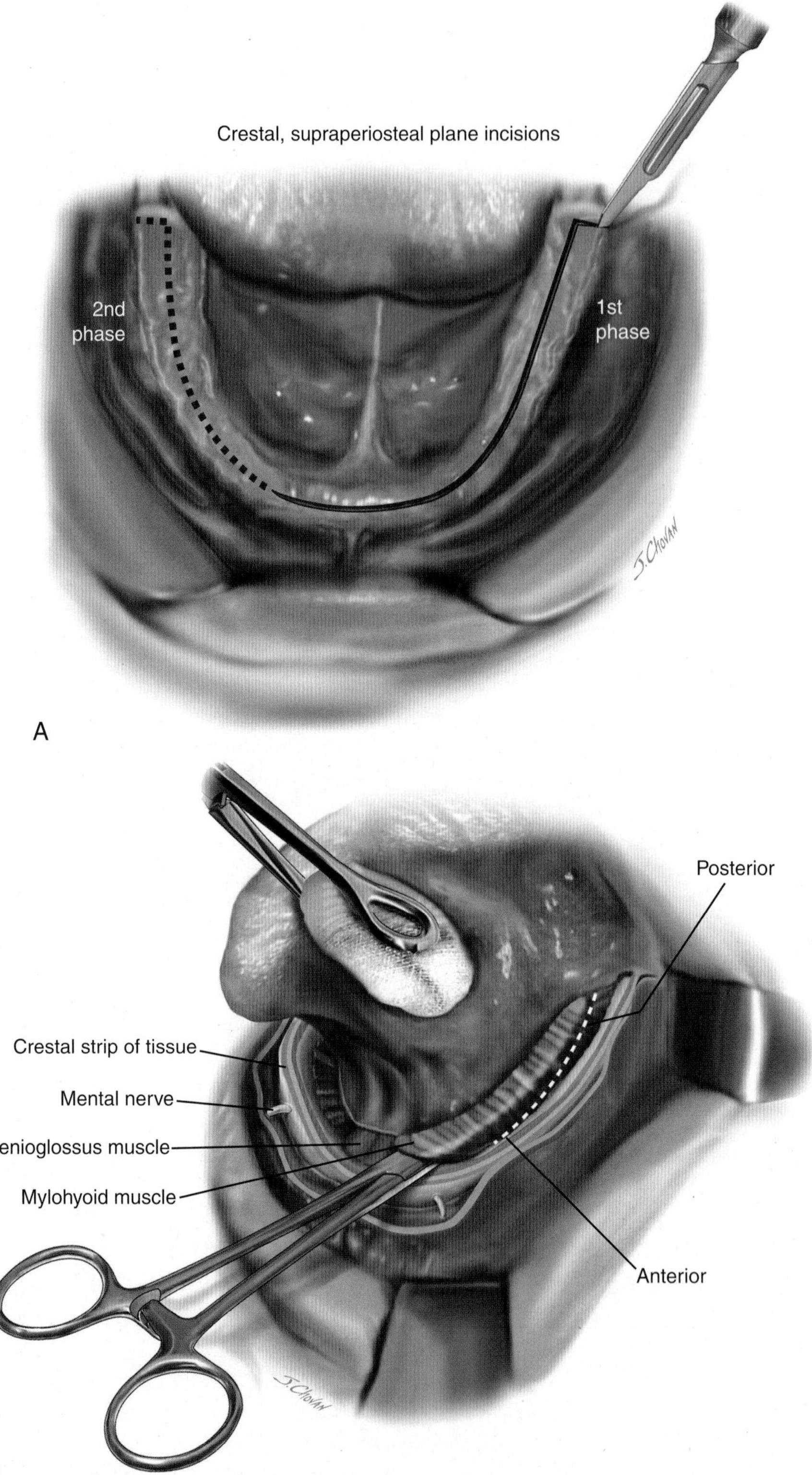

Figure 19.2 **A,** The continuous line indicates the initial incision in the supraperiosteal plane for the first phase of the dissection, and the dashed line shows the completion of the initial incision on the other side of the arch for the second phase of the dissection. **B,** A curved Kelly forceps is placed beneath the mylohyoid muscle to make the dissection of this structure from the lingual side of the mandible easier. Posterior: Division of the attachment of the mylohyoid muscle should occur slightly medial to the mandible to avoid the lingual nerve, which is lateral in this area. Anterior: Division of the attachment of the mylohyoid muscle should occur closer to the mandible to avoid the lingual nerve, which is more medial in this area.

TECHNIQUE: Vestibular Skin Grafting and Lowering of Floor of Mouth—cont'd

STEP 2: Floor of Mouth Dissection

If a floor of the mouth dissection is planned, local anesthesia with a vasoconstrictor is infiltrated in the submucosa, mylohyoid, and genioglossus regions. A gauze bolus in a forceps is placed in the sublingual region and rotated away from the crest of the ridge to provide retraction and visibility. The incision is started at the anterior border of the retromolar region at the margin of the fixed and free mucosa and carried to the midline. The incision should be quite shallow posteriorly to avoid damage to the lingual nerve, and as it is advanced, the entire depth of the mucosa is incised more anteriorly to the contralateral cuspid region. The same procedure is completed on the contralateral side until the incision is joined. Blunt dissection in an inferior direction is completed with a peanut sponge, periosteal elevator, or back or edge of a #15 blade to the level of the mylohyoid muscle. Posterior to the genial muscles, the mylohyoid is incised anteriorly from its attachments to the lingual mandible. After cutting the mylohyoid muscle anteriorly, the posterior limit of this structure is more easily identified by placing a curved Kelly hemostat under it and elevating it for identification before incising it. At the posterior limit of the mylohyoid attachment, care must be used to prevent cutting the muscle from its attachments to the mandible too close to prevent lingual nerve damage. After removal of the mylohyoid attachments, finger dissection is carried out in the submandibular region with care exercised not to go beneath the inferior border of the mandible. After bilaterally completing the previous steps, attention is directed more anteriorly where approximately half of the genioglossus can be sectioned. Overzealous removal of the genioglossus can result in difficulty swallowing postoperatively for several months[20] (Fig. 19.2B).

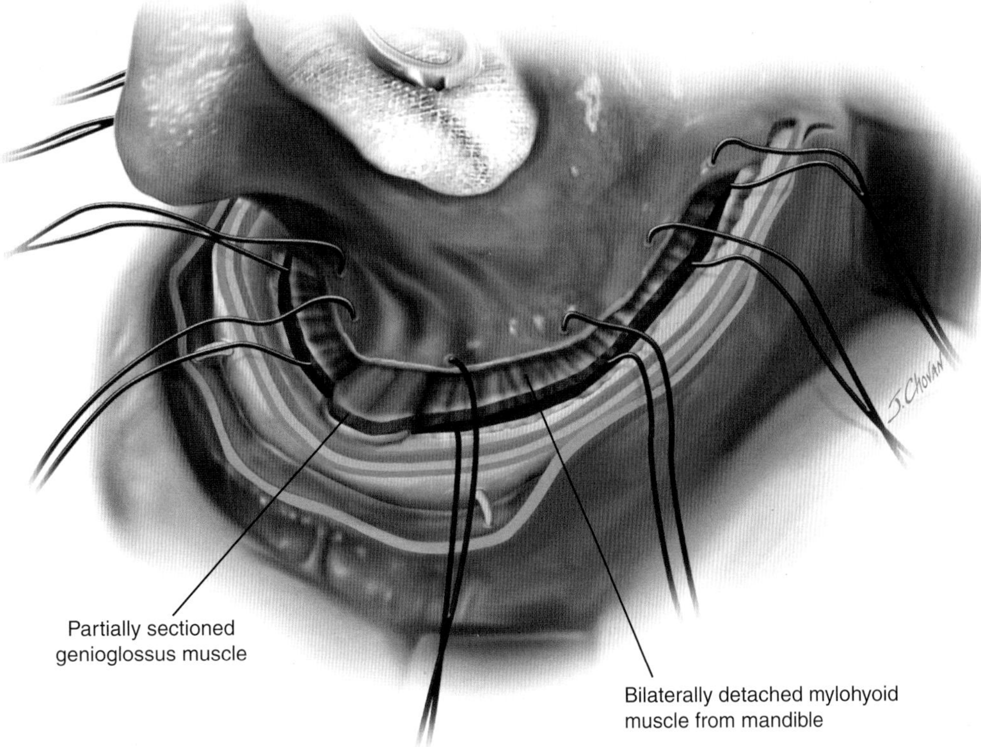

Figure 19.2, cont'd **C,** Six to eight sutures are passed through the lingual mucosa.

Continued

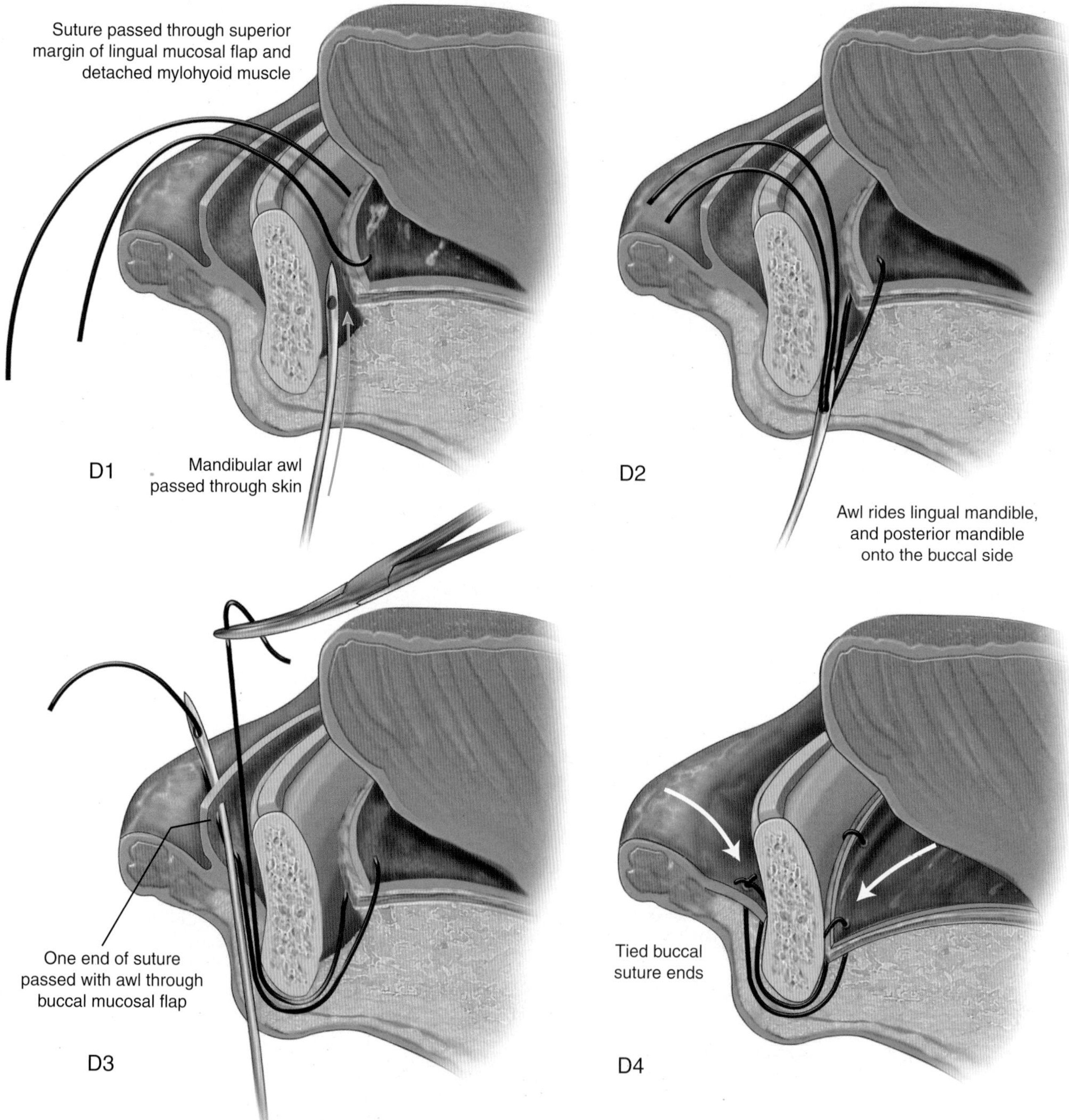

Figure 19.2, cont'd D1, A suture is passed in the superior margin of the lingual mucosal flap. A curved awl is passed from the skin to the lingual side of the mandible in close contact with the lingual surface of the lower jaw. **D2,** Both ends of the suture are passed through the eye of the awl. **D3,** One end of the suture is removed from the eye of the awl and grasped with a hemostat while the end remaining in the awl is passed through the buccal mucosa. **D4,** The two buccal suture ends are then tied to each other, retracting the buccal and lingual tissues inferiorly.

TECHNIQUE: Vestibular Skin Grafting and Lowering of Floor of Mouth—cont'd

STEP 3: Muscle Attachment Management

Sharp mylohyoid and genial attachments can be reduced with an osteotome and bone file if necessary, but this is typically avoidable as they will usually resorb adequately. Attention is then directed to the crestal tissues. If suturing the graft is planned, some crestal tissue must be left to suture the graft, but any loose tissue should be excised supraperiosteally with a #15 blade or Metzenbaum scissors. If there are any sharp bony projections, the soft tissue over these areas should be removed by meticulous sharp dissection and the periosteum sharply incised and minimally reflected, and the bone removed with a rongeur and smoothed with a small bone file.

STEP 4: Submandibular (Hammock) Sutures

It should be pointed out that the graft can be placed to cover lingual tissues if desired, but this area covered by an intact periosteum will granulate quite readily in about 2 weeks under a stent if not grafted. If the LFM procedure has been part of the surgery, submandibular sutures are applied after meticulous attention to hemostasis to avoid swelling in the floor of the mouth, which could cause airway embarrassment postoperatively. There are six to eight submandibular 2-0 resorbable or gut sutures that are initially passed through the lingual tissue dissection margin. After all are placed initially, a fine-gauge curved mandibular awl is utilized to carry both of the tag ends of the sutures from the lingual side of the mandible to the buccal aspect, where one of the ends is then passed through the buccal tissue dissection margin and then tied to the other tag end. As these sutures are tied, the lingual and buccal tissues are retracted inferiorly, completing the LFM as well as securing the buccal extension of the tissues in an inferior direction. If only the buccal tissues are to be treated, 3-0 catgut sutures can be utilized to suture the margins of the dissected buccal mucosa inferiorly to the intact periosteum in the inferior aspect of the newly created sulcus (Fig. 19.2C and D).

STEP 5: Graft Placement

In all cases the surgery is completed by application of the graft (mucosal, split-thickness skin, or AlloDerm) to the periosteal bed on the buccal surface and to the lingual surface if this is the surgeon's choice. Grafts can be trimmed and adapted closely to the graft bed and sutured prior to placement of the surgical stent, which has been border-molded with green compound (Kerr Dental, Orange, CA) and lined with Coe-Comfort reline material (GC America, Alsip, IL) to achieve a close adaptation of the graft. The graft can also be trimmed and adapted to the underside of the stent with care to place the epithelial surface to the splint and fixated to the stent with Dermabond (Ethicon, San Angelo, TX). In either case, the stent is then fixated to the mandible with three 26-gauge wire passes in a circummandibular fashion from the lingual to the buccal surface and tightened over the stent to secure the graft in close approximation to the graft bed. In the maxilla the surgical stent can be attached with a palatal screw of 2.7-mm diameter and appropriate length. Screws can also be utilized to fixate the mandibular stent to the ridge if adequate bone is available above the inferior alveolar bundle posteriorly. It is advisable to place a stainless steel washer in the stent at fabrication in the areas where screws are to be placed to help reinforce the holes drilled in the stent and prevent cracking of the stent when the screws are tightened. A pressure dressing similar to one used for a genioplasty can be utilized for mandibular procedures. The surgical stent should remain for 7 to 10 days, and circummandibular wires and nonresorbable sutures or screws can be removed under local anesthesia or with sedation as preferred. Prophylactic antibiotics are indicated for stent removal, and topical antisepsis of wires and sutures prior to removal is also advisable. After stent removal, frequent saline irrigation is advised, and the existing denture or stent can be modified and worn as a dressing until the prosthesis can be comfortably fabricated (Fig. 19.2E).

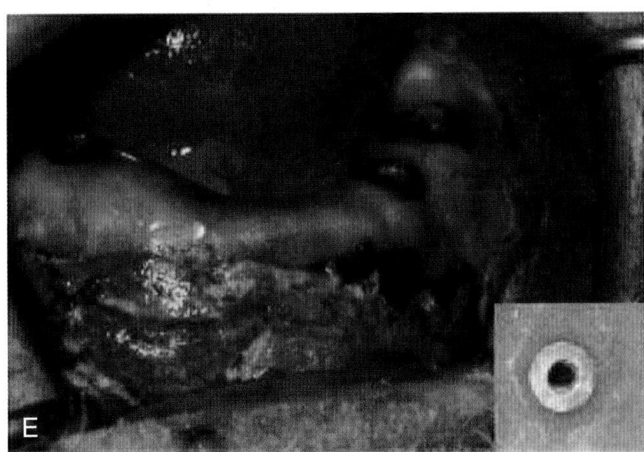

Figure 19.2, cont'd E, Mandibular stent affixed to the mandible using screws in the alveolar crest. Inset shows detail of washer-reinforced hole for the screw in the stent.

ALTERNATIVE TECHNIQUE 1: Maxillary Submucous Vestibuloplasty

Submucous vestibuloplasty was initially advocated in the mandible by Kazangian[5] but proved to be an unreliable surgery according to Obwegeser,[12] who did recommend and described the procedure for application in the maxilla. Submucous vestibuloplasty can be utilized for maxillary ridges where low tissue attachments in the bicuspid and anterior midline associated with generally loose flabby tissues buccally conflict with comfortable denture wear. The procedure can be performed under local or general anesthesia as preferred by the patient and the operator.

STEP 1: Initial Incision and Submucosal Dissection

After local anesthetic is infiltrated into the buccal soft tissues, a midline incision is made from the crest of the ridge to bone and extended superiorly about 15 mm.[1] Following this a small pair of Metzenbaum scissors is used to separate the mucosa from the submucosal layer as far posteriorly as is required to obtain adequate vestibular depth. It may be necessary occasionally to add bilateral vertical incisions more posteriorly to separate the mucosal and submucosal tissues completely (Fig. 19.3A).

STEP 2: Supraperiosteal Dissection

Attention is then redirected to the midline incision, where a second layer of dissection is created in a supraperiosteal plane with a periosteal elevator separating the intact periosteum from the tissues lateral to it (Fig. 19.3B).

STEP 3: Crestal Attachment Division

After this step is completed, a #15 blade or a pair of small scissors is introduced into the supraperiosteal pocket and the crestal attachment of the tissue between the periosteum and the mucosa is excised. When this dissection has been completed, the intermediate layer is retracted superiorly or can be excised with a wedge resection. This allows the mucosal layer to directly collapse to the periosteum (Fig. 19.3C).

STEP 4: Anterior Nasal Spine Reduction

Anteriorly the nasal spine should be removed with a rongeur and the mucosa closed with a figure-eight suture to the nasal septum to elevate the mucosa anteriorly.

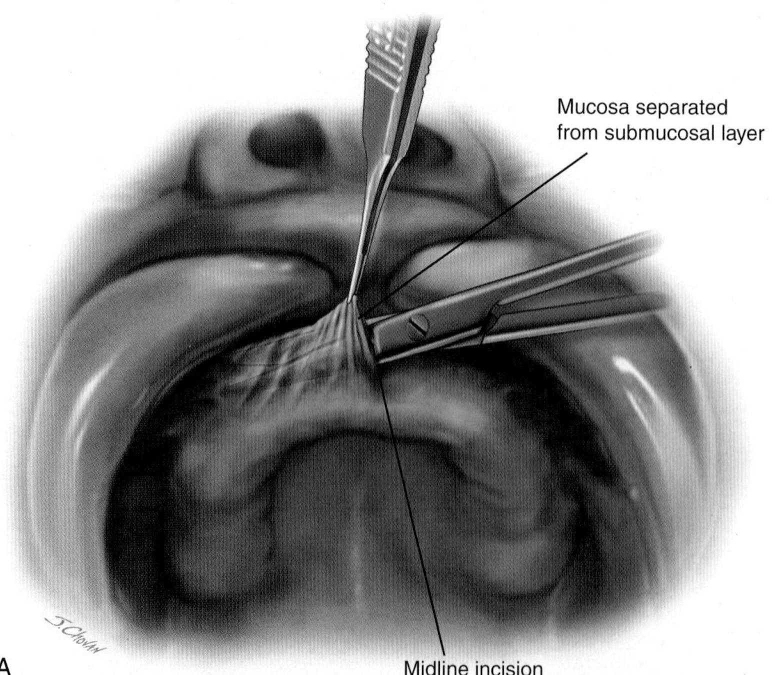

Figure 19.3 **A,** Small Metzenbaum scissors are used to separate the mucosa from the submucosa.

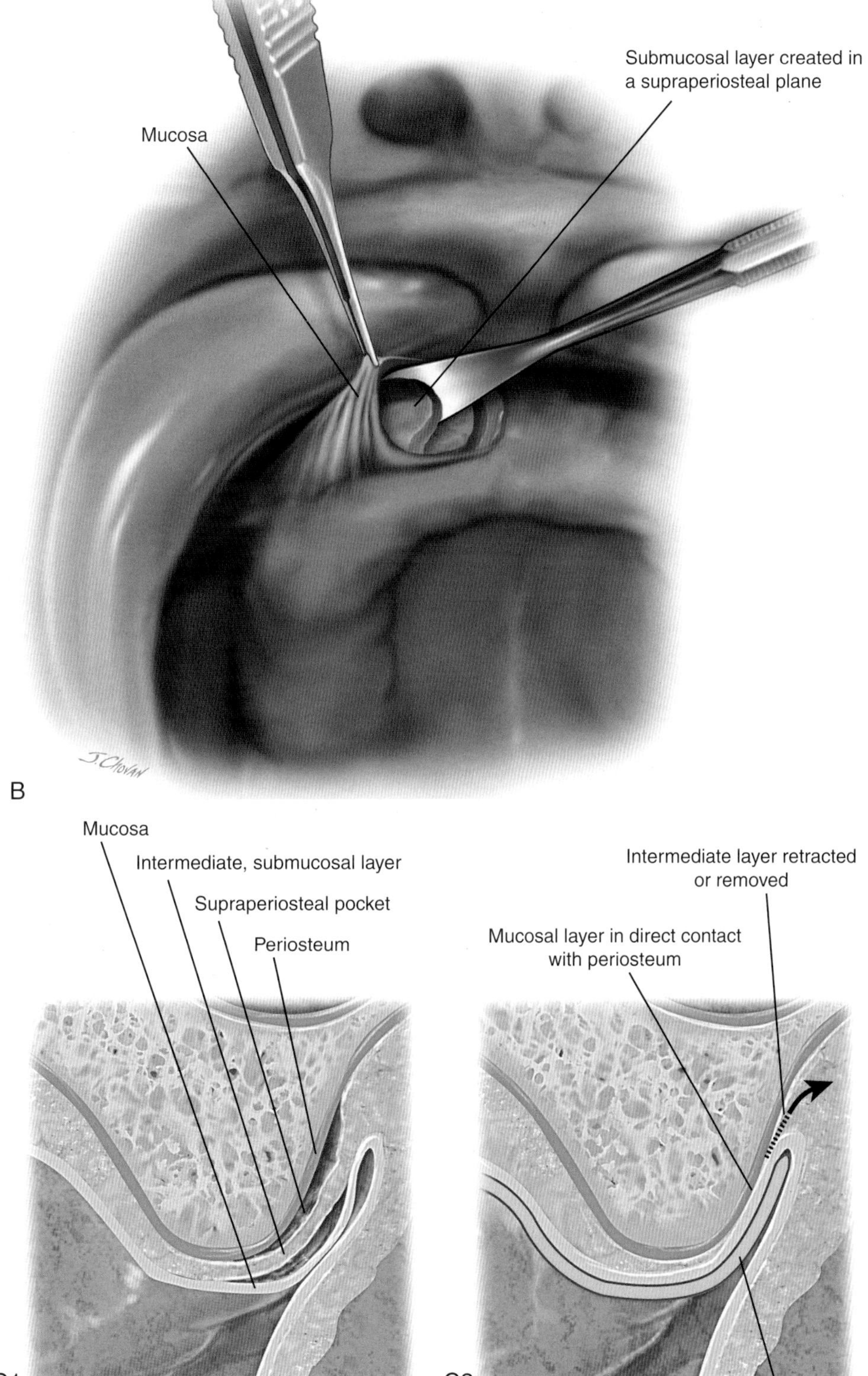

Figure 19.3, cont'd B, A second layer of dissection is created in a supraperiosteal plane with a periosteal elevator separating the intact periosteum from the tissues lateral to it. **C1,** A submucosal and a supraperiosteal pocket are developed. **C2,** After the intermediate layer is excised or cut and allowed to retract superiorly, the mucosa collapses against the periosteum.

Continued

ALTERNATIVE TECHNIQUE 1: Maxillary Submucous Vestibuloplasty—cont'd

STEP 5: Closure and Stent Placement

The mucosal incision and any other necessary incisions are then closed with 3-0 gut. The patient's denture or a prefabricated stent can then be border-molded with green compound, relined with a soft reline material, and fixated to the maxilla with 2.7-mm screws in the cuspid eminence bilaterally and in the palate to maintain the newly established sulcus. The stent must be very stable to prevent relapse and is left in place for 1 week and easily removed in an office setting with local anesthesia. Denture construction can commence as soon as the patient is comfortable, but the stent should be modified as needed and relined for wear until a definitive prosthesis has been completed to prevent relapse (Fig. 19.3D).

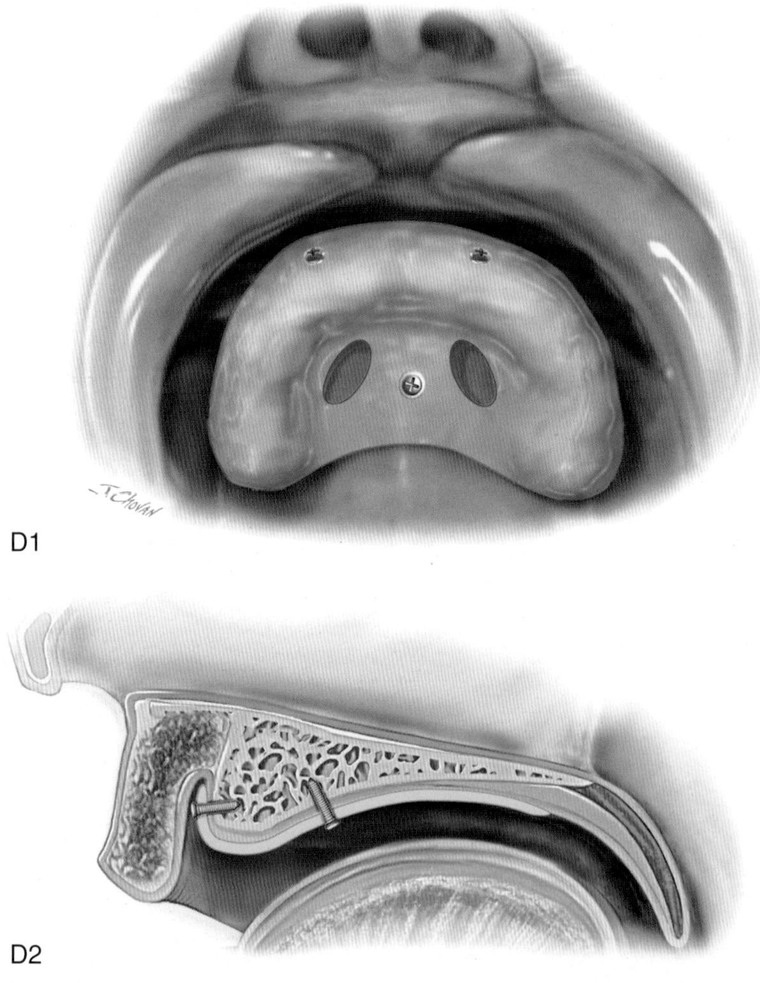

Figure 19.3, cont'd **D1,** Occlusal view of the palatal screw fixation of the stent. **D2,** Sagittal view of the stent showing palatal and cuspid eminence screw fixation options.

ALTERNATIVE TECHNIQUE 2: Maxillary Secondary Epithelialization

The maxillary secondary epithelialization technique can be utilized to manage the maxillary epulis fissuratum associated with alveolar bone loss and denture flange impingement. Obwegeser[21] described a predictable technique for this surgery, which still has appreciable application in the modern oral and maxillofacial practice of preprosthetic surgery. The epulis can be removed and denture wear prohibited until healing occurs before the secondary epithelialization is performed, or a full thickness of mucosa containing the lesion can be elevated and the lesion excised at the time of the secondary epithelialization procedure.

STEP 1: Initial Incision and Dissection

In either case, after instillation of local anesthesia with a vasoconstrictor, an incision starts bilaterally in the most posterior limit that is to be elevated and proceeds to the midline, creating a mucosal-submucosal flap and leaving intact periosteum over the maxillary buccal face. The flap is elevated by blunt dissection to a level slightly up the zygomatic buttress posteriorly and the nasal floor anteriorly (double skin hooks for tension on the flap help to keep tension on the flap throughout dissection). The nasal spine can be removed with a rongeur if needed.

STEP 2: Flap Retraction and Suturing

The elevated flap is retracted superiorly and sutured to the periosteum there with several 4-0 chromic catgut horizontal mattress sutures on a small ½ round needle. Anteriorly a figure-eight suture can be utilized to attach the most anterior portion of the flap to the nasal septum for maximum elevation of this portion of the incision. If the periosteum is left intact, a pseudomembrane will form rapidly and rapid reepithelialization will follow (Fig. 19.4).

STEP 3: Stent Placement

A firmly affixed stent (the patient's current denture or a laboratory prepared stent) can be useful, and it is border-molded with green compound, relined with a soft reline material, and fixated to the maxilla with screws as described earlier. It is also possible to leave the wound uncovered, but in this case dentures must not contact the tissues, as any movement will cause irritation resulting in granulation tissue excess. A scar band may be present for many months after this procedure and the denture flange extension should be limited to be short of this, but in time the band usually softens.

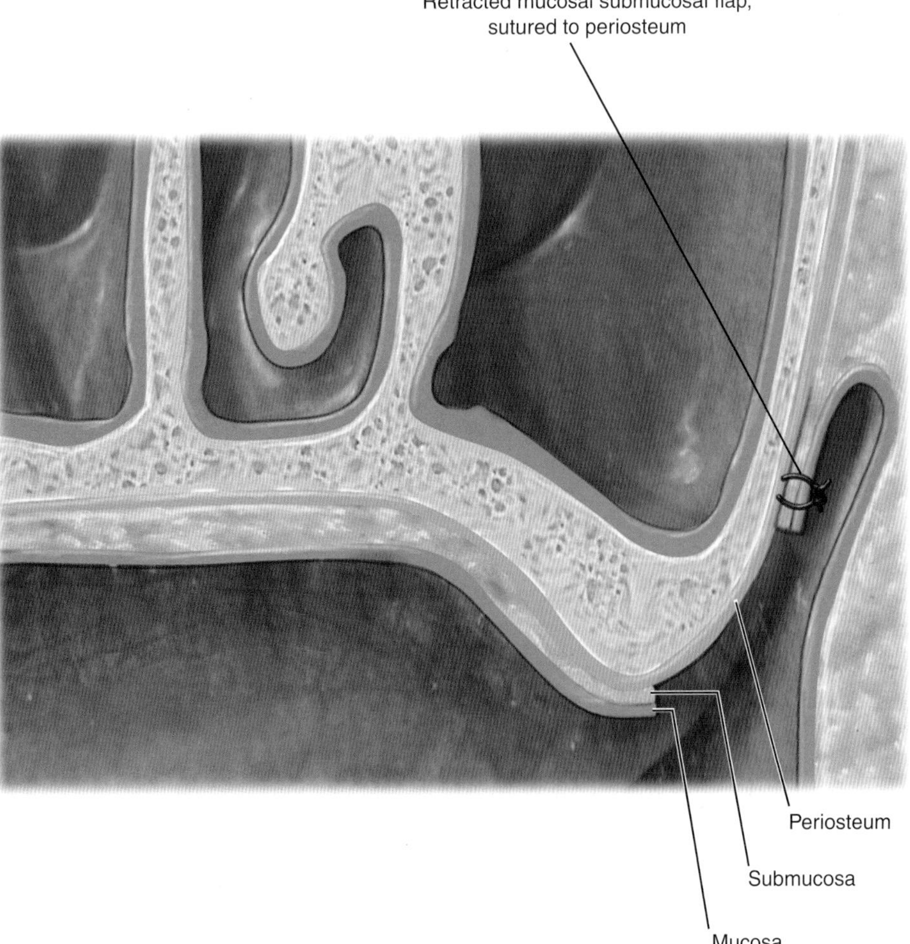

Figure 19.4 Horizontal mattress sutures are placed as high as possible in the vestibule to complete the secondary epithelialization procedure.

ALTERNATIVE TECHNIQUE 3: Crestally Pedicled Mucosal Graft (Lip Switch Myotomy) of the Mandible

A lip switch myotomy of the mandible can be a useful technique for obtaining additional lower denture retention/stability in a patient who is not healthy enough for a more major procedure such as VSG/LFM or cannot afford implant retained overdentures. The procedure was originally presented by Kazanjian[22] and modified by Godwin,[23] who presented the basis of the currently used technique for a crestally pedicled mucosal graft, and important modifications have been added by other authors[24–27] since his paper from 1947. This procedure lends itself well to local anesthesia or sedation and is initiated in either case by infiltration of a local anesthesia with a vasoconstrictor throughout the lower anterior vestibule.

STEP 1: Initial Incision and Dissection

An incision is marked medial to the area of the mental nerve on the inner surface of the lower lip, which should be about 1.5 times as long as the expected vestibular depth to be created. The incision is accomplished in the mucosa and elevated to be pedicled to the attached mucosa at the crest of the ridge (Fig. 19.5A and B).

STEP 2: Periosteal Incision

At the junction of the aforementioned flap and the periosteum of the mandible, an incision is made through the submucosa and periosteum horizontally superiorly and vertically bilaterally, mirroring the dimensions of the previously elevated pedicled flap and elevated from the mandible. The most inferior margin of the periosteum flap is also incised horizontally at the desired depth of the vestibule (Fig. 19.5C).

STEP 3: Flap Transposition

The superior edge of the periosteal flap is transposed anteriorly and its superior margin sutured to the incised lip mucosal margin as superiorly as is possible.

STEP 4: Closure

The pedicled flap is then placed in the created depth of the vestibule and sutured to the periosteum there with resorbable sutures (Fig. 19.5D).

STEP 5: Dressing

A pressure dressing similar to one that would be used in a genioplasty procedure is applied, to be left for 2 days or longer if possible. Denture construction can commence about a week after surgery is completed with the labiobuccal flange slightly underextended for several months (Fig. 19.5E).

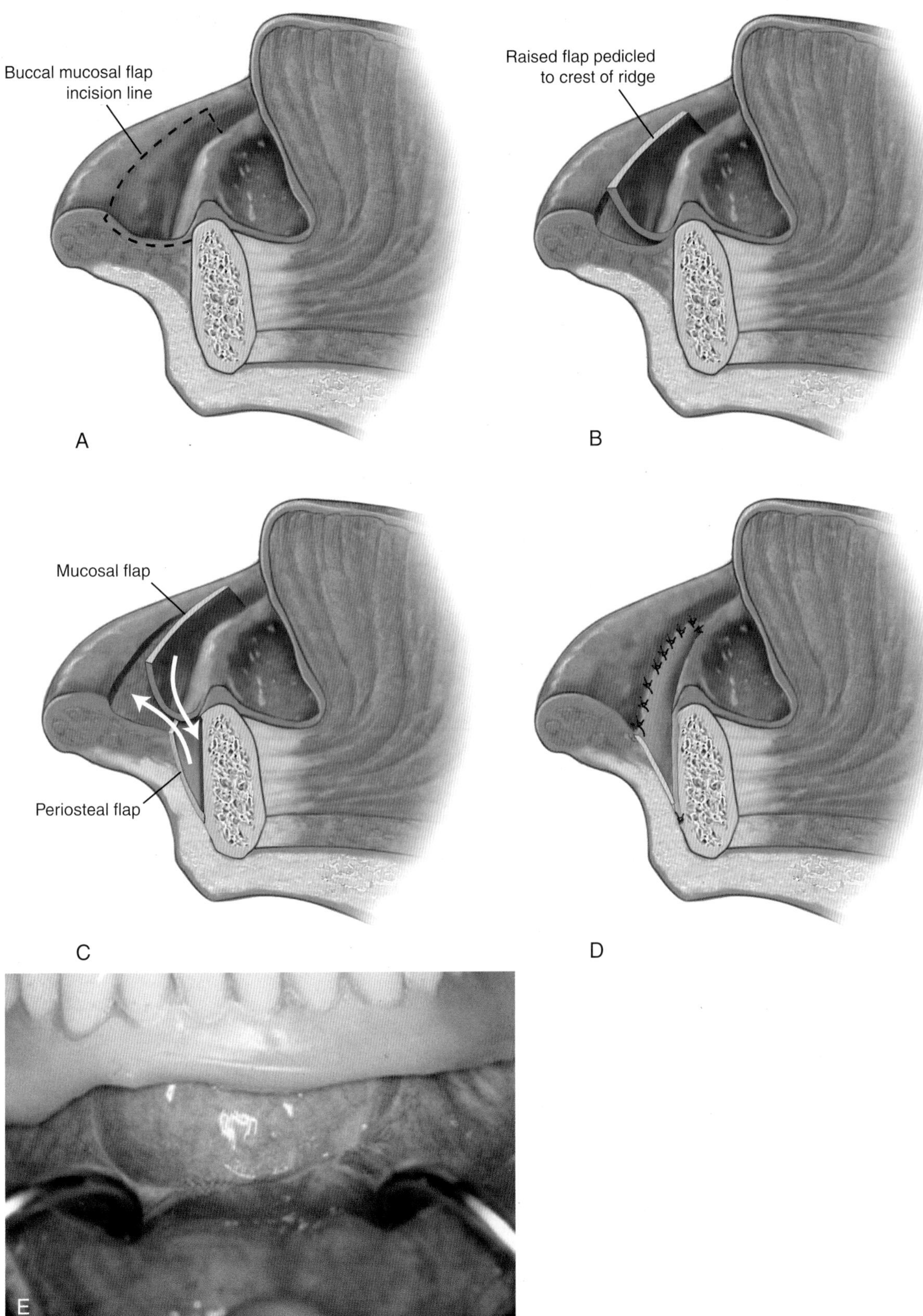

Figure 19.5 **A,** A mucosal flap one and a half times as long as the proposed depth of the vestibule is outlined on the inner surface of the lip medial to the mental nerves. **B,** A thin mucosal flap is elevated and pedicled from the crest of the ridge. **C,** The periosteum is incised superiorly at the crest of the ridge and laterally anterior to the mental foramina, reflected beyond the projected depth of the vestibule, and incised again just above the depth of the periosteal dissection, leaving a periosteal tag to which the mucosa can be sutured. **D,** The pedicled mucosa is sutured to the inferior periosteal margin and the superior periosteum margin is sutured to the margin of the lip mucosa. **E,** A patient who had a lip switch myotomy is wearing his existing denture showing how much additional flange extension is possible after this procedure.

ALTERNATIVE TECHNIQUE 4: Soft Tissue Drape Optimization in Osseous Reconstructed Jaws

If a jaw resection and osseous reconstruction (conventional or free flap osseous reconstruction) have been components of ablative tumor surgery or if osseous augmentation of the jaws has been performed, the soft tissue drape associated with such surgeries is frequently of a nature that prevents conventional dental prostheses as well as implant-based prosthetic rehabilitation. In such cases, the surgeon should modify the principles presented previously in this chapter with ingenuity to achieve a soft tissue architecture to which prosthetic appliances can be applied to complete structural and dental rehabilitation for the patient (Fig. 19.6). Skin, mucosa, and AlloDerm grafts fixated with surgical stents as described in the VSG and LFM sections can be modified according to case-specific needs to achieve favorable results.

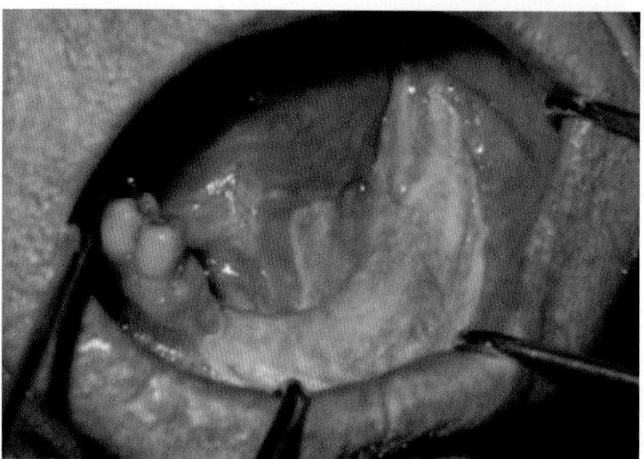

Figure 19.6 VSG and LFM procedures result in a patient who had an ablative procedure followed by osseous reconstruction, which resulted in an unfavorable soft tissue drape.

ALTERNATIVE TECHNIQUE 5: Implant Related Vestibuloplasty Procedures

Because implant-based restorations have become such an important component of restorative dentistry in modern times, it behooves the surgeon to be competent in managing soft tissue problems associated with this modality. Although fixed mucosa is not an essential requirement for successful implant restorations,[15–17] none would argue that if it is possible to obtain fixed mucosa where implant abutments and attachments emerge, it is preferable. Such a situation is frequently noted where implants are placed in a markedly atrophic mandible or maxilla anterior for overdentures, and soft tissue mobility around attachments utilized to fix the overdenture (bars or locator abutments) leads to irritation at the point of soft tissue and abutment contact. Soft tissue pull can be alleviated by vestibuloplasty procedures in a supraperiosteal plane and placement of skin, mucosal, or AlloDerm grafts. Ingenuity is again applicable here with stent usage, as frequently stents can be placed at such surgeries and retained by integrated or completely stable implants (Fig. 19.7).

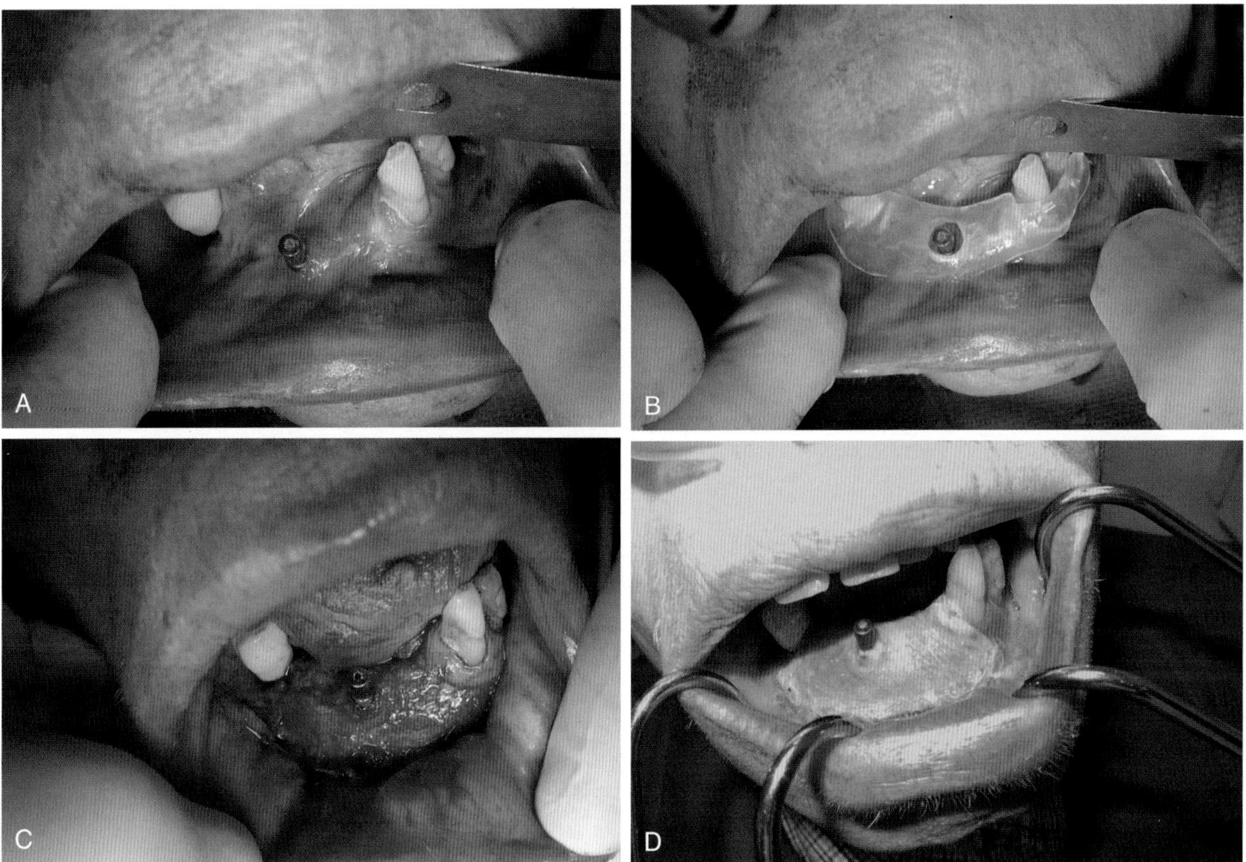

Figure 19.7 **A,** Poor soft tissue drape and lack of fixed mucosa around an implant fixture in a patient who had an en bloc anterior mandible resection followed by bone grafting. Prosthetic restoration requires improved gingival drape and additional implant fixtures. **B,** Surgical stent fabricated for surgery tried in the mouth for fit and adjustment. **C,** Supraperiosteal dissection for LFM and VSG procedures accomplished. **D,** Patient shown at 10 days postoperative after stent removal. Implants can be placed after skin graft is healed completely.

ALTERATIVE TECHNIQUE #6: Skin Graft Substitutes

As noted earlier in the chapter, several mucosal and skin substitutes have gained popularity in grafting to increase both the presence and width of keratinized gingiva.[28] Acellular dermis and resorbable collagen matrix are the commonly used substitutes. These substitutes are acellular and work by vascularization and ingrowth of epithelium and eventual replacement of the graft by keratinized oral mucosa. The clear advantages of using a skin graft substitute includes the lack of a skin harvest site and its morbidities, reduced operating time, and some predictable excellent healing.[29–31] Histopathologic studies have shown that graft substitutes may actually show reduced inflammation, fibrosis, and keratinization when compared with a skin graft.[32] The technique for a vestibuloplasty utilizing these substitutes does not differ from a classic approach as described earlier (Figs. 19.8A and B, and 19.9A and B).

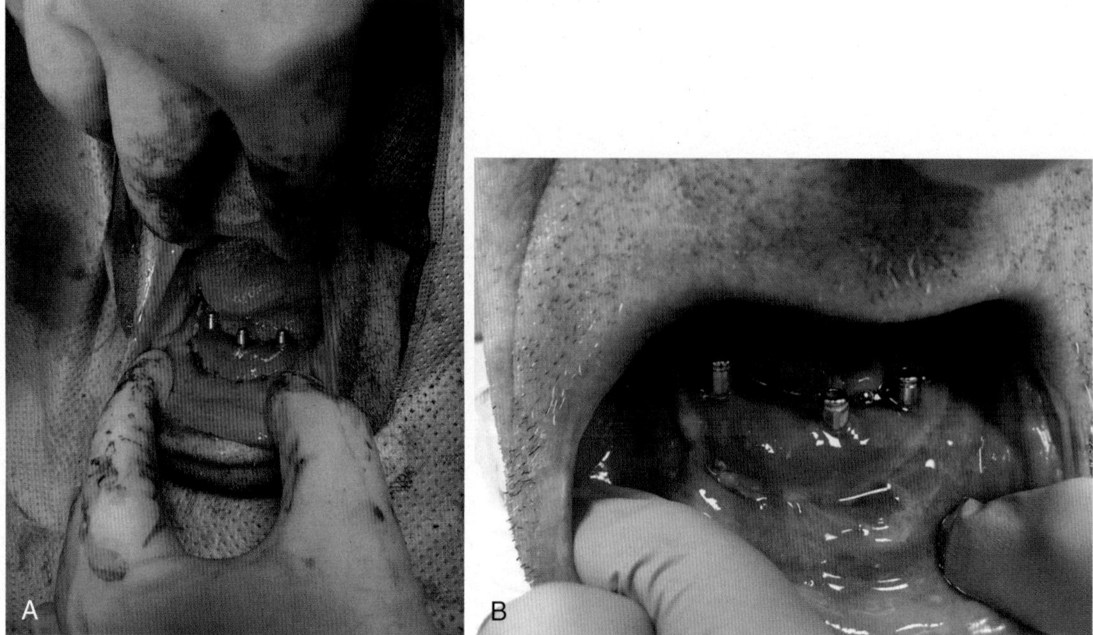

Figure 19.8 **A,** Acellular dermal matrix substitute vestibuloplasty, immediately postoperative. **B,** Acellular dermal matrix following 1 month of healing. (Courtesy of Stuart Lieblich DMD, Avon, CT)

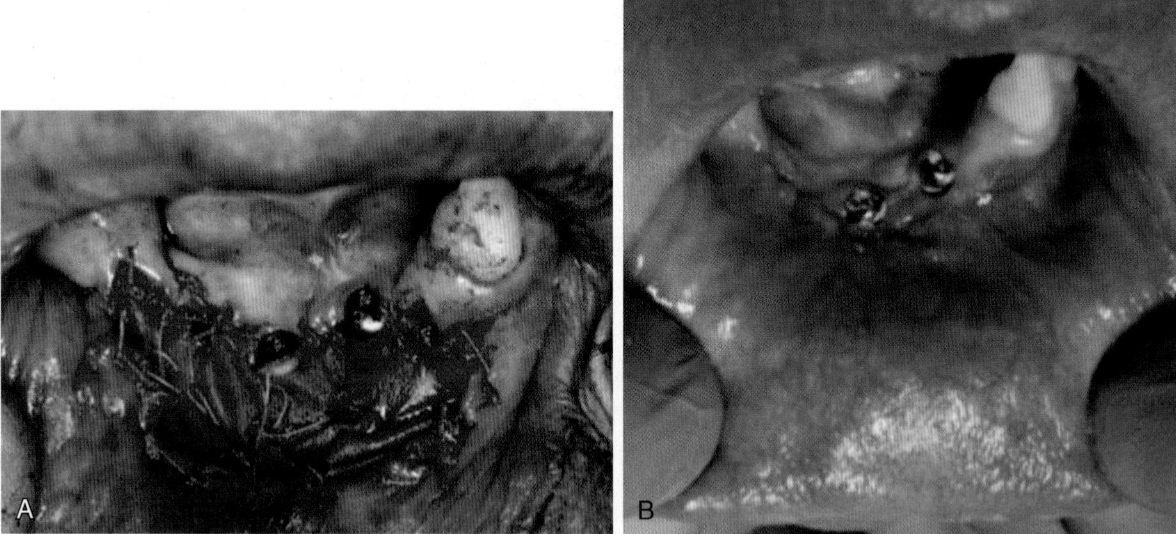

Figure 19.9 **A,** Collagen matrix substitute used to increase vestibular depth and keratinized tissue. **B,** Collagen matrix substitute well healed and incorporated into the vestibule increasing keratinized tissue and vestibular depth.

Avoidance and Management of Intraoperative Complications

Intraoperative complications are rare with vestibuloplasty techniques. With skin graft acquisition, care must be used to avoid grafts that are too thick, bleeding should be controlled prior to dressing with topical hemostatic agents, the graft should be carefully stored in moist gauze until utilized to avoid drying and rolling up, and the donor site should be dressed with Opsite (Smith & Nephew) or the equivalent, which allows moisture to escape; excess can be aspirated if desired. Care must be exercised to avoid mental nerve damage in the mandible and infraorbital nerve damage in the maxilla. Hemostasis must be meticulous, particularly in the floor of the mouth, to avoid airway embarrassment. Bony projections, which will interfere with the denture base, must be excised carefully. Stent construction and affixation are important complements to the procedure.

Postoperative Considerations

The patient should be adequately prepared for the level of pain and swelling that will accompany vestibuloplasty procedures, and they should be provided with a reliable analgesic. The patient should be informed that the wearing of dentures will be prohibited for about 2 to 3 weeks. Stents must remain well adapted to prevent loss of graft attachment. After stent removal, granulation tissue is frequently present and can be removed with cotton pliers and irrigation. Bone exposures will typically granulate without incident. Dentures can be constructed when the patient is ready, but most of the vestibuloplasty techniques employed are accompanied by shrinkage and relapse, so prosthetic intervention should be timely initiated.

References

1. Davis WH, Davis CL, Delo R, et al. Surgical management of soft tissue problems. In: Fonseca RJ, Davis WH, eds. *Reconstructive Preprosthetic Oral and Maxillofacial Surgery*. Philadelphia, PA: WB Saunders; 1986.
2. Weiser R. Ein jahr chirurgisch-zahnarztliche tatigkeit im kiererspital. *Z für Stomatol (1984)*. 1918;XVI:133.
3. Pickerill HP. Intra-oral skin grafting: the establishment of the buccal sulcus. *Proc R Soc Med*. 1919;12(Odontol Sect):17–22.
4. Kilner TP, Jackson T. Skin grafting in the buccal cavity. *Br J Surg*. 1921;9:148.
5. Kazanjian VH. In: Blair VP, et al., ed. *Essentials* of Oral *Surgery*. 3rd ed. St. Louis, MO: CV Mosby; 1944.
6. Pichler H, Trauner R. Die alveolarkammplastik. *Oest Z Stomatol*. 1930;25:54.
7. Wassmund M. Ueber chirurgische formgestaltung des atrophisen kiefers zum zwecke prothetischer versorgung. *Virrteljahreschrift Zahnheilkd*. 1931;47:305.
8. Trauner R. Alveoloplasty with ridge extensions on the lingual side of the lower jaw to solve the problem of a lower dental prosthesis. *Oral Surg Oral Med Oral Pathol*. 1952;5(4):340–346.
9. Obwegeser H. Die totale mundbodenplastik. *Schweiz Mschr Zahnheilkd*. 1963;73:565.
10. Mathis H. Einfache chirgische massnahmen zur sicherung von halt und stabilitat der prosthesen in der alltagspraxis. *Dtsch Zahnärztl Z*. 1951;6:44.
11. Schuchardt K. Die epidermistransplantation bie der mundvorrhofplastik. *Dtsch Zahnarztl*. 1952;7:364.
12. Obwegeser H. Die submukose vestibulumplaspik. *Dtsch Zahnärztl Z*. 1959;14:629.
13. Spagnoli DB, Nale JC. Preprosthetic and reconstructive surgery. In: Milaro M, Ghali GE, Larson PE, Waite PD, eds. *Peterson's Principles of Oral and Maxillofacial Surgery*. 3rd ed. Shelton, CT: People's Medical Publishing House; 2012.
14. Landesman HM, Davis WH, Martinoff J, Kaminishi R. Resorption of the edentulous mandible after a vestibuloplasty with skin grafting. *J Prosthet Dent*. 1983;49(5):619–622.
15. Geurs NC, Vassilopoulos PJ, Reddy MS. Soft tissue considerations in implant site development. *Oral Maxillofac Surg Clin North Am*. 2010;22(3):387–405 (vi-vii).
16. Kim BS, Kim YK, Yun PY, et al. Evaluation of peri-implant tissue response according to the presence of keratinized mucosa. *Oral Surg Oral Med Oral Pathol Oral Radiol Endod*. 2009;107(3):e24–e28.
17. Linkevicius T, Apse P, Grybauskas S, Puisys A. The influence of soft tissue thickness on crestal bone changes around implants: a 1-year prospective controlled clinical trial. *Int J Oral Maxillofac Implants*. 2009;24(4):712–719.
18. Hashemi HM, Parhiz A, Ghafari S. Vestibuloplasty: allograft versus mucosal graft. *Int J Oral Maxillofac Implants*. 2012;41(4):527–530.
19. Wei PC, Laurell L, Geivelis M, Lingen MW, Maddalozzo D. Acellular dermal matrix allografts to achieve increased attached gingiva. Part 1. A clinical study. *J Periodontol*. 2000;71(8):1297–1305.
20. Obwegeser H. Eine modification der lingualen alveolar klammplastiek nach R Trauner. *Schweiz Mschr Zahnheilkd*. 1953;63:788.
21. Obwegeser H. Co-report: surgical preparation of the mouth for full dentures. *Int Dent J*. 1958;8:252.
22. Kazanjian VH. Surgical operations as related to satisfactory dentures. *Dent Cosmos*. 1924:66.
23. Godwin JG. Submucous surgery for better denture service. *J Am Dent Assoc*. 1947;34(10):678–686.
24. Edlan A, Mejchar B. Plastic surgery of the vestibulum in periodontal therapy. *Int Dent J*. 1963;13:593.
25. Howe GL. Preprosthetic surgery in the lower labial sulcus. *Dent Pract Dent Rec*. 1965;16(4):119–124.
26. Kethley JL Jr, Gamble JW. The lipswitch: a modification of Kazanjian's labial vestibuloplasty. *J Oral Surg*. 1978;36(9):701–705.
27. Wessberg GA, Hill SC, Epker BN. Transpositional flap technique for mandibular vestibuloplasty. *J Am Dent Assoc*. 1979;98(6):929–933.
28. McLaurin WS, Krishnan D. Preprosthetic dentoalveolar surgery. *Oral Maxillofac Surg Clin North Am*. 2020;32(4):583–591.
29. Maiorana C, Pivetti L, Signorino F, Grossi GB, Herford AS, Beretta M. The efficacy of a porcine collagen matrix in keratinized tissue augmentation: a 5-year follow-up study. *Int J Implant Dent*. 2018;4(1):1.
30. Preidl RHM, Wehrhan F, Weber M, Neukam FW, Kesting M, Schmitt CM. Collagen matrix vascularization in a peri-implant vestibuloplasty situation proceeds within the first postoperative week. *J Oral Maxillofac Surg*. 2019;77(9):1797–1806.
31. Schmitt CM, et al. Long-term outcomes after vestibuloplasty with a porcine collagen matrix (Mucograft) versus the free gingival graft: a comparative prospective clinical trial. *Clin Oral Implants Re*. 2016;27(11):e125–e133.
32. Girod DA, Sykes K, Jorgensen J, Tawfik O, Tsue T. Acellular dermis compared to skin grafts in oral cavity reconstruction. *Laryngoscope*. 2009;119(11):2141–2149.

CHAPTER 20

Endosseous Dental Implants

R. Gilbert Triplett, Jorge Gonzalez, and Andrew Read-Fuller

Armamentarium (Fig. 20.1)

#9 Molt periosteal elevator
Adson tissue forceps with teeth
Appropriate sutures
Bone file
Calipers/ruler
Cheek retractors (self-retained)
Cotton pliers
Dean tissue scissors
Dental curettes
Disposal punch (for use with flapless technique) (sizes 4.0, 5.0, 6.0)
Gauze sponges
Hemostat
High-speed surgical handpiece/saw
Implant placement kit
Local anesthetic with vasoconstrictor
Minnesota retractor
Mouth mirror
Needle holder and suture
Periodontal probe
Rongeur
Scalpel handle, #15 or #12 blade
Seldin retractor
Suction tip and tubing
Torque wrench
Variable-speed implant drilling unit
Weider tongue retractor

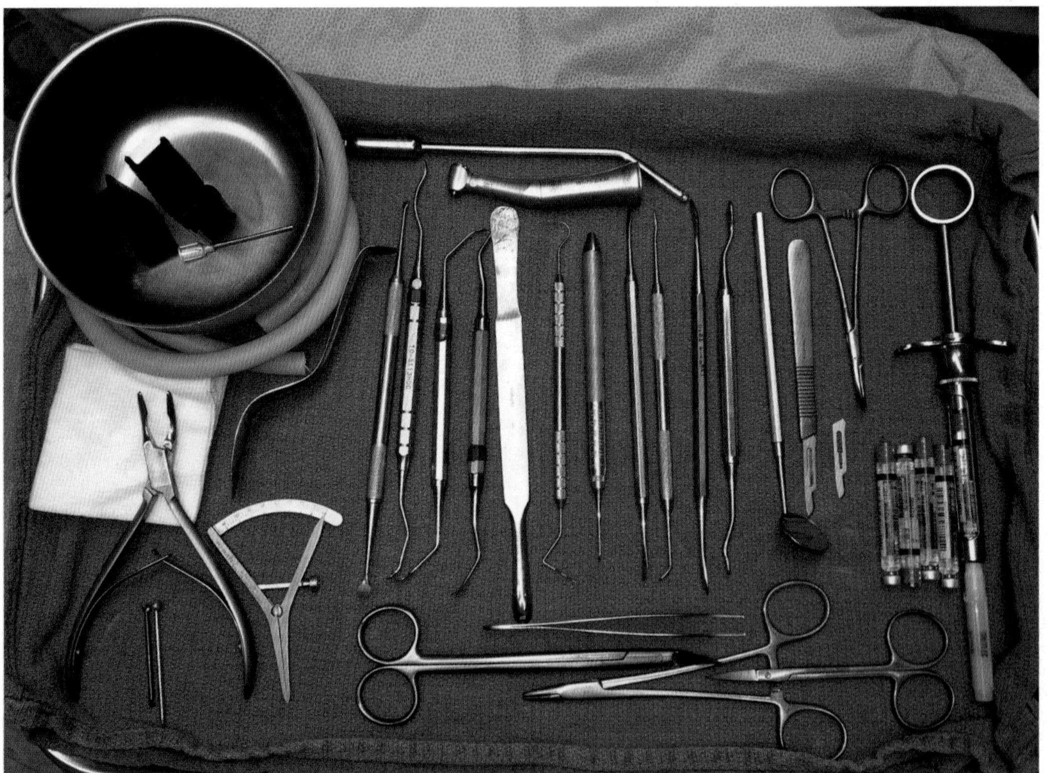

Figure 20.1 Instrument tray for exposure and closure of an implant site.

History of the Procedure

Dental implants are thought to date back to Mayan times, when seashells were trimmed and shaped before being hammered into the jaw to replace missing teeth. Numerous dental practitioners participated in advancing the art of dental implantology to solve the scourge of edentulism.[1] These clinicians worked with various materials, such as steel, chrome cobalt, and vitreous carbon, with varying results. Clinicians such as Linkow and Dorfman,[2] Roberts, Duke, Gershoff, Goldberg, Small,[3] and Tatum were visionaries and innovators dedicated to treating edentulism. However, it was Dr. Per-Ingvar Brånemark[4] who revolutionized the art and science of dental implantology with his discovery of the utility of titanium in 1952 while studying methods to improve orthopedic surgery. He discovered that bone would bond irreversibly to implanted titanium screw-shaped cylinders. He demonstrated, under carefully controlled conditions, that at the light microscopic level, titanium could structurally integrate with living bone. He further defined the surgical procedure for implantation, emphasizing careful technique, minimizing injury to bone by controlling overheating through the use of a series of increasingly larger drills with copious irrigation and then allowing a healing period for integration of bone with titanium bone cylinders. He further confirmed that this could be achieved with a high degree of predictability and without long-term soft tissue inflammation, fibrous encapsulation, or implant failure. Implant surface technology was advanced by Schroeder and Letterman, who developed a titanium plasma spray coating with a one-piece transmucosal screw.

These scientific advances, in addition to the recognition of the need for better techniques to replace missing dentition, have revolutionized dentistry in the 20th and 21st centuries.[1]

Indications for the Use of the Procedure

The placement of dental implants is indicated to support tooth replacements in edentulous and partially edentulous arches. Endosteal root form implants have been shown to support crown and bridge replacement for missing teeth in a very predictable manner, with low failure and complication rates. Implant and prosthetic design and service characteristics have improved success rates and shortened the osseointegration period before loading. Quantitative measures of torque and resonance frequency analysis (implant stability quotient [ISQ]) can be used to guide the timing for loading of an implant; torque values of 35 Ncm or higher and/or an ISQ of 70 or higher indicates implant stability sufficient to support immediate loading of the implant (Fig. 20.2).[5]

Patients who are missing teeth may be good candidates for an implant-supported prosthesis. Patients who are

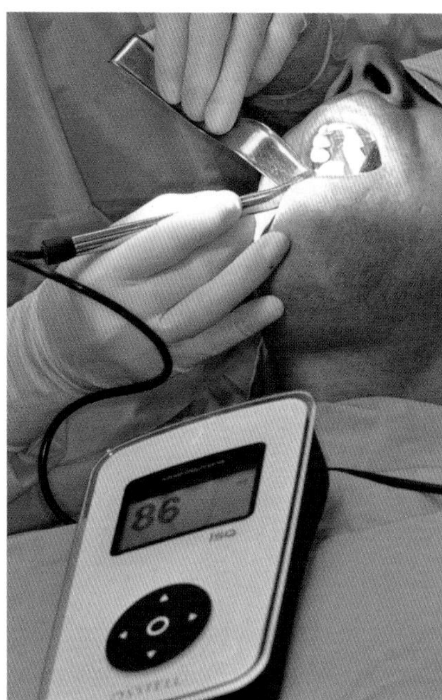

Figure 20.2 The Osstell ISQ (Osstell, Gothenburg, Sweden) analyzes resonance frequency measurements, providing a quantitative measurement of implant stability.

edentulous in the mandible, in particular, may not be able to comfortably manage a normal-textured diet because of the mobility of the denture. After tooth removal, the alveolar bone resorbs, and the bone loss in height and width causes a poor fit for the removable denture; in addition, dislodgement from the perioral musculature becomes greater than the retentive forces of the denture, which moves on the edentulous ridge, causing discomfort and dysfunction.[6] Dental implants provide excellent support for a prosthesis in an edentulous arch and improve the patient's ability to function and socialize. Likewise, the use of implants to support a prosthesis in partially edentulous patients may eliminate the need for crown prep on teeth adjacent to the edentulous space that will be used as bridge abutments.[6] This preserves dental structure and encourages healthier mouths. If removal of nonfunctioning or nonrestorable teeth is necessary, it is advisable to consider the best replacement choice for that particular patient; if an implant-supported prosthesis is indicated, extraction and immediate implant placement should be considered based on the diagnosis and treatment planning. This may minimize resorptive alveolar bone loss after extraction and allow for a less complex restoration.

Dental implants are indicated to support natural tooth replacements in both edentulous and partially edentulous sites and in minimally and severely resorbed alveolar bone because it has been shown that osseointegrated implant-supported restorations can arrest or minimize the natural progression of alveolar bone loss after tooth removal. Implant placement and function can minimize the morbidity of edentulism and improve function and quality of life for these patients.

Limitations and Contraindications

Inadequate or excessive vertical restorative space
Limited jaw opening and restricted interarch distance
Inadequate alveolar width for optimal buccolingual positioning

Medically Compromised Conditions

Uncontrolled diabetes mellitus
Long-term therapy with an immunosuppressant medication
Connective tissue disease (e.g., uncontrolled systemic lupus erythematosus or scleroderma) and autoimmune diseases
Blood dyscrasias and coagulopathies
Intraoral and perioral malignancies
Irradiation of the jaws that may lead to radiation necrosis
Intravenous bisphosphonate treatment for malignancy or osteoporosis
Severe psychological disorders
Alcohol and drug addiction
Prolonged use of corticosteroids

Relative Local Contraindications

Insufficient quantity or quality of bone
Uncontrolled periodontal disease
Severe bruxism
Unbalanced relationship between the maxilla and mandible (severe class II or class III malocclusion)
Poor oral hygiene

TECHNIQUE: Implant Placement in Edentulous (Healed) Alveolar Sites

Diagnosis and treatment planning are critical to the execution of implant placement and should be performed as part of a team effort. The process should include an examination, clinical and radiographic analysis, and laboratory aids and support as indicated.

STEP 1: Initial Evaluation
The examination should encompass the entire oral cavity, including the dentition and edentulous sites, jaw relationship, and occlusion. The edentulous areas should be evaluated for height, width, and length of the proposed operative site as well as available restorative space. The character of the gingival soft tissue and the amount and location of attached and unattached tissue should be assessed and recorded.[7] Remaining teeth should be free of decay and periodontally healthy.

STEP 2: Imaging
Inherent diagnostic limitations (e.g., distortion in conventional radiology) have been significantly improved by new technologies such as computed tomography (CT). CT allows for reformatting of a volumetric dataset in axial, coronal, and sagittal cuts and the building of multiple cross-sectional and panoramic views.[7,8] Such preoperative radiographic images can be uploaded into three-dimensional implant planning software to expand the indications for oral implant-based treatments. CT also enables protection of critical anatomic structures and provides the esthetic and functional advantages of prosthodontics-driven implant positioning.

STEP 3: Surgical Guide
Once implant treatment planning has been determined, usually by computer generated virtual surgery, the data can be sent to manufacturing facilities for a guide splint and prosthesis construction, or the implant team fabricates the guides with three-dimensional orienting. Some advantages of this technology are reduced operating time, minimal surgical trauma, more precise placement, and a shorter postoperative recovery period (Fig. 20.3A).[9]

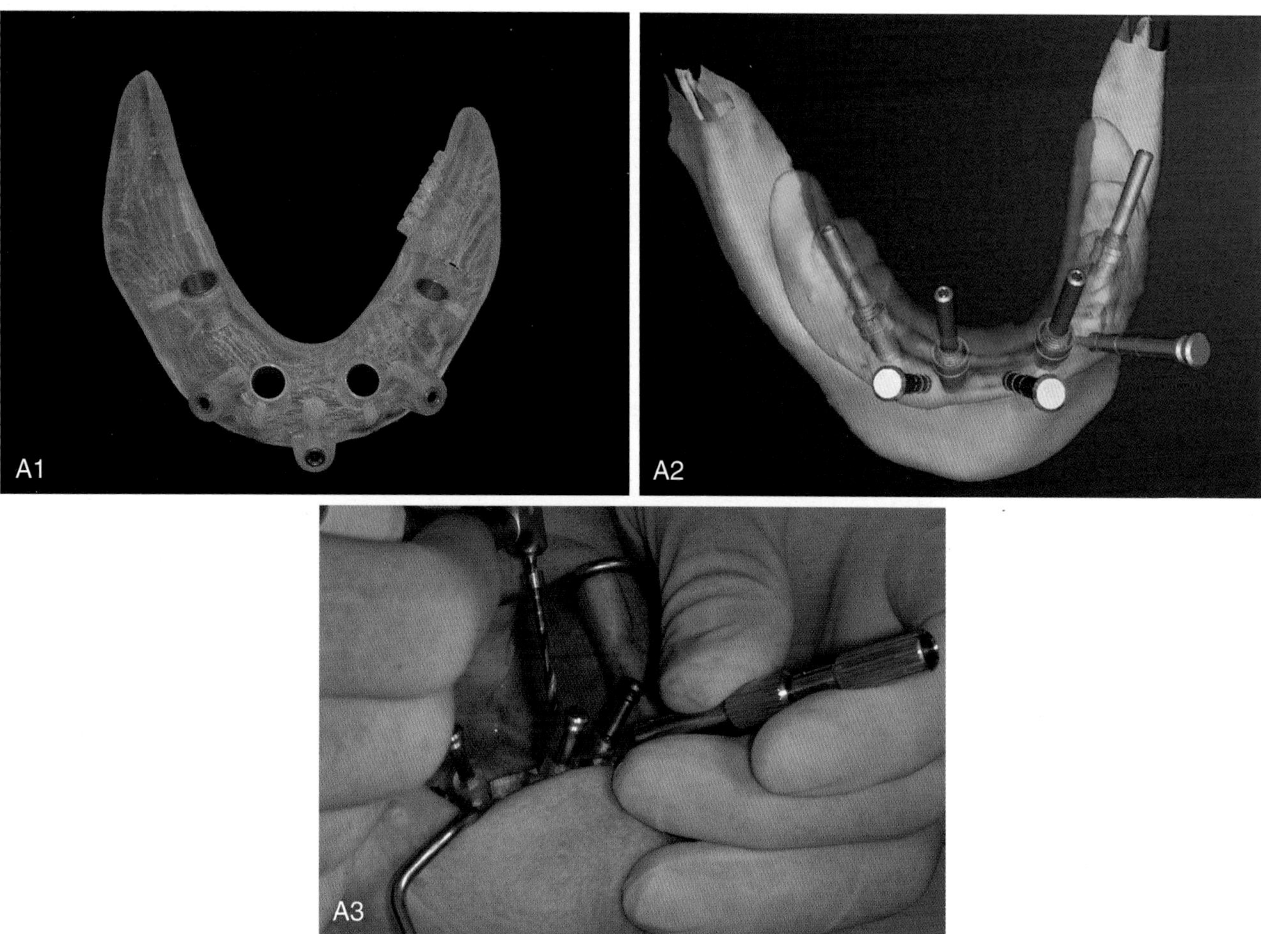

Figure 20.3 **A1,** Guide splint (from tissue site). **A2,** Computer image demonstrating stabilizing virtual pins and implants. **A3,** Drilling through guide sites. **B,** Drill sequence for site preparation and implant placement.

TECHNIQUE: Implant Placement in Edentulous (Healed) Alveolar Sites—*cont'd*

STEP 4: Implant Selection

A wide array of dental implants is available. Worldwide, approximately 600 different options can be chosen, although most are similar in form and surgical steps.[10] Most of the endosseous implant systems use a series of incrementally larger diameter drills. A good rule of thumb is to select the drills in increments of 0.5 to 1 mm; increasing the bur diameters gradually generates less heat and trauma to the osteotomy site.[6,7] Slow drilling, sharp burs, chilled irrigation, and light drilling pressure all minimize temperature elevation during bone site preparation (Fig. 20.3B).

STEP 5: Surgical Procedure

Standard local anesthetic blocks and infiltration may be supplemented with sedation. Both open mucoperiosteal flaps or flapless techniques may be used. If an open flap technique is selected, the flap design should be carefully planned to allow access and good visibility. An incision is made over the proposed implant site, and the mucoperiosteal flap is elevated to expose the underlying bone; this allows the surgeon to adequately identify and avoid vital structures and also to identify bony irregularities and undercuts. The ridge crest is assessed, and the surgeon determines whether osteoplasty is required before osteotomy site preparation. If a knife-edge ridge or bony irregularities are present, they can be removed, and the ridge is flattened with side-cutting rongeurs or a vulcanite bur and finished with bone files. Current imaging and planning are able to determine accurately the height and width of bone at selected sites. A customized, sterilized surgical template (guide) is positioned and stabilized.

Continued

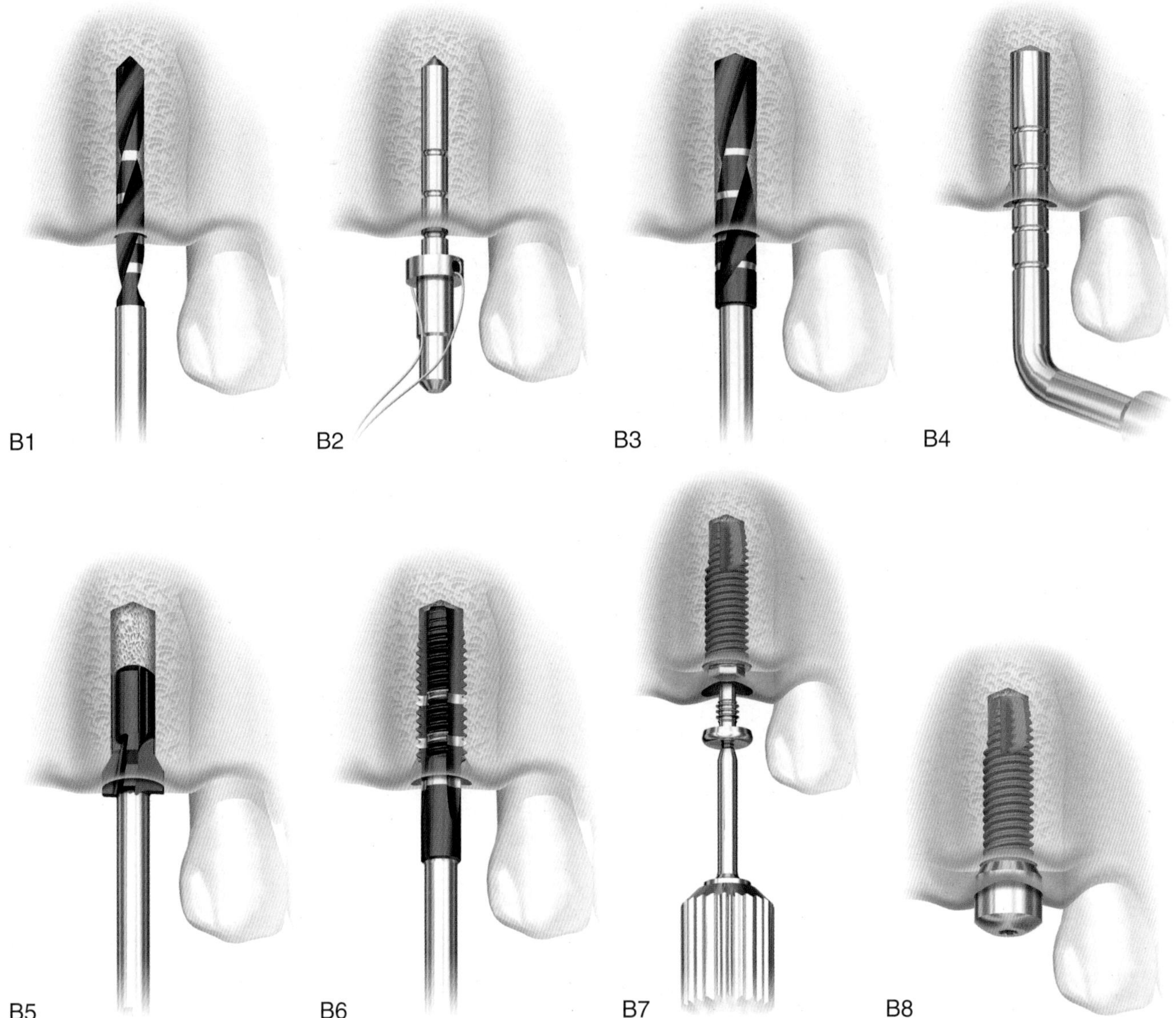

Figure 20.3, cont'd B1, 2-mm twist drill. **B2,** Direction indicator. **B3,** 3-mm twist drill. **B4,** Countersink. **B5,** Depth gauge. **B6,** Bone tap. **B7,** Cover screw. **B8,** Healing abutment.

TECHNIQUE: Implant Placement in Edentulous (Healed) Alveolar Sites—*cont'd*

STEP 6: Osteotomy Preparation, Orientation, and Sequence

The starter drill is used to prepare the osteotomy center of each proposed implant site with liberal use of an irrigant. A series of twist drills are used subsequently to expand the osteotomy depth, width, and position determined during surgical planning.

Because individual implant systems vary slightly, the surgeon should be familiar with the specifics of the instrumentation used for a particular system. Determination of implant position and angulation must be accomplished with a prosthetic design in mind; a stone model or computer software programs can help visualize the prosthetic-driven concept. Implant spacing is important for the prosthetic reconstruction and the patient's ability to maintain hygiene. It is recommended that implant margins be no closer than 2 mm to natural teeth and 3 mm to adjacent implants. The first twist drill (1.6 to 2.2, depending on the system) should be drilled to depth using irrigation (internal irrigation, external irrigation, or both). Drill guides should ensure proper angulation while preparing the osteotomy. However, if the surgeon is preparing the osteotomy without a guide splint, a paralleling guide pin is placed in the first osteotomy as a directional indicator. If the position is not satisfactory, correction can be made without jeopardizing the osteotomy site because only a small amount of bone has been removed.

TECHNIQUE: Implant Placement in Edentulous (Healed) Alveolar Sites—*cont'd*

When the surgeon is satisfied with the position of the initial implant site, additional implant sites are prepared in sequence, first using the smallest diameter twist drill, until all sites have been prepared to depth. The guide splint is extremely important for achieving the proper implant position and angulation. The drill should be turning at the requisite speed, which is based on the recommendations of the system used (usually 800 to 1200 revolutions per minute). The torque of the drilling motor, bone density, pressure applied, and sharpness of the drill all affect site preparation. During the drilling, the surgeon should "lock the wrist" and prepare the osteotomy with an in-and-out motion to assure accuracy of the osteotomy. If the wrist is flexed during the site preparation, an arc is created in the osteotomy site and it can be easily oversized.[6] In addition, the in-and-out drilling allows cooling irrigant to reach the depth of the osteotomy site and minimize heat to the walls and floor.

The drilling sequence is repeated for each of the drill sizes (e.g., 1.6, 2.5, and 3). In the parallel wall osteotomies used with some systems, a special guide drill is used that has a protruding tip 2 mm in diameter. This design guides the drill into the osteotomy site and minimizes trauma to the crestal bone. This is particularly helpful in narrow ridges. It allows the drill to enter the osteotomy site smoothly and enlarges the superficial portion of the osteotomy 2 to 3 mm. This is followed by a full length 3-mm drill. The system that uses a tapered design allows easy entry into the initial osteotomy site and eliminates the need for the guide drill.[6] For systems with larger diameter implants, the procedures continue at incremental increases in the drill size until the final drill for the selected implant is completed. The final drill should be at least 0.5 mm smaller than the implant diameter chosen. If the surgeon determines that the bone is very soft (bone quality type IV), the last drill may be eliminated. This choice is based on the surgeon's experience and skill. In many systems, countersink or profiling burs are used to accommodate a slightly larger coronal end of the implant (Fig. 20.3C and D).

Continued

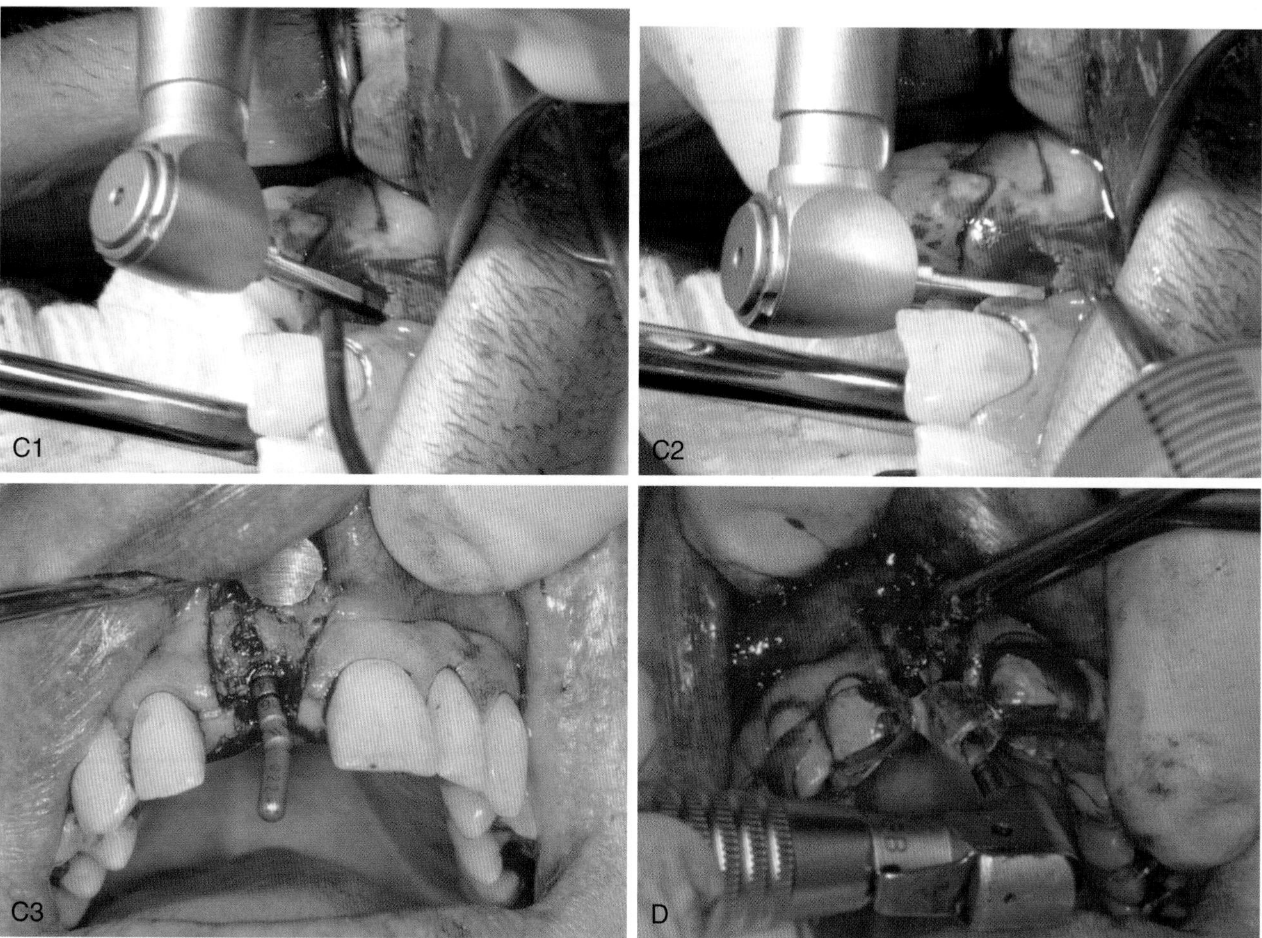

Figure 20.3, cont'd **C,** Sequence of site preparation and correction of initial osteotomy angulation. It is initially angulated too far labially (C1) and is corrected (C2 and C3). **D,** Demonstration of the final implant position in relationship to the guide splint.

TECHNIQUE: Implant Placement in Edentulous (Healed) Alveolar Sites—*cont'd*

STEP 7: Implant Placement

If the density of the bone is determined to be type I (very dense), the surgeon may choose to use a bone tap (drill) at slow speeds (18 to 20 revolutions per minute) prior to implant placement to avoid overtightening the implant. If an implant insertion torque exceeds 50 Ncm before the implant is completely seated, the surgeon should reverse the insertion direction of the implant and tap or enlarge the osteotomy site to prevent bone injury of the osteotomy, including microfracture, fracture of the alveolus, or fracture of the implant.

Once the implant has been successfully seated, it is advisable to measure the final insertion torque using a torque wrench. In addition, recording the resonance frequency analysis value provides a quantitative measure of initial primary implant stability. ISQ values at 55 or below indicate that too much lateral movement is possible, therefore compromising the expected osseointegration process of the fixture (Fig. 20.3E).

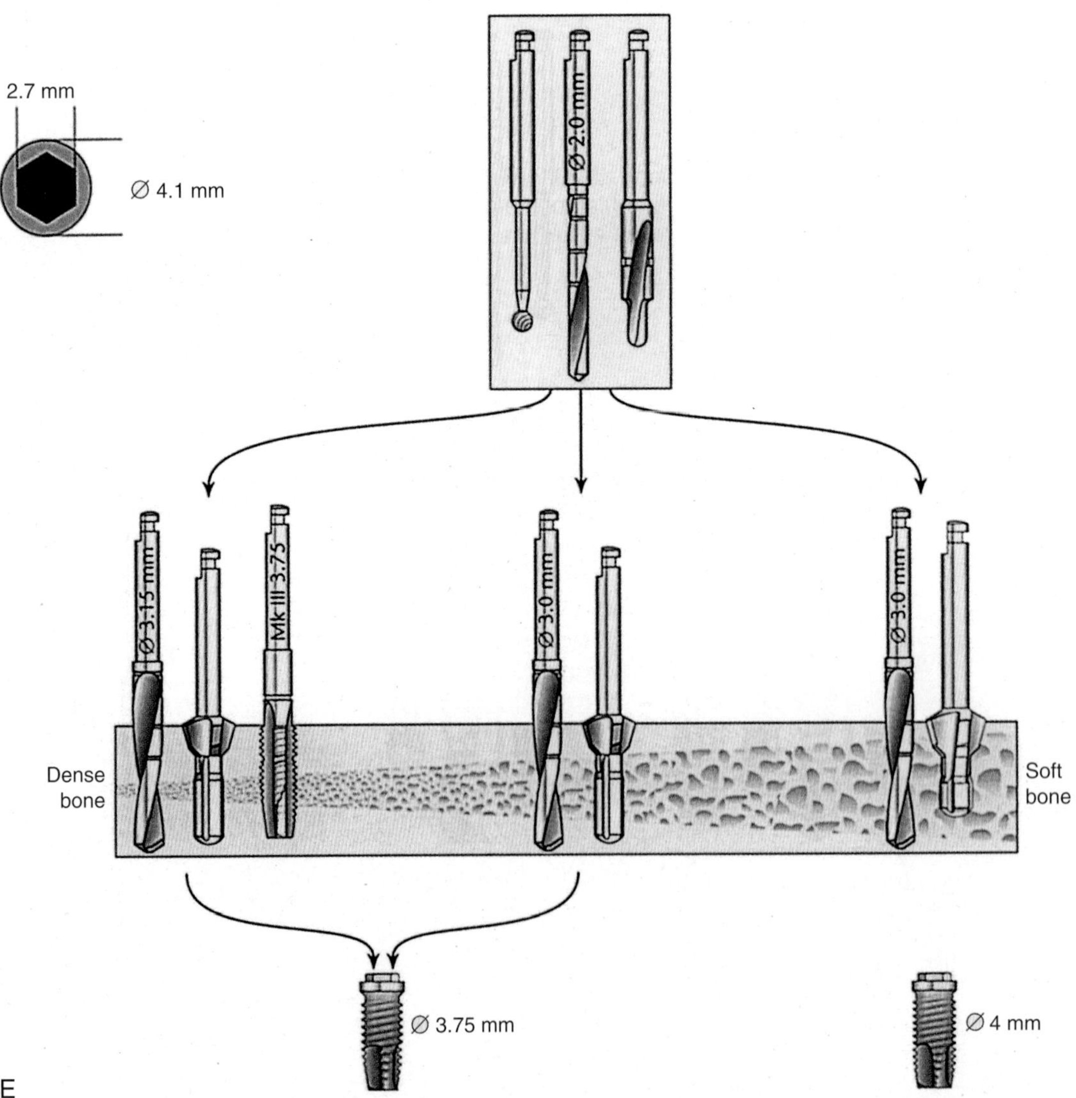

Figure 20.3, cont'd E, Drilling sequence in dense and soft bone. In the top panel, a special drill guide is shown to enlarge the osteotomy from 2 to 3 mm at the crest of the ridge. The drill tap can be used in very dense bone and eliminated in soft bone.

TECHNIQUE: Implant Placement in Edentulous (Healed) Alveolar Sites—*cont'd*

STEP 8: Soft Tissue Closure

The surgical wound is given a final inspection (irrigated and thoroughly cleaned) before soft tissue closure. If a submerged implant technique is chosen, a cover screw is now placed, any additional procedures required (e.g., guided bone regeneration) are performed, the wound is closed with interrupted or continuous sutures, and a screw provisional prosthesis is placed for function and esthetics. Although the closure technique seems routine, meticulous attention should be paid to accurate reapproximation of the wound margins. After closure, the surgeon is responsible for ensuring that any temporary prostheses are relieved and adjusted before placement and patient discharge. If a one-stage procedure has been chosen, the surgeon places the healing or final abutment and sutures the soft tissue around the abutment, assuring that the closure is complete and the flap does not creep occlusally.

It may be necessary to use an appropriate length abutment to prevent the flap from covering the coronal portion of the chosen abutment as the oral function is reestablished. Some implant systems have small plastic caps, resembling umbrellas, that can be placed on top of the abutment; these attempt to keep the flap compressed. The disadvantages of this technique are that a prosthesis may not be used with these caps and they are uncomfortable for the patient. Before discharge, the patient should be prescribed analgesics, antiinflammatory medications, and an antibacterial oral rinse. Antibiotic use is guided by the surgical findings and whether supplemental procedures (e.g., bone grafting, barrier membranes) were performed. Antibiotics are not indicated for routine implant placement into healed edentulous sites. A follow-up appointment is usually scheduled for 1 week later, and a team decision should be made regarding the loading protocol and timing. In a staged approach, integration time should be coordinated with the recommended loading times for the specific system regarding the arch, implant position, bone quality, presence or absence of augmentation procedures, torque value, and ISQ (Fig. 20.3F).

STEP 9: Uncovering Submerged Implants

Dental implants are ready to be uncovered and abutments connected after a period of bone healing and osseointegration (2 to 6 months), depending on the manufacturer's recommendation and the findings at initial implant placement. Second-phase surgery has two goals: (1) to allow the implant to pierce the mucosa and (2) to create a favorable soft tissue anatomy that results in a perimucosal contour and seal.[11] The site should be radiographed using standard panoramic and periapical films. The bone adjacent to the implant should appear to have normal trabeculation, without an intervening, radiolucent area of bone adjacent to the surface of the implant. Once it has been established that the implant appears to be integrated, the surgeon is ready to expose the implant, remove the cover screw, and place a healing abutment or final abutment. If a guide splint was used to place the implants, it can be used to precisely locate the site for the incision or tissue punch. Torque measurements or preferably ISQ should be measured and recorded and guide the implant team as to the probability of successful osseointegration

Second-phase surgery is usually accomplished with local anesthesia alone; however, this phase can be difficult, time-consuming, and challenging. After the sites have been identified, the patient is anesthetized and exposure is made. If the surgeon wishes to limit the amount of mucoperiosteal flap to be reflected, a small incision is made over the implant site with a #15 blade and the tissue is spread apart adequately to allow visualization of the cover screw or healing abutment. A decision is then made whether to use a tissue punch or further reflect the flap. If abundant keratinized gingival tissue overlies the implant, a tissue punch is a good choice; it minimizes soft tissue reflection and accelerates healing compared to the full-thickness mucoperiosteal flap. However, if minimal keratinized tissue is available, it is prudent to incise through the keratinized tissue, maintaining a keratinized band on each side of the abutment (buccal and lingual), or to use free palatal or connective tissue grafts. The flap should be adequately reflected with laxity to allow tight closure around the abutment. Usually this will be a healing abutment, but other options are available.

Continued

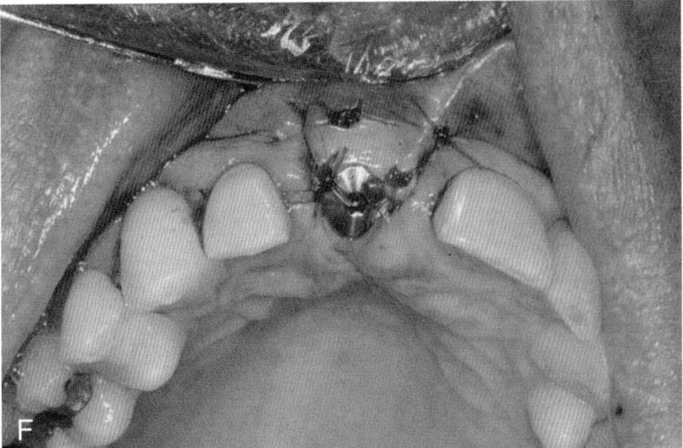

Figure 20.3, cont'd F, Modification of the mucoperiosteal flap to ensure proper tissue type and position after the healing abutment has been placed.

TECHNIQUE: Implant Placement in Edentulous (Healed) Alveolar Sites—*cont'd*

STEP 10: Abutment Selection and Placement

A final abutment is selected based on treatment needs and the planning of the implant team. If a temporary restoration will be placed over the site, the abutment length should be selected so that approximately 2 mm of abutment is exposed after flap closure. The kind of healing abutment used is based on the prosthetic goal for the specific implant restoration. This should be considered before the surgical uncovering and may require modification of the temporary prosthesis. In cases in which no provisional prosthesis is used (e.g., posterior edentulous areas or totally edentulous segments of the arch), it is prudent to choose an abutment length at least 4 mm occlusal to the soft tissue crest. This ensures that the abutment remains exposed postoperatively. It is not uncommon for swelling and inadequate readaptation on the flap margins to cover the entire abutment postoperatively, necessitating another surgical procedure. It is desirable to allow adequate soft tissue healing before final impressions or scans. If the surgeon simply will be uncovering an implant connection with minimal soft tissue reflection, 2 weeks is an adequate healing period before impressions or scans. However, in more complex, second-phase surgeries with extensive mucoperiosteal flap reflection and releases, a healing period of up to 4 weeks is required. To minimize conflicts and misunderstandings, patients should be advised of this healing period.

Releasing incisions may be required to achieve the desired tissue type around the abutment and a good adaptation of the soft tissue to the abutment. The modified margin of the flap should be meticulously sutured with small, tapered needles and 4-0 or 5-0 suture material.

Often, the inexperienced surgeon fails to realize how challenging it is to manage the soft tissue at the abutment connection when two or more adjacent implants are uncovered. It can be time-consuming and frustrating; therefore, it is particularly important to recognize the potential risk when only a small band of keratinized tissue (less than 4 mm) overlies the uncovered implant.

After closure of the tissues is complete, the temporary prosthesis is tried in and adjusted to minimize soft tissue irritation and trauma during healing (Fig. 20.3G).

ALTERNATIVE TECHNIQUE 1: Extraction of Teeth and Immediate Implant Placement

STEP 1: Tooth Removal

Immediate implant placement after an extraction eliminates postextraction waiting for primary healing of soft tissue and bone. However, if purulent exudate is present, placement of the implant should be delayed to improve predictability of outcomes.[12]

If the criterion for immediate placement is met, the tooth should be extracted with minimal trauma. Attempts to preserve all alveolar bone with instruments such as periotomes, a PowerTome, and root extraction systems all enhance alveolar bone preservation. Endodontically treated teeth are brittle and very tightly bound at the alveolar bone; therefore, supplemental aids to minimize bone loss are useful. The pneumatic PowerTome system and root retrieval devices have significantly improved our ability to remove difficult teeth and preserve bone.

STEP 2: Implant Placement After Extraction

In the anterior maxilla, it is desirable to orient the line of insertion through the palatal aspect of the socket beginning about halfway up the socket (on the palatal wall). At least two-thirds of the implant should be in contact with the host bone at the receptor site. The implant should be at least 2 mm longer than the socket, depending on the available basal bone.[6] It should be stable when placed before any bone graft material is placed into the socket to maximize the chance of achieving osseointegration. Any space around the implant greater than 2 mm should be grafted, and some strategies should be used to minimize graft washout and soft tissue migration into the space. Graft should be contained to achieve predictable results. Selection of the implants should be based on the size of the socket; large implants that engage the lateral socket walls are easier to stabilize, require less grafting, and have more predictability.[13] Numerous scientific reports regarding immediate implant placement demonstrate high success rates. The time to osseointegration depends on the size of the defects and the stability and status of the alveolar bone. Immediate loading is even possible in many extraction sites if the appropriate-size implants are chosen (Fig. 20.4). ISQ measurements are particularly valuable in these cases.

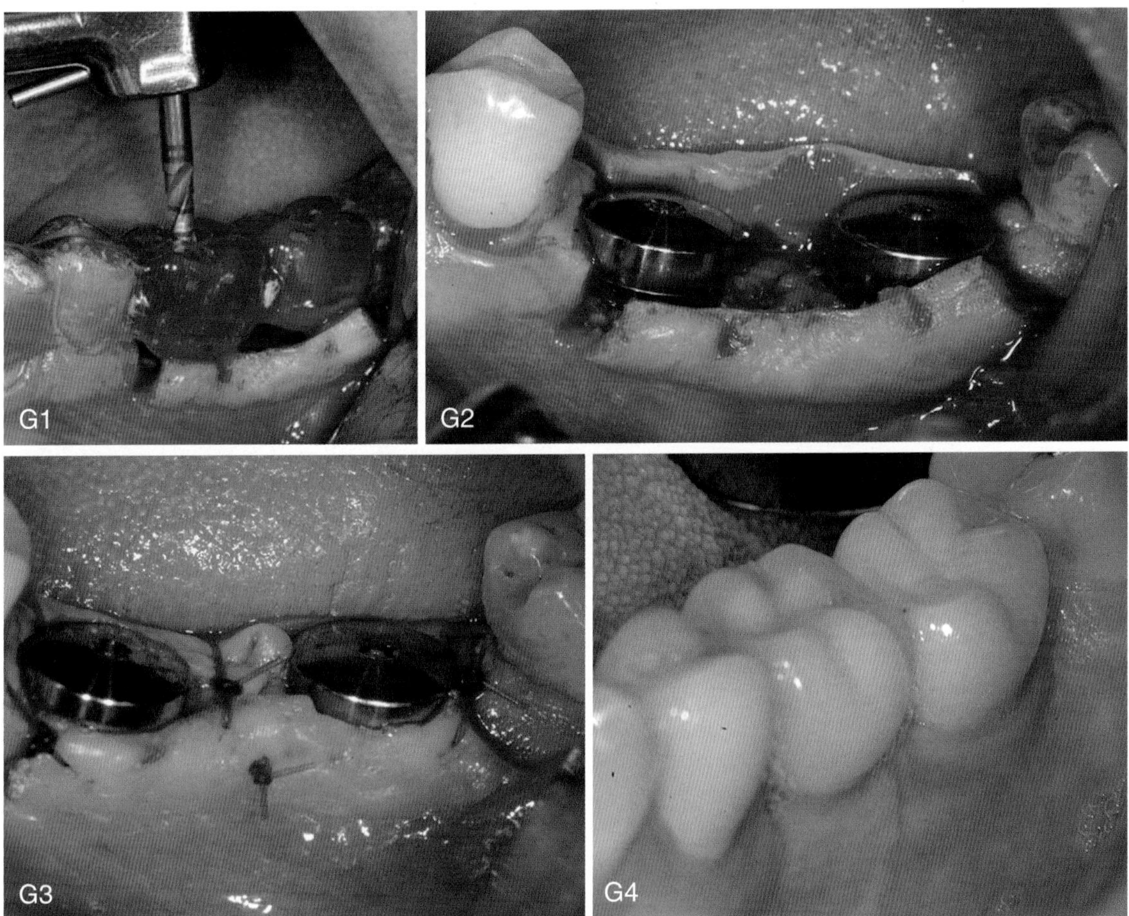

Figure 20.3, cont'd **G1,** Preoperative try-in of the surgical template indicated that the flapless approach was contraindicated at the first molar implant site. Nevertheless, during surgery, a round bur was used to mark the center of the implant osteotomy by penetrating through the soft tissues at the ridge crest before elevation of the abbreviated flap seen here. **G2,** The location of the soft tissue puncture clearly demonstrates that the use of a 6-mm tissue punch would have excised all the keratinized tissue buccal to the emerging first molar implant. Note that a tissue punch approach would have been feasible for the second molar site. **G3,** A simple interrupted suture was used to secure the abbreviated buccal flap mesial and distal to the emerging first molar implant, and a horizontal mattress suture was used to secure the lingual pedicles in the interimplant space without embarrassing their circulation. Note the 6-mm margin of apicocoronal keratinized tissue present on the buccal flap adjacent to the second molar implant. Resective contouring was performed at the second molar site with a 15c blade, and a simple interrupted suture was used to secure the flap distal to the second molar implant. **G4,** Three-year follow-up clinical photograph demonstrating a stable and self-cleansing periimplant soft tissue environment as a result of appropriate flap design and use of surgical maneuvers to create scalloped soft tissue contours that resist collection of food debris. (From Sclar AG. Guidelines for flapless surgery. *J Oral Maxillofac Surg*. 2007;65:20-32.)

Continued

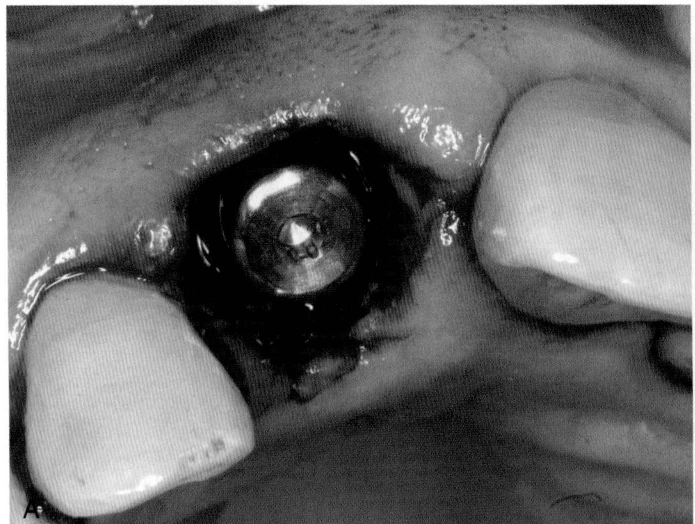

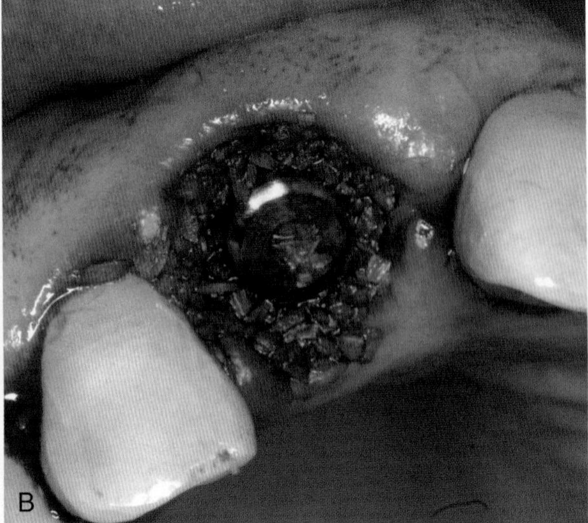

Figure 20.4 **A,** Implant placed in an extraction socket. The implant is stable, but there is 3 mm of space between the mesial palatal wall and the implant margin. **B,** A bone allograft was placed to eliminate dead space between the socket wall and the implant.

Avoidance and Management of Intraoperative Complications

Careful attention should be paid to details of the operative procedure, including utilizing copious irrigation while drilling, and following recommended manufacturer protocols regarding drilling speed in order to avoid overheating the surrounding bone, which can lead to necrosis and implant integration failure. Bone quality and cortical thickness vary based on anatomic location and patient-specific characteristics, and sometimes it is prudent to over or underprepare the osteotomy to ensure insertional torque falls within recommended ranges. Under torquing and implant can lead to reduced chance of successful integration while over torquing can lead to crestal bone loss or integration failure.

The most troublesome and avoidable complications occur as a result of inadvertent damage to adjacent structures during implant osteotomy or placement, especially to surrounding teeth or nerves. Careful preoperative planning is paramount in all cases, but in situations where there is limited space between adjacent teeth and the planned implant site, or from the alveolar crest to the inferior alveolar nerve or maxillary sinus, the surgeon should consider obtaining a cone beam CT imaging or using computer implant planning software, fabricating implant guides, or using shorter or narrower implants as necessary to accommodate anatomical limitations. Implants should be no closer than 2mm from the inferior alveolar nerve to minimize the risk of injury, and 5mm from the mental foramen given the potential for an anterior loop of the inferior alveolar nerve prior to exiting the foramen.

Postoperative Considerations

Following implant placement, the surgeon should plan for follow up within the first 1-2 weeks to ensure adequate soft tissue healing and assess any possible problems that can occur in the immediate postoperative period. Particular attention should be paid to excessive pain on palpation or percussion of the implant or mobility, all of which could indicate infection or implant failure. Reports of paresthesia or pain in adjacent teeth should also warrant additional imaging to ensure damage to surrounding structures did not occur.

During the integration phase, it must be emphasized to the patient not to load the implant in any way. The patient should be given detailed postoperative instructions such as avoiding chewing at the surgical site, particularly if a healing abutment or temporary restoration has been attached to the implant which can allow excessive forces to be transmitted to the implant and risk integration failure. Occasionally, a healing abutment or cover screw may come loose or fall out of the mouth, which can cause significant consternation to the patient who assumes the entire implant has failed, but a detailed clinical exam and replacement of the abutment as needed will solve the problem.

After adequate time for osseointegration has passed—typically 3-4 months—the patient should be evaluated one final time prior to fabrication and placement of the final restoration. This assessment should include obtaining a radiograph and periodontal probing to evaluate surrounding bone and the level of the alveolar crest, as bone loss could compromise the implant in the long term. A torque test and/or radio frequency analysis should be completed to ensure integration is successful. Finally, a healing abutment is placed if one is not already present to help create favorable gingival contours in anticipation of the definitive restoration.

References

1. Norton MR. The history of the dental implants. *US Dentistry*. 2006;9:24.
2. Linkow LI, Dorfman JD. Implantology in dentistry. A brief historical perspective. *N Y State Dent J*. 1991;57(6):31–35.
3. Small IA, Metz H, Kobernick S. The mandibular staple implant for the atrophic mandible. *J Biomed Mater Res*. 1974;8(4 Pt 2):365–371.
4. Brånemark PI, Hansson BO, Adell R, et al. Osseointegrated implants in the treatment of the edentulous jaw. Experience from a 10-year period. *Scand J Plast Reconstr Surg Suppl*. 1977;16:1–132.
5. O'Sullivan D, Sennerby L, Meredith N. Measurements comparing the initial stability of five designs of dental implants: a human cadaver study. *Clin Implant Dent Relat Res*. 2000;2(2):85–92.
6. Singh PP, Cronin AN. In: *Atlas of Oral Implantology*. 3rd ed. St Louis, MO: Mosby; 2009.
7. Schwarz MS, Rothman SL, Rhodes ML, Chafetz N. Computed tomography: part II. Preoperative assessment of the maxilla for endosseous implant surgery. *Int J Oral Maxillofac Implants*. 1987;2(3):143–148.
8. Schwarz MS, Rothman SL, Rhodes ML, Chafetz N. Computed tomography: part I. Preoperative assessment of the mandible for endosseous implant surgery. *Int J Oral Maxillofac Implants*. 1987;2(3):137–141.
9. Parel SM, Triplett RG. Interactive imaging for implant planning, placement, and prosthesis construction. *J Oral Maxillofac Surg*. 2004;62(9) (suppl 2):41–47.
10. Jokstad A, ed. *Osseointegration and Dental Implants*. Hoboken, NJ: Wiley-Blackwell; 2009.
11. Palacci P, ed. *Peri-implant Soft Tissue Augmentation Procedures in Esthetic Implant Dentistry*. Chicago, Illinois: Quintessence; 2001.
12. Babbush CA, Hahn JA, Krauser JT, Rosenlicht JL, eds. *Dental Implants: The Art and Science*. St Louis, Missouri: Saunders; 2011.
13. Balshi TJ, Wolfinger GJ, Wulc D, Balshi SF. A prospective analysis of immediate provisionalization of single implants. *J Prosthodont*. 2011;20(1):10–15.

CHAPTER 21

Implants in the Esthetic Zone

Waldemar D. Polido and Dean Morton

Armamentarium

Common to all procedures: #9
- **Molt periosteal elevator**
- Surgical loupes
- Chlorhexidine gluconate 0.12% (for preoperative rinse)
- Topical anesthesia
- Local anesthetic with vasoconstrictor
- Gauze (2 × 2 and 4 × 4)
- Metal dish
- Saline solution
- Irrigation syringe
- Disposable sterile drapes
- Sterile gloves
- Minnesota retractor
- Periodontal probe
- 15C Scalpel blade and handle
- Microsurgical handle and blades
- PP Buser periosteal elevator
- Mosquito hemostat
- Frazier tip suction (small) and tubing
- Delicate (Crile-Wood or similar) needle holders
- Tissue forceps (DeBakey or Gerald), no teeth
- Monofilament 4-0, 5-0, and 6-0 sutures (Prolene, Monocryl, e-PTFE)
- La Grange scissors
- Suture scissors

For implant placement:
- Implant drilling unit
- Contra-angle 20:1 reduction
- Implant surgical kit with direction indicators
- Prosthetically driven surgical template (analog or guided)
- ISQ measurement device (Osstell)

For extraction:
- Periotome
- Luxator SDI #3 and #1
- Root tip elevators
- Root tip forceps
- Vertical extraction devices
- Electric high-speed contra-angle for tooth sectioning
- 701 Drill (FG grip, for above mentioned contra-angle)

For bone graft:
- Bone graft materials of preference (autogenous, allograft, xenograft, xenograft + collagen, alloplast)
- Bone scraper
- Bone condenser (oval shaped, delicate, composite or amalgam dental plugger)
- Rongeur, delicate tip, double-hinge
- Fixation pins (tacks or screws)
- Barrier guided bone regeneration membranes (resorbable or nonresorbable)

For soft-tissue grafts:
- Microsurgical handle
- Microsurgical blades
- Kirkland gingivectomy knife
- Orban gingivectomy knife
- Langer universal curette, angled
- Langer universal curette, straight
- Soft-tissue substitutes

History of the Procedure

Dental implants were initially utilized in the rehabilitation of completely edentulous patients. With time, the indications for use expanded to partially edentulous areas and to single-tooth applications, inclusive of the esthetic zone, which can be defined objectively as any dentoalveolar segment that is visible at full smile, while subjectively it may be defined as any dentoalveolar area of esthetic importance to the patient.[1] Patients with missing teeth in the esthetic zone present with a unique set of challenges for the clinician beyond what may be considered routine to achieve a natural-looking outcome.

Any esthetic rehabilitation should be predictable and characterized by a reproducible and stable outcome in the short and long term. The ability to achieve this aim depends on the interaction between clinicians and technicians (experience) as well as biologic (anatomic factors, host response), surgical (procedures, materials, techniques), implant (dimensions, compositions, surface characteristics, designs), and prosthetic (techniques and materials) factors.[2] When one or more of these factors are compromised or not performed correctly, an esthetic disaster may occur.

The primary objectives of implant therapy in the esthetic zone include an optimal esthetic and functional treatment outcome with high predictability and a low risk of complication.[3] Esthetic outcomes in sites in which dental implants are utilized must be viewed with a mid- to long-term perspective, since the stability of the facial hard and soft tissues over time is critical.

Dental implant-assisted treatments in the esthetic zone are considered to be advanced or complex in difficulty, according to the International Team for Implantology's (ITI) straightforward, advanced, complex (SAC) classification. The increased degree of difficulty is the result of expectations of the patient and the desire for an outcome that resembles the natural adjacent teeth and surrounding tissues. Improved understanding of alveolar bone anatomy and the biology of tooth loss and its effects on the alveolar process have led to changes in how dental implants in the esthetic zone are utilized. The healing process following tooth extraction and its related dimensional hard- and soft-tissue alterations must be understood to make the appropriate clinical decisions and procedures.[4–7] Esthetic success requires hard- and soft-tissue architecture that resembles that present around the natural dentition, and the need for regeneration or preservation of this architecture is often a primary concern. The timing of implant placement can also directly influence the outcome, and so the decision to place an immediate, early, or delayed implant in the esthetic zone has to be carefully evaluated.[8,9]

The need for bone and/or soft-tissue augmentation to optimize tissue contour and obtain an acceptable esthetic outcome is a necessity in most instances. The use of narrow diameter implants made from improved materials maximizes the volume of bone surrounding implants for any given bone volume. Reduced diameter implants can also ensure maintenance of a gap between the implant and the buccal bone in immediate implant placement, facilitating application of grafting materials and maintenance of alveolar contour.

Implants with a butt-joint (coincident platform) connection have been for the most part replaced by a platform switch or horizontal offset type of connection. Implants with the platform switch connection have been associated with improved tissue stability around the implant neck.[10] Tapered body implants with more aggressive threads are widely used to optimize the primary stability achieved during implant placement. The vertical position of the implant is critical and should be restoratively driven, along with implant inclination and mesio-distal and buccolingual positioning.

Recent technological advances, including the use of cone beam computed tomography (CBCT) to assess bone and soft tissues and software for digital planning, guided implant surgery, and CAD/CAM restorative solutions, are now part of the daily planning and execution.[11,12]

Ceramic and titanium-zirconium alloy implants and zirconia restorative materials became available to optimize outcomes in patients with thin phenotypes.[13] In addition, a checklist approach to diagnosis and treatment planning, based on evidence-based techniques, is available, allowing less experienced clinicians to recognize difficulties and avoid complications.[14,15]

An appropriate restoratively driven plan and a correct three-dimensional implant position are mandatory to obtain an implant-supported restoration that blends in with the adjacent teeth and provides an esthetically satisfactory outcome. Success criteria must include several modifiers, such as the implant osseointegration, acceptable condition of the periimplant soft tissues, and the optimal quality of the restoration and its relationship with the adjacent dentition.[1,16]

Currently, the use of implants to replace missing teeth in the esthetic zone is widely used, and the advantages and risks should be well known by clinicians treating these patients.

Indications for Use of the Procedure

Indications for the procedure include replacement of single or multiple missing teeth in the esthetic zone using implant-supported restorations, and understanding that the factors that influence outcome in relation to the extraction and timing of implant placement is mandatory to define indications.

Timing for Implant Placement

Defining the most appropriate moment to place an implant in relation to a tooth extraction is a challenge and is unique to each site. In the esthetic area this decision may represent the difference between success and disaster.

A key prerequisite for optimal esthetic outcomes in the anterior maxilla is an adequate three-dimensional osseous volume of the alveolar ridge, including an intact facial bone wall of sufficient thickness and height in combination with correct restoration-driven implant positions.[16–18] Deficiencies in the facial bone anatomy have a negative impact on esthetics and are a critical causative factor for complications and failures.[2,16] It is important to not only evaluate the amount of bone at the time of extraction but also anticipate the response of bone to the extraction of the tooth and ultimately the volume of bone that will remain after healing.

Clinicians should understand the physiological and dimensional alterations of the ridge that occur following tooth extraction and implant placement in the anterior maxilla. According to Araujo and collaborators[6], there are four fundamental factors that should be considered based on current knowledge of the socket-healing process. First, a relatively thin buccal bone wall at the anterior maxillary region characterizes the alveolar socket, and this bony wall provides the framework for the outline of the buccal aspect of the alveolar process. Second, the buccal bone wall will be resorbed following tooth extraction as part of the natural healing process. Following resorption of the buccal bone, the soft tissue collapses into the socket, creating a ridge defect. Third, the immediate placement of an implant does not prevent buccal bone loss, nor does a socket graft with various biomaterials. Rather, bone grating into sockets limits the collapse of the soft tissues into the healing alveolar socket and, at the same time, supports bone formation. Thus, the preservation of ridge dimension occurs as a compensatory mechanism for the buccal bone loss. Finally, tooth extraction, once considered a simple and straightforward surgical procedure, should be performed with the understanding that ridge reduction will follow, and thus in addition to performing procedures with a minimum of trauma, further clinical steps should be considered to compensate for such a change when considering future reconstruction or replacement of the extracted tooth.

Clinical and imaging analysis of the soft tissues, as well as appropriate soft-tissue management, is also important in choosing the most appropriate moment to place an implant in the esthetic zone.[19,20] The terminology of immediate, early, and late implant placement post extraction has been widely adopted after the definition was published initially by Hammerle and colleagues[2] and refined by Chen and Buser.[3]

Based on current knowledge and evidence, the clinician should be able to identify the most suitable evidence-based approach to implant placement and loading, along with the most appropriate biomaterials.[16,8] Planning decisions, protocols, and biomaterial choices should, where practical, be decided prior to the extraction of teeth.[21,22]

Options for implant placement in relation to timing of tooth extraction include the following:

- Immediate implant placement where dental implants are placed in the same surgical session as the extraction. Possible advantages include the following:
  - Reduced trauma because treatment is provided in one procedure
  - Opportunity to utilize a flapless protocol
  - Possibility of immediate loading
- When immediate placement is being considered, important anatomic conditions should be evaluated. These conditions include the presence of a fully intact facial bone wall of adequate volume (with a minimum thickness of 1 mm) and the presence of a thick gingival phenotype with no evidence of recession. Possible disadvantages associated with immediate implant placement, particularly in the esthetic zone, include the complexity of the procedure. This procedure should therefore be undertaken with caution by less experienced clinicians, especially when implant placement and bone grafting are undertaken using a flapless approach. Lack of soft-tissue volume or an unfavorable phenotype, may lead to recession and there may be difficulty placing the implant with adequate stability.
- Early implant placement involves the implant being placed in a second procedure, usually 6 to 8 weeks after extraction of the tooth. Postponing the placement of the implant facilitates healing of the soft tissues after extraction. Soft-tissue healing improves both the quality and quantity of soft tissues around the implant, significantly improving the esthetic outcome. Disadvantages include the placement of the implant as a second procedure, most likely the use of an open flap and the need for use of a contour augmentation to manage resorption of the facial bone wall. There is usually a flattening of the cervical region, but the implant is usually placed within the alveolar bone contour.
- Early implant placement can be delayed until healing has resulted in partial filling of the extraction socket with bone. This requires additional time. It is important to note that while bone is observable in the apical region of the extraction during this period of healing, there is a concurrent flattening in the cervical or coronal region. This may lead to an inability to position an implant and the need for a staged bone graft approach. This procedure is described elsewhere in this book.
- Late implant placement, also described as conventional, is undertaken after complete postextraction healing of the alveolar bone. This requires between 4 and 6 months of healing after the extraction of the tooth or teeth. Late or conventional implant placement is often an intentional treatment alternative, when a graft is required at the time of extraction to facilitate future placement. This approach is described elsewhere in this book.

Limitations and Contraindications

Implant treatment is highly successful and is considered an evidence-based treatment modality. However, patients and clinicians should anticipate complications and make decisions that help to avoid them. In addition, clinicians should develop strategies for managing complications as they are inevitable. The functional and esthetic rehabilitation of missing teeth in the esthetic zone should be predictable. This implies treatment should be stable and reproducible in both the short and long term and satisfying to both the patient and the treatment team. Failure to achieve esthetic and functional outcomes with dental implants can be disastrous and often require additional surgical and restorative procedures in an attempt to correct the compromise. These procedures, undertaken in an effort to overcome complications, are often more susceptible to them.

Several factors can contribute to increased risk when providing treatment assisted by dental implants. Risk is elevated substantially when treatment is provided in the esthetic zone. In 2009, the ITI published the SAC classification. This textbook describes patient treatment indications (from a surgical and restorative perspective) based on their anticipated degree of difficulty, using objective pretreatment observations. The objective criteria were defined and agreed on at a 2007 consensus conference convened to consider the topic.[14] The SAC classification has been widely adopted by clinicians, teaching institutions, and dental organizations to aid in the diagnosis and planning for patients and pretreatment consideration of risk to outcome. In addition to patient-related factors and treatment difficulty, the education and experience of the clinician are considered.[14] In 2006, Martin et al.[23] published a study on esthetic risk assessment. The risk assessment table was designed to assist clinicians in the identification of patients who present with a greater risk of a negative outcome. Risk assessment considers an accurate diagnosis and sound treatment planning, ensuring the identification of clinical situations that elevate risk. The esthetic risk assessment was updated in 2017[24] and provides a checklist and a visual analog scale for the clinician and patient to utilize when determining the risk and limitations of implant treatment in the esthetic zone (Table 21.1).

Adjacent missing teeth with compromised three-dimensional space relationships, immediate implant placement in patients with a thin tissue phenotype, and the presence of extended combined vertical and horizontal bone and soft-tissue defects clearly add to the degree of treatment difficulty and elevate the likelihood of risk and a negative treatment outcome. The predictability of a prosthetically driven horizontal and/or vertical bone augmentation is influenced by many factors, specifically the expertise of the surgeon.[25,26] When larger alveolar bone defects are present, pink ceramics restorations may be considered.[27,28] As a result of both surgical and restorative factors influencing risk and outcome predictability, it is generally recommended that the esthetic risk assessment checklist be used in all instances where treatment of esthetic significance is undertaken.

Technique

Immediate Implant Placement

Immediate implant placement has, in theory, several distinct advantages for both the patient and the clinician. However, there is an increased risk of complications of esthetic significance. These include soft-tissue recession, implant malpositioning, implant loss, and the associated lack of an acceptable esthetic prosthesis.

According to Buser and Chen,[4] a detailed clinical assessment and a CBCT should be done before proceeding with the extraction, and a comprehensive plan should be developed prior to extraction of the tooth inclusive of all surgical and restorative interventions. In all cases, all options should be considered inclusive of maintaining the teeth, and after discussion with the patient, informed consent obtained. Anatomic structures to be examined include the following:

1. Thickness, height, and integrity of the facial bone wall
2. Height and thickness of the palatal bone wall
3. Crest width and height adjacent to the extraction site
4. Height and inclination of the alveolar ridge
5. Height of the alveolar bone at adjacent teeth
6. Location and extension of the nasopalatine canal
7. Bone volume available apically and palatal to the root
8. Mesio-distal size of the resulting single-tooth gap post extraction

Table 21.1 Esthetic Risk Assessment.

	LEVEL OF RISK		
Esthetic Risk Factors	**Low**	**Medium**	**High**
Medical status	Healthy, uneventful healing		Compromised healing
Smoking habit	Nonsmoker	Light smoker (≤10 cigs/day)	Heavy smoker (>10 cigs/day)
Gingival display at full smile	Low	Medium	High
Width of edentulous span	1 tooth (≥7 mm)[1] 1 tooth (≥6 mm)[2]	1 tooth (<7 mm)[1] 1 tooth (<6 mm)[2]	2 teeth or more
Shape of tooth crowns	Rectangular		Triangular
Restorative status of neighboring teeth	Virgin		Restored
Gingival phenotype	Low-scalloped, thick	Medium-scalloped, medium-thick	High-scalloped, thin
Infection at implant site	None	Chronic	Acute
Soft-tissue anatomy	Soft tissue intact		Soft-tissue defects
Bone level at adjacent teeth	≤5 mm to contact point	5.5–6.5 mm to contact point	≥7 mm to contact point
Facial bone wall phenotype*	Thick-wall phenotype, ≥1 mm thickness		Thin-wall phenotype, <1 mm thickness
Bone anatomy at alveolar crest	No bone deficiency	Horizontal bone deficiency	Vertical bone deficiency
Patient's esthetic expectations	Realistic expectations		Unrealistic expectations

*(Chappuis V., Martin W. 2017)
Chappuis V, Martin W. ITI Treatment Guide Vol 10: Implant Therapy in the Esthetic Zone: Current Treatment Modalities and Materials for Single-tooth Replacements. Berlin: Quintessence Publishing Co, Ltd, 2017.

Tooth extraction procedure

The trauma of tooth extraction should be limited by using minimally invasive surgical procedures.[29,30] These procedures prevent expansion of the socket housing and reduce the likelihood of fracture of the thin adjacent bony walls. Good surgical technique and minimizing trauma can reduce the need for more extensive bone augmentation. The use of forceps to luxate the tooth, and in particular the application of primary-drive forces that expand the socket and apply forces toward the buccal-palatal/lingual aspects of the socket, is not recommended. Likewise, forceps should not be used with rotational movements, as the asymmetric shape of most tooth roots will result in trauma. Extraction methodology has evolved to include technologies and instrumentation that promote minimally invasive tooth extraction and trauma reduction. Periotomes and vertical tooth extraction systems are the most frequently utilized examples. Periotomes are designed to sever the periodontal ligament fibers at the mesial and distal aspects of the socket and to expand the socket with a minimum of trauma and facilitate extraction. Vertical tooth extraction systems are designed to pull teeth or roots in a vertical direction and hence avoid any trauma to the socket walls caused by expansion. Both techniques result in no pressure being applied to the labial or buccal socket wall and are mostly indicated for the extraction of single-rooted teeth and are most efficient when roots are straight and conical. Where possible, elevation of a mucoperiosteal flap for the purpose of tooth extraction should be avoided. For immediate implant placement, every effort should be made to preserve the buccal bone and surrounding soft tissues during the extraction (Fig. 21.1).

Implant placement

After tooth extraction, a surgical template that communicates the preferred three-dimensional implant position based on the restorative plan is placed. The three-dimensional position of the implant is based in part on the concepts of "comfort and danger zones."[30] For this patient and implant choice, this represents an orofacial position of the implant shoulder around 1.5 mm palatal to the future point of emergence and a vertical distance of 3 to 4 mm from the implant shoulder to the future mucosal margin of the planned restoration at the midfacial point. In addition, maintaining a minimal distance of 1.5 mm from adjacent teeth on the mesial and distal aspects is important (Fig. 21.2A–D).

The use of a surgical template is considered mandatory. The template can be analog or digital (where the template is computer designed and fabricated). It is important that the cervical margin of the future crown is visualized or accounted for in any digital plan (Fig. 21.3).

Development of the osteotomy for the placement of a dental implant is initiated with a needle or small round bur. The preferred location for the initial purchase point is on the palatal wall, below the apex. After confirmation of the implant inclination and position with a direction indicator pin and the surgical template, final depth of preparation is undertaken according to the selected implant length and diameter. The implant shoulder should be positioned 3 to 4 mm apical to the planned midfacial mucosal margin of the prosthesis. Mesio-distal implant position is usually centered according to the planned restoration or slightly distal in the esthetic zone if space is ideal. The labial-palatal position in

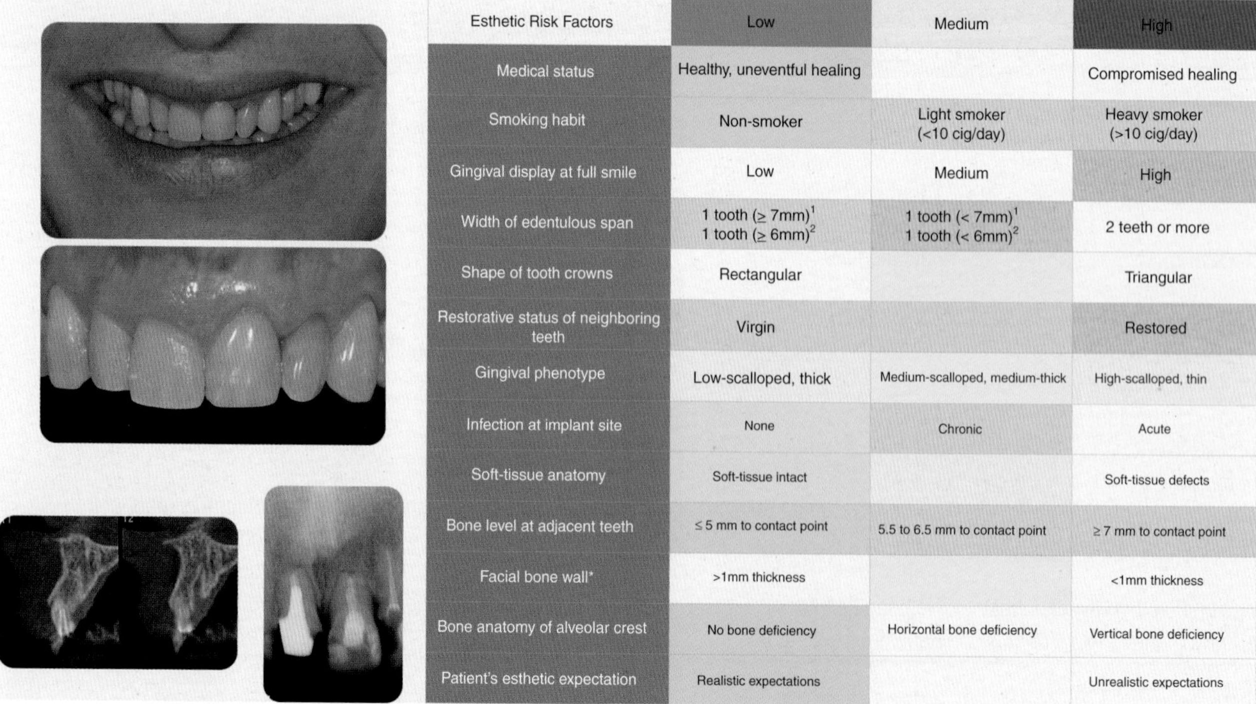

Esthetic Risk Factors	Low	Medium	High
Medical status	Healthy, uneventful healing		Compromised healing
Smoking habit	Non-smoker	Light smoker (<10 cig/day)	Heavy smoker (>10 cig/day)
Gingival display at full smile	Low	Medium	High
Width of edentulous span	1 tooth (≥ 7mm)[1] 1 tooth (≥ 6mm)[2]	1 tooth (< 7mm)[1] 1 tooth (< 6mm)[2]	2 teeth or more
Shape of tooth crowns	Rectangular		Triangular
Restorative status of neighboring teeth	Virgin		Restored
Gingival phenotype	Low-scalloped, thick	Medium-scalloped, medium-thick	High-scalloped, thin
Infection at implant site	None	Chronic	Acute
Soft-tissue anatomy	Soft-tissue intact		Soft-tissue defects
Bone level at adjacent teeth	≤5 mm to contact point	5.5 to 6.5 mm to contact point	≥7 mm to contact point
Facial bone wall*	>1mm thickness		<1mm thickness
Bone anatomy of alveolar crest	No bone deficiency	Horizontal bone deficiency	Vertical bone deficiency
Patient's esthetic expectation	Realistic expectations		Unrealistic expectations

Figure 21.1 Indicated clinical and imaging views for planning treatment in the esthetic zone, and esthetic risk assessment for potential implant placement on right maxillary central incisor.

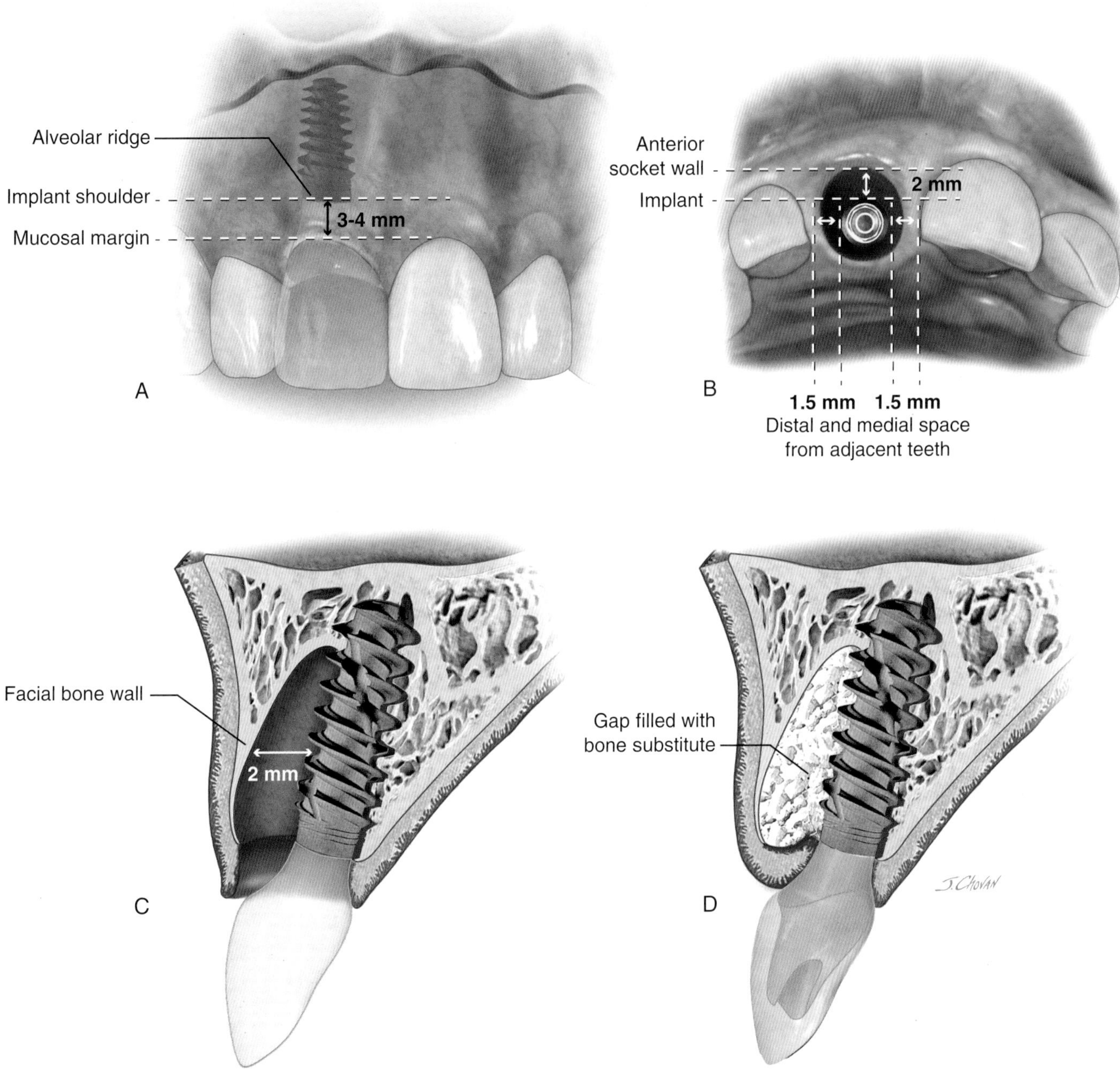

Figure 21.2 Ideal implant positioning, dictated by the prosthetic template. A, Mesio-distal and vertical (apico-coronal) position. **B,** Buccal-palatal position, occlusal view. **C,** Buccal-palatal position, sagittal view. **D,** Implant position in relation to future restoration, including gap filling with bone substitute, sagittal view.

conjunction with the long axis inclination should direct screw access for the planned restoration toward the cingulum.

For immediate implant placement a gap should be maintained between the implant body and a viable facial bone wall of adequate volume (greater than 1 mm). The gap can be filled with a bone substitute, which when combined with a stable implant (with an appropriate microroughened surface) and sound facial bone, can minimize the esthetic and volume impact of physiologic bundle bone resorption following extraction.

In sites characterized by a thin tissue phenotype, a soft-tissue graft (autogenous or substitute) can be utilized in a flapped or a flapless manner. A connective tissue graft can be harvested from the tuberosity or the palate in the region of the second premolar. Alternatively, a soft tissue substitute material can be used.[31]

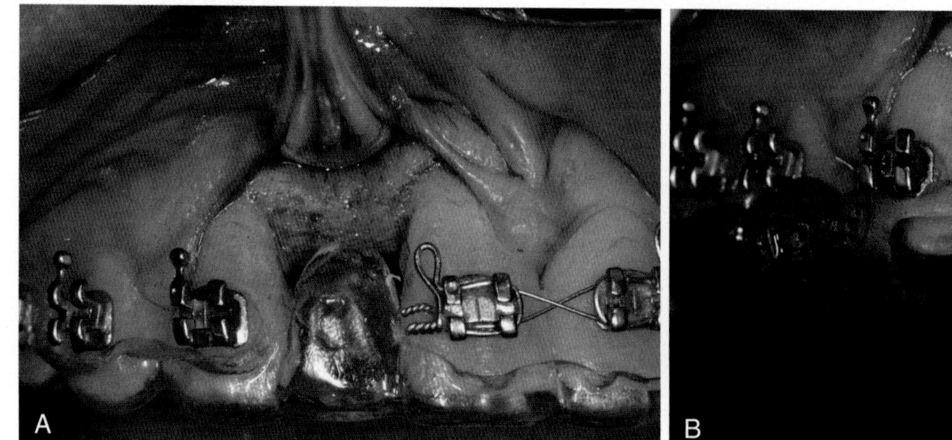

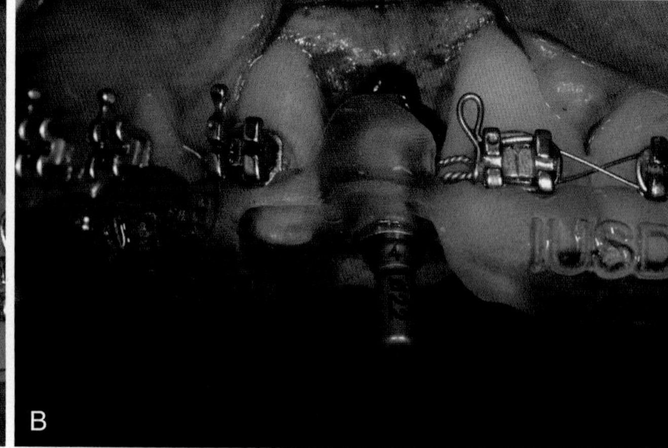

Figure 21.3 Prosthetic template with the gingival margin of the future restoration. A, Analog template. **B,** Static-guided template.

An immediate provisional or a custom designed (computer-aided design [CAD]/computer-aided manufacturing [CAM]) healing abutment can be used to assist in supporting the soft tissues and maintain its shape and configuration. After a period of healing (ranging from 8 weeks to 3–4 months, depending on implant used, primary stability, amount of grafting, and patient overall health and compliance), the provisional restoration or healing abutment can be removed, and the final restorative work can be initiated. In many clinical situations, adjunct dental esthetics work is needed to improve the outcome (Fig. 21.4).

Early Implant Placement

An extraction method that minimizes trauma, inclusive of a flapless technique, should be utilized when early implant placement is indicated. After extraction, a collagen plug may be considered to limit collapse of the soft tissues. A healing period of 6 to 8 weeks is required for soft-tissue healing, and a flattening of the buccal wall is expected, due to resorption of the bundle bone. To facilitate implant placement, an incision should be made slightly palatal to the midcrestal region of the edentulous area. Intrasulcular incisions on the buccal aspect of the adjacent teeth are preferred, although in many instances, there is a need for a unilateral or bilateral vertical releasing incision. Extending the flap to position releasing incisions out of the esthetically sensitive area should be considered. Careful attention should be maintained to minimize soft-tissue trauma when the flap is elevated. The tissue overlying the alveolar crest of the edentulous site is elevated labially to provide access, and this tissue can ultimately increase soft-tissue volume on the mucosal margin of the facial aspect of the proposed restoration.

The osteotomy for the dental implant is sequentially prepared using a template communicating the proposed three-dimensional implant position developed from the restorative plan. The comfort and danger zones must be carefully identified. The correct drilling sequence for the proposed implant of choice should be followed to ensure appropriate position and to optimize primary stability. When augmentation of the facial bone volume and contour is required, autogenous bone chips can be harvested from the area of the nasal spine or from the alveolus apical to adjacent teeth. After positioning of the implant and placement of a healing cap or healing abutment, the local bone contour augmentation can be performed using a guided bone restoration technique. A combination of the autogenous chips previously harvested, positioned immediately adjacent to the implant surface, and deproteinized bovine bone material reconstitutes the contour and volume of the missing facial bone. The graft material is covered with a double layer of a noncrosslinked collagen membrane. Horizontal mattress sutures are preferred over the alveolar crest, and interrupted sutures are preferred on the vertical releasing incisions and the papillae.

After 10 to 12 weeks of healing, the implant can be exposed. At reopening, there may be a need and an opportunity to use a soft-tissue graft to further enhance the tissue quality and thickness. Once implants are exposed, the prosthetic phase can be initiated. Tissue contouring and development of the emergence profile can be achieved with appropriately shaped and finished provisional restorations, which can be modified as required until the desired profile is achieved. Excellent laboratory and clinical phases are critical to obtain satisfactory results. Long-term outcomes have been demonstrated with the early placement approach[32] (Fig. 21.5).

Late Implant Placement

Late implant placement (>6 months after extraction) can be indicated depending on site and patient-specific conditions. Growing patients, medically compromised patients, and patients who require a standalone graft procedure to facilitate implant positioning are examples of late placement indications. When bone volume is inadequate to facilitate primary stability of an implant positioned in the correct three-dimensional restoration-driven position, late implant placement is indicated. This decision should be made prior to the extraction of the tooth so that grafting alternatives can be fully considered. These options can include socket grafting for alveolar ridge preservation or a more complex staged grafting of the alveolar ridge. Grafting options have the goal of providing the appropriate future bone volume capable of accepting an implant in the appropriate position. The detailed surgical technique of ridge preservation is described elsewhere in this book.

Surgical positioning of the implant according to a late placement protocol employs procedures similar to those described previously for immediate and early options. There may be a need for additional contour augmentation of the facial bone and/or soft-tissue augmentation (Fig. 21.6).

Considerations for Adjacent Missing Teeth in the Esthetic Zone

Ideal esthetic outcomes are less predictable when replacing adjacent missing teeth in the anterior maxilla, particularly, with implant-supported restorations. The bone volume is almost always deficient, and soft-tissue volume, in both the horizontal and vertical dimensions, is also compromised. These sites often require three-dimensional bone and soft-tissue augmentation. The larger the defect or defects, the more likely the efficacy and predictability of these procedures will be compromised, especially in the vertical dimension.[25,26]

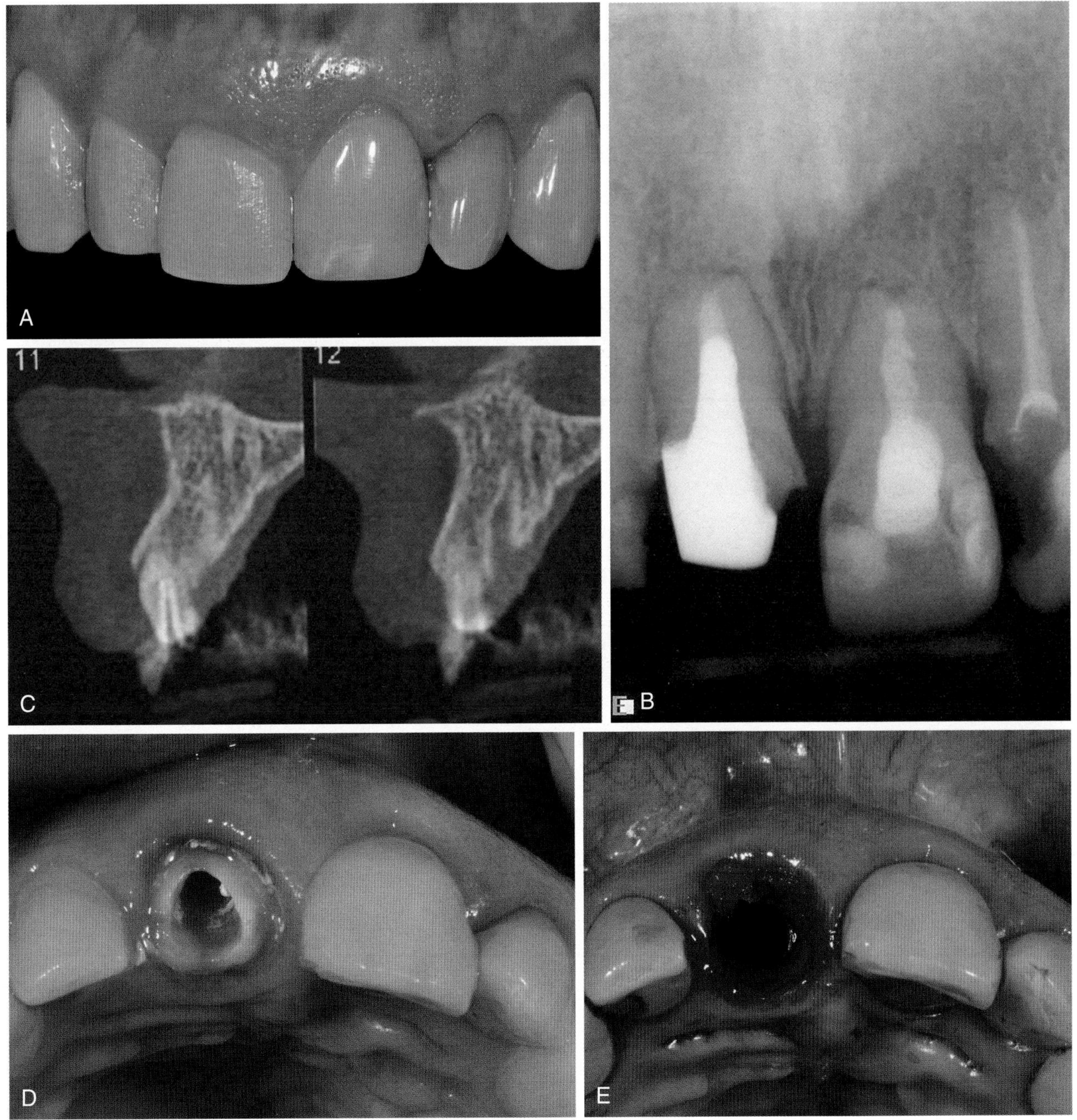

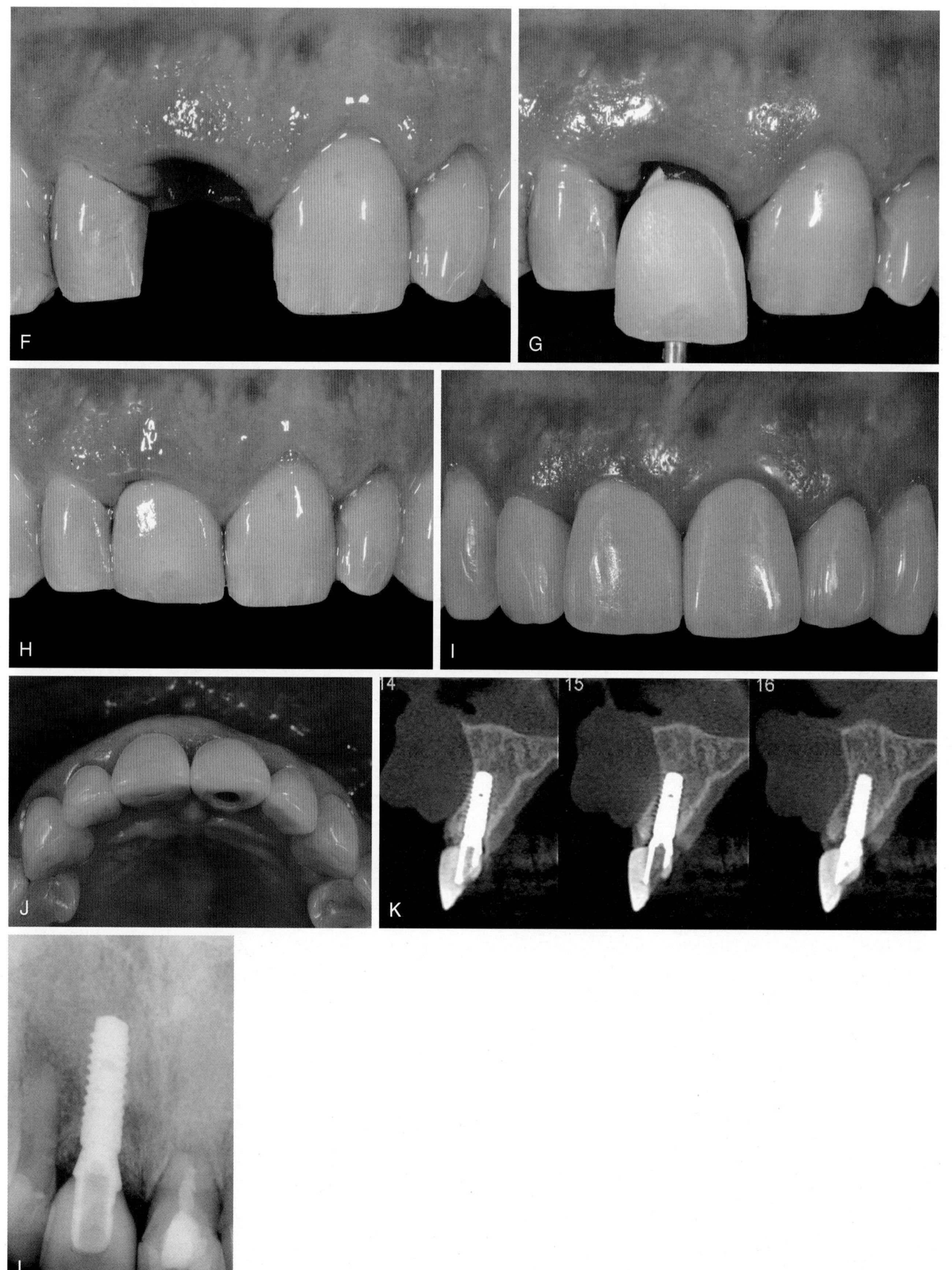

Figure 21.4 Clinical case. Immediate implant placement. A)Buccal view, tooth #8 to be exracted. Gingival margin lower than #9. B) Periapical radiograph, showing adequate proximal bone levels; C) CBCT of #8, showing favorable ridge height and widht for immediate placement; D) Occlusal view of #8 before extraction; E) Occlusal view, implant placed and graft on buccal gap; F) Buccal view, after implant placement; G) Immediate provisional being placed; H) Immediate provisional placed. I-L) Four years follow-up images; I)Buccal view, Note cosmetic dentistry on adjacet teeth, to optimize outcome; J) Occlusal view; K) CBCT; I) Periapical radiograph.

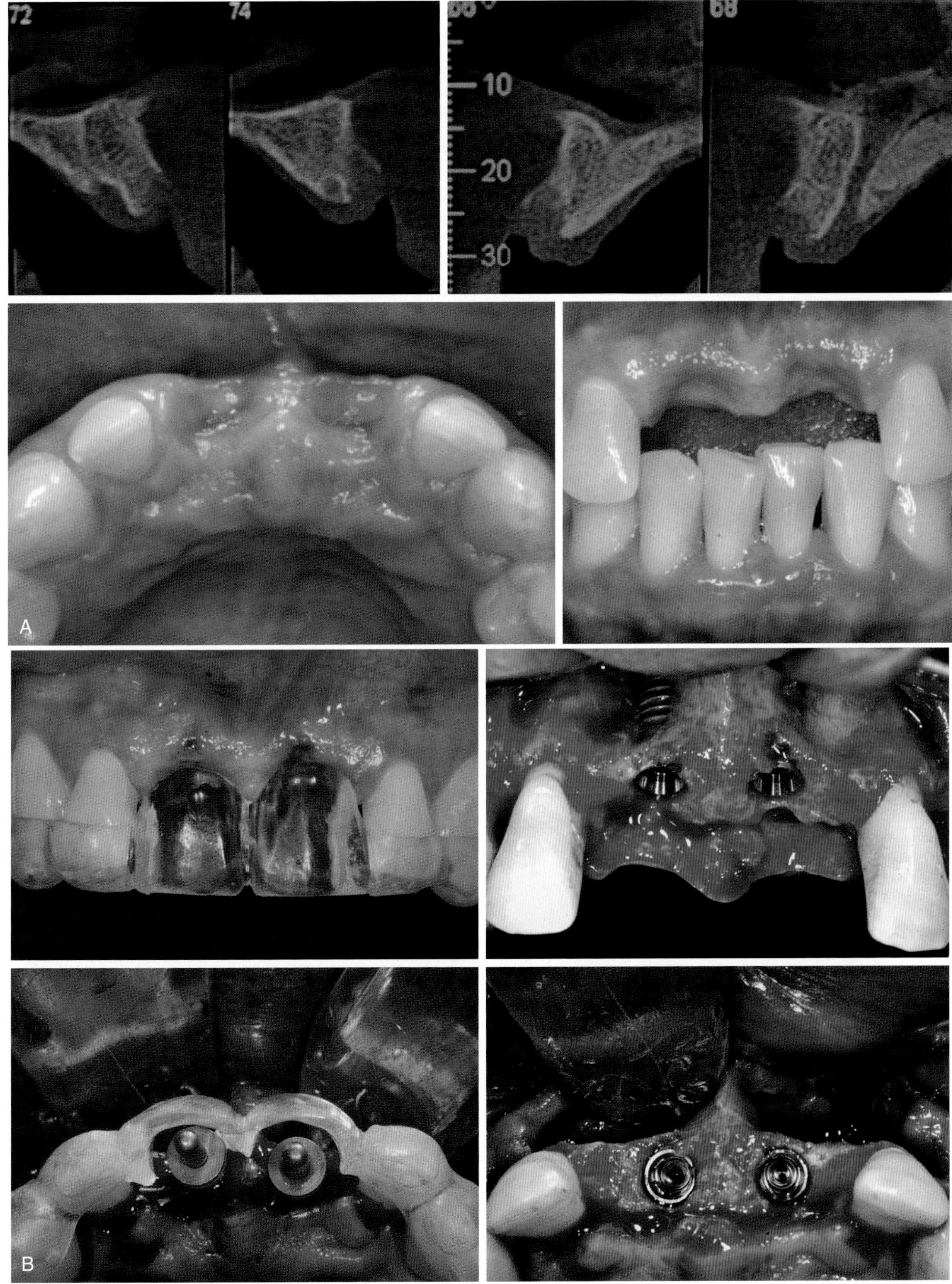
72
74
10
20
30
68
A
B

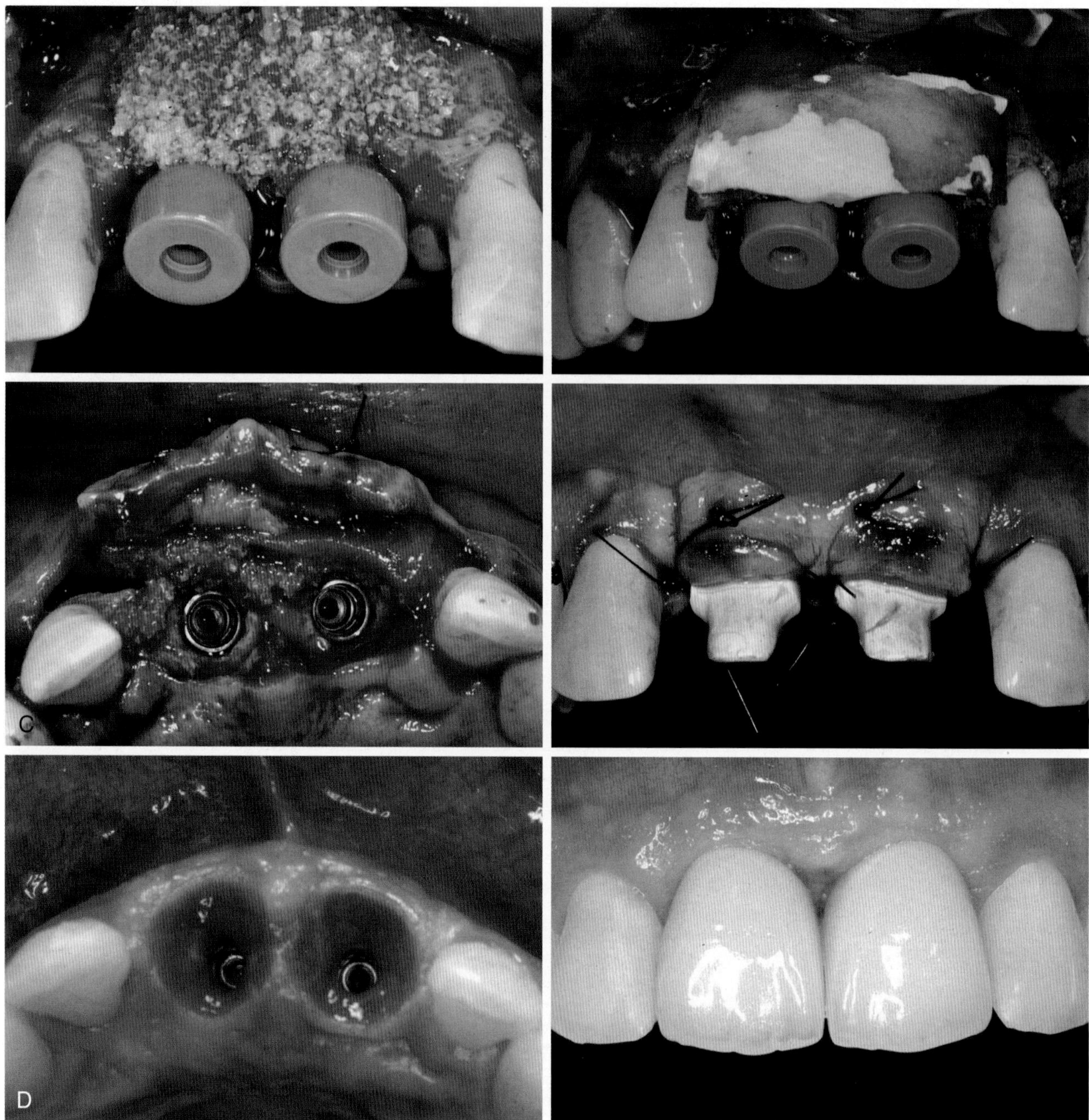

Figure 21.5 Early implant placement with guided bone regeneration procedure. A, Preoperative facial and occlusal views 8 weeks after extraction of maxillary central incisors, with complete soft-tissue healing. Note: On cone beam computed tomography (CBCT), the alveolar socket was not completely healed. **B,** Implants placed in the ideal restorative position according to restorative plan template. Exposed threads and lack of facial volume require the guided bone regeneration procedure. **C,** Intraoperative view showing use of particulate bone substitute and long-term resorbable membrane, in a dual-layer fashion, and soft-tissue graft. Closure obtained over custom healing abutments. **D,** Occlusal view before placing final restoration and facial view of final restoration. Restoration performed 4 months after implant placement.

These deficiencies lead to limitations in developing and maintaining bone and soft tissue between implants. Hence, a reduction of support for the papillae should be anticipated.

Inter-implant support for hard and soft tissues is unpredictable and is influenced by the implant and abutment design characteristics, in particular their diameter. Larger diameter implants and abutments encroach on the volume required for prostheses and surrounding tissues and can lead to increased periimplant crestal bone loss between two implants and consequent loss of soft-tissue dimension. In combination, this can lead to less-than-optimal esthetic outcomes, loss of tissue support, and the appearance of the so-called black triangle. Particular attention should be given when replacing adjacent, lateral, and central incisors or adjacent canines and

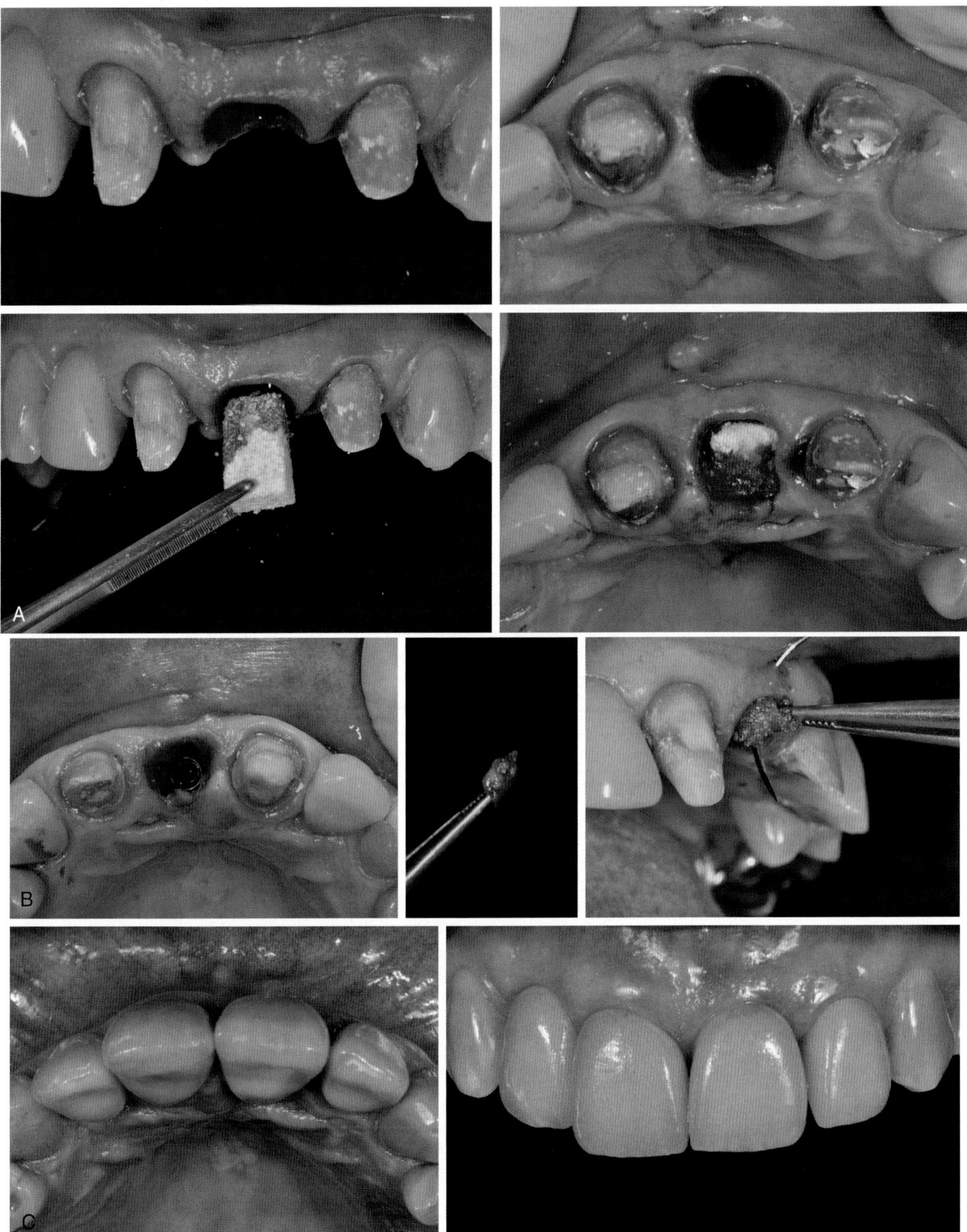

Figure 21.6 Alveolar ridge preervation utilizing deproteinized bovine bone matrix + collagen. Implant placement 5 months later in the healed ridge, with a simultaneous connective tissue graft.

lateral incisors, since the available space may be inadequate for the placement of two implants, and esthetic tissue contour is required to be asymmetric as a result of the tooth shape variations. Treatment options considering implant distribution, the need for cantilevers and contoured pontics, and the use of pink supplements to the restorations should be carefully evaluated.[27,28]

Avoidance and Management of Intraoperative Complications

While substantial improvements and innovations in implant dentistry have occurred in recent years, the complication rates remain high.[30,31] Complications lead to the emotional distress of the patient and can require multiple additional procedures and a longer treatment time. In many instances, complications can be impossible to correct in an optimal manner.

Esthetic complications can result from biologic, technical, or mechanical risk factors, alone or in combination. Most importantly, esthetic complications can be iatrogenic, the result of poor judgement. Complications are the result of inadequate assessment of preoperative risk, selection of an inappropriate treatment approach (timing in relation to the extraction), inaccuracy in three-dimensional implant positioning, inappropriate implant dimensions, or a poorly executed restorative phase.

Incorrect implant positioning (too deep and/or too labial) is the most common complication and negatively impacts the functional and esthetic outcome. Potential improvement of the esthetic outcome can often require implant removal, site enhancement, and placement of a new implant in the appropriate position (Fig. 21.7).

The use of a surgical template, being it analog or digitally manufactured, leads to a prosthetically driven implant and reduces the risk of a poor outcome. Oversized implants (diameter > 4.5 mm) should be avoided in the esthetic zone. Wider diameter implants increase the likelihood of facial mispositioning and often result in the placement of an implant outside of the alveolar bone envelope. As a rule, a regular or reduced diameter microroughened implant fabricated from improved materials and a reduced diameter platform are recommended in the esthetic zone. For implants fabricated from improved materials, diameters in the range of 3.5 to 4.1 mm can be considered for maxillary central incisors, canines and pre-molars, and reduced diameter implants and platforms in the 2.9 to 3.5 mm range are recommended for maxillary lateral incisors.

Lack of adequate volume and contour of soft tissues around the implant and restoration may also lead to inadequate esthetic outcomes and may require soft-tissue management procedures before, during, or after implant placement. Usually, soft-tissue procedures performed prior to or during the implant placement procedure result in the best outcomes.[31,33] When insufficient horizontal and vertical bone wall dimensions exist, preventing the placement of a stable implant in the correct three-dimensional position, use of a staged bone augmentation is indicated.

Postoperative Considerations

Immediate implant placement is usually partnered with the use of an immediately positioned provisional restoration (immediate loading). This requires good primary stability of the implant, and care should be taken by the restorative dentist to correctly adjust the emergence profile and occlusion of the provisional restoration.[34] It is recommended that the provisional restoration be screw-retained and not cemented.

When an early approach is taken, some swelling of the tissues should be anticipated. Care should be taken to ensure any interim prosthesis that is not implant supported does not apply pressure in the site of the surgery, particularly if the area is grafted. The use of postoperative antibiotics is generally recommended for at least 7 days after the procedure.

For the assessment of esthetic outcomes, objective criteria such as the pink and white esthetic scores have been proposed. These criteria do not reflect the patient's subjective opinion about the outcome of therapy. The clinician's objective evaluation and the patient's subjective opinion of a successful outcome may not agree but should be aligned as best possible when assessing treatment outcomes.[35–37]

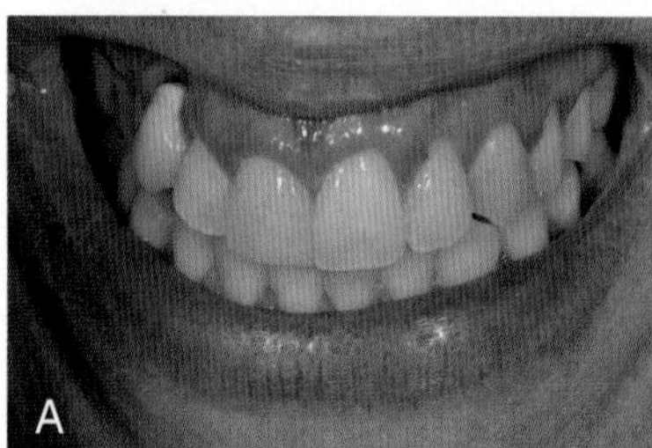

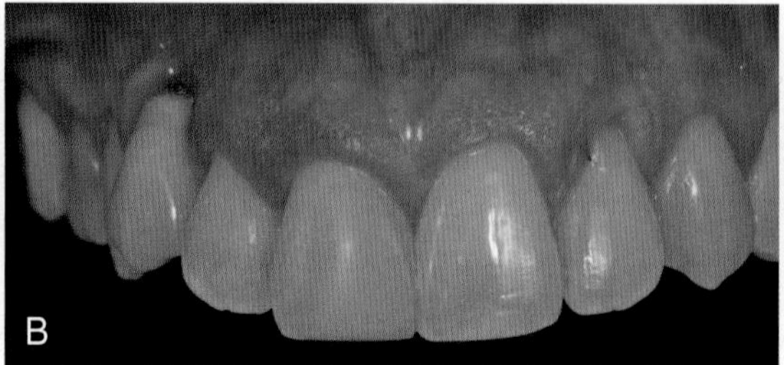

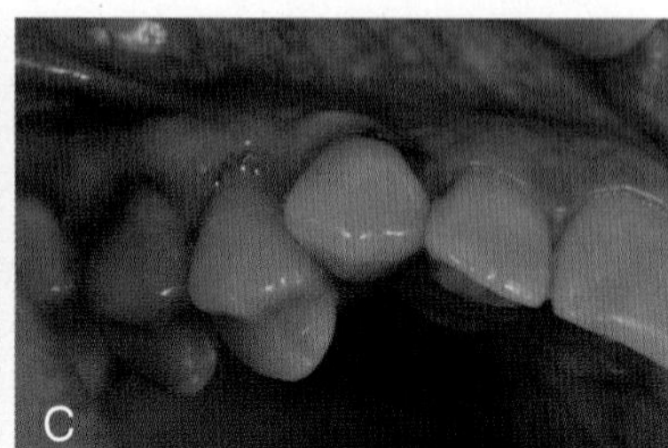

Figure 21.7 Esthetic complications. A, Patient with high lip line, classified as high esthetic risk. **B and C,** Implant in right canine is too wide, too buccal, and too deep, leading to unsatisfactory esthetic outcome.

References

1. Belser U, Buser D, Higginbottom F. Consensus statements and recommended clinical procedures regarding esthetics in implant dentistry. *Int J Oral Maxillofac Implants.* 2004;19(suppl):73–74.
2. Hämmerle CH, Chen ST, Wilson TG Jr. Consensus statements and recommended clinical procedures regarding the placement of implants in extraction sockets. *Int J Oral Maxillofac Implants.* 2004;19(suppl):26–28.
3. Chen ST, Buser D. ITI treatment Guide vol 3: implants in extraction sockets. In: Buser D, Belser U, Wismeijer D, eds. *Implants in Post-extraction Sites: A Literature Update.* Berlin, Germany: Quintessence Publishing Co, Ltd; 2008.
4. Buser D, Chen ST. Implant placement in post-extraction sites. In: *Buser D. 20 Years of Guided Bone Regeneration in Implant Dentistry.* 2nd ed. Chicago, Illinois: Quintessence Publishing Co., Inc.; 2009.
5. Januário AL, Duarte WR, Barriviera M, Mesti JC, Araújo MG, Lindhe J. Dimension of the facial bone wall in the anterior maxilla: a cone-beam computed tomography study. *Clin Oral Implants Res.* 2011;22(10):1168–1171.
6. Araújo MG, Silva CO, Misawa M, Sukekava F. Alveolar socket healing: what can we learn? *Periodontol 2000.* 2015;68(1):122–134. https://doi.org/10.1111/prd.12082.
7. Chappuis V, Engel O, Shahim K, Reyes M, Katsaros C, Buser D. Soft tissue alterations in esthetic postextraction sites: a 3-dimensional analysis. *J Dent Res.* 2015;94(suppl 9):187S–193S. https://doi.org/10.1177/0022034515592869.
8. Chappuis V, Araújo MG, Buser D. Clinical relevance of dimensional bone and soft tissue alterations post-extraction in esthetic sites. *Periodontol 2000.* 2017;73(1):73–83. https://doi.org/10.1111/prd.12167.
9. Buser D, Chappuis V, Belser UC, Chen S. Implant placement post extraction in esthetic single tooth sites: when immediate, when early, when late? *Periodontol 2000.* 2017;73(1):84–102. https://doi.org/10.1111/prd.12170.
10. Chappuis V, Bornstein MM, Buser D, Belser U. Influence of implant neck design on facial bone crest dimensions in the esthetic zone analyzed by cone beam CT: a comparative study with a 5-to-9-year follow-up. *Clin Oral Implants Res.* 2016;27(9):1055–1064.
11. Tahmaseb A, Wismeijer D, Coucke W, Derksen W. Computer technology applications in surgical implant dentistry: a systematic review. *Int J Oral Maxillofac Implants.* 2014;29(suppl):25–42.
12. Bornstein MM, Al-Nawas B, Kuchler U, Tahmaseb A. Consensus statements and recommended clinical procedures regarding contemporary surgical and radiographic techniques in implant dentistry. *Int J Oral Maxillofac Implants.* 2014;29(suppl):78–82.
13. Roehling S, Schlegel KA, Woelfler H, Gahlert M. Performance and outcome of zirconia dental implants in clinical studies: a meta-analysis. *Clin Oral Implants Res.* 2018;29(suppl 16):135–153. https://doi.org/10.1111/clr.13352.
14. Dawson A, Chen S, eds. *The SAC Classification in Implant Dentistry.* Chicago: Quintessence; 2009.
15. Correia A, Rebolo A, Azevedo L, Polido W, Rodrigues PP. SAC assessment tool in implant dentistry: evaluation of the agreement level between users. *Int J Oral Maxillofac Implants.* 2020;35(5):990–994. https://doi.org/10.11607/jomi.8023.
16. Chen ST, Buser D. Esthetic outcomes following immediate and early implant placement in the anterior maxilla—a systematic review. *Int J Oral Maxillofac Implants.* 2014;29(suppl):186–215.
17. Grunder U, Gracis S, Capelli M. Influence of the 3-D bone-to-implant relationship on esthetics. *Int J Periodontics Restorative Dent.* 2005;25(2):113–119.
18. Kan JYK, Roe P, Rungcharassaeng K, et al. Classification of sagittal root position in relation to the anterior maxillary osseous housing for immediate implant placement: a cone beam computed tomography study. *Int J Oral Maxillofac Implants.* 2011;26(4):873–876.
19. Januário AL, Barriviera M, Duarte WR. Soft tissue cone-beam computed tomography: a novel method for the measurement of gingival tissue and the dimensions of the dentogingival unit. *J Esthet Restor Dent.* 2008;20(6):366–373. https://doi.org/10.1111/j.1708-8240.2008.00210.x.
20. Kan JYK, Rungcharassaeng K, Morimoto T, Lozada J. Facial gingival tissue stability after connective tissue graft with single immediate tooth replacement in the esthetic zone: consecutive case report. *J Oral Maxillofac Surg.* 2009;67(s):40–48.
21. Gallucci GO, Hamilton A, Zhou W, Buser D, Chen S. Implant placement and loading protocols in partially edentulous patients: a systematic review. *Clin Oral Implants Res.* 2018;29(suppl 16):106–134.
22. Morton D, Gallucci G, Lin WS, et al. Group 2 ITI Consensus Report: prosthodontics and implant dentistry. *Clin Oral Implants Res.* 2018;29(suppl 16):215–223.
23. Martin W, Morton D, Buser D. Pre-operative analysis and prosthetic treatment planning in esthetic implant dentistry. In: Belser U, Buser D, Hämmerle C, et al., eds. *ITI Treatment Guide. Implant Therapy in the Esthetic Zone: Single-Tooth Replacements*; Vol. 1. Berlin, Germany: Quintessence; 2006.
24. Chappuis V, Martin W. In: *Implant Therapy in the Esthetic Zone:Current Treatment Modalities and Materials for Single-Tooth Replacements.* Vol. 10. Berlin: Quintessence Publishing Co, Ltd; 2017. ITI Treatment Guide.
25. Chiapasco M, Casentini P. Horizontal bone-augmentation procedures in implant dentistry: prosthetically guided regeneration. *Periodontol 2000.* 2018;77(1):213–240. https://doi.org/10.1111/prd.12219.
26. Rocchietta I, Ferrantino L, Simion M. Vertical ridge augmentation in the esthetic zone. *Periodontol 2000.* 2018;77(1):241–255. https://doi.org/10.1111/prd.12218.
27. Coachman C, Salama M, Garber D, Calamita M, Salama H, Cabral G. Prosthetic gingival reconstruction in a fixed partial restoration. Part 1: introduction to artificial gingiva as an alternative therapy. *Int J Periodontics Restorative Dent.* 2009;29(5):471–477.
28. Wittneben J-G, Weber HP. *Extended Edentulous Spaces in the Esthetic Zone. ITI Treatment Guide.* Vol. 6. Berlin, Germany: Quintessence; 2012.
29. Muska E, Walter C, Knight A, et al. Atraumatic vertical tooth extraction: a proof of principle clinical study of a novel system. *Oral Surg Oral Med Oral Pathol Oral Radiol.* 2013;116(5):e303–e310.
30. Buser D, Martin W, Belser UC. Optimizing esthetics for implant restorations in the anterior maxilla: anatomic and surgical considerations. *Int J Oral Maxillofac Implants.* 2004;19(suppl):43–61.
31. Deeb GR, Deeb JG. Soft tissue grafting around teeth and implants. *Oral Maxillofac Surg Clin North Am.* 2015;27(3):425–448. https://doi.org/10.1016/j.coms.2015.04.010.
32. Buser D, Chappuis V, Kuchler U, et al. Long-term stability of early implant placement with contour augmentation. *J Dent Res.* 2013;92(suppl 12):176S–182S. https://doi.org/10.1177/0022034513504949.
33. Chackartchi T, Romanos GE, Sculean A. Soft tissue-related complications and management around dental implants. *Periodontol 2000.* 2019;81(1):124–138. https://doi.org/10.1111/prd.12287.
34. Martin WC, Pollini A, Morton D. The influence of restorative procedures on esthetic outcomes in implant dentistry: a systematic review. *Int J Oral Maxillofac Implants.* 2014;29(suppl):142–154. https://doi.org/10.11607/jomi.2014suppl.g3.1.
35. Cooper LF. Objective criteria: guiding and evaluating dental implant esthetics. *J Esthet Restor Dent.* 2008;20(3):195–205.
36. Belser UC, Grütter L, Vailati F, Bornstein MM, Weber HP, Buser D. Outcome evaluation of early placed maxillary anterior single-tooth implants using objective esthetic criteria: a cross-sectional, retrospective study in 45 patients with a 2- to 4-year follow-up using pink and white esthetic scores. *J Periodontol.* 2009;80(1):140–151.
37. Vilhjálmsson VH, Klock KS, Størksen K, Bårdsen A. Aesthetics of implant-supported single anterior maxillary crowns evaluated by objective indices and participants' perceptions. *Clin Oral Implants Res.* 2011;22(12):1399–1403.

CHAPTER 22

All-on-Four Technique

David Knight Sylvester II and Daniel Joseph Pinkston

Armamentarium

#2 Molt elevator
#9 Periosteal elevator
#15 Blade and handle
Bone file
Cheek retractors
Curettes
Dean tissue scissors
Elevators
Forceps
Fox plane
Hemostats
High speed/torque surgical handpiece
Interocclusal bite registration
Implant system with multiunit abutments
Intraoral caliper
Minnesota retractor
Monojet syringe
Needle holder
Prosthetic driver kit
PVS bite registration material
Reduction bur
Right angle driver
Rongeur
Rubber dam
Seldin retractor
Self-curing PMMA
Slotted surgical guides
Sterile pencil
Suture
Temporary cylinders
Tissue forceps
Weider tongue retractor

History of the Procedure

Full-arch implant rehabilitation of the terminal dentition has undergone significant changes since the concept of osseointegration was first introduced. Controversy over the ideal number of implants, axial versus angled implant placement, and grafting versus graftless treatment modalities have been subjects of continuous debate and evolution.

Brånemark first demonstrated that a full-arch prosthesis could successfully be supported with only four implants placed at the cornerstones of the archform.[1] Concomitant research showed angled and axial implants had similar survival rates and marginal bone loss in the mandible and maxilla.[2–4] Maló demonstrated immediate loading of angled and axial implants in the mandible and maxilla.[5,6] Today, all-on-four is a common treatment modality utilized by clinicians all over the world for immediate, full-arch rehabilitation with high clinical success and supporting scientific evidence.[7–9]

Advantages of all on four:

- Avoidance of anatomic structures
- Decreased treatment time
- Avoidance of bone grafting and associated complications
- Decreased patient cost
- Bicortical stabilization is more easily achieved, resulting in greater primary stability
- Angled implants provide secondary resistance to vertical displacement by virtue of their nonaxial, oblique position in the archform, which is perpendicular to occlusal forces
- Distal cantilevers are minimized
- Anteroposterior (AP) spread is enhanced

Indications for Use of the Procedure

Patients with terminal dentitions and varying states of edentulism are ideal candidates. Systemic and local risk factors are the same as those for traditional implant placement.

Successful all-on-four rehabilitation is a complex, patient-tailored, and prosthetically driven treatment solution. Prosthetic material, teeth size, lip support, incisor positioning, teeth show at rest and animation, phonetics, orofacial musculature, bite force, parafunctional habits, and alterations to the occlusal vertical dimension are just some of the factors used to determine interarch prosthetic space. Many of these treatment planning parameters are beyond the scope of this chapter. In all cases, the final prosthetic design dictates the vertical position of the osteotomy, which, in turn, directs functional implant positions and angulations. The vertical position of the osteotomy after extractions and alveolar reduction is sometimes referred to as the "all-on-four shelf."[10,11]

At a minimum, 15 mm of vertical space per arch is needed to meet prosthetic requirements.[12] Less space weakens both the interim and final prostheses. Significant variability exists among candidates. Some require teeth removal and significant alveolar reduction. In other candidates, years of edentulism and progressive atrophy require little alveolar recontouring during surgery.

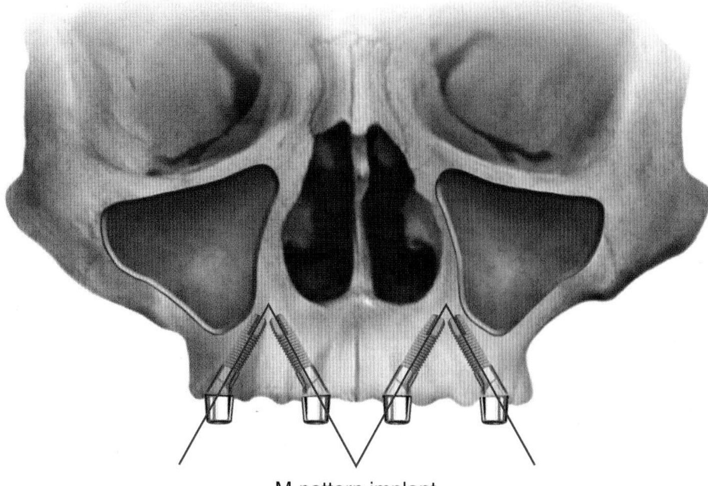

Figure 22.1 Implant placement strategy visualized at the vertical level of the proposed osteotomy. The implant "M-pattern" depicted maximizes AP spread while obtaining mechanical fixation at the paranasal bone.

It is equally important that the interface between the prosthesis and the residual ridge, often termed the "transition zone,"[13] be concealed when the patient's lip is at rest and during animation. Inadequate alveolar reduction can result in catastrophic esthetic outcomes.[14]

Limitations and Contraindications

Few absolute contraindications exist. Systemic and local risk factors that preclude general implant therapy should be considered.

Limitations imposed by variability in bone quality and quantity at the vertical level of the osteotomy are overcome by angling implants to avoid anatomic structures while maximizing mechanical fixation in cortical bone. Various classifications have been proposed to help the surgeon maximize the interimplant arch span and more predictably achieve sufficient insertion torque.[13,15] Quantitative limitations are generally due to increased pneumatization of the sinuses, crestal bone loss, cortical thinning, and the position of the inferior alveolar nerve. These are overcome by angling implants 30 to 45 degrees off-axis to avoid the anterior sinus wall and the anterior loop of the mental nerve while maximizing creative use of residual bone.[16–19] Qualitative limitations are overcome by achieving bicortical, mechanical fixation at the paranasal bone, midline nasal crest, and lingual/palatal cortical shelves. Surgical manipulation of the osteotomy via underpreparation of the implant site may be used to increase primary stability. A composite insertion torque of at least 120 Ncm is recommended to facilitate immediate loading[17,20] (Fig. 22.1).

Patient expectations are best managed prior to treatment. Unrealistic esthetic and functional expectations should be addressed. This is a rehabilitation of function with the best esthetics that can be reasonably achieved.[21] In cases of limited AP spread (less than 15 mm), the distal cantilever must be proportionally decreased.[22,23] All-on-four may not be appropriate for patients who rely on a flange for adequate lip support.[24] In cases of single-arch treatment, the occlusal plane and condition of the opposing arch must be carefully evaluated. Supraeruption of teeth/alveolar segments or malopposed teeth may impinge on restorative space and decrease predictability.

TECHNIQUE: All-on-Four Surgery (Figs. 22.2–22.12)

STEP 1: Initial Evaluation

Initial evaluation of the patient should include a thorough examination of remaining teeth, hard and soft tissues, and appropriate imaging (cone beam computerized tomography [CBCT] and full-mouth series [FMX]). Anticipated changes to the vertical dimension of occlusion, midline, incisal positioning, occlusal plane, overbite, and overjet must be determined prior to surgical planning. Restorative space parameters for dentate and some partially edentulous patients can be measured with CBCT viewing software. Partially and completely edentulous patients may require fabrication of wax rims and a record of their maxillomandibular relation to assess restorative space and determine osseous reduction needed (Fig. 22.2).

TECHNIQUE: All-on-Four Surgery (Figs. 22.2–22.12)—cont'd

STEP 2: Imaging and Splint Fabrication

CBCT is performed, and residual bone volume is quantitatively and qualitatively evaluated. Intraoral records and radiographic records are digitally overlayed. A surgical splint and bite registration are three-dimensionally printed. A trough is made at the proposed vertical level of the osteotomies. A second trough for abutment verification is placed lingual to the anterior dentition and extending through the central groves of the posterior teeth (Figs. 22.3–22.5).

STEP 3: Application of Local Anesthesia With Vasoconstrictor and Incision

Profound anesthesia is obtained via bilateral nerve blocks and local infiltration. A #15 blade is used to make a sulcular incision with bilateral, posterior releasing incisions. Care is taken to maintain keratinized tissue. A full thickness mucoperiosteal flap is elevated exposing bilateral mental nerves and the piriform rim.

STEP 4: Extraction of Teeth and Alveoplasty

A caliper and intraoral references (incisal edges or alveolar bone levels) are used to approximate bone reduction. Facial and interproximal bone are removed with a rotary bur. Teeth are extracted. Interdental papillae are excised with a second lingual incision. Lingual tissue is elevated with a periosteal elevator (Fig. 22.6).

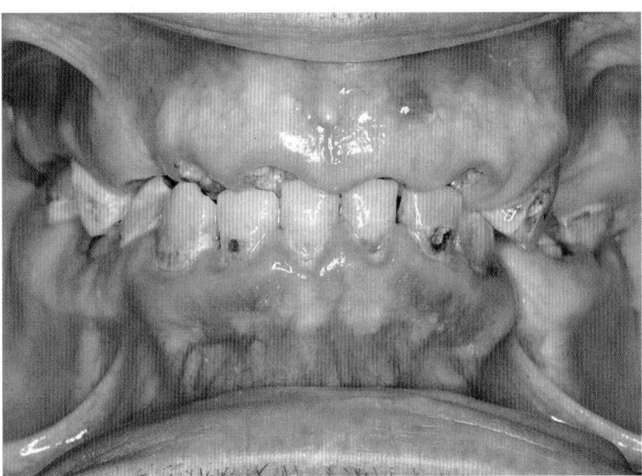

Figure 22.2 Intraoral photograph showing rampant dental caries, attrition, and significant loss of occlusal vertical dimension.

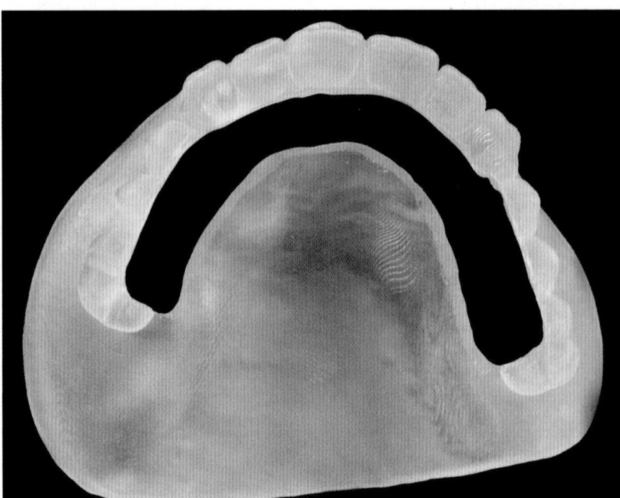

Figure 22.4 A lingual trough is placed in the surgical guide extending through the central grooves of the posterior teeth to determine ideal abutment positions.

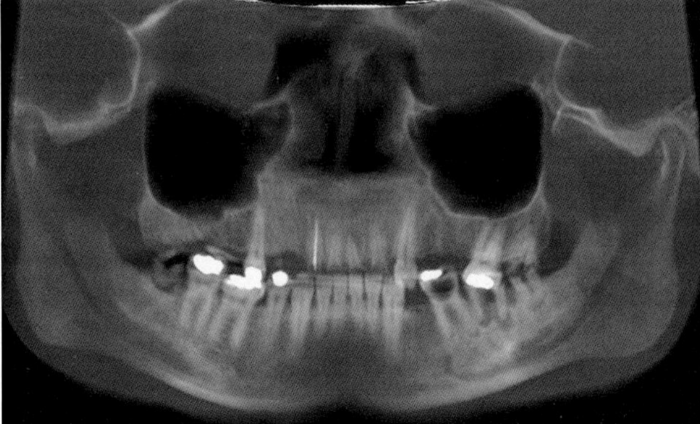

Figure 22.3 Panoramic reconstruction from a cone beam computerized tomography (CBCT). Residual anatomy is visualized at the level of the proposed vertical osteotomy. Implant placement strategies are selected to maximize anteroposterior (AP) spread and avoid vital structures.

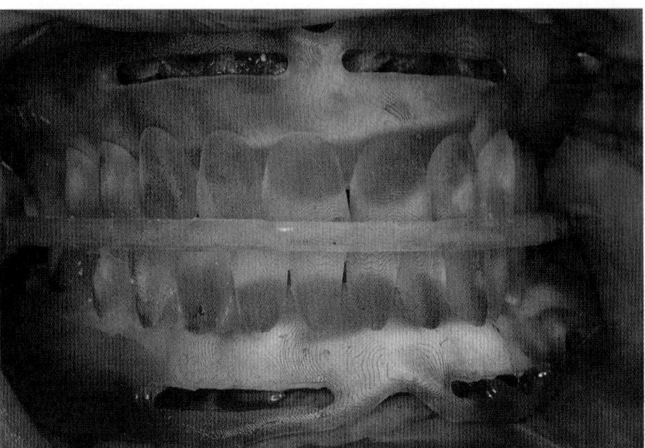

Figure 22.5 Maxillary and mandibular surgical guides appropriately seated with vertical windows indicating the level of the proposed osteotomy.

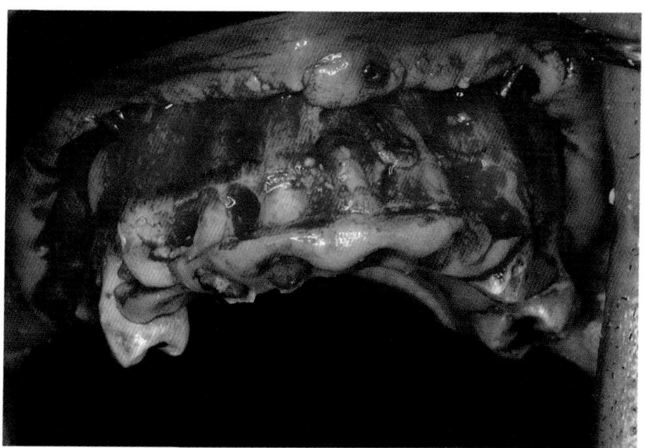

Figure 22.6 Facial and interproximal bone reduction performed to the proposed level of alveolar reduction facilitates easier extractions.

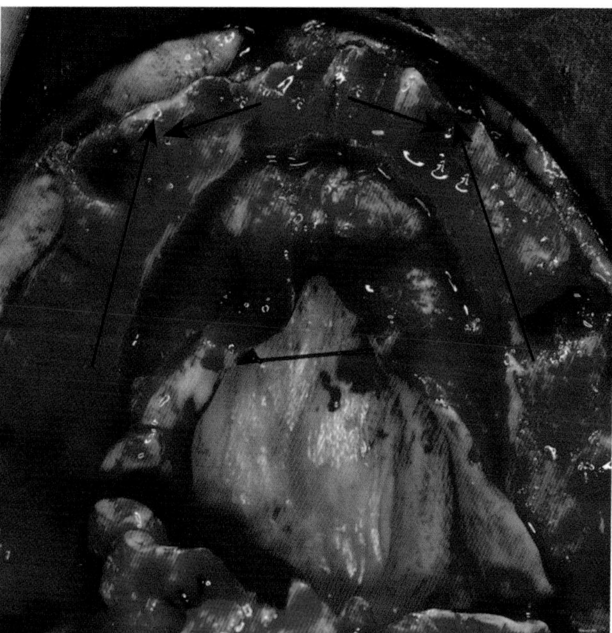

Figure 22.7 The all-on-four shelf. Primary stability can be obtained by grooving the palatal cortical bone. The implant trajectory is passed in an anterior, transalveolar direction and is apically fixated in piriform bone. Anterior implants enter at the lateral incisor region and are apically directed towards the piriform in cases of amble bone.

TECHNIQUE: All-on-Four Surgery (Figs. 22.2–22.12)—cont'd

STEP 5: Verification of Restorative Space and Creation of the All-on-Four Shelf

Surgical guides are placed using the palate, tuberosity, retromolar pads, and interocclusal bite registrations as stable reference points. The vertical position of the osteotomy is scribed on the residual alveolar ridge with a sterile pencil. Alveolar reduction is performed using an aggressive reduction bur or reciprocating saw. The all-on-four shelf is created parallel to the interpupillary line and Frankfort horizontal plane. Surgical guides and a fox plane are used to verify appropriate reduction. Granulation tissue is curetted from residual extractions sites. Alveolar smoothing is performed with a bone file. A rotary bur is used to bevel/smooth the facial and lingual contours of the shelf as these are common sources of postoperative discomfort (Fig. 22.5).

STEP 6: Determination of Primary and Secondary Implant Positions

Residual bone and patient anatomy dictate posterior implants positions. The anterior deflection of the sinus wall is appreciated via bilateral sinus fenestrations with a rotary bur and bone-sounding with a periodontal probe. Direct visualization of the mandibular foramen and consideration of the anterior loop determine posterior mandibular implant positions. Primary and secondary (fallback) implant positions are identified. Posterior implant sites are planned at 30 to 45-degree angles. Anterior implant sites are planned at the lateral incisor regions and may be axial or angled depending on residual anatomy (Fig. 22.7).

STEP 7: Osteotomy Preparation and Implant Placement

Sequential twist drills are used to prepare the implant osteotomies. If poor bone quality is immediately encountered, the trajectory is redirected. Crestal stability is obtained by grooving the lingual cortical plate. The trajectory then passes in a transalveolar fashion and obtains apical stability in the dense bone of the piriform or facial mandibular bone. Posterior implants are placed first. They are the primary determinants of maximum AP spread. Anterior implants are then placed (Fig. 22.7).

TECHNIQUE: All-on-Four Surgery (Figs. 22.2–22.12)—cont'd

STEP 8: Multiunit Abutment Placement

The surgical guide is secured. Multiunit abutments are tied-in. Any necessary implant and/or abutment rotation is performed to ensure implant access is lingual to anterior teeth and emerges through the occlusal/lingual aspects of posterior teeth (Fig. 22.8).

STEP 9: Soft Tissue Removal and Closure

Excess soft tissue is selectively undermined and removed with a #15 blade, scissors, or rotary tissue punch. Transalveolar osteotomies are made, and suturing is performed to immobilize and secure the soft tissue to underlying bone. A thick band of keratinized tissue is maintained around abutments shiftenter(Fig. 22.9).

STEP 10: Pickup and Conversion

Dentures are seated and articulated intraorally, relieving intaglio surfaces and flanges to allow complete seating on soft tissues. The midline, occlusal plane, and occlusal contacts are evaluated to confirm appropriate positioning and articulation. PVS bite registration material is injected on the distal aspect of the prosthesis to improve stability. Excess registration material is trimmed to allow clearance around anterior implants so they can be luted to the denture. The process of connecting temporary titanium cylinders to the denture base is known as the pickup. This can be done for all four implants or just the anterior implants as discussed here. Access holes are cut through the denture base to allow visualization and passage of the two temporary cylinders. Dental dam material should be placed around each seated cylinder at its base to protect soft tissue during the pickup (Fig. 22.10).

Self-cured methyl methacrylate resin is injected around each anterior cylinder to connect these cylinders to the denture base, leaving the access channels free of any resin. This process is similarly completed for the opposing arch. The occlusion is reevaluated. If reasonable occlusal contact is present, a centric relation record is made with PVS. Dentures and connected temporary cylinders are removed from the mouth. Direct impression copings are seated on all abutments, and an open tray impression is made with PVS material. The remainder of the conversion is completed by a laboratory technician. The interim prosthesis is then secured to the patient's implants, and occlusal adjustments are made (Figs. 22.11–22.13).

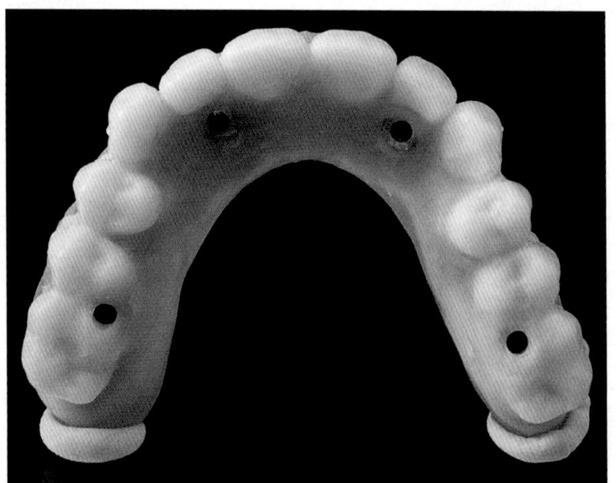

Figure 22.8 Interim prosthesis with access holes lingual to anterior teeth and through the palatal aspect of posterior teeth.

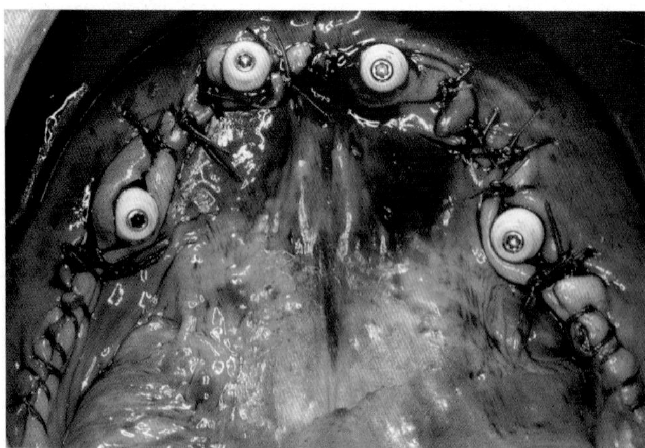

Figure 22.9 Soft tissue closure. Keratinized tissue is maintained around multiunit abutments. Soft tissue is immobilized and secured to the underlying alveolar bone via transalveolar osteotomies and suturing.

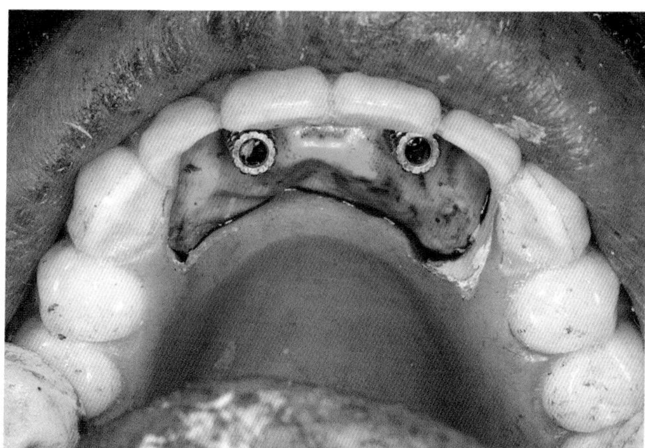

Figure 22.10 Occlusal view prior to pick up with rubber dam and temporary cylinder in place ready to inject self-curing PMMA.

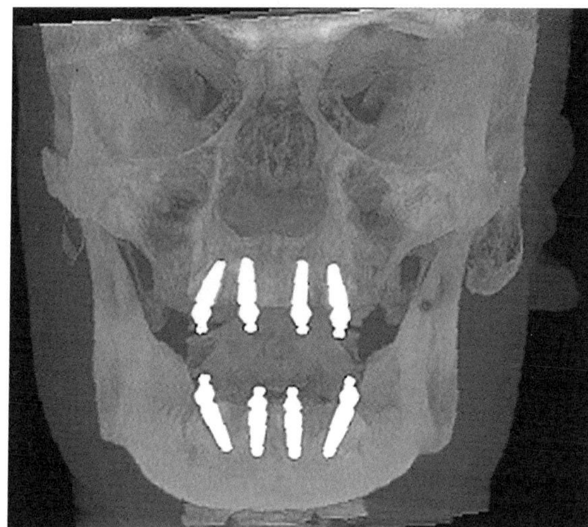

Figure 22.12 Postoperative radiograph.

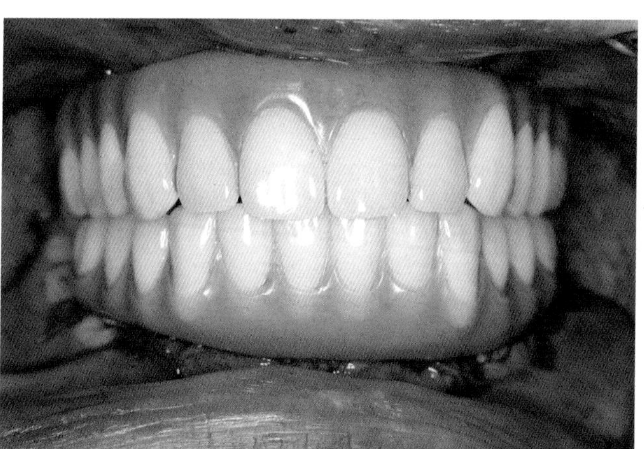

Figure 22.11 Immediate intraoral postoperative photo.

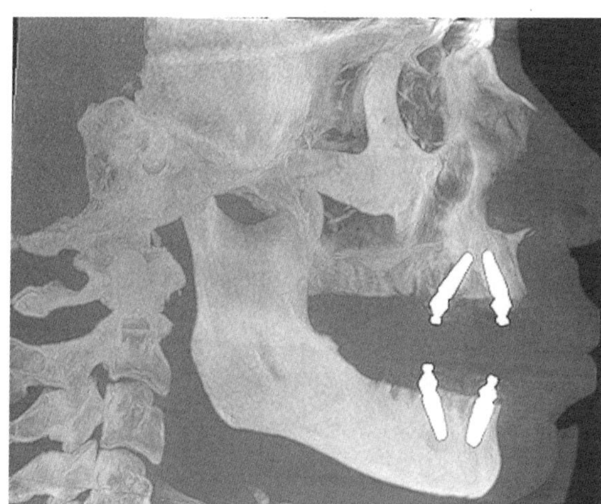

Figure 22.13 Postoperative radiograph.

ALTERNATIVE OR MODIFIED TECHNIQUE 1: Transsinus All-on-Four (Figs. 22.14 and 22.15)

Cortical thinning of paranasal bone, loss of subantral bone mass, and anterior pneumatization of the maxillary sinus may require transsinus placement of posterior implants. AP spreads in excess of 15 mm can be achieved. The all-on-four surgery is the same as previously outlined with minor exceptions. Following alveolar reduction, a small antrostomy is made at the anterior deflection of the sinus. This is usually just distal to the canine eminence. The sinus membrane is reflected. The piriform is exposed, and the soft tissue is elevated from the nasal floor and protected with a retractor. Posterior implant trajectories are started at the alveolar crest, passed anteriorly through the sinus, and are apically fixated in paranasal bone. Anterior implants enter at the lateral incisor position. They are angled up to 30 degrees and directed towards the midline nasal crest resulting in an inverted V-pattern when viewed on radiographs.[25–27]

Avoidance and Management of Intraoperative Complications

Low implant insertion torque is a common intraoperative encounter. In cases of poor bone quality, longer implants should be considered. D2/D3 bone responds well to more aggressive/compressive implant designs. Underpreparation of the osteotomy width is a common practice to allow compression of medullary bone and increase stability. Care should be taken to not underprepare the length of the osteotomy. This may result in good initial stability during implant insertion, which decreases when the implant apex encounters dense cortical bone. Redirection of the implant osteotomy to incorporate bicortical stabilization is a basic tenant of all-on-four surgery.[28]

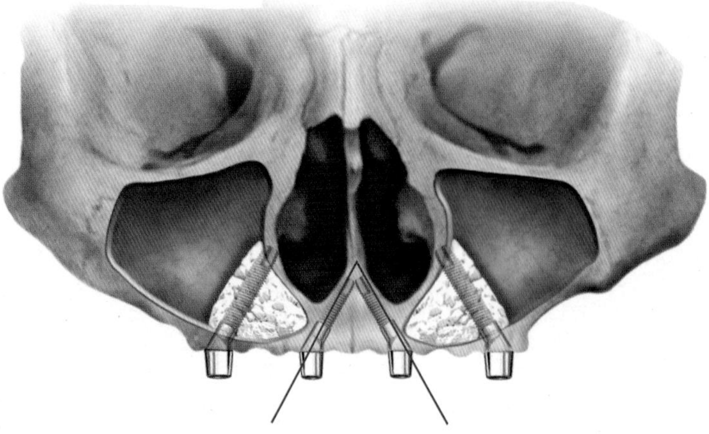

Figure 22.14 Anterior pneumatization of the maxillary sinuses and transsinus implant placement. Cortical thinning at the paranasal bone only permits apical fixation of a single implant. Anterior (vomer implants) are directed towards the midline nasal crest.

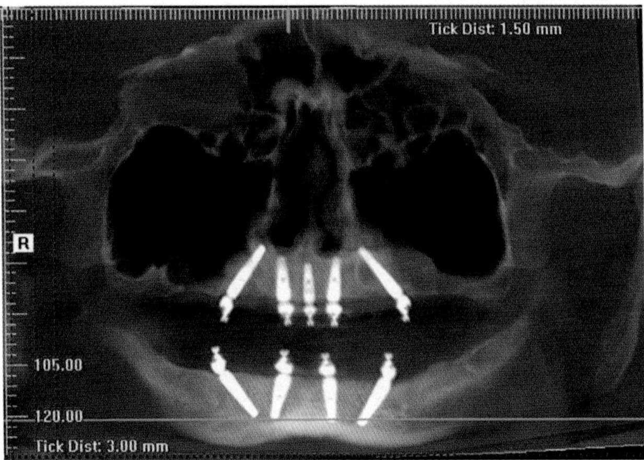

Figure 22.15 Panoramic radiograph depicting all-on-four surgery utilizing transsinus implants. A midline nasal implant is also depicted.

Perforation of nasal and sinus membranes at the time of implant placement has been shown to have comparable success with implants that did not perforate the membrane.[29] However, a slight decrease in implant success is observed when membrane perforation occurs in conjunction with sinus lift procedures and implant placement.[30] Underpreparation of the osteotomy width to allow an intentional greenstick fracture of the anterior sinus wall during placement is a technique that can be utilized to decrease the risk of membrane perforation.

Brittle alveolar bone and aggressive implant designs can result in greenstick fractures of the alveolar ridge. Mandibular fracture is a possible complication if implants are highly torqued in dense cortical bone.

Postoperative Considerations

Implants can exhibit signs of early and late failure throughout the healing phase. Postoperative considerations are primarily focused on prosthetic complications.

Fracture of the interim prosthesis has a multifactorial etiology that includes occlusal overload, prosthetic misfit, excessive cantilever, and an unbalanced, inappropriate occlusal scheme. Patient compliance with a soft diet is critical during the healing phase. Error introduced at the impression or conversion can result in a prosthetic misfit, making the prosthesis more prone to fracture.[31] Distal cantilevers should be minimized and not extend past distal access channels. Screw loosening and fracture commonly occurs with occlusal overload or misfit of the prosthesis. Posterior occlusion should be balanced with even, bilateral contacts that are easily reproducible in centric relation. Reprogramming of the patient's neuromusculature and calibration of the bite requires reassessment. Articulating paper is used to mark and evaluate occlusal contacts. Occlusal prematurities are relieved until even, bilateral contact is present on posterior teeth. The interim prosthesis should have no anterior contact when in centric relation. Anterior, occlusal prematurities will prevent occlusion of posterior teeth.[32]

A functional occlusion may present with lip, cheek, and tongue biting. Insufficient horizontal overlap of anterior teeth may result in lip biting, which can be corrected by relieving the incisal and facial aspects of the mandibular anterior teeth. Cheek biting can be addressed by relieving the buccal aspects of mandibular posterior teeth. Tongue biting may be due to lingual overjet and can be corrected by flattening the lingual cusps of the mandibular posterior teeth.[33]

References

1. Brånemark PI, Svensson B, van Steenberghe D. Ten-year survival rates of fixed prostheses on four or six implants ad modum Brånemark in full edentulism. *Clin Oral Implants Res.* 1995;6(4):227–231.
2. Mattsson T, Köndell PA, Gynther GW, Fredholm U, Bolin A. Implant treatment without bone grafting in severely resorbed edentulous maxillae. *J Oral Maxillofac Surg.* 1999;57(3):281–287.
3. Krekmanov L, Kahn M, Rangert B, Lindström H. Tilting of posterior mandibular and maxillary implants for improved prosthesis support. *Int J Oral Maxillofac Implants.* 2000;15(3):405–414.
4. Aparicio C, Perales P, Rangert B. Tilted implants as an alternative to maxillary sinus grafting: a clinical, radiologic, and periotest study. *Clin Implant Dent Relat Res.* 2001;3(1):39–49.
5. Maló P, Rangert B, Nobre M. "All-on-Four" immediate-function concept with Brånemark System implants for completely edentulous mandibles: a retrospective clinical study. *Clin Implant Dent Relat Res.* 2003;5(suppl 1):2–9.
6. Maló P, Rangert B, Nobre M. All-on-4 immediate-function concept with Brånemark System implants for completely edentulous maxillae: a 1-year retrospective clinical study. *Clin Implant Dent Relat Res.* 2005;7(suppl 1):S88–S94. s1.
7. Hopp M, de Araújo Nobre M, Maló P. Comparison of marginal bone loss and implant success between axial and tilted implants in maxillary All-on-4 treatment concept rehabilitations after 5 years of follow-up. *Clin Implant Dent Relat Res.* 2017;19(5):849–859.
8. Chrcanovic BR, Albrektsson T, Wennerberg A. Survival and complications of zygomatic implants: an updated systematic review. *J Oral Maxillofac Surg.* 2016;74(10):1949–1964.
9. Ata-Ali J, Peñarrocha-Oltra D, Candel-Marti E, Peñarrocha-Diago M. Oral rehabilitation with tilted dental implants: a metaanalysis. *Med Oral Patol Oral Cir Bucal.* 2012;17(4):e582–e587.
10. Jensen OT, Adams MW, Cottam JR, Parel SM, Phillips WR III. The All-on-4 shelf: maxilla. *J Oral Maxillofac Surg.* 2010;68(10):2520–2527.
11. Jensen OT, Adams MW, Cottam JR, Parel SM, Phillips WR III. The all on 4 shelf: mandible. *J Oral Maxillofac Surg.* 2011;69(1):175–181.
12. Carpentieri J, Greenstein G, Cavallaro J. Hierarchy of restorative space required for shiftendifferent types of dental implant prostheses. *J Am Dent Assoc 1939.* 2019;150(8):695–706.
13. Bedrossian E, Sullivan RM, Fortin Y, Malo P, Indresano T. Fixed-prosthetic implant restoration of the edentulous maxilla: a systematic pretreatment evaluation method. *J Oral Maxillofac Surg.* 2008;66(1):112–122.
14. Schnitman PA. The profile prosthesis: an aesthetic fixed implant-supported restoration for the resorbed maxilla. *Pract Periodontics Aesthet Dent.* 1999;11(1):143–151.
15. Jensen OT. Complete arch site classification for all-on-4 immediate function. *J Prosthet Dent.* 2014;112(4):741–751. e2.
16. Jensen OT, Adams MW, Butura C, Galindo DF. Maxillary V-4: four implant treatment for maxillary atrophy with dental implants fixed apically at the vomer-nasal crest, lateral pyriform rim, and zygoma for immediate function. Report on 44 patients followed from 1 to 3 years. *J Prosthet Dent.* 2015;114(6):810–817.
17. Jensen OT, Adams MW. Secondary stabilization of maxillary m-4 treatment with unstable implants for immediate function: biomechanical considerations and report of 10 cases after 1 year in function. *Int J Oral Maxillofac Implants.* 2014;29(2):e232–e240.
18. Jensen OT, Cottam J, Ringeman J. Avoidance of the mandibular nerve with implant placement: a new "mental loop." *J Oral Maxillofac Surg.* 2011;69(6):1540–1543.
19. Jensen OT, Adams MW. All-on-4 treatment of highly atrophic mandible with mandibular V-4: report of 2 cases. *J Oral Maxillofac Surg.* 2009;67(7):1503–1509.
20. Jensen OT, Adams MW. The maxillary M-4: a technical and biomechanical note for all-on-4 management of severe maxillary atrophy—report of 3 cases. *J Oral Maxillofac Surg.* 2009;67(8):1739–1744.
21. Roumanas ED. The social solution-denture esthetics, phonetics, and function. *J Prosthodont.* 2009;18(2):112–115.
22. Benzing UR, Gall H, Weber H. Biomechanical aspects of two different implant-prosthetic concepts for edentulous maxillae. *Int J Oral Maxillofac Implants.* 1995;10(2):188–198.
23. Jensen OT, Adams MW, Smith E. Paranasal bone: the prime factor affecting the decision to use transsinus vs zygomatic implants for biomechanical support for immediate function in maxillary dental implant reconstruction. *Int J Oral Maxillofac Implants.* 2014;29(1):e130–e138.
24. Galindo DF. The implant-supported milled-bar mandibular overdenture. *J Prosthodont.* 2001;10(1):46–51.
25. Jensen OT, Cottam J, Ringeman J, Adams M. Trans-sinus dental implants, bone morphogenetic protein 2, and immediate function for all-on-4 treatment of severe maxillary atrophy. *J Oral Maxillofac Surg.* 2012;70(1):141–148.
26. Jensen OT, Adams MW, Butura C, Galindo DF. Maxillary V-4: four implant treatment for maxillary atrophy with dental implants fixed apically at the vomer-nasal crest, lateral pyriform rim, and zygoma for immediate function. Report on 44 patients followed from 1 to 3 years. *J Prosthet Dent.* 2015;114(6):810–817.
27. Jensen OT, Cottam JR, Ringeman JL, Graves S, Beatty L, Adams MW. Angled dental implant placement into the vomer/nasal crest of atrophic maxillae for All-on-Four immediate function: a 2-year clinical study of 100 consecutive patients. *Int J Oral Maxillofac Implants.* 2014;29(1):e30–e35.
28. Sylvester DK, Sylvester DK, Jensen OT, Berry TD, Pappas J. Marillary all-on-four surgery: a review of intraoperative surgical principles and implant placement strategies. *SROMS.* 2018;25:4.
29. Brånemark PI, Adell R, Albrektsson T, Lekholm U, Lindström J, Rockler B. An experimental and clinical study of osseointegrated implants penetrating the nasal cavity and maxillary sinus. *J Oral Maxillofac Surg.* 1984;42(8):497–505.
30. Al-Moraissi E, Elsharkawy A, Abotaleb B, Alkebsi K, Al-Motwakel H. Does intraoperative perforation of Schneiderian membrane during sinus lift surgery causes an increased the risk of implants failure?: a systematic review and meta regression analysis. *Clin Implant Dent Relat Res.* 2018;20(5):882–889.
31. Slauch RW, Bidra AS, Wolfinger GJ, Kuo C-L.. Relationship between radiographic misfit and clinical outcomes in immediately loaded complete-arch fixed implant-supported prostheses in edentulous patients. *J Prosthodont.* 2019;28(8):861–867.
32. Kim Y, Oh T-J., Misch CE, Wang H-L.. Occlusal considerations in implant therapy: clinical guidelines with biomechanical rationale. *Clin Oral Implants Res.* 2005;16(1):26–35.
33. McCord JF, Grant AA. Identification of complete denture problems: a summary. *Br Dent J.* 2000;189(3):128–134.

CHAPTER 23

The Role of the Zygoma Implant in Maxillary Reconstruction

Edmond Bedrossian and Edmond Armand Bedrossian

Armamentarium

#15 Blade
3.0 Gut suture
Acrylic luting material
Conversion denture
Duplicated denture
Endosseous implants
Frazier tip suction
Implant motor and handpiece
IV Sedation armamentarium and medications
Local anesthetic with vasoconstrictor
Minnesota retractor
Needle holder
No. 7 toe-out retractor
Sterile water or saline irrigation
Straight and 17-degree screw-retained abutments
Surgical guide
Suture scissors
Titanium temporary cylinders
Zygoma drills
Zygoma implants

History of the Procedure

The zygoma implant has been used in the treatment of the edentulous maxillae for almost three decades.[1] This chapter presents and consolidates the principles described in the literature in regard to the biomechanical principles of the zygoma implant under load, the trajectory of the zygoma implant, the use of the zones of the maxillae, and the zygoma anatomic guided approach (ZAGA) for treatment planning in this group of patients.

The maxillary sinuses and the position of the nasal floor in the premaxillary region may limit the placement of implants in the edentulous maxillae. The superior, medial, and posterior resorption pattern of the edentulous maxilla limits the vertical as well as the horizontal bony volume necessary to house endosseous implants within the alveolar housing for the fabrication of a fixed implant-supported prosthesis.

Various grafting procedures to reconstruct bony volume in the edentulous maxilla have been reported in the literature by Adell et al., Breine and Branemark, and others.[2,4–6] Keller and Tollman have reported success rates ranging from 87% to 95% for implants and prosthetics, respectively, with grafting of the maxillae with delayed implant placement and delayed loading.[6–7] Autogenous onlay, onlay, and Le Fort I procedures reported by Rasmusson et al.[8] have success rates of 80% and 77% for grafting with delayed implant placement and for grafting with simultaneous implant placement, respectively. Extended treatment time, inability to wear a functional provisional implant during the various healing times, and the morbidity associated the various stages of the treatment limit the number of patients who choose to have reconstruction of their maxillae. The ability to use the zygoma implant in the posterior maxilla and avoiding grafting procedures allows for a higher case acceptance by patients.

Indications for the Use of the Procedure

The contemporary literature has described the use of tilted implants to avoid extensive bone grafting procedures for patients who have residual alveolar bone in the premaxilla and the bicuspid region.[9–11] However, for patients who have premaxillary alveolar bone but are lacking alveolar bony height in the bicuspid and the molar regions, the zygoma implant is considered to avoid bone grafting procedures. The zygoma implant is recommended when there is less than 2 to 3 mm of vertical alveolar bone in zones 2 and 3. The zygoma implant is unique in that it is quad-cortically stabilized at the maxillary crest, the floor of the maxillary sinus, the base of the zygoma bone, and the lateral cortex of the zygoma bone (Fig. 23.1). Placement of the zygoma implant with bony support at the implant platform should be attempted as occlusal loads will be better supported. The presence of bony support around the platform of the zygoma implant will also allow for better adaptation of the overlying soft tissues, isolating the implant platform from the oral cavity. However, in cases of less than 2 mm of crestal bone, under function and over time, the minimal crestal bone may resorb. However, it is prudent to use the ad modum Branemark technique to allow initial stabilization of the implant as well as better force distribution as described by Freedman et al.[12,13]

Limitations and Contraindications

Over the last two decades, the use of the zygomatic implant has been studied internationally, with reported success rates between 94% and 100%.[14–19] Potential contraindications for the reconstruction of the maxillae with the zygoma implant include patients with a history of chronic sinus infections, inadequate prosthetic, or surgical training of the implant team. Treatment of the edentulous maxillae with the zygoma implant is an advanced procedure requiring training and understanding of the anatomy as well as the physiology of the maxillofacial region.

Zones of the Maxilla

The intent of radiographic evaluation is to allow treatment planning of the maxilla with the graftless approach. Although sinus grafting is possible, it is not included in this chapter as immediate loading of grafted implants is not recommended.

Initial radiographic evaluation of patients begins with a panoramic X-ray. The maxillary alveolus is divided into three zones.[20] The premaxilla, from cuspid to cuspid, is referred to as zone 1. The premolar area is zone 2, and the molar region is zone 3 (Fig. 23.2). The presence or lack of zones determines the surgical treatment for the placement of implants.

In cases where all three zones are present, axial implants are distributed along the arch length.

In cases where only zones 1 and 2 are present, the tilted concept, which involves the tilting of the posterior implants beginning in the first or second molar area paralleling the anterior tilt of the maxillary sinus wall establishing posterior support for a fixed provisional prosthesis, is considered.

In cases where there is lack of bone in zones 2 and 3 and the presence of bone in zone 1, placement of the zygoma implant for posterior support in conjunction with two to four premaxillary implants is considered.

In cases of advanced maxillary hypoplasia or resorption or in cases where maxillectomy procedures were performed, the absence of all three zones of the maxilla lends for the clinician's consideration of the quad zygoma implant concept.

Zygoma Anatomy Guided Approach

To better understand the trajectory of the zygoma implant, in 2011, Aparicio[21] described the various relationships of the implant platform as well as the relationship of the middle portion of the zygoma implant with the lateral maxillary sinus wall (Fig. 23.3). In this anatomic description, the lateral maxillary sinus wall is described as "straight" or "concave." If the lateral maxillary sinus wall is convex, the middle portion of the zygoma implant will be inside the sinus, and bone surrounds the implant platform. However, if it is concave, a portion or the entire middle portion of the zygoma implant may be "outside" the maxillary sinus, and the implant platform may or may not have maxillary crestal bony support. The classification described by Aparicio[22] is ZAGA 0, which is straight lateral maxillary wall with the middle portion of the zygoma implant inside the sinus, through to ZAGA 4, which is the most extreme resorption of the maxillary sinus with a significant concavity of the lateral maxillary sinus wall placing the middle portion of the zygoma implant outside of the sinus with no bony support at the implant platform. Preoperative radiographic evaluation to determine the zones of the maxilla as well as the ZAGA classification is essential in understanding the position of the intended zygoma implant.

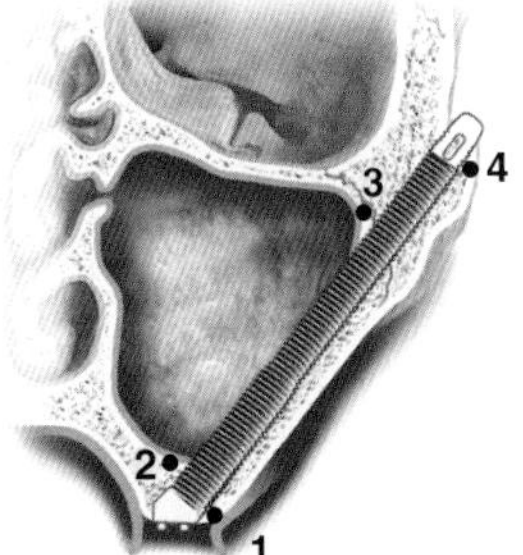

Figure 23.1 The zygoma implant is quad-cortically stabilized. Source: Edmond Bedrossian and E. Armand Bedrossian

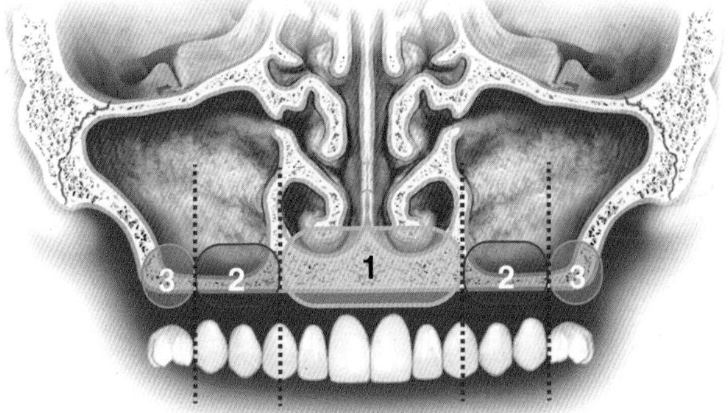

Figure 23.2 The presence or the lack of various zones of the maxilla influences the adoption of a particular surgical protocol. Source: Edmond Bedrossian and E. Armand Bedrossian

TECHNIQUE: Zygoma Anatomic Guided Approach 0–2

STEP 1: Planning

Three-dimensional radiographs allow the evaluation of the lateral maxillary wall contour (Fig. 23.4).

Using the radiographic findings, the surgeon visualizes and plans the path of the initial drill, which will establish the implant trajectory; the starting point of the osteotomy for the placement of the zygoma implant is at the first molar-second bicuspid area of the maxillary crest with the apex traveling through and perforating the lateral cortex of the zygoma bone.

STEP 2: Anesthesia

Intravenous sedation is generally used in conjunction with local anesthesia. Lidocaine (2%) with 1:100,000 epinephrine is used to establish the following bilateral nerve blocks: infraorbital, posterior superior alveolar, greater palatine, and inferior alveolar. Nasopalatine and circumferential maxillary vestibular infiltrations are also performed. Extraoral infiltrations over the zygoma bone blocking the lesser and greater zygomatic nerve, are recommended.

STEP 3: Incision

A crestal incision is made over the maxillary alveolus with three releasing incisions, in addition to midline and bilateral posterior hockey stick releasing incisions. The lateral wall of the maxillary sinus is exposed. It is recommended to expose one side at a time and complete the placement of the implant prior to exposing the contralateral side. The dissection is carried superiorly identifying the infraorbital nerve and carried laterally at the level of the inferior-orbital nerve, exposing the lateral cortex of the zygoma bone. The periosteal elevator is placed over the lateral wall of the zygoma bone with gentle advancement and elevation of the overlying soft tissues over the lateral cortex of the zygoma bone (blunt dissection/elevation) toward the fronto-zygomatic notch. The toe-out retractor is then placed in the fronto-zygomatic notch allowing the surgeon to visualize the anatomy form the maxillary crest, over the lateral maxillary wall, to the body zygoma bone to the fronto-zygomatic notch. It is very important to directly visualize the path of the zygoma implant to prevent complications, including a trajectory entering the orbit or a trajectory entering the infratemporal fossa (Fig. 23.5).

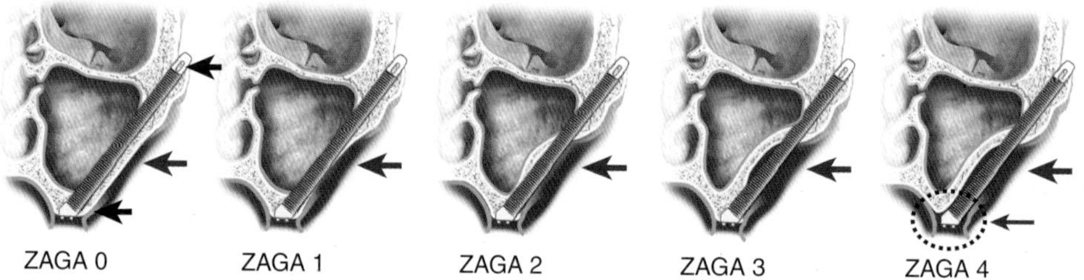

Figure 23.3 The zygoma-guided anatomy approach describing the contour of the lateral maxillary sinus wall. Source: Edmond Bedrossian and E. Armand Bedrossian

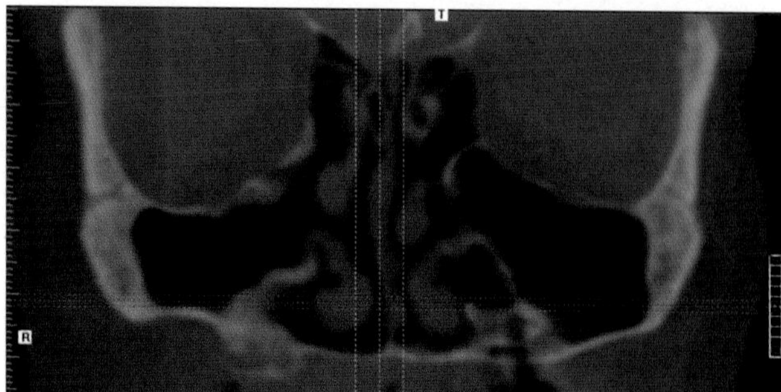

Figure 23.4 Frontal three-dimensional view of the bony volume of the zygoma bone, the anatomy of the sinus, and the ostiomeatal complex (OMC). Source: Edmond Bedrossian and E. Armand Bedrossian

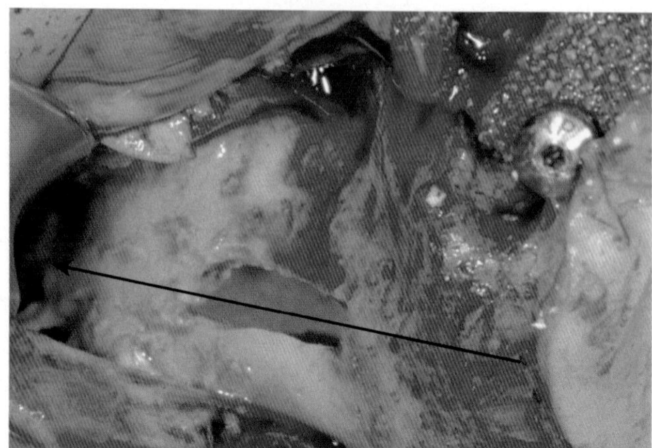

Figure 23.5 Direct visualization of the entire surgical field is necessary. Source: Edmond Bedrossian and E. Armand Bedrossian

TECHNIQUE: ZAGA 0–2—cont'd

STEP 4: Establishing the Trajectory

The posterior lateral corner of the maxillary sinus wall is identified, and its vertical distance from the base of the zygoma buttress to the maxillary crest is identified as the "black dotted line" (Fig. 23.6). A window is made through the lateral wall of the maxillary sinus wall, with the posterior wall of the window paralleling the black dotted line. The round zygoma drill enters the maxillary alveolus at the first molar-second bicuspid position, travels through the maxillary sinus parallel to the posterior wall of the sinus opening, and makes an indentation at the base of the zygoma bone in preparation for the next drill (Fig. 23.7). The indentation prevents the chattering of the subsequent 2.9-mm drill.

The 2.9-mm drill follows the same path as the round drill; it enters the base of the zygoma bone, travels through the zygoma bone, and exits at its lateral cortex approximately 2 to 3 mm prior to the fronto-zygomatic notch. The final drill is the 2.9 to 3.5 mm pilot drill, which creates a final osteotomy diameter of 3.5 mm both at the maxillary crest and through the zygoma bone.

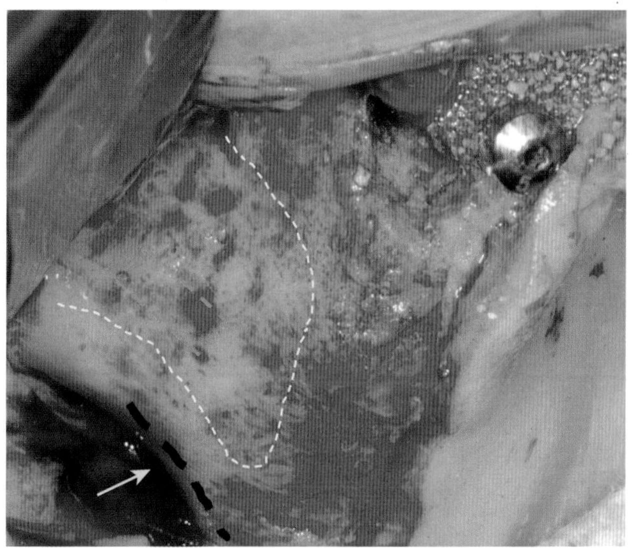

Figure 23.6 The "black dotted line" (*arrow*). Source: Edmond Bedrossian and E. Armand Bedrossian

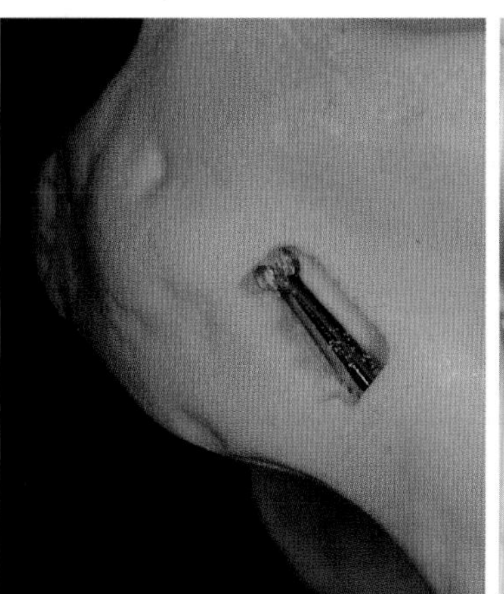

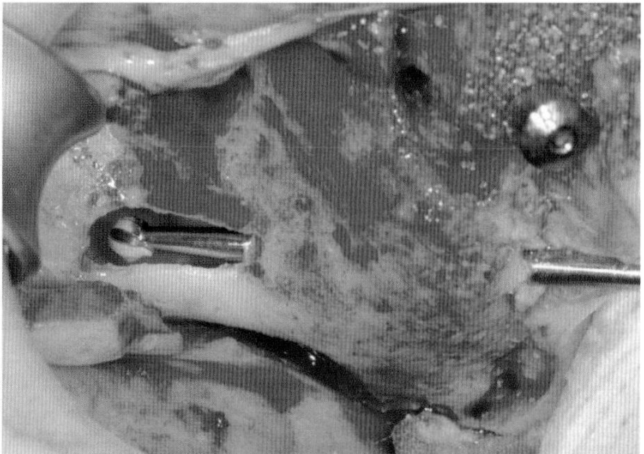

Figure 23.7 The round bur establishes the trajectory of the implant. Source: Edmond Bedrossian and E. Armand Bedrossian

TECHNIQUE: ZAGA 0–2—cont'd

STEP 5: Placement of the Implant

Prior to placement of the implant, the maxillary sinus is thoroughly irrigated with sterile irrigation fluid to remove gross debris created by the osteotomy preparation phase. The implant is removed sterilely from its container and enters the crestal osteotomy and travels with the posterior portion of the implant in intimate contact and parallel to the posterior wall of the window created through the lateral maxillary sinus wall (Fig. 23.8A and B). An insertion torque of 35 to 40 Ncm for each implant placed (the premaxillary axial implants and the bilateral posterior zygoma implants) is desired if immediate loading is considered.

It is important to note that prior to the removal of the toe-out retractor, the subperiosteal area must be irrigated to remove debris from the preparation of the osteotomy while avoiding potential subperiosteal accesses.

STEP 6: Placement of the Abutments and Direct Conversion

Upon completion of the placement of two or four premaxillary axial implants and the bilateral posterior zygoma implants, screw-retained abutments are secured and a torque of 35 Ncm is used in preparation for the conversion of the patient's denture to a fixed provisional hybrid prosthesis.

Protection caps are placed on the abutments before registering their positions for the conversion step. Registration paste is used to transfer the position of the abutments to the intaglio surface of the patient's denture (Fig. 23.9). Temporary titanium cylinders are placed onto the abutments, in preparation for the conversion steps, and the passive and complete seating of the patient's denture is confirmed prior to luting of the temporary titanium cylinders to the denture (Fig. 23.10).

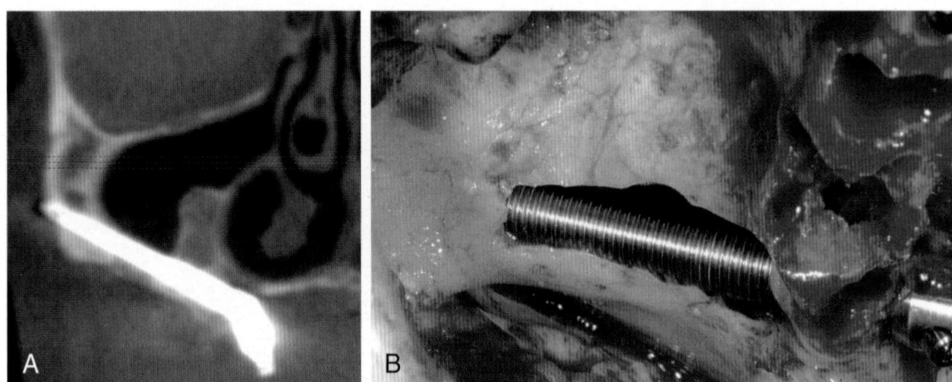

Figure 23.8 **A,** The implant is intimate contact with the lateral wall of the maxillary sinus. **B,** The posterior aspect of the implant is parallel to the posterior wall of the sinus window. Source: Edmond Bedrossian and E. Armand Bedrossian

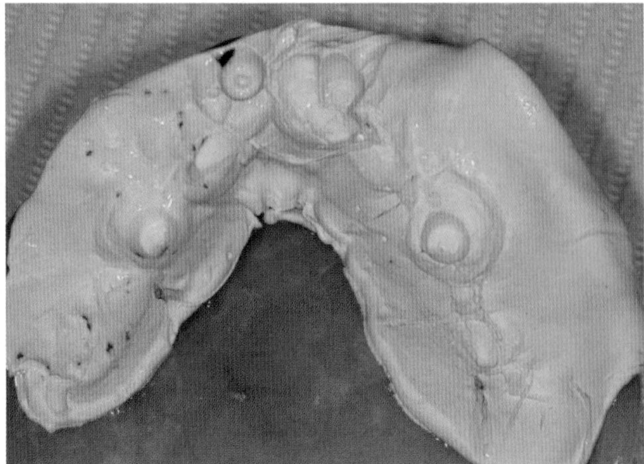

Figure 23.9 Registration paste indexes the position of the abutments to the denture base. Source: Edmond Bedrossian and E. Armand Bedrossian

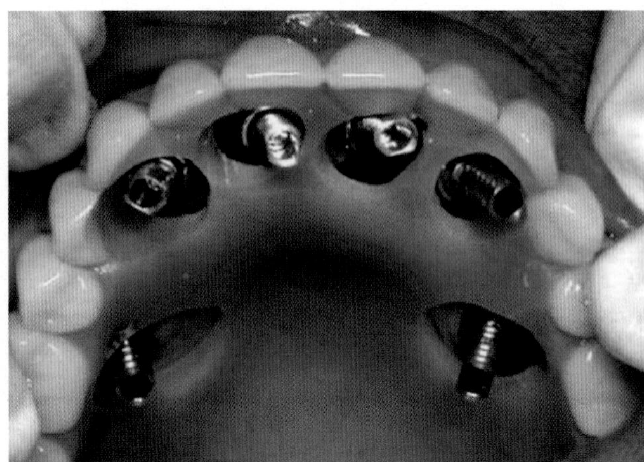

Figure 23.10 Passive and complete seating of the denture over the titanium cylinders. Source: Edmond Bedrossian and E. Armand Bedrossian

TECHNIQUE: ZAGA 0–2—cont'd

STEP 7: Delivery of the Immediate Load Prosthesis

After complete curing of the luting agent, the prosthesis is removed and the remaining voids between the titanium cylinders and the denture are filled. The palate and the flange of the denture are removed; the intaglio surface is filled with additional acrylic to ensure a flat surface for the proper seal of the transition space between the soft tissues and the intaglio surface of the prosthesis. Prosthetic screws connecting the fixed provisional prosthesis to the abutments are placed and tightened to 15 Ncm. Bilateral group function is the desired occlusal scheme for the full arch prosthesis (Fig. 23.11).

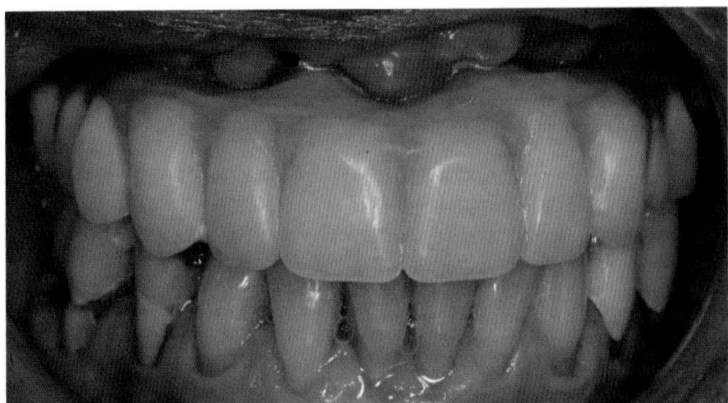

Figure 23.11 Completed provisional with bilateral group function. Source: Edmond Bedrossian and E. Armand Bedrossian

ALTERNATE TECHNIQUE: Zygoma Anatomic Guided Approach 3 and 4

The clinician should be aware of the influence of the contour of the lateral wall of the maxillary sinus as well as the degree of the posterior maxillary alveolar resorption. There is only one trajectory, the starting and ending points, of the zygoma implant. The so-called intrasinus or extrasinus zygoma is not a technique; rather, it is an observation of whether the implant is inside or outside the maxillary sinus, which is influenced by the concavity of the lateral maxillary sinus wall as well as the degree of maxillary alveolar resorption. In ZAGA 3 and 4 cases, the minimal available maxillary alveolar bone and a significant concavity of the lateral maxillary sinus wall only allow the stabilization of the zygoma implant within the zygoma bone.

STEP 1: Planning

Generally, in ZAGA 3 and 4 cases there is total loss of the maxillary alveolar bone, which necessitates the placement of two zygoma implants within each zygoma bone, that is, the quad zygoma concept. When planning ZAGA 3 and 4 cases, understanding the position of the apical portion of the two zygoma implants within the same zygoma bone is critical. The anterior zygoma implant is in the superior position, and the posterior zygoma implant is in the inferior position within the body of the zygoma bone (Fig. 23.12).

STEP 2: Anesthesia

The anesthesia is the same as the ZAGA 0–2 cases as described earlier.

STEP 3: Incision

The incision is the same as ZAGA 0–2 cases, with the exception of careful dissection exposing the inferior-lateral corner of the bony orbit. This landmark allows the surgeon to be aware of this border and to stay lateral to the orbital rim while establishing the trajectory of the implant with the initial round drill for the anterior zygoma implant.

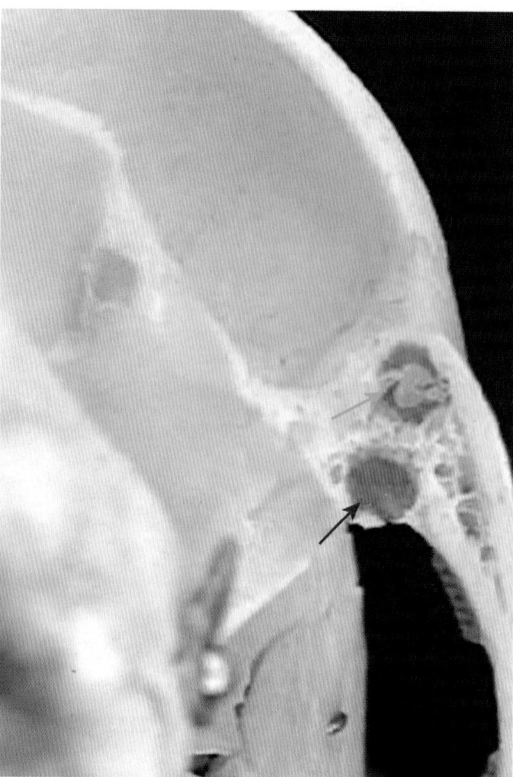

Figure 23.12 The anterior zygoma apex is in the upper position, and the posterior zygoma apex is in lower position within the zygoma bone. Source: Edmond Bedrossian and E. Armand Bedrossian

ALTERNATE TECHNIQUE: ZAGA 3–4—cont'd

STEP 4: Establishing the Trajectory

The posterior lateral corner of the maxillary sinus wall is identified, and the black dotted line, the vertical distance from the base of the zygoma buttress to the maxillary crest, is identified. A window is made through the lateral wall of the maxillary sinus wall, with the posterior wall of the window paralleling the black dotted line. Since two zygoma implants are planned, the window through the maxillary wall is extended 90 degrees parallel and inferior to the infraorbital rim allowing the surgeon to better visualize the base of the zygoma bone (the roof of maxillary sinus) before using the round bur (Fig. 23.13). For the anterior zygoma implant, the premaxillary dissection is extended superiorly exposing the inferior-lateral corner of the nasal aperture. The round bur is used to establish the trajectory of the anterior zygoma implant, marking the entry point of the drill at the corner of the nasal aperture with the apex of the implant in the "superior" portion of the zygoma bone under direct visualization. To maintain the proper distance between the apices of the implants and to establish the largest anterior-posterior distribution of the implant platforms, the two osteotomies are completed simultaneously (Fig. 23.14). For the posterior zygoma implant, the round zygoma drill enters the maxillary alveolus at the first molar-second bicuspid position, travels through maxillary sinus parallel to the posterior wall of the sinus opening, and makes an indentation at the base of the zygoma bone in preparation for the next drill. The 2.9-mm drill followed by the 2.9 to 3.5 mm pilot drill completes the preparation of the osteotomy. Because of the concavity of the lateral maxillary wall in the anterior position (Fig. 23.15), the drill and subsequently the anterior zygoma implant will be outside the maxillary sinus. At times, the posterior zygoma implant may not have maxillary crestal support, and the midportion will be outside the maxillary sinus. It is important for the surgeon to understand that the technique/trajectory of the site preparation is the same. There is only one trajectory of the zygoma implant. The variable is the contour of the lateral maxillary sinus wall (the ZAGA classification).

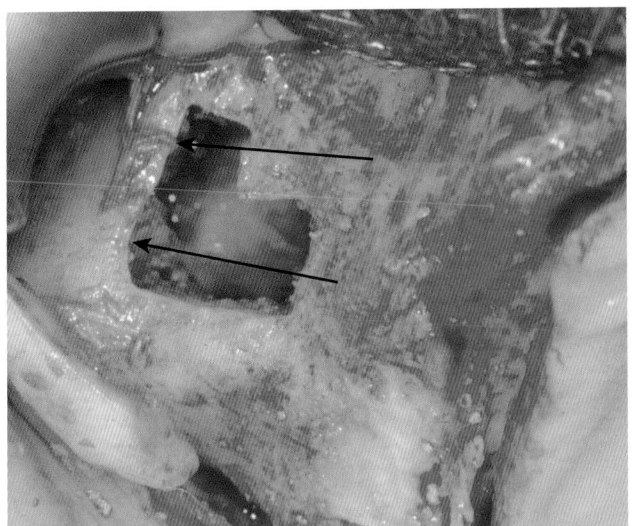

Figure 23.13 Direct visualization of the base of the zygoma bone in quad zygoma cases (*arrows*). Source: Edmond Bedrossian and E. Armand Bedrossian

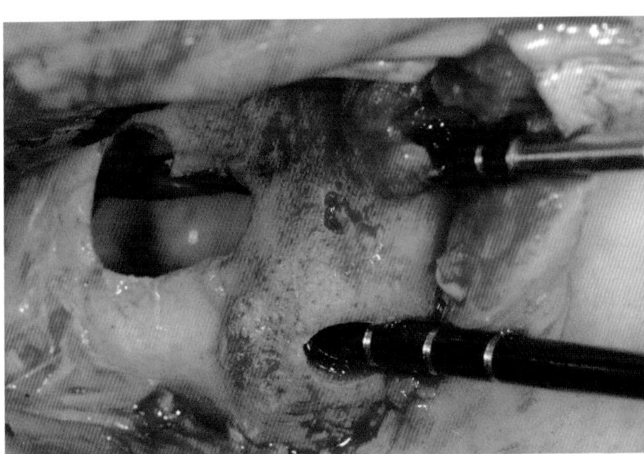

Figure 23.14 Simultaneous preparation of the osteotomies. Source: Edmond Bedrossian and E. Armand Bedrossian

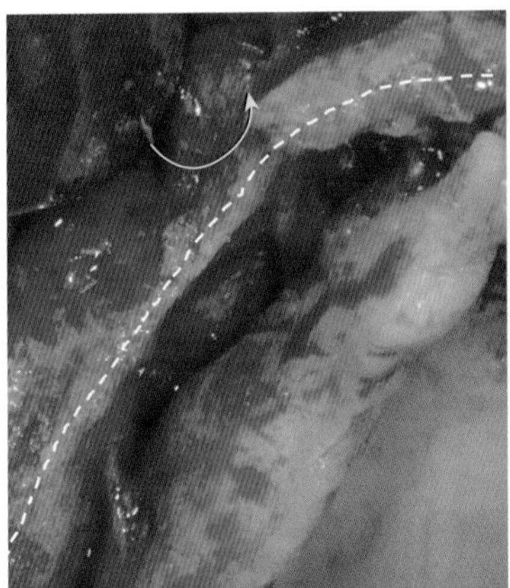

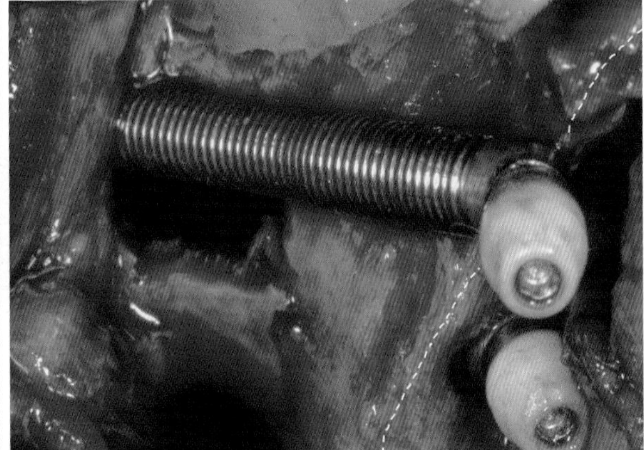

Figure 23.15 Concave ZAGA 3 and 4 contour of the anterior maxillary sinus wall (*arrow*). Source: Edmond Bedrossian and E. Armand Bedrossian

ALTERNATE TECHNIQUE: ZAGA 3–4—cont'd

STEP 5: Placement of the Implant

Prior to placement of the posterior zygoma implant, the maxillary sinus is thoroughly irrigated with sterile irrigation fluid to remove gross debris created by the osteotomy preparation phase. For the anterior implants, the surgeon must be aware of anatomic landmarks and ensure the placement of the implant is in the same trajectory as the drills used to prepare the osteotomy. The implants are removed sterilely from their container and placed using an insertion torque of 35 to 40 Ncm if immediate loading is considered.

STEP 6: Placement of the Abutments and Direct Conversion

The same aforementioned protocol is used.

STEP 7: Delivery of the Immediate Load Prosthesis

The delivery of the final prosthesis follows the same protocol as mentioned in the ZAGA 0–2 technique. It is imperative to educate patients to maintain a soft diet and report immediately if the prosthesis feels loose or is mobile.

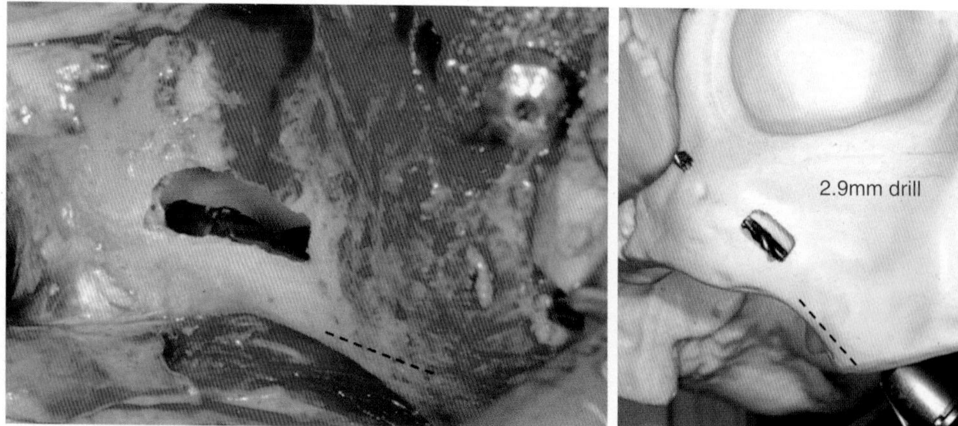

Figure 23.16 Direct visualization of the apex of the 2.9-mm drill. Source: Edmond Bedrossian and E. Armand Bedrossian

Avoidance and Management of Intraoperative Complications

The prevention and treatment of potential complications with the zygoma implant were reported by Bedrossian and Bedrossian in 2018.[22] However, it is prudent to highlight potential complications.

1. Avoiding the orbit
2. Fracture of the zygoma implant
3. Management of failed zygoma implants
4. Etiology and the management of sinus infections

Avoiding the orbit: As mentioned earlier in this chapter, the trajectory of the zygoma implant is from the maxillary alveolar crest through the maxillary sinus through the zygoma bone, with the termination point being through the lateral cortex of the zygoma bone with the 2.9-mm drill. Direct visualization of the path of the drill is a must, specifically, the direct visualization of the tip of the 2.9-mm drill exiting through the lateral cortex of the zygoma bone, before proceeding to the next drill (Fig. 23.16). If the drill tip cannot be visualized, the trajectory could be in the bony orbit or in the infratemporal fossa (Fig. 23.17). If the apex of the drill cannot be visualized, at this point the clinician must stop, reevaluate the surgical site and correct the drill trajectory. To underscore the need for direct visualization of the drill, it is imperative for the clinician to understand that to determine the length of the zygoma implant needed, the depth gauge follows the same path as the drills entering the osteotomy at the maxillary crest, traveling through the maxillary sinus and zygoma bone, with the final exit at the lateral cortex of the zygoma bone. The tip of the depth gauge must be visualized for the accurate determination of the implant length. By following the aforementioned surgical path, iatrogenic placement of the zygoma implant is readily avoided.

Fracture of the zygoma implant: As described in the literature,[23] the majority of occlusal forces are supported by the implant platform as the first 2 to 3 mm of the implant threads. The same is true for the zygoma implant as reported by Freedman et al. Fractures due to overload usually occur at or 2 to 3 mm apical

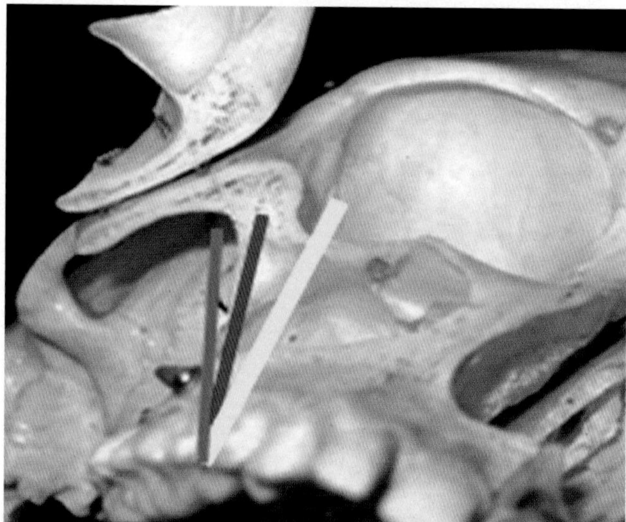

Figure 23.17 The red arrow simulates the proper trajectory of the zygoma implant. Source: Edmond Bedrossian and E. Armand Bedrossian

to the implant platform (Fig. 23.18). Therefore, the presence of bone around the implant platform is recommended specially in ZAGA 0–3 cases. In ZAGA 4 cases where it is not possible to secure the implant platform in bone, maintaining cross arch splinting of the implants with the prosthesis is extremely important. If cross arch stabilization is interrupted by either a loose prosthetic or abutment screw, the resultant metal fatigue will lead to the fracture of the screws or the fracture of the zygoma implant below its platform. In cases of implant fracture, if possible, the fractured implant is removed by counterclockwise rotation. If the implant is osseointegrated, cutting of the fractured implant at the base of the zygoma bone is recommended as excessive counterclockwise pressure to remove the implant may fracture the body of the zygoma bone. The placement of a new zygoma implant through the same crestal opening but with the apex of the implant above the fracture implant within the zygoma bone (Fig. 23.19) allows for the immediate replacement of the fractured zygoma implant, known as the "rescue concept."[24]

Management of failed zygoma implants: In cases where the zygoma implant fails, the removal of the implant and

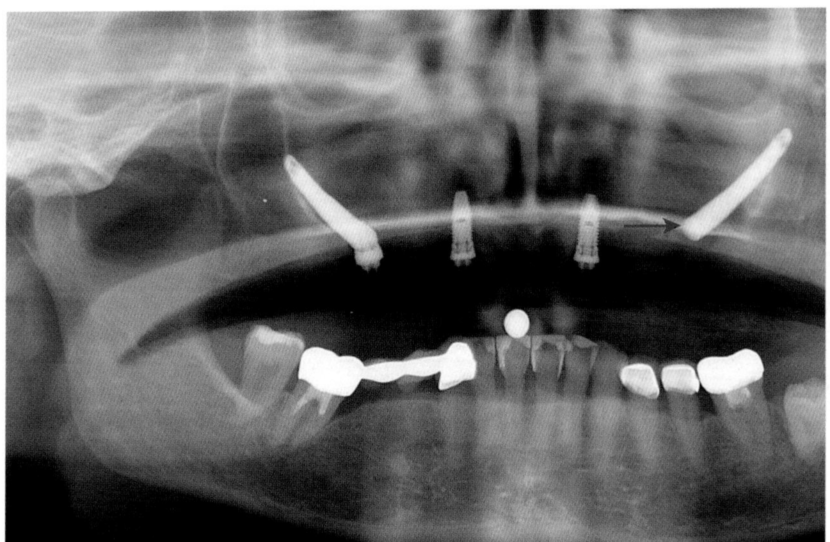

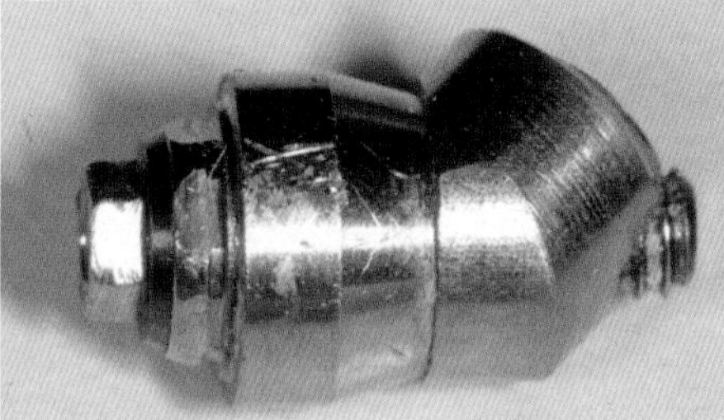

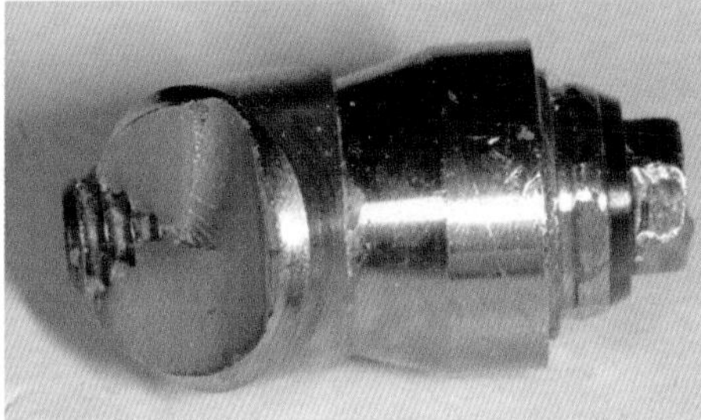

Figure 23.18 Zygoma fractures occur 1 to 2 mm apical to the implant platform. Source: Edmond Bedrossian and E. Armand Bedrossian

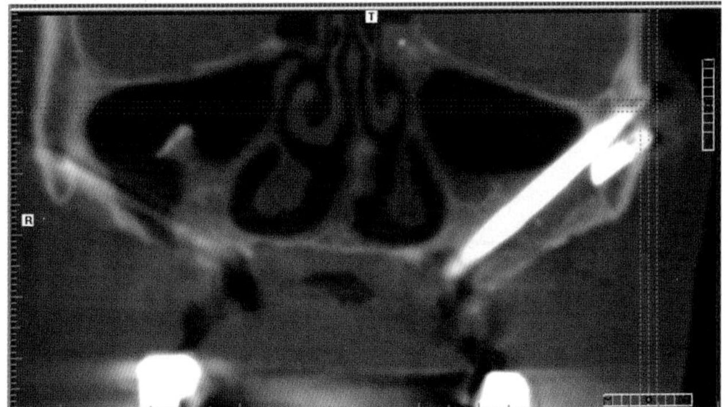

Figure 23.19 The new zygoma implant has the same crestal platform position. Source: Edmond Bedrossian and E. Armand Bedrossian

reorientation of the trajectory of the osteotomy, as described in the management of the fractured implant, are recommended. Evaluation of adequate space above the failed implant apex is determined by cone beam imaging (Fig. 23.20). When possible, the failed implant is removed and the new implant is placed, and the position of the new implant is connected to the provisional prosthesis and allowed to heal for an additional 6 months before fabrication of the final prosthesis.

Etiology and the management of sinus infections: Sinus infections in patients with bilateral zygoma implants are generally unilateral (Fig. 23.21). Acute sinusitis usually responds to oral antibiotics and associated palliative treatments. However, chronic sinusitis is generally due to the blockage of the osteomeatal complex (OMC) and recurs once oral antibiotics are discontinued. Titanium within the maxillary sinus does not cause a foreign body response.[25–27] If palliative treatment including humidified air treatment and chemotherapy including pseudoephedrine (Sudafed), guaifenesin (Mucinex), and antibiotics is not effective, functional endoscopic sinus surgery to increase the opening of the OMC and to allow the sinus to drain, leading to the resolution of the sinusitis, is recommended (Fig. 23.22).

Postoperative Considerations

The surgical procedure is usually performed in the office setting under intravenous sedation. Prophylactic use of 2 g of amoxicillin or 600 mg of clindamycin (Cleocin) in penicillin-allergic patients 1 hour before the surgical procedure is recommended. The continuation of the antibiotics for 1 week postoperatively is recommended. Analgesics are taken as needed. No specific decongestant or any special nasal or maxillary sinus lavage or care is routinely advocated.

Patients are advised to report any motion of the provisional prosthesis immediately as the loss of cross arch stabilization may lead to the lack of osseointegration of the implants. A soft diet is advocated during the osseointegration period and after the delivery of the final prosthesis. The authors still advocate a soft diet for the patients who undergo quad zygoma treatment.

Having a clear view of the path of the instruments needed in establishing the osteotomy and visualizing the path of the implants during their insertion prevents disorientation and potential complications associated with placement of the zygoma implants. It is critical to visualize the path of the drills and the zygoma implant from the premolar area to the base of the zygoma as well as the lateral cortex of the zygoma bone 2 to 3 mm below the fronto-zygomatic notch. Extensive knowledge of the anatomy and physiology of the maxillofacial region in conjunction with proper surgical training allows for predictable outcomes using the zygoma concept.

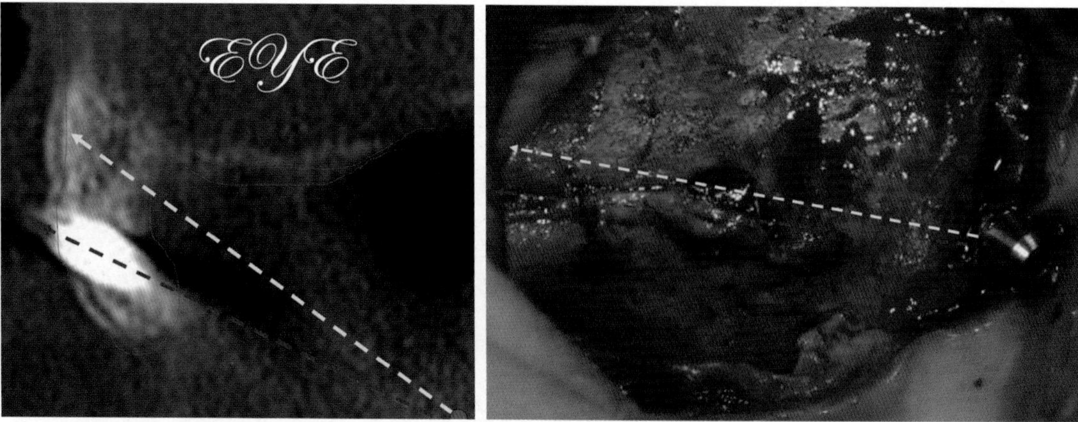

Figure 23.20 Preoperative evaluation of a failed zygoma implant for immediate replacement. Source: Edmond Bedrossian and E. Armand Bedrossian

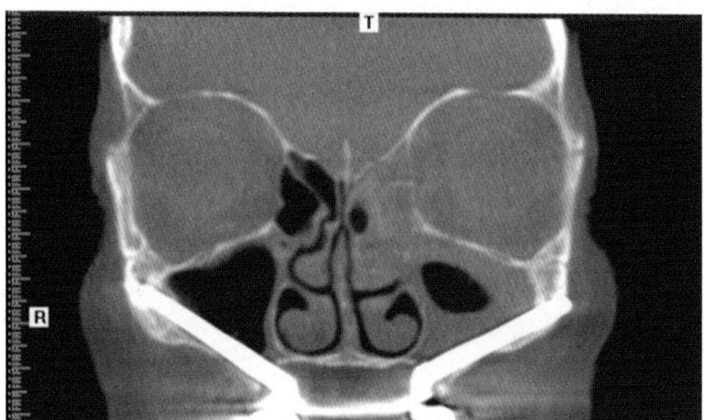

Figure 23.21 Unilateral infection of the maxillary sinus. Source: Edmond Bedrossian and E. Armand Bedrossian

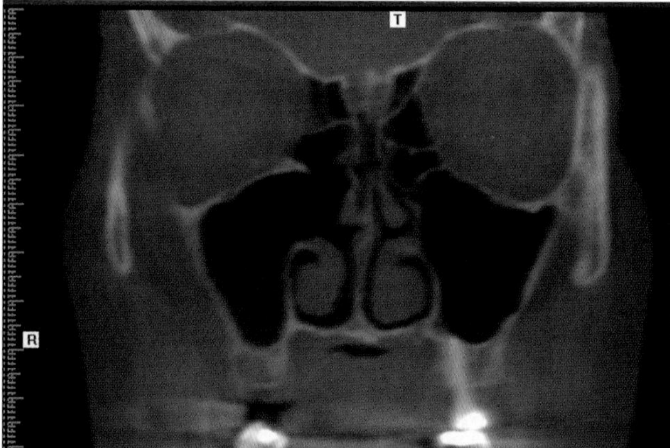

Figure 23.22 Postoperative view of a functional endoscopic sinus surgery procedure performed in the patient's right sinus. Source: Edmond Bedrossian and E. Armand Bedrossian

References

1. Breine U, Brånemark PI. Reconstruction of alveolar jaw bone. An experimental and clinical study of immediate and preformed autologous bone grafts in combination with osseointegrated implants. *Scand J Plast Reconstr Surg*. 1980;14(1):23–48.
2. Adell R, et al. A 15-year study of osseointegrated implants in the treatment of the edentulous jaw. *Int J Oral Surg*. 1981;10:387–416.
3. Issaksson S, et al. Early results from reconstruction of severely atrophic (class VI) maxillas by immediate endosseous implants in conjunction with bone grafting and Lefort I osteotomy. *J Oral Maxillofac Surg*. 1993;22:144–148.
4. Adell R, Lekholm U, Gröndahl K, Brånemark PI, Lindström J, Jacobsson M. Reconstruction of severely resorbed edentulous maxillae using osseointegrated fixtures in immediate autogenous bone grafts. *Int J Oral Maxillofac Implants*. 1990;5(3):233–246.
5. Isaksson S, Alberius P. Maxillary alveolar ridge augmentation with onlay bone-grafts and immediate endosseous implants. *J Cranio-Maxillo-Fac Surg*. 1992;20(1):2–7.
6. Tolman DE. Reconstructive procedures with endosseous implants in grafted bone: a review of the literature. *Int J Oral Maxillofac Implants*. 1995;10(3):275–294.
7. Keller EE, Tolman DE, Eckert SE. Maxillary antral-nasal inlay autogenous bone graft reconstruction of compromised maxilla: a 12-year retrospective study. *Int J Oral Maxillofac Implants*. 1999;14(5):707–721.
8. Rasmusson L, Meredith N, Cho IH, Sennerby L. The influence of simultaneous versus delayed placement on the stability of titanium implants in onlay bone grafts. A histologic and biomechanic study in the rabbit. *Int J Oral Maxillofac Surg*. 1999;28(3):224–231.
9. Fortin Y, Sullivan RM, Rangert BR. The Marius implant bridge: surgical and prosthetic rehabilitation for the completely edentulous upper jaw with moderate to severe resorption: a 5-year retrospective clinical study. *Clin Implant Dent Relat Res*. 2002;4(2):69–77.
10. Krekmanov L, Kahn M, Rangert B, Lindström H. Tilting of posterior mandibular and maxillary implants for improved prosthesis support. *Int J Oral Maxillofac Implants*. 2000;15(3):405–414.
11. Aparicio C, Perales P, Rangert B. Tilted implants as an alternative to maxillary sinus grafting: a clinical, radiologic, and periotest study. *Clin Implant Dent Relat Res*. 2001;3(1):39–49.
12. Freedman M, Ring M, Stassen LFA. Effect of alveolar bone support on zygomatic implants: a finite element analysis study. *Int J Oral Maxillofac Implants*. 2013;42(5):671–676.
13. Freedman M, Ring M, Stassen LFA. Effect of alveolar bone support on zygomatic implants in an extra-sinus position—a finite element analysis study. *Int J Oral Maxillofac Implants*. 2015;44(6):785–790.
14. Stevenson ARL, Austin BW. Zygomatic fixtures—the Sydney experience. *Ann R Australas Coll Dent Surg*. 2000;15:337–339.
15. Higuchi KW. The zygomaticus fixture: an alternative approach for implant anchorage in the posterior maxilla. *Ann R Australas Coll Dent Surg*. 2000;15:28–33.
16. Bedrossian E, Stumpel III L, Beckely ML, Indresano T. The zygomatic implant: preliminary data on treatment of severely resorbed maxillae. A clinical report. *Int J Oral Maxillofac Implants*. 2002;17(6):861–865.
17. Malevez C, Abarca M, Durdu F, Daelemans P. Clinical outcome of 103 consecutive zygomatic implants: a 6–48 months follow-up study. *Clin Oral Implants Res*. 2004;15(1):18–22.
18. Brånemark PI, Gröndahl K, Ohrnell LO, et al. Zygoma fixture in the management of advanced atrophy of the maxilla: technique and long-term results. *Scand J Plast ReConstr Surg Hand Surg*. 2004;38(2):70–85.
19. Aparicio C, Ouazzani W, Garcia R, Arevalo X, Muela R, Fortes V. A prospective clinical study on titanium implants in the zygomatic arch for prosthetic rehabilitation of the atrophic edentulous maxilla with a follow-up of 6 months to 5 years. *Clin Implant Dent Relat Res*. 2006;8(3):114–122.
20. Bedrossian E, Bedrossian EA. Systematic treatment planning protocol of the edentulous maxilla for an implant-supported fixed prosthesis. *Compend Contin Educ Dent*. 2019;40(1):20–25.
21. Aparicio C. A proposed classification for zygomatic implant patient based on the zygoma anatomy guided approach (ZAGA): a cross-sectional survey. *Eur J Oral Implantol*. 2011;4(3):269–275.
22. Bedrossian E, Bedrossian EA. Prevention and the management of complications using the zygoma implant: a review and clinical experiences. *Int J Oral Maxillofac Implants*. 2018;33(5):e135–e145.
23. Pierrisnard L, Renouard F, Renault P, Barquins M. Influence of implant length and bicortical anchorage on implant stress distribution. *Clin Implant Dent Relat Res*. 2003;5(4):254–262.
24. Bedrossian E. Rescue implant concept: the expanded use of the zygoma implant in the graftless solutions. *Oral Maxillofac Surg Clin North Am*. 2011;23(2):257–276, vi.
25. Petruson B. Sinuscopy in patients with titanium implants in the nose and sinuses. *Scand J Plast ReConstr Surg Hand Surg*. 2004;38(2):86–93.
26. Jung JH, Choi BH, Zhu SJ, et al. The effects of exposing dental implants to the maxillary sinus cavity on sinus complications. *Oral Surg Oral Med Oral Pathol Oral Radiol Endod*. 2006;102(5):602–605.
27. Davó R, Malevez C, López-Orellana C, Pastor-Beviá F, Rojas J. Sinus reactions to immediately loaded zygoma implants: a clinical and radiological study. *Eur J Oral Implantol*. 2008;1(1):53–60.

CHAPTER 24

Pterygomaxillary Implants

David Knight Sylvester II and Daniel Joseph Pinkston

Armamentarium

#15 Blade and handle
#2 Molt elevator
#9 Periosteal elevator
Weider tongue retractor
Seldin retractor
Suture
Tissue forceps
Needle holder
Dean tissue scissors
Minnesota retractor
Elevators, Forceps
Intraoral caliper
Cheek retractors
Curettes
Bone file
Sterile pencil
Rongeur
High speed/torque surgical handpiece
Drill extender or long implant drills
Reduction bur
Hemostats
Slotted surgical guides
Straight osteotomes
Implant system with multiunit abutments
Right angle driver

History of the Procedure

Quantitative and qualitative challenges inherent to the posterior maxilla have made implant rehabilitation a controversial topic. Structural support for implant fixation and maintenance is further complicated by increased occlusal forces present in the posterior maxilla. Quantitative bone changes are the result of predictable patterns of bone resorption. Disuse atrophy results in facial and crestal alveolar bone loss with concomitant pneumatization of the maxillary sinuses. Qualitatively, the region has minimal cortical bone and is dominated by poorly mineralized cancellous bone. The posterior maxilla is often classified as Cawood and Howell IV-VI and Lekholm and Zarb III/IV.[1,2]

The natural maxillofacial buttresses represent the sites of residual bone most resistant to resorption due to ongoing functional demands. A pillar of dense cortical bone routinely present at the pterygomaxillary buttress is an opportunistic extramaxillary site for implant fixation (Fig. 24.1). Tulasne first described the use of pterygoid bone for implant anchorage.[3] Surgical steps with rotary burs and retrospective studies by Graves, Balshi, and Venturelli further detailed and validated Tulasne's success.[4–6] Site preparation with cylindric osteotomes in addition to rotary burs was proposed by Valerón and Velazquez to decrease potential surgical risks, particularly hemorrhage.[7] Long-term follow-up studies have shown that pterygoid implants have high survival rates and high degrees of predictability. Ten-year success rates average 94.85%.[8–13]

Indication for Use of the Procedure

In the application of fixed, full-arch implant rehabilitation, pterygomaxillary implants have many advantages (Box 24.1). As an alternative to augmentation procedures, they are associated with deceased costs, morbidity, and treatment times. They represent a treatment alternative for patients who are not candidates for sinus grafting or zygomatic implants. Alternatively, they can be incorporated with zygomatic and angled anterior implants in cases where maximum anteroposterior (AP) spread is desired. In cases of severe atrophy, the combined use of two zygomatic and two pterygoid implants may obviate the need for a quad-zygoma, thereby preserving zygomatic bone for future use. The implants can be placed quickly and utilized as a rescue implant when high composite torque is not achievable during conventional all-on-four surgery. This allows immediate loading of a provisional prosthesis.[14]

Apical implant fixation is possible in the pterygomaxillary region due to the fusion of three cortical structures: the posterior maxillary wall, the pyramidal process of the palatal bone, and the medial pterygoid process of the sphenoid bone (Fig. 24.2). A thick pillar of cortical bone is found 3 to 4 mm medial to the alveolar crest. On average, this measures 6 to 6.7 mm on axial view of cone beam computerized tomography (CBCT) (Fig. 24.3). Engagement of this bone at an oblique angle allows residual bone volume to be maximized and high insertional torque obtained.[5,6,11,15] The AP and buccopalatal angles recommended to maximize apical bone fixation have been described differently in the literature. Early studies advocated a 45-degree AP angulation using the occlusal plane as a reference.[5,6] More

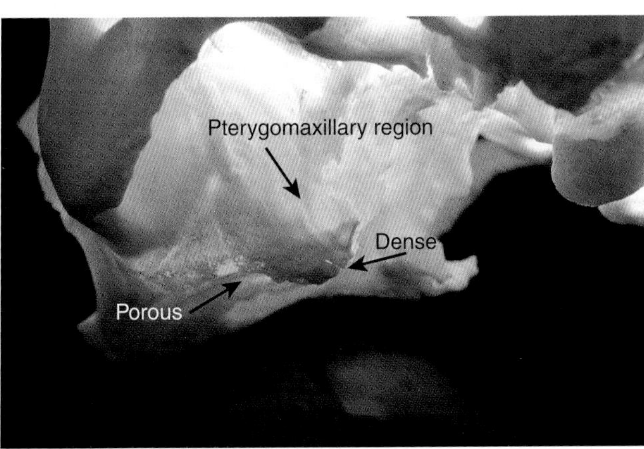

Figure 24.1 Transillumination of an edentulous skull highlights distinct qualitative differences between the porous alveolar tuberosity and the dense fixating bone of the pterygomaxillary fusion. (Clinical Photos - David Knight Sylvester II, Daniel Joseph Pinkston)

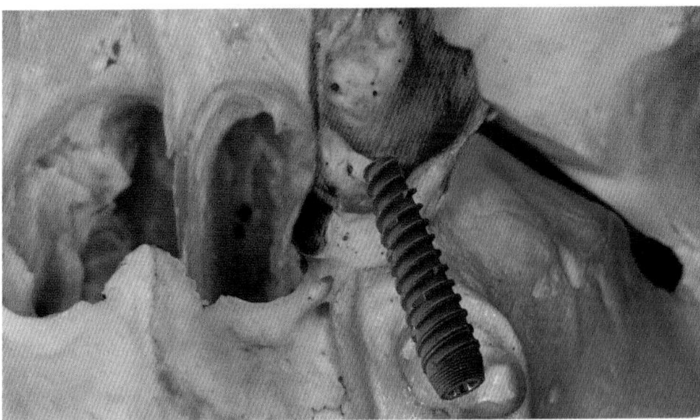

Figure 24.2 The fusion of the posterior maxillary wall (green), the pyramidal process of the palatal bone (blue), and the medial pterygoid plate (red) constitute a dense pillar of bone routinely available for implant fixation. The neurovascular bundle of the greater palatal foramen is in direct line with the hamular process, an easily palpable intraoral reference mark. Contrary to common implant practices and concepts, pterygomaxillary implants are not directed within the long axis of the ridge. They must be medially oriented to bisect and maximize residual bone as depicted in this image.

BOX 24.1 Pterygomaxillary Implant Advantages

Fast procedure
Obviates need for sinus graft
Predictable success rates
Maximizes anteroposterior spread (no distal cantilever)
Decreased postoperative pain, swelling, and infection
Shorter healing times
Excellent primary stability for immediate loading

recent studies have recommended a more vertical angulation of 72 degrees using Frankfort horizontal as the reference plane.[16–18] At this angulation, the average bone column measured from the alveolar crest to the base of the pterygomaxillary fissure is 22.5 ± 4.8 mm. This suggests that appropriate fixation requires a minimum implant length of 13 mm and average implant lengths of 15 to 18 mm.[16,19] Buccopalatal angulation is 10 to 15 degrees directed medially. In all cases, variability in patient anatomy dictates the angle necessary to bisect the maximum bone volume. Trajectories that are less oblique may require longer implants. The pterygoid fossa is void of vital structures and primarily occupied with the origin of the medial pterygoid muscle.

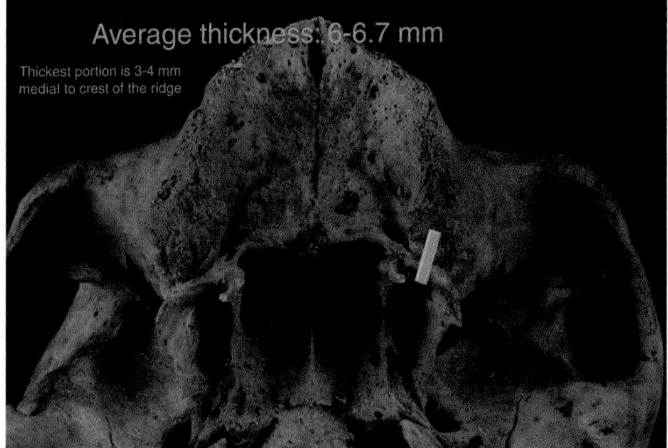

Figure 24.3 Inferior view of an edentulous skull depicting the average cortical bone thickness in the pterygomaxillary region ranging from 6 to 6.7 mm.

Limitations and Contraindications

The relatively blind nature of the procedure requires a steep surgical learning curve. Surgical access can be challenging in patients where incisal opening is limited. Implant preparation and placement require the use of long drills or drill extenders. The osteotomies and implants are in close proximity to vital structures. The presence of impacted third molars and the lack of adequate bone may preclude placement.

TECHNIQUE

STEP 1: Initial Evaluation

Preoperative imaging is obtained and evaluated to determine the quantity and quality of residual subantral bone. The posterior deflection of the sinus wall determines the AP entry point and angulation of the anticipated trajectory (Fig. 24.4). The fusion of the posterior maxillary wall, the pyramidal process of the palatal bone, and medial pterygoid plate constitute a dense, radiopaque pillar of bone on imaging (Fig. 24.5). Implant lengths and approximate angulations needed to bisect these structures are noted. Restorative space at the location of implant emergence should be evaluated. A minimum of 7.5 mm of space is recommended. This portion of the prosthesis is often not in occlusion with the opposing arch and serves as an extension of the prosthesis connecting anterior functional components to distal implant fixtures.

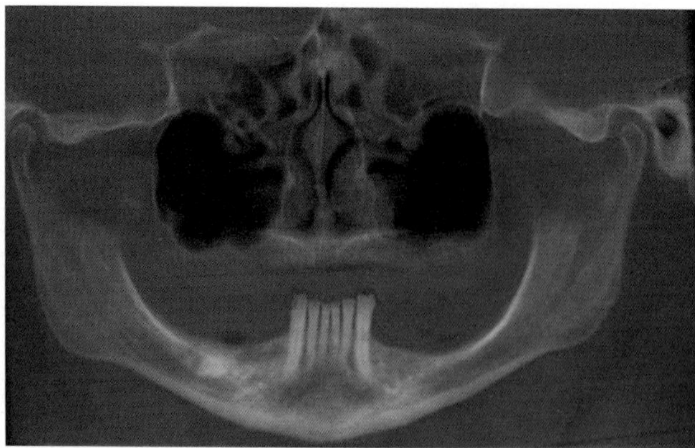

Figure 24.4 Preoperative imaging of a pterygomaxillary implant candidate. Thirty years of edentulism with progressive bone resorption has resulted in bone confined to the intercanine region with limited subnasal bone.

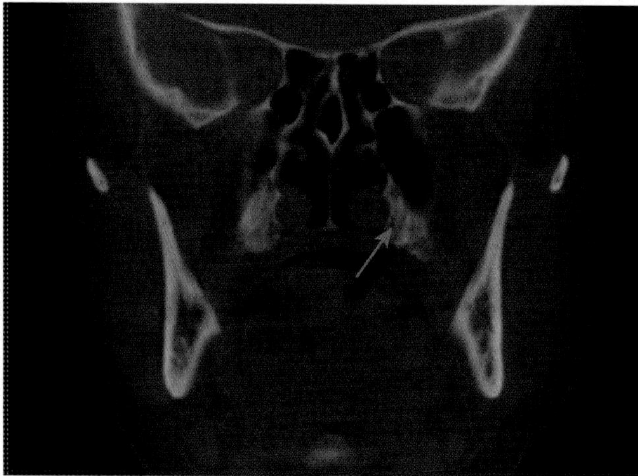

Figure 24.5 Coronal view of cone beam computerized tomography (CBCT). The *arrow* indicates the dense pillar of cortical bone found in the pterygomaxillary region.

TECHNIQUE—*cont'd*

STEP 2: Administration of Local Anesthesia and Incision

The patient is anesthetized with 2% lidocaine with 1:100,000 epinephrine by way of local nerve blocks and infiltration. An incision is made 2 to 3 mm medial to the alveolar crest and extends along the posterior aspect of the tuberosity. A small distobuccal releasing incision can be made. A full thickness mucoperiosteal flap is elevated buccally and palatally exposing the tuberosity and extending to the lateral pterygoid plate.

STEP 3: Preparation for Initial Osteotomy

The entry point is patient-specific and anatomically determined. In cases of amble residual bone, the entry point is approximated with a caliper using the distal aspect of the tuberosity as a reference. This entry point is often at the second or third molar position. Alternatively, a small crestal window can be made with an osteotome anterior to the anticipated entry point, and the sinus membrane elevated with a curette. Residual subantral bone can be sounded and explored to ensure an intraosseous trajectory.

STEP 4: Obtain Buccopalatal Trajectory

The hamular process is palpated. The location of the neovascular bundle is assessed. The densest pillar of pterygomaxillary bone is found 4 to 5 mm lateral to the hamular process. Osteotomes and twist drills should be apically directed to this point. The clinical reproduction of this angle is challenging. It has been described differently utilizing different reference markers.[5,16] Most importantly, the trajectory must be medially oriented by 10 to 15 degrees. This corresponds to a buccopalatal angulation of 81.3 ± 2.8 degrees relative to the Frankfort horizontal plane. The hamular process should be repeatedly palpated during the procedure to maintain ideal buccopalatal implant orientation.

Continued

TECHNIQUE—*cont'd*

STEP 5: Determine Anteroposterior Trajectory

The occlusal or Frankfort horizontal plane serve as AP reference points. Average trajectories are ≥45 degrees to the occlusal plane and 72 ± 4.9 degrees to the Frankfort horizontal plane.[5,16,19,20] Again, these are dictated by patient anatomy and variability.

STEP 6: Implant Site Preparation

A narrow-diameter straight osteotome is used to establish the implant trajectory. The osteotome advances with minimal resistance, condensing the cancellous bone of the posterior maxilla until the dense pillar of pterygomaxillary bone is tactically and audibly encountered. A series of twist drills on an extender are used to carefully prepare the implant bed. Significant resistance is encountered as the drill obliquely passes through the pterygomaxillary bone. Sequential osteotomes may be used in conjunction with twist drills to verify implant trajectory and decrease surgical risk. A decrease in resistance during apical advancement indicates the osteotomy has reached the pterygoid fossa. Due to the density of the bone in this region, underpreparation of the osteotomy in width is generally not recommended.

STEP 7: Implant Placement

A depth gauge is used to explore the surgical site and determine implant length. This length is almost always more than 13 mm. A depth less than this may indicate the implant is not oriented medially or deep enough. An extender is generally required to place the implant. High torque values in excess of 60 Ncm are routinely encountered (Figs. 24.6 and 24.7).

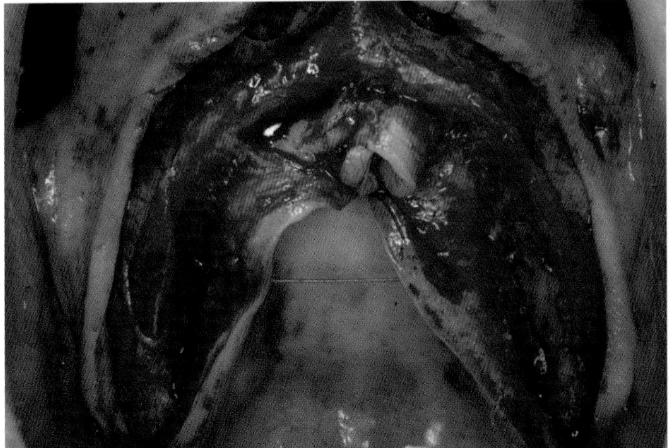

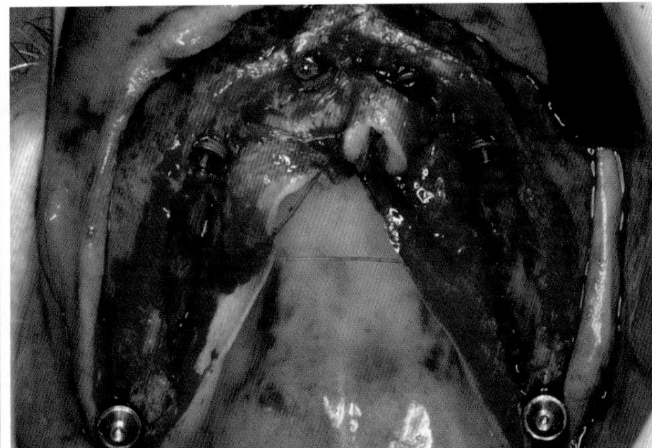

Figure 24.6 Occlusal view of a narrow residual ridge with exposure of the piriform and elevation of the nasal floor *(left)*. Limited anteroposterior spread obtainable with anterior implants is overcome with the incorporation of pterygomaxillary implants *(right)*.

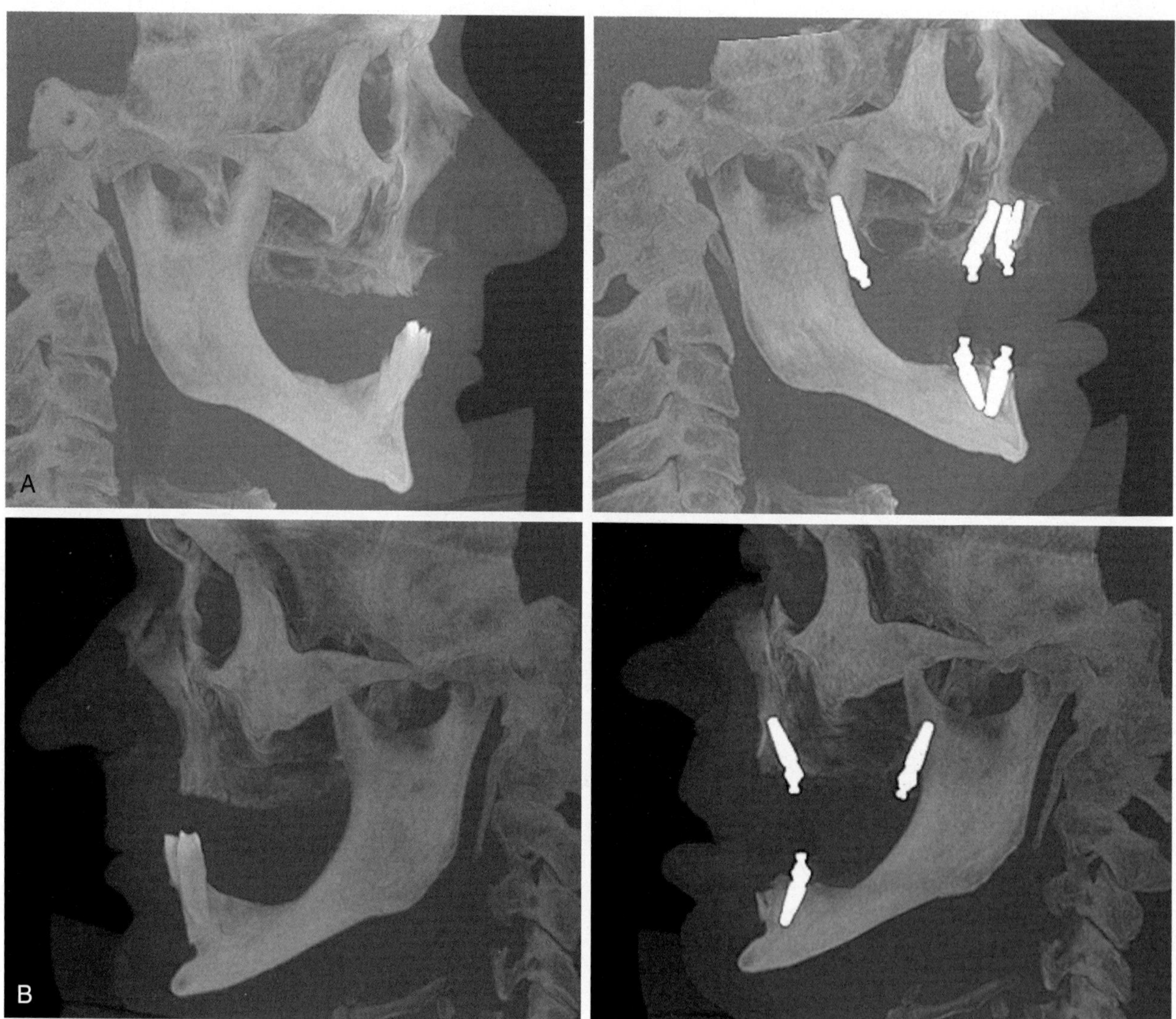

Figure 24.7 **A,** Preoperative and postoperative lateral cephalad. Note the posterior position and angulation of the pterygomaxillary implants. **B,** Preoperative and postoperative lateral cephalad. Note the posterior position and angulation of the pterygomaxillary implants.

Continued

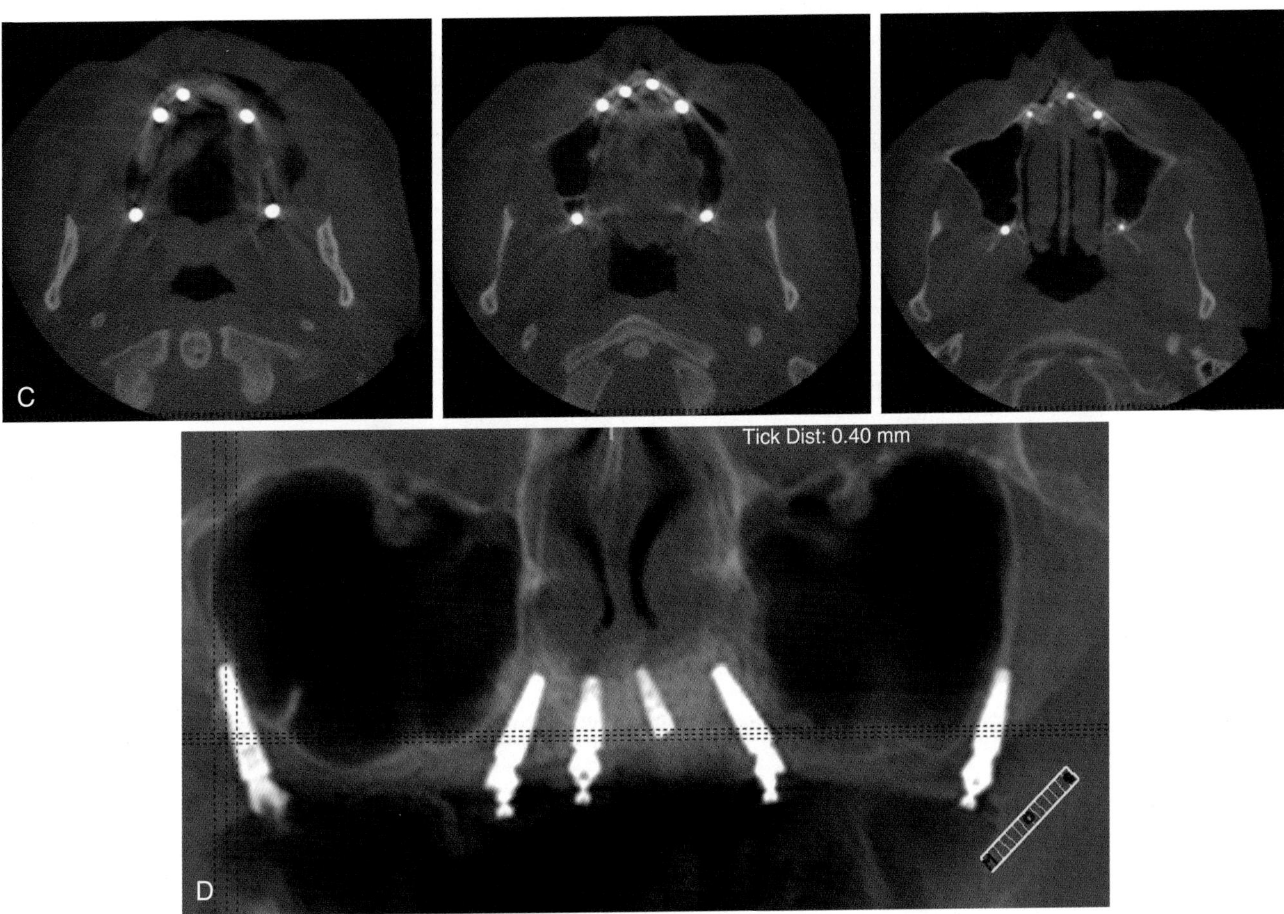

Figure 24.7, cont'd **C,** Postoperative axial views depicting ideal implant placement in residual pterygomaxillary bone. Axial slices move in a superior direction from left to right. **D,** Panoramic reconstruction showing 4.3 × 18 mm implant *(right)* and a 4.3 × 16 mm implant *(left)*. The implants are fixated in residual bone and extend to the base of the pterygomaxillary fissure.

TECHNIQUE—*cont'd*

STEP 8: Abutment Selection

A slotted surgical guide is placed and used to select multiunit abutments. Because of the buccal-palatal trajectories, tall 17-degree multiunit or straight abutments are generally selected. These abutments allow for a passive prosthetic fit via the rotational path of insertion. Access channels are commonly found posterior to the maxillary dentition resulting in no distal cantilever.

STEP 9: Soft Tissue Closure

Wedge excision of the fibrous tuberosity in conjunction with tall abutments are often required to facilitate abutment access. Soft tissue is closed with resorbable suture (Fig. 24.8).

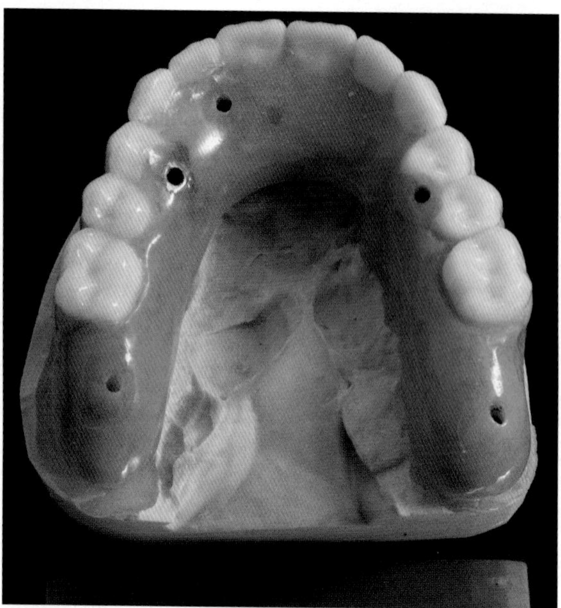

Figure 24.8 Interim prosthesis. Note the posterior position of the distal access holes.

TECHNIQUE—*cont'd*

STEP 10: Interim Prosthesis

Fabrication of a hygienic interim prosthesis with an ovate intaglio surface is imperative to permit cleaning and periimplant health. Accessibility can be challenging because of the distal implant emergence positions (Fig. 24.9).

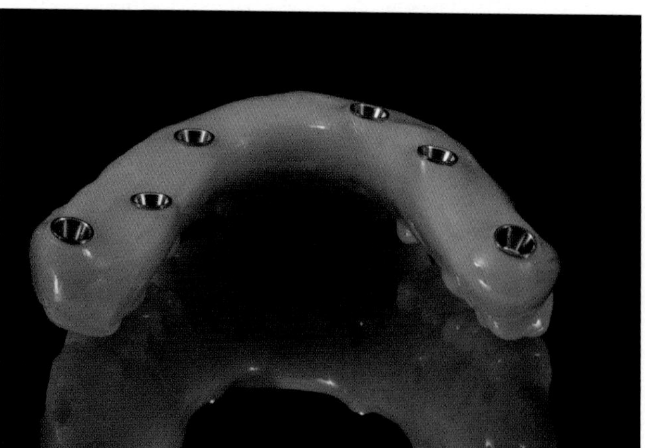

Figure 24.9 Ovate and cleansable intaglio surface of an interim prosthesis.

Avoidance and Management of Intraoperative Complications

A recent systematic review and meta-analysis reviewed 1893 pterygomaxillary implants placed in 634 patients.[12] No major complications were reported. Hemorrhage is a common concern with emphasis placed on the pterygoid plexus, descending palatal artery, and internal maxillary artery as potential sources of bleeding. The average height of the pterygomaxillary suture is 15 mm. The internal maxillary artery courses an average of 10 mm above the base of the pterygomaxillary suture for an average distance of 25 mm above any proposed implant entry point[21] (Fig. 24.10). On average, the descending palatal artery is 2.9 mm medial to the most inferior point of the pterygomaxillary fissure.[18,22] The greater palatal artery is in line with the hamular process at the level of the alveolus and can be repeatedly palpated during surgery. Bleeding was the most common complication reported in the literature. All bleeding resolved with implant placement and was likely due to muscle bleed from the medial pterygoid muscle.[9,19,20]

Low insertion torque is generally the result of inadequate implant length or inadequate buccopalatal positioning. Repeated studies have supported 13 mm as the minimum length needed to engage fixating bone, with implant lengths of 13 to 20 mm commonly used.[15,16,18] A tendency to place the implant parallel with the alveolar ridge results in an insufficient buccopalatal angle. The dense bone is more medial, and the trajectory should be redirected.

Displacement into the sinus is possible and requires retrieval. Displacement into the pterygoid space is a rare complication that has been reported in the literature.[23]

Postoperative Considerations

Postoperative palatal paresthesia and pain have been reported.[9,19] The few instances of mild trismus reported were likely due to the drill passing beyond the pterygoid fossa and impinging on the medial pterygoid muscle. All cases were resolved with physiotherapy and muscle relaxers.

Patients must be able to clean any implant-supported prosthesis (Fig. 24.11). This requires a reasonable level of manual dexterity and compliance. Any convex or flat intaglio surface that allows access for floss-threaders or a water flosser can be enhanced using sluiceway cuts. These channels are placed on the buccogingival aspect of the prosthesis mesial and distal to abutments and may aid in cleanability (see Box 24.1).

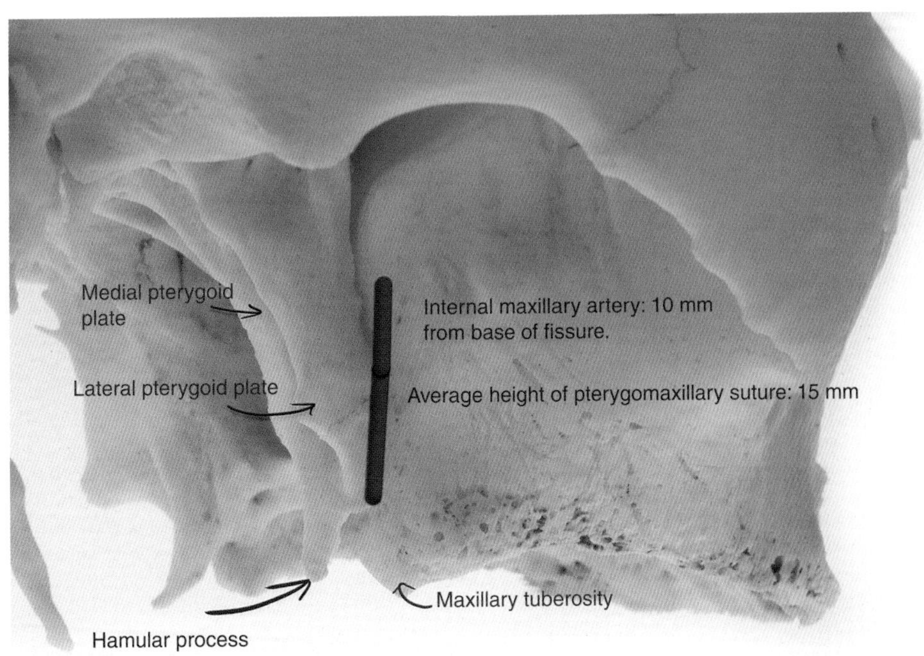

Figure 24.10 Photograph of edentulous skull. Relevant anatomy is labeled. Note the height of the pterygomaxillary fissure and average distance to the internal maxillary artery.

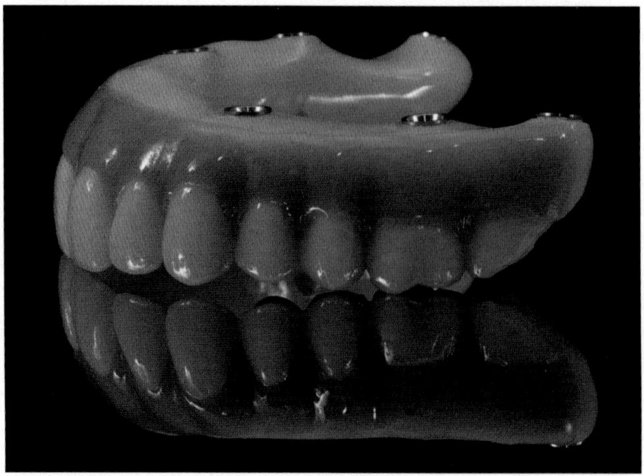

Figure 24.11 Photograph of a titanium/acrylic final prosthesis incorporating pterygomaxillary implants.

References

1. Lekholm U, Zarb GA. Patient selection and preparation. In: Brånemark PS, Zarb GA, Albrektsson T, eds. *Tissue-Integrated Prosthesis: Osseointegration in Clinical Dentistry*. Chicago, Illinois: Quintessence; 1985.
2. Cawood JI, Howell RA. A classification of the edentulous jaws. *Int J Oral Maxillofac Surg*. 1988;17(4):232–236.
3. Tulasne JF. Osseointegrated fixtures in the pterygoid region. In: Worthington P, Branemark PI, eds. *Advanced Osseointegration Surgery: Applications in the Maxillofacial Region*. Chicago, Illinois: Quintessence Publishing; 1992.
4. Balshi TJ, Lee HY, Hernandez RE. The use of pterygomaxillary implants in the partially edentulous patient: a preliminary report. *Int J Oral Maxillofac Implants*. 1995;10(1):89–98.
5. Graves SL. The pterygoid plate implant: a solution for restoring the posterior maxilla. *Int J Periodontics Restorative Dent*. 1994;14(6):512–523.
6. Venturelli A. A modified surgical protocol for placing implants in the maxillary tuberosity: clinical results at 36 months after loading with fixed partial dentures. *Int J Oral Maxillofac Implants*. 1996;11(6):743–749.
7. Valerón JF, Velázquez JF. Placement of screw-type implants in the pterygomaxillary-pyramidal region: surgical procedure and preliminary results. *Int J Oral Maxillofac Implants*. 1997;12(6):814–819.
8. Peñarrocha M, Carrillo C, Boronat A, Peñarrocha M. Retrospective study of 68 implants placed in the pterygomaxillary region using drills and osteotomes. *Int J Oral Maxillofac Implants*. 2009;24(4):720–726.
9. Valerón JF, Valerón PF. Long-term results in placement of screw-type implants in the pterygomaxillary-pyramidal region. *Int J Oral Maxillofac Implants*. 2007;22(2):195–200.
10. Balshi TJ, Wolfinger GJ, Slauch RW, Balshi SF. A retrospective comparison of implants in the pterygomaxillary region: implant placement with two-stage, single-stage, and guided surgery protocols. *Int J Oral Maxillofac Implants*. 2013;28(1):184–189. https://doi.org/10.11607/jomi.2693.
11. Bidra AS, Huynh-Ba G. Implants in the pterygoid region: a systematic review of the literature. *Int J Oral Maxillofac Implants*. 2011;40(8):773–781. https://doi.org/10.1016/j.ijom.2011.04.007.
12. Araujo RZ, Santiago Júnior JF, Cardoso CL, Benites Condezo AF, Moreira Júnior R, Curi MM. Clinical outcomes of pterygoid implants: systematic review and meta-analysis. *J Cranio-Maxillo-Fac Surg*. 2019;47(4):651–660. https://doi.org/10.1016/j.jcms.2019.01.030.
13. American College of Prosthodontists. Position statement: use of implants in the pterygoid region for prosthodontic treatment https://www.prosthodontics.org/about-acp/position-statement-use-of-implants-in-the-pterygoid-region-for-prosthodontic-treatment-/. Accessed January 31, 2019.
14. Jensen OT, Adams MW. Secondary stabilization of maxillary m-4 treatment with unstable implants for immediate function: biomechanical considerations and report of 10 cases after 1 year in function. *Int J Oral Maxillofac Implants*. 2014;29(2):e232–e240. https://doi.org/10.11607/jomi.te59.
15. Lee SP, Paik KS, Kim MK. Anatomical study of the pyramidal process of the palatine bone in relation to implant placement in the posterior maxilla. *J Oral Rehabil*. 2001;28(2):125–132. https://doi.org/10.1046/j.1365-2842.2001.00741.x.
16. Rodríguez X, Rambla F, De Marcos Lopez L, Méndez V, Vela X, Jiménez Garcia J. Anatomical study of the pterygomaxillary area for implant placement: cone beam computed tomographic scanning in 100 patients. *Int J Oral Maxillofac Implants*. 2014;29(5):1049–1052. https://doi.org/10.11607/jomi.3173.
17. Rodríguez X, Lucas-Taulé E, Elnayef B, et al. Anatomical and radiological approach to pterygoid implants: a cross-sectional study of 202 cone beam computed tomography examinations. *Int J Oral Maxillofac Implants*. 2016;45(5):636–640. https://doi.org/10.1016/j.ijom.2015.12.009.
18. Uchida Y, Yamashita Y, Danjo A, Shibata K, Kuraoka A. Computed tomography and anatomical measurements of critical sites for endosseous implants in the pterygomaxillary region: a cadaveric study. *Int J Oral Maxillofac Implants*. 2017;46(6):798–804. https://doi.org/10.1016/j.ijom.2017.02.003.
19. Rodríguez X, Méndez V, Vela X, Segalà M. Modified surgical protocol for placing implants in the pterygomaxillary region: clinical and radiologic study of 454 implants. *Int J Oral Maxillofac Implants*. 2012;27(6):1547–1553.
20. Curi MM, Cardoso CL, Ribeiro K de CB. Retrospective study of pterygoid implants in the atrophic posterior maxilla: implant and prosthesis survival rates up to 3 years. *Int J Oral Maxillofac Implants*. 2015;30(2):378–383. https://doi.org/10.11607/jomi.3665.
21. Turvey TA, Fonseca RJ. The anatomy of the internal maxillary artery in the pterygopalatine fossa: its relationship to maxillary surgery. *J Oral Surg*. 1980;38(2):92–95.
22. Rodriguez X, et al. Anatomical study of the pterygomaxillary area for implant placement: cone beam computed tomographic scanning in 100 patients. *Int J Oral Maxillofac Implants*. 2014;29(5):1049–1052.
23. Dryer RR, Conrad HJ. Displacement of a dental implant into the pterygoid fossa: a clinical report. *J Prosthodont*. 2019;28(9):1044–1046. https://doi.org/10.1111/jopr.13126.

CHAPTER 25

Site Preservation and Ridge Augmentation

Tara Aghaloo, Joan Pi-Anfruns, and Danny Hadaya

Armamentarium

#9 Periosteal elevator
#15 Scalpel blade
#701 Bur
Appropriate sutures
Barrier membranes (resorbable/nonresorbable)
Bone graft substitutes (allograft, xenograft, alloplast, or autogenous bone)
Bone scraper
Collagen plug
Elevators
Fixation pins (tacks or screws)
Forceps
Local anesthetic with vasoconstrictor
Minnesota retractor
Needle holder
Periotomes
Tissue forceps
Woodson elevator

History of the Procedure

Changes that occur after tooth extraction have been well documented since the early 1900s. Both animal and human studies have examined the healing mechanisms and pattern of alveolar ridge resorption after a tooth is extracted. In 1923, Euler examined the healing process of extraction wounds in dogs and determined that there were seven distinct phases.[1] Clafin, the first to report on dogs and humans, noted that healing was slower in humans than in dogs.[2] In 1967, Pietrokovski and Massler published a study on the morphologic changes taking place after tooth extraction on duplicate study casts; they concluded that the buccal plate showed greater resorption than the lingual plate, both in the maxilla and the mandible.[3] These findings were later confirmed in a histologic study by Araújo and Lindhe.[4] The term *socket preservation,* attributed to Cohen, involves the placement of a filler into a fresh extraction socket with the objective of minimizing bone remodeling after tooth extraction.[5] A number of materials have been studied for this purpose, and they have shown comparable results.[6]

By definition, a socket is a cavity. Therefore to preserve the socket means to maintain the socket intact, as a cavity. The term *socket augmentation* best describes the goal of the procedure, which is to fill a cavity by generating new bone. Several augmentation procedures have been proposed to compensate for ridge deficiencies. The basic principles for guided tissue regeneration were established by Melcher, who described the need to protect the healing sites from unwanted cells to allow for regeneration of the desired tissues.[7] Since the introduction of the first barrier membranes in the early 1980s, research in the field of guided bone regeneration (GBR) for ridge augmentation has grown exponentially. Barrier membranes play a key role in successful outcomes for GBR.[8,9] Their biocompatibility, ability to maintain space, occlusivity, and manageability dictate bone regeneration. Both resorbable and nonresorbable membranes have been used in GBR procedures. Resorbable barriers can be made of natural or synthetic materials, such as collagen, polyglycolide, and polylactic acid. Nonresorbable membranes usually are made of polytetrafluoroethylene (PTFE) and titanium mesh.[10,11] During the 1990s, GBR was proven to be a successful and viable technique for ridge augmentation[12–14] and continues to be one of the most commonly performed grafting procedures in implant dentistry.[15]

An array of grafting materials has been investigated for use in GBR. Autogenous bone is the gold standard material that possesses osteogenic, osteoinductive, and osteoconductive properties. Although a donor site is required and supply is limited, an autogenous graft is the only material where osteocompetent cells are transplanted to the recipient site and continue to stimulate new bone formation.[16] For most GBR procedures, intraoral sources of autogenous bone can be utilized. These include using a bone scraper to collect 2- to 3-mm shavings of cortical or cancellous bone from the local surgical site or a secondary minimally invasive site such as the tuberosity or the mandibular external oblique ridge. Combining autogenous bone with other "off-the-shelf" materials can decrease the bone graft healing time and improve the remodeling and turnover of the composite graft. Allografts, both mineralized and demineralized, have advantages and disadvantages. Demineralized allografts contain picogram concentrations of bone morphogenetic protein (BMP) that may provide minimal osteoinductive properties. However, clinically relevant doses of BMP-2 to promote the chemotaxis of undifferentiated mesenchymal stem cells to the recipient site and stimulate osteoblast differentiation and subsequent bone formation are in milligram concentrations. This difference in BMP dose leaves little use for demineralized allografts, as they are primarily osteoconductive without the mineralized structure to provide support to overlying soft tissue. Mineralized allografts and xenografts possess osteoconductive properties and have a calcified structure to be utilized both in socket augmentation and GBR procedures. Mineralized allografts generally resorb in 3 to 4 months, which provide a recipient site similar to native bone if implants are placed during that time frame. In implant dentistry, allografts, xenografts, alloplasts, and growth factors have been used alone or in combination to promote bone regeneration and have generally shown comparable results. To date, the data are insufficient to prove the superiority of one material over another. An ideal graft material should remain in place to provide a scaffold for bone formation and to prevent the volume reduction that occurs over time. Resorption time, volume stabilization, and soft tissue support contribute to the popularity of xenografts for grafting procedures. Other than autogenous bone, xenografts, especially bovine hydroxyapatite, are the most well-studied osteoconductive graft material to support implant survival and success, in both the long and short term.[15,17] Bone grafting materials continue to be developed and modified to improve outcomes and prevent the need for autogenous harvesting. As new materials become available, predictability, ease of use, and cost are some of the most important factors.

Indications for the Use of the Procedure

Changes in alveolar ridge dimensions occur in well-defined patterns. If not corrected, these alterations can lead to unfavorable functional and esthetic results. Ridge augmentation procedures and site preservation are intended to correct such deformities so as to maximize the functional and esthetic outcome of dental implant therapy.

Socket Augmentation

The main indication for socket augmentation is to minimize the remodeling of hard and soft tissue that occurs after tooth extraction. Placement of a graft material into a socket allows for stability of the blood clot and provides a scaffolding for new bone formation.[18] Unfortunately, remodeling of the socket occurs even if the site is grafted because the bundle bone present in the crest and inner portion of the socket is resorbed and replaced by woven bone.[4]

Socket augmentation has been shown to decrease the amount of horizontal and vertical bone loss, implant marginal bone loss, and esthetic soft tissue support when compared to no augmentation in both anterior and posterior sites.[19–22] When a simple socket augmentation is performed, there is no need to obtain primary closure or use a resorbable collagen membrane. When the buccal bone is missing, the four-wall defect is now a three- or two-wall defect, which will require a collagen membrane to promote GBR and prevent soft tissue ingrowth.[23–26]

Guided Bone Regeneration for Vertical and Horizontal Defects

Remodeling after tooth extraction can have devastating effects on the contours of the alveolar ridge and may prevent dental implant placement. In some instances, to achieve optimal functional and esthetic outcomes, regeneration of the defects must be accomplished. GBR, in association with dental implant procedures, can be used to augment deficient alveolar ridges, to cover implant fenestrations and dehiscences, to allow immediate implant placement in residual osseous defects and postextraction sites, and to treat peri-implant disease.[13,27–29] These defects may be localized to a single tooth or may extend to multiple teeth. If the defect is horizontal, it may lead to thread exposure, dehiscence, or fenestration. Ideally, the residual ridge width should be no less than 6 mm for a 4-mm diameter implant.[30] If the defect is vertical, it may lead to the placement of shorter implants than desired, long clinical crowns, and unesthetic results. Net bone gain reports after GBR procedures are scarce. For vertical GBR, bone augmentation can range from 2 to 7 mm, and for horizontal GBR, from 2 to 4.5 mm.[31]

Autogenous or alloplastic block grafts may be used in place of particulate bone. Although studies show no difference in bone gain between the two, autogenous block grafting may have additional risks and disadvantages such as donor site morbidity or increased chair time, and are more technique-sensitive.[32] In recent years, autologous platelet concentrates have been introduced and utilized for several oral reconstructive procedures, including socket, ridge and maxillary sinus augmentation. Although data on platelet concentrates to improve outcomes in bone gain are minimal, evidence seems to support its ability to enhance soft tissue closure and reduce postoperative discomfort.[33]

Limitations and Contraindications

With any surgical procedure, limitations are determined by biology itself. The healing mechanisms after injury (in this case, ridge augmentation procedures) are very similar from patient to patient. The difference is in the individual's ability to heal. Age, certain systemic diseases, medications, social habits, and oral hygiene habits play key roles in the individual's healing potential. Clinicians should consider these factors before recommending treatment for their patients. In addition, some limitations apply to the procedure itself. Socket augmentation does not prevent remodeling after tooth extraction, but it may minimize it. GBR procedures are limited in the amount of bone that can be generated. When GBR alone cannot fulfill the requirements of the defect, an alternative technique should be selected, such as distraction osteogenesis or an interpositional graft.

No matter which grafting technique is utilized, soft tissue management is the key to successful bone regeneration. An adequate zone of keratinized mucosa and tension-free closure of the flap margins minimize or prevent wound dehiscence. Soft tissue should be examined carefully before GBR procedures are initiated. In some instances, it may be necessary to improve the quality and quantity of soft tissue before regenerative procedures are performed. If the patient has significant medical problems, is a smoker, or has a previously failed graft or implant, vascularity is likely compromised and longer healing times may be required. In cases where multiple procedures are required, they should be performed one at a time to make sure that appropriate healing takes place.

Wound dehiscence and infection are the most common complications in GBR and can lead to partial or total graft loss.

TECHNIQUE: Socket Augmentation

STEP 1: Tooth Extraction

After administration of a local anesthetic, the tooth should be removed with as little trauma as possible. To achieve this, a periotome can be used to carefully luxate the tooth (Fig. 25.1A). The periotome should be used only in the interproximal spaces to prevent buccal plate damage. A gentle but firm rocking movement in the buccal-lingual direction should be applied to widen the periodontal ligament space. If needed, an elevator can be used to further luxate the tooth. After adequate luxation, a pair of forceps can be used to remove the tooth. For maxillary anterior teeth, apical pressure and careful rotation allow for successful extraction, maintaining an intact buccal plate. If teeth fracture or cannot be removed intact with a pair of forceps, a small fissure bur can be used to remove part of the root and create space for the periotome or small elevator. Once the tooth has been removed, the socket should be cleared of any remaining granulation tissue with an excavator and thorough irrigation.

STEP 2: Graft Placement

The selection of the graft material is at the surgeon's discretion. The material should be evenly distributed in the socket and lightly condensed. Care must be taken not to crush the material because this may alter its properties. It is important not to fill the extraction socket above the bone level because this will prohibit the placement of the collagen plug and cause more difficulty with suturing.

STEP 3: Closure

A resorbable cellulose or collagen plug can be used as a dressing to facilitate wound closure and prevent extrusion of the graft material. A figure-eight 4-0 chromic gut suture is placed to secure the graft and dressing (Fig. 25.1B). In the anterior maxilla or a very thin gingival biotype, a 5-0 chromic gut suture on a small needle can be utilized. When the buccal plate is missing from the extraction socket or it is traumatized during the extraction procedure, it becomes a GBR procedure. A Woodson or periosteal elevator is used to reflect the periosteum and gingiva from the underlying buccal bony walls adjacent to the extraction socket (Fig. 25.2A). A resorbable collagen membrane is trimmed to fit the buccal defect, making sure the edges overlap the bony margins anterior and posterior to the buccal socket defect (Fig. 25.2B). The particulate bone graft material can then be lightly packed inferior and buccal against the membrane (Fig. 25.2C). The graft will still come to the level of bone on the adjacent teeth and allow adequate space for the collagen plug as a dressing over the graft material (Fig. 25.2D).

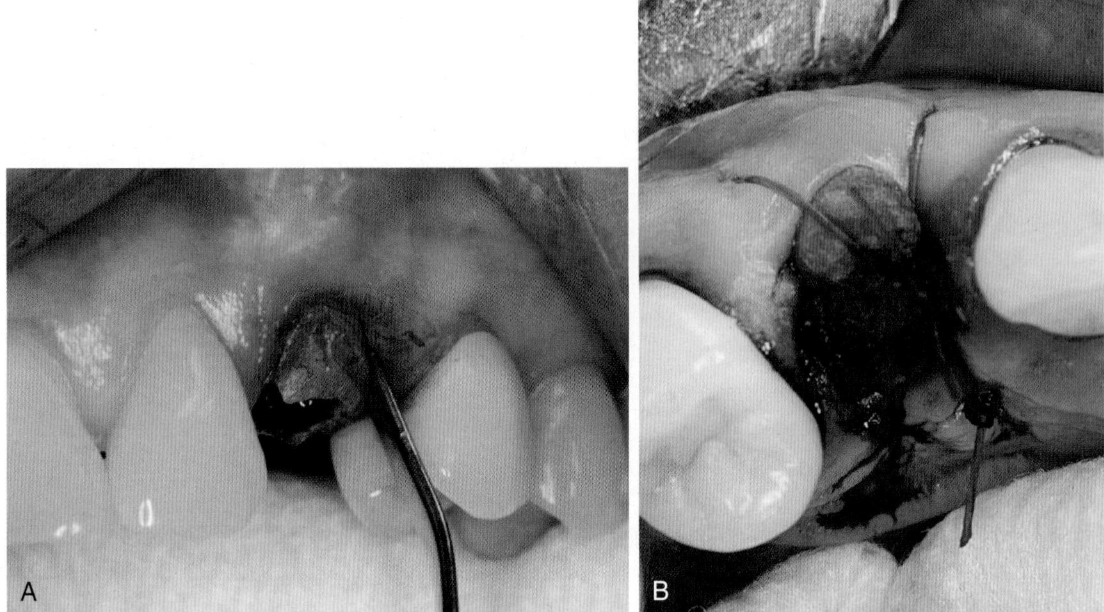

Figure 25.1 **A,** A periotome is used interproximally to carefully luxate the tooth. **B,** A collagen plug and figure-eight suture are used to contain the graft material.

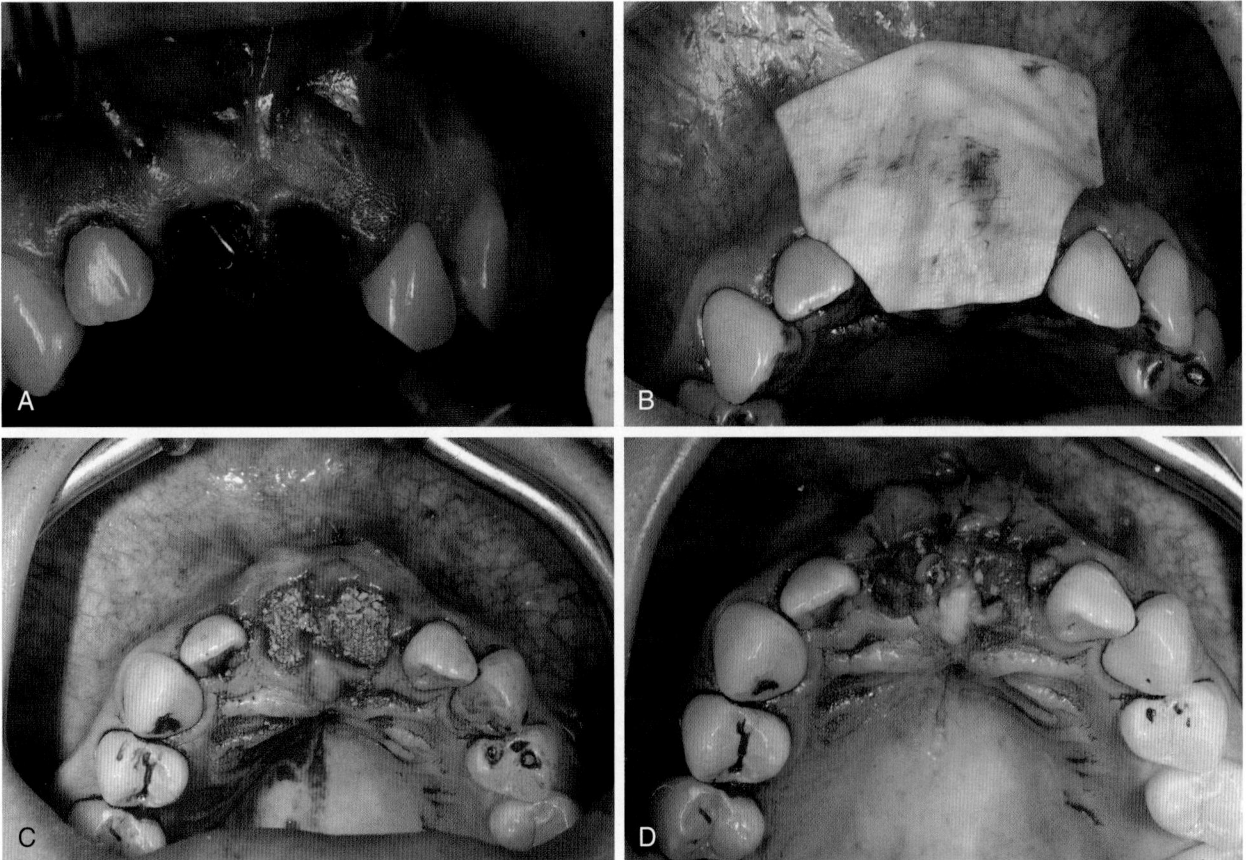

Figure 25.2 **A,** Subperiosteal dissection to identify buccal bone margin. **B,** Contouring collagen barrier membrane. **C,** Particulate grafting material in sockets. **D,** Collagen plug and crestal sutures.

TECHNIQUE: Guided Bone Regeneration for Horizontal Defects

STEP 1: Flap Design

Before surgery, careful consideration should be given to the flap design. As mentioned, a key factor for successful bone regeneration in ridge augmentation procedures is primary closure. In anticipation of the augmentation, the flap should have enough laxity to allow tension-free closure. Similarly, blood supply plays a key role in wound healing and should be taken into consideration. For that purpose, a trapezoid-shaped flap with a wide base is recommended.

STEP 2: Incision

After administration of a local anesthetic, a full-thickness crestal incision is made within the keratinized gingiva. The incision is carried out in a sulcular fashion, extending to at least one adjacent tooth on either side of the defect or to the distal end in an edentulous space. Vertical releasing incisions are made at the mesial-buccal and distal-buccal line angles or at the distal aspect of the crestal incision in an edentulous space. In esthetic areas, papilla-sparing incisions can be made to prevent interproximal soft tissue loss around existing full-coverage restorations (Fig. 25.3A). Next, elevation of the flap begins with a Woodson elevator at the crest and mesial and distal line angles, followed by release of the periosteum with a periosteal elevator. Care should be taken not to damage adjacent vessels or nerves or the flap itself.

STEP 3: Creation of Vascular Channels

Providing vascular channels from the recipient bed is the key to ensuring an adequate flow of nutrients to the graft. A bone-scraping instrument can be used to decorticate the recipient bed and collect autogenous shavings that can be mixed with the graft material. Next, a #701 fissure bur can be used to create vascular channels. The distribution of these channels should provide the maximum blood supply to the graft. Again, care should be taken not to damage adjacent teeth, vessels, or nerves or the flap itself (Fig. 25.3B).

STEP 4: Graft Delivery

The graft should be delivered in small quantities to allow for appropriate placement and to prevent extrusion of any graft particles into the flap. Loose particles within the confines of the flap can trigger an inflammatory reaction that could be detrimental to the healing process. The graft material should be mildly condensed; however, as mentioned, care must be taken to avoid crushing the particles because this may alter their properties (Fig. 25.3C).

STEP 5: Securing the Membrane

Fixation of the membrane allows better containment of the graft material. The membrane should be trimmed so that it adapts to the recipient bed, and the surgeon must make sure the edges do not come in contact with the vertical releasing incisions. The edges of the membrane should be 2 mm from such incisions. Fixation pins, tacks, or screws can be used to prevent movement of the membrane during the healing period. The number of fixation pins used depends on the size and design of the membrane. Larger membranes may require three to five pins, whereas two or three pins may suffice for smaller membranes (Fig. 25.3D). For the regeneration of large defects, a rigid structure may be required to maintain the space. This can be achieved with nonresorbable structures like titanium mesh (Fig. 25.4) or nonresorbable, titanium-reinforced PTFE membranes (Fig. 25.5).

STEP 6: Wound Closure

Adequate wound closure is of utmost importance for optimal outcomes. Tension-free closure should be achieved to prevent wound dehiscence and infection. For this purpose, periosteal releasing incisions can be made, taking into account adjacent vessels or nerves. A modified release via the tunnel approach may be used to eliminate the risk of nerve damage and significantly improve flap mobility and wound closure (Fig. 25.6).

Then, 4-0 Vicryl or chromic sutures are placed on the crestal portion of the flap in a horizontal mattress or an interrupted fashion to allow for adequate approximation of the flap edges. Vertical releasing incisions can be closed with single interrupted or continuous locking 5-0 chromic sutures. Small-caliber sutures in the unattached mucosa can help with postoperative discomfort (Fig. 25.3E).

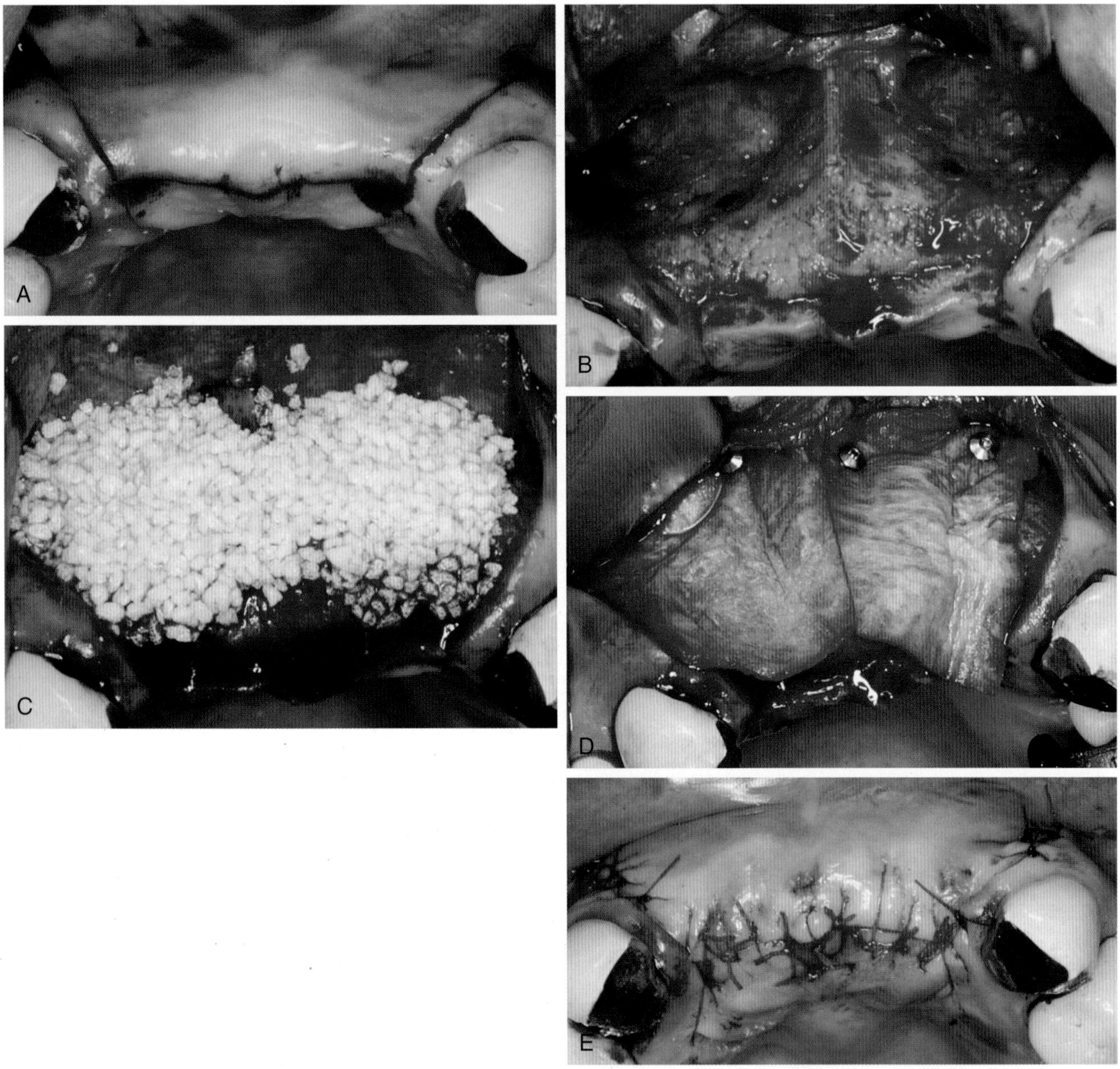

Figure 25.3 **A,** Midcrestal and papilla-sparing incisions with vertical releases extending to the vestibule. **B,** Vascular channels created with a #701 bur to provide nutrients to the graft. **C,** Graft material in place. **D,** Two resorbable membranes have been secured with fixation pins to contain the graft material. **E,** Closure is obtained with 4-0 Vicryl sutures in a horizontal mattress fashion and 4-0 and 5-0 interrupted chromic sutures.

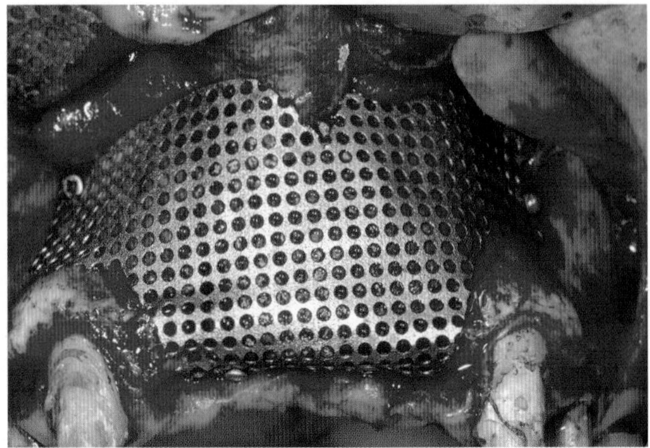

Figure 25.4 Titanium mesh in place, fixated with screws superiorly on the buccal aspect, and on the palatal or crestal bone to prevent movement and dehiscence.

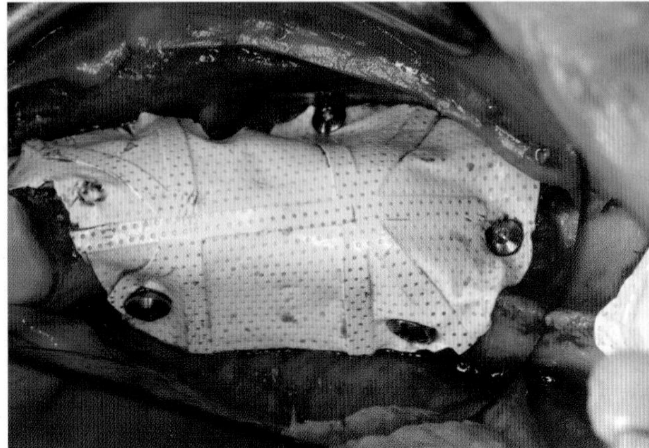

Figure 25.5 Nonresorbable, titanium-reinforced polytetrafluoroethylene (PTFE) membrane to maintain space for vertical augmentation or large horizontal augmentation.

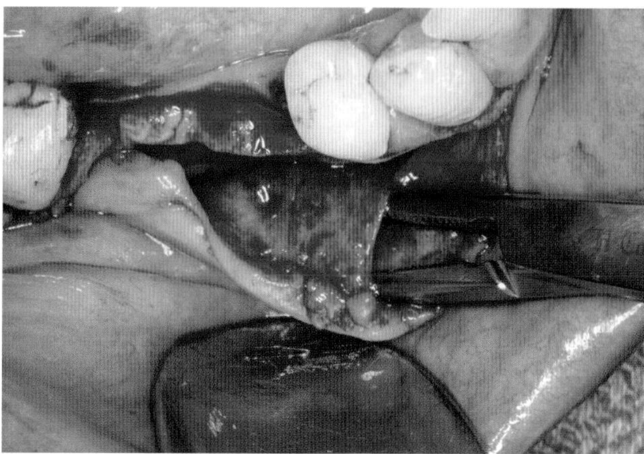

Figure 25.6 Periosteal releasing incision via dissection through a vertical incision on the inner surface of the flap. This avoids multiple small incisions and inadvertent trauma to vital structures (such as the mental nerve).

ALTERNATIVE TECHNIQUE 1: Guided Bone Regeneration for Vertical Defects

GBR for vertical defects may be needed when vital anatomic structures may limit the placement of implants of adequate length. This can lead to unfavorable crown-to-implant ratios and unesthetic results. GBR for vertical augmentation can be achieved alone or simultaneously with implant placement. The same principles described in steps 1, 2, and 3 can be used for this modification. For vertical regeneration, a tenting effect is required to provide space for new bone formation, which prevents the membrane from collapsing due to the pressure exerted by the soft tissue. This can be achieved either by the implant itself (providing supracrestal placement for a tenting effect) or by tenting screws (Fig. 25.7).

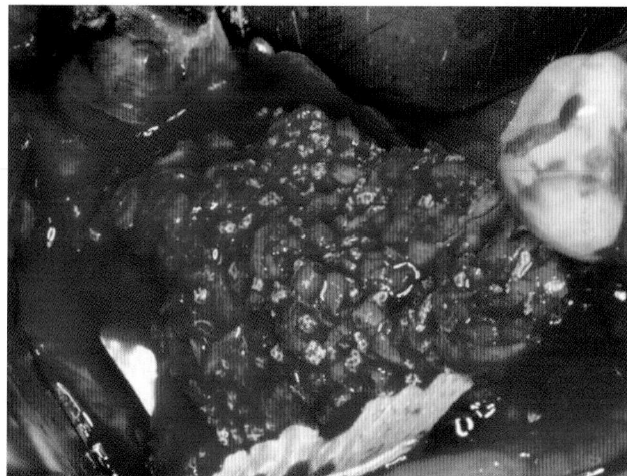

Figure 25.7 Vertical guided bone regeneration (GBR). Implants have been placed to provide a tenting effect. The site is grafted with a combination of autogenous bone and an alloplastic material.

ALTERNATIVE TECHNIQUE 2: Guided Bone Regeneration With Implant Placement

GBR can also be achieved simultaneously with implant placement. To determine whether these two procedures can be combined, the surgeon must assess the residual ridge. If primary stability of the implant cannot be achieved, a staged approach should be used. Vascular channels should be created before implant placement to prevent damage to the implant itself. Primary wound closure is a requirement for successful regeneration; therefore, a two-stage approach should be considered. It has been recommended that augmentation of the defect be performed in two layers.[34] For optimal long-term results, the layer in direct contact with the implant surface should be composed of autogenous bone harvested from the local site; the layer on top of this should be composed of the bone substitute of choice (Fig. 25.8). A barrier membrane (resorbable or non-resorbable) should be utilized in these cases to prevent soft tissue migration.

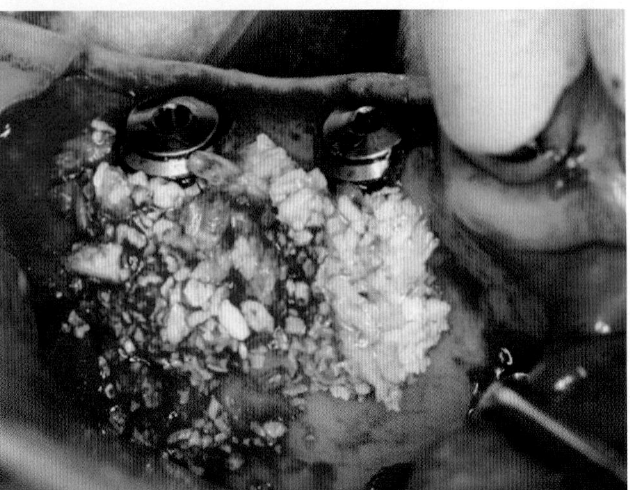

Figure 25.8 Implant placement and simultaneous guided bone regeneration (GBR). Autogenous bone shavings obtained from a bone scraper are placed in contact with the exposed implant surface. A xenograft is placed on top to provide long-term stability.

Avoidance and Management of Intraoperative Complications

The most important factor in achieving predictable outcomes with GBR is primary closure of the wound. Wound dehiscence is the most commonly reported complication.[35] To prevent wound dehiscence, a number of preoperative, intraoperative, and postoperative factors must be considered.

Preoperative Factors

Some systemic diseases, such as diabetes and chronic corticosteroid therapy, radiation therapy, and antiresorptive medications, may jeopardize wound healing. Social habits such as smoking, excessive alcohol consumption, and recreational drug use also can interfere with the wound healing process. Adequate oral hygiene habits before surgery can help minimize plaque accumulation and bacterial contamination.

Intraoperative Factors

As with any other surgical procedure, adequate flap design and clean, sharp incisions should be considered. Adequate muscle and flap release should allow sufficient flap elongation to achieve tension-free closure. Soft tissues should be handled with kindness, and special care should be taken when releasing the buccal tissues in the lower jaw to avoid nerve injury. Adequate barrier fixation and mattress sutures prevent displacement of the membrane and wound dehiscence.

Postoperative Factors

Instructing the patient in proper oral hygiene habits can help minimize plaque accumulation and bacterial contamination during the postoperative period. Antibiotic and antiinflammatory medications can decrease the chances of infection and reduce wound tension. Removable prostheses should be avoided to prevent membrane exposure.

Postoperative Considerations

Oral antibiotics and pain medication should be prescribed to prevent infection and to manage postoperative pain. Postoperative edema, hematoma, and bleeding are common with these procedures, and patients should be advised accordingly. Patients also should be advised not to use a toothbrush around the wound for at least 1 week to prevent wound dehiscence. Rinses with a bacteriostatic/bactericidal agent are recommended to minimize bacterial accumulation on sutures. A nonchewing diet should be recommended.

Use of a removable prosthesis over the grafted site is strongly discouraged. Unless otherwise indicated, follow-up visits should be scheduled for 1 week and 2 weeks after surgery for monitoring of wound healing. Sutures should not be removed before 1 week, and it is recommended that they be left in place for 2 weeks whenever possible. If resorbable sutures, such as Vicryl are utilized, they should dissolve in less than 2 to 3 weeks.

References

1. Euler H. Die heilung von extraktionswunden. *Deut Mschr Zahnk.* 1923;41:685.
2. Clafin R. Healing of disturbed and undistrubed extraction wounds. *J Am Dent Assoc.* 1936;23:945.
3. Pietrokovski J, Massler M. Alveolar ridge resorption following tooth extraction. *J Prosthet Dent.* 1967;17(1):21–27.
4. Araújo MG, Lindhe J. Dimensional ridge alterations following tooth extraction. An experimental study in the dog. *J Clin Periodontol.* 2005;32(2):212–218.
5. Cohen E. Socket preservation. In: Cohen E, ed. *Atlas of Cosmetic and Reconstructive Periodontal Surgery.* Philadelphia, PA: Lippincott, Williams, and Wilkins; 1988:347–363.
6. Vignoletti F, Matesanz P, Rodrigo D, Figuero E, Martin C, Sanz M. Surgical protocols for ridge preservation after tooth extraction. A systematic review. *Clin Oral Implants Res.* 2012;23(suppl 5):22–38.
7. Melcher AH. On the repair potential of periodontal tissues. *J Periodontol.* 1976;47(5):256–260.
8. Nyman S, Lindhe J, Karring T, Rylander H. New attachment following surgical treatment of human periodontal disease. *J Clin Periodontol.* 1982;9(4):290–296.
9. Urban IA, Monje A. Guided bone regeneration in alveolar bone reconstruction. *Oral Maxillofac Surg Clin North Am.* 2019;31(2):331–338.
10. Naung NY, Shehata E, Van Sickels JE. Resorbable versus nonresorbable membranes: when and why? *Dent Clin North Am.* 2019;63(3):419–431.
11. Rakhmatia YD, Ayukawa Y, Furuhashi A, Koyano K. Current barrier membranes: titanium mesh and other membranes for guided bone regeneration in dental applications. *J Prosthodont Res.* 2013;57(1):3–14.
12. Dahlin C, Lekholm U, Linde A. Membrane-induced bone augmentation at titanium implants. A report on ten fixtures followed from 1 to 3 years after loading. *Int J Periodontics Restorative Dent.* 1991;11(4):273–281.
13. Simion M, Trisi P, Piattelli A. Vertical ridge augmentation using a membrane technique associated with osseointegrated implants. *Int J Periodontics Restorative Dent.* 1994;14(6):496–511.
14. Buser D, Dula K, Belser U, Hirt HP, Berthold H. Localized ridge augmentation using guided bone regeneration. 1. Surgical procedure in the maxilla. *Int J Periodontics Restorative Dent.* 1993;13(1):29–45.
15. Aghaloo TL, Moy PK. Which hard tissue augmentation techniques are the most successful in furnishing bony support for implant placement? *Int J Oral Maxillofac Implants.* 2007;22(suppl):49–70.
16. Fillingham Y, Jacobs J. Bone grafts and their substitutes. *Bone Joint Lett J.* 2016;98-B(1)(suppl A):6–9.
17. Elnayef B, Porta C, Suárez-López Del Amo F, Mordini L, Gargallo-Albiol J, Hernández-Alfaro F. The fate of lateral ridge augmentation: a systematic review and meta-analysis. *Int J Oral Maxillofac Implants.* 2018;33(3):622–635.
18. Cardaropoli G, Araújo M, Hayacibara R, Sukekava F, Lindhe J. Healing of extraction sockets and surgically produced—augmented and non-augmented—defects in the alveolar ridge. An experimental study in the dog. *J Clin Periodontol.* 2005;32(5):435–440.
19. Marconcini S, Giammarinaro E, Derchi G, Alfonsi F, Covani U, Barone A. Clinical outcomes of implants placed in ridge-preserved versus nonpreserved sites: a 4-year randomized clinical trial. *Clin Implant Dent Relat Res.* 2018;20(6):906–914.
20. Lim HC, Shin HS, Cho IW, Koo KT, Park JC. Ridge preservation in molar extraction sites with an open-healing approach: a randomized controlled clinical trial. *J Clin Periodontol.* 2019;46(11):1144–1154.
21. Nevins M, Camelo M, De Paoli S, et al. A study of the fate of the buccal wall of extraction sockets of teeth with prominent roots. *Int J Periodontics Restorative Dent.* 2006;26(1):19–29.
22. Iasella JM, Greenwell H, Miller RL, et al. Ridge preservation with freeze-dried bone allograft and a collagen membrane compared to extraction alone for implant site development: a clinical and histologic study in humans. *J Periodontol.* 2003;74(7):990–999.
23. Castro AB, Meschi N, Temmerman A, et al. Regenerative potential of leucocyte- and platelet-rich fibrin. Part B: sinus floor elevation, alveolar ridge preservation and implant therapy. A systematic review. *J Clin Periodontol.* 2017;44(2):225–234.
24. Sun DJ, Lim HC, Lee DW. Alveolar ridge preservation using an open membrane approach for sockets with bone deficiency: a randomized controlled clinical trial. *Clin Implant Dent Relat Res.* 2019;21(1):175–182.
25. Sharma A, Ingole S, Deshpande M, et al. Influence of platelet-rich fibrin on wound healing and bone regeneration after tooth extraction: a clinical and radiographic study. *J Oral Biol Craniofac Res.* 2020;10(4):385–390.
26. Faria-Almeida R, Astramskaite-Januseviciene I, Puisys A, Correia F. Extraction socket preservation with or without membranes, soft tissue influence on post extraction alveolar ridge preservation: a systematic review. *J Oral Maxillofac Res.* 2019;10(3):e5.
27. Rocchietta I, Simion M, Hoffmann M, Trisciuoglio D, Benigni M, Dahlin C. Vertical bone augmentation with an autogenous block or particles in combination with guided bone regeneration: a clinical and histological preliminary study in humans. *Clin Implant Dent Relat Res.* 2016;18(1):19–29.
28. Benic GI, Eisner BM, Jung RE, Basler T, Schneider D, Hämmerle CHF. Hard tissue changes after guided bone regeneration of peri-implant defects comparing block versus particulate bone substitutes: 6-month results of a randomized controlled clinical trial. *Clin Oral Implants Res.* 2019;30(10):1016–1026.
29. Wessing B, Lettner S, Zechner W. Guided bone regeneration with collagen membranes and particulate graft materials: a systematic review and Meta-Analysis. *Int J Oral Maxillofac Implants.* 2018;33(1):87–100.
30. Buser D, Martin W, Belser UC. Optimizing esthetics for implant restorations in the anterior maxilla: anatomic and surgical considerations. *Int J Oral Maxillofac Implants.* 2004;19(suppl):43–61.
31. Chiapasco M, Zaniboni M, Boisco M. Augmentation procedures for the rehabilitation of deficient edentulous ridges with oral implants. *Clin Oral Implants Res.* 2006;17(suppl 2):136–159.
32. Dasmah A, Thor A, Ekestubbe A, Sennerby L, Rasmusson L. Particulate vs. block bone grafts: three-dimensional changes in graft volume after reconstruction of the atrophic maxilla, a 2-year radiographic follow-up. *J Cranio-Maxillo-Fac Surg.* 2012;40(8):654–659.
33. Dai Y, Han XH, Hu LH, Wu HW, Huang SY, Lü YP. Efficacy of concentrated growth factors combined with mineralized collagen on quality of life and bone reconstruction of guided bone regeneration. *Regen Biomater.* 2020;7(3):313–320.
34. Buser D, Chappuis V, Bornstein MM, Wittneben JG, Frei M, Belser UC. Long-term stability of contour augmentation with early implant placement following single tooth extraction in the esthetic zone: a prospective, cross-sectional study in 41 patients with a 5- to 9-year follow-up. *J Periodontol.* 2013;84(11):1517–1527.
35. Lim G, Lin GH, Monje A, Chan HL, Wang HL. Wound healing complications following guided bone regeneration for ridge augmentation: a systematic review and meta-analysis. *Int J Oral Maxillofac Implants.* 2018;33(1):41–50.

CHAPTER 26

Distraction Osteogenesis for Height, Width, or Repositioning of the Alveolar Process

Ole T. Jensen, Zvi Laster, Amir Laviv, and Nardy Casap

Armamentarium

#9 Periosteal elevator
#15 Scalpel blade
Appropriate sutures
Bidimensional crest distracter
Bidimensional distracter driver
Bone graft substitutes (allograft, xenograft, alloplast, or autogenous bone)
Crest widener
Local anesthetic with vasoconstrictor
Minnesota retractor
Needle holder
Osteotomes
Piezosurgery knife
Thin tungsten bur
Tissue forceps
Titanium wire
Woodson elevator

History of the Procedure

Closely related to the principles of posttraumatic osseous repair, the development of distraction osteogenesis (DO) is an outstanding contribution from the work of Ilizarov.[1] The Russian surgeon developed innovative devices for skeletal fixation and osteotomy techniques that deliver minimal trauma to the periosteum and the bone marrow. His landmark set of clinical experiments led to the discovery of the biologic basis of osteodistraction, the Ilizarov effects, which suggest that gradual traction applied on living tissues can stimulate and maintain regeneration and active growth and that the mass and shape of bones and articulations depend on their blood supply and their functional burden. His studies later determined the technical protocols for DO and are still used as a basic reference for studies in this field.

Applications in craniofacial surgery were first seen in 1973, when Snyder et al.[2] applied the approach to mandibular lengthening in a canine animal model. Almost 20 years passed before McCarthy et al.[3] in 1992 published the first report of mandibular lengthening in children with congenital mandibular deficiency. Thereafter, the role of DO rapidly expanded to the midface and to nearly all classic approaches to craniofacial reconstruction. In humans, DO has been used for surgical palatal expansion,[4] mandibular symphysis elongation,[5] correction of congenital facial abnormalities,[6] treatment of cleft conditions,[7] repair of continuity defects of the mandible, alveolar crest augmentation,[8] and mandible reconstruction after tumor resection.[8,9]

Since the first case report on alveolar DO in the literature by Chin and Toth,[10] numerous case series[11–16] and clinical investigations,[17–19] in addition to two prospective clinical studies,[20,21] have been published. In addition, the idea of moving an entire edentulous jaw by distraction to reposition the alveolar process for definitive alveolar reconstruction is currently being addressed in the literature.[22,23,24]

Indications for the Use of the Procedure

After dental extractions, a rapid process of buccal plate resorption occurs. As result, very often the oral and maxillofacial surgeon encounters a ridge that has sufficient crestal bone height but is too narrow for implant insertion. In addition to augmentation by alveolar ridge split, onlay block, or guided bone regeneration, DO can be used to gain width for the alveolus.[22–26] The advantage of this technique is the *distraction histogenesis* of associated soft tissues, which provides sufficient keratinized tissue coverage of the increased volume of the expanded crest.[26]

Resorption of the alveolar crest takes place in all dimensions, yet can generally be thought of as bidimensional—vertical and horizontal.[27–29] In general, vertical bone loss seldom occurs strictly without considerable loss of bone in the horizontal dimension, with a resultant shift of alveolar bone mass to the lingual side.[30] Frequently, for both the maxilla and the mandible, a loss of buccal bone mass occurs initially, including the buccal crest. With further resorption, the lingual crest is lost and alveolar vertical bone loss develops. When vertical loss is 5 mm or more, vertical distraction is indicated.[10,31,32] However, because of vector control problems, vertical distraction of a typical alveolar segment further shifts the alveolar bone mass lingually.[33–35] Therefore, unidirectional distraction may improve crestal height, but it compromises alveolar position, preventing ideal implant placement. During the course of distraction, traction from the lingual/palatal periosteum, muscles, and attached gingiva prevents maintenance of an axial vector. One solution to this technical problem is to use a bidirectional device that moves the segment both vertically and buccally.[35]

The use of small, low-profile devices, which can be used without substantially interfering with the occlusal and esthetic functional requirements, enables the surgeon to manipulate small segments of osteotomized bone into more ideal positions for dental implant installation.[36] A bidirectional device, the bidimensional crest distracter (2DCD; Surgi-Tec, Bruges, Belgium), was designed to enable both vertical and horizontal distraction.[35] The device works in sequence, first by vertical distraction and then by horizontal distraction, to correct horizontal deflection.

Limitations and Contraindications

Total edentulous maxillary distraction, including full mandibular horseshoe alveolar distraction and maxillary Lefort I, has been used to gain vertical height and improve horizontal position, but these procedures have largely been supplanted by local osteotomies done either in the posterior or anterior part of the mouth to avoid major surgery.[37–40]

The surgeon must understand that alveolar form in the ablated condition is never ideal; therefore, the use of alveolar distraction is an intermediate step toward achieving orthoalveolar form. After DO, the alveolar process will likely need further reconstruction with bone graft material or sometimes soft tissue to be made suitable for dental implants.[31] Most often, bone grafting can be done at the same time as implant placement; however, in some cases the distraction is done in preparation of the soft-tissue envelope for a definitive grafting procedure.[41]

Once used extensively, alveolar distraction has declined in popularity with the development of osteoperiosteal flap procedures, particularly the alveolar split (book bone flap) and the sandwich osteotomy (interpositional graft) procedure.[42,43] The use of bone morphogenetic protein-2 (BMP-2) has increased the capability of both fixed osteoperiosteal flaps and those using bone transport achieved by DO. However, the fixed osteoperiosteal flap interpositional space is highly vascular and the use of conductive material such as xenograft has been shown to be highly successful.[44,45,46]

TECHNIQUE: Alveolar Width Distraction

A 67-year-old male was referred for bone augmentation of the upper left maxilla. Examination of a computed tomography (CT) scan reveals a residual ridge 2.6 mm wide. A horizontal distraction device or crest widener (e.g., Laster Crest Widener; M.I.S., Shlomi, Israel) is used to expand the alveolar crest. The crest widener consists of four associated arms, each couplet moving apart to separate the bone when activated. The advantage of the crest widener is that the periosteum is not stripped; thus, the blood supply to the distracted segment is not impaired (Fig. 26.1A–C).

STEP 1: Flap Design and Incision

Under local anesthesia, three transmucosal incisions are made—two vertical and a crestal cut 1 mm palatal to the peak of the crest—which define the borders of the buccal segment to be distracted (Fig. 26.1D).

STEP 2: Bony Cuts

A very thin tungsten bur is used to make bony cuts through the mucoperiosteal incisions without stripping the periosteum; the cuts are made halfway through the width of the crest. At the crest, an alveolar split vertical cut may extend up to 10 mm. These bony cuts may also be made using a piezo knife (Fig. 26.1E).

STEP 3: Buccal Plate Out-Fracture

An osteotome is used to split the buccal plate in an incomplete blowout fracture (book flap) (Fig. 26.1F).

STEP 4: Insertion of Crest Widener

The crest widener is inserted into the split crest and secured by a titanium safety wire ligated to an adjacent tooth (Fig. 26.1G).

STEP 5: Wound Closure

Tension-free closure should be achieved to prevent wound dehiscence and infection. Sutures (4-0 chromic), made in a horizontal mattress or interrupted fashion, are placed at the releasing incisions and, where possible, at the crestal (distracter) portion of the flap to allow for adequate approximation of the flap edges. Vertical releasing incisions can be closed with single interrupted or continuous locking 5-0 chromic sutures.

Continued

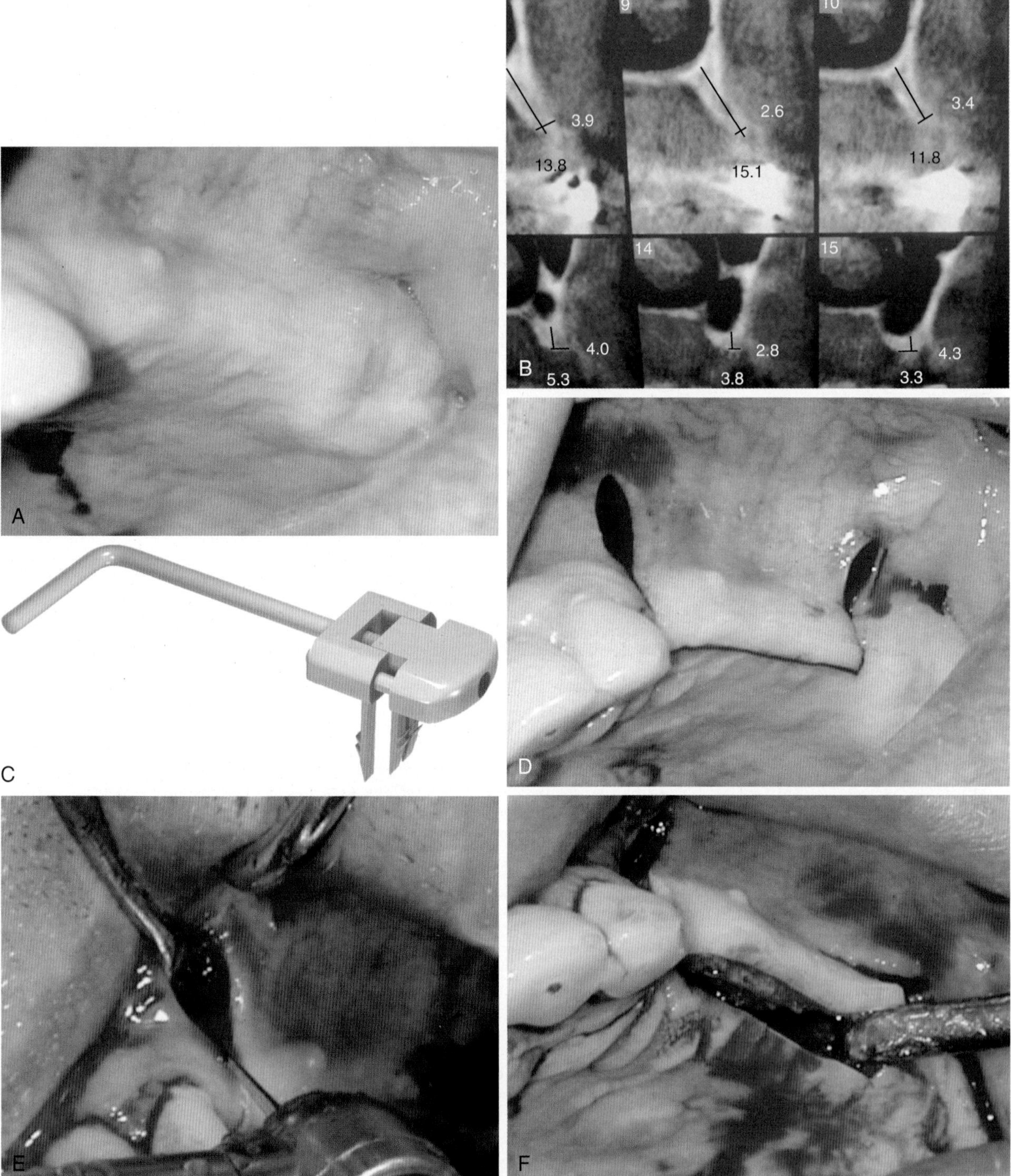

Figure 26.1 **A,** Preoperative clinical findings indicate a narrow ridge form. **B,** Examination of the computed tomography (CT) scan reveals a 2.6-mm width of the residual ridge. **C,** Crest widener. (Courtesy Cortex Dental Implants Industries, Ltd.) **D,** Three incisions define the buccal segment to be distracted. **E,** Bone cuts are made using a thin tungsten bur. **F,** Incomplete fracture of the buccal plate.

TECHNIQUE: Alveolar Width Distraction—cont'd

STEP 6: Latency and Activation Periods

After a latency period of 1 week, the patient is instructed to start activating the distracter one-quarter turn (0.3 mm) a day. After achieving sufficient width within 14 days, the activation is stopped (Fig. 26.1H).

STEP 7: Consolidation Period

Activation is stopped for a 2-week consolidation period. The crest widener is then removed under local anesthesia, and the soft tissue is left to heal for an additional 2 weeks (Fig. 26.1I).

STEP 8: Postoperative Assessment

The patient is referred for a postoperative CT scan before dental implant placement. The scan should reveal a wide crest with the facial plate pushed buccally and a still uncalcified callus in between (Fig. 26.1J–L).

STEP 9: Implant Placement

The expanded crest is now wide enough for transmucosal insertion of 4.2-mm dental implants. An indirect sinus floor intrusion is performed at the same time. Eight months later, the final restoration is finished (Fig. 26.1M–O).

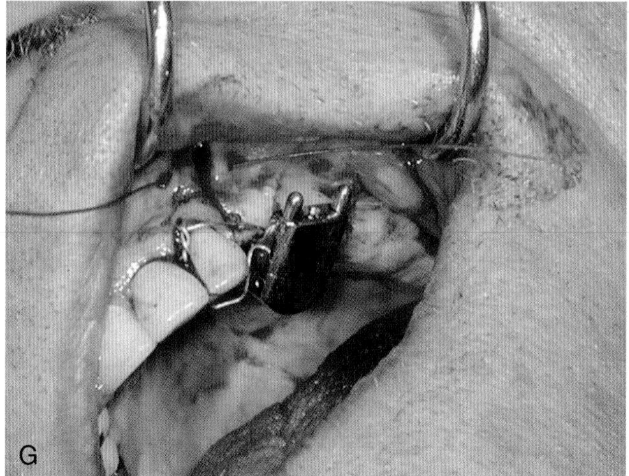

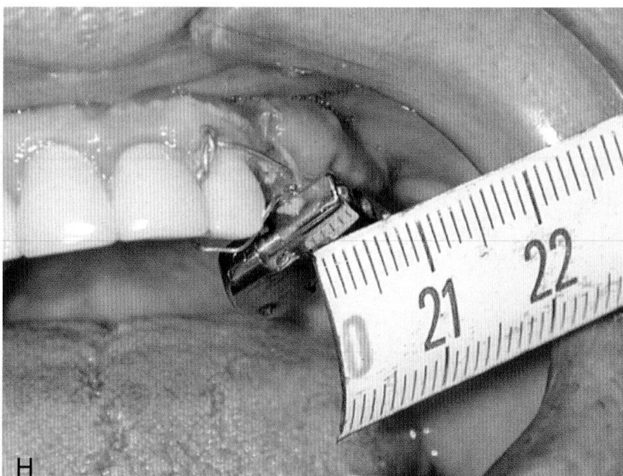

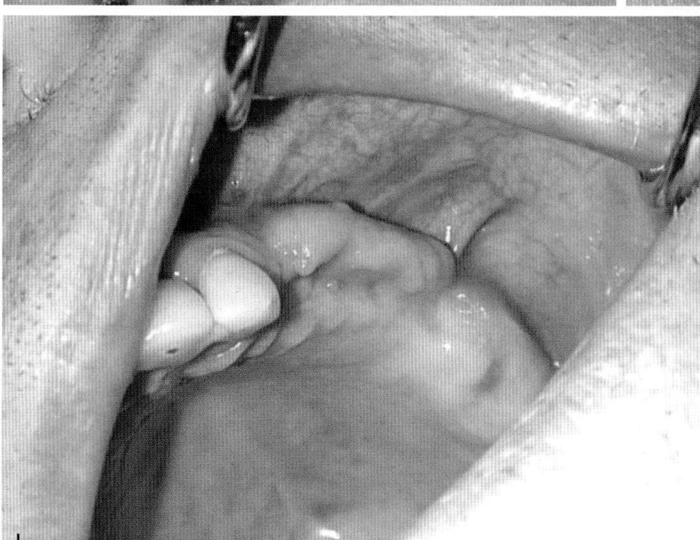

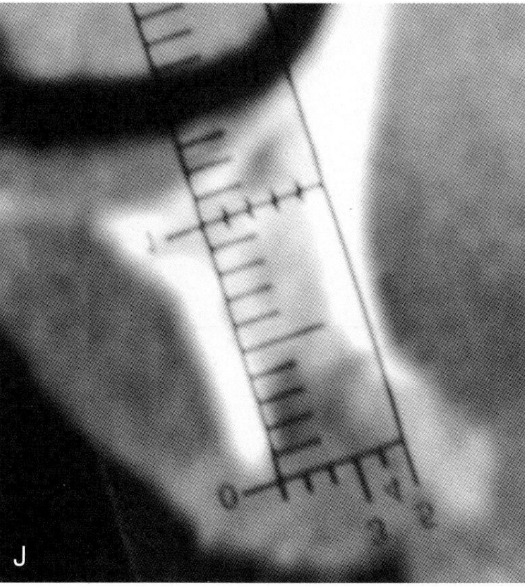

Figure 26.1, cont'd **G,** The crest widener is inserted and secured with a titanium wire to an adjacent tooth. **H,** Sufficient width is achieved within 14 days. **I,** Distracted site at 2 weeks after device removal. **J,** CT scan of the widened alveolar crest.

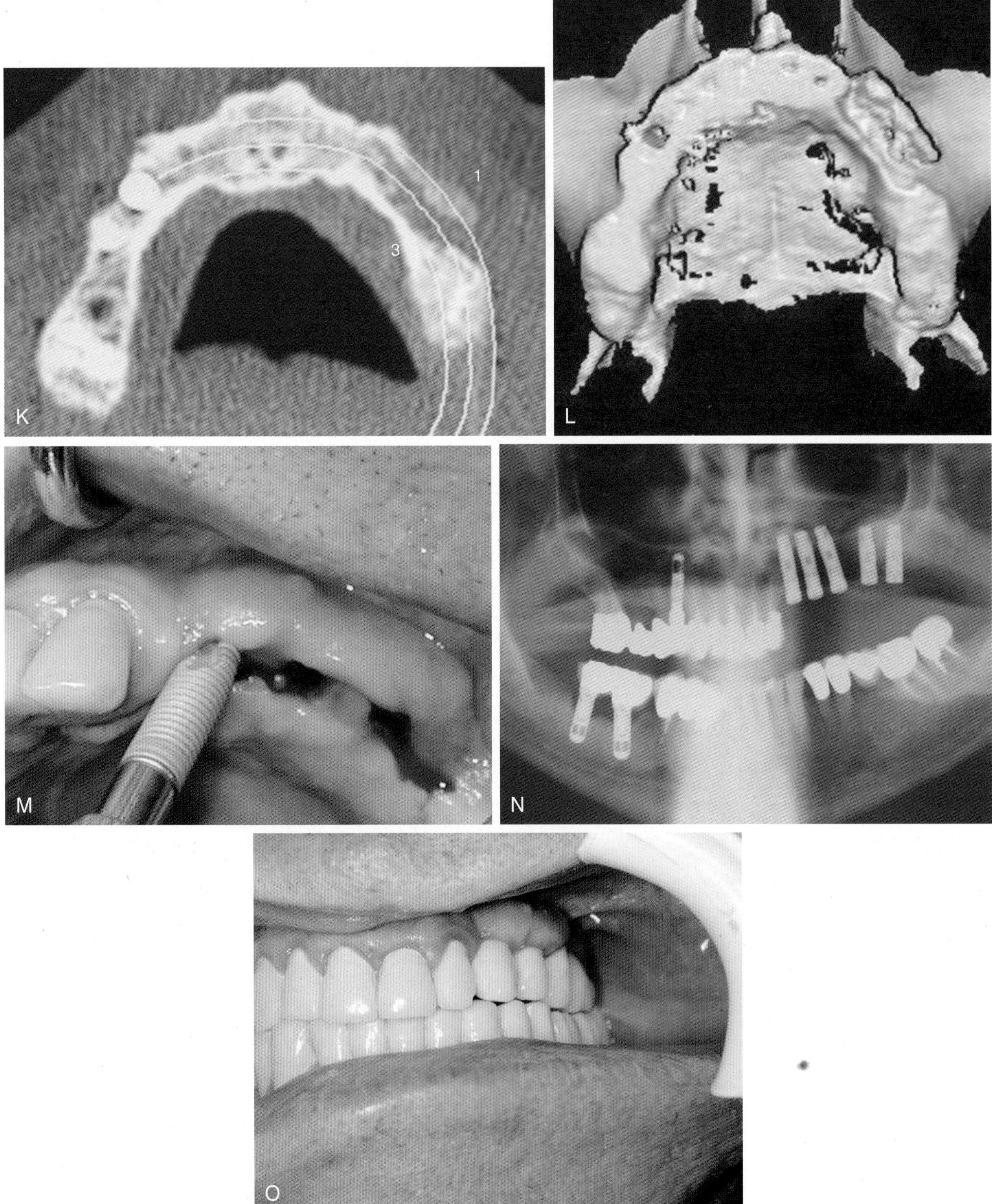

Figure 26.1, cont'd **K,** Axial CT scan shows the expanded crest. **L,** Three-dimensional reconstruction shows the distracted buccal plate with uncalcified woven bone in between. **M,** Implants 4.2 mm in diameter are inserted to the expanded crest. **N,** Radiograph taken after implantation and sinus lifting. **O,** Final restoration. (Ole T. Jensen, Zvi Laster, Amir Laviv, Nardy Casap)

MODIFIED TECHNIQUE: Bidimensional Distraction

A 35-year-old male is referred after two failed attempts to augment the missing alveolar crest resulting from a motor vehicle accident. The soft tissue has twice broken down over the graft site, indicating that an important reason for graft failure is the lack of viable soft tissue. DO is selected as the optimal choice for treatment of this highly compromised situation (Fig. 26.2A).

STEP 1: Osteotomy and Distracter Placement

Under general anesthesia, a segmental osteotomy is performed through a vestibular incision, and a bidirectional distracter (Surgi-Tec, Bruges, Belgium) is assembled and screwed into place. The device has a driver that is inserted through a hole at the top of the device. One full turn of the driver is equal to 0.8 mm of vertical distraction. The nuts on the screws that fix the distal segment, when tightened, move the segment buccally (Fig. 26.2B).

STEP 2: Latency Period

After a 1-week latency period, a panoramic radiograph is taken (Fig. 26.2C).

STEP 3: Vertical Activation Period

The distracter is then activated at a rate of 0.8 mm a day (one full turn). After 18 days of activation, nearly 15 mm of vertical height has been achieved (Fig. 26.2D).

Continued

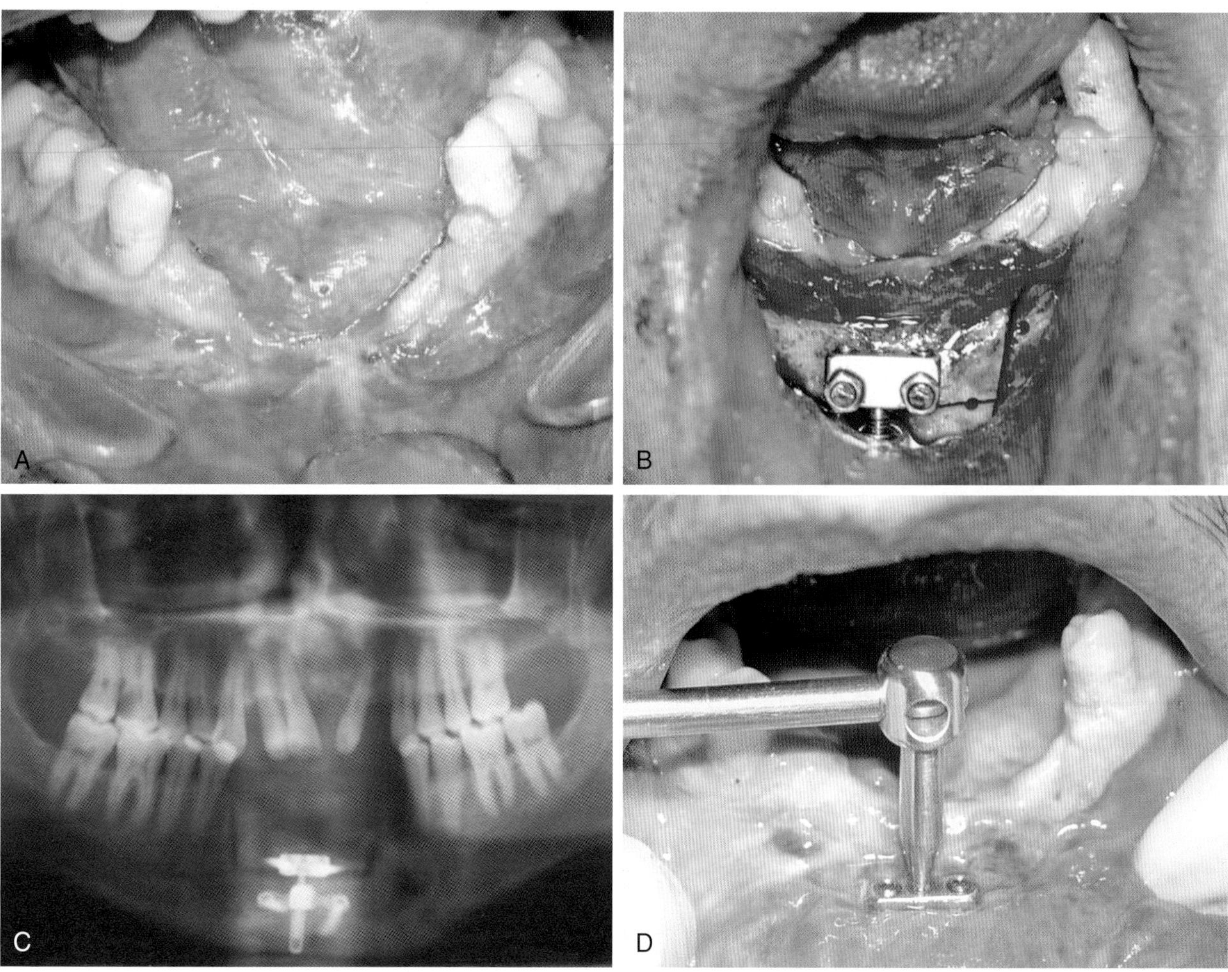

Figure 26.2 **A,** Preoperative findings demonstrate a vertical bone deficit greater than 10 mm and deficient and scarred soft tissues. **B,** Bidirectional distracter is assembled and placed on the buccal side. **C,** Panoramic radiograph showing the start position for segmental distraction. **D,** Horizontal distraction.

MODIFIED TECHNIQUE: Bidimensional Distraction—cont'd

STEP 4: Horizontal Activation Period

Because of lingual traction, the segment is then distracted facially (horizontally) by rotating the horizontal nuts on the fixation screws over a 5-day period. Sufficient alignment is achieved within 23 days of activation. A postdistraction panoramic radiograph is then obtained (Fig. 26.2E–G).

STEP 5: Consolidation Period

After 2 months of consolidation, the distracter is removed under local anesthesia. Three weeks later, implants are inserted, and the patient is sent back to the dentist for fabrication of the final restoration (Fig. 26.2H).

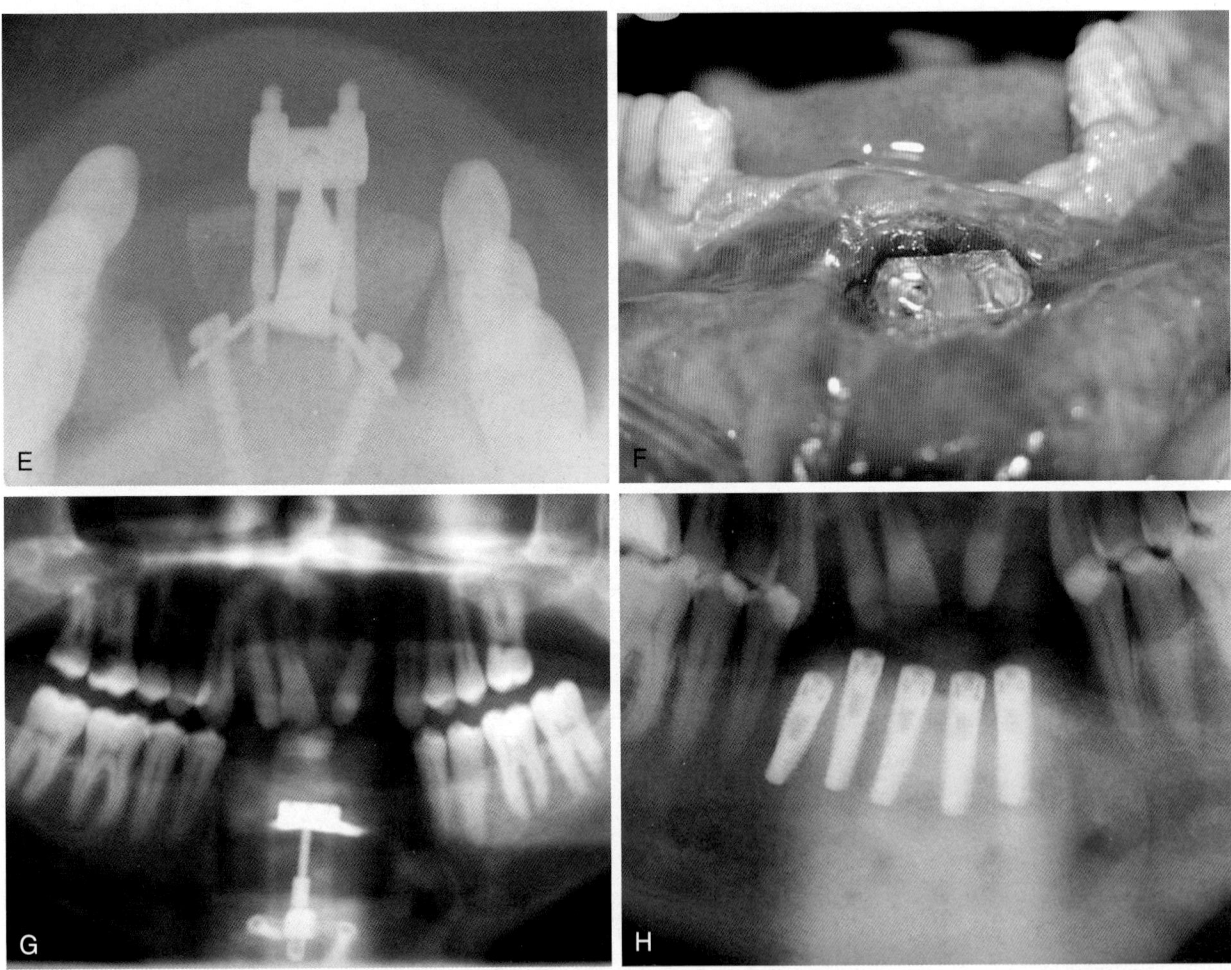

Figure 26.2, cont'd **E,** Vertical activation of the distracter halfway through treatment. **F,** Sufficient alignment is achieved within 23 days of activation. **G,** Panoramic radiograph showing that maximum height has been achieved. **H,** Five implants are inserted through the bone transport. (Ole T. Jensen, Zvi Laster, Amir Laviv, Nardy Casap)

Avoidance and Management of Intraoperative Complications

It is important not to strip mucosa from the residual alveolar crest or lingual mucosa during performance of the osteotomy or placement of the distraction device.[35,43,46] Also, it is important to avoid rents in the lingual mucosa when the osteotomy cuts are made; rents in the lingual pedicle are less likely if a sagittal saw is used. Although the piezo knife can cut bone well and is atraumatic to soft tissues, deeper bone cuts may actually burn the bone as a result of inadequate irrigation of the device at such depth.[47] One approach is to use the piezo knife to define the outer cut, then make deeper bone cuts with a saw or drill, and, finally, complete the separation with osteotomes.[48]

Postoperative Considerations

Extensive discussion on how and when to activate the distraction device is necessary to ensure the proper timing and direction of the distraction. Patients should understand that they will experience slight soreness in the region after activation. Oral antibiotics and pain medication should be prescribed to prevent infection and manage postoperative pain. Postoperative edema is common for these procedures, and patients should be advised accordingly. Patients should be advised not to use a toothbrush around the wound for at least 1 week to prevent wound dehiscence. Rinses with a bacteriostatic/bactericidal agent are recommended to minimize bacterial accumulation on the device. Unless otherwise indicated, follow-up visits should be scheduled for 1 week and 2 weeks after surgery for monitoring of wound healing.

One additional distraction procedure that should be mentioned is the idea to move an alveolus into position, usually horizontally. This can be achieved segmentally such as might be done with a segmental advancement osteotomy with interpositional bone graft or by a total alveolar approach such as repositioning an edentulous maxilla by DO. This is important because, in select cases, it may be the most conservative and least invasive method to achieve orthoalveolar form.

Fig. 26.3A–E shows the surgical technique for Lefort I edentulous maxilla in a younger patient who lost horizontal alveolar bone mass following dental extractions and placement of an immediate denture restoration. Here, the maxilla was subsequently distracted forward about 7 or 8 mm into an idealized position three-dimensionally, and then implants were placed later trans gingivally without additional hard or soft-tissue grafting. A late-term follow-up report found these procedures to be stable 13 years after DO surgery.[38,49,50]

In summary, the clinician should consider alveolar modification by DO to gain vertical height, width, or improved alveolar position. The use of traditional grafting methods sometimes has limitations that can more easily be overcome by the use of DO. In general, the use of any bone augmentation method should consider a method that is most likely to achieve the desired result using the least invasive approach possible, which sometimes will be alveolar DO.

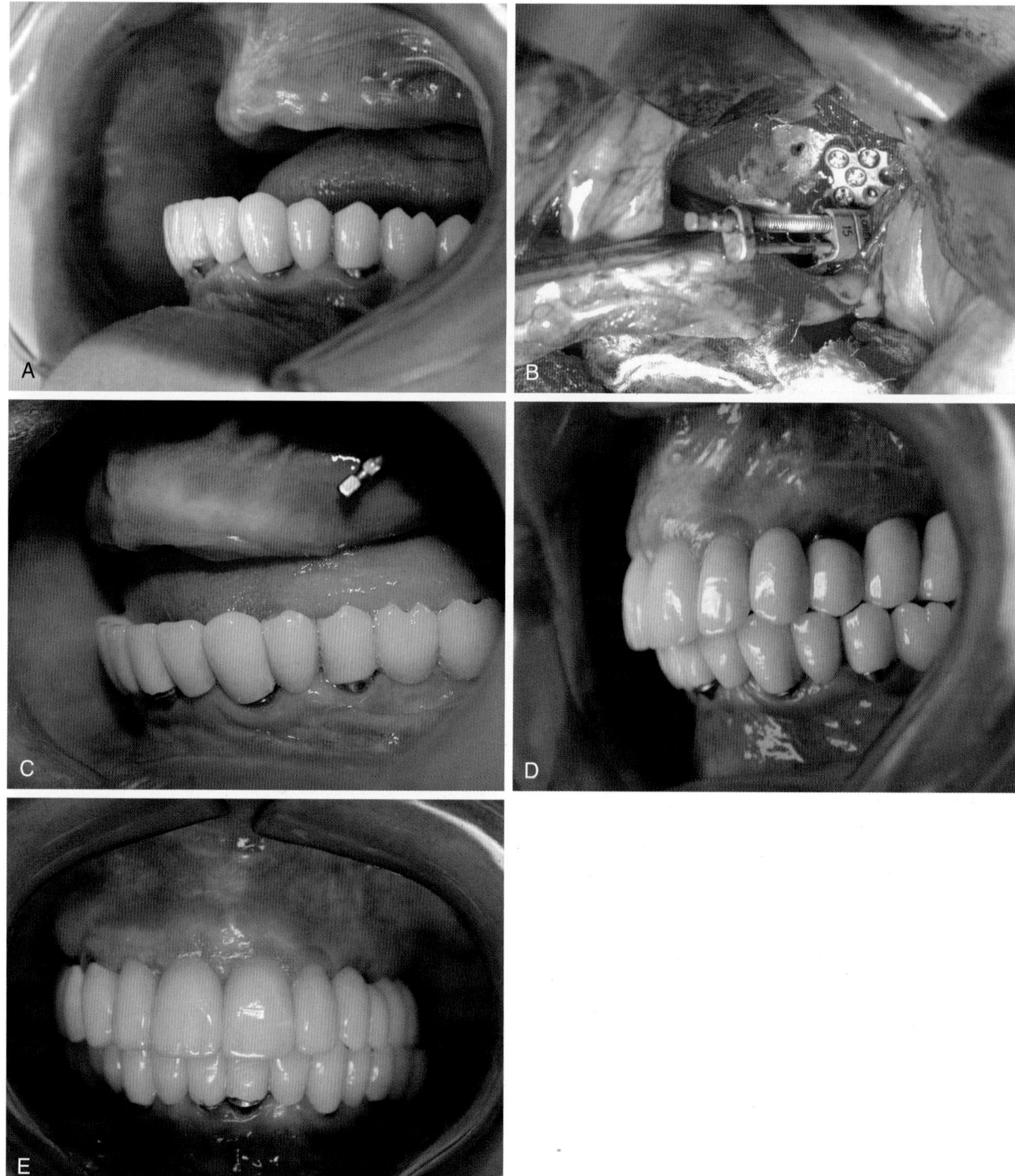

Figure 26.3 **A,** The preoperative retro-displaced maxilla in a younger female edentulous patient. **B,** The placement of a horizontal distractor (bilaterally) to move the maxilla forward and down. **C,** Postdistraction, about 2 weeks later, shows the maxilla in vertical alveolar alignment with the mandible. **D,** The postimplant restoration from a lateral view. **E,** The postimplant restoration from a frontal view showing emergence profile esthetics and orthoalveolar form. (Ole T. Jensen, Zvi Laster, Amir Laviv, Nardy Casap)

References

1. Ilizarov GA. The principles of the Ilizarov method. *Bull Hosp Jt Dis Orthop Inst.* 1988;48(1):1–11.
2. Snyder CC, Levine GA, Swanson HM, Browne Jr EZ. Mandibular lengthening by gradual distraction. Preliminary report. *Plast Reconstr Surg.* 1973;51(5):506–508.
3. McCarthy JG, Schreiber J, Karp N, Thorne CH, Grayson BH. Lengthening the human mandible by gradual distraction. *Plast Reconstr Surg.* 1992;89(1):1–8.
4. Bell WH, Epker BN. Surgical-orthodontic expansion of the maxilla. *Am J Orthod.* 1976;70(5):517–528.
5. Bell WH, Harper RP, Gonzalez M, Cherkashin AM, Samchukov ML. Distraction osteogenesis to widen the mandible. *Br J Oral Maxillofac Surg.* 1997;35(1):11–19.
6. Chin M. Distraction osteogenesis in maxillofacial surgery. In: Lynch SE, Genco RJ, Marx RE, eds. *Tissue Engineering: Applications in Maxillofacial Surgery and Periodontics.* Chicago, Illinois: Quintessence; 1999.
7. Wen-Ching Ko E, Figueroa AA, Polley JW. Soft tissue profile changes after maxillary advancement with distraction osteogenesis by use of a rigid external distraction device: a 1-year follow-up. *J Oral Maxillofac Surg.* 2000;58(9):959–969.
8. Chiapasco M, Brusati R, Galioto S. Distraction osteogenesis of a fibular revascularized flap for improvement of oral implant positioning in a tumor patient: a case report. *J Oral Maxillofac Surg.* 2000;58(12):1434–1440.
9. Fukuda M, Iino M, Yamaoka K, Ohnuki T, Nagai H, Takahashi T. Two-stage distraction osteogenesis for mandibular segmental defect. *J Oral Maxillofac Surg.* 2004;62(9):1164–1168.
10. Chin M, Toth BA. Distraction osteogenesis in maxillofacial surgery using internal devices: review of five cases. *J Oral Maxillofac Surg.* 1996;54(1):45–53.
11. Zaffe D, Bertoldi C, Palumbo C, Consolo U. Morphofunctional and clinical study on mandibular alveolar distraction osteogenesis. *Clin Oral Implants Res.* 2002;13(5):550–557.
12. McAllister BS. Histologic and radiographic evidence of vertical ridge augmentation utilizing distraction osteogenesis: 10 consecutively placed distractors. *J Periodontol.* 2001;72(12):1767–1779.
13. Rachmiel A, Srouji S, Peled M. Alveolar ridge augmentation by distraction osteogenesis. *Int J Oral Maxillofac Surg.* 2001;30(6):510–517.
14. Uckan S, Haydar SG, Dolanmaz D. Alveolar distraction: analysis of 10 cases. *Oral Surg Oral Med Oral Pathol Oral Radiol Endod.* 2002;94(5):561–565.
15. Raghoebar GM, Liem RS, Vissink A. Vertical distraction of the severely resorbed edentulous mandible: a clinical, histological and electron microscopic study of 10 treated cases. *Clin Oral Implants Res.* 2002;13(5):558–565.
16. Kunkel M, Wahlmann U, Reichert TE, Wegener J, Wagner W. Reconstruction of mandibular defects following tumor ablation by vertical distraction osteogenesis using intraosseous distraction devices. *Clin Oral Implants Res.* 2005;16(1):89–97.
17. Enislidis G, Fock N, Millesi-Schobel G, et al. Analysis of complications following alveolar distraction osteogenesis and implant placement in the partially edentulous mandible. *Oral Surg Oral Med Oral Pathol Oral Radiol Endod.* 2005;100(1):25–30.
18. Mazzonetto R, Serra E Silva FM, Ribeiro Torezan JF. Clinical assessment of 40 patients subjected to alveolar distraction osteogenesis. *Implant Dent.* 2005;14(2):149–153.
19. Gaggl A, Schultes G, Kärcher H. Vertical alveolar ridge distraction with prosthetic treatable distractors: a clinical investigation. *Int J Oral Maxillofac Implants.* 2000;15(5):701–710.
20. Jensen OT, Cockrell R, Kuhike L, Reed C. Anterior maxillary alveolar distraction osteogenesis: a prospective 5-year clinical study. *Int J Oral Maxillofac Implants.* 2002;17(1):52–68.
21. Chiapasco M, Consolo U, Bianchi A, Ronchi P. Alveolar distraction osteogenesis for the correction of vertically deficient edentulous ridges: a multicenter prospective study on humans. *Int J Oral Maxillofac Implants.* 2004;19(3):399–407.
22. Jensen OT. Distraction osteogenesis and its use with dental implants. *Dent Implantol Update.* 1999;10(5):33–36.
23. Khojasteh A, Behnia H, Shayesteh YS, Morad G, Alikhasi M. Localized bone augmentation with cortical bone blocks tented over different particulate bone substitutes: a retrospective study. *Int J Oral Maxillofac Implants.* 2012;27(6):1481–1493.
24. Block MS, Ducote CW, Mercante DE. Horizontal augmentation of thin maxillary ridge with bovine particulate xenograft is stable during 500 days of follow-up: preliminary results of 12 consecutive patients. *J Oral Maxillofac Surg.* 2012;70(6):1321–1330.
25. Jensen OT, Ellis III E. The book bone flap: a technical note. *J Oral Maxillofac Surg.* 2008;66(suppl):43.
26. Langer B, Langer L, Sullivan RM. Planned labial plate advancement with simultaneous single implant placement for narrow anterior ridges followed by reentry confirmation. *Int J Periodontics Restorative Dent.* 2012;32(5):509–519.
27. Sun Z, Herring SW, Tee BC, Gales J. Alveolar ridge reduction after tooth extraction in adolescents: an animal study. *Arch Oral Biol.* 2013;58(7):813–825.
28. Farmer M, Darby I. Ridge dimensional changes following single-tooth extraction in the aesthetic zone. *Clin Oral Implants Res.* 2014;25(2):272–277.
29. Vera C, De Kok IJ, Chen W, Reside G, Tyndall D, Cooper LF. Evaluation of post-implant buccal bone resorption using cone beam computed tomography: a clinical pilot study. *Int J Oral Maxillofac Implants.* 2012;27(5):1249–1257.
30. Barone A, Ricci M, Tonelli P, Santini S, Covani U. Tissue changes of extraction sockets in humans: a comparison of spontaneous healing vs. ridge preservation with secondary soft tissue healing. *Clin Oral Implants Res.* 2013;24(11):1231–1237.
31. Jensen OT, Cockrell R, Kuhlke L, Reed C. Anterior maxillary alveolar distraction osteogenesis: a prospective 5-year clinical study. *Int J Oral Maxillofac Implants.* 2002;17(1):52–68.
32. Jensen OT, Block M. Alveolar modification by distraction osteogenesis. *Atlas Oral Maxillofac Surg Clin North Am.* 2008;16(2):185–214.
33. Chiapasco M, Romeo E, Casentini P, Rimondini L. Alveolar distraction osteogenesis vs. vertical guided bone regeneration for the correction of vertically deficient edentulous ridges: a 1-3-year prospective study on humans. *Clin Oral Implants Res.* 2004;15(1):82–95.
34. Chin M. Distraction osteogenesis for dental implants. *Atlas Oral Maxillofac Surg Clin North Am.* 1999;7(1):41–63.
35. Gaggl A, Schultes G, Kärcher H. Distraction implants: a new operative technique for alveolar ridge augmentation. *J Cranio-Maxillo-Fac Surg.* 1999;27(4):214–221.
36. Stucki-McCormick SU, Moses JJ, Robinson R, et al. Alveolar distraction devices. In: Jensen OT, ed. *Alveolar Distraction Osteogensis.* Chicago, Illinois: Quintessence; 2002.
37. Soares M, Bauer J. Increase of the mandibular alveolar ridge with internal distraction osteogenesis device. *Int J Oral Maxillofac Surg.* 1999;28(suppl):43.
38. Jensen OT, Leopardi A, Gallegos L. The case for bone graft reconstruction including sinus grafting and distraction osteogenesis for the atrophic edentulous maxilla. *J Oral Maxillofac Surg.* 2004;62(11):1423–1428.
39. Jensen OT, Kuhlke L, Bedard JF, White D. Alveolar segmental sandwich osteotomy for anterior maxillary vertical augmentation prior to implant placement. *J Oral Maxillofac Surg.* 2006;64(2):290–296.
40. Jensen OT, Cottam JR. Posterior maxillary sandwich osteotomy combined with sinus grafting with bone morphogenetic protein-2 for alveolar reconstruction for dental implants: report of four cases. *Oral Craniofac Tissue Eng.* 2011;1:227.
41. Block MS, Baughman DG. Reconstruction of severe anterior maxillary defects using distraction osteogenesis, bone grafts, and implants. *J Oral Maxillofac Surg.* 2005;63(3):291–297.
42. Jensen OT, Kuhlke L. Maxillary full arch alveolar split osteotomy with island osteoperisoteal flaps and sinus grafting using morphogenetic protein-2 and retrofitting for immediate loading with a provisional: surgical and prosthetic procedures and case report. *Oral Craniofac Tissue Eng.* 2011;1:50.
43. Jensen OT, Ringeman JL, Cottam JR, Casap N. Orthognathic and osteoperiosteal flap augmentation strategies for maxillary dental implant reconstruction. *Oral Maxillofac Surg Clin North Am.* 2011;23(2):301–319 (vi).

44. Laviv A, Jensen OT, Tarazi E, Casap N. Alveolar sandwich osteotomy in resorbed alveolar ridge for dental implants: a 4-year prospective study. *J Oral Maxillofac Surg*. 2014;72(2):292–303.
45. Rachmiel A, Aizenbud D, Peled M. Enhancement of bone formation by bone morphogenetic protein-2 during alveolar distraction: an experimental study in sheep. *J Periodontol*. 2004;75(11):1524–1531.
46. Jensen OT. Sandwich osteotomy bone graft in the anterior mandible. In: Jensen OT, ed. *The Osteoperiosteal Flap*. Chicago, Illinois: Quintessence; 2010.
47. Laster Z, Rachmiel A. Alveolar distraction osteogenesis. In: Jensen OT, ed. *The Osteoperiosteal Flap*. Chicago, Illinois: Quintessence; 2010.
48. Jensen OT, Bell W, Cottam J. Osteoperiosteal flaps and local osteotomies for alveolar reconstruction. [review] *Oral Maxillofac Surg Clin North Am*. 2010;22(3):331–346 (vi).
49. Jensen OT. Alveolar segmental "sandwich" osteotomies for posterior edentulous mandibular sites for dental implants. *J Oral Maxillofac Surg*. 2006;64(3):471–475.
50. Jensen OT. Lefort I distraction osteogenesis for orthoalveolar form. A 12 year follow-up report. *Oral Maxillofac Surg Clin North Am*. 2019:339–349. Dental Implants Part I, Reconstruction. Jensen OT.

CHAPTER 27

The Maxillary Sinus Lift

Patrick J. Louis

Armamentarium

#15 Scalpel blade
Appropriate sutures
Implant drill kit
Implant osteotomes
Local anesthetic with vasoconstrictor
Minnesota retractor
Needle holder
Periosteal elevator
Sinus curettes of various sizes
Surgical handpiece with round bur (3 mm)
Tissue forceps

Alternative Instruments

Piezoelectric handpiece with round cutting tip
Piezoelectric handpiece with sinus elevation curettes
Piezoelectric handpiece with sinus floor elevator

History of the Procedure

The sinus lift procedure is a technique of bone reconstruction along the maxillary sinus floor. It is designed to increase the vertical posterior maxillary alveolar dimension for placement of dental implants. O. Hilt Tatum[1] proposed the first sinus lift procedure in 1976 at an implant meeting in Birmingham, Alabama.[2,3] However, in 1980, Boyne and James[4] were the first to publish this surgical technique, followed by Tatum[1] also in 1980. The sinus lift technique has undergone numerous modifications since its introduction. These procedures are routinely performed on an outpatient basis, without a hospital stay.

With the evolution of predictable sinus lift methods, this technique has become one of the primary surgical options allowing placement of dental implants in the posterior maxilla. The principles of the sinus lift procedure are simple; however, a number of anatomic variations and techniques should be considered to achieve reliable outcomes.

The apex of the sinus extends to the zygomatic process of the maxilla. The floor of the maxillary sinus is approximately 1 cm below the nasal floor in dentate adults.[5] The base of the pyramid contributes to the lateral wall of the nasal cavity. The three sloped walls of the pyramid are formed by the orbital floor and the anterior and lateral walls of the maxillary sinus. The sinuses are theorized to reduce the weight of the skull, provide resonant function, regulate the inhaled air humidity, and pneumatize with age.[6,7] Adult males have larger maxillary sinuses than females.[8,9] The approximate dimensions of the maxillary sinus in adult males are 21 to 29 mm in width, 39 to 49 mm in height, and 36 to 43 mm in length. In adult females, these dimensions are 19 to 27 mm in width, 35 to 45 mm in height, and 33 to 41 mm in length. Maxillary sinus volume is approximately 5 to 35 mL, depending on the referenced literature.[9–11]

The maxillary sinus is lined with ciliated columnar epithelial cells, which clear secretions toward the ostia. This thin membrane is also called the *Schneiderian membrane.* The medial wall of the sinus has an opening (ostia) that connects the sinus with the nose. The opening is in the hiatus semilunaris, which drains into the middle meatus of the nasal cavity. Gosau et al.[11] reported that the location of the semilunar hiatus ranges from approximately 18 to 35 mm (mean, 25.6 mm) above the nasal floor. The orbital floor of the maxilla contains blood vessels and the infraorbital nerve. The maxillary sinus receives its blood supply from branches of the internal maxillary artery, including the infraorbital, sphenopalatine, greater palatine, and alveolar arteries.[12]

Indications for the Use of the Procedure

The primary indication for the sinus lift procedure is pneumatization of the maxillary sinus, which prevents the placement of dental implants in the posterior maxilla. Poor bone quality that prevents adequate initial stability during implant placement is another indication. Dental extraction in the posterior maxilla appears to be partly responsible for pneumatization in elderly patients. The alveolar process forms the sinus floor, which is situated below the nasal floor level. The curved sinus floor conforms to the conical root apices of posterior maxillary teeth. McGowan and James[5] explained the pneumatization of the maxillary sinuses with respect to dental extraction and age. Sharan and Madjar[13] reported that sinus pneumatization occurred in an inferior direction after extraction of maxillary posterior teeth.

Preoperative planning is essential for successful management of the patient. It includes a careful history and physical exam, in addition to preoperative radiologic investigation, which could include conventional sinus radiographs, an orthopantomogram, and/or a computed tomography (CT) scan to evaluate the sinus+ and rule out any contraindication to the sinus lift procedure.

Limitations and Contraindications

Conditions blocking the ventilation and clearance of the maxillary sinus are the main contraindication to the sinus lift procedure. Many of these causes are reversible and should be treated before the sinus lift procedure.[14,15] Questions designed to elicit risks for sinus obstruction should be asked as part of the preoperative assessment. These risks may include a history of smoking; allergic rhinitis; previous nasal surgery or trauma; a history of chronic and/or recurrent sinusitis (the former defined as a sinus infection lasting more than 4 weeks and the latter as at least four episodes of acute sinusitis in the previous 12 months or at least three episodes in the previous 6 months); chronic use of nasal steroids and/or vasoconstrictors; chronic nasal obstruction and/or rhinorrhea; chronic hyposmia and/or hypogeusia; previous treatment for head and neck neoplasms; and comorbidities, particularly systemic diseases and pathologies that interfere with mucosal composition or ciliary movements (e.g., primary or secondary immunodeficiencies, cystic fibrosis, Kartagener and Mounier-Kuhn syndromes, dehydration, ciliostatic drugs, peripheral hypereosinophilia, asthma, chronic pulmonary disease, and acetylsalicylic acid hypersensitivity).[14]

The maxillary sinus cavity is frequently interrupted with septa and bony ridges. The incidence of maxillary sinus septa was reported to be 14% to 33%.[11,16–20] The main location of the septa was the region of the first and second molars.[11,17] When septa were identified in one maxillary sinus, there was a 66% to 70% chance of the same sinus configuration on the contralateral side.[17,21] This may make it difficult to perform a sinus lift. A preoperative cone beam CT scan can be helpful in planning the surgery and determining whether a lateral or transalveolar approach would be the better choice.

The size of the maxillary sinuses substantially affects the sinus wall thickness. If the sinus is large, the walls may be thin, and the converse also is often true. Small sinuses also may have thick osseous lamellae. Yang et al.[22] reported that the lateral wall of the maxillary sinus emerges as a thick cortical plate at the first premolar area, becomes thinner in the posterior direction, and then increases in thickness to the first molar area in dentate skulls. Zijderveld et al.[23] reported that 78% of lateral sinus walls were thin, and 48% of maxillary sinuses had septa. The mean thickness of the maxillary sinus ranged from 0.5 to 2 mm.[22] Amin and Hassan[24] and Yang et al.[22] showed that there were no significant differences in the thickness of the lateral wall according to patient age. These results also suggest that lateral pneumatization is not age related, contrary to the findings of Lee et al.,[25] who described a gradual increase in volume of the paranasal sinuses with age.

If the lateral sinus wall is thick, the entire sinus window should be thinned out to assist the elevation of the Schneiderian membrane and avoid perforation. The Schneiderian membrane should be kept intact to contain the graft material and provide a vascular bed. Clinical evaluation of the lateral sinus wall can provide valuable information during surgery. If the lateral sinus wall is thin and looks grayish blue, the outline of the sinus can be determined easily. Transpalatal illumination can also help determine the location of the sinus.

TECHNIQUE: Sinus Lift—Lateral Approach

STEP 1: Incision

A crestal or slightly palatal incision is made over the alveolar crest through the keratinized oral mucosa. The remainder of the incision is dictated by the presence or absence of teeth. When the ridge is edentulous and bilateral sinus lifts are planned, the crestal incision extends anteriorly, crossing the midline to the opposite side. Releasing incisions are made posterior to the tuberosity. When teeth are present or when a unilateral sinus lift is planned, the crestal incision extends over the posterior edentulous region, with a releasing incision that begins anterior to the anterior extent of the sinus, usually in the canine region. The posterior extent is to the tuberosity region, with a releasing incision posterior to the tuberosity. This trapezoidal flap, which is designed to be broad based, allows minimal disturbance of the blood supply, sufficient coverage of the surgical wound, and adequate access for the lateral sinus osteotomy, with graft placement and simultaneous implant placement if indicated.

STEP 2: Exposure

The full-thickness flap is elevated, exposing the lateral wall of the maxillary sinus (Fig. 27.1A). The infraorbital neurovascular bundle is usually identified anteriorly and superiorly and protected.

TECHNIQUE: Sinus Lift—Lateral Approach—cont'd

STEP 3: Osteotoamy

The osteotomy of the lateral sinus wall is created as a curved window, following the floor and anterior wall of the maxillary sinus. The posterior aspect of the osteotomy extends to the molar region, turning vertically. The superior aspect of the osteotomy can be a complete or interrupted horizontal line. The window is designed with a wide cranial hinge, base, and rounded corners. It is prepared initially with a 3-mm round bur or piezoelectric handpiece with a round tip. The preparation of the sinus lift window should be wide enough to easily accommodate the sinus lift instruments (Fig. 27.1B and C).

STEP 4: Elevation of the Sinus Membrane

Elevation of the Schneiderian membrane begins at the inferior aspect of the window. After initial elevation of the membrane along the inferior, anterior, and posterior aspects, the bone window is luxated inward and upward into the maxillary sinus with gentle pressure and the fracture at the superior aspect acting as a hinge. The sinus lift instruments are used to carefully elevate the membrane while bringing the trapdoor into a horizontal position (Fig. 27.1D and E).

Continued

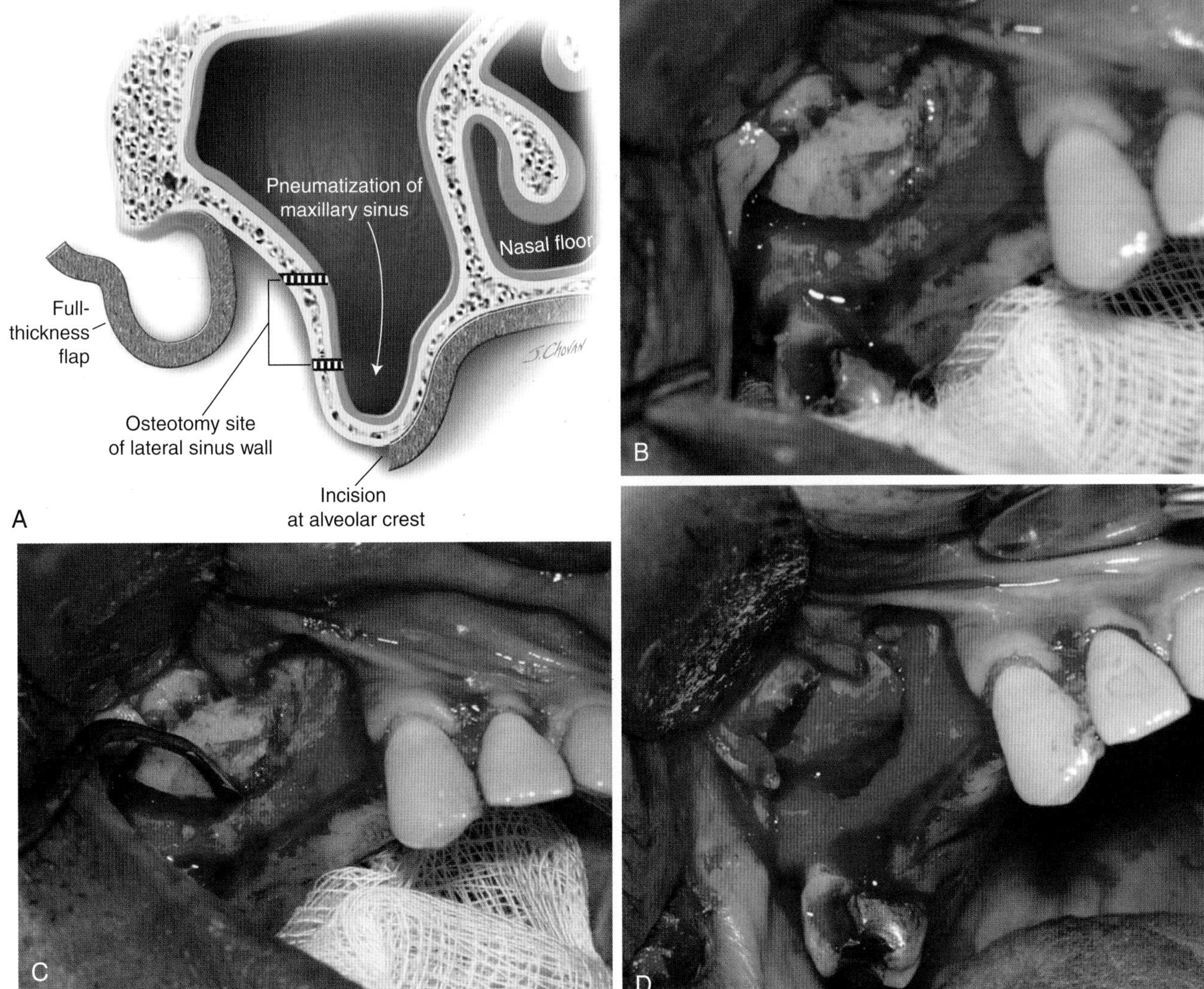

Figure 27.1 **A,** Coronal cross section through the maxillary sinus; lateral maxillary sinus lift, showing a crestal incision and lateral osteotomy. **B,** Creation of an osteotomy along the lateral aspect of the right maxillary sinus wall. **C,** Sinus curette in place, beginning the elevation of the sinus membrane. **D,** The sinus membrane has been elevated, and the lateral window has been infractured.

Continued

TECHNIQUE: Sinus Lift—Lateral Approach—cont'd

STEP 5: Grafting

The space beneath this lifted door and sinus mucosa can be filled with graft material. Multiple studies have shown that autogenous bone, allogeneic bone, and xenogenic bone graft materials work well along the sinus floor.[26–28] Alternatively, biologics, such as bone morphogenic proteins, have also been successful (Fig. 27.1F and G).

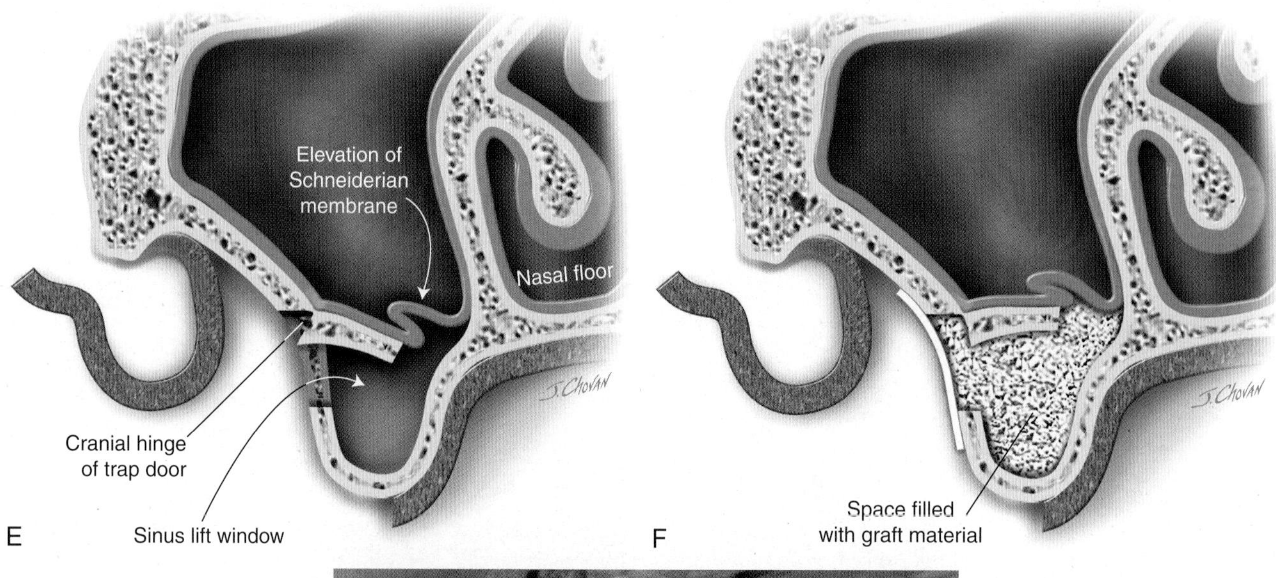

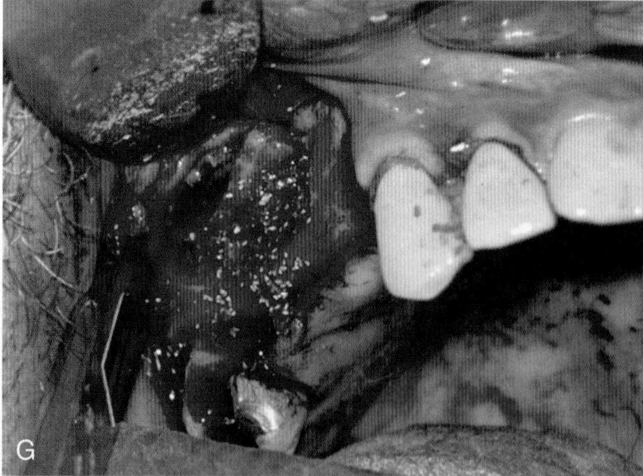

Figure 27.1, cont'd **E,** Infracture of the lateral sinus window with sinus membrane elevation. **F,** Particulate bone graft in place. **G,** Particulate allogeneic bone graft was placed along the sinus floor of the right maxillary sinus. This was performed bilaterally.

TECHNIQUE: Sinus Lift—Lateral Approach—cont'd

STEP 6: Implant Placement

The decision whether to insert the implant simultaneously with the sinus lift procedure or in a second-stage procedure depends on the ability to achieve primary stability of the implant. Sufficient bone quantity and quality are essential for dental implant placement. Resorption of alveolar bone in the posterior maxilla and pneumatization of the maxillary sinus often compromise the ability to place dental implants. Implants can be placed in the posterior maxilla with or without bone grafting as long as bone height is sufficient for stability (greater than 4 mm).[29] The primary stability of a dental implant might not be adequate if the bone height is less than 4 mm. A dental implant can be inserted in the second phase, after sinus floor grafting, in 4 to 6 months.[30–33] The width of the alveolar crest is also important for the longevity and stability of dental implants. If the alveolar width is less than 5 mm, augmentation should be considered or a ridge-split technique may be used (Fig. 27.1H–J).[34]

STEP 7: Wound Closure

Wound closure is performed with resorbable suture.

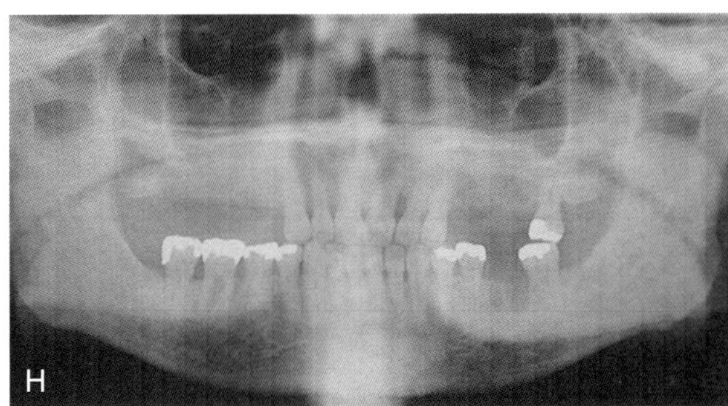

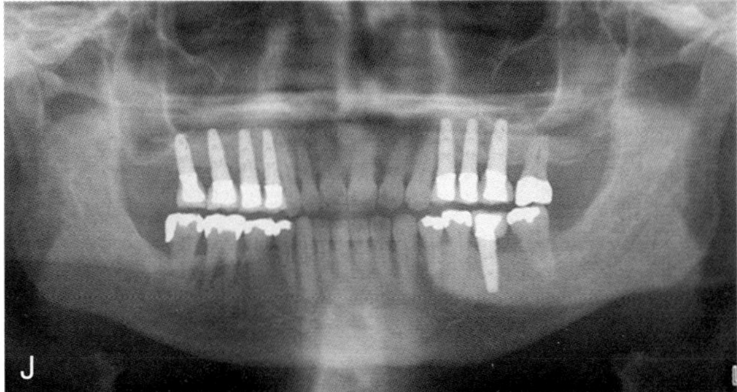

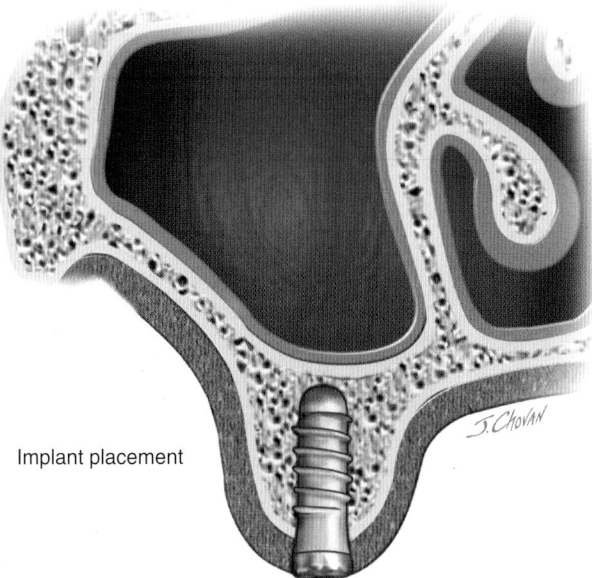

Figure 27.1, cont'd **H,** Panoramic radiograph approximately 6 months after removal of tooth #2 and 8 months after the sinus lift. Note the excellent bone in the posterior maxilla bilaterally. **I,** Second-phase surgery with mature bone graft and implant in place. **J,** Postoperative panoramic radiograph showing implants in good position. The patient was 5 years postop and had a stable result. (Clinical photos: Patrick J. Louis. Illustrations: Joe Chovan).

ALTERNATIVE TECHNIQUE 1: Sinus Lift—Transalveolar Approach

Sinus floor elevation using the transalveolar approach (Summers or Cosci technique) can be performed if the alveolar crest width is sufficient and the initial bone height is 5 mm or more.[35,36] Endosinus bone can be increased about 4 to 6 mm with the transalveolar sinus lift.[37] Primary implant stability is a requirement for this technique. In the many variations of the Summers technique, sequential osteotomes are used to push the sinus floor upward.[38] In the Cosci technique, sequential atraumatic drills are used to elevate the sinus floor.[39] Alternatively, reverse-cutting drills can be used to preserve bone and elevate the sinus membrane.[40]

STEP 1: Incision and Flap Elevation

A midcrestal incision should be performed for flap elevation without vertical releasing incisions (Fig.27.2A).

STEP 2: Pilot Hole

Cortical bone marking for site positioning is started with a 1.4-mm pilot drill. The depth of the osteotomy is 2 mm below the maxillary sinus floor (Fig. 27.2B).

STEP 3: Osteotomy

The transalveolar osteotomy is continued with sequential pilot drills or osteotomes of increasing diameters and elevating the sinus floor. The final osteotomy diameter is undersized to ensure implant stability (Fig. 27.2C).

STEP 4: Grafting

Particulate graft material is gradually placed in the osteotomy site and pushed upward to elevate the sinus floor with the osteotome or reverse-cutting drill.

STEP 5: Implant Placement

The implant is inserted into the undersized osteotomy site (Fig. 27.2D).

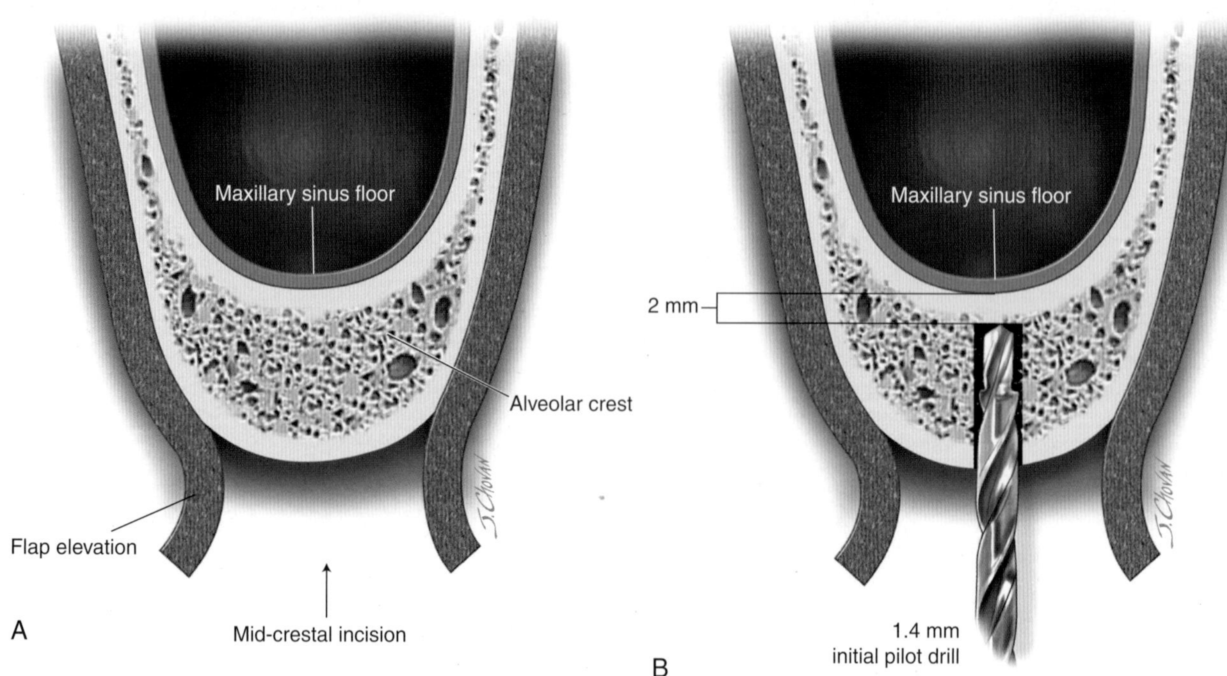

Figure 27.2 **A,** Coronal cross section through the maxillary sinus; transalveolar maxillary sinus lift, showing that a crestal incision was made and buccal and palatal flaps were elevated. **B,** Pilot drill stopped about 2 mm below the maxillary sinus floor.

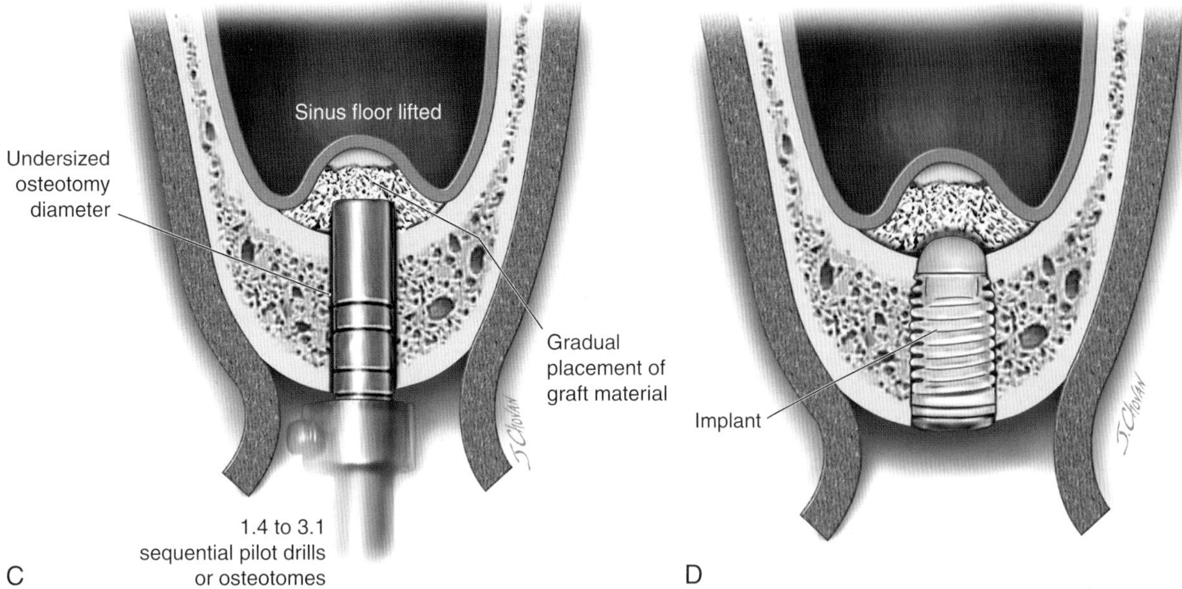

Figure 27.2, cont'd **C,** The final osteotome, which is undersized to ensure initial implant stability, is used to tap the sinus floor up. This can also be done with allogeneic bone by placing the graft material in the osteotomy and tapping it upward to begin to elevate the sinus floor. **D,** The implant is placed and used to elevate the sinus floor about 3 to 5 mm to help tent the sinus membrane superiorly. (Illustrations: Joe Chovan).

ALTERNATIVE TECHNIQUE 2: Ridge-Split Transalveolar Approach

When both alveolar width and alveolar height are deficient, a modified transalveolar approach may be used. This technique involves creating a ridge-split osteotomy, after which the principles and sequence of the transalveolar approach are followed. Ridge splitters, expanders, or chisels are inserted through the crestal cut to expand gently and mobilize laterally the buccal bone plate while elevating the sinus floor with osteotomes. The bone graft is then applied internally, with or without immediate implant placement (Fig. 27.3).

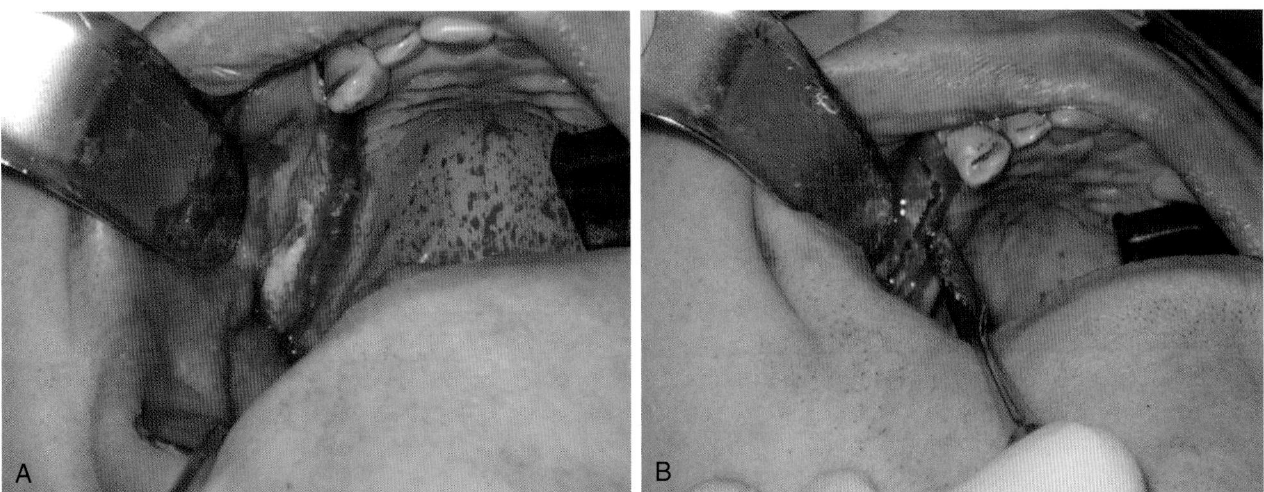

Figure 27.3 **A,** Crestal incision with minimal elevation of the flap. **B,** A spatula osteotome is used to deepen the osteotomy but staying about 2 mm below the maxillary sinus floor.

Continued

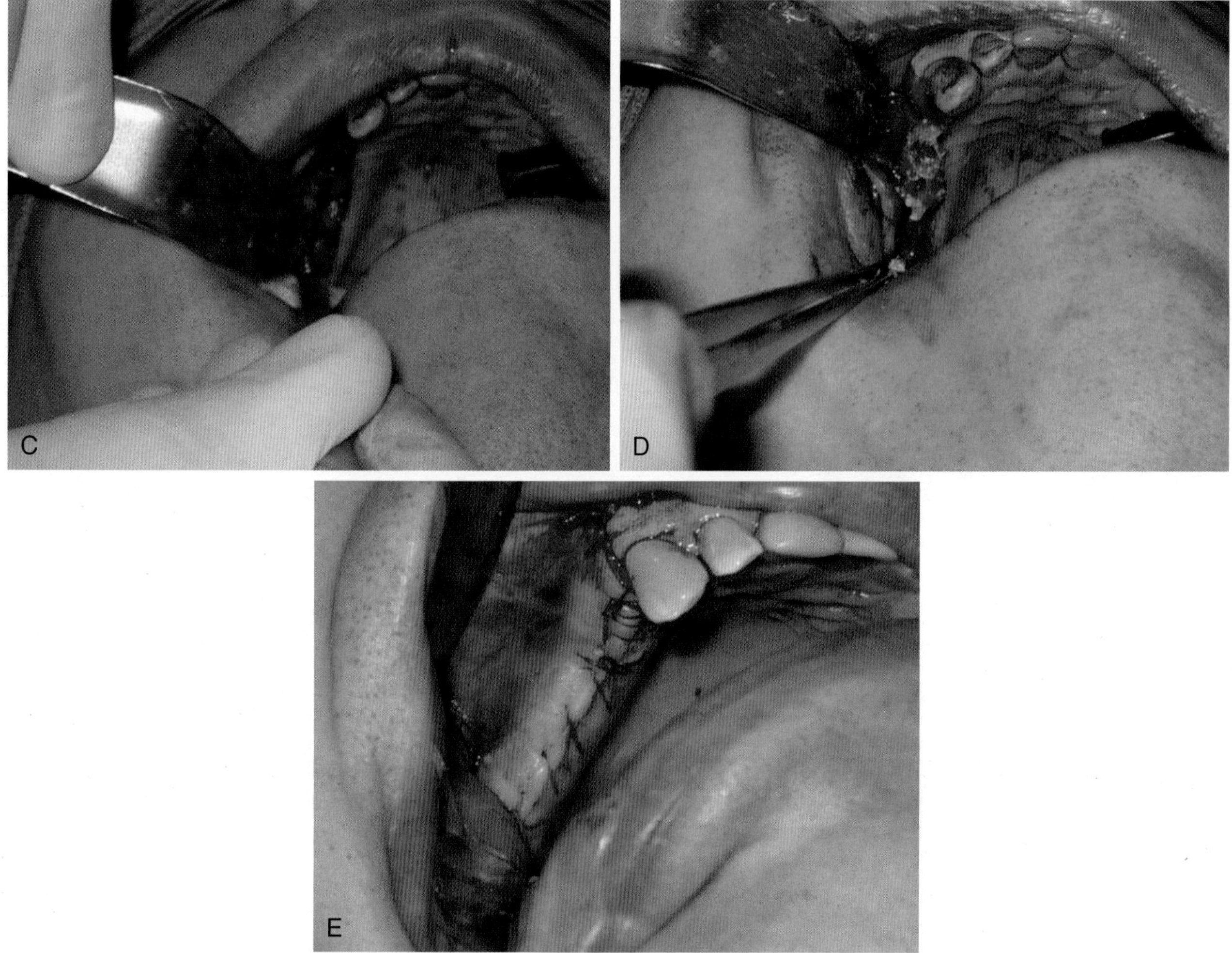

Figure 27.3 **C,** An osteotome is used to begin widening the ridge and elevate the sinus floor. **D,** Bone graft is placed and packed into the osteotomy site. **E,** Wound closure; note the increase in ridge width. (Clinical photos: Patrick J. Louis).

ALTERNATIVE TECHNIQUE 3: Graftless Sinus Elevation

According to the principle of guided tissue regeneration, bone formation is created by the elevated sinus membrane and maintained by the implant placement. Sinus membrane elevation without the use of additional graft material is found to be a predictable technique for bone augmentation of the maxillary sinus floor. Palma et al.[41] reported no difference in the amount of augmented bone tissue in the maxillary sinus after 6 months of healing after sinus membrane elevation with or without adjunctive autogenous bone grafts. However, this technique is difficult to manage if the sinus membrane is perforated. When membrane perforation is less than 4 mm of protruding implants, the membrane can heal uneventfully.[42] A large sinus perforation may need to be treated with the lateral sinus lift approach.

Several studies have shown great potential for healing and bone formation in the maxillary sinus without the use of additional bone grafts or bone substitutes.[29,37,43–46] Sul et al.[47] reported that dental implants placed into the sinus cavity and used alone to elevate the sinus membrane, without the addition of any graft material, appeared to have little influence on the histologic characteristics of the sinus membrane.

Avoidance and Management of Intraoperative Complications

Maxillary sinus floor elevation with or without graft material has proven to be a reliable method that enables the insertion of endosseous implants in patients with a severely resorbed maxilla. The complications of maxillary sinus floor elevation procedures include perforation of the sinus membrane, loss of implants, local wound dehiscence, intraoperative hemorrhage, graft infection, postoperative maxillary sinusitis, and loss of graft.[23,48,49] A thorough preoperative evaluation is important to evaluate the maxillary sinus for any pathology.

Perforation of the Schneiderian membrane is a complication that threatens the coverage of the bone graft (Fig. 27.4). Inadvertent tearing of the sinus membrane with extrusion of graft material into the antrum can initiate chronic sinusitis in reaction to the particulate graft material. Timmenga et al.,[50] Bhattacharyya,[51] and Jensen et al.[52] reported that sinus mucosa perforation represents the most common complication, with a prevalence of approximately 35%. These perforations are most likely to occur at sharp edges and maxillary sinus septa.[2]

If the perforation of the sinus membrane is not large and near the elevated mucosal fold, it can be covered with a resorbable material (e.g., membrane and bioglues) to prevent loss of the graft. The sinus membrane should be carefully elevated and released from the sinus walls around the perforation. This can reduce the size of the sinus perforation. The biodegradable membrane can be shaped and contoured to cover and reinforce the membrane defect. Graft material can be simultaneously placed and retained in this sinus lift repair. When the perforation is very large in an unfavorable area, delayed sinus lift should be considered. Reentry sinus lift should be delayed for 6 to 8 weeks after the first surgical attempt.[2,34]

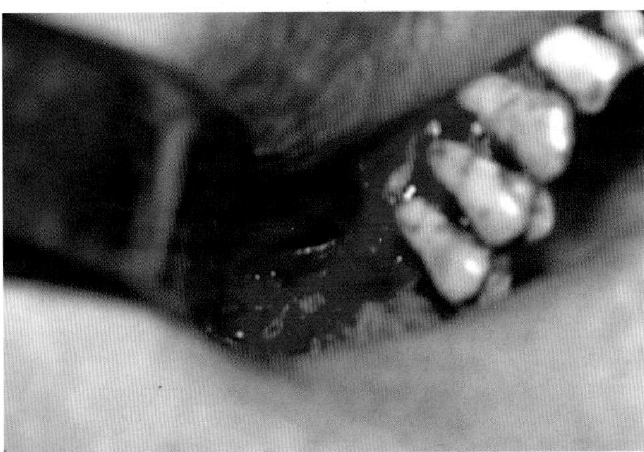

Figure 27.4 Perforation of the maxillary sinus membrane. (Clinical photos: Patrick J. Louis).

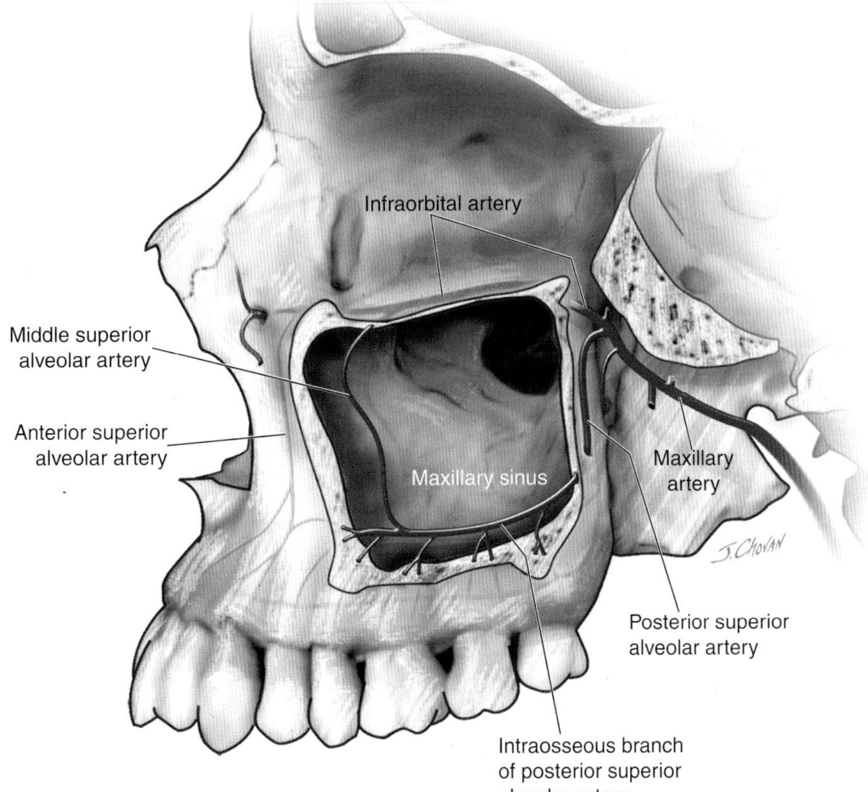

Figure 27.5 The intraosseous branch of the posterior superior alveolar artery or the middle superior alveolar artery can be encountered during a lateral approach to the maxillary sinus. (Illustration: Joe Chovan).

Maximum diameters of the posterior superior alveolar and infraorbital arteries may reach 2 and 2.7 mm.[53] The risk of bleeding during the sinus lift procedure is greater when larger vessels are present. Ronsano et al.,[12] Solar et al.,[53] and Traxler et al.[54] reported an endosseous anastomosis between the posterior superior alveolar and infraorbital arteries in 100% of cadavers. In a CT study,[55] the artery was detected at a mean distance of 18 mm (±4.9) from the alveolar ridge. In anatomic studies in cadavers, this distance was 18.9 to 19.6 mm.[50,51] Therefore, this structure is more likely to be encountered in atrophic ridges because the superior osteotomy line is placed more caudally than in a dentate ridge (Fig. 27.5).[55,56] Bleeding can usually be controlled by pressure with a saline-moistened gauze pad; electrocautery should be avoided because of the risk of perforating the Schneiderian membrane.

Postoperative Considerations

Patients are placed on antibiotics and chlorhexidine mouth rinse, postoperatively. Sinus precautions are recommended (e.g., no nose blowing, use of nasal decongestants). Postoperative sinusitis should be evaluated with a CT scan to evaluate the patency of the ostium of the maxillary sinus. Medical management is recommended first (antibiotics, decongestants, and saline nasal spray). If this is unsuccessful, nasal or sinus surgery should be considered.

References

1. Tatum H Jr. Maxillary and sinus implant reconstructions. *Dent Clin North Am.* 1986;30(2):207–229.
2. Chanavaz M. Maxillary sinus: anatomy, physiology, surgery, and bone grafting related to implantology—eleven years of surgical experience (1979–1990). *J Oral Implantol.* 1990;16(3):199–209.
3. Chanavaz M, Francke JP, Donazzan M. [The maxillary sinus and implantology]. *Chir Dent Fr.* 1990;60(519):45–54.
4. Boyne PJ, James RA. Grafting of the maxillary sinus floor with autogenous marrow and bone. *J Oral Surg.* 1980;38(8):613–616.
5. McGowan DA, Baxter PW, James J. *The Maxillary Sinus and its Dental Implications.* Oxford, UK: John Wright; 1993.
6. Ritter FN. *The Paranasal Sinuses: Anatomy and Surgical Technique.* St Louis, Missouri: Mosby; 1978.
7. Blanton PL, Biggs NL. Eighteen hundred years of controversy: the paranasal sinuses. *Am J Anat.* 1969;124(2):135–147.
8. Uthman AT, Al-Rawi NH, Al-Naaimi AS, Al-Timimi JF. Evaluation of maxillary sinus dimensions in gender determination using helical CT scanning. *J Forensic Sci.* 2011;56(2):403–408.
9. Ikeda A. [Volumetric measurement of the maxillary sinus by coronal CT scan]. *Nippon Jibiinkoka Gakkai Kaiho.* 1996;99(8):1136–1143.
10. Ariji Y, Kuroki T, Moriguchi S, Ariji E, Kanda S. Age changes in the volume of the human maxillary sinus: a study using computed tomography. *Dentomaxillofac Radiol.* 1994;23(3):163–168.
11. Gosau M, Rink D, Driemel O, Draenert FG. Maxillary sinus anatomy: a cadaveric study with clinical implications. *Anat Rec.* 2009;292(3):352–354.
12. Rosano G, Taschieri S, Gaudy JF, Del Fabbro M. Maxillary sinus vascularization: a cadaveric study. *J Craniofac Surg.* 2009;20(3):940–943.
13. Sharan A, Madjar D. Maxillary sinus pneumatization following extractions: a radiographic study. *Int J Oral Maxillofac Implants.* 2008;23(1):48–56.
14. Torretta S, Mantovani M, Testori T, et al. Importance of ENT assessment in stratifying candidates for sinus floor elevation: a prospective clinical study. *Clin Oral Implants Res.* 2013;24(suppl A100):57–62.
15. Pignataro L, Mantovani M, Torretta S, Felisati G, Sambataro G. ENT assessment in the integrated management of candidate for (maxillary) sinus lift. *Acta Otorhinolaryngol Ital.* 2008;28(3):110–119.
16. Rosano G, Gaudy JF, Chaumanet G, Del Fabbro M, Taschieri S. [Maxillary sinus septa. Prevalence and anatomy]. *Rev Stomatol Chir Maxillofac.* 2012;113(1):32–35.
17. Rosano G, Taschieri S, Gaudy JF, Lesmes D, Del Fabbro M. Maxillary sinus septa: a cadaveric study. *J Oral Maxillofac Surg.* 2010;68(6):1360–1364.
18. Krennmair G, Ulm CW, Lugmayr H, Solar P. The incidence, location, and height of maxillary sinus septa in the edentulous and dentate maxilla. *J Oral Maxillofac Surg.* 1999;57(6):667–671.
19. Velásquez-Plata D, Hovey LR, Peach CC, Alder ME. Maxillary sinus septa: a 3-dimensional computerized tomographic scan analysis. *Int J Oral Maxillofac Implants.* 2002;17(6):854–860.
20. Kim MJ, Jung UW, Kim CS, et al. Maxillary sinus septa: prevalence, height, location, and morphology. A reformatted computed tomography scan analysis. *J Periodontol.* 2006;77(5):903–908.
21. Ella B, Noble RC, Lauverjat Y, et al. Septa within the sinus: effect on elevation of the sinus floor. *Br J Oral Maxillofac Surg.* 2008;46(6):464–467.
22. Yang HM, Bae HE, Won SY, et al. The buccofacial wall of maxillary sinus: an anatomical consideration for sinus augmentation. *Clin Implant Dent Relat Res.* 2009;11(suppl 1):e2–e6.
23. Zijderveld SA, van den Bergh JP, Schulten EA, ten Bruggenkate CM. Anatomical and surgical findings and complications in 100 consecutive maxillary sinus floor elevation procedures. *J Oral Maxillofac Surg.* 2008;66(7):1426–1438.
24. Amin MF, Hassan EI. Sex identification in Egyptian population using Multidetector Computed Tomography of the maxillary sinus. *J Forensic Leg Med.* 2012;19(2):65–69.
25. Lee DH, Shin JH, Lee DC. Three-dimensional morphometric analysis of paranasal sinuses and mastoid air cell system using computed tomography in pediatric population. *Int J Pediatr Otorhinolaryngol.* 2012;76(11):1642–1646.
26. Froum SJ, Tarnow DP, Wallace SS, Rohrer MD, Cho SC. Sinus floor elevation using anorganic bovine bone matrix (OsteoGraf/N) with and without autogenous bone: a clinical, histologic, radiographic, and histomorphometric analysis—part 2 of an ongoing prospective study. *Int J Periodontics Restorative Dent.* 1998;18(6):528–543.
27. Hallman M, Hedin M, Sennerby L, Lundgren S. A prospective 1-year clinical and radiographic study of implants placed after maxillary sinus floor augmentation with bovine hydroxyapatite and autogenous bone. *J Oral Maxillofac Surg.* 2002;60(3):277–284.
28. Hising P, Bolin A, Branting C. Reconstruction of severely resorbed alveolar ridge crests with dental implants using a bovine bone mineral for augmentation. *Int J Oral Maxillofac Implants.* 2001;16(1):90–97.
29. Lundgren S, Andersson S, Gualini F, Sennerby L. Bone reformation with sinus membrane elevation: a new surgical technique for maxillary sinus floor augmentation. *Clin Implant Dent Relat Res.* 2004;6(3):165–173.
30. Misch CE. Maxillary sinus augmentation for endosteal implants: organized alternative treatment plans. *Int J Oral Implantol.* 1987;4(2):49–58.
31. ten Bruggenkate CM, van den Bergh JP. Maxillary sinus floor elevation: a valuable pre-prosthetic procedure. *Periodontol 2000.* 1998;17:176–182.
32. van den Bergh JP, ten Bruggenkate CM, Krekeler G, Tuinzing DB. Sinusfloor elevation and grafting with autogenous iliac crest bone. *Clin Oral Implants Res.* 1998;9(6):429–435.

33. Hirsch JM, Ericsson I. Maxillary sinus augmentation using mandibular bone grafts and simultaneous installation of implants. A surgical technique. *Clin Oral Implants Res.* 1991;2(2):91–96.
34. van den Bergh JP, ten Bruggenkate CM, Disch FJ, Tuinzing DB. Anatomical aspects of sinus floor elevations. *Clin Oral Implants Res.* 2000;11(3):256–265.
35. Chen ST, Beagle J, Jensen SS, Chiapasco M, Darby I. Consensus statements and recommended clinical procedures regarding surgical techniques. *Int J Oral Maxillofac Implants.* 2009;24(suppl):272–278.
36. He L, Chang X, Liu Y. Sinus floor elevation using osteotome technique without grafting materials: a 2-year retrospective study. *Clin Oral Implants Res.* 2013;24(suppl A100):63–67.
37. Nedir R, Nurdin N, Szmukler-Moncler S, Bischof M. Osteotome sinus floor elevation technique without grafting material and immediate implant placement in atrophic posterior maxilla: report of 2 cases. *J Oral Maxillofac Surg.* 2009;67(5):1098–1103.
38. Summers RB. A new concept in maxillary implant surgery: the osteotome technique. *Compendium.* 1994;15(2):152.
39. Cosci F, Luccioli M. A new sinus lift technique in conjunction with placement of 265 implants: a 6-year retrospective study. *Implant Dent.* 2000;9(4):363–368.
40. Salgar N. Osseodensified crestal sinus window augmentation: an alternative procedure to the lateral window technique. *J Oral Implantol.* 2020;10:1563. [Published online ahead of print, July 14, 2020].
41. Palma VC, Magro-Filho O, de Oliveria JA, Lundgren S, Salata LA, Sennerby L. Bone reformation and implant integration following maxillary sinus membrane elevation: an experimental study in primates. *Clin Implant Dent Relat Res.* 2006;8(1):11–24.
42. Jung JH, Choi BH, Zhu SJ, et al. The effects of exposing dental implants to the maxillary sinus cavity on sinus complications. *Oral Surg Oral Med Oral Pathol Oral Radiol Endod.* 2006;102(5):602–605.
43. Hatano N, Sennerby L, Lundgren S. Maxillary sinus augmentation using sinus membrane elevation and peripheral venous blood for implant-supported rehabilitation of the atrophic posterior maxilla: case series. *Clin Implant Dent Relat Res.* 2007;9(3):150–155.
44. Sohn DS, Lee JS, Ahn MR, Shin HI. New bone formation in the maxillary sinus without bone grafts. *Implant Dent.* 2008;17(3):321–331.
45. Nedir R, Bischof M, Vazquez L, Nurdin N, Szmukler-Moncler S, Bernard JP. Osteotome sinus floor elevation technique without grafting material: 3-year results of a prospective pilot study. *Clin Oral Implants Res.* 2009;20(7):701–707.
46. Schlegel A, Hamel J, Wichmann M, Eitner S. Comparative clinical results after implant placement in the posterior maxilla with and without sinus augmentation. *Int J Oral Maxillofac Implants.* 2008;23(2):289–298.
47. Sul SH, Choi BH, Li J, Jeong SM, Xuan F. Histologic changes in the maxillary sinus membrane after sinus membrane elevation and the simultaneous insertion of dental implants without the use of grafting materials. *Oral Surg Oral Med Oral Pathol Oral Radiol Endod.* 2008;105(4):e1–e5.
48. Ziccardi MH. *Complications of Maxillary Sinus Augmentation: The Sinus Bone Graft.* Chicago, IL: Quintessence; 1999.
49. Wannfors K, Johansson B, Hallman M, Strandkvist T. A prospective randomized study of 1- and 2-stage sinus inlay bone grafts: 1-year follow-up. *Int J Oral Maxillofac Implants.* 2000;15(5):625–632.
50. Timmenga NM, Raghoebar GM, Boering G, van Weissenbruch R. Maxillary sinus function after sinus lifts for the insertion of dental implants. *J Oral Maxillofac Surg.* 1997;55(9):936–939.
51. Bhattacharyya N. Bilateral chronic maxillary sinusitis after the sinus-lift procedure. *Am J Otolaryngol.* 1999;20(2):133–135.
52. Jensen J, Sindet-Pedersen S, Oliver AJ. Varying treatment strategies for reconstruction of maxillary atrophy with implants: results in 98 patients. *J Oral Maxillofac Surg.* 1994;52(3):210–216.
53. Solar P, Geyerhofer U, Traxler H, Windisch A, Ulm C, Watzek G. Blood supply to the maxillary sinus relevant to sinus floor elevation procedures. *Clin Oral Implants Res.* 1999;10(1):34–44.
54. Traxler H, Windisch A, Geyerhofer U, Surd R, Solar P, Firbas W. Arterial blood supply of the maxillary sinus. *Clin Anat.* 1999;12(6):417–421.
55. Güncü GN, Yildirim YD, Wang HL, Tözüm TF. Location of posterior superior alveolar artery and evaluation of maxillary sinus anatomy with computerized tomography: a clinical study. *Clin Oral Implants Res.* 2011;22(10):1164–1167.
56. Mardinger O, Abba M, Hirshberg A, Schwartz-Arad D. Prevalence, diameter and course of the maxillary intraosseous vascular canal with relation to sinus augmentation procedure: a radiographic study. *Int J Oral Maxillofac Surg.* 2007;36(8):735–738.

CHAPTER 28

Endosseous Craniofacial Implants

Sabine C. Girod

Armamentarium

#15 blade
#9 periosteal elevator
3-0 Polyglactin suture
5-0 Polilecaprone suture undyed
EO implant
EO profile drill for implant 2.8 mm
EO stop drill for implant 2.8 mm
Hand piece and motor unit
Healing cap
Implant inserting device
Local anesthetic with vasoconstrictor
Mayo scissors
Needle electrocautery
Parallel gauge
Ratchet with torque control device
Round bur 2.3 mm
SCS screw driver
Skin retractors
Tweezers with and without titanium plasma coated tips

History of the Procedure

Traditionally, craniofacial prostheses have been used to cover facial defects in cases when surgical reconstruction is not an option. As early as 1965, subperiosteal implants were suggested for the fixation of extraoral prostheses.[1] Due to local inflammation and loosening, the clinical application of these devices was unpredictable and largely unsuccessful.

In 1969, Per-Ingvar Branemark and colleagues were the first to report the long-lasting direct contact of bone with a metallic implant under functional loading.[2] In the years following, endosseous implants in the oral cavity revolutionized the treatment of the edentulous jaw.[3] Based on this work, the first clinical trials with skin-penetrating implants in the mastoid process began in 1977. Five years later, favorable results and a low complication rate for percutaneous endosseous implants as retention elements for facial prostheses were reported.[4,5] Since then, multiple publications and case reports have demonstrated the successful craniofacial rehabilitation and improved quality of life of patients who are not only confronted with a deadly disease but also have to cope with a potentially disfiguring treatment.[6–9]

Indications for Use of the Procedure

Microsurgical techniques have overcome many of the traditional problems in craniofacial reconstructive surgery, and, whenever possible, surgical reconstruction is the treatment of choice. However, in some cases, primary reconstruction of soft tissue and bone defects is likely to fail or not be desirable or feasible. Generally, older age in connection with age-related health problems is a limiting factor for extensive surgical reconstructions, as the risks associated with anesthesia increase, and postoperative immobilization and rehabilitation become a problem. In these cases, secondary reconstruction, including endosseous craniofacial implants, is the preferred option. In some cases, such as in ablation of the auricle or in certain orbital defects where the upper and lower lid are missing, implant-supported prostheses may be the only option or can provide simpler, safer, and esthetically superior results than plastic reconstructive surgery.

The successful rehabilitation of patients with craniofacial defects depends on the motivation of the patient, careful preoperative planning, interdisciplinary cooperation, and adequate surgical and prosthodontic techniques. Ideally, the surgeon, the prosthodontist, and the anaplastologist should discuss all therapeutic options, including surgical and implant-based reconstruction, before any surgery. If craniofacial endosseous implants and rehabilitation with a prosthesis are considered (e.g., before removal of an auricle), an impression of the auricle can be taken and used to model the prosthesis. Furthermore, the tissue bed can be prepared for extraoral implants during ablative surgery. When possible, bone can be preserved or reconstructed in areas crucial for later placement of endosseous implants; in some cases, immediate implantation can be considered. The soft tissue can also be prepared for implantation; for example, transplantation of split-thickness skin grafts can be performed to create an area of thin and hairless skin at the intended implantation site.[10]

For each individual case, the repair of craniofacial defects using endosseous implants should be uniquely planned, with implants being placed wherever bone is available. In general, the temporal bone, the supraorbital rim, the zygoma, the piriform aperture, and the pterygoid process provide sufficient bone for the anchorage of implants.

Preoperative Planning

Functional and esthetic reconstruction of craniofacial defects requires thorough preoperative planning and preparation, with careful evaluation of the unique clinical situation. The thickness and mobility of the soft tissue at the margins of the defect are especially important for the esthetic result, as the appearance of an extraoral prosthesis is usually limited in areas where the surrounding tissue is mobile due to muscle movements in the face (e.g., in the cheeks). Therefore, ideal indications are for the replacement of the ear, eye, and nose. At the implantation sites, the thickness and mobility of the skin are even more important. An area of thin and hairless skin should be created around the implants to avoid inflammatory reactions and loss of the implants.[11]

Assessment of the bone available for implantation is essential during preoperative planning. The introduction of improved imaging such as computed tomography (CT) allows for the visualization of the precise anatomical extent of craniofacial hard and soft tissue defects and the structure and thickness of the bone available prior to implant placement.[12–14] Recently, surgical navigation has been introduced into dental implantology. A substantial advantage of navigation is precise preoperative planning, which is optimized by taking into consideration anatomic and prosthetic aspects. Using this technology, a plastic template of the ideal position of the implants is made using radiopaque markers, and the patient is scanned with the template (Fig. 28.1A). The available bone can then be assessed, and implant placement can be planned such that damage to critical anatomic structures is avoided, improving intraoperative safety (Fig. 28.1B).[15,16] For example, in cases when the external ear, the mastoid process and its air-cell system are replaced, the position of the sigmoid sinus and the level of the middle cranial fossa can be determined to avoid penetration during implantation.

If no bone has been removed during surgery, computed tomography (CT) of the temporal bone is not required. However, if an orbital, nasal, or midface prosthesis is planned, a CT scan is necessary to select the ideal implantation site with respect to the amount and quality of bone available. Furthermore, implants in the orbital rim are difficult to position, as they need to point internally into the orbit and sufficient bone needs to be available. CT scans and surgical navigation allow for the precise planning of the implantation site and the angulation of the implants necessary for camouflage by the prosthesis later on.

Prosthodontic Methods in Endosseous Craniofacial Implants

The prosthetic requirements of treatment with extraoral or complex combination devices differ greatly from intraoral prostheses. In all cases of craniofacial defects following tumor surgery, the surgical and prosthodontic team should discuss the approach to rehabilitation. General guidelines comparable to intraoral rehabilitation are difficult to establish because of the high number of interindividual differences in defect size and location, the amount of bone available and bone quality, and the thickness and mobility of the soft tissue. Accordingly, the number and site of implants to be placed vary greatly and largely depend on the individual situation. For example, for the retention of an auricular prosthesis, two implants may be sufficient, whereas in extended midface defects, as many implants as possible should be placed to distribute the load. If necessary, craniofacial defects secondary to malignant tumor surgery can be minimized with plastic surgery techniques without obstruction of potential implantation sites (Fig. 28.2A–D).

Prosthodontic assessment of the implantation sites should take a number of fundamental principles into account. First, the retention and support for the prosthesis should fall within the peripheral extension of the device. Preferably, the margins of the prosthesis should extend in areas of limited mobility of the bordering tissue bed. Overextension of a prosthesis, especially in the midface, is therefore limited.

Implants should be angulated such that they point internally, which may be particularly difficult in the orbit. External placement can cause difficulties in masking the necessary abutments and implants. The anchorage system also needs to be placed deep enough to allow for sufficient thickness of the prosthetic material. A transparent template is helpful to assess the dimensional relationship between the surface of the prosthesis and the intended implantation point. The attachment system should be designed according to the individual requirements, either firm and rigid, flexible, or a combination of both, depending on the size and location of the defect and the areas to be covered. Flexible devices have the advantage that they can be extended in undercuts for additional stability.

In principle, mechanical or magnetic attachments or a combination of both can be used for retention of the prosthesis. A greater dimension is needed for magnetic attachments than for mechanical devices, and they require less force upon removal of the prosthesis, thereby minimizing the stress on the implants.

The support system should be designed such that stress concentration is avoided and forces are distributed uniformly to ensure long-term survival of the implants. While this does not pose many problems in auricular, orbital, or simple midface prostheses, difficult design problems can occur in combined intra-/extraoral defects. Individually designed open bar systems can fulfill these engineering requirements. In these cases, angulation and direction of the implants are secondary, as the custom-designed retention system can compensate for these issues. It is of greater importance to place many implants in the remaining skeleton to distribute the load and achieve maximum rigidity. In combined defects where the maxilla is missing, the primary goal is restoration of masticatory and phonetic function.[17] For integration of maxillary prostheses, it is important to establish a horizontal anchorage

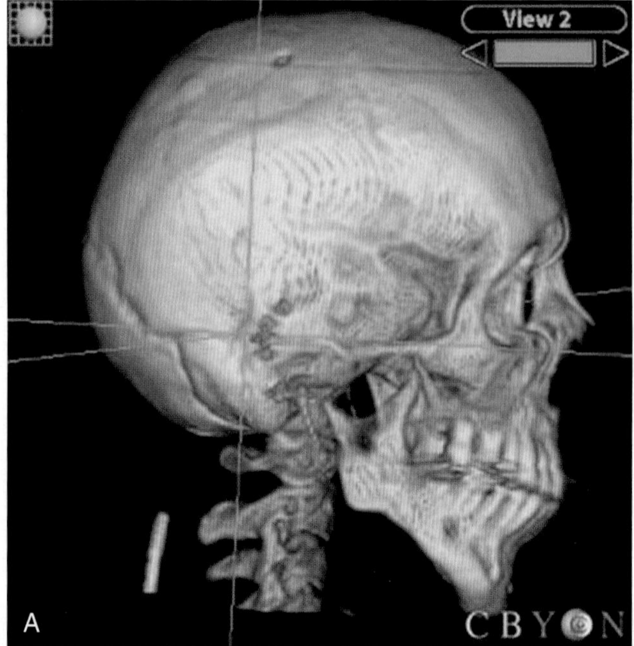

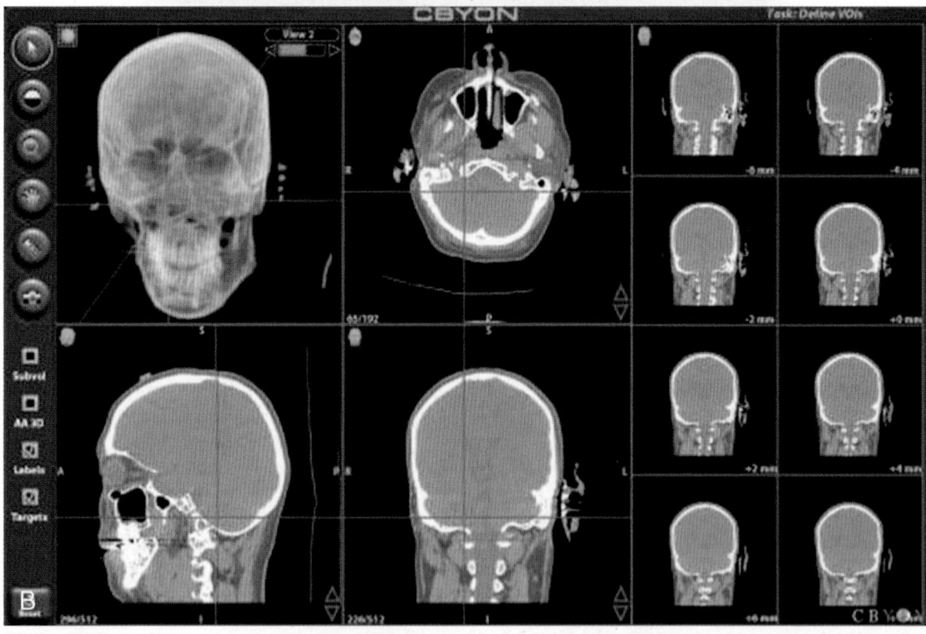

Figure 28.1 **A,** Preoperative planning CT for surgical navigation. **B,** Multiplanar views allow the assessment of bone available for implantation. The position of plastic ear models with radiopaque markers is visible in all views. (Sabine C. Girod)

system; vertical bars can then be used to support the facial part of the prosthesis.

Limitations and Contraindications

The placement of endosseous implants for the rehabilitation of craniofacial defects is limited by three factors: the availability of bone, the extension of the prosthesis, and the quality of the recipient site. The primary challenge in the construction of a prosthesis based on endosseous implants is the availability of bone suitable for the placement. In addition, the prognosis of osseointegration may be impaired in patients who have undergone radiation therapy, for example, after tumor ablation.[18–20] After irradiation, the bone gradually becomes ischemic due to an arteritis that consequently leads to the loss of the end arteries. This process is accompanied by histological changes such as osteolysis and infiltration of fibrous tissue. Although osseointegration is possible in radiated bone, a higher rate of osseointegration failure is expected. In addition,

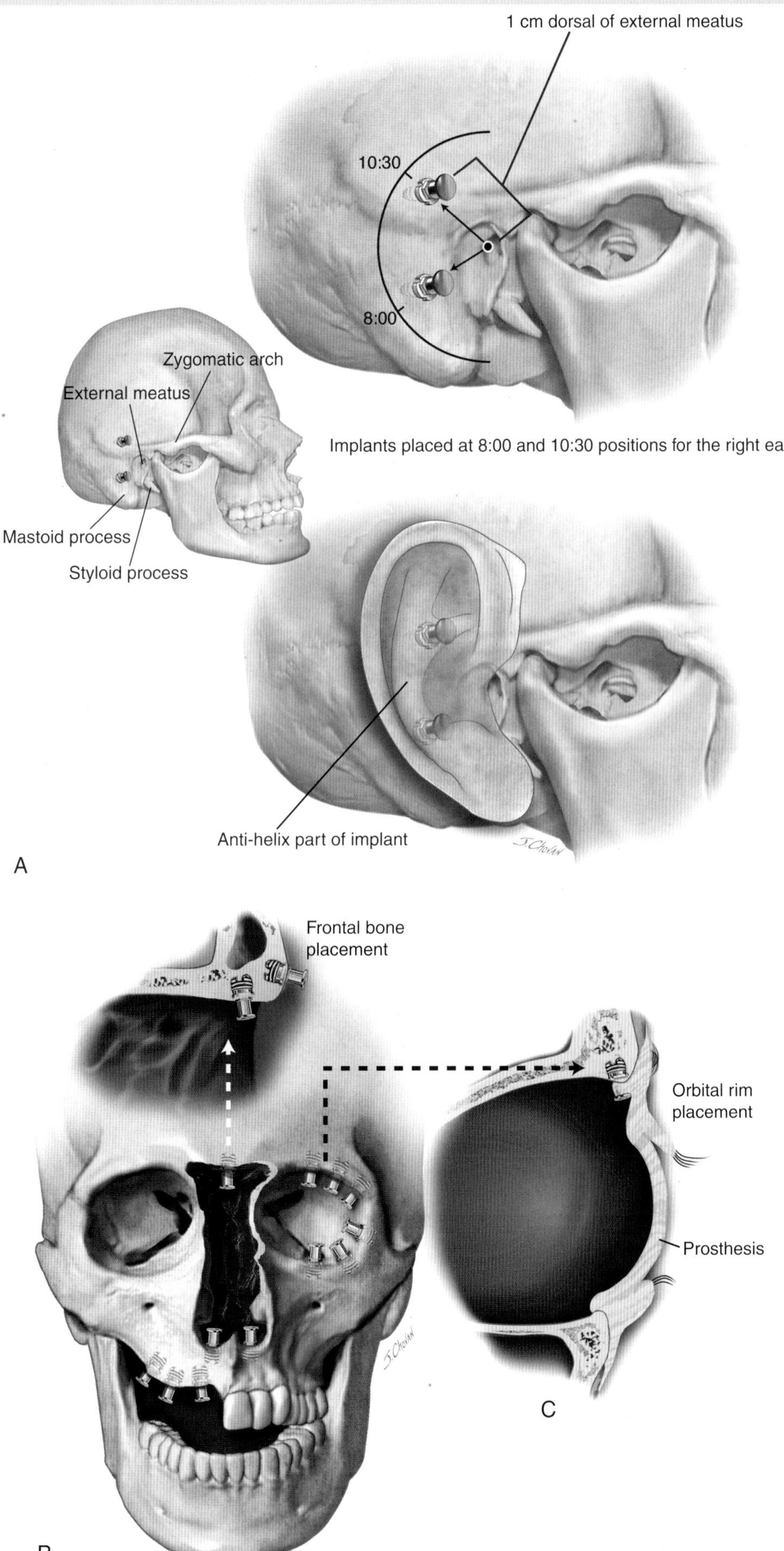

Figure 28.2 **A,** For an auricular prosthesis, two to three implants are inserted into the temporal bone, approximately 1 cm dorsal of the external meatus. Ideally, the implants should be placed in a semilunar fashion. Placement of implants into the frontal bone **(B)** and the orbital rim **(C)**.

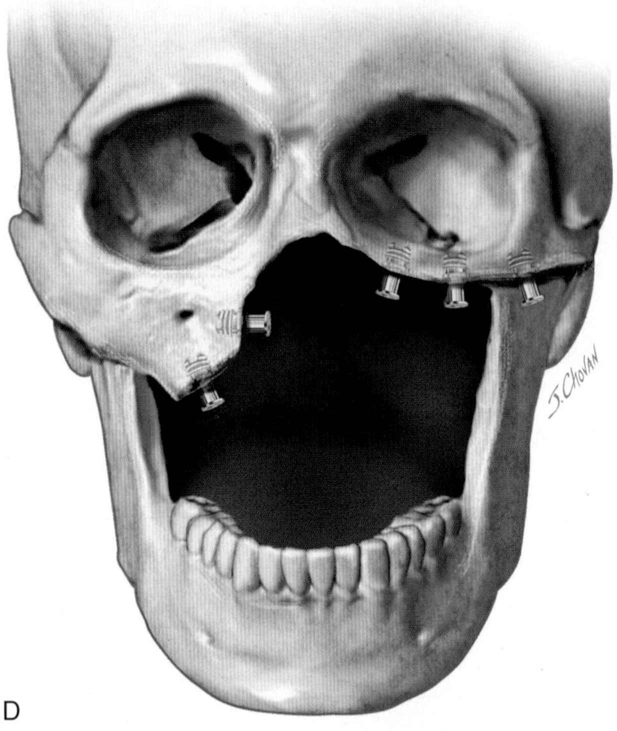

Figure 28.2, cont'd **D,** Areas suitable for implantation of implants in combined intra-/extraoral defects. (Sabine C. Girod)

the failure rate is especially high when implant placement is performed immediately following radiation therapy. There is still insufficient clinical and biological information to suggest an established timetable for the implantation of endosseous implants in irradiated bone because the bone-healing capacity can vary depending on the period of irradiation, the site, and the addition of chemotherapy.[21] Preoperative hyperbaric oxygen (HBO) can be considered as an adjuvant therapy to improve oxygenation and neovascularization of the irradiated bone. Recent studies have shown that the long-term survival of craniofacial implants placed in irradiated bone in patients treated with HBO was dramatically improved compared to patients without HBO treatment.[22–26]

TECHNIQUE: Endosseous Craniofacial Implants

The prerequisite for implant-based retention of orbital, auricular, or midface prostheses is the establishment of osseointegration.[2] For stable anchorage of extraoral prostheses, specially designed titanium implants are available in short lengths (e.g., 3 and 4 mm). A flange is designed for these implants to avoid dislocation into interior compartments (Fig. 28.3). Using these implants, many of the former limitations of prostheses designed to cover defects after tumor ablation in the face have been eliminated. Extraoral prostheses can now be directly anchored to the underlying bone with functional and esthetic improvements and long-lasting results.

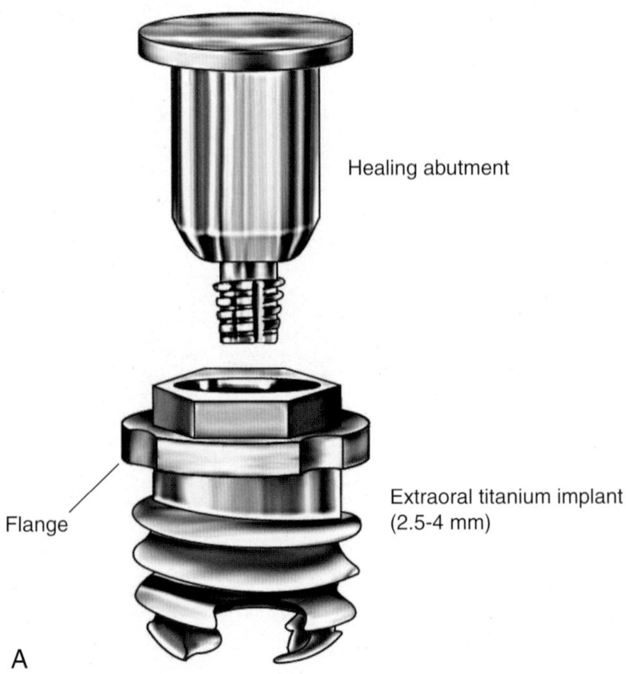

Figure 28.3 **A,** Extraoral implants and healing cap.

TECHNIQUE: Endosseous Craniofacial Implants—cont'd

STEP 1: Positioning of Implants

To position the implants, it is helpful to sculpture a wax replica of the prosthesis, which can also be used to fabricate a template for surgery.[27] In auricular prostheses, the external meatus can be incorporated into the template and used as a reference point during surgery. If no template is used, the position of the implants should be marked prior to surgery with a pen or needle, as the optimal implantation sites are difficult to determine in the operating room when the patient is dressed for surgery, due to a lack of visible landmarks (Fig. 28.1A).

STEP 2: Preparation of the Implant Site

In order to place the craniofacial implants, the implant sites are exposed by reflection of a full thickness skin flap with the incision line safely away from the intended implant sites.[28] Sharp bone edges or slopes should be avoided or smoothed. It is important to use sharp drilling instruments and sufficient irrigation to avoid thermal trauma to the bone and to optimize bone healing.

STEP 3: Implant Insertion

For the insertion of craniofacial implants, a guide drill is first used to give the depth and position of the implantation site, and a spiral drill is then used to give the final exact diameter and direction of the implant. For implantation into the temporal bone, the widened hole is threaded with a titanium tap. In other craniofacial locations, pretapping is not required because of the lower bone density. Finally, the implant is inserted gently, preferably with a low insertion torque. A cover screw is placed into the implant to prevent ingrowth of soft tissue during the healing period.

Conventionally, a two-stage procedure is used. The implants can be exposed after a healing interval of 3 to 4 months. In irradiated bone, a longer healing period is recommended. The implants are not exposed until 6 to 12 months after the installation, especially in the midface and orbital regions because of lower survival rates of osseointegrated implants in these areas.

STEP 4: Reduction of Subcutaneous Tissue

The most crucial step in the second-stage procedure is the reduction of the subcutaneous tissue. Ideally, the skin 10 mm around the abutment should be free of hair follicles and immobile; in addition, thinned and fat-free skin is required to prevent granulation tissue formation that leads to a higher implant failure rate.[8] In skin-penetrating abutments, it is important that the abutment/gold interface is at least 2 mm and a maximum of 5 mm above the tissue surface.[29] Subdermal margins and flange exposure can potentially lead to inflammation and loss of the implant. When the implants are uncovered, if the surrounding tissue is too thick and mobile resulting in chronic irritation, then surgical revision needs to be considered. This goal can also be achieved by the transplantation of hairless skin grafts, which can be combined with the second-stage procedure when the abutments are attached. For extraoral locations, split skin grafts with a 7 to 8 mm thickness can be harvested behind the ear, where the skin is thin, the texture is ideal, and the scar is not visible. Alternatively, a split skin graft can be taken from the thigh or the inside of the upper arm, which is usually more convenient for the patients. For intranasal or intraoral locations, mucosal skin grafts (e.g., from the hard palate) are preferred, as the risk of inflammation is smaller than for skin grafts. The tissue can be harvested paramarginally with a scalpel or a small mucotome. The thickness of the mucosal flap should be 0.5 to 1 mm. In the donor area, wound healing by free granulation of the tissue is usually rapid.

STEP 5: Impressions

Impressions of craniofacial defects are taken with the patient in an upright, sitting position. In combined intra-/extraoral or nasal prostheses, the defect should be carefully packed with gauze to prevent the impression material from flowing down into the throat. Copings are mounted on each abutment cylinder in order to ensure the correct transfer into the master impression. Alginate impression material is poured over the defect around the impression copings. Gauze is placed on the alginate surface for retention, and the impression is supported with fast-setting plaster and turned. Often, impressions need to be taken in several sections and then reassembled again. A master cast is produced with brass replicas in the correct position and used for fabrication of the retention structure.

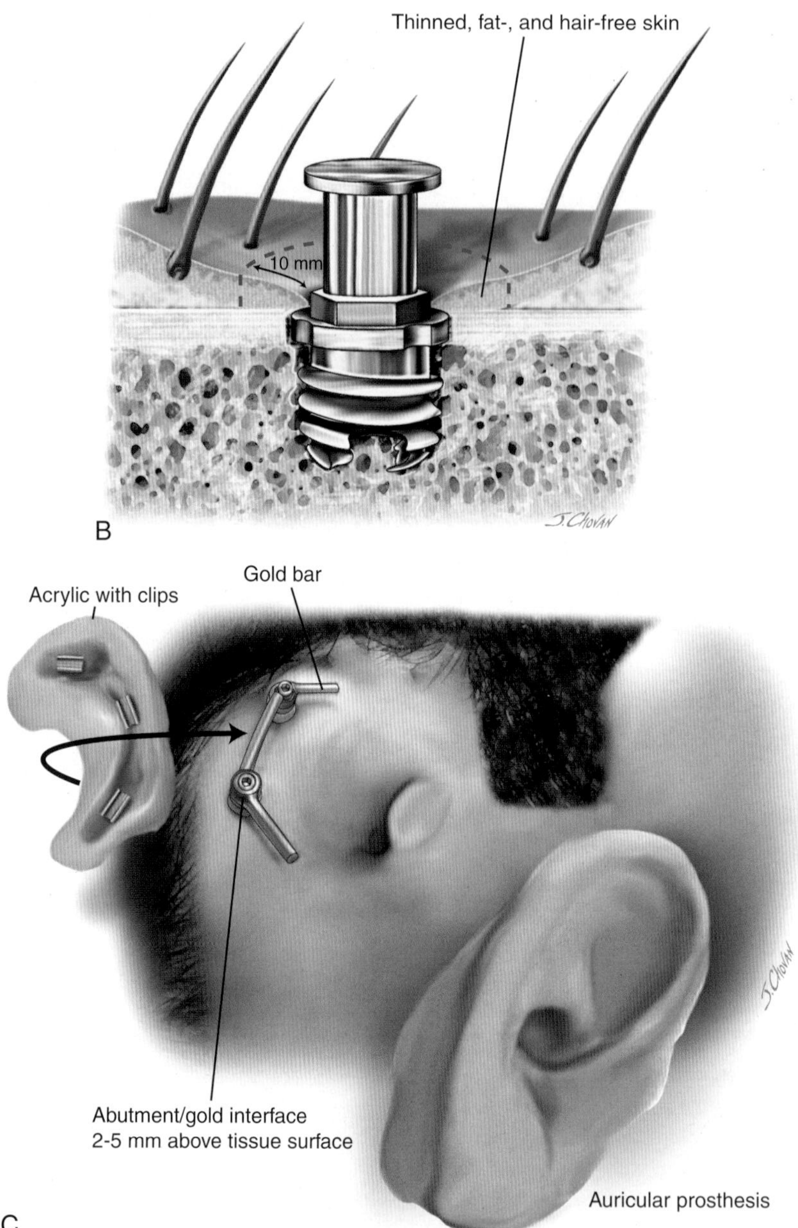

Figure 28.3, cont'd **B,** Reduction of the subcutaneous tissue. **C,** With skin-penetrating abutments, it is important that the abutment/gold interface is at least 2 mm and a maximum of 5 mm above the tissue surface. (Sabine C. Girod)

Avoidance and Management of Intraoperative Complications

Long-term success of a facial, orbital, or auricular prosthesis depends on the maintenance of anchorage function. The viability of all components of the prosthesis should be assessed by clinical evaluation of the implants and the anchorage system at least every 6 months. X-rays do not need to be performed routinely, as a right-angle projection, which allows assessment of the implant-bone interface, is not usually possible for extraoral implants. Clinical evaluation of the stability of the implant and the status of the surrounding tissues is crucial. The integrity of the prosthesis and the surgical follow-up should initially be scheduled in an alternating manner, so that the patient is seen every 3 months. Later, both appointments can be combined in a semiannual review.

The survival rates of extraoral implants depend on the site of implantation, ranging from 73.2% to 78.8% in irradiated bone and 95.2% in nonirradiated bone after 5 years.[7,30–32] The highest failure rates are observed in the frontal bone, zygoma, mandible, and nasal maxilla. The lowest implant failure rates are observed in the oral maxilla.[33] The failure rate of extraoral implants placed into irradiated bone appears to be even higher and also depends on the retention system of the prostheses. Fixed-retention systems have the highest implant survival rate, whereas removable retention systems, which are the combination of clips and magnets on cantilever extensions, have the lowest implant survival rate.[34] The time of the second-stage surgery, when the skin-penetrating abutments are attached to the implant, needs to be adjusted accordingly to allow for sufficient bone healing. In the mastoid, where the success rate of osseointegrated implants is high, the second-stage procedure is performed after 3 to 4 months. Alternatively, a one-stage procedure can be used. In all other craniofacial locations and in irradiated bone, a healing period of 6 months is advised, as clinical experience has shown that osseointegration appears to be slower, likely due to differences in bone quality. In general, the intervals for implantation and prosthetic restoration can be shortened in patients with a poor tumor prognosis, for maximal improvement of quality of life.[35]

Soft-tissue inflammation and ingrowth of soft tissue may lead to the loss of an extraoral implant and can be avoided in most cases by proper preparation of the implant site and adequate postoperative care. Inflammation can be caused by surrounding tissues that are too thick and mobile. It is therefore favorable for the skin mucosa to be thin and firmly attached to the underlying bone. To achieve this goal, the skin can be thinned out in the area where the implant is inserted at the time of implantation.

Ingrowth of soft tissue can also cause the loss of an implant. To avoid this problem, it is important to check the implant-bone-soft tissue interface regularly during follow-up. If ingrowing soft tissue is detected, it has to be carefully removed; it is not sufficient to excise the skin surrounding the implant. In these situations, transplantation of a split-thickness skin graft should be performed as a secondary procedure, as the implants are already in place. If skin grafts are performed in the nasal or oral cavity, mucosa transplants should be used for transplantation. In general, it is better to avoid such problems by preparing the implant site several weeks prior to implantation with a skin graft, in cases where the locally available soft tissue does not provide an adequately thin and immobile surrounding for the implant.

In addition, there appears to be a direct correlation between the level of hygiene and inflammatory soft tissue reactions of the skin at extraoral implantation sites. After tumor surgery and a radical neck dissection, the patient may be impaired in their movements, or the implant sites may not be visible to the patient. Orbital implants are most difficult to clean for the patient, and the failure rate is the highest among all facial locations. The floor of the nose is the easiest to clean and has the lowest rate of soft-tissue reactions leading to loss of the implant. With proper hygiene, the soft-tissue reaction can be influenced favorably. Patient follow-up should therefore be adjusted to individual needs. If soft-tissue reactions are found and the patient is unable to clean the implant sites, a daily recall may be necessary until the inflammation subsides.

Postoperative Considerations

A craniofacial prosthesis requires a lifetime commitment and cooperation by the patient. For the survival of endosseous craniofacial implants, it is especially important that the patient is willing and physically able to clean the skin around the implants daily. In general, patients with physical disabilities may have problems cleaning the implant sites. After a stroke or after tumor surgery with radical neck dissection, the mobility of one arm and the head can be impaired. In addition, implants in the temporal bone and the orbit are difficult to visualize for cleaning purposes. Patients should be informed that prostheses need to be replaced at certain intervals, as the color and the material, and therefore the esthetic appearance of the appliance, changes due to sunlight, air pollution, or loss of flexibility of the material. Patients may also require different prostheses as their skin color changes due to different degrees of suntan.

References

1. Köle H. Erfahrungen mit Gerüstimplantaten unter der Sdchleimhaut und Haut zur Befestigung von Prothesen und Epithesen. *Fortschr Kiefer Gesichtschir*. 1965;10:76.
2. Brånemark PI, Hansson BO, Adell R, et al. Osseointegrated implants in the treatment of the edentulous jaw. Experience from a 10-year period. *Scand J Plast Reconstr Surg Suppl*. 1977;16:1–132.
3. Branemark PI, Adell R, Breine U, Lindström J, Ohlsson A. Intra-osseous anchorage of dental prosthesis. *Scand J Plast Reconstr Surg*. 1969;3(2):81–100.
4. Brånemark PI, Albrektsson T. Titanium implants permanently penetrating human skin. *Scand J Plast Reconstr Surg*. 1982;16(1):17–21.
5. Tjellström A, Rosenhall U, Lindström J, Hallén O, Albrektsson T, Brånemark PI. Five-year experience with skin-penetrating bone-anchored implants in the temporal bone. *Acta Otolaryngol*. 1983;95(5–6):568–575.
6. Ariani N, Visser A, van Oort RP, et al. Current state of craniofacial prosthetic rehabilitation. *Int J Prosthodont (IJP)*. 2013;26(1):57–67.
7. Visser A, Raghoebar GM, van Oort RP, Vissink A. Fate of implant-retained craniofacial prostheses: life span and aftercare. *Int J Oral Maxillofac Implants*. 2008;23(1):89–98.
8. Curi MM, Oliveira MF, Molina G, et al. Extraoral implants in the rehabilitation of craniofacial defects: implant and prosthesis survival rates and peri-implant soft tissue evaluation. *J Oral Maxillofac Surg*. 2012;70(7):1551–1557.
9. Nemli SK, Aydin C, Yilmaz H, Bal BT, Arici YK. Quality of life of patients with implant-retained maxillofacial prostheses: a prospective and retrospective study. *J Prosthet Dent*. 2013;109(1):44–52.
10. Neukam FW, Scheller H, Schmelzeisen R. Perkutane verankerung von Gesichtsepithesen. In: Haneke E, ed. *Fortschritte der Operativen Dermatologie*. Berlin, Germany: Springer; 1988.
11. Reyes RA, Tjellström A, Granström G. Evaluation of implant losses and skin reactions around extraoral bone-anchored implants: a 0- to 8-year follow-up. *Otolaryngol Head Neck Surg*. 2000;122(2):272–276.
12. Schwarz MS, Rothman SL, Rhodes ML, Chafetz N. Computed tomography: part I.

Preoperative assessment of the mandible for endosseous implant surgery. *Int J Oral Maxillofac Implants*. 1987;2(3):137–141.
13. Schwarz MS, Rothman SL, Rhodes ML, Chafetz N. Computed tomography: part II. Preoperative assessment of the maxilla for endosseous implant surgery. *Int J Oral Maxillofac Implants*. 1987;2(3):143–148.
14. Andersson L, Kurol M. CT scan prior to installation of osseointegrated implants in the maxilla. *Int J Oral Maxillofac Surg*. 1987;16(1):50–55.
15. Girod SC, Rohlfing T, Maurer CR Jr. Image-guided surgical navigation in implant-based auricular reconstruction. *J Oral Maxillofac Surg*. 2008;66(6):1302–1306.
16. Thimmappa B, Girod SC. Principles of implant-based reconstruction and rehabilitation of craniofacial defects. *Craniomaxillofac Trauma Reconstr*. 2010;3(1):33–40.
17. Neukam FW, Schmelzeisen R, Schliephake H, Scheller H. Epithetische und defektprothetische Versorgung mit osteointegrierten Implantaten als Halteelementen zur funktionellen und ästhetischen Rehabilitation nach Tumorresektion. In: Rahmanzadeh R, Scheller EE, eds. *Alloplastische Verfahren und mikrochirurgische Maßnahmen*. Reinbek, Germany: Einhorn; 1994.
18. Jacobsson M, Tjellström A, Thomsen P, Turesson I. Integration of titanium implants in irradiated bone. Histologic and clinical study. *Ann Otol Rhinol Laryngol*. 1988;97(4 Pt 1):337–340.
19. Chrcanovic BR, Nilsson J, Thor A. Survival and complications of implants to support craniofacial prosthesis: a systematic review. *J Cranio-Maxillo-Fac Surg*. 2016;44(10):1536–1552.
20. Elledge R, Chaggar J, Knapp N, et al. Craniofacial implants at a single centre 2005–2015: retrospective review of 451 implants. *Br J Oral Maxillofac Surg*. 2017;55(3):242–245.
21. Jegoux F, Malard O, Goyenvalle E, Aguado E, Daculsi G. Radiation effects on bone healing and reconstruction: interpretation of the literature. *Oral Surg Oral Med Oral Pathol Oral Radiol Endod*. 2010;109(2):173–184.
22. Granström G. Placement of dental implants in irradiated bone: the case for using hyperbaric oxygen. *J Oral Maxillofac Surg*. 2006;64(5):812–818.
23. Larsen PE. Placement of dental implants in the irradiated mandible: a protocol involving adjunctive hyperbaric oxygen. *J Oral Maxillofac Surg*. 1997;55(9):967–971.
24. Granström G, Bertsröm K, Tjellström A, Branemark PI. A detailed analysis of titanium implants lost in irradiated tissues. *Int J Oral Maxillofac Implants*. 1994;9:653.
25. Niimi A, Fujimoto T, Nosaka Y, Ueda M. A Japanese multicenter study of osseointegrated implants placed in irradiated tissues: a preliminary report. *Int J Oral Maxillofac Implants*. 1997;12(2):259–264.
26. Franzén L, Rosenquist JB, Rosenquist KI, Gustafsson I. Oral implant rehabilitation of patients with oral malignancies treated with radiotherapy and surgery without adjunctive hyperbaric oxygen. *Int J Oral Maxillofac Implants*. 1995;10(2):183–187.
27. Ciocca L, Mingucci R, Bacci G, Scotti R. CAD-CAM construction of an auricular template for craniofacial implant positioning: a novel approach to diagnosis. *Eur J Radiol*. 2009;71(2):253–256.
28. Tjellström A. Osseointegrated system and their applications in the head and neck. *Adv Otolaryngol Head Neck Surg*. 1989;3:39.
29. Petrovic L, Schlegel KA, Wiltfang J, Neukam FW, Rupprecht S. Preclinical animal study and clinical trail of modified extraoral craniofacial implants. *J Plast Reconstr Aesthet Surg*. 2007;60(6):615–621.
30. Toljanic JA, Eckert SE, Roumanas E, et al. Osseointegrated craniofacial implants in the rehabilitation of orbital defects: an update of a retrospective experience in the United States. *J Prosthet Dent*. 2005;94(2):177–182.
31. Subramaniam SS, Breik O, Cadd B, et al. Long-term outcomes of craniofacial implants for the restoration of facial defects. *Int J Oral Maxillofac Implants*. 2018;47(6):773–782.
32. Balik A, Ozdemir-Karatas M, Peker K, et al. Soft tissue response and survival of extraoral implants: a long-term follow-up. *J Oral Implantol*. 2016;42(1):41–45.
33. Granström G. Osseointegration in irradiated cancer patients: an analysis with respect to implant failures. *J Oral Maxillofac Surg*. 2005;63(5):579–585.
34. Granström G. Craniofacial osseointegration. *Oral Dis*. 2007;13(3):261–269.
35. Karayazgan B, Gunay Y, Atay A, Noyun F. Facial defects restored with extraoral implant-supported prostheses. *J Craniofac Surg*. 2007;18(5):1086–1090.

CHAPTER 29

Implant Rehabilitation and Maxillomandibular Free Flap Reconstruction

Devin Joseph Okay and Daniel Buchbinder

Armamentarium

#9 Molt periosteal elevator
#15 Bard-Parker scalpel
0.9% Normal saline
Appropriate sutures
Dean scissors
Dental implant kit
Dental implant power drill set
Dental implants
Implant cover screws
Implant healing abutments
Local anesthetic with vasoconstrictor
Needle holder
Patient-specific computer-aided designed and manufactured (CAD-CAM) surgical guides
Planning software
Ruler

History of the Procedure

The goals of reconstruction in head and neck oncology may vary from patient to patient due to comorbidities involved with surgical reconstruction and patient motivation. Microvascular free tissue transfer has revolutionized the way surgeons address composite defects from ablative surgery of large tumors in a single-stage procedure. Furthermore, contemporary management of the patient with head and neck cancer integrates these surgical reconstructive techniques with prosthetic rehabilitation to optimize function and esthetics.[1–3] The biology of the disease and the wound healing properties of the recipient site from prior therapy further affect the plan for reconstruction.

The complexity of rehabilitation for patients with maxillomandibular defects reconstructed with vascularized bone free flaps makes it necessary to devise treatment strategies that meet the patient's expectations in terms of function, esthetics, and psychological and social aspects. Edentulous cancer patients who do not achieve oral rehabilitation after cancer surgery can exhibit significant functional and psychological morbidity.[4] Major advances in surgical reconstructive techniques and new approaches to maxillomandibular defects effectively provide a more conventional setting for prosthetic reconstruction of the dentoalveolar arch and surrounding structures.

Indications for the Use of the Procedure

Composite free flaps from the fibula, iliac crest, and scapula regions are designed and harvested to address tissue volumetric loss to restore mandibular continuity and to separate the oral cavity from sinonasal cavities.[5–8] Soft-tissue defects involving the overlying skin, mucosal defects involving the lip or cheek, and sensory and motor nerve deficits all define which reconstructive option is best for functional recovery. Preservation of tongue motion and the restoration of tongue volume are critical in obtaining a favorable functional outcome if tumor extension involves a significant portion of the tongue or floor of the mouth.[9] Vascularized bone–containing free flaps (VBFF) either restore continuity defects of the mandible or reproduce the stable base of the maxilla. Vascularized bone flaps from the fibula or iliac crest donor sites provide good to excellent bone volume and quality, which are required for osseointegration to enhance prosthetic rehabilitation. Composite free flaps from the scapula are selected when the soft-tissue requirements of the defects are significant or when the use of the fibula donor site is contraindicated due to poor vascular runoff in the lower extremity or advanced age of the patient. However, this bone flap has a comparatively poor bone volume for osseointegration (Table 29.1). If it is selected, two to four implants, no more than 10 mm in length, can be placed along the medial aspect of the angular tip for a removable prosthesis.[10,11] Orientation of this area as a denture-bearing surface may prove challenging. Subsequent debulking of the overlying soft-tissue will most likely be needed.

The fact that a bone–containing free flap has its own blood supply offers additional strategies for implant-assisted prosthetic rehabilitation of acquired defects resulting from the treatment of large benign and malignant tumors of the jaws. One such strategy is to take advantage of the rich vascular bed

Table 29.1 Comparison of Donor Site Attributes for Reconstruction of Maxillomandibular Defects

	Fibula[a]	Iliac Crest	Scapula	Radius
Bone volume	++++	+++++	+++	+
Osseointegration	++++	++++	++	
Soft tissue	+++	++++[b]	+++++	+++
Donor site morbidity	++	++++	++	+

[a]The overall favorable characteristics of the fibular donor site makes this composite free flap the workhorse for jaw reconstruction compared to other donor sites.
[b]With the internal oblique muscle.

for osseointegration before the delivery of adjuvant radiation therapy. Implant placement at the time of the initial reconstructive procedure also shortens the overall treatment time to a definitive prosthetic restoration. Once the bone has been fixed to the reconstruction plate and the anastomosis of recipient vessels is complete, implant placement can be performed before the insetting of the soft-tissue used to restore the intraoral defect. After primary implant placement, the restorative team must allow 12 to 16 weeks for undisturbed healing and osseointegration of the fixtures.[12] When the patient has completed radiation therapy after reconstruction and primary implant placement, the fixtures are uncovered once the soft-tissue reaction from the radiation treatment has subsided. At that time, soft-tissue modification (e.g., flap debulking or vestibuloplasty procedures) can also be performed. A surgical stent can be used and secured to the implants for healing purposes before the fabrication of the definitive prosthesis. The surgical stent can be made with or without teeth, depending on the clinical situation and the patient's wishes. The stent promotes undisturbed healing, maintains vestibular height, and improves the function and appearance of the lips and mouth.

Primary implant placement is the key to developing a comprehensive approach to ablative surgery, subsequent reconstruction, and prosthodontic rehabilitation with adjunctive radiation. This also holds true for implant placement into native bone at the time of tumor resection to optimize prosthetic rehabilitation without additional surgical reconstructive procedures. Primary implant placement can circumvent the need for hyperbaric oxygen before secondary placement of fixtures in patients who will receive radiation therapy after the reconstruction.[13] In addition, primary implant placement minimizes time with an unstable prosthesis and compromised function in the edentulous patient. In 1998, the authors reported the success of implants placed into VBFF as the primary setting and subsequently irradiated as 86% (n = 81 implants). This information was part of a patient cohort of 210 cases using microvascular composite flaps for oromandibular reconstruction.[14]

Limitations and Contraindications

If a patient has received radiation therapy to the head and neck region, review of the simulation plan, including dosimetry and fields, is necessary to determine whether native bone or the VBFF has been affected, resulting in a compromised situation for osseointegration. Patients who undergo a hyperbaric oxygen protocol[15,16] do so to enhance the vascularity of the surgical bed (soft tissue) before implant surgery. Hyperbaric oxygen has been reported as beneficial to postirradiated native mandible[17,18] and fibula free flaps.[19,20]

The decision for fixed or removable prosthetic restorations depends on clinical factors such as bone availability, the number and position of implants to assist or support the restoration, and the hygiene maintenance and manual dexterity of the patient. In addition to these clinical factors, other considerations, such as comfort and psychosocial implications, affect prosthetic design. When addressing the reconstruction of the dental arch with osseointegrated fixtures, our preference is to provide patients with a fixed implant-supported restoration. When the remaining arch is edentulous and a lateral mandibular free flap reconstruction is performed, the fixtures should be placed in the anterior native mandible. This is an ideal location for implant placement in patients undergoing lateral jaw resection for posterior alveolar, floor of the mouth/lateral tongue, or tonsillar primary tumors because this area is usually spared radiation. A minimum of four or five implants, with the greatest anterior-posterior spread to minimize cantilever forces of the distal extension of the prosthesis, is recommended to restore the total dental arch. Posterior placement of the distal implant on the contralateral side of the mandible is potentially limited by the inferior alveolar neurovascular bundle and mental nerve. These landmarks must be identified, and care must be taken to avoid injuring them. Three or four implants placed into VBFF are recommended for unilateral maxillomandibular defects. As the defect crosses the midline, more implants are necessary to support the prosthesis. At the very least, four but usually up to six implants are required to support a fixed restoration.[21]

Issues regarding periimplant soft-tissue maintenance also arise. When muscle from the free flap is used for lining the oral cavity, the neomucosa around the implants might require repeated surgical débridement of hyperplastic inflammatory tissue around the transmucosal abutments. This problem may require excision and simple repair to possible split-thickness skin grafting if repeated robust growth of this unwanted tissue continues to be a problem.

TECHNIQUE: Mandible Reconstruction

The placement of dental implants in a VBFF is not substantially different in principle or method from the placement of implants in the native bone of the maxilla and mandible. The reader is encouraged to review Chapter 19 for technical information on the actual sequencing and implant placement details. Relevant differences in surgical technique and planning for implant placement in VBFF reconstructions of mandibular and maxillary defects are reviewed in the following sections.

STEP 1: Incision Design

For microvascular flaps with an intraoral skin paddle, the incision should be placed at the junction between the native oral mucosa and the skin of the free flap.

STEP 2: Flap Retraction

The dissection plane should be advanced to the level of the underlying bone. The surgeon should remain cognizant of the location of the perforating blood vessels to the free flap. Doppler ultrasound may be helpful in finding the location of these vessels.

STEP 3: Implant Placement

Implant placement is as previously described (see Chapter 19).

STEP 4: Closure and Soft-Tissue Management

In cases of maxillofacial free flap reconstruction, secondary soft-tissue procedures such as debulking or deepithelialization of the skin paddle often must be performed, along with implant placement, to facilitate a more favorable tissue emergence of the dental implants. These adjunctive procedures may need to be performed in advance of dental implant placement to obtain appropriate soft-tissue contour.

The advantages of the fibula free flap have made this a "workhorse" flap for mandibular reconstruction of discontinuity defects. The length of the bone that can be harvested allows for near total mandibular reconstruction (from condyle to condyle). The low donor site morbidity and its distance for the primary surgical field allow for a two-team approach, which reduces overall surgical time and associated morbidity. Additionally, there is good to excellent bone stock for osseointegration. The bicortical nature of the fibula offers approximately 12 to 15 mm of bone height for endosteal implant placement.[22] Unlike the scapula or iliac crest free flaps, which are monocortical in terms of implant fixation, implants placed into the fibula should engage both cortices to improve initial stability, osseointegration, and the ability to resist forces.[23]

The fibula is tubular and triangular in cross section, and the three surfaces have dedicated characteristics. One surface has cutaneous perforators arising from the peroneal artery and vein, another surface is where the vascular pedicle runs, and the lateral aspect is used for internal fixation hardware that will secure the flap in position to allow for undisturbed healing of the osteotomized fibula and union to the remaining native mandibular stumps. Orientation of skin will determine whether the base or apex of the triangle is oriented as the neo-ridge of the maxilla or mandible.[24] These factors have significant implications for whether implants can be placed in the immediate setting at the time of the surgical reconstruction.

The use of fibula rather than iliac crest donor sites can present a geometric challenge for prosthetic reconstruction. As mentioned, the fibula is best positioned at the inferior border of the mandible to reproduce contours of the lower third of the face. This may lead to an intraoral height discrepancy with the native mandible. Additionally, because the alveolus is naturally positioned lingual to the inferior border, a neomandible created by placing bone at the inferior border can result in subsequent implants placed facial to the dentition in the opposing arch. In such cases, an implant-assisted, removable overdenture can be constructed so that lip and cheek support and oral competence are promoted. The use of a bar framework positioned lingual to implants can overcome the height discrepancy and facial position. The overdenture has small fenestrations at the base of the facial flange, thereby overcoming the facial position of the implants. The contours of the mandibular prosthesis can provide support to the lower lip to restore projection and symmetry to the lower face. The loss of motor function from injury of the marginal mandibular branch of the facial nerve can be ameliorated with this means of lip support.

The restoration of bilateral occlusal contacts, where occlusal guidance and protection schemes are restored to that of a fully dentate individual, is a critical step to optimal functional rehabilitation. The position of the mandible is determined for both condyles by elements and by the dental occlusion. Reconstruction of the mandibular continuity defect with VBFF allows for both condylar determinants to function normally. The condition of the occlusion and dentition has an effect on function. The non-sensate nature of the VBFF reconstruction, other sensory deficits, and potential motor nerve to the lip and cheek make occlusal rehabilitation a restorable variable. A distinction is made between tissue-supported occlusal contacts and implant-supported tooth contacts and functional outcome. A further distinction is made between fixed and removable implant restorations. Rehabilitation with a fixed dental prosthesis (FDP) has better results for chewing capacity and esthetics and results in less physiologic discomfort and psychological disability than do removable prosthetic counterparts.[25–28] The rigidity of an FDP and replacement of teeth with

Continued

TECHNIQUE: Mandible Reconstruction—*cont'd*

surrounding alveolus is a "near normal" design without the daily reminder of a removable prosthesis. These restorations are screw retained where the prosthesis is retrievable rather than a cemented restoration. This design consideration is an important factor in case direct visualization of tissue is necessary.

Treatment planning involves more implants rather than a minimum number for support of a fixed restoration. In the event of an implant failure, prosthetic success is still achievable with a shorter restoration of the dental arch or an implant-assisted overdenture, without added time or surgery.

Other approaches have been used to overcome this height discrepancy of fibula free flap reconstruction of the mandible. One is to position the fibula more superior and use the reconstruction plating system to reproduce contours of the inferior border. Another is the double barrel technique, in which the fibula is folded to increase the bone height and reduce the discrepancy between the occlusal plane and reconstruction.[29,30]

Another surgical technique is distraction osteogenesis of the fibula to overcome the height discrepancy. One study reported a mean vertical bone height of 13.58 mm in five patients receiving 22 implants and dental restorations. However, infection of the distraction rod was mentioned as a potential complication.[31]

The authors recently reported a retrospective case series (n = 28 patients) in which inclusion criteria for all patients were VBFF reconstruction and computer-assisted planning (CAP) for FDP restoration in preparation for implant surgery. Implant success with immediate load, provisional, and definitive FDP restorations in VBFF was reported for the first time in a patient cohort. Patients were evaluated for implant success, computed tomography (CT)-derived surgical templates, immediate provisional restorations, and prosthodontic framework design.

Ninety-nine of 116 osseointegrated implants placed were used for prosthetic restorations, achieving an 85.4% success rate. One hundred two implants achieved osseointegration (87.1%). Twenty-five of 28 patients (89.3%) received definitive implant FDP restorations. Two patients received removable implant-assisted restorations, and one patient was unable to complete rehabilitation due to implant failure. Thirteen of 28 patients received immediate or early-loaded fixed restorations at stage 1 implant surgery. The success rate for implants in the immediate restoration group was 89.3% (50/56). All 13 patients with immediate restorations had CT-derived surgical templates for their implant surgeries. Twelve of 13 immediate restorations were successful. Functional recovery for patients who undergo maxillomandibular reconstruction with VBFF is potentially more attainable with computer-assisted implant rehabilitation. Although the overall treatment time may be similar to that for patients without immediate restorations, we found the potential to provide patients with fixed provisional restorations during time for osseointegration and definitive FDP fabrication (Fig. 29.1).[32]

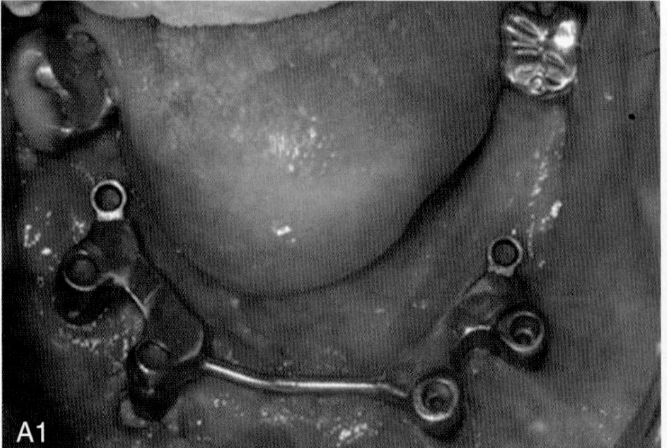

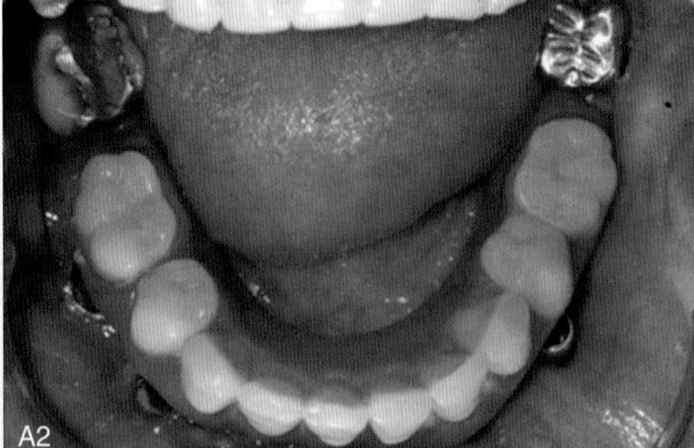

Figure 29.1 As part of the geometric puzzle for mandibular reconstruction, the dental arch sits anatomically within the mandibular arch. The design of the implant bar framework for a removable dental prosthesis negotiates this difference. **A1,** Implant support is centered for occlusal rehabilitation by positioning the bar lingual to the fibula and implants. **A2,** Fibula free flap reconstruction of the mandible creates a significant height discrepancy between native mandible and fibula if the inferior border and outline form of the lower third of the face are restored.

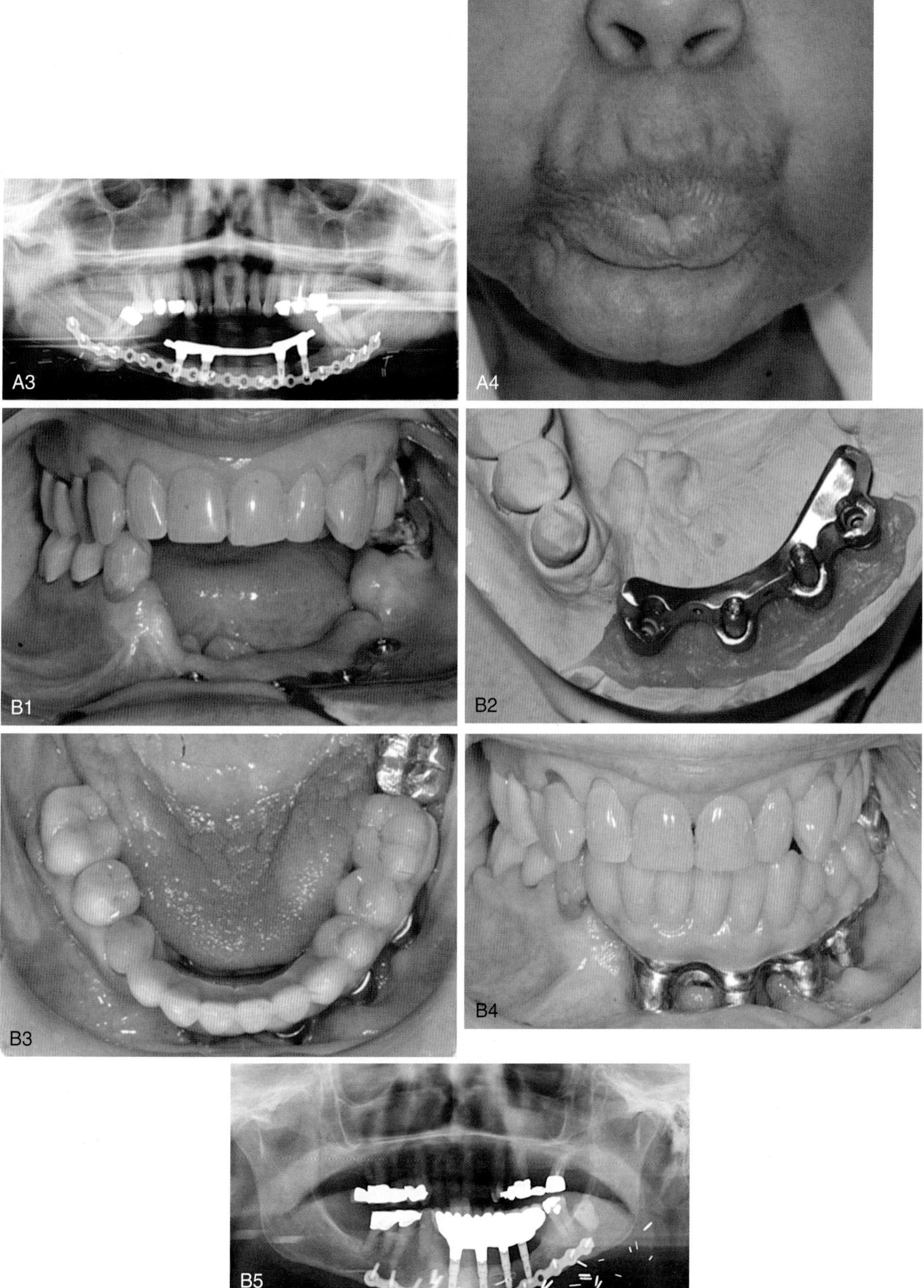

Figure 29.1, cont'd **A3,** Implant framework and prosthetic design are critical to achieve lip and oral competence (**A4**). **B1,** Frontal view of the height discrepancy between native mandible and occlusal plane to the fibula free flap reconstruction and implants. **B2,** The facial implant position and large height discrepancy are overcome with a cast titanium mesostructure connecting the implants and milled to the corresponding superstructure of the fixed dental prosthesis. **B3,** In this case, a ceramic-metal system is used for the superstructure and is retained by lingual set screws. **B4,** Function and esthetics are optimized through the thoughtful prosthodontic design considerations of this fixed restoration. **B5,** Panoramic radiographic view.

ALTERNATIVE TECHNIQUE: Palatomaxillary Reconstruction

Surgical reconstruction of palatomaxillary defects has also evolved over the past decade to emerge as a viable option for patients undergoing resection of large tumors resulting in significant arch defects. Although the use of soft-tissue flaps for the closure of large palatomaxillary defects can provide closure of the oral cavity, problems are encountered with large soft-tissue flaps occupying the functional space over the tongue that are not amenable to dental reconstruction. Obturators can provide a safe and effective way to successfully restore the defects, and these remain a standard of maxillofacial prosthetic rehabilitation because as defects get larger, nasal escape can compromise speech and swallowing. These side effects also can influence comfort and psychosocial interaction, making surgical reconstruction of palatomaxillary defects an approach that achieves optimal functional rehabilitation.[33,34]

The use of vascularized bone free flaps to reconstruct large palatomaxillary defects provides surgical closure, restores the alveolar defect, and provides a platform for the placement of osseointegrated fixtures.

Our classification system essentially addresses the size and location of palatomaxillary defects and considers the biomechanical properties that contribute to prosthetic instability and compromised function.[35] The remaining dental arch and palatal shelf and other components for anatomic retention, such as scar band formation with a split-thickness skin graft, have been useful prognostic factors for treatment algorithms and, in particular, the indications for VBFF reconstruction. As the remaining dental arch shortens and the palatal surface decreases, prosthetic instability is more likely to occur. Three defect classifications describe the horizontal nature of palatal defects. If an orbital defect is in combination with a maxillectomy defect, surgical reconstruction should address the separation of the combined defect. Maxillectomy defects have subscripts *o* (orbital floor) and *z* (zygoma) to address these areas in the restorative decision-making process. The class I defect is the subtotal maxillectomy defect, in which there is loss of the posterior alveolus to the canine tooth. This type of defect is characterized by sufficient remaining retentive and stabilizing components. Class I defects, therefore, are amenable to either prosthetic obturation or surgical reconstruction with a radial forearm free flap or palatal island flap. The remaining dental arch and palate are used to provide restoration to the dental arch with a tissue-borne prosthesis. Implants in the remaining native maxilla are necessary if the dentition is hopeless or if the patient is edentulous for rehabilitation. A class II defect is a hemimaxillectomy defect extending to the midline. In class II defects, the increased size of the defect and the loss of the ipsilateral canine and molar dentition make the use of a VBFF reconstruction important if the surgeon and prosthodontist decide not to use an obturator. This approach optimizes function and addresses the shortcomings of an obturator.

The anatomic complexity of the maxilla is related to its three-dimensional (3D) construct, a latticelike structure that is supported by three separate buttresses. These buttresses, which form as an adaptation to the vertical forces of mastication, are the nasomaxillary, zygomaticomaxillary, and pterygomaxillary buttresses. The integrity of these structures is essential to providing a stable occlusal surface for the mandible. Furthermore, they allow for an even distribution of forces across the skull base.[36,37] A possible challenge to reconstruction of the dental arch arises when the nasomaxillary and zygomaticomaxillary buttresses are used to fixate underlying vascularized bone. The position of the fibula should not be used for final projection and support of the lip; that role is given to the definitive prosthesis and tooth replacement. VBFF plating to the nasomaxillary buttress is positioned just beneath the anterior nasal spine, the piriform aperture, and the nasal sill. The maxillary anterior teeth are facial to this area such that implant placement would then be favorable for a prosthetic restoration. If a fibula free flap is used, there is a tendency for bone availability to be more lateral as the reconstruction moves posterior toward the zygoma. This may lead to implants in a facial position to the dental arch, surrounded by movable cheek mucosa, becoming poor candidates for prosthetic rehabilitation. CAP with a radiographic scanning appliance can improve implant position to overcome this relationship. Vascularized bone offers the ability to reestablish the bony dental arch for the placement of osseointegrated implants. This allows for the distribution of masticatory forces across an intact maxillary arch and thereby reestablishes a favorable biomechanical condition to the maxilla.

The preference for fixed dental prostheses is evident in this classification. Surgical reconstruction with fibula or iliac crest free flaps and implant-supported fixed dental prostheses replace analogous structures of a stable palatomaxillary complex. An FDP restoration for a class II defect reconstructed with VBFF leaves remaining palatal mucosa exposed over the tongue, promoting lingual-palatal feedback during function. Furthermore, the VBFF permits the primary reconstruction of the orbital rim and the prominence of the zygomatic body with autologous tissue. Class II defects are perhaps best reconstructed and rehabilitated by VBFF to optimize function.[38]

A class III defect extends beyond the midline. The defect involves both canines and ipsilateral molar dentition, resulting in a bilateral defect with a poor prosthodontic prognosis that severely compromises speech and swallowing. Class III defects are best restored with a VBFF, patient factors allowing. As a maxillectomy defect increases in size and the remaining dentition and palate decrease in size, a VBFF is clearly preferred over a fasciocutaneous free flap for functional recovery. Although soft-tissue reconstruction of a class III defect serves to effectively partition the oral cavity from the sinonasal cavities, orodental rehabilitation is not addressed with a soft-tissue flap. VBFF reconstruction, osseointegration, and a FDP can restore stable dentoalveolar structures and occlusal contacts to optimize speech and swallowing functions (Fig. 29.2).

Avoidance and Management of Intraoperative Complications

CAP is a next-generation tool in surgical reconstruction and implant placement. In our clinical setting, its application is considered routinely for patients with VBFF surgical reconstruction of maxillomandibular defects. In the absence of postoperative irradiation, secondary placement of implants with CAP is a progressive approach in prosthodontic rehabilitation. CAP can be accurately used 4 to 6 weeks after VBFF reconstruction. Plate screws can be avoided with virtual implant surgery, or a decision can be made to modify internal fixation hardware that may interfere with the placement of a sufficient number of implants for a fixed restoration. In this situation, implant surgery is performed once bony union of the VBFF osteotomies has been established, approximately 6 to 8 weeks after surgical reconstruction. Advances in the reconstruction and rehabilitation treatment of patients with head and neck cancer involve application of computer planning software with computer-aided design and computer-aided manufacturing (CAD-CAM). This approach has ushered in a new way of thinking about implant-assisted prosthetic rehabilitation.

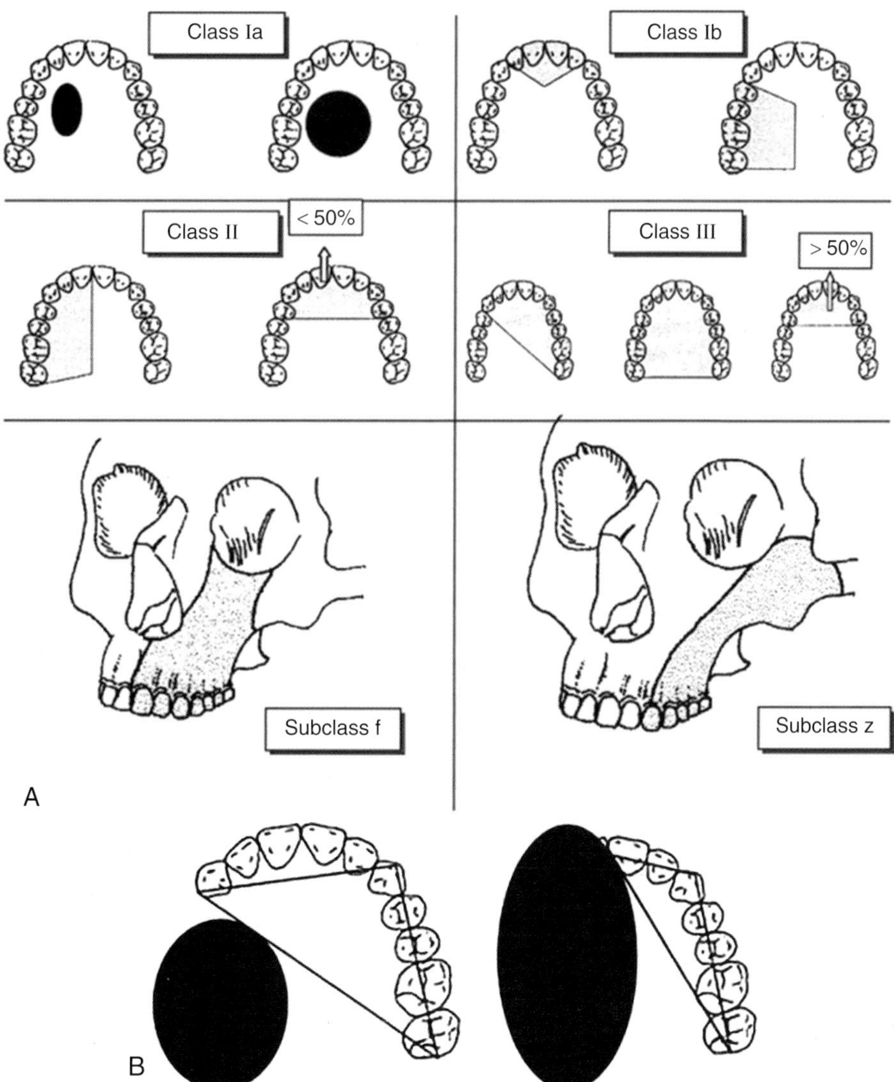

Figure 29.2 **A,** Classification of horizontal and vertical components to a maxillectomy defect. Palatal defects of increasing size in the horizontal plane are classified I, II, and III. **B,** Potential for prosthetic stability decreases as the size of the defect increases and the remaining dental arch with palatal surface area diminishes. The ability to stabilize the fulcrum line of a prosthetic removable partial denture framework is diminished and possibly problematic. Side effects such as hyper-nasal speech and leakage (this does not belong here) into the sino-nasal cavity become more likely under these circumstances. These physical parameters are critical to restorative decision making between class I and class II defects. Where class I defects are amenable to surgical reconstruction with soft-tissue flaps, surgical reconstruction and the import of vascularized bone for an implant-supported fixed dental prosthesis optimize functional recovery of class II and III defects.

Continued

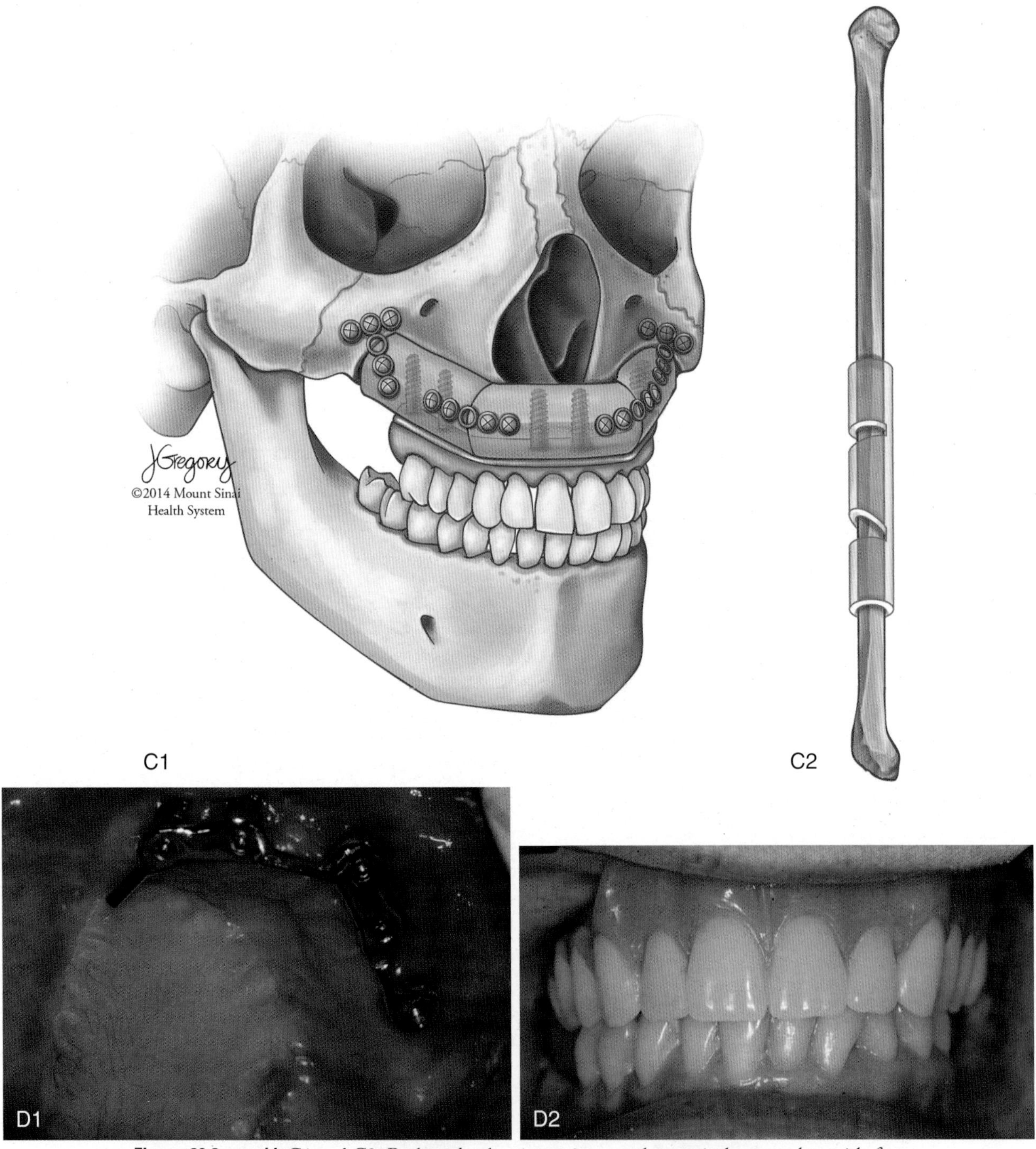

Figure 29.2, cont'd **C1** and **C2,** Backwards planning, microvascular surgical approaches with free fibular flaps, and sound treatment concepts for prosthodontic rehabilitation become the basis for computer-assisted surgical (CAS) planning. Artist rendering of class III defect reconstructed with fibula and implants (**C1**) using CAS planning and guides (**C2**). **D1** and **D2,** Class Ib paloto-maxillary defect reconstructed with a radial forearm free flap in an edentulous patient. Implants placed at the time of reconstruction allow for an osseointegrated removable dental prosthesis promoting function and cosmesis.

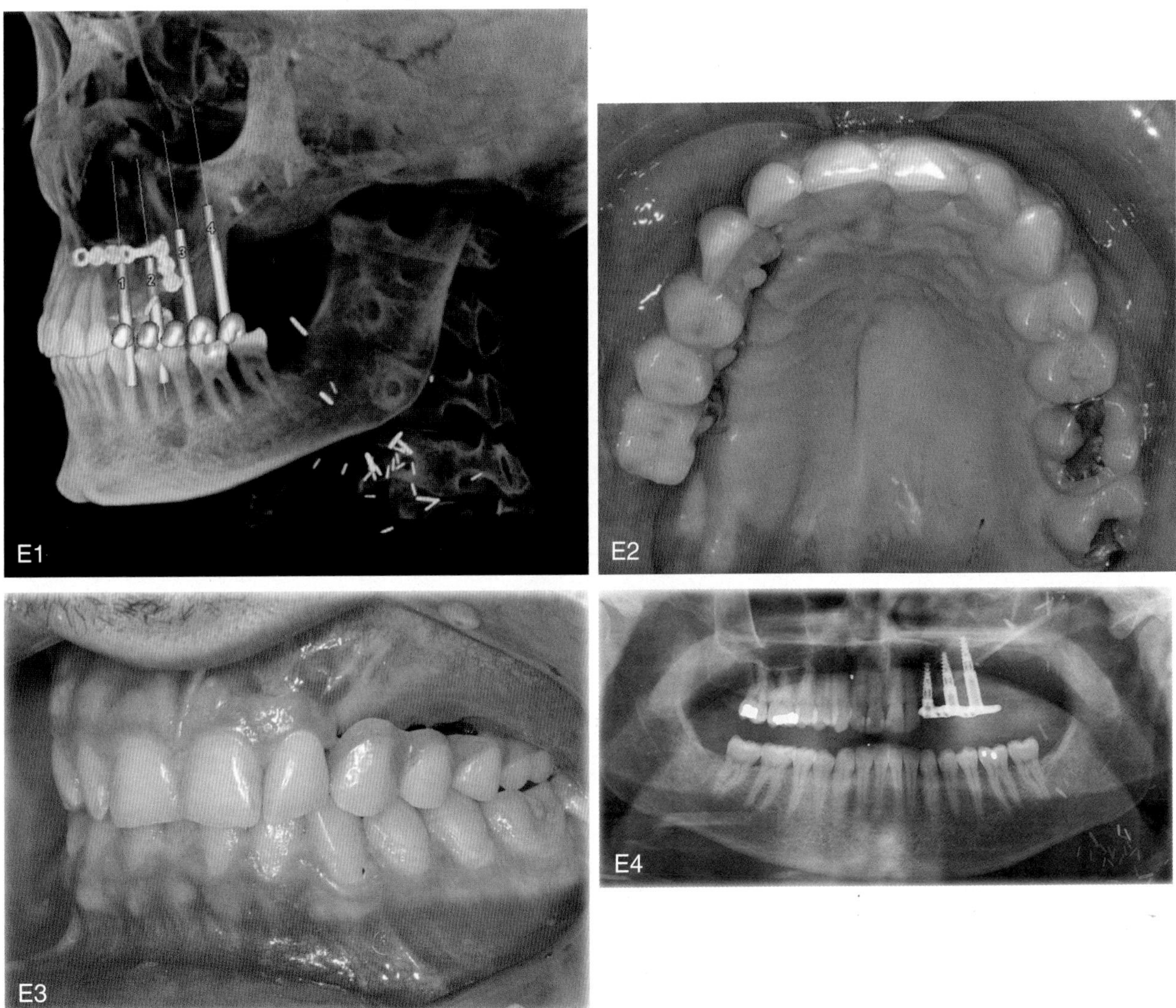

Figure 29.2, cont'd **E1,** Computer-assisted three-dimensional (3D) reformation after virtual implant placement into the fibula free flap reconstruction of a class II maxillary defect. **E2** and **E3,** Screw-retained fixed dental prosthesis is seen in occlusal and side views, restoring occlusal contacts and form to the dental arch. Panoramic radiograph of vascularized bone–containing free flaps (VBFF) reconstruction of implant rehabilitation with screw-retained fixed dental prosthesis. The outcome resembles the computer planning with the exception of the virtual fourth implant which is unnecessary, difficult to access, and can present soft-tissue problems. **E4,** Fibula free flap reconstruction of the mandible with double barrel segment fixation with miniplate and precontoured fixation plate seen in blue.

Continued

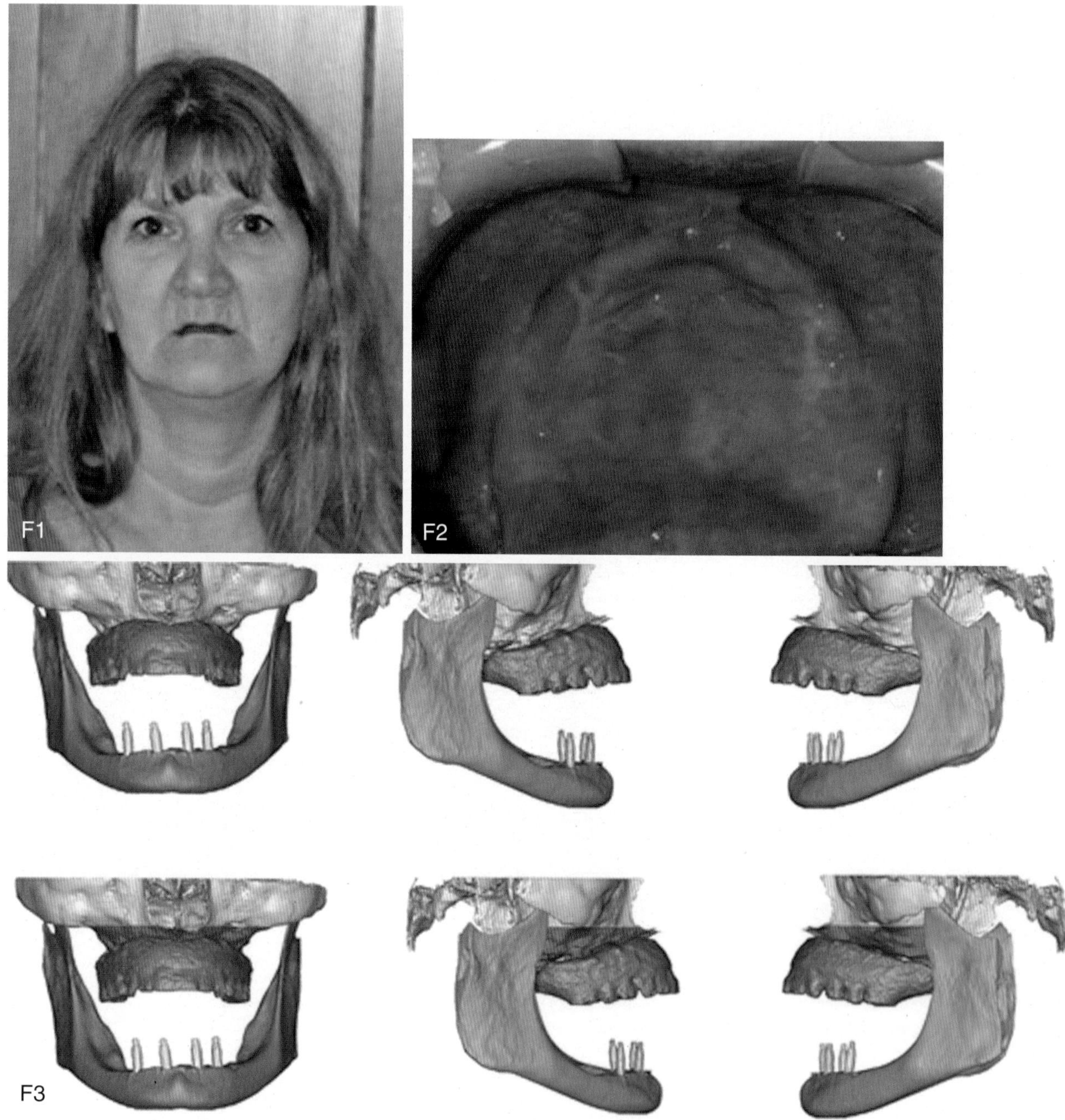

Figure 29.2, cont'd **F1** and **F2,** Preoperative views of a patient with severe maxillary atrophy after repeated failures of free bone grafts (over 20 attempts). **F3,** Computer planning with existing complete denture duplicated into barium scanning appliance for diagnostic purposes. Vertical space for fibula free flap reconstruction is created with an infrastructure maxillectomy (Le Fort I) and resulting class III defect.

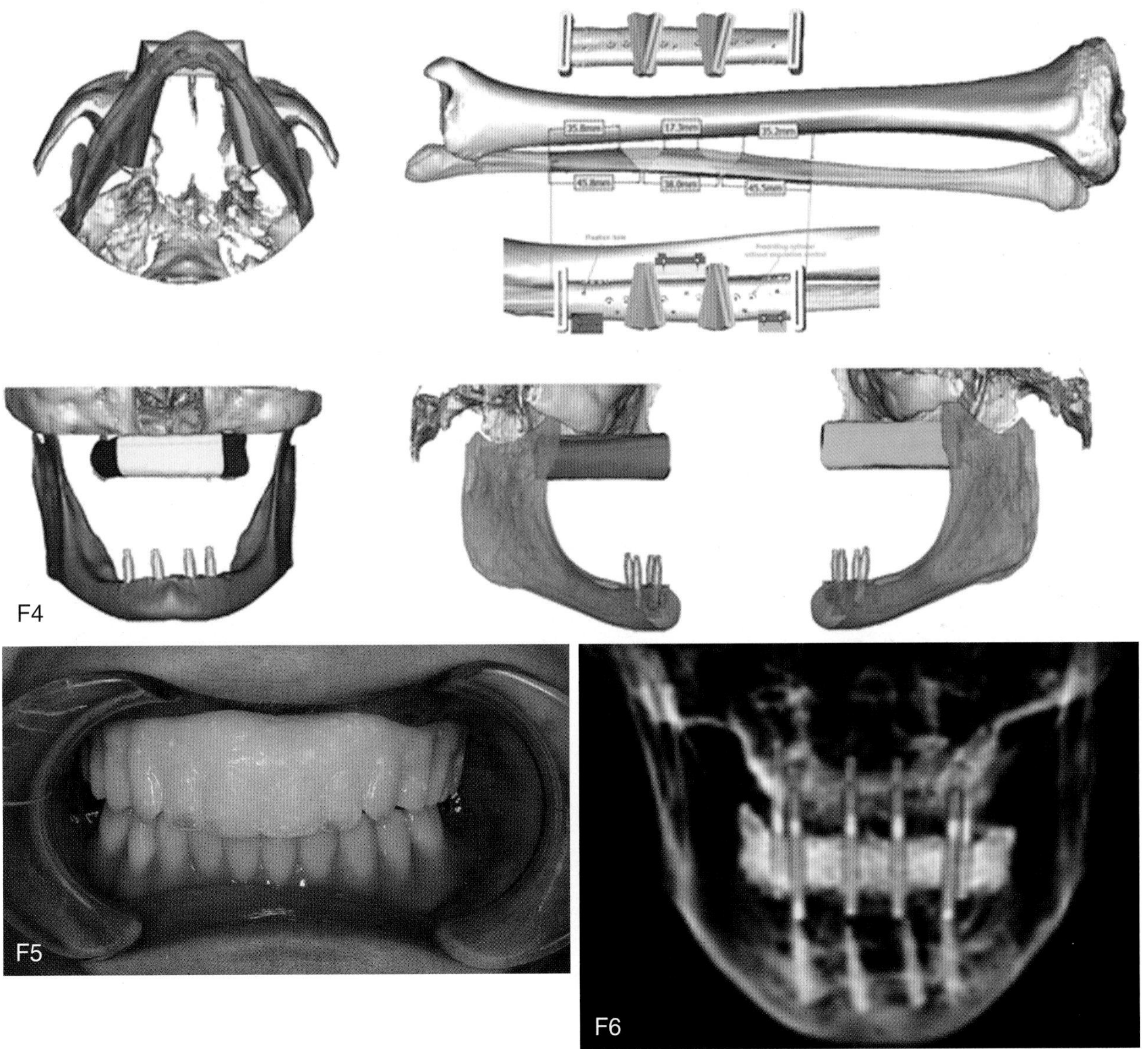

Figure 29.2, cont'd **F4,** CAS ostectomy guides are virtually planned with fibula free flap reconstruction visualized into a favorable, horizontal, and anterior-posterior position. **F5** and **F6,** Clinically verified radiographic scanning appliance is fabricated 8 weeks postsurgical reconstruction and registered on 3D planning software prior for virtual stage 1 implant surgery.

Continued

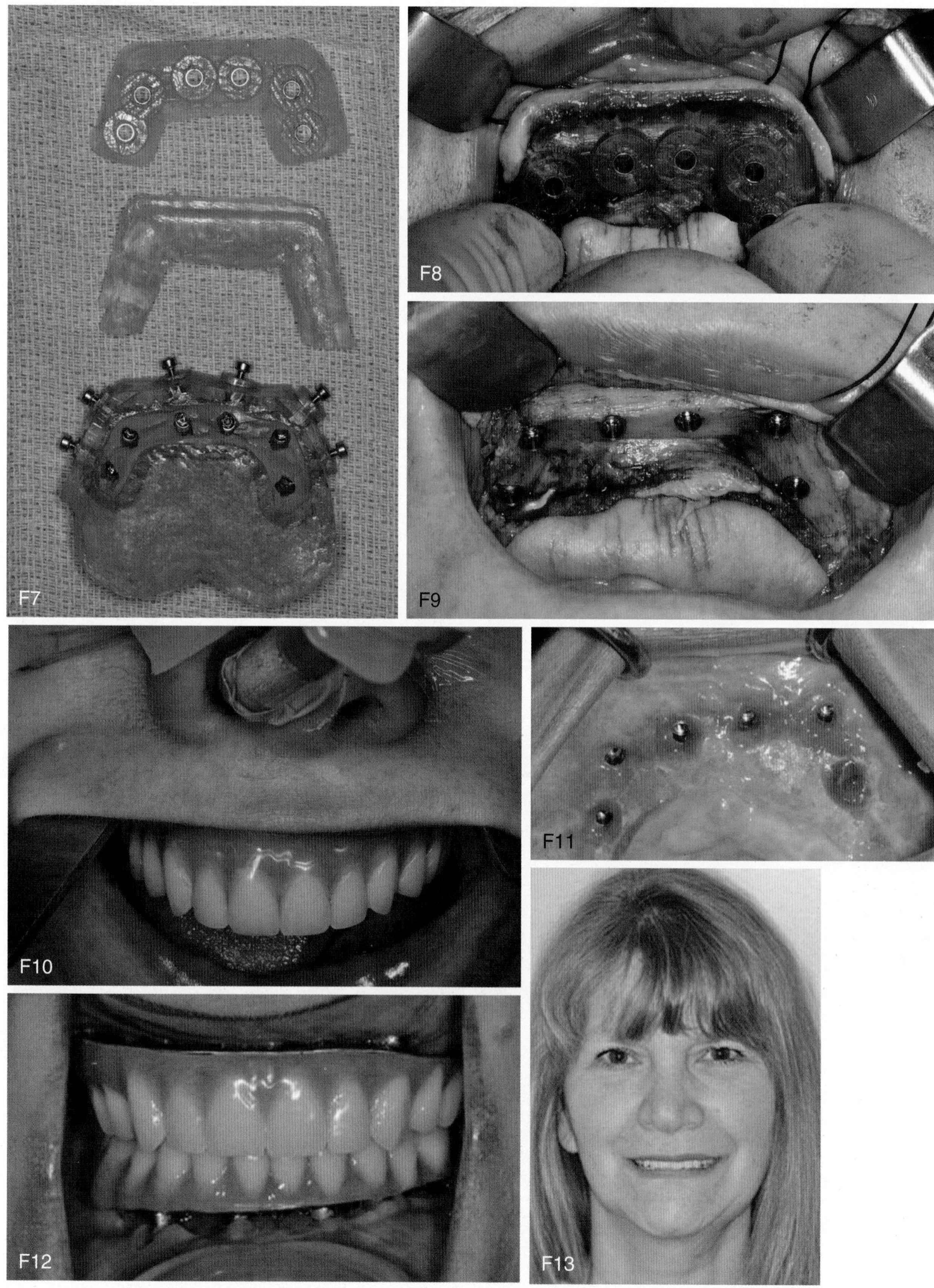

Figure 29.2, cont'd **F7,** Computer planning for implant placement and immediate restoration is performed with the aid of computer-aided designed and manufactured (CAD-CAM) models and surgical guide. **F8** and **F9,** Implant surgical guide is positioned onto the fibula free flap for osteotomy preparation and implant placement. **F10,** Connection of clinically verified immediate fixed dental prosthesis achieved with abutment screws. **F11** and **F13,** Clinical views of implants after definitive reconstruction with CAD-CAM titanium framework fixed dental prosthesis.

Rapid prototyping is an automated process in which construction is accomplished with a 3D printer or stereolithography (laser-driven polymerizing) machines. Digital technology can create accurate models from 3D imaging data or can be applied to the fabrication of surgical templates with the aid of software programs. The software programs allow for virtual surgery in preoperative planning, and then this data are translated to the surgery via the template. For implant placement, this approach is prosthodontic driven, whereas a CT study is made with a radiographic scanning appliance in place. The appliance is fabricated so that the position of the dentition and their occlusal surfaces are captured in the CT scan. The scanning appliance is processed with a radiopaque material or with fiducials. 3D software provides panoramic, axial, and horizontal planes to perform accurate virtual implant placement according to bone availability and tooth position.[39] The angulation of the fixtures is such that their screw access is confined to the occlusal surface, rather than perforating esthetic facial surfaces, which is desirable for a screw-retained restoration.

CT-derived surgical templates can reduce operating time and improve the accuracy of implant placement.[40,41] However, the use of CT-derived surgical templates, although helpful, does have shortcomings. The guides can be fixated to the jaw, rest on the edentulous ridge, or be supported by the teeth. If the guide is fixed, examination of the osteotomy is not possible until its completion before implant placement. Checking the preparation sequence of the osteotomy may be useful with a removable surgical template. Bicortical stabilization is critical to the success of implant placement in the fibula, and bone volume is limiting. Direct visualization of the implant osteotomy is sometimes necessary for verification and should remain an option during surgery.

Clinical studies have described virtual planning for maxillomandibular reconstruction at the fibula donor site and recipient site by using ostectomy guides and rapid prototype modeling for the adaptation of the reconstruction plates.[42,43] This reconstruction approach relies heavily on CAP and stereolithography techniques before ablative and reconstructive procedures. CAD-CAM technology and rapid prototype modeling have the potential to save operative time and improve the accuracy of surgical reconstruction. This approach may be particularly useful for cases in which the original architecture of the mandible has been distorted or destroyed by extension of the tumor beyond the cortical margin of the mandible.[44] There is potential for the bone flap reconstruction to be contoured and plated with implants placed at the donor site before transfer, anastomosis, and fixation to the recipient site. Further advancement of techniques can also provide CAD-CAM implant restorations in conjunction with this approach before transfer in the immediate setting.[45]

The implant bearing surface is almost perpendicular to the plating system such that implants can be placed either primarily or secondarily and can be incorporated into the ostectomy guide. Connection of a provisional fixed prosthetic restoration to the implants at the time of fibula free flap reconstruction requires in-depth virtual planning,[46,47] additional CAD-CAM technique, and careful consideration to patient selection.

Postoperative Considerations

A misconception about prosthetic rehabilitation and fibula free flap reconstruction of the mandible is that the large lever forces resulting from the high vertical dimension of an implant-supported prosthesis may lead to overloading of the implants and endanger their longevity. The authors have found this not to be the case and the height discrepancy can also be addressed through prosthetic design.

Excessive height discrepancy of the fibula to the occlusal plane can be overcome by using a cast mesostructure-superstructure design for a screw-retained fixed restoration. The mesostructure is milled so that the implant support is centralized over the mandibular neo-ridge, and the corresponding superstructure acts as a fixed partial denture set with screws into the mesostructure. This type of prosthetic restoration allows the significant height discrepancy from the implant head to the occlusal plane to be negotiated by two corresponding milled framework structures. The framework design also overcomes limited intermaxillary distance on opening and instrumentation to fabricate an FDP. A prosthodontic framework design with the use of Computer assisted planning (CP) improves the predictability of implant rehabilitation after VBFF surgical reconstruction. Implant position and angulation are determined from CT scans, in which the tooth position is visualized (Fig. 29.3).

Prosthetic design considerations are part of the computer planning stage because the tooth position is visualized. A CAD-CAM surgical template is fabricated by stereolithography and rapid prototyping techniques. Implant surgical templates can be designed to be tooth, mucosa, or bone supported. Confidence in the accuracy and position of the implants also allows for their placement without elevation of the periosteum (flapless). Clinically, the fact that the periosteal blood supply does not need to be disturbed with this transmucosal approach is very important in patients who have undergone radiation therapy. In addition, postoperative pain and swelling can be minimized with this less invasive surgery.[48] If the angulation and position of the implants are accurate, an immediate restoration can be fabricated for prosthetic reconstruction, provided the restoration is protected from any occlusal forces and the primary implant stability exceeds 20 Ncm.[49–53] This procedure can be performed because of the absence of a bloody field and the predetermined implant angulation oriented to the denture teeth. Patient selection is critical to success; patients with questionable bone quality or availability subsequent to free flap reconstruction should not be chosen for this procedure.[54–56]

Guide Design – Resection

Mandible resection guide:

- Slot width: 1 mm
- Diameter fixation holes: 2.2 mm (suitable for 1.5 mm drill, 2.0 mm screws)
- Fixation holes are intended for temporary fixation of the guide

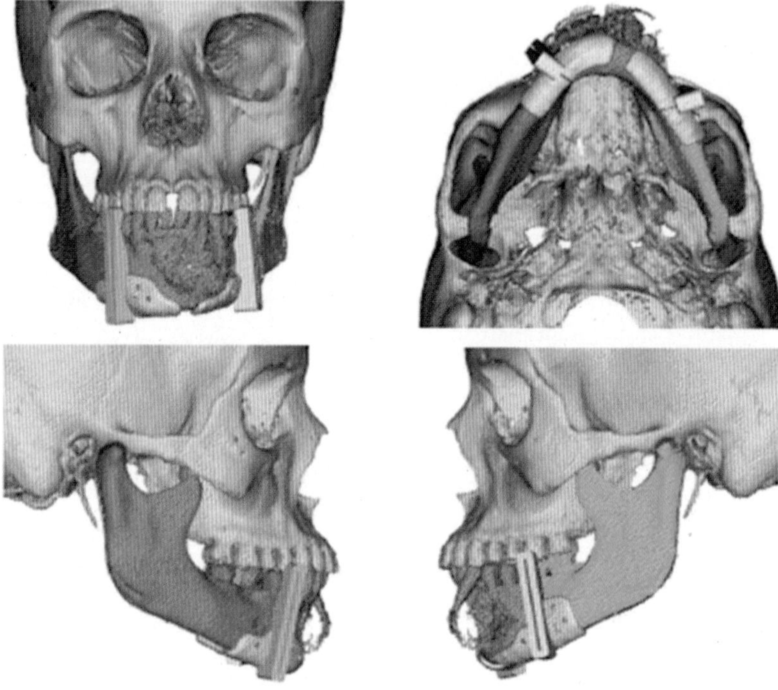

A1

Guide Design – Fibula Graft

Fibula guide:

- Slot with: 1 mm
- Diameter fixation holes: 2.2 mm (suitable for 1.5 mm drill, 2.0 mm screws)
- Fixation holes are intended for temporary fixation of the guide

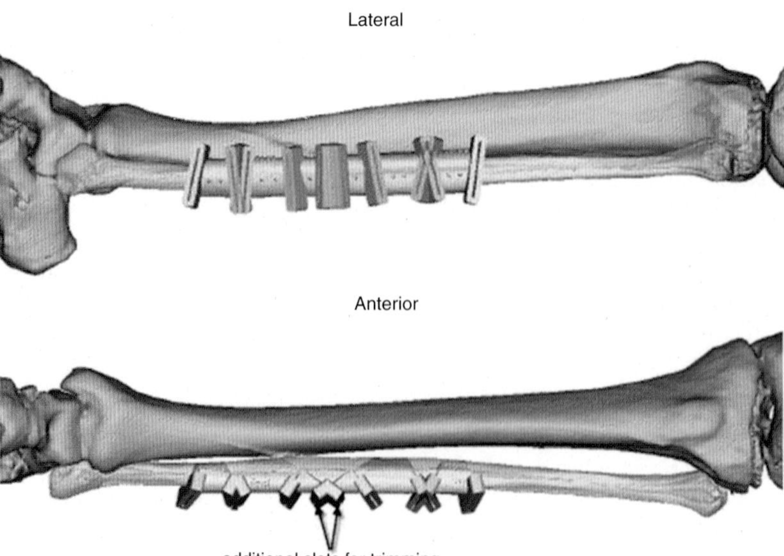

A2

Figure 29.3 **A1,** Computer-assisted surgical plan of a 24-year-old patient with ameloblastoma outlined in red. Mandibular cutting guides (resection guides) are planned through the body of the mandible, bilaterally allowing for a good margin on either side of the tumor and resulting in a segmental resection. **A2,** Fibula free flap reconstruction and patient-specific fibula ostectomy guides are virtually planned by registering a computed tomography (CT) angiography scan into dedicated software. This stage of planning can incorporate predictive holes for bicortical and monocortical fixation screws of a milled computer-aided designed and manufactured (CAD-CAM) or three-dimensional (3D) printed mandibular reconstruction plate. Guide cylinders can also be incorporated into the ostectomy guide for immediate implant placement at the time of the primary reconstructive procedure.

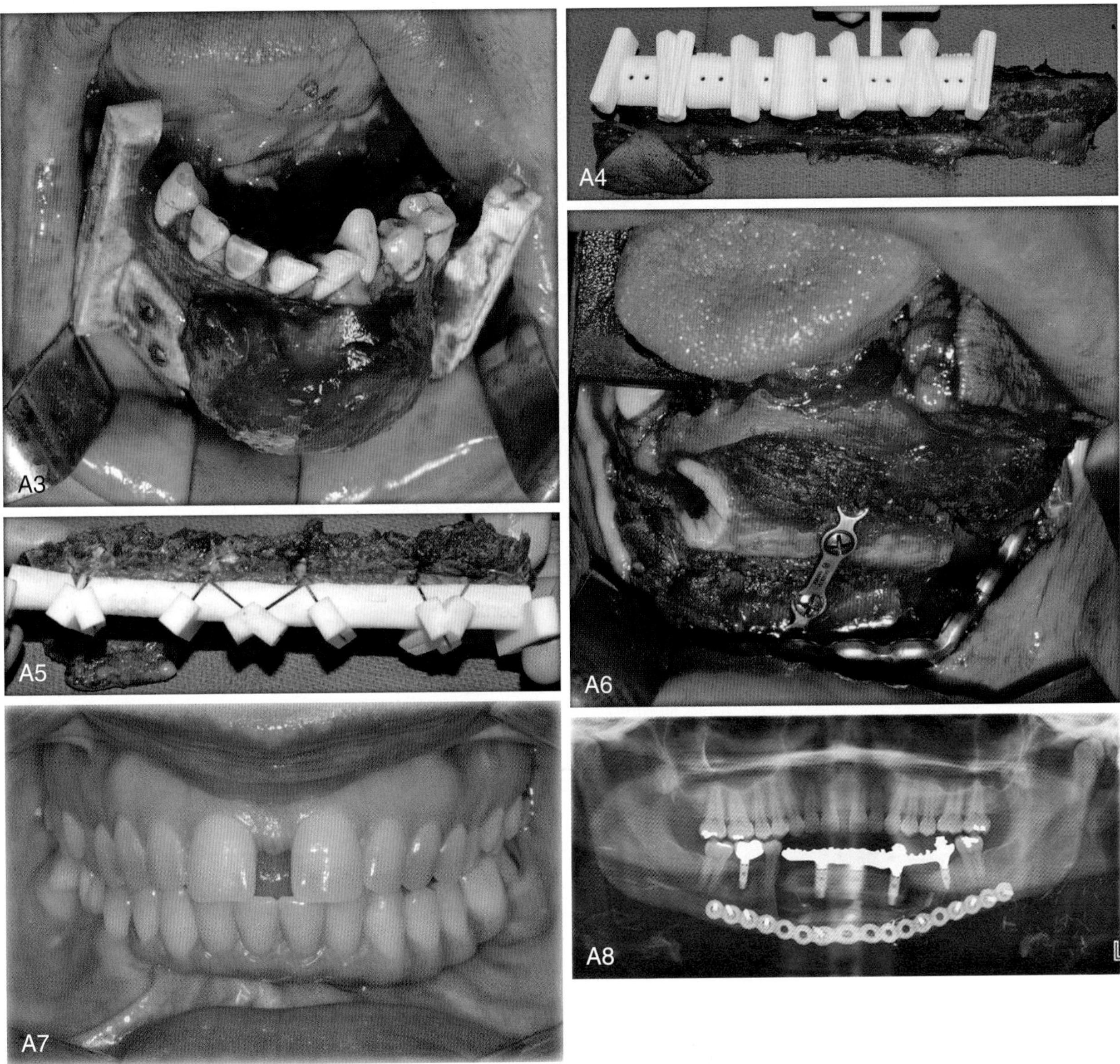

Figure 29.3, cont'd **A3,** Cutting guide set into position with fixation screws for right and left osteotomies of the mandible with an en bloc delivery of the tumor. **A4** and **A5,** Ostectomy guide in position at fibula donor site prior to contouring of the bone flap. **A6,** The multifunctional fibular guide that incorporates not only the slots to aid in the contouring of the flap but also predictive hole drilling cylinders for the monocortical screw to fixate the fibula to the patient-specific plate and drill guides for the precise placement of the dental implants (blue cylinders). **A7,** Definitive prosthodontic rehabilitation with fixed dental prosthesis. **A8,** Superior fibula segment for alveolar process reconstruction and implant placement surgically addresses vertical height discrepancy of native mandible.

Continued

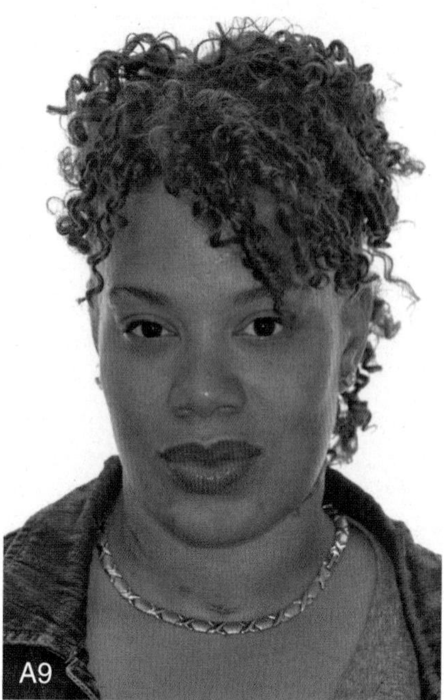

Figure 29.3, cont'd **A9,** Transoral surgical approach provides absence of facial scarring in a patient with known history of keloid formation.

References

1. Urken ML, Buchbinder D, Weinberg H, et al. Functional evaluation following microvascular oromandibular reconstruction of the oral cancer patient: a comparative study of reconstructed and nonreconstructed patients. *Laryngoscope.* 1991;101(9):935–950.
2. Leung AC, Cheung LK. Dental implants in reconstructed jaws: patients' evaluation of functional and quality-of-life outcomes. *Int J Oral Maxillofac Implants.* 2003;18(1):127–134.
3. Schmelzeisen R, Neukam FW, Shirota T, Specht B, Wichmann M. Postoperative function after implant insertion in vascularized bone grafts in maxilla and mandible. *Plast Reconstr Surg.* 1996;97(4):719–725.
4. Rogers SN, McNally D, Mahmoud M, Chan MF, Humphris GM. Psychologic response of the edentulous patient after primary surgery for oral cancer: a cross-sectional study. *J Prosthet Dent.* 1999;82(3):317–321.
5. Urken ML, Bridger AG, Zur KB. The scapular osteofasciocutaneous flap: a 12-year experience. *Arch Otolaryngol Head Neck Surg.* 2001;c127:862.
6. Hidalgo DA. Fibula free flap: a new method of mandible reconstruction. *Plast Reconstr Surg.* 1989;84(1):71–79.
7. Brown JS. Deep circumflex iliac artery free flap with internal oblique muscle as a new method of immediate reconstruction of maxillectomy defect. *Head Neck.* 1996;18(5):412–421.
8. Futran ND, Wadsworth JT, Villaret D, Farwell DG. Midface reconstruction with the fibula free flap. *Arch Otolaryngol Head Neck Surg.* 2002;128(2):161–166.
9. Genden EM, Wallace D, Buchbinder D, Okay D, Urken ML. Iliac crest internal oblique osteomusculocutaneous free flap reconstruction of the postablative palatomaxillary defect. *Arch Otolaryngol Head Neck Surg.* 2001;127(7):854–861.
10. Frodel JL Jr, Funk GF, Capper DT, et al. Osseointegrated implants: a comparative study of bone thickness in four vascularized bone flaps. *Plast Reconstr Surg.* 1993;92(3):449–455.
11. Urken ML, Weinberg H, Vickery C, Buchbinder D, Lawson W, Biller HF. Oromandibular reconstruction using microvascular composite free flaps. Report of 71 cases and a new classification scheme for bony, soft-tissue, and neurologic defects. *Arch Otolaryngol Head Neck Surg.* 1991;117(7):733–744.
12. Brånemark PI. Osseointegration and its experimental background. *J Prosthet Dent.* 1983;50(3):399–410.
13. Urken ML, Buchbinder D, Weinberg H, Vickery C, Sheiner A, Biller HF. Primary placement of osseointegrated implants in microvascular mandibular reconstruction. *Otolaryngol Head Neck Surg.* 1989;101(1):56–73.
14. Urken ML, Buchbinder D, Costantino PD, et al. Oromandibular reconstruction using microvascular composite flaps: report of 210 cases. *Arch Otolaryngol Head Neck Surg.* 1998;124(1):46–55.
15. Marx RE. A new concept in the treatment of osteoradionecrosis. *J Oral Maxillofac Surg.* 1983;41(6):351–357.
16. Granström G, Jacobsson M, Tjellström A. Titanium implants in irradiated tissue: benefits from hyperbaric oxygen. *Int J Oral Maxillofac Implants.* 1992;7(1):15–25.
17. Arcuri MR, Fridrich KL, Funk GF, Tabor MW, LaVelle WE. Titanium osseointegrated implants combined with hyperbaric oxygen therapy in previously irradiated mandibles. *J Prosthet Dent.* 1997;77(2):177–183.
18. Granström G, Tjellström A, Brånemark PI. Osseointegrated implants in irradiated bone: a case-controlled study using adjunctive hyperbaric oxygen therapy. *J Oral Maxillofac Surg.* 1999;57(5):493–499.
19. Barber HD, Seckinger RJ, Hayden RE, Weinstein GS. Evaluation of osseointegration of endosseous implants in radiated, vascularized fibula flaps to the mandible: a pilot study. *J Oral Maxillofac Surg.* 1995;53(6):640–644.
20. Salinas TJ, Desa VP, Katsnelson A, Miloro M. Clinical evaluation of implants in radiated fibula flaps. *J Oral Maxillofac Surg.* 2010;68(3):524–529.
21. Buchbinder D, Okay D, Urken M. Oromandibular reconstruction. In: Urken M, ed. *Multidisciplinary Head and Neck Reconstruction: A Defect-Oriented Approach.* New York, NY: Lippincott Williams & Wilkins; 2010.
22. Moscoso JF, Keller J, Genden E, et al. Vascularized bone flaps in oromandibular reconstruction. A comparative anatomic study of bone stock from various donor sites to assess suitability for enosseous dental implants. *Arch Otolaryngol Head Neck Surg.* 1994;120(1):36–43.
23. Rohner D, Meng CS, Hutmacher DW, Tsai KT. Bone response to unloaded titanium im-

plants in the fibula, iliac crest, and scapula: an animal study in the Yorkshire pig. *Int J Oral Maxillofac Surg*. 2003;32(4):383–389.

24. Futran N, Urken M. Fibula free flap. In: Urken M, ed. *Atlas of Regional and Free Flaps for Head and Neck Reconstruction*. 2nd ed. New York: Wolters Kluwer/Lippincott Williams & Wilkins; 2012.
25. Brennan M, Houston F, O'Sullivan M, O'Connell B. Patient satisfaction and oral health-related quality of life outcomes of implant overdentures and fixed complete dentures. *Int J Oral Maxillofac Implants*. 2010;25(4):791–800.
26. Roumanas ED, Garrett N, Blackwell KE, et al. Masticatory and swallowing threshold performances with conventional and implant-supported prostheses after mandibular fibula free-flap reconstruction. *J Prosthet Dent*. 2006;96(4):289–297.
27. Raoul G, Ruhin B, Briki S, et al. Microsurgical reconstruction of the jaw with fibular grafts and implants. *J Craniofac Surg*. 2009;20(6):2105–2117.
28. Smolka K, Kraehenbuehl M, Eggensperger N, et al. Fibula free flap reconstruction of the mandible in cancer patients: evaluation of a combined surgical and prosthodontic treatment concept. *Oral Oncol*. 2008;44(6):571–581.
29. Bähr W, Stoll P, Wächter R. Use of the "double barrel" free vascularized fibula in mandibular reconstruction. *J Oral Maxillofac Surg*. 1998;56(1):38–44.
30. He Y, Zhang ZY, Zhu HG, Wu YQ, Fu HH. Double-barrel fibula vascularized free flap with dental rehabilitation for mandibular reconstruction. *J Oral Maxillofac Surg*. 2011;69(10):2663–2669.
31. Chenping Z, Min R, Liqun X, et al. Dental implant distractor combined with free fibular flap: a new design for simultaneous functional mandibular reconstruction. *J Oral Maxillofac Surg*. 2012;70(11):2687–2700.
32. Okay DJ, Buchbinder D, Urken M, Jacobson A, Lazarus C, Persky M. Computer-assisted implant rehabilitation of maxillomandibular defects reconstructed with vascularized bone free flaps. *JAMA Otolaryngol Head Neck Surg*. 2013;139(4):371–381.
33. Rieger JM, Wolfaardt JF, Jha N, Seikaly H. Maxillary obturators: the relationship between patient satisfaction and speech outcome. *Head Neck*. 2003;25(11):895–903.
34. Rieger J, Wolfaardt J, Seikaly H, Jha N. Speech outcomes in patients rehabilitated with maxillary obturator prostheses after maxillectomy: a prospective study. *Int J Prosthodont*. 2002;15(2):139–144.
35. Okay DJ, Genden E, Buchbinder D, Urken M. Prosthodontic guidelines for surgical reconstruction of the maxilla: a classification system of defects. *J Prosthet Dent*. 2001;86(4):352–363.
36. Larabee WF, Makielski KH. *Surgical Anatomy of the Face*. New York, NY: Raven Press; 1993.
37. Yamamoto Y, Kawashima K, Sugihara T, Nohira K, Furuta Y, Fukuda S. Surgical management of maxillectomy defects based on the concept of buttress reconstruction. *Head Neck*. 2004;26(3):247–256.
38. Genden EM, Okay D, Stepp MT, et al. Comparison of functional and quality-of-life outcomes in patients with and without palatomaxillary reconstruction: a preliminary report. *Arch Otolaryngol Head Neck Surg*. 2003;129(7):775–780.
39. Di Giacomo GA, Cury PR, de Araujo NS, Sendyk WR, Sendyk CL. Clinical application of stereolithographic surgical guides for implant placement: preliminary results. *J Periodontol*. 2005;76(4):503–507.
40. Cassetta M, Stefanelli LV, Giansanti M, Calasso S. Accuracy of implant placement with a stereolithographic surgical template. *Int J Oral Maxillofac Implants*. 2012;27(3):655–663.
41. Soares MM, Harari ND, Cardoso ES, Manso MC, Conz MB, Vidigal GM Jr. An in vitro model to evaluate the accuracy of guided surgery systems. *Int J Oral Maxillofac Implants*. 2012;27(4):824–831.
42. Roser SM, Ramachandra S, Blair H, et al. The accuracy of virtual surgical planning in free fibula mandibular reconstruction: comparison of planned and final results. *J Oral Maxillofac Surg*. 2010;68(11):2824–2832.
43. Foley BD, Thayer WP, Honeybrook A, McKenna S, Press S. Mandibular reconstruction using computer-aided design and computer-aided manufacturing: an analysis of surgical results. *J Oral Maxillofac Surg*. 2013;71(2):e111–e119.
44. Hanasono MM, Skoracki RJ. Computer-assisted design and rapid prototype modeling in microvascular mandible reconstruction. *Laryngoscope*. 2013;123(3):597–604.
45. Rohner D, Guijarro-Martínez R, Bucher P, Hammer B. Importance of patient-specific intraoperative guides in complex maxillofacial reconstruction. *J Craniomaxillofac Surg*. 2013;41(5):382–390.
46. Williams FC, Hammer DA, Wentland TR, Kim RY. Immediate teeth in fibulas: planning and digital workflow with point-of-care 3D printing. *J Oral Maxillofac Surg*. 2020;78(8):1320–1327.
47. Qaisi M, Kolodney H, Swedenburg G, Chandran R, Caloss R. Fibula jaw in a day: state of the art in maxillofacial reconstruction. *J Oral Maxillofac Surg*. 2016;74(6).
48. Okay D, Buchbinder D. Implant assisted prosthetic reconstruction after tumor ablation. In: Bagheri S, Bell RB, Khan H, eds. *Current Therapy in Oral and Maxillofacial Surgery*. St Louis, MO: Saunders; 2012.
49. Nkenke E, Eitner S, Radespiel-Tröger M, Vairaktaris E, Neukam FW, Fenner M. Patient-centred outcomes comparing transmucosal implant placement with an open approach in the maxilla: a prospective, non-randomized pilot study. *Clin Oral Implants Res*. 2007;18(2):197–203.
50. Luongo G, Di Raimondo R, Filippini P, Gualini F, Paoleschi C. Early loading of sandblasted, acid-etched implants in the posterior maxilla and mandible: a 1-year follow-up report from a multicenter 3-year prospective study. *Int J Oral Maxillofac Implants*. 2005;20(1):84–91.
51. Vanden Bogaerde L, Pedretti G, Dellacasa P, Mozzati M, Rangert B, Wendelhag I. Early function of splinted implants in maxillas and posterior mandibles, using Brånemark System Tiunite implants: an 18-month prospective clinical multicenter study. *Clin Implant Dent Relat Res*. 2004;6(3):121–129.
52. Cornelini R, Cangini F, Covani U, Barone A, Buser D. Immediate loading of implants with 3-unit fixed partial dentures: a 12-month clinical study. *Int J Oral Maxillofac Implants*. 2006;21(6):914–918.
53. Schincaglia GP, Marzola R, Scapoli C, Scotti R. Immediate loading of dental implants supporting fixed partial dentures in the posterior mandible: a randomized controlled split-mouth study—machined versus titanium oxide implant surface. *Int J Oral Maxillofac Implants*. 2007;22(1):35–46.
54. Del Fabbro M, Testori T, Francetti L, Taschieri S, Weinstein R. Systematic review of survival rates for immediately loaded dental implants. *Int J Periodontics Restorative Dent*. 2006;26(3):249–263.
55. Odin G, Balaguer T, Savoldelli C, Scortecci G. Immediate functional loading of an implant-supported fixed prosthesis at the time of ablative surgery and mandibular reconstruction for squamous cell carcinoma. *J Oral Implantol*. 2010;36(3):225–230.
56. Chiapasco M, Gatti C. Immediate loading of dental implants placed in revascularized fibula free flaps: a clinical report on 2 consecutive patients. *Int J Oral Maxillofac Implants*. 2004;19(6):906–912.

CHAPTER 30

Implant Salvage Procedures

Christian A. Loetscher

Armamentarium

#15 Scalpel
#9 Periosteal elevator
4-0 and 3-0 chromic gut suture
Adson pick-up with teeth
Bone dish
Citric acid
Cotton pellets
Irrigation syringes
Local anesthetic with vasoconstrictor
Minnesota retractor
Mosquito hemostat
Mx-Grafter bone harvester
Platelet-rich fibrin
Platelet-rich plasma
Titanium rotary brushes
Titanium scalers
Tongue retractor
Woodson elevator

History of the Procedure

Since the introduction of osseointegrated dental implants into dentistry began in Europe in the 1960s and North America in the 1980s, dental implants have enjoyed phenomenal success.[1] However, in the past decade it has become evident that the same periodontal disease processes that affect teeth also affect dental implants.

Periimplantitis is defined as an inflammatory process affecting the tissues around an osseointegrated implant that results in loss of the supporting alveolar bone.[2,3] Clinically it is defined when three situations exist: radiographic evidence of bone loss exceeding the typical anatomic remodeling, pocket depths greater than 5 mm, and bleeding or suppuration on probing (Figs. 30.1 and 30.2A and B). The precursor to periimplantitis is termed periimplant mucositis (Fig. 30.3), which is periimplantitis without concomitant bone loss and may be reversible with proper treatment. Some have estimated that after 5 years, nearly 50% of implant sites may develop periimplant mucositis.[4] Periimplant mucositis typically is treated nonsurgically, with curettage, chlorhexidine mouth rinse, and antibiotics. With the increased use of screw retained prosthetics, versus cement retained prosthetic, the incidence of periimplantitis and perimucositis appears to be decreasing.

Procedures to salvage dental implants are presently evolving. Roos-Jansåker's[5] study in 2006 revealed a 12% incidence of periimplantitis after 10 years in a European population. Recent studies have confirmed the undeniable prevalence of this problem.[2] In a review of the epidemiology of periimplantitis, Mombelli et al. states the prevalence of periimplantitis is 10% for implants and 20% for patients after 5 to 10 years.[6] Most studies also conclude that smoking and a history of periodontitis significantly affect a patient's predisposition toward developing periimplantitis.[7]

Periimplantitis results in the loss of supporting bone and soft tissue. Its treatment ranges from removal of the implant (deplantation) to debridement procedures and regenerative procedures in conjunction with debridement. In the 1990s and early 2000s, many of the studies on periimplantitis were performed in the canine model using ligature-induced periimplantitis.[8] However, in the past decade enough implants exist in the general population, allowing studies utilizing implants in patients.

It has been shown that reosseointegration can occur on a repaired surface.[9,10] Reintegration may consist of soft tissue reattachment, osseous reattachment, or a combination of both. Regenerative procedure protocols are evolving, ranging from allogeneic bone graft materials and autogenous bone graft materials to commercially available tissue engineering products such as recombinant human bone morphogenic protein and recombinant platelet-derived growth factor (rhPDGF). Success rates vary depending upon the anatomy and amount of preexisting bone loss, and typically are in the 60% to 70% range.[11,12] When an ideal repair situation exists, success rates approach 100%.[11] In 2012, Heitz-Mayfield and coworkers reported a 47% elimination of bleeding when probing and a 92% level of resolution of bone loss after 12 months with antiinfective treatment combined with open debridement.[13]

The etiology of the periimplantitis is multifactorial. One of the most common causes of periimplantitis is retained cement from prosthesis cementation.[14,15] When inflammation develops within weeks and months following crown cementation, surgical exploration for retained cement is indicated (Fig. 30.4A–C). Another common cause is periodontally compromised teeth elsewhere in the mouth.[16] This cause is often overlooked during treatment planning. Studies have conclusively shown that pocket depths around teeth of 6 mm or more cause the seeding of implants with periodontal pathogens, with the periimplantitis presenting itself with a lag time of approximately 2 to 3 years following pocket development.[17] Presently, considerable research is underway looking at the genetic component underlying the individual susceptibility to implant loss.[18] The interleukin-1 and interleukin-6 genes have been studied and may explain the clustering phenomenon where upon certain individuals appear to be susceptible to chronic periodontitis and periimplantitis, resulting in an increased incidence of implant loss.[18,19]

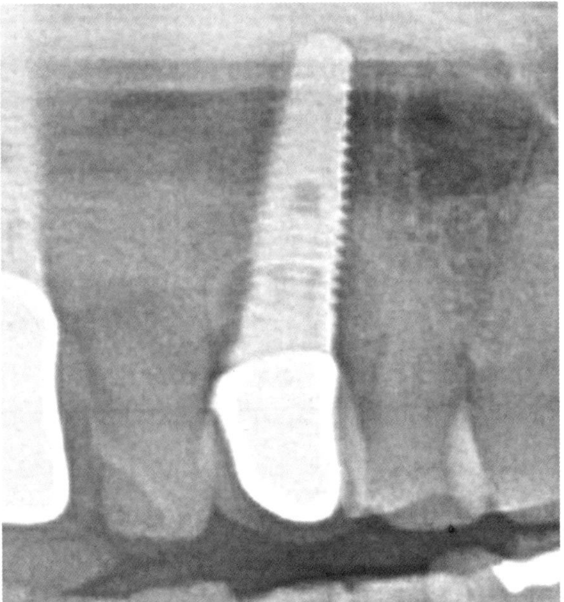

Fig. 30.1 Periimplantitis bone loss.

Placement of an implant into a site with inadequate buccal plate thickness may result in loss of the buccal plate, resulting in gingival recession and loss of attached tissue. This, in time, results in a high predisposition to periimplantitis.

Other common causative factors include poor prosthesis design inhibiting hygiene, inadequate attached tissue, endodontic defects on adjacent teeth, and systemic issues such as smoking and diabetes.[20] These issues need to be addressed and eliminated when possible before the repair is undertaken.

It is interesting to note that when Branemark and colleagues originally presented their 15-year success rates, their long-term success rates were high, and periimplantitis was not a major issue in their patient population. This is likely because the vast majority of their original patients were edentulous and had screw retained prosthesis. Their protocol thereby eliminated the two most common causes of periimplantitis: retained cement and periodontal pathogens associated with periodontally compromised natural teeth.

Prevention of periimplantitis starts with proper implant site development, obtaining optimized bone and soft tissue, and subsequent ideal implant placement. Prevention of periodontal disease elsewhere in the mouth, proper prosthesis design for adequate hygiene, prevention of retained cement, and regular hygiene recall for early detection of periimplantitis are all necessary to minimize periimplant disease.

Indications for Use of the Procedure

Once the diagnosis of inflammation with bone loss is made, one must determine if the implant is treatable. Unlike teeth, when implants are removed, they typically leave a sizable non-four-walled defect. The resultant osseous regeneration often is minimal and typically requires aggressive bone grafting to

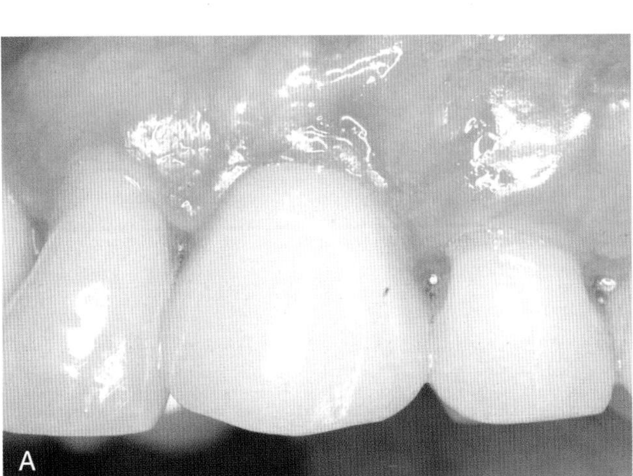

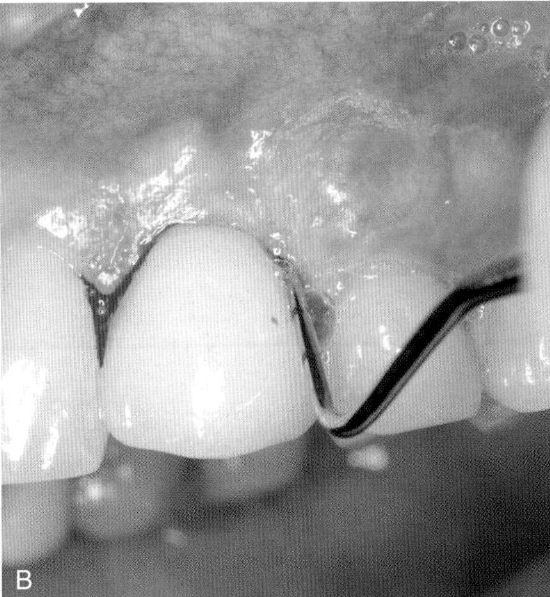

Fig. 30.2 **A** and **B,** Periimplantitis.

regenerate the site for a new implant. For this reason, undergoing an implant salvage procedure is often in the patient's best interest.

Typically, osseous defects of 5 to 6 mm or less vertically along the implant are amenable to treatment. Larger defects may be treated if the implants are critical in support of the prosthesis, and removal may result in complete loss of a significant prosthesis. Fig. 30.5A and B illustrates an example where implant #10 was vital to the prosthesis, and a repair was carried out, in the presence of greater than 50% bone loss. The most treatable defects appear to be the circumferential crater-type lesions found caused by retained cement, closely mimicking a three- or four-walled periodontal defect (Figs. 30.6A–E and 30.7A and B).

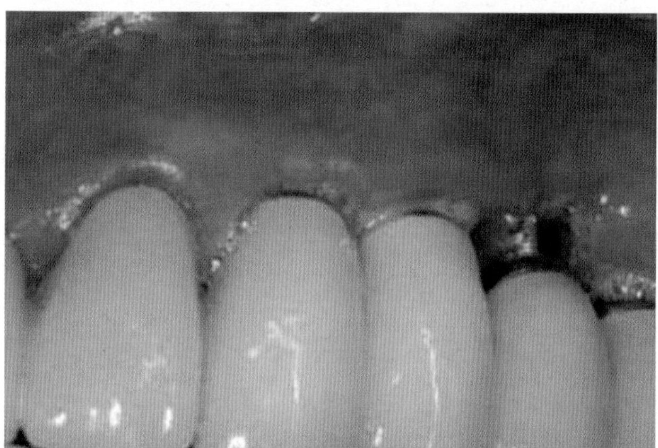

Fig. 30.3 Periimplant mucositis.

Limitations and Contraindications

The treatment and resolution of the inflammation associated with periimplant disease will often result in some degree of gingival recession. In the esthetic zone, this becomes a major concern, where just a slight amount of gingival recession may adversely affect dental esthetics. In these esthetically demanding situations, the best treatment results esthetically and functionally are obtained when the prosthesis is removed, cover screws are placed, and treatment is performed 8 to 10 weeks later. The 8 to 10 week wait period prior to osseous regeneration allows time for resolution of the infection and inflammation, some to complete soft tissue coverage, and improved surgical success. This may leave the patient in provisional prosthetics for 3 to 9 months. For this reason, prevention of periimplant disease in the first place of course is ideal,

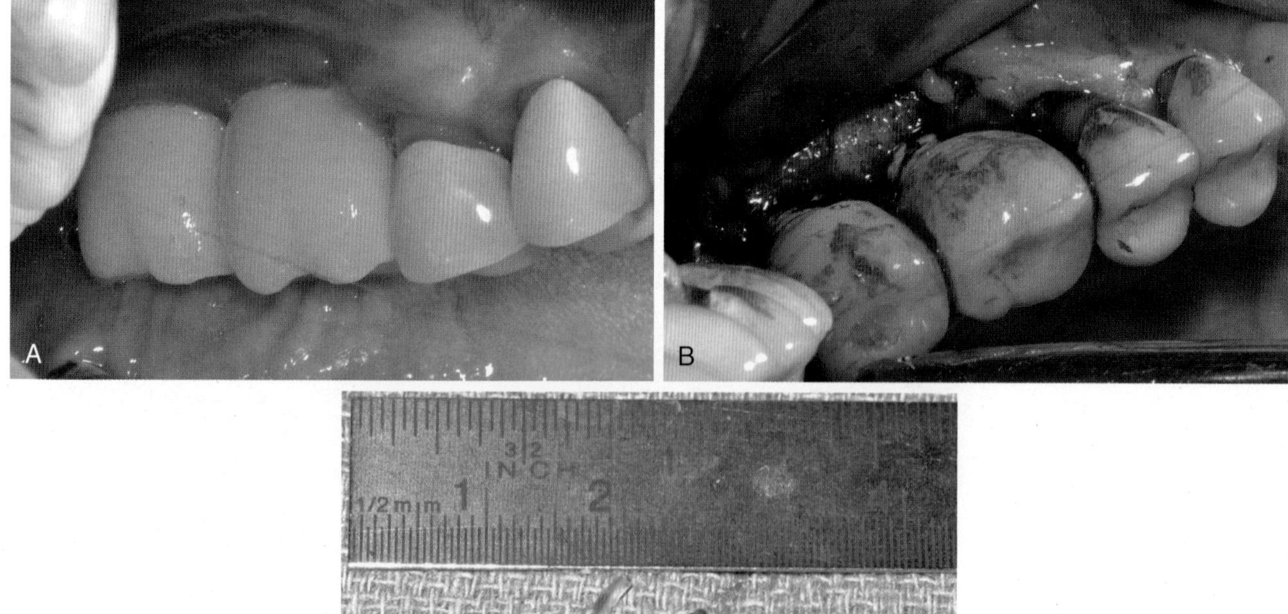

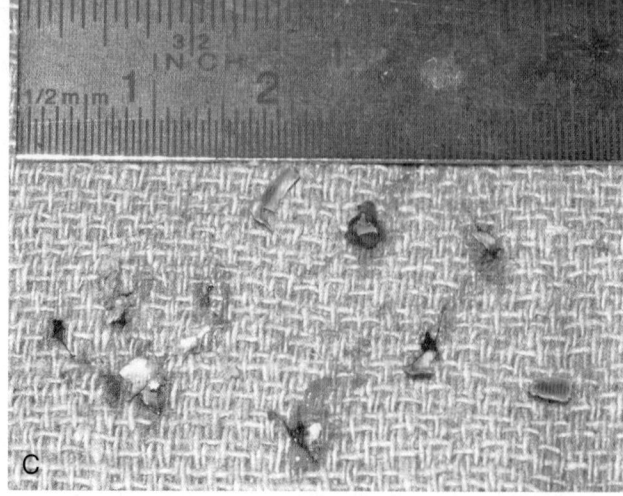

Fig. 30.4 **A–C,** Surgical exploration for retained cement.

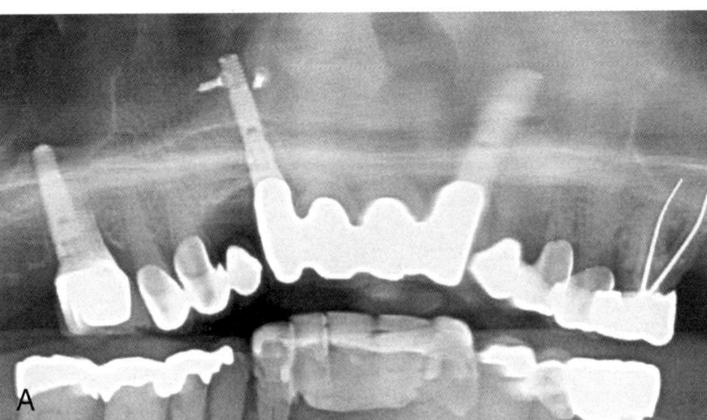

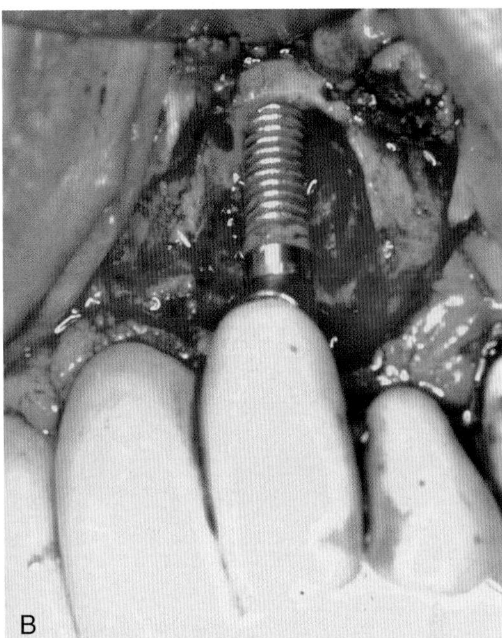

Fig. 30.5 A and B, Periimplantitis affecting an implant key to survival.

but when it occurs, treatment should be initiated as soon as the diagnosis is made.

When there is less than 2 to 3 mm of supporting bone around the implant, or the implant is mobile, the implant should be removed. Typically, when bone loss approaches 50% of the implant length, implant removal should be seriously considered. Exceptions can be made if the implant is a key abutment to a prosthesis and the clinician feels the tissue health can be restored, especially with longer implants.

The cause of the periimplantitis also needs to be addressed prior to initiating therapy. If it is a poorly designed prosthesis, causing the inability to clean, it needs to be redesigned. Intaglio surface concavities and buccal flange regions of the prosthesis are often culprits and need to be addressed. If the periimplantitis is due to bacterial seeding from periodontally involved teeth elsewhere in the mouth, they need to be treated or removed.

Implants presently being placed have roughened surfaces to enhance osseointegration. In theory, they are designed so the roughened surface is always within the osseous crest and does not become exposed to the oral environment. However, as patients age and periimplant disease progresses, these roughened surfaces and screw threads become exposed, either within the pocket or visibly. This contributes to the difficulty in removing the adherent bacterial plaque and biofilm.[21] Debridement techniques must take this into consideration.

The inflammation associated with periimplantitis causes a secondary loss of attached tissue. Often when periimplantitis has been left untreated for extended period of time, the attached tissue is completely lost due to inflammation. An adequate band of keratinized tissue is necessary for long-term maintenance of periimplant health. This must be addressed surgically either simultaneously with the repair or following the repair. The inflammation present in the host tissue bed prevents successful grafting of keratinized tissue prior to an implant repair.

Technique for Implant Salvage

Salvage and repair of dental implants requires first the removal of the infected granulomatous soft tissue and removal of the biofilm on the infected implant (surface decontamination), followed by regenerative procedures when the defect anatomy allows. Microorganisms or foreign body material initiate periimplant disease, and their removal and prevention of reattachment are essential to the success of the repair and regeneration of attachment.

There are two categories of implant salvage and repair procedures.

Nonregenerative Debridement Therapy

This technique is indicated in nonesthetic areas for implants exhibiting an osseous dehiscence defect and lacking an osseous multiwalled defect that can contain bone graft material. It consists of debriding and cleansing the implant site, implant surface decontamination, and pocket elimination via either gingivectomy or apically repositioned flaps.

Regenerative Therapy

Regenerative therapy can be carried out when two or more wall defect exists, allowing containment of the graft material.

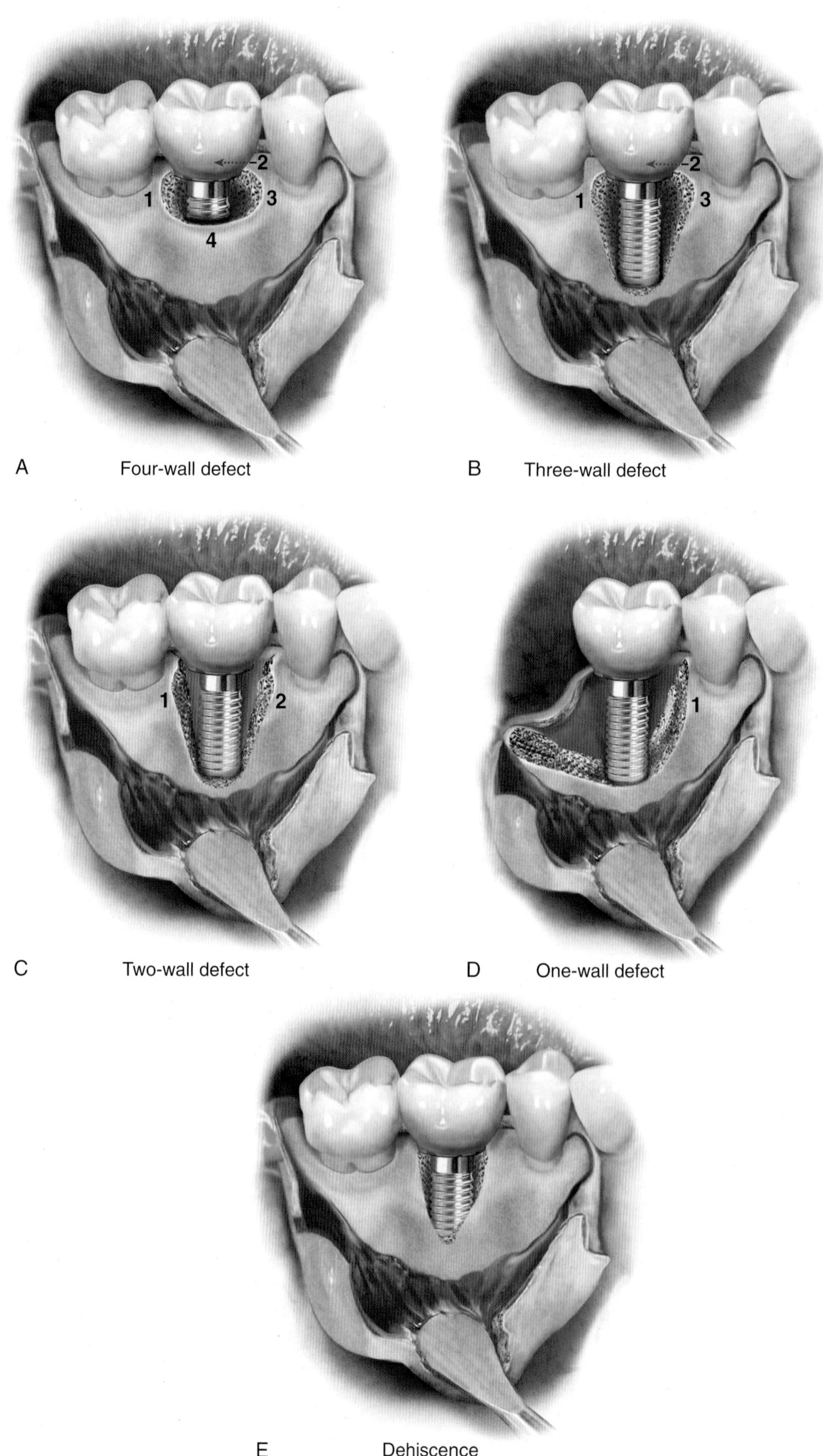

Fig. 30.6 A–E, Examples of defects.

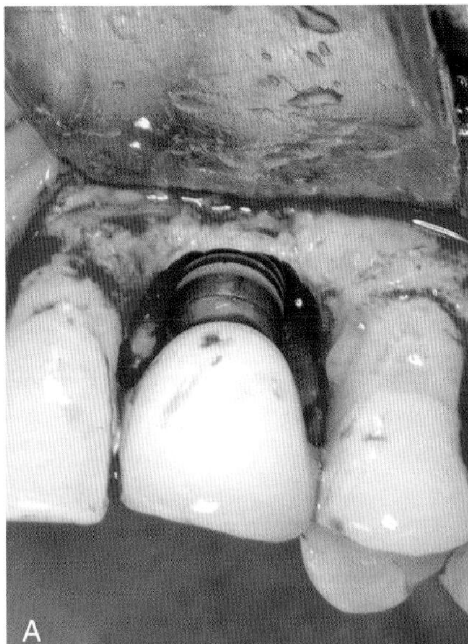

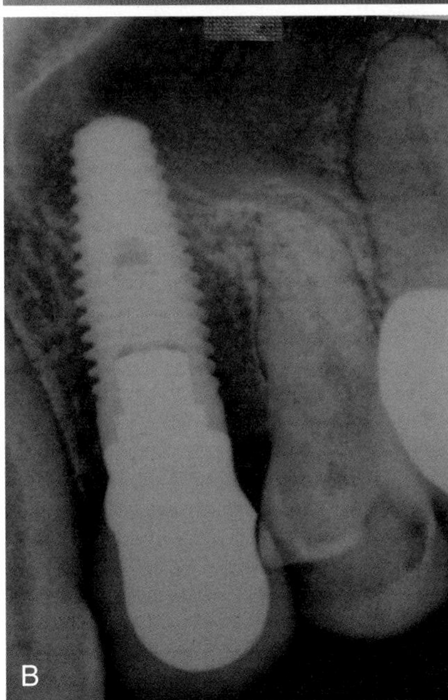

Fig. 30.7 **A** and **B,** Four-wall crater defect of periimplantitis.

Typically, this is the ideal treatment in the most common periimplantitis type defect—the crater-type defect surrounding the implant. Parma-Benfenati et al.[22] categorized this type of vertical bone defect into two morphologies: A contained infrabony defect (funnel or three-wall defect) or a uncontained one—two-to-wall defect. Parma-Benfenati's technique for the uncontained defect utilizes a membrane to contain graft material (see following section).

In this technique, the implant site is treated similar to that of the nonregenerative and debridement technique, with the addition of grafting bone to the area. The goal is to obtain osseous and soft tissue reattachment along the implant surface, decreasing the pocket depth, obtaining a maintainable hygienic situation.

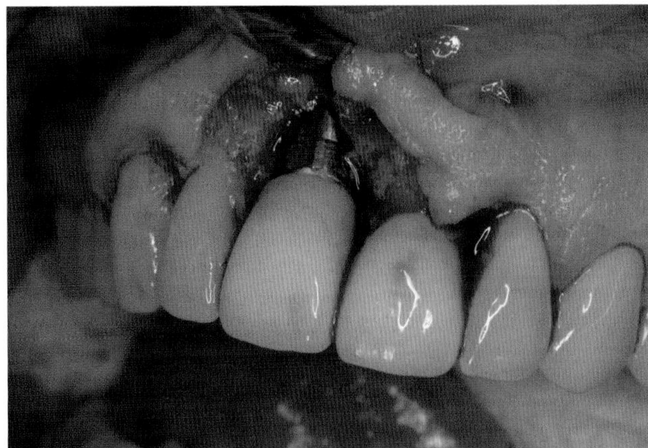

Fig. 30-8 A careful reflection of the flap, exposing the periimplantitis defect.

In both treatment categories, the addition of soft tissue grafting to facilitate adequate keratinized tissue may be used as a simultaneous surgical procedure.

1. Preoperative chemotherapy regimen. Control of the infection is begun 2 days prior to the salvage procedure. An antibiotic regimen to control both the common periodontal pathogens, as well as anaerobes, is initiated. Amoxicillin/clavulanic acid 500 mg (Augmentin) TID and metronidazole 500 mg TID are initiated 2 days preoperative for a 14-day course. Chlorhexidine mouthwash (0.12%) BID is also initiated 2 days preoperatively for a 14-day course. Substitutions such as cephalexin 500 mg QID or clindamycin 300 mg TID may be substituted for amoxicillin/clavulanic acid when a penicillin type allergy exists.
2. After administering proper sedation and/or general anesthesia along with local anesthesia, the patient is prepped with a Betadine facial scrub and the application of sterile drapes around the oral cavity. A #15 blade is used to make a sulcular incision around the crown of the implant tooth, extending one tooth on either side. Full-thickness mucoperiosteal flaps are reflected to obtain full visualization buccal and lingually of the defect. Occasionally a release incision will be made distal to provide better access (Fig. 30.8). During this step, careful reflection of the flap is needed to avoid tearing, due to the weakened state of the tissue from long-term inflammation.
3. The defect is visualized. Full access to the infected portion of the implant is necessary. Granulation tissue is typically found and is removed with curettes and scalers. Titanium or carbon fiber instruments are preferred. Rotary titanium brushes (Salvin Dental) are useful (Fig. 30.9A and B). The goal is to remove the bacterial biofilm, debride and clean the implant and osseous defect of plaque, calculus, cement, or other foreign body material. The biofilm is composed of attached microbial cells encased within a matrix of extracellular polymeric secretions, which surround and protect cells. Failure to remove the biofilm decreases treatment success. Mechanical debridement can also be facilitated

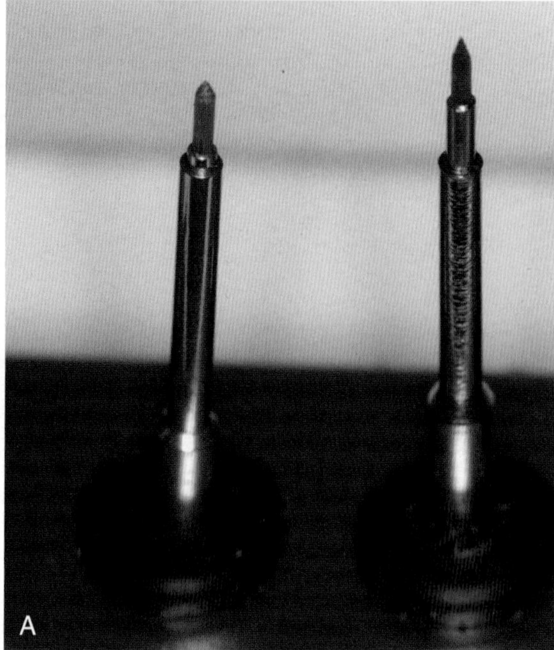

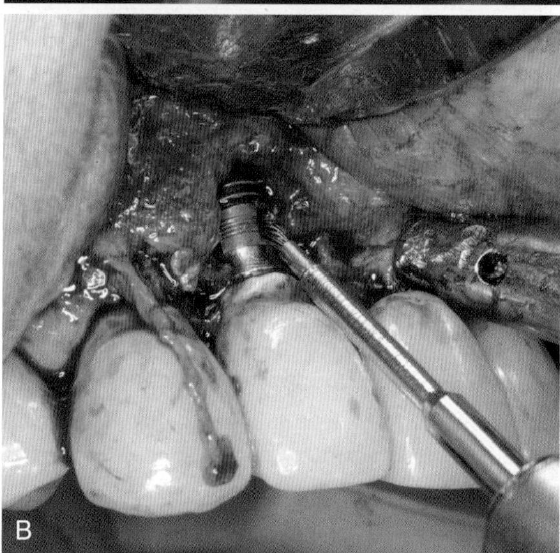

Fig. 30.9 **A,** Latch-type titanium brushes–Salvin Dental. **B,** Titanium brushes mechanically removing biofilm.

utilizing #8 round burs and air abrasion with bicarbonate powder using a prophy-jet.

4. Chemical decontamination of the implant surface is performed. The goal is to remove the biofilm from the exposed implant surface. Cotton pellets soaked in citric acid are rubbed onto the surface and allowed to sit for 5 minutes (Fig. 30.10).

The cotton pellets are counted prior to placing and after removing to avoid leaving a foreign body in the wound. The site is then thoroughly irrigated with sterile saline. Consideration can also be given to irrigating with 0.12% chlorhexidine mouth rinse as well.

Studies have shown equal debridement efficacy with reintegration when comparing citric acid, sandblasting, and laser/

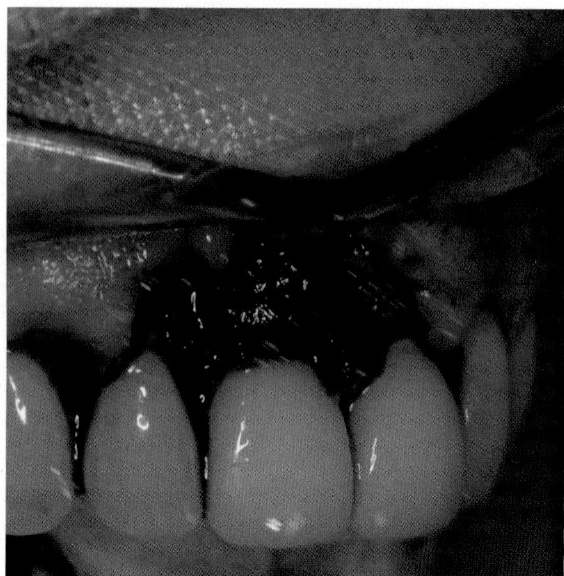

Fig. 30.10 Citric acid-soaked pellets for chemical debridement of biofilm.

photodynamic therapy.[23,24] Photodynamic therapy utilizing the Er:Yag, Nd:Yag, and CO_2 lasers have all been shown to be effective in removing bacterial contamination from infected implants without damaging the implant surface.[25,26] The diode laser has been shown to reduce bacterial contamination but not completely eliminate it.[26] From a practical standpoint, lasers are not widely available in the office setting, and citric acid treatment following mechanical debridement of the biofilm appears to be effective.

5. When regenerative therapy is being carried out, autogenous bone is harvested. A 1.5-cm incision is made along the mandibular external oblique ridge and ascending ramus, exposing the lateral mandible. A total of 1 to 2 cc of bone is harvested utilizing a bone scraper (KLS Martin). This is mixed with previously harvested platelet-rich plasma (PRP) (Fig. 30.11A–C).

The mandibular donor site is thoroughly irrigated with sterile saline. The donor site is closed with a mid-incision interrupted 3-0 chromic suture, followed by a running 3-0 chromic sutures. (The addition of a single interrupted suture will significantly reduce wound breakdown or dehiscence during the initial healing period.)

6. The site is now grafted with bone, densely packing the material into the defect. PRP is sprayed into the wound and bone graft as well. Alternative graft materials include mineralized freeze dried allografts, bovine bone, bone morphogenic protein (BMP-2, Medtronics), or a product sold as Gem 21S, a mixture of beta tricalcium phosphate and recombinant human platelet-derived growth factor (rhPDGF-BB, Gem 21S, Osteohealth). Studies comparing one bone graft material with the other are lacking at this point. Therefore, with the osseoinductive properties present only in autogenous bone and BMP-2, one of these two materials is recommended.

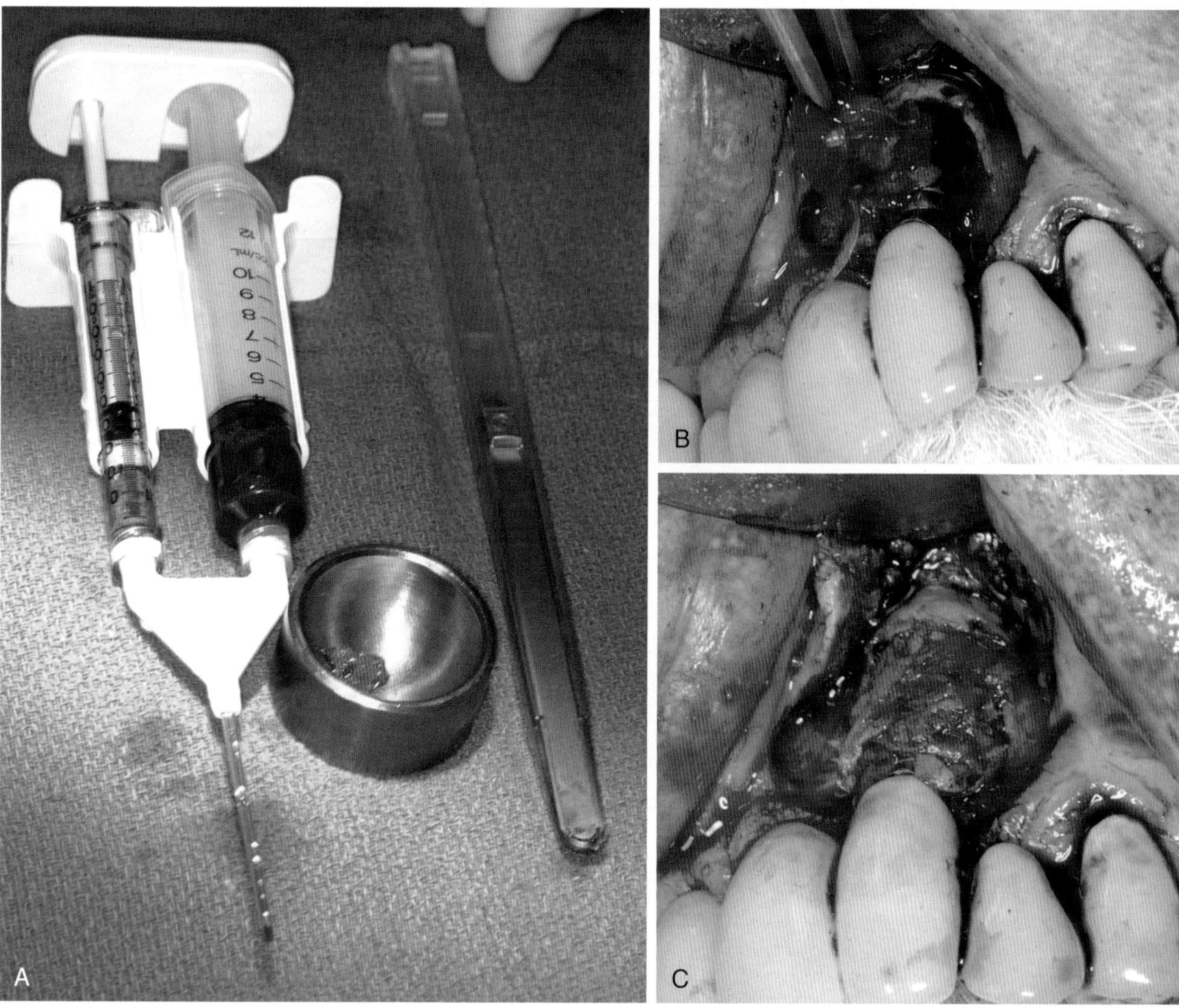

Fig. 30.11 A–C, Regenerative therapy.

7. As an alternative to use of autologous bone, Fig. 30.12A shows periimplantitis that is secondary to retained cement presence 5 years after crown placement. The sites were mechanically and chemically debrided, and a crown on #14 was removed. A cover screw was placed on #14. Human cancellous allograft soaked in platelet-rich fibrin (PRF) plasma was packed around the implant (Fig. 30.12B). PRF membranes were placed over this graft prior to closure (Fig. 30.12C).
8. The site is then closed using 4-0 chromic vertical mattress sutures. Alternatively, 5-0 Vicryl on a tapered needle works well, removing it at 2 to 3 weeks, or Gortex sutures.

Fig. 30.13A–C shows a circumferential defect around implant #30 repaired with autogenous bone 11 months after repair.

MODIFIED TECHNIQUE #1—REGENERATIVE APPROACH IN A ONE-WALLED DEFECT: Graft Containment via Membrane

A regenerative approach for a one-walled defect is indicated when the osseous anatomy does not allow for graft containment, and debridement with an apically repositioned flap results in esthetically unacceptable exposed implant threads.

The prosthesis is removed, and cover screws are placed. The same regenerative repair technique as above is carried out. However, guided bone regeneration is carried out using a particulate bone graft material over the implant, covered by a membrane—either resorbable or nonresorbable. The area is allowed to consolidate 6 to 9 months, depending upon the graft material.[22] This technique is biologically challenging due to the use of a membrane in inflamed tissue, and subsequently will be less predictable. This should be discussed with the patient preoperatively. Removing the prosthesis, debriding the periimplantitis site, and placing a cover screw on the affected implants 8 weeks prior to the regenerative procedure will improve the chance for successful salvage.

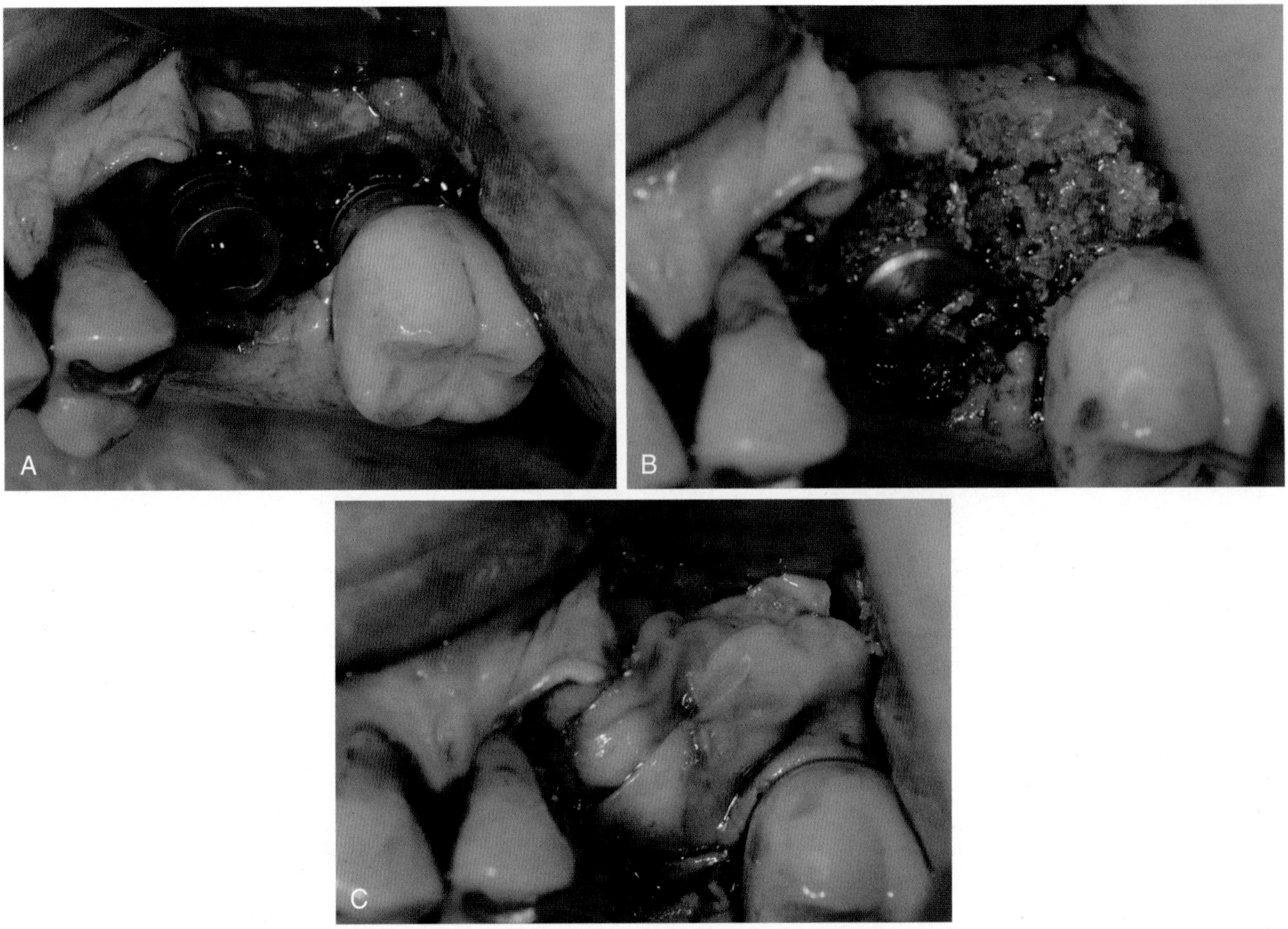

Fig. 30.12 **A,** Periimplantitis that is secondary to retained cement presence 5 years after crown placement. **B,** Human cancellous allograft soaked in platelet-rich fibrin (PRF) plasma was packed around the implant. **C,** PRF membranes were placed over this graft prior to closure.

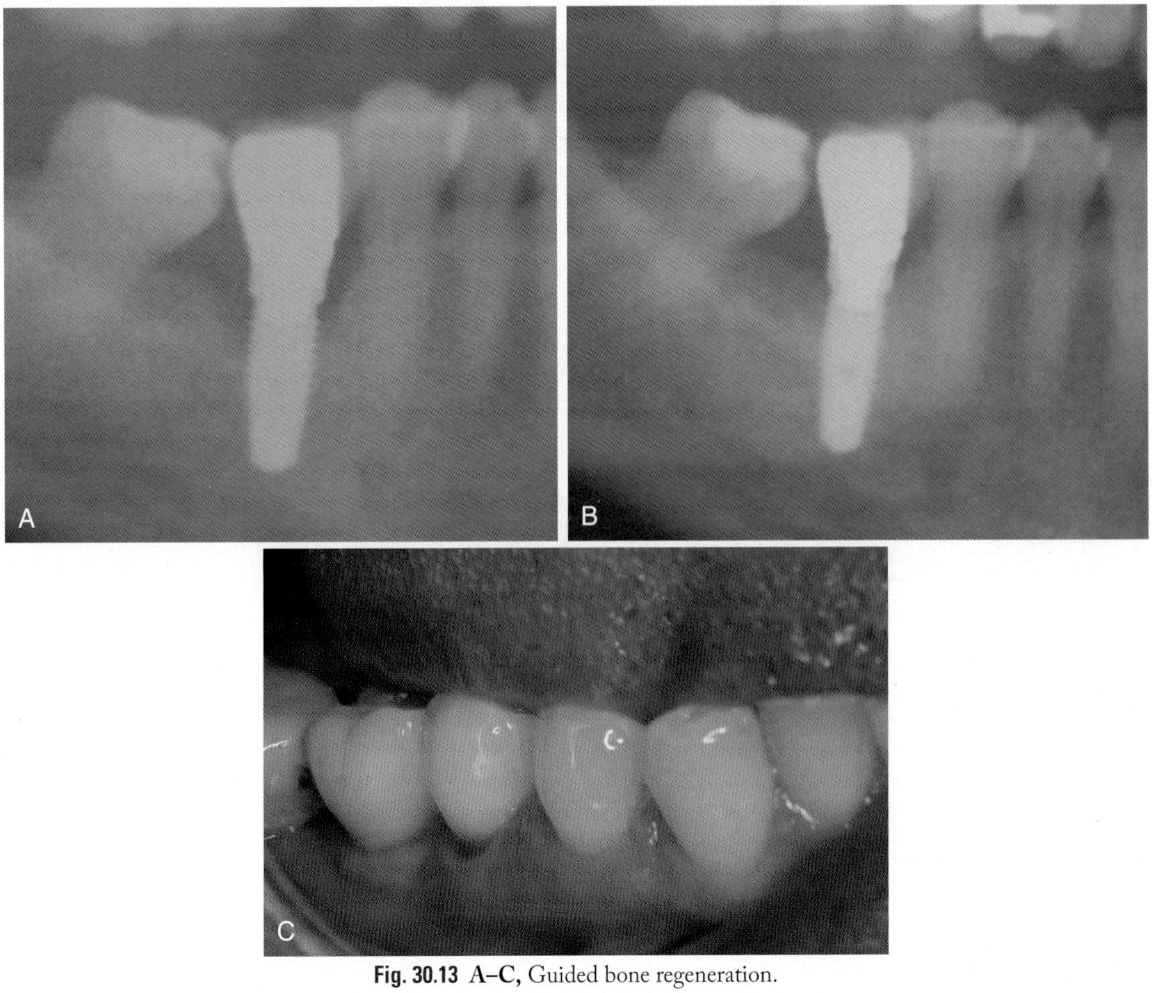

Fig. 30.13 **A–C,** Guided bone regeneration.

MODIFIED TECHNIQUE #2—DEBRIDEMENT WITH SOFT TISSUE GRAFTING

Apically repositioning a flap with free gingival grafting is indicated in nonesthetic areas and implant sites where crater-type walled defects are not present to contain bone graft material. The addition of free gingival grafting is performed when loss of attached tissue exists.

Debridement without osseous regenerative procedures is indicated when the anatomy consists mostly of bone loss, without a walled defect to contain the graft material therefore not amenable to bone grafting regenerative procedures. The goals include apically repositioning a flap, eliminating pockets, and improving accessibility for hygiene, and grafting attached tissue to provide protection to the periimplant soft and hard tissues when attached tissue is missing.

The tissue is moved apically along the implant to decrease pocket depth, leaving the implant surface exposed. In the maxilla, palatal gingivectomies can be performed to decrease pocket depth on the palate as well. Free gingival grafts or subepithelial connective tissue grafts can be placed to provide an increase in the width of keratinized tissue. Alternatively, allograft connective tissue grafts can be used.

Fig. 30.14A and B illustrates a 19-year-old hybrid prosthesis. A nonsalvageable infected implant is present in site #11, with advanced periimplantitis having extensive bone loss throughout the remaining six implants. The chronic inflammation throughout the maxillary arch has resulted in atrophy of much of the attached tissue, leaving mostly mucosa adjacent to the implant sites.

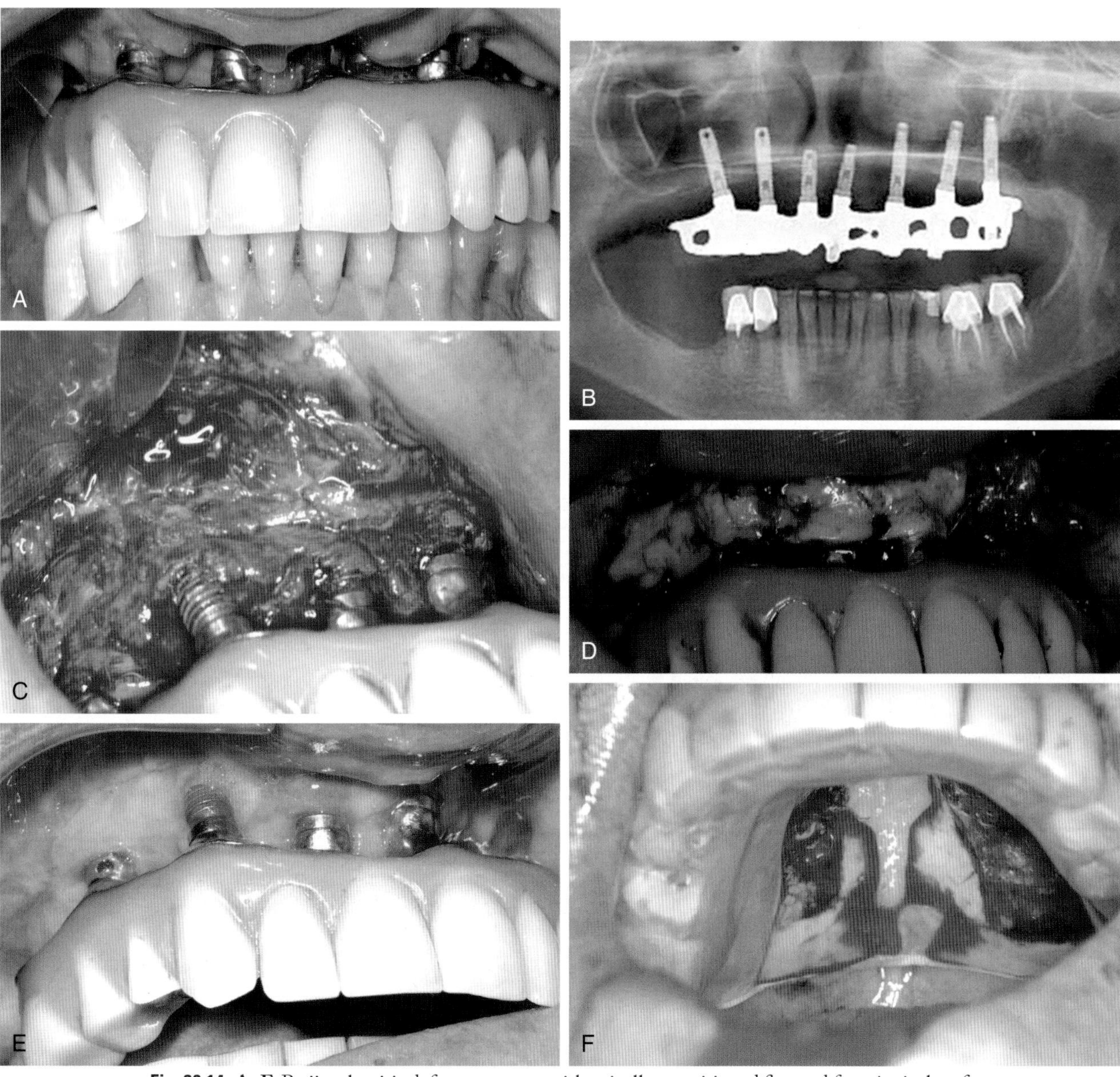

Fig. 30.14 A–F, Periimplantitis defect treatment with apically repositioned flap and free gingival graft repair.

A combination flap is made. This consists of sulcular incisions around the implant and mid-crestal incision, staying subperiosteal until the extent of the exposed threads is reached (Fig. 30.14C). This is followed by a supraperiosteal dissection taken an additional 8 to 10 mm apically. This 8 to 10 mm supraperiosteal dissection sets up a host bed for a free gingival graft to gain attached tissue. Posterior buccal release incisions are made; they are typically minimal with a combination flap.

Free gingival grafts are harvested from the palate and sutured into place with 4-0 or 5-0 chromic sutures, 4 to 5 mm apart (Fig. 30.14D). Once suturing is done, firm pressure with moistened gauze is held over the graft site for 10 minutes to obtain the initial clot, adherence to the periosteum, and minimize hematoma formation. The graft will initially survive by plasmatic circulation. Eight weeks later the tissue should be healthy, free of inflammation, and an adequate band of attached tissue. Note, that the free gingival margin has receded, exposing the implant body secondary to the apically repositioned tissue (Fig. 30.14E).

Postoperative palatal coverage splints, made from 0.020-inch polypropylene sheets, function as a palatal adhesive bandage (Fig. 30.14F). They are worn full time for the first week, except to be removed for hygiene. These palatal splints aid in hemostasis and significantly reduce postoperative discomfort, making the donor site very tolerable.

Avoidance and Management of Intraoperative Complications

When possible, it is ideal to have the prosthesis removed, and consideration for placing a cover screw on the implant 6 to 8 weeks prior to the repair. This will allow better access and improved soft tissue health at the time of the repair procedure.[9] Often, however, the prosthesis is cement retained and difficult to remove, or removing it may destroy part or all of the prosthesis. In these cases, one must work around the prosthesis, which is technically more demanding.

Donor site complications include bleeding from either the palatal soft tissue donor site (greater palatine artery) or the mandibular bone graft donor site (long buccal artery). In either case, use of electrocautery may be necessary to obtain adequate hemostasis. Paresthesia of the buccal mucosa may also occur due to disruption of the long buccal nerve from the access incision during bone graft harvesting along the lateral surface of the mandible. The patient should be warned of this potential complication as well.

Postoperative Considerations

Postoperative antibiotics and chlorhexidine mouthwash are utilized for 10 to 12 days. A soft nonabrasive diet is also necessary to avoid trauma to the closure site. Periodontal dressings have not typically been used. By the 6-month follow-up appointment, one can typically gauge the success of the procedure.[12] The regenerative surgeon should follow the patient until they have been disease-free for 9 to 12 months.

The 14-day course of aggressive antimicrobial therapy may have some adverse effects in some patients. The most common one will be gastrointestinal disturbances. This should be discussed with the patients preoperatively, and a course of action planned in the event they arise (such as the discontinuance of a specific antibiotic), depending upon the adverse event.

Access surgery and flap reflection will result in 1 mm of tissue recession or more.[13] This is an obvious issue in the esthetic zone and should be discussed preoperatively with the patient. When osseous recontouring and implant-plasty are also performed, the recession can be much greater. In addition, apically repositioned flaps and palatal gingivectomies often distort normal tissue contours underneath the prosthesis, and patients will report food collecting in the areas. With time, 6 to 12 months, much of this will remodel, somewhat helping to self-correct this issue. However, if food entrapment remains a problem, the prosthesis may need to be redesigned and refabricated.

Patient Hygiene

Postsurgically, the patient's oral hygiene habits must be established to prevent recurrence of periimplant disease. Communication with the patient's restorative dentist and hygienist is important for follow-up care, maintenance of the repair, and being observant for signs of recurrence.

Treatment Planning for Prevention

Present day digital treatment planning allows surgeons to plan implant reconstructions with preventative techniques. With the large volume of all-on-x full arch treatments being performed, this is even more critical. Techniques that are helpful in prevention of periimplantitis include the following:

1. Designing and utilizing surgical guides that will allow the subsequent implant prosthetics to be screw retained. This can eliminate retained cement as a causative factor in periimplantitis.
2. Placing screw access openings on full arch prosthetic cases into nonesthetic areas. This allows the removal of a prosthesis during recall examinations to assess hygiene, clean the prosthesis, and educate the patient on how to improve their hygiene (Fig. 30.15).
3. Designing a multitooth prosthesis with grooves and notches (Fig. 30.16A and B) so patients know where to insert hygiene devices in between implants, such as floss and proxybrushes.
4. Making sure all intaglio surfaces of the prosthesis have only convex surfaces, with no hidden concavities that would cause plaque accumulation.
5. Setting up a proper recall system for implant restorations.

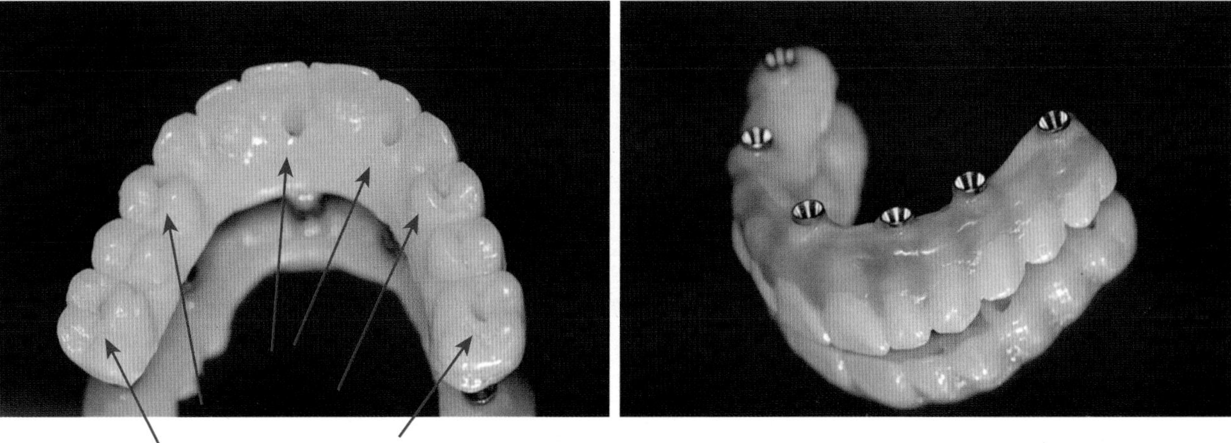

Fig. 30.15 Placing screw access openings on full arch prosthetic cases into nonesthetic areas.

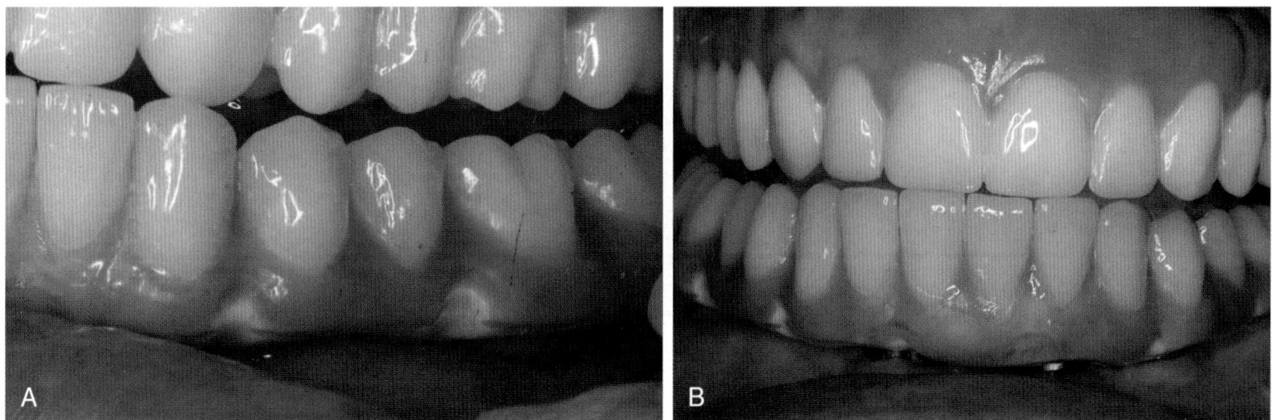

Fig. 30.16 **A** and **B,** Designing a multitooth prosthesis with grooves and notches.

A recent report on the prevalence of periimplantitis in full arch four-implant supported restorations illustrates the importance of incorporating preventative techniques when possible. Francetti et al.'s study of 96 full arch rehabilitations revealed an implant periimplantitis rate of 13%.[26] A total of 39% of their patients had at least one implant with a periimplantitis defect over a 10-year period. This study and others emphasize the importance of ongoing vigilance for longevity factors in our surgery and prosthetics.

References

1. Adell R, Lekholm U, Rockler B, Brånemark PI. A 15-year study of osseointegrated implants in the treatment of the edentulous jaw. *Int J Oral Surg*. 1981;10(6):387–416.
2. Zitzmann NU, Berglundh T. Definition and prevalence of peri-implant diseases. *J Clin Periodontol*. 2008;35(suppl 8):286–291.
3. Albrektsson T, Isidor F. Consensus report: implant therapy. In: Lang NP, Karring T, eds. *Proceedings of the 1st European Workshop on Periodontology*. Berlin, Germany: Quintessence; 1994.
4. Pjeturrson, et al. A systematic review of the survival and complication rates of fixed partial dentures (FPD'S) after at least 5 years. *Clin Oral Implants Res*. 2004a;15:625–642.
5. Roos-Jansåker AM, Lindahl C, Renvert H, Renvert S. Nine- to fourteen-year follow-up of implant treatment. Part II: presence of peri-implant lesions. *J Clin Periodontol*. 2006;33(4):290–295.
6. Mombelli A, Müller N, Cionca N. The epidemiology of peri-implantitis. *Clin Oral Implants Res*. 2012;23(23 suppl 6):67–76.
7. Heitz-Mayfield LJA. Peri-implant diseases: diagnosis and risk indicators. *J Clin Periodontol*. 2008;35(suppl 8):292–304.
8. Schwarz F, Herten M, Sager M, Bieling K, Sculean A, Becker J. Comparison of naturally occurring and ligature-induced peri-implantitis bone defects in humans and dogs. *Clin Oral Implants Res*. 2007;18(2):161–170.
9. Kolonidis SG, Renvert S, Hämmerle CHF, Lang NP, Harris D, Claffey N. Osseointegration on implant surfaces previously contaminated with plaque. An experimental study in the dog. *Clin Oral Implants Res*. 2003;14(4):373–380.
10. Renvert S, Polyzois I, Maguire R. Re-osseointegration on previously contaminated surfaces: a systematic review. *Clin Oral Implants Res*. 2009;20(suppl 4):216–227.
11. Froum SJ, Froum SH, Rosen PS. Successful management of peri-implantitis with a regenerative approach: a consecutive series of 51 treated implants with 3- to 7.5-year follow-up. *Int J Periodont Restor Dent*. 2012;32(1): 11–20.

12. Serino G, Turri A. Outcome of surgical treatment of peri-implantitis: results from a 2-year prospective clinical study in humans. *Clin Oral Implants Res*. 2011;22(11):1214–1220.
13. Heitz-Mayfield LJA, Salvi GE, Mombelli A, Faddy M, Lang NP. Anti-infective surgical therapy of peri-implantitis. A 12-month prospective clinical study. *Clin Oral Implants Res*. 2012;23(2):205–210.
14. Wilson TG Jr. The positive relationship between excess cement and peri-implant disease: a prospective clinical endoscopic study. *J Periodontol*. 2009;80(9):1388–1392.
15. Wadhwani C, Piñeyro A, Hess T, Zhang H, Chung KH. Effect of implant abutment modification on the extrusion of excess cement at the crown-abutment margin for cement-retained implant restorations. *Int J Oral Maxillofac Implants*. 2011;26(6):1241–1246.
16. Roccuzzo M, Bonino F, Aglietta M, Dalmasso P. Ten-year results of a three arms prospective cohort study on implants in periodontally compromised patients. Part 2: clinical results. *Clin Oral Implants Res*. 2012;23(4):389–395.
17. Cho-Yan Lee J, Mattheos N, Nixon KC, Ivanovski S. Residual periodontal pockets are a risk indicator for peri-implantitis in patients treated for periodontitis. *Clin Oral Implants Res*. 2012;23(3):325–333.
18. Dirschnabel AJ, Alvim-Pereira F, Alvim-Pereira CC, Bernardino JF, Rosa EAR, Trevilatto PC. Analysis of the association of IL1B(C-511T) polymorphism with dental implant loss and the clusterization phenomenon. *Clin Oral Implants Res*. 2011;22(11):1235–1241.
19. Casado PL, Villas-Boas R, de Mello W, Duarte ME, Granjeiro JM. Peri-implant disease and chronic periodontitis: is interleukin-6 gene promoter polymorphism the common risk factor in a Brazilian population? *Int J Oral Maxillofac Implants*. 2013;28(1):35–43.
20. Moy PK, Medina D, Shetty V, Aghaloo TL. Dental implant failure rates and associated risk factors. *Int J Oral Maxillofac Implants*. 2005;20(4):569–577.
21. Renvert S, Giovnnoli JL. Treatments. In: *Peri-Implantitis. Paris, France*: Quintessence International; 2012.
22. Parma-Benfenati S, Roncati M, Tinti C. Treatment of peri-implantitis: surgical therapeutic approaches based on peri-implantitis defects. *Int J Periodont Restor Dent*. 2013;33(5):627–633.
23. Ntrouka V, Hoogenkamp M, Zaura E, van der Weijden F. The effect of chemotherapeutic agents on titanium-adherent biofilms. *Clin Oral Implants Res*. 2011;22(11): 1227–1234.
24. Kreisler M, Kohnen W, Marinello C, et al. Bactericidal effect of the Er:YAG laser on dental implant surfaces: an in vitro study. *J Periodontol*. 2002;73(11):1292–1298.
25. Yamamoto A. *Predictable treatment of peri-implantitis using erbium laser micro-explosion. In: 11th International Symposium on Periodontics and Restorative Dentistry*; 2013. Boston.
26. Francetti L, Cavalli N, Taschieri S, Corbella S. Ten years follow-up retrospective study on implant survival rates and prevalence of Peri-implantitis in implant-supported full-arch rehabilitations. *Clin Oral Implants Res*. 2019;30(3):252–260.

CHAPTER 31

Prosthodontic Temporization Procedures in Implant Dentistry

Edward R. Schlissel

Armamentarium

Appropriate sutures
Diagnostic tooth arrangement
Implant analogs
Intraoral radiographs
Local anesthetic with vasoconstrictor
Materials for impressions (irreversible hydrocolloid or polyvinyl siloxane)
Provisional implant abutments
Provisional restorative material
Teflon tape
Torque device with driver tips

History of the Procedure

The earliest noted use of dental implants occurred in the Mayan culture. Specimens have been found with seashell fragments inserted into the alveolar processes. Modern prosthetic replacement of the dentition emerged with the creation and evolution of dental materials, notably vulcanite, acrylic, gold, and porcelain. Many types of materials are used in contemporary restorative implant dentistry. The material chosen depends on a number of factors, including cost, esthetics, durability, and function, which must be taken into consideration along with the patient's preference.

Indications for the Use of the Procedure

Implant restorations may be used to replace single teeth or multiple teeth or to restore complete dental arches. With appropriate occlusal design and osseous support, these restorations can provide functional and esthetic outcomes that satisfy the patient and have long-term clinical success.[1,2] Provisional restorations can be an important part of the process; they satisfy esthetic and functional needs during healing and provide a template for the final prosthesis.[3,4]

Fixed provisional restorations on implants provide a scaffold for the development of soft-tissue contours and are a valuable aid in communication with the dental laboratory. Although not necessary for every case, provisional restorations are very helpful in areas of high esthetic demand and should be strongly considered as part of the plan when the scope and sequence of treatment are developed.[5–7]

Provisional restorations may also be made as removable prostheses. Although they can meet cosmetic and functional needs, they are seldom assets in developing soft tissues for the final restorations. Dentists should be familiar with these prostheses and their limitations because circumstances may prevent the use of fixed provisional restorations during the healing phase after implant placement.

Provisional restorations may always be placed on implants after integration is completed. In the traditional sequence, this is between 2 and 6 months. The length of time to integration depends on the site, healing capacity of the patient, presence or absence of graft materials, and nature of the implant surface. The surgeon must provide guidance in this area to the restorative team.

In some circumstances, it is possible to deliver a provisional restoration at the same time as the implant.[8] An individual temporary restoration may be placed on an implant that has a high insertion torque level, indicating good primary stability. There should not be any contact in centric occlusion or during excursive movements of the mandible. Although the restoration may not have contact in centric occlusion, it is possible to generate significant force on a bolus of food. Therefore, the patient must be instructed to refrain from chewing on that side until integration is complete.

Multiple implants (typically four or more, which can be connected across the midline) may also be restored provisionally at the time of placement. These restorations may be used immediately in function; however, the patient should be advised to eat a soft diet until integration is complete.

If all the criteria for immediate placement of a fixed provisional restoration are not met, the dentist and the patient must decide whether to use a removable prosthesis during implant integration. If no provisional restoration is used, a vacuum-formed orthodontic retainer is helpful for preventing tooth movement during the healing phase. It is easy to

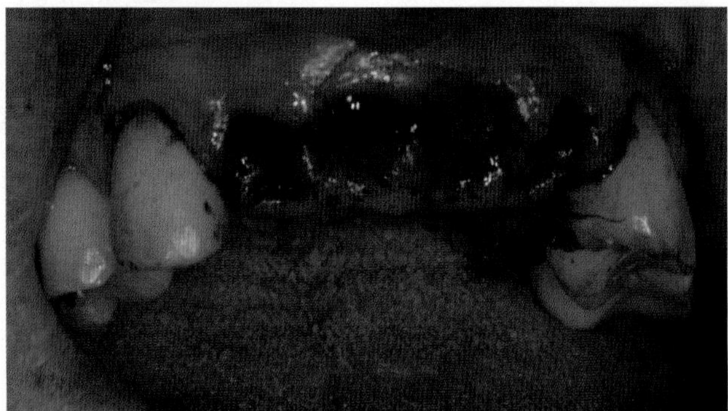

Figure 31.1 Surgical site immediately after extractions.

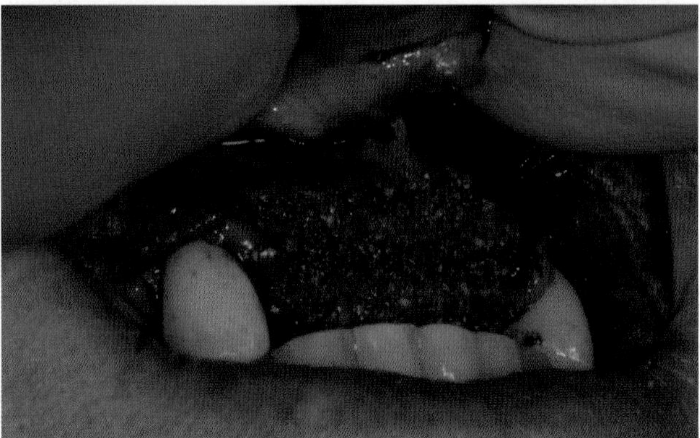

Figure 31.2 Graft material in place.

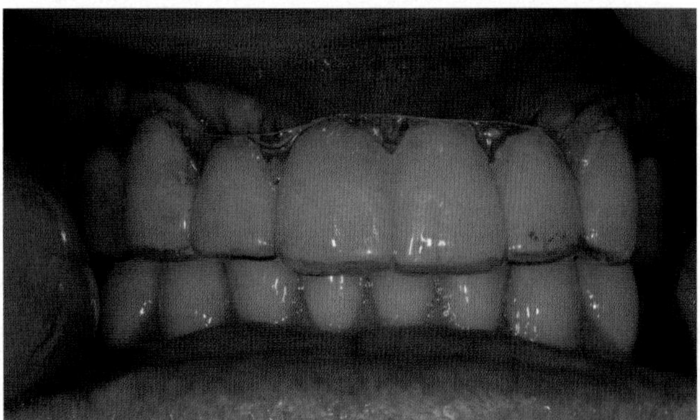

Figure 31.3 Provisional in place, no tissue contact.

include a prosthetic tooth in this appliance. An advantage of this type of appliance is the full support offered by the remaining teeth; an occlusal load is never transferred to the surgical site (Figs. 31.1–31.3).

Alternatively, a provisional prosthesis may be a traditional acrylic removable partial denture ("flipper"), although flexible materials such as Valplast (Valplast International, Long Beach, New York) or Flexite (Flexite, Mineola, New York) may be easier for the patient to insert and remove (Figs. 31.4 and 31.5). Care should be taken to avoid pressure on the tissue immediately over the site of surgery.

It is also possible to use a provisional fixed partial denture (FPD) with adjacent natural teeth as retainers. A disadvantage

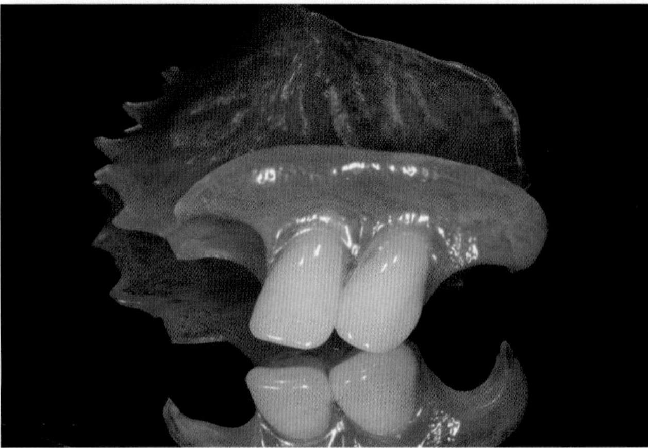

Figure 31.4 Removable partial denture (RPD) as provisional (buccal aspect).

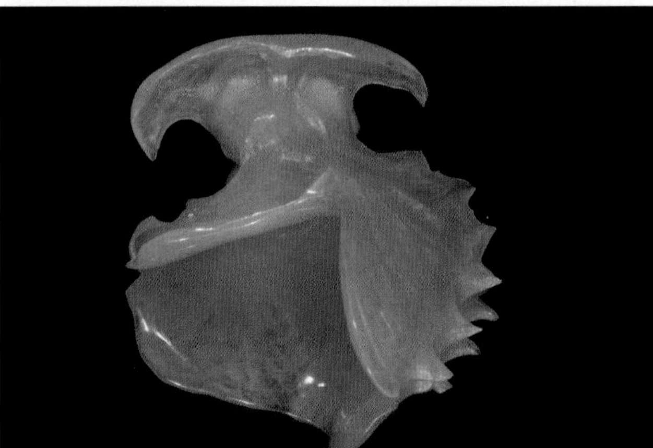

Figure 31.5 Removable partial denture (RPD) as provisional (tissue aspect).

of this procedure is the need to prepare the adjacent teeth for restorations that may not be otherwise indicated. A Maryland-type FPD may be used as a provisional; however, it requires removal during the restorative phase and is often associated with damage to the adjacent teeth during debonding and widening of the restorative space of the implant.

Limitations and Contraindications

Provisional restorations on individual implants are contraindicated at the time of implant placement if the forces of occlusion cannot be eliminated or if patient compliance is not likely. Provisional restorations on multiple implants are contraindicated at the time of implant placement if any of the potential implants supporting the prosthesis do not have sufficient primary stability and if there is no cross-arch stabilization.

Although the benefits of same-day immediate implant provisional restorations are appealing to many patients and dentists, they have significant costs that often limit their use. The laboratory and professional fees associated with these

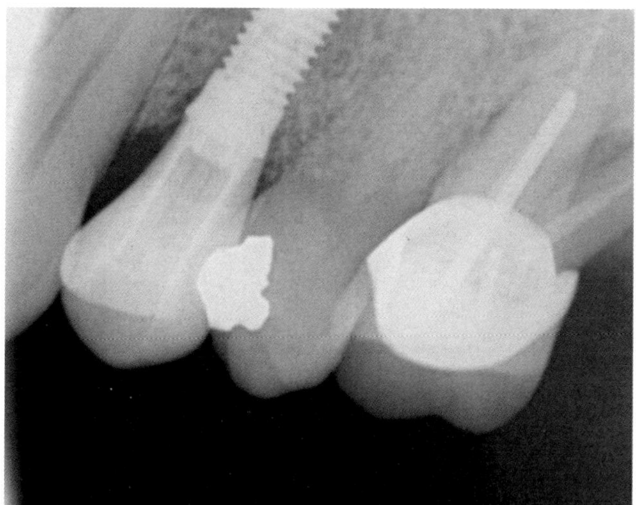

Figure 31.6 Radiograph of provisional with titanium cylinder.

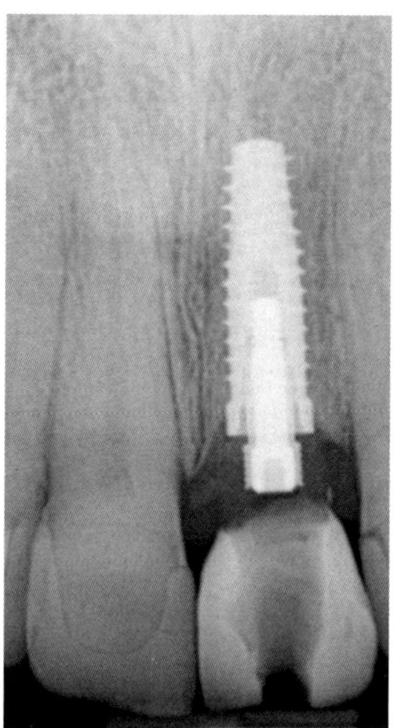

Figure 31.7 Radiograph of provisional with polyether ether ketone (PEEK) cylinder.

procedures can be substantial and must be considered during the treatment planning process.

If the surgeon or restorative dentist is inexperienced in the process of making implant provisional restorations, this can be a limiting factor. The problem can be overcome by obtaining proper support from a qualified dental laboratory and by performing meticulous advance planning. The significant benefits of using provisional implant restorations in the esthetic zone make this collaboration extremely worthwhile.

Abutments for temporary restorations may be made of titanium or polyether ether ketone (PEEK). Both materials have intaglio surfaces that mate well with implant platforms and provide adequate stability. PEEK abutments are approved for intraoral use for up to 6 months. Titanium cylinders may be preferable if the restoration is expected to be in place for a longer period. PEEK abutments are minimally radiopaque, making it difficult to use radiographs to evaluate full seating. If this is a concern, titanium may be preferred (Figs. 31.6 and 31.7).

TECHNIQUE: Procedure Performed Directly on Implant at the Time of Implant Placement (Immediate Provisional)

STEP 1: Implant Assessment

After implant placement is complete, primary stability is assessed. If deemed to be sufficient, a provisional abutment with antirotational features is placed on the implant. Full seating of the temporary abutment must be evaluated visually or radiographically. Occasionally, if the implant platform is below the crest of alveolar bone, it is necessary to use a bone profiler to create room for the emergence profile of the prosthetic part. The screw is tightened by hand. The length of the temporary abutment is adjusted until it is just free of occlusal contacts in centric occlusion and excursive movements (Fig. 31.8A).

STEP 2: Abutment Preparation

Titanium abutments may be cut with diamond instruments in a high-speed handpiece using copious water spray. When titanium abutments are adjusted in the mouth, care must be taken to use irrigation and suction to minimize heat transfer and to prevent inadvertent tissue tattooing. If substantial reduction is necessary, it may be easier to mark the extent of the reduction needed on the abutment, remove it from the mouth, place it on an implant replica, and then make the modifications. PEEK abutments are easily modified with carbide finishing burs in a high-speed handpiece or a green stone in a low-speed handpiece.

Continued

Technique: Procedure Performed Directly on Implant at the Time of Implant Placement (Immediate Provisional)—cont'd

STEP 3: Temporization

After adjustment, the access opening over the screw should be closed provisionally with a material that is easily removed. Teflon tape should be packed gently over the screw; then, wax or a light-cured provisional material (e.g., Fermit, Ivoclar Vivadent, Amherst, New York) is placed and cured. If a resin-based material is used, the clinician should lightly lubricate the provisional covering with a petroleum-based material before proceeding to make the temporary crown; this prevents adhesion to the inner surface of the provisional crown and facilitates uncovering of the screw access opening.

STEP 4: Provisionalization

The provisional crown may be made with a preformed crown shape (e.g., Protemp; 3M, Minneapolis, Minnesota) or a vacuum-formed template and resin. The crown is joined to the provisional abutment with resin. The connection is mechanical and depends on the surface area and roughness of the provisional abutment. Before the curing process is complete, it is advisable to make an opening in the provisional crown to reach the screw access opening (Fig. 31.8B and C).

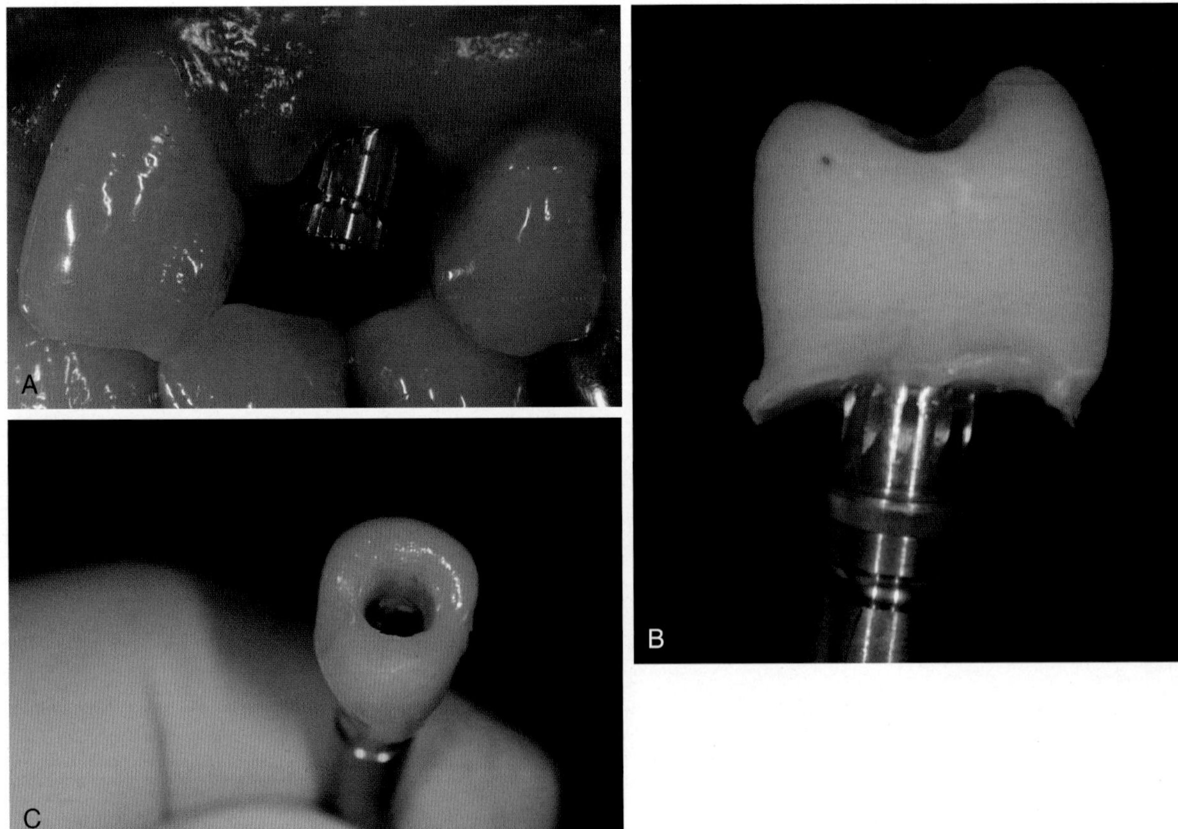

Figure 31.8 **A,** Titanium cylinder, reduced to freedom from contact. **B,** Provisional secured to titanium cylinder. **C,** Provisional restoration, showing occlusal access to abutment screw.

Technique: Procedure Performed Directly on Implant at the Time of Implant Placement (Immediate Provisional)—cont'd

STEP 5: Crown Placement

After the crown has been polymerized, the block-out material and Teflon tape are removed from the screw access opening. The screw is removed and the abutment and crown are removed in one piece. After cleaning with water spray and drying, the emergence profile is completed. The subgingival walls should be smooth and gently contoured. Flowable composite resin may be used for this step (Fig. 31.8D). Autopolymerizing polymethyl methacrylate (PMMA) may be used but care must be taken to minimize porosity.

STEP 6: Adjustment

The crown, including surfaces that will contact soft tissue, must be polished to a high gloss. Interproximal contacts should be adjusted to the desired location and strength. Occlusal contacts should be removed.

STEP 7: Final Seating

The provisional restoration is replaced on the implant and seating is verified (see Fig. 31.6). The screw is tightened by hand, not with a torque control device. Teflon tape is compacted over the screw, and restorative resin is placed in the cavity. If esthetic demands permit, it is advantageous to select a shade for the opening that is slightly different from that of the crown; this makes identification of the screw access opening during removal easier in the future.

At the time of implant placement, screw-retained provisional restorations are preferable to cement-retained temporaries. It is very challenging to prepare the margins of the abutment and develop good adaptation of the provisional in a surgical field. Additionally, there is the concern of leaving excess cement below the margins. It has been shown that leaving cement in the vicinity of the implant platform has extremely undesirable consequences.

Having a traditional healing abutment available during the process is helpful. Whenever the provisional abutment is removed, the healing abutment should be placed and tightened gently; this prevents the collapse of soft tissue over the implant platform.

Continued

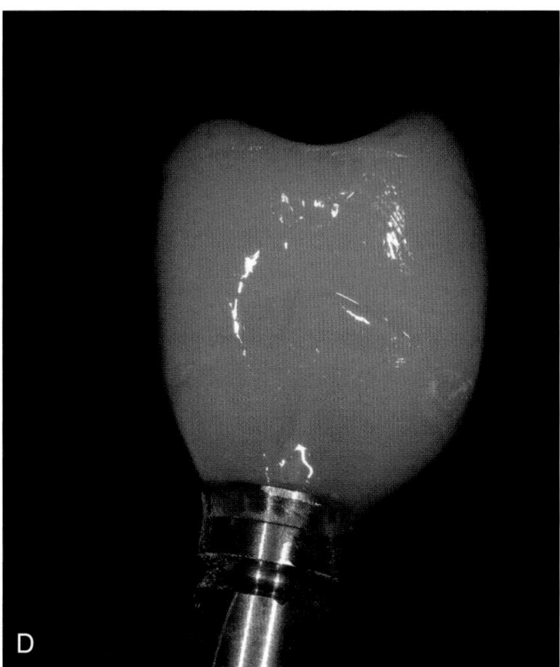

Figure 31.8, cont'd D, Provisional restoration, contoured.

ALTERNATIVE TECHNIQUE 1: Implant Index at the Time of Surgery: Placement of Provisional After Integration

STEP 1: Abutment Considerations

If traditional implant timing is selected, the provisional restoration still may be prefabricated. This technique offers an additional, significant advantage in the esthetic zone. Because the angulation of the implant is commonly different from the desired path of insertion for the final restoration, an angled abutment may be needed. With traditional techniques, the surgeon would place a healing abutment, which the restorative dentist would remove to make the impression and place the restoration. When angular correction is necessary, very often in the esthetic zone, this results in loss of tissue on the facial aspect of the implant. With this modified technique, the provisional, with correction of the angle, is ready at the time of uncovering. The surgeon may place it at the uncovering appointment, preserving facial soft-tissue. The benefits can be significant.

STEP 2: Model Preparation

Before the uncovering, it is necessary to have study models of both arches. If changes in tooth shape or position are needed, they should be made on a duplicate model. A vacuum-formed template of the tooth to be restored is made and trimmed to include several adjacent teeth. The anticipated surgical site is modified on a copy of the model. A cutout is made, removing the area of the model that corresponds to the location into which the implant will be placed. The space should be significantly wider and deeper than the dimensions of the implant to be used.

STEP 3: Indexing

After placement of the implant and evaluation of primary stability, an implant impression coping designed for the open-tray technique is placed on the implant. Seating is verified visually or radiographically. An incisal index that captures the impression coping and several adjacent teeth is made with fast-setting polyvinyl siloxane (PVS) bite registration material. These products typically have a working time of 90 seconds and a setting time of less than 2 minutes. After setting, the impression coping is unscrewed and removed as one piece with the index. A healing abutment or cover screw is placed on the implant during the integration period. The provisional restoration may be fabricated during this phase, which may last 2 to 6 months.

STEP 4: Impression Preparation

The incisal index is disinfected and an implant analog is connected to the impression coping. During this process, care must be taken to avoid rotating the impression coping. This is accomplished by using a hand driver in the screw of the impression coping while holding the implant analog; this avoids torque on the PVS (Fig. 31.9A).

STEP 5: Index Transfer

The incisal index, with implant analog attached, is placed gently on the model that was prepared before the procedure. The index should fit passively, with no contact between the implant analog and the model. If seating is not possible, the index should be removed, the model examined and modified as needed, and seating reattempted. Bubbles on the model, which are not present in the index, may also prevent seating. They should be removed (Fig. 31.9B).

STEP 6: Analog Connection

When the incisal index seats passively, the analog should be connected to the model with a fast-setting gypsum product. A plaster that is a different color from the model should be used because this allows inadvertent placement to be identified and corrected. As an alternative to gypsum product, self-curing resin may be used to join the analog and model. If this is chosen, care must be taken to monitor the results of polymerization contraction.

STEP 7: Provisional Restoration

After the analog has been secured, the provisional abutment is contoured and the restoration is made. Any technique may be used, as long as care is taken to maintain the screw access opening. The restoration is polished, disinfected, and returned to the treatment room for placement. The healing abutment is removed and the provisional restoration is delivered. The provisional is an asset in the development of soft-tissue contours. It makes an esthetic final restoration possible (Fig. 31.9C–G).

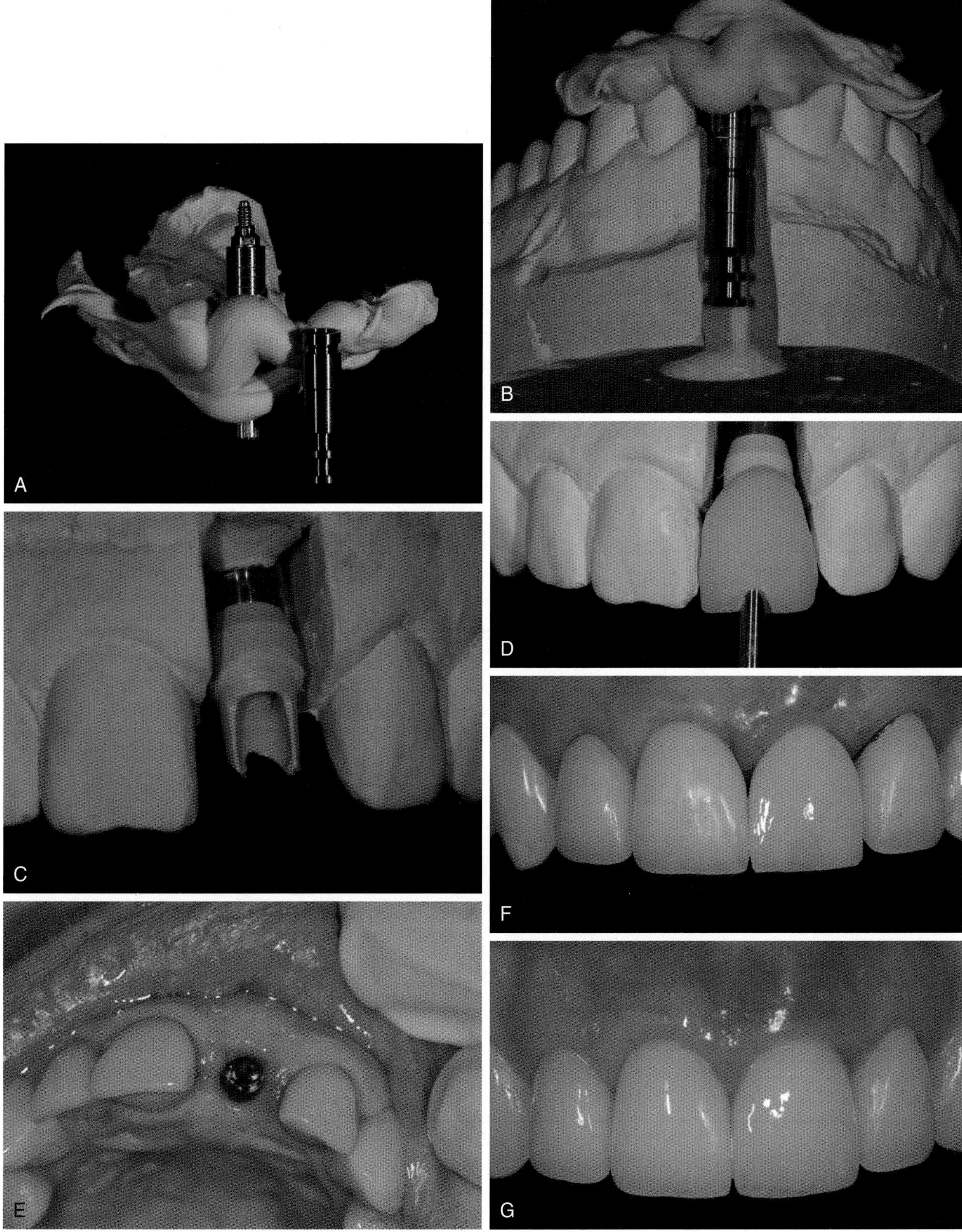

Figure 31.9 **A,** Surgical index and implant analog. **B,** Surgical index and analog on modified study model. **C,** Polyether ether ketone (PEEK) temporary abutment after contouring. **D,** Provisional restorations on model, with driver tip in place. **E,** Implant platform after surgical exposure and removal of healing cap. **F,** Provisional restoration at the time of placement. **G,** Final restoration, 2 months after placement of provisional restoration.

ALTERNATIVE TECHNIQUE 2: Placement of Provisional at Time of Implant Placement, Fabricated Indirectly

It may be more convenient for the dentist and surgeon to make an immediate provisional restoration outside of the mouth. This is easily accomplished and offers the advantage of allowing fabrication to be done away from the surgical field. Contamination of the implant site is less likely, there is no interference with the setting of the restorative materials, and the patient may rest comfortably during the procedure. Additionally, the dentist, laboratory technician, or dental assistant may make the provisional restoration in a setting more comfortable for the procedure. Planning in advance of the surgical appointment makes this process efficient and accurate.

The clinical steps in this procedure are the same as those described in the Alternative Technique 1 section. The index and provisional are made according to the same steps, except that delivery must be completed within 24 hours.

Avoidance and Management of Intraoperative Complications

Screw-retained provisional restorations are more desirable than the cemented type. If cemented restorations are used, care must be taken to ensure that no excess cement is left apical to the margins and below the implant platform. The use of radiopaque materials makes this task easier. A posttreatment radiograph should be taken to verify removal of all excess material.

If the provisional restoration is made in the mouth at the time of implant placement, blood and saliva may interfere with the polymerization of some restorative materials. Composite resins, especially those that harden on exposure to light, may not be satisfactory. Self-curing materials, such as acrylics (e.g., PMMA), are less susceptible to moisture contamination problems. For this reason, many clinicians prefer an indirect technique, even though it may take slightly longer to complete.

If the patient is receiving a full-arch provisional restoration, it may be beneficial for the dental laboratory to send a technician to the surgeon's office. Modification of a large provisional restoration can be time-consuming and technically challenging for dentists or their staff. It is often worthwhile to have a technical specialist available for this task.

Postoperative Considerations

If a provisional restoration is placed the same day as the implant, the patient should be seen the next day. Home care instructions include the use of dental floss, toothbrush, and dentifrice. If a bruxism splint or night guard has been made, it should be delivered with instructions for use.

References

1. Tarnow DP, Magner AW, Fletcher P. The effect of the distance from the contact point to the crest of bone on the presence or absence of the interproximal dental papilla. *J Periodontol.* 1992;63(12):995–996.
2. Tarnow D, Elian N, Fletcher P, et al. Vertical distance from the crest of bone to the height of the interproximal papilla between adjacent implants. *J Periodontol.* 2003;74(12):1785–1788.
3. LeSage BP. Improving implant aesthetics: prosthetically generated papilla through tissue modeling with composite. *Pract Proced Aesthet Dent.* 2006;18(4):257–263.
4. Santosa RE. Provisional restoration options in implant dentistry. *Aust Dent J.* 2007;52(3):234–242.
5. Priest G. Esthetic potential of single-implant provisional restorations: selection criteria of available alternatives. *J Esthet Restor Dent.* 2006;18(6):326–338.
6. Touati B, Guez G, Saadoun A. Aesthetic soft tissue integration and optimized emergence profile: provisionalization and customized impression coping. *Pract Periodontics Aesthet Dent.* 1999;11(3):305–314.
7. Neale D, Chee WW. Development of implant soft tissue emergence profile: a technique. *J Prosthet Dent.* 1994;71(4):364–368.
8. Lemongello GJ. Customized provisional abutment and provisional restoration for an immediately-placed implant. *Pract Proced Aesthet Dent.* 2007;19(7):419–424.

Soft Tissue Augmentation Surgery for Dental Implants

Meaghan Bradley and Hussam Batal

Armamentarium

Appropriate sutures
Buser elevator
Dean scissors
Dental mirror
Gauze: 2 × 2
Keratome blades or microblades
Local anesthetic with vasoconstrictor
Minnesota retractor
Needle holder
Palatal stent (if needed)
Periodontal probe
Scalpel blades: #15 or #15C
Surgical suction tip
Tissue forceps or cotton pliers
Tunneling instruments
Woodson elevator

In the last 30 years, there has been a paradigm shift in implant dentistry relative to concepts, especially for the anterior esthetic zone. The objective has shifted from obtaining a functional restoration to a functional restoration that fully blends with the surrounding teeth and hard and soft tissue structures. Adequate quality and quantity of soft tissue provide the best periimplant environment. Attached tissue around dental implants increases soft tissue stability and decreases the incidence of periimplant mucositis. Recent data suggest that adequate height of attached tissue of ideally 2.5 mm or more decreases the incidence of bone remodeling around the dental implant. Adequate band and thickness of soft tissue in the esthetic zone are needed to provide the much needed optimal esthetic outcome that allows the final restoration to seamlessly blend with the surrounding dentition.

Esthetic outcomes in implant dentistry strongly correlate with the patient gingival biotype. Two distinct gingival biotypes have been described by Olsson et al.[1]: the thin scalloped biotype and the thick flat biotype. There are three key areas of variation between the two biotypes: soft tissue, bone, and teeth morphology. Patients with the thin gingival biotype usually require more aggressive grafting in conjuncture with implant placement.[1–3]

History of the Procedure

The use of an autogenous soft tissue graft that did not include the epithelial layer was first reported in 1974 by Alan Edel. Edel[4] secured the tissue onto a connective tissue recipient bed, similar to a free gingival graft technique, and left it exposed to the oral environment to increase the width of keratinized tissue. Langer and Calagna[5] first introduced the term *subepithelial connective tissue graft* (SCTG). They harvested autogenous connective tissue from the palate and placed it underneath a partial-thickness flap to esthetically rehabilitate soft tissue irregularities and concavities of resorbed edentulous ridges. During the 1980s, many authors attempted to develop soft tissue grafting techniques that could improve anterior esthetics in edentulous areas, providing a natural emergence profile for pontics of fixed partial dentures.

It was not until the mid-1990s that the SCTG was used in conjunction with dental implant cases to improve esthetics.[6] Since then, numerous publications have verified the predictability of autogenous soft tissue grafts around implants, including their excellent clinical results and long-term stability. Clinicians who practice implant dentistry should consider aiming higher than just osseointegration of the implant to achieve an esthetically successful outcome.[7] The esthetic success of an implant case lies in attention to fine details, through which adequate connective tissue can (1) provide a natural emergence profile for the restoration through healthy periimplant gingiva, (2) create a labial profile over the bone and implant body similar to the root prominence of a natural tooth, and (3) support papillae, fill interdental embrasures, and hide the restorative components of the implant restoration.

Indications for the Use of the Procedure

Practically every implant placement, especially in the esthetic region, constitutes an indication for soft tissue grafting. The inevitable alteration of the alveolar ridge dimensions that follows every tooth extraction results in the placement of the implant in a site that has undergone a reduction in tissue volume in comparison to neighboring dentate sites.[8–10] This discrepancy is more pronounced in single-implant sites where a concavity is formed between the edentulous site and the root prominence of the neighboring dentate sites. SCTGs can be used in those cases to reconstruct the gingival dimensions of the site, create the illusion of root prominence, and increase the width of the crestal periimplant gingiva, providing sufficient tissue for a restoration that closely resembles a natural tooth.

The long-term stability of pink esthetics around a dental implant prosthesis has been strongly correlated with an adequate soft tissue thickness around the implant, a thick periimplant biotype.[11,12] When a thin biotype is diagnosed, a SCTG can be used to prevent potential long-term recession of the facial mucosa margin.[13–15]

Factors that should be considered when evaluating the need for soft tissue grafting include the following:[16,17]

1. The level of clinical attachment on adjacent teeth to support papillary height
2. The thickness of the coronal soft tissue margin to ensure a proper emergence profile
3. The thickness of labial soft tissue to simulate root eminence and prevent transillumination of underlying metallic structure
4. The position of the mucogingival junction and amount of keratinized tissue, which should allow harmonious blending with that of the adjacent teeth

Factors that should be considered when deciding on a technique for soft tissue grafting include the following:

1. Type of augmentation needed thickness versus attached tissue
2. Need for implant temporization at the time of placement
3. Dental arch in which the procedure is being performed
4. Size and morphology of the defect
5. Need for bone grating at the time of soft tissue graft placement

The flow chart below ("Implant site evaluation algorithm") illustrates different graft indications based on the clinical indications, the need for bone augmentation, the size of the defect, timing of implant placement, and the need for temporization.

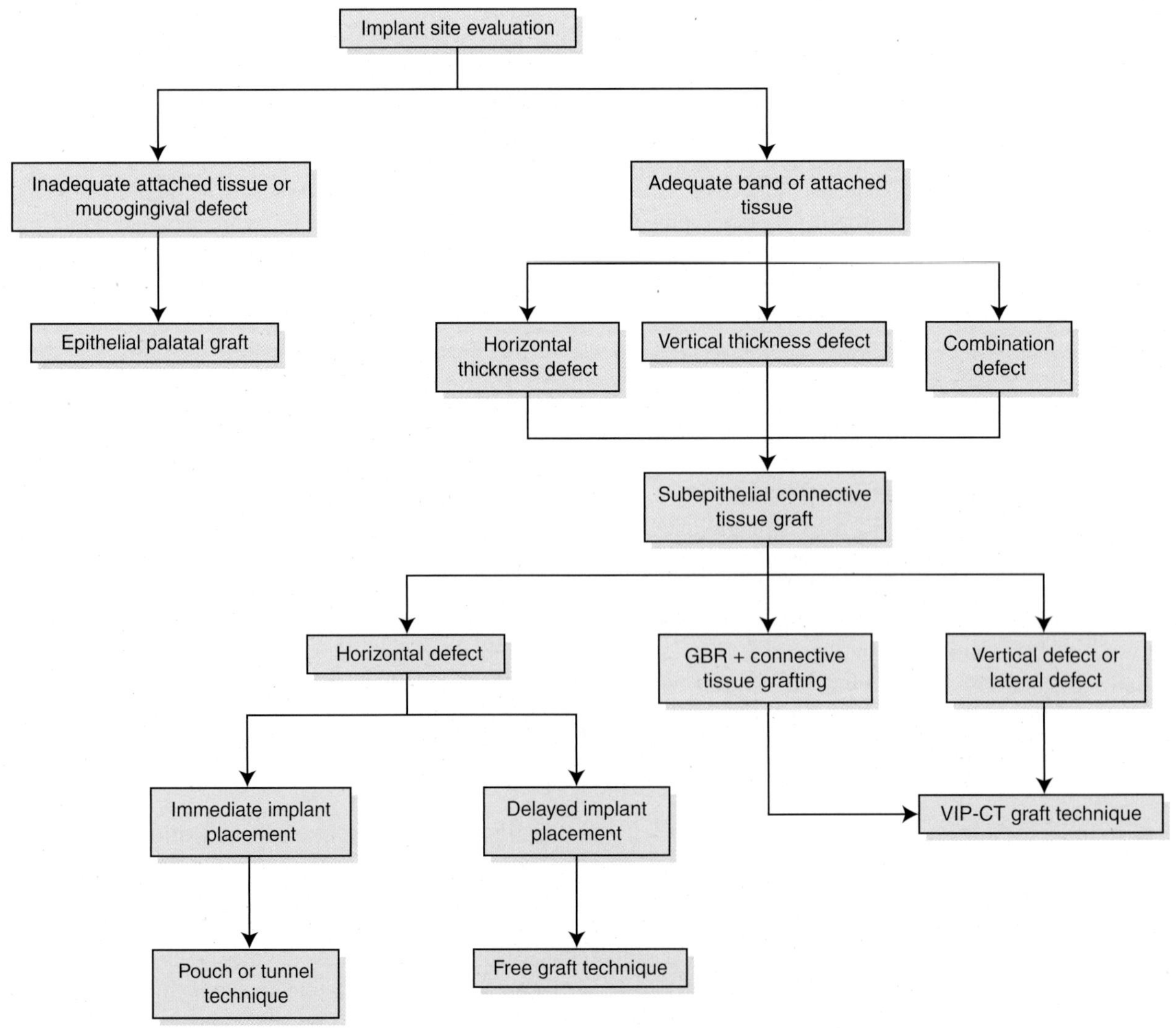

Implant site evaluation algorithm

Limitations and Contraindications

General and specific limitations apply to the use of this soft tissue augmentation technique around dental implants. Underlying medical conditions that present as contraindications to surgical intervention are general contraindications. Medical conditions associated with collagen disorders, such as erosive lichen planus or pemphigoid, may pose a risk to the viability of autogenous connective tissue grafts placed on a recipient bed that exhibits a pathologic healing mechanism. There is no published evidence to support the use of this technique in such cases.

A key determinant in the success of this technique is revascularization of the graft. Heavy smoking can have a deleterious effect on the survival of grafted soft tissue by producing gingival vasoconstriction that often results in necrosis of the soft tissue graft.[18] Nicotine-associated vasoconstriction, in combination with lack of adherence of the fibroblasts[18] and an alteration in immune response,[19,20] diminishes the chance for a successful outcome. Preoperative assessment should attempt to identify such patients, and the clinician must inform the patient of the potential adverse effects associated with smoking. Ideally, the surgeon should have the patient first participate in a smoking cessation program and then return later for surgery. However, in clinical reality, this is not always an option. The surgeon must make the final decision on whether to proceed with a delicate procedure in a smoker, bearing in mind that proper patient selection is imperative to achieving the desired treatment outcome. Preoperative interruption of the smoking habit, followed by a smoke-free period during the critical stages of initial revascularization, and adjunctive measures (e.g., use of nicotine patches) should be the minimum precautions taken before subjecting a smoker to soft tissue grafting. Local factors that may also limit patient selection include lack of adequate tissue thickness at the palatal donor site and restricted surgical access to intraoral donor sites, such as the posterior aspect of the hard palate or tuberosity.

Connective Tissue Autografts

A variety of intraoral donor sites have been described for connective tissue grafts. The most commonly used source is the hard palate. Other possible donor sites are the maxillary tuberosity and retromolar pad area. Although the greatest thickness of tissue is usually present in the maxillary tuberosity area, the maximum volume of tissue obtainable is from the palate.

Types of connective tissue that are harvested from intraoral sites can be divided into epithelial connective tissue grafts, SCTGs, and a combination of epithelial and SCTGs.

Subepithelial Connective Tissue Grafts

There are different graft techniques that can be used for a variety of clinical situations. Technique selection depends on clinical situations and the need for temporization. Please see flow chart "Implant site evaluation algorithm". Three techniques are described:

1. Pouch or tunnel technique
2. Free subepithelial graft
3. Vascularized interpositional periosteal—connective tissue (VIP-CT) graft

Pouch or Tunnel Technique

The pouch technique is commonly used for the augmentation of soft tissue in the buccal area. The technique is ideal for augmentation of buccal soft tissue at the time of immediate implant placement, or correction of soft tissue defects around the nonsubmerged implant or a restored implant. Two variations of the technique are described. The variation depends on if the pocket is developed in a supraperiosteal or subperiosteal fashion. The supraperiosteal variation is more technique sensitive but offers the advantage of a dual supply from the periosteum and overlying tissue. Both techniques have excellent success rates. The advantage of these techniques is that immediate temporization can be performed, and no releasing incisions are needed.[17,18]

STEP 1: Creation of Pouch
Subperiosteal Pouch

After extraction of the tooth and the placement of the dental implant and grafting of the gap, a Buser or a Woodson elevator is inserted under the free gingival margin in the mid-buccal area. The elevator is used to dissect the soft tissue in a plane between the periosteum and the buccal plate. Attention should be made not to reflect the papilla and extend the pouch into the midbuccal area. The dissection is then extended laterally to allow for increased blood supply to the graft. The dissection should be extended beyond the mucogingival junction, as this will facilitate subsequent tunneling of the graft (Fig. 32.1A). Once the pouch is completed, a periodontal probe is used to estimate the pocket's size.

STEP 2: Harvest of the Subepithelial Connective Tissue Graft
Harvesting the SCTG

The two most commonly used intraoral donor sites and types of harvest for obtaining connective tissue grafts include the single incision (deep palatal) harvest and the tuberosity harvest.

Continued

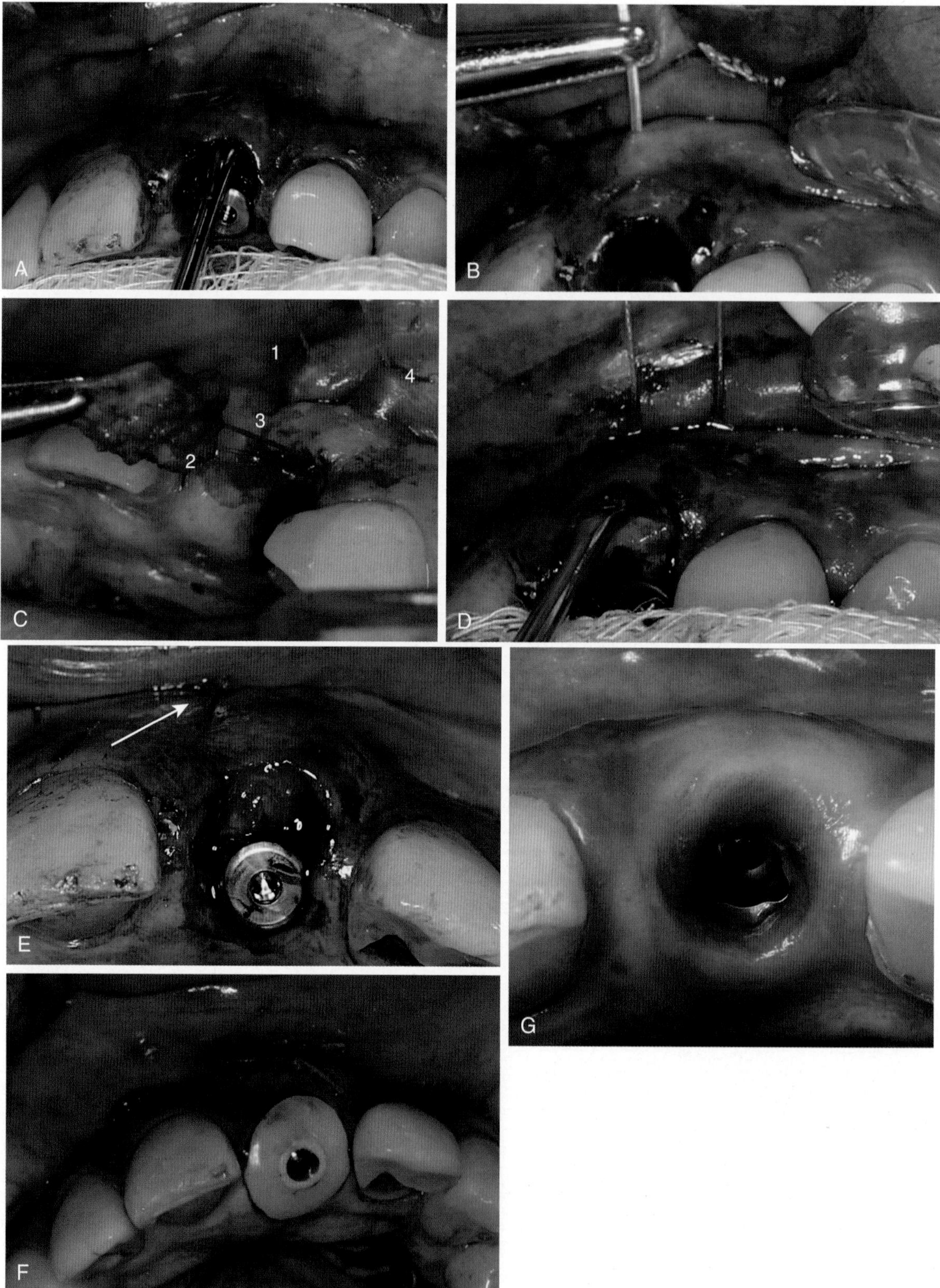

Figure 32.1 **A,** Creation of a subperiosteal pouch with a Woodson elevator. Note how the papilla is left intact and dissection is carried in the midbuccal area down past the mucogingival junction. **B,** After creation of the pocket, a suture is passed from the depth of the pocket and exists in the socket. **C,** Sequence of passing the suture from the mucogingival junction out though the socket (1). The suture is then passed through the graft from an inferior to superior direction (2) and then back through the graft from superior to inferior direction (3), and then through the socket and out at the mucogingival junction (4). **D,** The suture is used to pull the graft in the pocket, and an instrument is used to push the graft in the pocket. **E,** The apically positioned suture is used to prevent the graft from migrating coronally. **F,** Graft is secured coronally using horizontal mattress sutures, and a custom healing abutment is placed. **G,** A 4-year follow-up showing excellent buccolingual soft tissue thickness that will prevent show through of implant component and simulate root convexity.

STEP 2A: Single Incision (Deep Palatal) Harvest

Gingival grafts are commonly harvested from the palate from an area between the palatal root of the first molar and the canine tooth. The tissue tends to be thickest in this region. During the harvesting procedure, careful attention should be given not to injure the greater palatine artery. According to Reiser's study[21], the greater palatine artery enters the palate in the greater palatine foramen area. It travels across the palate anteriorly in the direction of the incisive foramen. The greater palatine foramen is most commonly located at the junction of the horizontal and vertical shelf of the palatine bone in an area corresponding to the position between the second and third molar teeth. The neurovascular bundle is located 7 to 17 mm from the cementoenamel junction of the teeth, with an average of 12 mm. The distance is shorter in patients with a shallow palatal vault and longer in patients with a higher palatal vault. Injury to the greater palatine artery closer to the foramen can cause extensive bleeding when compared with iatrogenic vasculature damage to the anterior palatal area. Limiting the dissection to 8 mm in height will limit the risk of bleeding in most patients.[22]

The palatal soft tissue is composed of three layers: epithelium, subepithelial connective tissue, and submucosa. In the anterior palatal area, especially in the palatal raphe area, the subepithelial layer is rich in fat. After the graft harvest, the fat layer is removed with scissors prior to suturing. This will decrease subsequent mobility of the graft. Moreover, it will allow the graft to be uniform in size and optimize its adaptation to the host recipient bed. It is advisable to keep the harvested and prepared graft in saline or saline-soaked sponges for temporary storage to maintain vitality. One should always aim to harvest a SCTG with attached periosteum, as this makes handling easier and decreases secondary shrinkage and contraction of the graft.

After local anesthetic infiltration, a split-thickness incision is made 2 to 3 mm away from the cementoenamel junction of the teeth. The incision extends from the mesial aspect of the first molar to the canine (Fig. 32.2A). A split-thickness flap is developed within the first incision with a #15 blade. The direction of dissection is parallel to the palatal tissue (Fig. 32.2B). The flap should be a least 1 mm thick to decrease the chances of sloughing and necrosis that could cause postoperative pain and discomfort. This incision also determines the thickness of the tissue that will be harvested. The dissection is carried on with sharp instruments to the height of approximately 8 mm. This usually corresponds to the cutting portion of the #15 scalpel blade. A properly carried out dissection should create a rectangular pouch. Later, a second horizontal incision is made within the pocket all the way down to bone 1 to 1.5 mm apical to the initial incision (Fig. 32.2C). This variation leave a 1 mm ledge of connective tissue that can be sutured to the epithelial flap with the aim to increase the potential for primary healing and to decrease chances of dehiscence and failure. Once the pouch is created, an anterior incision is made inside the pouch at the most anterior aspect all the way down to bone to the desired depth (Fig. 32.2D). Next, an incision is made in a similar fashion at the posterior aspect (Fig. 32.2E). A Woodson or similar a periosteal elevator is used to elevate the graft in a subperiosteal plane. The partially elevated graft is held with issue pickups, and an incision is made at the most apical aspect (Fig. 32.2F). Using tissue forceps and gentle traction, the graft is harvested. Once the connective tissue graft has been obtained, it should be stored between two saline-soaked gauze squares to prevent dehydration. The donor site flap is sutured closed at this time, with a continuous interlocking running suturing technique.

STEP 2B: Harvesting the SCTG: Tuberosity Harvest

On the distal aspect of the tuberosity, a single, crestal, beveled incision is made from the mucogingival junction to the distal-facial line angle of the most distal tooth. The incision is located on the buccal aspect of the ridge crest, rather than midcrestal, and is connected to the distal surface of the most posterior tooth by a sulcular incision. Use of an Orban knife enhances the access for this sulcular incision. At this point, the palatal flap is raised until the distal-palatal surface of the most distal tooth is exposed. Subsequently, a new #15C blade is used to meticulously dissect the connective tissue from the flap and the underlying periosteum. Tissue forceps and the suction tip should be used delicately during procurement of the graft to minimize trauma to the donor tissue and to make sure the graft is not lost down the suction, respectively (Fig. 32.2G and H). Once the connective tissue graft has been obtained, it should be stored between two saline-soaked gauze squares to prevent dehydration while the recipient bed is prepared. The donor site flap is sutured closed at this time, preferably with 4-0 chromic gut placed with a continuous interlocking running suturing technique.

STEP 3: Passing the Suture Through the Pouch

Appropriate suture material (e.g., 3-0 Vicryl suture on PS2 needle) is passed from an area beyond the mucogingival junction though the pocket out into the socket, leaving enough suture to facilitate tunneling (Fig. 32.1B).

STEP 4: Passing the Suture Through the Graft

The suture is passed through one end of the graft from an inferior to superior direction.

STEP 5: Passing the Suture Through the Graft

The suture is passed through the other end of the graft from a superior to inferior direction.

Continued

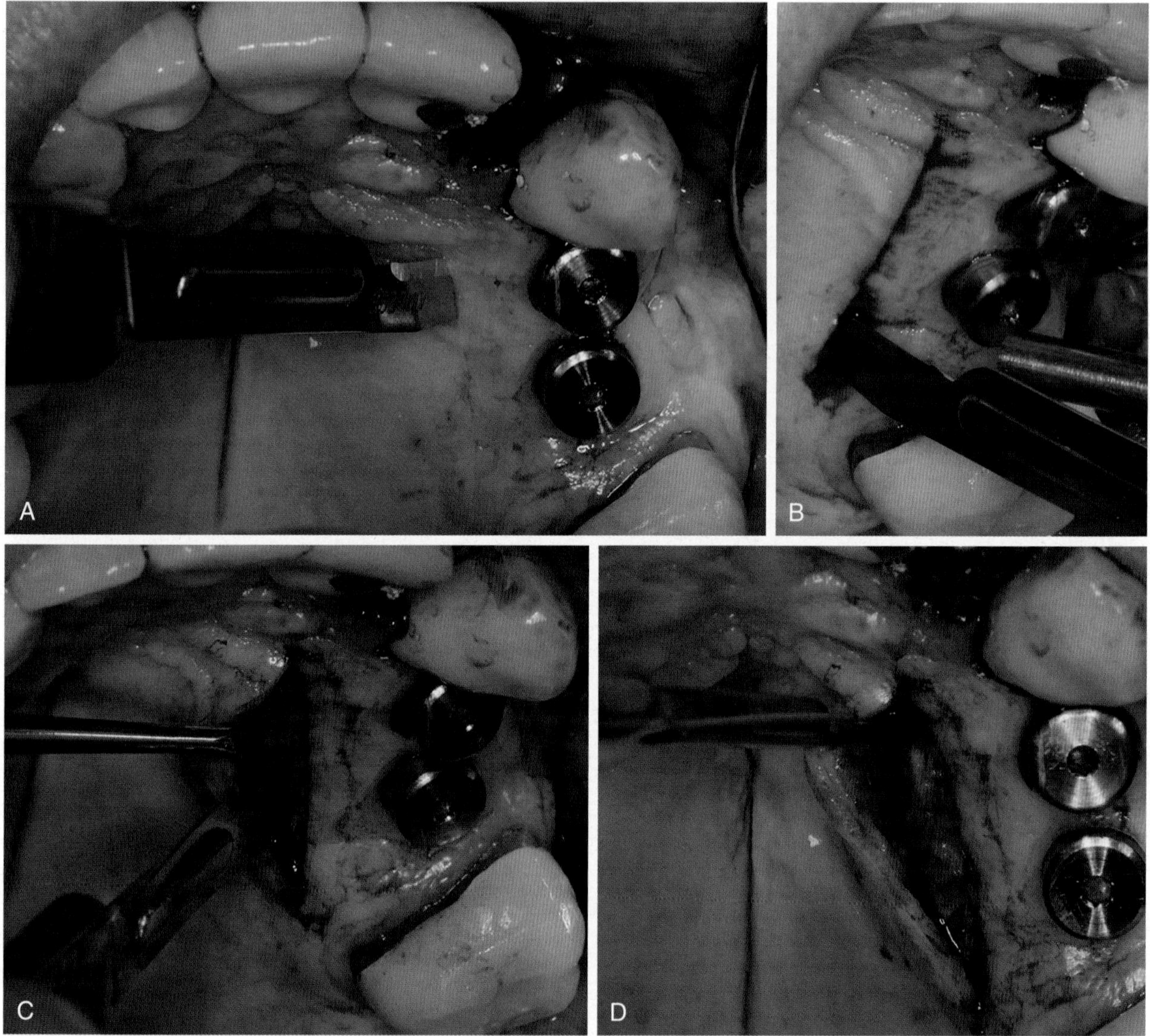

Figure 32.2 **A,** Initial partial-thickness palatal incision from canine to first molar. **B,** Development of a split-thickness flap within the initial incision. **C,** Second horizontal incision within the pocket, placed 1 to 1.5 mm apical to the initial incision. Incision should extend down to bone.

STEP 6: Passing the Suture Through the Pouch
The suture is passed back through the pouch out past the mucogingival junction (Fig. 32.1C).

STEP 7: Pushing the Graft Through the Tunnel
The needle part of the suture is removed. The graft is then tunneled manually by pulling both ends of the suture with a hemostat on one end and pushing the graft with a Woodson on the other end into the pocket simultaneously (Fig. 32.1D).[23]

STEP 8: Securing the Graft Apically
Once the graft is placed in the desired position, the suture used to tunnel the graft is tied to prevent the graft from migrating apically (Fig. 32.1E).

STEP 9: Securing the Graft Coronally
The graft is further adapted to the free gingival margin coronally and secured with a horizontal mattress suture at the coronal aspect. Then pressure is applied to the area for 5 to 10 min (Fig. 32.1F and G).

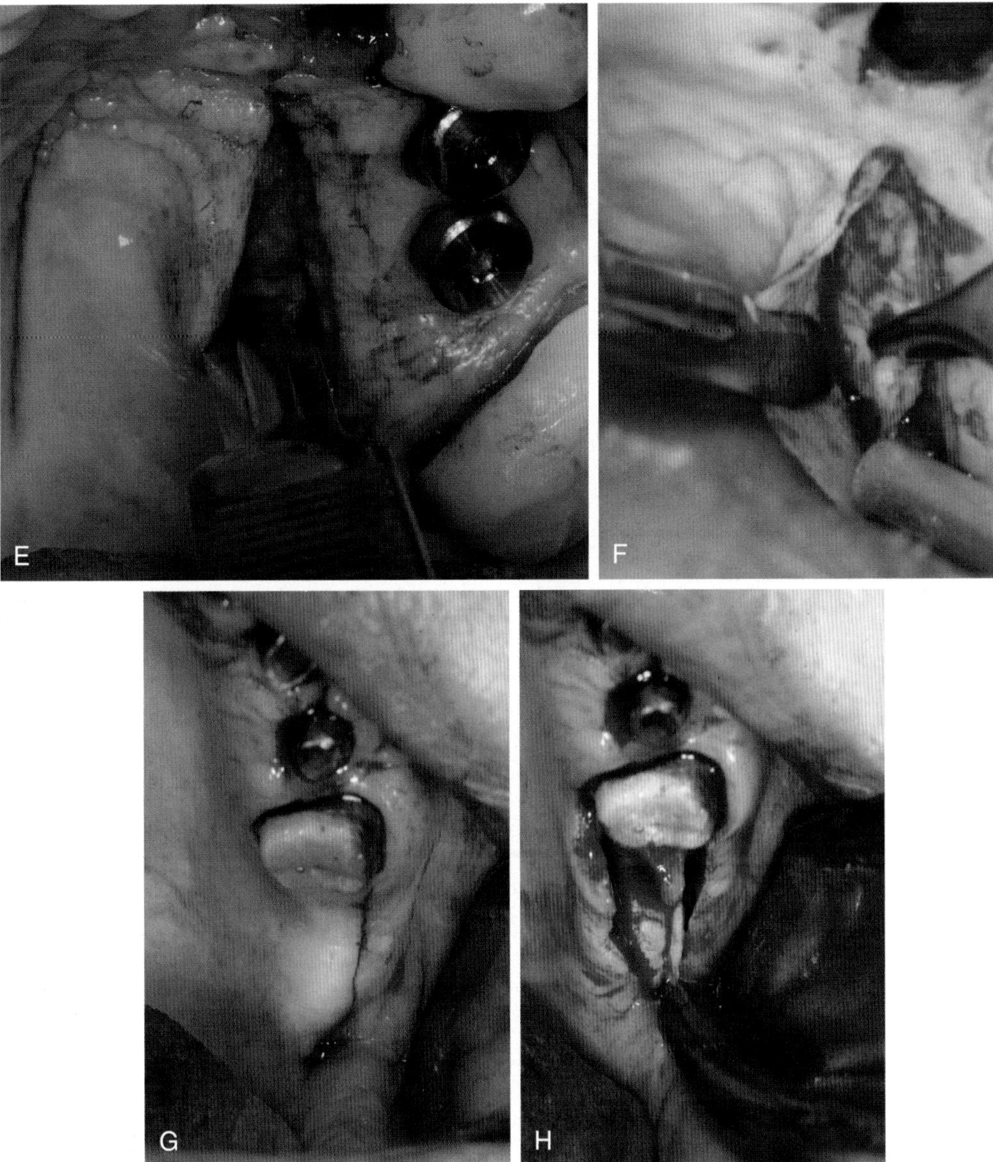

Figure 32.2, cont'd **D,** Incision at the anterior aspect of the pouch, extending down to bone. **E,** Incision made at the posterior aspect of the pouch, extending down to bone. **F,** Incision made at the most apical portion of the graft. **G** and **H,** A subepithelial connective tissue graft (SCTG) is harvested from the tuberosity using a crestal incision at the distal surface of the most posterior tooth.

TECHNIQUE: Vascularized Interpositional Periosteal—Connective Tissue (VIP-CT) Flap

Sclar described this flap for the augmentation of large soft tissue defects.[22] This technique involves rotation of a pedicled finger flap to the anterior maxillary area. The blood supply to the flap is a random-pattern blood supply. One of the main advantages of the vascularized interpositional periosteal—connective tissue (VIP-CT) flap is its ability to be effective during simultaneous hard and soft tissue augmentation. The VIP-CT flap allows for superior soft tissue augmentation in both the vertical and horizontal directions compared with conventional free soft tissue grafts. Practitioners can expect increased graft stability with decreased secondary shrinkage when using these flaps. It is also an ideal graft to use when the tissue bed is compromised (e.g., extensive scarring at the recipient site with decreased blood supply to the area) after administration of local anesthesia in both the recipient and donor site.

STEP 1: Preparation of the Recipient Site

A curvilinear, full-thickness papilla-sparing incision is used and extended to the palatal aspect of the ridge. Then a horizontal full-thickness incision is placed on the palatal ridge to connect the two papilla-sparing incisions. This will allow for complete exposure of the alveolar ridge and increase vertical soft tissue thickness at the end of the procedure (Fig. 32.3A).

Continued

STEP 2: Palatal Full-Thickness Incision

Papilla-sparing incisions are extended palatally. The mesial papilla-sparing incision is extended 3 mm into the palate in a curvilinear fashion. Also, a full-thickness incision from the distal papilla-sparing incision is extended posteriorly to the first molar area. The incision is placed around 3 mm from the free gingival margin (Fig. 32.3B).

STEP 3: Development of Partial-Thickness Palatal Flap

A split-thickness palatal incision is initiated at the first molar area and extended anteriorly in a split-thickness manner to the palatal incision area. As the dissection is carried anteriorly, the flap becomes harder to develop, especially in the palatal rugae area (Fig. 32.3C). Maintaining a good thickness of the flap (at least 1 mm) and starting the dissection from posterior to anterior facilitates flap development.

STEP 4: Completion of Partial-Thickness Flap Development

Partial-thickness dissection is started in the edentulous ridge palatal area and extended posteriorly toward the posterior partial-thickness palatal flap. This will facilitate the development of the flap in the palatal rugae area (Fig. 32.3D). It is recommended that the flap's split-thickness portion be entirely developed at this stage (Fig. 32.3E).

STEP 5: Development of the Posterior Aspect of Finger Flap

A vertical incision is made in the distal aspect of the second premolar. The incision is carried down to the bone and extended as far as apically as possible without damage to the greater palatine artery (Fig. 32.3F).

STEP 6: Development of the Horizontal Aspect of Finger Flap

A second horizontal incision is next made at the most apical aspect of the previous vertical incision. The incision is made parallel to the previous horizontal incision extending to the mesial of the first premolar curving toward the midpalatal area. The incision should not extend past the mesial aspect of the first premolar in order not to interrupt the blood supply to the flap (Fig. 32.3G).

STEP 7: Reflection of the Flap in a Subperiosteal Fashion

A Woodson or similar elevator is used to reflect in a subperiosteal plane, starting at the most distal aspect in the second premolar area and extending anteriorly to the midpalatal area (Fig. 32.3H and I). The more anterior the desired final resting position of the VIP-CT flap, the longer the graft's arc of rotation and more anterior and medial dissection is required. For severe cases, a reverse cutback may be needed.

STEP 8: Rotating and Securing the Graft

After releasing the pedicled finger flap, it is secured to the recipient site with the use of 4-0 chromic gut sutures (Fig. 32.3J). It is usually beneficial to keep the periosteal aspect of the graft facing the bone as this takes advantage of the osteoblastic potential of the flap. On occasion, when the increased height of soft tissue thickness is needed, the flap can be rotated with the periosteum facing away from the bone. This will allow for the increased augmentation of soft tissue height. After securing the flap, collagen or hemostatic dressing is placed in the area where the graft was harvested, and the area is closed with overlying resorbable sutures.

STEP 9: Closure Over the Pedicle Graft and Donor Site

After securing the flap, collagen or hemostatic dressing is placed in the area where the graft was harvested, and the area is closed with overlying resorbable sutures.

The buccal flap is then approximated to the palatal flap using standard suturing techniques. On occasion, primary closure might not be achieved, and small areas of the pedicle may remain exposed; usually, these areas will epithelize over the pedicle without loss of any of the graft.

The use of removable partial denture (flipper) is not recommended, given that it may put pressure on the palatal pedicle, thereby compromising its inherent blood supply. Moreover, dentists will frequently encounter considerable difficulty adjusting the denture to fit the space because of the grafted tissue volume on the palate. The author prefers the use of an Essex type of retainer instead of a conventional denture in these cases.

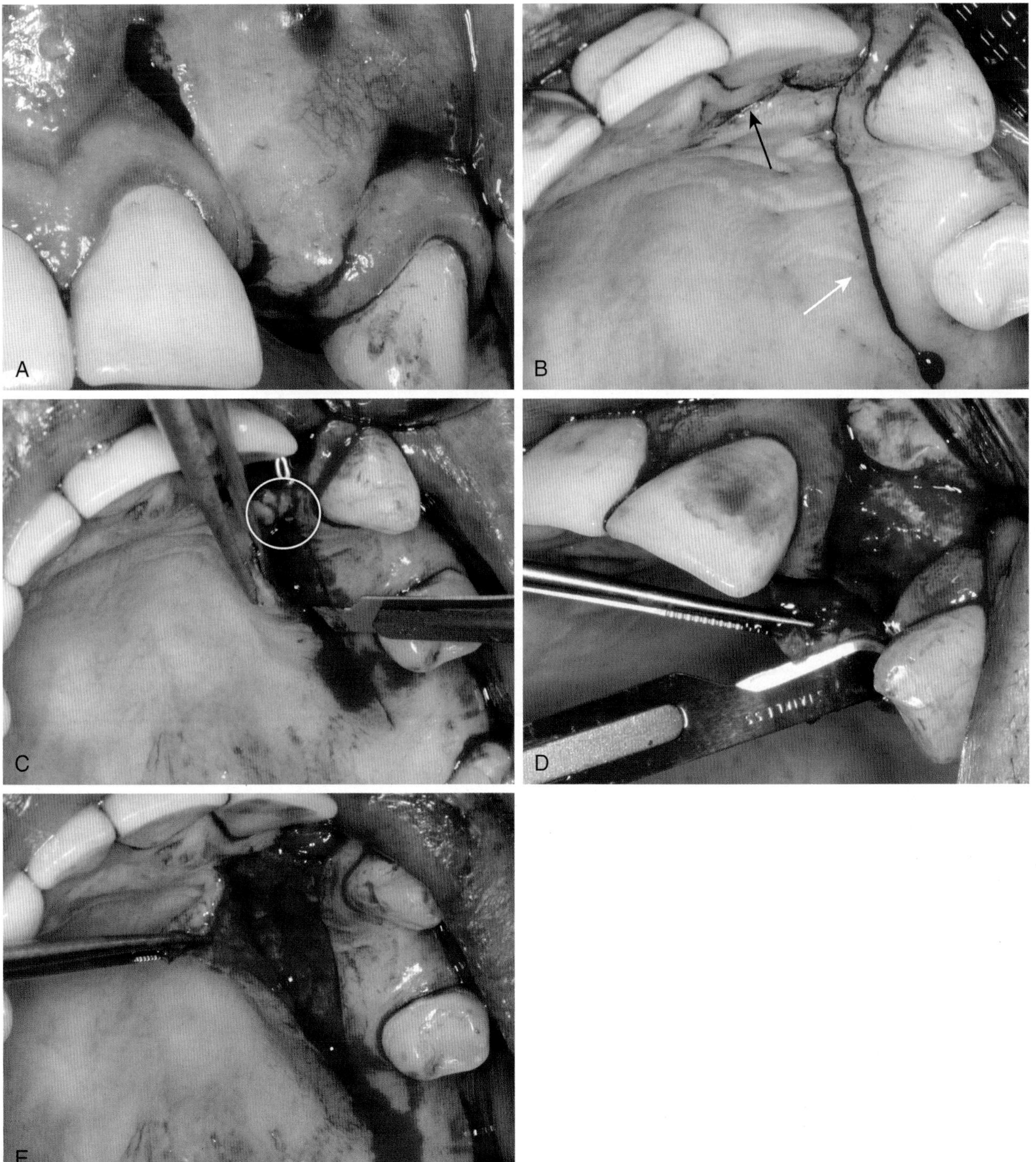

Figure 32.3 **A,** Papilla-sparing incisions on the mesial and distal of the edentulous space, with the crestal incision on the palatal aspect of the ridge. **B,** Papilla-sparing incisions are extended palatally. The mesial papilla-sparing incision is extended 3 mm into the palate in a curvilinear fashion (*black arrow*). Also, a full-thickness incision from the distal papilla-sparing incision is extended posteriorly to the first molar area. The incision is placed approximately 3 mm from the free gingival margin (*white arrow*). **C,** Split-thickness incision is created. The dissection is started posteriorly and extended anteriorly. The anterior area is the last area to be dissected (*white circle*). **D,** Extension of the split-thickness incision anteriorly to the edentulous space. **E,** Reflection of the split-thickness incision palatally.

Continued

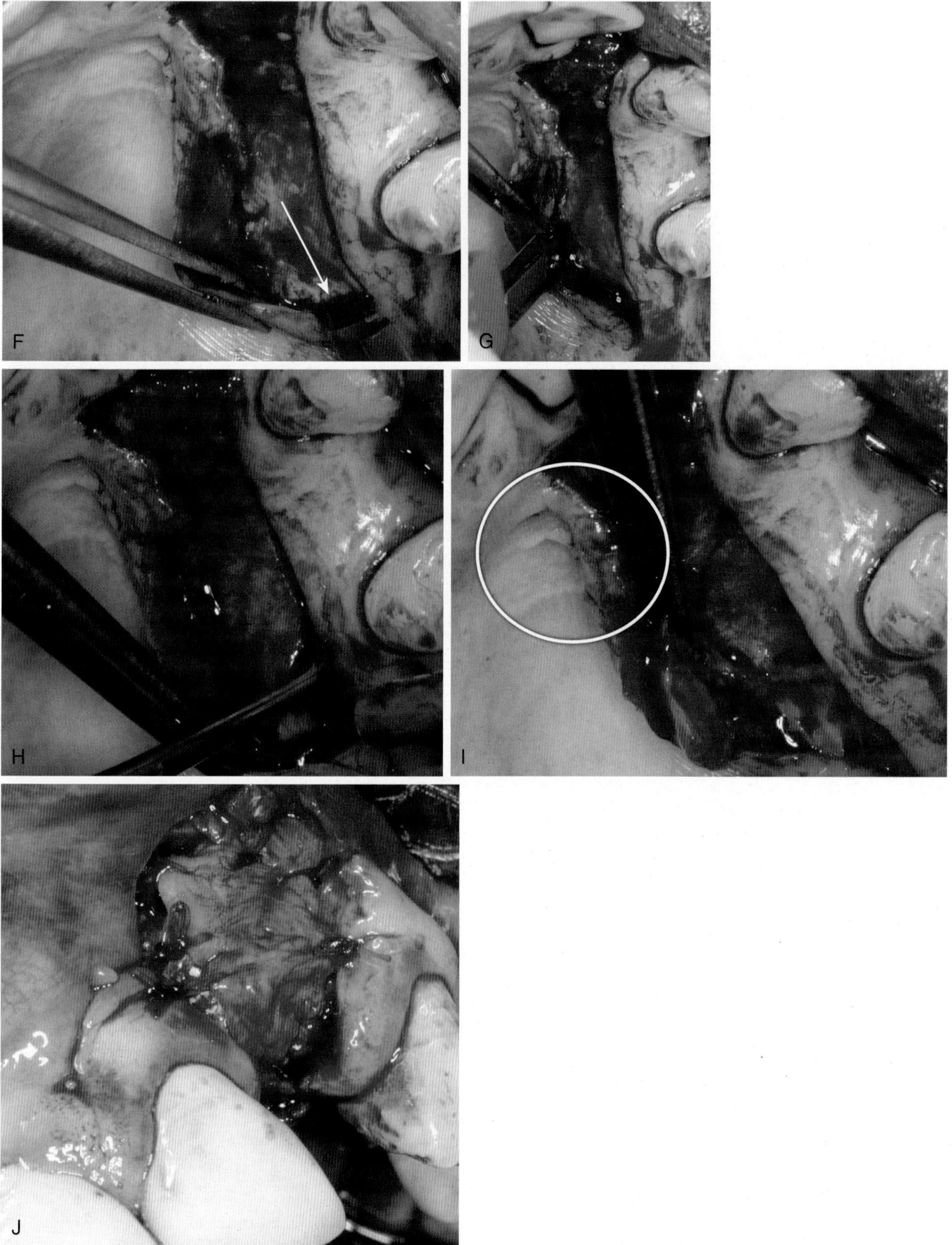

Figure 32.3, cont'd **F,** White arrow pointing to vertical incision made at the distal aspect of the second premolar, carried down to bone. **G,** Incision is curved toward the midpalatal area. And extended to the area of the first premolar. **H,** Elevator is used to elevate the tissue in a subperiosteal plane. **I,** After reflection of the posterior aspect, subperiosteal dissection is carried anteriorly and medially (white circle). This will free and allow rotation of the finger flap anteriorly. **J,** Securing the graft with sutures.

TECHNIQUE: Free Subepithelial Connective Tissue Graft

Another variation of soft tissue grafts around dental implants is the use of free subepithelial connective tissue. This technique is commonly used when an implant is placed in an edentulous ridge and a flap is being reflected. The preparation of the recipient site depends on the timing of the soft tissue graft.

STEP 1: Preparation of the Recipient Site

A split- or full-thickness flap is reflected in the edentulous ridge area. Usually a dental implant is placed.

STEP 2: Harvest of the Subepithelial Connective Tissue Graft

The graft is harvested similar to the technique described earlier using the single incision technique.

STEP 3: Planning Location of Augmentation

The graft is trimmed and adapted inside the buccal flap. The location that needs to be augmented is verified by holding the graft and flap with a pickup simultaneously (Fig. 32.4A and B).

STEP 4: Securing the Graft

While holding the graft against the buccal flap, a resorbable suture such as 4-0 Vicryl is used to secure the graft to the buccal flap using one or multiple horizontal mattress sutures. The flap is sutured, and this closure will automatically secure the graft in place (Fig. 32.4C–E).

An alternative option is to develop a supraperiosteal dissection and secure the graft to the recipient periosteal bed first and then suture the buccal flap over to cover the connective tissue graft (Fig. 32.4F and G).

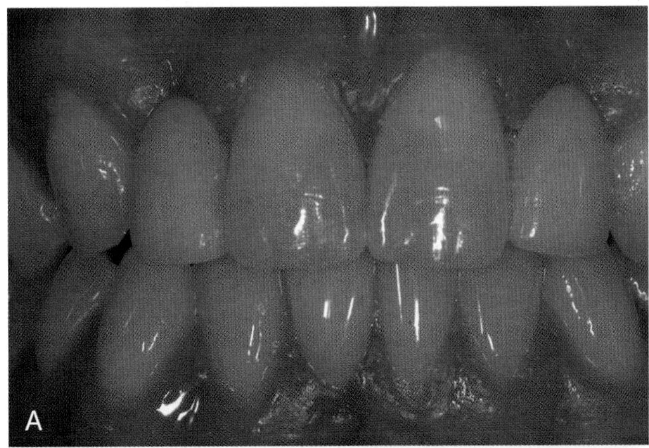

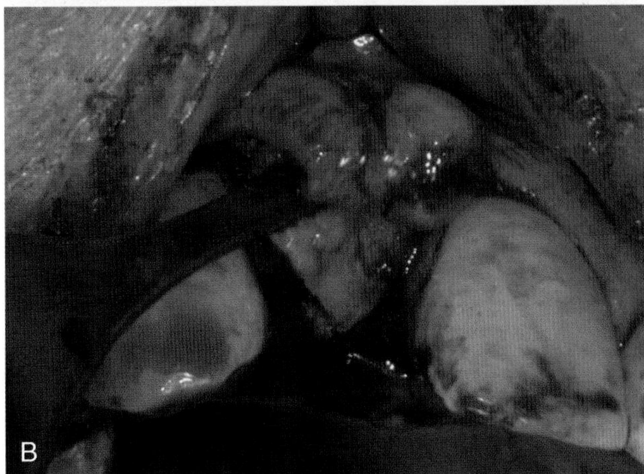

Figure 32.4 **A,** Congenital missing lateral with clefting of the soft tissue. **B,** Location of the augmentation needed is verified by holding the subepithelial connective tissue graft against the buccal flap.

Continued

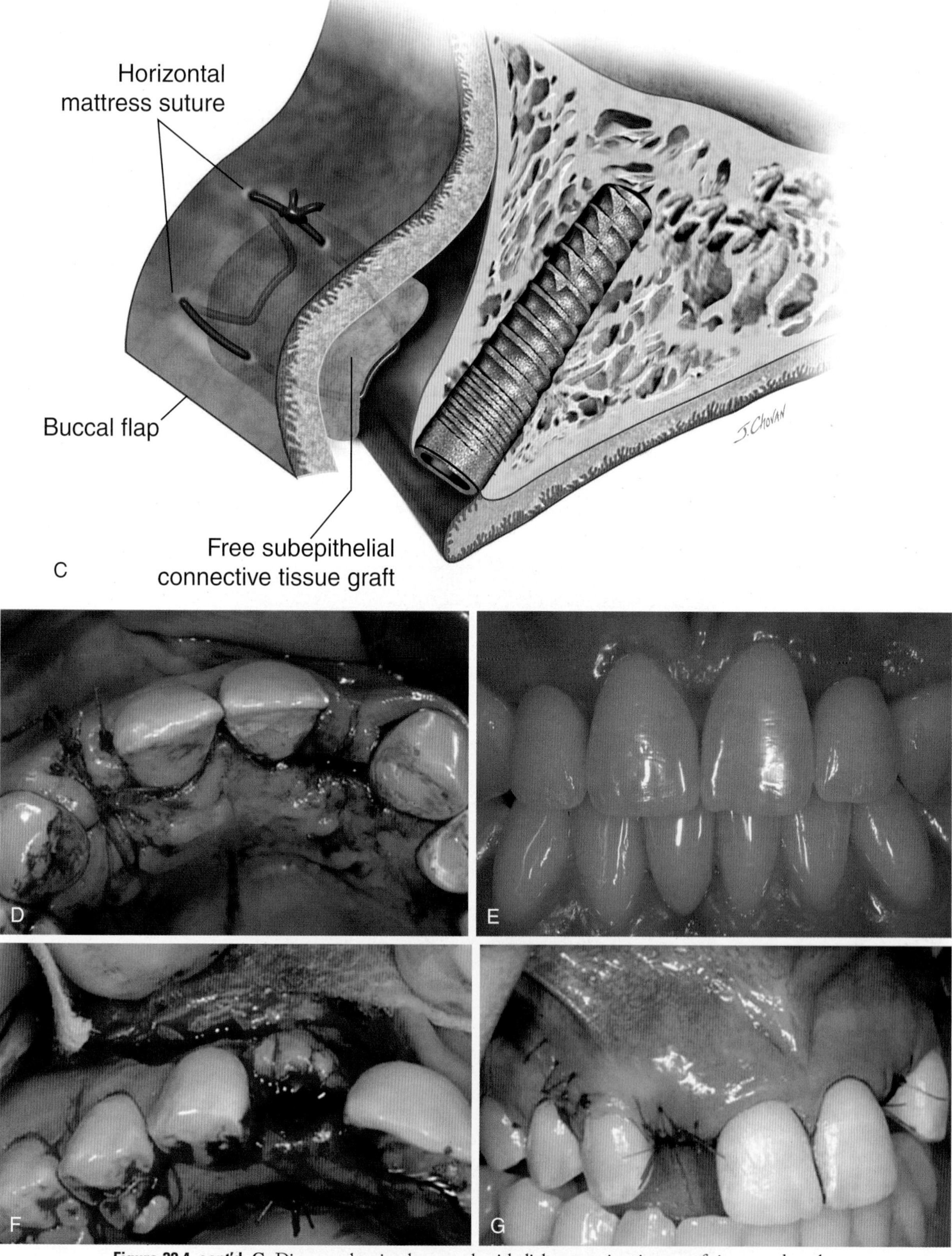

Figure 32.4, cont'd **C,** Diagram showing how a subepithelial connective tissue graft is secured to the buccal flap using a horizontal mattress suture. **D,** Area 7 grafted and flap closed compared with area 10, which has not been grafted. Note how the soft tissue defect has been corrected buccolingually. **E,** Final restoration. **F,** Subepithelial connective tissue graft secured to existing periosteal bed. The trimmed triangular conical piece of SCTG is sutured at the coronal margin and apical base to simulate the profile of a root prominence. **G,** The graft is secured in place using the buccal flap to cover the grafted tissue.

Avoidance and Management of Intraoperative Complications

Complications involving bleeding may occur during the surgery or in the acute postoperative period. Firm pressure should be applied first. If the pressure application does not slow the bleeding, cautery may be used if the bleeding source can be identified. If the bleeding source cannot be identified, over suture the greater palatine artery area to apply further pressure. Local anesthesia with epinephrine may also be injected to help slow the bleeding and find the source.

Postoperative Considerations

Dehiscence is a common complication of soft tissue grafts and should be managed conservatively. The exposed area will granulate in and heal by secondary intention. Patients should be instructed to keep the area clean. Complete or even partial loss of the soft tissue graft is an uncommon complication. If it occurs any necrotic tissue should be carefully removed. Patients should be closely followed, and good oral hygiene maintained.

References

1. Olsson M, Lindhe J, Marinello CP. On the relationship between crown form and clinical features of the gingiva in adolescents. *J Clin Periodontol.* 1993;20(8):570–577.
2. Olsson M, Lindhe J. Periodontal characteristics in individuals with varying form of the upper central incisors. *J Clin Periodontol.* 1991;18(1):78–82.
3. Shah R, Sowmya NK, Thomas R, Mehta DS. Periodontal biotype: basics and clinical considerations. *J Interdiscip Dent.* 2016;6:44–49.
4. Edel A. Clinical evaluation of free connective tissue grafts used to increase the width of keratinised gingiva. *J Clin Periodontol.* 1974;1(4):185–196.
5. Langer B, Calagna L. The subepithelial connective tissue graft. *J Prosthet Dent.* 1980;44(4):363–367.
6. Silverstein LH, Kurtzman D, Garnick JJ, Trager PS, Waters PK. Connective tissue grafting for improved implant esthetics: clinical technique. *Implant Dent.* 1994;3(4):231–234.
7. Garber DA, Belser UC. Restoration-driven implant placement with restoration-generated site development. *Compend Contin Educ Dent.* 1995;16(8):798–802. 796 ,804.
8. Pietrokovski J, Massler M. Alveolar ridge resorption following tooth extraction. *J Prosthet Dent.* 1967;17(1):21–27.
9. Farmer M, Darby I. Ridge dimensional changes following single-tooth extraction in the aesthetic zone. *Clin Oral Implants Res.* 2013. (Epub ahead of print).
10. Schropp L, Wenzel A, Kostopoulos L, Karring T. Bone healing and soft tissue contour changes following single-tooth extraction: a clinical and radiographic 12-month prospective study. *Int J Periodontics Restorative Dent.* 2003;23(4):313–323.
11. Geurs NC, Vassilopoulos PJ, Reddy MS. Soft tissue considerations in implant site development. *Oral Maxillofac Surg Clin North Am.* 2010;22(3):387–405. (vi-vii).
12. Fu JH, Lee A, Wang HL. Influence of tissue biotype on implant esthetics. *Int J Oral Maxillofac Implants.* 2011;26(3):499–508.
13. Kan JY, Rungcharassaeng K, Lozada JL, Zimmerman G. Facial gingival tissue stability following immediate placement and provisionalization of maxillary anterior single implants: a 2- to 8-year follow-up. *Int J Oral Maxillofac Implants.* 2011;26(1):179–187.
14. Hsu YT, Shieh CH, Wang HL. Using soft tissue graft to prevent mid-facial mucosal recession following immediate implant placement. *J Int Acad Periodontol.* 2012;14(3):76–82.
15. Cosyn J, Hooghe N, De Bruyn H. A systematic review on the frequency of advanced recession following single immediate implant treatment. *J Clin Periodontol.* 2012;39(6):582–589.
16. Nisapakultorn K, Suphanantachat S, Silkosessak O, Rattanamongkolgul S. Factors affecting soft tissue level around anterior maxillary single-tooth implants. *Clin Oral Implants Res.* 2010;21(6):662–670.
17. Lai HC, Zhang ZY, Wang F, Zhuang LF, Liu X, Pu YP. Evaluation of soft-tissue alteration around implant-supported single-tooth restoration in the anterior maxilla: the pink esthetic score. *Clin Oral Implants Res.* 2008;19(6):560–564.
18. Tipton DA, Dabbous MK. Effects of nicotine on proliferation and extracellular matrix production of human gingival fibroblasts in vitro. *J Periodontol.* 1995;66(12):1056–1064.
19. Cheung WS, Griffin TJ. A comparative study of root coverage with connective tissue and platelet concentrate grafts: 8-month results. *J Periodontol.* 2004;75(12):1678–1687.
20. Saadoun AP. Current trends in gingival recession coverage—part I: the tunnel connective tissue graft. *Pract Proced Aesthet Dent.* 2006;18(7):433–438. quiz 440.
21. Reiser GM, Bruno JF, Mahan PE, Larkin LH. The subepithelial connective tissue graft palatal donor site: anatomic considerations for surgeons. *Int J Periodontics Restorative Dent.* 1996;16(2):130–137.
22. Zuhr O, Hurzler M. *Plastic-Esthetic Periodontal and Implant Surgery a Microsurgical Approach.* Quintessence Publishing; 2012.
23. Sclar A. *Soft Tissue and Esthetic Considerations in Implant Therapy.* Quintessence Publishing; 2003.

CHAPTER 33

Computer Planning for Orthognathic Surgery

Stephanie Joy Drew

Armamentarium

Bite registration material
DICOM data acquisition: cone-beam or medical CT
Facial photographs
Facial soft tissue measurements—mm ruler
Laser level
Documentation of natural head position
Radiographic skin markers
Stone models vs. intraoral scanner to register dentition and occlusion: STL files computer to upload to create the composite model and plan surgery

History of the Procedure

Medical modeling and simulation have improved over the past 20 years by software engineers partnering with health care professionals to enable the transfer of clinical information to computer-based planning programs and then translating this information back to the operating room. The technologic advances have allowed health care professionals to be more precise, to become better teachers, and to improve the care of the general public. This technology is used not only in oral and maxillofacial surgery but also in many other surgical specialties, such as neurosurgery and otolaryngology.

In 2003 Gateno et al.[1,2] published two papers on the use of three-dimensional (3D) surgical planning for jaw surgery, in addition to the techniques for creating a composite 3D virtual skull model. In 2007 these same researchers published work on feasibility studies for using computer-assisted surgical simulation systems in the treatment of dentofacial deformities.[3] In 2013 Hsu et al.[4] published data from three teams in a multicenter study evaluating the accuracy of computer-aided design for corrective jaw surgery and found that the protocols and procedures produced accurate results.

Use of a digital platform for planning and executing skeletal facial movements has quickly become a routine methodology of treatment. However, despite its rapid acceptance, this technology is not a substitute for a thorough clinic exam and diagnosis to provide a sound platform for virtual treatment planning. The analysis of the clinical exam findings along with the incorporation of the surgeon's understanding of jaw function, long-term stability, and facial esthetics will enable the virtual planning session to be efficient and accurate. All of these factors must be included in the treatment planning process, regardless of whether the surgeon uses traditional model surgery planning techniques or a digital model surgery platform.

Indications for the Use of the Procedure

Computer planning and design are used in oral and maxillofacial surgery to plan osteotomies for orthognathic surgery, distraction surgery, tumor debulking, and resection/reconstructive surgery and total joint replacement. Computer planning is also used to create stereolithic models for planning and machine-generated occlusal splints to use in the operating room to guide the surgeon to achieve the digitally planned result. Today, computer planning has evolved to include the fabrication of cutting guides, drill guides, and patient-specific (custom) plating based on the digital plans. In addition, computer planning is used in stereotactic surgery, for navigation during difficult 3D movement, or in reconstructive surgery.[5–23]

Limitations and Contraindications

There are no known contraindications to computer planning. However, financial constraints may be a factor. These financial issues include the purchase of the necessary equipment, including hardware and software, and fees for processing the information and fabrication of the models and splints and custom plates.

Unless a proper quality digital imaging and communications in medicine (DICOM) data set is sent to the modeling company, an accurate model and surgical guides cannot be fabricated. All cone-beam computed tomography (CBCT) machines are not alike, and it is best to ask the virtual planning company which settings to use for the specific machines to get the best scan. A medical grade CT scan can also be used for planning orthognathic surgery.

Clinical records also must be excellent to transfer the data and "mount" the case in the computer in the natural head position (NHP). This mounted head position is the basis for which all cephalometric and movement measurements are made during the planning session. It is the "home base." The engineers use skeletal landmarks, the clinical measurements, and facial photos to help them align the skull into the best X, Y, and Z orientation close to the NHP.

In addition, proper cephalometric analysis and the diagnosis of skeletal, soft tissue, and dental issues need to be performed before a planning session can begin. The 3D nature of these sessions allows the surgeon to better visualize all changes in the frontal view and submentovertex view; however, lateral movements can be determined with cephalometric values as a starting point, including anterior-posterior (A-P), vertical, and adjustment of the occlusal plane based upon both clinical and cephalometric values.

The virtual planning software may provide cephalometric analysis tools; however, it will only work well if the patient's natural (or adjusted) head position is correct. Having a basic understanding of cephalometric norms is essential to planning orthognathic surgery.

TECHNIQUE: The Correct Bite and Head Position—Data Acquisition

STEP 1: Bite Registration

Find the centric relation (CR) bite registration with either a blue mouse or pink baseplate wax. Take care to have only the dentition covered with the material. Have the teeth in CR occlusion and check the posterior region thickness of the material so as not to rotate the bite open on the scan; otherwise, this will distort the condylar position. Also, the bite material should have minimal distortion (Fig. 33.1). Note, practice with the patient until you are confident of first contact of the occlusion. A centric relation-centric occlusion (CO-CR) shift will change the position of the condyle and may lead to inaccuracies in planning and execution of the surgery.

The bite may also be registered with an intraoral scanner. This will create a rendered stereolithographic (STL) model file to be uploaded to create a digital bite.

Continued

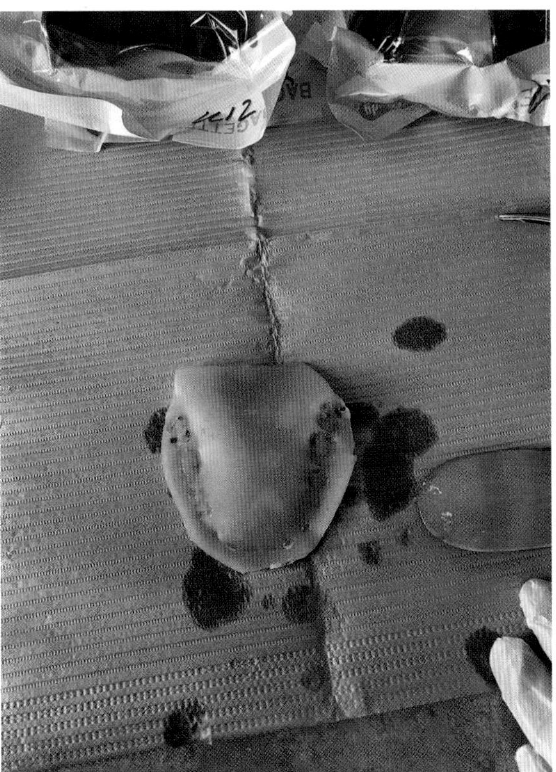

Figure 33.1 Wax bite.

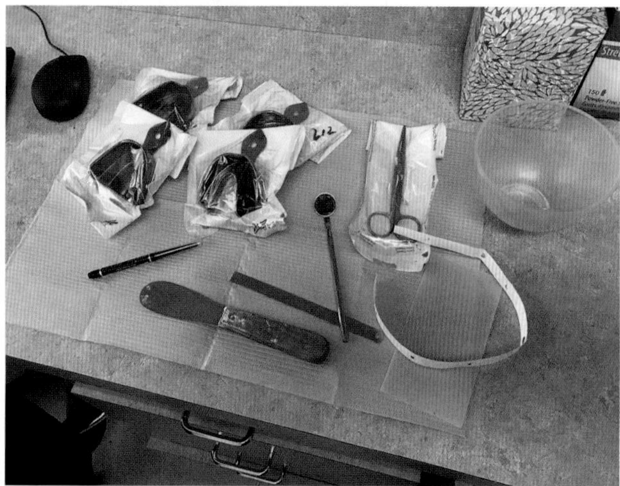

Figure 33.2 Supplies needed for workup.

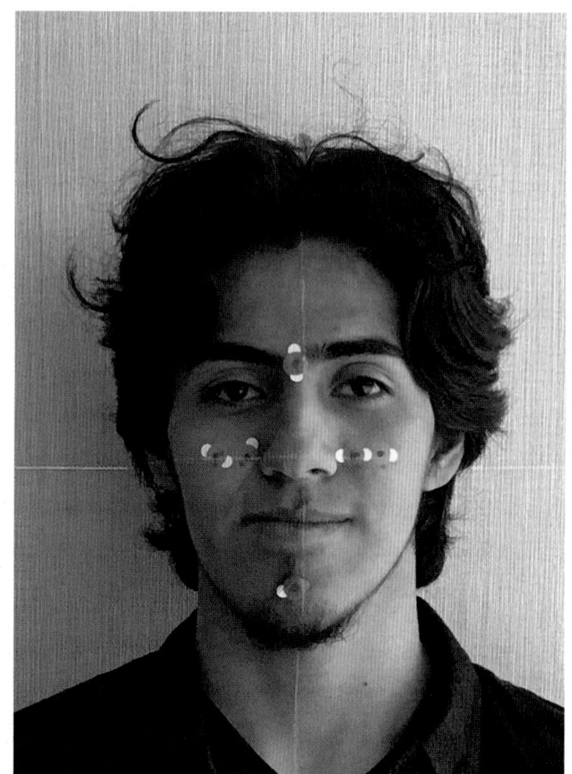

Figure 33.3 Laser lines with radiographic markers in place.

TECHNIQUE: The Correct Bite and Head Position – Data Acquisition—*cont'd*

STEP 2: ESTABLISHING THE PATIENT'S NHP

For the NHP registration, the head position is actually an adjusted NHP. The author uses three items to achieve this: a mirror, laser level, and an eyeliner pen (black for light skin and white for darker skin) (Fig. 33.2). Placement of radiographic marker stickers (dots) on the vertical midline and horizontal plane help the engineers orient the scans.

Register the NHP with a laser level; this will take time in the beginning. Practice by having the patient look into their eyes in the mirror for you to visually register position laterally. (Photograph this with lips in repose to use for reference). Next, have the laser level from the frontal plane shine on the vertical and mark the soft tissue facial midline. (You should have recorded your dental midline of the maxilla. This laser line should be placed on the skeletal midline. If they are coincident, then the laser line will align with the maxillary dental midline.) Once confirmed, place a radiographic sticker on the soft tissue nasion and soft tissue pogonion.

Next mark the horizontal plane. This position should look the same as when you were looking into their eyes laterally. Have them go into that position and then place the radiographic fiducial markers on the face along the horizontal line. Place four stickers across the head position, placing two on either side of the nose marking any facial cant (Fig. 33.3). (Note this is similar to using the Frankfort horizontal plane.) Using a black eyeliner pen for light skin and white liner for darker skin works well when marking the line. Place the fiducial stickers on the line once marked. If you try to place the stickers on while trying to maintain NHP, the patient will keep moving; just mark with the makeup pencil and then place the stickers.

When the markers are in place and the laser lines have been drawn, a photo can be taken. Do not use a flash. It is also helpful to have the patient bite on a tongue blade to photograph canting from the frontal view.

While this NHP marking is not mandatory for virtual planning software, it is quite helpful in the clinical examination of the soft tissues, especially in asymmetry cases.

STEP 3: CT Scanning: Digital Imaging and Communications in Medicine Data

Take a CT scan with the CR bite in the patient's mouth and with the fiducial markers of the skin to accomplish your digital facebow (Fig. 33.4).

Different CT scan machines require different protocol settings to acquire these scans. These protocols should be investigated ahead of time to ensure adequate digital information capture (Fig. 33.5).

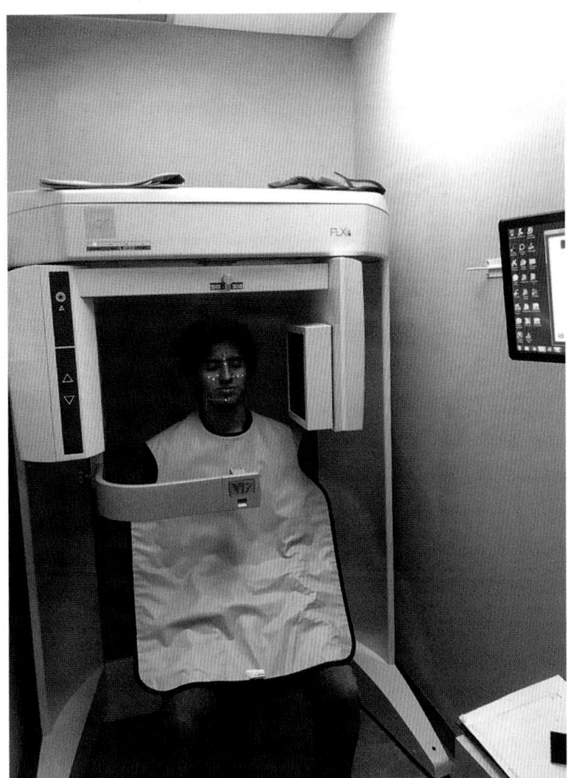

Figure 33.4 Patient in CT scanner aligning with facial markers.

Recommended Protocol for CT Scanners

Acquisition:	Helical
FOV:	20.0 - 25.0 cm
Gantry tilt:	0°
Scan spacing:	0.5 -1.0 mm
Slice thickness:	0.5 -1.0 mm
Algorithm:	Standard (not bone or detail)
Pitch:	1:1

Patient Positioning & Area of Interest

Area of Interest

Image Plane

Figure 3: CT Scanners

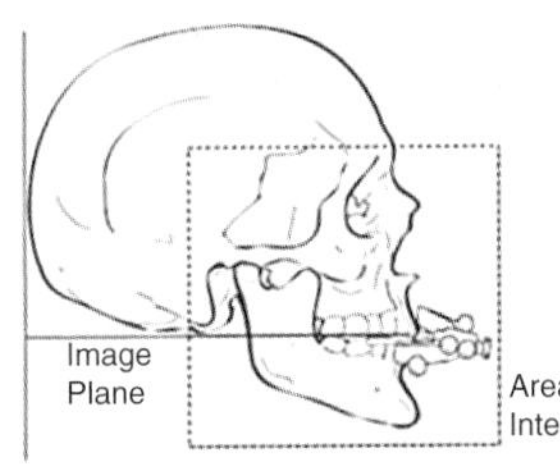

Figure 4: CBCT Scanners

Recommended Protocol for CBCT Scanners

Scanner	Scan Time	Voxel Size	Field of View
Classic i-CAT®	40 sec	0.4 mm	16 cm (d) × 13 cm (h) (Preferred) Extended FOV: 16 cm (d) × 22 cm (h)
Next Generation i-CAT®	26.9 sec	0.4 mm	16 cm (d) × 13 cm (h) (Preferred) Extended FOV: 23 cm (d) × 17cm (h)
Iluma Ultra Cone Beam CT™	40 sec	0.4 mm	[Portrait] 14 cm (w) × 18 cm (h) (Preferred) [Portrait] Extended FOV: 16.4 cm (d) × 18 cm (h)
Other CBCT Scanners	Longest Available	0.3 - 0.5 mm	Largest Available

Shipping Information ***DICOM Internet Transfer***

Figure 33.5 Protocols for different scanners. *CBCT*, Cone-beam computed tomography. (Courtesy Medical Modeling/3D Systems)

TECHNIQUE: The Correct Bite and Head Position – Data Acquisition—*cont'd*

STEP 4: Facial Measurements (Clinical Examination and Recording)
Take facial soft tissue measurements and record them. These are used to make the diagnosis and then the surgical plan, along with cephalometric analysis norms, before the computer model surgery session. The engineers also need to see this data to make "digital mounting" more accurate.

STEP 5: Initial Surgical Plan Data Transmission to Engineers
Record the initial preliminary surgical plan from your cephalometric analysis and send it to the engineers when you upload the DICOM data. This is based on the surgeon's initial clinical examination and cephalometric analysis and diagnosis, the process for which depends on the individual's treatment planning and philosophy. For example, the preliminary plan may state "Le Fort I forward 5 mm, up 2 mm at incisor and 4 mm at first molar. Rotate the midline to right 3 mm. Bilateral sagittal split osteotomy (BSSO) back at incisor 5 mm. No genioplasty." If necessary, this can be changed if necessary as the model surgery is planned, once online.

STEP 6: Impressions and Stone Models
With stone models, take two sets of impressions of the maxilla and mandible. These stone models are sent to the engineers to laser surface scan the teeth and make a composite model. First, put the models in final occlusion and mark them. Then photograph them in the final occlusion in right and left lateral and frontal views. Save these images for reference during the planning call. If the occlusion must be adjusted, mark the spots and photograph them as well. Next, create a bite (blue mouse or baseplate was) in the final occlusion to send along with the models (see Step 8) (Figs. 33.6 and 33.7). The engineers will turn the scanned models into a digital image that will be married to the DICOM creating a composite model.

Intraoral Scanner
Digital impressions or scanning the dentition with an intraoral scanner creates a digital model of the occlusal surfaces and the preoperative bite. Here too the engineers must create a digital composite model by marrying the digital STL file to the DICOM of the skull. The files are aligned to best fit just like the stone models.

Next, the final occlusion must be set virtually. Typically, an algorithm is used to create the ideal occlusion and then the images are adjusted to best avoid significant collisions (i.e., where we may need to adjust occlusion).[21] The order in which the virtual occlusion should be set is to simply follow the steps by first aligning the dental midlines of the maxilla and mandible, and then adjust the Overjet to have the mandible incisors be 2 mm behind the maxillary incisors. Next, adjust the overbite so that there is 2 mm of bite depth. The yaw is then rotated about the dental midline to align the arch width. The pitch is next to adjust for posterior collision of the molar and premolar teeth (overlap); again, the midline is the point of rotation. Finally, the roll around the midline is adjusted for even vertical contact. Remember to have a goal of at least a tripod occlusal pattern for stability post operatively. Notably, segmental surgery can also be created with virtual models.

Remember the occlusion is set before the skeleton is moved.

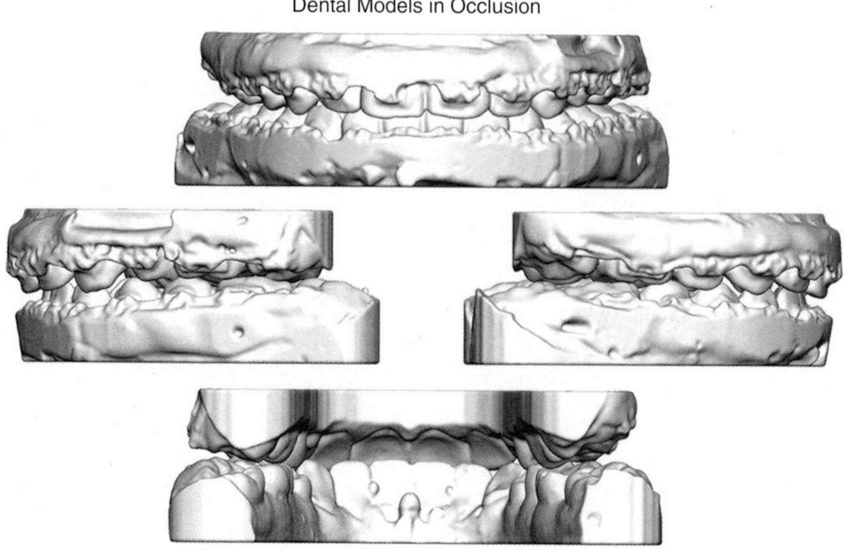

Figure 33.6 Virtual models set in final occlusion.

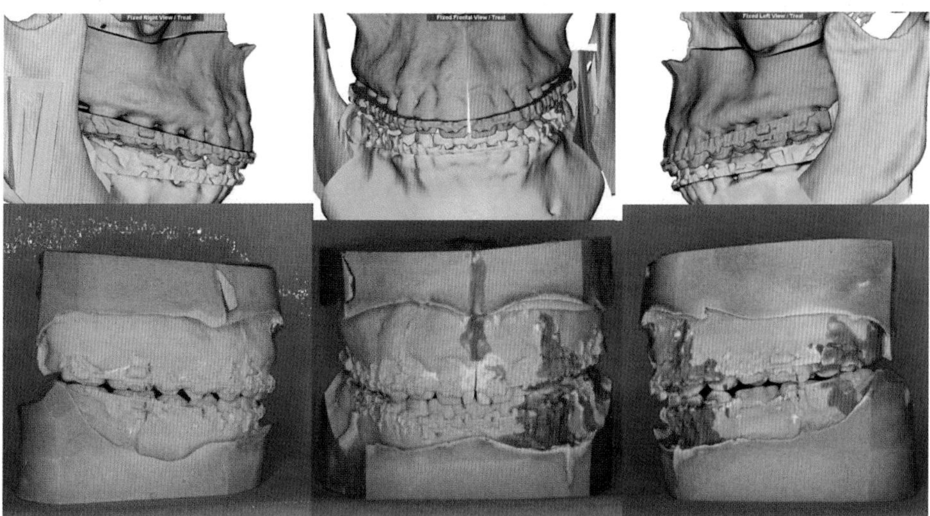

Figure 33.7 Image of cases compared with virtual models in occlusion.

TECHNIQUE: The Correct Bite and Head Position – Data Acquisition—*cont'd*

STEP 7: Special Consideration for Stone Models and the Segmental Maxilla

NECESSARY LABORATORY WORK FOR SEGMENTAL CASES ONLY WITH STONE MODELS

If segmental surgery of the maxilla is to be done, some laboratory work is required to establish the final occlusion. Therefore, both a cut and an uncut maxilla (or mandible) must be sent. For the cut maxilla (or mandible), the final occlusion should be marked and photographed. This allows the engineers to create the width changes and torqueing of the segments accurately.

STEP 8: Establishing the Final Occlusion With Stone Models

Set the final occlusion with stone models and photograph the bite. If possible, adjust the occlusion on the models before sending them. When mailing the models, use a stiff registration material to establish the desired final bite so that the software engineers can see the desired final result.

STEP 9: Information and Materials to Be Sent to the Modeling Company

Send the DICOM data of the patient scan by computer, including photographs of the patient, NHP photos, and a frontal photo with a bite stick if there is a cant and initial plan. Send the models with the preoperative bite and registered final bite by mail. Please note that you can use CBCT to scan your models as well and send the scans as a digital DICOM file to create the composite models. This technique saves time and obviates the need for expensive mailing costs. Ask the engineers how to set your scanner to get the best DICOM files for these models (see Step 11).

STEP 10: Make a Diagnosis

CEPHALOMETRIC ANALYSIS AND PLANNING OF SURGICAL MOVEMENTS

Develop your diagnosis from the cephalometric analysis and soft tissue analysis. The initial treatment planning of the surgical movements will be recorded here. Make an appointment for the virtual model surgery online meeting. Please note that if you want to use a patient-specific plating technique, more lead time ahead of surgery will be necessary. Plan to do this at least 3 weeks prior to surgery, which means the orthodontist has to be done moving teeth well before these records are taken.

STEP 11: The DICOM Data

Several scans must be taken to send all of the data completely digitally to the modeling company. However, only one scan of the patient is done. This eliminates the need for mailing the models and speeds up the process of getting data to the modeling company.

PATIENT AND STONE MODEL DICOM IMAGING

First, take the patient scan with the skin markers and base plate wax bite in the mouth in CR. The CT protocol depends on the type of machine used and the model company's request. Make sure the patient condyles are located in the fossa before you send them out (see Step 3).

Next, the stone models should be scanned to obtain three different files:

1. Scan the models with the CR bite between them (preop occlusion) using a wax bite or blue moose bite. This way, the software engineers can align the teeth with the CT scan to create the composite model in the preoperative bite.

Continued

TECHNIQUE: The Correct Bite and Head Position – Data Acquisition—*cont'd*

2. Scan the models apart to see each model at same time; this lets the engineers see the surfaces of the teeth and the bases of the models. This makes the splints more accurate and easier to create the composite model. Make sure the entire base of each model is visible and not cut off.
3. Scan the models with the bite in final occlusion.

Photograph the final bite on the models and send the photographs to the engineers. Then, upload all data files digitally to the planning engineers.

Now that the engineers have all of your data and have created a digital composite model in NHP and you have your initial plan ready, it is time to do your digital model surgery. Please note that if the maxilla is segmented, a fourth DICOM scan should be sent (the cut maxilla alone).

TECHNIQUE: Digital Model Surgery

STEPS OF THE VIRTUAL PLANNING SESSION

Online meetings should be organized to follow a series of steps. In this way, as the model surgery is done virtually, the participants can track movements and look at vital anatomy as osteotomy segments are repositioned to the final result. The treatment plan from the cephalometric analysis and clinical information should be finalized before this online session. All movements are tracked from a "home," or zero, position (NHP) and measured (Fig. 33.8A–D). In addition, the surgeon can visualize the soft tissues by asking the software engineers to show them as the movement is completed. The author prefers to move the maxilla into position first and then bring the mandible to it and make final adjustments for yaw and pitch to maximize esthetics and for the ease and accuracy of surgery.

CAUTION: Always recheck the position of the condyles on the scans before you begin your session to reconfirm that they are correctly positioned in the fossa (Fig. 33.9).

STEP 1: Osteotomy Lines

For the adjustment of osteotomy lines, the engineers will have prepared the segments for the osteotomy types the surgeon sent as the preliminary plan (Fig. 33.10A–D). These can be adjusted before you begin or after you move into position.

STEP 2: Width Movements

If segmental surgery is to be done, adjust the width and check the movements. Check the torque of the segments to see the geometry of the movements superiorly. Often width changes are not straight and create tipping or torqueing of the osteotomy.

STEP 3: Checking Photographs of Model Final Bite Against the Virtual Bite

Before moving on, check the final occlusion on the virtual model against the photographs of the stone models or the actual models if scanned (modified workup 2). If stone models are not being used, check your intraoral preoperative scan and planned occlusion.

It is important to note that with intraoral scanning you will need to establish a final virtual bite at this time.

Now it is time to move the segments, starting by moving the maxilla into position.

STEP 4: Cant Adjustment

Correct the occlusal cant (i.e., the roll movement). Level according to the surgical plan (Fig. 33.11). The goal is to have the maxillary canines as close to level as possible.

STEP 5: Midline Adjustment

Correct the maxillary midline (Fig. 33.12).

STEP 6: Anterior-Posterior Adjustment

Move the maxilla to the determined A-P position (Fig. 33.13). This should have been determined by your cephalometric tracings.

STEP 7: Vertical Movement

Move the maxilla vertically at the incisor. Examine the soft tissue changes and the position of the pogonion (Fig. 33.14). This should have been determined by your clinical exam.

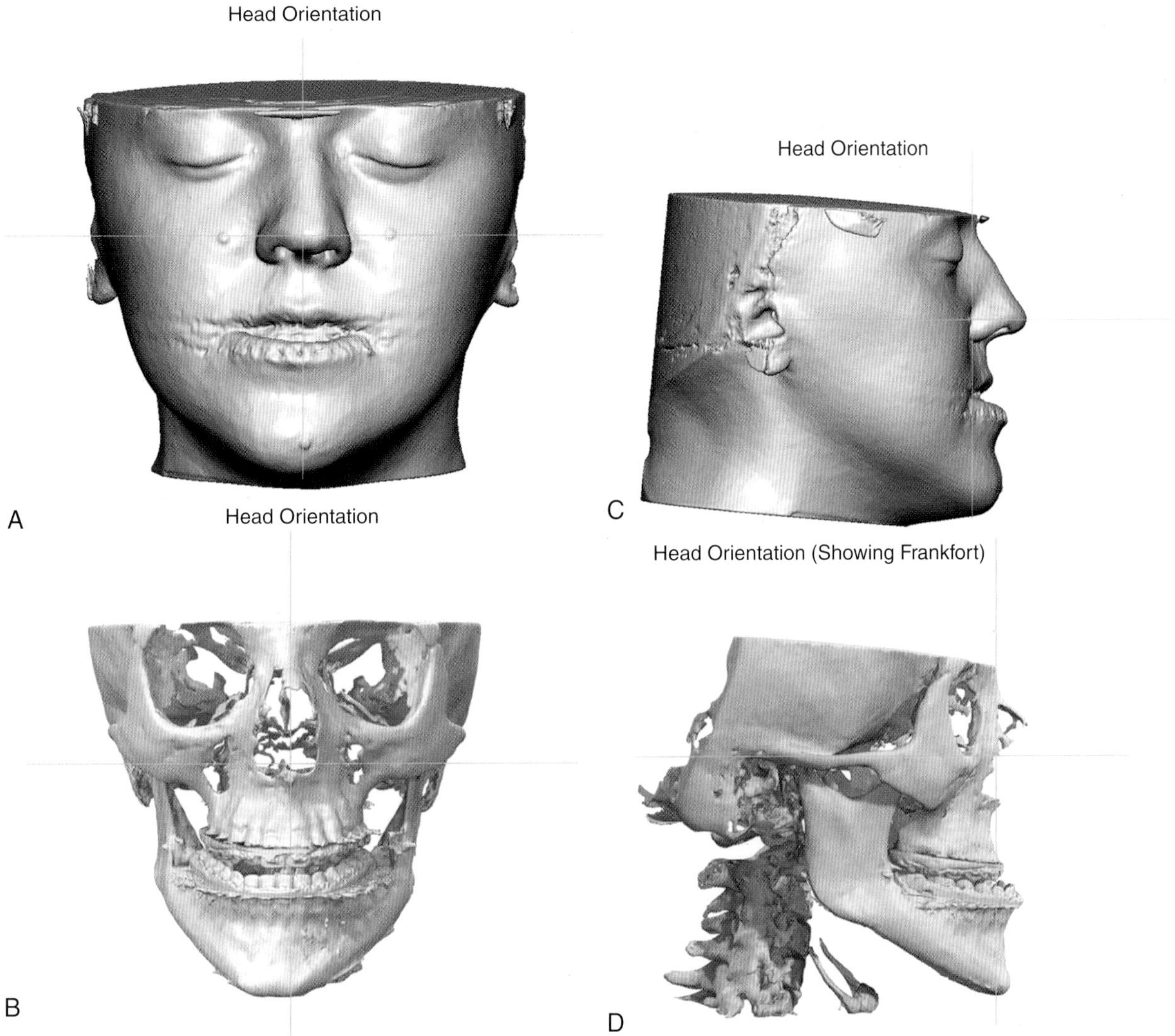

Head Orientation

A

Head Orientation

B

Head Orientation

C

Head Orientation (Showing Frankfort)

D

Figure 33.8 **A,** Head orientation soft tissue with markers frontal. **B,** Head orientation skeleton. **C,** Head orientation lateral soft tissue. **D,** Head orientation to Frankfort HP skeleton lateral.

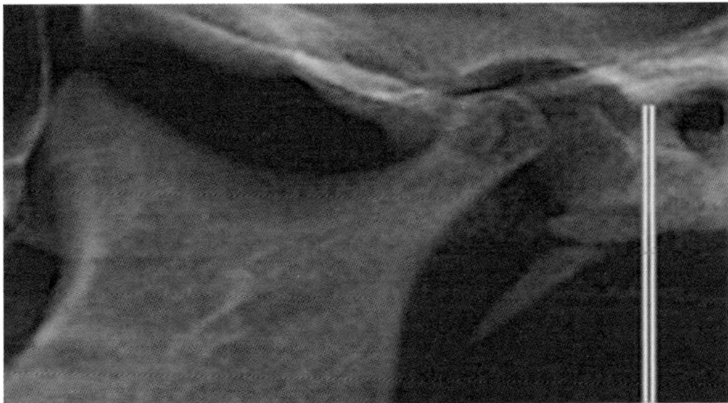

Figure 33.9 Temporomandibular joint out of fossa, as seen on cone-beam computed tomography (CBCT) image.

TECHNIQUE: Digital Model Surgery—*cont'd*

STEP 8: Occlusal Plane: Pitch

Change the pitch (i.e., alter the occlusal plane). Clockwise or counterclockwise rotations are performed now. The midline of the incisor is now the point of rotation for all remaining movement. The posterior maxilla may be impacted to steepen the occlusal plane angle (Fig. 33.15). This will bring back pogonion and soften the lower third of the face. If the maxilla is rotated counterclockwise, the pogonion will become more prominent bringing the chin further forward.

Continued

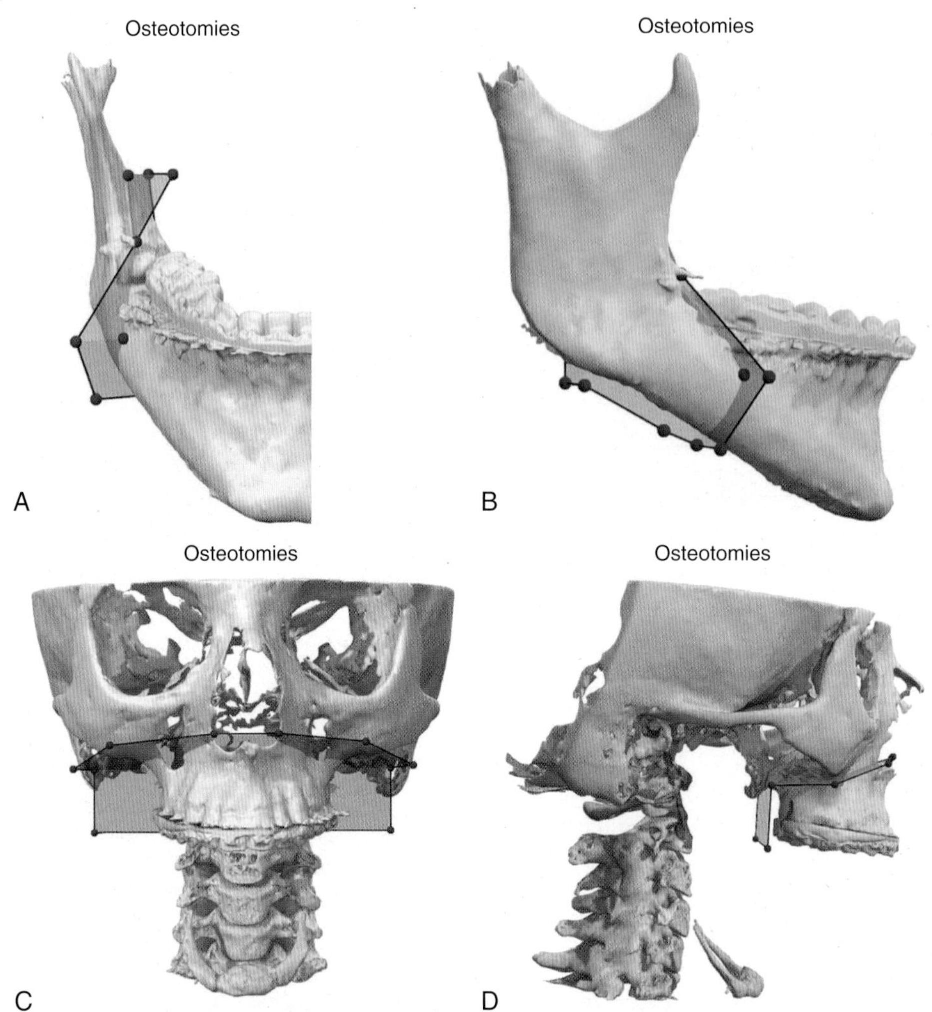

Figure 33.10 **A,** Bilateral sagittal split osteotomy (BSSO) design frontal. **B,** BSSO design lateral. **C,** Define LeFort osteotomy cut. **D,** Define LeFort osteotomy lateral.

TECHNIQUE: Digital Model Surgery—*cont'd*

STEP 9: Yaw

The maxilla is now almost completely set. Put the mandible into final occlusion and examine the yaw movements at the ramus. The maxillary incisor's midline should be in the final position, and all movements should be rotated around this point (this is similar to how you create the virtual dental occlusion). Adjust the mandibular yaw to correct for the torque of the mandibular ramus osteotomy segments. Once this has been done, check the yaw at the maxillary canines. Remember as little as a 2-mm discrepancy can be seen as abnormal by the human eye. This includes the midline, the roll, and the A-P position of the canines in the maxillary occlusal scheme.

All of the midlines should be correct at this point except perhaps the genial region. This depends on the severity of asymmetry (Figs. 33.16A–D and 33.17).

In asymmetry cases, once the maxillary yaw is correct, one can then determine several things about the mandible surgery. Do we need an implant to fill out contour? Do we need to do an osteoplasty to take away bone? Which osteotomy will accommodate the movements of the ramus: bilateral sagittal split osteotomy (BSSO), inverted L, or intraoral vertical ramus osteotomy? What you initially thought can be modified easily in the planning session to compare different osteotomies.

STEP 10: Proximal Segments of the Mandible

Adjust the proximal segments of the mandible (Fig. 33.18). This is done in both the vertical and transverse dimensions. Determine the osteotomy segment contact and condylar position. Collisions will be noted and marked for contouring or shimming as needed. The osteotomy design of the mandible can be changed if necessary (Fig. 33.19).

STEP 11: Genioplasty (if needed)

Plan a genioplasty, if needed. The osteotomy design can be modified if a complicated movement is needed. Cutting jigs and repositioning splints can be fabricated to improve the accuracy of the digital translation to the operating room.

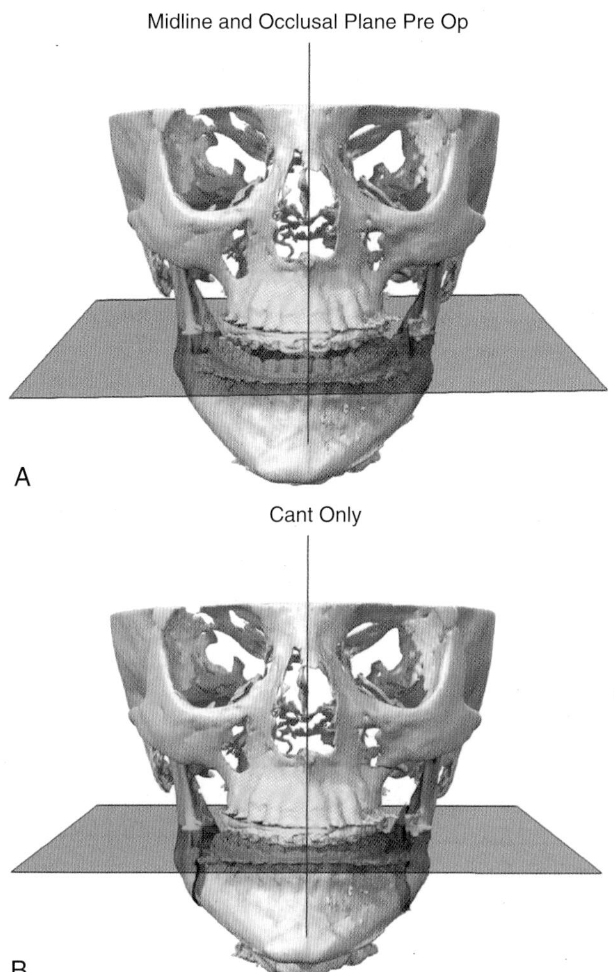

Figure 33.11 **A,** Midline and occlusal plane preoperative. **B,** Cant leveled.

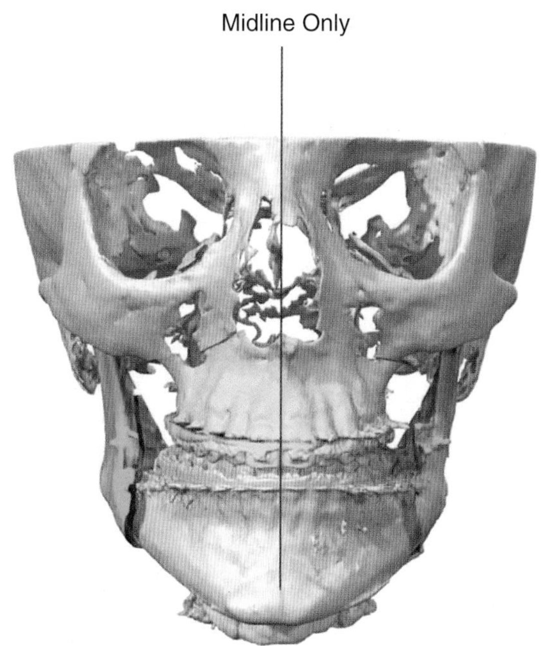

Figure 33.12 Midline corrected only.

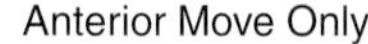

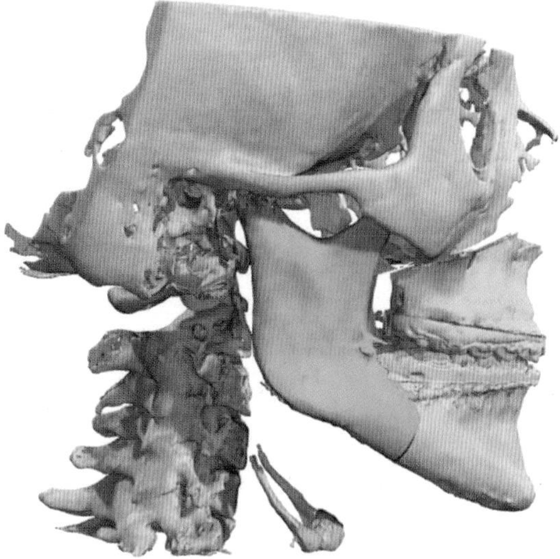

Figure 33.13 Anterior move.

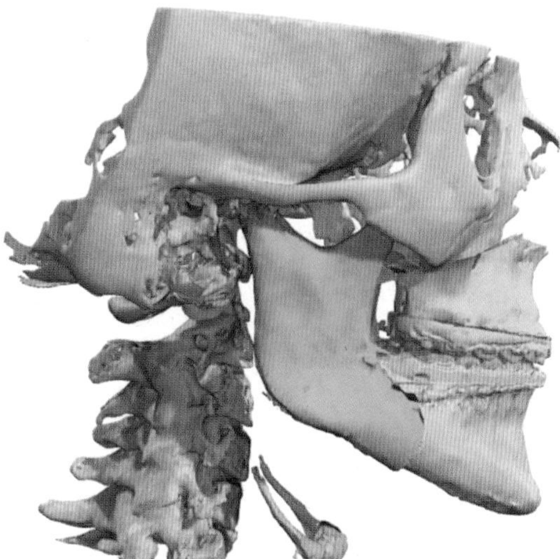

Figure 33.14 Anterior plus vertical move.

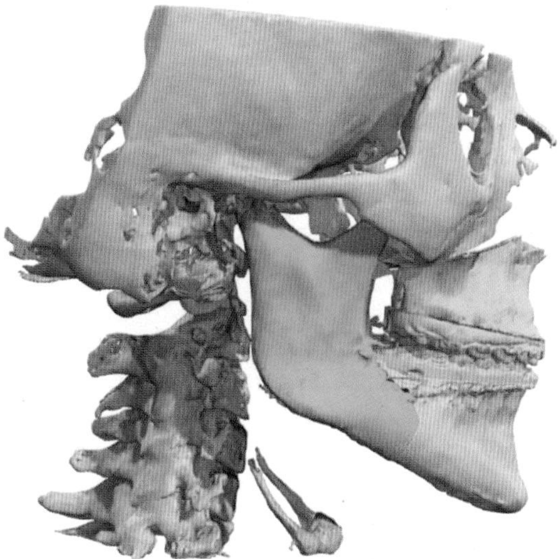

Figure 33.15 Lateral view of pitch change.

TECHNIQUE: Digital Model Surgery—*cont'd*

STEP 12: Plan Review

Review the final measurements, occlusion, and any vital anatomy. If patient-specific plates are to be used, then the plate design should be discussed (Fig. 33.20). For instance, in the maxilla a two-plate (single plate on each side) versus a four-plate (one at the alar region and one on the buttress on each side) design may be considered. The cutting/drill guides can also be discussed, including the potential need of interdental cutting guides or guides as an example to recontour the inferior border (Fig. 33.21). The degree of surgical movements will be summarized by the planning software for reference (Tables 33.1 and 33.2).

Ask for critical measurements you may want to use during surgery, for instance, the location of the lingula or the location of the inferior alveolar nerve at the area of your anterior cut of a BSSO. Ask to see where interferences will be occurring in the maxilla. Look for root height and length if needed for your cuts.

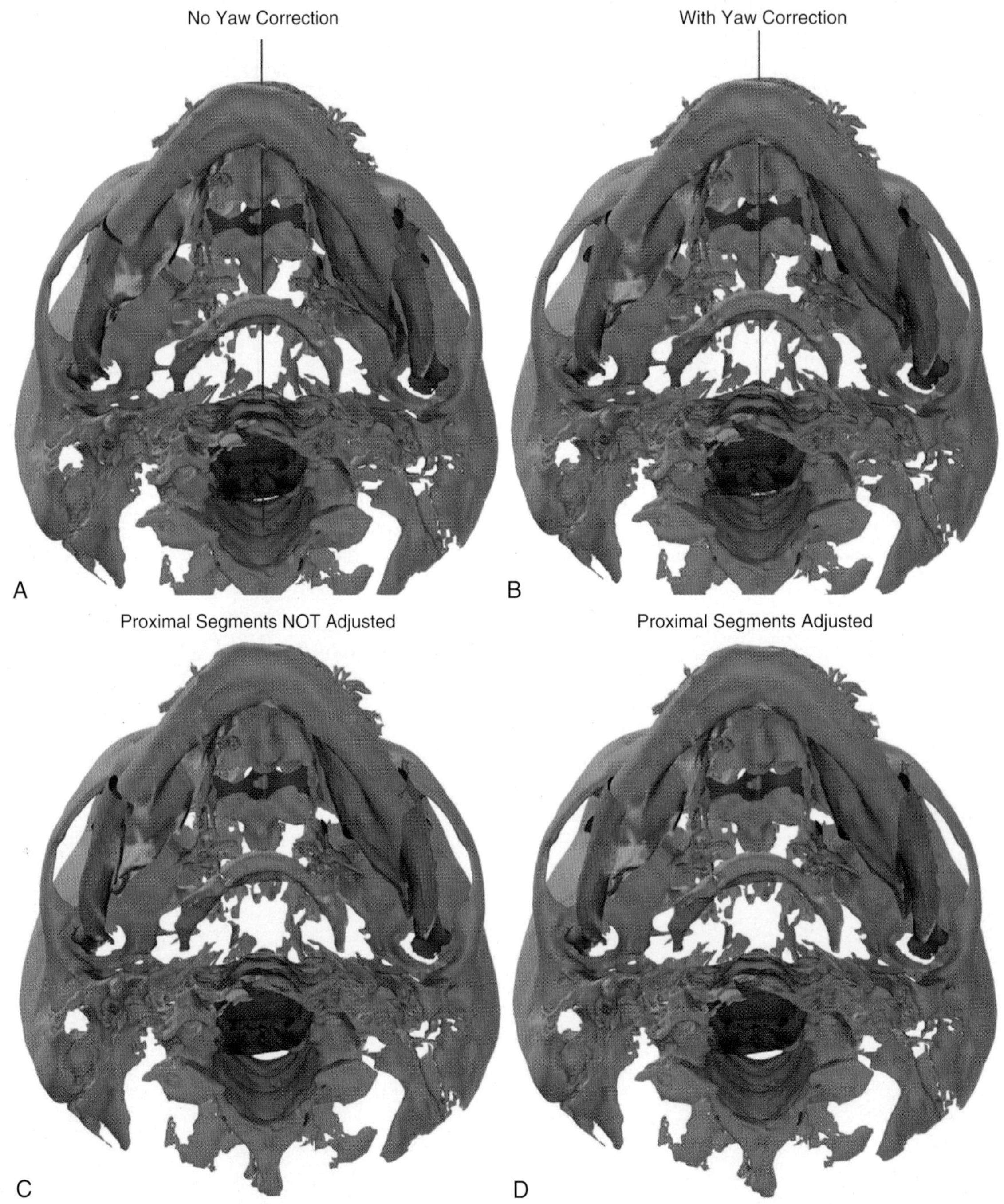

Figure 33.16 **A,** SMV no yaw correction. **B,** SMV with yaw correction. **C,** SMV yaw corrected proximal segments not adjusted. **D,** SMV yaw corrected proximal segments.

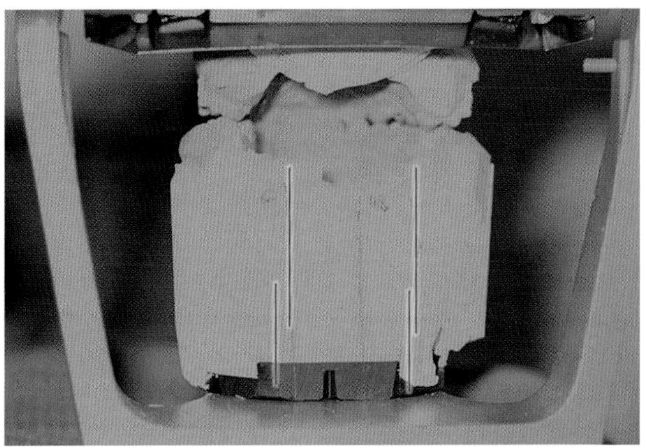

Figure 33.17 Evaluate yaw of mandible first and adjust around midline upper incisors, and then check the maxillary canine.

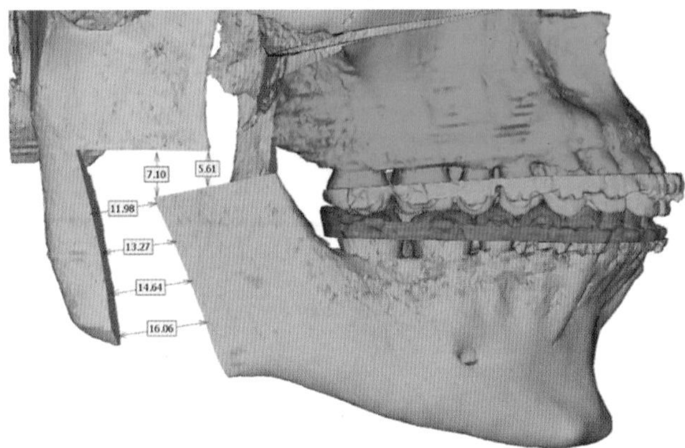

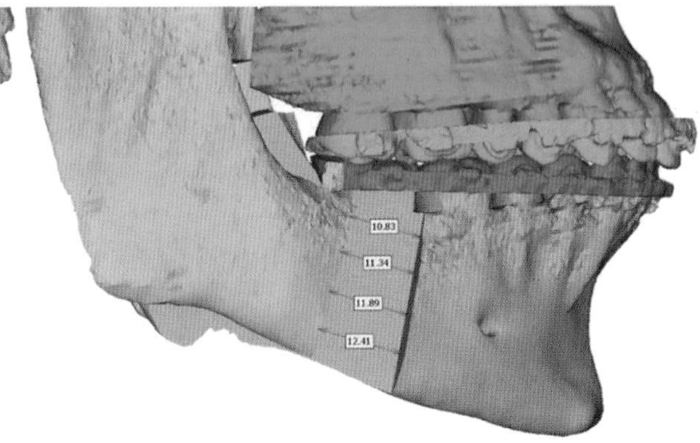

Figure 33.18 Compare different osteotomies if needed.

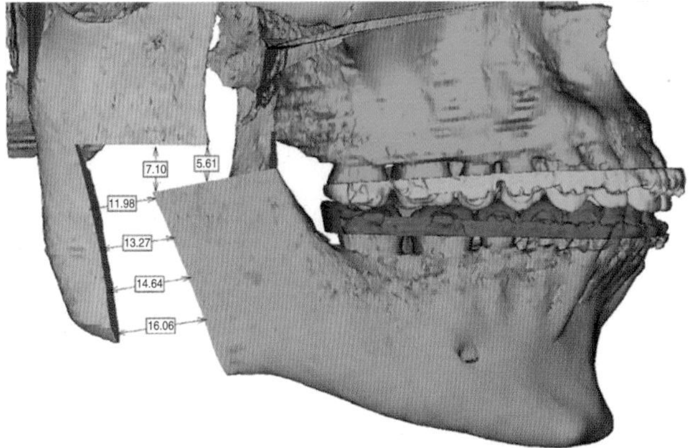

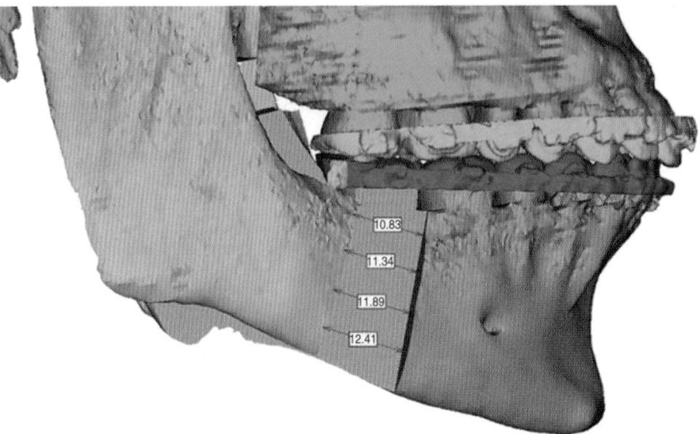

Figure 33.19 Which osteotomy you choose will be base on the desired outcome.

Precise measurements for inferior border osteotomy

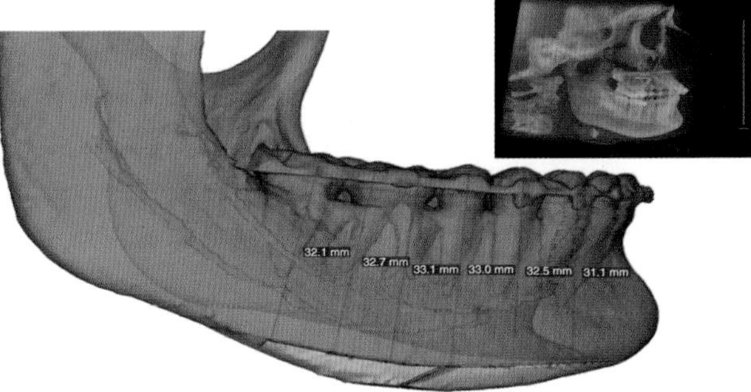

Figure 33.20 Precise measurements can be obtained to compare asymmetries.

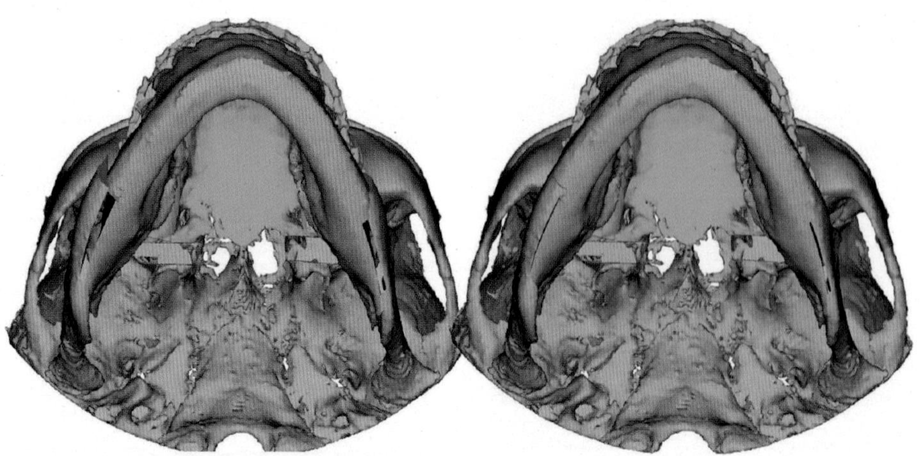

Figure 33.21 Adjust proximal segments of mandibular cuts.

Table 33.1 Example Cephalometric Chart

Point	Landmark	Anterior-Posterior	Right-Left	Down-Up	Final Distance From Midline
ANS	Anterior nasal spine	7.3 mm anterior	1.4 mm left	01. mm down	–
A	A-Point	7.0 mm anterior	1.3 mm left	0.1 mm up	–
UI (m)	Upper incisor midpoint	6.0 mm anterior	1.0 mm left	0.0 mm	0.0 mm
UC (l)	Upper canine cusp left (U3L)	6.0 mm anterior	1.0 mm left	0.2 mm up	16.0 mm left
UC (r)	Upper canine cusp right (U3R)	6.0 mm anterior	1.0 mm left	0.7 mm up	16.6 mm right
Umcusp (l)	Upper molar cusp left (U6LO)	6.2 mm anterior	1.1 mm left	0.7 mm up	22.2 mm left
Umcusp (r)	Upper molar cusp right (U6R)	6.1 mm anterior	1.1 mm left	1.3 mm up	22.8 mm right
LI (m)	Lower incisor midpoint	3.6 mm posterior	3.8 mm left	3.9 mm up	0.2 mm right
Lmcusp (l)	Lower molar cusp left (L6L)	5.3 mm posterior	2.3 mm left	2.8 mm up	21.6 mm left
Lmcusp (r)	Lower molar cusp right (L6R)	2.3 mm posterior	2.3 mm left	2.3 mm up	22.9 mm right
B	B-Point	2.7 mm posterior	3.8 mm left	3.7 mm up	–
Pog.	Pogonion	1.5 mm posterior	4.2 mm left	3.8 mm up	–
Men.	Menton	1.3 mm posterior	3.9 mm left	3.5 mm up	–

Table 33.2 Example Cephalometric Chart

Cephalometric Measurement	Preoperative Value	Postoperative Value	Change
SNA	75.6 deg	83.3 deg	+7.7 deg
SNB	79.5 deg	77.9 deg	-1.6 deg
Occlusal plane cant	1.4 deg CCW	0.5 deg CCW	0.9 deg CW
Occlusal plane pitch	7.4 deg CW	10.1 deg CW	2.7 deg CW
Upper canine cusp left (U3L) vertical distance from orbitale	43.2 mm	43.1 mm	0.1 mm up
Upper canine cusp right (U3R) vertical distance from orbitale	43.7 mm	43.1 mm	0.6 mm up

CCW, counterclockwise; *CW*, clockwise.

Avoidance and Management of Intraoperative Complications

Temporomandibular Joint Position on the CT Scan

Confirm the condylar position on the final scan before discharging the patient during the presurgical workup appointment (see Fig 33.9). Posturing of the mandible during CR bite registration can be a concern and will induce an error in surgical execution if not using patient-specific plating. This happens especially when the maxilla is operated first in two jaw surgery.

Bite

The bite can be challenging if too much registration material is used. This causes the condyles to rotate open and may

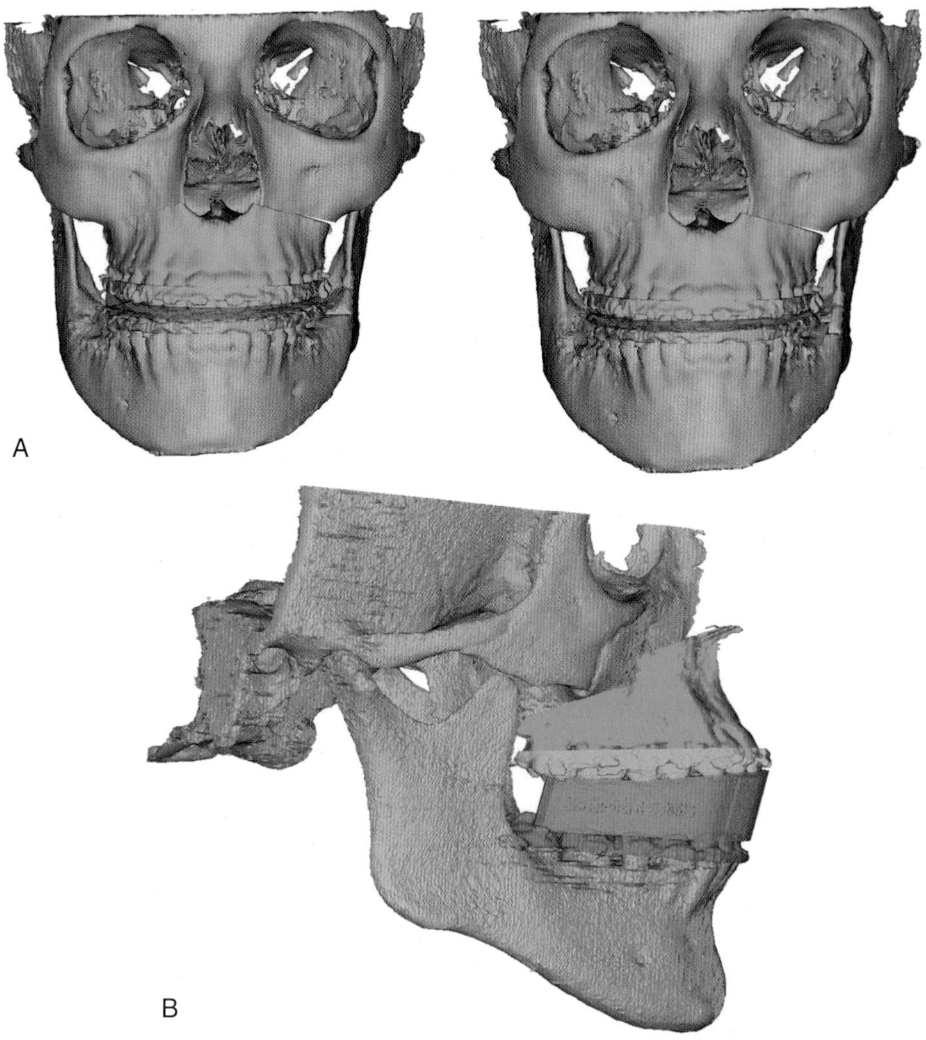

Figure 33.22 A and B, Final and intermediate splint and splint that is too large.

change the position of the TMJ so that the intermediate position of the segment is incorrect intraoperatively. The bite registration should be as thin as possible and lock in the anterior teeth.

CR Registration and Splint Design Pearls

If pink base plate wax is used, it is important to trim it back to allow visualization of the actual occlusion. Confirm that the bite is accurate and does not affect the condylar position.

Bulky splints lead to difficulty seating the dentition during surgery (Fig. 33.22). Struts can be made for additional palatal stability if desired for segmental cases. Confirm the intermediate position of the osteotomies during the planning session online. Thinner splints (if possible) can allow for more accurate seating of the dentition. The larger the space, the thicker the splint, and this may drive your decision as to which jaw to operate on first, such as when the jaw will have a large counterclockwise rotation. Perhaps doing the mandible first will be more advantageous.

Clear Aligner Considerations

While patient-specific plating may take the need for intermediate splints out of the equation, it is difficult to establish intraoperative maxillomandibular fixation (MMF) unless you are using MMF screws. Innovative techniques in splint fabrication have made the establishment of occlusion with clear aligners more accurate.[22]

Patient-Specific Plating Considerations

Using the plating technique with custom plates and guides may make the surgery more accurate; however, there is a learning curve to get the technique down. The plates align perfectly if the osteotomies are cut correctly with the guides and all bone interferences are removed. Having the cutting and drill guide printed with tabs to help with alignment makes it more predictable and accurate. The author finds it helpful to place an intermediate splint in to stabilize the maxilla and not freehand this alignment while securing the custom plates (Fig. 33.23).

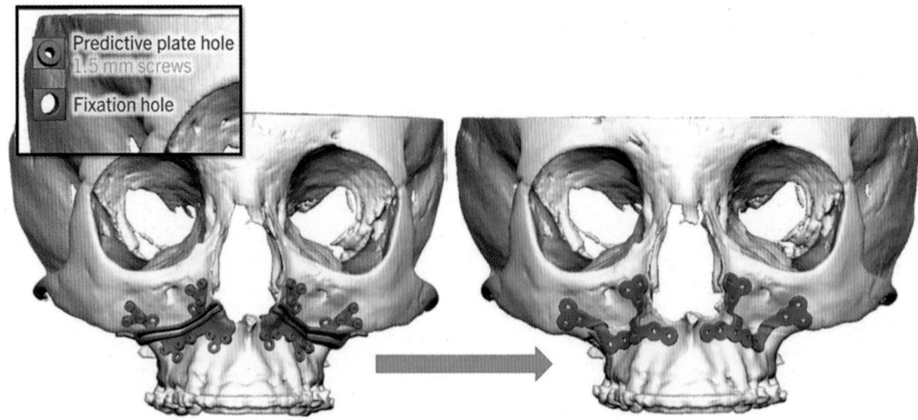

Figure 33.23 Patient-specific guides and plates.

Postoperative Considerations

Malocclusion

Unless hardware failure is confirmed, malocclusion is created either by not setting the bite correctly in the treatment planning session or by not controlling the occlusion in the operating room. The virtual planning session allows for confirmation of the final occlusion before the digital plan is accepted. Photographs of the final occlusion also assist the virtual planner with accuracy before the segments are moved.

Splints

Several materials are used in splint fabrication. Each material has variable characteristics that may alter the length of time they may be left in the patient's mouth. Selection of the appropriate material by the surgeon is necessary and should take into account the length of time the splint will be used postoperatively.

Confirm splint accuracy preoperatively, especially if segmental surgery is not planned. Orthodontic bracket interference with the splint requires adjustment.

Time

Although the incorporation of digital technology reduces surgeon chair time labor, timing remains an important consideration. This technology requires at least 2 to 3 weeks of lead time, especially with the patient-specific plating technique. Thus, orthodontic surgical wires should be in place with stable dental position for at least 1 month before the planned date of surgery. The surgeon must ensure that models are not damaged or lost when sent through conventional mail.

Software engineers usually require several days to accurately prepare the CT data that are sent to make the digital information useable for the virtual planning sessions. They contact the surgeon once the materials are all in the database and make an appointment for the session. The digital planning session should occur no later than 2 to 3 weeks before the actual date of surgery.

Bringing Virtual Surgical Planning (VSP) and 3D Printing In-House

The advent of personal 3D printing technology may allow us to eventually bring the fabrication of splints back in-house once the final plans are established. The planning can either be done by you or you can work with the planning engineers. The plan can be sent to your 3D printer and the splints or guides can fabricated at your office or institution.

If you decide to do the whole VSP in-house you will need several pieces of hardware and software. The initial costs may be high, ultimately leading to a cost savings if nothing goes wrong. Do not forget that licenses need to be paid for and the machines need to be maintained and upgraded. Software also needs to be updated and supported.

Potential list of what you need to do:

1. CBCT to create a DICOM image of the skull. These eventually get converted to STL files (separate software application needed). Your accuracy of 3D printing depends upon the accuracy of the CBCT. Slices need to be thinner than 1 to 2 mm.
2. Intraoral scanner to capture the dentition into an STL file. (This gives us accurate topography of the dentition.)

Note you can also scan the models using CBCT and have a DICOM file of the teeth.

3. Software to combine the STL files of the skull and the teeth to create a composite model.

You can also combine the DICOM data of the skull with the DICOM of the models. Combining the skull and dental models is typically part of the planning software.

4. Now you will need software to segment out what you want to move and perform your VSP. This is where the VSP modeling companies have their strength for us at this time. To use this technology properly will take a great deal of practice. Remember, if it is wrong, the jaw winds up in the wrong position or the splints and guides may not fit.

5. Once you save the final plan you will need to make splints and guides. These are typically from STL files. A 3D printer is needed to either do this by additive manufacturing or by subtractive manufacturing (extremely expensive technology not for the private sector) depending upon the machine chosen and materials utilized.
   1. The type of material is very important for precision and ensuring that there are no deformities. Do not use what you buy from a local hobby or home improvement shop. Material approved by the FDA is available at a reasonable price. The manufacturers have biocompatibility testing done, and this material must be used per the FDA recommendations.
   2. Not all printers are alike. Again you need a precision printer nozzle of at least 0.4 mm, and the printing profile accuracy needs to be close to 0.1 to 0.06. This is considered fine/ultra-fine.
   3. Most planning software will put out a basic splint; however, it is never a finalized splint, and some work needs to be done to clean it up. Holes will also need to be placed if you want to wire it in, perhaps palatal straps for width changes and sandwich features for intermediate splints.
   4. Cutting guides have to be designed in a separate software program adding additional costs and a great deal of expertise in CASS software. This software is not typically available to the private sector. One solution in the beginning would be to let the modeling company do the designs and then they would be sent to your in-house printer. This would make the design requirements by the surgeon easier and more predictable.

Please note that the FDA has been recently looking into the in-house fabrication of medical devices such as splints and guides. The modeling companies have all been vetted. The FDA has also approved the use of the software for the manufacturing of surgical guides.

1. Custom titanium plates and cutting/drill guides cannot be made in-house without the appropriate type of printers and materials. At this time titanium is too costly for the individual practitioner.

References

1. Gateno J, Xia J, Teichgraeber JF, Rosen A. A new technique for the creation of a computerized composite skull model. *J Oral Maxillofac Surg*. 2003;61(2):222–227.
2. Gateno J, Xia J, Teichgraeber JF, Rosen A, Hultgren B, Vadnais T. The precision of computer-generated surgical splints. *J Oral Maxillofac Surg*. 2003;61(7):814–817.
3. Xia JJ, McGrory JK, Gateno J, et al. A new method to orient 3-dimensional computed tomography models to the natural head position: a clinical feasibility study. *J Oral Maxillofac Surg*. 2011;69(3):584–591.
4. Hsu SS, Gateno J, Bell RB, et al. Accuracy of a computer-aided surgical simulation protocol for orthognathic surgery: a prospective multicenter study. *J Oral Maxillofac Surg*. 2013;71(1):128–142.
5. Song KG, Baek SH. Comparison of the accuracy of the three-dimensional virtual method and the conventional manual method for model surgery and intermediate wafer fabrication. *Oral Surg Oral Med Oral Pathol Oral Radiol Endod*. 2009;107(1):13–21.
6. Tucker S, Cevidanes LH, Styner M, et al. Comparison of actual surgical outcomes and 3-dimensional surgical simulations. *J Oral Maxillofac Surg*. 2010;68(10):2412–2421.
7. Gateno J, Xia JJ, Teichgraeber JF, et al. Clinical feasibility of computer-aided surgical simulation (CASS) in the treatment of complex cranio-maxillofacial deformities. *J Oral Maxillofac Surg*. 2007;65(4):728–734.
8. Orentlicher G, Goldsmith D, Horowitz A. Applications of 3-dimensional virtual computerized tomography technology in oral and maxillofacial surgery: current therapy. *J Oral Maxillofac Surg*. 2010;68(8):1933–1959.
9. Xia JJ, Gateno J, Teichgraeber JF, et al. Accuracy of the computer-aided surgical simulation (CASS) system in the treatment of patients with complex craniomaxillofacial deformity: a pilot study. *J Oral Maxillofac Surg*. 2007;65(2):248–254.
10. Kaipatur N, Al-Thomali Y, Flores-Mir C. Accuracy of computer programs in predicting orthognathic surgery hard tissue response. *J Oral Maxillofac Surg*. 2009;67(8):1628–1639.
11. McCormick SU, Drew SJ. Virtual model surgery for efficient planning and surgical performance. *J Oral Maxillofac Surg*. 2011;69(3):638–644.
12. Swennen GR, Mollemans W, Schutyser F. Three-dimensional treatment planning of orthognathic surgery in the era of virtual imaging. *J Oral Maxillofac Surg*. 2009;67(10):2080–2092.
13. Xia JJ, Gateno J, Teichgraeber JF. Three-dimensional computer-aided surgical simulation for maxillofacial surgery. *Atlas Oral Maxillofac Surg Clin North Am*. 2005;13(1):25–39.
14. Schatz EC, Xia JJ, Gateno J, English JD, Teichgraeber JF, Garrett FA. Development of a technique for recording and transferring natural head position in 3 dimensions. *J Craniofac Surg*. 2010;21(5):1452–1455.
15. Xia JJ, Phillips CV, Gateno J, et al. Cost-effectiveness analysis for computer-aided surgical simulation in complex cranio-maxillofacial surgery. *J Oral Maxillofac Surg*. 2006;64(12):1780–1784.
16. Bell RB. Computer planning and intraoperative navigation in orthognathic surgery. *J Oral Maxillofac Surg*. 2011;69(3):592–605.
17. Bell RB. Computer planning and intraoperative navigation in cranio-maxillofacial surgery. *Oral Maxillofac Surg Clin North Am*. 2010;22(1):135–156.
18. Xia JJ, Gateno J, Teichgraeber JF. A new paradigm for complex midface reconstruction: a reversed approach. *J Oral Maxillofac Surg*. 2009;67(3):693–703.
19. Xia JJ, Gateno J, Teichgraeber JF. New clinical protocol to evaluate craniomaxillofacial deformity and plan surgical correction. *J Oral Maxillofac Surg*. 2009;67(10):2093–2106.
20. Swennen GR, Mollemans W, De Clercq C, et al. A cone-beam computed tomography triple scan procedure to obtain a three-dimensional augmented virtual skull model appropriate for orthognathic surgery planning. *J Craniofac Surg*. 2009;20(2):297–307.
21. Ho CT, Lin HH, Lo LJ. Intraoral scanning and setting up the digital final occlusion in three-dimensional panning of orthognathic surgery: its comparison with the dental model approach. *Plast Reconstr Surg*. 2019;143(5):1027e–1036e.
22. Caminiti M, Lou T. Clear aligner orthognathic splints. *J Oral Maxillofac Surg*. 2019;77(5):1071.e1–1071.e8.
23. Elnagar MH, Aronovich S, Kusnoto B. Digital workflow for combined orthodontics nd orthognathic surgery. *Oral Maxillofac Surg Clin North Am*. 2020;32(1):1–14.

CHAPTER 34

Genioplasty

Ron Caloss

Armamentarium

#9 Periosteal elevator
#15 Blade handle
#701 Bur
1/4-inch paper tape
24-Gauge wire
2-0 or 3-0 Vicryl suture
3-0 or 4-0 chromic gut
Appropriate sutures
Aufricht retractor
Cobb elevator
Double skin hooks
Fixation plate and screw set
Large Tegaderm dressing
Lidocaine with epinephrine
Local anesthetic with vasoconstrictor
Mastisol
Needle tip electrocautery
Obwegeser retractors
Self-retaining cheek retractors
Thin reciprocating saw blade
Wire driver

History of the Procedure

Genioplasty using a sliding osteotomy via an intraoral approach was introduced more than 50 years ago. Trauner and Obwegeser[1] and Converse and Wood-Smith[2] described the technique for correction of microgenia in 1957 and 1964, respectively. These events occurred along with the development of maxillary and mandibular osteotomies for orthognathic surgery. Later, attention was turned to slight modifications, such as performing an ostectomy for correction of macrogenia. In the 1980s, plate and screw fixation was introduced, which was an improvement over previous wire fixation for segment stabilization.[3]

Genioplasty using alloplastic implants became an alternative method for increasing chin projection as various people published studies on this technique from the 1970s through the 1990s. Several implant biomaterials were introduced. They included solid silicone (Silastic), porous polyethylene (Medpor), mesh polymers (Dacron, Mersilene, Supramid), polytetrafluoroethylene and carbon fibers (Proplast), expanded polytetrafluoroethylene (Gore-Tex), and hydroxyapaptite.[4–6] Silicone and porous polyethylene preformed implants are the main ones used today. In the future, tissue engineering may offer the ability to generate contoured facial implants composed of immunocompatible cells and a matrix construct.[6]

Two- and three-dimensional digital imaging and planning programs have been developed (e.g., Dolphin Imaging). This technology enhances the surgeon's ability to plan treatment and communicate with the patient. The surgeon performs the virtual treatment objective on a computer, and the patient views his or her morphed profile photograph. As the patient views the simulated profile change, he or she can appreciate and participate in treatment choices. More recently, virtual surgical planning software programs have been developed that allow for planning virtual osteotomies and surgical cutting guides and repositioning guides using CAD-CAM technology.

Indications for the Use of the Procedure

Genioplasty is performed to improve facial balance and/or rejuvenate the lower facial third. Evaluation of the chin in three dimensions is important for proper diagnosis and treatment planning. From the frontal view, the chin and inferior border of the mandible should be well defined and provide separation of the lower third of the face from the neck. The chin width should be in balance with the bizygomatic and bigonial facial widths. A narrow chin or a person with jowling and disruption of a smooth jaw line would benefit from lateral augmentation with an alloplast implant.[7]

The chin's vertical dimension influences vertical facial balance. The middle facial height (glabella to subnasale) and the lower facial height (subnasale to soft tissue menton) should be approximately equal. The lower third can be further subdivided. The upper lip length (subnasale to stomion superius) should be approximately one-half the lower lip length (stomion inferius to soft tissue menton). The normal lower lip length is 40 mm (± 2) in females and 44 mm (± 2) in males. The normal hard tissue length of the chin or anterior dental height is measured from the mandibular incisor tip to the inferior border of the mandible. The average height is 40 mm (± 2) in females and 44 mm (± 2) in males.

If there is excessive lower facial height (in the presence of normal vertical maxillary position), a vertical reduction genioplasty with an ostectomy may be indicated. Conversely, if there is deficient vertical height, vertical augmentation of the chin may be indicated with an osteotomy and interpositional bone graft. Asymmetry of the vertical height may require the combination of ostectomy on the excessive side and the use of the removed bone as a graft on the deficient side.[8]

Chin projection should be in balance with the entire profile. The anteroposterior chin position can be assessed with cephalometric analysis. The bony chin position can be assessed with NB:pogonion and A:pogonion relationships to the lower incisor. The lower incisor tip and pogonion relationship to the NB line should be 2:1 to 1:1. The lower incisor tip should be on or 1 to 2 mm posterior to the line through A:pogonion. These analyses assume that the maxilla and mandible are in the proper anterior-posterior relationship to one another and that the lower incisor inclination is normal. Subnasale perpendicular can be used to assess the soft tissue chin position. Soft tissue pogonion should be 3 mm (± 3) behind this line. Generally, a stronger chin is considered masculine, and a retrusive chin is considered feminine.[7,8]

These cephalometric analyses provide only some guidance. It is important to assess chin projection with other factors, such as chin shape, depth of the labiomental fold, lower lip position, and mandibular anteroposterior position. Cultural differences and trends are also important to keep in mind. For instance, a well-defined chin and jaw line with stronger projection often is seen as esthetic for females in Western culture. A weaker chin is generally considered more esthetic in Asian cultures.[8]

An osteotomy is more versatile than a stock alloplast implant in altering the three-dimensional position of the chin. It can manage a sagittal and vertical deficiency or excess. It can also correct an asymmetric chin, such as that seen in hemifacial hyperplasia. An osteotomy is more commonly used as an adjunct to orthognathic surgery.[9] If bimaxillary surgery is being performed, chin projection can be influenced by clockwise or counterclockwise rotation of the maxillomandibular complex. This may help avoid a genioplasty procedure altogether, especially in a patient with good chin shape to begin with.

Stock alloplast implants are limited to the correction of a sagittal and/or transverse chin deficiency. However, custom-designed and fabricated implants using CAD-CAM technology enhance the ability to correct three-dimensional deformities including asymmetries. Implants offer several advantages, including ease of placement, cosmetic enhancement in chin projection and lateral jaw line contour (by effacing the prejowl sulcus), and structural stability. It is technically easier to widen the chin with an implant rather than an osteotomy and bone graft. Alloplast augmentation typically is used in the context of facial cosmetic surgery. For instance, an implant can be used to augment a deficient chin, at the same time a nasal dorsal hump reduction is performed. The extended prejowl genial implant can be used for rejuvenation of the lower third of the face, either alone or as an adjunct to rhytidectomy, platysma plication, or neck liposuction. An implant improves structural support to the overlying lax or ptotic soft tissue. This has the effect of improving chin-neck esthetics and effacing a deep prejowl sulcus (Fig. 34.1).[4,7]

Limitations and Contraindications

Anatomic, physiologic, and psychological limitations should be considered when assessing a patient for genioplasty.

The locations of the inferior alveolar nerve and canine root apices, in addition to the vertical height of the chin, need to be assessed when an osteotomy is planned. Low-lying inferior alveolar nerves, long canine roots, and a vertically short chin make it more difficult to perform an osteotomy and have a decent-sized genial segment to advance. A sliding osteotomy can lead to notching of the inferior border of the mandible in these situations.[10] In older individuals with prominent jowls, a sliding osteotomy also may deepen the prejowl sulcus and worsen the effects of aging in this area. An implant with a prejowl extension is likely a better choice in these situations.

In certain situations implants may not be a good choice. In younger individuals, an implant may contribute over time to resorption of the underlying bone. Patients with labial incompetence and lip strain or hyperactive chin musculature may be more prone to bone resorption under the implant or displacement of the implant due to excessive forces. This is more likely if the implant is not properly fixated or if the implant has a short length. Underlying bone resorption is less likely when an extended chin implant is used because of the increased surface area of coverage. Some believe that a large augmentation is better served by osteotomy rather than an implant.[5,11,12]

Medical conditions that can contribute to complications should be considered. The immunocompromised patient may not be a candidate for elective surgery. Diabetic control should be optimized before proceeding. If the patient is anticoagulated, this may pose a problem if medication cannot be safely discontinued before surgery. Tobacco use may complicate healing and should be discontinued. Surrounding soft tissue, odontogenic, or periodontal infection should be treated beforehand.

With any elective surgery, the patient's chief complaint must be fully understood and addressed. The risks of the procedure and alternatives to care should be discussed and informed consent obtained. If the patient is mentally or emotionally unstable, they may not be a candidate for surgery. Also, if an adolescent does not have adequate family support and is poorly motivated for care, the procedure should not be performed.

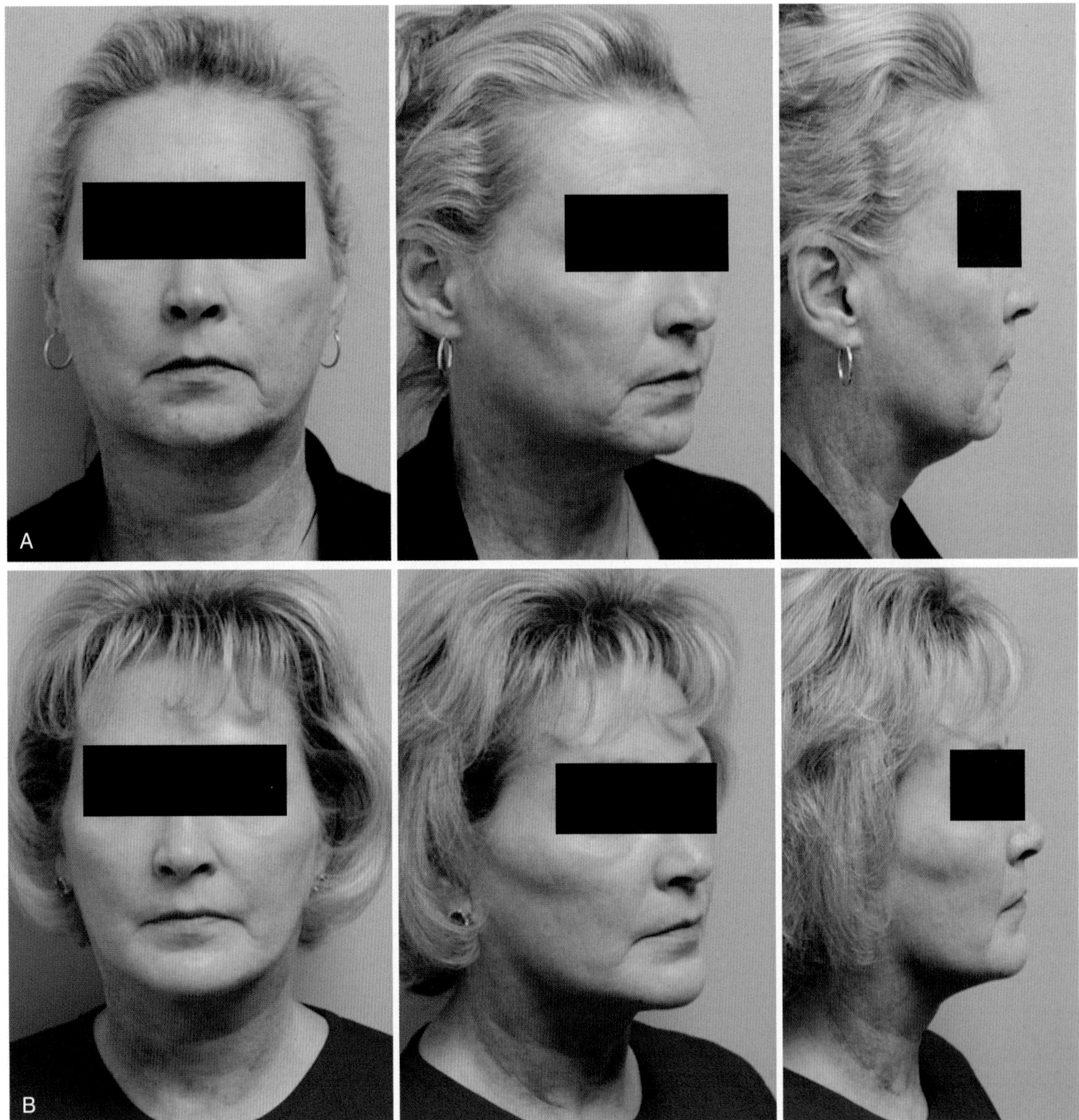

Figure 34.1 Preoperative (A) and postoperative (B) photographs of a patient who underwent a mini-facelift, submental liposuction, and placement of a silicone extended genial implant. In addition to improving chin projection, the implant improved support of the lax soft tissue and the definition of the lateral border of the mandible.

TECHNIQUE: Advancement Sliding Osteotomy

STEP 1: Incision and Dissection

A local anesthetic with a vasoconstrictor is infiltrated into the submucosal tissue of the chin. It is helpful to place the patient in maxillomandibular fixation with elastics to stabilize the mandible during the procedure. Double skin hooks are used initially to retract the lower lip. A self-retaining cheek retractor is useful for lip retraction as well.

After vasoconstriction has occurred, an incision is made through the lip mucosa from canine to canine, halfway between the depth of the vestibule and the wet-dry line, using a #15 blade and/or needle point electrocautery. The incision should traverse the mentalis muscle at an oblique angle so that an adequate portion attached to the mandible is maintained for muscle resuspension on closure.

Subperiosteal dissection is performed with a #9 periosteal or larger Cobb elevator to fully expose the symphysis down to the inferior border. Elevate the periosteum and muscle overlying the incisor roots on the anterior mandible to make resuspension of the muscle easier when closing. Subperiosteal dissection is then carried posteriorly into the molar region, keeping the elevator along the inferior border well below the mental nerve. The dissection is finally carried superiorly to identify and expose the mental nerve where it exits the foramen. Avoid excessive dissection along the inferior border. It is important to maintain adequate soft tissue attachment for blood supply to the advanced genial segment. This should hopefully minimize long-term bone resorption (Fig. 34.2A and B).

STEP 2: Marking the Midline

A #701 bur is used to score the facial cortex at the symphyseal midline above and below the intended osteotomy. This helps keep the repositioned genial segment oriented to the midline. Stand directly above the patient's head when scoring the cortex to help maintain midline orientation. It is easier to first make a series of indentations with the bur tip and then connect them in a straight vertical line (Fig. 34.2C).

Continued

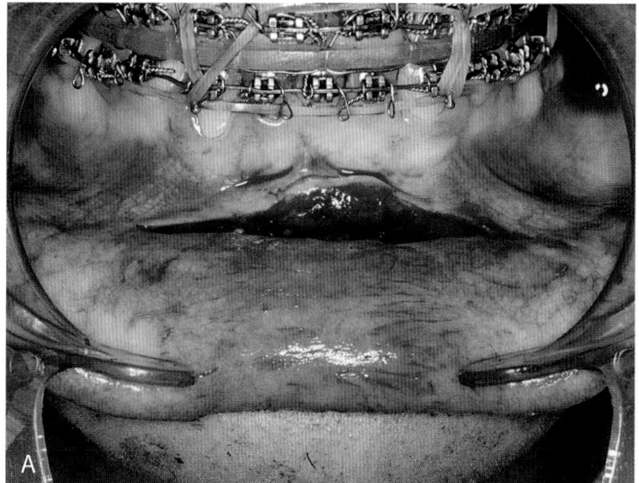

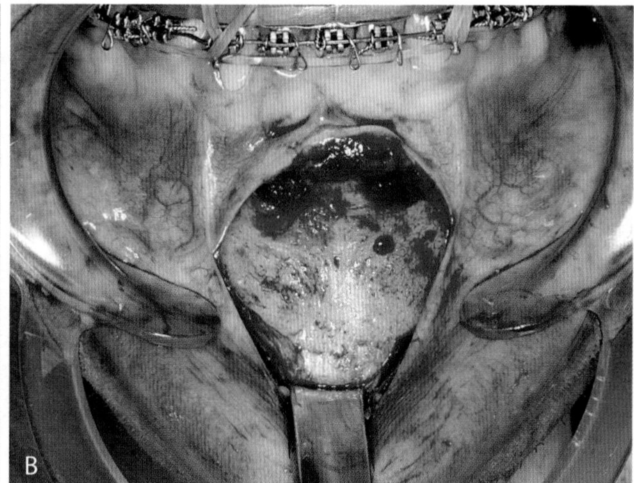

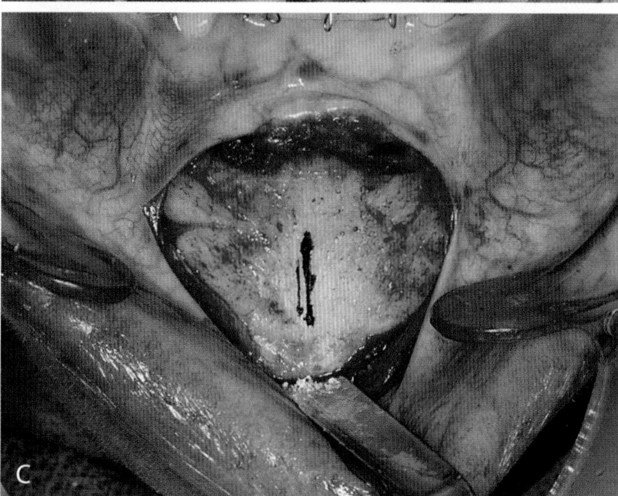

Figure 34.2 **A,** The incision is made through the mucosa from canine to canine, halfway between the depth of the vestibule and the wet-dry line of the lip. **B,** Subperiosteal dissection is carried down to the inferior border. **C,** The midline is marked by scoring a vertical line in the facial cortex with a #701 bur. The line is highlighted with a surgical marker.

TECHNIQUE: Advancement Sliding Osteotomy—cont'd

STEP 3: Osteotomy

Careful consideration should be given to the placement and angulation of the osteotomy. The osteotomy should be at least 5 mm below the apices of the canine teeth and 6 mm below the mental foramen. This is to avoid devitalization of the teeth and injury to the nerve that can run anterior and inferior to the foramen. Another important aspect is to angle the osteotomy so that it extends posteriorly into the first molar region. This prevents excessive notching of the inferior border and reduction in chin height with advancement of a foreshortened genial segment. Typically, the osteotomy will be approximately 12 mm above the inferior border at the midline. However, in a patient with a low-lying mental foramen or a short anterior chin height, the osteotomy can lie closer to the inferior border.

Obwegeser retractors can be used by the assistant to retract and protect the soft tissue of the lip during the osteotomy. An Aufricht retractor can be used by the surgeon to help retract soft tissue and orient the reciprocating saw blade properly. The retractor is held by the index finger and thumb in the surgeon's nondominant hand and brought into the wound. The tip of the retractor is placed at the inferior border in the first molar region and palpated with the ring finger. The reciprocating saw blade is brought into the wound, and the tip is palpated, along with the retractor blade tip at the inferior border. The retractor blade and reciprocating saw are aligned together, ensuring proper angulation of the osteotomy, as previously noted.

The osteotomy is made perpendicular to outer cortical bone. It is initiated posteriorly through both cortices of the inferior border. As the saw is advanced anteriorly, it should be upright, ensuring that the blade is cutting through both cortices. The saw should be oriented 90 degrees to the mandible by the time the midline is reached. Avoid overinsertion of the blade to minimize trauma to the mylohyoid and genioglossus muscles and to prevent excessive bleeding. When the midline is reached, the saw is removed, and the same osteotomy is carried out on the opposite side.

If the genial segment is not easily mobilized, the osteotomy should be rerun with the saw to ensure that both cortices have been fully cut. This prevents an irregular edge of bone from fracturing off along the osteotomy border, which most commonly occurs on the posterior lingual aspect of the genial segment. Any sharp or irregular edges can be smoothed with an egg-shaped bur so that the segment sits flush and even when advanced. Care should be taken to retract and protect the soft tissues in the floor of mouth when performing this action (Fig. 34.2D and E).

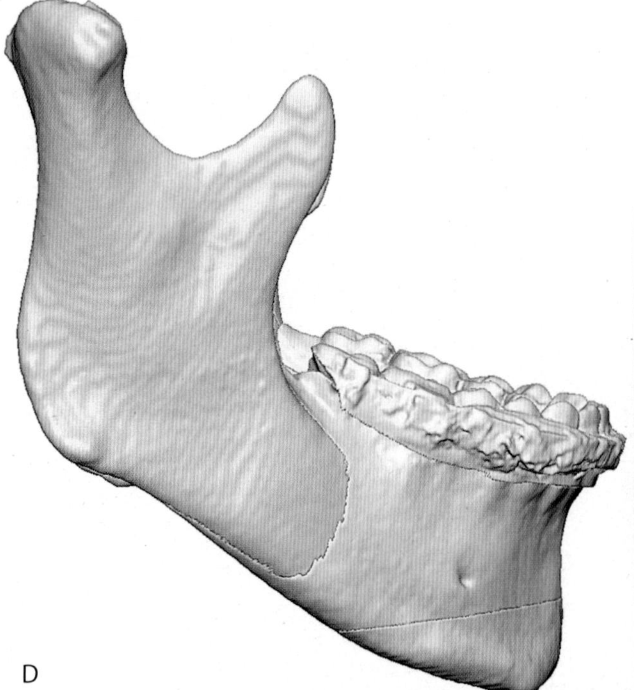

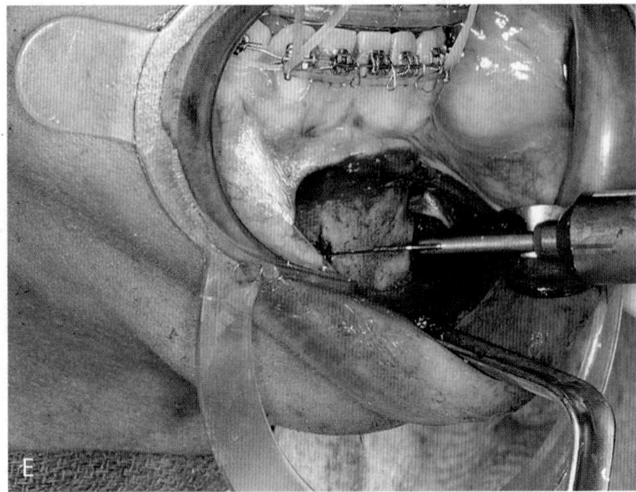

Figure 34.2, cont'd **D,** The osteotomy should be angled such that it extends posteriorly into the first molar region and lies 6 mm below the mental foramen. **E,** An Aufricht retractor can be used to retract soft tissue and help orient the reciprocating saw blade at the proper angle, as shown here.

TECHNIQUE: Advancement Sliding Osteotomy—cont'd

STEP 4: Advancement and Fixation

The genial segment is advanced straight forward, keeping proper alignment of the midline mark previously made. The lingual cortex of the genial segment should not be advanced beyond the facial cortex of the mandibular body to ensure stability and union. There should be minimal space between the advanced segment and mandibular body. If there is a small osteotomy gap, it can be grafted with autogenous and/or allogeneic bone.

Various prebent genioplasty plate designs are available for genial segment fixation. They typically come in 2-mm size increments and are fixated with 2- or 1.5-mm screws. The author prefers the H-shaped design. It allows easy visualization and alignment of the genial segment midline mark because the two prebent arms are off-centered from the plate midline.

A positioning wire can be used to help advance and stabilize the genial segment while the fixation screws are placed. A hole is placed obliquely through the edge of the facial cortex at the midline mark. A 24-gauge straight wire is then placed through the hole and twisted with a wire driver. It is important to make the hole far enough away from the osteotomy edge so that the wire does not pull through the bone.

The appropriate-size plate (based on the preoperative virtual treatment objective) is chosen. Changing the amount of advancement may be appropriate based on the esthetic assessment on the table. All four wings of the plate are bent to the appropriate contour of the underlying bone. The superior wings of the plate are secured first to the body of the mandible. If a positioning wire is used, it is brought through the middle of the two arms of the plate. The genial segment is then advanced and stabilized with the wire. It is also important to palpate and manually stabilize the wings of the advanced genial segment to ensure that they are symmetrically positioned on both sides. Screws are finally placed through the inferior wing holes to stabilize the genial segment. Typically, screws 10 to 12 mm long are used (Fig. 34.2F–H).

Continued

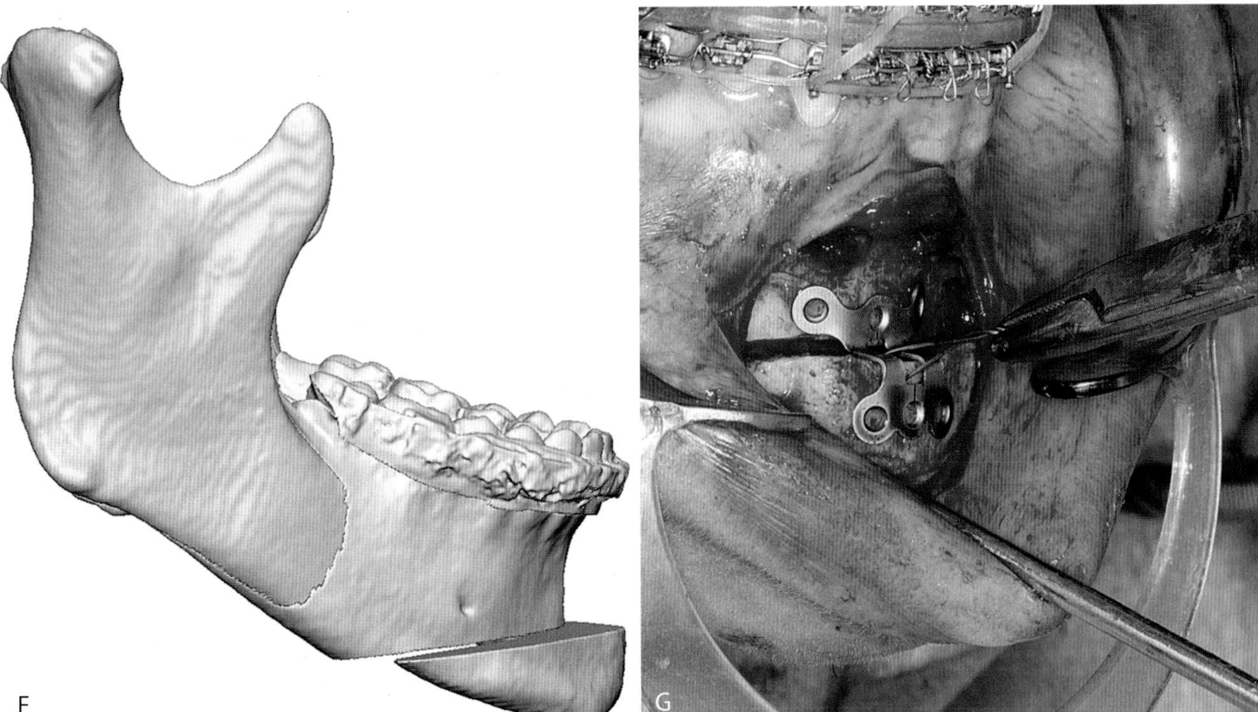

Figure 34.2, cont'd **F,** Straight genial advancement with minimal space in the osteotomy gap. **G,** The positioning wire helps advance the genial segment and stabilize it while fixation screws are placed.

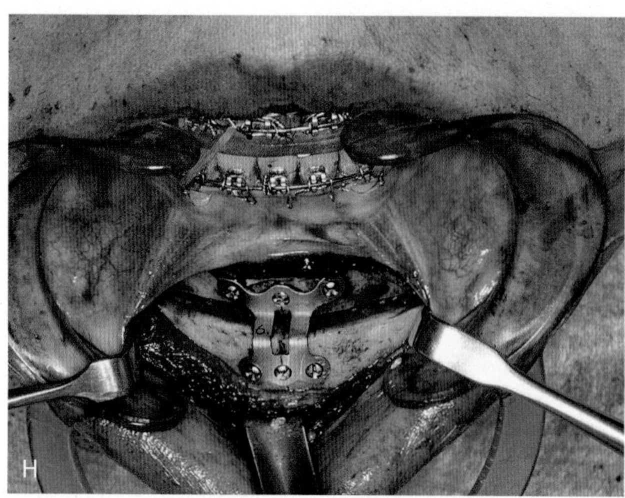

Figure 34.2, cont'd **H,** Segment advanced and stabilized with a prebent H-shaped genioplasty plate.

TECHNIQUE: Advancement Sliding Osteotomy—cont'd

STEP 5: Closure

The wound is closed in two layers. The mentalis muscle is resuspended using three interrupted 3-0 Vicryl sutures. This is important to maintain soft tissue contour to the chin and avoid chin ptosis. The mucosa is then closed in continuous fashion with 4-0 chromic gut. A surface pressure dressing is placed to further support the soft tissue envelope, minimize edema, and prevent hematoma formation. Mastisol adhesive is applied to the skin in the submental and chin region. Then, strips of 1/4-inch brown paper tape are applied vertically and horizontally across the chin in three layers. A Tegaderm occlusive dressing is then placed to minimize soiling of the tape. The dressing can be removed in 5 to 7 days (Fig. 34.2I–K).

Fig. 34.2L shows postoperative radiographs of a patient who underwent a Le Fort I posterior impaction and mandibular autorotation to close an anterior open bite and a concomitant advancement genioplasty.

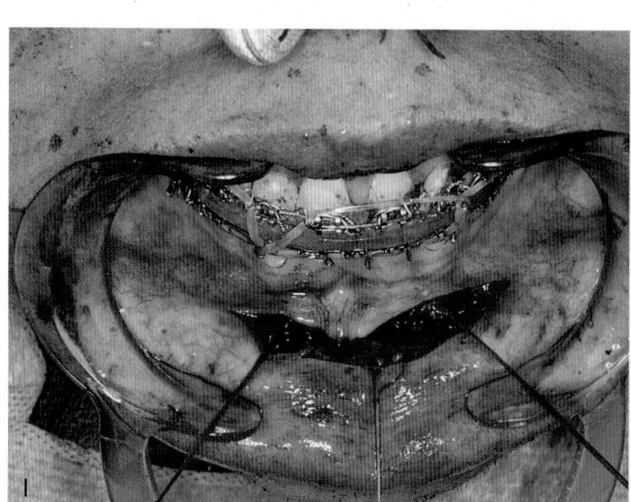

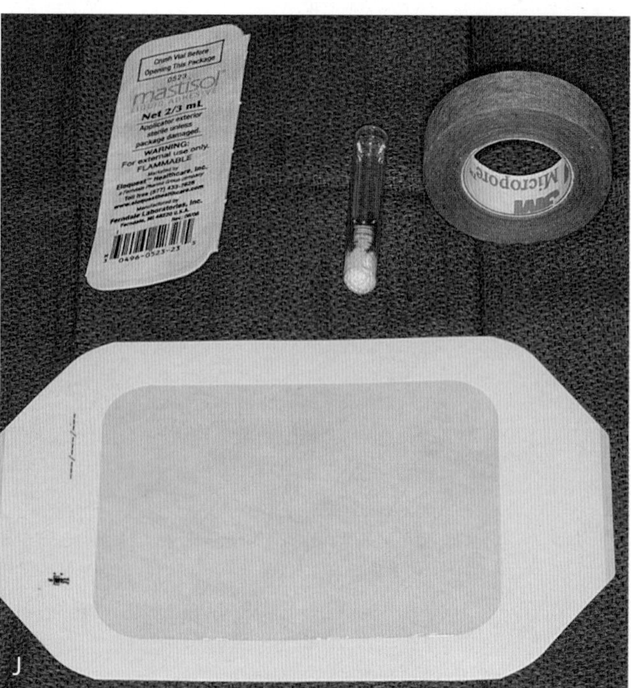

Figure 34.2, cont'd **I,** The mentalis muscle is resuspended with Vicryl sutures to help prevent soft tissue ptosis. **J,** Mastisol, 1/4-inch brown paper tape, and Tegaderm are used for a chin dressing.

Continued

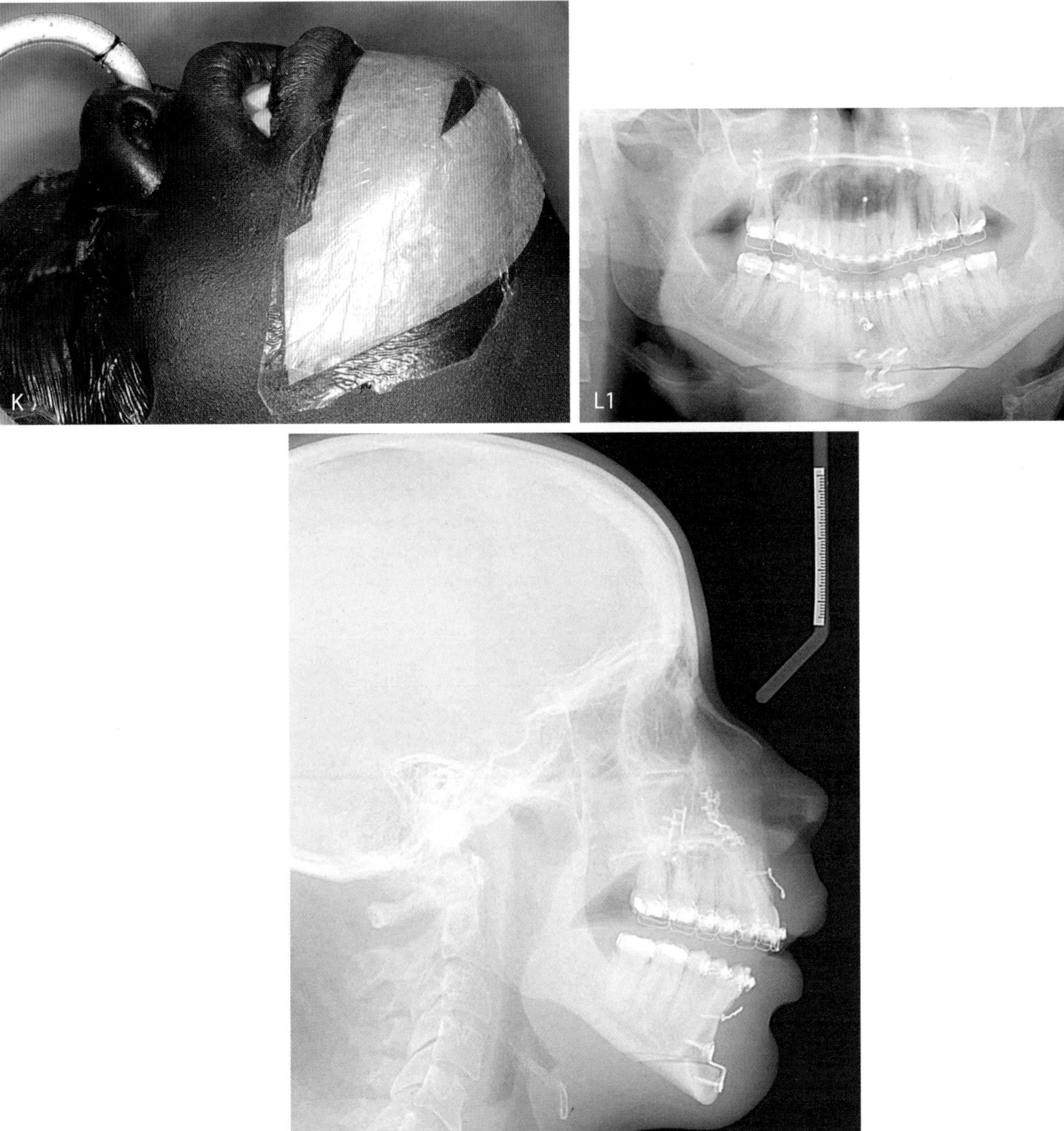

Figure 34.2, cont'd **K,** Three layers of tape are crisscrossed in a vertical and horizontal fashion. **L,** Postoperative Panorex and lateral cephalogram after an advancement sliding osteotomy. The osteotomy extends posteriorly to the first molar. A 6-mm prebent H-shaped plate was used.

ALTERNATIVE TECHNIQUE 1: Vertical Alteration

The chin can be vertically augmented or reduced to improve esthetic facial balance. This includes correction of asymmetry in a patient with hemimandibular hyperplasia.

For augmentation, the osteotomy is performed as previously described, and the genial segment is mobilized. If a concomitant advance is performed, a prebent genioplasty plate can be used. Otherwise, two straight plates placed off the midline are used with two holes superior and two holes inferior to the osteotomy. The posterior wings of the genial segment are maintained in contact with the body of the mandible for stability as the anterior portion is down-grafted the desired amount and fixated in place. Autogenous and/or allogeneic bone graft should be placed into the osteotomy defect to aid bony union of the segment. Block grafts are preferred if a bigger gap exists. Particulate grafts are easier to place in smaller defects (Fig. 34.3A).

For reduction, two osteotomies must be completed. An inferior osteotomy is performed first as previously described. A second superior osteotomy is performed to carry out the appropriate ostectomy/bone reduction as planned on the virtual treatment objective. It is important to carry out the inferior osteotomy first so that the ostectomy is not performed on a freely mobile genial segment. It is important to stay at least 5 to 6 mm below the canine roots and mental foramina when planning the position of the superior osteotomy. Either a prebent genioplasty plate or two straight plates placed off the midline are used to fixate the genial segment (Fig. 34.3B).

For vertical chin asymmetry that occurs with hemifacial hyperplasia, mark the midline of the chin (genial segment) and separately mark the facial midline of the mandible above the osteotomies. The inferior osteotomy is performed first, parallel to the inferior border of the chin. A second superior osteotomy is performed parallel to the true horizontal. Ostectomy of the asymmetric bone segment is performed. It can be rotated 180 degrees and placed on the opposite side as a free graft or maintained pedicled to muscle. The genial segment is aligned to the facial midline and then rigidly fixated (Fig. 34.3C).

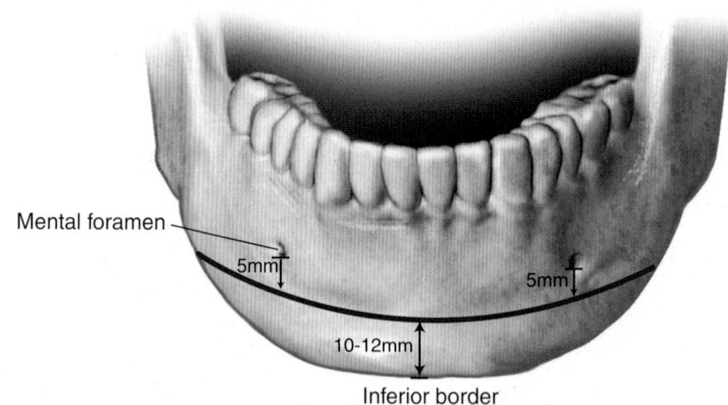

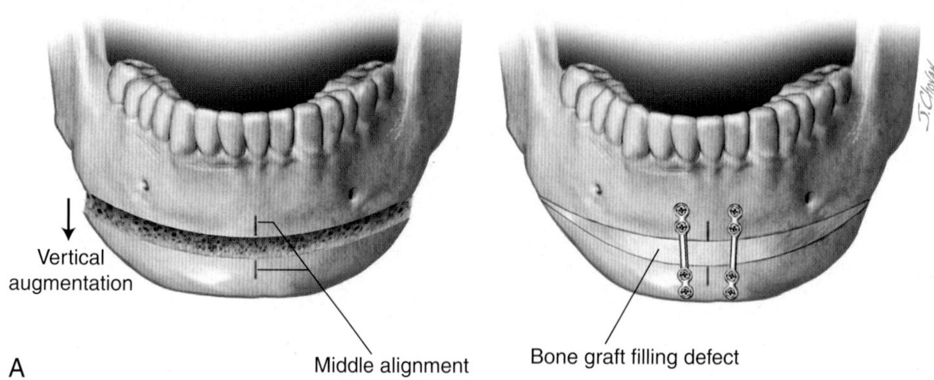

Figure 34.3 A, Vertical increase of the chin. The osteotomy gap is grafted with autogenous and/or allogeneic bone.

Continued

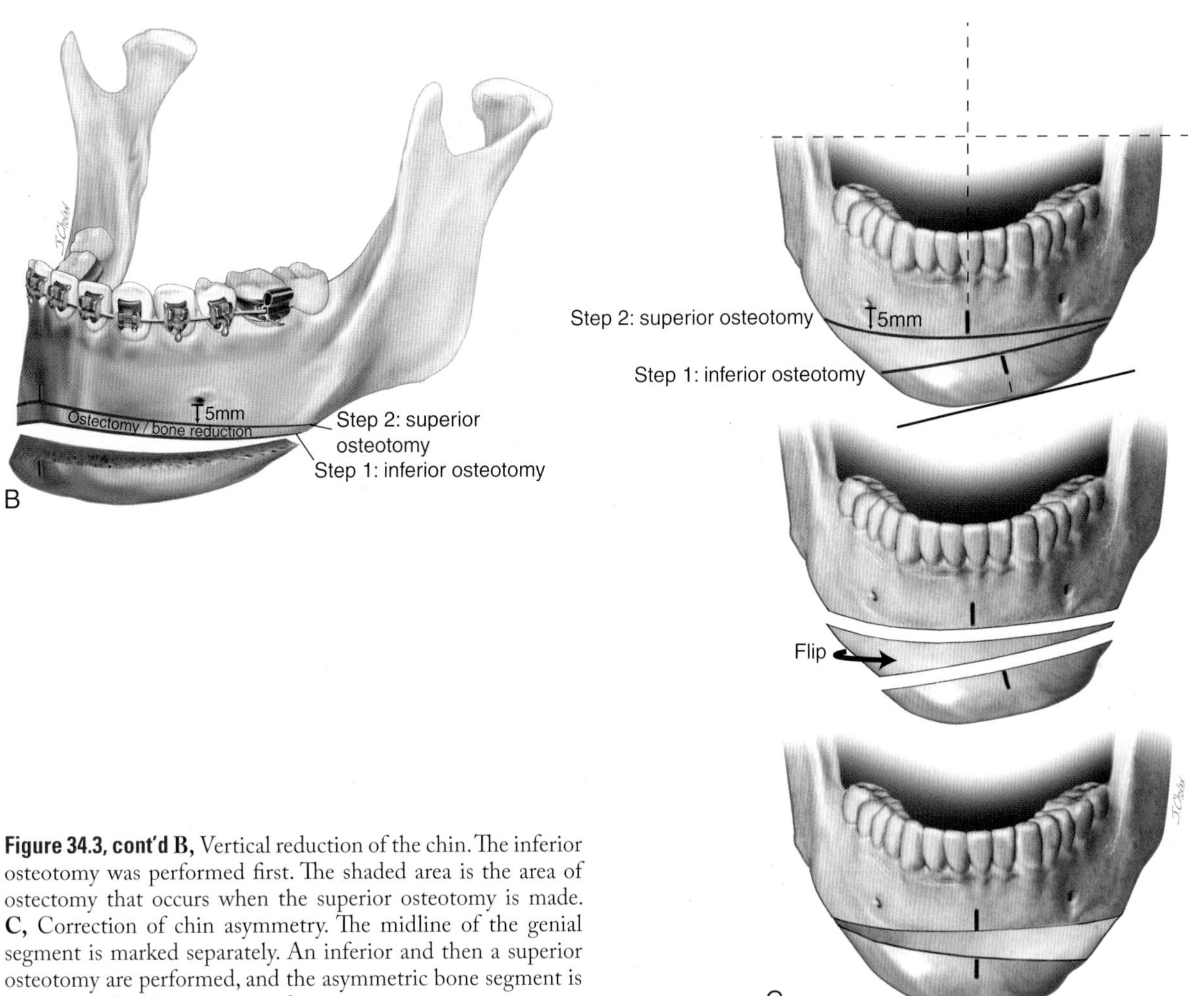

Figure 34.3, cont'd B, Vertical reduction of the chin. The inferior osteotomy was performed first. The shaded area is the area of ostectomy that occurs when the superior osteotomy is made. **C,** Correction of chin asymmetry. The midline of the genial segment is marked separately. An inferior and then a superior osteotomy are performed, and the asymmetric bone segment is repositioned to the opposite side.

ALTERNATIVE TECHNIQUE 2: Alloplastic Implant Augmentation

Genial augmentation with alloplastic implants can be performed under local anesthesia and intravenous sedation. Silicone extended preformed implants are a common material and design. They create a subtle increase in lateral fullness to augment the prejowl sulcus in addition to increasing chin projection (Fig. 34.4A and B). Preformed implants come in small, medium, and large sizes that primarily vary in the amount of anterior augmentation. They are typically placed in conjunction with other cosmetic procedures, such as rhytidectomy and neck liposuction (see Fig. 34.1).

Access for implant placement can be obtained through an intraoral approach in the same fashion as that described for a sliding osteotomy. An extraoral submental approach is ideal if a concomitant neck rejuvenation procedure is performed. The author prefers this approach. The soft tissue chin midline is marked to aid correct implant positioning. Paramidline marks can also be made, corresponding to the posterior extent of the implant and dissection. A 2- to 2.5-mm incision is marked just posterior to the submental crease. This prevents deepening of the crease with scar contracture. Bilateral inferior alveolar nerve blocks are performed using 2% lidocaine with 1:100,000 epinephrine. The submental incision is infiltrated with the local anesthetic. If a concomitant submittal liposuction/lipectomy or platysmal plication is performed, tumescent anesthesia is administered in the neck region (Fig. 34.4C). Approximately 10 minutes should be allowed after infiltration for vasoconstriction to occur.

The incision is made through skin and subcutaneous tissue. A short skin flap is raised to the inferior border superficial to the platysma muscle. Electrocautery is used to incise through periosteum just anterior to the platysma muscle attachment in the symphysis region (Fig. 34.4D). This minimizes intraoperative bleeding and potential postoperative hematoma formation. A #9 periosteal elevator is then used to dissect in a subperiosteal plane along the inferior border on each side. The dissection proceeds superiorly onto the facial aspect of the symphysis and body. Care is taken to identify the mental nerve and avoid overmanipulation. The pocket must be large enough to allow the implant to sit passively along the facial aspect of the inferior border, but not overextended, to ensure

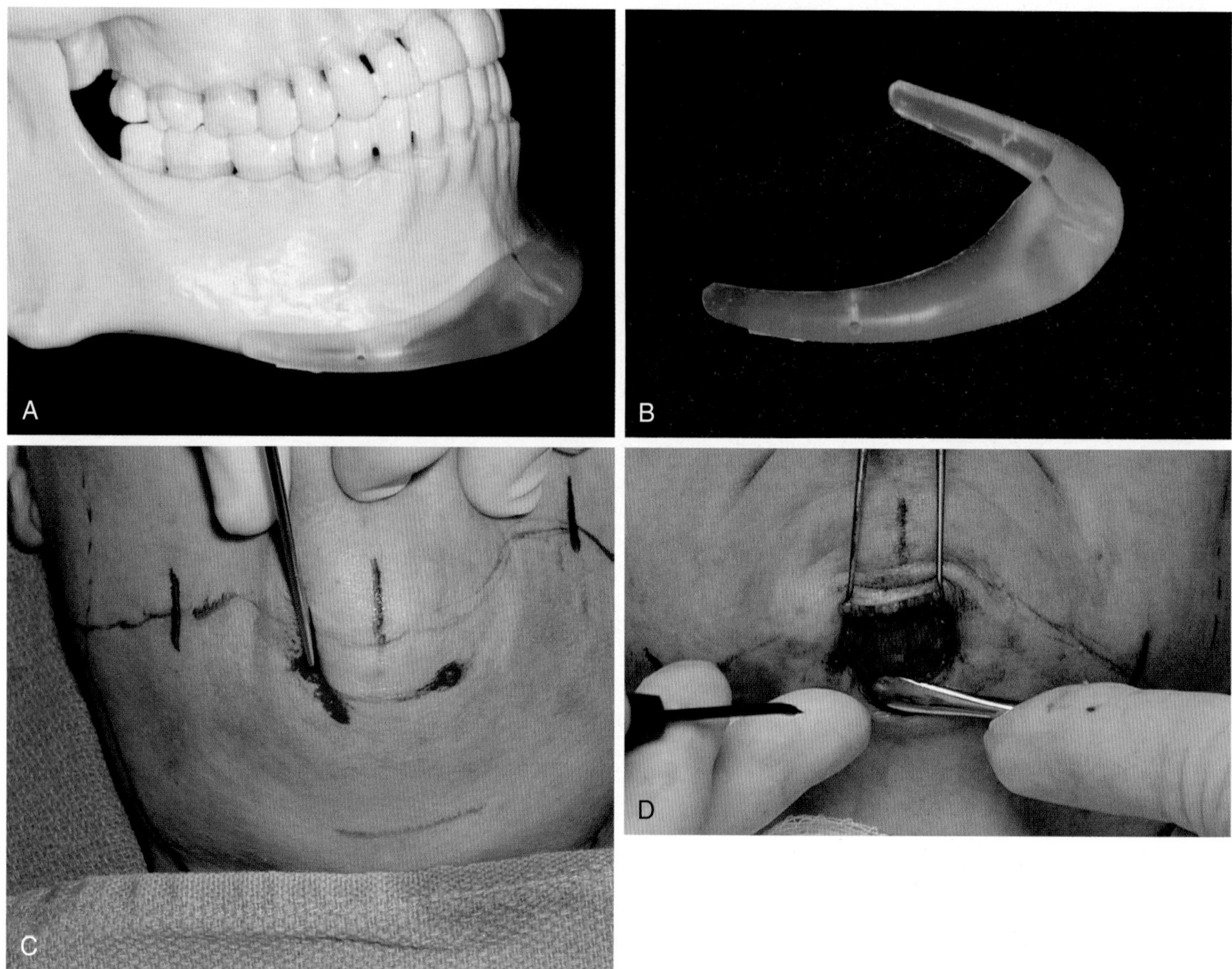

Figure 34.4 **A** and **B,** Silicone extended genial implant (Mittelman Pre Jowl Chin implant; Implantech, Ventura, CA). **C,** Markings for submental crease incision, inferior border of mandible, and facial midline. Tumescence is administered in this case for concomitant neck liposuction or lipectomy. **D,** Subperiosteal dissection is carried out along the facial aspect of the inferior border.

precise implant positioning. A sizer set corresponding to the actual preformed implant sizes (i.e., small, medium and large) can be used to help determine the best size. If a virtual treatment objective was performed, it also can aid the selection of the appropriate size. Minor implant contouring can be performed with sharp scissors or a #10 blade.

After insertion of the appropriate-size implant, the marked midline of the implant is aligned with the patient's previously marked soft tissue chin midline. The implant should sit passively along the facial aspect of the inferior border with no impingement on the mental nerve. Once the proper position has been verified, the implant should be fixated to prevent displacement. Stable fixation may minimize long-term mobility and bone resorption. Two monocortical 1.5- or 2.0-mm screws are placed off the midline to secure the implant in place. Two screws are necessary to prevent rotational movement. Alternatively, the implant can be sutured to the periosteum with a 3-0 polydioxanone suture. Eventually a capsule develops around a silicone implant to help further stabilize it in place. Tissue ingrowth occurs into a porous polyethylene implant. The wound is irrigated with sterile saline and then closed in layers. The periosteum is closed with 3-0 Vicryl. The subcutaneous layer is closed with 4-0 Monocryl. Finally the skin is closed with 5-0 or 6-0 fast-absorbing gut. Steri-Strips can be placed across the incision site. A multilayered pressure dressing is applied, as previously described (see Fig. 34.2K). A more extensive submental and neck pressure dressing can be placed if a neck procedure also was performed. The patient shown in Fig. 34.1 had an extended silicone genial implant placed in conjunction with a facelift and submental liposuction.

Avoidance and Management of Intraoperative Complications

Genioplasty involving an osteotomy is technically more challenging than an implant and thus has the potential for more complications. A common problem is foreshortening of the osteotomy by not extending it far enough posteriorly. When the foreshortened genial segment is advanced, it leaves a greater defect along the inferior border that disrupts a smooth inferior jaw line (Figs. 34.5 and 34.6). It can also deepen the prejowl sulcus with remodeling and aging. To avoid this problem, the osteotomy should extend posteriorly to the first molar, as previously described. If the osteotomy is inadvertently foreshortened, consider decreasing the forward genial segment advancement or grafting particulate hydroxyapatite along the inferior border defect at the time of surgery (Fig. 34.7).

Inferior alveolar nerve injury is another potential intraoperative complication. This can occur if the nerve runs low

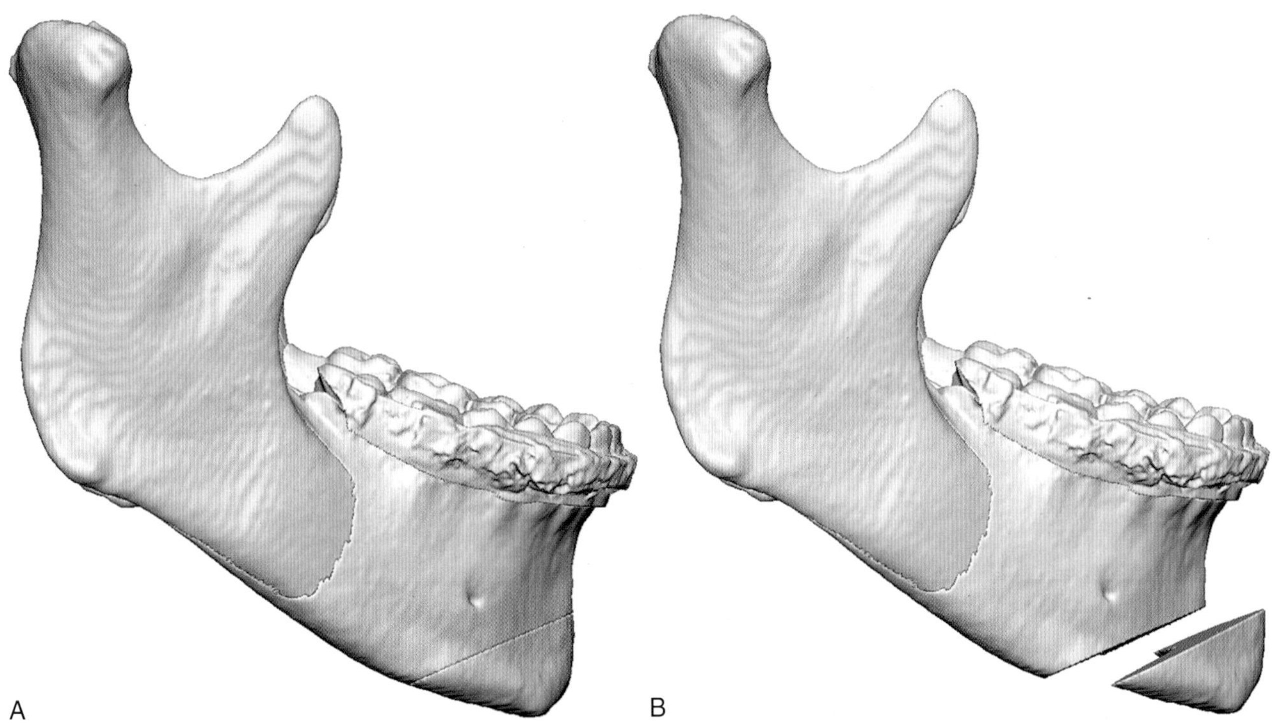

Figure 34.5 **A,** A foreshortened osteotomy that does not extend back into the first molar area. **B,** It depicts the segment relationship with a straight forward advancement. If the chin segment is then positioned superiorly for bony contact, it creates an unesthetic contour defect along the inferior border and reduction of chin height.

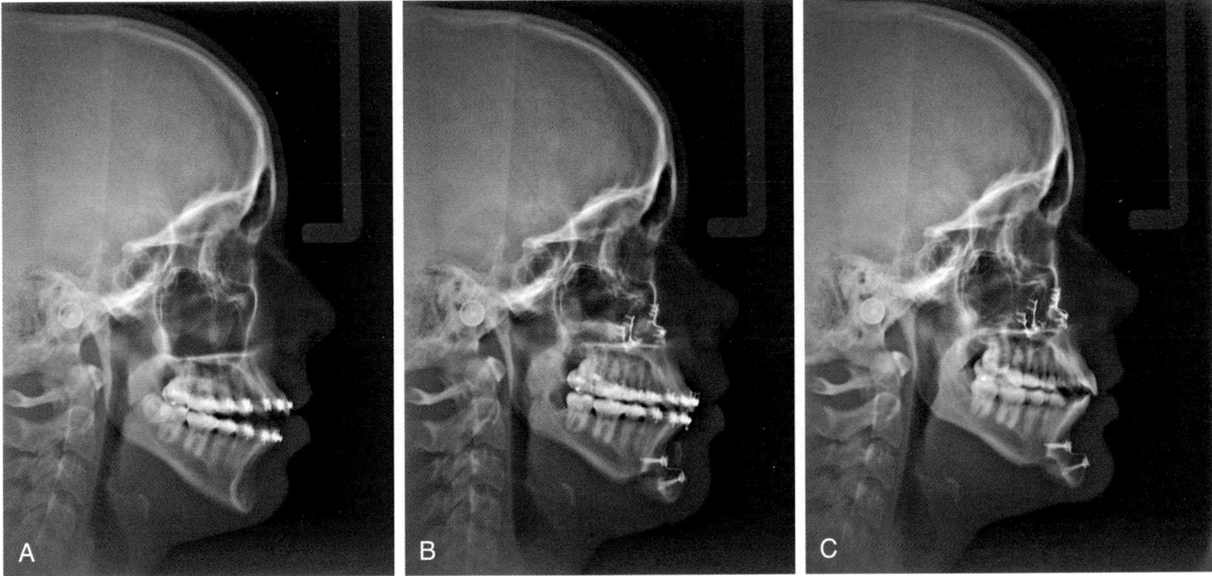

Figure 34.6 **A,** This osteotomy is foreshortened; it does not extend back into the first molar region. **B** and **C,** Immediate and 1-year postoperative X-rays, respectively.

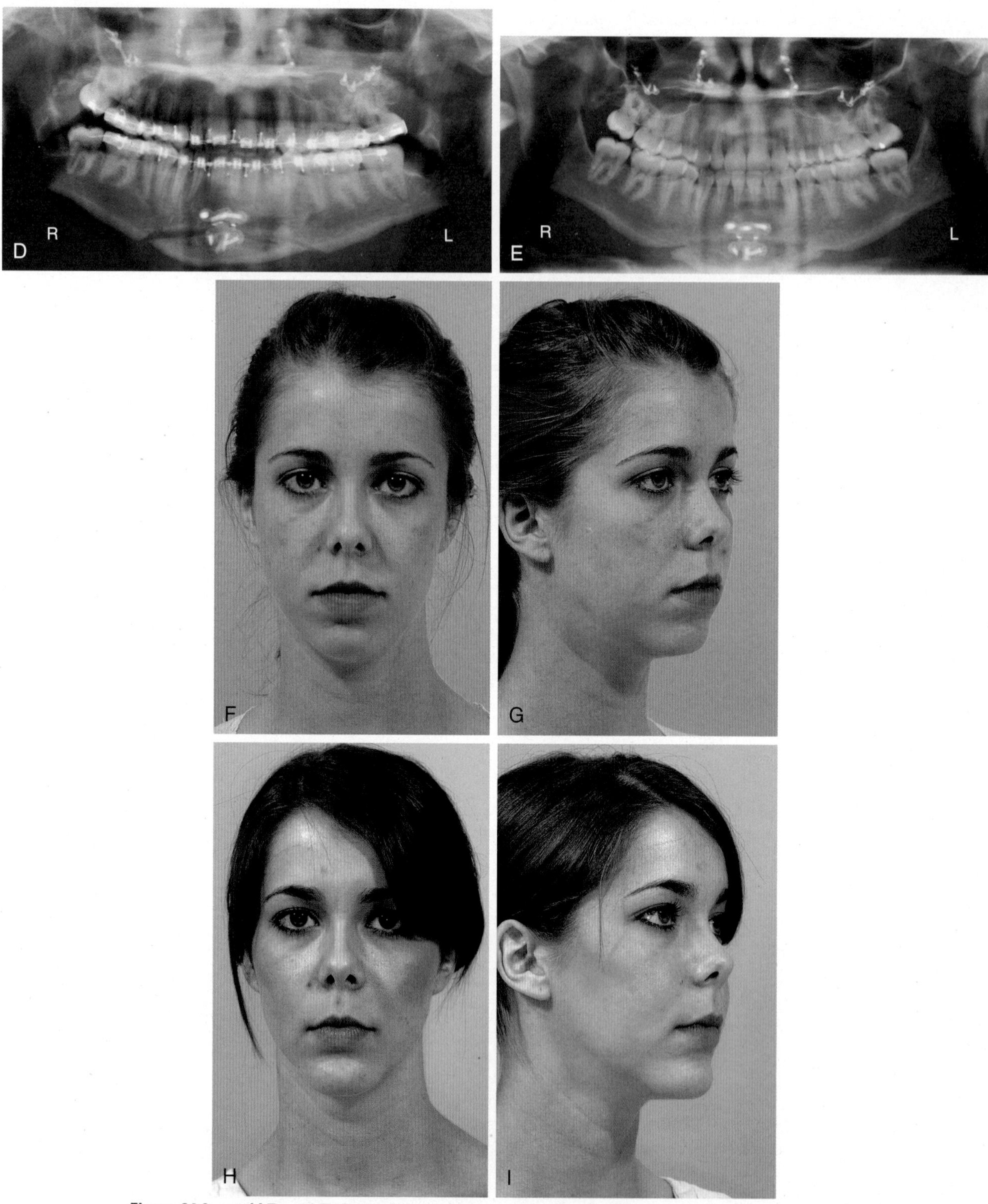

Figure 34.6, cont'd **D** and **E,** Immediate and 1-year postoperative Panorex radiographs, respectively. Note the resorption of the posterior wings of the genial segment over time, which contributes to the notching of the inferior border of the mandible. Preoperative photographs (**F** and **G**) and 1-year postoperative photographs (**H** and **I**) showing an inferior border contour defect due to the foreshortened osteotomy.

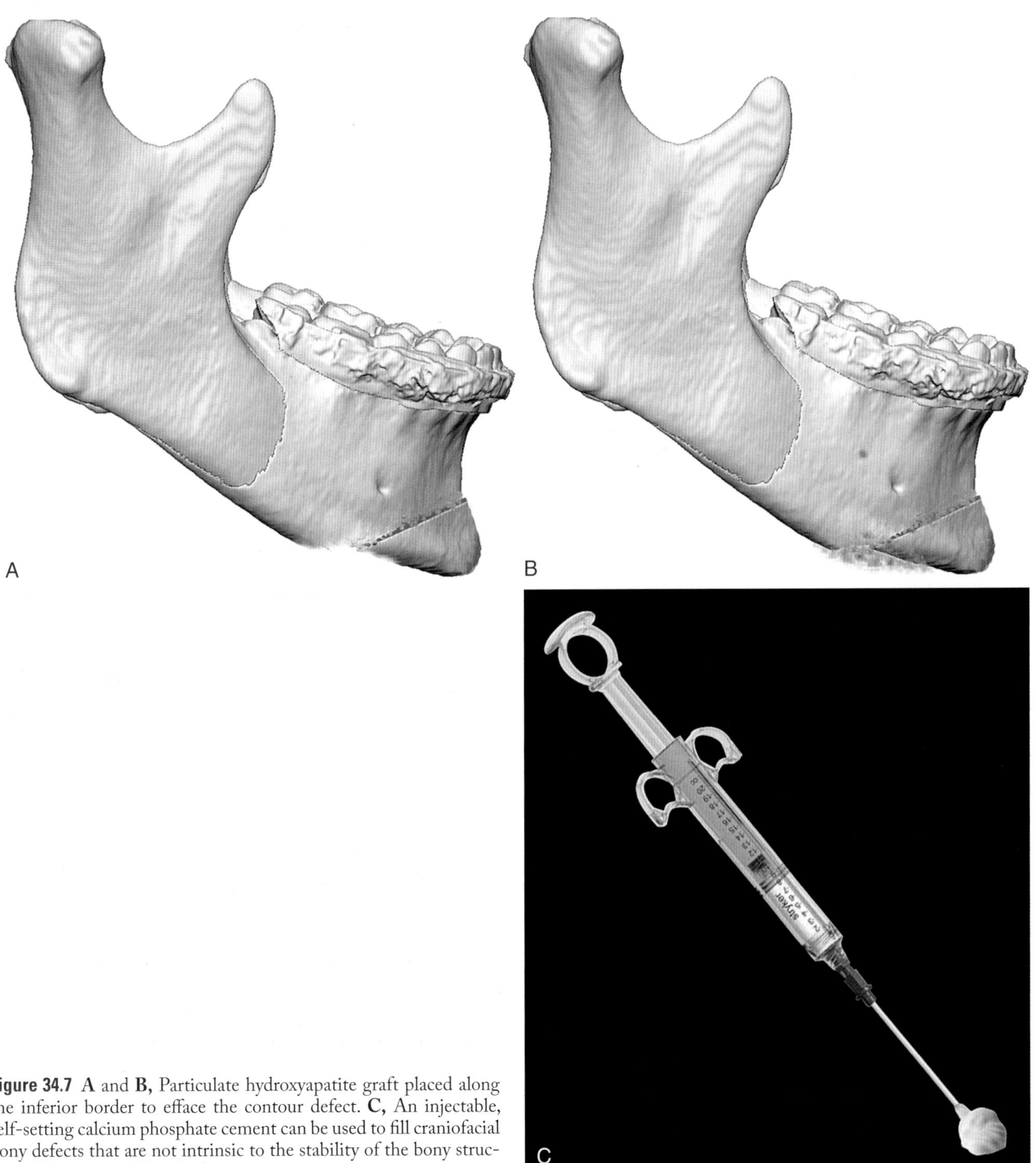

Figure 34.7 A and B, Particulate hydroxyapatite graft placed along the inferior border to efface the contour defect. C, An injectable, self-setting calcium phosphate cement can be used to fill craniofacial bony defects that are not intrinsic to the stability of the bony structure. (C, courtesy of Stryker.)

in relation to the inferior border of the mandible posterior to the mental foramen and it is not appreciated preoperatively and adjusted for during surgery. A chin that is vertically short also can contribute to the problem. It is important to review radiographs carefully before surgery to assess the position of the nerve. To minimize the risk of nerve transection, the osteotomy should be 6 mm below the mental foramen because of the inferior course of the nerve.[13,14] If the nerve is transected, a neurorrhaphy procedure using 7-0 Nurolon or Prolene suture can be attempted. However, it can be difficult to free enough of the proximal and distal segments for passive reapproximation. It may be most feasible to simply position the transected ends in close approximation to one another along the bony canal.

A hematoma on the floor of the mouth is a rare intraoperative complication.[4] It can occur with undue trauma to the floor of the mouth muscles during osteotomies.

Also, the patient may be taking anticoagulation medication (e.g., aspirin) or herbals (e.g., garlic, ginkgo). The patient also may have an undiagnosed coagulopathy. It is important to obtain a thorough history preoperatively. Also, the surgeon must avoid overinsertion of the reciprocating saw through the lingual cortex. If a hematoma is noted, it should be evacuated and the source of bleeding should be controlled. Injection of a local anesthetic with vasoconstrictor or placement of a hemostatic agent (e.g., Surgicel) is helpful for controlling bleeding. A drain also may be placed. Close postoperative airway monitoring is indicated.

To avoid chin ptosis or a "witch's chin" deformity, the surgeon should avoid excessive stripping of the mentalis muscle. Time should be taken to adequately reapproximate the mentalis muscle when closing.[15] In addition, an appropriate chin dressing should be placed as previously described to support soft tissue overlying the chin.

Postoperative Considerations

Prophylactic antibiotics and steroids are typically given preoperatively. Continued postoperative antibiotics and steroids can be considered for a short period. The patient should maintain a soft, nonchew diet for 1 to 2 weeks and then advance as tolerated. The chin dressing can be removed in 5 to 7 days.

Neurosensory deficit should be monitored and documented in a standard fashion. Testing should include two-point discrimination, static light touch, brush directional stroke, pin prick, and thermal discrimination. If there is persistent anesthesia, hyperesthesia/dysesthesia, or troublesome hypoesthesia, the patient should be offered referral for microneurosurgical repair.[16] Unless the patient has a dysesthesia, repair may offer little benefit.

Bone resorption of the posterior wing of the genial segment contributes to notching of the inferior border. One study found notching of the inferior border in 72.5% of patients.[10] If this creates an unacceptable cosmetic result, it can be corrected by grafting or implant placement. Hydroxyapatite is a good grafting material because of its biocompatibility and structural stability. HydroSet is an injectable hydroxyapatite bone substitute that can be used (see Fig. 34.7). A prejowl implant can also be placed. These are available in both silicone and porous polyethylene (Fig. 34.8). Avascular necrosis also has been reported when the chin is advanced as a free graft.[17,18] It is important to maintain as much soft tissue attachment as possible to the advanced genial segment to minimize such complications.

Pain secondary to infection or incomplete union at the osteotomy site is rare. It can occur with hardware failure or scar tissue formation along the osteotomy gap. A Panorex and/or computed tomography scan should be obtained for diagnostic purposes. Surgery should be performed to remove failed hardware. If there is incomplete union of the osteotomy gap with associated pain, reoperation may be indicated to explore the wound, debride soft tissue, and bone graft the defect. To avoid this complication, the genial segment should not be advanced beyond the point where its lingual cortex overlaps the facial cortex of the mandible. A larger osteotomy gap should be grafted to help prevent incomplete union.

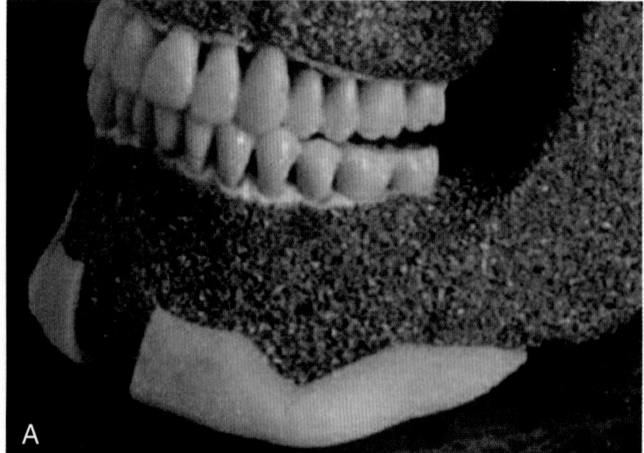

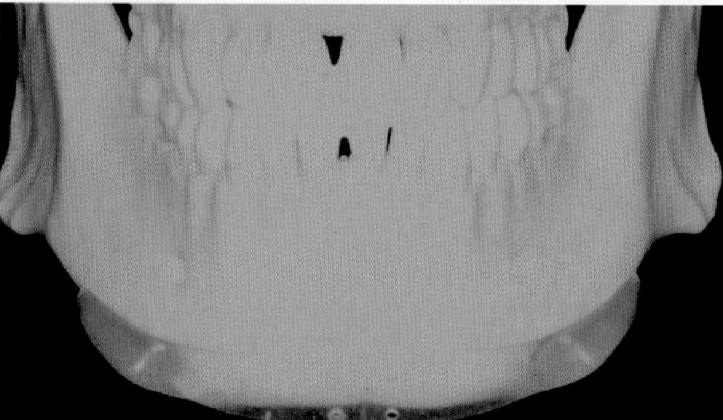

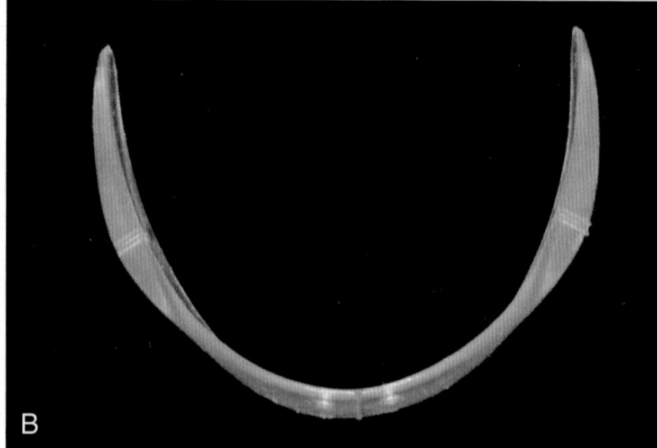

Figure 34.8 A, Medpor geniomandibular groove implant placed along the inferior border to efface a contour defect. **B,** The Mittelman Pre Jowl implant augments the prejowl sulcus without increasing chin projection. Both implants can correct a lateral inferior border contour defect of the mandible.

Alloplastic implants also can develop problems over time. These include displacement of the implant, resorption of underlying bone, and infection. Such problems can result from poor surgical technique or implant design. For instance, if the implant is not secured at the inferior border by either suturing to the periosteum or securing with bone screws, it is more prone to displace off the thicker inferior border and cause bone resorption at the superior aspect. It is also important to maintain a confined dissection and pocket along the inferior border. Resorption was more commonly seen in the past with the use of a chin button design in which the implant overlaid just the symphysis. It seems to occur less often today, with the commonly used extended chin implant design. This may be due to greater stability from wider surface distribution.[4]

Infection associated with alloplastic implants is rare. Local wound care and aggressive antibiotic therapy usually are not successful in resolving this problem because of biofilm formation on the implant surface. In most situations the implant must be removed.[3] It is important to counsel patients on the need for proactive treatment of surrounding skin infections or odontogenic infections, which, if left untreated, could eventually compromise the implant.

References

1. Trauner R, Obwegeser H. The surgical correction of mandibular prognathism and retrognathia with consideration of genioplasty. I. Surgical procedures to correct mandibular prognathism and reshaping of the chin. *Oral Surg Oral Med Oral Pathol.* 1957;10(7):677–689.
2. Converse JM, Wood-Smith D. Horizontal osteotomy of the mandible. *Plast Reconstr Surg.* 1964;34:464–471.
3. Strauss RA, Abubaker AO. Genioplasty: a case for advancement osteotomy. *J Oral Maxillofac Surg.* 2000;58(7):783–787.
4. Reed EH, Smith RG. Genioplasty: a case for alloplastic chin augmentation. *J Oral Maxillofac Surg.* 2000;58(7):788–793.
5. Binder WJ, Kamer FM, Parkes ML. Mentoplasty—a clinical analysis of alloplastic implants. *Laryngoscope.* 1981;91(3):383–391.
6. Binder WJ. Aesthetic facial implants, in cosmesis of the mouth, face and jaws. In: Guttenberg SA, ed. *Cosmesis of the Mouth, Face and Jaws.* West Sussex, UK: Wiley-Blackwell; 2012.
7. Epker BN. Alloplastic esthetic facial augmentation. In: Miloro M, ed. *Peterson's Principles of Oral and Maxillofacial Surgery.* 2nd ed. Hamilton, Ontario: Decker; 2004.
8. Reyneke JP. Systematic patient evaluation. In: Reyneke JP, ed. *Essentials of Orthognathic Surgery.* 2nd ed. Hanover Park, Illinois: Quintessence; 2010.
9. Reyneke JP. Surgical technique: genioplasty. In: Reyneke JP, ed. *Essentials of Orthognathic Surgery.* 2nd ed. Hanover Park, Illinois: Quintessence; 2010.
10. Lindquist CC, Obeid G. Complications of genioplasty done alone or in combination with sagittal split-ramus osteotomy. *Oral Surg Oral Med Oral Pathol.* 1988;66(1):13–16.
11. Matarasso A, Elias AC, Elias RL. Labial incompetence: a marker for progressive bone resorption in silastic chin augmentation. *Plast Reconstr Surg.* 1996;98(6):1007–1014.
12. McKinney P, Cunningham BL. *Aesthetic Facial Surgery.* New York, New York: Churchill Livingstone; 1992.
13. Ousterhout DK. Sliding genioplasty, avoiding mental nerve injuries. *J Craniofac Surg.* 1996;7(4):297–298.
14. Ritter EF, Moelleken BR, Mathes SJ, Ousterhout DK. The course of the inferior alveolar neurovascular canal in relation to sliding genioplasty. *J Craniofac Surg.* 1992;3(1):20–24.
15. Rubens BC, West RA. Ptosis of the chin and lip incompetence: consequences of lost mentalis muscle support. *J Oral Maxillofac Surg.* 1989;47(4):359–366.
16. Ghali GE, Epker BN. Clinical neurosensory testing: practical applications. *J Oral Maxillofac Surg.* 1989;47(10):1074–1078.
17. Ellis III E, Dechow PC, McNamara Jr JA, Carlson DS, Liskiewicz WE. Advancement genioplasty with and without soft tissue pedicle: an experimental investigation. *J Oral Maxillofac Surg.* 1984;42(10):637–645.
18. Mercuri LG, Laskin DM. Avascular necrosis after anterior horizontal augmentation genioplasty. *J Oral Surg.* 1977;35(4):296–298.

CHAPTER 35

Mandibular Subapical Osteotomies

Paulo Jose Medeiros and Fabio G. Ritto

Armamentarium

#15 Scalpel blade
Appropriate sutures
Bite block
Chisels (thin spatula and large ones)
Curved hemostats
Dietrich tissue forceps
Electrocautery
Frasier suction tip
Handpiece, #701, #702, #703 burs
Kocher's forceps
Local anesthetic with vasoconstrictor
Mallet
Metzenbaum scissors
Minnesota retractor
Needle holder
Obwegeser channel retractor
Obwegeser retractors (up, down, and ramus)
Periosteal elevator
Smith spreader
Weider retractor
Wire cutter
Wires (24 and 26 gauge)

History of the Procedure

Surgeries of the alveolar segments were probably the first techniques described to correct occlusal deformities. Kostecka[1] and Wassmund[2] were the pioneers of the technique, and other surgeons, such as Bell and Dann[3] and Kent and Hinds,[4] established details regarding indications and management. Most important, Bell and Levy,[5] Castelli et al,[6] and Hellem and Ostrup[7] studied the blood supply to the osteotomized segment. Epker[8] also pointed out important details that must be taken into consideration to avoid tooth loss and avascular necrosis, which he considered the most devastating complications.

Hofer[9] and Köle[10] were likely the first to describe the mandibular subapical osteotomy technique. They recommended operating on the models before actual surgery to achieve favorable occlusion and to fabricate the surgical splint. Hofer[9] proposed a technique to treat the prognathism with the incision located in the buccal gingiva. Harming the mental nerve was not a concern, and correction of the occlusion was limited to tilt the alveolar segment. Conversely, Köle[10] positioned the anterior incision in the vestibule so that the mobilized segment remained covered by mucosa and the nerve remained sound. The posterior portion of the incision was placed over the alveolar ridge and along the lingual gingival margin to the retromandibular triangle, with vertical extension provided medially. According to the author, this extensive incision permitted elongation of the mobilized mucosa, allowing for protrusion, and not merely tilting, of the osteotomized bone.

In 1974 MacIntosh[11] was the first to describe the total mandibular subapical osteotomy. MacIntosh recommended an extraoral approach to perform the vertical bone cut behind the last molar in cases of micrognathia complicated by limited mouth opening. In 1980 Epker and Wolford[12] described considerable improvements on this technique, combining a sagittal osteotomy with the total mandibular subapical osteotomy.

Indications for the Use of the Procedure

Mandibular subapical osteotomies are not the most common choices to treat patients with dentofacial deformity. However, the anterior subapical osteotomy is a very versatile technique that allows the osteotomized segment to be moved in different directions. It is possible to set the anterior segment backward, forward, upward, and downward, depending on the need. Also, this type of osteotomy may be performed along with a bilateral sagittal split osteotomy. According to Bell and Legan[13] and Wolford and Moenning,[14] the mandibular anterior subapical osteotomy may be indicated to (1) level the occlusion, (2) produce anteroposterior changes of the osteotomized segment, (3) correct crowding in the lower anterior arch, (4) correct anterior dentoalveolar asymmetries, (5) alter the axial inclination of the anterior teeth, (6) reduce treatment time, and (7) improve treatment stability.

As described by MacIntosh[11] in 1974, the total subapical osteotomy of the mandible was indicated primarily to treat infantile apertognathia. Other indications pointed out by MacIntosh[11] included treatment of retrognathia due to relapse of a previous ramus surgery and treatment of condylar agenesis/hypogenesis. Currently, the main indication for this technique is to correct a dentoalveolar retrusion in a "normal" mandible. With this technique, it is possible to correct an overjet discrepancy without affecting the position of the pogonion. However, the technique is extremely harmful to the inferior alveolar neurovascular bundle, often leading to dysesthesia and paresthesia. Furthermore, it poses a threat to the blood supply of the osteotomized bone.[14]

Finally, the posterior mandibular subapical osteotomy presents the single indication of repositioning an extruded posterior segment into proper relationship with the remaining occlusion, creating adequate space for esthetic and functional restoration. In the past, this osteotomy had also been indicated to close a dentoalveolar space, in the absence of a molar or premolar tooth, by advancing the mobilized segment. However, with the advance of dental implants, these absences are best treated with implant rehabilitation. Because it is necessary to detach most of the buccal mucosa to expose the bone and because of the tenacious mucosa that lies in the lingual bone in this region, there is a high risk of avascular necrosis. For these reasons, this technique should be mostly avoided.

Limitations and Contraindications

All segmental osteotomies in the maxillary bones share some potential complications, which may be mild, moderate, or severe. As proposed by Epker,[8] mild complications include periodontal defects, pulp necrosis, infection, and delayed union. Moderate complications may include infection, delayed union, and malunion. Severe complications include nonunion and tooth and/or bone loss.

Because the mandible presents a thick cortical bone, the blood supply may be threatened after soft tissue detachment. Therefore, osteotomies that involve small segments of bone, with one or two teeth mobilized, should be discouraged. Also, because the soft tissue pedicle attached to the mobilized segment is the exclusive blood supply, the more it is mobilized or manipulated surgically and the further it is repositioned, the greater the potential for detachment of the pedicle and thus compromise of its vasculature.[14]

The anterior subapical osteotomy is mostly contraindicated when the anterior mandible is short in height. In some cases, the apices of the anterior teeth, especially the canines, are close to the inferior border of the mandible, impeding the performance of the osteotomy. Even if enough space is available to complete the osteotomy, at least 1 cm of basilar bone should remain to ensure the integrity of the mandible.

TECHNIQUE: Anterior Subapical Osteotomy

STEP 1: Incision

Before the incision is made, the surgeon should inject a local anesthetic with a vasoconstrictor. This reduces both stimulus to the patient and bleeding during surgery. The incision begins toward the lip and usually extends from canine to canine, leaving at least 15 mm of mucosa attached to the gingiva. When the mentalis muscle is reached, the muscle is sectioned and the incision is directed to the bone, leaving part of the mentalis muscle attached to the mandible. This permits suturing of the muscle to avoid lip ptosis.

STEP 2: Mucoperiosteal Dissection

Bone is exposed according to how far posteriorly the osteotomy will be extended. Only enough bone to complete the osteotomy is exposed, keeping as much soft tissue attached as possible. This minimizes the risk of avascular complications. In some cases it might be necessary to expose and dissect the neurovascular bundle so that it is best protected. This can be accomplished by detaching the mucoperiosteum from around the mental foramen and making longitudinal incisions on the periosteum surrounding the nerve.

STEP 3: Osteotomy

It is essential to study the patient's tomograms carefully before performing the osteotomies. The horizontal osteotomy is made at least 5 mm below the teeth apices and should go deep enough to leave just a thin layer of bone in the lingual cortex. Care must be taken not to violate the lingual mucosa. A chisel is then used to finish the osteotomy. These distances can all be measured in the tomogram and then transferred to the surgery. If the vertical osteotomy is performed without tooth extraction, the orthodontist must separate the roots adjacent to the cut before surgery. Like the horizontal osteotomy, the vertical cuts should leave a thin layer of bone in the lingual cortex, and the final separation is achieved with a thin chisel. If the mental foramen is close to the osteotomy cut, it may be necessary to reposition the neurovascular bundle (Fig. 35.1A).

If extractions are planned and the space is closed with posterior positioning of the anterior segment (Fig. 35.1B–E), special care must be taken not to remove excessive bone. After the anterior segment has been mobilized and placed to the occlusal splint, final bone interferences are removed. Spending time removing interferences at this time is safer than trying to remove large amounts of bone initially. Absence of bone between teeth may result either in periodontal defect or in poor bone contact, which may jeopardize bone healing and affect stability.

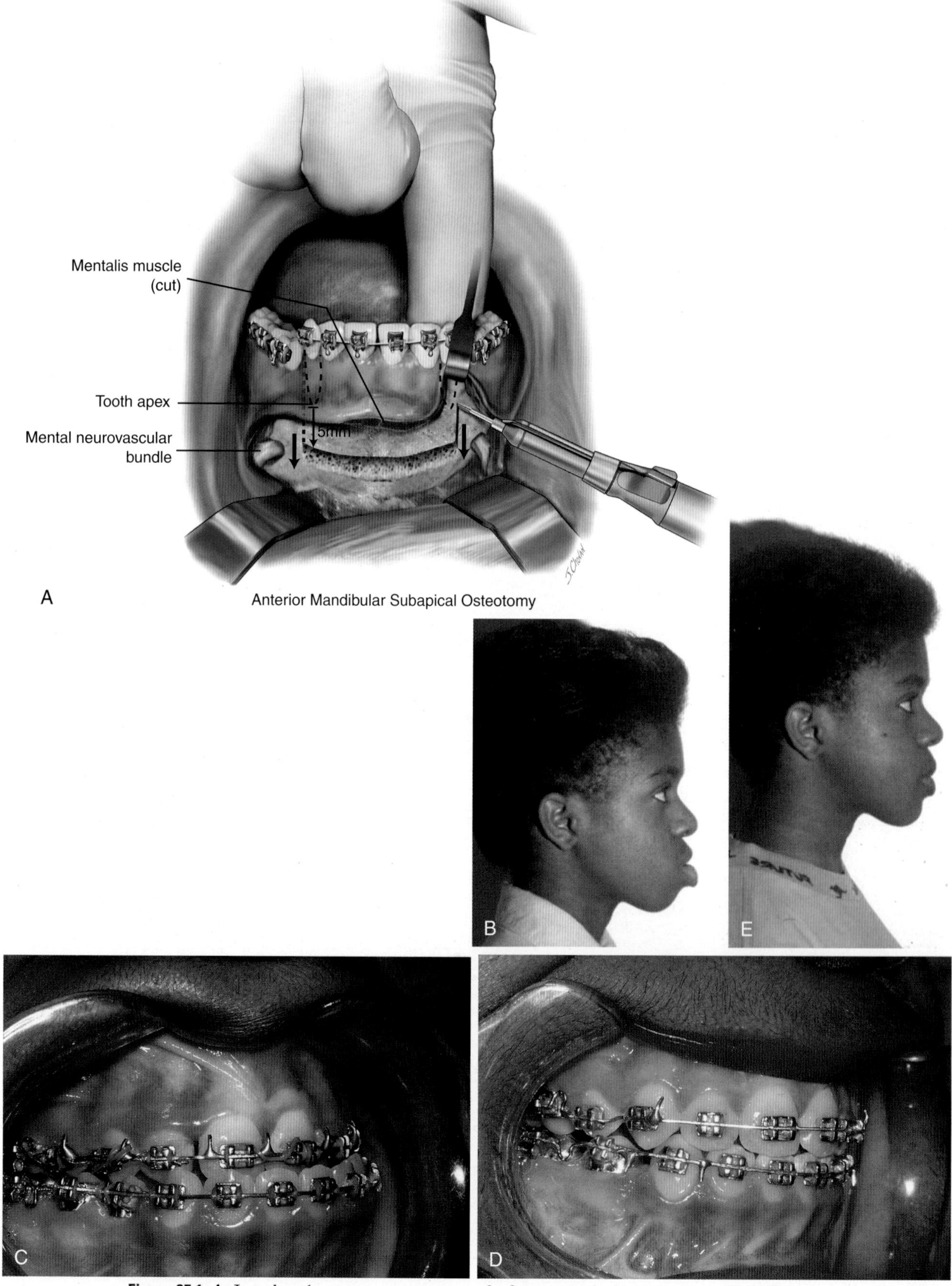

Figure 35.1 **A,** Interdental osteotomy positioning of a finger over the lingual mucosa. **B–E,** The patient underwent an anterior subapical osteotomy for posterior repositioning of the anterior segment of the mandible.

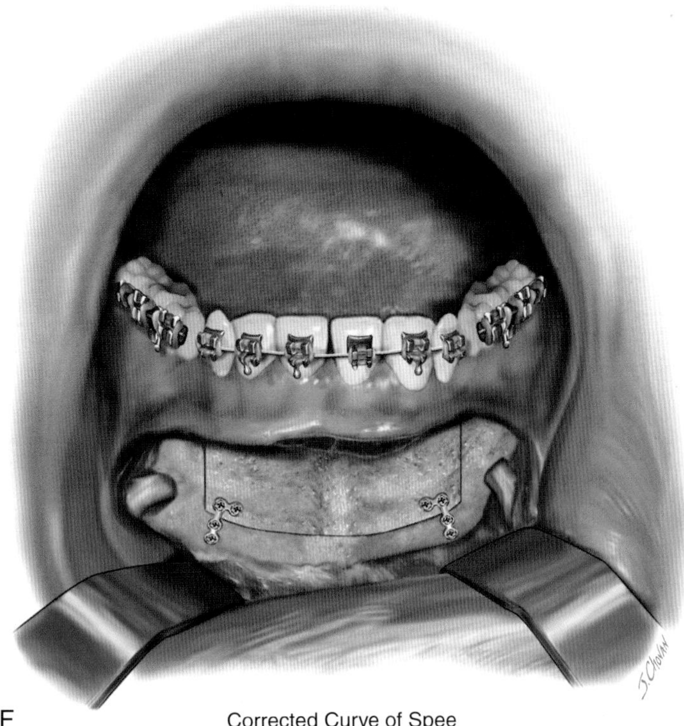

Figure 35.1, cont'd F, Fixation of the osteotomy with two L-shaped plates.

TECHNIQUE: Anterior Subapical Osteotomy—cont'd

STEP 4: Fixation

Although it may be easy to accomplish the anterior subapical osteotomies, fixating the anterior segment to its new position can be quite challenging. This happens because it may be necessary to remove large amounts of interference, especially when the purpose of the surgery is to correct the curve of Spee. After all bone interference has been removed, a prefabricated occlusal splint is placed to recompose the inferior arch. Fixation is then accomplished with two L-shaped titanium plates of the 1.6-mm system (Fig. 35.1F). In most cases it also is advisable to position a 26-gauge bridle wire around the teeth adjacent to the osteotomy in the cervical region. This controls the tension over the osteotomized segment and allows early removal of the acrylic splint. Removal of the acrylic splint makes the occlusion easier to control and facilitates oral hygiene.

STEP 5: Suture

Closure begins in the muscular layer with suturing of the mentalis muscles. This is very important to avoid labial ptosis. At least three sutures are placed in the muscular tissue. Suturing of the mucosa must begin by reapproximating the midline to avoid creating labial asymmetries. The remnant mucosa then is closed with continuous suture. A pressure dressing is applied to hold the lip and soft chin up and is kept in place for 5 to 7 days.

TECHNIQUE: Total Subapical Osteotomy

STEP 1: Incision

Before the incision is made, a local anesthetic with a vasoconstrictor should be injected. This reduces both stimulus to the patient and bleeding during surgery. The anterior part of the incision is the same as described previously for the anterior subapical osteotomy. This incision is extended posteriorly to the middle of the ascending ramus bilaterally.

STEP 2: Mucoperiosteal Dissection

After the symphysis has been exposed, dissection continues posteriorly to expose the whole body of the mandible. The mental neurovascular bundle is detached from the periosteum with longitudinal incisions through the periosteum. The coronoid process is almost fully exposed with the aid of a ramus Obwegeser retractor, and the medial periosteum is exposed to reveal the lingula; in this way, the mandibular foramen can be located. As much soft tissue as possible should be kept attached to the lateral part of the ramus.

STEP 3: Osteotomy

Before the osteotomy is performed, it is important to register a vertical reference from the pogonion to a landmark in the maxilla. The whole alveolar process with teeth will be mobilized; therefore, the surgeon must know the vertical position of the mandible so that the final facial height is the same as planned. Careful analysis of the tomogram also is important to measure the height of the inferior alveolar neurovascular bundle in the body of the mandible. In some cases there is a comfortable distance between the nerve and the basilar bone, and the horizontal osteotomy can be performed with minimal risk to the nerve. However, in most cases it is advisable to expose the bundle by removing the external cortex along the canal. This exposure can be safely performed with a #701 bur. One linear osteotomy is made superior and one inferior to the alveolar inferior canal, from the retromolar region to the mental foramen anteriorly. These lines should be parallel to each other and deep enough to cut the buccal cortex. After completion, the osteotomy lines are united with perpendicular ostectomies anteriorly and posteriorly, also through the buccal cortex. Additional perpendicular lines can be made to facilitate the removal of the buccal cortical bone with a chisel to expose the neurovascular bundle (Fig. 35.2A). All the bone removed from the lateral cortex must be kept in a physiologic solution in case grafting is necessary after the segment has been positioned.

When the exposure is complete, the bundle should be released from the canal only if it is in the path of or very close to the osteotomy. Horizontal osteotomies can then be performed either with a bur or a saw, beginning anteriorly in the symphysis and proceeding to the last molar. At least 1 cm of bone should remain in the inferior border to minimize the risk of fracture. While performing the horizontal cut, the surgeon must place a finger in the floor of the mouth to feel the lingual cortical bone so that the bone can be cut without harming the lingual mucosa. Final osteotomy of the lingual cortex may be accomplished with a chisel (Fig. 35.2B).

Ramus osteotomy begins in the lingual cortex with a horizontal osteotomy, similar to the sagittal ramus osteotomy. After detachment of the coronoid process is complete, a Kocher forceps is used to keep soft tissue retracted. A periosteal elevator is placed subperiosteally to expose the lingula, and a reciprocating saw is used to cut the medial cortex of the ramus just superior and posterior to the lingula and parallel to the occlusal plane. It is important to position the saw at a 45-degree angle to the medial surface of the ramus so that it will be easier to cut only the lingual cortex, preserving the buccal cortex. This sagittal cut runs until it meets the subapical cut.

A large chisel is used to lever the distal segment and complete the subapical osteotomy. Excessive force must be avoided so that the inferior border of the mandible remains sound. In the medial ramus, the split may be completed with the aid of a sagittal split Smith spreader. After the distal segment has been mobilized, additional mobilization may be necessary to complete the desired movement. Once the split is complete, a prefabricated acrylic splint is placed to guide the movement.

When this technique was first described by MacIntosh,[11] the posterior osteotomy was performed just posterior to the last molar, in a vertical direction. However, this vertical osteotomy carries greater risk to the inferior alveolar neurovascular bundle, either during the bone cut or after mobilization of the segment.

STEP 4: Fixation

After intermaxillary fixation has been performed, with or without a final splint in position, the vertical reference measured at the beginning of the procedure is checked to see whether it matches the preplanned position. Mandibular condyles must be seated in the glenoid fossa without extreme force. This can be accomplished with a tripod support, with the surgeon's thumb positioned over the patient's chin, and the first and second fingers over the mandibular angle bilaterally; the surgeon then pushes the mandible backward and upward until it reaches the preplanned vertical height (Fig. 35.2C).

In a total subapical osteotomy, it is advisable to use a 2-mm plate system because the whole mandible must be secured. One double-T-shaped plate is placed in each side of the mandibular body, posterior to the mental foramen, and one L-shaped plate is placed on each side, between the mental foramina (Fig. 35.2D).

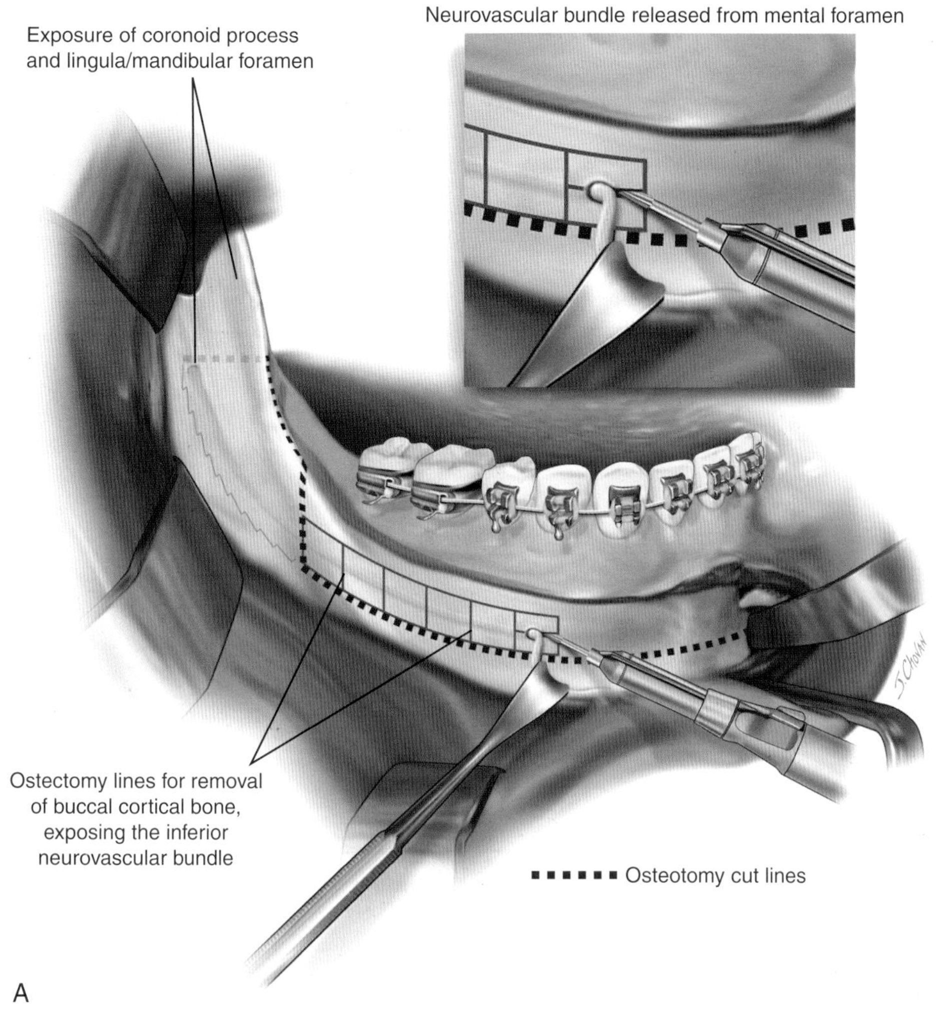

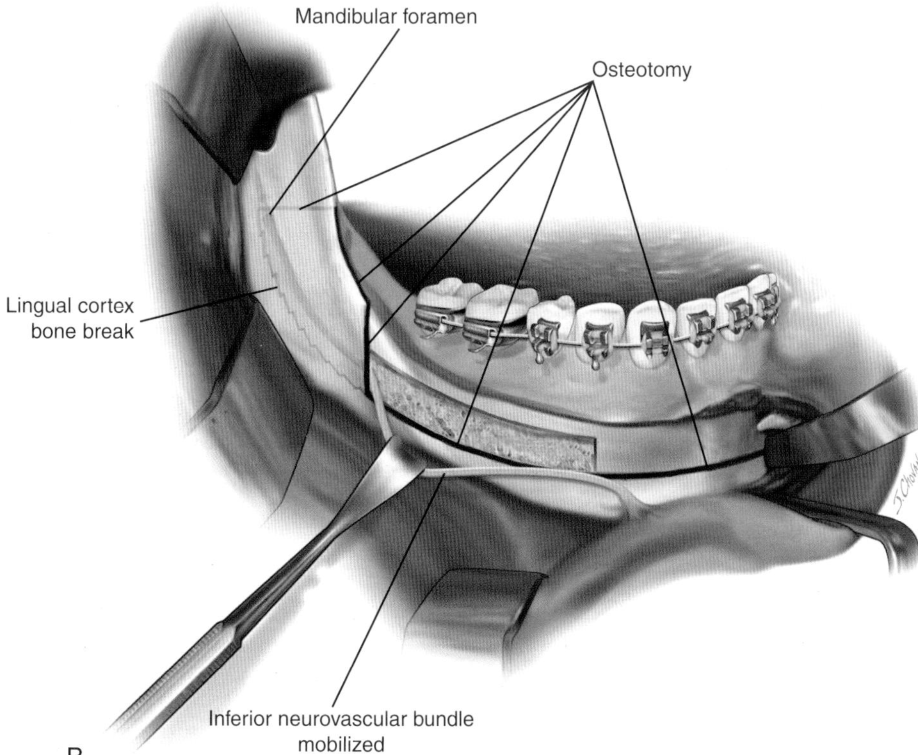

Figure 35.2 **A,** Removal of the labial cortex to visualize the nerve. **B,** Dissection of the nerve out of the canal.

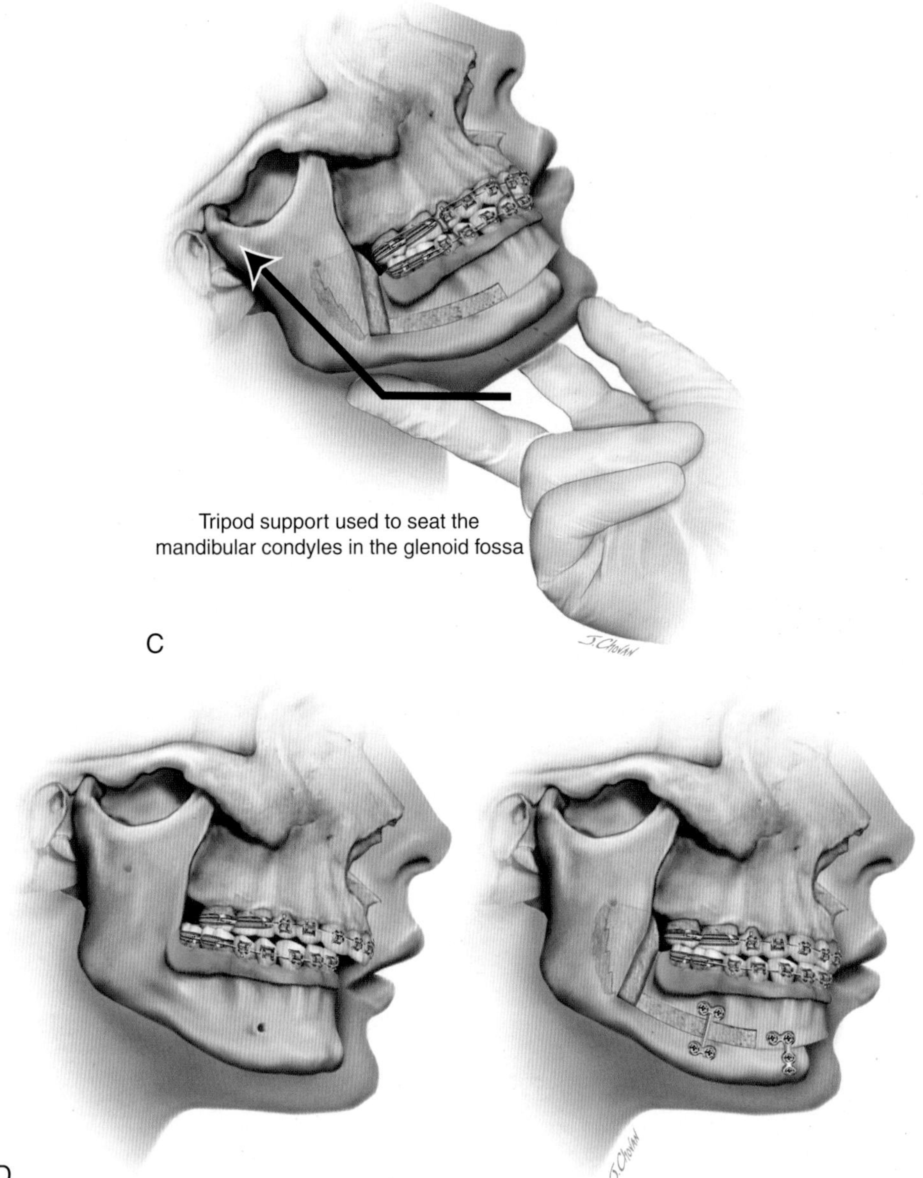

Figure 35.2, cont'd C, Positioning of the proximal segment, which involves gently pushing the condyles upward and backward. **D,** Fixation and profile changes.

TECHNIQUE: Total Subapical Osteotomy—cont'd

STEP 5: Suture

Closure begins in the muscular layer with suturing of the mentalis muscles. This is very important to avoid labial ptosis. At least three sutures are placed in the muscular tissue. Suturing of the mucosa must begin with reapproximation of the midline to avoid creating labial asymmetries. The remnant mucosa is then closed with continuous suture. If a graft is used, a two-plane suture should be performed, beginning in the muscular layer and finishing with a continuous suture of the mucosa. A pressure dressing is applied in the anterior region to hold the lip and soft chin up and is kept in place for 5 to 7 days.

TECHNIQUE: Posterior Subapical Osteotomy

STEP 1: Incision

Before the incision is made, a local anesthetic with vasoconstrictor should be injected. This reduces both stimulus to the patient and bleeding during surgery. The incision begins in the mucosa below the gingiva, leaving at least 10 mm of soft tissue attached to the segment to be mobilized. The incision should be extended anteriorly enough to expose the mental neurovascular bundle and posteriorly enough to expose the nerve posterior to the last molar.

STEP 2: Mucoperiosteal Dissection

Care must be taken to avoid unnecessary soft tissue detachment from the mobilized segment. This minimizes the risk of avascular complications. The mental foramen and the inferior border of the mandible are exposed.

STEP 3: Osteotomy

It is essential to study the patient's tomograms carefully before performing the osteotomies. The horizontal osteotomy is made approximately 5 mm below the teeth apices and should go deep enough to leave just a thin layer of bone in the lingual cortex to avoid violating the lingual mucosa. A chisel is then used to finish the osteotomy. These distances can all be measured in the tomogram and then transferred to the surgery. If the vertical osteotomy is performed without extraction of teeth, the orthodontist must separate the roots adjacent to the cut before surgery. Like the horizontal cut, the vertical osteotomy should leave a thin layer of bone in the lingual cortex. The final separation is achieved with a thin chisel.

The position of the inferior alveolar neurovascular bundle, determined previously by computed tomography (CT) scan, determines whether the horizontal osteotomy is performed superior or inferior to the canal. In a few cases, enough space is available below the apices to perform the horizontal osteotomy above the canal without risk to the nerve. In most cases, however, it is advisable to expose the neurovascular bundle by removing the lateral cortex. This removal is initiated with a bur, to cut the lateral cortex, and it should be completed with chisels. The cut usually is extended a few millimeters posterior to the last molar to facilitate the procedure. All the bone removed from the lateral cortex must be kept in a physiologic solution in case grafting is necessary after positioning of the segment.

After this window has been opened and the bundle dissected out of the mandible, the horizontal osteotomy can be performed safely. While making the horizontal cut, the surgeon must place a finger in the floor of the mouth to feel the lingual cortical bone to ensure that it is cut without harming the lingual mucosa. The final osteotomy of the lingual cortex may be accomplished with a chisel.

An anterior vertical cut is made between the roots of adjacent teeth either with a #701 bur in a handpiece or with a sagittal saw. Adjacent teeth must have been previously separated by orthodontic mechanics. A posterior vertical osteotomy is performed at least 5 mm posterior to the last molar. This keeps a large amount of soft tissue attached to the mobilized segment and prevents periodontal defects around the last molar.

The final split may be accomplished by levering the segment with a chisel; care must be taken not to break the inferior border by using excessive force. An additional osteotomy is performed in the fixed portion to accommodate the necessary movement of the mobilized segment (Fig. 35.3).

STEP 4: Fixation

Making the posterior subapical osteotomy cut may be difficult, and fixating the mobilized segment in its new position may be even more difficult. This is because interference must be removed to accommodate the segment in its new position because the main purpose of this procedure is to intrude the posterior segment. After all bone interference has been removed, a prefabricated occlusal splint is placed to recompose the inferior arch. The fixation is then accomplished with one X-shaped plate of the 2-mm system.

STEP 5: Suture

Suturing may be performed in either one or two planes. If a graft is used, it is preferable to perform two-plane suturing, beginning in the muscular layer and finishing with a continuous suturing of the mucosa.

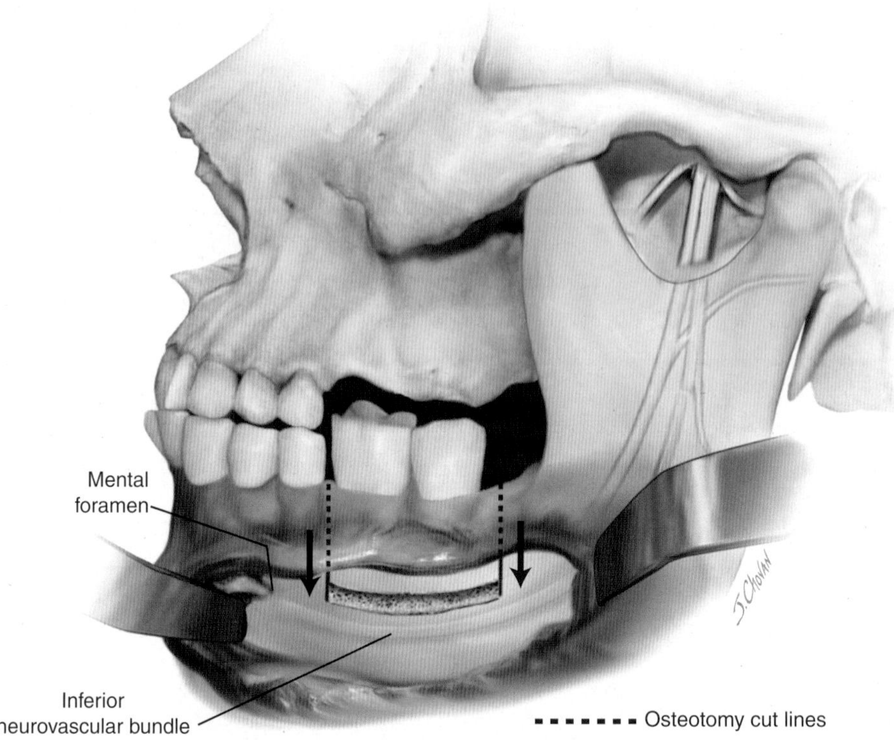

Figure 35.3 Posterior subapical osteotomy to intrude the segment.

ALTERNATIVE TECHNIQUE: Combined Sagittal Split Osteotomy and Reduction Genioplasty

Total mandibular subapical osteotomy has a very specific indication, which is to position the alveolar segment anteriorly while keeping the pogonion in the same position. However, this is a very sensitive technique that poses considerable risk to the inferior alveolar neurovascular bundle. Therefore, in some cases, especially when the inferior alveolar nerve is positioned close to the mandibular inferior border, it is best to perform a sagittal split osteotomy of the mandible for advancement, combined with a genioplasty to set the chin back. This approach maintains the pogonion in its original position. Some may argue that a setback genioplasty produces an excess of tissue in the submental region, which may be unesthetic. This is not always true, as shown in Fig. 35.4, because the pogonion is not retruded in these cases, but rather kept in the presurgical position. If the procedure results in an unesthetic excess of tissue in the submental region, liposuction can be performed to resolve this issue.

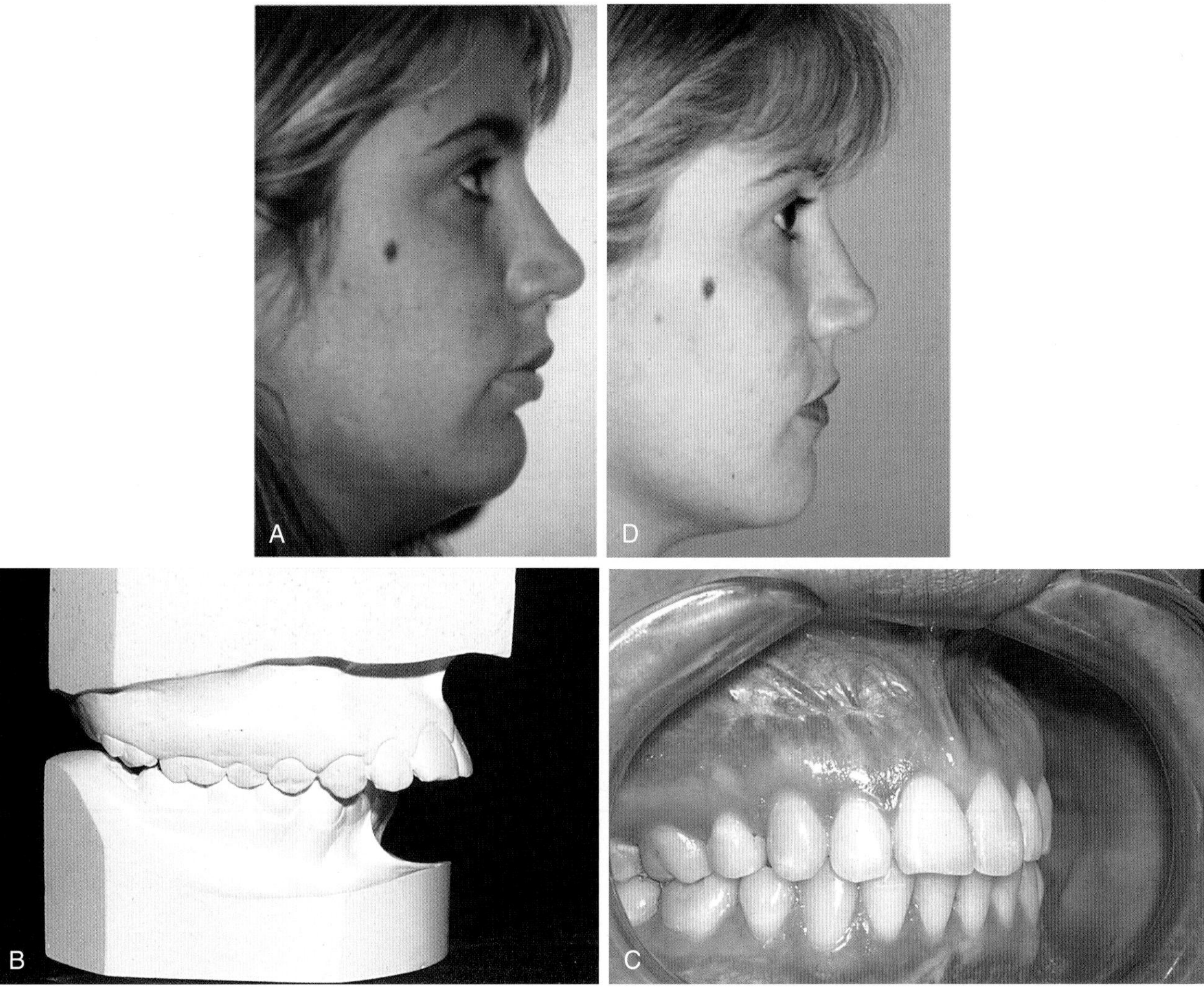

Figure 35.4 **A–D,** A class II patient underwent a bilateral sagittal split-ramus osteotomy to advance the mandible, in addition to genioplasty to retrude the chin.

Avoidance and Management of Intraoperative Complications

Several intraoperative complications can arise with mandibular subapical osteotomies.

- Tooth damage. There must be adequate space between roots to perform the interdental osteotomy safely. The orthodontist must separate the teeth by 2 to 3 mm, and only a fine chisel should be used in the crestal bone. Also, at least 5 mm of sound bone should be left between teeth apices and the inferior horizontal osteotomy.
- Nerve damage. Dissection of the mental nerve from the periosteum facilitates visualization and permits moving of the nerve anteriorly or posteriorly to protect it from the bur during the osteotomy. It is of outmost importance to study the CT scan and measure the distance to the inferior alveolar neurovascular bundle along the path of the osteotomy. It is also important to observe the proximity of the neurovascular bundle to the buccal or lingual cortical bone during its intraosseous path.
- Fracture of the inferior border of the mandible. Although rare, this fracture may occur when the teeth apices are close to the inferior border. Reconstruction plates are best applied to fixate the fractured segments and recompose the inferior border continuity. After repair, surgery continues in the usual sequence.

Postoperative Considerations

Early removal of the occlusal splint should always be the goal. This facilitates oral hygiene and allows more reliable occlusal control by the surgeon. With anterior subapical osteotomies, this can be safely accomplished by using the bridle wire in the tension zone and also by early placement of a continuous orthodontic wire.

References

1. Kostecka F. Surgical correction of protrusion of the lower and upper jaws. *J Am Dent Assoc.* 1928;12:362.
2. Wassmund M. *Frakturen und Luxationen des Gesichtsschgdels.* Leipzig, Germany: Hermann Meusser; 1927.
3. Bell WH, Dann JJ. Correction of dentofacial deformities by surgery in the anterior part of the jaws. *Am J Orthod.* 1973;64(2):162–187.
4. Kent JN, Hinds E. Management of dental facial deformities by anterior alveolar surgery. *J Oral Surg.* 1971;29(1):13–26.
5. Bell WH, Levy BM. Revascularization and bone healing after anterior mandibular osteotomy. *J Oral Surg.* 1970;28(3):196–203.
6. Castelli WA, Nasjleti CE, Díaz-Pérez R. Interruption of the arterial inferior alveolar flow and its effects on mandibular collateral circulation and dental tissues. *J Dent Res.* 1975;54(4):708–715.
7. Hellem S, Ostrup LT. Normal and retrograde blood supply to the body of the mandible in the dog. II. The role played by periosteo-medullary and symphyseal anastomoses. *Int J Oral Surg.* 1981;10(1):31–42.
8. Epker BN. Vascular considerations in orthognathic surgery. I. Mandibular osteotomies. *Oral Surg Oral Med Oral Pathol.* 1984;57(5):467–472.
9. Hofer O. Operation der prognathie und mikrogenie. *Deutsche Zahn Mund Kieferh.* 1942;9:121.
10. Köle H. Surgical operations on the alveolar ridge to correct occlusal abnormalities. *Oral Surg Oral Med Oral Pathol.* 1959;12(3):277–288.
11. MacIntosh RB. Total mandibular alveolar osteotomy. Encouraging experiences with an infrequently indicated procedure. *J Maxillofac Surg.* 1974;2(4):210–218.
12. EpkerBN,WolfordLM.eds.Mandibularosteotomies. In: Dentofacial Deformities: Surgical-Orthodontic Correction. St Louis, Missouri: Mosby; 1980.
13. Bell WH, Jacobs JD, Legan HL. Treatment of class II deep bite by orthodontic and surgical means. *Am J Orthod.* 1984;85(1):1–20.
14. Wolford LM, Moenning JE. Diagnosis and treatment planning for mandibular subapical osteotomies with new surgical modifications. *Oral Surg Oral Med Oral Pathol.* 1989;68(5):541–550.

CHAPTER 36

Intraoral Vertical Ramus Osteotomy

Samuel J. McKenna and James B. Lewallen

Armamentarium

#9 Periosteal elevator
Curved Freer elevator
#15 Scalpel blade
28-Gauge wire
Appropriate sutures
Bauer retractors
Langenbeck retractors
Laryngeal/mirror or 30-degree endoscope
Local anesthetic with vasoconstrictor
Oscillating saw, 11.5 × 7-mm blade
Ramus-measuring instrument
Rotary handpiece, 4-mm round bur
Kerrison rongeur

History of the Procedure

Efforts to shorten the mandible to correct mandibular excess and/or mandibular asymmetry have produced a variety of osteotomy designs and surgical instrumentation. Limberg[1] described the oblique subcondylar osteotomy in 1925. Subsequently, Moose[2–4] and others described intraoral procedures for mandibular reduction. The vertical ramus osteotomy popularized in 1954 by Caldwell and Letterman[5] required an extraoral approach. The sagittal split ramus osteotomy (SSO) described by Trauner and Obwegeser[6] in 1957 was the first intraoral ramus osteotomy that permitted mandibular reduction. In 1968, Winstanley[7] reported the first intraoral vertical ramus osteotomy (IVRO), performed with a dental drill. A significant advance in the IVRO technique was reported by Herbert et al.[8] in 1970 with the use of the motorized oscillating saw. The work of Hall et al.[9] and Hall and McKenna[10] in the 1970s further popularized the procedure, and Hall's work in the 1980s helped quantify clinical outcomes and proposed technique refinements to minimize proximal segment "sag." Usually described without internal fixation with the advent of right-angle instrumentation transoral internal fixation of IVRO is a straightforward modification when indicated.

Indications for the Use of the Procedure

IVRO is indicated for the management of horizontal mandibular excess.[11] Small distal segment advancement (less than 2 mm) and mandibular asymmetry may also be managed with IVRO.[12]

For symptomatic temporomandibular disorder, IVRO may be preferred over SSO because the condyle is passively positioned, with little opportunity to place the condyle in an unphysiological position. Experience with modified mandibular condylotomy suggests that IVRO may actually improve joint symptoms.[13–17] Importantly, this benefit may not be realized with internal fixation of IVRO. Temporomandibular symptoms should be considered in the decision to internally fixate IVRO. For the patient whose livelihood depends on normal lower lip sensation (e.g., professional use of a wind instrument) IVRO has a distinct advantage over SSO because of the very low incidence of inferior alveolar nerve dysfunction.[18,19]

Limitations and Contraindications

Early critics of IVRO highlighted unpredictable stability. Hall and McKenna[10] described "condylar sag" caused by stripping of the masseter and medial pterygoid muscles, which led to a 14% incidence of open bite at the time of maxillomandibular fixation (MMF) release. Subsequently, these researchers described a modification of the IVRO technique to preserve medial pterygoid attachment to the condylar segment.[10] IVRO should be used cautiously when vertical ramus lengthening is planned. Vertical ramus lengthening, as with two-jaw surgery and counterclockwise rotation of the maxillomandibular complex, creates a distracting force on the proximal segment predisposing to condylar sag and skeletal instability. When used for small mandibular advancement, distal segment advancement is less likely to result in condylar sag with simultaneous vertical ramus shortening. Vertical ramus shortening encourages condylar seating (and forward rotation of the proximal segment). Concerns regarding condylar sag from excessive medial pterygoid stripping or vertical ramus lengthening can be managed with internal fixation if the proximal segment is of sufficient size to accommodate screw placement.

In general, up to 10 mm of mandibular setback is possible with IVRO. If the posterior movement of the distal segment exceeds the width of the medial pterygoid attachment, there will be little or no remaining proximal segment medial pterygoid attachment. This promotes condylar sag and even condylar subluxation due to unopposed lateral pterygoid activity. This scenario can be managed with internal fixation, providing the proximal segment width is sufficient for plate and screw application. Conversely, if insufficient medial pterygoid muscle is stripped from the proximal segment, backward rotation of the segment occurs as the distal segment is positioned into the new posterior position, predisposing to postoperative forward relapse. Greater mandibular setbacks require more proximal segment trimming to obtain close and passive apposition of the overlapping segments. For this reason, SSO may be preferable for the larger mandibular setbacks. Finally, with larger setbacks, collision between the coronoid process and the proximal segment may require coronoidectomy.

Although readily achievable with a right-angle drill and screw systems, internal fixation is more technically sensitive with IVRO than SSO. This is particularly true in cases where the ramus curves medially at the posterior border and is more difficult to visualize. Successful internal fixation is dependent on creating a proximal segment of sufficient width to accommodate 2-mm screws. Without internal fixation, IVRO requires 2 to 3 weeks of MMF followed by 3 to 4 weeks of training elastic use.

Finally, with two-jaw surgery where the surgeon elects to perform mandibular surgery first, SSO may provide superior osteotomy stability due to the likely greater load-sharing nature of SSO internal fixation than IVRO internal fixation. In general, adherence to the above principles permits good long-term stability with IVRO.[19–22]

TECHNIQUE: Intraoral Vertical Ramus Osteotomy

STEP 1: Incision/Subperiosteal Dissection

Nasoendotracheal intubation is required. Local anesthetic with epinephrine is infiltrated in the region of the external oblique ridge. Access to the ramus is through a ramus-exposing incision positioned 3 to 5 mm lateral to the mucogingival junction extending from the level of the occlusal plane anteriorly to the first molar. A generous subperiosteal pocket is developed, exposing the antegonial notch, inferior border, and lateral ramus to the level of the sigmoid notch. The periosteal flap is further released by stripping the temporalis tendon from the anterior border of the mandible. If internal fixation is not planned, the posterior ramus periosteum and the most tenacious attachment of the masseter muscle at the angle should be preserved. Use of the Levasseur-Merrill retractor is discouraged because placement requires posterior border stripping. A Bauer retractor is placed into the sigmoid notch. A second Bauer retractor may be placed at the inferior border, although a single Bauer retractor is sufficient. If the subperiosteal pocket is so tight that the Bauer retractor cannot be rotated to expose the lateral ramus, additional stripping of the temporalis tendon will provide greater laxity of the pocket.

STEP 2: Determination of the Osteotomy's Location

Once exposed, the lateral ramus is inspected. A useful landmark is the antelingular prominence, the lateral bony protuberance that approximates the position of the lingula.[23,24] Using the oscillating saw and the 11.5 × 7-mm blade, a trial osteotomy in marked 7 to 8 mm anterior to the posterior border of the mandible at the level of the mandibular foramen. If the osteotomy is within or anterior to the antelingular prominence, the mandibular foramen or canal may be violated (Fig. 36.1A). The osteotomy position is verified with a ramus-measuring instrument or severely curved freer. Direct visualization of the osteotomy and ramus measuring instrument is not often possible, and visualization with a laryngeal mirror or 30-degree endoscope is often necessary. With preoperative computed tomography (CT) imaging, the distance from the posterior border of the mandible to the mandibular foramen can be measured allowing placement of the osteotomy as far anterior as possible. Finally, with virtual surgical planning and 3D printing, a custom cutting guide can be fabricated to facilitate optimal osteotomy placement.

STEP 3: Completion of the Superior Osteotomy

With the location of the osteotomy confirmed, the oscillating blade is reinserted into the trial osteotomy and the osteotomy is extended through medial cortex. If the 11.5 × 7-mm blade is too short to complete the osteotomy through the medial cortex, the trial osteotomy is likely too far anterior and the anterior-posterior position should be reconfirmed. The cutting edge of the blade is then directed cephalad with the shaft of the blade resting against the lateral ramus. Alternatively, the inferior osteotomy can be completed first. The cutting teeth of the saw should be lightly applied, with back-and-forth rotations of the motor shaft resulting in "chattering" of the blade. As the sigmoid notch is approached, the blade depth is decreased to accommodate the thinning ramus and minimize trauma to structures medial to the ramus.

TECHNIQUE: Intraoral Vertical Ramus Osteotomy—cont'd

STEP 4: Completion of the Inferior Osteotomy

Without removing the blade from the osteotomy, the blade is repositioned and directed toward the inferior aspect of the superior osteotomy. The upper Bauer retractor is removed and the lower Bauer is inserted at the inferior border of the mandible. The osteotomy may be performed with both Bauer retractors in place; however, the oscillating saw handpiece/motor adequately retracts the flap as the inferior osteotomy is developed. Because of the slight outward flare of the oscillating blade there is a tendency for the inferior osteotomy to migrate posteriorly. Therefore, as the osteotomy progresses, the distance from the blade to the posterior border is monitored. It is important to preserve as much proximal segment width as possible. This will preserve medial pterygoid attachment when internal fixation is not planned, and sufficient proximal segment width for plate/screw placement when internal fixation is planned. One of the most common technical errors is a posteriorly directed inferior osteotomy creating a narrow and short proximal segment with little medial pterygoid attachment and insufficient bone stock for internal fixation. When determining whether sufficient medial pterygoid attachment will be preserved, it is important to consider the amount of planned setback and segment overlap. Virtual planning methods are helpful for visualizing the magnitude of overlap. The greater the setback, the more anterior the inferior osteotomy should be directed. Greater setback/overlap also requires more proximal segment trimming which may leave insufficient bone stock for internal fixation. If the inferior osteotomy trajectory is too posterior, the blade should be re-directed more anteriorly (Fig. 36.1B).

Once the inferior osteotomy is complete, the surgeon verifies that the osteotomy is complete by confirming that the proximal segment can be moved lateral to the distal segment for the entire length of the osteotomy. The most common area for an incomplete osteotomy is at the sigmoid notch and/or mid-ramus. If the 11.5 × 7-mm blade is too short to complete the osteotomy at the mid-ramus region, the 11.5 × 12-mm blade can be used cautiously to complete the medial cortex osteotomy. Great care should be taken with the longer blade to avoid injury to structures medial to the ramus (Fig. 36.1B).

Continued

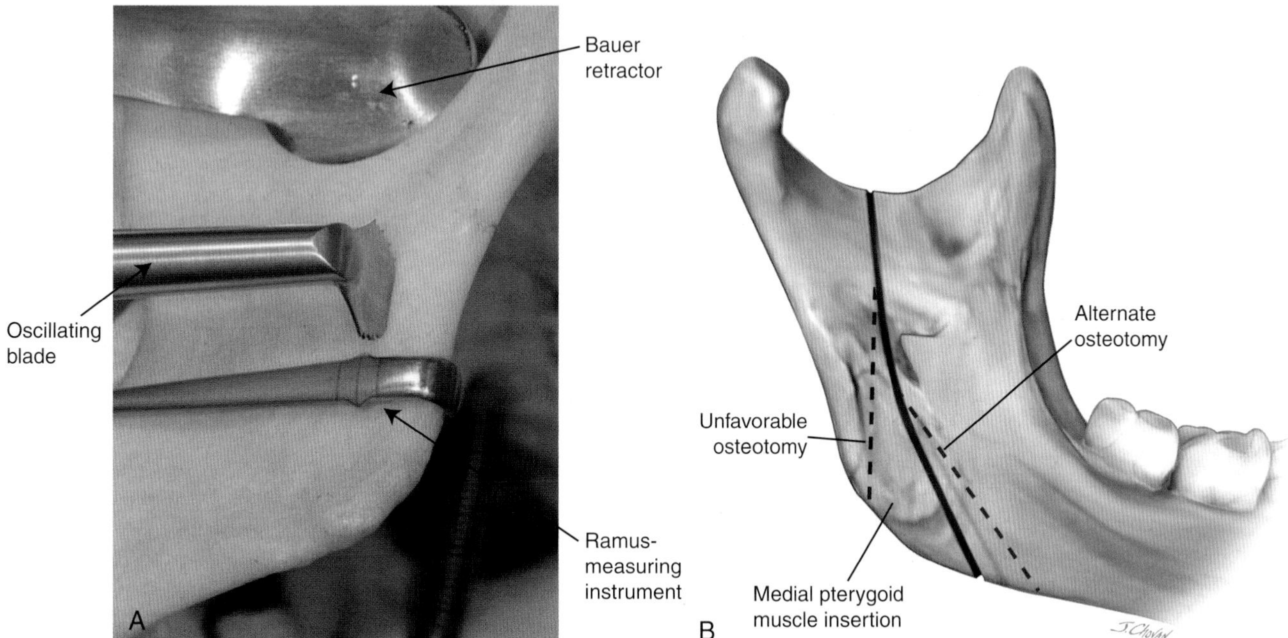

Figure 36.1 **A,** Ramus measuring instrument to locate the osteotomy 7 to 8 mm anterior to the posterior border of the ramus. **B,** Medial view of the osteotomy preserving the medial pterygoid insertion. An unfavorable osteotomy compromises the medial pterygoid insertion. Anteriorly directed osteotomy optimizes proximal segment muscle attachment in larger setbacks.

TECHNIQUE: Intraoral Vertical Ramus Osteotomy—cont'd

STEP 5: Preliminary Proximal Segment Trimming

Depending on the amount of overlap, the medial aspect of the condylar segment is trimmed with a rotary instrument and round bur to create a rabbet. A large Freer elevator is used to retract the proximal segment laterally and protect medial soft tissue. With mandibular surgery for class III deformity there is usually some counterclockwise rotation of the distal segment resulting in greater overlap and necessary superior trimming. The proximal segment should not be rotated posteriorly as this may predispose to forward relapse. In the case of a small advancement or clockwise rotation of the mandible, premature inferior contact is expected (Fig. 36.1C).

STEP 6: Establishing Maxillomandibular Fixation and Verifying Proximal Segment Position

After the osteotomies have been completed, the planned occlusion is established and MMF is placed. The osteotomies are evaluated for close, passive lateral positioning of the proximal segment. With condylar seating force applied to the proximal segment, the inferior aspect of the osteotomy is inspected. An inferior gap is addressed with additional judicious trimming superiorly (see Alternative Technique 2 later in the chapter). If the proximal segment tip is readily palpable in the submandibular region, it can be trimmed with a Kerrison rongeur. The incisions are irrigated and closed with running chromic suture.

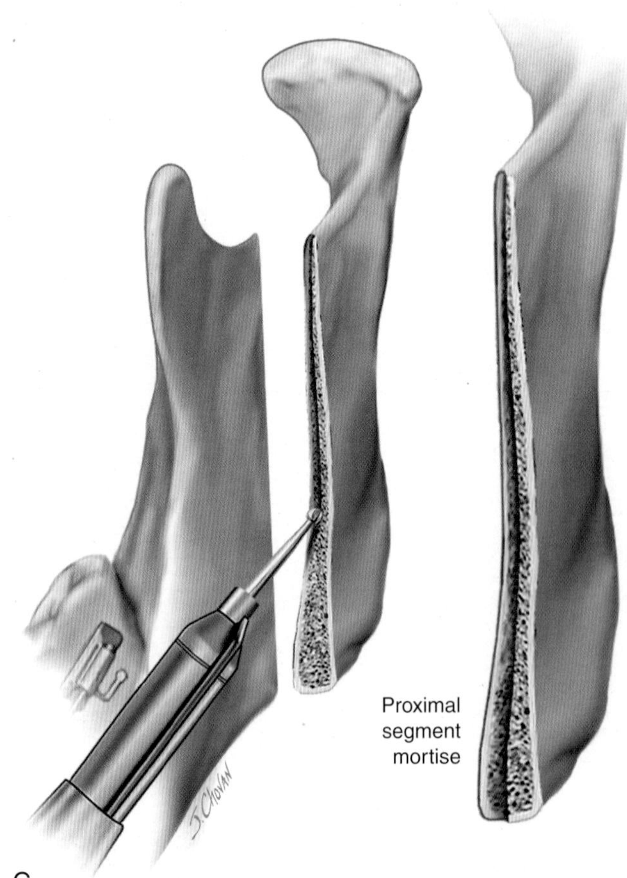

Figure 36.1, cont'd C, Medial edge of the proximal segment trimmed with a rotary instrument to ensure passive overlap of segments.

ALTERNATIVE TECHNIQUE 1: Simultaneous Coronoidectomy

In large mandibular setbacks (e.g., 10 mm), the coronoid process may collide with the proximal segment. This can be addressed with coronoidectomy. Advocates of this modification cite less bony interference, improved visibility of the sigmoid notch, and better postoperative stability.[25,26]

ALTERNATIVE TECHNIQUE 2: Modification of the Distal Segment for Superior Interference

Correction of horizontal mandibular excess with isolated mandibular surgery is usually associated with counterclockwise rotation of the distal segment and greater bony interference at the level of the sigmoid notch. In two-jaw surgery, if counterclockwise rotation of the maxillomandibular complex is planned, interference at the superior aspect of the IVRO is anticipated. Failure to address this superior interference results in backward rotation of the proximal segment and a gap inferiorly. In lieu of additional trimming of the proximal segment, a small triangular segment of distal segment may be excised superior by creating a second osteotomy with the oscillating saw (Fig. 36.2).

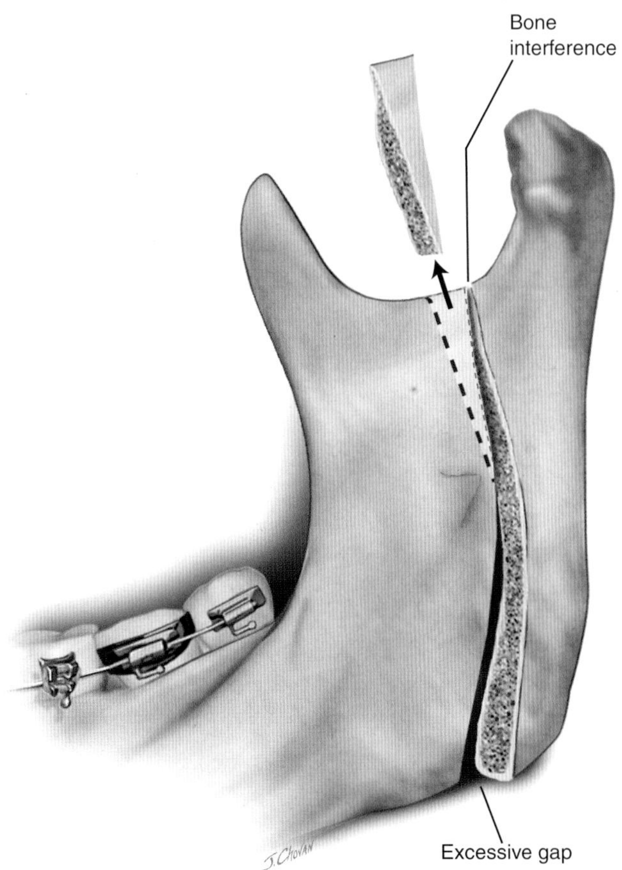

Figure 36.2 Superior interference from counterclockwise rotation of distal segment relieved with distal segment wedge excision.

ALTERNATIVE TECHNIQUE 3: Modification of the Distal Segment for Inferior Interference

In two-jaw surgery with clockwise rotation of the maxillomandibular complex, premature contact is anticipated at the inferior aspect of the IVRO. This may also occur when there is a small amount of mandibular advancement, and premature contact inferiorly as the proximal segment is rotated anteriorly to establish contact with the distal segment. This interference can be addressed with a second osteotomy to remove a small triangle of distal segment, avoiding additional medial pterygoid stripping and proximal segment trimming (Fig. 36.3).

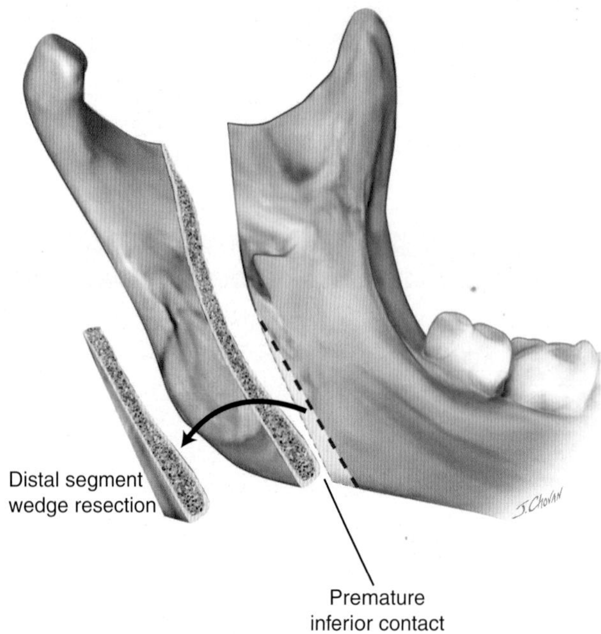

Figure 36.3 Inferior distal segment wedge excision to remove inferior interference and obviate additional medial pterygoid stripping and proximal segment trimming.

ALTERNATIVE TECHNIQUE 4: Internal Fixation

Vertical ramus osteotomy as originally described was performed without internal fixation. With a poorly designed osteotomy and a narrow and/or short proximal segment with little or no medial pterygoid attachment, condylar sag and even subluxation can occur.[27] Ramus lengthening and/or slight distal segment advancement will also promote condylar sag. With creation of a long proximal segment and preservation of medial pterygoid attachment, condylar seating is facilitated, but MMF is required. Proximal segment width of at least 7 to 8 mm allows for internal fixation. Stable internal fixation can be readily accomplished with two 0.8 mm thick L-shaped plates. With MMF established, the inferior plate position is determined and the plate adapted. The plate should be removed to drill the first hole to improve visibility and confirm that the first hole is equidistant from the osteotomy and posterior border. A laryngeal mirror is very helpful to confirm hole placement. A 30-degree endoscope may be used to visualize this area.[28] The plate is applied and the first screw placed. The remaining proximal segment screws are placed assuring placement in adequate bone. With the condyle seated and proximal segment stabilized, the distal segment screws are placed. The process is repeated to place a superior plate. Alternatively, with sufficient overlap of the proximal and distal segments, internal fixation can be achieved with transoral placement of at least two positioning screws (Fig. 36.4). MMF is released and occlusion evaluated.

Avoidance and Management of Intraoperative Complications

Risks of IVRO include injury to the inferior alveolar, lingual and facial nerves, condylar sag, condylar subluxation, skeletal relapse, bleeding, infection, and fibrous union. Whereas at least temporary inferior alveolar nerve sensory alteration is a consequence of SSO, any sensory alteration, even transient, is uncommon with IVRO.[18,19,29,30] With careful assessment of the osteotomy position relative to the posterior border of the mandible, inferior alveolar nerve injury can be avoided. Preoperative CT assessment of the mandibular foramen can be used in conjunction with the ramus measuring instrument or for fabrication of a cutting guide to further manage the risk of nerve injury.

Another source of inferior alveolar nerve injury, which occurs in approximately 3% to 8% of IVRO cases, is medial displacement of the proximal segment.[21,22] Muscle action will rotate the proximal segment anteriorly, with impingement on the inferior alveolar nerve at the mandibular foramen. In the authors' experience, medial displacement of the proximal segment is extremely uncommon with any amount of mandibular setback, well below the reported 3% incidence. Should this occur, proximal segment repositioning should be undertaken promptly to avoid long-term sensory alteration.

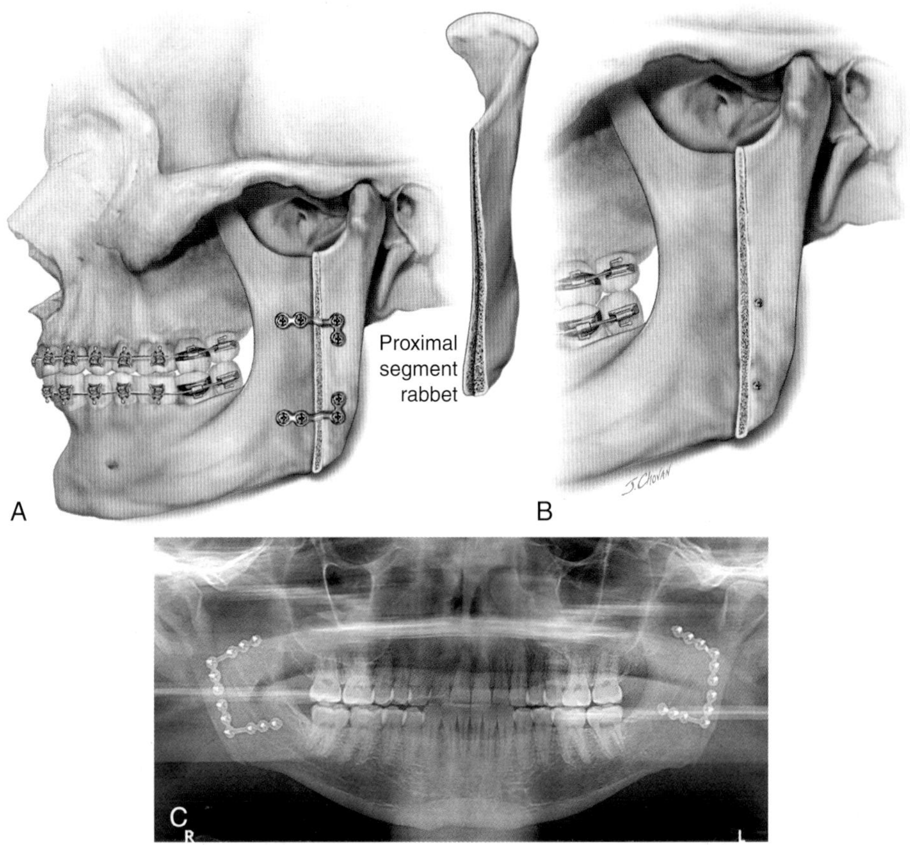

Figure 36.4 **A,** Internal plate fixation. **B,** Internal positioning or lag-screw fixation. **C,** Radiographic image of internal plate fixation.

Condylar sag and subluxation can be prevented by preservation of medial pterygoid attachment with the creation of a long osteotomy and wide proximal segment. A poorly executed osteotomy that passes through the posterior border of the mandible sacrifices medial pterygoid attachment. Constant vigilance is required to avoid this error as the inferior portion of the osteotomy is developed. In the worst-case scenario, a short proximal segment with little medial pterygoid attachment is subject to unopposed lateral pterygoid action and condylar subluxation. Should this be recognized at the time of surgery, the proximal segment should be internally fixated to ensure condylar seating and resist unopposed lateral pterygoid muscle activity. The concern for condylar sag with IVRO can be effectively addressed with transoral internal fixation.

Extraordinary bleeding can occur during IVRO, with injury to the contents of the sigmoid notch (e.g., masseteric artery) or vascular structures medial to the ramus. A properly positioned Bauer retractor minimizes injury to vascular structures at the sigmoid notch. If the 11.5 × 7-mm blade is too short to complete the lingual portion of the osteotomy at the level of the antelingular prominence (typically the thickest portion of the ramus), the surgeon should confirm that the osteotomy is not too far anteriorly. The 11.5 × 12-mm blade should be used very cautiously because of the greater risk of injury to medial structures.

Injury to the facial and inferior alveolar arteries and retromandibular vein is rare with proper technique. Injury to the marginal mandibular branch of the facial nerve can occur as the inferior limb of the IVRO is completed. The periosteum should be elevated from the inferior border to minimize the risk of soft tissue trauma from the oscillating blade. Lingual nerve injury may result from the use of a forked ramus retractor. Fibrous union is extremely uncommon, even without internal fixation.[31–33] MMF is necessary in the absence of internal fixation.

Postoperative Considerations

The position of the proximal segment should be confirmed with postoperative imaging if internal fixation has not been used. Mild condylar sagging can be effectively addressed with clenching exercises during the first 2 weeks. If ample medial pterygoid muscle has been preserved, muscle activity will promote physiologic condylar seating. Similarly, if a gap is noted at the inferior border, this often closes with postoperative clenching exercises. If internal fixation is not used, 2 to 3 weeks of MMF is recommended. This is followed by 3 to 4 weeks of a nonchewing diet and 22 hour/day training elastics. Active range-of-motion exercises are initiated during the fourth postoperative week. Patients may resume a normal diet after the sixth week.

References

1. Limberg A. Treatment of the open bite by means of plastic oblique osteotomy of the ascending rami of the mandible. *Dent Cosm.* 1925;67:1191.
2. Moose SM. Correction of abnormal mandibular protrusion by intra-oral operation. *J Oral Surg (Chic).* 1945;3:304–310.
3. Moose SM. Surgical correction of mandibular prognathism by intraoral subcondylar osteotomy. *J Oral Surg Anesth Hosp Dent Serv.* 1964;22:197–202.
4. Moose SM. Surgical correction of mandibular prognathism by intraoral sub-condylar osteotomy. *Br J Oral Surg.* 1964;1:172–176.
5. Caldwell JB, Letterman GS. Vertical osteotomy in the mandibular raml for correction of prognathism. *J Oral Surg (Chic).* 1954;12(3):185–202.
6. Trauner R, Obwegeser H. The surgical correction of mandibular prognathism and retrognathia with consideration of genioplasty. I. Surgical procedures to correct mandibular prognathism and reshaping of the chin. *Oral Surg Oral Med Oral Pathol.* 1957;10(7):677–689.
7. Winstanley RP. Subcondylar osteotomy of the mandible and the intraoral approach. *Br J Oral Surg.* 1968;6(2):134–136.
8. Hebert JM, Kent JN, Hinds EC. Correction of prognathism by an intraoral vertical subcondylar osteotomy. *J Oral Surg.* 1970;28(9):651–653.
9. Hall HD, Chase DC, Payor LG. Evaluation and refinement of the intraoral vertical subcondylar osteotomy. *J Oral Surg.* 1975;33(5):333–341.
10. Hall HD, McKenna SJ. Further refinement and evaluation of intraoral vertical ramus osteotomy. *J Oral Maxillofac Surg.* 1987;45(8):684–688.
11. Ghali GE, Sikes JW Jr. Intraoral vertical ramus osteotomy as the preferred treatment for mandibular prognathism. *J Oral Maxillofac Surg.* 2000;58(3):313–315.
12. McKenna SJ, King EE. Intraoral vertical ramus osteotomy procedure and technique. *Atlas Oral Maxillofac Surg Clin North Am.* 2016;24(1):37–43.
13. Bell WH, Yamaguchi Y, Poor MR. Treatment of temporomandibular joint dysfunction by intraoral vertical ramus osteotomy. *Int J Adult Orthodon Orthognath Surg.* 1990;5(1):9–27.
14. Nickerson JW, Veaco NS. Condylotomy in surgery of the temporomandibular joint. *Oral Maxillofac Clin North Am.* 1989;4:303.
15. Hall HD, Navarro EZ, Gibbs SJ. One- and three-year prospective outcome study of modified condylotomy for treatment of reducing disc displacement. *J Oral Maxillofac Surg.* 2000;58(1):7–17.
16. Al-Moraissi EA, Wolford LM, Perez D, Laskin DM, Ellis E III. Does orthognathic surgery cause or cure temporomandibular disorders? A systematic review and meta-analysis. *J Oral Maxillofac Surg.* 2017;75(9):1835–1847.
17. Jung HD, Jung YS, Park HS. The chronologic prevalence of temporomandibular joint disorders associated with bilateral intraoral vertical ramus osteotomy. *J Oral Maxillofac Surg.* 2009;67(4):797–803.
18. Zaytoun HS Jr, Phillips C, Terry BC. Long-term neurosensory deficits following transoral vertical ramus and sagittal split osteotomies for mandibular prognathism. *J Oral Maxillofac Surg.* 1986;44(3):193–196.
19. Al-Moraissi EA, Ellis E III. Is there a difference in stability or neurosensory function between bilateral sagittal split ramus osteotomy and intraoral vertical ramus osteotomy for mandibular setback? *J Oral Maxillofac Surg.* 2015;73(7):1360–1371.
20. Schilbred Eriksen E, Wisth PJ, Løes S, Moen K. Skeletal and dental stability after intraoral vertical ramus osteotomy: a long-term follow-up. *Int J Oral Maxillofac Implants.* 2017;46(1):72–79.
21. Choi SH, Cha JY, Park HS, Hwang CJ. Intraoral vertical ramus osteotomy results in good long-term mandibular stability in patients with mandibular prognathism and anterior open bite. *J Oral Maxillofac Surg.* 2016;74(4):804–810.
22. Kung AYH, Leung YY. Stability of intraoral vertical ramus osteotomies for mandibular setback: a longitudinal study. *Int J Oral Maxillofac Implants.* 2018;47(2):152–159.
23. da Fontoura RA, Vasconcellos HA, Campos AE. Morphologic basis for the intraoral vertical ramus osteotomy: anatomic and radiographic localization of the mandibular foramen. *J Oral Maxillofac Surg.* 2002;60(6):660–665.
24. Monnazzi MS, Passeri LA, Gabrielli MF, Bolini PD, de Carvalho WR, da Costa Machado H. Anatomic study of the mandibular foramen, lingula and antilingula in dry mandibles, and its statistical relationship between the true lingula and the antilingula. *Int J Oral Maxillofac Implants.* 2012;41(1):74–78.
25. Epker BN, Wolford L. *Dentofacial Deformities: Surgical-Orthodontic Correction.* St Louis, Missouri: Mosby; 1980.
26. Talesh KT, Motamedi MH, Yazdani J, Ghavimi A, Ghoreishizadeh A. Prevention of relapse following intraoral vertical ramus osteotomy mandibular setback: can coronoidotomy help? *Oral Surg Oral Med Oral Pathol Oral Radiol Endod.* 2011;111(5):557–560.
27. Yamauchi K, Takenobu T, Takahashi T. Condylar luxation following bilateral intraoral vertical ramus osteotomy. *Oral Surg Oral Med Oral Pathol Oral Radiol Endod.* 2007;104(6):747–751.
28. González-García R. Endoscopically-assisted subcondylar and vertical ramus osteotomies for the treatment of symmetrical mandibular prognathism. *J Craniomaxillofac Surg.* 2012;40(5):393–395.
29. Westermark A, Bystedt H, von Konow L. Inferior alveolar nerve function after mandibular osteotomies. *Br J Oral Maxillofac Surg.* 1998;36(6):425–428.
30. Takazakura D, Ueki K, Nakagawa K, et al. A comparison of postoperative hypoesthesia between two types of sagittal split ramus osteotomy and intraoral vertical ramus osteotomy, using the trigeminal somatosensory-evoked potential method. *Int J Oral Maxillofac Surg.* 2007;36(1):11–14.
31. Rokutanda S, Yamada S, Yanamoto S, et al. Comparison of osseous healing after sagittal split ramus osteotomy and intraoral vertical ramus osteotomy. *Int J Oral Maxillofac Implants.* 2018;47(10):1316–1321.
32. Blinder D, Peleg O, Yoffe T, Taicher S. Intraoral vertical ramus osteotomy: a simple method to prevent medial trapping of the proximal fragment. *Int J Oral Maxillofac Implants.* 2010;39(3):289–291.
33. Tuinzing DB, Greebe RB. Complications related to the intraoral vertical ramus osteotomy. *Int J Oral Surg.* 1985;14(4):319–324.

CHAPTER 37

Inverted L Mandibular Osteotomy

Joseph E. Van Sickels

Armamentarium

The inverted L osteotomy can be performed either extraorally or intraorally. The equipment for these two options is slightly different. For the purposes of this chapter, the instruments for the extraoral approach are listed first and followed by the separate instruments used for the intraoral procedure.

Extraoral Approach

#9 Molt periosteal elevators (two)
#15 Scalpel blade
#703 Bur
Adson with teeth or Cushing/bone forceps
Appropriate sutures
Langenbeck retractors (toe in and toe out)
Local anesthetic with vasoconstrictor
Metzenbaum scissors
Minnesota retractor
Needle electrocautery
Nerve stimulator
Plating system of surgeon's choice
Rake retractors
Reciprocating/oscillating saw
Senn retractors
Tonsil hemostat (one or more)
Wire drivers and cutters

Intraoral Approach

#9 Molt periosteal elevators (two)
Appropriate sutures
Bauer retractor (optional)
Coronoid notch retractor
J-strippers
Kelly clamp
Kocher with umbilical tape
LeVasseur Merrill retractor
Local anesthetic with vasoconstrictor
Minnesota retractor
Needle electrocautery
Oscillating saw
Plating system of surgeon's choice
Reciprocating saw

History of the Procedure

According to Steinhauser,[1] the inverted L osteotomy (ILO) was first described by Trauner in 1955. In 1957 and 1958, Schuchardt and then Immenkamp suggested the use of an autogenous corticocancellous bone graft between the proximal and distal segments. The extraoral technique described by Spiessl[2] in his 1989 textbook is very similar to what is used today.

In 1990, Van Sickels et al.[3] discussed the rigid fixation of the intraoral ILO. Although this was not the first report of the intraoral ILO, it appears to have been the earliest report of the use of rigid fixation with the ILO, which reduced the need for longer periods of maxillary-mandibular fixation. The rigid fixation technique described by Van Sickels et al.[3] was used for mandibular setbacks. It used a condylar positioning device to control the proximal segments during surgery.[3] In 1999, McMillan et al.[4] published a paper on the intraoral ILO and referenced a 1993 conference in Australia, where the technique was presented.[4] In addition, the technique was presented as an option to advance the mandible.

Indications for the Use of the Procedure

The ILO may be the operation of choice for large advancements (greater than 12 mm) with counterclockwise rotation or for large setbacks (greater than 10 mm).[5] It is also a good choice for reoperations resulting from altered ramal morphology and in patients with masseter hypertrophy with dense underlying cortical bone.

Extraoral Approach

The extraoral ILO (and its near cousin, the arching C osteotomy) can be used for advancements or setbacks. However, today it generally is used for large complicated advancements either because an alternative intraoral procedure is not feasible or because the mandibular anatomy is unusual (e.g., a thin ramus or a severely deficient mandibular posterior body height).[6] Frequently, a gap is created between the segments, requiring an autogenous or allogenic graft to fill the void created by the amount of movement. Selective cases of significant mandibular asymmetries may be managed better with an extraoral vertical ramus or ILO than an intraoral osteotomy.

Intraoral Approach

The major advantage of the intraoral approach over the extraoral approach is avoidance of a skin incision; this eliminates facial scarring and greatly reduces the risk of injury to the marginal mandibular branch of the facial nerve. The intraoral ILO involves a number of considerations.[3,4,7,8] These include whether to perform both medial and lateral dissection, deciding how much of a bevel to use between the medical and lateral sides, and choosing the best types of rigid fixation to fix the segments.[3,4,7,8] The intraoral ILO can be used for small mandibular setbacks and for large setbacks in selected cases. As with the extraoral osteotomy, it can be used for mandibular asymmetries and advancements. Several authors have advocated its use for either advancements or setbacks when the risk of damage to the inferior alveolar nerve is a particular concern.[3,4] It may be equally advantageous for cases in which the preoperative computed tomogram shows a thin ramus.

Limitations and Contraindications

There are only a few limitations and contraindications for the use of an ILO. The extraoral approach includes a skin incision, which may result in an unsightly scar and possible damage to the facial nerve. Injury to the inferior alveolar nerve is much less likely with the vertical ramus procedure than with bilateral sagittal split osteotomy (BSSO), but it is still possible.[9,10] Kobayashi et al.[10] compared neurosensory disturbances in patients undergoing either an ILO or a BSSO. They concluded that the long-term prognosis for resolution of postsurgical neurosensory disturbances was better for the patients who underwent the ILO. They also noted that the width of movement between the segments influenced postsurgical neurosensory disturbances immediately after the ILO but the relationship diminished with time.

Additional limitations and contraindications may apply for mandibular advancements without bone grafting. This technique may be less stable and may result in nonunion if the bone gap is too large. Grafting choices are autogenous or alloplastic.

TECHNIQUE: Extraoral Inverted L Osteotomy

STEP 1: Soft Tissue Incision and Dissection

A standard submandibular incision or Risdon approach is used to gain access to the lateral ramus of the mandible. Once the skin and subcutaneous tissues have been incised, a nerve stimulator is used to prevent injury to the marginal mandibular branch of the facial nerve. The masseter muscle is incised and retracted, and the sigmoid notch, anterior ramus, and posterior border of the mandible are identified (Fig. 37.1A).

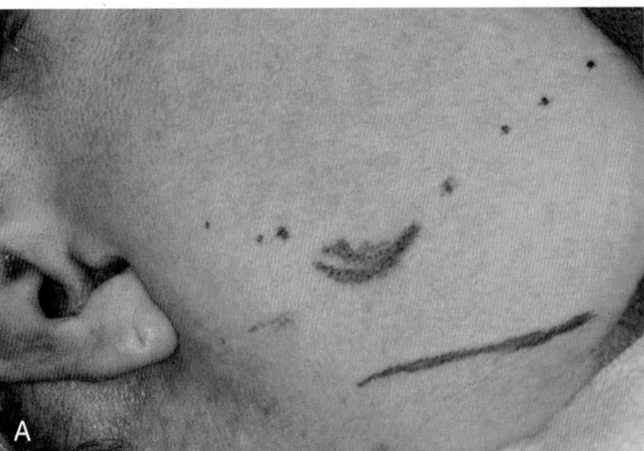

Figure 37.1 A, Outline of skin incision.

TECHNIQUE: Extraoral Inverted L Osteotomy—*cont'd*

STEP 2: Bony Osteotomy

A bony cut is made with a #703 bur or reciprocating saw from the ascending ramus to a point slightly posterior and superior to the estimated location of the mandibular foramen. From this point, the osteotomy is extended inferiorly in a vertical direction to the inferior border of the ramus. Usually a fine chisel is used to gently separate the segments. The procedure is then performed on the opposite side (Fig. 37.1B).

STEP 3: Application of Plates and Screws

The teeth are placed in occlusion or into the surgical splint. The segments are fixed with plates and screws. Typically, the plate is affixed first to the proximal segment. Then, while the condyle is placed into the fossa and the preplanned gap between the segments is maintained, the distal segment is fixed (Fig. 37.1C).

STEP 4: Placement of Grafting Material

Autogenous, allograft, or synthetic bone graft material may be placed into the gap created in the segments to bridge the osseous void and help with stability (Fig. 37.1D).

Continued

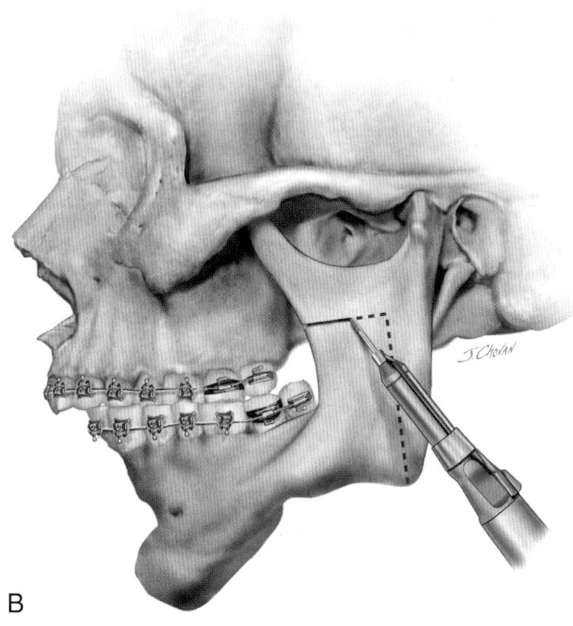

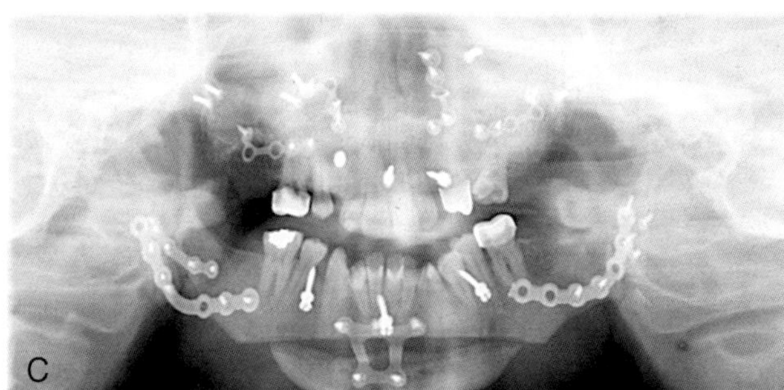

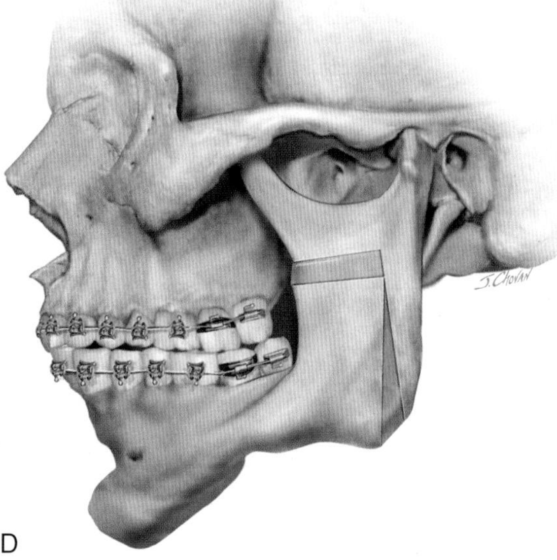

Figure 37.1, cont'd **B,** Projected extraoral osteotomy. **C,** Postoperative panoramic radiograph showing plates in place in a large mandibular advancement. **D,** Placement of bone graft to fill void.

TECHNIQUE: Extraoral Inverted L Osteotomy—*cont'd*

STEP 5: Use of Maxillomandibular Fixation
Maxillomandibular fixation (MMF) may or may not be needed, depending on the stability of the plates.

STEP 6: Completion of the Procedure
The extraoral wounds are closed (Fig. 37.1E).

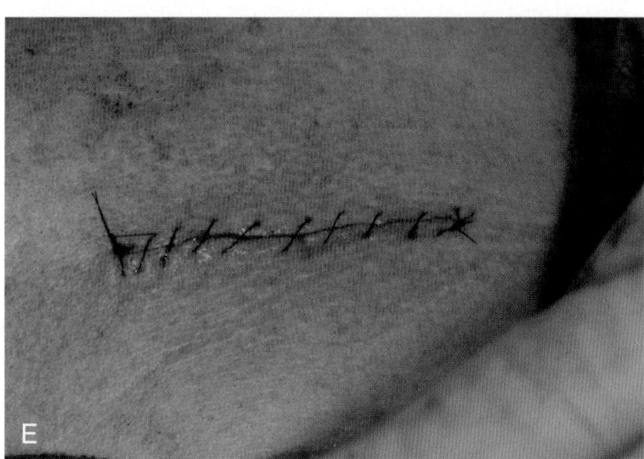

Figure 37.1, cont'd E, Closure of the wound.

ALTERNATIVE TECHNIQUE 1: Intraoral Inverted L Osteotomy

STEP 1: Soft Tissue Incision
An intraoral incision is made along the external oblique ridge, similar to the traditional BSSO incision. Subperiosteal dissection is performed up the ascending ramus to expose the coronoid process. A Kocher clamp with umbilical tape is placed at the tip of the coronoid to aid in retraction.

STEP 2: Dissection on the Lateral Aspect of the Mandible
With periosteal elevators, dissection is continued laterally to the posterior border of the mandible. A J-stripper, placed at the posterior border midway between the angle and condylar process, is used to strip the periosteal and muscular attachment off the posterior border. A LeVasseur Merrill retractor is placed to ensure adequate visualization of the lateral aspect of the ramus. It is then removed.

STEP 3: Dissection on the Medial Aspect of the Mandible
Dissection is then continued on the medial aspect of the mandible with a periosteal elevator in a similar fashion to that used with a BSSO. The periosteal elevator is extended posterior to lingual to the entrance of the inferior alveolar nerve.

STEP 4: Initial Osteotomy on the Medial Aspect of the Mandible
With a reciprocating saw, a horizontal cut is made above the lingula, beveling from medial to lateral and going through and through to the lateral surface from the ascending ramus to just posterior to the nerve (Fig. 37.2).

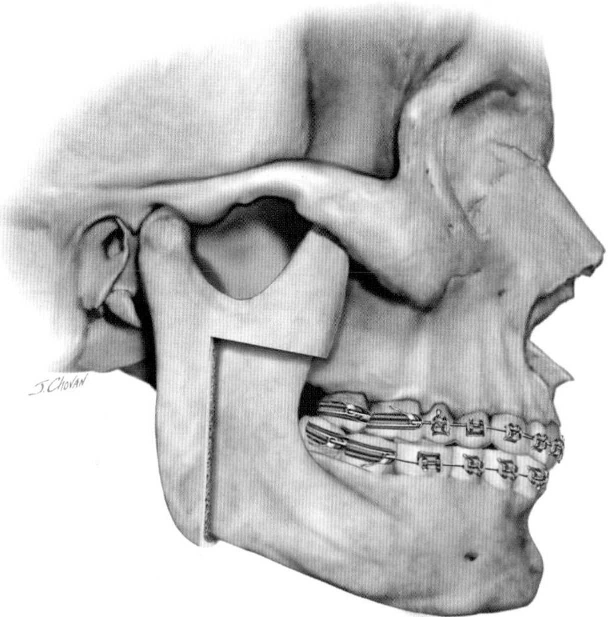

Figure 37.2 Osteotomy completed, before plating.

ALTERNATIVE TECHNIQUE 1: Intraoral Inverted L Osteotomy—*cont'd*

STEP 5: Osteotomy on the Lateral Aspect of the Mandible

The LeVasseur Merrill retractor is replaced, and an oscillating saw is used, connecting with the through-and-through bone and extending to just anterior to the mandible. The segments are then separated. The procedure is repeated on the opposite side.

STEP 6: Alignment of the Segments

The teeth are placed into MMF. The proximal segment is manipulated to lie lateral to the distal segment; any interferences between the segments can be reduced with a bur. (It is important to note that posterior open bites are indicative of interferences.) A number of different fixation schemes can be used. McMillan et al.[4] used two L plates to secure the segments. One is placed at the anterior border of the distal segment and the other at the inferior border. Van Sickels et al.[3] placed a single seven-hole, right-angled plate near the anterior aspect of the distal segment. Zhu et al.[11] placed two four-hole miniplates with an iliac crest bone graft, one at the anterior border and the other at the angle using a transbuccal approach. Their intraoral technique was very similar to that used by Van Sickels, Tiner, and Jeter,[3] except that they felt a positioning plate was not necessary when advancing the mandible.

STEP 7: Placement of Plates and Screws

With the single seven-hole plate technique, the most anterior hole on the proximal fragment is the first hole drilled. A trocar is used to achieve perpendicular screw placement. Next, the plate with a screw in the most anterior-superior hole is positioned, and the screw is engaged with a screwdriver and partially tightened. The inferior aspect of the plate is then manipulated on the distal fragment to achieve the best position. Then, a hole is drilled in the most convenient position, and a bicortical screw is placed (a monocortical screw may be placed if the location is close to the inferior alveolar nerve canal). All other screw holes are drilled, and the screws tightly placed.

STEP 8: Completion of the Procedure

After the procedure has been completed on both sides, the wounds are closed. Short class III elastics frequently are used after surgery for 4 to 6 weeks.

Continued

ALTERNATIVE TECHNIQUE 2: Positioning Plates Used With the Inverted L Osteotomy

A positioning plate may be helpful for securing better control of the segments.

STEP 1: Placement of Control Plate
The patient is placed in MMF after the horizontal cut is made in the mandible. Before the vertical cut is complete, a nine-hole, curved plate is placed from the coronoid process above the horizontal cut to the zygomatic buttress of the maxilla. This plate maintains control of the proximal segment and ensures that the condyle remains seated. To attach the positioning plate to the maxilla, a maxillary vestibular incision is made and the zygomaticomaxillary buttress is exposed bilaterally (Fig. 37.3A).

STEP 2: Placement of Positioning Plate
Trocar access is required transfacially to place the screws perpendicular to the coronoid. Two screws are placed into the coronoid process and two screws into the maxilla on each side. It is important to provide enough room between the horizontal osteotomy and this plate to allow room for an additional plate to be placed to secure the segments.

STEP 3: Placement of Plate to Fix the Segments
The vertical cut of the ramus is completed. The distal segment is moved posteriorly, and interferences are addressed. Then the seven-hole plate is applied bilaterally (Fig. 37.3B).

STEP 4: Removal of Positioning Plate
The temporary nine-hole plate is removed, and the wounds are irrigated and closed with 3-0 Vicryl suture.

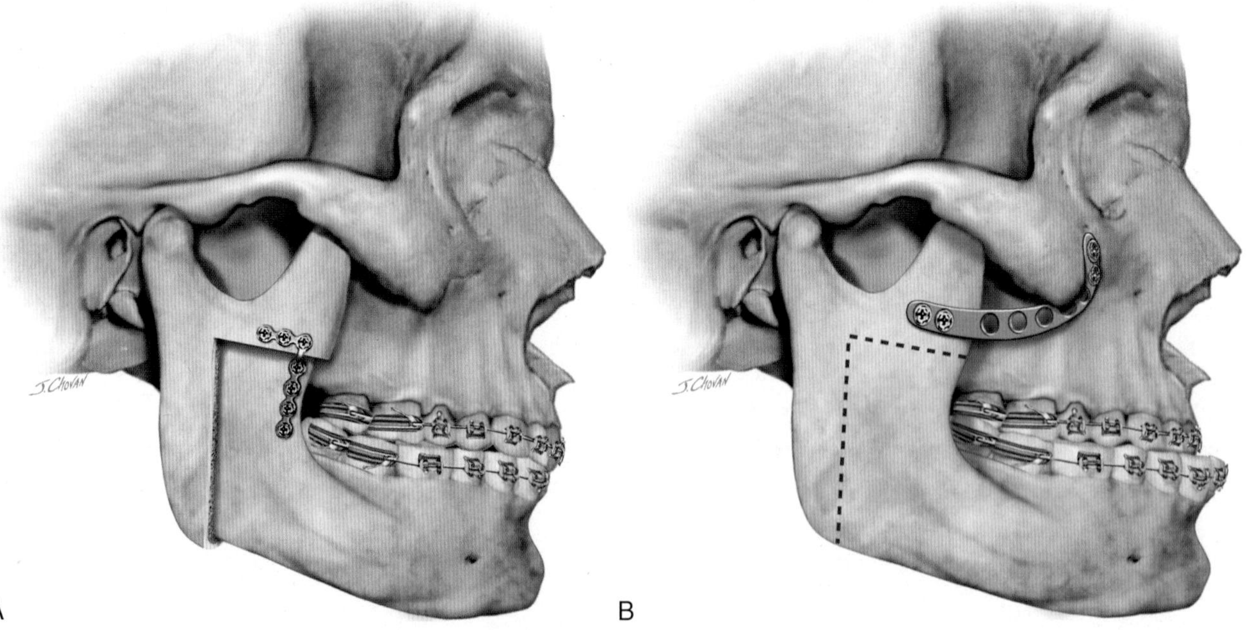

Figure 37.3 **A,** Plating of an intraoral inverted L osteotomy. **B,** Use of a positioning plate.

Avoidance and Management of Intraoperative Complications

A number of intraoperative complications are possible.

- Unfavorable osteotomy. If the horizontal osteotomy is extended too far posteriorly, there is a risk of fracturing the condylar process with both the intraoral and extraoral approaches. This complicates the surgery by making internal fixation much more challenging.[12]
- Sensory nerve injury. If the horizontal osteotomy is too short in the anteroposterior dimension, the vertical osteotomy that connects with the posterior aspect of this osteotomy is likely to injure the inferior alveolar neurovascular structures. This is especially true with the extraoral approach because there are no good guidelines to indicate where the inferior alveolar nerve is in relation to the lateral surface of the mandible.[13–15]
- Motor nerve injury. With the extraoral approach, there is a risk of injury to the marginal mandibular branch of the facial nerve, although this risk can be reduced with use of the nerve stimulator.
- Bleeding. Intraoperative brisk bleeding can occur and usually results from the transection of the inferior alveolar, masseteric, or maxillary artery. If bleeding occurs, it can usually be controlled with tamponade (packing). The masseteric artery is only 8 mm from the sigmoid notch.[16]

Postoperative Considerations

Some postoperative complications include excessive swelling, hemorrhage or hematoma, postoperative nausea and vomiting (N/V), infection, mandibular dysfunction, and relapse.

Postoperative swelling is related to the type and duration of surgery, patient-specific factors, and the medications administered. The dreaded result of excessive swelling is airway compromise. Unless contraindicated, preoperative and postoperative doses of dexamethasone (tapered over 24 hours) can be used, in addition to a universal pressure head wrap, to prevent swelling and hematoma.

Postoperative hematoma is possible but usually a minor issue. This sequela can be prevented by thorough control of intraoperative bleeding and the use of pressure dressings for 24 hours. Most often, postoperative bleeding is related to the retromandibular vein. However, profuse arterial bleeding is possible and may require external carotid artery ligation or embolization.[12]

Postoperative N/V and dehydration can occur for many reasons. Some triggers of N/V include anesthetic agents, pain, narcotic analgesics, and ingestion of blood. The administration of antiemetic drugs is an important tool in the management of this complication.[12]

Infection is a risk with any surgery, particularly when the surgeon is working in the oral cavity and performing transcutaneous techniques. The prevention of infections after orthognathic surgery is affected by factors such as the patient's age and immune status and the surgeon's experience (which affects the duration of the procedure and tissue handling). Routine use of perioperative intravenous antibiotics for 24 hours and postoperative antibiotics should minimize this complication.

Stability has not been studied in large series, but it is believed to be similar to a sagittal split.

References

1. Steinhäuser EW. Historical development of orthognathic surgery. *J Craniomaxillofac Surg.* 1996;24(4):195–204.
2. Spiessl B. *Internal Fixation of the Mandible: A Manual of AO/ASIF Principles.* Berlin, Germany: Springer-Verlag; 1989.
3. Van Sickels JE, Tiner BD, Jeter TS. Rigid fixation of the intraoral inverted "L" osteotomy. *J Oral Maxillofac Surg.* 1990;48(8):894–898.
4. McMillan B, Jones R, Ward-Booth P, Goss A. Technique for intraoral inverted "L" osteotomy. *Br J Oral Maxillofac Surg.* 1999;37(4):324–326.
5. Medeiros PJ, Ritto F. Indications for the inverted-L osteotomy: report of 3 cases. *J Oral Maxillofac Surg.* 2009;67(2):435–444.
6. Booth PW, Schendel SA, Hausamen JE. 2nd ed. *Maxillofacial Surgery.* Vol. 2. St Louis, Missouri: Churchill Livingstone; 2007.
7. Muto T, Akizuki K, Tsuchida N, Sato Y. Modified intraoral inverted "L" osteotomy: a technique for good visibility, greater bony overlap, and rigid fixation. *J Oral Maxillofac Surg.* 2008;66(6):1309–1315.
8. Aymach Z, Nei H, Kawamura H, Van Sickels J. Evaluation of skeletal stability after surgical-orthodontic correction of skeletal open bite with mandibular counterclockwise rotation using modified inverted L osteotomy. *J Oral Maxillofac Surg.* 2011;69(3):853–860.
9. Karas ND, Boyd SB, Sinn DP. Recovery of neurosensory function following orthognathic surgery. *J Oral Maxillofac Surg.* 1990;48(2):124–134.
10. Kobayashi A, Yoshimasu H, Kobayashi J, Amagasa T. Neurosensory alteration in the lower lip and chin area after orthognathic surgery: bilateral sagittal split osteotomy versus inverted L ramus osteotomy. *J Oral Maxillofac Surg.* 2006;64(5):778–784.
11. Zhu S-S, Feng G, Li JH, Luo E, Hu J. Correction of mandibular deficiency by inverted-L osteotomy of ramus and iliac crest bone grafting. *Int J Oral Sci.* 2012;4(4):214–217.
12. Fonseca RJ, Marciani RD, Turvey TA. 2nd ed. *Oral and Maxillofacial Surgery.* Vol. 3. St Louis, Missouri: Saunders; 2009.
13. Hogan G, Ellis III E. The "antilingula"—fact or fiction? *J Oral Maxillofac Surg.* 2006;64(8):1248–1254.
14. Aziz SR, Dorfman BJ, Ziccardi VB, Janal M. Accuracy of using the antilingula as a sole determinant of vertical ramus osteotomy position. *J Oral Maxillofac Surg.* 2007;65(5):859–862.
15. Monnazzi MS, Passeri LA, Gabrielli MF, Bolini PD, de Carvalho WR, da Costa Machado H. Anatomic study of the mandibular foramen, lingula and antilingula in dry mandibles, and its statistical relationship between the true lingula and the antilingula. *Int J Oral Maxillofac Implants.* 2012;41(1):74–78.
16. Hwang K, Kim YJ, Chung IH, Song YB. Course of the masseteric nerve in masseter muscle. *J Craniofac Surg.* 2005;16(2):197–200.

CHAPTER 38

The Bilateral Sagittal Split Ramus Osteotomy

Johan P. Reyneke and Steven M. Sullivan

Armamentarium

0.018-inch Ligature wire
#701 Fissure bur
#703 Fissure bur
Austin retractor
Castroviejo callipers
Cheek retractor
Drill
Epker osteotome, straight
Howarth elevator
Langenbeck retractors
Large vulcanite bur
Lightweight mallet
Mosquito forceps
Mouth prop
Obwegeser channel retractor
Obwegeser periosteal elevator, flat
Obwegeser periosteal J-stripper
Obwegeser ramus retractor (notched retractor)
Obwegeser splitting osteotomes
Optional instruments
Reyneke condylar positioner
Reyneke intraoral trochar/extraoral trochar
Reyneke sagittal split separator (large)
Reyneke sagittal split separator (small)
Scalpel
Tessier osteotome
Tongue depressor
Wire cutter
Wire twister

History of the Procedure

The specific anatomy of the human mandible is unique and lends itself to splitting the ramus in a sagittal plane. In 1957, Trauner and Obwegeser[1] described a basic surgical design to reposition the mandible by means of a sagittal split of the mandibular ramus. This technique was later modified by Dal Pont,[2] further refined by Hunsuck[3] in 1968, and later by Epker[4] in 1977. It is currently the surgical technique of choice for repositioning of the mandible in most cases. The ingenuity of the surgical design, development of special instruments, improvement of surgical skills, and surgeon experience have made it now possible to achieve our treatment goals relatively quickly and atraumatically. With the introduction of internal rigid fixation by Spiessl[5] in 1974, stability was increased, and because no intermaxillary immobilization was required, the safety of the procedure increased. The sagittal split ramus osteotomy (SSO), however, remains a technique sensitive and challenging procedure.

Indications for the Use of the Procedure

The SSO is an extremely versatile procedure and allows the surgeon to advance the mandible, set it back, and perform vertical and asymmetric mandibular corrections.[6–8] The belief that counterclockwise rotation of the distal tooth-bearing segment has poor postoperative stability, has been proven to be misunderstood. The Epker modification allows counterclockwise rotation to be performed without increasing the ramus height, eliminating muscle interference. Counterclockwise rotation of the distal segment allows for the surgical correction of anterior open bite malocclusions and counterclockwise rotation of the maxillomandibular complex.[9,10]

The authors believe that presurgical removal of impacted third molar teeth has several advantages, and when possible, the teeth should be removed 9 months before orthognathic surgery (see Step 9).

Limitations and Contraindications

There are numerous factors that can affect surgical results of a bilateral sagittal split osteotomy. Including the potential for relapse related to the magnitude and direction of movement. In addition, a variety of medical comorbidities that relate to anesthetic risk and compromised bone healing must be considered pre-operatively by the surgeon. Although performed as necessary for specific reasons, relative contraindications may include the skeletally immature patient and the potential development of obstructive sleep apnea with setback procedures in select patients.

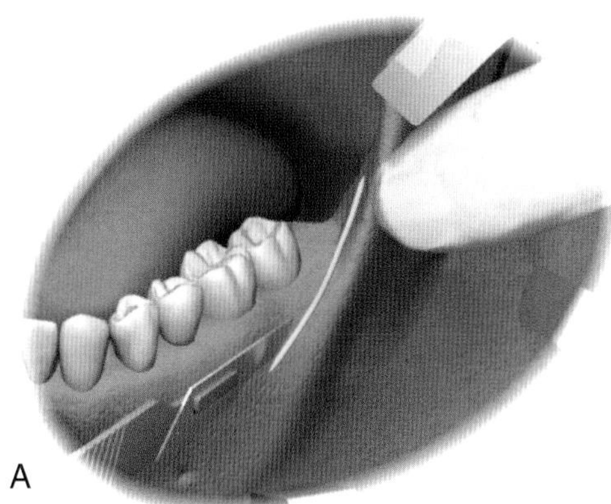

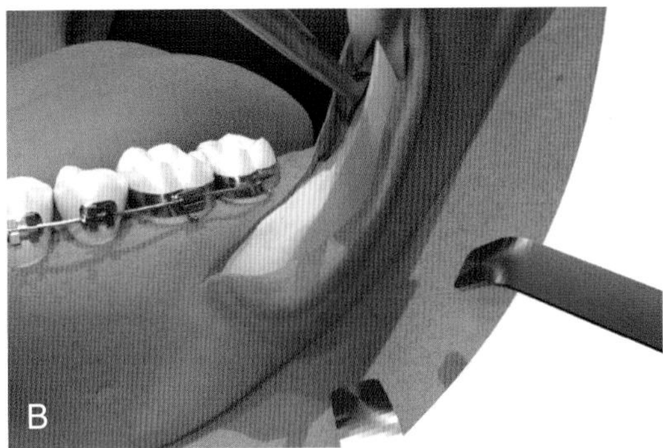

Figure 38.1 **A,** The soft-tissue incision. The incision is started from above, just lingual to the external oblique ridge (*arrow i*) and carried downward to mesial of the second molar. **B,** Buccal subperiosteal dissection down to the lower border of the mandible, vertical subperiosteal dissection removing the lower attachment of the temporal muscle, and medial subperiosteal dissection exposing the lingula.

TECHNIQUE: Surgical Technique[11]

STEP 1: Infiltrate the Area of Soft Tissue Dissection With a Vasoconstrictor

The area of the soft-tissue incision and dissection is infiltrated with a local anesthetic containing a vasoconstrictor (epinephrine in a concentration of 1:100,000), 10 minutes before commencement of surgery.

Keep a lubricant with steroid ointment handy as the lips should be kept lubricated throughout the surgical procedure. The surgical assistant should, throughout the procedure, take care to carefully retract the lips with the vermilions rolled out. This will prevent tearing and/or irritation of the skin of the lips and reduce postoperative swelling and morbidity.

STEP 2: Soft Tissue Incision

The incision is made through mucosa, muscle, and periosteum. Start the incision superior from halfway up the mandibular ramus, just lingual to the external oblique ridge downwards to mesial of the second molar.

It is important to leave at least 5 mm of nonkeratinized mucosa buccally at the lower end of the incision for ease of suturing later (Fig. 38.1A).

STEP 3: Soft Tissue Dissection of the Mandible

a. *Buccal subperiosteal dissection* (Fig. 38.1B): Use a periosteal dissector and strip the periosteum from the body of the mandible in the first and second molar area down to the lower border to allow for adequate visualization and placement of the channel retractor. There is no need to dissect the entire masseter muscle. One of the main aims of the procedure is to control the proximal segment of the mandible and to maintain the muscle and condyle relationship. Total detachment of the muscle will result in dead space and encourage swelling and hematoma formation.
b. *Superior subperiosteal dissection* (see Fig. 38.1B): Reflect the periosteum from the anterior border of the ramus and detach the lower fibres of the temporalis muscle. Place a swallowtail (notched or forked) retractor over the anterior border and retract the soft tissue superiorly. Now, dissect the periosteum from the internal oblique ridge down to the retromolar area.
c. *Expose the lingula* (see Fig. 38.1B): Dissect the periosteum from the lingual aspect of the mandibular ramus, starting from superior and move downward to visualize the lingula. The fossa superior to the lingual foramen can be located with the tip of the periosteal dissector and is usually a good guide.

Perforation of the periosteum in the area may cause brisk venous hemorrhage. This is usually from the medial pterygoid muscle; however, it often subsides spontaneously. Do not attempt to control the hemorrhage by either forcing a gauze into the area or by means of cautery, as that may damage the lingual and/or the inferior alveolar nerves.

Continued

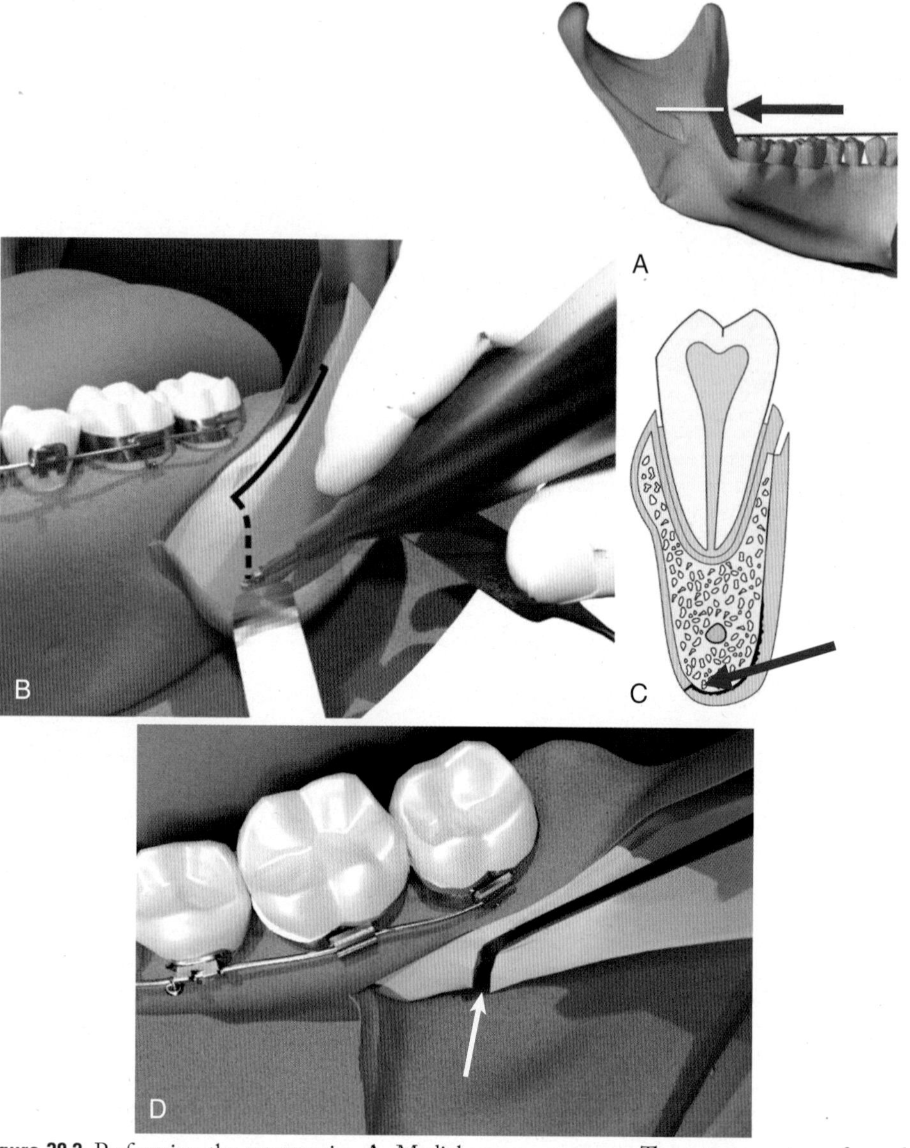

Figure 38.2 Performing the osteotomies. **A,** Medial ramus osteotomy. The osteotomy is performed parallel to the mandibular occlusal plane (*arrow i*) and carried backward to just posterior of the lingula and into the fossa (*arrow ii*). **B,** Sagittal osteotomy: The osteotomy is started superiorly from the medial horizontal osteotomy and carried inferiorly to mesial of the second molar. Stay just medial to the buccal cortex (*arrow i*). **C,** Vertical osteotomy: The osteotomy is started at the lower border and carried superiorly to meet the vertical osteotomy. Ensure that the lingual cortex is included at the lower border (C). **D,** Angulate the cut slightly backward (*arrow*).

TECHNIQUE: Surgical Technique—cont'd

STEP 4: Performing the Osteotomies

a. *Medial ramus osteotomy:* Position a suitable periosteal elevator into the medial dissection, with the tip of the instrument into the fossa superior to the mandibular foramen and visualize the lingula. Use a Lindeman or #701 fissure bur, and aim at the notch of the lingula and angle the osteotomy parallel to the mandibular occlusal plane as depicted by the red arrow in Fig 38.2A. In cases when proper visualization of the lingula is obscured by the convexity of the internal oblique ridge, the convexity can be reduced using a reduction bur.

Perforate the lingual cortex only and terminate the osteotomy into the fossa just posterior of the foramen as depicted by the white line. If the osteotomy is terminated short of the fossa, the osteotomy will split anterior to the foramen, leaving the foramen and superior aspect of the bony canal containing the inferior alveolar nerve still attached to the proximal segment (see Fig. 38.2A) (see Bad Split Type 3).

b. *Sagittal osteotomy:* Using a reciprocating saw or a #701 fissure bur, start the osteotomy at the medial horizontal osteotomy superiorly and complete the cut inferiorly

TECHNIQUE: Surgical Technique—cont'd

on the buccal side, to about mesial of the second molar tooth where the vertical or buccal osteotomy will be performed. Stay just medial to the buccal cortex and ensure that the osteotomy is made through the cortex (about 5 mm) (Fig. 38.2B). The presence of an impacted third molar tooth may interfere with the osteotomy at the retromolar area; however, the tooth should be treated as bone, and the osteotomy is performed through the tooth. The authors prefer to have impacted third molar teeth removed at least 9 months before surgery. The presence of an impacted third molar tooth may cause a fracture of the retromolar segment during splitting (see Bad Split Type 4).

c. *Buccal (vertical) osteotomy of the mandibular body:* Remove the notched retractor. To visualize the lower border and protect the soft tissue, place a channel retractor at the lower border of the mandibular body. Visualization of this area is improved by removing the mouth prop and rotating the mandible closed. The position of the vertical osteotomy is dependent on two factors[1]: By positioning the osteotomy more anterior, the split will be longer, increasing the area of bone contact and allowing for large advancements; however, it will increase the intersegmental bone defects with setback procedures or correction of mandibular asymmetriess.[1] Some surgeons prefer to position the osteotomy more posterior for ease of splitting and managing bone defects[2] (see Fig. 38.2B).

When completing the osteotomy, it is paramount that the cortex of the lower border is included in the cut (Fig. 38.2C). The actual start of the split should be at the lower border, including the lingual cortex (see Step 7). The authors prefer to use a #701 fissure bur and feel the bur perforate the buccal cortex only, taking care not to damage the inferior alveolar nerve. Angle the osteotomy slightly postero-medially to assist with the initiation of the split (Fig. 38.2D) (also see Step 7). The authors prefer to refine this osteotomy using a #703 fissure bur allowing the Reyneke splitters adequate purchase when starting the split.

STEP 5: Place Positioning Holes, Reference Marks, and Holding Wire Holes

The most important and critical step of an orthognathic procedure is positioning the condyle in the glenoid fossa, and it should be performed as a separate step prior the placement of rigid fixation of the jaws. To assist with the condylar positioning maneuver, the author (Johan P. Reyneke) prefers to use a holding wire, whereas the author (Steven M. Sullivan) prefers a specially designed clamp. Both allow the surgeon to accurately position the condyle in the fossa as a separate step (Figs. 38.3 and 38.4) (see Step 15). The condyle/fossa relationship is maintained by the wire while the rigid fixation is applied. Although this step is optional, it is recommended.

a. *Preparation for a holding wire:* The holes for the positioning wire are drilled in the retromandibular area in such a way that the wire has a vector supporting the proximal segment posteriorly and the occlusion anteriorly (see Fig. 38.3A). The ideal distance between the holes after repositioning the segments should be 4 mm.
Geometry–example 1: For a mandibular advancement of 6 mm the holes should be drilled 10 mm apart (the posterior hole on the distal segment). After an advancement of 6 mm, the holes will be 4 mm apart with a class II vector (see Fig. 38.4A).
Geometry–example 2: For a setback procedure of 6 mm, the holes should be drilled 2 mm apart (the anterior hole on the distil segment). Once the mandible is setback by 6 mm, the holes will be 4 mm apart with a class II vector (Fig. 38.4B).

b. *Place reference marks:* Reference marks are placed on the buccal cortex on either side of the vertical osteotomy. Ensure that the line on the proximal segment is made longer for setback procedures as a segment of bone will be removed from this part of the bone (see Fig. 38.3). These lines will assist in proximal segment control and lower border alignment of the segments (see Fig. 38.3B).

c. *Drill a purchase hole for the condylar positioner:* The purchase hole is drilled on the buccal cortex of the proximal segment close to the lower border and angled posteriorly (see Fig. 38.3C) (see Step 11).

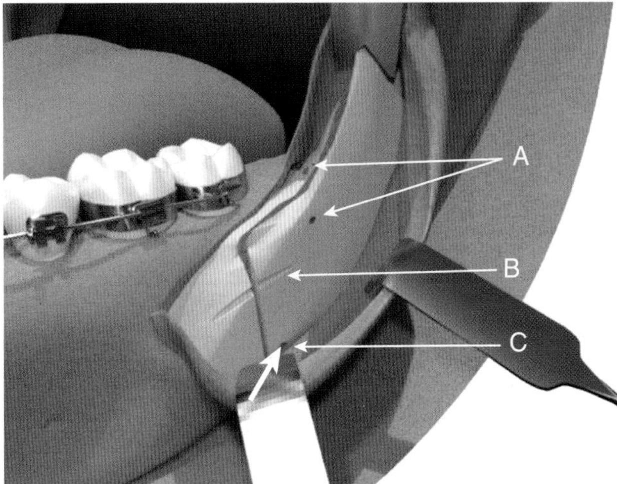

Figure 38.3 **A,** The holes for the holding wire. **B,** Reference line across the vertical osteotomy. **C,** Purchase hole angulated posteriorly (*arrow*) for the condylar positioner.

Continued

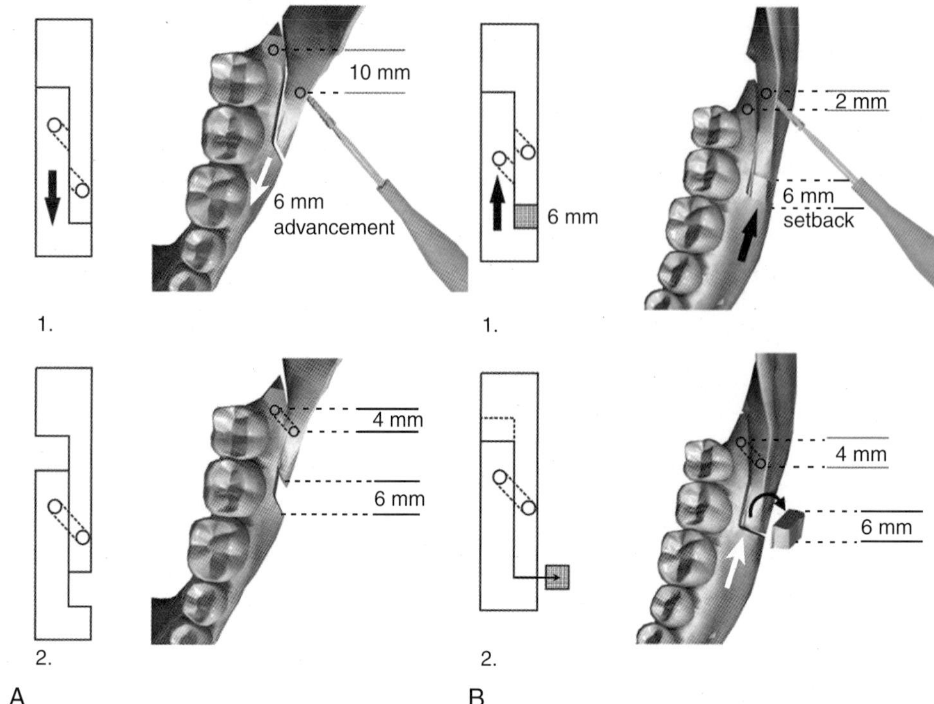

Figure 38.4 **A,** An example of a 6-mm mandibular advancement. 1. The holes are drilled 10 mm apart, the medial hole posteriorly through the distal segment and the buccal hole anterior through the proximal segment. 2. Following a 6-mm advancement, the holes are 4 mm apart. The holding wire will support the proximal segment posteriorly and the distal segment anteriorly. **B,** An example for a 6-mm mandibular setback. 1. The holes are drilled 2 mm apart. 2. Following a 6-mm setback the holes are 4 mm apart. The holding wire will support the proximal segment posteriorly and the distal segment anteriorly.

TECHNIQUE: Surgical Technique—cont'd

STEP 6: Lavage

Once the osteotomy cuts have been completed, it is recommended that the osteotomies on the contralateral side be completed (if indicated) before proceeding to split the mandible. The surgical area is now washed with saline solution and then a small sponge is gently place in the surgical site.

STEP 7: Splitting the Mandible

During this step, the mandible should be supported by the channel retractor (around the lower border) and digital pressure by the assistant to protect the temporomandibular joint and the contralateral hard- and soft-tissue structures (if already split).

The actual splitting of the ramus can be divided into two stages:

First stage:

a. The osteotomy lines are first initiated by tapping a 10-mm osteotome along the sagittal osteotomy line from the medial osteotomy above, downwards to the buccal osteotomy below (Fig. 38.5A).
b. Tap a large 10-mm Obwegeser osteotome superiorly into the sagittal osteotomy line and place a small Reyneke splitter into the buccal osteotomy line to engage the lower border of the mandible (Fig. 38.6).
c. Rotate the instrument gently but firmly and visualize that:
   1. The lower border of the mandible splits towards the proximal segment.
   2. The neurovascular bundle is intact and separates from the proximal segment.

Second stage:

a. Rotate the instruments further while observing that the lower border continues to split towards the proximal segment and the neurovascular bundle detaches from the proximal segment. In the case of excessive resistance to this maneuver, it should be stopped. By applying more force to the segments at this stage, it will lead to a bad split (see Bad Splits). The osteotomy lines should be revised before continuing with the procedure.
b. Proceed with the split. The Obwegeser osteotome is replaced by a larger osteotome and the small Reyneke splitter by a larger splitter; the split can now be completed.
c. The neurovascular bundle may occasionally remain attached to the proximal segment. This phenomenon is more prone to occur in mandibular anteroposterior excessive or asymmetric cases (excessive side), in the presence of an impacted third molar, and when there is unilateral condylar hyperplasia (excessive side). As soon as the surgeon identifies an unfavorable nerve separation,

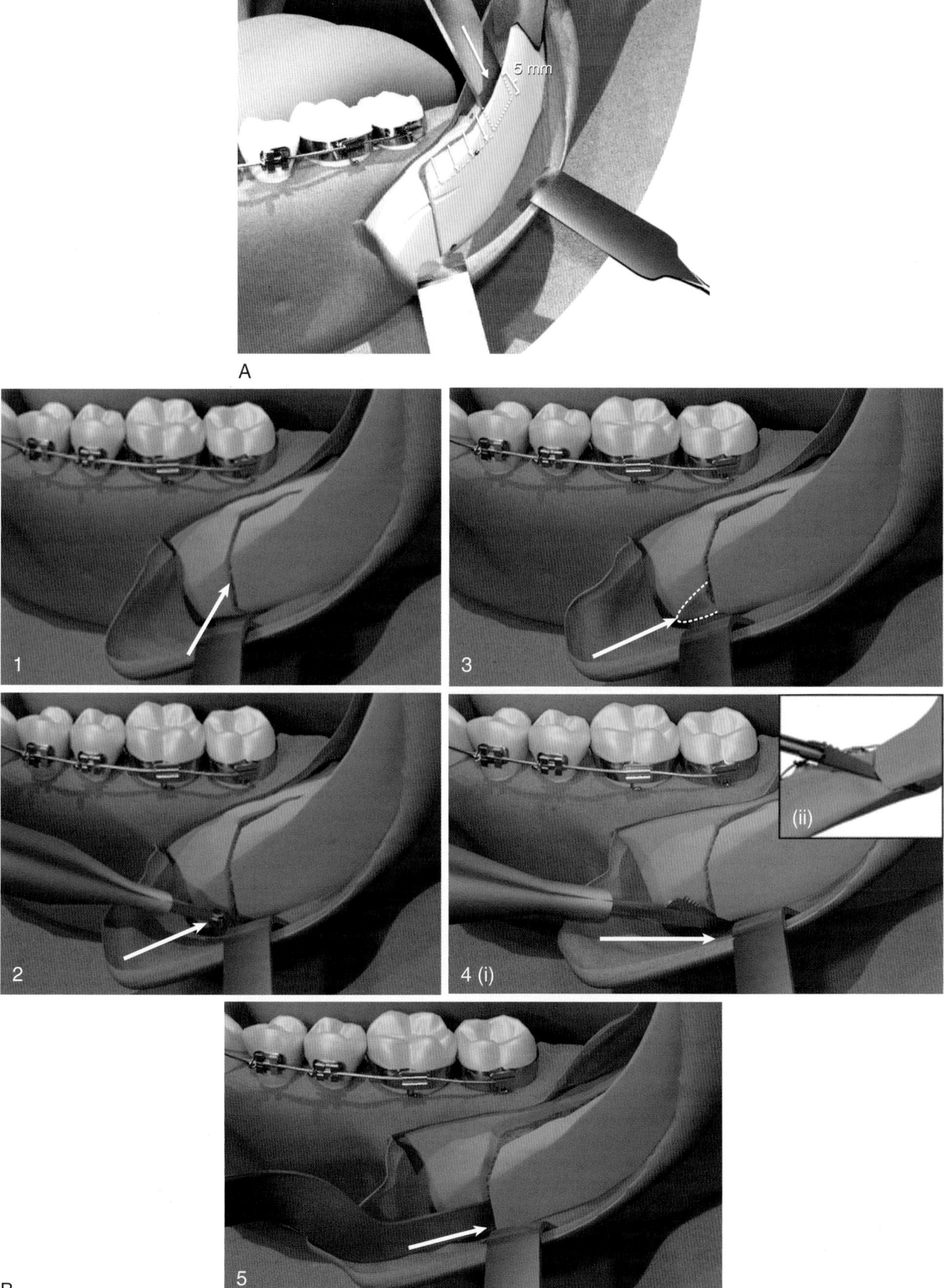

Figure 38.5 **A,** Initiating the split. An Obwegeser osteotome is tapped about 5 mm into and along the vertical osteotomy (*arrows*) to initiate the sagittal split and to ensure that the split starts favorably. **B,** Additional method to initiate and facilitate a safe split. 1. The angulated vertical osteotomy (*arrow*). 2. Use a 4-mm reduction bur to create a bevel on the distal segment (*arrow*). 3. The bevel (*dotted line*) will allow a purchase and angle to the reciprocating saw to ensure a safe start along the center of the lower border of the mandible (*arrow*). 4(I) The saw blade in position at the lower border of the mandible (*arrow*). 4(ii) The posision of the saw at the lower border of the mandible. 5. A Jeter inferior border osteotome is now placed low down in the osteotomy line to initiate the split down the center of the inferior border. A Reyneke or Smith splitter is then used as previously described (see Fig. 38.6).

Continued

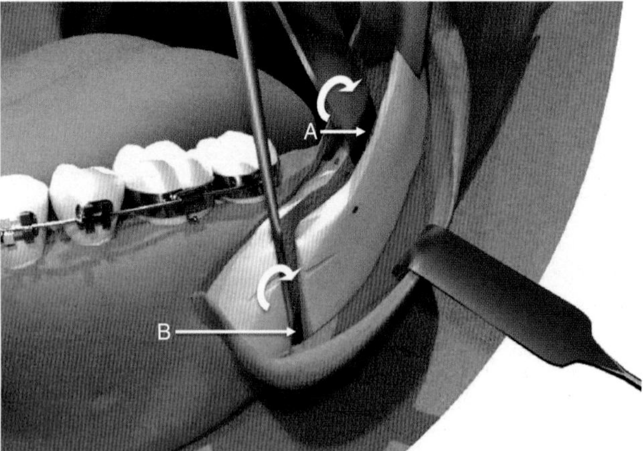

Figure 38.6 Splitting the ramus. **A,** A large Obwegeser osteotome or Smith separator is placed superior into the vertical osteotomy (*arrow a*) and a Reyneke splitter placed low down into the buccal osteotomy (*arrow*). **B,** The osteotomes are now gently but firmly rotated.

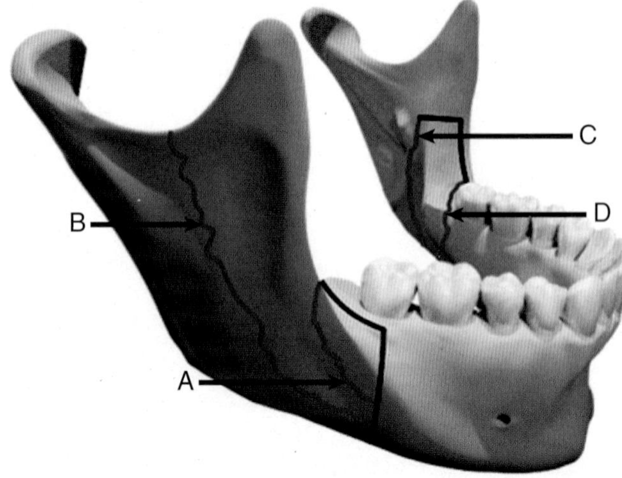

Figure 38.7 Typical patterns of unfavorable splits of the mandibular ramus. **A,** Buccal cortex fracture. **B,** Buccal cortex and coronoid fracture. **C,** Fracture short of the lingula. **D,** Retromolar fracture.

TECHNIQUE: Surgical Technique—cont'd

the split should be stopped and the bundle carefully detached from the proximal segment using a (Howarth) dissector.

The inferior alveolar bony canal may split towards the proximal segment side. The canal should be carefully detached using a small osteotome. Some clinicians are of the opinion not to release the bundle or dissect the canal to release the bundle.

An additional step to enhance the lower border split (Fig. 38.5B):

The surgeon may, in addition to the above steps and prior to the initiation of the split, consider using a reciprocating saw to start the lower border split along the lower border.

Use a 4-mm reduction bur to create a bevel on the distal segment along the buccal osteotomy. The bevel will allow a reciprocating saw to enter the lateral parallel to the buccal cortex. A Jeter osteotome is then inserted and gently tapped to start the split in the center of the lower border of the mandible encouraging a favorable lower border split. The Reyneke splitter (or Smith splitter) can now be placed low down in the osteotomy line to complete the split.

The Bad Split

The human mandibular ramus lends itself to the sagittal split procedure. The anatomical shape and form of the jaw certainly differ among individuals and are influenced by genetics, sex, age, and race, and it may be significantly congenitally deformed.

When surgeons meticulously adhere to the basic surgical technique, most surgeries will come together quietly to make the effort occur smoothly and successfully. However, unfavorable ramus splits do occur, and an understanding of the surgical design and its relationship with the mandibular anatomy will enable the surgeon to identify the start of a bad split early. Early diagnosis will ease salvaging the procedure.

If the surgeon suspects the split not to be proceeding favorably, they should stop and identify the problem under good vision. Unfavorable splits tend to follow a pattern linked to a specific technical maneuver[12–15] (Fig. 38.7).

Type 1. Fracture of the buccal cortex of the mandibular body (Fig. 38.7A).

Early diagnosis: The buccal cortex starts splitting; however, the lower border remains attached and a small fracture line can be observed on the buccal segment.

Solution: Use a #703 fissure bur and redefine the vertical buccal osteotomy, especially at the lower border. Place the Reyneke splitter low down into the osteotomy line and recapture the bone to split with the buccal cortex of the proximal segment. Proceed with the split.

Late diagnosis: The buccal plate fractures and separates completely from the mandible. Remove the segment and store in a moist sponge. Redefine the remaining vertical osteotomy at the lower border and take care not to damage the inferior alveolar neurovascular bundle. Replace the Reyneke splitter or use a small straight osteotome to engage the lower border to complete the split. Replace the separated bone segment and fixate it with a lag screw while the nonfractured segments can be fixated with either bicortical screws or bone plates.

Type 2. Fracture of the buccal cortex involving the ramus and coronoid process (Fig. 38.7B).

Early diagnosis: A fracture line occurs on the buccal cortex running superiorly towards the coronoid notch while the lower part remains attached to the distal segment. Stop and redefine the lower part of the vertical osteotomy, including the lower border. Replace the Reyneke splitter and ensure that the whole buccal segment separates from the distal segment, and then complete the split.

TECHNIQUE: Surgical Technique—cont'd

Late diagnosis: The buccal cortex, including the coronoid process separates from the mandibular ramus. The segment remains attached to the temporalis muscle and should not be removed. The proximal and distal segments are still attached, and every effort should be made to salvage the lower attachment of the proximal buccal cortex. Redefine the vertical osteotomy, and use a Reyneke splitter or small straight osteotome to carefully capture the segment to split towards the proximal segment. There will be limited bone contact between the segment, and one should use bone plate fixation or combination of plate and bicortical fixation.

Type 3. Fracture anterior to the inferior alveolar foramen (Fig. 38.7C).

Early diagnosis: This complication usually occurs when the medial horizontal osteotomy is stopped short of the lingula (see Step 4a). Early diagnosis is imperative to prevent inferior alveolar nerve damage. Carefully extend the osteotomy past the lingula into the fossa under good vision. Use a small osteotome and release the foramen and nerve from the proximal segment.

Late diagnosis: The split is now completed; however, the lingula, foramen, and inferior alveolar nerve are still attached to the proximal segment. Carefully extend the osteotomy posteriorly and release the bone and nerve from the proximal segment.

Type 4. Fracture of the retromolar aspect of the distal segment (Fig. 38.7D).

Early diagnosis: This part of the distal segment is often fragile, especially, with the presence of an impacted third molar tooth. Take care not to wedge against this area when performing the split. Carefully remove the tooth and use plate fixation.

Late diagnosis: Remove the tooth and take care not to damage the lingual or inferior alveolar nerves.

STEP 8: Stripping the Medial Pterygoid Muscle and Pterygomasseteric Sling

a. Use a curved periosteal elevator (J-stripper) and strip the muscle attachments from the lower border of the distal segment.
b. Use a straight periosteal elevator and strip the medial pterygoid muscle and stylomandibular ligament attachments from the medial aspect of the mandibular angle (tooth-bearing, proximal segment) (Fig. 38.8A). This is especially important in mandibular setback procedures and counterclockwise rotations where the muscle and ligament attachments in this area will interfere with free repositioning of the distal segment. The authors also believe that proximal segment control and postoperative stability are improved by removing these attachments (Fig. 38.8B).[16]

STEP 9: Removal of Third Molars

The authors are in favor of the removal of impacted third molars at least 9 months before orthognathic surgery. It will, however, subject the patient to a second surgery. The disadvantages of the presence of an impacted third molar at the time of orthognathic surgery should be considered (Fig. 38.9).[12]

a. The presence of an impacted third molar during the SSO will often interfere with ideal intersegmental bone contact (Fig. 38.9A).
b. A third molar will weaken the retromolar aspect of the distal segment leading to fracture of the segment during removal or even postoperatively (see Bad Split Type 4).
c. An unerupted tooth is often in very close relationship the inferior alveolar nerve, making the nerve more vulnerable during removal (see Fig. 38.9B).
d. The presence of an impacted tooth (or tooth socket) will jeopardize the placement of internal rigid fixation (see Fig. 38.12).
e. An impacted tooth (or tooth socket) will increase the risk of postoperative infection.

STEP 10: Smooth the Intersegmental Contact Areas and Note the Neurovascular Position

Use a reduction bur and smooth the contact areas between the segments, at the same time ensuring space for the neurovascular bundle. Take special care to protect the inferior alveolar neurovascular bundle and not to damage this important structure when using the bur. Also, take this opportunity to note the inferior alveolar neurovascular bundle position. This mental note will come in handy during placement of rigid fixation.

STEP 11: Place the Holding Wire

Feed a 0.018-inch stainless steel wire (or 25 gauge) through the holes drilled in Step 5.

STEP 12: Mobilize the Bone Segments

This important step is performed to ensure that the distal segment is totally mobile for adequate repositioning and not limited by soft tissue (periosteum, muscles and/or gingiva) or small bone intersegmental attachments. The proximal segment is supported by the index finger while the distal segment is gently but firmly pulled forward.

STEP 13: Position the Teeth Into the Planned Occlusion and Place Intermaxillary Fixation

When single jaw surgery is performed, the use of a final splint is optional.

In two-jaw surgery, an intermediate splint is used when mandibular surgery is performed first. However, when the mandibular surgery is performed second, the use of a final splint is optional. Fixate the teeth into occlusion using 0.014-inch (or 28-gauge) wires.

STEP 14: Removal of Bone From the Distal Segment in Class III Setback Cases (Fig. 38.10A–C)

With the teeth wired into occlusion, the channel retractor is placed in position and the distal segment pushed gently posteriorly (Fig. 38.10A). The bone segments will overlap at the vertical osteotomy. The overlap should coincide with the intended amount of setback (Fig. 38.10B). Remove enough bone from

Continued

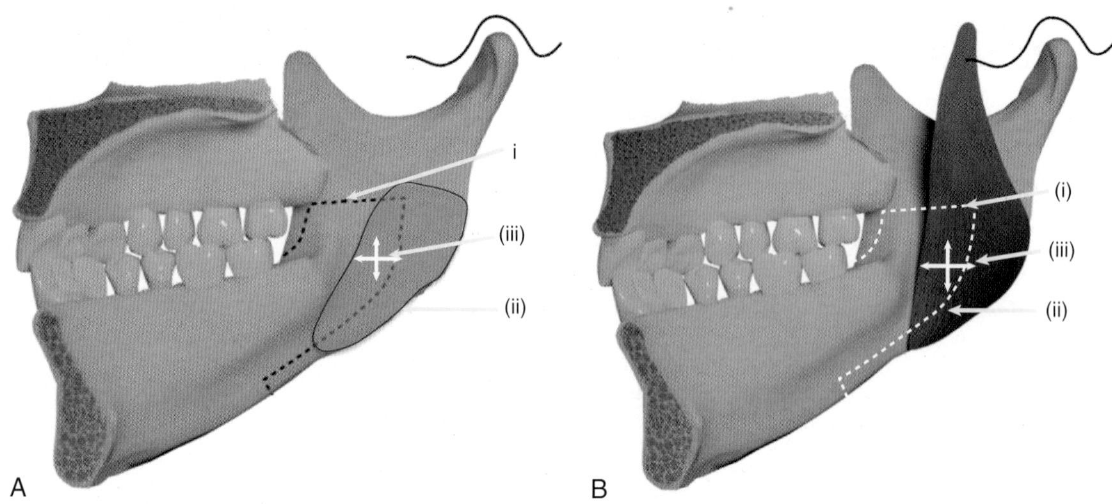

Figure 38.8 Stripping the medial pterygoid muscle off the medial aspect of the mandibular angle. **A,** The dotted line indicates the osteotomy line on the medial side of the mandible (*arrow i*) and the area of muscle attachment (*arrow ii*). Note the interference of the medial pterygoid muscle attachment on the surgical movements of the distal segment (*arrow iii*). **B,** The medial pterygoid muscle and its relation to the medial aspect of the mandibular angle (*arrow i*).

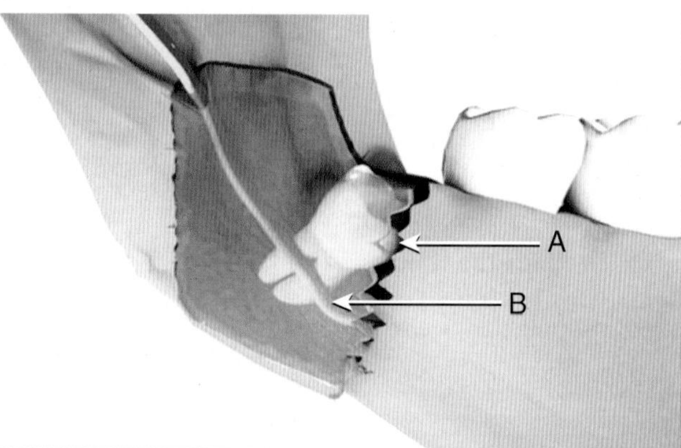

Figure 38.9 A, An unfavorable retromolar fracture as a result of the presence of an impacted third molar tooth (Bad Split Type 4). **B,** Note the vulnerable relationship of the inferior alveolar neurovascular bundle and the fractured segment.

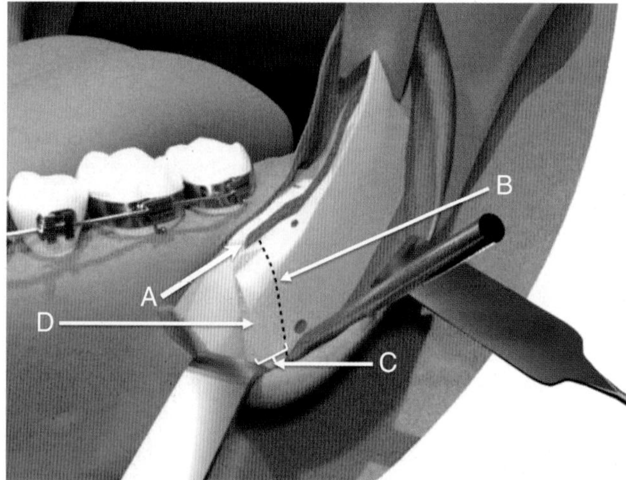

Figure 38.10 Remove overlapping bone in mandibular setback procedures (*arrow*). **A,** The overlap represents the amount of mandibular setback (B). Remove slightly more bone to allow free positioning of the proximal segment and condyle (C).

the distal segment to allow free repositioning (Fig. 38.10C). Do not force the segment into the defect as it will influence condylar positioning by pushing it backwards in the glenoid fossa. The bone removed may be used as a free graft elsewhere (Fig. 38.10D).

STEP 15: Condylar Positioning (Fig. 38.11)

The method of condylar positioning describe here has been developed after performing over 6000 sagittal split osteotomies over a period of 41 years.[17,18] It is a challenging maneuver and certainly the most important step of the procedure. Superb surgery followed by improper positioning of the condyle will fail.

a. Place the fork tail (notched) retractor on the ramus and the channel retractor at the lower border of the mandibular body.
b. Engage the Reyneke condylar positioner into the purchase hole drilled in Step 5, while the angle of the mandible is supported by extraoral digital pressure (Fig. 38.11A).
c. Apply gentle pressure with a posterior vector, and at the same time apply superior and slightly anterior digital pressure on the angle. Note the vector of forces in (Fig. 38.10). This will give the surgeon an awareness of the anatomical relationship between the condyle and the fossa (Fig. 38.11B).
d. Now, use the reference lines placed in Step 5c to gently rotate the distal segment to align the buccal reference lines to ensure proper alignment of the segments at the lower border of the mandible.
e. The assistant can now tighten the holding wire, taking care not to force the segments together in an attempt to close small intersegmental defects. The teeth are in the planned occlusion and the surgeon has poisoned the condyle in the glenoid fossa as described above. Excessive

TECHNIQUE: Surgical Technique—cont'd

force on the positioner and overtightening of the wire to close any intersegmental defects will displace the condyle in the fossa and lead to peripheral (distal, medial or lateral displacement) condylar malpositioning (Fig. 38.11C).

f. As an alternative to the holding wire a bone clamp may be used to maintain the condyle/fossa relationship while rigid fixation is placed. Take care not to force the segments together using the clamp. Clamps such as the Sullivan BSSO (Biomet Microfixation, Jacksonville, FL, USA) clamp are designed to preclude condylar torque if used judiciously.

STEP 16: Placement of Rigid Fixation

Placement of the trochar:

Intraoral approach—This approach is influenced or often limited by the position of the inferior alveolar nerve and second molar tooth roots (Fig. 38.12A), the presence and position of an impacted third molar tooth (Fig. 38.12B), and adequate access to appropriately orientate the screws (Fig. 38.13).

Extraoral approach—This approach gives the surgeon more flexibility when placing bicortical screws or plate fixation (Fig. 38.14). An extraoral stab incision is made through the skin only, about 10 mm below the lower border of the mandible (Fig. 38.14A). The extraoral trochar is now inserted through the stab perforating the soft tissue, periosteum, and mucosa intraorally. To avoid unnecessary force against the bone at this stage, the trochar should be aimed superiorly and the mucosa supported intraorally (Fig. 38.14B).

Bicortical screw fixation:

Several principles should be considered and adhered to during placement of rigid fixation (see Fig. 38.14).

a. The position of the inferior alveolar neurovascular bundle (noted in Step 10) (see Fig. 38.12).
b. The distal root of the second molar tooth (see Fig. 38.12).
c. The combined thickness if the bone segments to estimate the length of the screws (a depth gage may be helpful).
d. Ensure that the bur perforates both cortexes; however, do not push the bur further through the medial segment than required. This will avoid damage to the lingual nerve.
e. Configure the position of the screws to enable stable fixation.
f. Use enough screws for adequate fixation (3 to 4 screws are usually sufficient).

Guidelines to improve safety and efficiency during placement of bicortical screws:

a. Use a sharp bur and apply light pressure when drilling the bicortical holes. Excessive force by the trochar or bur on the bone segments may displace the segments, the occlusion, or the condyle.

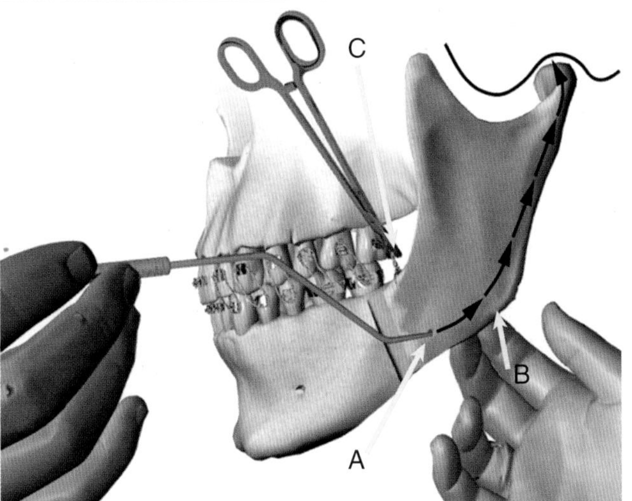

Figure 38.11 Condylar positioning. Place the Reyneke condylar positioner into the purchase hole drilled in Step 5. Push the proximal segment carefully posteriorly using the condylar positioner (A), and with superior digital pressure on the mandibular angles (B), the condyles are positioned into the fossae. The holding wire (C) can now be carefully tightened. Note the two vectors of force.

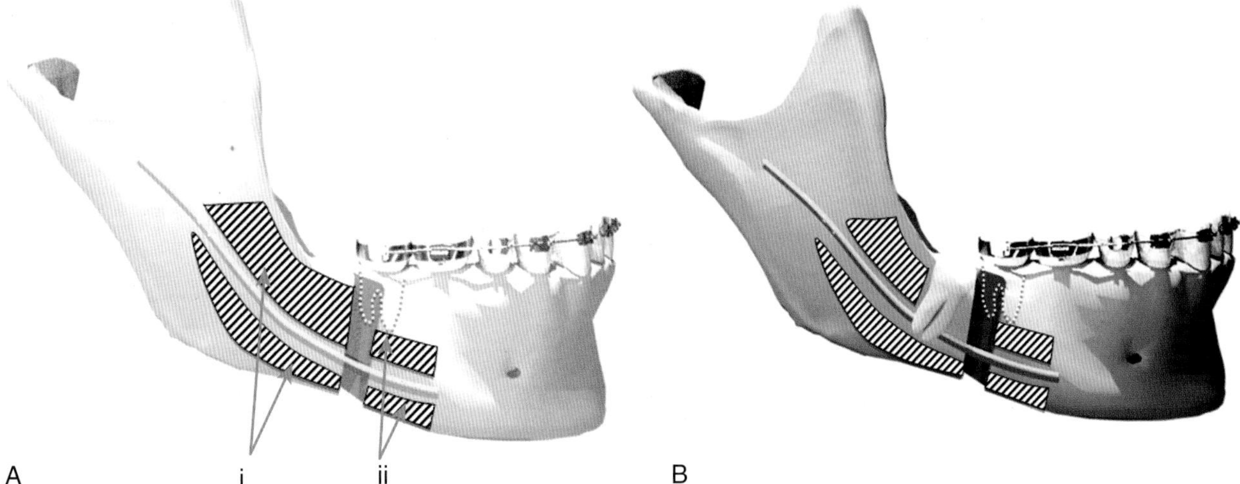

Figure 38.12 **A,** The patterned areas indicate safe positioning of bicortical screws and areas of placing unicortical screws, avoiding the neurovascular bundle and roots of the molar teeth in the absence of a third molar tooth. **B,** The presence of an impacted third molar (or tooth socket following removal) limits placement of bicortical screws and unicortical screws.

Continued

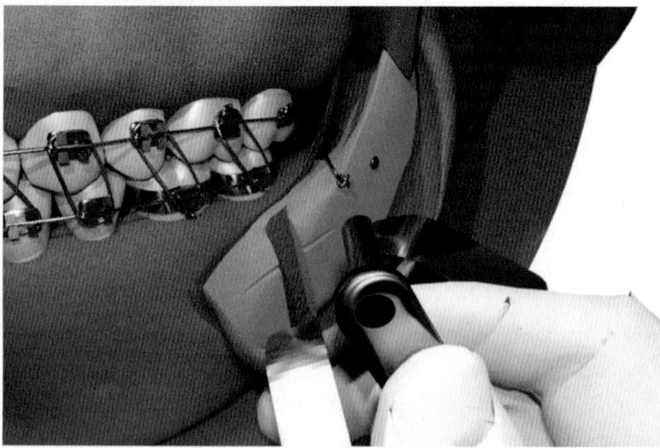

Figure 38.13 Placement of bicortical screw internal rigid fixation. The mandible is advanced. The teeth are wired into the planned occlusion (with or without a surgical splint). The first bicortical screw is placed through a Reyneke intraoral trochar, while the holding wire maintains the condyle in position.

b. Use copious water cooling on the trochar tube to prevent heat generation. The heat may burn the skin and subcutaneous tissue in contact with the tube of the trochar.
c. Angle the screws slightly posterior to support the condyle and repositioned segment.
d. For smooth placement of the screw, the assistant should have a screw with appropriate length ready for placement. An automatic screwdriver is a handy instrument at this time.
e. While applying the screw, observe the distal segment carefully to ensure that the lingual cortex is engaged without any displacement.
f. The bicortical screws are self-tapping and only require rotation to engage. Do not apply force as it may displace the segments and/or occlusion.
g. It is essential that the segments should not be forced together in an attempt to close intersegmental defects. By closing defects, the condyle will be displaced resulting in peripheral sag (see Condylar sag).
h. Small bone defects should be grafted.

Plate fixation:

Some surgeons prefer to use plate fixation routinely as method of fixation following SSO (Fig. 38.15). The principles discussed above will also apply when using this method of fixation.

a. Select an appropriate 2.0-mm plate to allow for placement of at least two screws on each segment. One or two plates may be used; however, some surgeons prefer to use two plates or one plate and one or two screws behind the second molar.
b. The plate should be bent to fit the segments accurately and allow for at least two screws on each side of the vertical osteotomy.
c. Place the screws on the proximal segment first (unicortical or bicortical screws may be used if avoiding teeth and the inferior alveolar nerve). When utilizing the holding wire or clamp (Step 15), this step is simplified

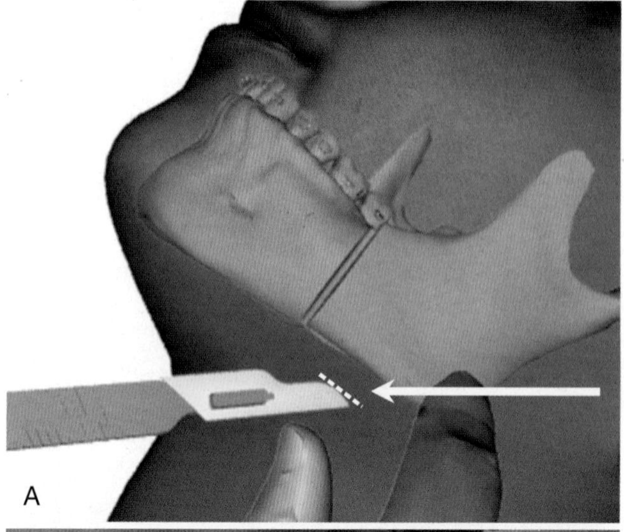

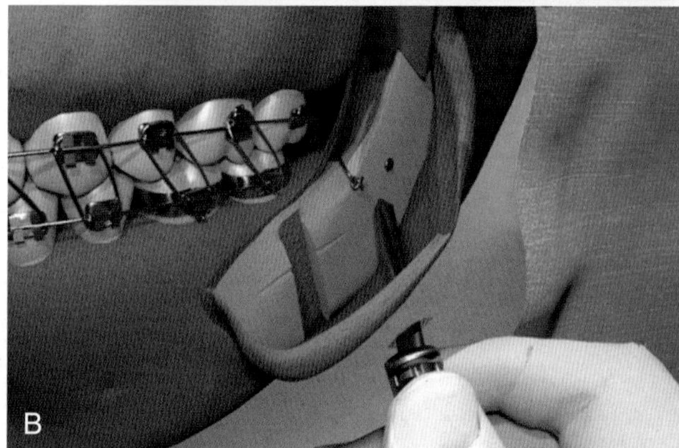

Figure 38.14 This approach gives the surgeon more flexibility when placing bicortical screws or plate fixation. An extraoral stab incision is made through the skin only, about 10 mm below the lower border of the mandible (A). The extraoral trochar is now inserted through the stab perforating the soft tissue, periosteum, and mucosa intraorally. To avoid unnecessary force against the bone at this stage, the trochar should be aimed superiorly and the mucosa supported intraorally (B).

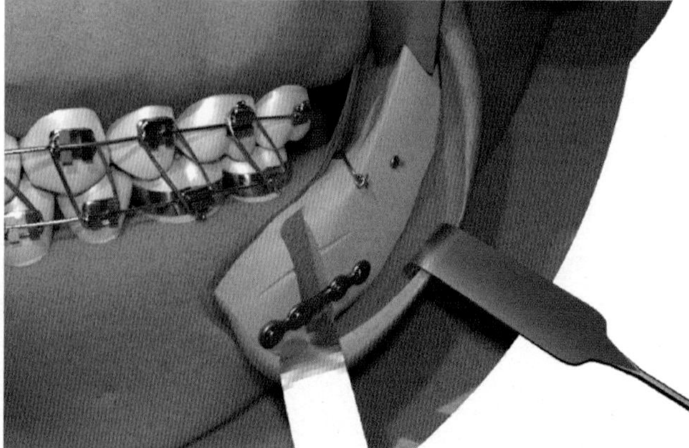

Figure 38.15 Placement of plate internal rigid fixation. The mandible is advanced. The holding wire maintains the condyle in position. One bicortical screw is placed to assist with fixation. Note the reference lines assisting with alignment and a four-hole plate as fixation.

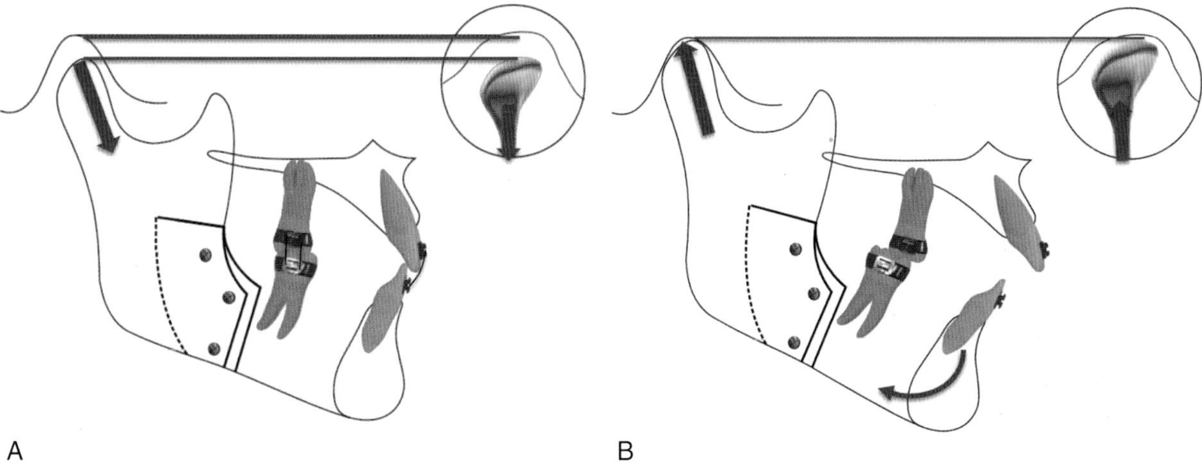

Figure 38.16 Central sag type 1. **A,** The condyle is inferiorly displaced in the fossa without any bone contact. Once the intramaxillary fixation is removed, the condyle moves superiorly into the fossa leading to a class II occlusion and an anterior open bite (B).

TECHNIQUE: Surgical Technique—cont'd

as the relationship between the segments, occlusion, and condyle has already been established and secured.

d. Unicortical screws engaging the distal segment can now be placed while the proximal segment (condyle) is held in place by either the holding wire or a positioning instrument. Avoid damage to the roots of the molar teeth by using unicortical screws.

STEP 17: Removal of Intermaxillary Fixation and Check the Occlusion

To ensure that the condyles were positioned correctly in the fossa, the occlusion should not be checked immediately, following removal of intermaxillary fixation (IMF).[14] Wait a few minutes, and then gently open and close the mouth and slowly translate the jaw to the left and right. With light finger pressure on the chin, close the mouth and check the occlusion. The occlusion should be exactly as planned or fit into the final surgical splint. Resist the temptation to force the teeth into occlusion. The authors are not in favor of a final splint in most cases, as it may hide small occlusal discrepancies, which will only be noticed once the splint is removed weeks after surgery.

STEP 18: Intraoperative Assessment of the Occlusion[19]

It is mandatory that once the IMF is removed, the mandible is carefully opened, translated, and transversely manipulated. The mandible is then slowly closed into occlusion (or surgical splint) and the occlusion assessed. The differential diagnosis of a malocclusion following intraoperative removal of IMF includes the following:

a. Failure of fixation
b. Displacement of the occlusion during placement of rigid fixation
c. An inaccurate surgical split
d. Intracapsular edema or hemarthrosis. These problems may only become apparent postoperatively
e. Incorrect positioning of the condyle(s) (condylar sag)

Condylar malposition or various forms of sag are a complication when performing the sagittal split osteotomy that can result in an immediate or delayed malocclusion. It is also a complication that is relatively easy to detect intraoperatively. The best time to diagnose and correct a malocclusion as a result of condylar sag is intraoperatively following removal of IMF. It is inappropriate to attempt correction of a malocclusion as result of condylar malpositioning by orthodontic means. In 2002, Reyneke and Ferretti in 2002[19] described the geometry of the different types of condylar malpositioning and proposed a straightforward method to identify the different forms of condylar malpositioning following intraoperative removal of IMF.

Central condylar sag: Central sag type 1: Central sag is defined as inadequate seating of the condyle, leaving the condyle inferiorly positioned in the glenoid fossa without any bone contact (Fig. 38.16A). This form of sag is detected upon release of maxillo-mandibular fixation and results in a class II malocclusion and an open bite (Fig. 38.16B). This form of sag may occur bilaterally in which case the dental midline is unaffected or unilateral in which case there is movement of the mandibular dental midline towards the affected side. This type of complication simply requires identifying the side(s) affected, reapplying the IMF, removal of the fixation on the affected side(s), reseating the condyle(s), reapplication of rigid fixation, and verification that the occlusion has been corrected.

Central sag type 2: Excessive posterior force during condylar positioning will push the condyle posteriorly in the fossa, sliding the condyle inferiorly on the posterior fossa surface. Following removal of IMF, the condyle will slip anteriorly and superiorly into the fossa, leading to an anterior open bite and a slight tendency to class II occlusion (Fig. 38.17A and B).

The other two forms of condylar malposition are referred to as peripheral condylar sag.

Peripheral condylar sag type 1

Type 1 peripheral sag occurs when an intersegmental defect (Fig. 38.18A, C) is surgically closed by forcing the segments together (Fig. 38.18B and C). The condyle is then moved

Continued

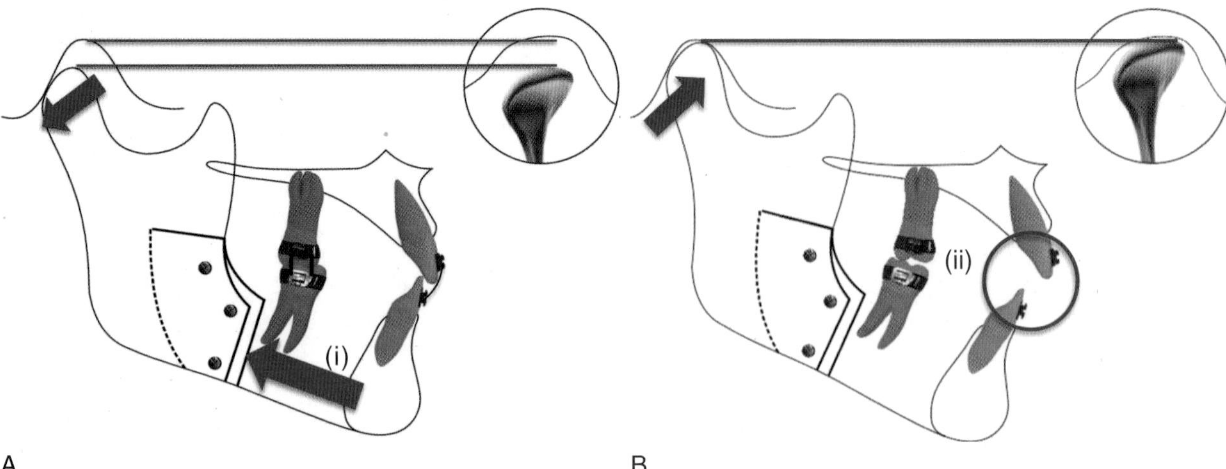

Figure 38.17 Central sag type 2. Due to excessive force applied by the condylar positioner (*arrow i*), the condyle is forced posteriorly in the fossa and will slide inferiorly along the posterior fossa surface (*arrow ii*) (A). Once the IMF is removed, the condyle will slide anteriorly and superiorly into the fossa (*arrow i*), leading to an anterior open bite and a slight class II relationship (*arrow ii*) (B).

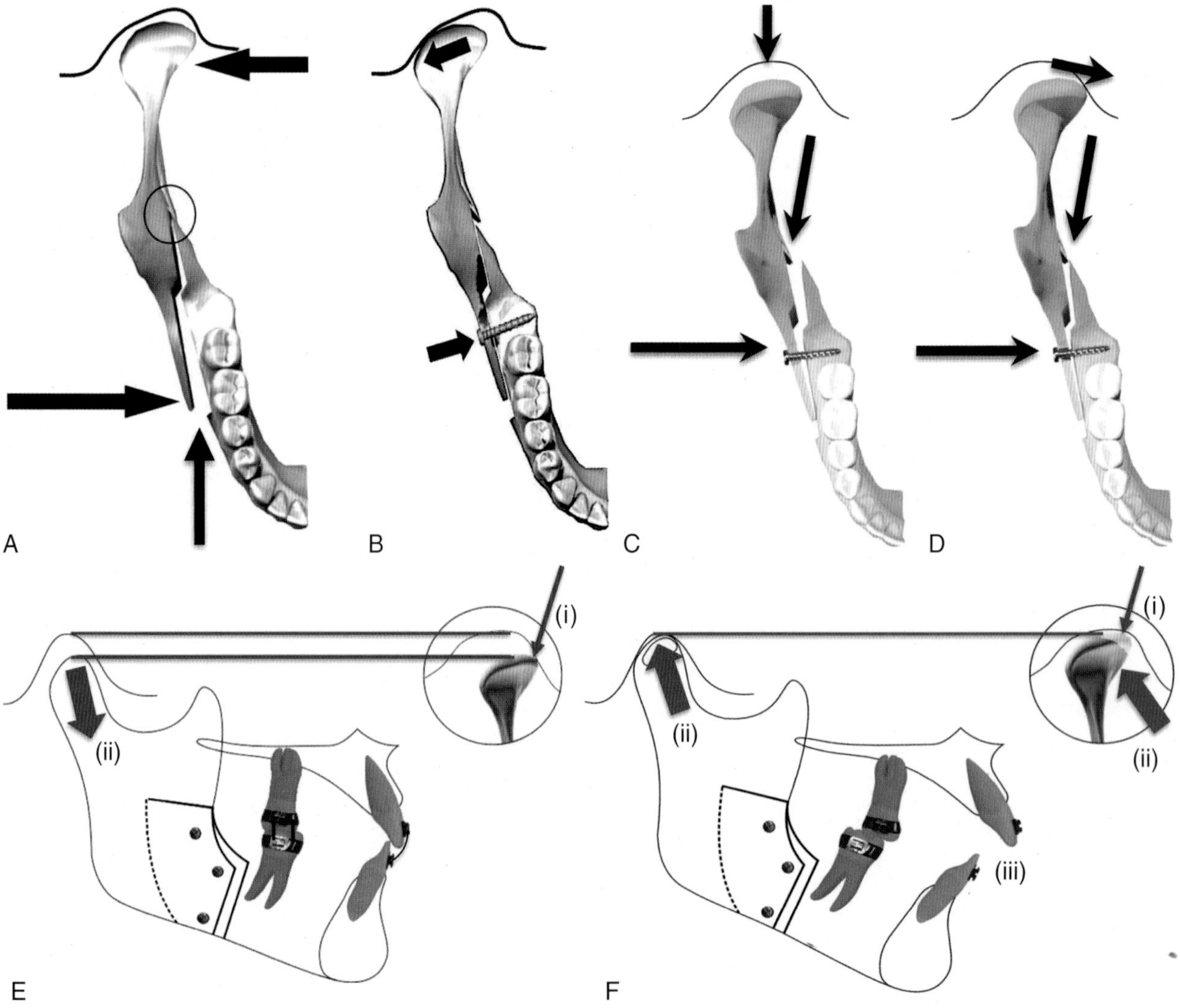

Figure 38.18 Peripheral sag type 1. In an attempt to close the intersegmental bone defect and achieve intersegmental bone contact, the segments are forced together (A), forcing the condyle laterally (B) or medially (C) and (D), and inferiorly in the fossa in the direction of the arrows. Positioning screws will maintain the defect and the condyle in position (C). The disadvantage of lag screws forcing the segments together will displace the condyle as demonstrated in (D). The condyle is displaced inferiorly with contact on the glenoid fossa wall (*arrow*). The contact area will support the articulation following removal of the intermaxillary fixation (IMF) (E). Postoperative condylar resorption in the contact areas will allow the condyle to slide superiorly into the fossa (F) leading to late occlusal relapse.

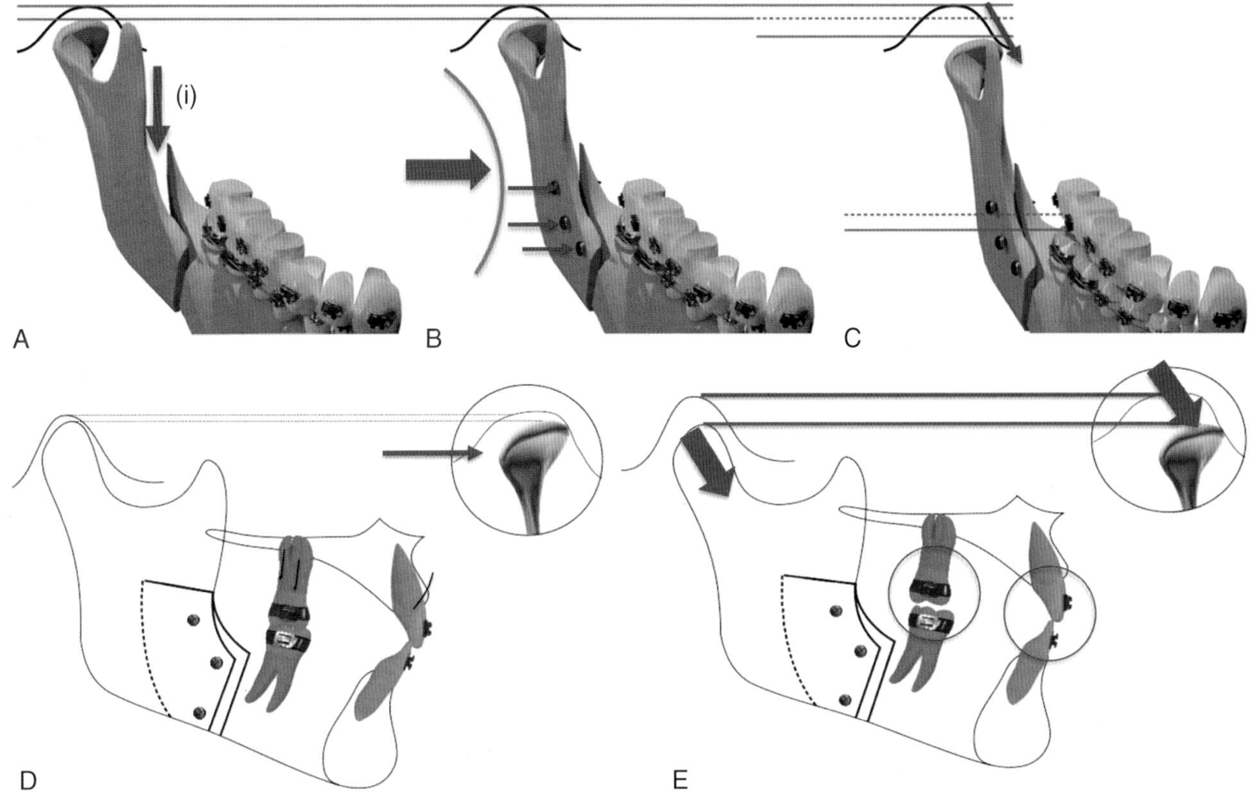

Figure 38.19 Peripheral sag type 2. Following advancement of the proximal segment, a defect is created between the segments (A). The defect is closed by the rigid fixation; however, a torquing force is placed on the condyle and ramus (B and D). After removal of the IMF, the condyle slides inferiorly along the medial (or lateral) wall of the fossa (C), leading to a posterior open bite and an edge-to-edge incisor relationship (E).

TECHNIQUE: Surgical Technique—cont'd

laterally (Fig. 38.18B) or medially (Fig. 38.18D) and will slide inferiorly along the fossa wall. Due to the fact that the condyle now articulates at a contact area, the articulation is supported by the bone contact making intraoperative diagnosis impossible (Fig. 38.18E). The contact in the fossa will maintain the occlusion until such time as resorption and remodeling of the condyle has occurred and will seat inferiorly in the fossa leading to delayed occlusal changes (Fig. 38.18F).

Peripheral condylar sag type 2

Type 2 peripheral sag occurs when the position of the condyle is vertically correct in the fossa; however, a medial force is placed on the condyle and ramus when rigid fixation is applied. The condyle is being torqued due to forceful apposition of the proximal and distal segment in an attempt to achieve bone contact (Fig. 38.19A and B). Once the IMF is removed, the tension is released, and the condyle then slides inferiorly along the medial wall of the fossa (Fig. 38.19C and D), creating a posterior open bite on the affected side and an edge-to-edge incisor relationship (Fig. 38.19E). There are often also sagittal changes leading to a tendency to a class III occlusion on the affected side and a lower dental midline shifts to the opposite side.

To avoid reoperation, condylar sag can be diagnosed intraoperatively and should be addressed at the time. Only peripheral sag type 1 cannot be diagnosed intraoperatively. Elastics are not recommended for the correction of any form of condylar sag.[19]

STEP 19: Place Intra- and Extraoral Sutures

Resorbable sutures are used intraorally in a continuous fashion. Nonresorbable suture are used extra orally and removed 2 days after surgery and replaced with Steri-Strips.

STEP 20: Place Intermaxillary Elastics

The purpose of the elastics is to override the proprioception and not an attempt to correct an incorrect occlusion.

Use 4-oz. 0.25-inch elastics and place one elastic on each side in a triangular fashion in the canine regions. The direction of the vectors should support the surgical movement (i.e., class II vector for mandibular advancements and class III vector for mandibular setbacks).

STEP 21: Apply a Pressure Bandage

The authors use a Surgifoam dressing designed to cover the surgical areas. The pressure bandage is removed 1 day after surgery and physiotherapy is then commenced.

Continued

Avoidance and Management of Intraoperative Complications

No matter how accurate the diagnosis and meticulous the surgical technique, complications will occur as with any other surgery. Risks and complications specific to the sagittal split ramus osteotomies include the following:

The bad split: The mandibular split may not occur according to the "classical" way as described in the text. The four typical unfavorable patterns of bad splits are described and solutions for each undesired split are suggested in Step 7.[12–14]

Condylar sag: Positioning the condyle into the glenoid fossa, once the planned occlusion is established, is mandatory. Tips regarding accurate condylar positioning (Step 15) and intraoperative occlusal diagnosis of a malpositioned condyle (incorrect condyle/fossa relationship) are discussed in Step 18.[19]

Inferior alveolar nerve damage: Loss or altered sensation may occur over the long term as a result of mandibular nerve damage. Posnick et al.[20] reported a residual subjective awareness of sensory alteration along the distribution of the mental nerve in 29% after 1 year. When the BSSO was combined with an osseous genioplasty, 67% of patients experienced varying degrees of subjective loss of sensation in the chin and lower lip area. Turvey[21] reported a 5.5% incidence of intraoperative laceration of the inferior alveolar nerve. Tay et al.[22] reported nerve laceration in 4 out of 240 patients who underwent SSO. The nerves underwent immediate repair; however, the postoperative sensory return proved not to be significantly better than expected after the simple approximation of the nerve endings within the ramus of the mandible. They described the anterior and inferior aspect of the osteotomy along the buccal shelf between the first and second molar as a "danger zone" for nerve damage.

Infection: Infection can occur and is most often due to an infected hematoma in the area. An intraoral incision and drainage frequently can manage this problem. In some cases, it may be necessary to remove the plates and screws that were placed. Alpha et al.[23] noted that they had a 6.5% incidence of hardware infections that required removal of the plates and screws in their series.

Significant bleeding: In current practice, significant hemorrhage is rarely encountered at the time of SSO. The vessels to consider include the inferior alveolar artery and maxillary artery and its branches, the retromandibular vein, and the facial artery and vein.[24]

Postoperative Considerations

Patients should be placed on a short course of oral antibiotic medication and be instructed to maintain a soft diet until initial bony union of the mandible occurs. The use of intermaxillary fixation with elastics is helpful in management of the occlusion during the early healing period. Coordination with postsurgical orthodontic care and appropriate surgical follow-up is mandatory.

References

1. Trauner R, Obwegeser H. Zur Operationstechnik bei der Progenia und anderen Unterkieferanomalien. *Dtsch Zahn Mund Kieferhlkd.* 1955;23:1–4.
2. Dal Pont G. Retromolar osteotomy for the correction of prognathism. *J Oral Surg Anesth Hosp Dent Serv.* 1961;19:42–47.
3. Hunsuck EE. A modified intra oral sagittal splitting technique for correction of mandibular prognathism. *J Oral Surg.* 1968;4:250–253.
4. Epker BN. Modifications in the sagittal osteotomy of the mandible. *J Oral Surg.* 1977;35(2):157–159.
5. Spiessl B. [Osteosynthesis in sagittal osteotomy using the Obwegeser-Dal Pont method]. *Fortschr Kiefer Gesichtschir.* 1974;18:145–148.
6. Reyneke JP. Basic guidelines for the surgical correction of mandibular anteroposterior deficiency and excess. *Clin Plast Surg.* 2007;34(3):501–517.
7. Blomquist DS, Lee JJ. Mandibular orthognathic surgery. In: Miloro M., Ghali G.E., Larson P., Waite P., eds. Peterson's Principles of Oral and Maxillofacial Surgery. Vol 2, 3rd ed. 2012:1317–1392, chap 57.
8. Reyneke JP, Ferretti C. The bilateral sagittal split mandibular ramus osteotomy. *Atlas Oral Maxillofac Surg Clin N Am.* 2016;24:27–37.
9. Reyneke JP, Ferretti C. Anterior open bite correction by Le Fort I or bilateral sagittal split osteotomy. *Oral Maxillofac Surg Clin N Am.* 2007;3:321–338.
10. Reyneke JP. Rotation of the Maxillomandibular Complex. In: Naini FB, Daljit SG, eds. *Orthognathic Surgery, Principles, Planning and Practice.* Oxford, UK: Wiley Blackwell; 2017:530–554.
11. Reyneke JP. *Johan P Reyneke's Techniques, Tips, Tricks and Traps: Volume 1: The Bilateral Sagittal Split Mandibular Ramus Osteotomy.* Vol. 1. Gainesville, FL: RA Education LLC Publ; 2019.
12. Beukes J, Reyneke JP, Becker PJ. Variations in the anatomical dimensions of the mandibular ramus and the presence of third molars: its effect on the sagittal split ramus osteotomy. *Int J Oral Maxillofac Implants.* 2013;42(3):303–307.
13. Steenen SA, van Wijk AJ, Becking AG. Bad splits in bilateral sagittal split osteotomy: systematic review and meta-analysis of reported risk factors. *Int J Oral Maxillofac Implants.* 2016;45(8):971–979.
14. Steenen SA, Becking AG. Bad splits in bilateral sagittal split osteotomy: systematic review of fracture patterns. *Int J Oral Maxillofac Implants.* 2016;45(7):887–897.
15. Tsakiris Reyneke JP, Becker PJ. Age as a factor in the complication rate after removal of unerupted/impacted third molar teeth at the time of mandibular sagittal split osteotomy. *J Oral Maxillofac Surg.* 2002;60:654–659.
16. Beukes J, Reyneke JP, Becker PJ. Medial pterygoid muscle and stylomandibular ligament: the effect on postoperative stability. *Int J Maxillofac Surg.* 2013;1:43–48.
17. Reyneke JP. *The Bilateral Sagittal Split Ramus Osteotomy, Techniques, Tips Tricks and Traps.* Gainesville, Fl: RA- Education, LLC Publ; 2019.
18. Reyneke JP. *Ch. 5, Surgical technique in: Essentials in Orthognathic Surgery.* 2nd ed. Chicago: Quintessence Pupl; 2013.
19. Reyneke JP, Ferretti C. Intraoperative diagnosis of condylar sag after bilateral sagittal split ramus osteotomy. *Br J Oral Maxillofac Surg.* 2002;40(4):285–292.
20. Posnick JC, Al-Qattan MM, Stepner NM. Alteration in facial sensibility in adolescents following sagittal split and chin osteotomies of the mandible. *Plast Reconstr Surg.* 1996;97(5):920–927.
21. Turvey TA. Intraoperative complications of sagittal split osteotomy of the mandibular ramus: incidence and management. *J Maxillofac Surg.* 1985;43:594.
22. Tay AB, Poon CY, Teh LY. Immediate repair of transected inferior alveolar nerves in sagittal split osteotomies. *J Oral Maxillofac Surg.* 2008;66(12):2476–2481.
23. Alpha C, O'Ryan F, Silva A, Poor D. The incidence of postoperative wound healing problems following sagittal ramus osteotomies stabilized with miniplates and monocortical screws. *J Oral Maxillofac Surg.* 2006;64(4):659–668.
24. Acebal-Bianco F, Vuylsteke PLPJ, Mommaerts MY, De Clercq CA. Perioperative complications in corrective facial orthopedic surgery: a 5-year retrospective study. *J Oral Maxillofac Surg.* 2000;58(7):754–760.

CHAPTER 39

The Anterior Segmental Maxillary Osteotomy

Dror M. Allon and Neeraj Panchal

Armamentarium

#9 Periosteal elevator	Bone hook	Malleable retractors
#15 Scalpel blades	Curved Mayo scissors	Needle electrocautery
#701 Bur	Double-guarded nasal septal osteotome	Obwegeser retractors
24- and 26-gauge wire	Fixation devices (P&S)	Reciprocating saw and/or piezosurgical saw
Appropriate sutures	K-wires	Seldin retractor
Arch bars	Local anesthetic with vasoconstrictor	Straight osteotomes

History of the Procedure

The first anterior segmental maxillary osteotomy (ASMO) was reported at the beginning of the 20th century. Günther Cohn-Stock tried to surgically "correct a marked overjet and overbite of the central maxillary teeth."[1] In his pioneering article in 1921, he described the evolution of his idea to perform an osteotomy of the anterior segment of the maxilla while preserving the vestibular pedicle and, in a later design, the palatal artery.[1]

Cohn-Stock presented two surgical cases performed under local anesthesia in his Berlin practice in May and June 1920. In his definitive version, "Cohn III," he described a transverse palatal wedge ostectomy palatal to the anterior teeth, performed through a subperiosteal tunnel, and then a manual manipulation to create a greenstick fracture at the ostectomy site to retract the anterior maxilla. Contemporary authors suggest that Cohn-Stock's greenstick fracture method resulted in significant relapse after removal of the fixation splint because the anterior maxilla was not adequately mobilized.

After Cohn-Stock's original report, three variations of the procedure were developed by Wassmund,[2] Wunderer,[3] and Cupar.[4] These variations were designed to maintain sufficient blood supply to the maxilla while giving adequate access for instrumentation.[5,6]

In 1927 Wassmund[2] improved Cohn-Stock's design by creating a direct approach to the labial premaxillary cortex using three vertical incisions and subperiosteal tunneling for completion of the labial osteotomy without the reflection of the labial or palatal flaps. Both the labial and palatal blood supply is maintained; however, the osteotomy is performed in a relatively blind fashion. This method may be indicated for closure of multiple interdental spaces[6] and for anteroposterior repositioning of the premaxilla.[7] It was found to maintain the best vascularity of the repositioned segment in comparison to all other ASMO methods.[8]

In 1954 Cupar[4] described a different approach for downfracture of the anterior maxilla: exposure of the labial aspect of the maxillary bone by a vestibular circumferential cut and labial flap to facilitate the labial osteotomy under direct vision. A palatal osteotomy was performed through a tunnel, maintaining the palatal blood supply. This technique is indicated for superior repositioning of the anterior maxilla in cases of vertical maxillary excess.

In 1963 Wunderer[3] advocated reflection of a palatal flap with out-fracturing of the anterior maxilla and maintenance of the labial blood supply. Direct access for the palatal osteotomy is the main advantage of this technique, especially if posterior segments of the premaxilla must be removed. Therefore, this technique may be indicated for setback of the anterior part of the maxilla. Blood flow studies have demonstrated that the transpalatal approach causes the greatest decrease in blood supply to the anterior maxilla.[9] However, transpalatal soft tissue incision and labial osteotomies impair blood supply to the anterior maxilla from the greater palatine vessels and the superior alveolar vessels, respectively, leaving the labial collaterals as the sole blood supply to the anterior maxilla.[10]

In 1977 Epker modified the Cupar technique for downfracture of the anterior maxilla. He used only labial flaps and vertical tunnels labial to the teeth to be extracted, which were usually premolars on both sides (this technique is described in detail later in the chapter).[11] Epker's modification enables repositioning of the anterior maxilla superiorly, posteriorly, and inferiorly. The main advantages of the Epker modification include preservation of the palatal pedicle, ease of placement of internal fixation, access to the nasal septal structures to prevent buckling of the nasal septum with superior repositioning of the maxilla, and a direct approach for removal of palatal bone. When required, bone grafting for stabilization of an inferiorly positioned anterior maxilla may also be performed using this method.

Indications for the Use of the Procedure

1. Anterior vertical maxillary excess in cases with acceptable posterior occlusion
2. Sagittal maxillary excess with acceptable posterior occlusion
3. Maxillary anterior protrusion of anterior teeth with normal incisor axial inclination to bone and acceptable posterior occlusion
4. Excessive proclination of anterior teeth
5. Dentoalveolar bimaxillary protrusion when an acceptable posterior occlusion is performed in association with a mandibular subapical osteotomy
6. Anterior open bite without vertical maxillary excess and normal posterior occlusion
7. When retraction of anterior teeth is indicated but cannot be accomplished with conventional orthodontic treatment (e.g., because of root resorption as a result of previous orthodontic treatment, tooth ankylosis, malpositioned dental implants)
8. Reduction of upper lip prominence relative to the nose and lower face
9. Maxillary excess combined with wide interdental spaces (malformed teeth, oligodontia)
10. Preprosthetic procedure: augmentation and repositioning of anterior edentulous atrophic maxillary ridge for dental implants
11. Dental crowding and anterior maxillary hypoplasia

Limitations and Contraindications

The same principles for every orthognathic procedure apply to the ASMO. Most authors advocate postponing the surgery until the craniofacial skeleton reaches full maturity. Orthodontic consultation and treatment should be scheduled well in advance (typically 9 to 12 months) to prepare the occlusion for the planned postoperative position of the anterior segment and the interdental or extraction sites. A useful application to accomplish this is the three-dimensional manipulation of the computed tomography scan, which can be used to predict orthodontic movement of teeth, subsequent segmental repositioning, and soft tissue changes.

Patient cooperation and compliance in the maintenance of good periodontal condition during the preoperative orthodontic treatment are crucial. Dental neglect, gingivitis, and periodontitis must be well controlled before the operation. Failure to do this is a relative contraindication and adversely affects the quality of the final outcome. Local factors and habits, such as tongue thrust and finger sucking, also impair treatment results if not diagnosed and addressed before intervention.

Other considerations include bone quality, anterior maxillary anatomy, palatal vault structure, nasal septum, and conchae (when maxillary impaction is planned). The choice of surgical technique depends on treatment objectives and the direction of the anterior maxillary repositioning movement. In selected cases with an anterior open bite, the anterior segment is rotated clockwise and downward after interdental osteotomies. In these cases, the down-fracture method is preferred. Conversely, if extraction of premolars is planned for setback of the anterior maxilla, direct visualization of the palatal osteotomy is required, and the Wunderer technique should be considered. The advantage is a transverse palatal incision, which allows direct instrumentation; the main disadvantage is compromised perfusion by the intact labial soft tissue pedicle.

TECHNIQUE: Anterior Segmental Maxillary Osteotomy

STEP 1: Intubation

A hypotensive general anesthetic is administered via nasoendotracheal intubation with a reinforced tube that exits superiorly across the face. The tube is secured with a drape and small sponge to the forehead. Because intraoperative intermaxillary fixation is necessary to establish the postoperative position of the anterior maxilla, oral intubation is less desirable and should be avoided. The length of the endotracheal tube must be sufficiently below the level of the vocal cords to prevent unintended dislodgement during premaxillary manipulation.

STEP 2: Preparation

The maxillary vestibule and palatal mucosa are infiltrated with 3.6 cc of local anesthetic solution (lidocaine 2% with adrenaline 1:100,000) for vasoconstriction and minimal intraoperative bleeding. The face, head, and oral cavity are then prepared with Betadine scrub. The entire operative field is straight, exposing the oral cavity, nose, and forehead.

TECHNIQUE: Anterior Segmental Maxillary Osteotomy—cont'd

STEP 3: Exposure

A horizontal incision is made by diathermy or a #15 scalpel blade in one strike to the bone in the depth of the buccal vestibule, circumferentially from the right to left second premolar. Next, the periosteum is reflected superiorly to expose the entire canine fossa and piriform aperture bilaterally. Inferiorly, care should be taken to avoid unnecessary periosteal stripping to maximize blood supply to the osteotomized maxilla. The alveolar mucoperiosteum should be undermined to the crestal bone only at preplanned osteotomy or ostectomy sites. The nasal mucoperiosteum should be carefully separated from the nasal cavity floor to prevent intraoperative bleeding, postoperative oronasal communication, and fistula formation. The cartilaginous nasal septum is separated from the nasal groove of the maxilla to facilitate its manipulation later.

STEP 4: Extractions and Horizontal Osteotomies

If indicated, one or two maxillary premolars are extracted on each side. Then, a reciprocating saw or piezosurgical saw is used to perform horizontal osteotomies. These bone cuts should run posteriorly from each side of the piriform rim, including the lateral maxillary walls and the lateral nasal cavity walls; the nasal mucosa is protected with a curved periosteal elevator. Care should be taken to avoid injury to the infraorbital nerve during retraction of the upper mucoperiosteal flap. The posterior limit for these osteotomies is the planned vertical osteotomy/ostectomy, usually the first or second premolar (Fig. 39.1A–B).

Continued

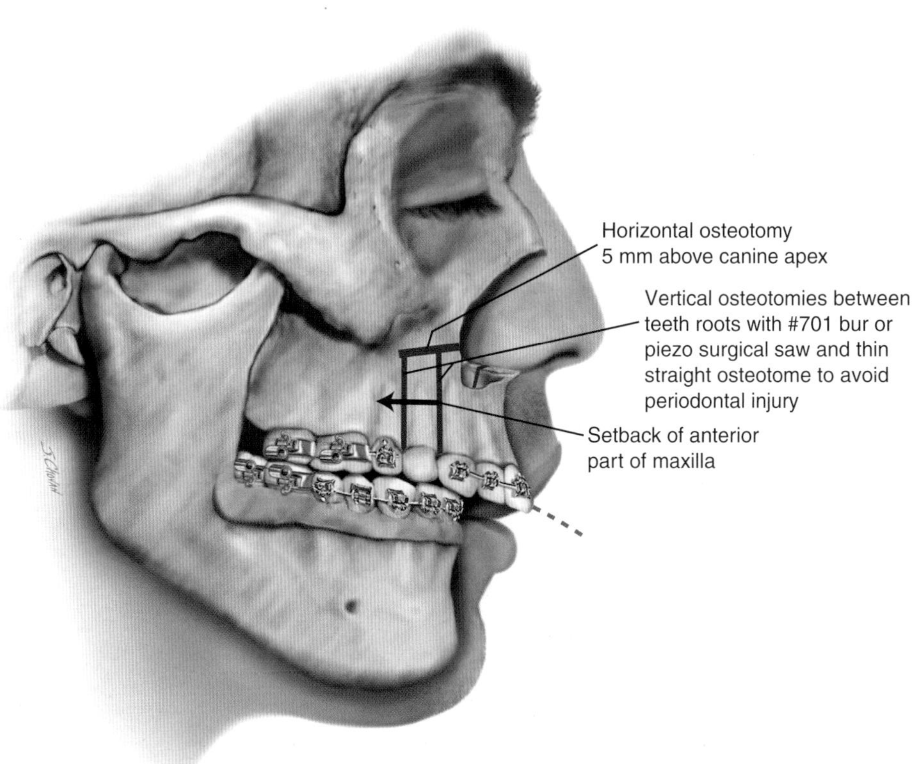

Figure 39.1 Epker's modification of Cupar's down-fracture anterior maxillary osteotomy. **A** and **B**, Horizontal osteotomies are performed using a #701 bur or piezosurgical saw.

Continued

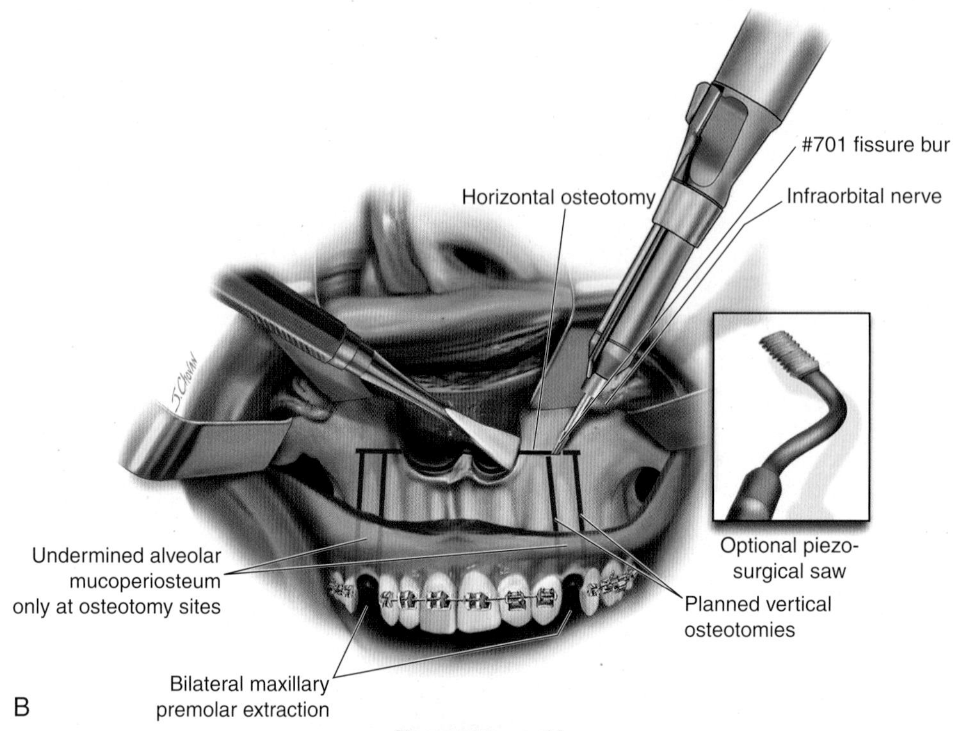

Figure 39.1, cont'd

TECHNIQUE: Anterior Segmental Maxillary Osteotomy—cont'd

STEP 5: Vertical Osteotomies/Ostectomies

Precise bone removal should be done to ensure an accurate post-operative position and sufficient intersegmental bony contacts. Meticulous tissue handling is of paramount importance at this stage. Failure to preserve buccal mucosa may lead to an impaired blood supply to the down-fractured maxilla or establishment of an oroantral fistula, in addition to periodontal compromise of the adjacent teeth (Fig. 39.1C–E).

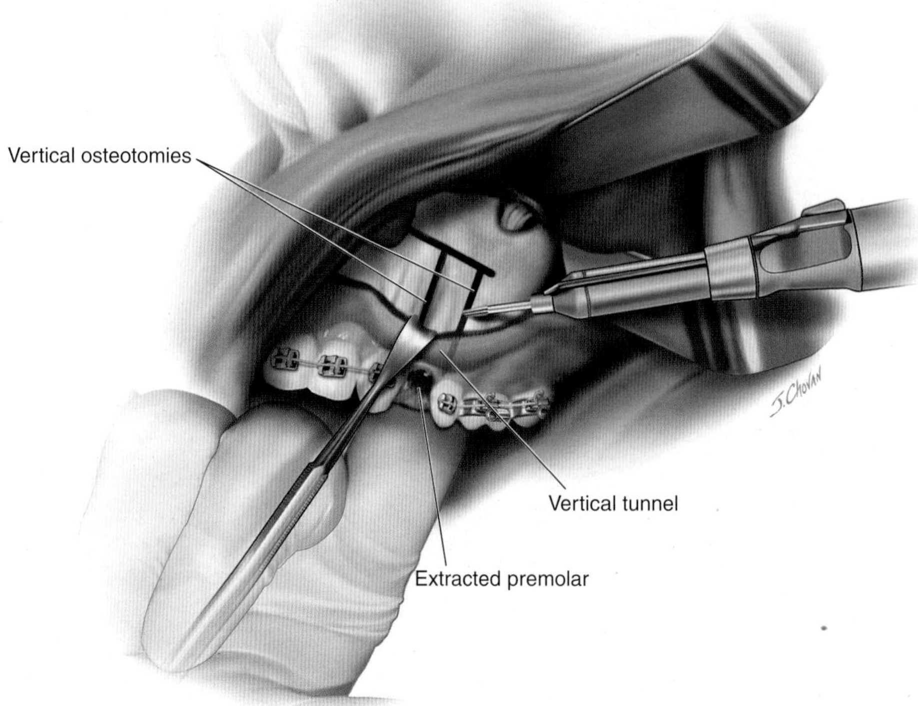

Figure 39.1, cont'd C–E, Care should be taken when performing vertical osteotomies and ostectomies.

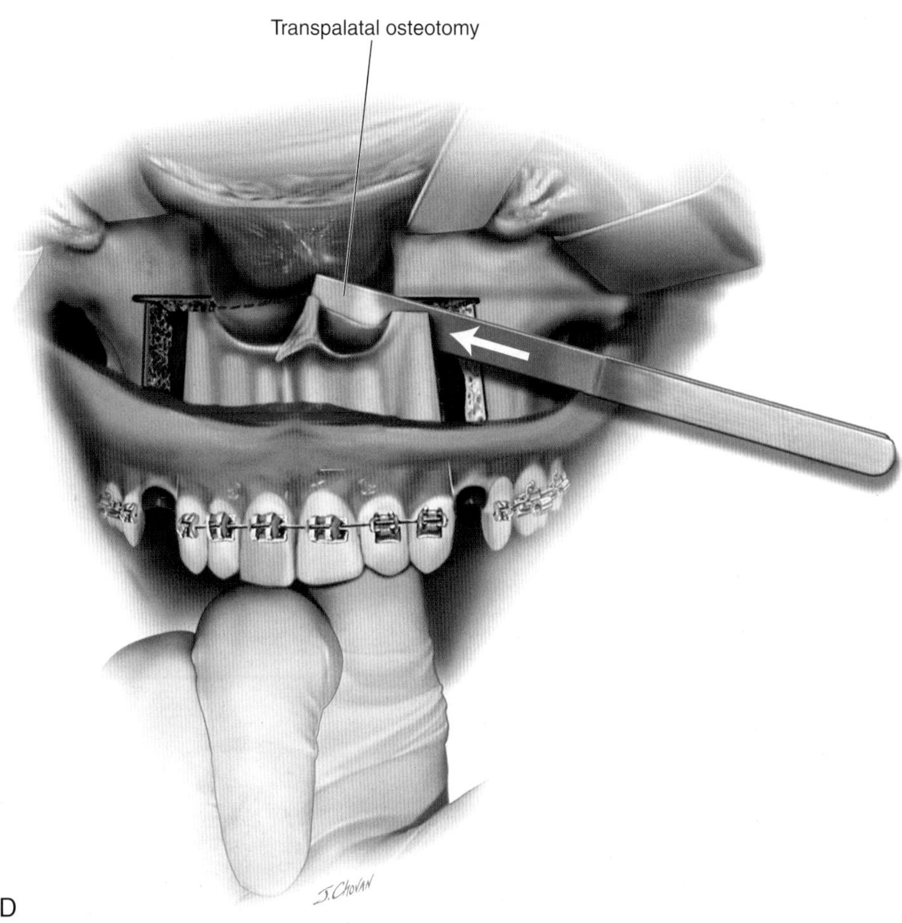

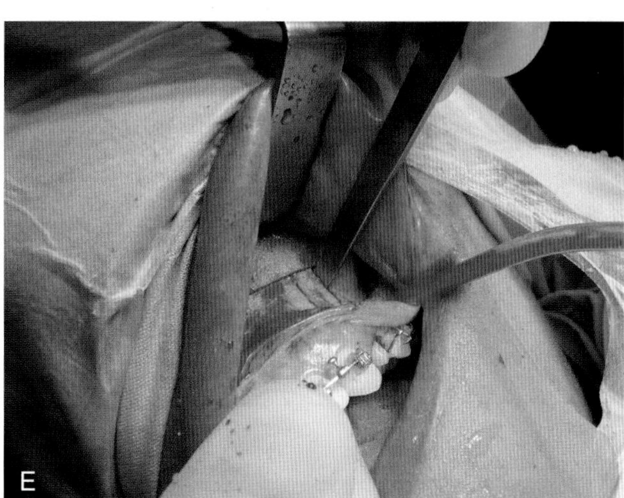

Figure 39.1, cont'd

Continued

TECHNIQUE: Anterior Segmental Maxillary Osteotomy—cont'd

STEP 6: Final Osteotomy and Down-Fracture of the Premaxilla

After completion of the planned osteotomies and ostectomies under direct visualization, the final osteotomy is performed using an osteotome. Neither a palatal incision nor mucosal undermining is done at this stage. A palpating finger is placed on the palatal mucosa, and the transpalatal osteotomy is completed with an osteotome. Down-fracture of the premaxilla is accomplished with a bone hook.

Additional transpalatal and nasal ostectomies may be necessary at this stage and should be finalized under direct access gained to the nasal aspect of the down-fractured premaxilla. Careful separation of the mucoperiosteum from the posterior segment of the palate facilitates setback of the anterior segment and prevents it from becoming detached from the anterior segment, compromising the blood supply (Fig. 39.1F).

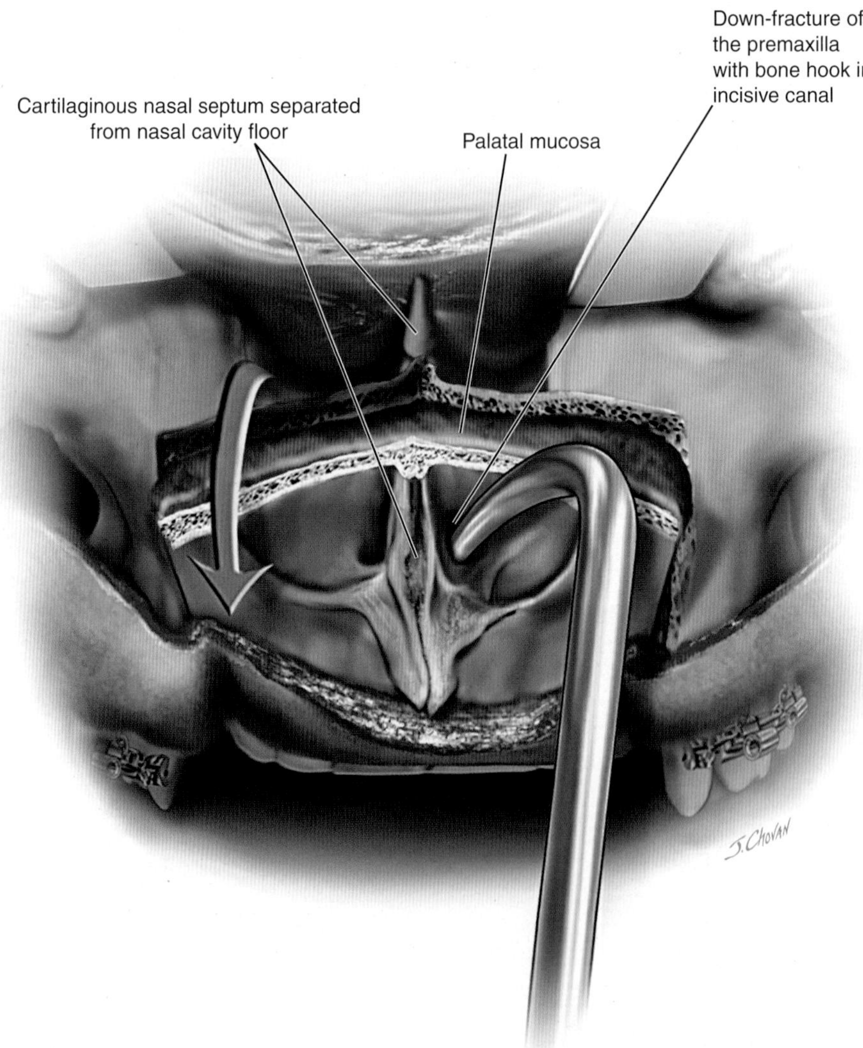

Figure 39.1, cont'd F, Final osteotomy and down-fracture of the premaxilla.

TECHNIQUE: Anterior Segmental Maxillary Osteotomy—cont'd

STEP 7: Midpalatal Osteotomy
If indicated for transverse widening or narrowing of the premaxilla or closure of a diastema, a midpalatal osteotomy is performed with an osteotome or piezosurgical saw (Fig. 39.1G).

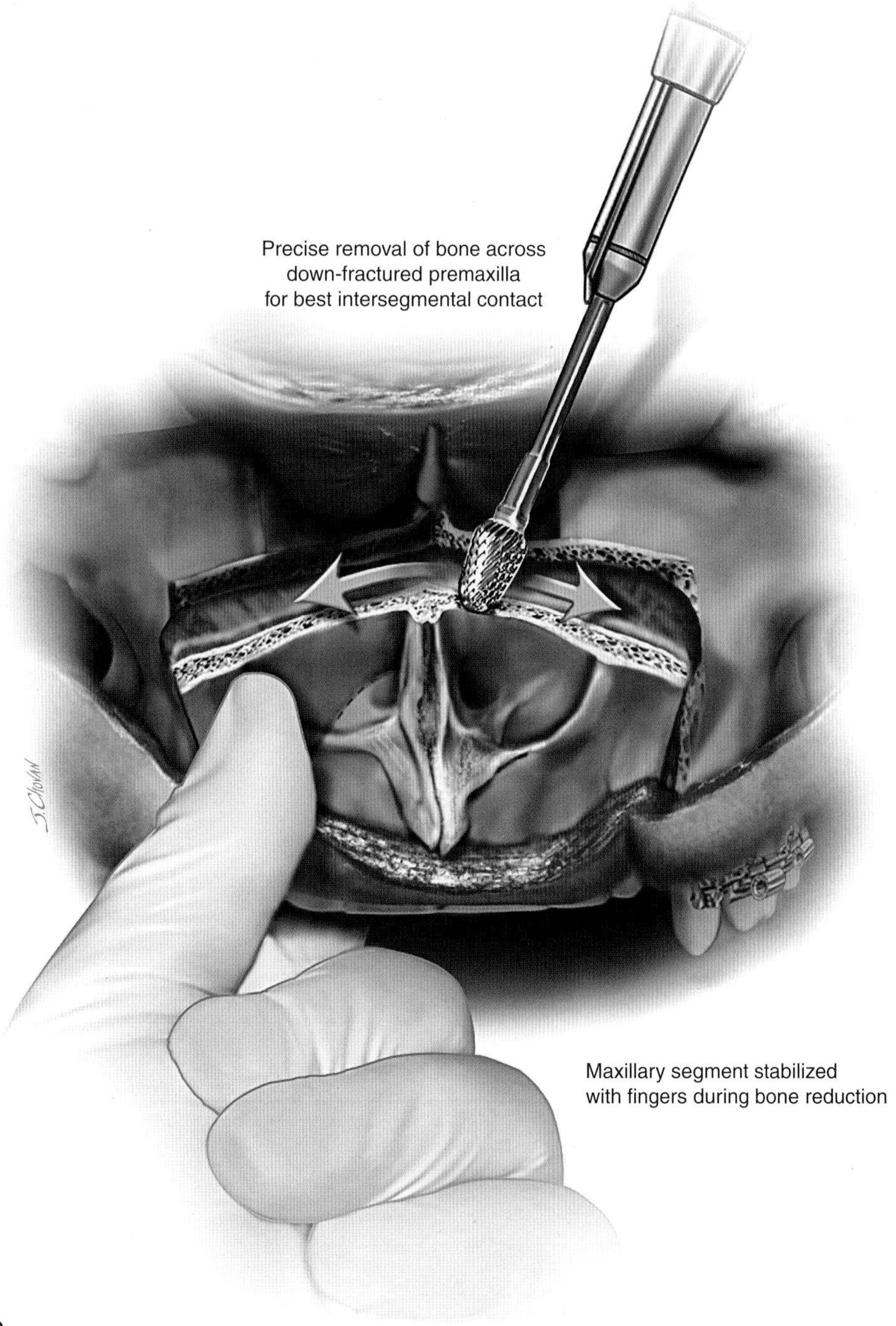

Figure 39.1, cont'd **G,** A midpalatal osteotomy is performed with an osteotome or piezosurgical saw.

Continued

TECHNIQUE: Anterior Segmental Maxillary Osteotomy—cont'd

STEP 8: Fixation

After completion of the ostectomies, maxillary teeth are placed into a preformed acrylic occlusal splint, and the splint is wired to the maxillary dentition. Temporary intermaxillary fixation then is performed, and a standard 1.5 or 2.0 maxillary plating system is used at the maxillary buttresses to fixate the bone segments in their planned postoperative position (Fig. 39.1H and I).

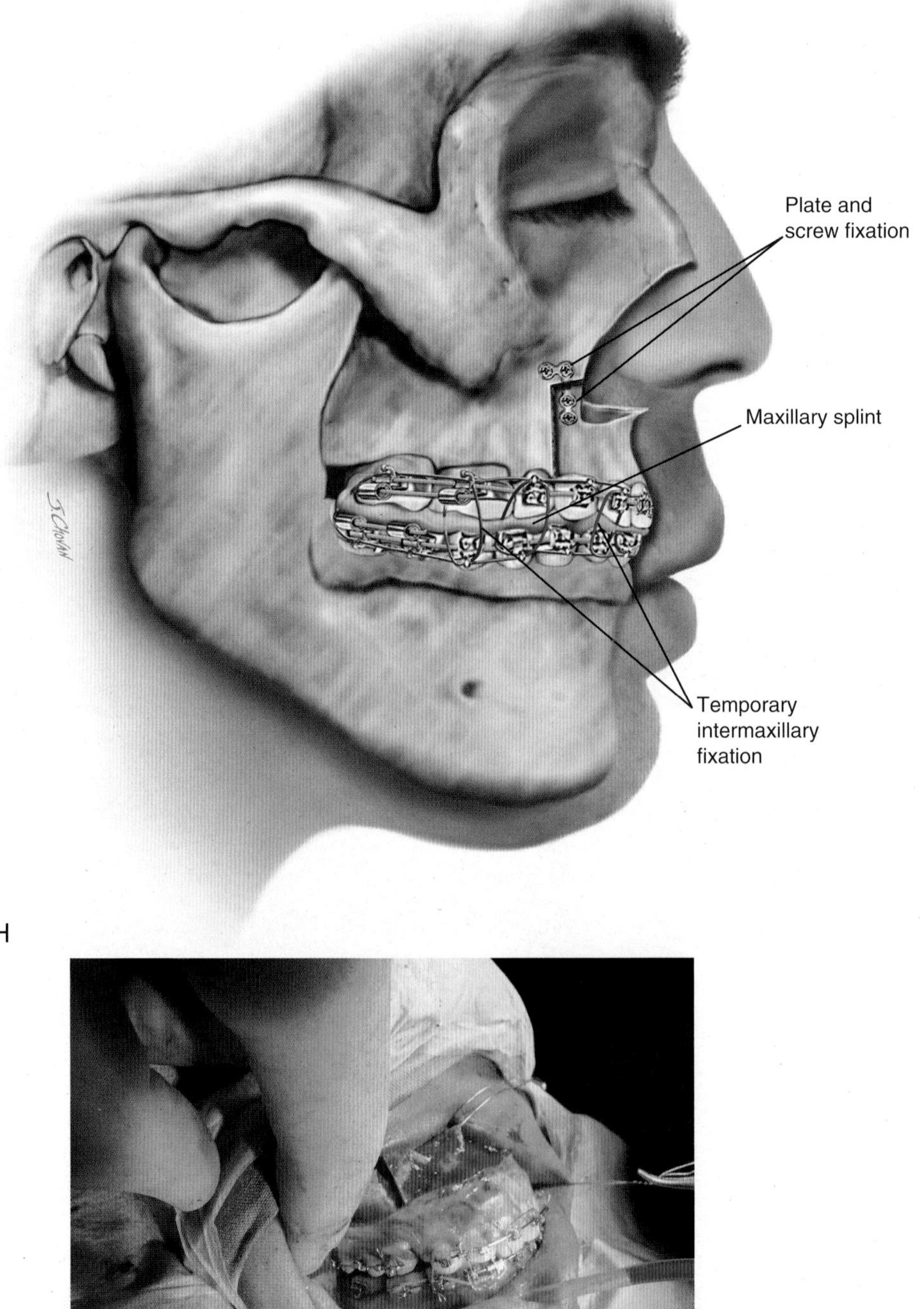

Figure 39.1, cont'd **H,** Maxillary teeth are placed into a preformed acrylic occlusal splint, and the splint is wired to the maxillary dentition. **I,** Intraoperative photograph of intermaxillary fixation.

TECHNIQUE: Anterior Segmental Maxillary Osteotomy—cont'd

STEP 9: Closure

After thorough irrigation of the surgical site with saline, the mucosal incisions are closed with 3-0 chromic suture. If indicated, alar cinch and VY closure of the buccal incision are performed at this stage. Intermaxillary fixation can be removed at the end of the procedure. The maxillary splint should be kept in place for 6 weeks for additional stability of the maxillary segments and occlusal guidance (Fig. 39.1J and K).

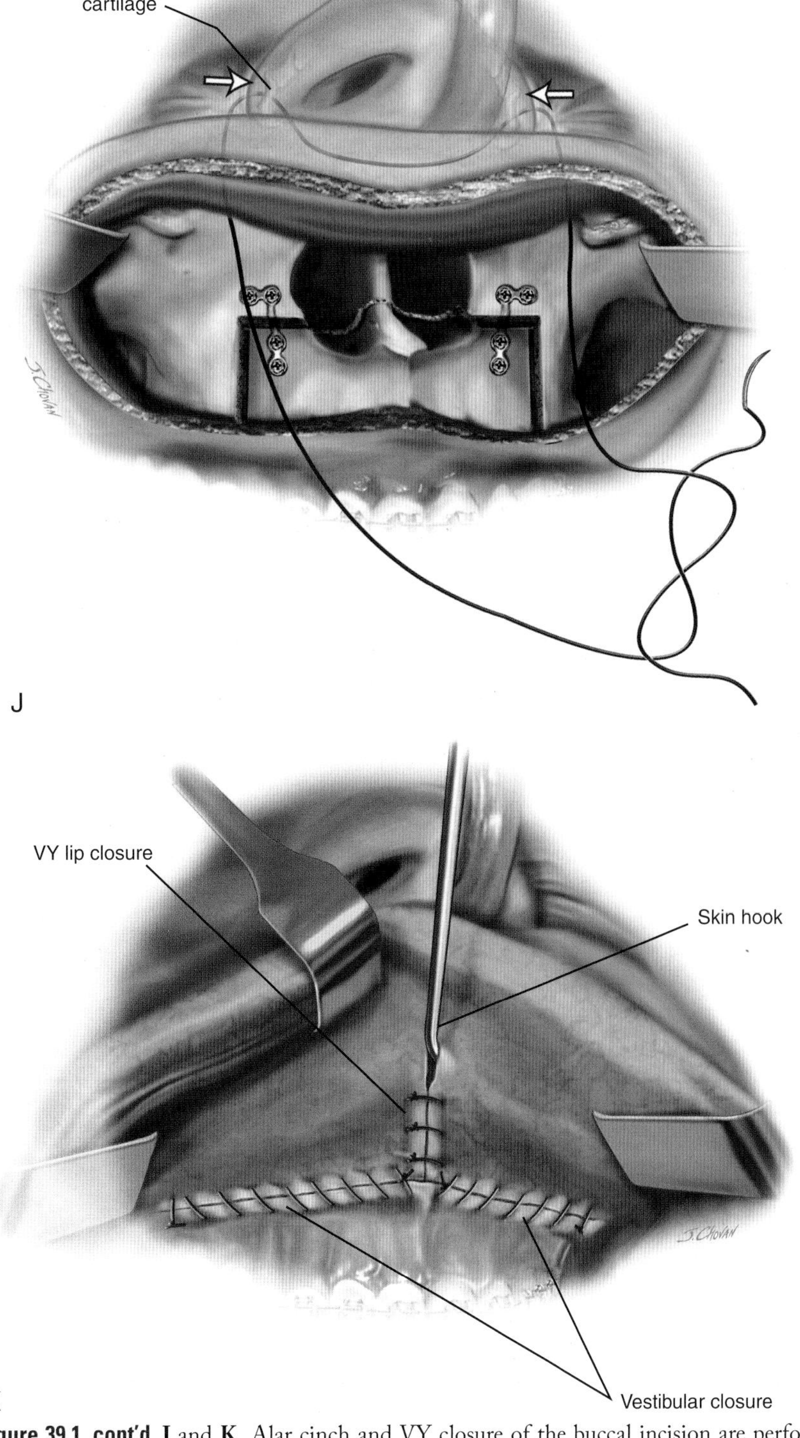

Figure 39.1, cont'd **J** and **K,** Alar cinch and VY closure of the buccal incision are performed using 3-0 chromic suture.

Avoidance and Management of Intraoperative Complications

Complications of ASMO may be divided between airway issues, mechanical difficulties, bleeding, vascular complications, and soft tissue injuries. Unlike the original case reported by Cohn-Stock[1] mentioned earlier in this chapter, most ASMO procedures are performed under general anesthesia using nasoendotracheal intubation. Drilling of the palatal bone, which is performed according to some modifications through a tunnel from either the palatal or the buccal side, may perforate the tube.[7] Caution should be practiced by the surgeon during this relatively blind approach. The anesthesiologist should be prepared for the possibility of an intraoperative tube exchange.

Mechanical difficulties include difficult down-fracture[7] due to insufficient bone release, especially in the palatal osteotomy. Excessive application of force to down-fracture an unreleased maxillary segment may result in an uncontrolled fracture line.

Excessive intraoperative bleeding is extremely rare in ASMO. Various studies have analyzed intraoperative bleeding and the need for blood transfusions. In one study, the mean overall blood loss was found to be 250 cc.[12]

Dental complications include hypersensitivity of teeth on the anterior maxillary segment, a lower threshold in electric pulp testing,[7] and direct damage to teeth in the osteotomy site ("shaving").[13] Periodontal consequences of interdental osteotomies include slightly decreased osseous support and width of attached gingiva adjacent to the osteotomy sites. No significant changes in the periodontal structures should be expected,[14] as long as interdental osteotomies are performed at a proper distance (at least 5 mm) apical to the involved teeth (special attention should be given to the canine area) and in respect to the periodontal ligament of the teeth adjacent to the vertical osteotomy. As in any other orthognathic surgery, the orthodontist should be aware of the surgical plan and prepare the interdental osteotomy site by diverting the adjacent roots. The most common complication encountered in one study was soft tissue injury.[7] In that particular study, 11 of 103 patients experienced an injury to the soft tissue. Laceration of the palatal mucosa may be caused by palatal tunneling or may occur during the osteotomy as a result of traumatic instrumentation by an osteotome, a bur, or a saw. An oroantral or oronasal fistula may be established if the laceration is located over the osteotomy site, especially in advancement cases, but this is rare (reported in one series in only 1 case out of 1133 ASMO procedures).[13] Every effort should be made not to perforate the palatal mucosa when segmentalizing the maxilla. Significant horizontal palatal perforations definitely seem to compromise the already tenuous blood supply to the anterior maxilla.[15] Partial necrosis of the soft tissue at the osteotomy site may result either from aggressive retraction of the buccal flap or from poorly located vertical releasing cuts, and these should be avoided if at all possible. When required, vertical releasing cuts should not be done directly over the planned vertical osteotomy sites or the tooth to be extracted. Hematomas are common, resolve spontaneously, and should not be considered a complication.

Postoperative Considerations

Nonunion and delayed union of segments is much less common in recent publications, as the routine use of internal fixation devices has become more widespread. Proper fixation (preferably, 1.5- to 2-mm screws, 1-mm-thick miniplates), intersegmental bone interface, aggressive use of bone grafts in cases of downward repositioning of the mobilized anterior maxillary segment, adequate postoperative use of a surgical splint when necessary, and a gradual return to a normal chewing diet all contribute to rapid, uninterrupted bone healing.

Three cases of postoperative aseptic necrosis of the anterior maxilla as a result of ASMO were reported by Lanigan et al.[15] Blood flow in the down-fracture technique has been studied and has been found to be better than that in the Wassmund and Wunderer procedures.[9] In all three cases, failure to preserve the integrity of the palatal mucosa led to partial necrosis in the anterior segment after 5 to 10 days. Mobility of teeth, sloughing of gingiva, and rapid bone resorption were the most common findings. Treatment consisted of conservative débridement and necrotic bone removal until bleeding occurred, extraction of mobile teeth, and later, repair of antral and nasal fistulas with local flaps.

The most devastating reported complication of ASMO is total necrosis of the anterior maxilla. This complication was observed in a 13-year-old male 3 months after the procedure.[16] Consequently, the entire segment had to be removed. However, in this rare case, obvious deviations from the usual methods described in this chapter occurred; the blood supply was not preserved (buccal and palatal flaps were reflected using a periodontal approach), and rigid fixation was not used.[17]

Although very popular in the early years of orthognathic surgery, ASMO has been slowly phased out. For the most part, this is due to advances in the capabilities of the orthodontic-surgical team and better results with planned Le Fort osteotomies. Although seldom used, with proper planning, execution, and follow-up care, ASMO is a reliable, safe, and predictable procedure. With complete mobilization of the anterior segment with good vascular viability, proper design, and achievable surgical objectives, ASMO should be part of the maxillofacial surgeon's treatment of selected dentofacial deformities (Figs. 39.2–39.4).

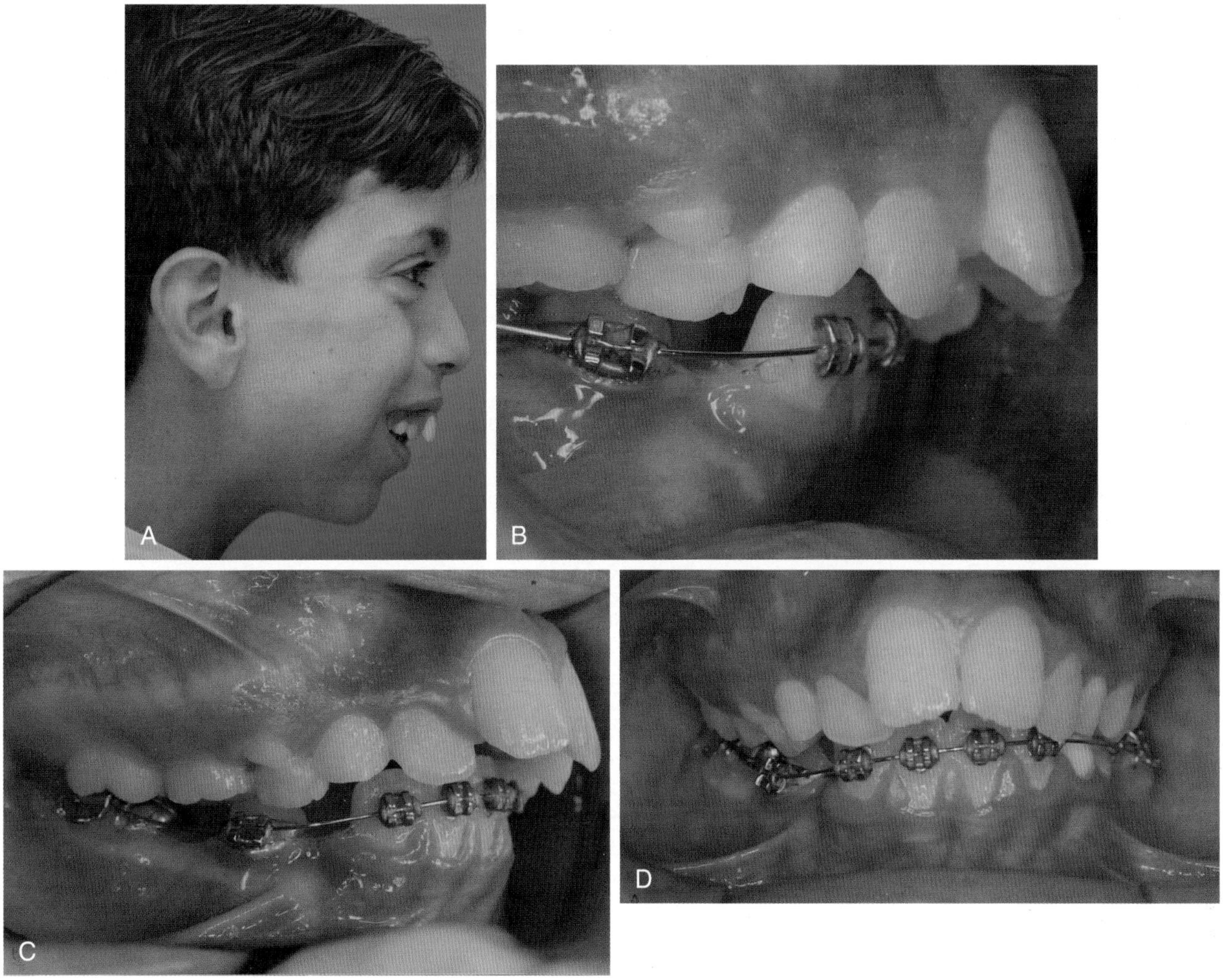

Figure 39.2 Early orthodontic treatment of an 11-year-old patient.

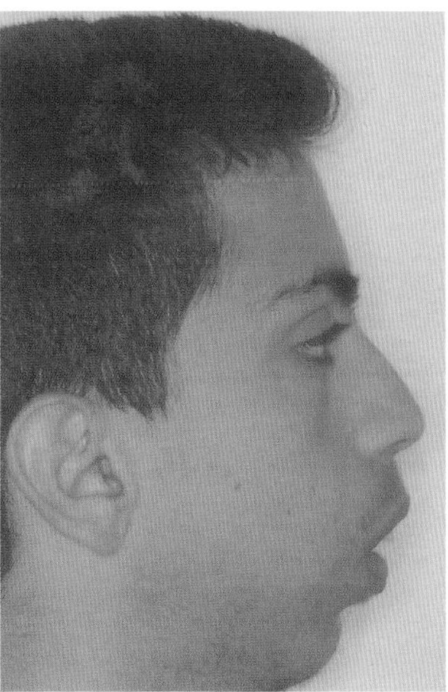

Figure 39.3 Before surgery on an 18-year-old patient.

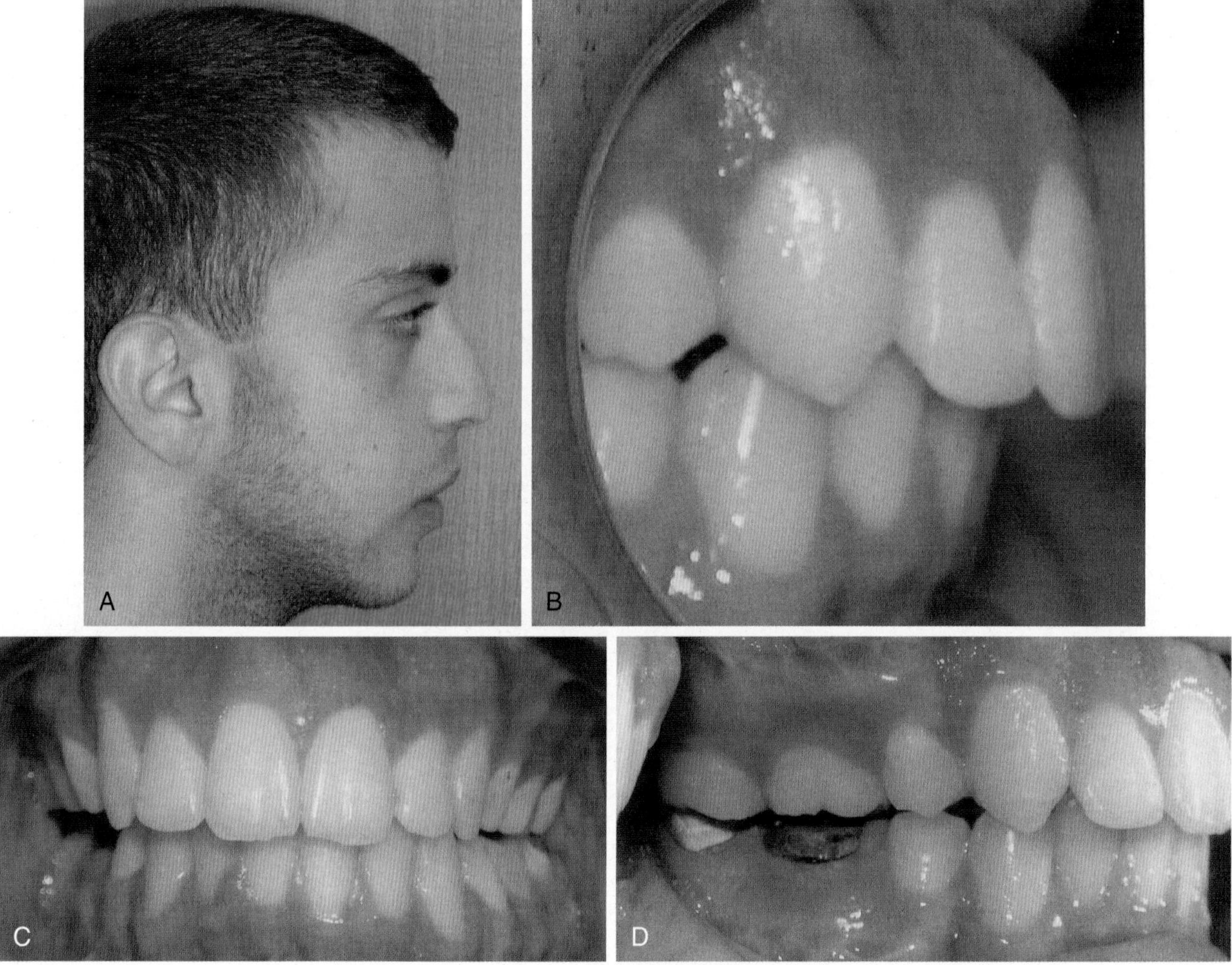

Figure 39.4 Three years after surgery on a 21-year-old patient.

References

1. Cohn-Stock G. Die Chirurgische Immediatregulierung der Kiefer, Speziell die Chirurgische Behandlung der Prognathie. *Vjschr Zahnheilk*. 1921;37:320.
2. Wassmund M. *Frakturen und luxationen des gesichtsschadels*. Leipzig, Germany: Meusser; 1927.
3. Wunderer S. Erfahrungen mit der Operativen Behandlung Hochgradiger Prognathien. *Dtsch Zahn-Mund-Kieferheilkd*. 1963;39:451.
4. Cupar I. Die chirurgische Behandlung der Form- und Stellungsveränderungen des Oberkiefers. *Osterr Z Stomatol*. 1954;51(11):565–577.
5. Bell WH. Revascularization and bone healing after anterior maxillary ostectomy. *J Oral Surg*. 1969;27:249.
6. Bell WH. Correction of maxillary excess by anterior maxillary osteotomy. A review of three basic procedures. *Oral Surg Oral Med Oral Pathol*. 1977;43(3):323–332.
7. Gunaseelan R, Anantanarayanan P, Veerabahu M, Vikraman B, Sripal R. Intraoperative and perioperative complications in anterior maxillary osteotomy: a retrospective evaluation of 103 patients. *J Oral Maxillofac Surg*. 2009;67(6):1269–1273.
8. Rosenquist B. Anterior segmental maxillary osteotomy. A 24-month follow-up. *Int J Oral Maxillofac Surg*. 1993;22(4):210–213.
9. Meyer MW, Cavanaugh GD. Blood flow changes after orthognathic surgery: maxillary and mandibular subapical osteotomy. *J Oral Surg*. 1976;34(6):495–501.
10. Epker BN. Vascular considerations in orthognathic surgery. II. Maxillary osteotomies. *Oral Surg Oral Med Oral Pathol*. 1984;57(5):473–478.
11. Epker BN. A modified anterior maxillary ostectomy. *J Maxillofac Surg*. 1977;5(1):35–38.
12. Yu CN, Chow TK, Kwan AS, Wong SL, Fung SC. Intra-operative blood loss and operating time in orthognathic surgery using induced hypotensive general anaesthesia: prospective study. *Hong Kong Med J*. 2000;6(3):307–311.
13. Sher MR. A survey of complications in segmental orthognathic surgical procedures. *Oral Surg Oral Med Oral Pathol*. 1984;58(5):537–539.
14. Kwon HJ, Pihlstrom B, Waite DE. Effects on the periodontium of vertical bone cutting for segmental osteotomy. *J Oral Maxillofac Surg*. 1985;43(12):952–955.
15. Lanigan DT, Hey JH, West RA. Aseptic necrosis following maxillary osteotomies: report of 36 cases. *J Oral Maxillofac Surg*. 1990;48(2):142–156.
16. Parnes EI, Becker ML. Necrosis of the anterior maxilla following osteotomy. *Oral Surg Oral Med Oral Pathol*. 1972;33(3):326–330.
17. Poulton DR. Surgical orthodontics: maxillary procedures. *Angle Orthod*. 1976;46(4):312–331.

Surgically Assisted Rapid Palatal Expansion

Andrew Henry and Pushkar Mehra

Armamentarium

#15 Scalpel	Double-guarded nasal septal osteotome	Reciprocating saw
#9 Molt periosteal elevator	Local anesthetic with vasoconstrictor	Sagittal saw or side cutting carbide bur, 1 mm
Appropriate sutures	Mallet	Scissors (e.g., Mayo and/or Dean)
Bone rongeurs	Maxillary expansion appliance and activation key	Single skin hook
Curved Freer elevators	Needle electrocautery	Spatula osteotome
Curved pterygoid osteotome	Obwegeser retractors	Woodson elevator

History of the Procedure

The procedure for transverse maxillary expansion by opening the midpalatal suture using an orthodontic appliance was first described by Angell more than a century ago.[1] This concept was initially met with skepticism but later was repopularized through the works of several clinicians, including Issacson and Ingram[2] and Haas,[3] as a viable method of treating maxillary transverse deficiency. It was noted that palatal expansion may result in a forward and downward movement of the maxilla due to resistance not entirely from the midpalatal suture, as was thought initially, but also from surrounding bony structures, such as an intact zygomatic buttress, the pterygoid plates, and the piriform aperture. The findings on the increased facial skeletal resistance to expansion at the zygomaticotemporal, zygomaticofrontal, and zygomaticomaxillary articulations have led to a better understanding of the anatomic barriers to expansion beyond the midpalatal suture[2,4] (Fig. 40.1).

Identification of the areas of resistance in the facial skeleton prompted the development of various maxillary osteotomies to expand the maxilla in conjunction with the use of orthodontic expansion devices. An earlier surgical technique, a midpalatal split, was described by Brown.[5] Steinhauser[6] reported a maxillary expansion osteotomy without the use of distraction but with placement of iliac crest bone graft in the expansion gap. In 1999, bone-borne transpalatal distraction was introduced, suggesting that bone-borne devices may overcome some potential disadvantages of tooth-borne devices, such as undesirable movements of the abutment teeth during expansion.[7]

Over the years, various technical modifications have been introduced, with an emphasis on procedures that can be performed with predictable outcomes and as an ambulatory surgical procedure.[8] Some surgeons advocated complete separation of all maxillary articulations and areas of resistance,[9] whereas others advised against separation at the pterygomaxillary junction to avoid potential pterygoid plate fracture and ensuing complications.[8,10] Those in favor of leaving the pterygoid plates intact base their stance on two principles: (1) surgical separation at the pterygoid plates has not been shown to improve the expandability of the maxilla or prevent relapse in a consistent manner, and (2) surgically assisted rapid palatal expansion (SARPE) with pterygoid plate (and nasal septal separation) significantly increases the risk of hemorrhage and thus necessitates hospital-based surgery under general anesthesia with a secure airway. Consensus regarding the least invasive SARPE technique to produce consistent and stable maxillary expansion in adults continues to remain controversial, and thus other procedural variations have been proposed.[11,12] Regardless of which surgical modification is used, based on the surgeon's training and preference, SARPE has become an important treatment modality for the management of maxillary transverse deficiency in adult patients.

Indications for the Use of the Procedure

The main indication for SARPE is transverse maxillary deficiency in skeletally mature patients. These patients frequently have a clinical picture with excessive display of buccal

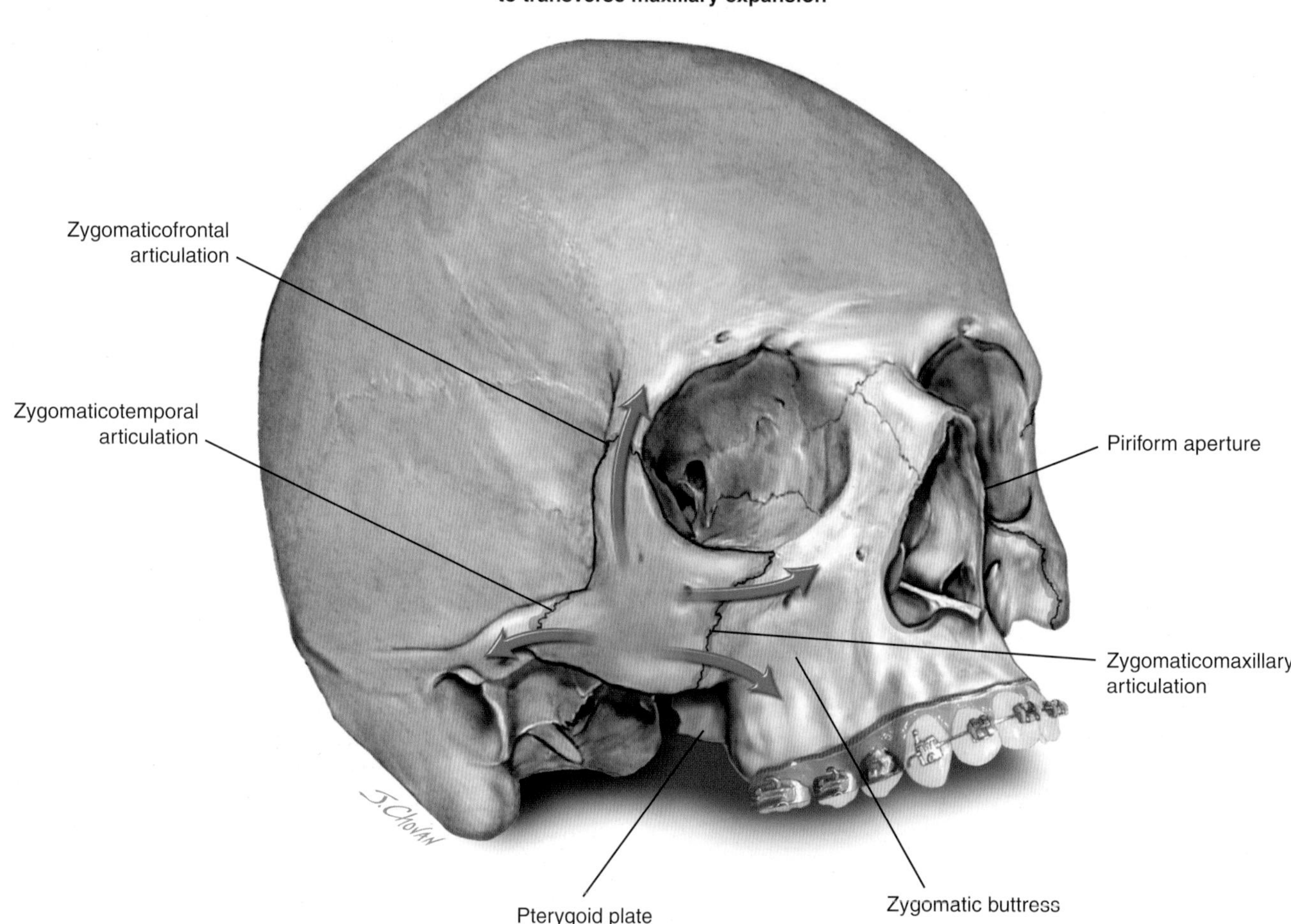

Figure 40.1 Areas of resistance in the facial skeleton.

corridors when smiling and anterior dental crowding, often with a V-shaped maxillary arch. Any clinical situation in which nonsurgical orthodontic expansion has failed should be evaluated for potential sutural resistance to expansion. For many clinicians, the patient's age and the degree of skeletal maturity are the basis for considering nonsurgical expansion rather than SARPE. It has been shown that ossification of the midpalatal suture has wide variations in various age groups.[13] In general, SARPE is always recommended for patients over 15 years of age.[14] Nonsurgical expansion can be a reasonable consideration for patients younger than 12 years of age. However, for patients over the age of 14, surgical corticotomies are essential to address the areas of resistance to expansion.[7] SARPE is also indicated as phase 1 surgery in the early stage of orthodontic arch alignment and in preparation for future maxillary osteotomies for other vertical and anterior-posterior discrepancies. In addition, it may help obviate the need for complex segmentation of the maxilla and hence avoid complications associated with segmental osteotomies. Indications for SARPE include the following:

1. Increasing the maxillary arch perimeter so as to correct unilateral or bilateral posterior crossbite, with or without additional surgical procedures for other discrepancies
2. Increasing the maxillary transverse width, especially when the transverse discrepancy is greater than 5 mm
3. Alleviating dental crowding when bicuspid extractions are not indicated
4. Reducing excessively prominent and visible buccal corridors when smiling
5. Overcoming resistance at the sutures and bony articulations when nonsurgical orthodontic maxillary expansion has failed

The determination of maxillary transverse discrepancy is based on the identification of the problem as absolute or relative. An absolute transverse discrepancy is a true horizontal width deficiency in the maxilla, whereas a relative transverse discrepancy is a result of the discrepancy in the maxilla or both jaws in the anterior-posterior plane. Placing diagnostic models in class I occlusion can be helpful for differentiating between absolute and relative transverse discrepancy. It also can yield valuable information about the location and nature of a maxillary transverse constriction.

To diagnose maxillary hypoplasia accurately, a detailed clinical examination is performed and appropriate measurements taken. In addition, posterior-anterior cephalometric radiographs can be used to identify transverse skeletal discrepancies between the maxilla and the mandible.[15] With the advent of three-dimensional imaging techniques and the availability of cone beam computed tomography in surgery offices, clinicians now routinely evaluate the actual dimensions of apical bases at different levels of the alveolar ridge in the maxilla. A radiographic survey, clinical examination, model analysis using diagnostic casts held in class I occlusion, and a detailed arch length analysis provided by orthodontists can provide the means to quantify the parameter for expansion.

Nonsurgical maxillary expansion in skeletally mature patients may lead to undesirable effects on the surrounding hard and soft tissues, in addition to unstable dental compensations due to tipping, not to mention total failure of expansion. Additional adverse sequelae of this nonsurgical approach include gingival recession and periodontal compromise since teeth roots are often moved to unstable positions outside the bony envelope. Therefore, it is prudent to determine the patient's skeletal maturity and to monitor the initial response to an orthopedic expansion and force application. A prompt decision must be made to proceed with surgically assisted expansion if resistance to expansion due to skeletal maturation is suspected.

Preoperative Considerations, Limitations, and Contraindications

There is no absolute contraindication to SARPE. Most relative contraindications relate to the general systemic status of patients and their ability to safely undergo the procedure under the planned anesthetic (monitored anesthesia care/intravenous sedation vs. general anesthesia). Some specific disorders where the procedure may be relatively contraindicated include patients with significant coagulopathy because of the risk of hemorrhage and conditions such as immune compromise or uncontrolled diabetes mellitus and inherent bone diseases that could compromise healing. Just as with any surgical procedure, measures should be taken to optimize the patient's medical condition before surgery. Patients with generalized periodontal disease and a heavy smoking habit should be informed about local and regional complications related to the soft and hard tissue architecture of the alveolus. This includes potential loss of gingival attachment in the maxillary anterior region in the area of the interdental osteotomy. Patient selection is important in determining the type of anesthesia to be used (i.e., intravenous sedation or general anesthesia); the osteotomy design (pterygoid and/or nasal septum osteotomy) may also influence the decision for a type of anesthesia that is appropriate for the procedure.

SARPE has been reported to have a wide relapse rate, between 5% and 28%,[7,8,16,17] and hence, some overexpansion should be considered to account for this relapse. Advocates of the bone-borne transpalatal distractor suggest that overexpansion is not necessary because their study showed no relapse at the time of follow-up, a finding they attributed to the direct application of distraction forces to the skeletal base.[7] However, further studies are necessary to substantiate the efficacy and superiority of the bone-borne transpalatal distractor over tooth-borne devices, which still remain as the most popular type of appliance for SARPE.

TECHNIQUE

STEP 1: Prepping and Positioning

The patient is induced with either general anesthesia or intravenous sedation. If the surgeons are going to be performing a pterygoid disjunction, it is recommended that general anesthesia with a controlled airway is utilized due to the increased risk of hemorrhage. If general anesthesia is utilized, the patient can be intubated with either a nasoendotracheal tube or an oral Ring-Adair-Elwin (oral-RAE) tube. The patient is then prepped and draped in the traditional fashion in the supine position, preferably in a reverse Trendelenburg position to help maintain controlled hypotension with an aim to decrease intraoperative blood loss.

STEP 2: Surgical Exposure

Local anesthesia with vasoconstrictor is infiltrated labially and buccally from the pterygoid plate region, forward to the midline bilaterally. A horizontal incision is made with a #15 blade or needle-tip electrocautery, extending from the area of the first molar to the contralateral first molar, 3 to 4 mm above the mucogingival junction. Retraction is maintained with down-turned Obwegeser retractors, and the superior mucoperiosteal flap is elevated with a #9 Molt periosteal elevator. The anterior nasal spine, piriform rim, infraorbital foramen, lateral maxillary wall, and zygomaticomaxillary junction are exposed. Exposure of the posterior maxillary wall and pterygomaxillary junction is then performed with a Molt periosteal elevator, placed parallel to the maxillary teeth, and advanced posteriorly below periosteum until the pterygomaxillary junction is encountered. The nasal/septal mucosal dissection is performed after the bilateral maxillary osteotomies have been completed and involves elevation of the nasal mucosa with a curved freer elevator or a Woodson elevator to the posterior palatine bone.

Continued

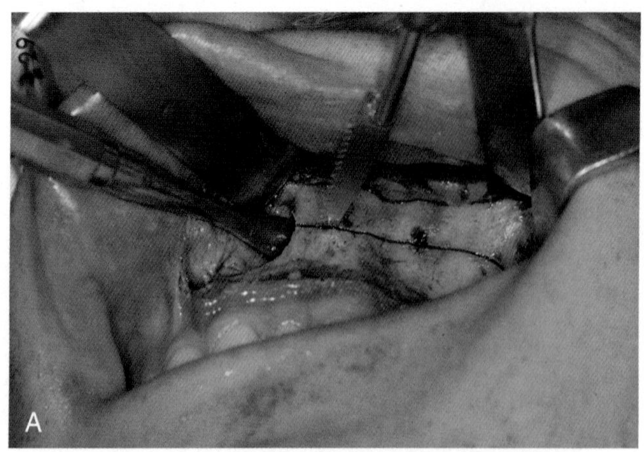

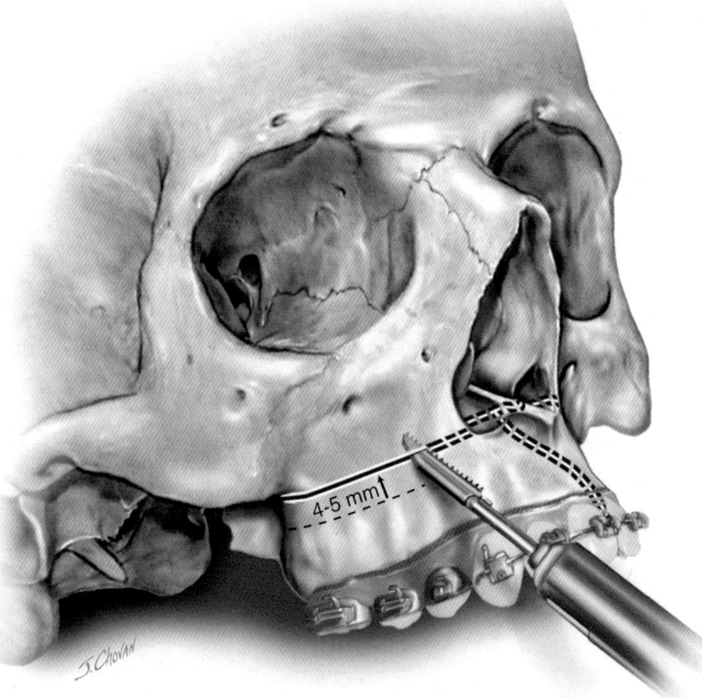

Figure 40.2 **A** and **B,** A buccal osteotomy is made from the pterygomaxillary junction to the piriform rim anteriorly, using a reciprocating saw.

TECHNIQUE—*cont'd*

STEP 3: Bony Osteotomies

A reciprocating saw or a 1-mm side cutting carbide bur (e.g., 701) is used to create the lateral maxillary osteotomy from the lateral nasal rim to the zygomaticomaxillary junction. An Obwegeser toe-up retractor is used to protect the buccal pedicle during this approach. The osteotomy starts 4 to 5 mm above the nasal floor and is carried to the depth of the maxillary sinus, back to the pterygomaxillary junction (Fig. 40.2A and B). Cuts are made at least 5 mm above the roots of the teeth and can be made higher as necessary. Attention is then directed toward the midline osteotomy and bone rongeurs are used to trim the anterior nasal spine, which is often sharp and may make the interdental cut difficult to precisely control. Next, the gingiva between the two central incisors is elevated inferiorly using a Woodson elevator and retracted using a curved freer with care taken to avoid damage to the tissue. Care should be taken not to reflect the gingiva too much laterally beyond the interdental area between the central incisors to avoid subsequent gingival retraction and periodontal defects. A sagittal saw or a 701 bur is used to begin the osteotomy in a vertical fashion. A spatula osteotome is then used to complete the midline osteotomy with a finger on the inner surface of the palate to palpate when the osteotome has reached the end of the hard palate (Fig. 40.3A and B). A fine osteotome or similar instrument can be placed in the midline osteotomy to gently mobilize the osteotomized areas. It is critical to visualize separation of the right and left sides of the maxillary bone and central incisor teeth as individual segments during this maneuver.

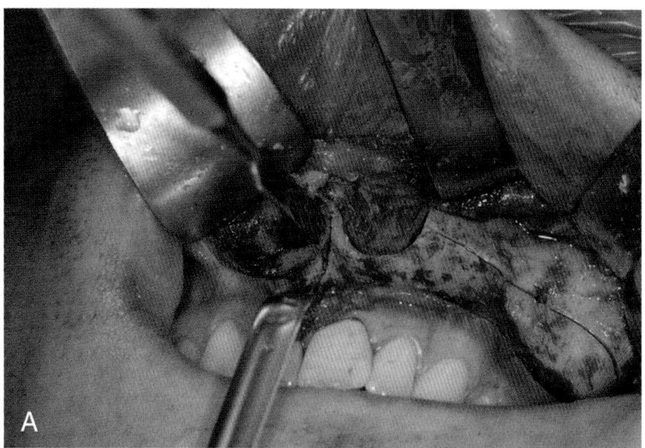

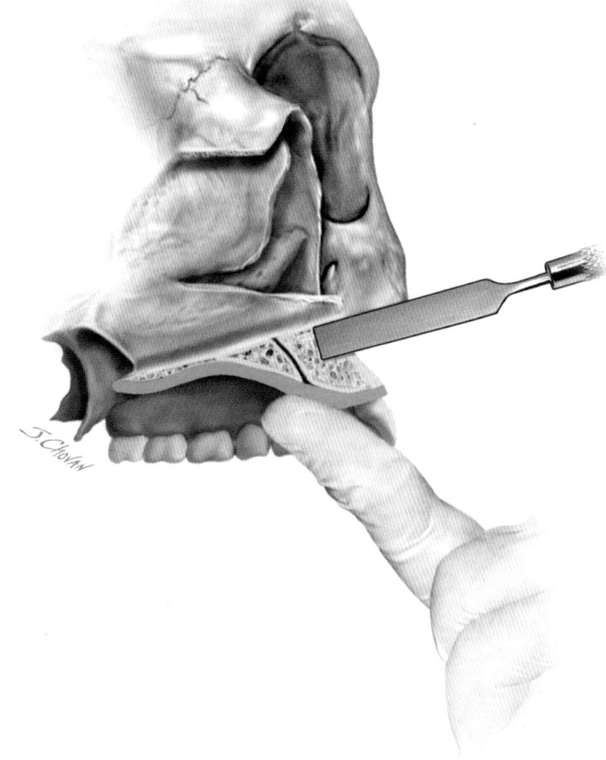

Figure 40.3 **A** and **B,** A midline osteotomy is made using a fine spatula osteotome. The osteotome is driven posteriorly to the midpalatal suture.

TECHNIQUE—*cont'd*

Pterygoid Plate Separation

A 6- to 8-mm wide, curved osteotome (pterygoid osteotome) is placed in the pterygomaxillary junction, with the leading edge angled inferior, medial, and anterior. It is positioned in the junction with the horizontal osteotomy centered over the middle of the osteotome. A finger can be placed palatally at the junction of the hamulus with the tuberosity, and the mallet is used to drive the chisel through the junction. The end of the osteotome should be palpated on the palatal side as it comes through the junction, but it should not penetrate the palatal tissue. There should be minimal resistance to separation, and if significant resistance is encountered, the osteotome position should be evaluated and repositioned (Fig. 40.4A and B). There is some debate over whether this step is necessary. In the authors' opinion, this is the preferred method.

Continued

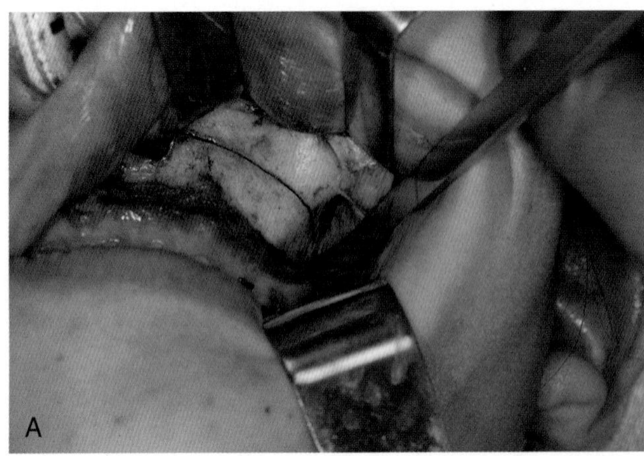

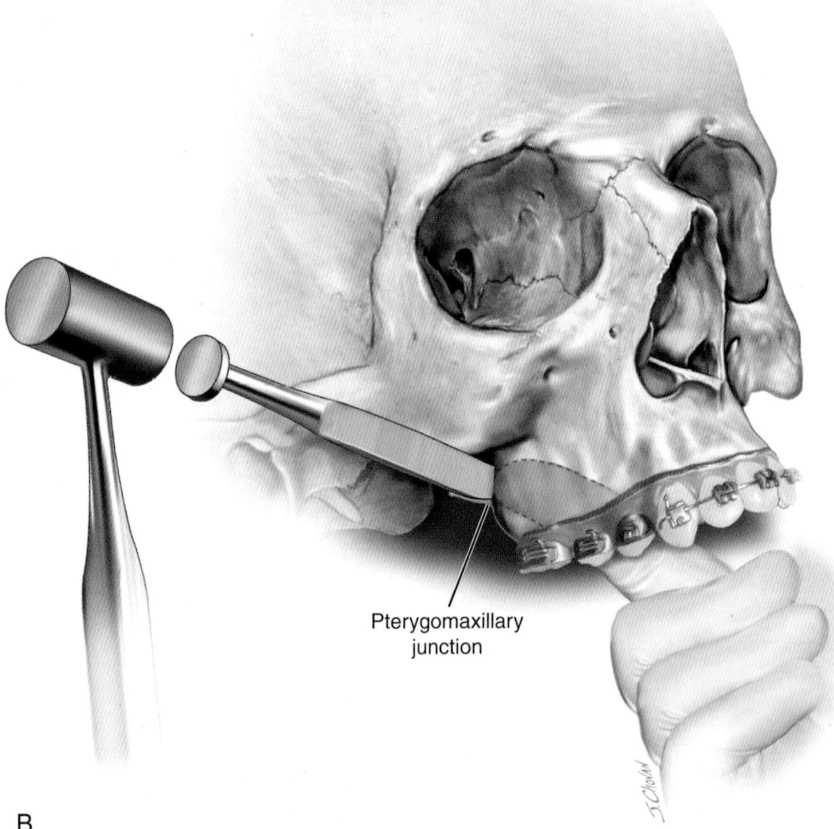

Figure 40.4 A and B, A curved osteotome may be used to separate the pterygomaxillary junction.

TECHNIQUE—*cont'd*

Lateral Nasal Wall and Septal Osteotomies

Two separate #9 Molt periosteal elevators or curved freer elevators are placed submucosally in the piriform rim area to protect the nasal mucosa, and a pair of curved Mayo scissors are used to further dissect under the mucosa and then cut through the cartilaginous septum. Extensive nasal mucosal dissection in the area of the nasal floor is not required in these procedures unlike a formal Le Fort 1 osteotomy where down-fracture and mobilization of the osteotomized maxilla is required. The scissors are removed and replaced with a double-guarded osteotome that is then driven in an inferior and posterior direction to ensure separation of the maxilla and palatine bone from the vomer and remainder of the nasal septum (Fig. 40.5A and B).

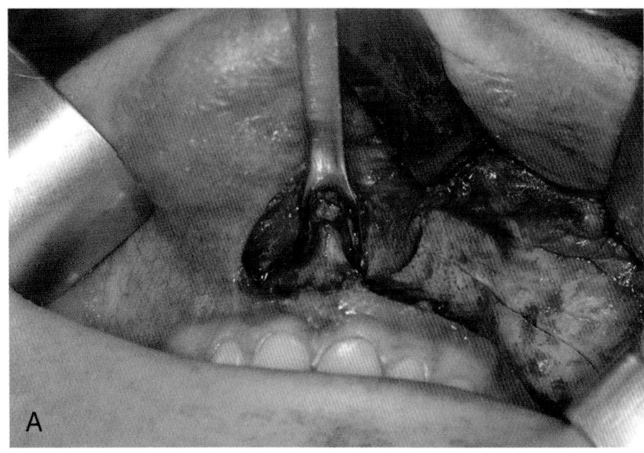

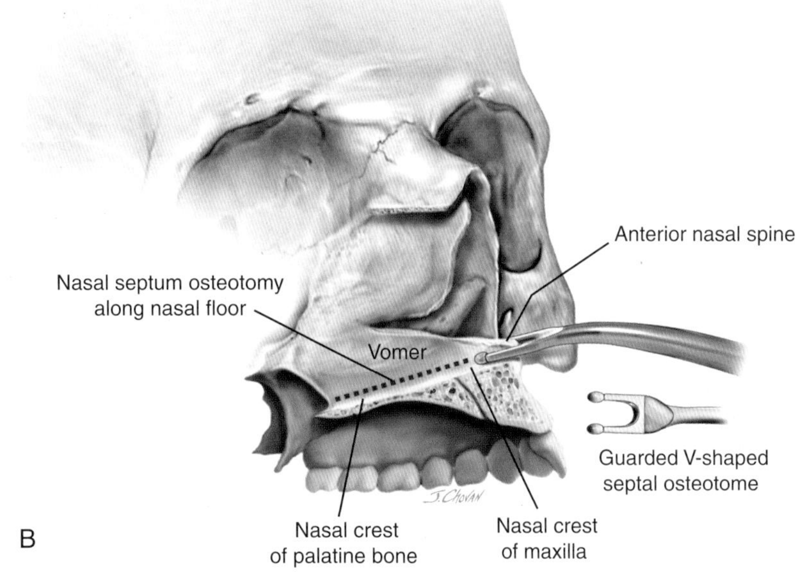

Figure 40.5 **A** and **B,** A double-guarded osteotome is used to separate the nasal septum.

TECHNIQUE—*cont'd*

A small spatula osteotome or a single guarded osteotome is then inserted along the piriform rim and driven in a posterolateral direction, following the natural divergence of the lateral nasal wall. There is less pressure required on the mallet during these perinasal osteotomies than is required during the pterygoid disjunction. The process is then completed on the contralateral side (Fig. 40.6A and B).

STEP 4: Activation of the Appliance

Next, the Hyrax or other type of maxillary expansion device should be activated to ensure expansion bilaterally. This can be done by inserting the activation key and rotating through two to three turns while watching for the formation of a midline diastema. There should be no resistance to the activation. If there is, it is paramount that the surgeon reassesses all osteotomies to avoid an asymmetric expansion. Many clinicians recommend that the appliance be returned back to its original starting position at this time by reversing the turns made earlier.

Continued

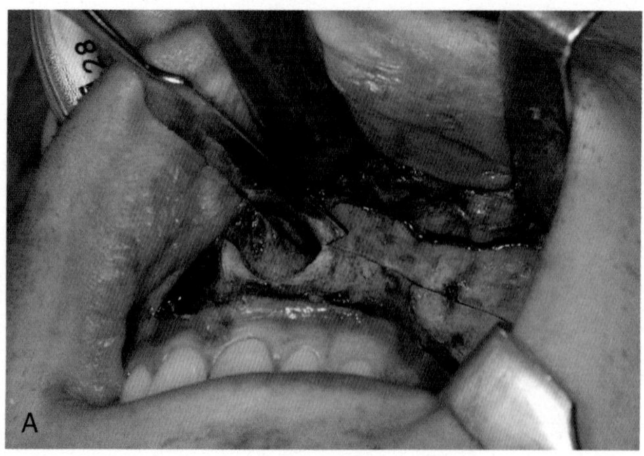

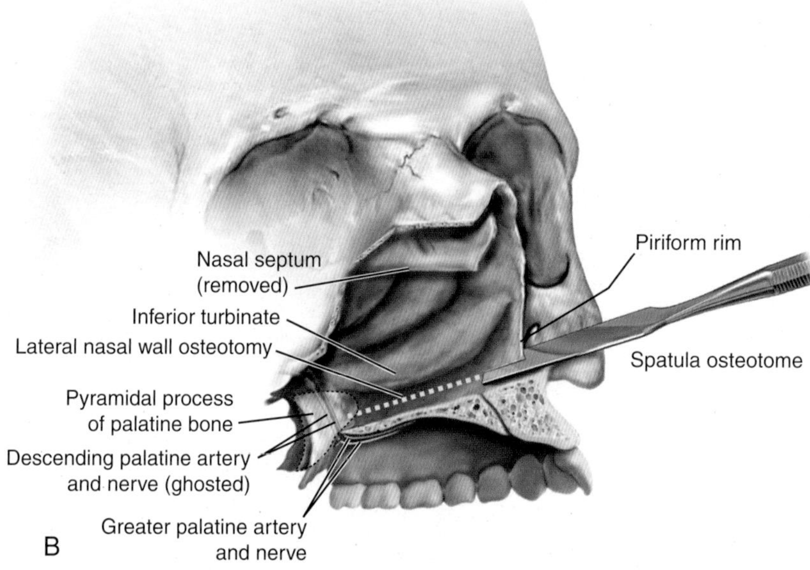

Figure 40.6 **A** and **B,** A straight osteotome is used to separate the lateral nasal walls.

TECHNIQUE—*cont'd*

STEP 5: Wound Closure (Fig. 40.7)

After verifying hemostasis, the wound is irrigated with copious amounts of normal saline solution.

Similar to the separation of the pterygoid plates, there is some debate over whether an alar cinch suture or a VY closure is necessary for a SARPE. Once again, in the authors' view, these sutures result in enhanced postoperative esthetics. The alar cinch suture provides appropriate repositioning of the perinasal musculature that has been dissected during the procedure. This is accomplished by using a slowly resorbable suture (e.g., 2-0 polyglycolic acid) placed from an intraoral approach through the nasalis muscle bilaterally. When completed correctly, this should tighten the alar base to an equal or even slightly narrower width than the preoperative measurement.

The VY closure is an advancement technique performed to counteract the upper lip's tendency to scar and shorten. This is completed by placing a single skin hook at the midline and pulling superiorly. A resorbable suture (e.g., 4-0 chromic gut) is then used to create a 1-cm vertical limb in the midline. The remaining vestibular incision is closed with the same resorbable suture in a running continuous fashion.

Miscellaneous Considerations

In the authors' experience, it is best to have the appliance fabricated with bands on the molars since they ensure greater stability. We also recommend that the orthodontist cement the maxillary expansion appliance prior to surgery. This makes the patient familiar with the appliance itself and also with the activation mechanism prior to surgery. If this is not possible for any reason, then the surgeon must cement the appliance after intubation and prior to starting the surgical procedure using an appropriate bonding

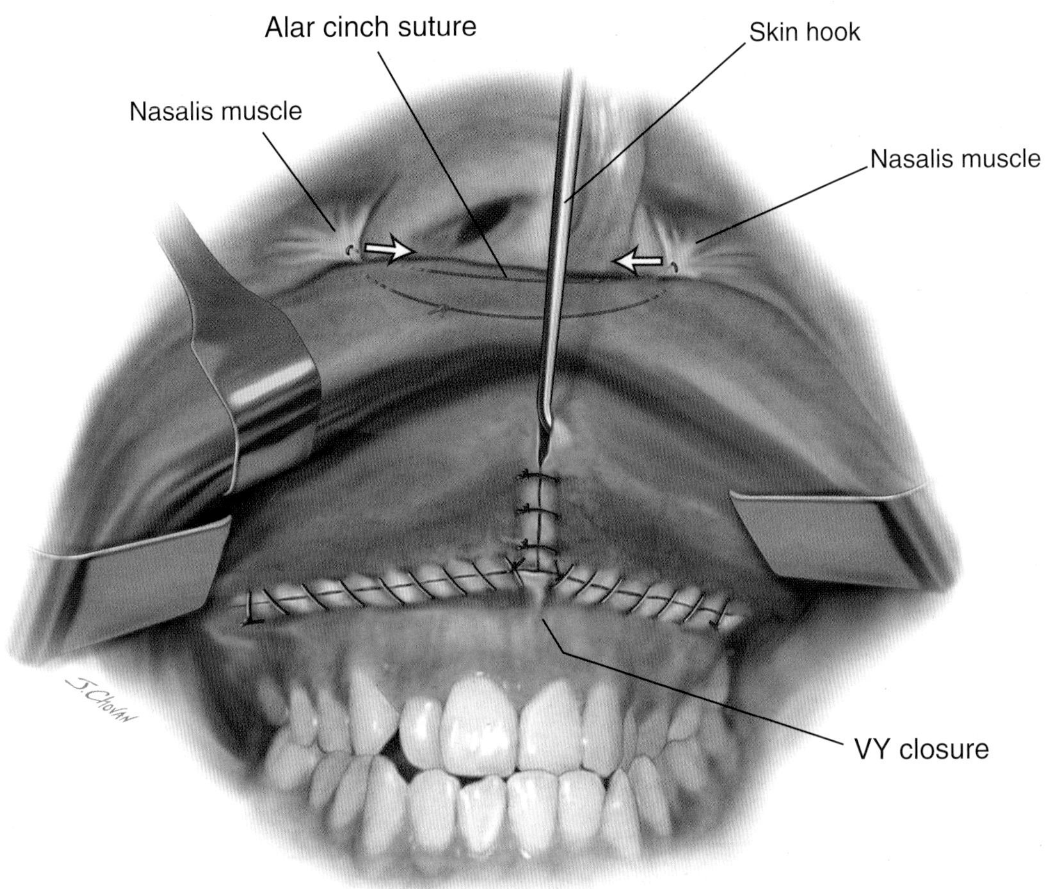

Figure 40.7 Closure is completed using an alar base suture as well as a VY closure to prevent shortening of the lip.

TECHNIQUE—*cont'd*

technique and cement. Bone-borne expanders may have to be similarly placed by the surgeon after the patient is sedated or intubated at the start of the procedure because of patient comfort.

Depending on the surgeon's preference and experience, the duration of the latency period prior to the activation of expansion can range between 0 and 7 days. The authors recommend initiating the expansion approximately 5 days after surgery in most patients. Shorter latency periods are used for younger individuals while longer periods may be indicated for older patients, those with specific bone or wound healing considerations, or if increased "surgical trauma" was encountered intraoperatively. Special consideration may be required for patients with very little interseptal bone and those with a thin gingival papilla between the maxillary central incisors. When less than ideal periodontal support is a factor, a longer latency period and slower activation may be more beneficial than immediate activation and/or the routine expansion rate of 1 mm per day.

ALTERNATIVE TECHNIQUES

1. **Avoidance of Pterygoid Plate Separation**: As previously mentioned, some practitioners do not advocate performing this step. Their rationale is that similar expansion predictability and relapse can be encountered without pterygomaxillary separation thereby minimizing risk of severe bleeding and making it easier to perform the surgery in an ambulatory setting under intravenous sedation.
2. **Unilateral Expansion**: If the patient has a unilateral transverse maxillary deficiency, unilateral SARPE can be used. A vertical interdental osteotomy is made at the anterior border of the segment to be expanded, using a spatula osteotome driven through the midpalatal suture. A horizontal buccal osteotomy is made to connect to the vertical osteotomy on the side to be expanded.

3. **Surgically Assisted Orthodontics:** Surgically assisted or surgically facilitated orthodontic treatment (also known in the literature as accelerated orthodontics, corticotomy, Wilckodontics, and periodontal accelerated osteogenic orthodontics [PAOO]) has been used as an outpatient, office-based oral surgical procedure. In addition to having the advantage of reducing the duration of orthodontic therapy, it has the potential to expand the existing alveolar base, thereby allowing for dental crowding resolution without extractions. The traditional procedure requires full-thickness mucoperiosteal flap elevation followed by particulate bone grafting on the labial and buccal aspects of the alveolus and rapid expansion of the dental arch with or without an expansion appliance to correct crowding and transverse deficiency.[18]
4. **Palatal Incision and Paramedian Palatal Osteotomies**: This technique has been described in the literature but is not commonly practiced, at least not in the United States. A midline incision is made over the midpalatal suture, extending from the posterior aspect of the incisive canal to near the posterior edge of the hard palate. The palatal mucosa is reflected and a reciprocating saw is engaged to make a palatal cut approximately 2 mm lateral to the midpalatal suture, all the way to the point just posterior to the incisive canal. On the contralateral side, a second similar bony osteotomy is made 2 mm lateral to the midpalatal suture. The two cuts are joined in the midline at a point posterior to the incisive canal.

Avoidance and Management of Intraoperative Complications

Failed expansion and a subsequent return to the operating room can cause great distress for all parties, and thus, it cannot be overemphasized that adequate mobility of the operated maxilla and confirmation of device activation before the completion of surgery are of prime importance. The midline cut between the maxillary central incisors should be made with the utmost care to ensure adequate separation within the interseptal bone without jeopardizing the viability of root structure. Use of an ultra-fine spatula osteotome or sagittal saw is recommended. Extra care should be taken when the interseptal bone between two roots is of minimal thickness. Asymmetric and/or inadequate expansion is the most common surgical complication (13.3%), whereas gingival recession is the most frequent tissue complication (8.3%). If the interdental bone cut impinges on dental root structure and does not leave some residual bone on either side of the tooth, gingival retraction and loss of soft tissue in the papilla region can occur. Although devastating periodontal defects with loss of teeth and bone have been reported, they are seen much less often than in segmental Le Fort I osteotomies.[19]

Postoperative Considerations

SARPE may result in complications such as bleeding, infection, buccal tipping of posterior teeth, gingival recession, attachment loss in the midline papilla between the maxillary central incisors, oronasal fistula, palatal tissue necrosis, expansion failure, unintended asymmetric expansion, and pain. Pain after surgery is easily managed with oral medications. V2 distribution paresthesia is common and should resolve within the first month. An oronasal fistula is rare even with an iatrogenic perforation during surgery. If a perforation is encountered during surgery, a slightly longer latency period may be indicated. Small oronasal communications tend to close spontaneously without further surgical repair. Minor nose bleeding is not uncommon after surgery, but significant bleeding should be managed with the placement of nasal packs, proper control of blood pressure, and judicious injection of a local anesthetic with vasoconstrictor. Recurrent and severe epistaxis may require further diagnostic or therapeutic interventions. Swelling after SARPE, is typically moderate and starts to subside in a week or so. Infection after maxillary surgery is uncommon and most are easily treated with antibiotics, rinsing or incision and drainage procedures. The patient is instructed, preferably at the presurgical visit, in the proper use of the activation key and the appropriate activation schedule. At the conclusion of the expansion, the device should be left in place for at least 12 weeks as a retention device (consolidation period). Fibrous or nonunion is extremely rare, and some degree of relapse is to be expected. An example of a patient who successfully underwent surgically assisted maxillary expansion is depicted in Fig. 40.8A–G.

Patients are advised to keep the head of the bed elevated to approximately 45 degrees after surgery. This aids in swelling dissipation and reduces the nasal and sinus congestion. Patients are usually placed on universal sinus precaution instructions including short-term oral decongestants. A full liquid diet is recommended for the first few days followed by advancing to a soft mechanical diet with minimal chewing to allow for adequate healing.

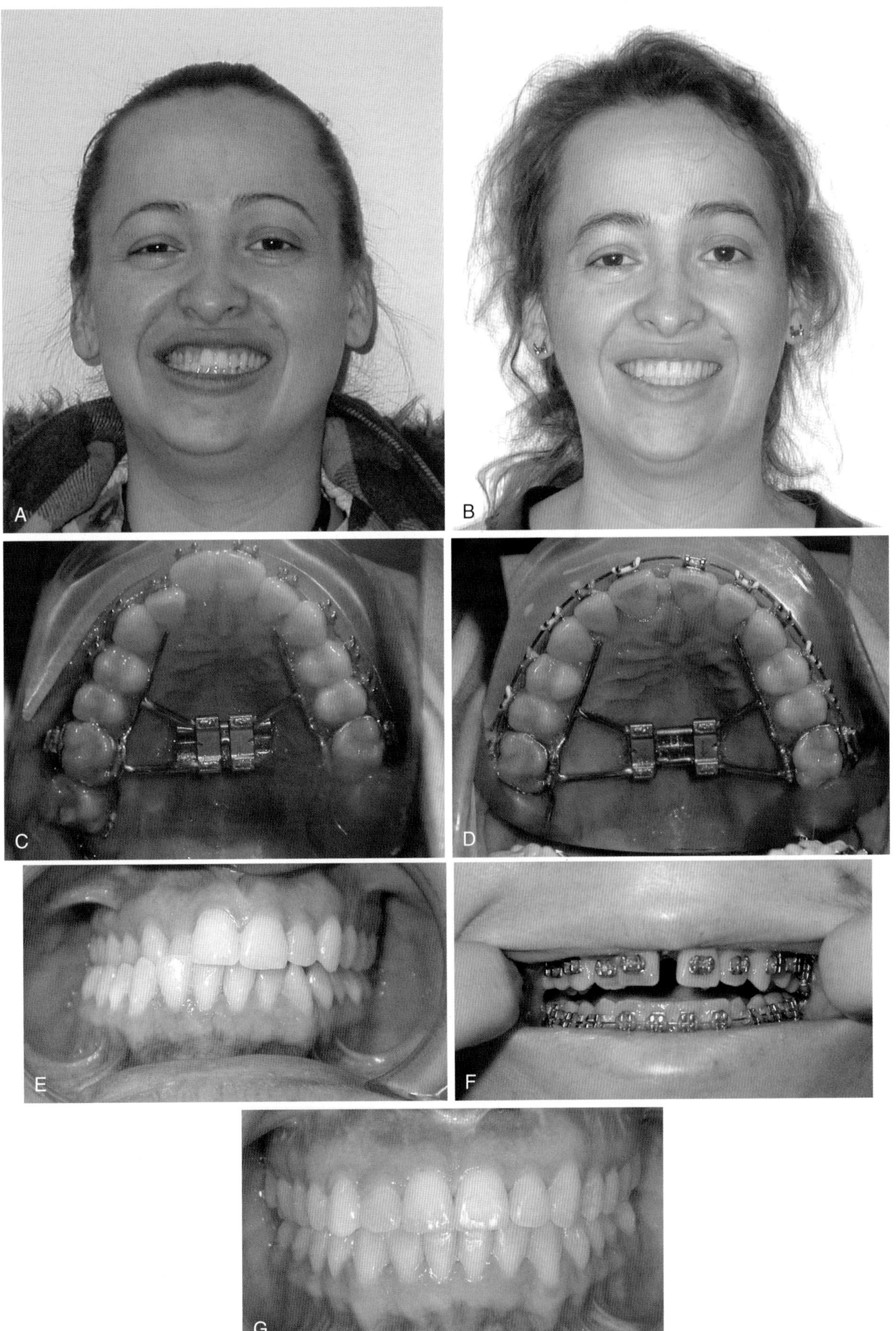

Figure 40.8 Adult patient prior to surgery (A, C, E) and postoperatively (B, D, F, G).

References

1. Angell EH. Treatment of irregularity of permanent adult teeth. *Dent Cosmos*. 1860;1:540.
2. Issacson R, Ingram A. Forces produced by rapid maxillary expansion: forces present during treatment. *Angle Orthod*. 1964;34:256.
3. Haas AJ. The treatment of maxillary deficiency by opening the midpalatal suture. *Angle Orthod*. 1965;35:200–217.
4. Bell WH, Epker BN. Surgical-orthodontic expansion of the maxilla. *Am J Orthod*. 1976;70(5):517–528.
5. Brown GVI. *The Surgery of Oral and Facial Diseases and Malformations*. 4th ed. London, UK: Lea & Febiger; 1938.
6. Steinhauser EW. Midline splitting of the maxilla for correction of malocclusion. *J Oral Surg*. 1972;30(6):413–422.
7. Mommaerts MY. Transpalatal distraction as a method of maxillary expansion. *Br J Oral Maxillofac Surg*. 1999;37(4):268–272.
8. Bays RA, Greco JM. Surgically assisted rapid palatal expansion: an outpatient technique with long-term stability. *J Oral Maxillofac Surg*. 1992;50(2):110–113.
9. Betts NJ, Ziccardi VB. Surgically assisted maxillary expansion. In: Fonseca RJ, ed. *Oral and Maxillofacial Surgery*. Philadelphia, PA: Saunders; 2000.
10. Marin C, Gil JN, Lima SM Jr. Surgically assisted palatine expansion in adult patients: evaluation of a conservative technique. *J Oral Maxillofac Surg*. 2009;67(6):1274–1279.
11. Bierenbroodspot F, Wering PC, Kuijpers-Jagtman AM, Stoelinga PJ. [Surgically assisted rapid maxillary expansion: a retrospective study]. *Ned Tijdschr Tandheelkd*. 2002;109(8):299–302.
12. Pogrel MA, Kaban LB, Vargervik K, Baumrind S. Surgically assisted rapid maxillary expansion in adults. *Int J Adult Orthodon Orthognath Surg*. 1992;7(1):37–41.
13. Persson M, Thilander B. Palatal suture closure in man from 15 to 35 years of age. *Am J Orthod*. 1977;72(1):42–52.
14. Epker BN, Wolford LM. *Transverse Maxillary Deficiency Dentofacial Deformities: Integrated Orthodontic and Surgical Correction*. St Louis, MO: Mosby; 1980.
15. Betts NJ, Vanarsdall RL, Barber HD, Higgins-Barber K, Fonseca RJ. Diagnosis and treatment of transverse maxillary deficiency. *Int J Adult Orthodon Orthognath Surg*. 1995;10(2):75–96.
16. Berger JL, Pangrazio-Kulbersh V, Borgula T, Kaczynski R. Stability of orthopedic and surgically assisted rapid palatal expansion over time. *Am J Orthod Dentofacial Orthop*. 1998;114(6):638–645.
17. Chamberland S, Proffit WR. Short-term and long-term stability of surgically assisted rapid palatal expansion revisited. *Am J Orthod Dentofacial Orthop*. 2011;139(6):815–822.e1.
18. Brugnami F, Caiazzo A, Mehra P. Can corticotomy (with or without bone grafting) expand the limits of safe orthodontic therapy? *J Oral Biol Craniofac Res*. 2018;8(1):1–6.
19. Williams BJD, Currimbhoy S, Silva A, O'Ryan FS. Complications following surgically assisted rapid palatal expansion: a retrospective cohort study. *J Oral Maxillofac Surg*. 2012;70(10):2394–2402.

CHAPTER 41

The Le Fort I Osteotomy

Steven M. Sullivan

Armamentarium

Appropriate sutures
#15 Bard–Parker scalpel blades
Bone rongeurs
Bovie with Colorado tip
Burton palatal retractor
Burton pterygoid osteotome
Calipers
Double-guarded nasal septal osteotome
24-gauge and 28-gauge stainless steel wire
Internal fixation kit (midface)
K-wire
Local anesthetic with vasoconstrictor
1.5-mm Wire passing bur
#9 Molt periosteal elevator
Nasal freer
Nasal mucosa retractor
Notched right-angle retractor
Obwegeser retractors
Oscillating saw
Oval side cutting carbide bur, 4 mm
Reciprocating saw with 33-mm blade
Periotome and spatula osteotome
Rowe disimpaction forceps
Side cutting carbide bur, 1.1 mm (#701)
Single-guarded lateral nasal wall osteotome
Single skin hook
Suture or Dean scissors
Vestibular retractor

History of the Procedure

Introduction

The desire to mobilize the maxilla through an osteotomy dates back 150 years. Langenbeck[1] discussed the utilization of a maxillary osteotomy to facilitate nasal polyp removal in 1859. In 1876, Cheever[2] similarly discussed down-fracture of the hemi-maxilla for clearing the nasal cavity of an obstructing lesion. The concept or desire for movement and repositioning of the maxilla was not Langenbeck's or Cheever's goal; however, the thought process of freeing the maxilla from a fixed position was described.

In 1901, Le Fort[3] helped to bring clarity to the natural cleavage planes of the facial skeleton. By defining the level I cleavage plane of the maxilla from the cranial base, predictable manipulation of the maxilla could be planned for treatment of a malpositioned maxilla. In fact, in 1927, Wassmund[4] discussed the technique for mobilization of the maxilla but did not include separation of the pterygoid plates. Schuchardt,[5] in 1942, reported the successful advancement of the maxilla via separation from the pterygoid plates and complete down-fracture after an unsatisfactory attempt without pterygoid plate separation.

By the late 1960s and early 1970s, Bell[6] capitalized on the ability to mobilize the maxilla and he discussed segmentalization for the facilitation of orthodontic treatment goals as well as the vascular supply, which permitted these surgical movements. In the 1980s, continued refinement of the Le Fort I osteotomy procedure focused on techniques to facilitate postoperative stability. Kaminishi et al.[7] discussed carrying the osteotomy cut high into the dense cortical bone of the zygomatico-maxillary buttress to facilitate postoperative stability and internal fixation. Bennett and Wolford[8] further advocated the step osteotomy of the maxilla to avoid unwanted vertical movement from an angulated nonstepped osteotomy of the maxilla. Their design kept the anterior and posterior maxillary osteotomies parallel to one another with the step at a right angle near the buttress.

Reyneke and Masuriek,[9] somewhat conversely, advocated a sloped osteotomy for inferior anterior maxillary repositioning, with the goal of improved bony contact during inferior repositioning of the maxilla.

The versatility of the Le Fort 1 osteotomy to correct maxillary deformities is unquestioned. As a result, the osteotomy design has undergone modification to enhance the ability of the surgeon to accuratcly reposition the maxilla and to improve bony contact and the initial stability of the mobilized jaw until healing takes place. The technique described here further enhances bony contact by increasing bony surface area while decreasing osteotomy gaps along the buttress and posterior maxilla.

Indications for the Use of the Procedure

The Le Fort I osteotomy is indicated when repositioning of the maxilla will aid in the correction of hard- or soft-tissue deformities or functional disorders of the maxillomandibular complex. The various abnormalities include maxillary excess, maxillary deficiency, and maxillary asymmetry, all of which can result in a broad range of functional issues including malocclusion, difficulty with eating and swallowing, speech disorders, myofascial pain dysfunction, temporomandibular joint dysfunction, obstructive sleep apnea, dental/periodontal disease, and psychosocial issues.

Maxillary dentofacial abnormalities can generally be broken down into disorders of vertical or transverse dimension, disorders of horizontal position, and abnormalities relating to symmetry and the combination of these various problems. Vertical disorders of the maxilla may include both vertical hyperplasia and hypoplasia and require upward or downward movement of the maxilla. Transverse disorders commonly include transverse deficiency and on occasion transverse excess. In these cases, the maxilla will require widening and sometimes narrowing. Most horizontal deficiencies involve maxillary hypoplasia and require advancement surgery. Maxillary disorders often occur in multiple planes, including the pitch, roll, and yaw, and will thereby have a corresponding disorder in the mandible. An example of this is a high mandibular plane angle, class II asymmetry, with or without an open bite.

Limitations and Contraindications

There are many factors that can affect surgical outcome. They include surgical technique, bone quality and buttressing, the type of fixation, and the magnitude of surgical repositioning.

Specific surgical movements are known to have a higher degree of relapse (e.g., anterior maxillary down-grafting and transverse widening) than others such as superior movement or advancement. Aside from well-known general medical comorbidities that relate to anesthesia management and bone healing issues (uncontrolled diabetes mellitus, immune compromise, bone and joint disease, etc.), specific contraindications of the Le Fort I osteotomy may also include skeletal immaturity. A relative contraindication in the skeletally immature patient includes the Le Fort I osteotomy performed in a growing patient, in which antero-posterior (A-P) growth of the maxilla ceases postoperatively due to nasal septal separation from the upper jaw.[10] Vertical growth of the maxilla and A-P and vertical growth of the mandible continue postoperatively, and though may be small, it can possibly result in a secondary malocclusion, especially in class III horizontal growing patients.

TECHNIQUE: Le Fort I Osteotomy

Execution of the surgical procedure is best done with controlled hypotension and nasotracheal intubation. It is important that the smallest endotracheal tube that meets the necessary length requirement to pass through the vocal cords without impingement of the balloon on the cords be used. Typically a size 6.5 to 7 is adequate. It is important, especially at the termination of the case when closing, to be able to control the diameter of the nares as well as alar base as the tube size can play a role in creating asymmetry if it is too large and dilates the nares more so than its natural size.

The endotracheal tube should be passively secured in such a way that there is no upward or cephalad traction on the nose causing distortion that would impact the ability to get an appropriate recapitulation of the nasal base or alter it in cases where it is excessively wide, narrow, or asymmetric.

The surgeons preferred sterile draping is completed with the patient in a supine position, preferably in a slight reverse Trendelenburg position. Hypotensive anesthesia with the systolic blood pressure below 100 mm Hg is recommended, and the administration of 10 mg/kg tranexamic acid can also be given to aid in hemostasis. Preoperative medications such as antibiotics and a steroid such as Decadron should be administered 1 hour in advance of surgery. A throat pack is inserted, and the oral cavity is prepped with chlorhexidine or a suitable disinfectant. Adjustment of any dental prematurities noted during model surgery are made with a round diamond bur at this time. Local anesthesia with vasoconstrictor is infiltrated bilaterally, labially, and buccally from the second molar region forward to the midline and including a second division block via the greater palatine approach. Typically, 10 cc of 0.25% bupivacaine with 1:200,000 epinephrine is administered.

STEP 1: Reference Point

External reference markers are advised, as they have been shown to be more accurate than internal markers.[11] A stable extraoral reference point is established with a 0.045-inch K-wire placed in the nasal bridge approximating nasion. The wire is drilled until stable or up to 1 cm in depth and then shortened to 10 mm above the skin surface to allow for near parallel measurements. A Marchac or suitable caliper is used to measure the vertical distance from the K-wire to the arch wire or brackets of the central incisor teeth, and these measurements are recorded (Fig. 41.1).

STEP 2: Surgical Exposure

A horizontal incision is made with needle-tip electrocautery, extending from the first molar to the contralateral first molar, 4 to 5 mm above the mucogingival junction. A #15 blade is used to incise the periosteum. Bear in mind that the soft tissue will retract somewhat, so a generous collar of soft tissue should be accounted for. The entire maxilla is exposed with a mucoperiosteal elevator and retracted anteriorly with Minnesota retractors and with Obwegeser curved-out right-angle retractors being inserted behind the buttress and engaging the pterygomaxillary juncture (Fig. 41.2). To facilitate the

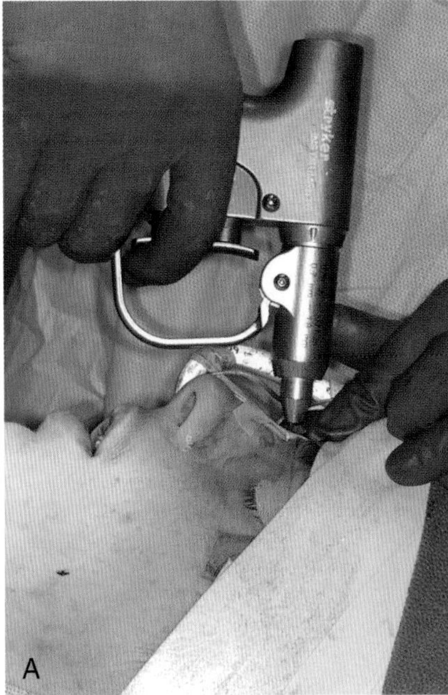

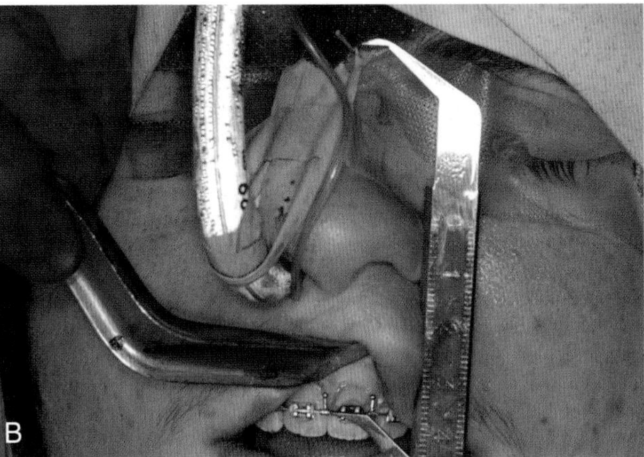

Fig. 41.1 **A** and **B,** External reference pin placed in the bridge of the nose. A preoperative measurement is recorded. External measurements are more accurate than internal measurements and more reproducible.

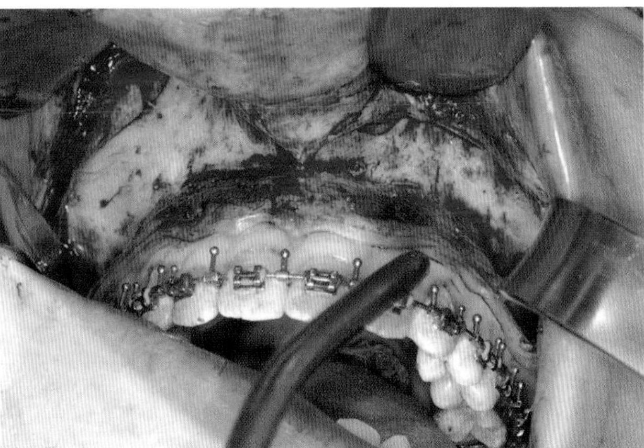

Fig. 41.2 The maxilla is degloved to facilitate complete visualization.

TECHNIQUE: Le Fort I Osteotomy—*cont'd*

reflection of the nasal mucosa the author finds that the disarticulation of the septum from the anterior nasal spine if most helpful. The nasal septum can be easily disarticulated by the use of a right-angle notched retractor by engaging the septum at the junction of the anterior nasal spine. Using cephalad and slight posterior traction, the septum will disarticulate from the maxillary crest and anterior nasal spine and initiate the elevation of the mucoperiosteum from the anterior floor of the nasal cavity (Fig. 41.3). A nasal freer is then used to complete the remaining reflection of the nasal mucosa. It is important that the mucoperiosteum be reflected from the entire lateral nasal wall, nasal floor, and off the septum bilaterally. This will minimize tears to the nasal mucosa during the osteotomies. Utilizing this technique often will preclude the need for any nasal mucosa repair following down-fracture (Fig. 41.4).

STEP 3: Bony Osteotomies

The proposed geometry of the Le Fort I osteotomy now can be clearly visualized and even premarked using a sterile pencil so that there is symmetry, appropriateness in the height bilaterally, and location of the buttress cut such that tooth roots can be avoided (Fig. 41.5).

A nasal mucosa retractor is then inserted at the piriform rim between the base of the rim and the inferior turbinate to protect

Continued

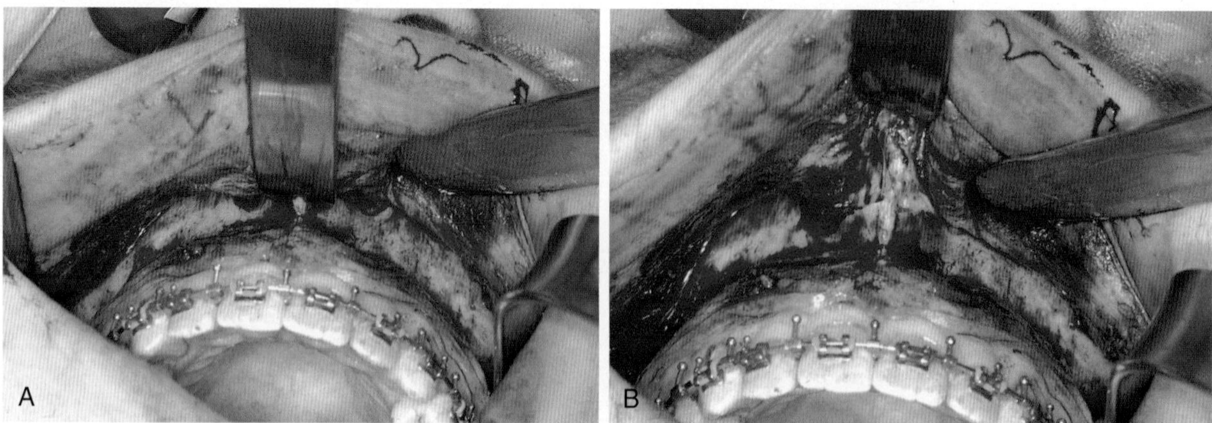

Fig. 41.3 A and B, The nasal septum is easily disarticulated with a notched right-angle retractor by engaging the caudal edge and applying firm upward pressure. The disarticulation will also initiate the reflection of the nasal mucosa and facilitate its further reflection from the nasal cavity and septum.

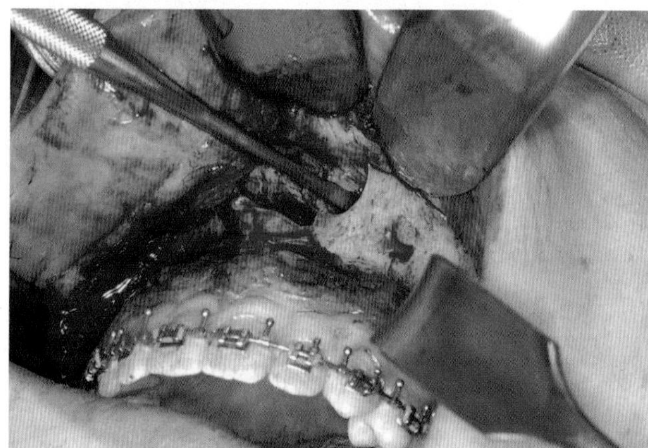

Fig. 41.4 The nasal mucosa should be completely reflected from the nasal cavity bilaterally and septum to preclude damage to the turbinates and maintain the nasal mucosal integrity during osteotomy and down-fracture.

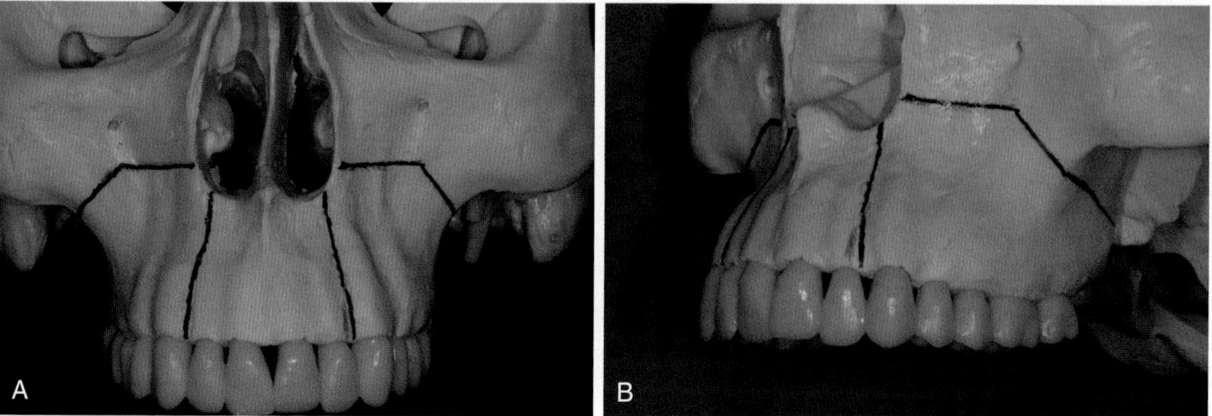

Fig. 41.5 A and B, The osteotomy design is a modification of the Wolford-Bennett design and facilitates the application of fixation in more dense bone and along the distribution of forces. It is more angular in nature to improve bone contact.

TECHNIQUE: Le Fort I Osteotomy—*cont'd*

the turbinate from the reciprocating saw, which is used to make the anterior maxillary wall and the lateral nasal wall cut. A reciprocating saw will easily pass through the thin maxillary bone. As it is swept medially, the lateral nasal wall will also be osteotomized. Often, this method precludes the use of other osteotomes prior to down-fracture (Fig. 41.6).

The buttress and posterior maxillary cut has been modified from how it has been previously described in the literature. Historically, a right-angle stepped buttress cut has been utilized; however, that leaves a very precarious area of the thin bone at the buttress, which makes it challenging to place bone plates along the lines of force distribution. With this in mind, a modified osteotomy is done at a 45-degree angle to the anterior maxillary cut and 90 degrees to the buttress with a bevel 45 degrees from lateral to medial and making the terminus of the cut at the lower one-third of the pterygoid plates (Fig. 41.7).

This procedure creates an osteotomy angled in all three dimensions. The resulting sagittal bevel through the buttress facilitates excellent bone-to-bone contact. The 45-degree angle cut to the anterior maxillary osteotomy facilitates bone plates being placed 90 degrees to the buttress and parallel to the direction of force distribution. The contralateral osteotomies are then completed (Fig. 41.8).

If the maxilla is being impacted, this is an appropriate time to estimate the amount of anterior maxillary bone removal that will be required to facilitate the superior repositioning. With impactions greater than 5 mm, removal of this bone at the time of the initial anterior maxillary osteotomy can be done with a lesser amount being removed at the buttress. Because the maxilla will rotate superiorly, one should remove less bone than the actual amount of impaction initially and refine the vertical dimension prior to fixation. If the maxilla is also being advanced, be very cautious with the initial bone removal as every millimeter of advancement can diminish the amount of necessary bone removal for impaction by the same amount due to the rotation. It is for this reason that vertical bone removal with maxillary advancement and impaction may be best done when determining the vertical dimension prior to fixation (Fig. 41.9).

Continued

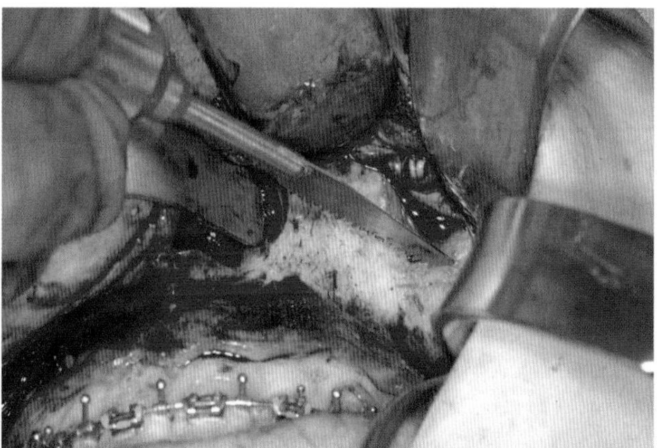

Fig. 41.6 A nasal mucosa retractor is inserted to the depth of the nasal cavity to protect the turbinates and a reciprocating saw is used to make a horizontal osteotomy parallel to the maxillary occlusal plane. The lateral nasal wall can be cut simultaneously by sweeping the saw medially after the saw penetrates the anterior maxillary wall.

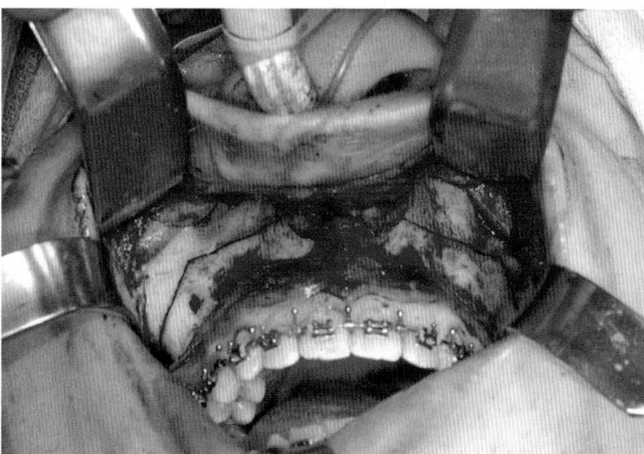

Fig. 41.8 The completed osteotomies should be symmetrical.

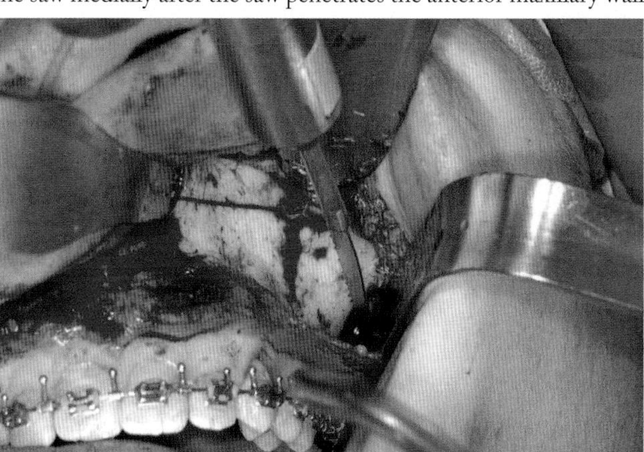

Fig. 41.7 The buttress is osteotomized by angling the saw 90 degrees to the buttress, 45 degrees to the horizontal osteotomy, and 45 degrees inferiorly toward the lower third of the pterygoid plates as shown in Fig. 41.5.

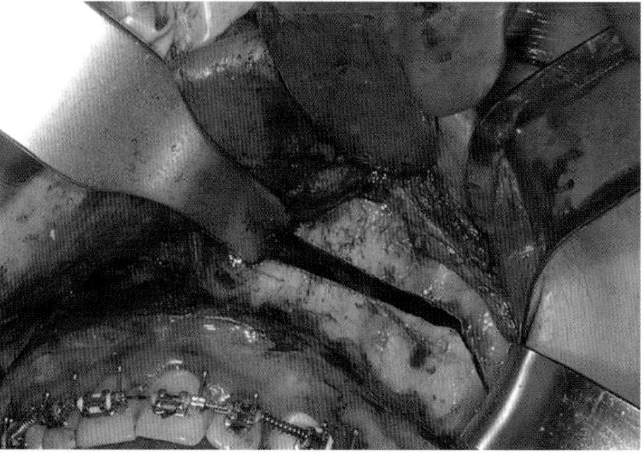

Fig. 41.9 Anterior bone removal can be done prior to down-fracture if large impactions are being done, or judicially and incrementally removed, as the maxilla is being repositioned.

TECHNIQUE: Le Fort I Osteotomy—*cont'd*

SEPTAL AND LATERAL NASAL WALL OSTEOTOMIES

A double-guarded osteotome is then used to separate the nasal septum from the maxilla (Fig. 41.10). When using the technique previously described, it is unusual to osteotomize the lateral nasal walls as a separate step. In the event it is felt that this was not accomplished with the saw, a single-guarded osteotome can be used by inserting it at the confluence of the anterior wall osteotomy and piriform rim and gently advancing with a mallet until resistance is met.

PTERYGOID PLATE SEPARATION

A 10-mm Burton curved osteotome is placed in the pterygomaxillary junction, with the leading edge angled inferior, medial, and anterior. It is positioned such that the superior edge of the osteotome is level with the posterior maxillary osteotomy. The index finger of the operating assistant can be placed palatally at the junction of the hamulus with the tuberosity, and the mallet is used to drive the chisel through the junction. The separation of the pterygoid plates is palpable on the palatal side as the osteotome passes through the junction, but it should not be allowed to penetrate through the palatal tissue. Little resistance is usually encountered; however, if significant resistance is felt, the osteotome position should be evaluated and repositioned (Fig. 41.11).

STEP 4: Down-Fracture and Mobilization

Once the osteotomy cuts have been completed, some mobility should be readily evident. Down-fracturing should typically not require much downward pressure and be easily done with manual digital pressure on the anterior maxilla. Slowly separate the maxilla by pushing the anterior portion inferiorly. If significant resistance is encountered, it is best to determine where the resistance is occurring and verify completeness of the osteotomies again. The most common site for resistance is at the posterior aspect of the lateral nasal walls and pterygoid plates. Once the down-fracture is completed, it is advised to further mobilize the maxilla. Judicious use of Rowe disimpaction forceps accomplishes this very nicely

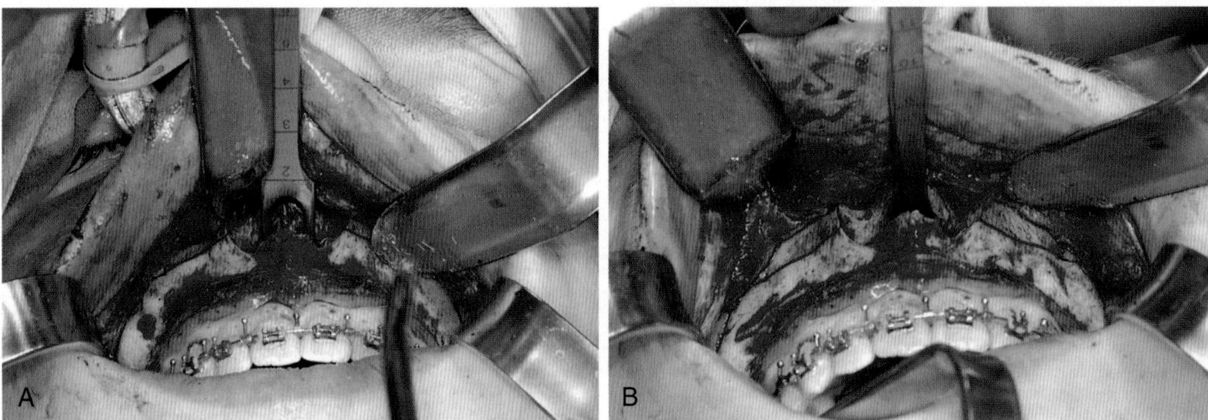

Fig. 41.10 **A** and **B,** The septum is osteotomized using a double-guarded osteotome.

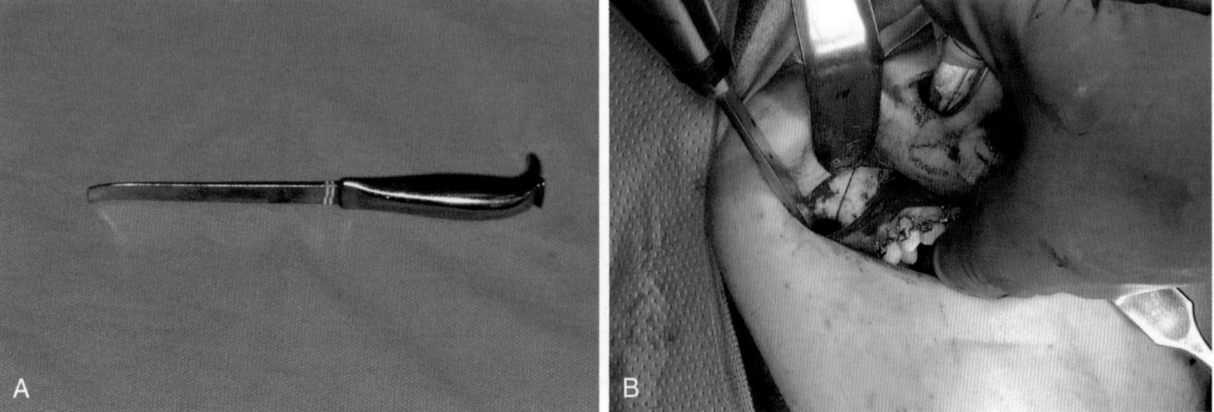

Fig. 41.11 **A** and **B,** A curved Burton osteotome is inserted low on the maxilla at the pterygoomaxillary junction. The assistant surgeon's index finger is placed intraorally in the region of the hamulus. The osteotome is advanced with a mallet until the posterior maxilla is separated. The assistant will feel the separation and preclude perforation of the osteotome intraorally.

TECHNIQUE: Le Fort I Osteotomy—*cont'd*

and with a high degree of directional control. Gentle traction and rotation of the down-fractured maxilla will fully mobilize it from its attachments (Fig. 41.12A and B).

It has been suggested that for large advancements, freeing the tissue from the nasal side of the posterior maxilla in the soft palate area will provide significantly more forward mobility and prevent soft-tissue tears. It is imperative that the maxilla have sufficient mobility to passively couple with the mandible. In revision maxillary surgery, one will spend a considerable amount of time attaining appropriate mobility.

STEP 5:

After complete mobilization, a 1.5-mm wire passing bur is used to make a hole at the base of the anterior nasal spine, and then a 24-gauge wire is passed and tightened to facilitate downward traction (Fig. 41.13). This hole will also be used at the time of closure so that there is anchoring of the soft tissues. This will be described later.

The use of a double-bladed palatal retractor facilitates visualization of the down-fractured maxilla and enhances visibility during instrumentation (Fig. 41.14).

Double-action rongeurs are then used to remove residual components of the nasal septum and lateral nasal wall, with great care being taken to minimize trauma to the descending palatine vessels (Fig. 41.15). It is often not necessary or advantageous to immediately ligate or cauterize the descending palatine vessels but that is an option.

Often, in the tuberosity region at the terminus of the buttress cut, there will be a small triangle of bone that needs to be removed. Once this interference has been completed, it is essential that any potential bony interference around the greater palatine vessels and pterygoid plates be removed so that passive repositioning of the maxilla, especially if it is moving superiorly, can be accomplished (Fig. 41.16). The maxillary crest is reduced and a septal groove is placed to allow the cartilaginous septum to fit passively into it (Fig. 41.17).

If the decision to segment the maxilla has been made preoperatively, segmentation can be achieved very quickly with the maxilla

Continued

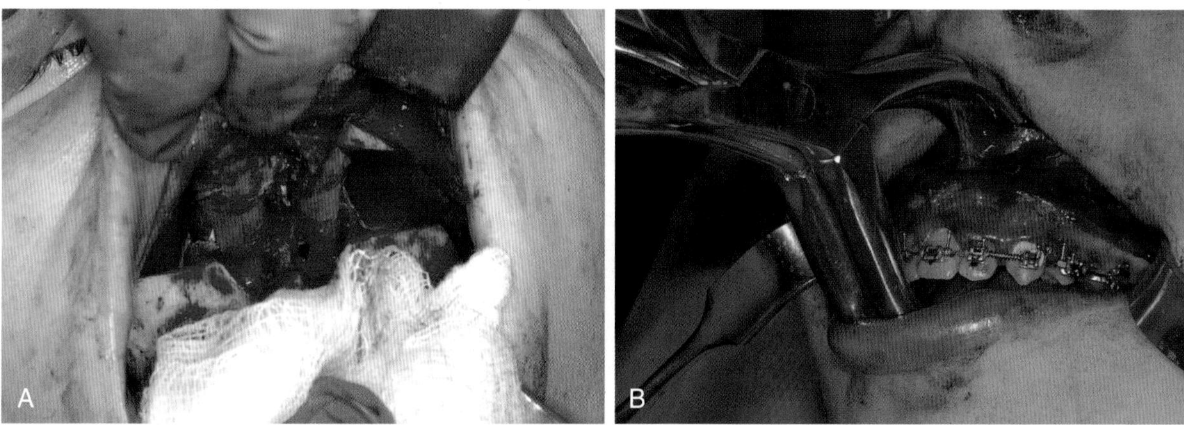

Fig. 41.12 **A** and **B,** The maxilla can be down-fractured with digital pressure. The maxilla must be completely mobilized. Rowe disimpaction forceps are being used in this case.

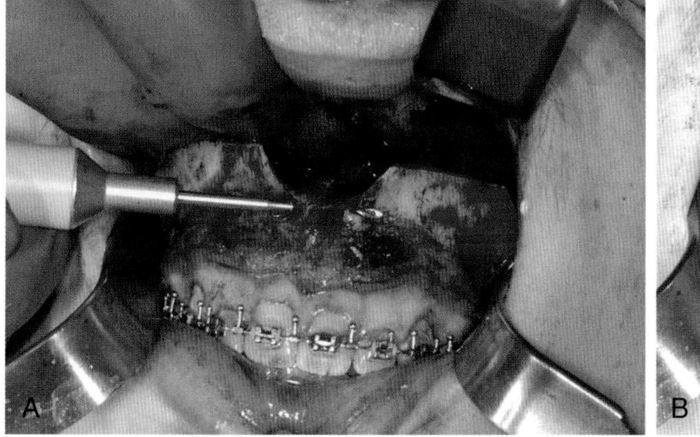

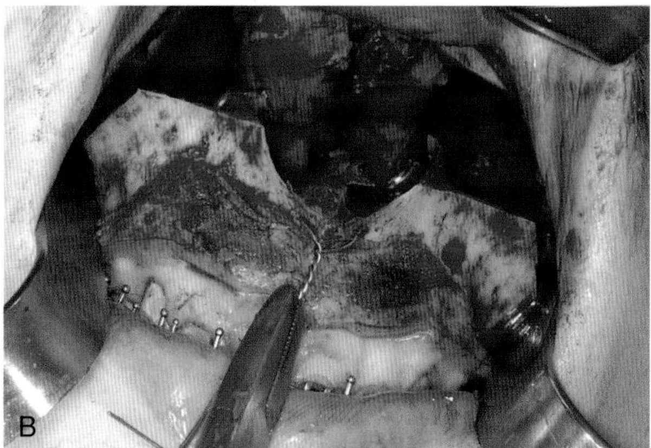

Fig. 41.13 **A** and **B,** A hole is drilled the anterior nasal spine to facilitate placement of a retraction wire and later to anchor the nasal septum and alar cinch.

TECHNIQUE: Le Fort I Osteotomy—*cont'd*

in a down-fracture position. It is rare that segmentation takes place anywhere other than between the lateral and canine teeth. The rationale for this is the three-dimensional changes in the dentition typically are in the posterior teeth, and inclusion of the canine allows one to alter canine width, account for Bolton discrepancies with the segmentation, and effect changes in the pitch and roll of the posterior segments independent of one another. The four-tooth anterior segment is considered the esthetic unit, and vertical changes that are skeletal in nature can then be accomplished, such as partial closure of open bites and improvement of the smile line. Reangulation of the incisors skeletally, rather than orthodontically, can also be done. Segmentation behind the canine is usually reserved for cases in which there is a step in the occlusal plane occurring at that point, which is not often experienced unless preplanned.

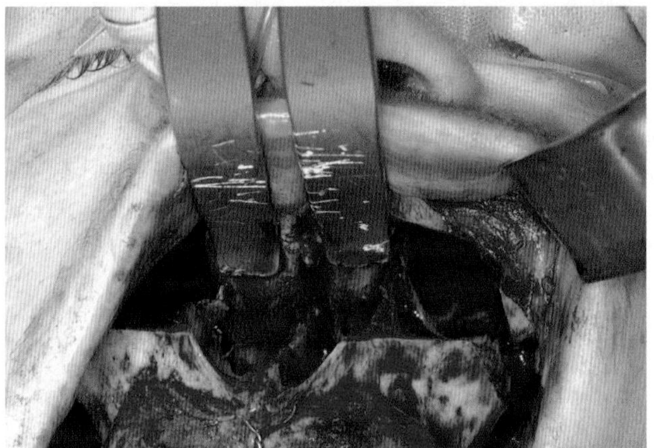

Fig. 41.14 A double-bladed Burton palatal retractor greatly enhances visualization for bony reductions and segmentation.

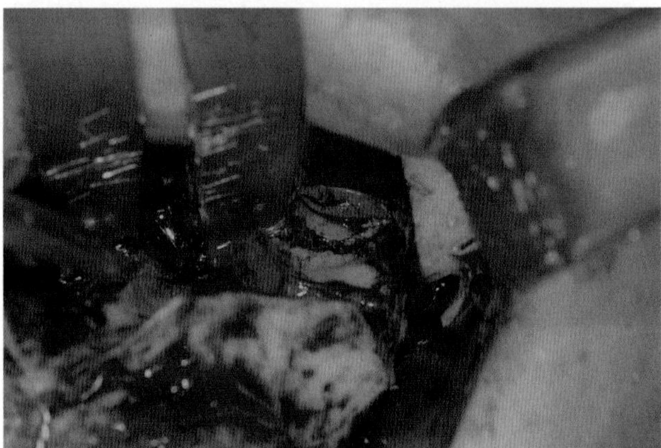

Fig. 41.16 It is important that the posterior maxilla be free of interferences.

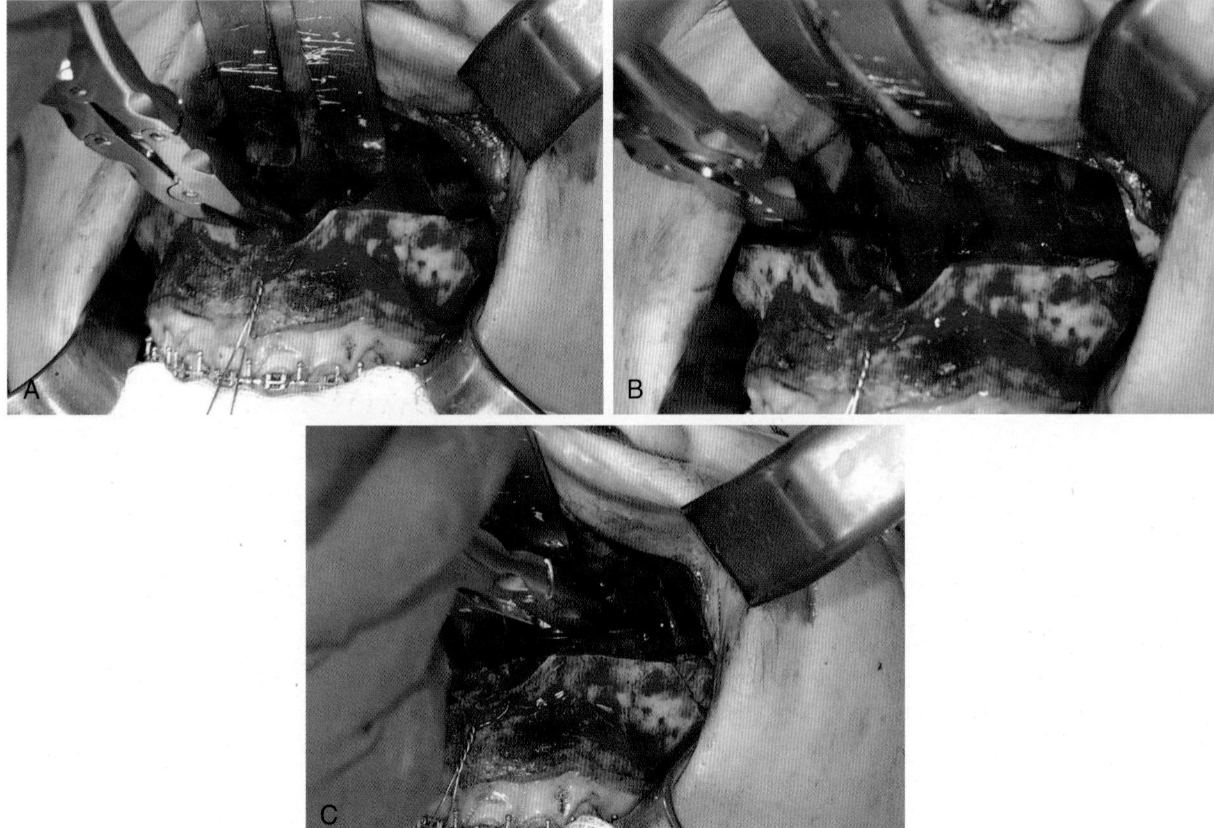

Fig. 41.15 A–C, The nasal septum and lateral nasal walls are carefully reduced.

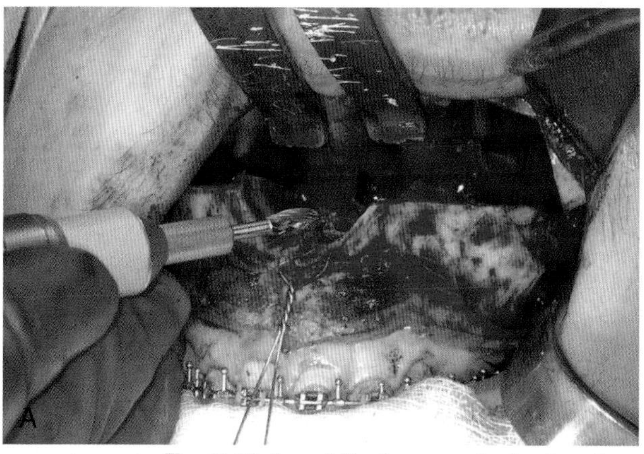

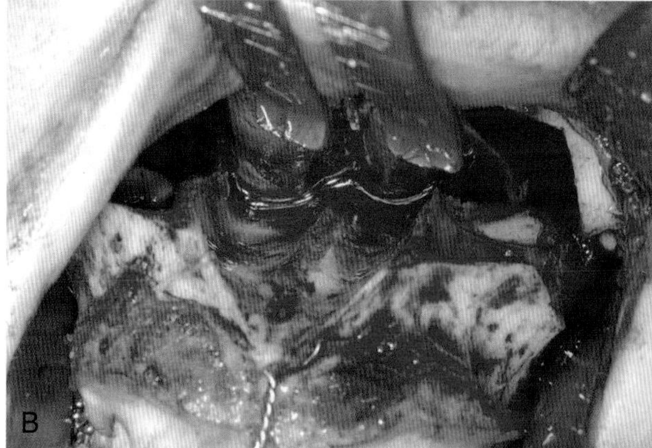

Fig. 41.17 **A** and **B,** A groove is developed on the maxillary crest to facilitate positioning of the septum when the maxilla is repositioned.

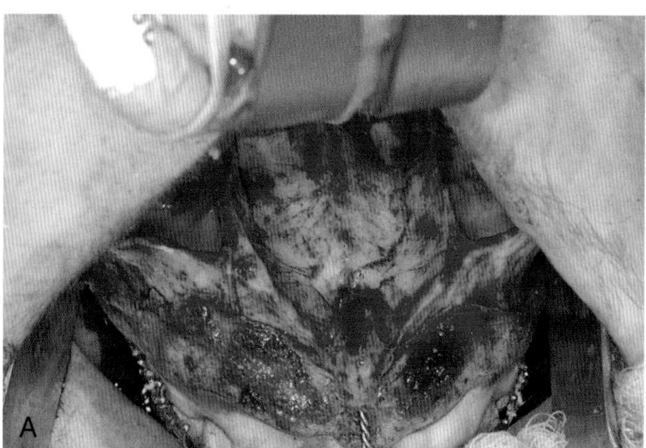

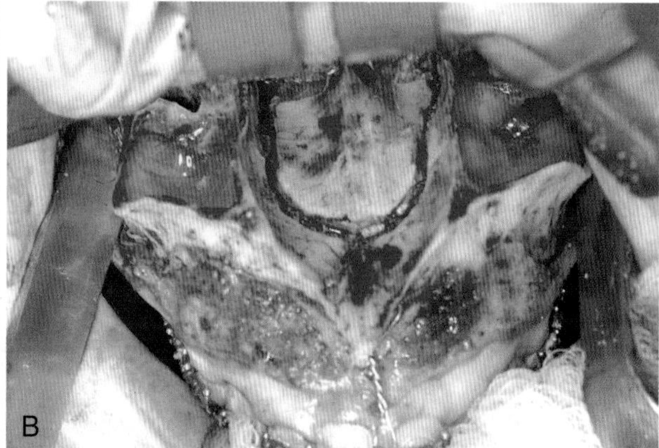

Fig. 41.18 **A** and **B,** A horseshoe osteotomy is used for most segmentation requiring 5 mm or less of transverse change.

TECHNIQUE: Le Fort I Osteotomy—*cont'd*

Though some surgeons prefer to segment before down-fracture, the orientation of the osteotomy cuts are far easier to visualize in the down-fractured state and can be accomplished very quickly and efficiently, often requiring less than 10 minutes. Changes in the width of the maxilla will dictate the osteotomy design that is used for the palatal osteotomy. If there is less than 5 to 6 mm in width change, a horseshoe osteotomy is accomplished with a #702 bur with the anterior aspect of the osteotomy coming forward to no closer than about 10 to 15 mm from the piriform rim. This is done to ensure a good bony pedicle for the anterior segment (Fig. 41.18).

Width changes greater than 6 mm will be accomplished with a midline osteotomy after a lateral palatal releasing incision with reflection of the palatal mucosa.

A sterile pencil can be used to mark the roots of the teeth and then draw out the proposed interdental osteotomies directly on bone to ensure proper angulation. A #701 bur is then used to make a cortical kerf in the bone above the apices of the teeth. Once this has been accomplished bilaterally and the arch wire cut, a small oscillating saw with a rounded end blade can then be used to complete the osteotomy through the lateral piriform rim, joining the osteotomy in the nasal cavity in a converging direction. A periotome is used to initiate the segmentation between the teeth and to create an initial osteotomy in the bone, which is not full thickness in nature. Because of its flexibility, it will minimize the possibility of root damage. The periotome osteotomy extends from the coronal one-third of the root superiorly to the full-thickness osteotomy, which is above the apices of the root. A spatula osteotome is then used to facilitate splitting of the alveolus from the mid root area superiorly to the full-thickness osteotomy and is completed with wood handle osteotome gently mobilizing the anterior segment to ensure that they have been appropriately separated (Fig. 41.19A–D).

A Turvey palatal spreader is then used to ensure that the posterior dento-alveolar components have been separated from the nasal floor. A palatal splint can be inserted and ligated to the teeth to aid in the maintenance of transverse changes. Once the segmentation is complete, three-dimensional changes in the maxilla are easily effected (Fig. 41.20).

If the superior movement of the maxillary is more than 6 or 7 mm, a partial inferior turbinectomy may be indicated to allow a

Continued

TECHNIQUE: Le Fort I Osteotomy—*cont'd*

passive impaction. The nasal mucosa is incised with Colorado tip electrocautery along its inferior surface in the posterior to anterior direction. The inferior portion, but less than half, of the turbinate is grasped with a curved hemostat, and a Dean scissors is used to excise this portion. Complete removal of the inferior turbinate should be avoided and can result in untoward clinical side effects such as atrophic rhinitis and, in the worst case scenario, empty nose syndrome. Electrocautery is used to coagulate the incised edge of the turbinate to minimize bleeding. The nasal mucosa is then sutured with a running 4-0 chromic gut suture.

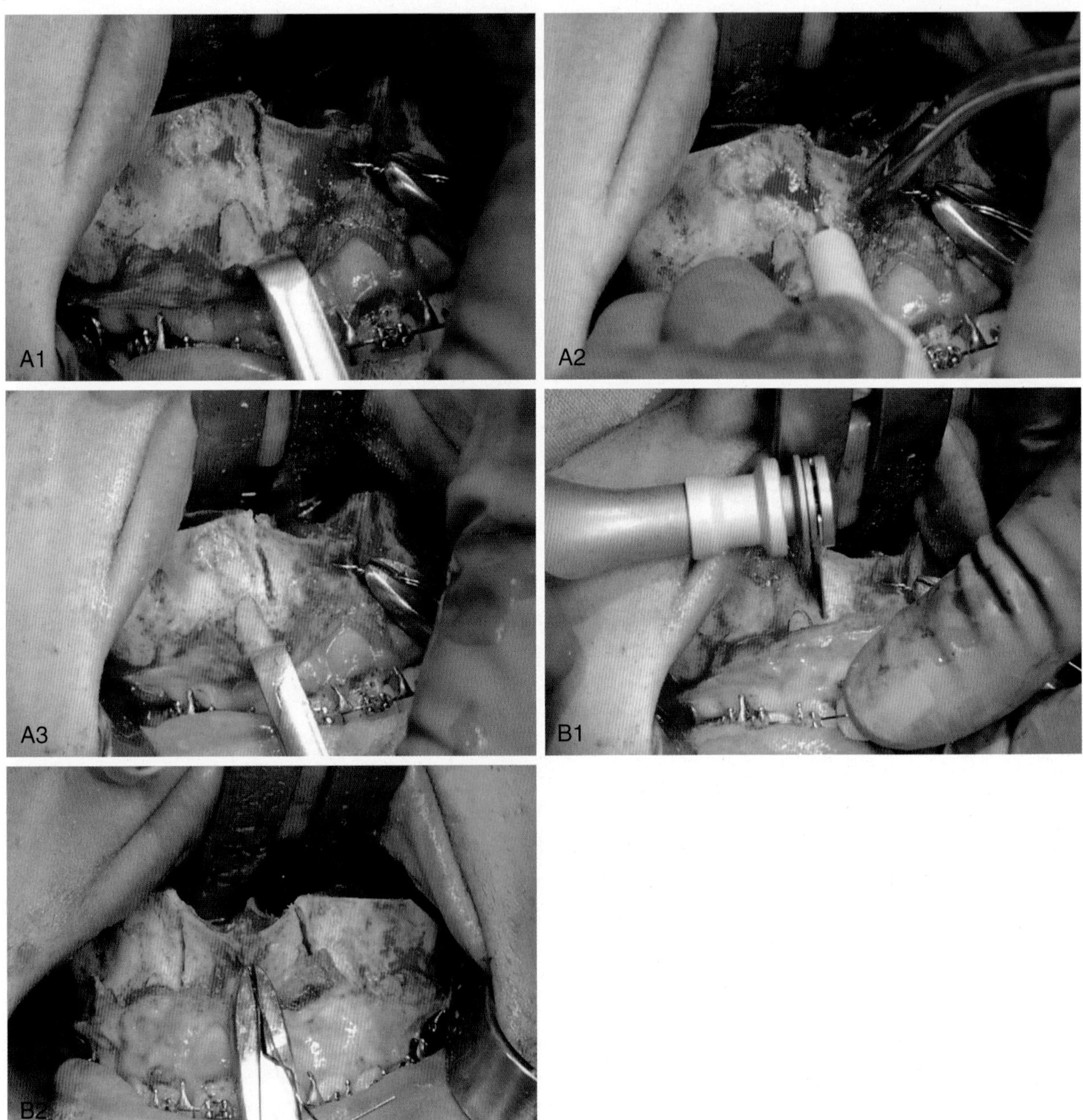

Fig. 41.19 **A1** and **A3,** The initial interdental osteotomies are done after identifying the roots and near or above the root apices. Angular orientation is better with the maxilla down-fractured. **B1** and **B2,** An oscillating saw is used to complete the osteotomy and joins the palatal horseshoe osteotomy and should converge posteriorly.

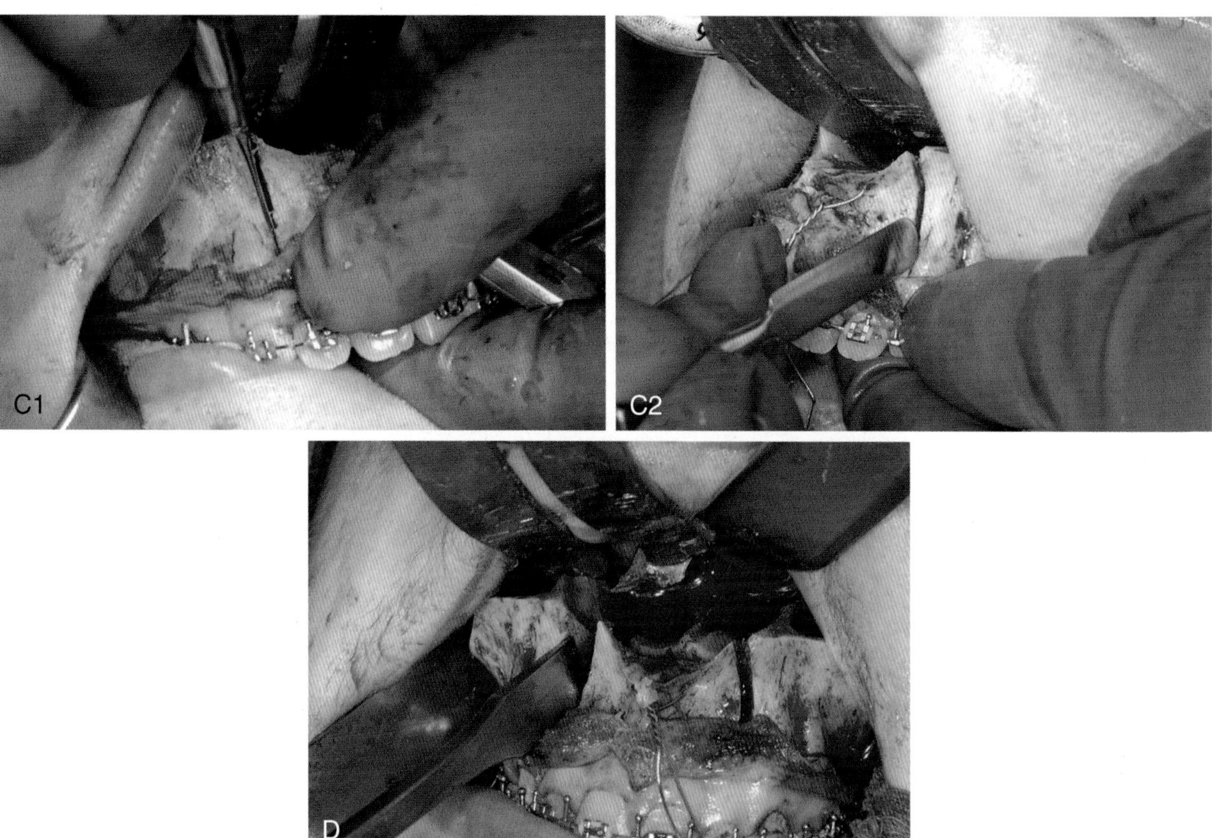

Fig. 41.19, cont'd **C1** and **C2,** A periotome is used to initiate the segmentation between the roots and is only 2 to 3 mm in depth. A spatula osteotome is then used to complete the segmentation. **D,** A wood-handled osteotome is used to gently complete the separation.

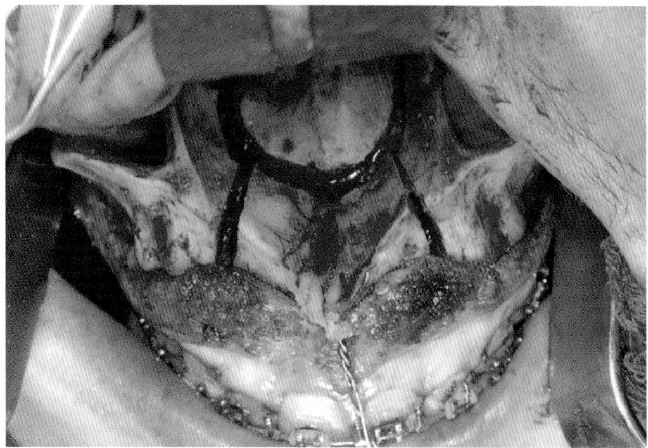

Fig. 41.20 The segmentation will allow for the segments to move three dimensionally without interference.

TECHNIQUE: Le Fort I Osteotomy—*cont'd*

STEP 6: Placement of Surgical Guide

If the maxillary osteotomy is being performed as an isolated procedure and the occlusion is acceptable, then tooth-to-tooth occlusion is preferred over the use of a prepared surgical guide with occlusal coverage. If the case involves operating on the mandible, an appropriate intermediate splint taking into consideration the surgeons preferred sequencing, mandible first or maxilla first, will be fabricated in advance and used. The guide is generally ligated to the upper teeth with 28-gauge wire. The upper and lower teeth are then wired together with 28-gauge wire.

Continued

TECHNIQUE: Le Fort I Osteotomy—*cont'd*

STEP 7: Removal of Anterior Interferences

With the maxillo-mandibular complex secured in mandibulomaxillary fixation, the maxilla is rotated into position with posterior and superior pressure on the mandible. It is imperative that the maxillo-mandibular complex be properly rotated upward. Upward pressure is applied at the gonial notches, and the thumb exerts a slight posterior pressure (Fig. 41.21). This method ensures full seating of the condyles during mandibular rotation and maxillary positioning. Upward rotation is stopped as soon as the first contact is detected and the vertical dimension measured. If the vertical dimension is more than desired, this interference is reduced accordingly. If adequate reduction in the posterior was completed as described in Step 5, this contact will likely be anterior and easily visualized. Anterior interferences can be easily reduced with a reduction bur. The caliper is used to check the vertical distance from the anterior orthodontic brackets to the K-wire and interferences are reduced accordingly (Fig. 41.22). Closely observe the nasal septum for early inferences and deviation. When all the bony interferences have been completely removed, the maxillo-mandibular complex should be easily rotated up into a stable reproducible position, with the condyles fully seated. If this is the case, you may begin the process of maxillary fixation.

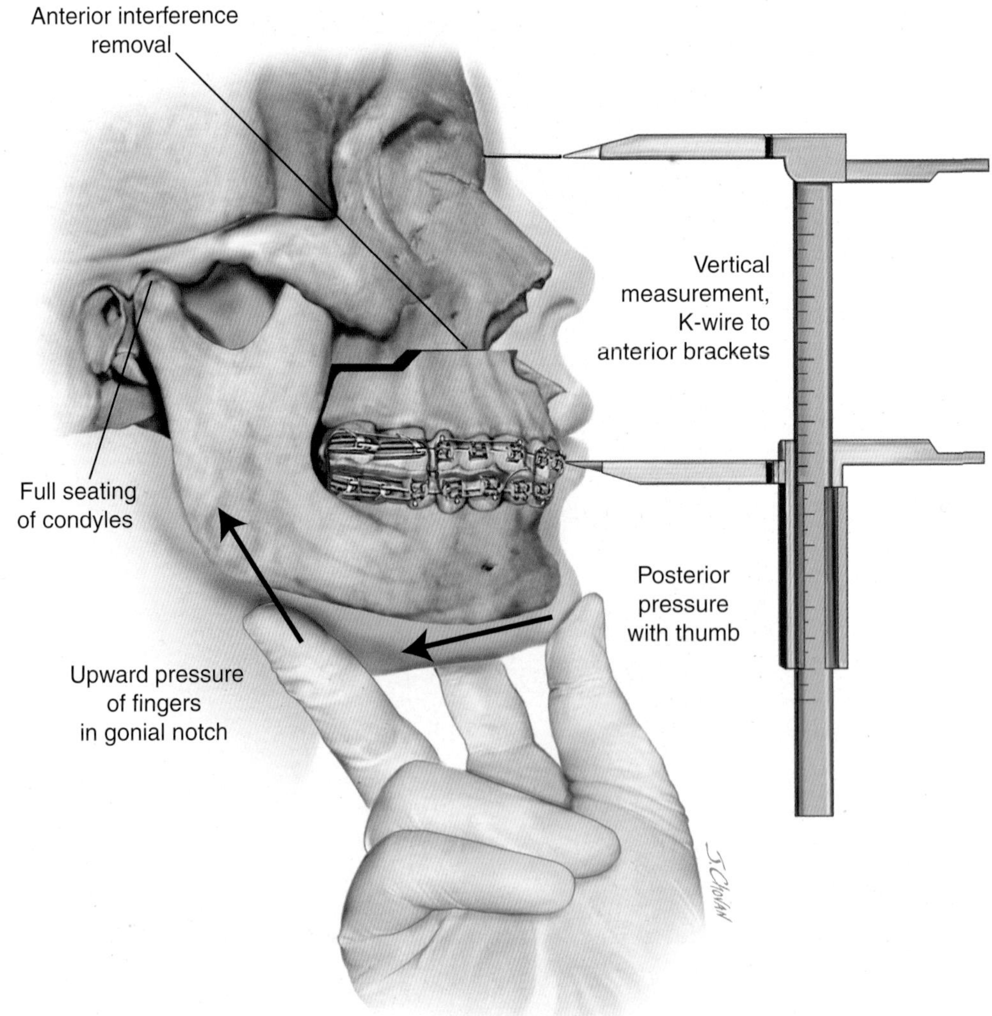

Fig. 41.21 Interferences in repositioning the maxilla are usually posterior near the pterygoid plates and passive repositioning is essential.

TECHNIQUE: Le Fort I Osteotomy—*cont'd*

STEP 8: Fixation, Grafts, and Final Measurements

With the maxilla positioned, four miniplates are bent to passively fit across the osteotomy in the piriform and zygomatic buttress areas of the maxilla. If the maxilla has been segmented, it is helpful to incorporate the anterior segment into the fixation plate. Typically, there are two fixation holes in the plate above and below the osteotomy and in each segment anteriorly to allow for placement of four to six screws per plate (Fig. 41.23). Thin bone or large bone gaps may require more fixation screws in each plate or even require additional plates. Bone grafts or alloplasts can be adapted or applied over or into the osteotomy gaps. Structural grafts can be either press-fit into position, or rigidly fixed if necessary.[12] Once the fixation has been competed, final measurements with calipers are made to confirm proper vertical placement.

STEP 9: Check Occlusion

Once the maxillary fixation is completed, the intermaxillary fixation is released. With the condyles seated, the tongue manipulated out of the way and the cheeks and lips retracted, the mandible is passively rotated into the maxillary dentition or splint if one is being used. Any premature dental contacts should be noted as well as any unexpected changes in the dental midlines or opening of the bite anteriorly. If the preplanned occlusion is different that what is observed then you must ascertain the reason, remove the rigid fixation, address it, and then replace the bone plates. Most often it is an unexpected posterior interference on or around the pterygoid plates that is causing condylar displacement at the time of seating and during the rotational closure of the maxillo-mandibular complex to the desired vertical position.

STEP 10: Closure

Proper closure occurs in four steps.

NASAL SEPTAL SUTURE

Suturing of the nasal septum back to the maxillary crest will help maintain the septum in its proper position and often preclude its inadvertent displacement during extubation. A 2-0 polyglycolic suture is passed through the anterior caudal edge and then through the hole drilled through the base of the anterior nasal spine where it is then tied (Fig. 41.24).

ALAR BASE SUTURE[13]

With the necessary exposure of the maxilla, the paranasal musculature is reflected and retracted so its accurate reapproximation is

Continued

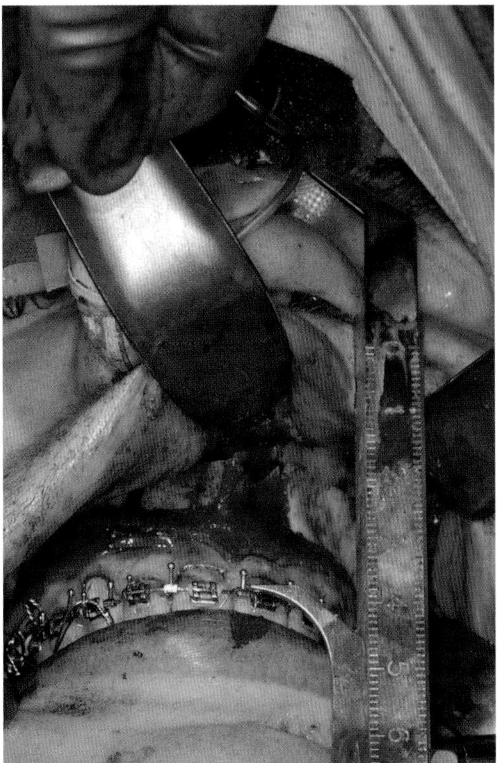

Fig. 41.22 With the maxilla in occlusion and repositioned, the planned vertical change is verified.

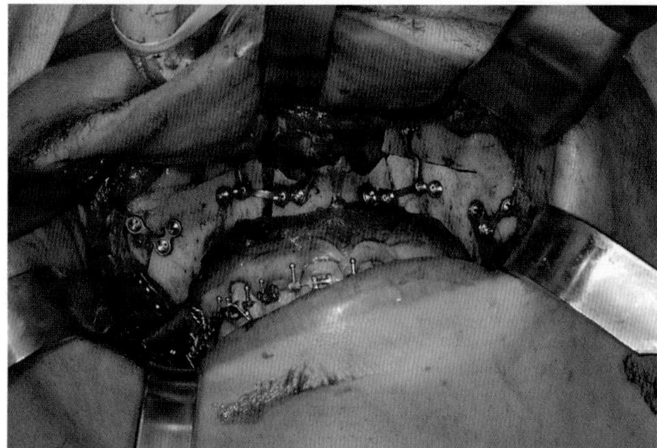

Fig. 41.23 The maxilla is plated with 1.5 mm system. A specially designed anterior segmental plate is used to secure the incisor tooth and posterior segments. Posterior plates are placed 90 degrees to the buttress osteotomy as a result of the osteotomy geometry.

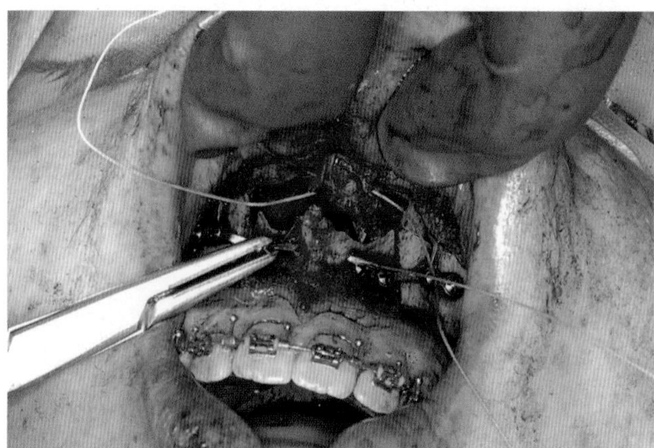

Fig. 41.24 The nasal septum is reapproximated to the anterior nasal spine. The suture is passed through the anterior nasal spine hole and tied.

TECHNIQUE: Le Fort I Osteotomy—*cont'd*

imperative. The alar base suture provides the appropriate repositioning of the soft tissue at the base of the nose to minimize postoperative nasal base widening. A slowly resorbing suture (e.g., 2-0 polyglycolic acid) is placed from an intraoral approach into the alar base bilaterally. The alar base is palpated and the curved needle should be passed from lateral to medial at a 45-degree angle inferiorly. Once domed bilaterally, pulling the suture should result in the alar bases being pulled medially toward each other. If the desired effect has been attained, then the suture is passed through the hole in the anterior nasal spine then the suture is tightened and tied. If properly done, tightening should result in an equal or shorter alar base width when compared with the preoperative width. If properly done, it should result in the projection and definition of the philtrum with a well-defined nasal base that recapitulates the natural nasal base anatomy and dimensions (Fig. 41.25).

ZYGOMATICUS MUSCLE AND V-Y CLOSURE[14]

The normal healing of the circumvestibular incision can result in lip shortening, lip thinning, and decreased vermillion show. The muscular and V-Y closure is done to minimize these undesirable effects. The zygomaticus muscles are reflected during the course of the surgical exposure so reestablishment of their orientation and approximation is important so as to not flatten the upper lip and to provide definition to the nasolabial creases. A 2-0 polyglycolic suture is passed lateral to medial in the premolar region the muscular layer of the vestibular incision and tied through the anterior nasal spine hole or as a sling under it. It should be snug enough to passively bring the margins of the vestibular incision together but also provide some depth and definition to the nasolabial creases and pouting of the lip and a small amount of eversion. It is common to see more vermillion display and thickness with this maneuver (Fig. 41.26).

The V-Y closure can now be done. With the use of a skin hook, the tissue of the midline vestibular incision is grasped and gently pulled superiorly. The length of the vertical limb will vary with each patient but can be easily ascertained by simply digitally bringing the vestibular incisions that are now approximated by the muscle suture, medially until they touch. The assistant holding the skin hook will release tension to facilitate this. Using a 5-0 resorbable suture (e.g., 5-0 fast absorbing polyglycolic acid), the base is approximated first and then the remaining vertical limb with interrupted or a continuous suture (Fig. 41.27).

VESTIBULAR CLOSURE

The remaining vestibular closure continues from the posterior portion of the incision medially with the same suture material and in a running fashion.

Avoidance and Management of Intraoperative Complications

The Le Fort I osteotomy is a procedure that is not difficult to accomplish and is typically a safe and effective treatment for the vast majority of maxillary deformities. Because mandibular orthognathic procedures often have long-term postoperative problems, such as neurosensory deficits, swelling, and range of motion issues, maxillary procedures are associated with more severe intraoperative complications. The Le Fort I osteotomy has been associated with severe hemorrhage, blindness, and death; however, those are extremely rare. It is imperative that the surgeon be cognizant of the local anatomy and perform the procedure with the utmost care and precision.

A common and avoidable problem of the vestibular incision is making it too short, causing tears with retraction and even during the down-fracture. The lateral and posterior vascular pedicle can be compromised by incisions that are too long. Separation of the pterygomaxillary junction above the horizontal osteotomy will have no benefit, so care muse be

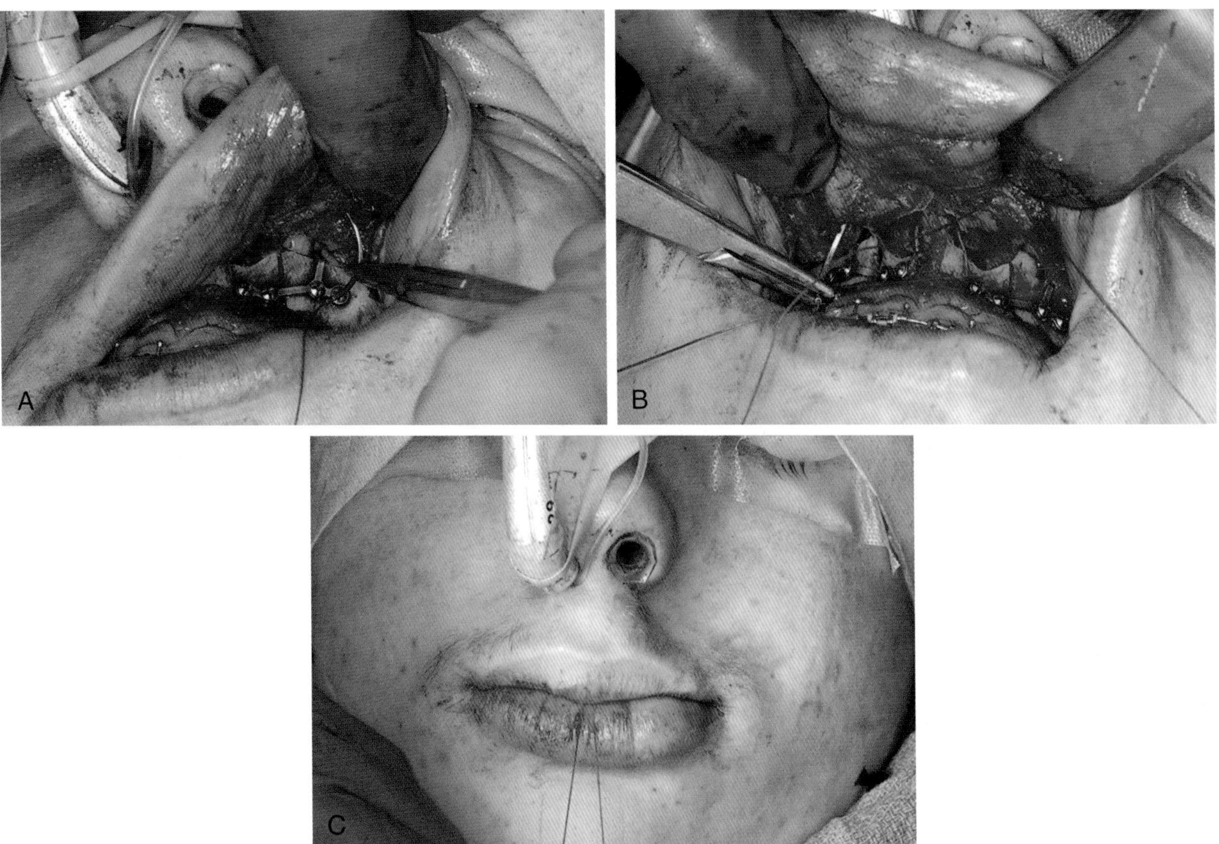

Fig. 41.25 A–C, An alar base suture is passed from left to right and symmetry is verified with gentle traction and secured by passing the suture through the anterior nasal spine hole. A nasal trumpet equally sized to the endotracheal tube helps maintain symmetry.

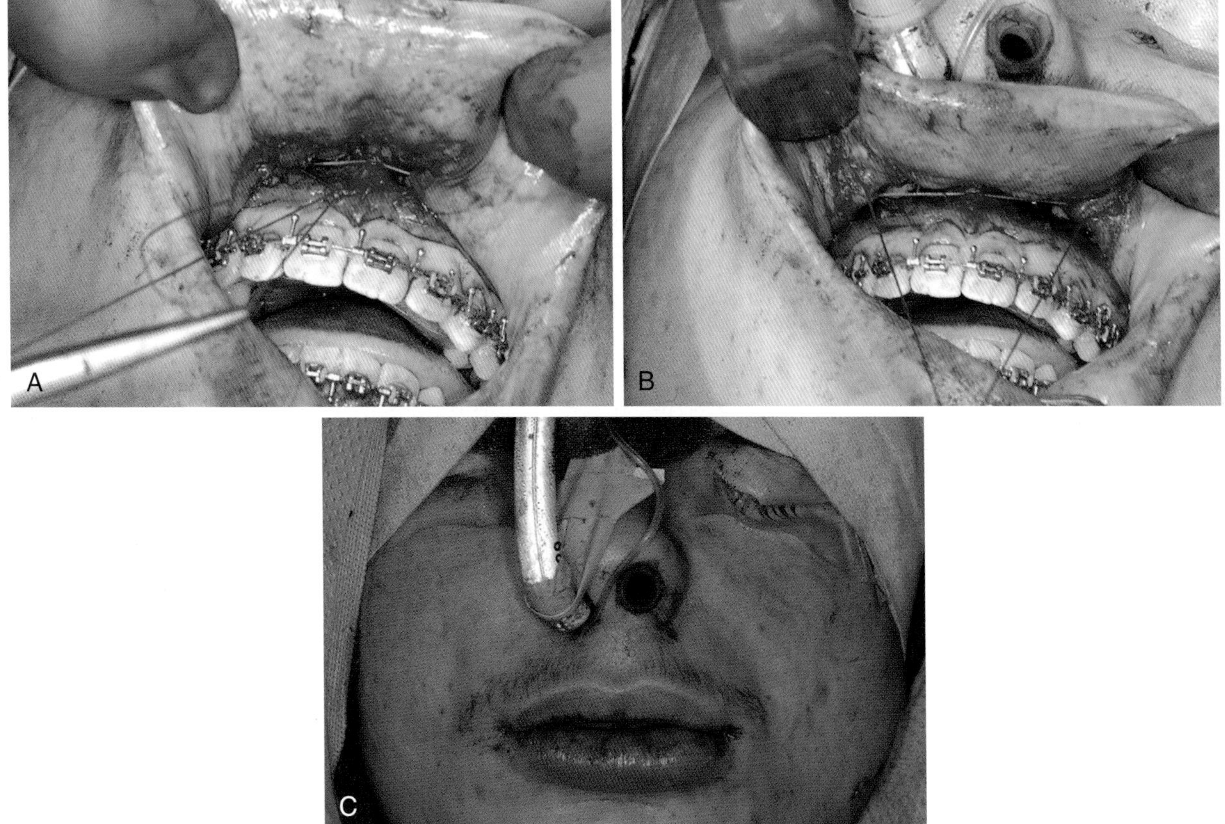

Fig. 41.26 A–C, A suture through the approximate location of the reflected zygomaticus muscles adds definition to the nasolabial folds and bolsters the alar base suture.

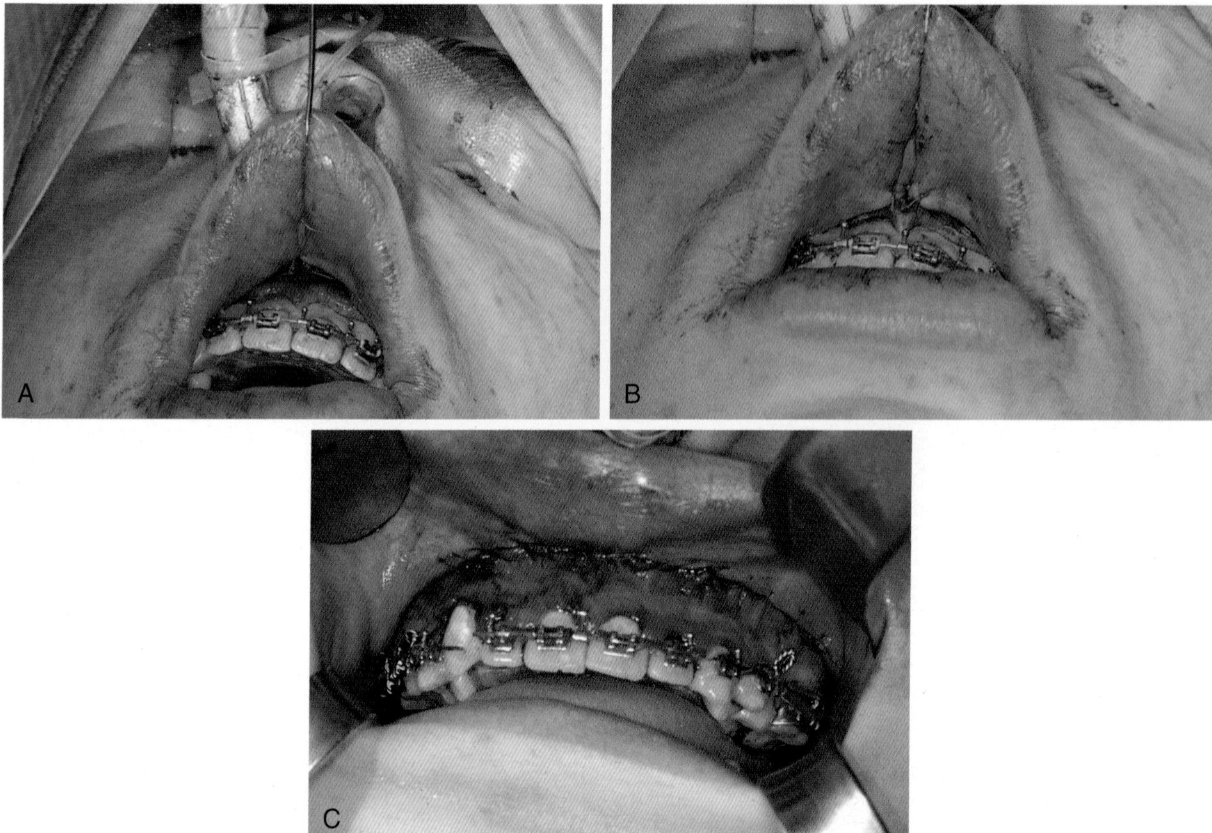

Fig. 41.27 **A–C,** V-Y and vestibular closure.

taken to ensure separation in the lower third of the pterygoid plates, otherwise you increase the risk for bleeding and the creation of added bony interferences that can complicate repositioning. The internal maxillary artery courses approximately 25 mm superior to the base of the junction of the pterygoid plate and maxilla so keeping instrumentation and the maxillary separation low are important.[15] The descending palatine (usually found 30 to 35 mm posteriorly) can be injured during the lateral nasal wall osteotomy if extended further posteriorly through the pyramidal process, which can also cause significant hemorage.[16]

Resistance to down-fracture will occur most commonly in the pyramidal process of the palatine bone or pterygomaxillary junction. If resistance is encountered, the surgeon should repeat those steps to ensure completeness. In the lateral nasal wall area, a thin spatula osteotome can be placed through the anterior wall osteotomy and the pyramidal process can be engaged from the lateral side and gently tapped with a mallet a few more millimeters posteriorly and rotated to help the separation of the pyramidal process. If there is resistance at the pterygomaxillary junction, the surgeon should insert the curved Burton osteotome into the junction and then gently strike with a mallet until it is palpated with a finger in the palatal area. The handle should be rotated down to encourage separation. It is critical that the down-fracture is completed with as minimal force as possible. Excessive force during down-fracture is encouraged by incomplete osteotomy and then the use of certain instruments, such as the Rowe maxillary forceps, Tessier bone hooks, and Smith bone spreaders. Excessive force and incomplete osteotomies during down-fracture can be associated with unfavorable maxillary, orbital, and skull base fractures. Previous Le Fort I surgery or surgically assisted maxillary expansion may result in unusual bony healing in the posterior maxilla, especially in the pterygoid plate and pyramidal process areas making down-fracture more difficult. Extra care must be taken in those cases to ensure adequate separation prior to down-fracture, or one risks the added possibility of complications and inadvertent fracture patterns.[17]

When establishing the vertical position of the maxilla, it is imperative that superior pressure is not exerted only at the chin because this will often, if a posterior interference is present, lead to a fulcrum effect and distraction of the condyles and a post fixation open-bite malocclusion. Gentle upward pressure at the angles of the mandible and simultaneous rotation of the maxillo-mandibular complex will disclose posterior interferences that can be relieved to preclude maxillary malpositioning. Anterior open-bite tendencies with early posterior contacts most likely are the result of improper seating of the condyles. In these cases, the fixation should be removed, interferences relieved, and the fixation reapplied. Lastly, inaccurate fixation placement, such as poorly adapted plates, can lead to a postoperative malocclusion. The osteotomy design should also keep plates and screws well away from the tooth roots.

In the author's view, there is no role for a final occlusal splint when doing Le Fort I osteotomies. A splint will never be superior to tooth-to-tooth contact; therefore, they are not necessary, especially if you have good coupling of the dentition with your dental models. If not, segmentation of the maxilla will often yield a far better occlusal coupling, and as a result virtually all of the author's Le Fort I osteotomies are three-piece segmentations. Segmental maxillary surgery may need a palatal splint to maintain width and arch form, but a good post operative occlusion without occlusal coverage will allow far better monitoring of the occlusion and allow for minor adjustments in the postoperative period. Guiding inter-arch elastics are placed for maintenance of occlusion, and patients are instructed on their use and replacement.

Postoperative Considerations

Intravenous antibiotics and steroids are always recommended preoperatively, and they can be continued postoperatively in certain situations such as extensive bone grafting or for other medical necessities and depending on the surgeon's preference. Routine cases are typically extubated in the operating room and will have a nasogastric tube place. Following their recovery in the post anesthesia care unit, they are transferred to a standard hospital room for overnight observation. Head-of-bed elevation to 45 degrees is recommended. Oral intake is encouraged immediately following nasogastric tube removal with a clear liquid diet, and a full liquid diet is prescribed for approximately 2 weeks. Patients should be instructed on routine oral hygiene care with daily tooth brushing and frequent saline rinses. Chlorhexidine oral rinses (0.12%), two to three times daily, are also used as an adjunct. Sinus precautions include use of a systemic oral decongestant and saline nasal sprays as needed, judicious use of local nasal decongestant sprays for 3 days, and instructions to open-mouth sneeze and avoid nose blowing and thereby prevent subcutaneous air emphysema. Patients are closely followed as outpatients and reevaluated at postoperative weeks 1, 3, and 6 or more often if needed. The palatal splint is removed at week 6 and prior to resuming orthodontic treatment.

References

1. Langenbeck BV. Beitrage zur Osteoplastik—die osteoplastische Resektion des Oberkeifers. In: Goshen A, ed. *Deutche Klinik*; 1859.
2. Cheever DW. Naso-pharyngeal polypus, attached to the basilar process of the occipital and body of the sphenoid bone successfully removed by a section, displacement, and subsequent replacement and reunion of the superior maxillary bone. *Boston Med Surg J*. 1867;8:162.
3. LeFort. Fractures de la machoire superieure. *Rev Chir*. 1901:4360.
4. Wassmund M. *Frakturen und Luxationen des Gesichtsschadels*. Meusser; 1927.
5. Schuchardt K. Ein Beitrag zur chirurgischen Kieferorthopade unter Berucksichtgung iher Bedeutung Fur die Behandlung angeborener und erworbner Kieferdeformitaten bei Soldaten. Dtch. Zahn-Mund- un. *Kieferheilk*. 1942;9:73.
6. Bell WH. Le Forte I osteotomy for correction of maxillary deformities. *J Oral Surg*. 1975;33(6):412–426.
7. Kaminishi RM, Davis WH, Hochwald DA, Nelson N. Improved maxillary stability with modified Lefort I technique. *J Oral Maxillofac Surg*. 1983;41(3):203–205.
8. Bennett MA, Wolford LM. The maxillary step osteotomy and Steinmann pin stabilization. *J Oral Maxillofac Surg*. 1985;43(4):307–311.
9. Reyneke JP, Masureik CJ. Treatment of maxillary deficiency by a Le Fort I downsliding technique. *J Oral Maxillofac Surg*. 1985;43(11):914–916.
10. Wolford LM, Karras SC, Mehra P. Considerations for orthognathic surgery during growth, part 2: maxillary deformities. *Am J Orthod Dentofacial Orthop*. 2001;119(2):102–105.
11. Hörster W. Experience with functionally stable plate osteosynthesis after forward displacement of the upper jaw. *J Maxillofac Surg*. 1980;8(3):176–181.
12. Mehra P, Hopkin JK, Castro V, Freitas RZ. Stability of maxillary advancement using rigid fixation and bone grafting: cleft lip versus non-cleft patients. *Int J Adult Orthodon Orthognath Surg*. 2001;16:193.
13. Muradin MS, Seubring K, Stoelinga PJ, vd Bilt A, Koole R, Rosenberg AJ. A prospective study on the effect of modified alar cinch sutures and V-Y closure versus simple closing sutures on nasolabial changes after Le Fort I intrusion and advancement osteotomies. *J Oral Maxillofac Surg*. 2011;69(3):870–876.
14. Peled M, Ardekian L, Krausz AA, Aizenbud D. Comparing the effects of V-Y advancement versus simple closure on upper lip aesthetics after Le Fort I advancement. *J Oral Maxillofac Surg*. 2004;62(3):315–319.
15. Turvey TA, Fonseca RJ. The anatomy of the internal maxillary artery in the pterygopalatine fossa: its relationship to maxillary surgery. *J Oral Surg*. 1980;38(2):92–95.
16. Li KK, Meara JG, Alexander A Jr. Location of the descending palatine artery in relation to the Le Fort I osteotomy. *J Oral Maxillofac Surg*. 1996;54(7):822–825.
17. Kramer FJ, Baethge C, Swennen G, et al. Intra- and perioperative complications of the LeFort I osteotomy: a prospective evaluation of 1000 patients. *J Craniofac Surg*. 2004;15(6):971–977.

Model Surgery Planning

Joseph J. Fantuzzo

Armamentarium

Acrylic bur
Acrylic liquid (pink, clear) and powder
Alginate
Bite fork
Caliper (facial measurements)
Centric relation (wax) bite
Dental stone
Die saw
Erickson model table
Face-bow
Hot glue gun
Lab knife
Lab wax
Lathe
Marking pens (black and red)
Model grinder
Petroleum jelly
Plaster
Pumice and Acrilustre
Scissors
Semi-adjustable hinge articulator
Straight or round bur (for 1-mm splint holes)

History of the Procedure

Since the first mandibular osteotomy (Hullihen, 1849), orthognathic surgical techniques have developed into the standard surgical approach for the correction of the majority of craniomaxillofacial deformities. The application of orthognathic surgical techniques has always involved complex three-dimensional movements that require thoughtful preoperative planning. Early on, surgeons relied solely on their clinical and surgical experience to carry out osteotomies of the mandible (Hullihen, 1849; Blair, 1907)[1,2]. In 1935, Wassmund planned surgery by fabricating silver alloy splints from handheld segments of sectioned dental models.[3] The use of the arbitrary face-bow transfer gained support after Schallhorn[4] demonstrated that the arbitrary intercondylar hinge axis is within a 5-mm radius of the true hinge axis. In the 1960s and early 1970s, Obwegeser used a combination of handheld and mounted models on articulators to prepare for bimaxillary osteotomies. Lockwood[5] developed a key spacer system for model surgery that used a plane line hinge articulator. Hohl[6] advocated the use of an anatomic articulator and face-bow transfer in segmental maxillary surgery. Model surgery measurements using handheld millimeter rulers gave way to the Erickson model surgery table (Great Lakes Orthodontics, Tonawanda, NY), allowing for more accurate model planning. Heggie[7] challenged the accuracy of model surgery alone and encouraged the use of a calibrator (modified Vernier caliper) to register the distance between the nasion (rhinion) and an arbitrary point on the nose and midline incisor tip to assess the vertical maxillary position during surgery.

The traditional sequencing of bimaxillary orthognathic surgery, more commonly used by orthognathic surgeons, repositions the maxilla first, using the uncut mandible as a template. The mandible is then repositioned into occlusion with the repositioned maxilla. Contrary to established practice, Lindorf and Steinhauser,[8] Buckley et al.,[9] Cottrell and Wolford,[10] and Posnick[11] suggested altering the sequence of bimaxillary model surgery planning and the step-by-step operative procedure for specific indications. Their modified "reverse" approach repositions the mandible first, and the maxilla is then placed into the most ideal occlusal relationship with the mandible. Only the vertical incisor position needs to be set, based on presurgical clinical decision making, at the surgical repositioning of the maxilla. This sequence reduces laboratory time and avoids potential displacement of the repositioned maxilla during mandibular surgery, especially in cases where unreliable centric relation (CR) stops exist due to malformed or absent mandibular condyle (or condyles), and in large mandibular advancements, maxillary segmentation, and/or with thin maxillary walls.[9–11]

Both traditional and reverse planning methods depend on the demands of the clinical problem, in addition to the surgeon's knowledge, training, experience, and personal preferences, to achieve an outstanding outcome. Standard model surgery planning, although time consuming in the laboratory, is still a predictable and reliable method for achieving accurate surgical repositioning in the operating room. More recently, computed tomography-based, virtual model surgery planning has gained popularity, and proponents have shown it to be an efficient and accurate alternative to standard model surgery planning.[12] The learning curve and cost of virtual planning technology may be limiting factors. Certainly, an accurate clinical examination must be performed, and a thoughtful surgical plan developed, before computer software planning can be effectively employed.

Indications for the Use of the Procedure

Craniomaxillofacial deformities involve both hard and soft tissues in all three planes of space. Prediction tracings provide an estimate of the amount and direction of maxillary and/or mandibular movement, but only in two dimensions and from a profile view. Definitive model surgery provides a more accurate assessment of planned surgical movements designed to establish an ideal, functional occlusion, with the condyles properly seated in the fossae, and with simultaneous repositioning of the jaws, in all three planes of space, to enhance facial aesthetics.[13,14] Model surgery planning ultimately allows the surgeon to apply these goals, based on clinical and radiographic evaluation, to the operating room. Reasons for performing model surgery include (1) determining the magnitude and direction of skeletal movement; (2) assessing the position of planned osteotomies, especially interdental ones; (3) confirming the surgical plan and the final occlusion; (4) allowing fabrication of surgical splints, to be used at the time of surgery, based on occlusion and condylar function; and (5) providing a comparative reference to the occlusal result actually achieved after the release of intermaxillary fixation.[15]

Face-bow transfer and articulator mounting are not necessary in surgery of the mandible alone. In isolated mandibular surgery, the mandible is repositioned into occlusion with the maxilla. The surgeon has determined that the maxilla is ideally positioned. Therefore, the maxilla is used as a template. Mandible-only surgical planning can easily be performed on a hinge (Galetti) articulator. Only a single (final) splint is required, which is fabricated from the planned ideal occlusal relationship.

Model surgery is especially important in the planning of bimaxillary surgery. When bimaxillary surgery is planned, accurate repositioning of the maxilla is critical because the maxilla must be ideally repositioned based on clinical and radiographic examination and using the current mandibular position as a template.[16]

Occlusal splints make intraoperative surgical repositioning of the maxilla and mandible relatively simple, fast, accurate, and predictable.[17,18] Given the three-dimensional complexity of maxillary repositioning, the intermediate splint accounts for anteroposterior and mediolateral positioning, in addition to pitch, roll, and yaw. Only the vertical position of the maxillary incisors needs to be planned for and addressed at surgery. The incisor vertical position is based on the presurgical clinical evaluation. Although model surgery planning and the fabrication of splints are time consuming, they allow the surgeon to enter the operating room with confidence in the surgical plan.

Limitations and Contraindications

Although model surgery planning can provide consistently reliable results during surgery, there are many steps along the way. Each step has the potential to introduce inaccuracies that could ultimately affect the final outcome.[19,20] Lapp[20] outlined a number of arguments against model planning and splint fabrication, such as the distortion of alginate impressions, inaccurate face-bow transfer, improper mounting of study models, dimensional distortion of acrylic splints, and a thin or overly thick intermediate splint acting as a potential factor in mandibular repositioning. A thin intermediate splint made without keeping a neutral pin position on the articulator leads to overreliance on condylar autorotation. A splint that is too thick can cause condylar distraction during maxillary repositioning. Lapp suggests that model planning and splint fabrication give the surgeon a "false sense of security."[21]

TECHNIQUE: Model Surgery Planning

STEP 1: Presurgical Planning: Clinical and Radiographic Evaluation and Records

A full history and clinical examination should always be obtained. Facial measurements (in millimeters) are recorded and include the maxillary dental midline to facial midline, mandibular dental midline to facial midline and to maxillary dental midline, presence or absence of maxillary cant, and maxillary incisor vertical position relative to the upper lip in repose and in posed smile.[22] The surgeon must assess and plan for changes in the maxillary transverse dimension (buccal corridors), maxillary anteroposterior position, and maxillary and mandibular plane (pitch rotation). Maxillofacial plane rotation can have a positive influence on consonance of the maxillary incisors to the lower lip, incisor inclination, A-B point relationship, and nasolabial and profile esthetics.

A series of radiographs should be obtained (lateral cephalometric, posterior-anterior cephalometric, and panoramic radiographs or computed tomography with panoramic and lateral cephalometric reformatting). Cephalometric analyses should be performed using manual or computer software tracings. These should be available, if only as a guideline, at the time of clinical examination and planning.

The preferred repositioning of the maxilla, mandible, and chin is determined according to the patient's desires and the surgeon's preference based on the overall clinical assessment (i.e., the patient's objectives, the assessment of facial and smile esthetics, morphologic skeletal and dental limitations, and the cephalometric analysis).

Continued

TECHNIQUE: Model Surgery Planning—cont'd

STEP 2: Centric Relation Bite

As defined in the Glossary of Prosthodontic Terms,[22] centric relation (CR) is the maxillomandibular relationship in which the condyles articulate with the thinnest avascular portion of their respective disks with the complex in the anterior-superior position against the shapes of the articular eminencies. This position is independent of tooth contact.[23] CR is clinically discernible when the mandible is directed superiorly and posteriorly. It is restricted to a purely rotary movement about the transverse horizontal axis. To record the CR bite, place soft wax on the maxillary occlusion. Then register the patient's maxillary occlusion into the soft wax. It is important that the surgeon be able to reproduce this CR bite with the patient in a neutral head position and the jaw relaxed. The CR bite is a bite the surgeon must accurately reproduce with the patient asleep on the operating table (Fig. 42.1A and B).[24–30]

STEP 3: Face-Bow Transfer to Articulator

An accurate face-bow transfer allows for registration of important points for the establishment of accurate relationships between the condyles, maxilla, and the skull base.[31–NaN] First, place the upper side of the bite fork, with green foil-reinforced wax, into the maxillary occlusion, taking care to center the bite fork between the maxillary central incisors. The ear prongs of the "bow" portion are then placed in each ear canal and held by the patient at the temporal extensions to ensure even pressure medially, superiorly, and forward in each ear canal. Next, insert the bite fork (with the wax registered into the patient's maxillary teeth) into the face-bow apparatus. In profile, adjust the face-bow temporal extensions to match the Frankfurt horizontal. In frontal view, adjust the face-bow to parallel with the pupils or other predetermined horizontal in the case of clinically significant orbital dystopia. The nasal portion should rest passively at the nasion (rhinion). Tighten the face-bow thumbscrew and tighten the screw to secure the bite fork to the vertical portion of the face-bow apparatus. After confirming the three points of reference, release the ear prongs by loosening the screw at the temporal extensions and remove the face-bow from the patient (Fig. 42.1C–E).

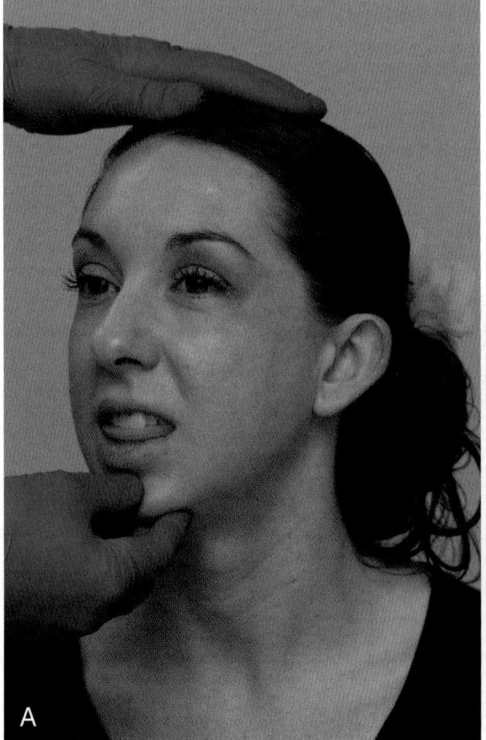

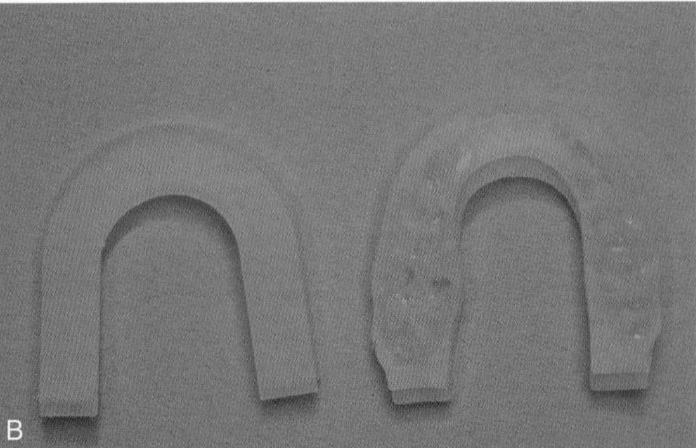

Figure 42.1 **A,** Capturing the centric relation wax bite. **B,** Centric relation wax bite.

TECHNIQUE: Model Surgery Planning—cont'd

STEP 4: Mounting Models

As part of the presurgical record, alginate impressions of the maxillary and mandibular dental arches are obtained. The alginate impressions are poured up in dental stone. Be sure to remove all occlusal blebs. In addition, it is helpful to incorporate an adequate base using base formers, measuring from molar cusp tip to base and canine cusp tip to base. The models are trimmed precisely using a dental model grinder. Next, mount the maxillary cast on the articulator with white plaster using the face-bow and bite fork support piece to prevent sagging of the maxillary cast. It is helpful to place a thin (dime-sized) coat of petroleum jelly on the center of the base of the maxillary cast before adding the plaster base; this helps facilitate separation later. When hot glue is used during model planning, the plaster should be allowed to dry overnight. After drying, articulate the mandibular cast to the mounted maxillary cast in CR, using the CR wax bite, and secure the current occlusion into position with hot glue. Next, mount the mandibular cast on the articulator with white plaster. Once the plaster is dry, trim each maxillary and mandibular cast mounted with mounting plaster, all as one unit. Let the plaster used to mount the mandibular cast dry overnight (Fig. 42.1F).

Continued

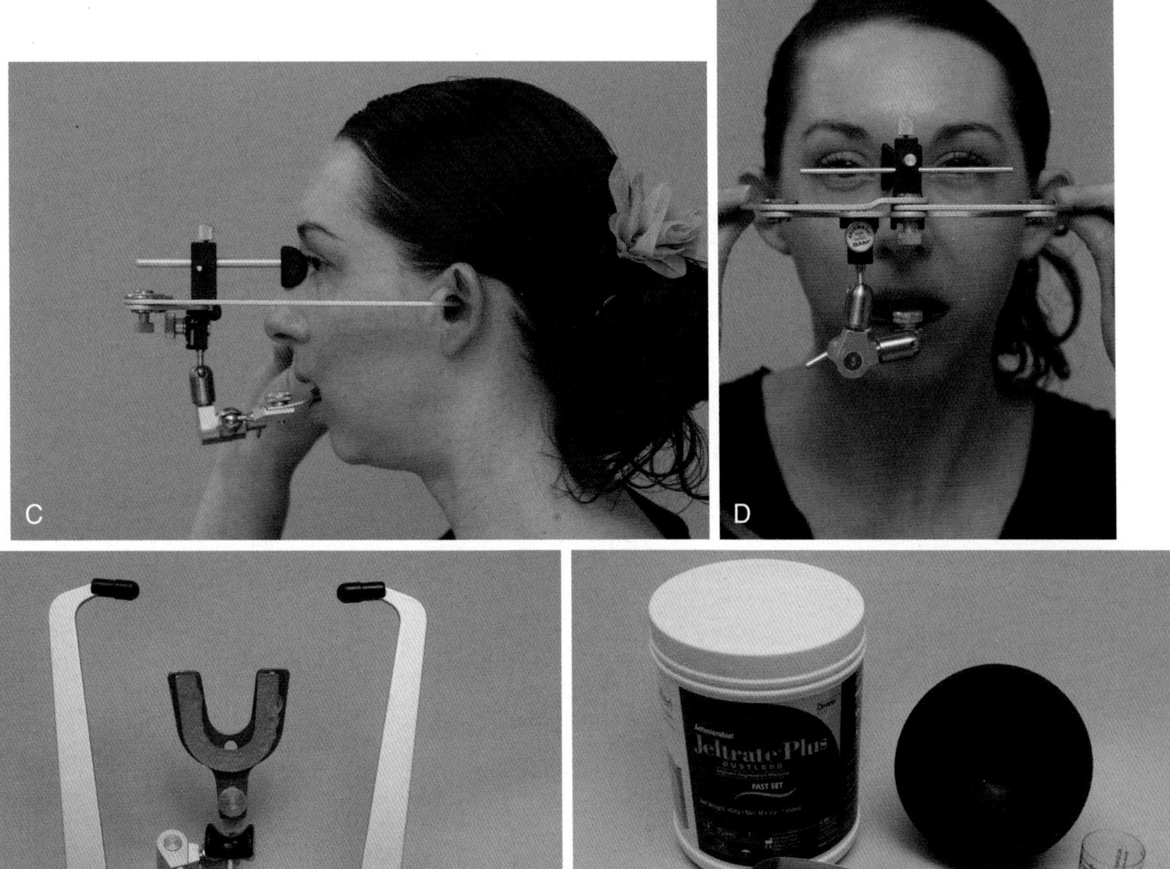

Figure 42.1, cont'd **C** and **D,** Face-bow transfer (side and frontal views). **E,** Face-bow ready for articulator. **F,** Alginate impressions.

TECHNIQUE: Model Surgery Planning—cont'd

STEP 5: Reference Lines/Marking Casts

After the mounted models have dried overnight, use a black marking pen to mark two horizontal circumferential reference lines on the maxillary unit. Place the first horizontal line entirely in green stone. Then measure and place the second horizontal line entirely in white plaster. The reference lines are marked with a 20-mm separation. Next, mark the vertical reference lines at the mesiobuccal groove of each first molar, between the central incisors (at the dental midline), from each canine cusp tip and at the posterior tuberosity/retromolar area (mid ridge) bilaterally. These reference lines allow for easy visualization of the changes achieved during the model surgery. Using a black marking pen, place a dot at the mesiobuccal cusp tip of each maxillary first molar, each maxillary canine, and at the midpoint of the incisal edge of each maxillary central incisor (Fig. 42.1G–I).

STEP 6: Use of the Erickson Model Table

Record (in millimeters) the preoperative measurements taken from the Erickson model table. Measure the current vertical with the model block on its base. The model table is used to measure the distance (in millimeters) at the marked maxillary incisal edge of each maxillary central incisor and marked mesiobuccal cusp tip of each maxillary molar and canine. Next, measure the current anterior-posterior (horizontal) with the model block on end. The caliper is used to measure the distance (in millimeters) at the marked incisal edge of each maxillary central incisor. Next, measure the current transverse width (marked mesiobuccal cusp of maxillary molar to maxillary molar and canine to canine) and maxillary midline with the model block on each side. The current maxillary position, based on these measurements, is recorded on the model planning worksheet (Fig. 42.1J).

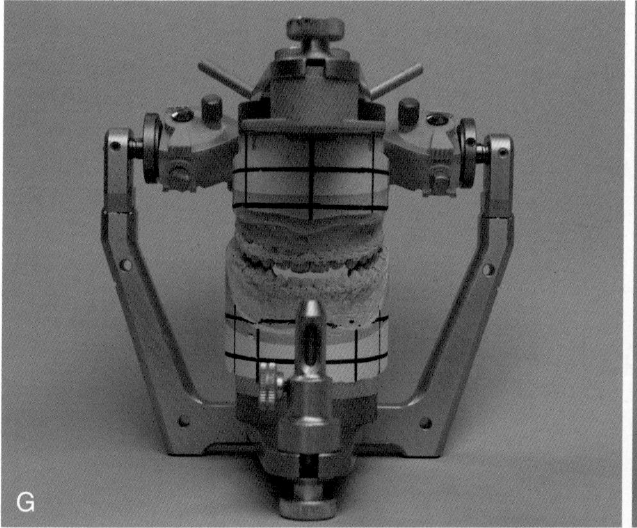

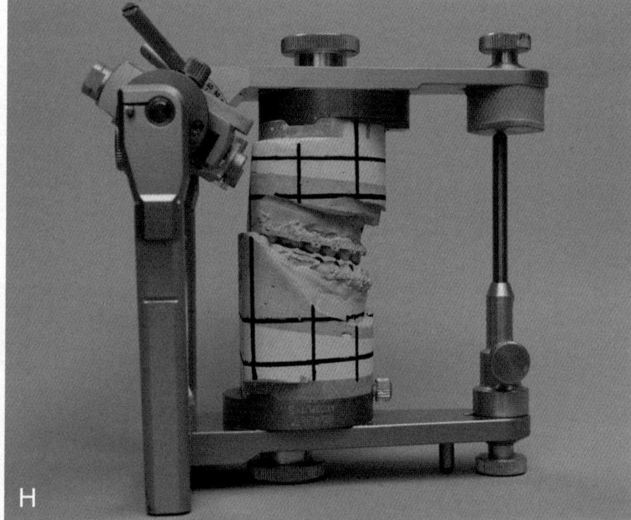

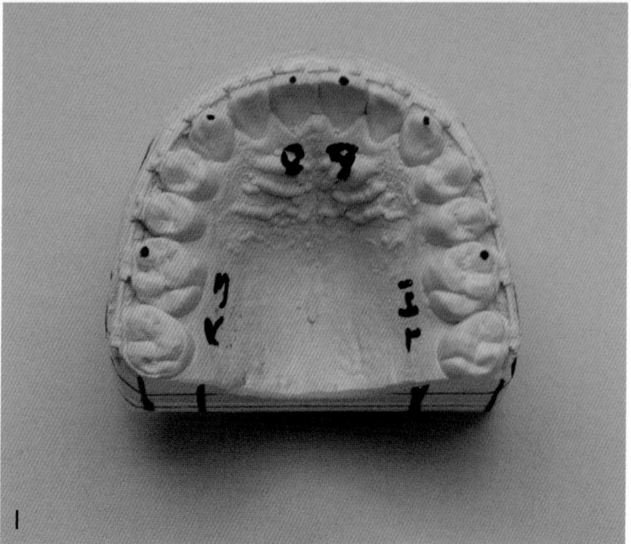

Figure 42.1, cont'd **G** and **H**, Mounted and referenced (uncut) models. **I**, Marked and referenced model (occlusal view).

TECHNIQUE: Model Surgery Planning—cont'd

STEP 7: Setting the Occlusion and Repositioning the Maxilla

To reposition the maxilla, remove the mounted maxilla from the articulator and separate the maxillary cast from the plaster base over a protective surface using a die saw and lab knife. Using a handheld technique, determine the planned occlusion. Segment the maxilla into two or three pieces, if indicated, using the die saw as planned. Next, align the maxilla (or maxillary segments) over the mandibular arch into the ideal occlusion. If adjustments are required to the cusps of teeth (enameloplasty), to help establish a more ideal occlusion, this can be performed on the models by removing green stone where indicated using the lab knife. Where cusps are reduced on the green stone, mark these areas with a red pencil, for future reference and reproduction in the operating room. If segmentation was required, create a one-piece maxilla by securing the maxillary segments together in the planned occlusion with hot glue. Take the maxillary cast back to the articulator. The maxilla is repositioned as determined during the clinical and radiographic examination performed with the patient present. The final maxillary position is determined according to plan using the Erickson model table (anterior-posterior, vertical, and transverse). Maintaining the articulator pin in a neutral position, use wax to facilitate repositioning of the maxillary cast to the mounted plaster base on the articulator. Next, secure the maxillary cast in the final position to the plaster base with hot glue (Fig. 42.1K and L).

Continued

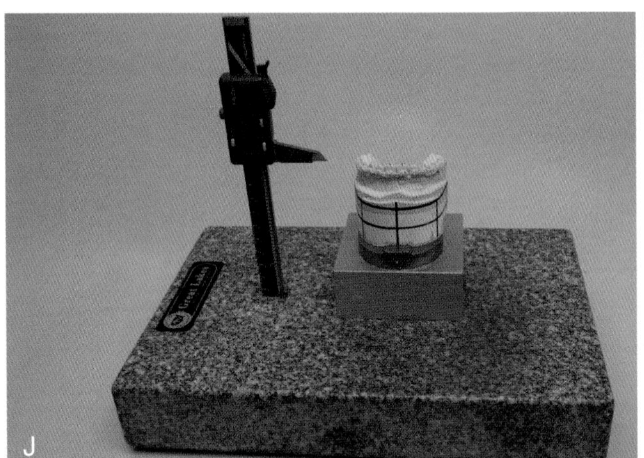

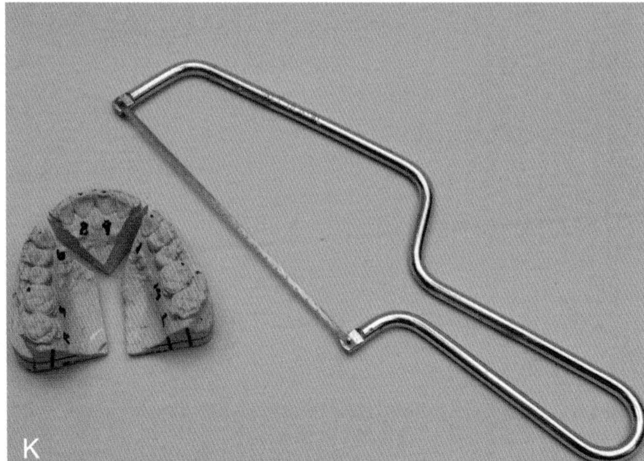

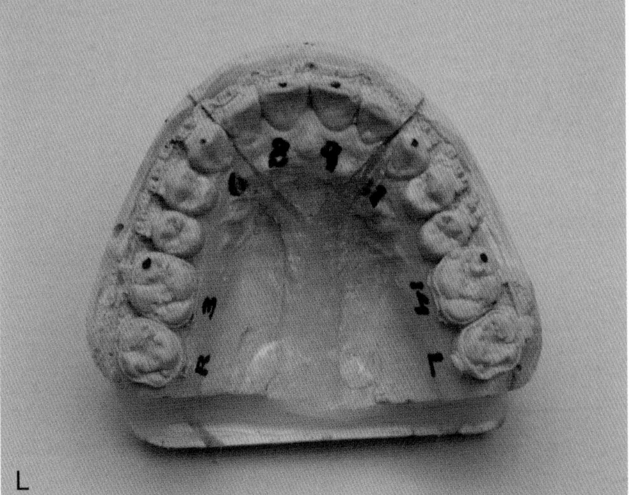

Figure 42.1, cont'd **J,** Erickson model surgery table. **K,** Model cut in segments. **L,** Three-piece model set in planned occlusion.

TECHNIQUE: Model Surgery Planning—cont'd

STEP 8: Intermediate Splint Construction and Maintenance of Neutral Pin Position

Now that the maxilla has been placed in the planned position and without change in the mounted mandibular model, construct the intermediate splint. To ensure that the acrylic does not stick to the teeth of the stone models, apply a thin coat of petroleum jelly to the maxillary and mandibular teeth using a toothbrush. Using pink acrylic liquid and white powder, mix acrylic until the mass does not slump. A thickness of acrylic can be rolled out on a wood cutting board and trimmed to approximate the occlusion. Apply petroleum jelly to your hands and adapt the mass to the maxillary occlusal surface. Close the articulator until the pin touches; this results in an imprint of the occlusion on each side. To avoid undercuts in the acrylic, maintain the level of the acrylic below the level of the base of the maxillary orthodontic brackets and above the base of the mandibular orthodontic brackets. Use sharp scissors to remove any excess acrylic as necessary. To help ensure that no undercuts remain, open and close the articulator into the intermediate occlusion until the acrylic finally sets. Once the acrylic intermediate splint has hardened, use a lathe with an acrylic bur to trim the excess. To prevent a lingual ramping effect, remove excess acrylic in the region of the mandibular teeth in a manner that prevents interferences that occurs during opening and closing due to the arc of rotation of the mandible.

STEP 9: Repositioning the Mandible

To reposition the mandible, first mark the vertical and horizontal reference lines on the mounted mandibular casts as for the maxilla with a black marking pen. The current position of the mandibular cast can be referenced and documented similar to that for the maxillary cast, using the Erickson model table. Separate the mandibular cast from the plaster base, as was done for the maxillary cast, and place the mandibular cast into the preferred "final" occlusion with the maxilla and secure with hot glue. Align the mandibular cast hot-glued into the final occlusion with the mounted maxillary cast to the plaster base with the articulator pin maintained in a neutral position. Then remove any interference in the plaster base. Next, secure the mandibular cast to the plaster base with hot glue. Remove the glue securing the maxillary and mandibular casts in occlusion and confirm that the final occlusion is as preferred. The new mandibular position can be determined by measuring it on the Erickson model table and documenting the result in millimeters (Fig. 42.1M and N).

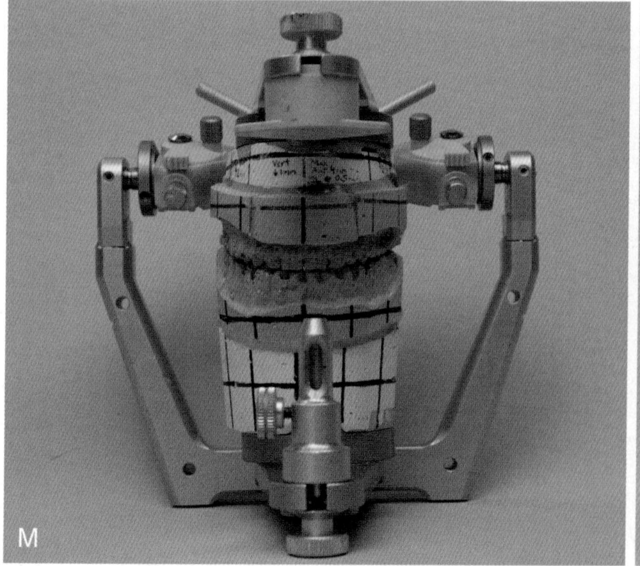

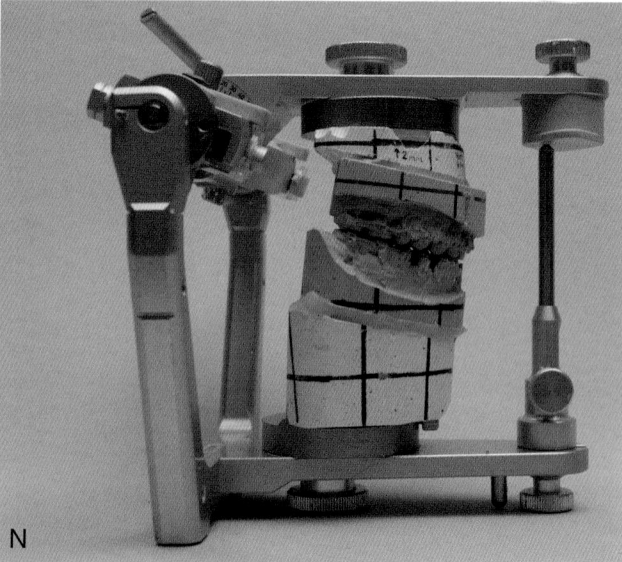

Figure 42.1, cont'd **M** and **N,** Final models marked and mounted; model surgery completed.

TECHNIQUE: Model Surgery Planning—cont'd

STEP 10: Final Splint Construction

The final splint is fabricated as was done for the intermediate splint. Prevent the acrylic from sticking to the models by reapplying petroleum jelly to the maxillary and mandibular teeth using a toothbrush. Then mix clear acrylic liquid and white powder until there is no slumping. Apply petroleum jelly to your hands and roll the acrylic into a log. Roll out a flat piece of acrylic on a wood cutting board and pretrim the acrylic, approximating the occlusal surface of the teeth. Next, adapt and readapt the acrylic as for the intermediate splint. Trim the final splint as was done for the intermediate splint. Once the acrylic has hardened and cooled, place the splint on the maxillary cast, and to allow easy passage of wires used intraoperatively to secure the splint to the maxillary orthodontic brackets, mark the ideal location and direction of interdental holes with a pencil. Drill 1-mm holes in both the intermediate and final splints, and then polish the splints on a lathe with a cloth buffing wheel using pumice and Acrilustre (Fig. 42.10).

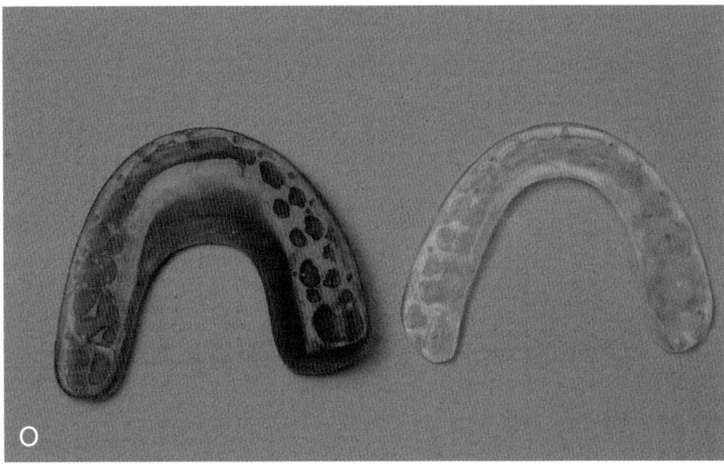

Figure 42.1, cont'd O, Intermediate and final splints.

Avoidance and Management of Intraoperative Complications

Taking care to ensure that important steps are performed along the way confirms accuracy and helps reduce the risk of complications. The occlusal splints determine the final position of the maxilla and mandible at surgery. Only the vertical position of the maxillary incisor, determined during the preoperative clinical examination, is set during surgery, somewhat independently of model surgery planning. Therefore, precise model planning is critical. The importance of recording a reproducible CR wax bite and accurate face-bow record cannot be overstated. Consider having the patient return to the office after model planning and before surgery for a final preoperative visit. The accuracy of model planning and the overall surgical plan can be confirmed at this time. This allows for a "measure twice, cut once" approach.

When proper repositioning of the maxilla and mandible is attempted, intraoperative complications can occur as a result of failure to seat the condyles properly into the fossae, inadequate removal of bony interferences, inaccurate vertical repositioning, and incomplete seating of the occlusion into the occlusal splints.

When the maxilla is repositioned, measuring from a vertical point of reference is important to avoid inadequate removal of bony interferences and inaccurate vertical positioning. The use of an external reference (e.g., a Kirschner wire placed in the bony nasal bridge or measuring from the fixed medial canthus to the incisal midline) has been shown to be more accurate and dependable during vertical maxillary repositioning than the use of intraoral reference points.[34]

Before applying fixation to the maxilla at the time of Le Fort I repositioning, be sure to check the midlines and overall maxillary position for unintended midline, cant (roll), or arch rotation (yaw) deformity. The maxillary and mandibular positions should be rechecked after mandibular repositioning to ensure that no midline discrepancy, occlusal cant, or arch rotation error has been introduced. A "yaw deformity" occurs with oscillation of the maxilla along the long axis in a horizontal plane. Paying attention to change at the posterior vertical reference lines placed on the dental models can help prevent unintentional rotation of the maxilla at maxillary repositioning during model planning. A yaw deformity in the maxilla also leads to a secondary mandibular repositioning error. Asymmetry and/or unintended prominence of the angle of the mandible on one side can result.

After repositioning and fixation of the maxilla and the mandible, confirm that the condyles are properly seated in each fossa by checking the occlusion. If the occlusion is not found to be reproducible as planned into the splints, the surgeon must remove the fixation and repeat repositioning and fixation, in stepwise fashion, until the planned occlusion is achieved. If this is not performed, the result is inaccurate repositioning of the jaws and malocclusion.

Transverse widening of the maxilla is inherently unstable. When segmental maxillary osteotomies are planned, the final occlusal splint is used to maintain the transverse expansion postoperatively during initial healing (4 to 6 weeks). The transverse width gained at surgery must be retained by the orthodontist using a transpalatal appliance or heavy arch wire. Typically, the final splint is fixed to the maxillary dentition with straight wires that are inserted through predrilled holes and tightened around the orthodontic brackets. Therefore, the splint must have adequate durability and stiffness, but at the same time be smooth and not bulky (thin) for patient tolerance (comfort) during the postoperative recovery phase (initial healing period). Because this can reduce the overall strength, the final splint should be reinforced with a stainless-steel wire or paperclip. Splint fracture can be an intraoperative nuisance; if it occurs in a delayed fashion, it can result in the relapse of the transverse maxillary expansion and compromise of the final occlusion.

Postoperative Considerations

It is important that the patient maintain good oral hygiene during the postoperative phase. Regular postoperative visits are arranged so that the surgeon can monitor activity level and encourage hydration, caloric intake, and hygiene. At each postoperative visit, the surgeon must watch for postoperative concerns, monitor healing, and check the reproducibility of the patient's occlusion. Postsurgical "guiding" elastics are maintained throughout the initial healing period. Diet, hygiene, and activity level instructions are reviewed and advanced as appropriate. A liquid (blenderized) diet must be tolerated during the initial weeks after surgery. Within 3 to 6 weeks, the patient may move on to a mechanical soft diet and eventually return to a regular diet.

The models created during the presurgical model planning workup should be kept as part of the patient record. Facial and occlusal photographs are taken to document the patient's progress before a return to the orthodontist for orthodontic treatment. The surgeon must remain available should concerns arise and to monitor the stability of the orthodontic and surgical result.

References

1. Hullihen S. Case of elongation of the underjaw and distortion of the face and neck, caused by a burn, successfully treated. *Am J Dent Sci.* 1849;9:157.
2. Blair VP. Operations on the jaw bone and face. *Surg Gynecol Obstet.* 1907;4:67.
3. Wassmund J. Lehrbuch der praktischen Chirurgie des Mundes und der Kiefer. vol 1. Leipzig: Meusser; 1935:p282.
4. Schallhorn RG. A study of the arbitrary center and the kinematic center of rotation for facebow mountings. *J Prosthet Dent.* 1957;7:162.
5. Lockwood H. A planning technique for segmental osteotomies. *Br J Oral Surg.* 1974;12(1):102–105.
6. Hohl TH. The use of an anatomic articulator in segmental orthognathic surgery. *Am J Orthod.* 1978;73(4):428–442.
7. Heggie AA. A calibrator for monitoring maxillary incisor position during orthognathic surgery. *Oral Surg Oral Med Oral Pathol.* 1987;64(6):671–673.
8. Lindorf HH, Steinhäuser EW. Correction of jaw deformities involving simultaneous osteotomy of the mandible and maxilla. *J Maxillofac Surg.* 1978;6(4):239–244.
9. Buckley MJ, Tucker MR, Fredette SA. An alternative approach for staging simultaneous maxillary and mandibular osteotomies. *Int J Adult Orthodon Orthognath Surg.* 1987;2(2):75–78.
10. Cottrell DA, Wolford LM. Altered orthognathic surgical sequencing and a modified approach to model surgery. *J Oral Maxillofac Surg.* 1994;52(10):1010–1020.
11. Posnick JC, Ricalde P, Ng P. A modified approach to "model planning" in orthognathic surgery for patients without a reliable centric relation. *J Oral Maxillofac Surg.* 2006;64(2):347–356.
12. Anwar M, Harris M. Model surgery for orthognathic planning. *Br J Oral Maxillofac Surg.* 1990;28(6):393–397.
13. Bamber MA, Harris M, Nacher C. A validation of two orthognathic model surgery techniques. *J Orthod.* 2001;28(2):135–142.
14. Epker BN, Fish LC. Definitive model surgery and surgical occlusal splint construction. In: Epker BN, Stella JP, Fish LC, eds. *Dentofacial Deformities: Integrated Orthodontic and Surgical Correction.* Vol. 1. St Louis, Missouri: Mosby; 1995.
15. Marko JV. Simple hinge and semiadjustable articulators in orthognathic surgery. *Am J Orthod Dentofacial Orthop.* 1986;90(1):37–44.
16. Ellis III E. Bimaxillary surgery using an intermediate splint to position the maxilla. *J Oral Maxillofac Surg.* 1999;57(1):53–56.
17. Bouchard C, Landry PÉ. Precision of maxillary repositioning during orthognathic surgery: a prospective study. *Int J Oral Maxillofac Implants.* 2013;42(5):592–596.
18. Ellis III E. Accuracy of model surgery: evaluation of an old technique and introduction of a new one. *J Oral Maxillofac Surg.* 1990;48(11):1161–1167.
19. Ellis III E, Tharanon W, Gambrell K. Accuracy of face-bow transfer: effect on surgical prediction and postsurgical result. *J Oral Maxillofac Surg.* 1992;50(6):562–567.
20. Lapp TH. Bimaxillary surgery without the use of an intermediate splint to position the maxilla. *J Oral Maxillofac Surg.* 1999;57(1):57–60.
21. Bell W, Proffit W, White R. Treatment planning for dentofacial deformities. In: Bell W, ed. *Surgical Correction of Centofacial Deformities.* Vol. 1. Philadelphia, Pennsylvania: Saunders; 1980.

22. The glossary of prosthodontic terms. *J Prosthet Dent*. 2005;94(1):10–92.
23. Jasinevicius TR, Yellowitz JA, Vaughan GG, et al. Centric relation definitions taught in 7 dental schools: results of faculty and student surveys. *J Prosthodont*. 2000;9(2):87–94.
24. Keshvad A, Winstanley RB. An appraisal of the literature on centric relation. Part I. *J Oral Rehabil*. 2000;27(10):823–833.
25. Keshvad A, Winstanley RB. An appraisal of the literature on centric relation. Part II. *J Oral Rehabil*. 2000;27(12):1013–1023.
26. Keshvad A, Winstanley RB. An appraisal of the literature on centric relation. Part III. *J Oral Rehabil*. 2001;28(1):55–63.
27. Campos AA, Nathanson D, Rose L. Reproducibility and condylar position of a physiologic maxillomandibular centric relation in upright and supine body position. *J Prosthet Dent*. 1996;76(3):282–287.
28. Hellsing G, McWilliam JS. Repeatability of the mandibular retruded position. *J Oral Rehabil*. 1985;12(1):1–8.
29. Tarantola GJ, Becker IM, Gremillion H. The reproducibility of centric relation: a clinical approach. *J Am Dent Assoc*. 1997;128(9):1245–1251.
30. Adrien P, Schouver J. Methods for minimizing the errors in mandibular model mounting on an articulator. *J Oral Rehabil*. 1997;24(12):929–935.
31. O'Malley AM, Milosevic A. Comparison of three facebow/semi-adjustable articulator systems for planning orthognathic surgery. *Br J Oral Maxillofac Surg*. 2000;38(3):185–190.
32. Mayrink G, Sawazaki R, Asprino L, de Moraes M, Fernandes Moreira RW. Comparative study between 2 methods of mounting models in semiadjustable articulator for orthognathic surgery. *J Oral Maxillofac Surg*. 2011;69(11):2879–2882.
33. Stanchina R, Ellis III E, Gallo WJ, Fonseca RJ. A comparison of two measures for repositioning the maxilla during orthognathic surgery. *Int J Adult Orthodon Orthognath Surg*. 1988;3(3):149–154.
34. Bamber MA, Harris M. The role of the occlusal wafer in orthognathic surgery; a comparison of thick and thin intermediate osteotomy wafers. *J Cranio-Maxillo-Fac Surg*. 1995;23(6):396–400.

CHAPTER 43

Bimaxillary Orthognathic Surgery

Vincent J. Perciaccante and Deepak G. Krishnan

Armamentarium

#9 Molt periosteal elevators (two)
#15 Bard–Parker scalpel blades
A series of chisels and one curved chisel
Appropriate sutures
Bipolar electrocautery (if necessary)
Bone rongeurs
Calipers
Coronoid notch retractor
Curved Kocher forceps with umbilical tape
Dean suture scissors
Double-guarded nasal septal osteotome
Fissure burs if third molars are present
Hargis retractor
Internal fixation kit (mid-face)
J strippers
Jeter–Van Sickels bone clamp
Kelly hemostat
K-wires
Local anesthetic with vasoconstrictor
Minnesota retractor
Needle electrocautery
Obwegeser retractors
Oval side cutting carbide bur (ZB-136)
Pear-shaped bur or a round bur if the mandible is to be set back
Pterygoid chisel
Reciprocating rasp
Reciprocating saw
Seldin retractor
Side cutting carbide bur, 1 mm (#701)
Single skin hook
Spatula osteotomes
Weider retractor
Wire pushing instrument ("pickle fork")

The armamentarium for bimaxillary orthognathic surgery is essentially the combination of the armamentaria for maxillary and mandibular orthognathic procedures. However, the need for precise, accurate preoperative records is magnified by the fact that both jaws are being repositioned at one sitting, and therefore when the second jaw is repositioned it is indexed by the newly positioned other jaw. If the new position of the first operated jaw is slightly off in any of the three planes of space that may not be clearly apparent at the time, this may result in a completely unsatisfactory placement of the second jaw. The preoperative three-dimensional examination (Fig. 43.1), cephalometric study (Fig. 43.2), bite registration, and articulator mounting (Fig. 43.3) all play a more crucial role in completing the two-jaw surgery satisfactorily. A note of caution: Preoperative photos do not take the place of a good, in-person clinical examination to evaluate critical areas such as tooth-lip relationship (repose and functioning), cants, and midlines.

History of the Procedure

The history of simultaneous maxillary and mandibular orthognathic surgery is unclear. It is likely that two-jaw surgeries were performed many years before any published reports were made.[1,2] Subapical segmental surgeries such as that reported by Hullihen in 1849 were probably combined with subapical surgery of the anterior maxilla for the treatment of bimaxillary protrusion and anterior openbite.[3,4]

Indications for the Use of the Procedure

Bimaxillary orthognathic surgery is indicated under the following conditions:

- The magnitude of movement for single-jaw orthognathic surgery is unrealistic.
- Asymmetries necessitate three-dimensional repositioning of both jaws (generally, maxillary dental midline deviation of 1.5 to 2 mm or less from the facial midline is considered acceptable; however, the decision as to whether or not to operate on the maxilla must be made with the advice and consent of the patient, family, and orthodontist[5]).
- There is a significant cant to one or both jaws.
- Telegnathic surgery is being performed for obstructive sleep apnea syndrome.
- Mandibular surgery is needed and maxillary transverse dimension requires widening, and surgically assisted rapid maxillary expansion is not indicated.

Limitations and Contraindications

Bimaxillary orthognathic surgery is contraindicated when an acceptable surgical result can be achieved with single-jaw surgery, when medical factors limit the duration of general anesthesia, when a hemorrhagic disorder precludes multiple surgical procedures, and when potential blood transfusions are refused or contraindicated.

Orthognathic Physical Exam Database			
Transverse	Date:	Date:	Date:
Maxilla to Face			
Mand to Max			
Chin to Max			
Occlusal Plane			
Mand Angles			
Arch Width			
Vertical			
Crown Length			
Upper Lip Length			
Upper Lip—Rest			
Upper Lip—Speech			
Upper Lip—Smiling			
Openbite / Overbite			
Anterior—Posterior			
Overjet			
Nasolabial Angle			
Nasal Contour			
Labiomental Fold			
Chin			

Figure 43.1 Sample of a simple clinical orthognathic database that includes essential measurements in three planes.

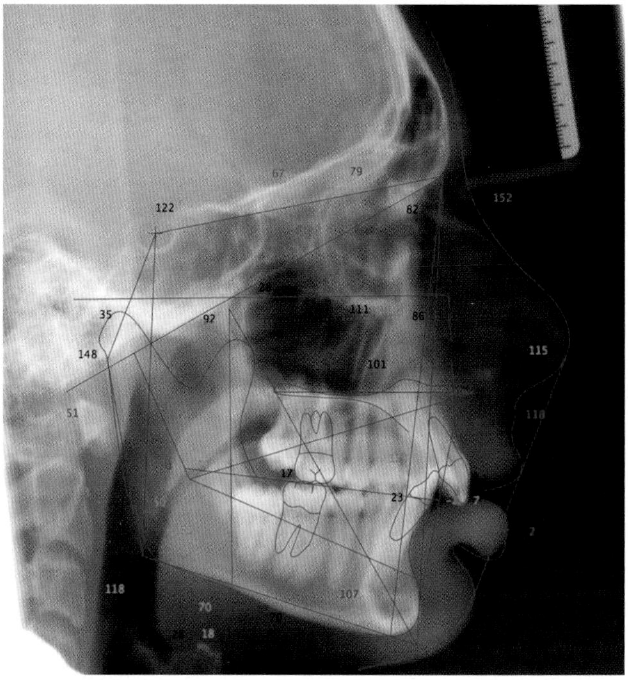

Figure 43.2 Cephalometric radiograph and analysis.

TECHNIQUE: Bimaxillary Orthognathic Surgery

In the initial patient evaluation before any treatment, it is necessary to predict the possible need for two-jaw surgery. If it is obvious that only mandibular surgery is necessary, then no further considerations may be required at this early stage. However, if maxillary surgery is considered, mock surgery is necessary to evaluate the impact of that maxillary surgery on the mandibular autorotation position and subsequently new maxillary position. Although clinical and cephalometric evaluations are important, model surgery or computerized virtual surgery on centric relation mounted models is the only accurate method to determine the autorotation of the mandible after maxillary repositioning. This exercise may reveal that the maxilla will be drawn more posterior than desired or that the maxilla will be deflected laterally when condyles are seated. In such cases, two-jaw surgery may be the only alternative to correct all of the discrepancies. This knowledge is important to properly plan the combined orthodontic-surgical treatment with the orthodontist and to inform the patient of the anticipated treatment plan.

STEP 1: Presurgical Assessment

Preoperative assessment is vital in all orthognathic surgeries. Preparation for bimaxillary orthognathic surgery needs to be more detailed than that for isolated maxillary or mandibular orthognathic surgery because mobilizing both jaws provides more freedom in three-dimensional positioning. With more freedom in this positioning, there is a greater need for detailed preoperative measurements to achieve the desired outcome position. Standard radiographic assessment includes lateral cephalometric radiographs and analysis, anteroposterior (AP) cephalometric radiographs and analysis, and a panoramic radiograph (see Fig. 43.2). Cone-beam computed tomography is rapidly becoming a radiographic standard for corrective jaw surgery as virtual planning becomes more and more prevalent. Facial database gathering must include evaluation of the vertical, AP, and transverse dimensions as well as the dental occlusion (see Fig. 43.1).

STEP 2: Establishment of Rough Movement Goals

Based on the findings of the preoperative assessment, one must set goals and establish the moves of the initial treatment plan. This will be modified as needed during surgical simulation. Regardless of the intended surgical sequence, the movement goals start with the maxilla. Although much has been written about vertical measurements, the most important value is the tooth-lip relationship. Because there are no hard and fast rules to follow

Continued

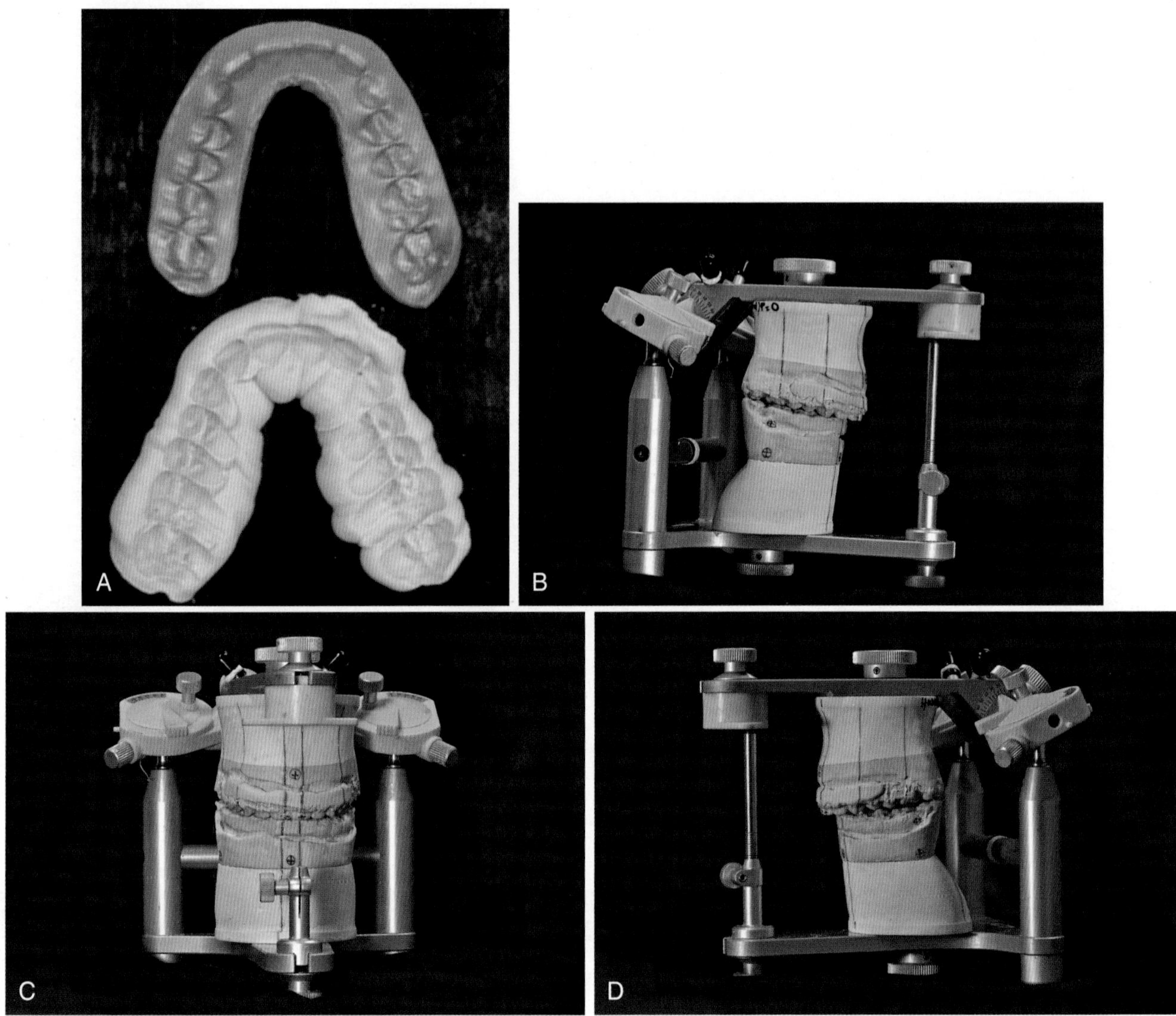

Figure 43.3 **A,** Centric relation bite registration in wax and polyvinylsiloxane. **B–D,** Surgical models mounted in centric relation on a semi-adjustable articulator. (**A,** From Steed MB, Bays RA, Perciaccante VJ. Model surgery and virtual planning for orthognathics. In: Miloro M, Larsen P, Ghali G, Waite P, eds. *Peterson's Principles of Oral and Maxillofacial Surgery*. 3rd ed. Shelton, CT: People's Medical Publishing House; 2012.)

TECHNIQUE: Bimaxillary Orthognathic Surgery—*cont'd*

here, our clinical experiences recommend always erring on the side of too much tooth show, and because most orthognathic surgery is performed on young people, one should allow for facial soft tissue sagging with age (i.e., tooth show decreases with age). Also, when there is a conflict between repose and smiling, repose should prevail. If the tooth show is favorable in repose but excessive gingiva shows during function, the repose position should be honored. Lip length must be considered as well. A patient with a short upper lip may show excessive tooth display in repose yet a pleasing tooth display when smiling, so vertical changes in this scenario can prematurely age a patient or make for an unesthetic smile line.

The AP position of the maxilla is determined by the clinical and cephalometric analysis as well as patient concerns. Midlines and cants are corrected with an eye for their effect on the final position of the mandible (described later).

STEP 3: Determination of Surgical Order

Bimaxillary surgery can be performed by first operating the maxilla or the mandible. Though there are certain advantages to performing either maxillary or mandibular surgery first, this decision is largely based on personal preference.[6,7]

TECHNIQUE: Bimaxillary Orthognathic Surgery—*cont'd*

MAXILLA FIRST

Advantages of performing maxillary surgery first may include completion of the osteotomy with the expected, more significant blood loss first, in cases where intermaxillary fixation (IMF) is planned after mandibular surgery (e.g., an intraoral vertical ramus osteotomy without rigid fixation). Another advantage of performing maxillary surgery first relates to mitigation of the impact of a potential unfavorable split of the mandible when performing a sagittal split osteotomy, which may necessitate IMF.

MANDIBLE FIRST

Advantages of performing mandibular surgery first include decreased critical nature of preoperative bite registration. When performing maxillary surgery first, the preoperative bite registration is critical. Because splints fabricated against an unoperated mandible will dictate the position of the operated maxilla, an exact interarch registration in centric relation is necessary. Performing mandibular surgery first eliminates this as a critical factor. Certain situations lend themselves to more simplicity when performing mandibular surgery first. Counterclockwise rotation of the maxillomandibular complex is one such situation. When performing a counterclockwise rotation, the intermediate splint can be cumbersome when maxillary surgery is performed first. Another situation where mandibular surgery before maxillary surgery may be prudent is when orthognathic surgery is being performed after concomitant temporomandibular joint (TMJ) surgery. This eliminates the variability caused by a change in mandibular position from TMJ surgery. Another published rationale for performing mandibular surgery first involves cases where the maxillary surgery will be segmental and therefore the rigidity of its stabilization more questionable.

As a convention, the authors most often perform maxillary surgery first. However, this is decided on a case-by-case basis determined by the merits of the individual case. Historically, in cases beginning with maxillary positioning, the mandible was begun to the point of corticotomies and then finished after the completion of maxillary surgery. With rigid, stable fixation of the maxilla, this seems like an unnecessary step that leaves the mandibular wound open for a longer period of time (Fig. 43.4A).

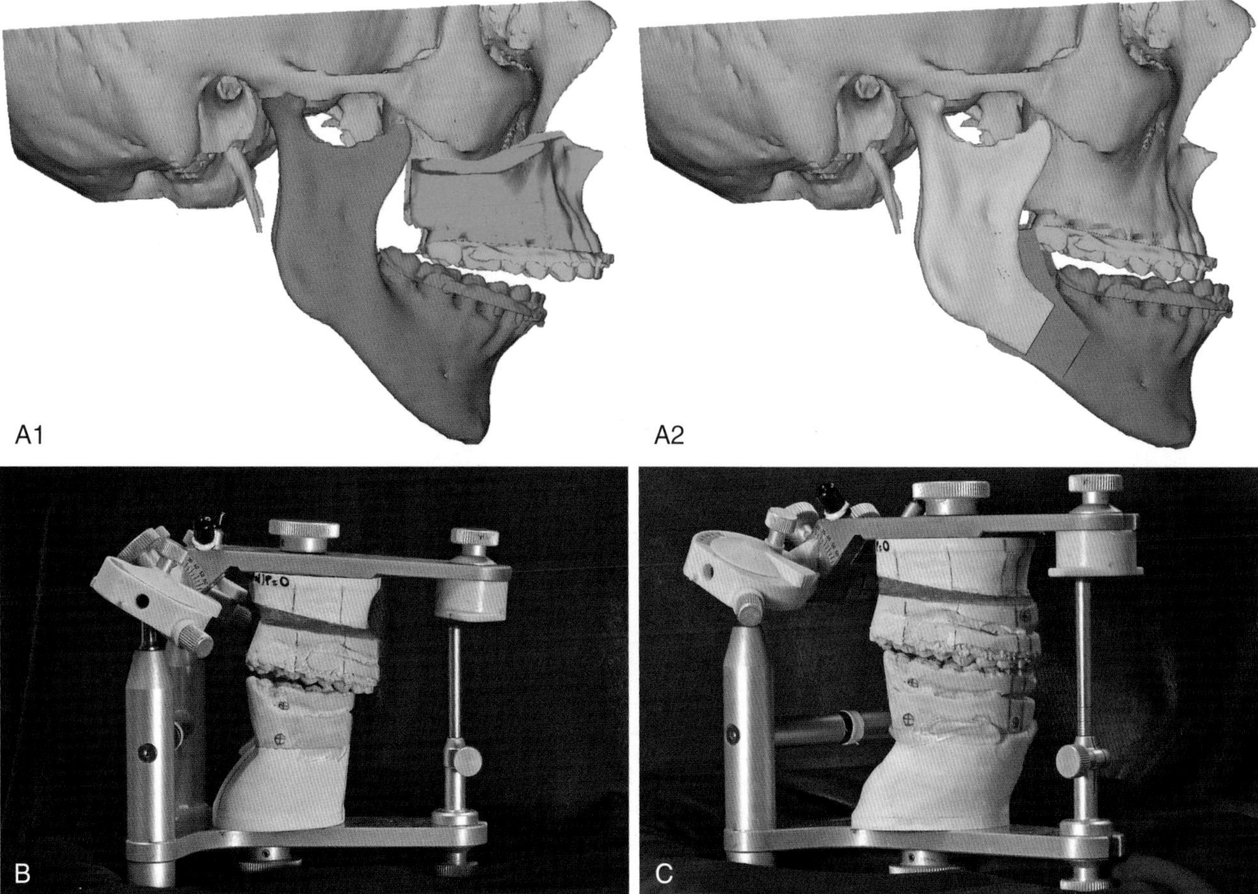

Figure 43.4 Surgical planning for 10-mm bimaxillary advancement with counterclockwise rotation for treatment of obstructive sleep apnea. **A1,** Intermediate position if the maxillary surgery is done first. **A2,** Same case. Intermediate position if the mandible is done first. **B,** Bimaxillary case in intermediate position after positioning the maxilla. **C,** Bimaxillary case in final position after positioning both jaws.

Continued

TECHNIQUE: Bimaxillary Orthognathic Surgery—*cont'd*

STEP 4: Surgical Simulation

Surgical simulation for splint fabrication can be performed via either traditional analytic model surgery or computer-based virtual surgical planning.[8]

TRADITIONAL MODEL SURGERY

Maxillary and mandibular models must be marked according previously described methods (see Chapter 37) so that any movements made can be evaluated in all three planes. Also, a mechanism must be planned to return the jaw (model) that will be operated on second to its preoperative position for fabrication of an intermediate splint.

MAXILLA FIRST

The maxillary model is moved into the desired position and fixed to the base. The mandibular model is then moved to the desired occlusion and temporarily fixed to the base. If this position renders the mandibular model in a slightly undesirable position, both models can be fixed together in the final occlusion and adjusted as one unit until they are both in an ideal position. The final splint is constructed. It is handy to have a second mandibular base or mounted model so that the mandible can be returned to the preoperative position for intermediate splint construction. In cases where segmental maxillary surgery is planned as part of a bimaxillary case and maxillary surgery is performed first, the intermediate splint must be a "piggyback" splint within the final splint. Because the maxillary surgical positioning will depend on the accuracy of this intermediate position, the articulator mounting must be as precise as possible.

MANDIBLE FIRST

The maxillary model is moved first into the desired position as described previously and fixed to the base. The mandibular model is then moved to the desired occlusion and the final splint is constructed. The maxillary model is then moved back to the preoperative position through the use of a second base or mounted model, and the intermediate splint is constructed. There is no need for a piggyback splint.

Though splints for segmental maxillary surgery must be rigid, such as those made with acrylic, polyvinylsiloxane can be used for both intermediate and final splits for surgeries involving single jaws or for the piggyback splint in a segmental case.

COMPUTER-BASED VIRTUAL SURGICAL PLANNING

When computer-based virtual surgical planning and splint fabrication are performed, it is not necessary to have a final decision as to which jaw will be operated first until completion of the surgical simulation and prior to splint generation (Fig. 43.4B–J).

STEP 5: Blood Management

Management of intraoperative blood loss is more important with two-jaw surgery over one-jaw surgery, due to the potential for greater blood loss.[9] Hypotensive anesthesia, at least for the maxillary portion of the procedure, is recommended with a mean arterial pressure of approximately 60 mm Hg as well as patient positioning into a reverse Trendelenburg "lawn chair" type position.[10–12] Other preparations that have been suggested include preoperative donation, donor-directed donation, and acute normovolemic hemodilution. The literature on the subject does not seem to support preoperative donation.[13] Perioperative donation does not eliminate the risk of clerical error or contamination of the blood, which are common sources of transfusion-related complications.[13] Acute normovolemic hemodilution is likely a better choice in cases of great concern for major blood loss, as the blood products do not significantly degrade over time and the products do not leave the operating room; however, its benefit may be questionable.[14] Typically, the authors' blood management involves hypotensive anesthesia, appropriate patient positioning, and expeditious surgery with careful technique. It has also been suggested that administration of tranexamic acid (10 mg/kg) may be of benefit in helping to minimize blood loss.

STEP 6: Osteotomy

The actual technique for performing the osteotomies is well described elsewhere in this text (see Chapters 31, 32, 33, and 38).

ALTERNATIVE TECHNIQUE 1: Splint-less or Wafer-less Surgery and Patient-Specific Fixation

Modern advances in surgical simulation and computer-based virtual surgical planning have given rise to options including cutting guides and patient-specific fixation, which can allow splint-less intermediate positioning and fixation. The technique involves utilization of patient-specific cutting guides and fixation guides and often custom fixation hardware that can accurately and predictably aid in segment positioning during orthognathic surgery.[15] Contrary to conventional orthognathic surgery where the position of the maxilla may be dictated by surgical splints and reference lines, the positioning of the maxilla in splint-less surgery is predetermined by preoperative virtual planning. Custom cutting guides will ensure that the osteotomy is replicated as per the virtual plan. Patient-specific hardware is then used to move the maxilla into a preplanned appropriate position. The ability to avoid key anatomic structures in three dimensions based on preoperative imaging is of particular advantage in this technique. Further, hardware can be designed to fit at the most ideal position on the bone, avoiding nerves, roots, and thin bone (Figs. 43.5A and B, 43.6, 43.7A and B).

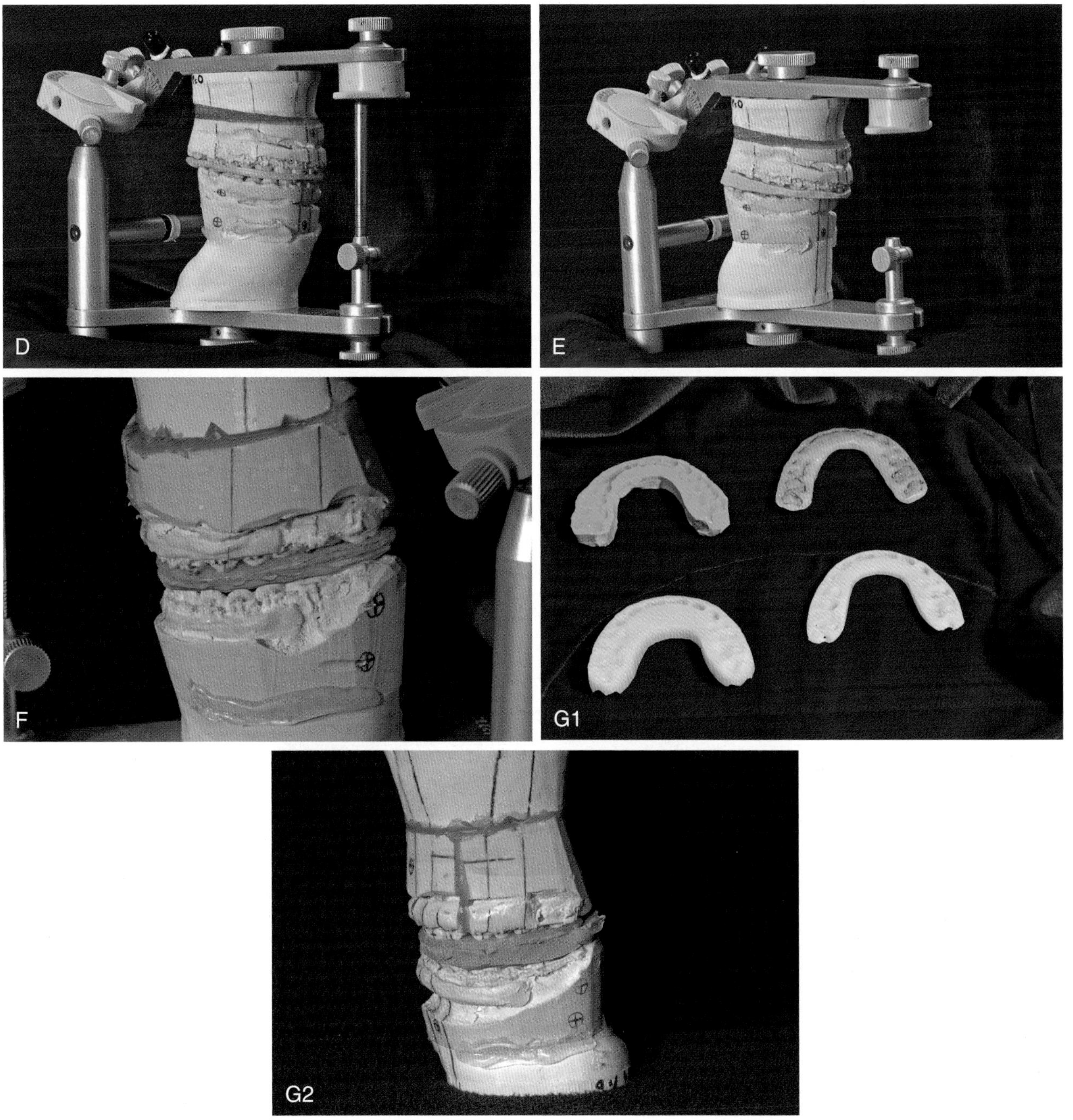

Figure 43.4, cont'd **D,** Models with fabricated acrylic final splint. **E,** Models with fabricated polyvinylsiloxane intermediate splint. **F,** Bimaxillary case with segmental maxilla showing "piggyback" splints. Pencil marks on split to delineate the final splint *(blue)* and the intermediate piggyback splint *(red)*. **G1,** Splints for the case first pictured in Fig. 43.3. Traditional model surgery *(top)*. Computer-based virtual surgical planning *(bottom)*. Traditional intermediate splint is polyvinylsiloxane, final is acrylic. Computer-planned splits are computer-aided design and computer-aided manufacturing generated. **G2,** Bimaxillary case with segmental maxilla showing piggyback splints. The final splint is acrylic, and the intermediate piggyback splint is polyvinylsiloxane.

Continued

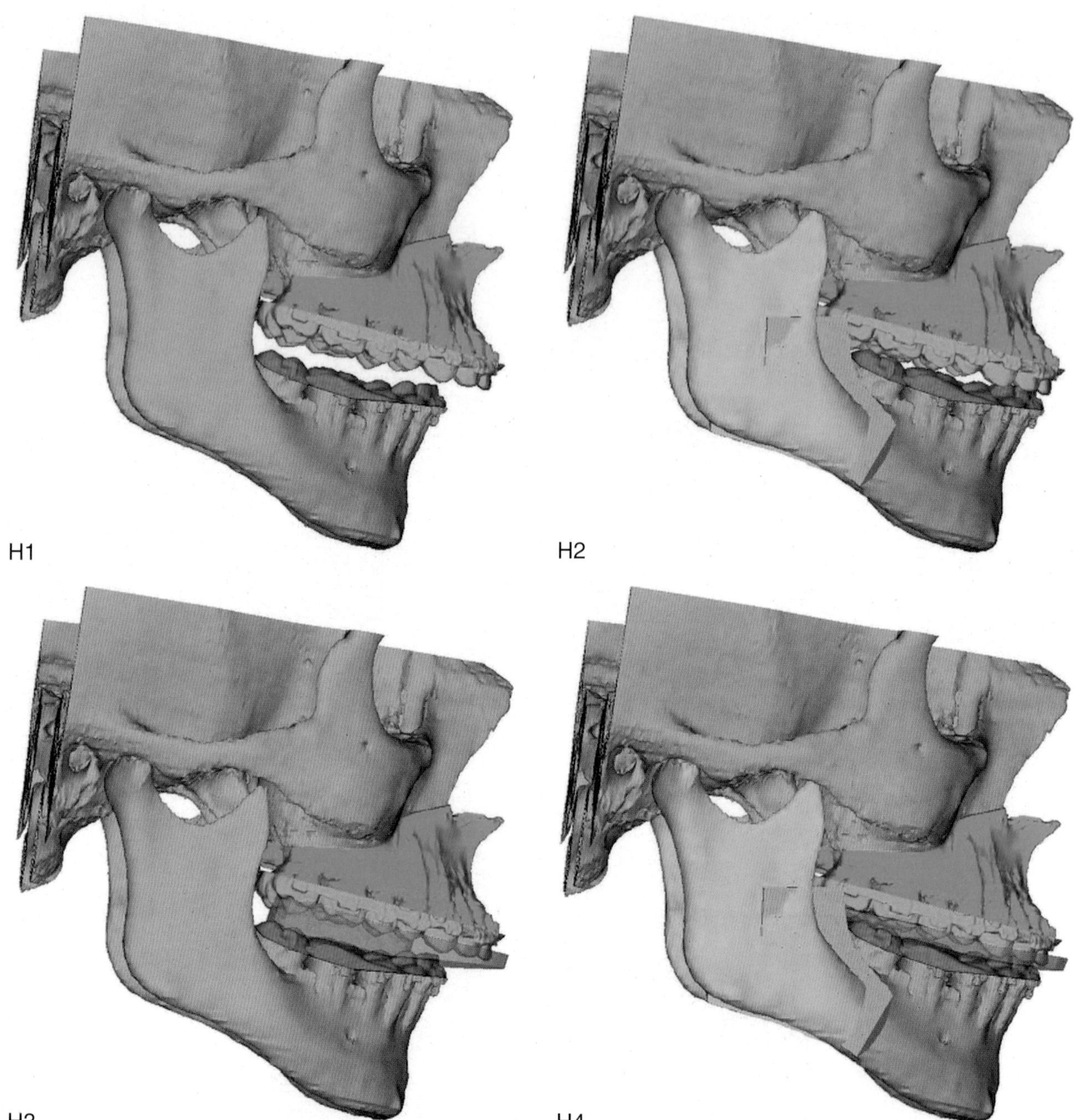

Figure 43.4, cont'd **H1–H4,** Bimaxillary case from Fig. 43.3 worked up with computer-based virtual surgical planning. **I1–I3,** Computer-based virtual surgical planning for a bimaxillary case with a three-piece maxilla. Final position; intermediate position with intermediate CAD splint in place; final position with final CAD splint in place.

Continued

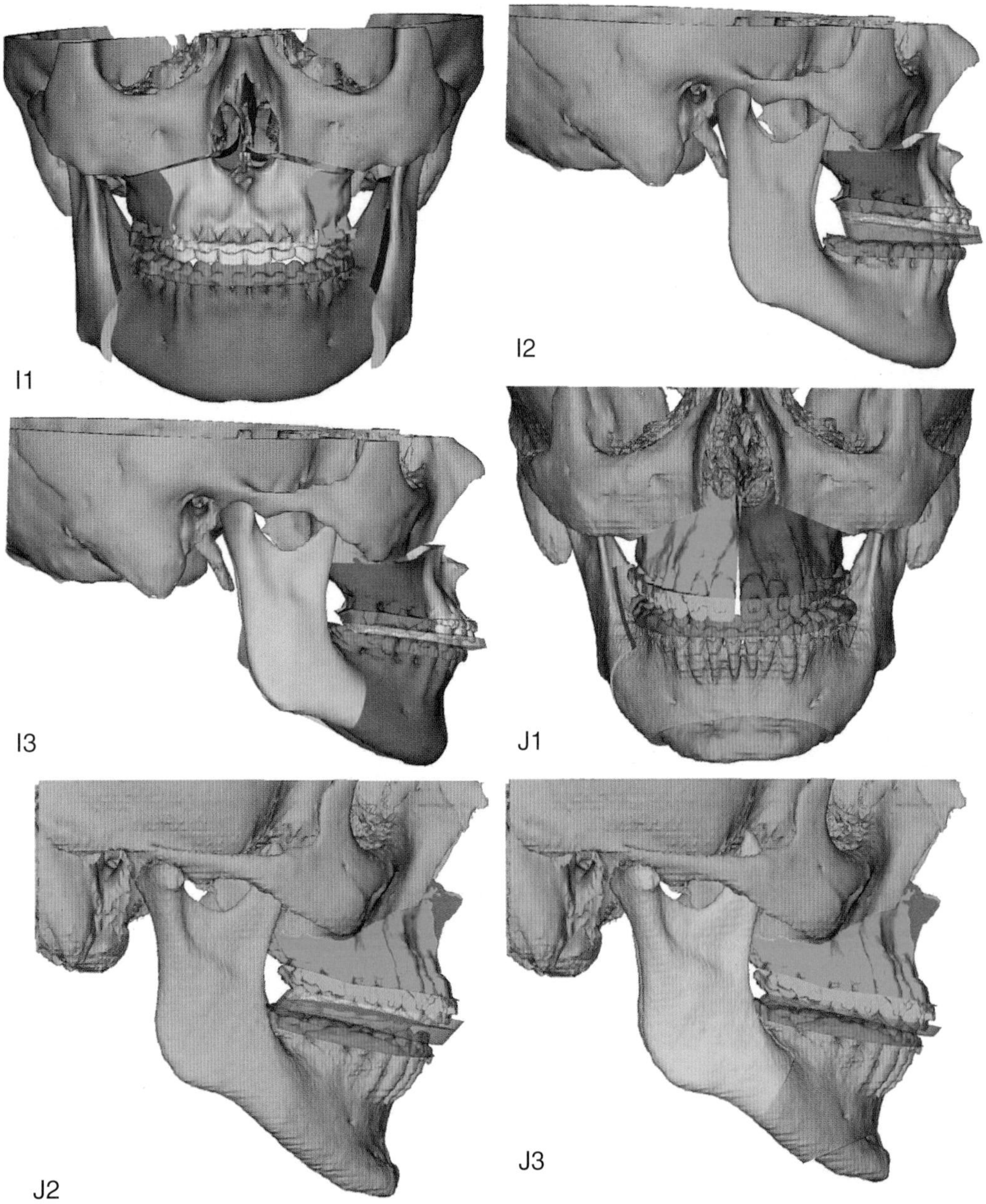

Figure 43.4, cont'd J1–J3, Computer-based virtual surgical planning for a bimaxillary case with a two-piece maxilla. Final position; intermediate position with intermediate CAD splint in place; final position with final CAD splint in place. (**F and G2** From Steed MB, Bays RA, Perciaccante VJ. Model surgery and virtual planning for orthognathics. In: Miloro M, Larsen P, Ghali G, Waite P, eds. *Peterson's Principles of Oral and Maxillofacial Surgery*. 3rd ed. Shelton, CT: People's Medical Publishing House; 2012.)

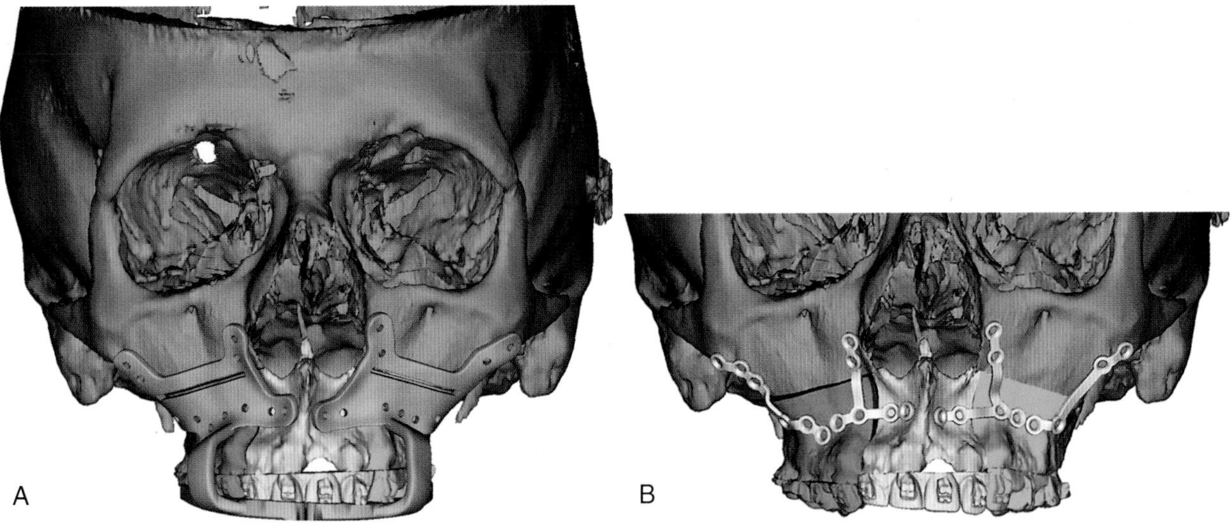

Figure 43.5 A, Cutting guides for splint-less Le Fort I maxillary osteotomy. **B,** Custom maxillary hardware for the same patient. The holes outlined in red are predicted by the guide and incorporate the proposed maxillary movements.

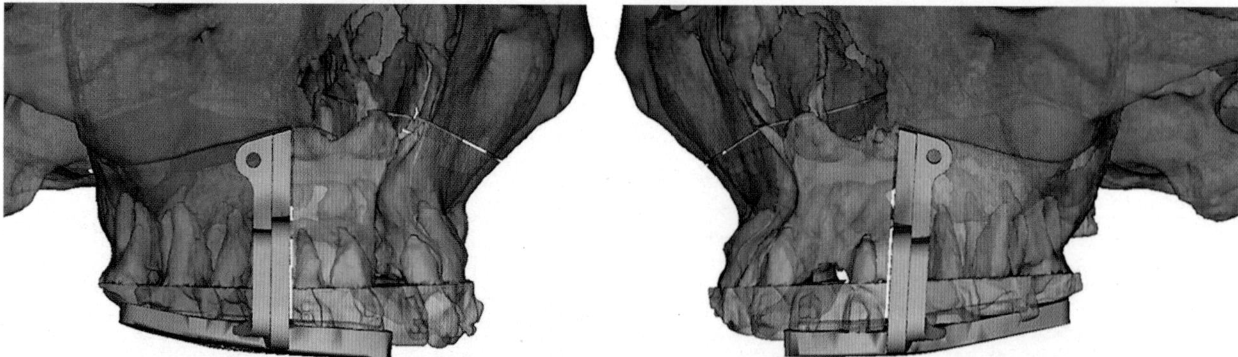

Figure 43.6 When employing a segmental maxillary osteotomy with the splint-less technique, precision of the segments is controlled by employing cutting guides for the segments. Presurgical planning permits safe cutting avoiding the teeth roots in all planes.

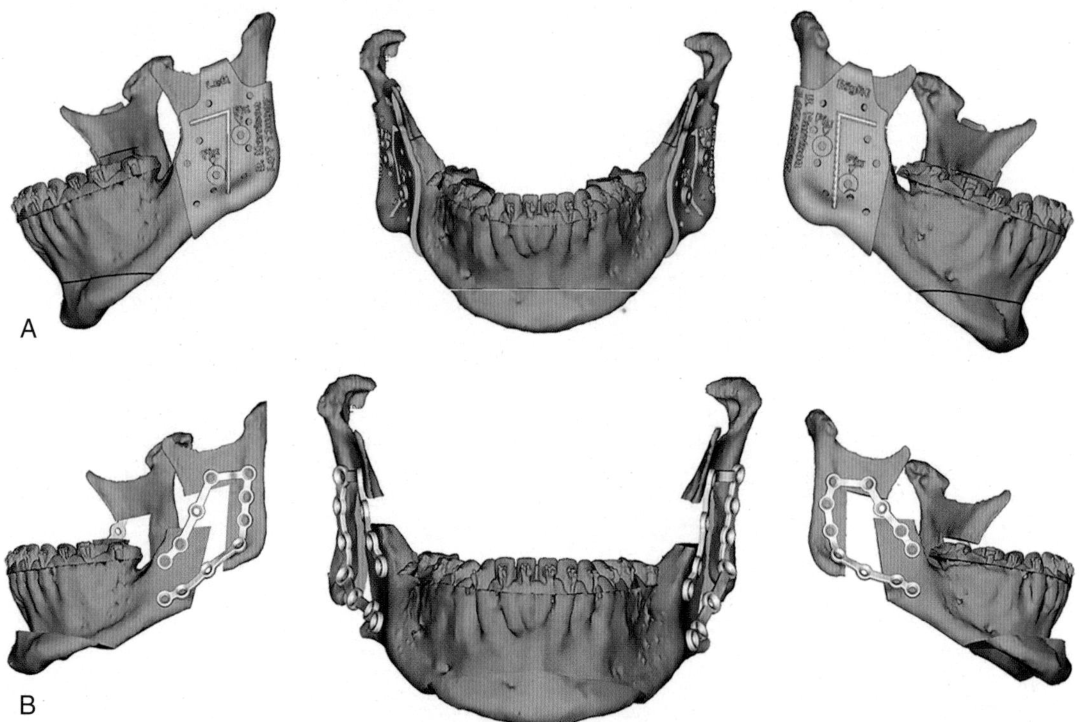

Figure 43.7 **A,** Splint-less surgery and custom hardware can be employed in mandibular movements as well. Patient-specific cutting guides can be employed to ensure precision osteotomies avoiding the inferior alveolar nerves. **B,** Custom hardware allows for precise mandibular positioning, negating the need for a splint.

Avoidance and Management of Intraoperative Complications

Most intraoperative complications associated with bimaxillary surgery mirror those of single-jaw surgery. Intraoperative malpositioning of the two jaws is the result of preoperative errors of database measurements, errors in model surgery measurements or positioning, and errors in bite registration. The occlusion may be perfect, but both jaws are malpositioned as a result of these preoperative planning errors. Meticulous preoperative planning using measurements that are checked and verified in the data gathering phase must be performed so that it is almost always a poor decision to make an intraoperative change in plans. If preoperative measurements and mock movements are meticulously made and checked, apparent deviations from the plan are more likely attributable to issues such as deviation of the nasal tip or lip caused by the nasoendotracheal tube.

Postoperative Considerations

Postoperative care for bimaxillary orthognathic surgery is largely a combination of that for the individual procedures.

Patients undergoing bimaxillary surgery have usually undergone more extensive surgery with greater blood loss and experience greater discomfort and swelling than single-jaw patients, and therefore the intensity of recovery is greater. Duration of recovery is generally unchanged or slightly elongated. Most bimaxillary patients can still be discharged from the hospital or surgical center after a 23-hour observation.

The stability of orthognathic surgical procedures has been shown to follow a predictable hierarchy. That hierarchy has been well described elsewhere.[16,17] It is notable how combined upper and lower jaw procedures that fall within this hierarchy compare to their similar single-jaw counterparts. For example, a combined maxilla forward and mandible backward surgery is more stable than mandible back alone, but it is less stable than maxilla forward alone.

References

1. Gross BD, James RB. The surgical sequence of combined total maxillary and mandibular osteotomies. *J Oral Surg*. 1978;36(7):513–522.
2. Epker BN, Turvey T, Fish LC. Indications for simultaneous mobilization of the maxilla and mandible for the correction of dentofacial deformities. *Oral Surg Oral Med Oral Pathol*. 1982;54(4):369–381.
3. Hullihen SP. Case of elongation of the under jaw and distortion of the face and neck, caused by a burn, successful treated. *Am J Dent Sci*. 1849;9(2):157–165.
4. Wassmund M. *Frakturen und Lurationen des Gesichtsschadels*; 1927.
5. Cardash HS, Ormanier Z, Laufer BZ. Observable deviation of the facial and anterior tooth midlines. *J Prosthet Dent*. 2003;89(3):282–285.
6. Perez D, Ellis E III. Sequencing bimaxillary surgery: mandible first. *J Oral Maxillofac Surg*. 2011;69(8):2217–2224.
7. Turvey T. Sequencing of two-jaw surgery: the case for operating on the maxilla first. *J Oral Maxillofac Surg*. 2011;69(8):2225.
8. Steed MB, Bays RA, Perciaccante VJ. Model surgery and virtual planning for orthognathics. In: Miloro M, Larsen P, Ghali G, Waite P, eds. *Peterson's Principles of Oral and Maxillofacial Surgery*. 3rd ed. Shelton, CT: People's Medical Publishing House; 2012.
9. Kretschmer W, Köster U, Dietz K, Zoder W, Wangerin K. Factors for intraoperative blood loss in bimaxillary osteotomies. *J Oral Maxillofac Surg*. 2008;66(7):1399–1403.
10. Choi WS, Samman N. Risks and benefits of deliberate hypotension in anaesthesia: a systematic review. *Int J Oral Maxillofac Surg*. 2008;37(8):687–703.
11. Rohling RG, Zimmermann AP, Biro P, Haers PE, Sailer HF. Alternative methods for reduction of blood loss during elective orthognathic surgery. *Int J Adult Orthodon Orthognath Surg*. 1999;14(1):77–82.
12. Gong SG, Krishnan V, Waack D. Blood transfusions in bimaxillary orthognathic surgery: are they necessary? *Int J Adult Orthodon Orthognath Surg*. 2002;17(4):314–317.
13. Kessler P, Hegewald J, Adler W, et al. Is there a need for autogenous blood donation in orthognathic surgery? *Plast Reconstr Surg*. 2006;117(2):571–576.
14. Ervens J, Marks C, Hechler M, Plath T, Hansen D, Hoffmeister B. Effect of induced hypotensive anaesthesia vs isovolaemic haemodilution on blood loss and transfusion requirements in orthognathic surgery: a prospective, single-blinded, randomized, controlled clinical study. *Int J Oral Maxillofac Implants*. 2010;39(12):1168–1174.
15. Heufelder M, Wilde F, Pietzka S, et al. Clinical accuracy of waferless maxillary positioning using customized surgical guides and patient specific osteosynthesis in bimaxillary orthognathic surgery. *J Craniomaxillofac Surg*. 2017;45(9):1578–1585.
16. Proffit WR, Turvey TA, Phillips C. Orthognathic surgery: a hierarchy of stability. *Int J Adult Orthodon Orthognath Surg*. 1996;11(3): 191–204.
17. Proffit WR, Turvey TA, Phillips C. The hierarchy of stability and predictability in orthognathic surgery with rigid fixation: an update and extension. *Head Face Med*. 2007;3:21.

CHAPTER 44

Combined TMJ and Orthognathic Surgery

Larry M. Wolford and Reza Movahed

Armamentarium

#15 Scalpel blades
#703, #701, #699 Burs
60-Degree curved Freer elevator
Appropriate sutures
Bone plates/screws
Channel retractor
Curved pterygoid osteotome
Dean scissors
Inferior border retractor
Inferior border saws
Large reciprocating rasp
Local anesthetic with vasoconstrictor
Mallet
Minnesota retractor
Mitek mini anchor kit
Nasal septal osteotome
Needle electrocautery
Needle holders
Obwegeser retractors
Patient-fitted total joint prosthesis
Periosteal elevators
Reciprocating saw blade
Selden retractor
Short Lindemann bur
Skin hooks
Spatula osteotome
Tenotomy scissors
Wire twisters
Wolford TMJ retractors
Z-plates

History of the Procedure

The first known combined temporomandibular joint (TMJ)-orthognathic surgery was performed by Wolford in 1976 on a 16-year-old patient. The procedure involved removal of an osteochondroma from the right TMJ accompanied by bilateral sagittal split osteotomies and maxillary osteotomies. Numerous techniques have been used during the years to treat TMJ pathologies, many with adverse outcomes. In 1992, Dr. David Hoffman became the first surgeon to use an internal condylar "cleat" as a stabilizing device to support an artificial ligament to attach to the articular disk. In 1992, Wolford introduced the Mitek mini anchor, which used two artificial ligaments to stabilize the articular disks and was used in combination with double jaw orthognathic surgery. In 1989, Techmedica (TMJ Concepts, Ventura, CA) introduced TMJ total joint prostheses patient-fitted for a patient's specific anatomic requirements. In 1990, Wolford performed the first TMJ reconstruction with the custom-fitted total joint prosthesis in combination with orthognathic surgery.

Indications for the Use of the Procedure

The TMJs are the foundation for jaw position, facial growth and development, jaw function, occlusion, facial balance, oropharyngeal airway patency, and comfort. If the TMJs are not stable and healthy, patients requiring orthognathic surgery may have unsatisfactory outcomes relative to function, aesthetics, occlusal and skeletal stability, and pain.[1–3] TMJ disorders and pathologic conditions and dental facial deformities commonly coexist. The TMJ pathology may be the causative factor for the jaw deformity or may develop as a result of the jaw deformity, or the two entities may develop independent of each other. Patients with these conditions may benefit from corrective surgical intervention, including TMJ and orthognathic surgery.[1–3]

Condylar Hyperplasia

Condylar hyperplasia (CH) is a generic term describing enlargement of the condyle caused by a number of different pathologies. The following sections present the classification system used by the authors to differentiate the etiology of these conditions.

Condylar Hyperplasia Type 1

CH type 1 develops during puberty as an accelerated and prolonged growth aberration of the normal condylar growth mechanism, causing mandibular prognathism. Growth is self-limiting, but the mandible can continue to grow into the mid-20s and can occur bilaterally (CH type 1A) or unilaterally (CH type 1B). These patients may have a class I occlusion at the beginning of puberty and develop a mandibular prognathism and class III occlusion, or they may begin with a class III skeletal and occlusal relationship but develop a worse class III. Not all prognathic mandibles are caused by CH, only those demonstrating accelerated, excessive mandibular growth continuing beyond the normal growth years.[4–7] Both CH type 1A with an asymmetric rate of condylar growth and CH type 1B can cause progressive deviated mandibular prognathism, facial asymmetry, TMJ articular disk dislocations, TMJ pain, headaches, masticatory dysfunction, and so on.[1,2,4–7]

The treatment protocol for active CH type 1 includes (1) high condylectomy, through removal of the top 4 to 5 mm of the condylar head to arrest mandibular growth; (2) TMJ disk repositioning over the remaining condyle with the Mitek anchor technique; (3) bilateral mandibular ramus osteotomies to reposition the mandible; (4) maxillary osteotomies, if indicated, to maximize function and facial balance; and (5) any indicated ancillary procedures, such as turbinectomies, septoplasty, genioplasty, rhinoplasty, and removal of third molars. Our studies[4–7] have shown that this protocol stops mandibular growth and provides highly predictable and stable skeletal and occlusal outcomes with normal jaw function and good esthetics.

Condylar Hyperplasia Type 2

CH type 2 is caused by an osteochondroma, which can develop at any age, although two-thirds of these cases arise in the teenage years. CH type 2 causes a unilateral vertical enlargement of the mandibular condyle, neck, ramus, and body, with compensatory unilateral maxillary vertical downgrowth, resulting in a transverse cant in the occlusal plane. It is not self-limiting. The condyle can grow predominately vertically (CH type 2A) or with additional horizontal exophytic growth extensions (CH type 2B). In the more progressive tumors, a posterior open bite develops on the ipsilateral side.[1,2] The overgrowth on the ipsilateral side loads the contralateral TMJ, causing disk displacement in 75% of cases.

The treatment protocol for CH type 2 includes (1) low condylectomy, which preserves the condylar neck; (2) recontouring of the condylar neck to function as a new condyle; (3) repositioning of the articular disk over the condylar stump and repositioning of the contralateral disk, if displaced, with the Mitek anchor technique; (4) bilateral mandibular ramus osteotomies to reposition the mandible; (5) maxillary osteotomies, if indicated; (6) vertical reduction of the inferior border of the mandible on the ipsilateral side, if indicated, to improve vertical facial balance, with preservation of the inferior alveolar nerve; and (7) any indicated ancillary procedures. Studies[8,9] have shown that this technique is highly predictable for eliminating the TMJ pathology, maintaining long-term skeletal and occlusal stability, and optimizing facial balance.

Condylar Hyperplasia Type 3 and Type 4

CH type 3 is benign, and CH type 4 is a malignant condition that can cause condylar enlargement. They are not discussed in this chapter.

Articular Disk Dislocation

The most common TMJ pathologies are anteriorly and/or medially displaced articular disks. These conditions can initiate a cascade of events, leading to TMJ arthritis.[1,6] Less commonly, the disks can become laterally and, in rare cases, posteriorly displaced. A magnetic resonance imaging (MRI) study can show the direction of disk displacement, progression of arthritic and degenerative changes, mobility of the joint components, and so on. Once the disk becomes displaced, there is generally a 4- to 6-year window during which the disks remain salvageable for repositioning, with highly predictable outcomes using the Mitek anchor technique. If the disks become nonreducing, the degenerative process proceeds more rapidly.

In patients in whom the TMJ condition has been present for longer than 6 years, significant TMJ degeneration is present, multiple other joints are involved, other systemic diseases are present, or the patient has a history of recurrent infections (e.g., urinary tract, gastrointestinal tract, and respiratory tract). These factors may indicate that a total joint prosthesis may provide a more predictable treatment outcome. If the disks meet the requirements for salvage, the treatment protocol is (1) TMJ articular disk repositioning and ligament repair with Mitek anchors; (2) bilateral mandibular ramus osteotomies to reposition the mandible; (3) multiple maxillary osteotomies, if necessary; (4) and any indicated ancillary procedures.[1,3,10,11] When displaced disks are repositioned, the condyle and mandible usually are displaced downward and forward, and in patients with class I occlusions to begin with, this displacement can create posterior open bites and an end-on incisor relationship. Mandibular ramus osteotomies may be indicated to maintain a good occlusion and allow the mandibular ramus and condyle to move inferiorly and forward to accommodate the repositioned articular disk within the joint space.

Adolescent Internal Condylar Resorption

Adolescent internal condylar resorption is one of the most common TMJ conditions seen in teenage females (8:1 female to male ratio). This hormonally mediated condition is initiated as the adolescent enters the pubertal growth phase, usually between the ages 11 and 15 years.[1,12–15] Our hypothesis is that the female hormones released during pubertal growth stimulate female hormonal receptors in the TMJ tissues. This results in a hyperplasia of the synovial cells, which produce chemical substrates that break down the ligaments supporting the disks in place, allowing the disks to become anteriorly displaced. The tissue then surrounds the condyle, and the chemical substrates cause the condyle to resorb; however, the fibrocartilage on the condyle and fossa remains intact as the condyle shrinks. At least 25% of these patients have no symptoms, but they nevertheless have a pathologic condition that causes the condylar resorption. These cases are best treated within 4 to 5 years after the onset of the TMJ pathology. The condition usually occurs bilaterally.

The treatment protocol for salvageable disks is (1) bilateral TMJ articular disk repositioning and ligament repair with Mitek anchors; (2) bilateral mandibular ramus osteotomies to advance the mandible in a counterclockwise direction; (3)

multiple maxillary osteotomies to advance the maxilla in a counterclockwise rotation; (4) ancillary procedures if indicated, such as genioplasty, turbinectomies, septoplasty, rhinoplasty, and removal of third molars. This treatment protocol produces highly stable and predictable results.[12–15] If the disks are nonsalvageable, patient-fitted total joint prostheses are indicated (these are discussed later in the chapter).

Reactive Arthritis (Seronegative Spondyloarthropathy)

Reactive arthritis is an inflammatory process that can occur in TMJs with or without displaced articular disks and with or without condylar resorption. It usually is related to bacterial or viral pathology. The condition is most commonly seen in females and does not usually begin until the late teenage years or later. Preliminary studies have identified bacterial species from the *Chlamydia* and *Mycoplasma* families.[16,17] These bacteria live and function as viruses, stimulating the production of substance P, cytokines, and tumor necrosis factor, which are pain modulators and contribute to the degenerative process in the TMJs. Other bacterial and viral elements also may be causative factors. An MRI may show displaced disks, inflammation, and progression of disk and condylar degeneration. Patients with localized TMJ reactive arthritis with displaced but salvageable disks may respond to joint débridement, articular disk repositioning with Mitek anchors, and appropriate orthognathic surgical procedures to correct the coexisting dental facial deformity. In more aggressive forms of the disease or with polyarthropathy, TMJ patient-fitted total joint prostheses with fat grafts may be indicated.

TMJ Ankylosis

TMJ ankylosis usually develops as a result of trauma, inflammation, sepsis, and/or systemic diseases, resulting in severely limited jaw function, oral hygiene, and nutritional problems. When this condition occurs during the growing years, it can severely affect jaw growth and development, resulting in significant dentofacial deformities, malocclusion, and airway compromise.[1,7]

The most predictable treatment protocol is (1) release of the ankylosed joint and removal of the heterotopic and reactive bone with thorough débridement of the joint and adjacent areas; (2) reconstruction of the TMJs with a patient-fitted total joint prosthesis (and, if indicated, advancement of the mandible)[1,2,18,19]; (3) coronoidectomy if the ramus is significantly advanced or vertically lengthened with the prosthesis; (4) autogenous fat graft harvested from the abdomen or buttock and packed completely around the articulating area of the prosthesis[19–21]; (5) additional orthognathic procedures, if indicated, such as a contralateral sagittal split osteotomy and/or maxillary osteotomies; and (6) any indicated ancillary procedures. In these cases, it is vital to place fat grafts around the articulating portion of the prosthesis to prevent the recurrence of heterotopic and reactive bone.

Congenitally Deformed/Absent TMJ (Hemifacial Microsomia, Treacher Collins Syndrome)

Hundreds of congenital syndromes can cause facial deformity. Hemifacial microsomia is one of the more common syndromes and may present with features such as unilateral hypoplasia or aplasia of the mandibular condyle, ramus, and body and hypoplasia of the maxilla, zygomatic orbital complex, and temple bone, with decreased ipsilateral facial height, a retruded mandible deviated toward the ipsilateral side, class II malocclusion with a transverse cant to the occlusal plane, and significant ipsilateral soft tissue deficiency. The treatment protocol for these patients includes (1) ipsilateral mandibular ramus and TMJ reconstruction with a patient-fitted total joint prosthesis; (2) contralateral disk repositioning if the disk is displaced; (3) contralateral sagittal split osteotomy; (4) maxillary osteotomies to advance and transversely level the maxilla; (5) placement of fat grafts around the TMJ prosthesis; and (6) any indicated ancillary procedures.[1,22] It is best to perform these procedures in females at the age of 15 and in males at the ages of 17 to 18 to prevent adverse effects of growth from the normal side. If done earlier, secondary orthognathic surgery may be indicated.[6,23–26]

Connective Tissue and Autoimmune Diseases

Connective tissue and autoimmune (CT/AI) diseases can affect the TMJs. Such diseases include juvenile idiopathic arthritis (JIA), rheumatoid arthritis, psoriatic arthritis, ankylosing spondylitis, Sjögren syndrome, systemic lupus erythema, scleroderma, mixed connective tissue disease, and others. Multiple systems are usually involved, although with JIA, occasionally only the TMJ joints are involved. Peripheral joints are usually symmetrically inflamed, resulting in progressive destruction of articular structures. Facial deformity can occur with involvement of the TMJs.[1,27] In growing patients, clinical and radiographic features include a retruded mandible, maxillary anteroposterior and posterior vertical hypoplasia, progressively worsening facial and occlusal deformity, high occlusal plane angle facial morphology, class II occlusion, anterior open bite, decreased oropharyngeal airway, sleep apnea, and TMJ symptoms, such as noise, pain, and jaw dysfunction.[7,27] MRI features include loss of condylar vertical dimension, significant mediolateral condylar narrowing, possible anteroposterior widening of the condyles, and resorption of the articular eminence. Articular disks usually are in position but are surrounded by a reactive pannus that eventually destroys the disk and also causes condylar and articular eminence resorption.

The treatment protocol for these conditions is (1) bilateral TMJ reconstruction and mandibular counterclockwise advancement with patient-fitted total joint prostheses; (2) bilateral coronoidectomies; (3) harvesting of autogenous fat grafts from the abdomen or buttock and packing of these grafts around the articulation aspect of the prostheses; (4) maxillary osteotomies to advance the maxilla in a counterclockwise direction; and (5) additional adjunctive procedures if indicated.[1,27,28] For one-stage surgery, it is best to treat females at 14 years and males at 17 years, when most of the normal facial growth is complete.[1,23–26]

Other End-Stage TMJ Pathology

Other TMJ end-stage conditions may include (1) advanced reactive arthritis or osteoarthritis; (2) neoplasms; (3) multiply operated TMJs; (4) failed TMJ alloplastic implants; and (5) failed autogenous tissue grafts. Patients with these TMJ pathologies would benefit from TMJ reconstruction and, when indicated, mandibular advancement using patient-fitted total joint prostheses and other indicated orthognathic surgical procedures.[1,18,28–30]

Limitations and Contraindications

TMJ surgeries should not be performed if infection is present. The Mitek anchor technique should not be used in patients who have had two or more previous TMJ surgeries or who have alloplastic implants in the joints, advanced arthritis, polyarthritis, known or suspected CT/AI disease, or significantly deformed and degenerated (nonsalvageable) disks. The technique should be used with caution in patients whose disks have been out of place for longer than 4 to 5 years or who have a history of chronic infections of the urinary tract or respiratory or gastrointestinal systems. In these cases, the patient-fitted total joint prosthesis is the preferred method of treatment. Use of a total joint prosthesis may be contraindicated if the patient has known hypersensitivities to any of the materials used in the device, but prostheses can be manufactured excluding the offending metals.

TECHNIQUE: Mitek Anchor Procedure

STEP 1: Access to the TMJ

After patient preparation, a Tegaderm dressing is placed over the mouth and nose to isolate them from the TMJ surgical areas. An endaural or preauricular incision is made to provide TMJ access. When dissection to the lateral capsule has been performed, 1.5 mL of local anesthetic is injected into the superior joint space. A #15 blade is used to open the superior joint space, and the lateral capsule is released along the articular eminence. An incision is made just above the lateral pole of the condyle and extended posterior to enter the lower joint space.

STEP 2: Disk Repositioning

Excessive bilaminar tissue covering the top of the condyle is excised forward to the posterior border of the articular disk. The disk is mobilized by freeing up the anterior attachment along the anterior slope of the articular eminence and elsewhere, as required; the disk then is repositioned passively over the condyle. The lateral pterygoid muscle attachment generally is maintained to provide anterior stability to the disk (Fig. 44.1A).

STEP 3: Mitek Anchor Insertion

The Mitek anchor drill is used to make a hole in the posterior condylar head lateral to the midsagittal plane and 8 mm from the top of the condyle. A Mitek anchor is double threaded with #0 Ethibond suture and inserted into the posterior head of the condyle with the special insertion device (Fig. 44.1B and C).

STEP 4: Disk Plication

Starting toward the medial aspect of the disk, three throws of the first set of artificial ligaments are passed through the posterior medial aspect of the posterior band of the disk. Then three throws with the second suture are passed more vertically and slightly lateral. The sutures are tied to secure the disk in place. A suture can be placed through the lateral ligaments up through the lateral disk to help stabilize it in position. The joint is irrigated, and the incision is closed (Fig. 44.1D).

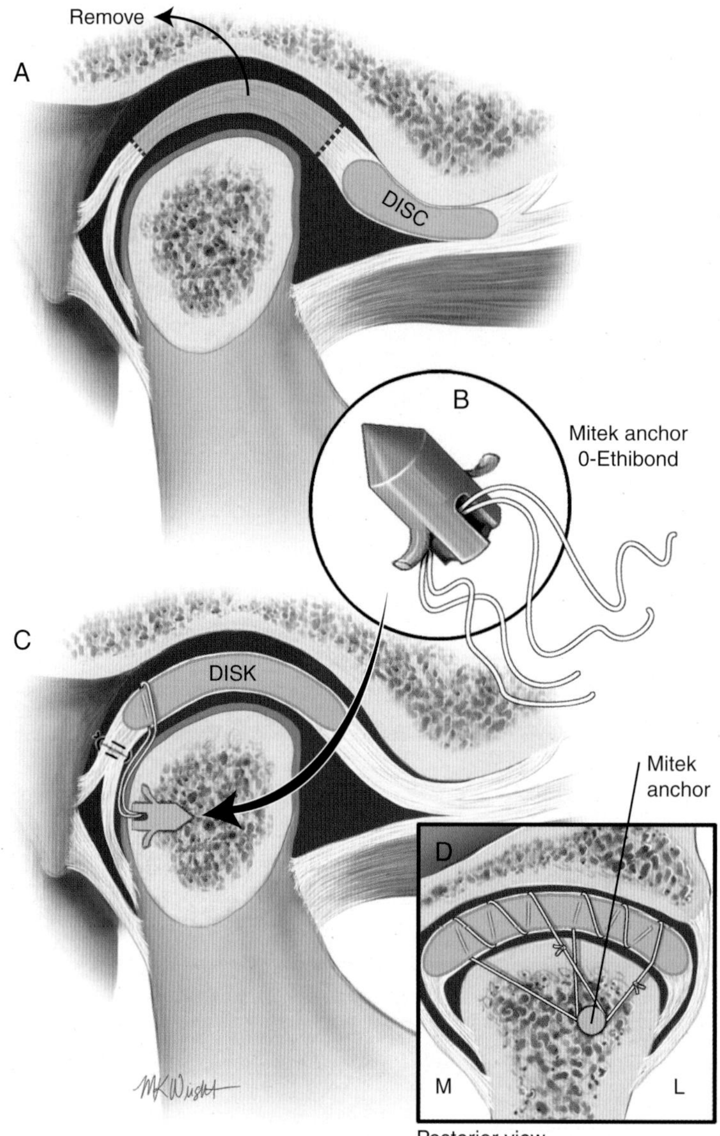

Figure 44.1 **A,** Excessive bilaminar tissue covering the top of the condyle is excised forward to the posterior border of the articular disk. The Mitek anchor drill is used to place a hole in the posterior condylar head lateral to the midsagittal plane and 8 mm from the top of the condyle. **B,** A Mitek anchor is double threaded with #0 Ethibond suture, and (C) inserted into the posterior head of the condyle with the special insertion device. **D,** Three throws of the first set of artificial ligaments are passed through the posterior medial aspect of the posterior band of the disk. Three throws of the second artificial ligament set are passed through the mid and lateral part of the posterior band.

TECHNIQUE: High Condylectomy

The superior and inferior joint spaces are entered as described previously. A #701 bur is used to cut off and remove the top 4 to 5 mm of the condylar head, including the medial and lateral poles. The articular disk is repositioned over the remaining condylar stump and secured with the Mitek anchor technique (Fig. 44.2).

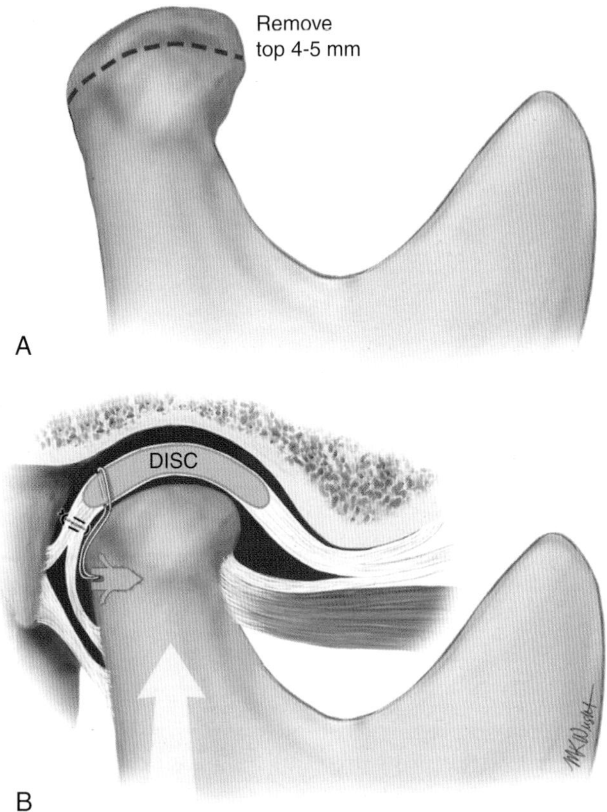

Figure 44.2 **A,** A #701 bur is used to cut off the top 4 to 5 mm of the condylar head and removed, including the medial and lateral poles. **B,** The articular disk is repositioned over the remaining condylar stump and secured with the Mitek anchor technique.

TECHNIQUE: Low Condylectomy

The superior and inferior joint spaces are entered as described previously. A #701 tapered fissure bur is used to make a bone cut at the junction of the condylar head and neck, and the condyle and tumor are removed. The condylar neck is recontoured to function as a new condyle, and the articular disk is repositioned over the condylar stump with the Mitek anchor technique (Fig. 44.3).

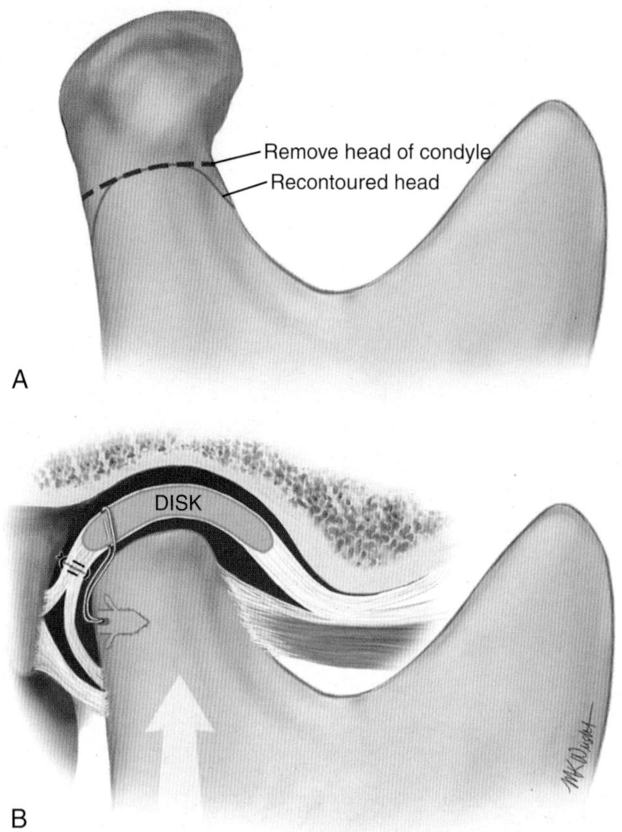

Figure 44.3 **A,** A #701 tapered fissure bur is used to perform a bone cut at the junction of the condylar head and neck, and the condyle and tumor removed. **B,** The condylar neck is recontoured to function as a new condyle and the articular disk repositioned over the condylar stump with the Mitek anchor technique.

TECHNIQUE: Mandibular Ramus Sagittal Split Osteotomy

The techniques for mandibular ramus sagittal split osteotomy are described in Chapter 38. Concomitant orthognathic surgery and TMJ surgery, including disk repositioning as well as high and low condylectomies, results in cutting of the capsular ligaments that normally provide vertical support to the condyle. Severing these ligaments can result in condylar sag affecting post-surgery mandibular stability. Condylar sag can be avoided by properly repositioning the condyle into a stable position in the fossa prior to rigid fixation application. Following completion of the osteotomies with separation of the distal and proximal segments, the patient is placed in the intermediate surgical splint and intermaxillary fixation applied. The proximal segment is gently pushed posteriorly from the intraoral approach, and externally, gently pushed upward at the angle of the mandible to seat the condyle into the fossa. Rigid fixation is then applied.

TECHNIQUE: Maxillary Osteotomies

The techniques for performing maxillary osteotomies are described in Chapter 41 and are not included here.

TECHNIQUE: Total Joint Prosthesis

STEP 1: Incisions and Condylectomy

An endaural or preauricular incision and a submandibular incision are required to place the total joint prosthesis. A condylectomy is performed, the condyle is removed, and the fossa is debrided. If required, a coronoidectomy is performed through this incision. Bone from the condyle and coronoid can be used to graft the maxillary osteotomies. Sometimes additional bone must be resected from the superior aspect of the ramus to make room for the patient-fitted TMJ prosthesis; a distance of 20 mm is required between the fossa and the ramus to accommodate the joint prosthesis.

STEP 2: Muscle Dissection

A submandibular incision is made to access the angle and ramus of the mandible. The masseter muscle is dissected off the lateral ramus. The medial pterygoid is reflected off only if the mandible will be significantly advanced forward in a counterclockwise direction or vertically lengthened. The lateral aspect of the ramus is recontoured, if necessary, and the mandible is mobilized. An intermediate splint and intermaxillary fixation are applied.

STEP 3: Component Placement

The fossa component is placed and stabilized with four 2-mm diameter, 6-mm length bone screws. The mandibular component is placed through the submandibular incision into the fossa, and the condyle is set against the posterior phalange of the fossa component. Commonly, eight bone screws, usually 8 to 12 mm long, are placed in the mandibular component. For the superior screws, a small stab incision is made about 1 cm below the earlobe, and a trocar is passed through the skin and soft tissues to drill holes and insert screws into the superior holes of the prosthesis (Fig. 44.4).

STEP 4: Muscle Suturing

The surgical area is irrigated. Three to four holes are made through the inferior border of the angle, and 2-0 polydioxanone suture is used to secure the masseter muscle to the inferior border of the angle with a running suture technique. The incisions are closed in layers.

STEP 5: Closure

Fat is harvested from the abdomen (either through a suprapubic or a periumbilical incision) or from the buttock. Good hemostasis is obtained, a drain is placed if necessary, and the incision is closed. The fresh fat is packed around the articulating area of the prosthesis anteriorly, medially, posteriorly, and laterally. The incision is closed in two layers.

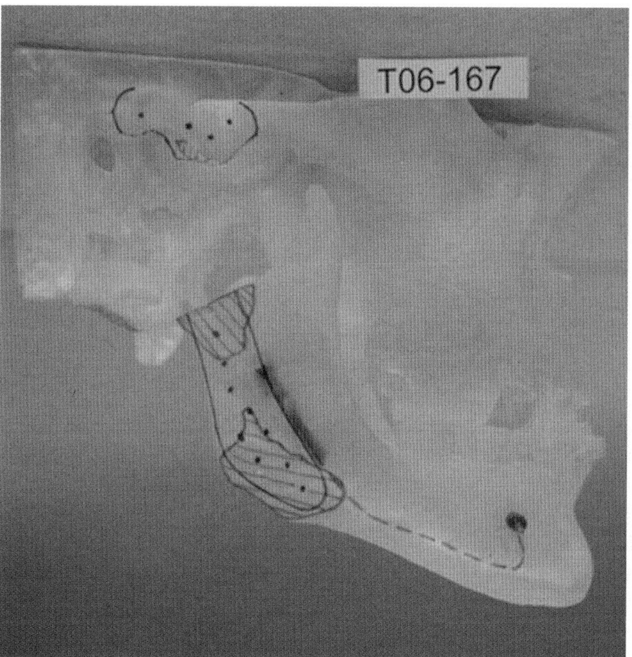

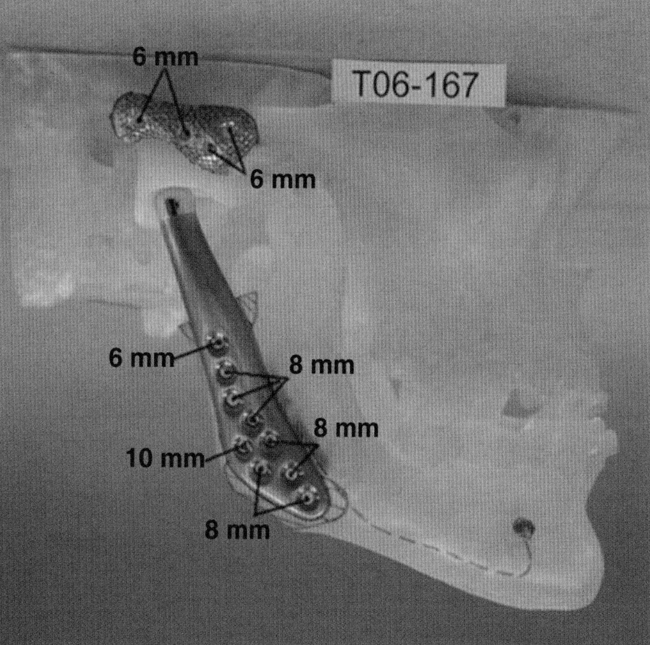

Figure 44.4 Place the fossa component and stabilize with four 2-mm diameter, 6-mm length bone screws. Place the mandibular component through the submandibular incision into the fossa and set the condyle against the posterior phalange of the fossa component. Eight bone screws are placed to stabilize the mandibular component.

TECHNIQUE: Ankylosis

The size and involvement of the ankylosis can be determined from CT scans and three-dimensional modeling before surgery. If the case is unilateral, the level at which the release of the ankylosis should be performed can be determined by measuring the height of the zygomatic arch and lateral rim of the fossa on the normal side and transferring the measurements to the ankylotic side. The bone cut can then be made through the outer cortical plate of the ankylotic bone. A curved osteotome can be used to separate the condyle and heterotopic bone from the base of the skull and fossa area. If the ankylosis extends some distance medially, a more careful approach is required, with removal of the buccal cortex and then removal of the deeper bone, with medial protection until the mass has been removed. The horizontal osteotomy at approximately the level of the sigmoid notch aids in removal of the inferior component of the heterotopic bone. Once the bone has been removed, the fossa is debrided with bone removal, as necessary, to return to the original structure of the fossa. If the mandible remains in its original position or if all of the reactive bone is not removed from the fossa, additional bone may require removal as outlined in red to provide 20 mm of clearance to accommodate the prosthesis. The prosthesis then is placed as previously described (Fig. 44.5).

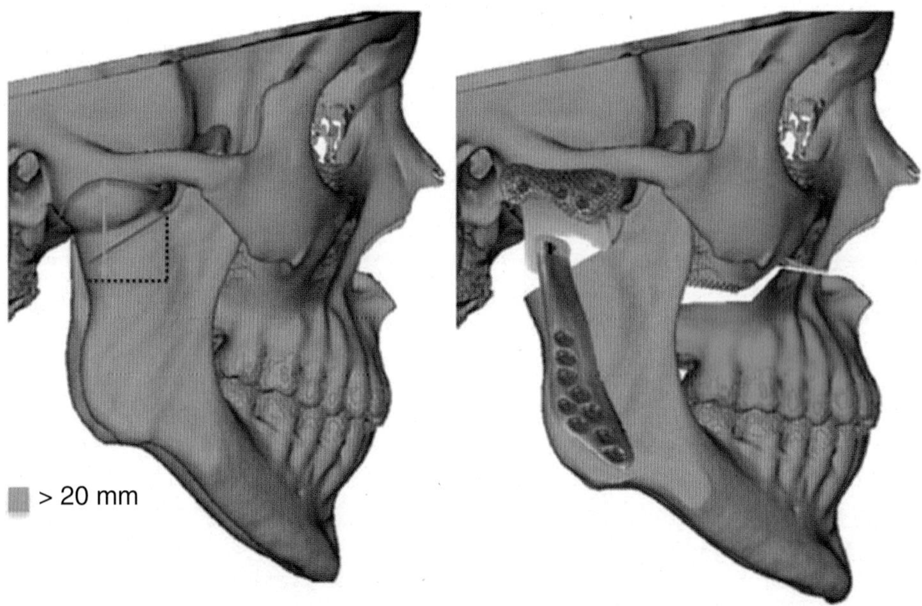

Figure 44.5 The size and involvement of the ankylosis can be determined from CT scans and three-dimensional modeling before surgery.

Avoidance and Management of Intraoperative Complications

TMJ surgery can involve branches of cranial nerves V and VII, so diligent care is necessary to minimize injury. The inferior alveolar, mental, and infraorbital nerves are localized in the osteotomy areas. Using the inferior border saw reduces inferior alveolar nerve injury. Entrapment of the inferior alveolar nerve in the proximal segment with the traditional sagittal split techniques increases the risk of temporary or permanent nerve damage. Likewise, the infraorbital nerve can be damaged by retraction or direct trauma.

Infection is a potential risk, but the risk can be reduced by the use of intraoperative antibiotics, thorough irrigation of the surgical sites with saline, a final irrigation with Betadine solution, and watertight closure of the incisions.

If an infection occurs around the total joint prosthesis, the incisions must be opened and the prosthesis thoroughly scrubbed with Betadine. Intravenous (IV) antibiotics are administered for about 4 to 5 days, and antibiotic irrigation at the site is performed every 4 hours to preserve the prosthesis. The patient is discharged on oral medications for an additional 3 to 4 weeks.[31] For infections of the sagittal split area, genioplasty, or maxillary osteotomy areas, irrigation with saline and antibiotic therapy usually resolve the problem without requiring removal of the bone plates and screws.

There is a potential risk for bleeding problems that could require a transfusion. If a patient is healthy and has a normal hemoglobin and hematocrit and the surgery is done appropriately, there is a very minimal risk of a transfusion being required, although the patients will be somewhat anemic after surgery. Using hypotensive anesthesia can significantly reduce blood loss. The use of IV steroids helps reduce swelling. Controlling IV fluids (i.e., to 1 L, or no more than 1500 cc for combined TMJ and orthognathic surgery) also significantly reduces the requirement for transfusion and diminishes postoperative edema.[32]

After surgery, the patient must be monitored carefully. No intermaxillary fixation is required, but inner arch elastics are usually helpful, particularly in TMJ-related surgeries, because disk repositioning tends to cause edema within the joint, which can result in some shifting of the mandible and the occlusion after surgery. Placing appropriate elastics with vertical and anteroposterior vectors (3 1/2-ounce elastics) usually works quite well. When the maxilla is segmentalized, the authors prefer to use a palatal splint which, depending on the amount of expansion between the segments, may have to remain in place for 6 weeks to several months.[32]

With properly planned surgery, the airway should remain the same; with counterclockwise advancements, it will be significantly improved for sleep apnea patients.[33–35] Patients are maintained on antibiotics for the Mitek anchor and orthognathic surgery techniques for approximately 5 to 7 days. With total joint prostheses, the patient should remain on appropriate antibiotics for 7 to 10 days. The diet usually is restricted to pureed food for the first week and then progresses to soft foods (e.g., pastas, soft fish, and other, similar consistencies) for the first 4 months, until the initial healing phase is over. Complete healing takes a full year, but by 4 months, almost all of the new bone growth that will occur in the upper jaw and mandibular osteotomy sites is complete, and the remaining healing time is for maturation of the new bone.[32]

Patients should not use straws or blow the nose for approximately 2 weeks after surgery. They will be quite tired for the first month after surgery and then should begin regaining their customary energy level. If the patient had preexisting sleep apnea, he or she should recognize a significant airway improvement with the counterclockwise rotation of the maxillomandibular complex.

Postoperative Considerations

Postoperative patient management is a critical factor for ensuring quality treatment outcomes. Three primary areas requiring emphasis include occlusion management, jaw exercises, postsurgical orthodontics, and retention.

Occlusion Management

Since the TMJ capsule is cut during surgery and joint effusion or edema may develop, condylar sag can occur, which affects the occlusion and jaw position. Therefore, immediate postsurgical elastics are usually necessary to keep the condyles seated and occlusion fitting together. Light elastics (3/16 inch and 3-1/2 ounce) can be used for occlusion control and may include elastic application for class III and vertical force vectors for 1 to 2 week or longer if needed until the edema decreases, the capsule begins to heal, and the occlusion is stable.[32]

Jaw Exercises

TMJ surgery usually results in an incisal opening that increases or remains the same as before surgery, but excursive movements may decrease. Self-administrated jaw exercises for excursions and incisal opening will maximize postsurgical jaw function and can be initiated 1 to 2 weeks after surgery or sooner and applied for 6 to 9 months.[32]

Postsurgical Orthodontics

Although immediate postsurgical occlusion management with elastics is usually necessary, active orthodontics can be reinitiated 4 to 6 weeks after surgery. Teeth move more rapidly following surgery for the first 6 to 9 months. The orthodontist must see the patient more frequently than usual to maximize the advantage of the increased tooth movement. The palatal splint can stabilize the maxilla transversely in segmental surgery. If minimal expansion and segment manipulation have been incorporated, then the splint can usually be removed in 6 weeks, and placement of a solid continuous arch wire can be accomplished. If a large expansion is made, then the palatal splint may be required for 3 to 6 months. A transpalatal arch bar may be indicated through the healing process.[32]

Postsurgical Retention

The orthodontic appliances should not be removed for at least 4 to 6 months after surgery to get through the initial healing phase. Fixed retainers for the mandibular arch from cuspid to cuspid usually work adequately. In the maxillary arch, Hawley or wrap-around retainers are recommended. Avoid Essex-type retainers or other devices that cover the occlusal surfaces because these can create posterior open bites in orthognathic and TMJ surgery patients.[32]

References

1. Wolford LM, Cassano DS, Goncalves JR. Common TMJ disorders: orthodontic and surgical management. In: McNamara JA, Kapila SD, eds. *Temporomandibular Disorders and Orofacial Pain: Separating Controversy from Consensus, Volume 46, Craniofacial Growth Series*. Ann Arbor, Michigan: University of Michigan; 2009.
2. Wolford LM. Facial asymmetry: diagnosis and treatment considerations. In: Fonseca RJ, Marciani RD, Turvey TA, eds. *Oral and Maxillofacial Surgery*. Vol. 3. 2nd ed. St Louis, Missouri: Saunders; 2008.
3. Wolford LM, Karras S, Mehra P. Concomitant temporomandibular joint and orthognathic surgery: a preliminary report. *J Oral Maxillofac Surg*. 2002;60(4):356–362.
4. Wolford LM, Mehra P, Reiche-Fischel O, Morales-Ryan CA, García-Morales P. Efficacy of high condylectomy for management of condylar hyperplasia. *Am J Orthod Dentofacial Orthop*. 2002;121(2):136–150.
5. Wolford LM, Morales-Ryan CA, García-Morales P, Perez D. Surgical management of mandibular condylar hyperplasia type 1. *Proc - Bayl Univ Med Cent*. 2009;22(4):321–329.
6. Wolford LM, Movahed R, Perez DE. A classification system for conditions causing condylar hyperplasia. *J Oral Maxillofac Surg*. 2014;72(3):567–595.
7. Wolford LM, Rodrigues DB. Temporomandibular joint (TMJ) pathologies in growing patients: effects on facial growth and development. In: Preedy VR, ed. *Handbook of Growth and Growth Monitoring in Health and Disease*. New York: Springer; 2012.
8. Wolford LM, Mehra P, Franco P. Use of conservative condylectomy for treatment of osteochondroma of the mandibular condyle. *J Oral Maxillofac Surg*. 2002;60(3):262–268.
9. Wolford LM, Movahed R, Dhameja A, Allen WR. Low condylectomy and orthognathic surgery to treat mandibular condylar osteochondroma: a retrospective review of 37 cases. *J Oral Maxillofac Surg*. 2014;72(9):1704–1728.
10. Mehra P, Wolford LM. The Mitek mini anchor for TMJ disc repositioning: surgical technique and results. *Int J Oral Maxillofac Surg*. 2001;30(6):497–503.
11. Goncalves JR, Cassano DS, Wolford LM, et al. Postsurgical stability of counterclockwise maxillomandibular advancement surgery: effect of articular disc repositioning. *J Oral Maxillofac Surg*. 2008;66(4):724–738.
12. Wolford LM, Cardenas L. Idiopathic condylar resorption: diagnosis, treatment protocol, and outcomes. *Am J Orthod Dentofacial Orthop*. 1999;116(6):667–677.
13. Wolford LM. Idiopathic condylar resorption of the temporomandibular joint in teenage girls (cheerleaders syndrome). *Proc - Bayl Univ Med Cent*. 2001;14(3):246–252.
14. Wolford LM, Galiano A. Adolescent internal condylar resorption (AICR) of the temporomandibular joint, part 1: a review for diagnosis and treatment considerations. *Cranio*. 2019;37(1):35–44.
15. Galiano A, Wolford L, Gonçalves J, Gonçalves D. Adolescent internal condylar resorption (AICR) of the temporomandibular joint can be successfully treated by disc repositioning and orthognathic surgery, part 2: treatment outcomes. *Cranio*. 2019;37(2):111–120.
16. Henry CH, Hughes CV, Gérard HC, Hudson AP, Wolford LM. Reactive arthritis: preliminary microbiologic analysis of the human temporomandibular joint. *J Oral Maxillofac Surg*. 2000;58(10):1137–1142.
17. Henry CH, Pitta MC, Wolford LML. Frequency of chlamydial antibodies in patients with internal derangement of the temporomandibular joint. *Oral Surg Oral Med Oral Pathol Oral Radiol Endod*. 2001;91(3):287–292.
18. Wolford LM, Cottrell DA, Henry CH. Temporomandibular joint reconstruction of the complex patient with the Techmedica custom-made total joint prosthesis. *J Oral Maxillofac Surg*. 1994;52(1):2–10.
19. Wolford L, Movahed R, Teschke M, Fimmers R, Havard D, Schneiderman E. Temporomandibular joint ankylosis can be successfully treated with TMJ concepts patient-fitted total joint prosthesis and autogenous fat grafts. *J Oral Maxillofac Surg*. 2016;74(6):1215–1227.
20. Wolford LM, Karras SC. Autologous fat transplantation around temporomandibular joint total joint prostheses: preliminary treatment outcomes. *J Oral Maxillofac Surg*. 1997;55(3):245–251.
21. Wolford LM, Cassano DS. Autologous fat grafts around temporomandibular joint (TMJ) total joint prostheses to prevent heterotopic bone. In: Shiffman MA, ed. *Autologous Fat Transfer*. Berlin, Germany: Springer-Verlag; 2010.
22. Wolford LM, Bourland TC, Rodrigues D, Perez DE, Limoeiro E. Successful reconstruction of nongrowing hemifacial microsomia patients with unilateral temporomandibular joint total joint prosthesis and orthognathic surgery. *J Oral Maxillofac Surg*. 2012;70(12):2835–2853.
23. Riolo ML, Moyers RE, McNamara JA, Hunter WS. *An Atlas of Craniofacial Growth: Cephalometric Standards from the University School Growth Study*. Ann Arbor, Michigan: University of Michigan; 1974.
24. Wolford LM, Karras SC, Mehra P. Considerations for orthognathic surgery during growth, part 1: mandibular deformities. *Am J Orthod Dentofacial Orthop*. 2001;119(2):95–101.
25. Wolford LM, Karras SC, Mehra P. Considerations for orthognathic surgery during growth, part 2: maxillary deformities. *Am J Orthod Dentofacial Orthop*. 2001;119(2):102–105.
26. Wolford LM, Rodrigues DB. Orthognathic considerations in the young patient and effects on facial growth. In: Preedy VR, ed. *Handbook of Growth and Growth Monitoring in Health and Disease*. New York: Springer; 2012.
27. Mehra P, Wolford LM, Baran S, Cassano DS. Single-stage comprehensive surgical treatment of the rheumatoid arthritis temporomandibular joint patient. *J Oral Maxillofac Surg*. 2009;67(9):1859–1872.
28. Dela Coleta KE, Wolford LM, Gonçalves JR, Pinto AS, Pinto LP, Cassano DS. Maxillo-mandibular counter-clockwise rotation and mandibular advancement with TMJ concepts total joint prostheses: part I—skeletal and dental stability. *Int J Oral Maxillofac Implants*. 2009;38(2):126–138.
29. Pinto LP, Wolford LM, Buschang PH, Bernardi FH, Gonçalves JR, Cassano DS. Maxillo-mandibular counter-clockwise rotation and mandibular advancement with TMJ concepts total joint prostheses: part III—pain and dysfunction outcomes. *Int J Oral Maxillofac Implants*. 2009;38(4):326–331.
30. Mercuri LG, Wolford LM, Sanders B, White RD, Giobbie-Hurder A. Long-term follow-up of the CAD/CAM patient fitted total temporomandibular joint reconstruction system. *J Oral Maxillofac Surg*. 2002;60(12):1440–1448.
31. Wolford LM, Rodrigues DB, McPhillips A. Management of the infected temporomandibular joint total joint prosthesis. *J Oral Maxillofac Surg*. 2010;68(11):2810–2823.
32. Wolford LM, Rodrigues DB, Limoeiro E. Orthognathic and TMJ surgery: postsurgical patient management. *J Oral Maxillofac Surg*. 2011;69(11):2893–2903.
33. Wolford LM, Perez D, Stevao E, Perez E. Airway space changes after nasopharyngeal adenoidectomy in conjunction with Le Fort I osteotomy. *J Oral Maxillofac Surg*. 2012;70(3):665–671.
34. Mehra P, Downie M, Pita MC, Wolford LM. Pharyngeal airway space changes after counterclockwise rotation of the maxillomandibular complex. *Am J Orthod Dentofacial Orthop*. 2001;120(2):154–159.
35. Coleta KE, Wolford LM, Gonçalves JR, Pinto AS, Cassano DS, Gonçalves DA. Maxillo-mandibular counter-clockwise rotation and mandibular advancement with TMJ concepts total joint prostheses: part II—airway changes and stability. *Int J Oral Maxillofac Implants*. 2009;38(3):228–235.

CHAPTER 45

Endoscopic and Strip Craniectomy

David A. Koppel and Jaime Grant

Armamentarium

Standard craniotomy or craniofacial instrument set
#15 and #10 scalpel blades
Needle-cutting diathermy
Bipolar electrocautery
Selection of sharp and blunt periosteal elevators
Selection of malleable brain retractors
Selection of artery and other clips
Jansen and Lexcell bone cutters
Bone shears
Kerrison rongeurs
Power tools: neurosurgical perforator and drill handpiece with matchstick bur
Neurosurgical craniotome
Hemostatic agents: Surgicel, Floseal, or similar
Bone wax
Appropriate sutures

History of the Procedure

Strip craniectomy for craniosynostosis (suturectomy) has a relatively long history in the management of craniosynostosis. Although craniosynostosis was identified by Hippocrates,[1] the term was coined by Virchow in 1851.[2] Virchow postulated that the prematurely fused suture restricted skull growth at 90 degrees and that compensatory growth occurred elsewhere in the skull, producing the characteristic skull shapes of the different types of craniosynostosis. This observation led to the development of surgical procedures to "release" the fused suture in the belief that this would allow normal skull growth. The first suturectomies were reported by Lannelongue (1890)[3] in Paris and Lane (1892)[4] in San Francisco. Later, Jacobi[5] reviewed 33 operated suturectomy cases that had an alarming mortality of almost 50%. Contributing to the mortality problem was the inability to differentiate between microcephaly and craniosynostosis. In the early 1920s, there was a revival of the procedure, and Mehner reported more successful outcomes.[6] Faber and Towne managed to improve results, and by the 1940s, the procedure was becoming more common.[7–8]

During this period, early intervention was advocated in children younger than 2 months, but reossification and the need for reoperation were becoming more common. Over the ensuing years, simple suturectomy and the creation of a neoartificial suture were not completely effective, with resynostosis being a common place and an increase in less-than-ideal aesthetic outcomes. These developments led to a more extensive open calvarial remodeling procedures we know today.[9,10] In addition to the increased complexity of the remodeling, attempts were made to reduce the chances of resynostosis with the use of a variety of silicone, plastic, or metal materials wrapped around the bone edges forming the neosuture.[11]

In more modern times, the isolated suturectomy became a rare event and was only used in very young children, often those with pan-synostosis and raised intracranial pressure. More often than not, it only formed a small part of a more complex skull remodeling procedure.[12]

In the 1990s, there was a move toward surgical procedures with decreased access in an attempt to reduce the length of the procedure, minimize the length of hospitalization, and limit blood loss. These techniques often utilized endoscopic or minimal access incisions combined with suturectomy and osteotomies of the adjacent cranial vault bones. These techniques are then commonly combined with the use of postoperative helmet molding or distraction devices/springs across the neosuture.[13]

Indications for Use of the Procedure

Craniosynostosis and increased intracranial pressure are common indications. As outlined above, the main indications for a suturectomy are part of a wider skull remodeling procedure or a limited access procedure with postoperative helmet therapy or distraction osteogenesis. Endoscopic procedures are generally used in infants under 5 months of age.

Limitations and Contraindications

Isolated suturectomies have limited value in older infants above the age of 5 months. This is secondary to the limited rapid growth potential of the underlying brain, which permits cranial remodeling and the increasing stiffness of the calvarium as the infant ages.

Open Technique

1. Positioning

For anterior sutures the child is placed supine in a gel head ring; however, for posterior procedures, the prone position is utilized using a neurosurgical horseshoe padded headrest. In the prone position, care must be taken to ensure there is no pressure on the eyes, and that during the procedure, the head is elevated for pressure relief for 60 seconds every 30 minutes.

2. Marking and skin prep

A stealth zigzag incision is used for access to the calvarium. It is marked with a small strip of hair shaved on either side of the marked wound and infiltrated with 1% lidocaine/1:200,000 epinephrine diluted up to 20 mL in a dose appropriate for the weight of the child (maximum dose 7 mg lidocaine/kg). Other appropriate weight-based local anesthetic solution with a vasoconstrictor may be used.

3. Incision and scalp elevation

The marked skin is scored with a #10 scalpel blade, and at one point off the midline, it is deepened to the subgaleal supraperiosteal plane (loose areolar tissue). Next, utilizing needle electrocautery and advancing from inside out, the scalp incision is completed on the coagulation setting. Skin hooks are placed on the wound edges by the surgeon, and the assistant maintains tension across the wound, which facilitates further separation across the plane of dissection. Additional hemostasis is achieved with bipolar cautery as needed. The subgaleal plane is opened, further utilizing scissors as needed, and the scalp is elevated. As the scalp is peeled backward or forward, needle diathermy is used to assist in dissection and hemostasis. Moist sponges are applied to the scalp to ensure the dissected flap tissue does not dry out and to assist with hemostasis.

Once the scalp has been elevated, the periosteal flaps are incised and elevated, taking care not to inadvertently cut through any skull defect or the often very thin cranium. The periosteal layer is elevated, and this may, particularly in children with raised intracranial pressure, cause significant hemorrhage. This bleeding should be controlled with bone wax, pressure, and moist sponges as necessary. The surgeon must exercise care when the exposure of large calvarial defects with underlying venous lakes occurs, as this may result in an air embolus. Sealing these exposed areas with bone wax or another hemostatic agent should be done promptly and is mandatory.

4. Bur hole placement/elevation of dura intracranially

Access into the inside of the cranial cavity can be achieved by dissecting carefully around the open fontanelle(s). A Mitchell trimmer is particularly useful for this technique. Alternatively, drilling of a bur hole can also be performed. This is usually accomplished with either a neurosurgical perforator or a matchstick bur (side but not end cutting bur, minimizing the chances of dural injury). Once access to the dura has been achieved, the bur hole can be enlarged using a Kerrison rongeur. The dura can then be safely elevated from the inner table of the skull, and this should be done using a periosteal or Penfield elevator. If the midline or a venous sinus needs to be crossed, the surgeons may either choose to widen the bur hole directly over the site of the sinus or place bur holes on either side and subsequently connect them. The extent of the dural elevation depends on the case, the position of the osteotomies, the ease of elevation, and whether other sutures are to be crossed. The dura is usually particularly adherent underneath sutures, and additional care must be taken to prevent dural tears (Figs. 45.1–45.3).

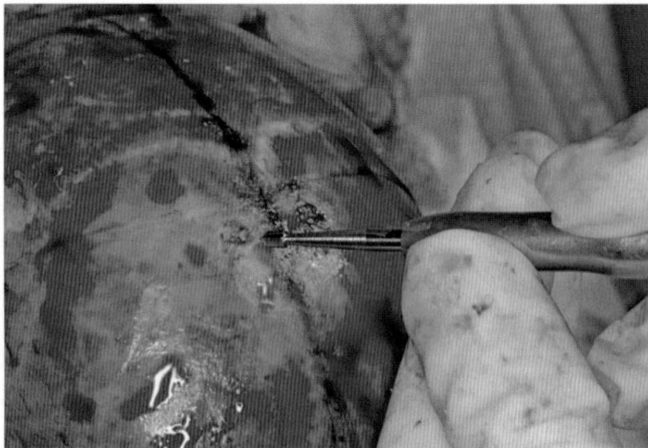

Figure 45.1 Matchstick bur to create bur hole.

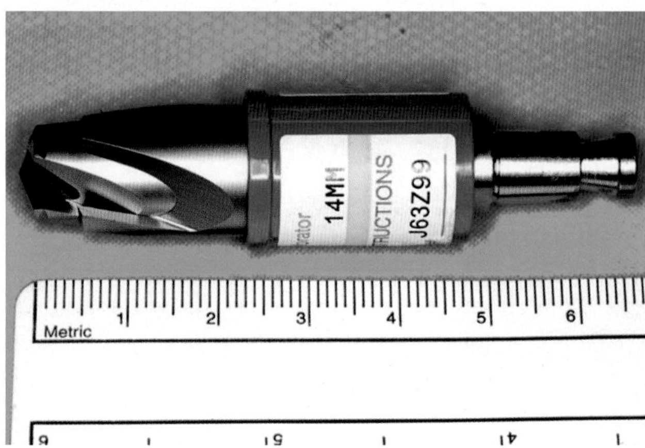

Figure 45.2 Pediatric-sized perforator.

5. Craniotome cuts

Once the dura has been partially elevated, a craniotome can be introduced and the bone cuts made safely with the footplate of the craniotome minimizing the chances of dural injury. In very young infants, the bone cuts can be completed with a pair of bone scissors or bone shears. With all power instruments, the instrument and surrounding tissue should be irrigated copiously to avoid overheating the bone (Fig. 45.4).

6. Elevation and removal of affected suture

After the bone flap osteotomies are complete, the bone often separates slightly but is still held by the dura being adherent to the inner table. In those cases where raised

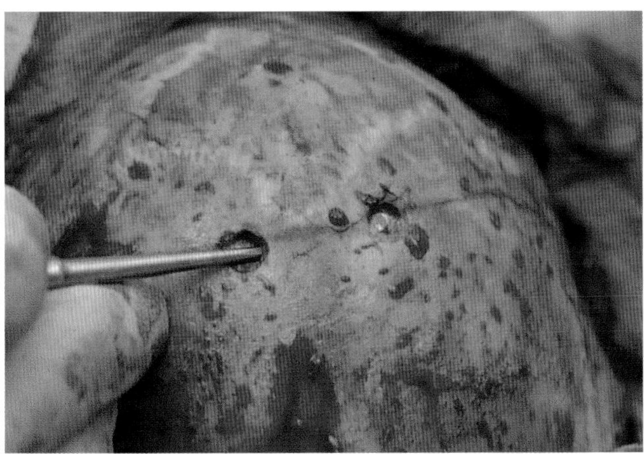

Figure 45.3 Bur holes completed. The periosteal elevator is used to strip dura away from inner table of bone, in this case crossing the midline and sagittal sinus.

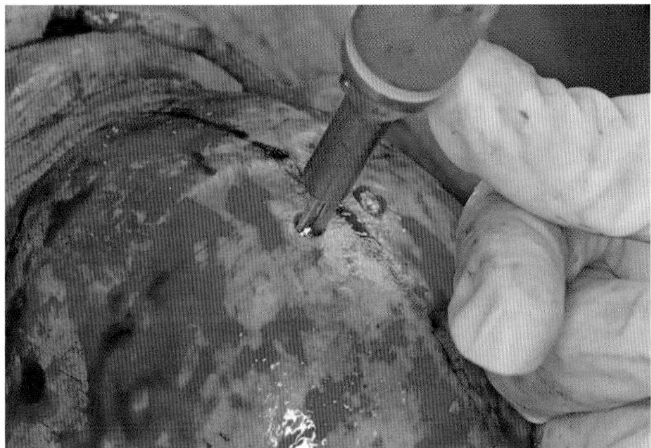

Figure 45.4 Craniotome is introduced into the bur hole prior to making the bone cuts.

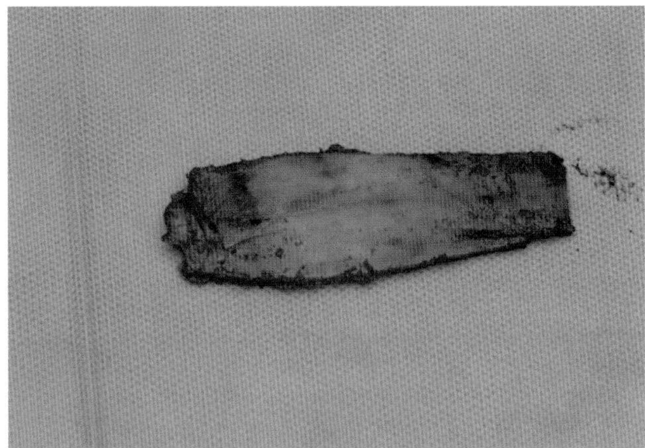

Figure 45.5 Portion of fused sagittal suture, outer surface up.

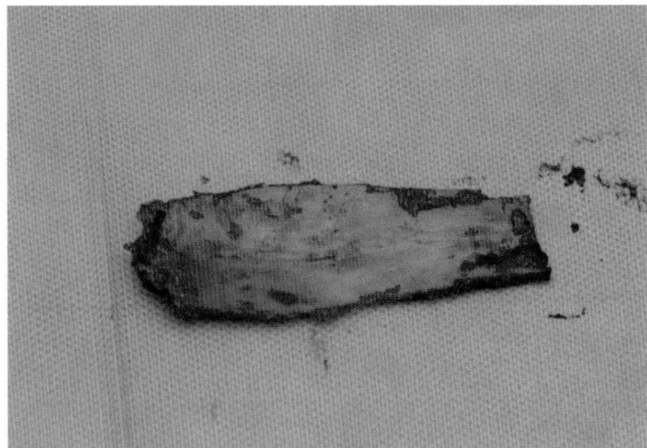

Figure 45.6 Portion of fused sagittal suture, inner surface up.

intracranial pressure is an issue, this widening at the cuts can be dramatic, and release of the pressure often reduces blood loss. Bone flap elevators are then used to lift the bone flap, and periosteal elevators are used to strip off the dura. Care must be taken around any venous sinuses because, on occasion, these sinuses can form grooves or channels in the bone and are prone to tearing at these points. It is important to note that while it is often called a simple suturectomy, the removal of the suture is performed in combination with other calvarial osteotomies such as lateral barrel staving to decrease the resistance to expansion in the biparietal dimension in sagittal synostosis (Figs. 45.5–45.7).

7. Debridement hemostasis

After the fused suture has been removed, attention must now be paid to the dura and sinuses. First, a check must be made to ensure there are no dural tears or areas of thinning, and then any bleeding is dealt with by judicious use of the bipolar diathermy. Particular care must be taken with the venous sinuses as overuse of bipolar cautery may damage the sinus wall. The bone edges should be checked for bleeding and diathermy, and bone wax can be used. Despite these maneuvers, if the dural surface continues to bleed, Surgicel, Floseal, or similar hemostatic agents should be used.

Any dural tears that occur during the procedure should be repaired either by direct suturing or with a small pericranial patch intraoperatively.

8. Closure

Once hemostasis has been achieved, the whole surgical area should be irrigated copiously with saline. The pericranium is repositioned and can be loosely opposed with absorbable 4-0 suture. It rarely stretches to allow for complete closure, which is unnecessary. A vacuum drain is used, secured to the skin, and positioned to lie in the subgaleal plane. The galeal layer is closed with a continuous 2-0 absorbable braided suture. We use a 3/4 round multipurpose needle to facilitate closure of this layer. The skin is closed with 4-0 absorbable monofilament suture.

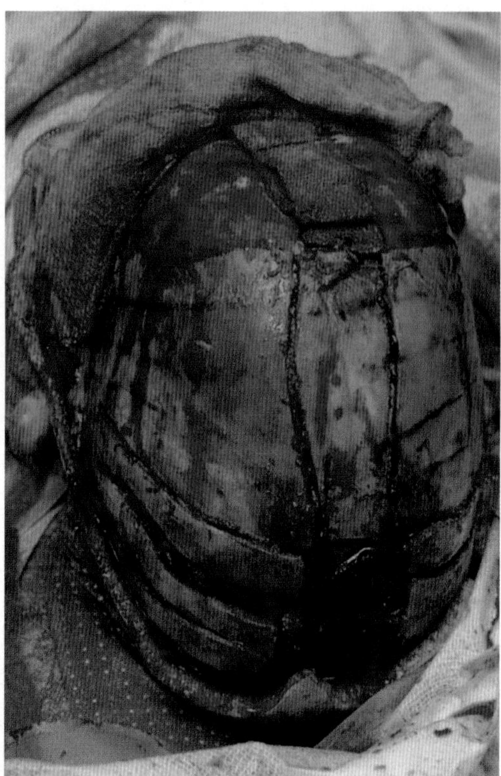

Figure 45.7 Image taken partway through total vault remodeling. Here, the posterior sagittal suture has been removed, with posterior parietal barrel staves osteotomized. The midportion of fused sagittal suture is yet to be removed, and the bifrontal craniotomy is completed. Lateral anterior barrel staves are marked.

ALTERNATE OR MODIFIED TECHNIQUE #1

A modification of this technique involves a minimal access approach utilizing smaller skin incisions at the anterior-posterior limits of the affected suture. In the case of sagittal synostosis, these incisions are positioned just forward of the anterior fontanelle and just behind the posterior fontanelle. The osteotomies are then facilitated with the assistance of an endoscope to increase visual access in the tunnel created between the two incisions. This procedure can be more easily achieved when the calvarial bone is still very malleable, typically prior to 3 months of age. In skilled hands, this procedure can also be combined with lateral cuts of the bilateral parietal bones after appropriate dural dissection is completed. Postoperative helmet therapy follows the operative procedure and is aimed at utilizing the rapid brain growth of the young infant to facilitate a resultant improvement in the shape.[13]

Avoidance and Management of Intraoperative Complications

Excessive Scalp Bleeding

Care must be taken when raising the cranial flaps to reduce blood loss by taking the time to adequately bipolar/monopolar dissect the tissues and vessels. In some centers the pericranium is left on the calvarium and taken down as a separate layer. Advocates of this method state that the vessels can be more easily identified by adding this step, and bipolar cautery at the interface between the loose areolar tissue and the pericranium lessens the bleeding caused by tearing the vessel from its bony fissure. If preoperative imaging is available, then large bridging veins can be identified and should be sought proactively.

The craniotome can be difficult to maneuver across sutures as the bony tissue remains soft at this age. In this case the Kerrison rongeur may be used. Alternatively, a broader dural dissection underneath the area of proposed osteotomy can be undertaken to allow for osteotomy with the placement of a malleable retractor underneath for dural/brain protection.

Dural tears can be avoided by careful use of the craniotome and/or matchstick bur with adequate irrigation and vision of the underlying tissues where possible. If the craniotome feels as if it is not readily advancing, pulling back with readvancement of the craniotome will reduce the chances of pulling the dura further and tearing it. If it still does not readily advance, it is better to try from the opposite side or create a further bur hole. Any dural tears should be repaired as described above.

Dural venous sinus tears are the most dreaded of complications and can be life threatening. Although it may seem counterintuitive, the patient should be placed in a head down position to avoid air embolus and the sinus repaired or ligated as dictated by the position and extent of the tear. A nonabsorbable vascular suture should be used for this purpose with immediate pressure over the area of bleeding with application of absorbable collagen thrombin-soaked sponges.

Postoperative Considerations

Postoperatively cerebrospinal fluid (CSF) may leak from unrecognized, unrepaired, or incompletely repaired dural tears. This may result in CSF leakage from the wound or into the surrounding tissues. On occasion this necessitates imaging and subsequent repair. Alternatively, it can be managed with relief of pressure through the placement of a lumbar drain or a combination of the two.

Excessive postoperative bleeding should be ameliorated in the initial surgical insult by meticulous operative technique; however, excessive postoperative bleeding may still occur. The authors advocate for the previously described subgaleal drain to monitor for this occurrence in almost all cases. In addition, the patient's hemoglobin should be checked the evening of the operation and again the next morning, with attention being paid to clotting ability and the proactive addition of clotting factors to the management of blood loss.

It is important to note that these techniques are only useful in young infants and are limited in the scope of their correction. In older infants and young children, these techniques are of little effective use. Strip craniectomy harnesses the resultant increase in growth at 90 degrees to the fused suture during the early rapid brain growth of the maturing infant. Therefore, it should follow that for infants older than 5 to 6 months of age and young children (who have achieved most of their growth potential), a more extensive open remodeling procedure addressing the resultant deformity (e.g., frontal bossing and occipital bulleting as seen in scaphocephaly) may be required. There is little to be done except reoperation with a more extensive procedure in the case of restenosis without improvement.

References

1. Kyutoku S, Inagaki T. Review of past reports and current concepts of surgical management for craniosynostosis. *Neurol Med Chir (Tokyo)*. 2017;57(5):217–224.
2. Virchow R. Uber den Cretinismus, namentlich in Franken, und uber pathologische Schadelformen. *Verh Phys Med Gesell Wurzburg*. 1851;2:230–271.
3. Lannelongue M. De la craniectomie dans la microcéphalie. *C R Seances Acad Sci*. 1890;50:1382–1385.
4. Lane LC. Pioneer craniectomy for relief of mental imbecility due to premature sutural closure and microcephalus. *J Am Med Assoc*. 1892;18:49–50.
5. Jacobi A. Non nocere. *Med Rec*. 1894;45:609–618.
6. Mehner A. Beiträge zu den Augenveränderungen bei der Schädeldeformität des sog: turmschädels mit besonderer Berücksichtigung des Röntgenbildes. *Klin Monatsbl Augenheilkd*. 1921;61:204.
7. Faber HK, Towne EB. Early craniectomy as a preventive measure in oxycephaly and allied conditions: with special reference to the prevention of blindness. *Am J Med Sci*. 1927;173:701–711.
8. Faber HK, Towne EB. Early operation in premature cranial synostosis for the prevention of blindness and other sequelae. Five case reports with follow-up. *J Pediatr*. 1943;22:286–307.
9. Mehta VA, Bettegowda C, Jallo GI, Ahn ES. The evolution of surgical management for craniosynostosis. *Neurosurg Focus*. 2010:1;29(6):E5.
10. Vollmer DG, Jane JA, Park TS, Persing JA. Variants of sagittal synostosis: strategies for surgical correction. *J Neurosurg*. 1984;61(3):557–562.
11. Keener EB. Experimental observations on the use of rubber in the treatment of craniosynostosis. *J Neurosurg*. 1958;15(6):642–652.
12. Clayman MA, Murad GJ, Steele MH, Seagle MB, Pincus DW. History of craniosynostosis surgery and the evolution of minimally invasive endoscopic techniques: the University of Florida experience. *Ann Plast Surg*. 2007;58(3):285–287.
13. Jimenez DF, Barone CM. Endoscopic craniectomy for early surgical correction of sagittal craniosynostosis. *J Neurosurg*. 1998;88(1):77–81.

CHAPTER 46

Fronto-Orbital Advancement and Anterior Cranial Vault Reconstruction

Ramon L. Ruiz, Paul S. Tiwana, and David C. Trent

Armamentarium

#1, #3, and curved #4 Penfield elevators
#2 Pencil
#9 Molt periosteal elevator
#15 BP scalpel
5-mm osteotome and mallet
Appropriate sutures
Bone wax
CMF power surgical handpiece with reciprocating saw blade and drill capability
Colorado needlepoint electrocautery tip
Cushing temporal retractor
Electric hair clipper
Eye lubrication ointment
Gelfoam with topical thrombin
Local anesthetic with vasoconstrictor
Marking pen
Mayfield U-shaped headrest with padding
Neurosurgical power surgical handpiece with bur hole and craniotome capability
Power scissors
Resorbable plates/screws system
Seldin elevator/retractor
Small/medium/large malleable brain ribbon retractors
Tessier bone bender
Tessier periosteal elevator
Two #12 Frazier suction tips
Two wide double skin hooks

History of the Procedure

The first recorded approaches for surgical management of craniosynostosis were documented in 1890 and 1892 by Lannelogue and Lane, respectively.[1,2] Their papers described the classical elements of what we understand today to be a strip craniectomy. In this procedure, the affected fused suture was excised in an attempt to limit brain compression or intracranial hypertension. As time progressed, modifications of the strip craniectomy were made in an attempt to also improve residual skull shape after surgery with the assistance of brain growth. Then, as now, improvements to the skull shape were limited.

Tessier accomplished a major breakthrough in 1967 when he described the transcranial approach to the upper orbits through the skull base. This revolutionized thinking about craniofacial surgery and formed the technical underpinning of many of the approaches in modern use today, especially in patients with craniofacial dysostosis. Rougerie expanded on this approach and included remodeling of the anterior cranial vault simultaneously.[3] Hoffman and Mohr described the lateral canthal advancement procedure in 1976, and in 1977, Whitaker and colleagues proposed more extensive anterior cranial vault remodeling with orbital advancement.[4,5] In 1979, Marchac and Renier described the floating forehead technique, in which the bandeau segment was loosely attached to the remaining orbits accompanied by vault reshaping.[6] They argued that the principal advantage of this technique was that it allowed brain growth to push further forward the upper face in a symmetric fashion. Unfortunately, this advantage failed to materialize for most patients postoperatively. Most recently, the incorporation of resorbable fixation as a method of providing stability to the orbits and forehead to limit relapse has been widely successful and has eliminated the risk of transcranial screw migration in infants.[7] Gaining popularity as a method of treatment for craniosynostosis is the limited access/endoscopic technique, which, ironically, is essentially an extended strip craniectomy.[8]

Indications for the Use of the Procedure

Craniosynostosis is defined as the premature fusion of one or more of the cranial vault sutures. Virchow first described the sequence of events that adversely affect skull growth in the presence of craniosynostosis. Growth is arrested in a direction perpendicular to the fused suture, whereas there is a compensatory amount of overgrowth at the sutures that remain open (Virchow's law).[9] This disrupted growth pattern creates a characteristic dysmorphology and a bilateral deformity.

If the rapid brain growth that normally occurs during infancy is to proceed unhindered, the cranial vault and base sutures must remain open and expand during phases of rapid growth, resulting in marginal ossification. In craniosynostosis, premature fusion of the suture causes limited and abnormal skeletal expansion in the presence of continued brain growth. Depending on the number and location of prematurely fused sutures, the growth of the brain may be restricted. In addition, abnormal cranial vault and midfacial morphology occurs as determined by Virchow's law. If the affected sutures are not surgically released and reshaped to restore a more normal intracranial volume and configuration, decreased cognitive and behavioral function is likely to result.[10,11]

Elevated intracranial pressure (ICP) is the most serious functional problem associated with premature suture fusion. Untreated craniosynostosis with elevated ICP will cause papilledema and eventual optic nerve atrophy, resulting in partial or complete blindness. If the orbits are shallow (exorbitism) and the eyes are proptotic (exophthalmus), as occurs in the craniofacial dysostosis syndromes, the cornea may be exposed and abrasions or ulcerations may occur. An eyeball extending outside of a shallow orbit is also a risk for trauma. If the orbits are extremely shallow, herniation of the globe itself may occur, necessitating emergency reduction followed by tarsorrhaphies or urgent orbital decompression.[12,13]

Some forms of craniofacial dysostosis result in a marked degree of orbital hypertelorism, which may compromise visual acuity and restrict binocular vision. Divergent or convergent nonparalytic strabismus or exotropia occurs frequently and should be considered during the diagnostic evaluation. It may be the result of congenital anomalies of the extraocular muscles themselves. Paralytic or nonparalytic unilateral or bilateral upper eyelid ptosis also occurs with greater frequency than what is encountered in the general population.[14,15]

Hydrocephalus affects as many as 10% of patients with a craniofacial dysostosis syndrome. Although the etiology is often not clear, hydrocephalus may be secondary to a generalized cranial base stenosis with constriction of all the cranial base foramina, which impacts the patient's cerebral venous drainage and cerebrospinal fluid flow dynamics.[16,17]

The surgical management of craniosynostosis involves the release of the fused suture and dismantling of the fused and dysmorphic skeletal components via craniotomy followed by reconstruction to reassemble those structures into a more normal anatomic position. As a result, the reconstructive approach must address the orbital deformity. Correction generally involves the creation of a fronto-orbital bandeau that is reshaped as part of the overall reconstruction.

Fronto-orbital advancement with anterior cranial vault reshaping is ideally reserved for the management of patients who have a diagnosis of isolated craniosynostosis or craniofacial dysostosis (syndromic craniosynostosis) involving the metopic, sagittal, unilateral coronal, or bilateral coronal sutures (Fig. 46.1). Additionally, it can be utilized as a selected surgical technique in unique skull base pathologies (i.e., craniofacial fibrous dysplasia).

Establishing the normal position of the forehead is critical to overall facial symmetry and balance. The forehead may be considered as two separate esthetic components: the supraorbital ridge–lateral orbital rim region and the superior forehead. The supraorbital ridge–lateral orbital rim region includes the glabella and supraorbital rim extending inferiorly down each frontozygomatic suture toward the infraorbital rim and posteriorly along each temporoparietal region. The morphology and position of the supraorbital ridge–lateral orbital rim region are key elements of upper facial esthetics. In a normal forehead, at the level of the frontonasal suture, an angle ranging from 90 degrees to 110 degrees is formed by the supraorbital ridge and the nasal bones when viewed in profile. Additionally, the eyebrows, overlying the supraorbital ridge, should be anterior to the cornea. When the supraorbital ridge is viewed from above, the rim should arc posteriorly to achieve a gentle 90-degree angle at the temporal fossa with a center point of the arc at the level of each frontozygomatic suture. The superior forehead component, about 1.0 to 1.5 cm up from the supraorbital rim, should have a gentle posterior curve of about 60 degrees, leveling out at the coronal suture region when seen in profile.[18–23]

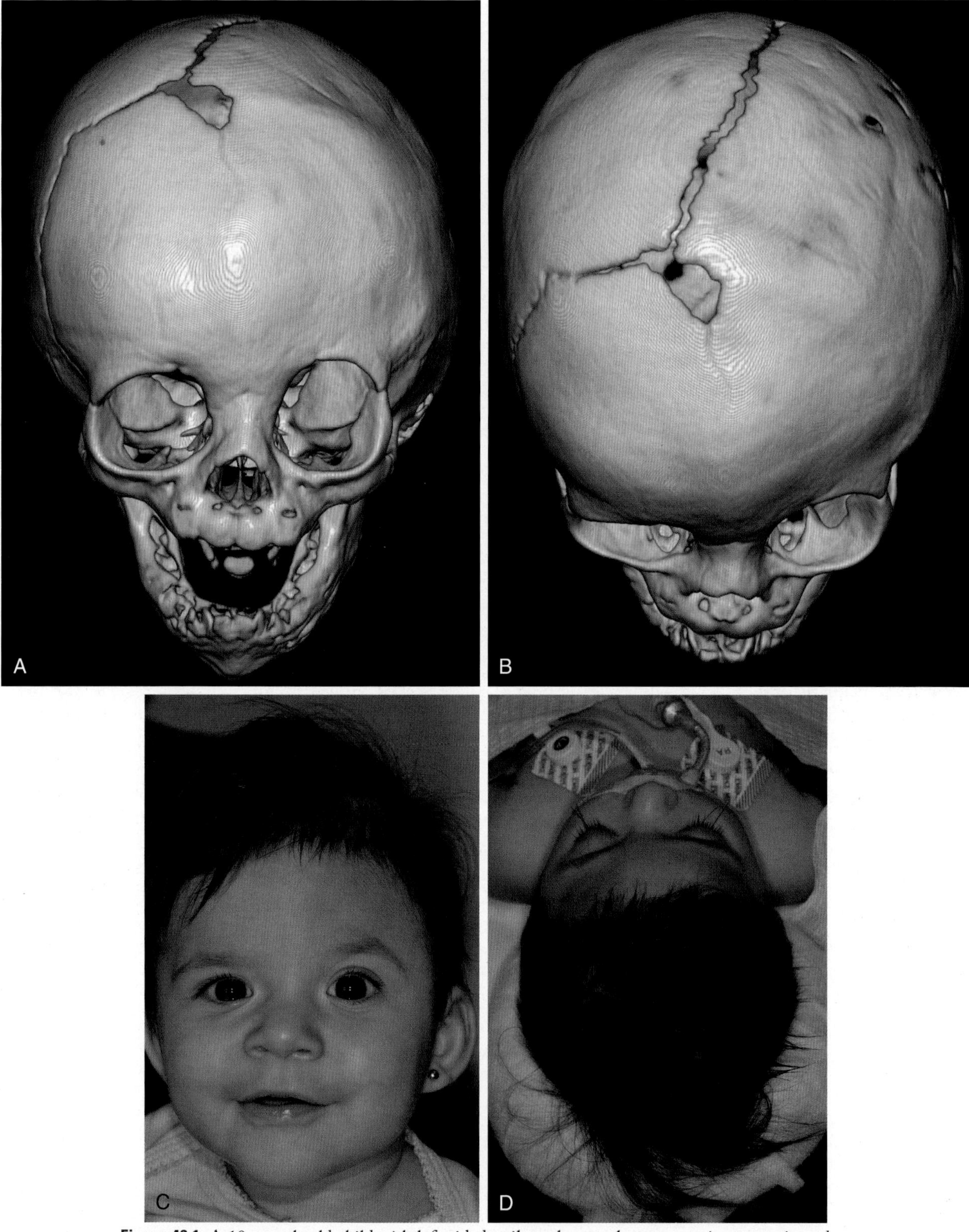

Figure 46.1 A 10-month-old child with left-sided unilateral coronal suture craniosynostosis undergoing fronto-orbital advancement and anterior cranial vault reconstruction/reshaping. **A** and **B,** Preoperative computed tomography scan demonstrating the absence of the left coronal suture. **C** and **D,** Preoperative frontal facial and bird's eye views demonstrating anterior plagiocephaly with flattening of the anterior cranial vault on the affected side, orbital dystopia, nasal asymmetry, and ipsilateral zygomatic hypoplasia.

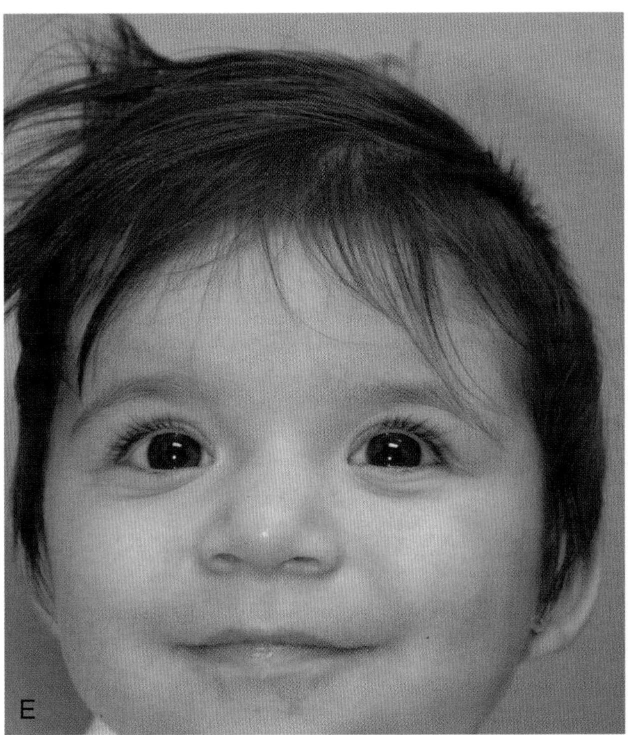

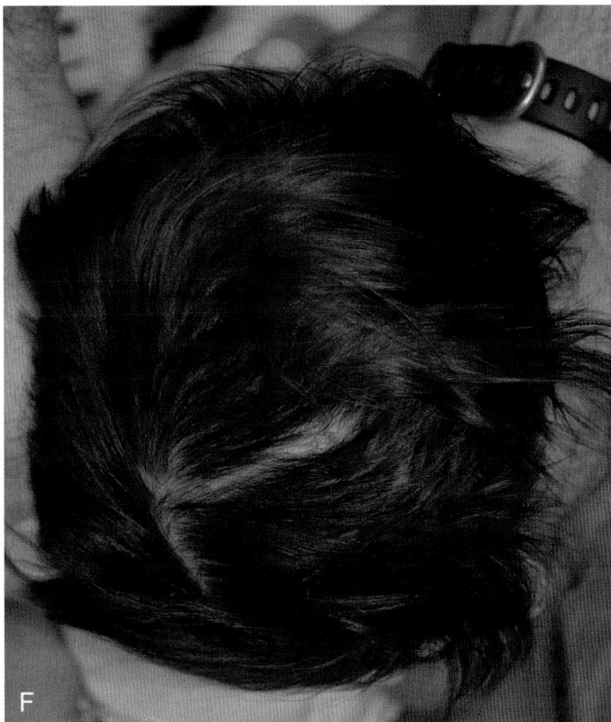

Figure 46.1, cont'd E and F, Postoperative appearance of the patient following release of the affected sutural region and skeletal reconstruction.

TECHNIQUE: Fronto-Orbital Advancement and Anterior Cranial Vault Reshaping

STEP 1: Patient Preparation

General anesthesia is induced with the placement of an oral (reinforced) endotracheal tube. The tube is generally secured in the midline.

The anesthetic team carries out placement of venous access (two peripheral venous lines or one central venous line) and an arterial line for intraoperative blood pressure monitoring. A Foley catheter is placed.

STEP 2: Tarsorrhaphy

Temporary tarsorrhaphy sutures are placed for corneal protection during the surgical procedure. The upper eyelid is gently retracted with a finger and held in place. A 5-0 silk suture on a noncutting (tapered) needle is passed through the gray line (canthal line) of the eyelid. The finger being used to retract the eyelid is kept in place until the needle driver recaptures the needle (this prevents movement of the eyelid, which can cause the needle to injure the cornea). The suture is passed through the lower eyelid in similar fashion, again with the index finger used to hold the position of the eyelid until the needle is recaptured safely.

The operating room table is then turned 90 degrees from the anesthesia team, and the patient is positioned with the head in a horseshoe-shaped Mayfield-type head holder, and all pressure points are padded. During positioning, maintenance of the cervical spine in a neutral position is confirmed (Fig. 46.2A and B).

STEP 3: Incision Design

A coronal scalp flap allows for broad access to the cranio-orbital region while concealing the surgical incision/scar within the hair-bearing scalp. The authors prefer a postauricular coronal scalp incision. A small strip of hair is clipped and a surgical pen is used to mark the postauricular coronal scalp incision. A curvilinear incision is outlined. The area is infiltrated with 0.5% lidocaine with 1:200,000 epinephrine for hemostasis.

Continued

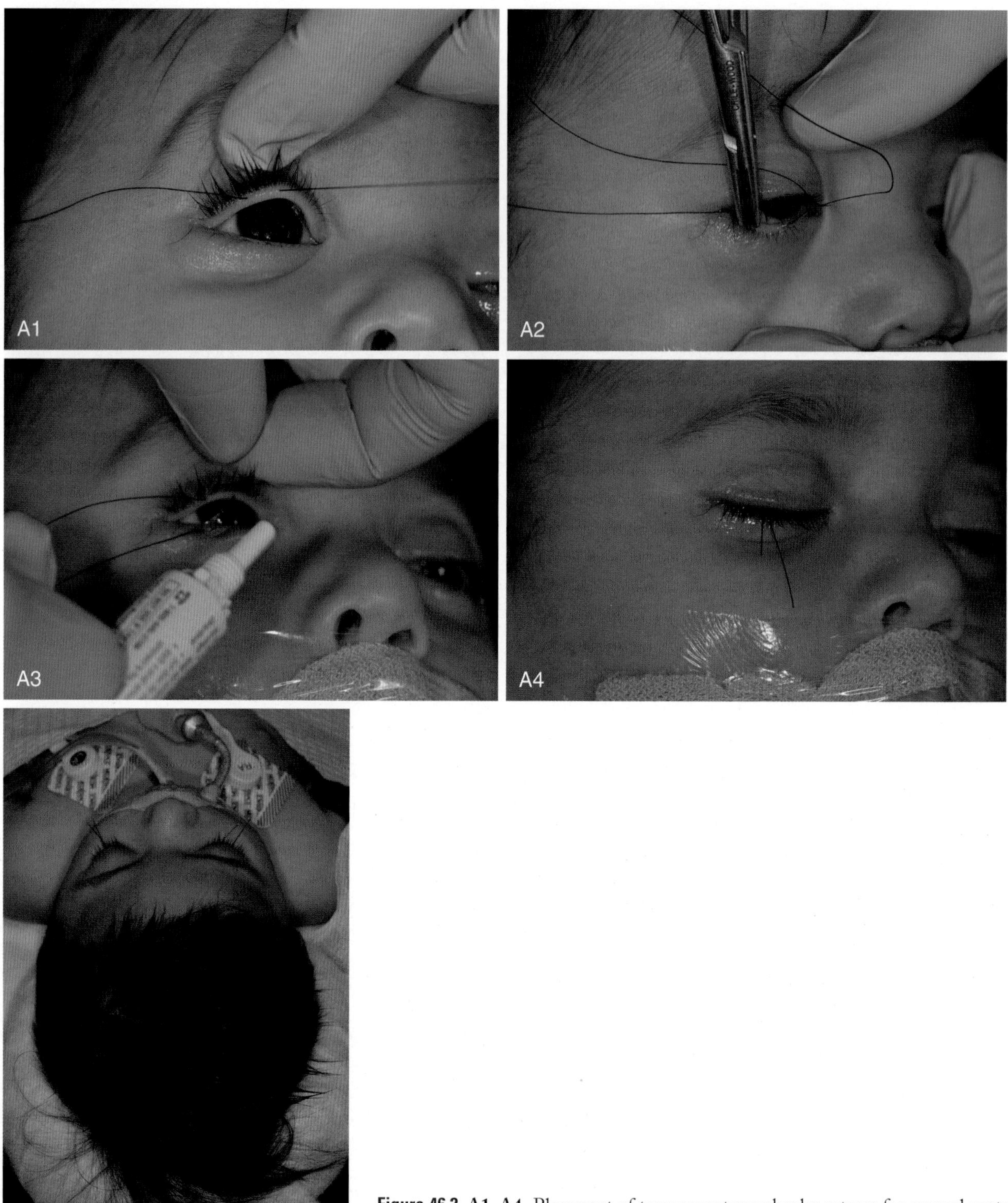

Figure 46.2 **A1–A4,** Placement of temporary tarsorrhaphy sutures for corneal protection during the procedure. **B,** Patient undergoing fronto-orbital advancement placed in the supine position within a Mayfield-type horseshoe-shaped headrest.

TECHNIQUE: Fronto-Orbital Advancement and Anterior Cranial Vault Reshaping—cont'd

The patient's face and head are then prepped with Betadine solution. The ears are prepped entirely, as they are usually within the sterile field. The face and head are then draped in a sterile fashion. After prepping the region with Betadine solution and paint, two sterile towels and base drape are placed underneath the head. One of the sterile towels is wrapped around the patient's head posterior to the coronal incision and secured with staples.

Using a #15 blade, the surgeon initially creates an incision at the vertex of the head, and sharp dissection is continued through the dermis. Double-prong skin hooks are placed at both edges of the incision and are retracted superiorly and away from the center of the incision. The dissection through the subdermal tissues and galea aponeurotica is then continued using a Colorado needle with the monopolar electrocautery on low-energy settings (typically cut of 8 and coagulation of 10). This approach allows for the initial development of a flap at the subgaleal/suprapericranial level.

The coronal flap is developed initially at the vertex, using the approach described earlier, and then continues toward the right and left sides along the temporal regions. Once the incision and initial subgaleal dissection have been carried out along the length of the incision, dissection proceeds rapidly and bloodlessly along the subgaleal/suprapericranial plane. The loose areolar connective tissue in this space is easily divided using blunt finger dissection or a combination of blunt and sharp dissection using a pair of scissors or electrocautery. The flap is turned and dissection continues anteriorly to a level approximately 2 cm behind the superior orbital rim.

Pericranial flaps are then elevated as a separate layer. Right temporoparietal, left temporoparietal, and anterior periosteal flaps are elevated. During this process, sterile bone wax and thrombin-soaked collagen sponge (Gelfoam) are used to control bleeding from the cranial vault. The prompt elimination of oozing from venous lakes not only decreases overall blood loss but is important in order to minimize the risk of a venous air embolism. Subperiosteal dissection continues until the entire frontal bone, nasofrontal junction, and upper three-fourths of the orbits are exposed. The infratemporal fossa is exposed laterally by elevating the temporalis muscles bilaterally (Fig. 46.2C and D).

STEP 4: Osteotomy Marking

Following adequate exposure of the cranio-orbital skeleton, a ruler and marking pen or pencil are used to mark the fronto-orbital bandeau. The upper half of the orbit is included, and tenon extensions are created bilaterally to facilitate the advancement and subsequent fixation. Next, the bifrontal craniotomy is outlined. Although the posterior extent of the craniotomy varies, in general, the bone segment should extend far enough to include the entire dysmorphic region. As described above, most patients with unilateral coronal craniosynostosis require surgical correction, which involves a bilateral orbital bandeau (Fig. 46.2E and F).

STEP 5: Craniotomy

Bur holes are created to allow for stripping of the dura from the overlying cranium in preparation for craniotomy. Craniotomy is then carried out using a protected drill bit with footplate. The bifrontal cranial bone flap is removed and placed in cool saline (Fig. 46.2G and Fig. 46.2E1).

Continued

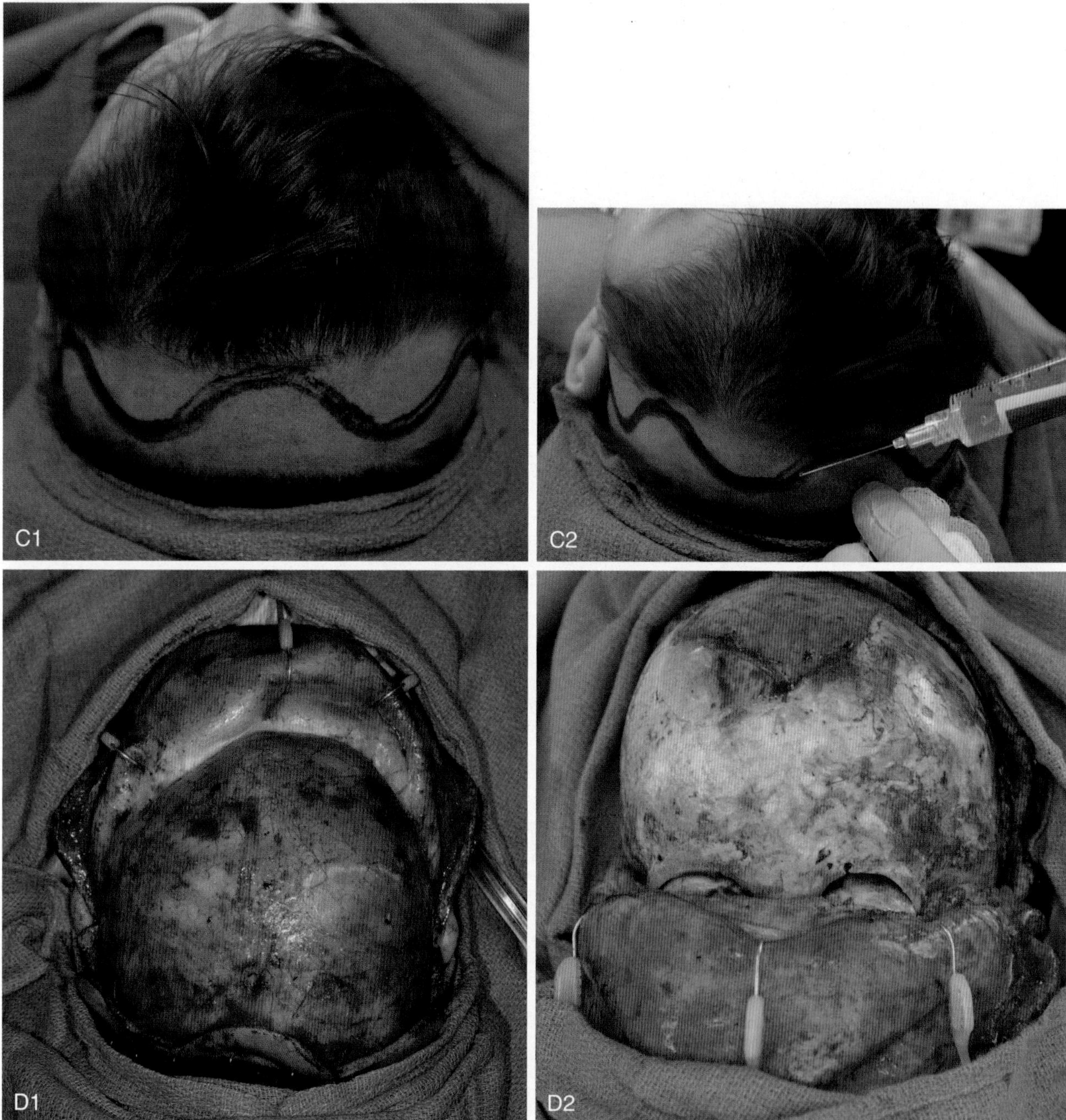

Figure 46.2, cont'd **C,** Marking of the postauricular coronal scalp flap incision. **C1,** A small area of hair is clipped. The incision is marked with a surgical pen. **C2,** The region is infiltrated with local anesthetic containing vasoconstrictor in order to aid with hemostasis. **D,** Coronal scalp incision and flap development. The incision is initially created at the vertex of the head and deepened to the subgaleal level with a combination of sharp and blunt dissection. The incision is continued along both temporal regions until complete. **D1,** Blunt dissection proceeds rapidly and bloodlessly in the subgaleal/supraperiosteal plane. **D2,** Pericranial flaps are developed as a separate layer. Subperiosteal dissection is continued below the temporalis musculature. Exposure of the cranio-orbital region including the upper three-fourths of the orbits and the nasofrontal region is accomplished easily through a coronal scalp flap.

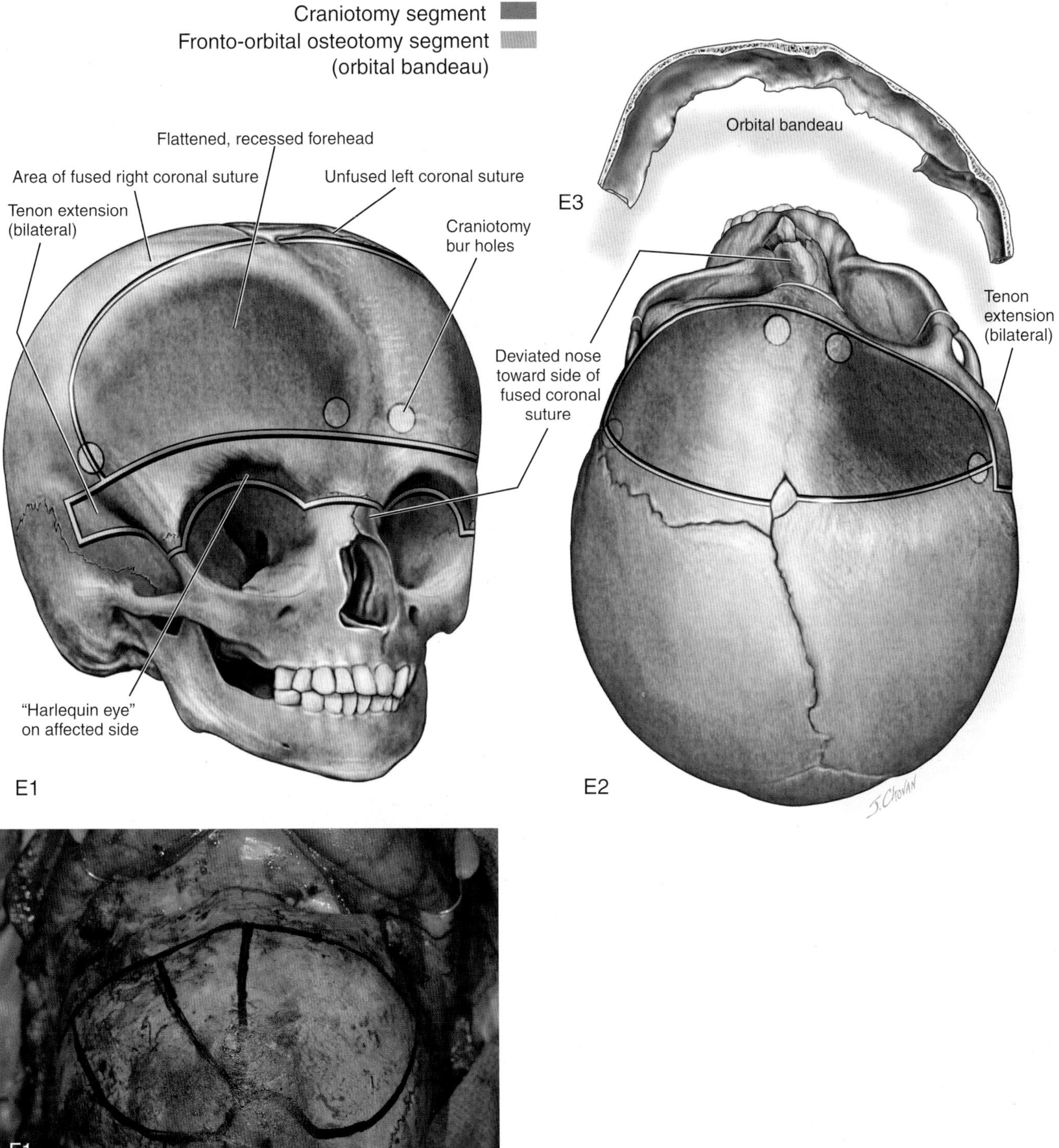

Figure 46.2, cont'd **E,** Illustration of the fronto-orbital advancement procedure markings for a patient with unilateral coronal craniosynostosis. **E1,** Markings for a fronto-orbital advancement procedure include the bandeau segment *(blue)* and bifrontal craniotomy *(purple)*. **E2,** Bird's-eye view. **E3,** Orbital bandeau segment. **F1,** Bird's eye view of planned craniotomy.

Continued

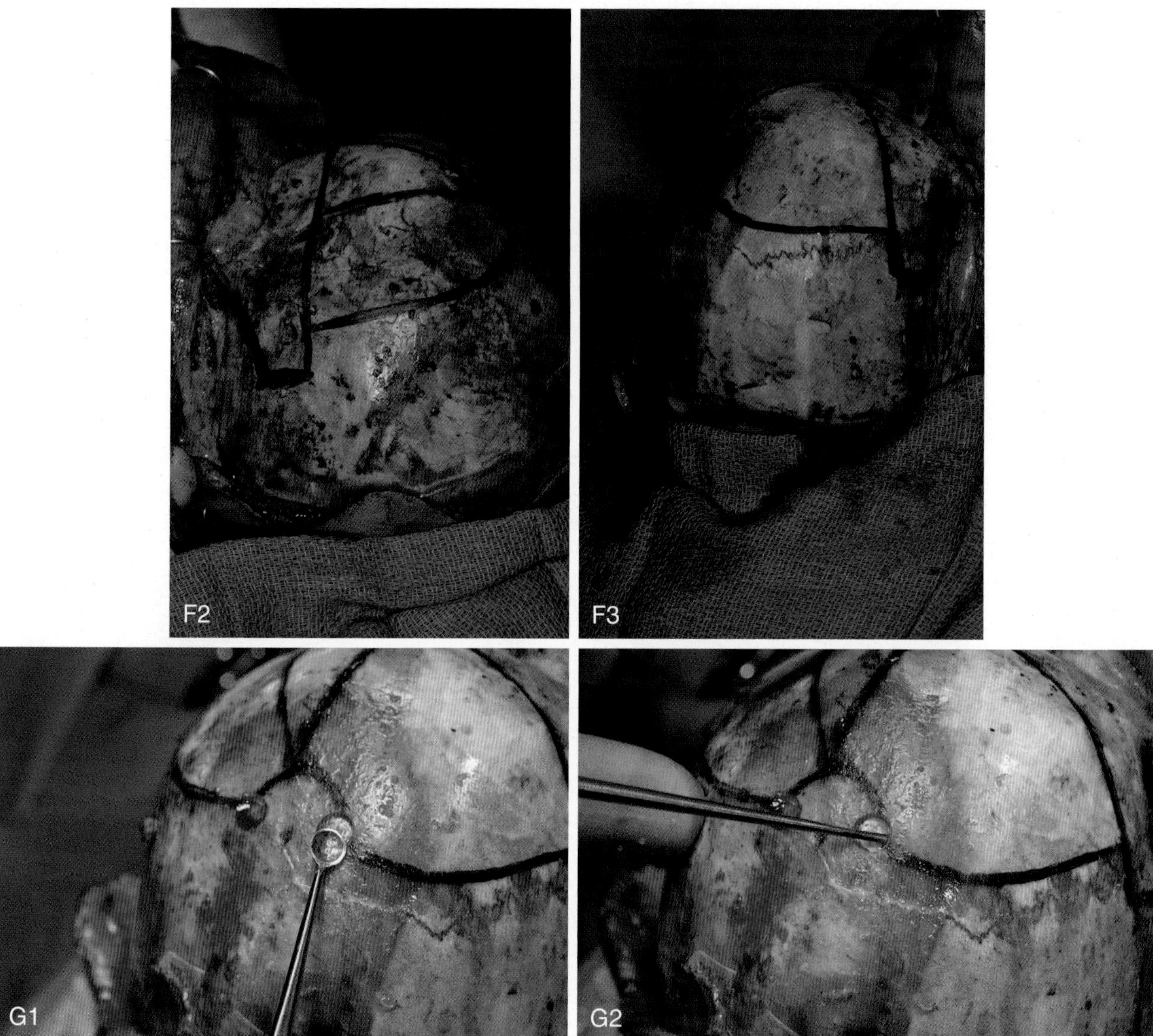

Figure 46.2, cont'd **F2** and **F3,** Side views of orbital bandeau tenon extensions. **G1** and **G2,** Bur holes are created to allow access to the epidural space. The dura is then separated from the overlying bone using a Penfield #1 elevator initially. A curved Penfield #4 elevator is also useful for stripping the dura from the overlying cranial vault. This minimizes the risk of dural tear during the craniotomy procedure.

TECHNIQUE: Fronto-Orbital Advancement and Anterior Cranial Vault Reshaping—cont'd

STEP 6: Fronto-Orbital Osteotomy

An osteotomy is started through the lateral orbital rim at the inferior extent of the bandeau. In general, the inferior extent of this cut is placed approximately half of the distance of the lateral orbital rim. In children less than 6 months of age, the inferior position of this bone cut is located at the zygomaticofrontal suture. The osteotomy is then carried superiorly along the lateral orbital wall and orbital roof. The osteotomy is continued along the tenon extension.

Next, the osteotomy is continued through the orbital roof. A reciprocating saw is used to continue the osteotomy from its lateral extent and it is carried, through a transcranial approach, across the roof to the medial orbital wall.

The exact procedure is then carried out for the contralateral orbit. Care is taken to maintain symmetric osteotomies for the construction of a symmetric orbital bandeau.

The final osteotomy in completion of the bandeau is a nasofrontal osteotomy. This connects the two medial orbital wall oste-

TECHNIQUE: Fronto-Orbital Advancement and Anterior Cranial Vault Reshaping—cont'd

otomies and allows for dismantling/removal of the bandeau segment. The reciprocating saw is placed at the inferior extent of the previous medial orbital wall osteotomy on one side (right or left) and then used to create an osteotomy across the nasofrontal area to the contralateral medial orbital wall osteotomy. This completes the bandeau and allows it to be removed as one bony segment (Fig. 46.2H and I).

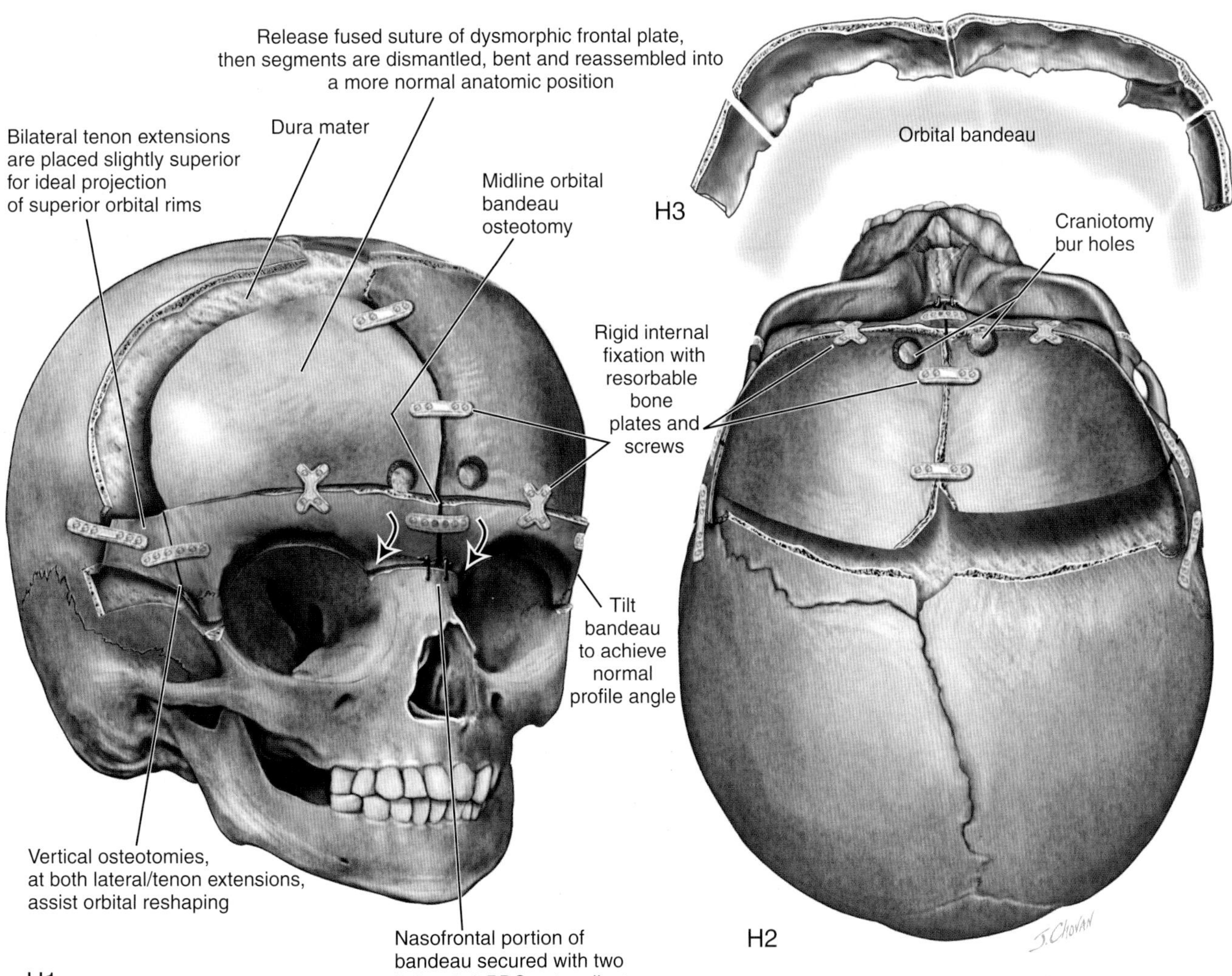

Reconstruction of Unilateral Coronal Synostosis
Craniotomy segment
Fronto-orbital osteotomy segment (orbital bandeau)
Release fused suture of dysmorphic frontal plate, then segments are dismantled, bent and reassembled into a more normal anatomic position
Dura mater
Bilateral tenon extensions are placed slightly superior for ideal projection of superior orbital rims
Midline orbital bandeau osteotomy
Orbital bandeau
H3
Craniotomy bur holes
Rigid internal fixation with resorbable bone plates and screws
Tilt bandeau to achieve normal profile angle
Vertical osteotomies, at both lateral/tenon extensions, assist orbital reshaping
Nasofrontal portion of bandeau secured with two 2-0 or 3-0 PDS suture ligatures
H1
H2

Figure 46.2, cont'd **H1** and **H2,** Illustration of the fronto-orbital advancement procedure reconstruction and rigid internal fixation for a patient with unilateral coronal craniosynostosis. Fixation for a fronto-orbital advancement procedure. Bird's-eye view of skeletal movements. Osteotomies and reshaping of bandeau segment. *PDS*, Polydioxanone.

Continued

TECHNIQUE: Fronto-Orbital Advancement and Anterior Cranial Vault Reshaping—cont'd

STEP 7: Orbital Reshaping

The orbital bandeau segment is then taken to a sterile back table where it is measured, cut, and contoured into a more normal anatomic shape. Osteotomies are generally carried out at the midline and may be combined with additional vertical osteotomies at each lateral orbital/tenon extension. This further dismantling of the dysmorphic skeleton allows for advancement of the orbital structures on the affected side (Fig. 46.2J and Fig. 46.2H3).

STEP 8: Bandeau Placement

The bandeau is then placed into final position. The lateral tenon extensions are placed slightly superior to their original position in order to achieve ideal projection of the superior orbital rims. Rigid internal fixation is applied at each lateral tenon extension with resorbable bone plates and screws. In addition, the nasofrontal portion of the bandeau is secured with wire or suture ligatures to prevent superior displacement when the coronal scalp flap is resuspended. The authors prefer to use two 2-0 or 3-0 polydioxanone sutures passed through the bandeau and secured to the nasal bones (Fig. 46.2K).

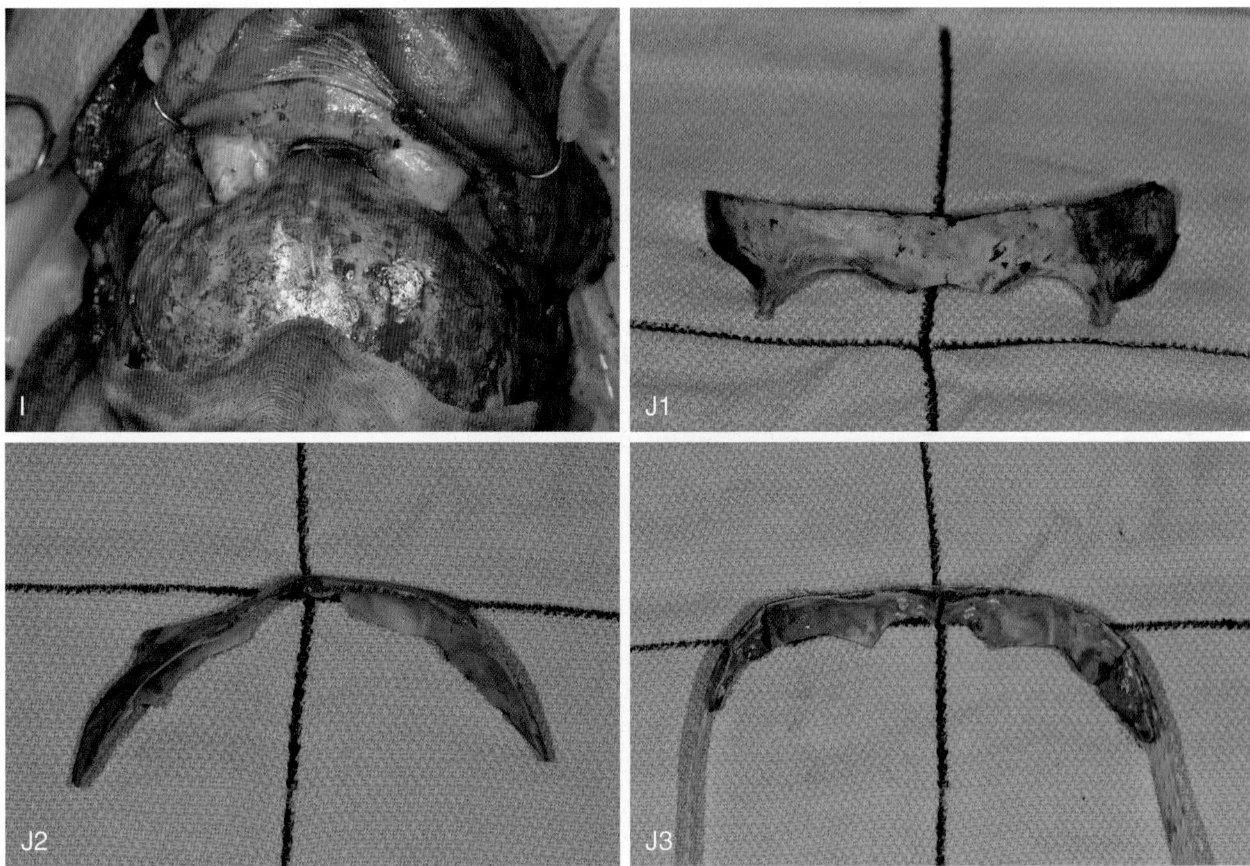

Figure 46.2, cont'd **I,** Dysmorphic skeletal components (e.g., frontal bone and bilateral orbital bandeau segment) have been dismantled. **J1–J3,** The orbital bandeau is taken to a sterile back table where it is further osteotomized, contoured with bone benders, and reconstituted into a more normal anatomic morphology. Resorbable rigid fixation is applied to the bony segments.

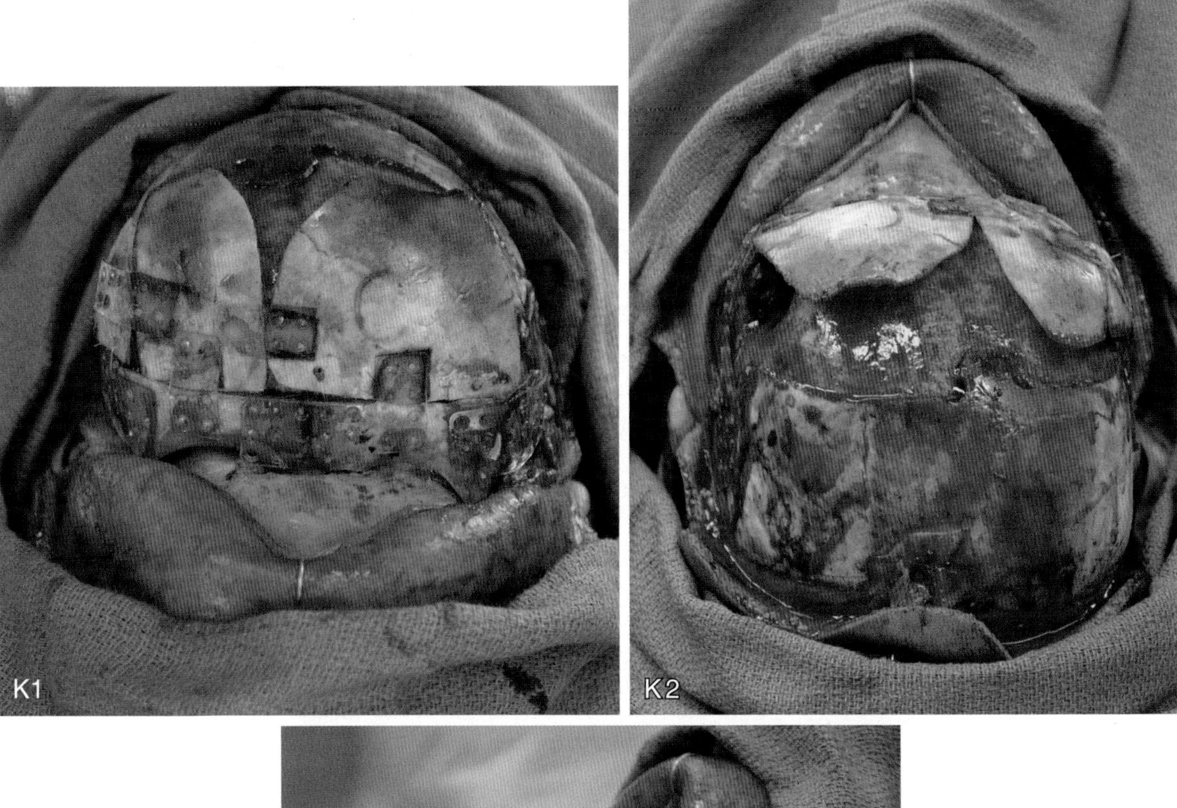

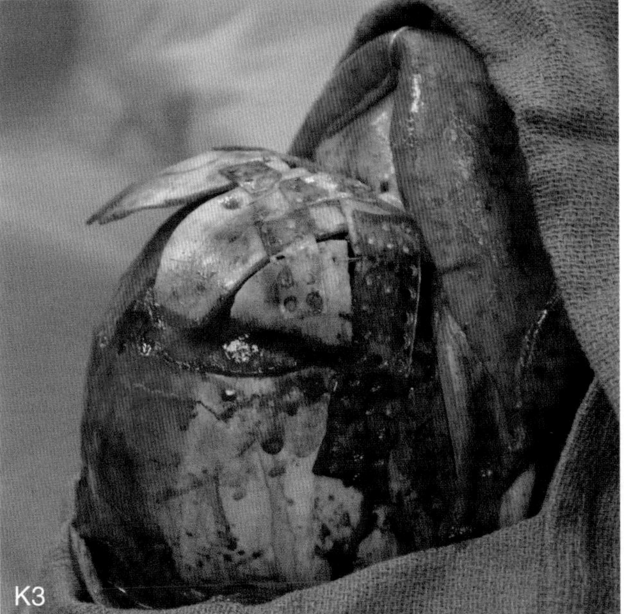

Figure 46.2, cont'd **K1–K3,** The reconstructed bandeau is then placed into final anatomic position and stabilized before the frontal bone segments are further osteotomized, contoured, and fixated in a corrected anatomic position. Intraoperative views of the fixated bandeau with resorbable fixation along the tenon extensions and suture stabilization at the nasofrontal junction, and anterior cranial vault reshaping.

Continued

TECHNIQUE: Fronto-Orbital Advancement and Anterior Cranial Vault Reshaping—cont'd

STEP 9: Frontal Bone Reshaping

The bifrontal craniotomy bone flap is then further osteotomized, contoured with bone-bending forceps, and reassembled into a more normal anatomic contour and position. The degree of morselization depends on the degree of asymmetry and the extent of the deformity, and it is customized for each patient. Additional mesh, bone plates, and monocortical screws from the resorbable rigid fixation system are used to secure the reconstructed frontal bone segments. Care must be taken when utilizing a drill during reconstruction of the anterior vault. A malleable retractor should be inserted under the bone flaps being secured to prevent inadvertent brain/dural injury during drilling/tapping for screw insertion.

STEP 10: Closure

The reconstructed bones and operative field are then irrigated thoroughly with normal saline. Closure is initiated with the pericranial flaps, which are loosely approximated/suspended and secured with interrupted 3-0 Vicryl sutures. The coronal scalp flap is replaced, and the galea and subcutaneous tissues are closed with additional 3-0 Vicryl sutures placed in an inverted, interrupted fashion. Skin closure is generally carried out with 4-0 Vicryl Rapide or 5-0 Monocryl placed in a continuous fashion.

At the completion of the procedure and closure, blood will have accumulated within the potential space created from subgaleal dissection. Subgaleal oozing from the flap and bone edges is usually limited and resolves quickly. Edema may contribute to the fluctuant appearance of the flap and periorbital swelling, both of which tend to peak at approximately 48 hours following the procedure. Subgaleal drains may be placed and passed out through the posterior edge of the coronal flap, but they are optional. The authors do not place drains routinely when carrying out fronto-orbital advancement for coronal or metopic suture craniosynostosis.

The hair and scalp are washed with a gentle shampoo and warm saline at the conclusion of surgery, and a circumferential Kerlix head dressing may be placed if desired (Fig. 46.2L).

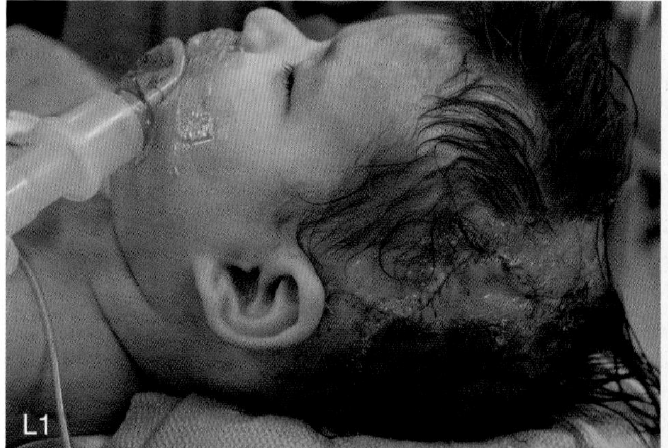

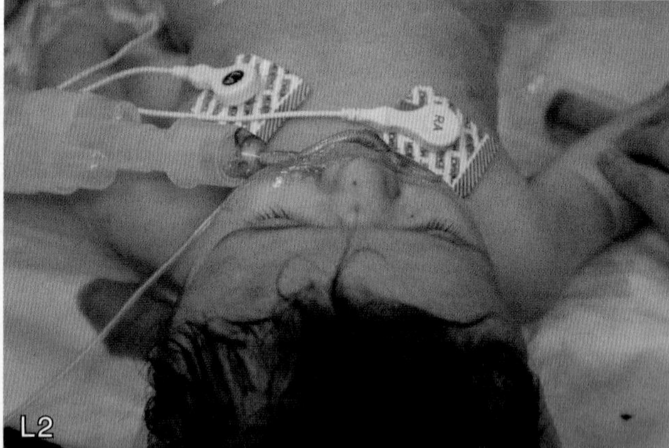

Figure 46.2, cont'd **L1** and **L2,** Closure of the coronal scalp flap. The wound is irrigated with copious amounts of antibiotic-containing normal saline. The pericranium is loosely approximated with air knot sutures of 3-0 Vicryl. The scalp is approximated, and closure is carried out using inverted interrupted 3-0 Vicryl sutures for repair of the galea and subcutaneous tissues and a finer, resorbable suture for the skin placed in continuous fashion. The hair is washed with a gentle shampoo, and antibiotic ointment is applied to the incision line.

TECHNIQUE: Fronto-Orbital Advancement and Anterior Cranial Vault Reshaping—cont'd

Metopic Suture Craniosynostosis

Fronto-orbital advancement and anterior cranial vault reconstruction are carried out in a manner similar to the above description for patients with metopic suture craniosynostosis. Patients with fusion of the metopic suture present with a characteristic dysmorphology that is the result of arrested development perpendicular to the metopic suture and compensatory overgrowth at the coronal sutures, which remain open. This creates a trigonocephalic skull shape, orbital hypotelorism, and horizontally retrusive lateral orbital rim segments. Successful correction requires bifrontal craniotomy, similar osteotomies for dismantling and reshaping of the orbital bandeau segment, and anterior cranial vault reconstruction (Fig. 46.2M and N).

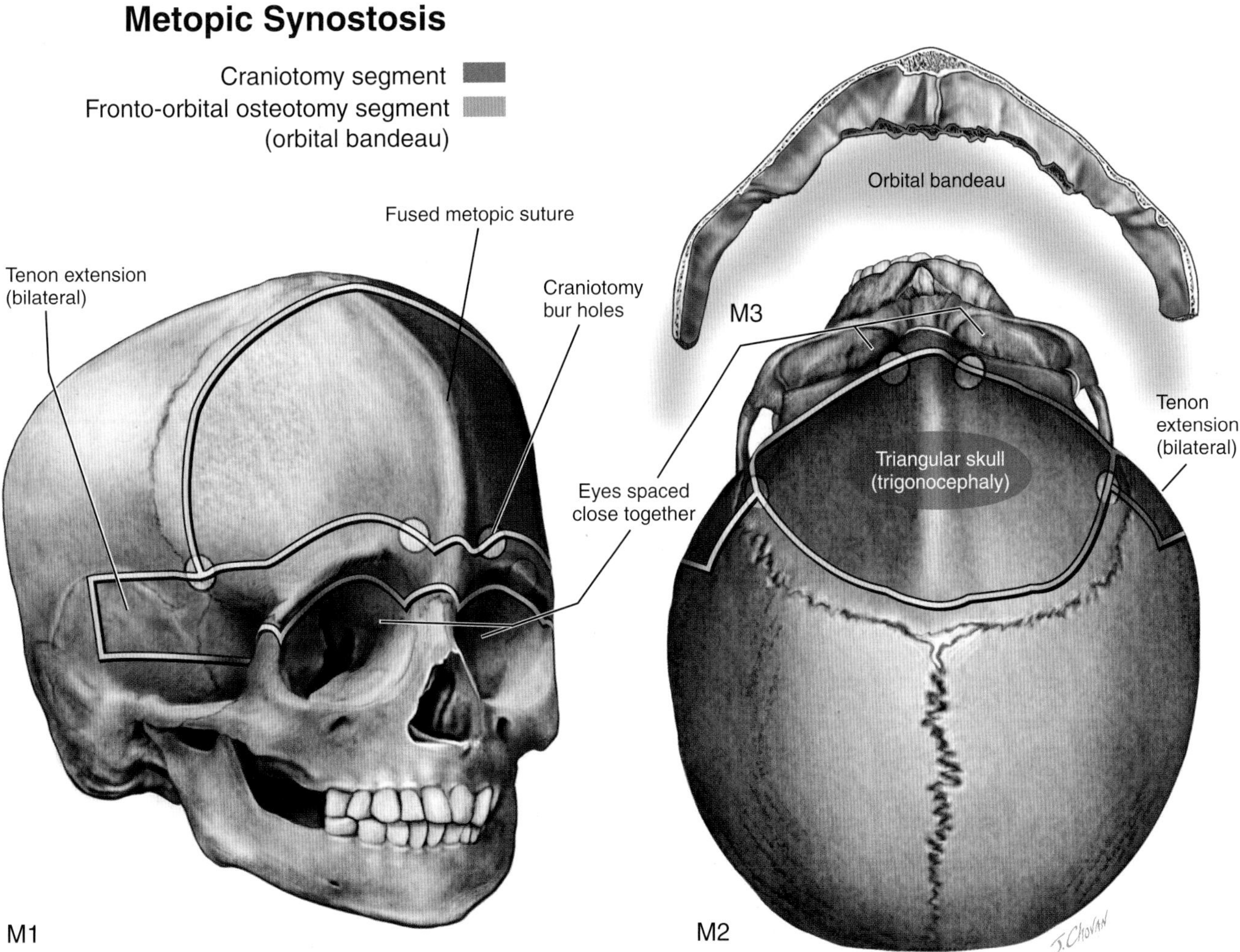

Figure 46.2, cont'd M, Illustration of the fronto-orbital advancement procedure for a patient with metopic craniosynostosis. **M1,** Markings for a fronto-orbital advancement procedure include the bandeau segment *(blue)* and bifrontal craniotomy *(purple)*. **M2,** Bird's-eye view. **M3,** Orbital bandeau.

Continued

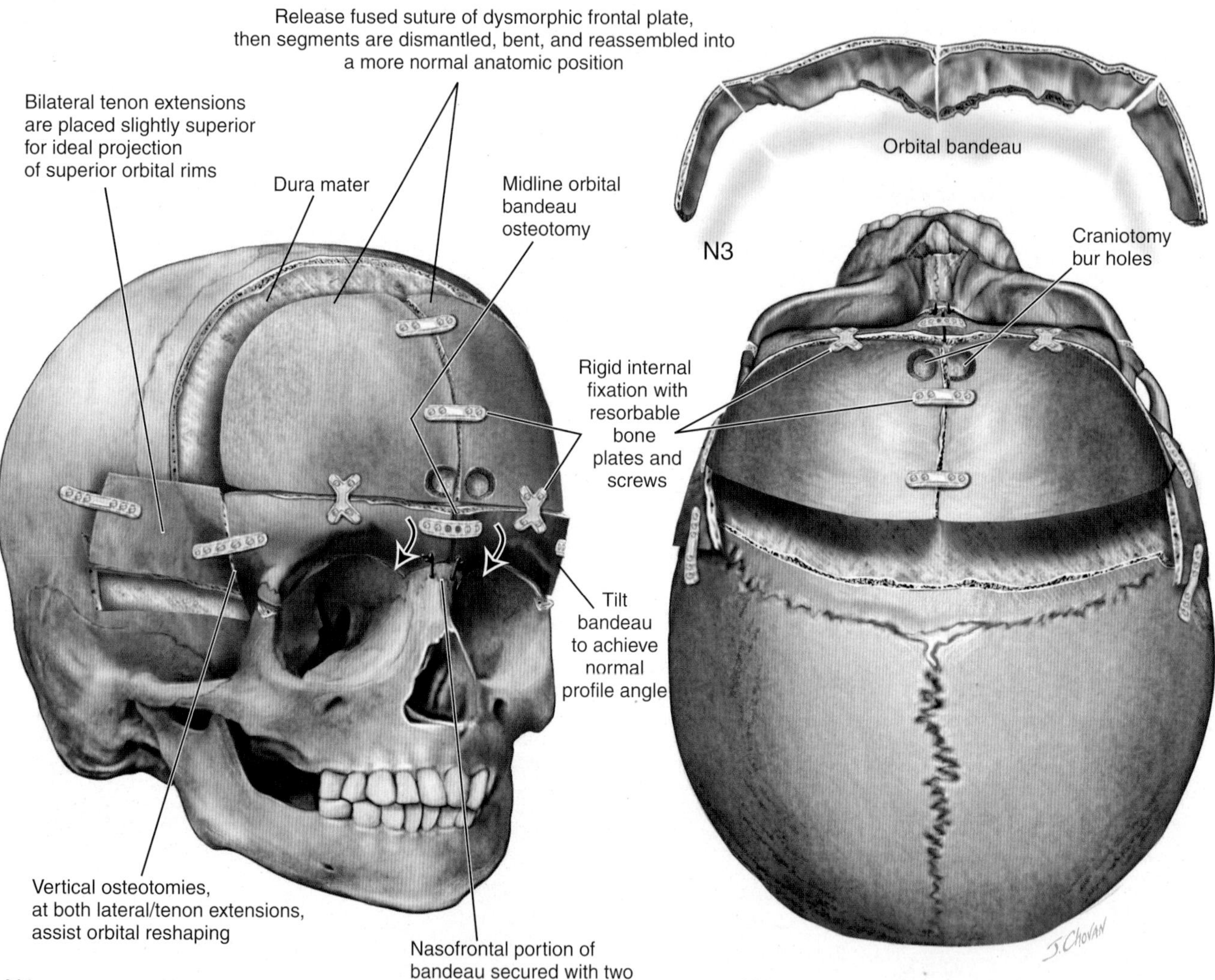
Reconstruction of
Metopic Synostosis
Craniotomy segment
Fronto-orbital osteotomy segment
(orbital bandeau)
Release fused suture of dysmorphic frontal plate, then segments are dismantled, bent, and reassembled into a more normal anatomic position
Bilateral tenon extensions are placed slightly superior for ideal projection of superior orbital rims
Dura mater
Midline orbital bandeau osteotomy
Orbital bandeau
N3
Craniotomy bur holes
Rigid internal fixation with resorbable bone plates and screws
Tilt bandeau to achieve normal profile angle
Vertical osteotomies, at both lateral/tenon extensions, assist orbital reshaping
Nasofrontal portion of bandeau secured with two 2-0 or 3-0 PDS suture ligatures
N1
N2
J. Chovan

Figure 46.2, cont'd **N,** Illustration of the fronto-orbital advancement reconstruction for a patient with metopic craniosynostosis. **N1,** Osteotomies and rigid internal fixation for a fronto-orbital advancement procedure include the bandeau segment *(blue)* and bifrontal craniotomy *(purple)*. *PDS*, Polydioxanone. **N2,** Bird's-eye view of skeletal movements and rigid internal fixation. **N3,** Osteotomies and reshaping of trigonocephalic bandeau segment.

ALTERNATIVE TECHNIQUE 1: Hemi-Bandeau

Modifications of the fronto-orbital advancement include two specific methods. First, although not routinely recommended, instead of removing the entire fronto-orbital unit, the osteotomy may proceed unilaterally on the affected side. In this case, the surgeon stops the osteotomy of the bandeau in the midline and, using a reciprocating saw with brain protection, proceeds to make a vertical osteotomy from the superior para-midline aspect of the bandeau to the para-midline side of the nasofrontal junction on the affected side. The affected unilateral bandeau is then removed as described earlier, and reshaping and replacement proceed as previously described. The authors note with caution that craniosynostosis is a bilateral problem even if a unilateral suture is affected. This is secondary to the compensatory change that occurs on the unaffected side secondary to growth. This technique is best reserved for minimal cases of compensatory overgrowth in unilateral coronal craniosynostosis or when the technique is used for the management of unilateral pathologic lesions affecting the skull base or orbital roof.

ALTERNATIVE TECHNIQUE 2: Modified Lateral Canthal Advancement

Some surgeons will decide to not disarticulate the fronto-orbital unit from the nasofrontal junction. This has the advantage of not allowing superior rotation of the bandeau with redraping of the scalp flap. As described previously, the preferred method for managing this problem is to use suture to secure this area when the bandeau is replaced after being completely removed. This allows for a more precise reshaping of the dysmorphology when the bandeau is completely disarticulated.

If the bandeau is to be left attached to the nasofrontal junction, the surgeon does not cross the midline of the anterior skull base and ends the osteotomy after leaving the medial orbital wall, stopping just short of the crista galli with the reciprocating saw. In the infant with relatively "soft" bone, bone-bending forceps are then used to advance each side of the bandeau forward. The segments are effectively "greenstick"-fractured. There is a risk of completely fracturing the bandeau as this is carried out, and force must not be applied disproportionately. If this occurs, resorbable fixation is used to secure the segments back together before proceeding. After this process has been carried out, the bandeau appears as a "gull wing" shape from above with extension of the tenon segments laterally from the temporal bone. The surgeon next utilizes bone-bending forceps or makes an osteotomy at the most anterior portion of the tenon extension where it meets the lateral orbital rim and repositions the tenon segments posteriorly back into the tenon groove. Each side of the bandeau is independently advanced and secured to achieve the necessary advancement and symmetry of the fronto-orbital unit.

ALTERNATIVE TECHNIQUE 3: Endoscopic or Limited Access

Limited access techniques for suture craniectomy have gained popularity among some craniofacial surgeons for cases involving metopic and coronal suture craniosynostosis. Although release of the involved cranial vault suture is possible using an endoscopically assisted method, the technique does not allow any access to the cranial base, and there is no dismantling of the dysmorphic orbital structures. Instead, there is a limited amount of improvement in the morphology as a result of subsequent brain growth, which drives postoperative remodeling.

When an endoscopic approach is used, the surgical procedure is carried out to release the fused suture, and a custom cranial orthosis (band or helmet) is then used during the postoperative period to reshape the dysmorphic fronto-orbital structures. Because cranial orthotic devices work best when there is rapid brain growth, endoscopic procedures are usually carried out earlier in life, typically prior to 4 months of age. Patients are placed into a cranial orthotic device within 2 weeks of surgery, and the correction may require the use of three or four helmets used over a 9- to 12-month period.

The authors' preferred approach for metopic and coronal suture craniosynostosis involves formal reconstruction using a fronto-orbital advancement and anterior cranial vault reconstruction, as this allows for complete access to the affected skull base, dismantling of the involved skeletal components, and adequate repositioning/reshaping in one surgical procedure. We have found the application of endoscopically assisted procedures to be more appropriate and predictable in cases where the sutures of the posterior cranial vault (sagittal or lambdoid) are affected.

Avoidance and Management of Intraoperative Complications

In addition to the general complications (e.g., swelling, infection, pain) that may be associated with any craniofacial procedure, there are a number of specific complications, intraoperative challenges, and complications particularly relevant to fronto-orbital advancement and anterior cranial vault reconstruction.

Safe craniosynostosis surgery requires that the surgical and anesthetic team pay particular attention to the management of intraoperative blood loss. Because surgery is carried out prior to the first year of life, the infant's total blood volume is relatively small. Appropriately typed and cross-matched units of blood must be available in the operating room prior to commencing surgery. Strict attention to opening the scalp in layers and the placement of bone wax or Gelfoam with topical thrombin can also limit blood loss. Additionally, these maneuvers also minimize the risk of air embolus.

Significant attention must be directed to protecting the eyes. In addition to the possibility of corneal abrasions, the surgeons must also defend the orbital contents during osteotomy. An assistant must be assigned with a malleable retractor to both protect the eye during osteotomy and to guide the surgeon, who is working transcranially, to the appropriate saw blade position and saw blade depth during the osteotomy across the skull base. Inordinate amounts of pressure by the surgeon or the assistant retracting on the eye can instigate the oculocardiac reflex. The resultant bradycardia in an infant with surgically induced hypervolemia can be disastrous if not managed aggressively. Likewise, the brain must also be protected during the osteotomy from above to prevent dural tearing and brain injury. Special consideration must be given to patients with craniofacial dysostosis, especially with Apert syndrome. In this select group of patients, herniation of the temporal lobe can occur forward into the orbital space. As a result, the lateral orbit in these children can be extremely shallow, and temporal lobe injury can occur if not adequately dissected and retracted posteriorly during osteotomy.[24–38]

Postoperative Considerations

The postoperative care of the infant who has undergone fronto-orbital advancement with anterior cranial vault reconstruction is similar to that of the age-matched patient undergoing craniotomy for any diagnosis.

Admission to the pediatric intensive care unit is mandatory. It is invaluable and necessary to also seek the assistance of the dedicated pediatric intensivist for postoperative care. Although the patients are routinely extubated at the conclusion of surgery, the potential for significant neurologic, respiratory, and cardiac events exists. Routinely, the patients should have both hemoglobin and serum sodium checked during the first 24 hours postoperatively. Intravenous antibiotics are given postoperatively for 48 hours following surgery. The stable postoperative craniosynostosis surgery patient usually can be transferred from the pediatric intensive care unit to the floor 24 hours postoperatively.

References

1. Lane LC. Pioneer craniectomy for relief of mental imbecility due to premature suture fusion and microcephalus. *J Am Med Assoc.* 1892;18:49.
2. Lannelogue M. De la Craniectomie dans la Microcephalie. *C R Acad Sci.* 1890;110:1382.
3. Rougerie J, Derome P, Anquez L. Craniosténoses et dysmorphies cranio-faciales. Principes d'une nouvelle technique de traitement et ses résultats. *Neurochirurgie.* 1972;18(5):429–440.
4. Hoffman HJ, Mohr G. Lateral canthal advancement of the supraorbital margin. A new corrective technique in the treatment of coronal synostosis. *J Neurosurg.* 1976;45(4):376–381.
5. Whitaker LA, Schut L, Kerr LP. Early surgery for craniofacial dysostosis. *Plast Reconstr Surg.* 1977;91:977.
6. Marchac D, Renier D. "Le front flottant." Traitement précoce des facio-craniosténoses. *Ann Chir Plast.* 1979;24(2):121–126.
7. Eppley BL. Resorbable biotechnology for craniomaxillofacial surgery. *J Craniofac Surg.* 1997;8(2):85–86.
8. Jimenez DF, Barone CM. Endoscopic techniques for craniosynostosis. *Atlas Oral Maxillofac Surg Clin North Am.* 2010;18(2):93–107.
9. Virchow R. Uber den cretinismus, nametlich in Franken, under uber pathologische. *Schadelformen Verk Phys Med Gesellsch Wurszburg.* 1851;2:230.
10. Turvey TA, Gudeman SK. Nonsyndromic craniosynostosis. In: Turvey TA, Vig KWL, Fonseca RJ, eds. *Facial Clefts and Craniosynostosis: Principles and Management.* Philadelphia, Pennsylvania: WB Saunders; 1996.
11. Renier D. Intracranial pressure in craniosynostosis: pre- and postoperative recordings. Correlation with functional results. In: Persing JA, Jane JA, Edgerton MT, eds. *Scientific Foundations and Surgical Treatment of Craniosynostosis.* Baltimore, Maryland: Williams & Wilkins; 1989.
12. Renier D, Sainte-Rose C, Marchac D, Hirsch JF. Intracranial pressure in craniostenosis. *J Neurosurg.* 1982;57(3):370–377.
13. Siddiqi SN, Posnick JC, Buncic R, et al. The detection and management of intracranial hypertension after initial suture release and decompression for craniofacial dysostosis syndromes. *Neurosurgery.* 1995;36(4):703–708.
14. Turvey TA, Ruiz RL. Craniosynostosis and craniofacial dysostosis. In: Fonseca RJ, Baker SB, Wolford LM, eds. *Oral and Maxillofacial Surgery.* Philadelphia, Pennsylvania: WB Saunders; 2000.
15. Posnick JC. Craniofacial dysostosis syndromes: a staged reconstructive approach. In: Turvey TA, Vig KWL, Fonseca RJ, eds. *Facial Clefts and Craniosynostosis: Principles and Management.* Philadelphia, Pennsylvania: WB Saunders; 1996.
16. Golabi M, Edwards MSB, Ousterhout DK. Craniosynostosis and hydrocephalus. *Neurosurgery.* 1987;21(1):63–67.
17. Hogan GR, Bauman ML. Hydrocephalus in Apert's syndrome. *J Pediatr.* 1971;79(5):782–787.
18. Gorlin RJ, Cohen MM Jr, Levin LS. In: *Syndromes of the Head and Neck.* 3rd ed. New York, New York: Oxford University Press; 1990.
19. Enlow DH, McNamara JA Jr. The neurocranial basis for facial form and pattern. *Angle Orthod.* 1973;43(3):256–270.
20. Friede H, Lilja J, Andersson H, Johanson B. Growth of the anterior cranial base after craniotomy in infants with premature synostosis of the coronal suture. *Scand J Plast Reconstr Surg.* 1983;17(2):99–108.

21. Marsh JL, Vannier MW. The "third" dimension in craniofacial surgery. *Plast Reconstr Surg.* 1983;71(6):759–767.
22. Marchac D. Radical forehead remodeling for craniostenosis. *Plast Reconstr Surg.* 1978;61(6):823–835.
23. Marchac D, Renier D, Jones BM. Experience with the "floating forehead." *Br J Plast Surg.* 1988;41(1):1–15.
24. Posnick JC. The craniofacial dysostosis syndrome: current reconstructive strategies. In: current concepts in craniofacial surgery. *Clin Plast Surg.* 1994;21:585.
25. Kreiborg S. Crouzon syndrome. A clinical and roentgencephalometric study. [Thesis (Disputats)]. *Scand J Plast Reconstr Surg.* 1981;18(suppl):198.
26. Posnick JC, Farkas LG. The application of anthropometric surface measurements in craniomaxillofacial surgery. In: Farkas LG, ed. *Anthropometry of the Head and Face.* New York, New York: Raven Press; 1994.
27. Whitaker LA, Munro IR, Salyer KE, Jackson IT, Ortiz-Monasterio F, Marchac D. Combined report of problems and complications in 793 craniofacial operations. *Plast Reconstr Surg.* 1979;64(2):198–203.
28. David DJ, Cooter RD. Craniofacial infection in 10 years of transcranial surgery. *Plast Reconstr Surg.* 1987;80(2):213–225.
29. Posnick JC. Craniosynostosis: surgical management in infancy. In: Bell WH, ed. *Orthognathic and Reconstructive Surgery.* Philadelphia, Pennsylvania: WB Saunders; 1992.
30. Posnick JC. Brachycephaly: bilateral coronal synostosis without midface deficiency. In: Posnick JC, ed. *Craniofacial and Maxillofacial Surgery in Children and Young Adults.* Philadelphia, Pennsylvania: WB Saunders; 2000.
31. Posnick JC. Crouzon syndrome: evaluation and staging of reconstruction. In: Posnick JC, ed. *Craniofacial and Maxillofacial Surgery in Children and Young Adults.* Philadelphia, Pennsylvania: WB Saunders; 2000.
32. Posnick JC, Ruiz RL. The craniofacial dysostosis syndromes: current surgical thinking and future directions. *Cleft Palate Craniofac J.* 2000;37(5):433.
33. Tessier P. Ostéotomies totales de la face. Syndrome de Crouzon, syndrme d'Apert: oxycéphalies, scaphocéphalies, turricéphalies. *Ann Chir Plast.* 1967;12(4):273–286.
34. Tessier P. Dysostoses cranio-faciales (syndromes de Crouzon et d'Apert): osteotomies totales de la face. In: *Transactions of the Fourth International Congress of Plastic and Reconstructive Surgery.* Amsterdam, Netherlands; 1969.
35. Cohen MM Jr. Transforming growth factor beta s and fibroblast growth factors and their receptors: role in sutural biology and craniosynostosis. *J Bone Miner Res.* 1997;12(3):322–331.
36. Posnick JC. Apert syndrome: evaluation and staging of reconstruction. In: Posnick JC, ed. *Craniofacial and Maxillofacial Surgery in Children and Young Adults.* Philadelphia, Pennsylvania: WB Saunders; 2000.
37. Posnick JC. Craniofacial dysostosis. Staging of reconstruction and management of the midface deformity. *Neurosurg Clin N Am.* 1991;2(3):683–702.
38. Cohen MM Jr, ed. *Craniosynostosis: Diagnosis, Evaluation, and Management.* New York, New York: Raven Press; 1986.

CHAPTER 47

Posterior Cranial Vault Remodeling

Douglas P. Sinn, Rahul Tandon, and Paul S. Tiwana

Armamentarium

#9 Periosteal elevator
#10 and #15 blade scalpel
Appropriate sutures
Bipolar electrocautery
Craniotome/perforator
Fine spatula osteotome
Local anesthetic with vasoconstrictor
Malleable retractors
Mayfield horseshoe headrest
Needle electrocautery
Raney clips
Reciprocating saw/blade
Resorbable plate and screw fixation system
Rib bender
Rongeurs

History of the Procedure

Posterior cranial vault remodeling is used primarily to treat infants and children with cranial deformities secondary to sagittal or lambdoid synostosis. Virchow first defined the term craniosynostosis in 1851. In its most basic form, craniosynostosis is a malformation in which one or more sutures of the cranial vault are prematurely fused. Virchow noted that this synostosis of the skull restricted growth perpendicular to the direction of the involved suture and promoted compensatory cranial overgrowth parallel to it.

The earliest recorded surgical attempts to treat craniosynostosis were performed by Lannelongue[1] in Paris in 1890 and shortly thereafter, in 1892, by Lane[2] in San Francisco. Strip craniectomies were performed on fused sagittal sutures to alleviate compression within the cranial vault. Synostosis treatment evolved considerably over the ensuring year and was revolutionized by the innovative techniques introduced by Tessier et al.[3,4] in 1967. Later, in 1972, Rougerie et al.[5] applied Tessier's concepts of simultaneous suture release and cranial vault reshaping in infants, and in 1977, Whitaker et al.[6] described a more formal anterior cranial vault remodeling and orbital reshaping procedure for unilateral coronal synostosis.

The current treatment for infants and children with moderate to severe deformities secondary to synostosis revolves around comprehensive open treatment with suture release, in conjunction with cranial remodeling to allow the brain to grow without restriction and to establish more normal contours of the craniofacial complex. In most cases, an intracranial approach is used to perform cranial vault and orbital osteotomies, which are reshaped and advanced to establish an ideal age-appropriate morphology.

Indications for the Use of the Procedure

Posterior cranial vault remodeling is indicated for correction of cranial malformation associated with sagittal suture synostosis or lambdoid suture synostosis. When planning the time and type of surgical intervention, the surgeon must take into account future craniofacial growth and development and the maintenance of a normal appearance. Diagnosis of craniosynostosis is based on clinical and radiographic evaluation. The clinical examination involves palpating the skull for any areas of movement, ridging, and the presence or absence of the anterior or posterior fontanelles. A high-resolution computed tomography scan and three-dimensional reconstruction of the craniofacial complex are routinely used to evaluate the extent and location of involved sutures and to plan any surgical treatment (Fig. 47.1).

In patients with sagittal suture synostosis, the skull typically has an anterior-posterior elongation with a compensatory narrowing in the transverse dimension (Fig. 47.2). This is the most common form of cranial vault synostosis, accounting for approximately 50% of cases of nonsyndromic, single-suture synostosis in the United States.[7] Children show different degrees of cranial deformity, depending on the extent of sutural involvement. They present with involvement of the anterior, posterior, or entire sagittal suture. When the posterior half of the sagittal suture is synostosed, the posterior two-thirds of the cranial vault is reshaped with the patient in the prone position. If the entire sagittal suture is synostosed, the child usually is treated in a staged manner, first undergoing posterior vault reconstruction and then anterior vault and orbital reconstruction 6 to 8 weeks later.

Lambdoid synostosis results in flatness of the affected ipsilateral parietal-occipital region. Clinically, the location of the ear canal and external ear are more posterior and inferior on the ipsilateral side than the contralateral side. This is more noticeable when the patient is examined from the superior aspect and relatively inconspicuous from fontal or profile views. Posterior plagiocephaly secondary to lambdoid synostosis must not be mistaken for positional or deformational plagiocephaly secondary to infant positioning or molding. With positional plagiocephaly, the ipsilateral ear and forehead are positioned anteriorly, and the ear is not inferiorly displaced, as it is with true lambdoid fusion. The overall incidence of true unilateral lambdoid synostosis cases is less than 3% of all isolated cases in the United States, with some studies demonstrating an incidence of less than 1 in 40,000 live births.[8,9] In the surgical treatment of this deformity, the patient's dysmorphic posterior vault is remodeled bilaterally, with the patient in the prone position, to a more symmetric and ideal age-appropriate shape.

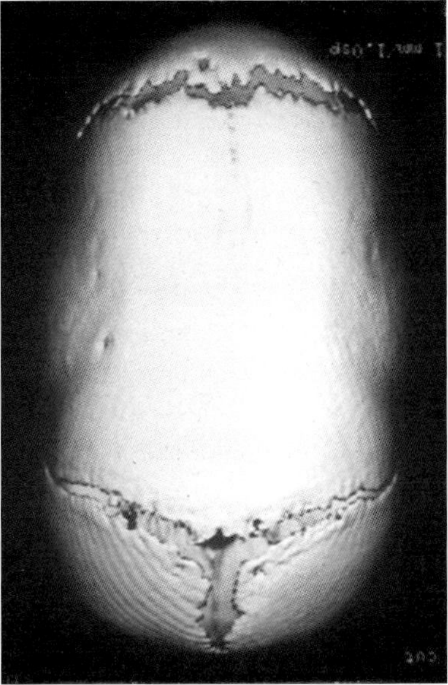

Figure 47.1 Three-dimensional computed tomography reconstruction of a child with sagittal synostosis.

Brain volume expansion in the normally developing child almost triples during the first year of life. If unimpeded brain growth is to occur, open sutures at the level of the cranial vault must expand outward during this phase of growth. When premature suture closure is combined with continued development, the growth potential of the brain may be physically limited. Surgical intervention, with suture release and cranial vault reshaping, is undertaken to restore normal intracranial volume.

Restricted cranial volume secondary to craniosynostosis can also result in elevated intracranial pressure (ICP). Normal ICP is defined as 0 to 15 mm Hg; elevated ICP occurs when the pressure exceeds 15 mm Hg. Renier et al.[10,11] measured the ICP in 121 children and found that elevated ICP occurred in 42% of children with multisuture involvement and in 13% with single-suture involvement. They also noted a decrease in ICP after corrective surgery. If elevated ICP goes untreated for a prolonged period, detrimental effects on brain function may result; therefore, increased ICP is an important indicator for surgical treatment. Children should also be monitored for additional ophthalmologic sequelae. Untreated elevated

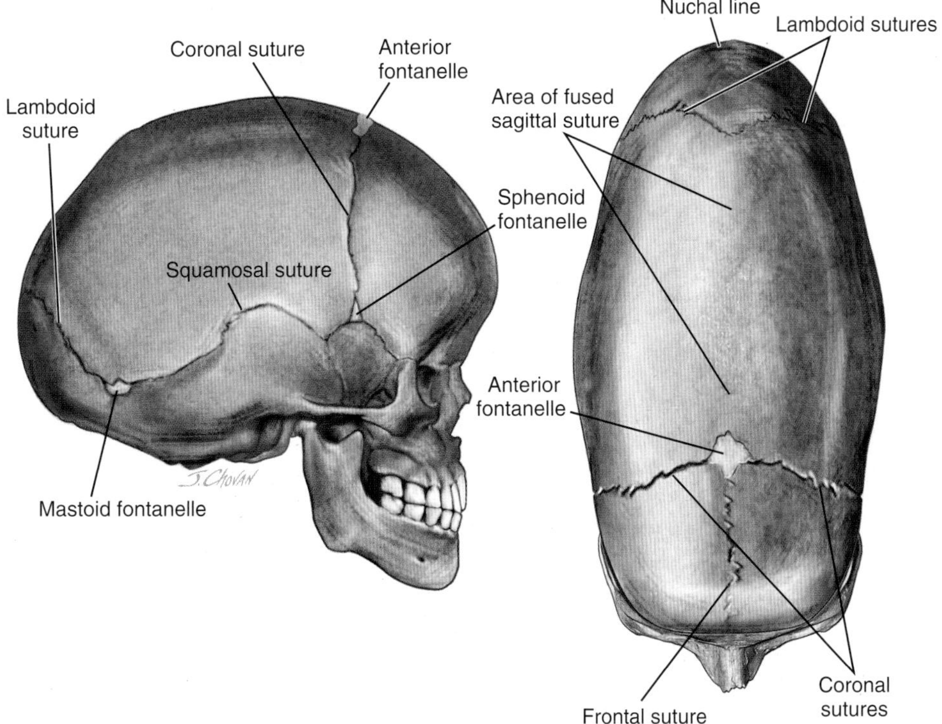

Figure 47.2 Lateral and superior views of scaphocephaly characteristic of sagittal synostosis.

ICP can lead to papilledema and optic nerve atrophy, possibly resulting in complete or partial loss of vision.

The timing of surgical treatment varies among surgeons and centers. Infants in the neonatal period who have been diagnosed with sagittal synostosis have been successfully treated with an open or endoscopic-assisted strip craniectomy of the sagittal suture. In the older infant with scaphocephaly, treatment with formal cranial vault remodeling is undertaken at 6 to 8 months of age, while the cranium is still highly malleable and easier to recontour. Early intervention also allows rapid brain growth to drive the expansion of the newly remodeled cranium. Bone gaps and residual defects at the sites of osteotomy are more likely to heal rapidly and reossify completely in children under 12 months old. When considering the benefits of early surgical intervention, one must also take into consideration possible positive effects on future craniofacial growth and the degree to which additional deformities may be diminished.

Limitations and Contraindications

Vault remodeling to treat craniosynostosis has few absolute contraindications. In most cases, surgery is the primary form of treatment. Children who are medically unstable or deemed unable to tolerate general anesthesia are not candidates for vault remodeling.

TECHNIQUE: Posterior Cranial Vault Remodeling

Vault remodeling is best carried out in dedicated pediatric centers, which provide access to experienced physicians, nursing staff, and pediatric intensive care units and also are well accustomed to treated pediatric patients. Well-coordinated multidisciplinary team care is also advocated in the case of patients undergoing craniofacial procedures; successful vault remodeling involves the combined care of a pediatric anesthesiologist, craniofacial surgeon, and pediatric neurosurgeon.

STEP 1: ANESTHESIA

The safe use of craniofacial techniques in pediatric surgery requires collaboration with an anesthesiologist well versed in infant physiology, neuroanesthesia, and pediatric neurosurgical critical care. Controlled hypotensive anesthesia is routinely used during craniofacial cases unless it is contraindicated because of existing cardiovascular, neurologic, or renal disease.[12]

Oral endotracheal intubation is preferred, and the tube is adequately secured in place because tube displacement can occur with head movement during the procedure. Two intravenous catheters and an arterial catheter are customarily used for vascular access. The patient is positioned prone with the head secured in a padded Mayfield horseshoe headrest, with care taken to prevent orbital pressure. Packed red blood cells are prepared and "in room" for use during the procedure. Preoperative antibiotics and steroids are administered before incision.

STEP 2: CRANIAL APPROACH

The patient's hair is parted, and a coronal incision is marked ear to ear across the vertex, with Z-plasty release bitemporally. Ten minutes before incision, the site is infiltrated with 0.25% lidocaine with 1:400,000 epinephrine to facilitate hemostasis. A scalp incision is made with a #10 blade scalpel, and hemostasis is carefully achieved with judicious use of low-level bipolar electrocautery and Raney clips.

The pericranium then is incised. Subpericranial dissection with a blunt periosteal elevator is carried anteriorly, exposing the bilateral coronal sutures, and posteriorly past the nuchal line. Laterally, the temporalis muscle is elevated to expose the bilateral squamosal sutures (Fig. 47.3A–D).

STEP 3: CRANIOTOMY

Bur holes are made by the pediatric neurosurgeon posterior to the coronal sutures on either side of the sagittal sinus and above the squamosal sutures bilaterally. Bur holes also are made anterior to the lambdoids on either side of the sagittal sinus and above the squamosal suture bilaterally. Next, the dura is carefully dissected off the overlying skull, and a craniotomy is performed to remove cranial portions A, B, C, and D. Craniotomy is also performed to remove bandeau segment E/F. Hemostasis is achieved, the dura and bone margins are inspected, and any bleeding is immediately addressed. The dura is carefully examined, and any tears are repaired, if necessary. The dura is kept moist with lap sponges while any bone work is performed on the back table.

STEP 4: BANDEAU RECONSTRUCTION

Next, the harvested bandeau segment E/F is split at the midline. A bone graft is harvested from the inner table of segment A or B in a predetermined width and length. The graft is inserted into the split bandeau and fixated in place with resorbable plates and screws. This segment is stabilized, thus expanding the cranium in the lateral dimension and reducing its vertical dimension of height. This sets the stage for final cranial bone positioning (Fig. 47.3E).

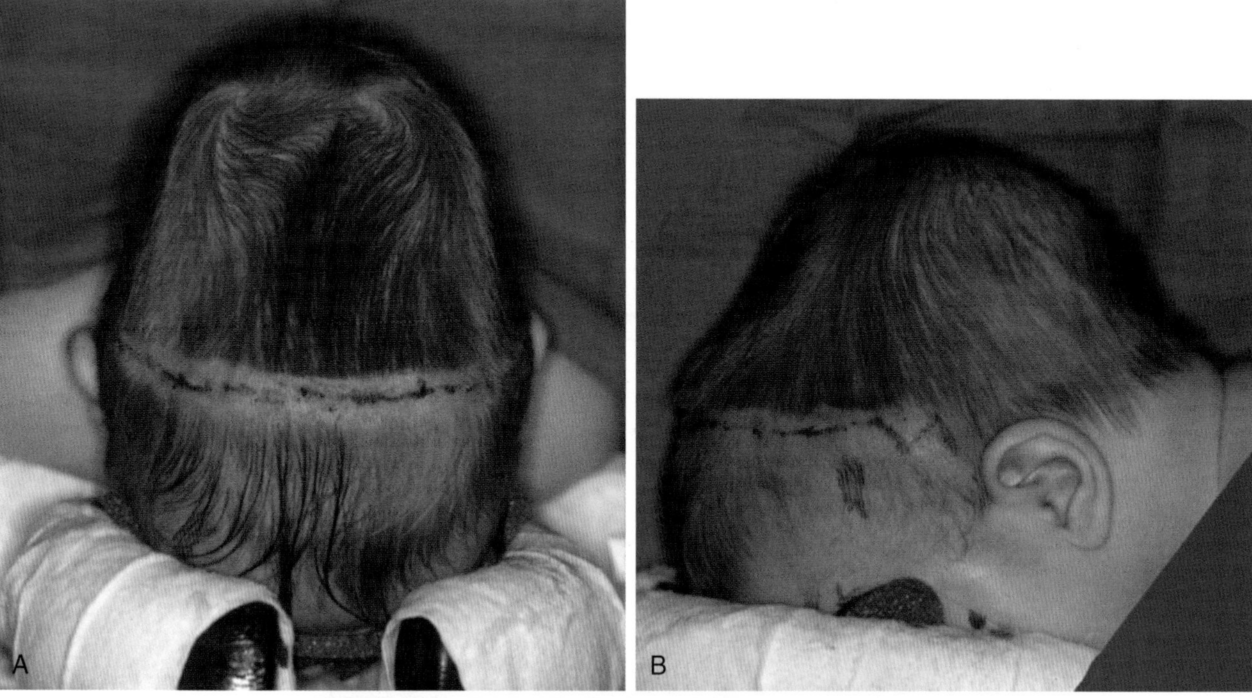

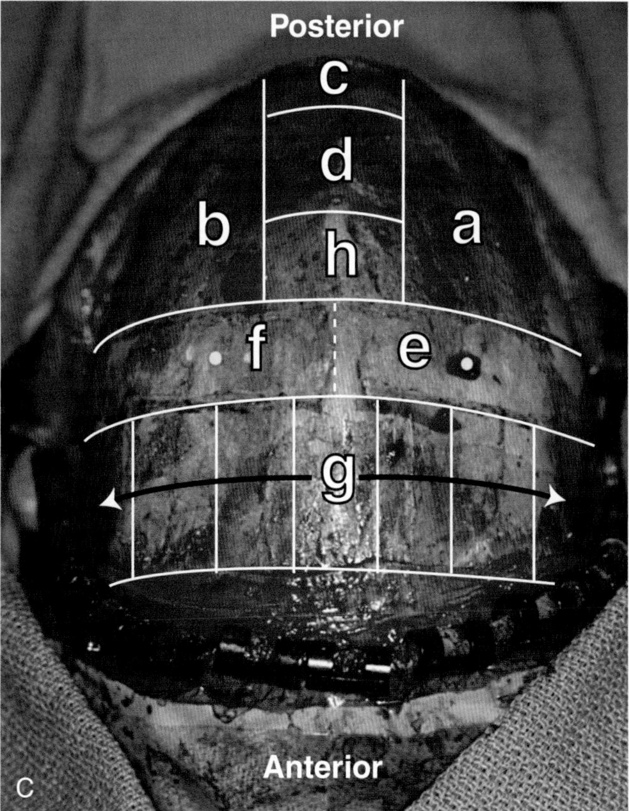

Figure 47.3 **A** and **B**, The patient is positioned prone with the head secured in the Mayfield horseshoe headrest, and the coronal incision is marked. **C**, Exposed cranial vault with osteotomy sites marked.

Continued

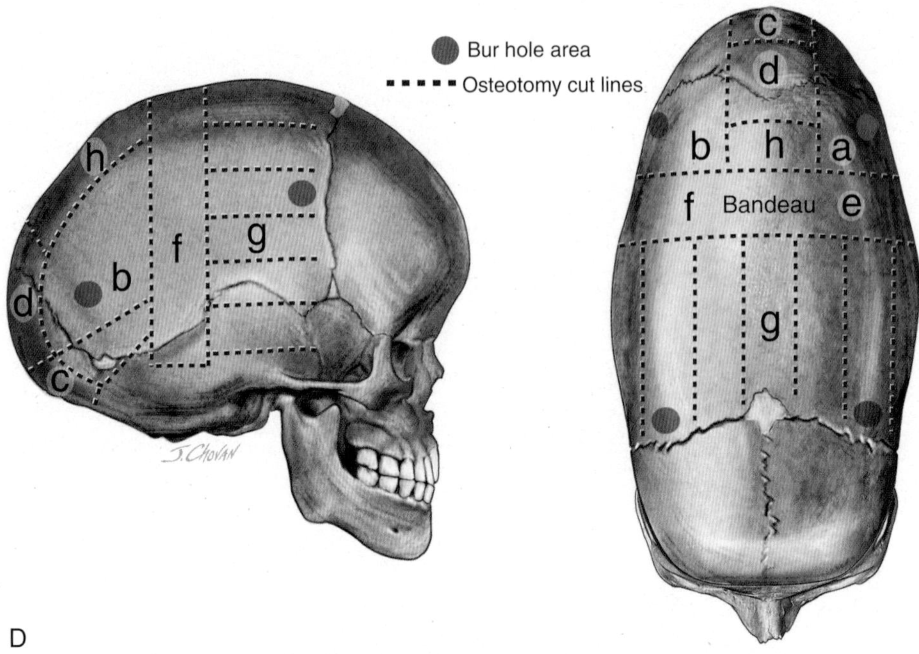

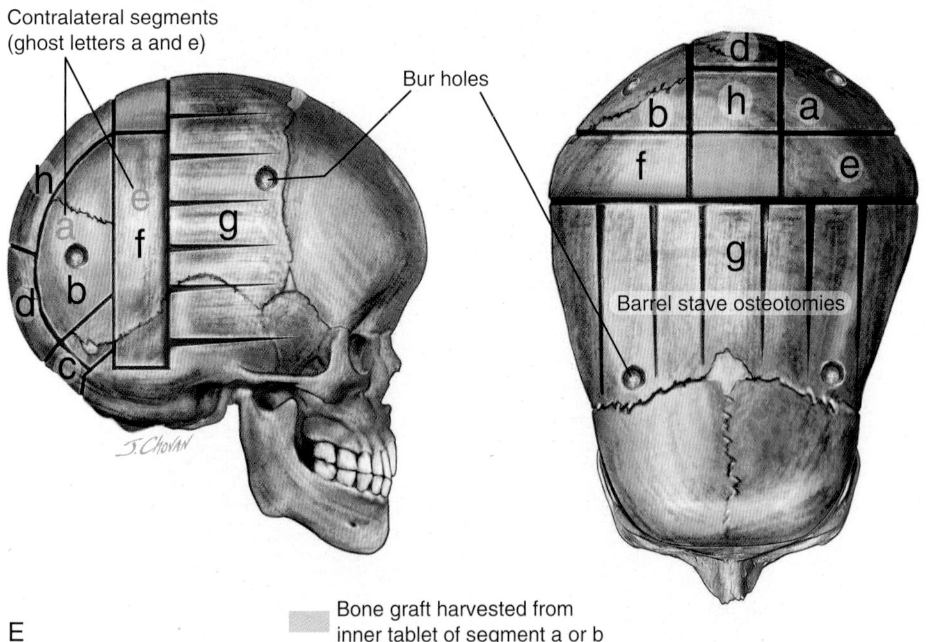

Figure 47.3, cont'd **D,** Schematic illustrations of planned vault remodeling. **E,** Bandeau segment is split and grafted to expand the cranium in the lateral dimension.

TECHNIQUE: Posterior Cranial Vault Remodeling—cont'd

STEP 5: CRANIAL VAULT ASSEMBLY

Biparietal segments A and B are inverted and inserted to adjust for the new cranial length and height. These segments are then secured using resorbable fixation anteriorly to bandeau E/F and medially to segment H, which remains attached to the dura. Cranial segment D is then fixated to segments A and B. Cranial segment C is replaced and stabilized in position (Fig. 47.3F).

STEP 6: BARRELL STAVE OSTEOTOMIES

Barrel stave osteotomies are then cut in the posterior portion of the anterior cranium to allow for expansile cranial width correction and to create a smooth transition with the anterior cranium.

STEP 7: CRANIAL BONE GRAFTING

With the cranial vault reconstructed and fixated in its newly remodeled configuration, any remaining osseous defects are grafted with previously harvested autogenous split calvarial grafts and collected bone dust from the cranial osteotomies (Fig. 47.3G).

STEP 8: CLOSURE

Hemostasis is assessed again, the pericranium and temporalis muscles are resuspended, a small subgaleal suction drain is routinely placed, and the scalp is closed in layered fashion using 3-0 Monocryl suture in the subgaleal layer and 4-0 Vicryl Rapide in the hair-bearing skin. The patient's incision is dressed, and the head is wrapped with soft head wrap.

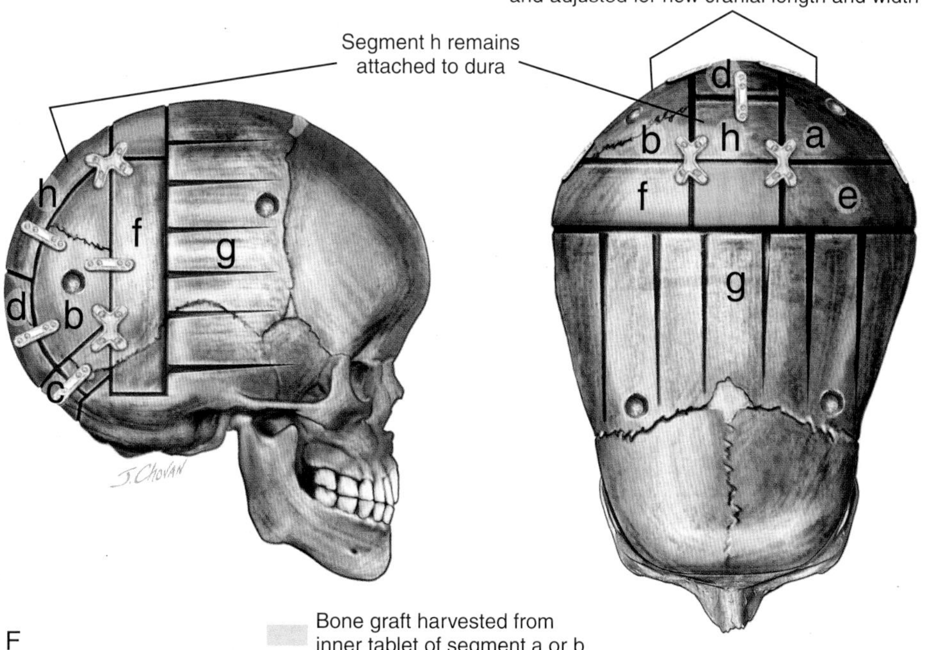

Figure 47.3, cont'd F, Posterior vault assembly.

Continued

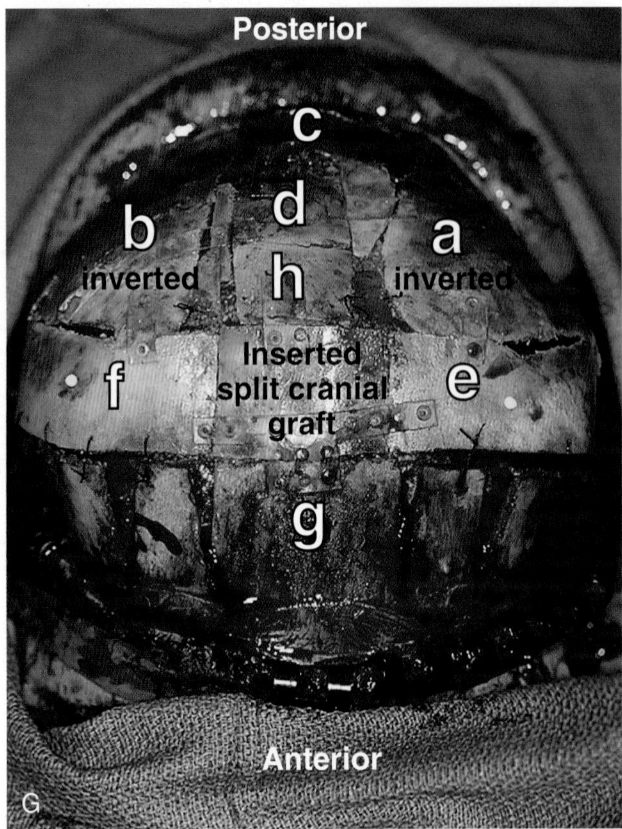

Figure 47.3, cont'd G, Remodeled posterior vault before closure.

Avoidance and Management of Intraoperative Complications

Communication and cooperation between the anesthetic and surgical teams before and throughout the procedure are necessary to facilitate a successful surgical outcome. Acute intraoperative complications associated with cranial vault remodeling are primarily related to blood loss. Careful attention to hemostasis is crucial throughout the procedure. Pressing absorbable bone wax or thrombin-soaked Gelfoam into the cut bony edges can control bleeding from the osteotomies. On rare occasions, significant bleeding may occur with tearing of a venous sinus or major cortical vein. Blood products should be used in the operating room before any osseous work is performed, and intraoperative transfusions should be performed as necessary while hemostasis is achieved.

Venous air emboli also are a possible complication in patients undergoing craniotomy for craniosynostosis repair. A head position above the level of the heart and exposed noncollapsible veins open to air, coupled with decreased central venous pressure, can result in a net pressure gradient favoring venous air entry. The incidence of venous air entry has been reported to be as high as 83%, although clinically significant embolic events are thankfully rare.[13] Early recognition of venous air emboli is possible with intraoperative precordial Doppler and end-tidal carbon dioxide monitoring. If hemodynamic instability develops, the patient's table can be tipped into the Trendelenburg position, the field flooded with sterile saline, and bone wax applied to cut cranium edges to prevent further entrapment of intravascular air.

Dural tears also may be encountered after the craniotomy portion of the procedure. These should be evaluated and repaired by the neurosurgical team to prevent cerebrospinal fluid leakage.

Postoperative Considerations

After cranial vault remodeling, patients are admitted to the pediatric intensive care unit for 24-hour observation. Preoperative intravenous antibiotics and steroids are administered at the start of the case and continued for 48 hours postoperatively. It is not uncommon for some blood loss to continue into the postoperative period from oozing dura or bone. Serial hemoglobin/hematocrit determinations are evaluated, and the subgaleal drain output is followed; losses may necessitate transfusion replacement therapy after surgery. Patients are also monitored closely for proper fluid and serum electrolyte balance, and abnormalities are corrected as needed.

Despite dramatic alteration of the cranial vault, surgery usually does not involve significant manipulation of the brain. Accordingly, postoperative issues involving intracranial hypertension, cerebral edema, bleeding, or other sequelae of major intracranial surgery are rare. Nonetheless, frequent neurologic checks are performed to monitor the patient's status during the immediate postoperative period.

Fever is to be expected in these patients postoperatively. In a series of 126 patients who underwent craniofacial procedures involving a transcranial component, postoperative fever was noted in 92% of patients under 2 years of age. Only 4 of 126 patients were noted to have minor infections, and only one of these involved a wound related to surgery. Fever and leukocytosis in the immediate postoperative period need not be worked up further in these patients unless associated clinical indicators of infection are present.[14] Twenty-four hours after surgery, the head wrap and drain are discontinued and, if progressing well, the patient is routinely transferred to a step-down unit or surgical floor, where they spend another 2 to 4 days before discharge home.

Minor cranial asymmetries are occasionally encountered after surgery. These discrepancies are usually well accepted and seldom need to be addressed.

Late complications of treatment can be associated with impaired osseous healing and bone growth after surgery. In one series of 592 patients who had cranioplasty for synostosis, 5% of the patients had inadequate ossification after surgery.[15] In rare cases, major postoperative asymmetries or failure to adequately correct the primary deformity must be addressed with surgical remodeling at a later date. Reoperation rates approach 7%, with higher rates for syndromic versus nonsyndromic craniosynostosis (Fig. 47.4).[16,17]

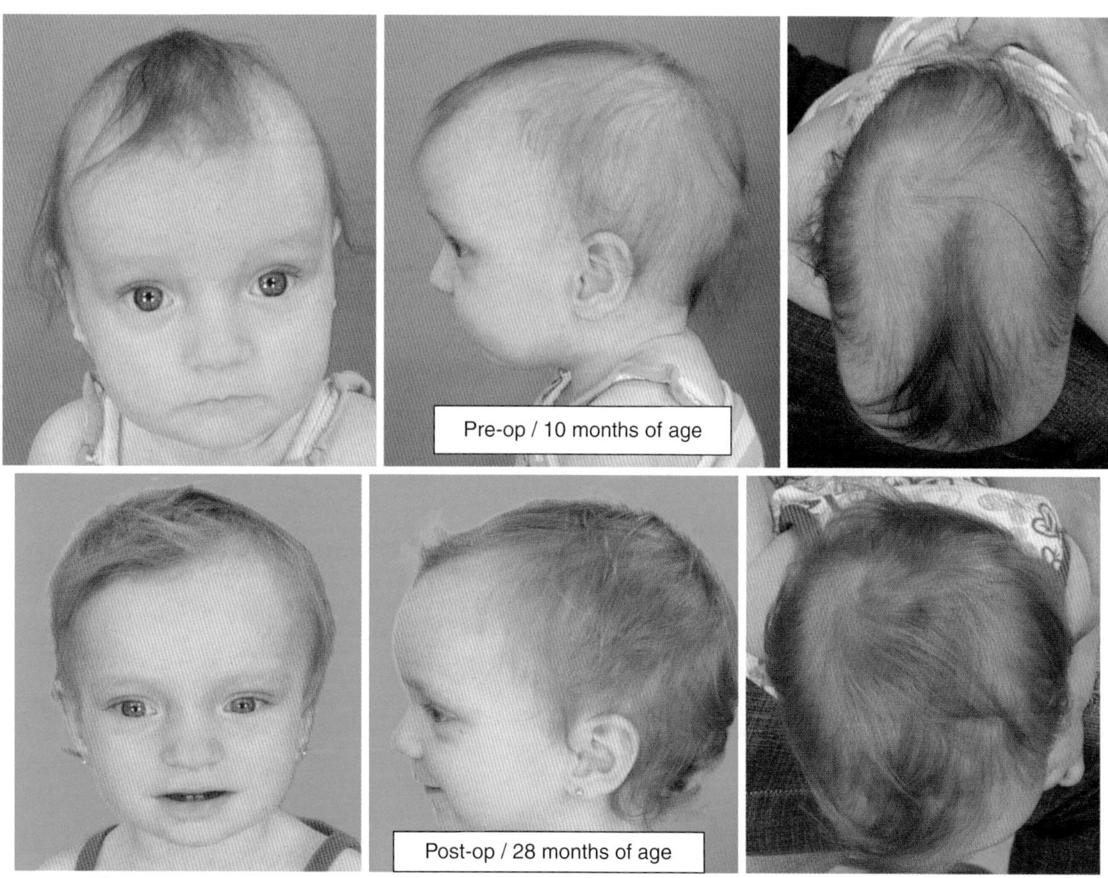

Figure 47.4 Preoperative and postoperative views (front, side, and superior) in a patient with sagittal synostosis.

References

1. Lannelongue M. De la cranietomie dans la microencephalie. *C R Acad Sci*. 1980;110:1382.
2. Lane LC. Pioneer craniectomy for relief of mental imbecility due to premature sutural closure and microcephalus. *J Am Med Assoc*. 1892;18:49.
3. Tessier P, Guiot G, Rougererie J, et al. Total facial osteotomy. Crouzon's syndrome, Apert's syndrome: oxycephaly, scaphocephaly, turricephaly. *Ann Chir Plast*. 1967;12:273.
4. Tessier P, Guiot G, Rougerie J, Delbet JP, Pastoriza J. Ostéotomies cranio-naso-orbito-faciales. Hypertélorisme. *Ann Chir Plast*. 1967;12(2):103–118.
5. Rougerie J, Derome P, Anquez L. Craniostenosis and cranio-facial dysmorphism. Principles of a new method of treatment and its results. *Neurochirurgie*. 1972;18(5):429–440.
6. Whitaker LA, Schut L, Kerr LP. Early surgery for isolated craniofacial dysostosis. Improvement and possible prevention of increasing deformity. *Plast Reconstr Surg*. 1977;60(4):575–581.
7. Lajeunie E, Le Merrer M, Bonaïti-Pellie C, Marchac D, Renier D. Genetic study of scaphocephaly. *Am J Med Genet*. 1996;62(3):282–285.
8. Huang MH, Gruss JS, Clarren SK, et al. The differential diagnosis of posterior plagiocephaly: true lambdoid synostosis versus positional molding. *Plast Reconstr Surg*. 1996;98(5):765–774.
9. Renier D, Sainte-Rose C, Marchac D, Hirsch JF. Intracranial pressure in craniostenosis. *J Neurosurg*. 1982;57:370.
10. Renier D. Intracranial pressure in craniosynostosis: pre- and postoperative recordings – correlation with functional results. In: Persing JA, Edgerton MT, Jane JA, eds. *Scientific Foundations and Surgical Treatment of Craniosynostosis*. Baltimore, Maryland: Williams & Wilkins; 1989.
11. Sinn DP, Ortega ME, Byrd HS, Sklar FH. Major craniofacial surgery. In: Levine D, Morriss F, eds. *Essential Guide to Pediatric Intensive Care*. St. Louis, Missouri: Quality Medical Publishing; 1990.
12. Faberowski LW, Black S, Mickle JP. Incidence of venous air embolism during craniectomy for craniosynostosis repair. *Anesthesiology*. 2000;92(1):20–23.
13. Hobar PC, Masson JA, Herrera R, et al. Fever after craniofacial surgery in the infant under 24 months of age. *Plast Reconstr Surg*. 1998;102(1):32–36.
14. Prevot M, Renier D, Marchac D. Lack of ossification after cranioplasty for craniosynostosis: a review of relevant factors in 592 consecutive patients. *J Craniofac Surg*. 1993;4(4):247–254.
15. Williams JK, Cohen SR, Burstein FD, Hudgins R, Boydston W, Simms C. A longitudinal, statistical study of reoperation rates in craniosynostosis. *Plast Reconstr Surg*. 1997;100(2):305–310.
16. Ghali GE, Sinn DP, Tantipasawasin S. Management of nonsyndromic craniosynostosis. *Atlas Oral Maxillofac Surg Clin North Am*. 2002;10(1):1–41.
17. Zubovic E, Woo AS, Skolnick GB, Naidoo SD, Smyth MD, Patel KB. Cranial base and posterior cranial vault asymmetry after open and endoscopic repair of isolated lambdoid craniosynostosis. *J Craniofac Surg*. 2015;26(5):1568–1573.

CHAPTER 48

Total Cranial Vault Remodeling

Andrew Alistair Heggie and Anthony David Holmes

Armamentarium

Mayo table
#15, #10 scalpel blades
Electrocautery: needle, blade, bipolar
Hall Surgairtome
Gelfoam patties/Surgicel fibrillar
Resorbable plating kit (sonic weld)
Langenbeck retractors
Tessier elevators
ModiVfied Freer elevator
Skin hooks
Cat paw retractors
Hot water bath
3/0 Vicryl, 4/0 Vicryl Rapide
5/0 PDS for dura as needed
Dressing gauze
2.5-cm Hypafix tape
Preparation trolley: elastics/shaver
Local anesthetic: epinephrine/steroid
Midas electric drill craniotome
Burs: flat fissure/pineapple
Bone wax
Howarth elevator
Penfield dural dissector
Stille-Listen bone cutter
Bone rongeurs: curved and straight
Resorbable plating kit (sonic weld)
2/0 PDS suture
5/0 BSS for eyelids
Jelonet
Medium Tegaderm
5-cm crepe bandage

History of the Procedures for Cranial Synostosis

Many techniques for remodeling the cranial vault have been proposed and range from simple suture removal to complete morphological alteration of the cranium. Isolated sagittal synostosis, the most frequently occurring form of nonsyndromic single-suture synostosis, varies in severity but may have a profound effect on the entire cranial shape. Similarly, craniosynostoses involving the coronal and metopic sutures may result in a brachycephalic/turricephalic deformity with a reverse pattern of calvarial field distortion. Strip craniectomies were undertaken over a century ago[1,2] to allow skull expansion, but due to poor results, further barrier techniques were applied to cover the osteotomized bony margins in order to prevent suture refusion,[3–5] but with limited success. With increasing recognition that the whole vault was affected, extended strip craniectomies[6] and total vertex craniectomies[7] were then performed. During this same period, total removal of the cranial vault and helmet protection was being advocated in parts of Europe with the goal of achieving a more normal skull morphology following reossification,[8] yet bony regeneration proved to be incomplete and unpredictable. Strip craniectomies are still widely practiced, usually in combination with helmeting, but there is evidence that a more comprehensive approach to remodeling yields superior results.[9–12] An additional procedure was introduced by the neurosurgeon, Jane, who described the "Pi" technique to reduce the frontooccipital dimension of the head by first removing a transverse strip of bone posterior to the coronal suture connected to parasagittal resections bilaterally. Posteriorly, the resected area extended laterally in front of the lambdoid sutures. Viewed from above, the resected bone resembled the shape of the Greek letter Pi.[13,14] The calvarium was then squeezed together in the anteroposterior direction with lateral displacement of the parietal segments. The frontal and occipital deformities were only partially addressed, and the risk of brain compression caused concern, with some neurosurgeons who recommended perioperative pressure monitoring. A similar technique utilizing gradual cranial compression after a modified bone resection using reverse distraction has been reported.[15] Others have recommended extensive posterior vault remodeling alone allowing the frontal bossing to self-correct.[16] An additional technique developed by Renier[17] with segment removal in an "H" pattern has been advocated for infants less than 6 months where retrocoronal and prelambdoidal segments are removed together with central segments over the sagittal suture. Spring-mediated cranioplasties[18] have also become popular at a young age, but again, the anterior and posterior phenotypical features are not corrected and rely on helmeting.

More recently, several studies of strip craniectomies using endoscopic techniques to treat scaphocephaly have been reported with good results.[19–21] These procedures are usually performed in infants, aged 3 to 6 months, and extended helmet therapy following this surgery is essential. This technique is more suitable for mild to moderate cases that present early. However, long-term results on the reoperation rates and assessing the aesthetic outcome together with intellectual function in the mature patients are not yet available. Patients older than 9 months and those with more severe deformities are usually considered unsuitable for this approach.

To correct the more severe deformities as well as cases presenting at a later age, a more radical approach was advocated.[22] It was dissatisfaction with multiple previous techniques that led to the development of the Melbourne technique of total calvarial remodeling, devised by the senior author (ADH) and our team.[23] The aims of the operation design were to have a single-stage procedure that corrected all the associated phenotypic deformities and simultaneously, significantly increased the cranial volume. It was also anticipated that no helmet therapy would be required. Since the inception of this technique in 1999 and subsequent to the first edition of this Atlas, a much larger number of patients have undergone correction, with further evaluation and minor modifications made to the Melbourne method. Of nearly 300 cases to date (2020), the overall reoperation rate has been approximately 1.5%. Four cases have required further biparietal expansion for raised intracranial pressure and these patients presented between the ages 6 and 10 years. The cranial index of all cases has remained within normal limits, and there has been no mortality nor major morbidity.[24] Those who have reached puberty or are postpubertal have retained a satisfactory head shape and are intellectually within the normal range of their cohort. The basic principles of our current approach to total calvarial remodeling are outlined in this chapter.

Indications for Total Cranial Vault Remodeling

The phenotypical deformities resulting from both the syndromic and nonsyndromic craniosynostoses have been better characterized in recent years with an ever-increasing understanding of the genetic basis of cranial suture fusion. There are differing views regarding the selection of procedures and the age that they can be undertaken. In general, the extent of the calvarial distortions and constrictions are proportional to the site and number of sutures that are fused, as is the risk of raised intracranial pressure. To fully correct the more severe deformities, a more comprehensive alteration of the shape of the total cranial vault is often required. The most common condition suitable for total cranial vault reconstruction is moderate to severe scaphocephaly. Modifications of the Melbourne technique can be useful in other severe synostoses, in particular multisutural synostoses causing turricephaly, oxycephaly, and cloverleaf skull. A reverse-type procedure can also be used to lengthen and lower the skull in severe brachycephaly resulting from coronal synostosis.

Scaphocephaly

In the scaphocephalic patient, the fusion of the sagittal suture causes narrowing of the bitemporal and biparietal dimensions with an elongated head and a higher vertex. The vertex is positioned anteriorly near the anterior fontanelle instead of posterior to the midline. There is an inferior sloping and posterior cranium constricting to a bullet-shaped occiput. The intracranial contents push anteriorly, causing compensatory frontal bossing. Partial fusion of the sagittal suture will lead to more localized adjacent transverse constrictions of the skull. There is also a tight constriction in the pterion region bilaterally, overlying the Broca area, which may explain why speech onset delay is commonly reported in this condition.

The diagnosis can be made clinically and confirmed with good plane film X-rays and three-dimensional computed tomography (CT). There is a low cranial index and usually an increased head circumference approximating the 90th percentile. Without treatment, the narrow head shape will persist, and any frontal bossing often remains evident. Patients with moderate to severe deformities over the age of 9 months constitute the strongest indication for this procedure as other therapies become less effective. The aim of the Melbourne procedure is to address all phenotypical features of the disorder and reconstruct the skull without any brain compression. In fact, the cranial volume is increased. By segmental repositioning, the sagittal suture is reshaped and placed in the normal adult position. The frontal bone is recessed and widened, along with the coronal suture. The occiput is elevated and widened to shorten the anteroposterior dimension and to position the vertex posteriorly. The biparietal diameter is markedly widened. The normal sutures are preserved as much as possible and repositioned, hopefully to allow the rest of the head to continue growing normally.[23] Our more recent modifications also expand the lateral supraorbital rim areas to match the widened frontal bone. The bony constriction at the pterion regions is resected, and at the same time, the remaining squamous temporal bones are barrel-staved out laterally to widen the cranial base.

Brachycephaly (Turricephaly/Oxycephaly)

Patients with more vertical deformities secondary to multisuture synostoses, such as Muenke syndrome, exhibit a variable reverse pattern of deformity to scaphocephaly. The anteroposterior dimension of the skull is foreshortened with raised, flattened frontal and occipital regions and an increase in bitemporal width. The head height may be spectacularly increased in syndromic patients with synostoses of the coronal ring that includes the coronal, frontosphenoidal, and frontoethmoidal sutures. The pattern of segment repositioning required is in reversal from that described above with lowering of the occiput by transferring a lower segment to increase the frontooccipital dimension and a narrowing of head width.

Precautions, Limitations, and Contraindications

Early raised intracranial pressure with scaphocephaly is exceedingly rare but must be excluded preoperatively. Increased pressure may be found in other more severe forms of synostosis. Later clinical signs of increased pressure may occur in any child with synostoses, and these patients must be kept under review. Usually, cranial vault expansion is expedited if there are signs of pressure, and this is done prior to insertion of a neurosurgical shunt to allow the brain to expand to fill the increased volume created by the surgery. Often, such expansion surgery may avert the need for shunting. In some forms of synostosis, especially those with associated base of skull abnormalities (Apert and Pfeiffer syndromes; severe brachycephaly), the posterior fossa may be constricted and a Chiari malformation with herniation of the cerebellar tonsils may be present. These patients may show prominent veins and venous markings indicating compromise of venous sinus drainage and incipient raised pressure. For these cases, it is prudent to consider early posterior fossa decompression, now usually performed by posterior vault distraction.

Total vault remodeling is a major procedure and requires an experienced craniofacial, neurosurgical, and anesthetic team. All children require an extensive medical work-up, including bleeding and clotting parameters, CT scan, neuropsychological assessment, and baseline three-dimensional photography. Fortunately, contraindications to surgery are rare.

TECHNIQUE: Total Calvarial Remodeling

SCAPHOCEPHALY

1. Preparation

Under general anesthesia via a well-secured, reinforced endotracheal tube, the patient is positioned supine with the head on a neurosurgical headrest. Only a small strip of hair overlying the incision is trimmed. A curvilinear incision is designed in the midcoronal plane from ear to ear. The whole head is prepared with nonalcoholic antiseptic after the eyelids have been sutured closed for protection. Draping is performed carefully to leave the head free to be turned completely side-to-side, thus allowing safe posterior access to the area inferior to the occipital prominence.

2. Coronal flap

After tumescent infiltration using local anesthetic with adrenaline,[25] the scalp flaps are dissected in the subperiosteal plane anteriorly to the supraorbital rims and posteriorly to well below the occipital prominence.

3. Osteotomies and frontal reconstruction

The pattern of the osteotomies is illustrated in Fig. 48.1. The supraorbital bar may be left intact, and a large precoronal frontal segment is removed and barrel-staved laterally and flattened slightly to increase the intertemporal width. It is rotated posteriorly to correct excess frontal bossing. The step created at the junction with the supraorbital bar is then burred to ensure even contour. Later modifications have been added to the original description in order to increase head width and volume. This has involved a lateral splaying of the supraorbital bar to match the expanded frontal bone, removal of bone over the pterion, and barrel-staving the lower squamous area. The coronal suture strip is undermined from the dura mater and detached laterally. The base of the coronal suture area bilaterally is always quite narrow and constrictive. The middle meningeal vessels are visible in this area on the surface of the dura mater and should be protected. The coronal suture strip is usually divided in the midline, separated and remolded, and then reconnected to the final frontal bone segment so as to widen the anterolateral parietal constriction.

Continued

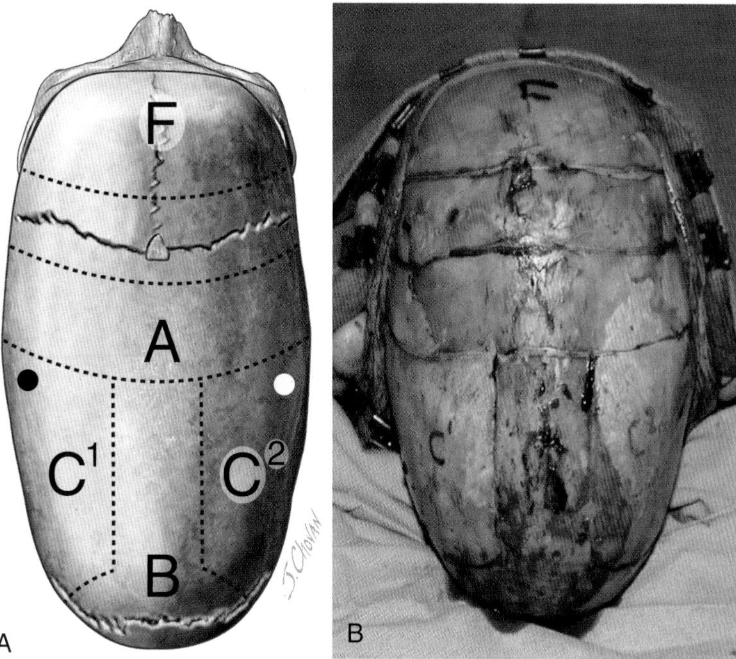

Figure 48.1 Pattern of intraoperative osteotomies marked out with accompanying diagrams: **A** and **B**, Superior view.

4. Osteotomies and posterior reconstruction

The strip of bone immediately posterior to the coronal strip (piece A in Fig. 48.1) is made 3 to 4 cm wide and then rotated and put back 90 degrees posteriorly to recontour the new lower occipital region. This is usually secured with bilateral resorbable plates to the squamous temporal region and resorbable polyglycolic monomer sutures through drill-holes in the bone posteriorly. The width of the A piece varies depending on the final height planned for the vertex. In general, the lower the slope of the original deformity, the wider the A piece. The original deformed occiput (including the lambdoid sutures) is raised in continuity with the fused sagittal suture (segment B). The parasagittal segment is approximately 3 to 4 cm wide. The posterior occipital aspect of this segment is then barrel-staved for expansion. The junction of the sagittal suture and the superior occiput is bent to form the new posterior vertex, and the sagittal suture fragment is straightened and reinforced on the inferior surface with a resorbable plate. The splayed occipital segment is then connected to the superior edge of the previously positioned A piece. Segment B is advanced anteriorly and fixed to the posterior margin of the frontal bone segment (coronal strip), thus considerably reducing the anteroposterior skull length. After the occipito-vertical elevation, there is a large space created in the new posteriorly positioned vertex area into which the brain may expand. There is no brain compression. The parietal pieces (C1 and C2) are reshaped and then replaced to broaden the biparietal region. A modification of the original pattern of osteotomies involves the postero-inferior parts of the C segments that are positioned on the outside of the anterior edge of the A segment and cannot collapse inwards before the brain has expanded to fill the new potential space (Fig. 48.2). Fixation is performed with resorbable sutures.

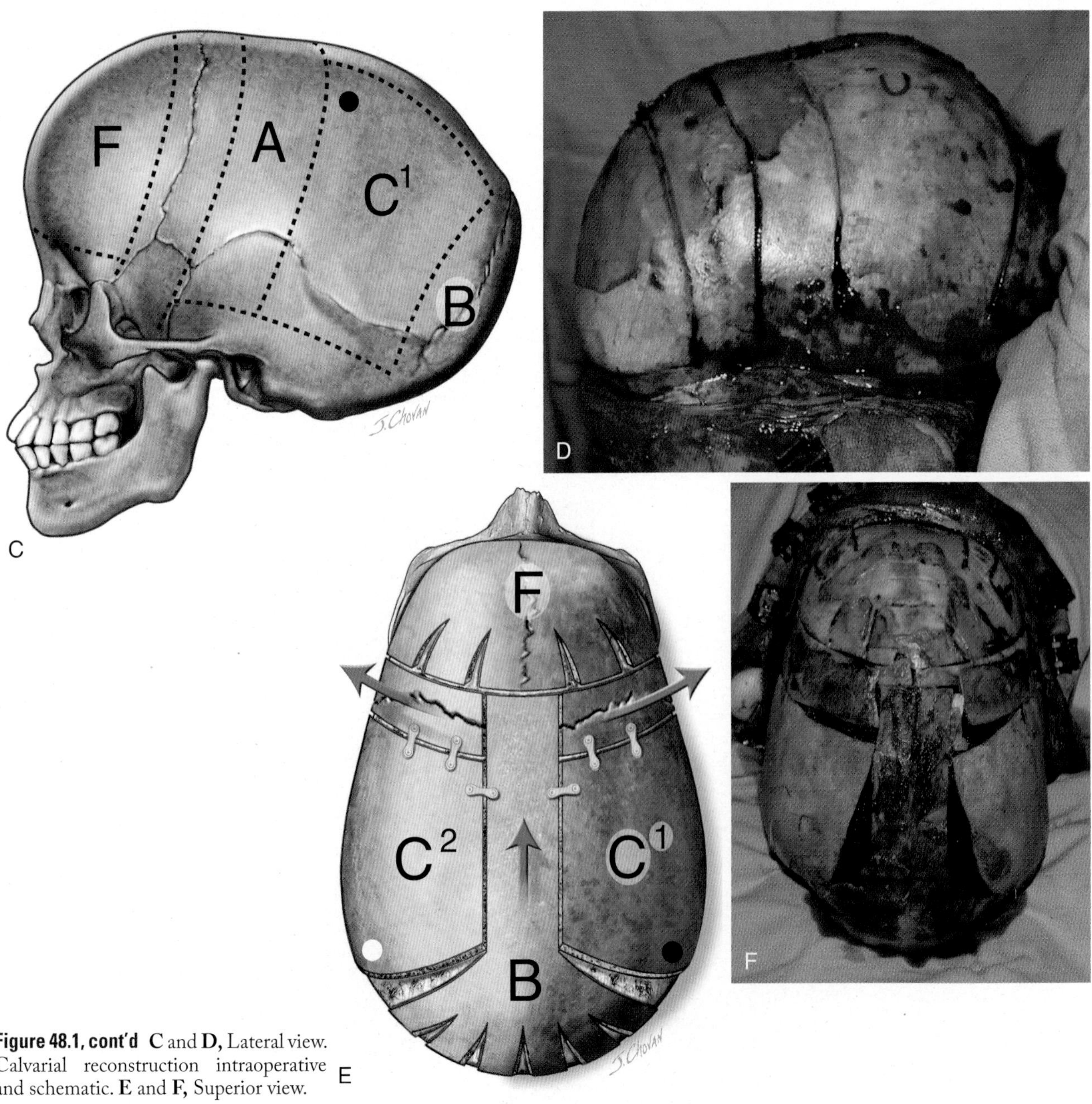

Figure 48.1, cont'd **C** and **D,** Lateral view. Calvarial reconstruction intraoperative and schematic. **E** and **F,** Superior view.

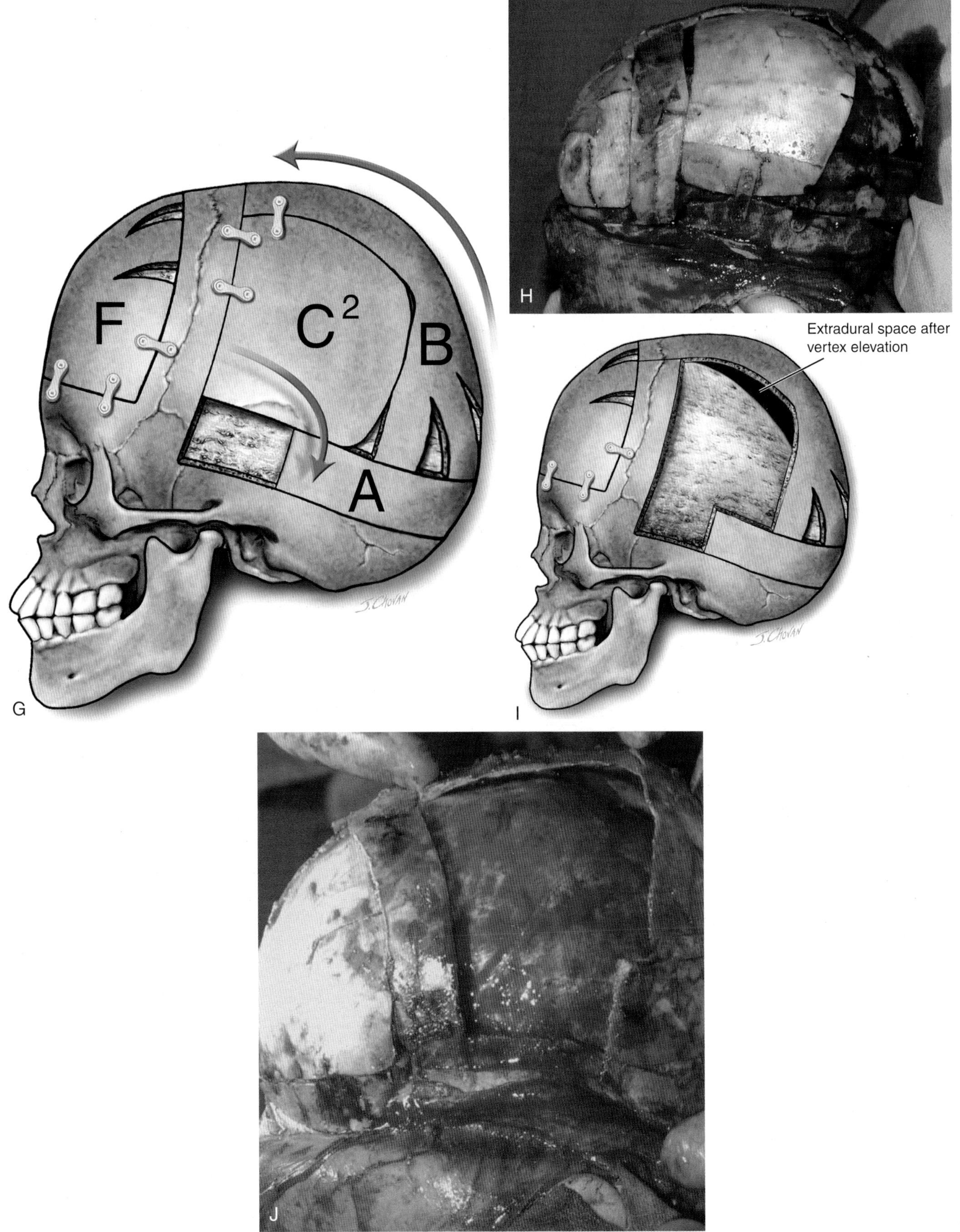

Figure 48.1, cont'd **G** and **H,** Lateral view. After reconstruction of the vertex, elevation of the occipital component gives a more normal posterior position by providing space for brain expansion to compensate for the radical anteroposterior shortening achieved and thereby avoid brain compression and the risk of raising intracranial pressure. **I** and **J,** Diagrammatic and corresponding intraoperative views.

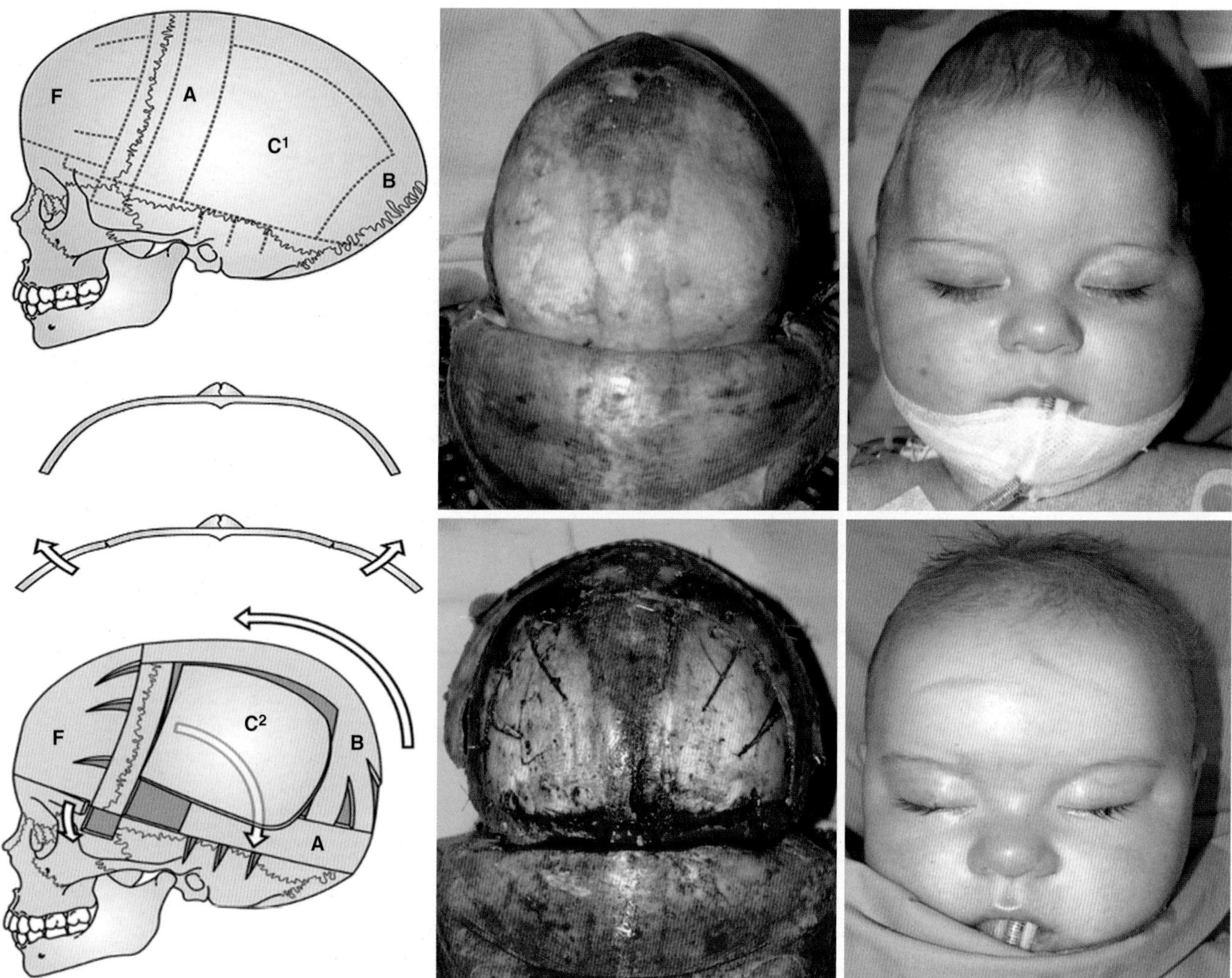

Figure 48.2 Modification of original osteotomy pattern: **A** and **B,** Schematic intraoperative and pre- and postoperative frontal views.

TECHNIQUE: Total Calvarial Remodeling—cont'd

5. Closure and dressings

The scalp is closed in layers, and usually no suction drainage is utilized. If there are any small, unrecognized dural breaches, suction can potentiate cerebrospinal fluid leakage. Dressings consist of paraffin gauze, cotton gauze, and 1-inch-thick foam padding over the occiput followed by double crepe bandages. Postoperatively, the child is nursed supine on the padded new occiput with the head held centrally. Illustrative cases are presented in Figs. 48.3 and 48.4.

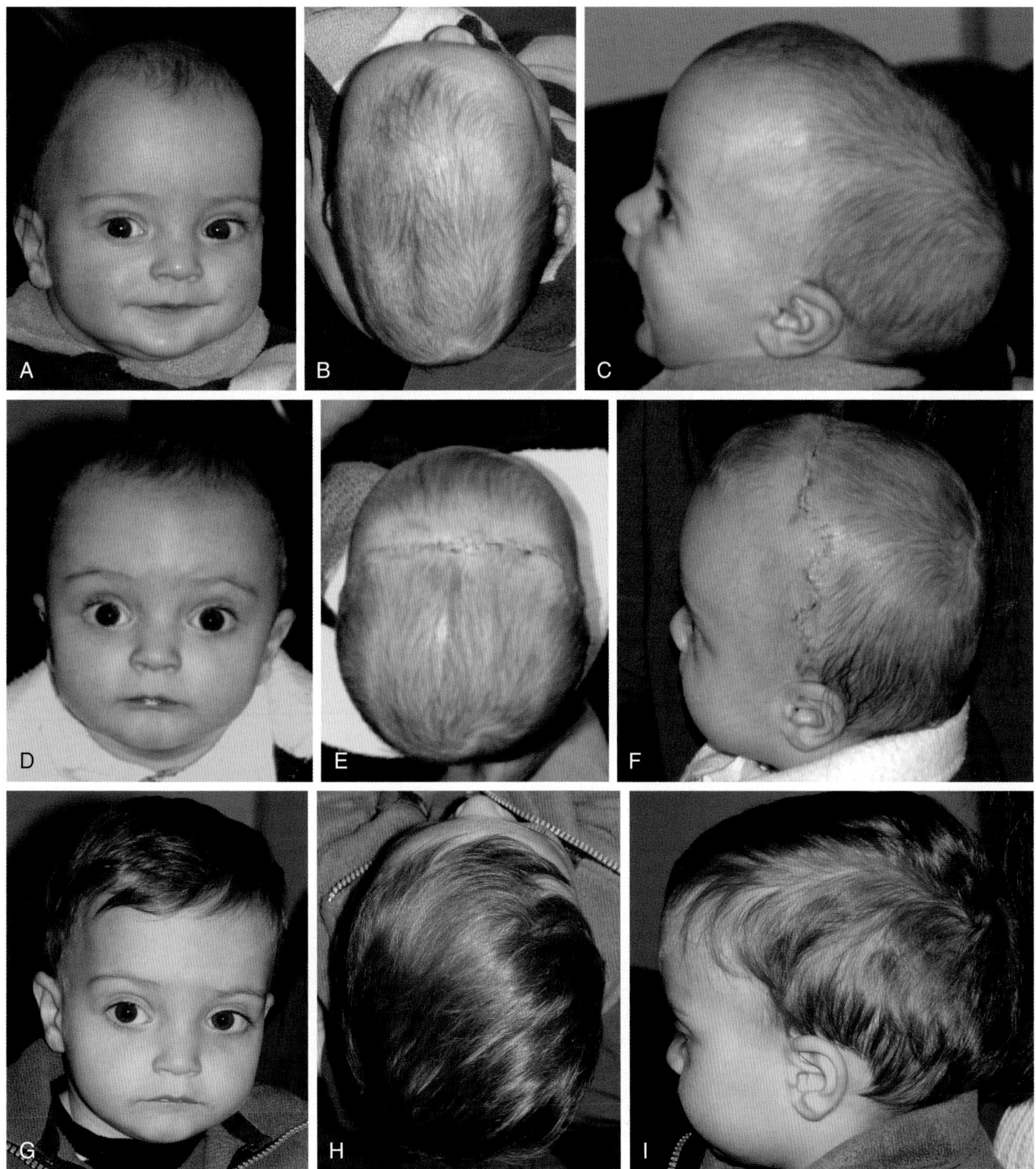

Figure 48.3 Male, 11 months, with scaphocephaly: Frontal, superior, and lateral views: **A–C,** Preoperative. **D–F,** Postoperative 1 week. **G–I,** Follow-up age 3 years.

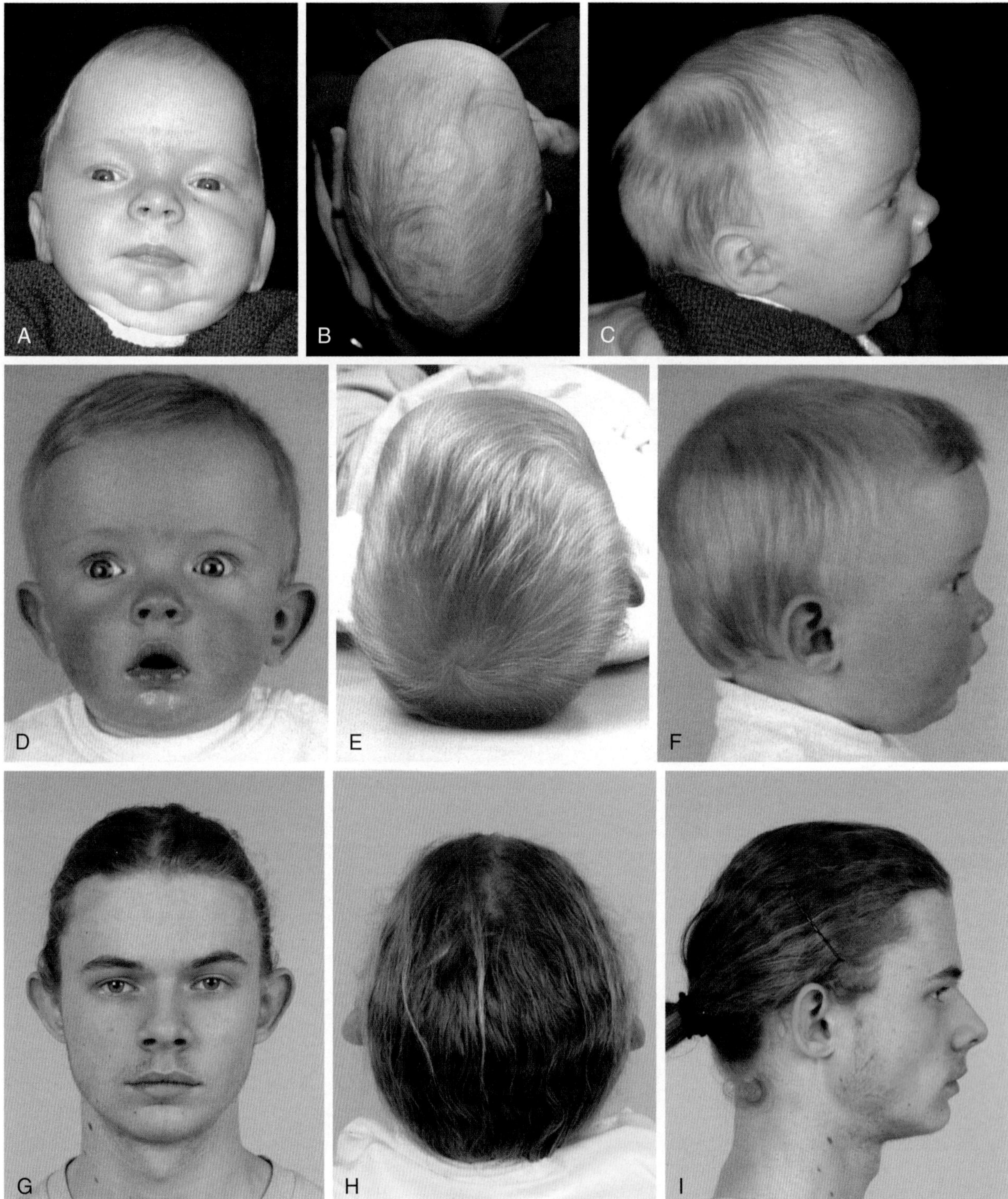

Figure 48.4 Male, 11 months, with scaphocephaly: Frontal, superior, and lateral views. **A–C,** Preoperative. **D–F,** Postoperative 12 months. **G–I,** Follow-up age 19 years.

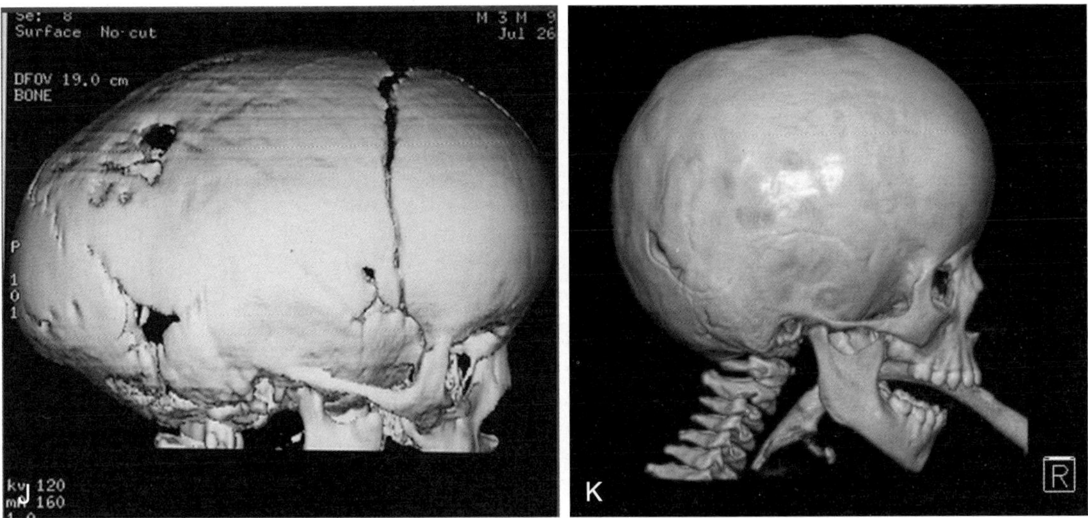

Figure 48.4, cont'd **J** and **K,** Lateral skull three-dimensional computed tomography; preoperative and postoperative 3 years.

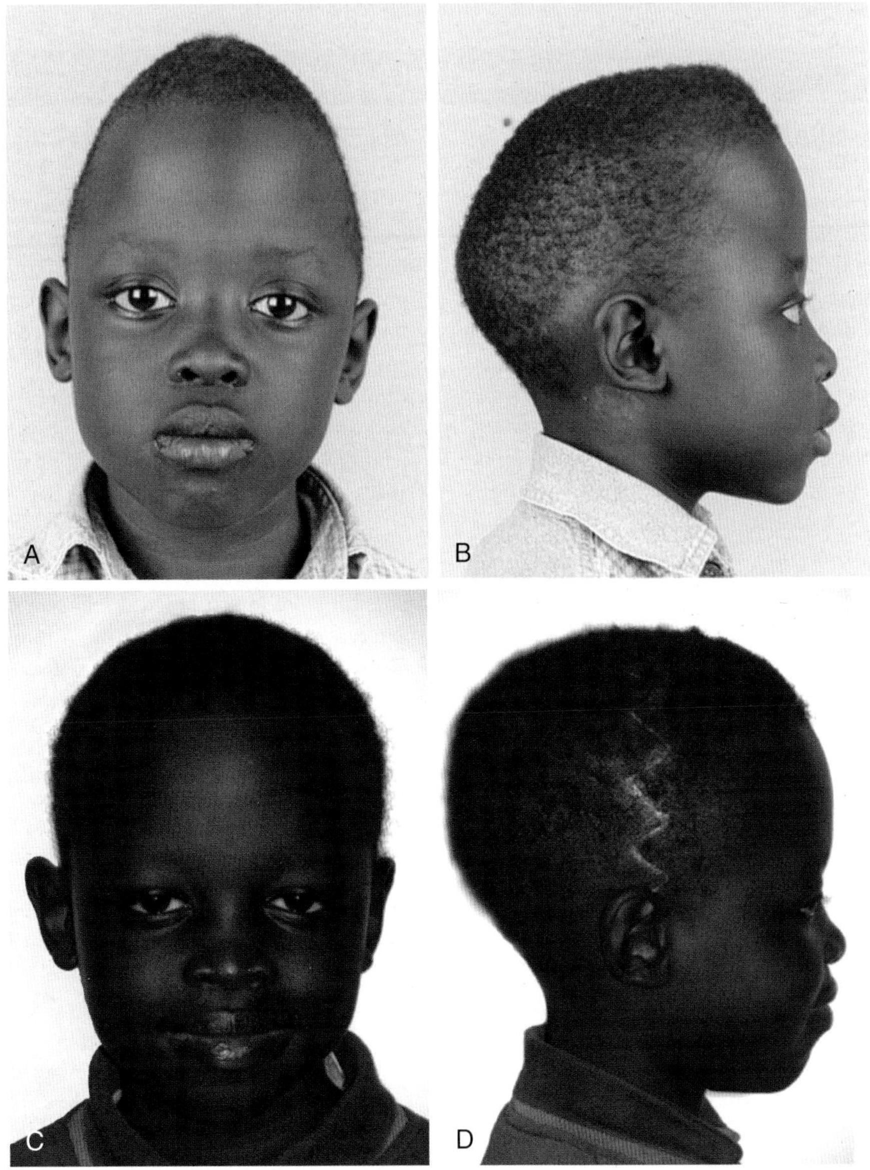

Figure 48.5 Male, 7 years, with delayed-onset oxycephaly: Frontal and lateral views. **A** and **B,** Preoperative. **C** and **D,** Postoperative 3 months.

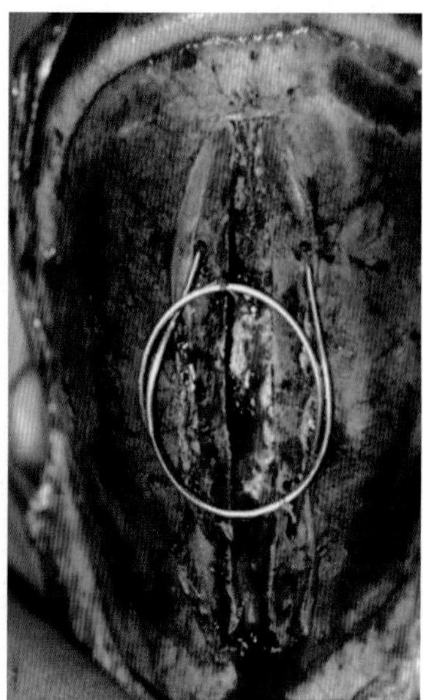

Figure 48.6 Spring cranioplasty for scaphocephaly in young infant.

TECHNIQUE: Total Calvarial Remodeling—cont'd

TURRICEPHALY AND BRACHYCEPHALY

To reduce head height and increase the frontooccipital dimension, the pattern of osteotomies above can be modified. For instance, the A piece in Fig. 48.1 may be removed from the high frontal region in a horizontal direction and turned 90 degrees to be inserted coronally behind a standard frontoorbital advancement procedure. This lengthens the antero posterior dimension of the head. The posterior B segment may need to be mobilized and pushed back depending on the severity of the individual deformity (Fig. 48.5). Alternatively, an A piece may be better harvested from the occipital region. The use of three-dimensional models to design these individual variations is recommended.

ALTERNATE OR MODIFIED TECHNIQUE

Other procedures to correct scaphocephaly include the release of the constrictive force of the fused suture to allow passive correction of head shape secondary to brain growth. These include strip craniectomies and extended strip craniectomies performed either endoscopically or with an open technique. Nearly all of these techniques require extended helmet therapy to improve the phenotypic features of scaphocephaly. The Pi procedure and its modifications, such as reverse distraction and spring-assisted cranioplasty (Fig. 48.6), combine active/passive forces either immediately or gradually to shorten the anteroposterior dimension.

Avoidance and Management of Intraoperative Complications

It is self-evident that major cranial vault reconstruction in young children requires the appropriate operative infrastructure and an experienced craniofacial, neurosurgical, and anesthetic team. During surgery, secure endotracheal intubation along with arterio-venous and temperature monitoring are essential. The two most dangerous complications are excessive bleeding and air embolism. Blood loss is anticipated, and the replacement of blood products is required in a preemptive manner to avert the serious consequences of a coagulopathy. The bleeding/clotting profile is continuously monitored throughout the procedure.[26,27]

Positioning of the patient is important. The patient is supine with little or no head flexion to avoid compromising venous drainage. Occipital access is gained easily by turning the head from side-to-side. The head should not be elevated to maintain a full venous circulation, thus lessening the possibility of air embolism. The risk of this complication is greatest during the bone segment removal phase, and a mild positive end-respiratory pressure also promotes a full venous circulation during this stage. All diploic veins are sealed with bone wax as they are dissected. With the patient in the supine position, it is easier to detect air embolism and to rapidly lower the head and treat if suspected.

Postoperative Considerations

Patients are normally returned to the ward for postoperative care and standard neurosurgical observation. Postoperative serology is performed for blood counts and electrolytes usually via the central intravenous line. Intravenous antibiotics are continued for 2 days. The head dressings are normally removed on the second or third postoperative day. In more active, older children and those who have started to walk, a soft noncompressive protective helmet is provided for 6 weeks postoperatively.

References

1. Lannelongue OM. De la craniectomie dans la microcephalie. *C R Acad Sci*. 1890;110:1382.
2. Lane LC. Pioneer craniectomy for relief of imbecility due to premature sutural closure and microcephalus. *J Am Med Assoc*. 1892;18:49.
3. McLaurin RL, Matson DD. Importance of early surgical treatment of crainosynostosis; review of 36 cases treated during the first six months of life. *Pediatrics*. 1952;10(6):637–652.
4. Ingraham FD, Alexander E Jr, Matson DD. Clinical studies in craniosynostosis analysis of 50 cases and description of a method of surgical treatment. *Surgery*. 1948;24(3):518–541.
5. Anderson FM, Johnson FL. Craniosynostosis; a modification in surgical treatment. *Surgery*. 1956;40(5):961–970.
6. Stein SC, Schut L. Management of scaphocephaly. *Surg Neurol*. 1977;7(3):153–155.
7. Epstein N, Epstein F, Newman G. Total vertex craniectomy for the treatment of scaphocephaly. *Childs Brain*. 1982;9(5):309–316.
8. Powiertowski H, Matlosz Z. [Effects of the treatment of craniostenosis with upper skull resection]. *Ann Chir*. 1970;24(21):1175–1180.
9. Kaiser G. Sagittal synostosis—its clinical significance and the results of three different methods of craniectomy. *Childs Nerv Syst*. 1988;4(4):223–230.
10. Marsh JL, Jenny A, Galic M, Picker S, Vannier MW. Surgical management of sagittal synostosis. A quantitative evaluation of two techniques. *Neurosurg Clin N Am*. 1991;2(3):629–640.
11. Maugans TA, McComb JG, Levy ML. Surgical management of sagittal synostosis: a comparative analysis of strip craniectomy and calvarial vault remodeling. *Pediatr Neurosurg*. 1997;27(3):137–148.
12. Panchal J, Marsh JL, Park TS, Kaufman B, Pilgram T, Huang SH. Sagittal craniosynostosis outcome assessment for two methods and timings of intervention. *Plast Reconstr Surg*. 1999;103(6):1574–1584.
13. Jane JA, Edgerton MT, Futrell JW, Park TS. Immediate correction of sagittal synostosis. *J Neurosurg*. 1978;49(5):705–710.
14. Jane JA Sr, Lin KY. Surgical management of scaphocephaly: pi-squeeze technique. *Tech Neurosurg*. 1997;3:179.
15. Greensmith AL, Furneaux C, Rees M, de Chalain T. Cranial compression by reverse distraction: a new technique for correction of sagittal synostosis. *Plast Reconstr Surg*. 2001;108(4):979–985.
16. Fearon JA, McLaughlin EB, Kolar JC. Sagittal craniosynostosis: surgical outcomes and long-term growth. *Plast Reconstr Surg*. 2006;117(2):532–541.
17. Di Rocco F, Knoll BI, Arnaud E, et al. Scaphocephaly correction with retrocoronal and prelambdoid craniotomies (Renier's "H" technique). *Childs Nerv Syst*. 2012;28(9):1327–1332.
18. Guimarães-Ferreira J, Gewalli F, David L, Olsson R, Friede H, Lauritzen CG. Spring-mediated cranioplasty compared with the modified pi-plasty for sagittal synostosis. *Scand J Plast ReConstr Surg Hand Surg*. 2003;37(4):208–215.
19. Jimenez DF, Barone CM, Cartwright CC, Baker L. Early management of craniosynostosis using endoscopic-assisted strip craniectomies and cranial orthotic molding therapy. *Pediatrics*. 2002;110(1 Pt 1):97–104.
20. Jimenez DF, Barone CM. Endoscopic technique for sagittal synostosis. *Childs Nerv Syst*. 2012;28(9):1333–1339.
21. Delye HHK, Borstlap WA, van Lindert EJ. Endoscopy-assisted craniosynostosis surgery followed by helmet therapy. *Surg Neurol Int*. 2018;9:59.
22. Hudgins RJ, Burstein FD, Boydston WR. Total calvarial reconstruction for sagittal synostosis in older infants and children. *J Neurosurg*. 1993;78(2):199–204.
23. Greensmith AL, Holmes AD, Lo P, Maxiner W, Heggie AA, Meara JG. Complete correction of severe scaphocephaly: the Melbourne method of total vault remodeling. *Plast Reconstr Surg*. 2008;121(4):1300–1310.
24. Holmes AD, Wray AC, Burge JA, Chong DK. The Melbourne method of total cranial vault reconstruction for scaphocephaly; a twenty-year overview. *Plast Reconstr Surg Glob Open*. 2019;7(8S-2):72.
25. Toma R, Greensmith AL, Meara JG, et al. Quantitative morphometric outcomes following the Melbourne method of total vault remodeling for scaphocephaly. *J Craniofac Surg*. 2010;21(3):637–643.
26. Choi WT, Greensmith AL, Chatdokmaiprai C, Holmes AD, Meara JG. Tumescent steroid infiltration reduces postoperative eye closure after craniofacial surgery. *Plast Reconstr Surg*. 2008;122(1):30e–32e.
27. Howe PW, Cooper MG. Blood loss and replacement for paediatric cranioplasty in Australia—a prospective national audit. *Anaesth Intensive Care*. 2012;40(1):107–113.

CHAPTER 49

The Le Fort III Osteotomy

Paul S. Tiwana and Timothy A. Turvey

Armamentarium

#9 Periosteal elevator
#10 and #15 scalpel blades
#701 Bur
Appropriate sutures
Arch bars and 24- and 26-gauge wire
Austin retractor
Bipolar electrocautery
Channel retractor
Curved Mayo scissors
Distraction osteogenesis devices
Double-guarded nasal septal osteotome
Fixation devices: P&S or internal/external
Hair elastics
K-wires
Local anesthetic with vasoconstrictor
Malleable retractors
Mayfield headrest
Needle electrocautery
Obwegeser retractors
Pterygoid chisel
Raney clips
Reciprocating saw
Rowe forceps
Seldin

History of the Procedure

The French anatomist René Le Fort published his classic treatise on the description of common fracture patterns in the middle facial third in 1901.[1] The ensuing engulfment of the World Wars produced horrendous mass casualties that steered facial reconstructive surgeons like Kazanjian[2] in their efforts to manage injuries to the middle third of the face. Building on the knowledge and skill born by these conflicts, Sir Harold Gillies, an otolaryngologist by training, was the first surgeon to publish an attempt at mobilization of the midface in the management of a patient with craniofacial dysostosis.[3] The procedure was unsuccessful, and Gillies later abandoned it. Subsequently, Longacre attempted reconstruction of the midface by autogenous rib grafting.[4] However, this procedure did nothing to address the functional impairments associated with total midface deficiency. In addition, the long-term stability of the reconstruction from an esthetic standpoint was questionable. In 1967, the pioneering efforts of Tessier revolutionized management of the patient with total midface deficiency.[5–13] His landmark presentations and publications concerning the mobilization of the entire middle face through the concept of combined intra- and extracranial approach in a safe and consistent manner were groundbreaking. Modifications and extensions of this concept by Tessier himself and others have produced surgical techniques that have provided relief of functional impairments and improved the stability of facial esthetics to the benefit of the patient with total midface deficiency. The first known performance of this surgery in the United States was by Robert V. Walker in 1967, shortly after Tessier's presentation in Rome.

Indications for the Use of the Procedure

Craniofacial anomalies, by their very nature, are repetitive patterns of deformity affecting the different functional and esthetic subunits of the facial hard and soft tissues. Perhaps their only common feature is the degree of variable expressivity of the deformity within each subtype of anomaly.[14–17] The surgical management of the full spectrum of craniofacial anomalies affecting the subcranial facial skeleton is beyond the scope of this chapter.

Craniofacial Dysostosis

The craniofacial dysostosis syndromes—Apert, Crouzon, Pfeiffer, and Saethre-Chotzen—are characterized by sutural involvement that not only includes the cranial vault but also extends into the skull base and midfacial skeletal structures.[18] Although the cranial vault and cranial base are thought to be the regions of primary involvement, there is also significant impact on midfacial growth and development. In addition to cranial vault dysmorphology, patients with these inherited conditions exhibit a characteristic "total midface" deficiency that must be addressed as part of the staged reconstructive approach. Although there is some similarity between the pattern of facial growth and development in these patients, there is a high degree of variable expressivity in each patient regardless of syndrome. This must be taken into account when planning and executing surgical correction of these deformities.[19–25]

Total Midface Deficiency

The role of the human face is significant in both a direct and an indirect fashion for reasons other than purely esthetic considerations. These are secondary to the highly evolved and specialized functions of the face in vision, breathing, speech production, smell, and hearing, among a few. In patients with craniofacial dysostosis, in addition to potential neurologic deficits, there is often variable fusion of the lesser sutures of the skull base.[26–28] This commonly results in abnormal ophthalmologic findings including exorbitism, exotropia, orbital dystopia, and ptosis secondary to a lack of orbital depth and diameter, as well as prolapse of the ethmoid sinuses through the medial orbital walls. The severe occlusal discrepancies found in this group of patients are characterized by generalized hypoplasia of the maxilla, transverse deficiency, class III malocclusion, and apertognathia. All of these abnormalities contribute to impair speech articulation and mastication. In addition, cleft palate, when present, can produce velopharyngeal incompetence. The severe retrusive position of the midface can also interfere with nasal breathing and produce chronic nasal obstruction. Varying degrees of orbital hypertelorism may or may not be present. The extent to which this condition is present strongly influences the type of surgical correction required for total midface deficiency (Fig. 49.1A–H).

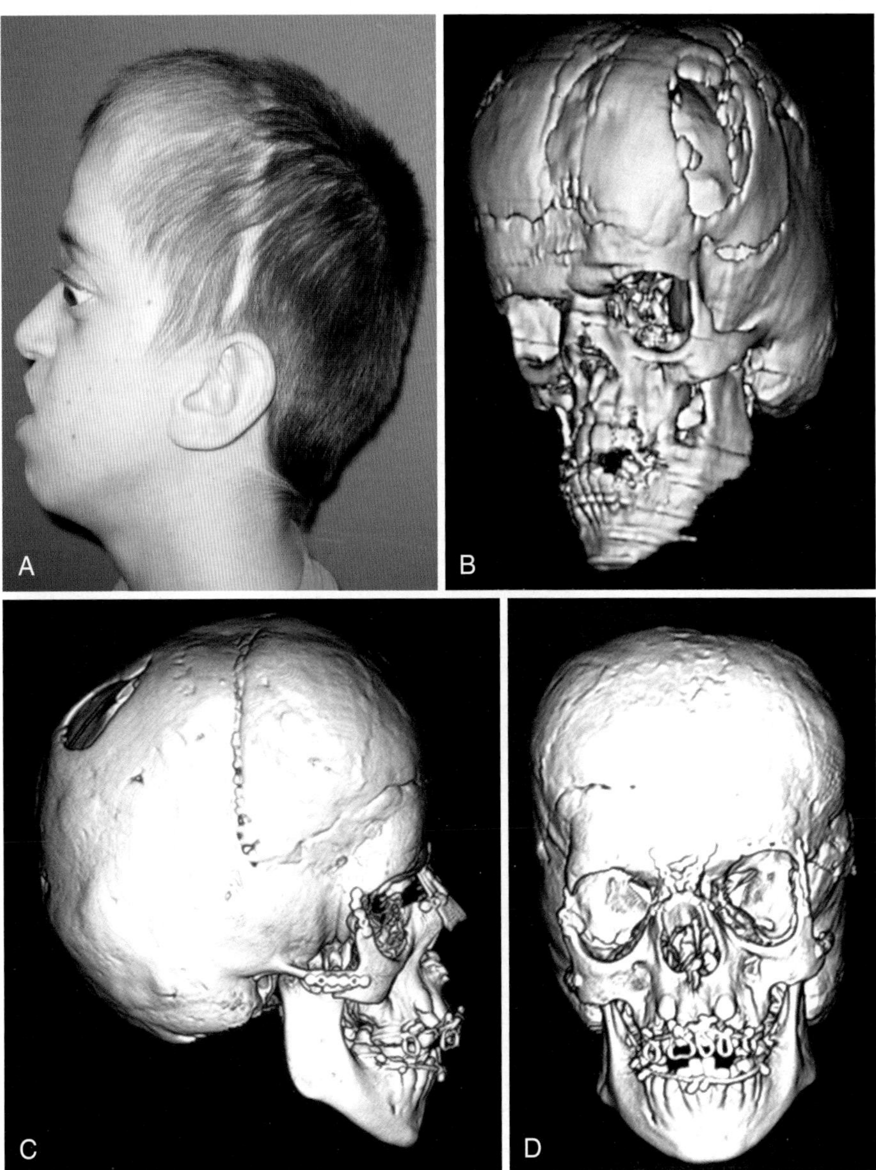

Figure 49.1 **A and B,** Facial and three dimensional (3D) computed tomography (CT) scan views prior to subcranial Le Fort III osteotomy. Note the skull defects from previous cranio-orbital decompression by another surgeon. **C and D,** 3D CT scans after subcranial Le Fort III osteotomy and repair of skull defects with resorbable mesh and bone cement.

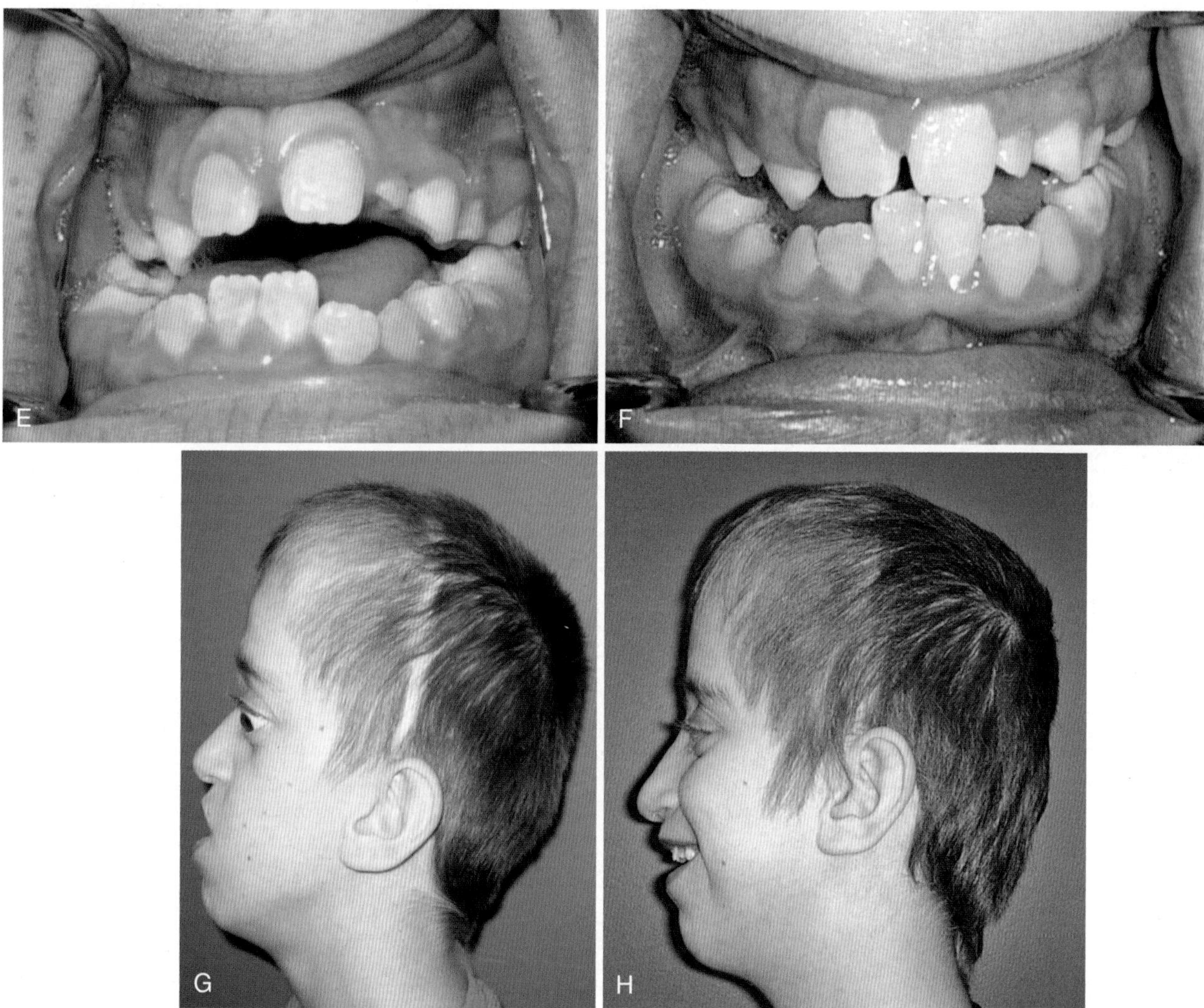

Figure 49.1, cont'd **E and F,** Pre- and postoperative occlusion at 6 months. **G and H,** Pre- and postoperative facial views at 6 months. (From Fonseca RJ, et al. *Oral and Maxillofacial surgery.* 2nd ed. Philadelphia, PA: Saunders, 2009).

The presence of total midface deficiency does not mitigate the coexistence of other facial skeletal abnormalities such as mandibular excess and retrogenia. In addition, there are often irregularities of the forehead as well as frontal bossing. Typically, the nasal length is short and projection is deficient. This gives rise to an exaggerated depression or flatness of the nasofrontal region. Because of the deficiency in orbital depth and diameter producing an exorbita, an excessive amount of scleral show may be present. Ptosis of the lids and lateral canthal dystopia are usually present. The nasolabial angle is commonly less than 90 degrees because of nasal deficiency and the overprojection of the maxillary teeth.

A more precise measurement of the degree of exorbitism can be obtained using the Hertel exophthalmometer or through computed tomography scan analysis of the position of the globe relative to the eye and the upper facial skeletal to normative values, as originally published by Posnick and colleagues.

Limitations and Contraindications

However, specific limitations apply to the use of this surgical maneuver. The bony structures of the middle facial third are in contiguity with the cranial base superiorly. Transgression of this natural barrier is called for in the surgical correction of some craniofacial anomalies. If the presenting deformity extends to excessive interorbital distance or there is significant aberration of the supraorbital/forehead subunit, consideration should be given to using a combined intra- and extracranial approach such as facial bipartition or monobloc osteotomy.[29] In addition, subcranial Le Fort III osteotomy does not address the three-dimensional vertical slanting of the facial halves or the convex arc of rotation of the face, as seen in some craniofacial dysostosis patients, which can only be adequately managed with facial bipartition osteotomy.[30]

The surgeon must give thoughtful consideration to addressing the presenting dysmorphology, with the intention of improving the overall esthetic and functional concerns of the patient while taking into account the potential complications and benefits inherent with the use of an intracranial approach. Management of the skeletally immature patient, as discussed later, requires surgical intervention based on the complex balance between the long-term stability of the correction and more immediate functional, psychological, and esthetic demands of each patient. As with all craniofacial procedures, patient selection is critical for a successful outcome.

TECHNIQUE: Le Fort III Osteotomy

STEP 1: Intubation

Nasoendotracheal intubation with a reinforced tube exiting inferiorly across the mouth, neck, and chest before returning to anesthesia is preferred. The tube is secured with suture to the membranous septum and columella. Because intermaxillary fixation is necessary to establish the projection of the middle face, oral intubation is less desirable and should be avoided unless the splint can be modified to accommodate the position of the tube. The length of the endotracheal tube must be sufficiently below the level of the vocal cords to prevent unintended dislodgment during midface disimpaction and advancement (Fig. 49.2A).

STEP 2: Tarsorrhaphy Suture

A tarsorrhaphy suture (6-0 silk) is used to secure the eyelids after ophthalmologic lubricant is placed. The hair is not shaved, rather it is parted and controlled with elastics along the proposed incision line in the scalp. The incision line is infiltrated with 2% lidocaine with 1:100,000 epinephrine to control bleeding during dissection. The scalp and upper forehead are infiltrated generously with injectable saline (approximately 100 cc) above the pericranium to aid in a blood-free dissection through the loose connective tissue just above the periosteum. The face, head, and oral cavity are then prepared with Betadine scrub. The entire operative field is straight, exposing the oral cavity, ears, and scalp posterior to the planned incision.

Continued

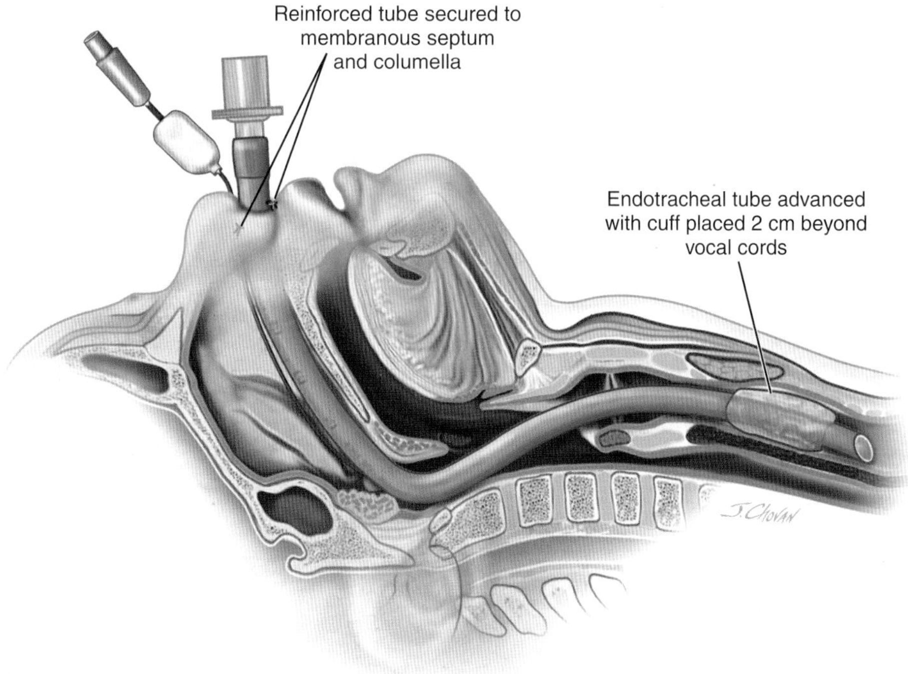

Figure 49.2 **A,** Endotracheal tube (through the nose) showing the endotracheal tube cuff extending at least 2 cm below the vocal cords.

TECHNIQUE: Le Fort III Osteotomy—*cont'd*

STEP 3: Incision

An incision is made from the midauricular area of the scalp across the top of the head to the opposite side. The incision is carried through the layers of the scalp to the pericranium. Hemostasis is achieved with bipolar cautery, and a flap is elevated in the bloodless supraperiosteal plane until a point approximately 2 cm behind the supraorbital rim is reached. At this point an incision is made through the periosteum and the dissection continues under the periosteum to expose the supraorbital rims, nasal bones, lateral orbital rims, zygomas, and infraorbital regions bilaterally. The supraorbital nerves are freed by releasing them from the supraorbital foramen bilaterally. Next, the periorbital dissection is performed subperiosteally, being careful not to detach the medial canthus and to dissect behind the lacrimal apparatus. Remaining under the periosteum during the facial dissection is critical to preserve facial nerve function. Once all of the tissues are dissected from the midfacial skeleton, the osteotomy commences (Fig. 49.2B).

STEP 4: Initial Osteotomy

The initial osteotomy is conducted vertically through the zygomatic arch with a reciprocal saw. The soft tissues are protected by placing a channel retraction below the zygomatic arch. The frontozygomatic suture is identified and an osteotomy is begun to separate the lateral orbital wall from the suture area inferiorly to the infraorbital fissure at a depth of approximately 1 cm from the orbital rim. A drill with a small fissure bur is then used to section the floor of the orbit from the infraorbital fissure medially and directed behind the lacrimal apparatus. The wound is then packed and attention is directed to the nasal frontal area (Fig. 49.2C).

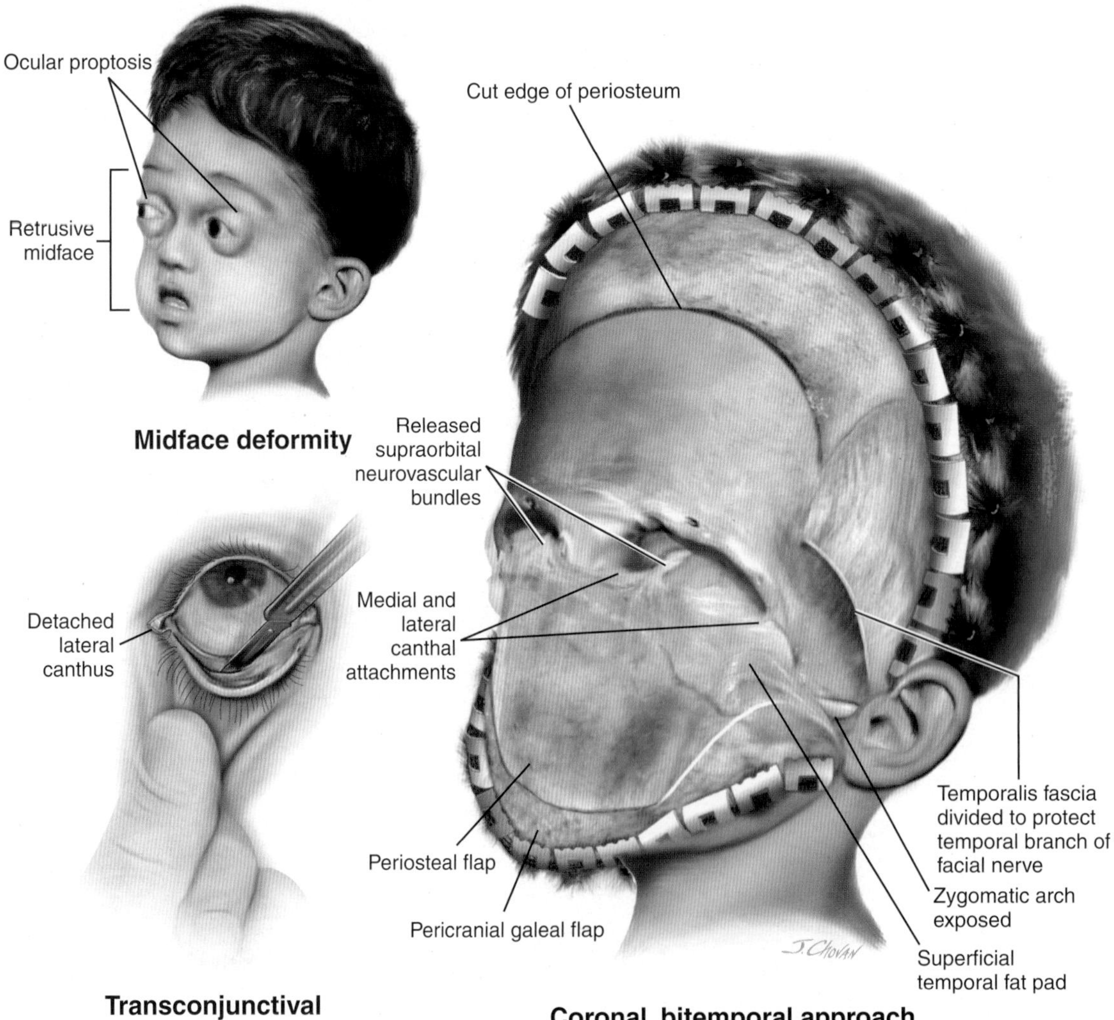

Figure 49.2, cont'd **B,** Coronal flap.

TECHNIQUE: Le Fort III Osteotomy—*cont'd*

STEP 5: Section of the Pterygoid Plate

Once this procedure is completed bilaterally, the wounds are packed and the scalp flap is returned to its original position. The oral cavity is entered and the tissue over the posterior maxilla is injected with 2% lidocaine with 1:100,000 epinephrine. The posterior wall of the maxilla and pterygoid plates are then approached through the two horizontal subperiosteal incisions. Subperiosteal dissection to the pterygoid plates and superior to the infratemporal fossa exposes the area of the midface, which must be sectioned next. The pterygoid plate is sectioned at the posterior maxillary wall junction from the pterygoid plate superiorly to the infraorbital fissure region. Remaining subperiosteal is critical to limit the possibility of hemorrhage from the internal maxillary artery and its terminal branches. These wounds are then packed, and the scalp flap is reflected again to expose the osteotomies from above (Fig. 49.2D).

STEP 6: Final Osteotomy

The final osteotomy is the separation of the vomer. This is done with a thin osteotome placed at the nasofrontal osteotomy and directed inferiorly and posteriorly. Care must be exercised to remain anterior to the skull base. Modified Rowe disimpaction forceps are then inserted in the nose and intraorally through the maxillary incision onto the bone of the nasal floor. Downward force with adequate head stabilization and care to minimize the risk of endotracheal tube displacement begins the process of mobilization (Fig. 49.2E).

STEP 7: Advance Middle Face

Once the middle face is adequately mobilized, it should be advanced to the predetermined position, using the prefabricated occlusal splint as a reference. A vertical reference should also be used to control the face height. Sometimes this requires the placement of a pin in the outer cortex of the frontal bone in the area of the frontal sinus. Intermaxillary fixation wires are then applied.

Continued

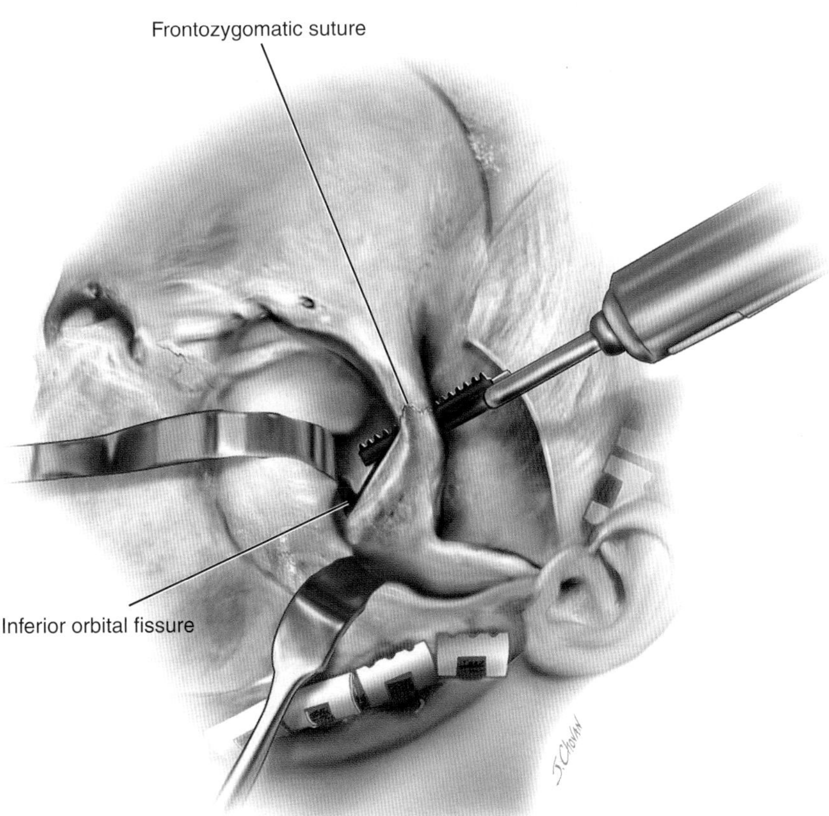

Figure 49.2, cont'd **C,** Reciprocating saw coming up through the inferior orbital fissure through the frontozygomatic suture.

TECHNIQUE: Le Fort III Osteotomy—*cont'd*

STEP 8: Bone Plate Stabilization

To stabilize the bone plate, biodegradable plates and screws are placed at the zygomatic and lateral orbital rim regions. Additional plating takes place at the nasofrontal region. Bone defects are filled with grafts harvested from the cranium or ileum. Additionally, autogenous bone is almost always used to further contour and refine the morphology of the facial skeleton. It is an exception for the authors to perform this operation and not use bone grafts to further contour the face. All bone grafts must be wedged or adequately stabilized with screws to prevent displacement and enhance revascularization (Fig. 49.2F).

STEP 9: Irrigation, Resuspension, and Closure of Scalp

All osteotomies are conducted with copious irrigation. At the completion of surgery, all surgical sites are thoroughly irrigated. The lateral canthus and temporalis muscle are resuspended with a 3-0 resorbable suture. Superior and posterior suspension of the deep layers of the flap should also be done with resorbable suture to minimize dead space and to encourage reattachment of the superficial musculoaponeurotic layer. Drains are usually not placed. The scalp is closed in two layers with 3-0 polyglycolate suture in deeper tissues and 3-0 chromic gut suture in the hair-bearing regions. The oral tissues and operative site are irrigated and closed with a 3-0 chromic gut suture (Fig. 49.2G).

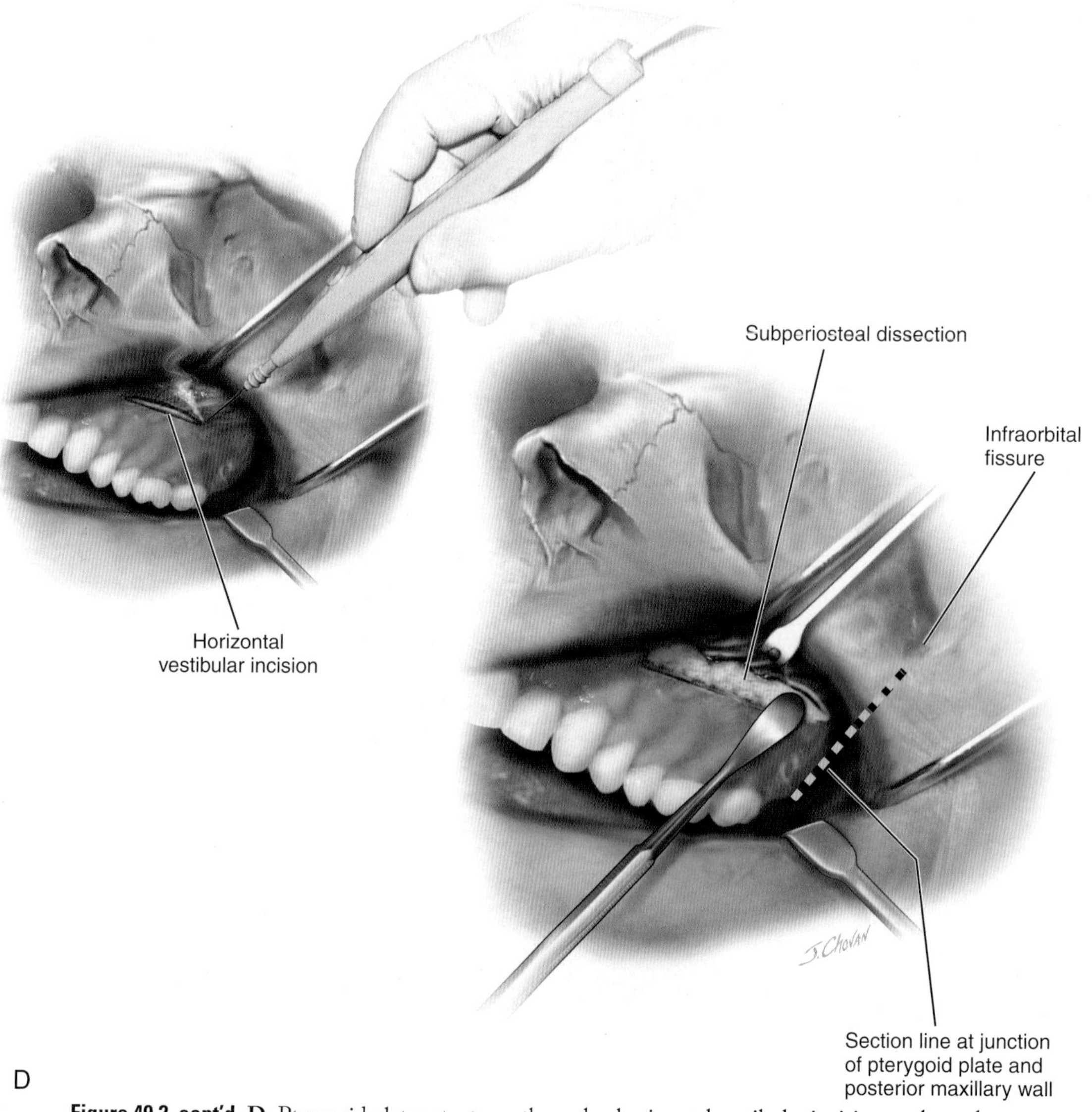

Figure 49.2, cont'd **D,** Pterygoid plate osteotomy through a horizontal vestibular incision or through the coronal flap.

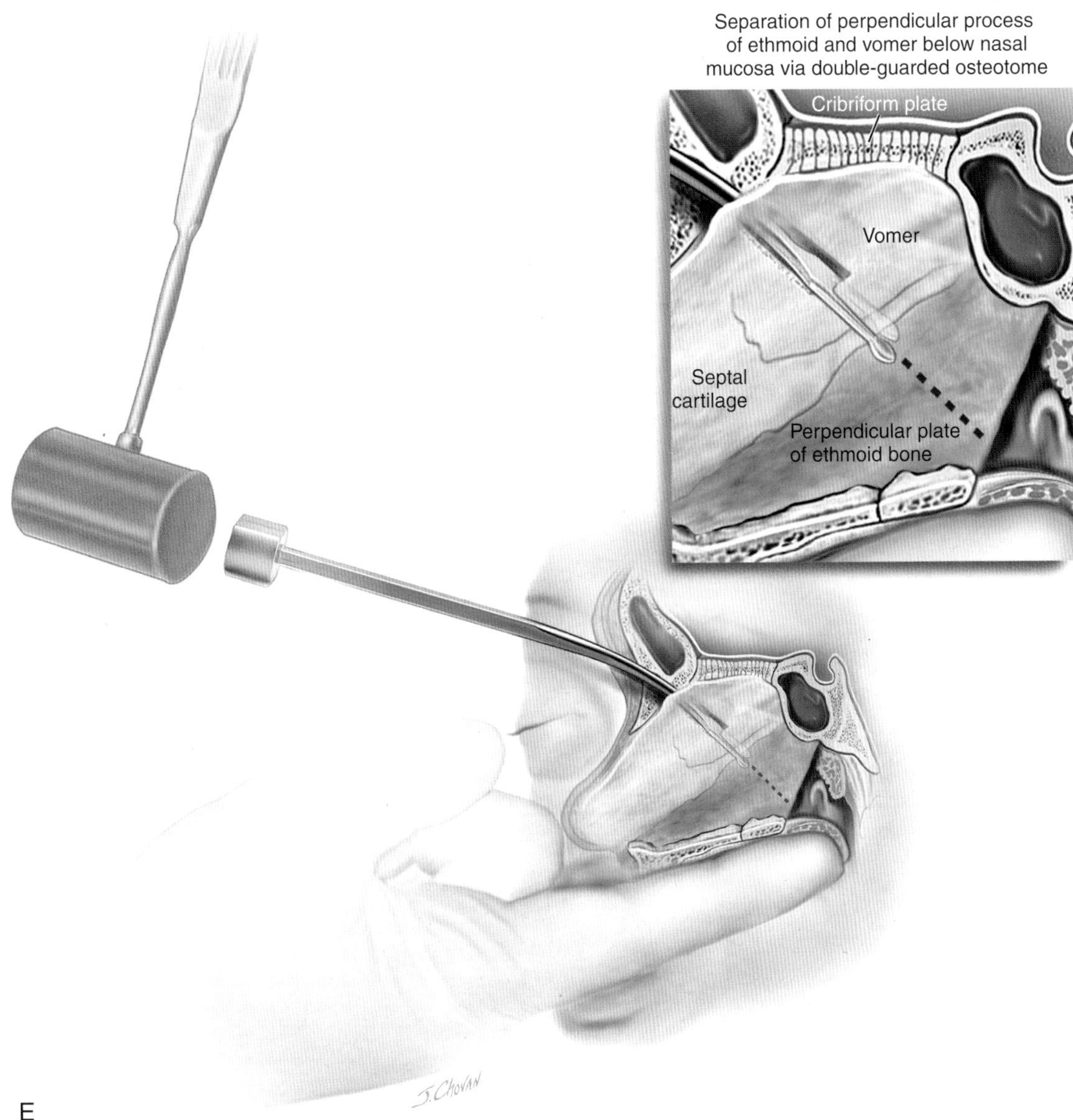

Figure 49.2, cont'd E, Nasofrontal osteotomy (chisel through the nasofrontal junction heading toward the posterior nasal spine with the surgeon's finger on the posterior nasal spine through the mouth).

TECHNIQUE: Le Fort III Osteotomy—*cont'd*

STEP 10: Removal of the Tarsorrhaphy Sutures

The tarsorrhaphy sutures are removed and forced duction of the globe is done bilaterally to assure eye mobility. A nasogastric tube is carefully inserted at the completion of surgery, and it is kept to low suction overnight. Extubation at the completion of surgery is common (see Fig. 49.1F–H).

ALTERNATIVE TECHNIQUE 1: Modifications of Le Fort III

Although numerous procedures exist for the management of the various craniofacial malformations in the middle third of the facial skeleton, only the subcranial Le Fort III osteotomy[31] addresses all of the functional and esthetic components of total midface deficiency, when considering an extracranial approach for surgical correction of the deformity. This is not to suggest that within the context of an extracranial procedure the Le Fort III osteotomy is inflexible; rather, the

Continued

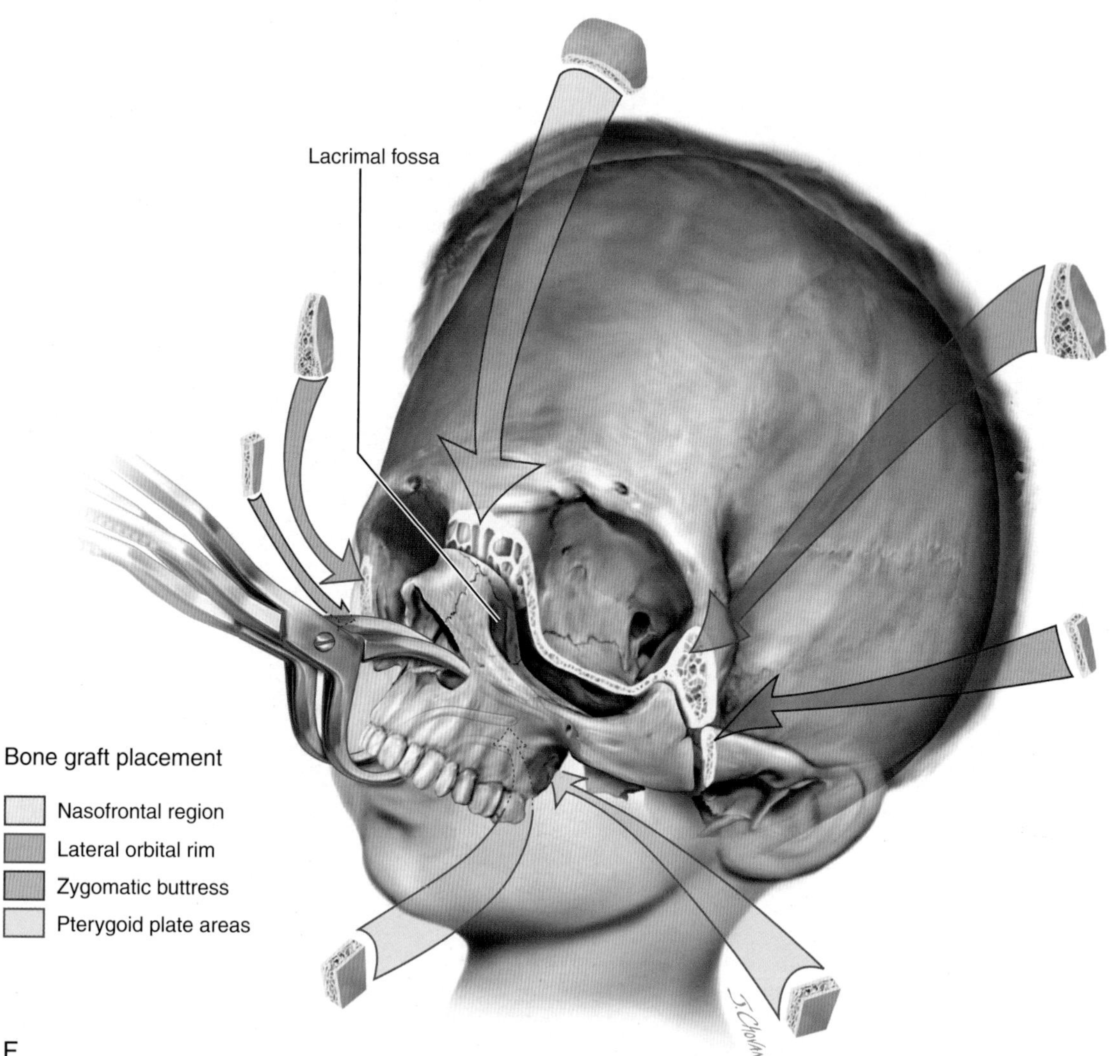

Figure 49.2, cont'd **F,** The Le Fort III osteotomy.

ALTERNATIVE TECHNIQUE 1: Modifications of Le Fort III—*cont'd*

opposite is true. Modifications of the Le Fort III osteotomy such as Kufner's operation are possible and can be utilized to address deformities that do not involve the nasal subunit.[32] In addition, the authors have documented the long-term stability of this procedure in both syndromal and nonsyndromal patients.[33,34] The orbital floor cuts are extended medially and inferiorly over the orbital rim toward the piriform aperture and enter the nasal cavity at the same height as a typical Le Fort I osteotomy. The separation of the septum and vomer is also the same as that typically seen during a Le Fort I osteotomy, as is separation of the lateral nasal wall (Fig. 49.3).

ALTERNATIVE TECHNIQUE 2: Simultaneous Le Fort III/I

The addition of simultaneous Le Fort I osteotomies can be helpful in the management of patients who have a specific disproportion between the deficiency of the Le Fort III level (inferior orbital rim) and the Le Fort I level (nasal base and anterior maxillary dentition).

If Le Fort I osteotomy is combined with the Le Fort III (or modified Le Fort III) procedure, it is done through two horizontal mucosal incisions, preserving an anterior pedicle to the independently mobilizing maxilla. Stabilization with bone plates and autogenous bone grafts is also used.

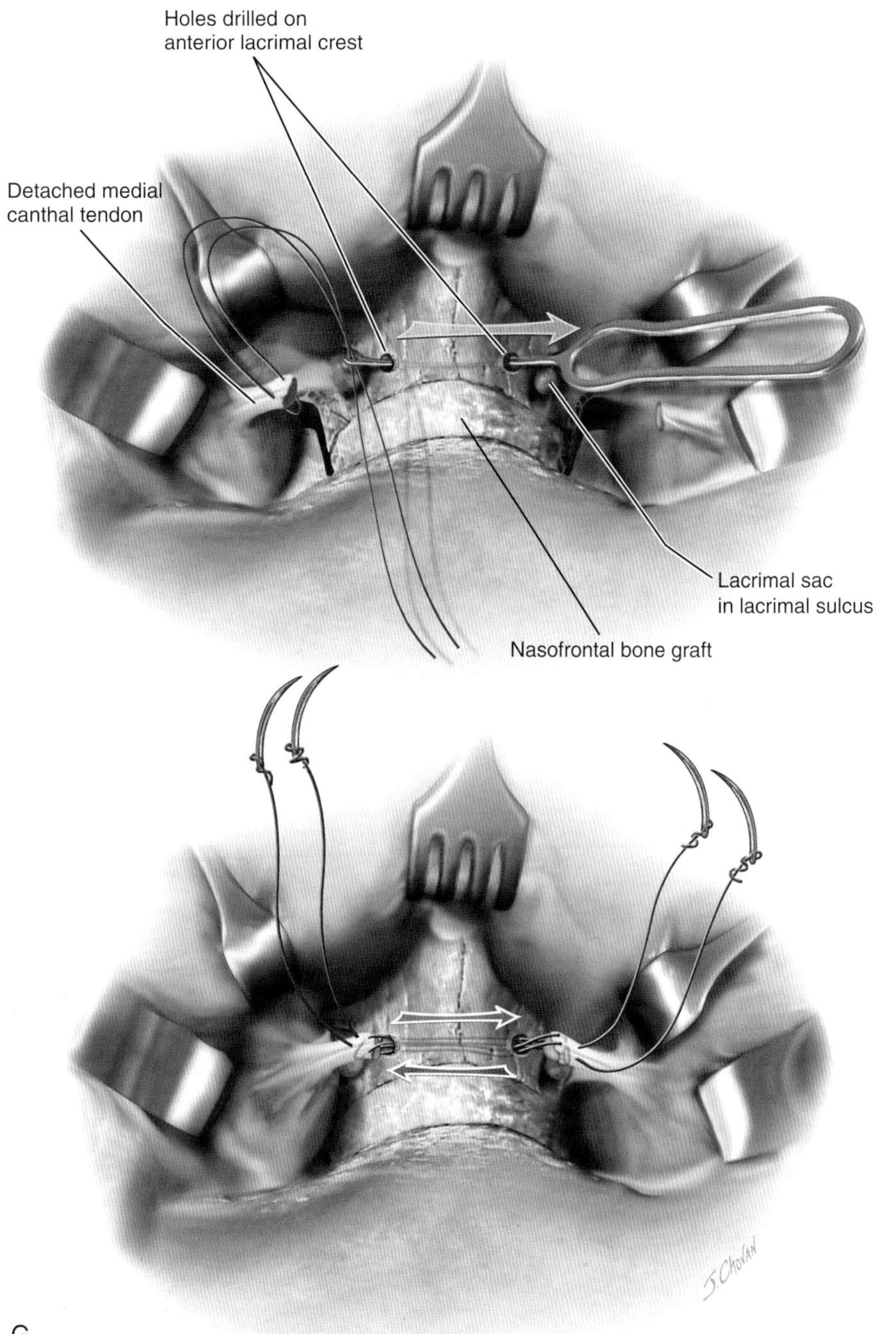

Figure 49.2, cont'd **G,** Medial canthopexy.

The addition of the Le Fort I osteotomy must be accomplished after stabilization of the upper area of the completed Le Fort III osteotomy. Usually, after total midface mobilization, a saw cut through the lateral and anterior maxillary wall is usually all that is necessary to mobilize the maxilla at the lower level. Two splint indexes are ideally utilized in this technique, the first to establish the position of the inferior orbital rim as the whole midface is anteriorly moved, and the second to establish the final occlusion at the Le Fort I level unless simultaneous mandibular osteotomies are also planned, in which case it becomes a second intermediate splint. Obvious considerations with regard to skeletal maturity and the eruption status of the permanent dentition must also be considered in planning the simultaneous Le Fort I osteotomy (Fig. 49.4).

ALTERNATIVE TECHNIQUE 3: Internal/External Distraction Osteogenesis of Le Fort III

Another technique that will assist with the advancement and fixation of the Le Fort III osteotomy is the use of distraction osteogenesis. External distraction at the Le Fort III level, first popularized by Polley and colleagues, has been utilized

Continued

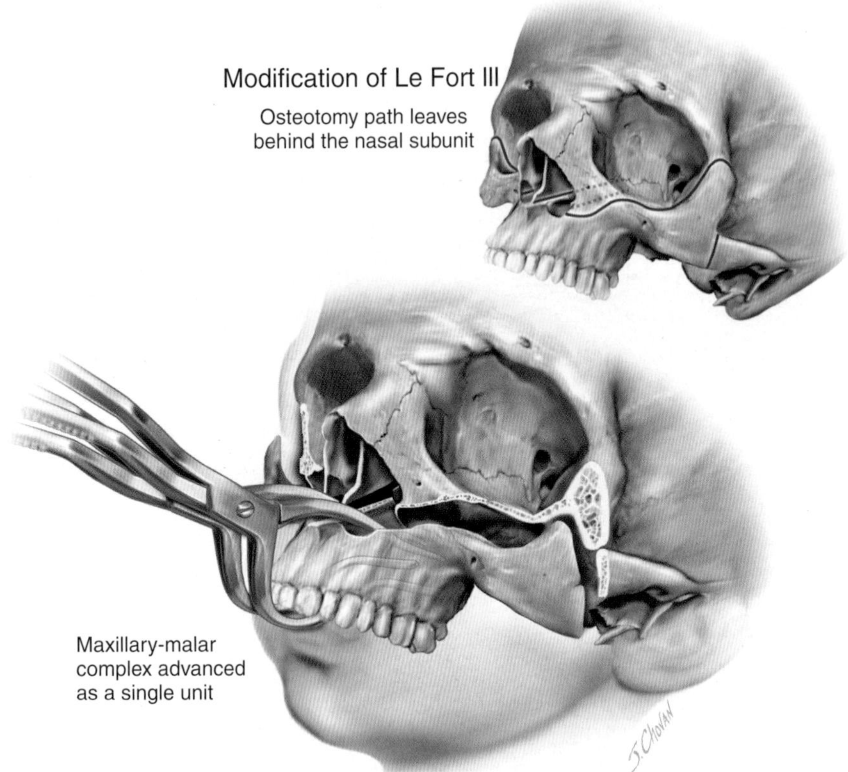

Figure 49.3 Bone grafts are used to improve the cheek and orbital rim contour.

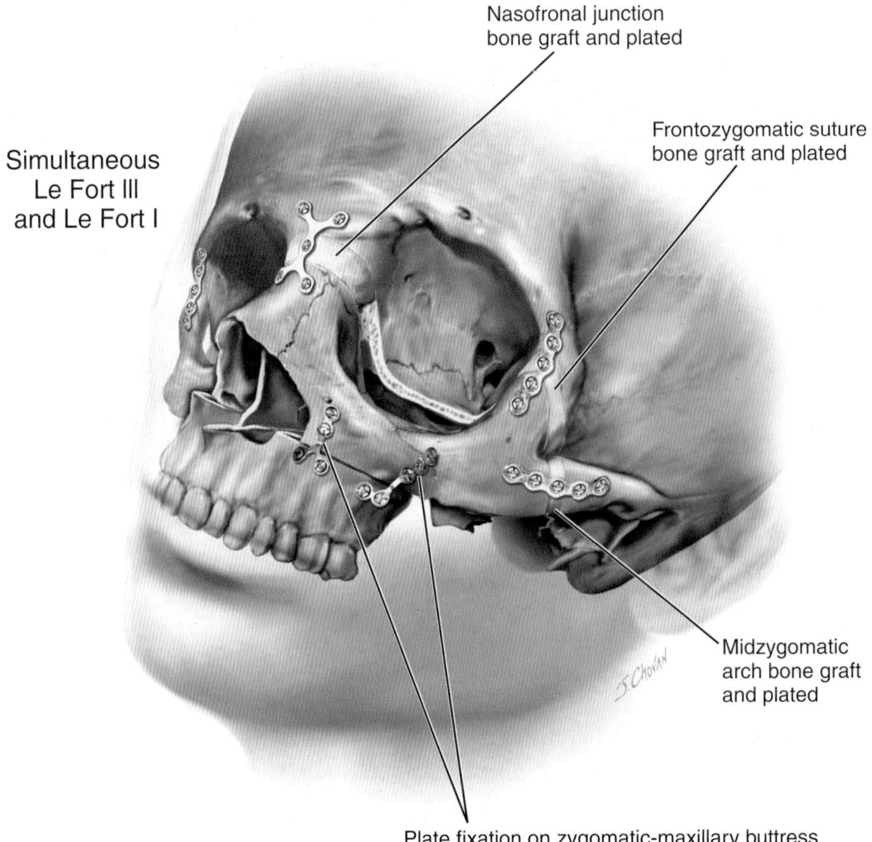

Figure 49.4 A Le Fort III osteotomy advanced and plated with a simultaneous Le Fort I osteotomy advanced and plated.

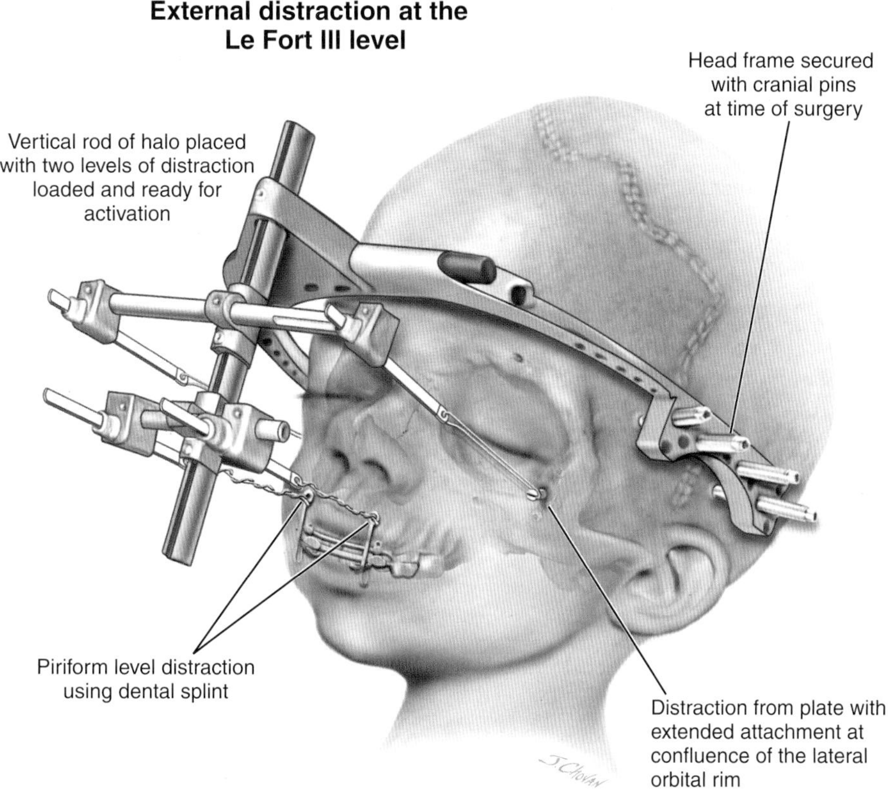
External distraction at the
Le Fort III level
Head frame secured
with cranial pins
at time of surgery
Vertical rod of halo placed
with two levels of distraction
loaded and ready for
activation
Piriform level distraction
using dental splint
Distraction from plate with
extended attachment at
confluence of the lateral
orbital rim

Figure 49.5 Le Fort III osteotomy with a halo (external distraction) appliance placed.

ALTERNATIVE TECHNIQUE 3: Internal/External Distraction Osteogenesis of Le Fort III—*cont'd*

extensively. The osteotomy must be carried out precisely as noted earlier and requires full mobilization of the segment to be distracted.

The head frame is carefully applied with the cranial pins at surgery (at least three on each side), taking care not to penetrate intracranially and to place the head frame as symmetrically as possible. The vertical rod is placed and the device is made ready for activation by loading the distractor at a minimum of two levels: the area of the zygoma and the piriform area. The fixation at the level of the zygoma is done with a bone plate and a transcutaneous wire to the distractor. At the Le Fort I level, two options exist, either the use of a bone plate with a transcutaneous wire in the piriform rim bilaterally or the use of a dental splint, which is greatly preferred. The use of bone plates can be problematic given the amount of continual force necessary during the distraction process to allow forward translation of the face. Stabilization with a dental splint to the permanent first molars with labial and palatal coverage allows for a more predictable outcome. The vector of distraction is counterintuitively at a more inferior angle to prevent formation of a large anterior open bite. Guiding elastics can also be of assistance in managing the occlusion during distraction. The distraction rhythm has been modified substantially by a number of individuals but, in the author's experience, usually a 0.5-mm bid is sufficient.

Yet another technique calls for the placement of internal distractors behind the step osteotomy of the zygoma bilaterally, with placement of additional distractors at the buttress Le Fort I level, if needed, or permitted by the eruption of the permanent teeth. These distractors are activated in a fashion similar to that previously described; however, little to no vector control is possible because the devices are buried. The occlusion can still be modified with elastics. A second procedure may be required to remove the devices as indicated. Lastly, the work of Padwa and colleagues describes use of the "push-pull" technique. In this application, a combination of internal and external distraction is used to advance the midface.

Distraction osteogenesis techniques have the advantage of allowing further advancement of the face than was traditionally possible with traditional osteotomy, with arguably an improvement in long-term stability. However, it is difficult to be precise because the vector adjustments become complex. The percutaneous wires cause unsightly facial scarring. In addition, a large stepoff in the nose is often seen after distraction. Lastly, the lateral canthi are often displaced inferiorly.

Although distraction osteogenesis has a place in the armamentarium of the surgeon for correction of severe deformities of the middle facial third, the distinct disadvantages of the inherent imprecision coupled with the obtrusive nature of the appliances to the patient/child make it suboptimal in some circumstances (Fig. 49.5).

Avoidance and Management of Intraoperative Complications

Adequate mobilization of the facial skeleton is critical for success. Downward, anterior, and rotary motion is necessary to completely free the face. Care that all osteotomy sites are moving similarly will reduce the chances of inadvertent fractures, especially of the orbits. Recutting areas of resistance is sometimes necessary and important.

The frontonasal suture is identified, and the level of the cribriform plate should be confirmed radiographically to be above the nasofrontal junction. If the plate is lower than this junction, the procedure should be modified to be certain that the osteotomy is inferior to the cribriform plate or consideration should be given to formal craniotomy to protect the intracranial contents. Similarly, the anterior extent of the temporal lobes should be identified radiographically before the lateral orbital rims are cut, especially in patients with Apert syndrome where the temporal lobes can be located more anteriorly within the lateral orbital rims.

During the mobilization process, the previously placed suture to secure the nasoendotracheal tube must be assigned an assistant to guard its position. Displacement of the endotracheal tube must be avoided during this critical process.

Postoperative Considerations

Steroids and antibiotics are always used with the first dose administered upon intubation and prior to this commencement of surgery. High-dose intravenous steroid is given intravenously every 4 hours throughout surgery and for the first 24 hours after surgery. Before the patient leaves the operating room, a further dose of intramuscular slow-release steroid is administered. A weight-appropriate dosage of cephalosporin is also administered intravenously every 4 hours during surgery and for the first 24 hours after surgery. Oral antibiotics are continued for 10 days.

Typically, the airway is improved as a result of surgery, and there is little reason for prolonged intubation following this surgery. Early during the postoperative course, ambulation and oral intake are encouraged. Although cerebrospinal fluid rhinorrhea may be suspected in some patients, prolonged bed rest is not encouraged. Nose blowing, Valsalva maneuvers, and the like are discouraged. Nasal packing is never performed, although drip pad usage is common. Nasal sprays with vasoconstrictors for congestion are used for 2 weeks. Diet is restricted to foods with a soft nonchew consistency for approximately 6 weeks. Guiding elastics are useful to reduce patient discomfort and control the occlusion.

Visual disturbance including diplopia is uncommon, although all patients must be warned prior to surgery. Anosmia is also uncommon, but informing the patient of this possibility is prudent. Altered sensation to the forehead, cheeks, lateral nose, gingiva, and palate is common, and patients must be counseled accordingly. Facial nerve injury should not occur, especially with subperiosteal dissection.

References

1. Converse JM, Kazanjian VH. *Surgical Treatment of Facial Injuries*. Baltimore, Maryland: Williams & Wilkins; 1949.
2. Le Fort R. Experimental study of fractures of the upper jaw: parts 1 and 2. *Rev Chir Paris*. 1902;23:208–360.
3. Gillies H, Harrison SH. Operative correction by osteotomy of recessed malar maxillary compound in a case of oxycephaly. *Br J Plast Surg*. 1950;3(2):123–127.
4. Longacre JJ, Destefano GA. Further observations of the behavior of autogenous split-rib grafts in reconstruction of extensive defects of the cranium and face. *Plast Reconstr Surg*. 1957;20(4):281–296.
5. Tessier P. Ostéotomies totales de la face. Syndrome de Crouzon, syndrme d'Apert: oxycéphalies, scaphocéphalies, turricéphalies. *Ann Chir Plast*. 1967;12(4):273–286.
6. Tessier P. The definitive plastic surgical treatment of the severe facial deformities of craniofacial dysostosis. Crouzon's and Apert's diseases. *Plast Reconstr Surg*. 1971;48(5):419–442.
7. Tessier P. Dysostoses cranio-faciales (syndromes de Crouzon et d'Apert): osteotomies totales de la face. In: *Transactions of the Fourth International Congress of Plastic and Reconstructive Surgery*. Amsterdam, Netherlands; 1969.
8. Tessier P. Relationship of craniosynostosis to craniofacial dysostosis and to faciosynostosis: a study with therapeutic implications. *Clin Plast Surg*. 1982;9:531.
9. Tessier P. Autogenous bone grafts taken from the calvarium for facial and cranial applications. *Plast Reconstr Surg*. 1971;48:224.
10. Tessier P. Total osteotomy of the middle third of the face for faciostenosis or for sequelae of Le Fort 3 fractures. *Plast Reconstr Surg*. 1971;48(6):533–541.
11. Tessier P. Traitement des dysmorphies faciales propres aux dysostoses craniofaciales (DGF), maladies de Crouzon et d'Apert. *Neurochirurgie*. 1971;17:295.
12. Tessier P. *Craniofacial Surgery in Syndromic Craniosynostosis: Craniosynostosis, Diagnosis, Evaluation and Management*. New York, NY: Raven Press; 1986.
13. Tessier P. Recent improvement in the treatment of facial and cranial deformities in Crouzon disease and Apert syndrome. In: *Symposium of Plastic Surgery of the Orbital Region*. St Louis, MO: Mosby; 1976.
14. Farkas LG, Posnick JC. Growth and development of regional units in the head and face based on anthropometric measurements. *Cleft Palate Craniofac J*. 1992;29(4):301–302.
15. Farkas LG, Posnick JC, Hreczko TM. Anthropometric growth study of the head. *Cleft Palate Craniofac J*. 1992;29(4):303–308.
16. Farkas LG, Posnick JC, Hreczko TM, Pron GE. Growth patterns in the orbital region: a morphometric study. *Cleft Palate Craniofac J*. 1992;29(4):315–318.
17. Cohen MM Jr. Sutural biology and the correlates of craniosynostosis. *Am J Med Genet*. 1993;47(5):581–616.
18. Cohen MM Jr. An etiologic and nosologic overview of craniosynostosis syndromes. *Birth Defects Orig Artic Ser*. 1975;11(2):137–189.
19. Whitaker LA, Munro IR, Salyer KE, Jackson IT, Ortiz-Monasterio F, Marchac D. Combined report of problems and complications in 793 craniofacial operations. *Plast Reconstr Surg*. 1979;64(2):198–203.
20. Posnick JC. Craniofacial dysostosis syndromes: a staged reconstructive approach. In: Turvey TA, Vig KWL, Fonseca RJ, eds. *Facial Clefts and Craniosynostosis: Principles and*

Management. Philadelphia, PA: WB Saunders; 1996.

21. Posnick JC, Ruiz RL. The craniofacial dysostosis syndromes: current surgical thinking and future directions. *Cleft Palate Craniofac J*. 2000;37(5):433.
22. Posnick JC. Craniofacial dysostosis. Staging of reconstruction and management of the midface deformity. *Neurosurg Clin N Am*. 1991;2(3):683–702.
23. Turvey TA, Gudeman SK. Nonsyndromic craniosynostosis. In: Turvey TA, Vig KWL, Fonseca RJ, eds. *Facial Clefts and Craniosynostosis: Principles and Management*. Philadelphia, PA: WB Saunders; 1996.
24. Renier D. Intracranial pressure in craniosynostosis: pre- and postoperative recordings: correlation with functional results. In: Persing JA, Jane JA, Edgerton MT, eds. *Scientific Foundations and Surgical Treatment of Craniosynostosis*. Baltimore, MD: Williams & Wilkins; 1989.
25. Gault DT, Renier D, Marchac D, Jones BM. Intracranial pressure and intracranial volume in children with craniosynostosis. *Plast Reconstr Surg*. 1992;90(3):377–381.
26. Hogeman KE, Willmar K. On le Fort III osteotomy for Crouzon's disease in children. Report of a four-year follow-up in one patient. *Scand J Plast Reconstr Surg*. 1974;8(1–2):169–172.
27. Epker BN, Turvey TA. The surgical correction of craniofacial synostosis and craniosynostosis. In: Peterson LJ, et al., eds. *Principles of Oral and Maxillofacial Surgery*. Philadelphia, PA: Lippincott-Raven; 1992.
28. Posnick JC. Craniofacial dysostosis: management of the midface deformity. In: Bell WH, ed. *Orthognathic and Reconstructive Surgery*. Philadelphia, PA: WB Saunders; 1992.
29. Ortiz-Monasterio F, del Campo AF, Carrillo A. Advancement of the orbits and the midface in one piece, combined with frontal repositioning, for the correction of Crouzon's deformities. *Plast Reconstr Surg*. 1978;61(4):507–516.
30. van der Meulen JC. Medial faciotomy. *Br J Plast Surg*. 1979;32(4):339–342.
31. Turvey TA, Hall DJ. In: *The Le Fort III Osteotomy: Surgical Correction of Dentofacial Deformities. Bell, Proffit, White*. Philadelphia, PA: WB Saunders; 1980.
32. Kufner J. Four-year experience with major maxillary osteotomy for retrusion. *J Oral Surg*. 1971;29(8):549–553.
33. Tiwana PS, Turvey TA, Ruiz RL. Long-term stability of subcranial Lefort III osteotomy in syndromic and non-syndromic patients. *J Oral Maxillofac Surg*. 2000;58(suppl):50.
34. Kaban LB, Conover M, Mulliken JB. Midface position after Le Fort III advancement: a long-term follow-up study. *Cleft Palate J*. 1986;23(suppl 1):75–77.

CHAPTER 50

Orbital Box Osteotomy

Likith Reddy

Armamentarium

#15 and #10 Scalpel blades and handle
24-gauge Wire
Appropriate sutures
Bipolar cautery
Bone rongeurs
Cottle, Freer, and #9 periosteal elevators
Curved Mayo or curved tenotomy scissors
Fine side-cutting fissure bur, 1.2 mm
Hair clippers and hair elastics
Local anesthetic with vasoconstrictor
Malleable retractors
Mayfield headrest
Midface titanium fixation devices
Needle electrocautery
Obwegeser retractors
Reciprocating saw
Sewall retractors
Smith spreaders
Tessier osteotomes

History of the Procedure

The orbital box osteotomies are used to correct vertical or horizontal malposition of the entire orbit and its contents. The orbital box osteotomy was first performed by Paul Tessier to correct hypertelorism.[1] He described osteotomies that separate the entire bony orbit from the skull and surrounding facial bones by combining both intracranial and facial approaches.[1,2] Converse and Wood-Smith described subcranial U-shaped orbital osteotomies to correct hypertelorism; however, these techniques produced limited results.[3] Schmid described circumferential orbital osteotomies to mobilize and translocate the orbits medially by an extracranial approach in patients with pneumatized frontal sinuses.[4]

Indications for the Use of the Procedure

The orbital box osteotomy is used to correct malpositions of the zygoma and the orbit and its contents in all planes.[5] It is primarily indicated to correct hypertelorism.[6] However, the box osteotomy can be used to correct vertical or horizontal dystopia due to congenital, pathologic, or traumatic abnormalities.[7]

Orbital hypertelorism is an abnormally increased distance between the orbits. In this condition, the distance between the medial canthi, medial, and lateral walls of the orbit and the pupils is greater than normal. This is different from telecanthus, where the distance between the medial canthi is greater than normal and the distance between lateral walls of the orbit and pupils is normal (Fig. 50.1).

Orbital hypertelorism is an anatomic condition associated with a heterogeneous group of congenital disorders. It can occur as an isolated sporadic anomaly or with conditions such as Edwards syndrome (trisomy 18), basal cell nevus syndrome, craniofrontonasal dysplasia, DiGeorge syndrome, Apert syndrome, and Crouzon syndrome. A heterogeneous collection of frontonasal malformations[8] is the group that most commonly displays hypertelorism (Fig. 50.2). The clinical findings in this group are usually symmetric hypertelorism, exaggerated widow's peak on the forehead, abnormal and wide-set eyebrows, down-slanting eyes, epicanthic folds, amblyopia, strabismus, a wide nose with a short philtrum, increased intrazygomatic distance, lateral and inferior positioned zygomas, median cleft lip, and a high arched palate.[8–10] Other congenital conditions associated with hypertelorism are frontal encephaloceles, craniofacial clefts, and craniofrontonasal dysplasia[11,12] (Fig. 50.3).

The other pathologic process for orbital dystopia is a slow-growing tumor, such as neurofibromatosis or frontal sinus mucocele. Also, some of the high-energy injuries or inadequate corrections can cause orbital dystopia in vertical or horizontal positions (Fig. 50.4).

The surgery to correct hypertelorism is usually performed when the patient is between 5 and 8 years of age. This timing addresses the psychosocial aspects of the developing child in the early school years. The physiologic reasons include the fact that the majority of the interzygomatic width is established by 6 years of age and there is adequate descent of tooth buds into the maxilla, providing space for an osteotomy below the infraorbital nerve. The disadvantages are that the orbital bones before 5 years of age are thin and fragile, and most patients who undergo correction of hypertelorism before the

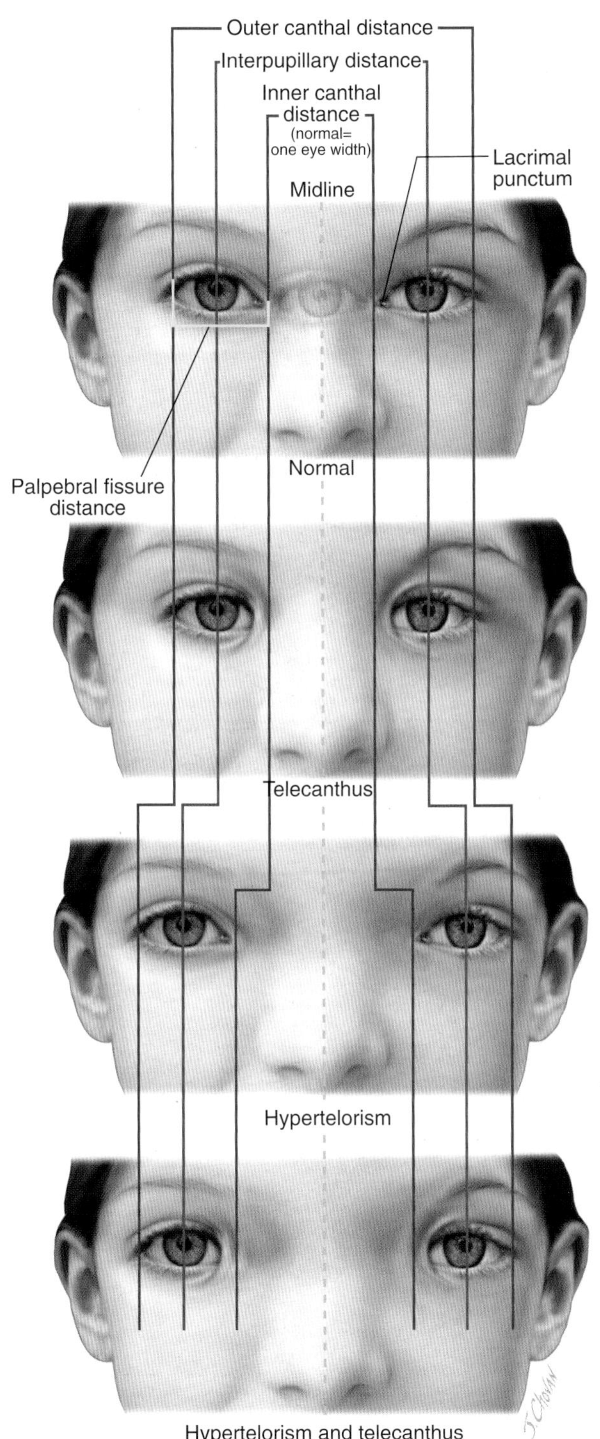

Figure 50.1 Normal and dysmorphic widths affecting the orbital bones and associated soft tissue attachments.

age of 8 by orbital osteotomies may require additional procedures for nasal correction in the future.[13–15] The best and most stable results for hypertelorism correction are in the adult or nongrowing patient. This could be because the orbital bones are thicker and allow for more stable skeletal fixation.[16]

The correction of orbital hypertelorism via box osteotomies should include correction of the nasal deformities. Bone and cartilage grafts may be necessary to create a nasal frame. Skin grafts may also be required for nasal coverage and can be accomplished with the use of local rotation flaps (i.e., forehead flaps) or advancement flaps.[17–19] In the presence of meningoceles, it is important to bone-graft the cranial base defect to minimize recurrence of the lesion.[20,21]

The preoperative planning for orbital box osteotomies should include evaluation by ophthalmology and neurosurgery specialists. These patients may have amblyopia or extraocular muscle dysfunction, or possibly develop binocular diplopia postsurgery. The surgical planning should include high-quality computed tomography (CT) scans with three-dimensional reconstructions. Stereolithographic models are also valuable for visualizing, marking, teaching, and understanding the osteotomies[22,23] (Fig. 50.5).

Limitations and Contraindications

No specific contraindication exists for the procedure. However, medical issues may mitigate the performance of this procedure due to significantly increased morbidity, especially in the patient with considerable congenital heart disease. One noteworthy limitation of the procedure is that the correction only occurs in the orbital region. Only the orbital width is corrected (narrowed). In patients who also have slanting of the facial halves or who require expansion of the transmaxillary width, a facial bipartition procedure is more ideally suited for correcting the entire facial deformity.

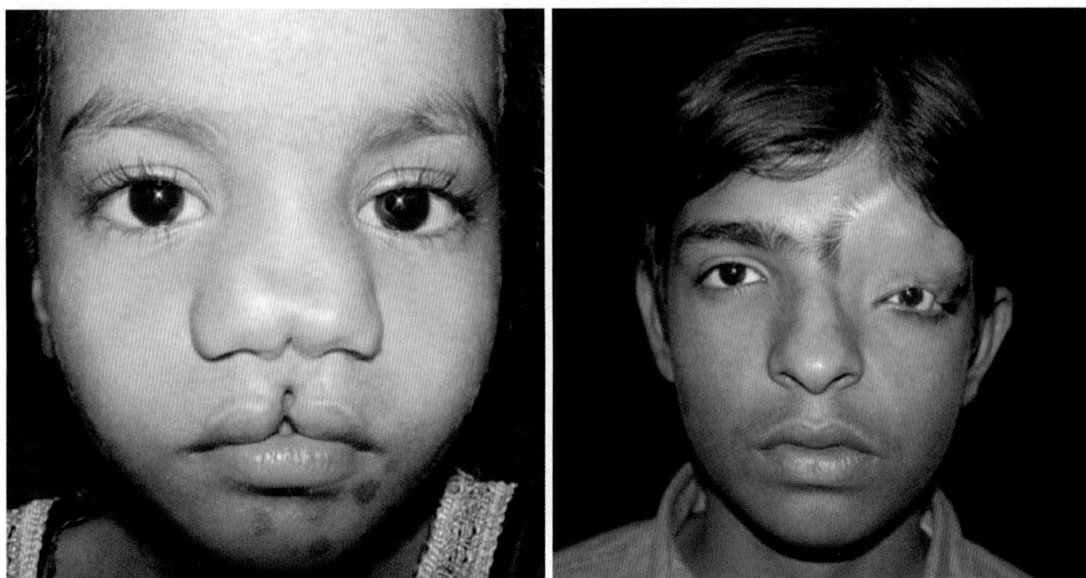

Figure 50.2 Orbital hypertelorism.

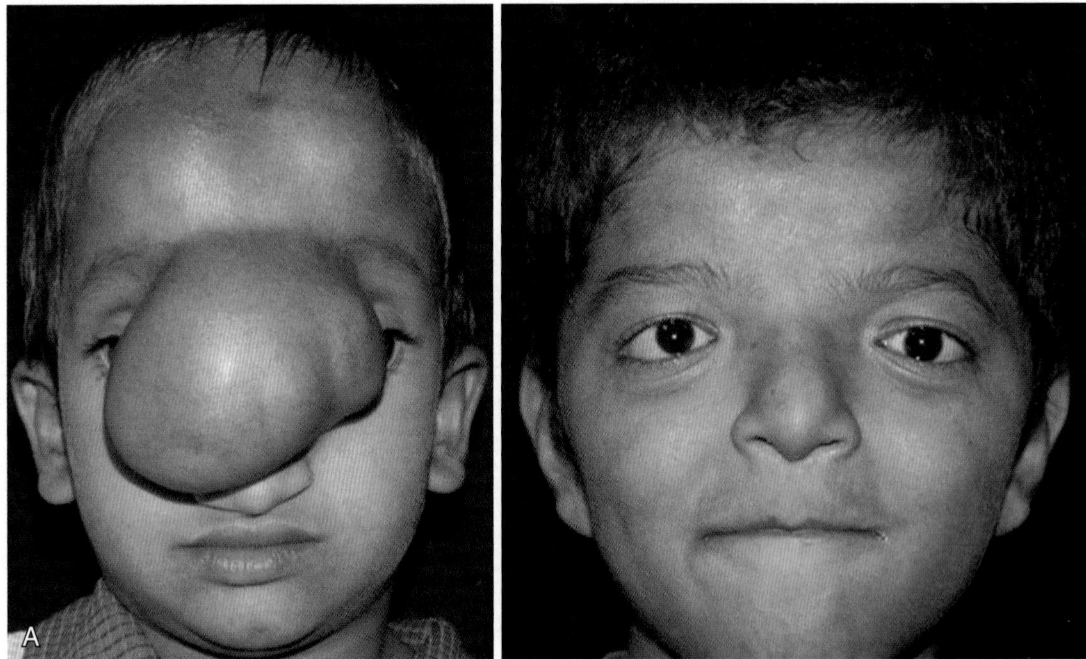

Figure 50.3 **A,** Other congenital conditions associated with hypertelorism are frontal encephaloceles, craniofacial clefts, and craniofrontonasal dysplasia.

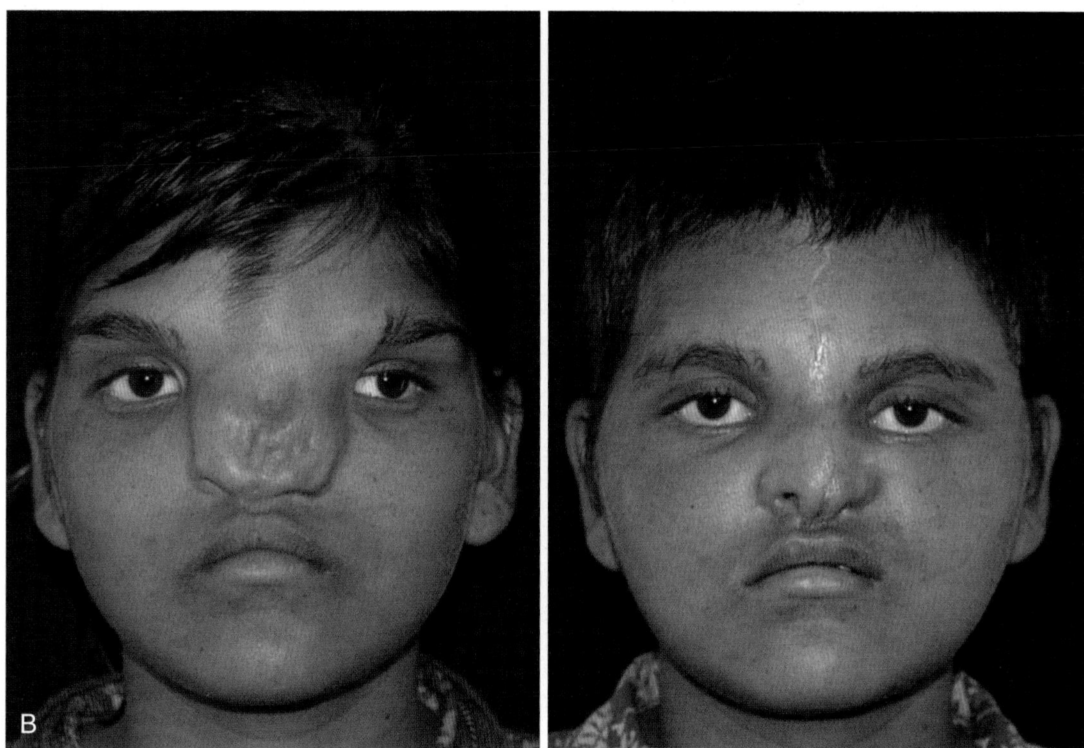

Figure 50.3, cont'd **B,** A heterogeneous group of frontonasal malformations[8] with hypertelorism.

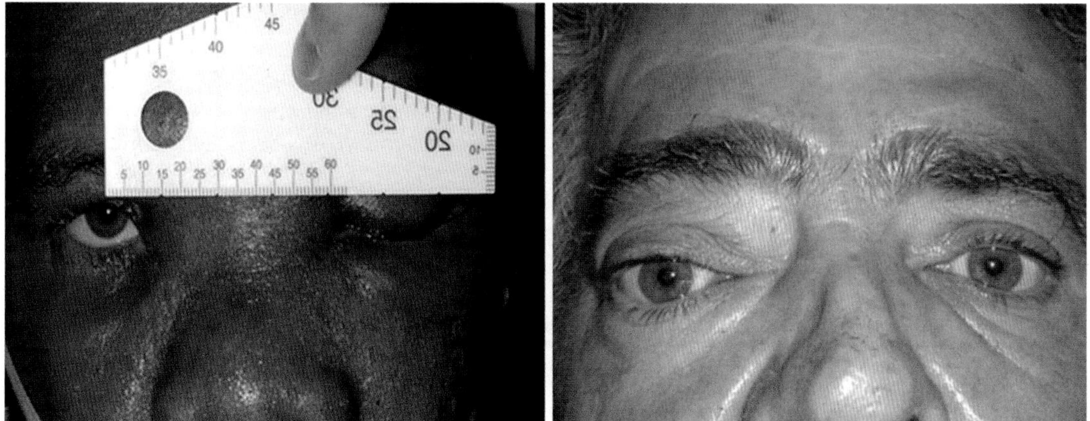

Figure 50.4 Orbital dystopia in vertical or horizontal positions.

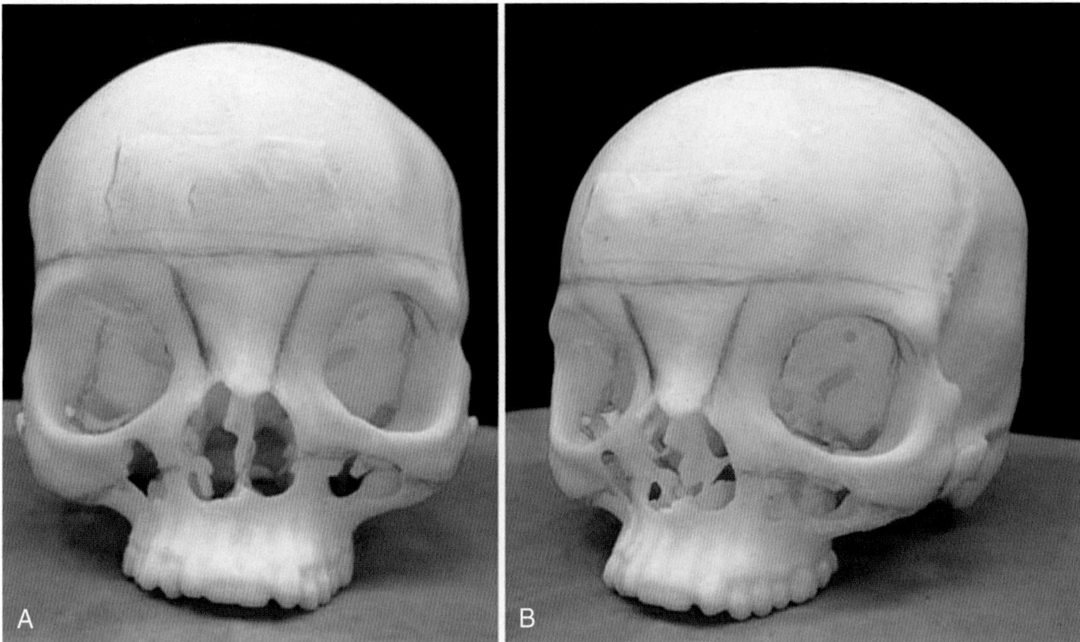

Figure 50.5 High-quality CT scans, and stereolithographic modeling (A) is also a valuable tool for visualizing, marking, teaching, and understanding the osteotomies (B).

TECHNIQUE: Orbital Box Osteotomy

STEP 1: Patient Positioning, Airway, and Corneal Protection

An oral Ring–Adair–Elwyn tube is used and secured to the midline by tape or to the lower two central incisor teeth using a 24-gauge wire. The upper and lower eyelids are sutured closed using a single horizontal mattress suture after placement of ophthalmic ointment to protect the cornea.

The coronal incision is marked, using a zigzag pattern, especially at the temporal region. A small 1-cm strip of hair is trimmed along the planned coronal incision.

A solution of 1% lidocaine with epinephrine or 0.25% Marcaine with epinephrine is injected along the planned coronal incision. Injection is also performed in the oral cavity along the maxillary vestibule and the dorsum of the nose. Afrin-soaked 1 × 3-cm neuropledgets are placed within the nose. The patient is placed in a Mayfield headrest and is prepped and draped with exposure of the entire face and the ears bilaterally.

STEP 2: Incision and Exposure

A coronal incision is made with a Colorado tip or microcautery tip usually set at 10 cut and 15 coagulation with blend mode. The incision on the scalp is performed with a cut mode, and the scalp is kept under constant tension during the incision. Once the incision is completed below the galea, the coagulate mode can be used with the edges being maintained under tension. A bipolar cautery is used judiciously to obtain complete hemostasis.

Subperiosteal dissection is carried out over the supraorbital rims. The supraorbital nerves are identified and carefully released if a foramen is present, using a 2-mm osteotome to make a V-notch to release the supraorbital nerve. The dissection is performed deeper to the temporoparietal fascia up to 1 cm above the zygomatic arch. Once the zygomatic arch is palpated, the incision is performed onto the zygomatic bone. This technique minimizes the chance of encountering the fat layer, which can result in subsequent fat atrophy. The temporalis muscle attachment is left intact, but the lateral rim attachment is released from the temporalis muscle. This provides access to the lateral rims and the bur holes for the craniotomy.

The periorbita is released circumferentially along the roof to 1 cm anterior to the optic nerve superiorly, laterally, medially, and the lateral one-third of the floor. The anterior and posterior ethmoidal arteries are identified and cauterized with bipolar cautery.

The bilateral zygoma, arches, superior orbital rims, superior aspect of the nasal dorsum, medial wall of the orbit, and the lat-

TECHNIQUE: Orbital Box Osteotomy—*cont'd*

eral one-third of the infraorbital rim are exposed. Meticulous dissection is performed anterior and posterior to the medial canthal attachment. It is critical to maintain the medial canthal tendon attachment.

A maxillary vestibular incision is made extending from the medial side of the first molar to the contralateral side. A subperiosteal dissection is performed exposing the nasal aperture, pyriform rims, and the zygomatic buttresses, infraorbital nerve, and the medial and middle thirds of the orbital rim. The nerve is skeletonized if needed for improved visualization. In midline cleft patients, the previous scar or the cleft can be used to access the medial aspects of the nose, pyriform rim, and the medial two-thirds of the orbital floor (Fig. 50.6A).

Continued

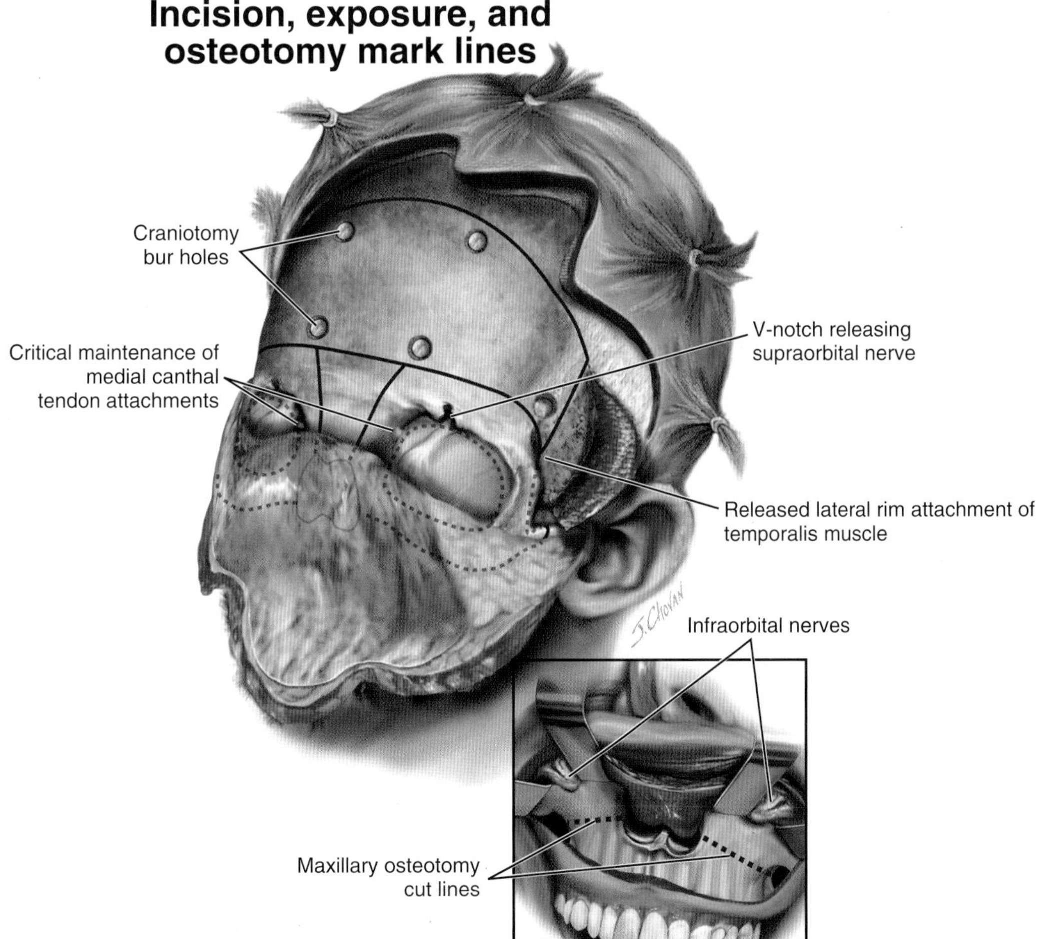

Figure 50.6 All the packings are removed, good hemostasis is obtained, and two-layer closure is obtained for the scalp.

TECHNIQUE: Orbital Box Osteotomy—*cont'd*

STEP 3: Frontal Craniotomy

The markings for the frontal craniotomy, V- or U-shaped ostectomy of the wide nasal bone, and the superior aspect of the orbital osteotomies are made with a sterile pencil or a #701 fissure bur. The design of the V- or U-shaped ostectomy of the nasofrontal junction and nasal dorsum is based on the desired movements of the orbits and zygoma. The neurosurgeon performs a frontal craniotomy as marked. The craniotomy bur holes are made in the pterional region only. The frontal bone flap is removed, providing access to the orbital roof, greater wing of the sphenoid laterally, and cribriform plates medially. The bleeding of minor vessels over the dura is controlled with meticulous bipolar cautery, gentle pressure, Gelfoam, and Surgicel as needed. If dural tears occur, they are identified and repaired with 4-0 Vicryl sutures (Fig. 50.6B).

STEP 4: Initial Facial Osteotomy

A reciprocating saw is used to osteotomize the lateral orbital wall, the lateral third of the orbital floor as far posterior as possible. Malleable retractors protect the periorbita and its contents. The brain is retracted to expose the anterior edge of the crista galli. The supraorbital and the upper third of the medial orbits osteotomies are performed transcranially. Throughout this period, malleable retractors protect both the brain and the periorbita.

The medial orbital osteotomy and the osteotomy for the medial two-thirds of the orbital floor are completed using a 3-mm osteotome. These osteotomies should be as posterior as possible. This is necessary to translocate the globes.

The remaining osteotomies, including those for the remaining zygoma and maxilla, are performed using a reciprocating saw. The maxilla osteotomy is made 5 mm inferior to the infraorbital nerve (Fig. 50.6C).

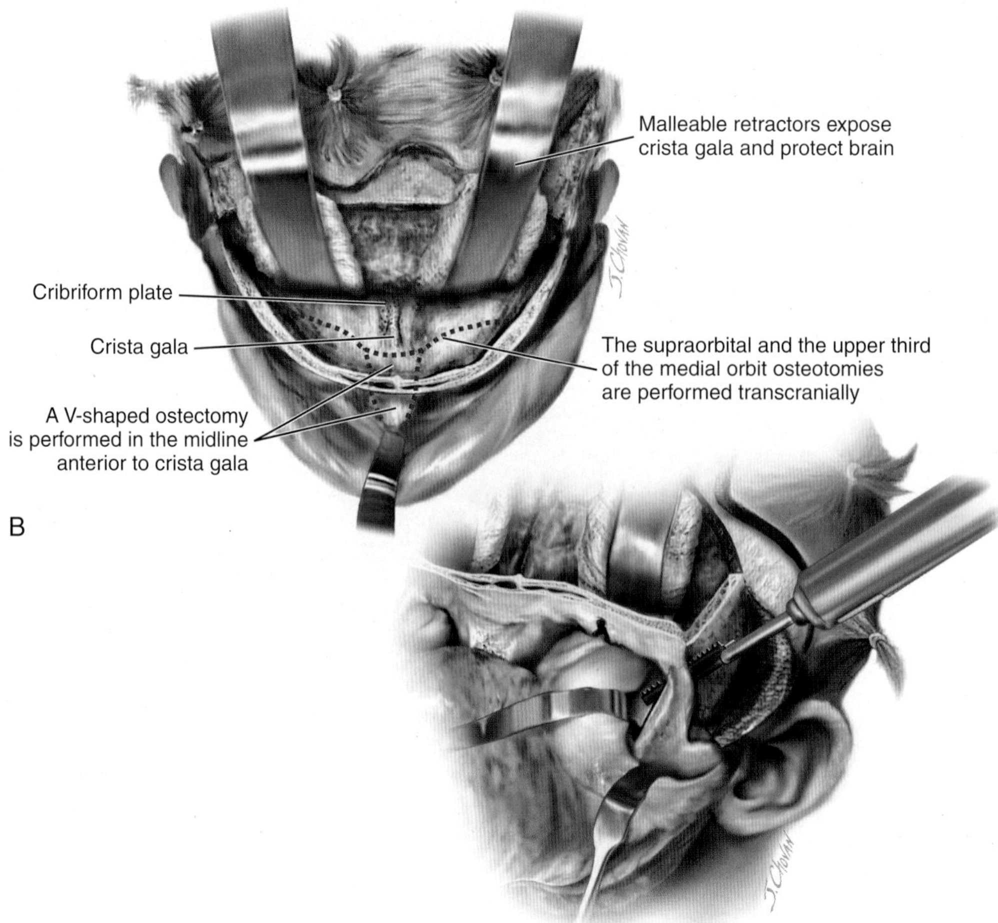
Malleable retractors expose
crista gala and protect brain
Cribriform plate
Crista gala
The supraorbital and the upper third
of the medial orbit osteotomies
are performed transcranially
A V-shaped ostectomy
is performed in the midline
anterior to crista gala
B
The lateral orbital wall,
lateral third of orbital floor, and zygoma
are cut with reciprocating saw
C

Figure 50.6, cont'd

TECHNIQUE: Orbital Box Osteotomy—*cont'd*

STEP 5: Final Osteotomy and Mobilization

A V-shaped ostectomy is performed in the midline, extending anterior to the crista galli. The shape and symmetry of the V vary based on the desired translocation of the orbit. The frontal bone, ethmoids, midline nasal dorsum, and superior part of the bony septum are removed. A rongeur is used to remove the ethmoidal air cells as needed. Thrombin- or Afrin-soaked neuropledglets are used to maintain good hemostasis during the removal of the ethmoids.

The orbits are methodically mobilized with Smith spreaders by placing them at the lateral orbital rim and walking them gently forward, making sure the orbits are moving. The area of the pyriform rims is often the most difficult region to mobilize. Attention should be directed to this region during the mobilization of the orbits. A triangle-shaped bone is removed at the pyriform region; this will facilitate visualization as well as remove the interferences that occur during the repositioning of the orbits. The orbits are translocated to the midline, and medial segments of the orbit should be passive to finger pressure. The translocation is not a pure medial translocation but involves superior rotation of the lateral orbital rims. The orbits are passively mobilized medially after the interferences are removed, and a 24-gauge wire is placed temporarily. The interorbital distance between the medial walls is measured by calipers and should be between 17 and 18 mm. Additional bone can be removed from the medial aspect if needed. For severe hypertelorism, about 3 to 5 mL of overcorrection is desired (Fig. 50.6D).

STEP 6: Skeletal Fixation

Rigid skeletal fixation is applied with titanium plates and screws in the midline, zygoma, and pyriform regions. The frontal bone flap is placed. The posterior wall and the sinus mucosa of the frontal sinus are removed; if the frontal sinus is present, it is cranialized by removing the posterior wall and mucosa. A triangular bone piece is removed from the frontal bone. These triangular bone pieces are wedged at the lateral orbital rim as bone grafts.

Continued

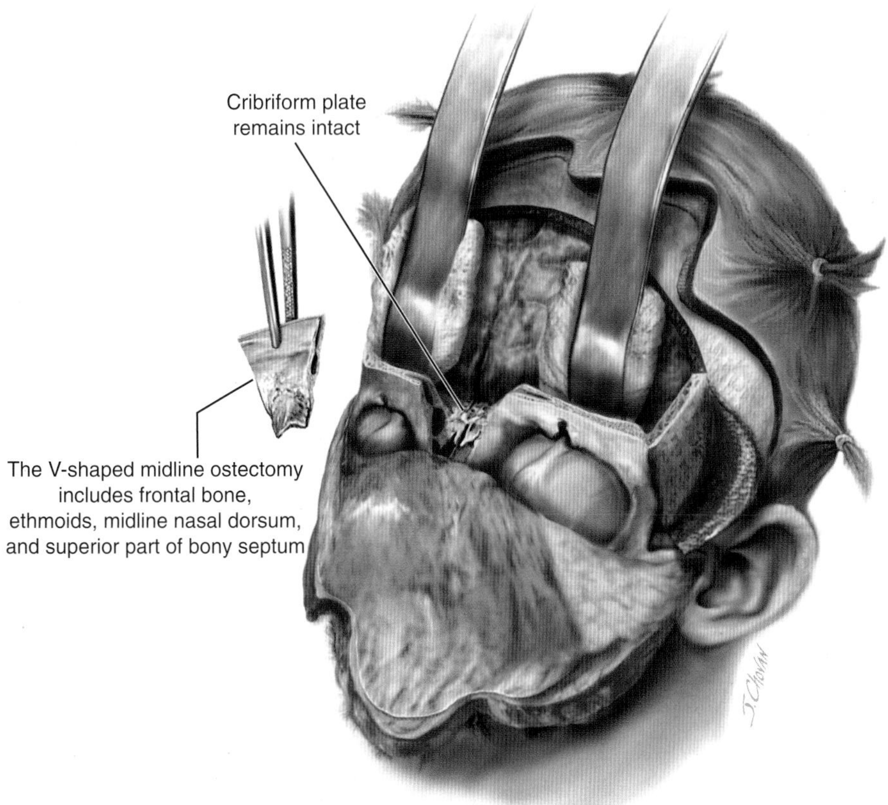

Cribriform plate remains intact
The V-shaped midline ostectomy includes frontal bone, ethmoids, midline nasal dorsum, and superior part of bony septum
D

Figure 50.6, cont'd

TECHNIQUE: Orbital Box Osteotomy—*cont'd*

STEP 7: Medial Canthal Reinforcement, Nasal Reconstruction

Bilateral medial canthal and soft tissue 2-0 braided nylon sutures are placed and tied posteriorly. This augments the medial canthal tendon and the surrounding soft tissue. The suture vector is posterior and superior to the medial canthal tendon attachments.

The temporalis muscle needs to be mobilized and moved anteriorly in large hypertelorism correction to prevent depression lateral to the lateral orbital rims. The wide cartilaginous septum is folded and sutured into an inverted V shape, effectively increasing the septal projection and decreasing the nasal width. A cranial bone graft to the nasal dorsum is placed to improve the nasal projection and length (Fig. 50.6E).

STEP 8: Closure

All the packings are removed, good hemostasis is obtained, and two-layer closure is obtained for the scalp. The oral layer is closed in a single layer. The soft-tissue refinements are made for the nasal reconstruction. The redundant subcutaneous tissue is debulked, and a horizontal mattress of subcutaneous 3-0 Vicryl stitches is placed. This causes bunching of the forehead skin, which settles down in a few months. However, large hypertelorism or facial clefts require the excess forehead skin to be removed and the eyebrow position to be corrected. The nasal skin is removed judiciously in rare cases; if so, it is performed with the incisions falling within the nasal aesthetic units.

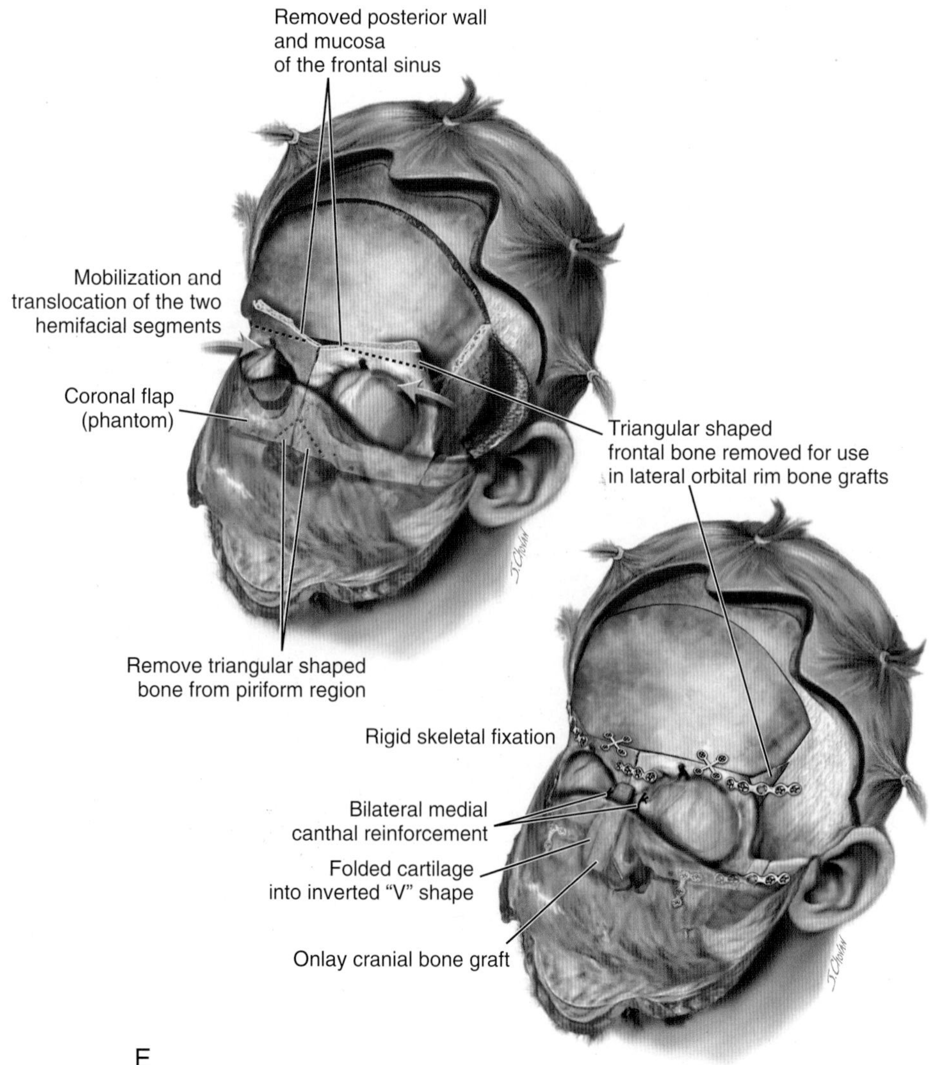

Figure 50.6, cont'd

ALTERNATIVE TECHNIQUE: Orbital Osteotomy With Frontal Bandeau

A frontal bandeau of approximately 1 cm is maintained between the frontal bone flap and the osteotomies of the supraorbital rim. The frontal band helps in positioning of the orbits and frontal bone flaps and avoids the possibility of creating frontal bossing due to unwanted forward positioning of the orbits and frontal bone flap. In addition, this band can be used for fixation. The frontal bar may decrease visualization of the crista galli region, increase brain retraction to improve visibility, and make it difficult to repair the dural tears if present. Also see Chapter 48 for a discussion of facial bipartition (Fig. 50.7). If the frontal bandeau is not removed, excessive retraction of the frontal lobes of the brain may be required. In addition, if dural tears are present, the presence of the unarticulated frontal bar may unnecessarily complicate dural repair.

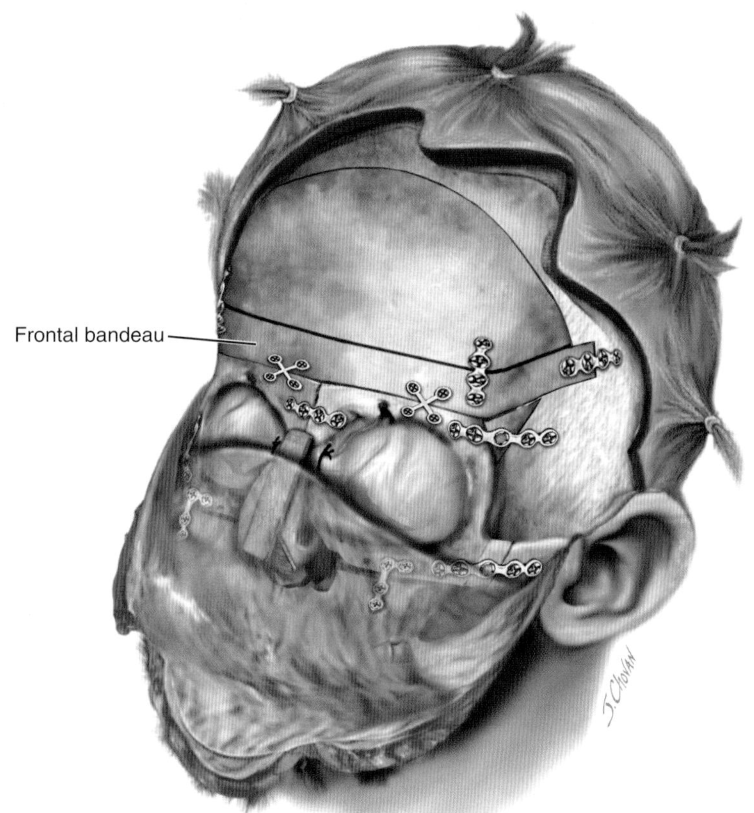

Figure 50.7 A frontal bandeau is maintained between the frontal bone flap and the osteotomies of the supraorbital rim.

Avoidance and Management of Intraoperative Complications

The complications in treatment of hypertelorism include excessive bleeding, risk of infection and cerebrospinal fluid leaks, and dural fistulas. Infections and leaks can be prevented by giving the patient perioperative antibiotics and identifying and closing any dural tears. Dural adhesions and bone spurs increase the risk of dural tears in repeat or secondary procedures. The risk of significant bleeding can be prevented by meticulous technique, and blood loss is compensated by transfusions. CT scans and magnetic resonance imaging as needed are critical for evaluating the cerebrovenous sinuses that are encountered in patients with a large meningocele. Maintaining hypotensive anesthesia can also reduce blood loss. Major eye injuries, including blindness, are rare. Visual disturbances can occur due to the eye muscle imbalance after orbital mobilization. Ptosis and diplopia can also occur postoperatively, but this usually self-corrects.

Delayed complications include relapse of the hypertelorism correction and canthal drifting, especially in patients younger than 5 years of age.[9,17,24] Stable skeletal fixation, bone grafting the gaps at the lateral orbital rims and zygoma will decrease the chances of relapse. The canthal drift is minimized by preserving the canthal tendon attachments during surgery and reinforcing further with transnasal braided nylon sutures or medial canthal tendon anchors in superior and posterior vector to the canthal attachments. Temporal hollowing is noted to some extent in all of the patients. Mortality is rarely seen in operative correction of hypertelorism by box osteotomies.[2,9,17]

Postoperative Considerations

All orbital box osteotomy patients need to be observed overnight in an intensive care unit setting postoperatively. The patient is monitored for increased intracranial pressure and intraorbital pressure due to bleeding. Most have significant periorbital and eyelid swelling. This can make the eye examination and the evaluation of extraocular muscles difficult. The swelling can be minimized by tight control of fluids, intraoperative and postoperative short-term steroids, and keeping the head of the surgical bed elevated during the first week after surgery. Steroids and antibiotics are always used with the first dose administered upon intubation and before commencement of surgery. A weight-appropriate dosage of antibiotics that cover staphylococcal bacteria can be given intravenously every 6 hours during surgery and for the first 24 hours. Oral antibiotics are continued for 7 days.

Postoperative CT scan imaging is critical to assess the new arrangement of the bony architecture of the nasal, orbital, and frontal regions. It would also help in assessing for intracranial hematoma formation in the frontal region and the assessment of the orbital soft tissue translocation and the optic nerve path. In addition, it serves as reference for further ongoing assessment.

Typically, the airway is not impacted, and there is little reason for prolonged intubation following this surgery. If cerebrospinal fluid rhinorrhea is suspected, elevating the head of the bed and short-term lumbar drain placement may be needed. Nose blowing and Valsalva maneuvers are discouraged. Doyle splints may be placed during surgery. However, no nasal packing should be placed. The use of external nasal splinting for a week is helpful to maintain the soft tissue adapted closely at the nasal and medial canthal tendon junction. Nasal sprays with vasoconstrictors for congestion are used for 1 to 2 weeks. Early postoperative ambulation and oral intake are encouraged.

Visual disturbance including diplopia is uncommon. Anosmia is also uncommon, but informing the patient of these possibilities is prudent. Patients with large hypertelorism may exhibit exotropia preoperatively, and it is unlikely this would be corrected with orbital surgery. These patients would benefit from strabismus surgery 3 months postoperatively.

References

1. Tessier P, Guiot G, Rougerie J, Delbet JP, Pastoriza J. [Cranio-naso-orbito-facial osteotomies. Hypertelorism]. *Ann Chir Plast.* 1967;12(2):103–118.
2. Tessier P. Experiences in the treatment of orbital hypertelorism. *Plast Reconstr Surg.* 1974;53(1):1–18.
3. Converse JM, Wood-Smith D. Craniofacial surgery for ocular hypertelorism and craniofacial stenosis. *Trans Am Acad Ophthalmol Otolaryngol.* 1973;77(5):ORL352–ORL367.
4. Schmid E. Surgical management of hypertelorism. In: Longacre JJ, ed. *Craniofacial Anomalies: Pathogenesis and Repair.* Philadelphia, Pennsylvania: JB Lippincott; 1968.
5. Whitaker LA, LaRossa D, Randall P. Structural goals in craniofacial surgery. *Cleft Palate J.* 1975;12(00):23–32.
6. Fearon JA, Bartlett SP, Whitaker LA. The skeletal treatment of orbital hypertelorism. *Neurosurg Clin N Am.* 1991;2(3):673–681.
7. Munro IR. Craniofacial surgical techniques for aesthetic results in congenital and acute traumatic deformities. *Clin Plast Surg.* 1981;8(2):303–316.
8. Tan ST, Mulliken JB. Hypertelorism: nosologic analysis of 90 patients. *Plast Reconstr Surg.* 1997;99(2):317–327.
9. De Ponte FS, Fadda T, Rinna C, Brunelli A, Iannetti G. Early and late surgical treatment of orbital dystopia in craniofacial malformation. *J Craniofac Surg.* 1997;8(1):17–22.
10. Ortiz-Monasterio F, Molina F. Orbital hypertelorism. *Clin Plast Surg.* 1994;21(4):599–612. Review.
11. van den Elzen ME, Versnel SL, Wolvius EB, et al. Long-term results after 40 years experience with treatment of rare facial clefts: part 2—symmetrical median clefts. *J Plast Reconstr Aesthet Surg.* 2011;64(10):1344–1352.
12. Kawamoto HK, Heller JB, Heller MM, et al. Craniofrontonasal dysplasia: a surgical treatment algorithm. *Plast Reconstr Surg.* 2007;120(7):1943–1956.
13. McCarthy JG. Discussion: hypertelorism correction: what happens with growth? Evaluation of a series of 95 surgical cases. *Plast Reconstr Surg.* 2012;129(3):728–730.
14. Wan DC, Levi B, Kawamoto H, et al. Correction of hypertelorbitism: evaluation of relapse on long-term follow-up. *J Craniofac Surg.* 2012;23(1):113–117.
15. Marchac D, Sati S, Renier D, Deschamps-Braly J, Marchac A. Hypertelorism correction: what happens with growth? Evaluation of a series of 95 surgical cases. *Plast Reconstr Surg.* 2012;129(3):713–727.
16. Raposo-Amaral CE, Raposo-Amaral CM, Raposo-Amaral CA, Chahal H, Bradley JP, Jarrahy R. Age at surgery significantly impacts the amount of orbital relapse following hypertelorbitism correction: a 30-year longitudinal study. *Plast Reconstr Surg.* 2011;127(4):1620–1630.
17. McCarthy JG, La Trenta GS, Breitbart AS, Zide BM, Cutting CB. Hypertelorism correction in the young child. *Plast Reconstr Surg.* 1990;86(2):214–225.
18. Sailer HF, Landolt AM. A new method for the correction of hypertelorism with preservation of the olfactory nerve filaments. *J Craniomaxillofac Surg.* 1987;15(3):122–124.
19. Miller PJ, Grinberg D, Wang TD. Midline cleft. Treatment of the bifid nose. *Arch Facial Plast Surg.* 1999;1(3):200–203.
20. Oucheng N, Lauwers F, Gollogly J, Draper L, Joly B, Roux FE. Frontoethmoidal meningoencephalocele: appraisal of 200 operated cases. *J Neurosurg Pediatr.* 2010;6(6):541–549.
21. Jackson IT, Tanner NS, Hide TA. Frontonasal encephalocele—"long nose hypertelorism." *Ann Plast Surg.* 1983;11(6):490–500.
22. Hidalgo HM, Romo GW, Estolano RT. Stereolithography: a method for planning the surgical correction of the hypertelorism. *J Craniofac Surg.* 2009;20(5):1473–1477.
23. Sailer HF, Haers PE, Zollikofer CP, Warnke T, Carls FR, Stucki P. The value of stereolithographic models for preoperative diagnosis of craniofacial deformities and planning of surgical corrections. *Int J Oral Maxillofac Surg.* 1998;27(5):327–333.
24. Mulliken JB, Kaban LB, Evans CA, Strand RD, Murray JE. Facial skeletal changes following hypertelorbitism correction. *Plast Reconstr Surg.* 1986;77(1):7–16.

CHAPTER 51

Monobloc and Facial Bipartition Osteotomies for the Reconstruction of Craniosynostosis Syndromes

Jeffrey C. Posnick and Paul S. Tiwana

Armamentarium

#15 Scalpel blades
Appropriate sutures
Arch bars (24- and 26-gauge wires)
Craniotome
Bipolar electrocautery
Bone-cutting instruments
Cottonoids, tissue glue, sutures (appropriate-sized needles and material)
Kocher clamps (straight and curved)
Local anesthetic with vasoconstrictor
Malleable retractors
Mayfield headrest
Nasomaxillary disimpaction forceps
Needle electrocautery
Oscillating saw (with appropriate blades)
Osteotomes (appropriate sizes)
Periosteal elevators (straight and curved)
Pterygomaxillary spreading forceps
Rotary drill (with appropriate burs)
Sagittal saw (with appropriate blades)
Scissors (Stevens, Metzenbaum, Mayo)
Titanium plate and screw fixation set (appropriate-sized plates and screws)
Wire cutters and twisters

History of the Procedure

Craniofacial surgeons use a variety of reconstructive approaches to correct the upper midface deformities observed in craniosynostosis syndromes, frontonasal dysplasias, midline cranio-orbital clefting, and isolated orbital hypertelorism. In 1971 Tessier described a single-stage frontofacial advancement in which the fronto-orbital band was advanced as a separate element in conjunction with the Le Fort III complex below and the frontal bones above.[1] Seven years later, Ortiz-Monasterio et al. developed the monobloc (MB) osteotomy to advance the orbits and midface as one unit, combined with forehead repositioning, to correct the deformity of Crouzon syndrome.[2,3] In 1979 van der Meulen described the "median fasciotomy" for the correction of midline facial clefting.[4] Van der Meulen split the MB osteotomy vertically in the midline, removed the central nasal and ethmoid bones, and then moved the two halves of the face together for correction of orbital hypertelorism. To correct the midface dysplasia and associated orbital hypertelorism in patients with Apert syndrome, Tessier refined the vertical splitting and reshaping of the MB segment, thus correcting the midline deformity in three dimensions, in a procedure now known as facial bipartition (FB).

Indications for the Use of the Procedure

Craniosynostosis, or premature fusion of cranial sutures, affects approximately 1 in 2500 children. Patients may present with a wide range of phenotypic and functional deformities that are etiologically heterogeneous and pathogenetically variable.[5] *Complex craniosynostosis,* defined as the fusion of multiple cranial sutures, occurs in about 5% of nonsyndromic cases.[6] *Cloverleaf skulls,* representing the extremes of phenotypic severity, are pathogenetically variable. Synostosis may involve the coronal, lambdoid, and metopic sutures, marked by bulging of the cerebrum through an open sagittal suture or, in some cases, through patent squamosal sutures. Isolated cloverleaf skull occurs in about 20% of cases. Apert syndrome is characterized by craniosynostosis, midface deficiency, symmetric syndactyly of the hands and feet, and other abnormalities.[7–24] Crouzon syndrome is characterized by craniosynostosis, maxillary hypoplasia, shallow orbits, and ocular proptosis.[4,19,25–48] Pfeiffer syndrome is characterized by craniosynostosis, midface deficiency, broad thumbs and/or great toes, brachydactyly, variable soft tissue syndactyly, and other anomalies.[49,50] Saethre-Chotzen syndrome is characterized by a heterogeneous phenotypic presentation involving craniosynostosis, a low-set frontal hairline, facial asymmetry, ptosis of the eyelids, deviated nasal septum, brachydactyly, partial soft-tissue syndactyly of the second and third fingers, and various skeletal anomalies.[51–54]

Morphologic Considerations

Examination of the patient's entire craniofacial region should be meticulous and systematic. The skeleton and soft tissues are assessed in a standard way to identify all normal and abnormal anatomy.[55–66] Specific findings tend to occur in particular malformations, but each patient is unique. The achievement of symmetry and normal proportions and the reconstruction of specific esthetic units are essential in forming an unobtrusive face in a child born with one of the craniosynostosis syndromes.

Frontoforehead Esthetic Unit

The frontoforehead region is dysmorphic in an infant with a craniosynostosis syndrome. Establishing the normal position of the forehead is critical for overall facial symmetry and balance. The forehead may be considered as two separate esthetic components: the supraorbital ridge–lateral orbital rim region and the superior forehead. The supraorbital ridge–lateral orbital rim unit includes the nasofrontal process and the supraorbital rims extending inferiorly down each frontozygomatic (FZ) suture toward the infraorbital rim and posteriorly along each temporoparietal region. The shape and position of the supraorbital ridge–lateral orbital rim region are key elements of upper facial esthetics. In a normal forehead, at the level of the nasofrontal suture, an angle ranging from 90 to 110 degrees is formed by the supraorbital ridge and the nasal bones when viewed in profile. Additionally, the eyebrows, overlying the supraorbital ridge, should be anterior to the cornea. When the supraorbital ridge is viewed from above, the rim should arc posteriorly to achieve a gentle 90-degree angle at the temporal fossa with a center point of the arc at the level of each FZ suture. The superior forehead component, about 1 to 1.5 cm up the supraorbital rim, should have a gentle posterior curve of about 60 degrees, leveling out at the coronal suture region when seen in profile.

Orbito-Naso-Zygomatic Esthetic Unit

In the craniosynostosis syndromes, the orbito-naso-zygomatic regional dysmorphology is a reflection of the cranial base malformation. In Crouzon syndrome, in which bilateral coronal suture synostosis is combined with skull base and midface deficiency, the orbito-naso-zygomatic region is dysmorphic and consistent with a short (anterior-posterior) and wide (transverse) anterior cranial base. In Apert syndrome, the nasal bones, orbits, and zygomas, like the anterior cranial base, are transversely wide from anterolateral bulging of the temporal lobes of the brain and horizontally short (retruded), resulting in a shallow, hyperteloric, "reverse curved" upper midface. Surgically advancing the midface without simultaneously addressing the increased transverse width and reverse curve will not adequately correct the dysmorphology.

Maxillary–Nasal Base Esthetic Unit

In the patient with a craniosynostosis syndrome and midface deficiency, the upper anterior face is vertically short (nasion to maxillary incisor), and there is a lack of horizontal (A-P) projection. These findings may be confirmed through cephalometric analysis, which indicates a deficient SNA angle and a short upper anterior facial height (nasion to anterior nasal spine). The width of the maxilla in the dentoalveolar region is generally constricted, with a highly arched palate. To normalize the maxillary–nasal base region, multidirectional surgical expansion and reshaping are generally required. The abnormal maxillary lip-to-tooth relationship and class III occlusion are improved through Le Fort I segmental osteotomies and orthodontic treatment as part of the staged reconstruction. The mandible and chin are frequently secondarily involved and benefit from surgical repositioning as part of the orthognathic correction.

Considerations in the Timing of Reconstruction

In considering both the timing and type of intervention, the experienced surgeon takes several biologic realities into account, including the natural course of the malformation (i.e., progressively worsening dysmorphology or a nonprogressive craniofacial abnormality), the tendency for growth restriction in operated skeletally immature bones (i.e., akin to the maxillary hypoplasia that occurs after cleft palate repair), the relationship between the underlying developing viscera (i.e., the brain) and the congenitally affected and/or surgically altered skeleton (i.e., brain compression if the cranial vault is not expanded), and the child's airway needs (i.e., midface deficiency resulting in obstructive sleep apnea [OSA]).

To limit impairment while simultaneously achieving long-term preferred facial esthetics and head and neck function, the surgeon must ask an essential question: During the course of craniofacial development, does the operated-on facial skeleton of a child with a craniosynostosis syndrome tend to grow abnormally, resulting in further distortions and dysmorphology, or are the initial positive skeletal changes achieved (at surgery) maintained during ongoing growth? Unfortunately, the proposed theory that craniofacial procedures carried out in early infancy "unlock growth" has not been documented through the scientific method.[58–60,67–73]

Limitations, Contraindications, and Alternatives

Management of the Upper Midface Deformity

Upper Midface Reconstruction Options

The approach selected to manage the upper midface deficiency/anomalies and residual cranial vault dysplasia in the child with a craniosynostosis syndrome should offer definitive corrections. The main objective of this phase of reconstruction is to "normalize" the orbits, zygomas, and cranial vault. Correction of the maxillomandibular deformity requires orthognathic surgery, including a separate Le Fort I osteotomy. The selection of an MB (with or without additional orbital segmentation), an FB (with or without additional orbital segmentation), or an extracranial Le Fort III osteotomy to manage the basic horizontal, transverse, and vertical upper and midface deficiencies/anomalies, should depend on the patient's specific morphology. The presenting dysmorphology is determined by the original malformation, the previous procedures carried out, and the effects of those procedures on growth (Figs. 51.1–51.3).

When evaluating the upper and midface morphology in the mixed-dentition child or young adult born with Crouzon syndrome, the surgeon should note (1) whether the supraorbital ridge is in good position when viewed from the sagittal plane (is the depth of the upper orbits adequate?), (2) whether the midface and forehead have an acceptable arc of rotation in the transverse plane (is the midface arc concave?), and (3) whether the root of the nose and orbits are of normal width (is there orbital hypertelorism?). If these structures are confirmed to have acceptable morphology, there is no need to further reconstruct the forehead and upper orbits. In those few patients with a craniosynostosis syndrome in whom the residual deformity is only in the lower half of the orbits, the zygomatic buttress, and the maxilla, an extracranial Le Fort III is likely to be an effective treatment.

If the supraorbital region, anterior cranial base, zygomas, the root of the nose (in addition to the lower orbits), and the maxilla all remain deficient in the sagittal plane (horizontal retrusion), an MB is indicated. In these patients, the forehead is also generally flat and retruded and requires reshaping and advancement. If upper midface hypertelorism (increased transverse width) with midface flattening (horizontal retrusion) and a concave facial curvature (reverse facial arc) is also present, the MB unit is split vertically in the midline (facial bipartition). A wedge of interorbital (nasal and ethmoidal) bone is removed, and the orbits and zygomas are repositioned medially while the maxillary arch is widened. An FB is rarely required in Crouzon syndrome, but the MB is. When an MB or FB osteotomy is carried out as the upper midface procedure, additional segmentation of the upper and lateral orbits may also be required to normalize the morphology of the orbital esthetic units.

For almost all patients with Apert syndrome, FB osteotomies combined with further cranial vault reshaping allow for better correction of the dysmorphology than can be achieved through any other upper midface procedure (i.e., MB or Le Fort III). When FB osteotomies are used, correction of the concave midface arc of rotation is also possible. This further reduces the stigma of the flat, wide, and retrusive facial appearance of Apert syndrome. The FB procedure allows the orbits and zygomas to shift to the midline (correction of hypertelorism) as units while the maxilla is simultaneously widened (i.e., relief of the V-shaped face). Horizontal advancement of the reassembled upper midface complex is then possible to improve orbital depth and zygomatic length. The forehead is generally flat, tall, and retruded, with a constricting band just above the supraorbital ridge. Reshaping of the anterior cranial vault is also simultaneously carried out. A Le Fort III osteotomy is virtually never adequate for an ideal correction of the residual upper midface anomalies documented in Apert syndrome.

A study by McCarthy confirms that the Le Fort III osteotomy is not effective as an esthetic option to manage the upper midface deformity in the majority of patients with craniosynostosis syndrome.[74] By anatomic design, the Le Fort III procedure prevents management of the whole orbital esthetic unit during one operative setting. Therefore, a major esthetic shortcoming of the Le Fort III osteotomy, when its indications do not fit the presenting dysmorphology, is the creation of irregular step-offs in the lateral orbital rims. This occurs even when only a moderate Le Fort III advancement is carried out. These lateral orbital stepoffs are visible to the casual observer as unattractive at conversational distance, and surgical attempts at modification performed later produce suboptimal results. Another problem with the Le Fort III osteotomy is the difficulty in judging an ideal orbital depth. This frequently results in either residual proptosis or enophthalmos. In addition, simultaneous correction of upper face (orbital) hypertelorism and the concave midface arc of rotation typical in Apert syndrome is not possible with the Le Fort III procedure. Excessive lengthening of the nose, accompanied by flattening of the nasofrontal angle, occurs if the Le Fort III osteotomy is selected when the skeletal dysmorphology favors an MB or FB procedure. Unfortunately, it is not possible to later correct the elongated nose or the flattened nasofrontal angle. Avoiding these shortcomings is not a matter of becoming more proficient at the Le Fort III osteotomy or simply managing the overlying soft tissues in a different way (i.e., canthopexies or midface lift). The Le Fort III osteotomy is not consistent with the presenting dysmorphology in most patients with craniosynostosis syndrome and therefore does not provide the opportunity to achieve the desired esthetic result. Nevertheless, the Le Fort III procedure often is considered the go-to approach by surgeons because (1) it is an extracranial procedure; (2) it requires less surgical skill and experience; (3) it is less likely to result in significant blood loss; and (4) it is less likely to result in perioperative complications (i.e., cranionasal fistula, intracranial abscess, bone resorption).

The osteotomy selected to manage the upper midface dysmorphology in the individual with a craniosynostosis syndrome (i.e., Le Fort III, MB, FB) should reflect the presenting skeletal deformities and provide a realistic opportunity for long-term esthetic enhancement of the upper midface (naso-orbito-malar) region.

In most patients with a craniosynostosis syndrome, a suboptimal esthetic result occurs if the surgeon attempts to simultaneously adjust the orbits and idealize the occlusion using the Le Fort III, MB, or FB osteotomy without completing a

Text continued on p. 9

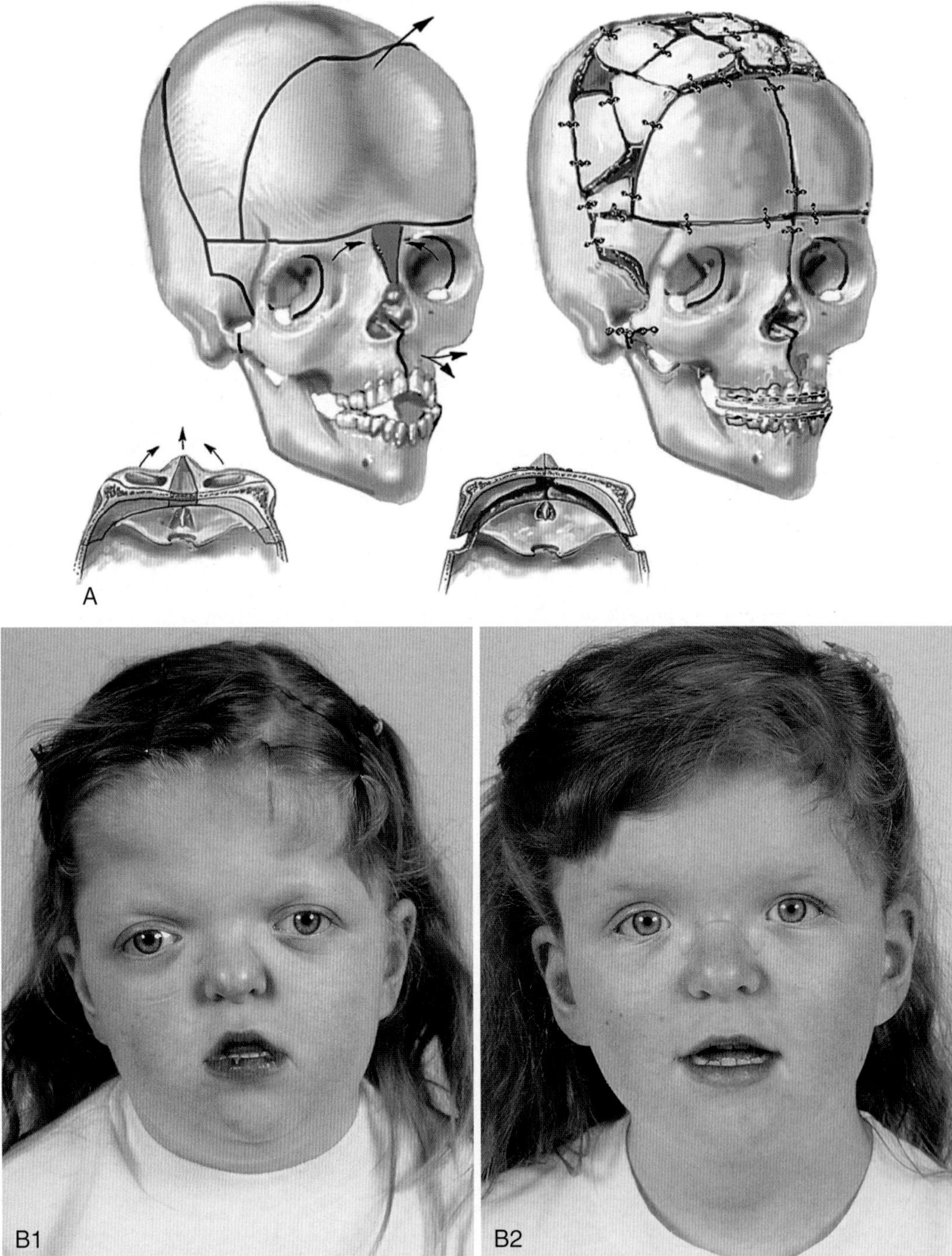

Figure 51.1 A 5-year-old girl with Apert syndrome who underwent lateral canthal advancements, performed by a neurosurgeon, at 6 months of age. She then presented with residual craniofacial deformities requiring anterior cranial vault and facial bipartition (FB) osteotomies with reshaping. She will require orthognathic surgery and orthodontic treatment in the teenage years to complete reconstruction. **A,** Illustration of preoperative craniofacial morphology. The planned cranial vault and FB osteotomies and reshaping are also shown. **B,** Frontal facial views before and after anterior cranial vault and FB reconstruction.

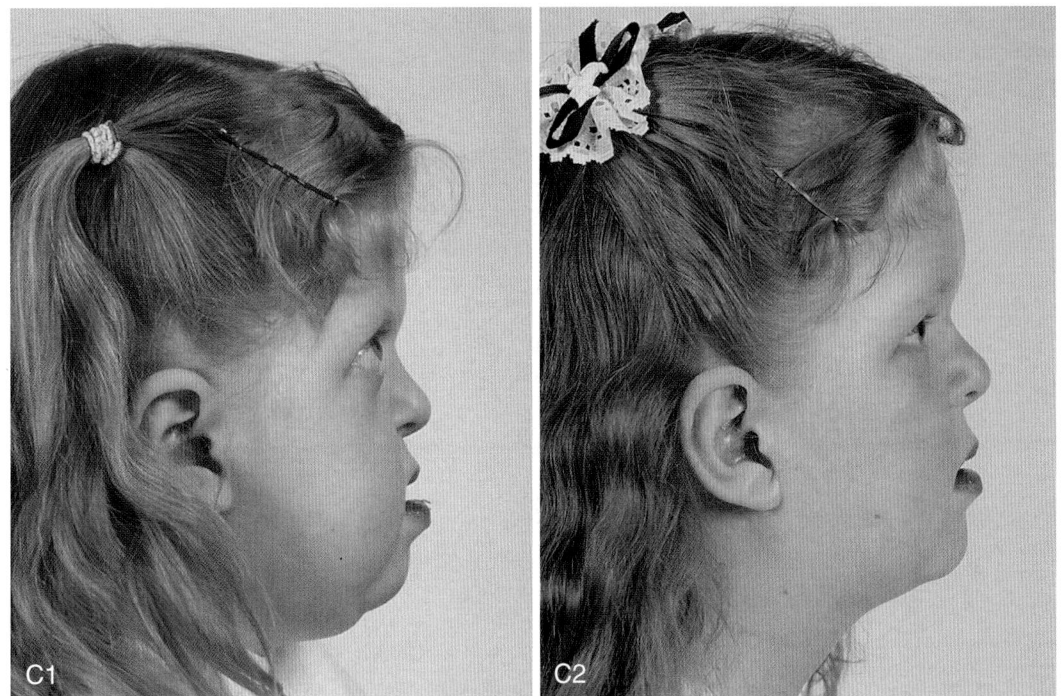

Figure 51.1, cont'd C, Profile views before and after FB reconstruction. (A and C1, From Posnick JC. Craniofacial dysostosis: staging of reconstruction management of the midface deformity—craniofacial disorders. *Neurosurg Clin North Am.* 1991;2:683. B1, B2, From Posnick JC. *Orthognathic Surgery: Principles and Practice.* St. Louis, Missouri: Saunders; 2014.)

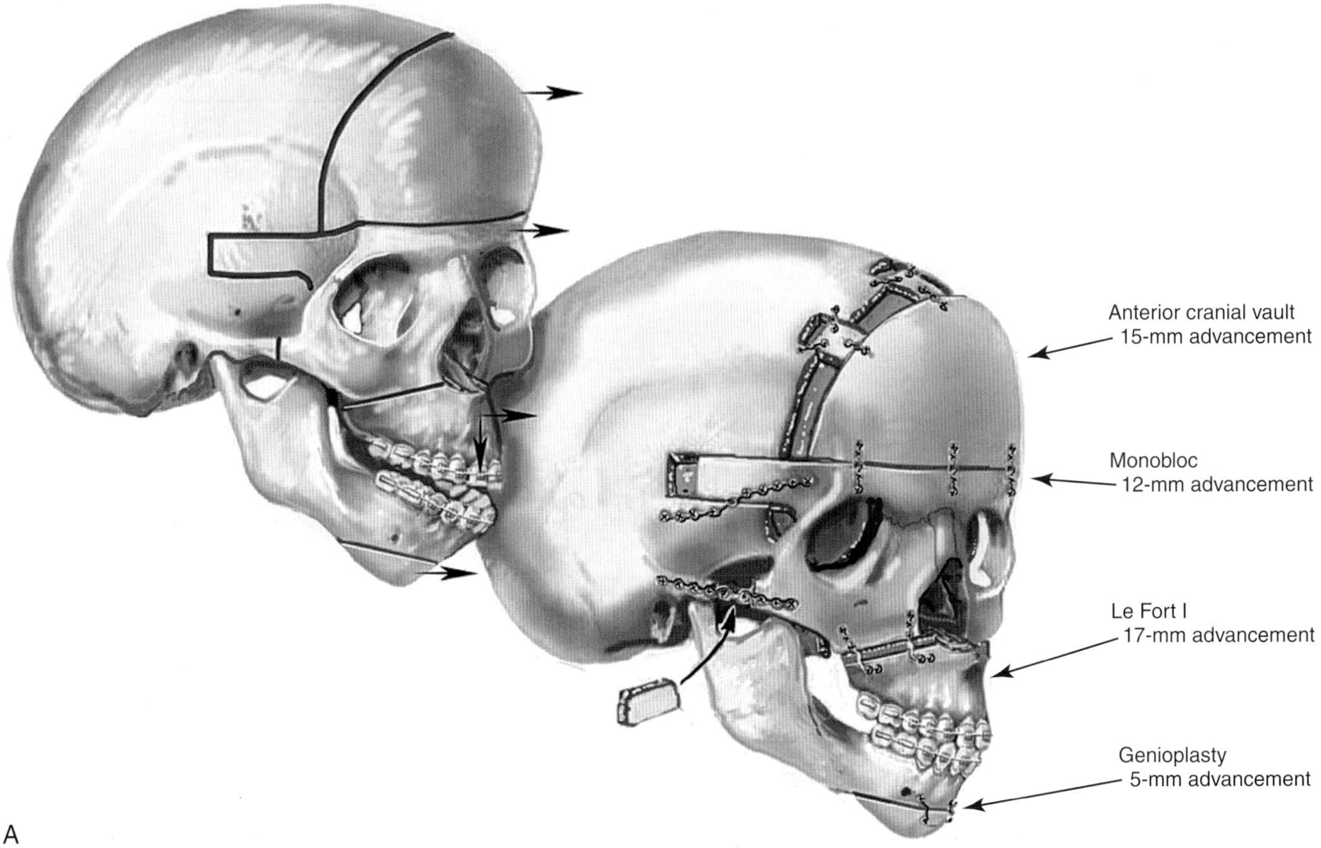

Anterior cranial vault
15-mm advancement

Monobloc
12-mm advancement

Le Fort I
17-mm advancement

Genioplasty
5-mm advancement

A

Figure 51.2 A child born with Crouzon syndrome who underwent bilateral coronal suture release at 3 months of age. Additional craniotomy and cranial vault reshaping were completed when she was 9 months old. At 2 years of age, she underwent a Le Fort III (midface) osteotomy and a forehead advancement procedure through an intracranial approach. She presented at the age of 14 years with residual deformities, for which she underwent simultaneous anterior cranial vault, monobloc (MB), Le Fort I, and chin osteotomies with differential advancement of each component. **A,** Illustration of planned and completed anterior cranial vault, MB, Le Fort I, and chin osteotomies.

Continued

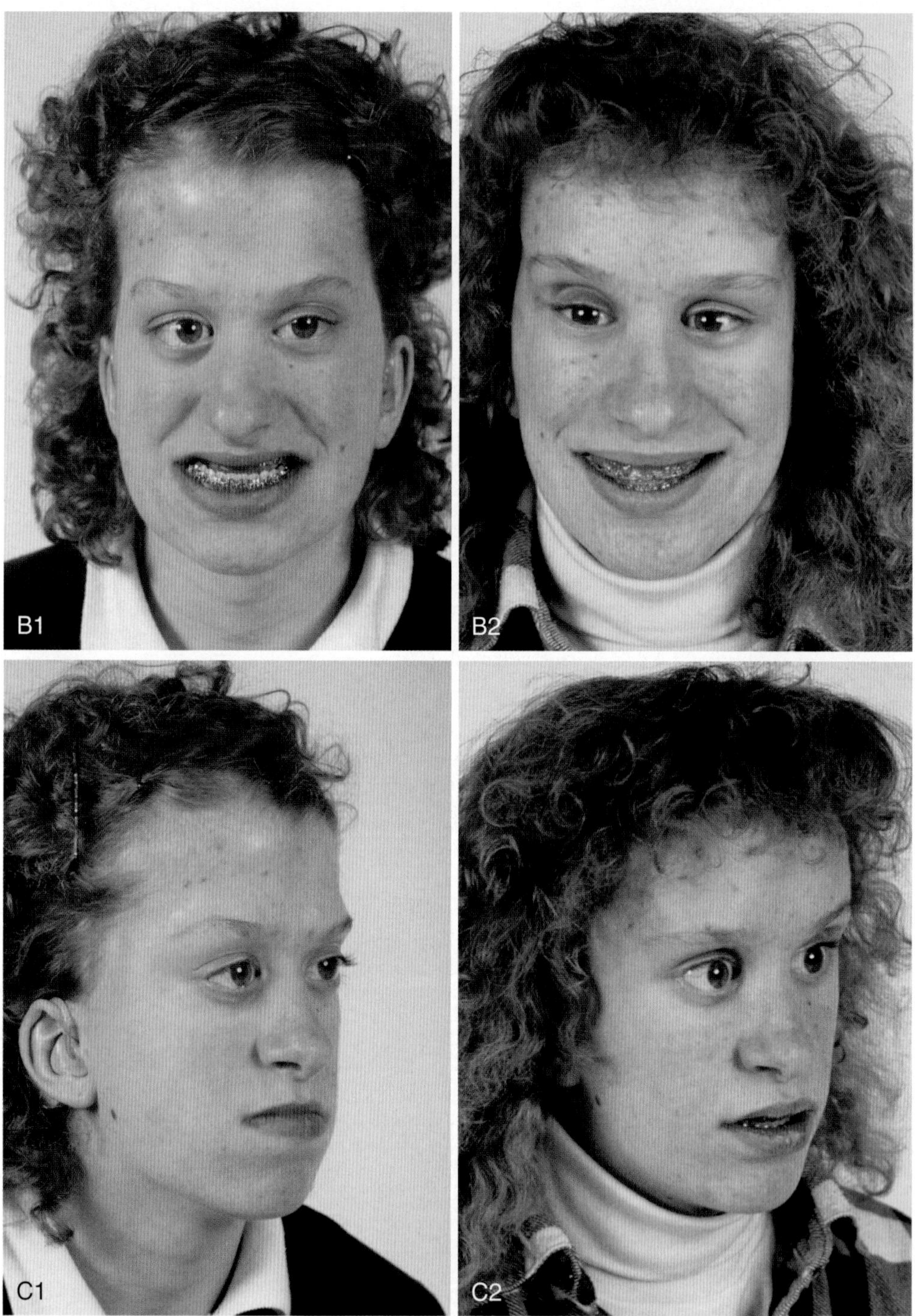

Figure 51.2, cont'd **B1–B2,** Frontal facial views before and after reconstruction. **C1–C2,** Oblique facial views before and after reconstruction.

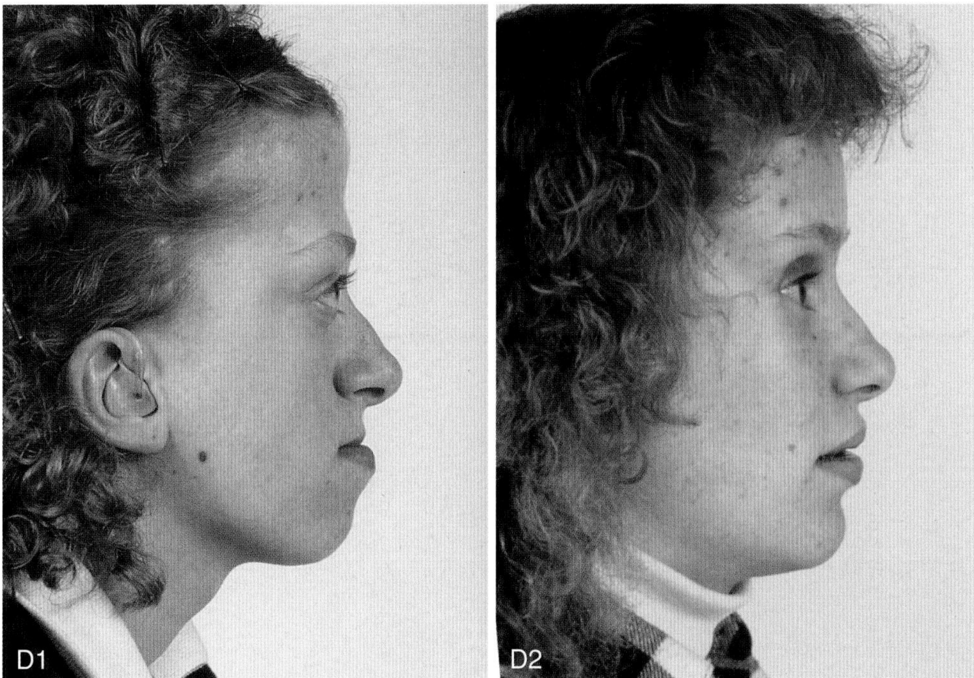

Figure 51.2, cont'd D1–D2, Profile views before and after reconstruction. (A, C1, C2, D1, and D2 from Posnick JC. Craniosynostosis: surgical management of the midface deformity. In: Bell WH, ed. *Orthognathic and Reconstructive Surgery,* Vol. 3. Philadelphia, Pennsylvania: Saunders; 1992; B1 and B2 from Posnick JC. *Orthognathic Surgery: Principles and Practice.* St. Louis, Missouri: Saunders; 2014.)

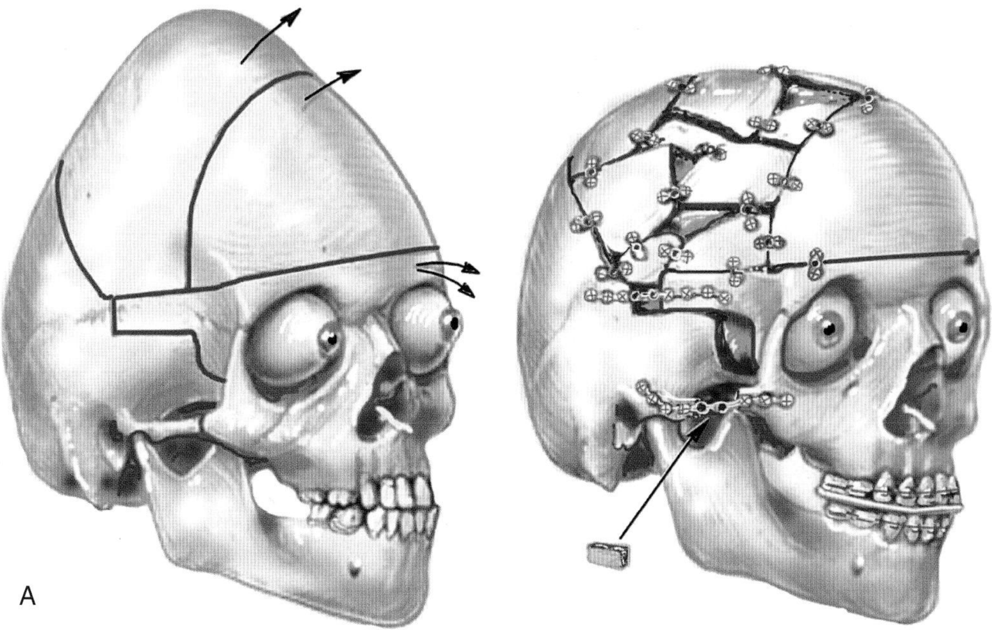

Figure 51.3 A 12-year-old boy with unrepaired Crouzon syndrome who was referred for evaluation. He underwent total cranial vault and MB osteotomies with reshaping and advancement. **A,** Illustrations of the patient's craniofacial morphology with planned osteotomy locations indicated. A second illustration is shown after osteotomies with reshaping and advancement.

Continued

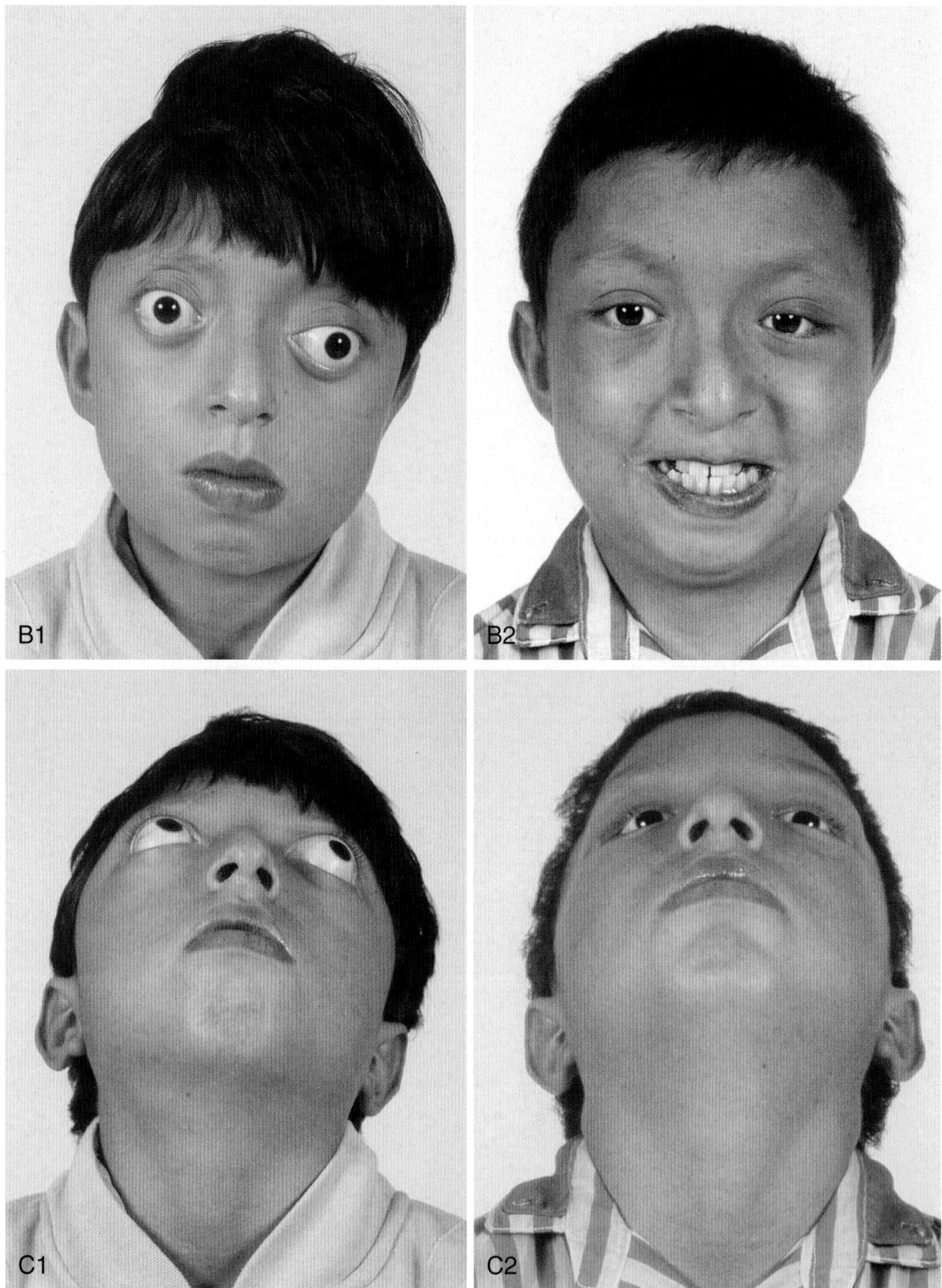

Figure 51.3, cont'd **B1–B2,** Frontal facial views before and after reconstruction. **C1–C2,** Worm's-eye views before and after reconstruction.

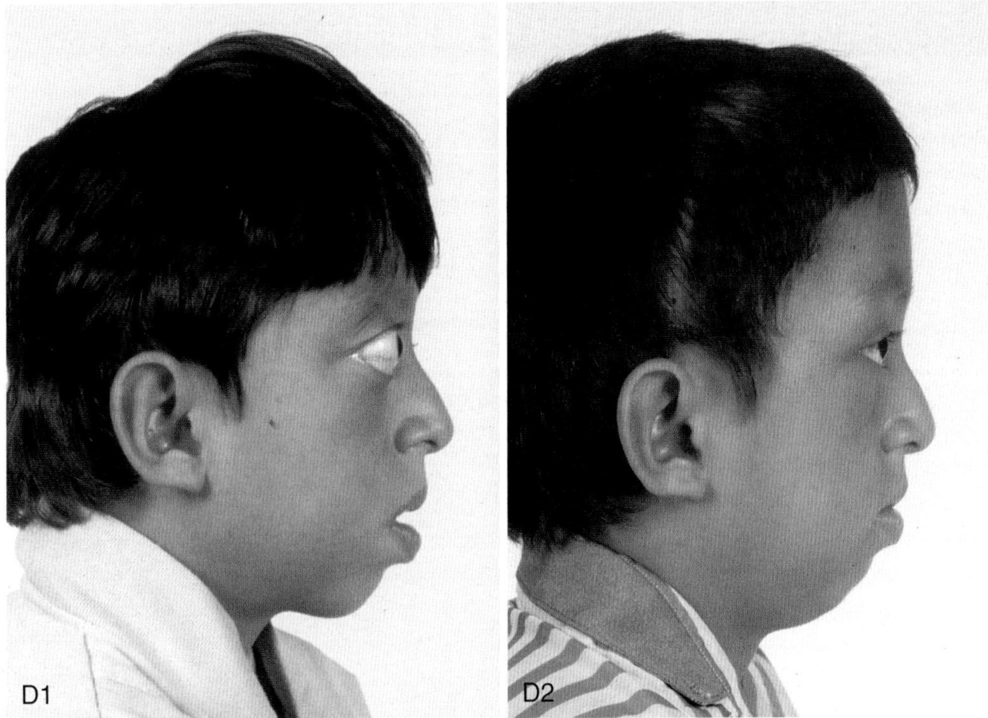

Figure 51.3, cont'd D1–D2, Profile views before and after reconstruction. (From Posnick JC. Craniosynostosis: surgical management of the midface deformity. In: Bell WH, ed. *Orthognathic and Reconstructive Surgery,* Vol 3. Philadelphia, Pennsylvania: Saunders; 1992.)

separate Le Fort I osteotomy. The degree of horizontal deficiency observed at the orbits and at the maxillary dentition is rarely uniform. If a Le Fort I osteotomy to separate the lower midface from the upper midface complex is not carried out, excess advancement at the orbits, with enophthalmos, is likely to occur as the surgeon attempts to achieve a positive overjet at the incisors. The Le Fort I osteotomy is generally not performed at the time of the upper midface procedure; it awaits skeletal maturity and is combined with orthodontic treatment. Until then, a degree of an angle class III anterior open bite negative overjet malocclusion remains. When the mature teenage or adult patient presents for surgical correction and requires both upper midface (i.e., naso-orbito-zygomatic) and lower midface (i.e., maxilla) management, the procedures may be carried out simultaneously.

Final reconstruction of the upper midface deformities in those born with a craniosynostosis syndrome can be managed as early as 7 to 10 years of age. By this age, the cranial vault and orbits normally attain approximately 85% to 90% of their adult size. Whenever feasible, waiting until the maxillary first molars have erupted is also preferred. When the upper midface reconstruction is carried out after approximately 7 years of age, the objective is to attain adult morphology in the cranio-orbito-zygomatic region, with the expectation of a stable result (no longer influenced by growth) once healing has occurred. Psychosocial considerations also support the age range of 7 to 10 years for the upper midface procedure. When a successful reconstruction is achieved at this age, the child may progress through school with an opportunity for a healthy body image and self-esteem.[38,75–116]

Monobloc and Facial Bipartition Osteotomies

The lack of consensus about the ideal timing and techniques for the management of complex upper midface malformations and deformities in craniosynostosis syndromes, reflects not only uncertainty about the potential results with any one approach to treatment but also confusion about how to perform these technically sensitive procedures.

The following section provides the surgeon with a step-by-step technical description of the MB and FB osteotomies.

TECHNIQUE: Monobloc and Facial Bipartition Osteotomies

STEP 1: Airway Management

Satisfactory airway management in a patient undergoing an MB/FB osteotomy is essential. The method the authors use is an orotracheal tube secured adjacent to the cusp edge of the mandibular central incisors with a circummandibular wire. After the MB/FB osteotomies and disimpaction are complete, a nasotracheal tube is placed, and the orotracheal tube is removed. Through this controlled approach, endotracheal tube injury (at completion of the osteotomies) and/or dislodgment (during disimpaction) are prevented. Also, direct contact between the maxillary and mandibular teeth can be achieved for improved control of the occlusion. The nasotracheal tube remains in place at the end of the procedure to allow for nasal mucosal stenting during the initial postoperative phase. Other approaches to manage the airway have been described and used effectively (i.e., tracheostomy, submental intubation, and orotracheal intubation without exchange) (Fig. 51.4A).

STEP 2: Nasolacrimal Tube Placement and Temporary Tarsorrhaphy

When feasible, placement of Crawford nasolacrimal tubes to protect the nasolacrimal apparatus during surgery is recommended. The puncta are dilated, and a probe is inserted through each punctum to confirm entrance into the nose. The Crawford tube is inserted through each punctum and pulled through the nose. Within the nose, the Silastic sheeting is stripped; the tubing is tied in the nose, and the excess is cut (in the nose with scissors).

Temporary tarsorrhaphies are placed with 6-0 nylon suture from gray line to gray line just lateral to the pupil of each eye. As an alternative, corneal shields may be used to protect the cornea, but this prevents direct examination of the pupils during surgery (Fig. 51.4B).

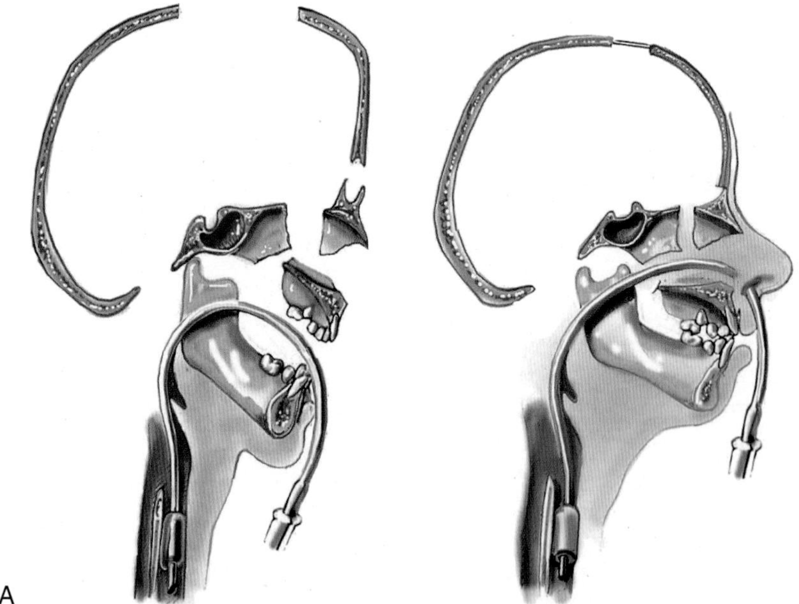

Figure 51.4 A, Endotracheal tube management during MB or FB osteotomy.

TECHNIQUE: Monobloc and Facial Bipartition Osteotomies—cont'd

STEP 3: Arch Bar Placement
Surgical arch wires are generally applied. A throat pack is placed, and the mouth is cleansed. Erich arch bars are applied to the maxillary and mandibular teeth. Circummandibular wires are placed to further stabilize the mandibular arch bar, and the orotracheal tube is secured with a wire to the symphyseal region of the surgical arch bar (Fig. 51.4C).

Continued

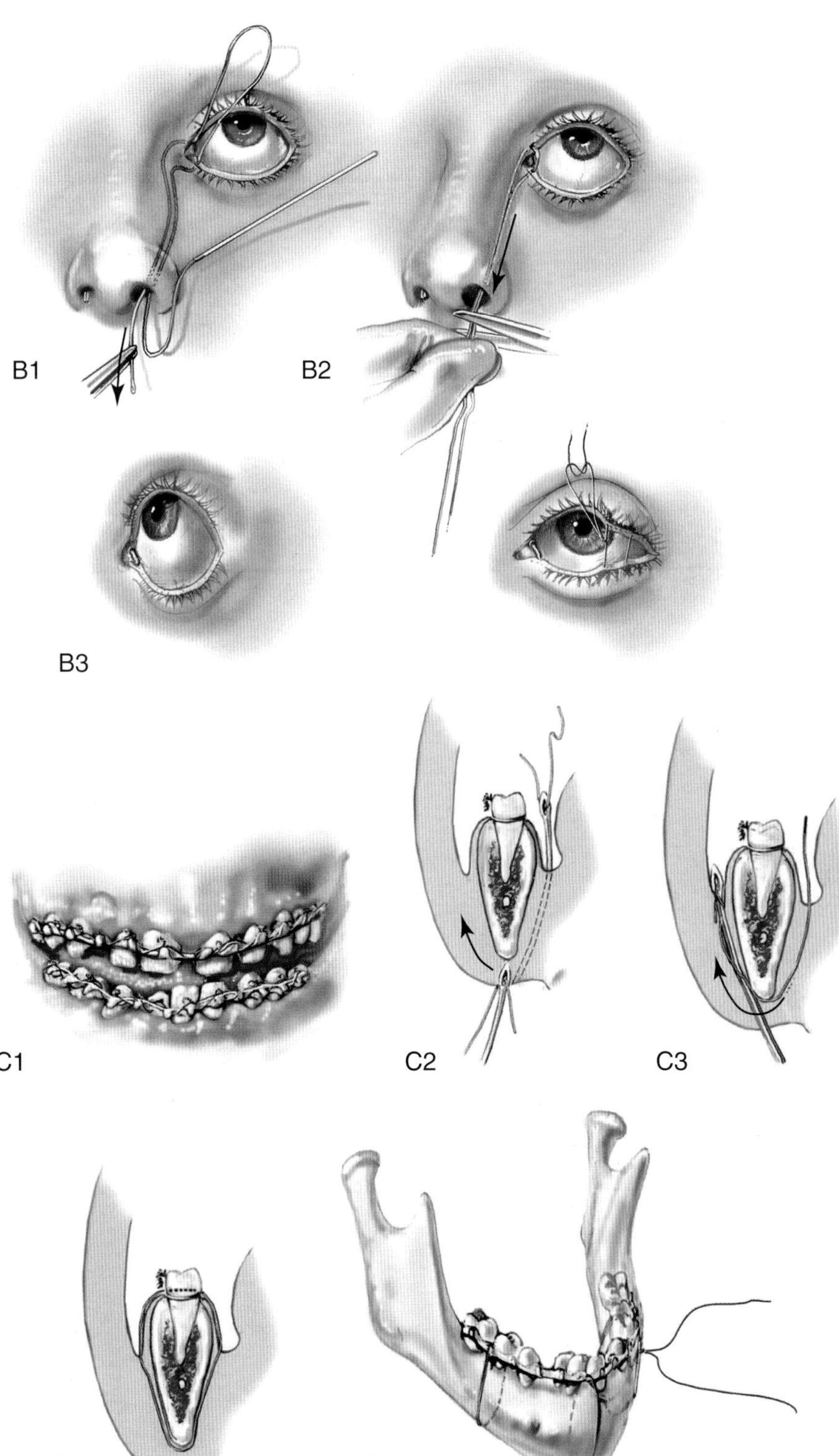

Figure 51.4, cont'd B1, Dilation and placement of Crawford nasolacrimal tubes coming through the nose. **B2,** Trimming of excess nasolacrimal tube length inside the nose. **B3,** Appearance of appropriately placed nasolacrimal tubes. **C1,** Placed Erich arch bars on the maxillary and mandibular dentition. **C2–C4,** Sequence of placement of a circummandibular wire using a mandibular awl from the lingual to the facial aspect of the mandible. **C5,** Securing and placement of circummandibular wires against the arch bar of the mandible.

TECHNIQUE: Monobloc and Facial Bipartition Osteotomies—cont'd

STEP 4: Patient Preparation

The patient is prepared and draped. The patient's head is placed in a Mayfield (horseshoe-shaped) head holder in the neutral neck position. The entire scalp is cleansed with povidone-iodine (Betadine) soap. The soap is then washed out with sterile water. Next, povidone-iodine solution is applied to the scalp, face, and neck. The surgical field is draped out to expose the neck down to the clavicles; the full face, including the external ears; and the anterior scalp back to the planned incision. Separation of the mouth/nose from the eyes/forehead is achieved with an additional sterile towel drape. This limits contamination of the intracranial cavity by oral and nasal flora.

STEP 5: Incision

A standard coronal (skin) incision is completed. The incision site is postauricular and posterior in the scalp. Other incision modifications have been described (e.g., Z-plasty in temporal regions). Lidocaine with epinephrine is injected to facilitate hemostasis (Fig. 51.4D).

STEP 6: Dissection

The anterior scalp flap is then elevated by remaining deep to the superficial layer of the deep temporal fascia over the temporalis muscles, subperiosteal over the midforehead region, subperiosteal down the lateral orbital rims, subperiosteal with exposure of the anterior maxilla, subperiosteal for exposure of the zygomatic arches, and subperiosteal over the dorsum of the nose. Elevation of the temporalis muscles off the squamous temporal bones is then carried out (Fig. 51.4E).

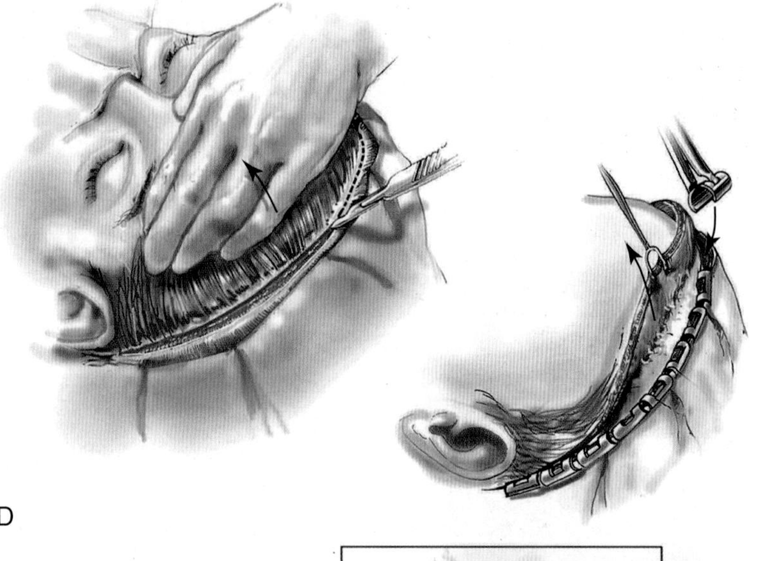

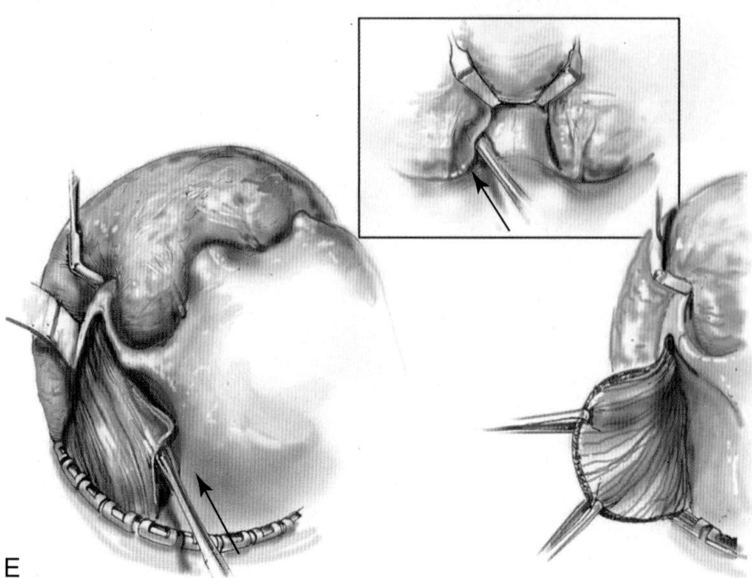

Figure 51.4, cont'd **D,** Postauricular scalp incision and placement of Raney clips for hemostasis. **E,** Nasal, orbital, and temporal muscle elevation and dissection.

TECHNIQUE: Monobloc and Facial Bipartition Osteotomies—cont'd

STEP 7: Craniotomy

Bifrontal craniotomy is completed. The craniotomy lines are drawn with a sterile pencil. Bur holes are made with a perforator as needed. The craniotomies are completed with a craniotome. The frontal bones are separated from the underlying dura and then removed. The frontal and temporal lobes of the brain are adequately retracted to safely accomplish osteotomies. The brain is protected with cottonoid pledgets (Fig. 51.4F).

STEP 8: Zygomatic Arch Osteotomy

Zygomatic arch osteotomies are performed. Retractors are placed, and an osteotomy is completed through the midzygomatic arch on each side with a sagittal (reciprocating) saw (Fig. 51.4G).

Continued

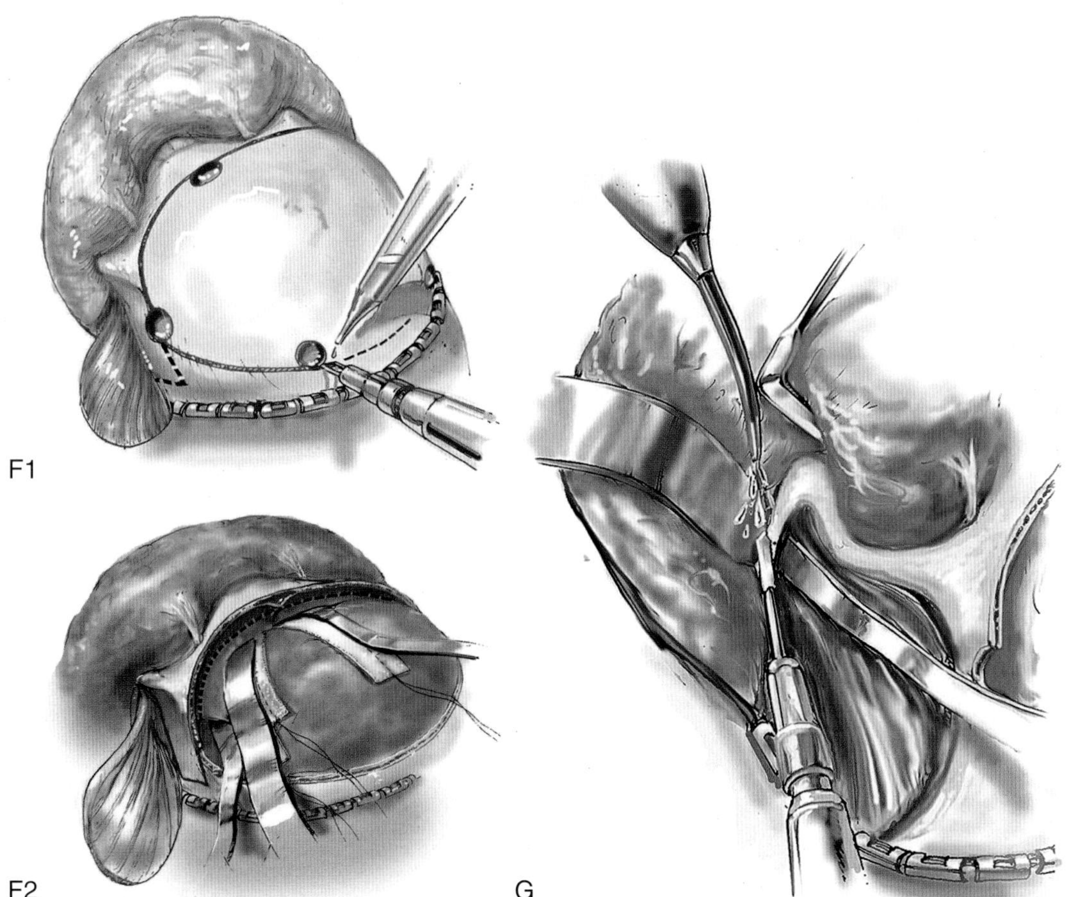

Figure 51.4, cont'd **F1,** Bifrontal craniotomy marked and performed with perforator and craniotome. **F2,** Dissection and retraction of the anterior cranial skull base contents. The brain is protected with cottonoid sponges. **G,** Midzygomatic arch osteotomy with reciprocating saw.

TECHNIQUE: Monobloc and Facial Bipartition Osteotomies—cont'd

STEP 9: Lateral Orbital Wall Osteotomy

With the sagittal saw the lateral orbital wall osteotomy is initiated into the inferior orbital fissure. The osteotomy is extended superiorly through the lateral orbital wall (Fig. 51.4H).

STEP 10: Skull Base Osteotomy

With continued use of the sagittal saw, the lateral tenon extension of the osteotomy through the squamous temporal bone and skull base is carried out (Fig. 51.4I).

STEP 11: Orbital Roof Osteotomy

The orbital roof osteotomy is completed with the sagittal saw through the anterior skull base (Fig. 51.4J).

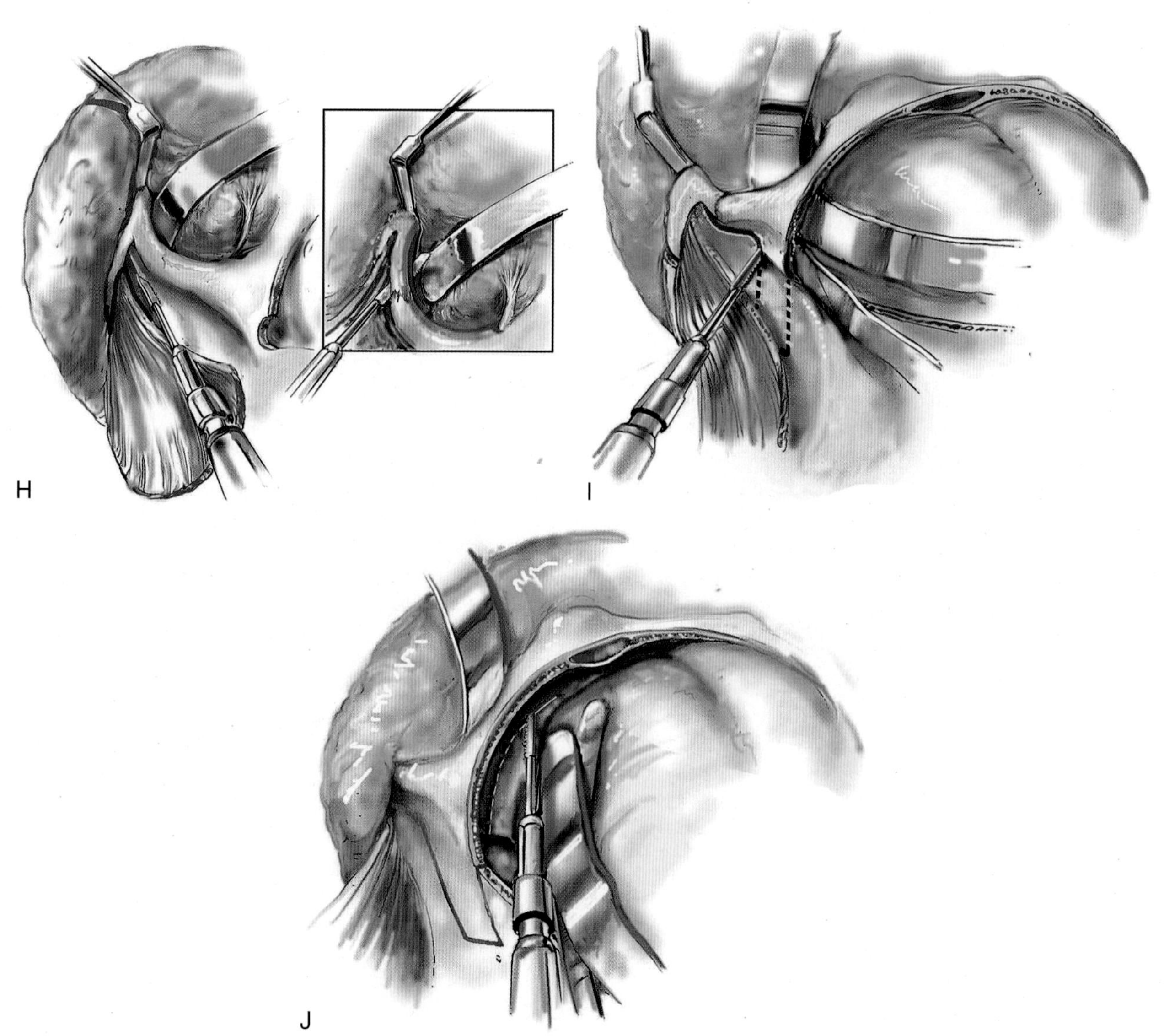

Figure 51.4, cont'd **H,** Lateral orbital wall osteotomy with reciprocating saw and protection of orbital contents. **I,** Continuation of the lateral orbital wall osteotomy into the tenon extension and protection of intracranial contents. **J,** Anterior skull base and orbital roof osteotomy.

TECHNIQUE: Monobloc and Facial Bipartition Osteotomies—cont'd

STEP 12: Lateral Skull Base Osteotomy

The orbital roof osteotomy continues laterally through the sphenoid wing. This osteotomy joins up with the previous tenon extension on each side (Fig. 51.4K).

STEP 13: Confirmation of Osteotomy

A thin chisel, placed through the anterior skull base, is used to confirm completion of the sphenoid wing osteotomy and continuity with the tenon extension (Fig. 51.4L).

Continued

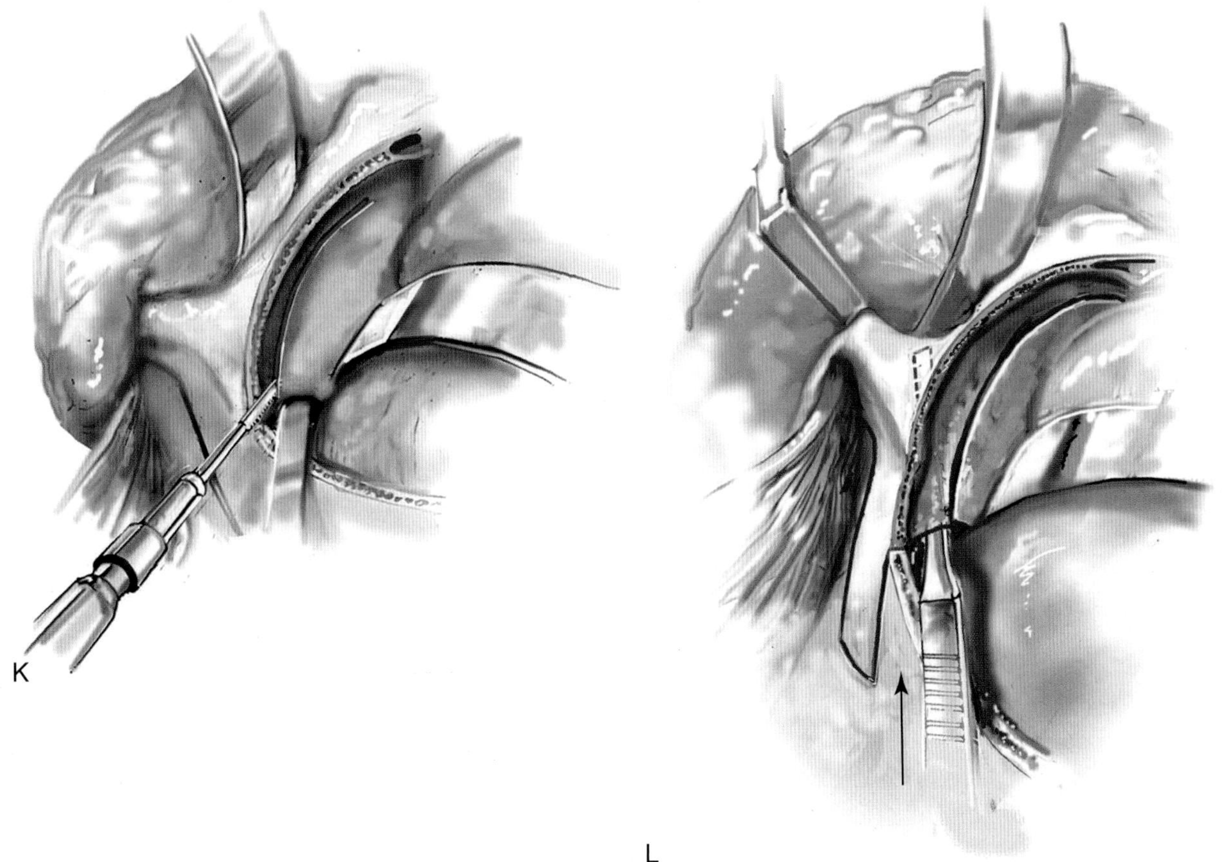

Figure 51.4, cont'd **K,** Extension of anterior cranial base osteotomy to the sphenoid wing and the previously made tenon osteotomy. **L,** Use of a thin osteotome to confirm separation at the sphenoid wing.

TECHNIQUE: Monobloc and Facial Bipartition Osteotomies—cont'd

STEP 14: Medial Orbital Wall Osteotomy

With a thin chisel and working through the skull base, the medial orbital wall osteotomy is completed posterior to the medial canthus and nasolacrimal apparatus and inferiorly into the inferior orbital fissure (Fig. 51.4M).

STEP 15: Nasal Septal Osteotomy

The anterior aspect of the nasal septum is separated from the cranial base. A straight chisel (15-mm wide), placed through the cranial base just anterior to the crista galli, is used to complete this osteotomy and further separate the midface (from the base of the skull) (Fig. 51.4N).

STEP 16: Pterygomaxillary Osteotomy

Separation of the pterygomaxillary sutures is completed. A long chisel (10-mm wide) is placed through the coronal incision and infratemporal fossa, to the pterygomaxillary suture. One hand (double-gloved) is placed in the patient's mouth, and the other hand is used to place the chisel through the coronal incision into the infratemporal fossa. A mallet is then used to separate the pterygomaxillary suture with the chisel. The success of the separation is confirmed with the pterygomaxillary spreader forceps (Fig. 51.4O).

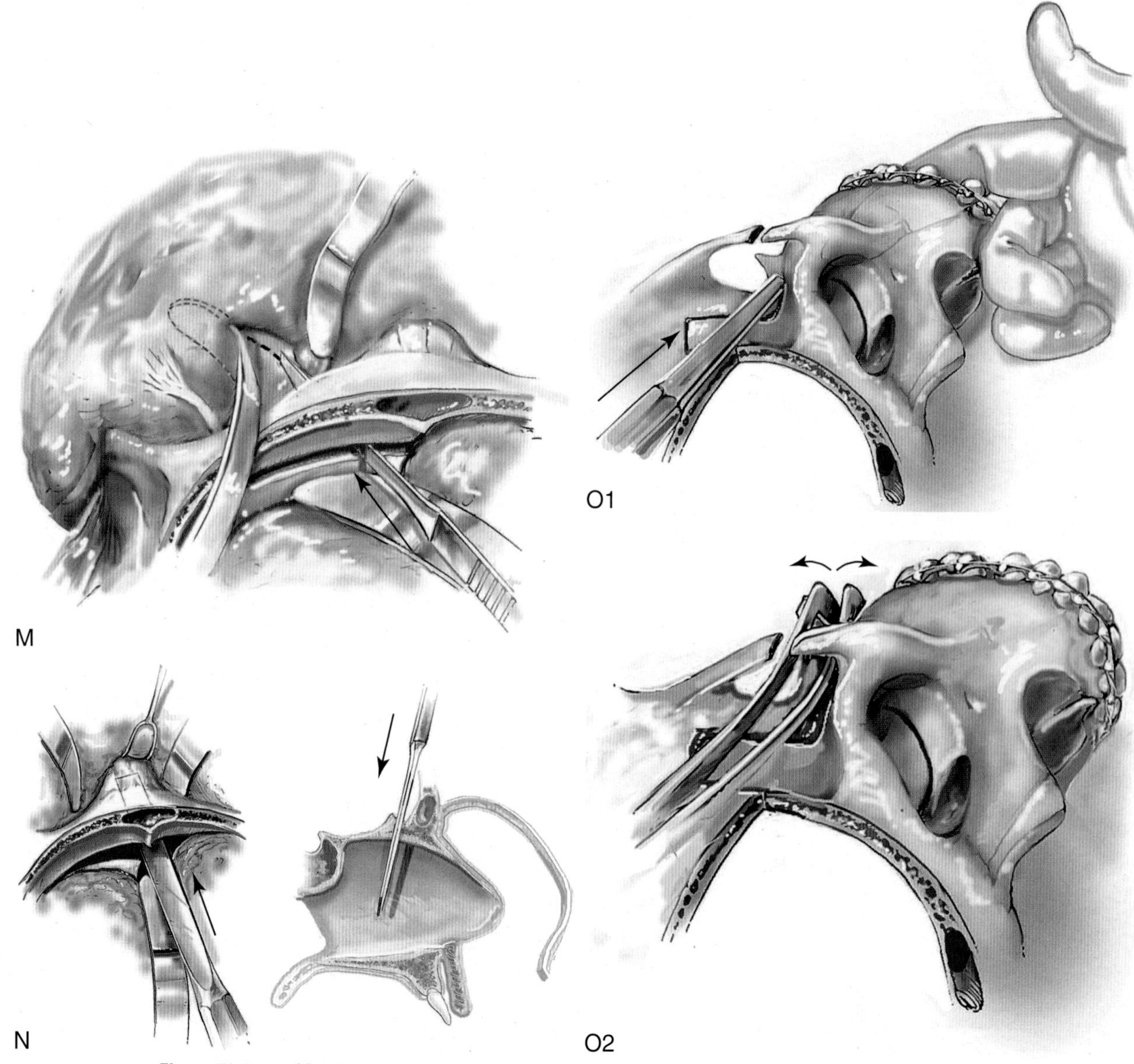

Figure 51.4, cont'd **M,** Medial orbital wall osteotomy using a thin osteotome behind the medial canthal tendon and lacrimal apparatus to the inferior orbital fissure, with protection of orbital contents. **N,** Nasoseptal osteotomy using a chisel anterior to the crista galli through the anterior cranial base. **O1,** Pterygomaxillary osteotomy through the scalp incision directed inferiorly. **O2,** Confirmation of pterygomaxillary dysjunction.

TECHNIQUE: Monobloc and Facial Bipartition Osteotomies—cont'd

STEP 17: Disimpaction

The midface (MB) is disimpacted with the use of two nasomaxillary forceps placed in the nose and mouth. Simultaneously, pterygomaxillary spreader forceps are placed through the coronal incision on each side. The midface is then disimpacted and stretched forward to confirm adequate advancement at the occlusal level. Next, the endotracheal airway exchange is completed. Additional sterile drapes are placed over the scalp and face/neck regions. The throat pack is removed. The surgeon places the nasotracheal tube through the nose and into the oropharynx. The anesthesiologist then removes the orotracheal tube and completes the insertion of the nasotracheal tube through the larynx, using the direct or GlideScope laryngoscopic technique. (For MB-only osteotomy, proceed to Step 21. For continuation of FB, proceed to Step 18) (Fig. 51.4P).

STEP 18: Midnasal Ostectomy

For FB, a midnasal osteotomy (ostectomy) is completed. Working through the coronal incision, the surgeon marks out the proposed midnasal osteotomy with caliper and pencil and then completes it with a sagittal saw. Once the ostectomy is complete, removal of portions of the underlying cartilaginous nasal septum is accomplished (Fig. 51.4Q).

Continued

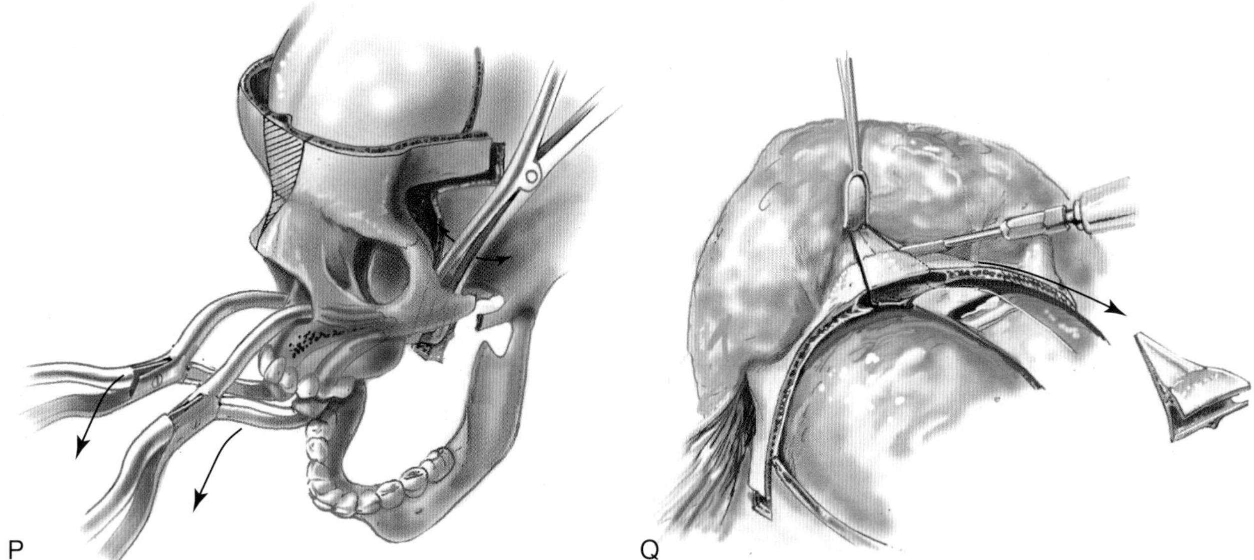

Figure 51.4, cont'd P, Midfacial and upper facial disimpaction completed as one unit with nasomaxillary forceps and bone spreaders placed in the pterygomaxillary junction. **Q,** Midnasal ostectomy.

TECHNIQUE: Monobloc and Facial Bipartition Osteotomies—cont'd

STEP 19: Inferior Maxillary Segmentation

For FB, separate sterile oral instruments are used to split off the maxilla into two segments. An intraoral maxillary vestibular incision is made, followed by subperiosteal exposure of the anterior maxilla, anterior nasal spine, and nasal floor. With a sagittal saw, a midline osteotomy is completed between the central incisors and then parasagittally down the hard palate (the palatal mucosa is left undisturbed). The segmental separation is completed with a thin chisel (5 mm wide) placed between the central incisors. The Erich arch bar also is cut between the incisors. Further separation of the posterior maxilla is completed with a spreader forceps as needed. The oral wound is closed. The intraoral instruments are discarded, and fresh gloves are put on (Fig. 51.4R).

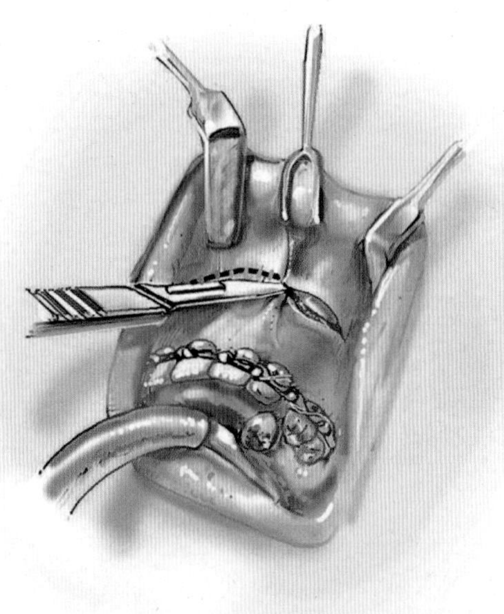

R1

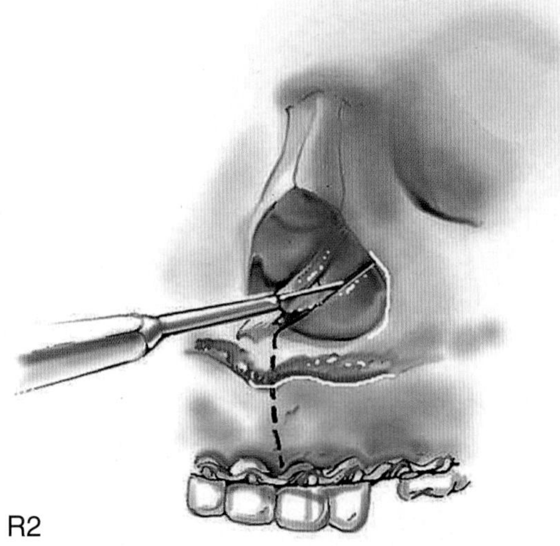

R2

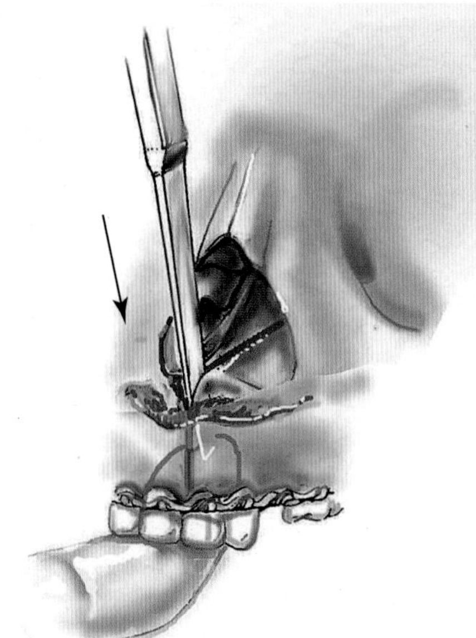

R3

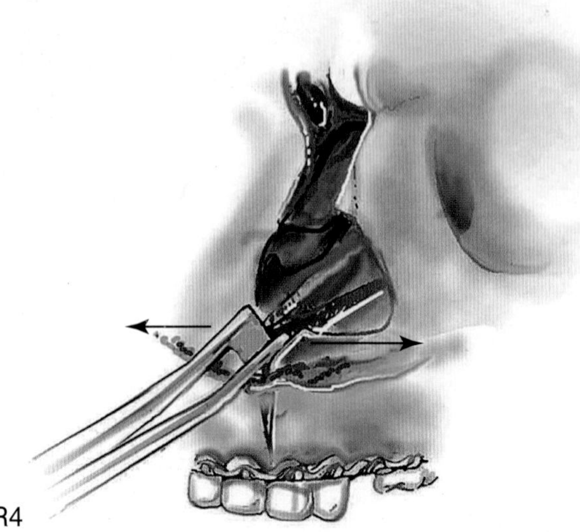

R4

Figure 51.4, cont'd **R1,** Anterior maxillary vestibular incision. **R2,** Parasagittal maxillary osteotomy with reciprocating saw. **R3,** Thin osteotomy to complete the interdental osteotomy between the central incisor dental roots. **R4,** Confirmation and expansion of the segmented maxilla.

TECHNIQUE: Monobloc and Facial Bipartition Osteotomies—cont'd

STEP 20: Facial Rotation

For FB, stabilization of the upper orbits and nasal bones is completed next. Repositioning of the facial halves medially with correction of the midface arc of rotation is completed; this requires refinement with a rotary drill. The upper orbits and nasal bones are fixed with a titanium plate and screws. A rotary drill also is used to cranialize the frontal sinus if needed (Fig. 51.4S).

STEP 21: Facial Advancement

Midface advancement at the level of the maxillary dentition is accomplished. Working through the coronal (scalp) incision, the primary surgeon advances the midface. Using separate sterile oral instruments, assistants wire the jaws together through the mouth (Fig. 51.4T).

Continued

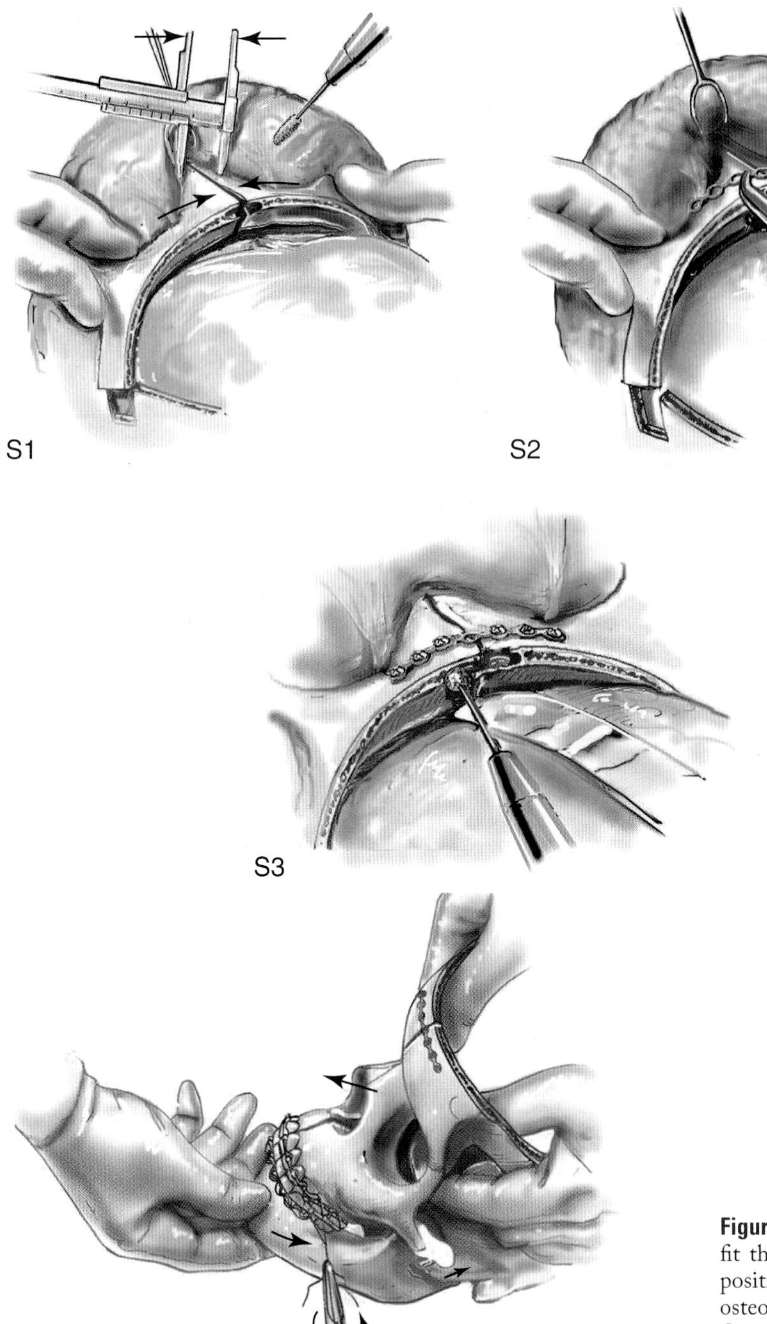

Figure 51.4, cont'd **S1,** Caliper and rotary drill used to adjust and fit the segmented upper facial unit medially to the preplanned position. **S2,** Application of titanium fixation across the midline osteotomy of the upper facial unit to secure its new position. **S3,** Cranialization of the remaining frontal sinus mucosa and posterior wall. **T,** Advancement of the entire facial unit and placement of the maxillomandibular fixation.

TECHNIQUE: Monobloc and Facial Bipartition Osteotomies—cont'd

STEP 22: Zygomatic Arch Fixation

Upper midface advancement is established at the zygomatic arches. The amount of advancement at each zygomatic arch is measured with a caliper. A titanium plate is conformed to extend from the anterior maxilla across the arch and surgical gap to the posterior zygoma on each side. The plate is secured with titanium screws (Fig. 51.4U).

STEP 23: Orbital Reshaping

Additional segmental osteotomies of the orbits are shown. Occasionally, the lateral superior orbits have further dysplasia and require segmental osteotomies with reshaping for reconstruction. If so, the lateral orbital segments are removed with a reciprocating saw. Additional segmental orbital osteotomies then are often completed with a reciprocating saw. The lateral orbital rim–superior orbital rim segments are further reshaped with a rotary drill. The segments are fixed with titanium plates and screws (Fig. 51.4V).

STEP 24: Tenon Extension Fixation

Stabilization of the midface advancement at the upper orbital (tenon) extension is accomplished. The desired advancement is measured with a caliper; a miniplate is adapted to bridge the gap between the tenon extension and posterior cranial vault. Titanium screws are used for plate stabilization (Fig. 51.4W).

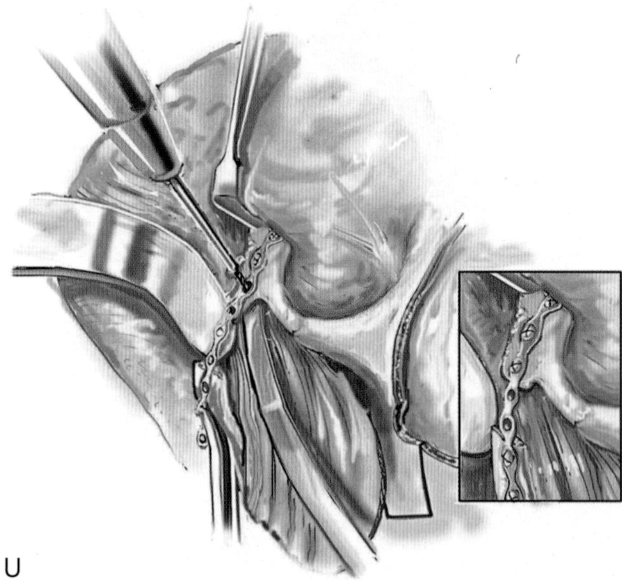

Figure 51.4, cont'd **U,** Advancement of the facial unit at the level of the zygomatic arch, with placement of titanium fixation (inset) to secure the preplanned advancement.

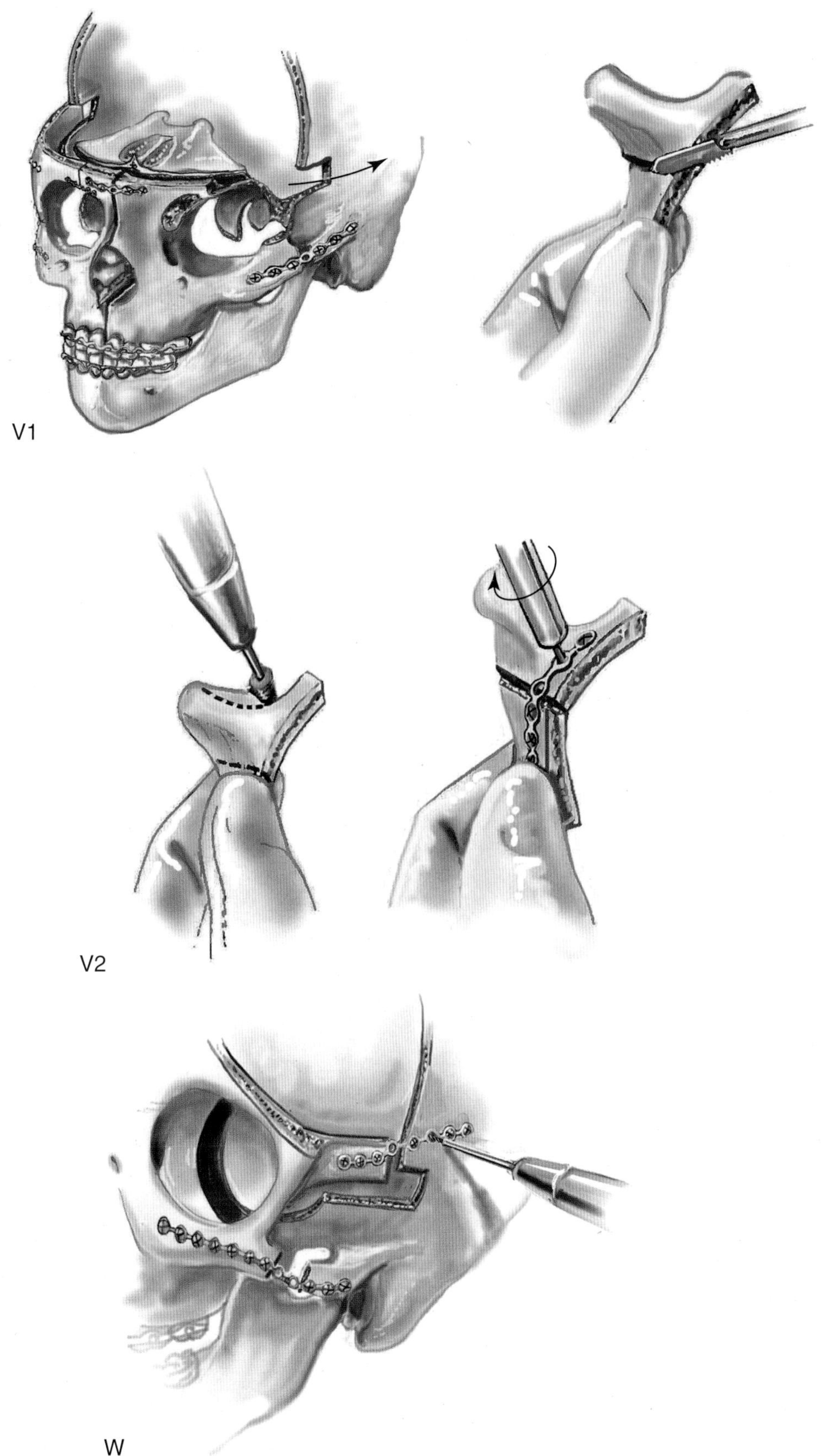

Figure 51.4, cont'd **V1,** *Left,* Removal of the upper orbital component to facilitate reshaping. *Right,* Osteotomy of the tenon extension to facilitate reshaping of the upper orbital unit. **V2,** *Left,* Rotary drill to reshape the upper orbital unit. *Right,* Titanium fixation to secure the newly reshaped orbital unit. **W,** Application of titanium fixation to secure the advancement of the upper orbital unit to the stable cranial vault across the tenon extension.

Continued

TECHNIQUE: Monobloc and Facial Bipartition Osteotomies—cont'd

STEP 25: Ethmoid Air Cell Management

Hyperplastic ethmoid air cells are debrided as needed in patients with orbital hypertelorism. With visualization through the anterior cranial base, rongeurs are used to débride hyperplastic ethmoid air cells and reduce midorbital hypertelorism (Fig. 51.4X).

STEP 26: Skull Base Management

The opening between the anterior cranial fossa and the nasal cavity is managed. The surgeon irrigates and suctions the intranasal cavity through the anterior cranial base exposure. A sheet of Gelfoam is applied to separate the opening between the two cavities. Fibrin glue is then injected over the Gelfoam to seal the separation. Other methods of managing the separation between the nasal cavity and anterior cranial fossa may be used, depending on the clinical circumstances (e.g., cranial bone grafts, soft tissue flaps) (Fig. 51.4Y).

STEP 27: Anterior Cranial Vault Reconstruction

The forehead (anterior cranial vault) is reshaped, advanced, and secured in place. With a reciprocating saw, osteotomies of the removed anterior cranial vault are completed. With a rotary drill, recontouring is accomplished to achieve the desired shape. Split- or full-thickness cranial bone graft is harvested and used as needed to fill in defects. Fixation is accomplished with plates and screws. A split-thickness cranial bone graft is also placed and fixed in the midzygomatic arch segmental defects (Fig. 51.4Z).

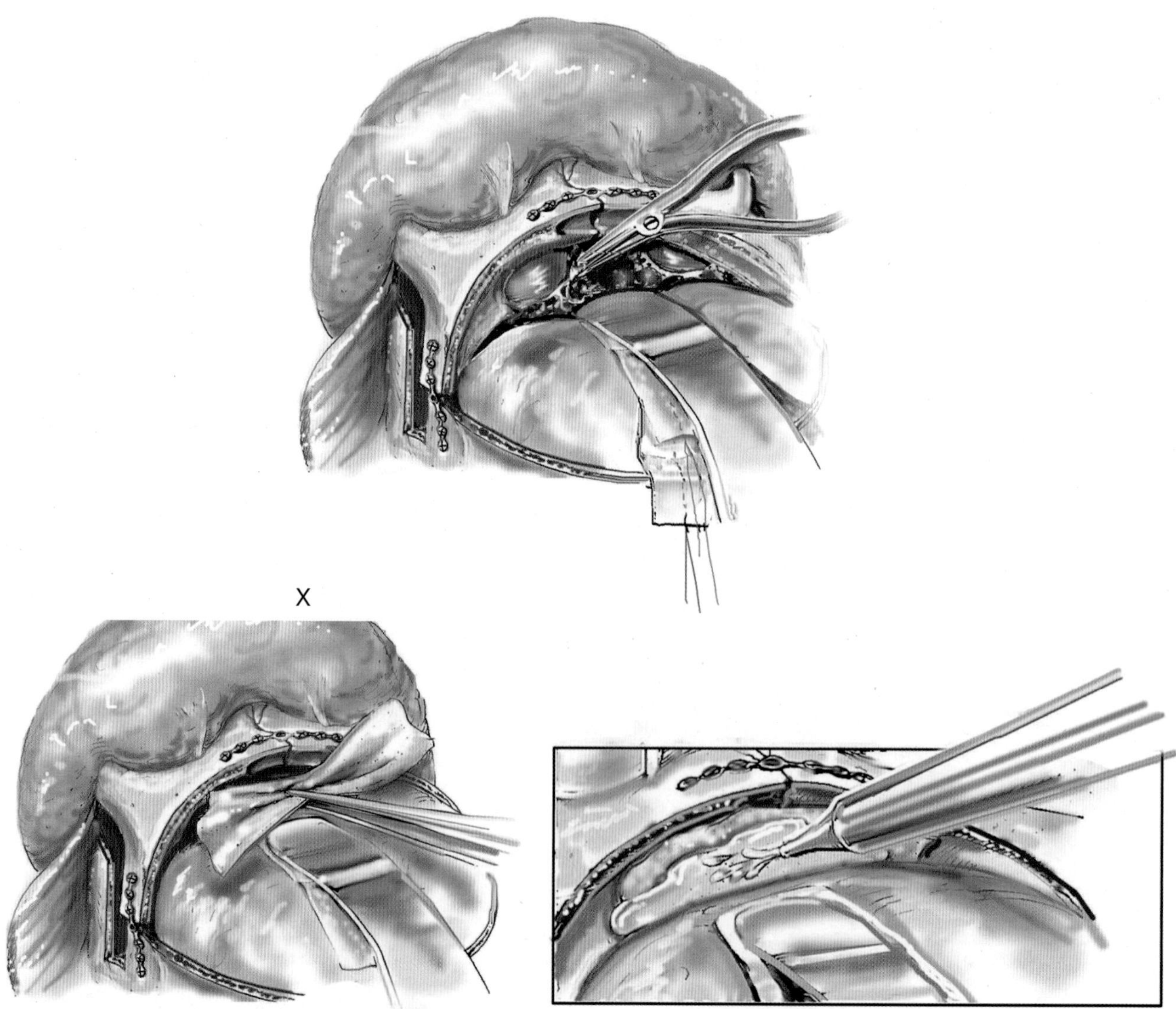

Figure 51.4, cont'd **X,** Débridement of excess ethmoid air cells through the anterior cranial base. **Y,** Application of Gelfoam and fibrin glue to seal the anterior cranial fossa from the nose.

TECHNIQUE: Monobloc and Facial Bipartition Osteotomies—cont'd

STEP 28: Lateral Canthus Suspension

Lateral canthopexies are completed. Two holes are drilled at each (new) FZ suture region. The lateral canthi are identified with a skin hook through the coronal incision. A figure-eight wire suture is placed through each lateral canthus (through the coronal incision). Each lateral canthus is fixed by passing the wire through the drill holes in the FZ suture (Fig. 51.4AA).

Continued

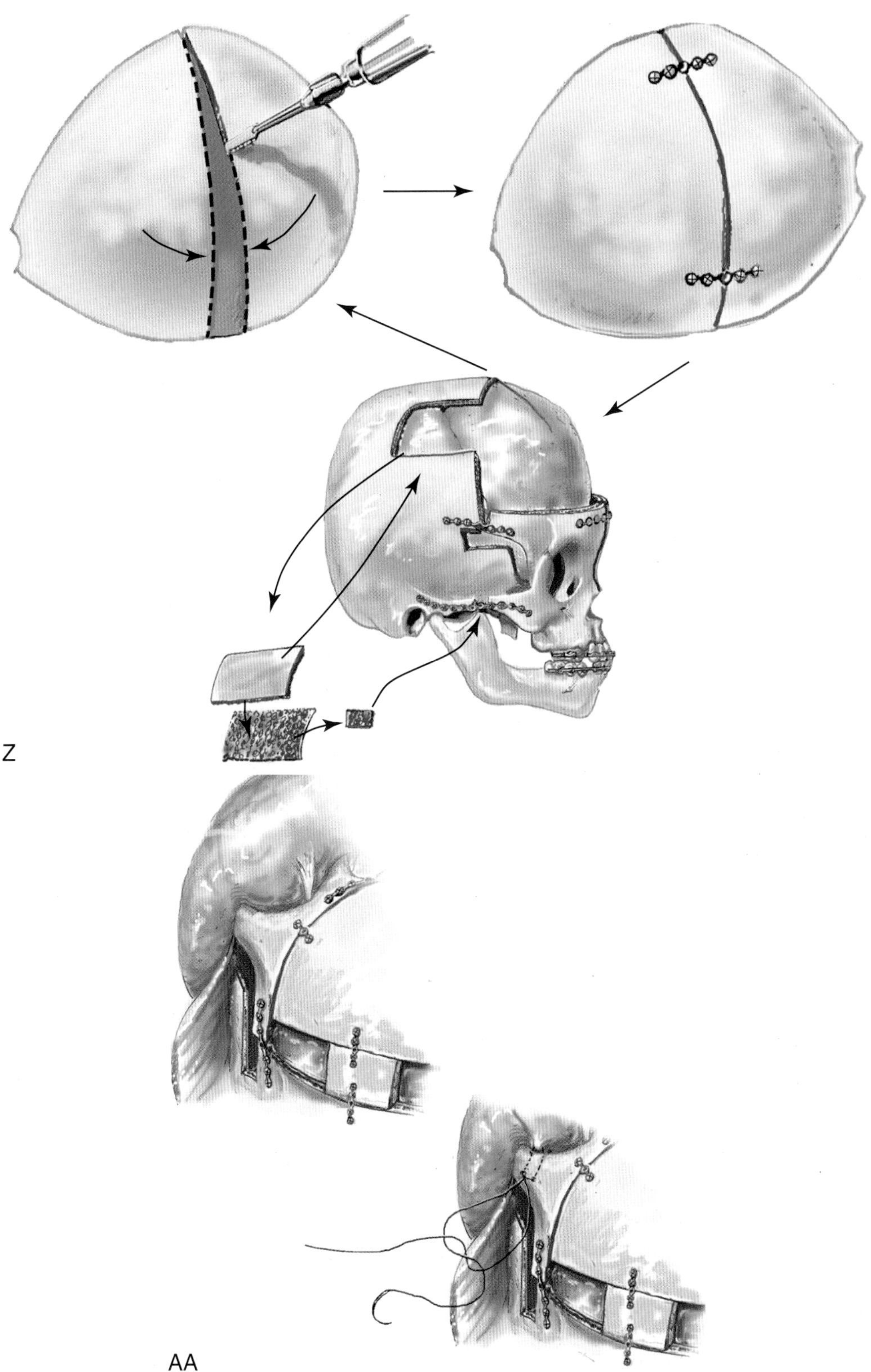

Figure 51.4, cont'd **Z,** Reshaping and fixation of the anterior cranial vault with placement of additional cranial bone grafts. **AA,** Resuspension of the lateral canthus to the advanced lateral orbital rim.

TECHNIQUE: Monobloc and Facial Bipartition Osteotomies—cont'd

STEP 29: Temporalis Muscle Reattachment

Each temporalis muscle is resecured to bone. The temporalis muscles are repositioned anteriorly and secured to the lateral orbital rims and temporal bones with interrupted sutures (Fig. 51.4BB).

STEP 30: Closure

The scalp wound is closed. Suction drains are placed through the posterior scalp flap (one on each side). One drain is placed under the anterior flap, and the other is placed below the posterior flap. The galea closure is completed with interrupted sutures. The skin layer closure is completed with staples or resorbable sutures, according to the surgeon's preference (Fig. 51.4CC).

An overview of the skeletal morphology is shown before and after FB osteotomies and anterior cranial vault reshaping/repositioning and stabilization. The locations of proposed osteotomies are indicated (Fig. 51.4DD).

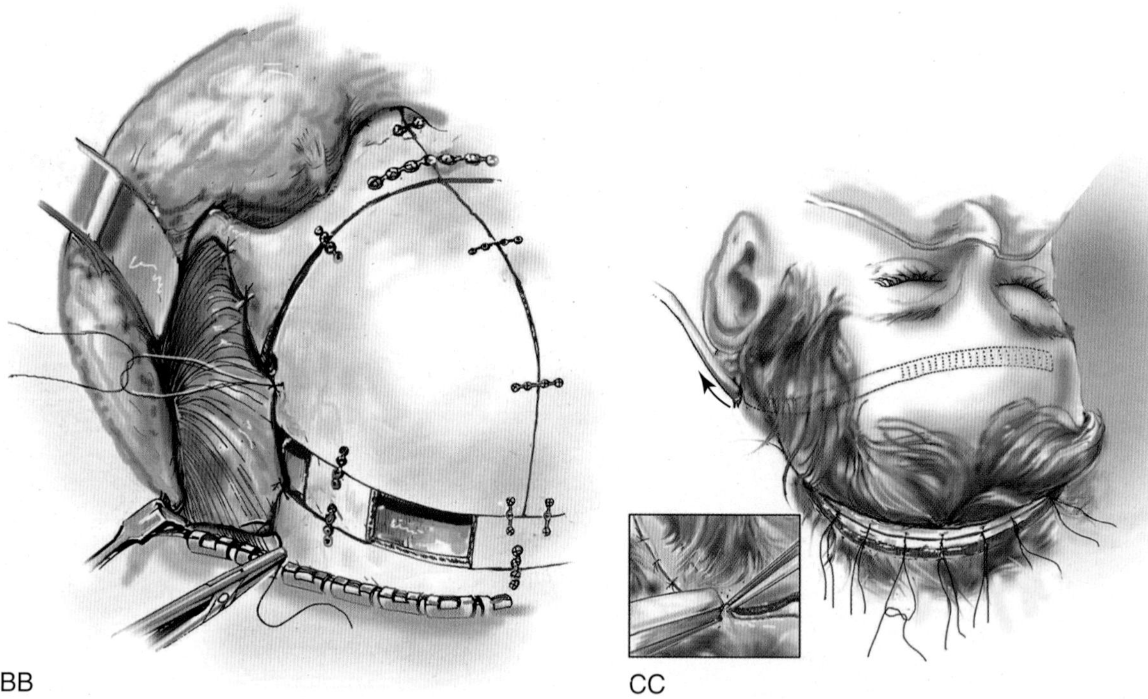

Figure 51.4, cont'd **BB,** Forward advancement and resuspension of the temporal muscles. **CC,** Drain placement and scalp closure.

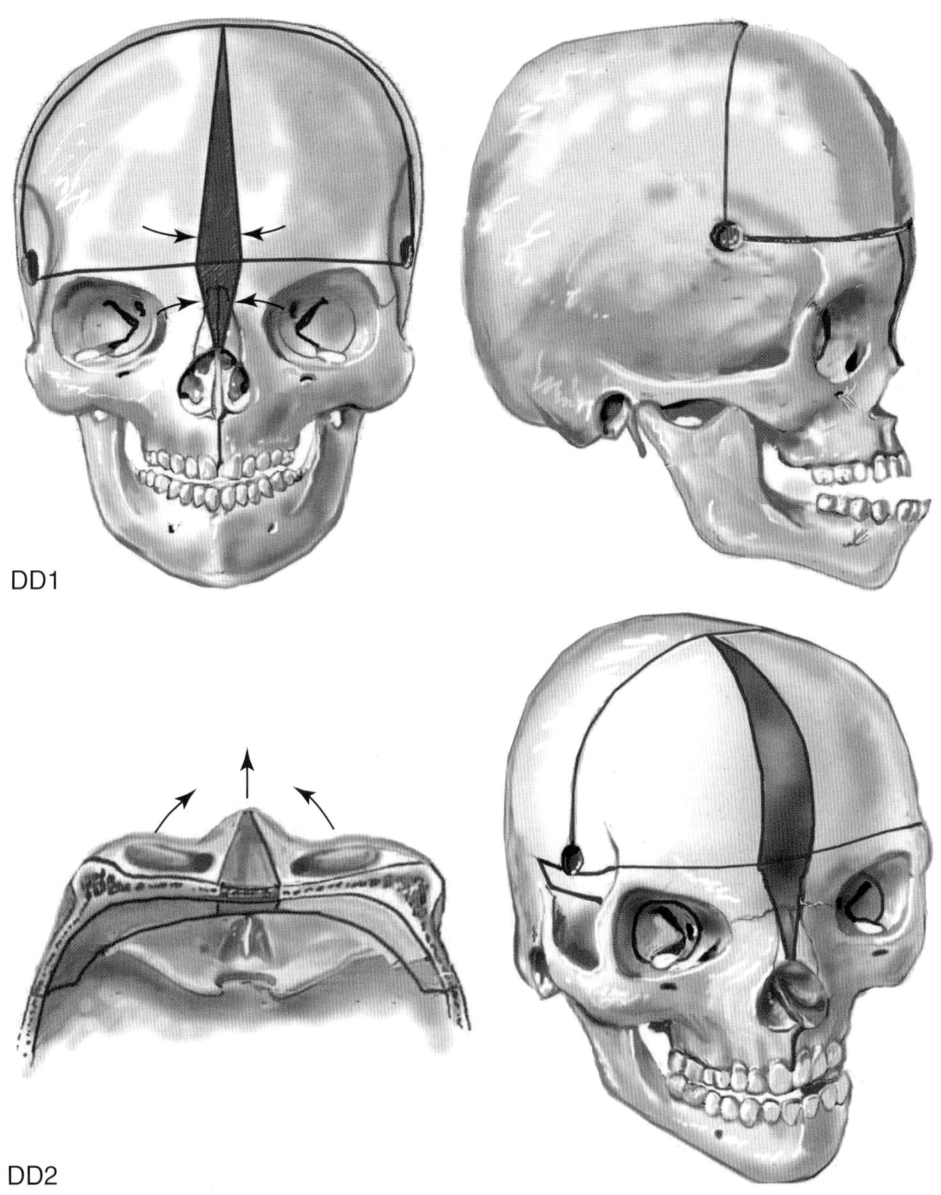

Figure 51.4, cont'd DD1–DD4, Overview of the skeletal morphology before and after facial bipartition osteotomy with repositioning and stabilization. (From Posnick JC. Orthognathic Surgery: Principles and Practice. St Louis, Missouri: Saunders; 2014.)

Continued

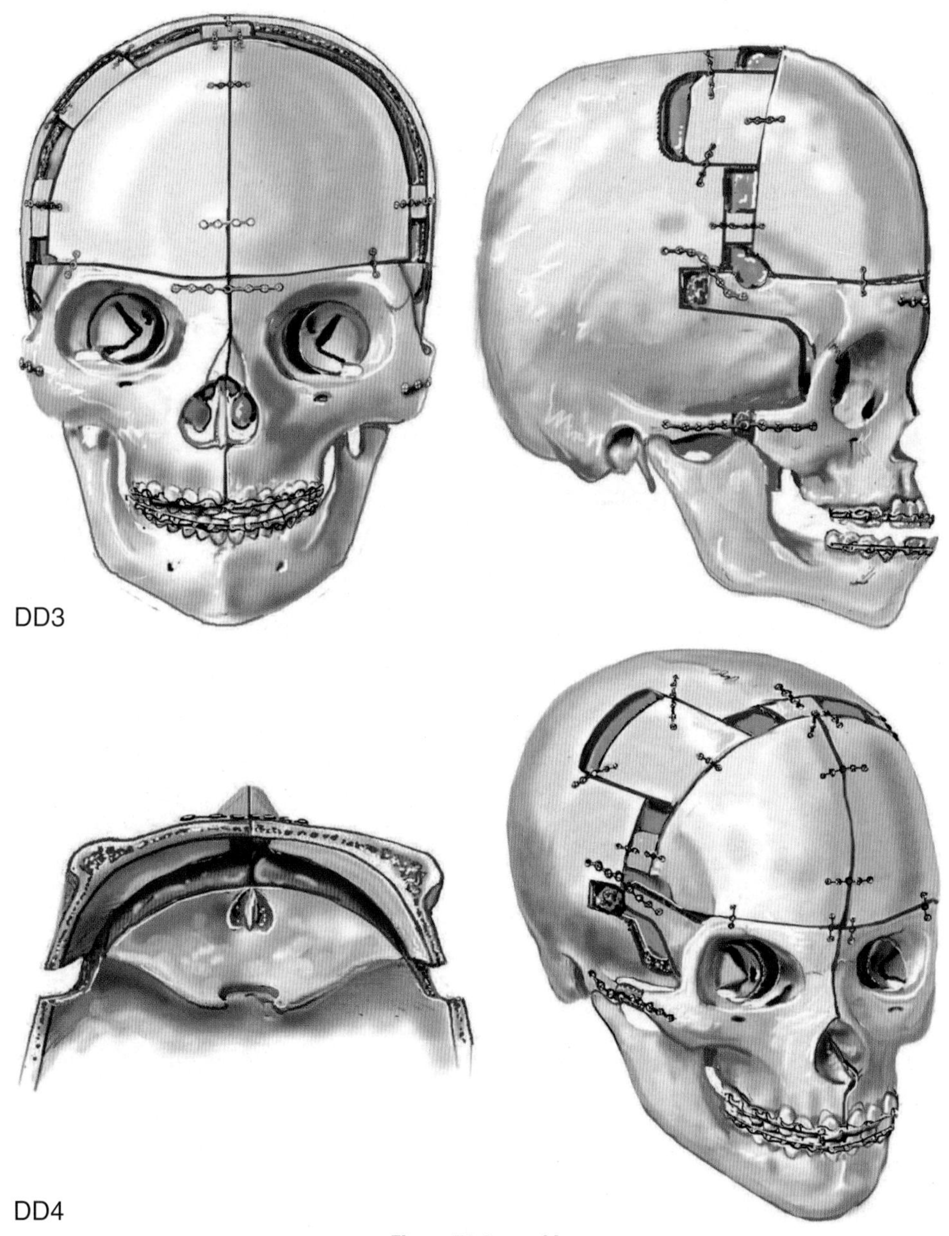

Figure 51.4, cont'd

Avoidance and Management of Intraoperative Complications

Cranial vault reconstruction in the child with a craniosynostosis syndrome should provide space for the compressed brain to expand. Immediately after the completion of cranial vault and MB or FB osteotomies with advancement, extradural (retrofrontal) dead space remains in the anterior cranial fossa above the skull base gap created by the osteotomy.[117] The skull base gap is in direct communication with the nasal cavity. Therefore, the postoperative recovery may be complicated by cerebrospinal fluid (CSF) leakage across the skull base gap and, subsequently, infection, fistula formation, and bone resorption in the glabella region. After frontofacial advancement by either MB or FB, the nasal cavity–cranial fossa communication must be managed to limit these potential complications. The most effective method remains unclear, but all agree that it is a critical aspect of a successful reconstruction.

Technical aspects of management include (1) gentle tissue handling, (2) achieving good hemostasis, (3) effective repair of dural tears, (4) avoidance of overadvancement, (5) maximum separation of the dura and nasal mucosal tissue planes (i.e., interposing tissue, such as bone grafts, tissue sealants, and flaps), (6) stable (plate and screw) fixation of the osteotomies and bone segments, (7) avoidance of pressure gradients across the opening to facilitate nasal mucosa healing, and (8) prevention of over or under ventriculoperitoneal shunting.

After cranio-orbital reconstruction in the infant with a craniosynostosis syndrome, rapid filling of the expanded intracranial volume by the previously compressed frontal lobes of the brain has been documented.[117] This has also been shown to occur after MB and FB advancement in children and young adults.[118] More gradual filling of the space is thought to occur in older adults. At the time of the MB or FB osteotomies, the nasal cavity can be sealed from the cranial fossa by (1) insertion of pericranial tissue, (2) placement of bone grafts to bridge the osteotomy gaps, and (3) use of tissue sealants. This provides time for reepithelialization (healing) of the nasal mucosa. Until the torn nasal mucosa heals, communication between the nasal cavity and anterior cranial fossa may result in the transfer of air, fluid, and bacteria, followed by infection and nasocranial fistula formation. Postoperative continuation of nasotracheal intubation for several days and nasopharyngeal tube placement after extubation have also proven useful in limiting pressure gradients across the communication. The avoidance of positive pressure ventilation, enforcement of sinus precautions, and restriction of nose blowing further limit the reflux of air, fluid, and bacteria early after surgery.

Four benchmark clinical studies clarify issues of morbidity related to MB or FB osteotomies for the reconstruction of an individual with a craniosynostosis syndrome. Posnick et al. studied the issues of retrofrontal dead space, communication across the skull base osteotomy gap, and associated morbidity in a consecutive series of mixed-dentition children and permanent-dentition young adults (n = 23) undergoing either MB or FB osteotomies combined with cranial vault expansion.[117] The procedures were carried out by a single craniofacial surgeon (Posnick) and one of three neurosurgeons during a 4-year period (1987 to 1991) at a single tertiary care hospital. The extradural (retrofrontal) dead space was measured from consistent computed tomography computed tomography scan images at specific postoperative intervals (immediate, 6 to 8 weeks, and 1 year). The study confirmed the presence of an immediate retrofrontal dead space that generally filled in with the expanding brain/dura by 6 to 8 weeks after surgery. Specific intraoperative maneuvers were undertaken by the surgeons to close (seal) the nasofrontal communication, including flaps, fibrin glue, bone grafts, and Gelfoam. After surgery, care was taken to limit a pressure gradient across the communication (repair of dural tears, sinus precautions, and nasal stenting), with the objective of providing time for nasal mucosal healing. The infection rate in this study group was limited to 2 of 23 patients (9%). In both patients who developed an infection, retrofrontal (extradural) fluid collection was noted, with drainage across the residual nasofrontal communication into the nose. Both patients healed without significant comorbidity (i.e., brain or eye injury), but they did require further reconstruction of resorbed portions of the anterior cranial vault and supraorbital ridges.

Wolfe completed a critical analysis of 81 MB advancements carried out over a 27-year period.[119] This was a retrospective chart analysis of a series of patients undergoing either MB (frontofacial) advancement (MFFA) or FB (MFFA plus FB). The surgeries were performed at seven different craniofacial centers and included 49 MFFA procedures and 32 MFFA plus FB procedures. The MFFA and MFFA plus FB osteotomies were either placed in their preferred location in the operating room (standard approach) or gradually distracted (distraction osteogenesis [DO] technique) with internal rather than external devices. Complications included two deaths (cardiac arrest in one patient and complications arising from hypovolemia in the other). One case was aborted due to large-volume blood loss; there were three infections/sequestrations; and one persistent CSF leak (no meningitis). Significant complications were documented in the distracted group, although fewer in the nondistracted group. Blood loss and operative time were equivalent for the standard and distraction techniques. Interestingly, the incidences of infection and CSF leakage were not diminished with the alternative distraction (DO) approach. The author also concluded that for most patients, the standard approach offered improved morphologic results. The authors then compared the morphologic results of the MMFA and MMFA plus FB to the extracranial Le Fort III option and concluded that the Le Fort III approach was less favorable. Regardless of the technique, all patients were thought to require orthognathic surgery (at the Le Fort I level) to complete the reconstruction.

Bradley et al. completed a single-center, retrospective study comparing differences in morbidity in a series of patients born with a craniosynostosis syndrome who underwent MB osteotomy for correction of upper and midface anomalies/hypoplasia.[120] They described three different sequential treatment approaches (groups) over a period of 23 years. Group I patients (1979 to 1989; n = 12) underwent MB without any special attention to the retrofrontal dead space or the communication through the skull base between the anterior cranial fossa and the nasal cavity. Group II patients (1989 to 1995; n = 11) underwent MB with varied attempts at closure of the skull base gap with pericranial flaps and fibrin glue. Group III patients (1995 to 2002; n = 24) underwent MB osteotomies without immediate advancement. An internal distraction device was placed across the osteotomized zygomatic arch on each side. After a 7-day latency period, advancement of the MB and forehead unit was initiated at 1 mm/day for approximately 2 to 4 weeks. The infection rate for group III patients was significantly lower (2 of 24 patients, or 8%) than for those in groups I and II. Neither of the two infections in group III resulted in bone loss. Group I patients, with limited fixation performed in the 1970s and 1980s, had the greatest morbidity.

As described by Bradley et al., the DO technique allows more time for the brain to expand into the retrofrontal dead space after completion of an MB osteotomy (i.e., delayed for 7 days) before advancement of the upper/midface.[120] In theory, this should facilitate early nasal mucosa healing and thereby limit communication of fluid, air, and bacteria across the surgically created skull base gap. This likely explains the reduction in the infection rates between group II and group III patients. The rate of infection in the group III patients (DO technique) essentially matches that described by Posnick et al. using a standard approach (8% and 9%, respectively).

Bradley et al. also described a greater advancement in group III patients (DO approach) than group I and group II patients.[120] Confounding variables may explain these differences, including increased surgical experience in the later years of the study (group III patients) and the impact of complications in the earlier years of the study (extremely high rate of infection in groups I and II), which likely resulted in relapse and limited the long-term midface advancement. More important, there was no correlation between the number of millimeters of MB advancement and either greater functional gains or enhanced facial esthetics.

With an MB osteotomy, as much esthetic damage is done by overadvancement (enophthalmos) as by underadvancement (residual eye proptosis). In addition, achievement of a "normal" occlusion is not usually a treatment objective at the time of MB advancement. Accomplishing an ideal occlusion without creating enophthalmos generally requires a separate Le Fort I osteotomy to differentially reposition the maxilla.

A fourth and more recent clinical study sheds further light on this subject. Ahmad et al. reported on a series of 12 children born with a craniosynostosis syndrome who suffered from multiple functional problems, including (1) raised intracranial pressure resulting from a diminished cranial vault volume, (2) exposure of the eyes (i.e., corneal irritation) resulting from shallow orbits, (3) airway obstruction from a reduced upper airway space (i.e., OSA), and (4) feeding difficulties.[121] Each of the study patients underwent frontofacial MB advancement using DO techniques. The mean age at surgery was 18 months (range, 4 to 30 months). The mean advancement was 16.6 mm at the forehead level and 17 mm at the midface level. Ocular protection and reduction of intracranial pressure (when raised) were achieved in all children. At least a degree of airway improvement was achieved in all but one child. The authors subjectively stated that there was marked improvement in every patient's appearance. Complications included CSF leaks (2 of 12 patients [16.6%]), pin site infections (3 of 12 patients [25%]), external DO device frame slippage requiring replacement (2 of 12 patients [16.6%]), and overadvancement with resulting enophthalmos (1 of 12 patients [8.3%]). One patient died 9 months after the procedure in conjunction with tracheal reconstruction. The published article was discussed by Hopper,[122] who recommended that clinicians consider a less extensive approach, accepting suboptimal esthetics to limit perioperative morbidity. His suggested approach includes (1) either anterior cranial or posterior cranial vault expansion without simultaneous midface advancement to relieve intracranial pressure; (2) extracranial Le Fort III advancement without simultaneous cranial vault expansion to open the upper airway; (3) tarsorrhaphies to protect the eyes from exposure rather than orbital expansion; and (4) continued tracheostomy for airway management rather than midface advancement.

The four reviewed studies and the discussion by Hopper demonstrate the variation in opinions on how best to reconstruct individuals with a craniosynostosis syndrome. In our opinion, for most of these children, only the MB or FB osteotomies offer a realistic opportunity both to achieve close to normal morphology and to enable the child to develop a healthy sense of self-esteem. Favorable craniofacial function follows the achieved enhanced facial form with cranial vault expansion (i.e., relief of intracranial pressure), orbital expansion (relief of proptosis and eye protection), and upper airway expansion (i.e., relief of OSA and improved breathing during the day). Gains in mastication, swallowing mechanism, speech articulation, breathing, vision, and cognitive function are also expected.

To achieve the most favorable facial harmony and head and neck function in the individual with a craniosynostosis syndrome, the surgeon needs both an esthetic sense and the technical expertise to execute effective upper and midface surgical procedures. Several key aspects of such expertise include the following:

1. The ability to remove, segment, reshape, and then stabilize the cranial vault
2. The ability to separate the orbits and midface as a unit (MB) from the skull base
3. The ability to segment and reshape the upper orbits of the MB, including interposing bone grafts as needed to reconstruct each orbital esthetic unit during a single operative setting
4. The ability to separate the MB into halves (FB) and then three-dimensionally reposition and stabilize the two facial halves (plate and screw fixation) to achieve the most favorable morphology in all three planes (i.e., pitch, roll, and yaw orientation). This often requires an increase in the maxillary width (i.e., arch expansion) and a decrease in the upper face width (i.e., correction of hypertelorism of the orbits, zygomas, and bitemporal regions). FB also provides the ability to correct the transverse facial arc of rotation such as changing the concave facial arc of rotation (i.e., yaw orientation) in Apert syndrome.

Postoperative Considerations

In current clinical practice, when either an MB or FB osteotomy is selected, the technique of distraction to gradually advance the upper/midface after closure of the wounds is frequently used. Any potential for reduced infection across the skull base using the DO technique should be considered in light of the limitations on achieving the aforementioned esthetic objectives (see points 1 to 4 in the preceding section). At the same time, clinicians must take into account the procedure-specific morbidity associated with the DO technique, including (1) pin tract infection; (2) soft tissue scarring; (3) hardware loosening, requiring reapplication; (4) brain trauma from the screw penetration; and (5) the need for device removal. In addition, effective DO technique depends on a continued commitment by the patient, family, and clinician to staying the course after surgery (approximately 4 months).

The hope for the future is that clinicians will both master the known surgical techniques and also find novel solutions to manage the potential for morbidity associated with MB/FB osteotomies (i.e., CSF leakage, intracranial abscess, and bone resorption), yet also be able to focus on the esthetic details so that individuals with a craniosynostosis syndrome can more commonly benefit from the procedures' inherent advantages.

The preferred approach to the management of the individual with a craniosynostosis syndrome is to stage reconstruction to coincide with craniofacial growth patterns, visceral functional needs, and psychosocial needs. Recognition of the advantages of a staged approach to reconstruction clarifies the objectives of each phase of treatment for the surgeon, the craniofacial team, and the family. For most of those born with a craniosynostosis syndrome, the preferred management of the upper midface deformity is either a MG or a FB osteotomy carried out in childhood.

References

1. Tessier P. The definitive plastic surgical treatment of the severe facial deformities of craniofacial dysostosis. Crouzon's and Apert's diseases. *Plast Reconstr Surg*. 1971;48(5):419–442.
2. Ortiz-Monasterio F, Fuente del Campo A. Refinements on the monobloc orbitofacial advancement. In: Caronni EP, ed. *Craniofacial Surgery*. Boston, Massachusetts: Little, Brown; 1985.
3. Ortiz-Monasterio F, del Campo AF, Carrillo A. Advancement of the orbits and the midface in one piece, combined with frontal repositioning, for the correction of Crouzon's deformities. *Plast Reconstr Surg*. 1978;61(4):507–516.
4. Tessier P. Total facial osteotomy. crouzon's syndrome, Apert's syndrome: oxycephaly, scaphocephaly, turricephaly. *Ann Chir Plast*. 1967;12(4):273–286.
5. Gorlin RJ, Cohen Jr MM, Levin LS. In: *Syndromes of the Head and Neck*. 3rd ed. New York: Oxford University Press; 1990.
6. Cohen Jr MM. No man's craniosynostosis: the arcana of sutural knowledge. *J Craniofac Surg*. 2012;23(1):338–342.
7. Apert E. De l'acrocephalosyndactlie. *Bull Mem Soc Med Hop Paris*. 1906;23:1310.
8. Kreiborg S, Barr Jr M, Cohen Jr MM. Cervical spine in the Apert syndrome. *Am J Med Genet*. 1992;43(4):704–708.
9. Bigot C. *L'acrocephalo-syndactylie (these pour le doctorat en medicine)*. Paris: Faculte de Medicine; 1922.
10. Cruveiller J. *La Maladie d'Apert-Crouzon (These Medicale)*. Paris, France; 1954.
11. Genest P, Mortezai MA, Tremblay M. Le syndrome d'Apert (acrocephalosyndactyly). *Arch Fr Pediatr*. 1966;23:887.
12. Gray TL, Casey T, Selva D, Anderson PJ, David DJ. Ophthalmic sequelae of Crouzon syndrome. *Ophthalmology*. 2005;112(6):1129–1134.
13. Green SM. Pathological anatomy of the hands in Apert's syndrome. *J Hand Surg Am*. 1982;7(5):450–453.
14. Harris V, Beligere N, Pruzansky S. Progressive generalized bony dysplasia in Apert syndrome. *Birth Defects*. 1977;14:175.
15. Kaloust S, Ishii K, Vargervik K. Dental development in Apert syndrome. *Cleft Palate Craniofac J*. 1997;34(2):117–121.
16. Kasser J, Upton J. The shoulder, elbow, and forearm in Apert syndrome. *Clin Plast Surg*. 1991;18(2):381–389.
17. Khong JJ, Anderson P, Gray TL, Hammerton M, Selva D, David D. Ophthalmic findings in apert syndrome prior to craniofacial surgery. *Am J Ophthalmol*. 2006;142(2):328–330.
18. Kreiborg S, Barr Jr M, Cohen Jr MM. Cervical spine in the Apert syndrome. *Am J Med Genet*. 1992;43(4):704–708.
19. Kreiborg S, Cohen Jr MM. The oral manifestations of Apert syndrome. *J Craniofac Genet Dev Biol*. 1992;12(1):41–48.
20. Kreiborg S, Prydsoe U, Dahl E, Fogh-Anderson P. Clinical conference I. Calvarium and cranial base in Apert's syndrome: an autopsy report. *Cleft Palate J*. 1976;13:296–303.
21. Mah J, Kasser J, Upton J. The foot in Apert syndrome. *Clin Plast Surg*. 1991;18(2):391–397.
22. Marsh JL, Galic M, Vannier MW. Surgical correction of the craniofacial dysmorphology of Apert syndrome. *Clin Plast Surg*. 1991;18(2):251–275.
23. McCarthy JG, Coccaro PJ, Eptstein F, Converse JM. Early skeletal release in the infant with craniofacial dysostosis: the role of the sphenozygomatic suture. *Plast Reconstr Surg*. 1978;62(3):335–346.
24. Peterson SJ, Pruzansky S. Palatal anomalies in the syndromes of apert and Crouzon. *Cleft Palate J*. 1974;11:394–403.
25. Atkins FRB. Herediatry craniofacial dysotosis or crouzon disease. *Med Press Circ*. 1937;195:118.
26. Baldwin JL. Dysostosis craniofacialis of Crouzon. A summary of recent literature and case reports with emphasis on involvement of the ear. *Laryngoscope*. 1968;78(10):1660–1676.
27. Carinci F, Pezzetti F, Locci P, et al. Apert and Crouzon syndromes: clinical findings, genes and extracellular matrix. *J Craniofac Surg*. 2005;16(3):361–368.
28. Crouzon O. Une nouvelle famille atteinte de dysostose craniofaciale hereditaire. *Arch Med Enfant*. 1915;18:540.
29. Crouzon O. Sur la dysostose craniofaciale hereditaire et sur les rapports avec l'acrocephalosyndactylie. *Bull Mem Soc Med Hop Paris*. 1932;48:1568.
30. Crouzon O. Les dysostose prechordales. *Bull Acad Med*. 1936;115:696.
31. DeGunten P. Contribution a l'etude des malformations de la face et des maxillaires dans la dysostose craniofaciale. *Ann Otolaryngol*. 1938;57:1056.
32. Devine P, Bhan I, Feingold M, Leonidas JC, Wolpert SM. Completely cartilaginous trachea in a child with Crouzon syndrome. *Am J Dis Child*. 1984;138(1):40–43.
33. Flippen Jr JH. Cranio-facial dysostosis of Crouzon; report of a case in which the malformation occurred in four generations. *Pediatrics*. 1950;5(1):90–96, illust.
34. Funato N, Nohtomi-Ohyama J, Ohyama K. Monozygotic twins concordant for Crouzon syndrome. *Am J Med Genet*. 2005;133A(2):225.
35. Garcin M, Thurel R, Rudeaux P. Sur en cas asole de dysostose craniofaciale (maladie de Crouzon) avec extradactylie. *Bull Soc Med Hop*. 1932;56:1458.
36. Golabi M, Chierici G, Ousterhout DK, et al. Radiographic abnormalities of Crouzon syndrome: a survey of 23 cases. *Proc Greenwood Genet Center*. 1984;3:102.
37. Gorry MC, Preston RA, White GJ, et al. Crouzon syndrome: mutations in two spliceoforms of FGFR2 and a common point mutation shared with Jackson-Weiss syndrome. *Hum Mol Genet*. 1995;4(8):1387–1390.
38. Gosain AK, Santoro TD, Havlik RJ, Cohen SR, Holmes RE. Midface distraction following Le Fort III and monobloc osteotomies: problems and solutions. *Plast Reconstr Surg*. 2002;109(6):1797–1808.
39. Grenet H, Leveuf J, Issac G. Etude anatomique de la maladie de Crouzon. *Bull Soc Pediatr*. 1934;32:343.
40. Juberg RC, Chambers SR. An autosomal recessive form of craniofacial dysostosis (the Crouzon syndrome). *J Med Genet*. 1973;10(1):89–94.
41. Kolar JC, Munro IR, Farkas LG. Patterns of dysmorphology in Crouzon syndrome: an anthropometric study. *Cleft Palate J*. 1988;25(3):235–244.
42. Kreiborg S. Crouzon Syndrome. A clinical and roentgencephalometric study. *Scand J Plast Reconstr Surg Suppl*. 1981;18(suppl):1–198.

43. Moretti G, Sraeffen J. Dysostose craniofaciale de Crouzon et syringomylie: association chez le frere et la soeur. *Presse Med*. 1959;67:376.
44. Reddy BSN, Garg BR, Padiyar NV, Krishnaram AS. An unusual association of acanthosis nigricans and Crouzon's disease—a case report. *J Dermatol*. 1985;12(1):85–90.
45. Regnault F, Crouzon O. Etude sur un cas de dysostose craniofaciale hereditaire. *Ann Med Enfant*. 1927;43:676.
46. Shiller JG. Craniofacial dysostosis of Crouzon; a case report and pedigree with emphasis on heredity. *Pediatrics*. 1959;23(1 Pt 1):107–112.
47. Seruya M, Oh AK, Boyajian MJ, et al. Long-term outcomes of primary craniofacial reconstruction for craniosynostosis: a 12-year experience. *Plast Reconstr Surg*. 2011;127(6):2397–2406.
48. Vuilliamy DG, Normandale PA. Craniofacial dysostosis in a Dorset family. *Arch Dis Child*. 1966;41:275.
49. Pfeiffer RA. Dominant erbliche akrocephalosyndaktylie. *Z Kinderheilkd*. 1964;90:301–320.
50. Robin NH, Scott JA, Arnold JE, et al. Favorable prognosis for children with Pfeiffer syndrome types 2 and 3: implications for classification. *Am J Med Genet*. 1998;75(3):240–244.
51. Anderson PJ, Hall CM, Evans RD, Hayward RD, Harkness WJ, Jones BM. The cervical spine in Saethre-Chotzen syndrome. *Cleft Palate Craniofac J*. 1997;34(1):79–82.
52. Chotzen F. Eine eigenartige familiare entwicklungsstorung. (Akrocephalosyndaktylie, dystosis craniofacialis und hypertelorismus). *Monatsschr Kinderheilkd*. 1932;55:97.
53. Cohen Jr MM. Saethre-Chotzen syndrome. In: Cohen Jr MM, MacLean RE, eds. *Craniosynostosis: Diagnosis, Evaluation and Management*. 2nd ed. New York: Oxford University Press; 2000.
54. Saethre H. Ein beitrag zum turmschadelproblem (pathogenese, erblichkeit und symptomatologie). *Dtsch Z Nervenheilkd*. 1931;117:533.
55. Farkas LG, Posnick JC. Growth and development of regional units in the head and face based on anthropometric measurements. *Cleft Palate Craniofac J*. 1992;29(4):301–302.
56. Farkas LG, Posnick JC, Hreczko TM. Anthropometric growth study of the head. *Cleft Palate Craniofac J*. 1992;29(4):303–308.
57. Farkas LG, Posnick JC, Hreczko TM. Growth patterns of the face: a morphometric study. *Cleft Palate Craniofac J*. 1992;29(4):308–315.
58. Posnick JC. Apert syndrome: evaluation and staging of reconstruction. In: Posnick JC, ed. *Craniofacial and Maxillofacial Surgery in Children and Young Adults*. Philadelphia, Pennsylvania: WB Saunders Co; 2000.
59. Posnick JC. Crouzon syndrome: evaluation and staging of reconstruction. In: Posnick JC, ed. *Craniofacial and Maxillofacial Surgery in Children and Young Adults*. Philadelphia, Pennsylvania: WB Saunders Co; 2000.
60. Posnick JC. Pfeiffer syndrome: evaluation and staging of reconstruction. In: Posnick JC, ed. *Craniofacial and Maxillofacial Surgery in Children and Young Adults*. Philadelphia, Pennsylvania: WB Saunders Co; 2000.
61. Posnick JC, Farkas LG. The application of anthropometric surface measurements in craniomaxillofacial surgery. In: Farkas LG, ed. *Anthropometry of the Head and Face*. New York: Raven Press; 1994.
62. Posnick JC, Farkas LG. Anthropometric surface measurements in the analysis of craniomaxillofacial deformities: normal values and growth trends. In: Posnick JC, ed. *Craniofacial and Maxillofacial Surgery in Children and Young Adults*. Philadelphia, Pennsylvania: WB Saunders Co; 2000.
63. Posnick JC, Lin KY, Jhawar BJ, Armstrong D. Crouzon syndrome: quantitative assessment of presenting deformity and surgical results based on CT scans. *Plast Reconstr Surg*. 1993;92(6):1027–1037.
64. Posnick JC, Lin KY, Jhawar BJ, Armstrong D. Apert syndrome: quantitative assessment by CT scan of presenting deformity and surgical results after first-stage reconstruction. *Plast Reconstr Surg*. 1994;93(3):489–497.
65. Waitzman AA, Posnick JC, Armstrong DC, Pron GE. Craniofacial skeletal measurements based on computed tomography: part I. Accuracy and reproducibility. *Cleft Palate Craniofac J*. 1992;29(2):112–117.
66. Waitzman AA, Posnick JC, Armstrong DC, Pron GE. Craniofacial skeletal measurements based on computed tomography: part II. Normal values and growth trends. *Cleft Palate Craniofac J*. 1992;29(2):118–128.
67. Posnick JC. Craniofacial dysostosis. Staging of reconstruction and management of the midface deformity. *Neurosurg Clin N Am*. 1991;2(3):683–702.
68. Posnick JC. Crouzon syndrome: basic dysmorphology and staging of reconstruction. *Tech Neurosurg*. 1997;3:216–229.
69. Posnick JC. The craniofacial dysostosis syndromes. Staging of reconstruction and management of secondary deformities. *Clin Plast Surg*. 1997;24(3):429–446.
70. Posnick JC. Brachycephaly: bilateral coronal synostosis without midface deficiency. In: Posnick JC, ed. *Craniofacial and Maxillofacial Surgery in Children and Young Adults*. Philadelphia, Pennsylvania: WB Saunders Co; 2000.
71. Posnick JC. Cloverleaf skull anomalies: evaluation and staging reconstruction. In: Posnick JC, ed. *Craniofacial and Maxillofacial Surgery in Children and Young Adults*. Philadelphia, Pennsylvania: WB Saunders Co; 2000.
72. Posnick JC, Ruiz RL. The craniofacial dysostosis syndromes: current surgical thinking and future directions. *Cleft Palate Craniofac J*. 2000;37(5):433.
73. Posnick JC, Ruiz RL, Tiwana PS. Craniofacial dysostosis syndromes: stages of reconstruction. *Oral Maxillofac Surg Clin North Am*. 2004;16(4):475–491.
74. Warren SM, Shetye PR, Obaid SI, Grayson BH, McCarthy JG. Long-term evaluation of midface position after Le Fort III advancement: a 20-plus-year follow-up. *Plast Reconstr Surg*. 2012;129(1):234–242.
75. Arnaud E, Marchac D, Renier D. Reduction of morbidity of the frontofacial monobloc advancement in children by the use of internal distraction. *Plast Reconstr Surg*. 2007;120(4):1009–1026.
76. Bachmayer DI, Ross RB. Stability of Le Fort III advancement surgery in children with Crouzon's, Apert's, and Pfeiffer's syndromes. *Cleft Palate J*. 1986;23(suppl 1):69–74.
77. Bachmayer DI, Ross RB, Munro IR. Maxillary growth following LeFort III advancement surgery in Crouzon, Apert, and Pfeiffer syndromes. *Am J Orthod Dentofacial Orthop*. 1986;90(5):420–430.
78. Bu BH, Kaban LB, Vargervik K. Effect of Le Fort III osteotomy on mandibular growth in patients with Crouzon and Apert syndromes. *J Oral Maxillofac Surg*. 1989;47(7):666–671.
79. Chin M, Toth BA. Le Fort III advancement with gradual distraction using internal devices. *Plast Reconstr Surg*. 1997;100(4):819–830.
80. Coccaro PJ, McCarthy JG, Epstein FJ, Wood-Smith D, Converse JM. Early and late surgery in craniofacial dysostosis: a longitudinal cephalometric study. *Am J Orthod*. 1980;77(4):421–436.
81. David DJ, Cooter RD. Craniofacial infection in 10 years of transcranial surgery. *Plast Reconstr Surg*. 1987;80(2):213–225.
82. David DJ, Sheen R. Surgical correction of Crouzon syndrome. *Plast Reconstr Surg*. 1990;85(3):344–354.
83. Chin M, Toth BA. Le Fort III advancement with gradual distraction using internal devices. [discussion]. *Plast Reconstr Surg*. 1997;100(4):819–830.
84. Fearon JA. The Le Fort III osteotomy: to distract or not to distract? *Plast Reconstr Surg*. 2001;107(5):1091–1103.
85. Fearon JA. Halo distraction of the Le Fort III in syndromic craniosynostosis: a long-term assessment. *Plast Reconstr Surg*. 2005;115(6):1524–1536.
86. Fearon JA, Whitaker LA. Complications with facial advancement: a comparison between the Le Fort III and monobloc advancements. *Plast Reconstr Surg*. 1993;91(6):990–995.
87. Fearon JA, Yu J, Bartlett SP, Munro IR, Chir B, Whitaker L. Infections in craniofacial surgery: a combined report of 567 procedures from two centers. *Plast Reconstr Surg*. 1997;100(4):862–868.
88. Gillies H, Harrison SH. Operative correction by osteotomy of recessed malar maxillary compound in a case of oxycephaly. *Br J Plast Surg*. 1950;3(2):123–127.
89. Hogeman KE, Willmar K. On le Fort III osteotomy for Crouzon's disease in children. Report of a four-year follow-up in one patient. *Scand J Plast Reconstr Surg*. 1974;8(1–2):169–172.

90. Hollier L, Kelly P, Babigumira E, Potochny J, Taylor T. Minimally invasive le Fort III distraction. *J Craniofac Surg*. 2002;13(1):44–48.
91. Iannetti G, Fadda T, Agrillo A, Poladas G, Iannetti G, Filiaci F. LeFort III advancement with and without osteogenesis distraction. *J Craniofac Surg*. 2006;17(3):536–543.
92. Jensen JN, McCarthy JG, Grayson BH, Nusbaum AO, Eski M. Bone deposition/generation with LeFort III (midface) distraction. *Plast Reconstr Surg*. 2007;119(1):298–307.
93. Kaban LB, Conover M, Mulliken JB. Midface position after Le Fort III advancement: a long-term follow-up study. *Cleft Palate J*. 1986;23(suppl 1):75–77.
94. Kaban LB, West B, Conover M, Will L, Mulliken JB, Murray JE. Midface position after LeFort III advancement. *Plast Reconstr Surg*. 1984;73(5):758–767.
95. Lee Y, Kim WJ. How to make the blockage between the nasal cavity and intracranial space using a four-layer sealing technique. *Plast Reconstr Surg*. 2006;117(1):233–238.
96. Mathijssen I, Arnaud E, Marchac D, et al. Respiratory outcome of midface advancement with distraction: a comparison between Le Fort III and frontofacial monobloc. *J Craniofac Surg*. 2006;17(4):642–644.
97. Matsumoto K, Nakanishi H, Koizumi Y, et al. Segmental distraction of the midface in a patient with Crouzon syndrome. *J Craniofac Surg*. 2002;13(2):273–278.
98. Mavili ME, Tunçbilek G, Vargel I. Rigid external distraction of the midface with direct wiring of the distraction unit in patients with craniofacial dysplasia. *J Craniofac Surg*. 2003;14(5):783–785.
99. McCarthy JG, Grayson B, Bookstein F, Vickery C, Zide B. Le Fort III advancement osteotomy in the growing child. *Plast Reconstr Surg*. 1984;74(3):343–354.
100. McCarthy JG, La Trenta GS, Breitbart AS, Grayson BH, Bookstein FL. The Le Fort III advancement osteotomy in the child under 7 years of age. *Plast Reconstr Surg*. 1990;86(4):633–646.
101. Meazzini MC, Mazzoleni F, Caronni E, Bozzetti A. Le Fort III advancement osteotomy in the growing child affected by Crouzon's and Apert's syndromes: presurgical and postsurgical growth. *J Craniofac Surg*. 2005;16(3):369–377.
102. Meling TR, Hans-Erik H. Per S, Due-Tonnessen BJ. Le Fort III distraction osteogenesis in syndromal craniosynostosis. *J Craniofac Surg*. 2006;17(1):28–39.
103. Mulliken JB, Godwin SL, Pracharktam N, Altobelli DE. The concept of the sagittal orbital-globe relationship in craniofacial surgery. *Plast Reconstr Surg*. 1996;97(4):700–706.
104. Murray JE, Swanson LT. Mid-face osteotomy and advancement for craniosynostosis. *Plast Reconstr Surg*. 1968;41(4):299–306.
105. Nout E, Cesteleyn LL, van der Wal KG, van Adrichem LN, Mathijssen IM, Wolvius EB. Advancement of the midface, from conventional Le Fort III osteotomy to Le Fort III distraction: review of the literature. *Int J Oral Maxillofac Surg*. 2008;37(9):781–789.
106. Ousterhout DK, Vargervik K, Clark S. Stability of the maxilla after Le Fort III advancement in craniosynostosis syndromes. *Cleft Palate J*. 1986;23(suppl 1):91–101.
107. Phillips JH, George AK, Tompson B. Le Fort III osteotomy or distraction osteogenesis imperfecta: your choice. *Plast Reconstr Surg*. 2006;117(4):1255–1260.
108. Polley JW, Figueroa AA. Management of severe maxillary deficiency in childhood and adolescence through distraction osteogenesis with an external, adjustable, rigid distraction device. *J Craniofac Surg*. 1997;8(3):181–185.
109. Posnick JC. The craniofacial dysostosis syndromes. Current reconstructive strategies. *Clin Plast Surg*. 1994;21(4):585–598.
110. Posnick JC. Craniofacial dysostosis syndromes: a staged reconstructive approach. In: Turvey TA, Vig KWL, Fonseca RJ, eds. *Facial Clefts and Craniosynostosis: Principles and Management*. Philadelphia, Pennsylvania: WB Saunders; 1996.
111. Posnick JC, Goldstein JA, Clokie C. Refinements in pterygomaxillary dissociation for total midface osteotomies: instrumentation, technique, and CT scan analysis. *Plast Reconstr Surg*. 1993;91(1):167–172.
112. Satoh K, Mitsukawa N, Hosaka Y. Dual midfacial distraction osteogenesis: le Fort III minus I and Le Fort I for syndromic craniosynostosis. *Plast Reconstr Surg*. 2003;111(3):1019–1028.
113. Shetye PR, Boutros S, Grayson BH, McCarthy JG. Midterm follow-up of midface distraction for syndromic craniosynostosis: a clinical and cephalometric study. *Plast Reconstr Surg*. 2007;120(6):1621–1632.
114. Shetye PR, Grayson BH, McCarthy JG. Le Fort III distraction: controlling position and path of the osteotomized midface segment on a rigid platform. *J Craniofac Surg*. 2010;21(4):1118–1121.
115. Shin JH, Duncan CC, Persing J. Monobloc distraction: technical modification and considerations. *J Craniofac Surg*. 2003;14(5):763–766.
116. Whitaker LA, Bartlett SP, Schut L, Bruce D. Craniosynostosis: an analysis of the timing, treatment, and complications in 164 consecutive patients. *Plast Reconstr Surg*. 1987;80(2):195–212.
117. Posnick JC, al-Qattan MM, Armstrong D. Monobloc and facial bipartition osteotomies for reconstruction of craniofacial malformations: a study of extradural dead space and morbidity. *Plast Reconstr Surg*. 1996;97(6):1118–1128.
118. Spinelli HM, Irizarry D, McCarthy JG, Cutting CB, Noz ME. An analysis of extradural dead space after fronto-orbital surgery. *Plast Reconstr Surg*. 1994;93(7):1372–1377.
119. Wolfe SA. *Critical Analysis of 81 Monobloc Frontofacial Advancements over a 27-year Period: Should They All Be Distracted, or Not? Abstract Presentation, 88th Annual Meeting*. California: American Association of Plastic Surgeons. Rancho Mirage; 2009:200–201.
120. Bradley JP, Gabbay JS, Taub PJ, et al. Monobloc advancement by distraction osteogenesis decreases morbidity and relapse. *Plast Reconstr Surg*. 2006;118(7):1585–1597.
121. Ahmad F, Cobb ARM, Mills C, Jones BM, Hayward RD, Dunaway DJ. Frontofacial monobloc distraction in the very young: a review of 12 consecutive cases. *Plast Reconstr Surg*. 2012;129(3):488e–497e.
122. Hopper RA. Discussion: frontofacial monobloc distraction in the very young: a review of 12 consecutive cases. *Plast Reconstr Surg*. 2012;129(3):498e–501e.

CHAPTER 52

Techniques for Skull Base and Cervical Spine Access

James B. Holton

Adaptations and improvements in maxillofacial osteotomies have changed the spectrum of skull base surgery. Imaging, endoscopic and open techniques, embolization, navigation, focused radiation therapy, and infection control have all improved the outcomes in surgery of the skull base. Certain tumors require an open approach. The expertise of maxillofacial surgeons in trauma, corrective, cosmetic, and reconstructive surgery of the craniofacial complex allows for expanded options in providing wide field exposure for skull base surgery. Many tumors of the skull base cross anatomic boundaries, as is seen with invasion of the orbit and frontal, ethmoid, and sphenoid sinuses. Creative planning and surgical exposure are imperative. The goals of treatment are to remove the tumor safely and to provide reconstructive options for the complex residual deformity. Endoscopic and minimum incision access can limit exposure for large, complex lesions in difficult anatomic locations. Common osteotomy techniques for maxillofacial procedures can easily be used for wide field cranial base access[1–4] (Fig. 52.1). These access osteotomies are related procedures that use the same instrumentation and can be used for multiple purposes, even in combination[5,6] (Fig. 52.2).

Transfrontal Approach: Access to the Anterior Cranial Fossa, Orbit, Cribriform Plate, and Accessory Sinuses

Armamentarium

#9 Periosteal elevator
#10 and #15 blades
1/2- and 1-inch cottonoids
Appropriate sutures
Avitene
Bipolar cautery
Bone burs
Bovine pericardium
Curettes
Curved Mayo scissors
DuraHooks
Evoked potential monitoring
Gelfoam with thrombin
Hair elastics
Hemoclips
Kerrison rongeur
Langenbeck periosteal elevator
Layla bar
Local anesthetic with vasoconstrictor
Malleable retractors
Mayfield head holder
Minnesota retractors
Nerve hook
Obwegeser retractors
Osteotomes
Pituitary forceps
Point electrocautery
Raney clips
Reciprocating saw
Seldin retractor
Skin closure clips
Small plates and screws
Tissue glue

History of the Procedure

The transfrontal approach, involving removal of the supraorbital bar combined with a bifrontal craniotomy, is used for multiple conditions, including congenital deformities, frontobasilar trauma, and tumors of the anterior cranial fossa.[1,4] The advantage of this method is the direct low approach, which limits the retraction of the frontal lobe.

Indications for the Use of the Procedure

The transfrontal approach is indicated for tumors and conditions of the anterior cranial fossa, including intracranial tumors involving the cribriform plate, paranasal sinuses, and supraorbital roofs (Fig. 52.3).

The most common pathologic conditions include the following[7]:

- Meningioma
- Fibroosseous lesions

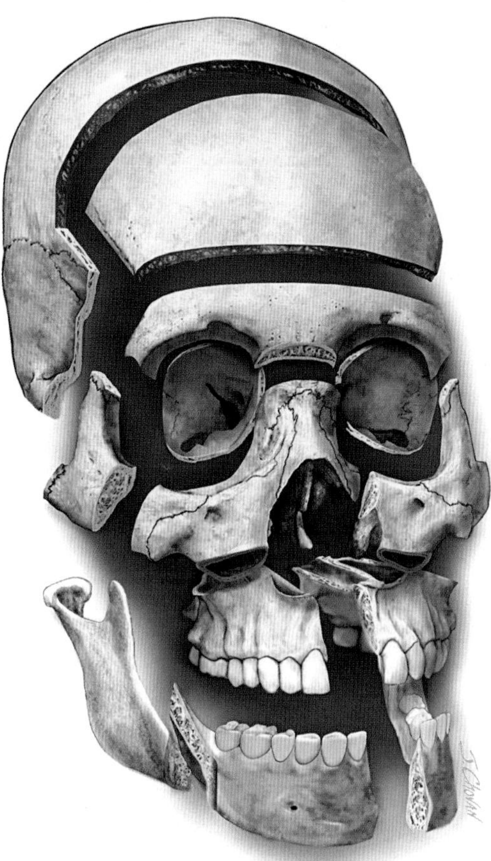

Figure 52.1 Common osteotomy techniques for maxillofacial procedures.

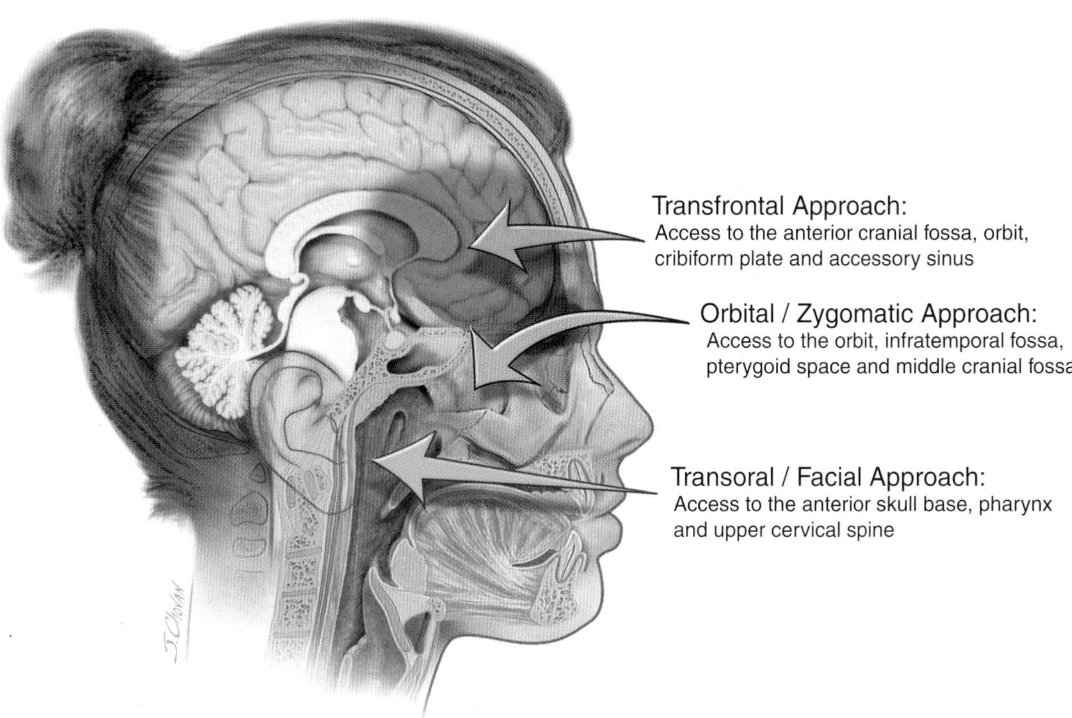
Transfrontal Approach:
Access to the anterior cranial fossa, orbit, cribiform plate and accessory sinus
Orbital / Zygomatic Approach:
Access to the orbit, infratemporal fossa, pterygoid space and middle cranial fossa
Transoral / Facial Approach:
Access to the anterior skull base, pharynx and upper cervical spine

Figure 52.2 These access osteotomies are related procedures that use the same instrumentation and can be used for multiple purposes, even in combination.

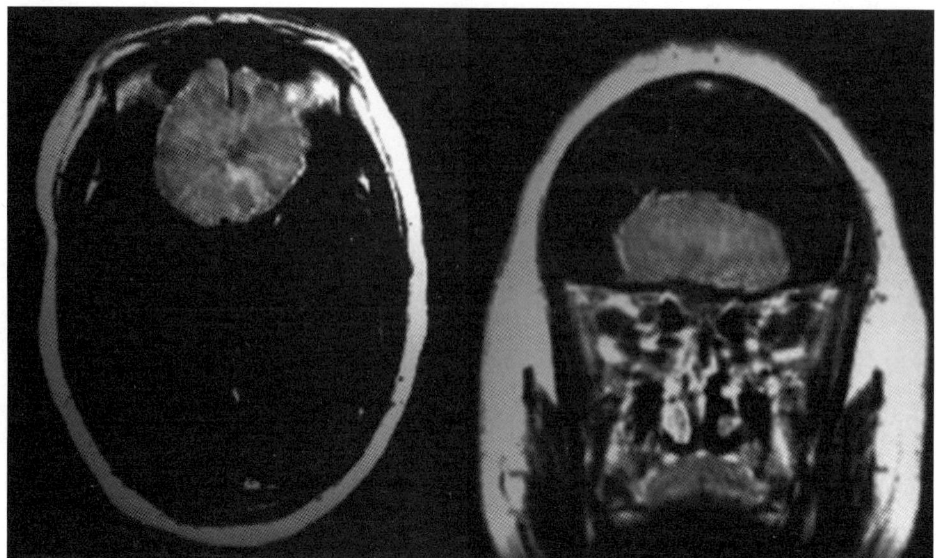

Figure 52.3 Tumor of the cribriform plate, requiring a transfrontal access approach.

- Traumatic loss of the cribriform plate
- Frontal/ethmoid mucocele
- Osteomas
- Dermoid/epidermoid tumors
- Neurofibroma
- Neural sheath tumors
- Pituitary adenoma
- Craniopharyngioma
- Sinonasal carcinoma
- Chordoma

Limitations and Contraindications

Compromised frontal soft tissue requires an alternative type of closure, which could include a rotational scalp flap or a free flap. Irradiated tissue can pose problems with healing. The vascularity of the bicoronal and pericranial flap allows coverage and closure after wide field exposure of the anterior cranial fossa.

TECHNIQUE: Transfrontal Approach

STEP 1: Incision

An extended bicoronal incision is used in combination with elevation of a full pericranial flap from the vertex to the supraorbital ridges (Fig. 52.4A).

STEP 2: Dissection

The supraorbital and supratrochlear nerves are freed as the subperiosteal dissection traverses over the supraorbital rim. A subperiosteal orbital dissection is carried out to the orbital apex.

STEP 3: Craniotomy

A bifrontal craniotomy is then performed to expose the anterior cranial fossa.

STEP 4:
Dural Elevation

The frontal lobe is elevated off the anterior cranial fossa as far back as necessary, even to the sella.

STEP 5: Osteotomy

The osteotomy of the frontal bar is accomplished under direct visualization, first with vertical osteotomies of the lateral orbital rims carried through the supraorbital bar approximately 1 cm into the orbital roof. This is accomplished bilaterally (Fig. 52.4B).

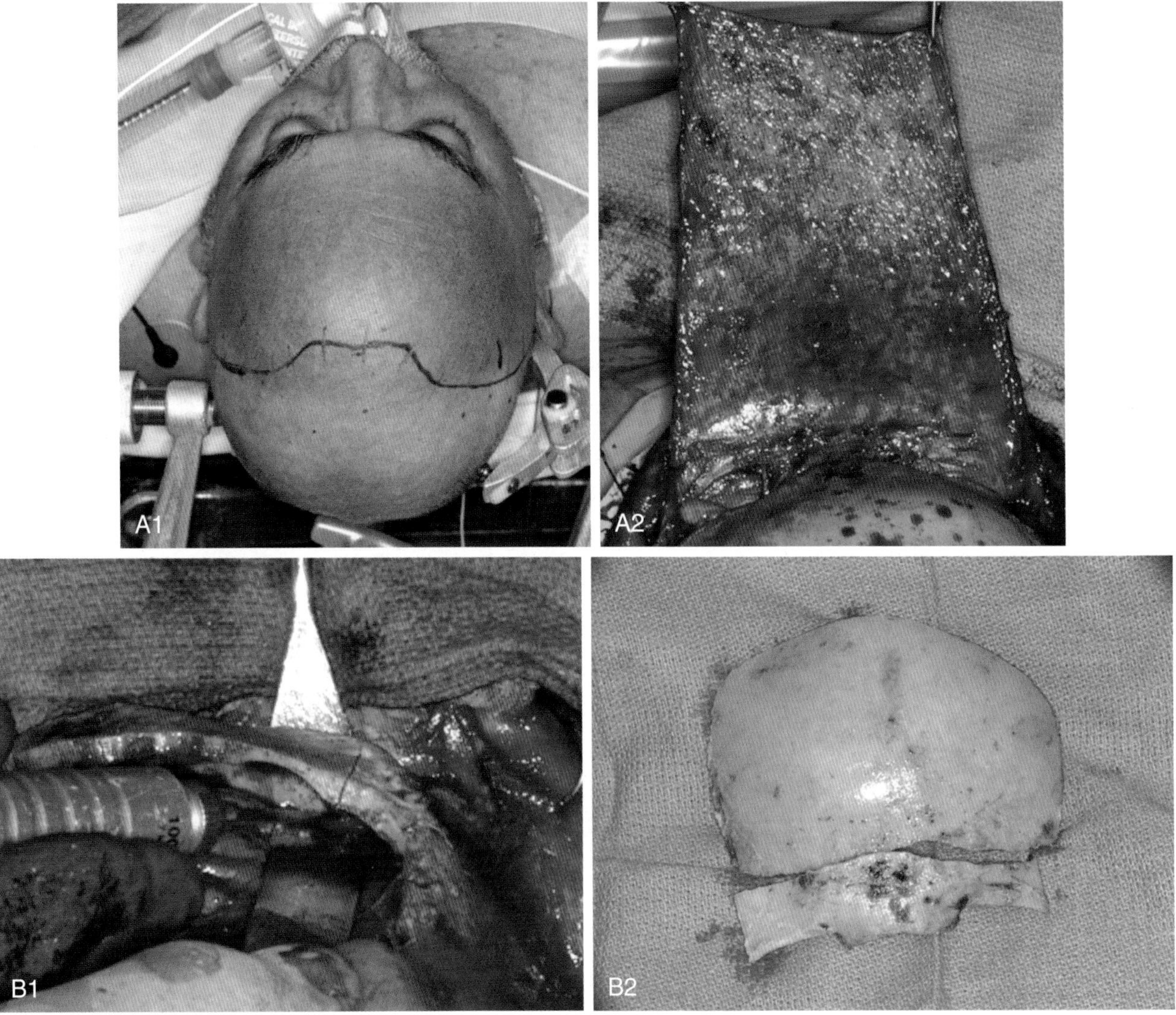

Figure 52.4 **A1** and **A2**, Mayfield head holder in place. Bicoronal and pericranial flaps raised. **B1**, Thin reciprocating saw for removal of the frontal bar. **B2**, Frontal and supraorbital bone flaps.

TECHNIQUE: Transfrontal Approach—cont'd

STEP 6: Frontoorbital Osteotomy

A reciprocating saw then is used to connect the vertical incisions traversing the frontal region at the level of the nasion. The reciprocating saw passes through the frontal sinus, which is obliterated as part of this procedure. The supraorbital bar is lifted off and placed in a saline sponge until reinsertion.

STEP 7: Cranialization

Cranialization of the frontal sinus is then performed. The posterior wall of the frontal sinus is removed using a combination of rongeurs and small bone burs. The sinus membrane is removed, and the nasal frontal ducts are imbricated, sutured primarily, or obliterated with thrombin Gelfoam sponges with tissue glue in preparation for pericranial flap closure (Fig. 52.4C).

Continued

TECHNIQUE: Transfrontal Approach—cont'd

STEP 8: Flap Insertion

After the interventional surgical procedure has been carried out, the pericranial flap is inserted under the supraorbital bar over the orbital roofs and attached to stable dura with 4-0 nylon sutures. If the supraorbital bar is not removed, the flap is brought over the bar. Tissue glue can also be used to aid in the stabilization of the pericranial flap. If pericranium is not available, fascia lata, temporalis muscle, or bovine pericardium can be used for barrier separation.[8]

STEP 9: Bone Grafting

Grafting of defects of the supraorbital roof is suggested to prevent pulsatile proptosis should the orbital roofs have to be removed. The supraorbital bar is then brought back to the surgical site and stabilized with small plates. The bifrontal craniotomy bone flap is reinserted and secured with plates (Fig. 52.4D).

STEP 10: Closure

The bicoronal incision is closed in two layers, Jackson-Pratt drains are inserted for 3 days.

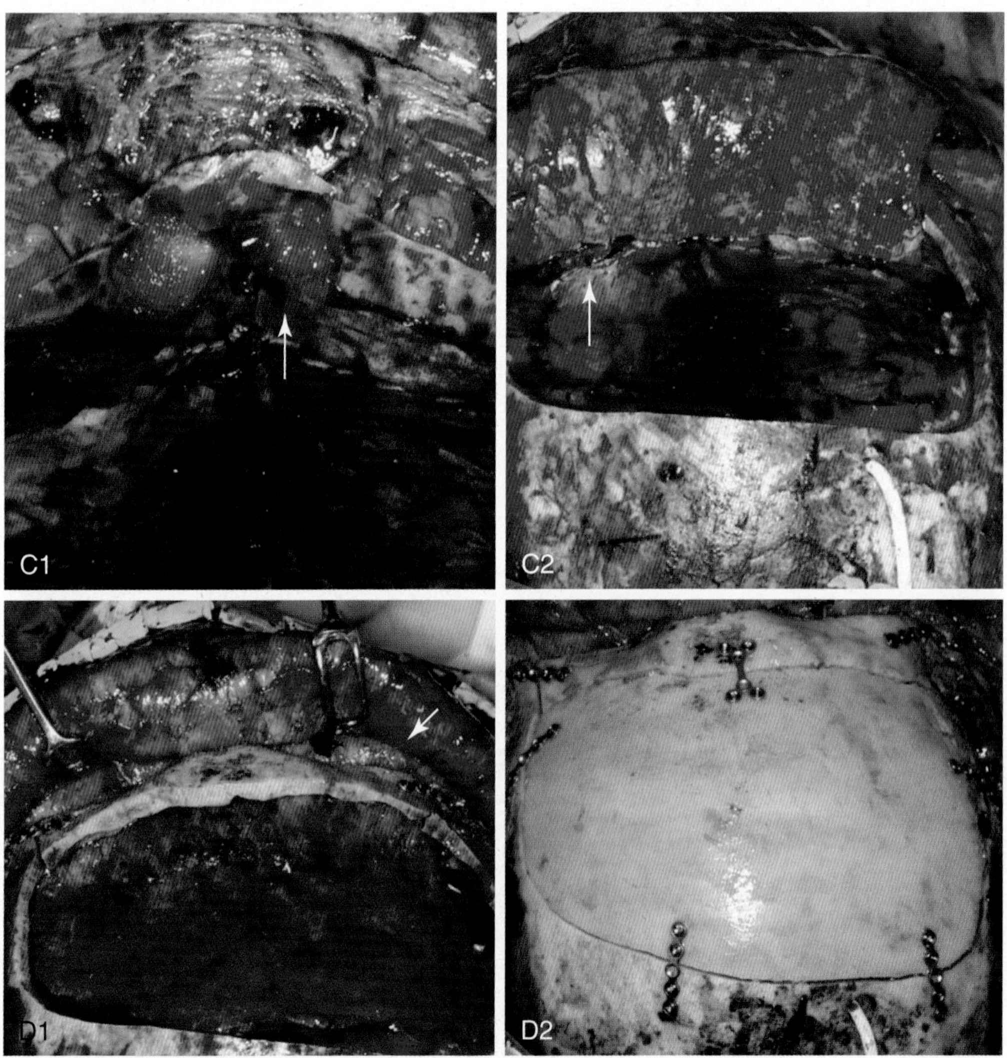

Figure 52.4 **C1**, cont'd Gelfoam/thrombin sponges in imbricated nasofrontal ducts (*arrow*). **C2**, Pericranial flap sutured to dura over the orbital roofs (*arrow*). **D1**, Pericranial flap over orbital roof under the supraorbital bar. **D2**, Bone flaps replaced.

Avoidance and Management of Intraoperative Complications

1. The design of the bicoronal flap and the necessity of obtaining a full pericranial flap need to be decided as part of the surgical planning procedure. The decision on how to deal with the nasofrontal ducts and the frontal sinus should be made in advance. Sealing the cribriform plate from the intranasal contents is the major consideration in the transfrontal approach. Fascia lata or bovine pericardium can be used if autologous tissue is unavailable.
2. Selective preoperative embolization of the tumor may be used.
3. Evoked potential monitoring is used to monitor intraoperative nerve function.

Postoperative Considerations

- Anosmia
- Cerebrospinal fluid (CSF) rhinorrhea (a lumbar CSF drain may be required)
- Meningitis
- Infection
- Loss of bone
- Cosmetic defect
- Antibiotics are used before and after surgery
- Neural deficits can occur, depending on the tumor's location

Orbital/Zygomatic Approach: Access to the Orbit, Infratemporal Fossa, Pterygoid Space, and Middle Cranial Fossa

Armamentarium

#9 Periosteal elevator
#10 and #15 blades
1/2- and 1-inch cottonoids
Appropriate sutures
Avitene
Bipolar cautery
Bone burs
Bovine pericardium
Curettes
Curved Mayo scissors
DuraHooks
Evoked potential monitoring
Gelfoam with thrombin
Hair elastics
Hemoclips
Kerrison rongeur
Langenbeck periosteal elevator
Local anesthetic with vasoconstrictor
Malleable retractors
Mayfield head holder
Layla bar
Minnesota retractors
Nerve hook
Obwegeser retractors
Osteotomes
Pituitary forceps
Point electrocautery
Raney clips
Reciprocating saw
Seldin retractor
Skin closure clips
Small plates and screws
Tissue glue

History of the Procedure

The orbital/zygomatic osteotomy is a versatile procedure that has been used for decompression of orbital proptosis and access to the infratemporal fossa.[6,9] The disarticulation of the lateral orbit and zygoma replicates a fracture of the zygomaticomaxillary complex and is familiar to the maxillofacial surgeon. This procedure maintains the origin of the masseter muscle rather than using en bloc removal of the zygomatic complex.

Indications for the Use of the Procedure

Wide field exposure is beneficial for tumors of the infratemporal fossa and orbit. Also, when combined with a frontal temporal craniotomy, it allows minimal retraction of the temporal lobe for conditions of the floor of the middle cranial fossa and sphenoid wing (Fig. 52.5A and B).

The most common pathologic conditions include the following[7]:

- Meningioma
- Pituitary tumors
- Craniopharyngioma
- Chondrosarcoma
- Endochondroma
- Cavernous sinus pathology
- Cholesteatoma
- Temporal bone tumors

Limitations and Contraindications

Previous radiation therapy or compromised tissue may be contraindications to this procedure.

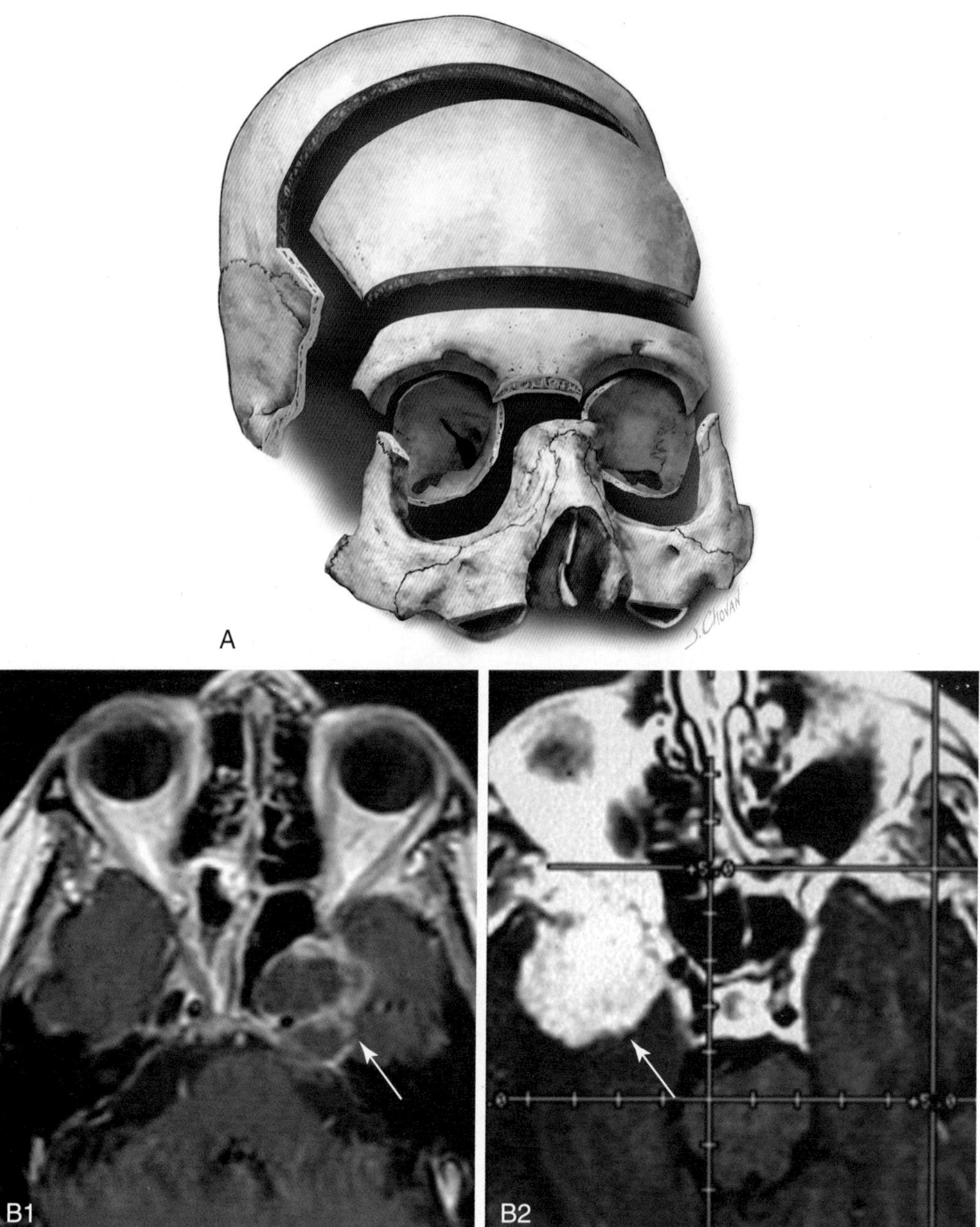

Figure 52.5 **A**, Cranial and facial osteotomies allowing for skull bone access. **B1** and **B2**, Typical sphenoid wing lesions *(arrows)* requiring a transorbital/zygomatic approach.

TECHNIQUE: Orbital/Zygomatic Osteotomy

STEP 1: Incision

A preauricular or postauricular bicoronal incision is used.

STEP 2: Dissection

The zygomatic complex from the supraorbital rim to the infraorbital rim to the base of the zygomatic arch is skeletonized. A subperiosteal orbital dissection is carried out from the supraorbital nerve to the infraorbital nerve to the orbital apex.

TECHNIQUE: Orbital/Zygomatic Osteotomy—cont'd

STEP 3: Muscle Retraction
The temporalis muscle is taken down, leaving a small portion of the origin at the temporal crest for suspension purposes. The muscle is reflected laterally and secured with DuraHooks.

STEP 4: Orbital Osteotomy
The inferior oblique fissure intraorbitally is first identified, and an osteotomy is accomplished with a small reciprocating saw, commencing at the lateral extent of the inferior oblique fissure and proceeding through the malar eminence under direct visualization.

STEP 5: Zygomatic Osteotomy
An osteotomy then is performed with a reciprocating saw at the zygomatic sphenoid junction, starting at the lateral aspect of the inferior oblique fissure and carried up and through the frontal zygomatic articulation. The saw is placed in the infratemporal fossa, and the orbital contents are retracted and protected under direct visualization. An oblique osteotomy is accomplished at the root of the zygomatic arch with a reciprocating saw.

STEP 6: Disarticulation
The orbital/zygomatic complex is then disarticulated and held laterally with DuraHooks and a Layla bar. The masseter muscle is not stripped (Fig. 52.5C).

STEP 7: Craniotomy
Access to the middle cranial fossa is facilitated by a sphenotemporal craniotomy.

STEP 8: Reconstruction
Once the cranial or orbital procedure has been performed, the zygomatic complex is reconstructed. Because there is no movement of the zygoma, it can be stabilized with positional screws to the oblique osteotomies or plates (Fig. 52.5D).

STEP 9: Closure
Closure of the temporalis fascia, suspension of the temporalis muscle to the temporal crest, and closure of the bicoronal incision are then carried out. The temporalis muscle can be suspended with nonresorbable sutures to the lateral orbital rim using purchase holes along the lateral orbital wall and/or calvarium (Fig. 52.5E).

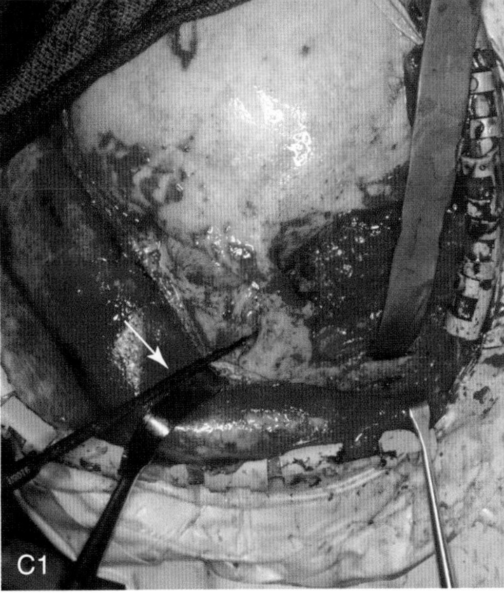

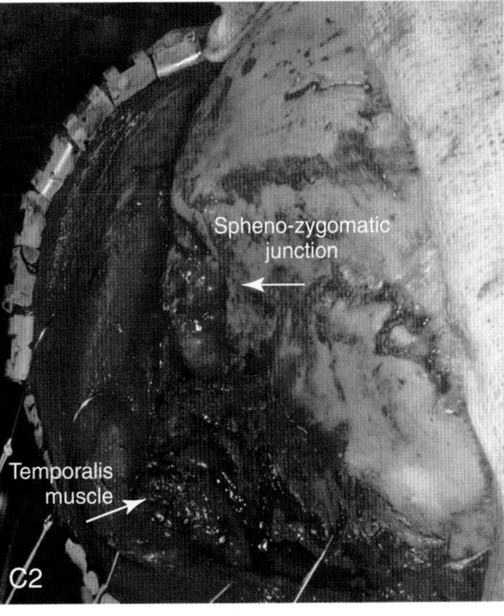

Continued

Figure 52.5, cont'd **C1**, Left zygoma skeletonized. Nerve hook in lateral inferior oblique fissure. **C2**, Left zygoma osteotomized and lateralized. Temporalis muscle detached.

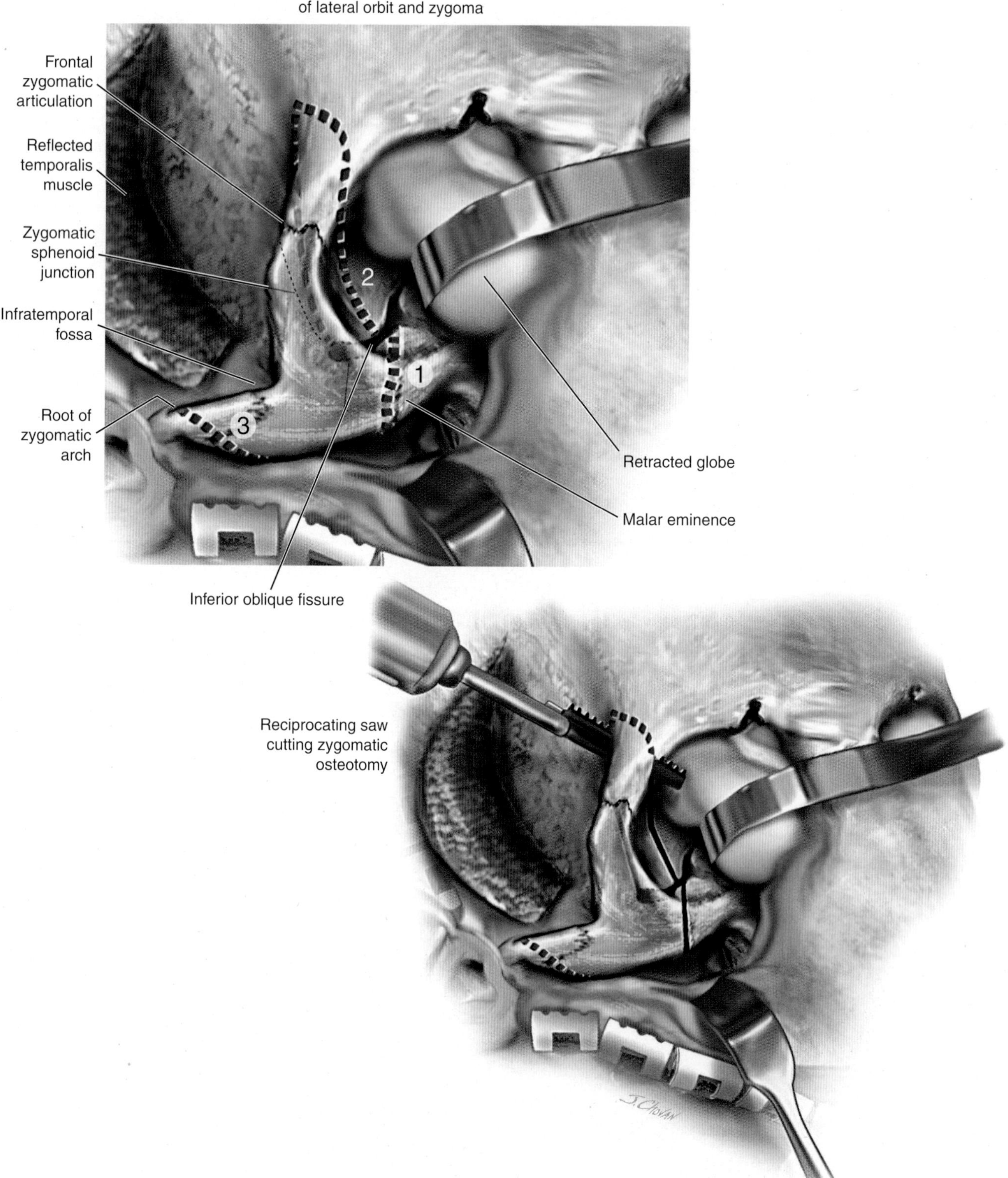

Figure 52.5, cont'd **C3,** Typical osteotomy pattern used for orbito-zygomatic approach.

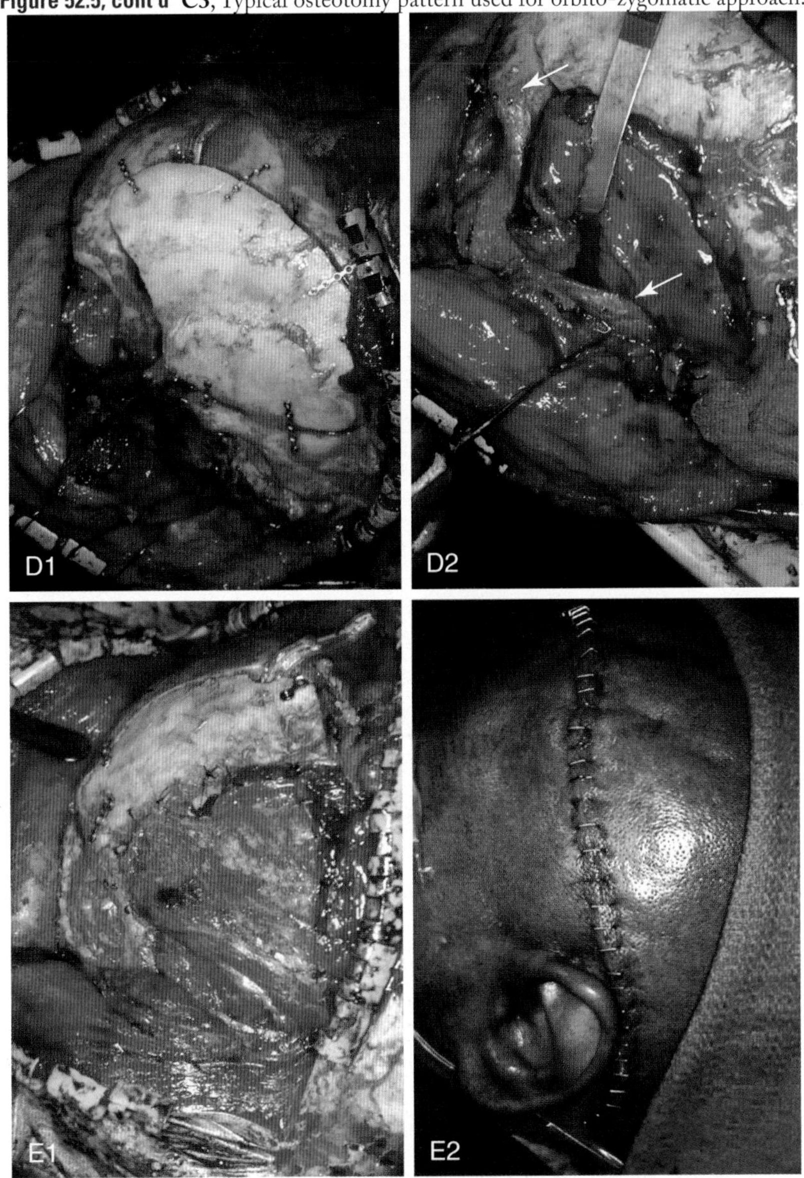

Figure 52.5, cont'd **D1**, Skull flap replaced. **D2**, Zygomatic complex replaced and stabilized with positional screws. **E1**, Wound closure with suspension of the temporalis muscle. **E2**, Postauricular bicoronal flap closure.

Avoidance and Management of Intraoperative Complications

1. Careful attention during skeletonization of the zygoma is imperative to avoid injury to the temporal branch of the facial nerve.
2. The most common complication is temporal wasting due to elevation of the entire temporalis muscle. Wasting can be lessened by resuspending the anterior margin of the temporalis muscle and its fascia to the lateral orbital rim and the temporal crest.
3. Evoked potential monitoring is used to monitor intraoperative nerve function.
4. If the frontal sinus is involved, a tissue barrier is used to seal the connection.
5. Selective preoperative embolization of the tumor may be used.

Postoperative Considerations

- Neural deficits can occur, depending on the tumor's location.
- Calvarial defects can be reconstructed immediately or delayed.
- Antibiotics are used before and after surgery.
- The care of the zygomatic osteotomy is similar to that for traumatic injuries and reconstruction of the zygoma, orbit, and frontal bone.

Transoral/Facial Approach: Access to the Anterior Skull Base, Pharynx, and Upper Cervical Spine

Armamentarium (Fig. 52.6)

#9 Periosteal elevator
#15 Blades
1/2- and 1-inch cottonoids
8-inch tenotomy scissors
8-inch vascular forceps
Appropriate sutures
Arch bars/ortho braces
Bipolar cautery
Bone burs
Cloward retractor
Curettes
Curved Mayo scissors
Evoked potential monitoring
Freer elevators
Gelfoam with thrombin
Hardy retractor
Hemoclips
Kerrison rongeur
Local anesthetic with vasoconstrictor
Malleable retractors
Minnesota retractors
Modified Dingman retractor
Nerve hook
Obwegeser retractors
Occlusal splint
Osteotomes
Pituitary forceps
Plates and screws
Point electrocautery
Pterygoid osteotome
Reciprocating saw
Rowe forceps
Seldin elevator
Thorek scissors
Tissue glue

History of the Procedure

The one-segment and multisegment maxillary osteotomy is a safe and effective procedure for treating multiple conditions of the maxillofacial skeleton. Kole[10] popularized the Le Fort osteotomy in 1959. The blood supply, as outlined by Bell[11] and Bell and Levy,[12] allows the security of downfracturing and mobilizing the maxilla even into multiple segments.

Indications for the Use of the Procedure

The transoral/transfacial osteotomy via Le Fort I with a midline split of both the hard and soft tissue of the palate allows direct access to the midline base of the skull from the clivus to the base of C3 (Fig. 52.7).[1,13–15]

The most common pathologic conditions include the following[7]:

- Clivus chordoma
- Vascular abnormalities

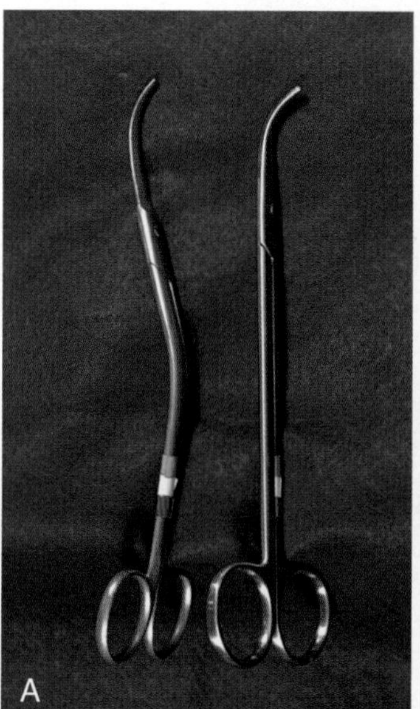

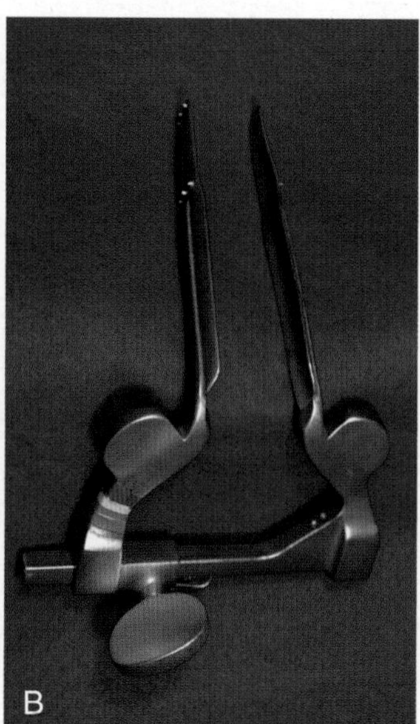

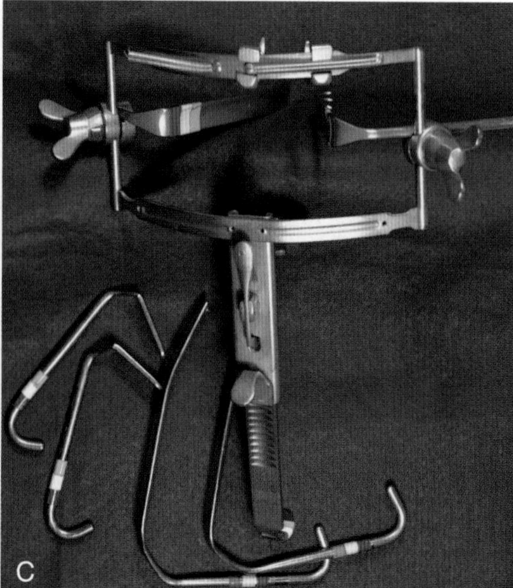

Figure 52.6 **A,** Angled Thorek scissors to raise pharyngeal flap. **B,** Cloward/Holton retractor to separate the maxilla and pharyngeal wall. **C,** Modified Dingman retractor with long blades to reach the posterior pharyngeal wall.

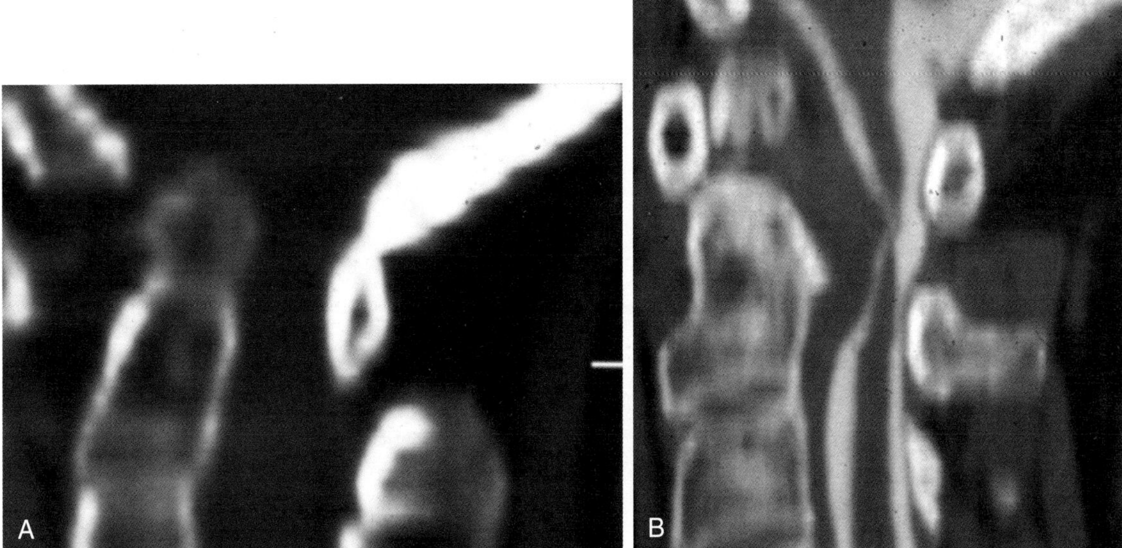

Figure 52.7 Images showing common pathology involving the odontoid process. **A**, Subluxation of the odontoid into the foramen magnum. **B**, Arthritic pannus compressing the brain stem.

- Basilar invagination
- Meningioma of the foramen magnum
- Pituitary tumors with sphenoid extension
- Odontoid process abnormalities
- Nasopharyngeal tumors

The general overall health of the patient must be considered. Often these patients have longstanding arthritis and have been taking medications such as methotrexate and prednisone for years. Furthermore, they frequently live a largely sedentary lifestyle and often smoke. The general nutritional status of the patient should be evaluated closely, and taking steps to implement nutritional control in the perioperative period is essential.

Most anterior transfacial approaches involve access through the posterior pharyngeal wall, prevertebral fascia, and/or clival base. The dura may be encountered, and the ablative procedure may leave a dural defect. Options for watertight closure are planned for in advance and include fascia lata, pericranium, and bovine pericardium. Protection of the oral and pharyngeal mucosa is essential.

Limitations and Contraindications

There are few limitations for this procedure. It has been performed safely on patients ranging in age from 16 to 85. However, previous radiation treatment for oral, pharyngeal, or laryngeal tumors likely will preclude this procedure.

The preoperative evaluation for transfacial access is similar to that for reconstructive patients requiring orthognathic surgery. The examination includes the following:

- An oral examination to identify and eliminate dental disease
- Anatomic models with an occlusal splint
- Radiographic examination, including Panorex and computed tomography, to evaluate the health of the maxillary and ethmoid sinuses, in addition to the midline and perimidline areas for osteotomy purposes

Often these patients undergo an anterior approach to the skull base combined with a posterior cervical fusion, especially if the odontoid process is involved. Long-term nutritional management with a percutaneous enteral gastrostomy (PEG) feeding tube is suggested. A tracheostomy allows precise airway and respiratory management. An armored oral endotracheal tube can be used and lateralized during the intermaxillary fixation phase if oral intubation is selected.

TECHNIQUE: Modified Le Fort I Osteotomy With Midline Split

STEP 1: Incision

A shortened vestibular incision is combined with a midline split of the soft palate, starting in the true midline of the uvula and progressing through the soft palate to the posterior nasal spine and then continuing into the midline through the hard palate, stopping at the incisive papillae. The palatal and pharyngeal incision should be made with a cold knife; electrocautery should be avoided as much as possible to prevent die-back of the wound margins.

STEP 2: Osteotomy

An osteotomy is accomplished with a small reciprocating saw from the piriform rim to the pterygoid plate bilaterally. Once this incision has been completed, fixation plates are brought to the field and adapted to the piriform rim and the zygomatic buttresses, and the drill holes are placed for reconstruction purposes. Because the maxilla will not be moved anteriorly, posteriorly, or laterally, prefabrication of the plates is helpful. The plates are marked, set on the back table, and placed at the end of the procedure. The nasal mucosa and septum are separated.

STEP 3: Down-Fracture

The maxilla is then down-fractured per normal technique, and a paramidline osteotomy is accomplished from a point lateral to the posterior nasal spine just off the midline into the alveolus and then through the alveolus and the anterior nasal spine, between the central incisors. This osteotomy is performed with a 1-mm reciprocating blade and completed with small osteotomes (Fig. 52.8A).

STEP 4: Palatal Incisions

The maxilla is brought into its up position. Then, 4-0 silk sutures are placed through the lateral portions of the uvula and a #15 blade is used to make an incision through the uvula and the soft palate to the posterior nasal spine in the true midline and brought up to the incisive papillae. Slight undermining of the soft tissue flap is carried out to join the osteotomy site, and the maxilla is separated in the midline. To gain access to the posterior pharyngeal wall up to the vomer base, horizontal lateral incisions are made through the nasal mucosa just above the posterior border of the maxilla (Fig. 52.8B).

STEP 5: Retractor Placement

The maxilla is mobilized, and the Dingman mouth prop is inserted; this holds the mouth open, yet allows retraction of the maxillary segments into a lateral position. The Dingman hooks, which normally are placed on the upper incisor teeth, are placed in the maxillary sinus at the piriform areas for stabilization. Appropriate retractors are then placed, specifically the Holton/Cloward retractor, to retract the lateral pharyngeal walls and expose the posterior pharynx from the vomer to the upper cervical spine. The tongue retractor engages the armored oral endotracheal tube (if used) as part of the retraction process (see Fig. 52.8B).

STEP 6: Pharyngeal Incision

For conditions of the clivus, a midline incision is made from the anterior lip of the foramen magnum up through the vomer; the soft tissue of the clivus can be dissected laterally and then retracted with appropriate retractors.

For conditions of the upper cervical spine below the foramen magnum, a superior-based pharyngeal flap is used to offset a midline incision in the area of the superior constrictor muscle, which tends to dehisce a midline incision (Fig. 52.8C).

STEP 7: Pharyngeal Closure

After the neurosurgical procedure has been completed, the wounds are closed. The midline incision of the clivus or the superior-based pharyngeal flap is closed with a combination of 3-0 chromic and 4-0 Vicryl sutures. The clivus area from the base of the vomer to the anterior lip of the foramen magnum is very thin, consisting of nasal pharyngeal mucosa, periosteum, and then the clivus. Careful dissection of this tissue is imperative because there is little room for error in closing this wound. Should a soft tissue defect occur, fascia lata is a good choice to aid in closure. A two-layer closure is preferable: first, the prevertebral fascia, and then the posterior pharyngeal wall, including the superior constrictor.

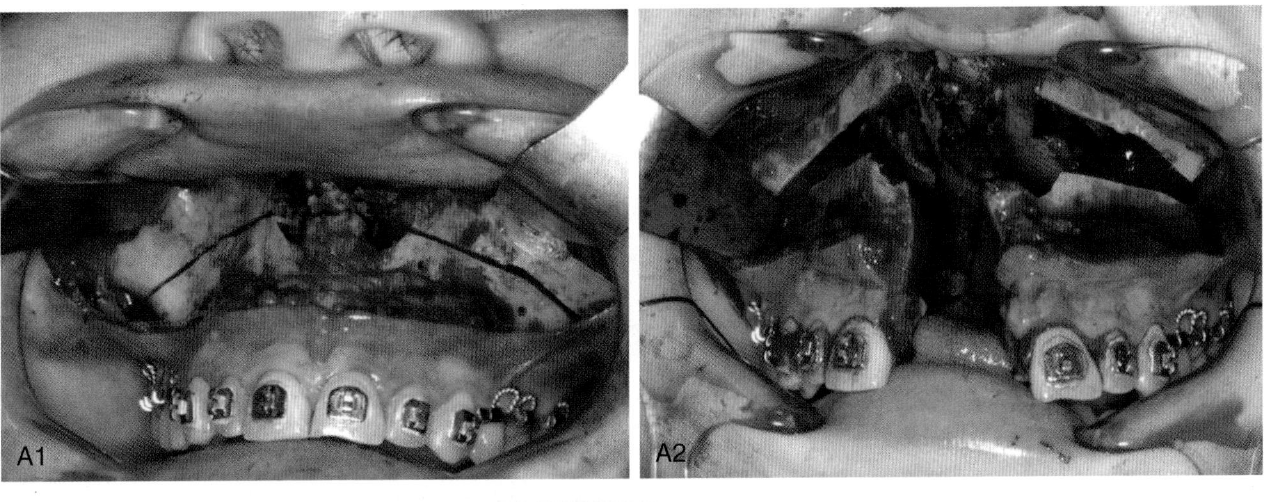

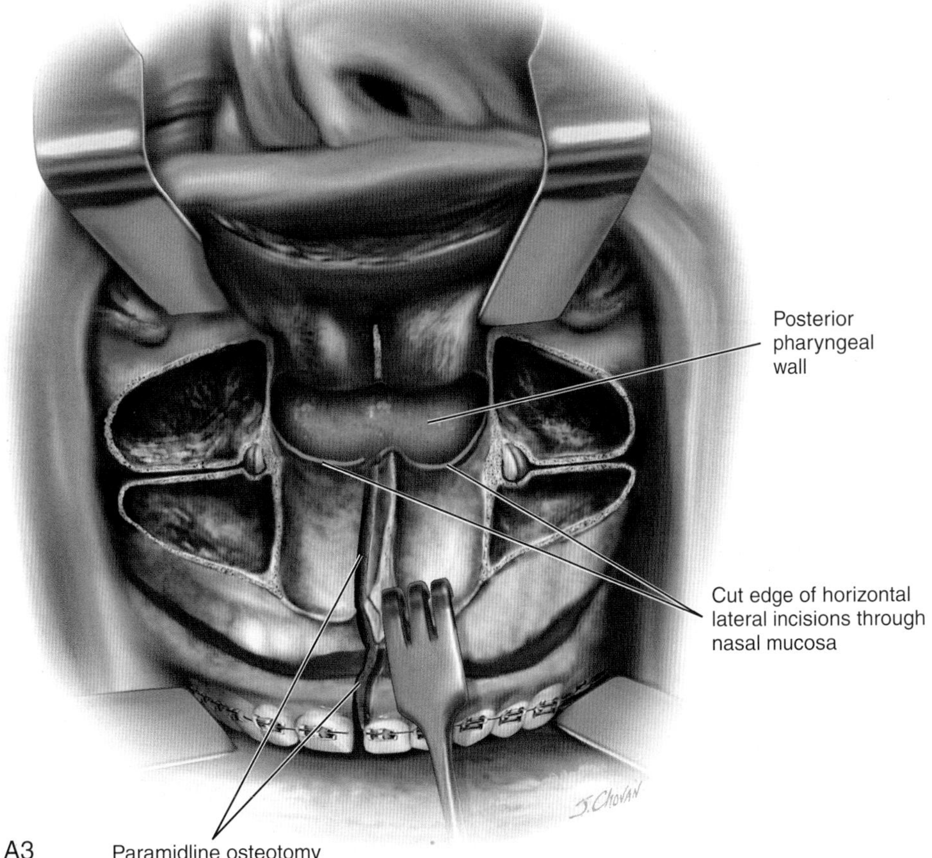

Figure 52.8 **A1**, and **A3**, Le Fort I osteotomy with midline split, including the hard and soft palates.

Continued

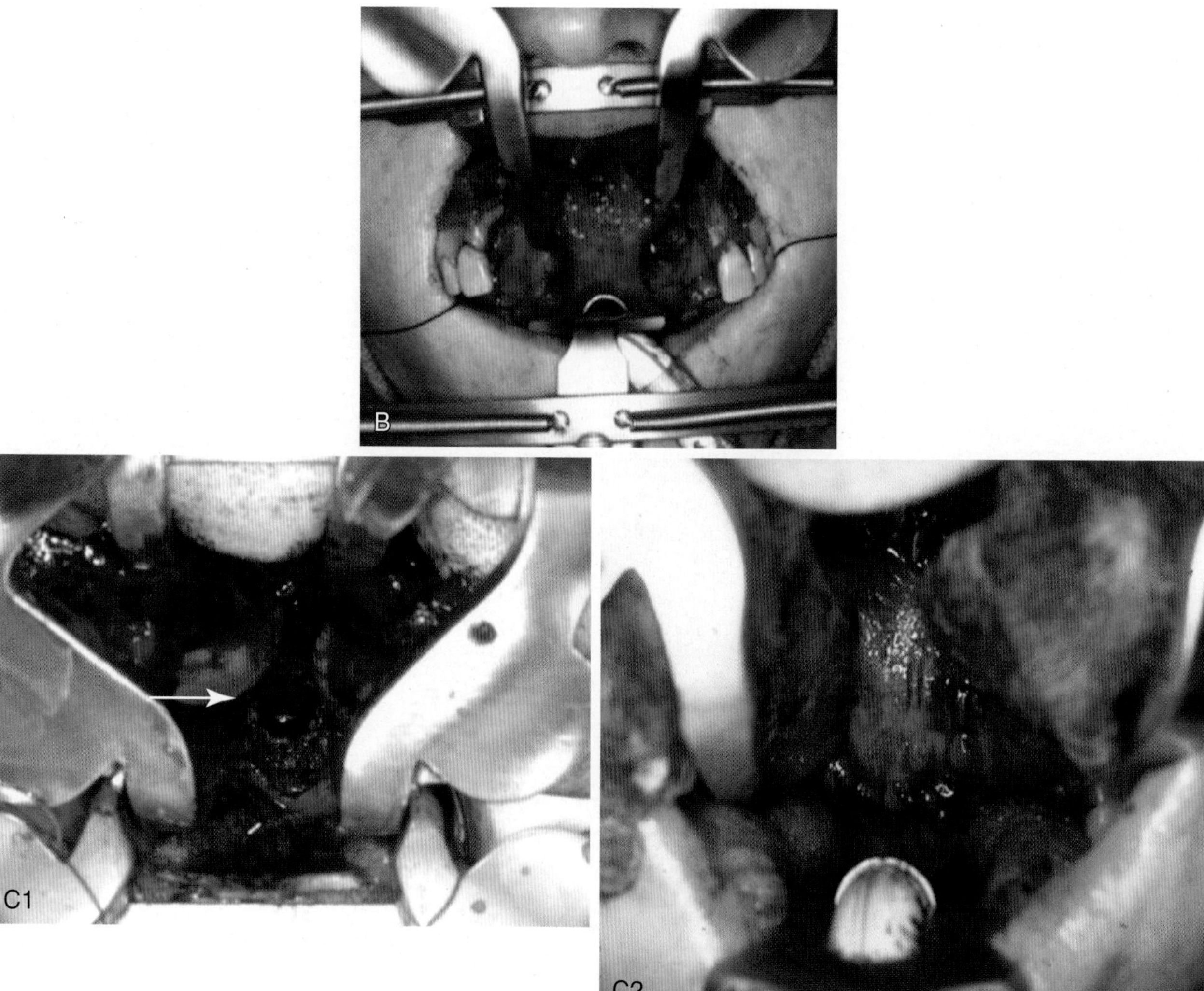

Figure 52.8, cont'd B, Le Fort I with midline split and retractors in place, showing access to the posterior pharyngeal wall. **C1**, Posterior wall defect after odontoid removal. **C2**, Closure of the superior-based pharyngeal flap.

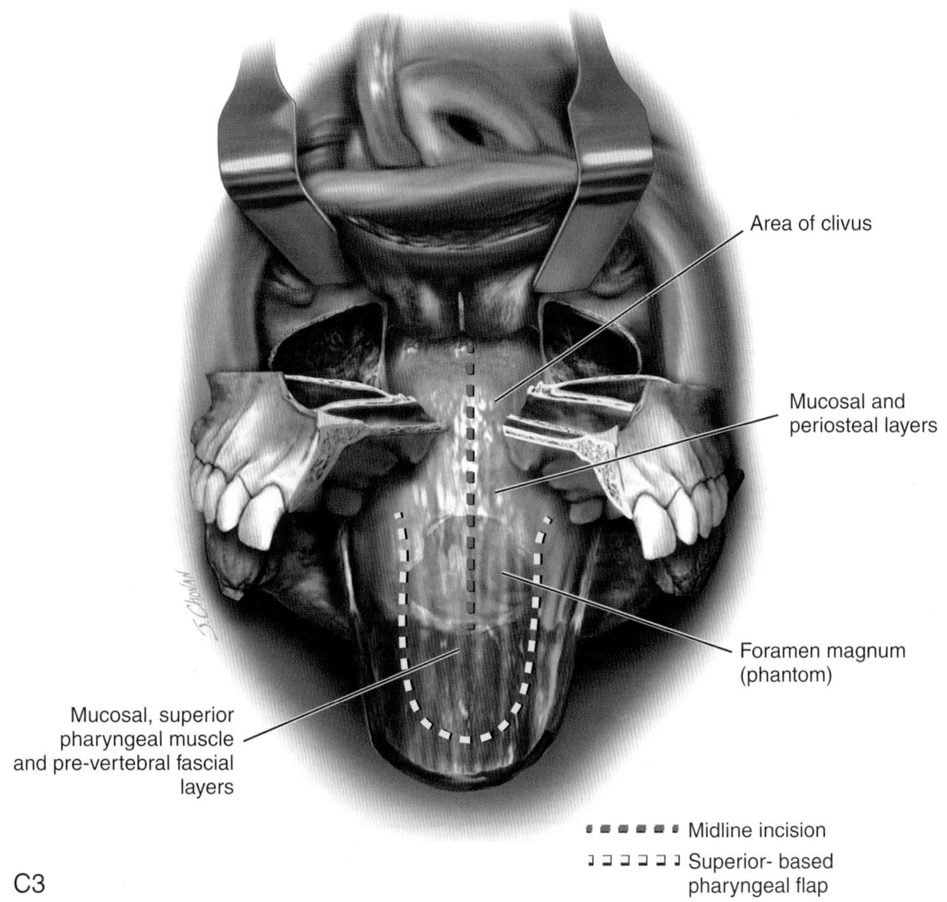

Figure 52.8, cont'd C3, Typical incision lines used for a midline and superior-based pharyngeal flap.

TECHNIQUE: Modified Le Fort I Osteotomy With Midline Split—cont'd

STEP 8: Palatal Closure

Once the posterior pharyngeal wall and/or clivus area has been closed, the soft palate is closed. The nasal portion of the soft palate is closed with interrupted 4-0 Vicryl sutures, and then the tip of the uvula is closed with 4-0 Vicryl sutures; finally, a two-layer closure of the soft palate to the posterior nasal spine is performed.

STEP 9: Maxillary Repositioning

The maxilla is then raised into its presurgical position. The arch bars or orthodontic appliances that have been placed on the maxillary teeth are engaged. A surgical splint can secure the occlusion. The patient is placed in intermaxillary fixation, and the maxilla is stabilized with the plates along the piriform rim and the zygomatic buttresses. Intermaxillary fixation is not routinely used postoperatively. The midline of the maxilla can be repaired with a positional screw across the midline at the anterior nasal spine area or with a small plate with four screws (Fig. 52.8D).

STEP 10: Closure

The hard palate is closed from the posterior nasal spine to the incisive papillae with 4-0 Monocryl sutures. The vestibular incision is then closed in two layers with 3-0 chromic suture. If extensive dissection along the nasal septum has been accomplished, Doyle splints are inserted and secured with transseptal 3-0 nylon sutures (Fig. 52.8E).

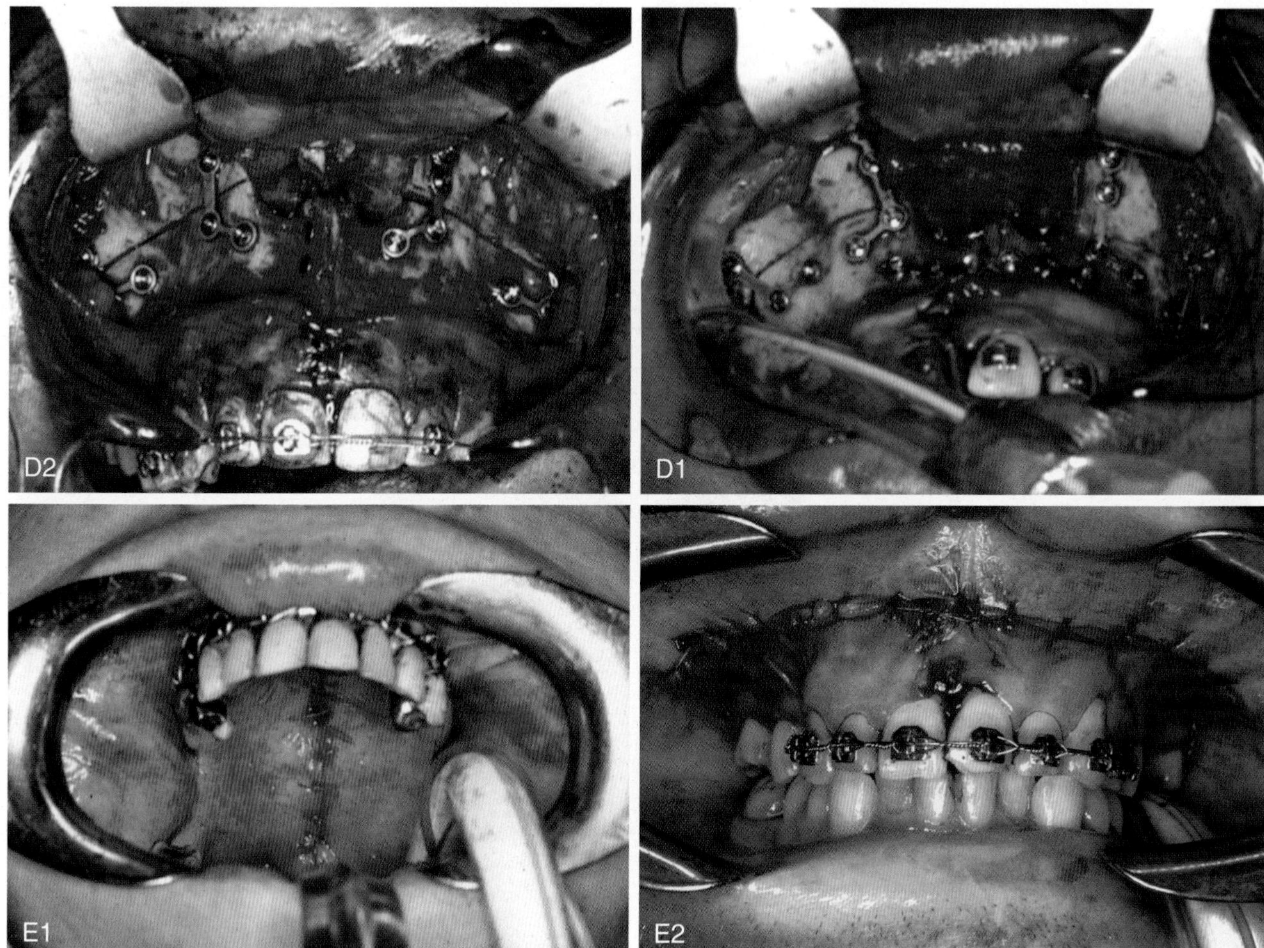

Figure 52.8, cont'd **D1** and **D2**, Rigid fixation and closure. Plate or positional screws across the midline. **E1** and **E2**, Soft tissue closure.

Avoidance and Management of Intraoperative Complications

1. Preoperative nasopharyngoscopy to evaluate both nasal passages and the posterior pharyngeal wall can identify potential access issues, such as enlarged adenoid masses or a torturous carotid artery loop
2. Limited use of electrocautery
3. Three-layer closure of the soft palate
4. Use of a superior-based pharyngeal flap for exposure below the foramen magnum
5. Use of a PEG feeding tube
6. Use of a tracheostomy
7. Evoked potential monitoring is used to monitor intraoperative nerve function
8. Eliminating oral or nasal tubes or devices that could abrade or cause pressure on the incision site is preferable.

Postoperative Considerations

- Dehiscence of the posterior pharyngeal wall
- Dehiscence of the soft palate
- Loss of tooth or bone structure
- Loss of gingival tissue
- Velopharyngeal incompetence due to loss of posterior wall volume can occur
- Antibiotics are used before and after surgery
- Neural deficits can occur, depending on the tumor's location
- Nasal and oral irrigations with saline, with visualization and suction, are advocated until healing has occurred

Surgery of the skull base presents many challenges. Careful planning and a thorough understanding of the pathologic condition can increase favorable outcomes. In many cases wide field exposure with self-retained retraction provides the best option for tumor ablation.

References

1. Grime PD, Haskell R, Robertson I, Gullan R. Transfacial access for neurosurgical procedures: an extended role for the maxillofacial surgeon. I. The upper cervical spine and clivus. *Int J Oral Maxillofac Surg*. 1991;20(5):285–290. review.
2. Grime PD, Haskell R, Robertson I, Gullan R. Transfacial access for neurosurgical procedures: an extended role for the maxillofacial surgeon. II. Middle cranial fossa, infratemporal fossa and pterygoid space. *Int J Oral Maxillofac Surg*. 1991;20(5):291–295.
3. Jackson IT. Craniofacial osteotomies to facilitate the resection of tumors of the skull base. *Neurosurgery*. 1996;2:1585.
4. Raza SM, Conway JE, Li KW, et al. A modified frontal-nasal-orbital approach to midline lesions of the anterior cranial fossa and skull base: technical note with case illustrations. *Neurosurg Rev*. 2010;33(1):63–70.
5. Holton J. Oral and maxillofacial surgical approaches for tumors and conditions involving the anterior cranial base and the middle cranial fossa. *Oral Maxillofac Surg Clin North Am*. 1997;9(2):451.
6. Holton J. *Modifications of the Le Fort I Osteotomy for Cranial Base Access*. OMS Knowledge Update; 1997.
7. Hankinson TC, Haque R, Bruce JN. *Skull Base Tumors*. eMedicine from WebMD; 2010. Available at: http://emedicine.medscape.com/article/250237-overview.
8. Abdullah J, Rushdan A, Hamzah M, Ariff AR, Rani A. Use of bovine xenograft in reconstruction of traumatic anterior cranial fossa bone defects involving the frontal sinus. *Ann Transplant*. 1999;4(3–4):28–31.
9. Melamed I, Tubbs RS, Payner TD, Cohen-Gadol AA. Trans-zygomatic middle cranial fossa approach to access lesions around the cavernous sinus and anterior parahippocampus: a minimally invasive skull base approach. *Acta Neurochir (Wien)*. 2009;151(8): 977–982.
10. Kole H. Surgical operations on the alveolar ridge to correct occlusal abnormalities. *Oral Surg Oral Med Oral Pathol*. 1959;12(3): 277–288.
11. Bell WH. Revascularization and bone healing after anterior maxillary osteotomy: a study using adult rhesus monkeys. *J Oral Surg*. 1969;27(4):249–255.
12. Bell WH, Levy BM. Revascularization and bone healing after posterior maxillary osteotomy. *J Oral Surg*. 1971;29(5):313–320.
13. James D, Crockard HA. Surgical access to the base of skull and upper cervical spine by extended maxillotomy. *Neurosurgery*. 1991;29(3):411–416.
14. Sandor GK, Charles DA, Lawson VG, Tator CH. Trans oral approach to the nasopharynx and clivus using the Le Fort I osteotomy with midpalatal split. *Int J Oral Maxillofac Surg*. 1990;19(6):352–355.
15. Rawlins JM, Batchelor AG, Liddington MI, Towns G. Tumor excision and reconstruction of the upper cervical spine: a multidisciplinary approach. *Plast Reconstr Surg*. 2004;114(6):1534–1538.

CHAPTER 53

Facial Translocation

Kaushik H. Sharma and Deepak Kademani

Armamentarium

9 Periosteal elevators
15 BP scalpel blades
Appropriate sutures
Army-Navy retractors
Bone rongeurs
Colorado tip needle
Cook-Swartz Doppler probe
Corneal shield
Curved Mayo scissors
Double prong wide skin hooks
Internal fixation kit (midface and orbit)
Freer elevators
Kerrison rongeurs
Lahey (if performing neck dissection)
Local anesthetic with vasoconstrictor
Malleable retractors
Minnesota retractors
Monopolar and bipolar electrocautery
Mouth prop
Nasal RAE or armored endotracheal tube or cuffed tracheostomy tube
Neurosurgical patties (1/4" × 3")
Obwegeser retractors
Osteotomes—straight and curved (4 to 6 mm)
Pterygoid osteotome
Reciprocating saw
Plastic cheek retractor
Senn retractor
Smith bone spreader
Surgical loupes
Topical decongestant for nasal packing
Volkmann bone hook

History of the Procedure

The facial translocation approach was first described by Janecka et al.[1] in 1990 for access to the cranial base. This approach included an inferiorly based cheek flap developed on the facial and labial vascular pedicles. The flap included the entire cheek soft tissue, lower lid, facial nerve, and the parotid gland.[2] Janecka et al. described the facial translocation approach in three steps. The first step was to develop a composite facial soft tissue flap, the second step was to perform planned osteotomies, and the third step was the reconstruction component.[3] In 1993 Forcada et al. concluded that facial translocation can be used in combination with the transcranial approach for safer care of the cephaloceles and to achieve better cosmetic results.[4] In 1995 Janecka classified the facial translocation approach to the skull base.[5] In 2002 Bales et al.[6] concluded that a combined craniofacial approach can be utilized for juvenile angiofibroma with intracranial extension. In 2002 Movassaghi and Janecka described a technique for optic nerve decompression via midfacial translocation approach for the patients with optic neuropathy, whose local anatomy and landmarks were distorted by the pathologic process.[7]

Anatomical Considerations[8]

The cranial base is considered one of the most complex anatomical regions, and it can be challenging during access for tumor ablation. This is due to its intimate relationship with the central nervous system and the cervical and facial regions.[3] The goal of any ablative surgery is complete tumor resection and to minimize blood loss and morbidity for the patient. In order to achieve this, the operator must possess a thorough understanding of the skull base anatomy and the spatial relationship of pathology in question (Figs. 53.1–53.3). The extracranial component of anterolateral skull base anatomy is discussed in this chapter.

Boundaries of Infratemporal Fossa

- Anterior: posterolateral wall of the maxillary sinus
- Posterior: the petro-occipital suture
- Medial: the lateral pterygoid plate
- Lateral: the squamous and petrous portions of the temporal bone, the mandibular ramus, and condyle
- Posteroinferior: the parapharyngeal space
- Superior: the greater wing of the sphenoid bone

Contents

The muscles of mastication and the internal maxillary artery. The internal maxillary artery provides blood supply to these muscles and should be preserved in case a temporalis flap is necessary to reconstruct skull base defects. Dissecting further in a medial direction reveals the cartilaginous eustachian tube and the tensor and levator veli palatini muscles.

Bony Surgical Landmarks

1. The root of the lateral pterygoid plate lies immediately posterior to the foramen rotundum and anterior to the

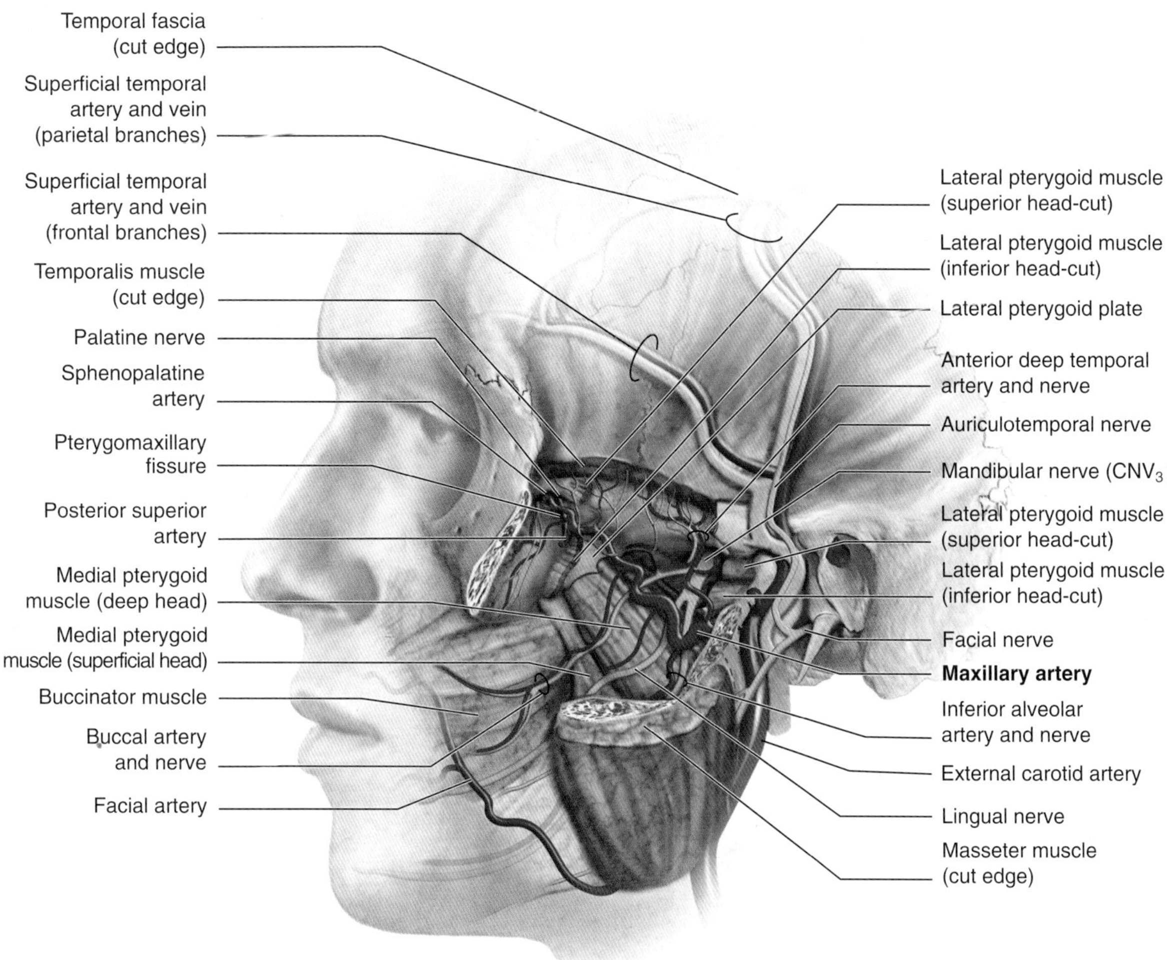

Fig. 53.1 Contents of the infratemporal fossa. Note the branches of the internal maxillary artery in close proximity to the anterolateral skull base.

foramen ovale. Once the foramen ovale is identified, the foramen spinosum is easily identifiable immediately posterior to the foramen.

2. The sphenoid spine helps in identifying the highest portion of the cervical internal carotid artery (ICA) and the carotid canal. It is located just medial to the glenoid fossa and posterolateral to the foramen spinosum.

Venous Drainage

Drainage of the external lateral skull base involves the internal and external jugular venous system and the retromandibular vein. The mastoid and occipital emissary veins can link the intracranial dural sinus system with the external circulation, namely, the branches of the occipital, postauricular, or retrofacial veins. The pterygoid venous system can be highly variable in this region.

Arterial Supply

The facial, superficial temporal, occipital, and postauricular branches of the external carotid artery provide arterial supply to the lateral skull base. The internal maxillary artery, with its deep temporal and middle meningeal branches, can be identified in the infratemporal fossa. The cervical portion of the ICA ascends vertically to enter the middle fossa medial to the sphenoid spine.

Important Structures/Relationships

The pterygomaxillary fissure transmits the maxillary artery to the pterygomaxillary fossa. The greater petrosal nerve joins the deep petrosal nerve to form the vidian nerve, which enters the fossa through the vidian or pterygoid canal enroute to the pterygopalatine ganglion. The maxillary nerve enters through the foramen rotundum to transmit sensory information from the face. Both nerves send branches to the parasympathetic sphenopalatine ganglion. The inferior orbital fissure is at the most anterior limit of the pterygomaxillary fossa and is continuous with the infratemporal fossa.

The deep lobe of the parotid gland with the facial nerve and its branches may be encountered in the lateral aspect of the extracranial skull base. The facial nerve exits the mastoid through the stylomastoid foramen and enters the substance of the parotid gland.

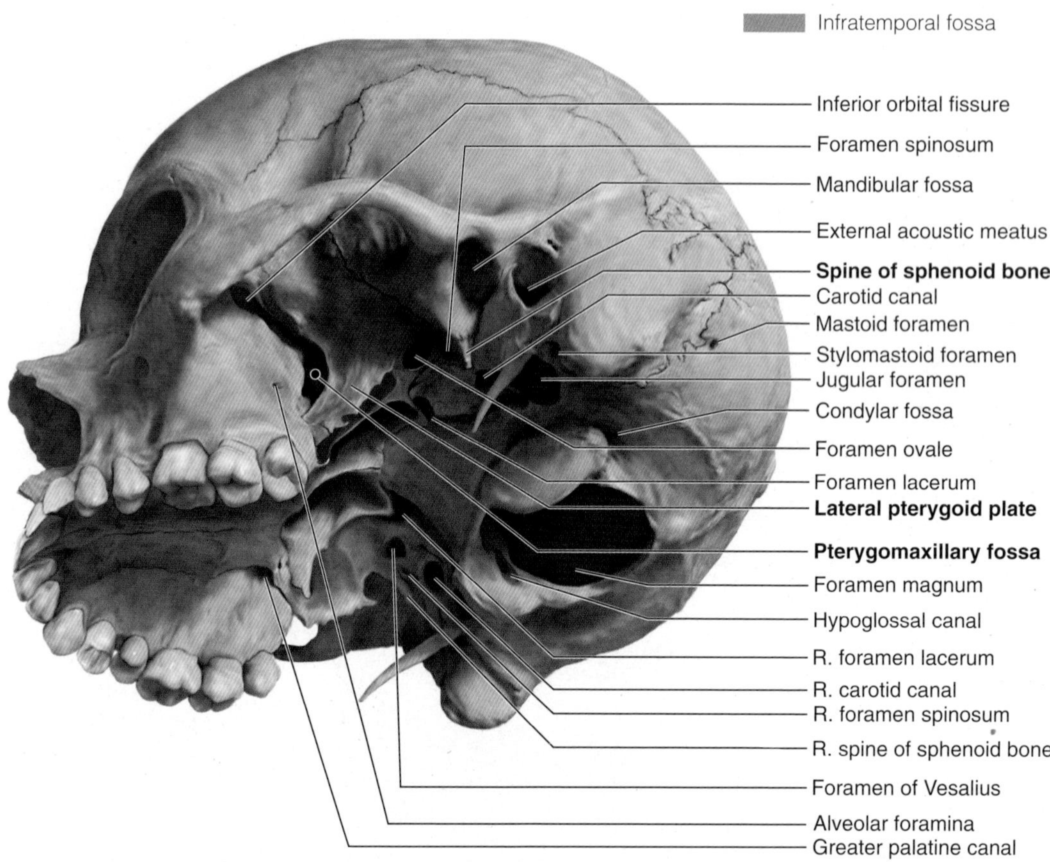

Fig. 53.2 Osteology of the skull base and the pterygomaxillary fossa. Note the lateral pterygoid plate and spine of sphenoid bone as the bony landmarks and their relationship to skull base foramina.

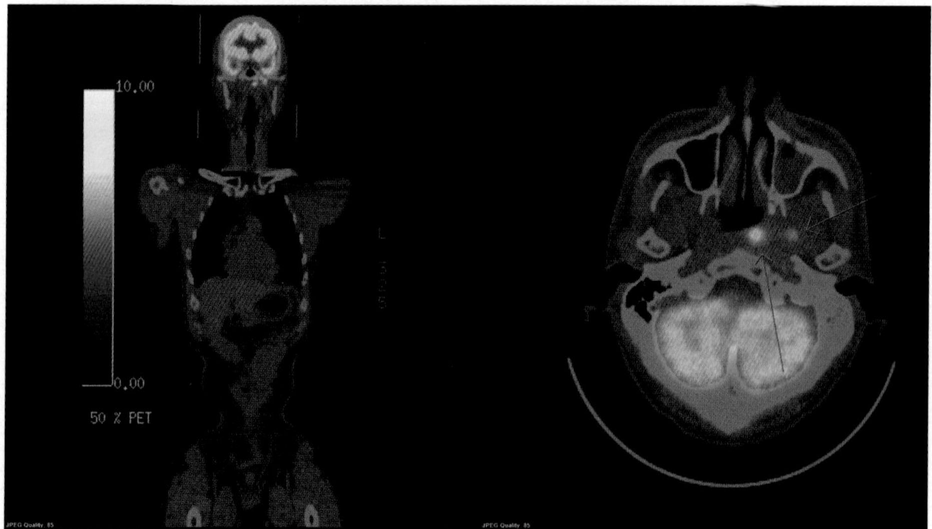

Fig. 53.3 Positron emission tomography scan demonstrating nasopharyngeal carcinoma. Note the proximity to skull base and the relationship to the pterygoid plates and mandibular left condyle.

The jugular foramen transports cranial nerves (CN) IX, X, and XI between the jugular process of the occipital bone and the jugular process of the petrous bone. In the extracranial aspect, its anterior border is the carotid canal, its lateral border is the styloid process sheath, and its medial borders are the hypoglossal foramen and canal. It lies posterolaterally in the lateral skull base and anteromedially to the mastoid tip. The jugular foramen can be divided into the pars nervosa anteriorly and the pars venosa posteriorly.

The sphenoid sinus can serve as an access route to the pituitary and the clivus. It is important to avoid disrupting the lateral wall during instrumentation, because the ICA and optic nerve are just lateral to a thin margin of bone. Dehiscence may be present in the lateral wall of the sphenoid, resulting in exposure of the carotid artery, optic nerve, or vidian nerve.

The nasopharynx lies posterior and inferior to the sphenoid sinus along the midline. Mucosa covers the medial surface of the medial pterygoid plate. The investing fascia (pharyngobasilar fascia) of the nasopharynx is suspended from the skull base and clivus located superiorly. The vertebrobasilar artery and the brainstem lie posterior to the clivus. The sphenoid sinus, the investing pharyngobasilar fascia, and the superior pharyngeal constrictor muscle help to form the lateral portion of the choana and part of the lateral portion of the nasopharynx.

The sinus of Morgagni is a weak point in the superolateral nasopharyngeal wall, which is created by the passage of the levator veli palatini and the cartilaginous eustachian tube through the superior constrictor muscle. This is a region for infections or tumor to potentially invade the skull base. Directly superior to the nasopharynx is the foramen lacerum and the ICA, just before its entry point into the cavernous sinus.

Skull Base Approaches

The choice of surgical approach depends upon the tumor, tumor bed vasculature, patient preference, and the surgical team experience. Endoscopic transnasal resection is reserved for small tumors limited to the nasopharynx, the nasal cavity, and the ethmoid and sphenoid sinuses, which provides minimal soft tissue and bony disruption.[9] However, endoscopic approaches offer restricted access and bleeding can obscure visibility. The transpalatal technique is indicated for tumors limited to the nasopharynx, nasal cavity, and sphenoid sinus, but the lateral exposure is very limited. The Le Fort I approach is indicated for tumors involving the nasopharynx, nasal cavity, paranasal sinuses, pterygopalatine fossa, infratemporal fossa, and the medial part of the cavernous sinus. The medial maxillectomy approach is useful to access tumors involving the nasopharynx, orbit, ethmoids, sphenoid sinus, pterygopalatine fossa, infratemporal fossa, and the medial part of the cavernous sinus.[10] Tumors involving the anterior skull base can be managed anterolaterally through the orbitozygomatic approach and the transzygomatic approach.[11] Some operators prefer the transmandibular approach in conjunction with the orbitozygomatic approach to access the anterolateral skull base. The facial translocation approach provides the most exposure of the nasopharynx, sphenoid sinus, pterygopalatine fossa, infratemporal fossa, and cavernous sinus.[10,12]

Classification (Janecka)[5]

The facial translocation approach to the cranial base is an invaluable technique in cranial base surgery and has undergone significant evolution since its original description in 1990 by Janecka et al. (Fig. 53.4).[1–3]

1. Mini facial translocation

   Central

   - Provides access to medial orbit, sphenoid and ethmoid sinus, and the inferior clivus[13]

   Lateral

   - Provides access to the infratemporal fossa
2. Standard facial translocation with palatal extension
   - Provides good access to the anterolateral skull base especially when the infratemporal fossa is also involved
3. Extended facial translocation—medial with palatal extension
   - Provides access to the ipsilateral infratemporal fossa and central and paracentral skull base bilaterally. The entire clivus, optic nerves, both precavernous internal carotid arteries, and the nasopharynx can also be accessed. The wide communication with the infratemporal fossa allows for the placement of the temporalis muscle flap for vascularized reconstruction of the skull base defect.
4. Extended facial translocation—medial and inferior
   - Provides a significant inferior and upper cervical surgical access. This involves lower lip incision with mandibular split osteotomy.
5. Extended facial translocation—posterior
   - Provides access to the anterior and posterior aspects of the temporal bone with control of the key neurovascular structures.
6. Bilateral facial translocation
   - Provides access to both infratemporal fossae, central and the entire paracentral skull base, both distal cervical internal carotid arteries, and clivus. The palatal split can provide access to the level of C2 to C3. If mandibular split osteotomy added, a vertical reach to the level of C3 to C4 is accomplished.

Indications for the Use of the Procedure

A successful oncologic operation depends on the technical ease of achieving clear surgical margins.[1] Using the facial translocation approach, the surgeon can access the anterior, middle cranial base, and related structures. The facial translocation approach offers wide and direct exposure, with a potential for immediate reconstruction of this complex region.[2] The surgical field can extend from the contralateral eustachian tube to the ipsilateral geniculate ganglion and from the superior orbital fissure/cavernous sinus area to the level of the hard palate.[1] The midface contains pneumatized cavities such as the oronasal and paranasal sinuses and the nasopharynx, which facilitate the relative ease of surgical access to the central skull base.[15,14] This approach facilitates direct approach to the nasopharynx, clivus, superior orbital fissure-cavernous sinus, infratemporal, and pterygopalatine fossae.[1] A lateral approach such as facial translocation with or without removal

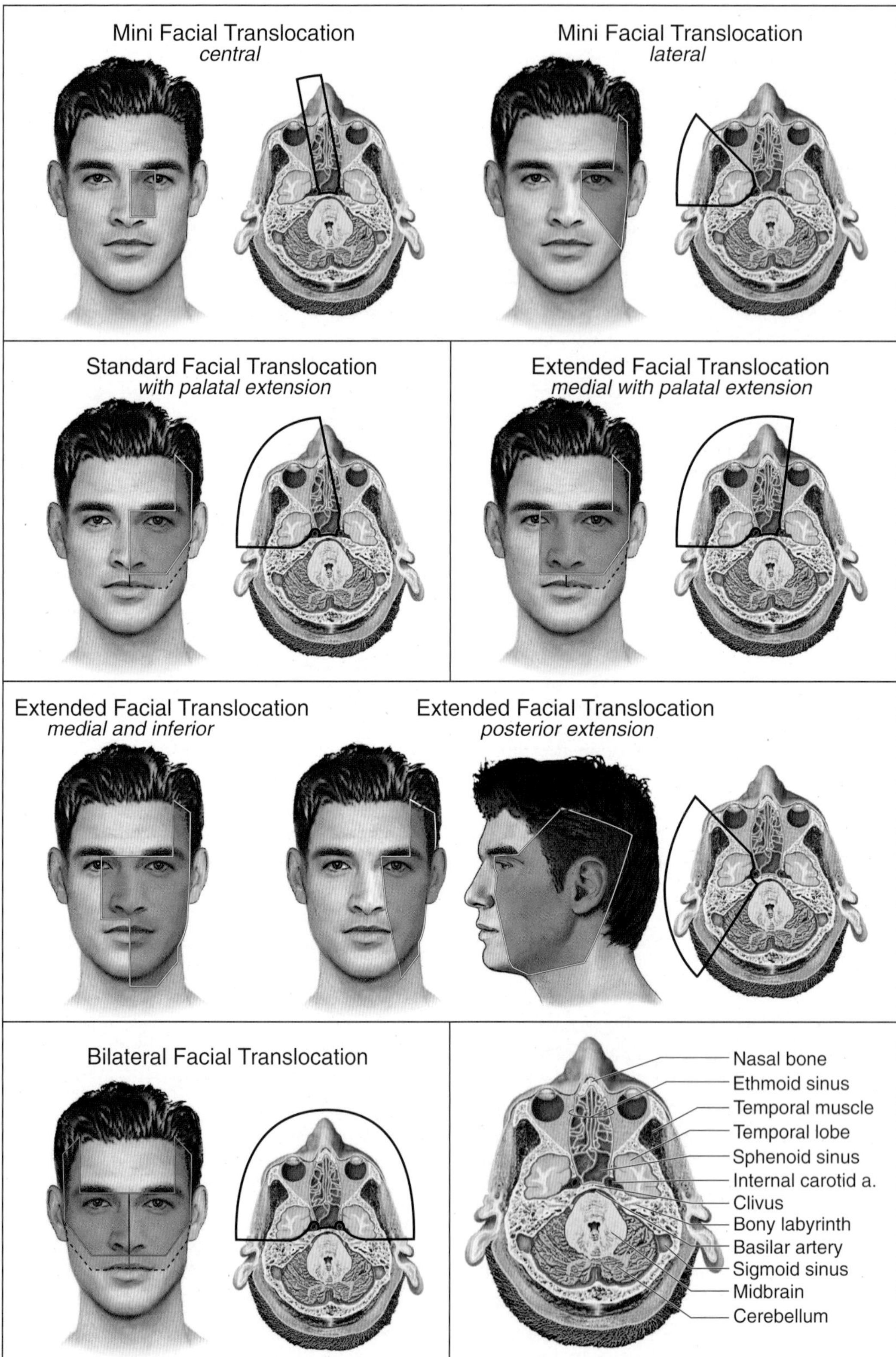

Fig. 53.4 Facial translocation classification as per Janecka.[5]

of the ICA offers the widest operative field for resection of nasopharyngeal tumor recurrence.[6,15] The contemporary principle of skull base approaches is to minimize brain retraction while maximizing skull base visualization.[5]

Limitations and Contraindications

Facial translocation approach has several disadvantages, including the need for facial incisions with subsequent scar development.[5] This can be of great importance for someone with a history of keloid or hypertrophic scar formation. The potential need for supplementary airway management including postoperative intubation and/or temporary tracheostomy should be assessed. Cerebrospinal fluid fistula can result if the dura mater is damaged during surgical intervention and not accessible at the time of surgery. A neurosurgical consult is warranted in this scenario. The standard facial translocation approach should be used with caution in growing individuals as extensive soft tissue dissection and multiple osteotomies are required, which may affect facial growth due to scar formation and may result in some facial asymmetry.[9] The complete encasement of the petrous ICA by the tumor is considered a contraindication to skull base surgery.[16]

TECHNIQUE

STEP 1: Preoperative Examimation and Photo Documentation

It is important to perform a thorough head-to-toe examination on the day of surgery with emphasis on CN I–XII functions. As illustrated in Fig. 53.5, the patient had a preexisting left upper eyelid congenital ptosis. Preoperative photo documentation from the frontal and lateral views should be completed at rest and in function.

STEP 2: Patient Positioning and Preparation

The patient is transferred to the operating room table in a supine position. An armored oral endotracheal tube or a contralateral nasal endotracheal tube can be used to secure the airway. A tracheostomy, if indicated, should be performed. Anesthetist should provide hypotensive anesthesia for the procedure to prevent excessive blood loss. An oxymetazoline intranasal (Afrin)-soaked neuropatty can be placed in the ipsilateral nasal cavity. A corneal shield with ophthalmic bacitracin or tarsorrhaphy suture must be used for globe protection if orbital preservation is planned.

STEP 3: Skin Incisions (Weber-Ferguson, Subciliary/Transconjunctival With Lateral Canthotomy, Preauricular)

Local anesthesia with epinephrine is administered to the planned incision sites. A #15 blade is used for an upper lip split incision starting at the crest of the ipsilateral philtral column of the lip and extending inferiorly up to the vermilion border. The incision is carried out medially up to the midline and then extended inferiorly through the vermilion of the lip, orbicularis oris, and labial mucosa. Alternatively, one can use an incision extending from the base of the columella inferiorly through the philtral groove and up to the white roll. A 3-mm lateral step-off incision up to the philtral ridge can be performed and carried inferiorly through the vermilion. The superior extent of the incision is carried out laterally and closely around the base of the nose and then turns medially to extend through the nasofacial groove, which ends inferior to the medial canthus. The authors prefer subciliary over the transconjunctival incision to access the infraorbital rim and orbital floor. The subciliary incision is placed 2 mm inferior to the lower eyelashes along the entire length of the eyelid and extended laterally to perform lateral canthotomy and cantholysis. A monopolar electrocautery can be used to deepen the incision through the subcutaneous, muscular, and periosteal layers to expose the bone. Extreme care should be taken to avoid excessive periosteal stripping to prevent devascularization of the edges of translocated bone segment. A full-thickness incision of the upper lip can be completed at this time (Fig. 53.6). Bipolar electrocautery can be used for hemostasis. Next, the patient's head is turned in the contralateral direction and attention is directed to the preauricular region. A 2-cm preauricular incision is carried through skin, subcutaneous tissue, superficial musculoaponeurotic system, temporalis fascia, and the periosteum to expose the zygomatic arch.

Continued

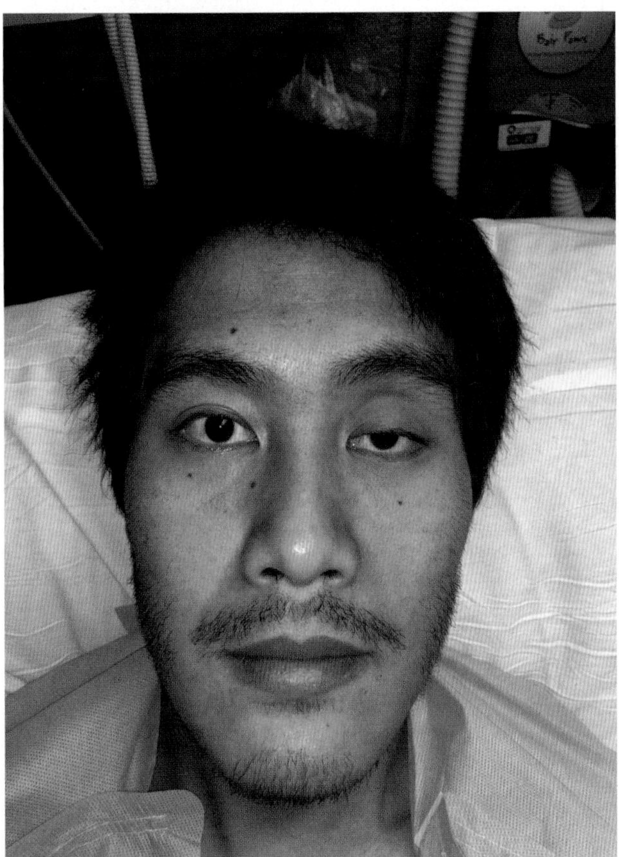

Fig. 53.5 Preoperative photo of the patient showing preexisting left upper eyelid congenital ptosis.

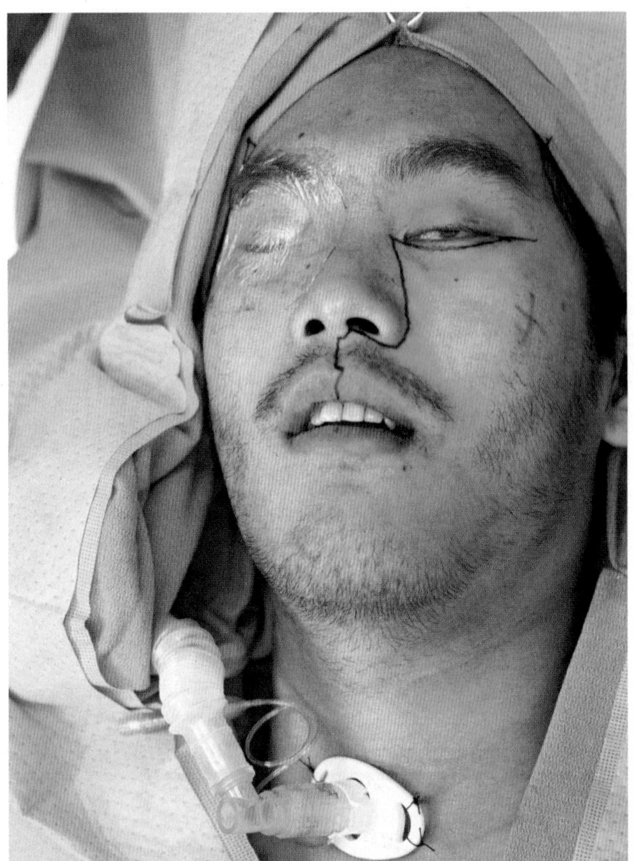

Fig. 53.6 Proposed skin incisions (Weber-Ferguson, subciliary with lateral canthotomy).

TECHNIQUE—*cont'd*

STEP 4: Oral Incisions (Vestibular)

The incision is extended through the labial frenum and interdental papilla between the maxillary incisors. A palatal sulcular incision extending from contralateral first molar to ipsilateral distal most erupted tooth and extended buccally into the buccal vestibule to access the ipsilateral pterygoid plates can be placed. Alternatively, a mid-palatal incision through hard and soft palate can be used also with a vertical incision placed in the buccal vestibule to access the ipsilateral pterygoid plates.

STEP 5: Preplating of the Proposed Osteotomy Sites With Minimal Soft Tissue Dissection

Midface miniplates can be contoured and secured using monocortical screws at the intermaxillary suture, nasomaxillary and frontozygomatic buttresses, and the zygomatic arch. Osteotomies can be indexed, and all the plates and screws are removed at this point (Fig. 53.7A–7B).

STEP 6: Osteotomies (Intermaxillary Suture, Nasomaxillary Buttress, Orbital Floor, Frontozygomatic Buttress, Zygomatic Arch, Pterygoid Plates)

A reciprocating saw under normal saline irrigation is used for osteotomies through intermaxillary suture, nasomaxillary buttress, orbital floor, and frontozygomatic buttress. One should take precaution to not cause any dental root damage during intermaxillary osteotomy. The superior extension of the nasomaxillary buttress osteotomy is extended posterolaterally to the infraorbital rim through the orbital floor to end into the inferior orbital fissure. The osteotomy is extended superolaterally from the inferior orbital fissure through the frontozygomatic suture. The infraorbital nerve is transected at this time. Attention is directed to perform a zygomatic arch osteotomy. The ipsilateral pterygoid plates can be separated using a mallet and a pterygoid osteotome. The nasal septum can be dissected away from the nasal crest of the maxilla and median palatine suture at this point. The remainder of the mid-palatal split can be achieved using a thin, straight osteotome and mallet to propagate the fracture posteriorly through the median palatine suture.

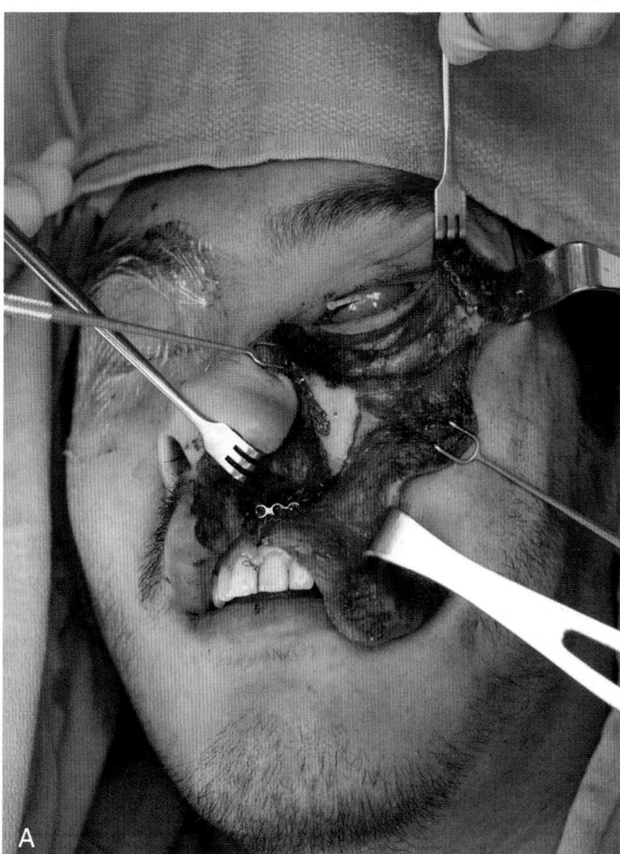

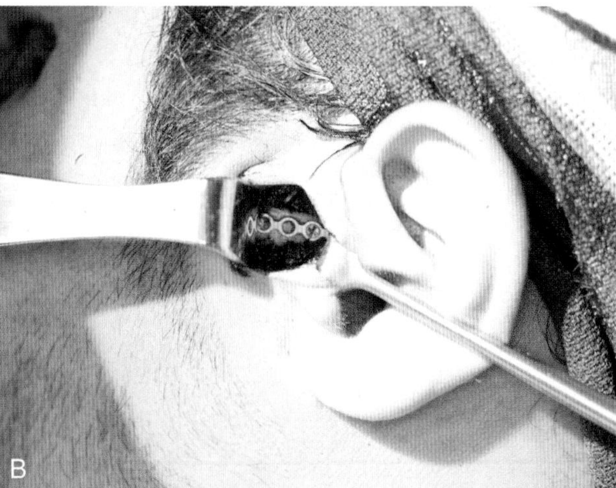

Fig. 53.7 **A,** Preplating of the proposed osteotomy sites with minimal soft tissue dissection. **B,** Preplating of the ipsilateral zygomatic arch via the preauricular approach.

TECHNIQUE—*cont'd*

STEP 7: Translocation of Osteotomized Facial Unit for Surgical Access

The facial translocation can be performed using gentle inferolateral displacement using a Smith bone spreader and Volkmann bone hook. Any bleeding should be controlled at this time. The translocated facial unit can be retracted inferolaterally and suspended using lone star elastic stays engaging the bony edges only. Extreme care should always be taken to avoid any periosteal stripping of the translocated facial unit (Fig. 53.8).

STEP 8: Ablation of the Tumor/Repair of Persistent Cerebrospinal Fluid Leak/Decompression of Optic Nerve

The ablative procedure is completed with wide access offered by facial translocation. The tumor's size and histology will dictate the ablative surgery. If the tumor extends posteriorly to skull base, one should be cautious to not inadvertently damage the ICA and internal jugular vein. This is especially true in the cases of salvage surgery status post chemoradiation therapy. In the cases of failed endoscopic repair of a cerebrospinal fluid leak and optic nerve decompression procedure, facial translocation can provide superior access.

STEP 9: Reconstruction

An ablative defect can be reconstructed using a pedicled temporalis, pericranial flaps, and/or a microvascular free flap, depending on the extent of the defect and the patient comorbidities (Fig. 53.9).

Continued

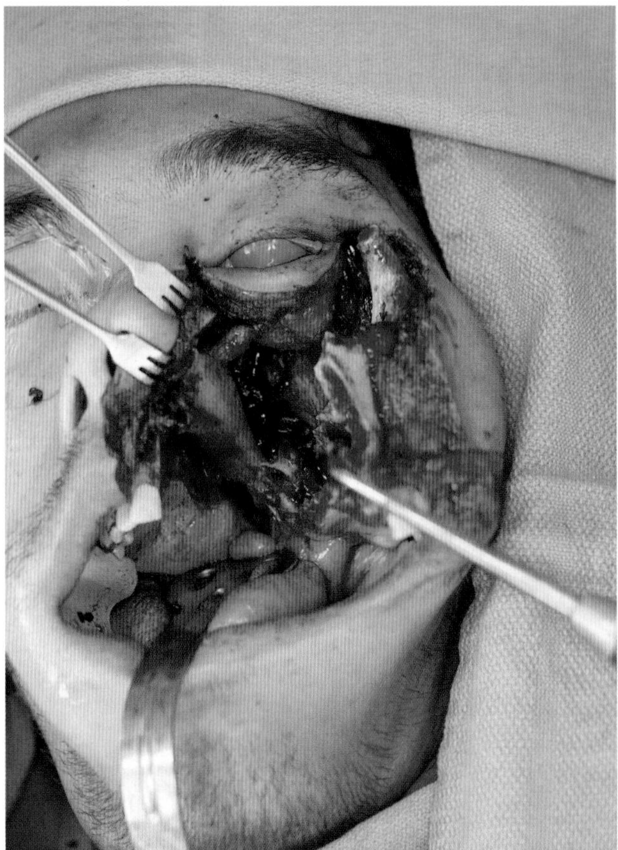

Fig. 53.8 Translocated composite facial bone graft allowing access to the nasopharyngeal carcinoma. Note the preservation of the nasal septum and minimal soft tissue dissection over the facial bone graft to preserve vascularity.

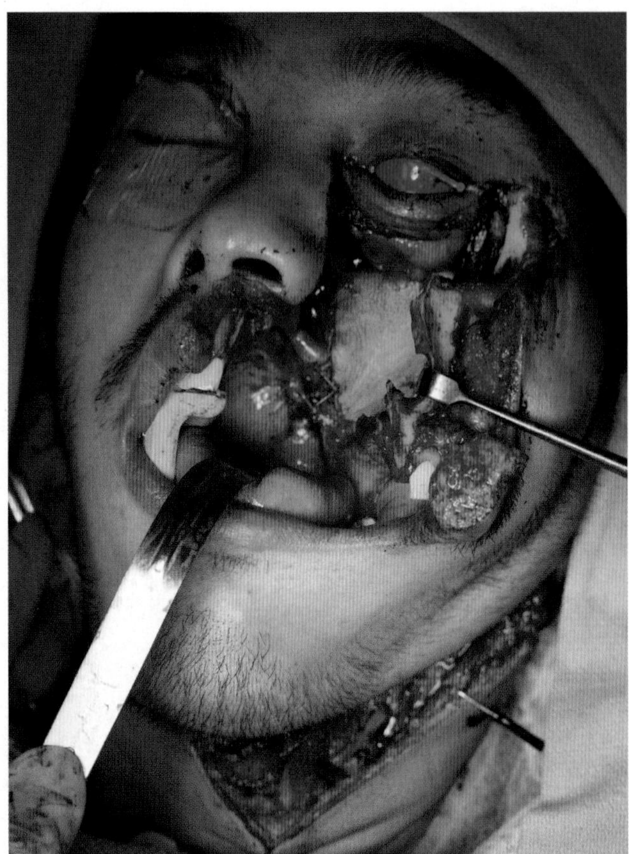

Fig. 53.9 Radial forearm free flap used for reconstruction of ablative defect.

TECHNIQUE—*cont'd*

STEP 10: Repositioning of Translocated Facial Unit and Fixation

Once the reconstruction is complete, the translocated facial unit can be repositioned and secured in place using the previously placed plates and screws. If a microvascular free flap reconstruction is used, an implantable Cook-Swartz Doppler probe can be useful for postoperative monitoring as the skin paddle may not be accessible for postoperative monitoring purposes.

STEP 11: Closure

The closure begins with resuspension of lateral canthus using 4-0 Vicryl suture. The facial incisions are approximated using 4-0 Vicryl for deep layers. Careful approximation should be used for the vermilion border incision. The oral incisions can be closed using 3-0 Vicryl or chromic gut sutures. If the incision extends from the mid-palatal region through the soft palate, layered closure is performed to avoid any velopharyngeal insufficiency. The skin layer can be approximated using 6-0 prolene suture in continuous or interrupted fashion (Fig. 53.10).

STEP 12: Adjunctive Procedures

Often, neck dissection is performed in cases of the malignant tumors. Careful consideration should be given to tracheostomy and feeding tube placement for airway protection and nutritional requirements, respectively, in the postoperative phase. The Valsalva maneuver should be performed prior to neck closure. Appropriate drains should be placed in the neck. A feeding tube can be passed through the contralateral nasal cavity if not violated or through the oral route.

STEP 13: Extubation

The patient is extubated during the postoperative intensive care unit phase to allow any airway edema to subside. If tracheostomy was performed, the patient can wean off the ventilator on postoperative day 1 as per the unit criteria.

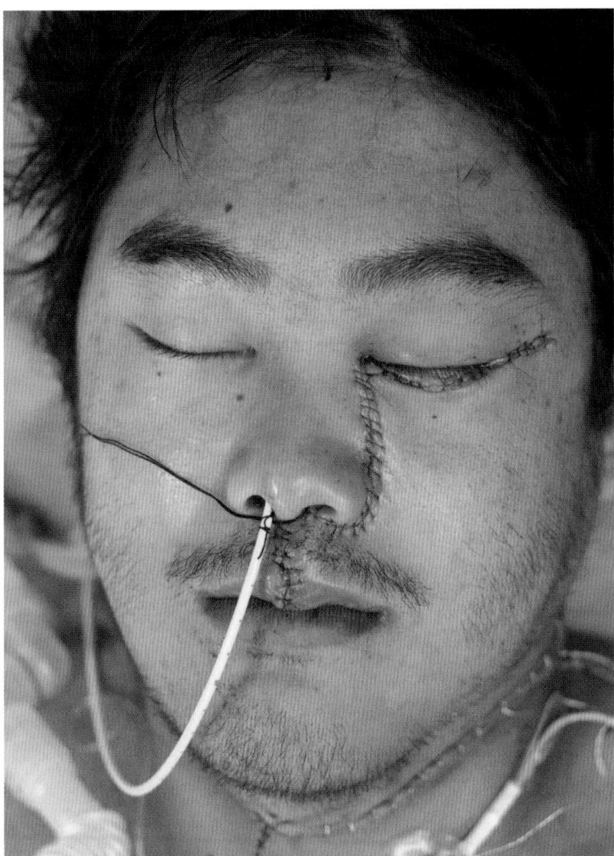

Fig. 53.10 Skin closure of the incision with lateral canthal suspension. Feeding tube for postoperative nutrition. An implantable Cook-Swartz Doppler probe is used for postoperative monitoring of the free flap.

ALTERNATIVE OR MODIFIED TECHNIQUE

Preservation of the integrity of the infraorbital nerve in facial translocation has been described by Ducic.[17] The craniofacial skeleton, except for the mandible, is directly supplied by periosteal perforators and muscular attachments.[18] These bones, unlike the mandible, have no intramedullary blood vessels. As a result, preservation of blood supply via the infraorbital artery can augment the redundant blood supply from the facial artery if the infraorbital nerve is released prior to translocating the facial unit. This will prevent traction injuries to the infraorbital nerve and minimize postoperative sensory disturbances. The operator can use subciliary incision instead of transconjunctival incision to avoid epiphora and entropion postoperatively.

Avoidance and Management of Intraoperative Complications

ICA blowout should be kept in mind if the patient has received more than 70 Gy irradiation, and if dissection is near the artery during surgery.[19] The surgeon may be better off removing the ICA to avoid the artery blowout. External carotid artery-internal carotid artery bypass should be considered in such instances to reduce the risk of cerebral ischemic stroke caused by resultant loss of blood supply due to the sacrifice of the ICA. Ducic described a technique to preserve the function of the infraorbital nerve, which improved access for facial translocation procedures.[17] This technique can be utilized if feasible to avoid any postoperative infraorbital sensory deficits.

Postoperative Considerations

1. The viability of translocated facial bone segment. In a retrospective review of 56 patients, Hao et al. noted that 12 patients (21.4%) had devitalized bone segment and required sequestrectomy. The incidence of devitalization was increased among the irradiated patients and was decreased in the patients whose paranasal sinuses defect was reconstructed with a vascularized flap.[20,21] The operator can secure the composite soft tissue flap to the translocated bone by using central and peripheral sutures to help early revascularization.[20] Hyperbaric oxygen therapy

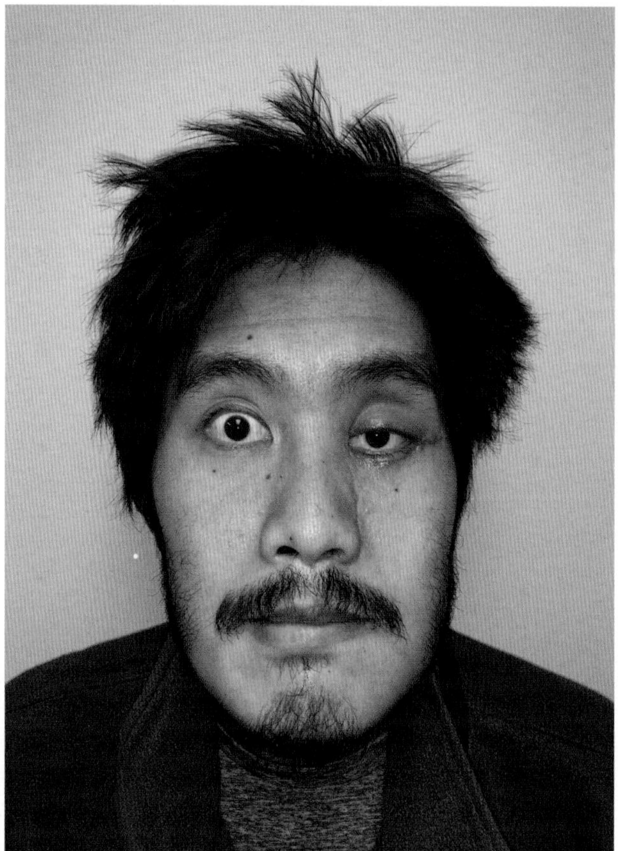

Fig. 53.11 Postoperative photo showing dystopia and enophthalmos due to increased orbital volume. Note the healing of the facial incision with minimal scarring.

is indicated in patients who have previous radiation history to the operative field and also in cases if the patient will be receiving postoperative radiotherapy after a facial translocation procedure.[11]

2. If the transcaruncular incision with medial canthal detachment is utilized instead of the subciliary incision, the reconstruction of the nasolacrimal system is indicated. Epiphora can be prevented by avoiding the transcaruncular incision. If the transcaruncular incision is used, Crawford tubes should be used for 6 to 8 weeks to allow lacrimal canaliculi repair.
3. Facial scarring can be minimized by carefully placing incisions in a natural skin crease or parallel to the resting skin tension lines.
4. Facial growth retardation can be prevented by selecting the infratemporal fossa approach instead of the facial translocation approach as this approach leaves the maxilla and midface undisturbed.[9] In contrast, Bales et al.[6] reported that none of the patients in their series demonstrated facial asymmetry at long-term follow-up.
5. Enophthalmos and dystopia may result if the orbital floor is inadvertently fractured due to the operator error intraoperatively or due to the tumor resection. This should be addressed immediately with evaluation of the orbital floor defect size and repaired with appropriate reconstructive material if indicated (Figs. 53.11 and 53.12).
6. If a free flap is used for reconstruction of skull base defect, Cook-Swartz internal Doppler should be used to allow arterial and venous monitoring of the vascular anastomosis as the skin paddle may not be accessed once the facial translocation unit is fixated.
7. Oronasal and/or oroantral fistula can result due to poor wound healing in some cases, especially in the cases of salvage surgery due to history of radiation exposure.
8. Osteoradionecrosis of the translocated facial bone graft or the skull base can occur due to higher radiation doses, which may result in postoperative infections and cerebrospinal fluid leak. The patients should be made aware of this complication, and hyperbaric oxygen therapy may be helpful in the preoperative and postoperative phases.[22,23]
9. Meningitis can result in the event of cerebrospinal fluid leak.[17] Adequate repair of dural tears using temporalis fascia, galeopericranial flap, fascia lata, and fat graft can prevent this complication if addressed at the time of facial translocation.[24]
10. ICA blowout is a frequent cause of death.[19,25]

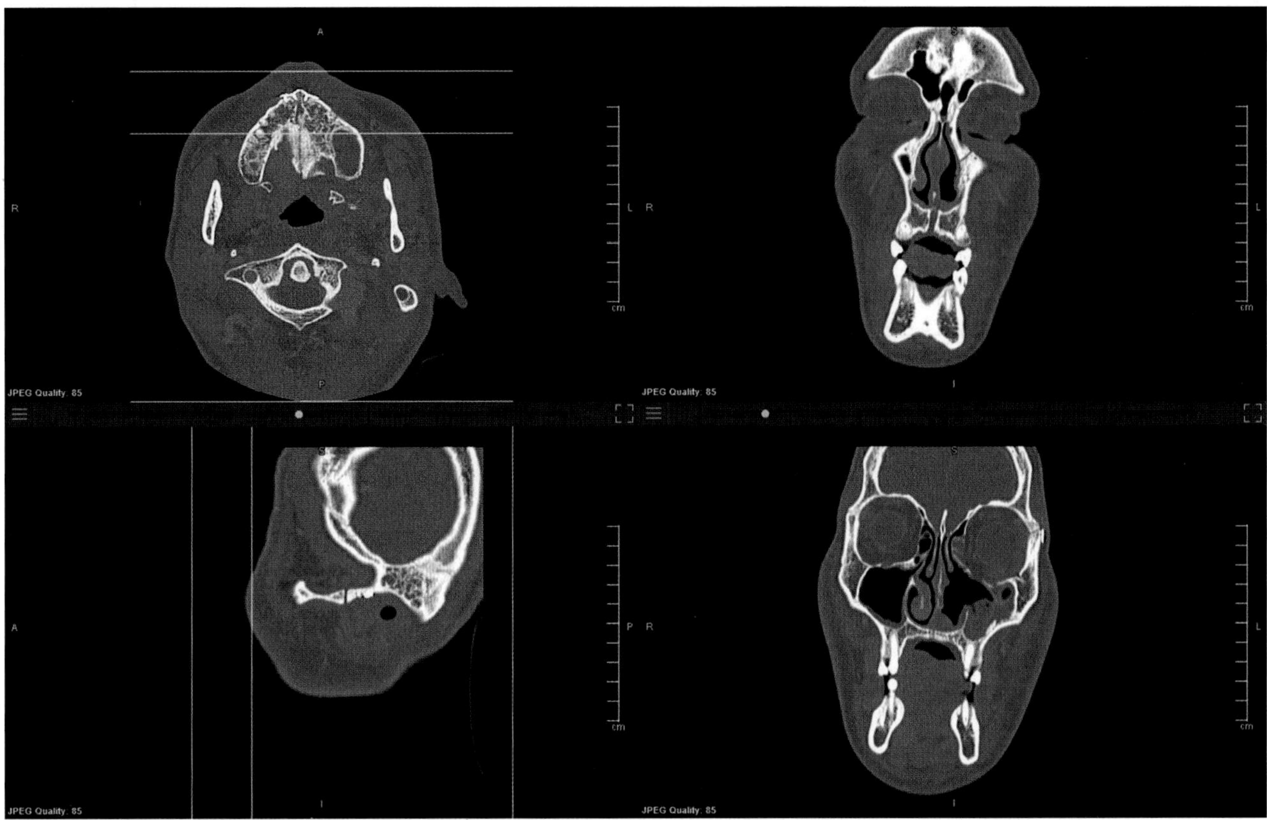

Fig. 53.12 Postoperative computed tomography images showing well-approximated osteotomy sites with intact hardware. A left inferior turbinectomy was performed at the time of facial translocation.

References

1. Janecka IP, Sen CN, Sekhar LN, Arriaga M. Facial translocation: a new approach to the cranial base. *Otolaryngol Head Neck Surg.* 1990;103(3):413–419.
2. Arriaga MA, Janecka IP. Facial translocation approach to the cranial base: the anatomic basis. *Skull Base Surg.* 1991;1(1):26–33.
3. Janecka IP, Sen CN, Sekhar LN, Nuss DW. Facial translocation for cranial base surgery. *Keio J Med.* 1991;40(4):215–220.
4. Forcada M, Montandon D, Rilliet B. Frontoethmoidal cephaloceles: transcranial and transfacial surgical treatment. *J Craniofac Surg.* 1993;4(4):203–209.
5. Janecka IP. Classification of facial translocation approach to the skull base. *Otolaryngol Head Neck Surg.* 1995;112(4):579–585.
6. Bales C, Kotapka M, Loevner LA, et al. Craniofacial resection of advanced juvenile nasopharyngeal angiofibroma. *Arch Otolaryngol Head Neck Surg.* 2002;128(9):1071–1078.
7. Movassaghi K, Janecka I. Optic nerve decompression via mid-facial translocation approach. *Ann Plast Surg.* 2005;54(3):331–335.
8. Netter F. In: *Atlas of Human Anatomy.* 6th ed. Elsevier; 2014.
9. Fagan JJ, Snyderman CH, Carrau RL, Janecka IP. Nasopharyngeal angiofibromas: selecting a surgical approach. *Head Neck.* 1997;19(5):391–399.
10. Dhirawani R, Asrani S, Pathak S, Sharma A. Facial translocation approach for management of invasive sinonasal aspergillosis. *J Maxillofac Oral Surg.* 2015;14(suppl 1):482–487.
11. Hao S-P, Tsang N-M, Chang C-N. Salvage surgery for recurrent nasopharyngeal carcinoma. *Arch Otolaryngol Head Neck Surg.* 2002;128(1):63–67.
12. Hussain A, Shakeel M, Vallamkondu V, Kamel M. Modified midfacial translocation for access to ventral skull base tumours. *J Laryngol Otol.* 2014;128(9):803–809.
13. de Mello-Filho FV, Mamede RCM, Ricz HMA, Susin RR, Colli BO. Midfacial translocation, a variation of the approach to the rhinopharynx, clivus and upper odontoid process. *J Cranio-Maxillo-Fac Surg.* 2006;34(7):400–404.
14. Hao S-P, Pan WL, Chang CN, Hsu YS. The use of the facial translocation technique in the management of tumors of the paranasal sinuses and skull base. *Otolaryngol Head Neck Surg.* 2003;128(4):571–575.
15. Chang K-P, Hao S-P, Tsang N-M, Ueng S-H. Salvage surgery for locally recurrent nasopharyngeal carcinoma—a 10-year experience. *Otolaryngol Head Neck Surg.* 2004;131(4):497–502.
16. Hao S-P, Tsang N-M, Chang K-P, Hsu Y-S, Chen C-K, Fang K-H. Nasopharyngectomy for recurrent nasopharyngeal carcinoma: a review of 53 patients and prognostic factors. *Acta Otolaryngol.* 2008;128(4):473–481.
17. Ducic Y. Preservation of the integrity of the infraorbital nerve in facial translocation. *Laryngoscope.* 2000;110(8):1415–1416.
18. Hao S-P. Modified facial translocation technique to prevent necrosis of bone graft. *Laryngoscope.* 2002;112(9):1691–1695.
19. Shu C-H, Cheng H, Lirng J-F, et al. Salvage surgery for recurrent nasopharyngeal carcinoma. *Laryngoscope.* 2000;110(9):1483–1488.
20. Hao S-P. Facial translocation approach to the skull base: the viability of translocated facial bone graft. *Otolaryngol Head Neck Surg.* 2001;124(3):292–296.
21. Suárez C, Llorente JL, Muñoz C, García LA, Rodrigo JP. Facial translocation approach in the management of central skull base and infratemporal tumors. *Laryngoscope.* 2004;114(6):1047–1051.
22. Sanger JR, Matloub HS, Yousif NJ, Larson DL. Management of osteoradionecrosis of the mandible. *Clin Plast Surg.* 1993;20(3):517–530.
23. Marx RE, Ames JR. The use of hyperbaric oxygen therapy in bony reconstruction of the irradiated and tissue-deficient patient. *J Oral Maxillofac Surg.* 1982;40(7):412–420.
24. Kuriakose MA, Trivedi NP, Kekatpure V. Anterior skull base surgery. *Indian J Surg Oncol.* 2010;1(2):133–145.
25. Chan JYW. Surgical management of recurrent nasopharyngeal carcinoma. *Oral Oncol.* 2014;50(10):913–917.

CHAPTER 54

Mandibular Distraction Osteogenesis in Craniofacial Deformities

Cesar A. Guerrero, Marianela Gonzalez, Elena Mujica, and Gisela Contasti-Bocco

Armamentarium

#9 Molt periosteal elevators (two)
#15 Scalpel blades
A series of chisels and one curved chisel
Allevyn Ag dressing
Appropriate sutures
Bipolar electrocautery (if necessary)
Cat paw retractors
Coronoid notch retractor
Curved Kocher with umbilical tape
Distraction kit and screwdriver
Fissure burs if third molars are present
Hargis retractor
"J" strippers
Jeter–Van Sickels bone clamp
Kelly hemostat
Langenbeck retractors
Local anesthetic with vasoconstrictor
Mallet
Mandibular pediatric distraction appliances
Metzenbaum scissors
Minnesota retractor
Mosquito forceps
Needle electrocautery
Needle electrocautery, bipolar
Osteotomes, fine
Pediatric gel horseshoe headrest and shoulder roll
Pear-shaped bur or a round bur if the mandible is to be set back
Periosteal elevators
Reciprocating saw
Steri-Strips
Surgairtome with fine bur (101)
Tegaderm dressing
Tenotomy scissors
Vari-Stim nerve stimulator
Wire pushing instrument "pickle fork"

History of the Procedure

Traditionally, patients with severe mandibular deficiency were treated with surgery alone or surgery combined with dental extractions and orthodontics.[1–5] Individuals who underwent major surgical movements showed limited results, severe relapse, condylosis, temporomandibular arthrosis, postoperative sleep apnea, and failures. The experienced surgeon knows the limitations of orthognathic surgery in multiple clinical situations, especially in large movements and particularly in patients with syndromic mandibles.

Another limiting issue is correcting the transverse dimension deficiencies. The orthodontist usually tries to increase the intercanine distance with mechanical methods, confronting either relapse or severe periodontal problems secondary to bringing the teeth outside the alveolar bone and producing secondary gingival recessions.[5] Extraoral distraction osteogenesis has been widely used to treat major mandibular deficiencies, but this method has led to facial scars and social inconveniences.[6] The latest technologies in intraoral distraction osteogenesis have evolved to offer a friendly and comfortable surgical technique.[7–13] The obstetrician, pediatrician, and pedodontist arc thc first practitioners to evaluate patients with severe three-dimensional mandibular deficiencies, with a severe class II malocclusion and anterior teeth crowding, with or without symmetry. They should manage this information to guide the patients according to the state-of-the-art technology.

Indications for the Use of the Procedure

This technology is indicated for patients who present with severe mandibular deficiency (more than 10 mm), temporomandibular arthritis, sleep apnea, previous failures in advancing the mandible, and inadequate anatomy (syndromic mandibles).[14,15]

Limitations and Contraindications

Intraoral distraction osteogenesis biology is based on sound surgical principles that depend on vascularity and bone quantity and quality. It should not be applied after radiotherapy or conditions involving very poor bone. Also, this technology requires patient and family collaboration.[14,15]

TECHNIQUE: Mandibular Widening

STEP 1: Incision and Dissection

The incision is made 4 to 6 mm labial to the depth of the mandibular vestibule through the orbicularis muscle. After the muscle is transected, the dissection is directed obliquely through the mentalis muscle until contact has been made with the mandibular symphysis. The periosteum is responsible for the distraction chamber healing and must be carefully reflected inferiorly to the lower border of the mandible; a small channel retractor is positioned to protect it throughout the osteotomy procedure.

STEP 2: Osteotomy

The osteotomy is carried out from the inferior border up to the apices with a reciprocating saw, the soft tissue between the mandibular central incisors is carefully reflected superiorly to the alveolar crest, and a skin hook is used to retract and protect the soft tissues while the interdental osteotomy is completed. The procedure is initiated with a 701 bur mounted in a straight handpiece; just the outer cortex and the sectioning are finalized with a straight chisel below the teeth, and the best anterior interdental space is selected for the osteotomy. A step may be necessary to start in the symphyseal midline and finish between the lateral and canine to avoid postsurgical chin asymmetry. Also, patients who need major widening (more than 8 mm) should have the genioplasty osteotomy performed simultaneously so as not to widen the lower part of the face, an undesirable feature in most women[16–18] (Fig. 54.1).

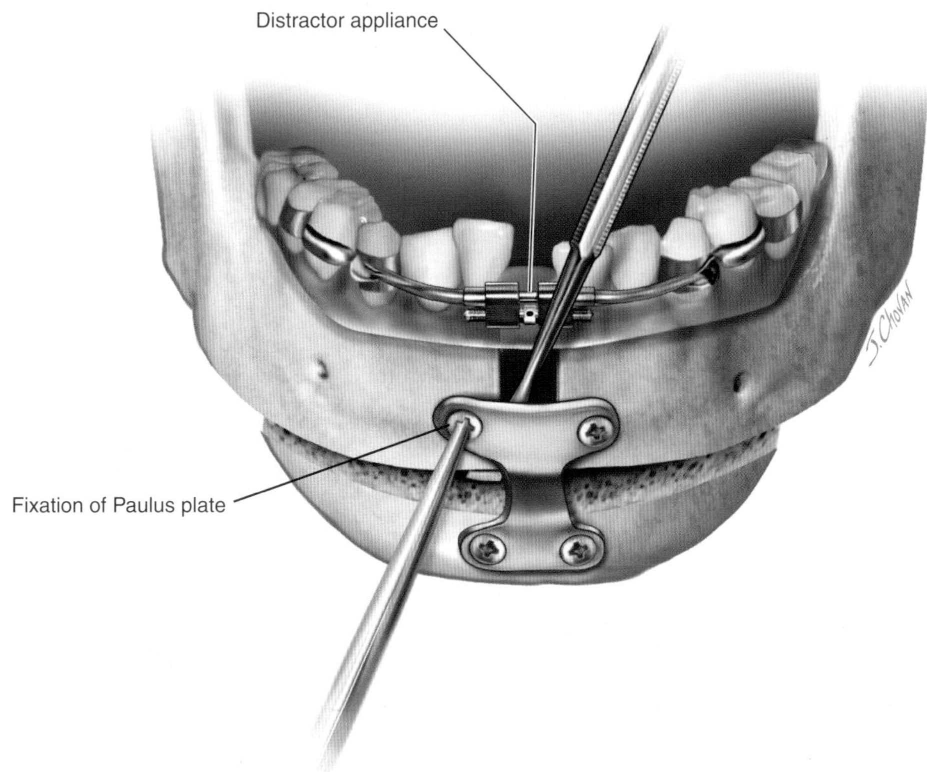

Figure 54.1 Mandibular widening with simultaneous genioplasty.

TECHNIQUE: Mandibular Widening—*cont'd*

STEP 3: Distractor Application

Tooth-borne appliances are commonly used because they are less expensive and time saving during surgery. If a bone-borne device is to be used, it must be fixed before the osteotomy is completed. The upper arms of the prebent bone-borne appliance are connected to the anchorage teeth with a 0.024-inch gauge wire, and a 2-mm transmucosal bicortical screw is used on each side to fixate the lower arms. Acrylic is placed over the wires around the teeth to provide more rigidity. The widening obtained is similar to that achieved with any distractor, but the tooth-borne distractor is easier to activate and remove.[11,15]

Most patients require an advancement genioplasty with vertical augmentation to ideally treat the three-dimensional deformity. This can be done simultaneously by acutely widening the mandibular basal bone with an instrument, fixating the chin segment, and then releasing the instrument from the osteotomy site.

At this point, a 0.026-inch gauge wire could be used to unite each central incisor to the consecutive lateral incisor or canine to prevent the teeth from "walking" into the distraction site secondary to transseptal fibers stretching during the activation period. Once the osteotomy and 2-mm activation have been performed, the periosteum, muscles, and mucosa wound layers are meticulously closed using a 3-0 chromic suture.

STEP 4: Distraction Protocol

The activation is initiated 7 days later, at a rate of 1 mm per day and a rhythm of once per day. Once the desired widening is obtained, acrylic is placed on the activation screw to stabilize it, and the patient is advanced to soft diet. The consolidation or mineralization stage usually lasts 60 days for every centimeter of distraction. Radiographs are used for confirmation, and then the surgeon removes the distraction device to follow orthodontic mechanics.[15,17,18] Following distraction removal, the orthodontist places a dental pontic or a plastic tooth, fixed with a bracket to the dental orthodontic arch. This maintains the open space for a few weeks as the teeth are brought together with slow movements of 1 mm per month per side, until there is complete closure. Faster movements into an unconsolidated bone area may create a periodontal defect and a gingival recession.

TECHNIQUE: Bilateral Mandibular Lengthening

Posterior Body Osteotomy

This osteotomy is designed for mandibular deficiencies that present ideal occlusal planes. Even though most patients with a severe class II show a steep curve of Spee with crowding, this secondary problem should be addressed by orthodontics, inferior-repositioning subapical osteotomy, or combining mandibular widening with advancement to correct the anterior crowding or transverse discrepancy. The treatment objective is to obtain an ideal canine and molar class I occlusion relation with a flat occlusal plane.[19,20]

The adequate positioning of the distraction is fundamental to achieve the correct distraction vector, and different variables are taken into consideration for adequate planning and fixation. The option of changing the distraction vector after surgery is sometimes employed for an ideal functional-aesthetic outcome.

The orthodontist and surgeon should plan the positioning of the distraction appliance based on photographs, radiographs, dental models mounted in an articulator, and clinical examination, sometimes requiring a three-dimensional model. The distractors need to be parallel to the occlusal plane to avoid developing a posterior or anterior open bite.[15]

Additionally, as the mandible is transversely wider in the posterior portion and narrower in the anterior portion, the distractor appliances need to be adjusted by creating a step of 5 to 8 mm in the anterior fixation arms, allowing the distractor's screw to be placed parallel to the axis of distraction to compensate for this important variation in mandibular width. If this is underestimated, the reciprocal forces exerted on the mandible by the appliance will advance the mandible, moving the proximal segment not only posteriorly (this could be overcome with the use of heavy class II elastics) but also laterally and exerting detrimental forces to the temporomandibular joint (TMJ), causing pain, dysfunction, and damage to the joints, as well as lateral torque force against the condyle, which can loosen the screws and bend the appliance.[20,21]

Mandibular advancement needs to be achieved by transporting the anterior segment anteriorly into an ideal class I occlusion and eliminating the posterior reciprocal forces with heavy class II elastics (8 to 12 ounces per side for 3 months).[15,20,21]

Continued

TECHNIQUE: Bilateral Mandibular Lengthening—*cont'd*

STEP 1: Incision and Dissection

A 2.5-cm full-thickness incision is made over the external oblique line, extending inferiorly over the alveolar ridge to the position of the first molar. A subperiosteal tunneling dissection is performed to expose the alveolar ridge and the buccal cortex down to the inferior border of the mandible between the second and third molars, where a small channel retractor is placed to protect the soft tissues during the osteotomy. The periosteum, muscles, and soft tissues are minimally detached, maintaining the best blood supply possible to the area.

STEP 2: Osteotomy

A reciprocating saw is used to section the inferior border of the mandible bicortically at a 45-degree angle to increase the bony surfaces, up to 3 mm away from the inferior alveolar nerve and continuing on the lateral mandibular cortex superiorly. A periosteal elevator is placed between the lingual soft tissues and the mandible to guard against lingual nerve injuries while the alveolar area is sectioned bicortically from the top toward the inferior alveolar nerve area 3 or 4 mm away, with the saw upside down and at a 45-degree angle. Abundant irrigation is used throughout the osteotomy to avoid bone overheating.

STEP 3: Distractor Application

At this point, the uncut bone is just 6 mm around the mandibular nerve, the flaps are sutured, and the distraction appliance is fixed with transmucosal bicortical screws above and underneath the nerve; an interdental wire could be used to avoid the need for interdental screws. A small incision is left open so that a torque movement can be applied with a chisel to complete the mandibular osteotomy, and a single mattress suture is placed to close the remnant of the flap; this maneuver ensures primary closure over the osteotomy, eliminating distraction chamber contamination and offering periosteum integrity. When the operation involves both sides, final sectioning of the ramus is deferred until the osteotomy of the opposite side has been completed. A sagittal split osteotomy could also be used to obtain a broader bone surface if adequate bone width is present; this approach is beneficial, in that it allows the surgeon to avoid pulling the mandibular nerve, especially in large advancements where the nerve is elongated 20% to 30% of its length, causing paresthesia[15,19–21] (Fig. 54.2).

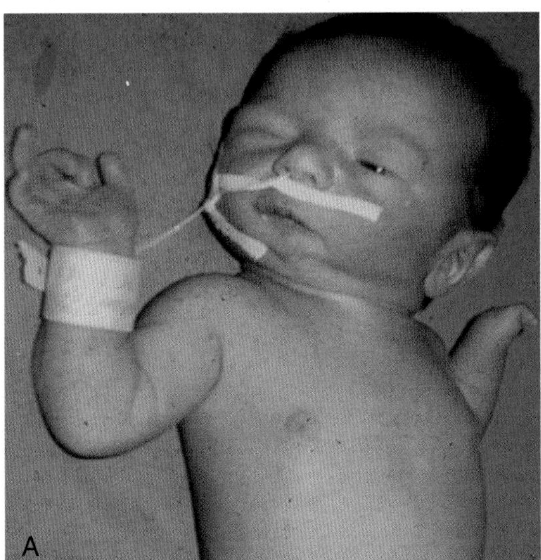

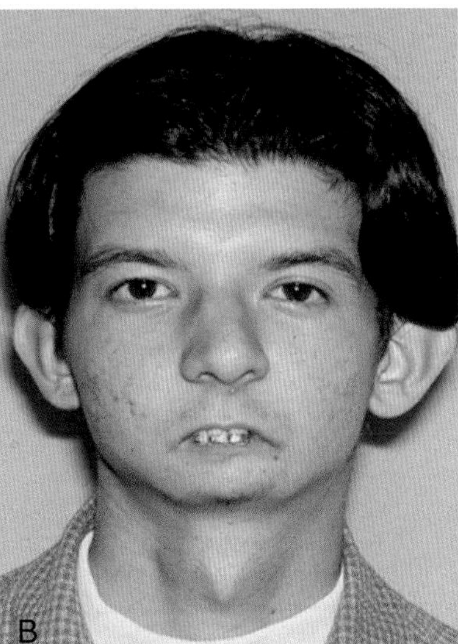

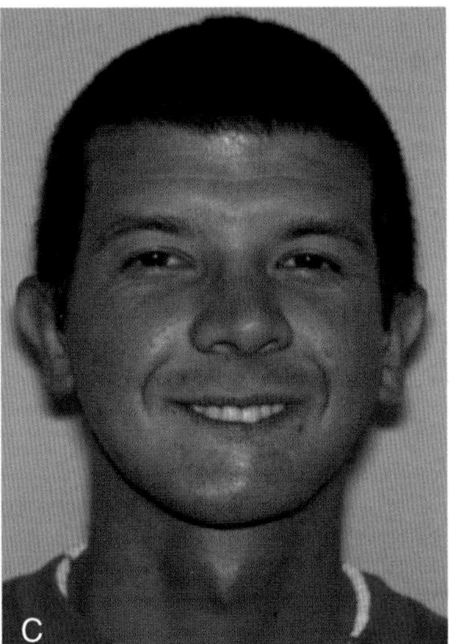

Figure 54.2 **A–O,** A hypoglossia-syndactyly syndromic patient underwent a two-stage intraoral mandibular widening and body lengthening with custom-made distractors to widen 20 mm and lengthen 15 mm. In a second stage, the appliances were removed, and vertical chin distraction of 9 mm was executed. A 10-year follow-up shows a stable occlusion, although many teeth were absent, and there were remarkable facial and dental changes. Combined maxillomandibular widening and body lengthening resulted before the commercial distractors were available. Auriculoplasties were also performed on the second surgical stage. This technology was not available when the patient was born, and traditional osteotomies only allowed minor movements.

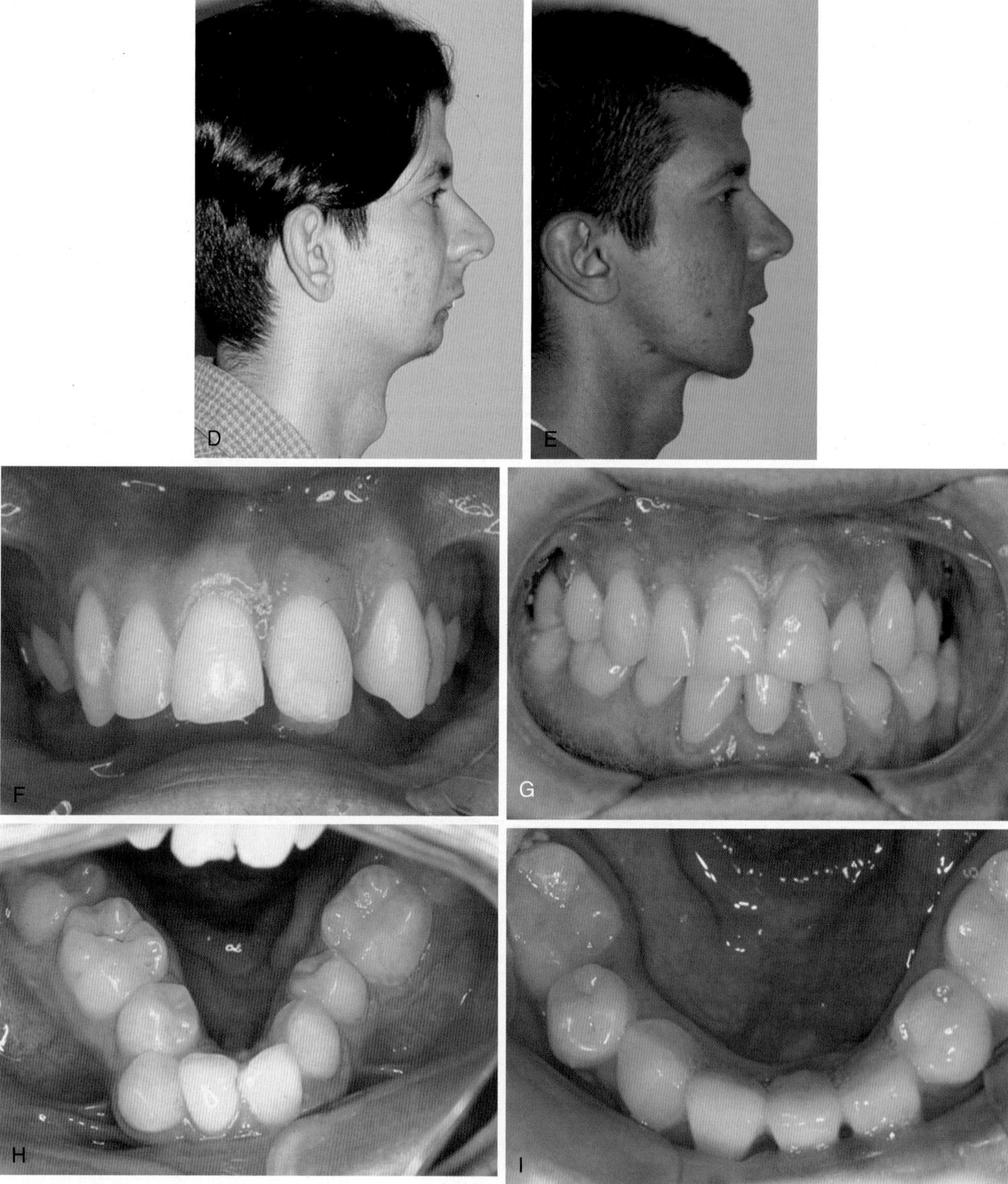

Figure 54.2, cont'd

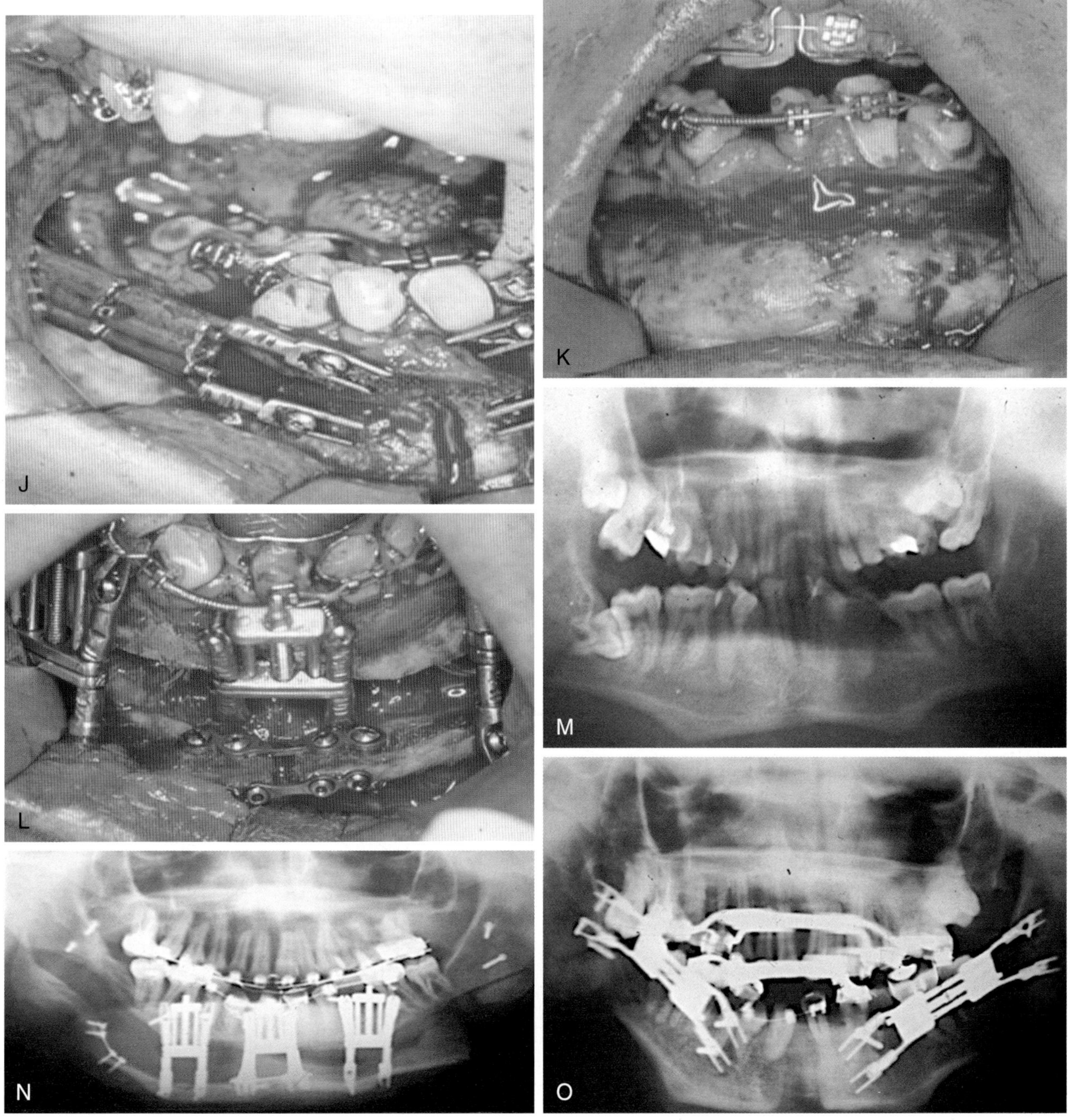

Figure 54.2, cont'd

ALTERNATIVE TECHNIQUE 1: Parasymphyseal Osteotomy

This option is indicated in patients with inadequate anatomy at the mandibular angle area region, who usually present with a severe anterior open bite and severe crowding. This mandibular area possesses the best bone stock, which has over 3 cm of height and 1 cm of basal bone width. It is an interdental osteotomy, which may require presurgical orthodontics to create an interdental space. The distraction gap is utilized to align and level the occlusion postsurgically, or dental implants could be inserted. This technique is also ideal for major movements, as it is anterior to the mental nerve and the mandibular nerve is not stretched or damaged.[15,19–21]

ALTERNATIVE TECHNIQUE 1: Parasymphyseal Osteotomy—*cont'd*

STEP 1: Incision and Dissection

A 3-cm incision is made 4 to 6 mm inferior to the attached gingiva, well above the mental nerve. A subperiosteum dissection is carried out, exposing the mental nerve and inferior border of the mandible to allocate a channel retractor.

STEP 2: Osteotomy

The osteotomy is executed from the inferior border to the level of the dental roots, under abundant irrigation to avoid bone overheating. Next, a 701 bur mounted in a straight handpiece is used to complete the outer cortex bone section between the teeth, and a straight chisel is used to complete the osteotomy.

STEP 3: Distractor Placement

The distractor is fixed with inferior bicortical screws, interdental wires are used around the teeth, and acrylic is applied on top to increase rigidity and to avoid damaging the roots with heat and screw placement.[15,19–21] Ideally, the wound is closed before the distractor is fixed so that there is a close distraction chamber without food and saliva contamination.

The distraction protocol is similar; however, as the distraction chamber enlarges, the open bite increases; this is determined in the planning and prediction phases. The patient requires a major advancement at the mandibular base and a few millimeters between the teeth, once most of the activation has been completed. The patient is taken to the operating room so that the surgeon can change the mandibular vector by eliminating the wires and acrylic from the anterosuperior distractor arm, keeping only a single inferoanterior bicortical screw; bilaterally, the mandible rotates counterclockwise, closing the open bite. It is important to have extra millimeters left in the distractor rod to accommodate the midline and make final adjustments in the occlusion.[15,19–21]

Children with first dentition requiring mandibular lengthening need Erich arch bars during surgery for class II elastics placement through the activation and consolidation phases and postsurgical occlusion control. The clinician needs to monitor the range of opening and avoid mandibular deviation during function; physiotherapy is mandatory to obtain at least a 40-mm opening in a vertical straight fashion.[15,19–21]

The surgeon rigidly fixates the distractors using bicortical screws, while avoiding teeth and the alveolar nerve. When a bicortical screw cannot be placed without damaging a dental structure, a 0.024-inch gauge wire can be used to fixate the distractor. A transcutaneous trocar could be used to place the distractor's posterior screws, especially in small children, patients with small oral commissures, or where the vertical osteotomy is located too far posterior.[15,19–21]

STEP 4: Distraction Protocol

A 7-day latency period follows surgery, which allows time for collagen type I fibers to develop, primary soft tissue to heal, and the initial surgical edema to reduce. Activation follows at a rate of 1 mm and a rhythm of once a day until the desired distraction is complete. While the patient is activating the distractors, close monitoring should take place to avoid midline deviations owing to inadequate counterclockwise or uneven activation of the distraction devices. If needed, asymmetric activation should be done to correct a midline discrepancy.[15,19]

An important issue is the TMJ. The presurgical orthodontic phase should include rectangular surgical orthodontic arches with welded vertical pins to apply class II elastics for 3 months after surgery until the muscles enlarge and adapt.

After total activation is accomplished, acrylic is placed over the distraction's rod for stabilization purposes, and the appliances are used throughout the consolidation period as a fixation system. Radiographs are taken to verify the distraction chamber ossification for appliance removal.

A liquid diet, including high-protein supplements, is recommended during the activation period, followed by a soft diet once the distractor is stabilized with acrylic until consolidation is achieved, typically between 2 and 12 months according to the magnitude of the movement[15,19,21] (see Fig. 54.2).

ALTERNATIVE TECHNIQUE 2: Unilateral Mandibular Lengthening

Patients with unilateral craniofacial microsomia, unilateral Treacher Collins syndrome, or other forms of unilateral micromandibulism may present with minimal bone stock in the postmolar and angle regions, compromising the possibility of performing either traditional surgery or distraction osteogenesis; frequently, these patients require major movements. In these clinical cases, it is advisable to plan the surgery along the body of the mandible between the premolars, anterior to the mental nerve, because of bone stock and to avoid lip paresthesia. Some patients benefit from vertical ramus and horizontal body lengthening performed simultaneously.[22,23]

TECHNIQUE: Ramus Lengthening Procedure

When the height of the mandibular ramus increases, the TMJ function is fundamental. The reciprocal forces exerted toward the glenoid fossa secondary to lengthening the pterygoid–masseteric sling will maintain a continuous pressure and provoke disk displacement, condylar resorption, and TMJ arthrosis. The process is similar to that used to lengthen the femur: the orthopedic surgeon places two rings in the femur with expansible screws and another ring across the tibia and fibula, with maintenance bars, in order to avoid detrimental forces into the knee, crushing the cartilages and producing arthrosis.[22–24]

There are three different scenarios for lengthening the mandibular ramus: a unilateral mandibular deficiency with a functional condyle, a unilateral mandibular deficiency with a gap between the malformed condyle and the glenoid fossa, and TMJ ankylosis. Each group should be treated differently to obtain a symmetric mandibular frame and a functional TMJ as determined by function, aesthetics, and stability in time. These are complicated patients, and many of them will present after numerous surgical failures. The clinician must perform all the surgical procedures in one stage, if possible, or perform as many as indicated in every surgical stage.[23,24]

TECHNIQUE: Ramus Procedure With a Functional Condyle

STEP 1: Incision and Dissection

A 3-cm incision is made in the lateral retromolar area to allow wide periosteal elevation of the lateral mandibular ramus up to the coronoid process.

STEP 2: Osteotomy Design

A horizontal osteotomy is performed above the antilingula to ensure there is no damage to the mandibular nerve and vessels. Before completing the cut, rigid fixation is placed from the body of the zygoma to the upper mandibular ramus segment to stabilize the cranium to the upper mandibular ramus segment. A horizontal incision in the maxillary molar area, followed by exposing the zygoma, allows at least three screws to be inserted into the body, and the remaining plate is inserted through the soft tissue into the lateral mandibular area; another three screws are inserted into the coronoid vicinity area.

STEP 3: Distractor Placement

The mandibular osteotomy is complete after the distractor has been fixed into both mandibular segments and a connector emerges extraorally through a 2-mm incision. The connector will allow activation and should be removed once the clinician has completed the objectives. The distraction appliances remain in place until adequate consolidation occurs; this can be observed radiographically. Once the patient has been placed under intravenous sedation or general anesthesia, the distractor is removed intraorally, and the rigid fixation plate is disconnected through the retromolar incision and the maxillary incision to get to the body of the zygoma (Fig. 54.3).

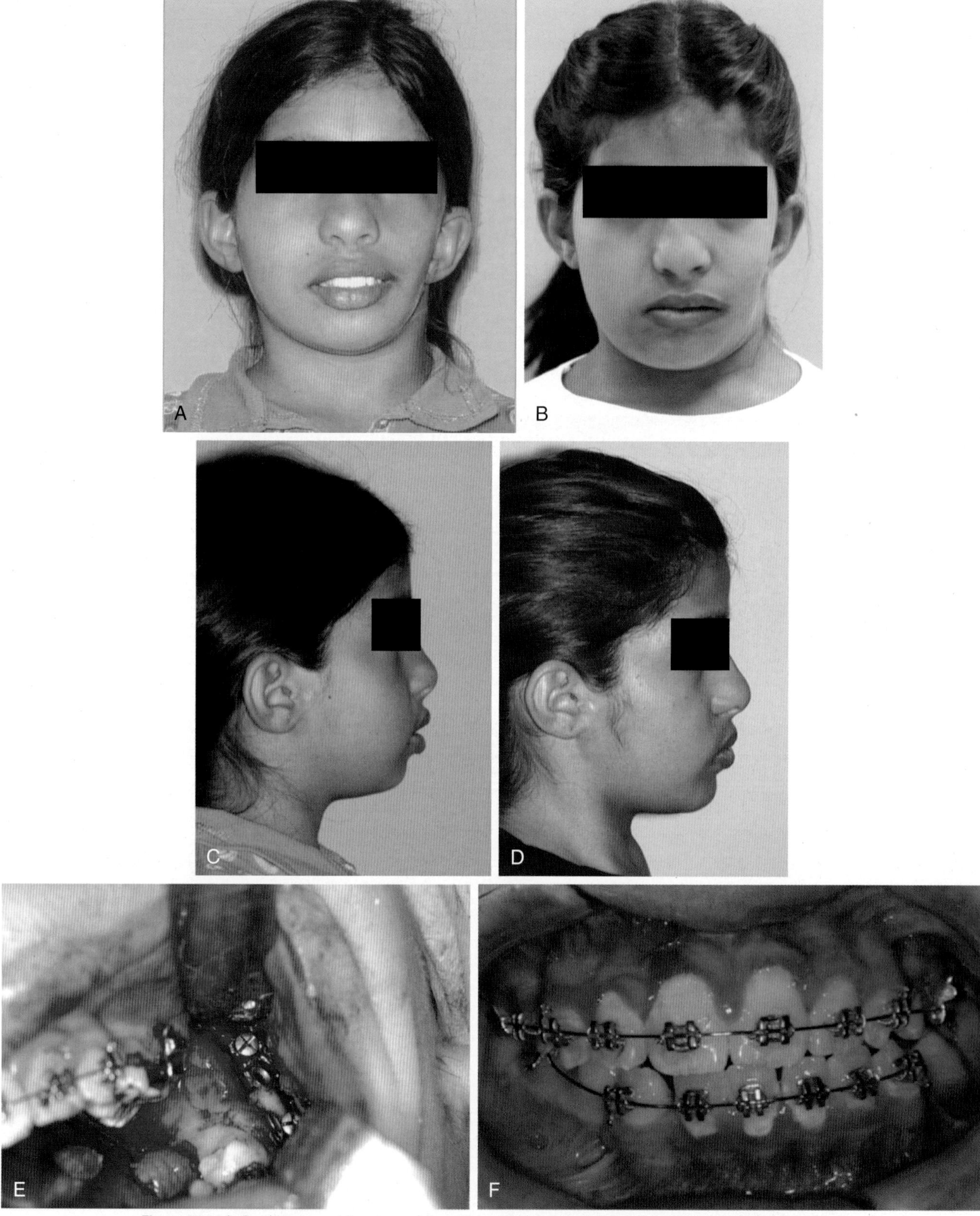

Figure 54.3 **A–L,** A 9-year-old patient with unilateral left craniofacial microsomia type II B treated by intraoral mandibular ramus lengthening. A zygoma to the superior mandibular fragment was rigidly fixated to avoid temporomandibular joint (TMJ) compression and damage. Once the distraction chamber healed, the distractor and the rigid fixation were removed, and orthodontic treatment was continued. An incision is made to expose the zygoma, the masseter muscle insertion to the zygomatic arch is cut and separated to allow fixation of a "Y" type 2.0 plate with 8-mm-long screws in the posterior zygoma body, and then the plate is connected to the coronoid process and screws inserted via the lateral mandibular ramus. Ramus lengthening continues with the use of an intraoral distractor with an external connector. This procedure is done intraorally, using only a stab incision to bring the connector out and allow it to be activated. Orthodontic treatment follows surgery. A soft tissue augmentation via free fat graft should be performed in the future.

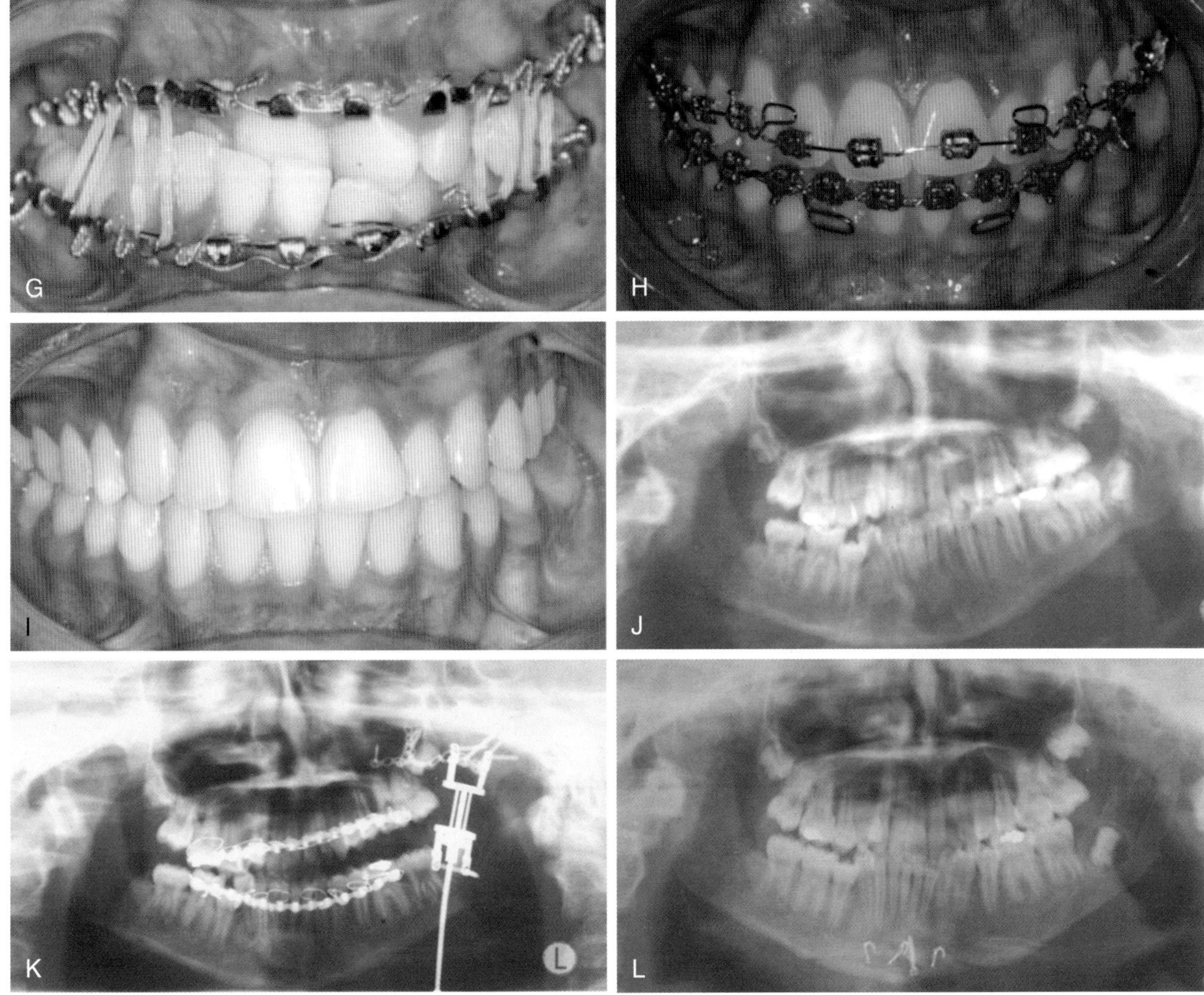

Figure 54.3, cont'd

TECHNIQUE: Condylar Bone Transport to Lengthen the Ramus and Close the Gap

After the patient's records have been carefully evaluated and three-dimensional models made, the distractors are cut to length, bent, and adapted to the clinical situation. The distractors are fixed to the model and acrylic section to simulate the actual surgery. The screws' length and positioning are selected, and they should be ready in the exact order needed for the surgical intervention. This is a timesaver maneuver that needs to be done carefully and meticulously to warrant the surgical outcome.

STEP 1: Incision and Dissection

A 3-cm incision is made at the lateral mandibular area, allowing exposure of the lateral mandibular angle and bone stump, and the medial and posterior soft tissues are left intact to ensure vascularization. This is a pedicle segment to be transported, not a free graft.

TECHNIQUE: Condylar Bone Transport to Lengthen the Ramus and Close the Gap—*cont'd*

STEP 2: Osteotomy

The osteotomy is performed with a reciprocating saw under abundant irrigation in a 15- to 20-degree angulation to increase the bone surface.

STEP 3: Distractor Placement

Before osteotomy has been completed, a 2-mm incision is made at the mandibular angle skin so as to insert the distraction's connector inside out and to localize the selected distractor, which is fixed with three screws (using the tripod concept) on either side of the osteotomy; then the section is completed.

A second distractor is usually placed in the body of the mandible for horizontal lengthening. This second distractor is placed after the ramus surgery has been concluded[22–24] (Fig. 54.4).

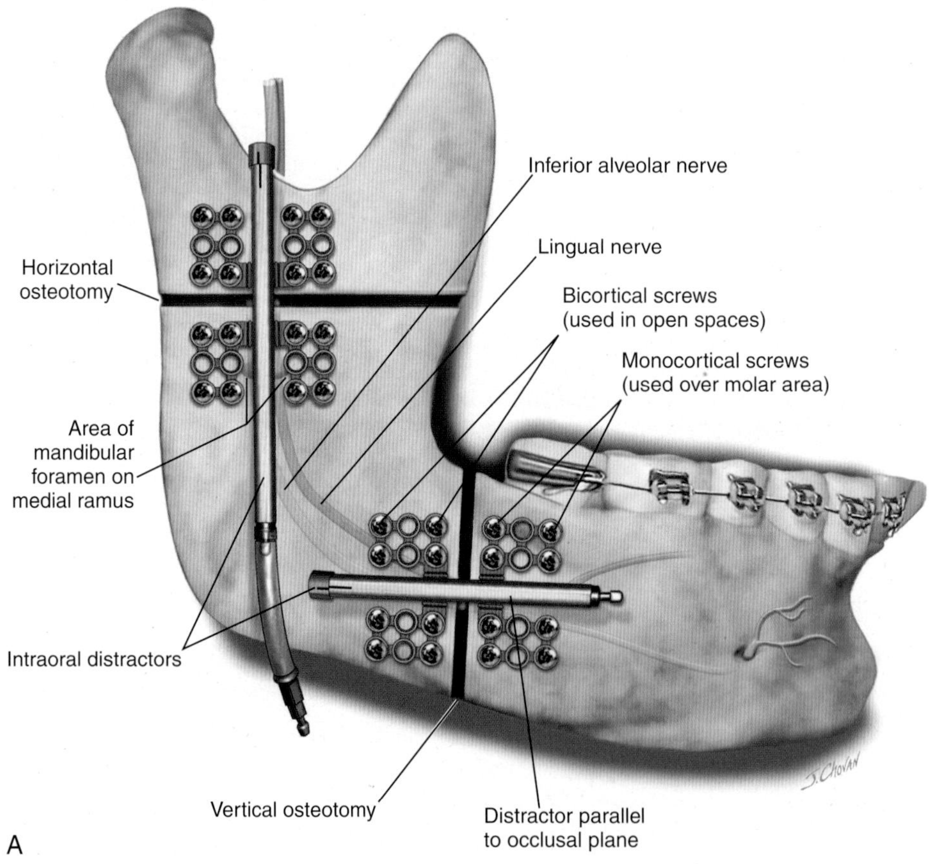

Figure 54.4 **A,** Horizontal and vertical osteotomies for distractor placement.

Continued

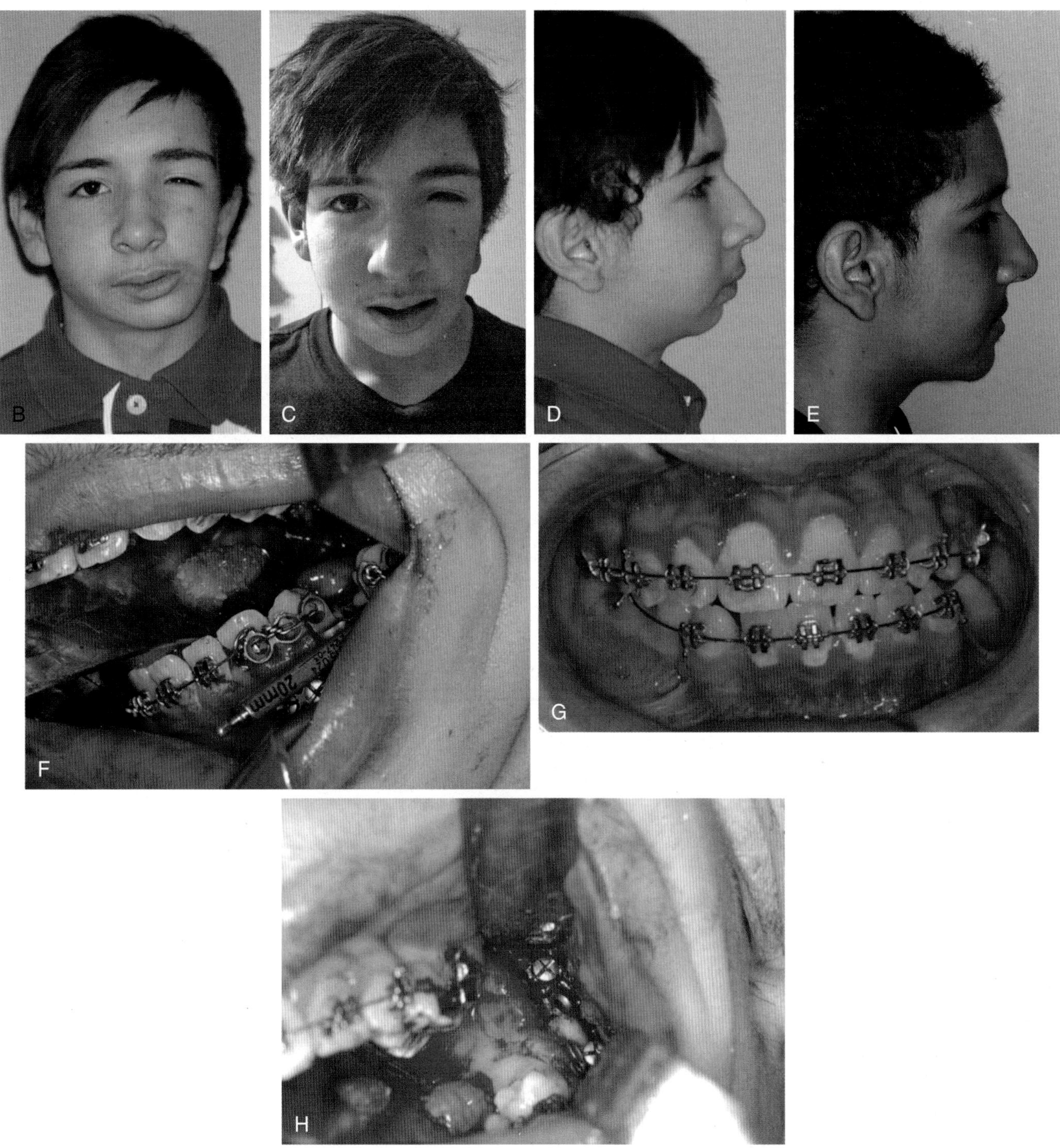

Figure 54.4, cont'd **B–O,** A severe left grade III craniofacial microsomia in a 12-year-old patient, with left mandibular body underdevelopment treated by orthodontics combined with simultaneous intraoral body and ramus mandibular distraction osteogenesis. A removable connector was used to activate the vertical appliance and allow bone transport toward the glenoid fossa. The bony segments were augmented to create symmetry with the contralateral side, the remaining occlusion was treated orthodontically, and the interdental space created in the right mandibular body was completed with dental implants.

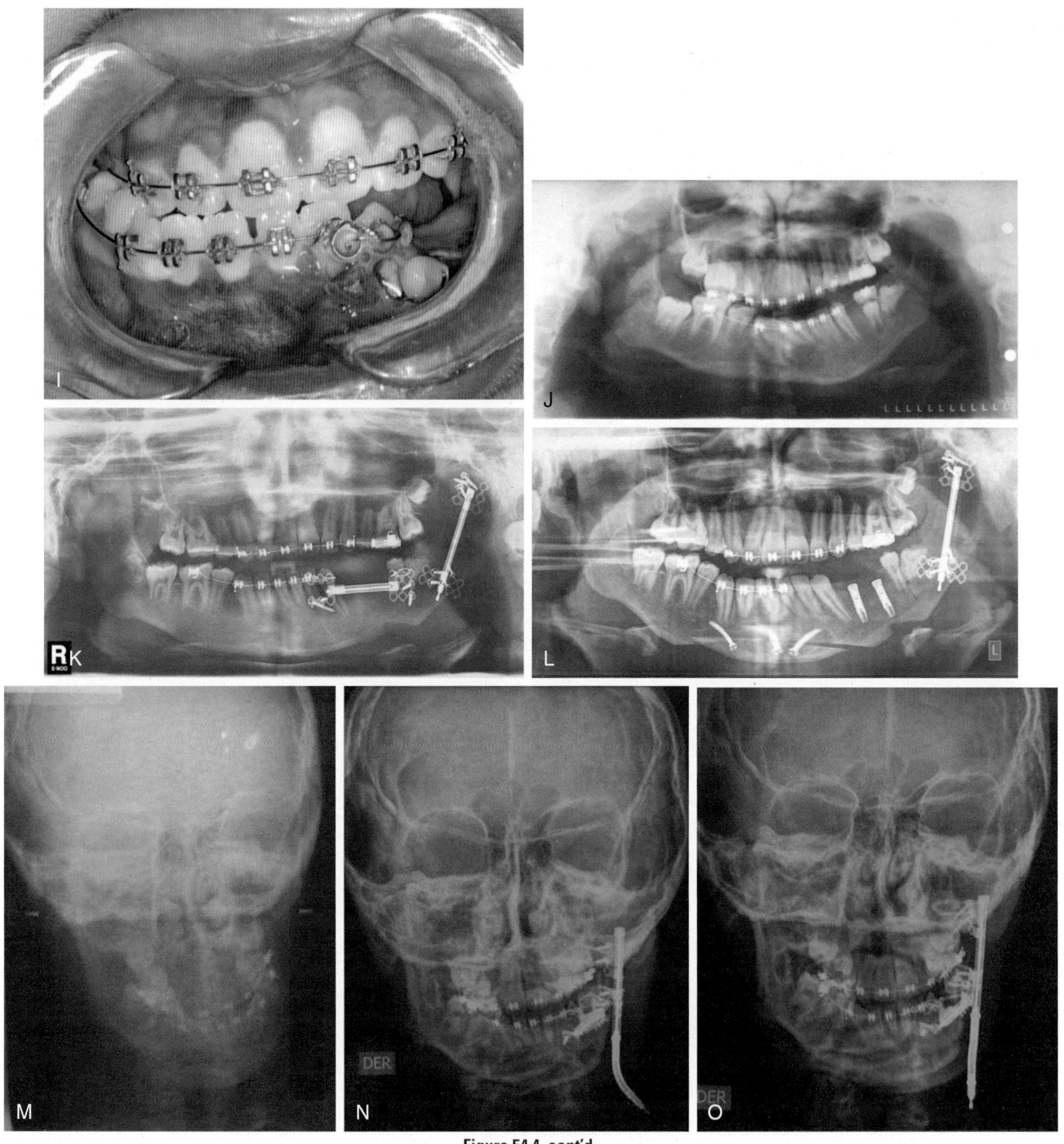

Figure 54.4, cont'd

TECHNIQUE: Ramus Lengthening in TMJ Ankylosis

Historically, long-term ankylosis in children involves severe mandibular growth arrest and sleep apnea. Most surgical procedures were wrongly planned to release the ankylosis first and in a secondary surgical stage improve the mandibular shape and size, frequently ending in reankylosis.[23]

The TMJ ankylosis patient will require two surgical stages and long-term physiotherapy to rehabilitate the joint. The first stage includes enlargement of the mandibular frame by lengthening the mandibular ramus and body, as well as a major genioplasty; these three procedures increase the mandible frame and lengthen the perimandibular muscles; the distractors are left in place until complete consolidation. There is no relapse because the muscles and bone have matured in a new position for longer than 6 months. In the second surgical stage, through the same Risdon approach, the distraction appliance is removed and TMJ arthroplasty is performed, continuing with either a maxillary Le Fort I or a partial maxillary osteotomy to close the lateral open bite and to eliminate the maxillary cant, if necessary (in younger children, orthodontic means are sufficient), and a secondary genioplasty is performed to obtain ideal anterior symmetry.

The secondary genioplasty is needed to reduce the muscles' push against the newly performed arthroplasty and to avoid ankylosis recurrence because increasing the mandibular frame in the first surgical stage will have created a stable muscle environment that allows for stability during second-stage osteotomies.

There may be a need for lateral ramus augmentation on the affected side. When required, this procedure is performed a year after facial muscles have healed and stabilized, the physiotherapy has been completed, and the orthodontics (braces) have been removed. A preformed mandibular angle prosthesis is indicated.[23]

TECHNIQUE: Ramus Lengthening in an Ankylosed TMJ Procedure

STEP 1: Incision and Osteotomy

Utilizing the submandibular Risdon approach, a 3-cm incision is made through the skin, platysma muscle, and periosteum. The mandibular angle and the ramus are exposed completely, the ankylosis area is identified, and a horizontal osteotomy is performed using a reciprocating saw, which protects the anterior and posterior soft tissues with channel retractors above the antilingula and avoids the mandibular bundle medially.

STEP 2: Distractor Placement

Once the segment is mobilized, the prebent, preshaped distraction appliance and measured screws from the three-dimensional model are installed. The surgeon carefully checks the distraction vector to ensure that it is similar to the unaffected side.

The internal distractor is provided with a connector to be exposed extraorally at the submandibular incision site. The area is copiously irrigated, and the wound is closed in layers. The appliance is activated intraoperatively 2 or 3 mm to avoid premature consolidation. This is probably the best distraction osteogenesis environment, as it involves a close chamber and the best blood supply with a wide bone contact, especially because the osteotomy is performed in a diagonal fashion (at a 15- to 25-degree angle), secondary to the inclination working from below through the Risdon incision (Fig. 54.5A–C).

STEP 3: Distraction Protocol

Seven days after surgery, the activation starts for 1 mm every day until the desired distraction is obtained. At that point, new radiographs are taken to measure the facial skeleton in detail, and then the patient is scheduled for connector removal. The connector is removed by twisting the screwdriver in the other direction (if the connector head has a double system, internal for the activation and external for removal), and it is released from the distractor or is cut off under the skin. Steri-Strips are placed over the small wound, and during the second surgical stage, the scar should be removed and a new cosmetic closure performed. The patient resumes regular activities without any limitations while wearing the internal distractor.[23]

Once adequate consolidation is observed in the radiographs, usually 8 to 12 months after the first surgical stage, the patient undergoes surgery to have the distraction devices removed, TMJ arthroplasty, and leveling Le Fort I osteotomy[2,22] (see Fig. 54.5).

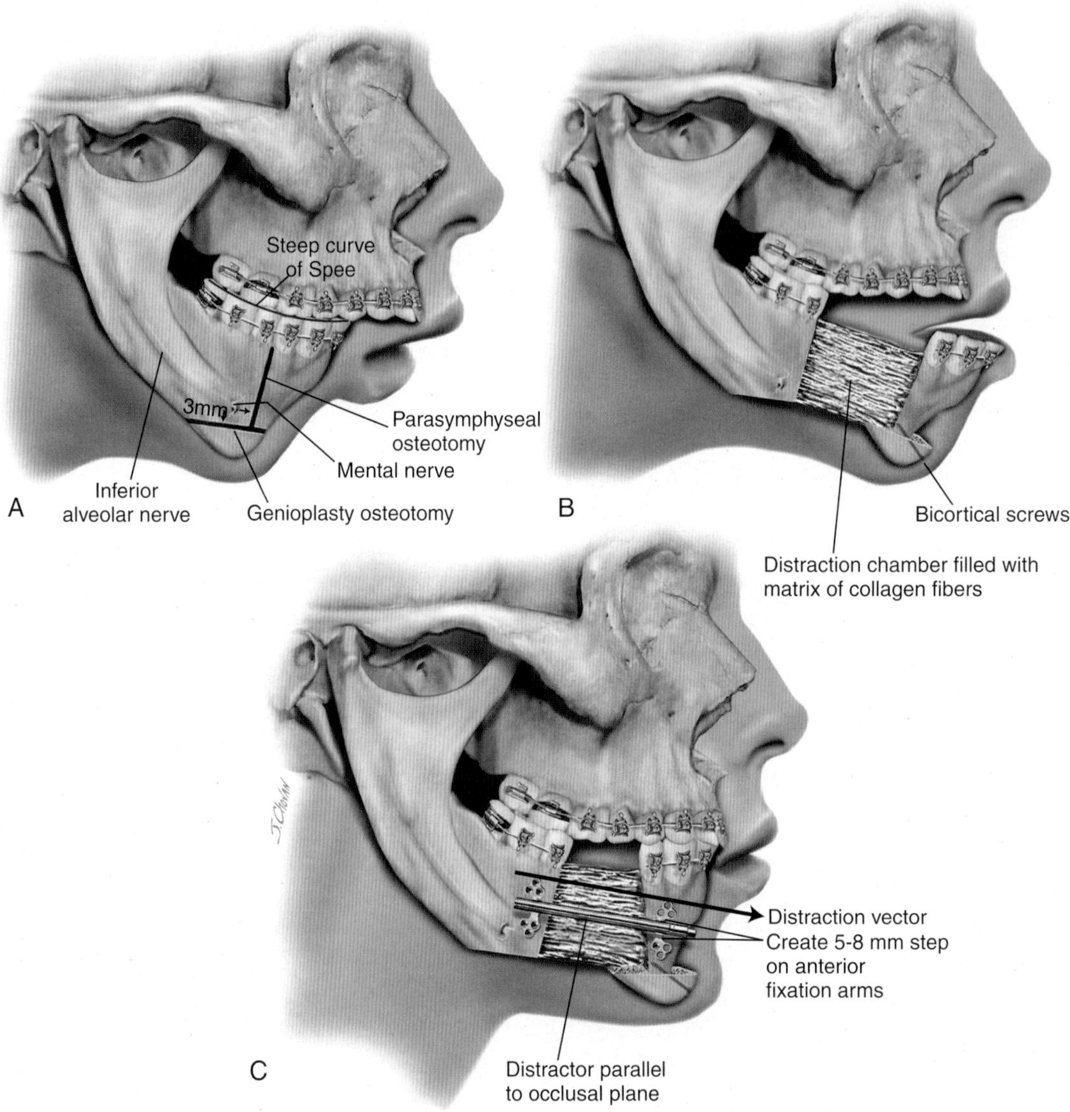

Figure 54.5 **A–C,** Mandibular-lengthening parasymphyseal osteotomy with genioplasty.

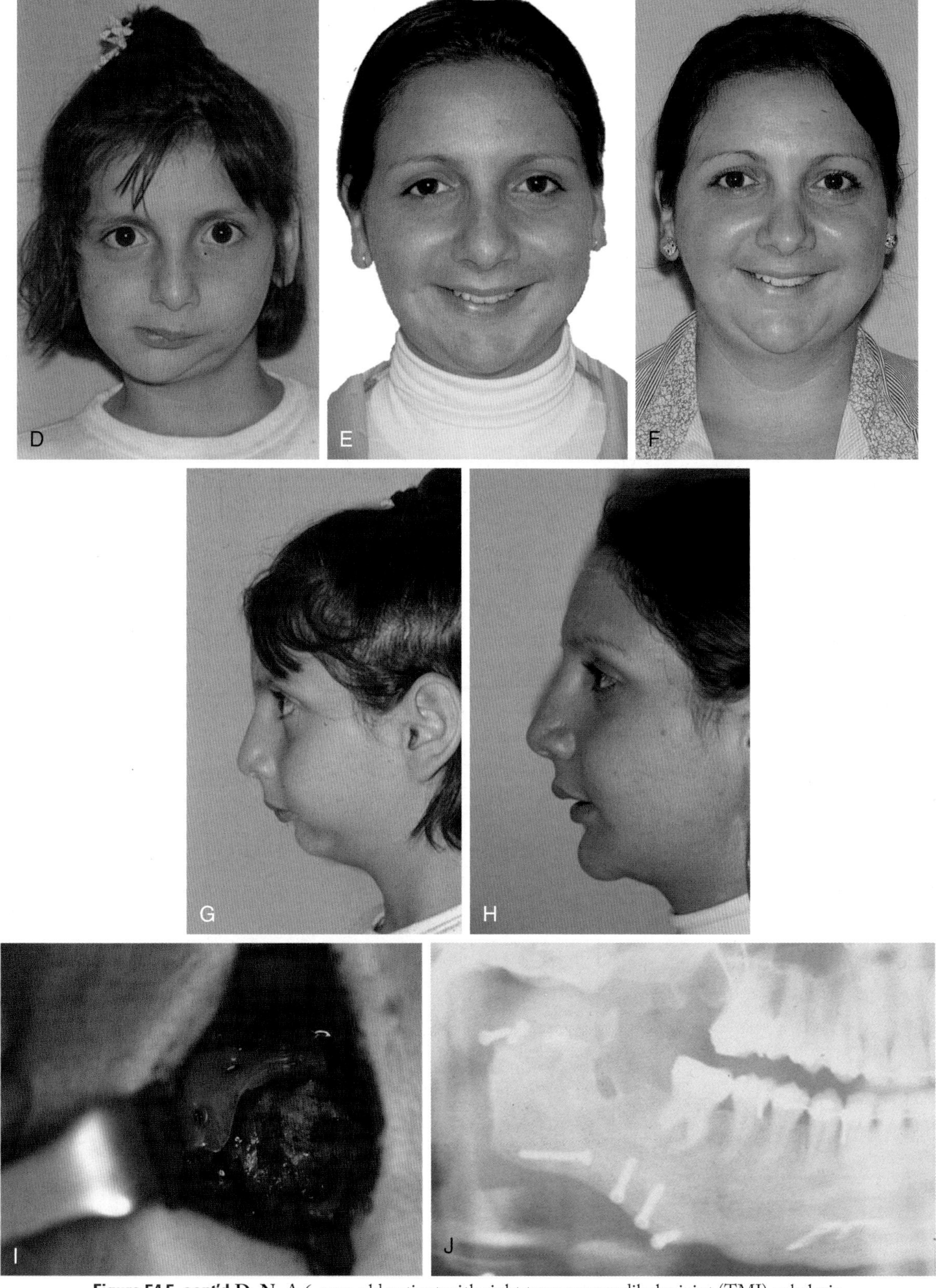

Figure 54.5, cont'd D–N, A 6-year-old patient with right temporomandibular joint (TMJ) ankylosis, after falling from a tree. She underwent two surgeries, orthodontics, and physiotherapy for mandibular rehabilitation. This is a 20-year follow-up. The first surgery was performed to lengthen the mandibular body and ramus with intraoral distractors, once the patient consolidated the distraction chambers; a second surgery was scheduled to correct the chin positioning and a gap arthroplasty with silicon fixed with bicortical screws. **O–R,** Before and after facial photographs and lateral cephalic radiographs.

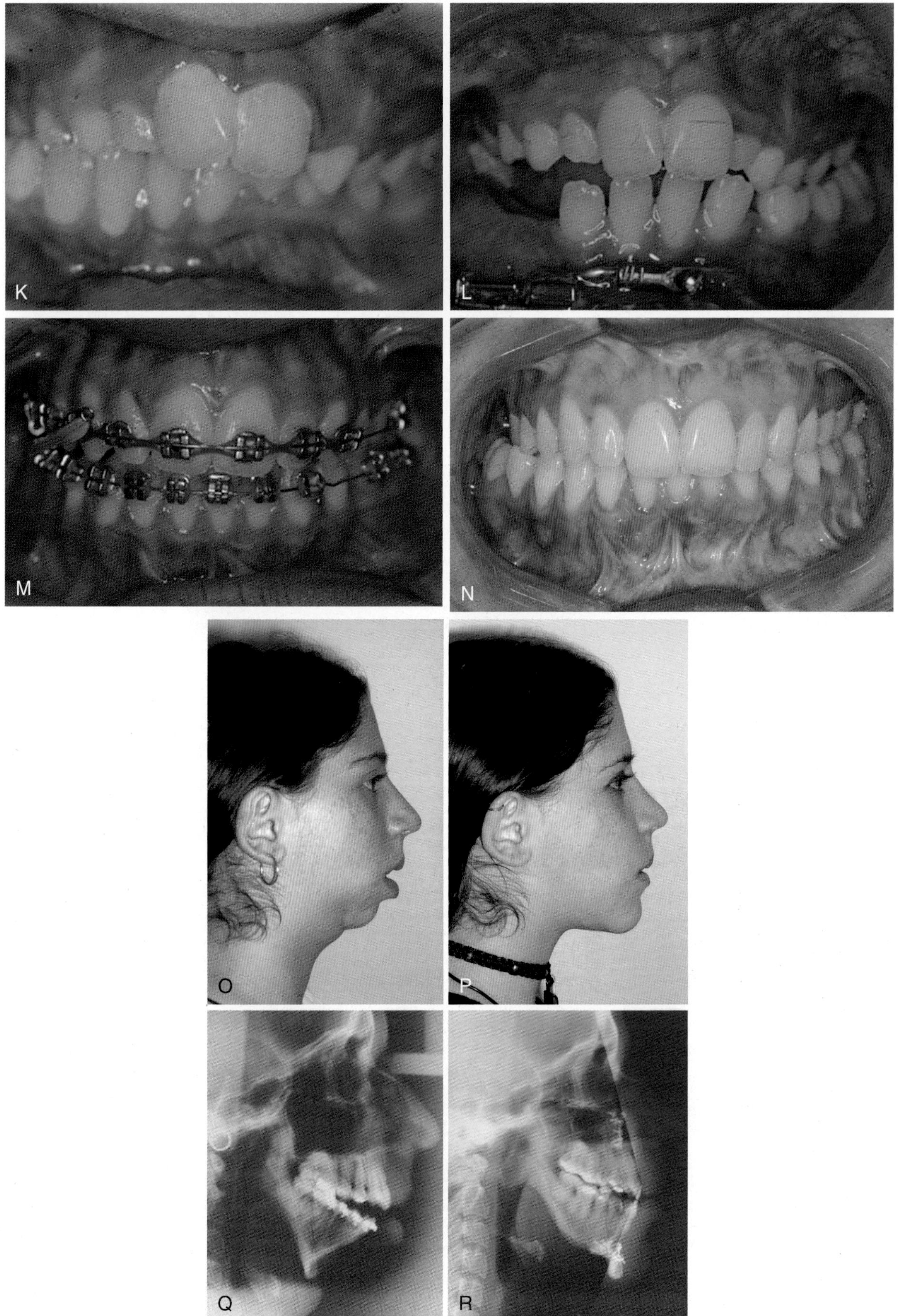

Figure 54.5, cont'd

Postoperative Considerations

The distractors should be removed after proper ossification has occurred, as confirmed by a radiographic evaluation and considering the different variables involved in the healing process, such as the age of the patient, amount of movement, quality and quantity of bone, infection, inadequate stability during consolidation, poor patient selection, and some systemic diseases.

If the clinician removes the appliances before adequate bone ossification, perimandibular muscles will force the segments away from the planned repositioning, with the consequent development of an open bite, anterior mandibular ramus rotation (proximal fragment counterclockwise rotation), disappearance of the mandibular angle projection, and TMJ pain and dysfunction. The use of maxillomandibular elastics to close the open bite is not indicated because extruding the superior incisors will cause the anterior open bite to relapse and prolong the postsurgical orthodontics, and the final occlusion will be unstable, leading to relapse and symptoms of TMJ dysfunction. Once the proper stabilization period has elapsed, usually 60 days for every centimeter of lengthening, the distractor is removed.[15,21]

Intraoral distraction osteogenesis allows mandibular lengthening with meticulous occlusal finishing in a predictable and stable manner that keeps the TMJ intact and conserves the preoperative anatomic characteristics. The surgical technique permits progressive augmentation of the hard and soft tissues into an ideal dental occlusion. The procedure requires that an orthodontist prepare the dentition presurgically into an ideal arch and fixate the dental positioning with heavy rectangular arches. This step will permit the use of heavy intermaxillary elastics during the early postsurgical period but will allow for complete joint unloading during the activation and consolidation phases.

References

1. Obwegeser H, Trauner R. Zur operationstechnik bei der progenie und anderen unterkieferanomalien. *Dtsch Zahn Mund Kieferheilkd.* 1955;23:1.
2. Bell WH, Epker BN. Surgical-orthodontic expansion of the maxilla. *Am J Orthod.* 1976;70(5):517–528.
3. Epker BN. Distraction osteogenesis for mandibular widening. *Atlas Oral Maxillofac Surg Clin North Am.* 1999;7(1):29–39.
4. Schendel SA, Wolford LM, Epker BN. Mandibular deficiency syndrome. III. Surgical advancement of the deficient mandible in growing children: treatment results in twelve patients. *Oral Surg Oral Med Oral Pathol.* 1978;45(3):364–377.
5. Little RM, Wallen TR, Riedel RA. Stability and relapse of mandibular anterior alignment-first premolar extraction cases treated by traditional edgewise orthodontics. *Am J Orthod.* 1981;80(4):349–365.
6. Little RM, Riedel RA, Artun J. An evaluation of changes in mandibular anterior alignment from 10 to 20 years postretention. *Am J Orthod Dentofacial Orthop.* 1988;93(5):423–428.
7. McCarthy JG, Schreiber J, Karp N, Thorne CH, Grayson BH. Lengthening the human mandible by gradual distraction. *Plast Reconstr Surg.* 1992;89(1):1–8.
8. Diner PA, Kollar EM, Martinez H, Vazquez MP. Intraoral distraction for mandibular lengthening: a technical innovation. *J Cranio-Maxillo-Fac Surg.* 1996;24(2):92–95.
9. Wangerin K, Gropp H. Die intraorale distraktionsosteotomie des mikrogenen unterkiefers zur beseitigung der atemwegsobstruktion. *Dtsch Z Mund Kiefer Gesichtschir.* 1994;18:236.
10. Chin M, Toth BA. Distraction osteogenesis in maxillofacial surgery using internal devices: review of five cases. *J Oral Maxillofac Surg.* 1996;54(1):45–53.
11. Guerrero C. Rapid mandibular expansion. *Rev Venez Ortod.* 1990;48:1.
12. Triaca A, Minoretti R, Dimai W, et al. Multiaxis intraoral distraction of the mandible. In: Samchukov ML, Cope JB, Cheraskin AM, eds. *Craniofacial Distraction Osteogenesis.* St. Louis, Missouri: Mosby; 2001.
13. Razdolsky Y, Dessner S, El-Bialy T. Correction of alveolar ridge deficiency using the ROD-5 distraction device: a case report. In: Samchukov ML, Cope JB, Cheraskin AM, eds. *Craniofacial Distraction Osteogenesis.* St. Louis, Missouri: Mosby; 2001.
14. Guerrero C, Bell W, Dominguez E. Intraoral distraction osteogenesis versus sagittal split osteotomy to lengthen the mandible. In: Arnaud E, Diner PA, eds. *Proceedings of the 4th International Congress of Maxillofacial and Craniofacial Distraction. Paris, France, July 2-5.* Vol. 133. Bologna: Monduzzi Editore; 2003.
15. Guerrero C, Figueroa F, Bell W, et al. Surgical orthodontics in mandibular lengthening. In: Bell W, Guerrero C, eds. *Distraction Osteogenesis of the Facial Skeleton.* Hamilton, Ontario, Canada: BC Decker; 2007.
16. Guerrero CA, Bell WH, Contasti GI, Rodriguez AM. Mandibular widening by intraoral distraction osteogenesis. *Br J Oral Maxillofac Surg.* 1997;35(6):383–392.
17. Guerrero C, Contasti G. Transverse mandibular deficiency. In: Bell WH, ed. *Modern Practice in Orthognathic and Reconstructive Surgery.* Philadelphia, Pennsylvania: WB Saunders; 1992.
18. Contasti G, Guerrero C, Rodriguez AM, Legan HL. Mandibular widening by distraction osteogenesis. *J Clin Orthod.* 2001;35(3):165–173.
19. Gonzalez M, Bell WH, Guerrero CA, Buschang PH, Samchukov ML. Positional changes and stability of bone segments during simultaneous bilateral mandibular lengthening and widening by distraction. *Br J Oral Maxillofac Surg.* 2001;39(3):169–178.
20. Guerrero C, Bell W, Gonzalez M. Mandibular remodeling: the fifth stage in distraction osteogenesis healing. In: Arnaud E, Diner P.A, eds. *Proceedings of the 3rd International Congress on Facial Distraction Processes, Paris, France.* Vol. 267. Bologna: Monduzzi Editore; 2001.
21. Guerrero C, Rivera H, Mujica E, et al. Principles of distraction osteogenesis. In: Bagheri S, Bell B, Khan H, eds. *Current Therapy in Oral and Maxillofacial Surgery.* St Louis, Missouri: Elsevier; 2012.
22. Gonzalez M, Guerrero CA, Figueroa F. Predictable mandibular ramus lengthening in TMJ ankylosis. In: Arnaud E, Diner PA, eds. *Proceedings of the 4th International Congress of Maxillofacial and Craniofacial Distraction, July 2, 2003, Paris, France.* Vol. 169. Bologna, Italy: Monduzzi Editore; 2003.
23. Gonzalez M, Egbert M, Guerrero CA, Van Sickels JE. Vertical and horizontal mandibular lengthening of the ramus and body. *Atlas Oral Maxillofac Surg Clin North Am.* 2008;16(2):215–236.
24. Stucki-McCormick SU. Reconstruction of the mandibular condyle using transport distraction osteogenesis. *J Craniofac Surg.* 1997;8(1):48–52.

CHAPTER 55

Maxillary Intraoral Distraction Osteogenesis

Cesar A. Guerrero, Marianela Gonzalez, and Mariana Henriquez

Armamentarium

#9 Molt periosteal elevators (two)
#15 Scalpel blades
A series of chisels and one curved chisel
Appropriate sutures
Basic oral surgery instruments
Bipolar electrocautery (if necessary)
Cat paw retractors
Distraction kit and screwdriver
Intraoral maxillary distraction osteogenesis instruments
Kelly hemostat
Langenbeck retractors
Local anesthetic with vasoconstrictor
Mallet
Metzenbaum scissors
Minnesota retractor
Mosquito forceps
Needle electrocautery
Needle electrocautery, bipolar
Obwegeser retractor
Osteotomes, fine
Orthognathic surgery set
Pear-shaped bur or a round bur if the mandible is to be set back
Pediatric gel horseshoe headrest and shoulder roll
Periosteal elevators
Reciprocating saw
Rigid fixation set
Surgairtome with fine bur (101)
Tenotomy scissors
Wire pushing instrument "pickle fork"

History of the Procedure

Three-dimensional maxillary deficiency may be present in a variety of craniofacial syndromes, clefts, and some idiopathic clinical situations. The deficiency may be present at different maxillary levels and must be treated accordingly. These levels may include Le Fort I, either low or high (Figs. 55.1 and 55.2), and quadrangular Le Fort I. This chapter covers only intraoral devices; it does not address the problem of total midface or frontofacial deficiency.

Traditional surgery has some limitations in terms of the amount of movement, the need for iliac crest bone grafts, and the stability and quality of bone. The soft tissues can also be a limitation, especially clefts and scar tissue from multiple surgeries. Intraoral distraction osteogenesis may be a better choice as an alternative method; it provides better stability and easier surgery (based on performing the osteotomies and fixing the appliances); no bone grafts are needed, and costs are reduced because the patient is discharged from the hospital earlier and is able to resume activities in a week's time. Through the years, two different approaches have been published for distraction osteogenesis in the craniofacial region: extraoral distractors or intraoral distractors. Extraoral distractors involve a semicircular metal structure fixed to the skull with multiple screws with a vertical bar connected to facial plates by wires and coils to exert the anteroposterior pressure and advance the midface.[1–5] There have been modifications and improvements to ensure skull stability and vector control, and attachments and connectors are available from various companies. Common problems associated with extraoral distractors are social inconvenience and facial scars, and more important, all patients have the distractors removed before completing the distraction consolidation phase (in large movements this would require up to a year); consequently, the stability is jeopardized.[2–5]

Internal maxillary distractors are based on a solid body with a barrel that is activated between anterior and posterior plates for bony fixation. Different designs have been published to improve bone anchorage, easier activation, and vector control and to facilitate removal. An understanding of biology and biomechanics is fundamental to predictably correct facial anomalies. The distraction protocol is based on the amount of movement, the age of the patient, and the quality and quantity of bone; minor or standard deformities are corrected with traditional surgery.[6–12]

To obtain optimal results, ideally ortho-dontics will be used in the correction of facial and occlusal discrepancies. The surgery must be planned in three-dimensional models to perform the model surgery; the distractors are prebent, preshaped, and activated to full movement, and the vector is planned to the objective movement. Once the appliances have been activated and perfect occlusion has been obtained in the model, the actual surgery is performed with proper vectors; the size of the distractors (e.g., 15, 20, 25 mm) and the length of the screws are measured and will be ready for surgery. All this work is done before the surgical intervention and must be supervised by the group expert and discussed with the orthodontist. The surgeon ensures that the final positioning of the midface is occlusally stable and must be maintained until bone rigidity occurs, after the distraction's consolidation phase. This may take 3 to 12 months, depending on the amount of movement, age of the patient, and quantity and quality of bone.[12,13] The distractor appliances are easy for the patient to use and can remain in place comfortably for a long time, with the patient resuming regular activities a few days after surgery.[12–14]

Some patients show divergences from the treatment plan, even though the appliances were prepared to obtain the best occlusion possible. In such cases, the surgeon needs to install a secondary method to make postoperative changes in the vector, such as circumferential vertical anterior suspension wires, or he or she must change the position of the anterior plate by changing the screws under intravenous sedation. Under no circumstances should the surgeon remove the distraction appliances and expect guiding elastics to improve or maintain the occlusion. The collagen fibers in the distraction chamber are under tension, awaiting mineralization in the consolidation stage; if the appliance's rigidity collapses or it is removed, the fibers contract, the segments become unstable, and complete recurrence results.[10,13,15]

Chin, Guerrero, Salyer, Wangerin, and Kessler were pioneers in developing internal devices and in using existing mandibular technology to advance the maxilla at different levels, following the true indications for distraction osteogenesis.[16–22]

Indications for the Use of the Procedure

Intraoral distraction osteogenesis is indicated for patients who have severe maxillary deficiency (over 10 mm), sleep apnea, previous failures in advancing the maxilla, inadequate anatomy for traditional surgery, and syndromic deficiency situations.

Limitations and Contraindications

Intraoral distraction osteogenesis is based on sound surgical principles that depend on vascularity and bone quality. It should not be used after radiotherapy or for conditions involving extremely poor bone quantity or quality. It also requires patient and family collaboration.

TECHNIQUE: Maxillary Le Fort I Level Advancement

Intraoral devices are ideal means to treat maxillary deficiencies in a two- or three-dimensional manner. In specific situations in which there is a lack of hard and soft tissues, different distraction osteogenesis techniques can be combined to solve deficiencies secondary to trauma or syndromes. This surgical approach eliminates the need for bone grafts or extraoral devices. Selection of the correct surgical timing and surgical technique avoids permanent surgical damage to the teeth, nerves, and lacrimal ducts.[12–14,23]

STEP 1: Patient Preparation

Either arch bars (in children) or full orthodontics (in mixed or adult dentition) are used to control the occlusion postoperatively. Once the dental objectives have been met in the presurgical phase, rectangular orthodontics are fixed to the orthodontics' braces. Training elastics are used after surgery to improve the dental occlusion.

Three-dimensional models may be used for planning, distraction device selection, and preadaptation. Also, an acrylic interdental splint may be fabricated for use after the maxillary down-fracture and intermaxillary fixation. The splint maintains the positioning while the distraction devices are securely fixed. The surgeon must ensure total mobilization of the maxilla at surgery; exerting too much pressure within the distractors and fixation screws to advance it may be detrimental for the device, disengage bone screws, create asymmetric movements, and cause instability.[23,24]

The patient is nasotracheally intubated after administration of general anesthesia with controlled hypotension. Local anesthesia is infiltrated as necessary.

STEP 2: Incision and Dissection

An incision is made from premolar to premolar through the mucosa, muscles, and periosteum. The tissues are elevated superiorly with two #9 Molt elevators anterior and posterior to the infraorbital nerve and posteriorly up to the pterygomaxillary junction through a tunnel, maintaining the lateral blood supply as much as possible.

STEP 3: Osteotomy and Down-Fracture

Calipers are used to measure the length of the canines and first molar, and 5 mm above them, the osteotomy is performed. The osteotomy design may vary depending on the individual clinical features. Careful medial dissection is performed, and a periosteal elevator is placed between the detached nasal mucosa and piriform rim. Reference lines are drawn in the maxillary lateral wall anterior and posterior, bilaterally. All soft tissues are meticulously reflected and separated to complete the osteotomy without tearing them. Langenbeck-Obwegeser retractors are placed anterior and posterior to the infraorbital nerves. Through the lateral wall osteotomy line, a spatula osteotome is used to weaken the maxil-

Continued

TECHNIQUE: Maxillary Le Fort I Level Advancement—*cont'd*

lary sinus medial wall to avoid irregular fractures up to the orbit. A second incision is made in the tuberosity area to place a curved chisel to section the tuberosity into the palatine bone; working through tunnels maintains the best blood supply, reduces edema, and improves bone healing.[12–14,23] The maxilla is down-fractured and released from the posterior maxillary union using a rough periosteal elevator. The nasal airway is approached and treated if necessary (e.g., septum, turbinates, deviations, cyst removal). The nasal mucosa is closed, and attention moves to placing the distractors.

STEP 4: Distractor Application

The positioning of the distractors is important. Either the distractors are placed into position before the down-fracture maneuver, with the screws placed to serve as a guide once the maxilla has been freed (the screws are not tightened to avoid loosening during final fixation), or the distractors are fixed after the maxillary mobilization, using references lines to avoid incorrect positioning. In either situation the surgeon must have a three-dimensional model to preshape, prebend, and adapt the distractor; measure the moving distance; and create the right vector of movement. The distractor is fixed with three or four screws in every plate, the upper and the lower, to ensure stability; the activation rods must be as parallel as possible. The distractors offer an excellent and secure way to advance the maxilla. In large movements, minimal discrepancies in the vertical fashion may create either an anterior or posterior open bite; the solution for many surgeons is to remove the distractor and place rigid fixation plates and screws, with the inconvenience of a second major surgery and also instability caused by the distraction chamber collapsing secondary to contraction of the immature callus formation.[15] An alternative solution is to create a secondary mechanism to control the distraction vector. The surgeon can place a 24-gauge wire from the nasal bone to the anterior maxilla, using a long bur to proceed transcutaneously at the nasal bone region from right to left. The wire is passed through the hole, and an Obwegeser passing owl needle is used from the anterior maxilla on the right side, emerging through the skin hole and repeating the maneuver on the left side. The wires emerge in the anterior maxilla and embrace the maxilla; this wire is loosely placed at the time of surgery but can be tightened or released in the event of open bite development, either anterior or posterior.[24]

STEP 5: Closure

The soft tissues are carefully closed by advancing the facial musculature anteriorly. A V Y lip closure is used after an adequate nasal cinch has been tightened.[25] Once there is radiographic evidence of mineralization, the distractor is removed, under intravenous sedation in the clinic, through small lateral maxillary incisions, and the screws are retrieved. The superoposterior plate can be cut and left in place. Resorbable sutures are used to close the wounds.[13]

TECHNIQUE: Maxillary Le Fort I Level Advancement in Clefts

Most cleft patients, after multiple surgeries, have a severe lack of three-dimensional maxillary growth. The surgeon confronting this problem must create a surgical-orthodontics plan that includes maxillary widening and vertical and anteroposterior movements.

The single most important aspect is to convert the two or three pieces of the maxilla (either a unilateral or a bilateral cleft) into a single unit. Once that is complete, the only remaining task is to place the maxilla in the best possible occlusion to follow postsurgical orthodontics. The surgeon must understand the principles of roll, yaw, and pitch to properly reposition the maxilla. The transverse correction must be addressed by surgical maxillary widening in a previous surgical stage, indicated for more than 4 mm of widening or immediate minor widening with the maxillary vertical and anteroposterior repositioning.[24,26–30]

After diagnosis and treatment planning, three-dimensional models are created, and distraction appliances are preshaped, prebent, and preadapted. A palatal splint is also fabricated, with multiple holes for interdental wires and an internal metal frame to avoid intraoperative splint fractures.[24] The splint is made from the model surgery and includes minor maxillary widening. The patient undergoes surgery, in which the same technique for a conventional Le Fort I osteotomy is used; the only difference is the need to create three flaps (nasal, palatine layer, and buccal layer) for alveolar bone grafts simultaneously with the maxillary repositioning. Patients with bilateral clefts need soft tissue management in the right and left side equally, but no incision is made in the premaxilla buccal area, which contains the only vascular supply. The nasal septum can be fractured or partially resected behind the premaxilla, but the premaxillary buccal blood supply must be maintained.

Once the two or three maxillary segments have been down-fractured and the three-dimensional alveolar graft sites have been prepared, the palatine and nasal layers are closed watertight. The maxillary pieces are carefully positioned into the acrylic splint with interdental wires, and a long, 2-mm-thick titanium plate is placed above the tooth level and fixed with 6- to 8-mm-long microscrews to create bone rigidity. The orthodontic rectangular arch, rigid fixation plate, and acrylic splint offer stable maxillary rigidity, creating a single-piece maxillary unit to be fixed to the upper midface with the

TECHNIQUE: Maxillary Le Fort I Level Advancement in Clefts—*cont'd*

maxillary distractors and anterior suspension 24-gauge wire around the nasal bones and anterior maxilla.[24] Bone grafts are placed into the alveolar clefts, and careful and meticulous soft tissue closure is obtained. Exposed dental roots next to the cleft may indicate the need for tooth removal to avoid bone graft contamination and loss; the periodontal ligament is a route for bacteria to infiltrate into the closed alveolar bone graft area.[13,24]

A 7-day period precedes appliance activation. Then, the maxilla is advanced 1 mm per day until class I canine and molar occlusion is obtained; there is no need for overcorrection. Complete mineralization must occur before the distraction devices are removed. Once the ideal positioning has been obtained, the midlines are carefully monitored; more activation on one side may be necessary to obtain the perfect positioning. If an anterior or posterior open bite develops, the anterior vertical suspension wire is adjusted to control the final vertical positioning (Figs. 55.1 and 55.2).

Distraction Protocol

A latency period of 7 days is followed by activation of 1 mm a day until distraction is complete; then, a consolidation period of 60 to 90 days for each centimeter distracted is indicated. One distractor may be activated more than the other to obtain symmetry and adequate midline positioning.

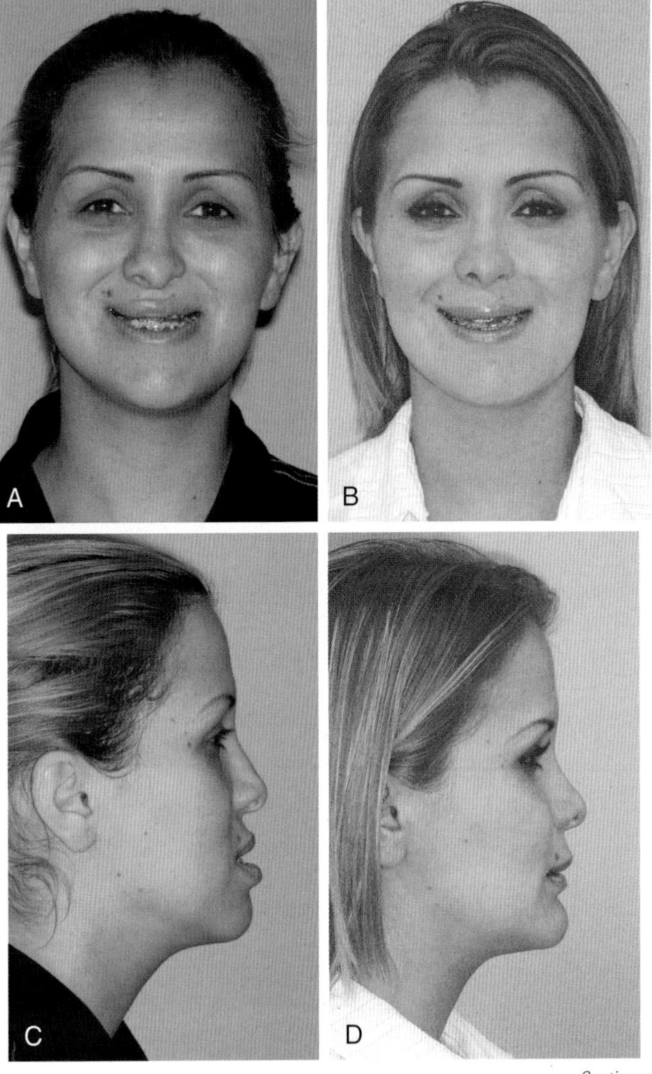

Figure 55.1 A–N, A 30-year-old patient after unilateral cleft lip and palate repair and maxillary hypoplasia. The patient was treated with intraoral maxillary advancement, mandibular subapical osteotomy, and orthodontics. Radiographs show intraoral distractors, the advancement vector, and anterior suspension wire to control vertical movement. A unilateral or bilateral cleft maxilla was converted into a single unit by fixing the two or three segments into an acrylic-metal palatal splint out of the model surgery with multiple interdental wires. The cleft maxilla is converted into a single unit through the use of a long, 2-mm-thick plate across the cleft, fixed with multiple screws above the tooth level; the plate had been prebent, preadapted, and premeasured in the three-dimensional model. An orthodontic surgical arch is fixated to the braces. The alveolar cleft could be simultaneously grafted with bone grafts into a three-layered flap chamber. The distractors were installed, and an anterior suspension wire controlled the vertical movement as the maxilla was advanced. A maxillary Le Fort I was performed, and the single-unit maxilla was advanced into occlusion progressively after a latency period of 7 days with activation of 1 mm once a day and a consolidation period of 6 months. To avoid velopharyngeal incompetence, a mandibular subapical osteotomy was performed, dividing the major discrepancy between the two jaws. In addition, a right posterior maxillary osteotomy was used to close the edentulous space. The patient was referred to the orthodontist for finishing and dental implant insertion in the alveolar bone graft site.

Continued

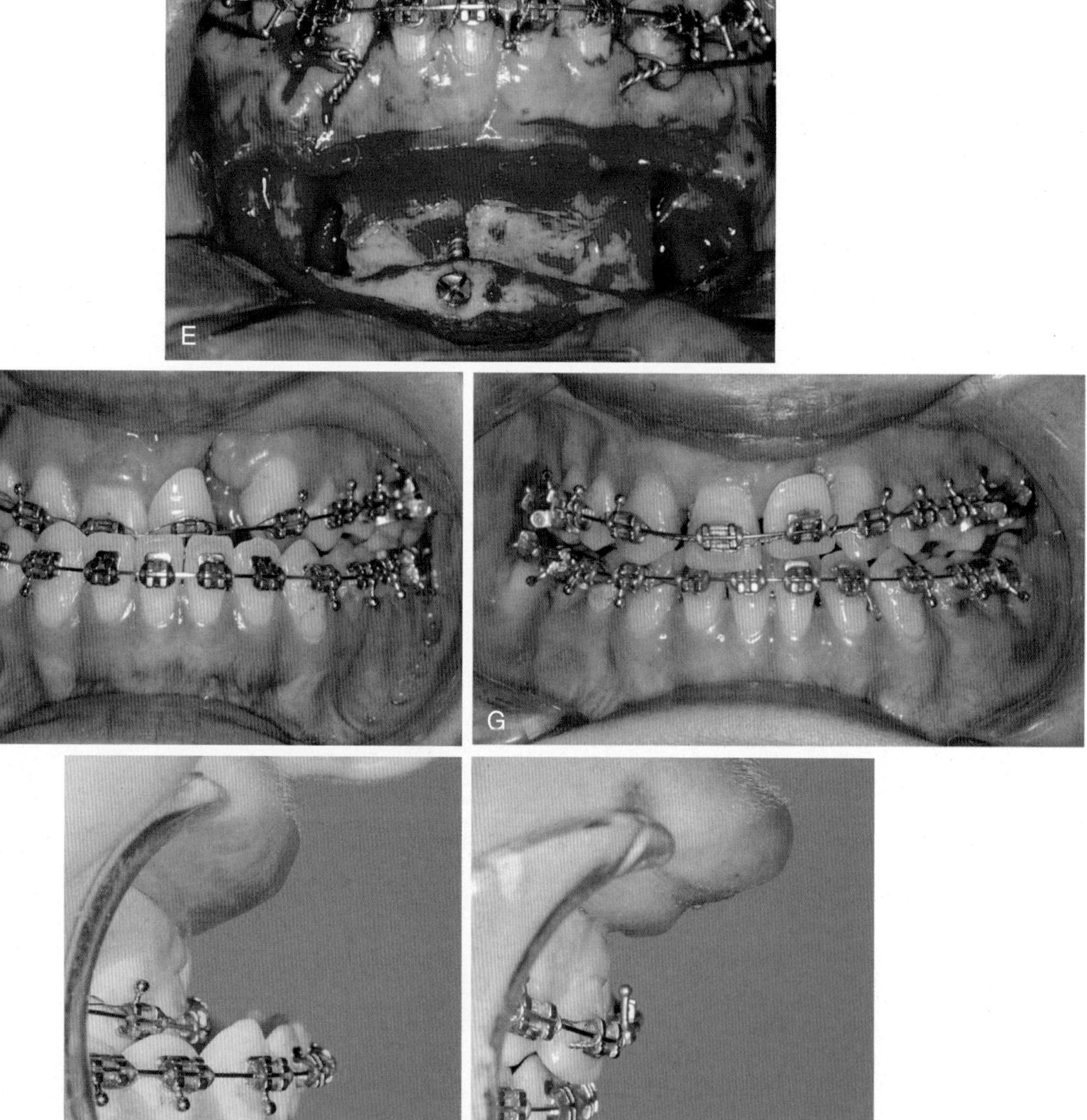

Figure 55.1, cont'd

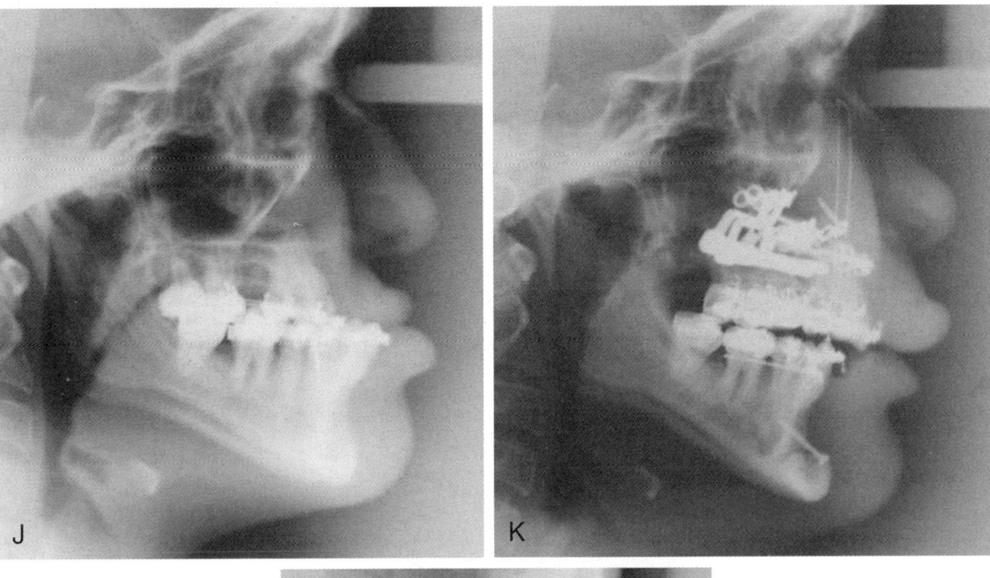

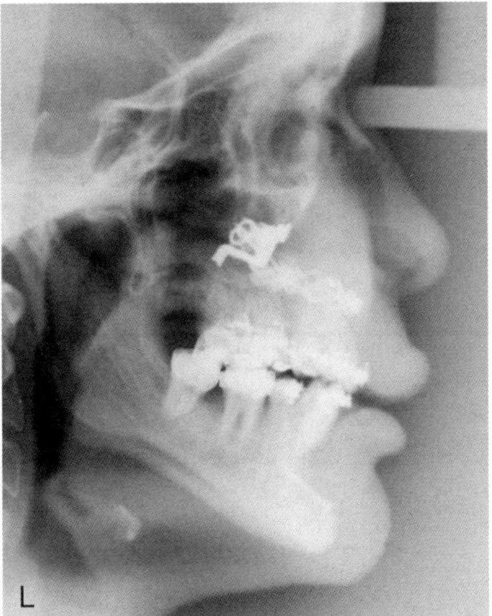

Figure 55.1, cont'd

Continued

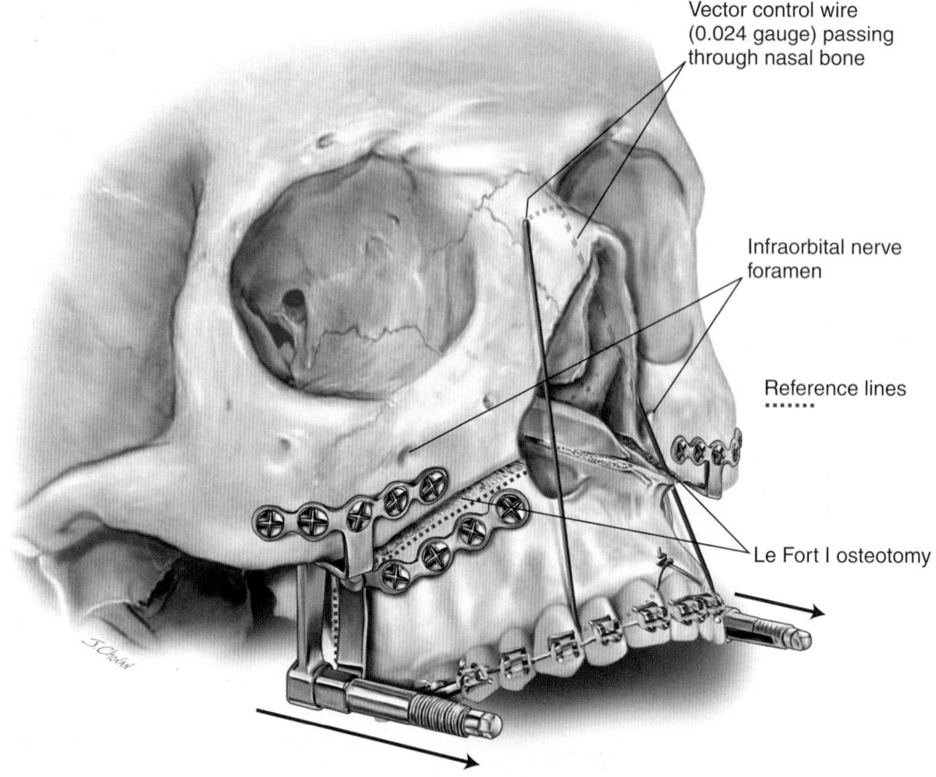

M

Intraoral Distraction Osteogenesis

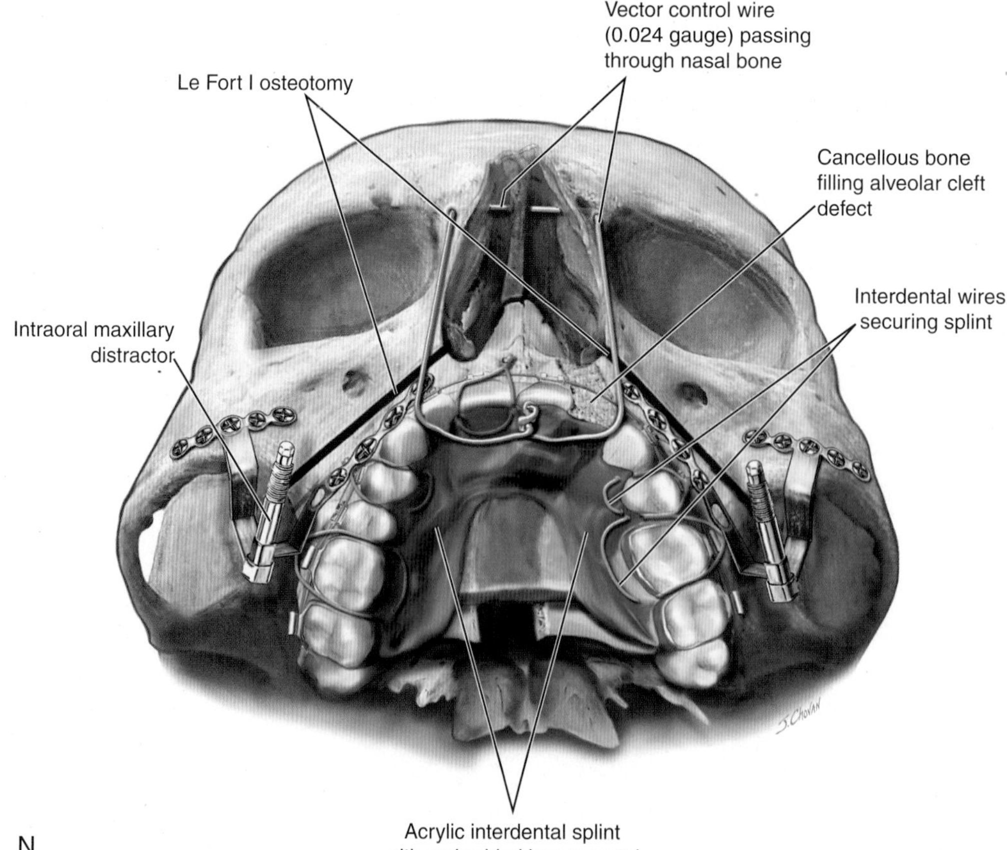

N

Figure 55.1, cont'd

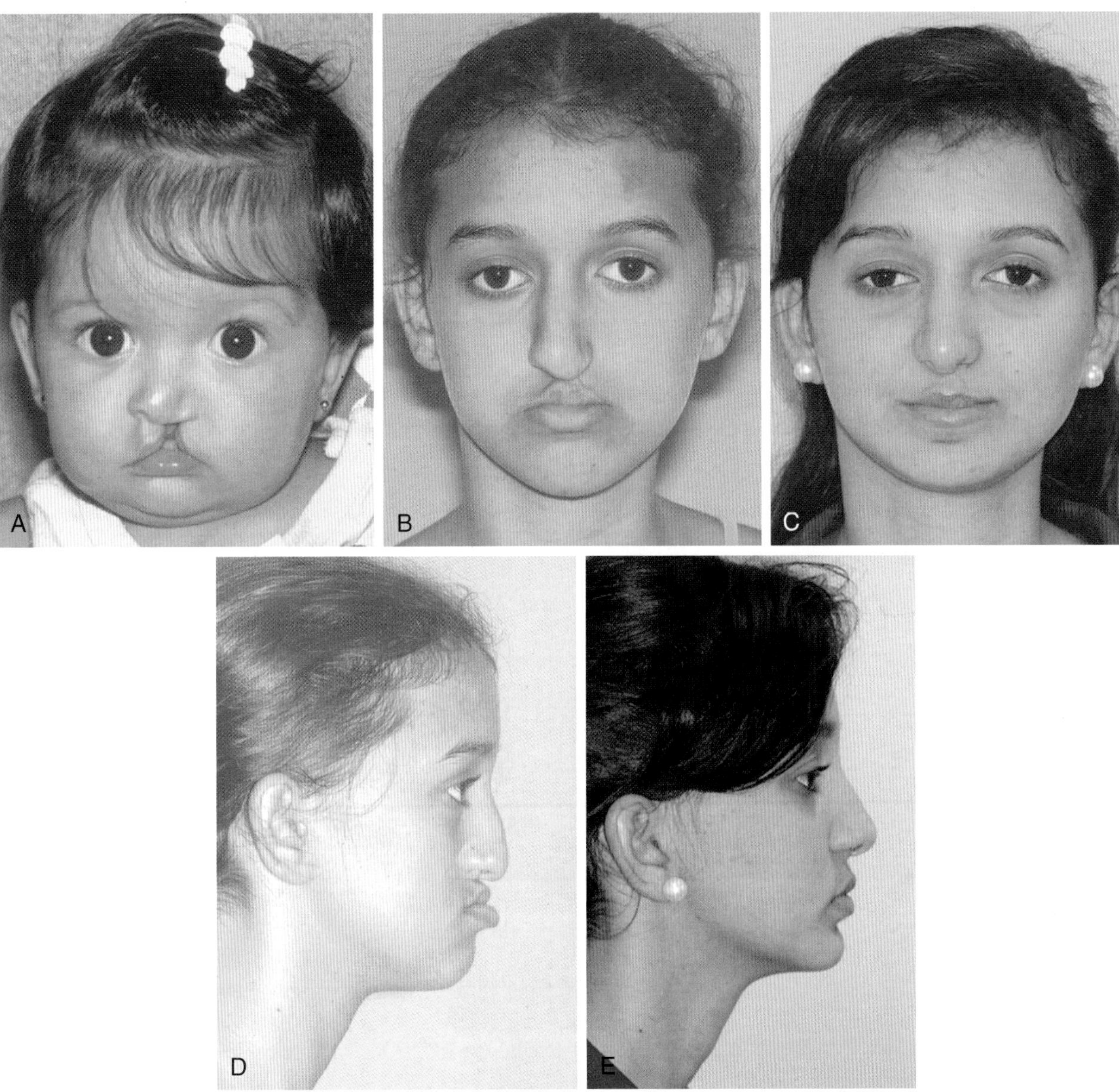

Figure 55.2 Long-term follow-up of 20 years in a patient with a unilateral cleft lip and palate. Treatment involved Millard's rotation and advancement cheiloplasty, followed by Veau's push-back palatoplasty. At the end of growth, the patient presented with a severe maxillary deficiency and occlusal compensations. She was then treated with a mandibular subapical osteotomy to level the occlusal plane and close the temporary tooth extraction spaces, allowing partial class III correction. In addition, maxillary advancement via internal distraction osteogenesis and widening were performed, followed by finishing orthodontics and lateral incisor dental implants. The rhinoplasty was performed when the internal distractors were removed. Note that the distractors were carefully fixated with the ideal vector; however, for postoperative control, a pyramidal vertical suspension 0.024-gauge wire was used to control the vertical final maxillary positioning. **A,** Four months of age. **B,** End of growth. **C,** After rhinoplasty. **D** and **E,** The osteotomy design included a high Le Fort I to project the perinasal areas, and the lower lip was improved by a posterior repositioning subapical osteotomy. Cephalic radiographic views.

Continued

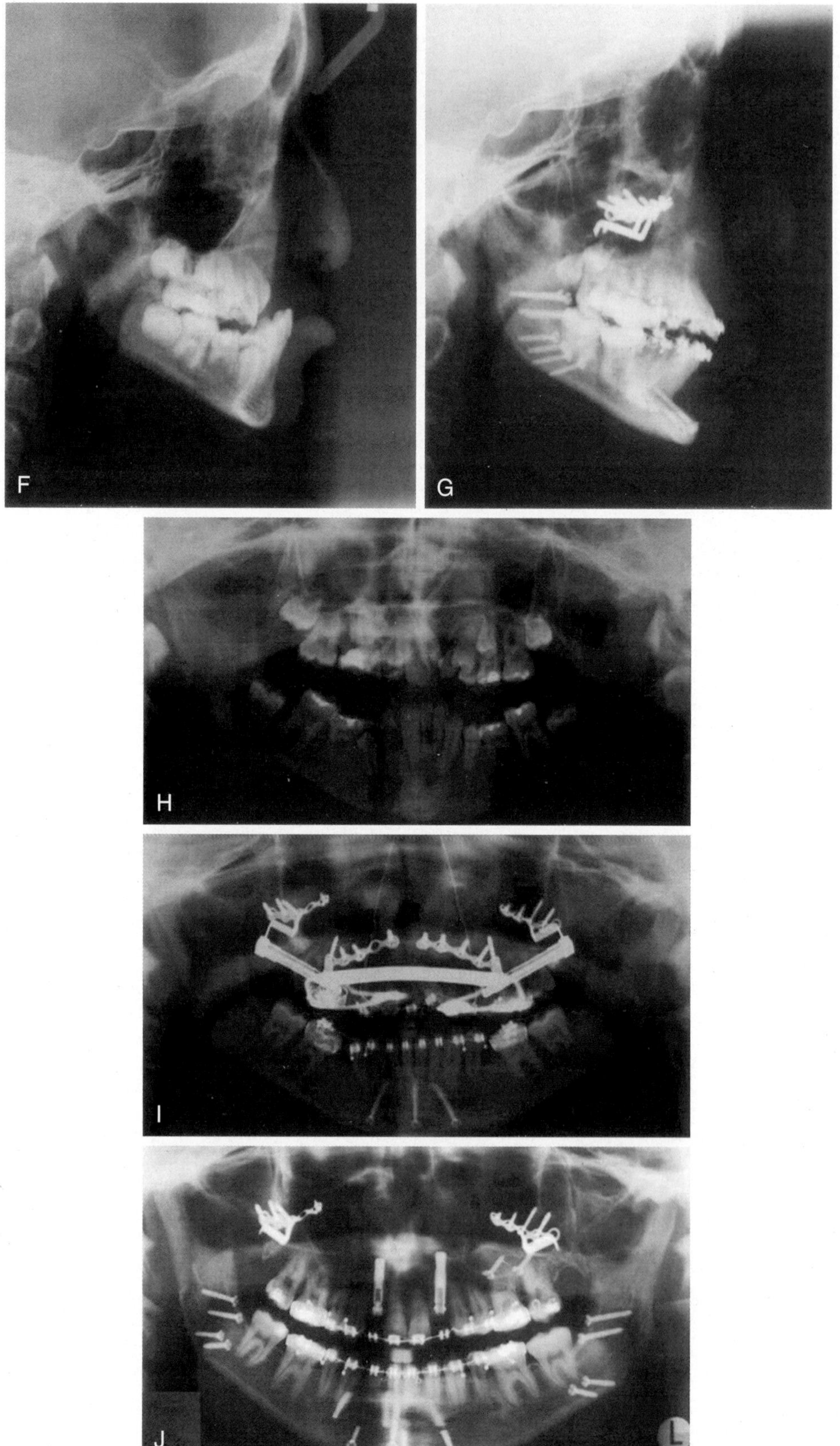

Figure 55.2, cont'd Preoperatively (**F**) and after the distractors were removed (6 months after surgery) (**G**). Panoramic views. Preoperatively (**H**), during distraction protocol (**I**), and 6 months after surgery with dental implants in position (**J**).

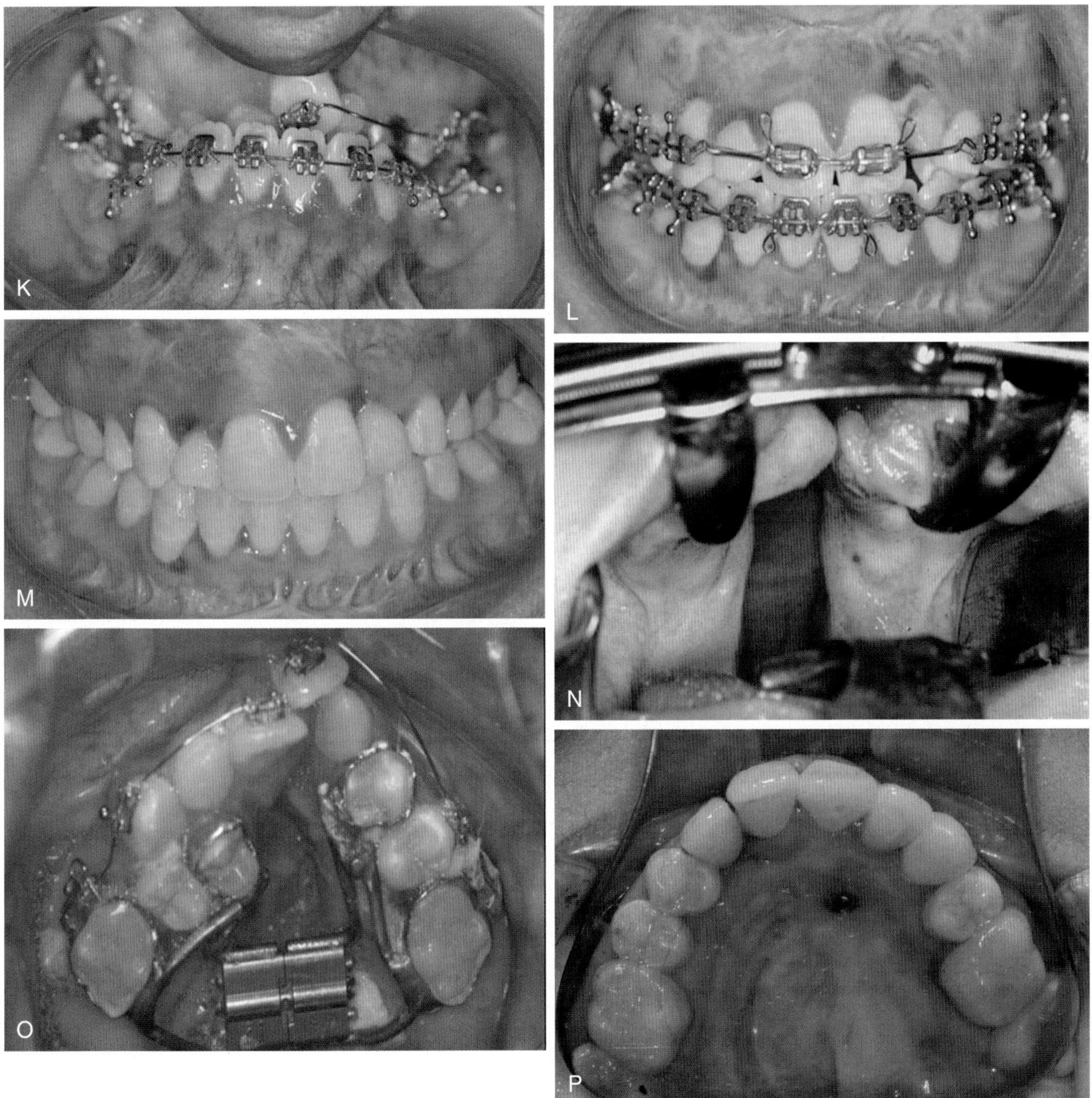

Figure 55.2, cont'd Intraoral views. Frontal views: before surgery (**K**), during orthodontic alignment (**L**), and final photograph after 20-year follow-up (**M**). Occlusal view: unilateral cleft lip and palate (**N**). **O,** After the end of growth, the patient presented severe transverse maxillary deficiency. **P,** After distraction osteogenesis and widening surgery.

Avoidance and Management of Intraoperative Complications

The intraoperative complications associated with intraoral distraction osteogenesis are no different from those noted for the previously described classic Le Fort I osteotomy. Significant attention must be paid to appropriate distractor placement to aid maxillary advancement.

Postoperative Considerations

The patient can resume regular activities a few days after surgery. Activation should be done in the morning, before going to school or work, and a liquid diet is indicated for the activation period. Once the midface is in the proper position and has been adjusted with the suspension wire or repositioned under intravenous sedation in the clinic, the patient's diet is improved to soft food. The blender is useful; anything the patient may want or the family is having should be passed through the triturating process, put in a glass or on a soup spoon, and given to the patient.

After total activation has been accomplished and the consolidation period is complete, radiographs are taken to verify the distraction chamber ossification. Once adequate radiopacity is observed, the patient is taken to the operating room and, under intravenous sedation, the appliances' anterior plates are disengaged by removing the multiple screws. Mobility is then checked, and the decision is made whether to continue removing the posterior plates and anterior suspension wire.

The distractors should be removed after proper ossification has occurred, confirmed by a radiographic evaluation and with consideration given to the different variables involved in the healing process, such as the age of the patient, amount of movement, quality and quantity of bone, infection, inadequate stability during consolidation, poor patient selection, and some systemic diseases.

Intraoral distraction osteogenesis allows maxillary advancement with meticulous occlusal finishing in a predictable and stable manner. The surgical technique permits progressive augmentation of the hard and soft tissues into an ideal dental occlusion. The orthodontist must have prepared the dentition presurgically into an ideal arch situation and fixated the dental positioning with heavy rectangular arches so that intermaxillary heavy elastics can be used during the early postsurgical period, still allowing complete joint unloading during the activation and consolidation phases.

References

1. Ilizarov GA. The tension-stress effect on the genesis and growth of tissues: part II. The influence of the rate and frequency of distraction. *Clin Orthop Relat Res*. 1989;239:263–285.
2. Polley JW, Figueroa AA. Maxillary distraction osteogenesis with rigid external distraction. *Atlas Oral Maxillofac Surg Clin North Am*. 1999;7(1):15–28.
3. Figueroa AA, Polley JW. Management of the severe cleft and syndromic midface hypoplasia. *Orthod Craniofac Res*. 2007;10(3):167–179.
4. Figueroa AA, Polley JW, Figueroa AL. Introduction of a new removable adjustable intraoral maxillary distraction system for correction of maxillary hypoplasia. *J Craniofac Surg*. 2009;20(suppl 2):1776–1786.
5. Wen-Ching Ko E, Figueroa AA, Polley JW. Soft tissue profile changes after maxillary advancement with distraction osteogenesis by use of a rigid external distraction device: a 1-year follow-up. *J Oral Maxillofac Surg*. 2000;58(9):959–969.
6. Ilizarov GA. The principles of the Ilizarov method. *Bull Hosp Jt Dis Orthop Inst*. 1988;48(1):1–11.
7. Ilizarov GA. The tension-stress effect on the genesis and growth of tissues. Part I. The influence of stability of fixation and soft-tissue preservation. *Clin Orthop Relat Res*. 1989;238:249–281.
8. Ilizarov GA. The tension-stress effect on the genesis and growth of tissues: part II. The influence of the rate and frequency of distraction. *Clin Orthop Relat Res*. 1989;239:263–285.
9. Samchukov M, Cherkashin A, Makarov M, et al. Muscle adaptation during single and double level tibial lengthening. In: Stein H, Suk S, Leung P, et al., eds. *SIROT 99 International Research Society of Orthopaedic Surgery and Traumatology*. Sydney, Australia: Tel Aviv; 1999 (Freund).
10. Samchukov M, Cope J, Cherkashin A. *Craniofacial Distraction Osteogenesis*. St Louis, Missouri: Mosby; 2001.
11. Bell W, Gonzalez M, Samchukov M, Guerrero C. Intraoral widening and lengthening the mandible by distraction osteogenesis and histogenesis. *J Oral Maxillofac Surg*. 1999;57:548.
12. Guerrero C, Bell W, Meza L. Intraoral distraction osteogenesis: maxillary and mandibular lengthening. *Atlas Oral Maxillofac Surg Clin North Am*. 1999;7(1):111–151.
13. Guerrero C, Gonzalez M, Dominguez E. Bone transport by distraction osteogenesis for maxillomandibular reconstruction. In: Bell W, Guerrero C, eds. *Distraction Osteogenesis of the Facial Skeleton*. Hamilton, Ontario, Canada: Decker; 2007.
14. Guerrero C, Bell W. Intraoral distraction. In: McCarthy JG, ed. *Distraction of the Craniofacial Skeleton*. New York: Springer-Verlag; 1999.
15. Guerrero C, Rivera H, Mujica E, et al. Principles of distraction osteogenesis. In: Bagheri S, Bell B, Khan H, eds. *Current Therapy in Oral and Maxillofacial Surgery*. St Louis, Missouri: Mosby; 2012.
16. Chin M, Toth BA. Le Fort III advancement with gradual distraction using internal devices. *Plast Reconstr Surg*. 1997;100(4):819–830.
17. Guerrero C. Rapid mandibular expansion. *Rev Venez Ortod*. 1990;48:1.
18. Wangerin K, Gropp H. Die intraorale Distraktionsosteotomie des mikrogenen Unterkiefers zur Beseitigung der Atemwegsobstruktion. *Dtsch Z Mund Kiefer Gesichtschir*. 1994;18:236.
19. Shokirov S, Wangerin K. Transantral distraction devices in correction of severe maxillary deformity in cleft patients. *Stomatologija*. 2011;13(1):25–32.
20. Kessler P, Wiltfang J, Schultze-Mosgau S, Hirschfelder U, Neukam FW. Distraction osteogenesis of the maxilla and midface using a subcutaneous device: report of four cases. *Br J Oral Maxillofac Surg*. 2001;39(1):13–21.
21. Cheung LK, Lo J. Distraction of Le Fort II osteotomy by intraoral distractor: a case report. *J Oral Maxillofac Surg*. 2006;64(5):856–860.
22. Gonzalez M, Guerrero C, Ding M. Distraction osteogenesis. In: Bagheri S, Bell B, Khan H, eds. *Current Therapy in Oral and Maxillofacial Surgery*. St Louis, Missouri: Mosby; 2012.
23. Guerrero C, Bell W, Gonzalez M, Meza L. Intraoral distraction osteogenesis. In: Fonseca RJ, ed. *Oral and Maxillofacial Surgery*. Philadelphia, Pennsylvania: Saunders; 2000.
24. Schendel S, Delaire J. Facial muscles: form, function and reconstruction in dentofacial deformities. In: Bell W, Proffit W, White R, eds. *Surgical Correction in Dentofacial Deformities*. Philadelphia, Pennsylvania: Saunders; 1984.
25. Guerrero CA. Intraoral bone transport in clefting. *Oral Maxillofac Surg Clin North Am*. 2002;14(4):509–523.
26. Guerrero C. Intraoral distraction osteogenesis. In: *Selected Readings in Oral and Maxillofacial Surgery*. Vol. 10. Dallas: University of Texas Southwestern Medical Center at Dallas; 2002:1.
27. Guerrero C, Bell W, Gonzalez M, Meza L. Intraoral distraction osteogenesis. In: Fonseca RJ, ed. *Oral and Maxillofacial Surgery*. Vol. 2. Philadelphia, Pennsylvania: Saunders; 2002.
28. Cohen SR, Burstein FD, Stewart MB, Rathburn MA. Maxillary-midface distraction in children with cleft lip and palate: a preliminary report. *Plast Reconstr Surg*. 1997;99(5):1421–1428.
29. Guerrero C, Bell W, Gonzalez M, Rojas A. Maxillary advancement combined with posterior palate reposition via distraction osteogenesis: a case report. In: Samchukov ML, Cope JB, Cherkashin AM, eds. *Craniofacial Distraction Osteogenesis*. St Louis, Missouri: Mosby; 2001.
30. Guerrero C. Maxillary intraoral distraction osteogenesis. In: Arnaud E, Diner PA, eds. *Proceedings of the Third International Congress on Facial Distraction Processes, June 14-16, 2001; Paris*. Bologna: Monduzzi Editore; 2001.

CHAPTER 56

Unilateral Cheilorhinoplasty–Delaire

David S. Precious and Jean-Charles Doucet

Armamentarium

Marking pen
25-gauge long needle (tattoo)
Local anesthetic with vasoconstrictor
Long scalpel blade handle, short scalpel blade handle
#15, #15c, #12, and #11 blades
#10 Suction tip
Molt periosteal elevator
Angled periosteal elevator
Woodson elevator
Bishop retractor
Cottle elevator
Double skin hooks
Single skin hooks
Adson forceps
Long fine forceps with teeth
Long fine forceps without teeth
Mosquitos
Small needle driver
Long fine needle driver
Straight scissors
Small curved scissors
Appropriate sutures
Koken nasal retainer

History of the Procedure

The earliest attempts at cleft management used simple coaptation of the margins of the cleft after they had been surgically exposed. The results obtained with these techniques were, unfortunately, consistently bad, for many reasons, but particularly because of poor surgical reconstruction of the labial musculature. It was on muscle reconstruction that Victor Veau concentrated in his book, *Cleft Lip, Clinical-Surgical Forms,* published in 1938.[1] Through the principles espoused by Veau and more recently by Delaire,[2] modern cleft management has come to recognize the importance of (and to incorporate into surgical approaches) (1) wide undermining of the muscles of the lip, nasal sill, and floor of the nose by surgical dissection, (2) detailed reconstruction of the mucoperiosteal plane on the nasal side of the primary palate, (3) solid anchorage of the muscles of the nasal floor and the nasal sill to the region of the anterior nasal spine, and (4) progressive and systematic suturing of the orbicularis muscles of the upper lip, which have been surgically defined on both sides of the cleft.[3]

Indications for the Use of the Procedure

Congenital labiomaxillary clefts result from the absence of fusion or from incomplete fusion of the maxillary and medial nasal processes. The superficial muscles of the face, which arise from the second branchial arch, migrate laterally and medially between the epidermis and subjacent ectomesenchyme and normally reach the midline in the week after fusion of the facial processes. In a complete labiomaxillary cleft, the muscles of the nasal floor and the upper lip cannot bridge the gap of the cleft, nor can they unite with their muscular counterparts on the noncleft side. The muscular integrity of the region is considerably disrupted, which has a profound effect on the underlying skeleton. Abnormal muscle architecture is present during bone formation, and virtually all bone formation in the cleft fetus takes place at the direction and under the influence of dissymmetric and distorted muscle forces. To achieve the proper midline position and attitude of the nasal septum, the surgeon must perform a wide subperichondrial dissection of the cleft side of the septum. This permits the creation of a watertight nasal floor while preserving the integrity of the maxillary labial frenum, which, as described previously,[4] is an important constituent of the septopremaxillary traction system. It is necessary to reconstruct the nasolabial muscles of the cleft so that the result is a symmetric influence on the nasal septum from both the cleft and noncleft muscles. Successful lip/nose repair must establish a straight nasal septum positioned in the facial midline; symmetric reconstruction of the nasolabial muscles; the absence of a vestibular oral-nasal communication; and a functional patent nostril on the cleft side, all of which are essential for good subsequent facial growth.

Limitations and Contraindications

There are no contraindications to this procedure save the general health of the baby. The most significant factor is the extent of the surgeon's knowledge of the relevant functional anatomy and subsequent facial growth.

TECHNIQUE: Functional Cheilorhinoplasty of Delaire

STEP 1: Surgical Approach

At the beginning of the operation, the surgeon must adopt a surgical approach that is based on functional anatomy. The surgeon must avoid following a geometric plan (Fig. 56.1A).

STEP 2: Incision Design

The incision design is that described by Delaire, in which no absolute measurements are made. The entire incision plan is based on the baby's existing anatomy (Fig. 56.1B).

STEP 3: Anatomic Landmarks

An imaginary line is drawn through the summit of each nostril, joining point A to A'. A second imaginary line is drawn parallel to the first through the junction of the columella and the philtrum at the medial base of the nostril (point B) and then extended to the cleft side at a point similar to that on the noncleft side (point 1) (Fig. 56.1C).

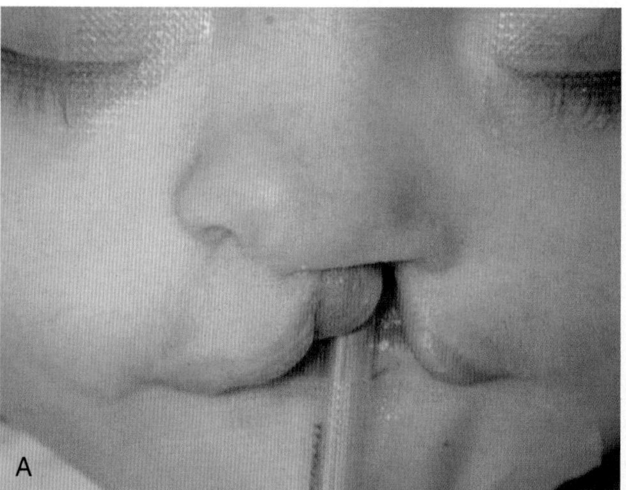

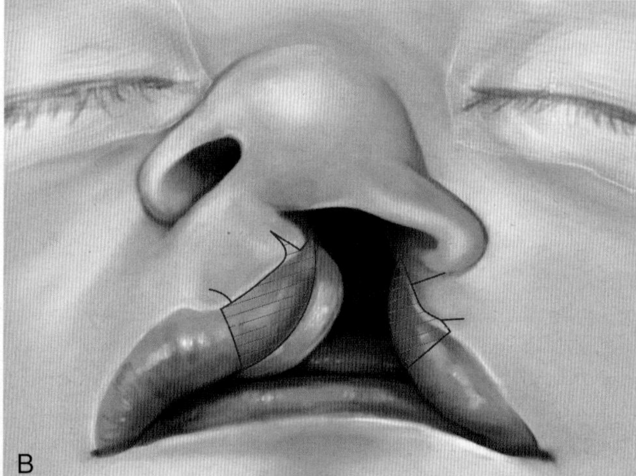

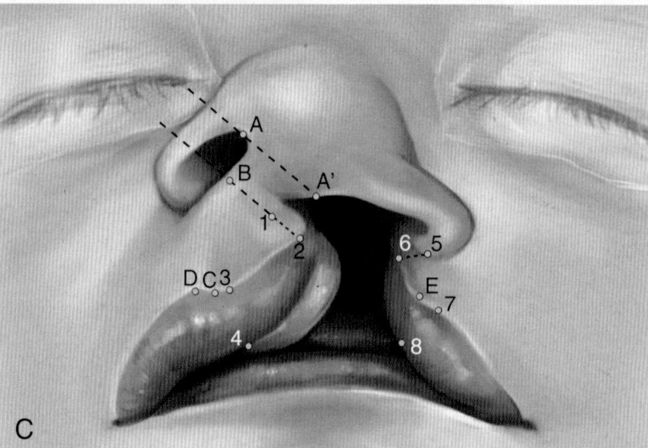

Figure 56.1 **A,** The surgeon must adopt a surgical approach that is based on functional anatomy. **B,** The incision design according to Delaire. **C,** Anatomic landmarks.

TECHNIQUE: Functional Cheilorhinoplasty of Delaire—*cont'd*

STEP 4: Incision Lines

A pen and ink line is now drawn from point 1 to point 2 as an extension of the inferior imaginary line, at the mucocutaneous junction. An arciform line is then drawn from point 1 to point 3, which is the future medial aspect of the cupid's bow. Note that the distance from point 3 to point C (the anatomic midline) is ever so slightly less than that between point C and point D (peak of cupid's bow on the noncleft side). A line is now drawn from point 3 to point 4 perpendicular to the junction of the wet and dry lip mucosae. The small triangular piece of mucosa lateral to the incision lines is ultimately resected.

On the lateral aspect of the cleft, a line is drawn from point 5 (the point of implantation of the nostril root) at right angles to the mucocutaneous junction (point 6). A line that is in skin but just above the mucocutaneous junction is extended to point 7, which is approximately 1.5 mm lateral to the disappearance of the white roll (point E). If the preoperative skin retraction is severe, a small equilateral triangular flap is marked just above the white roll and inserted into a 2- to 3-mm back-cut on the medial side of the cleft (which should never extend past the midline). A line is now drawn from point 7 to point 8 in a manner similar to that for the line drawn from point 3 to point 4. The small triangle of mucosa medial to the incision lines is also eventually resected. After a local anesthetic with vasoconstrictor has been injected into the lip on both sides, the relevant incisions are made, first on the medial side of the cleft and then on the lateral side (Fig. 56.1B and D).

STEP 5: Subperiosteal Dissection

On the lateral aspect of the maxilla, the mucosa is incised from the future deciduous molar area to the piriform aperture such that a very wide subperiosteal dissection can be made into the lateral part of the nasal cavity and over the entire facial surface of the maxilla, including the region of the infraorbital nerve. This is necessary so that all of the nasogenal muscles can be advanced at the time of suturing (Fig. 56.1E).

Continued

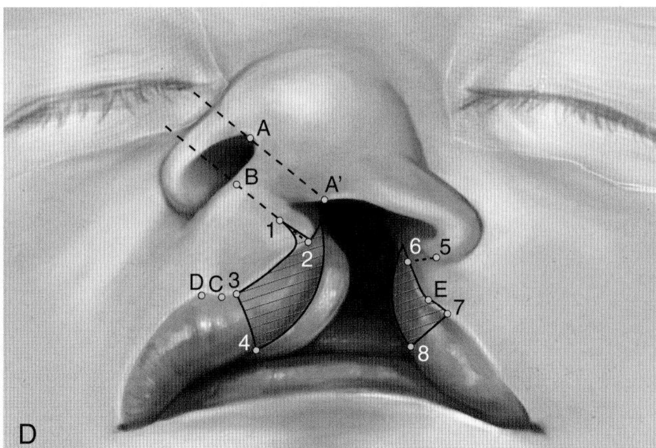

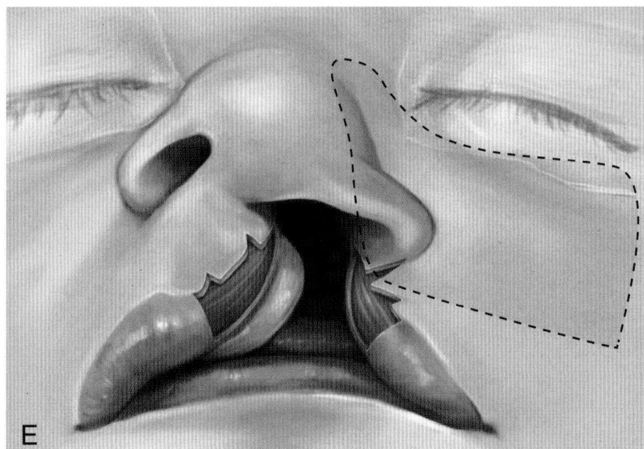

Figure 56.1, cont'd D, Details of the incision design showing the small amount of mucosal resection. **E,** The very wide subperiosteal dissection made into the lateral part of the nasal cavity and over the entire facial surface of the maxilla, including the region of the infraorbital nerve.

TECHNIQUE: Functional Cheilorhinoplasty of Delaire—*cont'd*

STEP 6: Perichondrial Dissections

Through the incision made from point 5 to point 6, which is now extended to meet the lateral maxillary intraoral incision, a supraperichondrial subcutaneous dissection is carried out over the lower lateral cartilage of the nose and extended superiorly to the midline between the medial crura. Similarly, through the same incision, a submucosal dissection is made on the medial aspect of the lower lateral cartilage and extended superiorly to meet the lateral dissection, thus completely freeing the lower part of the lower lateral cartilage (Fig. 56.1F).

STEP 7: Preparation for Suturing

An incision is now made carefully at the base of the nasal septum to include the perichondrium but no more. This incision is joined to that joining points 1 and 2 so that the nasal septum can be completely freed from the overlying perichondrium and soft tissue, allowing the surgeon to physically straighten the nasal septum in preparation for suturing. Through the same incision, a subcutaneous dissection frees the nasal septum from the columellar soft tissue; this represents the final preparatory freeing of the nasal septum (Fig. 56.1G).

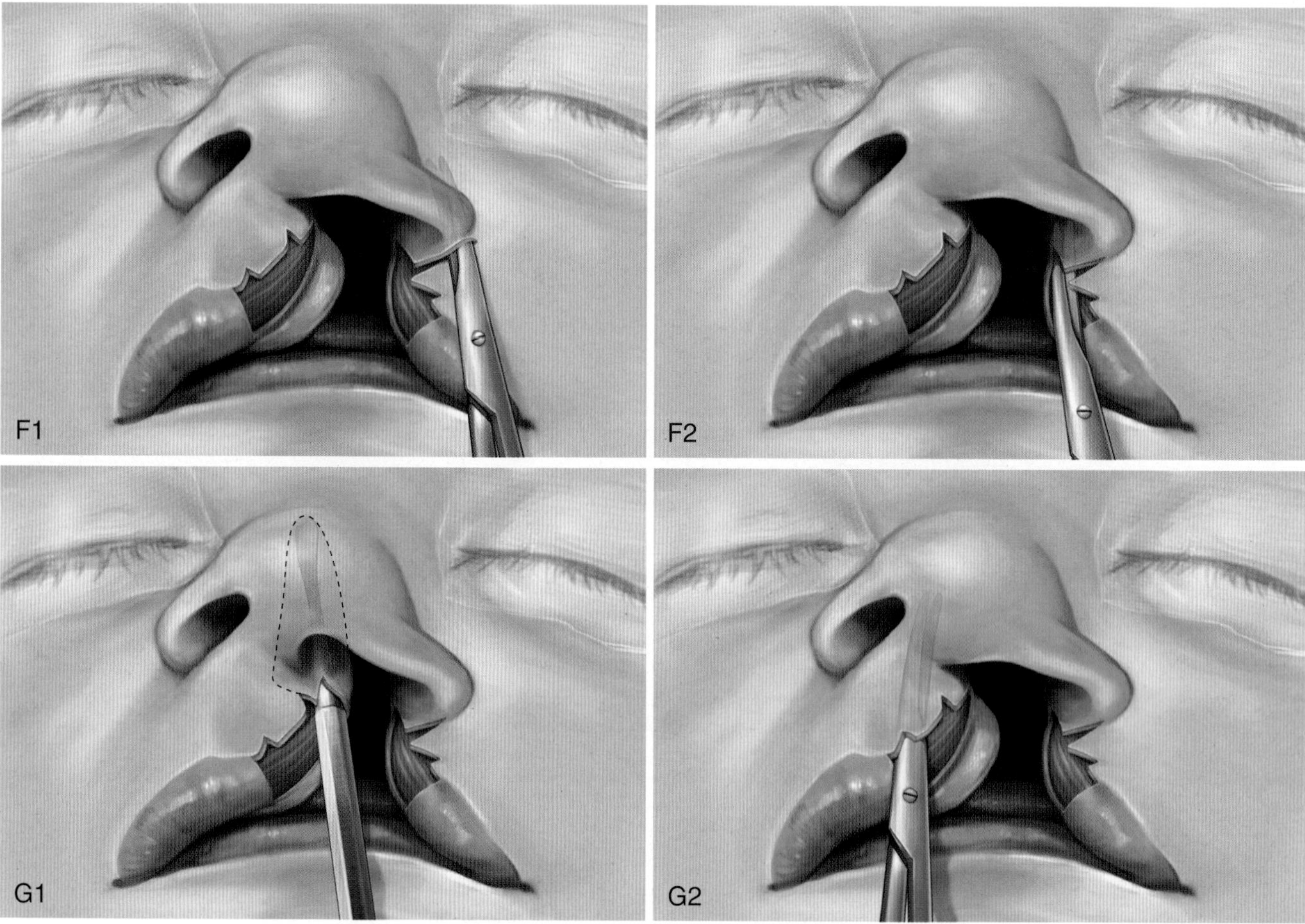

Figure 56.1, cont'd **F1,** Subcutaneous, supraperichondrial dissection on the lateral aspect of the nose. **F2,** Submucosal dissection on the medial aspect of the nose. **G1,** Subperichondrial dissection of the nasal septum. **G2,** Subcutaneous columellar dissection.

TECHNIQUE: Functional Cheilorhinoplasty of Delaire—*cont'd*

STEP 8: Suturing the Nasal Mucosa

Suturing begins from deep within the nostril floor and progresses until the nasal mucosa has a complete and watertight closure (Fig. 56.1H).

STEP 9: Suturing the Nasolabial Muscles

All the nasolabial muscles should now sutured with nonresorbable nylon sutures. This is done systematically in a progressive fashion, with the first suture being placed in muscle and periosteum such that the lateral aspect of the nose is elevated and brought medially to the midline at the level of the anterior nasal spine. Note that no skin sutures are placed until the muscular reconstruction is complete and the skin is lying passively coapted (Fig. 56.1I).

STEP 10: Skin Suturing

Finally, the 6-0 or 7-0 skin sutures are placed, and a nasal retainer is sutured in place for 1 week to support the almost perfect form of the newly constructed nostril. The parents are instructed to have the baby wear the nasal retainer for 1 year after surgery (Fig. 56.1J).

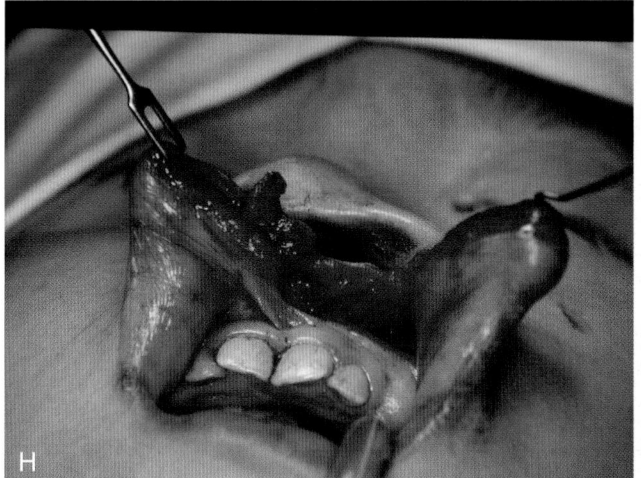

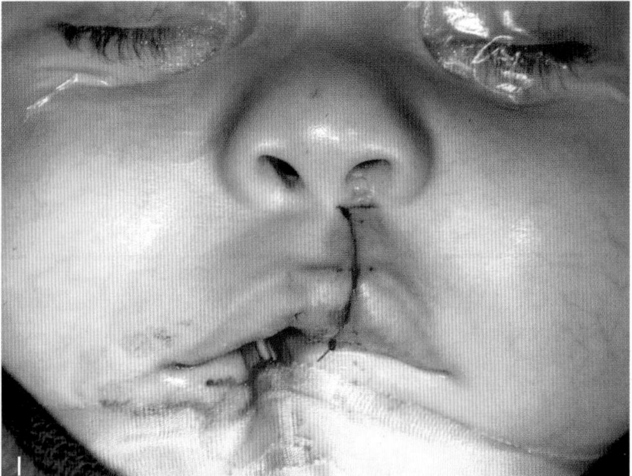

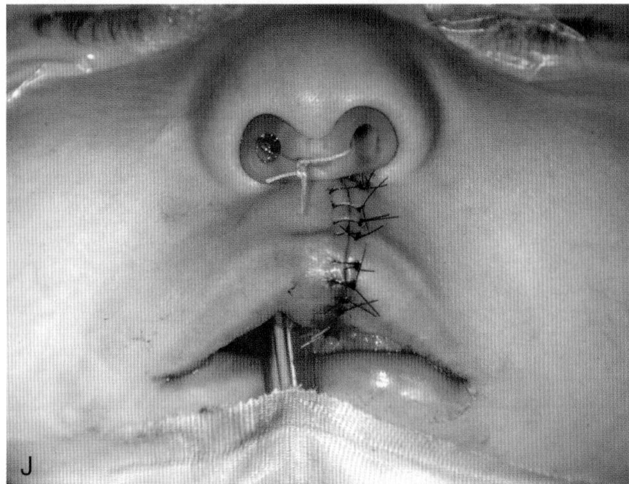

Figure 56.1, cont'd **H,** Complete and watertight closure of the nasal floor. **I,** Muscle surgery is more important than skin surgery. This photo shows good muscle reconstruction and passive coaptation of the skin. **J,** Final skin closure and placement of the nasal retainer.

ALTERNATIVE TECHNIQUE 1: Right Complete Unilateral Cheilorhinoplasty

The primary technique can be applied equally successfully to right complete unilateral cleft lip/nose. The principles are identical, but the surgery, of course, is reversed. Left unilateral cleft lip/nose (with or without cleft palate) is more common than the same deformity on the right side; therefore, some surgeons find that excellent results are more difficult to obtain on the right side. Equally good results can be achieved in both the right and left forms of the deformity by strictly applying the principles of functional anatomy and meticulously identifying the anatomic points on which the incision design is based (Fig. 56.2).

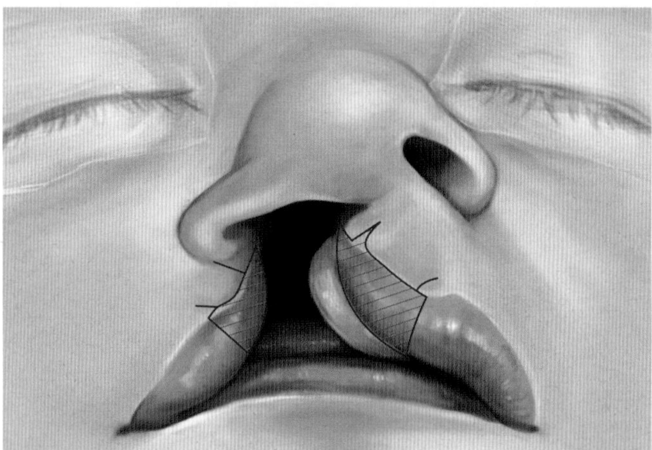

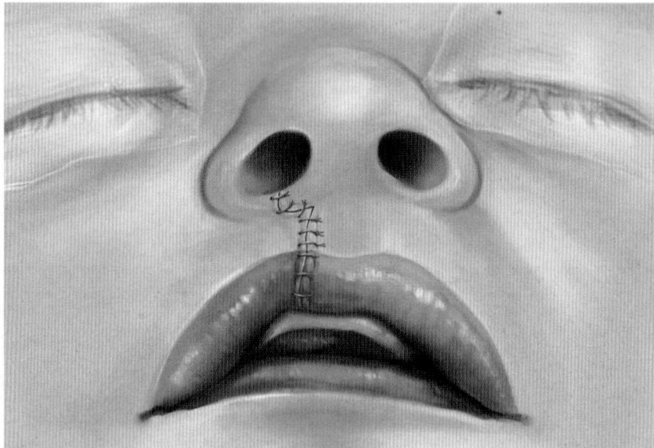

Figure 56.2 Complete unilateral right cleft lip before and after surgery.

ALTERNATIVE TECHNIQUE 2: Incomplete Unilateral Cheilorhinoplasty

Management of incomplete forms of unilateral cleft lip/nose requires special care because only a "complete" operation allows the surgeon to perform "complete" muscle reconstruction, without which the results will be disappointing. The parents of a baby with incomplete cleft lip/nose often believe that a partial operation with a "smaller scar" is all that is needed. The surgeon must explain to them, before the operation, that to achieve the best possible results, both functional and esthetic, the muscle reconstruction must be as perfect as possible (Fig. 56.3).

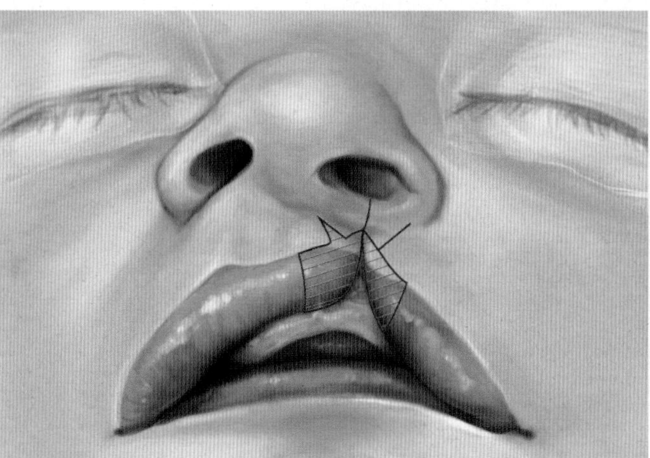

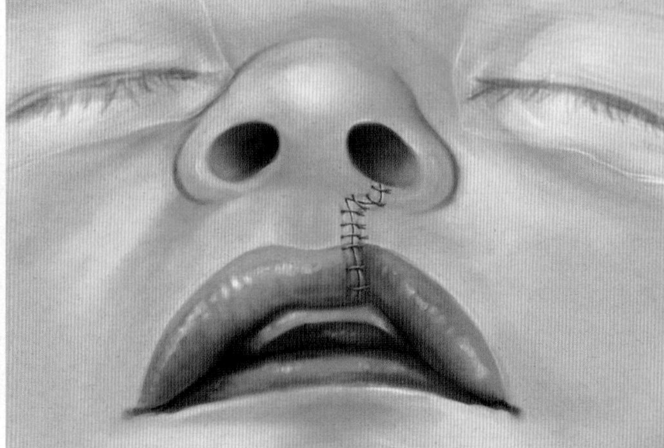

Figure 56.3 Incomplete unilateral cleft lip before and after surgery.

Avoidance and Management of Intraoperative Complications

Four principal intraoperative complications are possible, each of which affects subsequent facial growth.

1. Failure to achieve complete closure of the nasal floor in the alveolar portion of the premaxilla and maxilla. This results in an oral nasal fistula (ONF). This problem can be prevented through the use of adequate subperiosteal and subperichondrial dissections so that meticulous closure of the nasal mucosa is realized.
2. Failure to achieve a straight nasal septum at the completion of the operation. The surgeon should never adopt a strategy of dealing with this problem in a subsequent operation. The goal of primary surgery is to minimize the need for revision surgery.
3. Failure to achieve complete and symmetric nasolabial muscle reconstruction. The single biggest cause of this complication is preventable if the surgeon has a detailed knowledge of the functional anatomy and physiology of these muscles. The child never grows out of inadequate and inaccurate nasolabial muscle reconstruction; in fact, small dissymmetries simply become larger as the child grows.
4. Failure to achieve a functional patent nostril on the cleft side. Surgery creates the patent nostril, and the nasal retainer supports that creation. The nasal retainer can never create nasal patency in the absence of accurate surgery. The nasal retainer should be sutured in place at the end of the operation and remain in place for 1 week, after which the suture is removed. The parents must be carefully instructed to ensure that the baby wears the retainer as much as possible for 1 year after surgery.

Postoperative Considerations

Three assessments must be made as requisite follow-up to primary unilateral cheilorhinoplasty.

1. Presence of ONF. There are two types of ONF. Palatal ONF occurs between the palatal aspect of the premaxilla-maxilla and the nose. This condition is not so much a complication as it is the surgeon's failure to achieve the surgical objectives. Palatal ONF requires "re-do" palatal surgery at the time of alveolar bone grafting, at about 5.5 to 6 years of age. Vestibular ONF can be seen in the oral vestibule and represents, among other things, failure to adequately reconstruct the nasolabial muscles. Correction of vestibular ONF requires a secondary functional cheilorhinoplasty.
2. Deviation of the nasal septum to the noncleft side. This is proof that the nasal septum was inadequately positioned during primary cheilorhinoplasty; most frequently this finding is also related to failure to achieve symmetric nasolabial muscle reconstruction. Its correction requires a secondary functional cheilorhinoplasty.
3. Inability to symmetrically project the lips. This problem stems directly from poor and inadequate symmetric nasolabial muscle reconstruction during primary surgery. To correct this problem, "re-do" secondary functional cheilorhinoplasty is required.

References

1. Veau V. *Cleft Lip*. Clinical-Surgical Forms; 1938.
2. Markus AF, Delaire J. Functional primary closure of cleft lip. *Br J Oral Maxillofac Surg*. 1993;31(5):281–291.
3. Precious DS, Delaire J. Clinical observations of cleft lip and palate. *Oral Surg Oral Med Oral Pathol*. 1993;75(2):141–151.
4. Delaire J, Precious D. Influence of the nasal septum on maxillonasal growth in patients with congenital labiomaxillary cleft. *Cleft Palate J*. 1986;23(4):270–277.

CHAPTER 57

Rotation-Advancement Unilateral Cheilorhinoplasty

Suzanne Barnes, Suganya Appugounder, and Paul Kloostra

Armamentarium

Betadine paint
Moistened Ray-Tec sponge
Fine-tip marking pen
Castroviejo caliper
25-Gauge needle
Methylene blue
1% Lidocaine with 1:100,000 epinephrine
#11 Blade
#15c Blade
0.5 Adson forceps with teeth
Guthrie skin hook
Frazier tip suction tip
Guarded needle tip Bovie electrocautery
Curved iris scissors
#9 Periosteal elevator
5-0 Monocryl with TF needle
6-0 Fast gut with PC1 needle or 6-0 plain gut with TG-140 needle
5-0 Chromic gut with RB1 needle
7-0 Undyed Vicryl with P1 needle
4-0 PDS with RB-1 needle
Skin glue (i.e., Dermabond)
¼-inch Brown Steri-Strips
0.25% Marcaine with 1:200,000 epinephrine

History

The techniques of primary unilateral cheilorhinoplasty have evolved over time. Initial attempts focused simply on bringing the edges together with a straight line closure. Various modifications were developed over the centuries including LeMesurier's quadrilateral flap, Phipher's wavy lines, Tennison's triangular flap, and Millard's vertical repositioning of the triangular flap below the columella with emphasis on the downward rotation of the greater segment and advancement of the lesser.

Dr. Millard developed his technique while serving in the US Marine Corps in Korea in the 1950s. He presented his new design to his mentor, Sir Harold Gillies, and insisted on presenting it at the International Congress of Plastic Surgery in Stockholm, Sweden.[1]

Over 60 years later, many modifications have been developed by Millard and others. Because a procedure by any given name will be performed differently in the hands of any given surgeon, and the intended audience is the novice surgeon, the following chapter describes the basics of a Millard rotation-advancement technique incorporating modifications and multiple additional reference points not included in many descriptions.

Indications and Advantages

Cleft lip and palate arise from partial or complete failure of fusion of the medial nasal processes and the maxillary prominence of the first branchial arch. This results in a spectrum of manifestations, from microform to complete cleft lip and palate, resulting in a spectrum of involvement of the facial musculature, variability in the size and shape of the residual segments, and the degree of resulting nasal deformation. Therefore, each cheilorhinoplasty must be tailored to the specific patient's needs, with special attention to the facial subunits, underlying musculature, and nasal complex to provide a near symmetric reconstruction. The advantages of the rotation-advancement technique include allowing for good nasal access, discarding minimal tissue, camouflaging the suture line, and providing a flexible repair.[2]

Limitations and Contraindications

There are no absolute contraindications to performing a cheilorhinoplasty beyond the systemic health limitations of the child. However, limitations of the rotation-advancement technique have been noted: the tendency to overconstrict the affected nostril, wide repairs may be subject to considerable tension with associated scar widening or hypertrophy and vertical contraction, and the rhinotomy incision produces an unsightly scar in the alar crease and should be avoided.[2–4] Because of these limitations, the repair described here will not provide the best outcome for every cleft lip that a surgeon will encounter. A surgeon must be familiar with the various procedures and modifications available to develop the best possible outcome in every situation.

TECHNIQUE: Millard Rotation-Advancement

BASICS

More than the style of repair, a surgeon's soft tissue handling will have the greatest effect on the esthetic outcome.

In the months prior to surgery, simple forms of presurgical orthopedics can be applied. A skin barrier is helpful in preventing excess skin irritation.

STEP 1: Preparation

The patient is positioned with an oral RAE endotracheal tube taped at the midline, a small shoulder roll, and slight Trendelenburg position for optimal viewing from the head of the bed.

STEP 2: Markings

A cleft may occur on either side of the midsagittal plane. Many authors have used various conventions and in many cases interchanging them within the same article or chapter, leading to confusion when describing anatomical landmarks. To reduce confusion, we use the following conventions:

Greater and Lesser Segments: The cleft divides the lip into two asymmetric segments. The smaller of these may be referred to as the lesser segment, and the larger, which includes the columella and philtrum, may be referred to as the greater segment.

Cleft-Side and Contralateral: When bilateral structures appear on the greater segment, these may be differentiated by their proximity to the cleft. For example, the height of Cupid's bow closest to the cleft may be called the cleft-side height of Cupid's bow, while the other may be referred to as the contralateral height of Cupid's bow (Fig. 57.1).

Greater Segment Cupid's Bow: A fine-tip marking pen is used to demonstrate the following landmarks. It is helpful to start with marking the wet-dry line on both the greater and lesser segments with a light dotted line before the mucosa dries and becomes difficult to identify. The depth of Cupid's bow at the midline (point 1) and height of Cupid's bow on the contralateral side (point 2) are both marked. The distance from the depth of Cupid's bow (point 1) to the contralateral height of Cupid's bow (point 2) is measured, then transposed to identify the cleft-side height of Cupid's bow (point 3). The flat of the lip above the cleft-side height of Cupid's bow (point 4) is marked perpendicular to the white roll (Fig. 57.2A and B).

The Nose: The contralateral columellar base, the point angle at the junction of the columella, philtrum, and nasal sill, is marked (point 5). The greater segment subalare (the most inferior point of the alar base) is marked (point 6). Next the lesser segment alar base is identified by estimating its final position. Using the index finger, applying superomedial pressure, reposition the ala to approximate symmetry, then mark the subalare (point 7). Finally, the lesser segment height of the nasal sill is identified (point 8).

Lesser Segment Cupid's Bow: Appropriate design of the opening incision on the lesser segment is critical to creating a

Continued

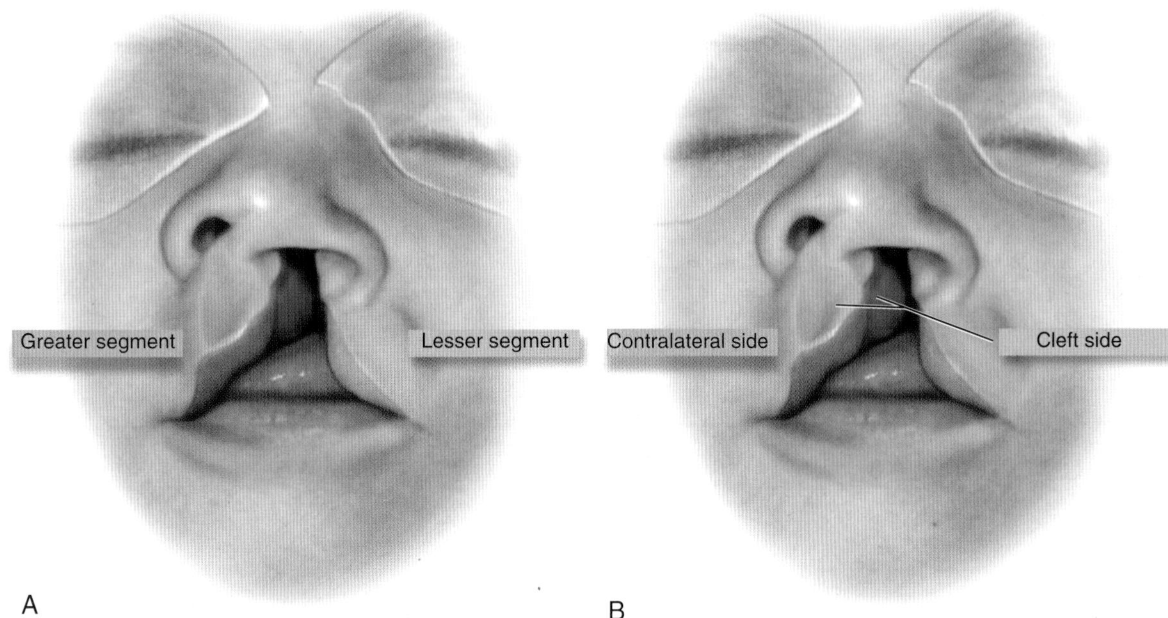

Fig. 57.1 **A,** Demonstration of the greater and lesser segments. **B,** Demonstration of the cleft and contralateral sides of the greater segment.

TECHNIQUE: Millard Rotation-Advancement—*cont'd*

natural appearing lip. If selected too far lateral, the lesser segment will be unnecessarily shortened. If too medial, the white roll will be diminutive and ill-defined, and the volume of the vermillion insufficient to create a symmetric tubercle. Noordhoff described this point in his article.[5] Noordhoff's point is most easily identified by holding a straight instrument perpendicular to the white roll, advancing from lateral to medial along the lesser segment, watching for where the white roll and wet-dry line begin to converge. This is the location of Noordhoff's point, which will later become the height of Cupid's bow. As a means of verifying correct selection, a Castroviejo caliper can be used to measure the height of the contralateral dry vermillion and verify the selected point is equal in height (Fig. 57.2C). Next, the point of the flat of the lip above Noordhoff's point, perpendicular to the white roll is marked (point 10), followed by the point on the wet-dry line below Noordhoff's point that is also perpendicular to the white roll (point 11).

Vermillion: Attention is then turned to the greater segment and the red line is marked perpendicular to the white roll below the contralateral side height of Cupid's bow (point 12) and the cleft-side height of Cupid's bow (point 13). To avoid flattening of the lip, often attributed to scar contracture, symmetric portions of the pars marginalis/tubercle of the lip will need to be brought together at closure. To achieve this, when marking the lesser segment flat of the lip (point 10), verify that the distance from the white roll to the flat of the lip on the greater segment (distance from point 3 to 4) is equal to its counterpart on the lesser segment (distance from point 9 to 10). The height of the dry vermillion is often deficient and can be augmented with a triangular flap that will insert to a back cut extending from point 13, just above the wet-dry line up to the midline, below the depth of Cupid's bow (point 14).

STEP 3: Incision Design

The skin incision of the greater segment consists of a gentle curve extending from the flat of the lip above the cleft-side height of Cupid's bow (Point 4) to the contralateral columellar base (point 5). The incision is further marked along the line from the flat of the lip above the cleft-side height of Cupid's bow (point 4) to the wet-dry line below. The design is then extended within the mucosa, to the depth of the vestibule paralleling the maxillary frenulum. Another incision line is marked out along the skin edge to separate mucosa and skin lateral to the height of Cupid's bow, extending into the nose and defines the C-flap (Fig. 57.3).

On the lesser segment, a preliminary incision design is marked extending from the flat of the lip above the Noordhoff point (point 10) to the lesser segment height of the nasal sill (point 8). Then along the line from the flat of the lip above the Noordhoff point through the wet-dry line, and as on the greater segment, brought through the oral mucosa to the depth of the vestibule. The traditional rotation-advancement technique includes a rhinotomy incision in the alar-facial crease to improve lateral advancement. If used, the incision should not extend beyond the lesser segment subalare. However, every effort should be made to avoid this incision all together, as it is not necessary, because it obliterates the natural crease and causes nasal distortion with hypertrophic scarring that is impossible to correct. If tempted to use this incision, stop and reassess your lesser segment maxillary and pyriform dissection, described below.

The surgeon is warned that the greater segment incision should be made before proceeding to the lesser segment, allowing modification of the incision design if needed.

SOLUTIONS

1. The cleft-side philtrum is lengthened utilizing the curved incision. When inferior rotation is not passive or easily attained, a back cut of 1 to 2 mm on the greater segment at the junction of the flat of the lip and the tubercle (point 4) can be incorporated to further level the height of Cupid's bow. If used, an equilateral triangular flap the size of the back cut will be incorporated in to the lesser segment incision design along the line from the Noordhoff point (point 10) to the height of the nasal sill (point 8) (see Fig. 57.3).
2. The cleft-side dry vermillion height (from point 3 to 13, Fig. 57.2) is often deficient relative to the contralateral (from point 2 to 12, see Fig. 57.2). However, the dry vermillion of the lesser segment, at the Noordhoff point (from point 9 to 11), provides sufficient bulk to create a symmetric Cupid's bow. The deficient dry vermillion of the cleft-side Cupid's bow can be compensated for and smoothly transitioned into the central tubercle by incorporating a dry vermillion isosceles triangular flap from the lesser segment, inserting to the cleft side dry vermillion, just above the wet-dry line. The width of the triangle will be determined by the difference between the height of the dry vermillion on the cleft side and the height of vermillion on the lesser segment. The length of the triangle will be determined by the distance from the planned incision on the greater segment, to the midline, along the wet-dry line (from point 13 to 14), which will also serve as the design for the back cut to receive the flap.

Dry Vermillion Triangle
Width = (9to11) - (3to13)
Length=13to14

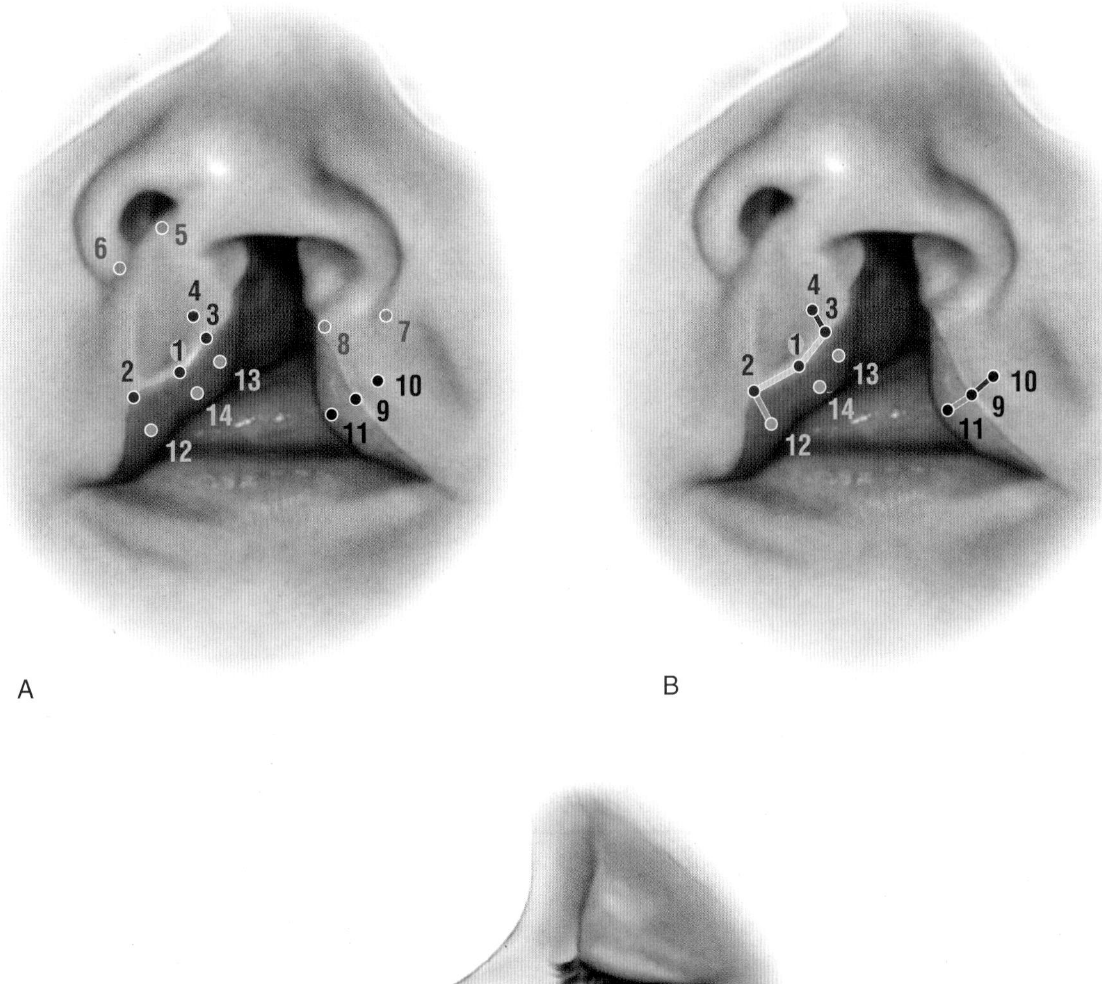

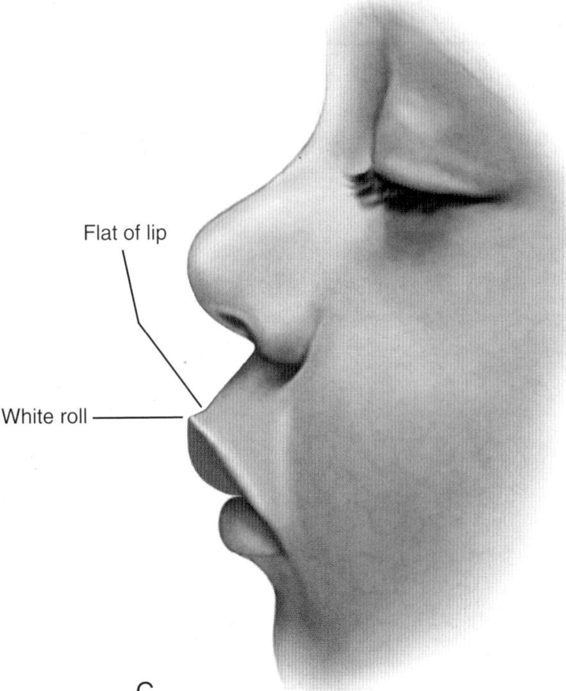

Fig. 57.2 Anatomical landmarks. **A,** Anatomical landmarks to assist with incision design. **B,** Key points of symmetry. **C,** Demonstration of the transition of the lip tubercle to the "flat" of the lip.

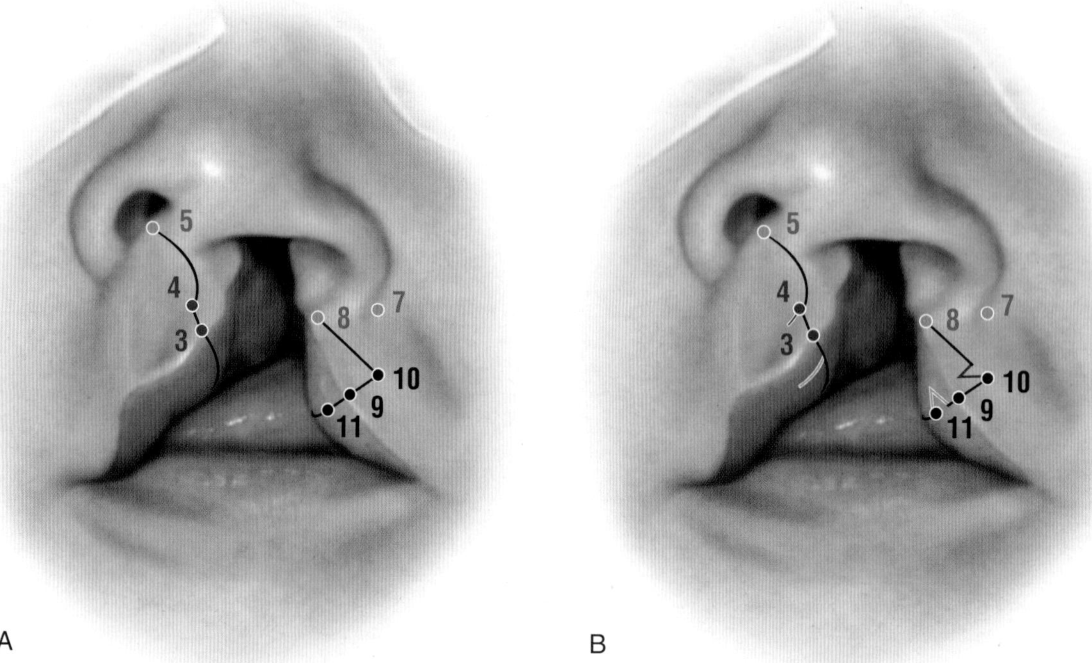

Fig. 57.3 Incision design. **A,** Basic incision design. **B,** Incision design with modifications. The incision design must resolve at least two problems that have resulted from the cleft:

1. The cleft-side philtral column is shorter than the contralateral side
2. The cleft-side dry vermillion is shorter than the contralateral side

TECHNIQUE: Millard Rotation-Advancement—*cont'd*

STEP 4: Tattoos

Key landmarks are tattooed with methylene blue and a 30-gauge needle.

STEP 5: Greater Segment Incision and Dissection

The skin is incised with a #11 blade taking care to create sharp corners and smooth continuous skin incisions. The incision on the mucosa is more easily achieved with a #15 or #15C blade. The hypoplastic tissue is dissected free from the underlying muscle and the C-flap is raised, separating skin from the orbicularis with curved iris scissors. The excess tissue is discarded. The skin is parsed from the orbicularis medially 1 to 2 mm with an iris scissors or #11 blade. Care should be taken not to extend inferiorly below the flat of the lip or release the philtral dimple at the depth of Cupid's bow. The orbicularis is then elevated off the premaxilla and anterior nasal spine (ANS) in a supraperiosteal plane. If the septum is displaced to the contralateral side, it is dissected free in the supraperichondrial plane and transposed to the cleft side. A freer can be run posteriorly to free the septum from the maxillary crest if needed. This will allow the nose to grow straight and prevent typical septal deviation associated with cleft lip and palate.

With the C-flap, skin edge, and orbicularis dissection complete, the cleft-side lip length is assessed with gentle inferior traction. If this does not easily produce a level Cupid's bow, additional modifications will be necessary. This may include extending the original incision on the philtrum with an additional back cut extending 45 degrees inferolateral but not extending any further than the contralateral philtral column. Alternatively, or in addition, a 1 to 2 mm back cut can be made at the inferior most part of the flat of the lip, extending medial from and perpendicular to the incision line at point 4 and addition of the equilateral triangle with its inferior most aspect approximating point 10 (as described above).

TECHNIQUE: Millard Rotation-Advancement—*cont'd*

STEP 6: Lesser Segment Incision and Dissection

With the extent of inferior rotation established on the greater segment, the incision design of the lesser segment should be adjusted as dictated by the needs of the greater segment. Again, sharp incision of the skin with a #11 blade. Similar to the greater segment, the incision crosses on to the dry vermillion perpendicular to the white roll. The dry vermillion triangle is incised, and then carried perpendicular across the wet-dry line into the free mucosa and into the height of the vestibule. A back cut at the height of the vestibule is incised with sharp or electrocautery dissection, just enough to allow access to the maxilla.

The orbicularis and transverse portion of nasalis are separated with an iris scissors. As with the greater segment, the orbicularis and the transverse portion of nasalis are lifted from the maxilla in a supraperiosteal plane as wide and superior as the infraorbital nerve. Electrocautery or sharp dissection is used to transition to a subperiosteal plane at the pyriform. The nasal mucosa is mobilized from the pyriform to allow medial advancement.

The junction of the oral and nasal mucosa along the primary and secondary hard palate is sharply separated on both segments. The greater segment incision starts at the height of the nasal sill and extends along the oral and nasal mucosal junction, which will often extend onto the vomer and may be extended to the posterior aspect of the hard palate for a primary uranoplasty as described by Sommerlad.[6] On the lesser segment, the separation of oral and nasal mucosa simply starts above the alveolus and extends posteriorly. Otherwise, a vertical back cut will be necessary to obtain passive closure. If used, the vertical release is generally placed somewhere below the inferior turbinate on the lesser segment.

The oral mucosa and minor salivary glands are lifted from the deep surface of the orbicularis, and if necessary, the back cut at the height of the vestibule is extended. The extent of the back cut and dissection is dictated by the width of the cleft and should provide sufficient laxity to advance the superomedial corner to the depth of the vestibule on the greater segment with minimal tension. Note, the inferior extent of the oral mucosa dissection should stop short of the orbicularis pars marginalis.

The skin of the lip is parsed from the orbicularis and carried lateral until the orbicularis can be brought across the cleft defect with relatively minimal tension. This can be carried as far lateral as subalare if necessary; again taking care not to extend onto the tubercle. If at this point any additional advancement is needed, carefully assess the point of greatest tension and revisit the subperiosteal and supraperiosteal dissections of the lesser segment. A back cut at the alar base (rhinotomy) of the lesser segment should only be used as an absolute last resort. The back cut should never extend past the subalare and should be placed 2 mm below the alar groove to preserve its natural shape.

Please note that microform and incomplete clefts with minimal advancement may not require much, if any, of the maxillary, pyriform, or mucosal dissection and may only require minimal parsing of the orbicularis from the skin of the lip.

STEP 7: Primary Rhinoplasty

Through the lesser segment incision, superior to the orbicularis, tenotomy scissors are used to dissect along the dorsal surface of the cleft-side lower lateral cartilage, extending over the middle crus into the interdomal ligaments. The caudal aspect of the medial foot plates and medial tip are approached through the greater segment incision just superior to ANS. The goal is to free the cleft-side lower cartilage from the overlying skin, allowing passive and independent movement as the ala and lip are set into their new position. The cartilage's new position will be further supported with transfixion sutures at the end of the procedure.

Please note that great care must be taken not to disrupt their integrity. Careless dissection can result in a soft, poorly projected ptotic tip and external nasal valve collapse.

STEP 8: Nasal Reconstruction

The nasal floor is closed by advancing the nasal mucosa of the lesser segment to the mucosa and septum and/or vomer flap. Closure proceeds from posterior to anterior with care, with simple interrupted 5-0 Vicryl on a TF or RB1, taking care to ensure that the points of nasal sill closure align. For a more complete discussion regarding nasal reconstruction, refer to Tse et al.[7]

STEP 9: Mucosal Closure

The superomedial corner of the lesser segment oral mucosa is advanced across the cleft defect and secured to the depth of the vestibule of the greater segment with an interrupted 5-0 chromic gut sutures on an RB1. A couple more interrupted sutures approximate the oral mucosa while leaving the mucosa overlying the pars marginalis free. Mucosal closure will be completed after setting the muscular, skin, and vermillion closures. This allows the surgeon the opportunity to critically inspect the symmetry of the vermillion and tubercle in three dimensions while adjusting the volume of mucosa prior to final closure.

Continued

TECHNIQUE: Millard Rotation-Advancement—*cont'd*

STEP 10: Muscular Reconstruction

The previously separated transverse portion of the nasalis muscle with its slightly different orientated fibers, when mobilized, will advance the ala. Care should be taken to position the ala appropriately in all three dimensions, securing its position with a 4-0 polydioxanone (PDS) within the periosteum of the premarital.

A temporary approximating suture is passed through the pars marginalis on its deep side with the tails passing deep to the orbicularis. Gentle inferior traction is then applied with a hemostat. This will help ensure appropriate muscular approximation for maximum lip length. The orbicularis is then closed with an interrupted 5-0 PDS.

STEP 11: Skin and Vermillion Closure

With the temporary suture at the pars marginalis still in place, the skin approximation is started. The C-flap is rotated and trimmed to provide skin for closure of the nasal sill. The subcutaneous tissue is approximated with buried 5-0 Monocryl. Care should be taken to prevent the suture from passing any more superficial than the deep dermal layer, to ensure the skin lays passively in its final position and prevent dimpling.

There is debate regarding the use of resorbable versus nonresorbable sutures for skin closure. While resorbable sutures and skin glue (i.e., Dermabond) are known to cause more inflammation, it is the authors' experience that there is no clinically significant difference in the resulting scar and use of nonresorbable sutures does not warrant the parental stress, traumatic in-office removal, or a second anesthetic. Close attention to passive approximation with ideal skin edge eversion is far more important in achieving an optimal esthetic outcome. We have previously utilized 6-0 fast gut, and recently started to explore outcomes with 6-0 plain gut on a TG-140 needle to provide a more ideal skin approximation with smaller puncture wounds, again with excellent results.

The dry vermillion is approximated with interrupted 7-0 Vicryl. Finally, the volume of mucosa is reassessed, noting that any redundancy or deficiency will not settle out over time. Therefore, care should be taken to obtain an even and symmetric lip margin, which may require reduction of the dry vermillion triangle or excision of excess oral mucosa.

STEP 12: Transfixion Sutures

The nasal cartilages are approximated with undyed 4-0 PDS transfusion sutures placed with a 22-gauge hypodermic needle. Four key sutures are placed: medial foot plates, interdomal, scroll, and alar groove.

1. The medial foot plates are approximated by passing the 22-gauge needle through he nasal mucosa, both foot plates, and contralateral nasal mucosa. The PDS is passed through the needle until extending out of the hub. The needle is then backed out of both cartilages, but not the first layer of nasal mucosa. The needle is redirected through both cartilages and back out the contralateral nasal mucosa. The suture is pulled through and tied. The remaining sutures are performed in a similar manner.
2. The domal suture is used to approximate the domal units and narrow the nasal tip.
3. The scroll of the upper and lower lateral cartilages is reconstructed by passing the 22-gauge needle through skin cephalic margin of the lower lateral cartilage and nasal mucosa. After passing the suture, the needle is backed out of the cartilage without exiting the skin, reoriented and reinserted through the caudal margin of the upper lateral cartilage. This suture should suspend the lower lateral cartilage, often mistaken for redundant web. This area should never be incised, as doing so will result in synechia, alar distortion, and obstruction.
4. The alar groove transfixion suture is passed through the skin of the lower alar groove and nasal mucosa, again, backed out and redirected to another point along the groove on the nasal mucosa. This suture will provide additional definition to the groove and obliterate dead space.

STEP 13: Dressing

Finally, dressings are applied with skin glue (i.e., Dermabond), which is then covered with ¼-inch Steri-Strips. The dressing remains in place for 2 weeks until autodiscontinued. Nostril retainers may be placed to assist with shaping the nostril; however, they are often unnecessary for microform or incomplete or narrow complete clefts. If placed, it is best to suture the nostril retainers in place to prevent extrusion or dislodgement, but take care not to allow the retainer to place pressure on the alar rim or soft triangle. Elbow immobilizers are applied before extubation.

ALTERNATIVE TECHNIQUE: Extended Mohler

Cutting described a modification of the rotation-advancement technique by omitting the back cut to the opposite philtral column. Instead, the curvilinear incision extends through the middle of the philtral dimple, then 1.5 to 2 mm up the columella, just to the contralateral side of midline, he notes this to be 4/7 the width of the columella. The back cut then extends back down the columella at a 45-degree angle to the contralateral philtral column. The C-flap is then used to back fill the columella and provide tissue for closure of the nasal sill, avoiding the dog ear often encountered in the classic rotation-advancement technique.[4]

Avoidance and Management of Intraoperative Complications

Thorough preoperative education for parents is a critical point for managing postoperative expectations. When parents are informed of what they will experience, their faith is returned in spades. An explanation after the fact is an excuse. Appropriate management of the nasal mucosa will prevent nasal stenosis. There is no reason to make an incision within the alar web. Never violate the cartilages during primary rhinoplasty. Disruption will result in an amorphous tip with poor projection. Appropriate selection of the Noordhoff point plays a crucial role in the appearance of the vermillion height. If the point is selected too medial, the volume of dry vermillion will be deficient. If the point is too lateral, too much lip tissue will be removed. Failure to incorporate the dry vermillion triangle will result in oral mucosa substitution, which will provide a poor esthetic substitute. Inadequate approximation of the pars marginalis will result in a whistle deformity.

Postoperative Considerations

The child is admitted to manage parental anxiety, pain, and IV maintenance until taking sufficient PO. The child is maintained on a liquid diet with elbow immobilizers for 2 weeks.

References

1. Millard DR. *Cleft Craft: The Evolution of its Surgery*. Boston: Little, Brown; 1977.
2. Ness JA, Sykes JM. Basics of Millard rotation-advancement technique for repair of the unilateral cleft lip deformity. *Facial Plast Surg*. 1993;9(3):167–176.
3. Fisher DM. Unilateral cleft lip repair: an anatomical subunit approximation technique. *Plast Reconstr Surg*. 2005;116(1):61–71.
4. Flores R, Cutting CB. Extended mohler unilateral cleft lip repair. In: *Comprehensive Cleft Care*. 2015;2:843–856.
5. Noordhoff MS, Chen Y-R, Chen K-T, Hong K-F, Lo L-J. The surgical technique for the complete unilateral cleft lip-nasal deformity. *Operative Tech Plast Reconst Surg*. 1995;2:167.
6. Sommerlad BC. Surgery of the cleft lip and nose—the GOStA approach. *B-ENT*. 2006;2(suppl 4):29–31.
7. Tse RW, Mercan E, Fisher DM, Hopper RA, Birgfeld CB, Gruss JS. Unilateral cleft lip nasal deformity: foundation-based approach to primary rhinoplasty. *Plast Reconstr Surg*. 2019;144(5):1138–1149.

CHAPTER 58

Unilateral Cheilorhinoplasty—Fisher

David Yates and Patrick Wong

Armamentarium

#9 Periosteal elevator
#11 Blade
#11 and #15 scalpels
#15 Blade
25-guage needle
Adson tissue forceps
Appropriate sutures:4-0 Polydioxanone (PDS) on P-3—alar base suture3-0 Nylon on PS-2—nasal stent suture4-0 Chromic gut on RB-1—mucosal suture5-0 Chromic gut on RB-1—mucosal suture4-0 Monocryl on RB-1—muscle suture5-0 Fast gut on PC-1—skin suture4-0 Vicryl on RB-1—deep suture5-0 Vicryl on TF—dermal suture
Bard Parker scalpel handle
Bishop Harmon forceps
Castroviejo
Calipers
Castroviejo forceps 0.5 mm
Curved iris scissors
Colorado tip Bovie
Dean scissors
Frazier tip suction, 8 Fr
Gillies dura and skin retractor local anesthetic with vasoconstrictor
Long 0.25-inch Steri-Strips
Mastisol
Nasal former size 3
Needle tip electrocautery
Ragnell retractor ×2
Straight iris scissors
Webster 5-inch needle holder

History of the Procedure

Early cleft lip repair dates as far back as 390 BC, when surgery was first performed to repair a cleft on a young 18-year-old Chinese soldier, Wey Young Chi. Legend tells of how his surgeon demanded he abstain from laughing or talking for 100 days after the surgery.[1] Throughout the centuries, cleft lip repair techniques have grown from simple straight line approximations to a multitude of repair techniques using rotational, advancement, and transpositional flaps. In the 1950s Ralph Millard championed a rotational-advancement technique that would become both a standard and a blueprint for the modern repairs utilized in the present day.[1]

One such modern technique was described in 2005 by Toronto-based cleft surgeon, David Fisher. Fisher trained under Daniel Marchac in Paris and M. Samuel Noordhoff in Taiwan. His technique pays homage to his former teachers by combining elements from each into a unique approach to the unilateral cleft lip deformity.[2] In the past two decades, the Fisher anatomic subunit repair has gained significant popularity and has represented a paradigm shift in modern cleft lip surgery.[3]

Indications for the Use of the Procedure

A fundamental understanding of both the relevant anatomy and embryology is critical to cleft repair as the aberrant anatomy in a cleft patient is a direct consequence of the anomalies that occur during fetal development. At 6 weeks in utero, fusion of the median nasal prominence with the maxillary prominences and lateral nasal prominences forms the nasal base, nostrils, upper lip, and primary palate. This fusion is mediated on a cellular level by a complex and only partially understood process involving cell migration, development, and apoptosis. Failure of this delicate process at any point can result in clefts of varying severity in the labiomaxillary unit.[4,5]

In complete labiomaxillary clefts, the musculature of both the nasal floor and upper lip is not only discontinuous but also abnormally arranged. This distorted muscle arrangement leads to dissymmetric and haphazardly arranged muscle forces resulting in profound defects in the underlying skeleton including the nasal septum. Successful repair of complete labiomaxillary clefts is predicated on closure of the nasal floor, establishment of a straight nasal septum positioned in the midline, reconstruction of the nasolabial musculature to a more physiologic arrangement, and formation of two patent nostrils. Furthermore, repair of the external upper lip should yield the best esthetic possible without stigmata of surgery.[4,5]

Fisher described repairing the lip and nose as closely to normal form and function as the chief goal of cleft repair. He believed this was best achieved by utilizing the “ideal line of repair.” Fisher described this line as extending from the cleft peak of the cupid’s bow to the base of the nose in a manner mirroring the noncleft philtral column and then continuing along the lip columellar crease.[2]

The underlying premise behind Fisher's technique was based on reestablishing lip height and aligning incisions along the anatomical subunits of the face. Fisher's technique uses 25 detailed surgical markings to align this repair. Because of the extensive markings and measurements, the appropriate lip length can be determined rather than estimated. Additional advantages include the technique's versatility regardless of cleft size, avoidance of an incision along the alar base of the affected side, particular attention toward reapproximation of the wet-dry line, and additional length built into the repair as needed.[3]

Some of the essential points of the Fisher repair include the following:

1. Incision line along the "ideal line of repair" emerging from the cleft side peak of the cupid's bow to the nasal base mirroring the noncleft side
2. A small cutaneous triangular flap above the white roll in cases where extra rotation is necessary, eliminating use of a Millard-style back cut
3. A laterally based triangular vermilion flap to address any central vermilion deficiency, similar to Noordhoff's technique
4. Eliminating the need for an alar base incision on the affected side
5. Primary nasal repair aimed at centralizing the columella, anterior repositioning the alar base, nostrils of equal circumference, and anteromedial advancement of the cleft side lateral crus and dome

Fisher originally described the use of an inferior turbinate flap, similar to that described by his mentor Noordhoff, for closure of the posterior lamella.[6,7] However, the authors of this chapter describe a variant of the technique using only medial and laterally based flaps without the use of a turbinate flap. The authors also advocate for a formal primary cheilorhinoplasty at the time of the repair.

Limitations and Contraindications

The main limitation to this procedure is the overall health of the baby. Timing of the cleft lip repair has historically been outlined by the "rule of 10s," suggesting that surgery be performed after the patient is at least 10 weeks old, 10 pounds in weight, and having a minimum hemoglobin of 10 dL/mg. Waiting until the patient is 10 to 12 weeks old allows for a more complete medical evaluation of the patient, is safer from an anesthetic perspective, and facilitates the surgery in that the child and their anatomical landmarks are larger and more easily defined. Currently, there seems to be little benefit to performing surgery earlier than 3 months of age.[4,5]

TECHNIQUE: Fisher Anatomic Subunit Reapproximation for Repair of Unilateral Cleft Lip

STEP 1: Intubation and Setup

The patient is placed in the supine position with a small shoulder roll for support. Broad spectrum antibiotics are administered intravenously for surgical prophylaxis. After intubation, the oral endotracheal tube is secured with tape to the chin in the midline (Fig. 58.1).

STEP 2: Surgical Markings: Medial Lip

The midline (1) and height of the noncleft philtral column (2) are marked at the columellar lip crease. The height of the cleft philtral column (3) is marked to mirror point 2. The upper lip midline (4) and peaks of the cupid's bow (5, 6) are marked along the vermilion-cutaneous junction (F).

Points 7 and 8 are drawn along lines perpendicular to the vermilion-cutaneous junction, just above the white cutaneous roll.

Continued

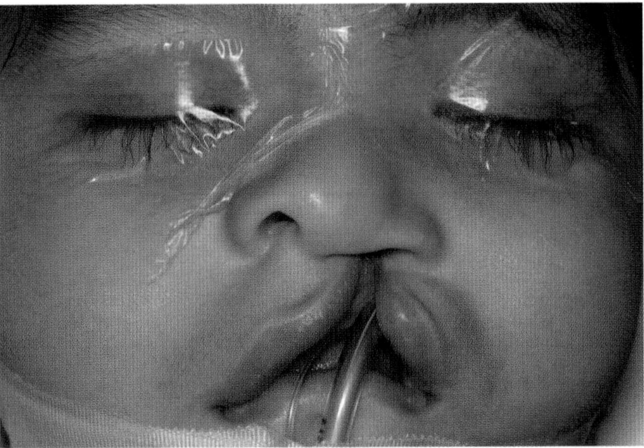

Figure 58.1 The patient is intubated with an oral endotracheal tube, which is then secured to the patient's chin. Sterile film dressings are then used to cover the patient's eyes. (Photo Courtesy Dr. David Yates.)

TECHNIQUE: Fisher Anatomic Subunit Reapproximation for Repair of Unilateral Cleft Lip—*cont'd*

A line is drawn connecting points 3 and 8 to mirror the noncleft philtral column. A line extending medially perpendicular to the philtral column (line 3-8) is drawn from point 8 terminating at point 9 (equal to length c). This line 8-9 (length c) represents the initial incision on the medial lip skin that corresponds to the back cut for the triangle formed by points 18, 20, and 22. The red line (mucovermilion junction) is marked in the midline (10), and below the peaks of the cupid's bow (11, 12). A line drawn through points 6, 8, and 12 should be perpendicular to the free margin of the upper lip. A line drawn from points 10 to 12 represents the initial incision in the red lip that will receive the lateral triangular vermilion flap. It should be just superior to the wet-dry line (Fig. 58.2).

STEP 3: Surgical Markings: Nose

The most inferior points of the alar-lip junction are marked bilaterally (13, 14). Point 14 (on the cleft side) is marked while holding digital pressure to reposition the ala in its predicted position.

Points 15 and 16 are variable, and their position depends on the amount of skin lateral to the cleft side columellar base and medial to the cleft side alar insertion. Point 16 is drawn along the columellar lip crease, representing the height of the lip at the site of proposed closure within the nostril sill on the cleft side. Point 15 is drawn on the noncleft side in a symmetric point, representing the noncleft nostril sill, which has a distinct convexity. The more available tissue medial to the alar insertion, the more medially placed point 16 will appear to be. The markings on the medial lip have little variation from case to case (Fig. 58.3).

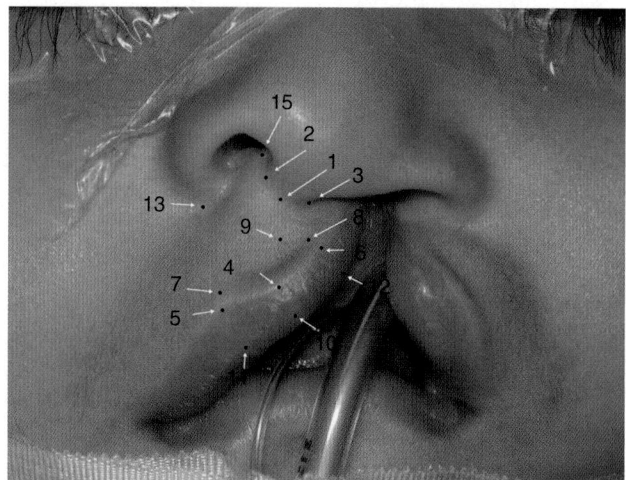

Figure 58.2 The medial lip and nasal landmarks are marked. (Photo Courtesy Dr. David Yates.)

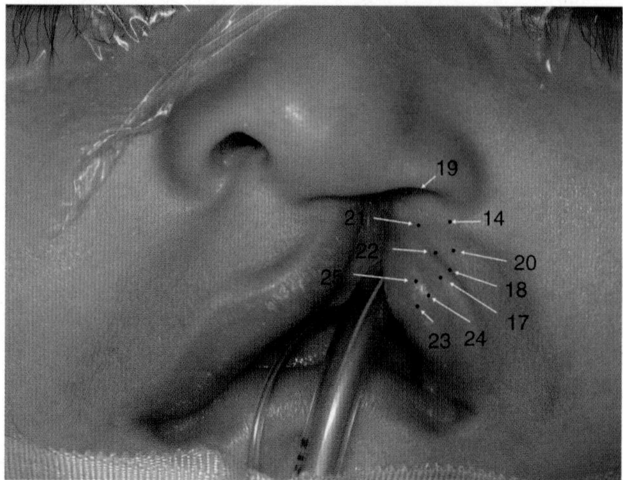

Figure 58.3 The lateral lip and nose landmarks are marked. Note: Point 16 will be marked within the cleft side nasal sill and is not visible in this photograph. (Photo Courtesy Dr. David Yates.)

TECHNIQUE: Fisher Anatomic Subunit Reapproximation for Repair of Unilateral Cleft Lip—*cont'd*

STEP 4: Anatomical Markings: Measurements and Calculations

The total lip height (line 2-7) is measured with the lip at rest. The greater lip height (line 3-8) is measured with gentle downward traction on the lip. The lesser lip height (width of the base of the inferior triangle on the cleft side) can be calculated using the following formula:

[a] Total Lip Height (line 2-7) – [b] Greater Lip Height (line 3-8) – 1 mm = [c] Lesser Lip Height (base of inferior triangle)

This lesser lip height, which corresponds to the base of the inferior triangle on the cleft side as well as the corresponding back cut on the medial lip, is variable. Fisher recommends not exceeding 2 mm for this length. In our experience, a longer length is sometimes required. Our results from these longer incisions are excellent and are not compromised in any way. The 1 mm accounted for in the equation is due to the Rose-Thompson effect, which accounts for one extra millimeter of lengthening. In cases of minor clefts, the need for an inferior triangle may be obviated (Fig. 58.4).

STEP 5: Surgical Markings: Lateral Lip

Point 17 is marked at Noordhoff's Point, the point along the vermilion-cutaneous junction where the cutaneous roll and cutaneous white roll and red line begin to converge medially. This point is where the vermilion height is the greatest. Point 18 is marked just above the white cutaneous roll on a line passing through point 17, perpendicular to the vermilion-cutaneous junction. Line 6-8 from the medial lip will be joined with point 17-18 on the lateral lip and should therefore be of equal length.

The superior and medial distances from point 15 to point 13 are then measured. A point (19) is drawn as far superior and medial to point 14 as the previously measured distances from point 15 to 13. This point (19) represents the point of predicted closure within the nostril sill and will eventually be joined with point 16. Therefore, point 19 should be positioned so that when it is joined with point 16, the cleft nostril circumference will be equivalent to that of the unaffected side. The vertical length of the lateral lip, indicated by the distance between points 18 and 19 will determine the position of the remaining markings.

The position of points 20, 21, and 22 are somewhat variable depending on the amount of vertical length needed. Line 20-21 is the same length as line 3-8 (this is essentially [b], the greater lip length). Point 22 forms the apex of the lateral triangle along the cutaneous white roll. It is placed such that its relationship with points 18 and 20 forms an isosceles triangle, with lines 18-22 and 20-22 being of equal length. The base of this triangle should be equivalent to [c], the lesser lip height.

It should be noted that the horizontal position of point 20 will vary depending on the amount of vertical lengthening effect needed. If more length of lip is needed on the lateral segment, the apex of the triangle (22) is rotated more superiorly. However, the position of point 21 should not be changed to accommodate the length of the lateral lip as this will compromise the final position of the alar insertion. If the lateral lip height is short, point 20 will be placed in a more lateral position rotating the point 22 of the triangle superiorly. The angle formed between points 21-20-22 will open, allowing for lengthening of the vertical height. Conversely, if the lateral lip is vertically long, point 20 will be rotated medially, which will place the point of 20 in a line connecting points 18 and 21. In the case that the lateral lip is still too long, a medially based wedge can be excised from the upper lip below point 19. This wedge has its upper limb positioned in the medial extent of the alar crease. The lateral extension of the wedge should not extend past point 14.

Continued

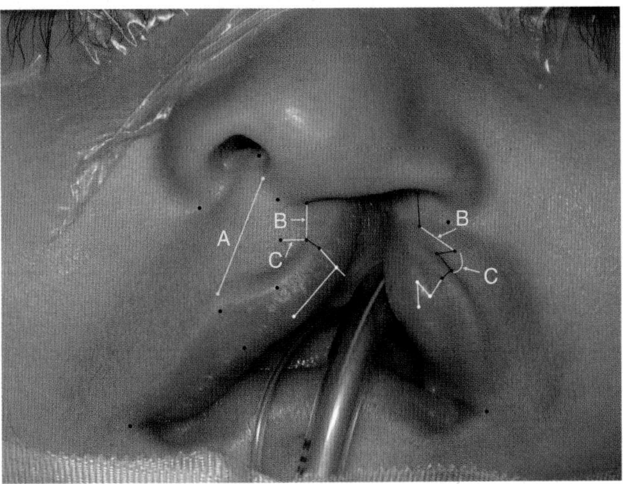

Figure 58.4 The lesser lip height (C) is equivalent to the base of the lateral cutaneous triangle (line 18-20). This length [C] can be found with the formula [A] - [B] -1 = [C]. Where [A] is the total lip length (line 2-7) and [B] is the greater lip length (line 3-8). (Photo Courtesy Dr. David Yates.)

TECHNIQUE: Fisher Anatomic Subunit Reapproximation for Repair of Unilateral Cleft Lip—*cont'd*

Point 21 should be placed so that the length of lines 21-19 and 21-20 are equivalent to the lengths of lines 3-16 and 3-8, respectively. The angle between points 19-21-20 should approximate that of 16-3-8. Point 21 is critical to have positioned correctly since this will come into contact with point 3. For the unexperienced, it is easy to inadvertently rotate the cleft side ala into the nose. Care must be taken to ensure that point 21, when brought into contact with point 3, is appropriately positioned with a good nasal esthetic. When needed, it is sometimes necessary to take a wedge between points 19-14-21 to avoid this (Fig. 58.5).

STEP 6: Surgical Markings: Mucosal Portion of Lip
Point 23 (the inferior point of the lateral triangle) is marked along the red (wet-dry) line below point 17. A line joining points 17 and 23, point 24 (the superior point of the lateral triangle) is marked such that the length of line 17-24 equals that of line 6-12. Lengths 23-25 and 24-25 are equal to the length of the initial incision superior to the red (wet-dry) line of the medial lip (line 10-12). It is important for the incision from 10-12 to still be just inside the wet-dry line of the lip. The base of the lateral triangle (line 23-24) should equal the amount of vermilion height augmentation required on the medial lip. The amount of vermilion height augmentation required can be calculated by subtracting the length of line 6-12 from line 5-11 (Fig. 58.6, Table 58.1).

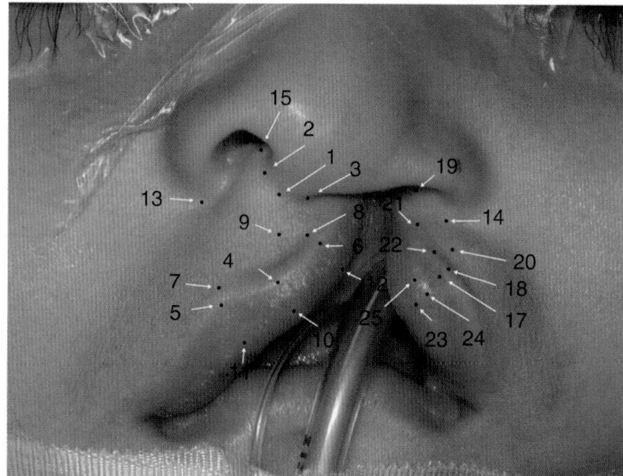

Figure 58.5 All 25 surgical landmarks are marked.

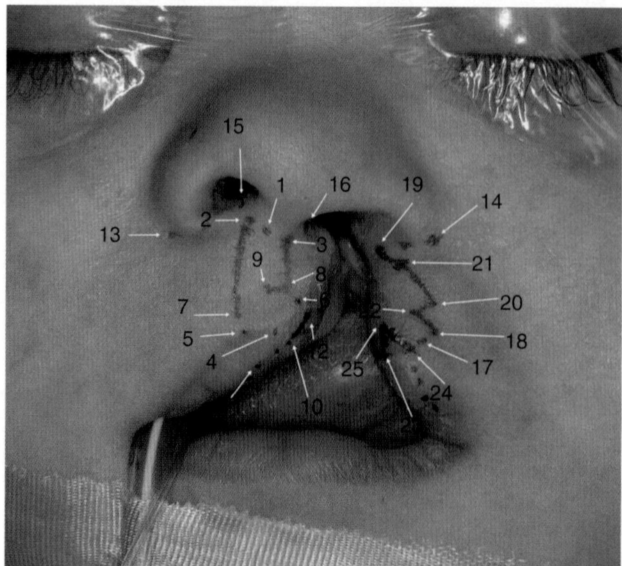

Figure 58.6 All 25 surgical landmarks are marked and then tattooed with methylene blue and a 30-gauge needle. The incisions lines are also drawn. Note: Line 2-7 is marked for calculation purposes only. No incision will be performed along this line. (Photo Courtesy Dr. David Yates.)

Table 58.1 Summary of Surgical Markings

Point	Location and significance
1	Superior midline of philtrum
2	Height on noncleft side philtral column
3	Height of cleft side philtral column (will be joined to point 21)
4	Midline of lip at vermilion-cutaneous junction
5	Peak of cupid's bow on unaffected side
6	Peak of cupid's bow on affected side
7	Just above peak of cupid's bow on unaffected side, superior edge of cutaneous white roll
8	Just above peak of cupid's bow on affected side, superior edge of cutaneous white roll
9	Medial extent of initial incision in medial lip, receiving point for lateral cutaneous triangle (will be joined to point 22)
10	Midline of red (wet-dry) line (muco-vermilion junction)
11	Just below peak of cupid's bow on unaffected side at red (wet-dry) line (muco-vermilion junction)
12	Just below peak of cupid's bow on affected side at wet-dry line (muco-vermilion junction)
13	Most inferior point of lip-alar junction (subalare) on unaffected side
14	Most inferior point of lip-alar junction (subalare) on affected side
15	Nasal sill of unaffected side, made symmetric to point 16
16	Point of proposed closure within nasal sill on affected side from medial lip element (will be joined to point 19), position variable depending on amount of available tissue medial to alar insertion
17	Point on lateral lip where vermilion height is greatest and wet-dry line and cutaneous white roll begin to converge medially (Noordhoff's Point)
18	Just above point 17 (Noordhoff's Point), superior edge of cutaneous white roll
19	Point of proposed closure within nasal sill on affected side from lateral lip element (will be joined to point 16)
20	Superior aspect of base of lateral cutaneous triangle (will be joined to point 8), position variable depending on lateral lip height (18-20 = c length)
21	Point of closure at cleft side philtral column from lateral lip element (will be joined to point 3), position determined based on calculation of greater lip height [b]
22	Apex of lateral cutaneous triangle (will be joined to point 9)
23	Inferior aspect of base of lateral vermilion triangle on wet-dry line (muco-vermilion junction)
24	Superior aspect of base of lateral vermilion triangle
25	Apex of lateral vermilion triangle (will be joined to point 10)

TECHNIQUE: Fisher Anatomic Subunit Reapproximation for Repair of Unilateral Cleft Lip—*cont'd*

STEP 7: Local Anesthesia and Tattooing

The patient's head is wrapped, the eyes are covered with sterile tegaderms, and a moist mouth pack is placed. The previous markings are tattooed with methylene blue dye and a 30-gauge needle. Local anesthesia is administered and includes bilateral infraorbital blocks and local infiltrations into the cleft side alar base, piriform rim, and inferior turbinate.

STEP 8: Medial Lip Dissection

Dissection begins with the initial incision in the mucosa approximately 5 mm superior to the mucogingival junction and approximately 1 cm toward the unaffected side. An incision is then made from the wet-dry line towards the initial mucosal incision with the #11 blade. Using a combination of the #15 and #11 blades, incise the cutaneous portion of the lip through the skin and subcutaneous tissue only. The marginal cleft tissue medial to the incision is saved and sometimes used as a mucosal flap to help decrease tension on the mucosal closure. In some instances, it is excised if not needed. The orbicularis muscle is then dissected from the overlying skin and underlying mucosa. Minimal dissection of the muscle is performed on the medial side in an attempt to preserve the philtral dimple. The orbicularis is then freed from its insertion within the columellar base and alveolar cleft. The deformed septum is then identified and dissected off the maxillary crest posteriorly approximately 1 cm using an iris scissor (Fig. 58.7).

Additionally, superficial dissection is performed along the medial crura up to the dome of the cleft side lower lateral cartilage. The lip and columella are then positioned into their predicted position and adequate rotation of the cleft cupid's bow (point 6) is verified. At this point any necessary changes to the lateral lip markings can be made.

Continued

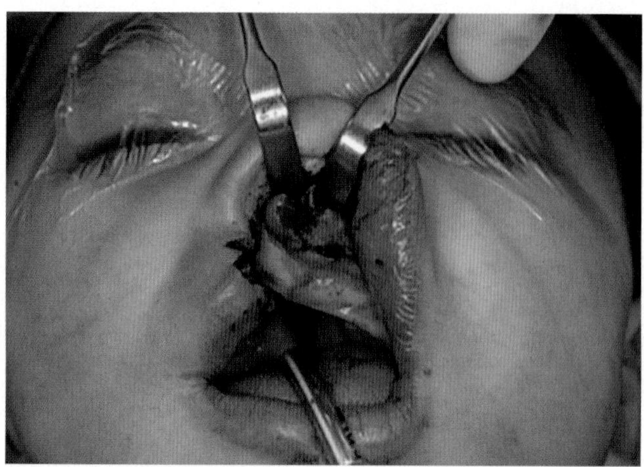

Figure 58.7 The nasal septum is identified and freed from the maxillary crest. (Photo Courtesy Dr. David Yates.)

TECHNIQUE: Fisher Anatomic Subunit Reapproximation for Repair of Unilateral Cleft Lip—*cont'd*

STEP 9: Lateral Lip Dissection: Mucosal Incision

For complete clefts, it is advantageous to start with the mucosal incisions first. The mucosal incision is made in the buccal vestibule starting from the superior extent of the mucosal incision traveling as far posterolaterally as necessary within the buccal sulcus at least 5 mm superior to the mucogingival junction. This will facilitate the release of the tethering effect of the lip from the alveolar cleft margin and piriform rim (Fig. 58.8).

STEP 10: Lateral Lip Dissection: Muscular Dissection

Similar to the medial incisions, the cleft marginal skin tissue is discarded. The mucosa is occasionally saved depending on the extent of the cleft and the vascularity of the flap. This can aid in mucosal closure by decreasing tension on the mucosa. The muscle is then dissected free of the overlying skin and underlying mucosa. However, the dissection between muscle and skin is more extensive on the cleft side. The orbicularis oris is dissected free from its insertion in the upper alveolar cleft margin as well as the alar base further laterally (Fig. 58.9).

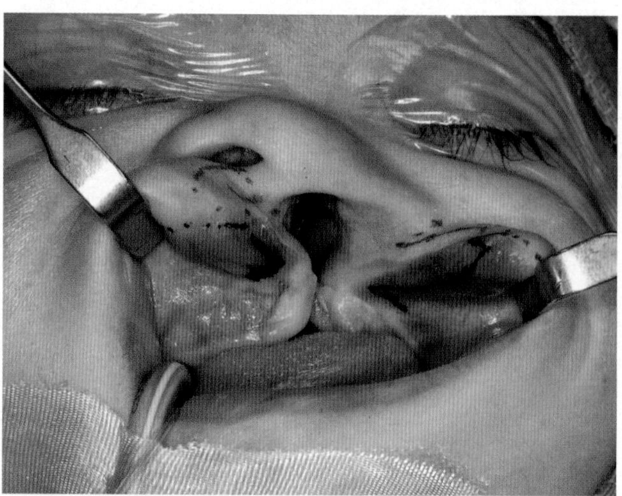

Figure 58.8 The intramural mucosal incisions are marked. (Photo Courtesy Dr. David Yates.)

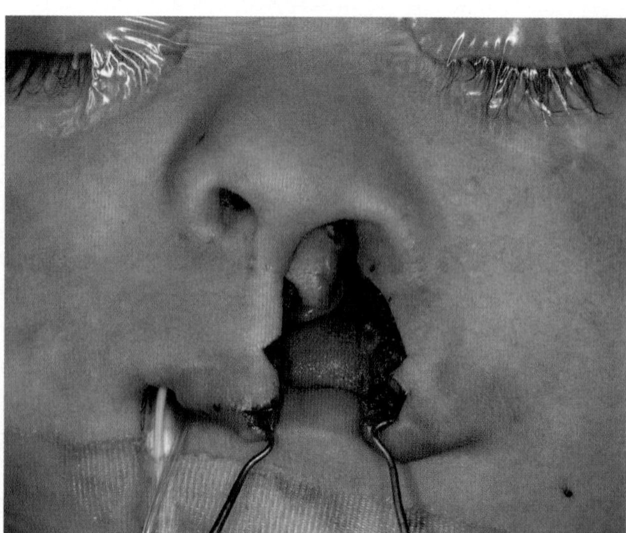

Figure 58.9 Following dissection, traction on the lip with skin hooks shows the downward rotation of the medial cleft segment. (Photo Courtesy Dr. David Yates.)

TECHNIQUE: Fisher Anatomic Subunit Reapproximation for Repair of Unilateral Cleft Lip—*cont'd*

STEP 11: Vestibular Web Dissection

Deep to the muscle, the alar base is dissected free from the maxilla in a supraperiosteal plane. The vestibular web, consisting of the caudal edge of the lateral crus of the lower lateral cartilage (LLC), accessory cartilages, and investing perichondrium, is released from the piriform rim. Once released from the piriform rim, the alar base can now be advanced anteromedially. The nasal dissection is then carried superior to point 19 along the nasal mucosa where the change from intranasal skin to mucosa occurs, where the vibrissae are first detected. This is essentially an intercartilaginous incision. This incision is carried circumferentially around the internal portion of the nare to the point where the cleft side LLC noticeably is weakened and classically crimped. The nasalis muscle is dissected out and identified, and a dissection superficial to the cleft side LLC is performed and joined to the point where the medial dissection had terminated. This results in the entire superficial surface of the LLC on the cleft side being dissected free (Figs. 58.10 and 58.11).

STEP 12: Posterior Lamella Closure: Medial and Lateral Flaps

The superior portion of the posterior closure is performed using up to two different components: a medial flap from the medial segment and a modified lateral flap from the lateral segment.

The medial flap is broadly based and consists of the tissue lateral to the incision along the medial lip (16-3-8-6-12) 5 mm superior to the mucogingival junction. There is usually an excess of mucosal tissue present so appropriate trimming is performed. The lateral flap consists of the tissue medial to

Continued

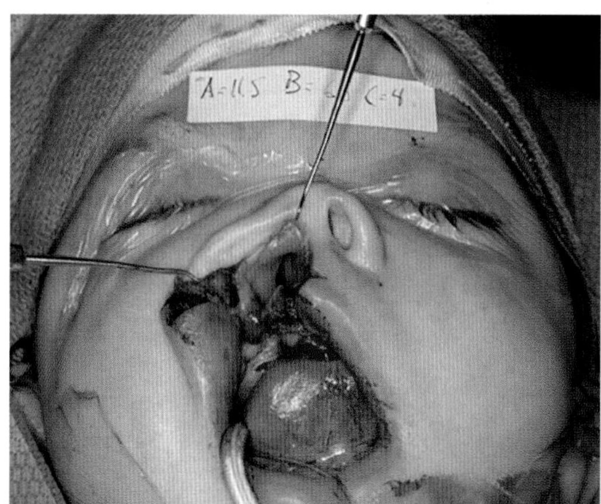
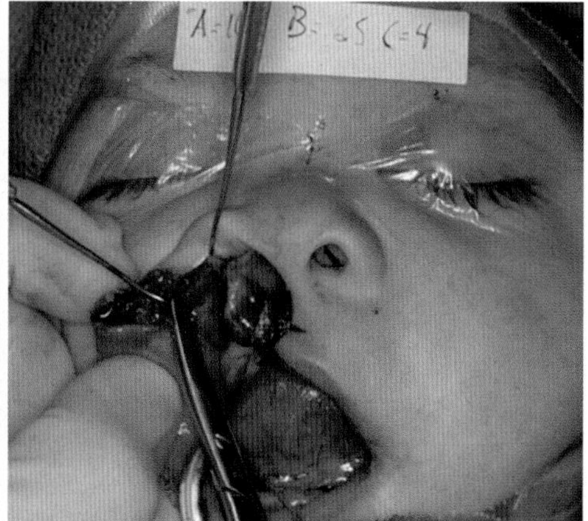

Figure 58.10 The initial nasal incision and superficial dissection are performed. (Photo Courtesy Dr. David Yates.)

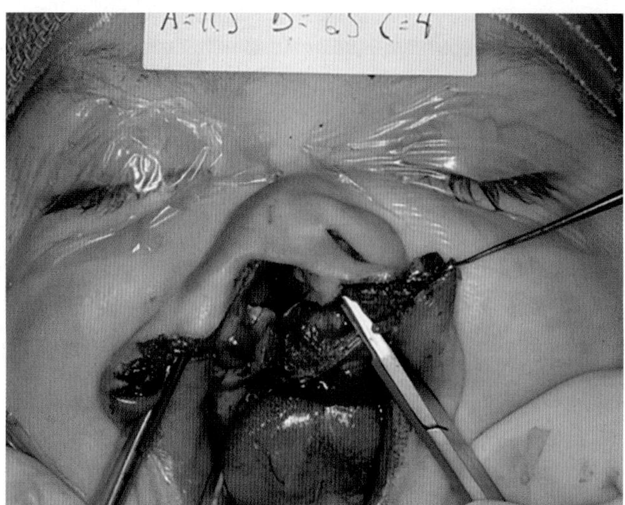

Figure 58.11 The complete dissection of the superficial surface of the lower lateral cartilage from both the medial and lateral aspect. (Photo Courtesy Dr. David Yates.)

TECHNIQUE: Fisher Anatomic Subunit Reapproximation for Repair of Unilateral Cleft Lip—*cont'd*

the incision along the lateral lip (19-21-20-22-18-17-24-25-23) 5 mm superior to the mucogingival junction. As with the medial flap described above, excessive mucosal tissue is usually present, so appropriate trimming is performed. The incisions are typically carried deeper into the nose superior to point 19 as previously described at the point where the intranasal skin becomes nasal mucosa.

Nasal floor closure is achieved by suturing the medial and lateral flaps to each other using 4-0 Vicryl suture. Care must be taken to not stenose the nasal aperture internally during this closure.

STEP 13: Posterior Lamella Closure: Putting It All Together

Once the floor of the nose and the medial and lateral flaps have been sutured, a stay suture is placed at the wet-dry line, which allows for the determination of the ideal position of the mucosa. The mucosa is then advanced from the medial lip and lateral lip segments to the most appropriate esthetic position and sutured along the vestibule using 4-0 Vicryl suture. The vertical closure of the mucosa is delayed until then end of the procedure (Fig. 58.12).

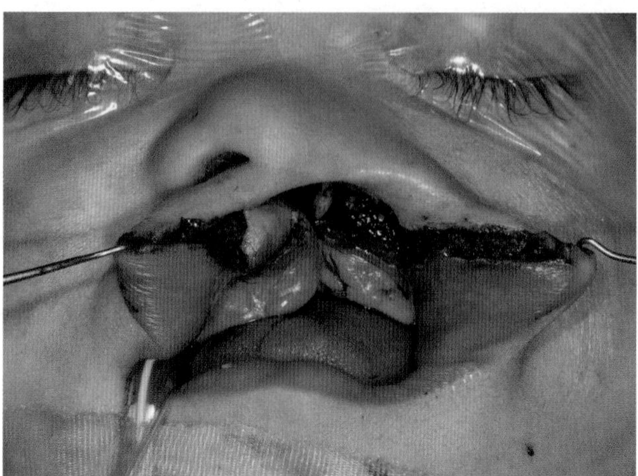

Figure 58.12 The posterior lamellar closure is performed by suturing together the medial and lateral flaps, thus forming the nasal floor. (Photo Courtesy Dr. David Yates.)

TECHNIQUE: Fisher Anatomic Subunit Reapproximation for Repair of Unilateral Cleft Lip—*cont'd*

STEP 14: Lower Lateral Cartilage and Alar Repositioning

An alar cinch suture is passed through the cleft side alar base to reapproximate the cleft ala to the detached portion of the anterior septum (4-0 polydioxanone [PDS])—usually two are placed. Care is taken to ensure that the columellar base and ala are at the same horizontal level.

STEP 15: Final Closure

The orbicularis oris muscle is then closed with a 4-0 Monocryl suture using a horizontal mattress stitch. The skin is closed first with deep dermal sutures (5-0 Vicryl or clear PDS on a TF) and then simple interrupted sutures (5-0 fast gut). The flap is then trimmed to the appropriate size and inset into the incision along the wet-dry line of the medial lip (line 10-12) (Fig. 58.13).

The cleft side dome (LLC) is then repositioned anteromedially and superiorly with forceps internally pushing up the affected side cartilage at the caudal margin of the upper lateral cartilage. This is performed using a 25-gauge needle and a 5-0 PDS suture. The needle is placed through the skin and into the nasal vestibule. The suture is manually threaded through the sharp end of the needle. Once the suture is obtained through the skin side, the surgeon holds onto the suture and retracts the needle till it almost is fully removed and then replunges the needle back into the nasal vestibule in the area where traction is desired. The suture end, which is still being held by the surgeon, is brought back through the nasal vestibule and sutured with the knot trapped intranasally. This is repeated around the affected side LLC until the desired shape is obtained (usually about four sutures) (Fig. 58.14).

These sutures serve not only as repositioning sutures but also as alar transfixion sutures to reattach the previously detached fibers connecting the LLC and overlying skin. This will obliterate any dead space created by the release of the vestibular web from the

Continued

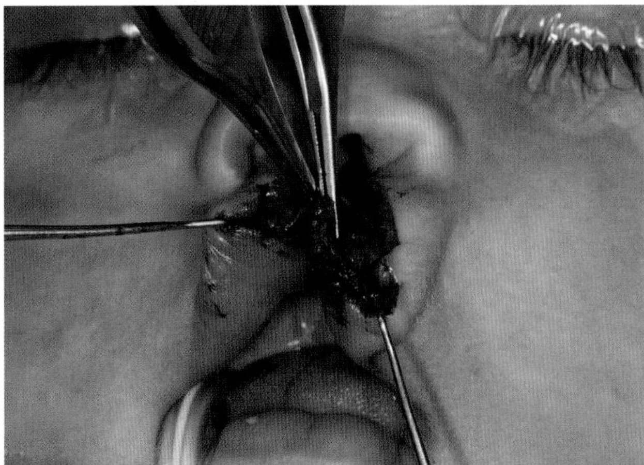

Figure 58.13 The orbicularis muscle is reapproximated. (Photo Courtesy Dr. David Yates.)

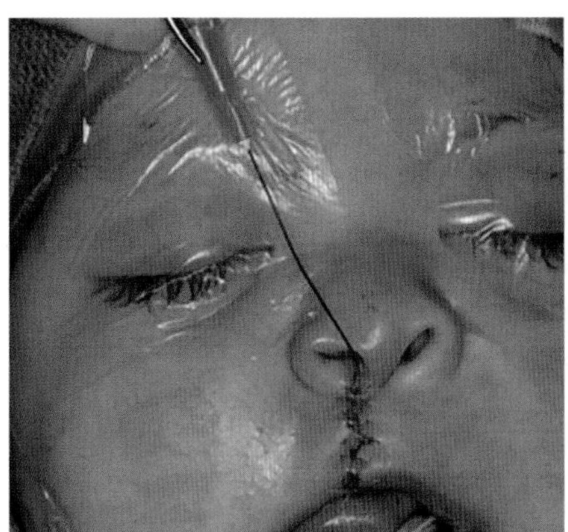

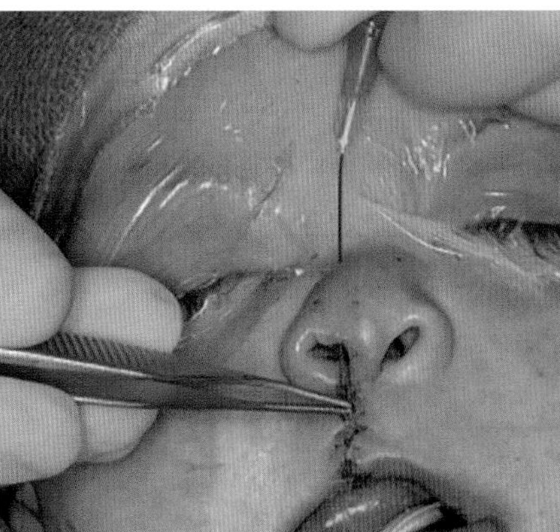

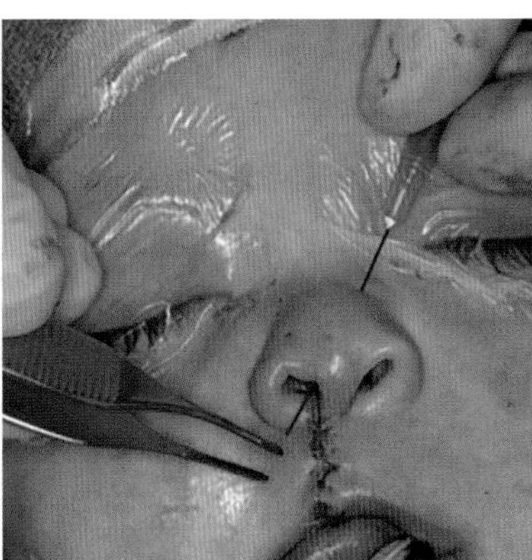

Figure 58.14 The cleft side dome is then repositioned using a 25-gauge needle and a 5-0 PDS suture. (Photo Courtesy Dr. David Yates.)

TECHNIQUE: Fisher Anatomic Subunit Reapproximation for Repair of Unilateral Cleft Lip—*cont'd*

piriform rim as well as hold the lateral crus in its newly advanced position (Fig. 58.15).

Antibiotic ointment is then applied to the closure and a silicone nasal former is trimmed and left in place and secured to the septum using a 3-0 nylon for a period of 4 months. Mastisol and Steri-Strips are then placed over the cleft to decrease tension on the wound during the first week of healing (Figs. 58.16 and 58.17).

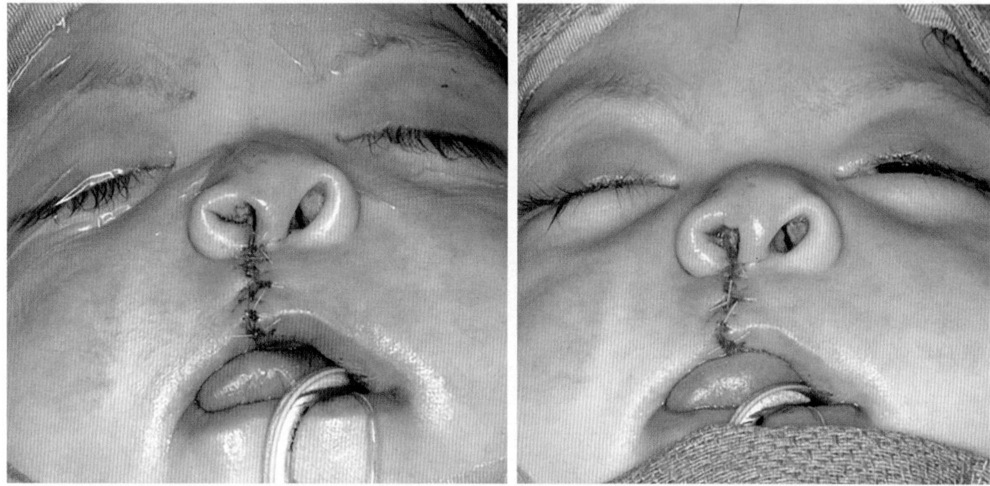

Figure 58.15 Nasal appearance before and after repositioning. (Photo Courtesy Dr. David Yates.)

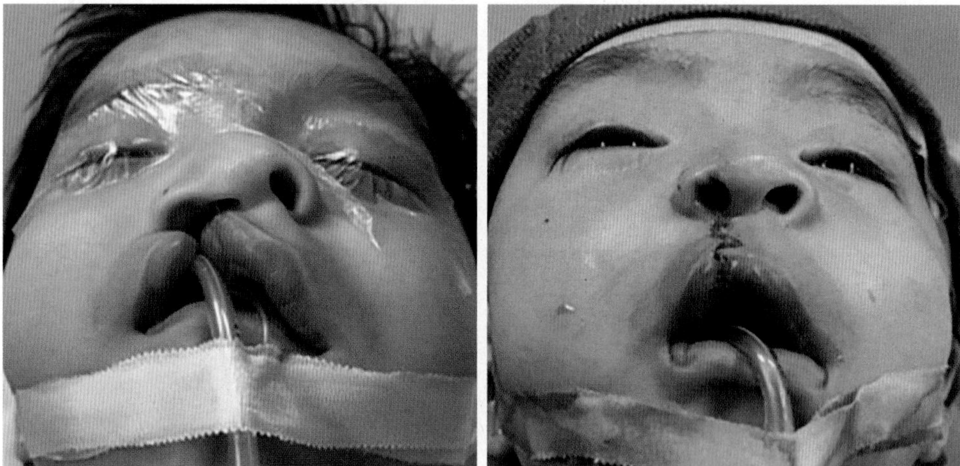

Figure 58.16 Immediate preoperative and postoperative photos of a complete unilateral cleft repaired using the described technique. (Photo Courtesy Dr. David Yates.)

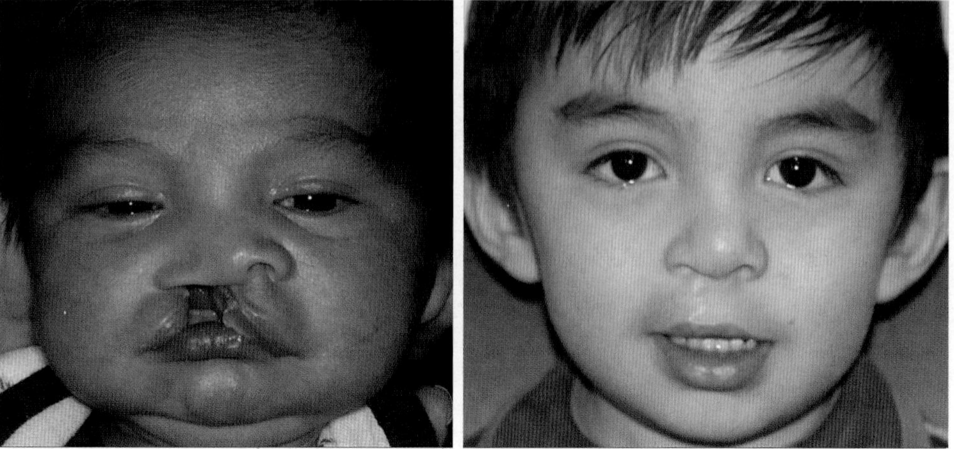

Figure 58.17 Preoperative and 6-month postoperative photos of the same patient pictured above. (Photo Courtesy Dr. David Yates.)

ALTERNATIVE TECHNIQUE: Incomplete Unilateral Cleft

In the case of an incomplete cleft, the cleft side is frequently elongated relative to the noncleft side. Thus, a wedge excision is commonly needed to allow for correct vertical positioning of the cleft side philtral column in relation to the noncleft side. This wedge excision is performed between points 14-x-21, where point x is a point about halfway between points 19 and 21 along the incision line. This wedge will extend into the nostril sill and consist of skin and mucosa from the cleft margins. The peak of the wedge must be above the cleft height (Fig. 58.18).

Particular care must be taken to handle the lateral triangle flaps delicately so as not to damage them. The vermilion flap is particularly delicate and cannot be pinched or traumatized.[2,6,7]

Avoidance and Management of Intraoperative Complications

One of the benefits afforded by the extensive markings of the Fisher subunit approximation is the reduced amount of guesswork required when estimating the lip length. Thus, a mentality of "measure twice, cut once" is imperative as the markings and measurements form the basis for the entire surgery.[2]

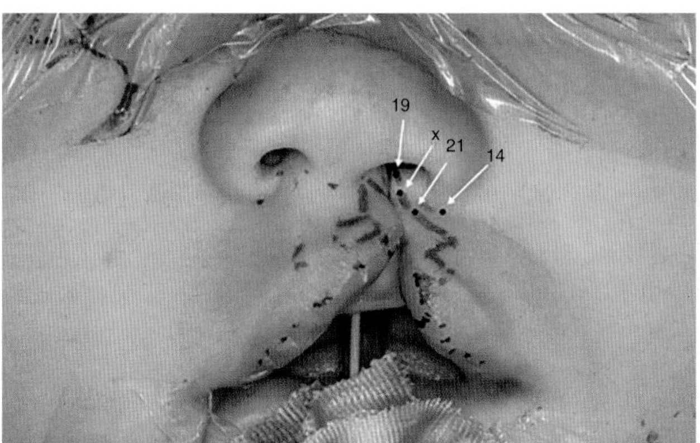

Figure 58.18 A small wedge excision in the superior aspect of the lateral lip element is often needed in incomplete clefts. (Photo Courtesy Dr. David Yates.)

Postoperative Considerations

Postoperative care is essential to achieve an overall excellent esthetic lip result. Patients are seen for follow-up on a weekly basis for the first 3 weeks and then on a monthly basis for the following 3 months.

The authors recommend syringe feeding via a 20-cc syringe with a connected red rubber catheter for 2 weeks postoperatively. Patients can resume bottle feeding after this period. Use of a pacifier is prohibited in the immediate postoperative period.

Mastisol liquid adhesive and Steri-Strip reinforced skin closures are placed immediately postoperatively to decrease tension on the wound for the first week. After 1 week, the dressing is removed, and the lip is cleaned using a 1:1 mixture of sterile water and hydrogen peroxide and cotton-tipped applicators. Caregivers are instructed to clean the patient's lip twice a day with warm water and soap using a gentle stroking motion along the incision line.

At 3 weeks caregivers can begin massaging the soft tissue along the scar during feedings. ScarAway silicone scar gel is placed once a day along the incision, and vitamin E cream is massaged into the wound twice a day. The nasal formers placed at the conclusion of the procedure are left in place for 4 months.

During the remodeling phase of wound healing (around 3 to 4 months postoperatively), it is not uncommon for patients to experience widening of the scar. If the widening is extensive, 10 to 20 mg of triamcinolone acetonide (Kenalog) injectable suspension can be injected directly into the scar. This has shown to be effective in limiting the unfavorable widening of the scars.

References

1. Santoni-Rugiu P, Sykes PJ. *A History Plastic Surg*. 1st ed. Springer; 2007.
2. Fisher DM. Unilateral cleft lip repair: an anatomical subunit approximation technique. *Plast Reconstr Surg*. 2005;116(1):61–71.
3. Roberts JM, Jacobs AD, Morrow M, Hauck R, Samson T. Current trends in unilateral cleft lip care: a 10-year update on practice patterns. *Ann Plast Surg*. 2020;84(5):595–601.
4. Michael M, McKeon M, Ackerman MB. In: *Peterson's Principles of Oral and Maxillofacial Surgery*. 3rd ed. 2011.
5. Kademani D, Paul S. *Tiwana. Atlas of Oral Maxillofacial Surg*; 2016.
6. Noordhoff MS, Millard D. Reconstruction of vermilion in unilateral and bilateral cleft lips. *Plast Reconstr Surg*. 1984;73(1):52–61.
7. Noordhoff MS, Chen YR, Chen KT, Hong KF, Lo LJ. The surgical technique for the complete unilateral cleft lip-nasal deformity. *Oper Tech Plast Reconstr Surg*. 1995;2(3):167–174.

CHAPTER 59

Unilateral Cheilorhinoplasty—Talmant Protocol

Jean-Charles Doucet and Jean-Claude Talmant

Armamentarium

8 and #10 Fraser tip suction
#15, #11, Beaver blades
0.5-mm Silicone sheet
Bishop retractor
Calipers
Castro needle holder curved
Cottle elevator
Crile-Wood needle holder short
Curved Ragnell scissors
Debakey forceps
Freer elevator
Fomon double blunt hook
Iris scissors
Joseph double skin hook 2 mm
Marking pen
Methylene blue with insulin syringe/needle (for tattoo)
Metzenbaum scissors
Micro-Adson forceps
Molt periosteal elevator #9
Mosquitos
Ragnell retractor
Scalpel handle round
Single skin hook
Sutures
Tissue forceps 0.5 mm
Woodson elevator

History of the Procedure

Victor Veau was right in his description of the cleft lip and palate deformity: "The normal structures are present on either side of the cleft, only modified by the presence of the cleft."[1] The deformity is mainly the result of displacement, deformation, and functional hypotrophy.[2] No true tissue hypoplasia exists except at the level of the "missing piece"—part of the premaxilla—where there is missing bone and a missing lateral incisor in 50% of the cases.[3,4] This "missing piece" changes the equilibrium of the facial envelope, changing its muscular organization and ventilation. This part of the premaxilla is not only important for our mastication but is also an important support for our nasal ventilation since it provides support to the pyriform aperture and nasal valve. The associated muscular breach also causes a sagging of the facial elements on the cleft side, causing the inferior portion of the nasalis muscle (myrtiformis muscle) to slide down and in front of lateral crus of the alar cartilage, leading to its rotation and deformation, and the creation of the nasal vestibular web[5] (Fig. 59.1A–C).

Victor Veau was again right when he said: "To put the normal structures on either side of the cleft into normal position is, by far, the best functional repair: no tissue importation is justified."[1] Behind these statements lie the key principles of a functional repair:

1. Restore a functional anatomy at the time of the primary surgery. This includes the restoration of a normal muscular function, speech, deglutition, and mastication but also the restoration of a normal nasal ventilation. This is especially important since any steps of the primary treatment threaten the nasal airway. The quality of this nasal airway depends on the residual deformity of the nostril (alar cartilage) and nasal septum but is also strongly influenced by the width of the nasal floor and the piriform orifice. Therefore scarring from healing by secondary intention of denuded areas (push back palatoplasty, single layer closure with a vomer flap) should be avoided to preserve the width of the nasal floor (hard palate). The width of the piriform orifice (alveolar cleft) should also be maintained by preserving the space of the lateral incisor with a good canine function.[5] If normal nasal ventilation is not restored, an oral breathing pattern develops with a low-lying tongue often leading to Class III anterior open bite dentofacial deformities.[5–7]
2. Minimize the negative effects of surgery including compression and contraction. The effects of compression, which can be orthopedic or surgical, will be worse in wide clefts, especially in early repairs.[7,8] To minimize these effects, the timing of the surgery should be reconsidered by delaying the lip repair until closer to 6 months of age. The delay will allow an increased ossification of the alveolus and maxilla, which will better resist compression.[5] It will also allow a safer and more complete dissection of the fragile nasal cartilages.[2] The effects of contraction, which promote fibrosis, retraction, stenosis, and restricted growth, will be worse with secondary scarring of denuded areas. To minimize them, the surgery should aim at leaving no open areas and close or draining any dead spaces.[5]

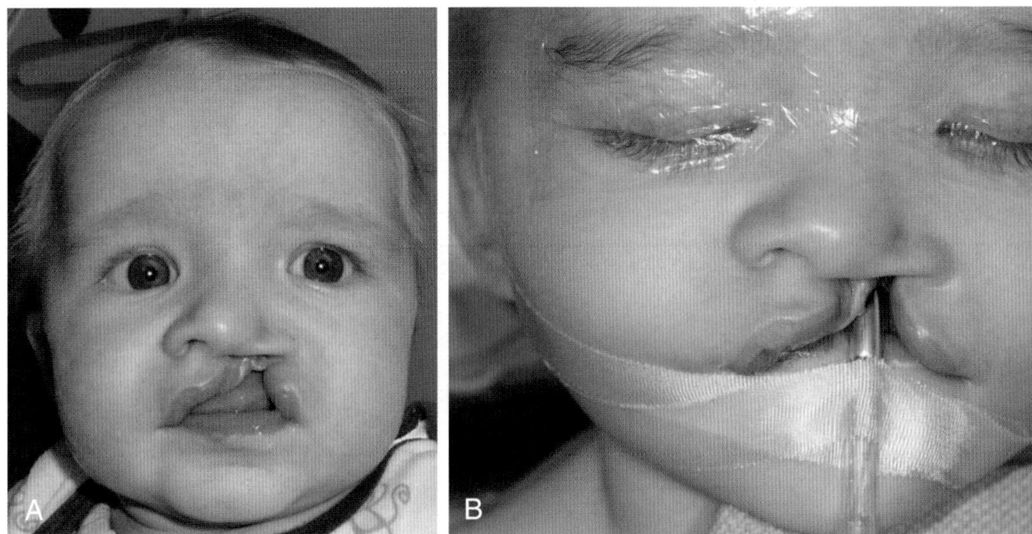

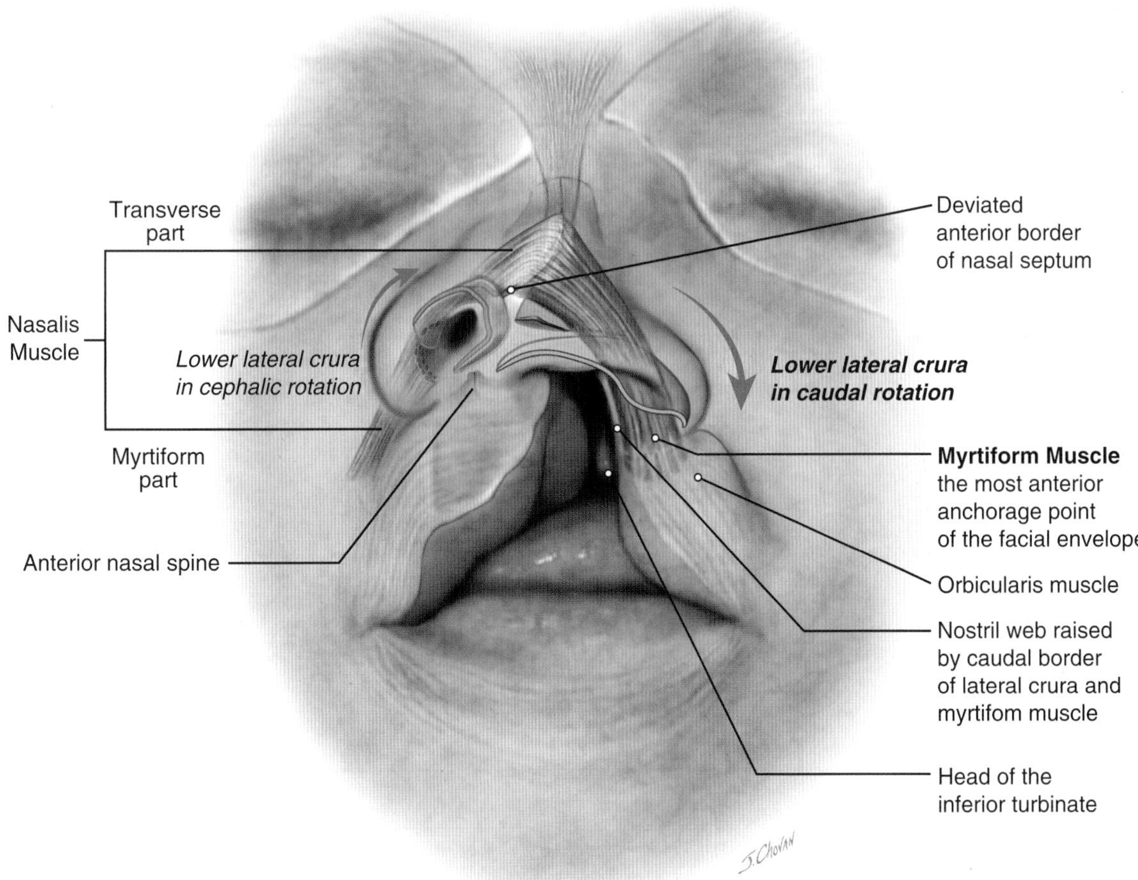

Figure 59.1 **A,** Unilateral cleft lip and nasal deformity. **B,** The disrupted muscular organization and nasal ventilation changes the equilibrium of the facial envelope, resulting in displacement, deformation, and functional hypotrophy. **C,** The inferior portion of the nasalis muscle is down and in front of the lateral crus of the alar cartilage, leading to its rotation and deformation, and the creation of the nasal vestibular web.

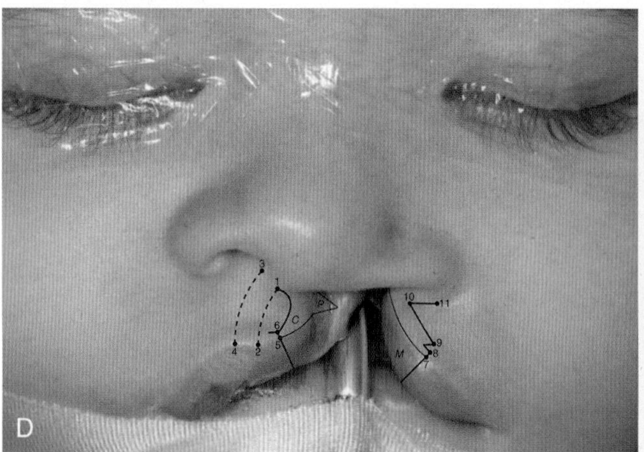

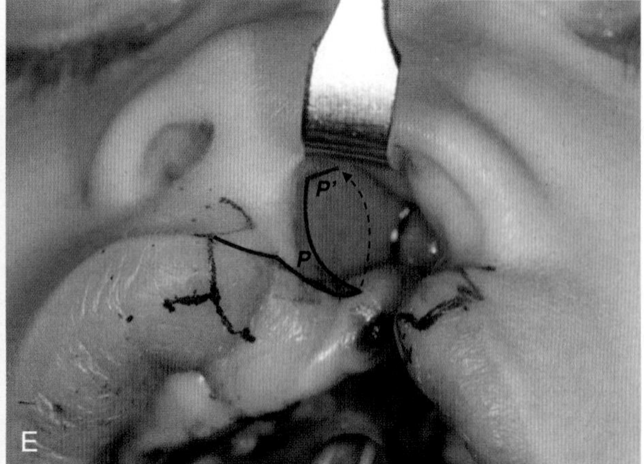

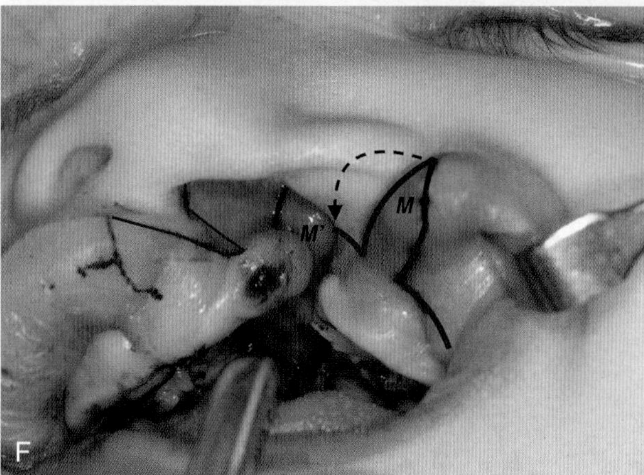

Figure 59.1, cont'd **D,** Incision design. **E,** Triangular P flap will be rotated into a back-cut P' of the septal mucosa. **F,** Mucosal flap M will be rotated into a back-cut M' following the piriform rim and ending in front of the inferior turbinate.

Indications for the Use of the Procedure

A unilateral cheilorhinoplasty is indicated in any form of congenital cleft affecting the primary palate. In children with complete unilateral cleft lip and palate, the approach aims at restoring form and function with a particular focus on restoring normal nasal ventilation at the time of the primary surgery. The procedure is performed without presurgical orthopedics, because it is essential not to prematurely close the alveolar cleft before having ensured a good intercanine maxillary width in relation to the intercanine mandibular width, which is the reference.[5] In addition, presurgical orthopedics has no capacity to restore the normal relationships of nasolabial muscles and cartilages, which can only be restored by extensive subperiosteal and subperichondrial dissections, the only ones to respect the growth potential of the bone and cartilage.[5] To achieve these goals, Dr. Jean-Claude Talmant developed the Nasal Breathing Approach protocol[5]:

1. At 6 months: the lip, nose, and soft palate are repaired simultaneously via a cheilorhinoplasty and Sommerlad intravelar veloplasty.[9] Nasal ventilation is restored and maintained with a nasal retainer for 4 months.
2. At 18 months: the hard palate is repaired without any denuded areas.
3. At 4 to 6 years: the alveolar cleft is repaired via an alveolar bone graft (harvested from the anterior iliac crest) before the eruption of the central incisors while maintaining a good canine function. If canine function is not adequate, an anterior maxillary expansion by quad helix should be performed.

Limitations and Contraindications

The procedure is limited by the surgeon's knowledge of the relevant anatomy and understanding of the goals required to achieve a functional result. The procedure is contraindicated in the very young patient (neonatal lip repair) or by significant comorbidities precluding the child's safety.

TECHNIQUE: Functional Cheilorhinoplasty of Talmant

STEP 1: Incision Design

The incision design respects the principle of rotation/advancement of Millard, which provides the best cutaneous distribution between the lip and nose.[10]

MEDIAL LIP DRAWINGS (FIG. 59.1D)

a. Draw the philtral groove by joining the midline of the columella (point 1) to the midline of the cupid's bow (point 2).
b. Draw the philtral column on the noncleft side by joining the top of the philtral column (point 3) to the top of the cupid's bow (point 4). The height of the philtral column is then measured with calipers.
c. Mark and tattoo the top of the cupid's bow on the cleft side (point 5). Points 2 and 5 should be equidistant to points 2 and 4, for an overall philtral width of 6 to 8 mm.
d. The incision through the mucocutaneous junction is perpendicular and extends from point 6 (located 1 mm above point 5) to the labial vestibule. From point 6, a 2 mm back-cut is planned just above the mucocutaneous junction to receive a small triangular flap from the lateral lip.
e. The medial lip incision is curvilinear and joins point 6 to point 1 and should respect the width of the philtrum.
f. The C flap is drawn by following the mucocutaneous junction from point 5 to the base of the alveolus (see Fig. 59.1D).
g. The triangular P flap is drawn using labial and premaxillary mucosa (see Fig. 59.1D and E). This flap will be transposed into a back-cut of the septal mucosa just under the upper lateral cartilage to adjust the columellar height and support the alar dome on the cleft side.

LATERAL LIP DRAWINGS (FIG. 59.1D)

a. Mark and tattoo the end of the white roll on the mucocutaneous junction of the lateral lip (point 7).
b. The incision through the mucocutaneous junction is again perpendicular and extends from point 8 (located 1 mm above point 7) to the labial vestibule.
c. A small triangular flap, with a 2 mm base (point 8 to point 9), is drawn just above point 8. This flap will be inserted into the back-cut on the medial lip to anchor the white roll and adjust the lip length. The axis of this flap can be rotated vertically to increase the lip length.[11]
d. The lateral lip incision is rectilinear and ascends obliquely toward the mucocutaneous junction to join point 9 to point 10. At the end of the procedure, the length of the lip on the cleft side should be 1 mm less than on the noncleft side due to the premaxillary remodeling (Rose-Thomson effect),[12,13] which lengthens the lip. The length of this lateral lip incision (point 9 to 10) is therefore adjusted based on the height of the philtral column on the noncleft side. For example, if the philtral column on the noncleft side is 11 mm, the lateral lip incision should measure 7 mm since the 3 mm length given by the small triangle will give a total of 10 mm.
e. The height of the lateral lip incision (point 10) is then joined to the alar base (point 11).
f. The mucosa medial to the lateral lip incisions will create a mucosal flap M (Muir flap), which will be rotated into a back-cut following the piriform rim (Fig. 59.1F). This flap M participates in the reconstruction of the nasal floor and vestibule.

TECHNIQUE: Functional Cheilorhinoplasty of Talmant—*cont'd*

STEP 2: Subperiosteal Dissection

a. A vestibular incision gives access to an extended subperiosteal dissection of the maxilla on the lateral aspect of the cleft. This dissection extends around the infraorbital nerve, anterior aspect of the zygoma, and nasal process of the maxilla, allowing a complete mobilization of the lateral facial elements, which is key to nasal and muscular reconstruction (Fig. 59.2A).
b. During this dissection, the nasalis muscle is disinserted from the medial margin of the small cleft segment and isolated with a suture (Fig. 59.2B).

STEP 3: Subperichondrial Dissection

a. Curved Ragnell scissors enter the base of the columella, ascend between the medial crura, and continue to dissect the superficial surface of the dome and lateral crus of the alar cartilage on the cleft side (Fig. 59.2C).
b. The anterior aspect of the septal cartilage is isolated through the hemitransfixion incision and both sides of the septal cartilage are dissected in the subperichondrial plane. The septal cartilage is also separated from the maxillary groove (with occasional conservative inferior

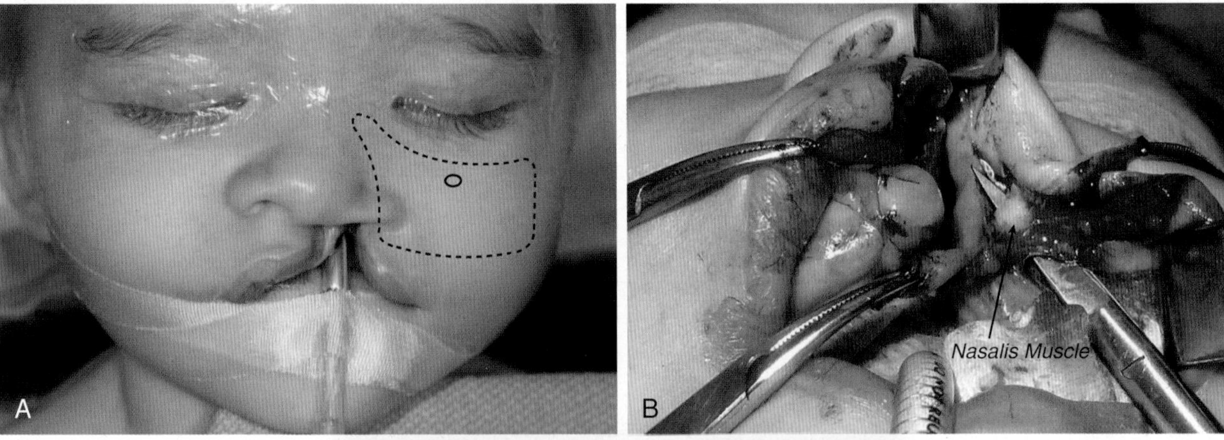

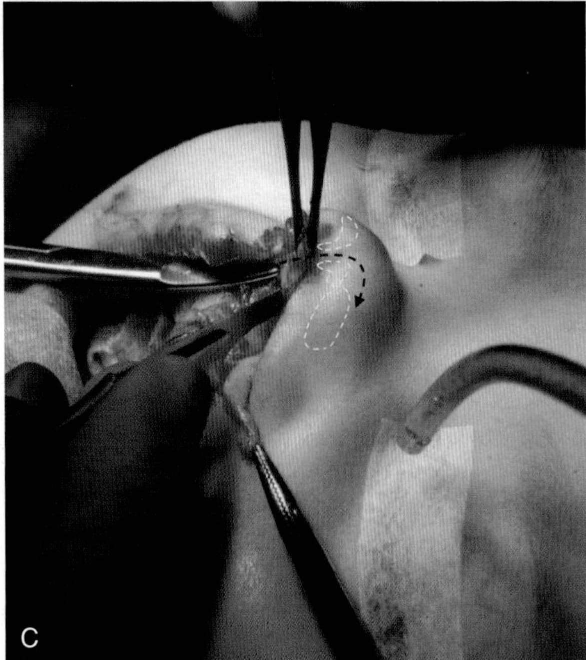

Figure 59.2 A, Wide subperiosteal dissection. B, Nasalis muscle is isolated. C, Dissection between the medial crura of the alar cartilages ascends toward the dome and lateral crus on the cleft side.

TECHNIQUE: Functional Cheilorhinoplasty of Talmant—*cont'd*

resection) to allow a midline repositioning (Fig. 59.2D, Video 59.1).

c. The Cottle elevator continues the septal dissection toward the deep surface of the nasal bone and rotates down to dissect the undersurface of the upper lateral cartilage in the subperichondrial plane.
d. The junction between the septal cartilage and upper lateral cartilage is then identified and curved Ragnell scissors continue the subperichondrial dissection toward the nasal bones and superficial surface of the upper lateral cartilage (Video 59.2). A Freer elevator is then used to connect this dissection with the maxillary subperiosteal dissection (see Fig. 59.2D).
e. This dissection completely separates the mucosa and nasal cartilages from the superficial muscular and cutaneous plane, allowing a proper repositioning of the nasal cartilages without the need for suspension sutures or grafting (Video 59.3).

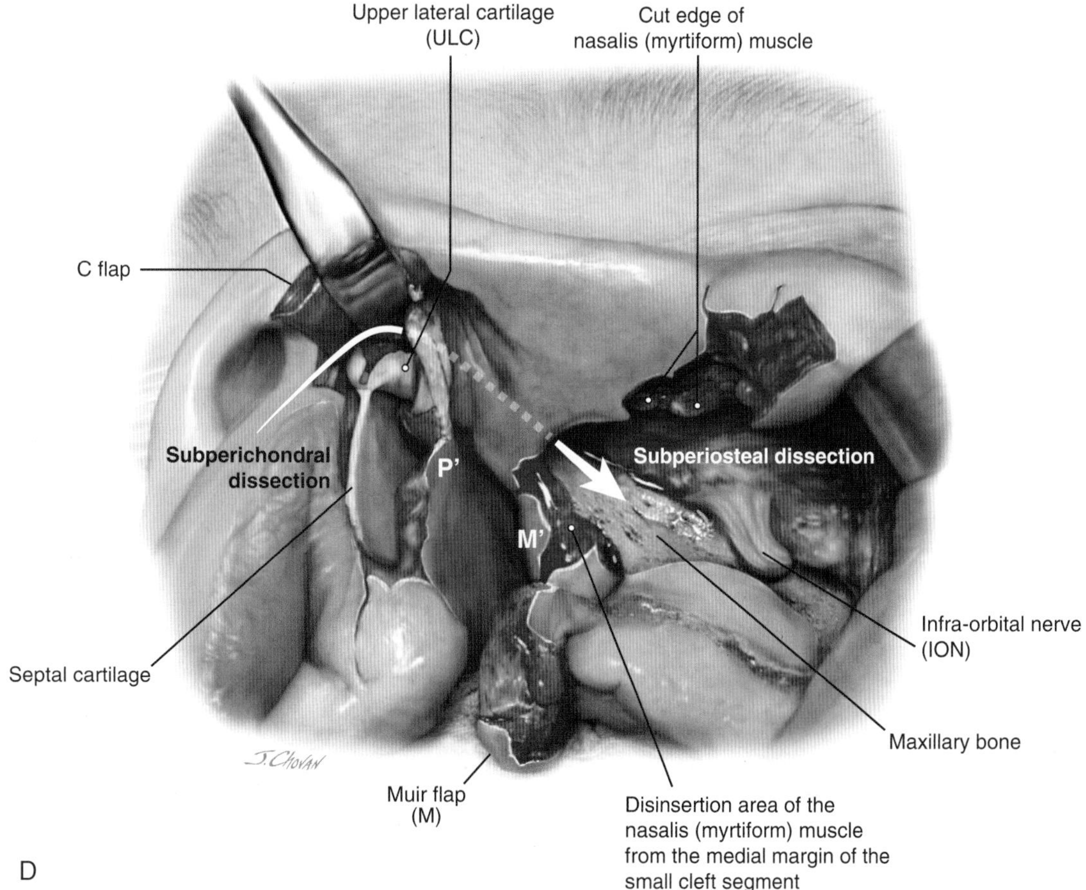

Figure 59.2, cont'd **D,** Subperichondrial dissection of the nasal septum and upper lateral cartilage (ULC) joins the vestibular subperiosteal dissection.

TECHNIQUE: Functional Cheilorhinoplasty of Talmant—*cont'd*

STEP 4: Mucosal Sutures

a. The P flap is sutured into a back-cut of the septal mucosa just underneath the upper lateral cartilage (Figs. 59.1E and 59.2F).
b. The Muir flap is sutured to the pyriform rim incision. The lateral border of the Muir flap is rotated and sutured to the premaxillary and septal mucosa to reconstruct the nasal floor (Figs. 59.1F and 59.2E).
c. The labial vestibular mucosa is advanced medially with a posterior release and sutured from posterior to anterior. The nasalis muscle suture (described in Step 5) should be passed but not tied before completely closing the vestibular incision.
d. The labial mucosa is closed while ensuring the proper alignment of the wet-dry junctions of the vermillion and symmetrical vestibular depth.

STEP 5: Muscular Sutures

a. The nasalis muscle suture is passed through the vestibular mucosa and its periosteum at the level of the future lateral incisor (Fig. 59.2F, *red point* and *white arrow*). This muscular suture should not be tied until the nasal retainer is in place. This muscular suture should also not be directed toward the anterior nasal spine since it would move the nasal vestibular web toward the septum, closing the nasal valve, and would insert the alar base superiorly, making the lip appear longer.
b. The perialar nasal muscles are resuspended to a point just underneath the anterior nasal spine (see Fig. 59.2F, *green points*). Attention must be paid to controlling the level of the alar base and preventing its elevation by the following ascending suture of the orbicularis oris muscle.
c. The superior aspect of the orbicularis oris muscle is resuspended to the anterior nasal spine (see Fig. 59.2F, *blue points*).
d. The deep and superior aspect of the orbicularis oris muscle is resuspended across the midline (beyond the noncleft philtral column and over the premaxillary periosteum) to the contralateral orbicularis oris muscle (see Fig. 59.2F, *yellow points*).
e. The rest of the orbicularis oris muscle is sutured along the philtral column, ensuring an adequate lip length and perfect alignment of the vermillion and white roll (see Fig. 59.2F, *purple points*).

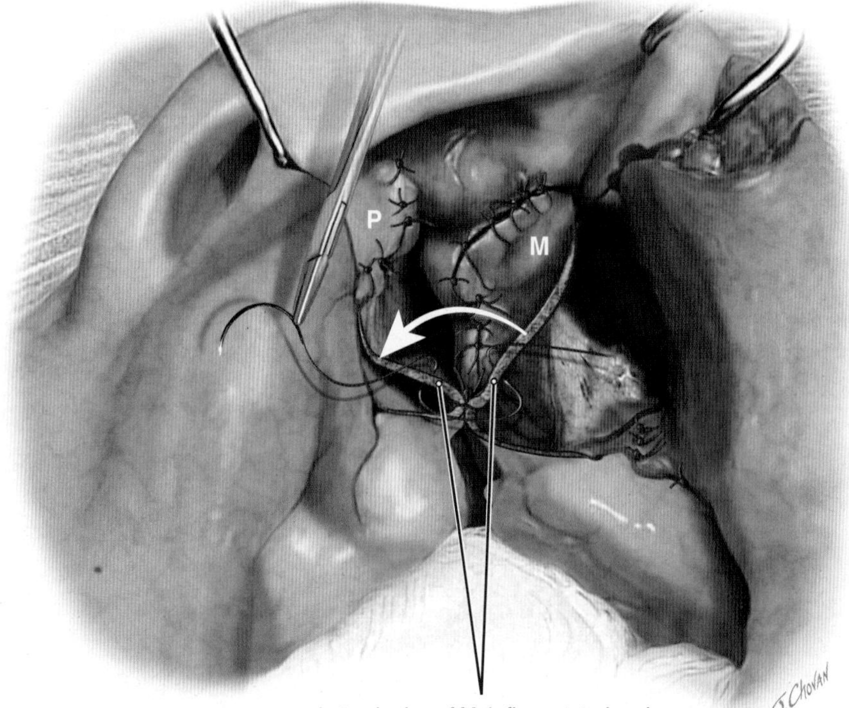
P
M
J. Chovan
E
Lateral edge of Muir flap rotated and
sutured to the premaxillary and septal mucosa

Figure 59.2, cont'd E, Triangular P flap inserted into back-cut P' and mucosal flap M inserted into back-cut M' and rotated to reconstruct the nasal floor.

TECHNIQUE: Functional Cheilorhinoplasty of Talmant—*cont'd*

STEP 6: Skin Sutures

a. The skin sutures complete the alignment of the vermillion and mucocutaneous junction (point 5 to point 7), the insertion of the small triangular flap (point 6 to point 8), and the superior lip (point 1 to point 10). At the end of the procedure, the length of the lip should be 1 mm shorter than the noncleft side (Fig. 59.2G).
b. The C flap is rotated superiorly (and trimmed as needed) to close the nasal sill.

STEP 7: Nasal Retainer

a. Intra- and extranasal retainers, made with 0.5 mm silicone sheets, are sutured to close the dead spaces preventing hematoma formation and eventual fibrosis and retraction. These sutures should be tied loosely (on top of a Cottle) to avoid skin necrosis.
b. The intranasal retainers are shaped (according to Fig. 59.2H and I), rolled into each nostril, and joined together with two 4-0 nylon sutures at the base and height of the columella.

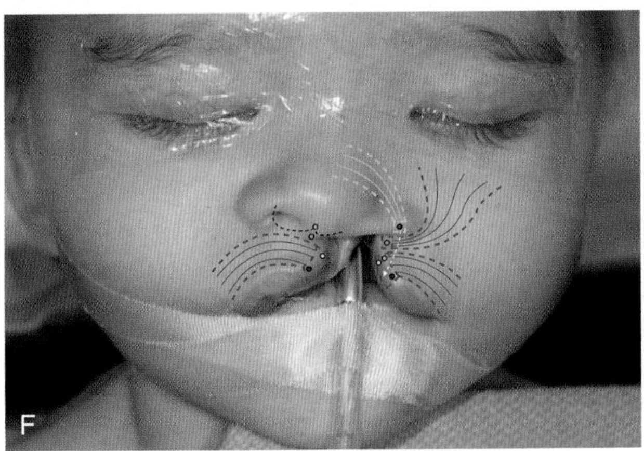

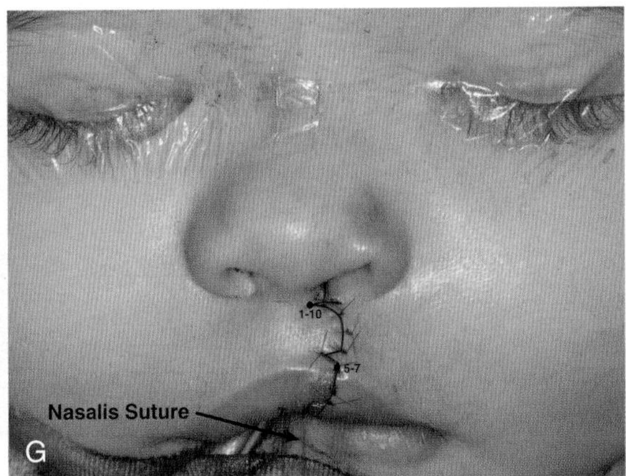

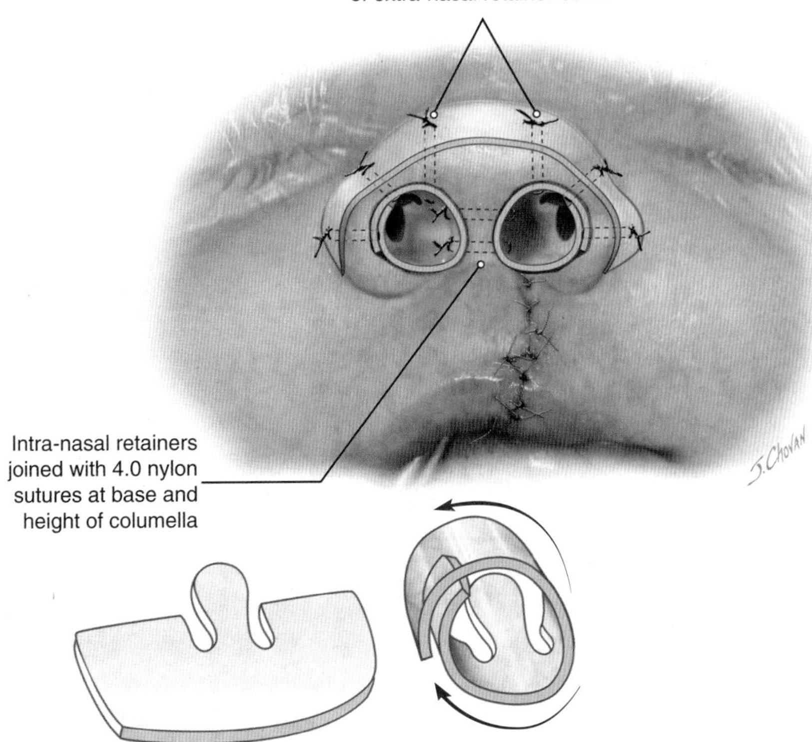

Figure 59.2, cont'd **F,** Functional muscular reconstruction brings the orbicularis oris to the anterior nasal spine, the perialar nasal muscles just underneath, and the nasalis muscle to the periosteum at the level of the future lateral incisor. **G,** Skin sutures. **H,** Intra- and extranasal retainers, made with 0.5-mm silicone sheets, are used to close the dead spaces.

TECHNIQUE: Functional Cheilorhinoplasty of Talmant—*cont'd*

c. The extranasal retainer is sutured to the intranasal retainers with transfixing sutures (see Fig. 59.2H and I, Video 59.4). While placing these sutures, the cutaneous and endonasal planes are sliding in opposite directions to lengthen the nose and deepen the nasal vestibule.

d. One week postoperatively, the skin sutures and nasal retainers are removed. A soft removable nasal retainer is then inserted and worn continuously (except for cleaning) for 4 months (Fig. 59.2J and K).

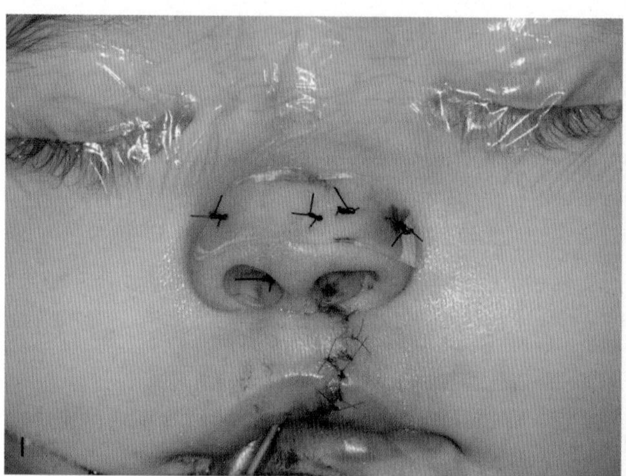

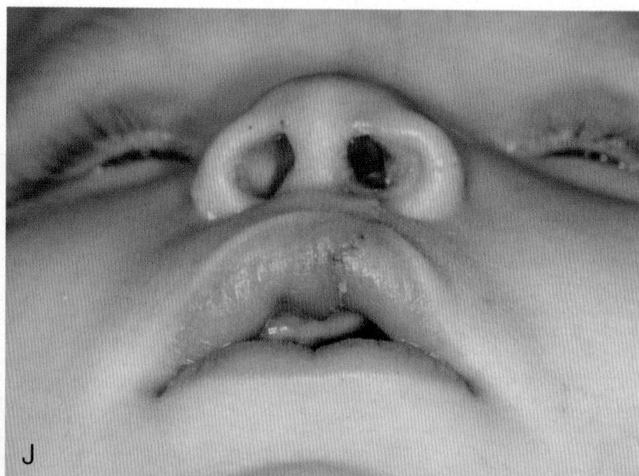

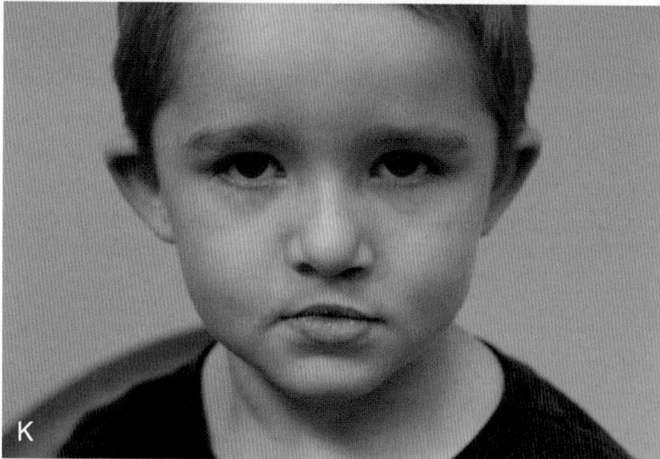

Figure 59.2, cont'd **I,** Intra- and extranasal retainers in place. **J,** Skin sutures and nasal retainers are removed 1 week postoperatively and a soft removable nasal retainer is worn for 4 months. **K,** Repaired unilateral cleft lip and nasal deformity at 5 years of age.

ALTERNATIVE TECHNIQUE: Vermillion Asymmetry

The width of the dry vermillion is often narrow on the medial side of the cleft. To balance the vermillion volume, when the width difference is greater than 2 mm (Fig. 59.3A), a triangular vermillion flap from the lateral lip (points 13 and 14) is inserted into a back-cut (point 12) following the wet-dry junction of the vermillion of the medial lip[11,14] (Fig. 59.3B and C).

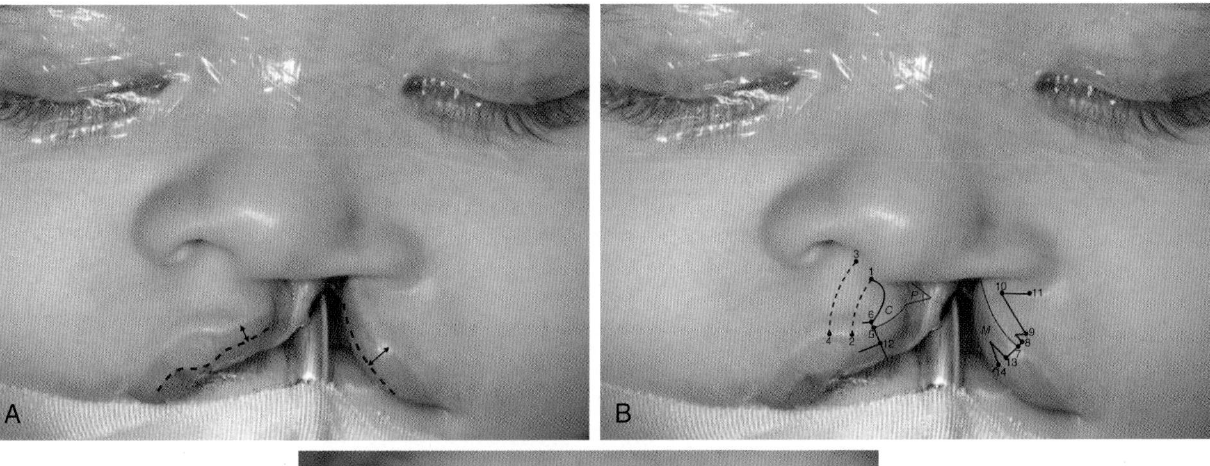

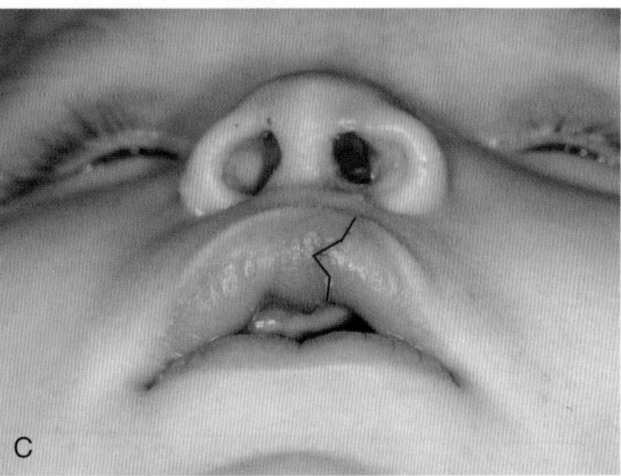

Figure 59.3 **A,** Difference in vermillion volume. **B,** Triangular vermillion flap from the lateral lip will be inserted into a back-cut following the wet-dry junction of the vermillion of the medial lip; the distance between points 7 and 13 should be equal to the distance between points 5 and 12. **C,** Triangular vermillion flap is inserted.

Avoidance and Management of Intraoperative Complications

The main intraoperative complications compromising the result of the functional repair include the following:

1. Failure to completely dissect and free the maxilla and nasal cartilages of their abnormal attachments will result in inappropriate repositioning or excessive tensions, resulting in the eventual relapse of the cleft deformity. A complete dissection should allow a symmetric nasal repositioning without the need for grafting or suspension sutures (see Video 59.3).
2. Failure to achieve a functional muscular reconstruction will result in residual asymmetries. The muscular reconstruction should "bring the lip up and bring the nose down" by repositioning the superior part of the orbicularis oris muscle to the anterior nasal spine, the perialar nasal muscle just underneath the anterior nasal spine, and the nasalis muscle to the vestibular periosteum at the level of the future lateral incisor. Redirecting all these muscles to the anterior nasal spine will lengthen the lip and compromise nasal ventilation by closing the nasal valve.
3. Failure to close open areas and close dead spaces or drain them will result in hematoma formation, fibrosis, retraction, stenosis, and restricted growth. The maxillary dissection area should be allowed to drain via the posterior release of the vestibular incision. The nasal vestibule and nasal floor are reconstructed with the Muir flap. Without this flap, the nasal vestibule and floor would be left to heal secondarily. The dead spaces of the nasal dissection are closed with the nasal retainer (see Video 59.4).

Postoperative Considerations

A functional reconstruction of the lip and nose should achieve the following goals.

1. A symmetric and functional upper lip with bilabial closure at rest. The lip should also be evaluated on animation to ensure adequate mobility and symmetry of facial expressions. Significant asymmetries of the lip length, vermillion alignment, alar base insertion, or any muscular diastasis require a complete secondary cheiloplasty. Residual nasal functional asymmetries can also be revised simultaneously

via a secondary rhinoplasty. The secondary functional cheilorhinoplasty should follow the same principles outlined in the primary functional repair.

2. A symmetric and functional nose with normal nasal ventilation. The internal and external nasal valves should be patent and oral breathing pattern absent. Any compromise in normal nasal ventilation should be addressed to prevent their sequelae, and early secondary nasal corrections can be planned 1 to 2 years after the alveolar bone grafting. Combined lip and nasal deformities can be addressed via a secondary functional cheilorhinoplasty. In the absence of significant lip deformity, the secondary rhinoplasty can be approached via a hemitransfixion incision on the noncleft side to reposition the nasal septum and via a marginal incision on the cleft side to expose the alar cartilage. The superficial perichondrium of the alar cartilage should be precisely excised to allow a convex dome and complete repositioning. An inferior turbinectomy on the noncleft side should be considered in case of hypertrophy. The dead spaces are closed and the nasal reconstruction is maintained again with the use of nasal retainers, which are applied in the same manner as with the primary repair. A removable nasal retainer is also used for 4 months postoperatively.

References

1. Veau V. Étude anatomique du bec-de-lièvre unilatéral total. *Ann Anat Pathol Anat Normale*. 1928;5:601–632.
2. Precious DS. Primary unilateral cleft lip/nose repair using the "Delaire" technique. *Atlas Oral Maxillofacial Surg Clin N Am*. 2009;17:125–135.
3. Tsai TP, Huang CS, Huang CC, See LC. Distribution patterns of primary and permanent dentition in children with unilateral complete cleft lip and palate. *Cleft Palate Craniofac J*. 1998;35:154–160.
4. Doucet JC, Delestan C, Montoya P, et al. New neonatal classification of unilateral cleft lip and palate part 2: to predict permanent lateral incisor agenesis and maxillary growth. *Cleft Palate Craniofac J*. 2014;51:533–539.
5. Talmant JC, Talmant JC, Rousteau G, Lumineau JP. Fentes labiales et palatines. Traitement primaire. In: Consulte EM, ed. *Techniques chirurgicales—Chirurgie plastique reconstructrice et esthétique*. Paris: Elsevier Masson SAS; 2018:45–580.
6. Warren DM. The nasal airway in breathing and speech. In: Berkowitz S, ed. *Cleft Lip and Palate, Perspectives in Management*. San Diego: Singular Publishing Group; 1996:61–73.
7. Meazzini MC. Maxillary growth impairment in cleft lip and palate patients: a simplified approach in the search for a cause. *J Craniofacial Surg*. 2008;19:1302–1307.
8. Ross RB. Treatments variables affecting facial growth in complete unilateral cleft lip and palate. *Cleft Palate J*. 1987;24:5–77.
9. Sommerlad BC. A technique for cleft palate repair. *Plast Reconstr Surg*. 2003;112:1542–1548.
10. Millard DR. Cleft craft: the evolution of its surgery. *The Unilateral Deformity*. vol. 1. Boston: Little, Brown; 1976.
11. Fisher DM. Unilateral cleft lip repair: an anatomical subunit approximation technique. *Plast Reconstr Surg*. 2005;116:61–71.
12. Rose W. *On Harelip and Cleft Palate*. London: HK Lewis; 1891.
13. Thompson JE. An artistic and mathematically accurate method of repairing the defect in cases of harelip. *Surg Gynaecol Obstet*. 1912;14:498.
14. Noordhoff MS. Reconstruction of vermilion in unilateral and bilateral cleft lips. *Plast Reconstr Surg*. 1984;73:52–61.

CHAPTER

60

Bilateral Cheilorhinoplasty

Ghali E. Ghali and Jennifer E. Woerner

Armamentarium

#9 Periosteal elevator
#11 and #15 Scalpel blades
Andrews-Pynchon suction
Appropriate sutures
Bard Parker scalpel blade handle
Bishop Harmon forceps with teeth
Castroviejo calipers
Castroviejo forceps 0.5 mm (2)
Freer double hooks (2)
French pattern osteotome
Jeter Baby-Dean scissors (2)
Local anesthetic with vasoconstrictor
Mayo scissors
Needle tip electrocautery
Salyer hooks, #2 (2)
Salyer hooks, #3 (2)
Webster needle holder

History of the Procedure

Throughout history, repair of the bilateral cleft lip deformity has been met with much controversy. The evolution of this technique has been slow, and many of the original techniques were based on the repair of a unilateral cleft lip deformity.[1] The fate of the prolabium has always been a concern. During the late 1600s, there was much debate as to whether the prolabium should be used in the final repair at all. An Englishman by the name of James Cooke was one of the first to advocate saving the prolabium. Even as late as the 1970s, there was still speculation over whether the prolabium could survive the surgical insult from the closure of both cleft sides during the same operation. At that time in the United States, cleft surgeons were divided, with 60% preferring to repair both sides at the same time and 40% advocating a staged technique repairing the more severe side first.[2] Even surgeons who preferred simultaneous closure based their designs on the idea that the prolabium had limited growth potential. With this in mind, the original techniques mainly relied on triangular flaps, rectangular flaps, or straight-line closure variants. Many of these techniques led to large philtral columns, abnormally long lips, or irregular scars, and none of these early repairs addressed the orbicularis oris muscle. During the latter part of the 20th century, reports began to emerge of the reconstruction of this muscle, and the technique was termed *functional cleft lip repair*.[1]

Indications for the Use of the Procedure

Prior to surgical repair of the bilateral cleft lip deformity, significant attention should be given to counseling of the family on how to care for a child with this condition, resolution of feeding issues, adequate weight gain, and the overall health of the newborn. Timing of the bilateral cleft lip repair has historically followed the "rule of 10s," requiring that the child be at least 10 weeks old, weigh at least 10 pounds, and have a minimum hemoglobin level of 10 mg/dL.[3] With the advancements in pediatric anesthesia and intraoperative monitoring, general anesthesia can be safely administered very early in life. Regardless of this ability, there has been no benefit to repairing the cleft lip deformity prior to 3 months of age.[4–6] Advantages to waiting until at least 10 weeks of age include improved ease of repair with slightly larger anatomic landmarks and adequate time for the primary care provider to evaluate the patient for other congenital abnormalities.[7] Advances in screening for comorbidities and the delivery of anesthesia make preoperative hemoglobin testing seldom necessary.

Limitations and Contraindications

The surgeon must be aware of medical concerns that may mitigate the ability to perform the procedure safely on the infant/child.

TECHNIQUE: Modified Millard for Bilateral Cleft Lip Repair

STEP 1: Intubation and Setup

The patient is placed in a supine position on the operating table with a small shoulder roll for support. A broad-spectrum antibiotic, typically a cephalosporin, is given before surgery as prophylaxis. Before the procedure, to reduce the postoperative inflammatory phase, a combination of short- and long-acting steroids is administered unless contraindicated. After induction, an oral endotracheal tube is secured to the patient's chin in the midline. After surgical preparation, the anatomic structures are palpated and marked with a sterile surgical pen.

STEP 2: Markings and Local Anesthetic

Anterior Lip

The design of the planned surgical incisions is marked, starting with the prolabium. At the level of the lip-columellar crease in the midline, two points are placed approximately 2 to 2.5 mm apart. The length of the philtral column is then established by marking a point 6 mm inferior to the lip-columellar crease. The widest point on the philtral column, established 1.5 mm superior to the inferior point, is 3 to 3.5 mm in width and forms the peaks of cupid's bow. These points are connected to produce the final design of the philtral column. The width of cupid's bow and the length of the philtral column are directly related to the age of the patient. Repairs in older patients have less of a tendency to widen over time. The measurements used to design the philtral column should be slightly enlarged in older patients to compensate for this decreased amount of growth potential (Fig. 60.1A–C).

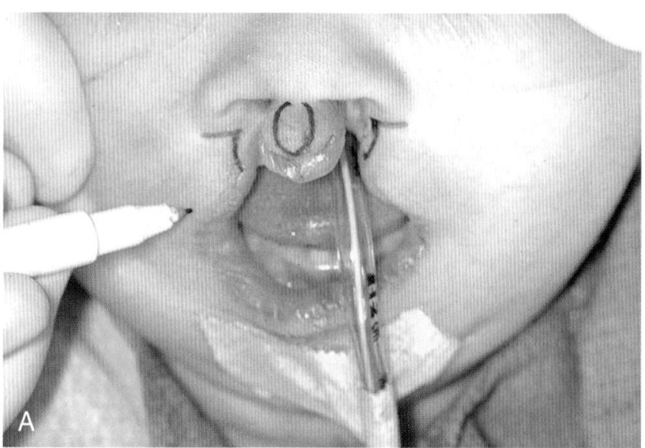

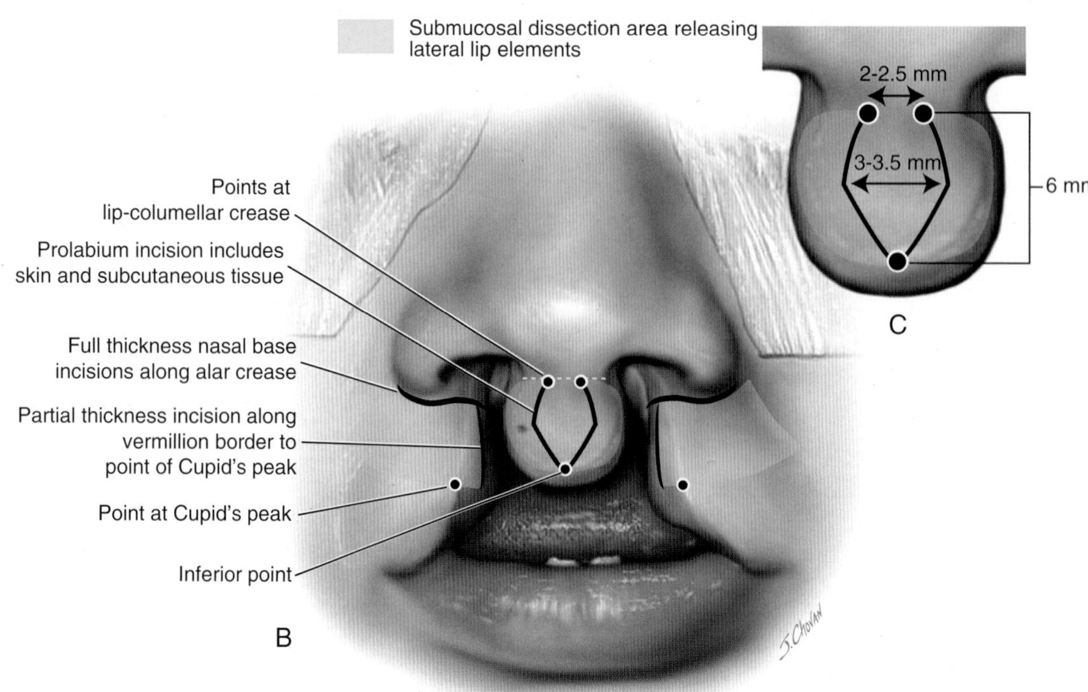

Figure 60.1 **A,** Intraoperative design for incision design. **B,** Design for prolabial, premaxillary, and lateral lip incisions. **C,** Preferred measurements for prolabium.

Technique: Modified Millard for Bilateral Cleft Lip Repair—*cont'd*

Lateral Lip

The nasal base incisions are first marked bilaterally, creating a curvilinear line along the alar crease. This forms the releasing incisions that aid in the advancement of the lateral lip elements. The peaks of cupid's bow are then marked and positioned at the vermilion-cutaneous border, where the vermilion border of the lip and the white roll begin to converge. The marks may then be adjusted to create an equal distance bilaterally from the commissure of the mouth to the marked points. A line perpendicular to the tangential line at the vermilion-cutaneous border is then marked through the vermilion. After markings, bilateral infraorbital nerve blocks are performed, and the anterior and lateral lips and alar bases are injected with 1% lidocaine and a 1:100,000 epinephrine mixture (Fig. 60.1D).

STEP 3: Incision

After placement of the moistened throat pack, the first incision is initiated on the prolabium. This incision includes skin and subcutaneous tissue. The flap should be raised from the philtral notch, elevating superiorly and gradually enlarging the thickness of the flap to preserve the columellar blood supply. The remaining vermilion and skin are reflected and turned intraorally as a flap based on the premaxilla. This tissue aids in the intraoral closure of the mucosal surface.

The alar bases are then freed from the lateral lip elements along the curvilinear line. The vermilion border is incised in a partial-thickness fashion to the point marking the peak of cupid's bow. Preservation of the lateral vermilion mucosal flaps inferior to the peak of cupid's bow is essential for reconstruction of the central lip region. The dissection to release the lateral lip elements from the maxilla is done with sharp scissors in a submucosal plane. The lateral lip elements must be completely separated from the intraoral mucosa. This dissection is usually performed at the malar prominences for adequate mobilization. The orbicularis oris is separated from the lateral lip flaps in the subdermal plane. The muscle bundles are separated from the anterior maxilla at the alar base to reorient the fibers in a horizontal direction. The nasovestibular web is released from its attachment at the piriform rim. This release allows advancement in an anteromedial direction, correcting the alar base width (Fig. 60.1E–I).

Continued

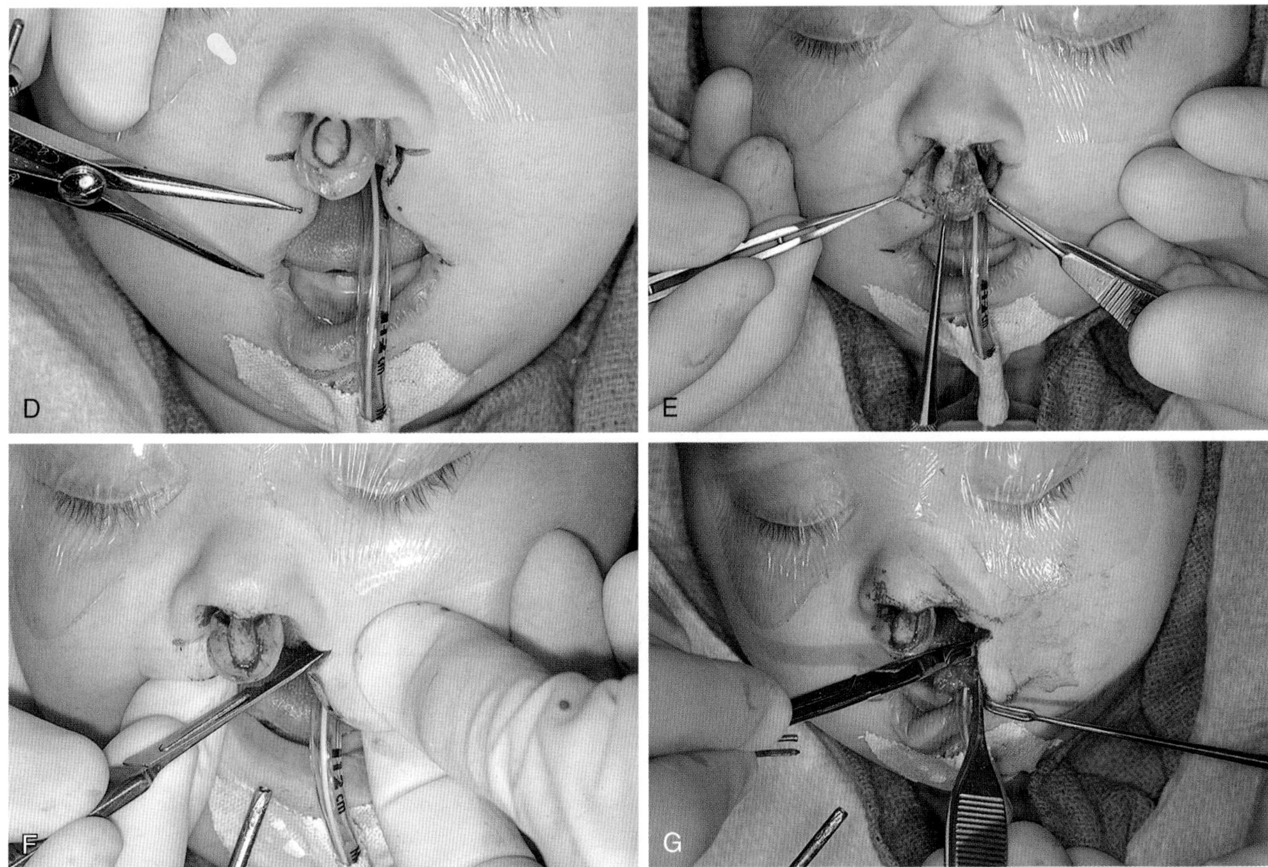

Figure 60.1, cont'd **D,** Calipers are used to ensure that the height of cupid's bow is equidistant from the commissures. **E,** Dissection of prolabium and demonstration of residual vermilion for mucosal closure. **F,** Full-thickness incisions along the alar base. **G,** The orbicularis oris is dissected circumferentially using sharp scissors.

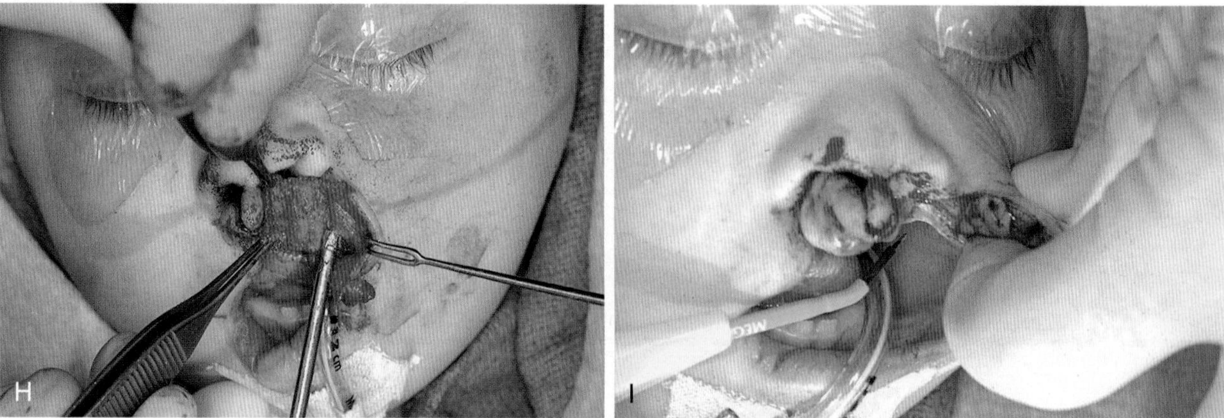

Figure 60.1, cont'd H, Orbicularis oris muscle dissection. **I,** Release of nasovestibular mucosa using the electrocautery.

Technique: Modified Millard for Bilateral Cleft Lip Repair—*cont'd*

STEP 4: Closure

The nasal floor is reconstructed from flaps created from the premaxilla and the released nasovestibular web. The edges of the vermilion border are approximated and temporarily sutured into position to aid in initial positioning. Once the vermilion border is in the correct position, mucosal closure begins. A slowly resorbing suture, such as 4-0 polyglactin 910, is recommended in these areas. The lateral lip mucosa is advanced and sutured to the premaxillary mucosa. It may be necessary to trim the edge of the lateral lip or premaxillary mucosa before suturing.

After the intraoral closures, attention is turned to construction of a continuous orbicularis oris muscle. The reoriented ends of the muscle are advanced horizontally and sutured into position using horizontal mattress sutures starting at the inferior edge and working superiorly. A slower resorbing 3-0 polyglactin 910 or polydioxanone suture on a tapered needle is recommended in this area. Once at the superior edge, the orbicularis muscle is sutured deep to the columellar base at the anterior nasal spine to maintain positioning.

The leading skin edges of the lateral lip are advanced after the newly created philtral column is inset. Closure is accomplished with a fine nonresorbable suture in a staggered fashion to prevent damage to the philtral flap. The remaining skin sutures at the alar bases complete the closure (Fig. 60.1J–O).

STEP 5: Postoperative Care

Sterile strips are applied after an adhesive application to reduce the tension placed on the closure. The patient is admitted for overnight monitoring and is routinely discharged home on postoperative day 1 or 2. The wound is kept dry for at least 48 hours, and the sterile strips are removed at the time of suture removal in 5 to 7 days. The patient is fed through a syringe during the early postoperative period, but most patients return to the use of a bottle by the first postoperative day (Fig. 60.1P).

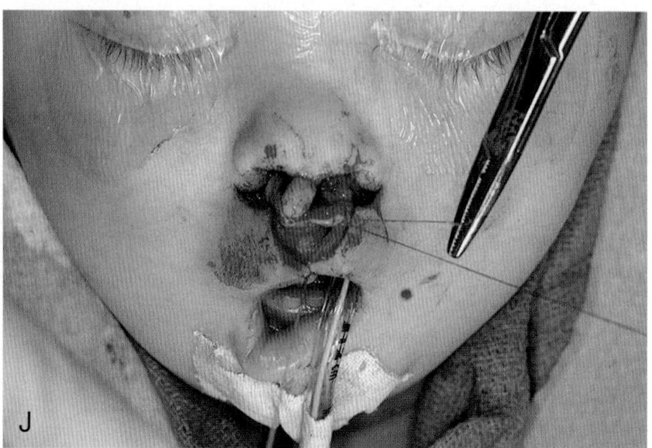

Figure 60.1, cont'd J, Suturing of lateral lip mucosa.

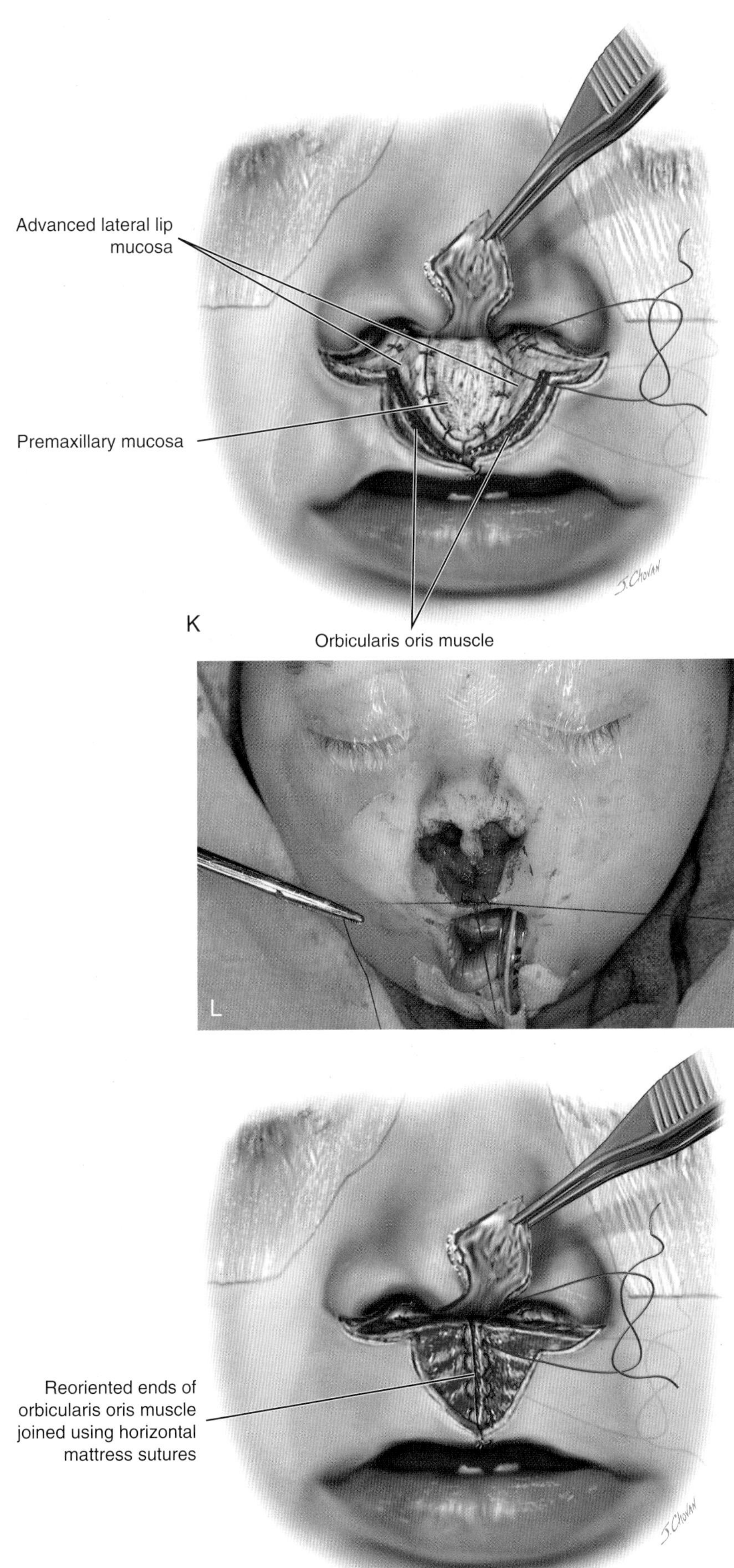

Figure 60.1, cont'd **K,** Diagram of advancement of lateral lip mucosa. **L,** Reconstruction of orbicularis oris. **M,** Diagram of muscle reconstruction.

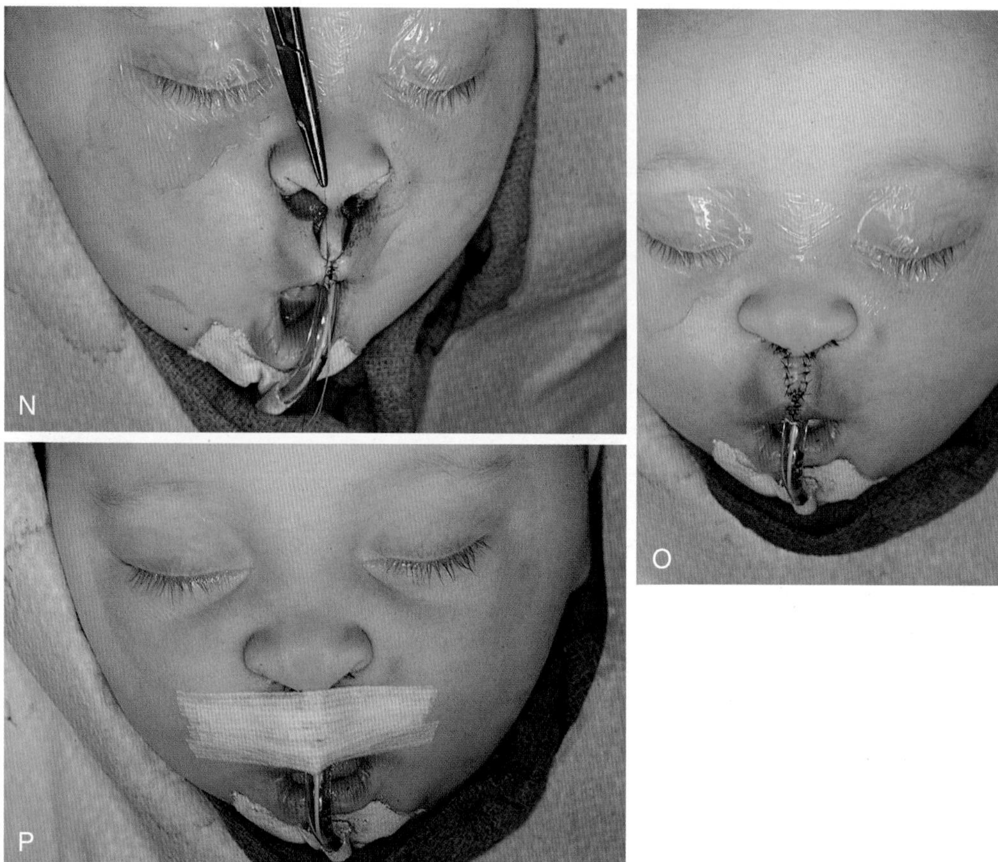

Figure 60.1, cont'd **N,** Inset of philtral column. **O,** Completion of skin closure. **P,** Wound is dressed with Mastisol and Steri-Strips. (A, D–J, L, N–P, from Ghali GE, Ringeman JL. Primary bilateral cleft lip/nose repair using a modified Millard technique. *Atlas Oral Maxillofacial Surg Clin North Am*. 2009;17:117.)

Avoidance and Management of Intraoperative Complications

There is little literature focused on the intraoperative surgical complications during cleft lip repair. Most of the major complications focus on morbidity and mortality due to general anesthesia, airway obstruction, or other congenital abnormalities. Prior to the mid-1950s, local anesthesia along with endotracheal intubation were not regularly employed; therefore, loss of airway and intraoperative hemorrhage were more common phenomena. The rule of 10s has helped to decrease many of the anesthetic complications previously encountered, especially in patients with other congenital abnormalities. Requiring the infant be at least 10 weeks old and of adequate weight reduces the incidence of difficult laryngoscopy, allows time for other congenital abnormalities or medical conditions to be identified, and reduces the percentage of intraoperative blood loss in comparison to total blood volume.[8] In a study performed by the University of Pittsburgh, researchers reviewed 585 cleft lip repairs performed from 1950 to 1964 and found that complications related to cleft lip repair were five times more prevalent when the rule of 10s was not strictly followed.[9]

Postoperative Considerations

Postoperative complications can range from minor issues directly related to the wound, such as hematoma formation, wound breakdown, and infection, to more serious sequelae such as airway obstruction, hospital-acquired infections, and devitalization of the prolabium. A majority of the literature reports hematoma formation as a rare complication occurring less than 1% of the time that can be easily treated with local compression and rarely requires reoperation.[10–12] It is important to ensure adequate hemostasis prior to closure in order to reduce this risk. Postoperative infection and wound breakdown are uncommon sequelae as well, with an incidence between 1% and 7.4%, and are more commonly found in cases of bilateral clefts.[10] Both of these complications can be minimized with the use of intravenous antibiotics prior to surgical start time, proper soft tissue handling, avoidance of tension on the skin closure, and adequate postoperative wound care.

In regard to a major complication such as airway obstruction, caution should be taken in children with large bilateral clefts of the lip and palate during the immediate postoperative period. These children may experience respiratory distress following closure of the lip alone. It should be communicated to the anesthesia team that adequate time should be allowed for full recovery from the volatile anesthetics and opioids administered prior to extubation. In our institution, large bilateral cleft lip repair patients are monitored in the pediatric intensive care unit for at least 24 hours postoperatively.

The rate of complications not directly related to the surgical repair itself, such as upper respiratory tract infections, pneumonia, or gastrointestinal infections, is often directly related to the length of hospital stay.[11,13] For this reason, it is important to minimize the infant's hospital stay if at all possible. At our institution, most patients are discharged within 24 to 48 hours of surgery as long as the child has adequate intraoral intake. This reduction in hospital stay minimizes the risk of hospital-acquired infections. The need for a detailed history and physical exam prior to surgery cannot be stressed enough. This ensures the patient does not have any early signs of infection that may further complicate the postoperative course.

Devitalization of the prolabium is a dreaded complication that has driven much debate throughout the history of bilateral cleft lip repair. As discussed previously, it was once thought that bilateral cleft lip repair required a staged closure because the prolabium could not withstand the surgical insult of a one-stage technique.[2] Though the true incidence is unknown, fear of prolabium necrosis still exists. When employing the surgical technique described in this chapter, the author cannot stress enough the importance of increasing the thickness of the prolabial flap as it is raised from the philtral notch and ensuring a final tension-free closure. If both of these conditions are met, the prolabium should remain viable with preservation of the columellar blood supply. The color, along with the capillary refill of the philtrum, should be checked throughout the procedure and during the postoperative period.

References

1. Ghali GE, Ringeman JL. Primary bilateral cleft lip/nose repair using a modified Millard technique. *Atlas Oral Maxillofac Surg Clin North Am*. 2009;17(2):117–124.
2. Millard DR. Cleft craft: the evolution of its surgery. In: Millard DR, ed. *Bilateral and Rare Deformities*. Vol. 2. Boston, Massachusetts: Little, Brown; 1977.
3. Thompson JE. An artistic and mathematically accurate method of repairing the defect in cases of harelip. *Surg Gynecol Obstet*. 1912;14:498.
4. Marsh JL. Craniofacial surgery: the experiment on the experiment of nature. *Cleft Palate Craniofac J*. 1996;33(2):1.
5. Eaton AC, Marsh JL, Pilgram TK. Does reduced hospital stay affect morbidity and mortality rates following cleft lip and palate repair in infancy? *Plast Reconstr Surg*. 1994;94(7):911–915.
6. Field TM, Vega-Lahr N. Early interactions between infants with craniofacial anomalies and their mothers. *Infant Behav Dev*. 1884;7:527.
7. Costello BJ, Ruiz RL. Cleft lip and palate. In: Miloro M, Ghali GE, Larsen P, Waite P, eds. *Peterson's Principles of Oral and Maxillofacial Surgery*. Vol. 2. Shelton, Connecticut: People's Medical Publishing House; 2012.
8. Fillies T, Homann C, Meyer U, Reich A, Joos U, Werkmeister R. Perioperative complications in infant cleft repair. *Head Face Med*. 2007;3:9.
9. Wilhelmsen HR, Musgrave RH. *Complications of Cleft Lip Surgery*. San Francisco, California: American Society of Plastic Surgeons; 1964.
10. Dingman RO, Ricker OL, Iob V. Blood loss in infant cleft lip and cleft palate surgery. *Plast Reconstr Surg*. 1949;4(4):333–336.
11. Holdworth WG. *Cleft Lip and Palate*. 2nd ed. London, UK: Heinemann; 1957.
12. Tempest MN. Some observations on blood loss in harelip and cleft palate surgery. *Br J Plast Surg*. 1958;11:34.
13. Oldfield MC. Modern trends in hare-lip and cleft palate surgery; with a review of 500 cases. *Br J Surg*. 1949;37(146):178–194, illustration.

CHAPTER 61

Cleft Palate—Modified Two-Flap Technique

Fabio G. Ritto, David Gailey, and Kevin Smith

Armamentarium

#7 Knife handle
#8 Frazier suction
Appropriate sutures
Beaver knife handle
Dean scissors
DeBakey forceps
Dingman mouth retractor
IMA needle holder
Local anesthetic with vasoconstrictor
PSC 4 fishhook needle
Scalpel blades (#11, #15C, #69 Beaver blade)
Sinus elevators (Tatum set, Lorenz)

History of the Procedure

The diagnosis of cleft lip and palate deformities dates back to ancient times. Archaeological evidence from ancient Schonwerda and Peruvian civilizations describes individuals who lived until adulthood with untreated cleft deformities.[1] Although the diagnosis of cleft lip and palate has existed for centuries, the treatment of such congenital defects has had little development until the modern age. It was during the Chin dynasty, in the 4th century AD, that the first description of surgical correction appears, and it addresses only the cleft lip.[2] Palatal clefts were left surgically unrepaired. Occluding the defect with rolls of cotton or metal plates made of silver or lead was the treatment for the palatal cleft. For many years the only treatment for palatal clefts involved the use of obturators because repair was a technically demanding procedure and adequate anesthesia was lacking.[3]

In 1764 French dentist Le Monnier performed the first surgical repair of a cleft velum. Le Monnier's technique involved three steps: approximating the cleft edges with suture, cauterizing the cleft edges, and then realigning the fresh edges.[4] The earliest successful repairs of the soft palate were reported by Von Graefe in 1816 and Philibert Roux in 1819.[5,6] The surgical techniques for cleft palate closure continued to evolve, with further developments contributed by various surgeons, including von Langenbeck[7] in 1861, who was the first surgeon to apply a periosteal elevator and perform subperiosteal dissection to correct a cleft palate.

In 1931 Veau[8] published his book condemning von Langenbeck's technique and proposed elevation of two palatal flaps. Veau's book recorded, using diagrams and description, 500 patients treated personally, with speech results analyzed by a speech therapist.[9] Six years later, in 1937, Kilner[10] and Wardill[11] independently published a modification of Veau's technique, which became known as the V-Y pushback technique, or Veau-Kilner-Wardill. There have been several modifications to the palatoplasty technique, and several names have been associated with each modification.

In 1967 Bardach described a two-flap technique with no attempt to pushback, but effort was concentrated on a solid, complete closure of the palatal defect, with two-layer closure of the hard palate. This involved obliteration of the dead space between the oral and nasal layers in the area of the hard palate, freeing up of the muscle attachment from the posterior edge of the hard palate, redirecting the muscles of the soft palate, and suturing them together to create a functional soft palate.[12]

Indications for the Use of the Procedure

The objectives of palatoplasty are the development of normal speech, separation of the oral and nasal cavities, creation of a functional swallowing mechanism, and improvement of eustachian tube function. The velum plays an essential role in all these functions. During speech, the levator palatine muscle elevates the soft palate to occlude on the posterior pharyngeal wall. This posterior movement, along with lateral pharyngeal constriction by the superior constrictor muscle, seals the oral pharynx from the nasal pharynx. Closure directs the flow of air from the larynx out the mouth. Speech is produced with the coordination of the larynx (specifically, the vocal cords), pharyngeal constrictors, velum, tongue, lips, and teeth. The process of speech development is a complex orchestration of muscles and hard and soft tissues that enables communication.

In the case of palatal clefts, the patient is unable to seal the oral pharynx from the nasal pharynx. Large volumes of air escape through the nasal passages, resulting in hypernasal speech, along with a multitude of secondary speech abnormalities. Controversy lingers with regard to the appropriate surgical timing of repair of the palatal cleft. Different studies have tried to determine the best time to perform palatoplasty. The advantage of performing it at around 6 months seems to be an improved speech function, while the disadvantage is that the scar tissue will form sooner on the palate, which may have a negative effect on maxillary growth. It is very difficult to perform long-term controlled trials to evaluate the effect of palatal surgery on growth, and the current systematic reviews are based on retrospective studies with very different methodologies and techniques. As of today, there is no consensus on the best time to perform the palatoplasty, as long as it is accomplished before 18 months.[13–16]

An intact velum is equally important for normal swallowing, which prevents nasal food regurgitation. Although nasal regurgitation can be a nuisance, the lack of intelligible speech is extremely detrimental to the patient. Eustachian tube dysfunction is almost universal in patients with cleft palate. The auditory canal is the only direct outlet to the middle ear. Pressure equilibration across the tympanic membrane occurs by this outlet. In patients with cleft palate, both the size and shape of the auditory canal, along with the muscular attachment to the cartilage, are abnormal. As a result, the middle ear is unable to equalize pressure differences across the tympanic membrane. The increase in middle ear pressure results in ear effusions, causing hearing loss.[4] Normal hearing is essential in normal speech development. Middle ear pressure differences are easily corrected with the surgical placement of myringotomy tubes. Patients with cleft palate should be closely followed for middle ear disease. Although all indications are important when treating patients with cleft palate, the development of adequate speech is the central objective in creating normal velar function.

The anatomy of the soft palate involves five muscle pairs that connect on the midline with its counterparts, interlacing their fibers at different proportions, and are essential for a normal function. They include the palatoglossus, palatopharyngeal, uvular, tensor veli palatini, and levator palatini muscles. Ideally, each muscle should be individually anastomosed on the midline during a palatoplasty, according to the proportion they connect in a noncleft person, but this is not feasible. It is important, however, that the muscle fibers are disinserted from their malattachments, mobilized, and reoriented to their correct directions towards the midline. This procedure is termed the intravelar veloplasty.[17]

Boorman and Sommerlad[18] studied the anatomy of the soft palate on adult cadavers and found that the average width of the levator at its insertion was 17 mm, and this corresponded to the intermediate 40% of the soft palatal length. Sommerlad[19] described a technique[19] of palatal closure that involves the radical dissection of the soft palate musculature, to disinsert all abnormally attached muscles and optimizing reorientation and anastomoses, which will be discussed in a separate chapter.

Some surgeons advocate early repair with a two-stage technique. This involves closing the soft palatal cleft at 4 to 6 months and delaying the repair of the hard palate until 15 to 18 months of age, allowing further facial development. The theory behind this approach is that closing the soft palate earlier will provide better velopharyngeal outcomes without compromising the maxillary growth, since the hard palate is not closed and bone is not exposed. This theory, however, has never been proven.[13,20]

The two-flap palatoplasty technique has an 80% to 90% success rate in obtaining palatal closure without secondary hypernasality.[21] It is very difficult to attribute a person's name to this technique since so many surgeons have contributed to the design, dissection, and closure of the presented palatoplasty. For instance, when Wardill described his four-flap palatoplasty, he idealized it as an improvement of Veau's two-flap palatoplasty by avoiding long flaps and overpressure on the vessels. Bardach revitalized the two-flap technique but did not emphasize the three-plane closure. Instead, the muscle layer was closed along with the oral mucosa layer. Kriens[17] provided a detailed description of the intravelar veloplasty but did not advocate too much muscle dissection, besides detachment from the posterior palate. Even the so-called von Langenbeck (1861) procedure came about after Dieffenbach (1826) recommended the separation of the mucosa covering the bony palate on each side and moving the flaps toward the midline.[22] The technique described below is a two-flap palatoplasty technique modified by the senior author (KSS) after 25 years of experience and more than 1000 palatoplasties performed.

TECHNIQUE: Two-Flap Palatoplasty

STEP 1: Intubation and Setup

After the oral tube is in place (either oral RAE or regular oral tube), the tube is positioned on the midline and fixed to the chin skin with tape or Tegaderm. The patient is appropriately positioned with the head at the edge of the operating table, a shoulder roll is used to achieve maximal neck extension, and the bed is placed in a mild Trendelenburg position to maximize visualization. Headlamps are strongly recommended, and most surgeons will use loupes. Sommerlad[23] advocates the use of a microscope.

Continued

TECHNIQUE: Two-Flap Palatoplasty—*cont'd*

STEP 2: Retractor Placement

The Dingman mouth retractor is placed in the patient's mouth for palatal visualization, taking care not to dislodge or kink the endotracheal tube. Care also must be taken to ensure that the anterior prongs are placed on the alveolar ridge and the upper lip is not pinched underneath, which would cause damage, and the tongue is constantly monitored for signs of congestion.

Once the Dingman mouth retractor has been positioned, 0.25% Marcaine with 1:200,000 epinephrine is injected into the hard and soft palate. This is done before prepping to allow the vasoconstrictor adequate time to take effect. The patient is then prepped, along with the retractor, and surgical drapes are placed, isolating the surgical site.

STEP 3: Incision

A pharyngeal throat pack is placed to maintain isolation of the oral cavity, and the mouth is rinsed with a chlorhexidine gluconate rinse. The surgical procedure is initiated using a # 11 blade to make an incision on the medial aspect of the palatal cleft beginning at the anterior aspect of the palatal cleft and extended distally toward the hemiuvula. The incision is made 1 to 2 mm lateral to the oral-nasal mucosal junction through mucosa and periosteum where bone is underneath. Care is taken to prevent inadvertent perforation of the nasal mucosa. A #15C blade is then used to make the lateral alveolar incision. The incision is initiated distal to the maxillary tuberosity. The incision at this point is carried only through the mucosa, allowing access to the space of Ernst. The incision is advanced anteriorly, curving around the tuberosity. Once the blade has been ensured to be over the hard palate, it is rotated perpendicular to the palate and the incision is carried through periosteum. The incision is made approximately 2 to 3 mm inferior to the base of the alveolar ridge and is carried anteriorly and medially, connecting with the medial incision (Fig. 61.1A). Use the tip of closed DeBakey forceps to help delineate the tuberosity pressure applied to the tissue posterior.

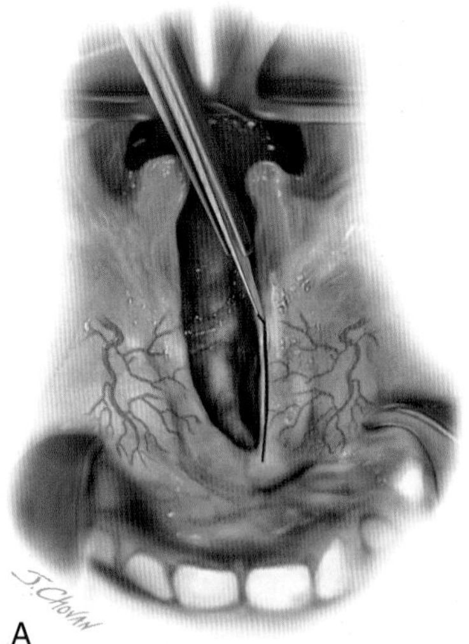

Figure 61.1 A, A #11 blade is used to make the mesial incision. The mucosal incision is made 1 to 2 mm lateral to the oral-nasal mucosal junction to allow adequate tissue for primary closure. The incision is initiated anteriorly and extends distally to the tip of the hemiuvula. The lateral mucosal incision is made using a #15C blade. The incision begins distal to the maxillary tuberosity and is made only through the oral mucosa in this area. It is then advanced anteriorly toward the alveolar ridge. Once over the bony hard palate, the incision extends full thickness to allow subperiosteal dissection.

TECHNIQUE: Two-Flap Palatoplasty—*cont'd*

STEP 4: Oral Mucoperiosteal Flap Elevation

The surgeon now elevates the mucosal flap in a subperiosteal plane. The 01-8269 sinus curette is inserted on the lateral aspect of the mucosal incision in a subperiosteal layer. The curette is advanced medially, exiting through the mucosal cleft incision. This ensures safe separation of the oral and nasal mucosal layers. The mucoperiosteal flap is elevated. Dissection continues posteriorly, with the sinus curette exposing and isolating the greater palatine neurovascular bundle. Bovie cautery is used to obtain hemostasis on the lateral aspect of the raised pedicle flap. The lateral aspect of the raised flap is the most common site of both intraoperative and postoperative bleeding (Fig. 61.1B and C).

STEP 5: Nasal Mucoperiosteal Flap Elevation

With the mucosal flap elevated, the surgeon now elevates the nasal mucosa. The curved 01-8269 sinus curette is carefully advanced on the medial aspect of the bony shelf in a subperiosteal plane, elevating the nasal mucosa. The dissection starts anteriorly, advances posteriorly between the nasal mucoperiosteal flap and the nasal floor, and once the posterior border of the hard palate is reached, the curette is maneuvered to disinsert the abnormally attached musculature on the distal aspect of the hard palate. Care must be taken to remove the muscular attachment while avoiding nasal mucosal perforations. The straighter 01-8264 sinus curette is used to dissect circumferentially around the neurovascular bundle and along the distal hard palate, distally on the lateral aspect into the space of Ernst for soft tissue release, and to dissect around the hamulus when necessary. Wider clefts require more aggressive dissection around the hamulus for further flap mobilization (Fig. 61.1D and E).

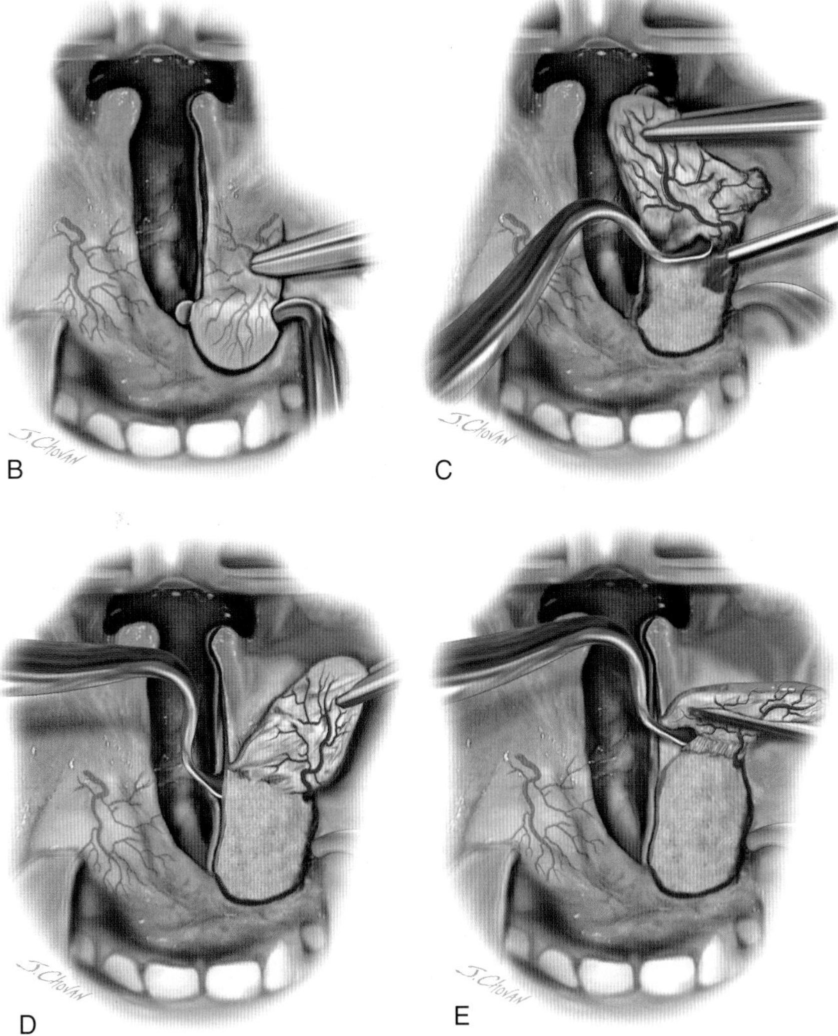

Figure 61.1, cont'd **B,** Mucosal incisions complete. A sinus curette is used to develop subperiosteal dissection. Dissection begins laterally and the curette is advanced medially, exiting through the mucosal cleft incision, ensuring safe separation of the oral and nasal mucosal layers. **C,** With various sinus curettes, the mucosal flap is elevated from anterior to posterior, exposing the greater palatine neurovascular pedicle. Care is taken during the dissection around the pedicle to avoid inadvertent damage. **D,** Once the mucosal flap has been elevated, the curette is used to dissect the nasal mucosa. The curette is carefully advanced on the medial aspect of the bony shelf, ensuring a subperiosteal plane. It is then advanced laterally and distally, obtaining adequate release of the nasal mucosa. **E,** The curette is advanced distally, removing the abnormally attached levator muscles from the hard palate. Muscle must be carefully removed. Inadvertent perforation of the nasal mucosa is most common during this stage of the dissection.

Continued

TECHNIQUE: Two-Flap Palatoplasty—*cont'd*

STEP 6: Palatal Musculature Dissection

Once the mucosal flap has been elevated and adequate mobilization has been obtained for medialization, a retraction suture is placed through the flap and secured to the Dingman retractor. Surgical dissection continues to mobilize the palatine musculature to allow for surgical reorientation. A right-angled Beaver blade is used to sharply dissect the muscles from the overlying mucosa. DeBakey forceps are used to grasp the oral mucosa. The Beaver blade is advanced in a sawing motion, sharply dissecting fibers of the glossopharyngeal and levator muscles from the oral mucosa. Extreme attention is dedicated to the oral mucosa while dissecting this plane with the Beaver blade because this is where most of oral perforations occur (Fig. 61.1F).

With the oral mucosa separated from the glossopharyngeal and levator, a #15C blade is used to dissect the muscles from the nasal mucosa. The white/blue colored nasal mucosa can be differentiated form the dark red musculature, indicating the plane of dissection. A cutting-pushing motion is used to free the muscle from the nasal mucosa. The glossopharyngeal muscle has flat aspect and is superficial to the more bundle shape levator. Again, care must be taken to prevent nasal mucosa perforation. Once the musculature has been adequately liberated from the posterior aspect of the palatal bone, from the oral mucosa, and from the nasal mucosa, it is possible to reorient the fibers in a more transverse and posterior position to perform the intravelar veloplasty. The procedure is repeated on the contralateral side. Once the dissection is complete bilaterally, the mouth is irrigated with saline and hemostasis is verified before closure (Fig. 61.1G).

STEP 7: Closure

Closure begins by medializing the elevated nasal mucosa toward the midline and applying single sutures from the anterior to the posterior aspect of the cleft. Several interrupted buried sutures are placed approximately 2 to 3 mm apart, using 4-0 Vicryl suture on a PS-4C needle. Once closure has been obtained distally, attention is turned to the reorientation of the muscles. The surgeon grasps the muscle layer and places two or three horizontal mattress sutures through it, performing a bilateral muscular anastomosis, and redirecting the muscles in the appropriate horizontal position across the soft palate (Fig. 61.1H and I).

The mucosal pedicle flaps are released by removing the retraction sutures from the Dingman mouth retractor. The uvula segments are reapproximated, with care taken that the tips are at equal levels, or one of the hemiuvulas is removed. Closure continues, following a posterior to anterior direction. Sutures are placed 3 to 4 mm apart, with every other suture including nasal mucosa to eliminate dead space between the mucosal flap and nasal mucosa. Once the mucosal flaps have been secured to each other at the midline, approximately four sutures are placed along the lateral aspect of the flap, securing it to the alveolar ridge and decreasing the amount of exposed bone (Fig. 61.1J).

The patient's mouth is again irrigated with saline, and hemostasis is verified. The pharyngeal throat pack is removed, along with the Dingman retractor. It is critical to remove the retractor with care not to prematurely extubate the patient on removal. It helps to hold the tube with the DeBakey forceps while the retractor is removed. The patient is turned over to the anesthesia team for extubation and recovery. Patients remain in the hospital overnight for airway evaluation and fluid management. Most patients can be discharged the next morning. Arm restraints are used for the first week after the surgery. Patients are fed with a bulb syringe for the first 3 days after repair and then transitioned to toddler feeding cups and type 2 baby foods. Patients are seen 1 week after the repair.

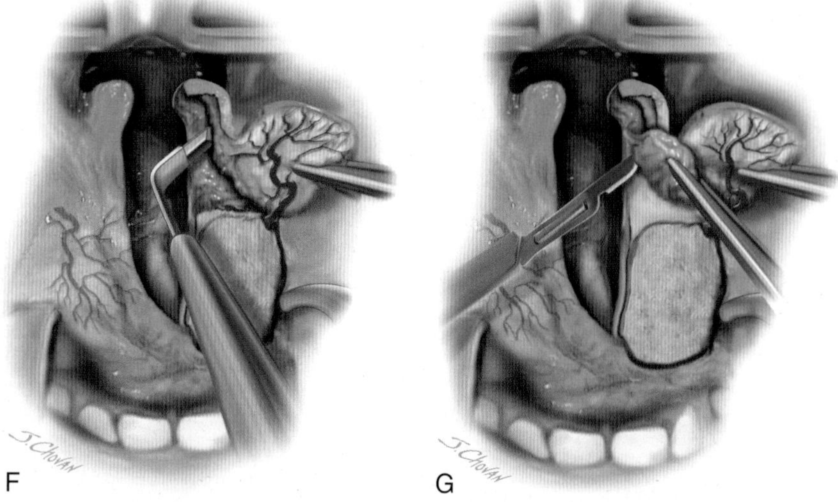

Figure 61.1, cont'd **F,** The levator muscle is sharply dissected from the overlying oral mucosa with a #69 Beaver blade used in a sawing motion. Careful dissection is vital during this stage due to the ease of oral mucosal perforation. **G,** A #15C blade is used to sharply dissect the levator muscle from the underlying nasal mucosa. With the belly of the blade, a pushing motion is used to release the muscle from the nasal mucosa to complete dissection.

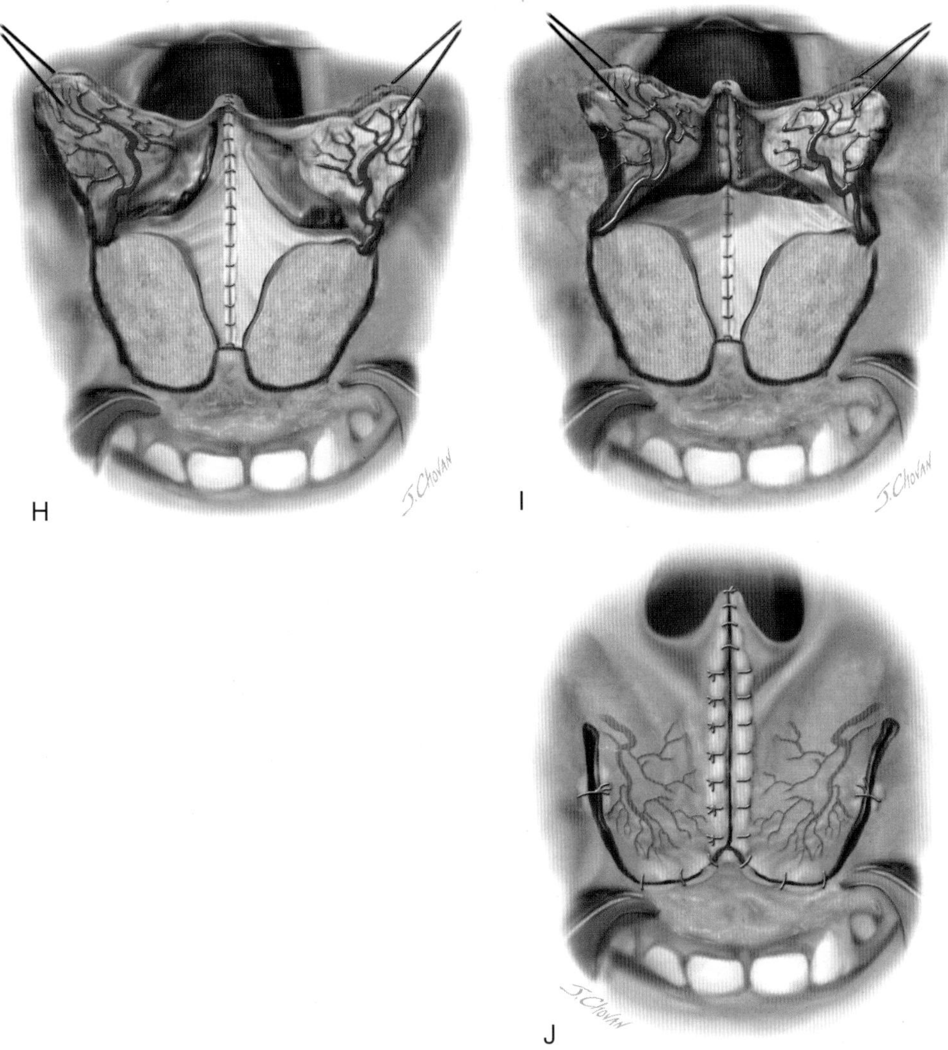

Figure 61.1, cont'd **H,** Completed dissection of bilateral mucosal flaps and levator muscles; also, primary closure of the nasal mucosa. **I,** The levator muscles are reoriented in a horizontal direction and sutured using a horizontal mattress technique, completing the intravelar veloplasty. **J,** The mucosal pedicle flaps are medialized to obtain primary closure and complete the closure of the palatal cleft. Lateral stay sutures are placed to secure the flaps to the alveolar ridge.

ALTERNATIVE TECHNIQUE 1: Vomer Flap

Cleft surgery can be very challenging because no two clefts are alike. This is one reason why the operating surgeon must have the experience and knowledge to modify techniques in order to achieve successful outcomes. In wide palatal clefts, the surgical incisions may need to be modified to obtain a tension-free closure. Some of the modifications that can be used to obtain increased mobility include dissection into the space of Ernst, tensor release, hamular in-fracture, a lateral nasal mucosa releasing incision, and the incorporation of a buccal fat pad between the oral and nasal mucosa. These modifications are frequently used to increase mobility, but few studies demonstrate the benefit, and some studies demonstrate increased morbidity associated with the maneuvers.[12,24]

A commonly used modification for wide anterior clefts is the development of the anterior vomerine flap. When the palatal cleft is wide enough that the nasal mucosa fails to span the cleft, the vomerine mucosa is used to split the cleft distance. This is accomplished by making superiorly based vomerine mucosal flaps (Fig. 61.2). A #15C blade is used to make a linear incision on the free vomerine ridge. A periosteal elevator is then used to dissect in a subperiosteal plane, elevating the vomerine mucosa. The mucosa is advanced laterally to the already elevated nasal mucosa from the medial cleft incisions. This releases the tension over the suture and decreases in the incidence of anterior oral-nasal fistulas.[15] As is typical in medicine, treatment plan decision making involves prioritizing certain aspects in detriment of others. Recent research suggests that exposure of the vomer bone may affect vertical maxillary growth.[25] The decision on whether a wide cleft will require a vomerine flap is made on a case-to-case basis.

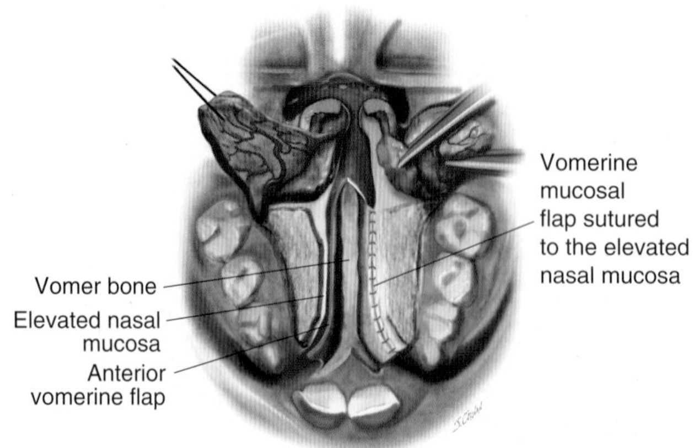

Figure 61.2 Making superiorly based vomerine mucosal flaps: the vomerine mucosa is used to split the cleft distance.

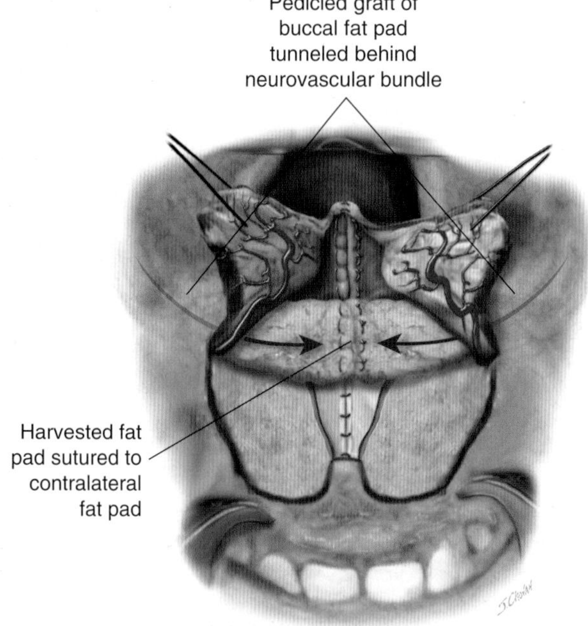

Figure 61.3 The pedicled graft of buccal fat pad can be used on of the nasal mucosa to add an extra layer of tissue.

ALTERNATIVE TECHNIQUE 2: Buccal Fat Pad

Originally described by Pinto and Debnath,[24] the pedicled graft of the buccal fat pad can be used on the nasal mucosa to add an extra layer of tissue (Fig. 61.3). Proponents of this technique claim that it reduces the fistula incidence. Harvesting the flap is initiated after closing nasal mucosa and muscle layer and before closure of oral mucosa. A tunnel may be created behind the neurovascular bundle to further aid on graft stabilization. Blunt dissection is performed on the most posterior aspect of the maxillary tuberosity through the previously made incision, and the tips of the hemostat are directed towards the fat pad, away from the bone. Suction can be inserted in the pocket created by the hemostat to start teasing out the fat, which is further pulled towards the midline behind the neurovascular bundle and is sutured to the contralateral fat pad flap. Finally, the oral mucosa is closed on a regular fashion.

Avoidance and Management of Intraoperative Complications

As with many other surgical procedures, the surgeon's experience is the key to avoiding and reducing the likelihood of intraoperative complications. However, even with a skilled, experienced surgeon, complications can occur. One of the most common complications is either oral or nasal mucosal perforations. Avoidance is ideal, but when perforations occur, they can be managed either by an attempt at suture closure or by placement of a collagen membrane over the perforation to help prevent fistula formation. Some surgeons recommend intentional perforation of the nasal mucosa in order to prevent hematoma formation, but this is not our preference.[19]

Postoperative Considerations

The most common postoperative complication in cleft palate repair is development palatal fistulas. This includes all techniques (including Z-plasty). Palatal fistula rates range from 12% to 45%, depending on the surgical technique and the surgeon's experience.[26] Fistula rates with the two-flap technique are much lower, ranging from 3.4% to 10%.[27] Fistulas are usually apparent early after repair and are a result of inadequate epithelialization over the cleft defect. Palatal fistulas may or may not be functionally problematic, depending on the size and location of the fistula and the extent to which it affects speech. Speech outcomes and velar function from the palatoplasty are not evident until much later in the child's growth. Velar function cannot be fully evaluated until the child reaches complete speech development, which is usually around the age of 4. Velopharyngeal insufficiency, resulting in complete velar closure and hypernasality, is reported in 6.4% to 10.9% of patients who undergo the two-flap technique.[18] Secondary speech surgeries, including pharyngeal flaps, are used to address this complication. A recent meta-analysis[28] suggested that the Furlow double-opposing Z-plasty is associated with decreased fistula rates when compared with the von Langenbeck and V-Y pushback techniques and decreased velopharyngeal insufficiency rates when compared with the Bardach technique.

References

1. Bill J, Proff P, Bayerlein T, Weingaertner J, Fanghänel J, Reuther J. Treatment of patients with cleft lip, alveolus and palate—a short outline of history and current interdisciplinary treatment approaches. *J Craniomaxillofac Surg.* 2006;34(suppl 2):17–21.
2. Boo-Chai K. An ancient Chinese text on a cleft lip. *Plast Reconstr Surg.* 1966;38(2):89–91.
3. Rogers BO. History of cleft lip and palate treatment. In: Grabb WC, ed. *Cleft Lip and Palate.* Boston, MA: Little, Brown; 1971.
4. Millard DR. *Alveolar and Palatal Deformities: Cleft Craft—The Evolution of its Surgery.* Vol 3. Boston, MA: Little, Brown; 1980.
5. McDowell F. The classic reprint: graefe's first closure of a cleft palate. *Plast Reconstr Surg.* 1971;47(4):375–376.
6. Roux PJ. Memoire sur la staphylorapphe, ou il sutre a loile du palais. *Arch Sci Med (Torino).* 1925;7:516.
7. von Langenbeck B. Die uranoplastic mittels ablösung des mukös-periostalen Gaumenüberzuges. *Arch Klin Chir.* 1861;2:205.
8. Veau V. *La Division Palatine.* Paris, France: Masson; 1931.
9. Calnan J. Palatorraphy V-Y pushback. In: Grabb W, Rosenstein S, Bzoch KR, eds. *Cleft Lipa and Palate.* London: J&A Churchill; 1971.
10. Kilner TP. Cleft lip and palate repair technique. *St Thomp Hosp Rep.* 1937;2:127.
11. Wadrill W. The technique of operation for cleft palate, BRIT. *J Surg.* 1937;25:117.
12. Bardach J, Salyer KE. *Surgical Techniques in Cleft Lip and Palate.* 2nd ed. St Louis, MO: Mosby; 1991.
13. Reddy RR, Gosla Reddy S, Vaidhyanathan A, Bergé SJ, Kuijpers-Jagtman AM. Maxillofacial growth and speech outcome after one-stage or two-stage palatoplasty in unilateral cleft lip and palate. A systematic review. *J Craniomaxillofac Surg.* 2017;45(6):995–1003.
14. Salgado KR, Wendt AR, Fernandes Fagundes NC, Maia LC, Normando D, Leão PB. Early or delayed palatoplasty in complete unilateral cleft lip and palate patients? A systematic review of the effects on maxillary growth. *J Craniomaxillofac Surg.* 2019;47(11):1690–1698.
15. Wong LS, Lu TC, Hang DTD, Chen PK. The impact of facial growth in unilateral cleft lip and palate treated with 2 different protocols. *Ann Plast Surg.* 2020;84(5):541–544.
16. Wlodarczyk JR, Brannon B, Munabi NCO, et al. A meta-analysis of palatal repair timing. *J Craniofac Surg.* 2021 Mar-Apr 01;32(2):647–651.
17. Kriens OB. Fundamental anatomic findings for an intravelar veloplasty. *Cleft Palate J.* 1970;7:27–36.
18. Boorman JG, Sommerlad BC. Levator palati and palatal dimples: their anatomy, relationship and clinical significance. *Br J Plast Surg.* 1985;38(3):326–332.
19. Sommerlad BC. A technique for cleft palate repair. *Plast Reconstr Surg.* 2003;112(6):1542–1548.
20. Kirschner RE, Randall P, Wang P, et al. Cleft palate repair at 3 to 7 months of age. *Plast Reconstr Surg.* 2000;105(6):2127–2132.
21. Salyer KE, Sng KW, Sperry EE. Two-flap palatoplasty: 20-year experience and evolution of surgical technique. *Plast Reconstr Surg.* 2006;118(1):193–204.
22. Dorrance GM. *The Operative Story of Cleft Palate.* Philadelphia: WB Saunders Company; 1933.
23. Sommerlad BC. The use of the operating microscope for cleft palate repair and pharyngoplasty. *Plast Reconstr Surg.* 2003;112(6):1540–1541.
24. Pinto PX, Debnath S. Use of pedicled graft of buccal fat pad to line a nasal defect in releasing pushback palatoplasty. *Br J Oral Maxillofac Surg.* 2007;45(3):249–250.
25. Xu X, Cao C, Zheng Q, Shi B. The influence of four different treatment protocols on maxillofacial growth in patients with unilateral complete cleft lip, palate, and alveolus. *Plast Reconstr Surg.* 2019;144(1):180–186.
26. Wilhelmi BJ, Appelt EA, Hill L, Blackwell SJ. Palatal fistulas: rare with the two-flap palatoplasty repair. *Plast Reconstr Surg.* 2001;107(2):315–318.
27. Murthy AS, Parikh PM, Cristion C, Thomassen M, Venturi M, Boyajian MJ. Fistula after 2-flap palatoplasty: a 20-year review. *Ann Plast Surg.* 2009;63(6):632–635.
28. Stein MJ, Zhang Z, Fell M, Mercer N, Malic C. Determining postoperative outcomes after cleft palate repair: a systematic review and meta-analysis. *J Plast Reconstr Aesthet Surg.* 2019;72(1):85–91.

CHAPTER 62

Cleft Palate—Furlow

Brent Golden and Michael Jaskolka

Armamentarium

#15 Blade
4-0 Vicryl suture on an RB1 needle
4-0 Vicryl suture on a TF needle
5-0 Vicryl suture on a TF needle
Bovie needle point electrocautery
Cleft mouth gag
Curved Freer elevator
Guthrie skin hooks
Hemostats
Oral RAE or oral reinforced tube
Periosteal elevator
Tenotomy scissors
Woodson elevator

History of the Procedure

Leonard Furlow presented his description of a double-opposing Z-plasty for the primary repair of the cleft palate in 1978 before officially publishing in 1986.[1] Following his description, his publication was preceded by the report and development of the technique by the Children's Hospital of Pennsylvania Unit.[2] His report stands out for uniting the concepts of careful muscle retropositioning and palatal lengthening. Although Kilner[3] and Schuchardt[4] reported using opposing Z-plasties of the oral and nasal mucosa decades before, Furlow deserves special credit for describing the technique in its modern form characterized by formal treatment of the cleft muscle (palatopharyngeus and levator veli palatini) with strategic inclusion in the posteriorly based flaps to maximize muscle retrodisplacement, transverse position, functional tension, tightening of the velopharyngeal port, and velar lengthening. Modification of Furlow's technique to routinely use lateral hard palate releasing incisions has been reported to decrease the risk of fistula formation.[5] The procedure was extended to include treatment of velopharyngeal dysfunction as a secondary procedure.[6]

Indications

The Furlow double-opposing Z-plasty is indicated for primary reconstruction of all cleft types including Veau I, II, III, IV, and submucous clefts.[5] It is also indicated for secondary palate surgery to revise the repaired cleft palate in patients with velopharyngeal dysfunction.[6]

Limitations and Contraindications

The Furlow double-opposing Z-plasty for primary repair has no absolute contraindications. A relative contraindication is the markedly wide cleft defect since increased tension of the tissues at the anterior soft palate is a feature of the repair. As the surgeon becomes more comfortable with the technique, wider cleft defects can be managed with predictable results.

When to employ the Furlow technique as a secondary procedure remains a topic for study, although guiding principles for the most predictable improvement are to use the procedure in patients with evidence of incomplete intravelar veloplasty exhibiting a small or moderate-sized residual velopharyngeal gap.[6]

TECHNIQUE: CLEFT PALATE REPAIR BY DOUBLE-OPPOSING Z-PLASTY

STEP 1: Preparation for Surgery

Myringotomy tube placement is often completed under mask anesthesia prior to intubation. Oral endotracheal intubation is subsequently performed; a wire reinforced tube is preferred to a standard oral RAE to minimize intraoperative compression by the cleft mouth gag. The tube is well secured in the midline and the eyes protected and padded. The patient is positioned with a shoulder roll to extend the neck. The surgeon works with loupe magnification and headlight illumination. Standard antibiotic prophylaxis is provided.

STEP 2: Placement of Cleft Mouth Gag

The cleft mouth gag is placed, taking care to select the proper tongue retractor size. The tongue and tube are ensured to be in a midline position prior to gag activation. Attention should be given to avoid injury to the upper lip, lower lip, or tongue when activating the gag. Confirmation of appropriate ventilation without excessive pressures should be performed just after activation. The cheek retractors should then be positioned.

TECHNIQUE: CLEFT PALATE REPAIR BY DOUBLE-OPPOSING Z-PLASTY—cont'd

STEP 3: Incision Design

The hard palate incision design is tailored to the cleft type while the soft palate incision design is consistently applied. For the purpose of this description, reconstruction of a Veau III complete cleft involving the alveolus is described.

Hard palate flaps are outlined extending from the anterior cleft margin to the retrotuberosity region bilaterally just inside the dental alveolar ridge. The flap incision medially is planned at the junction of the nasal and oral mucosa along the independent palatal shelf and along the vomerine-palatal junction contralaterally. Both planned medial incisions are continued posteriorly to the hemiuvula at the junction of the oral and nasal mucosa.

The patient's left side is by convention planned for the posteriorly based oral myomucosal flap (overlying the anteriorly based nasal mucosal flap). The anterior limb of this Z-plasty is drawn from the cleft margin at the posterior border of the hard palate posterior to the hamulus at an acute angle between 45 and 60 degrees.

The patient's right side is by convention planned for the anteriorly based oral mucosal flap (overlying the posteriorly based nasal myomucosal flap). The oral releasing incision is planned from the base of the hemiuvula toward the hamulus at a more oblique angle of 60 to 80 degrees (Fig. 62.1).

Continued

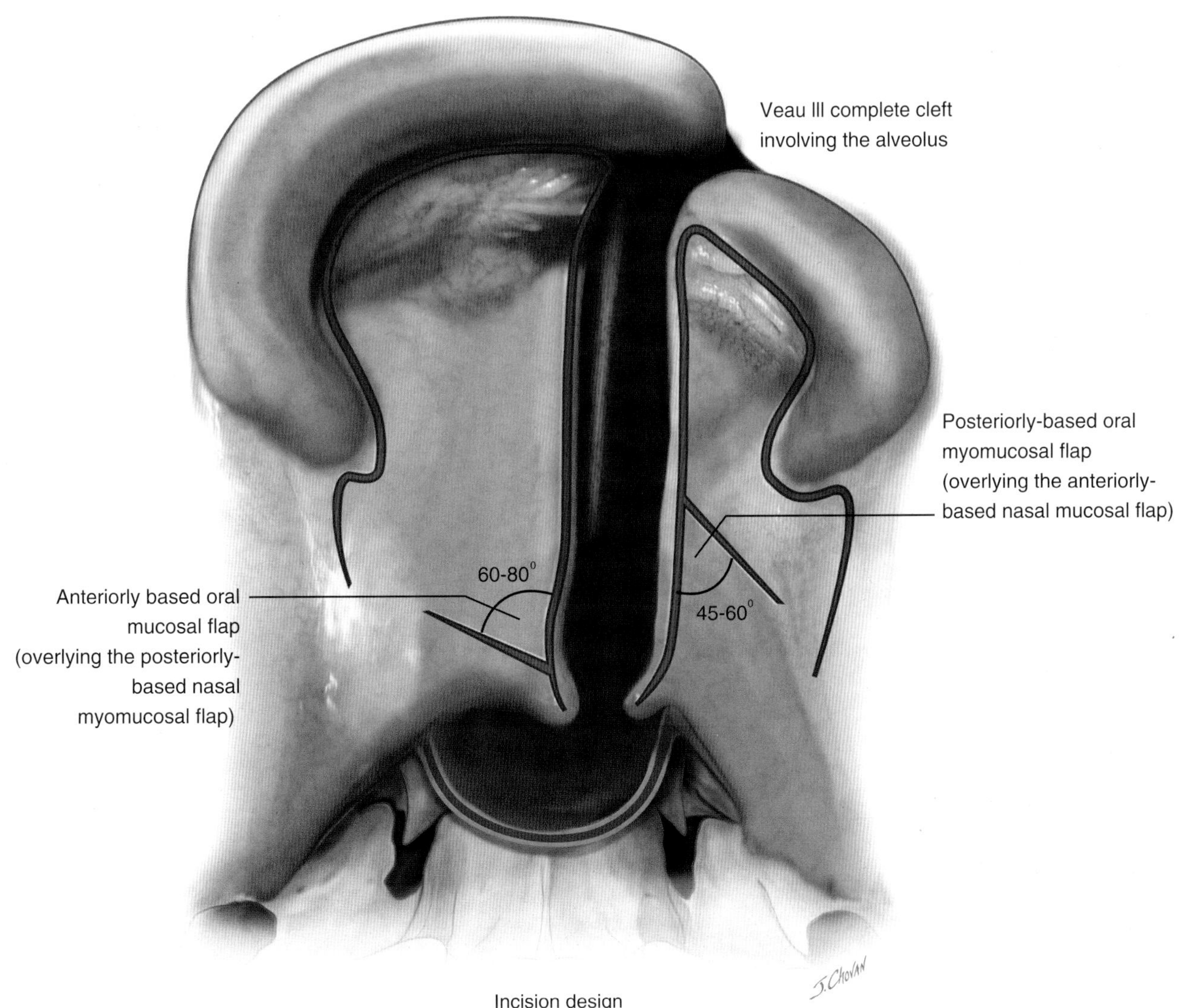

Figure 62.1

TECHNIQUE: CLEFT PALATE REPAIR BY DOUBLE-OPPOSING Z-PLASTY—cont'd

STEP 4: Local Anesthesia

Lidocaine with epinephrine is infiltrated throughout the soft and hard palate. Hydrodissection of the hard palate tissues can facilitate subperiosteal release. Several minutes are allowed for vasoconstriction. Release of the mouth gag during this time is prudent and should be carried out every 30 to 45 minutes during the procedure to minimize venous obstruction and reperfusion injury to the tongue.

STEP 5: Incisions

Just prior to incision, additional injectable saline or anesthetic can be delivered to the soft palate for increased turgor. Using a #15 blade, initial incisions are made bilaterally along the soft palate cleft margins at the junction of the oral and nasal mucosa from the hemiuvula to the anterior extent of the soft palate cleft. Tenotomy scissors are used to demucosalize the medial portion of each hemiuvula and begin the separation of the oral and nasal layers along the entire margin of the soft palate.

The lateral hard palate incisions are then made from the retrotuberosity to the anterior cleft margin bilaterally. A guarded needle tip cautery may be used to trace the incisions down to bone to minimize bleeding. In wider clefts, the incisions are extended posteriorly toward the retromolar region of the mandible to allow for tension-free medialization of the soft palate.

STEP 6: Elevation of Hard Palate Flaps

A Woodson or molt elevator is used to elevate the hard palate flaps in the subperiosteal plane from lateral to medial and anterior to posterior. The medial incision at the junction of the oral and nasal mucosa may need to be completed with Tenotomy scissors or #15 blade under direct visualization; adequate nasal mucosa must be left on the independent palatal shelf to facilitate closure later. Subperiosteal dissection is continued to the posterior hard palate until the greater palatine neurovascular bundles are identified. The hard palate flaps are tagged with a 4-0 Vicryl suture secured to hemostats.

STEP 7: Mobilization of the Neurovascular Bundle and Junction of the Hard and Soft Palate

Mobilization of the tissues associated with the neurovascular bundles and posterior hard palate attachment is a critical component of the procedure to allow for tension-free closure. Once the posterior margin of the hard palate is identified medially, a Woodson elevator can be used to lift the oral mucosa and attached minor salivary glands from the overlying tensor tendon and anterior insertion of the cleft muscles; this facilitates dissection of the greater palatine bundle.

The approach then proceeds from the lateral with subperiosteal dissection and continues in the subperiosteal plane at the retrotuberostiy region. There is a fibrous junction between the maxilla and pterygoid plate that should be released with a needle tip cautery. This allows the dissection to continue in the subperiosteal plane in an anteromedial direction posterior to the neurovascular bundle. This allows for complete circumferential dissection and release of the neurovascular bundle (Fig. 62.2A).

The tissue posterior to the neurovascular bundle is then retracted. The tensor tendon is identified crossing the medial aspect of the pterygoid plate and is cut using a needle tip cautery at this location. This tensor tenotomy is a critical maneuver to release tension for medial movement of the nasal tissues (Fig. 62.2B).

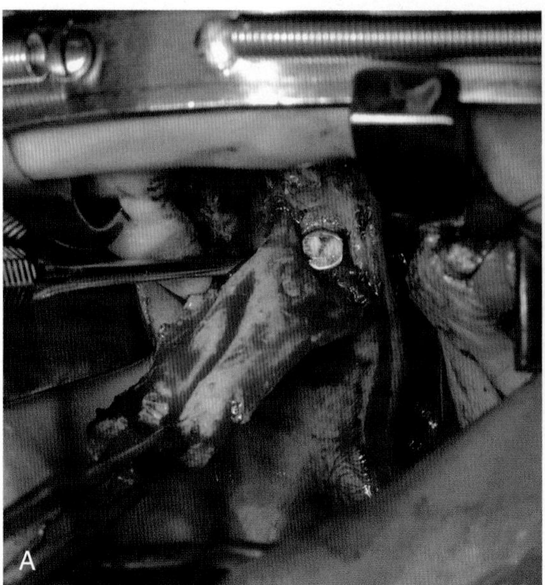

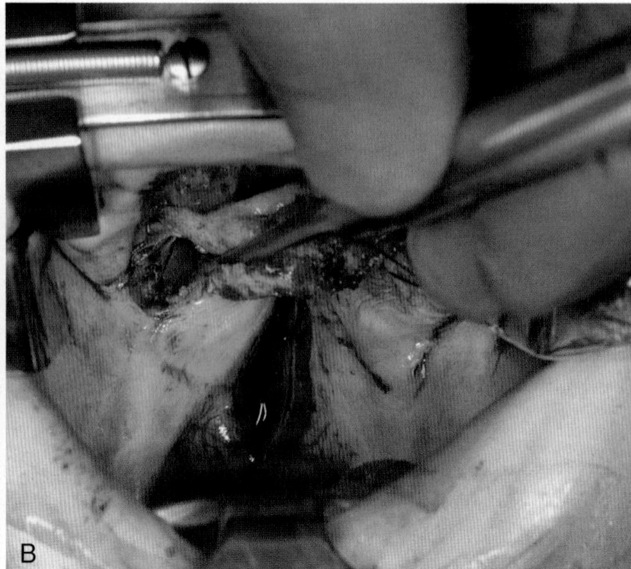

Figure 62.2

TECHNIQUE: CLEFT PALATE REPAIR BY DOUBLE-OPPOSING Z-PLASTY—cont'd

The procedure is repeated on the contralateral side. To provide the additional mobilization required for closure of wide clefts, more aggressive subperiosteal dissection is completed from this lateral approach along the medial aspect of the pterygoid plate extending to the nasal sidewall.

At this point, the nasal mucosa is elevated as widely as possible from the bony palatal shelves both from a posterior and medial approach. On the cleft side, this should continue to the alveolus anteriorly. On the noncleft side, nasal mucosal dissection may only continue to the vomerine junction, or as far as necessary to provide tension-free closure of the nasal layer.

STEP 8: Soft Palate Dissection

A general principle to be observed is that the muscle dissection will extend well beyond the mucosal incisions. This becomes more relevant the wider the cleft to allow for tension-free closure.

The posterior mucosal incision on the right is completed using a #15 blade, taking care to not violate the muscles deep to the incision. The mucosa is elevated with a combination of sharp and blunt dissection, taking care to preserve the glandular tissue on the oral flap. The flap is elevated in this way until it is in continuity with the identical plane developed during elevation of the hard palate flap. Blunt dissection along the lateral aspect of the cleft musculature at the tensor tendon easily separates the overlying mucosa where there is notably less interdigitation of the tissues and begins to define the loose plane adjacent to the superior constrictor (Figs. 62.3A and B).

At the posterior edge of the hard palate, the abnormal anterior insertions of the cleft muscle are sharply released from the nasal mucosa and the tensor tendon attachments using tenotomy scissors or a #15 blade combined with blunt dissection; the muscle release is only performed far enough posteriorly to allow the back-cut to be placed away from the hard palate facilitating closure. The muscle must be released fully from the tensor tendon until the levator tunnel is identified. During this approach, a small vein is frequently encountered and can be carefully cauterized if necessary.

The right-sided oral flap can be rotated and advanced to confirm the appropriate position of the left-sided oral myomucosal incision if desired. The anterior oral Z-pasty limb is incised and any significant glandular bleeding gently coagulated. The anterior portion of this flap has been elevated along with the hard palate flap. The loose plane overlying the tensor tendon and cleft musculature

Continued

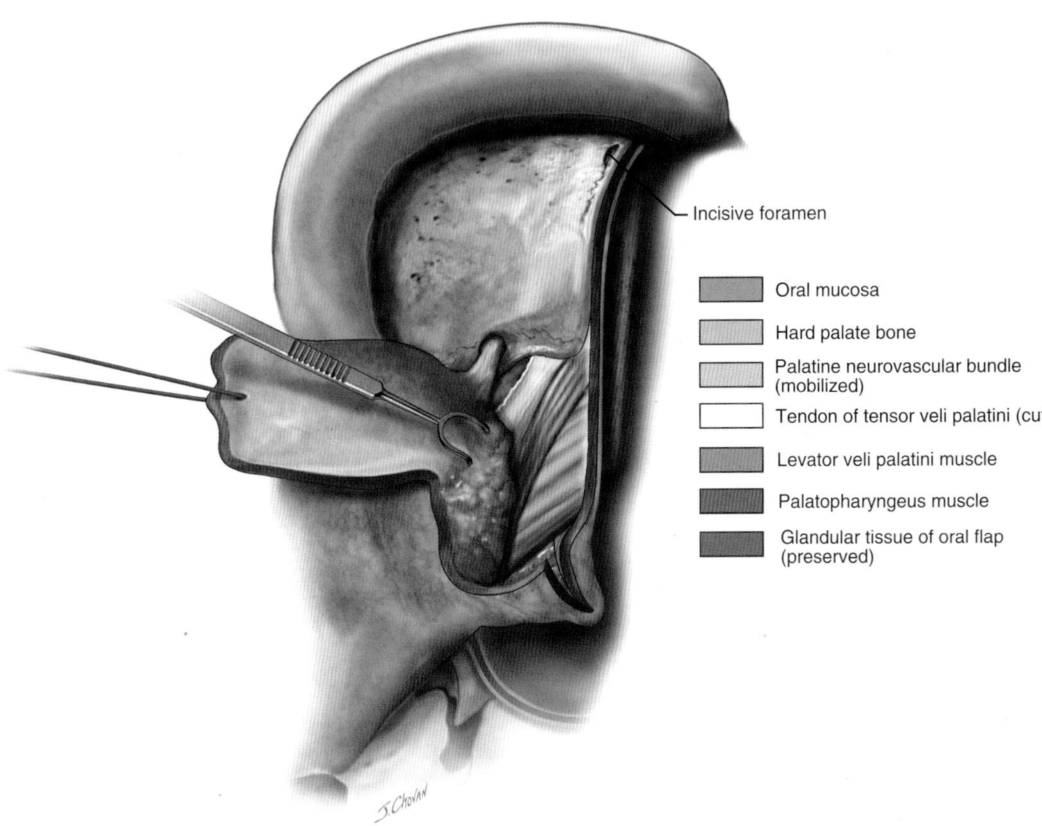

Figure 62.3

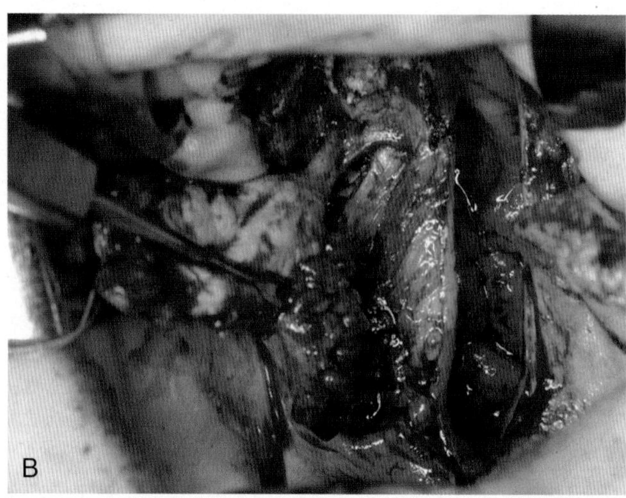

Figure 62.3, cont'd

TECHNIQUE: CLEFT PALATE REPAIR BY DOUBLE-OPPOSING Z-PLASTY—cont'd

is bluntly exposed. In a similar fashion to the right side, the abnormal attachments of the cleft muscle to the posterior hard palate are incised and elevated from the nasal mucosa. The tensor tendon is incised medially and the muscle is retrodisplaced until the levator tunnel is entered (Figs. 62.4A and B).

The left-sided dissection is extended along the nasal mucosa toward the base of the uvula and the cranial base. This mucosal flap is anteriorly based; the posterior nasal Z-plasty incision is made using a tenotomy scissor, understanding that the length of this incision will control the sphincter effect of the nasal closure (Fig. 62.5).

There is significant flexibility in the anteroposterior (AP) location of the right-sided nasal myomucosal incision; however, care must be taken not to place it too close to the hard palate to facilitate closure. The right-sided nasal myomucosal flap is released by an anterior Z-plasty incision also made with a tenotomy scissors. This incision is made just long enough to allow proper retrodisplacement and inset of the nasal myomucosal flap (Fig. 62.6).

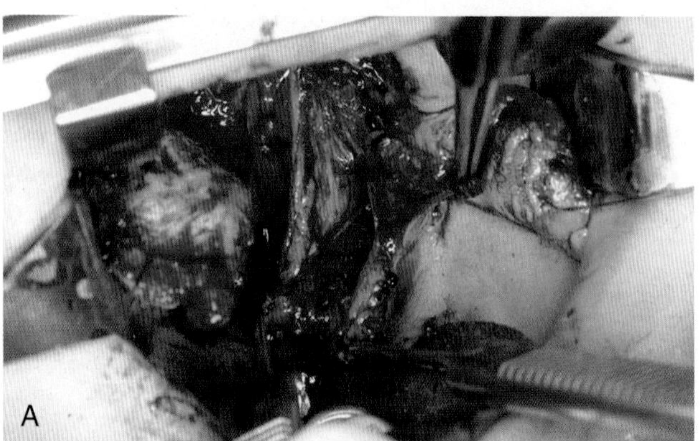

Figure 62.4

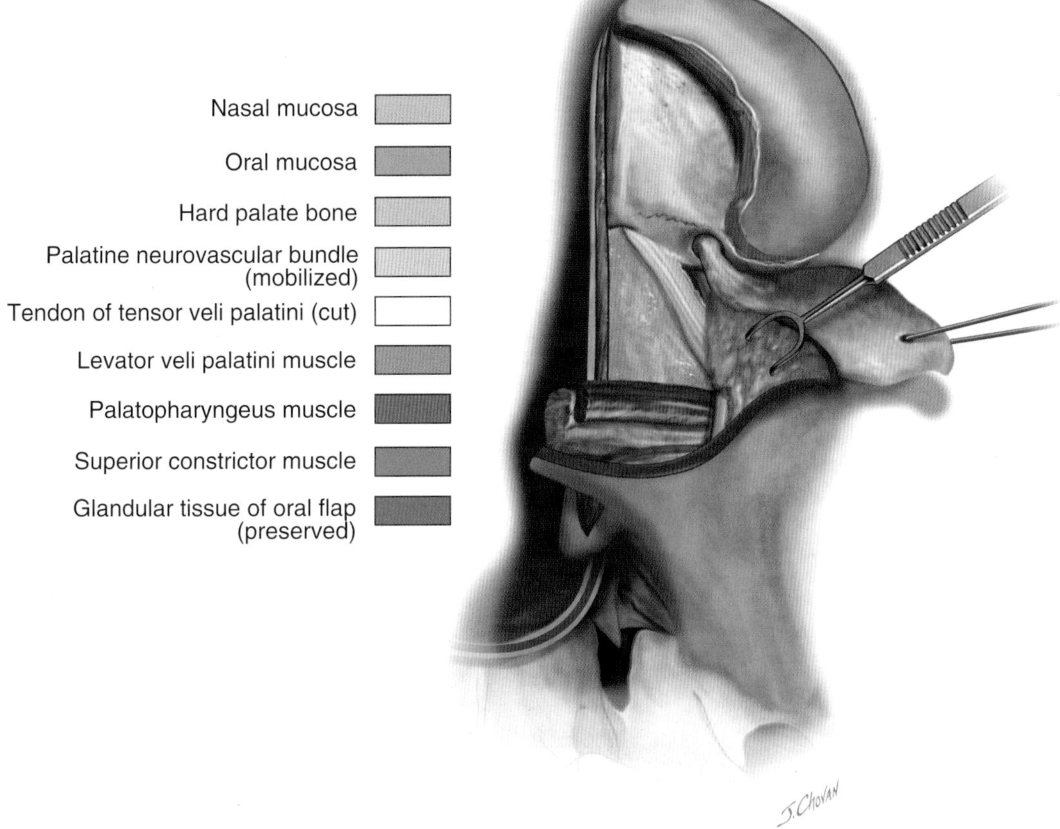
Nasal mucosa
Oral mucosa
Hard palate bone
Palatine neurovascular bundle (mobilized)
Tendon of tensor veli palatini (cut)
Levator veli palatini muscle
Palatopharyngeus muscle
Superior constrictor muscle
Glandular tissue of oral flap (preserved)
J. Chovan
B

Figure 62.4, cont'd

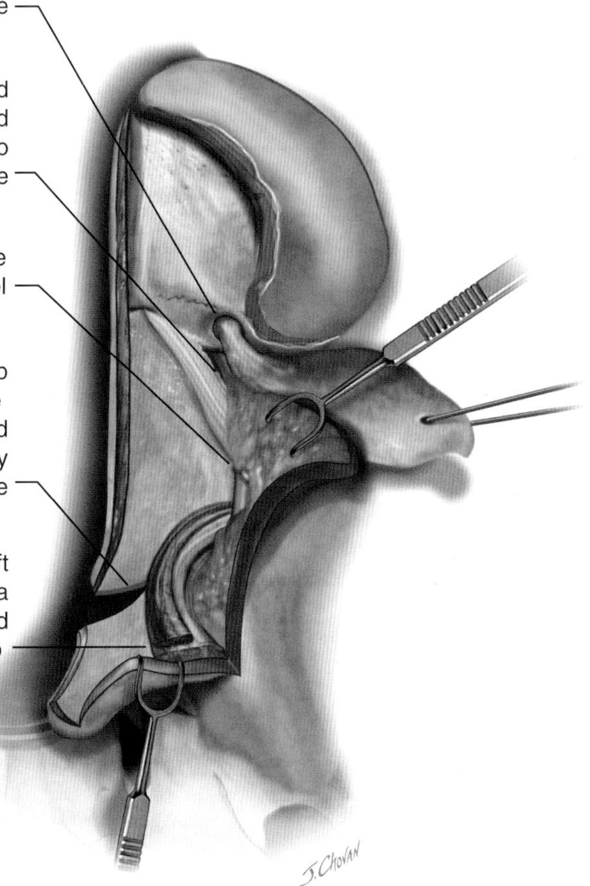
Circumferential dissection of the neurovascular bundle
The tensor tendon is cut and released from the medial pterygoid plate in the subperiosteal plane to facilitate nasal closure
The levator muscle is released from the tensor tendon fully into the levator tunnel
The back-cut for the nasal mucosal flap is placed posteriorly where the levator muscle is to be inserted- this release can extend all the way to the base of the skull laterally as needed to constrict the velopharyngeal aperture
The cleft musculature is left attached to the oral mucosa for the posteriorly-based myomucosal flap
J. Chovan

Figure 62.5

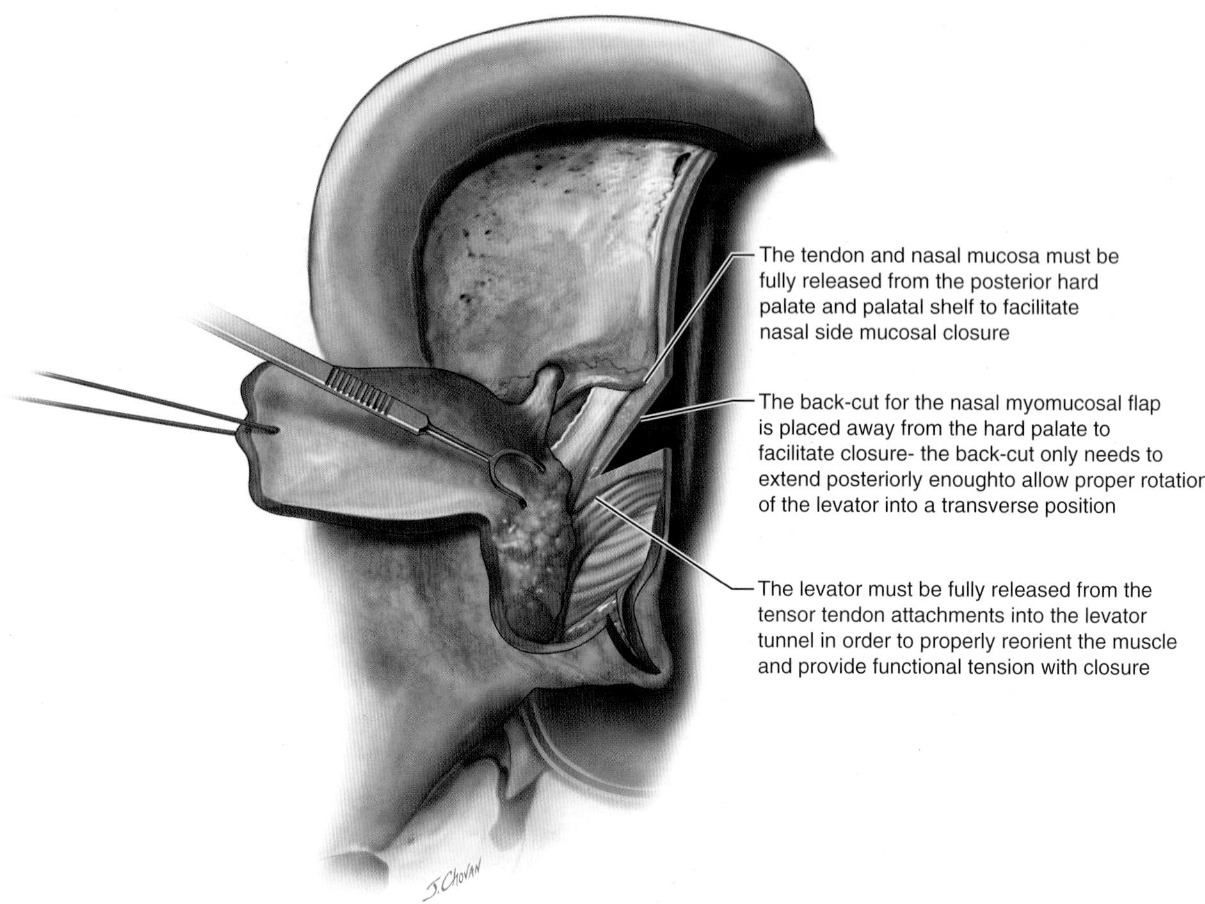
The tendon and nasal mucosa must be fully released from the posterior hard palate and palatal shelf to facilitate nasal side mucosal closure
The back-cut for the nasal myomucosal flap is placed away from the hard palate to facilitate closure- the back-cut only needs to extend posteriorly enoughto allow proper rotation of the levator into a transverse position
The levator must be fully released from the tensor tendon attachments into the levator tunnel in order to properly reorient the muscle and provide functional tension with closure
J. Chovan

Figure 62.6

TECHNIQUE: CLEFT PALATE REPAIR BY DOUBLE-OPPOSING Z-PLASTY—cont'd

STEP 9: Nasal Closure

The soft palate closure is aided by using noncutting needles given the delicate nature of the tissues (4-0 Vicryl with an RB1 needle). Nasal closure proceeds from anterior to posterior in the hard palate. The vomerine nasal mucosa is released posteriorly with a #15 blade or alternatively a guarded needle tip electrocautery. Posterior "Y" extension can be completed to allow for more release of the vomerine flaps, which are elevated with a Woodson elevator in the subperichondrial plane. Interrupted sutures are placed in an inverted fashion to close the nasal mucosa of the hard palate until the soft palate is reached.

Nasal soft tissue closure proceeds stepwise, starting with the uvula and the uvular base posteriorly, followed by insetting of the nasal myomucosal flap, and then finally reapproximating the nasal mucosal flap. Inset of the nasal myomucosal flap takes advantage of the more robust tissues posteriorly and laterally as the nasal mucosal flap anteriorly provides no significant structural support. Each intervening arm of the incision is then closed with interrupted or running resorbable suture (4-0 or 5-0 Vicryl on a tetralogy of Fallot [TF] needle). If the nasal mucosa anterior to the muscular repair is torn or inadequate, heroic efforts to gain closure are not pursued and pedicled buccal fat is placed for coverage (Fig. 62.7).

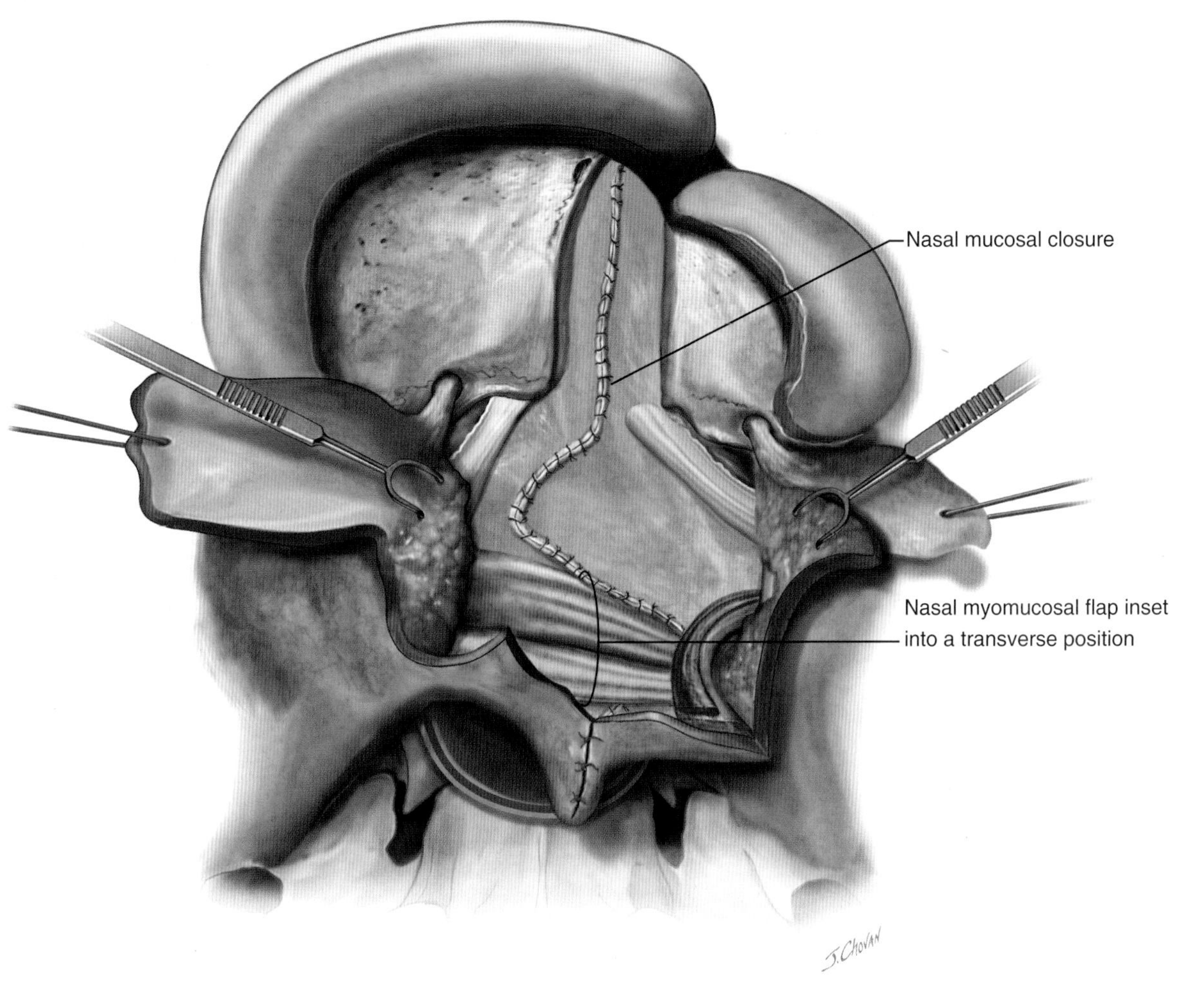

Figure 62.7

TECHNIQUE: CLEFT PALATE REPAIR BY DOUBLE-OPPOSING Z-PLASTY—cont'd

STEP 10: Pedicled Buccal Fat Pad Graft

A pedicled buccal fat graft is routinely used in double-opposing Z-plasty operations. The fat can be taken from either side or bilaterally. Routinely, one side is utilized.

A hemostat or tonsil clamp is bluntly inserted lateral and posterior to the maxillary tuberosity and the buccal fat is immediately encountered. Using a combination of tissue forceps and gentle suction, the fat is teased into the mouth. A hemostat is then opened posterior to the neurovascular bundle to enlarge the space just over the tensor tendon for delivery of the fat pad to the soft palate. The pedicled fat is secured to the nasal tissues using resorbable sutures. Often the contralateral tensor tendon is a good initial anchor point given the strength of the tissue (Figs. 62.8A and B).

STEP 11: Oral Closure

The oral closure then proceeds from posterior to anterior again using resorbable suture on a noncutting needle (4-0 Vicryl on an RB1 needle). The uvula has previously been reconstructed. The Z-plasty flaps are inset first with tacking sutures at the apex, followed by closure of the intervening limbs with interrupted or running suture. The midline hard palate is closed with interrupted resorbable suture. Several horizontal mattress sutures are prudent to ensure eversion at this location and minimize fistula risk. Capture of the fat pad here may be prudent to provide support for the thinner tissues in the event of wound breakdown. The hard palate flaps are inspected for

Continued

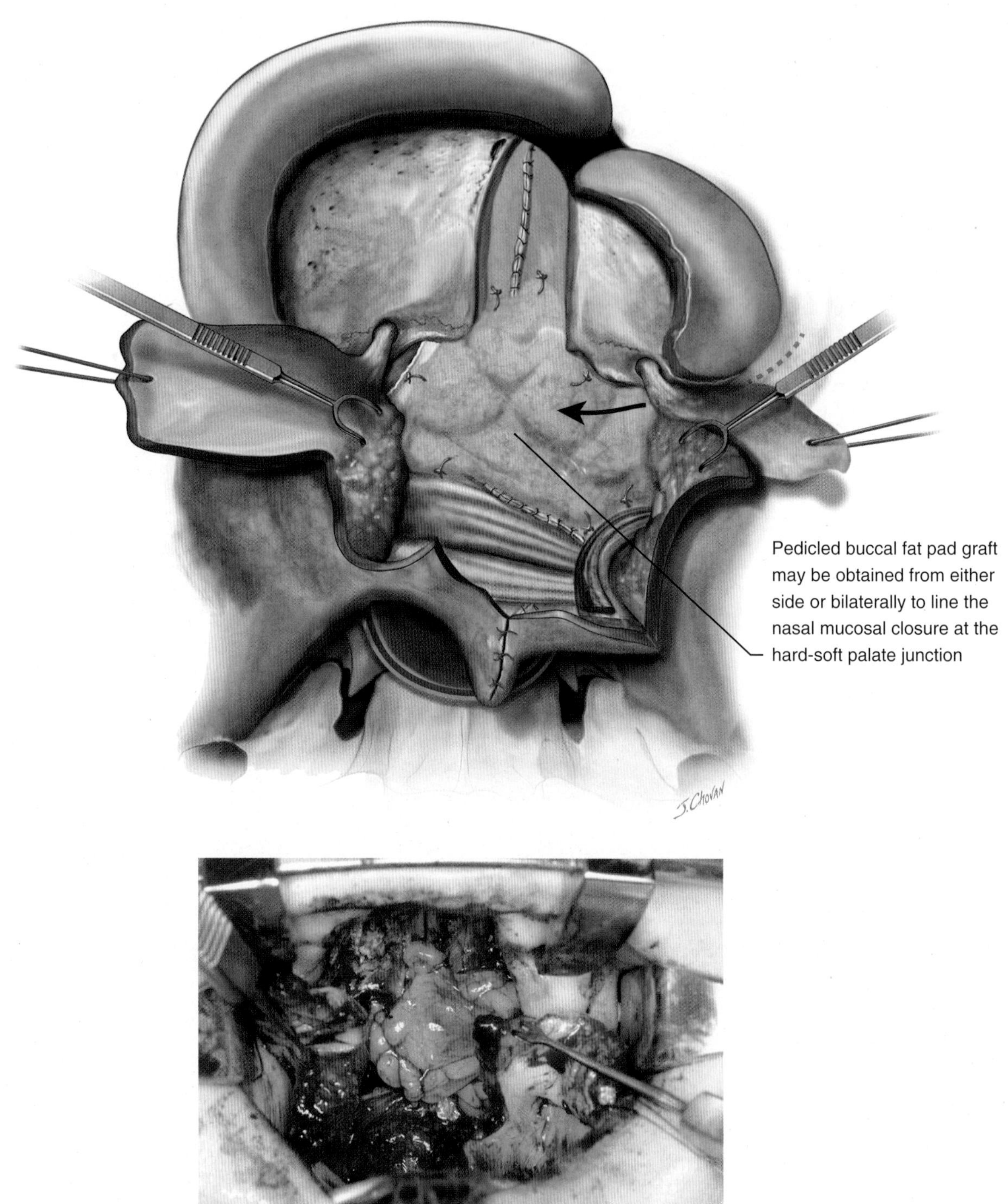
Pedicled buccal fat pad graft may be obtained from either side or bilaterally to line the nasal mucosal closure at the hard-soft palate junction
A
B

Figure 62.8

TECHNIQUE: CLEFT PALATE REPAIR BY DOUBLE-OPPOSING Z-PLASTY—cont'd

any active bleeding and all bleeding is controlled prior to final flap inset. Oral flap tacking sutures are removed. The flap is secured to the anterior alveolus with secure mattress sutures. The lateral wound is reapproximated with interrupted resorbable suture allowing for incomplete closure to relieve midline tension when necessary. Special attention is given to suturing over the buccal fat graft site to contain pedicled fat (Figs. 62.9A and B).

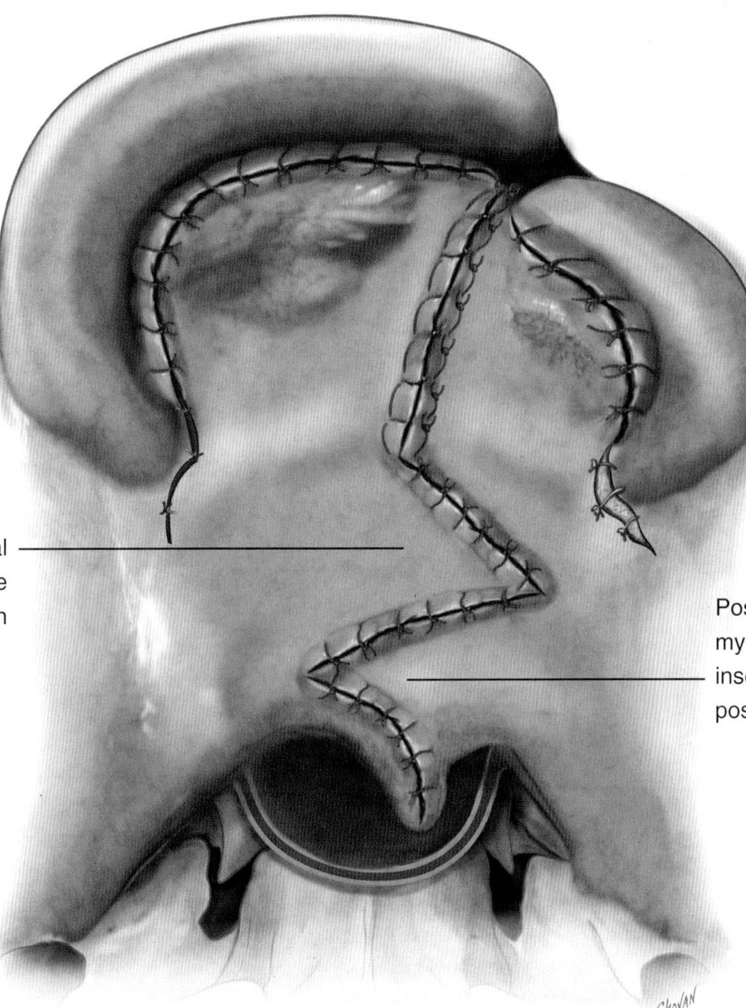
Anteriorly based oral mucosal flap inset anterior to the muscular reconstruction
Posteriorly based oral myomucosal flap inset into a transverse position
J. Chovan
A

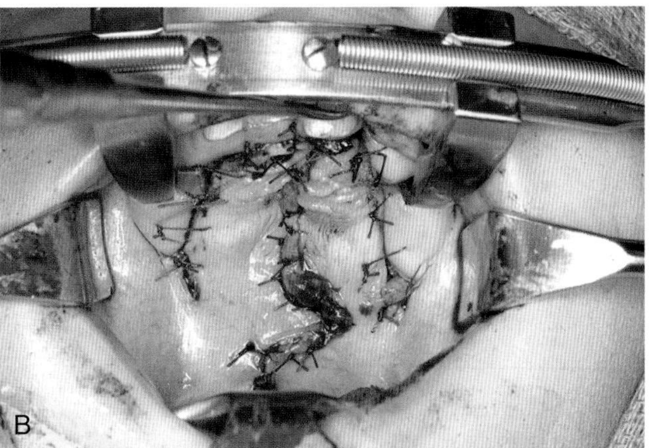
B

Figure 62.9

TECHNIQUE: CLEFT PALATE REPAIR BY DOUBLE-OPPOSING Z-PLASTY—cont'd

STEP 12: Extubation and Recovery

The patient's oropharynx is suctioned clean and a gastric tube passed by the surgical team to decompress the stomach. The patient is returned to the anesthesia team for emergence and extubation. Care is taken not to insert oral or nasal airways unless in an emergency to protect the wounds. Placement of a nasal trumpet may be used as an adjunct during recovery to facilitate airway management in select cases. Monitoring continues under anesthesia supervision in the proper anesthesia recovery unit.

ALTERNATE OR MODIFIED TECHNIQUE

The technique can be modified by eliminating the lateral hard palate releasing incisions when the closure can be completed without undue tension. This is more common when the hard palate cleft is not complete including surgery for Veau I, incomplete Veau II, and submucous clefts, as well as secondary conversion surgery.

The anterior soft palate repair, where the mucosal layers are thinnest and most likely to fistulize, has been managed in variable ways. This can be addressed with no additional reinforcement, with the addition of pedicled buccal fat unilaterally or bilaterally, with the addition of allogeneic dermis, or by layering gelfoam.

Avoidance and Management of Intraoperative Complications

Complications are best avoided with the fundamentals of good surgical technique. Dissection along the hard palate, nasal floor, and medial pterygoid should always be subperiosteal. Special care to promote gentle handling of the mucosal tissues of the soft palate is required. Skin hooks in deeper tissues are often superior to forceps for tissue retraction. Careful control of bleeding using vasoconstrictor, gentle electrocautery, and judicious use of hemostatic agents is prudent. Tears of the soft palate nasal mucosa do not lend themselves to repair and are typically managed by grafting with buccal fat. If there is excessive tension at closure, repeating the maneuvers described in the release of the midpalatal tissues is usually most productive. Closure should always utilize noncutting suture needles to protect delicate mucosal tissues.

Postoperative Considerations

Postoperatively, the patient should be monitored in the inpatient setting with close attention to airway patency, oral intake, and pain control. Level of care will vary depending on each center's experience and specialist availability. Pulse oximetry for the first night is prudent. Pain control is narcotic-sparing using scheduled acetaminophen and nonsteriodal antiinflammatory drugs (NSAIDs) with narcotic only for rescue. Antibiotic coverage postoperatively remains a matter of debate and will vary by center. The child may feed in the immediate postoperative period. If the child still feeds with a bottle, a cleft feeder is preferred. If the child uses a sippy cup, one that does not require suction is needed. No foods harder than stage 2 baby foods are allowed for a total of 3 weeks. Nothing hard is allowed in the mouth for 3 weeks. Sutures are allowed to fall out on their own, and temporary associated halitosis is not unusual.

In the immediate postoperative period, airway embarrassment and bleeding requiring intervention are the most troubling complications, although uncommon. Wound complications including infection, wound breakdown, hanging palatal flaps, or fistula formation appear to be the most commonly reported early complications. Hospital readmission for respiratory concerns or decreased oral intake may occur. In the long term, the need for secondary speech surgery is a significant measure of success. Growth disturbance is expected, although variable.[7–12]

Conclusion

The Furlow double-opposing Z-plasty is a contemporary procedure for cleft palate repair that takes advantage of both intravelar veloplasty for improved muscle positioning as well as palatal lengthening to achieve optimization of speech outcomes with a low rate of complications. Additional benefit may come from tightening of the velopharyngeal port, functional tension of the cleft muscle, and a nonlinear scar. The technique described can be used as a generalized description that leads to predictable success.

References

1. Furlow LT Jr. Cleft palate repair by double opposing Z-plasty. *Plast Reconstr Surg*. 1986;78(6):724–738. https://doi.org/10.1097/00006534-198678060-00002.
2. Randall P, LaRossa D, Solomon M, Cohen M. Experience with the Furlow double-reversing Z-plasty for cleft palate repair. *Plast Reconstr Surg*. 1986;77(4):569–576.
3. Champion R. Some observations on the primary and secondary repair of the cleft palate. *Br J Plast Surg*. 1957;9(4):260–264. https://doi.org/10.1016/s0007-1226(56)80049-0.
4. Schuchardt K. Operationen im Gesicht Teil des Kopfes. in Bier A, Braun H, Kummell H. C. Operationslehre; Vol. 2:605 Johann Ambrosius Barth, Leipzig.
5. Jackson O, Stransky CA, Jawad AF, et al. The Children's Hospital of Philadelphia modification of the Furlow double-opposing Z-palatoplasty: 30-year experience and long-term speech outcomes. *Plast Reconstr Surg*. 2013;132(3):613–622 https://doi.org/10.1097/PRS.0b013e31829ad109.
6. Chen PK, Wu JT, Chen YR, Noordhoff MS. Correction of secondary velopharyngeal insufficiency in cleft palate patients with the Furlow palatoplasty. *Plast Reconstr Surg*. 1994;94(7):933–943.
7. Chim H, Eshraghi Y, Iamphongsai S, Gosain AK. Double-opposing Z-palatoplasty for secondary surgical management of velopharyngeal incompetence in the absence of a primary Furlow palatoplasty. *Cleft Palate Craniofac J*. 2015;52(5):517–524. https://doi.org/10.1597/13-187.
8. Deshpande GS, Campbell A, Jagtap R, et al. Early complications after cleft palate repair: a multivariate statistical analysis of 709 patients. *J Craniofac Surg*. 2014;25(5):1614–1618. https://doi.org/10.1097/SCS.0000000000001113.
9. Schönmeyr B, Wendby L, Campbell A. Surgical complications in 1408 primary cleft palate repairs operated at a single center in Guwahati, Assam, India. *Cleft Palate Craniofac J*. 2016;53(3):278–282. https://doi.org/10.1597/14-206.
10. Mahboubi H, Truong A, Pham NS. Prevalence, demographics, and complications of cleft palate surgery. *Int J Pediatr Otorhinolaryngol*. 2015;79(6):803–807. https://doi.org/10.1016/j.ijporl.2015.02.032.
11. Nguyen C, Hernandez-Boussard T, Davies SM, Bhattacharya J, Khosla RK, Curtin CM. Cleft palate surgery: an evaluation of length of stay, complications, and costs by hospital type. *Cleft Palate Craniofac J*. 2014;51(4):412–419. https://doi.org/10.1597/12-150.
12. Meara JG, Hughes CD, Sanchez K, Catallozzi L, Clark R, Kummer AW. Optimal outcomes reporting (OOR): a new value-based metric for outcome reporting following cleft palate repair [published online ahead of print, 2020 Jun 18]. *Cleft Palate Craniofac J*. 2020. https://doi.org/10.1177/1055665620931708. 1055665620931708.

CHAPTER 63

Cleft Palate Repair—Intravelar Veloplasty

John Francis Caccamese Jr. and Max R. Emmerling

Armamentarium

#15 Blade with #5 and #7 (15.5 cm) scalpel handles
Appropriate sutures (5-0 Vicryl on a TF and TF-4 needle, 4-0 Vicryl)
Beaver (mini) blades #6600, #6700, and #6900 with V. Mueller scalpel handles
Castroviejo needle holders, curved and straight
Colorado-tip dissecting needle cautery
Guthrie double-prong skin hooks
Jeter or Sarot needle holders
Leibinger DeBakey forceps
Local anesthetic with vasoconstrictor
Metzenbaum scissors
Microbipolar cautery
Operating microscope or surgical loupes (minimum 2.5×)
Periosteal elevators and pickups (surgeon's preference)
Potts scissors
Schnidt tonsil forceps
Single-prong skin hook
Stevens scissors

History of the Procedure

Orofacial clefts are the most common congenital craniofacial malformation, with rates as high as 1 in 700 live births in the United States. Among these, cleft palate is seen in about four out of five cases, whether it presents alone or in combination with cleft lip.[1] For the cleft surgeon, cleft palate represents a particularly challenging clinical entity. Management of all cleft-related issues will have a long-term impact on both patients and their families, with implications related to oropharyngeal function, speech development, facial growth, and psychosocial health. The primary goal in any cleft repair should be to establish normal anatomy and function. Depending on the extent of the cleft, repair may involve restoration of anatomical structures in both the hard and soft palate and it is important that these two areas be considered individually. While hard palate repair is largely concerned with closure of the oral-nasal communication and maximizing growth, soft palate repair has been recognized for its importance in the development of normal speech. In particular, greater emphasis has been placed on restoring the anatomy and function of the soft palate musculature, primarily the levator veli palatini muscle. During normal speech, the elevating action of this muscle on the soft palate is responsible for creating an adequate velopharyngeal seal necessary for proper speech resonance. The inability to form this seal, or velopharyngeal dysfunction (VPD), is a potentially debilitating condition affecting between 5% and 40% of patients even after cleft palate repair.[2] These patients often require extensive speech therapy and sometimes one or more additional surgeries to improve or normalize their speech.

Abnormal insertion of the "cleft muscle" was originally highlighted by Veau in 1931.[3] However, it was not until 1969 that the concept of intravelar veloplasty (IVVP) was first described by Kriens.[4] This concept was further advanced with the introduction of the radical IVVP by Sommerlad[5] and Cutting et al.[6] This technique involves a more extensive dissection and mobilization of the levator muscle to facilitate appropriate posterior repositioning. An alternative technique for levator muscle repair and repositioning was proposed by Furlow, with the introduction of the double-opposing Z-plasty, which also serves to lengthen the soft palate.[7] Though there was some evidence that these procedures were associated with superior outcomes in regard to speech, controversy still remained. Much of this debate was likely due to significant variations in surgical technique and inconsistencies in terminology across different studies.[8–11] To better clarify what constitutes an IVVP, Andrades et al. described a classification system used to specify the degree of muscle dissection ranging from minimal to no dissection to radical IVVP (Fig. 63.1).[12] More recently, studies comparing speech outcomes for patients who underwent repair using the radical IVVP technique have demonstrated significantly superior results.[12–14]

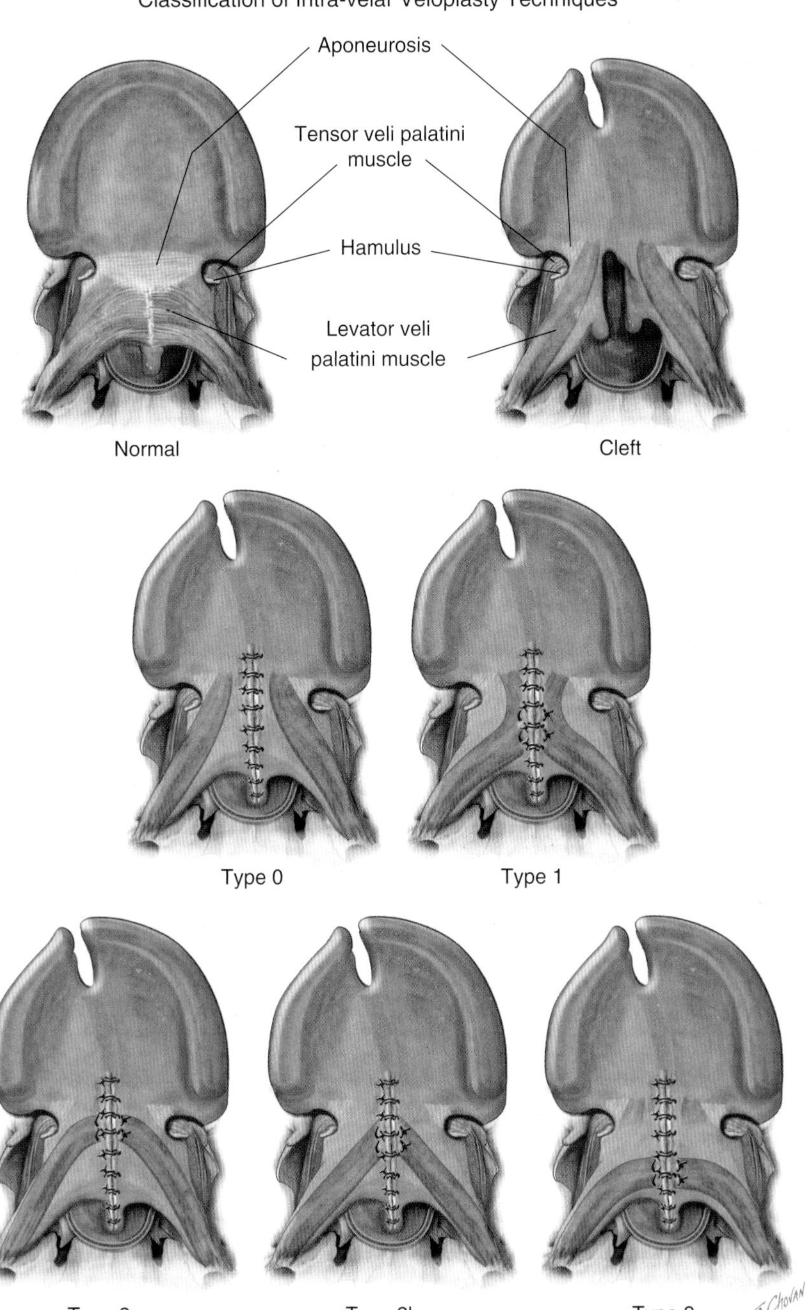

Figure 63.1 Classification of intravelar veloplasty techniques as proposed by Andrades et al. Higher numbers correspond with an increasing degree of dissection and retropositioning of the levator veli palatini muscle.[12] (Redrawn from Andrades P, Espinosa-de-los-Monteros A, Shell DHt, et al. The importance of radical intravelar veloplasty during two-flap palatoplasty. *Plast Reconstr Surg*. Oct 2008;122(4):1121–1130. https://doi.org/10.1097/PRS.0b013e3181845a21)

Indications for Use of the Procedure

The objectives of cleft palate repair should include closure of oral-nasal communication, creation of a dynamic and functional soft palate, minimization of growth impact, and the normal and timely development of speech. When addressing these objectives, it is important to consider the hard and soft palate as functionally separate units that are repaired using different techniques with differences in goals and timing. IVVP is indicated for any cleft palate patient with soft palate involvement resulting in abnormal insertion of the cleft muscle. This includes patients with submucous cleft palate, who may experience VPD in 5% to 10% of cases.[15] Restoration of normal muscle position is an important part of restoring the ability to create an adequate velopharyngeal seal and allow for the development of normal speech resonance. Along those lines, the timing of this procedure is predicated on minimizing interference with speech development while maximizing growth potential.

Most centers recommend repair at between 6 and 18 months of age; however, there remains significant controversy about both the timing and staging of repair. Those who advocate for early repair do so on the basis of improved speech development but may be risking maxillary growth restriction as a result.[16] Similarly, the order of operations regarding staging soft palate and hard palate repair represents a balancing act between these two outcomes. Early soft palate repair with delayed hard palate closure may be associated with favorable growth outcomes but can create problems with speech development.[17,18] For unilateral clefts, Sommerlad recommends single-layer repair of the hard palate using a vomerine flap at the time of lip repair, followed by definitive soft palate repair around 12 months of age with IVVP.[19] This technique facilitates soft palate repair by bringing the soft tissue edges closer together while minimizing growth restrictions due to the lack of intraperiosteal bone deposition associated with a single-layer repair.

IVVP has also been shown to be effective as a secondary surgery for correction of VPD in patients who have undergone previous palatoplasty without repositioning of the velar musculature. IVVP is more physiologic, with a lower incidence of sleep apnea and hyponasality and still leaves open the option for pharyngeal surgery if needed.[20,21] It may be possible to obtain records of the patient's previous surgery to determine the feasibility of palatal re-repair, or certain clinical findings such as anteriorly oriented muscles or a midline concavity in the nasal surface on nasoendoscopy can indicate that an IVVP has not been performed. Palate re-repair with IVVP has been shown to produce significant improvements in speech, including hypernasality and nasal emissions, and may eliminate the need for pharyngeal surgeries, which can be associated with significant morbidity.[21,22]

Limitations and Contraindications

Though timing is ideally determined on the basis of speech development, treatment may be limited by the patient's ability to tolerate surgery and general anesthesia. Compared to clefts involving the lip, cleft palate alone is more likely to present in association with other congenital anomalies or as part of a genetic syndrome.[23–25] Recognition of these associations is important in the assessment and treatment planning for these patients.[23] For patients with comorbidities, particularly those with congenital heart disorders or respiratory illness, it may be appropriate to delay repair until these conditions are optimized.

TECHNIQUE—Intravelar Veloplasty (see Video 63.1)

STEP 1: Setup and Positioning

The patient is intubated with an oral Ring-Adair-Elwyn (RAE) endotracheal tube and positioned supine on the operating room table. The oral cavity is rinsed with chlorhexidine gluconate or other oral prep. A shoulder roll is placed to allow for adequate extension of the neck. The bed may be placed in slight Trendelenburg to help maximize visualization. The patient is draped in a sterile manner. A cleft mouth gag is placed with care taken to avoid trauma to the lips or disruption of the endotracheal tube. Periodic relaxation of the retractor will help to prevent postoperative swelling of the tongue, which may lead to airway compromise. Local anesthesia is administered using 0.5% lidocaine with 1:200,000 epinephrine both as a greater palatine block and infiltration for hemostasis. Sommerlad advocates for the use of an operating microscope for enhanced comfort, superior lighting, and improved visualization of anatomy.[26] The authors use loupe magnification.

STEP 2: Incision and Nasal Mucosa Closure

After allowing sufficient time for the local anesthetic to take effect, a #6700 blade is utilized to create an incision along the cleft margin bilaterally extending from the apex at the anterior aspect of the cleft back to the tip of the uvula, and Potts scissors can be used to complete the uvular incision. A midline incision is carried on to the hard palate so that full-thickness flaps are developed to allow the posterior aspect of the hard palate to be dissected free from the tensor aponeurosis attachment as well as the abnormal insertion of the palatoglossus/pharyngeus and levator muscles. Subperiosteal dissection is then performed on the nasal side of the hard palate as well and carried over laterally toward the pterygoid plates. This is accomplished with the use of the Blair/hockey stick elevator and the angled #6600 Beaver blade (Fig. 63.2). With the nasal mucosa sufficiently released, this layer is then closed using simple interrupted sutures, placing the knots on the nasal side of the closure. This is accomplished using a 5-0 Vicryl suture, either on a TF or TF-4 needle (Fig. 63.3A).

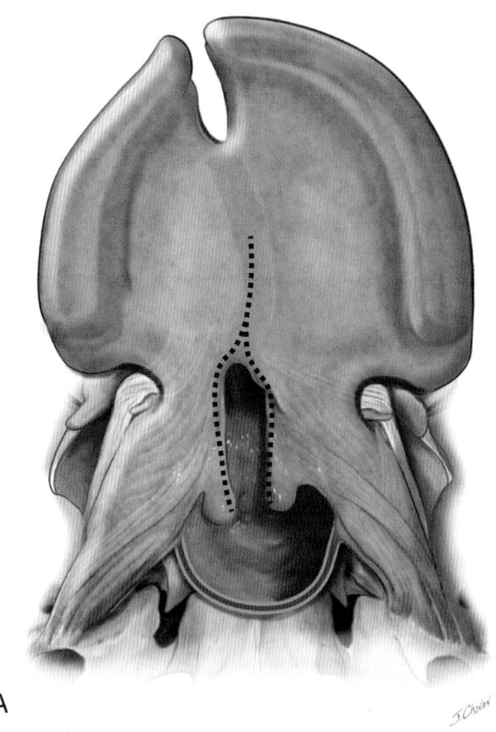

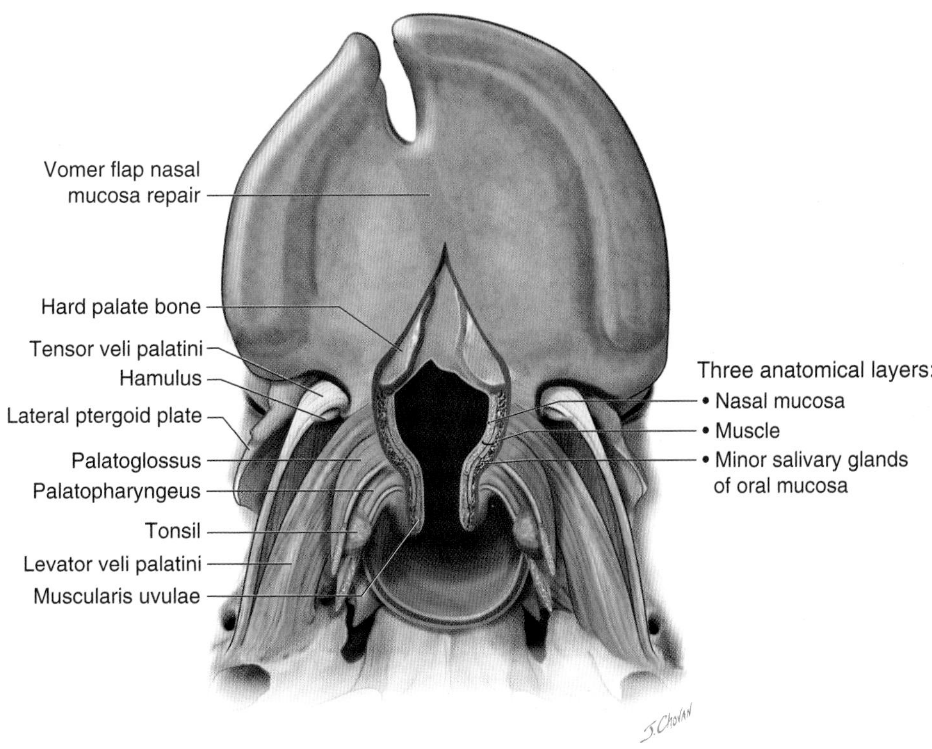

Figure 63.2 **A,** Prior to the administration of local anesthesia, the planned incision is marked along the cleft margin bilaterally, extending from the tip of the uvula forward to the apex at the anterior aspect of the cleft and onto the hard palate. **B,** After incision, full-thickness flaps are developed to allow the posterior aspect of the hard palate to be dissected free from the tensor aponeurosis attachment as well as the abnormal insertion of the palatoglossus/pharyngeus and levator muscles. The three anatomical layers are demonstrated, including the nasal mucosa, muscle, and the minor salivary glands, which distinguish the oral mucosa.

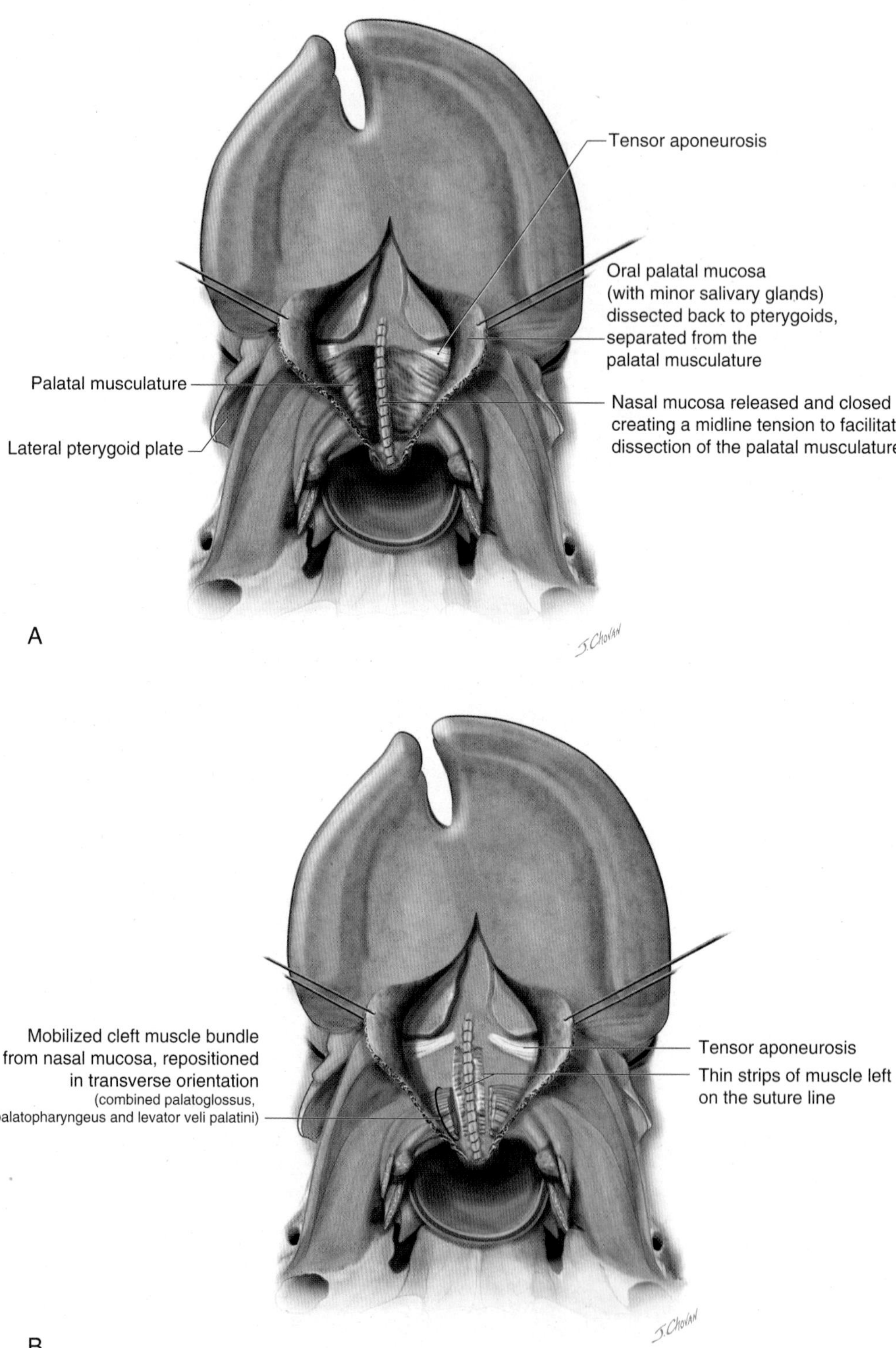

Figure 63.3 **A,** The nasal mucosa is closed at the midline to provide countertension to facilitate dissection of the musculature. Stevens tenotomy scissors are then used to dissect the cleft muscle laterally to the pterygoid plates and develop a plane between the oral mucosa and the muscle. **B,** Using a sharp #6900 Beaver blade, the muscle is then dissected off of the bluish nasal mucosa to allow it to be gently and freely repositioned posteriorly. A small cuff of muscle is left along the suture line of the nasal mucosal to maintain bulk and strength of the closure.

TECHNIQUE—Intravelar Veloplasty—cont'd

STEP 3: Cleft Muscle Dissection and Repositioning

Closure of the nasal mucosa provides midline tension to facilitate dissection of the palatal musculature. Stevens tenotomy scissors are used to separate the oral palatal mucosa, characterized by the presence of minor salivary gland tissue, from the palatoglossus, palatopharyngeus, and levator muscle laterally to the pterygoids and their junction with the tensor aponeurosis. This dissection is carried back toward the origin of the palatoglossus/pharyngeus at the pillars bilaterally (see Fig. 63.3A). With the oral mucosal flaps developed, a retraction suture may be placed through the flap margins bilaterally and held in place using the springs built into the cleft mouth gag. A #6900 Beaver blade is then used to sharply and carefully elevate the palatoglossus/pharyngeus and levator muscle bundle off of the thin bluish nasal mucosa as far back as the origin of the levator muscle as it can be seen emanating from its tunnel to the sphenoid bone. You should appreciate the muscle gliding freely through this tunnel with gentle repositioning tension in a setback motion. Small perforations in the nasal mucosa are not cause for concern and may be placed intentionally to prevent hematoma formation (Fig. 63.3B). Once the muscles are completely mobilized, they are repositioned posteriorly in a transverse orientation and closed in an overlapping fashion at the midline using 4-0 Vicryl horizontal mattressing sutures with the bulk of the muscle everted toward the nasal side. The overlap of the muscles should result in moderate tension across the sling. An additional single interrupted stitch is used to anchor the muscle posteriorly in the desired position, and to the nasal mucosa to prevent forward migration (Fig. 63.4A).

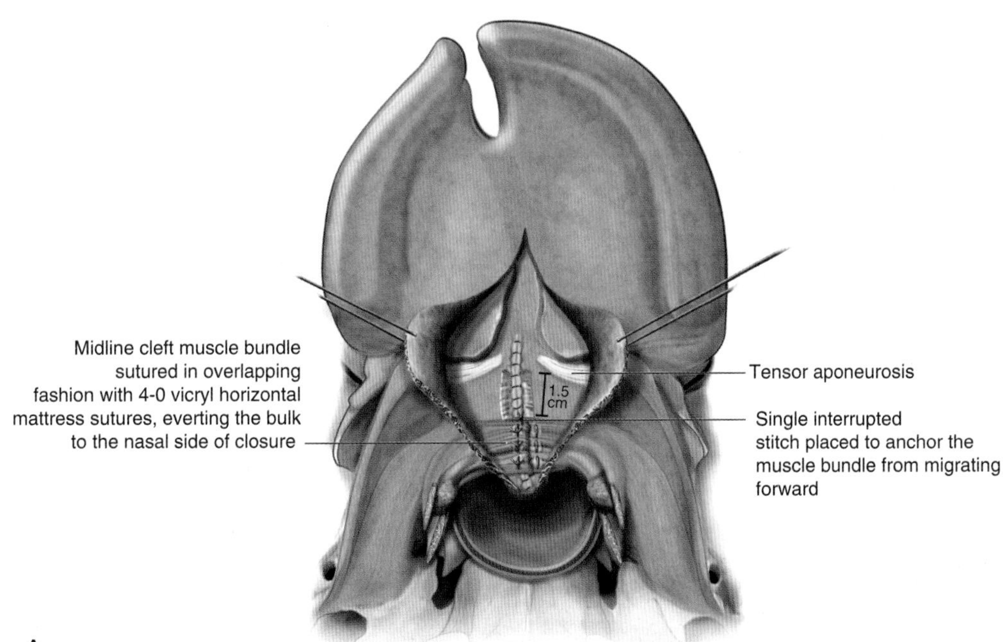

Figure 63.4 A, The muscle bundle is then sutured at the midline with mattress sutures in an overlapping fashion so as to create moderate tension across the sling. The bulk of the muscle should be everted to the nasal side of the closure.

Continued

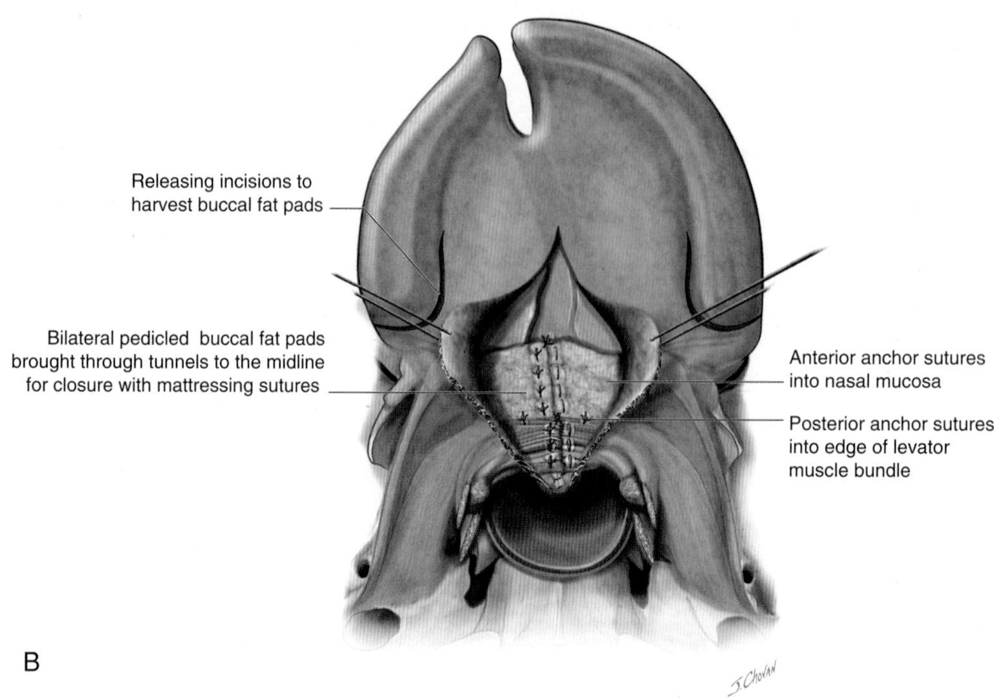

Figure 63.4 B, Buccal fat pad can be harvested bilaterally via releasing incisions along the hard palate and extending around the tuberosity to the vestibule. They are then inset into the wound via a submucosal tunnel to help eliminate dead space after intravelar veloplasty (IVVP).

TECHNIQUE—Intravelar Veloplasty—cont'd

STEP 4: Buccal Fat Pad Advancement

The IVVP leaves little bulk and considerable dead space at the hard palate-soft palate junction. This also happens to be the location of the majority of fistulae post palate repair. In order to mitigate the risk of fistula, as well as to provide tissue to close dead space, we use pedicled buccal fat in many of our repairs. With the IVVP completed, small releasing incisions are created using a #15 blade on either side of the hard palate, extending around the posterior of the maxillary alveolus with a small vestibular extension. A Schnidt tonsillar forceps is then used to access and release the buccal fat pads bilaterally through the vestibular incision. Tunnels are created under the palatal flaps to allow the fat pads to be brought into the midline of the closure site passively with minimal dissection. The buccal fat pads are joined in the midline using mattressing sutures and then anchored to both the anterior nasal mucosa and the leading edge of the levator muscle bundle posteriorly (Fig. 63.4B). The releasing incisions, along with skeletonization of the greater palatine neurovascular bundle, can also provide more laxity for the oral layer closure.

STEP 5: Z-Plasty and Mucosal Closure

Before final closure, the wound is irrigated with saline and hemostasis is confirmed. Based on the length of the palate, a Z-plasty may be incorporated into the oral mucosal closure to help create additional palate length.[13,14] Anterior and posterior triangular flaps are marked and incised through the mucosal layer. These flaps are then transposed into their final position and the mucosa is closed primarily, again, using 5-0 Vicryl (Fig. 63.5). The authors prefer to use locking vertical mattress sutures or looped mattress sutures, which have been shown to alleviate tension on the individual suture strands, leading to less tissue damage and better wound apposition (Fig. 63.6).[27] The vestibular and releasing incisions created for buccal fat pad advancement are closed primarily with simple interrupted sutures when possible. If not, the buccal fat will eventually mucosalize. Once closure is completed, the cleft mouth gag is removed and the patient is allowed to emerge from anesthesia prior to being extubated in the operating room. Patients will typically stay in the hospital for at least one night to monitor for airway concerns and issues with feeding. Arm splints are not utilized postoperatively as there is no strong evidence for their effectiveness.[28] Patients are started on a clear liquid diet for one night and then advance to a strict full liquid diet for 2 weeks until follow-up. Feeding is allowed through the use of the patient's preferred specialized cleft nipple and nonnutritive sucking is discouraged.

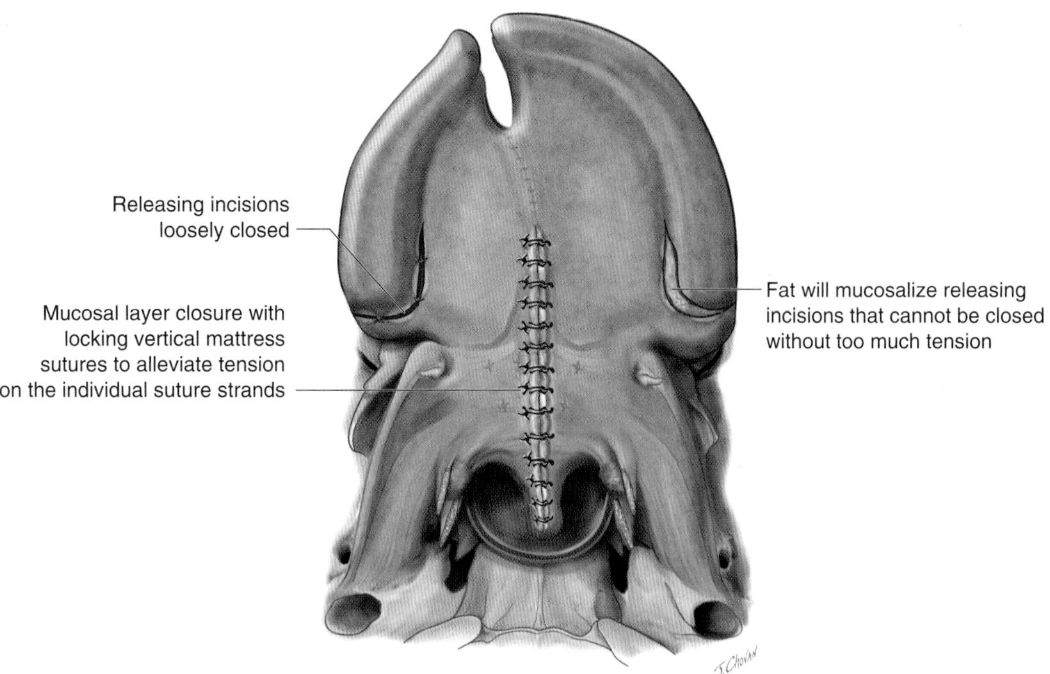

Figure 63.5 The mucosa is closed primarily at the midline utilizing locking vertical mattress sutures. If closure of the releasing incisions utilized for buccal fat pad harvest is not possible, these would heal via the mucosalization of the fat.

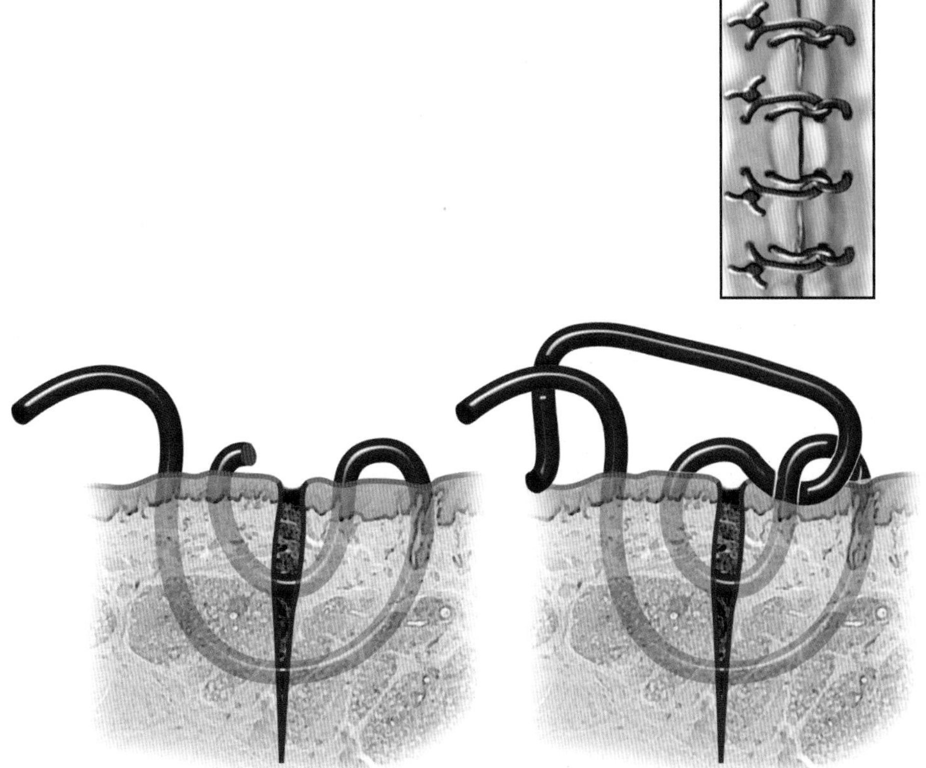

Figure 63.6 Illustration from Gault et al. that depicts the difference in technique between the nonloop and loop or locking vertical mattress suture. Utilization of this technique helps alleviate tension on the individual suture strands, leading to less tissue damage and better wound apposition.[27] (Redrawn from Gault DT, Brain A, Sommerlad BC, Ferguson DJP. Loop mattress suture. *BJS*. 1987;74(9):820–821. https://doi.org/10.1002/bjs.1800740922)

ALTERNATIVE TECHNIQUE: Woo Component Separation Palatoplasty

Woo et al. describe a variation in technique that involves the careful dissection and separation of the cleft muscle of Veau into its muscular subunits: tensor veli palatini, levator veli palatini, and the combined unit of the palatopharyngeus and palatoglossus muscles. Each muscular component must be dissected down to its origin in order to allow for adequate separation.[13] Following the pattern of the Andrades classification system, they designate their technique as a type IV IVVP. By performing this component separation, Woo believes that they can achieve maximal overlap and tightening of the levator muscle, resulting in significant improvements in speech outcomes when compared to other forms of IVVP.[14] The use of a Z-plasty in the closure of the oral mucosa is meant to position the oral mucosal incision away from the nasal mucosal incision in order to help prevent fistula formation.

Avoidance and Management of Intraoperative Complications

Potential intraoperative complications include bleeding, mucosal perforation, or dislodgment of the endotracheal tube. Most of these can be avoided with careful technique and special attention paid to inserting and removing the cleft mouth gag. As previously stated, small nasal mucosa perforations need not be repaired. Larger perforations of the nasal or oral mucosa can be primarily repaired at the time of surgery.

Postoperative Complications

Early postoperative complications may include bleeding and swelling, which may lead to airway obstruction. Patients should be carefully monitored in the hospital with continuous pulse oximetry over the first 24 hours. Periodic relaxation of the cleft mouth gag during the surgical procedure will help to reduce the risk of significant postoperative tongue swelling. Perioperative steroid administration over the first 24 hours has been shown to be effective in reducing the development of both airway distress and fever.[29] Infection is uncommon after surgery and patients do not require the use of extended perioperative antibiotics for surgical prophylaxis.

Fistula formation is difficult to predict and control for and may occur in 4.9% to 8.6% of patients, while some studies report an even higher rate of occurrence.[30,31] They may form as a result of wound breakdown secondary to excess tension, hematoma formation, trauma, or even infection. There is no convincing evidence that one technique of IVVP is superior to another; however, the severity of the cleft does appear to have a significant impact on fistula formation. Two systematic reviews demonstrated a significantly decreased incidence of fistula formation in patients with cleft palate alone (Veau I/II) compared to patients with cleft lip and palate (Veau III/IV).[30,31] A retrospective review of patients treated by IVVP showed a significantly higher rate of fistula formation in Veau II clefts and wide clefts.[32] The rate of fistula formation can potentially be reduced with adherence to careful diet restrictions and avoiding tension in the repair. The authors recommend a full liquid diet for at least 2 weeks with exclusive use of a specialized cleft nipple. Straws, spoons, and nonnutritive sucking should be avoided.

As previously discussed, VPD is a common long-term complication for many cleft palate patients. Though the use of IVVP has been shown to improve speech outcomes, a small percentage of these patients will go on to have some measure of VPD. Syndromic patients and patients with wider or more severe clefts involving the lip and palate may be at higher risk.[33] Speech therapy remains the mainstay of treatment for many patients; however, patients with dysfunction not amenable to therapy may require secondary surgeries with a sphincter pharyngoplasty or pharyngeal flap.

References

1. Mai CT, Cassell CH, Meyer RE, et al. Birth defects data from population-based birth defects surveillance programs in the United States, 2007 to 2011: highlighting orofacial clefts. *Birth Defects Res A Clin Mol Teratol.* 2014;100(11):895–904. https://doi.org/10.1002/bdra.23329.
2. Sell D, Grunwell P, Mildinhall S, et al. Cleft lip and palate care in the United Kingdom—the clinical Standards Advisory Group (CSAG) study. Part 3: speech outcomes. *Cleft Palate Craniofac J.* 2001;38(1):30–37. https://doi.org/10.1597/1545-1569_2001_038_0030_clapci_2.0.co_2.
3. Division palatine: anatomie—chirurgie phonétique. By Victor Veau, Chirurgien de l'Hôpital des Enfants assistés, with the collaboration of Mme. S. Borel. Large 8vo. Pp. 568 + viii, with 786 illustrations. 1931. Paris: Masson et Cie. Fr. 140. BJS (British Journal of Surgery). 1932/10/01 1932;20(78):355–355. doi:10.1002/bjs.1800207829
4. Kriens OB. An anatomical approach to veloplasty. *Plast Reconstr Surg.* 1969;43(1):29–41. https://doi.org/10.1097/00006534-196901000-00006.
5. Sommerlad BC. A technique for cleft palate repair. *Plast Reconstr Surg.* 2003;112(6):1542–1548. https://doi.org/10.1097/01.prs.0000085599.84458.d2.
6. Cutting CB, Rosenbaum J, Rovati L. The technique of muscle repair in the cleft soft palate. Article. *Operat Tech Plast Reconstr Surg.* 1995;2(4):215–222. https://doi.org/10.1016/S1071-0949(06)80035-1.
7. Furlow LT Jr. Cleft palate repair by double opposing Z-plasty. *Plast Reconstr Surg.* 1986;78(6):724–738. https://doi.org/10.1097/00006534-198678060-00002.
8. Dreyer TM, Trier WC. A comparison of palatoplasty techniques. *Cleft Palate J.* 1984;21(4):251–253.
9. Marsh JL, Grames LM, Holtman B. Intravelar veloplasty: a prospective study. *Cleft Palate J.* 1989;26(1):46–50.
10. Timbang MR, Gharb BB, Rampazzo A, Papay F, Zins J, Doumit G. A systematic review comparing Furlow double-opposing Z-plasty and straight-line intravelar veloplasty

methods of cleft palate repair. *Plast Reconstr Surg*. 2014;134(5):1014–1022. https://doi.org/10.1097/prs.0000000000000637.

11. Williams WN, Seagle MB, Pegoraro-Krook MI, et al. Prospective clinical trial comparing outcome measures between Furlow and von Langenbeck Palatoplasties for UCLP. *Ann Plast Surg*. 2011;66(2):154–163. https://doi.org/10.1097/SAP.0b013e3181d60763.
12. Andrades P, Espinosa-de-los-Monteros A, Shell DH, et al. The importance of radical intravelar veloplasty during two-flap palatoplasty. *Plast Reconstr Surg*. 2008;122(4):1121–1130. https://doi.org/10.1097/PRS.0b013e3181845a21.
13. Woo AS, Skolnick GB, Sachanandani NS, Grames LM. Evaluation of two palate repair techniques for the surgical management of velopharyngeal insufficiency. *Plast Reconstr Surg*. 2014;134(4):588e–596e. https://doi.org/10.1097/prs.0000000000000506.
14. Nguyen DC, Patel KB, Skolnick GB, et al. Progressive tightening of the levator veli palatini muscle improves velopharyngeal dysfunction in early outcomes of primary palatoplasty. *Plast Reconstr Surg*. 2015;136(1):131–141. https://doi.org/10.1097/prs.0000000000001323.
15. Sullivan SR, Vasudavan S, Marrinan EM, Mulliken JB. Submucous cleft palate and velopharyngeal insufficiency: comparison of speech outcomes using three operative techniques by one surgeon. *Cleft Palate Craniofac J*. 2011;48(5):561–570. https://doi.org/10.1597/09-127.
16. Ysunza A, Pamplona MC, Mendoza M, García-Velasco M, Aguilar MP, Guerrero ME. Speech outcome and maxillary growth in patients with unilateral complete cleft lip/palate operated on at 6 versus 12 months of age. *Plast Reconstr Surg*. 1998;102(3):675–679.
17. Nollet PJPM, Katsaros C, van't Hof MA, Semb G, Shaw WC, Kuijpers-Jagtman AM. Treatment outcome after two-stage palatal closure in unilateral cleft lip and palate: a comparison with Eurocleft. *Cleft Palate Craniofac J*. 2005;42(5):512–516.
18. Mølsted K, Brattström V, Prahl-Andersen B, Shaw WC, Semb G. The Eurocleft Study: intercenter study of treatment outcome in patients with complete cleft lip and palate. Part 3: dental arch relationships. *Cleft Palate Craniofac J*. 2005;42(1):78–82. https://doi.org/10.1597/02-119.3.1.
19. Sommerlad BC. Surgery of the cleft lip and nose—the GOStA approach. *B-ENT*. 2006;2(suppl 4):29–31.
20. Mchendale FV, Lane R, Laverty A, Dinwiddie R, Sommerlad BC. Effect of palate re-repairs and Hynes pharyngoplasties on pediatric airways: an analysis of preoperative and postoperative cardiorespiratory sleep studies. *Cleft Palate Craniofac J*. 2013;50(3):257.
21. Sommerlad BC, Mehendale FV, Birch MJ, Sell D, Hattee C, Harland K. Palate re-repair revisited. *Cleft Palate Craniofac J*. 2002;39(3):295–307. https://doi.org/10.1597/1545-1569_2002_039_0295_prrr_2.0.co_2.
22. Elsherbiny A, Amerson M, Sconyers L, Grant JH 3rd. Outcome of palate re-repair with radical repositioning of the levator muscle sling as a first-line strategy in postpalatoplasty velopharyngeal incompetence management protocol. *Plast Reconstr Surg*. 2018;141(4):984–991. https://doi.org/10.1097/PRS.0000000000004236.
23. Maarse W, Rozendaal AM, Pajkrt E, Vermeij-Keers C, Mink van der Molen AB, van den Boogaard MJ. A systematic review of associated structural and chromosomal defects in oral clefts: when is prenatal genetic analysis indicated? *J Med Genet*. 2012;49(8):490–498. https://doi.org/10.1136/jmedgenet-2012-101013.
24. Johnson CY, Honein MA, Hobbs CA, Rasmussen SA. Prenatal diagnosis of orofacial clefts, National birth defects prevention study. 1998–2004 *Prenat Diagn*. 2009;29(9):833–839. https://doi.org/10.1002/pd.2293.
25. Dixon MJ, Marazita ML, Beaty TH, Murray JC. Cleft lip and palate: synthesizing genetic and environmental influences. *Nat Rev Genet*. 2011;12(3):167–178. https://doi.org/10.1038/nrg2933.
26. Sommerlad BC. The use of the operating microscope for cleft palate repair and pharyngoplasty. *Plast Reconstr Surg*. 2003;112(6):1540–1541. https://doi.org/10.1097/01.prs.0000085598.26409.e3.
27. Gault DT, Brain A, Sommerlad BC, Ferguson DJP. Loop mattress suture. *BJS*. 1987/09/01 1987;74(9):820–821. https:// doi.org10.1002/bjs.1800740922
28. Jigjinni V, Kangesu T, Sommerlad BC. Do babies require arm splints after cleft palate repair? *Br J Plast Surg*. 1993;46(8):681–685. https://doi.org/10.1016/0007-1226(93)90200-U.
29. Senders CW, Di Mauro SM, Brodie HA, Emery BE, Sykes JM. The efficacy of perioperative steroid therapy in pediatric primary palatoplasty. *Cleft Palate Craniofac J*. 1999;36(4):340–344.
30. Hardwicke JT, Landini G, Richard BM. Fistula incidence after primary cleft palate repair: a systematic review of the literature. *Plast Reconstr Surg*. 2014;134(4):618e–627e. https://doi.org/10.1097/prs.0000000000000548.
31. Bykowski MR, Naran S, Winger DG, Losee JE. The rate of oronasal fistula following primary cleft palate surgery: a meta-analysis. *Cleft Palate Craniofac J*. 2015;52(4):e81–e87. https://doi.org/10.1597/14-127.
32. Yi CR, Kang MK, Oh TS. Analysis of the intrinsic predictors of oronasal fistula in primary cleft palate repair using intravelar veloplasty. *Cleft Palate Craniofac J*. 2020;57(8):1024–1031. https://doi.org/10.1177/1055665620915056.
33. Mahoney M-H, Swan MC, Fisher DM. Prospective analysis of presurgical risk factors for outcomes in primary palatoplasty. *Plast Reconstr Surg*. 2013;132(1):165–171. https://doi.org/10.1097/PRS.0b013e3182910acb.

CHAPTER 64

Techniques in Bone Grafting the Cleft Maxilla and Palate

Renie Daniel, Caitlin B. L. Magraw, and Timothy A. Turvey

Armamentarium

#15 Blade, scalpel handle
10-cc Syringe for bone graft transfer
Adson or Gerald forceps with teeth
Appropriate sutures
Cancellous bone, cortical strut
Cheek retractors
Iris scissors
Local anesthetic with constrictor
Metzenbaum scissors
Needle drivers (conventional and Castroviejo)
Periosteal elevator
Suture scissors
Tongue retractor
Woodson elevator

History of the Procedure

Bone grafting of the cleft maxilla was first described in 1901 by von Eiselsberg.[1–3] However, the technique did not gain popularity until the 1950s when Auxhausen challenged the maxillofacial surgical community by stating that obtaining bony continuity between the premaxilla and lateral segments was the final challenge facing cleft surgeons.[4] Patients who had not undergone bone grafting experienced oronasal fistulas recalcitrant to soft tissue closure, periodontal deterioration of teeth adjacent to the cleft, persistent stigmata of the cleft lip and palate attributable to insufficient bony support for the lip and nasal base, and challenging prosthetic rehabilitation that was prone to failure. Early responses to Auxhausen's challenge focused on primary bone grafting as described by Schmid.[4,5] As experience with the technique grew, reports emerged attributing significant adverse effects on midfacial growth. While a few centers have continued to perform bone grafting in infants, most centers worldwide have abandoned the procedure.[6–11]

Skoog introduced gingivoperiosteoplasty in the mid-1960s and demonstrated success at forming a bone bridge across the cleft towards the nasal side with soft tissue reconstruction only.[12] Presurgical orthopedic devices, ranging from the pin-retained Latham appliance to soft tissue-borne nasoalveolar molding appliances, were developed in an effort to align cleft segments so that gingivoperiosteoplasty could be performed with less subperiosteal dissection and presumably fewer negative effects on growth. Unfortunately, even when successful in creating bone, gingivoperiosteoplasty provides insufficient support for erupting dentition in the majority of patients. Consequently, additional grafting procedures are frequently required and the specter of negative effects on growth remains.[11–14]

In the 1970s Boyne and Sands[15,16] introduced secondary bone grafting or grafting during the mixed dentition. In actuality, what Boyne described was a primary attempt of placing a bone graft within the first decade of life but not within the first 18 months. He was highly aware of the anti-bone graft sentiment of the 1970s, and to distance his technique from the primary bone graft label, he called it secondary. The fact of the matter is that the concept of a secondary bone graft is one that is conducted after the first 5 to 6 years of life.[15–16] Their proposal was based on the concept that maxillary growth was 80% completed by 8 years of age and therefore, interventions after that time would lead to minimal growth disturbance but still provide the benefits touted by advocates of primary grafting. Because the goals of maxillary reconstruction are most comprehensively and predictably met with this technique, bone graft reconstruction at a developmentally appropriate time during the mixed dentition remains the procedure of choice in most centers.[7,17]

The best results are reported to occur when grafts are placed during the mixed dentition and before eruption of teeth adjacent to the cleft, with the success rate greater than 90% when this timing is used.[18,19] Initially, survival of the canine was the primary dental focus after grafting. Now, however, optimal timing is based on evaluation of all salvageable permanent teeth adjacent to the cleft, including not only the canine but also the lateral and central incisors.[20] Grafting is ideally performed when one-half to two-thirds of the root development is complete for the tooth in question. This degree of root formation permits eruption of the tooth through the graft in a timely manner, stimulating the graft and enhancing success. In addition, this should allow grafting to precede entry of the crown into the cleft because any graft placed adjacent to teeth with periodontal defects will always resorb to the level of the defect, compromising the final result.[21]

Despite the description of many bone sources for secondary bone grating of the cleft maxilla, including calvarium, mandibular symphysis, costochondral rib, tibia, allogeneic bone, and recombinant human bone morphogenetic protein-2 (rhBMP-2), cancellous bone from the ilium is the gold standard.[16,22,23]

Nomenclature

The cleft literature is replete with nomenclature that is layman-oriented and occasionally derogatory. For instance, "hare lip" was a slang term to describe the cleft lip, and the term was commonly used in the early literature. The terminology used to describe the timing of bone grafting is also prevalent. The terms primary, secondary, and tertiary in relation to bone grafts have developed in the cleft literature over the past 65 years to designate the timing in which the procedure takes place. Although Schmid described his technique as primary, he conducted it within the first 18 months of life. Indeed, it was a primary attempt at placing a graft. Because of the adverse growth effects of primary bone grafting, Boyne timed his surgery to occur between ages 8 and 12 to accommodate the dental development of the cuspid. To distinguish his technique from that of Schmid, Boyne called his technique "secondary." In actuality, it was a primary attempt to place the graft at a delayed age. A 2018 literature review by Kaura et al. highlights the confusion surrounding optimal timing of bone grafting as some practitioners rely on chronologic age, rather than dental development, to dictate the patient's readiness for surgery.[24] Alternatively, other centers describe the nomenclature as follows: primary bone grafting is that which has been done after lip repair but before palate repair, secondary bone grafting is that which takes place during the mixed dentition stage, and tertiary bone grafting occurs after the development of the permanent dentition. What confounds the terminology even further is that in typical surgical vernacular "primary" relates to the first attempt of the procedure, "secondary" relates to the second attempt, and "tertiary" relates to the third attempt. The authors prefer the use of the term "delayed bone grafting."

Another nomenclature controversy is related to bone graft reconstruction of the cleft maxilla and palate, referred to as alveolar bone grafting. Anatomically, all cleft lip and palate defects extend to the nasal floor, not just the alveolus. This is true even in cases of an incomplete cleft lip, and the cleft is always wider on the nasal side compared to the oral side. Although Boyne described his procedure as alveolar grafting, he recognized the importance of conducting the dissection to the level of the nasal floor. He also recognized the aesthetic benefit of grafting the entire cleft defect, not just the alveolus. When the alveolus only is grafted, the aesthetic benefit of enhancing lip and nasal symmetry is overlooked. The authors prefer the use of the term "bone graft reconstruction of the cleft maxilla and palate" rather than the term "alveolar bone grafting," which understates the procedure and is as inappropriate as the use of the term "hare lip."

Indications for the Use of the Procedure

Bone graft reconstruction of the cleft maxilla is a critical component of the staged reconstructive approach of patients with cleft lip and palate and serves multiple purposes.[15,19,20,25] First, it provides bone for the eruption of the permanent dentition as well as periodontal support and adequate attached tissue for teeth adjacent to the cleft defect. This is important for the long-term maintenance of the permanent dentition. Second, it allows for closure of the remaining oronasal fistula. Small anterior oronasal fistulas contribute to nasal regurgitation and may even contribute to altered speech. Furthermore, closure can improve upper respiratory tract hygiene. Third, bone grafting provides improved skeletal support of the nasal alar base and upper lip. Bony augmentation of the hypoplastic and dysmorphic maxilla is important for restoring the foundation and improving the aesthetic outcome of soft tissue cleft revision procedures in the future. Last, restoration of the bony continuity of the arch allows for orthodontic care and alignment as well as stabilization of the premaxilla in bilateral cleft cases.

Bone grafting that occurs before or at the time of lip repair has fallen out of favor, given the well-documented negative effects on facial growth and graft loss. Many of the patients who undergo primary bone grafting require additional grafting in the future. The majority of cleft centers follow delayed bone grafting protocols during the mixed dentition stage, whereby the periodontal health and development of the permanent dentition are the driving factors in the timing of surgery. If grafting is performed after the permanent canine on the affected side has fully erupted, the success rate is lower.[18] Consideration should be given to earlier grafting if there is evidence of viable permanent lateral incisors within the cleft site. Optimal timing of bone grafting takes into account the extent of root formation of the permanent dentition. Generally, grafting commences when the root of the permanent tooth to be preserved is one-half to two-thirds complete. Eruption of the permanent dentition through the graft site is critical to graft maturation. When determining the timing of the grafting, it is important to remember that any bone graft placed along the enamel or cemental surface of adjacent teeth will be lost to the level of existing bone. Interpositioned bone graft success is dependent on the health of the bone on either side of the defect. Bone grafts cannot attach to enamel or exposed cementum.

Many sources of autogenous donor bone have been described, including the ilium, which is considered the gold standard, plus calvarium, mandibular symphysis, costochondral rib, and tibia. There has been increasing interest in using rhBMP-2 as an alternative to autogenous bone, given its osteoinductive capacity. The main advantage of using rhBMP-2 is that it does not require a donor site and reduces surgical time. Use of rhBMP-2 requires a carrier sponge, and some surgeons prefer to mix it with allograft. A meta-analysis by Uribe et al. (2019) found promising results from the use of rhBMP-2 in bone volume formation; however, the authors recognized the low quality of evidence and risk of bias in the studies that met the inclusion criteria.[26] Controlled clinical trials are required to determine if rhBMP-2 or autogenous donor bone has better long-term outcomes. The authors prefer to use fresh autogenous anterior iliac crest because of its predictability with tooth eruption and orthodontic movement and known long-term success, especially with aesthetic outcome and contour. In the authors' experience, there is little morbidity with bone graft harvest in most children.

Preoperative Evaluation and Orthodontic Treatment

Thorough interdisciplinary evaluation of the patient must be undertaken by the cleft team, including the pediatric craniomaxillofacial surgeon, orthodontist, and pediatric dentist, prior to surgery. The surgeon must note the results of the lip and palate repairs, including the presence of residual palatal fistulas; the health of the dentition and periodontium; the presence of permanent, primary, and supernumerary teeth; arch form and length of the maxilla; the presence of traumatic occlusal contacts; and the degree of transverse dental arch discrepancy. In the case of the bilateral cleft, the position and stability of the premaxilla must also be evaluated.[27]

Almost all cleft patients will have transverse maxillary discrepancy with collapse of the alveolar segments given the lack of bony continuity of the maxilla and the effect of lip and palate scars. The decision to move forward with maxillary expansion before or after bone grafting varies by center and patient. Collapsed alveolar segments may limit surgical access to the oronasal fistula and residual palatal fistula if present. If surgical access is determined to be inadequate, the authors request a degree of maxillary expansion preoperatively. Ideally, the amount of expansion should be minimal to avoid an overly wide bony defect. Overexpansion requires additional grafting material and results in tension across the soft tissue closure over the graft, increasing the possibility of dehiscence and graft loss. During phase I orthodontic treatment, teeth adjacent to the cleft should not be moved or rotated into the defect as this creates periodontal defects recalcitrant to grafting.

In addition to the above, the orthodontist should remove traumatic occlusal contacts so that micromovement within the graft is minimized since this may lead to graft failure. This is most pronounced in the case of the bilateral cleft where the premaxilla is mobile and often traumatically occluding on the mandibular dentition. Options to eliminate micromovement include orthodontic movement of prematurely occluding teeth, fabrication of a maxillary stent to stabilize the premaxilla, and composite build-ups on posterior teeth to remove traumatic occlusion on the premaxillary segment. The surgeon should also coordinate with the orthodontist and pediatric dentist to determine which impacted supernumerary and/or dysmorphic teeth will need to be removed at the time of grafting. Supernumerary teeth that are already erupted may also require removal if their presence compromises soft tissue closure.[28]

Limitations and Contraindications

There are few absolute or relative contraindications to bone graft reconstruction of the cleft maxilla. If the patient is determined not to be a candidate to undergo general anesthesia for any reason, this would be an absolute contraindication. Immunocompromised status or a condition that impairs wound healing is a relative contraindication. In addition, smoking is a contraindication and tobacco cessation should be encouraged preoperatively. This is especially important since bone grafting the adult patient with permanent dentition is already associated with a lower success rate than during the mixed dentition stage.

TECHNIQUE: Bone Grafting of the Cleft Maxilla and Palate

The patient's airway is secured with an oral Ring-Adair-Elwin tube secured in the midline or nasoendotracheal intubation on the noncleft side. Antibiotics are administered per preoperative protocol, and intravenous steroids are also recommended. Local anesthetic with 1:100,000 epinephrine is used to infiltrate the surgical field. For the technical performance of the appropriate autogenous bone graft, see relevant chapters on mandibular, tibial, calvarial, costochondral rib, and iliac crest bone harvesting. The authors prefer the anterior iliac crest bone graft harvest for secondary reconstruction of the cleft maxilla in the mixed dentition.

Continued

TECHNIQUE: Bone Grafting of the Cleft Maxilla and Palate—*cont'd*

STEP 1: Incision

With a #15 blade, an incision is made along the cleft margin separating the attached gingival tissues from the mucosa of the cleft region. This incision is continued away from the cleft in a sulcular manner around the immediately adjacent teeth. The incision along the vertical cleft margin is made through the mucosa and periosteum medially and laterally but shallower (partial thickness) superiorly where there is no bone between the oral and nasal mucosal layers. The incision is continued palatally along the cleft margin with care taken so that the incision allows for adequate tissue to close the nasal layer (Fig. 64.1A and B).

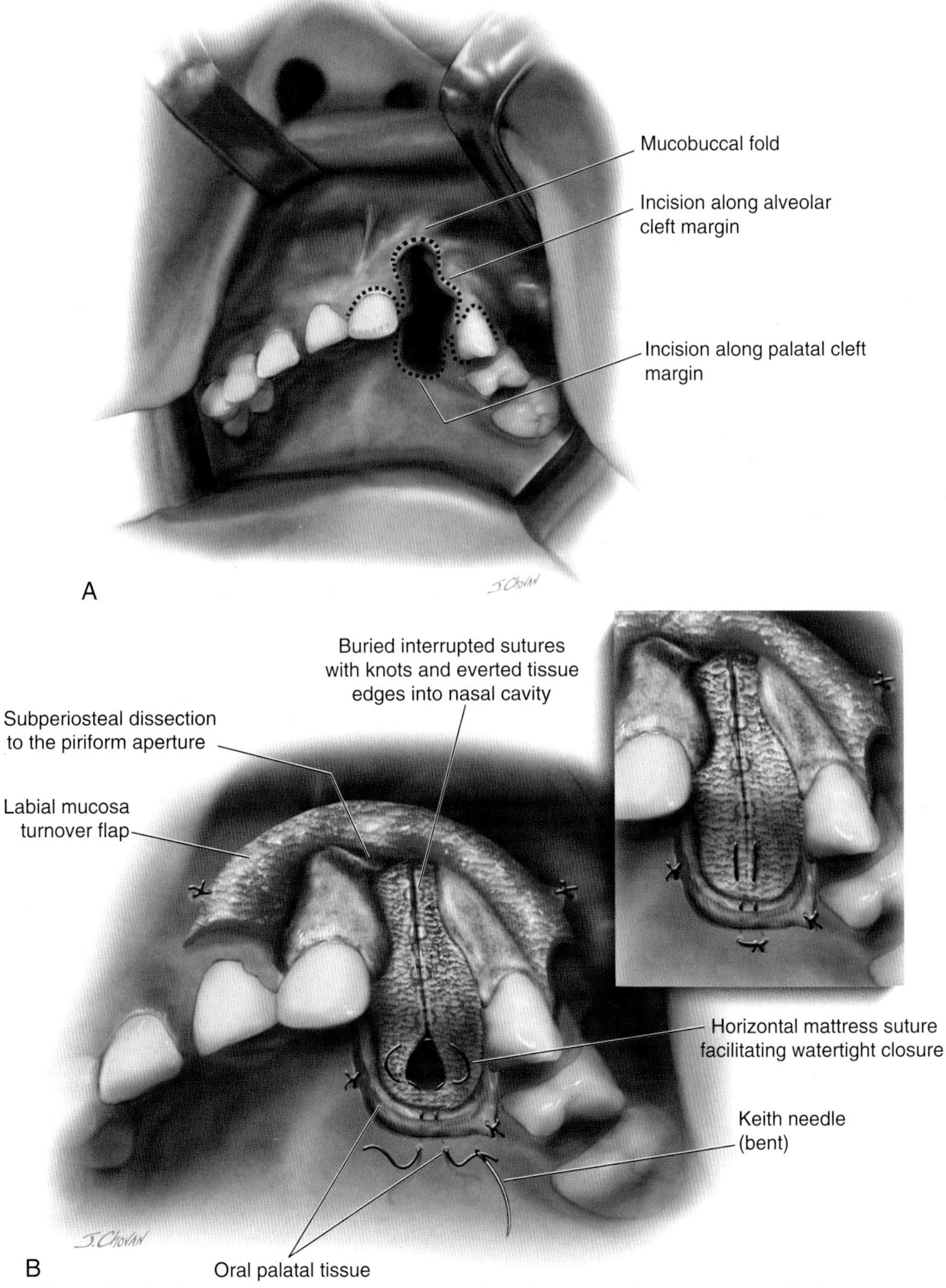

Figure 64.1 **A,** Planned incision to prepare the cleft site for bone graft reconstruction. **B,** The incision design must allow adequate tissue for nasal closure.

TECHNIQUE: Bone Grafting of the Cleft Maxilla and Palate—*cont'd*

STEP 2: Flap Elevation

Begin subperiosteal dissection at the crest of the alveolus. As the superior aspect of the incision is approached, the dissection is continued as a partial thickness flap using a combination of blunt and sharp dissection with iris or Metzenbaum scissors. The labial mucosa is dissected free from the residual oronasal fistula, and the nasal mucosa is closed as a turnover flap. It is important to expose the maxillary cleft to the level of the piriform aperture so that the nasal sill and floor may be reconstructed and so that an adequate recipient osseous bed is available. The palatal flaps are also elevated off the bony cleft margin.

STEP 3: Closure of the Nasal Layer and Palatal Flaps

Resorbable sutures on a small tapered needle are used to close the nasal layer anteriorly from the mucobuccal fold to the palatal portion of the cleft. The surgeon should ensure the soft tissue nasal layer is at or superior to the nasal floor of the noncleft side to allow for adequate bony nasal reconstruction. Knots should be placed within the nasal cavity with tissue edge eversion. A Castroviejo needle driver may be helpful to maneuver in this area since access is limited.

Sealing the posterior aspect of the nasal floor may be challenging. If the cleft continues posteriorly along the palate, a horizontal mattress suture passed through the nasal layer anteriorly to the palatal tissue posteriorly (posterior to the cleft margin) can facilitate watertight closure of the nasal layer in this region (Fig. 64.1C and D). A Keith needle can be custom bent to facilitate passage of this suture. The palatal flaps are then closed with resorbable sutures from posterior to anterior direction.

STEP 4: Placement of Bone Graft

With the bony margins of the cleft completely stripped of soft tissue and the anterior nasal spine, nasal floor and piriform rim exposed, the surgeon may elect to place a thin cortical graft at the nasal floor to support the newly constructed mucosal floor. The graft should be cut to size and perforated with a #701 bur to allow for vascular ingrowth to the cancellous bone, which will be placed adjacent to it.

The cancellous bone that was harvested (and ideally stored on ice to preserve its osteogenic potential) is then packed densely into the cleft defect beginning posteriorly and continuing anteriorly to ensure bone stock is placed along the entire cleft defect.[26]

Continued

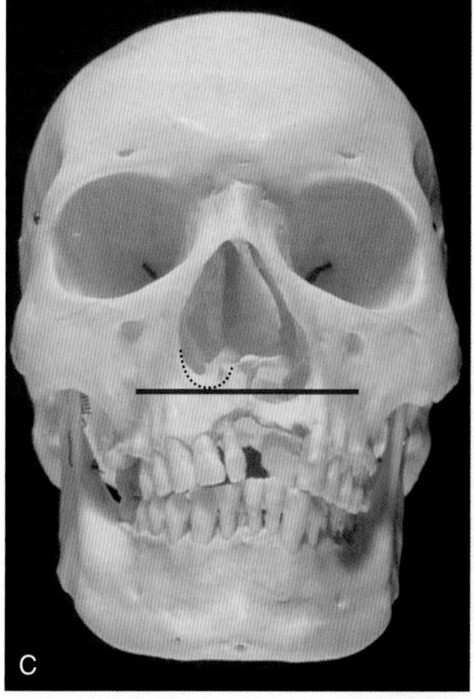

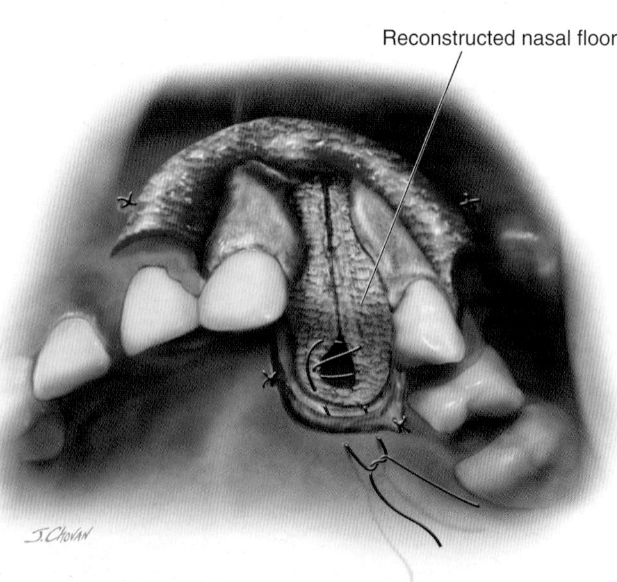

Figure 64.1, cont'd C, The nasal soft tissue closure must be at or superior to the noncleftedI nasal floor so that adequate bone construction is achievable. **D,** A traction suture may be passed through the reconstructed nasal floor to the palatal tissue to facilitate creation of a seal posteriorly.

TECHNIQUE: Bone Grafting of the Cleft Maxilla and Palate—*cont'd*

The surgeon should ensure there is well-packed graft at the level of the piriform rim. An additional strip of perforated cortical bone may be placed over the buccal surface of the cancellous graft spanning from anterior nasal spine to the lateral piriform rim. This provides support for the alar base. This cortical strut is usually self-retentive and does not require screw fixation (Fig. 64.1E and F).

STEP 5: Closure of the Maxillary Vestibule Mucosal Layer

It is imperative to close the oral layer in a tension-free manner to avoid both dehiscence and excessive graft resorption. The sliding buccal advancement flap is a frequently used technique. The sulcular incision that was initially created at the tooth adjacent to the cleft site is carried posteriorly to the first molar region. Here, a vertical releasing incision is extended in a superior and posterior direction to the mucobuccal fold. Subperiosteal dissection is then performed superiorly to the infraorbital rim with care to protect

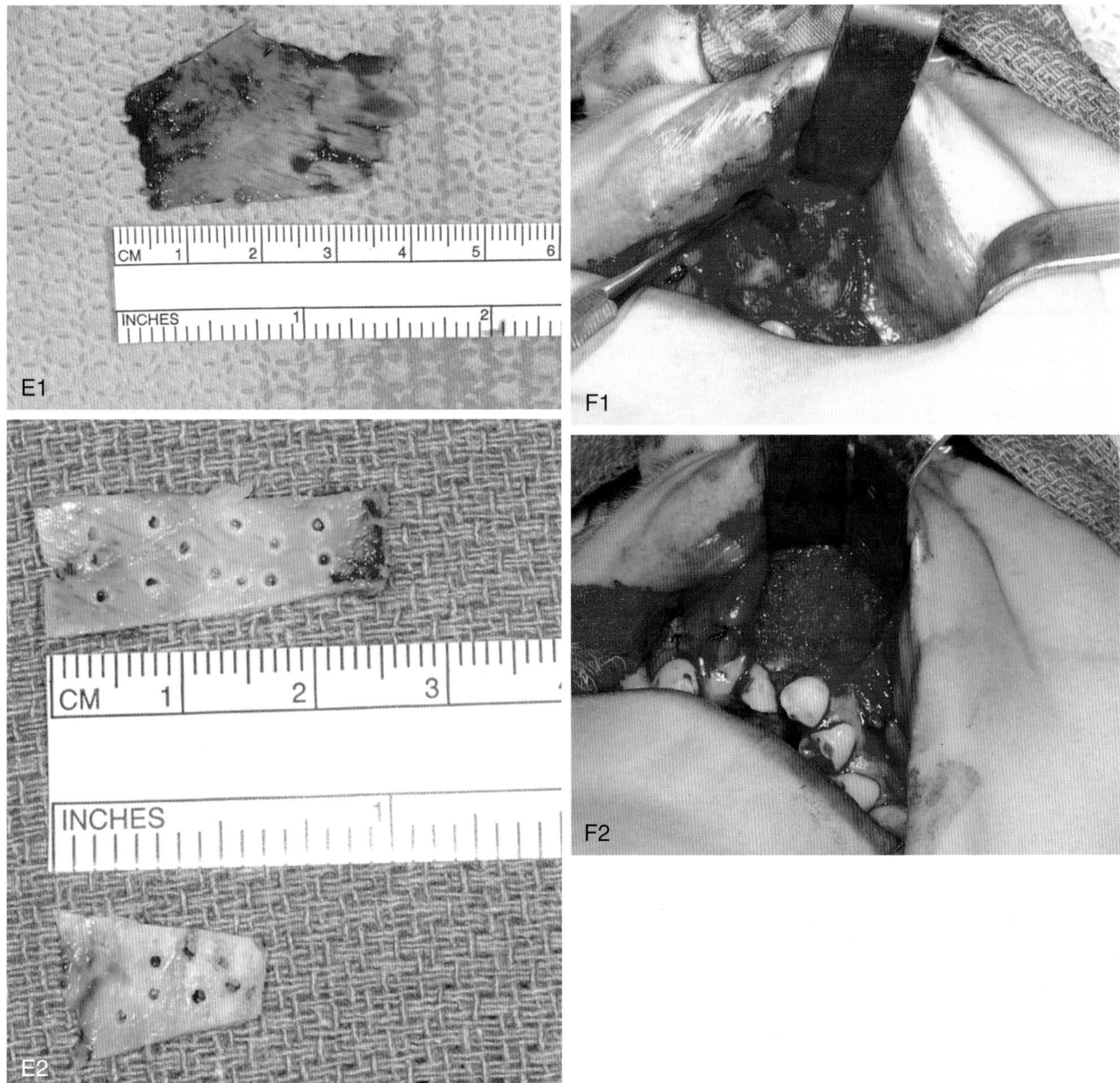

Figure 64.1, cont'd E1, Cortical strut harvested from the anterior iliac crest. **E2,** Perforated cortical strut. **F1,** Perforated cortical strut in place to construct the nasal floor. The cancellous side of the strut faces the defect. **F2,** Cancellous bone in place.

TECHNIQUE: Bone Grafting of the Cleft Maxilla and Palate—*cont'd*

the infraorbital nerve. The periosteum is scored with a #15 blade to allow for advancement of this flap, which is then secured to the oral mucosa on the noncleft side (or premaxillary segment) with interrupted resorbable sutures. As the flap is advanced, keratinized tissue is simultaneously brought forward for periodontal support.

The technical advantages of this flap include predictable blood supply and maintenance of attached gingiva anteriorly. However, there is a defect posteriorly that must heal by secondary intention. This combined with wide subperiosteal dissection inherent with the technique raises concern of further embarrassment to growth in the skeletally immature maxilla (Fig. 64.1G).

Continued

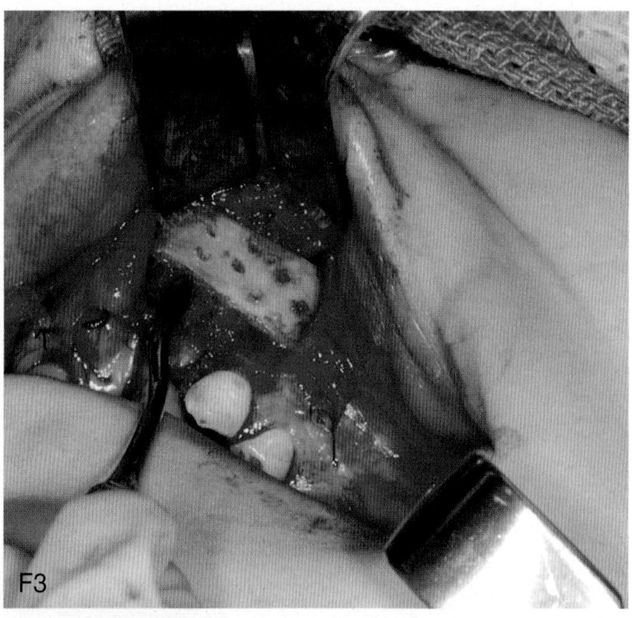

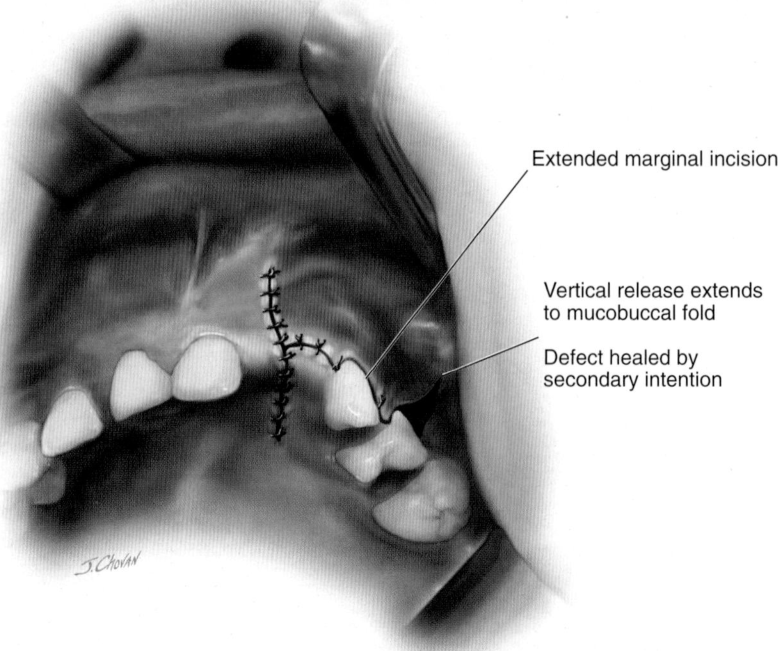

Figure 64.1, cont'd F3, Second cortical strut in place superficially to support the alar base. **G,** A sliding buccal gingival flap is advanced over the bone graft; tension-free closure is facilitated by periosteal release.

Alternative Techniques

1. Anterior Buccal Mucosal Rotational Flap

At the depth of the vestibule, parallel incisions are made, beginning at the superior portion of the cleft extending posteriorly in the buccal mucosa where they converge. The length of the flap should not exceed three times its width. The flap is elevated in the submucosal plane and the base is undermined to allow rotation into the defect. The flap is sutured into place with resorbable everting sutures beginning with a tacking suture at the tip to the palatal tissue. The advantages include minimal tension and avoidance of widespread subperiosteal dissection and its deleterious effects on maxillary growth. In addition, the flap may be advanced palatally to assist in closure of larger defects. Disadvantages include transfer of unattached mucosa to the cleft site, which may compromise periodontal health. This may be mitigated by elevating keratinized gingival flaps that may be closed over a deepithelialized mucosal flap.

2. Palatal Closure

Elevation of palatal flaps may be required to achieve adequate palatal coverage. This can be accomplished by creating a lateral releasing incision and may be all that is required to close the palatal portion of the oral wound. If the defect is of larger size, an incision is made several millimeters from the gingival margin from the first molar region to the cleft margin in a rotational flap design. A relaxing incision may be made with care to avoid the neurovascular bundle.

3. The Bilateral Cleft Maxilla

The technical execution of bone grafting of the bilateral maxilla is similar to unilateral cleft cases. Staging of bilateral clefts is not necessary and to do so places an unnecessary burden on the patient and family. Occasionally, in bilateral cases vomer mucosal elevations may be required to close the nasal floor. If this is performed, the bone graft must extend to the vomer. Premaxillary repositioning is performed orthodontically prior to surgery. Occasionally, the premaxilla must be surgically repositioned. An acrylic occlusal maxillary splint and a 0.036 buccal arch wire may be used to aid in stabilization of the premaxilla. Grafting is performed concomitantly with splint placement.

Premaxillary stabilization is a critical step to successful grafting of the bilateral cleft maxilla. If mobility or traumatic occlusion is present, the graft will be lost. Palatal and buccal flaps are completed as described above. The surgeon must avoid placing a horizontal incision across the soft tissue pedicle of the premaxilla to avoid compromising its vascularity. If a premaxillary osteotomy is necessary to position the segment, it is done as follows: a small vertical incision is made in the premaxillary facial soft tissue to allow for the placement of a small osteotome above the anterior nasal spine. The segment is then disarticulated from the septum and vomer (Fig. 64. 2). Alternatively,

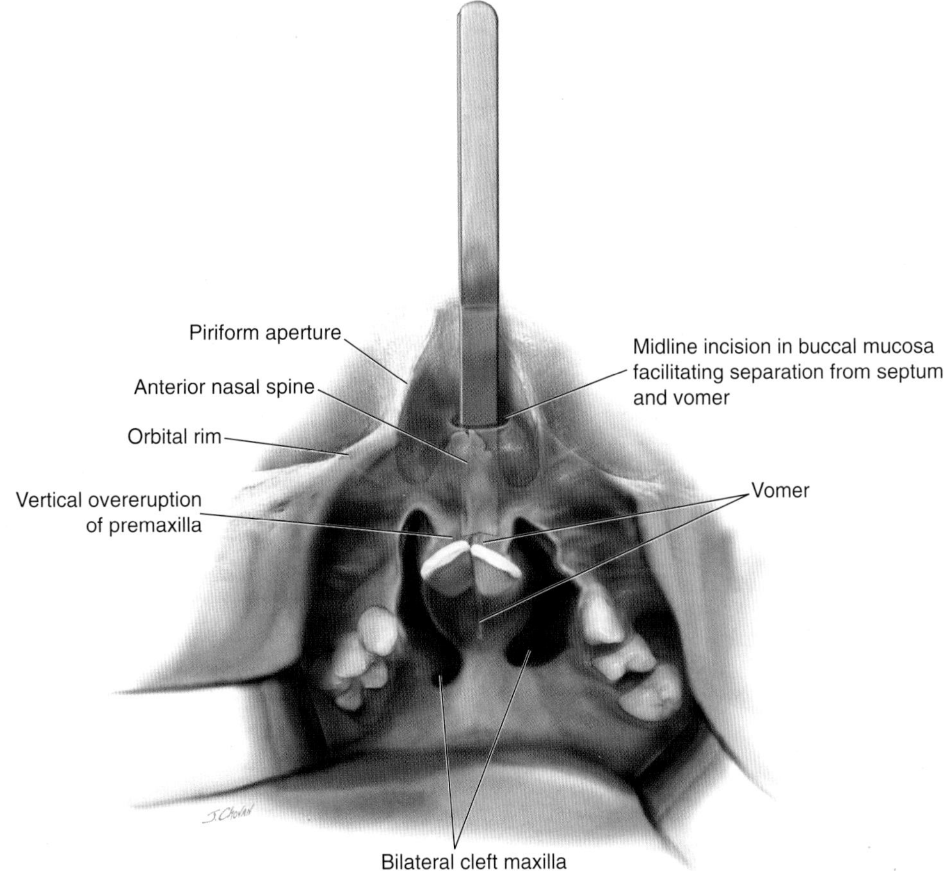

Figure 64.2 Osteotome separation of the premaxilla during surgical repositioning.

a small curved chisel can be used through the ungrafted cleft sites to section the premaxilla posteriorly from the vomer. The premaxilla is then out-fractured with digital pressure and the cartilaginous septum is freed from the premaxilla. The premaxilla is then positioned within the splint. This technique allows for the buccal mucosa soft tissue pedicle to remain intact.

4. Grafting in the Permanent Dentition

Grafting in the permanent dentition is less successful than in the mixed dentition. Patients experience increased root resorption, increased graft resorption, increased fistula rates, and decreased bony support.[18,29,30] There is often periodontal bone loss noted on teeth adjacent to the cleft site, and the cleft site is also often larger. As the final prosthodontic goal is usually endosseous implant placement with a prosthetic crown, a corticocancellous block is often used in this population.[16] The block can be stabilized with resorbable plates and/or screws so their removal is not required at the time of implant placement. Soft tissue closure is always completed with full thickness mucoperiosteal flaps. If simultaneous osteotomies are performed, the surgeon must ensure incisions and flaps are carefully designed to ensure adequate perfusion of the segments and revascularization of the grafts. Dental implants should be placed 6 months after grafting as resorption is predictable after this time period. To maximize success, the following principles should be considered.[17] Periodontal therapy should be performed 6 to 8 weeks before grafting to minimize inflammation in the region of surgery. Removal of periodontally compromised teeth adjacent to the cleft site is performed 2 months prior to grafting to allow for soft tissue healing and resolution of inflammation. The size of the bony defect may need to be reduced by osteotomies and advancement of the posterior tooth-bearing segment into the cleft. This procedure will also increase the feasibility of completing watertight nasal floor closure. This is accomplished via traditional segmental maxillary techniques, being certain to design soft tissue flaps to maintain vascularity to the mobilized segments.

Avoidance and Management of Intraoperative Complications

As with all surgery, meticulous handling of soft tissues is paramount to success. When planning incisions, it is important to ensure adequate soft tissue is available for nasal closure and no tension is present across suture lines. The importance of watertight nasal closure cannot be overstressed. Leakage of nasal fluid into the grafted area predictably reduces success.

It is also important to preserve the thin bone overlying the dental roots to avoid creation of periodontal defects or external root resorption. As mentioned previously, bone grafts should extend over the margins of the cleft to allow for proper contour of the alveolus and increased bone stock over areas of thin bone. The graft should fill the entire defect from the alveolus superiorly to the nasal sill and floor.

Postoperative Considerations

The surgeon should continue antibiotics for 7 to 10 days after surgery along with antibiotic mouth rinses up to 14 days. The patient and parents are instructed to maintain excellent hygiene, and good nutrition is encouraged. Patients should remain on a nonchew diet with special care to avoid hard and abrasive foods until cleared by the surgeon. Avoidance of the use of straws and forceful sucking, nose blowing, and forcing liquids through the cleft are discouraged.

Orthodontic tooth movement may begin as soon as 3 weeks after graft placement, as tooth movement through the graft site facilitates graft maturation. Postgraft expansion should be delayed until the mucosal wounds have matured (around 6 weeks after graft placement). Postgraft expansion also has a favorable effect on graft maturation; however, care should be taken not to expand excessively as it may lead to segmentation during maxillary advancement in a previously operated skeletal segment with inherent vascular and soft tissue compromise. Surgical exposure and orthodontic movement of unerupted teeth at the graft site are rarely indicated as the authors have observed spontaneous dental eruption through the graft almost always occurs.

Minor dehiscence and/or extrusion of small portions of graft may occur occasionally. In these cases, conservative debridement should be performed. Antimicrobial mouthwash, meticulous hygiene, and return to a soft diet are prescribed. Irrigation of the area must be gentle, and a short course of systemic antibiotics may be indicated. If large areas of dehiscence are present with graft extrusion, the patient may need more extensive debridement, but reclosure over a contaminated graft is not recommended.

Infection after grafting is rare and can be managed with local wound care and oral antibiotics. Conservative debridement may be indicated and consideration should be given to loose packing with petroleum gauze and daily irrigation using antimicrobial mouthwash. While buccal fistulas tend to remain closed after grafting, palatal fistulas may persist. These may be closed in subsequent procedures.

References

1. von Eiselsberg TW. Zur technik der uranoplastik. *Arch Klin Chir.* 1901;64:509–529.
2. Lexer E. Die verwendung der freien knochenplastik nebst versuchen uber gelenkversteifung und gelenentransplantation. *Acta Klin Chir.* 1908;86:939–954.
3. Drachter R. Die gaumenpalate und cherenoperative berandlung. *Dtach Zachr Chir.* 1914;134:2.
4. Koberg WR. Present view on bone grafting in cleft palate (a review of the literature). *J Maxillofac Surg.* 1973;1(4):185–193.
5. Schmid E. Die annaherung der kieferstumpfe bei lippen-kiefer-gaumenspalten: ihre schadlichen folgen und vermeidung. *Fortschr Kiefer Gesichtschir.* 1955;1:168–173.
6. Pruzansky S. Pre-Surgical Orthopedics and Bone Grafting for Infants With Cleft

Lip and Palate: A Dissent. Presented at the 1963 Convention of the American Cleft Lip and Palate Association, Washington DC. digital.library.pitt.edu/c/cleftpalate/pdf/e20986v01n2.03.pdf. Accessed July 23, 2020.

7. Berkowitz S. Gingivoperiosteoplasty as well as early palatal cleft closure is unproductive. *J Craniofac Surg*. 2009;20(suppl 2):1747–1758.
8. Pickrell K, Quinn G, Massengill R. Primary bone grafting of the maxilla in clefts of the lip and palate: a four year study. *Plast Reconstr Surg*. 1968;41(5):438–443.
9. Robertson NRE, Jolleys A. Effects of early bone grafting in complete clefts of lip and palate. *Plast Reconstr Surg*. 1968;42(5): 414–421.
10. Kuijpers-Jagtman AM, Long RE. The influence of surgery and orthopedic treatment on maxillofacial growth and maxillary arch development in patients treated for orofacial clefts. *Cleft Palate Craniofac J*. 2000;37:527–539.
11. Rehrmann AH, Koberg WR, Koch H. Long-term postoperative results of primary and secondary bone grafting in complete clefts of lip and palate. *Cleft Palate J*. 1970;7:206–221.
12. Skoog T. The management of the bilateral cleft of the primary palate (lip and alveolus). *Plast Reconstr Surg*. 1965;35:34–44.
13. Matic DB, Power SM. The effects of gingivoperiosteoplasty following alveolar molding with a pin-retained Latham appliance versus secondary bone grafting on midfacial growth in patients with unilateral clefts. *Plast Reconstr Surg*. 2008;122(3):863–870.
14. Grayson BH, Cutting C, Wood R. Preoperative columella lengthening in bilateral cleft lip and palate. *Plast Reconstr Surg*. 1993;92(7):1422–1423.
15. Boyne PJ, Sands NR. Secondary bone grafting of residual alveolar and palatal clefts. *J Oral Surg*. 1972;30(2):87–92.
16. Boyne PJ, Sands NR. Combined orthodontic-surgical management of residual palato-alveolar cleft defects. *Am J Orthod*. 1976;70(1):20–37.
17. Turvey TA, Ruiz RI, Tiwana PS. Bone graft construction of the cleft maxilla and palate. In: Losee JE, Kirschner RE, eds. *Comprehensive Cleft Care*. New York, NY: Mc-Graw-Hill; 2009:836–865.
18. Abyholm FE, Bergland O, Semb G. Secondary bone grafting of alveolar clefts. A surgical/orthodontic treatment enabling a non-prosthodontic rehabilitation in cleft lip and palate patients. *Scand J Plast Reconstr Surg*. 1981;15(2):127–140.
19. Turvey TA, Vig K, Moriarty J, Hoke J. Delayed bone grafting in the cleft maxilla and palate: a retrospective multidisciplinary analysis. *Am J Orthod*. 1984;86(3):244–256.
20. Precious DS. A new reliable method for alveolar bone grafting at about 6 years of age. *J Oral Maxillofac Surg*. 2009;67(10):2045–2053.
21. Horswell BB, Henderson JM. Secondary osteoplasty of the alveolar cleft defect. *J Oral Maxillofac Surg*. 2003;61(9):1082–1090.
22. Rawashdeh MA, Telfah H. Secondary alveolar bone grafting: the dilemma of donor site selection and morbidity. *Br J Oral Maxillofac Surg*. 2008;46(8):665–670.
23. Boyne PJ. Use of marrow-cancellous bone grafts in maxillary alveolar and palatal clefts. *J Dent Res*. 1974;53(4):821–824.
24. Kaura AS, Srinivasa DR, Kasten SJ. Optimal timing of alveolar cleft bone grafting for maxillary clefts in the cleft palate population. *J Craniofac Surg*. 2018;29(6):1551–1557.
25. Salyer KE, Jackson IT, Bardach J. Correction of skeletal defects in secondary cleft lip and palate deformities. In: Bardach J, Salyer KE, eds. *Surgical Techniques in Cleft Lip and Palate*. 2nd ed. St. Louis, Missouri: Mosby; 1991:297–333.
26. Hassanein AH, Greene AK, Arany PR, Padwa BL. Intraoperative cooling of iliac bone graft: an experimental evaluation of cell viability. *J Oral Maxillofac Surg*. 2012;70(7):1633–1635.
27. Bardach J, Salyer KE, Noordhoff MS. Bilateral cleft lip repair. In: Bardach J, Salyer KE, eds. *Surgical Techniques in Cleft Lip and Palate*. 2nd ed. St. Louis, Missouri: Mosby; 1991.
28. Dempf R, Teltzrow T, Kramer FJ, Hausamen JE. Alveolar bone grafting in patients with complete clefts: a comparative study between secondary and tertiary bone grafting. *Cleft Palate Craniofac J*. 2002;39(1):18–25.
29. Uribe F, Alister JP, Zaror C, Olate S, Fariña R. Alveolar cleft reconstruction using morphogenetic protein (rhBMP-2): a systematic review and meta-analysis. *Cleft Palate Craniofac J*. 2020;57(5):589–598.
30. Taylor HO, Sullivan SR. Alveolar bone grafting. In: Chang J, ed. *Global Reconstructive Surgery*. New York, NY: Elsevier; 2019.

CHAPTER 65

Pharyngoplasty for Velopharyngeal Incompetence

Bernard J. Costello and Ramon L. Ruiz

Armamentarium

#9 Periosteal elevator
#15C blade with long handle
Angled Beaver blade
Appropriate sutures
Arm restraints
Bipolar and monopolar cautery with needlepoint tip
Eye protection
Gerald forceps with teeth
Large curved Freer elevator
Local anesthetic with vasoconstrictor
Marking pen
Nasal trumpets
Peanut gauze on a tonsil forceps or Kitner forceps
Ratchet mouth retractor
Single skin hooks
Stevens tenotomy scissors
Woodson periosteal elevator

History of the Procedure

Problems with the velopharyngeal mechanism can greatly affect speech production and create varying degrees of difficulty with production of key speech sounds. The patients most often affected by this problem are those with cleft palates. The pharyngeal flap procedure is the most widely used surgical treatment for velopharyngeal insufficiency or incompetence (VPI). The procedure was first described by Schoenborn in 1876.[1–3] When randomly applied to patients with VPI, the superiorly based pharyngeal flap procedure is effective 80% of the time.[4] When the flap is applied using careful preoperative objective evaluations, success rates as high as 95% to 97% have been reported.[5,6] Shprintzen[4] and Shprintzen et al.[7] have advocated custom tailoring of the pharyngeal flap width and position based on the particular characteristics of each patient as seen on nasopharyngoscopy.

The high overall success rate and the flexibility to design the dimensions and position of the flap itself are advantages. The disadvantages of the pharyngeal flap procedure are primarily related to the possibility of severe nasal obstruction, resulting in mucus trapping, and postoperative obstructive sleep apnea. Inferiorly based pharyngeal flaps for the management of VPI were used in the past but are rarely performed today. Previous reports have documented increased morbidity without better speech outcomes associated with inferiorly based flaps.[8] In addition, inferiorly based flaps tend to cause downward pull on the soft palate after healing and contracture of the flap. The result may be a tethered palate with decreased ability to elevate during the formation of speech sounds.

The sphincter pharyngoplasty is another option for the surgical management of VPI. This procedure was described by Hynes in 1951 and has since been modified by a number of other authors.[9–14] Augmentation of the posterior pharyngeal wall has been attempted to facilitate closure of the nasal airway. Various autogenous and alloplastic materials have been used, including local tissue, rib cartilage, injections of Teflon, silicon, Silastic, Proplast, and collagen.[15,16] Improvement in speech after augmentation of the posterior pharyngeal wall is unpredictable. Difficulties with migration or extrusion of the implanted material and an increased rate of infection add to the problems of these techniques. For these reasons, pharyngeal wall implants are rarely used today.

Indications for the Use of the Procedure

The secondary palate is composed of a hard (bony) palate anteriorly and a soft palate, or velum, posteriorly. Within the soft palate, the levator veli palatini muscle forms a dynamic sling that elevates the velum toward the posterior pharyngeal wall during the production of certain sounds. Other muscle groups within the velum, the tonsillar pillar region, and the pharyngeal walls also affect resonance quality during speech formation. The combination of the soft palate and pharyngeal wall musculature forms what is described as the velopharyngeal mechanism (Fig. 65.1A). The velopharyngeal mechanism functions as a complex sphincter valve to regulate airflow between the oral and nasal cavities and creates a combination of orally based and nasally based sounds. By definition, children born with a cleft palate have a malformation that dramatically affects the anatomic components of the velopharyngeal mechanism. Clefting of the secondary palate causes division of the musculature of the velum into separate muscle bellies with abnormal insertions along the posterior

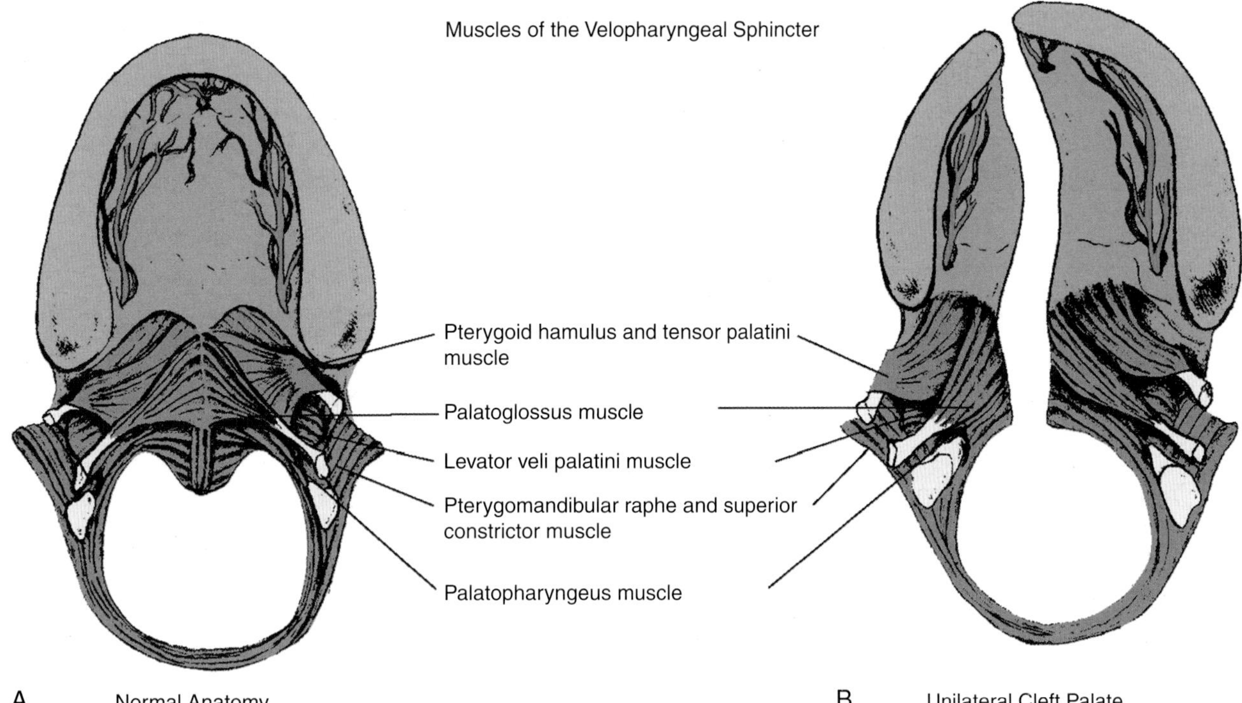

Figure 65.1 Anatomy of the palate and velopharyngeal valve mechanism. **A,** Normal anatomy. **B,** Unilateral cleft of the primary and secondary palate with associated anatomic abnormalities. (From Myers E, Operative Otolaryngology: Head and Neck Surgery. St. Louis: Saunders; 2009).

edge of the hard palate (Fig. 65.1B). The initial palatoplasty, as described earlier, is not simply carried out for closure of the palatal defect (oronasal communication) itself but is aimed at addressing the underlying muscular anatomic deformity. During two-flap palatoplasty, care must be taken to sharply separate the levator muscle bellies off the palatal shelves, realign them, and establish continuity to create a functioning palatal-levator muscle sling. Some describe this primary repair of the palatal musculature as an intravelar veloplasty. Although this description helps to articulate the importance of addressing the levator muscle, it may confuse some clinicians by suggesting that muscle repair, or intravelar veloplasty, is a separate procedure. The degree of aggressive retropositioning of the levator musculature can vary among surgeons. Regardless of the cleft palate repair technique used (e.g., von Langenbeck, Bardach, Furlow), meticulous release of abnormal levator muscle insertions with velar muscle reconstruction must be incorporated as a critical element of the surgical procedure.

Most children who undergo successful cleft palate repair during infancy (9 to 18 months) go on to develop speech that is normal or demonstrate minor speech abnormalities that are amenable to speech therapy. In a smaller segment of this patient population, the velopharyngeal mechanism does not demonstrate normal function despite surgical closure of the palate.[17,18] VPI is defined as inadequate closure of the nasopharyngeal airway port during speech production. The exact cause of VPI after "successful" cleft palate repair is a complex problem that remains difficult to define and quantify. Inadequate surgical repair of the musculature is one potential cause of VPI. The role of postsurgical scarring and its impact on muscle function and palatal motion are poorly understood. The theoretic advantages of using a Furlow double-opposing Z-plasty procedure for the initial palate repair include better realignment of the palatal muscles and lengthening of the soft palate. These benefits may be negatively balanced by a velum that demonstrates less mobility secondary to scarring associated with two separate Z-plasty incisions.

Even muscles that are appropriately realigned and reconstructed may fail to heal normally and function properly because of congenital defects having to do with their innervation. In addition, a repaired cleft palate is only one factor contributing to velopharyngeal function. Nasal airway dynamics and abnormalities related to vocal tract morphology and lateral and posterior pharyngeal wall motion may contribute to velopharyngeal dysfunction. Certainly, these other structures may also play a positive role in compensating for palatal deformity. For example, a short, scarred soft palate that does not elevate very well may be compensated for by recruitment and hypertrophy of muscular tissue within the posterior pharyngeal wall (activation of Passavant's ridge).[19–21] The audible nasal air escape that results in hypernasal speech associated with VPI is perhaps the most debilitating consequence of the cleft palate malformation. A variable number of children with VPI after palatoplasty go on to require management involving additional palatal and pharyngeal surgery.[18] The percentage is quite variable and not universally agreed on but generally is 15% to 40% for nonsyndromic patients. Patients with known and identifiable syndromes have higher rates of VPI, but these are generally due to other contributing factors, such as cognitive status or neural innervation. Other studies claim much lower rates of VPI, but measurement and reporting are neither uniform nor validated in these published studies. Without a truly objective measure of speech in this patient population, it is difficult to know the true incidence of VPI after repair.

Left untreated, nasal air escape-related resonance problems lead to other compensatory speech abnormalities and articulation errors. The aerodynamic demands theory proposed by Warren[22] provides the best explanation of what occurs with severe VPI. His theory states that nasal air escape due to inadequate velopharyngeal closure causes the patient to articulate pressure consonants at the level of the larynx or pharynx instead of within the oral cavity. These abnormal compensatory misarticulations further complicate problems with speech formation and reduce speech intelligibility in patients with cleft palate-related VPI.

Indications for and the Timing of Surgery

After the initial cleft palate repair, periodic evaluations are critical to assess the speech and language development of each child. Typically this involves a standardized screening examination performed by a speech and language pathologist as part of a visit to the cleft palate team. For patients with VPI, more detailed studies may be indicated, including the use of videofluoroscopy and nasopharyngoscopy. Videofluoroscopic studies are used to radiographically examine the upper airway with the aid of an oral contrast material. These techniques allow dynamic testing of the velopharyngeal mechanism with views of the musculature in action. In addition, details of the upper airway anatomy, including residual palatal fistulas, can be visualized and their contribution to speech dysfunction evaluated. For a videofluoroscopy study to be of diagnostic value, it must include multiple views of the velopharyngeal mechanism. The speech pathologist should be present to verbally test the patient in the radiology suite.

Nasopharyngoscopy using a small, flexible, fiberoptic endoscope is routinely used for the evaluation of patients with VPI. Nasopharyngoscopy allows for direct visualization of the upper airway, and specifically the velopharyngeal mechanism, from the nasopharynx. This technique avoids radiation exposure associated with videofluoroscopy but requires preparation of the nose with a topical anesthetic, skillful maneuvering of the scope, and a compliant patient. Once the endoscope has been inserted, observations of palatal function, airway morphology, and pharyngeal wall motion are made while the patient is verbally tested by the speech pathologist.[23] The opportunity for direct visualization of the velopharyngeal mechanism in action during speech formation provides information that is critical to clinical decision making related to secondary palatal surgery in cases of confirmed or suspected VPI. The pattern of closure and the characteristics of any abnormal closure patterns during certain speech sounds may help tailor treatment and tend to be valuable information to optimize speech.

Secondary palatal surgery in young children is indicated when VPI causes hypernasal speech on a consistent basis and is related to a defined anatomic problem.[24–26] The timing of surgery for VPI remains controversial. Recommendations typically range from 3 to 5 years of age. In young children, obtaining enough diagnostic information to make a definitive decision regarding treatment is often difficult. In such a young age group, variables such as the child's language and articulation development and a lack of compliance during the speech evaluation compromise the diagnostic accuracy of preoperative assessments.[27–29]

By the time a child reaches 5 years of age, compliance with nasopharyngoscopy is better, and there is enough language development to allow for a more thorough perceptual speech evaluation. These factors allow for more definitive conclusions regarding the status of velopharyngeal function or dysfunction in the child with a repaired cleft palate. It is also important to note that decisions regarding the advisability of surgery for VPI are usually made after close collaboration with an experienced speech and language pathologist. The surgeon and speech pathologist should make this decision together and try to tailor the treatment to that particular child's needs.

To solve this issue, the surgical maneuvers are directed at recruiting tissue by developing a superiorly based soft tissue flap from the posterior pharyngeal wall. The soft palate is then divided along the midsagittal plane from the junction of the hard and soft palates to the uvula, and the flap from the posterior pharyngeal wall is inset within the nasal layer of the soft palate. As a result, a large nasopharyngeal opening that cannot be completely closed by the patient's velopharyngeal mechanism is converted into two (right and left) lateral pharyngeal ports. Closure of these ports is easier for the patient to accomplish, as long as adequate lateral pharyngeal wall motion is present. The main advantage of the sphincter pharyngoplasty over the superiorly based flap is the perceived lower rate of complications related to nasal airway obstruction.[30–32] Despite this perceived advantage, there is no evidence that pharyngoplasty procedures achieve superior outcomes in the resolution of VPI.

VPI and hypernasal speech may also be encountered in older patients at the time of orthognathic surgery for treatment of cleft-related maxillary deformity. Approximately 25% of patients who have undergone cleft palate repair during infancy require additional surgery for treatment of midfacial deficiency during adolescence, when they are nearing skeletal maturity.[33] This usually involves midface advancement at the Le Fort I level with or without mandibular surgery to restore skeletal proportions, treat malocclusion, and improve facial balance. Advancements of the maxilla in patients with a repaired cleft palate may worsen existing

VPI or may be the cause of new-onset VPI.[34–36] A minority of patients with borderline velopharyngeal closure preoperatively develop hypernasal speech even after relatively small degrees of maxillary advancement. Because predicting exactly how each patient will respond to maxillary advancement is difficult, formal speech assessment and detailed counseling of the patient and family regarding the possible development of postoperative VPI is recommended before any cleft orthognathic surgery is undertaken. Fortunately, most patients who develop VPI after maxillary advancement recover adequate velopharyngeal closure without the need for additional palatal surgery within approximately 6 months of the orthognathic procedure. It is important to note that no significant difference in speech outcomes has been convincingly documented between use of distraction osteogenesis techniques for midface advancement and conventional orthognathic surgery.

Limitations and Contraindications

Procedures designed to provide more effective closure of the velum are not likely to help patients with neurogenic or other causes of velopharyngeal incompetence. These procedures are also highly coupled to carefully directed speech therapy. Patients with obstructive sleep apnea may not be candidates for procedures that further obstruct the airway tract. Patients with velocardiofacial syndrome or those with aberrant vasculature anatomy may have medially displaced carotid arteries that are at risk for injury with the typical incisions used in the pharyngeal flap and pharyngoplasty procedures. An appropriate workup is necessary in these patients to localize the vessels. This may include standard fluoroscopy-based angiography, computed tomography with angiography, or magnetic resonance imaging with angiography.

TECHNIQUE: Superiorly Based Pharyngeal Flap

STEP 1: Intubation

Oral and endotracheal intubation with an oral RAE tube is performed before a ratchet mouth prop is placed. The tube is taped in the midline with padding or protection for the anterior dentition in some cases. The ratchet mouth prop should be released approximately every 20 to 30 minutes to allow for both arterial inflow and venous outflow. If adequate time is not allowed for this throughout the course of the longer procedure, undue postoperative swelling in the tongue and pharyngeal structures can occur, obstructing the airway in some cases.

STEP 2: Incision Design

The surgical maneuvers used to recruit tissue for a superiorly based pharyngeal flap are directed at obtaining tissue from the posterior pharyngeal wall above the level of the prevertebral fascia (Fig. 65.2). The superior extent of these incisions is the highest point possible at or above the horizontal plane of the heart and soft palate junction. The lateral extent should allow for a broad-based flap that can be custom-tailored to the patient's needs. This allows for vertical incisions to be made in the lateral pharyngeal wall just inside the junction of the posterior pharyngeal wall in the beginning of the loose lateral pharyngeal wall tissues. Care is exercised to avoid involving the dissection near the great vessels deeper within these fascial planes. In certain syndromic conditions, these can be more superficial.

As such, the markings are placed in the posterior pharyngeal wall to avoid vital structures, and the flap is designed to be adequately long with a horizontal incision inferiorly that allows for dissection down to the level of the prevertebral fascia. The local anesthetic is injected into this area. Typically, 0.5% lidocaine with 1:200,000 epinephrine provides good anesthesia and adequate hemostasis for these areas. The injection is made in the prevertebral fascia area and then in soft tissue just superficial to this. The soft palate is also injected.

The incision line for the soft palate is typically made with a midline splitting incision, with slightly more dissection on the oral side than the nasal side with respect to the anterior extent of this incision. This allows for opening of the soft palate tissues for inset of the flap, once it has been raised from the posterior pharyngeal wall and permits easier placement of sutures. It is helpful to have a superior understanding of needle positioning skills when placing sutures in the posterior palate and pharynx.

The incision is made with a #15C blade, and a Gerald forceps with teeth is used to gently retract the tissue toward the medial. It is helpful to perform this procedure in an ambidextrous fashion. Once the additional mucosal incision has been made, long-handled Stevens tenotomy scissors can be used to bluntly and sharply dissect down to the level of the prevertebral fascia. Peanut gauze and a Kittner forceps are used to bluntly dissect this plane superficial to the prevertebral fascia inferiorly and superiorly, in addition to medially to connect the right side with the left side. The flap is divided at its inferior base with curved right-angle scissors or, if these are not available, Dean scissors. Once the flap has been elevated to its most superior position, hemostasis is gained with a bipolar electrocautery instrument set on a low to medium setting. Great care is taken to gain excellent hemostasis because postoperative bleeding can be a more common complication. The soft palate is then divided accordingly with a limited amount of dissection for inset of the flap. The posterior pharyngeal wall tissue at its most inferior aspect is sewn into the nasal side of the most anterior aspect of the divided palate with 4-0 polyglycolic acid suture placed with a RB-1 tapered needle. The remainder of the sutures are placed laterally in a mattress interrupted fashion. Once this is complete, the size of the port can be adjusted with the last couple of sutures; a nasal trumpet also can be helpful in

Continued

TECHNIQUE: Superiorly Based Pharyngeal Flap—*cont'd*

adjusting the size of the port. The further the divided soft palate is sewn along the lateral edge of the posterior pharyngeal flap, the smaller the port will be. The oral side is then closed over the top of this for primary closure. Polyglycolic acid mattress sutures are used in similar fashion.

In some instances, the posterior pharyngeal wall may be closed. Some surgeons prefer to allow this to granulate; others prefer to close it primarily. Interrupted 2-0 polyglycolic acid suture may be used. The tissue is quite mobile and easy to close without tension using a single-handed tie technique. Care should be taken not to take deep bites because the carotid vasculature is just lateral to the dissection field.

Once this is complete, irrigation is used to check for good hemostasis. The typical point of additional small capillary or arterial bleeding is along the superiorly based portion of the flap at the most superior extent of the lateral incisions. Monopolar cautery should not be used because the current may be transmitted along the flap.

A tongue stitch can be placed in patients who may have an issue with postoperative airway obstruction. One or two nasal trumpets are placed. If one is placed, the bevel should be placed toward the airway rather than the lateral pharyngeal wall. These are typically taped into position with ¼-inch Steri-Strips in the younger child to avoid dislodgement. The patient is checked for floor-of-the-mouth and tongue swelling before extubation.

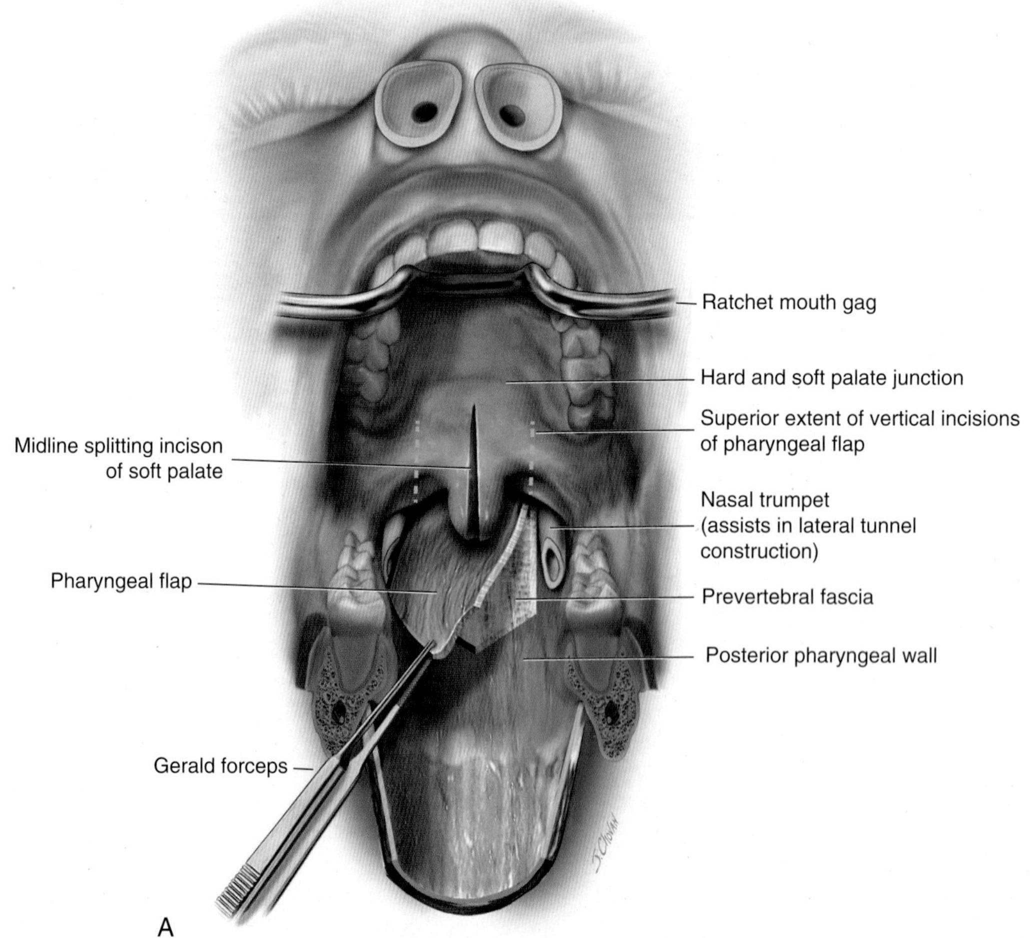

Figure 65.2 A, Elevation of a superiorly based pharyngeal flap with midline soft palate incision.

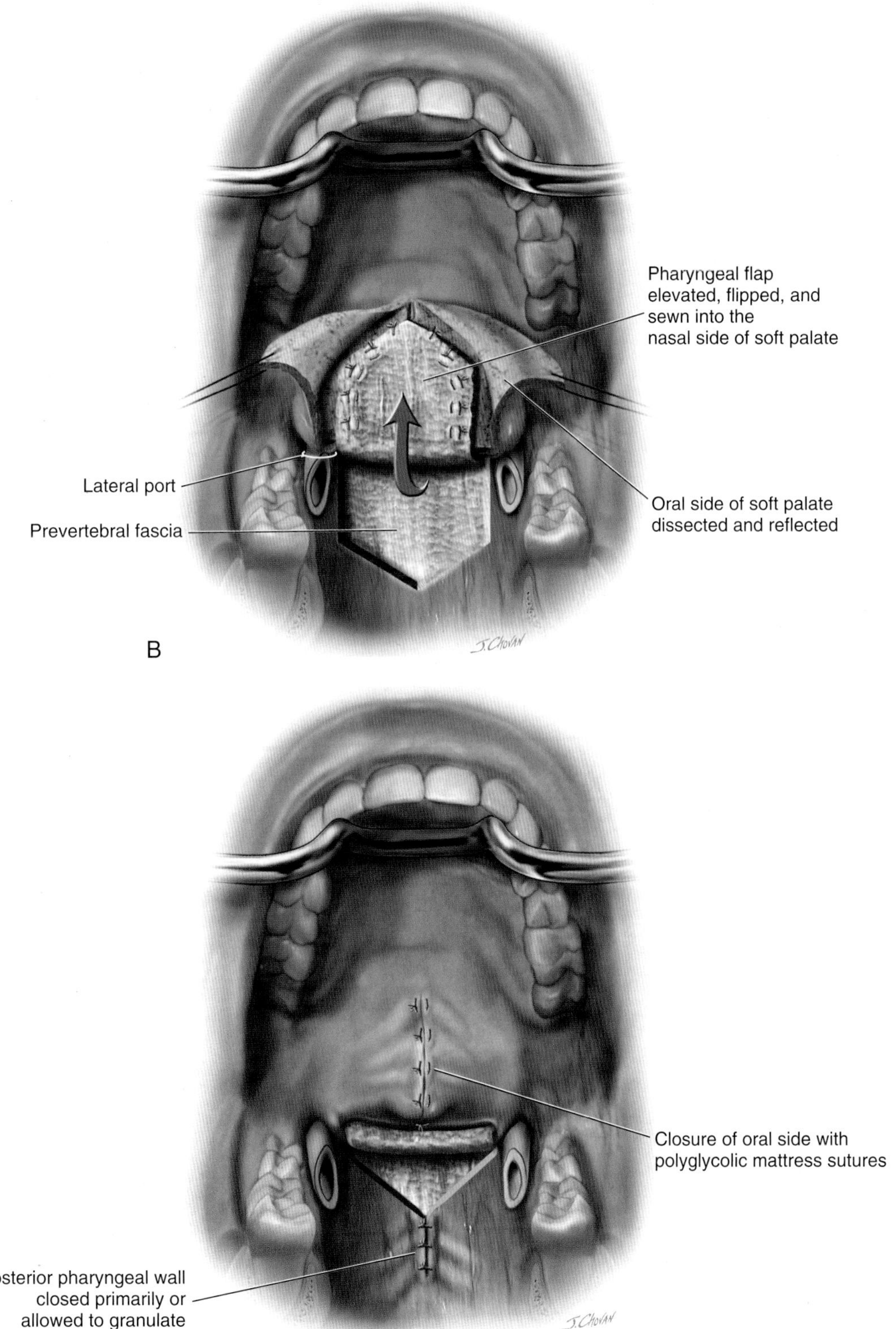

Figure 65.2, cont'd **B,** Inset of superiorly based flap to soft palate. **C,** Pharyngeal and soft palate closure.

Continued

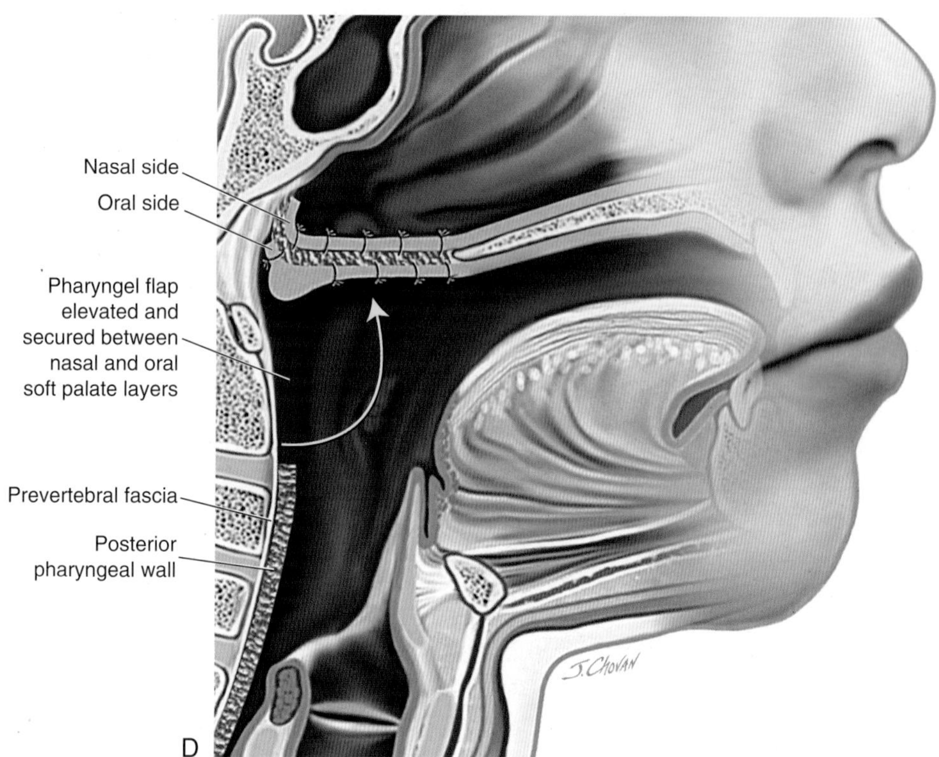

Figure 65.2, cont'd **D,** Lateral view demonstrating position of flap between the oral side and nasal side layers of the soft palate.

ALTERNATIVE TECHNIQUE 1: Pharyngoplasty

STEP 1: Intubation

Orotracheal intubation with an oral RAE tube is performed with the tube placed in the midline. Bilateral breath sounds are confirmed. The tube is held in place at the midportion of the chin with adhesive tape and occasionally an additional adhesive substance. The tube should be placed in the midline of the tongue so that it does not head down the lateral gutters on either the right or the left, and the patient should be positioned with a shoulder roll in place to allow for extension of the neck and visualization of the posterior pharynx.

STEP 2: Placement of the Ratchet Mouth Prop

Ratchet mouth props of several different varieties can be used, with the designed space for the endotracheal tube placed gently over this area. Occasionally, surgeons may use gauze or other protective material just over the lower incisor teeth to prevent soft tissue damage or kinking of the endotracheal tube underneath the ratchet mouth prop. This mouth prop is activated with the lateral cheek retractors in place and the superior maxillary positioning attachments off the central incisors to avoid subluxation of the teeth or damage to dental structures. The positioning attachments typically are placed to the lateral and the premolar area or on the alveolar ridge in the edentulous patient. The ratchet mouth prop should be released approximately every 20 minutes or so to allow for venous outflow and arterial inflow of the tongue and surrounding tissues. Adequate time should be allowed for this revascularization and venous outflow. Occasionally, significant tongue swelling can be seen if release of the tongue and pharyngeal tissues does not occur in the course of a longer procedure.

STEP 3: Making the Incision

The dynamic sphincter pharyngoplasty is an option for surgical management of velopharyngeal insufficiency. It involves the creation of two superiorly based mucosal flaps within each posterior tonsillar pillar (Fig. 65.3). These flaps are marked inferiorly with a marking pen, and the posterior pharyngeal wall is marked high or above the level of the soft palate in the horizontal plane. These areas are injected with 0.5% lidocaine with 1:200,000 epinephrine, with care taken to aspirate during this process. The solution is injected into the prevertebral fascial plane and the tissues just superficial to this for injection along the posterior pharyngeal wall. Once approximately 7 minutes have elapsed to allow the solution to take effect, the flap is elevated from inferior to superior, with care taken to include as much of the palatopharyngeal muscle as

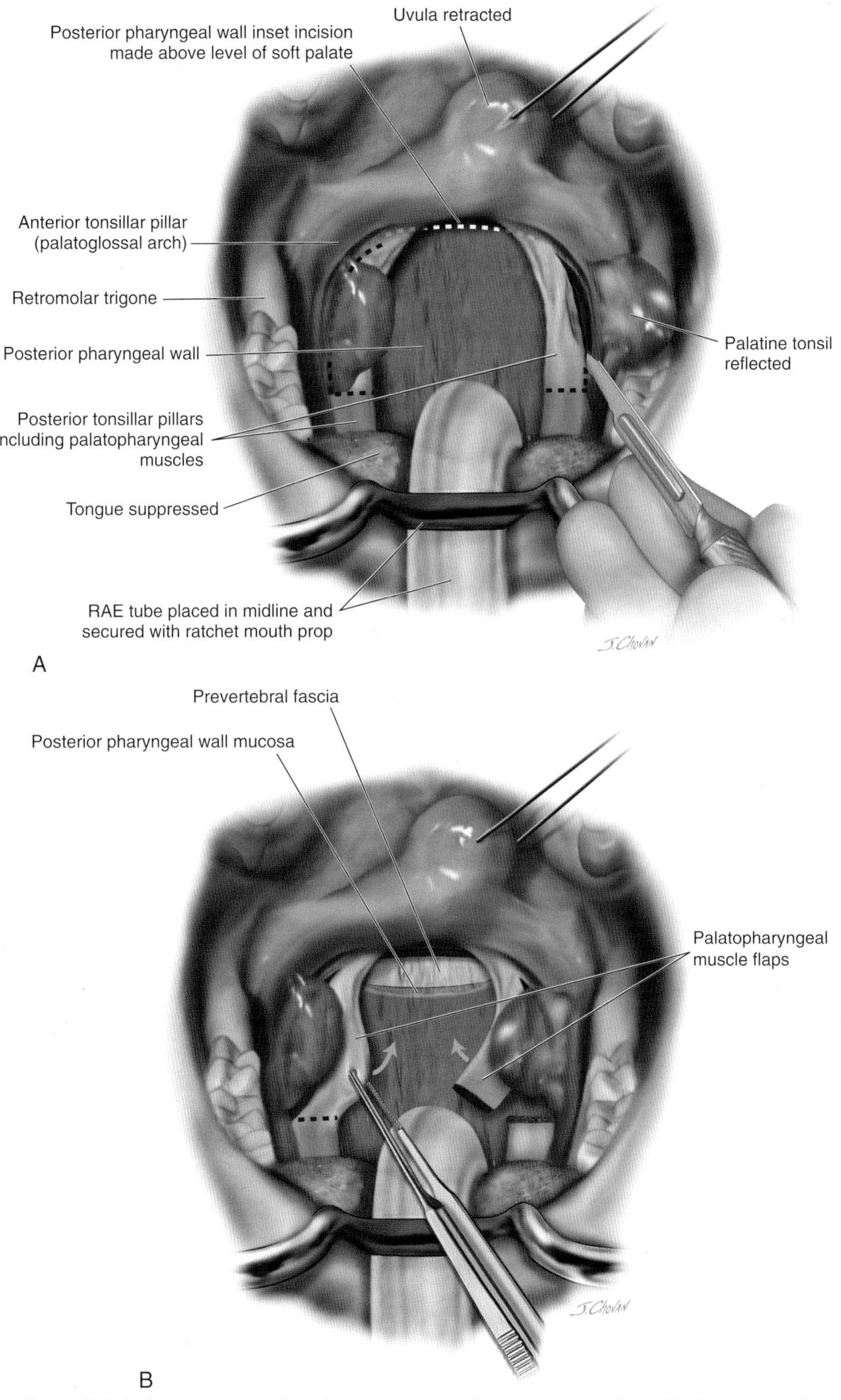

Figure 65.3 **A,** Incision design for sphincteroplasty in the posterior tonsillar pillar bilaterally and across the posterior pharyngeal wall. **B,** Elevation and medial rotation of flaps.

Continued

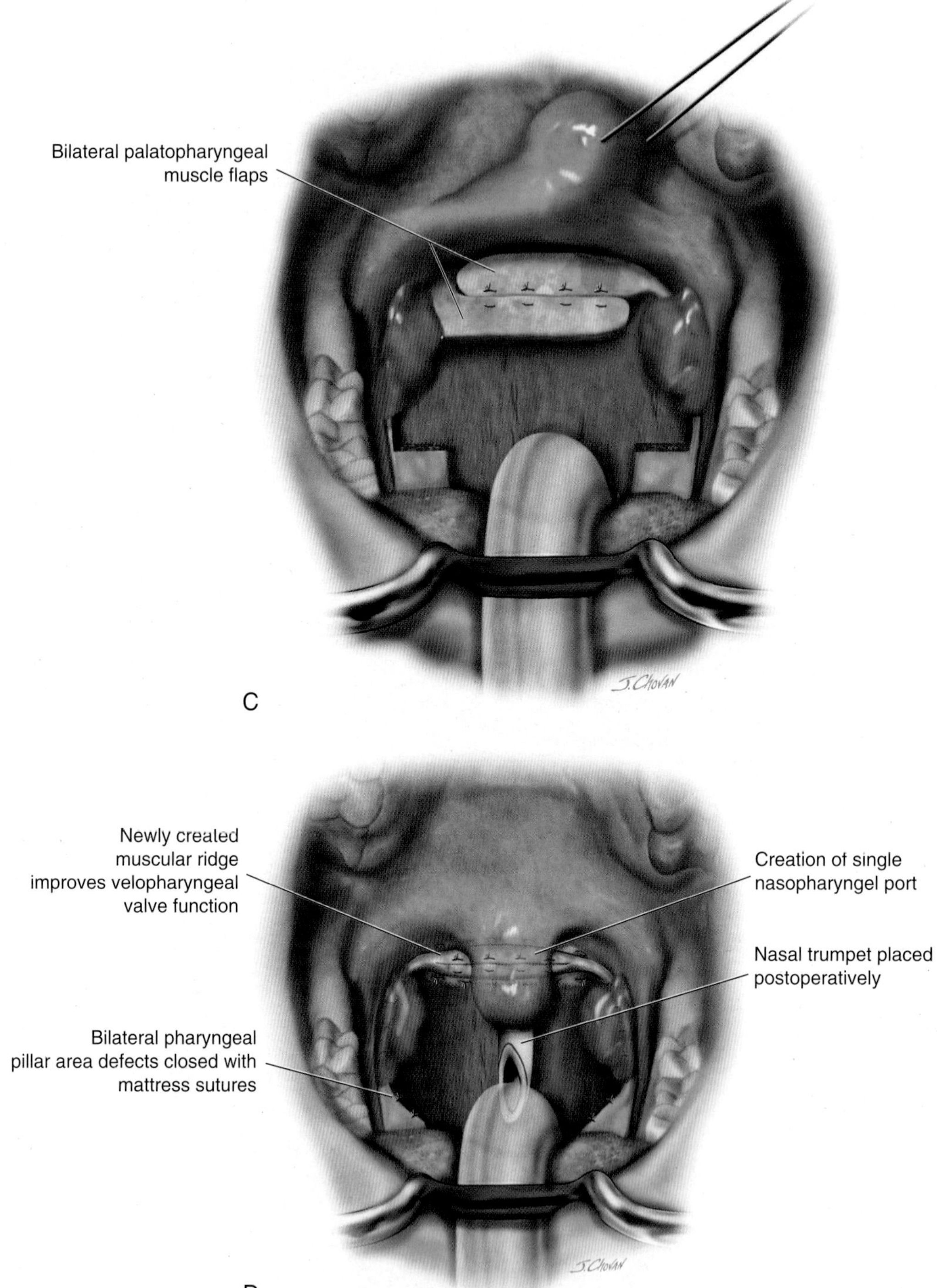

Figure 65.3, cont'd **C,** Flaps repositioned medially and superiorly to form sphincter. **D,** Creation of single nasopharyngeal port and closure of mucosal wounds.

ALTERNATIVE TECHNIQUE 1: Pharyngoplasty—*cont'd*

possible. The flaps are then attached in inset across the horizontal incision made high in the posterior pharyngeal wall. This is made to about the level of the prevertebral fascia and dissected slightly inferiorly and superiorly with a peanut and Kittner forceps to allow for inset of the flap. A bipolar electrocautery is used at a medium to low setting to obtain hemostasis. Care is taken to use a guarded bipolar electrocautery to avoid injuring the surrounding mucosal structures and oral commissure.

The goal of the inset of the flaps bilaterally is to cross over the musculature and create a single nasopharyngeal port instead of the two ports seen with a superiorly based pharyngeal flap. The ridge created posteriorly theoretically has the ability to contract and improve velopharyngeal valve function during closure for certain speech sounds. Thus, the aperture can be controlled by the length of the flaps and the particular inset of the flaps and is designed specifically for individuals with a velopharyngeal central defect, lateral defect, or other specific speech findings on preoperative nasopharyngoscopy or videofluoroscopy. The port is custom fit to allow for this placement. The flaps are inset with 4-0 polyglycolic acid sutures on a tapered needle; horizontal mattress sutures are preferred. The flaps can be tied end to end or crossover, based on the need for the particular port size. The defects left along the pharyngeal pillar areas can be closed with interrupted 0 mattress sutures, but good hemostasis should be ensured with the bipolar electrocautery instrument. A nasal trumpet can be placed postoperatively. Occasionally a tongue stitch may be used to facilitate tongue advancement in obtunded patients if this becomes a problem postoperatively.

ALTERNATIVE TECHNIQUE 2: Revision Palatoplasty

Some surgeons advocate the use of a revision palatoplasty instead of a pharyngeal flap or pharyngoplasty in the management of patients with VPI after cleft palate repair in infancy.[17] Some initial experience has shown this to be effective in a select group of patients who may have had incomplete or less aggressive muscular repairs. The technique can be performed using either a double-opposing Z-plasty or a two-flap palatoplasty with radical retropositioning of the levator musculature. Unfortunately, as yet, the anticipated benefits of these second palatoplasties have not been objectively established. The clinician must consider the disadvantages of this type of surgical procedure and weigh them against potential benefits. The double-opposing Z-plasty procedure requires a more aggressive dismantling of the palate than that required during a conventional pharyngeal flap procedure. The result may be a slightly longer palate but one with more extensive scarring and less physiologic movement. Another consideration is the significantly higher rate of fistula formation associated with this type of repair. This can be alleviated with the use of acellular dermal matrix as an interpositional graft material.

Avoidance and Management of Intraoperative Complications

Great care must be taken to avoid the great vessels that lie lateral and deep to the pharyngeal structures. In patients with certain syndromic diagnoses, these vessels may course more medially than expected. As such, the horizontal incision along the posterior wall should be made carefully in these individuals, and blunt dissection should be performed with the peanut gauze and Kittner forceps or Stevens tenotomy scissors to avoid injury to structures. Care should be taken to ensure hemostasis because postoperative bleeding is a relatively common complication.

Postoperative Considerations

Airway observation is important because airway problems can be a more common issue in patients who have undergone pharyngeal procedures. Steroids are often given to prevent airway problems; however, care must also be taken in ordering narcotic pain medications or other agents that may depress the respiratory system. Careful, regular assessments by the health care team and appropriate monitoring can help prevent respiratory depression episodes. Pain medication is used but must be carefully managed.

The patient should follow a liquid diet for approximately 2 weeks and should avoid strenuous or sports activities for 4 weeks. Speech therapy can resume within 1 to 3 months. A formal speech assessment should be performed at 3 to 6 months to evaluate progress.

References

1. Bernstein L. Treatment of velopharyngeal incompetence. *Arch Otolaryngol.* 1967;85(1):67–74.
2. Rosseli S. Divisione palatine 3 sua aura chirurgico. *Alu Congr Internaz Stomatal.* 1935;391.
3. Schoenborn D. Uber eine neue Methode der Staphylorraphies. *Arch Klin Chirurgie.* 1876;19:528.
4. Shprintzen RJ. The use of multiview videofluoroscopy and flexible fiberoptic nasopharyngoscopy as a predictor of success with pharyngeal flap surgery. In: Ellis F, Flack E, eds. *Diagnosis and Treatment of Palatoglossal Malfunction.* London, UK: College of Speech Therapists; 1979.
5. Argamaso RV, Levandowski GJ, Golding-Kushner KJ, Shprintzen RJ. Treatment of asymmetric velopharyngeal insufficiency with skewed pharyngeal flap. *Cleft Palate Craniofac J.* 1994;31(4):287–294.
6. Shprintzen RJ, Lewin ML, Croft CB, et al. A comprehensive study of pharyngeal flap surgery: tailor made flaps. *Cleft Palate J.* 1979;16(1):46–55.
7. Shprintzen RJ, McCall GN, Skolnick ML, Lencione RM. Selective movement of the lateral aspects of the pharyngeal walls during velopharyngeal closure for speech, blowing, and whistling in normals. *Cleft Palate J.* 1975;12(00):51–58.
8. Randall P, Whitaker LA, Noone RB, Jones WD. The case for the inferiorly based posterior pharyngeal flap. *Cleft Palate J.* 1978;15(3):262–265.
9. Hynes W. Pharyngoplasty by muscle transplantation. *Br J Plast Surg.* 1950;3(2):128–135.
10. Hynes W. The results of pharyngoplasty by muscle transplantation in failed cleft palate cases, with special reference to the influence of the pharynx on voice production; Hunterian lecture, 1953. *Ann R Coll Surg Engl.* 1953;13(1):17–35.
11. Orticochea M. Physiopathology of the dynamic muscular sphincter of the pharynx. *Plast Reconstr Surg.* 1997;100(7):1918–1923.
12. Orticochea M. Construction of a dynamic muscle sphincter in cleft palates. *Plast Reconstr Surg.* 1968;41(4):323–327.
13. Jackson I, Silverton JS. The sphincter pharyngoplasty as a secondary procedure in cleft palates. *Plast Reconstr Surg.* 1983;71:180.
14. Jackson IT. Sphincter pharyngoplasty. *Clin Plast Surg.* 1985;12(4):711–717.
15. Bluestone CD, Musgrave RH, McWilliams BJ. Symposium on synthetics in maxlloacial surgery. II. Teflon injection pharyngoplasty—status 1968. *Laryngoscope.* 1968;78(4):558–564.
16. Smith JK, McCabe BF. Teflon injection in the nasopharynx to improve velopharyngeal closure. *Ann Otol Rhinol Laryngol.* 1977;86(4 Pt 1):559–563.
17. Chen PK, Wu JT, Chen YR, Noordhoff MS. Correction of secondary velopharyngeal insufficiency in cleft palate patients with the Furlow palatoplasty. *Plast Reconstr Surg.* 1994;94(7):933–941.
18. Costello BJ, Ruiz RL, Turvey TA. Velopharyngeal insufficiency in patients with cleft palate. *Oral Maxillofac Surg Clin North Am.* 2002;14(4):539–551.
19. Glaser ER, Skolnick ML, McWilliams BJ, Shprintzen RJ. The dynamics of Passavant's ridge in subjects with and without velopharyngeal insufficiency—a multi-view videofluoroscopic study. *Cleft Palate J.* 1979;16(1):24–33.
20. Passavant G. On the closure of the pharynx in speech. *Archiv Heilk.* 1863;3:305.
21. Passavant G. On the closure of pharynx in speech. *Virchows Arch.* 1869;46:1.
22. Warren DW. Compensatory speech behaviors in individuals with cleft palate: a regulation/control phenomenon? *Cleft Palate J.* 1986;23(4):251–260.
23. Posnick JC. The staging of cleft lip and palate reconstruction: infancy through adolescence. In: *Craniofacial and Maxillofacial Surgery in Children and Young Adults.* Philadelphia, PA: Saunders; 2000.
24. Henningsson GE, Isberg AM. Velopharyngeal movement patterns in patients alternating between oral and glottal articulation: a clinical and cineradiographical study. *Cleft Palate J.* 1986;23(1):1–9.
25. Isberg A, Henningsson G. Influence of palatal fistulas on velopharyngeal movements: a cineradiographic study. *Plast Reconstr Surg.* 1987;79(4):525–530.
26. Lohmander-Agerskov A, Dotevall H, Lith A, Söderpalm E. Speech and velopharyngeal function in children with an open residual cleft in the hard palate, and the influence of temporary covering. *Cleft Palate Craniofac J.* 1996;33(4):324–332.
27. Shprintzen RJ, Bardach J. The use of information obtained from speech and instrumental evaluations in treatment planning for velopharyngeal insufficiency. In: *Cleft Palate Speech Management: A Multidisciplinary Approach.* St Louis, MO: Mosby; 1995.
28. Golding-Kushner KJ, Argamaso RV, Cotton RT, et al. Standardization for the reporting of nasopharyngoscopy and multiview videofluoroscopy: a report from an International Working Group. *Cleft Palate J.* 1990;27(4):337–347.
29. Warren DW, Dalston RM, Mayo R. Hypernasality and velopharyngeal impairment. *Cleft Palate Craniofac J.* 1994;31(4):257–262.
30. Guilleminault C, Stoohs R. Chronic snoring and obstructive sleep apnea syndrome in children. *Lung.* 1990;168(suppl):912–919.
31. Sirois M, Caouette-Laberge L, Spier S, Larocque Y, Egerszegi EP. Sleep apnea following a pharyngeal flap: a feared complication. *Plast Reconstr Surg.* 1994;93(5):943–947.
32. Ysunza A, Garcia-Velasco M, Garcia-Garcia M, Haro R, Valencia M. Obstructive sleep apnea secondary to surgery for velopharyngeal insufficiency. *Cleft Palate Craniofac J.* 1993;30(4):387–390.
33. Turvey TA, Ruiz RL, Costello BJ. Surgical correction of midface deficiency in cleft lip and palate malformation. *Oral Maxillofac Surg Clin North Am.* 2002;14(4):491–507.
34. Fonseca RJ, Turvey TA, Wolford LM. Orthognathic surgery in the cleft patient. In: Fonseca RJ, Baker SJ, Wolford LM, eds. *Oral and Maxillofacial Surgery.* Philadelphia, PA: Saunders; 2000.
35. Posnick JC, Tompson B. Cleft-orthognathic surgery: complications and long-term results. *Plast Reconstr Surg.* 1995;96(2):255–266.
36. Posnick JC, Ruiz RL. Discussion of management of secondary orofacial cleft deformities. In: Goldwyn RM, Cohen MM, eds. *The Unfavorable Result in Plastic Surgery: Avoidance and Treatment.* 3rd ed. Philadelphia, PA: Lippincott Williams & Wilkins; 2000.

CHAPTER 66

Cleft (Secondary) Rhinoplasty in the Adult Patient

Andrew Alistair Heggie

Armamentarium

#11, #15 Scalpel blades
¼-in. Steri-Strips/thermoplastic splint
4-0, 5-0 Chromic gut suture
5-0 Vicryl suture
6-0 Nylon suture
Adson-Brown dissector
Adson dissector, plain and toothed
Alar retractor
Angled cartilage scissors
Aufricht retractor
Blunt angled scissors
Caliper for measurement
Cartilage press
Cottle nasal retractors ×3
Curved mosquito artery forceps
Double-ended periosteal elevator (#9)
Double-ended rasp ×2
Double-guarded chisels ×4
Double-hook retractors ×2
Electrocautery, needle and bipolar
Fine long osteotome, 2 mm
Flat Padgett double-ended retractors ×3
Freer elevator
Hall Surgairtome drill/raspatory bur
Hollenback carver as cartilage dissector
Jayles dissector
Mallet
Metal grid for cartilage fragments
Nasal packing forceps, Kaltostat (rope)
Nasal saw
Needle holder, 6" fine
Rongeurs, small/single-action
Single-guarded osteotome
Single-hook retractor ×2
Straight mini-Metzenbaum scissor
Tenotomy scissors, fine
Tilley Henkel forceps

History of the Procedure

Rhinoplasty is one of the most commonly performed procedures in facial esthetic surgery and continues to generate an enormous amount of literature. From the early techniques of endonasal approaches to the sophisticated procedures of this century, there has been a transition to the open rhinoplasty technique, using a transcolumella approach, that delivers more predictable results. This open technique was described many decades ago in relation to the cleft nasal tip deformity.[1,2] For rhinoplasty procedures in general, the open approach has enabled a more direct manipulation of the osteocartilaginous framework allowing greater accuracy in resection, repositioning, and grafting of the associated hard and soft-tissue components for esthetic and functional improvement.

The secondary cleft nasal deformity is often the most prominent hallmark of an individual with a cleft anomaly and its correction is widely regarded as one of the most challenging procedures in which to achieve consistently good results. From the earliest descriptions of the features of the cleft nose,[3] more detailed analyses emerged describing the components of soft-tissue distortion and disproportionate bony anatomy.[4] Correction of the nasal tip asymmetry in the cleft patient has been advocated at the time of primary surgery[5–7] to minimize the future deformity, but the extent of nasal dissection advocated at this first stage remains controversial. The use of presurgical nasoalveolar molding has also been promoted as a method of improving nasolabial esthetics.[8] Some surgeons are prepared to further intervene with nasal procedures at any age if the deformity is deemed to be sufficiently severe from a functional or esthetic perspective. However, others have recommended that nasal surgery be delayed until adolescence, when growth is complete. At this stage, key anatomical defects, such as displacement of the lateral crus of the alar cartilage, are then stable and can be sculpted, reinforced, and definitively repositioned to a more normal position.[8] An analysis of the deformity and an appreciation of the action of the muscular forces associated with the cleft during development explain the malposition of the tissues observed. In unilateral cases, the septum deviates towards the side of the greater segment and there is lateral displacement of the lateral crus.[9] While the asymmetry of anatomical structures is well accepted, hypoplasia of tissues associated with the cleft is less accepted but has been observed at present in specific cases, thus compounding the extent of the deformity.[10]

It has been suggested that early correction of the lateral crus on the cleft side will minimize the degree of deformity manifesting in adolescence.[11] However, depending on the severity of the cleft deformity, all or some of the features seen in the primary nasal malformation may be present at the completion of growth. Definitive correction can then be undertaken, using any or a combination of accepted rhinoplasty techniques[6,12–16] that are adapted to the specific requirements of the secondary cleft nasal deformity.[17,18] Specific techniques have been developed for the cleft patient and are directed towards overcoming the anatomical soft-tissue distortions caused by the congenital deformity. A strong osseocartilaginous framework, augmented by cartilage grafts, is required.[19,20]

In the past decade, more attention has been directed towards outcome evaluation of secondary cleft rhinoplasty with respect to esthetics, quality of life, and the perceptions of success by both patient and surgeon.[21–25]

Indications for Use of the Procedure

At the completion of growth, a high percentage of cleft patients have a persistent nasal tip asymmetry, nasal dorsal disproportion, and unilateral or bilateral airway obstruction due to the commonly deviated and distorted nasal septum. The degree of the deformity is influenced by the type of surgical intervention undertaken at primary surgery and/or the effects of growth on the distorted and scarred nasal elements. Patients who undergo earlier correction of the cleft nasal component may have a lesser deformity at maturity due to the previous release of the lateral crus from the pyriform aperture, muscle closure across the nasal floor, and repositioning of the lateral alar cartilage.[26] Despite early attempts at correction of the malpositioned structures, the common features of the cleft nose deformity include the following: excess width of the bony dorsum, collapse of the alar cartilage on the cleft side with caudal displacement of the anterior edge, and lateral displacement of the lateral crus that often manifests an inward buckling just lateral to the dome. The alar base is often flared and the nasal sill widened on the affected side (Fig. 66.1A and B).

Deviation of the columella and septum to the non-cleft side is due to the angulation of the maxillary anterior nasal spine caused by the pull of the unopposed musculature during development at the margin of the cleft. This deviation of the antero-ventral cartilaginous septum to the non-cleft side is therefore a consistent finding. The septal deflection may extend posteriorly in continuity with the vomerine septum and result in a complete posterior obstruction. The markedly deviated nasal septum is also often accompanied by a hypertrophied turbinate on the concave side with relative obstruction on the convex side due the close proximity of the adjacent contralateral turbinate. This functional disability alone is a strong indication for a septorhinoplasty, whether aesthetic concerns are present or not. There is a varying degree of depression of the pyriform aperture on the cleft side that is influenced by the presence of an untreated or a poorly grafted alveolar cleft as the volume of bone remaining after remodeling may be markedly reduced. Compounding this lack of alar support is a more pronounced maxillary hypoplasia in some clefts on the affected side.

The bilateral cleft nasal deformity is usually more symmetrical. The nasal tip is drawn ventrally with a short columella and there is a lack of tip projection due to the depressed alar cartilages in addition to the flaring of the nasal alae that have a more horizontal orientation (Fig 66.2A and B). A congenital soft-tissue deficiency has been reported in the case of bilateral cleft deformities.[27] Many patients with a bilateral deformity have a “whistle notch” deformity due to the deficient central element of the lip. The short columella is very difficult to lengthen esthetically, and rhinoplasty procedures aim to strengthen the nasal tip in order to stretch the columella and to give sufficient projection. If an Abbé flap reconstruction is planned to lengthen the lip, the second stage of flap division is an opportunity to perform an open rhinoplasty to address the tip deformity.

Limitations and Contraindications

Patient expectations regarding the degree of improvement in esthetics may be unrealistic and counseling may be useful in preparing patients for a realistic outcome. When only minimal or no dissection of the alar cartilages has been performed at primary surgery, the tissue planes are likely to be more easily negotiated due to minimal scarring. However, for patients who have undergone several full nasal procedures during growth, a more difficult dissection should be anticipated. For patients who have had minimal intervention at primary surgery, the lateral crus of the alar cartilage on the affected side may be tethered to the piriform aperture and muscle may be absent under the nasal sill. Identification of these factors is important in determining how much additional dissection will be required to free and reposition the lower lateral cartilage as well as correct contour deformities that are reflected in the overlying skin distortion. In some cases, with a legacy of multiple procedures, little improvement may be gained esthetically due to the dense accumulation of scar tissue that blankets any change to the osseocartilaginous framework.

A further major challenge is the presence of nostril stenosis, due to a shortage of soft tissue on the cleft side, that may be severe. Achieving good nostril symmetry and bilateral airway patency may not be possible without further grafting techniques for additional lining as part of the treatment plan.

A considerable percentage of cleft patients have maxillary hypoplasia. This is a combination of an intrinsic deficiency in maxillary growth and the effects of palatal scarring from the primary surgery.[28,29] The degree of maxillary deficiency manifested in each individual with a cleft will vary, depending on their underlying genetically determined skeletal pattern. The relationship of the bony foundation of the maxilla to the nasal complex has a major impact on nasal morphology. During maxillary surgery, there is an opportunity to augment the deficient pyriform aperture and to reduce the often grossly deviated maxillary crest to better facilitate the subsequent nasal surgery. The alar base width is also influenced by a cinch suture that aims to return the alar bases to the preferred position

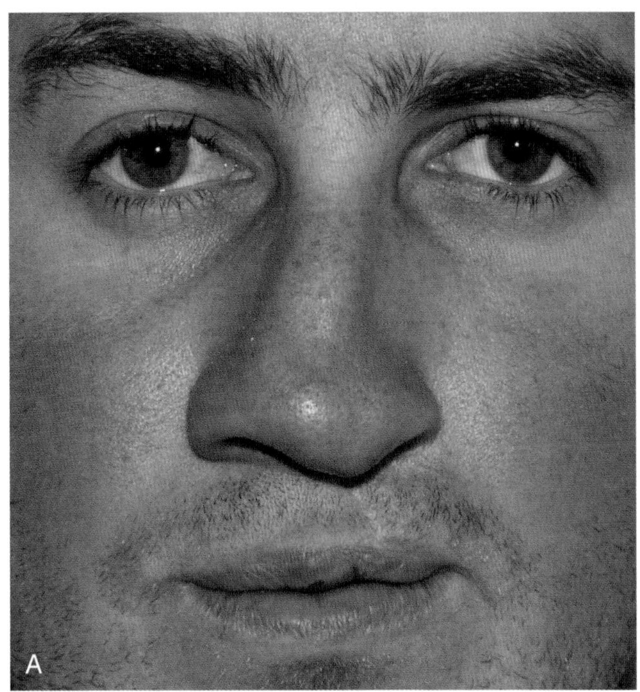

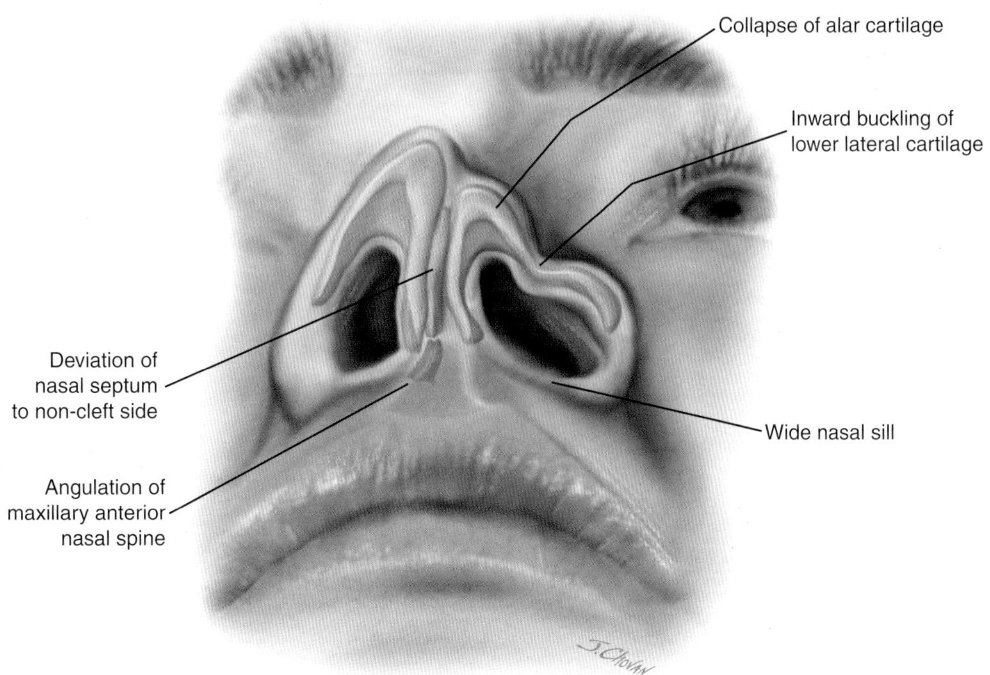

Figure 66.1 **A,** Unilateral secondary cleft nose deformity with slumping of cleft-side lower lateral cartilage. **B,** Schematic representation of lower lateral cartilages.

by reconstructing the circumoral muscular confluence onto the region of the anterior nasal spine.

Unless there are overwhelming psychological reasons for earlier treatment, nasal procedures during growth are best minimized. If orthognathic surgery is contemplated at the end of growth, lip revision and rhinoplasty should be delayed for at least 6 months to enable tissue maturity.[30] Hence, a definitive septorhinoplasty can be planned in females from around 15 to 17 years and in males from 17 to 19 years.

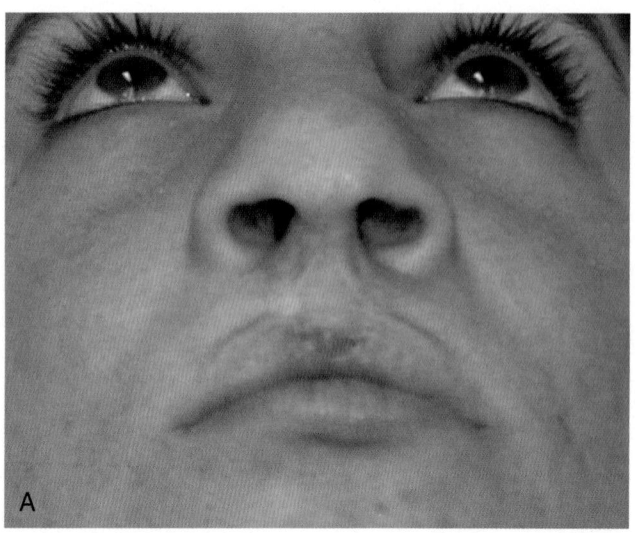

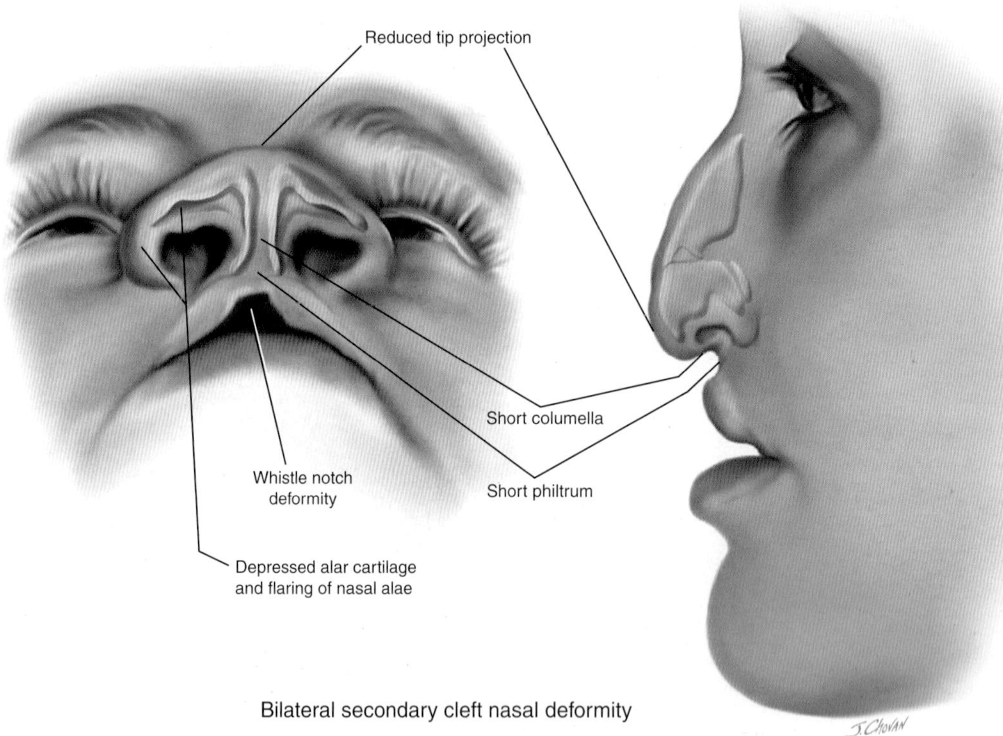

Figure 66.2 **A,** Bilateral secondary cleft nose deformity with collapse of tip and horizontal orientation of nares. **B,** Schematic representation of lower lateral cartilages.

TECHNIQUE: Secondary Cleft Rhinoplasty

STEP 1: Preparation

The patient is placed supine in a 15-degree raised head position. Preoperative intravenous dexamethasone (16 mg) and tranexamic acid (1 mg) are administered following intubation. Local anaesthetic is infiltrated (10 cc of 2% bupivacaine/ 1:100,000 epinephrine) with a 27-gauge needle into the nasal planes of dissection that should include the columella, dorsum, lateral crura, lateral nasal walls, and septal mucosae. Ribbon gauze soaked in 4 mL of 5%

TECHNIQUE: Secondary Cleft Rhinoplasty—cont'd

cocaine is then packed high into the superior nasal recesses of the nose, and the nasal vibrissae are trimmed. The eyes are protected with lubricating gel or taped shut allowing sufficient access to the inner canthal region. The nasal complex and surrounding area are then prepared with Betadine and routine draping applied.

STEP 2: Access

A "stair-step" transcolumellar incision with a #11 blade is made towards the base of the columella either just superior to the flaring of the medial crural footplates or through a previous access scar. Nasal rim incisions are then made with a #15 blade caudal to the edge of the lateral crura and are continued around to join the columella incision on each side. Using fine tenotomy scissors, the columellar flap is then carefully raised from the medial crura and over the alar domes taking care not to inadvertently damage the often thin, hypoplastic underlying cartilage. Cautery of the fine columella arteries may be required. The dissection is then developed beneath the fibromuscular/vascular layer to identify the cartilaginous septum and dorsum. The full extent of the lateral crura is exposed and any excess fatty tissue is removed between the domes (Fig 66.3A). The periosteum is then divided transversely over the bony dorsum and a subperiosteal pocket created over the nasal bones and laterally but leaving soft tissue attached at the line of the future "in-fracture". The inter-domal "ligament" is then divided to separate the lower lateral cartilages and to identify the caudal edge of the septum. Using sharp scissors or a #15 blade, the very thin subperichondrial plane is entered and elevated to expose the cartilaginous septum that has a faint bluish tinge. This plane is opened with a fine Freer elevator on each side of the septum to separate the nasal lining from the septum in the region of the internal valves to the perpendicular plate of the ethmoid (bony septum). With a #11 blade, the upper lateral cartilages are then separated bilaterally to reveal the septum (Fig. 66.3B).

STEP 3: Septoplasty

The goal for correcting a deviated nose and for providing sufficient structural support is the construction of a symmetrical robust septum. Depending on the complexity of septal distortion and/or deviation, either one or both sides are fully exposed via a subperichondrial plane. The dissection is continued down to the maxillary crest and posteriorly beyond the vomeris-cartilaginous junction in a subperiosteal plane. Care must be taken to avoid perforation, if possible, of the delicate nasal mucosa where the septal conformation deviates with sharp angles. A segment of the cartilaginous septum, leaving at least 10 mm of caudal and dorsal cartilage, is removed using a Hollenback carver that is useful as a cartilage dissector. The

Continued

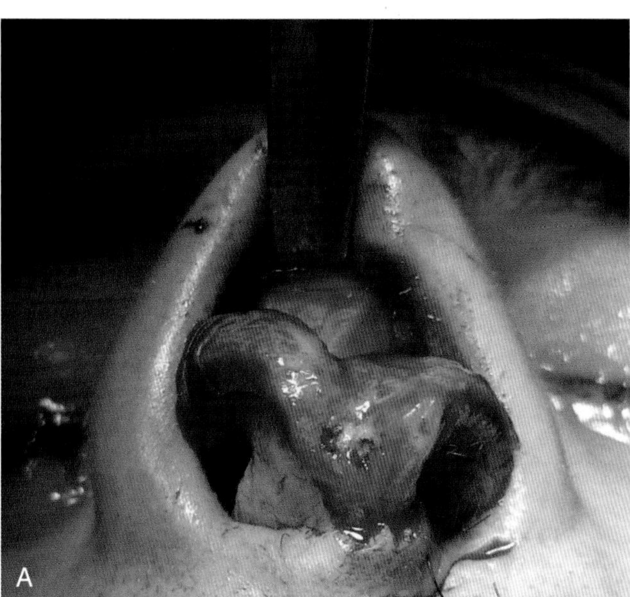

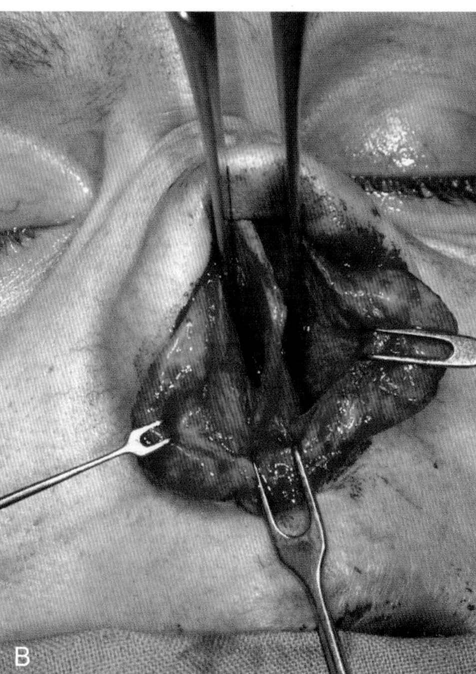

Figure 66.3 **A,** Full exposure of lower lateral cartilages. **B,** Subperichondrial dissection to expose the cartilaginous septum.

TECHNIQUE: Secondary Cleft Rhinoplasty—cont'd

harvested pieces are kept for potential use as a columella strut and for spreader grafts as required. At the region of the nasal crest, the inferior part of the septal cartilage may also require removal, together with the deviated nasal crestal bone that can be removed using a small square spatula osteotome. The anterior nasal spine is usually grossly deviated to the non-cleft side and requires reduction with an osteotome or rongeurs to free the septal connection. The septum should be able to be easily moved to either side of the midline. For a markedly deformed septum, scoring the surface or full division into strips may be necessary. In severe cases, extracorporeal reconstruction of the cartilaginous septum may be the only way to achieve a uniform construct. If there is turbinate hypertrophy compromising the nasal airways, then mucosal trimming, coblation, or lateral repositioning of the turbinate(s) may be indicated.

STEP 4: Dorsal Reduction

If reduction of a dorsal convexity is indicated, the cartilaginous septum is reduced the desired amount to the distal end of the nasal bones. With a bone file and/or nasal osteotome, the osteocartilaginous dorsal hump is then progressively reduced or removed. Minimal removal of the upper lateral cartilages is undertaken. Via intranasal stab incisions at the pyriform apertures, lateral osteotomies of the nasal bones are performed with an osteotome or sawed together with medial osteotomies to facilitate in-fracturing of the nasal bones. This is usually accomplished with finger pressure to close the "open roof" by greensticking the remaining cephalic connection at the nasofrontal articulation. However, if mobilization of a nasal plate is inadequate, a 2-mm osteotome can be introduced transcutaneously at this junction and "walked" across the area to be weakened to complete the reduction. The contour is then assessed, and any irregularities are removed with a rasp, either manually or using a raspatory handpiece.

STEP 5: Mid-Dorsum and Internal Valves

When the bony dorsal reduction is completed to the desired contour, further trimming of the septum is performed as required. The upper lateral cartilages can then be reattached to the septum with in-folding medially to preserve the internal valvular function. However, in the majority of cases this is either insufficient and spreader grafts are required to maintain the internal valves, and if indicated, to provide increased tip projection. Either septal cartilage grafts or costal cartilage is harvested and shaped into spreader grafts of approximately 2 cm in length and 3 to 4 mm in width to provide grafts of sufficient strength that together provide a uniform construct with no curvature. They are anchored between the upper lateral cartilages and the septum with 5-0 Vicryl or Monocryl sutures to maintain the integrity of the internal nasal valves and to provide a cantilever structure for tip strength (Fig 66.3C and D). A smooth transition between the bony dorsum and the mid-dorsum should be ensured.

STEP 6: Nasal Tip

The major aim in manipulating the structures that shape the nasal tip is to provide strength and stability. Depending on the support required, spreader grafts can be extended caudally and further strengthened by a columella strut that is sutured to the spreader grafts and placed in a pocket between the medial crura with or without anchorage to the anterior nasal spine by sutures or a K-wire (Fig 66.3E). This framework is then used as a support for elevating the lower lateral cartilages to the appropriate projection and/or rotation. There is a wide variation in the thickness and contour of the alar cartilages as well as asymmetry in orientation. The cleft-side lateral crus may remain tethered to the piriform aperture and it is not uncommon to observe buckles and folds in the malformed cartilage that must be dissected free before repositioning. If the non-cleft side cartilage is in a satisfactory position, then the contralateral cartilage is dissected from the underlying mucosa and rotated superiorly and sutured to match the morphology of its counterpart (Fig 66.3F). It is more common for both cartilages to require release from their soft-tissue attachments in order to shape them symmetrically against the columella strut/spreader grafts depending on the tip rotation desired. If the lateral crus is misplaced and/or short laterally, then batten grafts can be quilted to the existing cartilage and inserted into alar base soft-tissue pockets. This is often necessary to control the nostril "kink" on the cleft side. Excess tissue on the cleft side in the region of the soft triangle commonly results in nostril aperture asymmetry and despite attempts to fold in this tissue, differing nostril size often persists. A limited skin envelope of the tip together with a short columella may restrict an increase in nasal projection. More projection can be achieved by the attachment of shield grafts[16] that are carefully shaped and sutured to the junction of the domes. However, in patients with thin skin, onlay cartilage may become visible over years, so care in patient selection is important. In patients with bilateral clefts, there is less asymmetry, but often marked tip ptosis is present due to the collapsed lower lateral cartilages and a short columella. However, the principles of a strong framework to enable sufficient tip projection and support, as well as stretching of the overlying skin, remain the same.

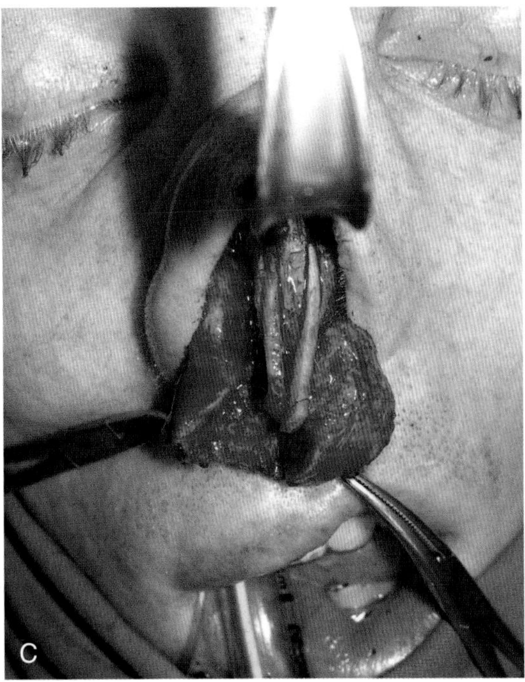

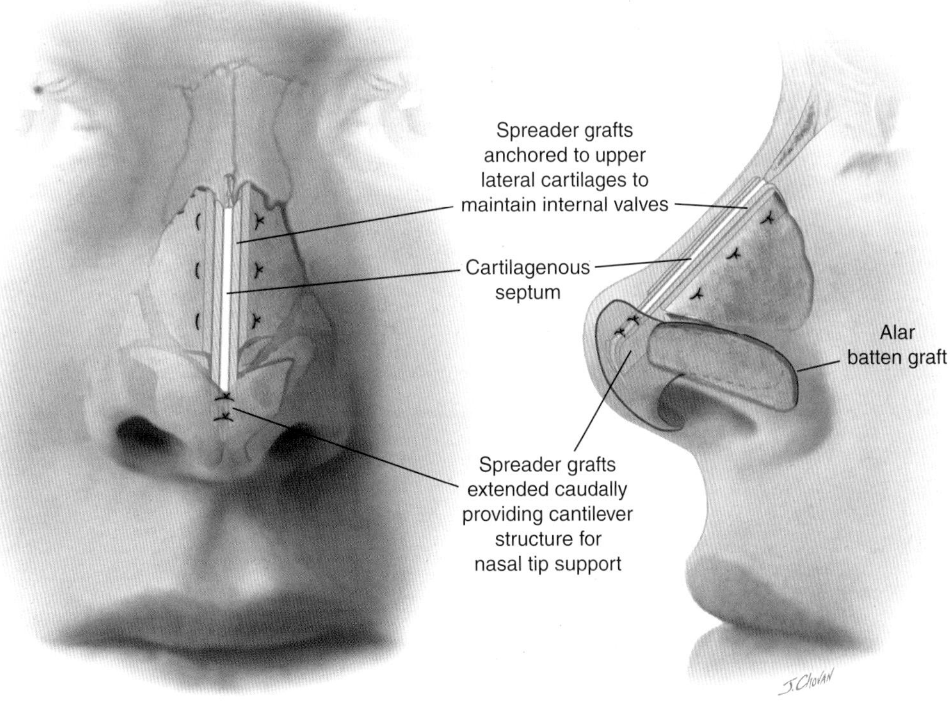

Figure 66.3, cont'd **C,** Spreader cartilage grafts to maintain internal valve function and to provide nasal tip support. **D,** Schematic diagram showing the correct orientation of spreader grafts.

Continued

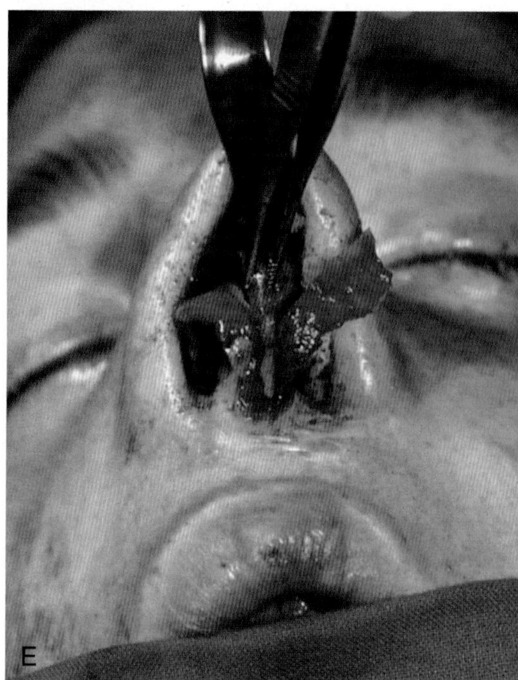

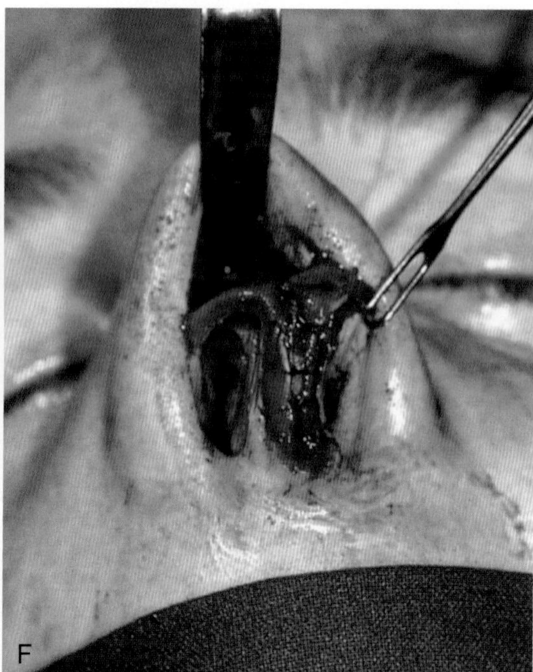

Figure 66.3, cont'd **E,** Insertion of columella strut to support the lower lateral cartilages. **F,** Repositioning and suturing of deficient alar cartilage on the cleft side.

TECHNIQUE: Secondary Cleft Rhinoplasty—cont'd

STEP 7: Wound Closure

When all maneuvers are completed, the osteocartilaginous framework is inspected for irregularities and asymmetries. If a subperichondrial layer remains, then it can be closed over the mid-dorsum. The columella incision is closed with interrupted 6-0 nylon sutures to the corner of the vestibules and 5-0 chromic catgut is used to close the internal wounds. If cartilage has been harvested, transseptal 4-0 chromic catgut quilting sutures are used to close the mucoperichondrial layer to the remaining septum and contralateral mucosa to eliminate dead space.

STEP 8: Alar Bases

If there is undesirable flaring of the nostrils, whether unilateral on the cleft side or bilateral, then alar base reduction is indicated via Weir incisions. The extent of tissue excision may need to be limited due to the potential reduction of the nasal aperture to maintain patent nasal airways.

STEP 9: Splints/Dressings

If further splinting of the septum is needed, silicon sheeting is trimmed into an ellipse and inserted on either side of the septum and sutured anteriorly for stability and later release. There are also preformed splints that permit airflow available. After application of a protective barrier wipe/adhesive across the nasal skin, 1/2-inch Steri-Strips are placed over the nasal dorsum to squeeze out and limit the accumulation of edematous fluid. They are extended to the nasal tip where further strips at right angles to shape the tip are added. A thermoplastic external splint is then applied over the Steri-Strips and supported by Elastoplast. Kaltostat "rope" is then packed into the nose to support the mucosa and a nasal gauze bolster is taped across the nares. Illustrative cases are shown in Figs. 66.4–66.6.

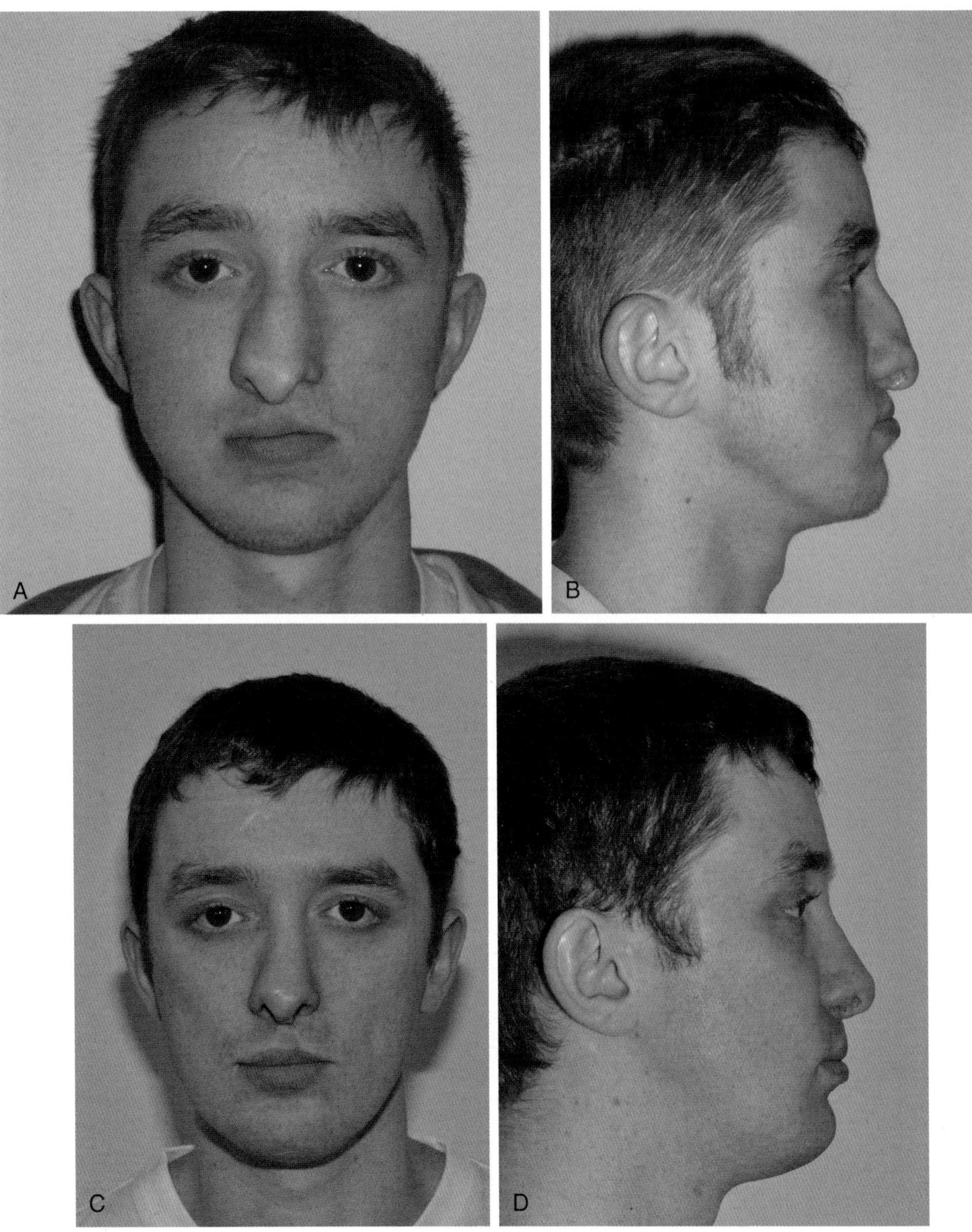

Figure 66.4 A 22-year-old male with left unilateral cleft lip and palate. Preoperative: **A,** Frontal facial view. **B,** Lateral facial view. **C,** Inferior view. Postoperative: **D,** Frontal facial view.

Continued

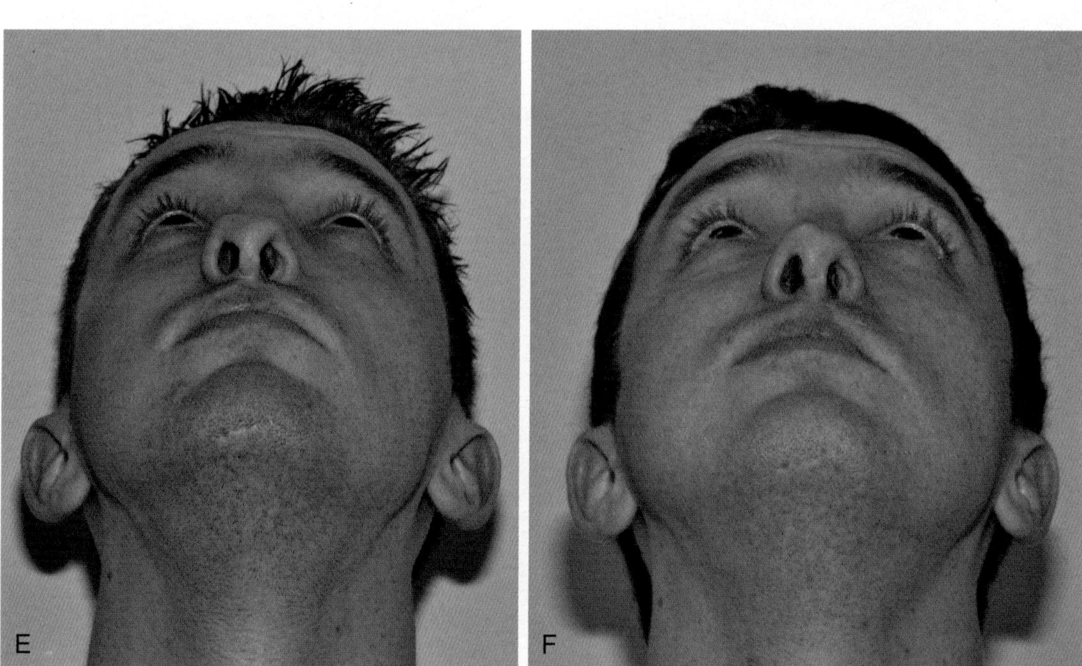

Figure 66.4, cont'd **E,** Lateral facial view. **F,** Inferior view.

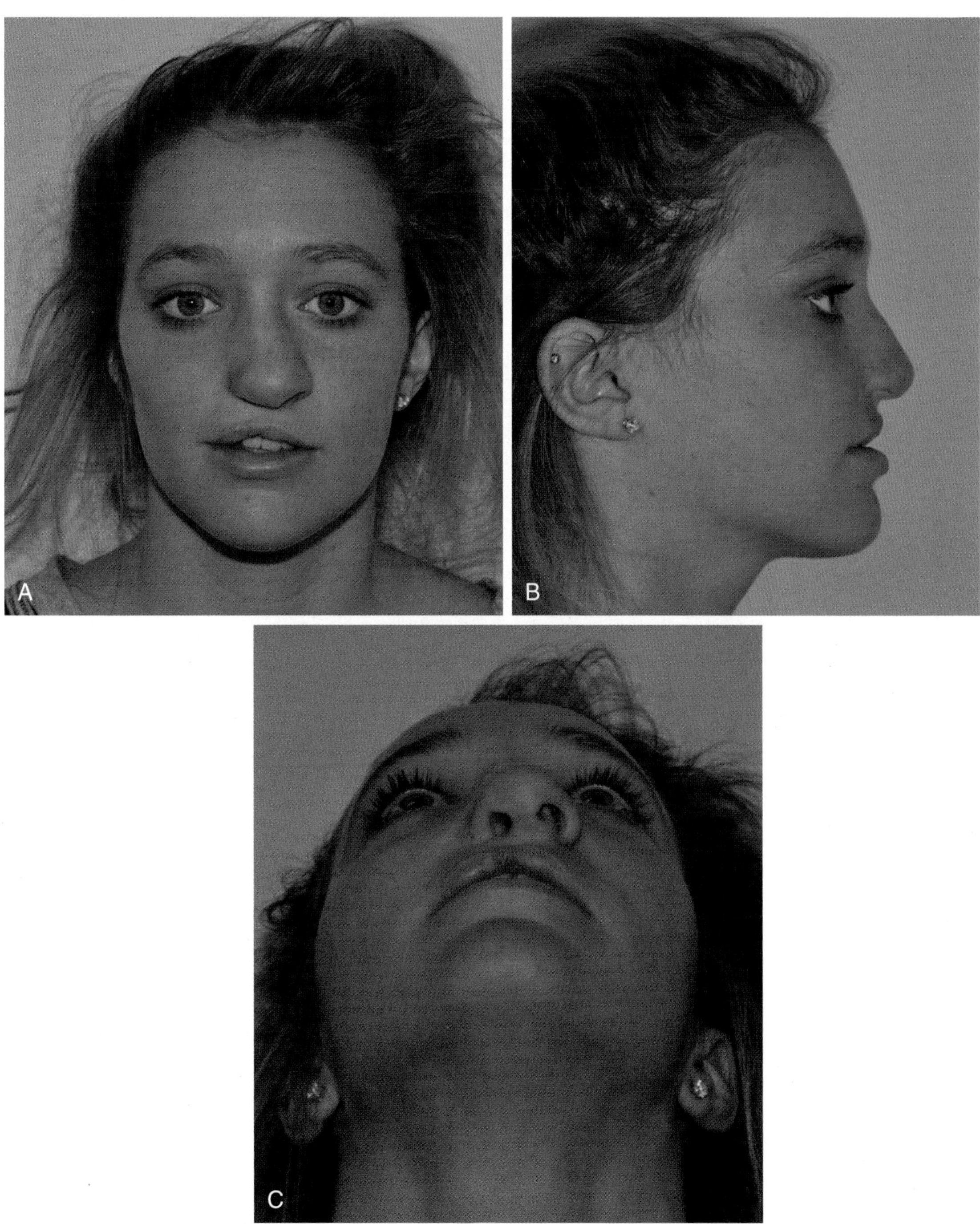

Figure 66.5 A 17-year-old female with right unilateral cleft lip and palate. Preoperative: **A,** Frontal facial view. **B,** Lateral facial view. **C,** Inferior view.

Continued

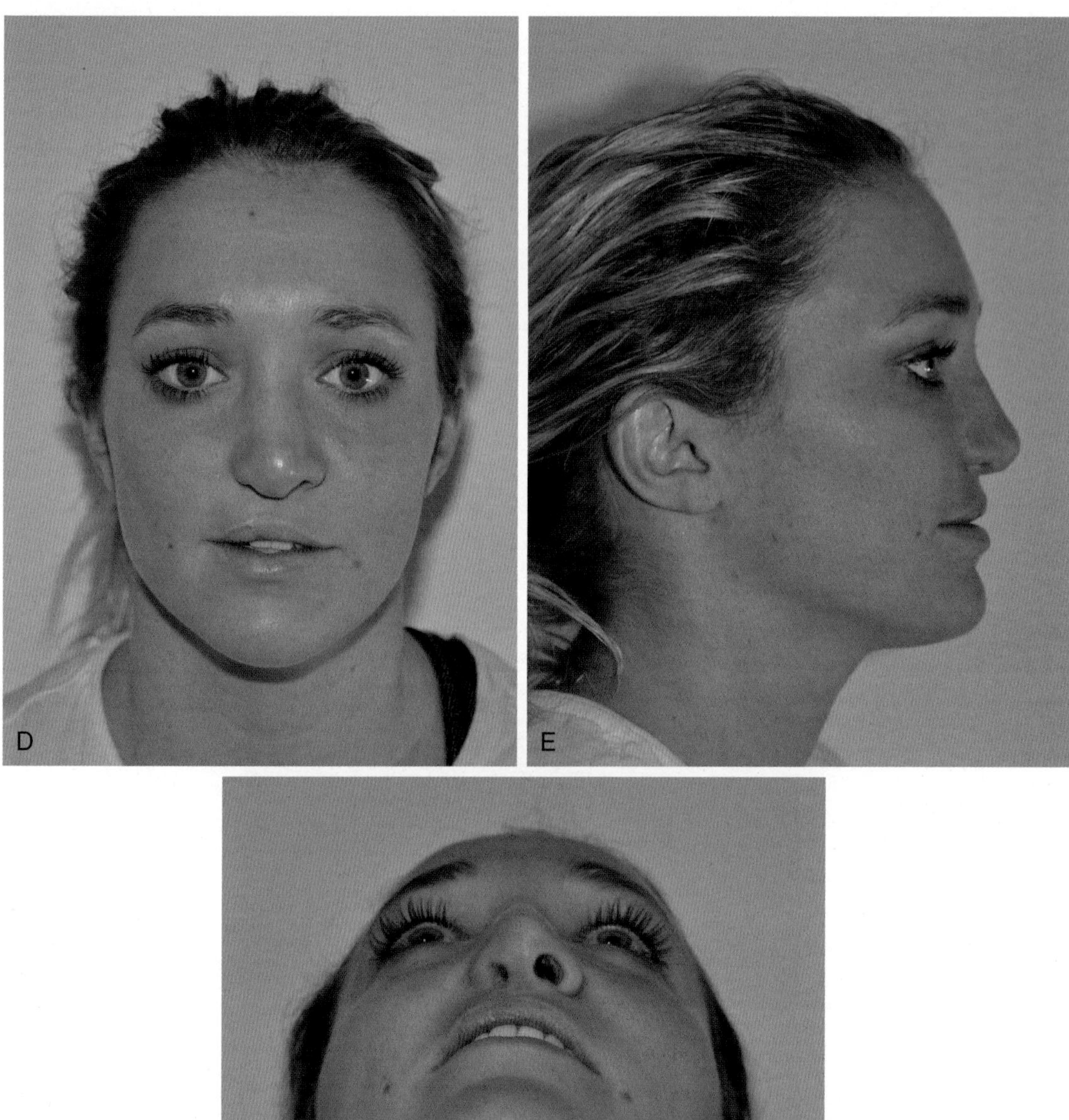

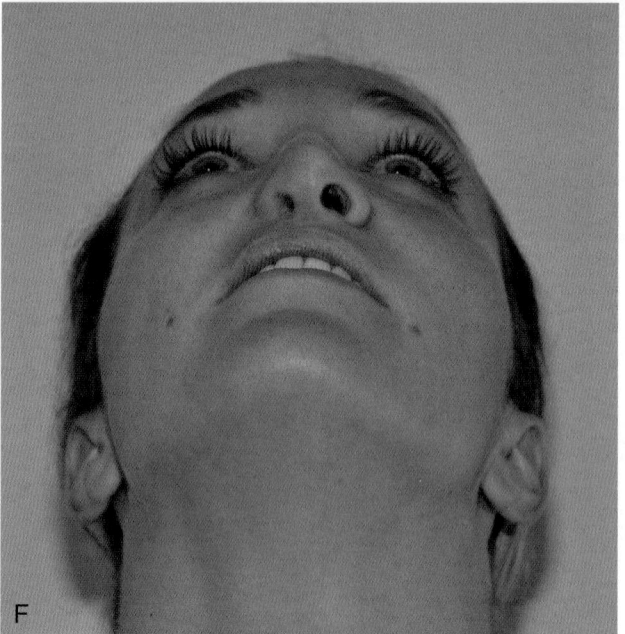

Figure 66.5, cont'd Postoperative: **D,** Frontal facial view. **E,** Lateral facial view. **F,** Inferior view.

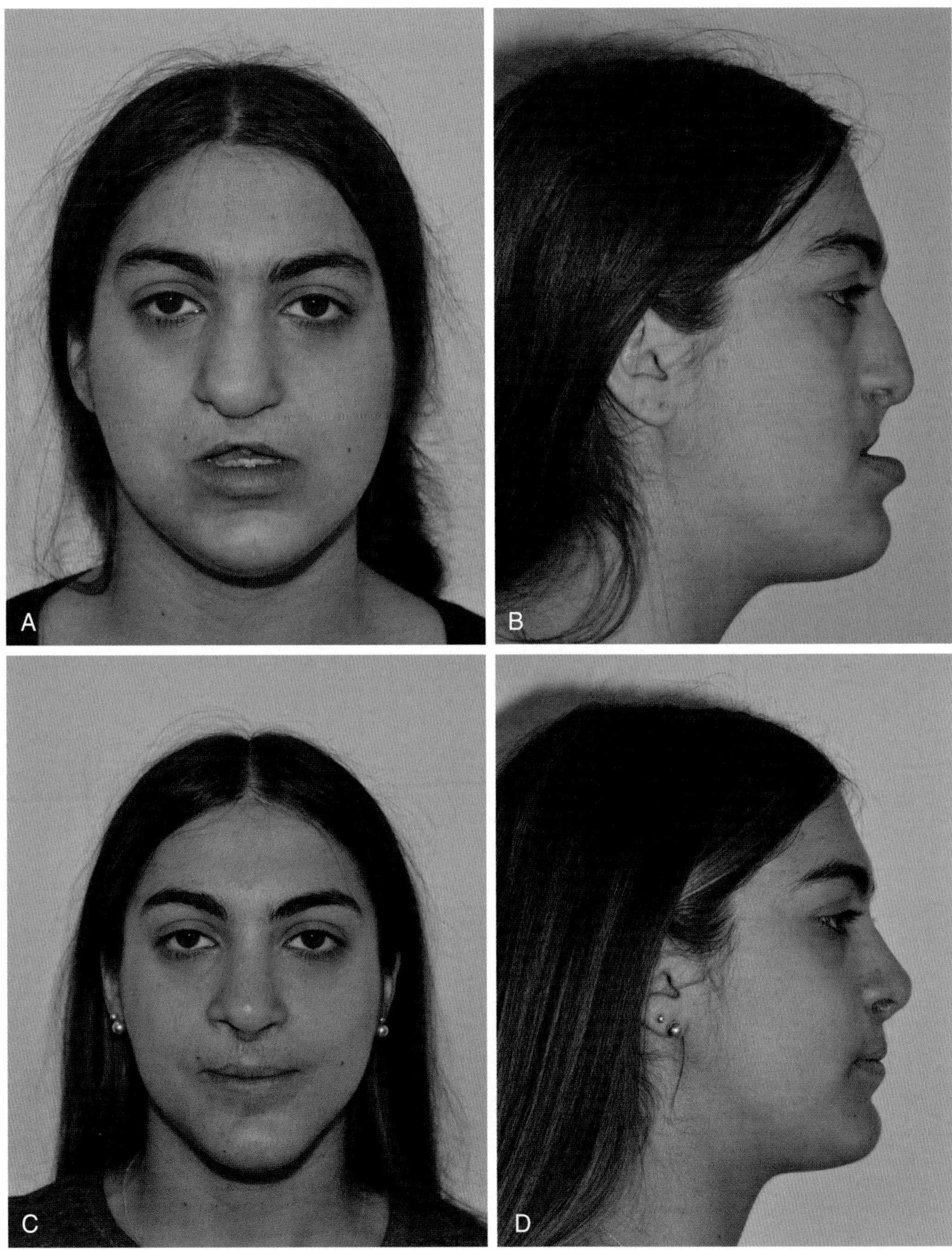

Figure 66.6 A 16-year-old female with bilateral cleft lip and palate following a two-stage maxillary advancement followed by an Abbé flap and septorhinoplasty. (The author wishes to acknowledge the involvement of Professor Tony Holmes in the management of this patient.) Preoperative: **A,** Frontal facial view. **B,** Lateral facial view. Postoperative: **C,** Frontal facial view. **D,** Lateral facial view.

Alternate Technique

Where the dorsum is low and the nasal tip is markedly ptotic due to weak lower lateral cartilages, a stronger cantilever rib graft is occasionally indicated. A segment from the 9th to the 11th rib, where the contour is straighter, is preferable and this is shaped to onlay the dorsum. This requires a degree of dorsal reduction to accommodate the bony portion to the nasofrontal junction. After ascertaining preoperatively that a frontal sinus is present, a tunnel into the frontal bone is prepared with a pineapple-shaped bur up to the sinus membrane. A peg shape is formed on the cephalic end of the graft after the length required is established for tip support. The graft is inserted as a dowel into the tunnel until sufficiently rigid and in a symmetrical position. The chondral end is then thinned to serve as the strut onto which the lower lateral cartilages are attached. The upper lateral cartilages can be attached to the periosteum remaining on the side of the rib. This is a powerful construct and very effective in projecting and straightening a collapsed tip complex but has the disadvantage if a rigid nose to the tip (Fig 66.7).

Avoidance and Management of Intraoperative Complications

There are very few intraoperative complications during rhinoplasty, but success is more dependent on good judgement of tissue repositioning, appropriate grafting, and judicious excision to achieve the desired morphology. Hemostasis is relatively easy to control with an open approach. Care must be exercised during the elevation of the columella skin from the

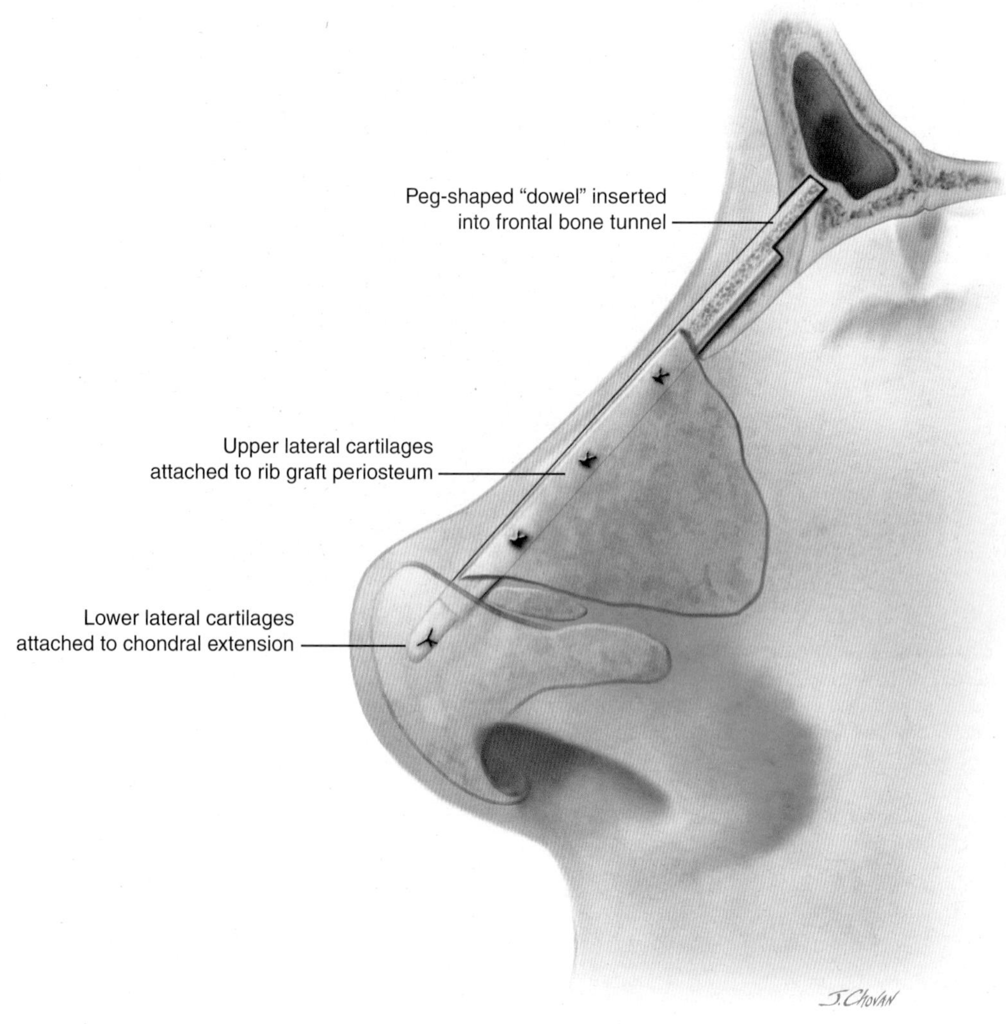

Figure 66.7 Schematic diagram of costo-chondral rib graft inserted as an inlay/onlay to provide more rigid support to the dorsum and nasal tip.

medial crura as damage to the lower lateral cartilages can easily occur. If inadvertently lacerated, the crura can be repaired with 5-0 Vicryl on a tapered needle. While the nasal skin is well perfused, care must be taken not to dissect the columella layer too superficially, particularly when scarring is present from previous surgery. Skin necrosis is a known complication, particularly with wide lateral dissection and loss of the lateral alar vessel perfusion.

It is important to maintain the plane deep to the fibromuscular/vascular layer when exposing the osteo-cartilaginous dorsum to reduce bleeding and subsequent scar formation. It may take time to locate the correct plane before elevating the mucoperichondrium cleanly to expose the septum for repositioning or harvesting a graft. Perforation of the septal mucosa may easily occur during elevation due to sharp contours of the septum, particularly in regions of scarring from previous trauma or surgery. It is difficult to close perforations intranasally, but repair can be attempted with fine needle holders and 4-0 chromic catgut.

Osteotomies of the nasal bones may result in avulsion of bony segments that may collapse and require additional intranasal splinting. Completion of lateral naso-maxillary bone in-fractures may be indicated using 2-mm transcutaneous osteotomes, particularly if a "rocker" deformity occurs. When increasing tip projection, it is important to redrape the soft tissues to determine if there is excessive skin blanching from tension over the lower lateral cartilages that may result in skin breakdown.

Postoperative Considerations

On return to the recovery room, the patient should remain in a head-up position, when conscious, with cold gauze packs placed over the eyes to reduce periorbital hematomas from the nasal osteotomies. Analgesia, antiinflammatory drugs, and a course of prophylactic antibiotic therapy are initiated. Nasal packing is normally removed on the first postoperative day with suture removal from the columella between 4 and 6 days. Patients are instructed to keep activity at a minimum for the first week and to clean their nostrils with cotton buds dipped in 3% hydrogen peroxide. Septal splints and the dorsal thermoplastic splint and Steri-Strips are removed at 7 to 10 days. Further, Steri-Strips are placed over the dorsum for an additional 5 to 7 days.

References

1. Rethi A. Uber die korrecktiven operationen der nasendeformitaten. I. *Die Hockerabtragung Chirurgie*. 1929;1:1103.
2. Potter J. Some nasal tip deformities due to alar cartilage abnormalities. *Plast Reconstr Surg*. 1954;13(5):358–366.
3. Blair VP. Nasal deformities associated with the congenital cleft of the lip. *J Am Med Assoc*. 1925;84:185.
4. Gorney MK. Cleft lip and nose. In: Stark RB, ed. *Plastic Surgery of the Head and Neck*. New York, NY: Churchill Livingstone; 1987.
5. McComb H. Primary correction of unilateral cleft lip nasal deformity: a 10-year review. *Plast Reconstr Surg*. 1985;75(6):791–799.
6. Trott JA, Mohan N. A preliminary report on one stage open tip rhinoplasty at the time of lip repair in bilateral cleft lip and palate: the Alor Setar experience. *Br J Plast Surg*. 1993;46(3):215–222.
7. Thomas C. Primary rhinoplasty by open approach with repair of unilateral complete cleft lip. *J Craniofac Surg*. 2009;20(suppl 2):1711–1714.
8. Bonanthaya K, Nayak T, Bitra S, Rachwalski M, Shetty PN. An assessment and comparison of nasolabial aesthetics in bilateral clefts using the anatomical subunit-based scale: a nasoalveolar moulding versus non-nasoalveolar moulding study. *Int J Oral Maxillofac Surg*. 2019;48(3):298–301.
9. Cronin TD, Denkler KA. Correction of the unilateral cleft lip nose. *Plast Reconstr Surg*. 1988;82(3):419–432.
10. McComb HK, Coghlan BA. Primary repair of the unilateral cleft lip nose: completion of a longitudinal study. *Cleft Palate Craniofac J*. 1996;33(1):23–30.
11. Musgrave RH. Surgery of nasal deformities associated with cleft lip. *Plast Reconstr Surg Transplant Bull*. 1961;28:261–275.
12. Byrd HS, Salomon J. Primary correction of the unilateral cleft nasal deformity. *Plast Reconstr Surg*. 2000;106(6):1276–1286.
13. Nolst Trenité GJ, Paping RH, Trenning AH. Rhinoplasty in the cleft lip patient. *Cleft Palate Craniofac J*. 1997;34(1):63–68.
14. Rohrich RJ, Hoxworth RE, Kurkjian TJ. The role of the columellar strut in rhinoplasty: indications and rationale. *Plast Reconstr Surg*. 2012;129(1):118e–125e.
15. Gunter JP, Friedman RM. Lateral crural strut graft: technique and clinical applications in rhinoplasty. *Plast Reconstr Surg*. 1997;99(4):943–952.
16. Tebbetts JB. Shaping and positioning the nasal tip without structural disruption: a new, systematic approach. *Plast Reconstr Surg*. 1994;94(1):61–77.
17. Sheen JH. Tip graft: a 20-year retrospective. *Plast Reconstr Surg*. 1993;91(1):48–63.
18. Salyer KE. Early and late treatment of unilateral cleft nasal deformity. *Cleft Palate Craniofac J*. 1992;29(6):556–569.
19. Guyuron B. MOC-PS(SM) CME article: late cleft lip nasal deformity. *Plast Reconstr Surg*. 2008;121(suppl 4):1–11.
20. Cuzalina A, Jung C. Rhinoplasty for the cleft lip and palate patient. *Oral Maxillofac Surg Clin North Am*. 2016;28(2):189–202.
21. Roosenboom J, Hellings PW, Picavet VA, et al. Secondary cleft rhinoplasty: impact on self-esteem and quality of life. *Plast Reconstr Surg*. 2014;134(6):1285–1292.
22. Gassling V, Koos B, Birkenfeld F, Wiltfang J, Zimmermann CE. Secondary cleft nose rhinoplasty: subjective and objective outcome evaluation. *J Craniomaxillofac Surg*. 2015;43(9):1855–1862.
23. Pausch NC, Unger C, Pitak-Arnnop P, Subbalekha K. Nasal appearance after secondary cleft rhinoplasty: comparison of professional rating with patient satisfaction. *Oral Maxillofac Surg*. 2016;20(2):195–201.
24. van Zijl FVWJ, Versnel S, van der Poel EF, Baatenburg de Jong RJ, Datema FR. Use of routine prospective functional and aesthetic patient satisfaction measurements in secondary cleft rhinoplasty. *JAMA Facial Plast Surg*. 2018;20(6):488–494.
25. Agochukwu-Nwubah N, Boustany A, Vasconez HC. Cleft rhinoplasty study and evolution. *J Craniofac Surg*. 2019;30(5):1430–1434.
26. Byrd HS, El-Musa KA, Yazdani A. Correction of secondary unilateral cleft lip and nose deformity. In: Losee JE, Kirschner RE, eds. *Comprehensive Cleft Care*. New York, NY: McGraw Hill; 2009.
27. Stark RB, Kaplan JM. Development of the cleft lip nose. *Plast Reconstr Surg*. 1973;51(4):413–415.
28. Liao YF, Mars M. Long-term effects of palate repair on craniofacial morphology in patients with unilateral cleft lip and palate. *Cleft Palate Craniofac J*. 2005;42(6):594–600.
29. Liao YF, Mars M. Long-term effects of clefts on craniofacial morphology in patients with unilateral cleft lip and palate. *Cleft Palate Craniofac J*. 2005;42(6):601–609.
30. Wolford LM. Effects of orthognathic surgery on nasal form and function in the cleft patient. *Cleft Palate Craniofac J*. 1992;29(6):546–555.

CHAPTER 67

Cleft Le Fort Osteotomy

Nabil Samman

Armamentarium

#15 and #10 Blades
Appropriate sutures
Calipers
Curved pterygoid osteotome
Double-guarded nasal osteotome
Freer double-ended elevator/retractor
Head ring
Langenbeck retractors
Local anesthetic with vasoconstrictor
Lindeman burs
Malleable retractors
Metzenbaum and curved Mayo scissors
Monopolar and bipolar diathermy
Obwegeser periosteal elevators
Plates and screws
Reciprocating saw
Rongeurs, double-action
Rowe forceps
Straight osteotomes 7 and 10 mm

History of the Procedure

Le Fort I osteotomy for the correction of maxillary hypoplasia in a cleft palate patient is reported to have been first performed by Axhausen in 1939, but the operation was improved by Schuchardt who added the posterior dysjunction procedure that enabled the necessary mobilization of the pedicled maxilla.[1] Scarring and possible obliteration of the greater palatine arteries as a result of earlier cleft palate repair gave rise to concerns about the blood supply of the down-fractured cleft maxilla through a buccal incision, but the seminal work of William H. Bell demonstrated the safety of the Le Fort I osteotomy.[2] Modifications of the Le Fort I technique were developed to enable differential movement of the maxillary segments and closure of dental gaps both in unilateral and bilateral clefts[3–6] and simultaneous grafting of the alveolar clefts.[7] When nasomaxillary hypoplasia is present, Henderson and Jackson proposed a Le Fort II osteotomy.[8]

Indications for the Use of the Procedure

A sizable proportion of repaired cleft lip and palate patients—unilateral cleft lip and palate (UCLP), bilateral cleft lip and palate (BCLP), and isolated cleft palate patients—present with variable degrees of maxillary growth deficiency or maxillary hypoplasia. Correction of these deformities by orthognathic surgery is a standard of care but is considered by many to be difficult to perform in terms of surgical movement due to scarring and in terms of risks to the blood supply of mobilized segments. This chapter addresses specific descriptions of the maxillary and midface surgery in cleft patients; however, considerations concerning the mandible in cases of bimaxillary skeletal corrections are beyond the scope of this chapter.

Maxillary Hypoplasia

The commonly encountered maxillary hypoplasia is a three-dimensional deformity: retrusion (horizontal plane), shortening (vertical plane), and collapse (transverse plane). Unilateral and bilateral alveolar clefts will be present in UCLP and BCLP, respectively, and may or may not have been bone grafted prior to orthognathic surgery. A Le Fort I osteotomy with relevant modifications is indicated.

Nasomaxillary Hypoplasia

In some patients, the nasal pyramid is deficient in length, projection, or both; this is in addition to the hypoplasia of the dentoalveolar complex. A Le Fort II osteotomy with modifications is indicated in such cases. When the anticipated correction of the nasal pyramid and dentoalveolar complex require differential movement to achieve the overall facial correction, a two-stage procedure is planned (Le Fort II followed some months later by Le Fort I).

Limitations and Contraindications

Surgical movement of the cleft maxilla after osteotomy is limited by a variable degree of tissue scarring in the repaired palate. Adequate mobilization of the maxilla is therefore essential and requires patience to achieve the maximum possible stretching of tissues without tearing. If the required surgical movement is extensive and considered beyond the reach of on-table achievement, a gradual distraction protocol of the Le Fort I may be planned[9] (description beyond the scope of this chapter).

Grafting of alveolar clefts in the mixed dentition permits arch alignment and elimination of interdental gaps orthodontically before orthognathic surgery.[10–11] If grafting results in an adequate bony bridge with good soft tissue coverage and no oronasal fistula, a standard Le Fort I down-fracture through a buccal incision is employed. However, if the result of such grafting is inadequate and a dental gap or fistula remains, osteotomy and differential segment movement to close or control the dimension of the dental gap with simultaneous alveolar cleft grating are possible in both unilateral and bilateral cleft situations.

If the bilateral alveolar clefts exhibit an inadequate bony bridge after grafting, or if a fistula is present palatally in association with the alveolar clefts, a maxillary down-fracture approach through a full buccal incision is contraindicated as a danger to the vascular supply of the premaxilla. Here a modification of technique is employed.

However, these osteotomies and simultaneous alveolar cleft grafts can only be done at the Le Fort I level. If the skeletal deformity requires a Le Fort II operation, alveolar cleft grafting is preferred before the procedure.

TECHNIQUE: Le Fort I Osteotomy—UCLP Ungrafted Alveolar Cleft

STEP 1: Incision

After infiltration of the mucosa with lidocaine (Xylocaine) and epinephrine, an incision is made in the upper labial mucosa to the level of the orbicularis muscle. The blade is then angled parallel to the muscle and taken through submucosal tissue and periosteum to bone. Incision extends from the second premolar to the contralateral equivalent but dips down in the alveolar cleft region to enable access to the bony edges of the cleft. Subperiosteal exposure of bone extends from one tuberosity to the other. The piriform aperture and the base of the nasal septum are exposed. The nasal mucosa is raised away from the alveolar cleft to expose the bony edges (Fig. 67.1A).

Continued

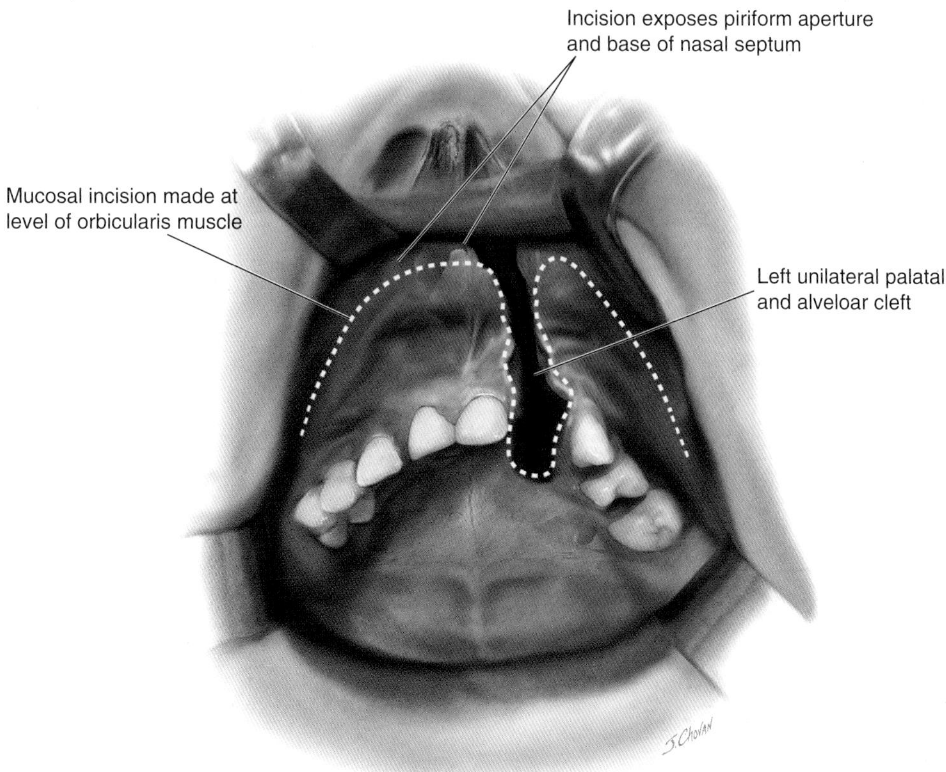

Figure 67.1 **A,** Mucosal incision from premolar to premolar dips down to the alveolar cleft to expose alveolar bony edges.

TECHNIQUE: Le Fort I Osteotomy—UCLP Ungrafted Alveolar Cleft—cont'd

STEP 2: Osteotomy

With the oscillating saw, a standard Le Fort I bone cut is made on the buccal bone surface of the major segment and minor segment. Lateral nasal wall osteotomies are completed with a 7-mm straight osteotome. The nasal septum is detached from the maxillary crest with the double-guarded nasal osteotome. Posterior tuberosity dysjunction is completed using the curved pterygoid osteotome (Fig. 67.1B).

STEP 3: Down-Fracture

The maxilla is down-fractured in two segments after sharp detachment of the repaired nasal mucosa from the palatal mucosa in the region of the deficient palatal bone shelves. Care is taken to ensure that the repaired palatal mucosa is not perforated (Fig. 67.1C).

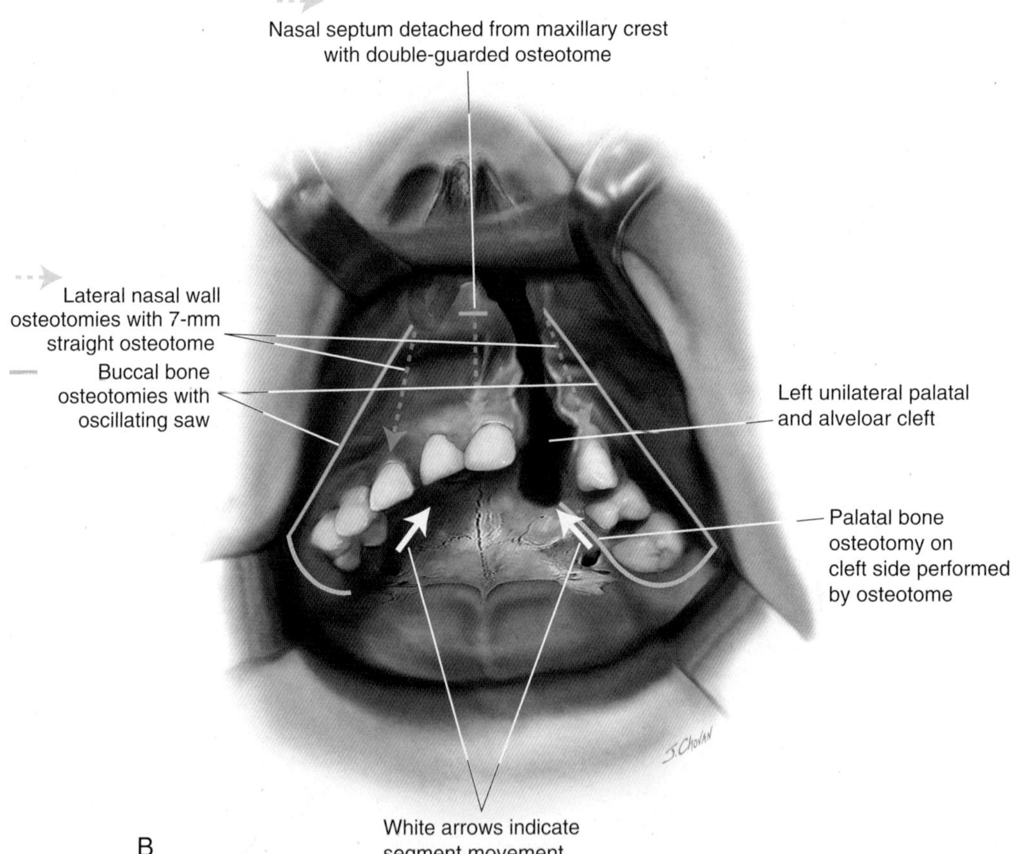

Figure 67.1,cont'd B, Maxillary osteotomies at Le Fort I level and base of septum.

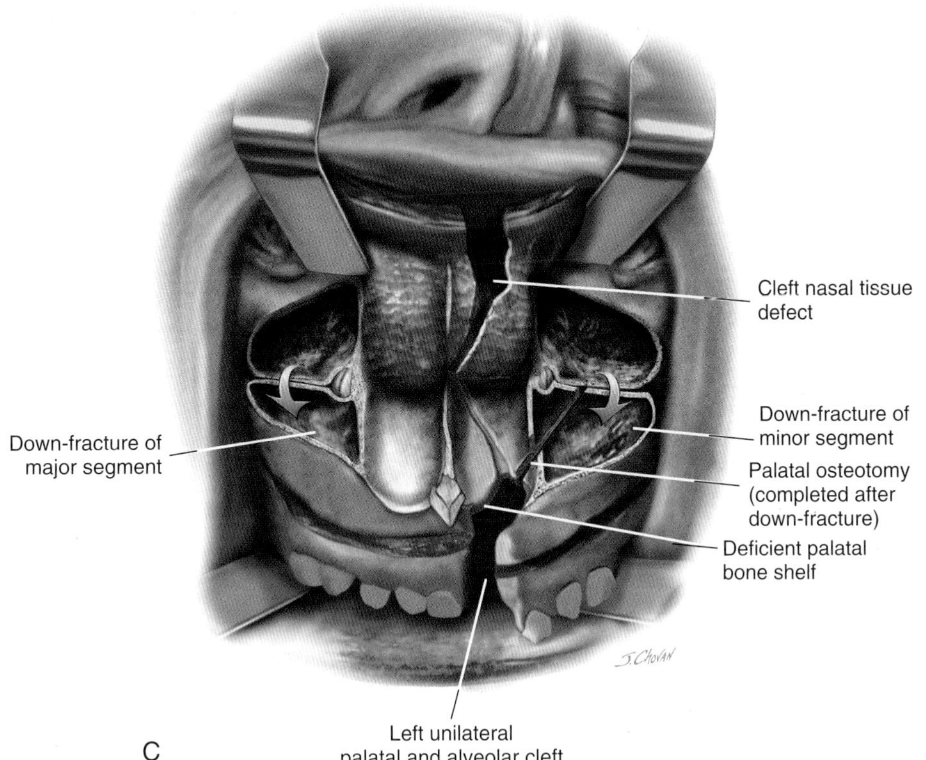

Figure 67.1,cont'd C, Maxilla down-fractured after carefully separating the nasal mucosa from the mucosa of the repaired palate.

TECHNIQUE: Le Fort I Osteotomy—UCLP Ungrafted Alveolar Cleft—cont'd

STEP 4: Mobilization

The curved pterygoid osteotome is inserted at the site of tuberosity disjunction with one hand while the thumb and the forefinger of the other hand are placed at the contralateral canine region. Force is applied through the curved osteotome forward and downward to stretch tissue and slowly mobilize the maxilla against the protective support of the fingers of the other hand. The action is repeated several times on each side until the required movement is achieved without tension. Rowe disimpaction forceps are seldom used because of the danger of tearing the palatal mucosa (Fig. 67.1D).

STEP 5: Fixation

Once the maxillary segments reach and fit into the occlusal wafer (splint), the nasal mucosa is sutured and temporary intermaxillary fixation enables plating the maxilla in the planned position.

STEP 6: Grafting and Closure

With the nasal mucosa closed and bony segments plated in position, the alveolar cleft is grafted with a suitable bone graft harvested from an autogenous site able to provide the required volume of graft. Mucosal closure is completed with attention given to covering the bone graft (Fig. 67.1E–G).

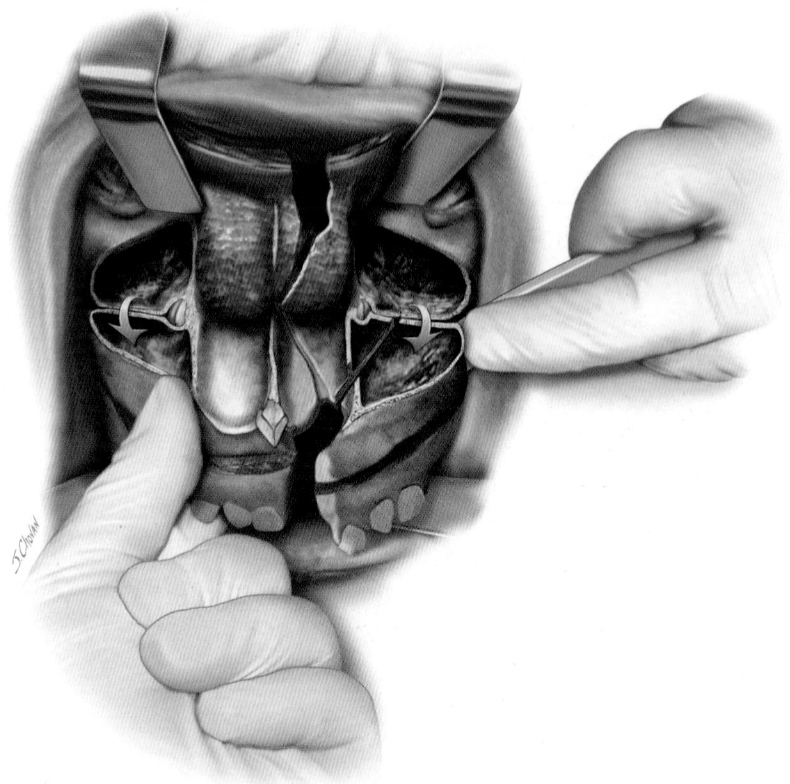

D

Plated bony segments

Closure of nasal mucosa

E

Autogenous bone graft of alveolar cleft

Maxillary segments fitted into occlusal wafer (splint)

Figure 67.1, cont'd D, Segment(s) mobilized slowly using the pterygoid (curved) osteotome posteriorly and the surgeon's fingers anteriorly to stretch the soft tissues.

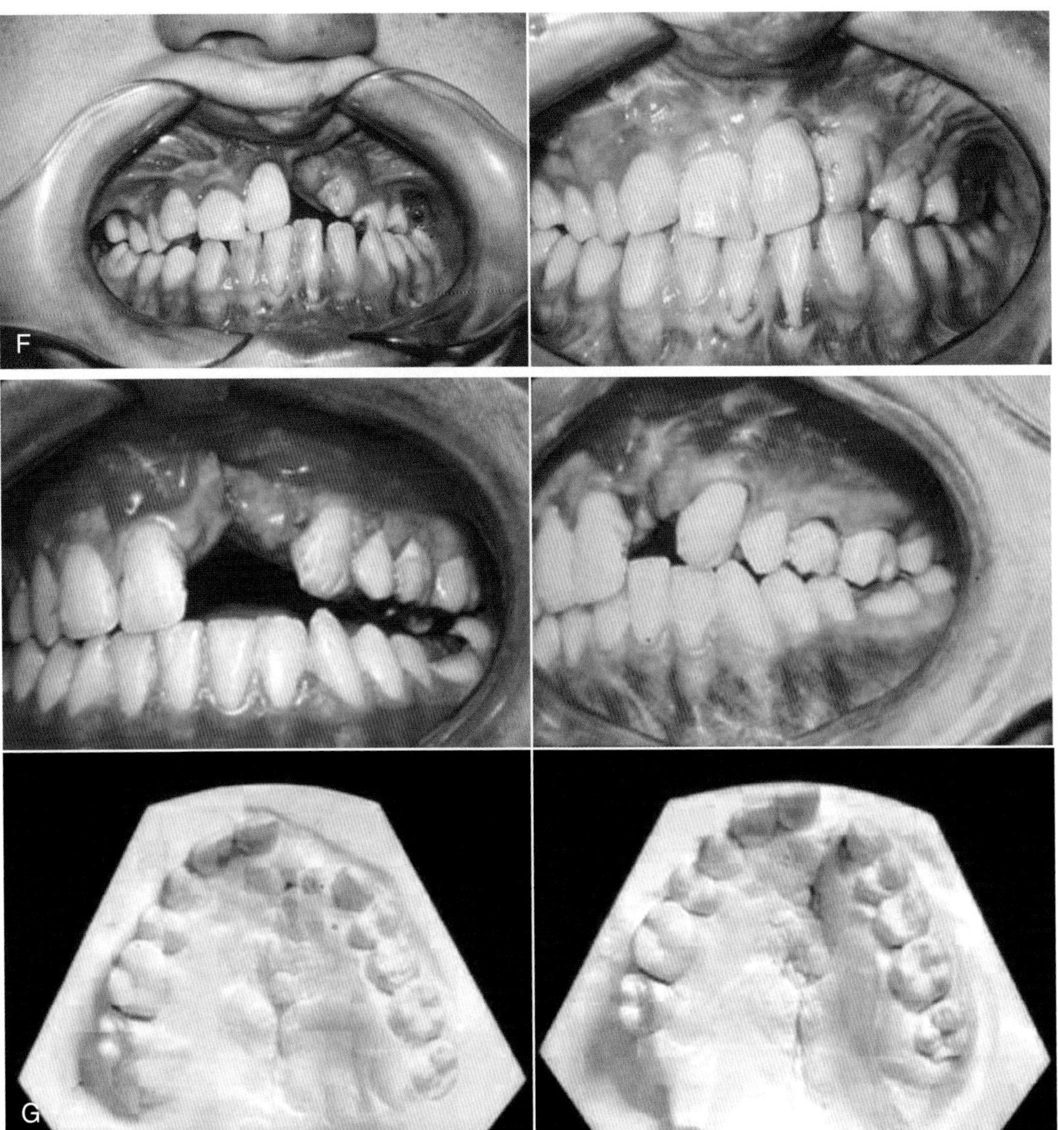

Figure 67.1, cont'd **E–G,** Differential movement of segments permits control of dental gap (complete closure or diminution).

TECHNIQUE: Le Fort I Osteotomy—BCLP Ungrafted Alveolar Clefts

STEP 1: Incision

Because the blood supply to the premaxilla from the palatal mucosa alone is likely to be inadequate, the previously described total buccal incision is taken palatally posterior to the premaxilla and continued on the contralateral buccal side instead of straight across the buccal aspect of the premaxilla. This ensures full attachment of the premaxilla to the buccal soft tissue pedicle (Fig. 67.2A).

STEP 2: Osteotomy

The premaxillary segment is out-fractured by a curved osteotome placed behind the incisive foramen area against the vomer bone and tapped at an angle to achieve a fracture of the premaxillary segment, which remains well pedicled on the buccal soft tissues. This segment is out-fractured and held out while the posterior segment osteotomies are completed on each side in a manner similar to that used for the lesser segment of the unilateral cleft (Fig. 67.2B).

Continued

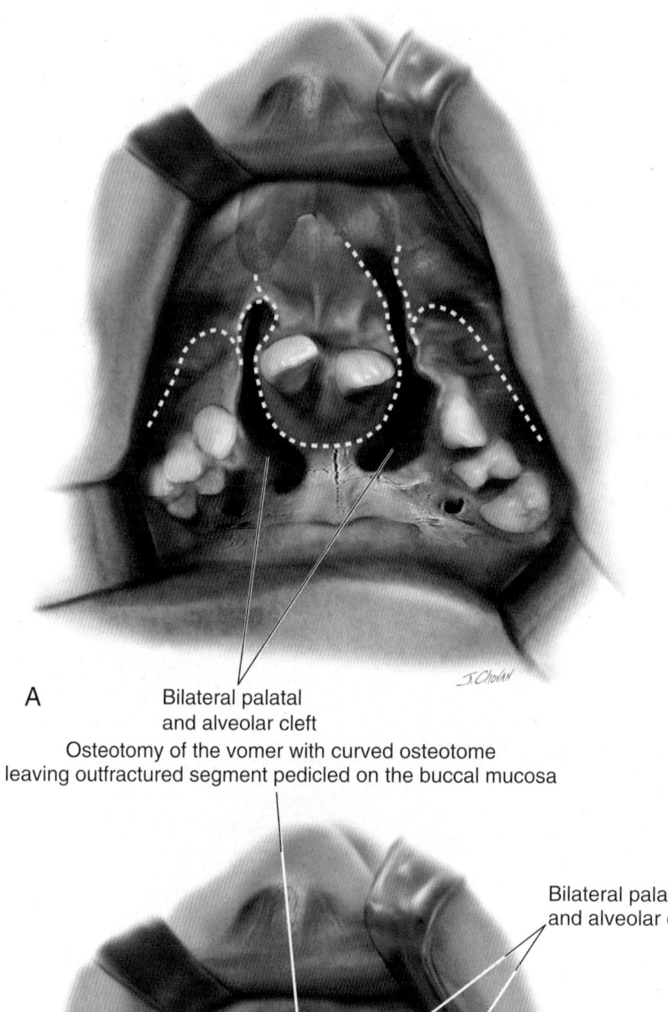

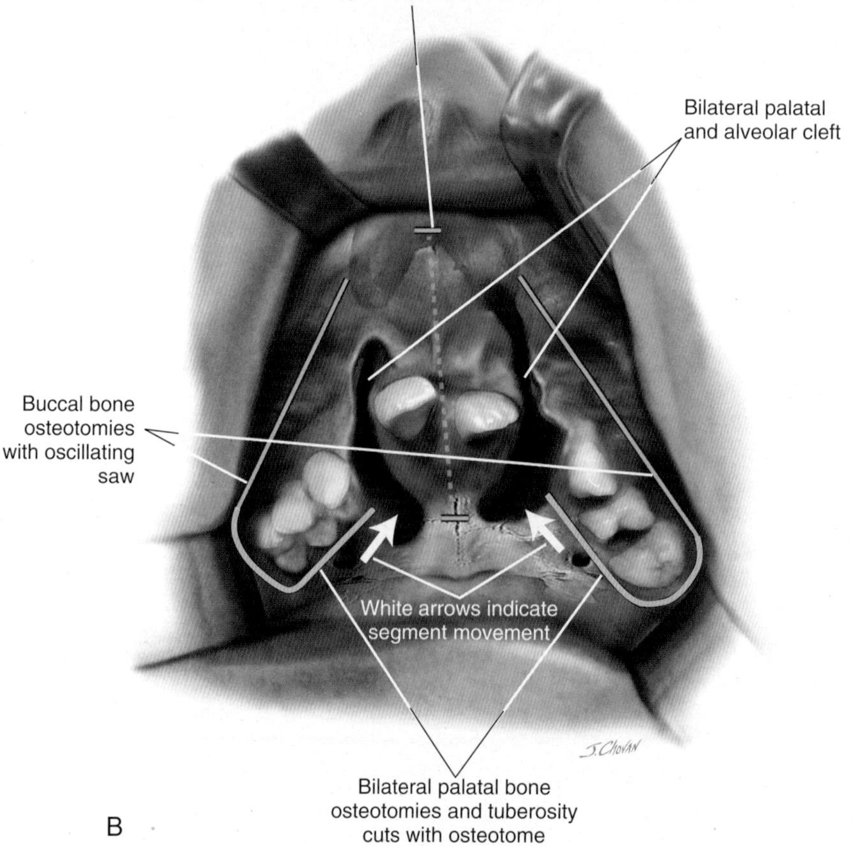

Figure 67.2 **A,** Soft tissue incision from second premolar to second premolar passing posterior (distal) to premaxilla to retain an intact buccal mucosal pedicle. **B,** Premaxillary osteotomy and outfracture retaining the buccal pedicle attachment of the premaxilla segment.

TECHNIQUE: Le Fort I Osteotomy—BCLP Ungrafted Alveolar Clefts—cont'd

STEP 3: Down-Fracture

With the premaxilla retracted upward, both posterior segments are down-fractured as previously described and mobilized separately into the desired position in the occlusal wafer (Fig. 67.2C).

STEP 4: Fixation

After suturing the nasal mucosa on both sides, the posterior segments are placed in the occlusal wafer and the premaxillary segment is brought back from its out-fractured position into the wafer to complete the arch. Posterior segments are plated; the premaxilla is not plated but rather fixed by attachment through brackets and arch wire to the occlusal wafer, which is ligated to the teeth and kept in situ for 4 to 6 weeks (Fig. 67.2D).

Continued

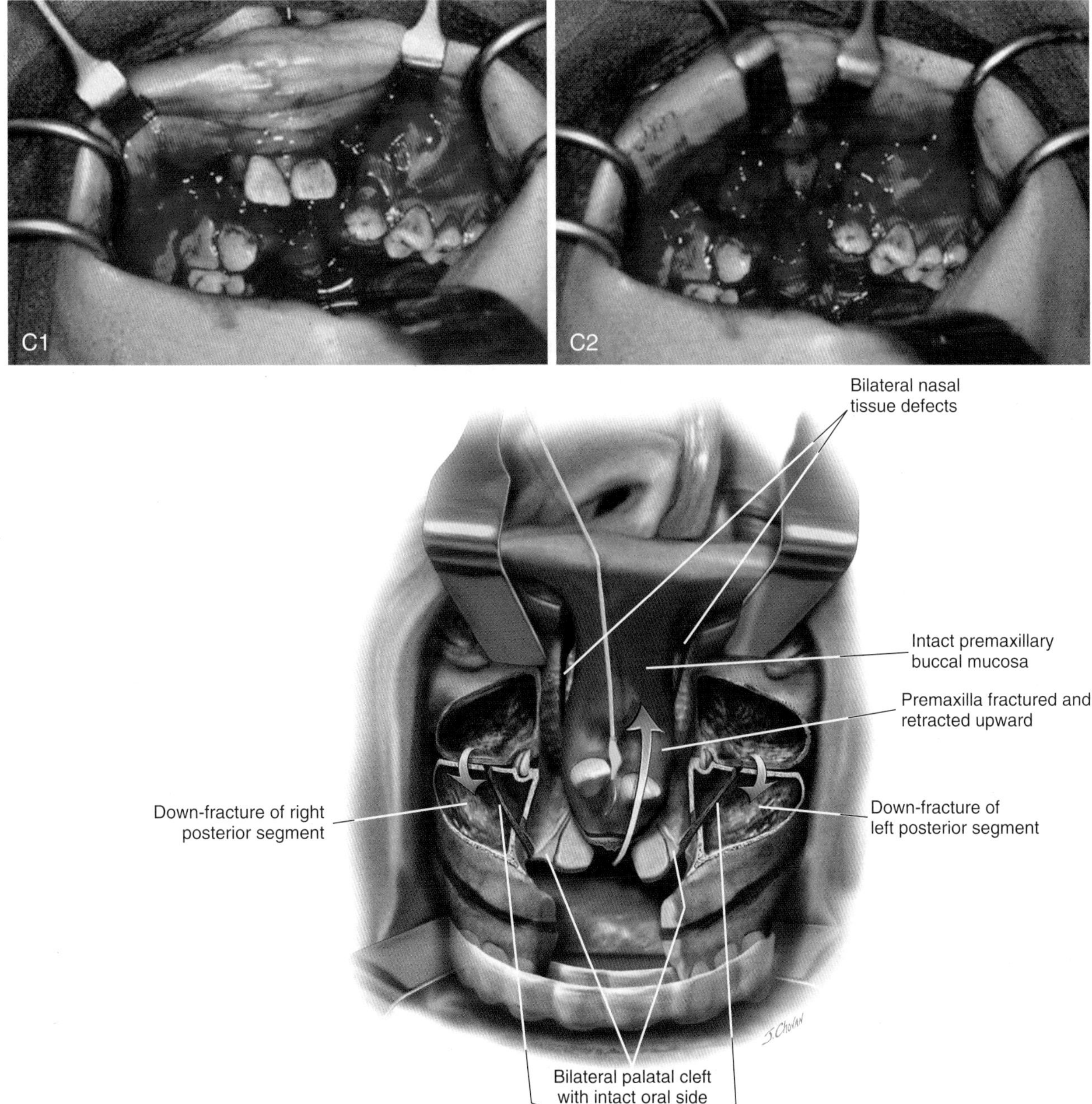

Figure 67.2, cont'd **C,** With the premaxilla retracted, the posterior segments are down-fractured and mobilized. **D,** Maxilla in three segments placed in the wafer (splint) and temporary intermaxillary fixation to enable plating.

TECHNIQUE: Le Fort I Osteotomy—BCLP Ungrafted Alveolar Clefts—cont'd

STEP 5: Grafting and Closure

With the nasal mucosa closed and the two lateral bony segments plated in position, the alveolar clefts are grafted with a suitable bone graft harvested from an autogenous site able to provide the required volume of graft. Mucosal closure is completed with attention given to covering the bone grafts (Fig. 67.2E and F).

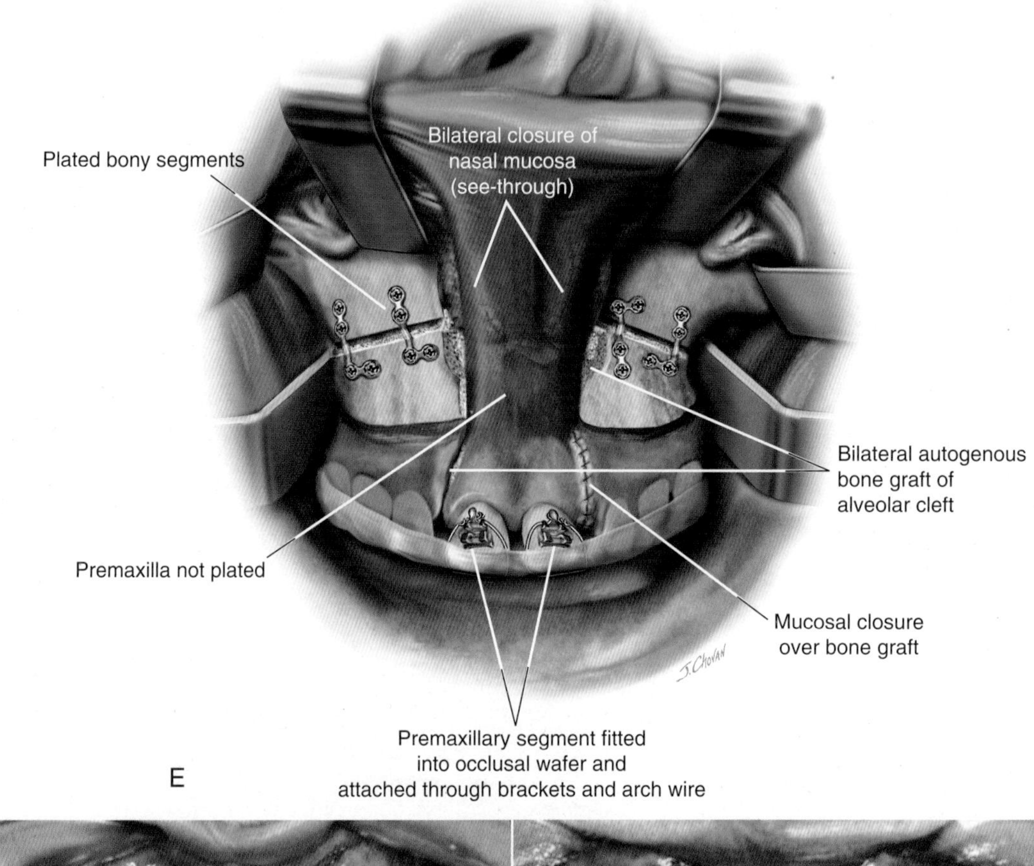

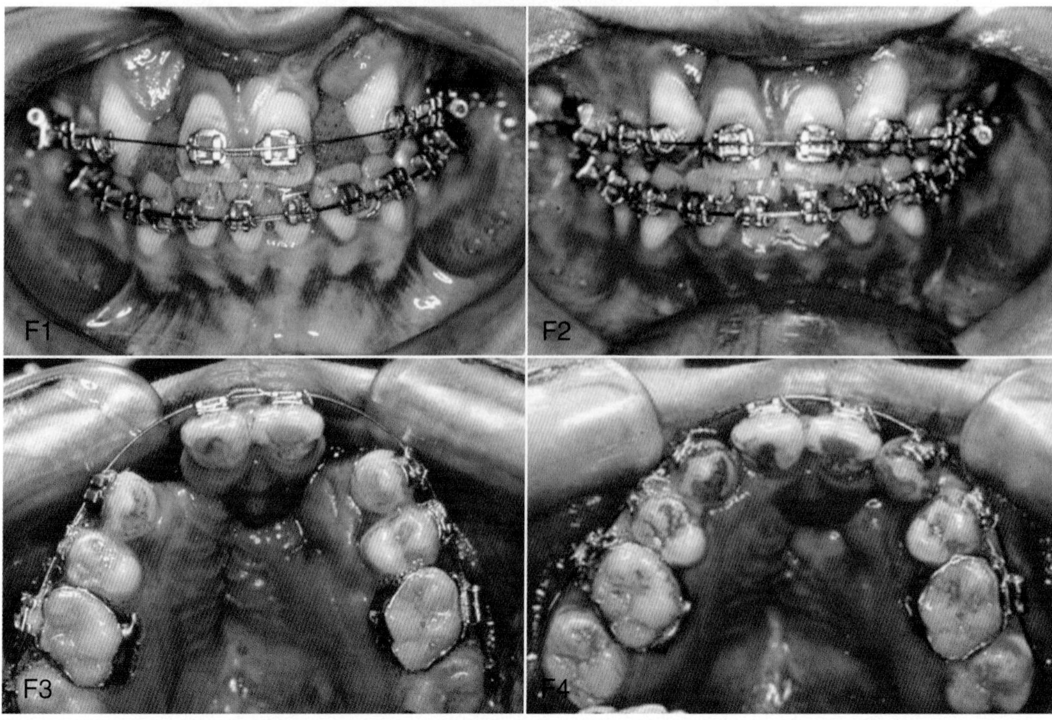

Figure 67.2, cont'd **E,** With the nasal mucosa already sutured, alveolar clefts are grafted with bone prior to closure of the oral incisions. **F,** BCLP with bilateral alveolar clefts before (**F1** and **F2**) and after (**F3** and **F4**) osteotomy and closure of the dental gap.

TECHNIQUE: Le Fort II Osteotomy—UCLP or BCLP Grafted Alveolar Clefts

STEP 1: Incision

A bicoronal incision is made, starting from the level of the top of the auricular area of one side and going over the forehead area well inside the hairline to reach the contralateral equivalent site of the auricular area. Dissection of the scalp proceeds down to the bloodless suprapericranial layer when the coronal flap is raised and taken down to the supraorbital region. About 2 cm above the superior orbital margins, the periosteum is divided with a knife and the flap raising proceeds subperiosteally to expose both superior orbital margins. The supraorbital nerves are released from their foramina to permit additional exposure of the frontonasal area and the subperiosteal dissection is extended to the medial aspect of each orbit and lacrimal sac region. The anterior limb of the medial canthal ligament is divided, and the lacrimal sac is retracted to enable later osteotomy.

After completing the osteotomies from the coronal approach, an intraoral incision is made in the lateral buccal sulcus. Subperiosteal dissection proceeds upward and medially to connect with the subperiosteal tunnel on the medial aspect of the orbit and laterally to the tuberosity region (Fig. 67.3A).

STEP 2: Osteotomy

A horizontal osteotomy is made with a Lindeman bur about 1 cm superior to the frontonasal suture. The direction of the bur is changed to a vertical osteotomy taken downward in the medial aspect of the orbital wall in the floor of the lacrimal fossa. This osteotomy is made with the lacrimal sac retracted posteriorly together with the intact posterior limb of the medial canthal ligament and globe of the eye. The osteotomy continues vertically across the inferior orbital margin medial to the infraorbital foramen and nerve. A long Lindeman bur is used to extend this osteotomy from the coronal flap side down along the maxillary bone to enable later access to the same bone cut from the intraoral incision below. The procedure is repeated on the contralateral side.

From the intraoral access, the osteotomy is continued posteriorly below the infraorbital nerve and foramen and laterally through the maxillary sinus to reach the tuberosity. The procedure is repeated on the other side. Pterygomaxillary dysjunction is achieved on both sides using the curved pterygoid osteotome.

Osteotomy and separation of the nasal septum are achieved using the double-guarded curved nasal osteotome inserted through the frontonasal osteotomy and angling the curved instrument in an inferoposterior direction and with a finger on the palatal surface aiming at the junction of soft and hard palate (Fig. 67.3B and C).

Continued

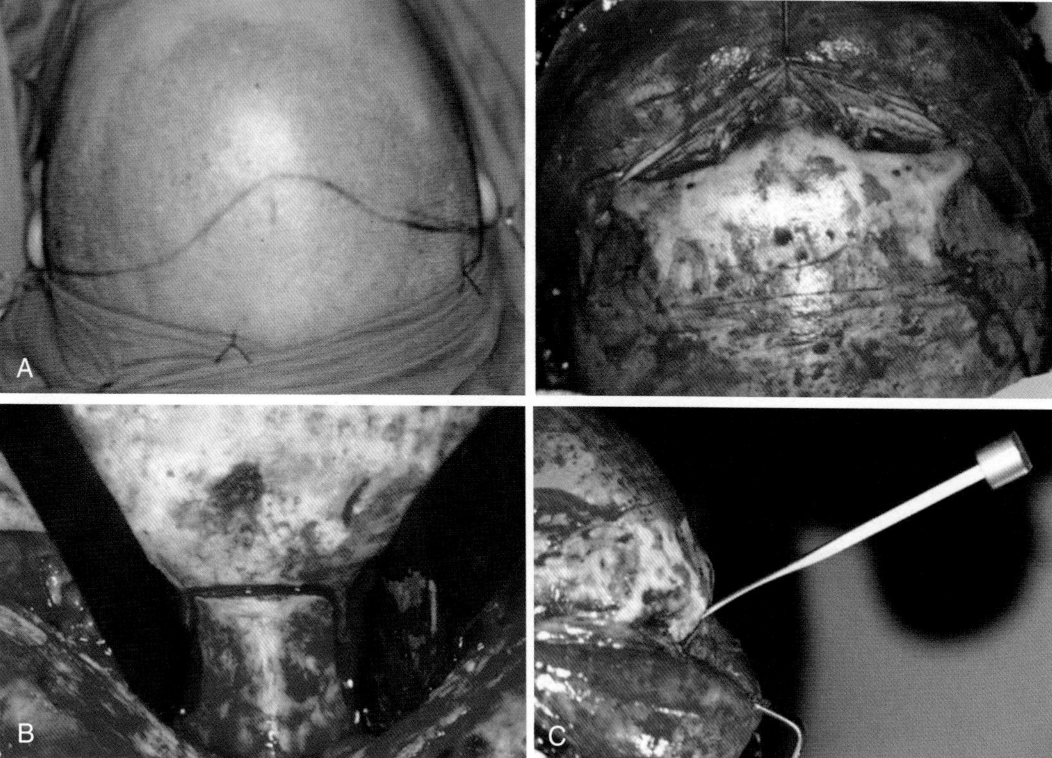

Figure 67.3 **A,** Coronal exposure focused on the medial aspect of the orbits and frontonasal area. **B,** Horizontal frontonasal bone cut is continued vertically down in the lacrimal fossa and across the lower orbital margin medial to the infraorbital foramen to reach the anterior maxillary sinus wall and enable further transoral osteotomy. **C,** Nasal osteotomy angled down in the direction of the junction of soft and hard palate.

TECHNIQUE: Le Fort II Osteotomy—UCLP or BCLP Grafted Alveolar Clefts—cont'd

STEP 3: Down-Fracture and Mobilization

The Rowe disimpaction forceps are used bilaterally and under adequate head stabilization to take a symmetrical action with both instruments to down-fracture the Le Fort II complex and mobilize forward and laterally to one side and then the other until the planned movement is achieved without tension. Temporary intermaxillary fixation is applied using prebent custom arch bars or existing orthodontic brackets (Fig. 67.3D).

STEP 4: Grafting and Fixation

Corticocancellous block and cancellous bone graft are required and are obtained from the anterior ilium for use in the frontonasal osteotomy and lateral maxillary wall osteotomies. An interpositional block is inserted at the frontonasal osteotomy to eliminate the step effect of the forward and downward movement of the midface complex. Further augmentation of the nasal dorsum by a block graft is undertaken if necessary for additional projection of the nose. Fixation by miniplate or screw is applied. An interpositional cancellous graft is placed in the lateral osteotomies before the two miniplates are fixed with screws on each side (Fig. 67.3E and G).

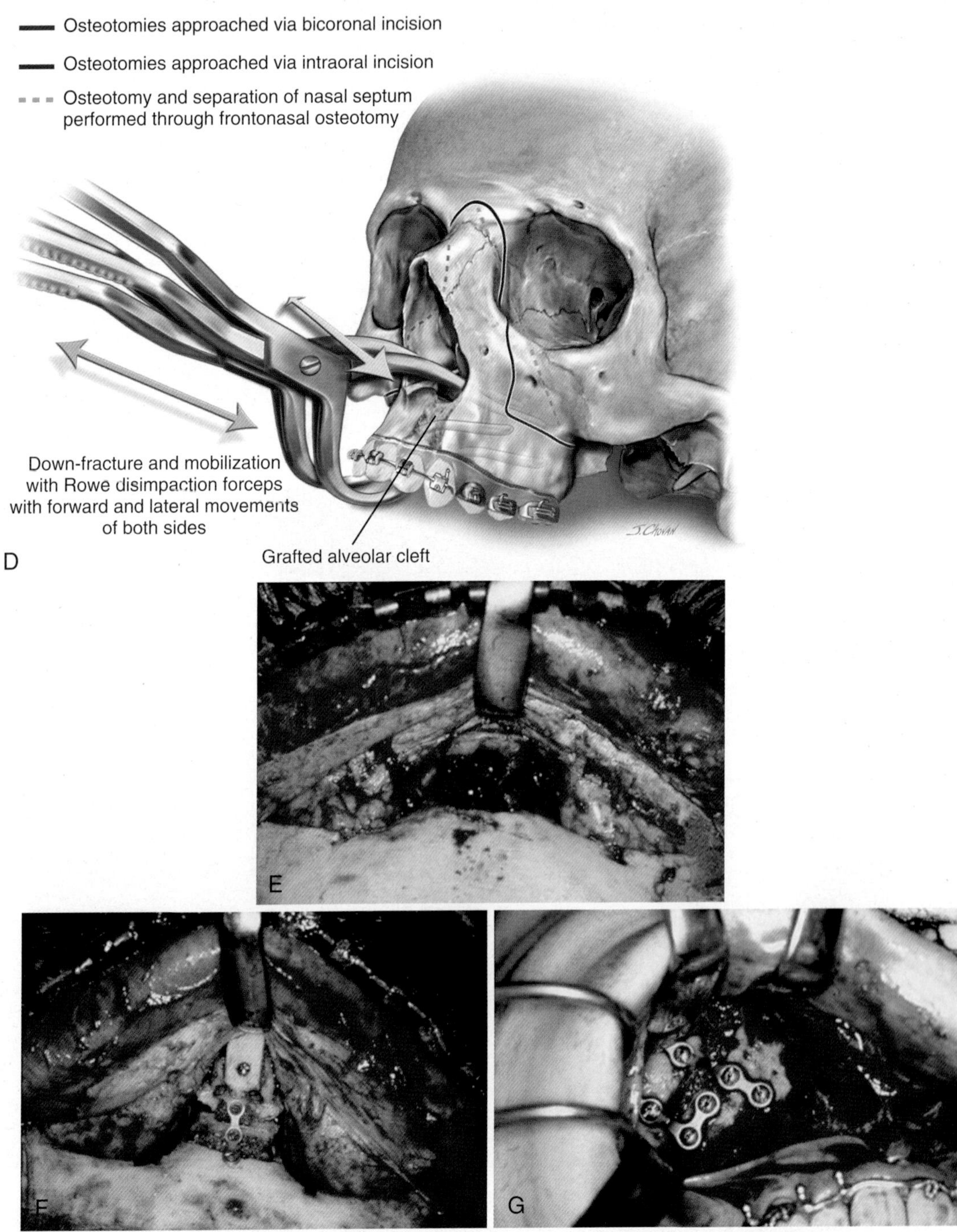

Figure 67.3, cont'd **D,** Rowe disimpaction forceps in place to mobilize Le Fort II segment. **E,** Bone gap created at the frontonasal area by surgical movement after mobilization of the Le Fort II (LF2) osteotomy. **F,** Interpositional and in this case also dorsal graft for added nasal projection fixed with plate and screws. **G,** Intraoral aspect of osteotomy with bony gap grafted and plate fixation applied.

ALTERNATIVE TECHNIQUE 1: Modified Le Fort I for UCLP

The changes concern the following steps.

The incision is modified on the side of the lesser segment by turning the knife upward at the level of the canine and extending the cut from the edge of the alveolar cleft upward to the sulcus. Subperiosteal tunneling is used to access the bone surface and reach the tuberosity. The incision and tunnel must enable safe and suitable access for both the osteotomy and the plating to follow while maintaining a wide buccal pedicle to the lesser segment (Fig. 67.4A).

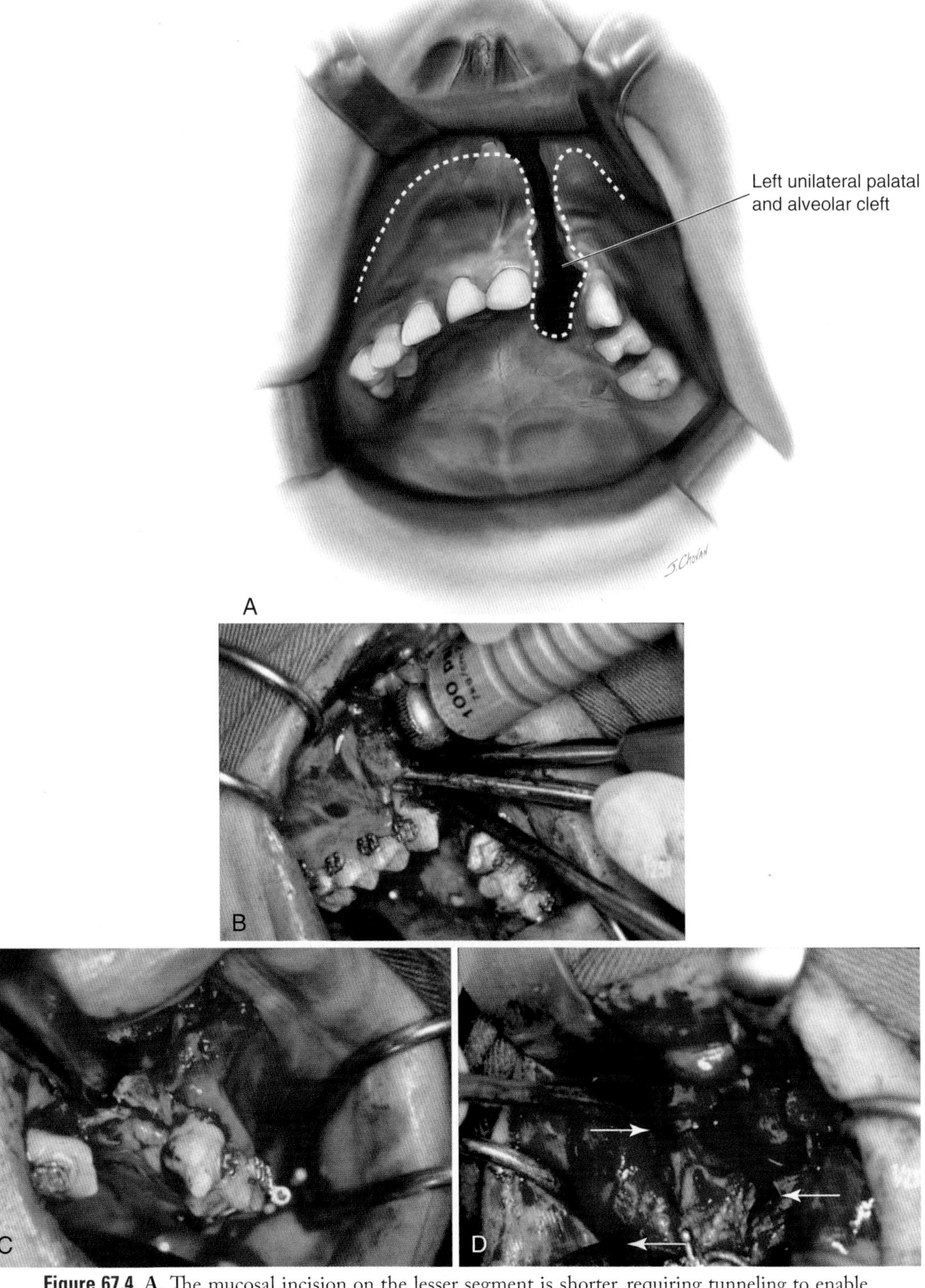

Figure 67.4 **A,** The mucosal incision on the lesser segment is shorter, requiring tunneling to enable osteotomy. Additional osteotomy is performed on the palatal aspect of the lesser segment through the palatal shelf lateral to the greater palatine foramen, enabling added freedom of movement of the lesser segment when required. **B,** Buccal osteotomy through a mucosal tunnel. **C,** Additional palatal shelf (sinus floor) osteotomy. **D,** Coronal view of segmental osteotomy showing buccal Le Fort I (LF1) bone cut *(white arrow)* and palatal shelf bone cut *(yellow arrow)*.

The modification concerns only the lesser segment. One additional osteotomy is made in the palatal shelf near its junction with the alveolar process and continued through the floor of the maxillary sinus lateral to the greater palatine foramen. This osteotomy is started with a bur cut at the anterior edge of the palatal shelf beside the canine tooth, and it is completed with a 7-mm straight osteotome with an index finger protecting the palatal mucosa while an assistant taps the mallet and supports the segment against the force of the osteotome. This additional osteotomy enables additional mobilization of the lesser segment if required for added differential surgical movement to close dental gaps (Fig. 67.4B and D).

The changes outlined in alternative technique 1 are applied bilaterally.

Avoidance and Management of Intraoperative Complications

Complications specific to cleft Le Fort osteotomies concern mobilization of segments and tearing of mucosal pedicles. Difficulty in mobilization is due to scarring, which is variable, and the effort required to achieve the desired movement would have to correspond to the difficulty encountered. In principle, the emphasis in mobilization must be on slow, deliberate, and repeated action using an appropriate instrument that allows stretching of tissue without tearing. Bone cuts may have to be revisited to ensure completeness before further tissue stretching is continued. As long as the planned movement is within the generally accepted range of feasibility (8 to 10 mm), patience is a key to safe and adequate mobilization. Movement beyond the 8- to 10-mm range is difficult to achieve and requires the use of a distraction protocol. This therefore needs to be recognized and planned preoperatively.

Postoperative Considerations

The use of perioperative steroids and prophylactic antibiotics is an accepted and useful practice. Dexamethasone is given intravenously for 48 hours starting when anesthesia is induced. A cephalosporin is chosen and used intravenously in a suitable dose starting when anesthesia is induced and continuing for 48 hours postoperatively. Extension of prophylactic antimicrobial coverage by oral administration for a week or 10 days is a controversial but common practice. A soft diet is prescribed for a week or 10 days. The use of guiding elastics is usually necessary, and this is started 5 to 7 days postoperatively when the needed osteolysis around the bone screws has begun, thus enabling the required elastic guidance.

References

1. Drommer RB. The history of the "Le Fort I osteotomy". *J Maxillofac Surg.* 1986;14(3):119–122.
2. Bell WH, Fonseca RJ, Kenneky JW, Levy BM. Bone healing and revascularization after total maxillary osteotomy. *J Oral Surg.* 1975;33(4):253–260.
3. Tideman H, Stoelinga P, Gallia L. Le Fort I advancement with segmental palatal osteotomies in patients with cleft palates. *J Oral Surg.* 1980;38(3):196–199.
4. Posnick JC, Tompson B. Modification of the maxillary Le Fort I osteotomy in cleft-orthognathic surgery: the unilateral cleft lip and palate deformity. *J Oral Maxillofac Surg.* 1992;50(7):666–675.
5. Posnick JC, Tompson B. Modification of the maxillary Le Fort I osteotomy in cleft-orthognathic surgery: the bilateral cleft lip and palate deformity. *J Oral Maxillofac Surg.* 1993;51(1):2–11.
6. Westbrook MT Jr, West RA, McNeill RW. Simultaneous maxillary advancement and closure of bilateral alveolar clefts and oronasal fistulas. *J Oral Maxillofac Surg.* 1983;41(4):257–260.
7. Samman N, Cheung LK, Tideman H. A comparison of alveolar bone grafting with and without simultaneous maxillary osteotomies in cleft palate patients. *Int J Oral Maxillofac Surg.* 1994;23(2):65–70.
8. Henderson D, Jackson IT. Naso-maxillary hypoplasia—the Le Fort II osteotomy. *Br J Oral Surg.* 1973;11(2):77–93.
9. Molina F, Ortiz Monasterio F, de la Paz Aguilar M, Barrera J. Maxillary distraction: aesthetic and functional benefits in cleft lip-palate and prognathic patients during mixed dentition. *Plast Reconstr Surg.* 1998;101(4):951–963.
10. Bergland O, Semb G, Abyholm FE. Elimination of the residual alveolar cleft by secondary bone grafting and subsequent orthodontic treatment. *Cleft Palate J.* 1986;23(3):175–205.
11. Posnick JC. Cleft lip and palate: bone grafting and management of residual oronasal fistula. In: Posnick JC, ed. *Craniofacial and Maxillofacial Surgery in Children and Young Adults.* Philadelphia, PA: WB Saunders; 2000.

CHAPTER 68

Secondary Surgery in Cleft Patients

John Francis Caccamese Jr., Patrick Byrne, Shaun C. Desai, and Mingyang Liu Gray

Armamentarium

#15 Blade with No. 3 and Dautrey (15.5 cm) scalpel handles
Adson forceps
Appropriate sutures
Beaver blades #67 and #69
Castroviejo caliper
Castroviejo 0.5-mm suturing forceps
Colorado-tip dissecting needle cautery
Guthrie double-prong skin hooks
Iris scissors
Leibinger DeBakey forceps
Local anesthetic with vasoconstrictor
Magee cleft palate retractor
Microbipolar cautery
Operating microscope or surgical loupes (minimum 2.5×)
Periosteal elevators and pickups (surgeon's preference)
Potts scissors
Single-prong skin hook
Stevens scissors
Universal mouth frame retractor with lateral blades (Dingman)
Webster needle holder

History of the Procedure

Revision cleft surgery can present unique reconstructive challenges that may be more difficult to treat than the initial cleft deformity. The surgeon is frequently asked to manage postsurgical problems, at times with little knowledge of any prior intervention. Additionally, if the lip and nose have been poorly positioned in infancy, growth can further compound the deformity. Palate surgery that results in large areas of denuded bone postoperatively can also result in growth restriction in both the sagittal and transverse planes. Improper muscle positioning or reconstruction in either the lip or palate repair can leave the patient with both esthetic and functional deficits that impair the individual's self-esteem. Cleft surgeons must be able to utilize a wide variety of procedures in order to meet the unique revision challenges posed by scarring and compromised blood supply in patients who have undergone previous surgery in cleft patients. This chapter provides an overview of problem-based techniques to address common challenges of secondary surgery in cleft lip and cleft palate repairs.

Indications

The indications for secondary cleft surgery are aggregated under esthetic and functional concerns related to a cleft lip and cleft palate. The appearance and function of the repaired lip and nose are largely determined by the primary repair during infancy. The reconstruction of functional nasal and labial muscles dictates the growth and development of the underlying facial skeleton and the appearance of the lip.[1,2] The esthetic form of the lip and nose is the result of a carefully designed skin incision, muscle and cartilage dissection, and both oral and nasal muscle repair during the initial surgery. The anatomic subunit repair and the advancement rotation technique, along with its modifications, most accurately replicate normal anatomic structures and are the most amenable to revision.[3-6] Another technique employs geometric triangular and quadrangular incisions that tend to violate the subunits of the upper lip. Additional disadvantages of the geometric techniques include the tendency to create a long lip and difficulty in converting the geometric incision to a more anatomically appropriate skin incision.

The repair of a cleft lip and/or palate consists of a series of procedures, the timing of which depends on chronologic and developmental milestones throughout life. Therefore, the lip and nose repair, which often is the first of many interventions, sets the tone for many of the procedures that follow. Much attention is paid to the lip in the primary repair; however, nasal positioning, especially the repositioning of the ala and nasal sill, may have broader implications for future revision efforts. It is also important to keep in mind that the staged reconstruction of these patients is a stepwise process, and careful consideration must be given to each procedure and its downstream effects on growth and subsequent procedures.

Analysis/problem list:

- Type of primary repair
- Underlying skeletal deficiency (bony cleft or maxillary hypoplasia)
- Soft tissue deficiency
- Presence of asymmetry
- Condition of the muscle
- Skin problems (soft tissue landmarks and scar assessment)
  - White roll
  - Wet-dry line
- Degree of nasal asymmetry

Limitations

Although the construction of the labial and nasal muscular rings guides the eventual appearance and symmetry of the lip and nose, the individual's innate ability to heal may also play a key role in the esthetic appearance of the repair.[1,2] Infection, postsurgical trauma, and medical comorbidities can all contribute to suboptimal results as well. The underlying skeletal platform must be considered when lip revision is planned because the presence or absence of a bony maxillary-alveolar cleft or maxillary hypoplasia greatly affects the appearance of the nasolabial structures as the child grows. Regardless of attempted soft tissue correction and camouflaging techniques, facial harmony can be accomplished only when the bony cleft and hypoplasia have been addressed. Therefore, depending on the age of the child and the degree of skeletal dysplasia, major soft tissue revisions should be deferred until bone grafting or a LeFort osteotomy has been accomplished, when possible. Occasionally, severe soft tissue problems and impaired self-esteem mandate earlier intervention, with the understanding that further revisional surgery may be required in the future.

When trying to determine whether a subtotal or total revision of the lip is required, the surgeon must have an understanding of the initial deformity and the goals of primary surgery. An understanding of the secondary deformity and its global functional and esthetic implications is also crucial. Tissue fillers (autologous, allogenic, and alloplastic) and scar revisions can be used to address minor height mismatches of the white roll, vermilion notching, or vermilion fullness when the muscle is otherwise functional and united across the cleft. If applied inappropriately, however, these "minor" procedures may accentuate the deformity, increase scarring, or leave the patient well short of a complete correction.

Total revision of the lip and nose should be considered if there are significant issues with lip or nasal asymmetry, substantial vermilion mismatches, or a dehiscent orbicularis oris. Reopening the lip may be advantageous in that it provides an excellent opportunity (and additional access) to address residual nasal and septal deformities or turbinate issues. In some cases, the total revision can be performed with maxillary bone grafting. When there is significant damage and scarring to the cleft adjacent tissue, especially with the bilateral cleft lip, the surgeon may need to recruit nearby tissue to reconstitute the philtrum and reconstruct the oral muscular ring.

Contraindications

Secondary cleft surgery is indicated in circumstances where the form and function of the lip and palate continue to be compromised despite prior procedures. Additional intervention is contraindicated in patients who are unstable or unable to tolerate intervention. The timing of secondary procedures depends on the individualized needs of the patient. Furthermore, certain patients are unable to tolerate the extent of surgery due to medical and social limitations.

TECHNIQUE: Problem-Based Surgical Management of the Cleft Lip

1. Unilateral cleft lip

The skin is marked in a manner similar to that for a primary repair. For this we favor Delaire's markings for a functional muscular repair.[3]

A—Superior internal angle of the noncleft nostril
A′—Superior internal angle of the cleft nostril
B—Base of the noncleft columella
B′—Base of cleft columella
C—Depth of cupid's bow
D—Noncleft peak of cupid's bow
E—End of the white roll on the cleft side
1—Medial aspect of nostril sill
2—Point from B-1 extended to the best skin adjacent to the scar (separates nasal skin from lip skin)
3—Point marks best lip skin adjacent to scar for the peak of the advancement flap
4—Back cut in the noncleft for lip for additional length as needed
5—Cutaneous dart/triangle to add length to the noncleft side of the lip
6—Point marks the best scar adjacent white roll on the noncleft side
7—Point marks the best scar adjacent white roll on the cleft side

Additional length in the repair can be obtained by creating a small triangular flap from the cleft side to be inserted into a linear release above the white roll. This should enable 1-3 to equal B-D in length.

Careful attention is given to dissecting and reconstructing the transverse nasalis and the orbicularis oris muscles. Wide subperiosteal undermining of the anterior maxilla, zygoma, and nasal bones should be performed as needed to facilitate advancement. Additional periosteal scoring may also be necessary. Every effort should be made to leave the skin closure without tension to minimize cutaneous scar widening (Fig. 68.1A and B).

1. Bilateral cleft lip

The skin is marked in a manner similar to that for a primary repair. For this we favor a modification of Millard's skin markings for functional oronasal muscular repair.[3] Care must be taken not to over resect and create an overly tight lip (Fig. 68.1C).

A—Junction of the alar base and lip

B—Line from A-B delineates the nasal skin from the lip skin

C—Extent of the back cut (C-D) superior to and including the best/thickest white roll (D); also lateral contribution to the peak of cupid's bow

D—Best/thickest white roll; also the lateral contribution to the depth of cupid's bow

E—Greatest width of wet-dry line, perpendicular from line D (these turndown flaps, C-D-E, form the lateral lip that will be used to reconstruct the central vermilion)

1—Point marks the best scar adjacent skin for the advancement flap of the lateral lip elements

2—Point marks the best scar adjacent skin at the base of the columella, leaving adequate blood supply. This should approximate the width of the columella itself

3—Point marks the best skin at the base of the philtrum/eventual peak of cupid's bow

4—Back cut in the cutaneous lip, above the white roll to develop musculomucosal turndown flaps to reconstruct the central lip/tubercle as well as reconstruct the lateral lip component of the cupid's bow peaks

5—Musculomucosal turndown flaps to reconstruct the central lip/tubercle. Take care to keep the cutaneous aspect of these flaps symmetric in height

6—Apex of philtrum/depth of cupid's bow

The muscular reconstruction, as with the vermilion, is accomplished via the lateral nasolabial elements. Again, wide subperiosteal undermining and periosteal scoring should be performed to facilitate this process (Fig. 68.1D).

2. Long upper lip

The long upper lip is infrequently seen with the predominance of advancement rotation repairs performed today. In fact, a short lip is far more common. Excessive lip length was primarily a problem of triangular and quadrangular repairs, but it can also be encountered with other techniques. The long lip can be a difficult problem to correct, requiring horizontal excision of tissue at the supravermilion level or in the subalar region. The scars left by these revisions can be camouflaged by the white roll and the alar crease, although they are less than optimal in appearance. The asymmetric long lip can be even more challenging, requiring a complete revision of the original repair, possibly along with one of the aforementioned tissue excisions applied unilaterally. The surgeon must also be sure that the appearance of a long upper lip is not actually hypoplasia of the maxilla with inadequate incisor display. In this instance, the solution lies not in a soft tissue revision, but rather in appropriate positioning of the maxilla by means of a LeFort osteotomy.

3. Excessive lip height

Subalar or supravermilion excisions can be used to adjust the height of the lip for excessive lip length. Either form of excision can be combined with philtrum modifications as needed. Both types generally require the removal of both skin and muscle. Subalar and supravermilion excisions can be designed symmetrically or asymmetrically to address specific length issues.

4. Deficient upper lip

The tight upper lip can be caused by overly aggressive soft tissue excision at the time of primary or secondary repair or a protuberant premaxilla. The appearance of tissue deficiency can be further accentuated by maxillary hypoplasia or a full lower lip. Further lip revision with soft tissue excision may serve only to compound the problem unless additional tissue is recruited in the form of an Abbe flap. This pedicled cross-lip flap, based on the inferior labial artery, adds width and appropriate bulk for improved harmony between the upper and lower lip. The Abbe flap may also be of value when the prolabial tissue has been severely damaged by scarring. It is important to establish the appropriate skeletal position of the maxilla or premaxilla prior to major lip reconstruction.

Abbe Flap

The Abbe flap is the preferred reconstructive option when the philtrum region has been affected by scarring or when there is a significant full-thickness tissue deficiency of the upper lip. The flap can be designed based on the inferior labial arterial pedicle of the lower lip. The flap and the inset defect can be customized based on the recipient site requirements for height and esthetics (Fig. 68.1E).[4]

- The upper lip incision can be designed to allow downward rotation of the lateral lip elements. It can involve a full-thickness excision of damaged or scarred tissue.
- A full-thickness shield, "W," or rectangular-shaped flap is designed in the lower lip, including the skin, vermilion, and mucosa.
- One side of the flap remains pedicled at the vermilion, based on the labial artery that runs within the muscle of the vermilion.
- The flap is rotated 180 degrees.
- Inset is accomplished by a three-layer closure (mucosa, followed by muscle and skin).
- The donor site is closed similarly.
- The pedicle is divided after 14 days, and the remainder of the flap is trimmed and inset.

1. Short upper lip

The short upper lip can occur for a number of reasons, including technical error in the primary lip repair. Most commonly, it is the result of scarring, an underrotated flap of the medial lip, improper and/or incomplete repair, a dehiscent orbicularis muscle, or an error in length planning when the lateral lip incision is designed. Additionally, the cleft width can contribute to this as well.

The short upper lip is often a full-thickness problem that requires a secondary repair of the lip. In this case, the original

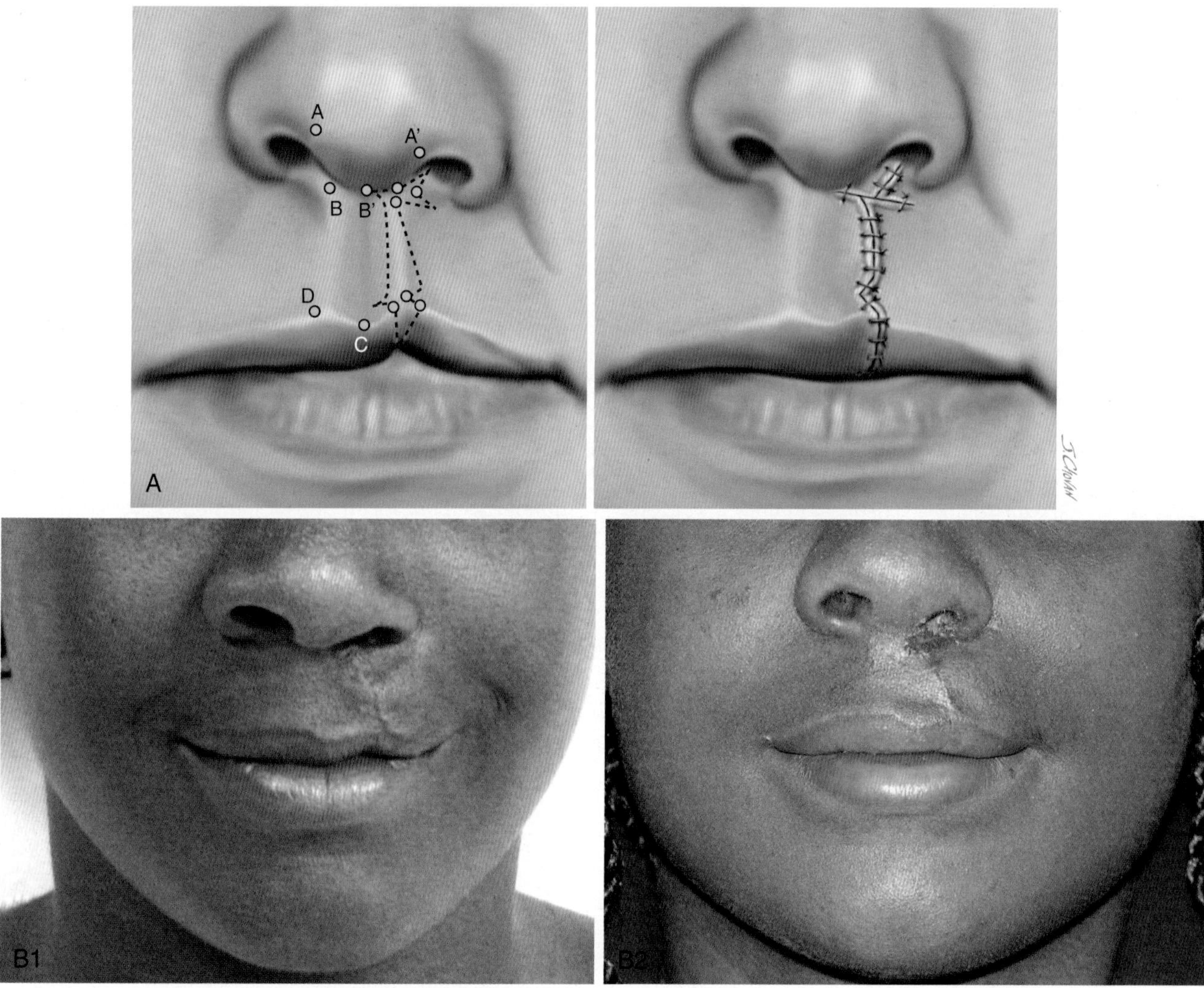

Figure 68.1 **A,** Unilateral cleft. **B,** Left unilateral cleft lip and palate. Note on the left, the slumping, deeply positioned ala, along with the vermilion notching, ill-defined cupid's bow peak, and inadequate fullness on the cleft side. The photograph on the right is post revision with functional nasal and lip muscle reconstruction only. A final reconstructive rhinoplasty can help with nasal tip definition and symmetry.

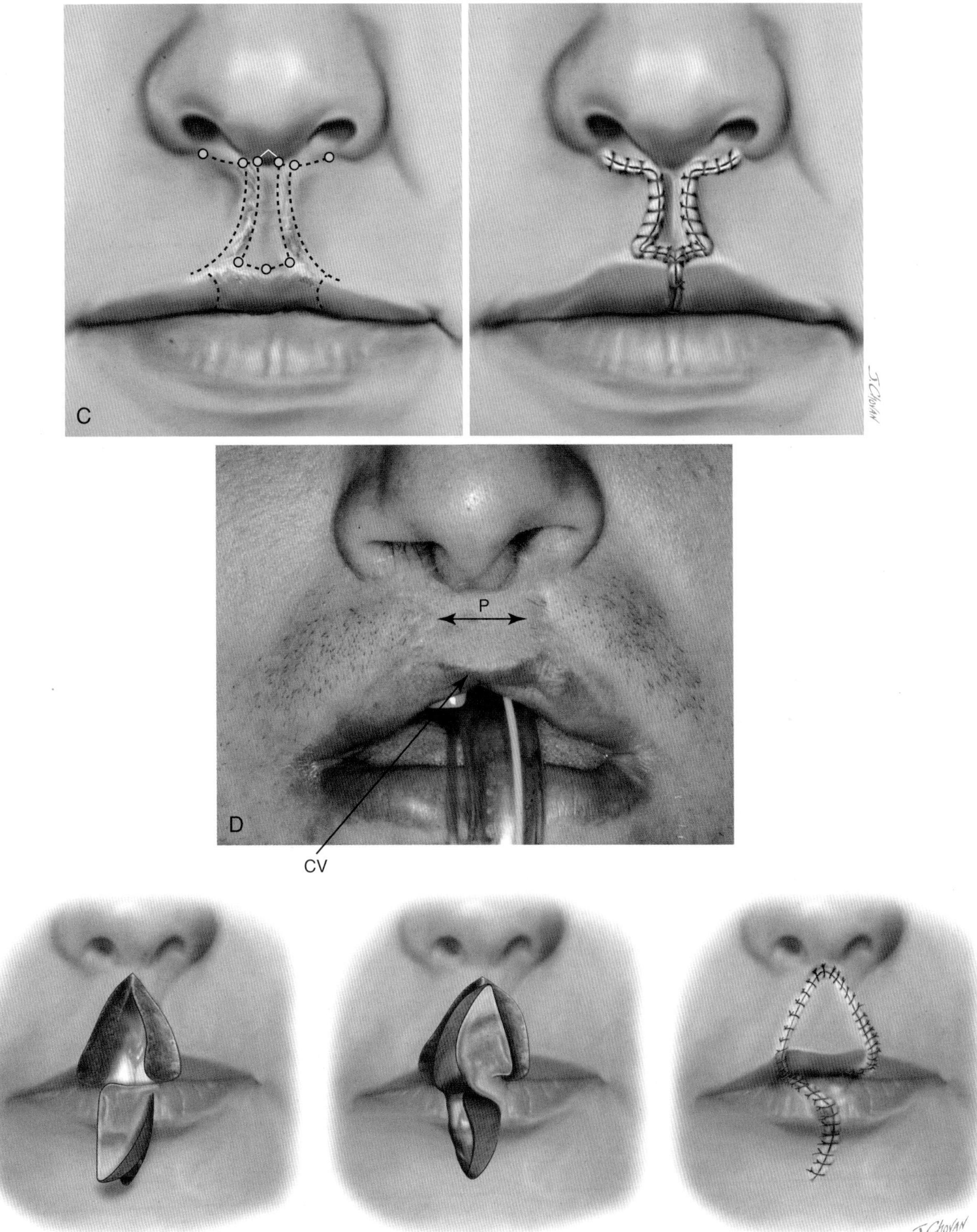

Figure 68.1, cont'd **C,** Bilateral cleft. **D,** Bilateral cleft lip and palate. In this case, the prolabial vermilion was used to construct the central vermilion *(CV)* of the lip; note the inadequate tissue volume and the whistle deformity. The philtrum *(P)* has also been left too wide. The slight bulge on either side of the repair likely indicates that the muscle has not been repaired in the midline. This requires a complete revision and reconstruction. **E,** Design and staging of Abbe flap upper lip reconstruction.

Continued

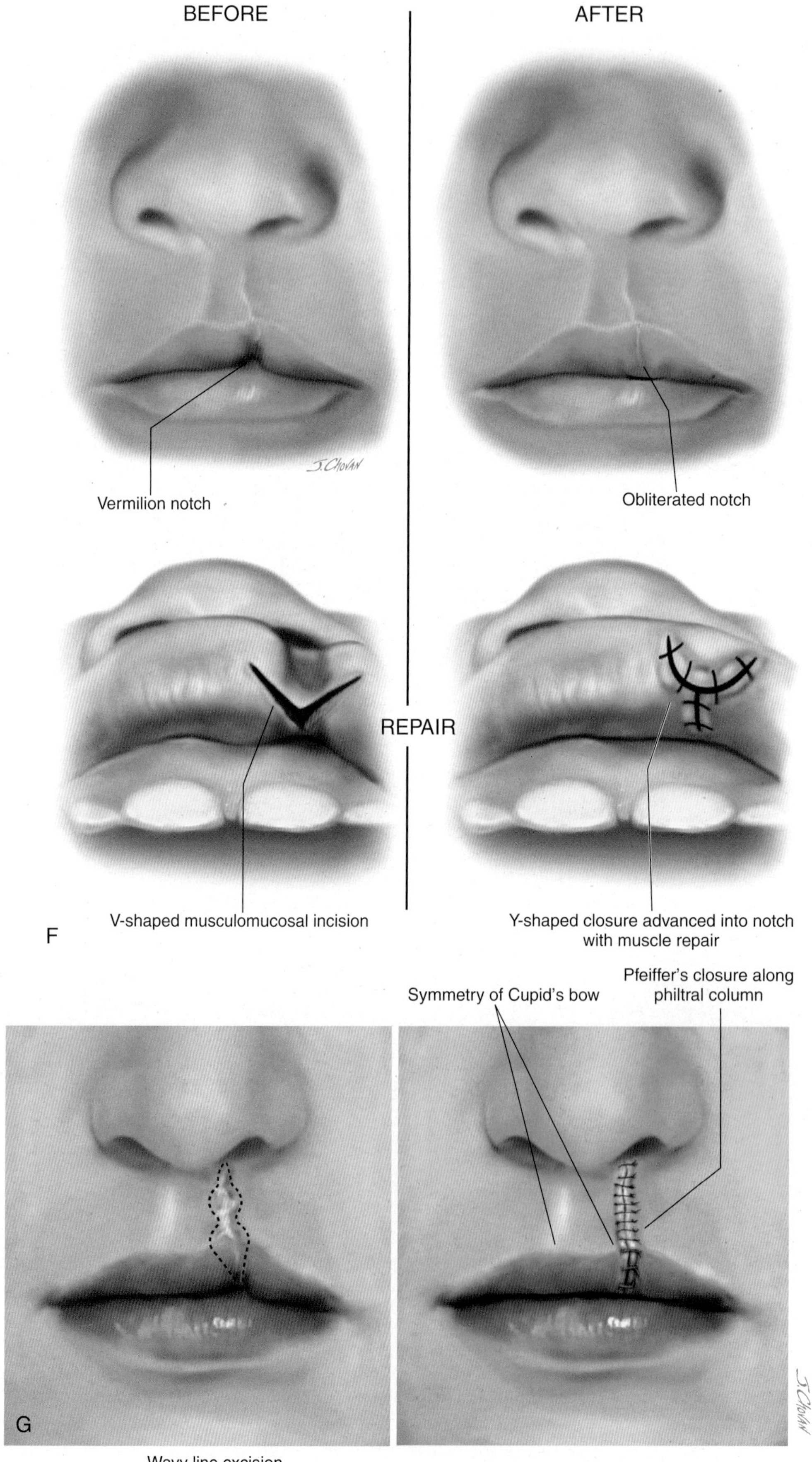

Figure 68.1, cont'd **F,** Vermilion VY plasty. **G,** Wavy line excision.

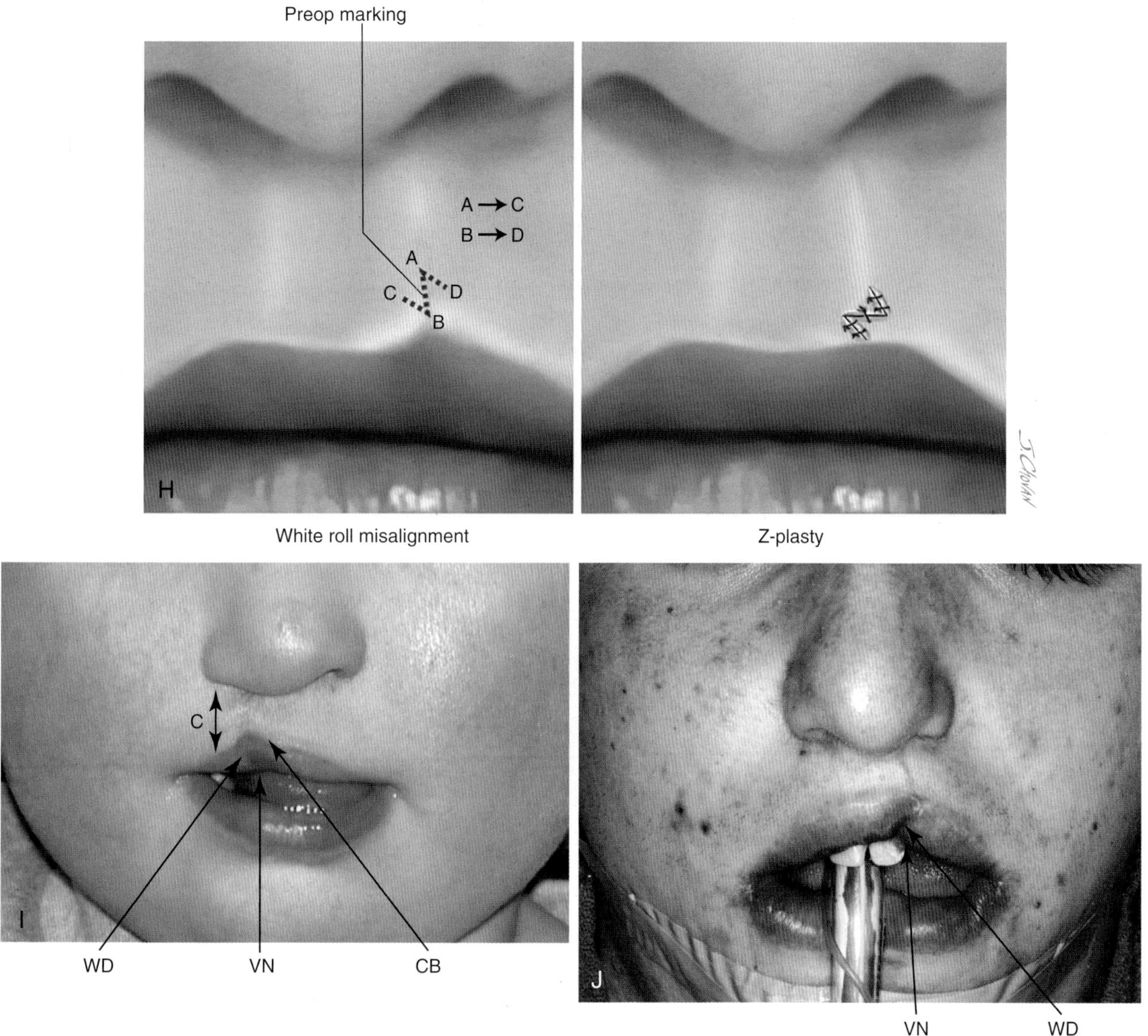

Figure 68.1, cont'd H, Z-plasty. **I,** Right unilateral cleft lip and palate. The vermilion-cutaneous junction is marked by a peaked cupid's bow *(CB)* on the cleft side. There is also a vermilion wet-dry mismatch *(WD)* and a short cutaneous *(C)* lip. Mild vermilion notching *(VN)* can be seen at the lip margin. This patient could benefit from a complete revision of the lip and nose. **J,** Left unilateral cleft lip. The entire lip is slightly short on the cleft side. There is notching of the vermilion *(VN)* and an elevated cupid's bow, despite a well-aligned white roll. There is also a mismatch of the wet-dry line *(WD)*. This would likely benefit most from a complete revision with further rotation of the medial segment and a dry vermilion flap/Z-plasty from the lateral element to better align the wet-dry line.

Continued

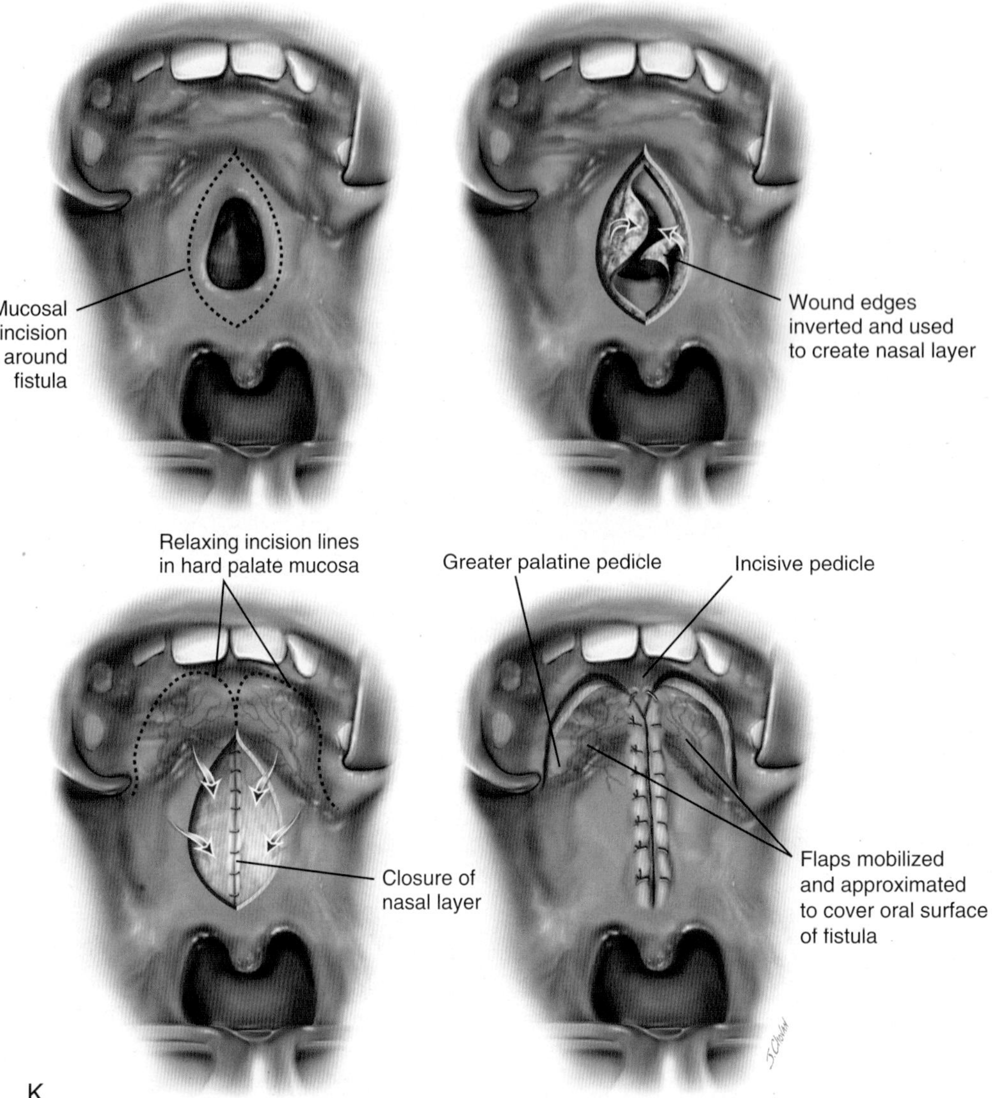

Figure 68.1, cont'd K, Midpalatal and junctional fistula repair.

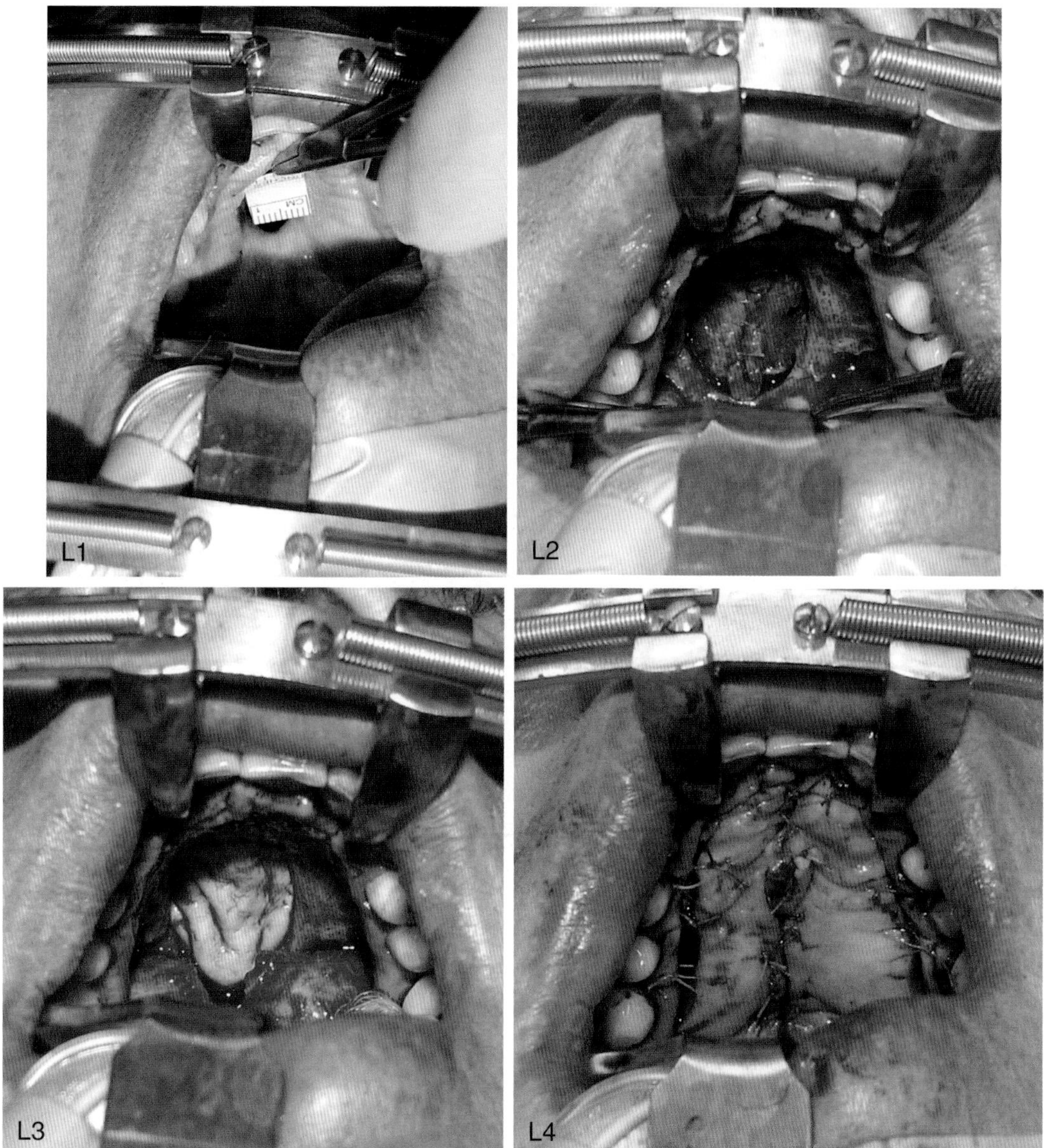

Figure 68.1, cont'd L, Closure of a hard palate oronasal fistula. **L1,** 9 × 12-mm hard palate fistula measured at the mucosa. **L2,** Considerably larger bony fistula once the edges have been defined and the nasal mucosa turned up and closed. **L3,** Placement of an interpositional acellular dermal graft tucked between the nasal floor and the bony palate. **L4,** Closure of the oral mucosa using a conventional two-flap palatoplasty technique.

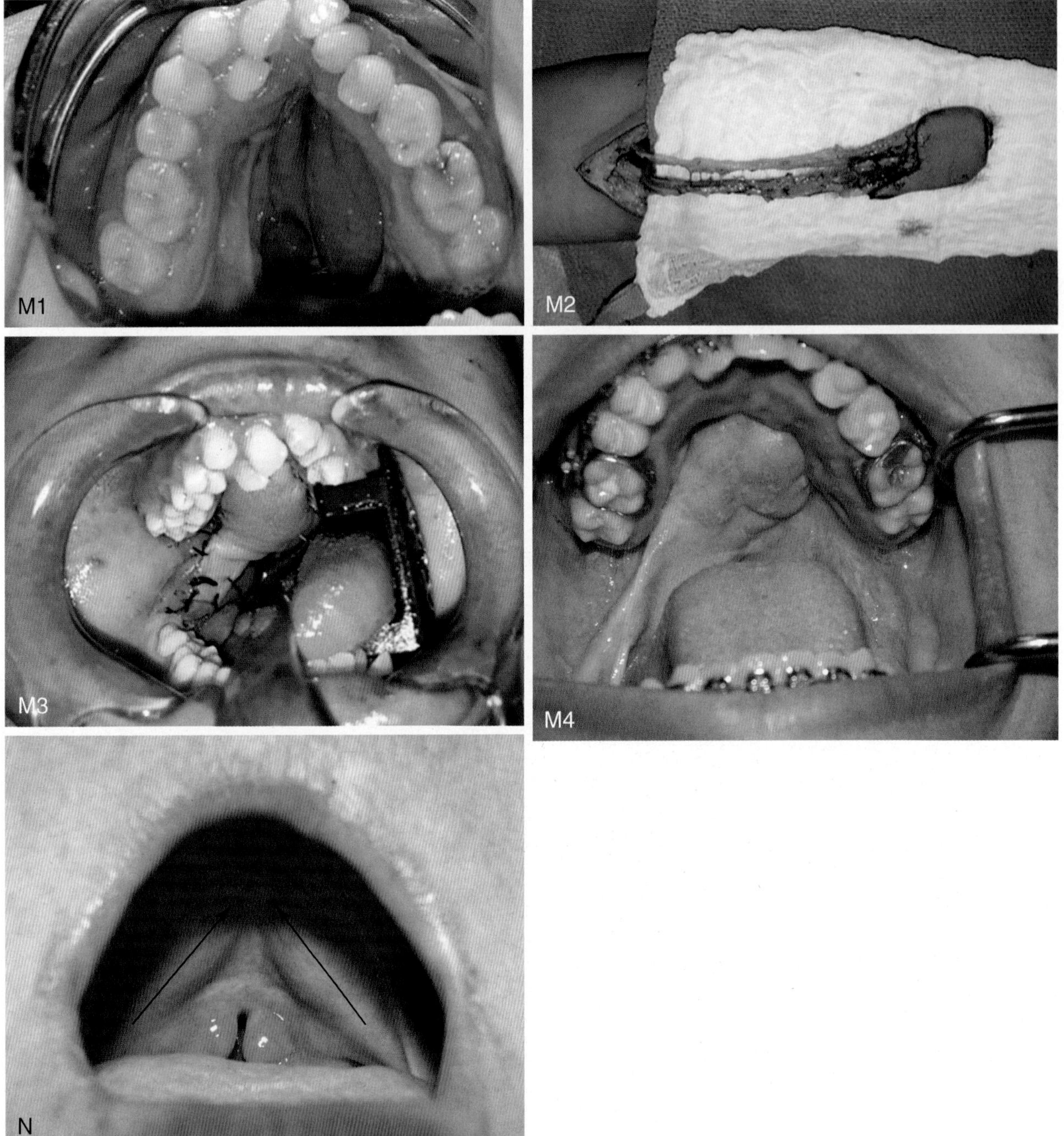

Figure 68.1, cont'd **M1,** Large secondary palate defect. **M2,** Radial forearm free flap harvested for secondary palate repair. **M3,** Inset of radial forearm free flap. **M4,** Long-term follow-up of repaired palate. **N,** Cleft palate repair without intravelar veloplasty. The muscle bundles have a sagittal orientation *(arrows).*

repair scar can be used to access the nasal and labial muscles for an exacting functional repair. If conversion to an advancement rotation from a geometric repair is feasible, it should be considered as it would place the cutaneous scars in a more natural position. Vertical scar contracture may also play a role in the short lip in straight-line lip repair designs.

In rare instances where the muscle is intact and symmetric, the height discrepancy or contracture can be corrected with a more limited cutaneous or musculocutaneous revision. This is appropriate when the area of concern involves only one aspect of the lip such as the vermilion or the vermilion-cutaneous junction.

2. Vermilion mismatch

Vermilion Z-Plasty

Vermilion muscle flaps are created at the site of the notch and transposed to fill the vermilion defect. Once the flaps have been raised, they can be transposed with skin hooks; the incisions then are more specifically extended or trimmed to fill the given defect.

Vermilion VY Plasty

A V-shaped musculomucosal intraoral incision is created approaching the vermilion notch with the apex of the V directed toward the maxillary vestibule. The incision then is closed as a Y, advancing the leading edge of the incision into the notch for added tissue volume (Fig. 68.1F).

Asymmetries and/or White Roll Misalignment

Wavy Line Excision

A wavy line excision of a scar can be used to create symmetry of the cupid's bow when it is peaked and there is otherwise no notch of the lip. This is based on the Pfeiffer wavy line lip closure, in which the wavy line helps to lengthen the skin of the lip along the philtral column (Fig. 68.1G).[7]

Diamond Excision

Similar to the wavy line, a diamond-shaped excision can be used to eliminate white roll misalignment and cupid's bow asymmetry, based on its geometry and ability to lengthen. Care must be taken not to create an unintentional bulge in the vermilion. This is closed as a straight line, however, and is itself susceptible to vertical contraction. A horizontal triangle or dart can be added above the vermilion for additional length or to break up the scar. This can also be performed in the vermilion if there is a wet-dry line mismatch.

Z-Plasty

When the defect simply involves a white roll misalignment, a simple Z-plasty can be performed to position the vermilion-cutaneous junction more favorably (Fig. 68.1H).

Complete Revision

For extensive misalignment, the cleft is recreated, and a complete muscular reconstruction and cutaneous revision are performed. Anatomic points are marked as they would be for a primary lip repair. Care is taken to define and reconstruct the nasal and perioral muscle groups to achieve anatomic accuracy and normal function of the nose and lip (Fig. 68.1I and J).

1. Philtrum defects

Loss of philtral dimple definition and cupid's bow asymmetries are occasionally seen after primary lip repair. A flattened cupid's bow is sometimes the result of a triangular repair in the unilateral lip, but it is more often seen in the bilateral repair. The philtral dimple can often be preserved in unilateral clefts and is best respected in the primary repair by minimally undermining the cutaneous wound edge of the noncleft side. Natural dimple contour is difficult to restore secondarily. Similarly, normal cupid's bow contour is a challenge to recreate. Conversely, scar widening in the philtral column position that occurs as a result of technical errors or poor wound healing at the initial repairs can often be treated by simple excision or skin surface treatments such as laser or dermabrasion.

The philtral column or columns are also often left flat at the site of the repair in both unilateral and bilateral clefts because dermal insertions of the orbicularis muscle cannot be surgically recreated. Therefore, the surgeon must provide surgical camouflage to raise the columns by using carefully everted skin edges, dermal grafts, or local subcutaneous, dermal, or muscular flaps.

2. Cutaneous irregularity

Isolated poor cutaneous lip scarring can be managed similarly to other facial scars with techniques such as excision or dermabrasion. Loss of volume can be augmented using injectable filler or fat grafting. The surgeon must keep in mind the orientation of the philtral column relative to other local lip structures. For example, the horizontal orientation of a running W-plasty may not suit this area as well as a wavy line excision to redefine the philtral column. The surgeon must also be mindful that the skin of the internal nose and the skin of the lip are of different quality. If the skin of the nose has bled down onto the skin of the upper lip (visible vibrissae) or, conversely, the skin of the vermilion has bled into the cutaneous lip, this must be considered as it will likely dictate subsequent steps in the revision.

TECHNIQUE: Problem-Based Surgical Management of the Cleft Palate

Speech and facial growth are the primary outcome measures of cleft palate surgery. Both are highly dependent on the type and timing of the initial repair as well as the width of the cleft and the presence of concomitant syndromes. Despite appropriate interventions at the correct time, maxillary hypoplasia, velopharyngeal dysfunction (VPD), and oronasal fistulas can occur. To identify those in need of revision surgery, patients should be followed and evaluated by an interdisciplinary team that provides interval evaluation of the palate, speech, dentition, and hearing. For the purposes of this chapter, the following discussion is limited to oronasal fistulas and VPD.

1. Oronasal fistula

Oronasal fistulas have been reported with a wide range of occurrence with reported rates up to 15%.[8] They are frequently left intentionally at the alveolus for repair at the time of secondary bone grafting. However, they can occur anywhere along the palatal closure and frequently occur in the middle of the hard palate or at the hard palate–soft palate junction. The chance of success in fistula repair declines with each unsuccessful attempt at revision due to scarring and tissue compromise. Many techniques for fistula repair have been described, including the application of local flaps, tongue flaps, pedicled flaps, free tissue transfer, and augmentation with acellular dermis.[9,10] The oronasal fistula reconstructive ladder is presented here as local flap, regional flap, and free flap.

Local Flap Reconstruction

For palatal fistula repair, raising the original hard palatal flaps and, if necessary, performing a functional revision of the soft palate muscle are most useful in most circumstances. In general, a two-layer closure is preferred over a single-layer closure. This technique is applicable for all but the largest fistulas. For large fistulas, acellular dermis or buccal fat can be useful as an additional intermediate layer and might facilitate healing in the eventuality of oral or nasal dehiscence (Fig. 68.1K and L). Otherwise, additional tissue must be recruited from the buccal mucosa, tongue, or distantly.

- Incisions are made in the mucosa around the fistula, and its edges are turned in toward the nasal side to allow creation of a nasal layer (wound edges everted and sutures tied to nasal side). Wide subperiosteal undermining should be performed to facilitate tension-free closure. This mucosal hinge flap creates the first layer of closure.
- 2-Flap (Bardach) or von Langenbeck palatal flaps are raised on the remaining hard palate mucosa. Release is performed laterally and around the neurovascular bundle as needed to mobilize the mucosa medially. The wound should be without tension at closure.
- Acellular dermis or pedicled buccal fat can be interposed and secured between the oral and nasal flaps as needed.
- The flaps are sutured in the midline.
- If the soft palate is to be included in the revision for VPD purposes and a muscular revision is performed, an intravelar veloplasty can be done according to the Sommerlad method or using the Furlow technique (discussed later).

Regional Flap Reconstruction

Large defects may not be closed using local tissue recruitment, particularly in the revision setting. Two possible choices for larger defects include the use of the facial artery musculocutaneous (FAMM) flap, buccal myomucosal flaps, and free tissue including the radial forearm or anterolateral thigh. First described in 1992, the FAMM flap was initially designed to close palatal fistulas.[11] In a comparison study between the FAMM flap and tongue flap, both were found to be adequate options for fistula closure, but the FAMM flap was more favorable with speech and swallowing outcomes.[8] The flap should be designed to be slightly bigger than the defect.[8,12] A superiorly based FAMM flap is preferable when the defect is near the alveolar ridge. An inferiorly based flap can be brought behind the maxillary tuberosity for patients with full dentition. The pedicle to the flap is traced using a Doppler intraorally prior to raising the flap, and care must be taken to avoid damaging the Stensen duct to the parotid gland. The donor site can be easily closed primarily in most cases with minimal functional deficit.

Free Flap Reconstruction

Larger defects, particularly in patients with prior failed attempts at closure, may require the use of free vascularized tissue. For these, we prefer the radial forearm free flap. This option is particularly favorable for patients who have had multiple procedures in the past and present with a large defect with minimal local tissue available for closurer.[13] The radial forearm is often hairless and can be prelaminated for nasal lining.[14] The long pedicle allows for anastomosis at the level of the facial artery and vein. The defect is completely closed, and the donor skin will mucosalize over time (Fig.68.1M–P) Any wound dehiscence or residual fistula can be closed at a later date with adjacent tissue transfer. Flap harvest technique and donor site management are outside the scope of this chapter. (See Chapter 127.)

1. Velopharyngeal dysfunction

Continuous perceptual speech evaluation is the primary tool for evaluating VPD. The longitudinal evaluation of speech intelligibility can begin after primary palate repair when the child can give an adequate speech sample. Early identification and correction of VPD helps avoid the development of compensatory misarticulations. It is important to determine whether the speech problem is the result of mislearning, velopharyngeal insufficiency, or velopharyngeal incompetence. Characteristics of VPD include hypernasal resonance, nasal escape, nasal turbulence, and inadequate intraoral air pressure.[15] In addition to perceptual speech evaluation, videofluoroscopy and nasal endoscopy might be used to identify the size and nature of the velopharyngeal defect.

Surgical treatment has most commonly consisted of three modalities: revision veloplasty, superiorly based pharyngeal flap, and sphincter pharyngoplasty. Recently, the use of interpositional buccal myomucosal flaps has been described with good success.[16] For minor insufficiency, fat grafting using a cannula injection technique can provide enough bulk for functional improvement. In general, the fat should be overinjected roughly 50% more than needed to account for some degree of fat necrosis. All are directed at either functionally lengthening the palate or partially obturating the velar port to improve speech.

Revision Veloplasty

Revision veloplasty restores functional continuity to the palatal muscles and length to the palate, especially in patients who have had little to no dissection of the velar muscles at the time of the initial repair. It is an effort to avoid the morbidity of pharyngoplasty in the appropriate surgical candidate. This is also a useful technique in patients with a submucous cleft palate. In these patients, the velar muscle bundles are oriented in a sagittal direction rather than transversely when observed intraorally. Techniques described for the treatment of this condition include radical intravelar veloplasty with retropositioning of the muscle sling and Furlow palatoplasty.[17-19] These revision procedures are thought to be more physiologic than pharyngoplasty and are best used for patients who demonstrate small to moderate anteroposterior gaps as viewed by nasoendoscopy or videofluoroscopy. If VPD persists after 6 to 12 months of additional speech therapy, pharyngoplasty is still an option. Thus, even in patients with a larger gap, it may be beneficial to reposition the muscles in order to perform a less obstructing pharyngoplasty to potentially reduce the risk of sleep-disordered breathing (Fig. 68.1Q).

Superiorly Based Pharyngeal Flap and Sphincter Pharyngoplasty

Both the pharyngeal flap and the sphincter pharyngoplasty have demonstrated value in the management of VPD. However, the size of the VP gap more so than the type of procedure performed will influence the clinical outcome of the operation. Despite multiple attempts in the literature to delineate the best operation for specific VP defects (coronal, sagittal, circular), recent randomized controlled comparisons of sphincter pharyngoplasty and pharyngeal flap for VPD demonstrated no difference in long-term speech outcomes.[15,20] Therefore, the surgeon must consider specific patient factors and the potential morbidities of the operation when selecting a VPD technique.

Superiorly Based Pharyngeal Flap

- The palate is divided in the midline a few millimeters from the hard palate through the uvula. Lateral incisions (nasal mucosa flaps) are made at the apex of the incision and extended toward the pharyngeal walls (these are T-shaped when viewed from the nasal side), and the nasal mucosal flaps are elevated off the muscle.
- A superiorly based pharyngeal flap is elevated at the depth of the prevertebral fascia approximately two-thirds the width of the posterior pharyngeal wall, long enough to reach the apex of the palatal incision without tension. The shape of the pharyngeal flap is an inverted chevron at its most distal aspect.
- The tip of the flap (the inverted chevron) is inset into the apex of the palatal incision, and the lateral aspect of the flap is sutured to the lateral edges of the soft palate flaps.
- The nasal flaps are closed over the raw surface of the pharyngeal flap.
- The palate is closed in the midline.

Modified Hynes Sphincter Pharyngoplasty[21]

- The palate is retracted superiorly with an instrument or by a suction catheter passed through the nose and sewn to the palate.
- Vertical incisions are made along the anterior aspect of the posterior tonsillar pillars in a cephalocaudad direction.
- A similar incision is made on the posterior aspect of the tonsillar pillars, capturing the palatopharyngeus muscle in a superiorly based flap.
- The flaps are transected as low as possible on the pillar near the tongue to allow tension-free apposition.
- The superior aspect of the posterior tonsillar incisions is joined transversely across the posterior pharynx at the depth of the prevertebral fascia and in a location where the genu, or "knee," of the velum has been determined to make contact with the posterior pharynx.
- The pillar flaps are transposed and sutured end-to-end or in an overlapping fashion side to side (to adjust the port size).
- The superior and inferior transverse incisions are closed.
- The tonsillar pillar defect is closed.

Postoperative Considerations

Perioperative antibiotics that cover oral and skin flora are routinely used for both lip and palate revision surgery, but administration stops at 24 hours except under unique circumstances. Topical antibiotics can be applied in cleft lip repair when the wound is left undressed to maintain a moist environment, prevent infection, and promote healing. Daily gentle cleansing of the wound is also encouraged. When the wound involves the nose, nasal saline can be used to moisten and irrigate the nostril, especially when a nasal conformer is left in place.

Fortunately, patients tend to be older at the time of revision and can more easily comply with postoperative instructions to ensure an optimal result. Nonabsorbable cutaneous sutures are removed at 5 days after surgery. Patients and parents are counseled about wound care and scar maturation, including massage and sun exposure. They also are informed that scar widening and hypertrophy are not uncommon in the growing child but should fade with time.

After palate surgery, a liquid or nonchewing diet is recommended. Nasal precautions are also enforced. Although some have advocated the use of arm restraints or cup feeding postoperatively for infants with cleft palate repairs, there is no evidence that either reduces the rate of complications.[22,23] Tongue swelling after prolonged use of the cleft mouth gag has been reported, and for that reason, patients who have undergone palate revision are routinely kept at least overnight for observation, especially those who are very young and cannot yet verbalize concerns or distress.[24]

References

1. Markus AF, Delaire J, Smith WP. Facial balance in cleft lip and palate. I. Normal development and cleft palate. *Br J Oral Maxillofac Surg*. 1992;30(5):287–295.
2. Markus AF, Delaire J, Smith WP. Facial balance in cleft lip and palate. II. Cleft lip and palate and secondary deformities. *Br J Oral Maxillofac Surg*. 1992;30(5):296–304.
3. Markus AF, Delaire J. Functional primary closure of cleft lip. *Br J Oral Maxillofac Surg*. 1993;31(5):281–291.
4. Millard D. *Cleft Craft: The Evolution of its Surgery*. Vol. I. Boston: Little Brown; 1976.
5. Millard DR Jr. A radical rotation in single harelip. *Am J Surg*. 1958;95(2):318–322.
6. Fisher DM, Sommerlad BC. Cleft lip, cleft palate, and velopharyngeal insufficiency. *Plast Reconstr Surg*. 2011;128(4):342e–360e.
7. Pfeifer G, Schmitz R, Herwerth Lenck M, Gundlach K.K.H, Pfeifer G (Ed). Craniofacial Abnormalities And Clefts Of The Lip, Alveolus And Palate: Interdisciplinary Teamwork: Principles Of Treatment, Long Term Results; 4th International Symposium, Hamburg, Germany, August 30-September 4, 1987 Xiii+490p Georg Thieme Verlag: Stuttgart, Germany; Thieme Medical Publishers, Inc: New York, New York, Usa Illus 239–245 1991.
8. Sohail M, Bashir MM, Khan FA, Ashraf N. Comparison of clinical outcome of facial artery myomucosal flap and tongue flap for closure of large anterior palatal fistulas. *J Craniofac Surg*. 2016;27(6): 1465–1468.
9. Kirschner RE, Cabiling DS, Slemp AE, et al. Repair of oronasal fistulae with acellular dermal matrices. *Plast Reconstr Surg*. 2006;118(6):1431–1440.
10. Eufinger H, Machtens E. Microsurgical tissue transfer for rehabilitation of the patient with cleft lip and palate. *Cleft Palate Craniofac J*. 2002;39(5):560–567.
11. Pribaz J, Stephens W, Crespo L, et al. A new intraoral flap: facial artery musculomucosal (FAMM) flap. *Plast Reconstr Surg*. 1992;90(3):421–429.
12. Shetty R, Lamba S, Gupta AK. Role of facial artery musculomucosal flap in large and recurrent palatal fistulae. *Cleft Palate Craniofac J*. 2013;50(6):730–733.
13. Chen HC, Ganos DL, Coessens BC, et al. Free forearm flap for closure of difficult oronasal fistulas in cleft palate patients. *Plast Reconstr Surg*. 1992;90(5):757–762.
14. Zemann W, Kruse AL, Luebbers HT, et al. Microvascular tissue transfer in cleft palate patients: advocacy of the prelaminated radial free forearm flap. *J Craniofac Surg*. 2011;22(6):2006–2010.
15. Abyholm F, D'Antonio L, Davidson Ward SL, et al. Pharyngeal flap and sphincterplasty for velopharyngeal insufficiency have equal outcome at 1 year postoperatively: results of a randomized trial. *Cleft Palate Craniofac J*. 2005;42(5):501–511.
16. Hens G, Sell D, Pinkstone M, et al. Palate lengthening by buccinator myomucosal flaps for velopharyngeal insufficiency. *Cleft Palate Craniofac J*. 2013;50(5):e84–e91.
17. Perkins JA, Lewis CW, Gruss JS, et al. Furlow palatoplasty for management of velopharyngeal insufficiency: a prospective study of 148 consecutive patients. *Plast Reconstr Surg*. 2005;116(1):72–80, discussion 81-84.
18. Sommerlad BC, Mehendale FV, Birch MJ, et al. Palate re-repair revisited. *Cleft Palate Craniofac J*. 2002;39(3):295–307.
19. Noorchashm N, Dudas JR, Ford M, et al. Conversion Furlow palatoplasty: salvage of speech after straight-line palatoplasty and "incomplete intravelar veloplasty." *Ann Plast Surg*. 2006;56(5):505–510.
20. Ysunza A, Pamplona C, Ramirez E, et al. Velopharyngeal surgery: a prospective randomized study of pharyngeal flaps and sphincter pharyngoplasties. *Plast Reconstr Surg*. 2002;110(6):1401–1407.
21. Hynes W. Observations on pharyngoplasty. *Br J Plast Surg*. 1967;20(3):244–256.
22. Kim EK, Lee TJ, Chae SW. Effect of unrestricted bottle-feeding on early postoperative course after cleft palate repair. *J Craniofac Surg*. 2009;20(suppl 2):1886–1888.
23. Michelotti B, Long RE, Leber D, et al. Should surgeons use arm restraints after cleft surgery? *Ann Plast Surg*. 2012;69(4):387–388.
24. Mukozawa M, Kono T, Fujiwara S, et al. Late onset tongue edema after palatoplasty. *Acta Anaesthesiol Taiwan*. 2011;49(1):29–31.

CHAPTER 69

Repair of Facial Lacerations

Neeraj Panchal and Hwi Sean Moon

Armamentarium

16- or 18-gauge angiocatheter
60-cc Syringe
Benzoin or Mastisol
Bishop-Harman tissue forceps
Hair clipper
Local anesthetic with vasoconstrictor
Needle holder
Needle monopolar or bipolar electrocautery
Normal saline solution irrigation
Single and double skin hooks
Single-toothed Adson tissue forceps
Steri-Strips
Suture materials
Suture scissors
Tegaderm film
Telfa nonadherent dressing
Tissue adhesives (surgical skin glue)
Topical external ointment

History of the Procedure

Wound management is one of the first surgical techniques ever known to mankind. The earliest documentation of wound care dates as early as 3500 BC in an ancient Egyptian manuscript later known as the Edwin Smith surgical papyrus. The document includes 48 cases, most of which highlight a specific laceration or penetrating wound of the face involving the scalp, forehead, eyebrow, cheek, nose, ear, or lip. Treatment was rudimentary, often in the form of applying honey, grease, or lint into wounds and bandaging with adhesives.[1] While the oldest sutures were first observed in ancient Egyptian mummies in 1100 BC, a detailed description of sutures and suturing techniques emerged from ancient India. The *Sushruta Samhita*, written between 1000 and 800 BC by Sushruta, was an ancient Sanskrit medical text that outlined a plethora of surgical techniques including suturing.[2] Suturing was described as one of eight key features of surgery and the manuscript illustrated over 125 surgical instruments, including various needles and suture types.[3]

The term "suture" was derived from the Latin term "sutura," a seam formed by sewing two edges together. The word was first used in the ancient Greco-Roman era by Hippocrates c. 400 BC. Hippocrates discussed that clean and well-approximated wounds healed better and faster.[4] At around 30 AD, Aurelius Cornelius Celsus wrote *De Medicina*, which classified wounds as straight, curved, contused, or avulsed. The book also described age, body habitus, physical strength, and the season at which the injury occurred as factors that influence wound healing potential.[5] Celsus was also the first to outline methods of wound hemostasis, recommending ligation of vessels that are difficult to control. Later, Galen of Pergamon in 150 AD described that a clean wound heals by primary intention and that a dirty wound requires drainage prior to healing.[4]

Principles of wound management have not changed significantly since its inception. For millennia, infection remained one of the major morbidities and mortalities associated with open wounds. In the late 19th century, Louis Pasteur's germ theory of putrefaction became a medical breakthrough that led to the understanding of microorganisms in disease pathogenesis including wound infection. Inspired by Pasteur, British surgeon Joseph Lister treated wounds with antiseptics, which became the standard for treating both traumatic and surgical wounds. Carbolic acid became one of the first antiseptics documented and catgut sutures were sterilized before use.[4,6] William Halsted introduced rubber gloves and a clean operating room environment. Sterilization of instruments began in the 1880s.[7] As such, these aseptic techniques along with the subsequent development of antibiotics helped control wound infections and decrease mortality.

The mass casualties of World War I brought great demands to increase suture production and improve existing suture technology. Scottish pharmacist George Merson began producing eyeless needled sutures where only one strand of suture is attached into the needle swage. Later, polyvinyl alcohol was used to develop the first synthetic absorbable sutures. In 1960, sutures were sealed in their packaging and then sterilized by irradiation using Cobalt 60 isotope, thus removing the challenges of aseptic transfers.[4] In the late 1960s and 70s, nonabsorbable (polypropylene) and absorbable (polyglycolic acid) synthetic sterile sutures were developed and became new suture prototypes. In 1998, the Food and Drug Administration (FDA) approved 2-octyl cyanoacrylate–derived wound adhesives as an alternative to skin closure with 5-0 superficial sutures

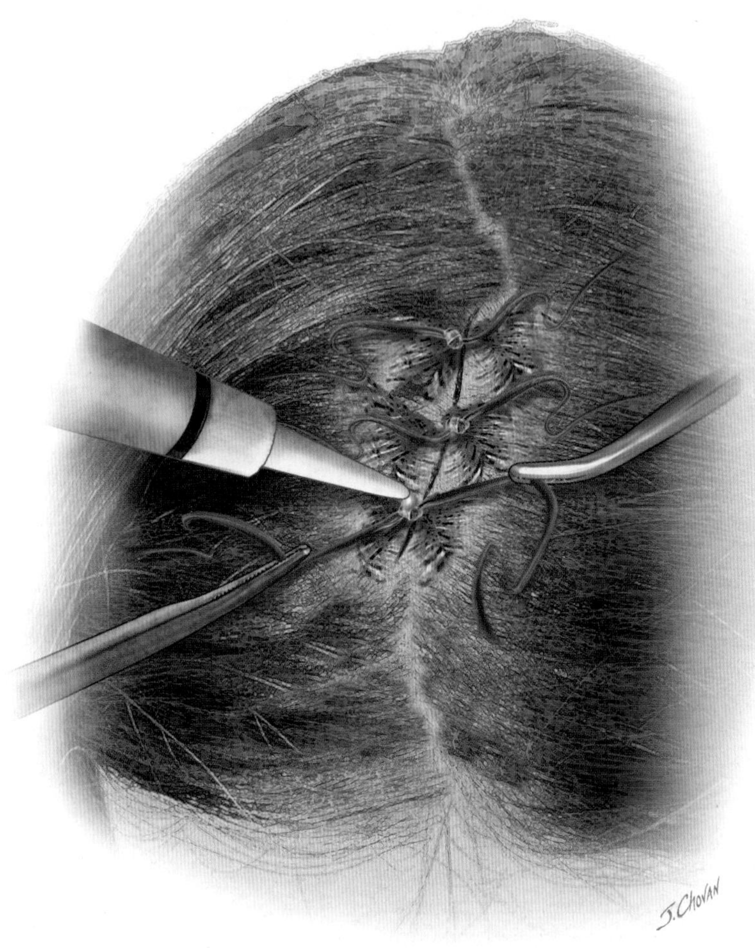

Figure 69.1 Simple scalp lacerations can be closed sequentially by braiding hair together from opposite sides of the wound and then using a skin glue adhesive to hold them in position.

or staples.[8] In 2002, the FDA approved triclosan-impregnated sutures, although there have been mixed reviews on the efficacy to reduce surgical site infections.[9] Today, the global surgical suture market is a multibillion-dollar industry owing to the wide variety of sutures and wound management products.

Indications

Wounds that are larger than 4 to 6 mm or esthetically or functionally critical require laceration closure. In instances where there is avulsion or necrosis of tissue, simple methods of laceration repair may not be sufficient. In such cases, adjacent tissue transfer, locoregional flaps, grafts, and/or distant flaps may be necessary for repair of the wound.

Anatomic Considerations

Scalp

Due to the substantial vascular network of the scalp with an arterial supply originating from three branches of the external carotid artery and two branches of the internal carotid artery, scalp lacerations are prone to significant hemorrhage and/or hematoma. Prompt hemostasis is an important consideration for scalp lacerations either via ligation, cautery, or closure of the wound. The scalp consists of five layers: ***S***kin, sub***C***utaneous tissue, ***A***poneurosis, ***L***oose areolar tissue, and ***P***ericranium/***P***eriosteum. Scalp lacerations most commonly separate at the level of loose areolar tissue. Conservative shaving of hair may be necessary to identify the extent of the laceration but should not be done routinely if adequate visualization is possible. Any depression or deformity of the skull may require additional imaging and neurosurgical workup. Lacerations involving just the dermis may be closed with staples with no difference in cosmesis as compared to suture closure.[10] In simple scalp lacerations with significant hair on both sides of the wound, an alternative method of closure known as the hair apposition technique can be used. Strands of hair are twisted on each side of the wound. Hair bundles from each side are interlocked or twisted together, resulting in the skin edges coming together. Tissue adhesive is then applied to the intertwined hair. This is repeated across the wound to close the length of the laceration[11] (Fig. 69.1). If a standard suturing technique is used, then sutures should ideally not be placed near a hair follicle to avoid a visible scar line from suture-related alopecia.

Forehead

Important anatomic considerations for forehead laceration repair are the frontalis muscle, resting skin tension lines (RSTLs), and eyebrow position. The frontalis muscle should be reapproximated appropriately to avoid worsening scars and abnormal depressions with movement of the forehead. Movement of the forehead may temporarily be reduced with the application of neurotoxin to the frontalis muscles. The heavy RSTLs often seen on the forehead must be appropriately aligned to avoid abnormal scar formation and forehead irregularity with movement. Closure of lacerations near the eyebrows necessitates appropriate alignment of the hair follicles, borders of the eyebrows, and symmetry with the contralateral eyebrow.

Eyelid

Lacerations involving the eyelid require appropriate ophthalmologic examination to rule out injury to the globe and any visual impairment. A ruptured globe must be ruled out as it is an ophthalmic emergency. The integrity of the opening and closing of the eyes must be assessed by checking the status of the orbicularis oculi and levator palpebrae muscles. Eyelid lacerations can be classified based on the severity and involvement of structures into simple eyelid lacerations, eyelid margin involving lacerations, canthal tendon involving lacerations, and canalicular lacerations.

Simple eyelid lacerations should be closed with 6-0 sized or small-diameter sutures due to the thin nature of the skin. Smaller bites of skin should be taken with minimal skin eversion. Knots should be tied without strangulating the adjacent skin.

Lacerations involving the eyelid margin require appropriate alignment of the gray line and tarsal plates on opposite sides of the wound to avoid notching deformities. Sutures are often placed at the gray line to gray line and tied in a delayed fashion. The tarsal plate is then aligned with resorbable suture and tied. Additional sutures are then placed along the eyelid margin and then the superficial eyelid skin.

Canthal tendon disinsertion is seen with rounding of the canthal angles or shortening of palpebral fissures and may require further investigation for bony injuries. Canthal disinsertion requires reconstruction of the periosteum in anatomic fashion based on the complex anatomy of the canthal tendon. In some cases, a titanium miniplate or transnasal wiring may be necessary to serve as an anchor for the tendon. Canalicular lacerations require identification of both upper and lower canalicular involvement (Fig. 69.2).

Any laceration medial to the puncta requires investigation. This is done by dilating the upper and lower puncta, probing the puncta to the sac, and irrigating to ensure no underlying blockage into the nose. If both puncta are involved, then a bicanilicular (Crawford) stent is placed and if one puncta is involved, then a monocanalicular (Monoka) stent is placed. For a bicanilicular stent, probes and attached stents are passed through the superior and inferior canaliculi and retrieved in the nose via a retrieval hook. The probes are then cut and the remaining stents are tied inside the nose. The monocanalicular stent is placed by advancing the stent through the punctum of the lacerated canalicular and out the distal aspect. The stent is then inserted into the canaliculus opening of the lacerated lateral edge. Anastomosis of the canaliculus is then performed with a small-diameter suture on a curved needle. The eyelid margin and superficial skin may be closed as described previously.[12]

Cheek and Facial Nerve

Soft tissue injuries to the cheek may potentially injure the main trunk of the facial nerve or its branches. Facial nerve injuries are evaluated and graded using the House Brackman scale (Table 69.1). When there is some distal function from the facial nerve, then the injury is often managed conservatively as this often means there is not a complete discontinuity of the nerve. Injuries to the facial nerve branches medial to the lateral canthus are also typically managed conservatively due to significant cross-innervation between the branches (Fig. 69.3). Complete paralysis often results in a worse prognosis and exploration is considered within 72 hours of the injury to prevent Wallerian degeneration. Both ends of the nerve injury are identified and microneurosurgical anastomosis of the nerve ends is performed with 8-0 or small nonabsorbable suture. When tension-free repair is not possible, then a cadaveric nerve graft/conduits or autogenous nerve grafts may be necessary.

Parotid Gland and Duct

Injuries to the parotid gland parenchyma warrant evaluation to rule out facial nerve injury. Parotid gland injuries will require oversewing of the parotid capsule, complete closure of the wound, and application of a pressure dressing. This should be done to avoid the complications such as sialadenitis or a sialocele.

Parotid (Stenson's) duct injuries are evaluated by massaging the parotid gland to identify salivary flow into the wound or into the oral cavity. The parotid duct can also be cannulated intraorally with a probe and the wound can be observed for the probe (Figs. 69.4A and B). When the two ends of the duct are identified, they may be microsurgically repaired over a silicone stent (Fig. 69.5). If the proximal portion of the duct is not identifiable, then the wound should be closed with the application of a pressure dressing and prescription antisialogogues. In some instances, neurotoxin may be injected to reduce salivary production from the parotid gland.

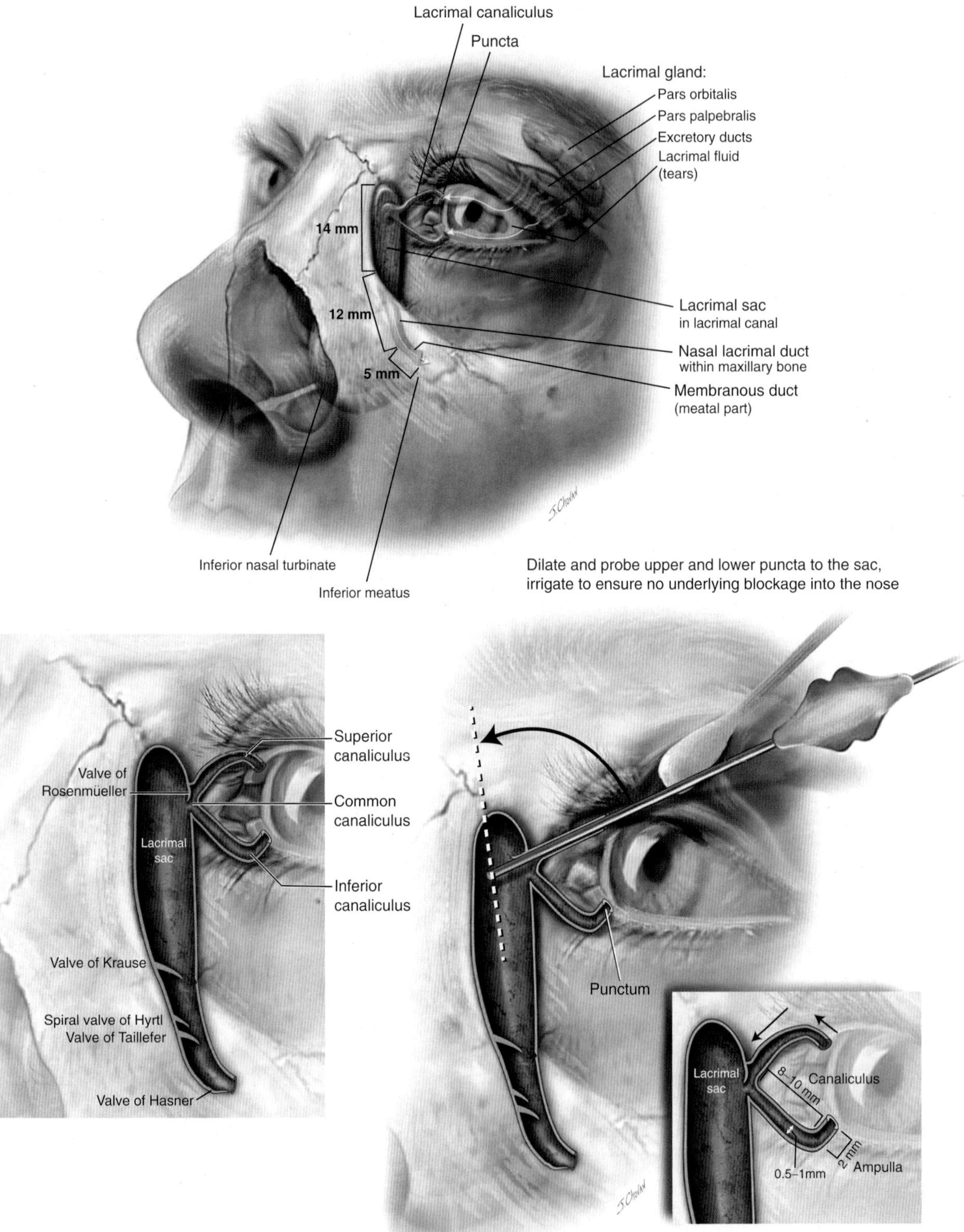

Figure 69.2 Relevant Canalicular System anatomy.

Table 69.1 House-Brackmann Facial Nerve Classification

Grade	Description	Characteristics
I	Normal	Normal facial function in all areas
II	Mild dysfunction	Slight weakness noticeable on close inspection, may have slight synkinesis
III	Moderate dysfunction	Obvious, but not disfiguring, difference between 2 sides, noticeable but not severe synkinesis, contracture, or hemifacial spasm, complete eye closure with effort
IV	Moderately severe dysfunction	Obvious weakness or disfiguring asymmetry; normal symmetry and tone at rest; incomplete eye closure
V	Severe dysfunction	Only barely perceptible motion, asymmetry at rest
VI	Total paralysis	No movement

From Radwan AM, Boxx C, Zuniga J. Post-traumatic injuries of the trigeminal and facial nerve. *Atlas Oral Maxillofac Surg Clin North Am.* 2019;27(2):127–133.

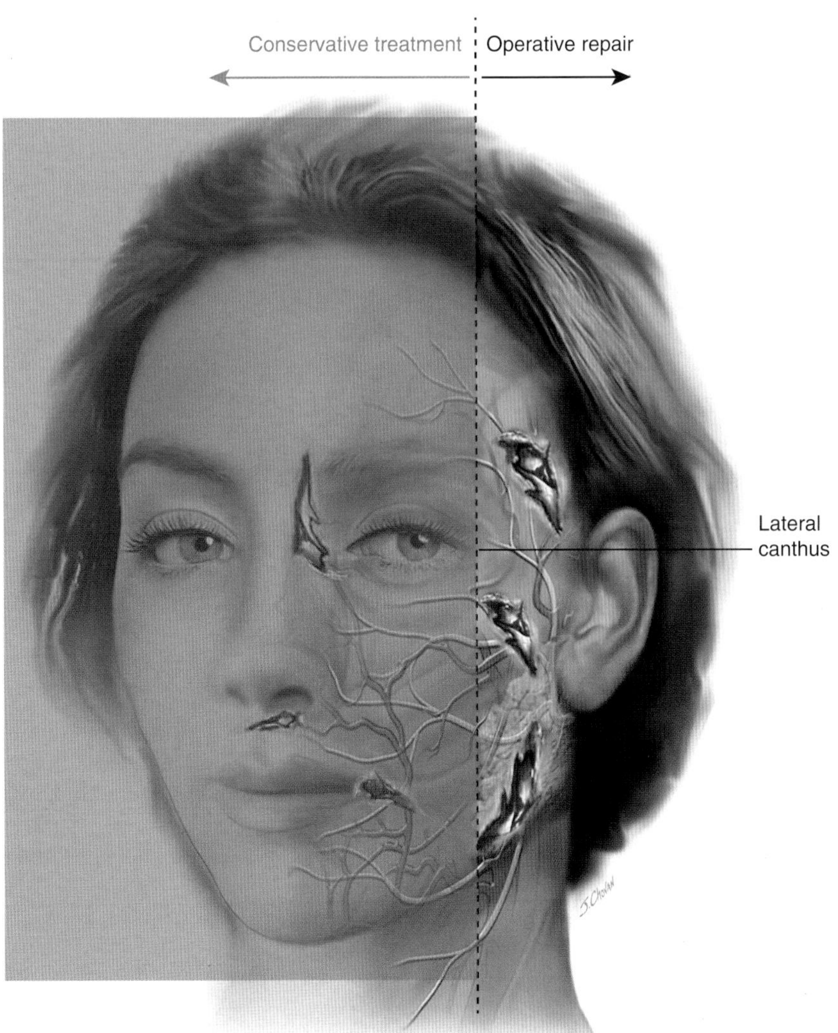

Figure 69.3 Demonstration of the line of arborization of the facial nerve.

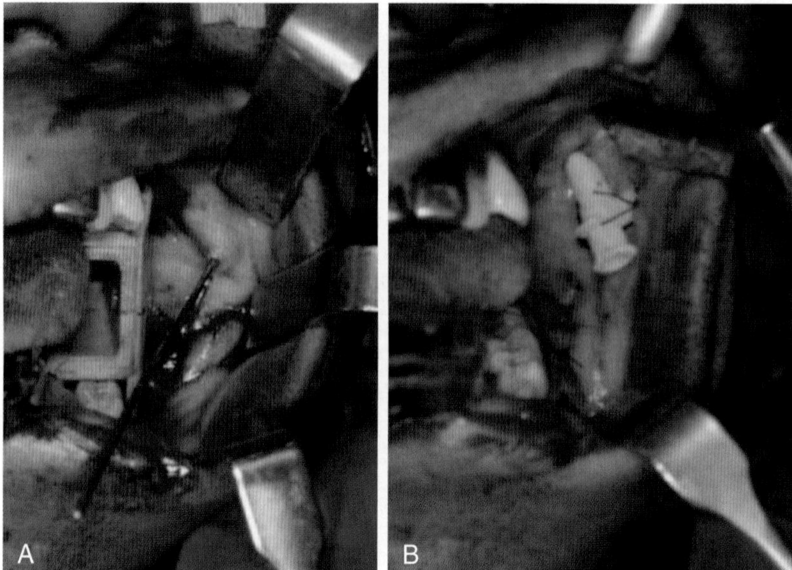

Figure 69.4 Cannulation of Stenson's Duct.

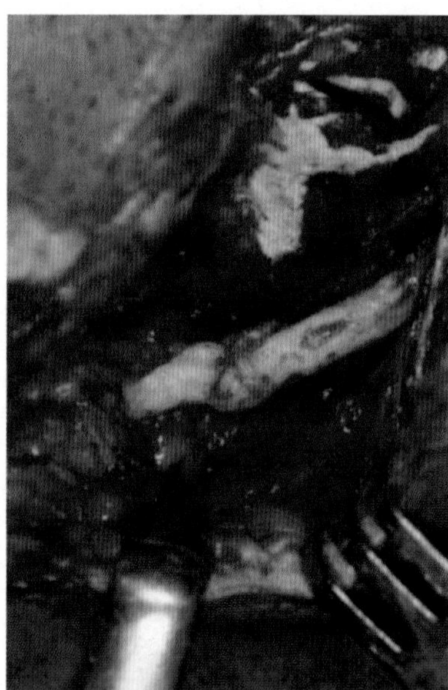

Figure 69.5 Suture anastomosis of Parotid Duct over silicone catheter.

Nose

Lacerations involving the nose are often associated with nasal bone fractures and further investigation must be performed to rule out nasal fractures. The nasal septum must also be evaluated for septal hematoma. Septal hematomas must be drained with the application of pressure dressings or Penrose drain to prevent reaccumulation. Lacerations of the nose must be closed to ensure appropriate definition of the nasal subunits. Adhesions and stenosis can occur due to injury to internal mucosal lining. The placement of intranasal stents can help reduce these complications.

Perioral

The lip and mouth are dynamic structures with defined anatomy requiring appropriate approximation. Specific landmarks that deserve the greatest attention include the philtral columns, cupid's bow, vermillion cutaneous border, and dry-wet line of the lips. These areas may often need to be marked prior to potential distortion with infiltration of local anesthetic. When repairing lacerations of the lip, it is important to ensure careful approximation of the orbicularis oris to avoid deformities with dynamic movement.

Ear

Ear lacerations can be challenging to repair due to the poor blood supply, complex anatomy of the cartilaginous structures, and differences in the thickness of the skin. Laceration involving the cartilage requires the cartilage to be reapproximated with a resorbable suture. Prevention of hematoma is critical to preventing cartilage necrosis, infection, and ear deformity. In some instances, the placement of a prophylactic bolster to prevent auricular hematoma is necessary. Significant lacerations of the ear canal may also require the placement of a stent to prevent stenosis.

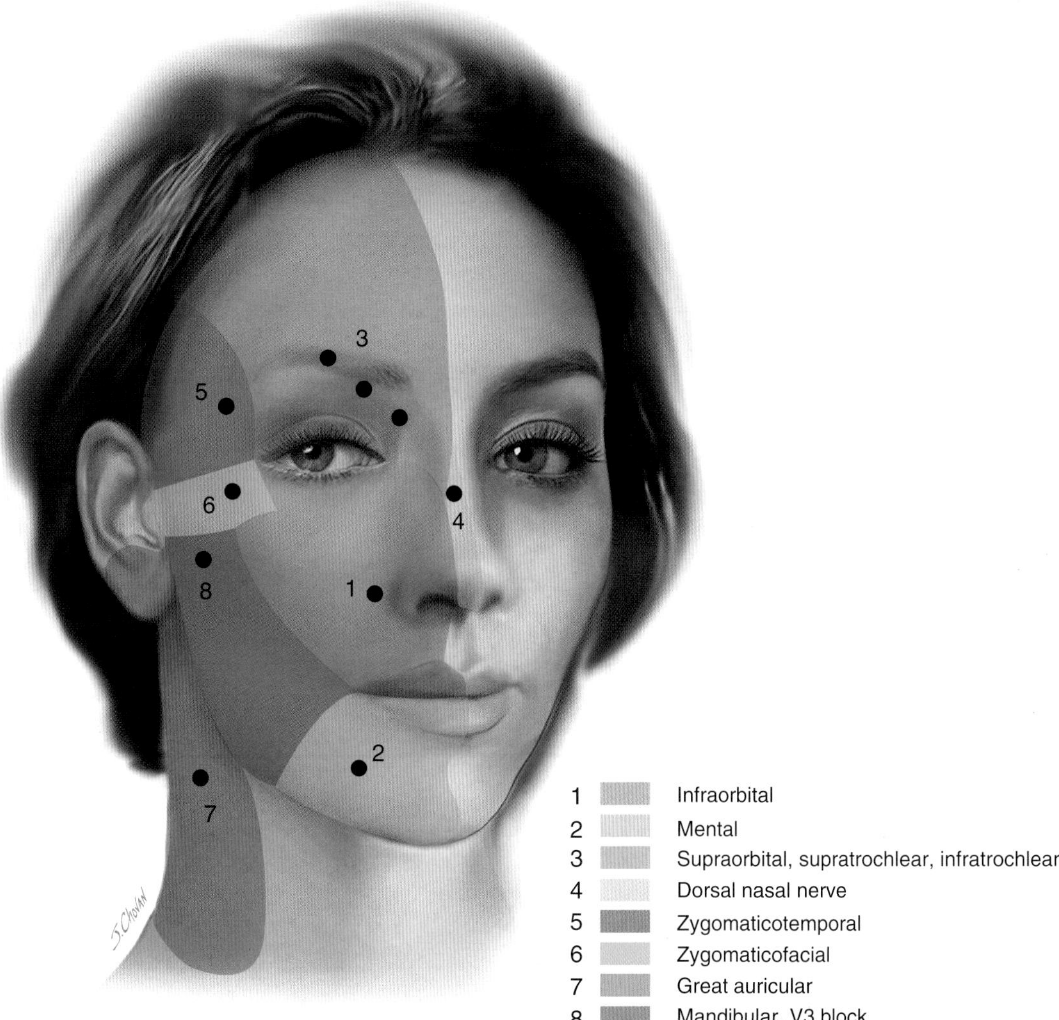

Figure 69.6 Injection points for specific areas of cutaneous anthesia.

TECHNIQUE: CLOSURE TECHNIQUE

STEP 1: Local Anesthesia

Local anesthesia should ideally be performed via nerve blocks of the face (Fig. 69.6). Infiltration of local anesthesia may be utilized if anatomic landmarks for approximation are not distorted. In the pediatric population, the usage of topical anesthetics may aid anesthetic comfort.

STEP 2: Irrigation and Hemostasis

The wound should be thoroughly irrigated with normal saline solution (NSS) or antibiotic-impregnated NSS and debrided to ensure no foreign material or debris is in the wound. Any devitalized tissue should be conservatively removed to preserve as much soft tissue as possible. Significant bleeding from the wound should be stopped with pressure, cautery, or vessel ligation.

STEP 3: Suture Selection

There are no significant differences in cosmetic outcome, wound infection, or wound dehiscence between absorbable (Table 69.2) and nonabsorbable sutures (Table 69.3). The smallest suture should be selected to give sufficient strength to reapproximate and support the laceration while it heals. Typically on the face, 3-0 or 4-0 absorbable sutures are used for deep sutures and 5-0 or 6-0 sutures are used for cutaneous sutures. If nonabsorbable sutures are selected, appropriate follow-up within 5 to 7 days should be scheduled for suture removal.

Table 69.2 Absorbable Suture Materials

Material	Structure	Tissue Reaction	Tensile Strength	Tissue Half-Life (Days)	Uses and Comments
Gut	Natural	++++	++	5–7	For mucosal closures, rarely used
Chromic gut	Natural	++++	++	10–14	For oral mucosal, perineal, and scrotal closures, can be annoying to patients because of stiffness
Polyglycolic acid (Dexon)	Braided	++	+++	25	For subcutaneous closure, coated version easier to use but requires more knots (Dexon-Plus)
Polyglactin 910 (Vicryl)	Braided	++	++++	28	Comes dyed and undyed, do not use dyed on face; irradiated polyglactin excellent for mucosal closures
Polyglyconate (Maxon)	Monofilament	+	+++++	28–36	For subcutaneous closure, less reactive and stronger than polyglycolic acid and polyglactin
Polydioxanone (PDS)	Monofilament	+	++++	36–53	For subcutaneous closures that need high degree of security, stiffer and more difficult to handle than polyglycolic acid or polyglyconate

From Trott AT. *Wounds and Lacerations-e-Book: Emergency Care and Closure.* 2012, Elsevier Health Sciences, pp. 102.

Table 69.3 Nonabsorbable Suture Materials

Material	Structure	Tissue Reaction	Tensile Strength	Knot Security	Uses and Comments
Silk	Braided	++++	++	++++	Easy to handle but has increased potential for infection
Nylon (Ethilon, Dermalon)	Monofilament	++	+++	++	Commonly used in skin closure but high degree of memory, requires several throws for secure closure
Polypropylene (Prolene)	Monofilament	+	++++	+	High degree of memory, low tissue adhesion, good for subcuticular pull-out technique
Dacron (Mersilene)	Braided	+++	++	++++	Easy to handle, good knot security, similar to silk but less risk to tissue for inflammation and infection
Polybutester (Novafil)	Monofilament	+	++++	++++	Excellent handling, strength, and security, expands and contracts with changes in tissue edema

From Trott AT. *Wounds and Lacerations-e-Book: Emergency Care and Closure.* 2012, Elsevier Health Sciences, pp. 104.

TECHNIQUE: CLOSURE TECHNIQUE—cont'd

STEP 4: Deep and Dermal Closure

Deep layers such as periosteum layers and muscle layers should be reapproximated with absorbable sutures. The dermal layer should be closed with buried knots such that the knot is away from the skin edges. This is performed by inserting the needle in the dermis directed toward the skin surface and exiting near the dermal-epidermal junction on the same side. Then the needle is inserted on the opposite side, near the dermal-epidermal junction, directly across from the point of exit toward the depth of the wound. The tip of the needle exits at the level of the dermis and the knot is tied. The dermal sutures should ensure that the skin edges are passively sitting against each other with a slight eversion of the skin (Fig. 69.7).

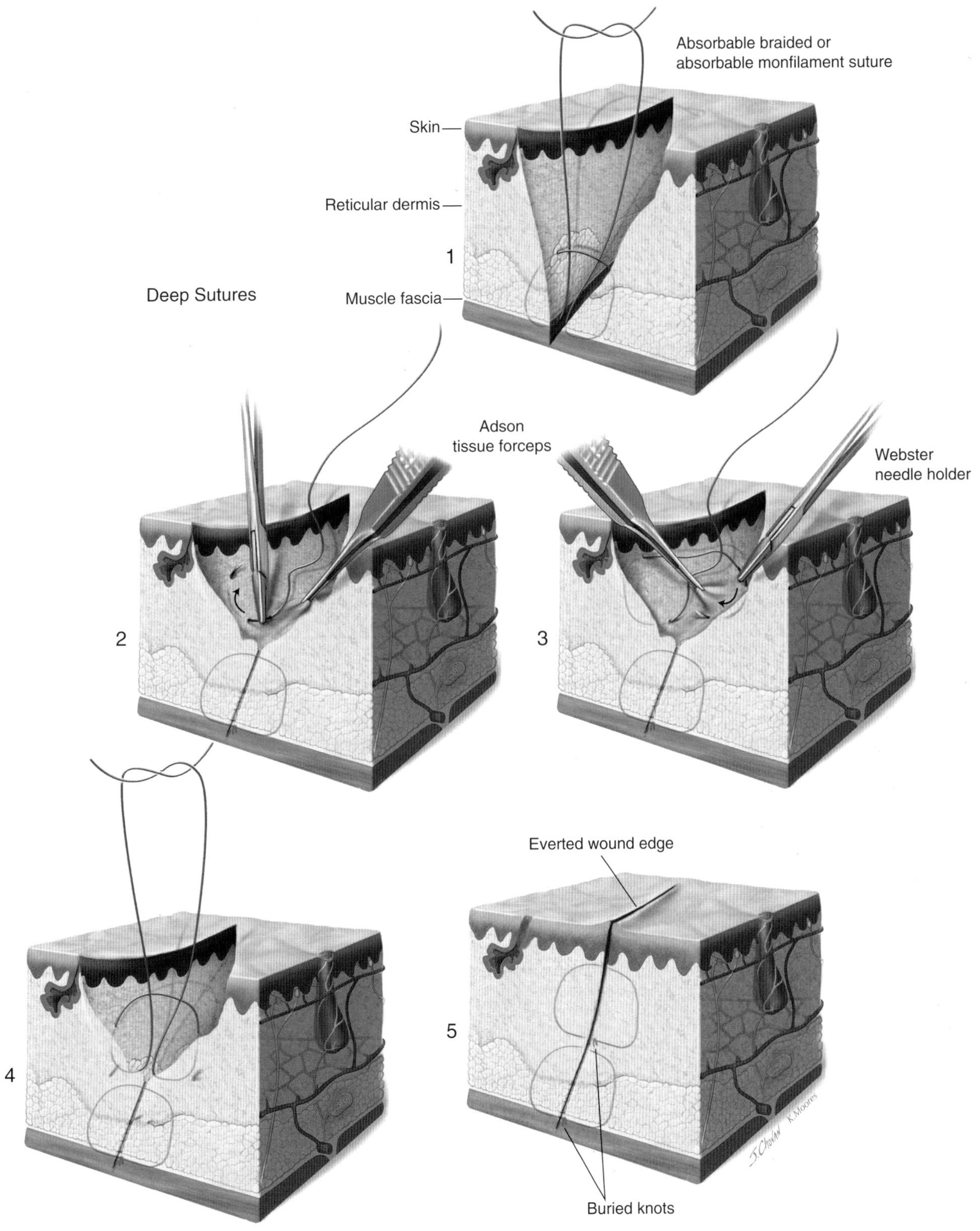

Figure 69.7 Deep wound closure.

TECHNIQUE: CLOSURE TECHNIQUE—cont'd

STEP 5: Skin Closure

The skin closure can be performed in a multitude of methods including tissue adhesive (surgical skin glue), simple interrupted sutures, percutaneous running, subcuticular running, vertical mattress, and horizontal mattress.

Tissue Adhesive: The skin layer may be closed with tissue adhesive if the skin edges passively sit together with a slight eversion. Tissue adhesive is often used for clean, minor lacerations in children or uncooperative patients. Ensure the skin edges are cleaned and dried from any blood or debris. Crush the vial of the tissue adhesive to begin the polymerization process. The tissue adhesive is then squeezed from the vial and applied to the skin edges. A thin layer of skin glue is applied by swiping the vial across the edges of the laceration. Allow the tissue adhesive to appropriately dry. An additional application may be necessary to ensure complete tissue adhesive coverage in larger wounds.

Simple Interrupted: The simple interrupted suture is one of the most common methods of skin closure. The needle is inserted through the skin at a 90-degree angle into the depth of the wound. On the opposite side, the needle is inserted at the same depth of the wound and exits at a similar point directly across from the initial insertion point. The knot is then tied on top of the skin. Simple interrupted sutures are placed at an appropriate distance such that skin edges across the entire laceration are in contact (Fig. 69.8).

Continuous Suture: The continuous or running suture is a method of suturing to allow for rapid closure of wounds with lower risks of infection. The technique creates an even distribution of tension along the length of the wound. The knot starts the same as a simple interrupted suture. Once the knot is tied, the free end of the suture is trimmed and then the needle is used to take repeated passes through the skin edges continuously. While taking repeated passes through the skin, the needle is angled at 45 degrees from one edge of the skin to the other to all for the crosses of the suture to be at 90 degrees on the skin edge. After completion of the final bite, the passed suture is left loose, acting as a free end to tie the knot.

Subcuticular Continuous: The subcuticular continuous suture is reserved for linear wounds with low risk of infection. The advantage of this suture is that it reduces the risk of postoperative track marks. Typically, a monocryl suture is anchored at one end of the laceration with a simple deep dermal stitch with only cutting the free end short. Then the needle is inserted from deep to superficial exiting at the epidermal-dermal junction on the apex of the laceration. The suture is then inserted at the epidermal-dermal junction and exits the epidermal-dermal junction further along the laceration on the same side. The needle is then inserted directly horizontal from its previous exit point into the opposite side of the laceration at the epidermal-junction. The needle exits further along the wound at the epidermal-dermal junction. The suture is brought back and forth from each side of the wound until the apex is reached. A knot is tied at the apex. The knot is buried deep into the wound by inserting the suture through the wound at the apex and taking a deep bite coming out of the skin. The suture is then cut flush with the skin surface (Fig. 69.9).

Vertical Mattress: The vertical mattress suture technique is beneficial in wounds with higher tension and skin edges that tend to invert. The first pass of the suture enters the skin on one side and goes through the deeper dermal layers of both sides of the wound and exits the skin on the opposite side. The needle is rotated 180 degrees and a small bite is taken entering the skin on one side, goes through the epidermal-dermal junction on both sides of the wound, and exits the skin. The knot is tied such that the knot sits on one side of the wound (Fig. 69.10).

Horizontal Mattress: The horizontal mattress technique is beneficial in high-tension wounds and is a water-tight method of closure. The needle is inserted through the skin at a 90-degree angle into the depth of the wound. On the opposite side, the needle is inserted at the same depth of the wound and exits at a similar point directly across from the initial insertion point. A second bite is taken approximately 4 to 7 mm from the first exit site and exits approximately 4 to 7 mm from the initial entry point. The knot is tied such that the knot sits on one side of the wound (Fig. 69.11).

STEP 6: Dressing

If no dressing is used, then the patient should be instructed to keep the wound moist with topical ointment to prevent scab formation. If a dressing is chosen, then Steri-Strips are applied across the wound with the aid of a tincture of benzoin or Mastisol for improved adhesion. Ointment may then be applied over the Steri-Strips. If the decision is made to cover the wound, a Telfa nonadherent dressing can be applied with a Tegaderm film to secure the Telfa.[13]

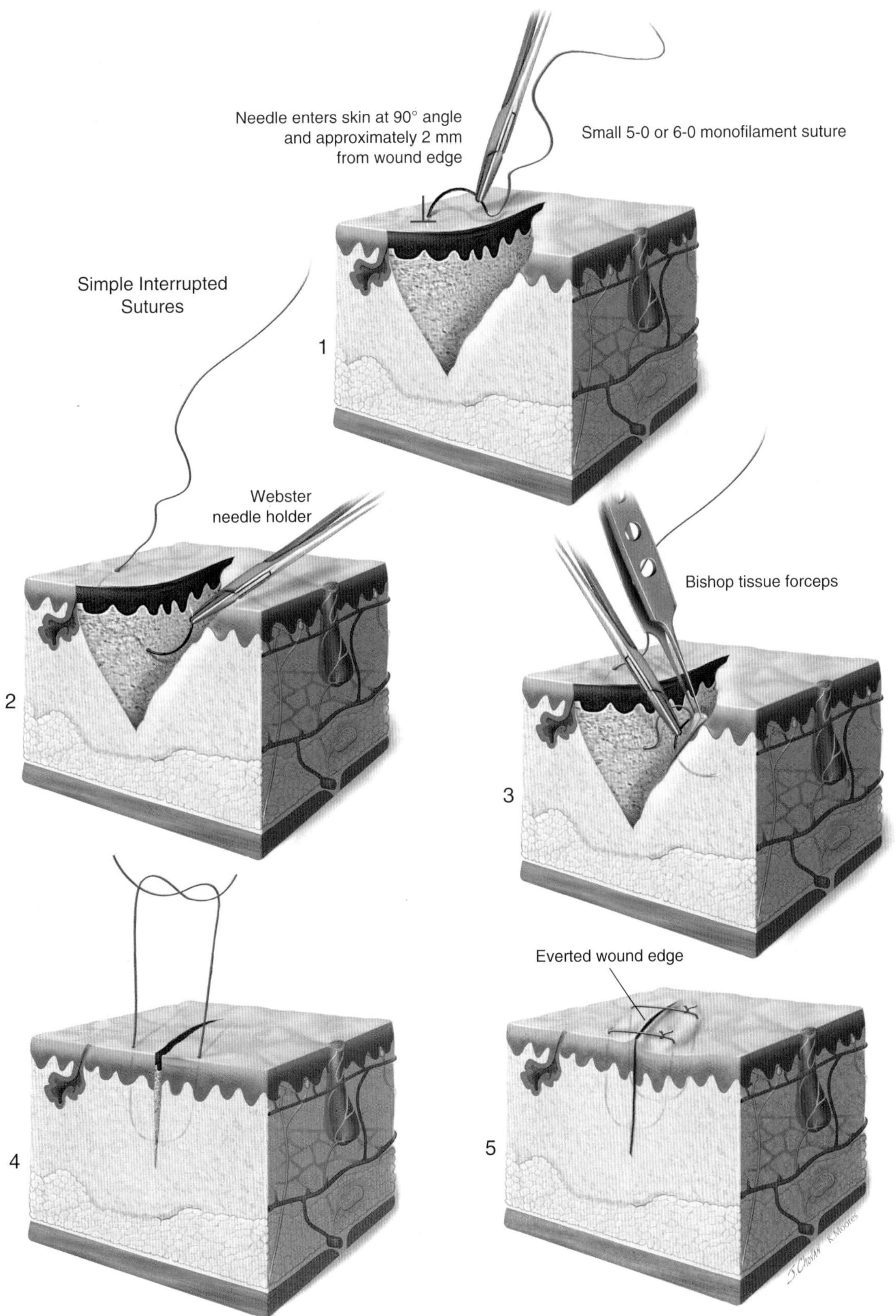

Figure 69.8 Simple interrupted skin closure.

Avoidance and Management of Complications

Repair of lacerations that parallel the RSTLs result in better cosmetic outcomes. The direction of traumatic facial lacerations does not necessarily parallel the RSTLs. Hypertrophic scarring can arise if lacerations cross RSTLs. To reduce the risk of hypertrophic scarring, appropriate eversion of the wound is critical. To ensure this, during wound closure, the deep layers must be approximated to allow for the skin edges to lie passively together prior to the application of cutaneous sutures. In some instances, early treatment with neurotoxin, steroids, and laser therapy will reduce scarring. Track marks from sutures can be avoided with the timely removal of nonabsorbable sutures within 5 to 7 days. Hypertrophic scars are often managed with injection of steroids, laser scar therapy, or surgical scar revision.

Infectious complications can be avoided by thorough irrigation and debridement of the contaminated wound. In some instances of highly contaminated wounds, delayed closure may reduce the risk of infectious complications. Wound infection of lacerations may require topical and systemic antibiotics. In some instances, sutures may need to be removed and the wound may need debridement.

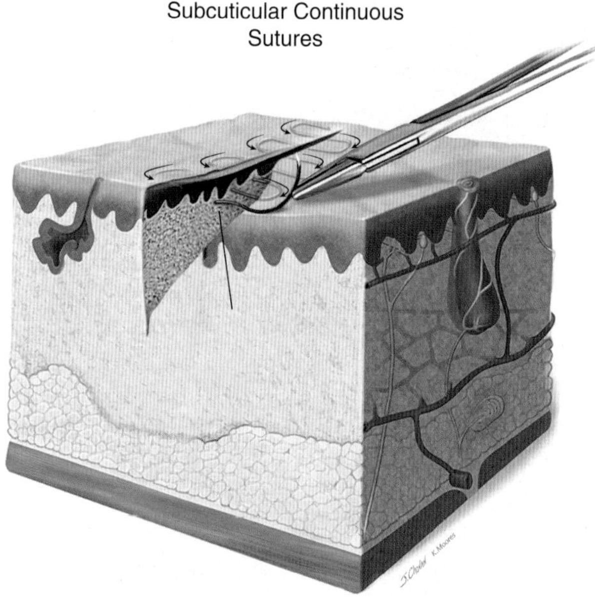

Figure 69.9 Subcuticular continuous suture.

Postoperative Considerations

Systemic antibiotics do not reduce the incidence of infections in simple lacerations.[14] However, antibiotics can be considered for significantly contaminated lacerations, immunocompromised patients, and smokers along with penetrating injuries, bite wounds, and lacerations involving the oral cavity.[13] Previous tetanus toxoid immunization history is important to elucidate and tetanus prophylaxis is administered as per appropriate immunization protocols. Bite wounds may also require rabies postexposure prophylaxis as per appropriate immunization protocols.

Lacerations may be cleansed in the shower after the first night. The wound should be kept moist for the first 2 days with topical antibiotic ointments and then nonantibiotic containing ointments afterward.[13]

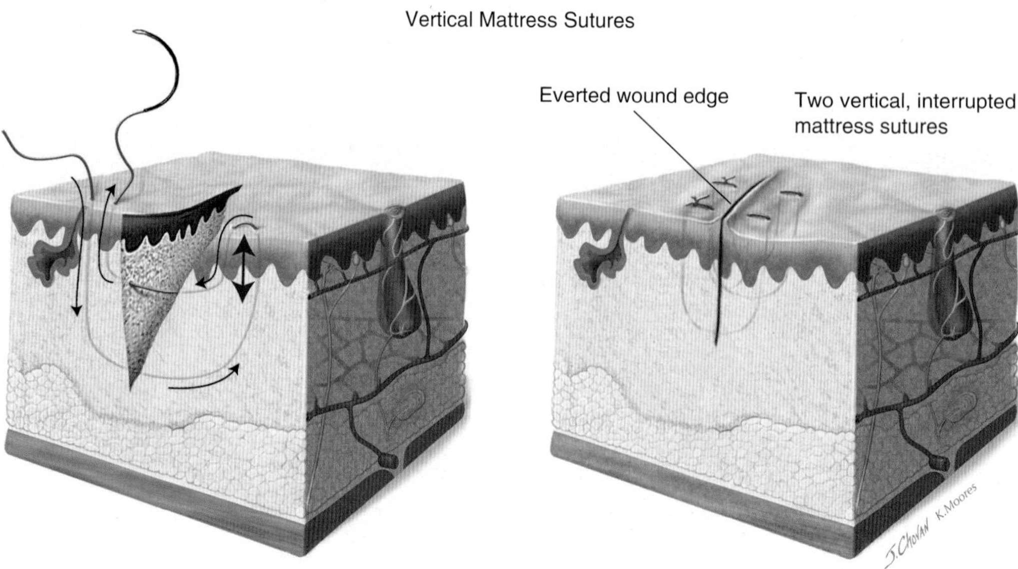

Figure 69.10 Vertical mattress suture.

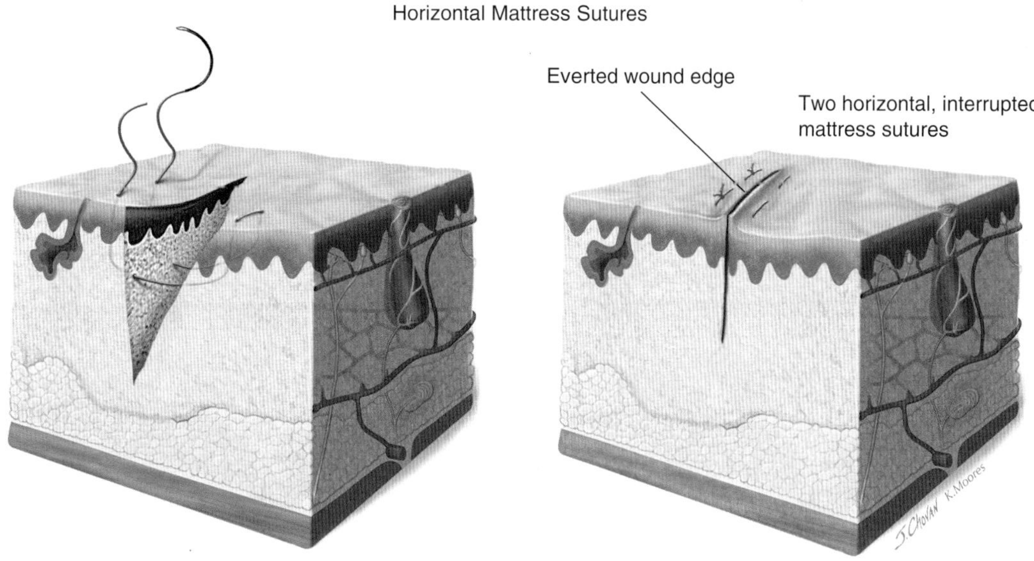

Figure 69.11 Horizontal mattress suture.

References

1. Meltzer ES, Sanchez GM. *The Edwin Smith Papyrus: Updated Translation of the Trauma Treatise and Modern Medical Commentaries.* ISD LLC; 2014.
2. Champaneria MC, Workman AD, Gupta SC. Sushruta: father of plastic surgery. *Ann Plast Surg.* 2014;73(1):2–7.
3. Bhishagratna KK. *An English Translation of the Sushruta Samhita*; 1911.
4. Mackenzie D. The history of sutures. *Med Hist.* 1973;17(2):158–168.
5. Broughton G 2nd, Janis JE, Attinger CE. A brief history of wound care. *Plast Reconstr Surg.* 2006;117(suppl 7):6S–11S.
6. Allen JG, Joseph L. A century of the antiseptic principle in the practice of surgery (Aug 12, 1865–Aug 12, 1965). *Arch Surg.* 1965;91(2):327–329.
7. Cameron JL. William stewart halsted. Our surgical heritage. *Ann Surg.* 1997;225(5):445–458.
8. Quinn J, Wells G, Sutcliffe T, et al. A randomized trial comparing octylcyanoacrylate tissue adhesive and sutures in the management of lacerations. *JAMA.* 1997;277(19):1527–1530.
9. Deliaert AE, Van den Kerckhove E, Tuinder S, et al. The effect of triclosan-coated sutures in wound healing. A double blind randomised prospective pilot study. *J Plast Reconstr Aesthet Surg.* 2009;62(6):771–773.
10. Khan AN, Dayan PS, Miller S, et al. Cosmetic outcome of scalp wound closure with staples in the pediatric emergency department: a prospective, randomized trial. *Pediatr Emerg Care.* 2002;18(3):171–173.
11. Hock MO, Ooi SB, Saw SM, et al. A randomized controlled trial comparing the hair apposition technique with tissue glue to standard suturing in scalp lacerations (HAT study). *Ann Emerg Med.* 2002;40(1):19–26.
12. Ko AC, Satterfield KR, Korn BS, et al. Eyelid and periorbital soft tissue trauma. *Facial Plast Surg Clin North Am.* 2017;25(4):605–616.
13. Medel N, Panchal N, Ellis E. Postoperative care of the facial laceration. *Craniomaxillofac Trauma Reconstr.* 2010;3(4):189–200.
14. Cummings P, Del Beccaro MA. Antibiotics to prevent infection of simple wounds: a meta-analysis of randomized studies. *Am J Emerg Med.* 1995;13(4):396–400.

CHAPTER 70

Techniques for Maxillomandibular Fixation

Duke Yamashita, Nam Cho, and Allen Huang

Armamentarium

#9 Molt periosteal elevator
24- and 26-gauge stainless steel wire
Appropriate sutures
Bite block
Dental syringe, needle, anesthetic
Erich-type arch bar
Heavy needle drivers (two)
Local anesthetic with vasoconstrictor
Minnesota or other cheek retractor
Wire cutters

History of the Procedure

The concept of immobilization for the treatment of skeletal fractures dates back to the days of ancient Greece as documented by Hippocrates.[1] Fixation methods have evolved over time through the use of the Barton bandage (Fig. 70.1) and Gunning splints.[2,3] Guglielmo Salicetti and Gilmer are thought to be among the first to make use of intermaxillary wires for the treatment of mandible fractures.[4] Although the introduction of rigid fixation has changed how surgeons are able to treat facial and skeletal fractures, the use of maxillomandibular fixation (MMF) remains an invaluable tool in the treatment of facial trauma.[5]

Indications for the Use of the Procedure

MMF is indicated when the dentition is able to assist in the reduction and realignment of the occlusion, which can often bring fractured bony segments closer together. MMF can be employed either as an aid to open reduction of mandible fractures or as definitive treatment for mandibular fractures not amenable to open reduction. These situations include minimally displaced fractures, grossly comminuted fractures, pediatric mandibular fractures, and intracapsular condylar fractures.[6] Although dentate jaws are ideal, MMF can also be accomplished for the edentulous arch through the use of Gunning splints or existing dentures. MMF is also indicated to reestablish occlusal relationships and restoration of the lower third of the facial skeleton during treatment of panfacial fractures. In addition, MMF is a useful treatment intermediary for orthognathic and other reconstructive procedures (Fig. 70.2).

Limitations and Contraindications

As with any other surgical procedure, MMF is not without its limitations. Prolonged immobilization of the maxillomandibular complex has been associated with trismus and decreased range of motion, often necessitating extensive physiotherapy and temporomandibular joint (TMJ) exercising in the postfixation period. Oral hygiene is also often difficult to maintain for many patients due to the presence of wires and arch bars. Ultimately, some patients, including the elderly, obtunded, developmentally delayed, and those with substance abuse issues, will be unable or unwilling to tolerate MMF for any period of time. Patients with a history of seizures or propensity towards nausea and vomiting are at risk for aspiration and may be best treated with other methods of fixation. Although edentulous patients can be treated with MMF through the use of splints, most surgeons prefer to treat edentulous fractures with rigid plates, forgoing the laborious and time-consuming task of either modifying existing dentures or fabricating Gunning splints.

Patients presenting with intracapsular condylar fractures should undergo only limited durations of MMF for pain relief, assuming the occlusion is stable and reproducible. TMJ ankylosis, though seldom seen, is a feared complication of prolonged MMF. Airway concern may also be a relative contraindication, especially in the obtunded trauma patient. A tracheostomy should be considered

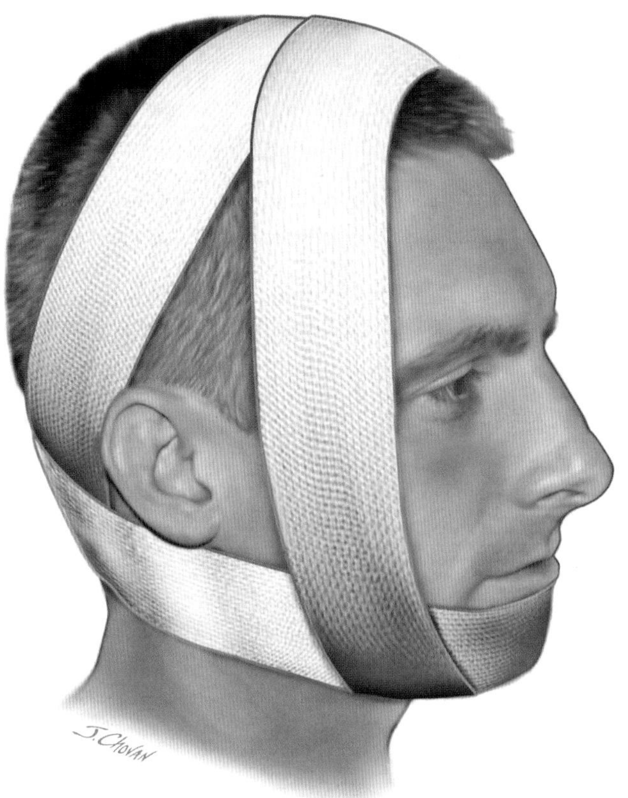

Figure 70.1 Barton bandage.

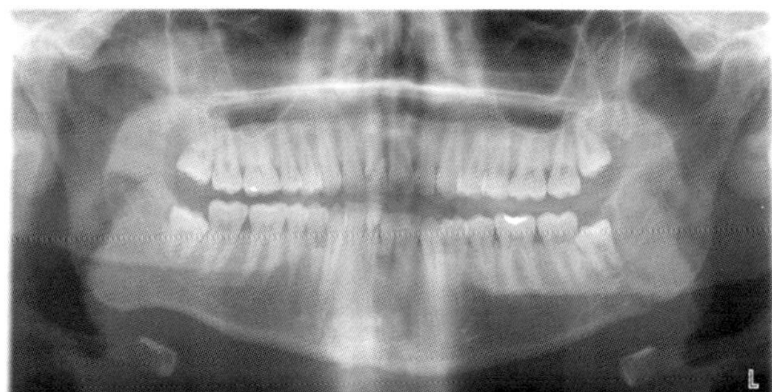

Figure 70.2 Orthopantogram showing mandible fractures of right parasymphysis and left angle.

to provide a secure airway in the polytrauma patient for whom an extended period of intubation is anticipated.

Mandible fractures in the pediatric patient deserve special mention. Tooth buds often preclude these fractures from rigid internal fixation and MMF is often the treatment of choice. In these instances, the duration of MMF should be shorter given their excellent healing and bone formation capacities. This is especially true for condylar fractures in children due to their propensity to grow heterotopic bone and undergo ankylosis.[7]

TECHNIQUE: Application of Erich Arch Bars

STEP 1: Intubation and Preparation

Erich arch bars should be trimmed to length, spanning any fractures occurring between teeth. Either 24- or 26-gauge wire should also be cut for interdental and interarch fixation. Once the hardware has been prepared, intermaxillary fixation can be completed using general anesthesia, IV sedation, or local anesthesia alone. Along with the soft tissue and dentition to be wired, the fracture sites should be anesthetized using local anesthesia with a vasoconstrictor, paying close attention to recommended maximum dosages.

STEP 2: Application of Arch Bar

Once adequately anesthetized, the arch bar can be fixed to each tooth using wires of appropriate length. The wire can be passed from labial to lingual on one side of the tooth and passed back from lingual to labial on the opposing surface. The wire should rest superior to the bar on one side and inferior to the bar on the other, effectively creating a loop, which can be tightened against the arch bar. This is repeated for all teeth within the span of the arch bar on both the mandible and maxilla. At this point, any teeth scheduled for removal should be extracted. The removal of teeth should be undertaken judiciously as torqueing forces can displace fractures and extractions may not improve outcomes[8] (Fig. 70.3A).

STEP 3: Management of Dentition

Teeth should be extracted if they are grossly carious or mobile, have a poor prognosis, have periodontal pathology, or interfere with the reduction of fracture segments. Fracture segments can be minimally manipulated at this point, especially in the angle area, to facilitate good bony apposition prior to MMF. Intermaxillary wires should be used to place the patient into centric occlusion. The posterior occlusion and anterior wear facets should be used as a guide to the patient's pretraumatic occlusion. Care should be taken to not over close the anterior-most wire as doing so can cause opening of the posterior occlusion.

The duration of MMF varies depending on host factors as well as the severity of injury.[9,10] The typical duration of immobilization has historically been 4 to 6 weeks. Prophylactic antibiotics should be used for compound fractures with penicillin being the agent of choice. For those unable to take penicillin, clindamycin should be used[11] (Fig. 70.3B).

Continued

TECHNIQUE: Application of Erich Arch Bars—*cont'd*

SPECIAL SITUATIONS

If there is a tooth missing within the span of the arch bar, each of the two adjacent teeth should be wired using two separate wires, to reinforce the fixation of the arch bar to the teeth. This can be done using an "over-under" technique, with the two wires in opposing orientation relative to the arch bar. Failure to do so could cause sagging or loosening of the arch bar when attempting to place intermaxillary wires.

For edentulous spans longer than a single tooth, a reinforced arch bar should be used. This is accomplished by securing an appropriate length of the stylet portion of an 18-gauge spinal needle against the arch bar using the lugs of the arch bar. This creates a rigid arch bar in the edentulous span that can be used during intermaxillary fixation. Care must be taken to adapt this rigid bar to the dentition because unwanted orthodontic forces could be generated (Figure 70.3C and D).

If a fracture in a dentate segment is proving difficult to reduce, it is often beneficial to leave a few of the wires loose on the teeth adjacent to the fracture site. The rest of the arch can be wired tightly and once the entire arch is in intermaxillary fixation against the opposing arch, tightening of the remaining loose wires may help in achieving a better reduction. Ultimately, the arch bar can also be segmented with later placement of a bridle wire once the arch form is established.

Le Fort I fractures displace in a predictable manner, creating what has classically been described as a posterior gag bite. The anterior maxilla typically intrudes while the posterior maxilla becomes inferiorly positioned. Patients treated in the acute posttraumatic stage usually present with a mobile and easily reduced maxilla. Patients with a longer delay in treatment may present with a maxilla that is difficult to mobilize and reduce. For these patients, arch bars and anterior guidance elastics can be used to aid in the mobilization and inferior repositioning of the maxilla. Once the anterior open bite is closed through the use of the elastic traction, the bands can be replaced with wires and definitive treatment can be pursued (Fig. 70.3E).

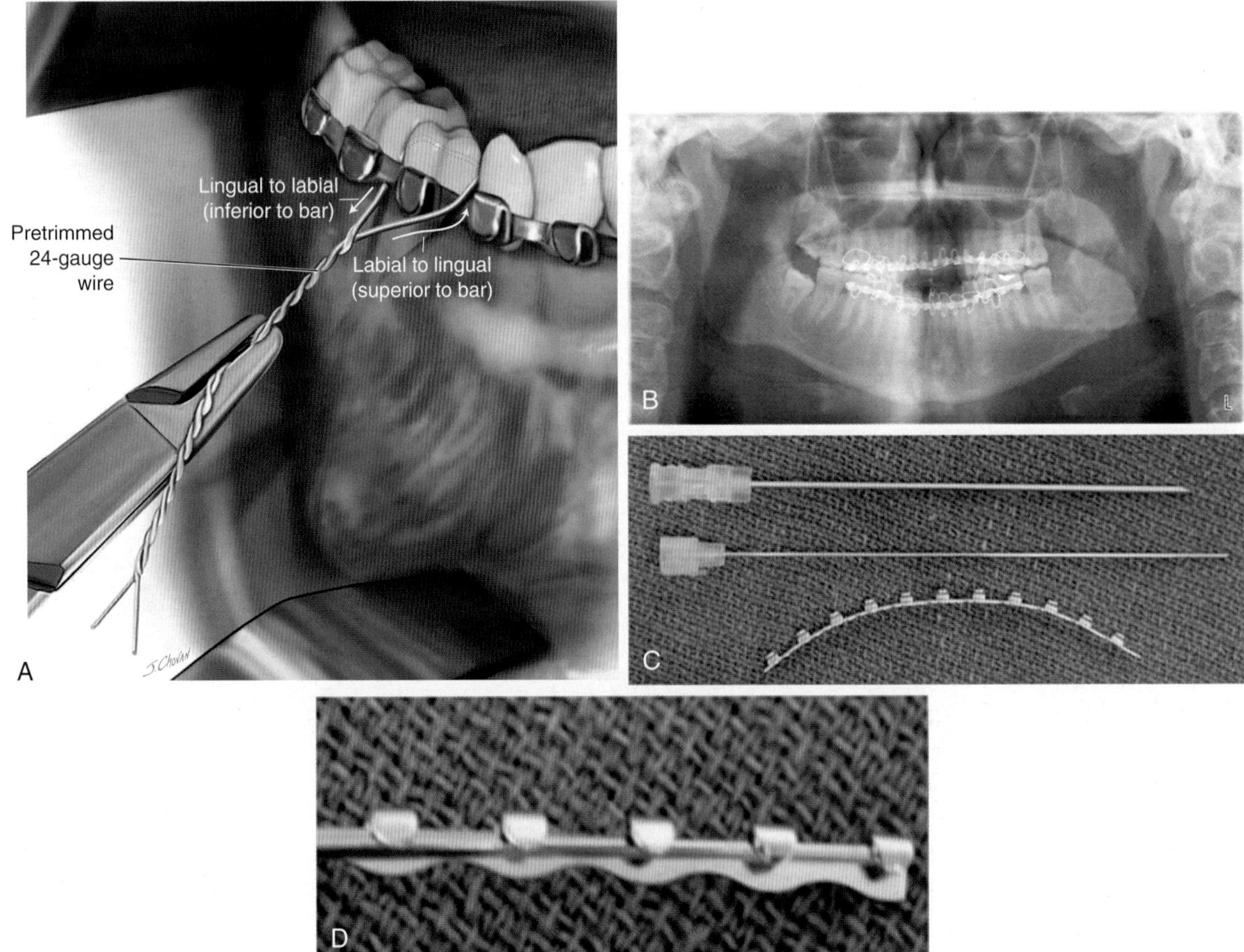

Figure 70.3 **A,** Applying Erich arch bar to dentition using wires. **B,** Postreduction orthopantogram. **C,** Spinal needle stylet and Erich arch bar. **D,** Stylet portion adapted to arch bar to create a reinforced arch bar.

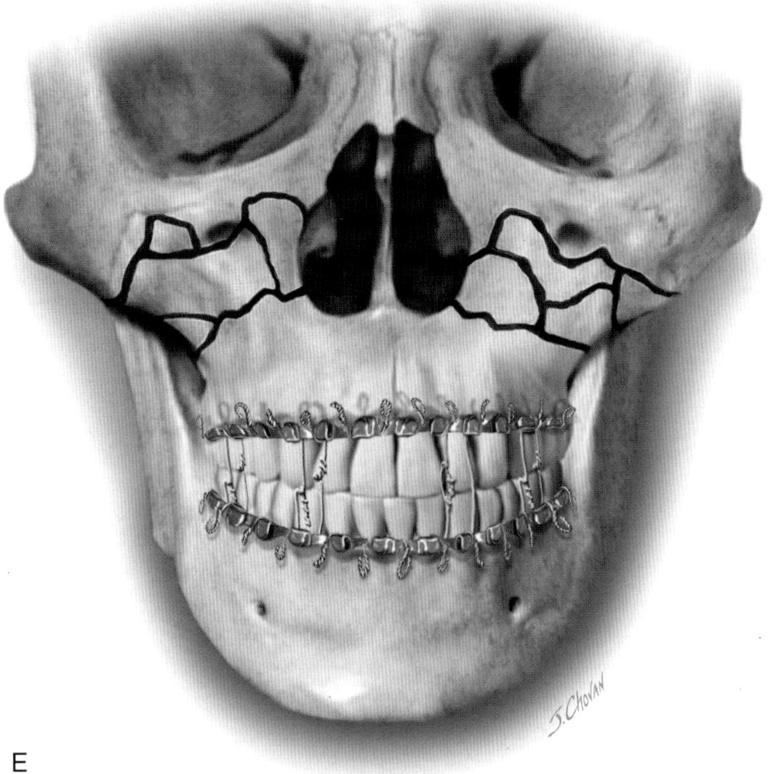

E

Figure 70.3, cont'd E, Reduced Le Fort I fracture.

ALTERNATIVE TECHNIQUE 1: Ivy Loops

Ivy loops can also be used in instances where there are only a few stable teeth within the arch or when the surgeon feels the use of arch bars are not necessary to maintain three-dimensional stability. Ivy loops should be prepared in advance. A 24-gauge stainless steel wire is bent in half and a small loop is created by tightly twisting the wire on itself for a few turns. A minimum of two wires should be used for each arch. The free ends of the loop are inserted from labial to lingual into the interproximal space between predetermined teeth. One free end is passed back to the labial one embrasure anterior while the other free end is passed back one embrasure posterior. The posterior free end is then passed through the preexisting loop, and the anterior and posterior ends are tightened. Once all of the ivy loops are placed and tightened, intermaxillary wires can be placed, making use of the loops for fixation (Fig. 70.4).

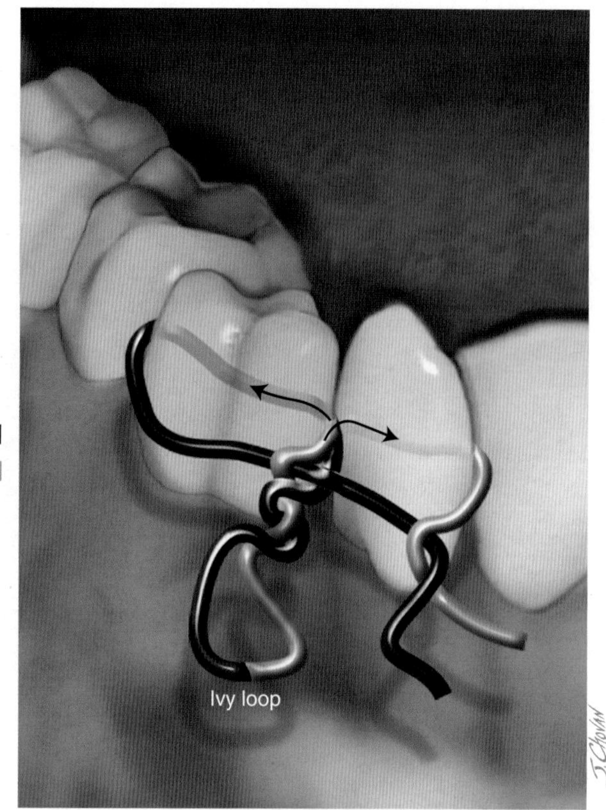

Figure 70.4 Ivy loop in place prior to intermaxillary fixation (IMF).

ALTERNATIVE TECHNIQUE 2: Intermaxillary Fixation (IMF) Screws

IMF screws are bone-borne anchorage screws used as fixation points for interarch fixation.[12] The screws are typically self-tapping and self-drilling, so power instrumentation is not needed. Care must be taken to avoid tooth roots and neurovascular structures. Although bone in the mandible and piriform area is dense and amenable to the use of these screws, bone over the antrum can be porous and provide little anchorage. Patient selection is of utmost importance because IMF screws are inappropriate for multiple segments due to their tendency to allow for independent segment rotation/displacement. IMF screws have also been known to loosen over time and may be a suboptimal choice for prolonged periods of MMF. Much like ivy loops, IMF screws also allow for only minimal elastic manipulation of the arches after fixation.

A minimum of two screws should be used for each arch. They are typically placed around the mucogingival junction with great care taken not to traumatize adjacent tooth roots. Once all of the screws are placed and noted to be stable, wires can be passed through the screw heads of opposing screws and tightened for fixation and immobilization. It is imperative that excellent hygiene be maintained due to the overgrowth of surrounding tissues over the screws and the potential for infection. Even with meticulous attention to hygiene, it is common for the soft tissue to grow over screw heads (Fig. 70.5A).

EDENTULOUS FRACTURES

For the completely edentulous patient with a mandible fracture, existing dentures can be wired to the maxilla and the mandible using circumzygomatic, piriform, and circummandibular wires. If the patient is without existing dentures or if they are unavailable, Gunning splints can be fabricated and used for IMF. Impressions of both jaws are taken, and acrylic baseplates can be created and used in a fashion similar to dentures. As previously mentioned, this is a time-consuming and labor-intensive process that has become less popular in favor of open reduction (Fig. 70.5B).

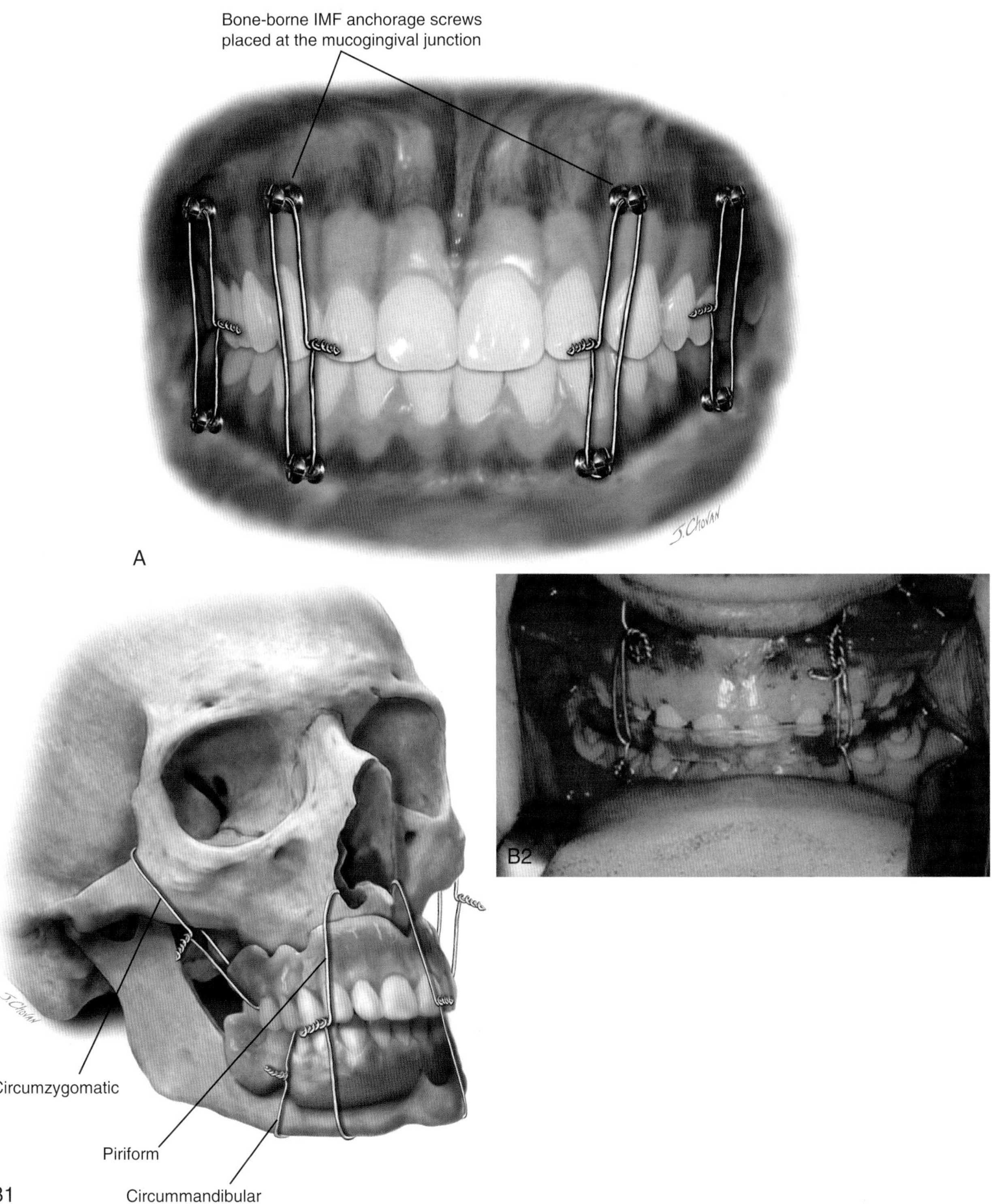

Figure 70.5 **A,** Intermaxillary fixation (*IMF*) screws used for reduction. **B1,** Dentures wired to maxilla and mandible. **B2,** Skeletal wire fixation securing interocclusal splint. (B2, Reprinted with permission from Myers E. *Operative Otolaryngology: Head and Neck Surgery.* 2nd ed. Philadelphia: Saunders; 2009.)

Avoidance and Management of Intraoperative Complications

The surgeon using MMF techniques should be cognizant of the need to avoid intraoperative soft/hard tissue and dental injuries. It also is important to note that intraoral wire placement poses a risk of needle stick injury between the patient and the operator. Wire cutting scissors should always accompany a patient with MMF in case fixation needs to be urgently removed, such as in cases of emesis in the postanesthetic state. Care must be taken to avoid the dental roots and nerve impingement during MMF screw placement. Attention should be given for the overall nutritional status of all patients with MMF.

Postoperative Considerations

Patients who have undergone MMF require close follow-up care to evaluate occlusion and range of motion. Patients presenting with persistent and worsening pain at the fracture site require further investigation both clinically and radiographically. Longer periods of MMF may be indicated, and elastics should be used to guide occlusion to overcome any occlusal discrepancies. Should the patient have persistent occlusal discrepancies, orthodontic therapy can be utilized for correction after bony consolidation. Importantly, maximum range of motion of the TMJ should be closely evaluated and maintained through the use of tongue blades, jaw exercises, or passive range-of-motion devices.

As surgeons, a general principle is to treat the underlying process by the simplest and least invasive method possible. For maxillofacial trauma, treatment of fractures through closed reduction proves to be a well-accepted and proven option with lower rates of postreduction infection when compared with open reduction.[13,14] Should a patient treated with closed reduction develop an infection, however, management principles remain the same with dependent drainage, further immobilization, and antibiotic therapy.

While MMF has been a time-tested treatment option for facial trauma, inadequate bony healing or nonunion, while infrequent, is a possibility. In fact, the lowest incidence of mandibular nonunion occurred for those fractures treated with MMF alone.[15] Patients with fractures complicated by nonunion usually need open treatment with the aid of bone grafts and large reconstruction plates.

References

1. Hippocrates. *Oeuvres Completes*. English translation by ET Withnington: Cambridge, MA; 1928.
2. Barton JR. A systemic bandage for fractures of the lower jaw. *Am Med Recorder Phila*. 1819;2:153.
3. Gunning TB. Treatment of fractures of the lower jaw by interdental splints. *Br J Dent Sci*. 1866;9:481.
4. Salicetti G (William of Saliceto): 125, Cirurgia.
5. Winstanley RP. The management of fractures of the mandible. *Br J Oral Maxillofac Surg*. 1984;22(3):170–177.
6. Barber HD, Bahram R, Woodbury SC, et al. In: Fonseca R.J., ed. St Louis, Missouri: Elsevier, Saunders; 2005. *Oral and Maxillofacial Trauma*. 3rd ed. 1.
7. Topazian RG. Etiology of ankylosis of the temporomandibular joint: analysis of 44 cases. *J Oral Surg Anesth Hosp Dent Serv*. 1964;22:227–233.
8. Ellis III E. Outcomes of patients with teeth in the line of mandibular angle fractures treated with stable internal fixation. *J Oral Maxillofac Surg*. 2002;60(8):863–865.
9. Maw RB. A new look at maxillomandibular fixation of mandibular fractures. *J Oral Surg*. 1981;39(3):187–190.
10. Amaratunga NA. The relation of age to the immobilization period required for healing of mandibular fractures. *J Oral Maxillofac Surg*. 1987;45(2):111–113.
11. Zallen RD, Curry JT. A study of antibiotic usage in compound mandibular fractures. *J Oral Surg*. 1975;33(6):431–434.
12. Karlis V, Glickman R. An alternative to archbar maxillomandibular fixation. *Plast Reconstr Surg*. 1997;99(6):1758–1759.
13. Terris DJ, Lalakea ML, Tuffo KM, Shinn JB. Mandible fracture repair: specific indications for newer techniques. *Otolaryngol Head Neck Surg*. 1994;111(6):751–757.
14. Leach J, Truelson J. Traditional methods vs rigid internal fixation of mandible fractures. *Arch Otolaryngol Head Neck Surg*. 1995;121(7):750–753.
15. Bochlogyros PN. Non-union of fractures of the mandible. *J Maxillofac Surg*. 1985;13(4):189–193.

CHAPTER 71

Surgical Correction of Injuries of the Nasolacrimal System

John Vorrasi and Radhika Chigurupati

Armamentarium

Appropriate sutures
Balanced sterile saline solution and fluorescein dye
Bard-Parker knife handle and blades (#15, #11, #12)
Bowman lacrimal probes
Corneal shield protectors
Cotton-tip applicators
Neuro cotton pads
Electrocautery (bipolar forceps)
Eye cannula with 3-cc syringe for irrigation
Fine directing hook
Kerrison bone rongeurs
Lacrimal punctal dilators
Local anesthetic with vasoconstrictor
Loupe magnification
Mitomycin C 0.5% solution
Nasal speculum
Ophthalmic Betadine 5% sterile solution
Oxymetazoline nasal spray (Affrin or 4% cocaine)
Periosteal elevators (Molt #9 and curved Freer)
Rotary instruments (round burs, Sonopet ultrasonic aspirator)
Senn retractors
Silicone tubing with stainless-steel probes (i.e., Crawford tubes) or Ritleng stent
Stevens tenotomy scissors
Westcott scissors

History of the Procedure

The correction of disorders of the nasolacrimal (NL) system dates back to the 1st century, when Cornelius Celsus (25 BC to AD 50) and Claudius Galenus (AD 130 to 200) described their original work on dacryocystorhinostomy (DCR) and NL obstruction.[1] It was not until 1904 that Addeo Toti, an Italian rhinologist, described the formal technique of external DCR. This surgical technique was subsequently modified and popularized by Dutemps, Bourguet, Ohm, and Iliff, making this procedure the gold standard for the treatment of chronic obstruction of the NL duct system.[1–4] In 1893, Caldwell first described the endonasal approach to the lacrimal sac; however, difficult access limited the use of this approach until recent advances in endoscopic surgical techniques. In 1989, McDonough and Meiring documented the first clinical series of studies on the intranasal endoscopic approach for DCR.[1,5] The instruments, stents, and tubes used to maintain patency of the NL duct system also have evolved. Henderson initially described the use of 1-mm polyethylene tubes for the management of lacrimal canaliculi strictures. Later, Gibbs introduced silicone tubes to maintain patency of the NL drainage system.[2,6] Crawford subsequently added the stainless-steel probe attachment to the silicone tubing, which is the most common design used currently. The Ritleng (FCI Ophthalmics, Marshfield Hills, MA) system uses the Seldinger technique to introduce a silicon tube to constricted or damage inferior or superior canaliculus, and it is secured at the punctum with a widened silicone flange preventing displacement. More recently, the neurosurgical ultrasound device (Sonopet OMNI; Stryker, Kalamazoo, MI), which uses both longitudinal and torsional motion of the tip, has been used for bone removal in surgical DCR procedures.[2] Endonasal endoscopic DCR procedures avoid any external incisions, and many studies have shown that they are as effective as external DCR procedures used in NL obstruction repair.[7–10]

Indications for the Use of the Procedure

The NL duct system, or the excretory component of the lacrimal apparatus, is composed of (1) the superior and inferior lacrimal puncta; (2) the superior and inferior canaliculi, with or without the common canaliculus; (3) the NL sac; and (4) the NL duct (Fig. 71.1A and B). The symptom of epiphora due to inadequate tear drainage is the most common indication for interrogation and/or surgical correction of the NL duct system. Pain, swelling, and mucopurulent discharge from the lacrimal puncta are other symptoms and signs that may indicate a need for these procedures. The timing of intervention and the choice of procedure to correct disorders of the NL duct system depend on several factors, such as the cause

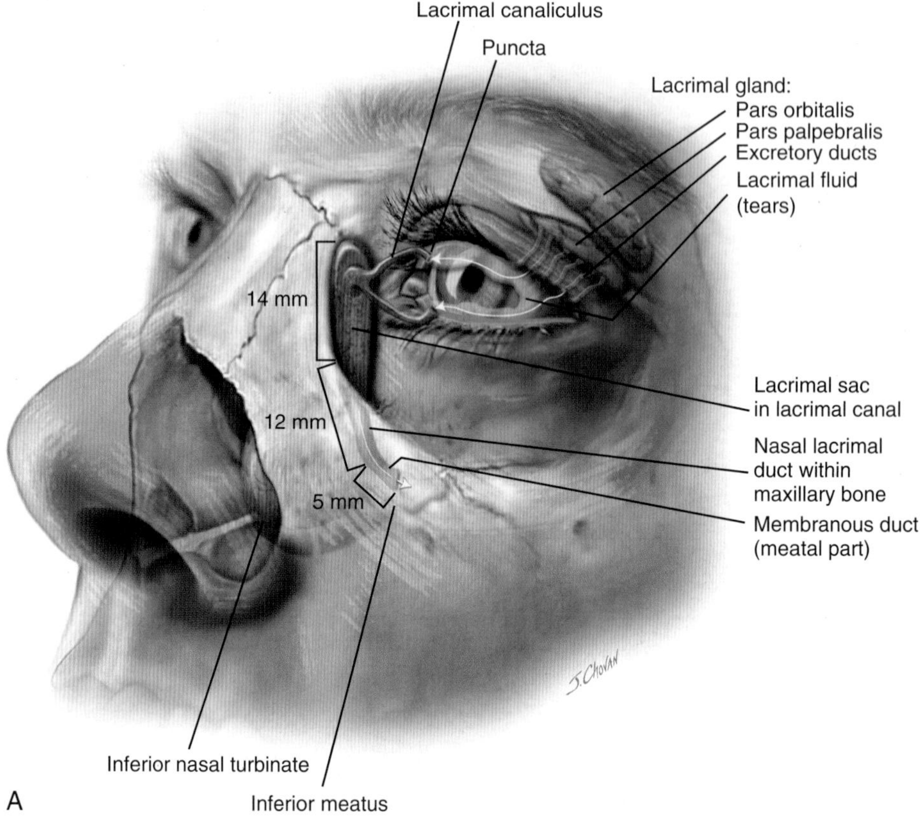

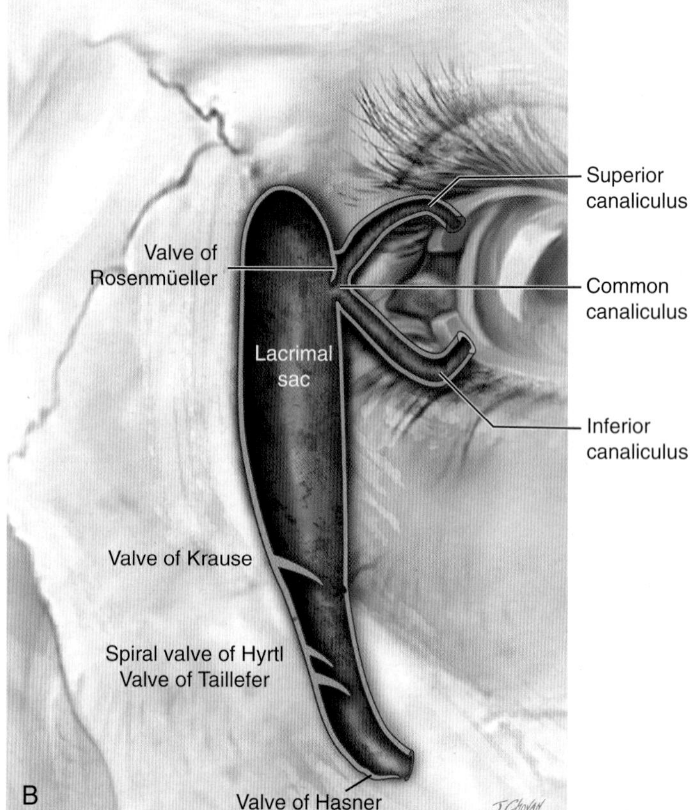

Figure 71.1 **A,** The lacrimal fluid or tears secreted by the lacrimal gland and accessory glands flow to the medial angle of the eye and enter the lacrimal canaliculi through the puncta. The canaliculi discharge into the lacrimal sac transmits the fluid into the nose through the nasolacrimal (NL) duct, which opens in the inferior meatus. The NL duct runs inferiorly encased in the maxillary bone for about 12 mm and then traverses as a membranous duct in a lateral and posterior direction before it exits beneath the bony horizontal ridge of the inferior meatus. **B,** Several membranous folds within the sac and NL duct function as valves to prevent retrograde tear movement. The valves can be points of stenosis or obstruction. The most superior valve of Rosen-müeller joins the sac with the common canaliculus. The inferior mucosal fold forms the valve of Hasner. The medial canthal tendon lies anterior to the canaliculi and attaches to the anterior lacrimal crest. The canaliculi are surrounded by fibers of the par lacrimalis (Horner muscle) of the orbicularis occuli, which compress the common canaliculus when the eyelid closes to facilitate tear drainage into the NL duct.

BOX 71.1 Causes of Obstruction of Nasolacrimal Duct System

- Aging
- Trauma
  - Blunt midfacial injuries: medial orbital wall, naso-orbito-ethmoid, and Le Fort II and III fractures
  - Thermal or chemical injury resulting in scarring
  - Facial soft tissue or lid lacerations (e.g., dog bites in children)
- Infection
  - Paranasal sinus or periorbital infections, dacryoliths
- Neoplasm
  - Lacrimal sac tumors
- Iatrogenic/surgery
  - Midfacial tumor resection (e.g., maxillectomy)
  - Craniofacial reconstructive surgery
- Idiopathic
  - Females more likely to develop obstruction of nasolacrimal duct
- Congenital or neonatal dacryocystitis

of the obstruction, the anatomic site of obstruction, and the duration of symptoms (Box 71.1). Common causes of obstruction of the NL duct system include congenital malformation or constriction, naso-orbito-ethmoid (NOE) fractures, facial soft tissue lacerations involving the eyelids, and periorbital or paranasal sinus infections (Fig. 71.2). Occasionally, the obstruction may be a consequence of reconstructive craniofacial surgery (e.g., frontal/midface osteotomies) or ablative surgery for midface tumor resection (e.g., maxillectomy).[11–14] Other infrequent causes of NL obstruction include lacrimal sac tumors and stenosis due to radiation therapy or thermal or chemical injury.[13,15]

The most common site of obstruction is the canaliculus, followed by the NL duct itself.[16] The inferior canalicular system is more commonly affected than the superior canaliculus, particularly in blunt force traumatic injuries of the midface. Timely treatment of fractures of the NOE complex can prevent scarring and bony interference of the NL drainage pathway.[11,17] Swelling and edema of midfacial soft tissues can cause transient obstruction of the NL duct system, which can be managed by close follow-up and may resolve with time. Intraoperative NL intubation during the management of NOE fractures has been reported and may be valuable in select cases.[18,19] Surgical intervention is indicated when there is obvious canalicular laceration, often seen in children with eyelid injuries due to dog bites.[20–22] NL duct system interrogation and ultimately DCR, with or without intubation, may be considered if symptoms of obstruction do not completely resolve with time after close follow-up.

Evaluation and Diagnostic Investigations

A thorough history and complete intranasal and ophthalmologic examination, including visual acuity, ocular motility, pupillary function, and slit-lamp examination of the eye, are recommended before surgical repair of disorders of the NL duct system. The application of pressure over the lacrimal sac, probing, and interrogation and irrigation of the lacrimal drainage system may relieve obstruction or help determine the exact anatomic site of obstruction. The most useful diagnostic investigations for evaluation of obstruction of NL duct system are the saline irrigation test and the Jones I and II tests using fluorescein dye. Imaging studies, such as computed tomography scans or magnetic resonance imaging, are helpful in the acute injury setting when edema and swelling may preclude the previously mentioned tests.[12,23] The Jones dye test is used to assess the functioning of the lacrimal drainage system. The test is designed as a two-part (primary and secondary) examination. Initially, 2% fluorescein dye is placed in the medial conjunctival fold area, and a cotton-tipped applicator is placed under the inferior turbinate. Recovery of the dye in the nose at 2- and 5-minute intervals is recorded. A positive test result (dye recovery) indicates a patent NL system and sufficient physiologic function. A positive primary Jones dye test in the presence of epiphora indicates hypersecretion by the lacrimal gland. If the primary test result is negative (dye is not recovered), a secondary Jones test can be performed to evaluate anatomic patency by irrigating the canalicular system with clear saline and instructing the patient to blow the nose into a tissue. Recovery of dye from the secondary test, after a negative primary test result, is consistent with gross patency but relative dysfunction or incomplete obstruction. In a negative secondary dye test result, undyed saline may be recovered from the inferior meatus; this indicates a punctual or canalicular obstruction. Both the inferior and superior canaliculi should be investigated. Table 71.1 presents a summary of the Jones dye tests.[24,25]

Nasolacrimal Interrogation

The canaliculi are interrogated for patency when there is a high index of suspicion for injury or obstruction. If surgery is required, canalicular dilation, probing, and irrigation may be helpful to identify components of the NL drainage system and assess the extent of the injury; in some cases, this may restore function. When the NL system is interrogated, care must be taken not to injure the canaliculi and duct or create a false passage. Procedures such as probing, irrigation, and intubation can be performed using a local anesthetic; however, more involved surgery, such as laceration repair or DCR, requires general anesthesia (Fig. 71.3A).

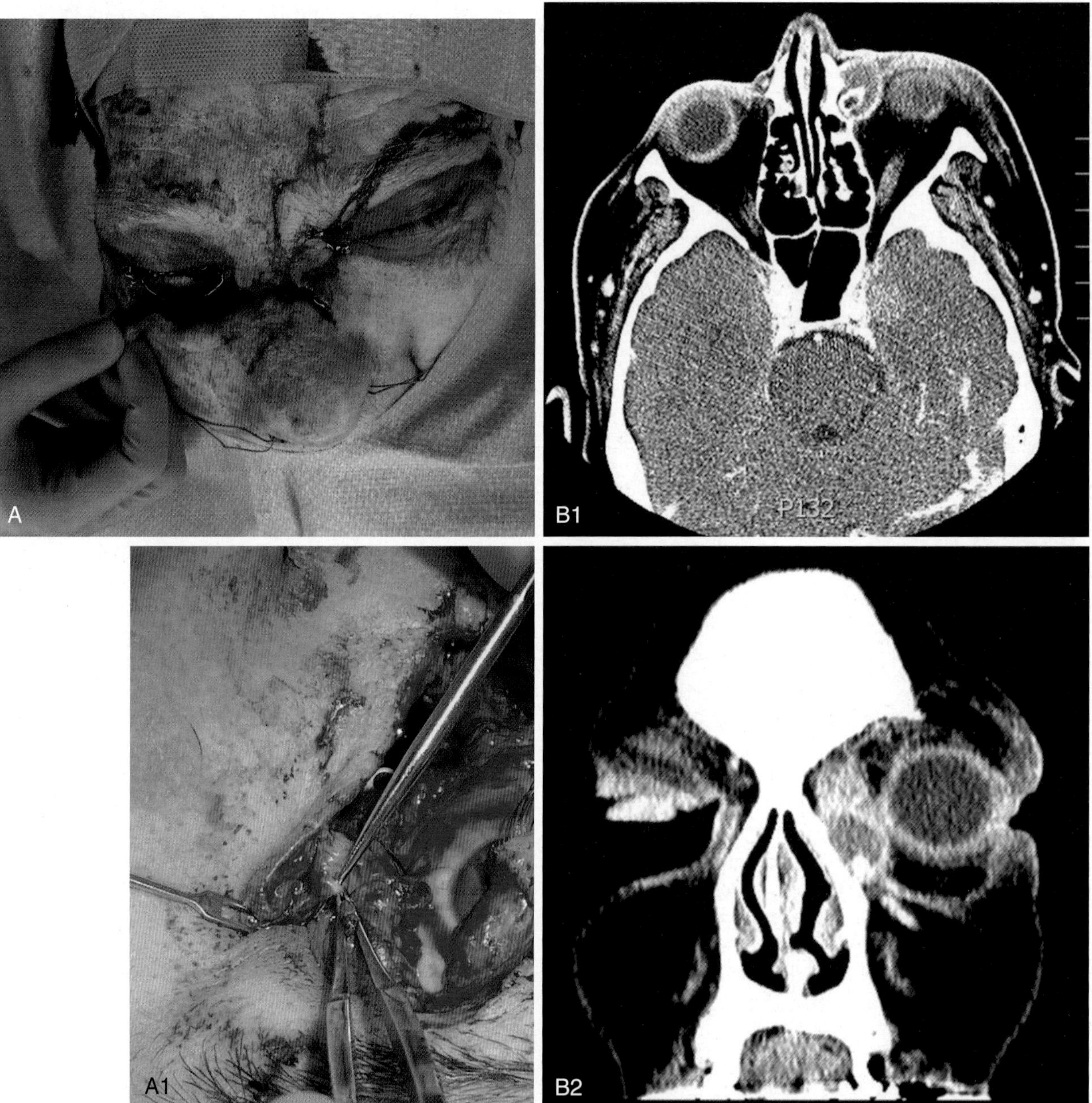

Figure 71.2 **A,** The medial canthal tendon and the inferior canaliculi may be disrupted in comminuted naso-orbito-ethmoid fractures, lower lid lacerations or orbital trauma, as shown here. In these injuries, the function of the pars lacrimalis of the orbicularis oculi, which facilitates the drainage of tears into the nasolacrimal (NL) duct may be disrupted. **A1,** Disrupted inferior canaliculus with dilator identification. **B1** and **B2** The axial and coronal images, respectively, of this computed tomography scan show periorbital cellulitis. The NL sac housed in the lacrimal fossa is enlarged and swollen. When unaffected, the NL sac is about 12 to 15 mm long and 6 mm wide, with a fundus portion superior to the entry of the common canaliculus. The computed tomography image shows the lacrimal fossa, which is formed by the lacrimal bone and frontal process of the maxilla. The medial wall of the lacrimal sac is adjacent to the most anterior part of the middle meatus of the nose and just below the middle concha. This relationship is important for cannulation of the sac with the endoscopic intranasal approach of dacryocystorhinostomy.

Table 71.1 Summary of Jones Dye Tests

Primary Jones Test	Secondary Jones Test	Results
+	(+)	Patent lacrimal system
–	+ saline, dye	Incomplete obstruction or dysfunction
–	+ saline, no dye	Punctal or canalicular obstruction
–	– no saline, no dye	Complete obstruction

(+) Assumed recovery of liquid, but not tested.
+ Liquid recovered on nasal swab.
– Unable to recover liquid on nasal swab.

NL intubation is performed mainly to reduce the risk of postoperative canalicular stenosis and adhesions.[26] The current evidence for performing intubation during DCR is controversial, although routine canalicular intubation during external and endoscopic DCR is common practice.[26–28] The presence of canalicular disease, previous acute dacryocystitis, a small sac, revision surgery, or poor mucosal flaps are reasons to perform intubation to reduce the risk of stenosis.[6,29] The silicone tubing may remain for approximately 6 weeks or longer (4 to 6 months), depending on the etiology and severity of the obstruction (Fig. 71.3B). If the NL stents must be left in place for prolonged periods or indefinitely, Pyrex glass tubes may be used. When intubation is performed to repair a canalicular laceration, both ends of the canaliculus should be identified. Interrupted sutures with 8-0 gut or 10-0 Prolene are placed to approximate the cut ends of the canalicular epithelium and the tarsus. The outer end of the tube can be anchored to the skin lateral to the punctum. The tube can be removed 10 to 14 days after injury.

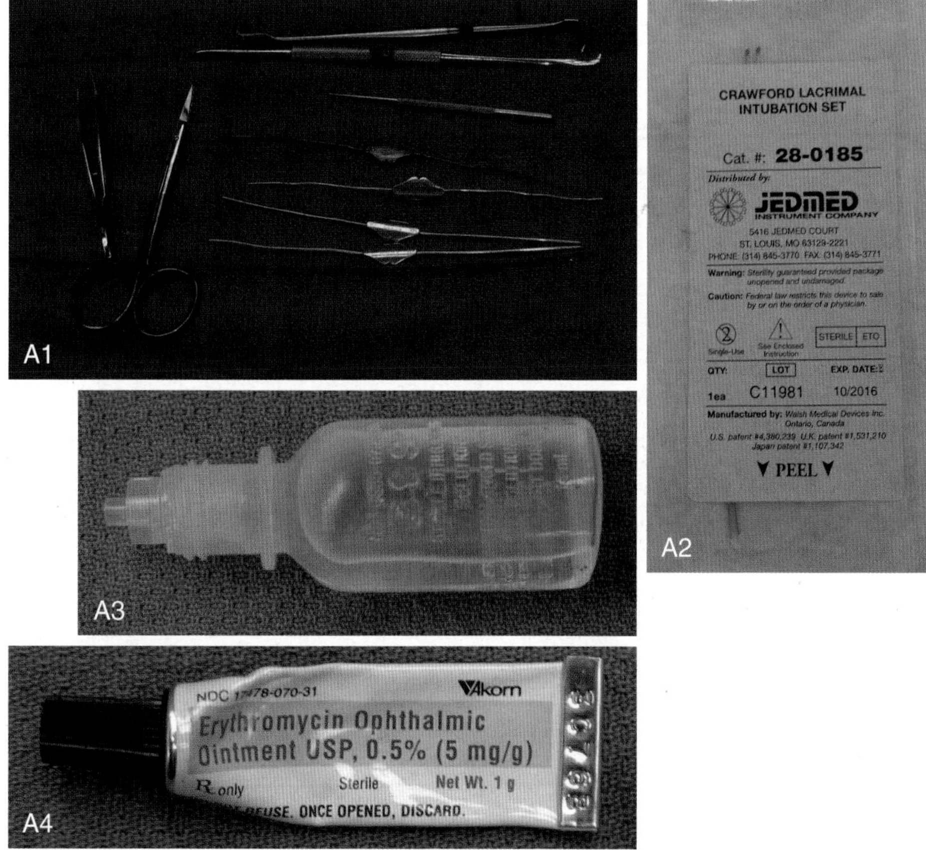

Figure 71.3 A1–A4, The essential armamentarium for nasolacrimal interrogation and intubation: lacrimal probe set, Crawford tubes, fluorescein dye, and ophthalmic ointment.

Continued

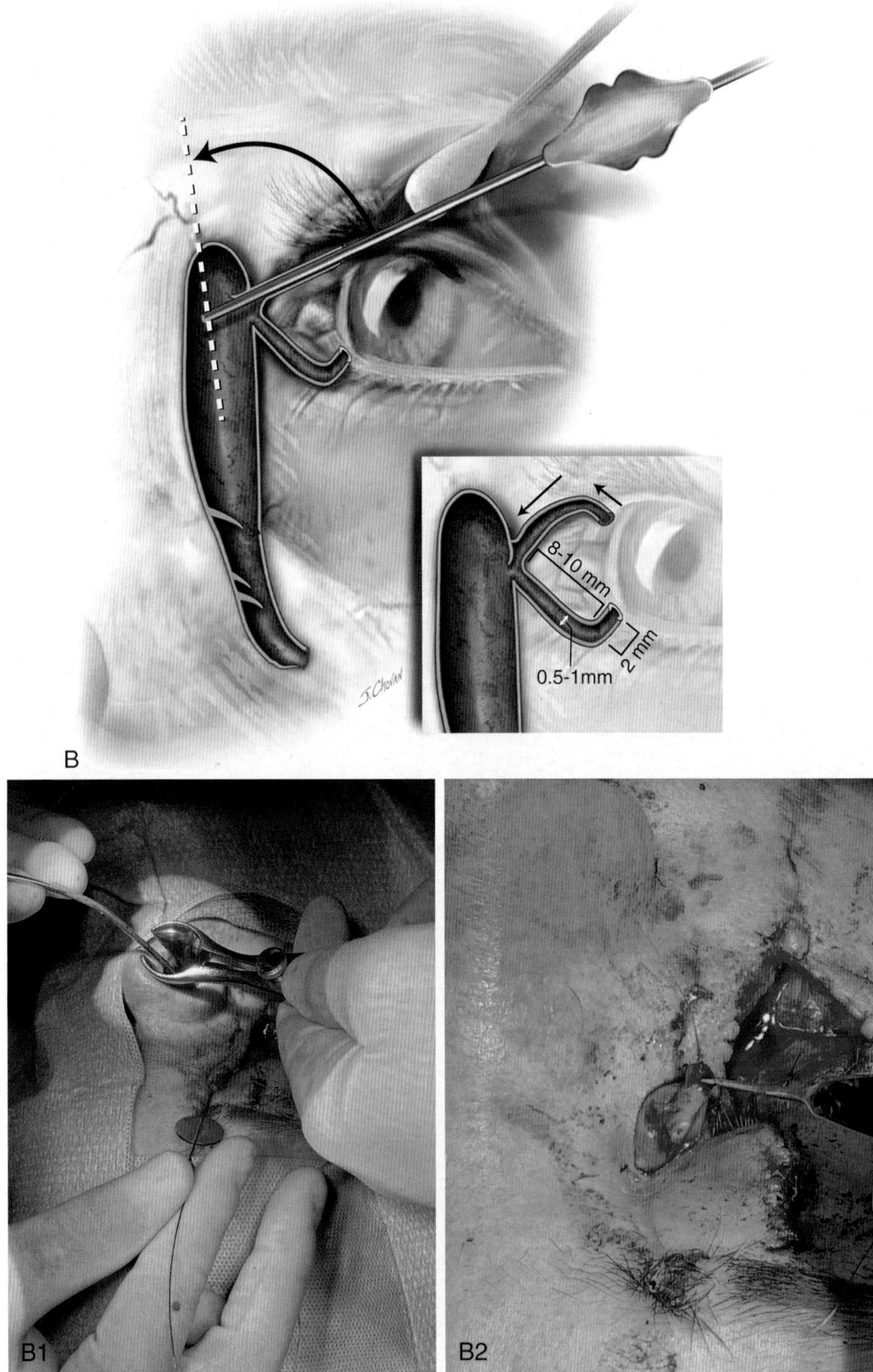

Figure 71.3, cont'd B, Schematic diagram showing the direction of probes and irrigation. Care should be taken when inserting the probes and irrigation syringes to avoid further injury to the canaliculi. The inferior and superior canaliculi extend vertically and perpendicular to the lid margin for 2 mm into the ampulla and then turn sharply medially to proceed in a horizontal direction parallel to the lid margin for 8 to 10 mm. The internal diameter of the canaliculi varies between 0.5 and 1 mm. **B1,** Introduction of Ritleng canaliculus stenting system and retrieval of stents below the inferior meatus of the inferior turbinate. **B2,** Resulting inferior canaliculus repair.

TECHNIQUE: Dacryocystorhinostomy[2,7]

External DCR via a skin incision is the most commonly used method. The surgery typically is performed with the patient under general anesthesia in the ambulatory setting (Fig. 71.4A–C).

STEP 1: Patient Preparation

The nose is prepared with a decongestant such as 0.04% oxymetazoline hydrochloride (Afrin) or 4% cocaine applied with cotton pads that are left in place for 10 to 15 minutes. The skin over the periorbital and paranasal areas is prepped sterile with ophthalmic Betadine solution. Local anesthetic injection (1% or 2% lidocaine (Xylocaine) with 1:100,000 epinephrine) may be used for infraorbital and supraorbital nerve blocks and infiltration at the nasomaxillary confluence.

STEP 2: Incision

A 1- to 1.5-cm curvilinear skin incision is made in a vertical direction about 4 mm lateral (nasal) to the medial commissure for access to the lacrimal sac. Blunt dissection of the subcutaneous and supraperiosteal tissues is performed with a hemostat and an iris or Stevens tenotomy scissors; care is taken to avoid laceration of or injury to the angular vessels.

Continued

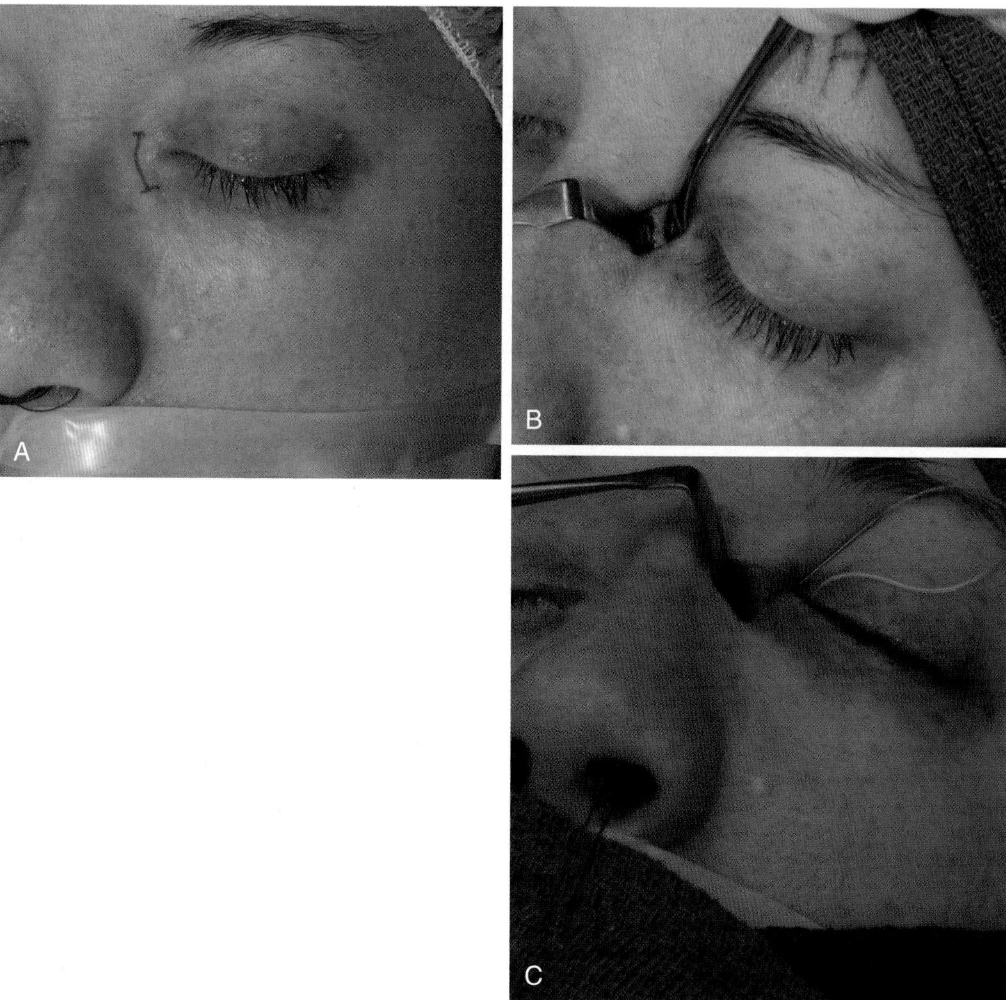

Figure 71.4 **A,** Dacryocystorhinostomy incision line. **B,** Elevation of the lacrimal sac from the fossa. **C,** Lacrimal intubation. (Courtesy Marc Hirschbein, Occuloplastic Surgeon, Sinai Hospital, Baltimore, MD).

TECHNIQUE: Dacryocystorhinostomy—*cont'd*

STEP 3: Dissection

The anterior attachment of the medial canthal tendon can be released from the nasal bone insertion to gain access, if necessary. The lacrimal sac is identified and elevated with a Freer elevator to expose the thin lacrimal bone.

STEP 4: Osteotomy

The thin bone of the lacrimal fossa is removed with a chisel or Kerrison rongeurs, carefully sparing the nasal mucosa. The extremely thin quality of the lacrimal bone allows easy access between the lacrimal fossa and nasal cavity during external and endoscopic approaches for DCR. High-speed rotary instruments may be used to remove the dense maxillary and nasal bone around the perforation in an inferomedial direction.

STEP 5: Lacrimal Sac Incision

The lacrimal sac is insufflated with a local anesthetic and then sharply incised to expose the full extent of the sac. If an inadequate opening is made in the sac, tear stasis may occur within the remaining sac, potentially acting as a nidus of infection.

STEP 6: Nasal Flaps

A precise incision is made in the nasal mucosa with a #11 blade to establish anterior and posterior flaps, which are sutured to the anterior and posterior flaps of the lacrimal sac lining.

STEP 7: Flap Closure

The posterior flaps of the lacrimal sac and nasal mucosa can be secured with 4-0 polyglactin (Vicryl) suture before patency is established through the NL duct.

STEP 8: Ductal Intubation

The canaliculi are then interrogated for patency. Punctal dilation is performed with the smallest size dilator and scaled to fit a 00 or 0 Bowman probe. Silicone tubing with steel probes (e.g., Quickert) can be inserted into the superior and inferior canaliculi to establish patency through the neolacrimal rhinostomy. Direct visualization through the external access confirms passage of the tubing through the lacrimal fossa and into nose.

STEP 9: Silicone Tubing Retrieval

A fine directing hook can then be used to retrieve the probes from the nose. A nasal septum may also assist in visualizing the probe. The ends of the tubing can be tied and tacked to the inner nasal mucosa using a nonresorbable 4-0 Prolene suture. This may need to be accessible for future removal.

STEP 10: Closure

The anterior flaps of the nasal mucosa and lacrimal sac are sutured with 5-0 polyglactin sutures. External access deep tissue (orbicularis oculi) closure can be achieved with interrupted 4-0 polyglactin sutures. Skin closure can be completed with 6-0 fast-absorbing plain gut.

ALTERNATIVE TECHNIQUE: Endoscopic DCR

Endoscopic DCR offers the advantage of evaluation and treatment of intranasal obstructive conditions, such as ethmoid sinus disease, enlarged middle turbinate, or adhesions or scar tissue in patients who have undergone previous surgery or radiation therapy. The other advantage is the elimination of a facial scar.[7,30,31] The challenges of the endoscopic technique include limited visualization to inspect the NL sac and duct, the need for meticulous hemostasis, and the need for costly, sophisticated surgical equipment and skilled ancillary personnel. This technique is contraindicated in patients with a neoplasm or when a neoplastic diagnosis cannot be excluded by initial clinical examination and investigations. The reported success rate for endoscopic DCR for revision cases ranges from 75% to 83%.[30] Sung et al. showed more failures in patients with eyelid laxity and more comorbidities.[9] A systemic review and meta-analysis of surgical endonasal and external DCR found similar outcomes in both groups.[10] Laser assistance was associated with worse functional outcomes when compared with rotary instrumentation in endonasal DCRs. A detailed description of this technique is outside the scope of this chapter but can be obtained from an atlas of endoscopic sinus surgery.

Limitations and Contraindications

One of the main limitations of DCR (external or endoscopic) is restenosis and loss of patency of the NL drainage system. NL intubation is often performed along with DCR to preserve the patency of the drainage system and avoid reoperation.[26] Although NL intubation can address this limitation to some degree, it is important to weigh the risks and benefits of intubation for each individual case. There have been several reports of iatrogenic injury resulting from improper probing and intubation. Another limitation of external DCR is facial scarring at the site of the access incision. A facial scar can be avoided by using endoscopic access in appropriate cases. The surgical anatomy of the region presents some challenges during the procedure. Intraoperative hemorrhage due to bleeding from the angular vessels can make creation and suturing of the mucosal flaps very difficult. Poor mucosal flap design and excessive use of cautery may result in scarring and loss of patency of the neo-ostium. Large intranasal polyps, an enlarged inferior turbinate, or an extremely deviated nasal septum in posttraumatic cases may present problems with creating the nasal opening during DCR. DCR is contraindicated in patients with acute dacryocystitis and in cases when the clinical or radiographic diagnosis indicates the presence of lacrimal sac tumors.

Avoidance and Management of Intraoperative Complications

Complications after DCR procedures can be categorized as immediate or delayed (Box 71.2). The most common adverse outcome of external and/or endonasal DCR is fistula stenosis and loss of patency. This may occur as early as 4 weeks or as late as 6 or 8 months. NL intubation and topical medications such as mitomycin C (MMC) have been advocated to maintain patency of the neorhinostomy. MMC, a potent DNA cross-linker, has been advocated to improve the outcomes of DCR by preventing fibrous obstruction and stenosis of the drainage pathway. The medication also has bacteriocidal properties to help prevent postoperative infections. In select high-risk patients (e.g., postirradiation, significant scarring, reduced canalicular length), Pyrex glass tubes can be inserted into the neolacrimal sac to ensure long-term patency. Excessive use of electrocautery should be avoided to reduce scarring and restenosis. Bleeding from the angular vein and nasal mucosa can make the surgical procedure challenging.[30]

Hemorrhage can be minimized with good local anesthetic technique and careful blunt dissection of the supraperiosteal tissues. Penetration or perforation of the cribriform plate may result in cerebrospinal fluid leakage. Consultation with an experienced neurosurgeon may be warranted. Perforation of the ethmoid air cells may be managed with local muscle patches such as with the orbicularis oculi. Surgical site infections usually can be treated with antibiotics and local débridement. Routine intubation of the NL ducts is not recommended. Some of the complications that may arise from NL intubation include punctual slitting, granuloma formation, corneal erosions, irritation of the nasal mucosa and nosebleeds, and superior displacement of tubes. When cannulating the duct, it is important to avoid the creation of a false passage and injury to the patent canaliculus. Prolapse of the tubing into the eye can be managed by tightly suturing the tubes into the mucosa of the nose. Failure to open the inferior portion of the lacrimal sac completely can result in lacrimal sump syndrome. The literature cites a lower failure rate with primary external DCR (5% to 10%) than with primary endoscopic DCR (10% to 33%).[8]

BOX 71.2 Complications with Dacryocystorhinostomy

Immediate (Perioperative) Complications

- Hemorrhage
- Cerebrospinal fluid leak
- Injury to the canaliculi from improper probing
- Corneal abrasions or other globe injuries from instruments
- Injury to lateral nasal mucosa due to improper bone removal
- Lacrimal sump syndrome

Delayed Complications

- Infection
- Incomplete improvement, persistent tearing
- Early loss or prolapse of silicone tube
- Hemorrhage
- Synechiae between the middle turbinate, nasal septum, or lateral wall
- Need for additional surgery

Postoperative Considerations

During the first 24 hours, a light pressure dressing over the surgical site may be used to minimize the postoperative risk of bleeding. Cold compresses over the eyelids and nasal bridge area during the first 48 hours after surgery help alleviate swelling and ecchymoses. Saline nasal spray two to three times daily for a week to reduce crusting around the tubes and ostium is recommended. Perioperative antibiotics (e.g., amoxicillin with a β-lactamase inhibitor [clavulanic acid]), which cover upper respiratory flora, may be prescribed, particularly in patients who have trauma or dacryocystitis and undergo open procedures. Sinus precautions are recommended to avoid air emphysema and soft tissue injury. Patients also are instructed to close the eyes when sneezing to avoid displacement of the canalicular tubes.

When canalicular intubation is performed to repair the lacrimal ducts. the tubes should be left in place until the tract has matured. The duration can range from 6 weeks to 6 months or longer if the tubes are well tolerated. Silicone tubes can cause granuloma formation as a result of a foreign body reaction if left in place for longer than 3 to 4 months. Pyrex glass tubes may be used to maintain patency for longer periods in patients with a high risk for recurrent stenosis or obstruction. For removal of the tubes, the loop is cut near the inner eyelid and the tube is removed from the nasal cavity.

References

1. Harish V, Benger RS. Origins of lacrimal surgery, and evolution of dacryocystorhinostomy to the present. *Clin Exp Ophthalmol.* 2014;42(3):284–287.
2. Yakopson VS, Flanagan JC, Ahn D, Luo BP. Dacryocystorhinostomy: history, evolution and future directions. *Saudi J Ophthalmol.* 2011;25(1):37–49.
3. Chandler PA. Dacryocystorhinostomy. *Trans Am Ophthalmol Soc.* 1936;34:240–263.
4. Iliff CE. A simplified dacryocystorhinostomy. 1954-1970. *Arch Ophthalmol.* 1971;85(5):586–591.
5. Watkins LM, Janfaza P, Rubin PA. The evolution of endonasal dacryocystorhinostomy. *Surv Ophthalmol.* 2003;48(1):73–84.
6. Madge SN, Selva D. Intubation in routine dacryocystorhinostomy: why we do what we do. *Clin Exp Ophthalmol.* 2009;37(6):620–623.
7. Lee DW, Chai CH, Loon SC. Primary external dacryocystorhinostomy versus primary endonasal dacryocystorhinostomy: a review. *Clin Exp Ophthalmol.* 2010;38(4):418–426.
8. Hartikainen J, et al. Prospective randomized comparison of endonasal endoscopic DCR and external DCR. *Laryngoscope.* 1998;108:1861.
9. Sung JY, Lee YH, Kim KN, Kang TS, Lee SB. Surgical outcomes of endoscopic dacryocystorhinostomy: analysis of age effect. *Sci Rep.* 2019;9(1):19861.
10. Huang J, Malek J, Chin D, et al. Systematic review and meta-analysis on outcomes for endoscopic versus external dacryocystorhinostomy. *Orbit.* 2014;33(2):81–90.
11. Becelli R, Renzi G, Mannino G, Cerulli G, Iannetti G. Posttraumatic obstruction of lacrimal pathways: a retrospective analysis of 58 consecutive naso-orbitoethmoid fractures. *J Craniofac Surg.* 2004;15(1):29–33.
12. Unger JM. Fractures of the nasolacrimal fossa and canal: a CT study of appearance, associated injuries, and significance in 25 patients. *AJR Am J Roentgenol.* 1992;158(6):1321–1324.
13. Ali MJ, Gupta H, Honavar SG, Naik MN. Acquired nasolacrimal duct obstructions secondary to naso-orbito-ethmoidal fractures: patterns and outcomes. *Ophthal Plast Reconstr Surg.* 2012;28(4):242–245.
14. Zapala J, Bartkowski AM, Bartkowski SB. Lacrimal drainage system obstruction: management and results obtained in 70 patients. *J Craniomaxillofac Surg.* 1992;20(4):178–183.
15. Lee-Wing MW, Ashenhurst ME. Clinicopathologic analysis of 166 patients with primary acquired nasolacrimal duct obstruction. *Ophthalmology.* 2001;108(11):2038–2040.
16. Fulcher T, O'Connor M, Moriarty P. Nasolacrimal intubation in adults. *Br J Ophthalmol.* 1998;82(9):1039–1041.
17. Gruss JS, Hurwitz JJ, Nik NA, Kassel EE. The pattern and incidence of nasolacrimal injury in naso-orbital-ethmoid fractures: the role of delayed assessment and dacryocystorhinostomy. *Br J Plast Surg.* 1985;38(1):116–121.
18. Iwai T, Yasumura K, Yabuki Y, et al. Intraoperative lacrimal intubation to prevent epiphora as a result of injury to the nasolacrimal system after fracture of the naso-orbitoethmoid complex. *Br J Oral Maxillofac Surg.* 2012.
19. Harris GJ, Fuerste FH. Lacrimal intubation in the primary repair of midfacial fractures. *Ophthalmology.* 1987;94(3):242–247.
20. Lee H, Ahn J, Lee TE, et al. Clinical characteristics and treatment of blow-out fracture accompanied by canalicular laceration. *J Craniofac Surg.* 2012;23(5):1399–1403.
21. Savar A, Kirszrot J, Rubin PA. Canalicular involvement in dog bite related eyelid lacerations. *Ophthal Plast Reconstr Surg.* 2008;24(4):296–298.
22. Kennedy RH, May J, Dailey J, Flanagan JC. Canalicular laceration. An 11-year epidemiologic and clinical study. *Ophthal Plast Reconstr Surg.* 1990;6(1):46–53.
23. Groell R, Schaffler GJ, Uggowitzer M, Szolar DH, Muellner K. CT-anatomy of the nasolacrimal sac and duct. *Surg Radiol Anat.* 1997;19(3):189–191.
24. Lang G. *Ophthalmology: A Pocket Textbook Atlas.* 2nd ed. Birmingham, UK: Thieme; 2007.
25. Cohen A, Mercandetti M, Brazzo B, eds. *The Lacrimal System: Diagnosis, Management and Surgery.* Springer Science; 2006.
26. Moscato EE, Dolmetsch AM, Silkiss RZ, Seiff SR. Silicone intubation for the treatment of epiphora in adults with presumed functional nasolacrimal duct obstruction. *Ophthal Plast Reconstr Surg.* 2012;28(1):35–39.
27. Saiju R, Morse LJ, Weinberg D, Shrestha MK, Ruit S. Prospective randomised comparison of external dacryocystorhinostomy with and without silicone intubation. *Br J Ophthalmol.* 2009;93(9):1220–1222.
28. Spinelli HM, Shapiro MD, Wei LL, Elahi E, Hirmand H. The role of lacrimal intubation in the management of facial trauma and tumor resection. *Plast Reconstr Surg.* 2005;115(7):1871–1876.
29. Connell PP, Fulcher TP, Chacko E, O' Connor MJ, Moriarty P. Long term follow up of nasolacrimal intubation in adults. *Br J Ophthalmol.* 2006;90(4):435–436.
30. Ben Simon GJ, Joseph J, Lee S, Schwarcz RM, McCann JD, Goldberg RA. External versus endoscopic dacryocystorhinostomy for acquired nasolacrimal duct obstruction in a tertiary referral center. *Ophthalmology.* 2005;112(8):1463–1468.
31. Kim DW, Choi MY, Shim WS. Endoscopic dacryocystorhinostomy with canalicular marsupialization in common canalicular obstruction. *Can J Ophthalmol.* 2013;48(4):335–339.

CHAPTER 72

Control of Facial Hemorrhage

Todd R. Wentland, Roderick Y. Kim, and Herman Kao

Armamentarium

#9 Periosteal elevator
#14 French Foley catheter
#15 Blade
1/2-inch Gauze strips
Antibiotic ointment
Appropriate sutures
Bayonet forceps
Frazier-tip suction
Freer elevator
Headlight
Hemostat
Local anesthetic with vasoconstrictor
Metzenbaum scissors
Nasal speculum
Needle electrocautery
Obwegeser retractors
Shoulder roll to extend the neck, sandbags to stabilize the head
Umbilical cord clamp
Vascular clamps
Vascular clips
Vascular loops

History of the Procedure

The first recorded ligation of a common carotid artery was performed by Ambroise Paré in 1551.[1] The earliest operations on the carotid arteries were ligations to control bleeding after trauma or surgical injury. In 1807, Amos Twitchell[2] was the first American surgeon to successfully ligate the common carotid artery of a soldier to stop hemorrhage from a bullet wound. In the next few decades, common carotid artery ligations were also used to treat aneurysms, arteriovenous fistulas, and bleeding neoplasms.[3] Unfortunately, ligation of the common carotid artery carried a high complication rate. In 1878, John Wyeth, an American surgeon, reported 898 cases of common carotid artery ligation with a mortality rate of 41%. On the other hand, he found a mortality rate of only 4.5% after external carotid artery (ECA) ligation.[1] In 1908, Barrett and Orr were among the earliest authors to report ECA ligation to treat postoperative nasal bleeding.[4] In 1963, Malcomson[5] also advocated early surgical ligation to arrest nasal bleeding. In addition to their use to arrest nasal hemorrhage, ECA ligation was performed as a presurgical procedure to reduce bleeding before composite resection of oral carcinomas.[6]

In the 1970s and 1980s, some authors advocated ligation of selective vessels to control epistaxis, such as the internal maxillary artery and the anterior ethmoidal artery.[7–10] Although this is consistent with the surgical principle of ligating the vessels nearest the bleeding site, it is technically difficult and may produce more complications.[11] Transantral ligation of the internal maxillary artery requires access through a Caldwell-Luc approach. Once the posterior maxillary wall has been removed, the internal maxillary artery is difficult to identify due to the many branches present in the pterygoid fossa. As interventional radiology techniques advanced in the 1980s, transcatheter arterial embolization (TAE) became a popular alternative to arterial ligation in controlling facial hemorrhages.[12] However, ligation of the ECA and/or its branches remains an important tool when other methods have failed.[13–16] Therefore, arterial ligation is an important emergency technique that all maxillofacial surgeons should know.

Indications for the Use of the Procedure

Massive facial hemorrhage is a rare but potentially life-threatening event. It is frequently associated with maxillofacial trauma or surgical injury, and the incidence ranges from 1.25% to 9.4%.[14,17] Some authors have attempted to classify the amount of blood loss to guide management[15,17]; however, the critical factor in effective control of massive facial hemorrhage is early recognition (Fig. 72.1).[18]

The main arterial supply of the maxillofacial region is the carotid artery, which branches in the neck at the level of hyoid bone and becomes the internal and ECA. Bleeding in the midface region is mainly from the branches of the ECA, especially the internal maxillary artery and its intraosseous branches.[14] In the upper face and the roof of the nasal cavity, bleeding also comes from branches of the internal carotid artery, such as the lacrimal arteries and the ethmoidal arteries.

Management of facial hemorrhage is largely dependent on the surgeon's ability to access the source of bleeding. Bleeding from superficial wounds is the result of injuries to end arterioles and the capillaries. Bleeding from deep vessels, such as the internal maxillary artery and its branches, are difficult to localize and treat. Bleeding from these deep vessels frequently funnels into the oral and nasal cavity.[19] Therefore, a significant amount of blood can be swallowed by the patient, and severe hemorrhage can be easily missed.

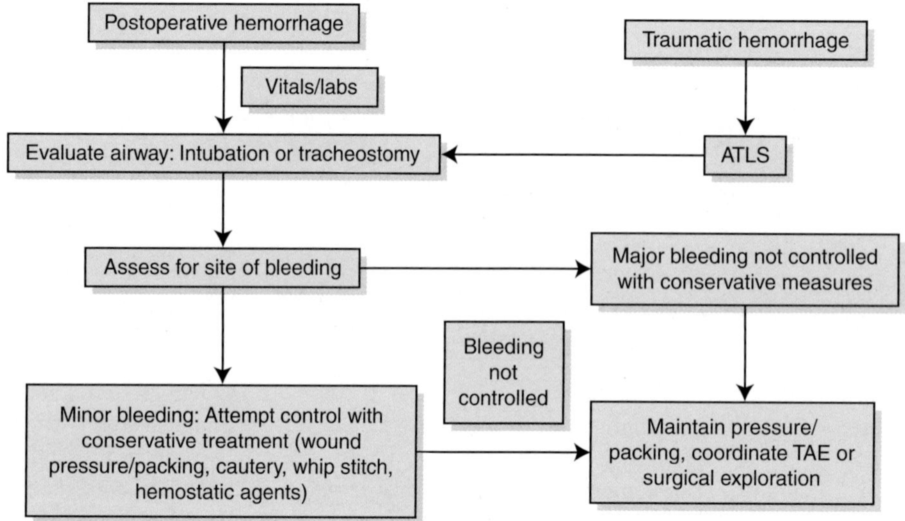

Figure 72.1 Comparison of types of hemorrhages. *ATLS*, Advanced trauma life support; *TAE*, transcatheter arterial embolization.

Various methods are used to treat massive facial hemorrhages from deep facial vessels. These include oronasal packing, early fracture reduction, TAE, and ECA ligation.[20] The decision whether to use TAE or ECA ligation has long been discussed in the literature. In the past, this choice often was determined more by the availability of a skilled interventional radiologist proficient in angiography and embolization and the ability of the surgeon to perform ligation of the ECA.12 However, due to increased availability of these practitioners and technical advances, authors now prefer TAE over arterial ligation when other noninvasive measures fail. This is largely due to the specificity and repeatability of TAE. Therefore, if a patient is stable and the bleeding is temporarily slowed by packing, TAE should be attempted first. If the bleeding cannot be controlled and the patient becomes unstable, immediate surgical arterial ligation should be considered. Ligation of the ECA is a relatively simple, low-risk procedure that can be performed quickly under general or local anesthesia. The surgical access to the ECA is straightforward compared with the internal maxillary artery. When dire conditions call for emergency control of facial hemorrhage, ligation of the ECA is a valuable tool in any maxillofacial surgeon's surgical armamentarium.

Here we describe the techniques for facial hemorrhage control, sequenced from the least invasive to the ECA ligation.

TECHNIQUE: Local Control of Non-Life-Threatening Hemorrhage

Prior to initiating care an assessment of the airway, breathing, and circulation needs to be conducted and addressed.

Often times holding hand pressure or packing with gauze will produce hemostasis for simple lacerations and nonpenetrating wounds. If the offending vessel is visualized and assessable, then vessel ligation with silk suture or vascular clip may be performed. Additionally, hemostatic agents and cautery may be used for local control of hemorrhage.

If the wound is more complex with significant hemorrhage, then a detailed evaluation of the wound needs to be undertaken with suction and irrigation. Assess the quality and quantity of the hemorrhage to determine if it is an arterial, venous, muscle bleed, etc. Once the source or site of bleeding is identified, hand pressure with gauze should be applied and held. If the wound is deep or penetrating and hand pressure is not easily applied, the wound should be packed tightly with gauze (4 × 4 or packing strips). Consideration to moisten the gauze with Afrin or local anesthetic containing epinephrine is an option to achieve hemostasis. Gauze impregnated with procoagulants has been shown to effectively aid in hemorrhage control,[21] and Surgicel (oxidized regenerated cellulose) is another consideration when packing sites of hemorrhage. Additionally, there are multiple hemostatic agents available that aid in preventing hemorrhage and maintaining hemostasis (Table 72.1).[22]

If there is a localized source of bleeding but no identified vessel, a whip stitch may be thrown. A whip stitch is meant to be a broad throw within the bleeding field in an attempt to capture the bleeding vessel or vessels upon cinching down and tying the suture.

If there is bleeding coming from fracture sites, an attempt to reduce the fracture should be made. In the maxillofacial region this can often be accomplished with bridle wires around teeth or with hand articulation until there is tamponade of the hemorrhage, with final fixation taking place in the operating room.

If attempts to control the hemorrhage fail, wound packing and pressure should be maintained while exploration in the operating room or TAE is arranged.

Table 72.1 A List of Common Topical Hemostatic Agents Used to Prevent and Maintain Hemostasis

Product	Indications	Contraindications
Gelfoam Porcine gelatin	Hemostatic device when conventional methods have failed	Do not: • use for closure of skin • use for intravascular compartments for risk of embolization
Surgicel Oxidized regenerated cellulose	Hemostatic device when conventional methods have failed	Do not: • place in bone defects as it may interfere with callus formation and cyst formation • use for control of large arterial bleeds
Evithrom Human thrombin	Aid for hemostasis from minor bleed when conventional methods have failed	Do not: • inject into circulatory system • use for patients with hypersensitivity to human blood products • use for severe or brisk bleeding
FloSeal Bovine gelatin and human thrombin	Adjunct to hemostasis when conventional methods have failed	Do not: • inject into vessels • apply in the absence of active blood flow • use for closure of skin incisions
Surgiflo Porcine gelatin and thrombin	Adjunct to hemostasis when conventional methods have failed	Do not: • use in intravascular compartments for risk of embolization • use in patients with porcine allergy • use for skin closure
Evicel Fibrin Sealant	Adjunct to hemostasis when conventional methods have failed	Do not: • inject into circulatory system • use in patients with hypersensitivity to human blood products • use for severe or brisk bleeding

TECHNIQUE: Controlling Anterior Nasal Hemorrhage

The nasal cavity is richly vascularized with arterial supply from the superior labial, anterior ethmoid, and posterior ethmoid arteries. The coalescence of these arteries form the Kiesselbach plexus and is a common source of nasal bleeds. However, nasal bleeds may be anterior, posterior, or both. A Foley catheter with 1/4-inch packing strips is a well-known and proven technique to tamponade both anterior and posterior nasal hemorrhage and is described later. However, there are multiple modalities to treat anterior nasal hemorrhage, which are discussed here. Most of these modalities are readily available in average emergency department.

Initial steps to control nasal hemorrhage include direct compression and the use of topical vasoconstrictors such as 0.05% oxymetazoline (Afrin), 0.5% phenylephrine hydrochloride, 1:1000 epinephrine, or 4% cocaine. If an oral and maxillofacial surgeon is consulted, these simple modalities have surely been exhausted.[23]

A thorough exam using nasal speculum, suction, and light source in an attempt to identify the source of bleeding needs to be performed. If the bleeding is anterior, an attempt to cauterize the area must be attempted first, prior to packing. This can be done with either electrical or chemical (silver nitrate) cautery,[23] and should not be performed bilaterally to avoid a septal perforation. If cautery fails, tranexamic acid (TXA)-soaked pledgets have been shown to be effective in controlling nasal hemorrhage.[24] The pledgets are lightly packed into the nose and left for 10 minutes, then removed. If bleeding still occurs, then nasal packing will be necessary. Commonly used and readily available products include polyvinyl acetyl polymer sponges, Merocel (Medtronic, Minneapolis, MN) and inflatable balloons, and Rapid Rhino (Smith & Nephew, Inc., Austin, TX). These nasal packing modalities work by applying direct pressure to the nasal mucosa. The Merocel packing will expand once placed, and the Rapid Rhino needs to be inflated with a 20-cc syringe until the cuff is firm. Both should be coated in petroleum jelly or topical antibiotic ointment prior to placement, and should remain for 24 to 72 hours.[23]

TECHNIQUE: Controlling Posterior Nasal Hemorrhage

Nasal packing is an effective way to control intractable epistaxis. If the anterior, posterior, or both nasal cavities are to be packed, a Foley catheter is used to pack the posterior nasal cavity first. The tip of the Foley catheter is trimmed to avoid pressure and ulceration of the posterior pharyngeal wall. The Foley catheter is lubricated with antibiotic ointment and then inserted along the floor of the nasal cavity until the tip is visible in the oropharynx. Then, 3 to 5 mL of normal saline is injected to inflate the balloon. The catheter is pulled back until the balloon occludes the nasopharynx just above the soft palate. Slight tension is applied to stabilize the position of the balloon, and an umbilical cord clamp is placed across the Foley catheter at the nostrils.

The anterior nasal cavity is packed in a layered fashion with 1/2-inch gauze strips impregnated with antibiotic ointment. Bayonet forceps are used to pass the tip of a gauze strip along the Foley catheter until the inflated balloon is reached. The forceps are removed, and a similar length of gauze strip is layered on top of the first. This continues superiorly until the anterior nasal cavity has been packed and the bleeding stopped. Next, sponge gauze is wrapped around the Foley catheter between the nostrils and the umbilical clamp to prevent pressure necrosis of the ala and columella. The remaining portion of the Foley catheter is taped to the patient's face to prevent accidental pulling (Fig. 72.2).

TRANSCATHETER ARTERIAL EMBOLIZATION

When conservative, nonsurgical treatment has failed to control hemorrhage, and when despite blood transfusion and medical treatment, the patient remains hemodynamically unstable, TAE should be the next treatment consideration.[25] Primarily performed by interventional radiologists, the procedure typically involves introducing diagnostic catheters into the femoral artery and then directing the catheter to the ECA under contrast guidance.[26] Gelatin sponges or microcoils are used to perform the embolization.[25] For life-threatening traumatic maxillofacial hemorrhage, TAE has been shown to have successful outcomes and decrease mortality.[27]

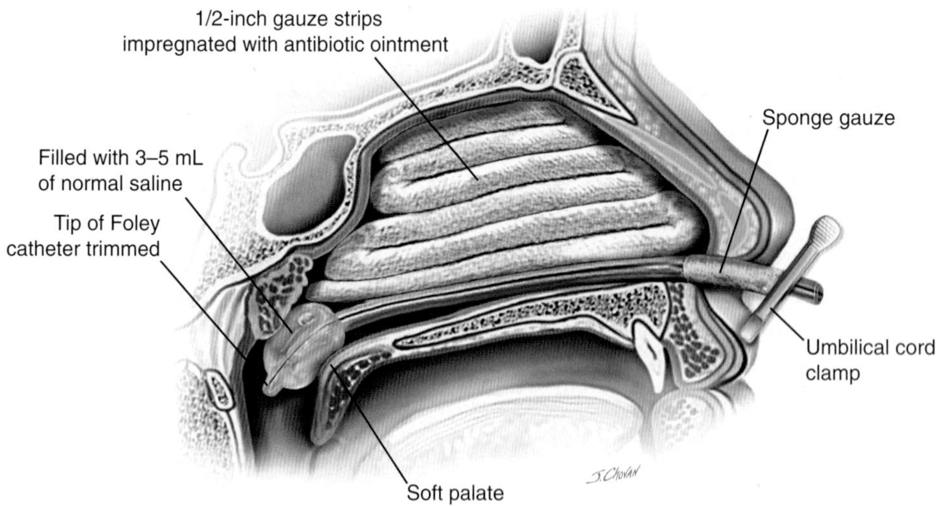

Figure 72.2 Placement of traditional anterior packing with Foley catheter in place.

TECHNIQUE: Ligation of the Anterior Ethmoidal Artery

The anterior ethmoidal artery branches from the ophthalmic artery. It courses through the anterior ethmoidal canal to supply the anterior and middle ethmoidal cells, the frontal sinus, and the lateral nasal wall. If there is significant bleeding from the roof of the nasal cavity, ligation of the anterior ethmoidal artery can be beneficial.

The anterior ethmoidal artery can be reached through a curvilinear incision over the superomedial orbital rim (Lynch incision). The incision is carried down to the anterior lacrimal crest. The dissection is taken posteriorly in the subperiosteal plane, and the superior portion of the lacrimal sac is reflected laterally from the lacrimal fossa. As the dissection continues posteriorly, the anterior ethmoidal artery can be found approximately 24-mm posterior to the anterior lacrimal crest. It can be seen piercing through the lamina papyracea and entering the orbital periosteum at the level of the pupils. A vascular clip is used to ligate the artery. The wound can be closed in a single layer at the skin (Fig. 72.3).

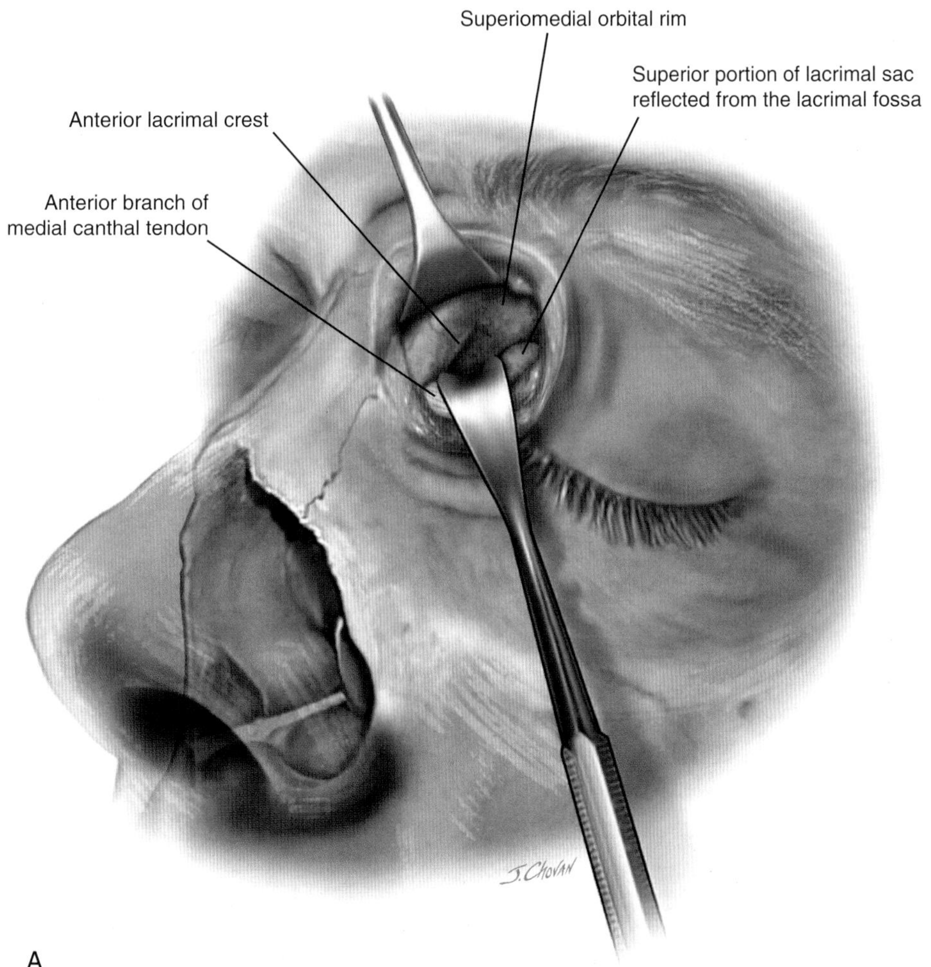

Figure 72.3 **A,** The anterior ethmoidal artery can be reached through a curvilinear incision over the superomedial orbital rim (Lynch incision).

Continued

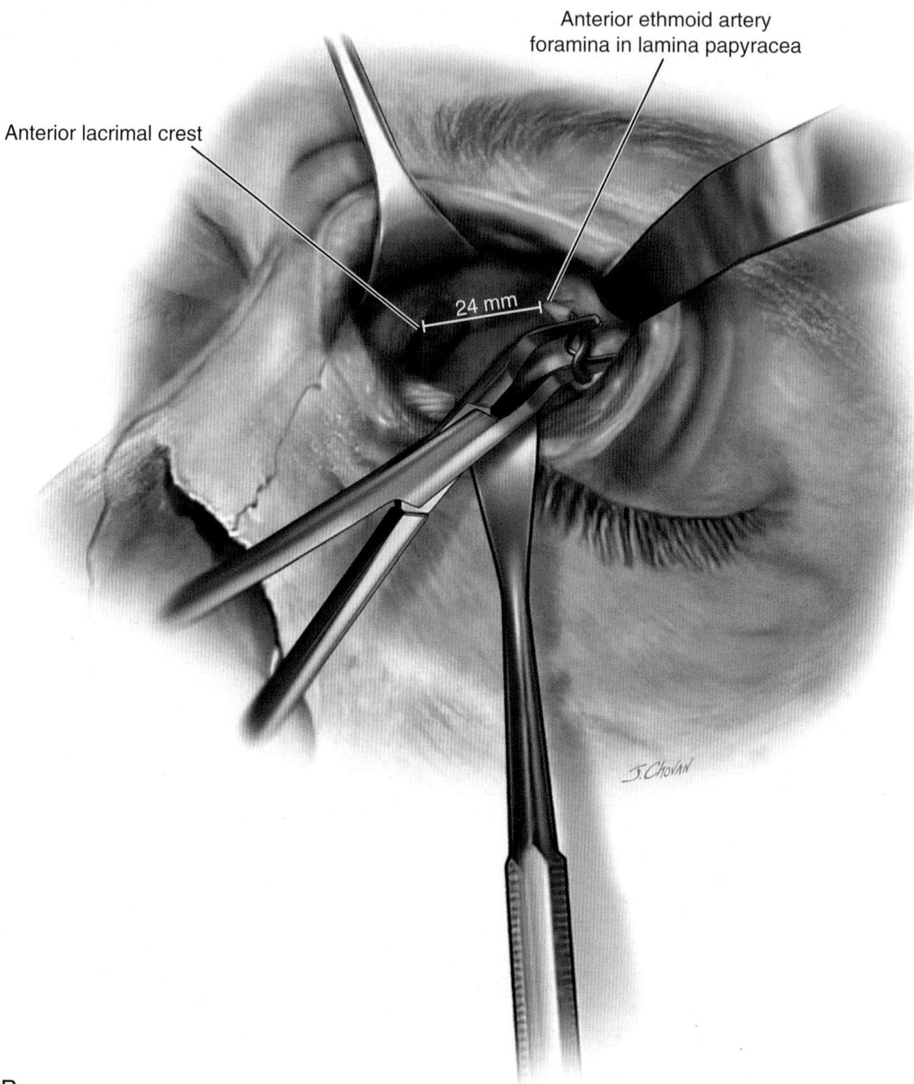

Figure 72.3, cont'd **B,** Vascular clipping and division of the ethmoidal artery.

TECHNIQUE: External Carotid Artery Ligation

STEP 1: Intubation and/or Surgical Airway

In a patient with significant facial hemorrhage, a secure airway is mandatory. For trauma patients, most endotracheal intubations occur in the field or in the emergency department.[28] There should be a low threshold for surgical airways because these patients often require multiple surgeries and prolonged hospital stays. A tracheostomy bypasses maxillofacial injuries, provides a secure airway, and simplifies facial fracture repair.

STEP 2: Positioning the Patient

The patient is placed in a supine position with a shoulder roll. The head is turned away from the side of the intended ECA ligation. This helps to accentuate the anterior border of the ipsilateral sternocleidomastoid muscle. Sandbags are placed on both sides of the neck to stabilize the head position.

TECHNIQUE: External Carotid Artery Ligation—*cont'd*

STEP 3: Incision

The anterior border of the sternocleidomastoid muscle is identified. A 5-cm horizontal skin incision is made 2 cm below and parallel to the inferior border of the mandible. The posterior one-third of the incision should be over the sternocleidomastoid muscle. This incision is carried through the subcutaneous tissue, the platysma muscle, and the investing layer of deep cervical fascia to reveal the sternocleidomastoid muscle (Fig. 72.4A and B).

STEP 4: Identifying the Carotid Sheath

The anterior edge of the sternocleidomastoid muscle is identified and retracted posteriorly. Blunt dissection is carried out in front of the sternocleidomastoid muscle with a hemostat, spreading parallel to the great vessels until the carotid sheath is identified. The internal jugular vein should be visible as it lies just inside the carotid sheath. The sternocleidomastoid muscle is dissected off the loose carotid sheath posteriorly.

STEP 5: Identifying the External Carotid Artery

The carotid sheath is entered bluntly to reveal the internal jugular vein. The common facial vein (or its branches) and the superior thyroid vein can be seen entering the internal jugular vein anteriorly and can be ligated and divided. The internal jugular vein is then gently retracted posteriorly, revealing the underlying common carotid artery. Once the common carotid artery has been isolated, further dissection is continued superiorly to reach the carotid bulb and the bifurcation of the internal and external carotid arteries. Care should be taken to identify and protect the hypoglossal nerve, which crosses the arteries just above the bifurcation. Note that the internal carotid artery lies posterior to the ECA and does not branch in the neck. Next, follow the ECA from the bifurcation and identify the first branch (superior thyroid artery) and the second branch (lingual artery) anteriorly (Fig. 72.4C).

STEP 6: Ligation of the External Carotid Artery

The ECA is double ligated between the first anterior branch (superior thyroid artery) and the second anterior branch (lingual artery) with 2-0 silk ties.[29] Ligation of the ECA at its root should be avoided to reduce the risk of proximal migration of a thrombus, which may enter the intracerebral circulation and result in a cerebrovascular accident (Fig. 72.4D).

STEP 7: Closure

The neck is closed in a layered fashion. The platysma is approximated with 3-0 Vicryl suture. The subcutaneous tissue is closed with interrupted 4-0 Monocryl sutures, and the skin is closed with running 5-0 Prolene suture. The wound is dressed with topical antibiotic ointment.

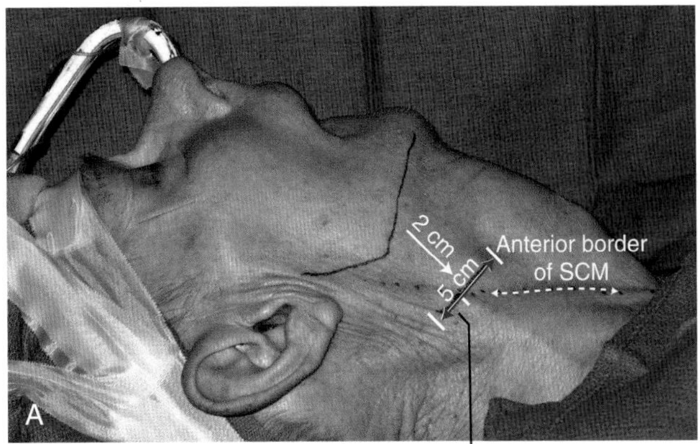

Figure 72.4 A, Patient positioning with incision lines marked.

Continued

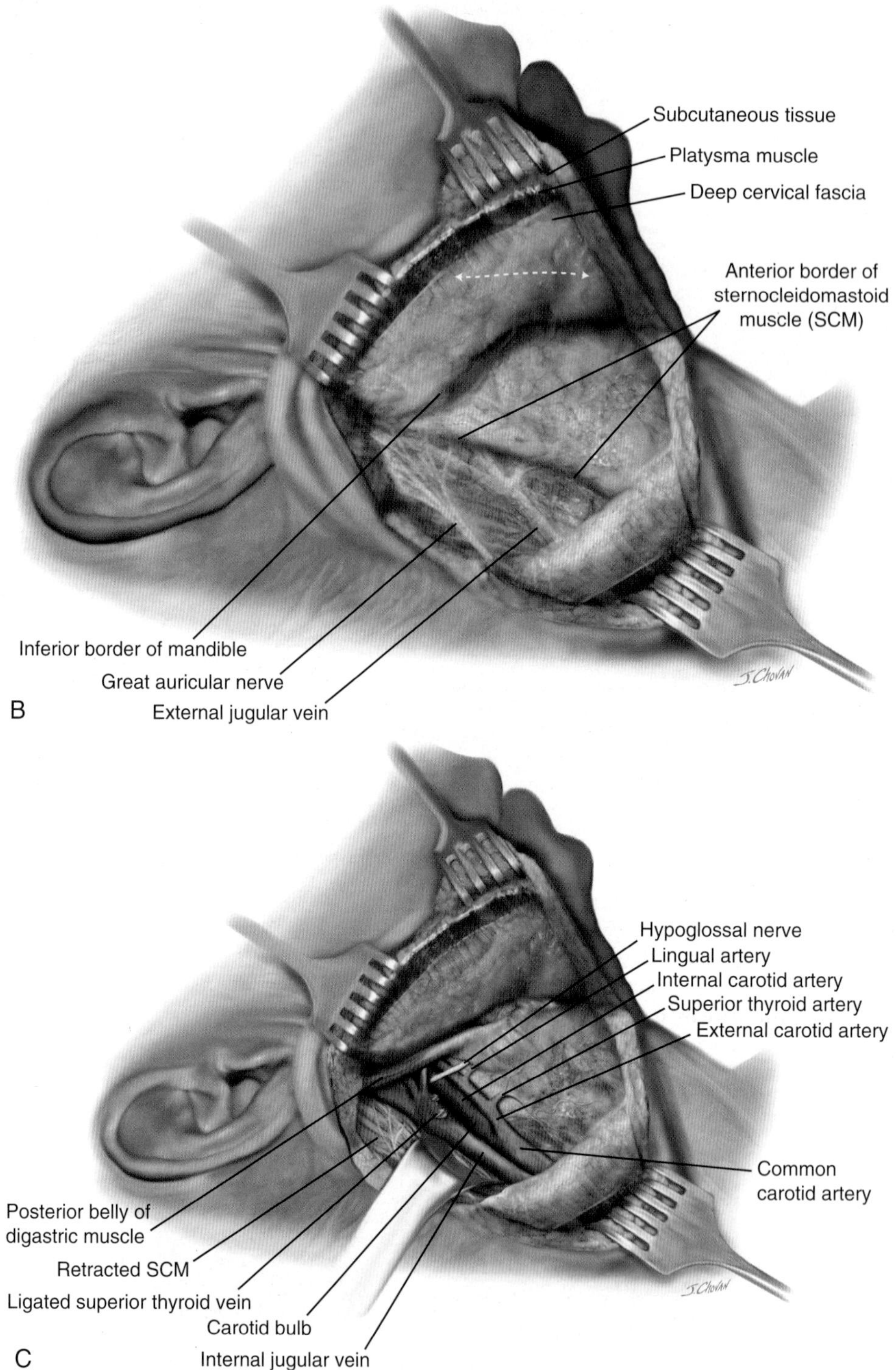

Figure 72.4, cont'd **B,** Horizontal skin incision. **C,** External carotid artery anatomy.

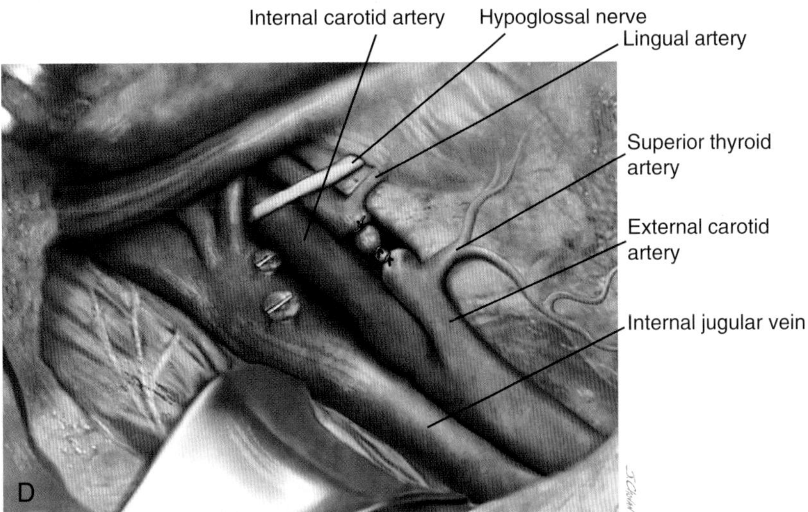

Figure 72.4, cont'd **D,** Ligation of the external carotid artery.

Avoidance and Management of Intraoperative Complications

During the initial skin incision to access the ECA, care must be taken to place the incision at least 2 cm below the mandibular border to avoid injury to the marginal mandibular nerve.

Once the common carotid artery has been identified, a vascular loop can be placed around the vessel. This can provide proximal control of the vessel in case of iatrogenic injury later.

During the dissection along the common carotid artery and the carotid bifurcation, the patient can become bradycardic due to the manipulation of the carotid bulb. If this occurs, plain 1% lidocaine can be injected into the carotid bulb adventitia.

When identifying the ECA, the surgeon must make sure that the anterior branches (e.g., the superior thyroid artery and the lingual artery) are present because the internal carotid artery does not branch in the neck. This prevents ligation of the internal carotid artery, which can have devastating consequences. It is also important to always identify and protect the hypoglossal nerve, which can traverse the ECA quite low near the carotid bifurcation.

Limitations and Contraindications

It is a well-known surgical axiom that a vessel should be ligated as close as possible to the point of hemorrhage to defeat anastomotic contributions to the vascular leak.[5] However, this is not always possible in the maxillofacial region due to the highly dense and critical structures in this area. The rich vascular network in this region ensures the vitality of tissue in the event of trauma or surgical injury. However, this extensive collateral blood supply diminishes the effectiveness and predictability of arterial ligation. The more distal the bleeding source, the more likely it has a collateral blood supply, from the ipsilateral side or even from the contralateral side. Therefore, ligation of the ECA is not always successful. If the bleeding involves the upper face and nasal cavity, contribution from the internal carotid artery via the ethmoidal arteries may necessitate a combined ligation of the ECA and the anterior ethmoidal artery. For the same reason, TAE can be more effective due to its ability to reach distant arteries, and it can be more selective. If TAE fails, ligation of the ECA is still an option. On the other hand, if the ECA is ligated first, the option to embolize through the same vessel no longer exists. Therefore, it is important to exhaust all other options before arterial ligation.

Postoperative Considerations

Postoperative complications related to ECA ligation are not well described in the literature. In 1985, Cooke described several complications in a series of 43 patients, including facial numbness, diplopia, hemiparesis, and gait disturbance.[11] However, his procedures included various combinations with transantral ligation of the internal maxillary arteries and ligation of the anterior ethmoidal arteries. The complications described were not correlated with the specific procedure.

If nasal packing is performed to stop epistaxis, it is prudent to ensure that the gauze strips are impregnated with antibiotic ointment. The packing should be removed in 3 days to avoid the risk of toxic shock syndrome secondary to *Staphylococcus aureus* infection.

Once the bleeding has been controlled and the patient stabilized, consideration should be given to the possibility of an underlying coagulopathy. A thorough medical history and physical examination should be performed. Further laboratory studies, such as liver function tests, factor levels, and platelet function tests, should be ordered if indicated. Prompt correction with transfusion of fresh-frozen plasma, vitamin K, platelets, or packed red blood cells can improve the patient's chances of survival. Hypertension, although seldom the single cause of massive facial hemorrhage, can make managing the bleeding difficult. Monitoring the patient's blood pressure before and during treatment is important to determine whether pharmacologic intervention is necessary to assist with control of hypertension.[11]

References

1. Bederson JB. *Treatment of Carotid Disease: A Practitioner's Manual.* Park Ridge, IL: The American Association of Neurological Surgeons; 1998.
2. Twitchell A. Gunshot wound of the face and neck: Ligature of the carotid artery. *New Engl Quart J Med Surg*. 1842;1:188–193.
3. Bryant III JD. Ligation of the external carotid artery, with remarks on the history of the operation. *Ann Surg*. 1887;6(2):115–126.
4. Hunter K, Gibson R. Arterial ligation for severe epistaxis. *J Laryngol Otol.* 1969;83(11):1099–1103.
5. Malcomson KG. The surgical management of massive epistaxis. *J Laryngol Otol.* 1963;77:299–314.
6. Martis C. Case for ligation of the external carotid artery in composite operations for oral carcinoma. *Int J Oral Surg*. 1978;7(2):95–99.
7. Chandler JR, Serrins AJ. Transantral ligation of the internal maxillary artery for epistaxis. *Laryngoscope*. 1965;75:1151–1159.
8. Hassard AD, Kirkpatrick DA, Wong FS. Ligation of the external carotid and anterior ethmoidal arteries for severe or unusual epistaxis resulting from facial fractures. *Can J Surg*. 1986;29(6):447–449.
9. Cooke ET. An evaluation and clinical study of severe epistaxis treated by arterial ligation. *J Laryngol Otol*. 1985;99(8):745–749.
10. Yin NT. Effect of multiple ligations of the external carotid artery and its branches on blood flow in the internal maxillary artery in dogs. *J Oral Maxillofac Surg*. 1994;52(8):849–854.
11. Viehweg TL, Roberson JB, Hudson JW. Epistaxis: diagnosis and treatment. *J Oral Maxillofac Surg*. 2006;64(3):511–518.
12. Sakamoto T, Yagi K, Hiraide A, et al. Transcatheter embolization in the treatment of massive bleeding due to maxillofacial injury. *J Trauma*. 1988;28(6):840–843.
13. Bouloux GF, Perciaccante VJ. Massive hemorrhage during oral and maxillofacial surgery: ligation of the external carotid artery or embolization? *J Oral Maxillofac Surg.* 2009;67(7):1547–1551.
14. Yang WG, Tsai TR, Hung CC, Tung TC. Life-threatening bleeding in a facial fracture. *Ann Plast Surg*. 2001;46(2):159–162.
15. Dean NR, Ledgard JP, Katsaros J. Massive hemorrhage in facial fracture patients: definition, incidence, and management. *Plast Reconstr Surg*. 2009;123(2):680–690.
16. Ardekian L, Samet N, Shoshani Y, Taicher S. Life-threatening bleeding following maxillofacial trauma. *J Craniomaxillofac Surg.* 1993;21(8):336–338.
17. Khanna S, Dagum AB. A critical review of the literature and an evidence-based approach for life-threatening hemorrhage in maxillofacial surgery. *Ann Plast Surg*. 2012;69(4):474–478.
18. Shuker ST. The immediate lifesaving management of maxillofacial, life-threatening haemorrhages due to IED and/or shrapnel injuries: "when hazard is in hesitation, not in the action". *J Craniomaxillofac Surg*. 2012;40(6):534–540.
19. Shimoyama T, Kaneko T, Horie N. Initial management of massive oral bleeding after midfacial fracture. *J Trauma*. 2003;54(2):332–336.
20. Ho K, Hutter JJ, Eskridge J, et al. The management of life-threatening haemorrhage following blunt facial trauma. *J Plast Reconstr Aesthet Surg*. 2006;59(12):1257–1262.
21. Granville-Chapman J, Jacobs N, Midwinter MJ. Pre-hospital haemostatic dressings: a systematic review. *Injury*. 2011;42(5):447–459.
22. Gabay M, Boucher BA. An essential primer for understanding the role of topical hemostats, surgical sealants, and adhesives for maintaining hemostasis. *Pharmacotherapy*. 2013;33(9):935–955.
23. Krulewitz NA, Fix ML. Epistaxis. *Emerg Med Clin North Am.* 2019;37(1):29–39.
24. Gottlieb M, DeMott JM, Peksa GD. Topical tranexamic acid for the treatment of acute epistaxis: a systematic review and meta-analysis. *Ann Pharmacother*. 2019;53(6):652–657.
25. Chen YF, Tzeng IH, Li YH, et al. Transcatheter arterial embolization in the treatment of maxillofacial trauma induced life-threatening hemorrhages. *J Trauma*. 2009;66(5):1425–1430.
26. Smith TP. Embolization in the external carotid artery. *J Vasc Interv Radiol.* 2006;17(12):1897–1912.
27. Matsumoto S, Akashi T, Hayashida K, et al. Transcatheter arterial embolization in the treatment of maxillofacial fractures with life-threatening hemorrhage. *Ann Plast Surg*. 2018;80(6):664–668.
28. Cogbill TH, Cothren CC, Ahearn MK, et al. Management of maxillofacial injuries with severe oronasal hemorrhage: a multicenter perspective. *J Trauma*. 2008;65(5):994–999.
29. Bailey BJ. *Atlas of Head and Neck Surgery: Otolaryngology*. 2nd ed. Philadelphia, PA: Lippincott Williams & Wilkins; 2001.

CHAPTER 73

Principles and Biomechanics of Rigid Internal Fixation of the Mandible

Michael R. Markiewicz and Mark Engelstad

Armamentarium

Essential to Fracture Repair
22-, 24-, and 26-gauge wire
Appropriate sutures
Arch bars
Bite blocks
Elastics
Intermaxillary fixation screws
hybrid IMF system
Wire director (pickle fork, gauze pusher, ligature tucker)
Wire twister and cutter

Osteosynthesis
Bone reduction forceps
Countersink
Depth gauge
Drill guides
Drills
Fissure bur
Local anesthetic with vasoconstrictor
Plate bending irons and forceps
Plate cutters
Plate-holding forceps
Plate templates
Plates
Screws
Screwdriver
Transcutaneous trocar with cannula, drill sleeve, and trocar retention clamp

History of the Procedure

Rigid internal fixation of the mandible, although technically described now for almost a century, has only recently been popularized. Traditional treatment of mandibular trauma has centered around the use of closed reduction and immobilization of the jaws. This allowed for secondary bone healing with callus formation, but it did not allow for convalescent jaw function and was susceptible to difficulty in achieving union and infection because of constant micromovement of the fracture site.

The first published descriptions of the use of internal fixation were by Lambotte, Warnekros, and Wassmund during the intervening years of the great world wars. However, it was not until the late 1960s and early 1970s when Luhr, Schilli, and Becker advocated for plate and screw fixation for mandibular trauma using bicortical screws at the inferior border of the mandible. In the late 1970s, further development of the concept of miniplate fixation with monocortical screws was developed by Champy.

Since these early reports, substantial research and refinement of the techniques and materials used today for contemporary internal fixation of the mandible have occurred. This has allowed for the routine and safe use of the techniques for the betterment of patient recovery and function during healing.

Instrumentation

Rigid fixation screws serve to secure plates to fractured bone or to compress bone fragments together. Screw holes are usually predrilled, and the size of the drill is equal to the inner diameter of the screw. The outer diameter of the screw is usually the basis for the sizing system of many fixation systems; for example, "2.0 system" might use a 1.8-mm-diameter drill and a screw with an inner diameter of 1.8 mm and an outer diameter of 2.0 mm (Fig. 73.1). The outer diameter of the screw is the thread width, which advances the screw and engages bone. The threading of bone by the screw is called "tapping," and it accounts for the feeling of torque resistance during initial screw placement. Some older fixation systems with non-self-tapping screws required an additional instrument to "tap" the drill hole, but contemporary sets are mostly metallic screws and are self-tapping. Threads engage the bone, transferring forces across the plate and bone, resisting dislodgement or "pull out" forces. Screws from different systems have different head shapes, screwdriver interfaces (i.e., hex, slot, cross), and pitch (the distance between the threads). Screws may require pretapping (biodegradable screws) or may be self-tapping (as described above) or self-drilling.[1]

The function of a plate is to stabilize adjacent bone fragments long enough to allow healing or "union." Various designs include *adaption* (round plate holes), *compression* (dynamic sloped, oval holes), *locking* (threaded holes), and *reconstruction* (wider, higher profile, stronger) plates. In addition, one or a combination of these designs may be seen. Compression plates have sloped holes designed to cause fragment movement (compression) when an eccentrically drilled screw head is tightened against the plate. Reconstruction plates are optimal for atrophic, comminuted, or mandibular

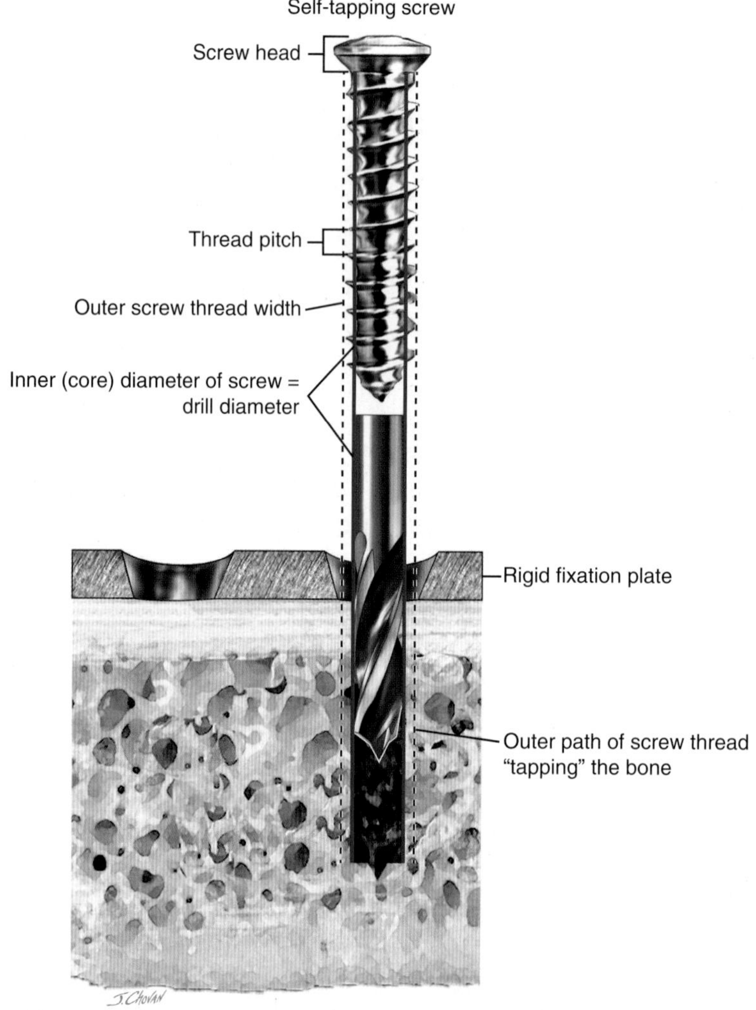

Figure 73.1 The drill diameter is equal to the inner diameter of the screw and defines the size of the plating set. The shaft of the screw has threads with a varying pitch. Because the drill diameter equals the diameter of the screw shaft, the threads engage bone, providing retention of the screw within bone.

fractures with defects in which little or no bone fragment buttressing exists.[2] Mandibular reconstruction plates are generally straight or longer curved plates designed to follow the contours of the mandibular inferior and posterior border. Each system includes smaller and larger profile sizes (plate depth and width), along with various configurations to adapt to specific areas such as the condylar and angle region.

Biomechanical Principles of Rigid Fixation

Definition

Internal fixation is a process of bone fragment stabilization achieved by internal (directly on bone) placement of implants, such as plates and screws. Rigid fixation is one type of internal fixation and has multiple definitions, including "a form of fixation applied directly to bones which is strong enough to prevent interfragmentary motion across the fracture when actively using the skeletal structure."[3] Another definition is, "any form of bone fixation in which otherwise deforming biomechanical forces are either countered or used as an advantage to stabilize the fracture fragments and to permit loading of the bone so far as to permit active motion."[4] Forms of fixation designated as rigid are generally stiff and resilient enough to prevent interfragmentary mobility during healing. Nonrigid fixation "stabilizes the fragments during function but may allow some interfragmentary motion."[4] Most forms of nonrigid fixation are functionally stable; that is, they do not prevent all interfragmentary motion, but rather create a plate-bone construct that is stable enough to allow some function during skeletal healing. For nonrigid fixation to succeed, the fracture itself must be carefully selected; it should be simple and have good interfragmentary fit and buttressing. The superior border miniplate technique of treating a mandibular angle fracture is a classic example of functionally stable fixation.

Materials

Although resorbable materials such as poly (L-lactide)/polylactic acid implants are available, titanium and its alloys remain the materials of choice in rigid fixation systems. (This chapter is limited to the discussion of nonresorbable fixation options.) Titanium is inert, nontoxic, and corrosion-resistant and has high tensile strength.[2,5,6] Most commercial internal fixation systems contain commercially pure titanium or titanium alloy plates and screws of various dimensions and strengths. Two of the greatest benefits of titanium are its high strength-to-weight ratio and its corrosion resistance. Because it is nonferromagnetic (i.e., safe for future magnetic resonance imaging) and resists all corrosion by bodily fluids, titanium has become and continues to be the implant material of choice for rigid fixation.

Osseointegration relies upon biocompatibility, and it plays a role in internal fixation. It allows bone to tolerate and stabilize metallic implants, such as screws. Titanium is one of the metals that promotes biocompatibility. Most plates are made from either commercially pure titanium or a titanium alloy consisting of mostly titanium and, to a lesser extent, a combination of aluminum, vanadium, nickel, chromium, iron, molybdenum, and niobium. Screws are usually made from commercially pure titanium, stainless steel, or a titanium alloy.

Principles of Fracture Healing

Mandibular bone is a composite of organic collagen and inorganic mineral. Mandibular collagen resists tensile forces, and the mineral component resists compressive forces.[7] Throughout life, mandibular bone is constantly remodeling in response to the functional loads created by the muscles of mastication.[8,9] In response to fracture, it heals by one of two processes: primary (contact or direct) healing or secondary (callus or gap) healing. An understanding of these processes will result in better treatment decisions (Fig. 73.2).[10,11] Primary bone healing occurs when the fractured bone fragments are well reduced and then stabilized in a way that allows minimal fragment mobility, usually by using a rigid form of osteosynthesis. Primary healing occurs in areas of good bone contact by direct remodeling of the haversian system with direct crossing of osteoclasts and osteoblasts across the fracture plane, with no callus formation. In contrast, secondary bone healing with a callus occurs when some mobility remains between the fractured fragments; for instance, when a fractured mandible is treated by intermaxillary fixation alone or when there is a gap leaving mobility between fragments. No callus is formed in primary bone healing. Secondary healing typically occurs when a fracture hematoma between bone fragments remodels into a callus. The callus evolves from granulation tissue to connective tissue, followed by mineralized cartilage and eventually compact bone formation.

Zones of Osteosynthesis and Screw Depth

The concept of lines of mandibular osteosynthesis were introduced by Michelet et al.[12] and later popularized by Champy; this concept is used mostly in miniplate osteosynthesis.[13,14] The lines represent regions of mandibular compressive or tensile forces, which can vary depending on muscle function and the location of the load.[14] It can be helpful to conceptualize these lines of osteosynthesis as strong, thick areas of the mandible that resist functional stresses and that also make ideal locations to place screws and smaller plates (miniplates) in fracture repair (Fig. 73.3).

In fractures of the angle and posterior body, most loading is anterior to the fracture site; therefore, the superior border is usually under tensile forces, whereas the inferior border undergoes more compressive forces. In fractures of the symphyseal region, these forces alternate between the superior and inferior border. When the surgeon uses nonrigid fracture fixation, miniplates and screws are placed along the lines of mandibular osteosynthesis. When miniplates and monocortical screws are used, the weakest portion of the entire construct is usually the plate itself; therefore, bicortical screws are not advantageous in nonrigid fixation (i.e., in dense bone the miniplate will fail before the monocortical screws). When larger reconstruction plates and screws are used correctly, they can stabilize the jaw under any force, no matter where they are placed along the mandible; however, because they gain additional durability when bicortical screws are used, they usually are placed along the inferior border to avoid tooth and nerve injury.

Indications for the Use of the Procedure

Internal fixation of the mandible is indicated for a variety of reasons, including biomechanical, functional reasons, and patient preference. Rigid internal fixation of the mandible is indicated when nonrigid fixation would not provide sufficient fragment stabilization to allow healing. In cases in which the probability of healing is equivalent, rigid forms of fixation may allow for more rapid return to function. It is important to understand that immobilization of the mandible through the use of arch bars and wire intermaxillary fixation (IMF) does not eliminate movement of fractured fragments; every time a patient swallows, the powerful muscles of mastication activate and move loose bone fragments, even when the patient is "wired shut." If the patient's behavior is a concern, rigid fixation techniques might be more appropriate than long periods of IMF because bony healing can occur independent of patient compliance. In addition, when a patient is put in IMF, respiratory function is diminished, which can be detrimental in older patients, those with serious medical comorbidities, and certain psychiatric patients.

Classifications of Rigid Fixation

Load Bearing and Load Sharing

Fracture treatment with rigid fixation also can be classified as either load bearing or load sharing. Load-bearing fixation uses high-strength rigid plates and screws, strong enough to bear the entire load of mandibular function for a period of months without any reliance on load sharing between bone fragments themselves; in other words, no buttressing is required for load-bearing constructs. An example of a load-bearing construct is a large reconstruction plate and screws spanning a comminuted fracture. In contrast, load sharing is a type of fixation in which the implants and the bone share

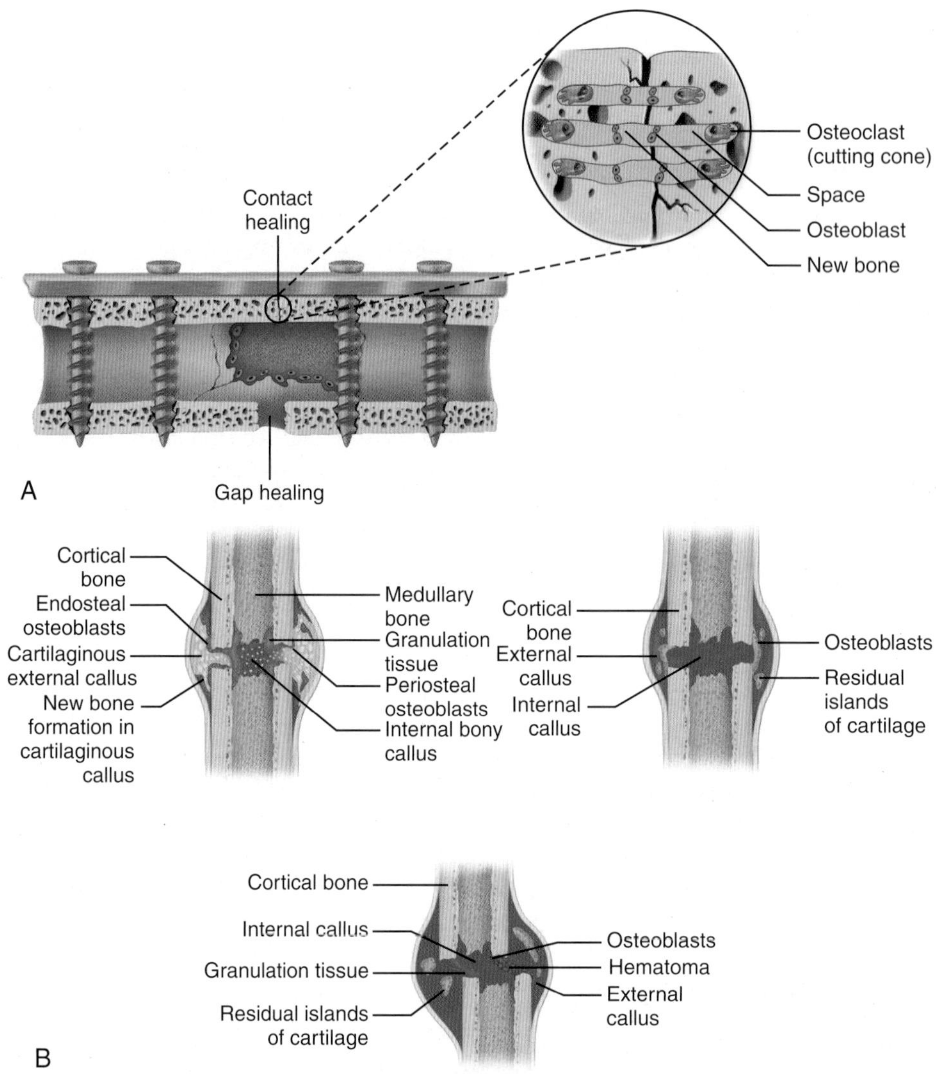

Figure 73.2 **A,** Primary bone healing occurs when the fractured bone fragments are reduced and then stabilized in a way that allows minimal fragment mobility. **B,** Secondary bone healing with a callus occurs when some mobility remains between the fractured fragments. (From Fonseca RJ, Barber HD, Walker RV, et al. Oral and Maxillofacial Trauma, 4th ed. St. Louis MO: Saunders; 2013).

functional loads. Load-sharing fixation can be used in simpler fracture types in which fragments are well buttressed against one another during healing and function. An example of load-sharing fixation is the superior border miniplate and screws across an angle fracture. Because load-sharing fixation relies on the fracture fragments to share forces by buttressing, it cannot be used in fractures that have little direct interfragmentary fit, such as old, comminuted, or atrophic fractures.

Locking and Nonlocking

Bone plating systems usually have both locking and nonlocking screw-plate interfaces, and it is important to understand the difference. Locking plates have holes that are threaded or shaped to allow the screw head to lock into the plate, creating a stiff plate-screw construct. Each locking screw has two attachment interfaces; one interface stabilizes the screw within the plate as mentioned, and the other anchors the screw to bone.[2] Because of these features, locking systems are more costly to manufacture, but they have important advantages.

- During screw tightening, the screw head locks into the plate instead of compressing the plate down against the bone surface, causing fragment distortion, as occurs in nonlocking systems. In a nonlocking system, a screw placed through an imperfectly adapted rigid plate pulls the mobile bone out of alignment toward the rigid plate, resulting in misalignment and malocclusion. Because the locking plate is not pulled against the bone surface, the adaptation (bending) of a locking plate does not have to be as precise as that of nonlocking plates A locking plate can be millimeters off the bone surface but still retain its structural integrity.
- The tight interface between plate and screw head reduces micromotion within the bone-screw-plate construct. In contrast, nonlocking systems depend on the bone-screw-plate friction to keep the construct stable (Fig. 73.4).

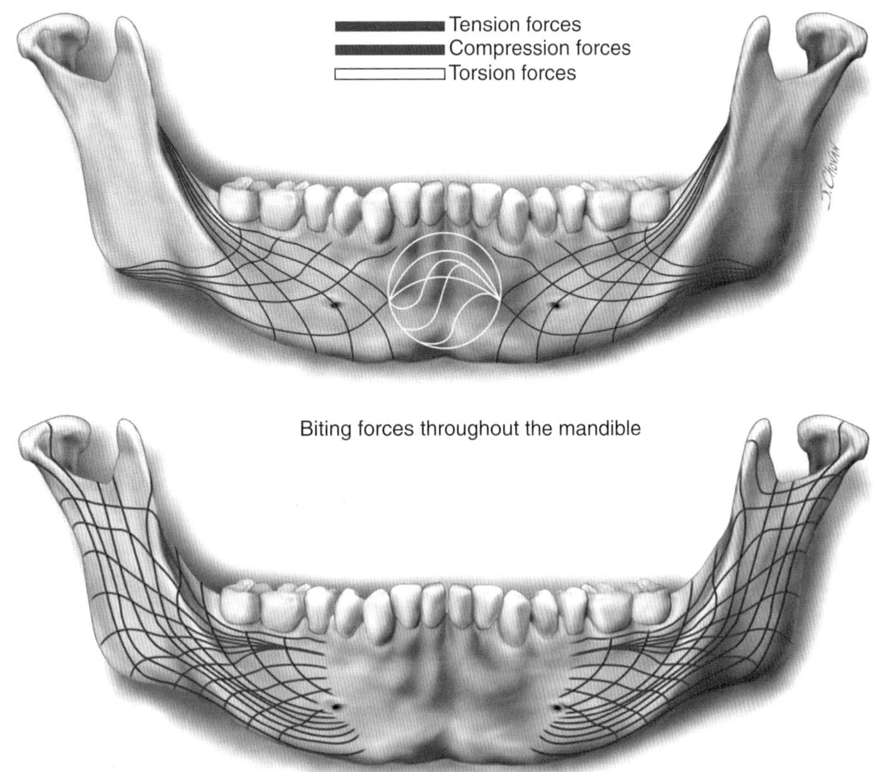

Figure 73.3 Zones of osteosynthesis.

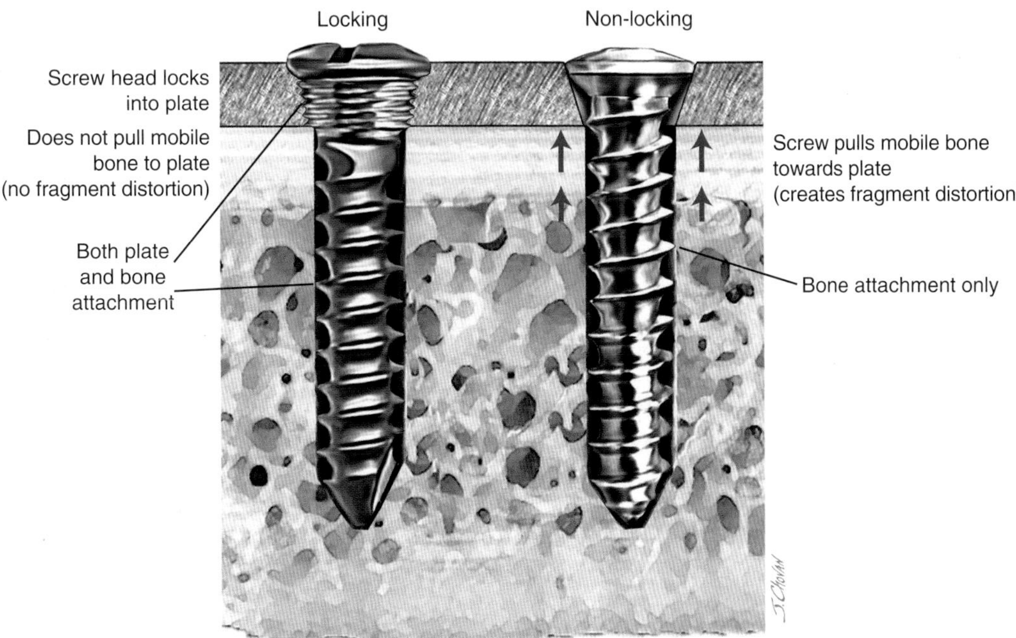

Figure 73.4 Screw-plate interfaces: locking and nonlocking.

Compression

Compression of bony segments can be achieved by specially designed drill guides, screws, and plates, or with lag screws alone. With the exception of lag screw compression in the mandibular symphysis or the occasional tangential body fracture, compression plating is not generally advantageous in craniomaxillofacial trauma and may be associated with higher postoperative morbidity, mostly because it is complicated and very technique sensitive.[15]

Lag screws are the simplest form of internal fixation. Their use in the mandible was popularized by Niederdellmann and Akuamoa-Boateng.[16] These screws provide a reliable and highly stable form of compression rigid fixation under the right conditions. Lag screw compression should be reserved for simple, noncomminuted fractures with good interfragmentary buttressing (e.g., a simple symphyseal fracture). It works similarly in all sites: a cortex of one fragment is engaged by the screw head but not by the screw threads (gliding hole), while a cortex of the other fragment is engaged by the distal screw threads (traction hole). Under these circumstances, with the right cortex alignments and good interfragmentary buttressing, turning the screw tightly compresses the two fragments against each other.

Limitations and Contraindications

The presence of developing permanent tooth buds or a very inferiorly positioned inferior alveolar nerve canal may contraindicate some forms of rigid fixation.

Rigid fixation of any type of surgical mandibular fracture occurs in four sequential steps: access, fragment reduction, internal fixation, and wound closure/healing. This chapter focuses on fragment reduction and internal fixation. The steps of reduction and internal fixation are discussed in the standard plate technique.

Recently, custom patient-specific plates have been utilized in patients undergoing orthognathic, craniofacial, head and neck, and reconstructive surgeries as well as other craniomaxillofacial procedures.[17,18] Their utility in these arenas has been reported by many. These types of implants have been advocated for use in the management of mandible and other facial fractures; however, their utility, cost-effectiveness, and superiority to traditional nonpatient specific implants is still an area of debate.

TECHNIQUE: Standard Plate Fixation

STEP 1: Approach

The approach to some fractures may be made easier by immobilizing the mandible first. Specific approaches are not discussed here because they are addressed elsewhere in this text. However, the surgical approach should allow visualization of enough of the fracture to verify ideal reduction; in the anterior mandible, for instance, the surgeon should always visualize the inferior border to ensure alignment.

In many intraoral approaches made through thin tissues, hardware placed too close to the level of incision can cause wound breakdown and plate exposure, necessitating an additional procedure or resulting in nonunion. In transoral approaches, a single stronger plate at the inferior border, well away from the incision site, may allow more reliable healing than a "simpler" two-miniplate configuration, in which the superior miniplate often becomes exposed, leading to delayed wound healing or nonunion (Fig. 73.5A).

STEP 2: Immobilization

Many fractures of the mandible require some form of short-term immobilization, either intraoperative only or intraoperative and postoperative. If no postoperative immobilization is required, there are forms of intraoperative IMF, such as embrasure wires, that are very inexpensive and take only minutes to apply.[19] When arch bars or IMF screws are used, wire IMF is non-self-tightening, intimidating, and a concern to patients; therefore, we recommend elastics for mandibular immobilization. With a jaw fracture, muscle strength is diminished considerably,[20] so just a few bilateral elastics provide very firm immobilization. Simple fractures can be repaired without IMF,[21] but what seems like a shortcut often results in malreduction or additional procedures.

STEP 3: Reduction

Finding and maintaining the correct occlusion while applying rigid fixation are critical because malreductions and malocclusions fixed with rigid plates often cannot be corrected with elastic dental traction. Whenever possible, fractures should be reduced by aligning the dentition and preloading the fracture using reduction forceps. Reduction forceps, when used correctly, help the surgeon obtain the best bony reduction possible. This is especially important in double fractures, in which even a minor malreduction of one fracture can make alignment of a second, distant fracture impossible. Reduction forceps are fairly simple to use when a few principles are followed. Two monocortical holes are drilled on both sides of the fracture, perpendicular to the fracture line. These holes should be drilled away from planned plate placement and as far from the fracture line as feasible (to prevent overclosing of the facial cortex and gapping at the lingual cortex). While the reduction forceps is closed, a periosteal elevator, along with digital manipulation, can be used to properly align and reduce the fracture line (Fig. 73.5B).

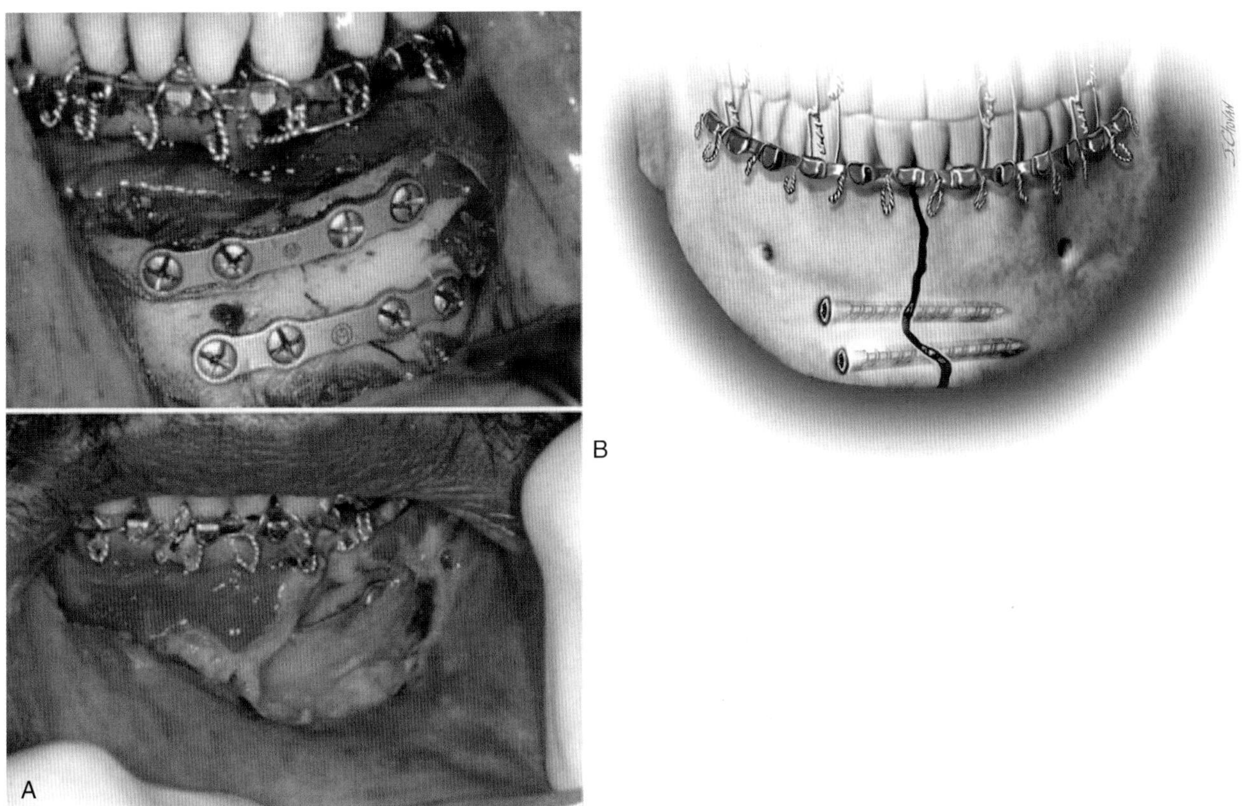

Figure 73.5 **A,** Incisions with hardware in the vicinity are more likely to break down *(A)*. Wounds heal better with solid bone underneath. **B,** Two monocortical holes are drilled on both sides of the fracture, perpendicular to the fracture line. The drill should enter and exit the bone at high speed to minimize bone burning, create the smallest hole possible, and prevent drill breakage. These holes should be drilled away from planned plate placement and as far from the fracture line as feasible (to prevent overclosing of the facial cortex and gapping at the lingual cortex). While closing the reduction forceps, the surgeon can use a periosteal elevator, along with digital manipulation, to properly align and reduce the fracture line.

TECHNIQUE: Standard Plate Fixation—*cont'd*

STEP 4: Plate and Screw Construct

Simple fractures of the mandibular symphysis and body with no bony defect or atrophy can be successfully repaired with several different plate-screw constructs: a single, more rigid plate along the inferior border, two smaller plates placed superiorly and inferiorly, lag screws, or even a combination of these (detailed elsewhere in this atlas).

A variety of forces affect the mandibular symphysis during function, so effective internal fixation should resist these forces. At the mandibular body there is less torsion, and only one line of osteosynthesis (running along the midmandible) is depicted in most illustrations. This is perhaps an oversimplification, and using Champy's lines as a guide for mandibular fracture treatment results in failure in many circumstances. This is because Champy's approach does not take into account the effects of other simultaneous mandibular fractures. For the isolated simple symphyseal fracture, many forms of fixation suffice. However, when that simple symphyseal fracture occurs along with one or two posterior mandibular fractures, more rigid forms of fixation (lag screw/reconstruction plate) must be used at the symphysis.

In general, fractures with more destabilizing elements (e.g., more than one fracture, low-quality bone, atrophy, poor buttressing, defects, comminution, infection) should be repaired with more rigid load-bearing construction. Fractures without these factors can be treated with less rigid, load-sharing constructs (Fig. 73.5C). For bicortical screws, a depth gauge ensures selection of the appropriate-length screws, which engage the deep cortex without endangering deeper structures. When locking screws are used, special drill guides are required to ensure precise fit of the locking screw into the plate. With few exceptions, screws should be placed perpendicular to the plate. To stabilize comminuted segments, such as a basal triangle, nonlocking screws may be preferable. Successful mandibular fracture repair with rigid fixation is highly correlated with experience[22] because each injury is unique and so many variables must be considered. Algorithmic approaches to fracture repair often fail. The appropriate drill is

Continued

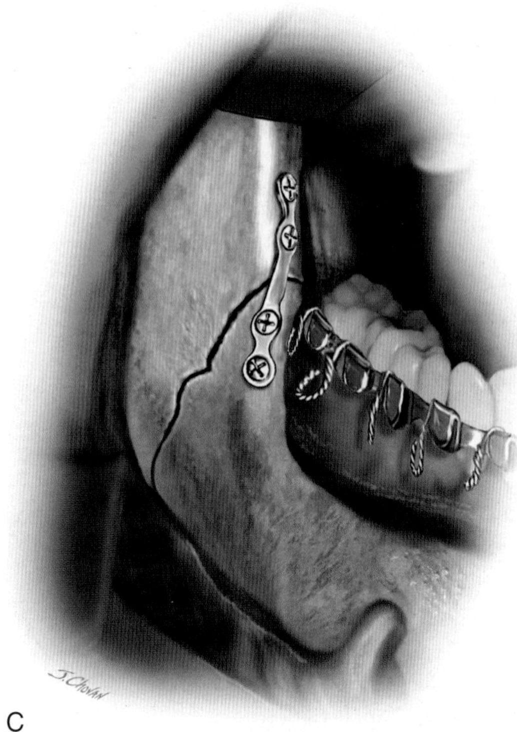

C

Figure 73.5, cont'd **C,** Examples of types of simple fractures appropriate for load bearing. Fractures with more destabilizing factors (e.g., more than one fracture, low-quality bone, atrophy, poor buttressing, defects, comminution, absence of infection) should be repaired with more rigidity in a more load-bearing construction. Fractures without these factors can be treated with less rigid, more load-sharing constructs.

TECHNIQUE: Standard Plate Fixation—*cont'd*

chosen (matching the core diameter of the screw to be used). When a longer drill is used, the drill should be stabilized with a drill guide. The drill guide and bone should be cooled so that the temperature remains below 47°C to minimize bone necrosis. Comminuted fragments should be reduced and temporarily stabilized with miniplates first, simplifying the fracture and preventing fragment mobility and making adaptation of large plates much easier and more reliable.

STEP 5: Quality Assurance

The quality of the dental occlusion is the most important indirect outcome assessment of mandibular fracture reduction and repair. IMF is removed, and while the condyles are seated into their fossa, the occlusion is checked for any gross discrepancies. Very minor "slides" (less than 1 mm) or malocclusions usually can be compensated for with postoperative guiding elastics. However, gross discrepancies warrant removal of hardware and improvement of bony reduction before replating. Malalignments and gross occlusal discrepancies (i.e., an open bite) are much easier to repair at the time of initial repair than in a later procedure.

STEP 6: Postoperative Function

If the repair is high quality and reliable (good bone quality, normal occlusion, advantageous biomechanics), the patient may not need postoperative immobilization or occlusal guidance. If there is any doubt, the reduction should be modified and improved or arch bars should be placed to allow for postoperative elastic traction. IMF screws can provide intraoperative immobilization, but because they are so far from the line of occlusion and often become covered with hypertrophic tissues, they are poor options for long-term postoperative immobilization and occlusal guidance.

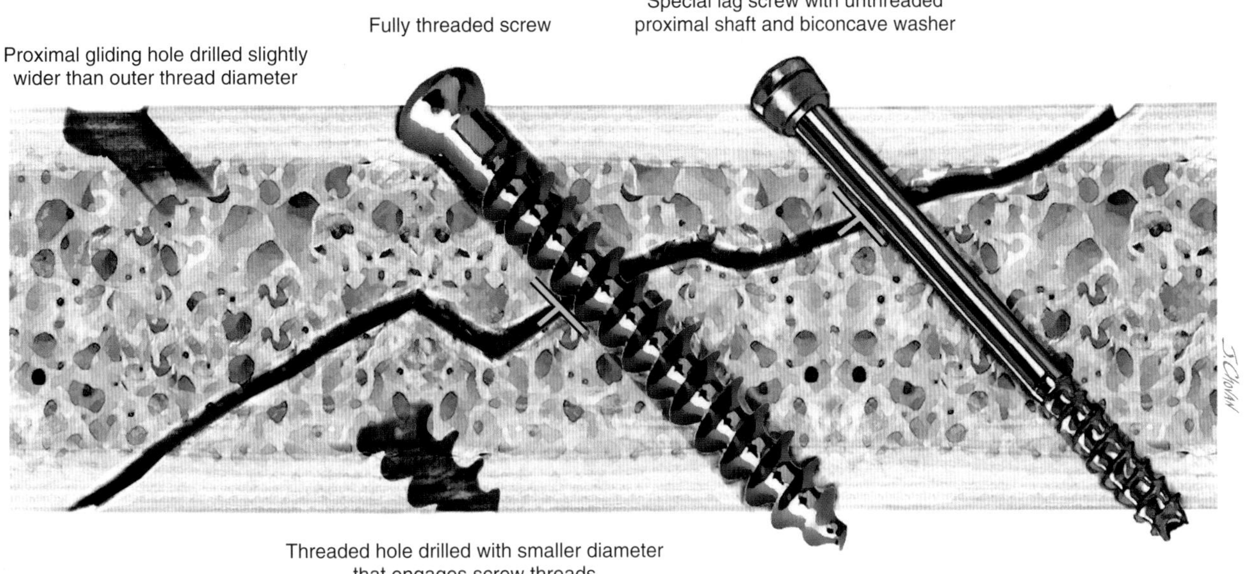

Figure 73.6 The lag screw should be placed perpendicular to the fracture with the gliding hole proximal and the screw threads engaging the distal cortex.

ALTERNATIVE TECHNIQUE 1: Lag Screw Fixation

The lag screw technique is a form of load-sharing osteosynthesis and may be used when any two solid, flat, bony surfaces must be approximated (Fig. 73.6). This technique is useful in oblique fractures, symphyseal fractures, fixation of bone grafts, and sagittal split osteotomies. Lag screws may be used in conjunction with a plate (this technique is not discussed here). They provide compression by engaging a cortex of one fragment with the screw head and a cortex from the other fragment with the screw threads. If proper drilling has been performed, screw tightening compresses these two fragments together.

Bone reduction forceps are applied, and the fracture is manipulated and reduced. The drill should enter and exit the bone at high speeds to minimize bone burning, create the smallest hole possible, and prevent drill breakage. The screw holes should be drilled as perpendicular to the fracture as possible to prevent telescoping or sliding with screw tightening. For sagittal fractures through the symphysis, lag screws are placed between the outer buccal cortices. For an oblique fracture through the symphysis or mandible, the lag screws are placed from buccal to lingual cortex to maintain perpendicular orientation to the fracture. A drill guide for both proximal and distal drills is needed to maintain concentricity between the segments. To prevent slippage of the drill on the outer cortex, a pilot hole is drilled first, perpendicular to the surface of the bone. The drill and guide are then reoriented so that they are perpendicular to the fracture. When fully threaded screws are used in the lag screw technique, the proximal or gliding hole is drilled slightly wider than the outer thread diameter. Next, the distal fragment or threaded hole is drilled with a smaller diameter drill that engages the screw threads. After both holes have been drilled, a depth gauge is used to measure screw length. Manufacturers also make special lag screws with an unthreaded proximal shaft and threaded distal tip. Alternatively, a less accurate way of drilling a lag screw is to drill both proximal and distal cortices with a drill matching the core diameter of the screw, then to overdrill the proximal gliding hole with a drill larger than the outer thread diameter of the screw. However, this may result in a less centrally located proximal hole relative to the distal hole and in drilling of the guiding hole too far into the distal segment.

For thick cortical bone in the proximal segment, a countersink hole should be drilled to allow full contact between the screw head and bone. The surgeon must beware of over coutersinking and removing too much cortical bone. The screw is then inserted; it will glide through the proximal hole and "grab" onto the distal threaded hole. Once the screw head engages the proximal segment, interfragmentary compression takes place. Two lag screws are often used to provide additional stabilization. The two lag screws may be placed with the screw heads on the same side or in opposite directions; this makes no biomechanical difference. If in doubt, the surgeon should confirm reduction at the lingual cortex.

ALTERNATIVE TECHNIQUE 2: Locking Reconstruction Plate Fixation

An extraoral approach is often needed for application of a locking reconstruction plate. After the fractures have been exposed and the patient has been placed in an IMF, a larger-sized locking reconstruction plate is selected. The fracture may be simplified by applying one to several small plates to the comminuted fragments. These plates may remain or may be removed after application of the reconstruction plate. The plate selected should be long enough to have a minimum of three or preferably four screws on each side of stable, noncomminuted fragments.

To improve outcomes and save money and time, plate bending should be practiced and perfected outside of the operating room. In general, large plates are bent in a certain sequence: in-plane bends first, followed by out-of-plane bends, followed by torquing or twisting bends (Fig. 73.7). Plate templates may be useful to achieve complex bends. Using the template as a guide, holes are then trimmed from the reconstruction plate using plate cutters. In-plane, out-of-plane bending, and torquing of the plate are then performed in a systematic manner to match the template. Frequent checking against the bone is recommended because the template itself is only a rough approximation. The plate is then adapted to the mandibular anatomy. The surgeon should keep in mind that locking plates do not have to be perfectly adapted; smaller gaps of 1 to 2 mm between plate and bone are tolerable.

The plate is then applied to the mandible with a plate-holding forceps or a drill guide screwed into the plate for use as a handle. While drilling the first few holes, the surgeon should carefully check reduction and occlusion because after more than two screws have been placed, any malalignments necessitate removal of all screws and replating. Locking screws are preferred but must be placed mostly perpendicular to the plate. If an angulated screw is required (to avoid a nerve or engage a distant bone fragment), nonlocking screws are advantageous because they can be placed at large angles to the plate. Modern screws are generally self-tapping, but in dense bone the surgeon may need to tap the hole; this is especially true in atrophic mandible fractures in older patients because the screw itself can create a new fracture if not tapped before placement. For drilling, a long or short drill guide with a threaded tip is screwed into the plate hole. A depth gauge is used to determine the screw length, and a screw of the appropriate size and length is inserted into the plate and bone. The screw stops turning once fully engaged with the plate; overtightening is not required and may be harmful.

Avoidance and Management of Intraoperative Complications

In the application of lag screws or any compression technique, two well-buttressed fragment faces must be compressed against each other. Therefore, the presence of comminution or any mobility after placement of lag screws should lead to an alternative approach. Although lag screws have the advantage of absolute stability and no plate bending, their placement must be precise, and the technique does not allow for

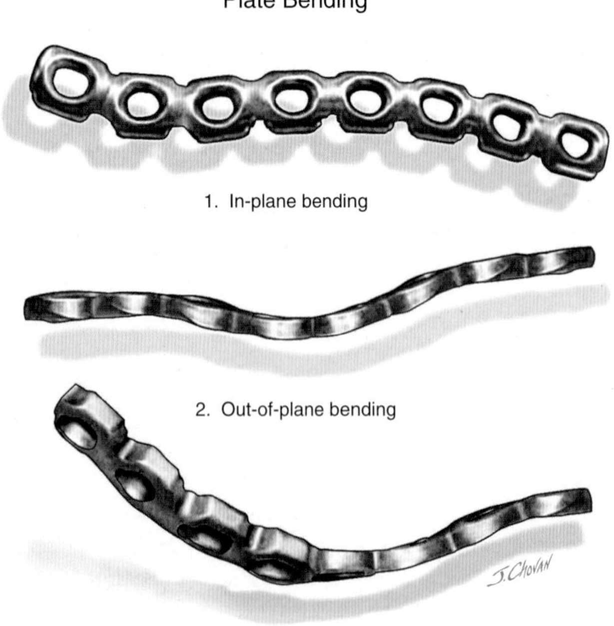

Figure 73.7 Plate bending should be performed in a specific sequence: in-plane bends, followed by out-of-plane bends, followed by torquing bends.

correction. When the threads in bone have been stripped or if a screw hole is drilled too large, an emergency/salvage screw, which is the next largest outer diameter screw, may be used.

Postoperative Considerations

Even with proper IMF and fixation placement, patients may experience residual malocclusion. Guiding elastics traction may be applied to arch bars or IMF screws to correct malocclusion. Unless the patient has a severe soft tissue injury that allows exposure of the fracture to the oral cavity and external environment, routine systemic postoperative antibiotics thus far have shown no improvement in outcomes.[23] Routine postoperative imaging is not absolutely required unless it is indicated clinically.

References

1. Baumgart FW, Cordey J, Morikawa K, et al. AO/ASIF self-tapping screws (STS). *Injury*. 1993;24(suppl 1):S1–S17.
2. Lekholm U, Adell R, Lindhe J, et al. Marginal tissue reactions at osseointegrated titanium fixtures. (II) A cross-sectional retrospective study. *Int J Oral Maxillofac Surg*. 1986;15(1):53–61.
3. Ellis E. Rigid skeletal fixation of fractures. *J Oral Maxillofac Surg*. 1993;51:163–173.
4. Allgower M, Spiegel PG. Internal fixation of fractures: evolution of concepts. *Clin Orthopaed Related Res*. 1979:26–29.
5. Bahr W, Stricker A, Gutwald R, Wellens E. Biodegradable osteosynthesis material for stabilization of midface fractures: experimental investigation in sheep. *J Craniomaxillofacial Surg*. 1999;27:51–57.
6. Dorri M, Nasser M, Oliver R. Resorbable versus titanium plates for facial fractures. *Cochrane Database Syst Rev*. 2009;1:CD007158.
7. Ascenzi A, Bonucci E. The tensile properties of single osteons. *Anat Rec*. 1967;158(4):375–386.
8. Moss ML. The primacy of functional matrices in orofacial growth. *Dent Pract Dent Rec*. 1968;19(2):65–73.
9. Moss ML, Rankow RM. The role of the functional matrix in mandibular growth. *Angle Orthod*. 1968;38(2):95–103.
10. Rahn BA, Gallinaro P, Baltensperger A, Perren SM. Primary bone healing. An experimental study in the rabbit. *J Bone Joint Surg Am*. 1971;53(4):783–786.
11. Reitzik M, Schoorl W. Bone repair in the mandible: a histologic and biometric comparison between rigid and semirigid fixation. *J Oral Maxillofacial Surg*. 1983;41:215–218.
12. Michelet FX, Deymes J, Dessus B. Osteosynthesis with miniaturized screwed plates in maxillo-facial surgery. *J Maxillofac Surg*. 1973;1(2):79–84.
13. Champy M, Lodde JP, Jaeger JH, Wilk A. [Biomechanical basis of mandibular osteosynthesis according to the F.X. Michelet method]. *Rev Stomatol Chir Maxillofac*. 1976;77(1):248–251.
14. Champy M, Loddé JP, Schmitt R, Jaeger JH, Muster D. Mandibular osteosynthesis by miniature screwed plates via a buccal approach. *J Maxillofac Surg*. 1978;6(1):14–21.
15. Ellis E, Sinn DP. Treatment of mandibular angle fractures using two 2.4-mm dynamic compression plates. *J Oral Maxillofacial*. 1993;51:969–973.
16. Niederdellmann H, Akuamoa-Boateng E. Internal fixation of fractures. *Int J Oral Surg*. 1978;7(4):252–255.
17. Wong A, Goonewardene MS, Allan BP, Mian AS, Rea A. Accuracy of maxillary repositioning surgery using cad/cam customized surgical guides and fixation plates. *Internatl J Oral Maxillofacial Surg*; 2020.
18. Johal M, Leinkram D, Wallace C, Clark JR. The Sydney Modified Alberta Reconstruction Technique (SM-ART) for dental rehabilitation following mandibulectomy or maxillectomy. *Int J Oral Maxillofac Surg*. 2020.
19. Engelstad ME, Kelly P. Embrasure wires for intraoperative maxillomandibular fixation are rapid and effective. *J Oral Maxillofacial Surg*. 2011;69:120–124.
20. Talwar RM, Ellis E 3rd, Throckmorton GS. Adaptations of the masticatory system after bilateral fractures of the mandibular condylar process. *J Oral Maxillofacial Surg*. 1998;56:430–439.
21. Cousin GC. Wire-free fixation of jaw fractures. *Br J Oral Maxillofac Surg*. 2009;47(7):521–524.
22. Kearns GJ, Perrott DH, Kaban LB. Rigid fixation of mandibular fractures: does operator experience reduce complications? *J Oral Maxillofacial Surg*. 1994;52:226–231, discussion 231–222.
23. Kyzas PA. Use of antibiotics in the treatment of mandible fractures: a systematic review. *J Oral Maxillofac Surg*. 2011;69:1129–1145.

CHAPTER 74

Dentoalveolar Trauma

Stone Thayer and Ravi Chandran

Armamentarium

#9 Periosteal elevator
Appropriate sutures
Cotton roll
Dental flowable composite
Dental handpiece and burs
Dental mouth mirror
Erich arch bars
Hemostats
Light cure unit
Local anesthetic with vasoconstrictor
Maxillofacial plating system
Minnesota retractor
Paper clip
Seldin retractor
Self-retaining cheek retractors
Stainless-steel wires (gauges 20 and 24)
Suction unit
Wire cutters
Wire drivers

History of the Procedure

Maxillofacial trauma includes fractures to the cranium, midface, mandible, and dentoalveolar structures. Isolated trauma to the dentoalveolar structures often requires the interplay between maxillofacial surgeons and various other dental practitioners. Injuries to these areas can result in fractured and displaced teeth, loss of dentition coupled with intraoral and extraoral soft tissue trauma, and fractures of the alveolar bone. A surgeon initially stabilizes such injuries, especially when soft tissue structures and supporting bone are involved. Subsequent reciprocal referral to other dental practitioners facilitates appropriate restoration of the dentition and evaluation of pulp vitality.

Injuries to the oral structures can have a deleterious impact on function, aesthetics, and the permanent dentition depending on the age of the patient. The father of medicine, Hippocrates of Greece, described the importance of the occlusal alignment and used gold dental wires to align the dentition and reduce mandibular fractures.[1]

Dentoalveolar injuries occur in all age groups. The prevalence and type of injury vary according to age, sex, and mechanism. Overall, emergency room visits resulting from trauma to the maxillofacial structures account for an estimated at 15%, and specifically, injuries to the dentoalveolar structures account for nearly 2%.[2] In the pediatric group, trauma to the oral structures has been reported to account for around 5% of all facial fractures.[3]

Mechanisms of Injury

Injuries to the dentition, its supporting structures, and surrounding soft tissue can occur because of falls, interpersonal violence and abuse, motor vehicle accidents, industrial accidents, contact sports, medical procedures, and penetrating objects.[4] Patients who suffer from seizure disorders and mental disabilities are also subject to an increased risk. Not surprisingly, males are twice as likely to be affected as females due to increased participation in contact sports and a greater tendency to engage in interpersonal violence. An increased incidence of oral/dental trauma has been correlated to increased participation in contact sports, and an increased frequency occurs during spring and summer.

Trauma can be sustained directly to the dental structures or occur secondarily, when the mandible is forcefully accelerated into occlusion against the maxilla. The anterior adult dentition is more prone to injury because of its prominent location.[5–7] Compounding factors include an increased overjet of greater than 4 mm, labially inclined incisors, and short upper lip, characteristics exemplified in a class II division I malocclusion.[3]

The pattern of injury and structural damage can vary between the pediatric and adult populations as a result of anatomical differences and degree of craniofacial development. The cranium is larger in relation to the midface and mandible in the pediatric population; hence, the dentoalveolar structures are more anatomically protected and subsequently sustain a smaller percentage of traumas. The lack of sinus pneumatization, higher cancellous-to-cortical bone ratio, and developing dentition within the facial skeleton tend to increase the elasticity of facial bones, making them less vulnerable to fractures.[8] Dental trauma in this population can adversely affect the development and eruption of permanent dentition by directly traumatizing the dental follicle and developing tooth. Traumatic forces inflicted on the primary dentition are transferred to the supporting structures, resulting in luxation type injuries, whereas the traumatic forces in the secondary dentition are transferred to the teeth themselves, resulting in crown and crown-root fractures.

Toddlers and young children usually suffer from falls due to poor coordination as they learn to coordinate skeletal movements with weight bearing and balance. There appears to be a bimodal distribution of injuries between ages 2 and 4, and 8 and 10, according to Andreasen.[9] Further, in this demographic, cuts and abrasions sustained to the lip and mental region are often accompanied by primary teeth subluxation or crown fracture of the permanent dentition. Children and young adolescents tend to have a higher incidence of injuries from falls and bicycle accidents.[10,11] Underlying suspicion of abuse should be considered when the pattern or degree of injury does not correlate with the mechanism of injury as explained by the supervising adult or caregiver. Trauma to the head and neck regions has been reported as high as 50% in cases of child abuse.[12] The highest incidence of oral-dental injuries is observed in the older adolescent and young adult demographic between the ages 18 to 23 years old, stemming from sports injuries and motor vehicle accidents.[13] Involvement in contact sports such as baseball, basketball, football, hockey, and wrestling can result in intraoral soft tissue injury and can be mitigated with use of mouth guards.

Classification of Injuries

Many classification systems have been proposed. The two most common systems are those developed by Ellis and Davey and Andreasen.[1,3,8,9]

Ellis Classification

The Ellis classification is a simple and practical dental injury classification system (Fig. 74.1):

Type I: Fractures within enamel

Type II: Fractures involving enamel and dentin

Type III: Fractures involving pulp

Type IV: Root fractures

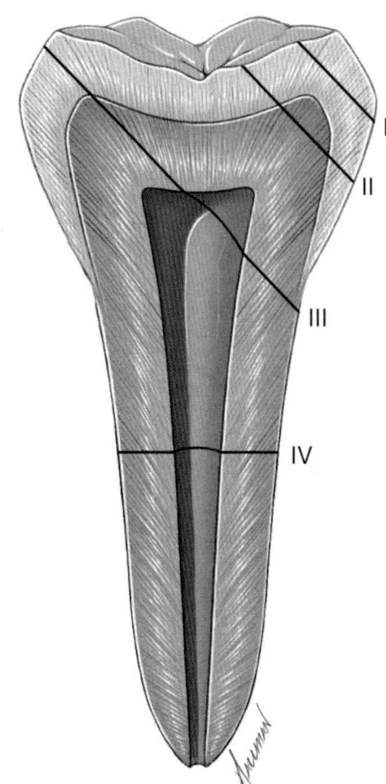

Figure 74.1 Ellis classification of dentoalveolar fractures.

Andreasen Classification

The classification devised by Andreasen and adopted by the World Health Organization system for disease classification is simple, comprehensive, and easy to communicate with the dentist or pediatric dentist. Injuries are divided into dental tissues and pulp, periodontal tissues, and supporting bones (Fig. 74.2).

Injuries to Dental Tissues and Pulp.

Crown infraction (craze lines without loss of tooth substance)

Complicated crown fracture producing a pulp exposure

Uncomplicated crown-root fracture without pulpal exposure

Complicated crown-root fracture with pulpal exposure

Root fractures (can be cervical, middle, or apical thirds and oblique root fractures)

Injuries to Periodontal Tissues

Concussion: Percussion sensitive without loosening of teeth

Subluxation: Tooth is loosened but not displaced

Luxation (lateral, intrusive, and extrusive luxations): Tooth is displaced without any fractures or comminution of the alveolar socket

Avulsion: Loss of teeth with or without supporting bone

Injuries to the Supporting Bone.

Fracture of a single wall of an alveolus

Comminution of the alveolar housing, seen with intrusive or lateral luxation

En bloc fracture of the alveolar process, the fracture line not necessarily extending through a tooth socket

Fracture involving the main body of the mandible or maxilla

Injuries to Gingiva or Mucosal Regions.

Abrasion

Contusion

Laceration

Indications for the Use of the Procedure

The common techniques used for stabilization of mobile dentoalveolar segments include acid etch/resin splints, Erich arch bars, and plating systems as discussed later. In general, subluxation and luxation injuries use a semirigid splint for a 2-week duration, whereas alveolar process fractures use rigid splinting for up to 6 weeks to allow bone healing.[1,9] Table 74.1 discusses the preferred management strategy for different types of injuries.

Limitations and Contraindications

The management of dentoalveolar fractures is time sensitive to achieve a successful outcome.[9,14] However, in the polytrauma

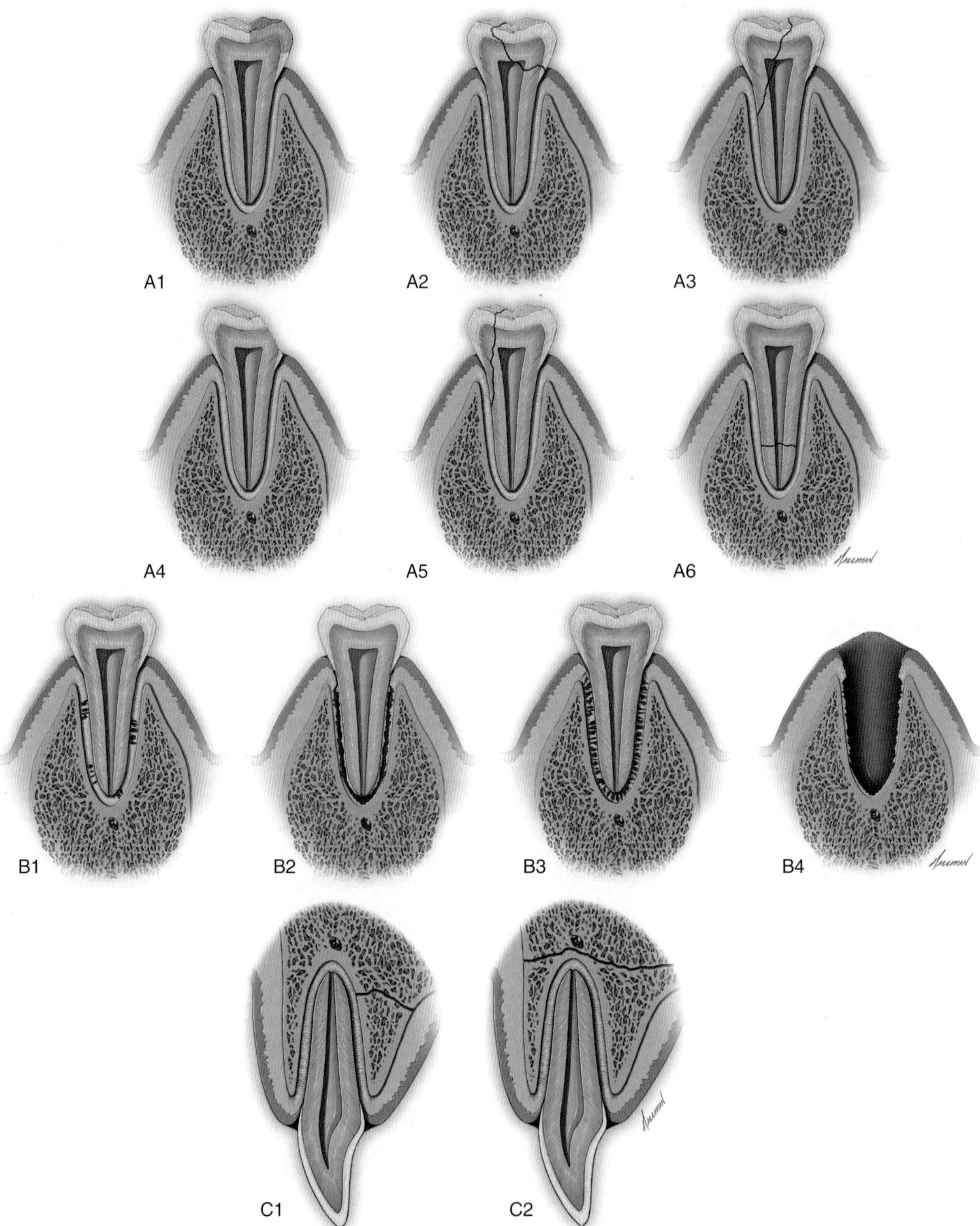

Figure 74.2 Andreasen classification of dental (A), periodontal (B), and alveolar injuries (C).

Table 74.1 Recommended Treatment for Dentoalveolar Injuries

Type of Injury/Indications	Recommended Treatment
Enamel fractures	Smoothen round edges; serial pulp testing
Uncomplicated crown fracture	Indirect pulp capping involving calcium hydroxide base, glass ionomer, dentin bonding agent, and composite cement
Complicated crown fracture (open apex)	Small pulpal exposures treated by direct pulp capping, larger exposures greater than 24 h treated by calcium hydroxide pulpotomy, followed by conventional root canal therapy at completion of root development
Complicated crown fracture (closed apex)	Small pulpal exposures treated by direct pulp capping; larger exposures greater than 24 h treated by conventional root canal therapy
Crown-root fracture	Most of these fractures will require extractions and socket preservation; however, conservative treatment in the form of orthodontic extrusions and crown lengthening can be used in select cases
Root fractures	Apical and middle third fractures if mobile needs rigid splint; cervical fractures poor prognosis, recommend extractions
Concussion	Relieve occlusion; soft diet
Subluxation	Similar to concussion; may need nonrigid splint if teeth mobile
Intrusion	Open apex: allow teeth to erupt; closed apex: reposition, stabilize, and treat root canal because of the high incidence of pulpal necrosis
Extrusion	Reposition, semirigid splint for 2–3 weeks, RCT prn
Lateral luxation	If coexisting alveolar process fractures, rigid splint for 2–8 weeks
Avulsions (<2 h)	Open apex: transport in Hank's balanced salt solution or milk, transfer to 1 mg/20 mL doxycycline bath, replant semirigid splint for 2 weeks; calcium hydroxide apexification if pathosis occurs Closed apex: same as above and endodontically treat at the time of splint removal
Avulsions (>2 h)	Same as above and surface treat with citric acid, 1% stannous fluoride, and endodontically treat at reimplantation
Alveolar fractures	Rigid splints for about a 6-week duration to achieve bony union

setting with multisystem injuries, the management of dental injuries is not a paramount concern. Delays in reduction and stabilization will likely lead to compromised vascularity. Arch bar fixation is contraindicated in subluxation injuries due to the inherent risk of extrusive force placed on the teeth during tightening of the interdental wire. In general, rigid or semirigid splints are contraindicated in cases of acute trauma, poor dental hygiene, compromised and grossly contaminated tissues, and other significant comorbidities.

TECHNIQUE: Closed Reduction of Dentoalveolar Fractures

Fractures of the alveolar process can involve one tooth or multiple teeth and can be associated with other facial fractures. Fractured bony segments usually occur in the incisor and premolar areas.

STEP 1: Preparation

Appropriate treatment of alveolar fractures requires, first, proper reduction and repositioning of segments and, second, adequate stabilization for 4 to 6 weeks to allow osseous healing.[15–17] At the time of stabilization, teeth that are considered nonsalvageable are usually retained because they help maintain space and help to reduce the fracture.

STEP 2: Manual Reduction

The closed technique reduction of dentoalveolar fractures entails using gentle pressure to reduce the fractured alveolus and dental segment back into the arch followed by splinting.

TECHNIQUE: Closed Reduction of Dentoalveolar Fractures—*cont'd*

STEP 3: Splinting

Splinting is accomplished with acid etch techniques that utilize a wire and composite material to splint the teeth or, alternatively, arch bars. Having the patient bite down on a tongue blade helps to reestablish the occlusion and may avoid postoperative occlusal adjustments.

STEP 4: Open Reduction

Open techniques are implemented when fractured segments are significantly displaced and cannot adequately be reduced via a closed technique. Hence, the open technique involves an incision for apical access and visualization of fractures to detect bony interferences. Subsequently, proper bony alignment and removal of bony interferences can then be facilitated. This is followed by stabilization with an application of a transosseous wire, arch bar, or a low-profile monocortical fixation plate.

SPECIAL CONSIDERATIONS

The splint should not be bulky or impinge on the gingiva to prevent caries or gingival disease, respectively. As such, the splint should also permit good oral hygiene and allow access for endodontic treatment.[14] Postoperatively, the patient must be placed on a soft diet during the healing process, and good oral hygiene must be maintained. Consideration for antibiotic coverage should be evaluated depending on the extent of the injury. Splinting can be achieved by acid etch, arch bars, or plating fixation if the fractures involve a large segment of bone.

COMPOSITE SPLINTING TECHNICAL CONSIDERATIONS

The acid etch technique requires restorative materials, adequate isolation of injury, and a dry environment for proper application of a composite/resin splint. Following thorough debridement and isolation of injury, the alveolar segment is reduced and the teeth are aligned. Digital pressure is used on the labial and lingual aspects initially to reduce the dentoalveolar segment, followed by having the patient bite down on a tongue blade to properly align the segment within the dental arch. Once the occlusion and alignment are reestablished, the resin splint can be applied to maintain the segment in position and allow for osseous healing. Soft tissue repair of the gingiva should precede the splinting of the teeth.

Fixation will require use of resin bonded to the teeth and paper clip or heavy (20-gauge) arch wire that will be attached to the resin. The splinting should be extended to at least two adjacent nondisplaced teeth on either side of the vertical fracture lines. The sequence entails cleansing of tooth surfaces, application of acid etch for 20 to 30 seconds, flushing the etch off the teeth, followed by drying of the tooth surface and application of a bonding agent, which is then light cured for 15 seconds. Next, the soft composite is applied to the selected teeth and the wire is attached onto the composite. Now the soft composite is light cured for 15 to 20 seconds to induce a photochemical reaction to convert the soft resin into a hard composite splint. The patient must bite down on the tongue blade to ensure that the occlusion is aligned; otherwise, prematurities in the occlusion will be encountered. A check for premature occlusal contacts is done, and high spots can be leveled with a dental bur. Additionally, the use of suction and cotton rolls to keep the area dry and isolated is key to achieving acceptable etching and bonding. Alveolar fractures can be typically fixated for 4 to 6 weeks and subsequently removed with a dental scaler or a dental bur (Fig. 74.3).

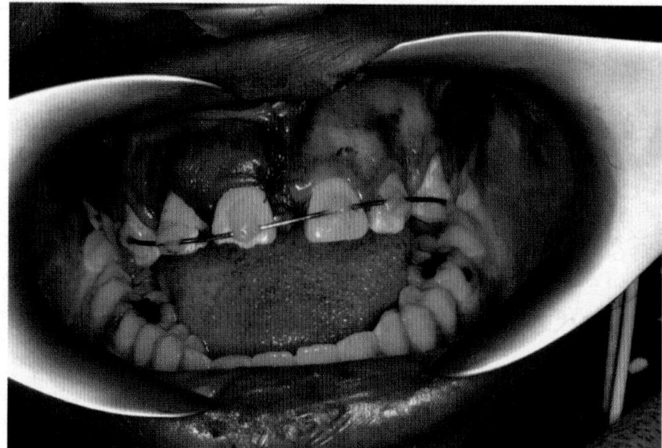

Figure 74.3 Acid etch composite splint technique for management of dentoalveolar injuries.

ALTERNATIVE TECHNIQUE 1: Erich Arch Bars

Dentoalveolar fractures can also be treated with the use of arch bars. Arch bars can reduce fractures in both the open and closed method of treatment modalities. They are often employed when dental equipment is not available or accessible (such as in the emergency room); dentoalveolar fracture accompanies other facial fractures with the need for intermaxillary fixation (IMF) or operator preference. With the closed technique, arch bars are fastened to the cervical portion of the dentition using 24-gauge wire that is twisted in a clockwise fashion after the fracture is reduced and aligned with digital pressure. They are usually placed across the entire arch but can also be used in shorter spans with the goal of achieving stability by tightening the wire, which is circumferentially placed around the cervical necks of the teeth, onto the arch bar to allow minimal mobility of the segment (Fig. 74.4).

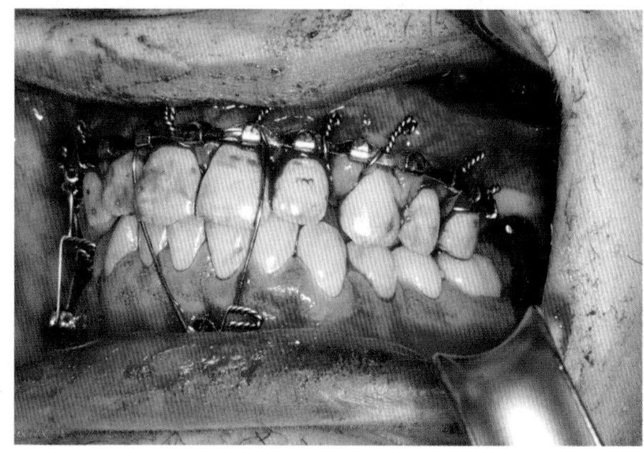

Figure 74.4 Reduction and arch bar fixation of posterior segmental maxillary alveolar fractures.

ALTERNATIVE TECHNIQUE 2: Plating/Fixation

The more extensive fractures often require open treatment and may need fixation with plates and screws in conjunction with arch bars or can employ arch bars independently. These techniques often are performed best in the operating room. The open technique allows access for visualization of the fracture and its reduction, especially when the closed method cannot reduce the fracture because of bony interferences. The fracture is exposed through either a marginal (envelope) incision or a vestibular incision and appropriate relaxation incisions in the vertical plane. After fracture segments are reduced, the patient is placed in IMF with either arch bars or IMF screws and 24-gauge wires to reestablish the habitual occlusion. Next, the fracture is plated with plates and screws. It is imperative to avoid tooth roots when drilling holes for screws. After fixation has been achieved, the patient is released from IMF and the occlusion is verified. The incisions are then closed (Fig. 74.5).

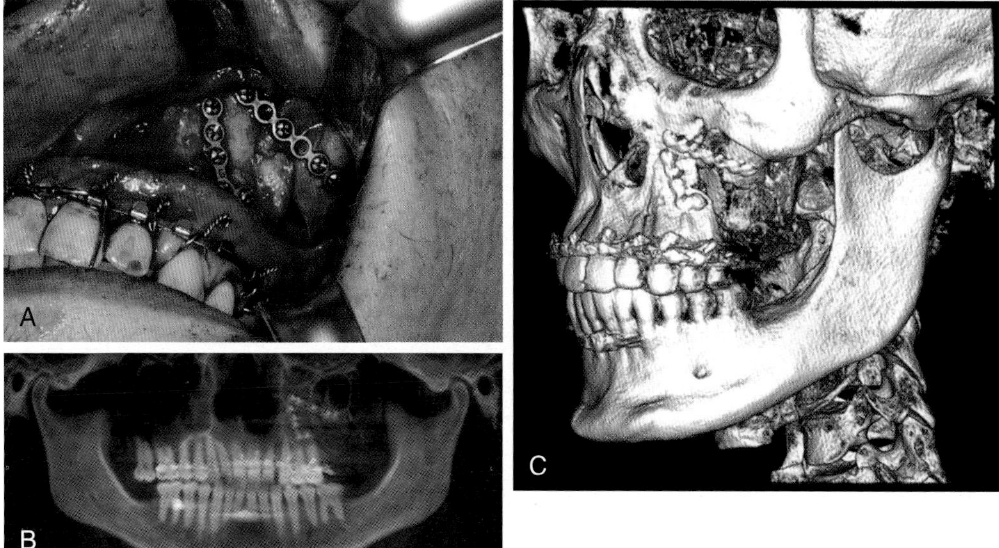

Figure 74.5 Comminuted alveolar and maxillary antral wall fractures managed by open reduction and internal fixation (A). Postoperative panoramic radiograph (B) and three-dimensional computed tomography reconstruction (C) showing good reduction and stable fixation of segments.

ALTERNATIVE TECHNIQUE 3: Bone Grafting and Dental Implant Restoration

When reconstructing the dentoalveolar complex for bony reconstruction with implants and/or dental prosthetics, adequate wound healing and revascularization of traumatized tissue are critical. As such, bone grafting and soft tissue grafting procedures should not be undertaken at the time of the initial trauma procedure. In cases requiring splinting of the dentoalveolar complex with composite splints or arch bars, adequate time has to be allotted for tissue healing. Bone structures that are fractured and subsequently stabilized require 6 weeks for initial bone healing. Bone healing involves primary phase that forms a callous and a secondary phase of ossification. Thereafter, bone continues to remodel every 6 weeks. The revascularization of the periosteum occurs due to new angiogenesis. Tissue injury leads to inflammation from the release of cytokines and secondarily a milieu of growth mediators initiates angiogenesis and differentiation of mesenchymal stem cells to form osteoblasts. Therefore, allowing for adequate healing time of the damage tissue is critical for its eventual reconstruction. A minimum of 12 weeks after the initial trauma stabilization is needed to reestablish vascularity for both soft and hard tissues. Early bone grafting to hard tissue injury usually leads to infection of the bone graft and subsequent failure due to tissue inability to vascularize the grafted tissue. If teeth are lost during the initial trauma, it is best to place bone morphogenic protein (BMP), or a collagen membrane in the sockets to form bone. Any combination of onlay block versus particulate grafting with or without scaffolding material will be needed to augment the lost bone volume in most situations. A fair amount of bone grafting can be performed in an acute setting during initial debridement as long as adequate soft tissue closure can be attained. In case of extensive trauma involving the basal maxillary or mandibular bone, it would be prudent to attain stable reduction and fixation of the fractured segments and delay bone grafting as a separate procedure (Fig. 74.6).

BMP may help with both soft and hard tissue healing but at the cost of robust swelling. Significant trauma such as

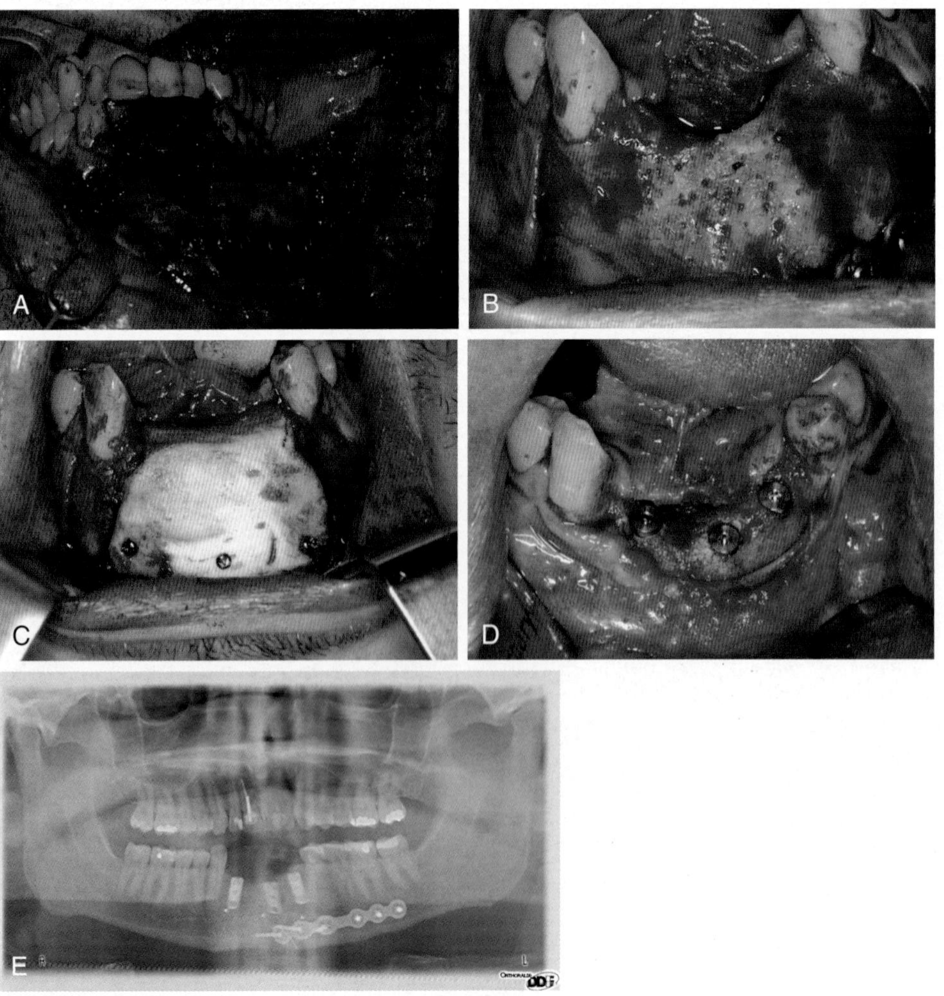

Figure 74.6 Extensive trauma with avulsion of dentoalveolar segments and mandible fracture treated by open reduction internal fixation (ORIF) of mandible (A). Site preparation and cancellous onlay grafting with scaffolding material fixation (B and C). Adequate volume of grafted bone allowing successful implant placement (D and E).

ALTERNATIVE TECHNIQUE 3: Bone Grafting and Dental Implant Restoration—*cont'd*

buccal wall fractures or continuity defects will require block bone grafting. Thus in the senior author's experience, it is best to bone graft after 12 weeks from the initial trauma surgery. This bone graft can vary due to the size of the defect, from socket preservation to block grafting utilizing BMP and human stem cells. Once bone grafting has been initiated at the second stage of dentoalveolar reconstruction, 6 months of healing time is necessary for subsequent placement of dental implants. This entails at least three cycles of bony remodeling after the initial 6-week healing phase. This enables the scaffolded/grafted bone to transform into native bone through consecutive resorption and remodeling modalities. Moreover, it is imperative to remember that grafted bone, if not loaded with implants, can start resorbing due to a lack of stimulation.

During temporizing the lost dentition with prosthetics after bone grafting, it is imperative to keep the temporary prosthetic from loading the soft and hard tissues. Loading the tissue can cause loss of the bone graft and traumatize the soft tissue by impairing the vascularity. This may lead to graft failure and wound dehiscence. Adequate follow-up and coordination with the restoring dental practitioner are paramount. Educating the patient on adhering to a full liquid and soft diet in the initial phases of healing is also of great importance.

Restoration of implants in the aesthetic zone can be challenging, requiring strict adherence to prosthodontics and periodontal principles. The patient's smile line, periodontal health, and medical issues are key components in the longevity and success of the reconstruction. Scarring, loss of attached tissue, and alteration of the vestibular depth are important considerations in soft tissue management. Consideration to soft tissue surgery with gingival grafting, connective tissue grafting, and vestibuloplasty can occur at the time of implant placement or in stages. Utilization of autogenous grafts or allogenic grafts depends on the size of defect and the practitioner's experience. Having 2 to 3 mm of attached tissue circumferentially around the implants is critical for optimum periodontal health and maintenance of the biological with. Space between the implants, space between implants and teeth, emergence profile of the implants, and height of crestal bone are key to the esthetic of restorations. Additionally, the height of the soft tissue spanning from the crestal bone to the contact point between the restorations is critical in forming the papilla. The use of preformed static surgical guides and computer-designed partial of fully guided static guides using computed tomography (CT) technology can ensure more predictable results especially in the esthetic zone. CT guided surgical navigation can also enhance the placement of dental implants with real-time data and predictability utilizing dynamic guides.

Avoidance and Management of Intraoperative Complications

Poor outcomes can be prevented by a thorough examination and an organized method for treating injuries. Radiographic imaging as an adjunct to a good examination will aid in diagnosing the extent of injury. Patient selection for such a procedure must take into consideration the degree of the injury and associated wounds, age of the patient, comorbid medical conditions, patient's ability to withstand the procedure, and other more serious injuries that, if present, may take precedence. For example, the condition of a small child who has been traumatized from her injuries with extensive alveolar fractures requiring splinting and closure of wounds will dictate treatment in a controlled environment such as an operating room. This is in contrast to an 18-year-old, suffering from a dentoalveolar fracture in the anterior maxilla after playing baseball, who can likely be treated with the application of a splint in the emergency room under a local anesthetic. The extent of resources available to the practitioner, such as splinting materials and dental equipment, a dental operatory, and an operating room, come into play when assessing whether or not one can adequately treat such injuries. Dentoalveolar fractures associated with mandible fractures and other facial injuries are usually best treated utilizing general anesthesia and a protected airway. This not only helps with patient immobility, need for site-specific isolation, adequate lighting, and other equipment, but the injuries can be treated efficiently and accurately in the operating room, thereby improving surgical outcomes. One cannot overemphasize the importance of an adequate examination, thorough exploration of wounds with debridement, proper splinting, and closure of wounds. Postoperative care is critical to evaluate healing and coordinate appropriate referral for dental prosthetic and endodontic needs.

Other complications that arise are usually due to improper reduction that can lead to malocclusion and mobility of the segments due to improper fixation. Improper reduction can be noted when the occlusion is not habitual and the alignment of the segment in the arch is poor. This will require repositioning and subsequent splinting. Smaller prematurities evident after stabilization can be adjusted with a dental bur. Poor alignment can lead to a malocclusion and may result in vascular compromise of the segment because it is now subject to trauma and mobility from the masticatory forces on the improper occlusion.

Postoperative Considerations

Due to the presence of splints or arch bars stabilizing the dentoalveolar segment, optimal oral hygiene is essential for a successful outcome. Meticulous tooth brushing, chlorhexidine mouth rinses, Proxabrushes, and other interdental aids are strongly recommended. This is especially important until the completion of gingival healing. Aftercare may include endodontic treatment of involved teeth that develop irreversible pulpitis or pulpal necrosis. During the follow-up visit, occlusion should be regularly checked as a sign of sufficient reduction and fixation.

Patients are encouraged to restrict themselves to a semisolid diet and avoid clenching and excessively overloading the previously traumatized alveolar segment for a period of 4 to 6 weeks postinjury. Further dental treatment may be required to restore tooth fractures, address tooth discolorations, and fabricate fixed prosthesis among others.

References

1. Miloro M. *Peterson's Principles of Oral and Maxillofacial Surgery*. Hamilton, ON: B C Decker Inc; 2004.
2. Andreasen JO, Andreasen FM, Skeie A, Hjørting-Hansen E, Schwartz O. Effect of treatment delay upon pulp and periodontal healing of traumatic dental injuries—a review article. *Dent Traumatol.* 2002;18(3):116–128.
3. Williams J. *Oral and Maxillofacial Surgery*. 2nd ed. London, UK: Churchill Livingstone; 1995.
4. Gassner R, Bösch R, Tuli T, Emshoff R. Prevalence of dental trauma in 6000 patients with facial injuries: implications for prevention. *Oral Surg Oral Med Oral Pathol Oral Radiol Endod.* 1999;87(1):27–33.
5. Berkowitz R, Ludwig S, Johnson R. Dental trauma in children and adolescents. *Clin Pediatr (Phila).* 1980;19(3):166–171.
6. Puelacher W, Toifl F, Röthler G, Waldhart E. [Sports-related maxillofacial trauma in young patients]. *Dtsch Stomatol.* 1991;41(11):418–419.
7. Moss SJ, Maccaro H. Examination, evaluation and behavior management following injury to primary incisors. *N Y State Dent J.* 1985;51(2):87–92.
8. Fonseca RM, Marciani RD, Carlson ER, Braun TW. *Fonseca's Oral and Maxillofacial Surgery*. 2nd ed. St. Louis, MO: Saunders Elsevier; 2009.
9. Andreasen JO. *Traumatic Injuries of Teeth*. 2nd ed. Philadelphia: W B Saunders co; 1981:19.
10. Judd PL. Paediatric dental trauma: a hospital survey. *Ont Dent.* 1985;62(6):19–20. 23.
11. Onetto JE, Flores MT, Garbarino ML. Dental trauma in children and adolescents in Valparaiso, Chile. *Endod Dent Traumatol.* 1994;10(5):223–227.
12. Bureau US. *National Child Abuse and Neglect Data System.* Summary of key findings from calendar year 2000. 2002.
13. Liew VP, Daly CG. Anterior dental trauma treated after-hours in Newcastle, Australia. *Community Dent Oral Epidemiol.* 1986;14(6):362–366.
14. Andreasen JO. *Essentials of Traumatic Injuries to Teeth*. 2nd ed. 2000:25.
15. Bernstein L, Keyes KS. Dental and alveolar fractures. *Otolaryngol Clin North Am.* 1972;5(2):273–281.
16. Kupfer SR. Fracture of the maxillary alveolus. *Oral Surg Oral Med Oral Pathol.* 1954;7(8):830–836.
17. Wagner WF, Neal DC, Alpert B. Morbidity associated with extraoral open reduction of mandibular fractures. *J Oral Surg.* 1979;37(2):97–100.

CHAPTER 75

Anterior Mandibular Fractures

Brian Bast and Stanley Yung-Chuan Liu

Armamentarium

#9 Periosteal elevator
#15 Scalpel blades
Antibacterial irrigant
Appropriate sutures
Elastic tape chin dressing
Erich arch bars, 24- and 26-gauge wire
Fixation device (plates, screws, lag screw)
Local anesthetic with vasoconstrictor
Minnesota retractor
Needle electrocautery
Obwegeser retractors (curved up and curved down)
Reduction forceps (screw retained)
Self-retaining cheek retractors

History of the Procedure

Until the 19th century, when new methods for internal and external fixation were introduced, treatment of mandibular fractures followed the original principles described by Hippocrates.[1] Hippocrates's method for treating fractures of the mandible by wiring the teeth and immobilizing the jaw with closed reduction remains timeless.[1,2] He addressed anterior mandibular fractures specifically in Chapter 34 of the voluminous *Hippocratic Collection*:

Anyone can treat separations of the symphysis at the chin. With the two ends of the bone forcefully separated, the protruding part is pushed inwards while the collapsed end is forced outwards … with completion of the reduction, the teeth are wired to each other … not only the two adjacent but several—using gold wire, or lacking that, linen thread until the bone has consolidated.

The next advance in the treatment of mandibular fractures came in the 19th century, when surgeons improved techniques for maxillomandibular fixation, especially in the design of various interocclusal splints, such as Hamilton's gutta-percha splint, Kingsley's apparatus, and the Gunning splint.[2] The predecessor to the current treatment plan of model surgery and arch bars is credited to London dentist Gurnell Hammond, a technique he devised in 1871. After realigning the displaced stone segments, a heavy iron wire was adapted to the teeth on the model. The bar was then subsequently wired to the patient's natural teeth.

With the development of osteosynthesis in modern traumatology, Bigelow described its first use for mandibular fractures in 1943. Michelet, Champy, and Lodde introduced miniplate osteosynthesis between 1973 and 1975. Of particular interest for anterior mandibular fractures is the lag screw technique, which was first published by Boateng in 1976, although it had been used by Brons and Boering since the early 1970s. As they described it, "When appropriate conditions are present, it is possible by lag screw osteosynthesis alone using two lag screws to achieve a functionally stable union of the lamellar fracture fragments by means of the interfragmentary pressure produced."[3] They did not specifically discuss the technique and results when used for anterior mandibular fractures. It was not until 1991 that Ellis and Ghali presented a series on lag screw technique specific to the anterior mandible and further championed its use for factures in this region, over plate osteosynthesis, as long as there was no comminution or bone loss in the fracture gap.[4]

Indications for the Use of the Procedure

Described in the AAOMS 2007 Parameters of Care, closed reduction is appropriate in cases of stable fractures, where adequate fixation is possible with maxillomandibular fixation, and where contraindications to open reduction are present. Additional indications for closed reduction may include atrophic edentulous mandibular fracture, loss of soft-tissue coverage over a fracture, and fractures in children. Closed reduction of fractures is most commonly achieved by applying Erich arch bars with circumdental soft stainless steel wires. Other closed reduction methods include Ivy loops, intermaxillary fixation bone screws, hybrid arch bars, and Gunning-type occlusal splints.[5]

For open reduction and internal fixation (ORIF), indications include unstable fracture, continuity defect, preference for early or immediate mobilization, injuries to associated soft or bony tissue, and need for vascular or neurologic exploration or repair.[6] In cases where there is delayed treatment with soft tissue in between the fracture, or malunion/nonunion of the fracture, ORIF is also recommended.[5] Semirigid internal fixation includes the use of miniplates, lag screw, or bicortical positioning screws. Rigid fixation includes the use of reconstruction plate (locking or nonlocking) and bicortical screws. With anterior mandible fractures, ORIF with lag screw fixation is uniquely favored due to the curvature of the anterior mandible, thickness of the bony cortices, and absence of anatomic hazards below apices of the teeth and between the mental foramina.[4]

The goals are the same for either treatment modality, which include the restoration of pretrauma occlusion, teeth, bone structure, and nerve function (motor and/or sensory).[6] There should also be the reestablishment of an adequate range of motion, facial and mandibular arch form, in the setting of pain-free function.[5]

Limitations and Contraindications

Although the type of fracture is the primary determinant of closed versus open treatment of anterior mandible fractures, certain patient and operative factors contribute to treatment planning. Open reduction is preferred in the care of noncompliant patients, patients who require early access to the oral cavity (ICU patients), patients with special nutritional needs (diabetic patients, alcoholic patients), and patients with seizure disorders.[7]

On the flip side, surgeons should be aware that HIV-infected patients have shown increased risk of postoperative infections especially after open treatment.[8] In comminuted fractures where residual mandibular fragments are associated with a tenuous blood supply, there is also support for closed reduction.[9] This is also a contraindication to the lag screw technique.[4]

In the era of managed care, cost-effectiveness also enters the consideration for choice of treatment. As an example, although closed reduction is cheaper, open reduction may yield better outcome in indigent populations for social reasons.[10] Nonetheless, outside of absolute contraindications to either open or closed treatment, it is the severity of the fracture and positive medical findings that contribute most to postoperative complications, after controlling for age, type of treatment, and time from injury to repair.[11]

TECHNIQUE: Open Reduction With Internal Fixation of Anterior Mandibular Fractures

STEP 1: Intubation

The preferred method is nasoendotracheal intubation with a nasal Ring-Adair-Elwyn (RAE) tube that exits superiorly across the forehead, allowing the tube to be secured to a head drape. The endotracheal tube is secured either with tape or with a nasal septal suture. Intermaxillary fixation is required to establish preinjury occlusion, and this makes oral intubation less desirable. If nasal intubation is not possible, submental intubation or tracheostomy should be considered.

STEP 2: Oral Prep

Once the airway has been secured, the patient is prepped and draped for surgery. The oral pharynx is suctioned and a throat pack is placed. Then, the oral cavity is cleansed with a chlorhexidine solution and suctioned. A local anesthetic with epinephrine then is injected. Dental extractions, if required, are completed at this point.

STEP 3: Maxillomandibular Fixation

Excellent treatment outcomes are critically dependent on accurate establishment of the preinjury occlusion maintained in firm maxillomandibular fixation. Many devices allow for the placement of maxillomandibular fixation. Intermaxillary fixation screws, Ivy loops, sharp free devices, and arch bar/screw hybrids all can be used to place a patient in maxillomandibular fixation. Erich arch bars secured with 24- and 26-gauge interdental wires are the gold standard to which all other methods should be compared. Arch bars allow for the initial reduction and stabilization of a fracture and provide a superior tension band across fracture segments. The arch bars hold the patient in the preinjury occlusion. Maxillomandibular fixation can be maintained with 26-gauge wire or heavy elastics.

STEP 4: Incision

The lower lip is everted and the area of planned incision is marked on the lip mucosa from canine to canine. The initial incision can be made with electrocautery or a scalpel, and it should be made through the lip mucosa only 1.5 to 2 cm from the mucogingival line. Gauze can be used to dissect submucosal tissue until the mentalis muscles are identified. Sharp dissection continues toward the mandible. A mucoperiosteal flap is developed to the inferior border of the mandible at the symphysis. Obwegeser curved-up retractors then can engage the inferior border and retract the soft tissue (Fig. 75.1A–C).

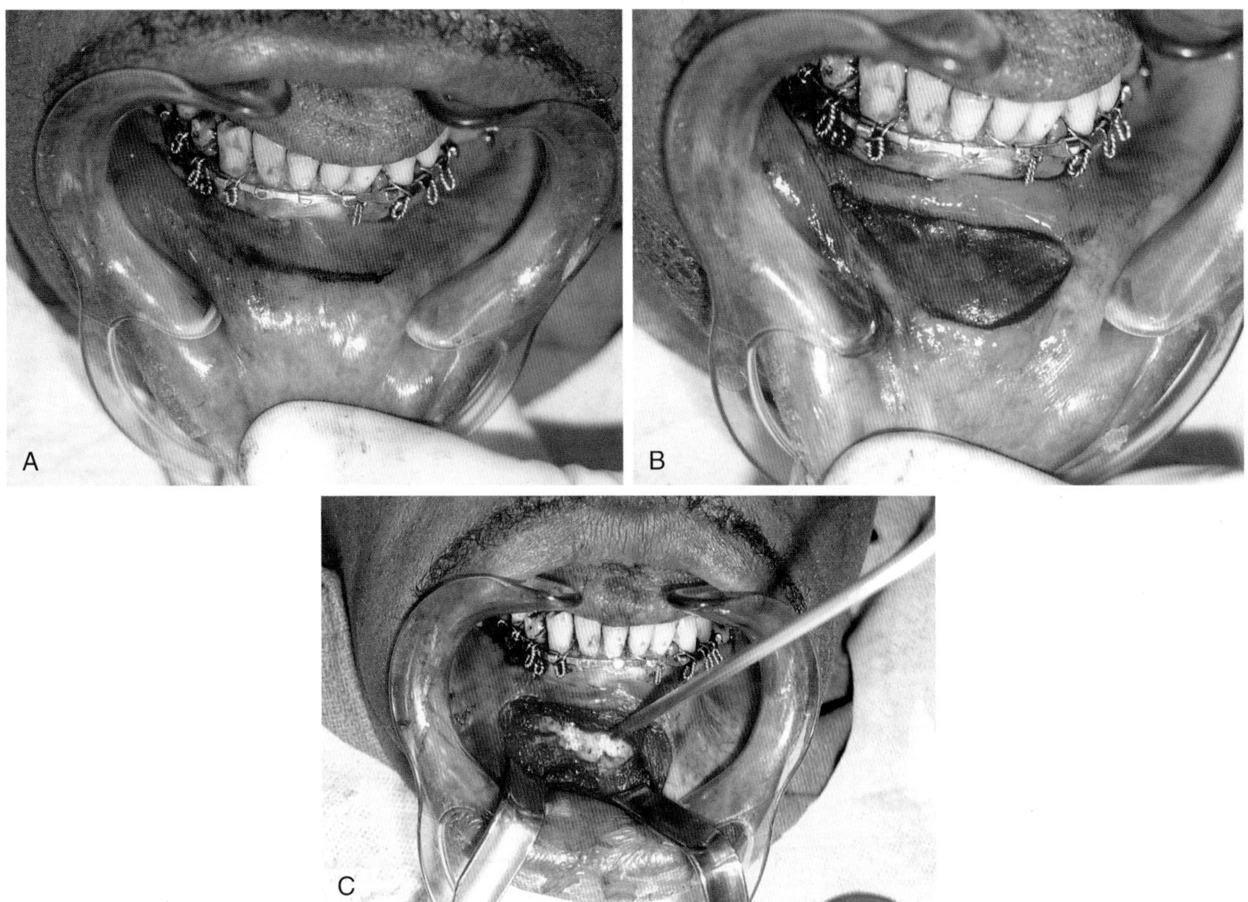

Figure 75.1 **A,** Planned initial lip incision. **B,** Submucosal dissection with exposure of mentalis muscle. **C,** Redirection of dissection with incision through muscle and periosteum.

TECHNIQUE: Open Reduction With Internal Fixation of Anterior Mandibular Fractures—cont'd

STEP 5: Identification of the Mental Foramen and Nerve

A #9 periosteal elevator is used to begin a subperiosteal dissection proximally just below the mucogingival junction. The soft tissue is elevated until the mental foramen and nerve are visualized. The mucosal incision then can be carried proximally above the foramen and nerve. The incision is carried proximally as needed to allow for exposure of the inferior border of the mandible. A scalpel or #9 periosteal elevator can be used to skeletonize the mental nerve. The nerve is skeletonized to relieve tension as the flap is reflected inferiorly. Adequate exposure allows access for placement of Obwegeser curved-up retractors at the inferior border both proximal and distal to the fracture (Fig. 75.1D–F).

STEP 6: Fracture Reduction

Fracture reduction is completed using reduction forceps. Parallel mandible reduction forceps are screw retained and allow for multiplane manipulation and reduction of the fracture (Fig. 75.1G).

Continued

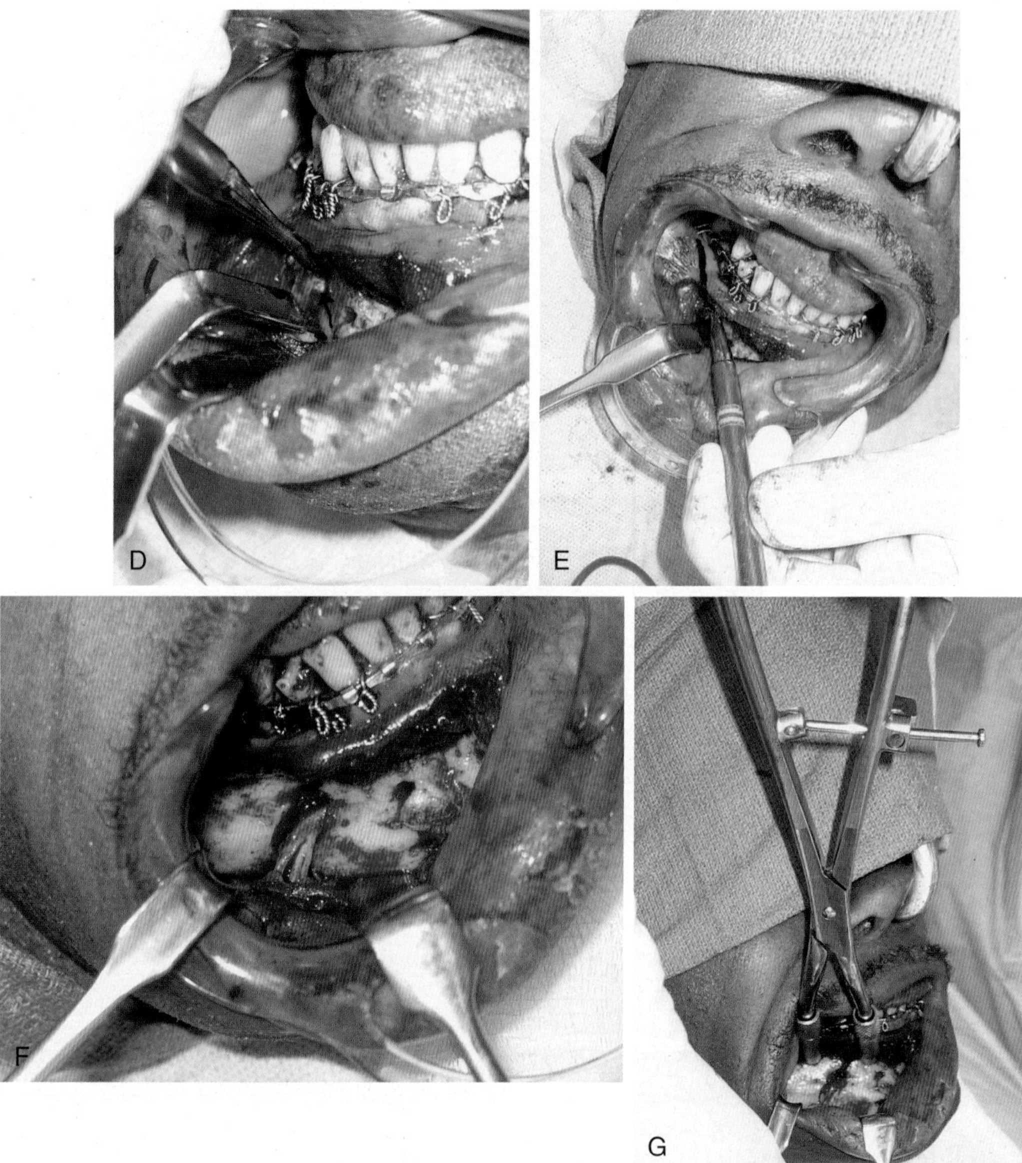

Figure 75.1 cont'd **D,** Exposure of mental foramen and nerve *(arrow)*. **E,** Planned incision above mental nerve. **F,** A scalpel or #9 periosteal elevator can be used to skeletonize the mental nerve. **G,** Fracture reduced with parallel mandible reduction forceps.

TECHNIQUE: Open Reduction with Internal Fixation of Anterior Mandibular Fractures—cont'd

STEP 7: Fracture Fixation

A fixation plate is selected that will ensure rigid fixation of the fracture. A 2.0 or 2.3 mandibular fracture plate with adequate length for three screw holes on both sides of the fracture provides rigid fixation. A malleable template of the selected plate can be used to capture the contour of the mandible. The bone plate should be positioned at the inferior border of the mandible below the level of the mental foramen. The template is used as a guide to bend the fixation plate. The fixation plate should rest passively when positioned on the mandible. When the contour and positioning of the plate have been confirmed, the plate is secured to the mandible with bicortical screws. Once the plate has been secured with three screws on both sides of the fracture, the reduction forceps is removed. The patient then should be taken out of maxillomandibular fixation to confirm the occlusion. If the occlusion is correct, the jaw is again immobilized and the wound is washed out with antibiotic-infused irrigation (Fig. 75.1H).

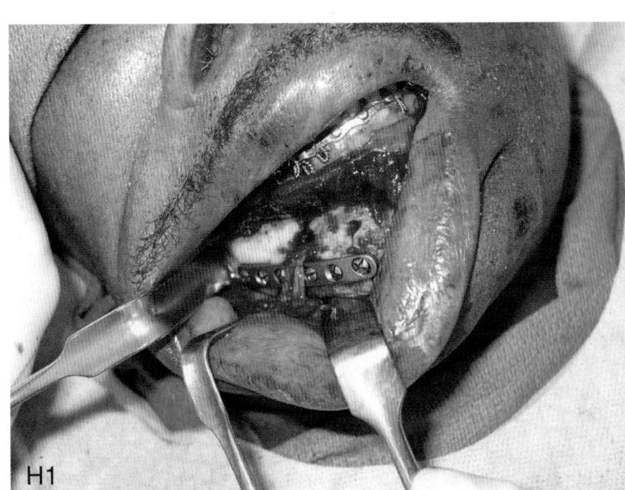

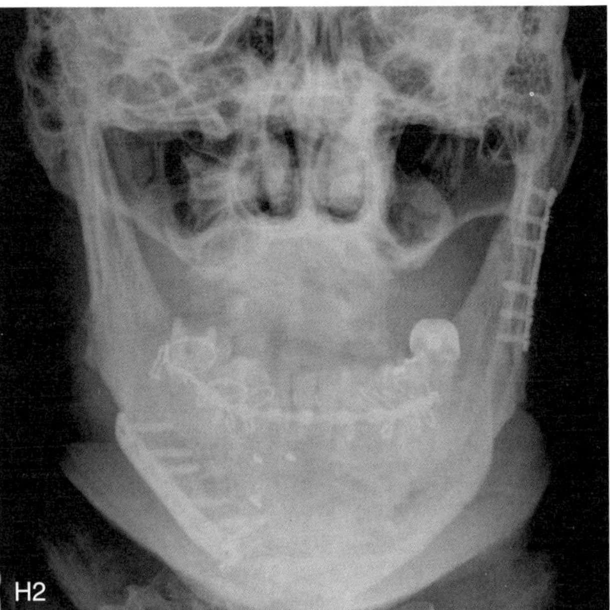

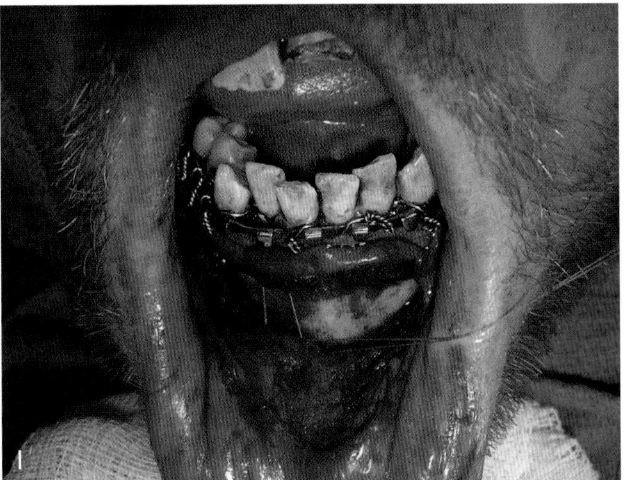

Figure 75.1 cont'd **H1,** Mandibular fracture plate secured with three bicortical screws on either side of the fracture. **H2,** Postoperative radiograph showing mandibular fracture plate at inferior border of the mandible. **I,** Resuspension of mentalis muscle using 3-0 horizontal mattress suture.

TECHNIQUE: Open Reduction with Internal Fixation of Anterior Mandibular Fractures—cont'd

STEP 8 : Wound Closure

Closure begins with resuspension of the mentalis muscles. The cut edges of the mentalis muscle are identified and reapproximated using 3-0 polyglactin sutures in a horizontal mattress fashion. A fibrous band of tissue between the two mentalis muscles can be reapproximated in a similar manner and provides additional support for the soft-tissue closure. The mucosa then can be sutured with 3-0 or 4-0 polyglactin suture in a running or running locking fashion. The patient is taken out of maxillomandibular fixation, the oral cavity is suctioned, and the throat pack is removed. An orogastric tube can be passed and the gastric contents evacuated. The patient is placed back in maxillomandibular fixation (MMF) using heavy elastics. An elastic chin dressing is applied and should remain in place for 1 week (Fig. 75.1I).

ALTERNATIVE TECHNIQUE: Lag Screw Fixation of Anterior Mandibular Fractures

The lag screw technique is a rigid form of fixation of anterior mandibular fractures that provides compression of fracture segments. With this technique, a large hole is created in the near plate of bone, and a smaller hole is created in the far plate of bone such that a screw passed through these two holes engages only the far cortex of bone. As the screw is tightened, it produces compression between the two segments of bone. Fractures of the anterior mandible are particularly suited for the lag screw technique for several reasons: the curvature of the mandible in this region allows for placement of lag screws perpendicular to the fracture line; the thickness of the cortical bone provides adequate strength for compression with tightening of the screws; and the lack of vital structures in this region ensures the safety of this technique. The forces that will act across fractures in the anterior mandible do require consideration. Mandibular function involves both shearing and torsional forces. Any form of fixation must be capable of resisting these forces to allow immobilization of the fracture segments. A single lag screw may still allow for torsional or twisting forces to produce rotation of the fracture segments. It is recommended that two lag screws be used to rigidly fixate fractures in this location.

Surgical access and fracture reduction are the same as for the ORIF technique, described previously. The lag screw armamentarium should be a component of any mandibular fracture fixation set (Fig. 75.2A). The lag screw set consists of a calibrated drill guide sleeve that can hold both 1.8-mm and 2.4-mm drill guides. Most sets have a gauge that attaches to the sleeve, allowing for an estimate of the exit point for the 1.8-mm drill bit. This allows the surgeon to hold the drill guide at the entry site of the near cortex and see an estimate of the exit point of the drill bit at the far cortex (Fig. 75.2B). The first lag screw to be placed is nearest the inferior border. The path of the screw should be perpendicular to the fracture line. First, a 2.4-mm bur is used to drill through the near cortex, aiming at the desired exit point on the far segment.

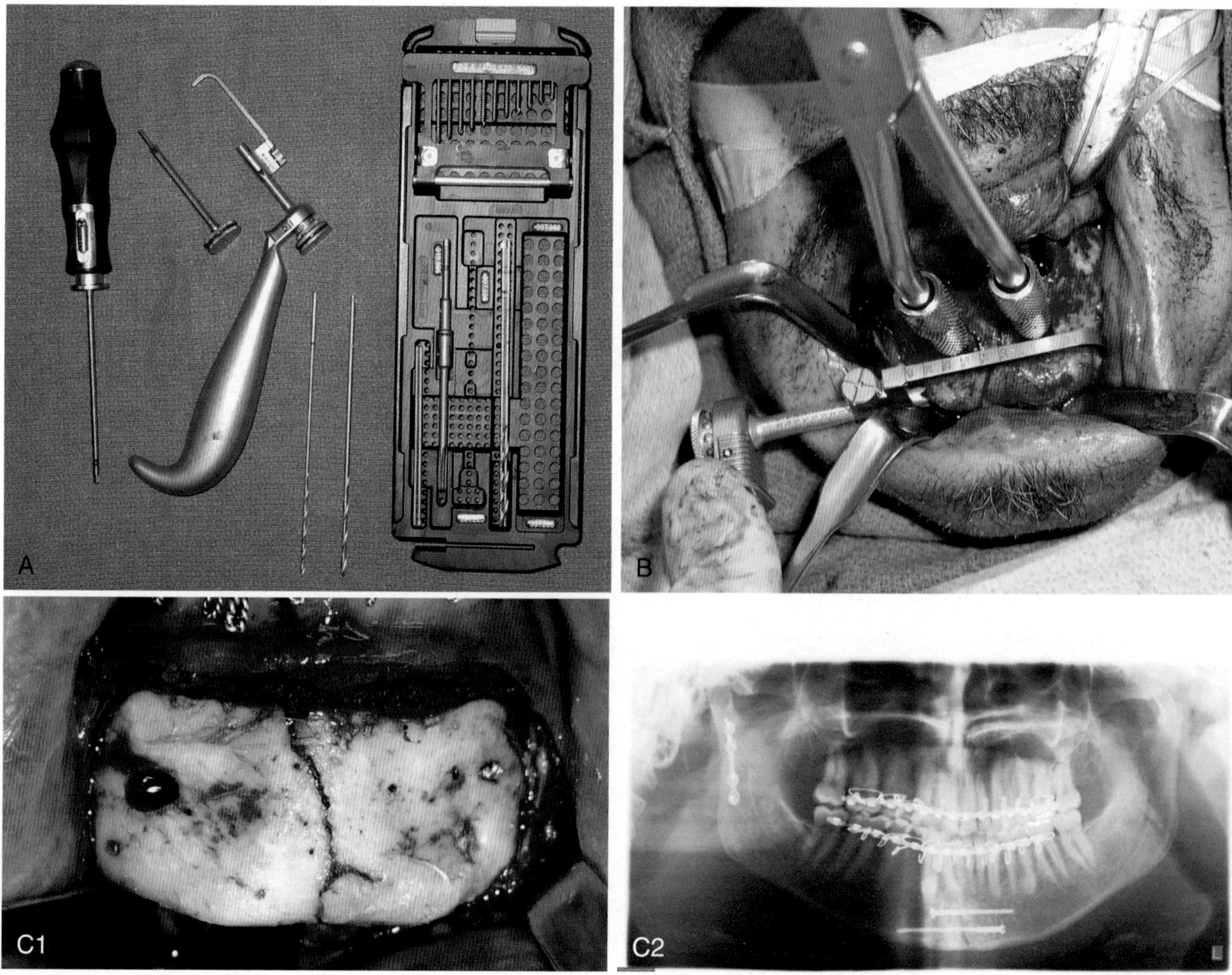

Figure 75.2 **A,** Lag screw armamentarium. **B,** Lag screw placement showing drill guide and position gauge. **C1,** Two lag screws in place in the anterior mandible. **C2,** Postoperative radiograph showing two lag screws in the anterior mandible.

The 2.4-mm drill goes only through the cortex of the near segment and continues to the fracture. Next, the 2.4-mm drill guide is removed, and a 1.8-mm drill guide is inserted into the sleeve. The tip of the 1.8-mm drill guide fits in the 2.4-mm drill hole. The 1.8-mm drill bit is used to continue this drill hole through the fracture and through the cortex of the far segment. Next, a countersink is used to create space in the near cortex for the screw head. Next, a depth gauge is used to measure the length of the screw hole and the correct length screw is inserted and tightened (Fig. 75.2C). Once the first lag screw has been firmly tightened, the reduction forceps are removed and the site for the second lag screw is selected. The second lag screw is positioned above and parallel to the first, below the dentition. Once the second lag screw is in place, the patient is taken out of MMF to confirm the occlusion. If the occlusion is accurate, the wound is irrigated and closed.

Avoidance and Management of Intraoperative Complications

Three common intraoperative complications can easily be avoided: inadequate maxillomandibular fixation, nerve injury, and immediate postfixation malocclusion.

MMF with tight control of the occlusion can easily be achieved with arch bars. Other forms of MMF may not provide tight control of the occlusion. This may not be recognized until attempts are made at fracture reduction and fixation.

Injury to the inferior alveolar nerve as it exits the mental foramen can occur during surgical exposure of the fracture or during retraction of the initial incision to expose the inferior border of the mandible. Limiting the initial incision to the lip mucosa between the mandibular canine teeth allows for careful reflection of the mucoperiosteal flap. In this way, the mental nerve and foramen can be identified and the incision safely carried posteriorly as needed. Once identified, the mental nerve can be skeletonized to relieve tension as the flap is retracted inferiorly to expose the inferior border of the mandible.

Rigid fixation plates must rest passively against the inferior border of the mandible. Rigid plates that do not correctly adapt to the mandible pull the bone toward the plate when bicortical screws are applied; this results in an immediate mandibular asymmetry and malocclusion. This problem can be avoided with careful adaptation of the fixation plate to the bony contour of the mandible.

Postoperative Considerations

Major postoperative complications for anterior mandibular fracture repair typically include infection, osteomyelitis, nonunion, malunion, delayed union, mental nerve paresthesia, and uniquely the "witch's chin deformity" consisting of ptosis of premental soft tissue with an accentuated submental crease.[12]

Besides proper surgical techniques as outlined in this chapter, prevention of infection and malunion should also take into consideration the social history of the patient. There is a significant correlation between illicit drug use and alcohol consumption with the development of postoperative complications.[12] In our level I trauma center with a high incidence of intravenous drug use and alcohol dependence, patients are placed on a 7- to 10-day course of antibiotics after surgery.

Follow-up is scheduled at a weekly basis after either open or closed reduction. MMF with elastics is maintained for 2 weeks postoperatively after ORIF, during which patients follow a full liquid diet. Sometimes volitional, patients return to clinic having removed the elastics, which may lengthen the period of MMF. Otherwise, patients are advanced to a mechanical soft diet with guiding elastics by week 3. By week 4, elastics are removed, but arch bars are maintained in place for one more week. There is usually significant gingival inflammation by the time arch bars are removed, and thus patients are strongly encouraged to receive dental cleaning.

Paresthesia of the mental nerve distribution is a common sequela of injury, although transient paresthesia can also result from open reduction procedures. Patients are appropriately counseled before surgery for the possibility of prolonged paresthesia. Directional sense is documented during weekly postoperative visits for signs of return to nerve function.

Prevention of the chin droop begins with the proper resuspension of the mentalis muscle to its appropriate high point as outlined earlier. The paired muscles of the mentalis consist of two parts: a horizontal upper part that originates below the attached gingiva and stabilizes the lip position; and an oblique part that elevates central lip, allowing pouting and tight labial competence. Resuspension to elevate the lip requires reinsertion of the upper muscles to just below the attached gingiva.[13] External chin dressing using Elastoplast is also applied postoperatively to assist in the prevention of iatrogenic chin ptosis.

References

1. Gahhos F, Ariyan S. Facial fractures: hippocratic management. *Head Neck Surg.* 1984;6(6):1007–1013.
2. Mukerji R, Mukerji G, McGurk M. Mandibular fractures: historical perspective. *Br J Oral Maxillofac Surg.* 2006;44(3):222–228.
3. Niederdellmann H, Schilli W, Düker J, Akuamoa-Boateng E. Osteosynthesis of mandibular fractures using lag screws. *Int J Oral Surg.* 1976;5(3):117–121.
4. Ellis III E, Ghali GE. Lag screw fixation of anterior mandibular fractures. *J Oral Maxillofac Surg.* 1991;49(1):13–21.
5. Chung W, Costello BJ. *Oral and Maxillofacial Surgery.* Hoboken, NJ: Wiley-Blackwell; 2010.
6. AAOMS Parameters of care. *J Oral Maxillofac Surg.* 2007;Version 4.0.
7. Dodson TB, Perrott DH, Kaban LB, Gordon NC. Fixation of mandibular fractures: a comparative analysis of rigid internal fixation and standard fixation techniques. *J Oral Maxillofac Surg.* 1990;48(4):362–366.
8. Schmidt B, Kearns G, Perrott D, Kaban LB. Infection following treatment of mandibular fractures in human immunodeficiency virus seropositive patients. *J Oral Maxillofac Surg.* 1995;53(10):1134–1139.
9. Ellis III E, Muniz O, Anand K. Treatment considerations for comminuted mandibular fractures. *J Oral Maxillofac Surg.* 2003;61(8):861–870.

10. Schmidt BL, Kearns G, Gordon N, Kaban LB. A financial analysis of maxillomandibular fixation versus rigid internal fixation for treatment of mandibular fractures. *J Oral Maxillofac Surg*. 2000;58(11):1206–1210.
11. Gordon PE, Lawler ME, Kaban LB, Dodson TB. Mandibular fracture severity and patient health status are associated with postoperative inflammatory complications. *J Oral Maxillofac Surg*. 2011;69(8):2191–2197.
12. Serena-Gómez E, Passeri LA. Complications of mandible fractures related to substance abuse. *J Oral Maxillofac Surg*. 2008;66(10):2028–2034.
13. Garfein ES, Zide BM. Chin ptosis: classification, anatomy, and correction. *Craniomaxillofac Trauma Reconstr*. 2008;1(1):1–14.

CHAPTER 76

Mandibular Body Fractures

Mark Stevens and Hany Emam

Armamentarium

#9 Periosteal elevator
#15 Scalpel blades
#701 Fissure bur
Ace bandage
Arch bars and 24- and 26-gauge wires
Antibiotic ointment
Army-Navy retractors
Bone clamps
Bone wax
Chromic gut suture 3-0
Dental extraction set
Dingman forceps
Hemostats (mosquito, tonsils, Kelly)
Kerlix gauze
Local anesthesia with vasoconstrictor
Malleable retractors
Mastisol
Mandible fixation trauma set
Metzenbaum scissor
Needle holders
Nerve stimulator
Needle electrocautery (Bovie)
Obwegeser retractors
Pickle fork
Proline suture 5-0
Seldin
Senn retractors
Silk ties 2-0, 3-0
Steri-Strips
Vicryl suture 3-0, 4-0
Wire cutters
Wire drivers

History of the Procedure

The earliest description of mandibular fracture was found in the Egyptian literature. The first described case was in 1650 BC and discussed the examination, diagnosis, and treatment of mandibular fractures.

Hippocrates was the first to describe reapproximation and immobilization through the use of circum-dental wires and external bandaging to immobilize the fracture. The importance of establishing proper occlusion first was described in a textbook written in Salerno, Italy, in 1180. Maxillomandibular fixation (MMF) first was mentioned in 1492, in an edition of the book *Cyrugia* printed in Lyons. Chopart and Desault used dental prosthetic devices to immobilize the fracture segments. Guglielmo Salicetti first accomplished the use of intermaxillary fixation. Orthodontic bands and arches were used for establishing the fixation. However, Glimer reformed the treatment of fractures when he fixed full arch bars on both the mandible and maxilla.[1]

Gordon Buck in the United States is credited with being the first to place an interosseous wire in mandibular fractures in 1847, just after the introduction of ether anesthesia.[2] The use of wire internal fixation in mandibular fractures was always supplemented with MMF. To overcome the lack of stability at the fracture site, the development of a more rigid hardware and technique evolved.

The use of external pin fixation became popular during the Second World War with compound, comminuted, and infected fractures. The major advantage of external fixation is that it did not require extensive dissection and stripping of soft tissues. A diminished role for external devices does not preclude the usefulness of these devices and the need of surgeons to be familiar with their placement. External pin fixation for maxillofacial applications has become synonymous with the term "the Joe Hall Morris appliance." The Joe Hall Morris appliance consisted of external pins with an acrylic bar apparatus used for closed reduction of mandibular fractures.[3]

Bone plates were originally introduced to maxillofacial surgery by Christiansen in 1945. He used tantalum plates to provide interfragmentary stability in mandibular fractures. The technique of rigid internal fixation was advanced and popularized by the Arbeitsgemeinshcft fur osteosynthesefragen/Association of the Study of Internal Fixation in Europe in 1970. Champy et al. (1978) developed the concept of adaptive osteosynthesis. He advocated transoral placement of small, thin, malleable miniplates with mono-cortical screws along the ideal lines of osteosynthesis in the mandible (Fig. 76.1). The locations of bone plate fixation should provide the most stable means of fixation. Arch bars or a plate placed along the superior border of the mandible provides the ideal position to resist tension forces in body fractures. The presence of teeth require this plate be mono-cortical. Additional fixation is still required to achieve the appropriate stability. Functional stable fixations with miniplate fixation remain controversial.[4] Large load-bearing plates are advocated in the treatment of mandibular fractures, especially in comminuted, continuity defects and/or infected fractures.

Locking Versus Nonlocking Plates

Locking plate/screw systems offer several advantages over the conventional one (Fig. 76.2):

1. Conventional plate/screw systems require precise adaptation of the plate to the underlying bone. The fixation screws "lock" to the plate, stabilizing the fracture segments without alteration of the reduction.
2. Theoretically they may also prevent disruption of the underlying cortical bone perfusion.
3. Screws inadvertently inserted into a fracture gap will not loosen since they are locked into the plate.

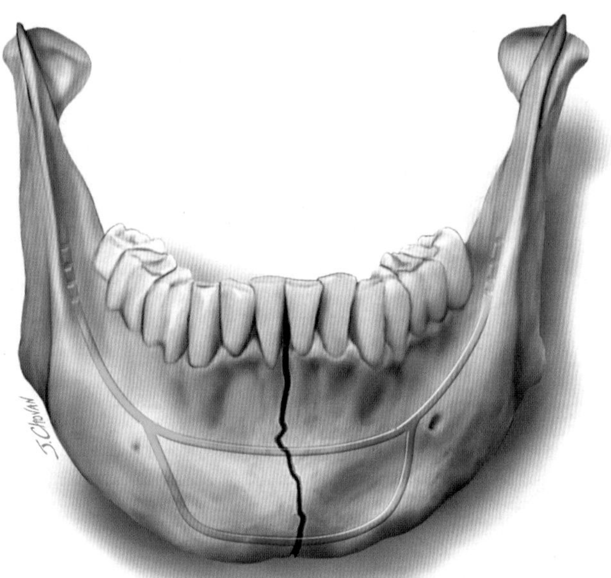

Figure 76.1 Ideal lines of osteosynthesis.

Mandibular Body Fracture

Definition

Body fractures occur between the distal aspect of the canines and a hypothetical line corresponding to the anterior attachment of the masseter muscle, corresponding to the distal aspect of the second molar.

Incidence

The mandible is involved in 70% of patients with facial fractures. The literature suggests the following mean frequency percentages based on location: body (29%), condyle (26%), angle (25%), symphysis (17%), ramus (4%), and coronoid process (1%).[5]

Biomechanics

Upon loading, the mandible exhibits the greatest tensile forces across the superior border and compression at the inferior border. The neutral zone lies approximately at the level of the inferior alveolar canal (Fig. 76.3).

Principles of Treatment

The principles of treating mandibular body fractures are the same as those for treating fractures in other parts of the body: reduction, fixation, and stabilization of the fractured segments to permit bone healing. Fractures of the mandible are treated by two major techniques: either closed or open reduction and fixation methods.[6]

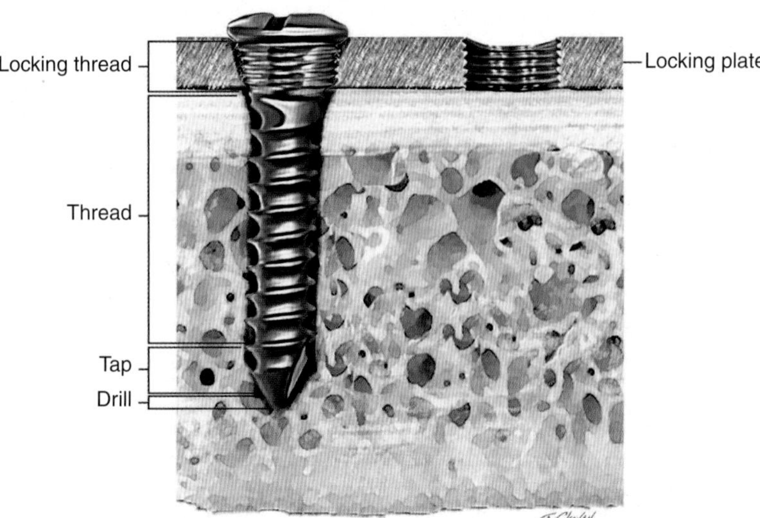

Figure 76.2 One type of locking screw mechanism.

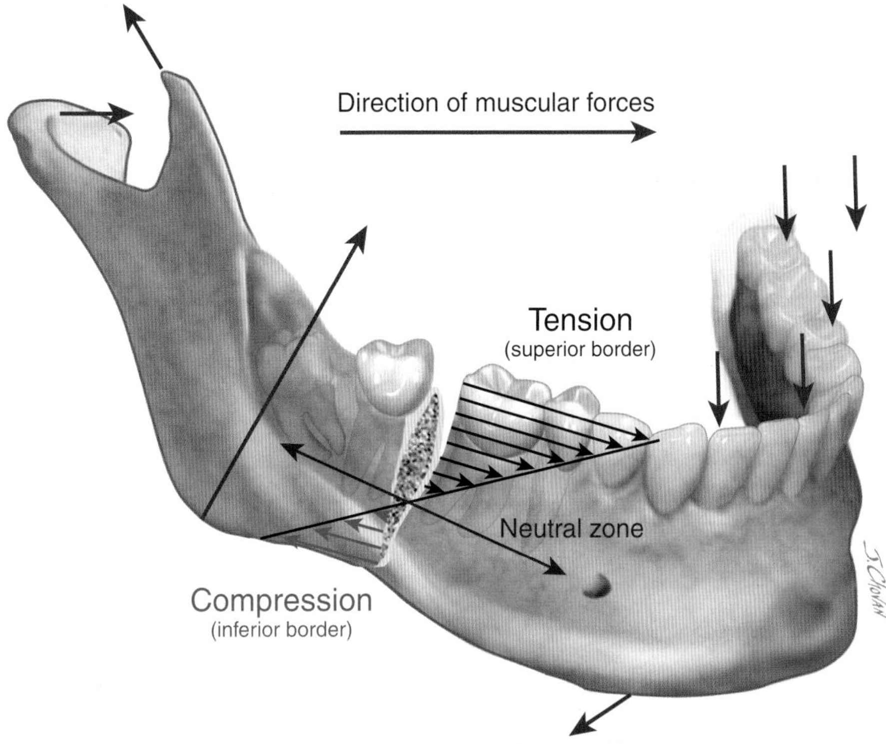

Figure 76.3 Biomechanics of the mandible.

TECHNIQUES

I Closed Reduction

INDICATIONS

1. Nondisplaced, favorable fracture
2. Grossly comminuted fracture
3. Fractures in children with developing dentition
4. Edentulous fractures (using a mandibular prosthesis)

Closed reduction is based on the idea that proper occlusion can act as a guide for reduction by using the intact maxilla as a fixed base (handle) to which the mandible is placed in a proper relationship (Figs. 76.4 and 76.5). Closed reduction techniques include the following:

1. Eyelet technique (Ivy loop-Robert H. Ivy 1881–1974)
2. Continuous loop (R.A. Stout 1892–1972)
3. Single double wire (Charles J. Essig 1841–1901)
4. Wire button (Varaztad Hovhanenes Kazanjian 1879–1974)
5. Twisted labial wire (E. Fulton Risdon 1880–1968)

I Open Reduction/Internal Fixation

INDICATIONS

1. Displaced, unfavorable fracture
2. Multiple facial fractures
3. Malunion
4. Special systemic condition contraindicating intramaxillary fixation as in seizures, psychiatric/neurologic problems, pulmonary disease, and gastrointestinal disorders
5. Delayed treatment with soft tissue interposition

TECHNIQUE: Extraoral Approach

STEP 1:

The skin incision is made 2 cm below the inferior border of the mandible within a relaxed skin tension line. The incision is carried down through the subcutaneous tissue to the level of the platysma muscle. Please note that the skin is undermined in a supraplatysmal plane in all directions to facilitate closure. Undermining also allows for movement of the access anteriorly or posteriorly increasing the exposure without the need to lengthen the skin incision (Fig. 76.6).

STEP 2:

Dissection and undermining of the platysma muscle is performed using a hemostat (Metzenbaum scissor can be used). Division of the muscle can be performed using a #15 blade or needle-tip Bovie as shown (Fig. 76.7).

Fig. 76.8 shows the superficial layer of the deep cervical fascia after the platysma muscle is sharply divided. The submandibular salivary gland and overlying capsule is visualized.

Continued

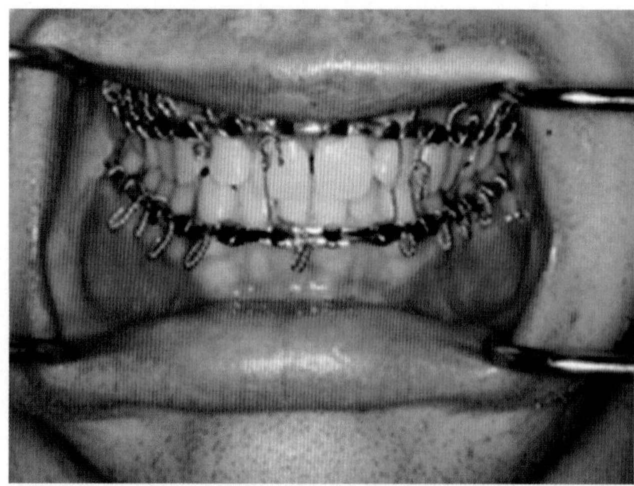

Figure 76.4 Photograph showing arch bars and intermaxillary fixation wires securing the occlusion.

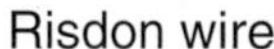

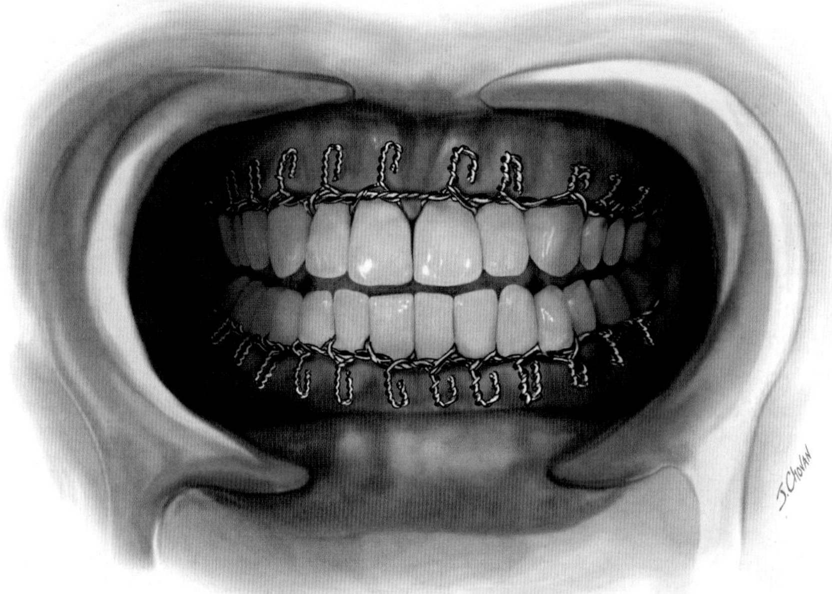

Figure 76.5 Risdon wire.

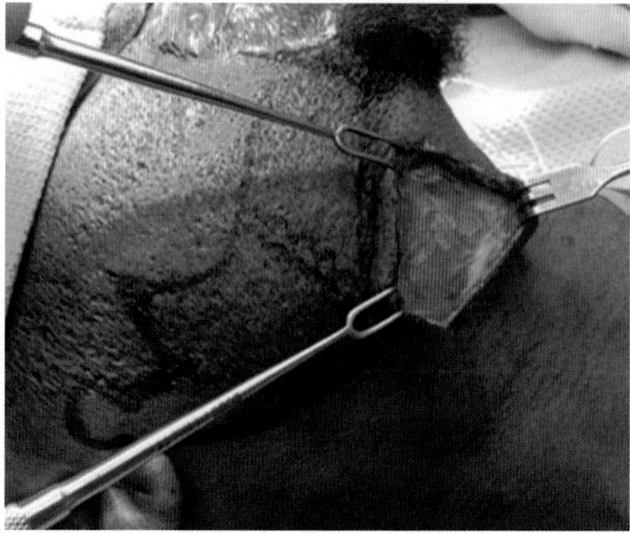

Figure 76.6 Dissection and undermining of the platysma muscle.

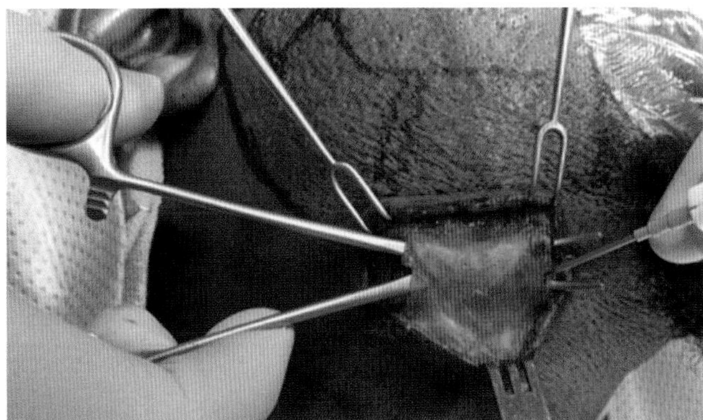
Figure 76.7 Division of the muscle.

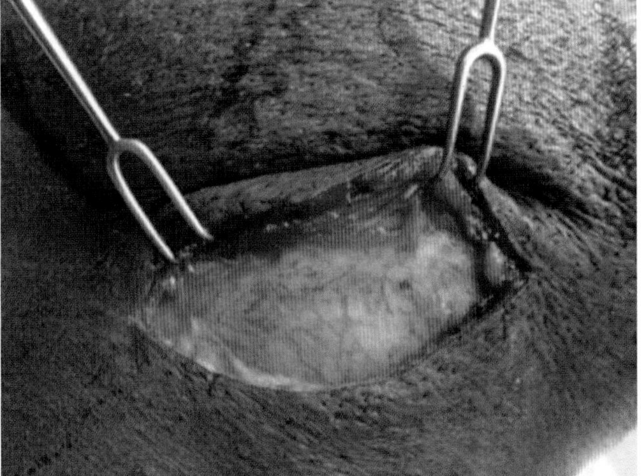
Figure 76.8 Visualization of the submandibular salivary gland and overlying capsule.

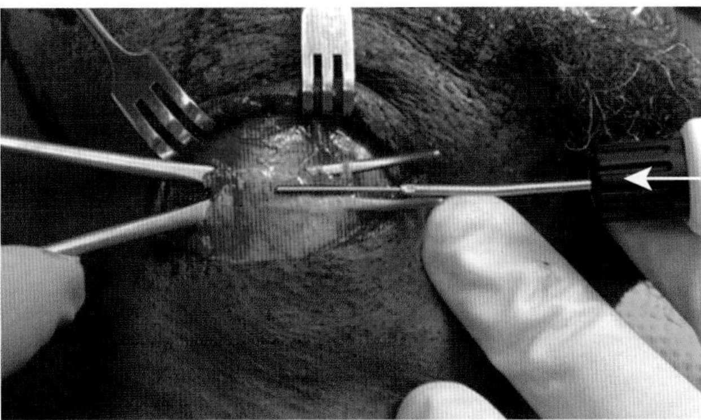
Figure 76.9 Superficial layer of the deep cervical fossa (SLDCR) is elevated.

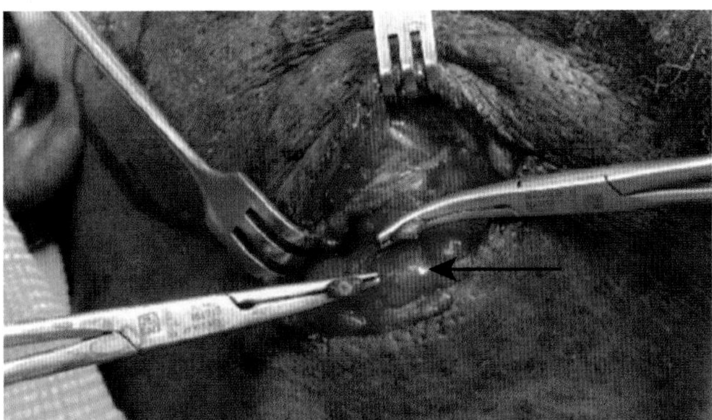
Figure 76.10 A bone compression clamp *(arrow)* is used to align and compress the fracture in place for anatomic reduction when possible.

EXTRAORAL APPROACH—*cont'd*

STEP 3:

Photo demonstrates the elevation of the superficial layer of the deep cervical fascia (SLDCF). The marginal mandibular branch of the facial nerve and facial vessels (artery and vein) are encountered when approaching the area of the premasseteric notch of the mandible. Use a nerve stimulator (arrow) to check the presence and avoid injury of the marginal mandibular branch of the facial nerve that can be within or just deep to the SLDCF. The level of the incision should be maintained near the lower third of the submandibular gland (Fig. 76.9).

Fig. 76.10 shows clamping and division of the facial artery to be ligated (2-0 silk ties are used for ligation). A submandibular lymph node (node of Stahr) is usually encountered; its presence alerts the surgeon to the facial artery just anterior to the node.

STEP 4:

Dissection is carried superiorly at the level between the inferior border of the mandible and the submandibular salivary gland reaching the periosteum of the mandible (anterior to the premasseteric notch) or the pterygomasseteric sling (posterior to the pterygomasseteric notch). Simultaneous retraction of the dissected tissues including the marginal branch superiorly in combination with inferior retraction of the submandibular gland with a malleable retractor allows for good visualization of the inferior border (Fig. 76.11).

STEP 5:

The pterygomasseteric sling/periosteum is sharply incised at the midinferior border, which is the most avascular portion of the sling. Incision can be done using scalpel blade or Bovie electrocautery (Fig. 76.12).

A sharp muco-periosteal elevator (#9) is then used to reflect the periosteum at the inferior border of the mandible. Stripping both the masseter laterally and medial pterygoid muscles medially is accomplished to expose the fracture site. Bovie cautery can aid in the severance of the tendinous muscle attachment to the bone (Figs. 76.13 and 76.14).

Continued

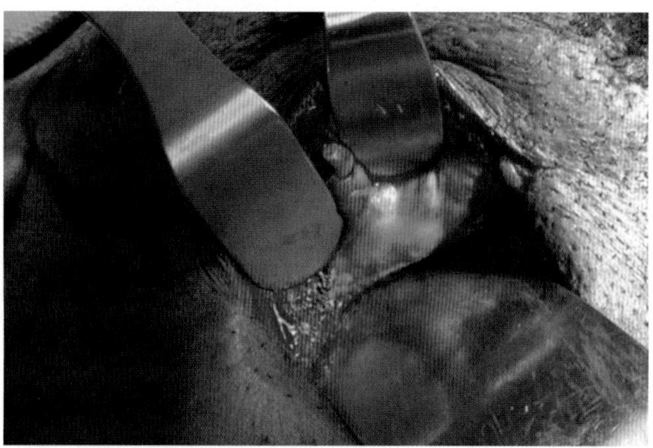

Figure 76.11 Retraction of the dissected tissues.

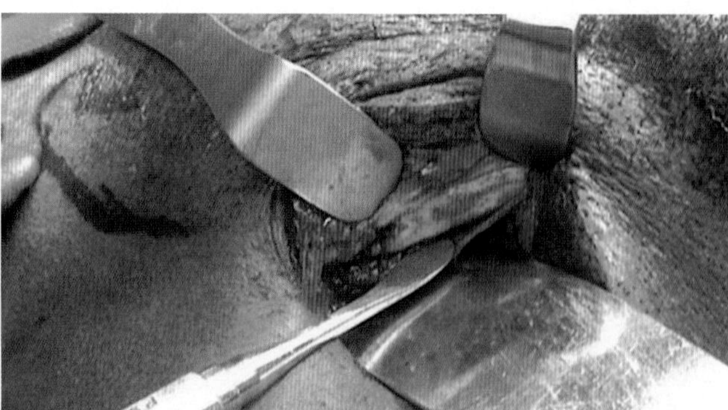

Figure 76.13 A sharp #9 mucoperiosteal elevator is used to reflect the periosteum at the inferior border of the mandible.

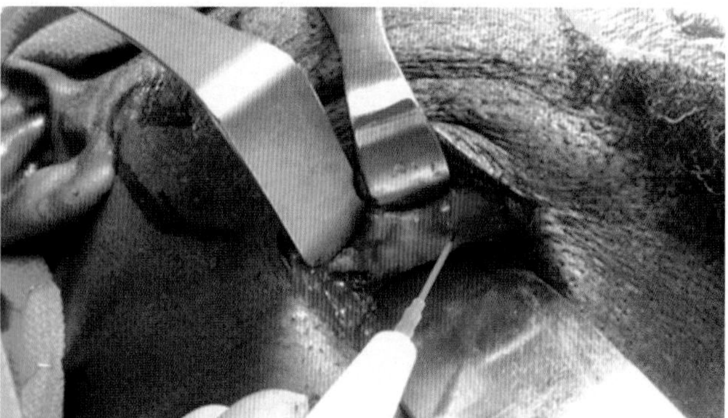

Figure 76.12 The pterygomasseteric sling/periosteum is sharply incised at the midinferior border.

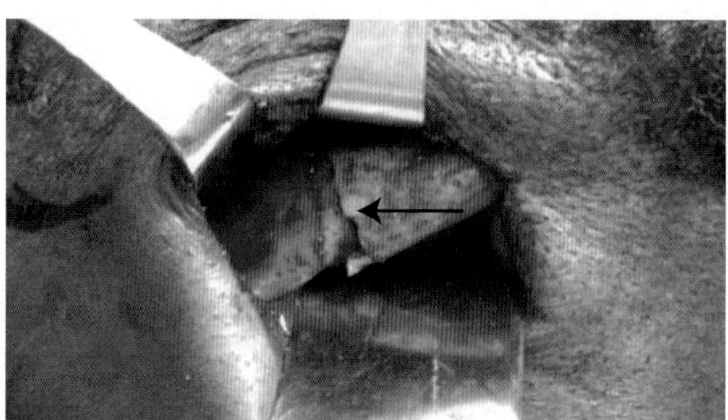

Figure 76.14 Exposure of fracture site.

EXTRAORAL APPROACH—*cont'd*

STEP 6:
Bone compression clamps are used to align and compress the fracture in place for anatomic reduction when possible. The clamp holes at the inferior border should be approximately 2 cm away from the fracture site. Two bur holes are created with the holes directed outwards using the #702 fissure bur. Rechecking of the patient occlusion is paramount following this step (Fig. 76.15).

TREATMENT OPTIONS: Fixation of Mandibular Body Fractures

Option 1: One-Plate Fixation

Fractures with good inter-bony buttressing after fracture reduction can be treated with one load-bearing bone plate at the inferior border using bicortical screws (Fig. 76.16).

Option 2: Two-Plate Fixation

Two-plate fixation is indicated when there is a gap at the fracture site after alignment. Interfragmentary bone buttressing is lost. Additional hardware placement is necessary to provide adequate rigidity/stability during fracture healing. Bone grafting of the fracture site depends on the size of the defect and soft tissue quality and availability (Fig. 76.17).

Option 3: Reconstruction Plate

A load-bearing reconstruction plate can be used to fix comminuted mandibular body fractures associated with fractures at other sites of the mandible (Fig. 76.18).

Closure

Deep layers: Vicryl 3-0 sutures (sometimes Vicryl 4-0 sutures are used for the subcutaneous layer)
Skin: Proline 5-0 suture in a continuous (running) fashion or Monocryl 5-0 in a subcuticular fashion

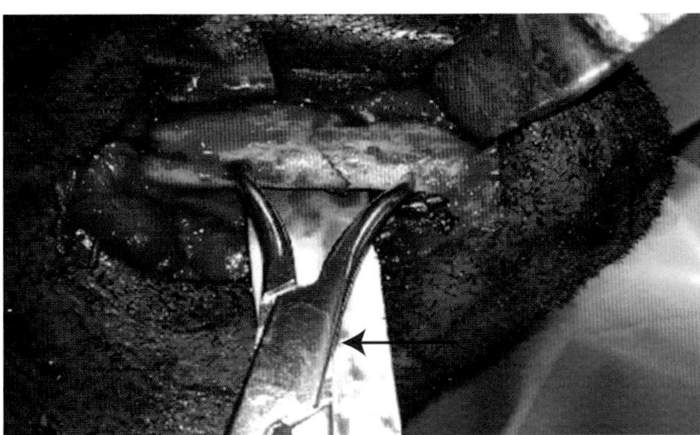

Figure 76.15 Bone compression clamps are used to align and compress the fracture in place for anatomic reduction when possible.

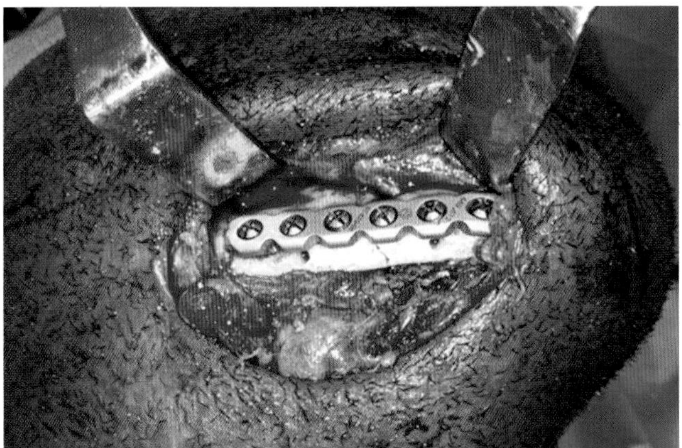

Figure 76.16 Fractures with good interbony buttressing after fracture reduction can be treated with one load-bearing bone plate at the inferior border using bicortical screws.

Transoral Approach

Indicated in minimally displaced, favorable mandibular body fractures. First, arch bars or a facsimile is placed. The mandible is placed into MMF. The incision is made approximately 5 mm below the mucogingival junction to periosteum to expose the fracture site. Care should be taken to avoid injuring the mental nerve. Proper reduction of the fractured segments should be confirmed. A transbuccal trocar is used to facilitate placement of the hardware across the fracture site with proper angulation during screw placement.

Closure: Mucosal closure achieved using chromic gut 3-0 suture.

Avoidance and Management of Intraoperative Complications

Whether extraoral or intraoral approaches were used for reduction and fixation of the fracture, MMF should be released to check the occlusion, which should be intact and reproducible. Malocclusion following fixation may denote improper reduction of the fractured segments with displacement of the condyle or the presence of concomitant fracture that should be addressed (e.g., subcondylar fracture).

The decision to remove or maintain the MMF after fixation will depend on the rigidity of fixation and the presence of concomitant injuries (e.g., in cases of subcondylar fractures that are not rigidly fixed, leaving the MMF for several weeks is warranted).

The authors prefer to use Mastisol, Steri-Strips, and antibiotic ointment to cover the extraoral incision. A pressure dressing in the form of Kerlix and an Ace bandage is applied and removed 48 hours following the surgery. Half-inch Penrose drains are used if the surgical wound has continuous oozing to prevent hematoma formation. Drains are removed when bleeding is minimal or usually on the second day.

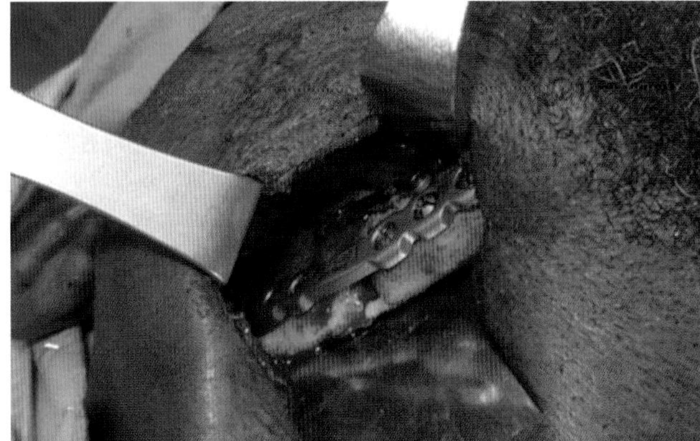

Figure 76.17 Photograph demonstrating placement of two plates, one on the inferior border (bicortical screws) and one on the superior border (mono-cortical screws) for fixation of mandibular body segment fracture.

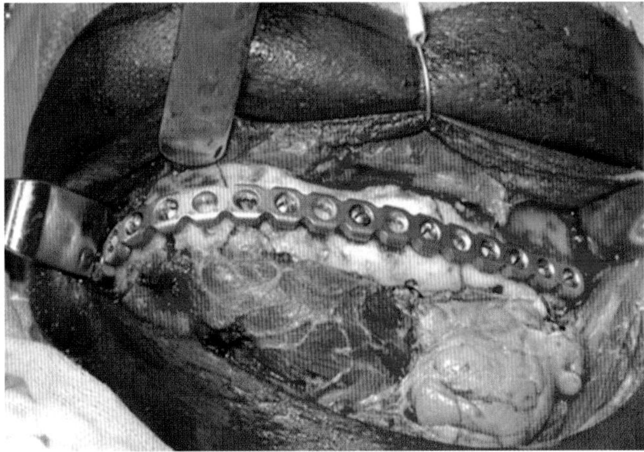

Figure 76.18 A load-bearing reconstruction plate can be used to fix comminuted mandibular body fractures associated with fractures at other sites of the mandible.

Postoperative Considerations

Following surgery, the patient must be maintained on a soft diet until bony union is achieved. It is imperative to counsel patients in the practice of good oral hygiene during convalescence from surgery. Regimented follow-up to ensure healing is necessary.

References

1. Leonard MS. History of treatment of maxillofacial trauma. *Oral Maxillofac Surg Clin North Am*. 1990;2:1.
2. Gordon SD. Wire suturing in the treatment of facial fractures. *Can Med Assoc J*. 1943;48(5):406–409.
3. Fonseca RJ, Marciani RD, Hendler BH. *Oral and Maxillofacial Surgery*. W.B Saunders; 2001.
4. Ellis E III, Walker LR. Treatment of mandibular angle fractures using one noncompression miniplate. *J Oral Maxillofac Surg*. 1996;54(7):864–871.
5. Fridrich KL, Pena-Velasco G, Olson RA. Changing trends with mandibular fractures: a review of 1,067 cases. *J Oral Maxillofac Surg*. 1992;50(6):586–589.
6. Chrcanovic BR. Open versus closed reduction: comminuted mandibular fractures. *Oral Maxillofac Surg*. 2013;17(2):95–104.

CHAPTER 77

Mandibular Angle and Ramus Fractures

Jayini Thakker, Rahul Tandon, Jason Rogers, and Meagan Miller

Armamentarium

#9 Periosteal elevators
#15 Blade
24-Gauge wire
Appropriate sutures
Bipolar cautery
Bone rongeurs
Fine side-cutting fissure bur (1.2 mm)
Local anesthetic with vasoconstrictor
Malleable retractors
Mandible titanium fixation devices
Metzenbaum or tenotomy scissors
Needle electrocautery
Nerve stimulator
Obwegeser retractors
Right angle screwdriver/drills
Senn retractors
Sigmoid notch retractor
TPS surgical drill
Transbuccal trocar

History of the Procedure

The treatment of mandibular fractures has a long, rich history that can be traced all the way back to Hippocrates. Immobilizing the fractured segment allowed him to wire adjacent teeth together. As such, Hippocrates initiated the key principles in treating such fractures.[1] Since that time, surgeons have established the importance of restoring appropriate occlusion and maintaining proper muscular balance.[2,3] Although those techniques now appear crude and antiquated, it is easy to understand the thinking and rationale behind them. Variations of bandages, appliances, splints, and wiring have been used to stabilize the jaws to ensure proper healing and restoration of function. Both bandages and external appliances appeared to be promising in the treatment of mandibular fractures; however, they both produced undesirable posterior directional forces, which could prove deleterious in treating angle and ramus fractures.[4,5] Splints were developed in the 19th century for both the maxilla and the mandible, providing stable IMF.[6] Gilmer popularized the use of wires, as he demonstrated excellent IMF through the wiring of arch bars.[7] With improved plating systems used to fixate mobile bony segments, only further refinement and more sophisticated technology were needed to produce the techniques seen today.

Indications for the Use of the Procedure

Any fracture of the mandible must be properly evaluated and thoroughly assessed, both clinically and radiographically. In fact, radiographic evaluation is of primary importance and the panoramic radiograph is one of the most valuable tools available, especially in ramus and angle fractures. However, a complete mandible film series should be ordered, and the included lateral oblique view can be used to also evaluate the ramus region, whereas the anteroposterior (AP) skull view is important for evaluating potential angle fractures. Currently, computed tomography (CT) scans have also become ubiquitous, and these allow for a more detailed view of mandible fractures as well as other concomitant facial injuries. Additionally, CT of the neck should be used to rule out more severe injuries such as cervical spine fractures, which occur nearly 10% of the time. These injuries, if not identified promptly, can lead to severe neurologic consequences, as C1 and C2 are most commonly involved vertebrae.

Mandibular angle and ramus fractures constitute less than half of the total number of mandibular fractures at 30% (25% for angle, 4% for ramus). Although ramus fractures remain relatively rare, angle fractures are the third most common and, as such, deserve greater attention. The cross-sectional area of the angle is relatively thin, and coupled with the presence of impacted third molars, it is a commonly fractured site. Statistical and literature reviews show that the majority of mandibular fractures occur in accidental or trauma-related incidents. However, when assault cases are further evaluated, it is found that angle fractures constitute a disproportionately high percentage. The general classification of mandibular fractures is comprehensive and discussed in chapters elsewhere; however, those that apply to these particular fracture patterns are addressed.

Angle fractures often occur in conjunction with other mandibular fractures, but the muscular attachments often dictate how the segments move in relation to one another. Angle fractures are classified according to their favorability and the direction of muscular force: vertically favorable or unfavorable and horizontally favorable or unfavorable[8] (Figs. 77.1–77.4). Favorable fractures tend to move the fragments toward each other, whereas unfavorable fractures tend to pull the segments apart (see Figs. 77.1 and 77.4). The masseter, temporalis, and medial pterygoid all play a role in the displacement of fractured segments. Fractures that are unfavorable will lead to displacement of the proximal segment upward and medially, while being impacted in the opposite direction during favorable fractures[8] (see Figs. 77.2 and 77.3). Due to the severity of forces that occur during a bilateral angle fracture, the patient may suffer from an obvious open bite (Fig. 77.5). Ramus fractures are typically classified as favorable due to the elevating forces of the muscles, whereas angle fractures are horizontally unfavorable due to the pull of the same muscles. This favorability of ramus fractures allows for treatment with maxillomandibular fixation (MMF). However, some studies have demonstrated that open reduction and internal fixation (ORIF) of ramus fractures provide adequate functional and anatomic reduction.[9]

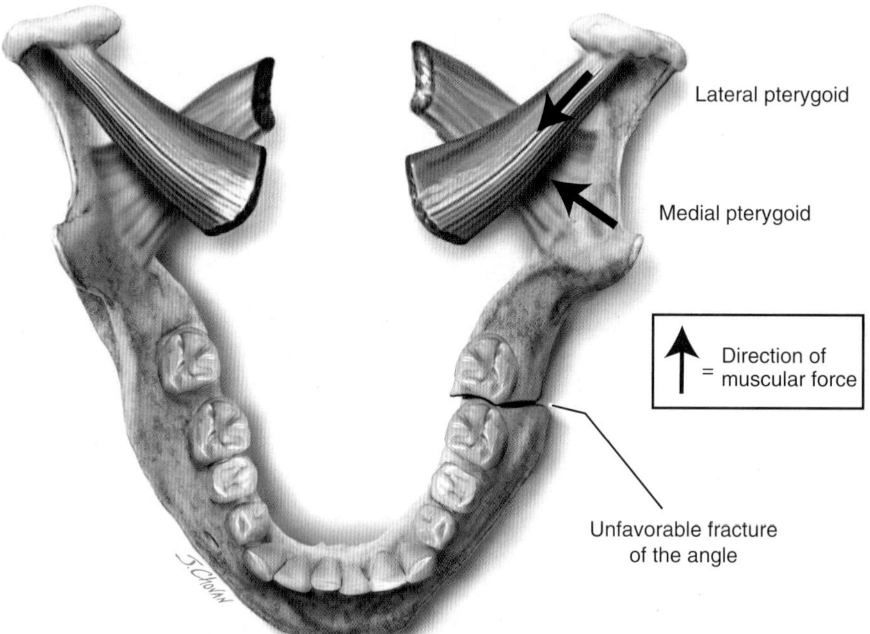

Figure 77.1 Vertically unfavorable fracture.

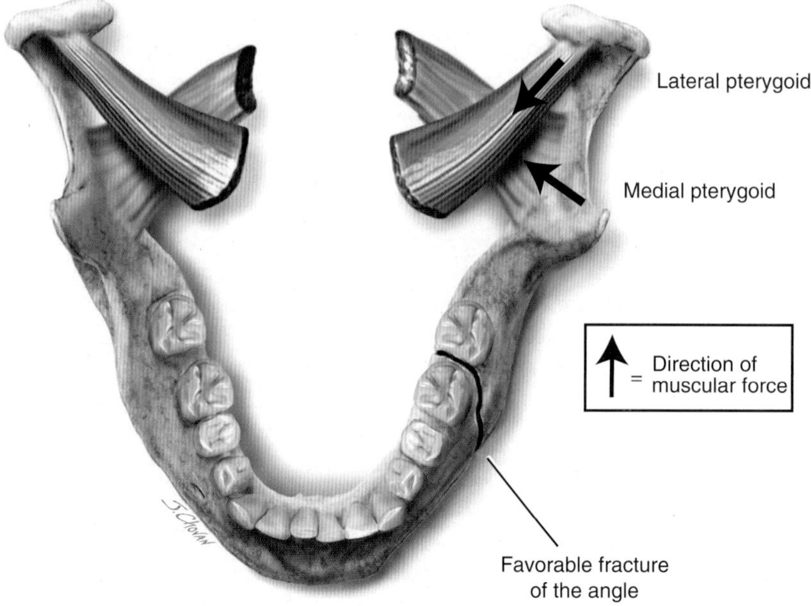

Figure 77.2 Vertically favorable fracture.

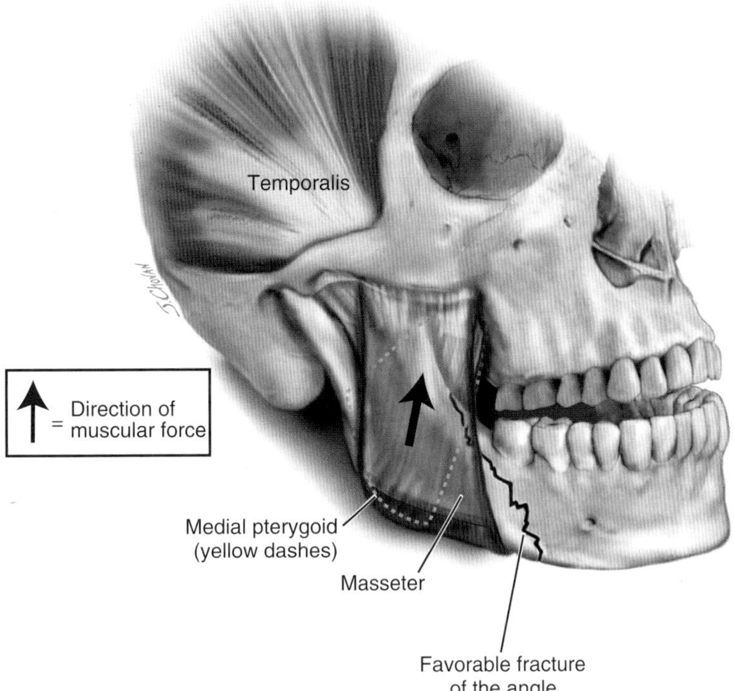

Figure 77.3 Horizontally favorable fracture.

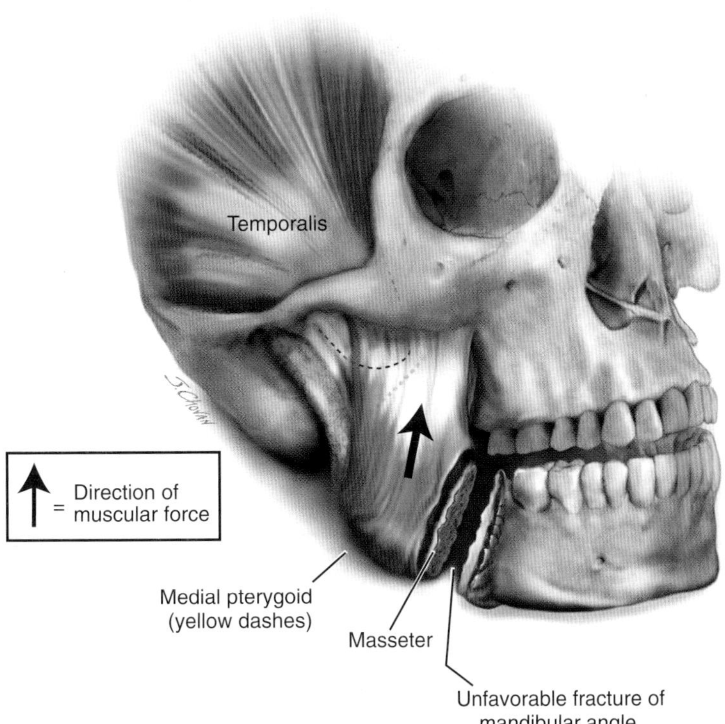

Figure 77.4 Horizontally unfavorable fracture.

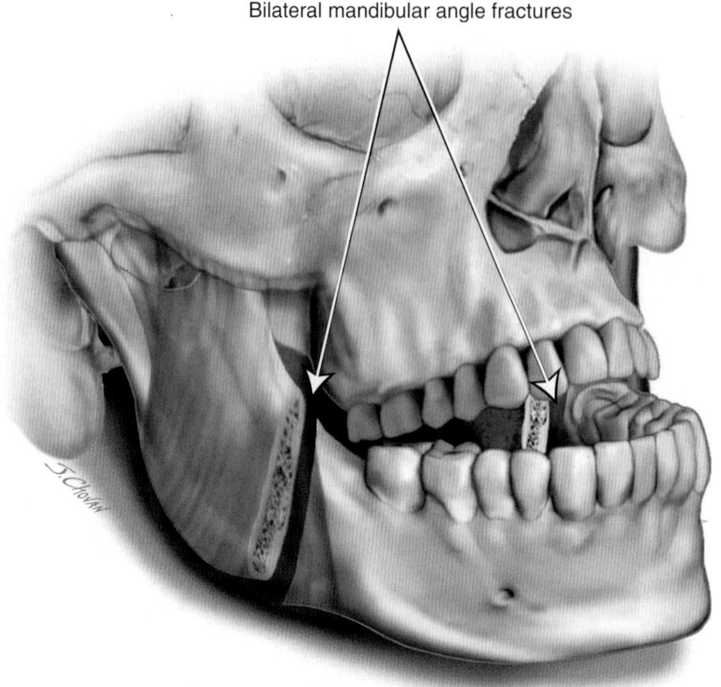

Figure 77.5 Bilateral angle fractures can lead to open bite.

Table 77.1 Summary of Techniques With Respective Advantages, Disadvantages, and Special Considerations With Indications and Contraindications.

	OPEN			
	INTRAORAL		EXTRAORAL	
	Champy or Single Lateral Border Plate	Superior and Inferior Border Plating	Risdon	Closed
Advantages	Minimal dissection	Tension and compression plating leads to greater stability/immobility of fracture segments	Excellent exposure for reduction	Conservative
Disadvantages	Best suited for straightforward cases, favorable fracture pattern	Requires more extensive, inferior, subperiosteal, dissection	Risk of damage to the marginal mandibular nerve, facial artery, and vein Extraoral scarring	Increased surgical time for placement/ removal of arch bars IMF screws may result in root injury, aspiration risk
Special considerations including indications/ contraindications	May be inadequate fixation for grossly comminuted fractures, atrophic mandibles, or concomitant facial injuries	May require transbuccal trocar use	Avoid neuromuscular blockade and local anesthetic administration with use of nerve monitoring	Must have proper occlusal reduction and stability

IMF, Intermaxillary fixation.

Limitations and Contraindications

Once the patient's history has been taken and the physical exam completed, the clinician should decide which diagnostic imaging method is most appropriate for visualizing the fracture (Table 77.1). Although the standard set includes a panoramic radiograph and a CT scan, both do have their limitations. Nevertheless, the clinician should supplement their radiologic findings with their clinical findings.

Open mandible fractures tend to have a higher risk of infection than closed fractures or midface fractures. Perioperative antibiotics are recommended and have been shown to significantly decrease the risk of infection. Extended periods of postoperative antibiotics, however, are not indicated and may actually be discouraged, especially in a hospital setting, where there is increased risk of *Clostridium difficile* infection. We prefer to use one to two doses of intravenous antibiotics preoperatively and one dose perioperatively (within an hour of incision). Also, the administration of oral chlorhexidine is useful for lowering the bacterial counts in the oral cavity when fractures are present; however, it can increase the staining of oral surfaces and alter the patient's taste perception for the duration of the medication's use.[10] When an extraoral approach is utilized, patients risk developing unsightly scars as well as potential injury to the marginal mandibular nerve.

TECHNIQUE 1: Intraoral Approach, Champy Technique

In the advent of rigid fixation with the use of titanium plates and screws, there has been an increasing trend toward ORIF. One of the most common techniques is the placement of a subapical four-hole miniplate at the tension band of the external oblique ridge. This technique was initially described by Champy and colleagues in 1978.[11] The efficacy of this technique is based on the placement of nonrigid or "functionally stable fixation" in an ideal line of osteosynthesis to counteract the muscular forces that tend to displace fractures in the angle region (Fig. 77.6A–C).

STEP 1: Surgical Site Preparation

The patient is prepped and draped in a sterile fashion. The patient is prepped for a potential transcervical approach to the mandibular angle in the instance of a difficult intraoral reduction. This will ensure that the ear, hairline, and neck region are visible, allowing for visualization of the muscles of facial expression if nerve stimulation is used as an adjunct. Other indications for a transcervical approach are grossly unfavorable fractures, comminuted fractures, atrophic mandible, and, in rare instances, a concomitant neck wound such as gunshot wound.

STEP 2: Local Anesthesia and Incision

One begins the procedure by placing the patient in intermaxillary fixation (IMF), using one of the following: arch bars, IMF screws, or any other acceptable technique. A solution of 1% lidocaine with epinephrine is administered via an inferior alveolar nerve block, lingual nerve block, long buccal nerve block, and local infiltration to provide appropriate hemostasis. A #15 blade or monopolar Bovie electrocautery with a Colorado needle tip is then used to make a buccal vestibular incision, leaving a 5-mm cuff of attached gingiva to allow for ease of closure after the procedure. The incision may be carried superiorly to the ascending ramus to allow for better visualization and carried as far anteriorly as needed for access, usually to the level of the mandibular first molar. The incision is carried down to bone and the periosteum is reflected to the inferior border of the mandible to allow adequate visualization and access to the fracture.

STEP 3: Reduction of the Fracture

It is important that the surgeon dissect appropriately to allow for reduction of the fragments, removal of any tooth fragments or debris, and placement of the fixation device. A toe-out Obwegeser retractor may be used to aid in reduction of the inferior border of the mandible. Third molars are often in the line of fracture, and they may be removed if they are loose, easily extracted, or do not allow for proper reduction. Alternatively, they may be left in place if they are fully impacted, not visible, or not hindering the reduction. Depending on the angulation of the fracture, fracture reduction can be facilitated by manual reduction or IMF.

Alternatively, a single superior lateral border plate may be used to immobilize the fracture. This provides a single vector of stability, so it is suited for more favorable fracture patterns, as the muscular pull in these cases aids in reduction and fracture stability.

STEP 4: Plating of the Fracture

A four-hole titanium miniplate is bent to allow for close adaptation to the bone. The proximal two holes lie medial to the external oblique ridge, and the distal two holes extend onto the buccal surface at the superior border of the mandibular body. The plate is thus bent in two planes to allow for optimal stability and resistance to forces. The plate is secured with four self-threading monocortical screws.

STEP 5: Wound Closure

Once acceptable stability has been achieved, the patient is taken out of MMF and the occlusion is verified to be stable and reproducible. The patient may be left in MMF if noncompliance is anticipated. However, Ellis, in 2010,[12] showed that this technique offered optimal outcomes with minimal morbidity, even when patients were not left in MMF. If the occlusion is stable, one can proceed with wound closure. The wound is thoroughly irrigated with 0.9% normal saline and the wound is closed with 3-0 Vicryl or 3-0 chromic gut in a running fashion.

Continued

TECHNIQUE 1: Intraoral Approach, Champy Technique—*cont'd*

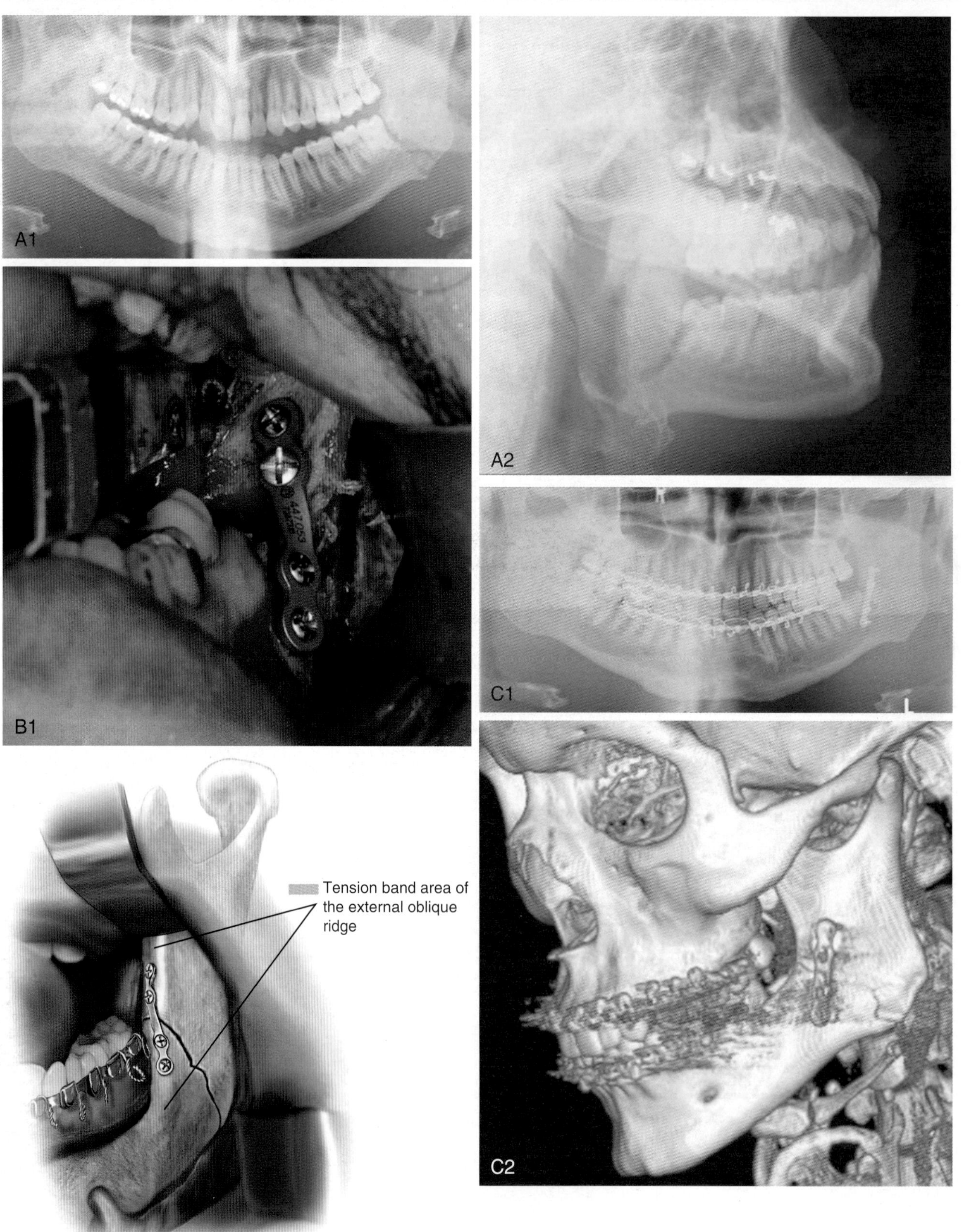

Figure 77.6 **A1** and **A2,** Panoramic and oblique radiographs indicating a displaced left angle fracture. **B1** and **B2,** Intraoperative photo of the Champy technique. Illustration of the Champy technique. **C1** and **C2,** Computed tomography three-dimensional reconstruction and panoramic radiograph demonstrating a reduced angle fracture through the use of the Champy technique.

ALTERNATIVE TECHNIQUE 1: Intraoral Approach, Superior and Inferior Border Plating Technique

Another commonly used technique involves the placement of two miniplates. The same technique for IMF is used, and a similar incision and dissection are employed to gain access to the fracture. However, this technique requires more extensive dissection down to the inferior border of the mandibular angle. This may be one of the reasons for somewhat less favorable outcomes, as demonstrated in some studies. Once the fracture is fully exposed and reduced, two four-hole miniplates are bent to adapt closely to the buccal cortex of the mandible. One is secured at the superior border using monocortical screws in order to avoid tooth roots. The second is placed at the inferior border, below the mandibular canal, and also secured with four screws. Due to limited access in this location, a transbuccal trocar approach may be required to gain inferior and posterior access to the fracture, thus allowing proper adaptation of the plating system and proper angle for screw placement (Fig. 77.7A–C). Use of a transbuccal trocar can carry risks due to the skin incision on the cheek/neck needed for insertion of the trocar. However, this incision is much smaller than a transcervical Risdon approach as full exposure of the fracture through the incision is not necessary. In a comparative, systematic review,[13] the transbuccal approach showed fewer complications than the extraoral approach.

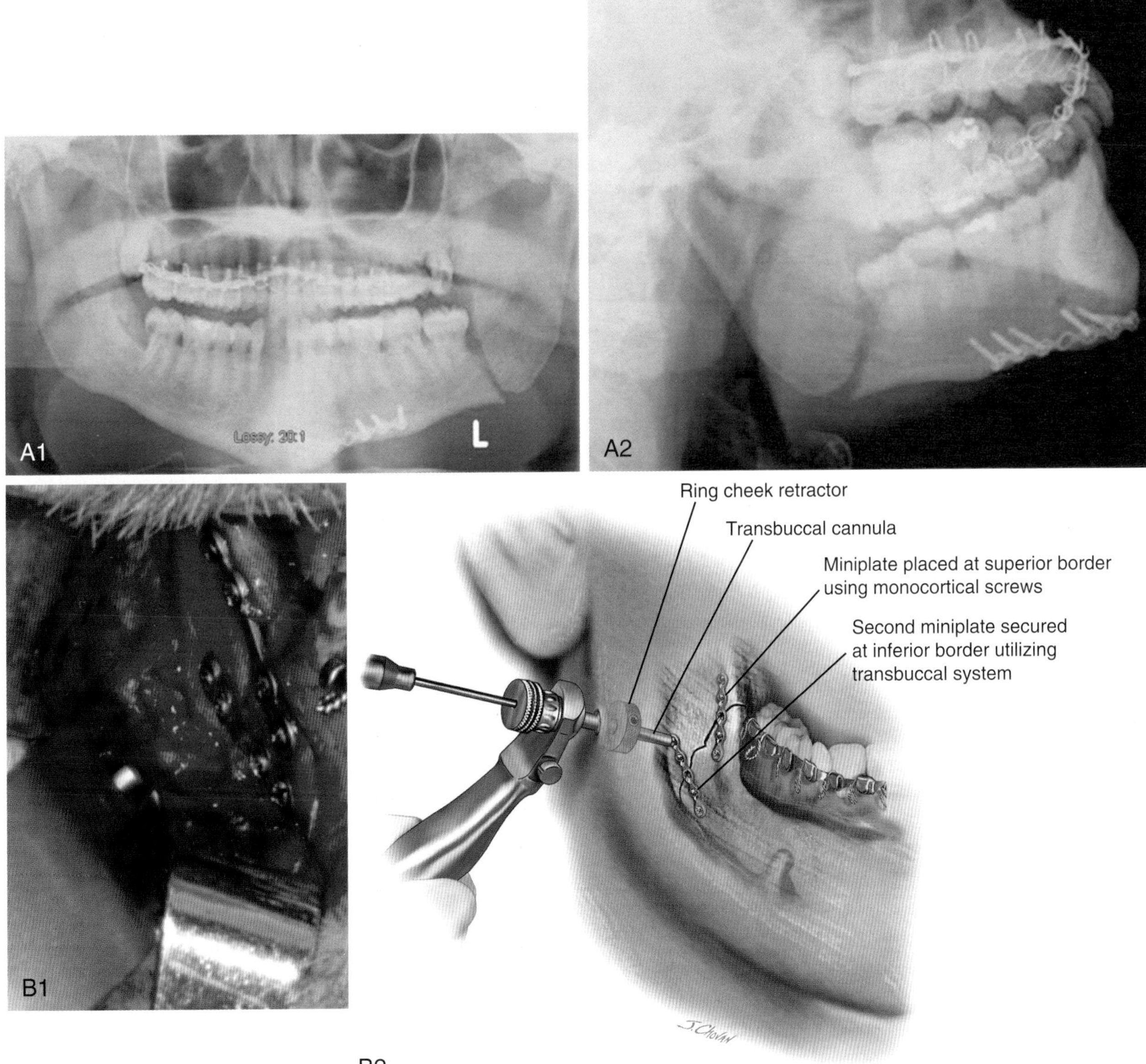

Figure 77.7 **A1** and **A2,** Panoramic and oblique radiographs demonstrating a displaced left angle fracture and a previously repaired left parasymphysis fracture. **B1** and **B2,** Intraoperative photo of the two-miniplate technique. Illustrations of the transbuccal trocar technique.

Continued

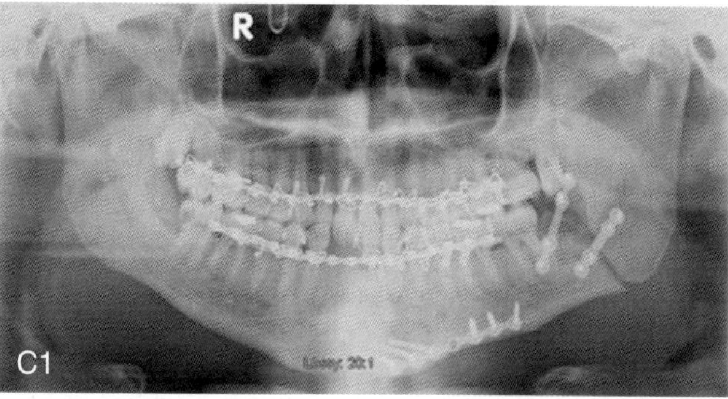

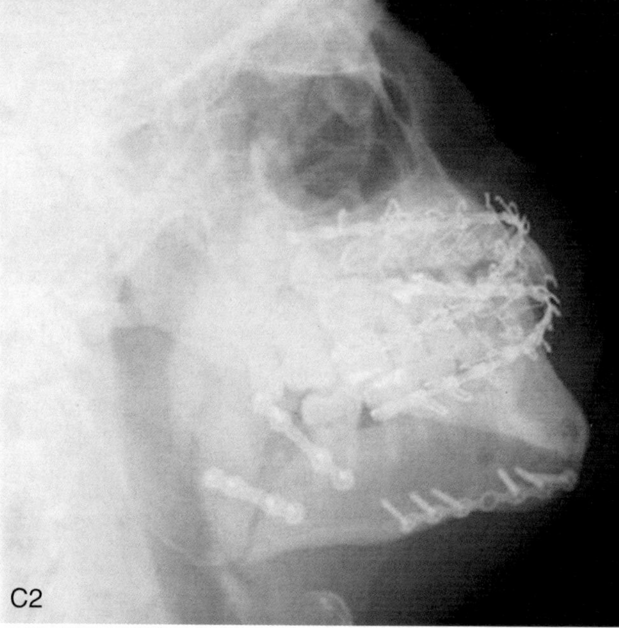

Figure 77.7 cont'd **C1** and **C2,** Postoperative panoramic and oblique radiographs indicating open reduction internal fixation through the use of the two-miniplate technique.

ALTERNATIVE TECHNIQUE 2: Submandibular/Transcervical (Risdon) Approach

The face and neck are prepped and draped, leaving the ear, inferior border of the mandible, neck, mouth, and lower lip open to visualization. A sterile marking pen is then used to outline the inferior border of the mandible, the course of the marginal mandibular branch of the facial nerve, and the proposed incision, which should stay approximately two fingerbreadths below the inferior border of the mandible and preferably within an existing skin crease to prevent inadvertent damage to the marginal mandibular nerve. The design of this incision is based on anatomic studies that mapped out the course of the mandibular nerve based on a series of prosections. Dingmann and Grabb showed that the nerve may travel up to 1 cm below the inferior border of the mandible, but it is always above the inferior border anterior to the facial artery.[14] Ziarah and Atkinson showed that the nerve extends up to 1.2 cm below the inferior border of the mandible and continues below the border as it courses anterior to the facial artery in a significant number of dissections.[15] Thus, we aim to keep the incision a safe distance below the expected course of the nerve. In addition, a facial nerve monitor may be used with the probes placed in the orbicularis oris muscle. If intraoperative nerve monitoring is used, one must inform the anesthesiologist not to paralyze the patient or to use a short-acting paralytic agent. In addition, one must be careful not to use local anesthetic below the platysma so as not to weaken neurotransmission of the marginal mandibular nerve.

An incision is then made through skin using a #15 blade followed by Bovie electrocautery for hemostasis. Superior and inferior subdermal flaps are elevated for 2 to 3 cm to improve adequate visualization. The platysma is then carefully divided. The next layer deep to the platysma is the superficial layer of the deep cervical fascia. The marginal mandibular nerve is located immediately superficial to this. Note that this layer is continuous with the submandibular gland capsule. Thus, the gland capsule is incised and subsequently elevated from inferior to superior, with the mandibular nerve being protected in the tissues immediately superficial to it. The facial artery and vein may be encountered during the dissection and can be ligated and divided if necessary. However, if the fracture is posterior to the submandibular gland, the facial vessels may not be encountered. Once the inferior border of the mandible is approached, the submandibular gland is retracted inferiorly and the muscles of the pterygomasseteric sling are sharply incised with either a #15 blade or electrocautery. The mandibular angle fracture should be easily identified at this point. The periosteum is stripped adequately, and the fracture can now be reduced manually or with a bone-reducing clamp. Plating with rigid internal fixation then proceeds preferably with a 2-0 locking system. Superior and inferior border plates may be placed at this point. If there is gross comminution, a reconstruction plate may be preferred to span the fracture.

The wound is thoroughly irrigated and closed in layers. We prefer to use 3-0 Vicryl sutures to close the platysma and deep dermal layer, and 4-0 or 5-0 Prolene or nylon sutures to close the skin. A subcuticular closure with 4-0 Monocryl is also an option. This obviates the need for suture removal.

ALTERNATIVE TECHNIQUE 3: Closed Reduction

Although open reduction internal fixation is appropriate and indicated in many situations, a more conservative approach can be just as effective. Much like open reduction, the closed reduction technique relies on the same principles of using MMF to restore form and function. Techniques most commonly used for these approaches include the placement of arch bars or IMF screws.

Placement of arch bars continues to be the most popular choice among surgeons when performing closed reduction with MMF. In this technique, the arch bars are fixed to the teeth and secured with circumdental wires. Once secured, the patient is then guided into the premorbid occlusion, which is then fixated with intra-arch wires. One advantage of using arch bars is that they help to reestablish segments of bone against one another. Furthermore, the arch bars allow placement of directing forces through wires or elastic, helping to guide the patient into occlusion during the postoperative period. However, the downfalls of using this technique include the increased surgical time for placement and subsequent removal. Arch bars can increase trauma to the periodontium, which can cause discomfort in the postoperative period as well as interfere with the patient's maintenance of good oral hygiene.

Use of IMF screws has begun to gain more attention as an alternative to using arch bars. The technique requires the placement of self-drilling screws into the periodontium, both proximally and distally to the fracture, ensuring adequate stabilization. The screws themselves are placed in a bicortical fashion at or near the mucogingival junction. Once the screws are in place, the patient is guided into the premorbid occlusion, which is then secured appropriately, either by elastics or wire. The advantage of this system includes reduced operating time, less risk of injury to the surgeon, and easy removal upon completion of the therapy. However, this procedure is not without its drawbacks: reported complications include root injury, screw loosening, and aspiration.

Avoidance and Management of Intraoperative Complications

Appropriate reduction and immobilization of fractured segments are critical to successfully treat these fractures. Injuries to the accompanying neurovascular bundles should be identified and immediately treated. Damage to the inferior alveolar artery and nerve can lead to profuse bleeding and possible neuropathy, respectively. If the artery is cut or severed, appropriate hemostasis should be achieved immediately. Damage to the nerve can be more difficult to identify initially and may only be realized after the patient has become aware of a loss of sensation on the treated side. Other complications include abscess formation, granulation tissue near the incision site with bone exposure, and loose hardware.[13] In the case of abscess formation, incision and drainage may be performed; with loose hardware and bone exposure, a second surgery may be required to remove the infected/loose piece of hardware. If there is fracture nonunion, the patient may be placed in MMF. A malunion may require reexploration, débridement of the area, and replacement of rigid fixation or IMF. Patients should be properly informed about possible complications prior to surgery to protect surgeon to patient rapport should complications arise.

Postoperative Considerations

Nearly all fractures of the mandible are considered open due to their communication with either skin or the oral cavity; however, those associated with the angle and ramus occur in non-tooth-bearing areas, reducing risks associated with other portions of the mandible. However, they have been described as having the highest postsurgical complication rate among the different types of mandibular fractures.[16] When initiating treatment of mandibular fractures, a tetanus booster may be indicated. Additionally, any preexisting nutritional deficiencies should be addressed and corrected to minimize any delay in healing. Although the timing of the reduction and fixation may vary, it is preferable to treat the fracture as soon as possible to reduce any patient discomfort. If the fracture cannot be reduced relatively quickly, there is not necessarily an increased risk of infection. However, when infection does occur, the pathogens involved include *Streptococcus, Staphylococcus,* and *Bacteroides*. Thus, the patient should be placed on antibiotic therapy with clindamycin or penicillin at the time of clinical presentation, with the therapy continued until the fracture is reduced. The patient should also be instructed on performing self-care with chlorhexidine oral rinses once discharged. Hardware placement requires a biweekly exam to assess the status of the hardware, the patient's occlusion, and the patient's nutritional status.

References

1. Hippocrates. *Oeuvres Completes.* English Translation by ET Withington. Cambridge, MA: Loeb Classical Library; 1928.
2. Brophy TW. *Oral Surgery: A Treatise on the Diseases, Injuries and Malformations of the Mouth and Associated Parts.* York, PA: Maple Press; 1915.
3. Chopart F, Desault PJ. *Treatment of Surgical Diseases.* Paris: Villiers; 1795.
4. Dorrance GM, Bransfield JW, eds. *The History of Treatment of Fractured Jaws.* ; 1941.
5. Schwartz L. The development of the treatment of jaw fractures. *J Oral Surg.* 1944;2:193.
6. Moon H. Mechanical appliances for treatment of fracture of the jaws. *Br J Dent Sci.* 1874;17:303.
7. Gilmer TL. Multiple fracture of the lower jaw with remarks on the treatment. *Arch Dent.* 1887;4:388.

8. Fonseca RJ, Walker RV, Barber DH, Powers MB. *Oral and Maxillofacial Trauma*. 3rd ed. vol. 1. St. Louis, MO: Saunders Elsevier; 2005.
9. Kale TP, Kotrashetti SM, Louis A, Lingaraj JB, Sarvesh BU. Mandibular ramus fractures: a rarity. *J Contemp Dent Pract*. 2013;14(1): 39–42.
10. Perez R, Oeltjen JC, Thaller SR. A review of mandibular angle fractures. *Craniomaxillofac Trauma Reconstr*. 2011;4(2):69–72.
11. Khouri M, Champy M. Results of mandibular osteosynthesis with miniaturized screwed plates. Apropos of 800 fractures treated over a 10-year period. *Ann Chir Plast Esthet*. 1987;32(3):262–266.
12. Ellis E III. Open reduction and internal fixation of combined angle and body/symphysis fractures of the mandible: how much fixation is enough? *J Oral Maxillofac Surg*. 2013;71(4):726–733.
13. Beza AB, Attia S, Ellis E, Omara L. Comparative study of transbuccal and extraoral approaches in the management of mandibular angle fractures: a systematic review. *Open Access Maced J Med Sci*. 2016;4(3): 482–488.
14. Dingman RO, Grabb WC. Surgical anatomy of the mandibular ramus of the facial nerve based on the dissection of 100 facial halves. *Plast Reconstr Surg Transplant Bull*. 1962;29:266–272.
15. Ziarah HA, Atkinson ME. The surgical anatomy of the mandibular distribution of the facial nerve. *Br J Oral Surg*. 1981;19(3):159–170.
16. de Melo WM, Antunes AA, Sonoda CK, Hochuli-Vieira E, Gabrielli MA, Gabrielli MF. Mandibular angle fracture treated with new three-dimensional grid miniplate. *J Craniofac Surg*. 2012;23(5):e416–e417.

CHAPTER 78

Mandibular Condyle Fractures

Likith Reddy and Andrew Read-Fuller

Armamentarium

#9 Periosteal elevators
#15 Scalpel blade
24-Gauge wire
Appropriate sutures
Bipolar cautery
Bone rongeurs
Fine side-cutting fissure bur (1.2 mm)
Local anesthetic with vasoconstrictor
Malleable retractors
Mandible titanium fixation devices
Metzenbaum and or tenotomy scissors
Needle electrocautery
Nerve stimulator
Obwegeser retractors
Senn retractors
Sigmoid notch retractor
Surgical drill

History of the Procedure

Fractures of the mandibular condyle comprise 25% to 35% of all mandible fractures. Classification and management of condylar fractures are controversial topics in maxillofacial trauma. This is due to the anatomic complexity of the condyle, the extensive attachments, and its contribution to the temporomandibular joint. Lindahl's classification of mandibular condyle fractures is a complex but commonly used system. It is based on the level of the fracture, the amount of displacement, and the relationship of the condylar head to the fossa (Fig. 78.1).[1] Lindahl classified the fractures based on the levels of the fracture: condyle head fracture, condyle neck fracture, and subcondyle fracture (Fig. 78.2). A condyle head fracture is located within the joint capsule; a condyle neck fracture is inferior to the joint capsule and inferior to the attachment of the lateral pterygoid muscle. A subcondyle fracture is inferior to the condyle between the sigmoid notch and the posterior aspect of the mandible. Spiessl identified six fracture types (1 to 6) that described the displacement of the fracture fragments and dislocation of the condylar head from the fossa.[2] The classifications are fracture with no dislocation, inferior condylar neck fracture with dislocation, superior condylar neck fracture with dislocation, inferior condylar neck fracture with luxation, superior condylar neck fracture with luxation, and intracapsular fracture.

Neff et al.[3] further classified condylar head fractures into three types. In this classification, type A is through the medial part of the condylar head, type B is through the lateral part of the condylar head, and type C is near the attachment of the lateral capsule. Bhagol et al.[4] developed a subcondylar fracture classification system based on ramus height shortening and the degree of fracture displacement. He recommended class I fractures (minimally displaced) be treated with conservative management. Class II fractures (moderately displaced) can be treated with conservative or surgical management, although functional outcomes in this group were slightly better in the surgically treated group. Class III fractures (severely displaced) are treated surgically. Loukota et al.[5,6] recently developed a subclassification of subcondylar fractures: high condylar neck, low condylar base, and dicapitular fractures. Ellis et al. further simplified condylar fractures into three groups: condylar head, neck, and base fractures.[7]

The management of condylar fractures is controversial and includes observation, closed treatment, and open reduction with or without endoscopic visualization by transfacial or intraoral approaches (Fig. 78.3). Studies published in the past decade are more favorable to open surgical management. The isolated intracapsular fracture is treated solely with physical therapy. Although these fractures can result in significant anatomic and radiologic changes in the appearance of the condyle itself, most patients do well if properly rehabilitated (Fig. 78.4). Singh et al.[8] recently published the largest blinded, randomized, controlled trial comparing surgical (open) techniques with closed management; they concluded that both treatment options yield acceptable results (Fig. 78.5). However, the surgically treated group was superior in all objective and subjective functional parameters except occlusion (Fig. 78.6). A recent meta-analysis, which contained 20 studies, including four randomized controlled trials, found that surgical management was as good as or better than conservative management (Fig. 78.7).[9]

The surgical approach to the condyle for open reduction and fixation is dictated by the level of the fracture, the surgeon's experience and skill level, the degree of fracture displacement or dislocation, the patient's desires, and the complication risk, among other factors. The retromandibular approach is the most versatile approach to the condylar head, neck, and ramus. There are two variations of this technique: transparotid and retroparotid. The transparotid technique described by Hinds[10] with modification by Ellis[11] provides the shortest

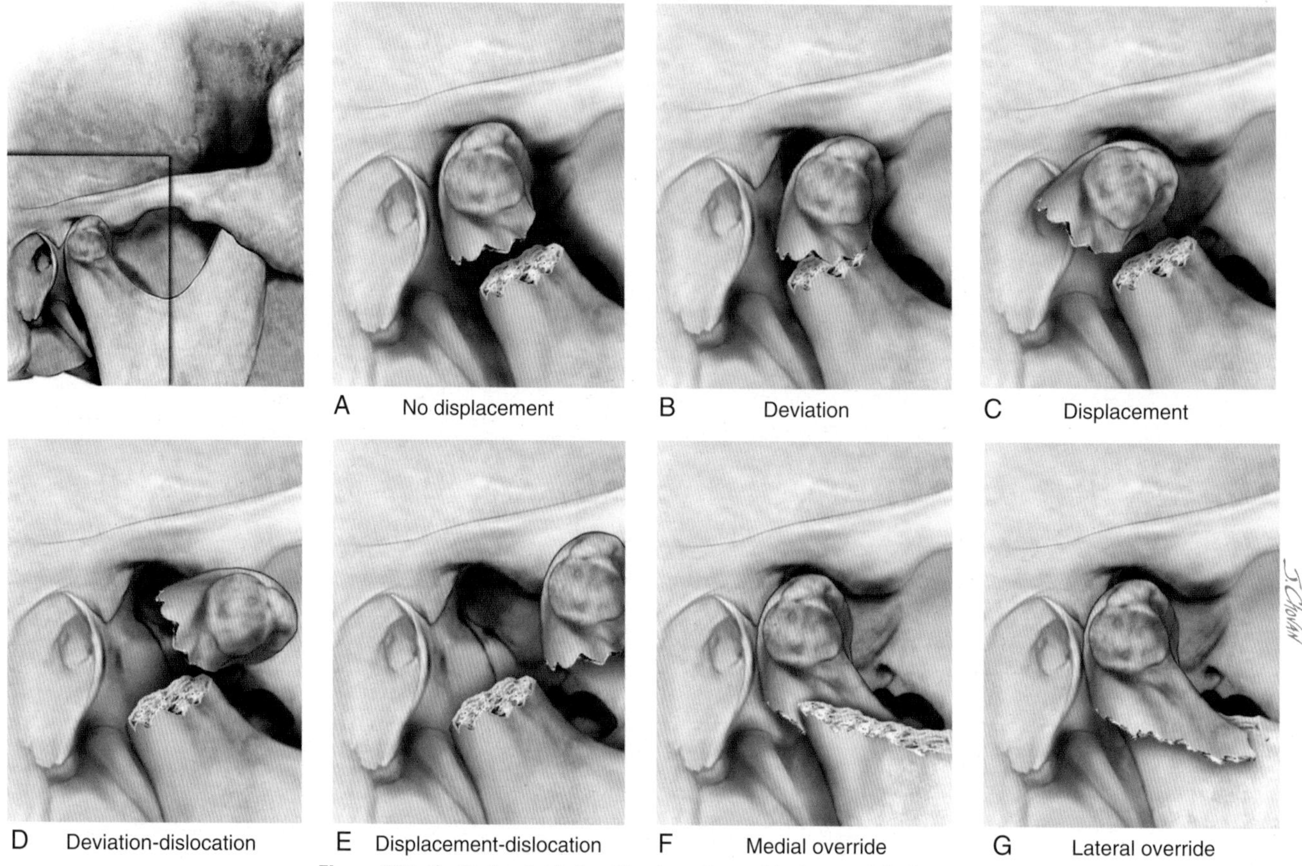

Figure 78.1 A–G, Lindahl classification of mandibular condyle fractures.

distance with quickest access from the skin to the mandible. The branches of the facial nerve are frequently encountered; however, complications with facial nerve weakness or injury seldom occur. The retroparotid technique requires an incision that is longer and is 2 cm posterior to the ramus, thus enabling dissection to proceed deep to the parotid gland and facial nerve. The disadvantage of this approach is the dissection and the working distance between the incision and the condyle.

Wire fixation, intramedullary pins, miniplates, and rigid compressive plates have been used to stabilize these fractures. However, a single rigid miniplate or two semirigid plates are the current treatments of choice (Fig. 78.8).

Indications for the Use of the Procedure

Zide and Kent[12] described absolute and relative indications for open reduction of mandibular condyle fractures. These have been revised by numerous authors, and the current absolute indications for open treatment are bilateral fractures, considerable dislocations, cases in which closed treatment does not reestablish occlusion, concomitant fractures of other areas of the face that compromise occlusion and for which rigid internal fixation will be used, foreign bodies (e.g., firearm projectiles), and dislocation of the condyle to the middle cranial fossa.[13–19] Others have proposed that condylar fractures with a deviation of more than 10 degrees or a shortening of the ramus greater than 2 mm should be treated with open reduction regardless of the fracture level.[20,21] Kellman suggested open reduction by endoscopic technique for significant angulation of the proximal segment (probably more than 30 degrees) and significant foreshortening of the ramus (probably more than 4 to 5 mm, or noticeable and bothersome to the patient).[22]

Open reduction and fixation of condylar fractures can be done by transfacial or intraoral approaches. The advantages of transfacial approaches are improved visualization and direct access to the fracture site, compared with intraoral techniques. The endoscopic technique allows for smaller incisions, less visible scarring, and less risk of facial nerve injuries than those seen with traditional approaches to condylar fractures.[22] The endoscopic technique can be performed intraorally or extraorally.[23–26]

Limitations and Contraindications

The retromandibular transparotid approach is used to safely approach fractures of the entire condylar neck, subcondyle,

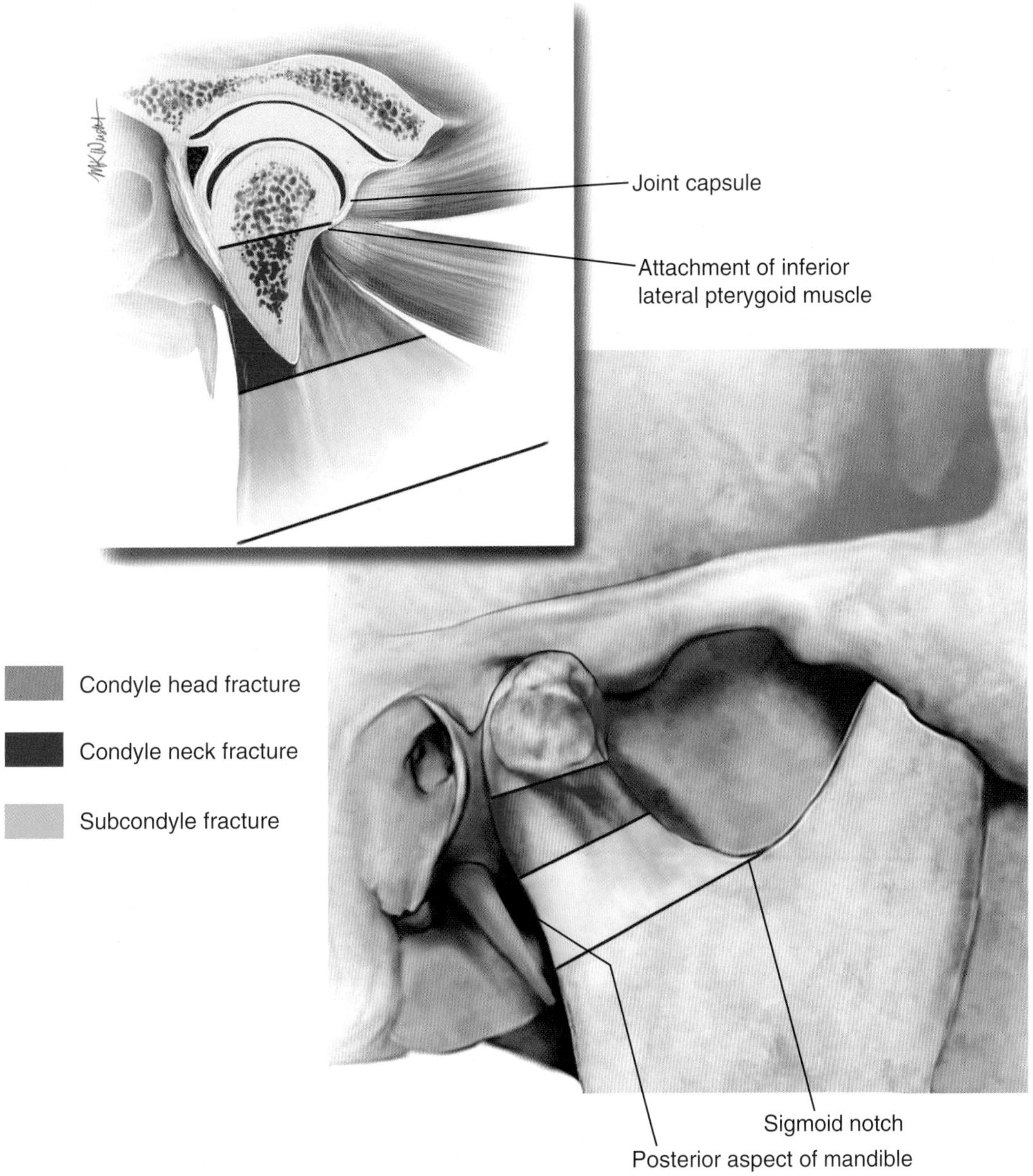

Joint capsule

Attachment of inferior lateral pterygoid muscle

Condyle head fracture

Condyle neck fracture

Subcondyle fracture

Sigmoid notch

Posterior aspect of mandible

Figure 78.2 Classification of condylar fracture according to anatomic fracture level.

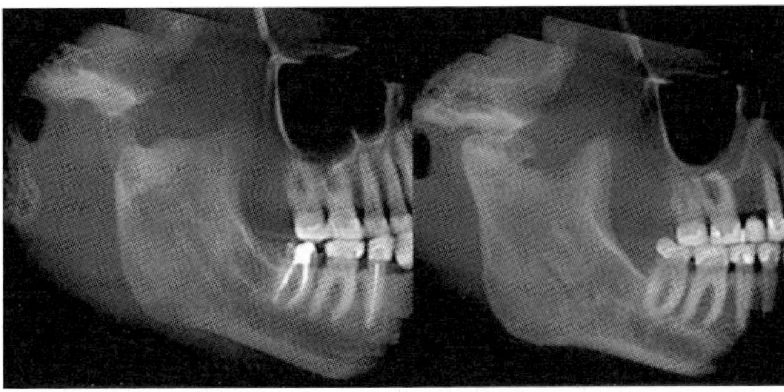

Figure 78.3 Sagittal computed tomography (CT) scan showing a fracture dislocation of the condylar head.

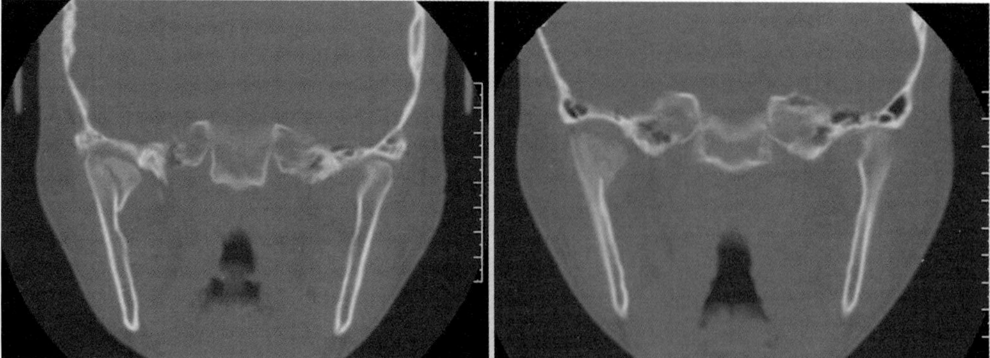

Figure 78.4 Coronal computed tomography (CT) scan showing an isolated intercapsular fracture of the right mandibular condyle.

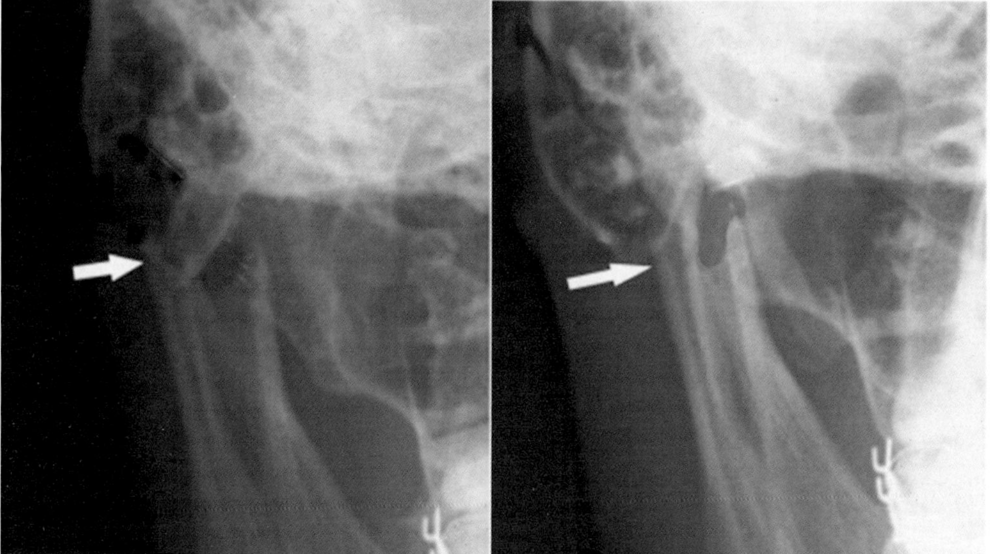

Figure 78.5 Plain coronal radiograph demonstrating a healed condylar fracture after rehabilitation (*arrows*).

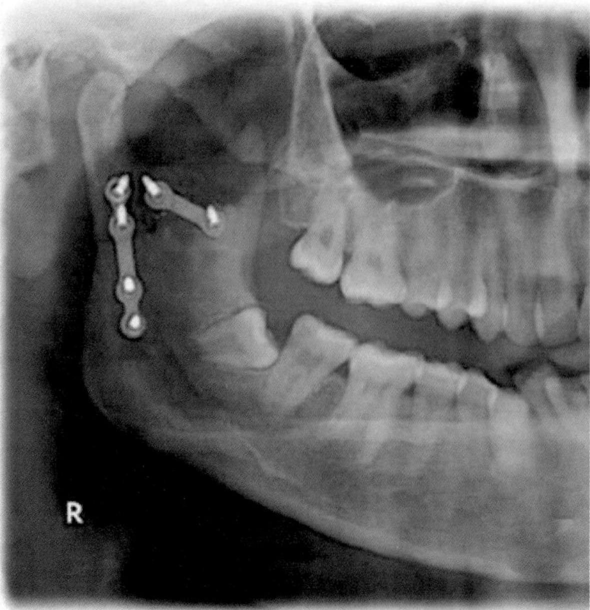

Figure 78.6 Panoramic radiograph showing fixation of a right mandibular condylar fracture.

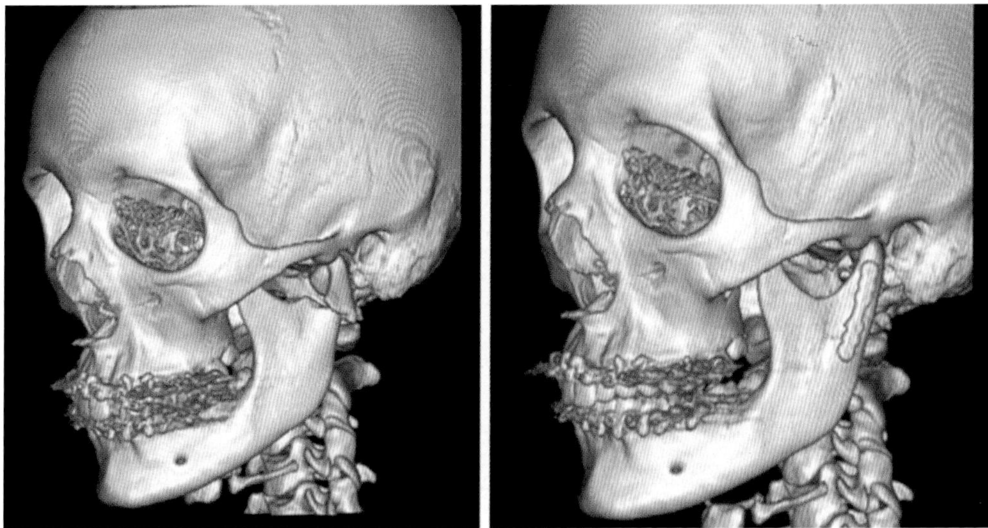

Figure 78.7 Three-dimensional computed tomography (CT) scan after reduction and internal fixation of the mandibular condyle.

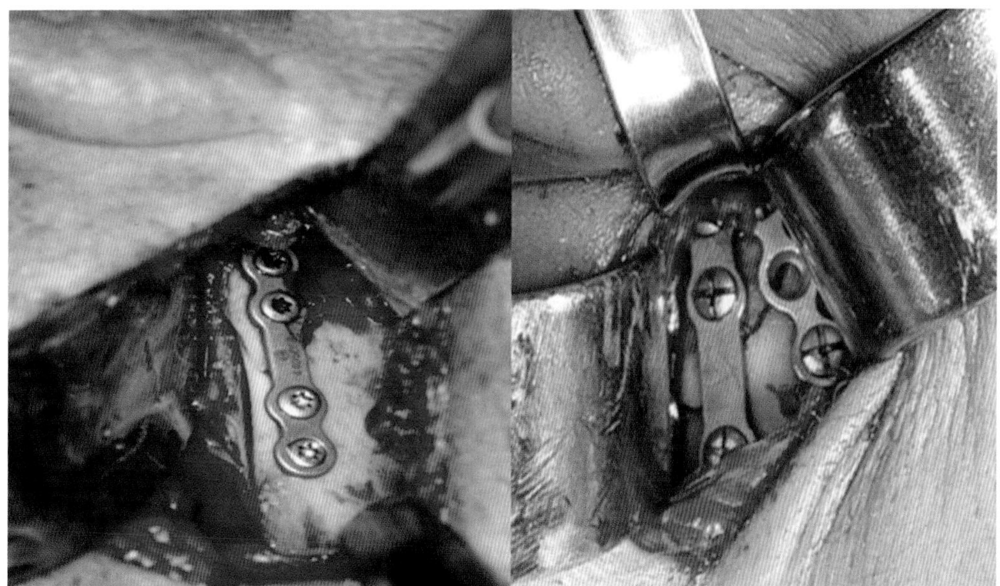

Figure 78.8 Intraoperative view of rigid fixation applied to a condylar fracture.

and ramus. However, visualization of the head of the condyle and the joint capsule is limited. The approach requires going through the parotid and frequently encountering one of the facial nerve branches. This approach is ideal for the vast majority of condylar fractures, including comminuted fractures of the condyle. Intracapsular fractures are best accessed by the preauricular approach. The submandibular approach is ideal for low subcondylar and ramus fractures. Significant traction or a trocar is needed to access the proximal condylar segment for reduction and fixation by submandibular access. This incision has a higher incidence of marginal mandibular weakness compared with retromandibular incision. The endoscopic approaches require additional training and skill (the learning curve can be steep) in addition to increased operating time. The endoscopic approach is contraindicated for comminuted fractures of the condyle-ramus complex. The preauricular access is appropriate for intracapsular and high condylar fractures. The trocar is needed often for fixation of hardware to the distal segment of the fracture by this approach.

TECHNIQUE: Retromandibular (Transparotid) Approach

STEP 1: Surgical Site Preparation

The patient is prepped and draped in a sterile fashion that ensures visibility of the entire ear, posterior hair line, and the lateral face from the forehead to the neck region. This exposure facilitates observation of the facial nerve stimulation. A sterile marking pen is used to mark the proposed incision site. A vertical 3- to 4-cm mark, beginning 0.5 cm below the earlobe, is placed at the posterior mandibular border. It is crucial that no paralysis be present before the facial incision is made (Fig. 78.9).

STEP 2: Local Anesthesia and Incision

A local anesthetic with vasoconstrictor is injected in a subcutaneous plane, staying superficial to the platysma. This avoids inadvertent anesthesia of the facial nerve. While the assistant provides countertraction, a #15 blade is used to incise through the skin and subcutaneous tissue to expose the platysma, which is scant in this region. Undermining the skin in a subcutaneous plane with Metzenbaum scissors at this point is critical to tensionless skin closure. Senn retractors are used to provide adequate retraction at this depth. Bovie electrocautery with a Colorado needle is used to provide hemostasis from bleeding subdermal vessels.

STEP 3: Dissection to the Parotid Capsule

A #15 blade is used to make a vertical incision to the parotid gland, parallel to the skin incision. The scant superficial musculoaponeurotic system (SMAS) layer and, finally, the parotid capsule are encountered; however, they are often confluent. Once the glandular, yellowish parotid tissue has been visualized, a finger sweep with moist gauze on the surface of the exposed gland improves exposure and confirms complete incision and release through the parotid fascia. Thorough hemostasis is obtained with a Colorado needle and Bovie cautery.

STEP 4: Dissection Through the Parotid Gland and Pterygomasseteric Sling

After encountering the parotid, the surgeon must be cognizant of the orientation of the facial nerve branches. Hemostats are used to bluntly dissect through the parotid, paralleling the direction of the branches of major facial nerves. Nerve stimulation should be used as needed in this plane, with close observation of the corner of the mouth and areas stimulated by branches of the marginal facial nerve. If encountered, it should be gently dissected free, at least for a short distance, to facilitate retraction, especially if retraction superiorly is planned. Most commonly, the dissection to the mandible is carried between the buccal branches and the marginal mandibular branch of the facial nerve. The dissection is continued to the pterygomasseteric sling, where the periosteum is sharply incised directly over the posterior mandibular border, thus avoiding the muscles themselves; this, in turn, minimizes bleeding, pain, and undue postoperative swelling. The retromandibular vein is commonly encountered in this area and retracted posteriorly. If necessary, it can be ligated with no significant consequence, just as the cervical branch of the facial nerve can be sacrificed with no adverse effect, to facilitate retraction. Subperiosteal dissection is carried out with a #9 periosteal elevator. A large toe-in with effortless tenting of the tissue facilitates exposure of the fracture site and minimizes nerve traction injury. A sigmoid notch retractor, Dingman clamp, or 24-gauge wire through the distal segment's inferior border can facilitate fracture site manipulation and reduction.

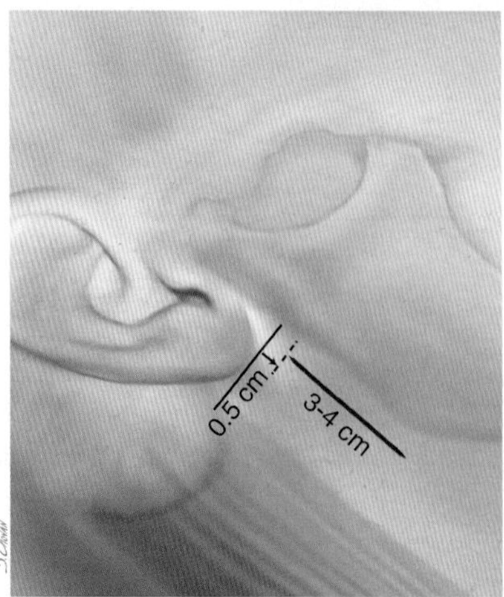

Figure 78.9 Modified retromandibular incision for exposure of the mandibular condyle.

TECHNIQUE: Retromandibular (Transparotid) Approach—cont'd

STEP 5: Paralysis of the Patient and Fracture Reduction

After the bony mandible is encountered, the anesthetist may administer a longer acting, nondepolarizing agent to facilitate manipulation and reduction of the fracture segments. The key to reducing these fractures is to counteract the muscle pull displacing the segments. If the fracture is easily reduced by a hemostat, a plate can be secured to the proximal segment while the distal segment is further manipulated into precise reduction by placement of intermaxillary fixation. A laterally overriding fracture is easier to reduce. However, the most common displacement of the condylar fragment is medial, by pull of the lateral pterygoid muscle. If the fragment is displaced medially, the surgeon must manipulate it and convert it into a lateral override situation. The plate can be fixed with one screw to the condylar fragment and is then centered over the long axis and supported by the underlying mandibular ramus. Using the plate as a handle, the condylar fragment can be reduced anatomically. When two plates are used, the anterior plate is used to reduce and initially stabilize the condylar fragment. The second plate is placed parallel to the posterior border of the ramus.

STEP 6: Hardware Selection and Fixation

The decision to place one or two plates is based on fracture morphology, the amount of bone available to hold plates and screws, and the surgeon's preference. The first screw should be placed in the plate hole adjacent to the fracture site of the proximal segment. This is critical in segment control, although often times at this point, if maxillomandibular fixation was used, reduction has already been established. A single heavier plate can be used if limited bone is available for plating. This plate is placed along the long axis of the condylar process. If two miniplates are used, they are applied in a triangular fashion with one plate below the sigmoid notch and one plate along the posterior border.

STEP 7: Closure of the Incision

Reapproximation of the pterygomasseteric sling is carried out with a slow-resorbing suture (e.g., 3-0 polyglactin) in an interrupted fashion. The same suture is then used in a running fashion to close the platysma, SMAS, and parotid capsule in a single watertight layer to prevent parotid fistula formation. Then, resorbable interrupted subcutaneous sutures are placed, followed by skin closure. Alternatively, a subcuticular stitch with Steri-Strips can be used.

ALTERNATIVE TECHNIQUE #1

RETROMANDIBULAR (RETROPAROTID) APPROACH

The retromandibular technique varies from the retromandibular transparotid technique in that the incision is about 1 cm posterior and follows the anterior edge of the sternocleidomastoid muscle. In addition, the parotid gland is lifted rather than dissected through. The exposure of the mandible is more posterior, and access to the anterior aspect of the ramus is difficult. An oblique incision is made through the SMAS. The posterior aspect of the parotid gland is identified and dissected forward, exposing the masseter muscle. An incision is made through the pterygomasseteric sling on the posterior aspect of the ramus, exposing the fracture site.

TRANSMASSETERIC (ANTEROPAROTID) APPROACH

The anteroparotid transmasseteric approach can be accomplished through a variety of incision designs including the submandibular (modified Risdon),[1] preauricular,[2] or rhytidectomy[3] approach[4]. The periangular approach—which, in and of itself, has several variations[5,6]—is advantageous in the ease of access it provides to low subcondylar fractures, while avoiding potential injury the facial nerve trunk.[5] This particular variation of the periangular approach is designed to place the incision and dissection in between the marginal mandibular and buccal branches of the facial nerve.

The incision is designed by measuring the distance from the tragus to the angle of the mandible, and dividing and marking that distance into thirds. The same distance is similarly marked and divided into thirds from the angle anteriorly along the inferior border of the mandible. The two markings closest to the angle are then connected in a curvilinear design to outline the skin incision. The superior skin edge is gently retracted superiorly (toward the fracture line). Using a nerve stimulator to check for the marginal mandibular branch, the SMAS and parotidomasseteric fascia are undermined and incised parallel and superior to the skin incision, exposing the masseter muscle, which should be just deep to the fascial layer. In the event that the marginal mandibular branch is located particularly superiorly, it is alternatively acceptable to divide the fascia below the nerve. In either case, the masseter is then bluntly divided with a hemostat exposing the fracture site.

PREAURICULAR APPROACH

The preauricular incision is made in the crease and is marked from the root of the helix to the lobule-facial junction; the surgeon must ensure that the incision is no farther anterior than 0.8 cm from the external auditory canal to avoid injury to the temporal branch of the facial nerve.[15] The dissection is then continued sharply through the temporoparietal fascia to expose the glistening superficial layer of temporalis fascia. The zygomatic arch is palpated, and the temporalis fascia is incised obliquely parallel to the frontal branch of the facial nerve, the zygomatic arch. The surgeon should then insert the periosteal elevator and enlarge the dissection, exposing the zygomatic arch, capsule of the temporomandibular joint, and the condylar neck inferiorly. Visualization of the neck and ramus is limited by this technique.

Continued

ALTERNATIVE TECHNIQUES #1—cont'd

SUBMANDIBULAR APPROACH

For the submandibular approach, a 4- to 5-cm incision is placed approximately 1.5 cm inferior to the mandible within the skin crease or parallel to resting skin tension lines to avoid damage to the marginal mandibular branch. A local anesthetic with a vasoconstrictor is injected in a subcutaneous plane, with care taken to stay superficial to the platysma and thus avoid inadvertent anesthesia of the facial nerve. Nerve stimulation typically should be done past the incision of the platysma, beginning on the deep surface of the platysma muscle and the superficial layer of the deep cervical fascia. Incision through the cervical fascia should be at the same level as the skin incision to avoid inadvertent damage to underlying neurovascular structures. At the premasseteric notch, the marginal mandibular branch of the facial nerve is often visualized passing superficial to the facial artery and vein. If encountered, facial vessels are isolated, clamped, and ligated. Needle electrocautery or a #15 blade is used to sharply incise through the avascular pterygomasseteric sling and periosteum on the inferior and posterior mandibular borders. This approach provides wide access to the ramus, angle, and condylar neck. Access to and hardware fixation of the proximal fracture segment are difficult using this technique and may require aggressive retraction for a brief period.

INTRAORAL APPROACH

For the intraoral approach, the incision is carried superiorly along the external oblique ridge to the level of the sigmoid notch. The long buccal nerve crosses the anterior region in this area and should be identified if further extension is necessary. Subperiosteal dissection is carried out to expose the lateral ramus and condylar process. Dissection should be carried to the posterior aspect of the distal and proximal segments to facilitate retractor placement and segment control. Lighted retractors or endoscopic visualization can be invaluable during the intraoral approach. Placement of a transbuccal trocar facilitates stabilization and fixation.

ALTERNATIVE ENDOSCOPIC TECHNIQUE #2

INTRAORAL APPROACH

A 2-cm incision is made on the external oblique ridge, similar to the traditional intraoral approach. Subperiosteal dissection is performed, exposing the lateral ramus, angle, and condylar process. The optical retractor is then placed and secured on the posterior mandibular border under direct visualization. A 4-mm, 30-degree endoscope is introduced. Numerous endoscopic hooks, straight and curved elevators, and a transbuccal mandibular angle screw can be used to assist in endoscopic fracture reduction. A transbuccal trocar or the right-angle screwdriver is used for the placement of screws for fixation.

EXTRAORAL APPROACH

For the extraoral approach, a 1.5-cm incision is made two fingerbreadths below the angle of the mandible, similar to the open submandibular incision technique. Once past the platysma, blunt dissection is carried to the inferior border of the mandible. A sharp incision is made through the pterygomasseteric sling with a cautery at the inferior border of the mandible using a #15 blade. The sharp dissection is continued down to the bone of the mandibular angle. A subperiosteal plane is established with suction-assisted endoscopic elevators; this helps create an optical cavity, which aids illumination and visualization. A 2.7-mm-diameter, 30-degree endoscope is placed through the incision and oriented parallel to the posterior border with direct access to the ramus condyle unit. A curved, long-handled retractor is placed to maintain the optical cavity. A long-handled, narrow-tipped clamp is used to grasp the condylar neck and position the condylar head in the fossa. After fracture reduction, the distracted mandible is released, wedging the two segments together. A five-hole, 2-mm plate is positioned, and the two proximal screws are placed percutaneously through a trocar.

Avoidance and Management of Intraoperative Complications

Meticulous dissection and maintaining the correct anatomic plane are critical to minimizing inadvertent neural or vascular injury. In the preauricular region, the temporal branch of the facial nerve crosses the zygomatic arch at a distance 8 to 35 mm anterior to the external auditory canal.[27] Incision through the superficial layer of temporalis fascia and periosteum at the root of the zygoma maintains a safe distance and avoids inadvertent nerve injury. Furthermore, the average distance from the inferior bony external auditory canal and facial nerve bifurcation is 2.3 cm.[27] This is the rationale for beginning the retromandibular incision 0.5 cm below the earlobe. Also in this region, the facial nerve crosses immediately lateral to the retromandibular vein. The retromandibular vein is located posterior to the mandibular ramus, just lateral to the external carotid artery and within or just deep to the parotid gland. If inadvertent injury to any of these major vessels occurs, isolation and ligation must be carried out. If intraoperative facial nerve injury is noted, primary repair should be undertaken. Gentle retraction and "tenting" of the tissues is vital to maximize visualization of the fracture segments and avoid neuropraxic injury. Using a trocar to place fixation screws is acceptable and at times necessary to avoid excessive tension on the tissues. When the periosteum and pterygomasseteric sling are closed, subperiosteal reflection of the medial pterygoid muscle a few millimeters facilitates closure and avoidance of inadvertent injury to major vessels nearby. Passing the suture needle parallel to the anticipated direction of the facial nerve minimizes inadvertent ligation of the facial nerve and the poor outcome of an operating room takeback. Watertight closure of the SMAS layer minimizes the chance of a salivary fistula forming. A well-placed pressure dressing kept on for 24 hours minimizes the chance of postoperative formation of a hematoma or sialocele.

Postoperative Considerations

The overall complication rates for the surgical management of condylar fractures are low. Ellis et al. found hypertrophic or wide scars in 7.5% of patients, most commonly in African American patients. He also noted that 17.2% of patients had facial nerve weakness at the 6-week point, but all had resolved by 6 months.[27] Facial asymmetry is a well-documented complication of closed treatment and should be discussed with patients before this management option is chosen. Hematomas occasionally occur postoperatively and are usually monitored and treated with direct pressure, although aspiration sometimes is required. If sudden neck expansion, a pulsatile mass, or airway compromise is evident, a return to the operating room is necessary for isolation and ligation of the source. Parotid fistulas develop in fewer than 3% of cases with the transparotid approach described previously. Clear, persistent serous drainage from the incision should alert the surgeon to this possibility. These cases typically resolve spontaneously or with the aid of an elastic pressure dressing. Botulinum toxin has been described recently for use with refractory parotid fistulas. Fortunately, Frey syndrome and postoperative infections are rare.

References

1. Lindahl L. Condylar fractures of the mandible. I. Classification and relation to age, occlusion, and concomitant injuries of teeth and teeth-supporting structures, and fractures of the mandibular body. *Int J Oral Surg.* 1977;6(1):12–21.
2. Spiessl B. Rigid internal fixation of fractures of the lower jaw. *Reconstr Surg Traumatol.* 1972;13:124–140.
3. Neff A, Kolk A, Deppe H, Horch HH. Neue Aspekte zur Indikation der operativen Versorgung intraartikulärer und hoher Kiefergelenkluxationsfrakturen. *Mund Kiefer Gesichtschir.* 1999;3(1):24–29.
4. Bhagol A, Singh V, Kumar I, Verma A. Prospective evaluation of a new classification system for the management of mandibular subcondylar fractures. *J Oral Maxillofac Surg.* 2011;69(4):1159–1165.
5. Loukota RA, Eckelt U, De Bont L, Rasse M. Subclassification of fractures of the condylar process of the mandible. *Br J Oral Maxillofac Surg.* 2005;43(1):72–73.
6. Loukota RA, Neff A, Rasse M. Nomenclature/classification of fractures of the mandibular condylar head. *Br J Oral Maxillofac Surg.* 2010;48(6):477–478.
7. Ellis E, Throckmorton GS. Celso Palmieri, Open treatment of condylar process fractures: assessment of adequacy of repositioning and maintenance of stability, *J Oral Maxillofac Surg.* 2000;58(1):27–34. ISSN 0278-2391, https://doi.org/10.1016/S0278-2391(00)80010-5.
8. Singh V, Bhagol A, Goel M, Kumar I, Verma A. Outcomes of open versus closed treatment of mandibular subcondylar fractures: a prospective randomized study. *J Oral Maxillofac Surg.* 2010;68(6):1304–1309.
9. Kyzas PA, Saeed A, Tabbenor O. The treatment of mandibular condyle fractures: a meta-analysis. *J Cranio-Maxillo-Fac Surg.* 2012;40(8):e438–e452.
10. Hinds EC. Correction of prognathism by subcondylar osteotomy. *J Oral Surg (Chic).* 1958;16(3):209–214.
11. Ellis J, Zide MF. *Surgical Approaches to the Facial Skeleton.* 2nd ed. Philadelphia, PA: Lippincott Williams & Wilkins; 2006.
12. Zide MF, Kent JN. Indications for open reduction of mandibular condyle fractures. *J Oral Maxillofac Surg.* 1983;41(2):89–98.
13. Mitchell DA. A multicentre audit of unilateral fractures of the mandibular condyle. *Br J Oral Maxillofac Surg.* 1997;35(4):230–236.
14. Banks P. A pragmatic approach to the management of condylar fractures. *Int J Oral Maxillofac Surg.* 1998;27(4):244–246.
15. Ellis E III, Simon P, Throckmorton GS. Occlusal results after open or closed treatment of fractures of the mandibular condylar process. *J Oral Maxillofac Surg.* 2000;58(3):260–268.
16. Brandt MT, Haug RH. Open versus closed reduction of adult mandibular condyle fractures: a review of the literature regarding the evolution of current thoughts on management. *J Oral Maxillofac Surg.* 2003;61(11):1324–1332.
17. Terai H, Shimahara M. Closed treatment of condylar fractures by intermaxillary fixation with thermoforming plates. *Br J Oral Maxillofac Surg.* 2004;42(1):61–63.
18. Davis BR, Powell JE, Morrison AD. Free-grafting of mandibular condyle fractures: clinical outcomes in 10 consecutive patients. *Int J Oral Maxillofac Implants.* 2005;34(8):871–876.
19. Tominaga K, Habu M, Khanal A, Mimori Y, Yoshioka I, Fukuda J. Biomechanical evaluation of different types of rigid internal fixation techniques for subcondylar fractures. *J Oral Maxillofac Surg.* 2006;64(10):1510–1516.
20. Schneider M, Erasmus F, Gerlach KL, et al. Open reduction and internal fixation versus closed treatment and mandibulomaxillary fixation of fractures of the mandibular condylar process: a randomized, prospective, multicenter study with special evaluation of fracture level. *J Oral Maxillofac Surg.* 2008;66(12):2537–2544.
21. Al-Kayat A, Bramley P. A modified pre-auricular approach to the temporomandibular joint and malar arch. *Br J Oral Surg.* 1979;17(2):91–103.
22. Kellman RM, Cienfuegos R. Endoscopic approaches to subcondylar fractures of the mandible. *Facial Plast Surg.* 2009;25(1):23–28.
23. Troulis MJ, Perrott DH, Kaban LB. Endoscopic mandibular osteotomy, and placement and activation of a semiburied distractor. *J Oral Maxillofac Surg.* 1999;57(9):1110–1113.
24. Schmelzeisen R, Cienfuegos-Monroy R, Schön R, Chen CT, Cunningham L Jr, Goldhahn S. Patient benefit from endoscopically assisted fixation of condylar neck fractures—a randomized controlled trial. *J Oral Maxillofac Surg.* 2009;67(1):147–158.
25. Troulis MJ, Kaban LB. Endoscopic approach to the ramus/condyle unit: clinical applications. *J Oral Maxillofac Surg.* 2001;59(5):503–509.
26. Iatrou I, Theologie-Lygidakis N, Tzerbos F. Surgical protocols and outcome for the treatment of maxillofacial fractures in children: 9 years' experience. *J Cranio-Maxillo-Fac Surg.* 2010;38(7):511–516.
27. Ellis E III, McFadden D, Simon P, Throckmorton G. Surgical complications with open treatment of mandibular condylar process fractures. *J Oral Maxillofac Surg.* 2000;58(9):950–958.

CHAPTER 79

Atrophic Edentulous Mandibular Fractures

Jeffrey S. Marschall, George M. Kushner, and Brian Alpert

Armamentarium

#15 Scalpel blade or monopolar electrocautery
Appropriate sutures
Army-Navy retractors
Autogenous bone grafting source with instrumentation
Dingman bone clamps
Freeze-dried bone allograft
Large rake retractors
Local anesthetic with vasoconstrictor
Nerve stimulation unit
Rigid fixation set with appropriate (2.3 or greater) locking and nonlocking plates, screws, and instrumentation
Vessel loops

History of the Procedure

Although it is estimated that 19% of adults aged 65 and over are edentulous in the US,[1] atrophic edentulous mandibular fractures are relatively uncommon,[2] representing 1% of all facial fractures.[3] These fractures are generally associated with long periods of edentulism and denture wearing. While usually associated with advanced age, mandibular atrophy is related more to actual time in dentures than actual age. As people retain their teeth longer (as a result of fluoride and other preventive measures), the prospect of edentulism and dentures will be delayed, so that encountering this particular fracture in the rapidly expanding elderly population will become less likely.

Atrophic edentulous mandibular fractures present unique challenges. Patients are often elderly or infirm.[4] The bone has less osteogenic potential and diminished healing capacity.[5,6] It is usually entirely cortical in nature, the character of porcelain. To be classified as atrophic, the remaining bone height must be 15 mm or less. Severely atrophic mandibular fractures are less than 10 mm in height.[7,8] Less bony height translates into less surface area for bony healing and buttressing.[9,10] These factors lead to an increased incidence of complications in the form of nonunion, malunion, recurrent fractures after repair, hardware failure, poor function with prolonged convalescence, and postoperative infection, osteomyelitis, and the need for additional reconstructive procedures. The incidence of these complications is 10% to 20%.[9–13]

Historical forms of treatment have all been directed toward fracture immobilization. Past techniques may be viewed as unnecessary or obsolete due to newer, more predictable techniques; however, there may be rare indications for their use. If a patient is unable to undergo general anesthesia or a long operative procedure, skeletal pin fixation techniques remain reasonable alternatives.

Gunning Splints

The Gunning splints technique is credited to Thomas Gunning, who used these splints to treat dentulous mandibular fractures as early as 1863. GV Black used maxillary and mandibular splints for edentulous patients. First, impressions are made of the patient's maxillary and mandibular ridges. The mandibular cast then is cut and realigned to correct the fracture displacement. Splints (one- or two-piece) are constructed that align the jaws in their correct position. As an alternative, when the patient has existing dentures, the dentures can be modified to function as splints. An opening is always made in the anterior region for food to be ingested. The splint or splints (or modified dentures) are retained with circummandibular/circumzygomatic/piriform aperture wires, which have significant comorbidities of their own. Later variations of these techniques used screws to retain the splints. Experience has shown that elderly, infirm patients do not tolerate maxillomandibular fixation (MMF) very well, and they deteriorate rapidly (Fig. 79.1).

Monomandibular Fixation/Circummandibular Wires Around a Preexisting Denture

When an existing mandibular denture that spans the fracture is available, it may be used with 22- or 24-gauge wire for fracture reduction and stabilization. An awl is passed percutaneously on the lingual surface of the mandible and introduced into the floor of the mouth. A wire is then introduced into the eyelet, and the awl is passed around the inferior border of the mandible and

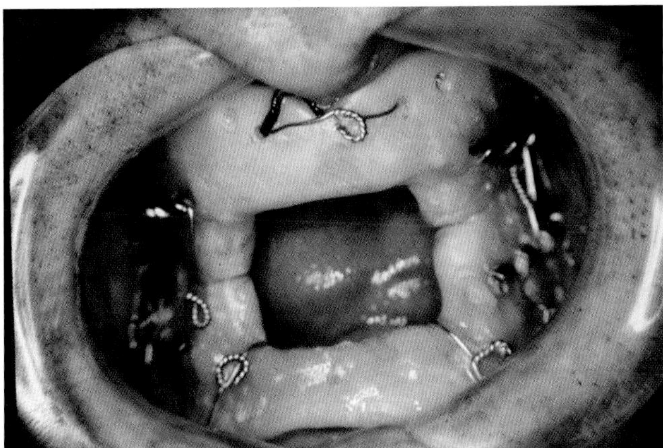

Figure 79.1 Gunning splints.

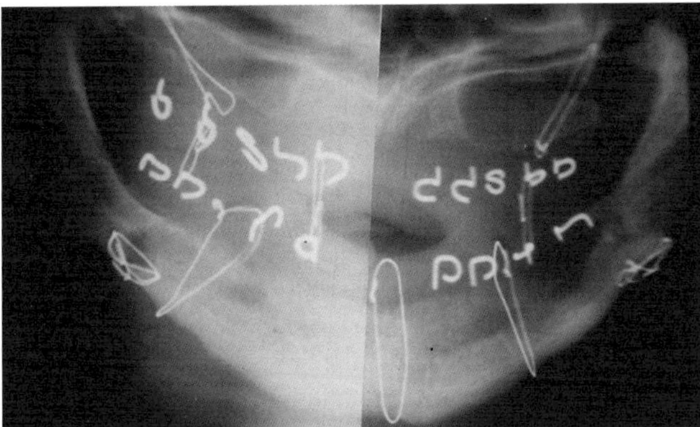

Figure 79.2 Radiograph of circummandibular wires securing a denture in place.

advanced into the buccal vestibule. This technique may be performed at several sites. The wire then is twisted down over the denture to immobilize the fracture. Caution must be exercised to avoid placing a wire into the fracture site, which would result in poor healing. This technique is easier in principle than in practice and has generally less-than-optimal results (Fig. 79.2).

External Fixator: Skeletal Pin Fixation

The most often cited external fixator is the biphasic connector described by Morris.[14] This technique relies on the placement of fixation pins in sound bone. After satisfactory reduction of the fracture with a first-phase metal frame, the pins are splinted with an acrylic bar that is placed over the fixation pins and metal framework and allowed to cure. The metal frame is removed, resulting in a simple, lightweight appliance. Pitfalls of the procedure include blind placement of the pins in the inferior alveolar nerve and inadequate pin stabilization due to fracture comminution or inadequate bone stock for pin placement (Fig. 79.3).

K-Wire Shish Kebab

For the K-wire shish kebab technique, a K-wire is driven into the medullary space while the fracture is held reduced. The fracture is exposed extraorally, and a K-wire 2- to 4-mm in diameter is driven through the distal fragment and out through the skin overlying the chin. The fracture is held in reduced position, and the K-wire (protruding through the skin) is driven back across the fracture into the proximal fragment. This procedure is done with essentially no periosteal dissection and could be considered a conservative approach. However, placement of the K-wire does not prevent rotational movement of the fracture segments and is extremely technique sensitive (Fig. 79.4).[15]

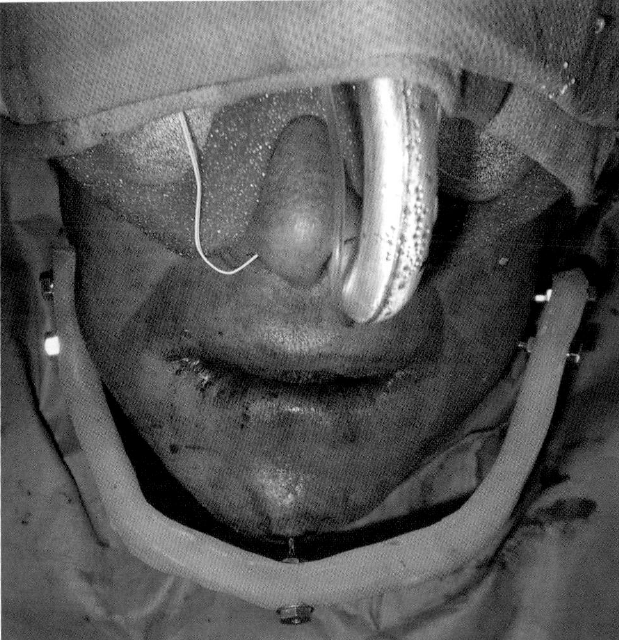

Figure 79.3 Joe Hall Morris biphasic appliance.

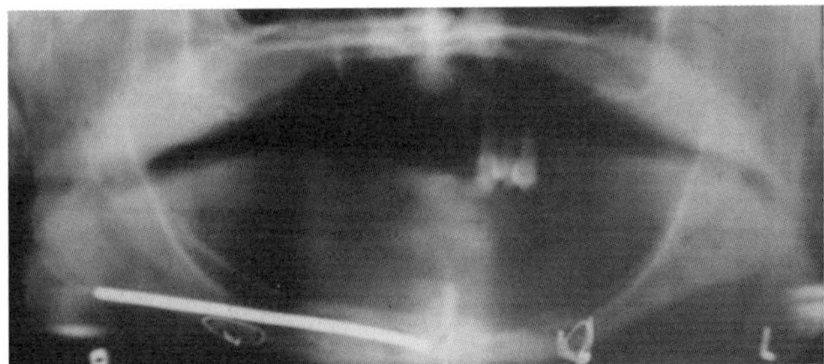

Figure 79.4 Radiograph of K-wire technique.

Split Ribs

Various approaches to gain increased buttressing or support of the bone at the fracture site have been advocated. Obwegeser used split ribs medially and laterally across the fracture, which were held in place with circummandibular wires. As rigid internal fixation was developing, the approach to both fracture management and mandibular reconstruction with either autogenous or freeze-dried rib grafts supplemented with autogenous marrow was advocated. This technique had some success, but the postoperative complications of pneumothorax were potentially devastating in elderly patients.[3,16,17]

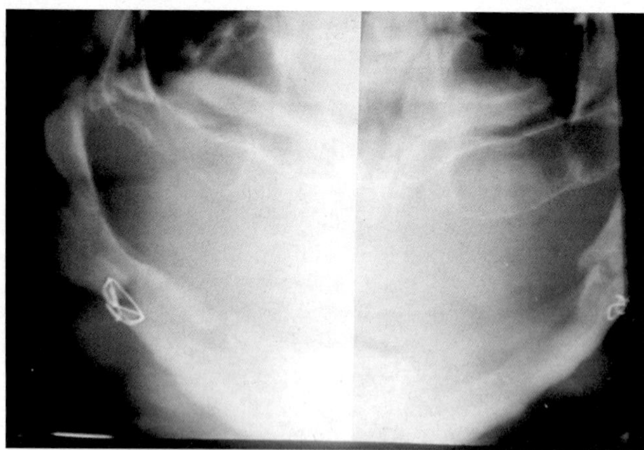

Figure 79.5 Radiograph of interior border wiring.

Mesh

Both vitallium and titanium mesh have been used for fixation of the fracture and as part of the reconstructive technique. After initial fracture reduction and stabilization, this technique has been used to gain rigid fixation and bulk. Generally, a titanium mesh is placed around the inferior and lateral borders of the atrophic mandible. Particulate (typically autogenous) bone from either the iliac crest or tibia is then placed under the mesh. More recently, this technique has been described using a resorbable mesh.[18] The advantage of the newer technique is that it should eliminate the need for a second surgery to remove the mesh once the graft has consolidated.

Wire Open Reduction

Before the use of plates and screws developed, this technique likely was the most common approach to fracture stabilization. In most cases it was used in addition to MMF with splints or dentures. The inferior border was approached, and stainless steel wires were passed through the inferior cortex and twisted to immobilize the fracture. This technique may still be used to temporarily immobilize the fracture while rigid internal fixation is placed with plates and screws (Fig. 79.5).

Conservative Approach: No Treatment

Although it does not seem like a reasonable option, minimally displaced fractures that are grossly stable on clinical examination may be managed nonoperatively. A dependable patient who is willing to adhere to a liquid diet and minimal function of the mandible would be a candidate for this approach. Likewise, this should be considered in patients unable to undergo a major surgical procedure.

Rigid fixation has resulted in improved fracture management and simplified convalescence. Although the treatment of atrophic mandibular fractures is not easy, rigid fixation has shortened the course of treatment, and outcomes have improved.[19]

Indications for the Use of the Procedure

Diagnosis of atrophic edentulous mandibular fractures is easily observed when bilateral mandibular bodies are fractured. This gives the patient a "bucket handle" fracture appearance (Fig. 79.6A). This is usually accompanied by facial or perioral ecchymosis (Fig. 79.6B). Generally, displacement and mobility of the fractures can be noted easily on bimanual clinical examination. Nondisplaced fractures and unilateral fractures can be more difficult to diagnose due to the dense cortical nature of the bone that remains in a mandible (Fig. 79.6C). Once a diagnosis has been made, the indications for the procedure include one or more of the following: radiographic and physical evidence of fracture, inability to function, airway compromise, gross mandibular mobility, poorly fitting denture, neurosensory disturbances, and pain secondary to fracture instability.

Limitations and Contraindications

Currently, there is inadequate evidence to support a single technique to manage atrophic edentulous mandibular fractures.[20] However, with modern fixation techniques, repair of these fractures is dictated by the surgical principle of doing what you know will work rather than what you hope will work. Atrophic edentulous mandibular fractures have inadequate surface area at the fracture to allow buttressing. Load-bearing osteosynthesis with a reconstruction plate (or locking reconstruction plate) provides a rigid construct for these debilitated and biomechanically compromised mandibles. This should be the treatment of choice.

The pencil-thin mandible is highly subject to muscle pull, resulting in a great deal of stress on any fixation system (Fig. 79.7A).

Much controversy exists regarding alternative and less invasive methods to repair these fractures, such as using miniplates. The argument that less periosteal stripping leads to improved osseous union is often cited. Also, because there is no occlusion, bite forces are much diminished, which reduces the need for absolutely rigid fixation, as long as the patient functions postoperatively on a soft diet. Additional arguments include ease of adaptation of the plates to bone and the ability to use smaller monocortical screws that lend themselves to placement in smaller bone areas.[21–24] However, displacement, comminution, lack of potential for load sharing, and muscle pull, which characterize these injuries, call for load-bearing osteosynthesis. In addition, the "wish boning" that occurs every time a person swallows leads to rapid work hardening and fracture of miniplates. Because of these anatomic and physiologic realities, miniplates are unpredictable in severely atrophic mandibular fractures.[25] Unless there is adequate buttressing to allow load sharing, they are contraindicated (Fig. 79.7B).

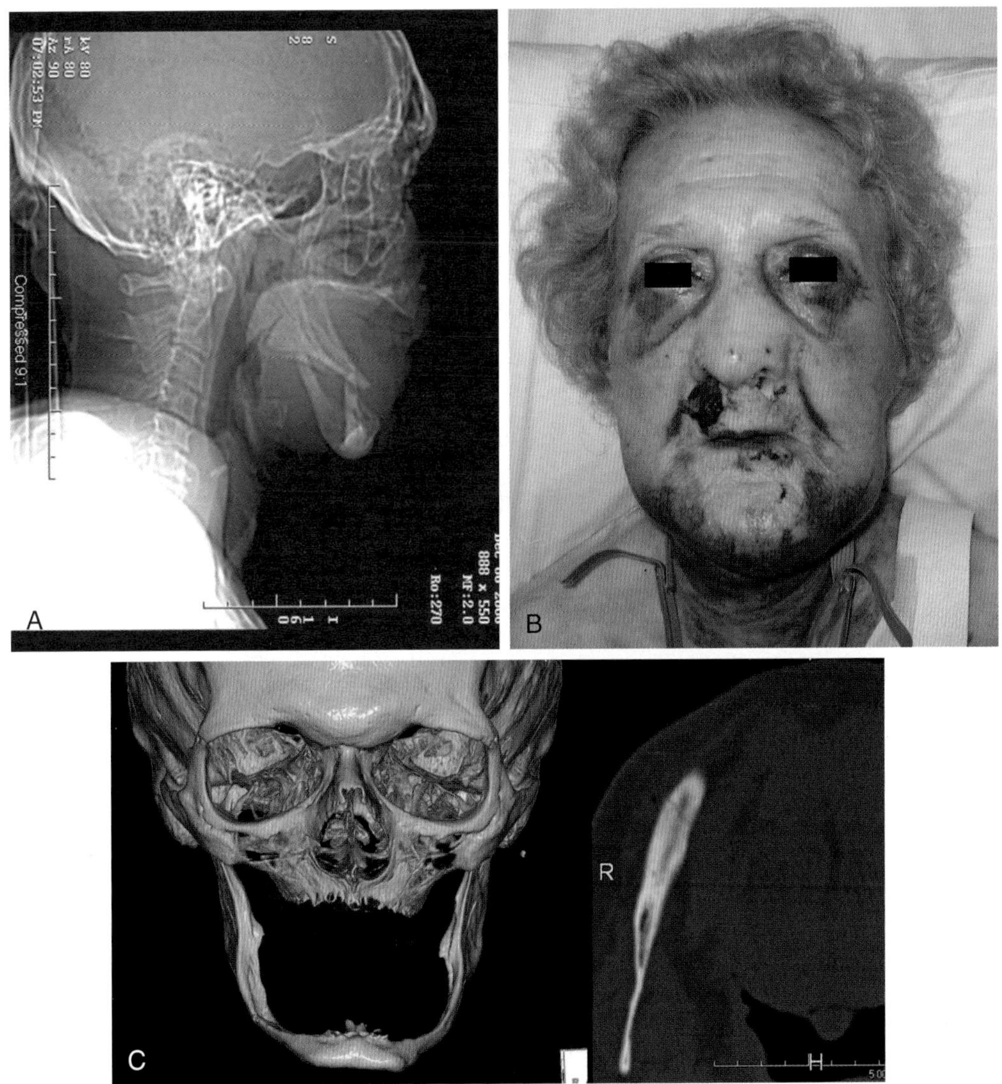

Figure 79.6 **A,** Radiograph of bilateral "bucket handle" body fractures. **B,** Facial ecchymosis associated with injury. **C,** Nondisplaced, unilateral fracture.

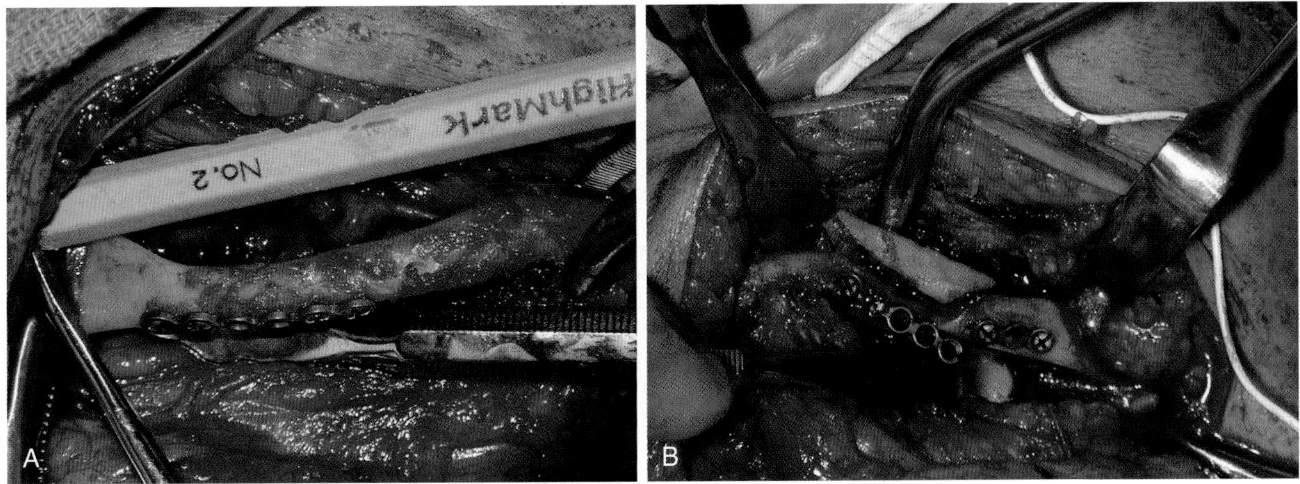

Figure 79.7 **A,** Photograph showing atrophy of the remaining bone. **B,** Fractured construct of miniplates.

TECHNIQUE: Transcervical Approach to the Atrophic Mandible

STEP 1: Incision Marking

Using a well-defined neck crease, mark a cervical apron-type incision that allows adequate exposure to the mandibular symphysis, bilateral mandibular bodies, and bilateral mandibular rami to approximately the region of the angles. Injection of a local anesthetic with a vasoconstrictor is preferred after the incision has been marked to avoid distorting the cervical anatomy during marking (Fig. 79.8A).

STEP 2: Incision

The incision is made with a #10 or #15 blade. It should be carried through the skin, into the supraplatysmal fat, and down to the platysma. Electrocautery may be used to control and superficial bleeding. The platysma is sharply divided, and the dissection is carried into the deep cervical fascia. A nerve stimulator may be used to identify the marginal mandibular branch of the facial nerve. If necessary, the facial artery and vein are identified, isolated, and ligated. Dissection is then carried to the inferior border of the mandible, where adequate exposure is crucial. The periosteum is sharply incised with a #15 blade, and the inferior and lateral borders of the mandible are exposed from angle to angle (Fig. 79.8B).

STEP 3: Mobilization/Reduction of Fracture

With Dingman bone clamps, the opposing ends of the fracture are mobilized and reduced. It usually is necessary to paralyze the patient to effect reduction, which often is difficult to maintain due to minimal buttressing. This often necessitates some form of temporary immobilization (Fig. 79.8C).

STEP 4: Immobilization

Temporary immobilization is accomplished using miniplates placed at the inferior border to maintain the reduction. An aluminum template is then placed along the lateral border and molded to the bony contours. A series of Kocher clamps may be used to closely coapt the template to the mandibular anatomy (Fig. 79.8D).

STEP 5: Locking Reconstruction Plate

With the template used as a guide, a 2.4 locking reconstruction plate is contoured to the anatomy of the lateral border of the mandible. An alternative is to use a smaller 2.0 locking reconstruction plate. Often small adjustments must be made due to the length of the plate (Fig. 79.8E).

STEP 6: Rigid Fixation

Once properly contoured, the plate is rigidly fixed to the areas where the most bone is encountered, at the symphysis and bilateral angle regions. The saddle areas of the body do not lend themselves to screws (Fig. 79.8F).

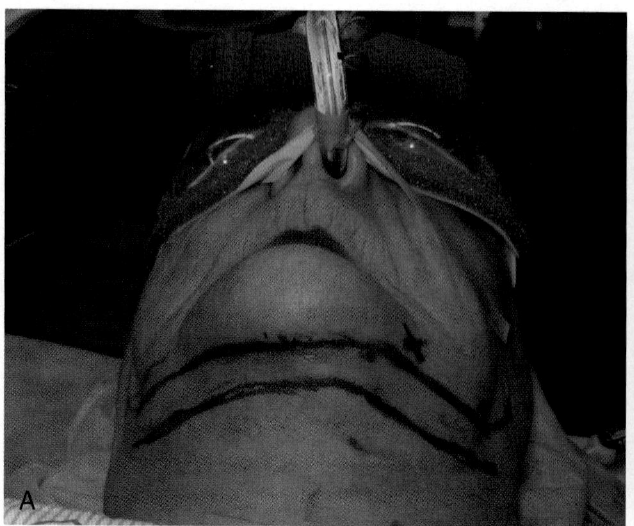

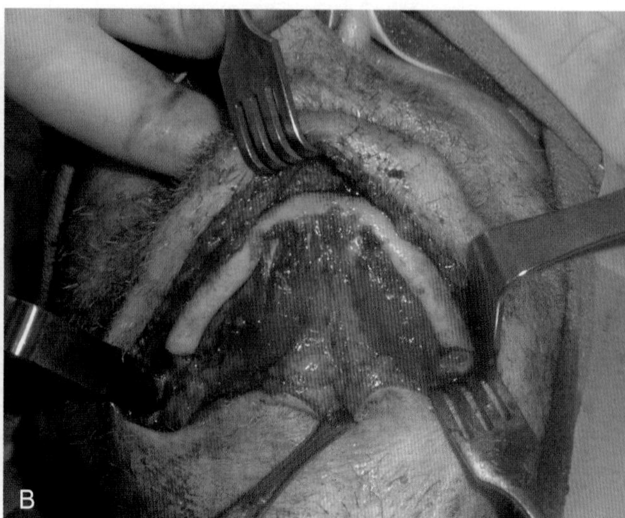

Figure 79.8 **A,** Marking the incision. **B,** Exposure of the mandible.

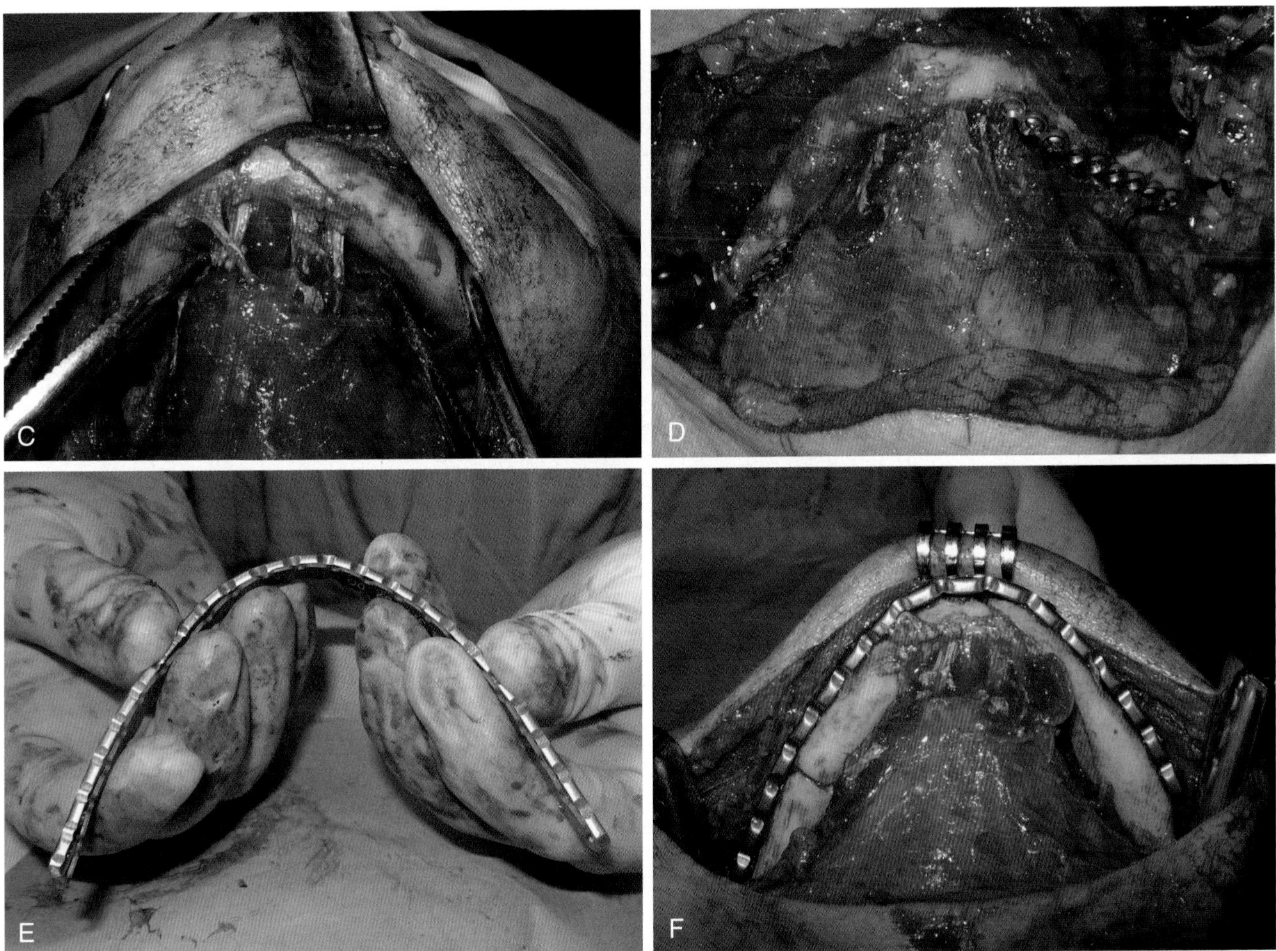

Figure 79.8, cont'd **C,** Mobilization and reduction of the fracture with bone clamps. **D,** Temporary immobilization with miniplates. **E,** Large locking reconstruction plate contoured to template. **F,** Locking reconstruction plate in place with screw fixation in symphysis and angle region.

TECHNIQUE: Transcervical Approach to the Atrophic Mandible—cont'd

STEP 7: Augmentation of Mandible

Once rigid fixation has been accomplished, the mandible may be augmented for either osteogenic potential or later implant reconstruction using grafting techniques. Autogenous grafting remains the gold standard. Tibial bone grafting may be easily accomplished with a second surgical team. In elderly patients who have vascular compromise of the lower extremities or a joint prosthesis, preventing tibial bone graft harvesting, banked allografts remain a viable option.[26] These grafts may be augmented using platelet-rich plasma and recombinant human bone morphogenetic protein-2[26] (Fig. 79.8G).

STEP 8: Closure

Once the mandible has been stabilized and augmented, careful attention is directed to closure. Ideally, periosteal closure over the graft and plate construct is performed first. Then, resuspension of divided musculature is accomplished. The platysma is reapproximated with interrupted sutures. The skin may be closed using a running 5-0 polypropylene suture. After skin closure, a compression dressing is placed (Fig. 79.8H).

Sequencing mandibular reconstruction is a decision that depends largely on experience and the patient's preference. Accomplishing rigid fixation is difficult, and the decision to proceed with additional grafting or prosthetic rehabilitation may be omitted due to anatomic compromises or health issues.[26] It has been well documented that, when more sophisticated options are available, fracture repair, bone grafting, and implant placement may be accomplished. Studies show predictable osseointegration of implants and good prosthetic rehabilitation (Fig. 79.9).[27–29]

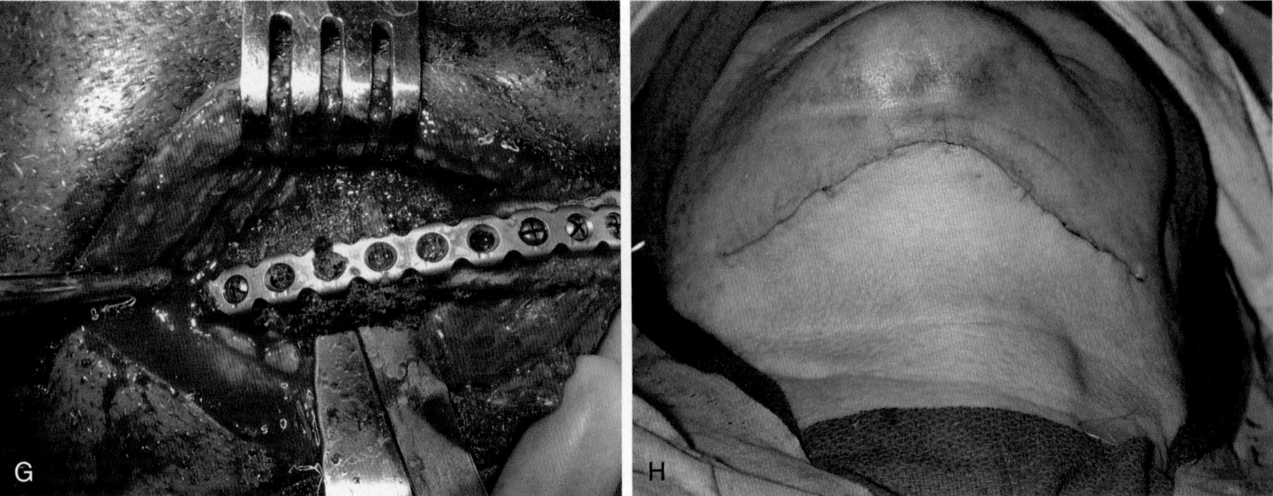

Figure 79.8, cont'd **G,** Autogenous graft around fracture. **H,** Final closure.

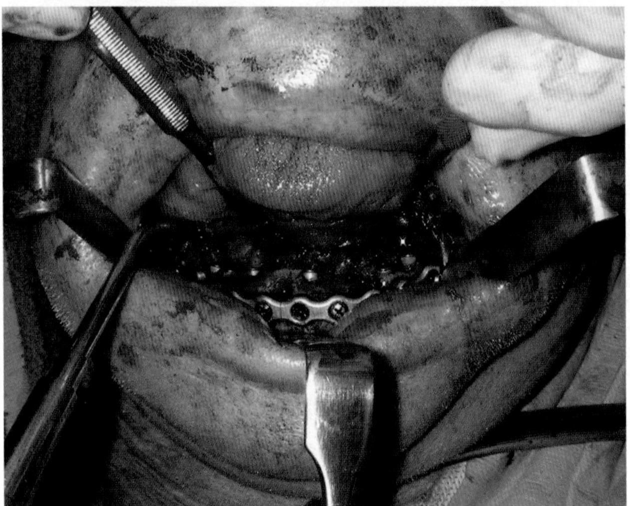

Figure 79.9 Simultaneous open reduction internal fixation, bone graft, and implant placement.

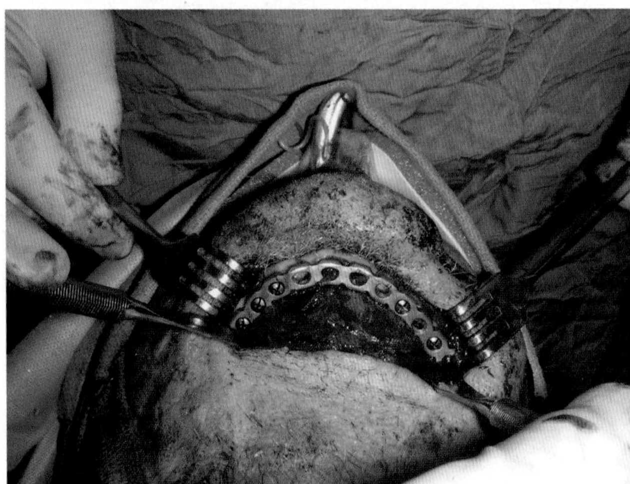

Figure 79.10 Inferior border plating technique.

ALTERNATIVE TECHNIQUE 1: Plating Inferior Border

Anatomic considerations play a big part in treatment planning of atrophic edentulous mandibular fractures. Comminuted segments, dental implants in sites where locking screws need to be placed, and shallow oral vestibules in patients who want to wear dentures must be considered. Often a large lateral border plate and a shallow vestibule make wearing a denture nearly impossible. Placement of a locking reconstruction plate at the inferior border can avoid some of these factors. The plate is contoured to the anatomy of the inferior border and then secured by locking screws in the standard fashion. In theory, this technique avoids intraoral plate dehiscence. It has been demonstrated that the biomechanics of a reconstruction plate placed on the inferior border of the mandible are similar to those of a reconstruction plate placed on the lateral border.[30] The patient may also continue to wear a prosthesis, which can further stabilize the fracture (Fig. 79.10).

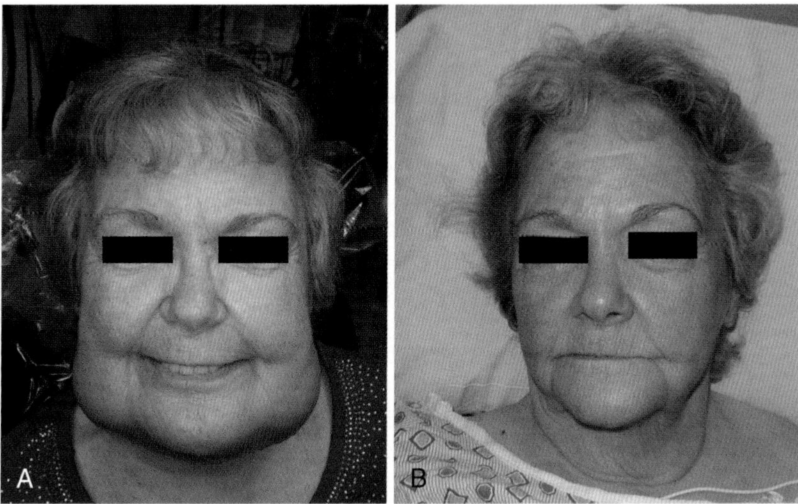

Figure 79.11 **A and B,** Postoperative swelling associated with bone morphogenic protein-2 (BMP-2).

Avoidance and Management of Intraoperative Complications

Intraoperative complications usually are related to anesthetic management and anatomic compromises. It is well known that geriatric trauma patients have higher anesthetic complications related to pulmonary and cardiac diseases. Preoperative studies should include an electrocardiogram, chest radiograph, complete blood count, and coagulation studies. Careful attention to hemostasis should prevent problematic blood loss during surgery, and our experience is that intraoperative transfusions are seldom needed.

Technology such as virtual surgical planning (VSP) and three-dimensional printing can also improve outcomes, decrease time in the operating room,[31] and help ameliorate complications such as malunion or nonunion. VSP sessions can be performed via a third party web meeting or performed in-house.[32] VSP allows for "virtual reduction" via mirror imaging of the contralateral noninjured side, or anatomic alignment of fractured segments. A milled plate can be manufactured, or alternatively, the mandible can be three-dimensionally printed and a stock reconstruction plate can be prebent using the model as a template. Surgeons should consider these technologies when encountering atrophic edentulous mandible fractures to help enhance surgical execution and help decrease surgical misadventures.

Some surgical intraoperative complications are related to the bony anatomy. Maintaining bony reduction is difficult and often requires chemical paralysis. Comminuted bony segments also make reduction more difficult. In cases of severe atrophy, additional fractures can occur during fracture manipulation and plating. Tapping of dense and/or brittle bone is often required before screw insertion. When additional procedures are attempted, such as simultaneous placement of implants, care should be taken to tap implant osteotomies also to avoid additional unnecessary stress to the remaining bone.

Postoperative Complications

Placement of patients into MMF complicates emergence from anesthesia, and the postoperative course is difficult for elderly patients. With rigid fixation, this is not as much of a concern. Although hospitalized, patients should be encouraged to ambulate as soon as possible. When a tibial bone graft has been harvested, the patient may ambulate and bear weight as tolerated on the lower extremities. In spite of the rigid construct, it is important that patients adhere to a soft diet and avoid stressing the fixation. When a reconstruction plate is placed from angle to angle with stable fixation in the symphysis, the patient is not likely to have any secondary fractures. If the plate is stopped short and terminates in the body region, the fixation may weaken the remaining bone, and the patient will develop a fracture proximal to the fixation. When bone morphogenic protein-2 is used, it is wise to advise the patient that significant postoperative swelling will occur and resolve over time (Fig. 79.11).

Balancing the complicated medical management of patients with atrophic edentulous mandibular fractures with anatomic considerations makes this fracture difficult to manage. Even though this fracture is uncommon, experience has shown that an aggressive initial approach is very effective. Extraoral open reduction with reconstruction plate fixation, in combination with particulate bone grafting, is the treatment plan of choice.[33]

References

1. Dye BA, Thornton-Evans G, Li X, Iafolla TJ. *Dental Caries and Tooth Loss in Adults in the United States, 2011–2012. NCHS Data Brief, No 197*. Hyattsville, MD: National Center for Health Statistics; 2015.
2. Ellis E III, Moos KF, el-Attar A. Ten years of mandibular fractures: an analysis of 2,137 cases. *Oral Surg Oral Med Oral Pathol*. 1985;59(2):120–129.
3. Newman L. The role of autogenous primary rib grafts in treating fractures of the atrophic edentulous mandible. *Br J Oral Maxillofac Surg*. 1995;33(6):381–386.
4. Marciani RD, Hill O. Treatment of the fractured edentulous mandible. *J Oral Surg*. 1979;37(8):569–577.
5. McGregor AD, MacDonald DG. Age changes in the human inferior alveolar artery—a histological study. *Br J Oral Maxillofac Surg*. 1989;27(5):371–374.
6. Friedman CD, Costantino PD. Facial fractures and bone healing in the geriatric patient. *Otolaryngol Clin North Am*. 1990;23(6):1109–1119.
7. Cawood JI, Howell RA, Howell RA. A classification of the edentulous jaws. *Int J Oral Maxillofac Surg*. 1988;17(4):232–236.
8. Cawood JI, Howell RA. Reconstructive preprosthetic surgery. I. Anatomical considerations. *Int J Oral Maxillofac Surg*. 1991;20(2):75–82.
9. Wittwer G, Adeyemo WL, Turhani D, Ploder O. Treatment of atrophic mandibular fractures based on the degree of atrophy—experience with different plating systems: a retrospective study. *J Oral Maxillofac Surg*. 2006;64(2):230–234.
10. Sikes JW Jr, Smith BR, Mukherjee DP. An in vitro study of the effect of bony buttressing on fixation strength of a fractured atrophic edentulous mandible model. *J Oral Maxillofac Surg*. 2000;58(1):56–61.
11. Bruce RA, Strachan DS. Fractures of the edentulous mandible by compression plating: a retrospective evaluation of 84 consecutive cases. *J Oral Maxillofac Surg*. 1996;54:254.
12. Bruce RA, Ellis E III. The second Chalmers J. Lyons Academy study of fractures of the edentulous mandible. *J Oral Maxillofac Surg*. 1993;51(8):904–911.
13. Luhr HG, Reidick T, Merten HA. Results of treatment of fractures of the atrophic edentulous mandible by compression plating: a retrospective evaluation of 84 consecutive cases. *J Oral Maxillofac Surg*. 1996;54(3):250–254.
14. Morris JH. Biphase connector: external skeletal splint for reduction and fixation of mandible fractures. *Oral Surg*. 1949;2:402.
15. Bisi RH. The management of mandibular fractures in edentulous patients by intramedullary pinning. *Laryngoscope*. 1973;83(1):22–38.
16. Woods WR, Hiatt WR, Brooks RL. A technique for simultaneous fracture repair and augmentation of the atrophic edentulous mandible. *J Oral Surg*. 1979;37(2):131–135.
17. Baker RD, Terry BC, Davis WH, Connole PW. Long-term results of alveolar ridge augmentation. *J Oral Surg*. 1979;37(7):486–489.
18. Louis P, Holmes J, Fernandes R. Resorbable mesh as a containment system in reconstruction of the atrophic mandible fracture. *J Oral Maxillofac Surg*. 2004;62(6):719–723.
19. Ellis E III, Price C. Treatment protocol for fractures of the atrophic mandible. *J Oral Maxillofac Surg*. 2008;66(3):421–435.
20. Nasser M, Fedorowicz Z, Ebadifar A. Management of the fractured edentulous atrophic mandible. *Cochrane Database Syst Rev*. 2007;24(1):CD006087.
21. Melo AR, de Aguiar Soares Carneiro SC, Leal JL, Vasconcelos BC. Fracture of the atrophic mandible: case series and critical review. *J Oral Maxillofac Surg*. 2011;69(5):1430–1435.
22. Clayman L, Rossi E. Fixation of atrophic edentulous mandible fractures by bone plating at the inferior border. *J Oral Maxillofac Surg*. 2012;70(4):883–889.
23. Sugiura T, Yamamoto K, Murakami K, et al. Biomechanical analysis of miniplate osteosynthesis for fractures of the atrophic mandible. *J Oral Maxillofac Surg*. 2009;67(11):2397–2403.
24. Mugino H, Takagi S, Oya R, Nakamura S, Ikemura K. Miniplate osteosynthesis of fractures of the edentulous mandible. *Clin Oral Investig*. 2005;9(4):266–270.
25. Madsen MJ, Kushner GM, Alpert B. Failed fixation in atrophic mandibular fractures: the case against miniplates. *Craniomaxillofac Trauma Reconstr*. 2011;4(3):145.
26. Van Sickels JE, Cunningham LL. Management of atrophic mandible fractures: are bone grafts necessary? *J Oral Maxillofac Surg*. 2010;68(6):1392–1395.
27. Marx RE, Shellenberger T, Wimsatt J, Correa P. Severely resorbed mandible: predictable reconstruction with soft tissue matrix expansion (tent pole) grafts. *J Oral Maxillofac Surg*. 2002;60(8):878–888.
28. Eyrich GK, Grätz KW, Sailer HF. Surgical treatment of fractures of the edentulous mandible. *J Oral Maxillofac Surg*. 1997;55(10):1081–1087.
29. Korpi JT, Kainulainen VT, Sándor GK, Oikarinen KS. Long-term follow-up of severely resorbed mandibles reconstructed using tent pole technique without platelet-rich plasma. *J Oral Maxillofac Surg*. 2012;70(11):2543–2548.
30. Madsen MJ, Haug RH. A biomechanical comparison of 2 techniques for reconstructing atrophic edentulous mandible fractures. *J Oral Maxillofac Surg*. 2006;64(3):457–465.
31. Castro-Núñez J, Shelton JM, Snyder S, Sickels JV. Virtual surgical planning for the management of severe atrophic mandible fractures. *Craniomaxillofac Trauma Reconstr*. 2018;11(2):150–156.
32. Marschall JS, Dutra V, Flint RL, et al. In-house digital workflow for the management of acute mandible fractures. *J Oral Maxillofac Surg*. 2019;77(10):2084.e1–2084.e9.
33. Tiwana PS, Abraham MS, Kushner GM, Alpert B. Management of atrophic edentulous mandibular fractures: the case for primary reconstruction with immediate bone grafting. *J Oral Maxillofac Surg*. 2009;67(4):882–887.

CHAPTER 80

Comminuted Mandibular Fractures

David B. Powers

Armamentarium

#9 Molt periosteal elevator
#15 Scalpel blades
Appropriate sutures
Bipolar electrocautery
Bone reduction forceps
Circular gel headrest
Comprehensive/clear radiographic studies, preferably with 3D reconstruction
Dental elastic bands
Erich arch bars
External fixator appliance
Hemostats
Local anesthetic with vasoconstrictor
Locking reconstruction plates
Mandibular trauma fixation set/plates
Miniplates (for simplification of fractures)
Minnesota retractor
Mouth props
Needle drivers
Needle-tip electrocautery
Percutaneous nerve stimulator
Pickle fork
Power equipment for drills
Saline irrigation
Self-retaining cheek retractors
Stainless steel surgical wire (24, 26, 28 gauge)
Suture scissors
Universal fracture plates
Vascular clips
Weider (sweetheart) retractor
Wire cutters
Wire drivers

History of the Procedure

Comminuted mandibular fractures occur when an excessive amount of force, and associated energy transfer, occurs to the osseous structures of the mandible. Frequently caused today by motor vehicle accidents or striking a rigid, nonmoveable structure, these fractures have been seen in Europe since the introduction of gunpowder and ballistic projectiles to warfare in the 14th century.[1] The historical treatment of comminuted mandibular fractures focused on the principle of closed management, used primarily to avoid stripping the periosteum and subsequent blood supply from the comminuted bony segments. A variety of surgical techniques, such as maxillomandibular fixation (MMF), surgeon-fabricated occlusal splints or Gunning splints, and extraoral skeletal pins, were used, with varying degrees of success and patient outcomes.[1–6] Kazanjian[7] was the first to challenge this notion, based on his observations of maxillofacial injuries sustained in World War I. He noted, "The majority of non-united fractures are due to inadequate immobilization of comminuted fragments of bone, and subsequent infection, rather than to the initial loss of bone." He believed that stabilization of the bony segments was the critical step in obtaining union and consolidation of the comminuted osseous fragments. Kazanjian's theories subsequently led to the development of numerous techniques for maintaining the reduced fracture segments in position, eventually leading to the current modality of open reduction and rigid internal fixation with surgical plates and screws.[8–16]

Indications for the Use of the Procedure

For craniomaxillofacial trauma surgeons, the current clinical presentation of comminuted mandibular fractures occurs secondary to a significant energy transfer to a localized region of the mandible, usually as the result of a motor vehicle accident, striking or being struck by an immoveable object, or a gunshot wound. As noted by Alpert et al.,[17] approximately 5% to 7% of all mandibular fractures present with comminution; therefore, the craniomaxillofacial trauma surgeon must be knowledgeable about the proper management of these conditions. The overwhelming majority of gunshot wounds encountered in the civilian trauma setting are caused by low-velocity, low-energy transfer handguns and do not display the characteristic soft-tissue changes seen in modern high-velocity/ultra-high-velocity ballistic injuries sustained in military conflicts (Fig. 80.1).[17,18] These injuries can produce debilitating soft-tissue avulsions, sequential necrosis, and loss of tissue over the course of several days after injury, which complicate both the short-term and long-term management of these patients.[18,19] The closest civilian corollary to these injuries is seen in patients who have attempted suicide, or been shot at close range (Sherman–Parrish class III), with a shotgun (Fig. 80.2).[20]

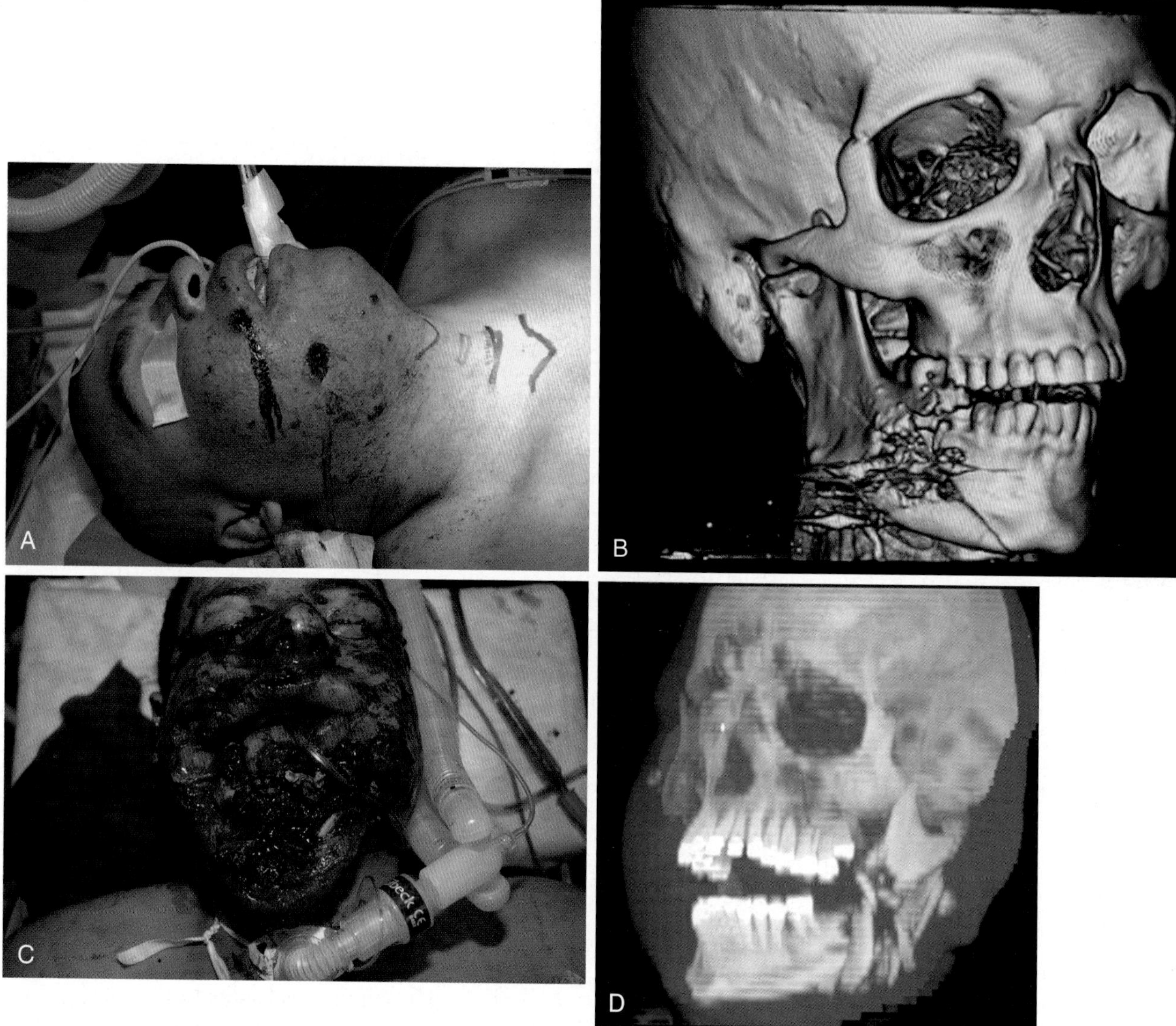

Figure 80.1 **A,** Typical clinical appearance of low-velocity–low-energy gunshot wound to the mandible. Note the lack of significant soft-tissue injury. **B,** Three-dimensional reconstruction of the computed tomography (CT) scan of the same patient. Note the localized area of comminution associated with this injury. **C,** Typical clinical appearance of a high-velocity–high-energy ballistic wound to the mandible and associated significant soft-tissue injury. **D,** Characteristic degree of comminution associated with a high-energy ballistic wound to the mandible. (A from Powers DB, Delo RI. Maxillofacial ballistic and missile injuries. In: Fonseca RJ, et al, eds. *Maxillofacial Trauma.* St Louis, MO: Mosby; 2012)

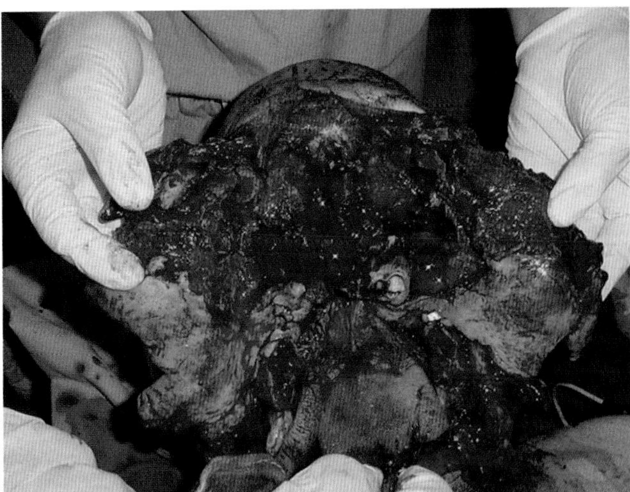

Figure 80.2 Clinical appearance of a patient who attempted suicide with a shotgun. Note the massive hard- and soft-tissue loss associated with this injury. (From Powers DB, Delo RI. Maxillofacial ballistic and missile injuries. In: Fonseca RJ, et al, eds. *Maxillofacial Trauma.* St Louis, MO: Mosby; 2012.)

Limitations and Contraindications

Avulsive tissue loss, with resultant exposure of any underlying surgical hardware, is an obvious limitation in the management of comminuted fractures. Definitive plans for reconstruction of the osseous skeleton must be coordinated with concurrent planning for recruitment of soft tissue to the site of tissue avulsion. If rigid internal fixation is the preferred management technique for a comminuted fracture, the fragmented portions of the mandible cannot be subjected to masticatory functional loads.[17,21] The surgeon must adhere to two basic tenets of treatment. First, the fixation must support the entire functional load (i.e., the principle of load-bearing osteosynthesis). The selected surgical plate must be of a sufficient size and strength to withstand the functional forces applied to it. Second, absolute stability of the reconstruction construct must be achieved. In comminuted fractures, the small bone fragments cannot take part of the functional load, as is seen in load-sharing osteosynthesis, nor can they be compressed due to risks of sequestration and devitalization.

TECHNIQUE: Surgical Treatment of the Comminuted Mandibular Fracture

STEP 1: Intubation and Induction of General Anesthesia

Coordination with the anesthesia team in the preoperative setting is an important component of therapy. Nasotracheal intubation affords the greatest flexibility to establish a functional occlusion and minimize the interference with the endotracheal tube commonly seen in conventional orotracheal intubation. If the patient is partially dentate or completely edentulous, consideration can be given to oral intubation, especially in the case of concurrent midfacial trauma and anesthesia concerns with potential nasal intubation. If the patient is completely dentate and has concurrent midfacial trauma that prevents nasotracheal intubation, consideration must be given to surgical tracheostomy or submental pull-through techniques. If the surgeon will be approaching the comminuted mandibular fracture via percutaneous incisions, communication regarding the use of neuromuscular blocking agents must occur before initiation of the surgical approach to allow for identification of the marginal mandibular branch of the facial nerve.

STEP 2: Application of Arch Bars and Establishment of a Functional Occlusion

After administration of a local anesthetic with a vasoconstrictor to establish hemostasis and for prolonged anesthesia, the establishment of arch bars is accomplished in the standard fashion with 24-, 26-, and/or 28-gauge stainless steel surgical wires. Use of the smaller-diameter wires increases the risk of fatigue fracture and wire breakage. Retraction of the cheeks can be facilitated with the use of either a Minnesota retractor or self-retaining plastic cheek retractors. Tightening of the wires is accomplished with wire drivers or needle drivers, based on the surgeon's preference, and rosettes at the terminal end of the wire are positioned with a pickle fork to prevent mucosal and labial trauma. Retraction of the tongue to gain access to the lingual borders of the mandible is accomplished with a Weider (sweetheart) retractor. The use of mouth props should be minimized to eliminate potential distraction/displacement of the fracture segments. Use of the newly marketed screw-retained arch bar systems is contraindicated in the mandible due to disruption of the occlusal table and comminution at the site of screw placement; however, these systems may be considered for use in an intact maxilla to expedite placement of fixation. MMF is established with either dental elastics or surgical wires through the lugs of the arch bars. Grossly unstable or nonsalvageable dentition should be removed at this time (Fig. 80.3A).

Continued

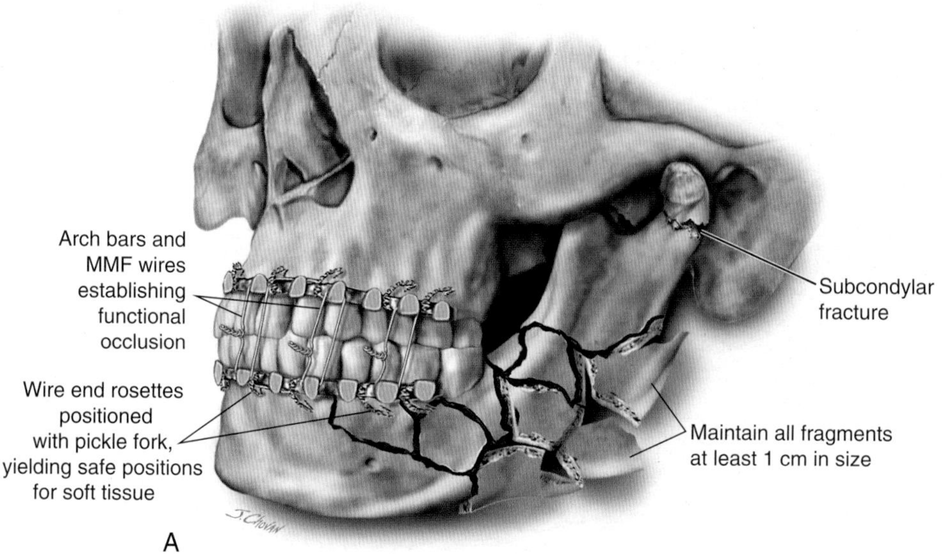

Figure 80.3 **A,** Proper application of maxillomandibular fixation (MMF), with Erich arch bars reestablishing a stable and functional occlusion.

TECHNIQUE: Surgical Treatment of the Comminuted Mandibular Fracture—cont'd

STEP 3: Surgical Access

After additional administration of any necessary local anesthetic with vasoconstrictor to establish hemostasis and prolonged anesthesia, an incision is made to access the area of fracture. Three classic approaches have been used to access the mandible: the transcervical or submental approach, the submandibular approach, and the intraoral degloving. The approach selected is determined by the surgeon's preference and experience and by the location and complexity of the fracture. Regardless of the technique chosen, all fractures must be exposed, explored, and reduced before stabilization begins.

The percutaneous incisions are made in an existing skin crease at least 2 to 3 cm below the inferior border of the mandible with a #15 scalpel blade. Hemostasis is obtained with electrocautery and/or bipolar cautery. Dissection proceeds bluntly through the superficial layer of the investing fascia, the platysma muscle, and superiorly to the inferior border of the mandible with hemostats. Evaluation of the marginal mandibular branch of the facial nerve is accomplished with a percutaneous nerve stimulator. The facial artery and vein can be separated and ligated with sutures or vascular clips if they interfere with access. The periosteum is incised with either the scalpel or needle-tip cautery and elevated superiorly with a #9 Molt periosteal elevator to gain access to the fracture site.

The intraoral approach proceeds with an incision anteriorly, initially through mucosa only, with a #15 scalpel blade or needle-tip cautery; the incision then is immediately redirected through the mentalis muscle and periosteum. Hemostasis is obtained with needle-tip cautery and/or bipolar cautery. Dissection proceeds in a subperiosteal plane inferiorly and posteriorly with a #9 Molt periosteal elevator; care is taken to identify and protect the mental nerve bilaterally. Once identified, the mental nerve is protected, and the remainder of the mucosal release occurs superiorly/posteriorly to the posterior border of the mandible with either the scalpel blade or needle-tip cautery.

Unless experienced and comfortable with the intraoral approach and associated soft-tissue restrictions and limitations on access, most surgeons have greater visualization of the sites of fracture with the percutaneous approaches and less difficulty in applying surgical plates. The tradeoffs for the percutaneous approaches are obvious: the creation of a visible external scar and the risk of permanent or temporary injury to the facial nerve (Fig. 80.3B–D).

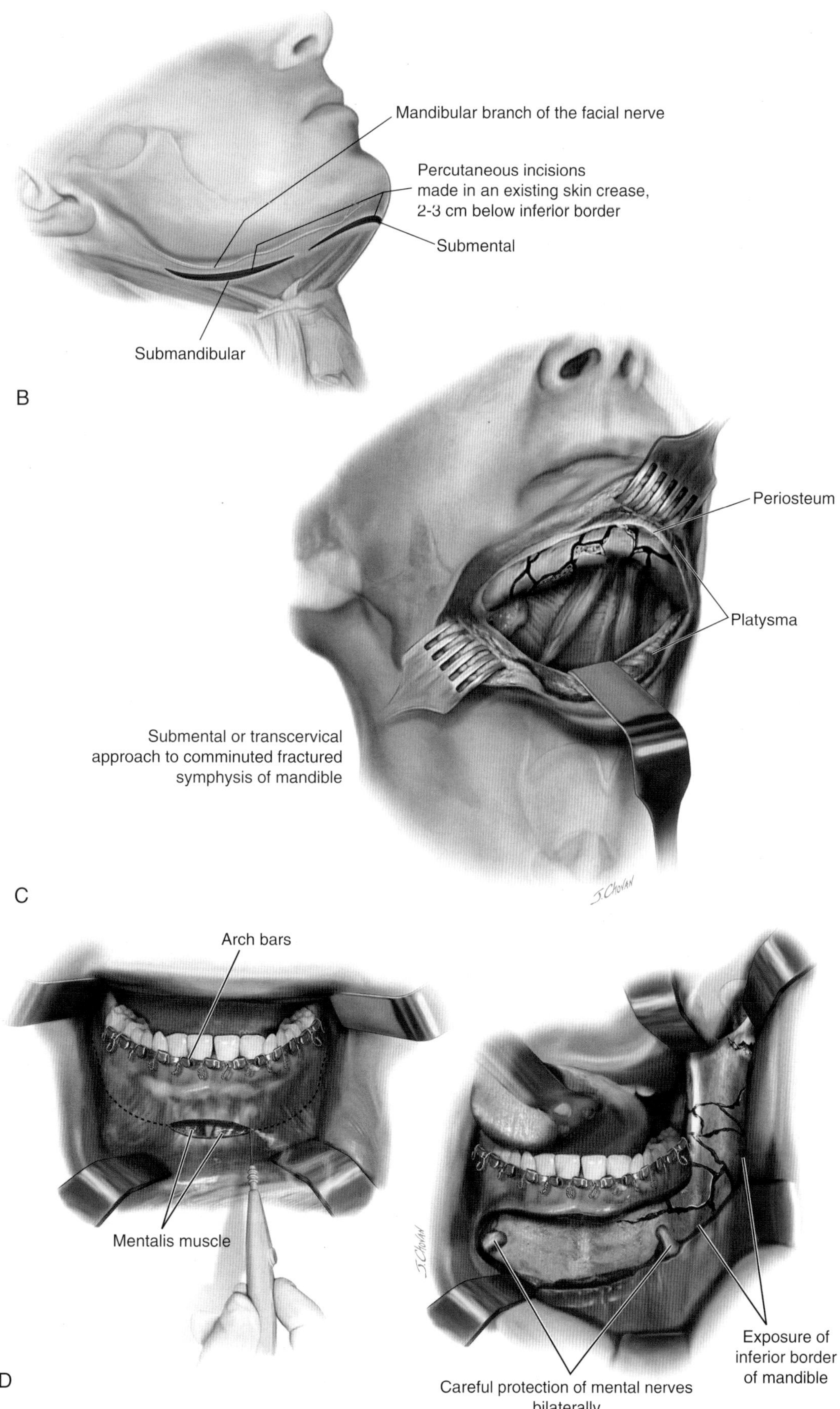

Figure 80.3, cont'd **B,** Submental, submandibular approach. **C,** Submental or transcervical approach to the mandible. **D,** Graphic representation of the intraoral degloving approach to the mandible.

Continued

TECHNIQUE: Surgical Treatment of the Comminuted Mandibular Fracture—cont'd

STEP 4: Evaluation of the Fracture Site

Bulb syringe irrigation with saline to assist with visualization and to dislodge grossly mobile fracture segments should be accomplished. Extreme caution is necessary if the surgeon uses a combination high-flow irrigation and suction device because the application of direct suction to comminuted fracture segments could result in excessive and unnecessary removal of bone fragments or detachment of the crucial lingual periosteum. A good clinical marker is to attempt to maintain all segments at least 1 cm in size. The condylar region of the mandible should be closely inspected because in cases of panfacial or bilateral facial fractures, a condylar/subcondylar fracture frequently exists. Simultaneous stabilization and fixation of the condylar fracture component should be accomplished to reestablish mandibular form and function (Fig. 80.3E and F).

STEP 5: Simplification of the Fracture

After identification of the fracture segments, surgical miniplates (1.3 to 1.5 mm) can be used in a monocortical fashion to initially reduce, or simplify, the fracture. A rotary handpiece/power source is used with a commercially available titanium surgical plating system to establish adaptation of the fracture segments. The larger segments should be reduced first and then the smaller segments. The concept is to take the numerous small, freely mobile components and sequentially connect them to each other in the proper anatomic position. Positioning an elevated small surgical screw within the fracture segments can allow for ease of reduction with the application of a hemostat to assist with control and movement of the segment. Care should be taken when placing the simplification plates so that their position does not compromise final placement of the load-bearing reconstruction plate (Fig. 80.3G).

STEP 6: Application of a Load-Bearing Reconstruction Plate

After stabilization and simplification of the fracture segment, the final reconstruction plate (2.4 to 2.7 mm) is positioned and secured with bicortical screws in the appropriate anatomic location and position to prevent iatrogenic injury to the inferior alveolar nerve and dentition. Verification of the proper anatomic form of the mandible after placement of the reconstruction plate is critical to assure proper future function of the mandible and mastication of food (Fig. 80.3H).

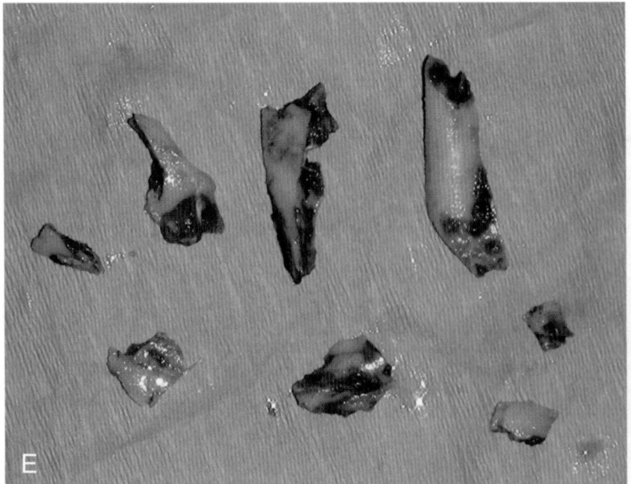

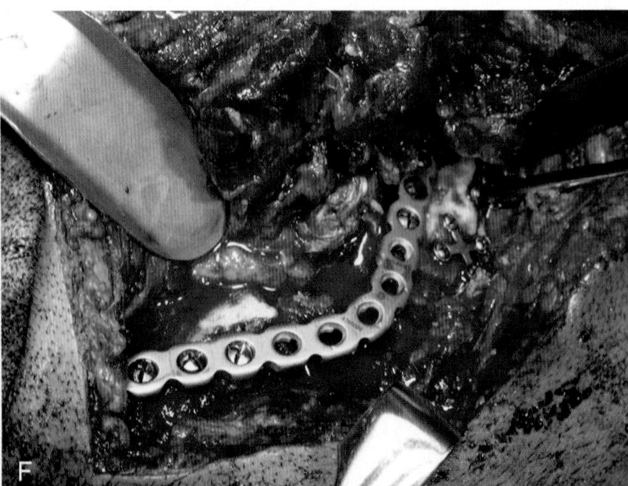

Figure 80.3, cont'd **E,** Representative removal of free-floating and nonviable fracture segments. Care should be taken during the removal of bony fragments to take only the areas of unsupported bone or small fragments completely disrupted from their periosteal supply. **F,** Note the presence of a left subcondylar fracture, which was treated at the same time as placement of the reconstruction bar for the comminuted left mandibular body fracture.

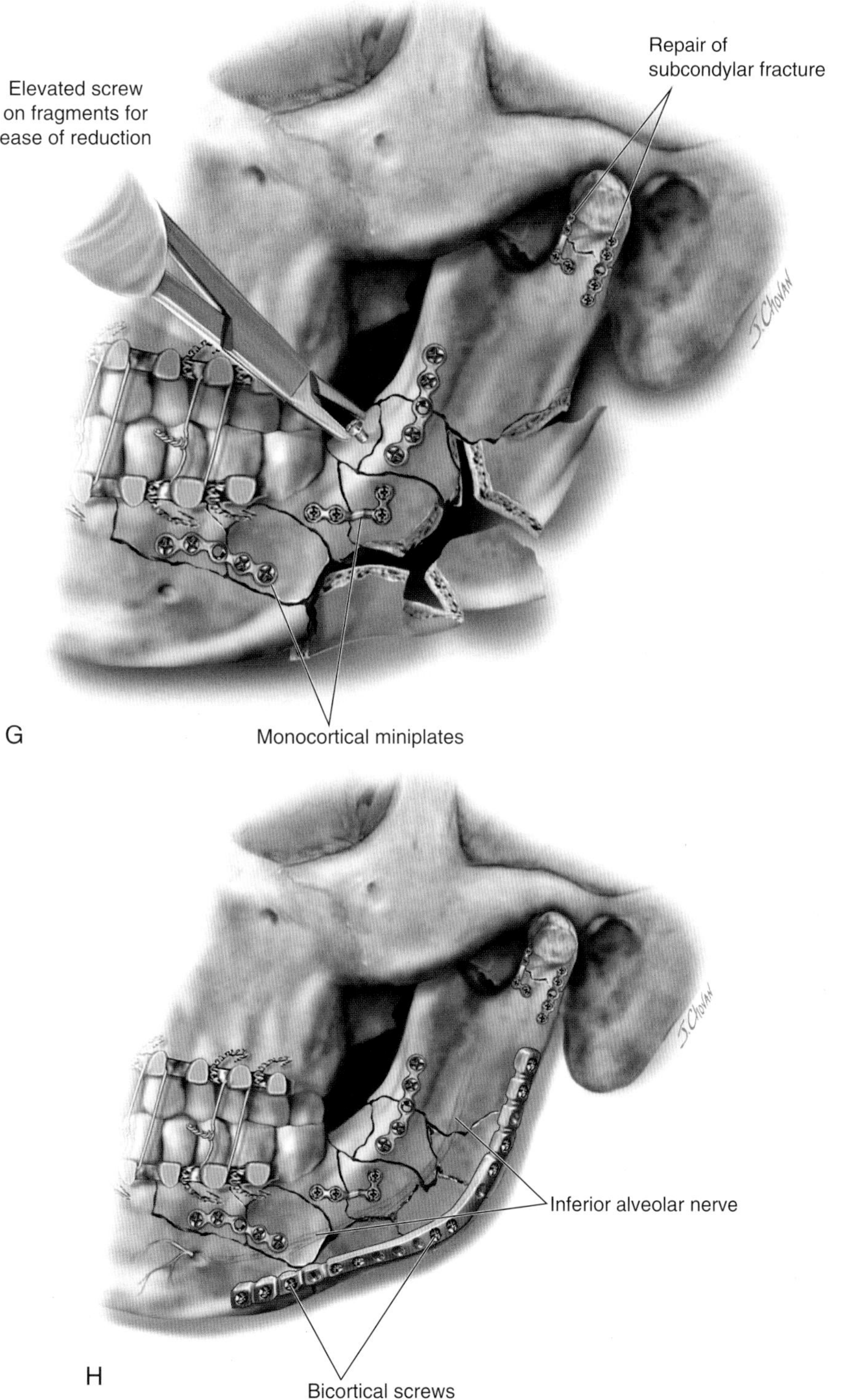

Figure 80.3, cont'd **G,** Graphic representation of the placement of a surgical screw in the comminuted bony segment to assist with mobilization and reduction of the fracture. Stabilization of the multiple fracture segments by the simplification technique. **H,** Properly adapted load-bearing reconstruction plate treating a comminuted mandibular body fracture with simplification plates.

TECHNIQUE: Surgical Treatment of the Comminuted Mandibular Fracture—cont'd

STEP 7: Evaluation of the Occlusion

After placement of the reconstruction bar, the patient should be released from MMF and the mandibular function verified to confirm correct positioning of the condyles and reestablishment of a stable functional occlusion. If the occlusion or function of the mandible is compromised, the surgeon should consider adjustment or replacement of the load-bearing reconstruction plate and also should investigate for any unrecognized additional facial fractures. If the occlusion is stable and reproducible, the decision either to remove or to retain the simplification plates is made at this time.

STEP 8: Evaluation of the Need for Potential Bone Grafting

Once the establishment of an anatomically correct and functional mandible has been accomplished, the possible need for bone grafting to osseous existing or resultant defects should be considered. With rigid fixation of the fracture sites, there is no micromovement to stimulate formation of a bony callus; consequently, any existing bone defect remains open and unfilled.[17,22] Bone grafting donor sites are dictated by the surgeon's preference but can include the anterior ileum, posterior ilium, tibia, or allogeneic sources. Cancellous bone is rapidly revascularized and has the added benefit of being a native material, which minimizes potential immune-mediated rejection at the site of already compromised healing due to the initial trauma. If soft-tissue viability or coverage of the defect is a concern, secondary bone grafting procedures can be accomplished at a later date, after primary healing has occurred.

STEP 9: Closure

The decision to return the patient to MMF or to allow him or her to function is based on an evaluation of the patient's compliance preoperatively, the degree of comminution or complication of the fracture management, and the presence of potential bone grafting materials. The use of materials such as platelet-rich plasma can be considered at this time as an adjunct to accelerate bone healing. For percutaneous approaches, reconstitution of the periosteum with 3-0 or 4-0 Vicryl sutures is critical. If the surgeon's preference is to place a drain postoperatively to prevent hematoma or seroma formation, the drain is positioned at this level. Closure continues in a multilayer fashion at the fascial and dermal layers with 3-0 or 4-0 Vicryl sutures. Any oral cavity involvement is closed with either 3-0 or 4-0 gut sutures or with 3-0 or 4-0 Vicryl sutures, based on the surgeon's preference. The skin is closed with 4-0 or 5-0 monofilament, and any percutaneous trocar access sites for screw placement are closed with either the monofilament or 6-0 fast-absorbing gut.

For the intraoral approach, resuspension of the mentalis muscle is vital and should be accomplished with 2-0 or 4-0 Vicryl sutures. The mucosal layer is then closed with either 3-0 or 4-0 Vicryl sutures or 3-0 or 4-0 chromic sutures in either a horizontal mattress fashion or a running locked technique, depending on the surgeon's preference. The surgeon should discuss with the patient the advisability of wearing an elastic jaw stocking postoperatively to relieve gravitational and functional stresses to the site of the mentalis muscle repair as a preventive measure against the development of a ptotic chin.

ALTERNATIVE TECHNIQUE 1: External Fixator

If a patient faces a long hospital course with questionable functional outcomes, such as an individual with a catastrophic neurologic injury, and the patient's overall medical condition does not allow a lengthy surgical procedure, or if a tenuous vascular supply remains to the injury site that could be further compromised or lost, the surgical team should consider the use of a closed technique, such as an external fixator appliance. Other scenarios in which external fixators can prove valuable include lack of remaining adequate dentition, proximal and distal to the comminuted fracture site, to establish the proper spatial relationship between the maxilla and mandible; low-velocity gunshot wounds; avulsive tissue loss that exposes the underlying surgical hardware; failed management with rigid internal fixation; or active osteomyelitis.[16,17,23] Historically, application of external fixation to the craniomaxillofacial skeleton was accomplished with the classic Joe Hall Morris (JHM) biphasic external fixator, using acrylic resin for the reconstruction bar.[6] Besides the obvious difficulty in mixing the acrylic resin, manufacturing the bar, and preventing iatrogenic thermal injury to the patient due to the exothermic reaction of the curing of the acrylic resin, the JHM set requires multiple specialized components for proper application to the patient. As a result of advances in modern metallurgic science, multiple external fixator sets now are commercially available that have eliminated the need for acrylic resin but have maintained the flexibility of the classic JHM assembly.

The establishment of MMF is accomplished as previously noted. Access to the mandibular body/symphyseal region is gained by a horizontal stab incision through the skin approximately the length of the #15 scalpel blade. The horizontal incision is preferred because it allows the skin of the face to be manipulated in a manner that minimizes "bunching" of the skin at the pin site, which creates an unsightly traction scar after removal. Any pin sites in the ascending ramus or condylar neck should be placed with a vertical stab incision, again to minimize scar tissue development secondary to pressure of the skin on the pin site. The surgical pins should be placed at least 1 cm from each site of fracture and obviously should not be positioned directly within the site of comminution. Ideally, the pins are placed approximately 5 mm above the inferior or posterior border of the mandible, preventing iatrogenic fracture of the inferior border or violation of the inferior alveolar complex (Fig. 80.4).

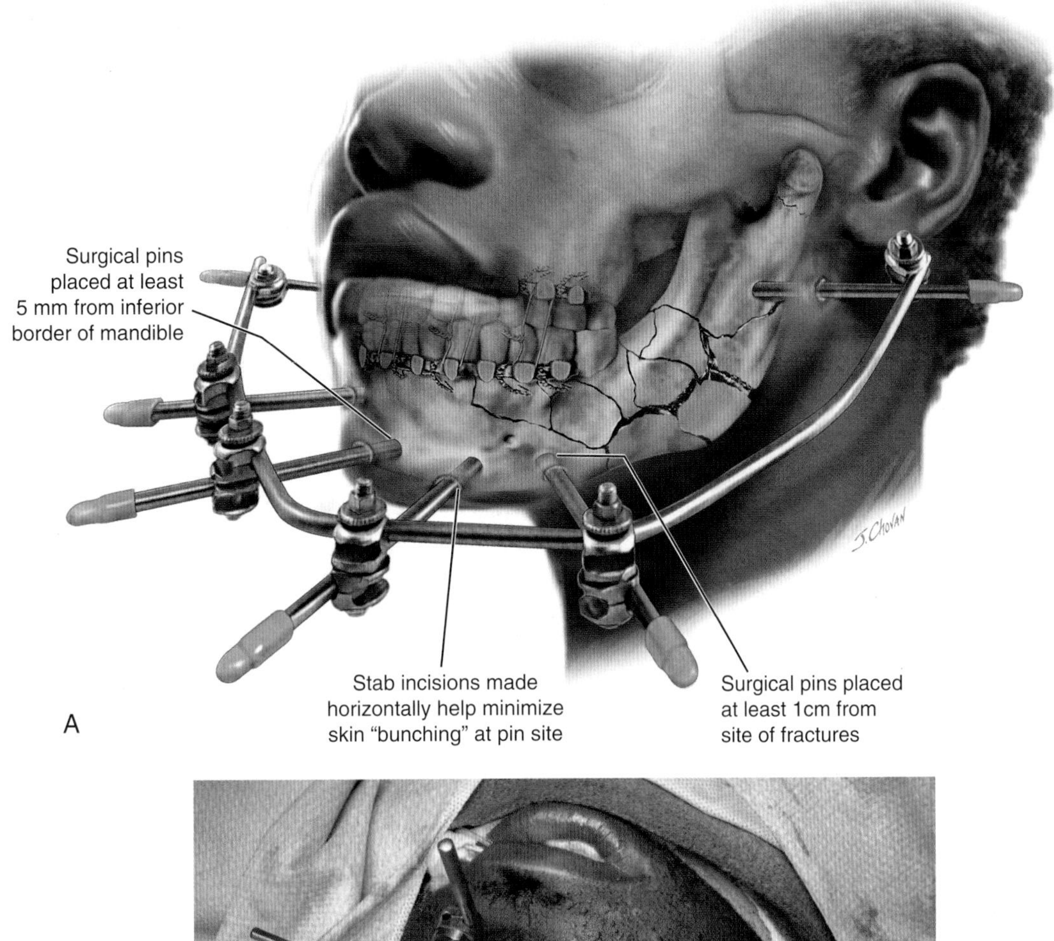

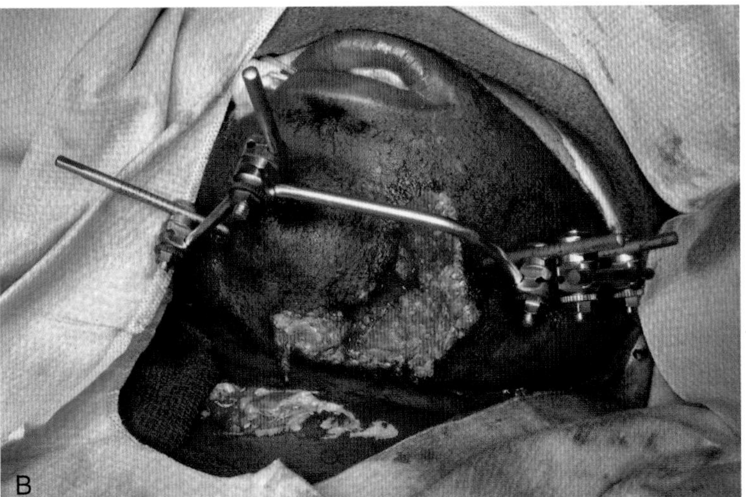

Figure 80.4 **A,** Graphic representation of the placement of an external fixator appliance for the treatment of a comminuted mandibular fracture. **B,** Clinical application of an external fixator for the treatment of a comminuted left mandibular gunshot wound. (B, from Powers DB, Delo RI. Maxillofacial ballistic and missile injuries. In: Fonseca RJ, et al, eds. *Maxillofacial Trauma.* St Louis, MO: Mosby; 2012.)

After stabilization of the fracture site with the external fixator, the patient is released from MMF to verify the occlusion and mandibular function. The need for return to MMF is based on the surgeon's preference, but patients historically have tolerated functioning with external fixators very well.

ALTERNATIVE TECHNIQUE 2: Maxillomandibular Fixation

In the circumstance of mandibular comminution with minimal or no loss of soft-tissue integrity, as is seen in blunt force trauma and some motor vehicle accidents, definitive treatment may be obtained with closed reduction and MMF exclusively (Fig. 80.3). Closed management with MMF should also be considered if the surgeon has inadequate experience with

Continued

ALTERNATIVE TECHNIQUE 2: Maxillomandibular Fixation—cont'd

the application of rigid internal fixation, limited personnel support in the operative theater, or is unable to obtain the appropriate surgical instrumentation to perform the operation. Finn[1] reported an exhaustive review of the historical data of comminuted mandibular fracture management with closed reduction and concluded that "the first steps in the management of any jaw fracture is the application of arch bars; establishment of the preinjury occlusion, facial symmetry, balance and form; and application of MMF. With comminuted mandible fractures, perhaps these should be the last steps in many instances."

Avoidance and Management of Intraoperative Complications

Virtually all intraoperative complications are the fault of the surgeon, through poor judgment and technique or improper application of the instrumentation, rather than of failure of the hardware itself. Box 80.1 presents a list of the most common intraoperative complications.

BOX 80.1 Common Intraoperative Errors

1. Lack of rigid stabilization of the fracture
2. Improper/nonanatomic reduction of the fracture sites
3. Positioning of the screws in the inferior alveolar canal
4. Positioning of the screws through the roots of the teeth
5. Iatrogenic avulsion of the inferior alveolar or mental nerves
6. Iatrogenic injury to the marginal mandibular branch of the facial nerve
7. Failure to recognize additional facial fractures, such as a concomitant subcondylar fracture
8. Inadequate reproduction of the occlusion with maxillomandibular fixation (MMF)
9. Application of compressive forces at the site of the comminuted fracture, leading to dislodgement of the fracture segments
10. Inadequate exposure to completely visualize all areas of the fracture site
11. Placement of screws in the lingual cortical component of an oblique fracture line
12. Failure to check the occlusion after placement of the load-bearing reconstruction bar
13. Repeated insertion/removal of screws in the same hole, leading to mobility of the hardware and potential movement of the bony component
14. Distraction of the condyles outside the articulating fossa during reduction

Postoperative Complications

Infection and the development of osteomyelitis are potentially devastating complications that must be recognized and addressed aggressively. Appropriate intervention with antibiotics, either orally or intravenously, should be started early in the clinical setting of infection of a comminuted mandibular fracture. However, the most important aspect of the management of a comminuted mandibular fracture is the surgeon's recognition that the most common cause of infection is instability of the fracture and loose surgical hardware. Definitive management requires surgical reexploration, stabilization of the fracture site, removal of any free-floating or nonviable bone fragments, and likely replacement of the load-bearing plate. Ideally, at least three bicortical screws should be placed in stable bone distal and proximal to the site of the comminuted fracture to minimize the potential for loss of stability of the reduction.

Malocclusion may be seen postoperatively as a result of inadequate or improperly performed MMF during surgery; lack of recognition of a malocclusion at the time of reconstruction; or loss of fixation of the surgical hardware, either through loosening of the screws or hardware failure. Minor malocclusions secondary to occlusal interference in the dentition can be managed with occlusal equilibration or, possibly, prosthodontic treatment of a localized site of irritation. Major occlusal disturbances can result in the possible need for orthodontic therapy, prosthodontic rehabilitation with multiple crowns and bridges, orthognathic surgery, or revision osteosynthesis. Neurosensory or motor disturbances to the trigeminal or facial nerves postoperatively may be due to neuropraxia or axonotmesis secondary to traction injury during exposure and treatment of the fracture site. Alternatively, these injuries may be iatrogenic due to improper positioning of the surgical screws through the inferior alveolar canal or lack of recognition of the facial nerve during surgery and subsequent neurotmesis.

Trismus or restricted mandibular opening may be seen after prolonged periods of immobilization due to scar contracture or muscular atrophy. Active range of motion exercises (the patient's own ability to open the mouth) should be instituted for essentially all patients once released from fixation. Passive range of motion exercises (physical therapy appliances or manual opening exercises) should be accomplished only after sufficient time has elapsed to allow for consolidation, maturation, and stabilization of the fracture site. The establishment of at least 30 to 35 mm of interincisal opening should be an achievable goal in the postoperative setting for patients with comminuted fractures.

A retrospective review of 198 comminuted mandibular fractures by Ellis et al.[24] confirmed the practicality of the three treatment modalities outlined in this chapter, including a low overall complication rate of 13%.[24] Specifically, these researchers noted a 35.2% complication rate with external fixation, a 17.1% rate with MMF, and a 10.3% rate with open reduction and internal fixation.[24] Although treatment selection criteria due to the severity of injury or concomitant injuries undoubtedly played a role in the specific complication rates, the overall low rate of complications (13%) should validate these treatment options. Rigid stabilization of the fracture segments is the key to successful treatment of comminuted mandibular fractures. Lack of adequate stabilization leads to chronic inflammation, which impairs the normal healing cascade, resulting in delayed union, fibrous union, malunion, or infection. Other critical factors in determining the success of the operative intervention are the mechanism of injury, the timing of initiation of treatment, and the skill of the surgeon.

References

1. Finn RA. Treatment of comminuted mandibular fractures by closed reduction. *J Oral Maxillofac Surg*. 1996;54(3):320–327.
2. Gillies HD. *War Injuries of the Face*. London, UK: Frowde; 1920.
3. Blair VP. Relation of the early care to the final outcome of major face wounds in war surgery. *Mil Surg (Wash)*. 1942;92:12.
4. Converse JM. War injuries of the face. *Trans Am Acad Ophthalmol*. 1942;46:250.
5. Ivy RH. Late results of treatment of gunshot wounds of the mandible. *J Am Med Assoc*. 1920;75:1316.
6. Morris JH. Biphase connector, external skeletal splint for reduction and fixation of mandibular fractures. *Oral Surg Oral Med Oral Pathol*. 1949;2(11):1382–1398, illust.
7. Kazanjian VH. Immobilization of wartime, compound, comminuted fractures of the mandible. *Am J Orthod Oral Surg*. 1942;28:551.
8. Kazanjian VH. An outline of the treatment of extensive comminuted fractures of the mandible (based chiefly on experience gained during the last war). *Am J Orthod Oral Surg*. 1942;28:265.
9. Walker RV, Frame JW. Civilian maxillofacial gunshot injuries. *Int J Oral Surg*. 1984;13(4):263–277.
10. Osbon DB. Intermediate and reconstructive care of maxillofacial missile wounds. *J Oral Surg*. 1973;31(6):429–437.
11. Buchbinder D. Use of rigid internal fixation in the treatment of mandibular fractures. *Oral Maxillofac Surg Clin North Am*. 1990;2:41.
12. Anderson T, Alpert B. Experience with rigid fixation of mandibular fractures and immediate function. *J Oral Maxillofac Surg*. 1992;50(6):555–560.
13. Assael LA. Results in rigid internal fixation in highly comminuted fractures of the mandible. *J Oral Maxillofac Surg*. 1989;47:119.
14. Smith BR, Teenier TJ. Treatment of comminuted mandibular fractures by open reduction and rigid internal fixation. *J Oral Maxillofac Surg*. 1996;54(3):328–331.
15. Li Z, Li ZB. Clinical characteristics and treatment of multiple site comminuted mandible fractures. *J Craniomaxillofac Surg*. 2011;39(4):296–299.
16. Futran ND. Management of comminuted mandible fractures. *Oper Tech Otolaryngol*. 2008;19:113.
17. Alpert B, Tiwana PS, Kushner GM. Management of comminuted fractures of the mandible. *Oral Maxillofac Surg Clin North Am*. 2009;21(2):185–192, v.
18. Powers DB, Delo RI. Characteristics of ballistic and blast injuries. *Atlas Oral Maxillofac Surg Clin North Am*. 2013;21(1):15–24.
19. Robertson BC, Manson PN. High-energy ballistic and avulsive injuries. A management protocol for the next millennium. *Surg Clin North Am*. 1999;79(6):1489–1502, xi.
20. Sherman RT, Parrish RA. Management of shotgun injuries: a review of 152 cases. *J Trauma*. 1963;3:76–86.
21. Spiessl B. Comminuted fractures. In: *Internal Fixation of the Mandible*. Berlin, Germany: Springer-Verlag; 1989.
22. Spiessl B. *New Concepts in Bone Surgery*. Berlin, Germany: Springer-Verlag; 1976.
23. Gibbons AJ, Mackenzie N, Breederveld RS. Use of a custom designed external fixator system to treat ballistic injuries to the mandible. *Int J Oral Maxillofac Implants*. 2011;40(1):103–105.
24. Ellis E III, Muniz O, Anand K. Treatment considerations for comminuted mandibular fractures. *J Oral Maxillofac Surg*. 2003;61(8):861–870.

CHAPTER 81

Pediatric Mandibular Fractures

Srinivas M. Susarla and Zachary S. Peacock

Armamentarium

Appropriate sutures
Arch bars (Erich, Risdon cable, or similar)
Dental cast models
Dental impression material (e.g., alginate)
Dental impression trays
Elastics
General anesthesia with nasotracheal intubation or tracheostomy (for severely injured patients)
Heavy needle drivers
Local anesthetic with vasoconstrictor
Mandibular fracture fixation kit (containing fracture plates, miniplates, and screws)
Oropharyngeal pack
Orthodontic acrylic
Orthognathic or craniofacial instrument kit
Pickle fork
Plastic double cheek retractor
Resorbable sutures
Retractors
Scalpel (#15) or needle-tip electrocautery
Stainless steel wire (24 and 26 gauge)

History of the Procedure

Mandibular fractures in children follow different patterns from those in adults.[1-11] In children, 80% of mandibular fractures involve the condyle or subcondylar region (up to 50%) or the mandibular angle.[1-4,10-11] Body fractures are relatively rare. Symphysis and parasymphysis fractures comprise approximately 20% of pediatric mandibular fractures.[1,8] Younger children (under 6 years of age) have thick, short condylar necks that fracture less often than those in older children. Young children have highly vascular condylar heads that are susceptible to crush injuries.[2,4] Treatment decisions must take into account the potential for mandibular growth and eruption of the primary and succedaneous teeth.[12] This has been a recognized tenet of management since the 1960s.[13,14] Since the advent of rigid fixation, there has been significant debate about its use in the growing mandible and also the use of resorbable materials for this purpose.[2,5,15-17] The goals of treatment in children are to obtain bony union, restore occlusion, and prevent and subsequently monitor for growth disturbances.[1-5]

Indications for the Use of the Procedure

Mandibular fractures in pediatric patients always require some form of treatment, ranging from observation with frequent follow-up examinations to open or closed reduction with or without maxillomandibular fixation (MMF).

Limitations and Contraindications

The presence of cranial, cervical spine, thoracoabdominal, or other injuries that may reduce the likelihood of survival should be assessed first. Although management of facial fractures is an important aspect of care of the traumatized pediatric patient, assessment generally occurs as part of the secondary survey and managed after life-threatening injuries. The practitioner should suspect additional injuries in any child with a mandibular fracture. Significant force is required to fracture the pediatric mandible, given its lower modulus of elasticity and tendency to greenstick rather than fracture completely.

Clinical and radiographic examinations are required for the diagnosis of pediatric mandibular fractures. The ability to elicit subjective complaints of malocclusion or inferior alveolar nerve dysfunction is limited in children, and imaging is often the best method of diagnosis. Plain films are often inadequate because they rely on cooperation from the child for accuracy. The short condyle-ramus unit in children leads to overlapping structures (e.g., skull base, cervical spine) in panoramic radiographs, and fractures can be missed. Computed tomography (CT) is needed to delineate this area and has become the standard in hospital settings due to its increased accuracy compared to plain films.[9]

Precise communication between the surgeon and parents, in addition to age-appropriate explanations to the patient, is required for full compliance with treatment. Although it was historically believed that children could not tolerate MMF, age is not a contraindication to MMF. The presence of significant medical conditions (e.g., epilepsy, coagulopathy) may be relative contraindications to a given approach (i.e., closed and open reduction).

TECHNIQUE: Closed Reduction With or Without Maxillomandibular Fixation

STEP 1: Overview

The procedure is most appropriately completed in younger children under general anesthesia with nasotracheal intubation. In adolescents, local anesthesia and/or intravenous sedation may be appropriate (Fig. 81.1A).

STEP 2: Reduction of Fracture

Once adequate anesthesia has been achieved, the fracture is reduced manually, based on the alignment of the mandibular dentition and occlusion with the maxillary teeth. Once this has been accomplished, arch bars or equivalent should be placed.[17]

STEP 3: Placement of Arch Bars

Placement of arch bars in dentate pediatric patients follows the same general principles as in adults: (1) tighten wires around the cervical aspect of the teeth below the height of contour with continuous tension; (2) direct apically when tightening the wires; (3) tighten all wires in a clockwise direction; (4) upon completion of tightening, turn one-half turn at a time; and (5) turn ends of wires down into embrasures. When arch bars cannot be placed because of traumatized or otherwise inadequate dentition, the fracture site can be immobilized with a Gunning or lingual splint (Fig. 81.1B). In such cases, impressions are taken with the patient (typically under general anesthesia), and the splint is fabricated on cast models. A separate anesthetic may be required for reduction and insertion of the splint.

Although arch bars generally can be placed in children, the short, bulbous crowns of primary teeth can limit their stability. Skeletal fixation in the form of circummandibular, circumzygomatic, or piriform aperture wires can be used to augment the fixation. Great care must be taken because skeletal wires tend to saw through the relatively soft bone in children. An additional option is the Risdon cable, which consists of a cable of twisted 24-gauge wires also secured (Fig. 81.1C) via circumdental wires. The advantage is that the cable is lower profile and can better adapt to the primary dentition.[17,18]

The arch bar or equivalent should be adapted closely to the involved dental segments; care must be taken to span well beyond the site of fracture when applicable (i.e., fractures through the body or symphysis) to ensure adequate immobilization. Among patients with minimal dental support, once the fracture has been reduced, an acrylic splint is inserted and fixed into place using circummandibular wires (one on either side of the fracture and at least two to stabilize the splint).

As an alternative, sutures (2-0 silk) may be used as ligatures placed through the embrasures in young children with fractures not involving the dentate portion of the mandible (e.g., ramus, subcondylar, or condylar fractures) (Fig. 81.1D). These sutures can be placed between any teeth and allow for short courses (<10 days) of MMF. The sutures can easily be removed by parents at home or in clinic without the use of anesthesia.

Continued

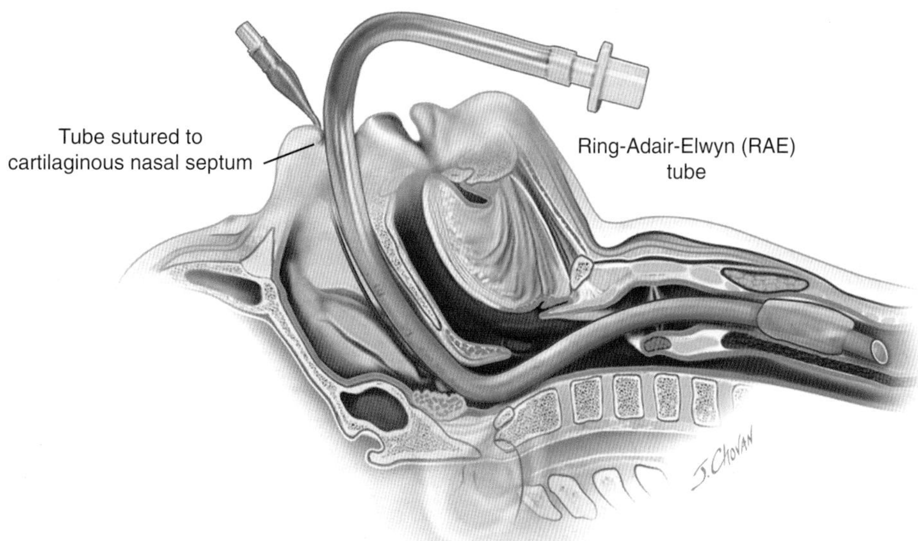

Figure 81.1 **A,** Schematic diagram for a nasotracheal intubation. Nasotracheal intubation is required for operative management of mandibular fractures to allow for the establishment of occlusion. It is our practice to use a nasal Ring-Adair-Elwyn (RAE) tube, secured to the cartilaginous nasal septum using a 2-0 dyed Vicryl suture.

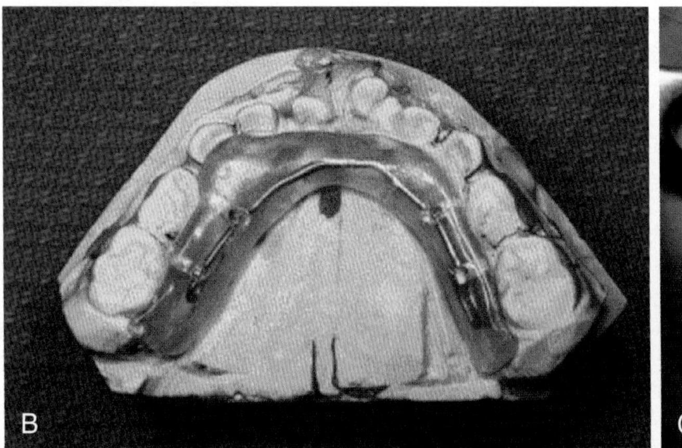

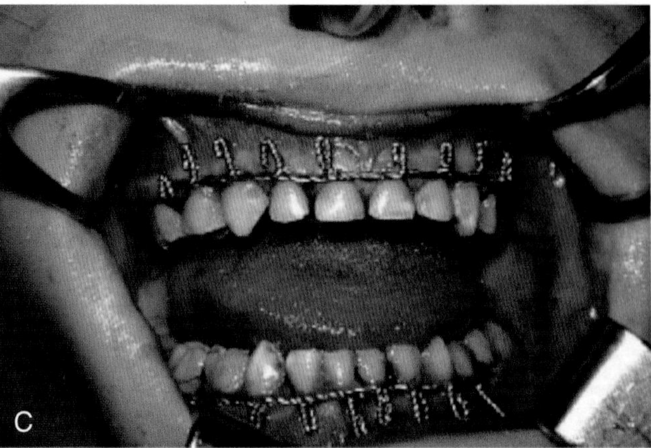

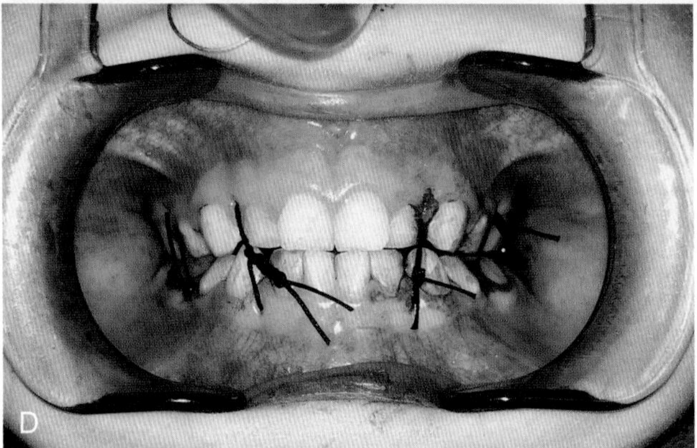

Figure 81.1, cont'd **B,** When the arch bars cannot be placed due to traumatized or otherwise inadequate dentition, the fracture site can be immobilized with a lingual splint. Dental impressions are taken using a fast-setting material (e.g., alginate). The models are then poured using dental stone. Model surgery is performed as necessary to realign any displaced segments of the mandibular arch. Once the final arch form has been constructed on the model, the splint can be fabricated using orthodontic acrylic. A 24-gauge stainless steel wire can be incorporated into the splint to help support the contour of the lingual splint, as seen here. The splint can be secured to several teeth on each side of the arch. **C,** The Risdon cable. A twisted 24-gauge wire is adapted to the cervical margins of the teeth across the dental arches and secured using interdental wires. This is a suitable alternative to arch bar placement in children and adolescents because its low profile is easier to adapt to the pediatric dentition. **D,** Suture ligatures for intermaxillary fixation. A heavy braided suture (e.g., 2-0 silk) is placed in the embrasures of the mandibular and corresponding maxillary teeth. The sutures are parachuted in the patient placed into occlusion and, with the occlusion held in place, the sutures are tied. This is an easy-to-use method for short periods of intermaxillary fixation in small children.[20] (B, From Zimmerman CE, Troulis MJ, Kaban LB. Pediatric facial fractures: recent advances in prevention, diagnosis and management. *Int J Oral Maxillofac Surg* 35:2, 2006. C, From Kushner GM, Tiwana PS. Fractures of the growing mandible. *Atlas Oral Maxillofac Surg Clin North Am.* 200917:81.)

TECHNIQUE: Closed Reduction With or Without Maxillomandibular Fixation—*cont'd*

STEP 4: Maxillomandibular Fixation

Once the arch bar or equivalent has been adapted and fixated, the patient can be placed into MMF, as needed, using 26-gauge wire loops or elastics. If MMF is required when an occlusal splint has been used, wires can be secured from the circummandibular wires to circumzygomatic or piriform wires.

STEP 5: Closure

Any lacerations (gingival or otherwise) should be irrigated thoroughly and closed with resorbable sutures.

STEP 6: Postoperative Imaging

After recovery from anesthesia, postoperative imaging is obtained (a panoramic radiograph, mandibular series, or cone beam computed tomography [CBCT]).

ALTERNATIVE TECHNIQUE 1: Open Reduction With or Without Internal Fixation

STEP 1: Overview

The procedure is most appropriately completed in younger children under general anesthesia with nasotracheal intubation. In adolescents, local anesthesia and/or intravenous sedation may be applicable in select cases.

STEP 2: Reduction of Fracture

Once adequate anesthesia has been achieved, the fracture is reduced manually, based on the alignment of the mandibular dentition and the occlusion. Once this has been accomplished, arch bars or equivalent should be placed, and the patient should be placed in MMF as in the preceding section either before or after fracture exposure.

STEP 3: Exposure of Fracture

For open reduction, the preferred approach is intraorally via vestibular mucosal incisions. The standard incision is marked several millimeters inferior to the mucogingival junction to allow an adequate cuff of tissue for closure. In the region of the mental nerves, the incisions can be stepped slightly superiorly to avoid the nerves. The technique then proceeds as follows:

1. Local anesthetic is infiltrated under the marked incision.
2. The incision is created with a #15 blade or electrocautery. The tissue is first incised perpendicular to the mucosal and submucosal tissues. The blade or needle tip is then reoriented so that it is perpendicular to bone, and the periosteal incision is created.
3. A subperiosteal dissection is completed, exposing the fracture and adequate proximal and distal bone for reduction and fixation. It is critical to expose the inferior border because internal fixation is most appropriately applied as close to the inferior border as possible, distant from the tooth buds and the inferior alveolar nerve (Fig. 81.2A1–A3).

STEP 4: Anatomic Reduction

The visualized fracture is reduced manually to the best anatomic alignment. Bone reduction forceps should be used with caution in the pediatric patient because they may injure developing tooth buds.

STEP 5: Fixation of Fracture

If adequate anatomic reduction is achieved and remains reduced with the mandibular arch bar, the arch bar can be acrylated for additional stability and the wound then closed. Alternatively, rigid fixation can be applied using fracture plates or miniplates with monocortical screws. Resorbable fixation also has been used in the pediatric population to avoid the potential long-term issues related to plate migration and to eliminate the risk of needing to remove hardware in the future (Fig. 81.2B and C).

ALTERNATIVE TECHNIQUE 2: Treatment of Mandibular Condylar/Subcondylar Fractures

The management of condylar and subcondylar fractures in children remains challenging because of the condylar growth center and the potential for growth disturbances and subsequent facial asymmetry or mandibular hypomobility. Fractures involving the condylar process can be classified as intracapsular or extracapsular, displaced or nondisplaced, and unilateral or bilateral. Although these descriptive terms are helpful in diagnosis, they have fewer implications for treatment. Treatment decisions should be based on the maximal interincisal opening, dental age (primary, mixed, or permanent dentition), occlusion, and level of pain.

In patients with a normal range of mandibular motion who have a stable, reproducible, age-appropriate occlusion and minimal pain, close observation and limiting the child to a blenderized diet is the treatment of choice.

Patients with a malocclusion require additional treatment. When the malocclusion is the result of mechanical obstruction from a displaced condylar segment, open reduction is indicated if closed manipulation is unsuccessful. If the occlusal discrepancy is minor and the patient can be guided into a stable occlusion, closed reduction with MMF using arch bars, Risdon cable, Ivy loops, stout wires, or embrasure sutures is preferable.[17,18] Skeletal screws should not be used for MMF because of the potential to damage the developing succedaneous dentition.

Patients with primary or mixed dentition who have unilateral subcondylar fractures can be treated with analgesics and a blenderized diet for 7 to 10 days. Minor malocclusions in this group are generally self-limited. Midline opening exercises are helpful for correction of deviation on opening. Short periods (7 to 10 days) of MMF are needed if there is severe pain or a significant malocclusion. This typically is followed by the use of guiding elastics for 4 to 6 weeks to reestablish the occlusion.

Continued

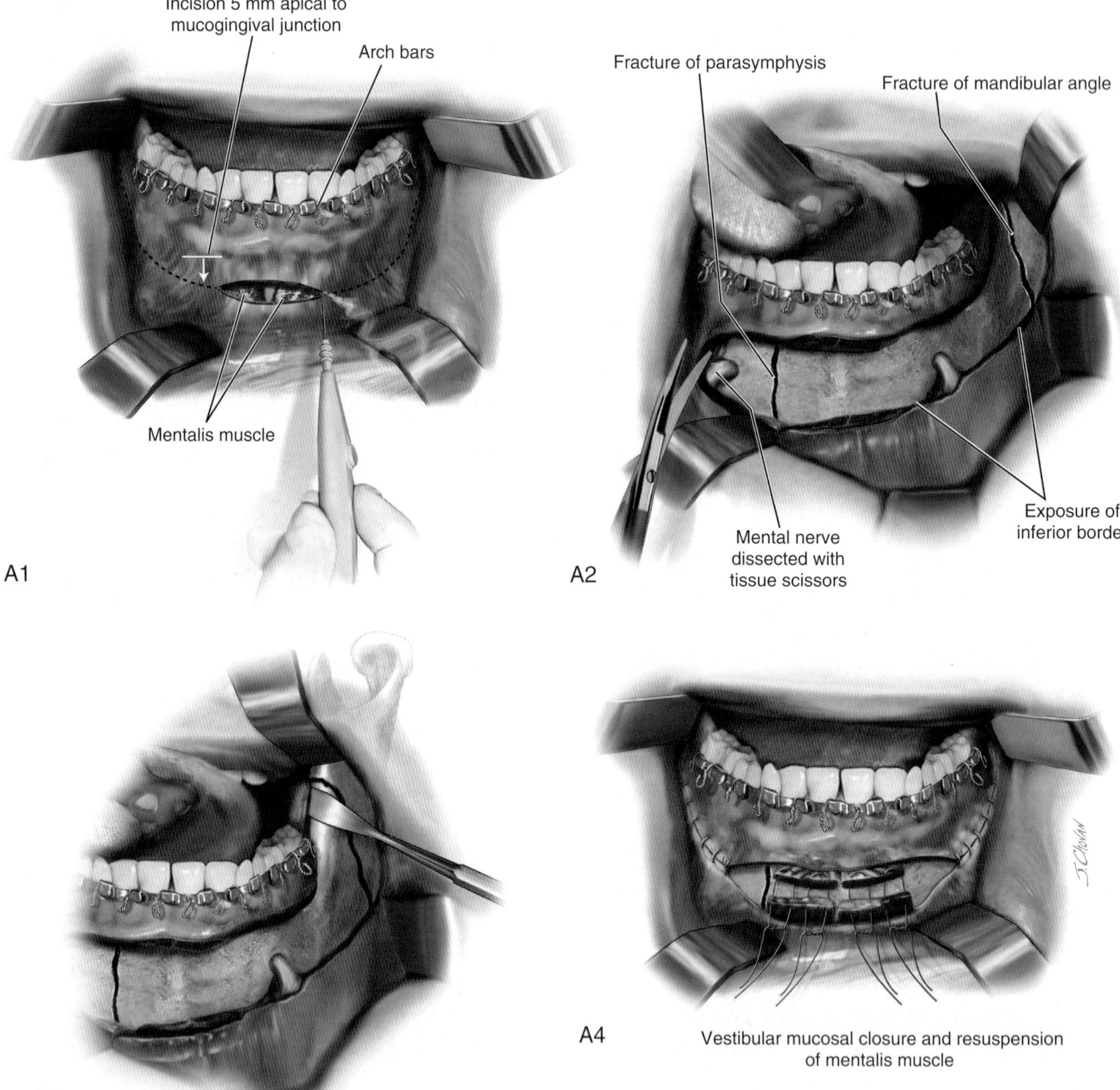

Figure 81.2 **A,** Surgical approach to the mandible via a vestibular incision. The incision is marked using a skin marker or brilliant green. The incision should be placed at least 5 mm apical to the mucogingival junction to allow an adequate cuff of tissue for closure. Local anesthetic is infiltrated for a vasoconstrictive effect. The incision is then made using Bovie electrocautery or a #15 blade, first with the orientation perpendicular to mucosa, then perpendicular to bone (A1). The mandible is skeletonized using Tessier or similar elevators (A2). If necessary, the mental nerves are carefully dissected using sharp dissection with tenotomy or other tissue scissors (A3). For closure, it is critical to resuspend the mentalis muscle (A4). It is our practice also to use a chin dressing to support the chin. The dressing is removed by the patient after 5 days.

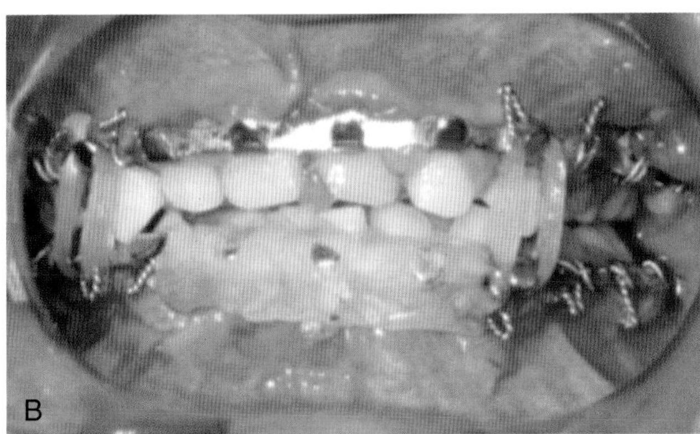

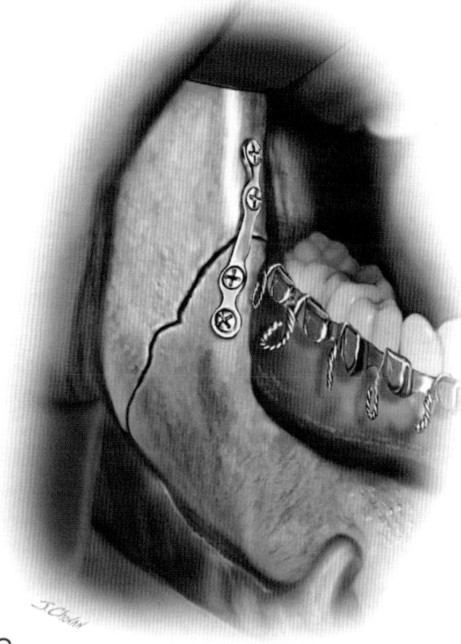

Figure 81.2, cont'd **B,** For additional stability, arch bars can be acrylated using orthodontic acrylic. **C,** Rigid fixation can be applied using miniplates and monocortical screws.

ALTERNATIVE TECHNIQUE 2: Treatment of Mandibular Condylar/Subcondylar Fractures—*cont'd*

Children with primary or mixed dentition who have bilateral subcondylar fractures with normal opening and stable occlusion can usually be treated with analgesics and a blenderized diet for 7 to 10 days. The diet can be advanced to soft foods after 10 days if tolerated by the patient. Any minor malocclusions resulting from such treatment resolve with growth and eruption of the permanent dentition.

Children with primary or mixed dentition with bilateral subcondylar fractures, with or without dislocation, who have an open bite malocclusion due to ramus height shortening should have MMF for 7 to 10 days. When the fixation is released, the patient should be placed in guiding elastics for 10 days and then reevaluated. If the malocclusion persists, further surgical intervention is warranted. However, the need for regimented follow-up in these cases cannot be overemphasized because delayed open reduction in children is extremely challenging. The need for delayed open reduction should be minimized by early recognition of malocclusion with correction via elastics or open reduction.

Children with permanent dentition who have unilateral or bilateral subcondylar fractures can be treated effectively with closed reduction, provided they have a stable and reproducible occlusion. Those who have a persistent malocclusion after 7 to 10 days of intermaxillary fixation and those whose fractures prevent a solid occlusion should undergo open reduction with or without internal fixation. This is an important adjunct to prevent progressive facial deformities. Adolescents have less capacity for bony remodeling, and ramus height may not be reconstituted. With the availability of minimally invasive methods for repair, which have lower attendant morbidity, open reduction should be used when appropriate.

Avoidance and Management of Intraoperative Complications

Careful planning is needed to avoid intraoperative complications. Discussion with the parents and the anesthesia team is critical to establish both the goals of treatment and the expectations for outcome. General anesthesia should be used whenever feasible, both for the patient's comfort and to assure adequate reduction and fixation. Given the small operative field in children, a pharyngeal pack should be placed to ensure that the airway remains free of debris and hardware. When MMF is used and removed intraoperatively, the surgeons should ensure that all wires are removed. Retained wires may not be noticeable around the narrow cervical region of primary teeth during postoperative visits or as the teeth erupt and the hardware becomes submerged. During manipulation, dissection, and placement of interosseous fixation, care should be taken to avoid damaging the unerupted tooth buds. The use of inferior border plates, monocortical screws and, whenever possible, closed reduction help avoid damage to tooth buds.

Postoperative Considerations

After the patient has recovered from general anesthesia, postoperative imaging is required. The most useful single study is the panoramic radiograph. If a panoramic image cannot be obtained because of lack of equipment or patient cooperation, a standard mandibular series is a reasonable alternative (right

Continued

and left lateral oblique, posterior-anterior, and Towne's views). Symphyseal and body fractures can also be assessed using occlusal radiographs. Condylar fractures can be adequately visualized using a Towne's view. In patients who are otherwise uncooperative, CBCT or medical grade CT may be useful. However, given the associated radiation exposure, practitioners are strongly advised to use plain films whenever possible, or a low-dose, limited-view CT protocol, when assessing reduction.

The need for a blenderized, nonchew diet should be emphasized with the parents and care providers (e.g., school, daycare staff). Consultations with a nutritionist can aid the parents in compliance.

For fractures not in the condylar head, MMF as primary treatment typically is maintained for 7 to 14 days for children with primary or mixed dentition. Three to 4 weeks typically is sufficient for older children and adolescents.

Serial clinical and radiographic examinations are recommended until growth completion to monitor for mandibular asymmetry or functional limitation, particularly with fractures of the condyle.[19]

References

1. Baumann A, Troulis MJ, Kaban LB. Facial trauma II: dentoalveolar injuries and mandibular fractures. In: Kaban LB, Troulis MJ, eds. *Pediatric Oral and Maxillofacial Surgery*. Philadelphia, PA: Saunders; 2004.
2. Myall RW. Management of mandibular fractures in children. *Oral Maxillofac Surg Clin North Am*. 2009;21(2):197–201. vi.
3. Posnick JC, Wells M, Pron GE. Pediatric facial fractures: evolving patterns of treatment. *J Oral Maxillofac Surg*. 1993;51(8):836–844.
4. Myall R. Condylar injuries in children: what is different about them? In: Worthington P, Evans J, eds. *Controversies in Oral and Maxillofacial Surgery*. Philadelphia, PA: Saunders; 1993.
5. Posnick JC. Management of facial fractures in children and adolescents. *Ann Plast Surg*. 1994;33(4):442–457.
6. Haug RH, Foss J. Maxillofacial injuries in the pediatric patient. *Oral Surg Oral Med Oral Pathol Oral Radiol Endod*. 2000;90(2):126–134.
7. Myall RWT, Dawson KH, Egbert MA. Maxillofacial injuries in children. In: Fonseca RJ, ed. *Oral and Maxillofacial Surgery*. 3rd ed. Philadelphia, PA: Saunders; 2000.
8. Zimmermann CE, Troulis MJ, Kaban LB. Pediatric facial fractures: recent advances in prevention, diagnosis and management. *Int J Oral Maxillofac Surg*. 2006;35(1):2–13.
9. Chacon GE, Dawson KH, Myall RW, Beirne OR. A comparative study of 2 imaging techniques for the diagnosis of condylar fractures in children. *J Oral Maxillofac Surg*. 2003;61(6):668–672.
10. Thorén H, Iizuka T, Hallikainen D, Lindqvist C. Different patterns of mandibular fractures in children. An analysis of 220 fractures in 157 patients. *J Craniomaxillofac Surg*. 1992;20(7):292–296.
11. Owusu JA, Bellile E, Moyer JS, Sidman JD. Patterns of pediatric mandible fractures in the United States. *JAMA Facial Plast Surg*. 2016;18(1):37–41.
12. Moss ML, Salentijn L. The primary role of functional matrices in facial growth. *Am J Orthod*. 1969;55(6):566–577.
13. MacLennan WD. Fractures of the mandible in children under the age of six years. *Br J Plast Surg*. 1956;9(2):125–128.
14. Rowe NL. Fractures of the jaws in children. *J Oral Surg*. 1969;27(7):497–507.
15. Eppley BL. Use of resorbable plates and screws in pediatric facial fractures. *J Oral Maxillofac Surg*. 2005;63(3):385–391.
16. Bos RR. Treatment of pediatric facial fractures: the case for metallic fixation. *J Oral Maxillofac Surg*. 2005;63(3):382–384.
17. Kushner GM, Tiwana PS. Fractures of the growing mandible. *Atlas Oral Maxillofac Surg Clin North Am*. 2009;17(1):81–91.
18. Morris C, Kushner GM, Tiwana PS. Facial skeletal trauma in the growing patient. *Oral Maxillofac Surg Clin North Am*. 2012;24(3):351–364.
19. Lund K. Mandibular growth and remodelling processes after condylar fracture. A longitudinal roentgencephalometric study. *Acta Odontol Scand Suppl*. 1974;32(64):3–117.
20. Farber SJ, Nguyen DC, Harvey AA, Patel KB. An alternative method of intermaxillary fixation for simple pediatric mandible fractures. *J Oral Maxillofac Surg*. 2016;74(3):582.e1–582.e8.

CHAPTER 82

Principles and Biomechanics of Rigid Internal Fixation (RIF) of the Midface and Upper Face

Sebastian Sauerbier, Rainer Schmelzeisen, and Robert Nadeau

Armamentarium

#10 and #15 scalpel blades
Appropriate sutures
Arch bars, 24- and 26-gauge wire
Bipolar electrocautery
Blakesley-Weil pliers (fragment or foreign body removal from maxillary sinus)
Curved Mayo scissors
Eschler retractors (two)
Fixation devices (miniplates and microplates)
Freer elevator
Gillies hooks
Hair elastics
Jackson-Pratt drain
Joseph elevator
Kocher clamp (with swab for blunt dissection of the periosteum)
Langenbeck retractors (two)
Local anesthetic with vasoconstrictor
Locklin scissors
Luniatschek pluggers (two) (to position fragments, plates, or wires)
Malleable orbital retractors
Needle electrocautery
Needle holder (Mathieu or Hegar-Mayo)
Raney clips
Rowe forceps
Skin stapler
Stromeyer hook
Surgical handpiece with sterile irrigation and motor
Toothed and anatomic forcep
Wassmund retractors
Wire scissors

History of the Procedure

The idea of plate osteosynthesis is more than 100 years old. In 1886, surgeon Carl Hansmann became the first to develop and present a procedure for subcutaneous fixation of bone fragments with a plate and screw system.[1] He therefore is regarded as the inventor of plate osteosynthesis. First, he surgically exposed the fracture, then he replaced and splinted the fragments with narrow, nickel-coated metal strips that had holes to receive screws. The steel screws were also nickel coated and had a conical screw thread, as do screws used in wood but not in metal. Both the plate and the screws stuck out of the wound and were removed 4 to 8 weeks later. Sir William A. Lane used screws and plates for fracture treatment in 1893. To gain a better fixation of the plates, he used conical screw heads, which fitted exactly into the conical holes of the plates. Two years later he reported corrosion of the material during the healing process.[2] The Belgian surgeon Albin Lambotte established the term *osteosynthesis*.[3] He is considered the father of modern internal and external splinting because he invented external fixation and various screws and plates made from aluminum, brass, copper, and silver. Sherman improved Lambotte's screws and plates by applying vanadium steel and self-tapping machine threads.[4] The screw tips received a cutting notch. Thus, the screw itself could cut a bone thread as it was inserted into the bone. This increased the screw's hold. These systems of osteosynthesis often showed severe corrosion, metallosis, broken plates, and loose screws. This resulted in impaired healing, which brought the whole procedure into question. The plates constructed by Lane and Sherman could not be substituted because there was no better material available.

Along with compression osteosynthesis, another procedure of plate osteosynthesis was established in the late 1960s. With miniplates, the path of static compression was avoided in favor of a dynamic compression. Plate osteosynthesis in the upper face and midface was not possible until the plates could be reduced in size to fit the maxillary structures.

Plate osteosynthesis is a breakthrough in maxillofacial surgery. The main advantage is that the patient does not need to undergo weeks of intermaxillary fixation. The introduction of noncorrosive materials, such as Vitallium and titanium, increased biocompatibility. The development of various system sizes, with screws as small as 0.8 mm in diameter, helps to extend the range of applications and patient convenience. Miniplate osteosynthesis in the upper face and midface was introduced by Champy and Loddé in 1976.[5]

Because of its biocompatibility and mechanical properties, titanium and titanium alloy is used as the standard material. Some disadvantages of titanium are a possible second surgery to remove the plates and screws, hot and cold irritation, bone growth inhibition in infants, migration and loosening of the screws, and interferences in imaging procedures. For these reasons, biodegradable osteosynthetic materials were developed more than 30 years ago.[6] Mechanical properties, biocompatibility, and degradation time vary from system to system. The amount of inserted material and the polymers themselves (i.e., their molecular weight and crystallinity) determine the material's in situ characteristics. The material most commonly used, besides polyglycolide, is polylactic acid, which exists in two enantiomers, L-lactic acid (PLLA) and D-lactic acid (PDLA). Increasing the amount of the D-form (PDLA) in a plate reduces crystallinity in a mix with PLLA, thus forming the amorphous poly-D,L-lactide (PDLLA). The degradation time of the available resorbable osteosynthesis systems ranges from 1 to more than 5 years.[7,8]

Today, three-dimensional (3D) implants and custom-made devices represent the next step in reconstruction of the midface and upper face.[9,10]

Indications for the Use of the Procedure

The aim in modern bone surgery is rapid reestablishment of form and function. The reduction of fractures of the midface and upper face must resemble the form in height, width, depth, and projection. The blood supply of the fragments and the surrounding tissue should be maintained or reestablished. Occlusion should be one of the primary additional functions sought along with nasal and form and function. Functionally stable internal fixation is indicated in multiple or comminuted fractures, panfacial fractures, defect fractures, wide open fractures, and dislocated midface fractures. A relative indication for internal fixation is patient noncompliance with conservative treatment. With polytrauma, patients absolutely need early fracture treatment. Sufficient stability prevents infection and secondary reconstructive surgery as there is an increased risk associated with mobility and exposure to sinus bacteria.

Due to the resorbable properties of osteosynthetic materials, the stiffness in particular is inferior to that of titanium plates. It is recommended that resorbable plates be used in non-load-bearing areas only, such as the cranium or midface. Therefore, they preferably are used for craniofacial surgery in growing patients.

Limitations and Contraindications

The level of stability needed depends on the fracture pattern. Adequate stability is not necessarily maximum stability. There are absolute and relative indications for the treatment of facial fractures. The decision to use conservative or surgical treatment depends on the fracture pattern and on the condition and situation of the patient. Stable, simple, and closed fractures can be treated conservatively.

Today, mostly self-tapping screws are used in fracture surgery, which saves the time-consuming extra step of cutting a thread into the bone but makes positioning the bone fragments of paramount importance. Self-drilling screws also are available. These are suited for bones with a thin cortical layer, which makes them useful in the upper facial and midfacial region. The fixation of large segments with self-drilling screws is possible. In trauma cases, it can be difficult to position self-drilling screws in small bone fragments without breaking the fragments.

The mechanical properties of resorbable osteosynthetic material contraindicate its use in most load-bearing areas.

TECHNIQUE: Rigid Internal Fixation of the Midface and Upper Face

The face is divided into upper and lower halves by the Le Fort I level. The upper face consists of the frontal unit and the upper midfacial unit. The lower midfacial unit reaches from the Le Fort I level to the occlusal plane. The frontal unit forms the upper face and contains the frontal and temporal bones, the supraorbital rims, the orbital roofs, and the frontal sinus. The midfacial unit consists of the maxilla, the zygomas, the nasoethmoid complex, the internal orbits, and the infraorbital rims. The facial skeleton is composed of a solid bone framework (Fig. 82.1A). Paper-thin bone stretches between its buttresses, which are stable enough for the fixation with miniplates with screws.

The principles of upper facial and midfacial trauma surgery have been developed from experience in orthopedic and craniofacial reconstructive surgery:

- Reestablishment of the occlusion
- Direct exposure of the buttresses
- Open reduction of the fracture while preventing of creating additional deficits during fracture reduction (i.e., orbital floor)
- Internal fixation of the buttresses with monocortical miniplates and the use of bone grafts to bridge bone gaps in the buttress that exceed 5 mm

The monocortical screws and miniplates are stable enough such that no external fixation is needed. The 3D stability of plate and screw osteosynthesis is better than that of wire fixation. The reduction aims at reestablishing the 3D form in height, width, and length, in addition to the function of the damaged region. Open reduction in combination with internal fixation has improved the quality of fracture treatment. The common methods for internal fixation are wire, K-wire, and plate osteosynthesis. The latter is the most rigid and most common in upper and midface fractures. Functional stability is sufficient in the midface. Therefore, miniplates should be applied along the buttress lines after the fracture has been reduced. Stable bone is found in the cranium, orbital rims and margins, and zygomatic bone, around the piriform aperture and in the zygomaticomaxillary buttresses (Fig. 82.1B).

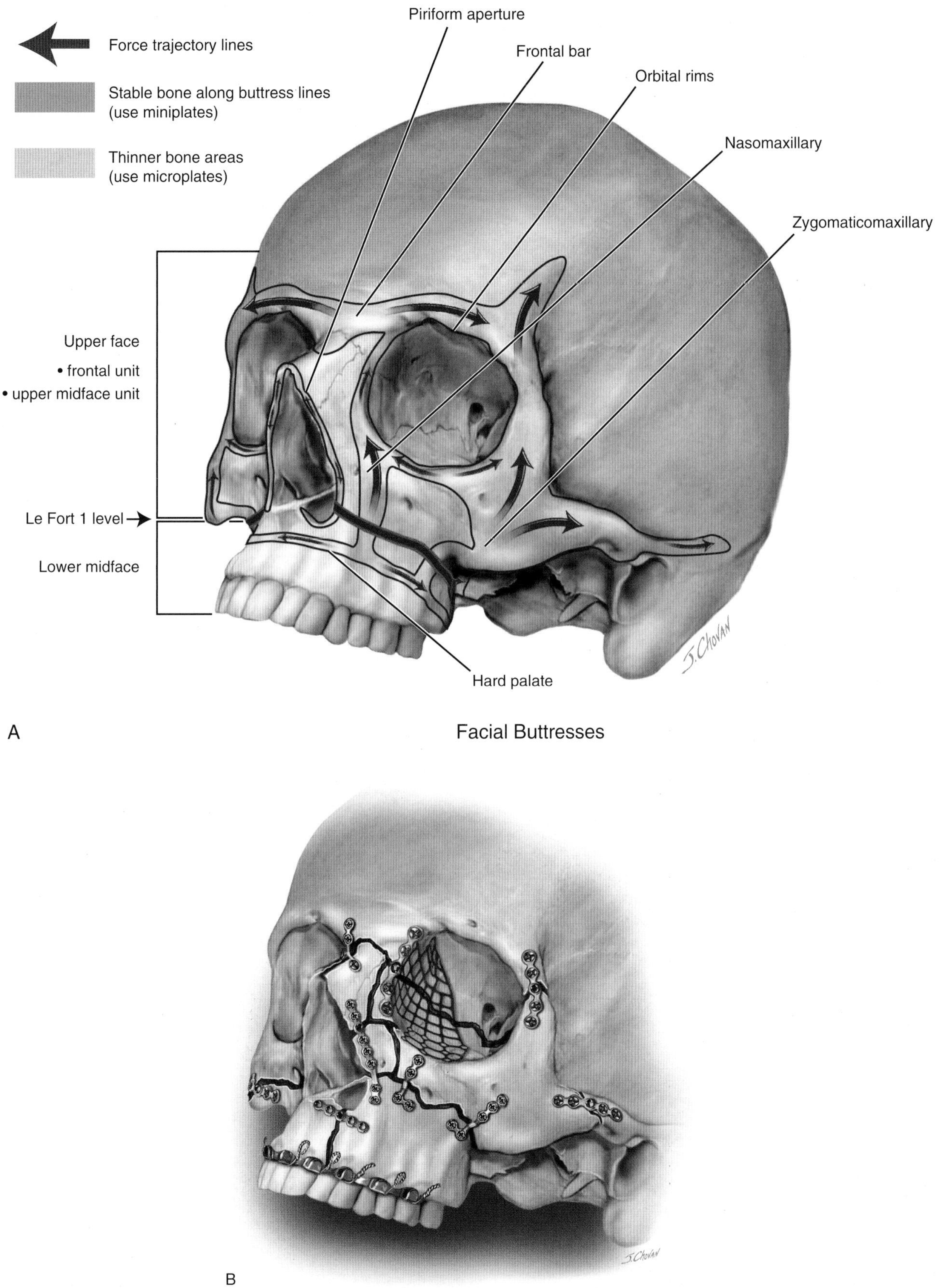

Force trajectory lines

Stable bone along buttress lines (use miniplates)

Thinner bone areas (use microplates)

Piriform aperture

Frontal bar

Orbital rims

Nasomaxillary

Zygomaticomaxillary

Upper face
• frontal unit
• upper midface unit

Le Fort 1 level

Lower midface

Hard palate

A

Facial Buttresses

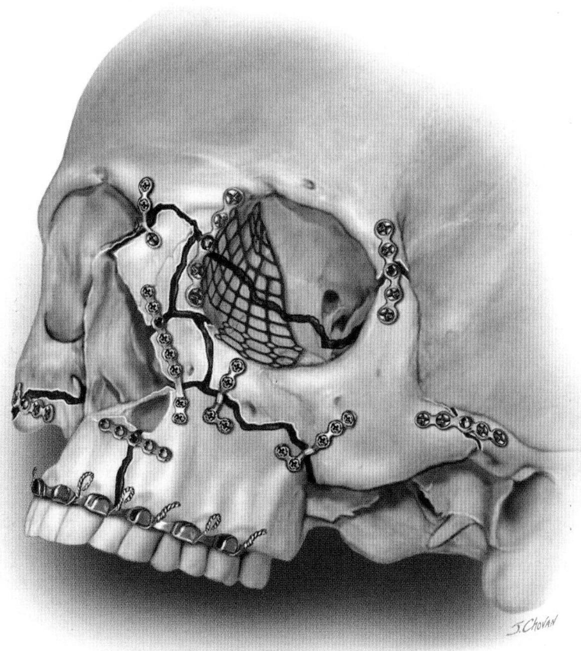

B

Figure 82.1 **A,** The trajectory lines in the upper face and midface run along the buttresses in which the forces are distributed. **B,** The framework is reestablished by the reduction of the fractures. In the buttress areas, the bone has sufficient thickness and strength to hold osteosynthesis screws and plates, which receive the forces and bridge the fractures.

TECHNIQUE: Rigid Internal Fixation of the Midface and Upper Face—*cont'd*

Microplates should be used for the thinner parts. The bone thickness should be considered when the length of the screws is chosen. The frontal bone is 4 to 9 mm thick. In the parietal aspect, screws should not exceed 3 mm in length, whereas in the area of the supraorbital rim, screws 6-mm long can be used. Drilling into the anterior cerebral fossa should be avoided. According to Champy, it is located 5 mm above an imaginary horizontal line through the superior orbital rim.[11] The inferior orbital rim also consists of thick bone. It is not affected by muscle pull and therefore does not necessarily need plating when the reduction alone is stable enough.

Essential for a secure and anatomically correct plate and screw osteosynthesis is the exact adaptation of the plates. An incongruent shape leads to dislocation of the bone fragments when the screws are tightened. Titanium plates can be bent without effort with bending pliers. After the plate has been adapted, holes are drilled, under irrigation with sterile saline solution, and the plate is fixed with screws. At least two screws should be inserted at each end of the plate for a total of four screws.

When resorbable osteosynthetic materials are used, the adaptation must be facilitated by heating the plates in a sterile water bath (depending on the system, the water temperature should be 45°C to 70°C). Air heating devices also are available. The heating and bending process can be repeated when necessary. A metal foil can be preadapted to form a bending template. At least two holes should be drilled into each of the fragments that are to be connected. The diameter of the drill depends on the screw core. With resorbable systems with screws, care must be taken not to twist off the screw heads. Fortunately, a new hole can be drilled through the broken screw for a new attempt. Ultrasonic pin fixation is easier to use.[12] After a hole has been drilled, the pin is melted into the bone's trabecular system and welded to the plate in one step. In frontal and midfacial fractures, the position of the resorbable plates is the same as for titanium plates. Of note, it is usually necessary to have wider access and exposure of the fractures needing fixation when using resorbable plates.

The surgical approaches for and treatment of particular types of midfacial and upper facial fractures are explained in detail in the corresponding chapters of this book.

STEP 1: Clinical Examination and Imaging

On clinical examination the surgeon should look for secure and unsecure fracture signs. Loss of projection and asymmetry are visible. In imaging, the preferred mode of viewing is via multiplanar reconstruction to evaluate the three planes in the skull. The examiner has to look for dislocations and loss of continuity. Malocclusion, sinus fluid levels, or hematomas are indirect fracture signs. The use of a contrast agent can help to visualize intracranial bleeding. Foreign bodies and emphysema are other possible pathologic findings. Rhinorrhea is a clinical sign of a cerebrospinal communication or fistula. This can be verified by beta-2-tranferrin or glucose testing. Intracranial air and fractures of the posterior sinus wall in the CT image should prompt a neurosurgical consult. Dural lesions should be treated together with a neurosurgeon (Fig. 82.1C).

STEP 2: Treatment Planning

For a patient with multiple facial fractures, the surgeon should develop a plan that leads to accurate anatomic positioning of the segments. Correct alignment of the fractures is achieved best when the facial buttresses are exposed, identified, reduced, and fixated. In panfacial fractures, it helps to develop the reduction from the intact cranium downward to the lower and the anterior face. The treatment of Le Fort and associated fractures should be embedded in this plan. The treatment plan prevents overdone soft tissue preparation and lays out the necessary surgical steps.

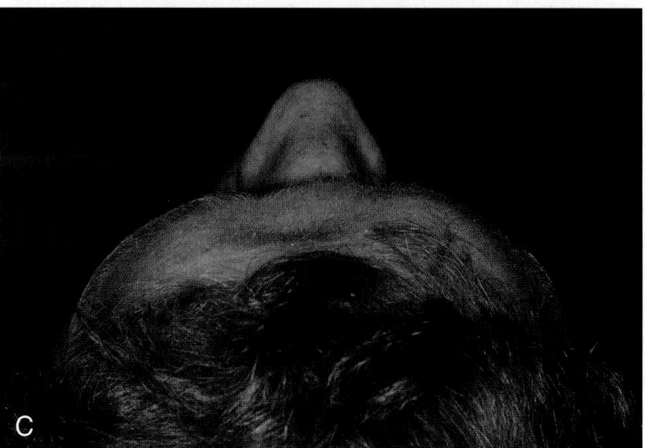

Figure 82.1, cont'd **C,** Loss of projection and asymmetry mark the clinical appearance of a frontal sinus fracture.

TECHNIQUE: Rigid Internal Fixation of the Midface and Upper Face—*cont'd*

STEP 3: Reestablishment of the Occlusion

If the occlusion is impaired, it can be secured by arch bars applied to the teeth of the maxilla and the mandible. Both the interdigitation of the teeth and the width of the dental arch must be aligned correctly. If the hard palate is fractured, it must be reduced and fixated with one or two miniplates in the roof before intermaxillary fixation is established. One consideration if unable to achieve adequate occlusion is the need to complete the Le Fort fracture to assess bony interferences that may prevent reduction.

STEP 4: Direct Exposition of the Fracture

The midface can be accessed via intraoral vestibular and upper and lower eyelid approaches. When the zygomatic arch is involved in complex fractures, it can be accessed via an extended coronal approach. In complex zygoma fractures, three pillars of the quadripod should be exposed. These are the zygomaticofrontal suture, the inferior orbital rim, and the zygomaticomaxillary buttress while not exposing the zygomatic arch and utilizing the zygomaticofrontal approach to monitor the sphenozygomatic suture for adequate reduction. With simple zygoma fractures, when intraoperative 3D imaging is available, the surgeon can determine whether exposure of only the inferior orbital rim and the zygomaticomaxillary buttress is sufficient.

The frontal bone is exposed by a coronal approach. A pulled-out gauze swab is wrapped around the wound edges and secured with Raney clips to obtain hemostasis. When the site is closed, the Raney clips can easily be removed by pulling off the gauze swab. Cauterization of bleeders should be done carefully because hair follicles can be damaged. The loss of hair can make the scar more visible in male patients. Releasing the supraorbital nerve and vessels from their foramen with osteotomes, a diamond burr, or piezo surgery allows enough retraction of the flap to enable the surgeon to reach the dorsum and tip of the nose after vertical relaxing incisions have been made in the pericranium over the dorsum nasi and after the upper and medial periorbita have been dissected. It might be necessary to cauterize and cut the anterior and posterior ethmoid neurovascular bundles (Fig. 82.1D).

STEP 5: Open Reduction of the Fracture

Removed segments are marked as they are detached. A digital camera helps document the prevention of creating additional deficits during fracture reduction (i.e., orbital floor) process and also aids later placement of the fragments. If the posterior wall of the frontal sinus is fractured, neurosurgical exploration is recommended. The supraorbital margin and the lower anterior frontal sinus form the so-called frontal bar and should be stabilized as the lower key landmark in frontal bone reconstruction.[13] Next, the temporal bones are reduced in correct width and length to establish the proper projection of the frontal bar. Smaller bone fragments then are fixated to the larger, already fixated frontal segments.

A nasoethmoid fracture is treated after the upper face. In case of traumatic detachment of the medial canthal tendon, the intercanthal distance can be reestablished by a transnasal wire (see Chapter 43). To achieve projection, the nasoethmoidal complex can be attached to the frontal bar. With a simple zygomatic fracture, the correct position can be confirmed after hook repositioning and provisional fixation in the intraoperatively made 3D image. In comminuted zygomatic fractures, the zygoma itself must be properly aligned with the infraorbital rim and the lateral orbit before the arch is reduced. The reduction begins at the stable posterior segment, and a plate is placed over the arch segments (Fig. 82.1E).

Continued

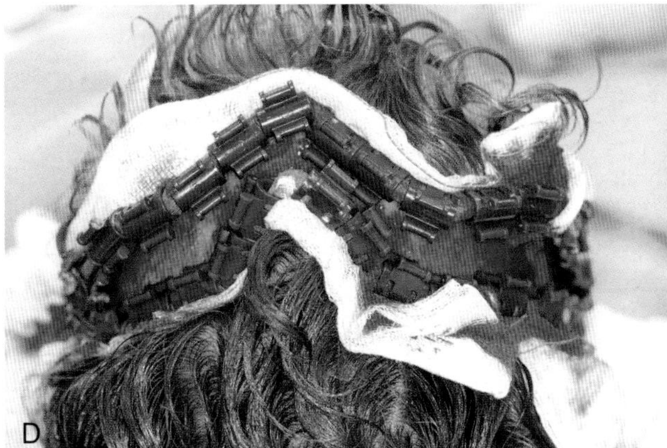

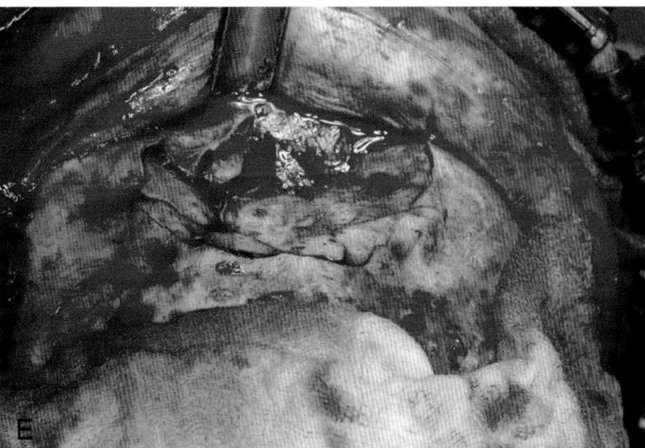

Figure 82.1, cont'd **D,** In a coronal approach, a pulled-out gauze swab is wrapped around the wound edges and secured with Raney clips to obtain hemostasis. When the site is closed, the Raney clips can easily be removed by pulling off the gauze swab. **E,** Open reduction of a frontal sinus fracture. A digital camera aids documentation and later placement of the fragments.

TECHNIQUE: Rigid Internal Fixation of the Midface and Upper Face—*cont'd*

STEP 6: Internal Fixation

Microplates and appropriate screws have been developed for the fixation of thinner bone in the midface or frontal area. In general, these plates span from stable bone to stable bone. The thin bone fragments are held in place by an elevator or Gillies hook and fixated to the bridging microplate. Another technique is to assemble the frontal bone segments on a separate table while neurosurgery is performed. In pediatric patients, titanium plates should not be applied because of their migration potential in the growing skeleton. Resorbable plate systems or resorbable suture material can be used to fixate bone fragments in children.

The buttress reconstruction prevents secondary deformation, collapse, and elongation of the midface. The miniplates are placed at the medial orbital rim to the frontal bone. Infraorbital rim fractures are reduced and fixated with a curved orbital plate. The anterior maxillary buttress, a key structure of the midface, should be reconstructed next. At the piriform aperture, the nasoethmoid segment is attached to the maxillary alveolus. Here the plates cross the fracture line in the Le Fort I level and follow the nasomaxillary buttress. This ensures the lower projection of the nasoethmoid. After the orbital frame has been reconstructed completely, the orbit itself must be reconstructed. In simple zygomatic fractures, a single L-plate at the zygomaticomaxillary buttress may be adequate (Fig. 82.1F–L).

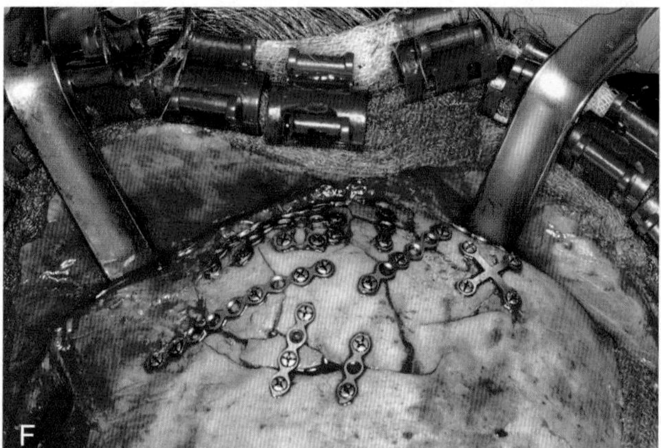

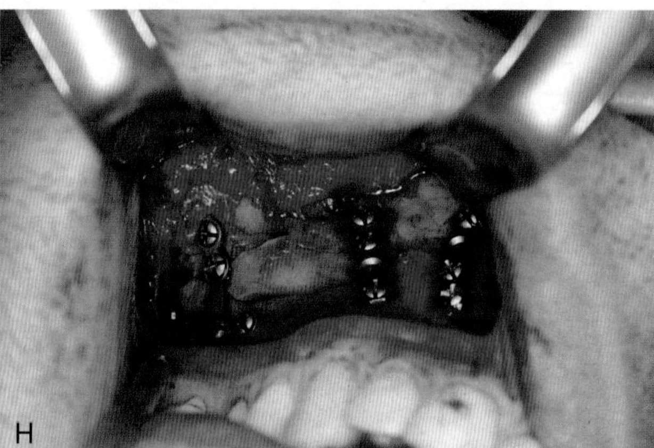

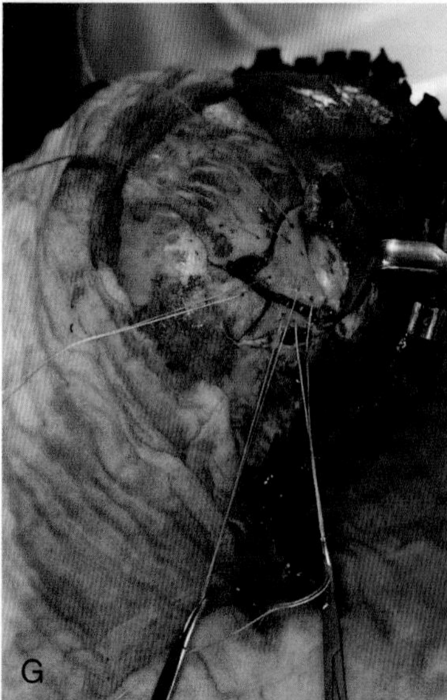

Figure 82.1, cont'd **F,** The plates span from stable bone to stable bone. The thin bone fragments are held in place by an elevator or Gillies hook and fixated to the bridging microplate. Another technique is to assemble the frontal bone segments on a separate table while neurosurgery is performed. **G,** In pediatric patients, titanium plates should not be applied because of their migration potential in the growing skeleton. Resorbable plate systems or resorbable suture material can be used to fixate bone fragments in children. **H,** In the Le Fort I level, the plates cross the fracture line and follow the nasomaxillary and zygomaticomaxillary buttresses.

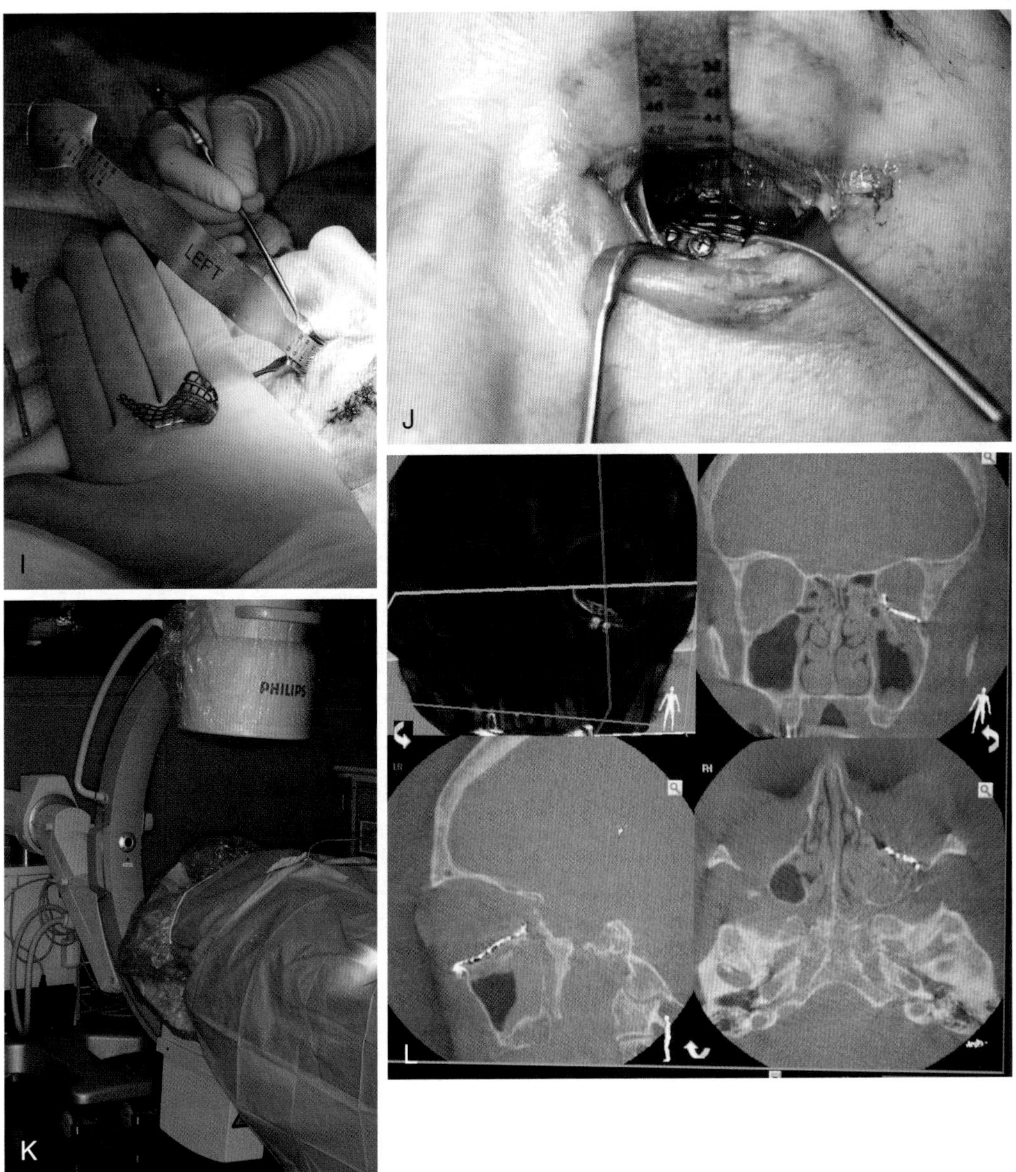

Figure 82.1, cont'd **I,** After the orbital frame has been reconstructed completely, the orbit itself must be reconstructed. If there is not enough "shelf" to support a resorbable membrane, a preformed titanium mesh can be used. **J,** A special malleable orbital retractor allows the surgeon to measure the needed size of the implant, which is fixated to the infraorbital rim with screws. **K** and **L,** The proper position of the implant can be verified by intraoperative three-dimensional imaging; this avoids a secondary surgery in case of a necessary correction.

Avoidance and Management of Intraoperative Complications

A proper physical examination and CT scan help set up the treatment plan. Significant nonfacial injuries must be evaluated before facial surgery is performed.

Airway protection by intubation or tracheostomy is mandatory. Fragment dislocation, swelling, and bleeding can impair nasal breathing in patients with midfacial trauma. Comminuted fractures of the midface can impede the insertion of a nasopharyngeal tube. A suspected skull base fracture is a contraindication to nasopharyngeal intubation. Oral intubation is feasible when the occlusion is not impaired. Otherwise, submental intubation is indicated.

To prevent infections, perioperative antibiotic treatment is recommended, and it is advised that preoperative antibiotics are tailored based on each institution's antibiogram.

Most facial trauma patients have soft tissue lacerations in addition to bone fractures. Fracture diagnostics should be performed before soft tissue wounds; in this way, already closed wounds do not have to be reopened for fracture treatment.

Definitive repair within 2 to 3 days is recommended to prevent scarring that hinders precise reduction of the fractures. A provisional intermaxillary fixation should be applied when the fracture treatment must be delayed.

Good reduction is easier when the fracture is exposed adequately. Other than in the peripheral skeleton, a direct approach is not favored in the exposed facial area. Attempts should be made to keep scars well hidden or have them blend into the environment. Therefore, the access often is distant from the area of interest. Major nerves and blood vessels must be retracted, particularly the facial nerve. Damage to this nerve not only impairs facial expression, it also can lead to corneal ulceration when shutting the eye is no longer possible. An electrical nerve stimulator should be at hand when the access is prepared. The relaxed skin tension lines should be followed. Trauma-related lacerations or preexisting scars can be used as access to avoid further scars. The incision line should be not too short, but rather as long as necessary.

When a coronal approach is closed, insertion of a flat suction drain (e.g., Jackson-Pratt drain) is recommended to prevent hematomas.

To shield the cornea when a transcutaneous approach through the lower eyelid is performed, tarsorrhaphy sutures can be applied or corneal shields utilized. An advantage of the subtarsal approach is the lower rate of scleral show and ectropion.[14] The retroseptal transconjunctival approach is favored in our treatment center because it allows the scar to be hidden, and it offers the possibility of extending the access some distance medially (transcaruncular) and laterally (canthotomy) when needed. The technique must be executed carefully to prevent the formation of an entropion and injury to the cornea. It is a rapid procedure because there is no need to dissect the skin or muscle of the eyelid. The lacrimal sac should not be injured when the transconjunctival approach is extended by the transcaruncular approach. Periosteal suturing is not necessary. It can be done if the access is wide enough. When a canthotomy has been performed, a canthopexy suture must be applied. The conjunctiva is closed with running 7-0 resorbable sutures. Submerged knots reduce postoperative irritation of the eye.

The eyebrow approach is a straightforward approach that is easy to perform. Because it runs parallel to the hair of the eyebrow, it is not suitable for patients whose eyebrows are not located laterally enough to reach the lateral orbital rim. The scar is sometimes noticeable, and for this reason, the authors prefer blepharoplasty.

In the maxillary vestibular approach, a local anesthetic with vasoconstrictor is injected vestibularly. Depending on the injury pattern, the access can be done on one side or bilaterally. The incision line is placed 5 mm from the fixated gingiva to ensure enough unattached gingiva for easier suturing. An incision line placed within the attached gingiva of a toothed patient can lead to postoperative suture dehiscence.

The Weber-Fergusson-Dieffenbach technique, another unilateral midfacial approach, offers a wider exposure. The scar is visible but blends into the esthetic units of the face. For trauma injuries, the authors prefer hidden approaches with concealed scars; they consider the Weber-Fergusson-Dieffenbach approach more suited to oncologic applications.

In some cases, the destroyed thin bone must be replaced by a titanium mesh or resorbable biomaterial sheets (e.g., Ethisorb fleece). In the past, calvarial bone also was used, but it had no long-term stability because of its substantial resorption.

Injury of teeth roots can be avoided by correct positioning of the screws. Drilling into a root does not necessarily lead to loss of the tooth. In a case of devitalization, the tooth should be treated endodontically after the osteosynthetic hardware has been removed. In the deciduous dentition, drill injuries to permanent tooth germs should be avoided.

In edentulous patients, the anteroposterior position of the maxilla is not easy to estimate. It is better established when the dentures are used as a splint for intermaxillary fixation. For better retention, the denture can be screwed onto the bone.

Postoperative Considerations

Complications in the upper facial and midfacial regions are less frequent than in the treatment of mandibular fractures. Common complications are impaired wound healing caused by infection, suture dehiscence, abscess, pseudarthrosis, and osteomyelitis. Infection can be caused by delayed treatment, omission of perioperative antibiotics, and unstable osteosynthesis of the fracture. Suture dehiscence can be caused by inappropriate placement of the incision line, poor oral hygiene, smoking, and mucosal disruption.

Postoperative major malocclusion as result of improper reduction necessitates reosteosynthesis. In cases with completed bone healing, minor malocclusion can be treated by selective grinding of the teeth; major discrepancies may require a reosteotomy. Some misalignments can be treated by an orthodontist, who also should be consulted when a reosteotomy is planned. To avoid emphysema and infection when a sinus is involved in a fracture, the patient should be instructed to avoid blowing the nose and to use decongestant nose spray for drug specific recommended length of use.

References

1. Hansmann C. A new method of fragment fixation in complicated fractures [title translated from German]. *Verh Dtsch Ges Chir.* 1886;15:134.
2. Lane WA. Some remarks on the treatment of fractures. *BMJ.* 1895;1(1790):861–863.
3. Lambotte A. *Le Traitement Des Fractures.* Paris, France: Masson; 1907.
4. Sherman WO. Vanadium steel bone plates and screws. *Surg Gynecol Obstet.* 1912;14:629.
5. Champy M, Lodde JP. Osteosynthesis of the external orbital cavity using screwed plates. Therapeutic indications and results. *Rev Otoneuroophtalmol.* 1976;48(4):243–248.
6. Kulkarni RK, Moore EG, Hegyeli AF, Leonard F. Biodegradable poly(lactic acid) polymers. *J Biomed Mater Res.* 1971;5(3):169–181.
7. Buijs GJ, Stegenga B, Bos RR. Efficacy and safety of biodegradable osteofixation devices in oral and maxillofacial surgery: a systematic review. *J Dent Res.* 2006;85(11):980–989.
8. Buijs GJ, van Bakelen NB, Jansma J, et al. A randomized clinical trial of biodegradable and titanium fixation systems in maxillofacial surgery. *J Dent Res.* 2012;91(3):299–304.
9. Metzger MC, Schön R, Zizelmann C, Weyer N, Gutwald R, Schmelzeisen R. Semiautomatic

procedure for individual preforming of titanium meshes for orbital fractures. *Plast Reconstr Surg*. 2007;119(3):969–976.

10. Strong EB, Fuller SC, Wiley DF, Zumbansen J, Wilson MD, Metzger MC. Preformed vs intraoperative bending of titanium mesh for orbital reconstruction. *Otolaryngol Head Neck Surg*. 2013;149(1):60–66 (Epub ahead of print).
11. Champy M, Lodde JP, Wilk A. Fronto-malar osteosynthesis by means of screwed plates [title translated from French]. *Rev Stomatol Chir Maxillofac*. 1975;76(6):483–488.
12. Eckelt U, Nitsche M, Müller A, Pilling E, Pinzer T, Roesner D. Ultrasound aided pin fixation of biodegradable osteosynthetic materials in cranioplasty for infants with craniosynostosis. *J Craniomaxillofac*. 2007;35(4–5):218–221.
13. Manson PN, Clark N, Robertson B, Crawley WA. Comprehensive management of pan-facial fractures. *J Craniomaxillofac Trauma*. 1995;1(1):43–56.
14. Bähr W, Bagambisa FB, Schlegel G, Schilli W. Comparison of transcutaneous incisions used for exposure of the infraorbital rim and orbital floor: a retrospective study. *Plast Reconstr Surg*. 1992;90(4):585–591.

Nasal Fractures

Shahrokh C. Bagheri and Behnam Bohluli

Armamentarium

1-cm Nasal tape
2-mm Osteotome
Appropriate sutures
Ash forceps
Boer elevator
Doyle internal splint
Freer elevator
Local anesthetic with vasoconstrictor
Mallet
Nasal speculum
Needle holder
Periosteal elevator
Scalpel blades (#11 and #15)
Thermoplastic external splint
Walsham forceps

History of the Procedure

The treatment of nasal fractures has been known since ancient times. Descriptions of nasal injuries and fractures can be found in the papyrus (circa 1600 BC) owned by Edwin Smith. In these cases, in addition to some usual magics and spells, a logical practical approach was followed. Reduction of nasal fractures was achieved by inserting tampons of linen saturated with oil and honey into the nostrils. This internal packing was externally reinforced by two stiff, splintlike rolls of linen, probably one on each side of the nose, which was then bandaged.[1]

The early documented reports on the management of nasal fractures date back to Hippocrates. He defined a simple classification for nasal injuries and proposed treatment modalities for each type of injury, and for a long time, these simple closed techniques were the gold standard for the treatment of nasal fractures.[2] In addition, many recent studies show that nasal fracture is not to be underestimated, and some of the simply reduced noses may end up in a complex septorhinoplasty procedure.[3–5]

Indications for the Treatment of Nasal Fracture

Esthetic deformities and functional changes are two main indications for the treatment of nasal fractures[3,4] A careful clinical examination, thorough interview, and sometimes precise analysis of preinjury photographs of the patient can help the surgeon discover any change of shape or any breathing pattern deformity that may have developed after nasal trauma. In some cases, nasal fractures without displacement or functional deformities may be best left untreated.[3–7]

Limitations and Contraindications

1. Excessive swelling and edema: Swelling may disturb clinical judgment and may lead to inadequate or improper reduction. The fractured nose may be treated before any considerable swelling develops (up to a few hours after trauma); otherwise, the procedure is best postponed until the swelling subsides (5 to 8 days after injury). Corticosteroid prescriptions and thermotherapy (cold compress for the first day and warm compress for the next 2 days) may be beneficial in shortening this period of delay.[8]
2. Panfacial fractures: Nasal fractures frequently occur with fractures of other facial bones. The treatment of multiple facial fractures follows a general rule: the fractures are reduced bottom up and from the outside in; the broken nose is the last to be addressed. Nasotracheal intubation may be a problem for nasal fracture repair. In such cases, after rigid fixation of all facial fractures, the nasotracheal tube is changed to oral intubation, and the nasal fracture then is treated as an isolated nasal fracture. The surgeon should never underestimate the importance of a nasal fracture even when focusing on other, seemingly more complex fractures; this mistake may never be compensated for subsequently, even with several revision operations.[9]
3. Naso-orbito-ethmoid (NOE) fracture: In NOE fractures, the nasal fracture is part of a more complex injury that requires special considerations. Inaccurate diagnosis may lead to undertreatment and several postoperative complications.[10]
4. Cerebrospinal fluid (CSF) leakage: CSF leakage is a possibility in severe nasal injuries. This leakage usually is controlled through conservative modalities, such as head position and diet. Some patients with resistant leakage that lasts several days may require endoscopic closure or open surgery. It is imperative that the treatments for the nasal fracture be done after neurosurgical clearance of the patient.[11]

TECHNIQUE: Closed Reduction of Nasal Fractures

EARLY MANAGEMENT

The proper technique to fix an acute nasal fracture greatly depends on the amount of displacement or depression of the nasal bones and the degree of septal involvement. Treatment varies, ranging from simple observation and prescription of antiinflammatory drugs to manual manipulation and reduction, to forceps reduction, to more complex open septorhinoplasty techniques.[5–8]

STEP 1: Anesthesia

A nasal fracture may be reduced using local or general anesthesia.[12,13] Local anesthesia may seem painful in an awake patient, and injection of even a few milliliters of a local anesthetic may distort the nose; it also may interfere with intraoperative judgments, the simplicity of the fracture, and the patient's cooperation. The surgeon's and the patient's desires are the main factors in the selection of the type of anesthesia. Local anesthesia usually involves anesthetic nasal packs (e.g., 4% cocaine packs) and injection of local anesthetics via infiltration and nerve blocks, usually using 1% lidocaine with 1:200,000 epinephrine as the drug of choice; 5 cc of this solution is dispersed around the nose and lateral sidewalls. A few drops of the local anesthetic is enough to block the infraorbital nerves on each side; the septum, internal mucosa, and subciliary block need another 3 cc.[12,13] It is important to bear in mind that in all cases, there is the possibility of an unacceptable reduction and the need for a much more complex procedure; therefore, the surgeon and the patient should be ready for a possible change from local to general anesthesia if a much more complex technique in that session. Alternatively, a second session may be scheduled for later to treat the patient under general anesthesia.[12,13]

STEP 2: Hand Manipulation

For hand manipulation, the direction of finger pressure is opposite the vector of injury and the direction of nasal displacement. Both hands hold the patient's head, and the thumbs are used to mobilize and reduce the nasal bones. The clinical appearance of the nose is checked precisely in case the reduction is not passive or an obvious deformity exists; in such cases, other steps may be required (Fig. 83.1A).[6–8]

Continued

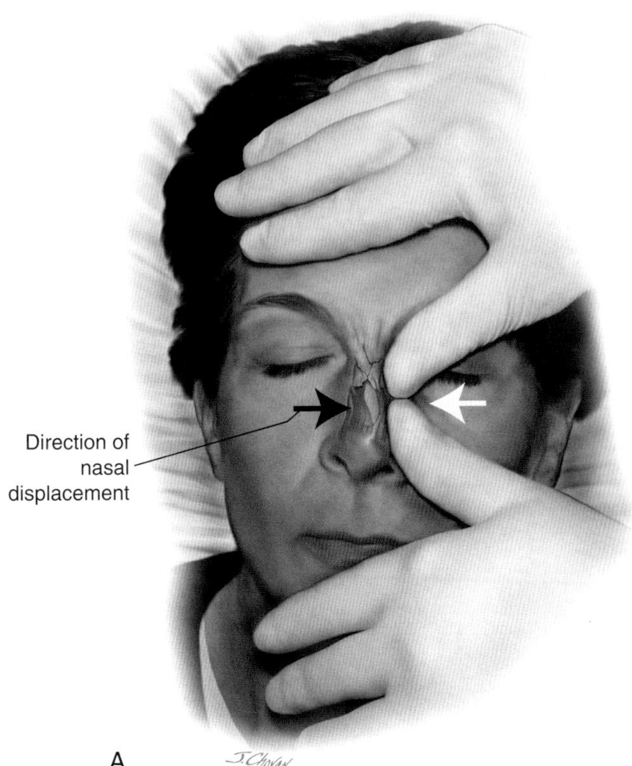

Figure 83.1 **A,** Hand manipulation of the nose. The direction of finger pressure is opposite the vector of injury and direction of nasal displacement.

TECHNIQUE: Closed Reduction of Nasal Fractures—*cont'd*

STEP 3: Nasal Bone Elevation

The fractured nose is held by the nondominant hand. A Boer elevator or any blunt instrument (e.g., a surgical knife handle) is inserted into the nose and gently passed inside the nostril. The fractured area is approached gradually, and the fractured bone is elevated. In some cases, the other (nondominant) hand may be used simultaneously to manually mold the nose. Finger palpation and visual observation are used to check the adequacy of reduction. The blunt instrument should be exactly beneath the fractured bone; this blind technique may be made more precise by adjusting the length of the instrument out of the nose (Fig. 83.1B–D).[6–8]

STEP 4: Forceps Reduction

Nasal forceps are specifically designed to grasp the displaced nasal tissue and move it in the desired direction. In nasal bone fractures, Ash forceps are opened, and one of the straight beaks of the forceps is inserted into the nose and gently moved forward until it is under the fracture site. The beaks then are gently closed, and the fracture site is held between one beak, which is inside the nose, and the other beak, which is placed over the skin. The fracture is reduced by gentle manipulation of the forceps handle.

In the case of a fractured or dislocated septum, the beaks of a Walsham forceps are passed into the nostrils, and the nasal septum is held by closing the beaks. The septum then is moved and reduced to its proper place. Walsham forceps may also be used to elevate a crushed and collapsed nose. In these cases, a hard stent is inserted into both nostrils and fixed by sutures to prevent collapse of the reduced structures (Fig. 83.1E and F).[6–8]

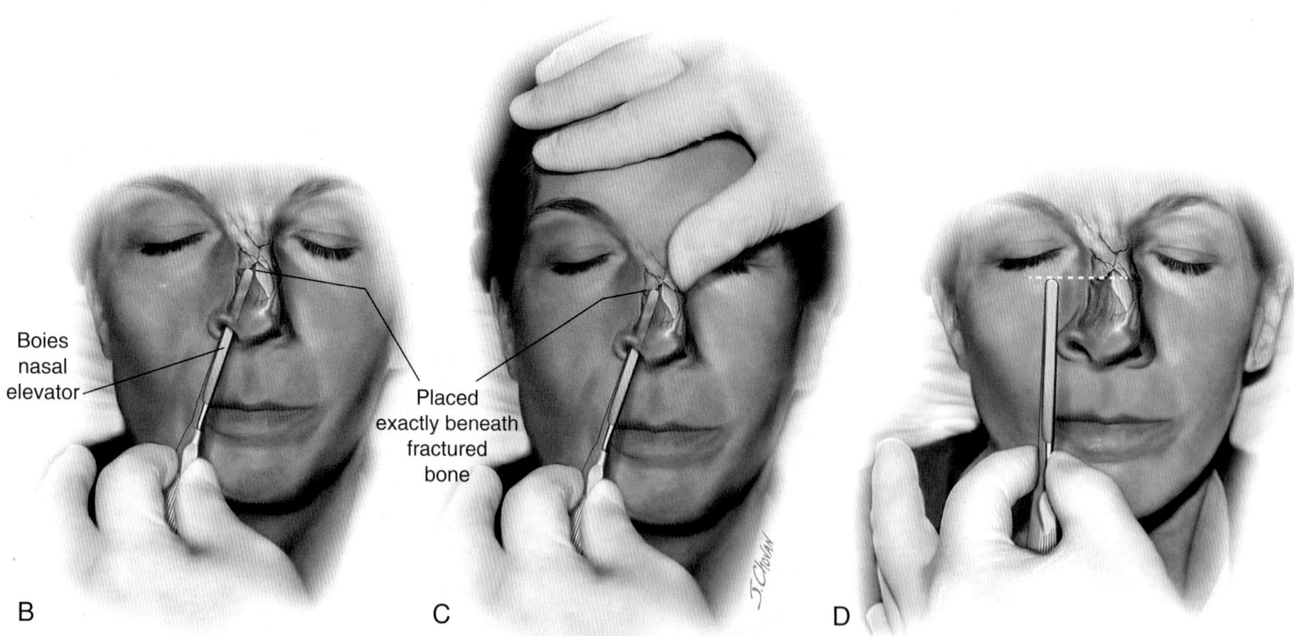

Figure 83.1, cont'd **B,** Insertion of nasal elevator to reduce fracture. **C,** Use of elevator with digital manipulation to reduce nasal fracture. **D,** The length of the elevator should be checked before nasal insertion so that the force applied for reduction is correctly placed.

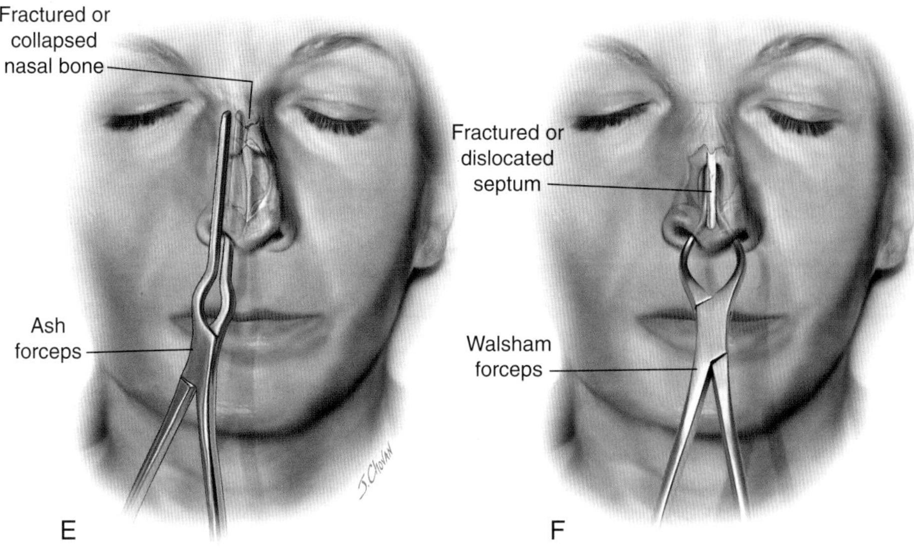

Figure 83.1, cont'd E, Walsham forceps may be used to reduce collapsed or crushed bone segments of the nose. F, Walsham forceps used to reduce and straighten a dislocated or fractured nasal septum.

TECHNIQUE: Closed Reduction of Nasal Fractures—*cont'd*

STEP 5: Internal Splints and Packs

After reduction of the nose, an internal splint or pack is used to hold the reduced parts in place and prevent hematomas or synechiae. Hard nasal splints (e.g., Doyle splints) have small tubes for breathing, so they are much more comfortable for patients. In a crushed nasal fracture, they may offer better control of fractured segments and may be left in the nose for a longer time postoperatively. Some surgeons prefer nasal packs impregnated with antibiotics; however, these packs are less tolerable and must be removed within a shorter period.[6–8]

STEP 6: Nasal Taping and External Splints

Small, narrow tape strips are used to redrape the skin on the nasal framework and to prevent edema formation. The tape also protects the skin from contact with hard external splints. A hard thermoplastic nasal splint is softened in warm water, trimmed and reshaped for the nose, and then placed over the taped nose. Light finger pressure is applied until the splint has cooled and is hardened by the application of cold water. External splints may remain for 5 to 7 days postoperatively (Fig. 83.1G).[6–8]

Continued

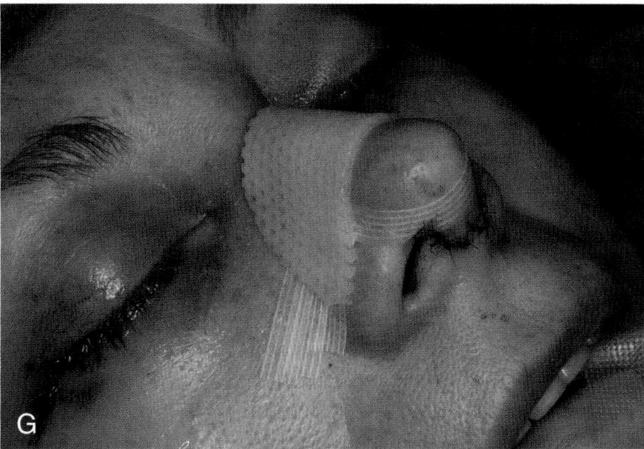

Figure 83.1, cont'd G, External nasal splinting to support and protect the nasal reduction.

ALTERNATIVE TECHNIQUES

Most nasal fractures are easily treated with the conservative techniques described, although some recent studies show many unfavorable results and complex sequelae in large series. It is logical to proceed with more advanced procedures in the early phases of treatment if any difficulty is encountered or inadequate reduction is assumed. These alternative techniques are usually undertaken to prevent postoperative functional and esthetic dissatisfaction.

ALTERNATIVE TECHNIQUE 1: Conventional Intubation and Submental Intubation

In multiple bone fractures of the face or panfacial trauma, the nasotracheal tube usually is changed to an orotracheal tube to enable work on a broken nose; however, sometimes concerns about edema and difficult reintubation may make the operating team consider other options.

The use of submental intubation has been frequently reported for simultaneous work on the jaws and nasal bones. In this technique, the surgeon injects a local anesthetic and makes an incision in the submental area. After creating an intraoral communication, the endotracheal tube is passed and orotracheal intubation is performed.[14]

ALTERNATIVE TECHNIQUE 2: Bone Reduction—Internal Approach Incisions and Access

For the internal approach, which is used for direct access to fractured bones, an intercartilaginous incision is made on the fracture side; then, using scissors for dissection, direct access to the fracture zone is obtained. Next, a Boer elevator is introduced through the dissected area, and broken bone is directly elevated and reduced. Some hold that this leads to a more precise reduction and repair in depressed nasal bones; however, the outcome depends on the surgeon's experience and the severity of the fracture.[15]

ALTERNATIVE TECHNIQUE 3: Bone Reduction—Use of an Osteotome

In some cases, the fractured bone segments are not passively reduced and may have resulting steps or palpable irregularities. An osteotomy with gentle manipulation may turn a greenstick fracture or locked bone fragments into a complete bone fracture; in this manner, passive reduction may be achieved.

In other scenarios, a nasal fracture may mimic an incomplete osteotomy in rhinoplasty. An external perforated osteotomy may easily help reduce this type of deformity. In this technique, a small stab incision is made in the skin on the lateral side of the nose. Then, with a 2-mm osteotomy and a few mallet strokes, the surgeon creates an accurate fracture in a well-designed line. The bone fragment is mobilized completely and reduced. The osteotomy site is gently palpated for bone spicules or irregularities, which are corrected if present.[16]

ALTERNATIVE TECHNIQUE 4: Septal Reduction—Septoplasty

Septal dislocation and fracture occur in many patients with nasal fractures. Early fibrosis and interlocked segments of cartilage and bones may preclude proper reduction of the septum; in these cases, a septoplasty with an intranasal approach may easily help the surgeon realign and reduce the septum.[17] A transfixion or Killian incision usually is made to gain access to the septum. The septum is exposed on both sides by subperichondrial dissection. Care is taken to preserve a strong L-shaped support of the septum. Interlocking segments then are released, resected, or reshaped. The anterior septal cartilage may be fixed to the anterior nasal spine (ANS) to prevent postoperative dislocation of the septum (Fig. 83.2).[18]

ALTERNATIVE TECHNIQUE 5: Delayed Rhinoplasty

With severely damaged noses (e.g., shattered nasal bones or saddle deformities), all efforts are made to obtain the best reduction and fixation, but the possible need for a late reconstructive rhinoplasty after a few months should be considered. For example, in three patients with severe nasal deformity after nasal fracture, all patients were treated with open septorhinoplasty several months after the original accident (Fig. 83.3).[18–20]

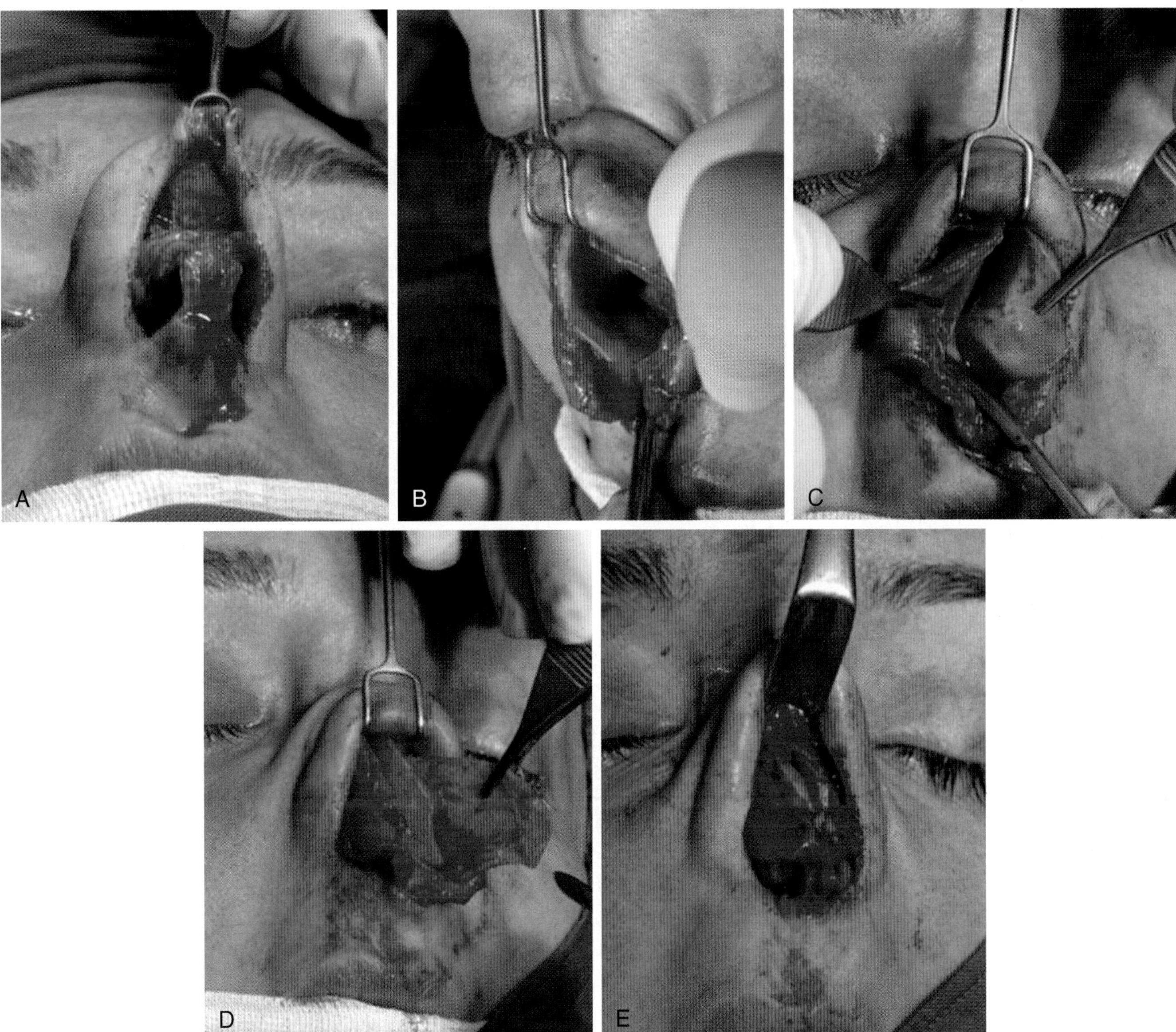

Figure 83.2 **A,** Columellar splitting incision to expose cartilaginous skeleton. **B,** Submucoperichondral dissection to expose nasal septum. **C,** Dissection completed bilaterally to complete exposure of the nasal septum. **D,** Removal of displaced or misshapen nasal septal cartilage. **E,** Septoplasty completed with stabilization of the previously divided lower lateral cartilages.

ALTERNATIVE TECHNIQUE 5: Delayed Rhinoplasty—*cont'd*

Late Management

After 2 weeks, fibrous bands around the dislocated septum and callus and around the displaced bones make it extremely difficult and sometimes impossible to properly treat the fractured nose by conservative methods. Therefore, in delayed treatment of a nasal fracture, the technique for managing the fractured nasal bone and septum poses a dilemma, requiring open approach septorhinoplasty. This procedure is performed to restore bone and septal cartilage and return the patient to the pretrauma appearance and function, provided the person does not want any esthetic changes. Late management of nasal fractures may be used for posttraumatic nose deformities that are 2 weeks to several months or years old.

Correction of Septal Deformities

With septal deformities, fibrotic tissue and healed deviated cartilages make restoration of esthetics and function a challenge. A wide approach to the septal dorsum may help the surgeon detect any subtle deformities. An open approach skeletonization is performed. Then the upper lateral cartilages are stripped from the septum; dissection is continued to the maxillary crest, and the septum is released from its base and relocated to its original position in the maxillary groove. The septum must be reduced passively. The nasal appearance is checked from all aspects; frontal and basal views may show any residual deformities. A long nasal speculum is passed through both nostrils to check airway patency. Many deformities are repaired in this stage;

Continued

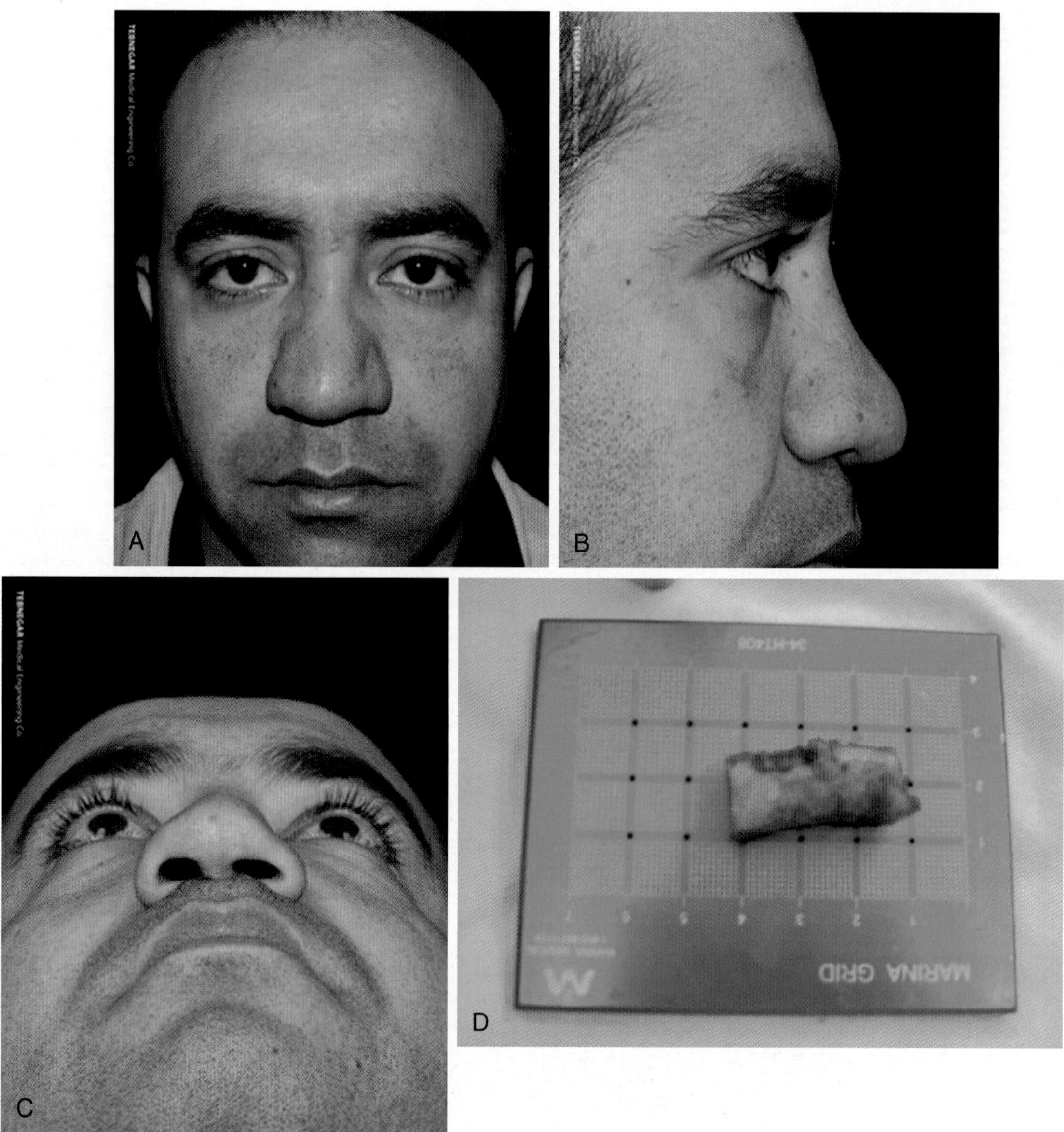

Figure 83.3 **A,** Frontal view of patient with a history of untreated nasal fracture. **B,** Lateral view of patient with a history of untreated nasal fracture. **C,** Worm's eye view of patient with a history of untreated nasal fracture.

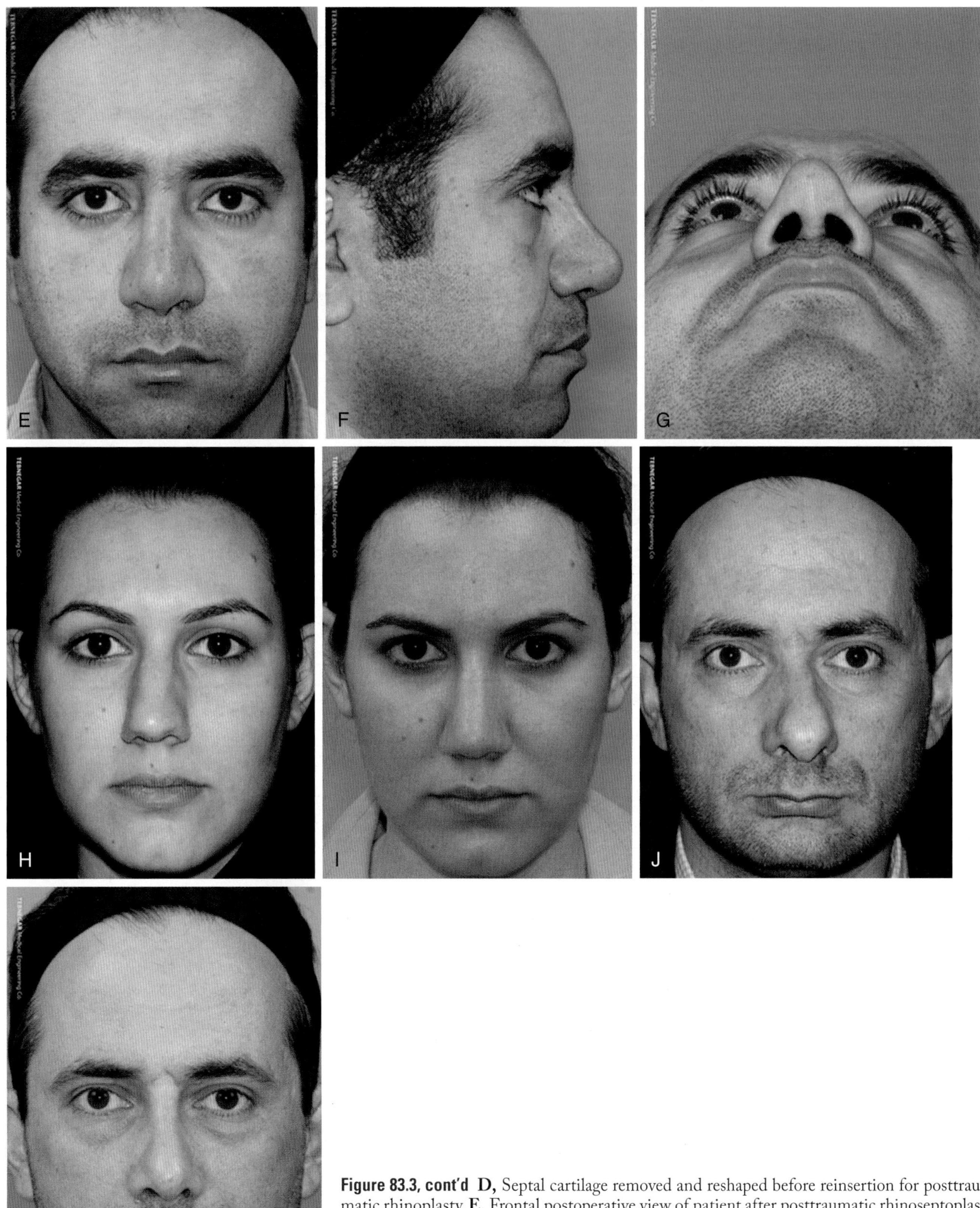

Figure 83.3, cont'd **D,** Septal cartilage removed and reshaped before reinsertion for posttraumatic rhinoplasty. **E,** Frontal postoperative view of patient after posttraumatic rhinoseptoplasty. **F,** Lateral postoperative view of patient after posttraumatic rhinoseptoplasty. **G,** Worm's eye postoperative view of patient after posttraumatic rhinoseptoplasty. **H,** Frontal preoperative view of patient after nasal fracture. **I,** Frontal postoperative view of patient after posttraumatic rhinoseptoplasty. **J,** Frontal preoperative view of patient after nasal fracture. **K,** Frontal postoperative view of patient after posttraumatic rhinoseptoplasty.

ALTERNATIVE TECHNIQUE 5: Delayed Rhinoplasty—*cont'd*

otherwise, further steps may be necessary later. Cartilage spurs are precisely trimmed, interlocking segments are conservatively resected, and major deviations in the dorsum are effectively straightened using unilateral or bilateral spreader grafts.[21,22]

Correction of the Bony Pyramid

In late management of the bony pyramid fracture, a lateral osteotomy can mobilize the lateral nasal walls, and a new, symmetric vault can be formed. A small stab incision is made in the skin in the lateral nasal wall, and a 2-mm lateral osteotome is used, with a few gentle strokes, to create a well-designed lateral osteotomy. In thick bone or widened bony vaults, a second stab incision is made just above the medial canthus and a lateral oblique osteotomy is made; the lateral nasal wall then is medialized with light finger pressure.[16]

ALTERNATIVE TECHNIQUE 6: Multiplane Lateral Osteotomy

When bone segments have started to heal in a new, malposed position, abnormal convexity and concavities and altered anatomy result. In some cases, a lateral osteotomy does not provide acceptable symmetric results. Osteotomies may be done in two or more planes, allowing fragmented bones to be molded to gain the best form. An external perforator osteotomy in two or more planes may create several greenstick fractures that can be shaped and molded by manual manipulation.[16,18]

ALTERNATIVE TECHNIQUE 7: Extracorporeal Septoplasty

Postfracture septal deformities in late treatment of nasal fractures are complicated. In extracorporeal septoplasty, the septal mucosa is completely dissected from the septum. The septum then is released from all its attachments to the maxillary crest, vomer, and ethmoid bones, and all ligamentous attachments to the medial crura are freed. The deformed septal cartilage is totally exposed. It is trimmed and reshaped outside of the nose; extremely curved or deviated segments may be resected. Crosshatching releases small deformities. After a stable and straight septal framework has been achieved, the septum is reimplanted in its original position and fixed to the nasal bones. The upper lateral cartilages are fixed to the dorsal septum, and the caudal border of the septum is fixed to the ANS. Intranasal splints help readapt the mucosa and stabilize the cartilage until it has healed in position (Fig. 83.4).[23,24]

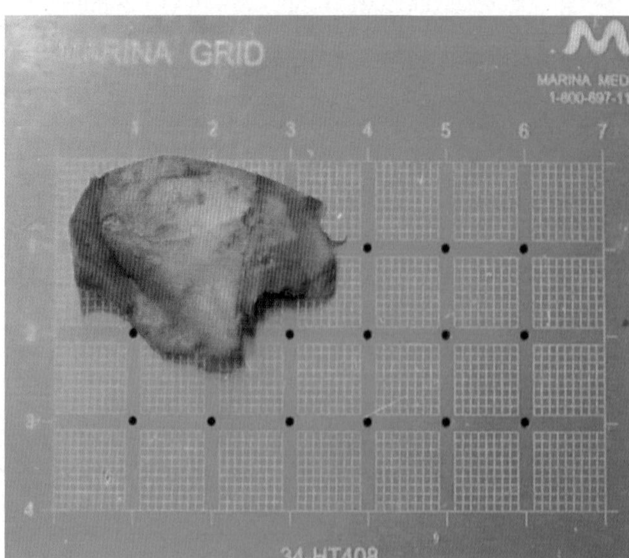

Figure 83.4 Nasal septum undergoing extracorporeal manipulation during posttraumatic rhinoseptoplasty.

ALTERNATIVE TECHNIQUE 8: Camouflage Grafts

With the camouflage grafts technique, instead of repositioning the fractured bones and cartilages, grafts are used to fill the depressed or collapsed nasal anatomy. The external approach rhinoplasty may provide the best access for precise graft placement and fixation. Septal cartilage, auricular cartilage, rib graft, temporalis fascia, and versatile types of alloplastic materials are recommended for this purpose. The amount of graft material required, the quality of the nasal skin, and the surgeon's experience and expertise are dominant factors in determining the best augmentation material for specific nasal regions. Table 83.1 presents some characteristics of augmentation materials.[18]

Sometimes subtle asymmetries and deformities remain; these nonfunctional defects are best restored by fillers or fat injections. A fat graft requires 3 to 5 cc of refined fat; therefore, 10 cc of fat is harvested from any donor site (e.g., thighs or abdomen) and purified by 3 minutes of centrifugation. The fat then is gently injected into depressed or asymmetric parts of the nose.

This technique may be an alternative to other augmentation techniques or may be used as an adjunct to other corrective surgeries. This technique may be used a few months after nasal fracture repair or simultaneously in late management of nasal fractures (Fig. 83.5).[25]

Table 83.1 Advantages and Disadvantages of Common Augmentation Materials Used in Revision Rhinoplasty

Material		Advantages	Disadvantages
Autogenous Grafts			
Fascia		Resistant to resorption Camouflages the sharp edge of grafts (e.g., crushed cartilage)	Donor site morbidity Patient compliance
Cartilage	Septal cartilage	The longitudinal characteristic of this cartilage makes it a favorable choice for spreader grafts	Usually consumed or scarred during primary rhinoplasty, especially the caudal portion
	Auricular cartilage	Excellent alternative for autogenous cartilage; the curved nature of auricular contours could be used for alar grafts and composite grafts. The remaining subcutaneous portion assists in fixation of the graft	Risk for hematoma inherent in anatomic curvatures Not suitable for crushing or morselizing
	Costochondral cartilage	First choice for massive reconstructions; an abundant amount of cartilage is available	Extensive surgery needed Risk of warping of cartilage and complications at the donor site
Allograft		Available in large quantities Lack of donor site morbidity	Risk of disease transmission Host immune reactions to the graft Resorption Warping
Alloplastic Grafts		Available in a range of sizes, volumes, and hardness Lack of donor site morbidity Easily contorted More favorable in dorsal augmentation	Foreign body reaction or chronic inflammation Infection Extrusion Expensive Unfavorable result in the lower third of the nose and function structures (e.g., strut, alar grafts, columella) Wound healing complications with subsequent nasal trauma Increased complications in younger patients

From Bagheri SC, Bell RB, Khan HA, eds. *Current Therapy in Oral and Maxillofacial Durger.* St Louis, MO: Mosby; 2011.

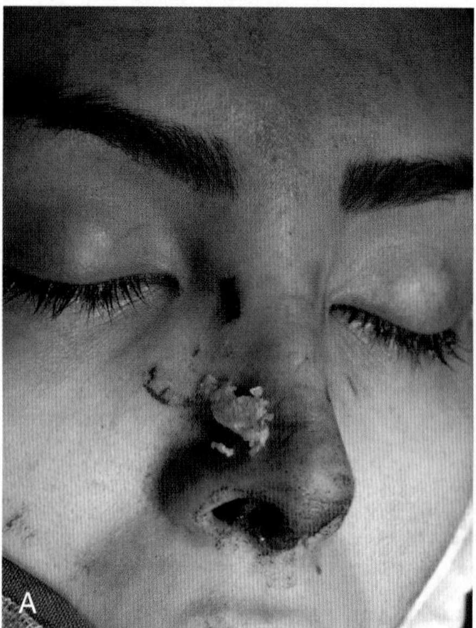

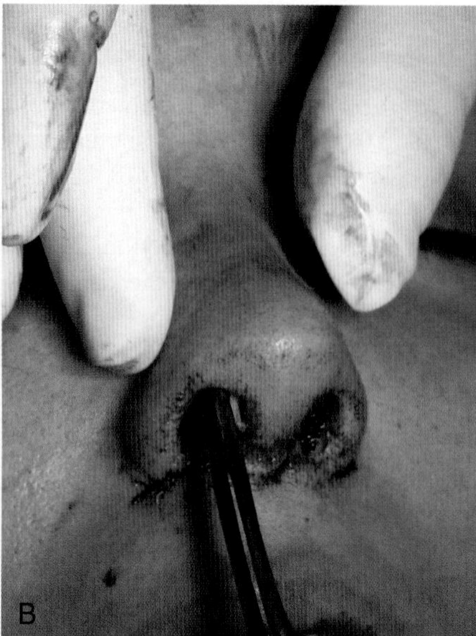

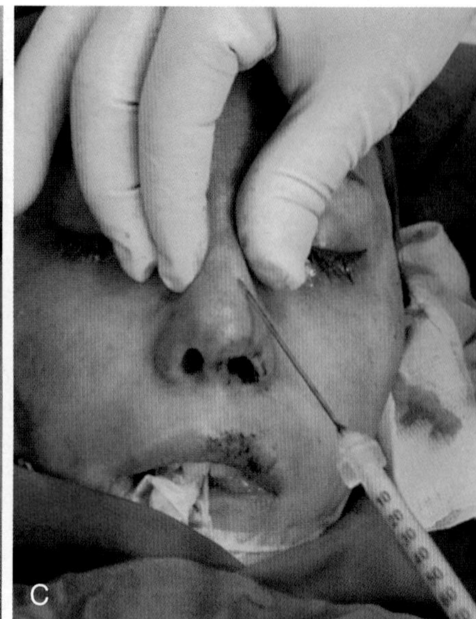

Figure 83.5 **A,** Morselized autogenous cartilage augmentation of defects during posttraumatic rhinoseptoplasty. **B,** Insertion of morselized autogenous cartilage for augmentation of defects during posttraumatic rhinoseptoplasty. **C,** Autogenous fat augmentation of defects during posttraumatic rhinoseptoplasty.

Avoidance and Management of Intraoperative Complications

Excessive Bleeding

Epistaxis may be seen immediately after any nasal trauma or during reduction procedures, especially when forceps are used. This bleeding often is self-limiting, or it may be controlled by anterior nasal packing. On rare occasions, when the nasoethmoid vessels are involved, severe bleeding may be encountered. Reduction of nasal fractures usually results in cessation of hemorrhage, although posterior packing and, in rare cases, ligation or embolization of the causative artery (anterior ethmoidal artery) may be necessary.[25,26]

Septal Hematoma

Septal hematoma is a relatively rare but critical complication. Blood accumulates between the septal cartilage and the perichondrium. This type of hematoma, if left untreated, leads to loss of the blood supply to the overlying mucosa. Necrosis and septal perforation are two devastating sequelae that may ensue within a few days. The diagnosis is generally based on clinical examination under direct observation with adequate light. The hematoma should be evacuated immediately. A small incision is made in the most dependent part of the hematoma, a delicate hemostat is inserted into the hematoma, and all the blood is drained. The incision is not usually closed to prevent reformation of the hematoma. Nasal packing and intranasal splints help redrape the mucosa over the septal cartilage. Septal hematomas are more frequently reported in children and adolescents, although they must be ruled out in all nasal trauma cases.[26]

Septal Perforation

A neglected septal hematoma and/or traumatic manipulations of the septum may result in septal perforation. As with most other complications, prevention and early diagnosis are essential. Septal hematoma is an emergency, and the hematoma should be drained as soon as possible. The septum and septal mucosa should be manipulated meticulously, with special attention to the integrity of the perichondrium. Numerous flap types and materials have been proposed for treatment of septal perforations, although the mainstay techniques are based on tension-free closure of wound edges in any type of flap or graft. Small defects may be repaired by wide dissection of mucosa on both sides and simple closure and suturing. In larger defects, local flaps can be used. Insertion of fascia, skin substitutes, and other types of grafts between two layers of mucosa may be a reasonable modality. Extremely large defects may be best left untreated.[24]

Dislodgement of Bone and Cartilaginous Segments

Vigorous manipulation and reduction maneuvers may pull out fractured segments and lead to iatrogenic collapse or defect. Each simple maneuver should be performed gently. If these are unsuccessful, subsequent, more complex maneuvers should be undertaken with minimal force and effort. Smaller incisions and dissections generally are advantageous for preserving ligament and attachments in the early treatment of nasal fractures. If a larger incision and direct access are needed, limited internal rhinoplasty approaches to the bones and septum may help prevent this type of complication. In late management of nasal deformities, the open approach with wide exposure may help the surgeon precisely address any existing deformities.

Collapse of Septum or Nasal Bones

In severe nasal injuries or during vigorous efforts to reduce a broken nose, fractured segments may lose their support and collapse. Collapsed septal cartilage is best repositioned by an open approach to the nose. After a wide skeletonization using this approach, the septum is completely exposed by separating the upper lateral cartilages and stripping off septal mucosa from the septum. The collapsed septal cartilage is then elevated, repositioned to its original location, and fixed at several points to the nasal bone, upper lateral cartilages, and ANS. A hard internal splint may be applied to stabilize the septum; this splint may be left inside the nose for several days to 1 month.

If collapse of the bone segments has occurred, they can be repositioned using the Ash forceps. In cases of instability during reduction, an open approach may help the surgeon reduce the segment and fix it using a narrow surgical wire.

For correction of the saddle nose deformity, the surgeon and patient should consider a delayed major reconstructive rhinoplasty.[18]

Postoperative Considerations

Routine postoperative care of the patient with nasal trauma should address analgesia, nausea, nutrition, antimicrobials, nasal hygiene, swelling, possible epistaxis, and, most important, postoperative visits and support of the patient during the healing process. We advocate frequent postoperative visits not only to reinforce wound healing, but also for emotional support, especially for the facial edema seen during the immediate postoperative period.

To reduce edema, the patient should be instructed to rest in bed with the head elevated and to frequently apply gentle cold compress for the first 24 hours, when possible. White gauze is taped or suspended at the nostrils to minimize the dripping of blood. Although significant postoperative hemorrhage is uncommon, most patients have minor epistaxis (especially with nasal osteotomies). Intranasal packings can accumulate blood clots and mucous secretions, significantly contributing to postoperative discomfort and pain. The intranasal septal packings and splints are sutured to the membranous septum to avoid displacement deeper into the nostril. We recommend placing the suture tie at an anterior and visible location for ease of removal.

Patients are encouraged to ambulate early and not to remain in bed. This helps to minimize edema and to reduce postoperative pulmonary complications and deep vein thrombosis. The nostrils can be gently cleansed with normal saline and coated with petroleum jelly. The sutures are removed at 7 to 9 days after surgery. Many patients present with significant anxiety related to the postoperative visit (removal of sutures or intranasal splints) and may require encouragement and support. Intravenous sedation can be used in select patients to reduce anxiety for suctioning of the nasal cavity and removal of old blood clots and sutures. With nasal osteotomies, the nasal cast is removed at 7 to 14 days. The patient is advised to avoid contact with the nasal structures. Postoperative systemic steroids can be used to reduce edema, although this may not be indicated in all patients. Steroids (triamcinolone) can be injected into the nasal tip in cases of prolonged nasal tip edema. We recommend at least three injections at 1-week intervals. Similarly, irregularities and depressions can be addressed with injectable fillers after several months have passed. Unfavorable results should be immediately addressed and acknowledged. Repair of subtle deformities may be done after several months. Extensive reconstruction in massive nasal trauma may be postponed for 6 months or longer after trauma.[3–6]

References

1. Skoulakis CE, Manios AG, Theos EA, Papadakis CE, Stavroulaki PS. Treatment of nasal fractures by Paul of Aegina. *Otolaryngol Head Neck Surg*. 2008;138(3):279–282.
2. Lascaratos JG, Segas JV, Trompoukis CC, Assimakopoulos DA. From the roots of rhinology: the reconstruction of nasal injuries by Hippocrates. *Ann Otol Rhinol Laryngol*. 2003;112(2):159–162.
3. Li K, Moubayed SP, Spataro E, Most SP. Risk factors for corrective septorhinoplasty associated with initial treatment of isolated nasal fracture. *JAMA Facial Plast Surg*. 2018;20(6):460–467.
4. Andrades P, Pereira N, Rodriguez D, Borel C, Hernández R, Villalobos R. A five-year retrospective cohort study analyzing factors influencing complications after nasal trauma. *Craniomaxillofac Trauma Reconstr*. 2019;12(3):175–182.
5. Basheeth N, Donnelly M, David S, Munish S. Acute nasal fracture management: a prospective study and literature review. *Laryngoscope*. 2015;125(12):2677–2684.
6. Hoffmann JF. An algorithm for the initial management of nasal trauma. *Facial Plast Surg*. 2015;31(3):183–193.
7. Park KS, Kim SS, Lee WS, Yang WS. The algorithm-oriented management of nasal bone fracture according to Stranc's Classification System. *Arch Craniofac Surg*. 2017;18(2):97–104.
8. Lanigan A, Lospinoso J, Bowe SN, Laury AM. The nasal fracture algorithm: a case for protocol-driven management to optimize care and resident work hours. *Otolaryngol Head Neck Surg*. 2017;156(6):1041–1043.
9. Curtis W, Horswell BB. Panfacial fractures: an approach to management. *Oral Maxillofac Surg Clin North Am*. 2013;25(4):649–660.
10. Pisano J, Tiwana PS. Management of panfacial, naso-orbital-ethmoid and frontal sinus fractures. *Atlas Oral Maxillofac Surg Clin North Am*. 2019;27(2):83–92.
11. Hiremath SB, Gautam AA, Sasindran V, Therakathu J, Benjamin G. Cerebrospinal fluid rhinorrhea and otorrhea: a multimodality

imaging approach. *Diagn Interv Imaging.* 2019;100(1):3–15.

12. Al-Moraissi EA, Ellis E III. Local versus general anesthesia for the management of nasal bone fractures: a systematic review and meta-analysis. *J Oral Maxillofac Surg.* 2015;73(4):606–615.
13. Kyung H, Choi JI, Song SH, Oh SH, Kang N. Comparison of postoperative outcomes between monitored anesthesia care and general anesthesia in closed reduction of nasal fracture. *J Craniofac Surg.* 2018;29(2):286–288.
14. Shetty PM, Yadav SK, Upadya M. Submental intubation in patients with panfacial fractures: a prospective study. *Indian J Anaesth.* 2011;55(3):299–304.
15. Kim HS, Suh HW, Ha KY, Kim BY, Kim TY. The usefulness of the endonasal incisional approach for the treatment of nasal bone fracture. *Arch Plast Surg.* 2012;39(3):209–215.
16. Bohluli B, Moharamnejad N, Bayat M. Dorsal hump surgery and lateral osteotomy. *Oral Maxillofac Surg Clin North Am.* 2012;24:75.
17. Arnold MA, Yanik SC, Suryadevara AC. Septal fractures predict poor outcomes after closed nasal reduction: retrospective review and survey. *Laryngoscope.* 2019;129(8):1784–1790.
18. Bohlouli B, Bagheri SC. Revision rhinoplasty. In: Bagheri SC, Bell RB, Khan HA, eds. *Current Therapy in Oral and Maxillofacial Surgery.* St Louis, MO: Mosby; 2011.
19. Bagheri SC. Primary cosmetic rhinoplasty. *Oral Maxillofac Surg Clin North Am.* 2012;24(1):39–48.
20. Bagheri SC, Khan HA, Jahangirnia A, Rad SS, Mortazavi H. An analysis of 101 primary cosmetic rhinoplasties. *J Oral Maxillofac Surg.* 2012;70(4):902–909.
21. Rohrich RJ, Hollier LH. Use of spreader grafts in the external approach to rhinoplasty. *Clin Plast Surg.* 1996;23(2):255–262.
22. Sheen JH. Spreader graft: a method of reconstructing the roof of the middle nasal vault following rhinoplasty. *Plast Reconstr Surg.* 1984;73(2):230–239.
23. Gubisch W, Hacker S, Neumann J, Haack S. 40 Years of total extracorporeal septal reconstruction—the past, the present and the future. *Plast Reconstr Surg.* 2020;146(6):1357–1367. Online ahead of print.
24. Bohluli B, Motamedi MHK, Varedi P, Malekzadeh M, Ghassemi A, Bagheri SC. Management of perforations of the nasal septum: can extracorporeal septoplasty be an effective option? *J Oral Maxillofac Surg.* 2014;72(2):391–395.
25. Bagheri SC, Bohluli B, Consky EK. Current techniques in fat grafting. *Atlas Oral Maxillofac Surg Clin North Am.* 2018;26(1):7–13. PMID.
26. Kasperek ZA, Pollock GF. Epistaxis: an overview. *Emerg Med Clin North Am.* 2013;31(2):443–454.

CHAPTER 84

Zygoma Fractures

Larry Cunningham Jr. and Blake Chaney

Armamentarium

#9 Periosteal elevator
#15, #11, #10 Blades
Adson forceps
Appropriate sutures
Balanced salt solution
Bite block
Carroll–Girard screw
Corneal shield
Desmarres retractors
Freer elevator
Joker elevator
Local anesthetic with vasoconstrictor
Malleable retractors
Manhattan forceps
Mayo scissors (curved)
Midface fixation kit (with drill and drill bits)
Needle-tip electrocautery
Obwegeser soft tissue retractors
Ophthalmic antibiotic ointment
Raney clips
Senn retractors
Stapler
Tenotomy scissors (curved)

History of the Procedure

The diagnosis and management of zygomatic fractures have undergone considerable development since they were originally described. Classification schemes that attempt to customize treatment according to the complexity of the fracture have been proposed by Keen, Knight and North, Manson et al., Gruss et al., Zingg et al., and Ellis and Kittidumkerng.[1–5] Fixation schemes have evolved from internal wire-pin stabilization[6] to internal fixation using miniplates.[7] Innovations in fixation technologies continue to emerge today.

Surgical approaches to zygomatic fractures have undergone significant development as well. Keen described an intraoral approach to the zygomatic arch for the first time in 1909. The approach still carries his name. In 1927, Gillies described a temporal incision that allows the surgeon to reduce zygomatic fractures. The incision is still widely used, especially in cases of isolated zygomatic arch fractures.[8]

Indications for the Use of the Procedure

Many zygomatic fractures do not require surgical intervention. The decision to proceed with surgical intervention should be made on a case-by-case basis, taking into consideration the patient's treatment expectations, comorbidities, and the severity of the injury. In their classic review of zygomatic fracture severity, Manson and colleagues divided the fractures into high-, medium-, and low-energy injuries.[2] Low-energy injuries may not require any surgical intervention, whereas medium- and high-energy injuries often require open reduction and internal fixation. Indications for surgical intervention are listed as follows.

Functional Indications

Impingement on the coronoid process of the mandible can occur following fractures of the zygoma. Impingement leads to pain upon mandibular function as well as restriction in the mouth opening (trismus). In these cases, reduction of the zygomatic fracture is necessary to restore the full range of motion of the mandible.

The unique three-dimensional position of the zygomatic bone supports the globe in its spatial orientation. Zygomatic fractures that cause a change in the volume of the orbit or in the position of the globe often produce visual disturbances. If binocular diplopia persists after the initial swelling has subsided, surgical treatment is required.

Although rare, entrapment of ocular muscles identified on clinical examination is an indication for immediate surgical intervention. Entrapment can occur in association with zygomatic fractures or in isolated orbital floor fractures.

Impingement on the second distribution of the trigeminal nerve (V2) is likely after zygomatic fractures. Anesthesia in the V2 distribution most often resolves following fracture reduction. However, patients should be advised of the possibility of an incomplete recovery of the sensory innervation.

Aesthetic Indications

Asymmetry of the malar projection, enophthalmos, orbital dystopia, and zygomatic arch depression are indications for repair. The surgeon's perception of an aesthetic problem should be in line with the patient's perception of the problem and the need for repair.

Limitations and Contraindications

Surgical treatment of fractures of the facial skeleton is rarely an emergency. Life-threatening injuries should be identified and treated prior to treatment of zygomatic fractures. Likewise, injuries to the globe (e.g., globe laceration, rupture, or hyphema) pose a significant problem. It may be necessary to delay treatment of a zygomatic fracture until the injury to the globe is treated or adequately controlled. This becomes critically important when the vision in the contralateral eye is affected. Even though the risk to the vision is minimal when repairing zygomatic fractures, the risk is still present. The decision to surgically repair the fracture in the presence of globe injury should be made with utmost care and in consultation with an ophthalmologist.

Delaying the treatment for 10 to 14 days to allow edema to resolve makes the surgical procedure easier and leads to better aesthetic outcomes. However, delaying the treatment longer than 2 weeks can complicate the surgical procedure. Fracture edge resorption can make reduction more difficult, and longer waiting times may lead to malunion. Bony osteotomies may be necessary. Soft tissue response to the delay is detrimental to the aesthetic result, and soft tissue resuspension techniques become necessary to achieve the best outcome.

TECHNIQUE: Maxillary Vestibular, Transconjunctival, and Lateral Canthotomy Approach

STEP 1: Intubation

An angled oral endotracheal tube is preferred. It can either be taped or sutured to the midline of the chin away from the surgical field. A regular oral endotracheal tube can be utilized but may interfere with the access to the oral cavity. Alternatively, a nasal tube may be utilized but is not necessary and may interfere with evaluation of the facial symmetry.

STEP 2: Forced Duction Test

Small Adson or Manhattan forceps are used to perform the forced duction test preoperatively. The conjunctiva in the inferior fornix is gently grasped with the forceps and the globe is then gently moved in all directions. If present, points of resistance are identified. Ease of globe movement preoperatively is also compared to that measured on a repeat test postoperatively; ease of globe movement should be identical (Fig. 84.1A and B).

STEP 3: Preparation and Draping

The oropharynx is thoroughly suctioned, and a moist throat pack is placed. Chlorhexidine is used to prepare the oral cavity. Corneal shields are lubricated with ophthalmic ointment and properly placed. The face is then prepared and draped in a way that includes both sides of the face for comparison purposes.

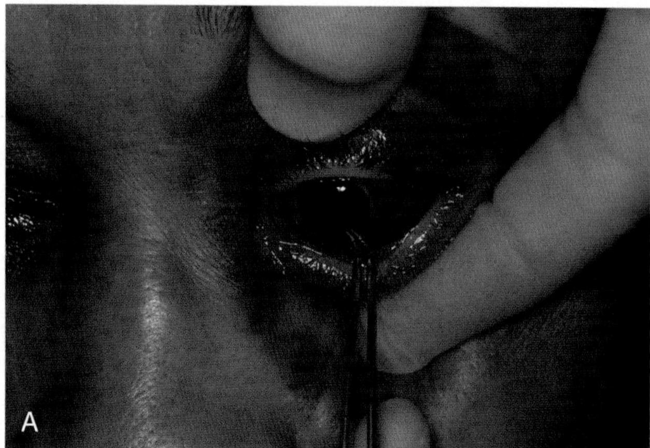

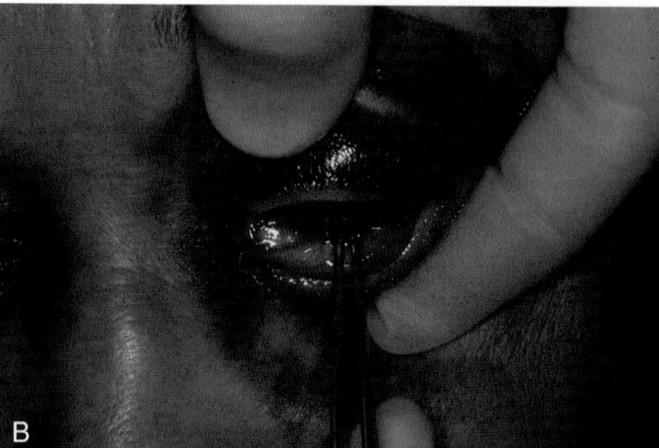

Figure 84.1 A and **B**, Forced duction test. Forceps grasping the conjunctiva in the inferior fornix and testing of the ease of movement of the globe.

TECHNIQUE: Maxillary Vestibular, Transconjunctival, and Lateral Canthotomy Approach—*cont'd*

STEP 4: Local Anesthesia

The surgeon's preferred local anesthetic with vasoconstrictor is injected in the maxillary vestibule, conjunctiva, and along the outline of the lateral canthotomy incision. It is preferable to mark the skin prior to the injection of local anesthesia. Alternatively, the incision for the lateral canthotomy is performed prior to injecting local anesthesia to avoid distortion caused by the volume of the anesthetic used. When injecting local anesthesia into the conjunctiva and the lateral canthus, the needle should be angled away from the globe.

STEP 5: Exposure of Fractures

Ellis and Kittidumkerng[5] have recommended exposure of all fracture sites using multiple approaches when a vestibular incision alone has failed to achieve the desired reduction or fixation. When preoperative imaging displays a severely comminuted fracture, multiple approaches will be necessary for treatment. The discussion that follows is meant to describe the techniques of various approaches. The authors do not recommend the use of all incisions for every zygoma fracture.

A maxillary vestibular incision (Keen approach) is made using needle-tip electrocautery. The incision should be of a sufficient length to allow access to the fracture without tearing. Typically, extension to the first molar tooth region is sufficient. About 5 mm of soft tissue is maintained on the buccal aspect of the teeth; this cuff is vital to prevent periodontal disease and for ease of suturing. The incision is carried through the oral mucosa, perioral musculature, and periosteum. A #9 periosteal elevator is then used for subperiosteal dissection superiorly and posteriorly to expose the fracture site. Extending the incision too far posteriorly, or dissection carried supraperiosteally, will lead to a cumbersome herniation of fat. The maxillary vestibular incision will expose the zygomaticomaxillary suture.

The infraorbital nerve is protected by identifying the neurovascular bundle and minimizing stretch injury to the nerve. The infraorbital foramen, which transmits the neurovascular bundle, can be palpated at 5 to 7 mm below the infraorbital rim and medial to the zygomaticomaxillary suture line.

The combination of a transconjunctival incision and a lateral canthotomy incision can provide access to the zygomaticofrontal suture, the zygomaticosphenoid suture, and the infraorbital rim. When combining the two incisions, performing the lateral canthotomy first can improve exposure and ease the access to the transconjunctival incision. The incision is 0.5 to 1 cm in length and extends from the lateral canthus temporally to the lateral orbital rim. The incision is made with a #15 blade in a natural skin crease through skin into the subcutaneous layer. Fibers of the orbicularis oculi muscle, orbital septum, and conjunctiva are then cut with the tenotomy scissors. The tips of the scissor then need to be directed vertically to release the lower lid completely from the lateral orbital wall. This action releases the lower eyelid from the anterior limb of the lateral canthal tendon.

Desmarres retractors can be used to retract the lower lid and expose the conjunctiva. Tenotomy scissors are then used to dissect bluntly posterior to the orbital septum. The same scissors are then used to make the transconjunctival incision in the already dissected plane halfway between the inferior margin of the tarsal plate and the inferior conjunctival fornix. Alternatively, an electrocautery can be utilized. The dissection is extended medially to the lacrimal punctum.

The orbital contents are then protected with a coated/insulated malleable retractor, and electrocautery is used to incise the periosteum exposing the orbital floor. Dissection in this plane is termed the *retroseptal approach* (incision is made in the orbital septum, exposing the periorbital fat). Some surgeons prefer a preseptal approach, in which the transconjunctival incision is made through the conjunctiva, dissection is carried out anterior to the orbital septum, and subperiosteal dissection is initiated anterior to the septum.

Different sizes of malleable retractors with the aid of freer elevators are used to achieve a wide exposure of the orbital floor (Fig. 84.1C–F).

Continued

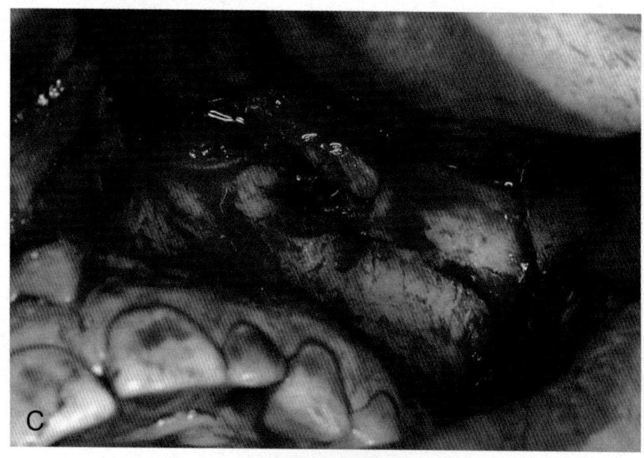

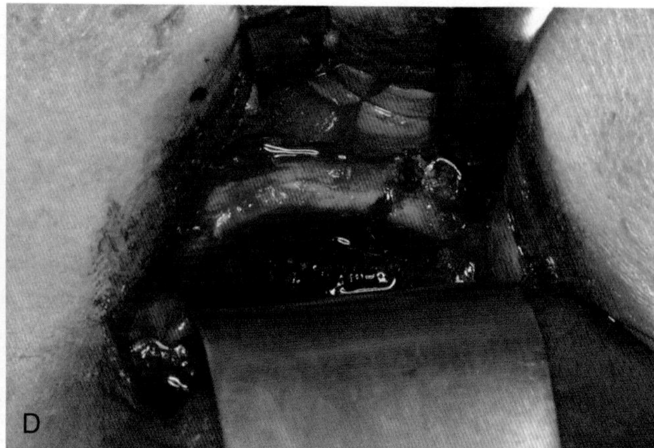

Lateral canthotomy

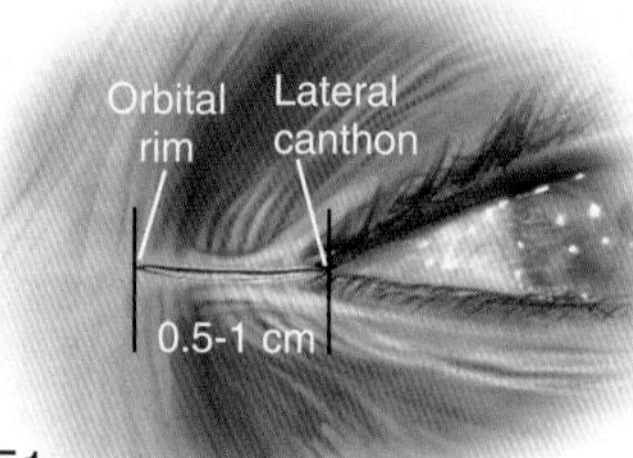

Skin/subcutaneous incision with #15 blade

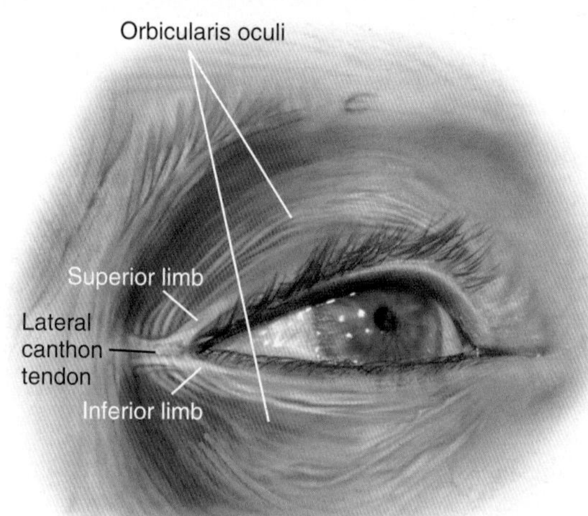

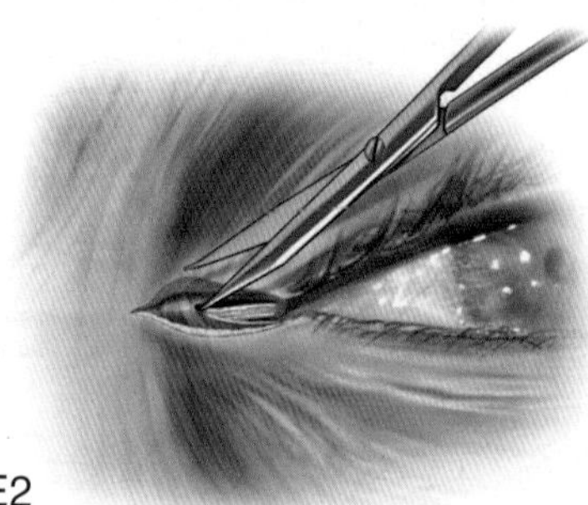

Fibers of orbicularis oculi, orbital septum, and conjunctiva cut with tenotomy scissors

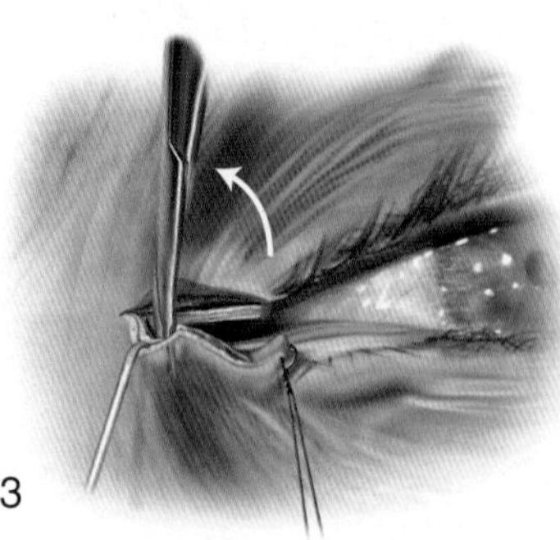

Vertical rotation of scissor tips to release lower lid from inferior limb of the lateral canthal tendon

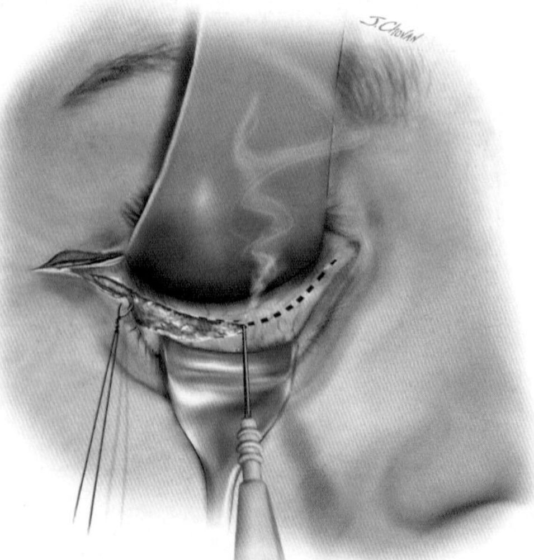

Transconjunctival incision made halfway between inferior margin of the tarsal plate and the inferior conjunctival fornix

Figure 84.1, cont'd **C,** Exposure of the zygomaticomaxillary buttress region using a vestibular incision. **D,** Infraorbital rim exposed using a combination of a lateral canthotomy incision and a transconjunctival incision. **E1,** Skin incision. **E2,** Scissors are used to cut the conjunctiva. **E3,** Vertical rotation of scissors. **E4,** Transconjunctional incision.

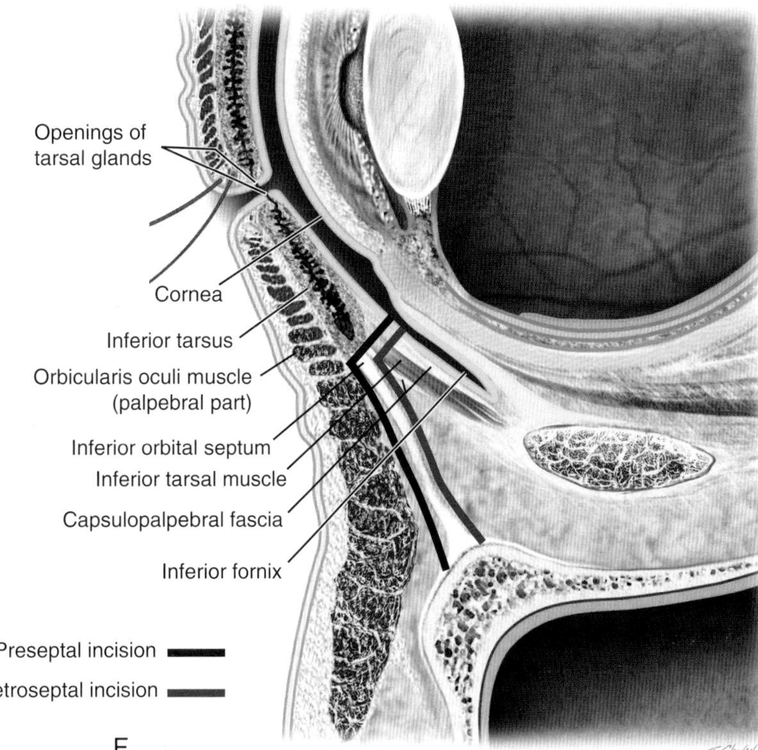

Figure 84.1, cont'd **F,** Sagittal view comparing the retroseptal and the preseptal incisions.

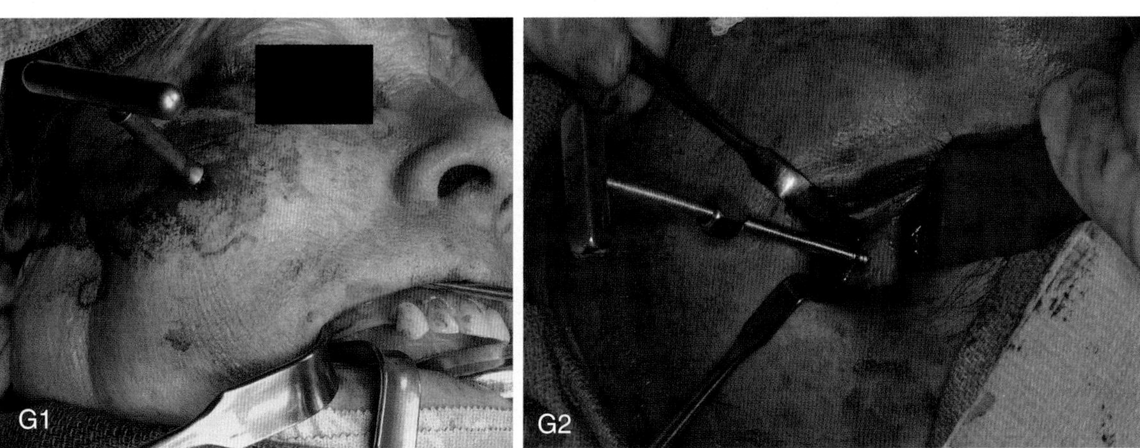

Figure 84.1, cont'd **G1** and **G2,** Carroll–Girard screw used to reduce the zygomatic fracture. Existing incisions may be used or additional transcutaneous access is made with a small incision placed in the malar eminence region using a #11 blade.

TECHNIQUE: Maxillary Vestibular, Transconjunctival, and Lateral Canthotomy Approach—*cont'd*

STEP 6: Reduction of the Fracture

A Carroll–Girard screw can be used to reduce the body of the zygoma. If exposure is sufficient to insert the screw with no additional skin incisions, then the screw is inserted onto the greatest convexity of the bone. If not, a small, 0.5-cm incision is made with a #11 blade in the skin overlying the malar projection. Dissection onto the malar projection is performed, and the screw is then inserted. Traction provided by this T-shaped screw can reduce the zygoma into its preinjury position.

The Joker elevator can also be used to elevate the zygomaticomaxillary complex. It is inserted from the maxillary vestibular incision and should be placed deep to the zygomaticomaxillary complex. This instrument makes it possible to reduce the zygomatic arch.

The adequacy of the reduction can be verified through inspection of the exposed fracture sites. Open reduction may be all that is needed to treat the fracture surgically. However, if the reduction does not provide stability, fixation plates should be used (Fig. 84.1G).

Continued

TECHNIQUE: Maxillary Vestibular, Transconjunctival, and Lateral Canthotomy Approach—*cont'd*

STEP 7: Fixation

Once reduction is achieved and the need for fixation is confirmed, the zygomaticomaxillary suture is plated. If stability of the complex is not achieved with one plate, additional plates are used in the zygomaticofrontal region and in the infraorbital rim region. If additional fixation is required to achieve stability, a wider exposure will be required (see the discussion presented under Alternative Technique 2).

In comminuted fractures and when the zygoma fracture is part of a panfacial fracture, plating the zygomaticofrontal suture first may prove most useful. The vertical strut is reconstructed, yet some rotation of the complex is still allowed for adjustment of malar projection.

Dierks and colleagues concisely described plate bending for the zygomaticomaxillary suture region.[9] An "L" plate is bent to fit the contour of the region. The zygomaticofrontal and the infraorbital rim fractures are fixated using curvilinear, low-profile plates. In most cases, only minimal bends are required (Fig. 84.1H–J).

STEP 8: Orbital Floor Reconstruction

Placing an orbital floor implant may be required at this point. If portable computed tomography (CT) scanning is available, the surgeon can determine with certainty the extent of the orbital floor defect. If an implant is required for reconstruction, the surgeon can choose from the multitude of the commercially available materials, such as preformed titanium mesh implants, titanium reinforced porous polyethylene (such as SynPOR by Depuy Synthes), porous polyethylene (such as MEDPOR by Stryker), or custom-made titanium mesh implants. Details of orbital floor repair can be found elsewhere in this book.

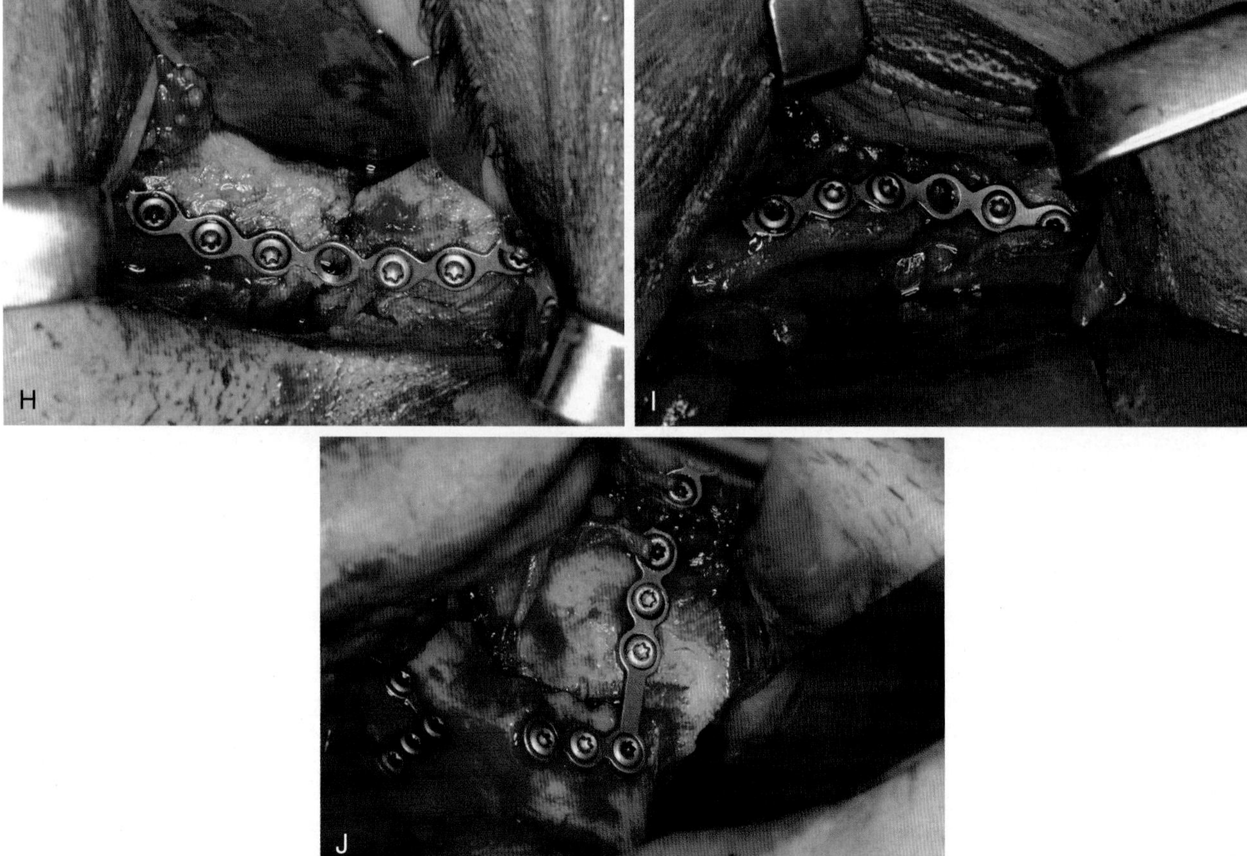

Figure 84.1, cont'd **H,** Curvilinear plate placed for fixation of the zygomaticofrontal region. **I,** Curvilinear plate placed for fixation of the infraorbital rim. **J,** An L-shaped plate for fixation of the zygomaticomaxillary buttress. (Note the need for an additional plate in the piriform rim region.)

TECHNIQUE: Maxillary Vestibular, Transconjunctival, and Lateral Canthotomy Approach—*cont'd*

STEP 9: Closure

It is necessary to irrigate the wounds with copious amounts of normal saline. At this point, the stability of the fractured zygoma is confirmed, and the alignment and symmetry are also confirmed. A postoperative forced duction test is repeated, and any restriction in the movement of the globe should be thoroughly investigated. Entrapment of periorbital tissue under the surface of the implant is possible and should be addressed prior to closure.

Closure of the maxillary vestibular incision is performed using 3-0 chromic gut sutures (or other resorbable sutures). If the incision extends past the midline, a V-Y closure prevents postoperative scarring and shortening of the upper lip.

Closure of the lateral canthotomy incision is performed using a 4-0 polydioxanone suture (or another slow resorbing suture). Reconstruction of the lateral canthus in its preincision position and contour is vital to prevent rounding of the canthus and soft tissue asymmetries. This is performed by grasping the lower lid tarsal plate and attaching it to the periosteum 0.5 cm posterior to the lateral orbital rim. If the periosteal attachment is not adequate in that region due to a prior dissection, a bur hole can be used to attach that suture. The suture is left untied until the transconjunctival incision is closed. We recommend a 6-0 fast-absorbing gut suture for transconjunctival incision closure. One suture with the knot buried is sufficient.

ALTERNATIVE TECHNIQUE 1: Maxillary Vestibular, Transconjunctival, and Upper Blepharoplasty Approach

The zygomaticofrontal suture can be accessed through an upper blepharoplasty incision. The incision can be used in conjunction with a maxillary vestibular incision and a transconjunctival incision. The upper blepharoplasty incision produces an inconspicuous scar and provides good visibility of the superior-lateral orbital rim and lateral orbital wall.

Preparation of the field prior to the incision is similar to that described previously. A corneal shield is inserted with ophthalmic ointment. An incision is marked on the upper eyelid prior to the injection of local anesthesia. The curvilinear incision is marked a minimum of 10 mm superior to the upper eyelid margin paralleling the tarsal crease.

The incision is carried through skin and orbicularis oculi muscle fibers. The skin muscle flap is then undermined to achieve access to the fracture site. Once the lateral orbital rim is identified, the periosteum is isolated and incised with a #15 blade or electrocautery with careful protection of the globe (Fig. 84.2).

Reduction and fixation are completed as is described in the previous section. Closure of this incision requires closure of the periosteum, orbicularis oculi muscle, and skin. A 3-0 polyglactin suture is used to close the periosteum, a 4-0 polyglactin suture is used to close the orbicularis oculi muscle, and a 6-0 fast-absorbing gut suture is used to close the skin.

ALTERNATIVE TECHNIQUE 2: Hemicoronal Approach for Severely Comminuted Zygomatic Fractures

Severely comminuted zygomatic fractures and severely depressed and comminuted zygomatic arch fractures can be addressed for reduction and fixation using a hemicoronal approach. A coronal approach may be necessary in cases of severely comminuted bilateral zygomatic fractures.

The incision marking is made from just past the midline (on the contralateral side of the fracture) to the helix of the ear. In most women and nonbalding men, the incision line can be curved anteriorly in the area of the vertex to be 4 to 5 cm within the hairline. If exposure of the zygomatic arch is required, a preauricular marking should be made as well. The preauricular incision should fall in a natural skin crease within 8 mm of the tragus.[10]

Corneal shields are placed, and preparation is performed as with the previously described approaches. Local anesthesia with a vasoconstrictor is injected in the subgaleal plane. The scalp has a rich blood supply, and the use of a vasoconstrictor reduces blood loss and improves visibility.

Crosshatches are made along the incision line to assist in the closure of the incision later. A #10 blade is used to incise through the skin, subcutaneous tissue, and musculoaponeurotic layer from the superior temporal line laterally to the end of the incision marking past midline medially.

Blunt finger dissection is performed in the subgaleal layer to allow the placement of Raney clips. Dissection also allows easier manipulation of the lateral aspect of the incision. Curved Mayo scissors are placed within the subgaleal plane medially and advanced toward the helix of the ear laterally to bluntly dissect that region. The incision is then made to the dissected depth. The previous action will place the incision superficial to the superficial layer of the temporalis fascia. The superficial layer of the temporal fascia appears as a glistening white fascial layer.

Additional Raney clips are used as needed. Blunt dissection or back cutting with a blade is performed to a point 3 to 4 cm superior to the supraorbital rims. The periosteum is then

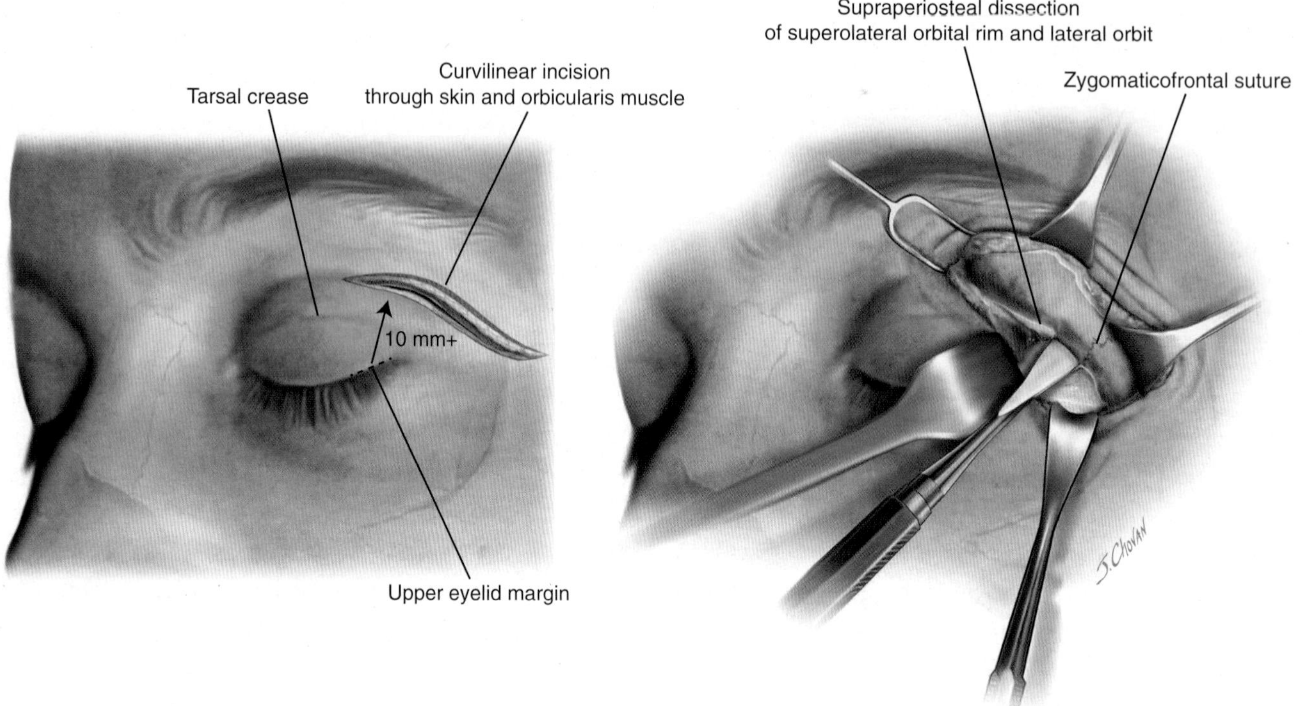

Figure 84.2 Access to the zygomaticofrontal region through an upper blepharoplasty incision.

ALTERNATIVE TECHNIQUE 2: Hemicoronal Approach for Severely Comminuted Zygomatic Fractures—*cont'd*

incised. The periosteal incision is performed from midline to the lateral aspect of the supraorbital rim.

If preauricular access is planned, the incision is carried through the skin and subcutaneous tissue using a #15 blade. A flap is developed anteriorly for a few centimeters. An incision is then made from the root of the zygomatic arch to the anterior-superior extent of the flap developed in the superficial layer of the temporalis fascia. This action will create a 45- to 60-degree angle incision. The zygomatic arch is then palpated, and the periosteal incision is performed as required to achieve adequate fixation.

Closure of the hemicoronal incision is performed in layers. A drain is placed in the hair-bearing region of the incision; it is removed in 24 to 48 hours. The musculoaponeurotic layer is closed using 3-0 polyglactin sutures. Soft tissue resuspension is beneficial and can be performed using a slow resorbing 3-0 suture (such as a polydioxanone suture). The subcutaneous layer is closed using a 3-0 polyglactin suture. Staples are used to close the skin in the hair-bearing region. In the preauricular region, the skin is closed using a 5-0 nylon suture.

Avoidance and Management of Intraoperative Complications

Testing for stability of the fracture intraoperatively is important. Lack of stable fixation may lead to fracture displacement and malunion, which can be difficult to treat and will require additional surgery. As with any other approaches in proximity to the globe, bradycardia may occur due to the oculocardiac reflex. The surgeon should be in communication with the anesthesia team and should be ready to stop manipulating the fracture if bradycardia occurs.

Intraoperative Imaging

Radiographic evaluation of fracture reduction prior to tissue closure and completion of surgery has been shown to prevent reoperation in patients with complex facial trauma including zygomaticomaxillary complex fractures.[11] Multiple modalities are currently available for imaging in the operating room including intraoperative CT (ICT), CT-based intraoperative navigation systems (INS), magnetic resonance imaging, and ultrasound. ICT and INS provide the best visualization of detailed bone anatomy and thus are the focus here.

The ICT technique is standard CT imaging except that it must be completed either inside the operating room or in a nearby setting capable of imaging an intubated patient under anesthesia while maintaining a sterile field. The use of INS provides real-time information to the surgeon to intraoperatively evaluate the status of fracture reduction. The navigation probe, preoperative imaging, and patient position are registered to each other using the navigation software prior to incision. Ideally this intraoperative evaluation is based

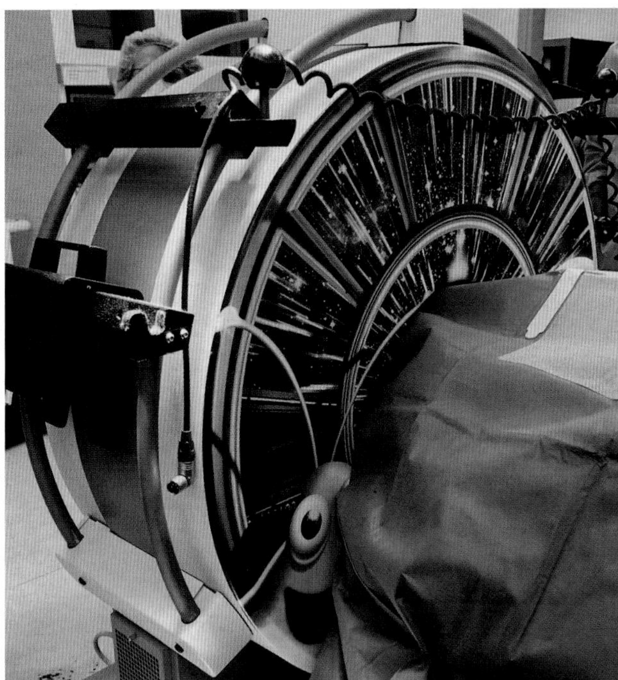

Figure 84.3 Intraoperative CT scanner.

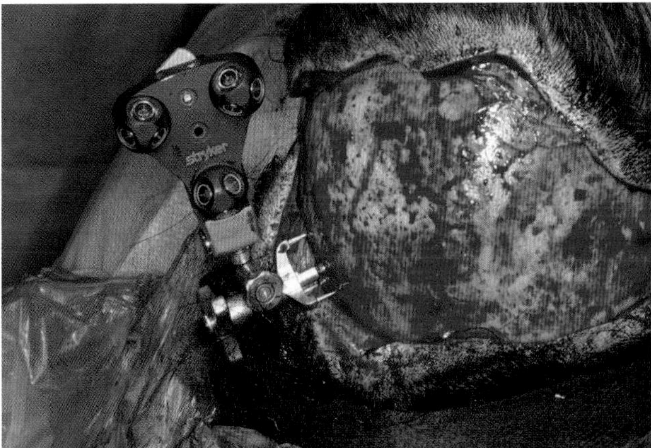

Figure 84.4 Intraoperative navigation fiducial markers secured to the cranial bone.

on preoperative planning. In the case of unilateral fractures, the diagnostic imaging of the contralateral side can used for comparison.[12]

Intraoperative CT

The logistics of ICT are relatively intuitive to maxillofacial surgeons since it is based on routine CT imaging; the only additional challenges are maintaining sedation and sterility of the field during imaging (Fig. 84.3). ICT is usually performed after fracture fixation and prior to wound closure. Confirmation of reduction on ICT imaging after fixation eliminates the need for postoperative imaging and may be referenced in the event of postsurgical complications such as failure of hardware, loss of fixation, or infection. ICT does not allow real-time evaluation, and it requires the surgical team to pause the procedure for image acquisition to be completed.

Intraoperative Navigation

The use of INS requires preoperative setup planning and additional equipment. Before surgery, preoperative CT imaging is uploaded into the navigation software. Once the patient is in position on the operating room table, fiducial markers are fixed to the patient registered in space using multiple stationary infrared cameras. Available markers include transcutaneous bone-born screws, custom dental occlusal splint with embedded markers, or premade patterns of markers attached to one another by a semirigid film secured to the skin with an adhesive backing (Fig. 84.4). For best accuracy, markers should be as close to the surgical field as possible while remaining unintrusive to surgery. Once the markers are registered to the INS, their position must be registered to the patient. This is accomplished by allowing the cameras to observe the probe touching standard areas of patient anatomy (e.g., infraorbital rim, glabella, anterior nasal spine) while a technician selects the same landmarks in the imaging platform. The surgeon can then touch anywhere in the field with the tip of the probe with simultaneous real-time tracking of its position on the imaging display.

Postoperative Considerations

Perioperative steroids are recommended when reducing and fixating zygomatic fractures. Perioperative antibiotics are administered prior to the procedure. No additional antibiotics are needed postoperatively. Postoperative analgesics are helpful. If eyelid incisions are made, ophthalmic ointments are recommended for patient comfort.

A Frost suture should be considered, particularly in older individuals with greater skin laxity. A single 4-0 silk suture placed at the gray line of the lower eyelid and fixed to the forehead skin, offering elevation of the lid during the initial healing phase, can decrease the risk of lid ptosis or ectropion (Fig. 84.5).

An eye patch or an oral airway can be taped onto the malar eminence as a reminder for the patient to avoid sleeping on that side. Pressure on the fractured side will most likely not cause any distortion of the fixation but may cause discomfort.

There are no dietary restrictions in the postoperative period. Patients should be encouraged to perform jaw physical therapy as early as 1 week postoperatively. Their progress should be monitored frequently. It is recommended that patients avoid contact sports during the initial postoperative period.

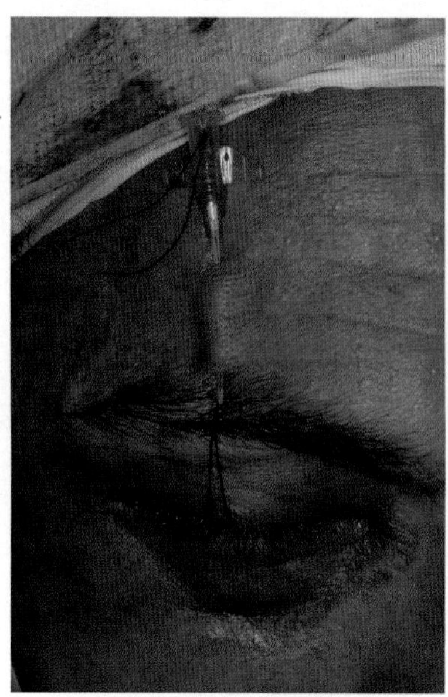

Figure 84.5 Frost suture.

References

1. Knight JS, North JF. The classification of malar fractures: an analysis of displacement as a guide to treatment. *Br J Plast Surg*. 1961;13:325–339.
2. Manson PN, Markowitz B, Mirvis S, Dunham M, Yaremchuk M. Toward CT-based facial fracture treatment. *Plast Reconstr Surg*. 1990;85(2):202–212.
3. Gruss JS, Van Wyck L, Phillips JH, Antonyshyn O. The importance of the zygomatic arch in complex midfacial fracture repair and correction of posttraumatic orbitozygomatic deformities. *Plast Reconstr Surg*. 1990;85(6):878–890.
4. Zingg M, Laedrach K, Chen J, et al. Classification and treatment of zygomatic fractures: a review of 1,025 cases. *J Oral Maxillofac Surg*. 1992;50(8):778–790.
5. Ellis E III, Kittidumkerng W. Analysis of treatment for isolated zygomaticomaxillary complex fractures. *J Oral Maxillofac Surg*. 1996;54(4):386–400.
6. Brown JB, Fryer MP, McDowell F. Internal wire-pin stabilization for middle third facial fractures. *Surg Gynecol Obstet*. 1951;93(6):676–681.
7. Michelet FX, Deymes J, Dessus B. Osteosynthesis with miniaturized screwed plates in maxillo-facial surgery. *J Maxillofac Surg*. 1973;1(2):79–84.
8. Gillies HD, Kilner TP, Stone D. Fractures of the malar zygomatic compound with a description of a new X ray position. *Br J Surg*. 1927;14:651.
9. Dierks EJ, Harper GA. The 4 cardinal bends of the zygomatico-maxillary buttress: technical note. *J Oral Maxillofac Surg*. 2009;67(5):1149–1151.
10. Al-Kayat A, Bramley P. A modified preauricular approach to the temporomandibular joint and malar arch. *Br J Oral Surg*. 1979;17(2):91–103.
11. Assouline SL, Meyer C, Weber E, et al. How useful is intraoperative cone beam computed tomography in maxillofacial surgery? An overview of the current literature. *Int J Oral Maxillofac Surg*. 2021;50(2):198–204.
12. Lübbers HT, Jacobsen C, Matthews F, Grätz KW, Kruse A, Obwegeser JA. Surgical navigation in craniomaxillofacial surgery: expensive toy or useful tool? A classification of different indications. *J Oral Maxillofac Surg*. 2011;69(1):300–308.

CHAPTER 85

Orbital Fractures

Paul S. Tiwana and Deepak Kademani

Armamentarium

Traditional Open Technique
Alloplastic implant or autogenous graft of choice
Appropriate sutures
Corneal shield
Desmarres eyelid retractor
Fine tissue forceps (Bishop–Harmon, Adson–Brown, Gerald)
Globe retractor
Local anesthetic with vasoconstrictor
Needle electrocautery
Osteosynthesis plating system
Periosteal elevator
Small malleable retractor
Tenotomy scissors

Endoscopic-Assisted Technique
0-degree and 30-degree 4-mm rigid endoscopes
Appropriate sutures
Blakesley nasal forceps
Cheek retractors
Corneal shield
Curved Freer elevator
Curved suction
Extra-thin alloplastic implant
Fine tissue forceps (Bishop–Harmon, Adson–Brown, Gerald)
High-speed handpiece with small round or fissure bur
Local anesthetic with vasoconstrictor
Needle electrocautery
Periosteal elevator
Pickle fork or wire director
Tenotomy scissors

History of the Procedure

The surgical management of orbital fractures continues to be a challenging field because no single approach or reconstruction material is suitable for all patients. In addition, the technical demands of the surgical repair and the related anatomy make precise repair difficult for the novice. The surgeon must ensure gentle tissue handling and careful globe retraction to allow for visualization of the fracture during operative repair.

Signs and symptoms of orbital fractures have been described throughout recorded human history. In 1957, Smith and Regan[1] coined the term *orbital blowout fracture* after they reproduced orbital floor and medial wall fractures in cadavers by hammering a hurling ball resting on the eye. In 1960, Converse and Smith[2] classified these fractures as "pure" (isolated floor) and "impure" (floor and rim). A year later, Converse et al.[3] discussed reconstruction of orbital floor fractures by coordinating graft volume replacement with orbital volume increase to avoid enophthalmos. In 1986, Manson et al.[4,5] suggested that the shape and position of the orbital graft/implant are more important than the orbital volume; they emphasized that the bony floor anatomy (bulge in the orbital floor) is instrumental in providing support to the globe.

More recently, several technologic advances have affected the surgical management of orbital fractures, such as virtual planning surgery, custom-made implants, navigation, and intraoperative computed tomography (CT) scanning.[6,7] The traditional technique uses either periorbital incisions or overlying lacerations. Orbital roof fractures may be directly accessed and repaired using a frontal craniotomy and brain retraction.

The initial use of endoscopic techniques in the diagnosis and management of orbital fractures can be traced to the 1970s, when Westphal and Kreidler[8] described sinusoscopy for the diagnosis of blowout fractures. However, the development of fine-cut CT scans for evaluation of these fractures obviated the need for this procedure in the ensuing years. In 1997, Saunders et al.[9] described the transantral approach for repair of orbital floor fractures, and in 1999, Chen et al.[10] described the endonasal approach for repair of medial wall fractures. A primary advantage of endoscopic repair is the avoidance of periorbital incisions, which may contribute to an unesthetic postoperative appearance and lid function problems.

Indications for the Use of the Procedure

Orbital fractures can be encountered in a number of clinical presentations, such as naso-orbito-ethmoid (NOE) fractures, orbitozygomaticomaxillary complex fractures, internal orbital fractures, and complex Le Fort II and III fractures. This chapter focuses on the surgical management of isolated internal orbital fractures; other types of fractures are described elsewhere in this text.

The bony orbit supports and protects the globe and allows for functioning of the eye. It is shaped like a pyramid, with the base making up the orbital rim. Seven bones form the orbit. The frontal bone and lesser wing of the sphenoid make up the orbital roof. The floor of the orbit is composed of the orbital portions of the maxillary and zygomatic bones. On the medial aspect of the orbit lies the lamina papyracea of the ethmoid, the frontal process of the maxilla, and the lacrimal and sphenoid bones. The lesser wing of the sphenoid and zygoma form the lateral wall. Any or all of these bones can be involved in orbital blowout fractures; however, usually either the floor or the medial wall is involved because these are the thinnest components (Fig. 85.1). Blow-in fractures are possible and most likely involve the orbital roof. Although outside the scope of this chapter, blow-in fractures of the orbital roof require special attention. They not only increase orbital volume and therefore are compressive on the orbital space, they also can involve herniation of the brain into the orbital space, with a characteristic pulsation felt by the patient. Neurosurgical consultation is warranted for these fractures.

Regardless of the clinical presentation, indications for surgery are divided into functional or esthetic reasons. Functional indications for surgery are related to either impingement by the fracture on the surrounding soft tissues or defects from fractures that are large enough to cause significant hypoglobus, dystopia, and enophthalmos resulting in visual changes. An ophthalmologist skilled in trauma care should evaluate all patients with orbital fractures, especially those with acute visual changes. Soft-tissue structures that maybe impinged upon or injured by the fracture can include the optic nerve, blood vessels, the second division of the trigeminal nerve, the motor nerves to the globe, muscles, and the periorbita itself. Although fortunately rare, both orbital apex syndrome and superior orbital fissure syndrome also can occur. Most functional issues are related to entrapment of the periorbita or rectus muscles by the fracture (Fig. 85.2). This may cause restriction of gaze, with resultant diplopia in the affected visual field. This can be clinically confirmed with a forced duction test of the affected muscle.

In most circumstances, orbital fractures with functional indications for repair should be considered urgent cases. Esthetic indications for repair are mostly due to globe malposition. In these cases, enophthalmos and hypoglobus are commonly encountered. The severity of these signs and symptoms dictate the need for either an observational period or early surgical repair. Occasionally, patients present with a large defect but are free of signs and symptoms. In these cases, surgery should still be considered because studies have shown a correlation between globe position and the size and location of the defect.[4,5,11–13] Most facial trauma surgeons agree that a 2 × 2 cm fracture defect behind the equator of the globe most likely will cause clinically significant enophthalmos (greater than 2 mm), and these patients are candidates for surgical repair. Special consideration should be given to orbital fractures in children with clinical or radiographic evidence of entrapment (also termed a *white-eyed blowout*). Clinically, these patients demonstrate entrapment and may also present with the ocular-cardiac reflex, which may cause significant bradycardia, heart block, and nausea and vomiting. The bony elasticity of the facial skeleton in children allows the orbital fracture to open and close back into position, tightly trapping periorbital soft tissues or muscles. Within 24 hours, involved muscle tissue may undergo avascular necrosis, with a resultant Volkmann's ischemic contracture. This causes permanent muscle imbalance and results in lifelong diplopia unless corrected surgically. Orbital entrapment in children is regarded as a surgical emergency and should be repaired immediately (Fig. 85.3).

Although the indications for endoscopic techniques are similar to those for the traditional approach, not all orbital fractures can be repaired endoscopically. In the authors' experience, small to medium-sized central orbital floor fractures with stable ledges are most suitable for endoscopic techniques. Because it involves minimal globe manipulation, the endoscopic approach may be appropriate in patients in whom traditional approaches are contraindicated, such as those with hyphema, retinal detachment, or globe injuries.

Limitations and Contraindications

Relative contraindications to repair of orbital fractures are mostly related to ocular injuries (e.g., hyphema, globe ruptures, retinal tears) and recent ophthalmologic surgery. Ophthalmologic evaluation and clearance are warranted in these cases before surgery is considered. Additional relative contraindications include patients who have vision only in the affected orbit/eye and life-threatening instability.

The same contraindications to the traditional approach apply to the endoscopic approach. However, an advantage of the latter is that endoscopic-assisted orbital repair surgery can be done earlier in some ocular injuries because the minimally invasive nature of the procedure requires less eye manipulation. Endoscopic repair of a large two-wall orbital defect is contraindicated because the implant is more difficult to stabilize.

As with any endoscopic approach, it is important to discuss with the patient the possibility that a traditional approach may have to be used if the endoscopic repair is unsuccessful.

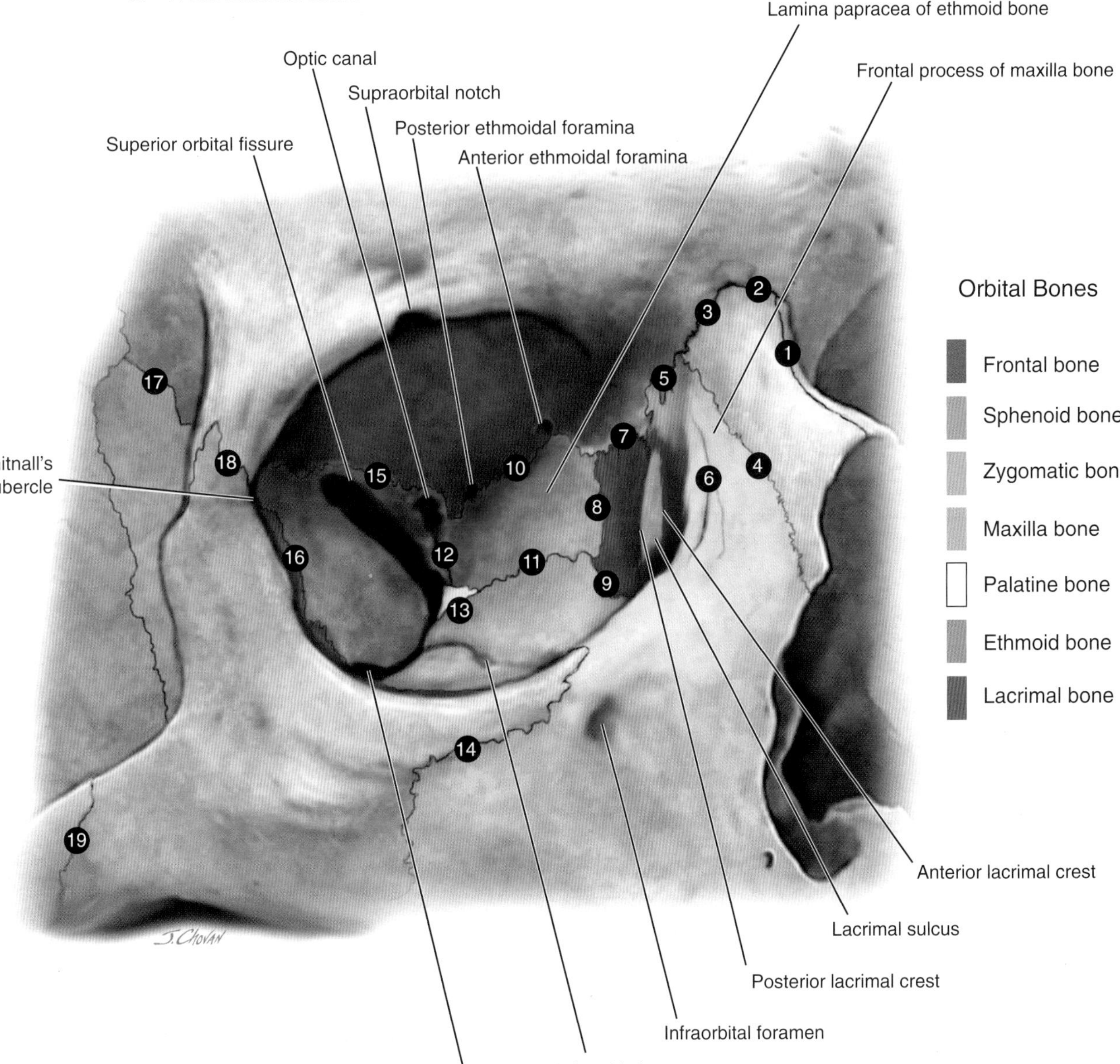
Orbital Sutures
1 Internasal suture
2 Nasion
3 Frontonasal suture
4 Nasomaxillary suture
5 Frontomaxillary suture
6 Sutura notha
7 Frontolacrimal suture
8 Ethmoidolacrimal suture
9 Lacrimomaxillary suture
10 Frontoethmoidal suture
11 Ethmoidomaxillary suture
12 Ethmoidosphenoidal suture
13 Palatomaxillary suture
14 Zygomaticomaxillary suture
15 Frontosphenoidal suture
16 Sphenozygomatic suture
17 Frontosphenoidal suture
18 Frontozygomatic suture
19 Temporozygomatic suture
Lamina papracea of ethmoid bone
Frontal process of maxilla bone
Optic canal
Supraorbital notch
Posterior ethmoidal foramina
Anterior ethmoidal foramina
Superior orbital fissure
Whitnall's tubercle
Orbital Bones
Frontal bone
Sphenoid bone
Zygomatic bone
Maxilla bone
Palatine bone
Ethmoid bone
Lacrimal bone
Anterior lacrimal crest
Lacrimal sulcus
Posterior lacrimal crest
Infraorbital foramen
Infraorbital groove
Inferior orbital fissure
J. Chovan

Figure 85.1 Anatomic representation of the bones that compose the orbit.

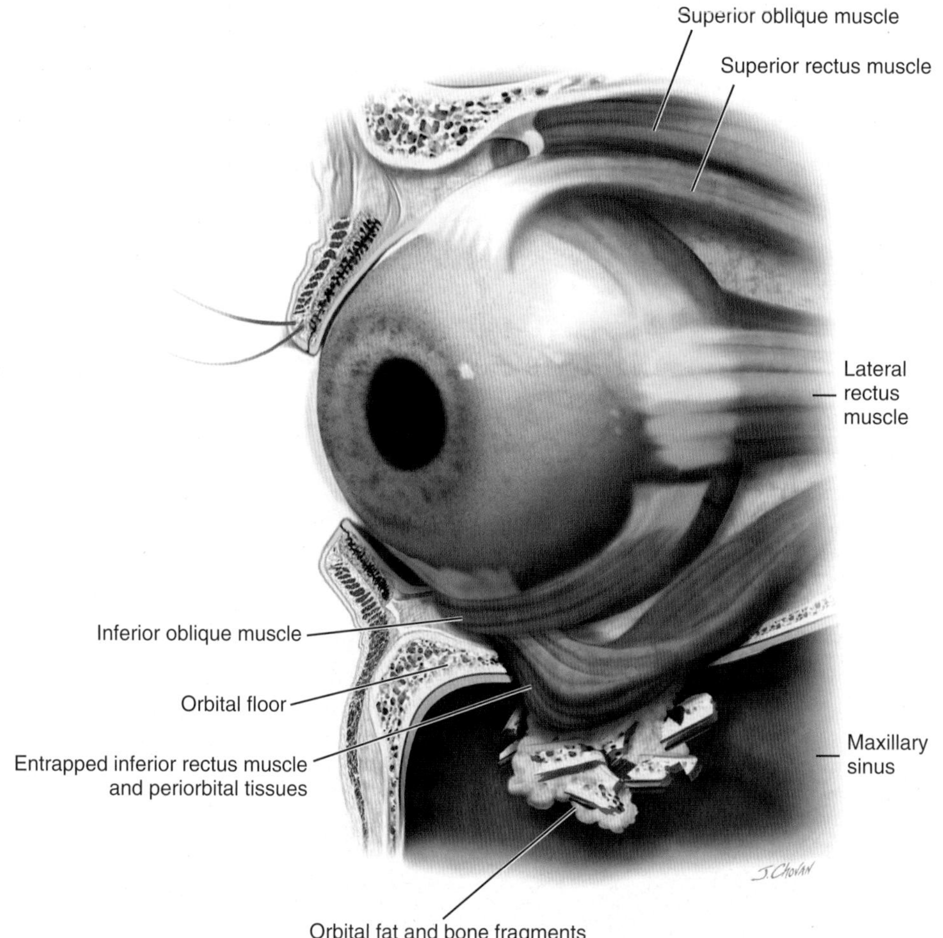

Figure 85.2 Orbital floor fracture with entrapment of the inferior rectus muscle.

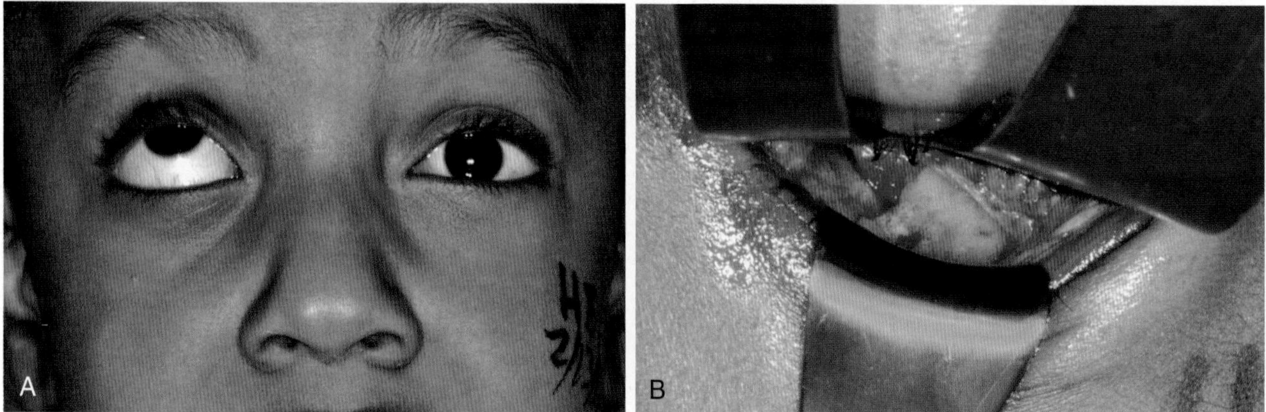

Figure 85.3 **A,** A 6-year-old child showing restriction of eye movement in the superior gaze after orbital fracture. **B,** The same child at the time of surgery showing entrapment of tissue in the orbital fracture.

TECHNIQUE: Isolated Orbital Wall Fractures

Step 1: Patient Preparation and Positioning

After intubation, the head of the table is turned away from the anesthesia equipment to allow for unrestricted access to the patient's head. Use of a radiolucent headrest should be considered if intraoperative CT scanning or imaging is to be performed. Application and registration of fiducial markers also can be done at this point if the use of intraoperative navigation is planned. Confirmation of which orbit is to be operated on is always prudent. A forced duction test is performed to assess any restriction of ocular motility in the affected orbit/eye. This test is performed by gently spreading the eyelids until the bulbar conjunctiva of the inferior portion of the eye is exposed. With a fine tissue forceps, a small portion of the conjunctiva is grasped close to the insertion of the inferior rectus muscle, allowing for eye manipulation in all directions. This maneuver also can be performed in the unaffected eye for comparison.

Corneal protection is imperative. This is achieved either by placement of a corneal shield with ample lubricant (if a transconjunctival approach is planned) or by a temporary tarsorrhaphy with 6-0 silk suture (if a lower eyelid skin incision is used). Lidocaine 2% with 1:100,000 epinephrine is infiltrated in the proposed incisions to control bleeding during dissection. Care should be taken to avoid distortion of the anatomy by applying excessive local anesthetic in the area (Fig. 85.4A).

STEP 2: Incision and Dissection

Surgical exposure of the orbit can be achieved through several approaches.[14] The choice of technique is based on the location and size of the orbital traumatic reconstruction and the surgeon's preference and experience. The options include the infraorbital, midlid, and subciliary incisions or the transconjunctival/transcaruncular approach.

The authors' preferred approach for the management of isolated orbital floor fractures is the transconjunctival approach. It provides adequate visualization of the orbital floor, and because of its versatility, if further exposure is required, it can be combined with a lateral canthotomy and/or transcaruncular extension for medial wall fractures. The approach is accomplished by placing a Desmarres and globe retractor to identify and isolate the tarsus and the inferior orbital rim. With the needle electrocautery on a low-power setting, a curved incision is made, either medial to lateral or lateral to medial, through the conjunctiva 1 to 2 mm below the inferior margin of the tarsus. Dissection can be done in either a preseptal or retroseptal fashion down toward the infraorbital rim (Fig. 85.4B–E).

STEP 3: Exposure of the Fracture and Repositioning of Herniated Periorbital Tissue

After the infraorbital rim has been exposed, subperiosteal dissection is carried out posteriorly. A periosteal elevator, in combination with a small malleable retractor and a globe retractor, is used to identify the margins of the fracture, to free an impinged muscle, and/or to reduce the herniated periorbital contents from the maxillary sinus. Care must be taken to avoid aggressively attempting to pull the tissue out of the fracture because this may cause bleeding further posteriorly in the orbit and may further injure the tis-

Continued

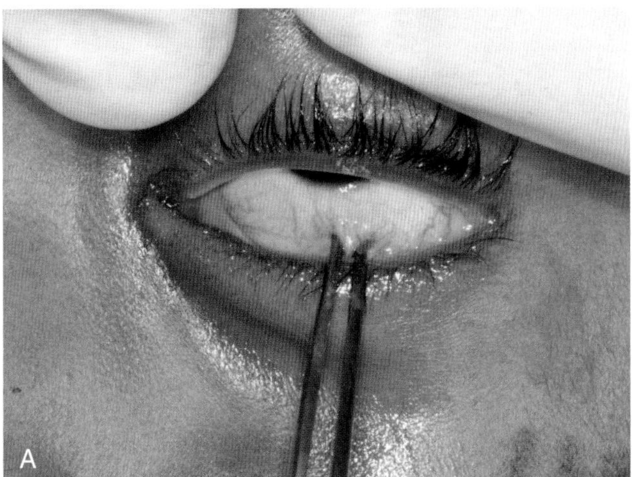

Figure 85.4 **A,** The same child as in Fig. 85.3 immediately after release of entrapped orbital contents during forced duction; no restriction of movement is seen with superior rotation.

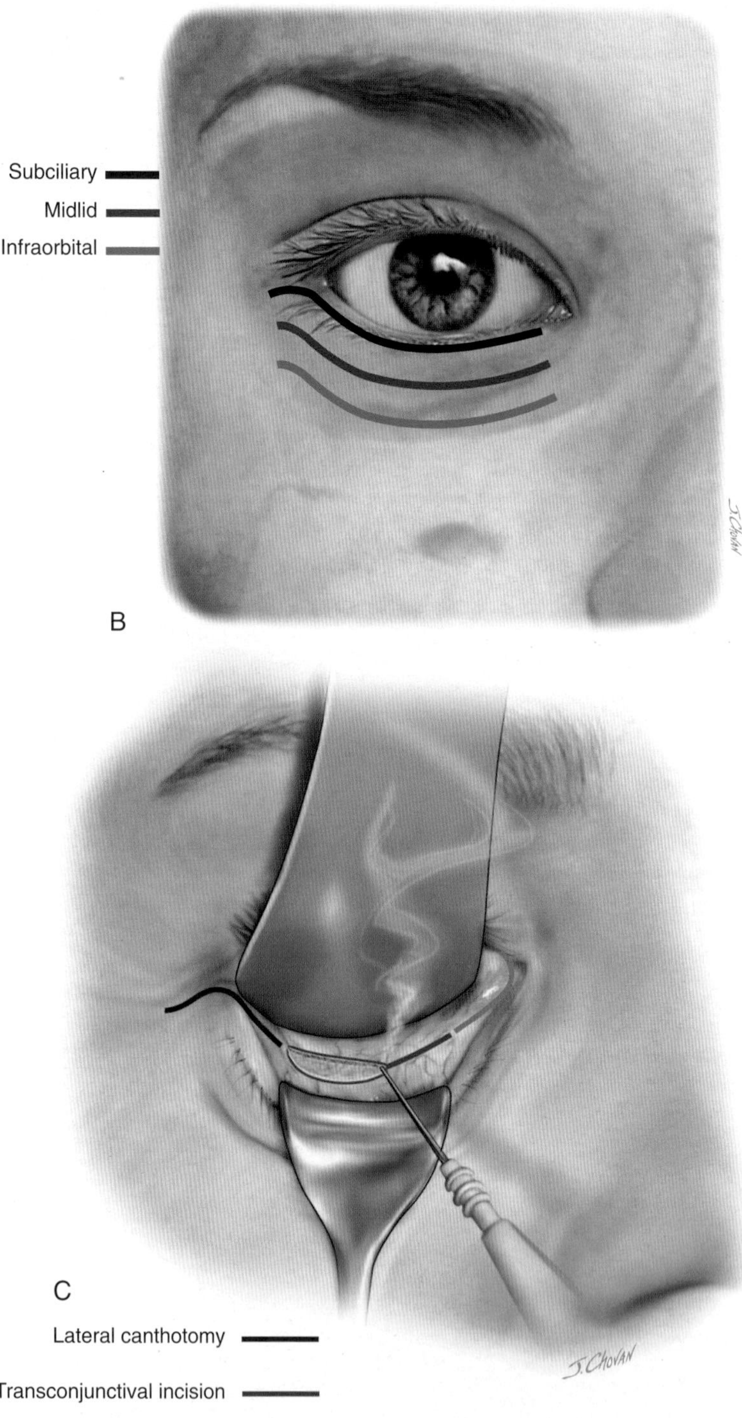

Figure 85.4, cont'd **B,** Skin incision placement for common approaches to the orbit floor. **C,** Transconjunctival approaches to the orbital floor. Transconjunctival incision either preseptal or retroseptal. Transcaruncular extension. Extension laterally through the skin with lateral canthotomy.

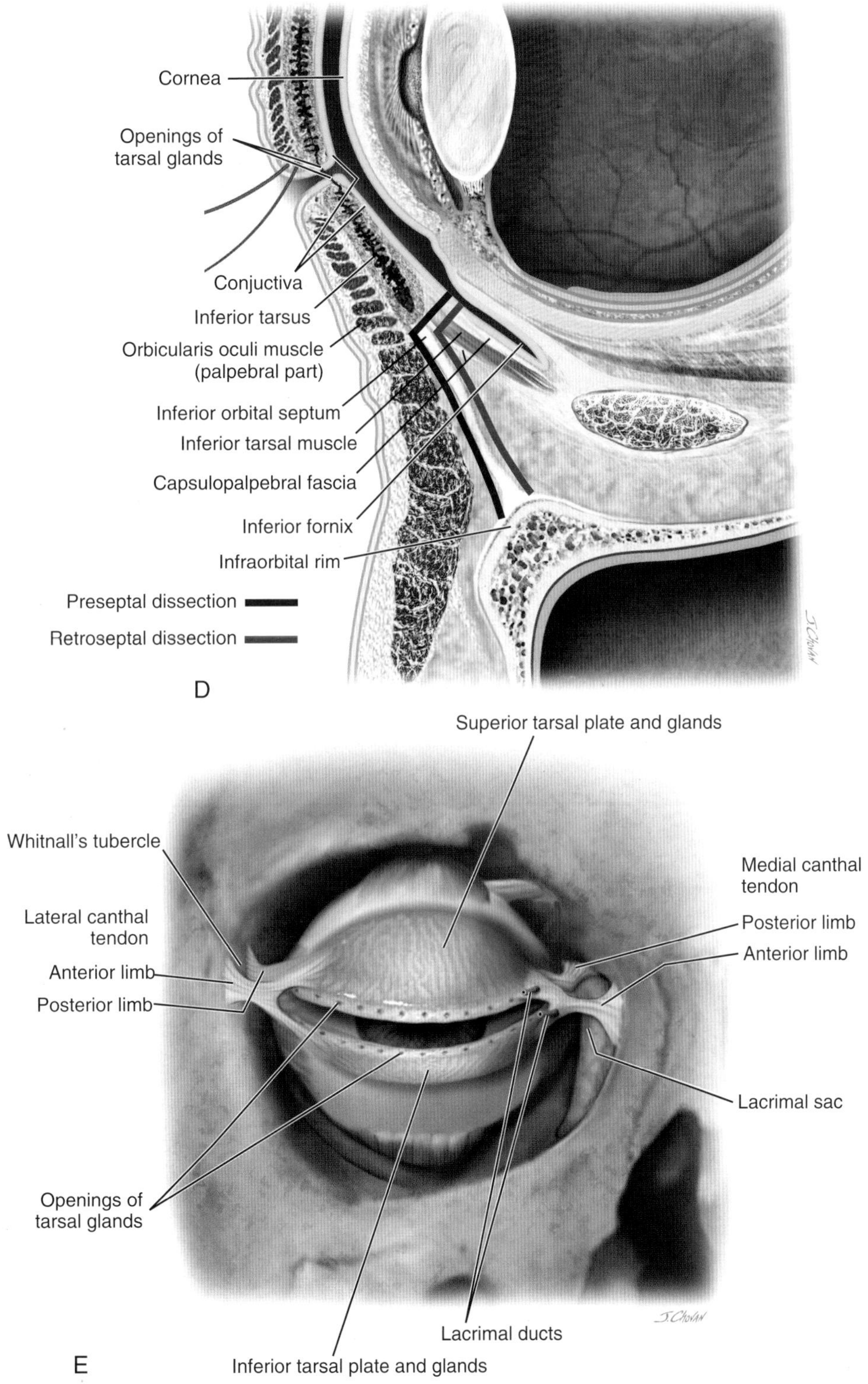

Figure 85.4, cont'd **D,** Surgical anatomy of the lower eyelid. Note the position of the orbital septum. **E,** Anatomy of the canthal tendons. The lateral canthal tendon attaches at Whitnall's tubercle and is composed of anterior and posterior limbs. The medial canthal tendon splits and attaches at the anterior and posterior lacrimal crest. The lacrimal sac sits in the lacrimal fossa between the anterior and posterior limbs of the medial canthal tendon.

Continued

TECHNIQUE: Isolated Orbital Wall Fractures—*cont'd*

sue; occasionally, it is necessary to enlarge the orbital defect to accomplish this tissue withdrawal atraumatically. As dissection proceeds further posteriorly along the floor or medial wall, the surgeon must be cognizant of the position of the orbital apex and the ethmoidal arteries, respectively. The end point of the dissection is reached when the surgeon has reduced all of the herniated tissue into the orbit and has exposed the bone of unfractured orbit floor/wall in a circumferential fashion.

STEP 4: Fracture Repair

Once the location, size, and shape of the defect have been recognized, a decision is made on the use of an autogenous graft or an alloplastic implant. Ellis[14] stated six principles for the reconstruction of an orbital fracture with either bone or biomaterials:

1. In large defects, a thin, rigid material should be used to maintain the orbital shape achieved during surgery.
2. Although all of the defect should be covered by the implant, the minimum size necessary should be used to avoid injury to the vital structures within the orbit.
3. Normal anatomy should be achieved by properly shaping the material before insertion.
4. Placement should be tension free to avoid trapping periorbital tissues that may restrict eye movement.
5. The material should be stabilized.
6. Orbital reconstruction should be verified for adequacy.

The authors' preference is to use a thin sheet of porous polyethylene in smaller defects. Larger defects, such as multiwall defects and fractures that extend farther posteriorly, may be better treated with a sheet of titanium-reinforced porous polyethylene secured with one or two screws just behind the anterior rim of the orbit. Considerable debate has arisen over which implant is preferred for internal orbital reconstruction. However, no clear scientific evidence indicates that one material is better than another. It should be noted that, in the growing orbit (before age 8), the surgeon should be cautious about using any material other than autogenous bone or resorbable material (Fig. 85.4F–I).

STEP 5: Irrigation and Closure

A forced duction test is repeated after the implant has been placed to ensure eye mobility. If intraoperative imaging is anticipated, it should be done before closure in case the implant requires repositioning.

The wound is inspected for hemostasis and then copiously irrigated. The periosteum is closed first at the orbital rim with suture, and primary closure then is achieved by grabbing small bites of the conjunctiva and placing two or three single 6-0 fast-absorbing gut sutures in a buried manner.

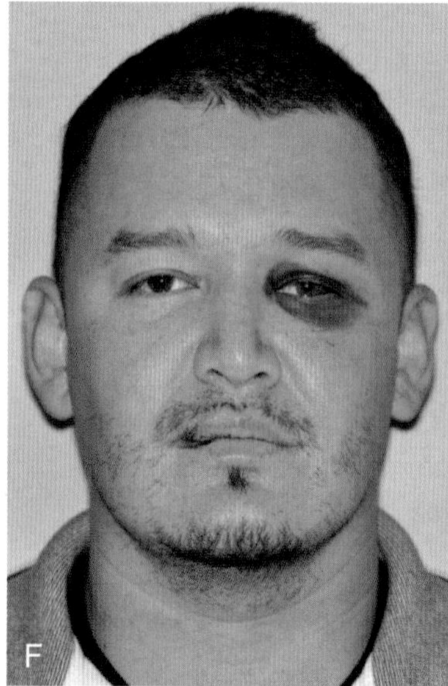

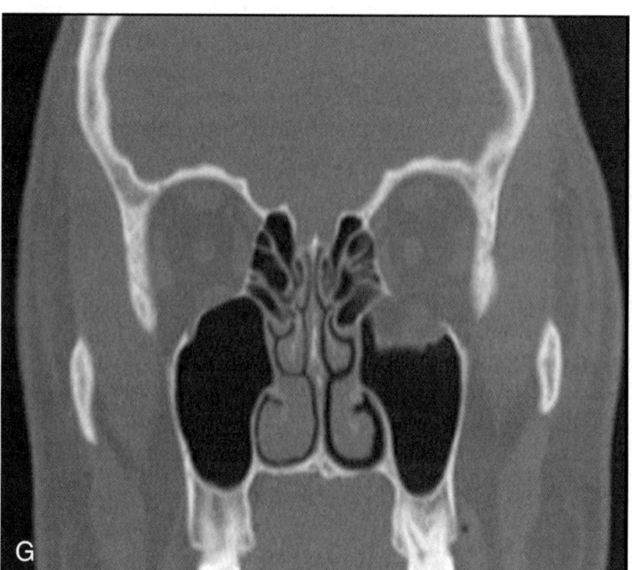

Figure 85.4, cont'd **F,** A 31-year-old male after an assault that resulted in an internal orbital fracture. **G,** Preoperative coronal computed tomography (CT) scan showing a large posterior orbital floor fracture with herniation of the orbital contents into the maxillary sinus.

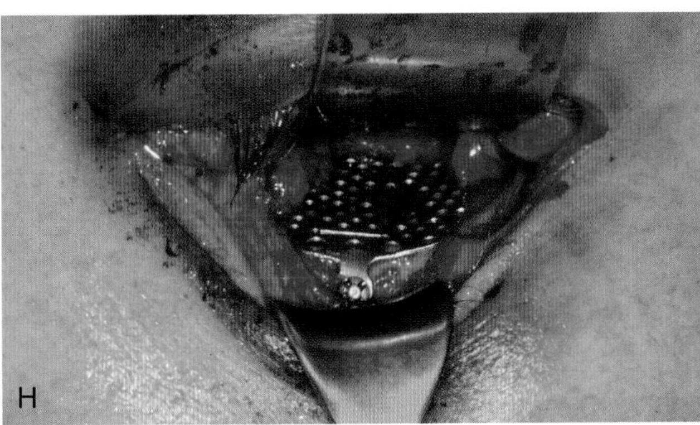

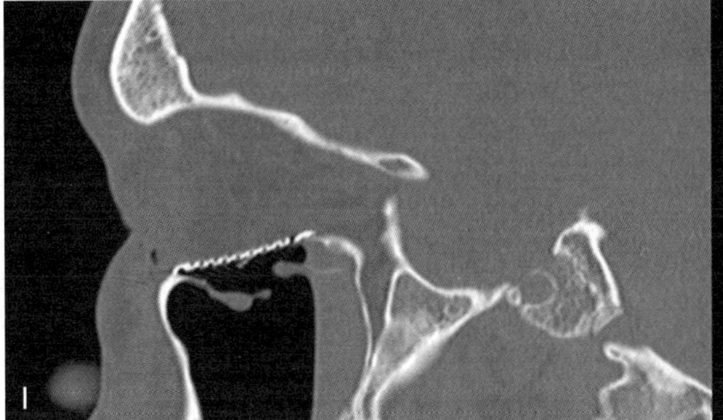

Figure 85.4, cont'd **H,** Intraoperative views of the placement of a titanium orbital plate with screw fixation to the orbital rim. **I,** Postoperative sagittal CT scan showing appropriate placement of the implant above the posterior orbital shelf.

ALTERNATIVE TECHNIQUE 1: Infraorbital Rim Involvement

Fracture of the infraorbital rim requires exposure until stable bone is found and must be repaired as the first step, before internal orbital repair. Once the broken pieces have been identified, they are reduced and fixated. When a single line of fracture exists, fixation is achieved with a small, low-profile, curved or straight osteosynthesis plate. Multiple lines of fracture through the orbital rim are better treated with a curved osteosynthesis plate. Once the infraorbital rim has been repaired, the orbital floor fracture reconstruction can proceed.

ALTERNATIVE TECHNIQUE 2: Lateral Orbital Canthotomy and Transcaruncular Extension

When further exposure is necessary, a lateral canthotomy may be indicated. Tenotomy scissors are placed at the palpebral fissure to the depth of the lateral orbital rim and angled at 45 degrees caudally. The conjunctiva, inferior limb of the lateral canthal tendon, orbital septum, orbicularis oculi, and skin are cut. The eyelid is retracted anteriorly, and a retroseptal plane is created with the tenotomy scissors from lateral to medial. The conjunctiva is then incised, allowing for dissection to the infraorbital rim. Once the orbit floor has been reconstructed, resuspension of the tendon is necessary. Usually, a buried suture can be placed through the edge of the tarsal plate and sutured back to the periosteum and intact superior limb of the lateral canthus. If the whole canthus was taken off during dissection, a hole is created in the lateral orbital rim with a fissure bur slightly above where the lateral canthus was originally inserted. A 3-0 Vicryl suture is passed through the hole, the superior and inferior eyelids are sutured toward each other to reestablish the palpebral fissure, and the lateral canthal tendon is resuspended. Primary closure is then achieved by layer closure of all the muscle and skin. The transconjunctival incision is then closed as described previously.

Transcaruncular extension is an esthetic and straightforward method of accessing the medial orbital wall. With traction sutures, the medial palpebral fissure is expanded and brought forward. Next, the lacrimal system and caruncle are identified. The transconjunctival incision is then extended medially and superiorly into the upper fornix, either through or behind the caruncle in the semilunar fold. Blunt scissor dissection then is carried out over Horner's muscle to a point behind the posterior lacrimal crest. Blunt dissection with the scissor tips on the medial orbital wall exposes the periosteum. An incision through the periosteum is then made, with subperiosteal dissection proceeding posteriorly along the medial wall. The anterior branch of the ethmoidal artery is encountered first and must be managed.

TECHNOLOGIC ADVANCES

Technologic advances have allowed the safe and predictable reconstruction of complex orbital fractures. Reestablishment of orbital contours and volumes can be obtained by virtual surgery planning with mirroring of the unaffected side and the fabrication of custom-made plates. Navigation-guided surgery and intraoperative CT scanning also assure accurate positioning of implant before the patient leaves the operating room.

TECHNIQUE: Transantral Endoscopic Repair of Orbital Wall Fractures

STEP 1: Patient Preparation

After the patient has been intubated, the head of the table is turned away from the anesthesia equipment to allow unrestricted access to the patient's head. Use of a radiolucent headrest should be considered if intraoperative CT scanning or imaging is to be performed. Application and registration of fiducial markers can

Continued

TECHNIQUE: Transantral Endoscopic Repair of Orbital Wall Fractures—*cont'd*

also be done at this point if intraoperative navigation is planned. Confirmation of which orbit is to be operated on is always prudent. A forced duction test is performed to assess any restriction on ocular motility in the affected orbit/eye. This is done by gently spreading the eyelids until the bulbar conjunctiva of the inferior portion of the eye is exposed. With a fine tissue forceps, a small portion of this conjunctiva is grasped close to the insertion of the inferior rectus muscle, allowing for eye manipulation in all directions. This maneuver can also be performed in the unaffected eye for comparison.

Corneal protection is imperative and is obtained by placement of a corneal shield with ample lubricant. The endoscopy towers should be situated so that the surgeon has a direct and unobstructed view of the monitor.[15]

STEP 2: Incision and Dissection

Lidocaine 2% with 1:100,000 epinephrine is infiltrated in the maxillary vestibule at the proposed incision site to control bleeding during dissection. Needle electrocautery is then used to make a 2- to 3-cm horizontal incision above the attached mucosa. Dissection is carried out subperiosteally to expose the anterior maxillary wall and the infraorbital nerve foramen.

STEP 3: Anterior Maxillary Sinus Wall Osteotomy and Placement of the Endoscope

Similar to a Caldwell–Luc access, a 15 × 15-mm window is created in the anterior maxillary wall with a fissure or round bur below the infraorbital foramen. A notch is made in the inferior border of this window to stabilize the endoscope (Fig. 85.5).[16]

STEP 4: Pulse Test

A pulse test is performed to facilitate identification of the fracture and periorbital tissues that have herniated into the maxillary sinus. The test consists of endoscopic visualization of the sinus roof while gentle pressure is applied on the eye.[16] A 0-degree or 30-degree endoscope can be used to perform this maneuver.

STEP 5: Removal of Sinus Membrane and Bone Fragments

Sinus membrane is removed with the aid of Blakesley nasal forceps to visualize the fracture margins. Care must be taken to identify the infraorbital nerve to prevent injury. All bony fragments are removed to prevent impingement of vital orbital contents at the time of implant placement.

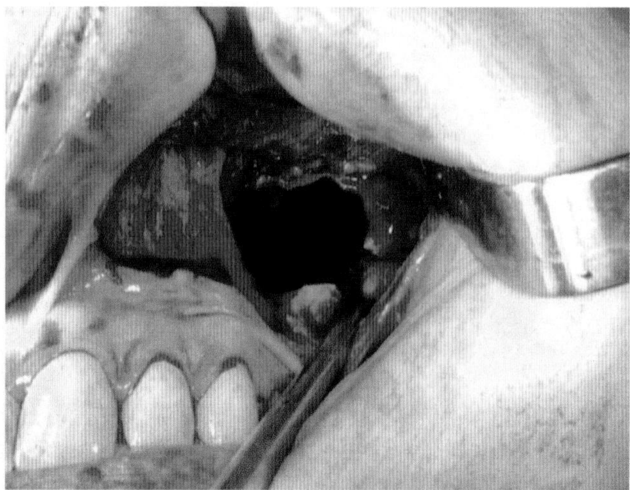

Figure 85.5 Canine fossa osteotomy.

TECHNIQUE: Transantral Endoscopic Repair of Orbital Wall Fractures—*cont'd*

STEP 6: Elevation of Periorbital Tissue Around the Fracture Margins

Once all the fracture margins have been identified, a 2- to 3-mm subperiosteal dissection is performed around the margins of the fracture, creating a space that allows placement of the implant.

STEP 7: Implant Placement

An extra-thin piece of porous polyethylene is trimmed a couple of millimeters larger than the defect. The implant is then rolled into the sinus. A pickle fork/wire director is used to manipulate the implant into position by pushing all the herniated tissues back into the orbit until the implant is secured around the bone ledges. The posterior dissection of the orbital defect to locate the posterior ledge of the sphenoid wing should be performed with care and should not ideally exceed 38 mm to avoid injury to the optic nerve.

STEP 8: Irrigation and Closure

Both the forced duction and pulse tests are repeated to ensure correct eye mobility and stability of the implant placement. The wound is inspected for hemostasis, and intraoral closure is performed with 3-0 absorbable suture.

ALTERNATIVE TECHNIQUE 3: Emergency Lateral Canthotomy

With acutely elevated intraocular pressure, emergency release of the lateral canthus can be a necessary and organ-preserving measure. This clinical presentation is usually the result of bleeding and hematoma formation posteriorly in the orbit, with the appearance of a tight or bulging orbit with or without acute visual changes. Imaging should not be performed to confirm the clinical diagnosis because the time delay may result in permanent injury.

This procedure can be performed in the emergency department, inpatient unit, or postanesthesia care unit. If a lateral canthotomy was done previously to aid in fracture repair, removal of the sutures usually is all that is necessary. Otherwise, adequate anesthesia is obtained by injecting lidocaine 1% to 2% with epinephrine into the lateral canthus. The tip of the needle should be directed toward the lateral orbit, touching bone.

A straight hemostat is used to compress the tissue at the lateral aspect of the palpebral fissure. The clamp is at the depth of the soft tissue, touching the bony lateral orbit. This is maintained for 60 to 90 seconds to aid hemostasis and mark the area. A forceps is used to grasp the tissue of the lateral orbit and elevate it laterally. Tenotomy scissors are then used to make a 1- to 2-cm incision extending laterally outward and in an inferior direction, with the tip of the scissors inside the lid, touching the orbital rim. The inferior lid is retracted downward, exposing the inferior aspect of the lateral canthal tendon if it was not released with the first scissor cut. The scissors are directed along the lateral rim, and with the tips pointed away from the globe, the anterior-inferior limb of the lateral canthus is cut. Despite high intraocular pressures, only a small amount of blood usually is expressed with evacuation of the hematoma.

Avoidance and Management of Intraoperative Complications

Complications from repair of orbital fractures are numerous and can include permanent loss of vision in the affected eye. A successful outcome requires meticulous surgical technique with gentle tissue handling. The surgeon must visually or tactilely confirm placement of the implant above the remaining orbital bone shelf and below the periorbita in a circumferential manner.

Intraoperative bleeding can obscure the surgical field, but most of the time it can be easily controlled by identification of the source and the use of bipolar or low-power electrocautery. The surgeon should be familiar with the anatomic boundaries of the orbital dissection to avoid damaging intraorbital vessels. Severe bleeding is rarely encountered. As discussed previously, aggressive traction on tissue may cause bleeding further posteriorly in the orbit and may lead to retrobulbar hematoma formation postoperatively. With any clinical indication that a retrobulbar hematoma has developed postoperatively in an orbital trauma patient, the condition should be managed immediately with lateral canthal release, medical treatment to lower intraocular pressure, and surgical reexploration of the affected orbit as necessary.

The ocular-cardiac reflex can be triggered during manipulation of the orbital contents, especially during deep orbital dissection, causing significant bradycardia. It is imperative that the surgeon discuss sudden intraoperative bradycardia with the anesthesia care team immediately. Usually, the removal of pressure from the orbital contents reverses the bradycardia, but occasionally anticholinergic drugs (atropine or glycopyrrolate) are needed.

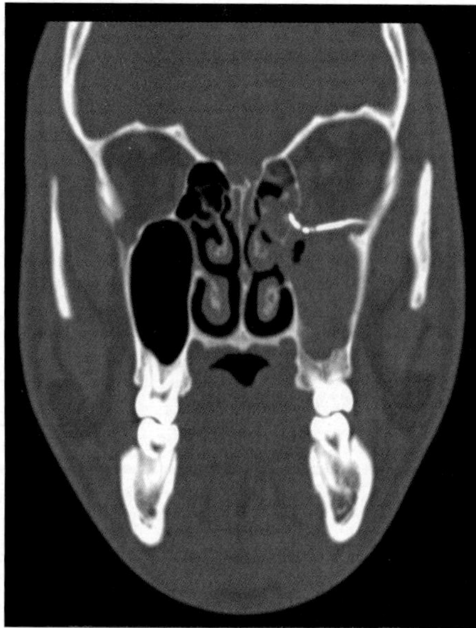

Figure 85.6 Preformed orbital implant placed too far medially into the ethmoid sinus.

Corneal abrasions are also possible if the globe is not adequately protected during surgery. Severe eye pain is usually seen in these patients postoperatively, and they should be seen by the ophthalmology service to document the clinical impression and provide supportive care for healing.

It is crucial to measure the depth of the dissection and the depth of implant insertion. Overdissection of the orbit posteriorly or overinsertion of the implant used for fracture repair can cause impingement on the orbital apex, possibly resulting in vision loss.

Confirming the placement of the implant, either through intraoperative scanning or postoperative imaging, is critical. It is not an uncommon error to insert an implant that either falls below the posterior lip of the orbital floor fracture or for the implant to extend too far medially into the ethmoid sinus in a patient with a medial wall fracture (Fig. 85.6). Strategies to assist the surgeon during surgery with finding the posterior orbital shelf can include temporary orbitotomy of the orbital rim or transantral osteotomy to visualize the fracture from below and confirm implant placement above the orbital shelf. In either scenario, revision of the orbital implant placement is indicated for an optimal outcome. A word of caution is appropriate regarding the use of preformed orbital reconstruction plates. These implants are constructed over anatomic averages, and patients rarely come in small, medium, or large. There is no substitute for accurate orbital reconstruction by the surgeon, either preoperatively using a custom computer design process or intraoperatively by manually bending or manipulating the orbital implant. Also, the use of preformed plates tends to provide a false sense of security regarding implant placement. Too often for comfort, postoperative imaging demonstrates that the implant is not closely adapted to the internal orbital walls in one or more areas. The use of preformed implants demands the same vigilance by the surgeon to ensure accurate placement as does the use of any other implant or technique. Any visual change after surgery must be documented, and immediate ophthalmology consultation is warranted.

Postoperative Considerations

The postoperative care of the orbital trauma patient is similar to that for any craniomaxillofacial surgical patient. Use of a Fox shield to protect the eye can be considered; the major drawback of this device, however, is that it hides the eye from casual observation by nurses or other care providers. Elevation of the head of the bed to 30 degrees is helpful for reducing edema in the postsurgical patient. Eye examinations for gross visual acuity and movement performed every few hours for the first 6 hours and then every shift can help detect any emerging postoperative complication. Any decrease in visual acuity with an increase in intraocular pressure and/or globe proptosis should prompt an immediate evaluation for a retrobulbar hematoma. Sinus precautions are recommended to avoid air emphysema, and patients should be instructed to sneeze with the mouth open. The use of postoperative medications, such as steroids, antibiotics, and nasal decongestants, can be considered. In rare cases, medications such as acetazolamide can be helpful in reducing intraocular pressure.

The adequacy of the orbital reconstruction is evaluated with a postoperative orbital CT scan unless intraoperative CT scanning or navigation-guided surgery was performed.

References

1. Smith B, Regan WF Jr. Blow-out fracture of the orbit; mechanism and correction of internal orbital fracture. *Am J Ophthalmol.* 1957;44(6):733–739.
2. Converse JM, Smith B. Blowout fracture of the floor of the orbit. *Trans Am Acad Ophthalmol Otolaryngol.* 1960;64:676–688.
3. Converse JM, Cole G, Smith B. Late treatment of blowout fracture of the floor of the orbit. A case report. *Plast Reconstr Surg.* 1961;28:183–191.
4. Manson PN, Clifford CM, Su CT, Iliff NT, Morgan R. Mechanisms of global support and posttraumatic enophthalmos: I. The anatomy of the ligament sling and its relation to intramuscular cone orbital fat. *Plast Reconstr Surg.* 1986;77(2):193–202.
5. Manson PN, Grivas A, Rosenbaum A, Vannier M, Zinreich J, Iliff N. Studies on enophthalmos: II. The measurement of orbital injuries and their treatment by quantitative computed tomography. *Plast Reconstr Surg.* 1986;77(2):203–214.
6. Schramm A, Suarez-Cunqueiro MM, Rücker M, et al. Computer-assisted therapy in orbital and mid-facial reconstructions. *Int J Med Robot.* 2009;5(2):111–124.
7. Markiewicz MR, Dierks EJ, Bell RB. Does intraoperative navigation restore orbital dimensions in traumatic and post-ablative defects? *J Craniomaxillofac Surg.* 2012;40(2):142–148.
8. Westphal D, Kreidler JF. Sinuscopy for the diagnosis of blow-out fractures. *J Maxillofac Surg.* 1977;5(3):180–183.
9. Saunders CJ, Whetzel TP, Stokes RB, Wong GB, Stevenson TR. Transantral endoscopic orbital floor exploration: a cadaver and clinical

study. *Plast Reconstr Surg*. 1997;100(3):575–581.
10. Chen CT, Chen YR, Tung TC, Lai JP, Rohrich RJ. Endoscopically assisted reconstruction of orbital medial wall fractures. *Plast Reconstr Surg*. 1999;103(2):714–720.
11. Ploder O, Klug C, Voracek M, Burggasser G, Czerny C. Evaluation of computer-based area and volume measurement from coronal computed tomography scans in isolated blowout fractures of the orbital floor. *J Oral Maxillofac Surg*. 2002;60(11):1267–1272.
12. Kolk A, Pautke C, Schott V, et al. Secondary post-traumatic enophthalmos: high-resolution magnetic resonance imaging compared with multislice computed tomography in postoperative orbital volume measurement. *J Oral Maxillofac Surg*. 2007;65(10):1926–1934.
13. Markiewicz MR, Bell RB. Traditional and contemporary surgical approaches to the orbit. *Oral Maxillofac Surg Clin North Am*. 2012;24(4):573–607.
14. Ellis E III. Orbital trauma. *Oral Maxillofac Surg Clin North Am*. 2012;24(4):629–648.
15. Fernandes R, Fattahi T, Steinberg B, Schare H. Endoscopic repair of isolated orbital floor fracture with implant placement. *J Oral Maxillofac Surg*. 2007;65(8):1449–1453.
16. Strong EB, Kim KK, Diaz RC. Endoscopic approach to orbital blowout fracture repair. *Otolaryngol Head Neck Surg*. 2004;131(5):683–695.

CHAPTER 86

The Naso-Orbito-Ethmoid Fracture

Mariusz K. Wrzosek and Stephen P. R. MacLeod

Armamentarium

#9 Periosteal elevator
#10 and #15 Bladed scalpel
#701 Fissure bur
Appropriate sutures
Asch septal forceps
Boies elevator
Canthal wire
Chisels, osteotome, mallet
Electrocautery (needle-tip and bayonet bipolar)
Flat, perforated drain
Local anesthetic with vasoconstrictor
Malleable retractors
Mayfield headrest
Metzenbaum scissor
Needle driver
Staple gun
Titanium miniplate system

History of the Procedure

Naso-orbito-ethmoid (NOE) fractures are complex injuries that affect the central midface. Fortunately, frontal bone and NOE complex injuries are relatively uncommon, accounting for approximately 15% of facial injuries. However, the intricate anatomy of the osseous and soft tissue components of this area makes surgical access and repair technically challenging. These injuries are typically a result of high-impact facial trauma and rarely occur in isolation. The most important factors in the repair of NOE complex fractures are the restoration of orbital shape, restoration of the medial canthal tendon (MCT) position, maintenance of appropriate intercanthal dimension, and maintenance of lacrimal system drainage.

The nomenclature, classification, and treatment techniques for these injuries have undergone transformation and refinement over the years. In 1970, Stranc[1] termed these injuries *naso-ethmoid* fractures, and in 1973, Epker[2] coined the term *naso-orbito-ethmoid* fracture, which is still the more popular term today. Classification of the fracture pattern has evolved since Stranc's initial attempt in 1970,[1] with Gruss[3] in 1985 and Markowitz et al.[4] in 1991 describing further classifications. The diagnostic classification by Markowitz and Manson is still widely used today.[4] This system is based on the fracture pattern and degree of comminution, and the status of the MCT disruption.[4] Injuries are further classified as unilateral or bilateral and extension into other anatomic locations. This classification has the advantage of helping to guide management options. The classification centers around the status of the MCT described as type I, II, or III (Fig. 86.1)[4]:

- Type I: Single-segment central fragment
- Type II: Comminuted central fragment with fractures external to the MCT insertion, with the MCT maintaining attachment to an adequate bone segment
- Type III: Comminuted central fragment with fractures extending into bone bearing the canthal insertion, and possible avulsion of the MCT

Before 1960, the treatment of NOE fractures involved the use of external splinting devices.[5] However, these methods failed to address the MCT and thus have fallen out of favor. Mustarde[6] in 1964 and Dingman[7] in 1969 both demonstrated superior results with open reduction and internal fixation using wire osteosynthesis. The development of internal fixation systems and advanced imaging techniques has led to the use of open reduction and internal fixation with plating techniques for these injuries, with improved functional and esthetic results. Thin-cut computed tomography (CT) imaging and three-dimensional reconstructions may be particularly helpful in these injuries.

Indications for an Open Procedure to Repair Naso-Orbital-Ethmoid Complex Fractures

It is necessary to distinguish between a nasal fracture and an unstable NOE fracture. A bimanual examination and the bowstring test can aide in the diagnosis of instability of the MCT. The bowstring test involves pulling the lateral canthus laterally while palpating the medial canthal area to detect movement of fracture segments, indicating instability. In the bimanual examination, an instrument is placed high into the nose, with the tip directly beneath the MCT, and gentle lifting and simultaneous digital palpation over the MCT externally allows for detection of movement and instability.

Indications for use of the procedure include the following:
Instability of canthal-bearing bone or avulsion of MCT
Loss of nasal projection and support
Comminution of medial orbital wall component

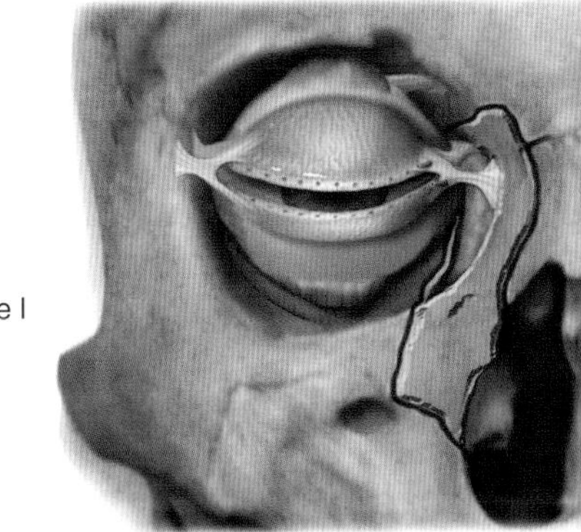
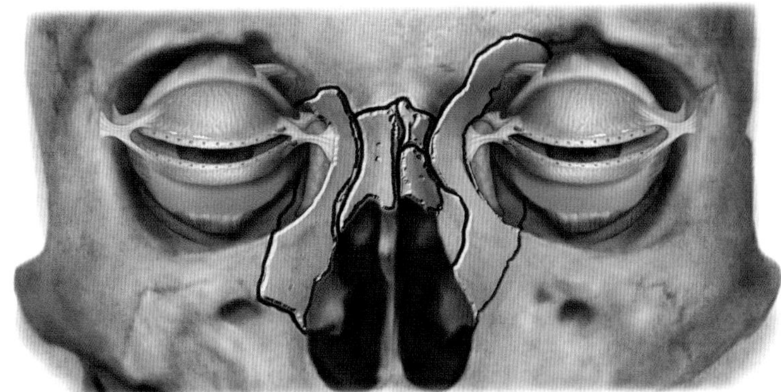

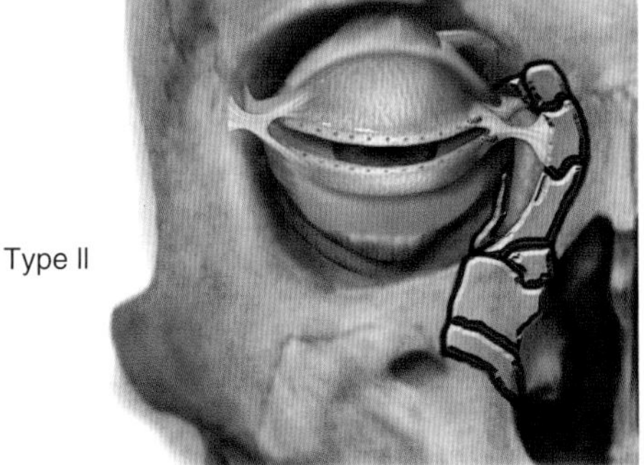
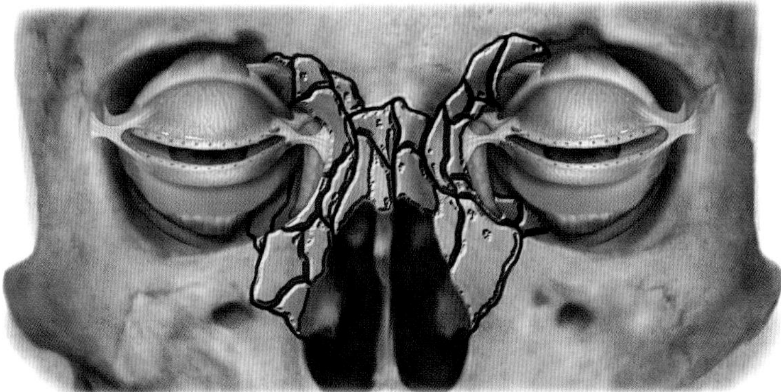

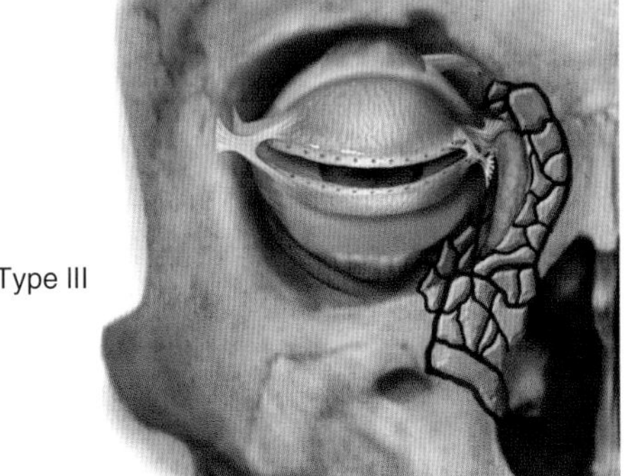
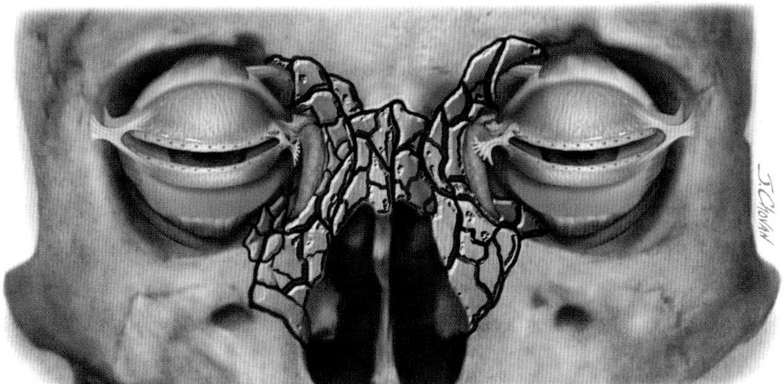

Figure 86.1 Classification of NOE fractures.

Interruption of lacrimal drainage
Concomitant facial fractures undergoing repair

Limitations and Contraindications

There are few strict contraindications to treatment of NOE fractures. Those that apply to any facial fracture include a hemodynamically unstable patient, acute neurologic hemorrhage, and pending demise. Contraindications that may apply specifically to an NOE fracture include an open globe injury and traumatic hyphema.

Limitations to open repair of the injuries depend principally on the ability to reduce and fixate the involved structures. In significant midfacial injuries, such as those with gross avulsion of tissue, such as in gunshot wounds, repair may be limited to soft tissue closure with minimal or no bony reduction and fixation being possible.

TECHNIQUE: NOE Fixation With Canthal Barb Suspension

A sequential approach to the repair of a NOE fracture is important so that all elements of the injury are addressed. The following sequential approach, provided by Ellis,[5] is widely used:

1. Expose fractures completely
2. Identify canthal-bearing bone or MCTs
3. Reduce or stabilize medial orbital rims
4. Reconstruct internal orbit
5. Perform transnasal canthopexy as required
6. Reduce septal fractures
7. Reconstruct bony dorsum
8. Perform soft tissue reduction

STEP 1: Exposing the Fracture

Type I fractures with minimal displacement may be addressed through an oral vestibular incision alone. Local anesthetic can be infiltrated in the maxillary vestibule from first molar to first molar. The incision begins through the mucosa and then is directed perpendicular toward bone. After the incision, elevation of the subperiosteal pocket from one zygoma to the other and up to the infraorbital rims is performed. Care in the identification of the piriform rim is important to avoid violating the nasal mucosa. The dissection can be carefully carried superiorly to the nasofrontal process of the maxilla, and infraorbital rim, identifying and preserving the infraorbital nerve. A large segment can be plated and rigidly fixed at the piriform.

Type II and type III fractures require coronal exposure. For adequate visualization during coronal exposure, it is recommended that the patient be positioned using a Mayfield headrest attachment on the operating room table. The table may be placed in a reverse Trendelenburg or lawn chair position to aid in correct positioning. Routine shaving is not required unless intracranial access is necessary in conjunction with a neurosurgeon.

With a marking pen, the surgeon marks a "lazy S" from the helical root of one ear to the contralateral ear approximately 4 cm behind the hairline. This curvature aids in postoperative camouflage of the incision. Lidocaine with 1:100,000 epinephrine is injected along the proposed incision in a subcutaneous plane. Midline and paramedian markings in the skin are made with the scalpel to aid reapproximation and correct aligning during closure. The incision is started with a #10 or #15 scalpel blade through skin, subcutaneous tissue, and galea until the periosteal layer is identified. Once the subgaleal plane has been identified, it may be bluntly dissected with a curved hemostat or Metzenbaum scissors toward one of the root helices. Maintaining the instrument in this plane, the surgeon continues the incision from skin down to the instrument. This incision is completed from ear to ear.

The flap may now be elevated in an anterior direction with finger dissection or a scalpel, remaining supraperiosteal to approximately 3 to 4 cm posterior to the supraorbital rim. At this point, an incision is made through the pericranium along the temporal crest bilaterally, and a connecting incision is made paralleling the supraorbital rim. It is important to note that in the scenario where a frontal sinus fracture is also being treated and a pericranial flap is necessary to line and obliterate the sinus, the pericranial flap may be started more posterior to the supraorbital rim. The subperiosteal plane is elevated until the supraorbital neurovascular bundles have been identified. If a notch is present, the bundles may be teased out and released. If a foramen is present, an osteotomy may be performed with a #701 fissure bur or a mallet and chisel. Freeing the bundle allows for significantly better exposure. The remainder of the flap can be elevated to sufficiently expose the nasal root and medial orbits.

In the case of panfacial trauma, exposure of all fracture sites should be completed before reduction or fixation of the individual components. In the setting of concomitant facial fractures, these fractures are treated first, to establish facial height and width, and NOE fractures are treated last (Fig. 86.2A and B).[8]

STEP 2: Identifying Canthal-Bearing Bone

Identification of the MCT can be challenging, with confirmation requiring visualization from above and below the coronal flap. Initial identification of the MCT is important because it is commonly still anchored to a fragment of bone.[5] The surgeon should avoid inadvertent avulsion of the MCT from this fragment if it is of sufficient size for plate fixation.[4]

STEP 3: Reducing or Fixating the Medial Orbital Rim

Fixation of the bony fragments must be addressed on a case-by-case basis. The degree of comminution dictates fixation patterns. The following is a rough guideline for these fractures. Fixation should proceed from areas of solid bone or fractures that have been adequately fixated to areas of instability and a higher degree of comminution. The frontal bone, piriform rim, and inferior orbital rim are the common points of stable fixation.

In type I fractures, minimal fixation is required and can be accomplished using a 1.5-mm miniplate spanning along the piriform from intact bone to the fractured segment. In type II and type III fractures, 1.2- or 1.5-mm miniplates are adapted to these sites. Comminuted bone fragments can then be secured to stable plates with screws or wire. Although the use of resorbable plates is attractive, they are more bulky and more difficult to contour, making titanium plates preferable (Fig. 86.2C and D).

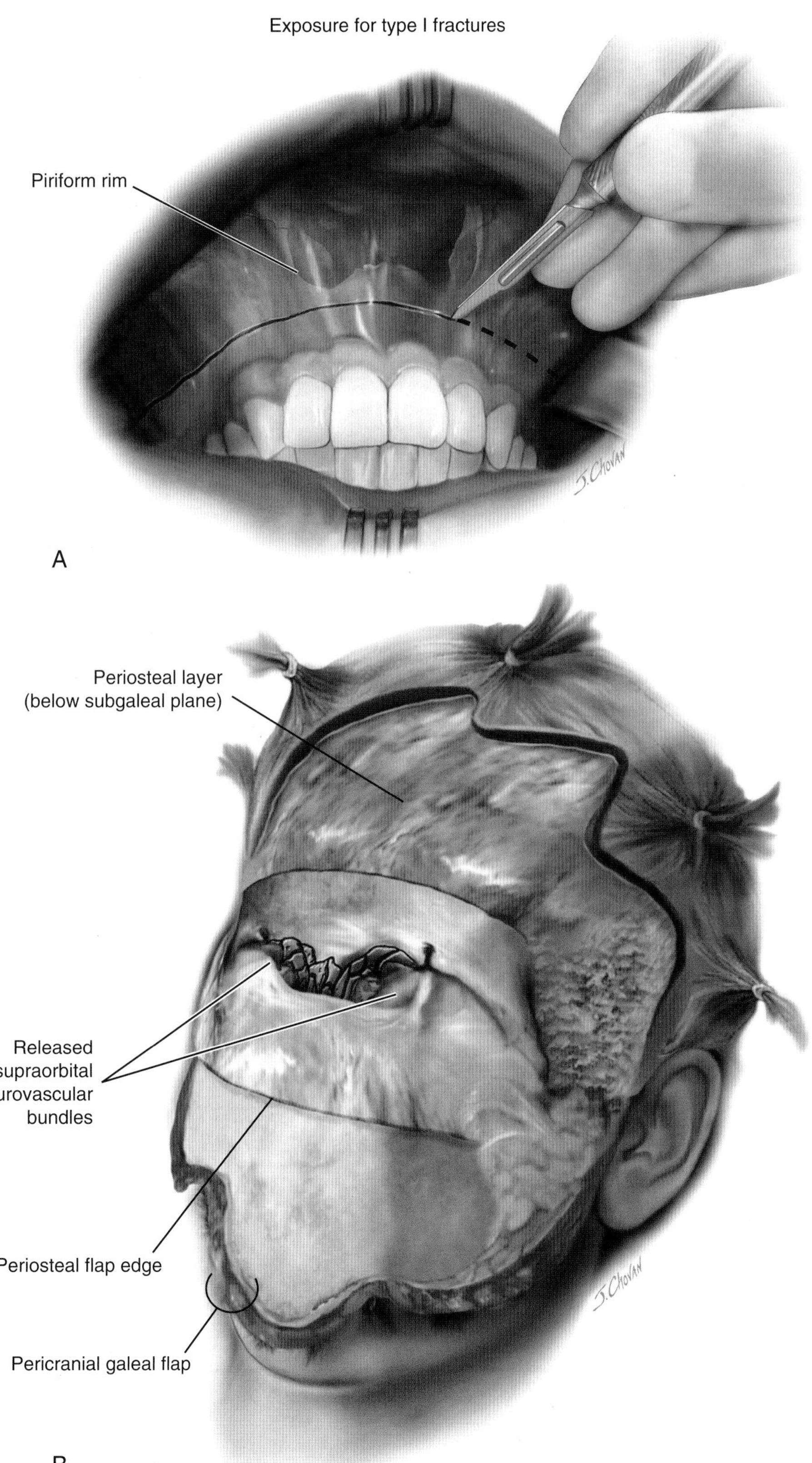

Figure 86.2 **A,** Maxillary vestibular. **B,** Coronal exposure.

Continued

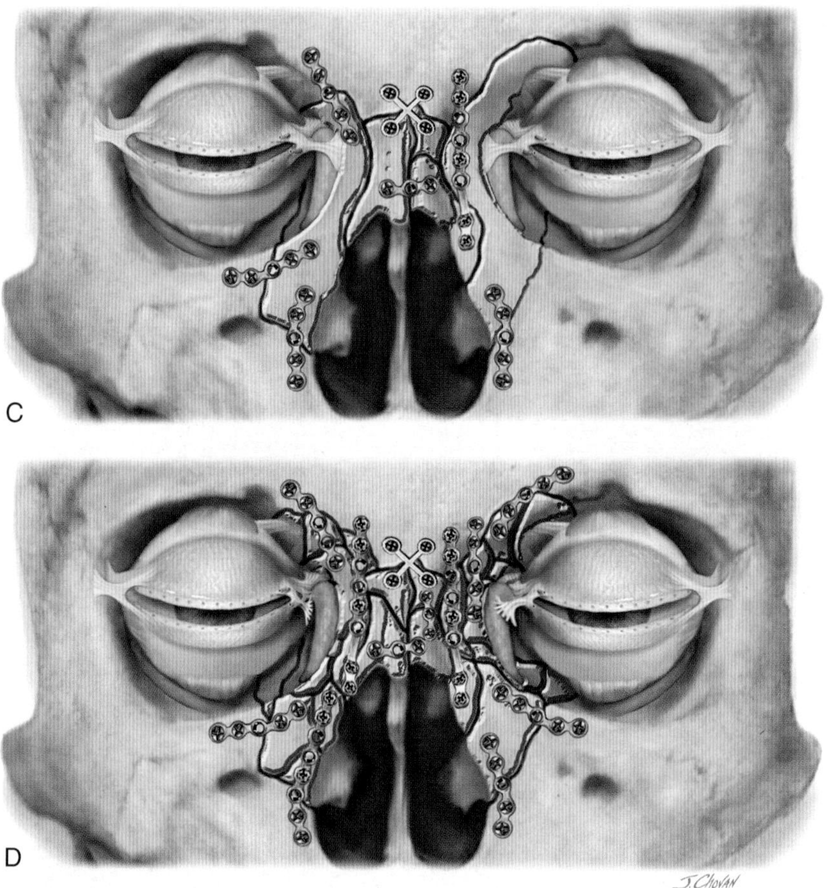

Figure 86.2, cont'd **C,** Examples of type I and type II fixation. **D,** Examples of type III fixation with and without avulsion.

TECHNIQUE: NOE Fixation with Canthal Barb Suspension—*cont'd*

STEP 4: Reconstructing the Internal Orbit

In type III fractures, the medial orbit may suffer considerable comminution.[8] Reconstruction of the medial wall is required to restore adequate orbital volume.[4] The first step in reconstruction is to determine what material to use. Available reconstructive materials include autogenous block graft harvested from the calvarium or anterior iliac crest, and synthetic options include porous polyethylene and titanium mesh.

The medial orbit should be sufficiently exposed using only the coronal flap. If there is involvement of the orbital floor or if the reconstruction material must span to this area for a stable margin, an inferior lid or subconjunctival approach may be required. A large segment of the nasofrontal process may also be plated inferiorly via an intraoral approach. Unnecessary bleeding may be prevented by avoiding, or cauterizing, the anterior and posterior ethmoidal vessels, found an average of 24 mm posterior to the lacrimal crest. Bayonet bipolar electrocautery is helpful because it allows increased visualization despite limited access.

Fixation of the reconstruction material is achieved with plate and screw fixation. Synthetic reconstructive materials are often fabricated with screw holes and can be easily adapted along an intact orbital rim. The further posterior the construct is placed along the medial wall, the more difficult fixation becomes.

STEP 5: Resuspending the Medial Canthal Tendon

The MCT is the confluence point where the upper and lower lids unite. It may be subdivided into a superficial part and deeper part, with the lacrimal sac found in between. The superficial part inserts into the frontal process of the maxilla, providing support of the eyelids and maintaining the palpebral fissure.

The canthal barb technique with use of miniplates in a pulley mechanism has shown promise.[9] A horizontal incision is made in the caruncle with iris scissors to facilitate passage of the barb. A needle is passed externally through this incision and located on the deep surface of the coronal exposure. The wire or suture is pulled through until the barb engages in the dense MCT tissue.

Once the MCT has been adequately identified and captured, the goal is to suspend the suture in an overcorrected posterior and superior vector. This establishes the appropriate palpebral shape and inclination. A four- to six-hole, 1.5-mm miniplate is adapted to

TECHNIQUE: NOE Fixation with Canthal Barb Suspension—*cont'd*

a stable area of the frontal bone, with the posterior plate holes positioned along the medial orbital wall. The needle is then passed through a posterior plate hole in a pulley fashion, and the suture or wire is wrapped around a lone screw secured in the frontal bone (Fig. 86.2E–I).

STEP 6: Reducing the Nasal Septum

The primary goal of septal management is to provide an unobstructed nasal airway.[5] An Asch septal forceps can be used to reduce the nasal septum. The beaks of the forceps are placed in each nare and directed posteriorly until the beaks are seated over the septum, with the deflection in the beaks positioned over the columella to avoid damage. The nasal septum is firmly grasped, and reduction is accomplished with manipulation to

Continued

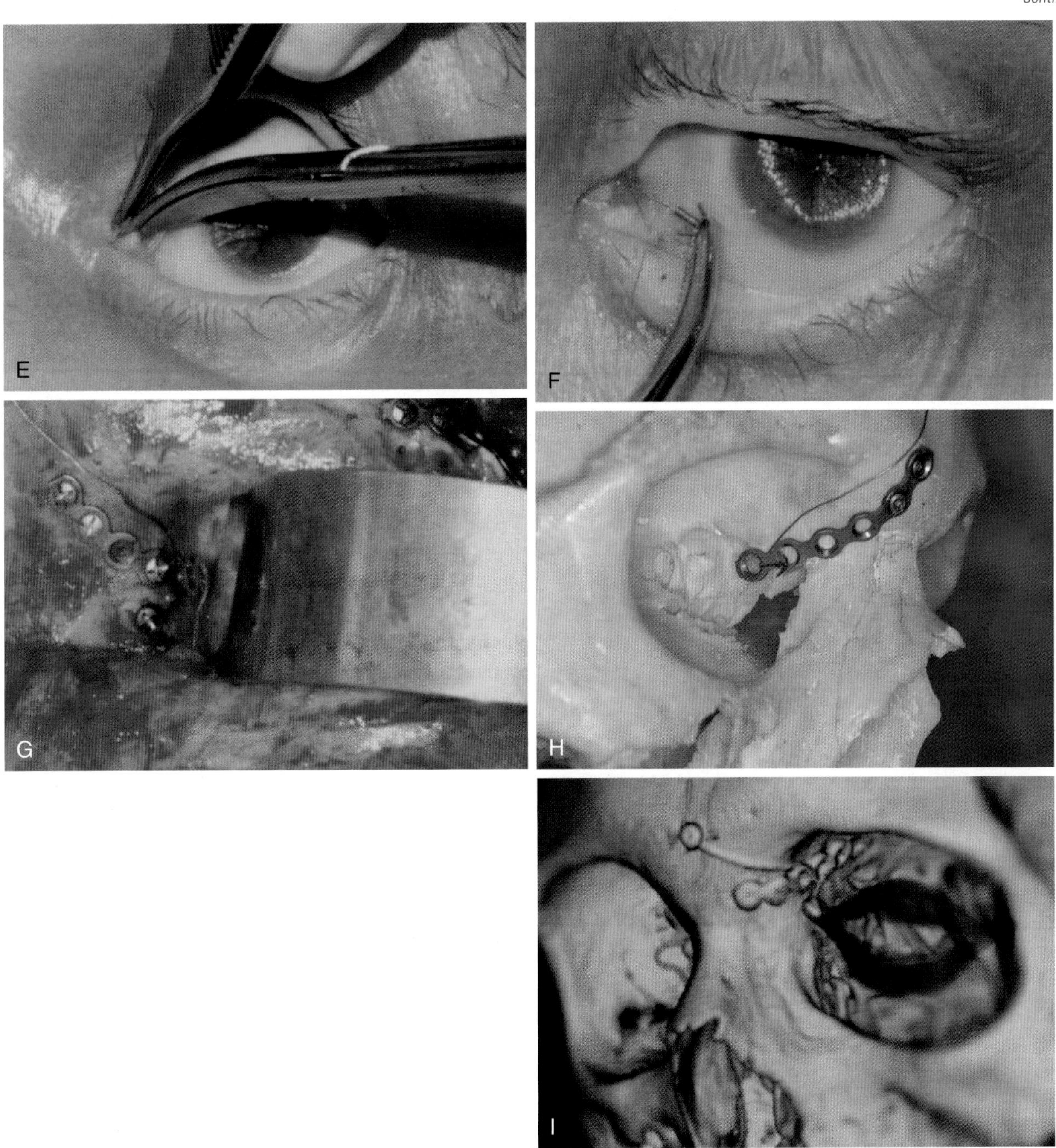

Figure 86.2, cont'd E, Horizontal incision trough caruncle. **F,** Passing a canthal barb through the incision of the caruncle. **G,** Suspension of the medial canthal tendon. **H,** Plate positioning with canthal barb. **I,** CT scan demonstrating fixation and resuspension of the medial canthal tendon.

TECHNIQUE: NOE Fixation with Canthal Barb Suspension—*cont'd*

the pretraumatic position. In severe cases, suturing of the septum to the anterior nasal spine may be indicated. Doyle splints may be placed at the end to provide stability in the initial healing period.

STEP 7: Reconstructing the Nasal Dorsum/Bone Grafting

In cases of significant comminution of the nasal root or septum, the loss of nasal projection may occur. In these cases, primary bone grafting has an important role in maintaining the soft tissue envelope and reestablishing nasal projection.[3–5] The best time for repair is at the time of primary exposure. If soft tissue contraction occurs in this area, it may be functionally impossible to fully correct this secondarily. Dorsal bone grafts are commonly required; Ellis reported grafting in 31% of his cases, and Markowitz et al. performed grafting in 42% of their cases.[4,5] Allogenic materials are available but can be a source of chronic inflammation.[10]

The calvarium is a preferred harvest site because it is commonly exposed for surgical access to the NOE region. The outer cortex can be harvested in block form from the parietal bone. This region provides the straightest and thickest bone. An outline of the bone graft is made with a round bur. The edges of the outline are beveled to facilitate osteotome placement. A thin fissure bur or a piezoelectric handpiece may be used to perform the osteotomy in the outer cortex. Osteotomes are then gently malleted around the periphery of the bone graft. The initial use of a curved chisel facilitates propagation in the correct plane. It is important to keep the chisel as parallel to the cranial surface as possible to avoid intracranial extension. Once the bone graft is free, it can be contoured with a bur into an elongated oval shape.

Soft tissue dissection is carried out on the dorsum of the nose to create a pocket for graft placement. This dissection can be carried out in a combined blunt and sharp technique with the use of Metzenbaum scissors. The bone at the nasion can be prepared with a bur to allow insetting of the graft.[8] There are multiple ways to fixate the graft. The authors' preferred method is to use a 1.5-mm Y-plate. The straight limb of the plate is fixated on the deep surface of the graft to prevent a palpable plate in a region where the overlying skin is thin. The opposite Y-end is fixated to the frontal bone. It is important to consider that nasal projection affects perceived intercanthal width,[5] and overcorrection is better tolerated than underprojection (Fig. 86.2J–L).[11]

STEP 8: Managing Soft Tissue Requirements

Adequate visualization of NOE fractures requires significant soft tissue dissection. It is important to ensure that the soft tissues are carefully resuspended, starting with reattachment of the MCT as previously described. Resuspension of the coronal flap near the frontozygomatic suture is required because failure to do so can lead to a prematurely aged appearance due to soft tissue sag, in spite of excellent repair of the fractures. This can be done with 4-0 Vicryl suture. Reapproximation of the pericranium is then performed. Next, a flat, perforated drain is placed under the coronal flap, with a percutaneous exit point in the postauricular region. Closure of the galeal layer of the coronal incision is best done with interrupted 4-0 Vicryl suture. Closure is finalized with staple placement or sutures, with staples allowing for easier removal in the clinic at 10 to 14 days. Any existing facial lacerations should be closed in a layered fashion after completion of remaining fracture reduction.

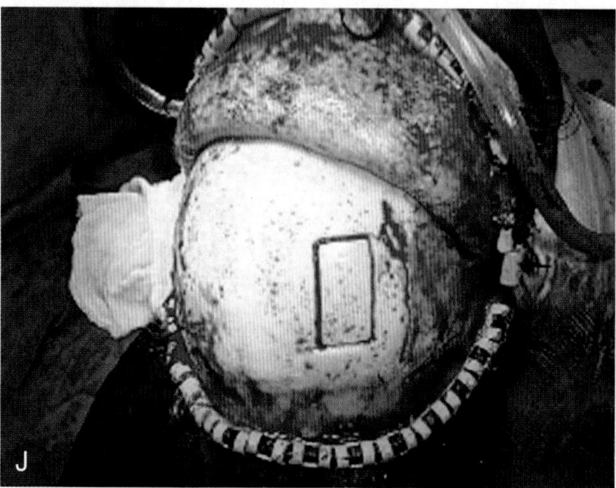

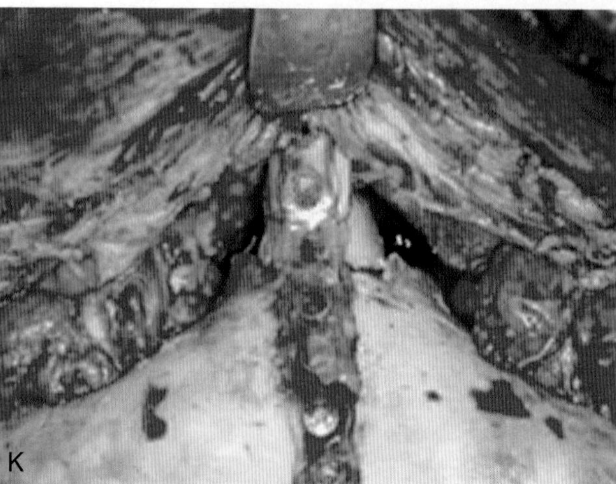

Figure 86.2, cont'd **J,** Harvesting of the outer table of the calvarium for nasal grafting. **K,** Fixation of the dorsal graft to the frontal bone.

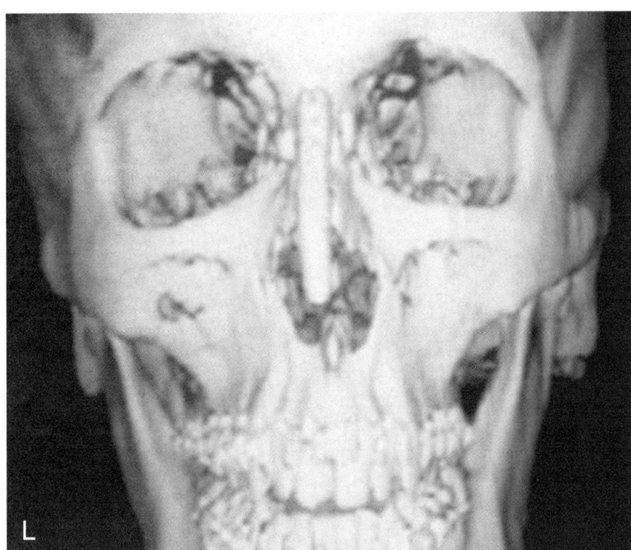

Figure 86.2, cont'd **L,** CT scan demonstrating fixation of a dorsal nasal graft using calvarium. (E, F, G, and I from Englestad M. Naso-orbito-ethmoid fractures. In: Bagheri S, Bell B, Khan H, eds. *Current Therapy in Oral and Maxillofacial Surgery.* St Louis, MO: Mosby; 2012; H, courtesy Mark Englestad; J, K, and L from Herford AS, Ying T, Bown B. Outcomes of severely comminuted [type III] nasoorbitoethmoid fractures. *J Oral Maxillofac Surg* 2005;63:1266.)

ALTERNATIVE TECHNIQUE: Transnasal Canthopexy

The main tenets of repair are the same in the treatment of NOE fractures. However, multiple methods have been described to address MCT resuspension. Transnasal wiring is the most commonly described technique for managing the disrupted MCT. After appropriate exposure of the fractures, a 2.0-mm-diameter long drill is used to drill a hole through the nasal cavity at a level that provides an adequate vector for MCT resuspension. The MCT is identified, and a suture or wire is passed through the transnasal pilot hole with an awl or a straight spinal needle. The suture or wire is tightened to provide adequate palpebral fissure shape and inclination. Repeated evaluation of the medial canthi position is done externally until adequate reduction and symmetry are achieved. A ruler or caliper should be used to measure the intercanthal distance. The normal distance in adult females is between 28.6 and 33 mm and in males between 28.9 and 34.5 mm. The medial intercanthal distance is also approximately equal to the length of the palpebral fissure of each eye. A disadvantage of this technique is that in highly comminuted cases, the bony architecture that is used for positioning of the transnasal canthopexy may not supply the structural support necessary to resuspend the MCT in an appropriate vector. Grafting may be required in these cases. This method works well if the contralateral segment is large enough.

Each of the canthopexy sutures is secured inside the orbital rim of the opposite orbit with a bone screw. If bilateral canthopexies are performed, each is secured independently within the contralateral orbital rim. Securing them together is not recommended[5]; if one were to loosen or pull free, both canthopexies would then fail (Fig. 86.3).

Avoidance and Management of Intraoperative Complications

Intraoperative complications can arise during the treatment of extensive midfacial trauma. It is important to perform a thorough clinical exam prior to the operation, particularly looking for cerebrospinal fluid leaks, especially in cases involving frontal sinus fractures. Fine-cut CT imaging and three-dimensional reconstruction may be especially helpful and should be carefully studied in preoperative planning. It is important to keep in mind, however, that the fractures may be worse in reality than the three-dimensional reconstruction suggests, since very thin nondisplaced fracture lines may not show up in the three-dimensional rendering algorithm.

During surgery, avoidance of iatrogenic trauma is of utmost importance. Damage to orbital contents, such as the globe, is possible with careless surgical technique. It is important to remain in a subperiosteal plane when elevating the tissues in this region. A malleable retractor can provide protection when passing a wire or suture or when drilling in the direction of orbital components.

The surgeon must be continually aware of location and direction during use of drills in the NOE region. It is important to recognize that the orbital roof and superior ethmoid spaces compose the floor of the anterior cranial fossa. This is of most concern when drilling transnasally during a canthopexy procedure. The frontoethmoidal suture on the medial wall of the orbit (level of the ethmoidal foramina) correlates with the level of the cribriform plate. This is a useful anatomic landmark to remain inferior to when drilling.

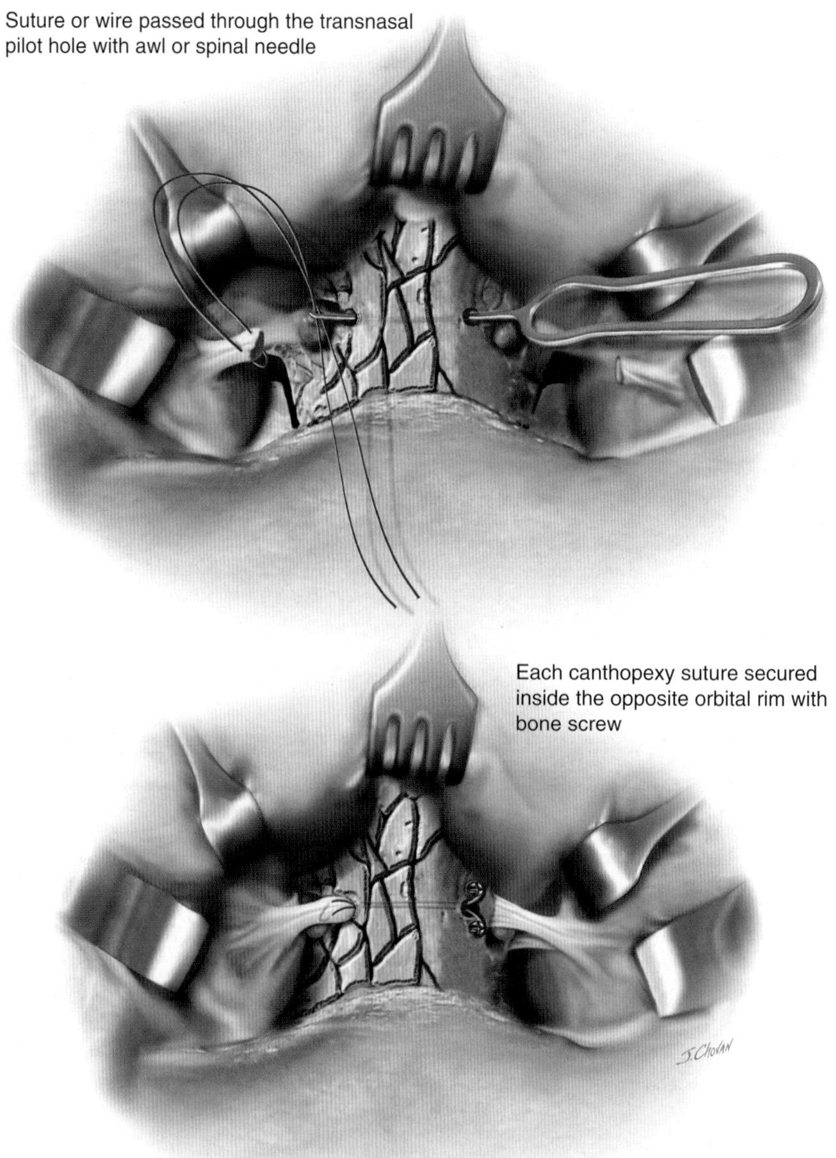
Suture or wire passed through the transnasal pilot hole with awl or spinal needle
Each canthopexy suture secured inside the opposite orbital rim with bone screw

Figure 86.3 Transnasal canthopexy.

If the MCT is anchored to a bony fragment of sufficient size for fixation, the surgeon should take care not to avulse it while dissecting along the medial orbital rim. Iatrogenic avulsion could transform a straightforward repair into a complicated resuspension procedure. If the medial canthal ligament is avulsed, the canthal barb technique, described previously, should be used to resuspend it.

Postoperative Considerations

Postoperative complications of NOE injury and repair can be functional or cosmetic in nature. Cosmetic defects, such as telecanthus, saddle nose deformity, or unsightly scarring, are generally the principal concern of both the patient and the surgeon. Telecanthus is defined as widening of the intercanthal distance beyond acceptable values. The average intercanthal distance is race- and sex-dependent but is generally 33 mm (±2 mm). Avoidance is best achieved by overcorrection during the canthal resuspension in both a superior and posterior direction. Transnasal wiring of the central fragment anterior to the medial canthal attachment results in postoperative telecanthus.[4] Measurement before closure of the coronal incision helps to confirm appropriate distance.

Saddle nose defects are the result of inadequate support to the nasal dorsum. Loss of this support is common with highly comminuted injuries. Dorsal bone grafting should be given significant consideration at the time of primary repair. Soft tissue contracts during healing, and secondary repair produces an unfavorable result.

Unsightly scars can be avoided by abandoning approaches such as the gull-wing incision and instead using the coronal incision. Placement of the coronal incision behind the hairline or near the vertex in men exhibiting male pattern baldness camouflages any resulting scar. Electrocautery should not be used in the initial incision and should be minimized in the dermal layer to avoid damaging hair follicles and minimize a noticeable scar. Raney clips have been historically used to help with hemostasis; however, there is some concern of injury to hair follicles as well. Adequate time after vasoconstrictor injection should help minimize bleeding from the scalp.

In cases with a significant orbital component, postoperative enophthalmos may present. Exploration of the defect and repair with an appropriate reconstruction material to restore preinjury orbital volume reduces the likelihood of enophthalmos. Intraoperative CT can be used to evaluate orbital reconstruction before closure of the incisions.

The nasolacrimal apparatus has an intimate relationship with the osseous and soft tissue components of the NOE region. Nasolacrimal injuries are most commonly accompanied by traumatic telecanthus.[12] Nasolacrimal dysfunction is reported in 5% to 17.4% of NOE injuries.[12] If needed, formal dacryocystorhinostomy is performed approximately 4 to 6 weeks later. NOE fractures may often occur in conjunction with frontal sinus fractures; therefore, it is also important to monitor the patency of the nasofrontal outflow tract since it is the most important factor in maintaining the health of the frontal sinus.[13,14]

Cerebrospinal fluid (CSF) leaks can occur with cribriform plate disruption. It has been reported that nearly 85% of CSF leaks resolve with observation only in a period of 2 to 10 days.[13] Those that do not resolve are treated with lumbar drainage or extracranial and intracranial procedures. CSF leaks warrant a consultation with neurosurgery, antibiotic coverage, and close follow-up to monitor resolution.

References

1. Stranc MF. Primary treatment of naso-ethmoid injuries with increased intercanthal distance. *Br J Plast Surg*. 1970;23(1):8–25.
2. Epker BN. Open surgical management of naso-orbital-ethmoid facial fractures. In: Kay L, ed. *Transactions of the IVth International Conference on Oral Surgery*. Munksgaard, Copenhagen: Munksgaard; 1973.
3. Gruss JS. Naso-ethmoid-orbital fractures: classification and role of primary bone grafting. *Plast Reconstr Surg*. 1985;75(3):303–317.
4. Markowitz BL, Manson PN, Sargent L, et al. Management of the medial canthal tendon in nasoethmoid orbital fractures: the importance of the central fragment in classification and treatment. *Plast Reconstr Surg*. 1991;87(5):843–853.
5. Ellis E III. Sequencing treatment for naso-orbito-ethmoid fractures. *J Oral Maxillofac Surg*. 1993;51(5):543–558.
6. Mustarde JC. Epicanthus and telecanthus. *Int Ophthalmol Clin*. 1964;4:359–376.
7. Dingman RO, Grabb WC, Oneal RM. Management of injuries of the naso-orbital complex. *Arch Surg*. 1969;98(5):566–571.
8. Herford AS, Ying T, Brown B. Outcomes of severely comminuted (type III) nasoorbitoethmoid fractures. *J Oral Maxillofac Surg*. 2005;63(9):1266–1277.
9. Englestad M. Naso-orbito-ethmoid fractures. In: Bagheri S, Bell B, Khan H, eds. *Current Therapy in Oral and Maxillofacial Surgery*. St Louis, MO: Mosby; 2012.
10. Papdopoulos H, Salib N. Management of naso-orbital-ethmoidal fractures. In: Laskin D, Abubaker OA, eds. *Current controversies in maxillofacial trauma, Oral Maxillofac Surg Clin North Am*. 2009;21(2):221.
11. Potter JK, Muzaffar AR, Ellis E, Rohrich RJ, Hackney FL. Aesthetic management of the nasal component of naso-orbital ethmoid fractures. *Plast Reconstr Surg*. 2006;117(1):10e–18e.
12. Gruss JS, Hurwitz JJ, Nik NA, Kassel EE. The pattern and incidence of nasolacrimal injury in naso-orbital-ethmoid fractures: the role of delayed assessment and dacryocystorhinostomy. *Br J Plast Surg*. 1985;38(1):116–121.
13. Bell RB, Dierks EJ, Homer L, Potter BE. Management of cerebrospinal fluid leak associated with craniomaxillofacial trauma. *J Oral Maxillofac Surg*. 2004;62(6):676–684.
14. Rodriguez ED, Stanwix MG, Nam AJ, et al. Twenty-six-year experience treating frontal sinus fractures: a novel algorithm based on anatomical fracture pattern and failure of conventional techniques. *Plast Reconstr Surg*. 2008;122(6):1850–1866.

CHAPTER 87

Le Fort Injuries

Justine Moe and Martin B. Steed

Armamentarium

#9 Periosteal elevator
#15 Scalpel blades
24- and 26-gauge wire
Appropriate sutures
Bipolar electrocautery
Bulldog retractors
Desmarres retractor
Erich arch bars
Fixation devices (plates and screws)
Local anesthetic with vasoconstrictor
Needle tip electrocautery
Obwegeser retractors
Rowe disimpaction forceps
Tenotomy scissors

History of the Procedure

The treatment of midfacial injuries was first described extensively in the 19th century. In 1823, von Graefe reported the first external splinting for a maxillary fracture.[1] In 1866, Guerin described the midfacial fracture pattern, noting involvement of the maxilla, the pyramidal part of the palatine bone, and pterygoid processes of the sphenoid bone. He noted an association with ecchymosis near the greater palatine foramen, which is termed *Guerin's sign*. In 1901, Rene Le Fort reported on his experiments on 35 cadaver heads that he subjected to various degrees of trauma.[2] His classification system of three patterns of maxillary fracture has been paramount in developing reconstructive strategies in trauma, craniofacial, and orthognathic surgery (Fig. 87.1).

Major advancements in the management of maxillary fractures in the 20th century coincided with times of war. During World War I, Fry and Gillies pioneered the treatment of maxillofacial injuries with collaboration between the anesthetist and surgeon.[1] During World War II, Le Fort fractures were treated by external fixation from metal splints to a headcap through rods and machined universal joints. In 1942, Adams introduced internal fixation for maxillary fractures, using suspension wires from the zygomatic process of the frontal bone, inferior orbital rim, or zygomatic bone.[3] The development of osteosynthesis heralded the advent of modern traumatology. Automatic compression plates were introduced by Luhr in 1968 and standardized by Spiessel in 1971.[4] The principles of monocortical miniplate fixation without axial compression that were proposed by Michelet and Moll (1971)[5] and Champy and Lodde (1976)[6] have been applied to the midface. Gruss (1982)[7] and Manson and colleagues (1985)[8] discussed the stabilization of buttresses with miniplates and proposed systematic approaches to the treatment of midfacial and panfacial fractures.

Indications for the Use of the Procedure

Maxillary fractures most frequently occur as a result of blunt trauma from assault, sporting injuries, and motor vehicle accidents. The Le Fort I fracture is a horizontal maxillary fracture resulting from a blow to the maxilla above the root apices. It involves the nasal septum, lateral nasal walls, anterior and lateral walls of the maxillary sinus, and pterygoid plates. The Le Fort II fracture pattern describes a pyramidal fracture resulting from blunt trauma to the infraorbital rim and nasofrontal junction. The central midface and maxilla are mobilized from the facial skeleton with the fracture line extending through the nasofrontal suture, frontal process of maxilla, lacrimal bone, inferior orbital rim, anterior wall of the maxillary sinus, and pterygoid plates. The Le Fort III fracture or craniofacial disjunction results from high-impact blunt trauma to the nasofrontal junction and upper lateral orbital rims. The facial skeleton is separated from the cranial base, with the fracture line extending medially through the perpendicular plate of the ethmoid, the vomer, and base of sphenoid, and laterally through the nasofrontal suture, medial orbital wall, orbital floor, zygomaticofrontal junction, and zygomatic arch. The continuum from Le Fort I to Le Fort III reflects an increasing severity of injury, increasing complexity of repair (with additional access requirements), and increasing likelihood for concomitant neurologic and ocular injury.

Ideally, surgical management of midfacial fractures should be completed as soon as the patient's medical status allows. Preoperative assessment includes clinical examination and radiographic evaluation with noncontrast computed tomography reformatted in three planes with a slice thickness of 1 mm or less (Fig. 87.2A and B). Goals of treatment include reestablishing premorbid occlusion and facial width, projection, and height. Failure to repair Le Fort fractures can result in midface retrusion, midface elongation, and anterior open bite due to the posteroinferior pull of the medial pterygoid on the posterior maxilla[8] (Fig. 87.2C). In addition, unrepaired orbital fractures of Le Fort II and III injuries can lead to enophthalmos, diplopia, and impaired lacrimal drainage. Early reconstruction allows for optimal restoration of the preinjury appearance as determined by the relationship between bone and soft tissue. Mobilization and reduction of osseous segments can be challenging in the delayed setting due to bone fragment impaction and soft tissue contraction. In addition, delayed reconstruction results in a second insult to the contused soft tissue and may increase subcutaneous fibrosis, rigidity, and hyperpigmentation.[9]

It should be emphasized that "pure" Le Fort fractures that follow the lines of Fig. 87.1 exactly are relatively uncommon in clinical settings. Le Fort injuries more often occur in a variety of permutations and combinations. For example, a patient may present with a left Le Fort I fracture and a right Le Fort II fracture (Fig. 87.2D). Unilateral or hemi–Le Fort injuries, comminuted fractures, and associated palatal fractures are also encountered.

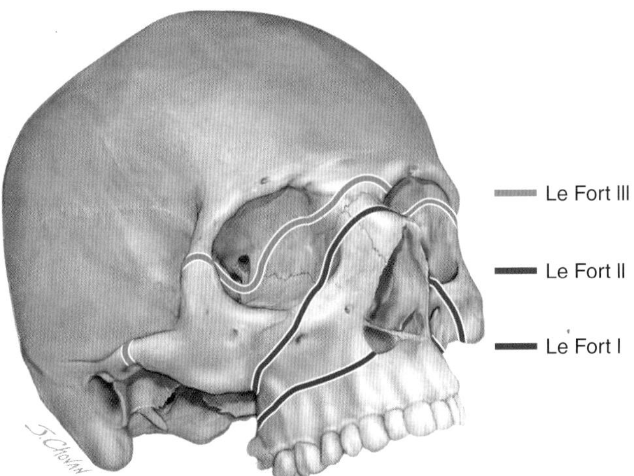

Figure 87.1 The Le Fort classification of maxillary fracture patterns.

Limitations and Contraindications

Le Fort injuries occur with high-impact force; as such, patients often have concomitant or life-threatening injuries. Initial management of patients with suspected maxillofacial fractures should follow the Advanced Trauma Life Support (ATLS) protocol. The primary survey includes airway and cervical spine stabilization, breathing and ventilatory support, circulation and hemorrhage control, disability and neurologic evaluation, and exposure and environment control (ATLS). Airway obstruction in Le Fort injuries mainly occurs secondary to hemorrhage into the upper airway from multiple sources, as well as altered airway anatomy with posteroinferior displacement of the midface into the oropharyngeal airway.[10] The incidence of life-threatening

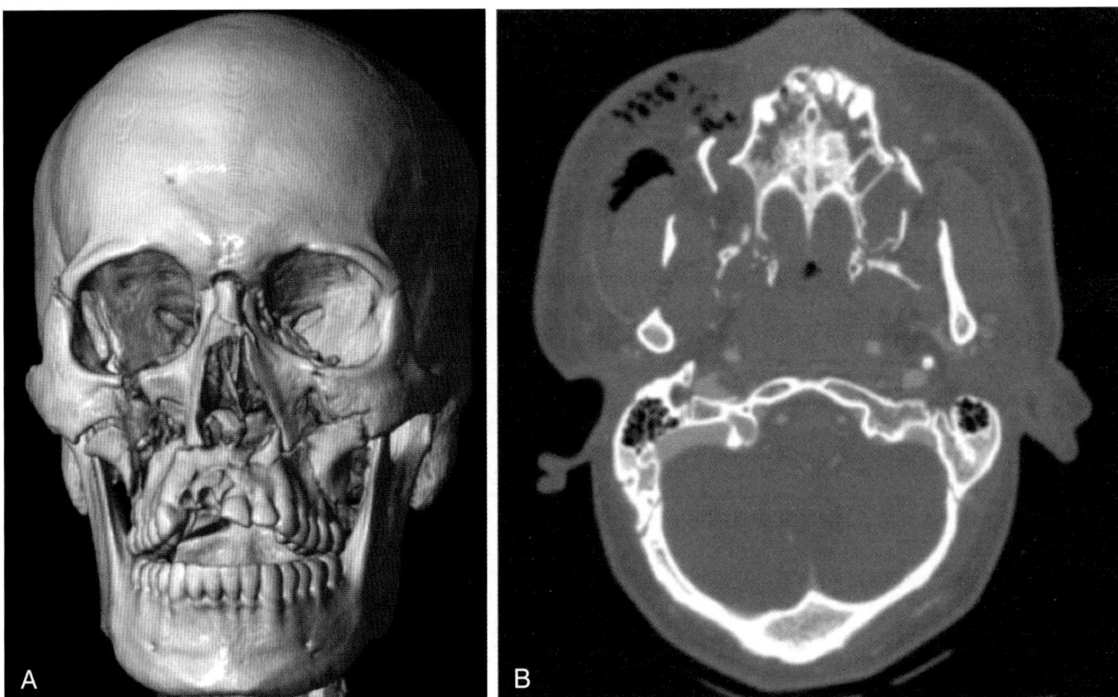

Figure 87.2 **A,** Three-dimensional computed tomography scan of multiple midfacial fractures including a Le Fort I level pattern. **B,** Computed tomography scan of axial cut bony window at the level of the maxilla demonstrating fracture of bilateral pterygoid plates—the hallmark of Le Fort fractures.

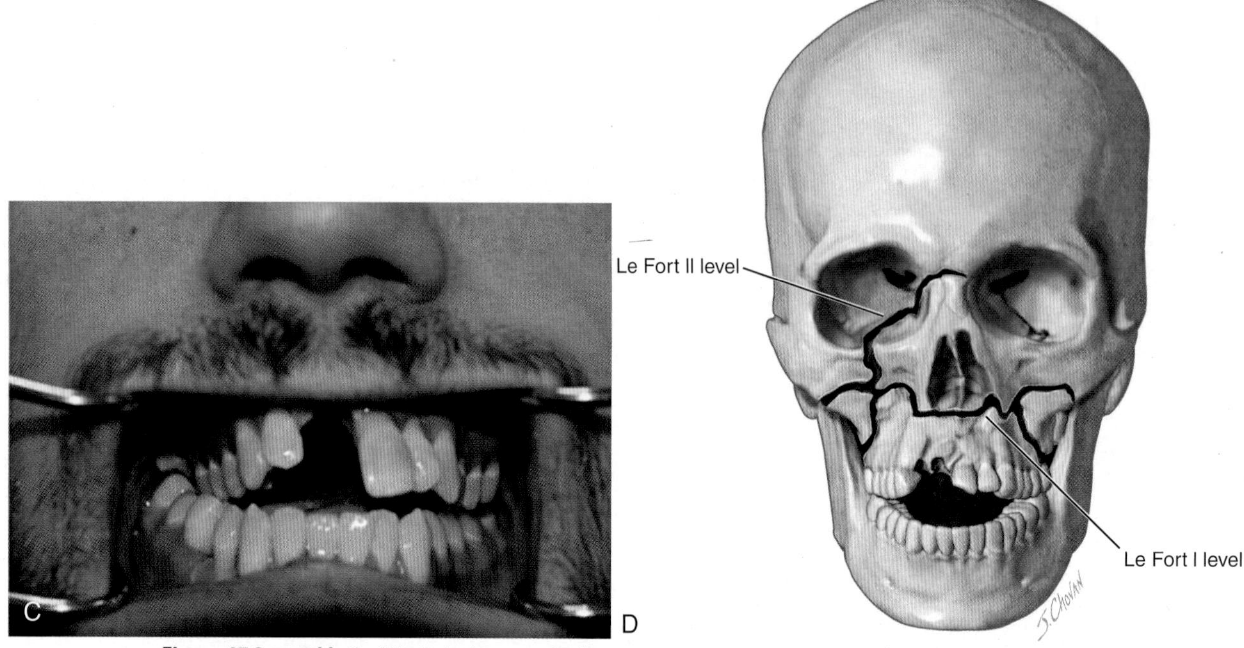

Figure 87.2, cont'd **C,** Clinical photograph demonstrating an anterior open bite as the result of a Le Fort fracture. This photo also demonstrates collapse of the maxillary width as a result of a palatal fracture component. **D,** Most midfacial fractures do not follow the classical "pure" Le Fort pattern. The fracture pattern on the patient's right reflects a Le Fort II pattern, whereas the fracture pattern on the patient's left is at the Le Fort I level.

hemorrhage in Le Fort II and III injuries is greater than that for all other facial injuries with rates of 5.5% as compared with 1.2%, respectively.[11] Airway protection and intubation should be considered in the setting of a significant pooling of blood in the oronasal cavity and a high risk of life-threatening aspiration and airway obstruction.[12] Up to one-third of Le Fort injuries may require emergent airway; therefore, clinicians treating midface trauma should be prepared to establish a surgical airway both acutely and in more controlled settings. Mild to moderate hemorrhage may be controlled with nasal packing or tamponade with a balloon catheter. However, severe hemorrhage that is not resolved with local measures may necessitate transcatheter arterial embolization.[13]

Le Fort fractures are also infrequently associated with cervical spine injury, with reported incidences of 1.5% to 2%.[14,15] In addition, midfacial fractures often present with traumatic brain injury with an incidence of 51%.[16] Le Fort fractures are more strongly associated with death from neurologic injury as compared with isolated mandible fractures.[17] The evaluation of maxillofacial fractures is part of the secondary survey and follows stabilization and resuscitation of the multisystem trauma patient. In Le Fort II and III fractures with orbital components, ophthalmologic evaluation of possible globe injury should be completed prior to surgery.

TECHNIQUE: Open Reduction and Internal Fixation of Le Fort Fracture

In general, the management of Le Fort fractures follows the principles of wide exposure and direct viewing of fracture segments, the use of vertical and horizontal buttresses of the face for alignment and fixation, and immediate bone grafting to reconstruct comminuted or avulsed bony structures.

STEP 1: Airway Management

Intra- and perioperative airway management should allow for safe anesthetic administration, optimal surgical access, and decreased morbidity. Nasoendotracheal intubation facilitates intraoperative maxillomandibular fixation (MMF) and is considered if extubation is expected at the completion of the procedure. Care must be taken in placing nasoendotracheal tubes in patients with midface fractures with basilar skull components as in Le Fort III fractures, as intracranial placement of endotracheal tubes, nasogastric tubes, and nasal catheters for epistaxis control have been reported with severe associated morbidity and high rates of mortality.[18] However, there is insufficient evidence to exclude nasotracheal intubation in the hands of skilled personnel.[19] Nasotracheal intubation may interfere with nasal septal correction.

Oral intubation is considered if the endotracheal tube may pass through an edentulous space to allow for MMF, or for conversion

TECHNIQUE: Open Reduction and Internal Fixation of Le Fort Fracture—*cont'd*

to submental intubation in which the endotracheal tube is passed through the anterior floor of the mouth and through a submental transcutaneous incision. Early tracheostomy is considered for severe midfacial fractures in which intubation is difficult and if prolonged postoperative intubation is expected.

STEP 2: Erich Arch Bar Application

Arch bars are secured to the teeth with circumdental 25-gauge wire. Care must be taken to apply the wires securely to the teeth without extruding mobile teeth. The arch bar can often help to reduce dentoalveolar components of the injury. Placement of the bar across larger fractures can preclude adequate reduction in which the bar may need to be placed segmentally (Fig. 87.3A).

STEP 3: Exposure of Fractures

Multiple surgical approaches are possible to access Le Fort fractures and are often used in combination. A maxillary transmucosal incision allows repair of Le Fort I fractures and is commonly required in Le Fort II and III fractures, as most require fixation at the lower maxillary level. It also provides access to the zygomaticomaxillary buttress and inferior orbital rim in Le Fort II fractures. The inferior orbital rim and orbital floor in Le Fort II or III fractures may be accessed by various transcutaneous approaches, including the lower lid, subtarsal and subciliary incisions, or transconjunctival incisions with or without lateral canthotomy and inferior cantholysis. For Le Fort III fractures, the coronal incision provides complete access and optimal visualization of the nasofrontal region, lateral orbital rim, and zygomatic arch. It is particularly advantageous for reduction and fixation of comminuted Le Fort III fractures. Releasing incisions in the coronal flap may be necessary to avoid intracranial monitoring devices including external ventriculostomy drains. The lateral brow and upper blepharoplasty or supratarsal fold incisions allow access to the nasofrontal and zygomaticofrontal buttress at the lateral orbital rim but not to the zygomatic arch. In rare cases, existing lacerations may be extended and used for access (Fig. 87.3B).

Continued

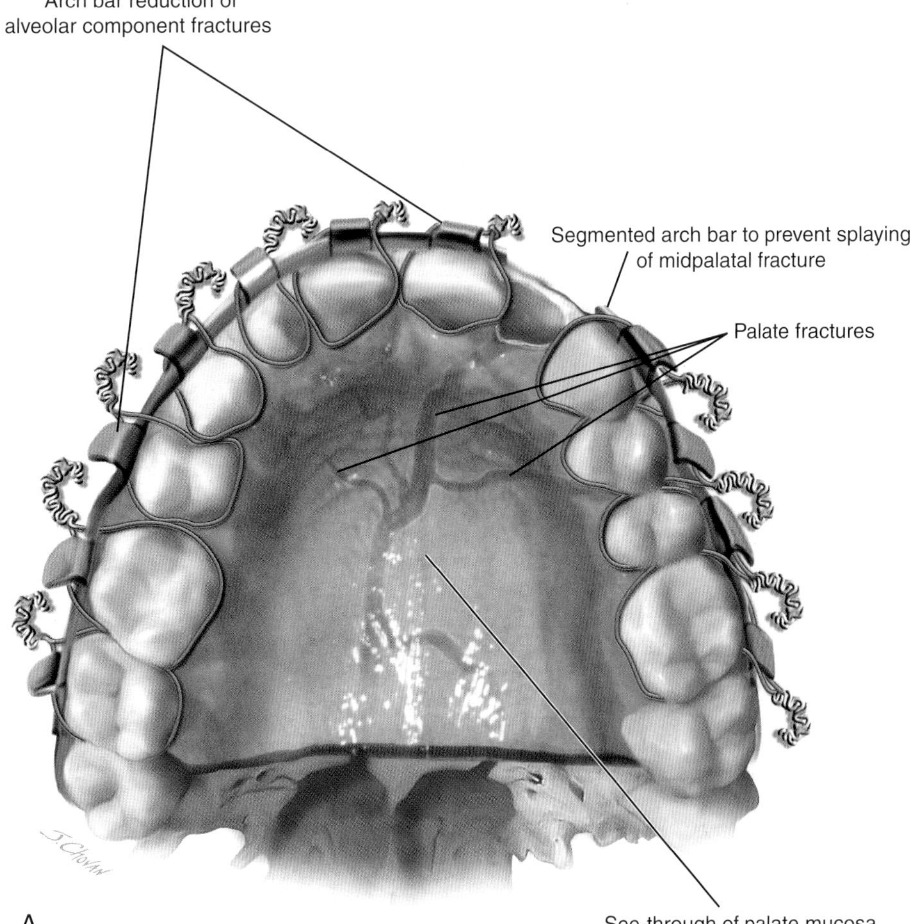

Figure 87.3 **A,** Palatal fractures may require a segmented arch bar to allow for proper reduction, preventing splaying, or collapse of a maxillary segment.

TECHNIQUE: Open Reduction and Internal Fixation of Le Fort Fracture—*cont'd*

STEP 4: Fracture Reduction

Following fracture exposure, the maxillary horizontal and vertical buttresses are anatomically aligned to restore normal midfacial height, projection, and width. Reduction should be achieved at the nasofrontal region, inferior orbital rim, and zygomaticomaxillary buttress in Le Fort II fractures and at the nasofrontal region, lateral orbital rim, and zygomatic arch in Le Fort III fractures. Reduction of the lower maxillary unit is critical in Le Fort I and in most Le Fort II and III fractures and may necessitate the use of a Rowe disimpaction forceps or a wire passed through the anterior nasal spine. If disimpaction cannot be achieved with these techniques and if the fracture pattern is above the Le Fort I level, a Le Fort I osteotomy can be completed unilaterally or bilaterally to mobilized and reduce the maxilla and dentate segment. An osteotomy should be considered only for noncomminuted maxillary fractures in which rigid fixation with adequate bone buttressing is possible. Passive positioning of the lower maxillary unit is necessary prior to fixation to prevent posterior relapse and may be achieved by overstretching the segment anteriorly (Fig. 87.3C and D).

STEP 5: Palatal Fracture Reduction

Concomitant palatal and maxillary alveolar fractures require reduction to establish transverse maxillary dimension and optimal occlusion. These fractures are often addressed prior to reduction at higher midfacial levels to allow the placement of MMF to guide reduction at the vertical buttresses. Although there is no general agreement for the ideal management of palatal fractures, several treatment modalities have been described, including surgical splints, MMF, transpalatal wiring, transmucosal or subperiosteal miniplate fixation, or a combination of techniques.[20,21] Palatal splints allow for proper occlusion, prevent maxillary segment rotation or collapse, and stabilize the maxillary segments if intermaxillary elastic traction is used.[22] Alveolar segments are stabilized with miniplate fixation placed through vestibular incisions, which should be placed judiciously so as not to jeopardize the vascular supply of the fractured segment (Fig. 87.3E).

STEP 6: Maxillomandibular Fixation

Establishment of dental occlusion is required in Le Fort fractures prior to internal fixation and is achieved most commonly with intraoperative MMF. In the setting of a stable mandible, the intact mandibular arc of rotation and mandibular ramus height are used to determine the correct reduction of the maxillary unit and to establish the height of the posterior buttress. MMF also guides reduction in the absence of direct visualization of fracture segments when closed reduction techniques are used and in severe comminution of the anterior maxillary buttresses. In the absence of an

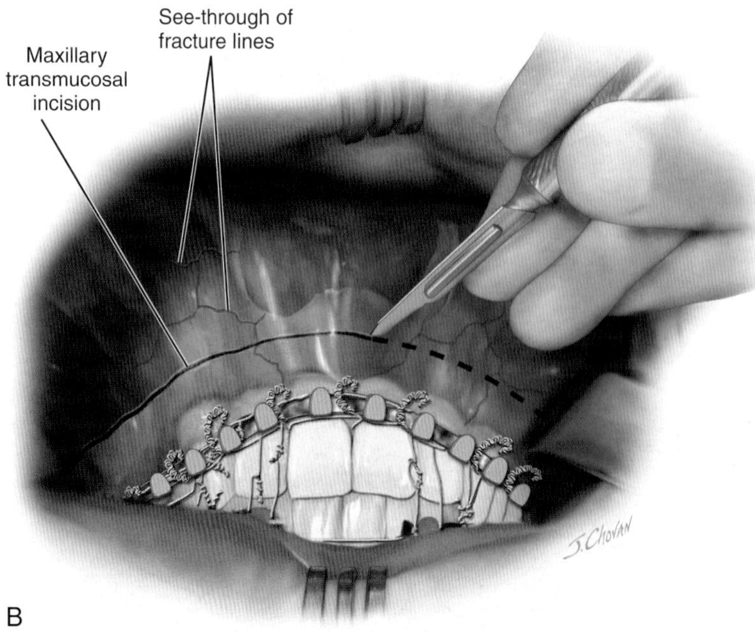

Figure 87.3, cont'd B, A maxillary vestibular incision made with a #15 blade through nonattached mucosa. The incision extends from left to right maxillary buttress. It is deepened at a right angle to the bone to allow for a robust tissue cuff to close to.

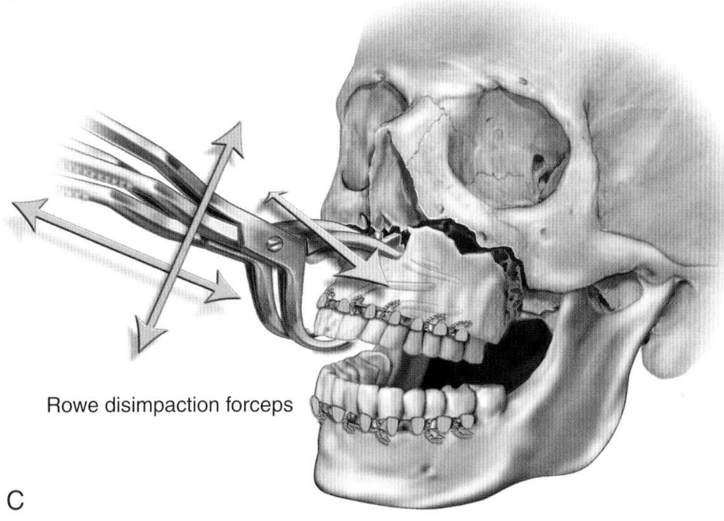

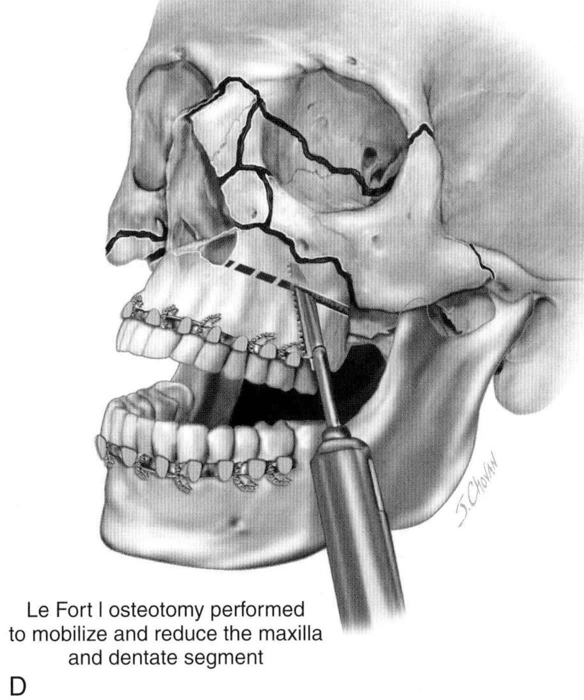

Le Fort I osteotomy performed to mobilize and reduce the maxilla and dentate segment
D

Figure 87.3, cont'd **C,** Demonstrates the use of the Rowe disimpaction forceps to mobilize the Le Fort I level fracture in multiple vectors to allow for proper reduction. **D,** Conversion of a high maxillary fracture to a more easily reduced level I fracture.

TECHNIQUE: Open Reduction and Internal Fixation of Le Fort Fracture—*cont'd*

intact dentition, dentures or gunning splints may be used to set the maxillomandibular relationship. In cases of an irreproducible dental occlusion or edentulous maxilla without an available denture or splint, or an unrepaired mandibular fracture, the treatment of midfacial fractures is dictated by anatomic reduction at the buttresses. However, buttress reconstruction is only a reference for maxillary height and not projection.[9]

Continued

TECHNIQUE: Open Reduction and Internal Fixation of Le Fort Fracture—*cont'd*

STEP 7: Internal Fixation

Rigid internal fixation using miniplate systems is completed following reduction of fracture segments. The location, amount, and size of the fixation depend on the severity of comminution and displacement, but in general, plates should be placed along the horizontal and vertical buttresses to allow for restoration of pretraumatic load paths.[23] It should be noted that only anterior buttresses are repaired at the Le Fort I level; the posterior or pterygoid buttresses are addressed indirectly with stabilization achieved by relating the maxilla to the intact mandible through MMF[9] (Fig. 87.3F–H).

STEP 8: Bone Grafting

Immediate or secondary bone grafting is infrequently required for osseous defects greater or equal to 5 mm, primarily for the reconstruction of unstable, comminuted, or missing buttresses.[24] Described donor sites include rib and ilium; however, autogenous calvarial bone graft through the coronal incision is favored, as it obviates the need for a second surgical site and the associated morbidity.

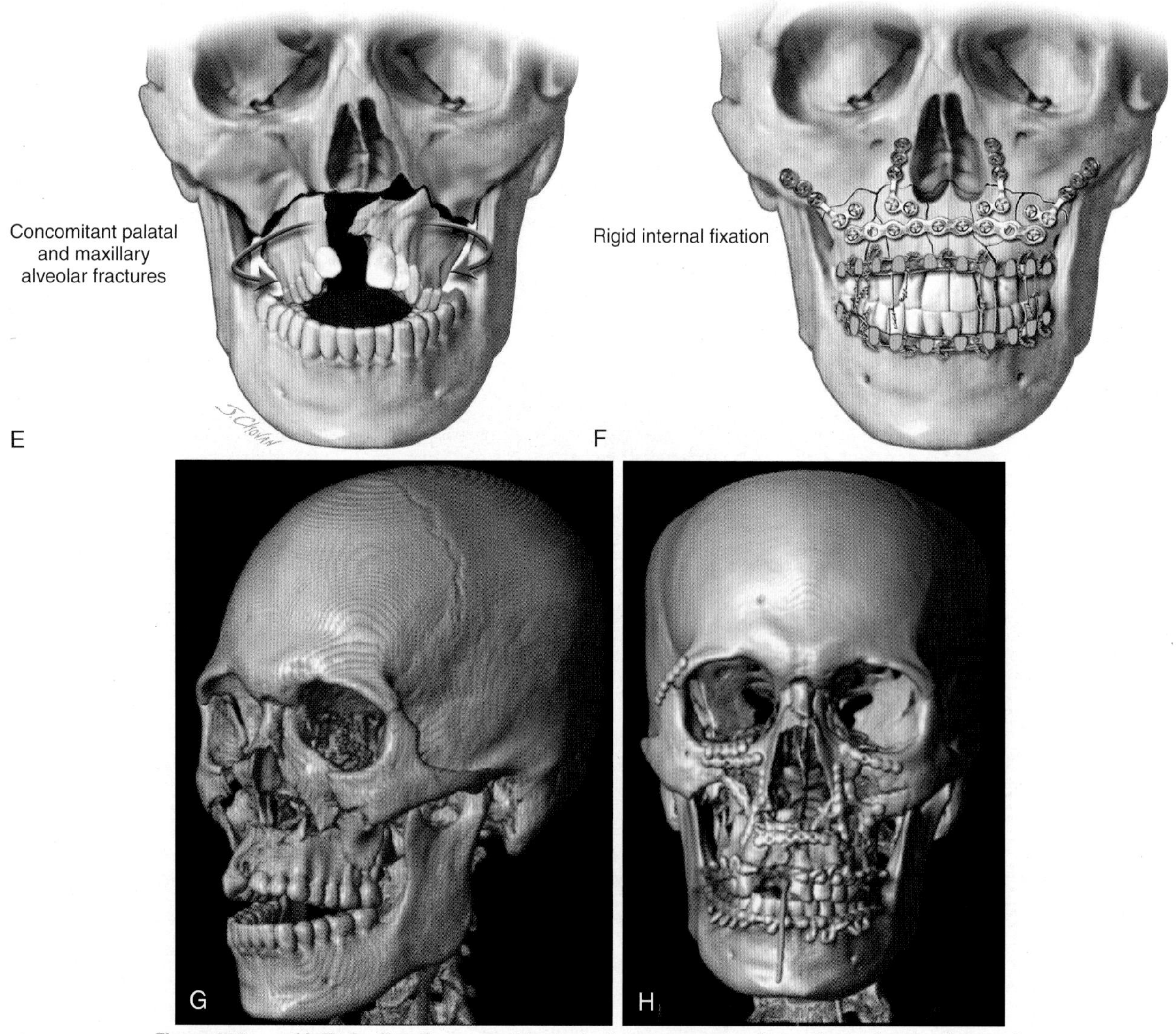

Figure 87.3, cont'd **E,** Le Fort fractures with a palatal component tend to collapse the maxillary arch transverse width at the level of the teeth by splaying superiorly. **F,** After proper occlusion has been established and the maxilla is properly reduced, the bones may be fixated with rigid internal titanium plates. The most inferior plate depicted here would require monocortical 5-mm screws to avoid injury to the maxillary teeth roots. **G,** Le Fort fracture prior to reduction and fixation demonstrating classic anterior impaction, posterior inferior displacement, and anterior open bite. **H,** After reduction and fixation.

TECHNIQUE: Open Reduction and Internal Fixation of Le Fort Fracture—*cont'd*

STEP 9: Soft Tissue Closure
Soft tissue closure is completed in layers to reapproximate anatomic components of the soft tissue envelope. Periosteal refixation is often necessary to prevent soft tissue sag postoperatively and to guide soft tissue readherence to the reconstructed craniofacial skeleton.[25-27] The surgical approaches for Le Fort fractures result in subtotal or total facial degloving and predispose to soft tissue dependent migration, ptosis, and thinning. As such, periosteal closure is considered at the zygomaticofrontal suture, inferior orbital rim, and deep temporal fascia.[26] Periosteal reattachment is considered at the malar eminence, inferior orbital rim, and medial and lateral canthi.[27] The temporalis fascia incision of the coronal approach should also be reattached or over suspended to allow for resuspension of fascia at the level of the arch.[9,27] Muscular layers are then approximated, and mucosa is closed in one or two layers in interrupted or continuing fashion.

ALTERNATIVE TECHNIQUE 1: Combination (Open and Closed Reduction) of Le Fort Fracture

Although visualization of fracture sites for reduction and fixation is generally desired, it is not always necessary to expose all components of Le Fort fractures. Techniques are generally categorized as open versus closed reduction, or a combination of the two. For example, adequate fixation at the bilateral inferior and lateral orbital rims of Le Fort II or III fractures, respectively, may preclude the need for fixation at the nasofrontal suture, thereby avoiding an additional incision for access. However, if the nasofrontal segment is unstable despite fixation at these buttresses, exposure of the nasofrontal area may be necessary using a variety of approaches as previously discussed. Initial closed reduction with disimpaction forceps and MMF may be completed for severely comminuted fractures prior to definitive treatment with open reduction and internal fixation after approximately 4 weeks.

ALTERNATIVE TECHNIQUE 2: Sequencing Alternatives for Le Fort Fractures

A variety of treatment sequences have been advocated for the treatment of Le Fort II and III–level fractures. The development of miniplate osteosynthesis has alleviated the need for external fixation and interfragmentary wiring, and it has allowed for greater flexibility in the sequence of repair. Fixation of comminuted Le Fort fracture patterns is often completed in a "stable to unstable" fashion. In particular, Le Fort III fractures usually present as a component of panfacial fractures rather than as isolated fractures. Several sequencing methods have been advocated for panfacial fracture management, including "bottom-up" and "outside-in."

Avoidance and Management of Intraoperative Complications

Intraoperative bleeding can occur as a result of damage to any number of vessels located in the vicinity, especially when significant disimpaction or an osteotomy is required to reduce maxillary fracture segments. Prevention is not always possible, but an understanding of vascular anatomy, protection of soft tissues during osteotomy, and relief of tension on visualized neurovascular bundles can help mitigate severe intraoperative hemorrhage. Potential sources of bleeding include the anterior and posterior superior alveolar, nasopalatine and descending palatine arteries, and, uncommonly, the internal maxillary artery. Packing, cauterization, and ligation are usually sufficient for achieving hemostasis in most situations. In cases in which hemorrhage cannot be controlled locally, external carotid artery ligation or transarterial embolization should be strongly considered.

Intraoperative malpositioning of the lower tooth-bearing maxillary segment can occur when the maxillomandibular complex is not seated passively at the time of fixation. This most commonly occurs when posterior maxillary bony interferences are not appropriately evaluated and application of digital pressure to the chin leads to reduction at the anterior buttresses while unintentionally displacing the mandibular condyles. Anterior open bite is evident at the time of MMF release. Prevention is best achieved by ensuring the full seating of mandibular condyles in the glenoid fossae prior to counterclockwise rotation of the maxillomandibular complex for lower maxillary reduction and fixation.

Maxillary hypoperfusion is uncommon but may occur with multiple segmental fractures or with soft tissue impingement from surgical splints. Hypoperfusion may be manifested intraoperatively by pale mucosa, prolonged or absent capillary refill, and later by mucosal sloughing, and in extremely rare cases it may lead to maxillary aseptic necrosis.[28] Prevention strategies include soft tissue incisions limited in length to allow visualization and treatment of fractures without compromising vascular supply to fracture segments. Subperiosteal dissection of severely comminuted maxillary fractures should be minimized. Occlusal splints should be fabricated to avoid impingement on the palatal soft tissues. Early reduction and stabilization with rigid internal fixation may also improve the outcome. Postoperative management with the use of hyperbaric oxygen has been suggested, but its benefits remain unclear.

Postoperative Complications

Early

Control of nasal bleeding can be obtained in the immediate postoperative period by using a variety of techniques for nasal packing. A speculum and a good light source are essential in order to determine an anterior versus posterior origin. If adequate control is not achieved, exploration in the operating room or interventional radiology for angiographic evaluation may be necessary.

Malocclusion can result from improper intraoperative maxillary positioning, early hardware failure, or undiagnosed mandibular or maxillary segmental fractures. Careful examination and appropriate imaging modalities help in discerning the etiology of malocclusion for surgical repositioning and refixation.

Infraorbital nerve paresthesia can result from nerve injury at the initial trauma, especially when fracture patterns extend through the infraorbital foramen, or from intraoperative traction or manipulation for adequate reduction. Nasal septal deviation can result from improper repositioning of the nasal septum onto the nasal crest of the maxilla, undiagnosed nasal septal injuries, or preoperative septal deformities. This can result in increased airway resistance, nasolacrimal obstruction, and esthetic complaints by the patient.

Loss of vision can result from an unfavorable fracture pattern of the maxilla or from the initial trauma, compounded by surgical manipulation of the segment during repositioning. The orbital process of the palatine bone makes up a portion of the bony orbit and has been hypothesized as possible cause (this is rare for Le Fort I fractures, but more common with Le Fort III injuries).

Early postoperative infection can result from foreign bodies, necrotic teeth, or bone segments but is also related to host factors (malnutrition, immunocompromised state, chronic alcohol use). Management should be directed at appropriate antibiotic selection, incision and drainage, and removal of any possible source.

Late

Malocclusion, if not addressed early, will typically present with an anterior open bite, posterior premature contacts, and an overall class III skeletal appearance. Once union has developed, small discrepancies can be treated with orthodontics, whereas larger ones will need to be addressed by orthognathic surgery.

Late postoperative bleeding (especially with an intermittent pattern) should be taken seriously. Pseudoaneurysm formation should be high on the differential diagnosis and can be evaluated by angiography.

Epiphora (excessive tearing) can result from damage or obstruction of the nasolacrimal duct (the nasolacrimal duct drains beneath the inferior turbinate 11 to 17 mm above the nasal floor and 11 to 14 mm posterior to the piriform aperture). Epiphora can be managed by a dacryocystorhinostomy procedure.

Nonunion or fibrous union will cause the maxilla to demonstrate mobility, which can often be subtle. Management should be directed at refixation of the maxilla with rigid internal fixation, skeletal fixation, extraskeletal fixation, or MMF.

References

1. Rowe NL. The history of the treatment of maxillo-facial trauma. *Ann R Coll Surg Engl.* 1971;49(5):329–349.
2. Le Fort R. Experimental study of fractures of the upper jaw. Parts I, II and II. *Rev Chir De Paris.* 1901;23(208):360–479.
3. Hausamen JE. The scientific development of maxillofacial surgery in the 20th century and an outlook into the future. *J Craniomaxillofac Surg.* 2001;29(1):2–21.
4. Luhr HG. [The development of modern osteosynthesis]. *Mund Kiefer Gesichtschir.* 2000;4(suppl 1):S84–S90.
5. Michelet FX, Moll A. [Surgical treatments of fractures of the corpus mandibulae without blockage, with diminutive screwed plates inserted via the endobuccal route]. *Rev Odontostomatol Midi Fr.* 1971;29(2):87–105.
6. Champy M, Lodde JP. [Mandibular synthesis. Placement of the synthesis as a function of mandibular stress]. *Rev Stomatol Chir Maxillofac.* 1976;77(8):971–976.
7. Gruss JS. Fronto-naso-orbital trauma. *Clin Plast Surg.* 1982;9(4):577–589.
8. Manson PN, Crawley WA, Yaremchuk MJ, Rochman GM, Hoopes JE, French JH Jr. Midface fractures: advantages of immediate extended open reduction and bone grafting. *Plast Reconstr Surg.* 1985;76(1):1–12.
9. Kelly KJ, Manson PN, Vander Kolk CA, et al. Sequencing LeFort fracture treatment (Organization of treatment for a panfacial fracture). *J Craniofac Surg.* 1990;1(4):168–178.
10. Ng M, Saadat D, Sinha UK. Managing the emergency airway in Le Fort fractures. *J Craniomaxillofac Trauma.* 1998;4(4):38–43.
11. Bynoe RP, Kerwin AJ, Parker HH III, et al. Maxillofacial injuries and life-threatening hemorrhage: treatment with transcatheter arterial embolization. *J Trauma.* 2003;55(1):74–79.
12. Chen CC, Jeng SF, Tsai HH, Liliang PC, Hsieh CH. Life-threatening bleeding of bilateral maxillary arteries in maxillofacial trauma: report of two cases. *J Trauma.* 2007;63(4):933–937.
13. Chen YF, Tzeng IH, Li YH, et al. Transcatheter arterial embolization in the treatment of maxillofacial trauma induced life-threatening hemorrhages. *J Trauma.* 2009;66(5):1425–1430.
14. Bagheri SC, Holmgren E, Kademani D, et al. Comparison of the severity of bilateral Le Fort injuries in isolated midface trauma. *J Oral Maxillofac Surg.* 2005;63(8):1123–1129.
15. Haug RH, Wible RT, Likavec MJ, Conforti PJ. Cervical spine fractures and maxillofacial trauma. *J Oral Maxillofac Surg.* 1991;49(7):725–729.
16. Haug RH, Prather J, Indresano AT. An epidemiologic survey of facial fractures and concomitant injuries. *J Oral Maxillofac Surg.* 1990;48(9):926–932.
17. Plaisier BR, Punjabi AP, Super DM, Haug RH. The relationship between facial fractures and death from neurologic injury. *J Oral Maxillofac Surg.* 2000;58(7):708–712.
18. Huang HM, Wei ST, Chen DC, Lin HL. Preventing iatrogenic injury from inadvertent intracranial migration of a urinary foley catheter while controlling profuse epistaxis after severe craniofacial trauma. *J Craniofac Surg.* 2011;22(2):748–749.

19. Bähr W, Stoll P. Nasal intubation in the presence of frontobasal fractures: a retrospective study. *J Oral Maxillofac Surg*. 1992;50(5):445–447.
20. Manson PN, Glassman D, Vanderkolk C, Petty P, Crawley WA. Rigid stabilization of sagittal fractures of the maxilla and palate. *Plast Reconstr Surg*. 1990;85(5):711–717.
21. Cienfuegos R, Sierra E, Ortiz B, Fernández G. Treatment of palatal fractures by osteosynthesis with 2.0-mm locking plates as external fixator. *Craniomaxillofac Trauma Reconstr*. 2010;3(4):223–230.
22. Manson PN, Shack RB, Leonard LG, Su CT, Hoopes JE. Sagittal fractures of the maxilla and palate. *Plast Reconstr Surg*. 1983;72(4):484–489.
23. Rudderman RH, Mullen RL. Biomechanics of the facial skeleton. *Clin Plast Surg*. 1992;19(1):11–29.
24. Gruss JS, Mackinnon SE. Complex maxillary fractures: role of buttress reconstruction and immediate bone grafts. *Plast Reconstr Surg*. 1986;78(1):9–22.
25. Dingman RO, Natvig P. *Surgery of Facial Fractures*. Philadelphia, PA: WB Saunders; 1964.
26. Phillips JH, Gruss JS, Wells MD, Chollet A. Periosteal suspension of the lower eyelid and cheek following subciliary exposure of facial fractures. *Plast Reconstr Surg*. 1991;88(1):145–148.
27. Manson PN, Clark N, Robertson B, et al. Subunit principles in midface fractures: the importance of sagittal buttresses, soft-tissue reductions, and sequencing treatment of segmental fractures. *Plast Reconstr Surg*. 1999;103(4):1287–1306.
28. Khan N, Memon W, Idris M, Ahmed M, Taufiq M. Post-traumatic near-complete aseptic necrosis of the maxilla: a case report and review of the literature. *Dentomaxillofac Radiol*. 2012;41(5):429–431.

CHAPTER 88

Pediatric Midface Trauma

Sean P. Edwards

Armamentarium

#9 Periosteal elevator
#15 Scalpel
26- and 28-gauge wire
Appropriate sutures
Ash forceps
Bipolar electrocautery
Bishop pickups
Bone hook
Carroll-Girard screw
Double skin hooks (two)
Erich arch bars
Local anesthetic with vasoconstrictor
Malleable retractors
Mayo scissors
Nasal and Doyle splints of choice
Needle electrocautery
Needle holders
Obwegeser retractors
Resorbable or titanium fixation set
Rowe forceps
Ruler
Senn retractors
Single skin hooks (two)
Tenotomy scissors
Vein retractors
Wire cutters
Wire drivers/twisters

History of the Procedure

Pediatric facial fractures have been the subject of many retrospective reviews. Most of these express some variation in terms of the demographics of the injuries seen. This is likely a reflection of the setting from which the dataset is drawn (e.g., urban versus suburban trauma centers). Imahara et al.[1] queried the National Trauma Data Bank of the American College of Surgeons from 2001 through 2005. This databank comprises inpatient data from more than 600 trauma centers. Over the period examined, 1.5 million patients were entered into the database, and roughly 19% of those were under 18 years of age. Approximately 4.6%, or 12,739, sustained a facial fracture. Motor vehicle accidents were the most common mechanism of injury. In the review, the incidence of fractures increased with the age of the injured patient. The lowest incidence was seen in infants and toddlers and the highest in teens. Also increasing with age was the number of fractures requiring operative intervention. Only 11% of toddlers required surgery, compared with 30% of those aged 15 to 18 years. The most common site of fracture was the mandible (32%). Midfacial injuries were next, with nasal fractures accounting for 30%, followed closely by the zygoma at 28.6%.

Scant instructive literature is available describing the incidence of growth attenuation after a midfacial injury. It would take a large sample size followed over a long period (years) to answer this question definitively because the effects of an injury and potentially any operative intervention are superimposed on a patient's premorbid growth pattern. For this reason, case reports and even small case series are of limited value in determining the growth consequences of a midfacial injury. Although the incidence is not known and experimental evidence is conflicting, there are reports of midface hypoplasia resulting after injuries to the midface. Injuries to the nasal and septal regions would seem to have the greatest potential for midface growth attenuation. Aizenbud et al.[2] studied a pair of identical twins, one of whom sustained Le Fort II and III fractures at the age of 2 years. The twin who sustained the fractures went on to develop a significant class III deformity that required surgical correction in late adolescence. This would seem to demonstrate the potential for growth attenuation resulting from nasomaxillary trauma; at the very least, it would suggest that some form of long-term growth observation is warranted in young injured patients. A similar observation in another set of twins, one of whom had minor septal surgery, by Grymer and Bosch,[3] seemed to confirm the importance of the nasal septum in driving maxillary growth.

This chapter focuses on injuries to the midface region in children. Rather than discussing in great detail the management steps of the various fractures encountered in the region, the chapter highlights where these injuries are different in children and the unique considerations involved.

Indications for the Use of the Procedure

Midface fractures are rare in children due to several anatomic differences. Craniofacial development proceeds in a cephalocaudal direction. Cranial volume to facial volume ratios at birth are roughly 8:1; at the completion of growth, this ratio is 2.5:1. As a result, the midface occupies a retruded and therefore protected position. Children also generally have an abundant layer of adipose tissue, a more elastic skeleton, and flexible suture lines. Pediatric fractures, therefore, are more often incomplete and minimally displaced and thus more often require no operative intervention.[4]

The typical fracture patterns seen in the midface of the adult skeleton require the presence of pneumatized paranasal sinuses. These act as weak points between the vertical and horizontal buttresses of the face. Sinus pneumatization begins around 4 years of age and continues through adolescence. For example, a typical zygomaticomaxillary fracture requires the presence of a maxillary sinus. When this is not present and a fracture occurs, it can be expected to propagate in a more atypical fashion. Orbital floor fractures also require the presence of a maxillary sinus; therefore, orbital roof fractures are more common in early childhood.[5]

The myriad of fixation options available for the adult trauma patient may also be safely applied to the pediatric skeleton, with some unique considerations. Rigid fixation can be safely applied to the craniomaxillofacial skeleton of the child, with due caution to avoid injury to vital structures such as developing tooth buds. The midface in the primary and mixed dentition stages is a crowded place. The sinuses are beginning their pneumatization, and the maxilla is full of tooth buds. In particular, the second molar and canine teeth sit relatively cranial, with only very thin overlying bone, which makes the application of hardware in these regions impossible.

Resorbable fixation has garnered a fair degree of enthusiasm in the management of pediatric facial fractures. The hope with these fixation systems was that the material would reduce the risk of growth attenuation, eliminate the potential for hardware migration into vital structures, and eliminate the need for hardware removal. These devices have gained a level of acceptance; however, in general, compared with titanium fixation systems, they are less rigid, have a thicker profile, and are technically more demanding to place.[6]

Limitations and Contraindications

Concomitant Injuries

Multisystem trauma is overall quite common in children who sustain facial fractures, with reported incidences ranging from 25% to 75%.[4,7] Brain injuries seem to be more common in children with facial injuries than in those without. In the review by Imahara et al.,[1] the difference was twofold. Cervical spine fractures are rarely encountered in pediatric patients with facial fractures. Imahara's review[1] found only a 1.4% incidence; this compares well with the series reported by Posnick et al.,[7] in which there were no reported cervical spine fractures, and that of Grunwaldt et al.,[8] who reported a 2.3% incidence.

Table 88.1 Average Percentage Growth Completion of Various Craniofacial Dimensions

	Average % of Growth Completed by Age 1	Average % of Growth Completed by Age 5	Average Age at Maturity in Years
Cranium	84–85	90–94	Males: 14 Females:16
Orbits	84–86	88–93	Variable
Zygoma	72	83	Males: 15 Females: 13
Maxilla	75–80	85	Males: 15 Females: 14
Mandible	60–70	74–85	Males: 16 Females: 14

From Costello BJ, Rivera RD, Shand J, et al. Growth and development considerations for craniomaxillofacial surgery. *Oral Maxillofac Surg Clin North Am*. 2012;24(3):377–396.

Growth Considerations

As mentioned, growth proceeds in a craniocaudal fashion. Table 88.1 highlights this progression, in which cranial growth is complete far in advance of mandibular growth. Of concern to surgeons, orthodontists, and parents are the growth consequences of the midfacial injury and its subsequent management. It is reasonable to expect that the impact of an injury and its operative correction would be proportional to the amount of growth remaining in that facial part. Understanding the differences in the timing of maturation of the different portions of the facial skeleton is critical in determining the potential for growth attenuation and for selecting fixation material.

TECHNIQUE: Zygomaticomaxillary Complex Fractures

As previously mentioned, the presence of a pneumatized maxillary sinus is required for the typical zygomaticomaxillary complex (ZMC) fracture to occur. Most ZMC fractures in children are nondisplaced or minimally displaced due to elasticity and the thick covering of adipose tissue. The greater tissue turgor and elasticity of the soft-tissue mask in children, compared with adults, are such that a greater degree of fracture displacement is needed to manifest malar flattening. Displacement of the lateral canthus is similar in children and adults.

Continued

TECHNIQUE: Zygomaticomaxillary Complex Fractures—cont'd

STEP 1: Incision and Dissection

When electing open reduction and internal fixation of a pediatric ZMC fracture, the surgeon must consider the surgical approach and the method of fracture stabilization. Common surgical approaches include the vestibular, transconjunctival with lateral canthotomy, and upper blepharoplasty methods, or combinations of these. Incorporation of a coronal incision can be helpful for severely comminuted zygomatic fractures. There is no significant difference between the execution of these approaches in children and their use in adults, although the surgeon must keep in mind the different anatomic distances in children, such as the shortened height of the piriform rim/zygomatic buttress to the orbital rim or from the orbital rim to the orbital apex. An appropriate, weight-based injection of a local anesthetic is administered before the incision is made.

STEP 2: Elevation and Reduction

Elevation of the displaced zygoma may be accomplished in several ways, including use of an elevator underneath the body/arch or use of a Girard screw or similar instrument. Care must be exercised not to inadvertently fracture portions of the sinus wall during elevation.

STEP 3: Open Reduction and Internal Fixation

The area of greatest interest is the line of fracture in the zygomatic buttress and its position relative to the second molar. Once this tooth has erupted, fracture management progresses as it would for an adult. However, if the second molar or its bud occupy the zygomatic buttress, fixation devices cannot be placed in this position, and the surgeon must rely instead on the periorbital buttresses for fixation. As in the adult patient, the surgeon applies as much fixation as is needed to maintain the three-dimensional position of the zygoma. Resorbable or titanium fixation may be used as discussed previously. Occasionally, the zygoma locks into place, obviating the need for fixation (Fig. 88.1).

STEP 4: Closure

Closure of the incisions proceeds as it normally would in an adult patient. However, wherever possible, consideration should be given to the use of resorbable suture material. The lateral canthus is resuspended if a cantholysis was performed. If orbital floor exploration or repair is performed simultaneously, a forced duction to document globe mobility should be performed at the end of the procedure.

TECHNIQUE: Orbital Floor Fractures

Orbital fractures represent approximately 20% to 30% of pediatric facial fractures.[4,7] Age is a prime determinant of fracture presentation. Orbital floor blowout fractures require a pneumatized maxillary sinus; as a result, they predominate in children older than 7 years. In children younger than 7 years of age, orbital fractures are rare and more typically involve the orbital roof. These orbital roof fractures are often transcranial injuries due to the absence of a significant frontal sinus.[5,9]

Trapdoor fractures are clinically more common in the pediatric population. This type of orbital floor fracture hinges open and then closes, entrapping and incarcerating orbital tissues. These tissues become ischemic as a result, and if left untreated, a permanent contracture occurs.[5] This type of fracture is one of the true pediatric trauma emergencies, and most surgeons elect to treat it within hours. Intraoperatively, the fracture is exposed and separated, and the incarcerated tissues

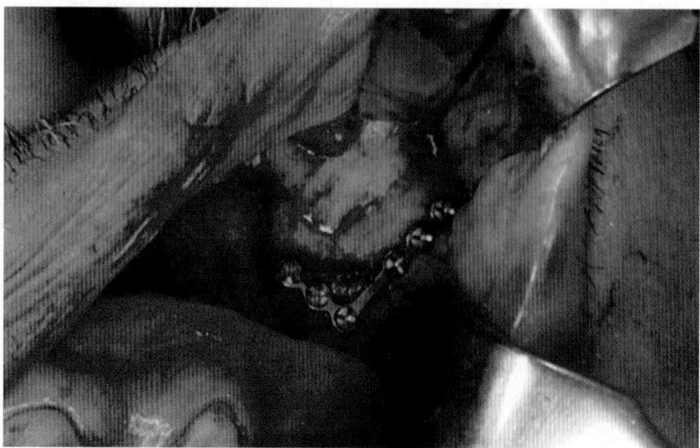

Figure 88.1 Care is taken to avoid injury to tooth buds when placing fixation devices on the zygomatic buttress.

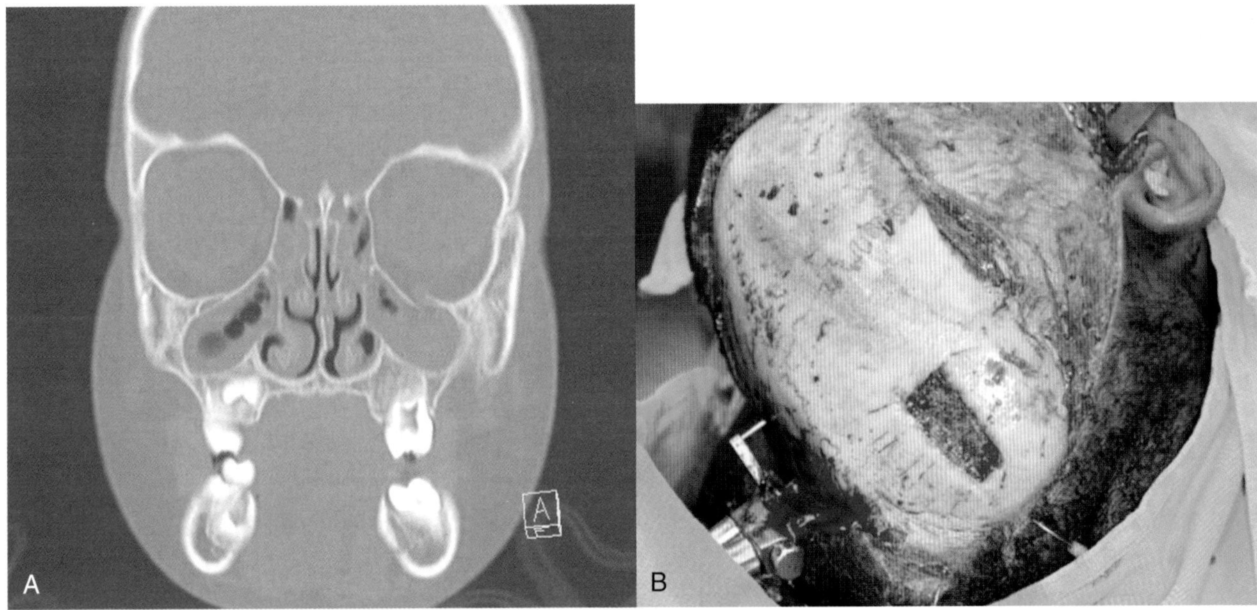

Figure 88.2 **A,** Coronal computed tomography (CT) scan demonstrating a trapdoor fracture with incarceration of the left internal oblique. Herniated fat can be appreciated as an area of low attenuation in the sinus adjacent to the fracture within the higher attenuation sinus hemorrhage. **B,** Outer table of the parietal bone harvested for orbital floor reconstruction.

TECHNIQUE: Orbital Floor Fractures—cont'd

are gently teased free. The fracture then is reconstructed as the size of the defect dictates.

Children with entrapment in addition to restricted gaze and diplopia are more likely to experience nausea and vomiting until this is reduced. Rare cases of bradycardia, as a result of the oculocardiac reflex, have also been reported.[9]

The indications for operative management of a pediatric orbital fracture are identical to those for adults:

- Mechanical limitation to globe movement
- Radiographic evidence of extensive fracture (greater than 50%)
- Enophthalmos or significant globe positional change
- Persistent diplopia not attributable to hematoma, edema, or neurogenic factors

Once a surgeon has made the clinical decision that an orbital floor fracture needs repair, the next steps in operative planning are the approach and the material to be used for orbital reconstruction (Fig. 88.2A).

STEP 1: Incision and Dissection

The surgical approaches to orbital fractures are identical to those used in adults. The eyelids of children are not as lax as those of older patients, and as a result, the transconjunctival approach more often necessitates a concomitant lateral canthotomy and inferior cantholysis for adequate access. Care must be exercised in young children to preoperatively measure the distance from the orbital rim to the orbital apex to prevent injury during dissection. An appropriate weight-based injection of local anesthetic is administered before the incision is made.

STEP 2: Elevation and Reduction

Elevation of herniated orbital contents proceeds in a fashion similar to that for the skeletally mature orbit. During elevation of the orbital contents from the sinus, care must be taken to gently reposition it back into the orbit. Excessive traction promotes bleeding, may cause further muscle injury, and further disrupts Lockwood's ligaments, which may increase the chance of postoperative enophthalmos. This may necessitate enlarging the floor defect to allow for atraumatic elevation of orbital contents from the sinus. At the conclusion of the reduction, the surgeon should be able to visualize the posterior lip of bone upon which the implant/graft will rest. The anesthesiologist should be alerted to the possibility of inciting the oculocardiac reflex, and if this occurs, the procedure should be halted until the baseline heart rate returns to normal before proceeding.

Continued

TECHNIQUE: Orbital Floor Fractures—cont'd

STEP 3: Open Reduction and Internal Fixation

As discussed previously, whatever material is chosen for repair should rest passively on the remaining shelf or lip of the posterior orbital floor. It should be measured before insertion so as not to cause embarrassment of the orbital apex. In addition, it should rest just behind the orbital rim so as not to be palpable. The decision on whether to fix the material in place depends on the material chosen and the surgeon's preference. In general, fixing the implant or graft in place prevents extrusion.

The materials most often selected for orbital repair in children include autogenous bone and alloplastic material, such as porous polyethylene. If significant growth remains in the orbit, autogenous bone should be selected. The calvarium is the optimal donor site for this. This bone can be harvested from the outer table of the skull in the parietal region of the skull or, when part of a combined maxillofacial-neurosurgical case, it can be harvested from the inner table of the craniotomy bone flap.

Development of the eye is the prime driver for development of the periorbital skeleton. Most of this growth is complete by age 7 years. As a result, a nonresorbable alloplastic material could be selected for orbital reconstruction after the age of 7, without fear of implant migration (Fig. 88.2B).

STEP 4: Closure

Closure of the incisions proceeds as in the adult patient. However, wherever possible, consideration should be given to the use of resorbable suture material. The lateral canthus is resuspended if a cantholysis was performed. A forced duction, to document globe mobility, should be performed at the end of the procedure.

TECHNIQUE: Maxillary Fractures

The classic Le Fort I, II, and III fracture patterns all require the presence of sinuses. These act as stress breakers, intervening between the vertical and horizontal buttresses of the face. The Le Fort fracture patterns rarely present as pure fractures in adults, and the complexity is only greater in children. Because of these anatomic realities, these patterns start to emerge only after age 7.

STEP 1: Incision and Dissection

When electing open reduction and internal fixation of a pediatric maxillary fracture, the surgeon must consider the surgical approach and the method of fracture stabilization. Common surgical approaches include the vestibular, transconjunctival with lateral canthotomy, and upper blepharoplasty methods, or combinations of these. Incorporation of a coronal incision can be helpful for severely comminuted or high midface fractures. There is no significant difference in the execution of these approaches between children and adults, although the surgeon must keep in mind the different anatomic distances, such as the shortened height of the piriform rim to the orbital rim, so as not to inadvertently injure the globe. An appropriate weight-based injection of local anesthetic is administered before the incision is made.

STEP 2: Elevation and Reduction

Once a patient is fully into the secondary dentition, maxillary fractures present and can be managed as in an adult. However, reduction and fixation of the maxilla in patients in the primary and mixed dentition stages, can be challenging for a variety of reasons. First, the fracture patterns can be quite unusual. Second, the dentition is often not amenable to circumdental and interdental wiring techniques. The Risdon cable technique can be helpful in the primary dentition.

For the maxilla, reduction of fractures is accomplished with digital pressure or the use of maxillary disimpaction instruments, such as Rowe forceps. If the fracture is comminuted or at a higher level through the orbits, elevation and reduction of individual fracture segments may be necessary (see relevant sections on other fractures/anatomic areas). Maxillomandibular fixation or skeletal fixation is achieved through whichever method is appropriate (Fig. 88.3).

STEP 3: Open Reduction and Internal Fixation

The bone quality in the maxilla is poor, and the bone typically overlies unerupted tooth buds. Also, the developing tooth buds of the canines and the second molars lie within the vertical buttresses of the midface, where the surgeon generally would elect to place fixation devices after fracture reduction. For these reasons, maxillary fractures in children often are treated with periorbital plating for high-level injuries and with suspension wiring techniques to manage the occlusion. After reduction, the maxilla is easily held in position with either or all of the following: circumzygomatic wires, piriform suspension wires, and infraorbital suspension wires. These are typically joined to the mandible with an additional wire.

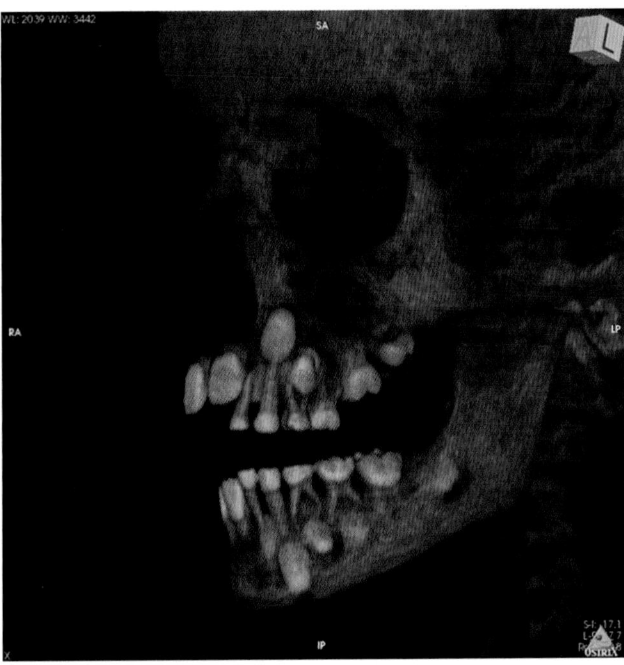

Figure 88.3 Three-dimensional image of a child in mixed dentition showing the presence of developing tooth buds in the piriform and zygomatic buttresses. The tooth buds would make rigid fixation difficult for a maxillary fracture in a child of this age.

TECHNIQUE: Maxillary Fractures—cont'd

Palatal fractures increase the complexity of fracture management in both adults and pediatric patients. These are best managed with fabrication of a palatal splint from models of a patient's corrected occlusion.

STEP 4: Wound Closure

Wound closure of the incisions proceeds in a routine fashion as in the adult. However, wherever possible, consideration should be given to the use of resorbable suture material. The lateral canthus is resuspended if a cantholysis was performed. A forced duction, to document globe mobility, should be performed at the end of the procedure.

TECHNIQUE: Naso-Orbito-Ethmoid Fractures

Fractures of the naso-orbito-ethmoid (NOE) complex are generally high-energy injuries. In younger children, in whom the sinuses have not yet developed, these often are transcranial injuries. Management goals include accurate repositioning on the medial canthal tendons, adequate support or reconstruction of the nasal dorsum, and protection of the dura and intracranial compartment from the nasal cavity when violated. Minimally displaced fractures maybe managed in a closed fashion with the assistance of nasal splinting.

STEP 1: Incision and Dissection

The surgical approaches used for NOE fractures are identical to those used in adults. They include coronal flaps, lid incisions (e.g., transconjunctival approach), and the transoral route. An appropriate weight-based local anesthetic is administered before the incision is made.

STEP 2: Elevation and Reduction

The increased osteogenic potential of children creates some additional challenges in the management of NOE fractures. First, accurate repositioning of small bony fragments in this region can be impaired by early bony healing; as such, these fractures need to be treated earlier in children than in adults. Second, elevation of the periosteum in this region often leads to additional bone deposition in the area, which can negatively affect the esthetic result in this region. Otherwise, elevation and reduction of the fragments proceed in the same fashion as for the adult patient. It is necessary to identify the status of the medial canthal tendon accurately (Fig. 88.4A).

Continued

TECHNIQUE: Naso-Orbito-Ethmoid Fractures—cont'd

STEP 3: Open Reduction and Internal Fixation

The NOE fracture classification of the central fragment and the status of the medial canthal tendon dictate the methods of fracture repair, as in the adult patient. Traditional techniques may be used, such as transnasal wiring, canthal barbs, or the use of plates and screws. Because growth in this region is mostly complete by age 7, titanium fixation devices can be used after that age. This is an advantage because titanium devices are the lowest profile hardware options available for use in this region, where the skin is also quite thin. The thinner skeleton of the pediatric patient may also lead to a greater degree of comminution in this region, to the point that adequate nasal dorsal projection cannot be achieved with simple fracture reduction and fixation. In these instances, the surgeon should not hesitate to graft the dorsum with either calvarial bone or rib. The former is generally preferred because it is predictable and avoids an additional wound for the donor site. The flat portion of the parietal bone is the ideal place for this graft to be harvested because it best mimics the natural nasal dorsum. If a craniotomy has been performed for a transcranial injury, this bone is easily harvested in full-thickness fashion and then split so that half becomes graft and the other half restores the calvarial contour (Fig. 88.4B–E).

STEP 4: Wound Closure

Wound closure of the incisions proceeds in a routine fashion, as in the adult. However, wherever possible, consideration should be given to the use of resorbable suture material. The lateral canthus is resuspended if a cantholysis was performed. A forced duction, to document globe mobility, should be performed at the end of the procedure.

A hematoma under a coronal flap may either ossify or may serve as substrate for a postoperative infection This can be prevented with meticulous attention to hemostasis and by supporting the soft tissues in the region with external wraps, drains, and/or splints.

ALTERNATIVE TECHNIQUE: Nasal Fractures

Nasal fractures are among the more common midfacial fractures in children. They are managed according to the same pragmatic guidelines applied to adults. Correction is undertaken for unsatisfactory cosmetic appearance and for nasal airway obstruction. Surgeons must be extra vigilant to detect nasal septal hematomas. These must be drained and bolstered because injury to the septal complex may be related to the development of midfacial hypoplasia. The approaches used for the management of nasal and septal fractures in children are identical to those used in adults.

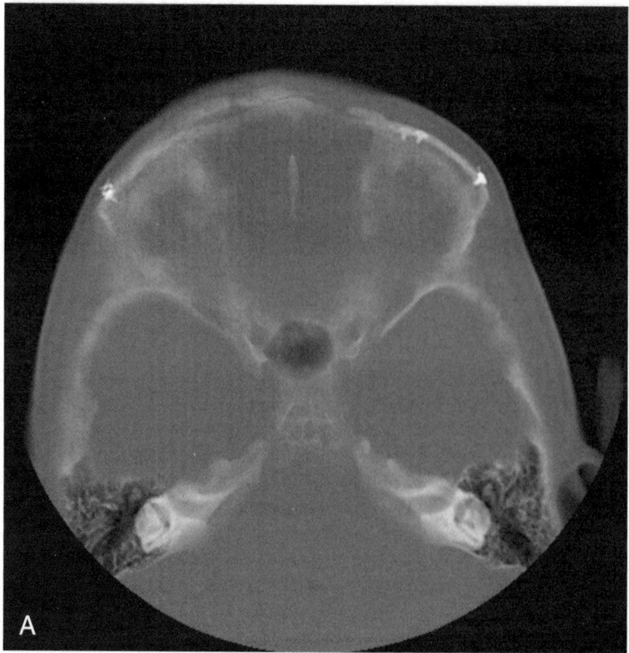

Figure 88.4 **A,** Axial computed tomography (CT) images several months after open reduction and internal fixation of an NOE fracture. Images demonstrate the deposition of additional bone on the surface of the calvarium.

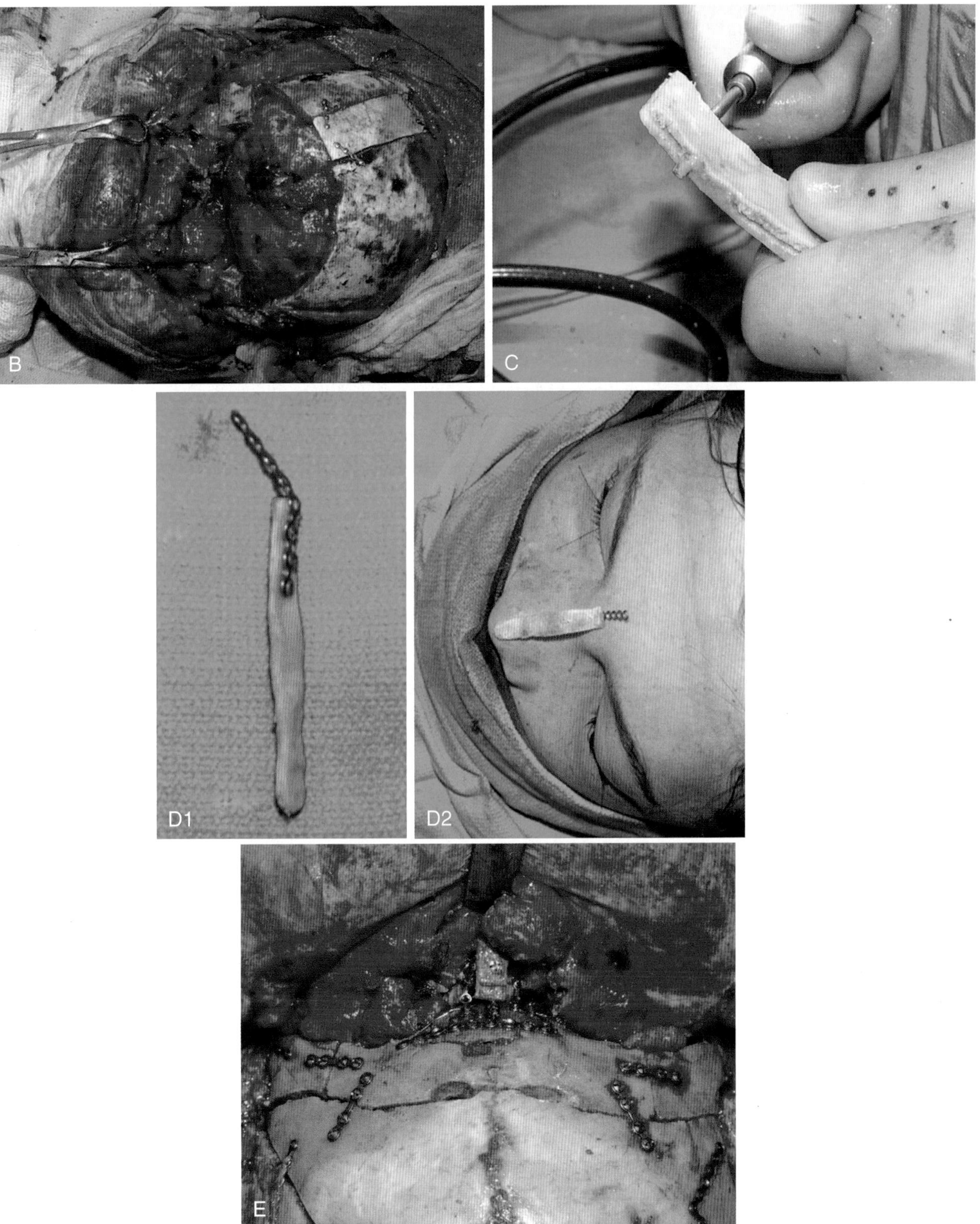

Figure 88.4, cont'd **B,** Site of harvest of calvarial bone in the right parietal bone for nasal dorsal onlay graft. The contour of the calvarium in this region is fairly straight, providing the desired shape of bone graft. **C,** Splitting of full-thickness calvarial graft to create dorsal onlay graft. **D1** and **D2,** Dorsal onlay graft prepared for insertion through the coronal approach. **E,** Graft inserted.

Avoidance and Management of Intraoperative Complications

Scant data are available that suggest that a retained rigid fixation device restricts facial growth.[10] The primary concern, therefore, is migration. This is a phenomenon in which surface apposition of bone leads to internal migration of the hardware and possibly impingement on a vital structure, such as a tooth bud. The likelihood of this occurring depends on the presence of a vital structure and the amount of remaining growth. Where a fracture involves a facial bone that is finished growing, it is difficult to justify the use of an inferior material for fracture fixation when the existing gold standard has such a good track record. The information provided in Table 88.1 can aid decision making about the appropriate use of resorbable fixation in midface trauma. Fixation of a periorbital, zygoma, or NOE fracture in a child under the age of 7 is a reasonable indication for the use of resorbable devices. In such situations use of titanium devices is also acceptable; these are lower in profile, and a plan is devised for their removal after healing is complete. Maxillary fractures require extra consideration because the maxilla in the primary and mixed dentition stages consists of thin bone covering multiple tooth buds. Regardless of the age of the patient, placement of fixation devices can be difficult in the infrastructure maxilla because the canine/piriform buttress is occupied by the permanent canine tooth bud, and the zygomatic buttress is occupied by the second molar bud. Once these teeth have erupted, the maxilla is treated as in an adult, with typical treatment protocols and fixation devices. In practice, it has been the author's experience that trauma cases that require resorbable fixation are rare.

Postoperative Considerations

Unlike adults, children are not tolerant of inappropriate fluid and drug administration. Care must be exercised in postoperative management to ensure that fluids and drugs are given in weight-based doses. In addition, the complication of hypovolemia is often underrecognized until late clinical findings are noted. In the young child or infant, the entire circulating blood volume can be lost through a coronal incision. Blood replacement for young children must be considered for the appropriate indications and should be initiated before complications arise. Significant attention must also be paid to nutritional status. When oral intake consistency is to be limited or if feeding takes place by gastrostomy tube in the young child postoperatively, the assistance of a registered dietitian can be helpful in maintaining the caloric intake necessary to achieve wound healing and prevent failure to thrive.

The late effects of midface trauma were covered earlier in the chapter. However, two particular issues of significance must be followed carefully in children with cranial/skull base or orbital injury. First, growing skull fracture is a particular phenomenon noted in young children in which herniation of the leptomeninges occurs through a skull or skull base fracture. This is thought to be secondary to a dural tear and rapid brain growth with pulsation. Second, the development of visual disturbance (i.e., diplopia) secondary to orbital trauma is a great concern in children. If resolution does not occur expediently after fracture repair, referral to a pediatric ophthalmologist is indicated. Midface injuries in children are uncommon and have many unique features and management considerations. Properly considered, these injuries can be well managed and good results can be expected.

References

1. Imahara SD, Hopper RA, Wang J, Rivara FP, Klein MB. Patterns and outcomes of pediatric facial fractures in the United States: a survey of the National Trauma Data Bank. *J Am Coll Surg*. 2008;207(5):710–716.
2. Aizenbud D, Morrill LR, Schendel SA. Midfacial trauma and facial growth: a longitudinal case study of monozygotic twins. *Am J Orthod Dentofacial Orthop*. 2010;138(5):641–648.
3. Grymer LF, Bosch C. The nasal septum and the development of the midface. A longitudinal study of a pair of monozygotic twins. *Rhinology*. 1997;35(1):6–10.
4. Zimmermann CE, Troulis MJ, Kaban LB. Pediatric facial fractures: recent advances in prevention, diagnosis and management. *Int J Oral Maxillofac Implants*. 2005;34(8):823–833.
5. Koltai PJ, Amjad I, Meyer D, Feustel PJ. Orbital fractures in children. *Arch Otolaryngol Head Neck Surg*. 1995;121(12):1375–1379.
6. Siy RW, Brown RH, Koshy JC, Stal S, Hollier LH Jr. General management considerations in pediatric facial fractures. *J Craniofac Surg*. 2011;22(4):1190–1195.
7. Posnick JC, Wells M, Pron GE. Pediatric facial fractures: evolving patterns of treatment. *J Oral Maxillofac Surg*. 1993;51(8):836–844.
8. Grunwaldt L, Smith DM, Zuckerbraun NS, et al. Pediatric facial fractures: demographics, injury patterns, and associated injuries in 772 consecutive patients. *Plast Reconstr Surg*. 2011;128(6):1263–1271.
9. Bansagi ZC, Meyer DR. Internal orbital fractures in the pediatric age group: characterization and management. *Ophthalmology*. 2000;107(5):829–836.
10. Dorri M, Nasser M, Oliver R. Resorbable versus titanium plates for facial fractures. *Cochrane Database Syst Rev*. 2009;21(1):CD007158.

CHAPTER 89

Management of Frontal Sinus Fractures

David A. Bitonti

Armamentarium

#9 Periosteal elevator
#10 and #15 Scalpel blades
#701 Bur
Appropriate sutures
Austin retractor
Bipolar electrocautery
Carroll–Girard screws
Channel retractor
Curved Mayo scissors
Curved tenotomy scissors
Diamond bur
Double-pronged skin hooks
Preferred endoscope
Fixation devices (plates and screws)
Hair elastics
Local anesthetic with vasoconstrictor
Malleable retractors
Mallet
Mayfield headrest
Molt curettes
Needle electrocautery
Obwegeser retractors
Outflow tract sealing material
Pear-shaped bur
Raney clips
Rotary handpiece
Round bur
Seldin retractor
Sinus obliteration material
Spatula osteotome
Sterile liquid for outflow tract evaluation
Suture skin staples

History of the Procedure

Frontal sinus fractures present a unique challenge in the management and treatment of craniomaxillofacial trauma. The earliest reports of frontal sinus fracture management involved the complete removal of the anterior table and, if involved, the posterior table. The forehead skin was then allowed to collapse down on to the posterior table if it remained, or it collapsed on to the dura if both tables had been removed. Although this effectively sealed the nasal cavity from the frontal sinus, it resulted in undesirable aesthetics and contour deformities. Modifications of this ablative procedure followed as surgeons attempted to improve cosmetic outcomes. In the 1950s, Bergara and Bergara described an approach that required an osteoplastic flap.[1] Their technique involved creating a window into the frontal sinus through the anterior table, which was hinged off an inferiorly based pericranial pedicle flap. After visualizing and removing damaged elements of the sinus, the bone flap was replaced, restoring forehead contour. Goodale and Montgomery later popularized the addition of frontal sinus obliteration with autologous fat,[2] thereby eliminating the functional sinus unit. In 1978, Donald and Bernstein described the cranialization procedure.[3] They advocated complete removal of the posterior sinus table and ablation of the sinus in cases involving significant comminution or displacement of the posterior table with a persistent cerebrospinal fluid (CSF) leak. Authors have emphasized the condition of the nasofrontal outflow tracts (NFOTs) as a major factor in management algorithms,[4–6] more recently, with consideration of observation as the treatment of choice.[7] Regardless of the treatment modality, the goal of frontal sinus fracture management continues to revolve around the restoration of the anterior table form, NFOT function, integrity of the posterior table, and prevention of complications.

Indications for the Use of the Procedure

Frontal sinus fractures rarely occur in isolation. Approximately 70% are associated with other maxillofacial injuries.[8] With motor vehicle accidents as the most common mechanism of injury, initial evaluation of the patient with a suspected frontal sinus fracture follows an advanced trauma life support protocol, and life-threatening injuries are addressed first. Patients with multisystem injuries and head trauma are often intubated and sedated. In these cases, a detailed history of the mechanism of injury and incident scene must be obtained from law enforcement officials and emergency medical services personnel, and the past medical history is contributed by the family of the patient. In one series, only 24% of patients were conscious, 42% were comatose, and 52%

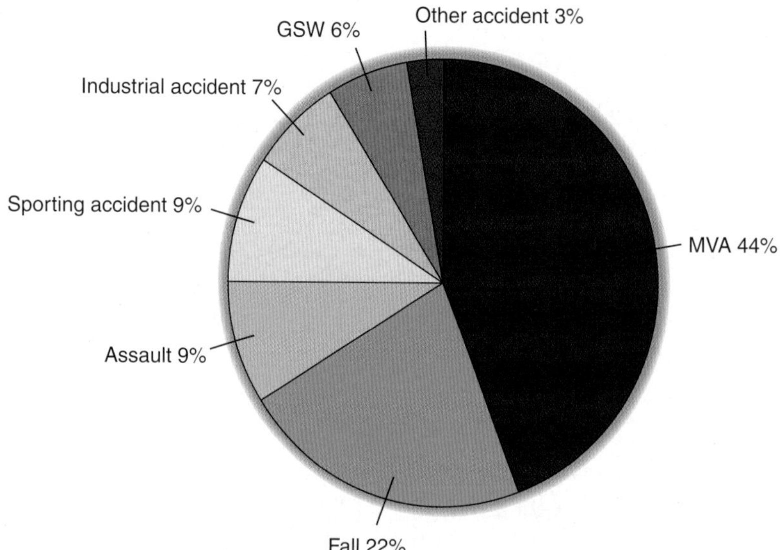

Figure 89.1 Mechanism of frontal sinus injuries. *GSW*, Gunshot wound; *MVA*, motor vehicle accident. (Data from Bell RB, Dierks EJ, Brar P, Potter JK, Potter BE. A protocol for the management of frontal sinus fractures emphasizing sinus preservation. *J Oral Maxillofac Surg*. 2007;65(5):825–839.)

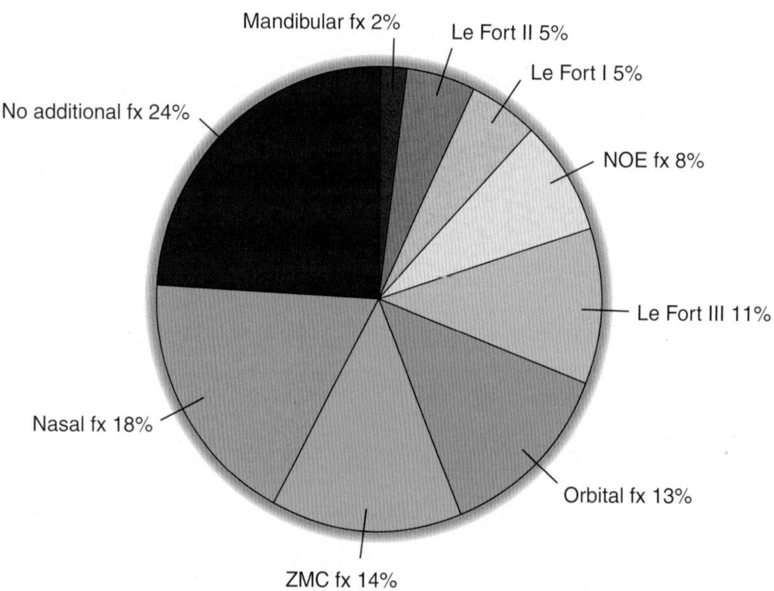

Figure 89.2 Concomitant maxillofacial fractures found with frontal sinus injury. *NOE*, Naso-orbito-ethmoid. (Data from Bell RB, Dierks EJ, Brar P, Potter JK, Potter BE. A protocol for the management of frontal sinus fractures emphasizing sinus preservation. *J Oral Maxillofac Surg*. 2007;65(5):825–839.)

had accompanying shock. A range of 800 to 2200 pounds of force is required to cause a frontal sinus fracture.[9] Bell and colleagues summarized the mechanism of injury and concomitant injuries found with frontal sinus fractures (Figs. 89.1 and 89.2).[10] Isolated anterior table injuries account for 43% to 61% of frontal sinus injuries, 0.6% to 6% are isolated posterior table injuries, and 19% to 51% have combined anterior and posterior table injuries.[11] Between 2.5% and 21% of frontal sinus injuries involve the NFOT.[11] Associated intracranial injuries range from 31% to 76%, and approximately 21% present with an associated ophthalmologic injury (Table 89.1).[10,12] As a testament to the significant force necessary to fracture the frontal sinus, following initial stabilization and subsequent frontal sinus fracture treatment, 25% of the patients succumbed due to concomitant injuries within 2 weeks of their initial surgery.

Evaluation and Diagnosis

When evaluating frontal sinus trauma, specific attention must be paid to potential intracranial injury. Specific clinical findings may include a palpable bony step, a contour deformity, crepitus, and mobility of bone segments. If the patient is conscious, discovery of a paresthesia or anesthesia of the

Table 89.1 Concomitant Injuries in Frontal Sinus Fractures

Injury	NFOT Uninjured	NFOT Injured
Orbital roof	13%	40%
Orbital wall	7%	13%
Orbital floor	2%	7%
NOE	12%	31%
Zygoma	8%	18%
Le Fort	2%	17%
Mandible	3%	5%
Intercranial	31%	76%
Cervical spine	7%	14%
Upper extremity fracture	15%	25%
Lower extremity fracture	13%	23%
Pneumothorax	12%	24%
Abdominal	7%	13%

NFOT, Nasofrontal outflow tract; *NOE*, naso-orbito-ethmoid.
From Stanwix MG, Nam AJ, Manson PN, Mirvis S, Rodriguez ED. Critical computed tomographic diagnostic criteria for frontal sinus fractures. *J Oral Maxillofac Surg.* 2010;68(11):2714–2722.

forehead and scalp may be present due to injury of the supraorbital nerves. Close attention should also be paid to the naso-orbito-ethmoid region for injuries that may contribute to sinus outflow tract dysfunction or obstruction. Rhinorrhea or otorrhea, when present, can have multiple causes and may indicate a CSF leak. The "halo" test can be used as a screening tool to detect the presence of CSF. When the fluid is placed on a piece of filter paper, gauze, or linen, a ring of clear CSF will surround a central component of blood. This is due to the differing diffusion rates of blood and CSF. Alternatively, the fluid can be tested for glucose and chloride in an attempt to differentiate among CSF, serum, and nasal secretions. In comparison to blood/serum and nasal secretions, CSF has a higher concentration of glucose and a lower concentration of chloride. This method has a low sensitivity and specificity for accuracy, so false-positive results lead to inconsistency in distinguishing among CSF, blood/serum, and nasal secretions. The most accurate confirmation of CSF is made by testing the fluid for β-2 transferrin. This laboratory test can take up to 4 days to process; therefore, it should not cause an unwanted delay in fracture diagnosis and treatment.[11] Reports exist of the presence of β-2 transferrin in aqueous humor[13] and the serum of patients with alcohol-related chronic liver disease.[14] This possibility must be considered, especially in cases of maxillofacial trauma and in the patient with a ruptured globe.

Ultrasound may be used as a screening tool when evaluating for frontal sinus fractures. It is most useful for visualization of the zygomatic arch and the anterior table of the frontal sinus. If a fracture is suspected following ultrasound screening, further imaging is indicated. Imaging via computed tomography (CT) in axial, coronal, and sagittal planes has revolutionized the diagnosis and management of frontal sinus injuries (Fig. 89.3). Whenever a frontal sinus injury is suspected, a high-resolution noncontrast CT scan with 1- to 1.5-mm cuts should be performed.[11] Axial slices will best evaluate the anterior and posterior tables of the sinus. The location of the fractures, amount of displacement, and degree of comminution are readily seen in this plane. Coronal slices are useful for evaluating the sinus floor, orbital roof, and anterior ethmoid cells, whereas sagittal slices provide valuable information about the NFOT. NFOT obstruction has been incorporated into several of the current treatment algorithms for fontal sinus injury.[4–6,7,11] NFOT injury or obstruction is typically assessed intraoperatively under direct visualization, with or without the use of a sterile colored fluid introduced into the NFOT system. Recently, the use of the endoscope and direct visualization of the NFOT has become more popular. It is suggested that it allows for the most accurate assessment of the actual functionality of the NFOT when compared with previously mentioned methods.[15–19] However, some authors have correlated CT evidence of NFOT injury findings directly into their treatment algorithm. Stanwix and coworkers[12] defined NFOT injury using at least one of the following criteria found on CT: fracture of the sinus floor, fracture of the medial aspect of the anterior table (anterior ethmoid cells), or outflow tract/duct obstruction (Fig. 89.4). Obstruction is defined as a segment of fractured bone lying partially or entirely within the outflow tract.

Limitations and Contraindications

The anatomic proximity of the frontal sinus to the brain, orbit, ethmoid sinus, and nasal cavity increases the potential morbidity and treatment complexity associated with treatment and repair of these injuries. Mismanagement, delayed treatment, or insufficient long-term follow-up can lead to serious, life-threatening complications including meningitis, mucocele pyocele, mucopyocele, pneumocephalus, vision changes, facial pressure, paresthesia, and brain abscess.[4,20–22] To date, there is no consensus on a single management algorithm.[4–6] This is largely due to the lack of prospective randomized clinical trials addressing different treatment modalities, which are neither feasible nor ethical.[11] Since the early 1900s, and despite the lack of consensus, there have been major advances in the treatment of frontal sinus injuries.

Classification schemes are helpful in that they offer a way to describe the specific characteristics of individual frontal sinus injuries. They are limited, however, in their ability to guide management and predict outcomes. Several authors have suggested specific treatment algorithms based on the classification or location of the fracture (anterior table, posterior table, combination anterior and posterior table), the degree of bone displacement, the presence of NFOT obstruction, and damage to intracranial structures (Figs. 89.5 and 89.6). A 2010 study analyzed data from 1907 cases and determined that NFOT involvement was critical to surgical management.[12] The authors did not find

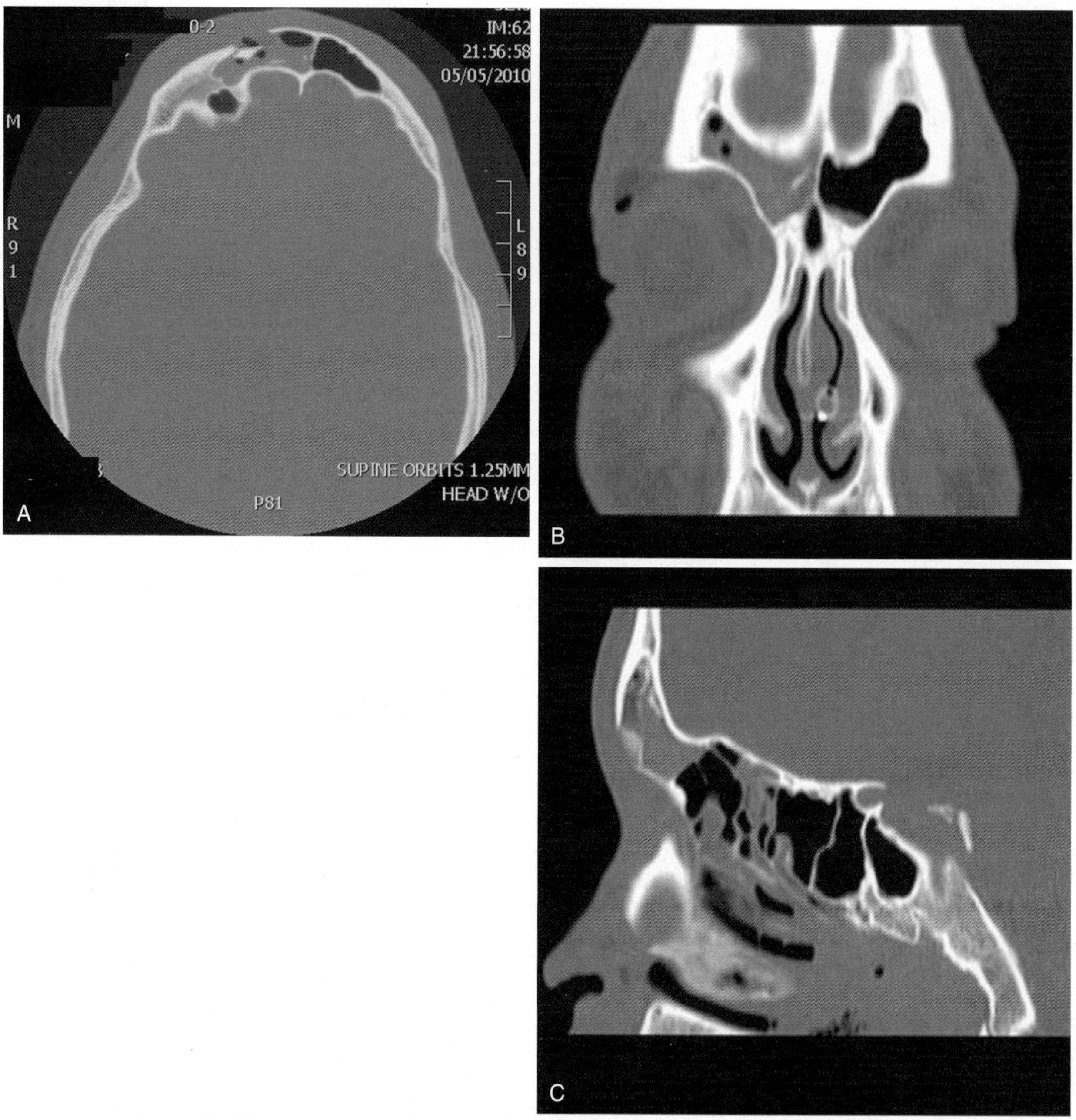

Figure 89.3 CT scan of patient with fracture of right anterior table of frontal sinus. **A,** Axial view. **B,** Coronal view. **C,** Sagittal view.

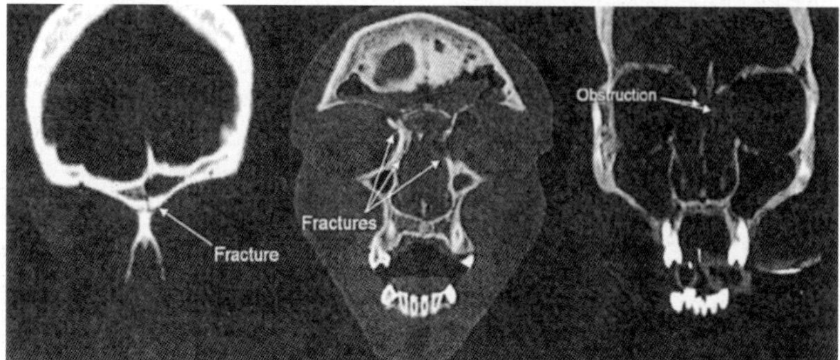

Figure 89.4 Computed tomography evaluation of the nasofrontal outflow tract. (From Stanwix MG, Nam AJ, Manson PN, Mirvis S, Rodriguez ED. Critical computed tomographic diagnostic criteria for frontal sinus fractures. *J Oral Maxillofac Surg*. 2010;68(11):2714–2722.)

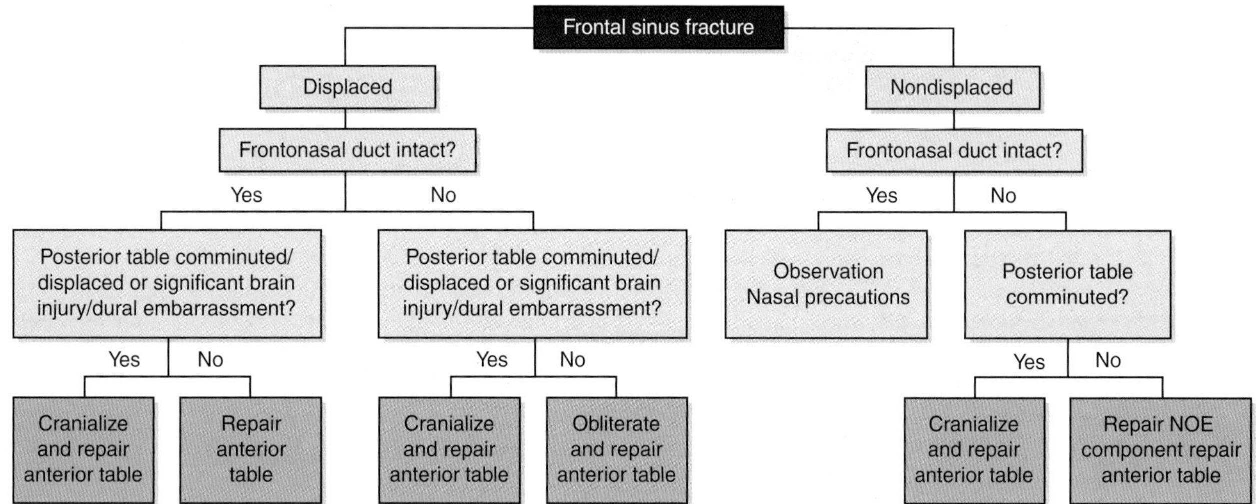

Figure 89.5 Algorithm for repair of frontal sinus fractures. *NOE*, Naso-orbito-ethmoid. (Data from Bell RB, Dierks EJ, Brar P, Potter JK, Potter BE. A protocol for the management of frontal sinus fractures emphasizing sinus preservation. *J Oral Maxillofac Surg*. 2007;65(5):825–839.)

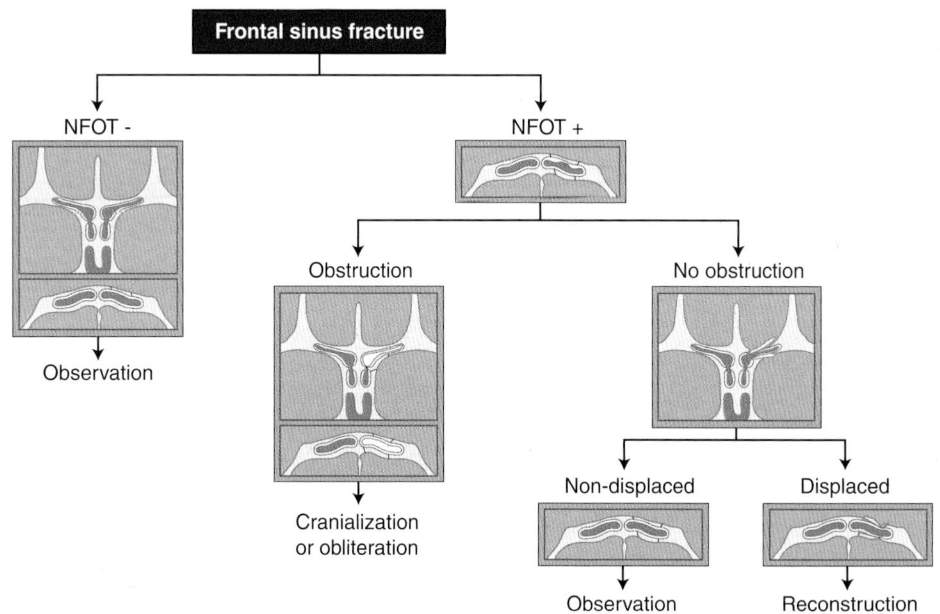

Figure 89.6 Frontal sinus fracture treatment algorithm. *NFOT*, Nasofrontal outflow tract. (Data from Stanwix MG, Nam AJ, Manson PN, Mirvis S, Rodriguez ED. Critical computed tomographic diagnostic criteria for frontal sinus fractures. *J Oral Maxillofac Surg*. 2010;68(11):2714–2722.)

other commonly used criteria for initiation and degree of surgical intervention (CSF leak, posterior table involvement, fracture comminution) to be statistically relevant or clinically powerful enough to play a role in their treatment algorithm. It must be noted that definitive proof of the superiority of one algorithm over another is lacking, and these algorithms are based primarily on clinical judgment, surgical experience, knowledge of sinus pathophysiology, and postsurgical complication potential. The fact remains that the literature lacks long-term data, and debate continues on this subject. The advent of and proficiency with minimally invasive surgery has also infused additional considerations and treatment options relative to frontal sinus injury. Ultimately, treatment should be performed based on the patient's clinical presentation, radiographic diagnosis, and complication potential if no intervention is rendered. Decisions on treatment modalities—endoscopic repair, open repair, obliteration material, technique, and plating system—are still largely based on surgical experience and provider preference.

TECHNIQUE: Anterior Table Reconstruction and Cranialization

Current literature describes many classification schemes based on fracture pattern and affected structures.[4,9–11,23,24] Classification may be as simple as differentiating two types of injuries based on skull base involvement or as detailed as the five types of injuries based on involvement of the anterior wall, posterior wall, naso-orbito-ethmoid (NOE) complex, orbital rim, dural injury or CSF leak, tissue or bone loss, and extent of displacement.[5,9,25,26] A useful classification based on anatomic location and fracture pattern has been described by Gonty and colleagues[23]:

Type I: Anterior table fracture
- a. Isolated to anterior table
- b. Accompanied by supraorbital rim fracture
- c. Accompanied by nasoethmoidal complex fracture

Type II: Combination anterior and posterior table fracture
- a. Linear fractures
  1. Transverse
  2. Vertical
- b. Comminuted fractures
  1. Involving both tables
  2. Accompanied by NOE fracture

Type III: Posterior table fracture

Type IV: Through and through frontal sinus fracture

In addition to addressing frontal sinus injuries in the pediatric population, there are other considerations relative to patient age, sinus development, nasal frontal outflow tract development, risks for complication, and others, which may lend itself to a more aggressive treatment.[27]

The primary goal of frontal sinus fracture management is to restore form and function while minimizing morbidity and complications. Management can be divided into two main categories: nonoperative observation and surgical intervention. Surgical management of frontal sinus fractures is reserved for cases involving a greater degree of bone displacement or damage to the NFOT. Cases involving a significant frontobasilar injury with a persistent CSF leak, or comminuted fractures of the region surrounding the NFOTs, are of particular concern.[8] Surgical management may involve one or more of the following:

- Anterior table reconstruction
- NFOT management
- Sinus obliteration
- Cranialization

STEP 1: Intubation

Orotracheal intubation with a reinforced tube is preferred; if traumatic injuries preclude this method or endoscopic surgery is not planned, nasoendotracheal intubation can be performed. The patient's accompanying injuries should be considered during this stage. The tube is secured in place with either tape, wire, or suture depending upon location, technique, and associated anatomy.

STEP 2: Incision

Surgical access can be achieved in several ways. The most common approach is with the use of the coronal flap. This provides excellent exposure of the frontal bone and NOE region. It also allows for a pericranial flap to be developed, if needed, and split-thickness calvarium bone graft to be harvested if necessary. Balding patients or those with a receding hairline should have the incision placed more posterior to avoid a noticeable scar. Existing lacerations may also be used, if broad enough, or they may be extended to accomplish sufficient exposure. The upper eyelid blepharoplasty, suprabrow, and endoscopic brow lift approaches have also been used.[28–32] Other options include the direct, open-sky, and gullwing approaches. These approaches are generally avoided to prevent unsightly scars (Fig. 89.7A).

STEP 3: Anterior Table Reconstruction

Displaced anterior table fractures without the involvement of the NFOT can be anatomically reduced and fixated with titanium mesh, titanium plates, or resorbable plates and the associated appropriate screws. Although no consensus exists, removal of the sinus membrane and obliteration of the sinus are not thought to be necessary in these cases.[4–6,10–12,23] Anatomic reduction of anterior table fractures prevents contour deformities that are unacceptable to the patient. Simple methods of fracture reduction include utilizing the end of a periosteal elevator or a Carroll–Girard screw to elevate the segments. If a bone segment has been lost, autogenous bone grafts can be used as necessary (Fig. 89.7B).

STEP 4: Cranialization

Frontal sinus fractures involving significant displacement or comminution of the posterior table often require cranialization to prevent devastating complications such as meningitis and mucoceles, pyoceles, and mucopyoceles.[4–6,10–12,20–23] Any injury where a suspicion of intracranial involvement is present warrants neurosurgical consultation. If there is a significant frontobasilar injury with a persistent CSF leak, exploration of the cranial base and dural repair are likely necessary. Cranialization is typically carried out after a neurosurgeon performs a bifrontal craniotomy. With the dura retracted and protected, the posterior table is removed with a rotary or hand instruments. The sinus mucosa is then removed, the nasofrontal duct is occluded, and a pericranial flap is utilized to separate the aerodigestive tract from the intracranial cavity. Finally, the anterior table is reconstructed as described earlier (Fig. 89.7C and D).

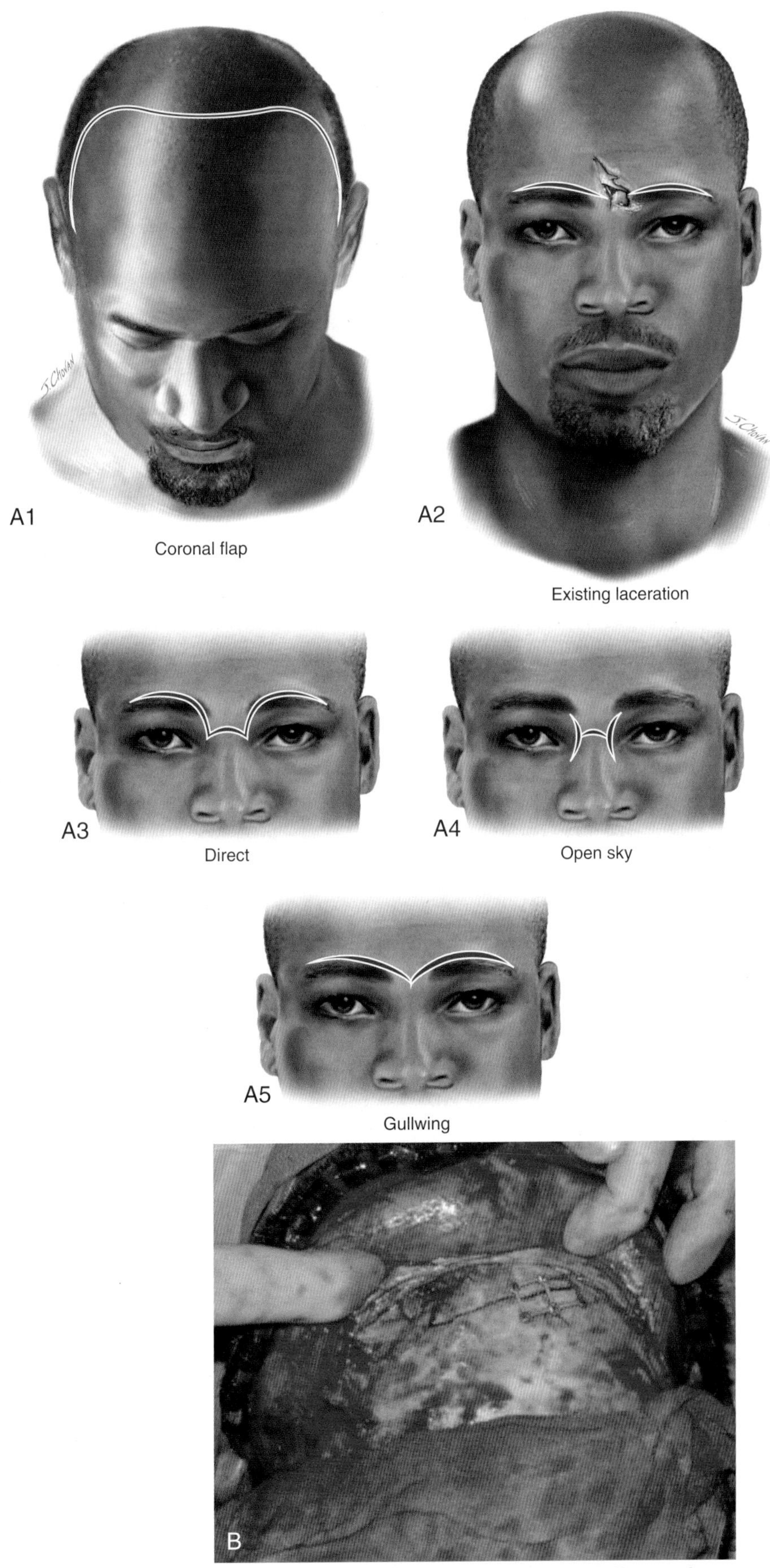

Figure 89.7 **A1–A5,** Surgical access and incision to the nasofrontal region. **B,** Repair of anterior table of frontal sinus.

Continued

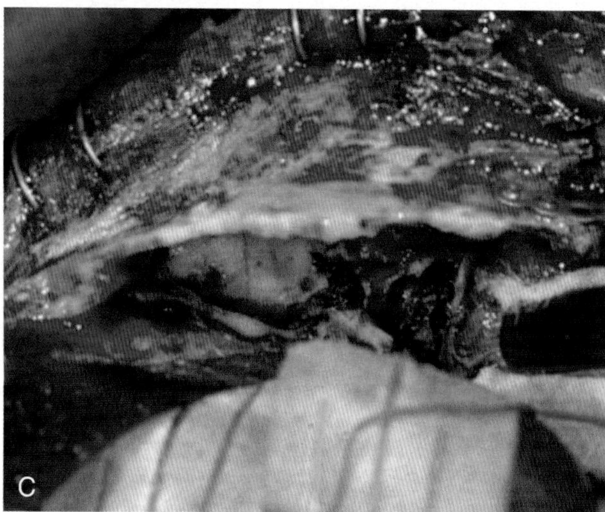

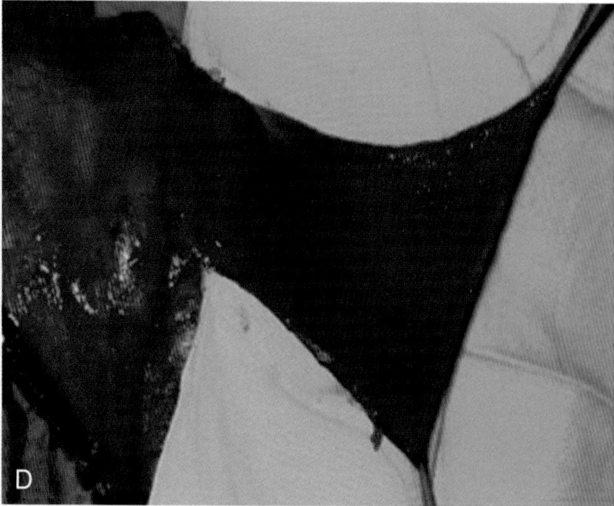

Figure 89.7, cont'd **C,** Cranialization of the frontal sinus. **D,** Pericranial flap. (B and C From Gentile MA, Tellington AJ, Burke WJ, Jaskolka MS. Management of midface maxillofacial trauma. *Atlas Oral Maxillofac Surg Clin North Am.* 2013;21(1):69–95.)

TECHNIQUE: Anterior Table Reconstruction and Cranialization—*cont'd*

STEP 5: Closure of Scalp

Following completion of surgery, thorough irrigation of the surgical sites is performed. The scalp is closed in layers. At a minimum, the galea aponeurotica and skin should be closed. The author prefers suturing the galea with 3-0 polyglycolate. The skin is then closed with 4-0 fast-resorbing polyglycolate or staples.

ALTERNATIVE TECHNIQUE 1: Obliteration

When there is damage to the nasofrontal and NOE region, an attempt can be made to assess the patency of the nasofrontal duct from above. A colored sterile liquid is injected into the duct, and its presence in the nose inferior to the middle turbinate is assessed. If drainage is delayed, poor, or absent, sinus obliteration should be considered. Sinus obliteration involves the following (Fig. 89.8A):

- Complete removal of sinus mucosa
- Permanent occlusion of the NFOT
- Obliteration of dead space

After surgical access elevation of the soft tissue, the anterior table is elevated and removed. Prior to removal, a technique to maintain orientation of the segments is recommended. One such technique involves the utilization of a 1.0 titanium universal plate (Fig. 89.8B). The anterior table must be removed next. A convenient technique for defining the perimeter of the frontal sinus utilizes Cushing forceps and a 701 tapered fissure bur (Fig. 89.8C). The sinus perimeter is initially outlined with perforations (holes) utilizing the bur, and the perforations are then connected so that the anterior table can be removed. The sinus mucosa is then meticulously removed with curettes, rotary instruments, or both. The nasofrontal duct can then be occluded. A commonly used technique involves the use of fibrin glue and temporal fascia. A pedicled pericranial flap can also be used for this purpose. Finally, the sinus is obliterated utilizing a variety of filler materials. Common fillers include abdominal fat, temporalis muscle, autologous bone, and alloplastic cement materials such as hydroxyapatite, calcium phosphate, and glass ionomer.[5] The anterior table is then reconstructed as described earlier.

ALTERNATIVE TECHNIQUE 2: Endoscopic Approaches

In addition to the open technique, endoscopic approaches are gaining popularity with many surgeons.[5,33,34] Defects of the anterior table, medial orbital wall, orbital floor, and frontal sinus posterior table may be addressed with the endoscope.[35,32,36] This technique is the preferred method for patients with a receding hairline or balding, as two to three conservative incisions of 3 cm in length may be needed to accommodate the endoscope ports. Fractures of the orbital floor, medial orbital wall, or frontal sinus posterior table are accessible via transantral and transnasal approaches, which

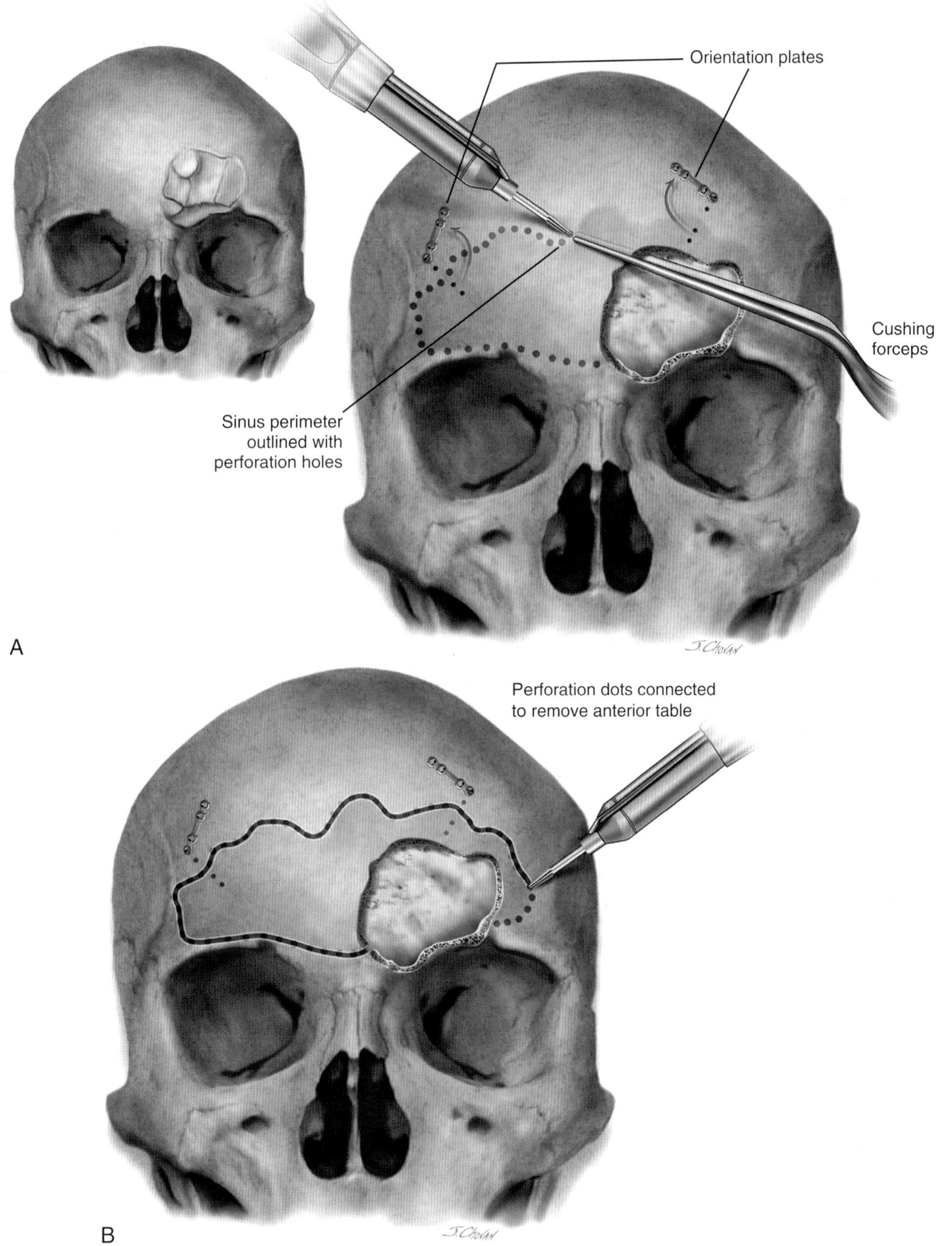

Figure 89.8 **A,** Use of a fissure bur and Cushing forceps to outline the extent of the frontal sinus in the anterior table through perforation. **B,** Fissure bur used to connect perforations to allow for safe elevation of the anterior table over frontal sinus.

Continued

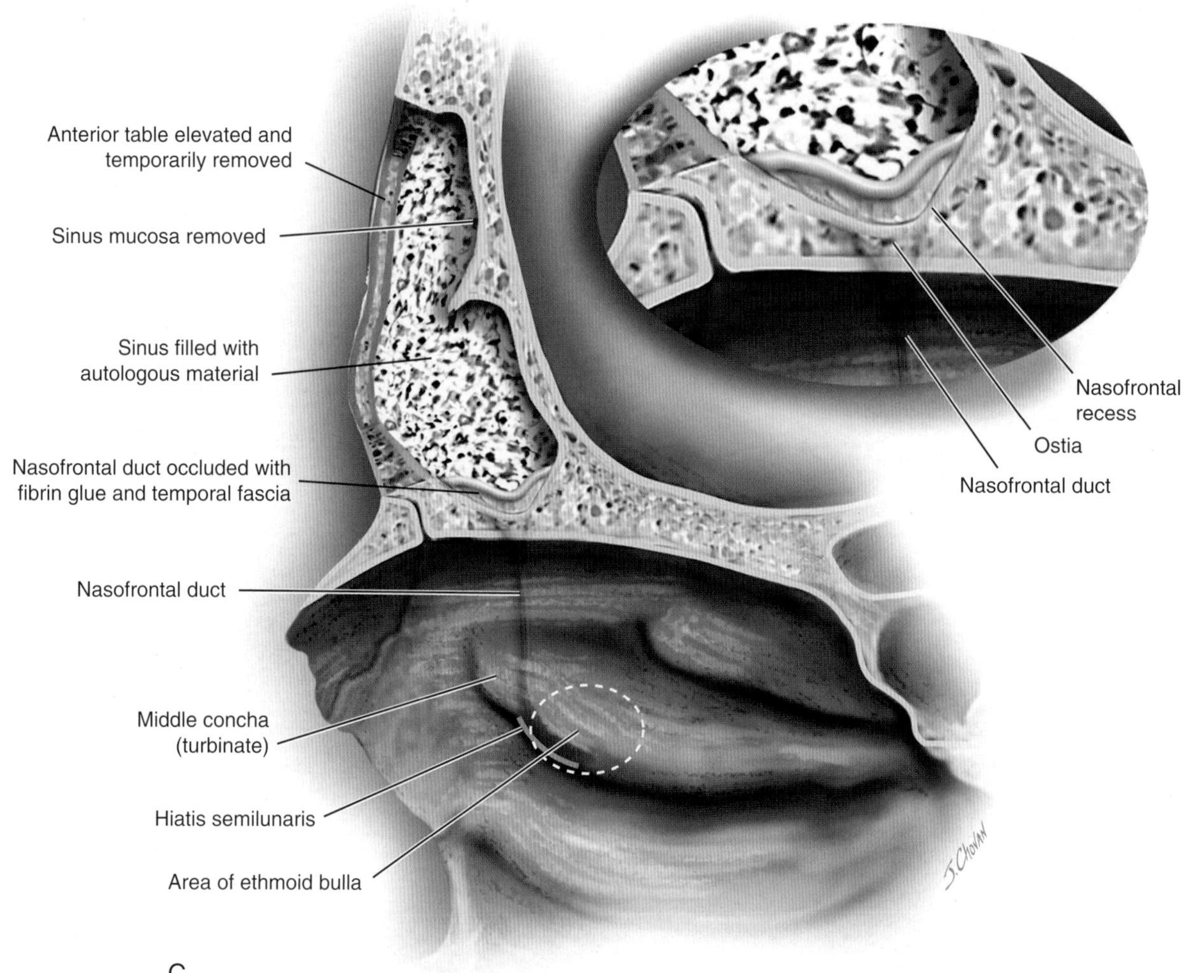

Figure 89.8, cont'd C, Frontal sinus filled with autologous bone after removal of mucosa and occlusion of the nasofrontal duct with temporal fascia.

do not require a single skin incision.[15–19,35] Alternatively, a transfacial type of incision may also be made. A prospective cohort study of 14 patients demonstrated treatment of frontal sinus posterior table fractures with Draf IIA, IIB, and III procedures to repair posterior table defects averaging 13 × 4.5 mm.[36] Typically, endoscopic management is case selective, being reserved for minimally displaced defects.[8] Compared with periodic imaging, the endoscopic technique also allows the practitioner to evaluate patients for mucocele formation utilizing further nasal endoscopy.[36] For more displaced fracture defects, other treatment approaches beyond endoscopy are necessary.

ALTERNATIVE TECHNIQUE 3: Nonoperative Observation

In general, most authors promote nonsurgical management in cases involving minimal displacement of the anterior and posterior tables with an intact NFOT.[4–6,10–12,23] One study included 154 patients and looked at anterior-posterior depth or displacement of the anterior table segment, measured from CT, and the resultant clinical soft tissue contour deformity to quantify parameters indicating the need for surgical intervention. No observable contour deformity was present with fracture depths of 4 mm or less. These patients were managed with observation only.[37] Another study following 857 patients for an average of 2.8 months demonstrated that NFOT obstruction played the most important role in complications (97%).[12] In this study, there was only one complication in a patient with NFOT injury who lacked outflow tract obstruction. Therefore, the authors recommend observation for frontal sinus fracture patients with intact NFOTs who lack intracranial injury and contour deformities. These patients should be followed at regular intervals for a long period of time, perhaps 10 years or more, to provide early detection of complications.[22]

Table 89.2 Effect of NFOT Injury and Type of Treatment Modality on Complication Rates

Treatment	NFOT	Number of Patients	Complications	Obstructed	Complication if Obstructed	Complications, Obstruction, and Other Criteria
Observation	–	222	0 (0%)			
	+	131	11 (8.4%)	16 (12%)	63%	100%
Reconstruction (sinus preserved)	–	15	1 (6.7%)			
	+	83	8 (9.6%)	11 (13%)	73%	100%
Osteoneogenesis	–	1	0 (0%)			
	+	21	9 (42.9%)	20 (95%)	45%	56%
Obliteration	–	7	0 (0%)			
	+	169	15 (8.9%)	164 (97%)	9%	10%
Cranialization	–	6	0 (0%)			
	+	202	17 (8.4%)	196 (97%)	9%	9%
NFOT	–	251	1 (0.4%)			
	+	606	60 (9.9%)	407 (67%)	14%	15%
Total		857	61 (7.1%)			

–, Absent; +, involved/injured; *NFOT*, nasofrontal outflow tract.

NOTE: There were 83 patients with NFOT injury treated by reconstruction, with 8 complications (9.6%). Eleven patients treated by reconstruction had a diagnosis of NFOT obstruction (13%). Of these patients with obstruction, 73% had a complication rate, and if a second criterion was used (anterior ethmoidal fracture or floor fracture), then there was a 100% complication rate. Thus, those with obstruction should not be treated by reconstruction (likewise for observation and osteoneogenesis).

From Stanwix MG, Nam AJ, Manson PN, Mirvis S, Rodriguez ED. Critical computed tomographic diagnostic criteria for frontal sinus fractures. *J Oral Maxillofac Surg.* 2010;68(11):2714–2722.

Avoidance and Management of Intraoperative Complications

Ideally, surgical correction of a frontal sinus fracture is to prevent complications from altered anatomy and restore function along with cosmesis. As stated previously, the literature supports anterior table reconstruction for depressed fractures larger than 4 mm to minimize contour changes of the skin that result in poor cosmesis.[38] Obliteration or cranialization of the frontal sinus in the presence of NFOT obstruction reduces the incidence of complications from 63% to 9% (Table 89.2).[12] However, surgical intervention comes with its own risks. Pseudoaneurysm of the superficial temporal artery, scarring, dehiscence, flap necrosis or loss, alopecia, scalp necrosis, facial nerve injury, decreased forehead sensation, and chronic pain are all related to the coronal incision and flap dissection.[37,39] Obliteration materials have also been linked to complications. Hydroxyapatite bone cement fails when in contact with blood, CSF, or other moist conditions, and removal of the degraded material can be challenging and problematic. Calcium phosphate bone cement is prone to degradation and chronic foreign body reaction when placed directly over dura. The long-term stability of glass ionomer is currently unknown.[5] The development of complications depends not only on the type of fracture pattern, anatomic structures involved, and surgical intervention performed, but also on the host flora at the site of injury. Altering drainage of the frontal sinus, or the typical flora at the site of injury, may promote sinusitis, mucocele, pyocele, or mucopyocele formation. A CSF leak in the area of sinus flora could lead to meningitis. Transnasal or transantral endoscopic treatment carries with it the inherent endoscopic risks, in addition to those listed above, including intracranial perforation.

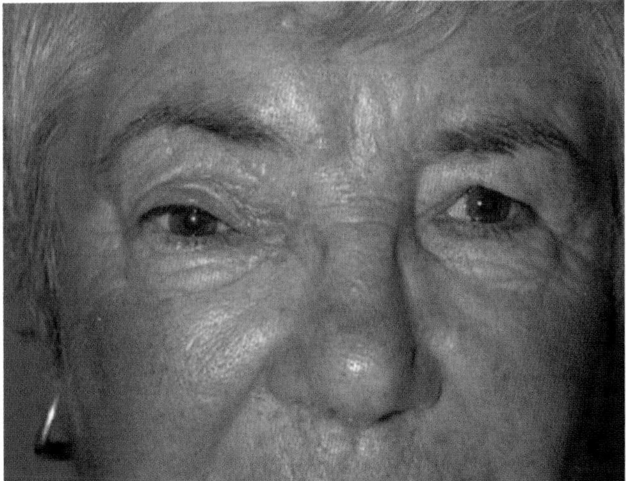

Figure 89.9 Clinical presentation of mucocele. (From Mourouzis C, Evans BT, Shenouda E. Late presentation of a mucocele of the frontal sinus: 50 years postinjury. *J Oral Maxillofac Surg.* 2008;66(7):1510–1513.)

Depending on the process of development, early complications may arise between 1 and 6 months following surgery, or late complications may arise greater than 6 months postsurgery.[4,10,40] Early complications include pain, headaches, CSF rhinorrhea, sinusitis, meningitis, brain abscess, osteomyelitis, residual aerodigestive communication, pneumocephalus, and contour irregularities. Late complications may include mucocele, pyocele, mucopyocele, osteomyelitis, and chronic pain (Figs. 89.9 and 89.10).

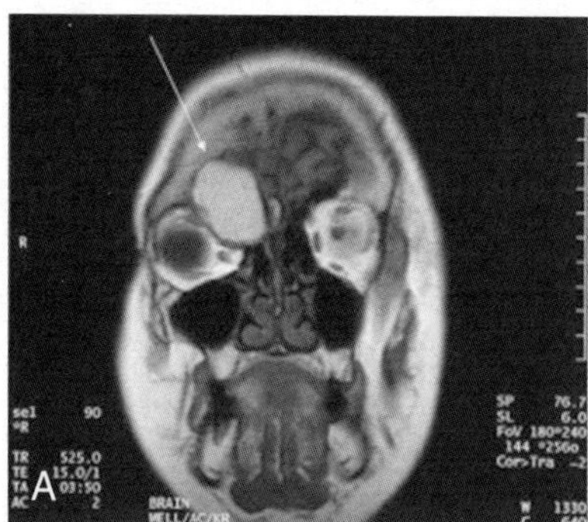
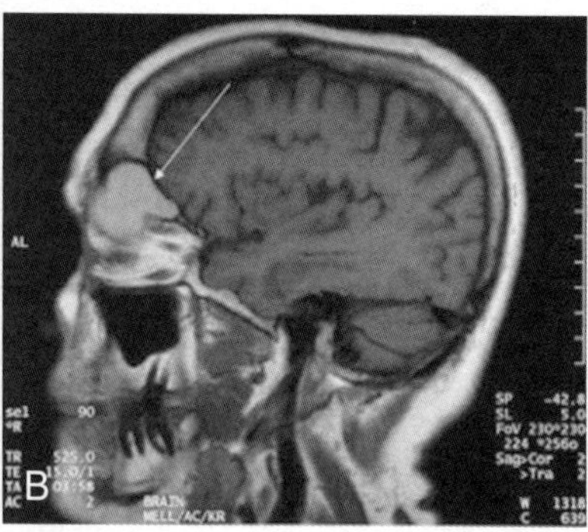

Figure 89.10 A and **B,** MRI presentation of mucocele in right frontal sinus. (From Mourouzis C, Evans BT, Shenouda E. Late presentation of a mucocele of the frontal sinus: 50 years postinjury. *J Oral Maxillofac Surg*. 2008;66(7):1510–1513.)

Postoperative Considerations

In the immediate postoperative period, a CT scan should be performed to evaluate the reconstruction and to acquire a baseline for comparison for future studies. Standard postoperative pain management techniques are used to control the patient's discomfort as necessary. Antibiotics should be used during the perioperative period to prevent infection. The use of additional antibiotics outside the perioperative time frame does not reduce the rate of postoperative infections; however, if the initial trauma created a contaminated wound, extending the antibiotic course for 7 to 14 days postoperatively is recommended.[41] Decongestants such as pseudoephedrine and oxymetazoline spray should be used judiciously in the postoperative period to maintain sinus patency for cases not involving occlusion of the NFOTs.

Long-term serial follow-up exams are critical for these patients due to the potential devastating late complications that can occur. The following strategy is recommended:

- Weekly up to 1 month
- Every 3 months up to 1 year
- Every year up to 5 years
- Every 5 years indefinitely

References

1. Bergara AR, Bergara C. Chronic frontoethmoidal sinusitis: osteoplastic method according to author's technique. *Ann Otorhinolaryngol*. 1955;5:192.
2. Goodale RL, Montgomery WW. Experiences with the osteoplastic anterior wall approach to the frontal sinus; case histories and recommendations. *AMA Arch Otolaryngol*. 1958;68(3):271–283.
3. Donald PJ, Bernstein L. Compound frontal sinus injuries with intracranial penetration. *Laryngoscope*. 1978;88(2 Pt 1):225–232.
4. Rohrich RJ, Hollier LH. Management of frontal sinus fractures. Changing concepts. *Clin Plast Surg*. 1992;19(1):219–232.
5. Bell RB. Management of frontal sinus fractures. *Oral Maxillofac Surg Clin North Am*. 2009;21(2):227–242.
6. Rodriguez ED, Stanwix MG, Nam AJ, et al. Twenty-six-year experience treating frontal sinus fractures: a novel algorithm based on anatomical fracture pattern and failure of conventional techniques. *Plast Reconstr Surg*. 2008;122(6):1850–1866.
7. Johnson NR, Roberts MJ. Frontal sinus fracture management: a systematic review and meta-analysis. *Int J Oral Maxillofac Implants*. 2021;50(1):75–82.
8. Gentile MA, Tellington AJ, Burke WJ, Jaskolka MS. Management of midface maxillofacial trauma. *Atlas Oral Maxillofac Surg Clin North Am*. 2013;21(1):69–95.
9. Doonquah L, Brown P, Mullings W. Management of frontal sinus fractures. *Oral Maxillofac Surg Clin North Am*. 2012;24(2):265–274, ix.
10. Bell RB, Dierks EJ, Brar P, Potter JK, Potter BE. A protocol for the management of frontal sinus fractures emphasizing sinus preservation. *J Oral Maxillofac Surg*. 2007;65(5):825–839.
11. Chuang SK, Dodson TB. Evaluation and management of frontal sinus injuries. In: Fonseca RJ, Walker R, Betts N, et al., eds. *Oral and Maxillofacial Trauma*. Vol 2. Philadelphia, PA: Saunders; 2004.
12. Stanwix MG, Nam AJ, Manson PN, Mirvis S, Rodriguez ED. Critical computed tomographic diagnostic criteria for frontal sinus fractures. *J Oral Maxillofac Surg*. 2010;68(11):2714–2722.
13. Tripathi RC, Millard CB, Tripathi BJ, Noronha A. Tau fraction of transferrin is present in human aqueous humor and is not unique to cerebrospinal fluid. *Exp Eye Res*. 1990;50(5):541–547.
14. Storey EL, Anderson GJ, Mack U, Powell LW, Halliday JW. Desialylated transferrin as a serological marker of chronic excessive alcohol ingestion. *Lancet*. 1987;1(8545):1292–1294.
15. Elkahwagi M, Eldegwi A. What is the role of the endoscope in the sinus preservation management of frontal sinus fractures. *J Oral Maxillofac Surg*. 2020;78(10):1811.e1–1811.e9.
16. Banks C, Grayson J, Cho DY, Woodworth BA. Frontal sinus fractures and cerebrospinal fluid leaks: a change in surgical paradigm. *Curr Opin Otolaryngol Head Neck Surg*. 2020;28(1):52–60.
17. Vincent A, Wang W, Shokri T, Gordon E, Inman JC, Ducic Y. Management of frontal sinus fractures. *Facial Plast Surg*. 2019;35(6):645–650.
18. Dedhia RD, Morisada MV, Tollefson TT, Strong EB. Contemporary management of frontal sinus fractures. *Curr Opin Otolaryngol Head Neck Surg*. 2019;27(4):253–260.
19. Ochs M, Chung W, Powers D. Trauma Surgery. *J Oral Maxillofac Surg*. 2017;75(8S):e151–e194.
20. Parish JM, Driscoll J, Wait SD, Gibbs M. Delayed traumatic tension pneumocephalus: A case report. *J Emerg Med*. 2020;59(6):e217–e220.

21. Firouzbakht PK, Mohiuddin IS, Varman RM, Heinrich MP, Saa L, Cordero J. Analysis of frontal sinus fracture management and resource utilization. *J Craniofac Surg.* 2020;31(8):2240–2242.
22. Jing XL, Luce E. Frontal sinus management and complications. *Craniomaxillofac Trauma Reconstr.* 2019;12(3):241–248.
23. Gonty AA, Marciani RD, Adornato DC. Management of frontal sinus fractures: a review of 33 cases. *J Oral Maxillofac Surg.* 1999;57(4):372–379.
24. Strong EB. Frontal sinus fractures: current concepts. *Craniomaxillofac Trauma Reconstr.* 2009;2(3):161–175.
25. Manolidis S. Frontal sinus injuries: associated injuries and surgical management of 93 patients. *J Oral Maxillofac Surg.* 2004;62(7):882–891.
26. Raveh J, Laedrach K, Vuillemin T, Zingg M. Management of combined frontonaso-orbital/skull base fractures and telecanthus in 355 cases. *Arch Otolaryngol Head Neck Surg.* 1992;118(6):605–614.
27. Lopez J, Pineault K, Pradeep T, et al. Pediatric frontal bone and sinus fractures: cause, characteristics, and a treatment algorithm. *Plast Reconstr Surg.* 2020;145(4):1012–1023.
28. Arnold MA, Tatum SA III. Frontal Sinus Fractures: evolving clinical considerations and surgical approaches. *Craniomaxillofac Trauma Reconstr.* 2019;12(2):85–94.
29. Kinzinger M, Steele TO, Chin O, Strong EB. Degree of frontal bone exposure via upper blepharoplasty incision: considerations for frontal sinus fracture. *Otolaryngol Head Neck Surg.* 2019;160(3):468–471.
30. Bourry M, Oliver C, Maalouf J, Corre P, Bertin H. Surgical approach of isolated fracture of the anterior wall of the frontal sinus: the upper eyelid incision. *J Stomatol Oral Maxillofac Surg.* 2019;120(3):240–243.
31. Hahn HM, Lee YJ, Park MC, Lee IJ, Kim SM, Park DH. Reduction of closed frontal sinus fractures through the suprabrow approach. *Arch Craniofac Surg.* 2017;18(4):230–237.
32. Fattahi T, Salman S. An aesthetic approach in the repair of anterior frontal sinus fractures. *Int J Oral Maxillofac Implants.* 2016;45(9):1104–1107.
33. Simmons O, Manson PN. Endoscopic management of orbital and frontal sinus fractures. *Craniomaxillofac Trauma Reconstr.* 2009;2(3):177–184.
34. Carter KB Jr, Poetker DM, Rhee JS. Sinus preservation management for frontal sinus fractures in the endoscopic sinus surgery era: a systematic review. *Craniomaxillofac Trauma Reconstr.* 2010;3(3):141–149.
35. Simmons O, Manson PN. Endoscopic management of orbital and frontal sinus fractures. *Craniomaxillofac Trauma Reconstr.* 2009;2(3):177–184.
36. Chaaban MR, Conger B, Riley KO, Woodworth BA. Transnasal endoscopic repair of posterior table fractures. *Otolaryngol Head Neck Surg.* 2012;147(6):1142–1147.
37. PD(1. Metzinger S, Metzinger R: complications of frontal sinus fractures. Craniomaxillofac Trauma Reconstr. 2009;2:27.
38. Kim DW, Yoon ES, Lee BI, Dhong ES, Park SH. Fracture depth and delayed contour deformity in frontal sinus anterior wall fracture. *J Craniofac Surg.* 2012;23(4):991–994.
39. Manzon S, Nguyen T, Philbert R. Bilateral pseudoaneurysms of the superficial temporal artery following reconstruction of the frontal sinus: a, case report. *J Oral Maxillofac Surg.* 2007;65(7):1375–1377.
40. Koudstaal MJ, van der Wal KG, Bijvoet HW, Vincent AJ, Poublon RM. Post-trauma mucocele formation in the frontal sinus; a rationale of follow-up. *Int J Oral Maxillofac Surg.* 2004;33(8):751–754.
41. Lauder A, Jalisi S, Spiegel J, Stram J, Devaiah A. Antibiotic prophylaxis in the management of complex midface and frontal sinus trauma. *Laryngoscope.* 2010;120(10):1940–1945.

CHAPTER 90

Panfacial Fractures

Alan S. Herford and Rahul Tandon

Armamentarium

#9 Periosteal elevator
#10 and #15 scalpel blades
#701 Bur
1.3 and 1.5 plating systems
Adson with teeth
Appropriate sutures
Arch bars and 24- and 26-gauge wires
Curved Mayo scissors
DeBakey pickups
Desmarres retractor
Jackson-Pratt drains
Local anesthetic with vasoconstrictor
Malleable retractors
Mayfield headrest
Needle electrocautery
Raney clips
Rowe forceps
Seldin retractor
Sinn rakes
Staples

History of the Procedure

Treatment of panfacial fractures poses unique challenges to the surgeon. These fractures are often complex in nature, and the treatment must be individualized for each patient. Many of these injuries are complicated by concomitant injuries that require immediate attention, which could delay early repair of the panfacial fractures. Important advancements have paved the way for more effective treatments, resulting in better prognoses and patient satisfaction.

Prior to the technologic amenities at a clinician's disposal, surgical exploration was used to analyze the extent of injuries caused by trauma, and plain radiographs provided limited information of bony involvement.[1,2] Advancements in technology have provided clinicians with the ability to identify areas of injury without more invasive exploration. The computed tomography (CT) scan has been one of the most significant gains in this area, as it identifies the location and exact fracture patterns in precise areas.[3] This was an important point in the history of treatments for panfacial injuries, as it allowed for better classification of facial injuries, thus enabling treating surgeons to better anticipate injuries and subsequent treatment. Ultrafast thin-section multidetector CT scanners now provide even more detail than those utilizing wider sections, thereby preventing clinicians from missing facial fractures that were unnoticed in previous years.[4–6] With these advances in radiographic imaging comes the responsibility to provide a more accurate interpretation as well as better preoperative planning and subsequent outcomes.[7,8] By combining CT scanned data with computer technology, the information can be viewed, analyzed, and manipulated in three dimensions, all without any invasive exploration.[9] Axial, coronal, and sagittal views are helpful, as well as three-dimensional views, especially in severely comminuted fractures. However, two-dimensional CT still displays some injuries more accurately, such as those involving the paranasal sinuses, orbital walls, and soft tissues.[10] The advantages of CT imaging are not just limited to diagnosis; they are also present in the surgical planning and treatment. This information is also readily transferable to a surgical navigation system that can be used intraoperatively.[11]

Other advances such as antibiotics and plate and screw fixation led to the improved treatment of facial fractures in general, especially panfacial fractures. The use of primary bone grafts was another advance that has impacted treatment of these fractures.

Standard Definition of Panfacial Fractures

Although there is no universally accepted definition for panfacial fractures, Markowitz and Manson defined it as a fracture that involves all three thirds of the face: upper, middle, and lower.[12] Because all three regions are affected, these fractures involve several skeletal structures: mandible, maxilla, zygomatic complex, frontal bone, and the naso-orbito-ethmoid (NOE) complex.[13] Severe panfacial fractures can lead to complex facial deformities, decreased facial movements, and malocclusion. The clinician should be aware of the soft tissue injuries often associated with these fractures, as well as other injuries (such as those that are intracranial, cervical, or vascular) that may be potentially life threatening.

Indications for the Use of the Procedure

Panfacial trauma poses several challenges for the treating surgeon, the most important of which is the complexity of injuries. The most serious injuries—which vary from case to case—should be quickly identified and addressed first. Mithani and colleagues reviewed 4786 patients treated for facial fractures and found that 9.7% had cervical spine injuries and 45.5% had associated head injuries.[14] These concomitant injuries should be investigated closely with distinct types of facial fractures.

Sound anatomic knowledge is necessary to ensure a successful long-term outcome for patients with few postoperative complications. Blunt force to the midface region may have devastating consequences to the orbital region, even if it is not directly involved. The zygoma articulates posteriorly with the greater wing of the sphenoid bone within the orbit, and anteriorly it attaches to portion of the orbicularis oculi muscle. Any significant change in the bony orbit volume may lead to enophthalmos, which if untreated could significantly delay or hamper future treatment. Blow-in fractures, which decrease the volume of the orbit, should likewise be considered.[15,16] The surgeon should also be aware of fragments of orbital bone directly damaging the globe itself, which would necessitate complete removal of the fragments.[17] Possible orbital injuries include proptosis, coronal displacement of the globe, globe rupture, superior orbital fissure syndrome, and optic nerve injury.[18]

There are situations in which the zygoma may not be involved directly, and instead a NOE injury may occur. The management of this type of injury may prove to be an arduous task for even the most-well trained surgeon, and it may require direct wiring and fixation of the fragmented and fracture sites with or without bone grafts.[19] For significant skeletal deformities, the use of bone grafts may prove to be essential. For some high-velocity/high-impact facial injuries, closed reduction of such comminuted fractures may lead to obvious bony collapse and soft tissue shrinkage, thus necessitating early exposure and treatment.[20,21] In severely comminuted fractures, such as those associated with significant bone loss or displacement in panfacial injuries, the use of primary bone grafting is often beneficial.[22] The use of the immediate bone graft to replace bone that is missing or damaged provides the surgeon with a better opportunity for successful reconstruction.[23–25] Immediate bone grafts provide several advantages such as decreased complications and reduced incidences of subsequent deformities that need additional surgical correction. However, an additional vascularized soft tissue flap might be needed to provide an adequate blood supply.[26]

The importance of integrity of the zygomatic arch for maintaining normal facial projection and prominence of the cheek has been well documented. The zygomatic bone articulates with several important structures: superiorly with the frontal bone, laterally with the zygomatic process of the temporal bone, and medially with the maxilla, and it forms the lateral wall of the orbit. The junction of the zygomatic bone with the sphenoid is often helpful to ensure accurate reduction of zygomaticomaxillary complex fractures. It also possesses important muscular attachments: zygomaticus minor and major attach anteriorly, whereas laterally the masseter muscle attaches. Any trauma that leads to a collapse of the zygomatic arch will lead to inadequate anteroposterior projection of the zygoma and subsequently an increase in facial width.[15] It is important to realize that when reconstructing the arch, it is rather straight and not "bowed." If it is not reconstructed properly, there can be increased facial width and decreased facial projection.

Complex facial fractures, however, may require more elaborate treatment than restoring facial projection. This includes addressing the facial width and vertical dimensions as well. These complex fractures often require reconstruction of the facial buttresses in order to restore facial height. The buttress system of the face absorbs and transmits forces and includes vertical and horizontal buttresses. Reconstructing panfacial fractures should proceed with particular attention to reconstructing these buttresses to provide the most stable result (Fig. 90.1). Three pairs of vertical structural supports, or buttresses, have been identified and, from anterior to posterior, are the following sites: nasal-maxillary, zygomaticomaxillary, and pterygomaxillary. The three horizontal buttresses, from superior to inferior, are superior orbital rims and the glabella, inferior orbital rims with the zygomatic arches, and the alveolar processes of the maxilla. Treatment of injuries to these areas, particularly in the anterior maxillary region, may require direct fixation of the medial and lateral buttresses combined with immediate bone graft support.[27] This may circumvent the need for multiple surgeries, as the reconstruction effort can be done in a single stage.

TECHNIQUE: Surgical Approaches

Adequate access to fracture sites is critical when treating panfacial injuries, and there are many approaches that are dependent on the area of treatment. Although there is debate among surgeons regarding which approach gives better access to sites in the lower and middle thirds of the face, the coronal approach is generally regarded as providing the widest exposure for fractures in the upper facial skeleton. Although this approach provides the best access, it does have some drawbacks: larger scars, peri-incisional hair loss, sensory deficits, frontalis nerve injury, and even corneal abrasion.[28] Nevertheless, the coronal approach has been the standard for Le Fort III and NOE fractures because it provides excellent exposure for reduction and fixation of the fractured sites.[29,30] The coronal approach also has the added benefit of allowing the surgeon to harvest a cranial bone graft for any fractures in the vicinity that may require an immediate bone graft.[31,32]

Continued

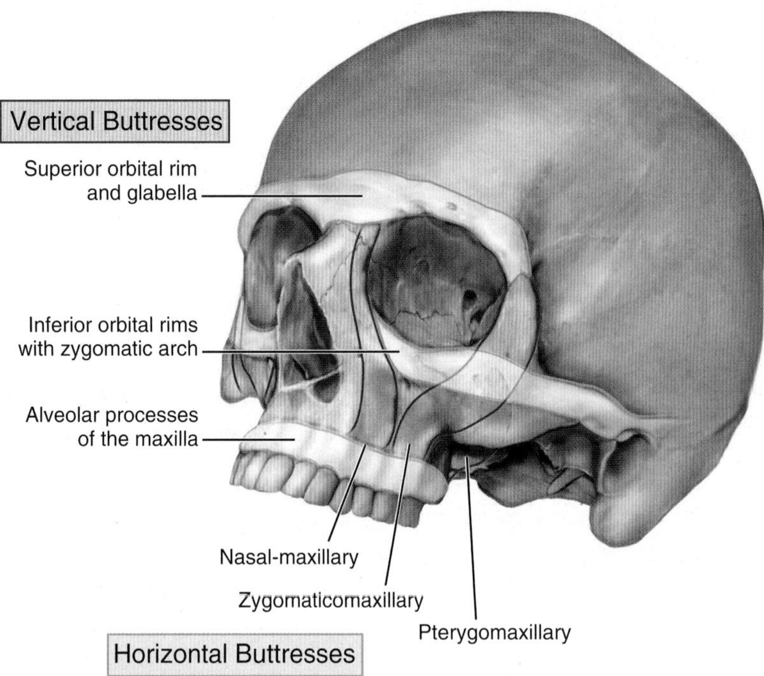

Figure 90.1 Vertical and horizontal buttresses of the facial skeleton.

TECHNIQUE: Surgical Approaches—*cont'd*

In those cases when the coronal incision is not required for adequate exposure other, less invasive, approaches may be used. One such method is the transconjunctival and upper blepharoplasty approach for orbital fracture repair and concomitant zygomaticomaxillary complex (ZMC) fractures.[33] The zygomaticosphenoid suture can be accessed, which aids in the evaluation for proper reduction of a ZMC fracture. This approach also offers the surgeon the option of using a lateral canthotomy. The need for this additional procedure varies depending on the goals of the surgeon: isolated orbital floor fractures can be treated without one, but those fractures that require a greater exposure may require it.[34]

In 1998, Garcia and colleagues introduced the transcaruncular extension of the transconjunctival approach, which provided excellent access and visualization of the medial orbital wall.[35] The transcaruncular approach is not as invasive as the traditional coronal approach, nor does it produce any significant visible external scars. Moreover, it has been used in the management of other pathologies such as frontoethmoid mucoceles.[36,37]

The zygoma and mandible are accessed through a gingivobuccal sulcus incision, which can be used to treat comminuted and malunited fractures. This approach allows for the visualization and reconstruction of important vertical buttresses.

SEQUENCING

Treatment of panfacial fractures can prove to be challenging for both experienced and inexperienced surgeons. As with any facial fracture, the goal of treatment is to restore both the facial contours (facial width, projection, and height) and function prior to the injury. Panfacial fractures involve all three regions of the face, so there are several sequencing algorithms at the surgeon's disposal: top to bottom, bottom to top, inside out, and outside in.[20,38]

BOTTOM-TO-TOP APPROACH (FIG. 90.2A)

Kelly and Manson advocated the bottom-to-top-to-middle approach, which begins with reconstruction of the mandible, including subcondylar fractures, and placement of maxilla-mandibular fixation.[39] Once the maxillomandibular complex is reconstructed, attention can then be focused on the frontal and temporal regions. The internal orbit is reconstructed following reconstruction of both the upper face and upper midface. Condylar fractures are a unique subset of mandibular fracture and may alter the prognosis of panfacial fractures. As opposed to isolated mandibular fractures, those sustained in panfacial fractures commonly affect the condylar neck rather than the subcondylar region.[2,40] Because the condyle plays an important functional role and maintains posterior facial height and mandibular position, reduction of these fractures is often helpful to restore posterior facial height. Aesthetically, by reducing the condyle, the surgeon can restore mandibular width and midface projection.[41] In the sequence of treatment, open reduction internal fixation of the condylar fracture should be performed first to reestablish sagittal position.[41] Once the sagittal positions of both the maxilla and the mandible have been reestablished, it is easier to identify the anterior height of the midface, as two of the vertical buttresses of the maxilla are aligned.[41,42] Securing these buttresses, in particular the zygomaticomaxillary, helps to prevent autorotation of the maxillomandibular complex.

TECHNIQUE: Surgical Approaches—*cont'd*

STEP 1: Incision

After general anesthesia has been administered and the patient appropriately prepared, a series of Erich arch bars are adapted to both maxillary and mandibular arches and secured with 24-gauge circumdental wires. An incision is made with Bovie electrocautery in the mandibular buccal vestibule to expose the mandibular fracture, which is subsequently débrided and irrigated (Fig. 90.2B).

STEP 2: Reduction of Mandibular and Maxillary Structures

Adapting two separate 2-0 plates to the superior portion of the fracture site and using two separate 2-mm screws, the surgeon fixates and stabilizes the plates, thereby reducing the fracture. A similar technique is used to reduce any other mandibular fractures. Although the plates and screws used may vary, it is important to reduce any and all mandibular fractures. Any maxillary fractures are then reduced, either manually or with fixation devices, and the patient's occlusion is stabilized with intermaxillary fixation (IMF) before proceeding (Fig. 90.2C–F).

STEP 3: Coronal Incision

Once the mandibular and maxillary fractures have been successfully reduced and the patient's occlusion is sufficiently stable, 10 cc of 1% lidocaine with 1:100,000 epinephrine is injected along the proposed line of the coronal incision to be made. After sufficient reduction of the infiltrative swelling (usually 5 minutes), a #15 blade is used to make the coronal incision, which is carried deep to the calvarium and carried to the temporal fascia laterally. A #9 periosteal elevator is used to create a full-thickness flap, exposing the calvarium, and then it is released all the way to the superior orbital rims on both sides.

STEP 4: Reduction of Zygomatic Fracture

At the lateral portions of the incision, the #15 blade is carried below the anterior layer of the deep temporal fascia; in the temporal fat pad, a #9 elevator is used to remove the overlying fascia off any fractured zygomatic arches. The fractured arch is then reduced appropriately with 1.5-mm plates (Fig. 90.2G and H).

Continued

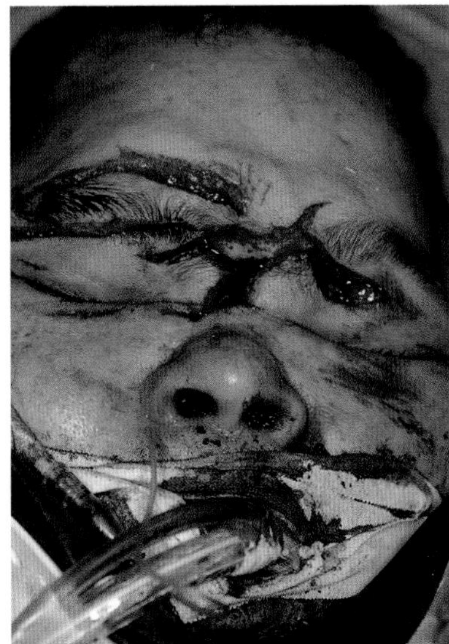

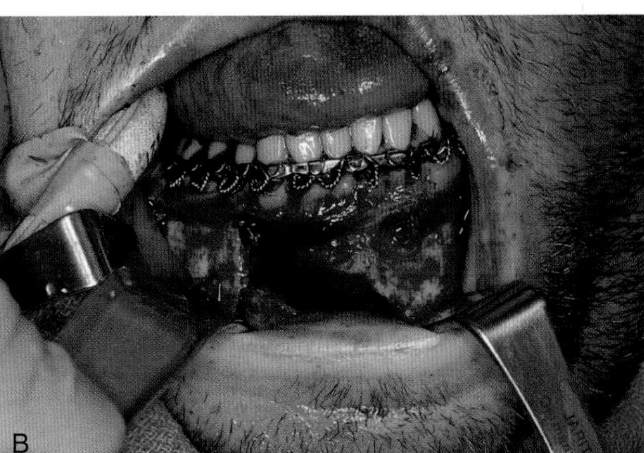

Figure 90.2 **A,** Patient initially presents intubated with multiple lacerations and facial fractures. **B,** Exposure of comminuted mandibular fracture.

TECHNIQUE: Surgical Approaches—*cont'd*

STEP 5: Repair of Orbital Fracture

Once either one or both zygomatic arches are reduced, attention can be directed toward any orbital fractures. Bilateral transconjunctival incisions are made with the Bovie electrocautery with concurrent lateral canthotomy incisions. Once the fractures have been isolated with a #9 elevator, they are reduced appropriately. If any other defects are noted in the orbital socket, such as a medial wall defect, a calvarial bone graft can be used from the exposed calvarium. Partial-thickness calvarial bone is removed using a cross-cut bur and osteotomes. The bone grafts are then placed in sterile saline and later adapted to any orbital defects. Inferior orbital defects are repaired with titanium meshes fixated anteriorly with screws and adapted to the full posterior orbit (Fig. 90.2I and J).

STEP 6: Repair of NOE Fractures

After reduction of any orbital fractures, NOE fractures can be addressed. Because the coronal flap has provided adequate exposure to the NOE site, a Y-type, 1.5-mm plate can reduce the NOE fracture bilaterally. Additional calvarial bone grafts can be obtained and used to contour a nasal strut graft and adapted with another Y-type plate, recreating any nasal defect incurred during the injury (Fig. 90.2K and L).

STEP 7: Closure of Incisions

Once all the panfacial fractures have been reduced and fixated, closure begins. Using multiple 3-0 Vicryl sutures for the muscular as well as subcutaneous layers, a Jackson-Pratt drain is placed under the patient's coronal flap and is sutured in place. The coronal portion is closed first with deep Vicryl pop-off sutures, followed by cutaneous closure with 4-0 Vicryl for the deep muscular and periosteal layers. The IMF loops are then cut and removed; however, the patient remains intubated. CT imaging confirms adequate reduction and fixation (Fig. 90.2M).

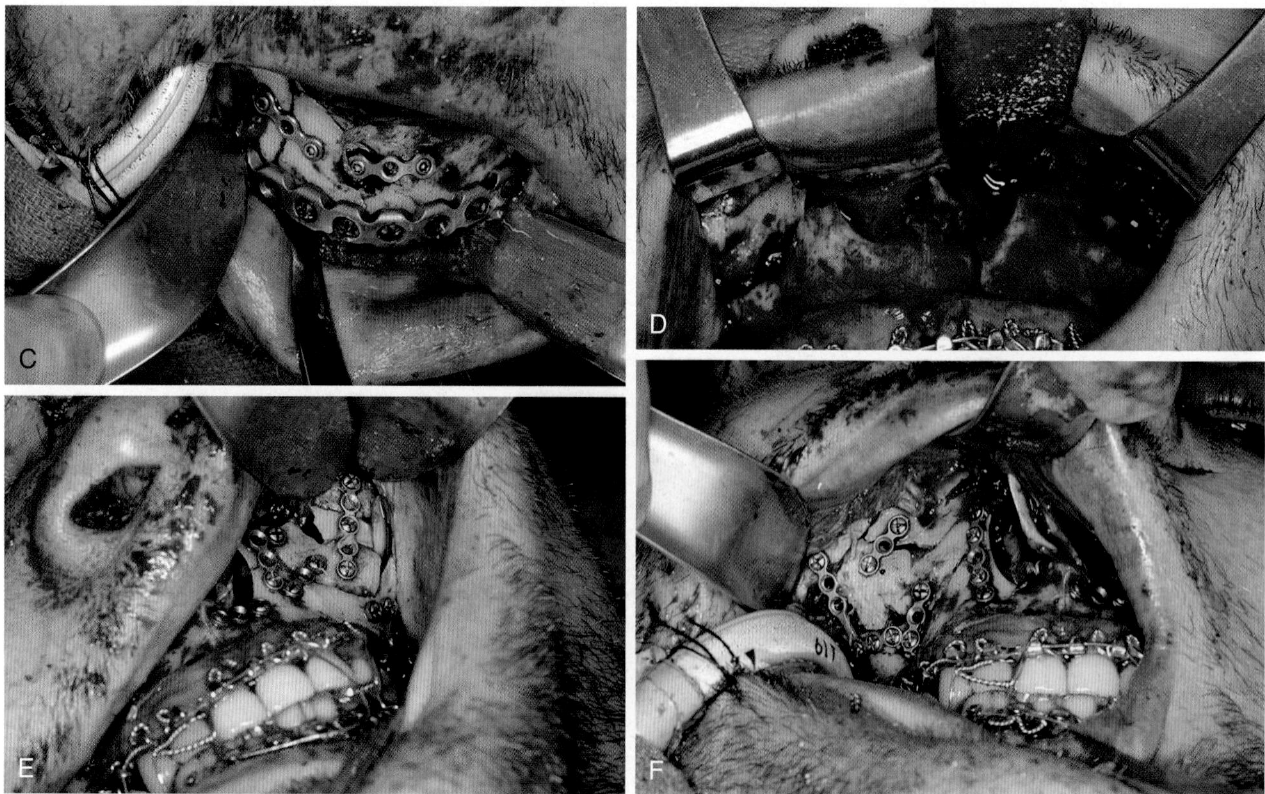

Figure 90.2, cont'd **C,** Reduction and fixation of mandibular fracture. **D,** Exposure of lower midface fractures. **E,** Reduction and fixation of midface fracture. **F,** Reduction and fixation of midface fracture; note the presence of a secured intubation tube.

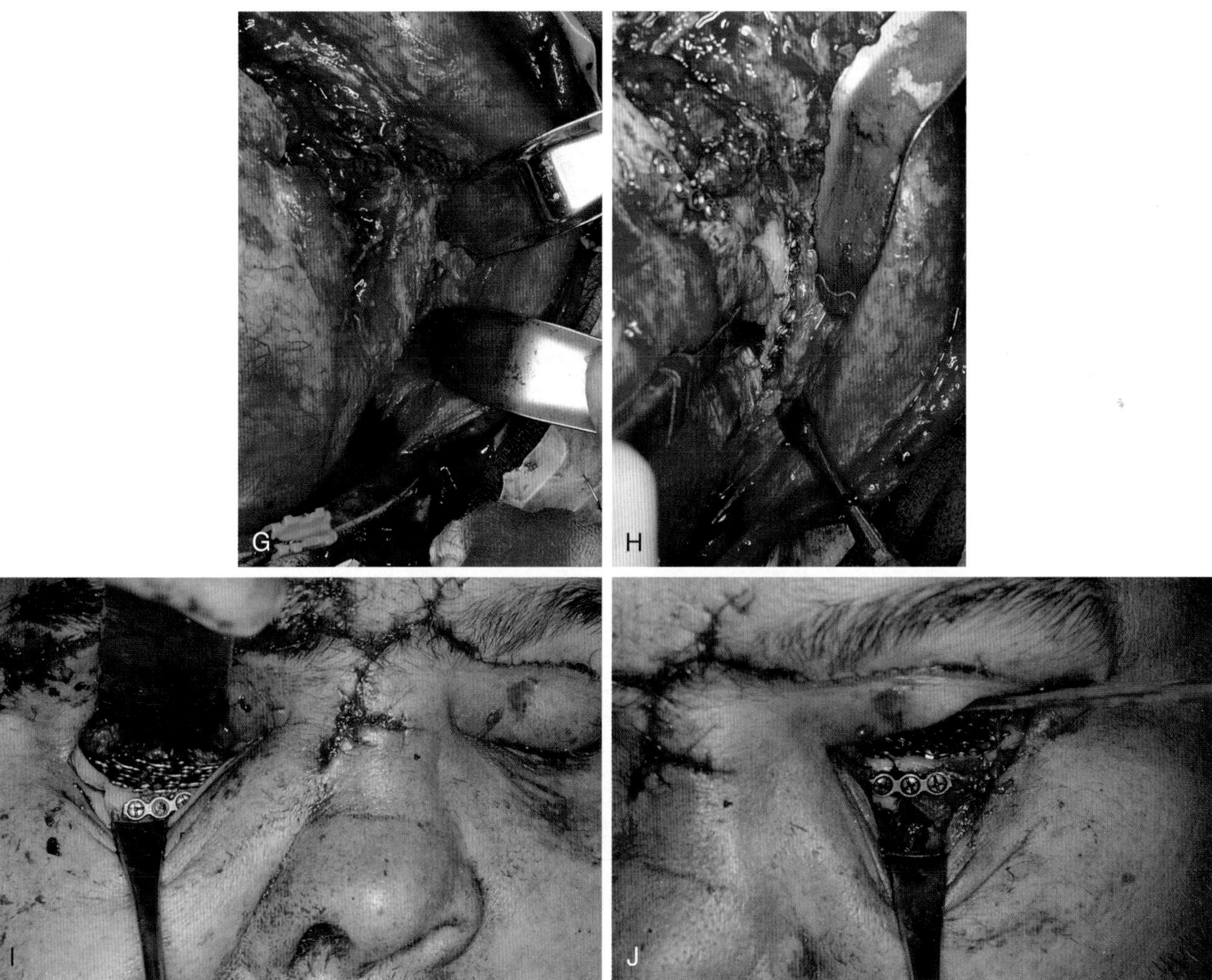

Figure 90.2, cont'd G and H, Zygomatic arch fracture and subsequent reduction. Note that the arch is relatively straight. **I,** Transconjunctival incisions allow proper visualization and access to orbital floor and orbital rim fractures. **J,** Orbital rim fractures reduced with plates and screws. Orbital floor reconstructed with titanium mesh.

TECHNIQUE: Surgical Approaches—*cont'd*

TOP-TO-BOTTOM APPROACH

Gruss and Phillips, however, promoted reducing the zygomatic arch and malar eminence, which would help to reestablish the outer facial frame.[20] They utilized plate and screw fixation and advocated reconstructing the outer facial frame beginning with the zygomatic arch, zygoma, and frontal bar. This was followed by reduction of the inner facial frame (the NOE complex), and finally the orbit was reduced and stabilized. In support of Gruss and Phillips, other authors also advocated this top-to-bottom approach if the NOE region was involved.[43] However, the lack of a reliable landmark in the NOE region may make orientation slightly more difficult than if another region were used.[44]

With the use of plates and screws for fixation, there is more flexibility in the order in which to treat panfacial fractures. Manson and colleagues stated in 1999 that "any [order of treatment] is satisfactory if one understands the anatomy, goals, and procedures."[45] Regardless of the approach used, early treatment of panfacial fractures reduces the risks of postoperative infection and maintains soft tissue integrity[34] (Fig. 90.3A–C).

Continued

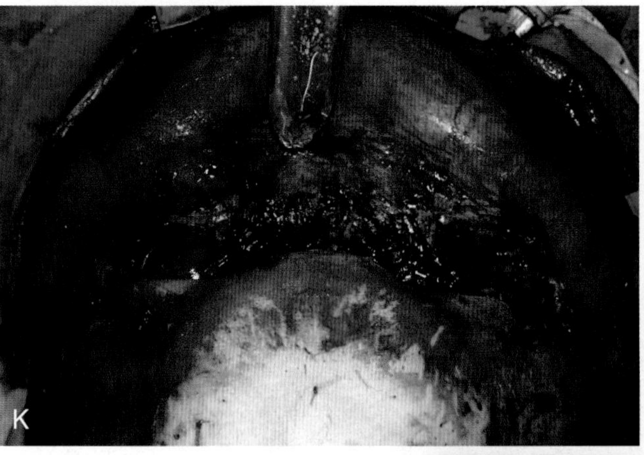

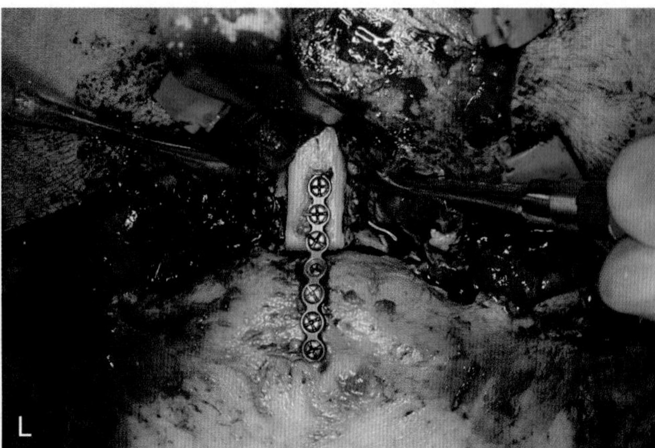

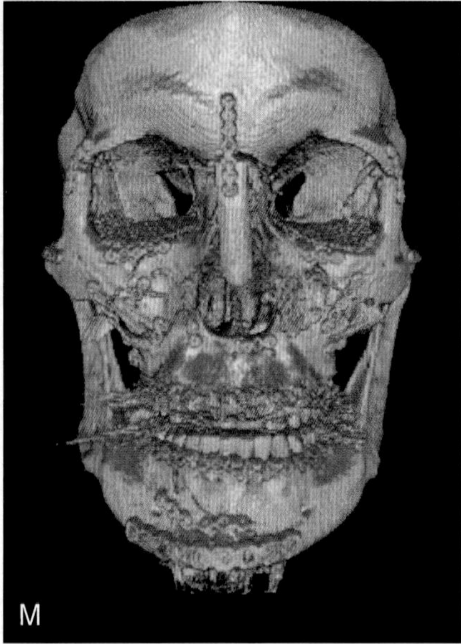

Figure 90.2, cont'd **K,** Exposure utilizing a coronal flap. Note the fractures of the frontal and nasal bones. **L,** Harvested calvarial partial-thickness bone graft used as a nasal strut graft to restore the dorsal portion of the nose. **M,** Final computed tomography (CT) image.

TECHNIQUE: Surgical Approaches—*cont'd*

STEP 1: Coronal Incision and Access to NOE Fractures

After administering general anesthesia and preparing the patient, Erich arch bars are placed on both dental arches and secured with interdental wiring. A full-thickness coronal incision is then made down to the periosteum. It is carried laterally until it approaches the temporalis muscle, and dissection is carried down on top of the temporalis fascia to protect vital vessels and nerves within the flap. The flap is elevated and extended to expose the superior orbital and NOE regions. Next, an incision is made through the anterior layer of the deep temporalis fascia. The dissection proceeds in this space, occupied by the temporal fat pad, down to the zygomatic arch. In this plane the facial nerve is protected. A #9 elevator is used to dissect the flap in a subperiosteal plane to the level of the orbits and NOE complex. The zygomatic frontal sutures are digitally reduced, and the sphenoid junctions are used to evaluate adequate reduction of the left and right zygoma (Fig. 90.3D).

STEP 2: Reconstruction of NOE Fractures

A monocortical bone graft is then harvested from the exposed calvarium and adapted to the nasal bone over the ethmoid region to ensure fit and provide projection of the nasal tip and the dorsum of the nose. The comminuted NOE fracture is reduced with the use of digital manipulation and repositioning the segmental fractures together. Using titanium plates, the fracture segments are fixated together. The cranial bone graft is then fixated to the nose to provide projection to the nose (Fig. 90.3E).

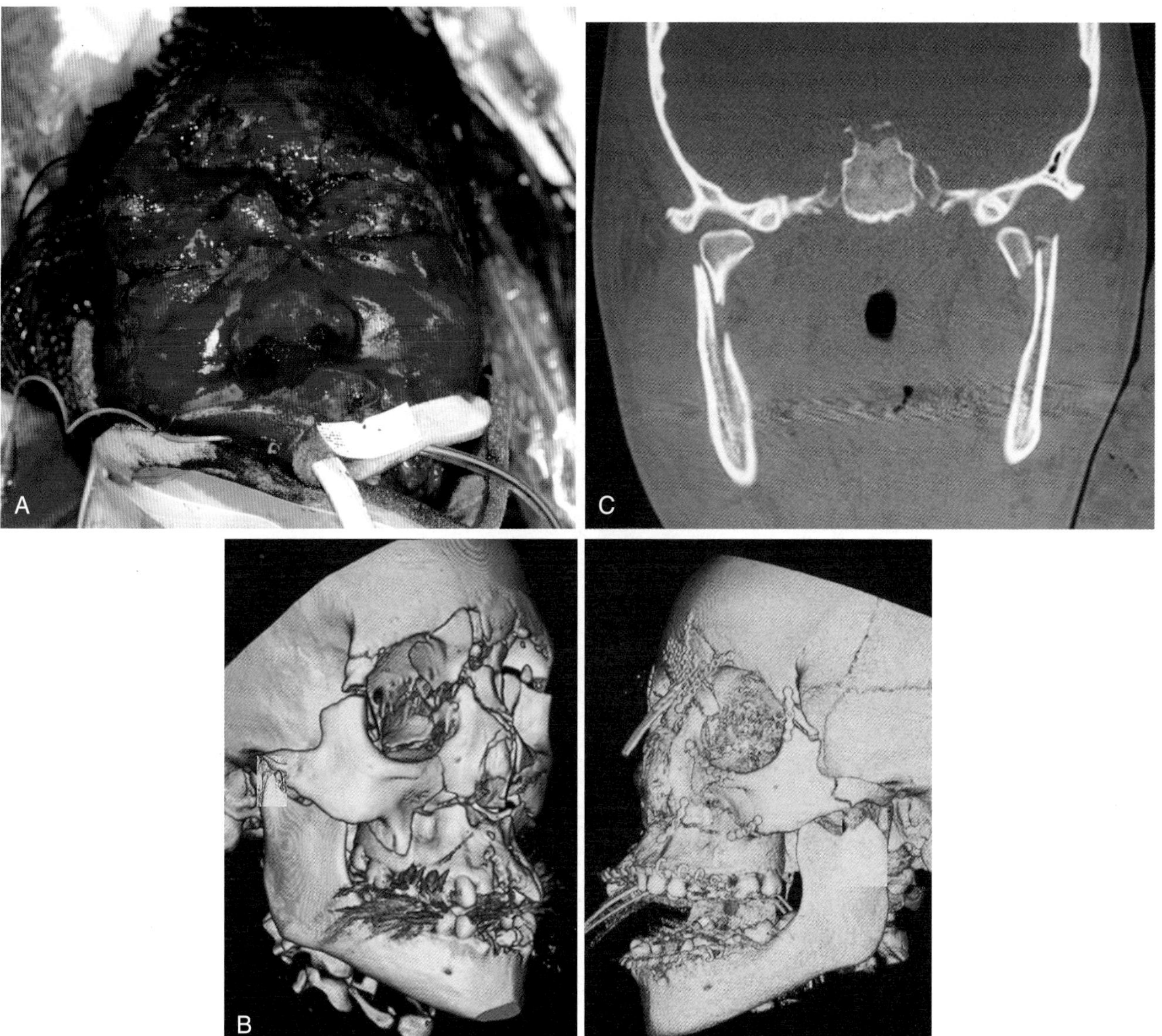

Figure 90.3 **A,** Initial presentation of panfacial trauma with extensive facial lacerations. **B,** Computed tomography (CT) imaging is important for visualizing fractures and fracture patterns. **C,** Radiographic images of bilateral condylar fractures.

TECHNIQUE: Surgical Approaches—*cont'd*

STEP 3: Reduction and Fixation of Zygomatic and Orbital Fractures

After fixation of the zygomatic and piriform fractures, attention can be turned toward any orbital fractures. Fractures of the infraorbital rim are accessed via transconjunctival incisions, and using a Desmarres retractor and a malleable retractor, the lid and suborbital contents are retracted. After the Bovie electrocautery is used to incise through the conjunctiva and to the infraorbital rim, a #9 periosteal elevator is used to explore the infraorbital rim to the medial portion. The fractures are fixated with titanium plates and screws (Fig. 90.3F and G).

Continued

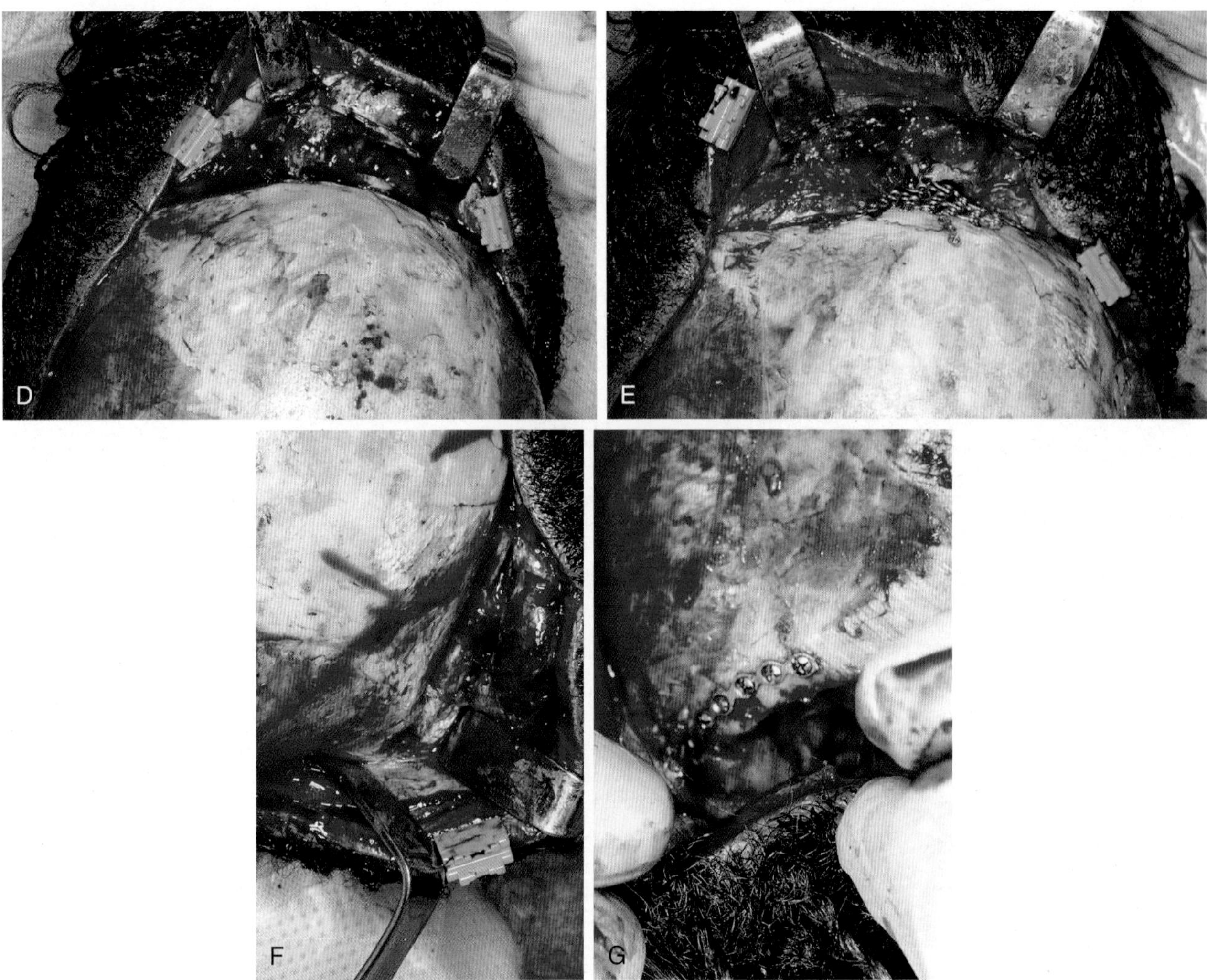

Figure 90.3, cont'd **D,** Coronal flap elevation for visualizing upper facial fractures (naso-orbito-ethmoid [NOE] fractures). **E,** Plated NOE fracture, which was accomplished first in the top-down approach. **F** and **G,** Fixation of the zygomatic fractures. Note visualization of the zygomaticosphenoid fracture to ensure proper reduction.

TECHNIQUE: Surgical Approaches—*cont'd*

STEP 4: Reduction of Any Maxillary and Mandibular Fractures

If a Le Fort fracture is present, it can be accessed through an incision in the maxillary vestibule and exposed with a #9 periosteal elevator. The fractures are reduced and titanium plates are placed along the zygomatic and piriform buttresses bilaterally. Finally, a period of maxillary-mandibular fixation may be considered. It is important to rehabilitate the condyle fractures if treated closed (Fig. 90.3H–J).

Avoidance and Management of Intraoperative Complications

Good surgical planning limits intraoperative or postoperative complications. Intraoperative CT scans as well as CT-guided navigation help to avoid damage to adjacent structures.

Postoperative Considerations

Postoperative imaging is helpful for determining whether adequate reduction was performed. Maxillomandibular fixation is not routinely necessary postoperatively, although some surgeons may prefer it. If, however, inadequate reduction or enophthalmos is noted postoperatively, early reoperation should be considered.

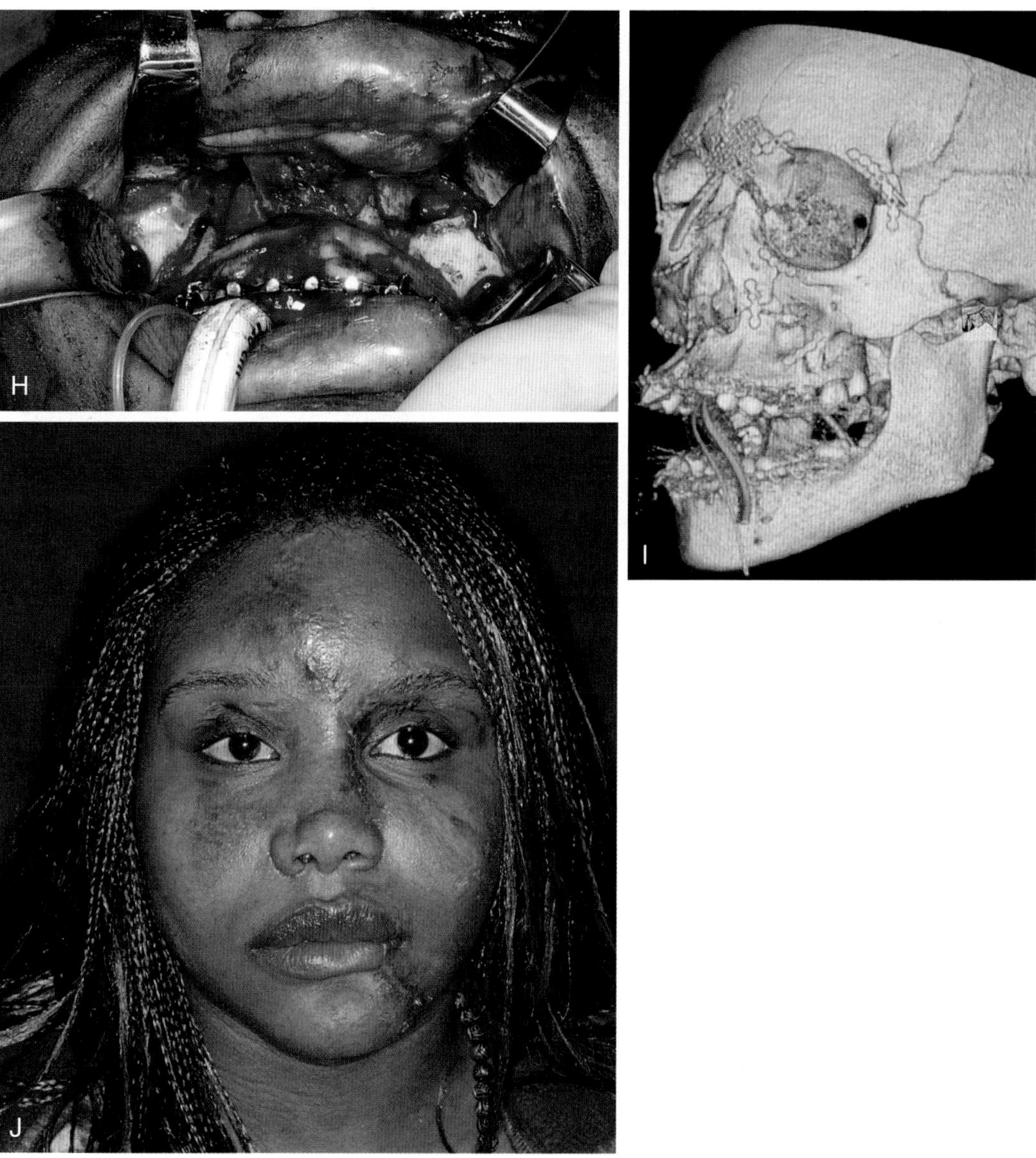

Figure 90.3, cont'd **H,** Access and visualization of the maxillary/midface fracture. **I,** Postoperative CT demonstrating reduction and fixation of panfacial fractures. **J,** Final photograph.

References

1. Bergara AR, Itoiz AO. Present state of the surgical treatment of chronic frontal sinusitis. *AMA Arch Otolaryngol.* 1955;61(6):616–628.
2. Donald PJ, Bernstein L. Compound frontal sinus injuries with intracranial penetration. *Laryngoscope.* 1978;88(2 Pt 1): 225–232.
3. Manson PN, Markowitz B, Mirvis S, Dunham M, Yaremchuk M. Toward CT-based facial fracture treatment. *Plast Reconstr Surg.* 1990;85(2):202–212.
4. Holmgren EP, Dierks EJ, Homer LD, Potter BE. Facial computed tomography use in trauma patients who require a head computed tomogram. *J Oral Maxillofac Surg.* 2004;62(8):913–918.
5. Kreipke DL, Moss JJ, Franco JM, Maves MD, Smith DJ. Computed tomography and thin-section tomography in facial trauma. *AJR Am J Roentgenol.* 1984;142(5):1041–1045.
6. Zimmerman RA, Bilaniuk LT, Gennarelli T, Bruce D, Dolinskas C, Uzzell B. Cranial computed tomography in diagnosis and management of acute head trauma. *AJR Am J Roentgenol.* 1978;131(1):27–34.
7. Hopper RA, Salemy S, Sze RW. Diagnosis of midface fractures with CT: what the surgeon needs to know. *Radiographics.* 2006;26(3):783–793.
8. Stanwix MG, Nam AJ, Manson PN, Mirvis S, Rodriguez ED. Critical computed tomographic diagnostic criteria for frontal sinus fractures. *J Oral Maxillofac Surg.* 2010;68(11):2714–2722.
9. Bui TG, Bell RB, Dierks EJ. Technological advances in the treatment of facial trauma. *Atlas Oral Maxillofac Surg Clin North Am.* 2012;20(1):81–94.
10. Mayer JS, Wainwright DJ, Yeakley JW, Lee KF, Harris JH Jr, Kulkarni M. The role of three-dimensional computed tomography in the management of maxillofacial trauma. *J Trauma.* 1988;28(7):1043–1053.
11. Bell RB. Computer planning and intraoperative navigation in cranio-maxillofacial surgery. *Oral Maxillofac Surg Clin North Am.* 2010;22(1):135–156.
12. Markowitz BL, Manson PN. Panfacial fractures: organization of treatment. *Clin Plast Surg.* 1989;16(1):105–114.
13. Yang R, Zhang C, Liu Y, Li Z, Li Z. Why should we start from mandibular fractures in the treatment of panfacial fractures? *J Oral Maxillofac Surg.* 2012;70(6):1386–1392.

14. Mithani SK, St-Hilaire H, Brooke BS, Smith IM, Bluebond-Langner R, Rodriguez ED. Predictable patterns of intracranial and cervical spine injury in craniomaxillofacial trauma: analysis of 4786 patients. *Plast Reconstr Surg.* 2009;123(4):1293–1301.
15. Gruss JS, Hurwitz JJ. Isolated blow-in fracture of the lateral orbit causing globe rupture. *Ophthal Plast Reconstr Surg.* 1990;6(3):221–224.
16. Fialkov JA, Phillips JH, Gruss JS, Kassel EE, Zuker RM. A stereotactic system for guiding complex craniofacial reconstruction. *Plast Reconstr Surg.* 1992;89(2):340–345.
17. Gruss JS, Hurwitz JJ. Isolated blow-in fracture of the lateral orbit causing globe rupture. *Ophthal Plast Reconstr Surg.* 1990;6(3):221–224.
18. Antonyshyn O, Gruss JS, Kassel EE. Blow-in fractures of the orbit. *Plast Reconstr Surg.* 1989;84(1):10–20.
19. Gruss JS. Fronto-naso-orbital trauma. *Clin Plast Surg.* 1982;9(4):577–589.
20. Gruss JS, Phillips JH. Complex facial trauma: the evolving role of rigid fixation and immediate bone graft reconstruction. *Clin Plast Surg.* 1989;16(1):93–104.
21. Antonyshyn O, Gruss JS. Complex orbital trauma: the role of rigid fixation and primary bone grafting. *Adv Ophthalmic Plast Reconstr Surg.* 1987;7:61–92.
22. Gruss JS, Antonyshyn O, Phillips JH. Early definitive bone and soft-tissue reconstruction of major gunshot wounds of the face. *Plast Reconstr Surg.* 1991;87(3):436–450.
23. Gruss JS. Naso-ethmoid-orbital fractures: classification and role of primary bone grafting. *Plast Reconstr Surg.* 1985;75(3):303–317.
24. Gruss JS. Complex nasoethmoid-orbital and midfacial fractures: role of craniofacial surgical techniques and immediate bone grafting. *Ann Plast Surg.* 1986;17(5):377–390.
25. Gruss JS, Mackinnon SE, Kassel EE, Cooper PW. The role of primary bone grafting in complex craniomaxillofacial trauma. *Plast Reconstr Surg.* 1985;75(1):17–24.
26. Gruss JS, Pollock RA, Phillips JH, Antonyshyn O. Combined injuries of the cranium and face. *Br J Plast Surg.* 1989;42(4):385–398.
27. Gruss JS, Mackinnon SE. Complex maxillary fractures: role of buttress reconstruction and immediate bone grafts. *Plast Reconstr Surg.* 1986;78(1):9–22.
28. Güven E, Uğurlu AM, Kuvat SV, Kanlıada D, Emekli U. Minimally invasive approaches in severe panfacial fractures. *Ulus Travma Acil Cerrahi Derg.* 2010;16(6):541–545.
29. Shaw RC, Parsons RW. Exposure through a coronal incision for initial treatment of facial fractures. *Plast Reconstr Surg.* 1975;56(3):254–259.
30. Shetty SK, Saikrishna D, Kumaran S. A study on coronal incision for treating zygomatic complex fractures. *J Maxillofac Oral Surg.* 2009;8(2):160–163.
31. Clauser L, Dallera V, Sarti E, Tieghi R. Frontobasilar fractures in children. *Childs Nerv Syst.* 2004;20(3):168–175.
32. Zhang QB, Dong YJ, Li ZB, Zhao JH. Coronal incision for treating zygomatic complex fractures. *J Craniomaxillofac Surg.* 2006;34(3):182–185.
33. Raschke GF, Rieger UM, Bader RD, Schaefer O, Guentsch A, Schultze-Mosgau S. Transconjunctival versus subciliary approach for orbital fracture repair—an anthropometric evaluation of 221 cases. *Clin Oral Investig.* 2013;17(3):933–942.
34. Martou G, Antonyshyn OM. Advances in surgical approaches to the upper facial skeleton. *Curr Opin Otolaryngol Head Neck Surg.* 2011;19(4):242–247.
35. Garcia GH, Goldberg RA, Shorr N. The transcaruncular approach in repair of orbital fractures: a retrospective study. *J Craniomaxillofac Trauma.* 1998;4(1):7–12.
36. Lai PC, Liao SL, Jou JR, Hou PK. Transcaruncular approach for the management of frontoethmoid mucoceles. *Br J Ophthalmol.* 2003;87(6):699–703.
37. Edgin WA, Morgan-Marshall A, Fitzsimmons TD. Transcaruncular approach to medial orbital wall fractures. *J Oral Maxillofac Surg.* 2007;65(11):2345–2349.
38. Kelly J. *War Injuries to the Jaws and Related Structures.* Washington, DC: US Government Printing Office; 1978.
39. Kelly KJ, Manson PN, Vander Kolk CA, et al. Sequencing LeFort fracture treatment (Organization of treatment for a panfacial fracture). *J Craniofac Surg.* 1990;1(4):168–178.
40. Zachariades N, Mezitis M, Mourouzis C, Papadakis D, Spanou A. Fractures of the mandibular condyle: a review of 466 cases. Literature review, reflections on treatment and proposals. *J Craniomaxillofac Surg.* 2006;34(7):421–432.
41. Tullio A, Sesenna E. Role of surgical reduction of condylar fractures in the management of panfacial fractures. *Br J Oral Maxillofac Surg.* 2000;38(5):472–476.
42. Rontal E, Hohmann A. Proceedings: external fixation of facial fractures. *Arch Otolaryngol.* 1973;98(6):393–396.
43. Merville L. Multiple dislocations of the facial skeleton. *J Maxillofac Surg.* 1974;2(4):187–200.
44. He D, Zhang Y, Ellis E III. Panfacial fractures: analysis of 33 cases treated late. *J Oral Maxillofac Surg.* 2007;65(12):2459–2465.
45. Manson PN, Clark N, Robertson B, et al. Subunit principles in midface fractures: the importance of sagittal buttresses, soft-tissue reductions, and sequencing treatment of segmental fractures. *Plast Reconstr Surg.* 1999;103(4):1287–1306.

Index

Note: Page numbers followed by "f" indicate figures, "t" indicate tables, and "b" indicate boxes.

B

C

F

J

M

N

P

Q

R

ATLAS OF ORAL AND MAXILLOFACIAL SURGERY

EDITION 2 VOLUME TWO

ATLAS OF ORAL AND MAXILLOFACIAL SURGERY

PAUL S. TIWANA, DDS, MD, MS, FACS, FACD

Francis J. Reichmann Professor and Chair
Division of Oral & Maxillofacial Surgery
College of Dentistry;
Professor
Department of Surgery
College of Medicine
The University of Oklahoma Health Sciences Center
Oklahoma City, Oklahoma
United States

DEEPAK KADEMANI, DMD, MD, FACS

President and Medical Director
Minnesota Oral & Facial Surgery
Fellowship Director
Oral/Head & Neck Oncologic and Reconstructive Surgery
Minneapolis, Minnesota
United States

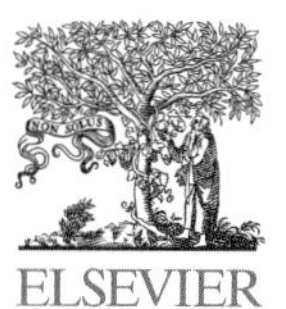

ELSEVIER

Elsevier
1600 John F. Kennedy Blvd.
Ste 1800
Philadelphia, PA 19103-2899

ATLAS OF ORAL AND MAXILLOFACIAL SURGERY, SECOND EDITION ISBN: 978-0-323-78963-9

Notice

Practitioners and researchers must always rely on their own experience and knowledge in evaluating and using any information, methods, compounds or experiments described herein. Because of rapid advances in the medical sciences, in particular, independent verification of diagnoses and drug dosages should be made. To the fullest extent of the law, no responsibility is assumed by Elsevier, authors, editors or contributors for any injury and/or damage to persons or property as a matter of products liability, negligence or otherwise, or from any use or operation of any methods, products, instructions, or ideas contained in the material herein.

Previous edition copyrighted 2016.

Senior Content Strategist: Lauren Boyle
Content Development Specialist: Deborah Poulson
Publishing Services Manager: Shereen Jameel
Senior Project Manager: Manikandan Chandrasekaran
Book Designer: Brian Salisbury

Printed in India

Last digit is the print number: 9 8 7 6 5 4 3 2 1

This book is dedicated to the following individuals:

To my family for all your love and support.

To my patients who have given me the privilege to care for them.

To students of our specialty in their quest for knowledge.

Deepak Kademani

This book is dedicated to the following individuals:

To my family; especially my wife Karen, and my daughters Jespreet (17), and Simran (15).

To my former residents and fellows.

Paul S. Tiwana

Section Editors

Richard Allen Finn, DDS
Professor
Oral and Maxillofacial Surgery Division
UT Southwestern Medical Center;
Chief
Oral and Maxillofacial Surgery
Veteran's Administration North Texas
Dallas, Texas
United States

Part I: Surgical Anatomy of the Head and Neck

Deepak G. Krishnan, DDS, FACS
Associate Professor—Surgery
Division of Oral Maxillofacial Surgery,
Department of Surgery
University of Cincinnati;
Oral Maxillofacial Surgeon
Cincinnati Children's Hospital and Medical Center
Cincinnati, Ohio
United States

Part II: Oral Surgery

Martin B. Steed, DDS, FACS
Professor and James B. Edwards Chair
Department of Oral and Maxillofacial Surgery
Medical University of South Carolina
James B. Edwards College of Dental Medicine
Charleston, South Carolina
United States

Part III: Implant Surgery

Steven M. Sullivan, DDS, FACS, FACD
Professor and Chair
Department of Surgical Sciences/Oral and Maxillofacial Surgery
University of Oklahoma College of Dentistry
Oklahoma City, Oklahoma
United States

Part IV: Orthognathic Surgery

Paul S. Tiwana, DDS, MD, MS, FACS, FACD
Francis J. Reichmann Professor and Chair
Division of Oral & Maxillofacial Surgery
College of Dentistry;
Professor
Department of Surgery
College of Medicine
The University of Oklahoma Health Sciences Center
Oklahoma City, Oklahoma
United States

Part V: Craniofacial Surgery

Ghali E. Ghali, DDS, MD, FACS, FRCS(Ed)
Director
Oral and Maxillofacial Surgery
Willis Knighton Health System
Shreveport, Louisiana
United States

Part VI: Cleft Lip and Palate

Alan S. Herford, DDS, MD
Chairman and Professor
Oral and Maxillofacial Surgery
Loma Linda University
Loma Linda, California
United States

Part VII: Craniomaxillofacial Trauma

Eric R. Carlson, DMD, MD, EdM, FACS
Professor and Kelly L. Krahwinkel Chairman
Department of Oral and Maxillofacial Surgery
University of Tennessee Graduate School of Medicine;
Director
Oral/Head and Neck Oncologic Surgery Fellowship
University of Tennessee Cancer Institute
Knoxville, Tennessee
United States

Part VIII: Benign Pathology

Deepak Kademani, DMD, MD, FACS
President and Medical Director
Minnesota Oral & Facial Surgery
Fellowship Director
Oral/Head & Neck Oncologic and Reconstructive Surgery
Minneapolis, Minnesota
United States

Part IX: Malignant Pathology

Brent B. Ward, DDS, MD, FACS, FACD
Professor, Chair and Fellowship Program Director
Oral and Maxillofacial Surgery
University of Michigan
Ann Arbor, Michigan
United States

Part X: Reconstructive Surgery

Gary F. Bouloux, MD, DDS, MDSc, FRACDS, FRACDS(OMS), FRCS (Eng), FACS
J. David Allen Family Professor
Division Chief
Oral and Maxillofacial Surgery
Department of Surgery
Emory University School of Medicine
Atlanta, Georgia
United States

Part XI: TMJ Surgery

Faisal A. Quereshy, MD, DDS, FACS
Professor/Program Director
Oral & Maxillofacial Surgery
Case Western Reserve University, Cleveland
Ohio
United States;
Medical Director
Facial Cosmetic Surgery
Visage Surgical Institute/V-Spa
Medina, Ohio
United States

Part XII: Facial Cosmetic Surgery

Joseph E. Cillo Jr., DMD, MPH, PhD, FACS
Division Chief and Program Director
Oral and Maxillofacial Surgery
Allegheny General Hospital;
Associate Professor
Oral and Maxillofacial Surgery
Allegheny General Hospital
Pittsburgh, Pennsylvania
United States

Part XIII: Obstructive Sleep Apnea

Contributors

A. Omar Abubaker, DMD, PhD
Professor and Chairman
Oral and Maxillofacial Surgery
VCU Medical Center
Richmond, Virginia
United States

Julio Acero, MD, DMD, PhD, FDSRCS, FEBOMFS
Full Professor Surgery
Alcala University;
Department Head
Oral and Maxillofacial Surgery
Ramon y Cajal University Hospital
Madrid, Spain

Ravi Agarwal, DDS
Program Director
Oral & Maxillofacial Surgery
Medstar Washington Hospital Center, Washington
District of Columbia
United States;
Chairman
Oral & Maxillofacial Surgery
Medstar Washington Hospital Center
Washington, District of Columbia
United States

Tara Aghaloo, DDS, MD, PhD
Professor
Oral and Maxillofacial Surgery
UCLA School of Dentistry
Los Angeles, California
United States

Maryam Akbari, DMD, MD, MPH
Oral and Maxillofacial Surgery
Mount Sinai
New York, New York
United States

Kyle P. Allen, MD, MPH
Tampa Bay Hearing and Balance Center;
Assistant Clinical Professor
Otolaryngology—Head and Neck Surgery
University of South Florida
Tampa, Florida
United States

Dror M. Allon, DMD
Director
Orthognathic and TMJ Surgery Unit;
Senior Lecturer
Oral and Maxillofacial Surgery
Tel Aviv University
Tel Aviv, Israel

Fernando Almeida, MD, PhD, DDS, FEBOMFS
Clinical Professor
Department of Surgery
Alcalá University (UAH);
Oral & Maxillofacial Surgeon
Department of Oral and Maxillofacial Surgery
University Hospital Ramón y Cajal
Madrid, Spain

Brian Alpert, DDS, FACS (Deceased)
Professor of Oral and Maxillofacial Surgery
University of Louisville School of Dentistry
Louisville, Kentucky
United States

Mehmet Ali Altay, DDS, PhD
Associate Professor
Oral and Maxillofacial Surgery
Akdeniz University, School of Dentistry
Antalya, Turkey

Felix Jose Amarista, DDS
Assistant Professor
Department of Oral and Maxillofacial Surgery
UT Health San Antonio
San Antonio, Texas
United States

Hatem Amer, MD
Associate Professor of Medicine
Division of Nephrology and Hypertension and
The William J von Liebig Center for Transplantation and
Clinical Regeneration
Mayo Clinic
Rochester, Minnesota
United States

Suganya Appugounder DMD, MS, FACS, MAJ, USAR, DC
Cleft and Craniofacial Surgery
Charleston Area Medical Center
Charleston, West Virginia
United States

Shyam Prasad Aravindaksha, BDS, MDS
Private Practice
Oral Maxillofacial Surgery
Greater Michigan Oral Surgeons
Flint, Michigan
United States

Sharon Aronovich, DMD
Clinical Associate Professor
Oral and Maxillofacial Surgery
University of Michigan
Ann Arbor, Michigan
United States

Leon Assael, BA, DMD, CMM
Professor Emeritus
Oral and Maxillofacial Surgery
Oregon Health & Science University
Portland, Oregon;
Affiliate Associate Professor
Public Health
University of California San Francisco
San Francisco, California
United States

Michael Awadallah, DDS, MD
Assistant Professor of Surgery
Weill Cornell Medicine
New York, New York
United States

Shahid R. Aziz, DMD, MD, FACS, FRCS (Ed)
Division Director
Oral & Maxillofacial Surgery
Hackensack University Medical Center;
Clinical Professor
Oral and Maxillofacial Surgery
Rutgers School of Dental Medicine
Newark, New Jersey;
Clinical Professor
Otolaryngology
Hackensack Meridian School of Medicine
Nutley, New Jersey
United States;
Visiting Professor
Oral and Maxillofacial Surgery
Update Dental College
Dhaka, Bangladesh

Shahrokh C. Bagheri, DMD, MD, FACS
Oral and Maxillofacial Surgeon
Georgia Oral and Facial Surgery
Atlanta, Georgia
United States

Jonathan Bailey, DMD, MD, FACS
Clinical Professor
Department of Surgery
Carle Illinois College of Medicine;
Associate Medical Director of Specialty Surgery
Division of Oral and Maxillofacial Surgery and Division of Head and Neck Cancer
Carle Foundation Hospital
Urbana, Illinois
United States

Andrew M. Baker, MD, DDS
Oral and Maxillofacial Surgery
Providence Cancer Institute
Portland, Oregon
United States

Karim Bakri, MBBS
Consultant
Division of Plastic Surgery
Mayo Clinic
Rochester, Minnesota
United States

Suzanne Barnes, DMD
Assistant Professor
Oral and Maxillofacial Surgery
University of Louisville
Louisville, Kentucky
United States

Brian Bast, DMD, MD
Professor and Chair
Oral and Maxillofacial Surgery
University of California, School of Dentistry
San Francisco, California
United States

Hussam Batal, DMD
Clinical Professor
Oral and Maxillofacial Surgery
Boston University Henry M. Goldman School of Dental Medicine
Boston, Massachusetts
United States

Dale A. Baur, DDS, MD
Professor and Chair, Vice Dean
Oral and Maxillofacial Surgery
Case Western Reserve University School of Dental Medicine;
Division Chief,
Oral and Maxillofacial Surgery
University Hospitals/Cleveland Medical Center
Cleveland, Ohio
United States

Edmond Bedrossian, DDS, FACD, FACOMS, FAO, FITI
Professor
Oral and Maxillofacial Surgery
University of the Pacific
San Francisco, California
United States

Edmond Armand Bedrossian, DDS
Private Practice
San Francisco, California
United States

R. Bryan Bell, MD, DDS, FACS, FRCS (Ed)
Physician Executive and Director
Division of Surgical Oncology, Radiation Oncology and Clinical Programs
Providence Cancer Institute;
Medical Director
Providence Head and Neck Cancer Program
Providence Cancer Institute;
Associate Member
Earle A. Chiles Research Institute
Providence Cancer Institute
Portland, Oregon
United States

David A. Bitonti, DMD
Clinical Associate Professor
Department of Surgery
F. Edward Hébert School of Medicine, Uniformed Services University of the Health Sciences
Bethesda, Maryland;
Dental Service Chief
Oral and Maxillofacial Surgeon
Hampton Veterans Affairs Medical Center
Hampton, Virginia
United States

Behnam Bohluli, DMD, FRCD(C)
Clinical Instructor
Oral and Maxillofacial Surgery
University of Toronto
Toronto, Ontario
Canada

Genevieve C. Bonin, BSc, MASc, DMD, FRCD(c), Dipl. ABOMS
Oral and Maxillofacial surgeon
Department of Oral and Maxillofacial Surgery
Verdun Hospital, University of Montreal
Montreal, Quebec
Canada

Gary F. Bouloux, MD, DDS, MDSc, FRACDS, FRACDS(OMS), FRCS (Eng), FACS
J. David Allen Family Professor
Division Chief
Oral and Maxillofacial Surgery
Department of Surgery
Emory University School of Medicine
Atlanta, Georgia
United States

Meaghan Bradley, DMD
Oral and Maxillofacial Surgery
Boston University
Boston, Massachusetts
United States

Omar Breik, BDSc (Hons) MBBS, MClinSc, FRACDS (OMS)
Consultant Maxillofacial/Head and Neck Surgeon
Department of Oral and Maxillofacial Surgery
Royal Brisbane and Women's Hospital;
Senior Lecturer
School of Dentistry/School of Medicine
University of Queensland
Brisbane, Queensland
Australia

Hans C. Brockhoff II, DDS, MD, FACS
Chief, Oral/Head and Neck Oncology and Microvascular Reconstructive Surgery
Oral and Maxillofacial Surgery
El Paso Children's Hospital, University Medical Center of El Paso;
Assistant Professor
Department of Surgery
Texas Tech University Health Sciences Center;
Program Director
El Paso Head & Neck and Microvascular Surgery Fellowship;
High Desert Oral & Facial Surgery
El Paso, Texas
United States

Daniel Buchbinder, DMD, MD
Professor and System Chief, Division of Maxillofacial Surgery
Department of Otolaryngology, Head and Neck Surgery
Icahn School of Medicine at Mount Sinai
New York, New York
United States

Tuan G. Bui, MD, DMD
Affiliate Assistant Professor
Oral and Maxillofacial Surgery
Oregon Health and Sciences University;
Head and Neck Surgical Associates
Portland, Oregon
United States

Patrick Byrne, MD, MBA
Chairman
The Head and Neck Institute
Cleveland Clinic
Cleveland, Ohio
United States

John Francis Caccamese Jr., MD, DMD, FACS
Professor and Vice Chairman
Oral-Maxillofacial Surgery
University of Maryland Dental School;
Clinical Professor
Pediatrics and Otorhinolaryngology
University of Maryland School of Medicine;
Co-Director
Randolph B. Capone Cleft Program at GBMC;
Adjunct Professor
Bioengineering
University of Maryland;
Baltimore, Maryland
United States

Ron Caloss, DDS, MD
Private Practice
Aligned Oral and Facial Surgery
Baptist Medical Center;
Professor
Oral and Maxillofacial Surgery
University of Mississippi Medical Center
Jackson, Mississippi
United States

Courtney Caplin, MD, DMD
Cosmetic Surgery Affiliates;
Clinical Assistant Professor
Oral and Maxillofacial Surgery
University of Oklahoma
Oklahoma City, Oklahoma
United States

Eric R. Carlson, DMD, MD, EdM, FACS
Professor and Kelly L. Krahwinkel Chairman
Department of Oral and Maxillofacial Surgery
University of Tennessee Graduate School of Medicine;
Director
Oral/Head and Neck Oncologic Surgery Fellowship
University of Tennessee Cancer Institute
Knoxville, Tennessee
United States

Nardy Casap, DMD, MD
Professor
Oral and Maxillofacial Surgery
Hebrew University-Hadassah Medical Center
Jerusalem, Israel

Carrie E. Cera Hill, MD, MBA
Pure Dermatology PLLC
Denver, Colorado
United States

Swagnik Chakrabarti, MBBS, MS, MCh
Chairperson
Chandan Cancer Institute
Lucknow, Uttar Pradesh
India

Ravi Chandran, DMD, PhD, FACS
Chairman and Residency Director
Oral and Maxillofacial Surgery/Pathology
University of Mississippi Medical Center
Jackson, Mississippi
United States

Blake Chaney, DDS, MD
Oral and Maxillofacial Surgery
University of Pittsburgh
Pittsburgh, Pennsylvania
United States

Allen C. Cheng, MD, DDS, FACS
Medical Director
Head and Neck Surgical Associates
Head and Neck Surgery;
Attending Surgeon
Providence Oral, Head and Neck
Providence Health;
Assistant Professor
Oral and Maxillofacial Surgery
Oregon Health Sciences University;
Medical Director
Oral/Head and Neck Oncology
Legacy Good Samaritan
Portland, Oregon
United States

Radhika Chigurupati, DMD, MS
Associate Professor
Oral and Maxillofacial Surgery
Boston University
Boston, Massachusetts
United States

Nam Cho, DDS, MD
Assistant Clinical Professor
Oral & Maxillofacial Surgery
Ostrow School of Dentistry
Los Angeles, California
United States

Joli Chou, DMD, MD
Associate Professor
Department of Oral and Maxillofacial Surgery
Sidney Kimmel Medical College
Thomas Jefferson University
Philadelphia, Pennsylvania
United States

Louis J. Christensen, DDS
Oral & Maxillofacial Surgery
HealthPartners;
Department of Oral & Maxillofacial Surgery
Regions Hospital
Saint Paul, Minnesota;
Assistant Clinical Professor
Division of Oral & Maxillofacial Surgery
University of Minnesota School of Dentistry
Minneapolis, Minnesota
United States

Joseph E. Cillo Jr., DMD, MPH, PhD, FACS
Division Chief and Program Director
Oral and Maxillofacial Surgery
Allegheny General Hospital;
Associate Professor
Oral and Maxillofacial Surgery
Allegheny General Hospital
Pittsburgh, Pennsylvania
United States

Scott T. Claiborne, DDS, MD
Minnesota Oral and Facial Surgery
Co-Fellowship Director
Oral/Head and Neck Oncologic and Reconstructive Surgery
Minneapolis, Minnesota
United States

David Collette, DMD, MD
Medical Director
The Oral Surgery Center Of Albuquerque
Albuquerque, New Mexico
United States

Gisela Contasti-Bocco, DDS
Assistant Professor
Orthodontics Department
Nova Southern University
Fort Lauderdale, Florida
United States

Bernard J. Costello, DMD, MD, FACS
Associate Dean for Faculty Affairs
Professor and Fellowship Program Director
Department of Oral and Maxillofacial Surgery
University of Pittsburgh, School of Dental Medicine;
Chief
Pediatric Oral and Maxillofacial Surgery Children's Hospital of Pittsburgh;
Professor and Fellowship Program Director
Department of Oral and Maxillofacial Surgery
University of Pittsburgh Medical Center Eye and Ear Institute UPMC
Pittsburgh, Pennsylvania
United States

Sebastian Cotofana, MD, PhD
Associate Professor of Anatomy
Department of Clinical Anatomy
Mayo Clinic
Rochester, Minnesota
United States

Marcus A. Couey, DDS, MD
Assistant Professor
Department of Oral and Maxillofacial Surgery
Boston University
Boston, Massachusetts
United States

Larry Cunningham Jr., MD, DDS
Professor and Chair
Oral and Maxillofacial Surgery
University of Pittsburgh School of Dental Medicine
Pittsburgh, Pennsylvania
United States

William J. Curtis, DMD, MD
Oral and Maxillofacial Surgery
Northern Nevada Oral & Maxillofacial Surgery
Reno, Nevada
United States

Angelo L. Cuzalina, MD, DDS
Cosmetic Surgery
Private Practice
Tulsa Surgical Arts;
Adjunctive Faculty
OSU Medical School
Otolaryngology Department
Tulsa, Oklahoma
United States

Rushil R. Dang, BDS, DMD
Maxillofacial Oncology and Reconstructive Surgery Fellow
Oral and Maxillofacial Surgery
Boston Medical Center and Boston University
Boston, Massachusetts
United States

Renie Daniel, MD, DMD, FACS
Assistant Professor
Department of Oral & Maxillofacial Surgery
The University of North Carolina
Chapel Hill, North Carolina
United States

David J. Dattilo, DDS
Director of Oral and Maxillofacial Surgery (Retired)
Allegheny Health System
Allegheny General
Hospital
Pittsburgh, Pennsylvania
United States;
Associate Professor of Surgery
Drexel University School of Medicine
Philadelphia, Pennsylvania
United States

Jeffrey S. Dean, DDS, MD, FACS
Oral and Maxillofacial Surgery
Dakota Dunes, South Dakota
United States

Shaun C. Desai, MD
Associate Professor
Facial Plastic and Reconstructive Surgery
Johns Hopkins University School of Medicine
Baltimore, Maryland
United States

Jasjit K. Dillon, MBBS, DDS, FDSRCS, FACS
Professor, Chief & Program Director
Oral & Maxillofacial Surgery
University of Washington
Seattle, Washington
United States

Jean-Charles Doucet, DMD, MD, MSc, FRCDC
Assistant Professor and Division Head of Oral and Maxillofacial Surgery
Oral and Maxillofacial Sciences
Dalhousie University;
Staff Surgeon
IWK Cleft Palate and Craniofacial Team
IWK Health Centre;
Staff Surgeon
Oral and Maxillofacial Surgery
QEII Health Science Centre
Halifax, Nova Scotia
Canada

Stephanie Joy Drew, DMD
Associate Professor
Emory School of Medicine
Atlanta, Georgia
United States

Donita Dyalram, DDS, MD, FACS
Associate Professor; Program Director/Associate Fellowship Director
Oral and Maxillofacial Surgery
University of Maryland Medical Center
Baltimore, Maryland
United States

Sean P. Edwards, DDS, MD
Clinical Associate Professor;
Director, Residency Program;
Chief, Pediatric Oral, and Maxillofacial Surgery
Oral and Maxillofacial Surgery/Hospital Dentistry
University of Michigan Health System
Ann Arbor, Michigan
United States

Hany Emam, BDS, MS, FACS
Associate Professor and Interim Chair
Oral and Maxillofacial Surgery
The Ohio State University College of Dentistry
Columbus, Ohio
United States

Max R. Emmerling, MD, DDS
Division of Oral and Maxillofacial Surgery
Cook County Health
Chicago, Illinois
United States

Mark Engelstad, DDS, MD, MHI
Associate Professor
Oral & Maxillofacial Surgery
Oregon Health & Science University
Portland, Oregon
United States

Helaman Erickson, DDS, MD, FACS
Oral and Maxillofacial Surgery
Permian Basin Oral Surgery and Dental Implant Center
Midland, Texas
United States

Maria Evasovich, MD
Associate Professor
Department of Surgery
University of Minnesota
Minneapolis, Minnesota
United States

Adam P. Fagin, DMD, MD
Private Practice
Peninsula Oral and Facial Surgery
San Mateo, California
United States

Christopher A. Fanelli, DDS, FRCD(C)
Private Practice
Interface—Centre for OMFS
London, Ontario
Canada;
Attending Surgeon—Consultant
Surgery—Oral Maxillofacial Surgery
London Health Sciences Centre, St Thomas Elgin General Hospital
St. Thomas, Ontario
Canada

Joseph J. Fantuzzo, MD, DDS, FACS
Clinical Associate Professor
Oral & Maxillofacial Surgery
University of Rochester Medical Center
Rochester, New York
United States

Tirbod Fattahi, DDS, MD, FACS
Professor and Chair
Department of Oral and Maxillofacial Surgery
University of Florida, College of Medicine
Jacksonville, Florida
United States

Rui P. Fernandes, MD, DMD, FACS, FRCS (Ed)
Professor
OMS, Neurosurgery, Orthopedic, Surgery
University of Florida College of Medicine
Jacksonville, Florida
United States

Richard Allen Finn, DDS
Professor
Surgery—Div OMFS
UTSWMC;
Chief
OMFS
Veteran's Administration North Texas
Dallas, Texas
United States

Peter B. Franco, DMD, FACS
Carolinas Center for Oral and Facial Surgery
Charlotte, North Carolina
United States

David Gailey, DDS, FACS
Surgical Cleft Director
Pediatric Surgery
Providence Children's Hospital;
President
Inland Oral Surgery
Spokane, Washington
United States

Pooja Gangwani, DDS, MPH
Assistant Professor
Oral and Maxillofacial Surgery
University of Rochester Medical Center
Rochester, New York
United States

Ghali E. Ghali, DDS, MD, FACS, FRCS(Ed)
Director
Oral and Maxillofacial Surgery
Willis Knighton Health System
Shreveport, Louisiana
United States

Waleed Gibreel, MBBS
Assistant Professor
Craniofacial Surgery
Division of Plastic Surgery
Mayo Clinic
Rochester, Minnesota
United States

Sabine C. Girod, MD, DDS, PhD, FACS
Professor Emeritus
Department of Surgery
School of Medicine, Stanford University
Stanford, California
United States

Brent Golden, DDS, MD, FACS
Fellowship Program Director
Pediatric Craniomaxillofacial Surgery
Orlando Health Arnold Palmer Medical Center
Orlando, Florida
United States

Jorge Gonzalez, DDS
Private Practice
Advanced Dental Implant Solutions
Fort Worth, Texas
United States

Marianela Gonzalez, DDS, MS
Clinical Associate Professor and Director
Oral and Maxillofacial Surgery
Texas A&M Health Science Center, College of Dentistry
Baylor University Dallas, Texas
United States

Eric J. Granquist, DMD, MD
Assistant Professor
Oral and Maxillofacial Surgery
University of Pennsylvania;
Director
UPenn Center For Temporomandibular Joint Disorders
Hospital of the University of Pennsylvania
Philadelphia, Pennsylvania
United States

Jaime Grant, MBChB, BDS (Hons), MRCS (Ed), FRCS (Ed) (OMFS)
Consultant Craniofacial/Maxillofacial Surgeon
Craniofacial/Maxillofacial Surgery
Birmingham Children's Hospital/Queen Elizabeth University Hospital
Birmingham, United Kingdom

Mingyang Liu Gray, MD, MPH
Resident Physician
Otolaryngology—Head and Neck Surgery
Icahn School of Medicine at Mount Sinai
New York, New York
United States

Cesar A. Guerrero, DDS
Private Practice
ClearChoice Houston
The Heights Hospital
Houston, Texas
United States

Danny Hadaya, DDS, PhD
Resident
Oral and Maxillofacial Surgery
UCLA School of Dentistry
Los Angeles, California
United States

David Hamlar, MD, DDS
Assistant Professor
Otolaryngology/Head and Neck Surgery
University of Minnesota Medical Center
Minneapolis, Minnesota
United States

Daniel A. Hammer, DDS, FACD, FACS
Vice Chair and Director of Research
Department of Oral and Maxillofacial Surgery and Dentistry
Naval Medical Center San Diego
San Diego, California;
Associate Professor of Surgery
Department of Surgery
Uniformed Services University
Bethesda, Maryland;
Voluntary Clinical Assistant Professor of Surgery
Department of Otolaryngology
UC San Diego School of Medicine,
San Diego, California
United States

Curtis Hanba, MD
Otolaryngology—Head and Neck Surgery
The University of Minnesota
Minneapolis, Minnesota
United States

Andrew Alistair Heggie, AM, MBBS, MDSc, BDSc, FRACDS (OMS), FFDRSC(I), FRCS (Ed)
Clinical Professor, Oral and Maxillofacial Surgery
Department of Plastic and Maxillofacial Surgery
Royal Children's Hospital of Melbourne
Parkville, Victoria
Australia

Mariana Henriquez, DDS
Santa Rosa Maxillofacial Surgery Center
Central University of Venezuela
Caracas, Venezuela

Andrew Henry, DMD, MD
Assistant Professor
Associate Director of Residency Training
Department of Oral and Maxillofacial Surgery
Boston University Goldman School of Dental Medicine
Boston, Massachusetts
United States

Alan S. Herford, DDS, MD
Chairman and Professor
Oral and Maxillofacial Surgery
Loma Linda University
Loma Linda, California
United States

Brandyn Herman, DMD
Assistant Professor
Oral and Maxillofacial Surgery
University of Kentucky College of Dentistry
Lexington, Kentucky
United States

David Hinkl, DMD
Oral and Maxillofacial Surgery
University of Oklahoma
Oklahoma City, Oklahoma
United States

Anthony David Holmes, AO, MB.BS, FRACS
Diplomate, American Board of Plastic Surgery
Clinical Professor, University of Melbourne
Dept. of Plastic and Maxillofacial Surgery
Royal Children's Hospital
Melbourne, Victoria
Australia

James B. Holton, DDS, MSD
Staff
Oral and Maxillofacial Surgery
UT Health Tyler
Tyler, Texas
United States

Mehran Hossaini-Zadeh, DMD
Professor and Chair
Oral and Maxillofacial Surgery
Temple University School of Dentistry
Philadelphia, Pennsylvania
United States

Reem H. Hossameldin, BDS, MSc, PhD
Associate Professor
Oral and Maxillofacial Surgery
Faculty of Dentistry, Cairo University
Cairo, Egypt

Tsung-yen Hsieh, MD
Assistant Professor
Department of Otolaryngology—Head & Neck Surgery, Division of Facial Plastic & Reconstructive Surgery
University of Cincinnati College of Medicine
Cincinnati, Ohio
United States

Allen Huang, DDS, MD
Assistant Professor
Oral and Maxillofacial Surgery
University of Southern California
Los Angeles, California
United States

Pamela J. Hughes, DDS
Oral and Maxillofacial Surgery
Kaiser Permanente
Portland, Oregon
United States

Tanisha Hutchinson, MD
Facial Plastic Surgery
Glasgold Group
Princeton, New Jersey
United States

Matthew R. Idle, BDS (Hons), MFDS, MBChB, FRCS (OMFS)
Consultant
Oral and Maxillofacial/Head and Neck Surgery
University Hospitals Birmingham
Birmingham, United Kingdom

Shyam Sunder Indrakanti, DDS, MD
Private Practice
Department of Oral and Maxillofacial Surgery
Parkland Memorial Hospital
Dallas, Texas
United States

Michael Jaskolka, DDS, MD, FACS
Director, Maxillofacial Surgery
Director, Cleft and Craniofacial Program
Physician Executive, Novant Health, Children's Institute, Coastal Region
Novant Health, New Hanover Regional Medical Center
Wilmington, North Carolina
United States

Jonathan James Jelmini, DDS, MD
Department of Oral and Maxillofacial Surgery
Oregon Health & Sciences University;
Resident
Trauma and Oral and Maxillofacial Surgery Service
Legacy Emanuel Medical Center
Portland, Oregon
United States

Ole T. Jensen, DDS, MS
Adjunct Professor
Department of Oral and Maxillofacial Surgery
School of Dentistry, University of Utah
Salt Lake City, Utah
United States

Ashok R. Jethwa, MD
Head and Neck Surgical Oncology/Microvascular Reconstruction
Otolaryngology
University of Minnesota
Minneapolis, Minnesota
United States

Baxter Jones, DDS
Resident
Department of Oral and Maxillofacial Surgery
Carle Foundation Hospital
Urbana, Illinois
United States

Deepak Kademani, DMD, MD, FACS
President and Medical Director
Minnesota Oral & Facial Surgery
Fellowship Director
Oral/Head & Neck Oncologic and Reconstructive Surgery
Minneapolis, Minnesota
United States

David R. Kang, MD, DDS
Medical Director
Surgery, Head & Neck Surgery
Methodist Dallas Medical Center
Dallas, Texas
United States

Herman Kao, DDS, MD
Vice Chairman
Oral and Maxillofacial Surgery
John Peter Smith Health Network;
Associate Professor
Surgery
TCU and UNTHSC Medical School
Fort Worth, Texas
United States

Vasiliki Karlis, DMD, MD, FACS
Associate Professor
Director OMS Training Program
Department of Oral and Maxillofacial Surgery
College of Dentistry
New York University
Bellevue Hospital Center
New York, New York
United States

Beomjune Kim, DMD, MD, FACS
Head and Neck/Microvascular Surgeon
Cancer Treatment Centers of America – Part of City of Hope
Newnan, Georgia
United States

D. David Kim, DMD, MD, FACS
Jack W. Gamble Endowed Chairman
Oral and Maxillofacial/Head and Neck Surgery
Louisiana State University Health Sciences Center Shreveport;
Edward and Freda Green Endowed Professor
Oral and Maxillofacial/Head and Neck Surgery
LSU Health Science Center Shreveport;
Fellowship Director, Head and Neck Oncology and Microvascular Reconstruction
Oral and Maxillofacial Surgery
LSU Health Science Center Shreveport
Shreveport, Louisiana
United States

Roderick Y. Kim, DDS, MD, MBA, FACS
Director of Research, Co-Fellowship Director, Vice Division Director
Oral and Maxillofacial Surgery
John Peter Smith Health Network;
Assistant Professor
Surgery
Texas Christian University
Fort Worth, Texas
United States

Paul Kloostra, DDS, MD
Fellowship Director
Cleft & Craniofacial Surgery
Charleston Area Medical Center
Charleston, West Virginia
United States

Antonia Kolokythas, DDS, MSc, MSed, FACS
Professor and Chair
Department of Oral and Maxillofacial Surgery
Augusta Univerity
Dental College of Georgia
Augusta, Georgia
United States

David A. Koppel, MB, BS, BDS, FDS, FRCS
Associate Professor
Faculty of Medicine/Faculty of Dental Medicine & Oral Health Sciences
McGill University
Montreal, Quebec
Canada

Deepak G. Krishnan, DDS, FACS
Associate Professor—Surgery
Division of Oral Maxillofacial Surgery, Department of Surgery
University of Cincinnati;
Oral Maxillofacial Surgeon
Division of Oral Maxillofacial Surgery
Department of Surgery
Cincinnati Children's Hospital and Medical Center
Cincinnati, Ohio
United States

Moni A. Kuriakose, MD, FRCS
Professor and Director
Surgical Oncology Chief Head and Neck Oncology
Mazumdar Shaw Cancer Center;
Director
Mazumdar Shaw Centre for Translational Research
Narayana Health Center
Bangalore, Karnataka
India

Li Han Lai, DDS
Oral and Maxillofacial Surgery
University of Washington
Seattle, Washington
United States

Zvi Laster, DMD
Maxillofacial Surgery Department
Poriya Governmental Hospital
Tiberias, Israel

Amir Laviv, DMD, MPH
Senior Lecturer
Department of Oral & Maxillofacial Surgery
Tel-Aviv University
Tel Aviv, Israel

Andrew W. C. Lee, MSc, DDS, MD, FRCD(C), FACS
Argyle Associates Oral & Maxillofacial Surgery
Department of Surgery
The Ottawa Hospital;
Lecturer
Faculty of Medicine
University of Ottawa
Ottawa, Canada

James B. Lewallen, DDS, MD, MSc
Private Practice
Southern Oral and Facial Surgery
Franklin, Tennessee
United States;
Affiliate Staff
Oral and Maxillofacial Surgery
Vanderbilt University Medical Center
Nashville, Tennessee
United States

Stanley Yung-Chuan Liu, MD, DDS, FACS
Associate Professor of Otolaryngology
And by Courtesy, of Plastic & Reconstructive Surgery
Director, Sleep Surgery Fellowship
Service Chief, Maxillofacial Surgery
Stanford University School of Medicine
Stanford, California
United States

Christian A. Loetscher, DDS, MS
Private Practice
Oral & Maxillofacial Surgery
Atlanta Oral & Maxillofacial Surgery, PC
Alpharetta, Georgia
United States

Patrick J. Louis, DDS, MD
Professor
Oral & Maxillofacial Surgery
University of Alabama at Birmingham;
Chairman
Oral & Maxillofacial Surgery
University of Alabama at Birmingham
Birmingham, Alabama
United States

Joshua E. Lubek, MD, DDS, FACS
Professor & Fellowship Director
Oral-Head & Neck Surgery/Microvascular Surgery
Marlene & Stewart Greenebaum Comprehensive Cancer Center &
Department of Oral & Maxillofacial Surgery
University of Maryland
Baltimore, Maryland
United States

Ricardo Lugo, DDS, MD
Assistant Clinical Professor
Department of Oral & Maxillofacial Surgery
University of California, San Francisco & Alameda Health System
Oakland, California
United States

Sofia Lyford-Pike, MD
Associate Professor
Otolaryngology Head and Neck Surgery
University of Minnesota
Minneapolis, Minnesota
United States

George M. Kushner, DMD, MD, FACS
Professor and Chairman
Oral and Maxillofacial Surgery
University of Louisville School of Dentistry
Louisville, Kentucky
United States

Colin MacIver, MBChB, FRCS, BDS, FDS, FRCS (Ed), FRCS (OMFS)
Consultant Maxillofacial/Head and Neck Surgeon
Maxillofacial Surgery
SSMC/Mayo Clinic Abu Dhabi;
Adjunct Professor
Department of Surgery
Khalifa University
Abu Dhabi
United Arab Emirates

Stephen P. R. MacLeod, BDS, MB ChB, FDSRCS (ED&ENG), FRCS (ED), FFSTRCS (ED), FACS
Joseph R and Louise Ada Jarabak Professor of Surgery
Oral and Maxillofacial Surgery
Loyola University Medical Center
Maywood, Illinois
United States

Caitlin B. L. Magraw, MD, DDS, FACS
The Head and Neck Institute
Head and Neck Surgical Associates;
Associate Clinical Professor
Oral and Maxillofacial Surgery
Oregon Health and Sciences University
Portland, Oregon
United States

Nicholas M. Makhoul, BSc, DMD, MD, FRCD(C), FACS Dip ABOMS
Chair, Associate Dean
Oral and Maxillofacial Surgery
McGill University;
Associate Professor
Faculty of Dentistry
McGill University
Montreal, Quebec
Canada

Ashley E. Manlove, DMD, MD, FACS
Residency Program Director
Oral and Maxillofacial Surgery
Carle Foundation Hospital;
Director Cleft Lip and Palate Team
Oral and Maxillofacial Surgery
Carle Foundation Hospital
Urbana, Illinois
United States

Samir Mardini, MD
Professor and Chair
Plastic Surgery
Mayo Clinic
Rochester, Minnesota
United States

Michael R. Markiewicz, DDS, MD, MPH, FAAP, FACS, FRCD(c)
Professor and Chair
School of Dental Medicine
Oral and Maxillofacial Surgery
Clinical Professor
Department of Neurosurgery and Department of Surgery
Jacobs School of Medicine and Biomedical Sciences
University at Buffalo
Co-Director
Craniofacial Center of Western New York
John R. Oishei Children's Hospital
Attending Surgeon
Department of Head & Neck and Plastic & Reconstructive Surgery
Roswell Park Comprehensive Cancer Center
Buffalo, New York
United States

Jeffrey S. Marschall, DMD, MD, MS
Pediatric Craniomaxillofacial Surgery
Arnold Palmer Hospital for Children
Orlando, Florida
United States

Nigel Shaun Matthews, BDS, FDS, MBBS, FRCS, FRCS (OMFS)
Clinical Professor and Chairman
Associate Dean for Hospital Affairs
Director, TMJ Institute
Department of Oral and Maxillofacial Surgery
Indiana University School of Dentistry
Indianapolis, Indiana
United States

Joseph P. McCain, DMD, FACS
Oral & Maxillofacial Surgery
Massachusetts General Hospital—Harvard
Boston, Massachusetts
United States

J. Michael McCoy, DDS, FACS
Professor
Oral and Maxillofacial Surgery;
Professor
Pathology;
Professor
Radiology;
Medical Director
In-Patient Hyperbaric Oxygen Therapy
University of Tennessee Graduate School of Medicine
Knoxville, Tennessee
United States

Samuel J. McKenna, DDS, MD, FACS
Professor and Chairman
Oral and Maxillofacial Surgery
Vanderbilt University Medical Center
Nashville, Tennessee
United States

Daniel J. Meara, MS, MD, DMD, MHCDS, FACS
Chair
Oral and Maxillofacial Surgery & Hospital Dentistry
Christiana Care Health System;
Director of Research
Oral and Maxillofacial Surgery
Christiana Care Health System
Wilmington, Delaware;
Affiliate Faculty
Physical Therapy
University of Delaware
Newark, Delaware
United States

Paulo Jose Medeiros, DDS, MS, PhD
Professor and Chairman
Oral and Maxillofacial Surgery
Rio De Janiero State University
Rio De Janiero, Brazil

Pushkar Mehra, BDS, DMD, MS, FACS
Professor and Chair
Oral and Maxillofacial Surgery
Boston University Medical Center
Boston, Massachusetts
United States

Louis G. Mercuri, DDS, MS
Visiting Professor
Orthopaedic Surgery
Rush University Medical Center
Chicago Illinois
United States;
Consultant
Clinical Affairs
TMJ Concepts
Ventura, California
United States

Brett A. Miles, DDS, MD, FACS
Professor and Chair
Otolaryngology/Head and Neck Surgery
Northwell Health/Lenox Hill/Manhattan Eye Ear Hospital
New York, New York
United States

Meagan Miller, DDS
Oral and Maxillofacial Surgery
Loma Linda University
Loma Linda, California
United States

Justine Moe, MD, DDS, FRCDC, FACS
Clinical Assistant Professor and Residency Program Director
Oral and Maxillofacial Surgery
University of Michigan
Ann Arbor, Michigan
United States

Hwi Sean Moon, MD, DDS
Cleft and Craniofacial Surgery
El Paso Children's Hospital
El Paso, Texas
United States

Marina Morante Silva, MD, FEBOMFS
Department of Oral and Maxillofacial Surgery
University of Florida, College of Medicine
Jacksonville, Florida
United States

Christopher Morris, DDS, MD, FACS
Private Practice
Katy Center for Oral and Facial Surgery
Katy, Texas
United States

Dean Morton, BDS, MS
Professor
Department of Prosthodontics
Director
Center for Implant, Esthetic and Innovative Dentistry
Indiana University School of Dentistry
Indianapolis, Indiana
United States

Reza Movahed, DMD, FACS
Clinical Assistant Professor
Department of Orthodontics
Saint Louis University
Saint Louis, Missouri
United States

Elena Mujica, DDS
Private Practice
Santa Rosa Maxillofacial Surgery
Caracas, Venezuela

Robert Nadeau, DDS, MD, FACS
Interim Division Director and Program Director for Oral and Maxillofacial Surgery
Department of Developmental and Surgical Sciences
University of Minnesota;
Surgical Service Lead, OMS
M Health Fairview Hospitals and Clinics
Minneapolis, Minnesota
United States

John M. Nathan, MD, DDS
Division of Oral and Maxillofacial Surgery
Mayo Clinic
Rochester, Minnesota
United States

Gregory M. Ness, DDS, FACS
Professor Emeritus—Clinical
Oral and Maxillofacial Surgery and Anesthesiology
The Ohio State University College of Dentistry
Columbus, Ohio
United States

Craig Norbutt, DMD, MD
Assistant Clinical Professor
Oral & Maxillofacial Surgery
Carle Foundation Hospital
Champaign, Illinois
United States

Erik Jon Nuveen, MD, DMD, FAACS
Director of Fellowship
Cosmetic Surgery Affiliates
Oklahoma City, Oklahoma and Jacksonville Beach, Florida;
Voluntary Assistant Professor
Oral and Maxillofacial Surgery
The University of Oklahoma College of Dentistry
Oklahoma City, Oklahoma
United States

George Obeid, DDS
Senior Attending
Oral and Maxillofacial Surgery
Medstar Washington Hospital Center
Washington, District of Columbia
United States

Devin Joseph Okay, DDS
Attending Faculty
Department of Otolaryngology Head and Neck Surgery
Mount Sinai Health System;
Director
Division of Prosthodontics and Maxillofacial Prosthetics
Mount Sinai Health System
New York, New York
United States

Petra Olivieri, DMD, MD
Clinical Assistant Professor
Case Western Reserve University
MetroHealth Hospital
Department of Oral and Maxillofacial Surgery
Cleveland, Ohio
United States

Robert Ord, MB, BCh (Hons), BDS, FRCS, FACS, MS, MBA
Professor and Chairman
Oral and Maxillofacial Surgery
University of Maryland;
Professor
Oncology Program
Greenbaum Cancer Center
Baltimore, Maryland
United States

Daniel Oreadi, DMD
Associate Professor
Oral and Maxillofacial Surgery
Tufts University School of Dental Medicine
Boston, Massachusetts
United States

Neeraj Panchal, DDS, MD, MA
Assistant Professor
Oral and Maxillofacial Surgery
University of Pennsylvania;
Section Chief
Oral and Maxillofacial Surgery
Penn Presbyterian Medical Center;
Section Chief
Oral and Maxillofacial Surgery
Philadelphia Veterans Affairs Medical Center
Philadelphia, Pennsylvania
United States

Sat Parmar, BChD, BMBS, BMedSci, FDSRCS, FRCS Mr
Oral and Maxillofacial Surgery
University Hospitals Birmingham
Birmingham, United Kingdom

Ashish A. Patel, MD, DDS, FACS
Fellowship Director
Head and Neck Surgical Oncology and Microvascular Surgery
Providence Cancer Institute;
Director of Reconstructive Microsurgery
Head and Neck Institute
Head and Neck Surgical Associates;
Medical Director
Cranio-Oral and Maxillofacial and Neck Trauma
Legacy Emanuel Medical Center
Portland, Oregon
United States

Zachary S. Peacock, DMD, MD, FACS
Associate Professor of Oral and Maxillofacial Surgery
Massachusetts General Hospital
Harvard School of Dental Medicine
Boston, Massachusetts
United States

Karl Pennau, DDS
Oral & Maxillofacial Surgery
Oral Surgery Associates of Colorado Springs
Colorado Springs, Colorado
United States

Vincent J. Perciaccante, DDS, FACS
Adjunct Associate Professor
Department of Surgery, Division of Oral & Maxillofacial Surgery
Emory University School of Medicine
Atlanta, Georgia
United States;
Private Practice
South Oral and Maxillofacial Surgery
Peachtree City, Georgia
United States

Jon D. Perenack, MD, DDS
Adjunct Associate Clinical Professor and Director of Fellowship in Facial Cosmetic Surgery
Oral and Maxillofacial Surgery
Louisiana State University;
Medical and Surgical Director
Williamson Cosmetic Center and Perenack Esthetic Surgery
Baton Rouge, Louisiana
United States

Yuliya Petukhova, DDS
Oral and Maxillofacial Surgery Resident
Oral and Maxillofacial Surgery
Mayo Clinic
Rochester, Minnesota
United States

Laurence D. Pfeiffer, MD, DDS
Oral and Maxillofacial Surgeon
Department of Dentistry
Bassett Medical Center
Cooperstown, New York
United States

Matthew H. Pham, DMD, MD
Private Practice
Carolina's Center for Oral & Facial Surgery
Columbia, South Carolina
United States

John N. Phelan, PhD
Associate Professor (Retired)
Cell Biology
UT Southwestern Medical School
Dallas, Texas
United States

Joan Pi-Anfruns, DMD
Assistant Clinical Professor
Oral and Maxillofacial Surgery/Restorative Dentistry
UCLA School of Dentistry
Los Angeles, California
United States

Brendan H. G. Pierce, MD
Otolaryngology
Palo Alto Medical Foundation
Palo Alto, California
United States

Daniel Joseph Pinkston, DDS
ClearChoice Dental Implant Centers
St. Louis, Missouri
United States

Waldemar D. Polido, DDS, MS, PhD
Clinical Professor
Oral and Maxillofacial Surgery
Co-Director
Center for Implant, Esthetic and Innovative Dentistry
Indiana University School of Dentistry
Indianapolis, Indiana
United States

Jeffrey C. Posnick, DMD, MD, FRCS(C), FACS
Adjunct Professor
Plastic and Reconstructive Surgery
Johns Hopkins School of Medicine
Baltimore, Maryland
United States;
Professor Emeritus
Plastic and Reconstructive Surgery and Pediatrics
Georgetown University;
Professor
Oral and Maxillofacial Surgery
Howard University College of Dentistry
Washington DC, Washington
United States;
Professor of Orthodontics
University of Maryland
Baltimore College of Dental Surgery
Baltimore, Maryland
United States

David B. Powers, MD, DMD, FACS, FRCS (Ed)
Professor of Surgery
Director, Duke Craniomaxillofacial Trauma Program
Fellowship Director, Craniomaxillofacial Trauma and Reconstructive Surgery Fellowship
Vice Chair, Division of Plastic, Maxillofacial and Oral Surgery
Department of Surgery
Duke University Medical Center
Durham, North Carolina
United States

Janine Prange-Kiel, PhD
Associate Professor and Chief of Section of Anatomy
Department of Surgery
University of Texas Southwestern Medical Center
Dallas, Texas
United States

Prav Praveen, FRCS, MRCS, MBchBFDSRCS, FFDRCSI
Consultant Oral and Maxillofacial Surgeon
Oral and Maxillofacial Surgery
University Hospitals Birmingham NHS Trust
Birmingham, West Midlands
United Kingdom

David S. Precious, CM, DDS, MSc, FRCDC, FRCS, Dhc
Dean Emeritus and Professor
Oral and Maxillofacial Surgery
Dalhousie University
Halifax, Nova Scotia
Canada

Faisal A. Quereshy, MD, DDS, FACS
Professor/Program Director
Oral & Maxillofacial Surgery
Case Western Reserve University
Cleveland Ohio
United States;
Medical Director
Facial Cosmetic Surgery
Visage Surgical Institute/V-Spa
Medina, Ohio
United States

Peter D. Quinn, DMD, MD
Chief Executive Physician
University of Pennsylvania Health System
University of Pennsylvania;
Schoenleber Professor of Oral & Maxillofacial Surgery
University of Pennsylvania
School of Dental Medicine
Philadelphia, Pennsylvania
United States

Matthew Radant, MD, DDS
Assistant Clinical Professor
Department of Oral and Maxillofacial Surgery
The University of Oklahoma
Oklahoma City, Oklahoma
United States

Christopher K. Ray, DDS
Eastern Oklahoma Oral and Maxillofacial Surgeons;
Clinical Assistant Professor Department of Oral and Maxillofacial Surgery
The University of Oklahoma
Oklahoma City, Oklahoma
United States

Andrew Read-Fuller, DDS, MD, FACS, FACD
Clinical Assistant Professor and Graduate Program Director
Oral & Maxillofacial Surgery
Texas A&M University School of Dentistry
Dallas, Texas
United States

Likith Reddy, MD, DDS, FACS
Professor, Department Head
Oral and Maxillofacial Surgery
Texas A&M University School of Dentistry;
Section Chief
Oral & Maxillofacial Surgery
Baylor University Medical Center;
Clinical Professor
Texas A&M University School of Medicine
Dallas, Texas
United States

Shravan Renapurkar, BDS, DMD, FACS
Associate Professor
Oral and Maxillofacial Surgery
Virginia Commonwealth University
Richmond, Virginia
United States;
Program Director
Oral and Maxillofacial Surgery
Virginia Commonwealth University
Richmond, Virginia
United States

Johan P. Reyneke, B ChD, M ChD, FCMFOS (SA), PhD
Director
Centre for Orthognathic Surgery
Cape Town Mediclinic;
Extraordinary Professor
Maxillofacial and Oral Surgery
University of the Western Cape
Cape Town, South Africa;
Clinical Professor
Oral and Maxillofacial Surgery
University of Oklahoma
Oklahoma City, Oklahoma;
Clinical Professor
Oral and Maxillofacial Surgery
Florida University
Gainesville, Florida
United States

Fabio G. Ritto, DDS, MD, MS, PhD
Professor and Program Director
Oral and Maxillofacial Surgery
The University of Oklahoma Health Science Center
Oklahoma City, Oklahoma
United States

Carrie E. Robertson, MD
Associate Professor of Neurology
College of Medicine
Mayo Clinic
Rochester, Minnesota
United States

Jason Rogers, DDS
Oral and Maxillofacial Surgeon
Private Practice
Santa Rosa and Rohnert Park Oral Surgery
Santa Rosa, California
United States

Brian Louis Ruggiero, MD, DMD
Oral and Maxillofacial Surgery
University of Michigan
Ann Arbor, Michigan
United States

Ramon L. Ruiz, DMD, MD
Director
Pediatric Craniomaxillofacial Surgery
Arnold Palmer Hospital for Children;
Associate Professor
Department of Surgery
University of Central Florida College of Medicine
Orlando, Florida
United States

Mary Ann C. Sabino, DDS, PhD
Oral and Maxillofacial Surgery
Hennepin County Medical Center;
Adjunct Clinical Professor
Oral and Maxillofacial Surgery
University of Minnesota
Minneapolis, Minnesota
United States

Sepideh Sabooree, MD, DMD
Georgia Oral and Facial Reconstructive Surgery
Atlanta, Georgia
United States

Andrew Salama, MD, DDS, FACS
Chief
Oral and Maxillofacial Surgery
Northwell Health—Long Island Jewish Medical Center
New Hyde Park, New York
United States

Thomas J. Salinas, DDS
Professor
Dental Specialties
Mayo Clinic;
Professor
Department of Dental Specialties
Mayo Clinic
Rochester, Minnesota
United States

Nabil Samman, FRCS, FDSRCS
Formerly Professor of Oral and Maxillofacial Surgery
University of Hong Kong, Hong Kong
China

Sebastian Sauerbier, PhD, MD, DDS
Associate Professor
Department of Craniomaxillofacial Surgery
University Medical Center Freiburg
Freiburg, Germany

Thomas Schlieve, DDS, MD, FACS
Associate Professor
Residency Program Director
Department of Surgery, Division of Oral and Maxillofacial Surgery
UT Southwestern Medical Center
Parkland Memorial Hospital
Dallas, Texas
United States

Edward R. Schlissel, DDS, MS
Emeritus Professor
General Dentistry
School of Dental Medicine, Stony Brook University
Stony Brook, New York
United States

Rainer Schmelzeisen, MD, DDS, PhD, FRCS (London)
Medical Director Center of Dental Medicine
Department of Oral and Maxillofacial Surgery
University Medical Center Freiburg
Freiburg, Germany

Jocelyn M. Shand, MBBS (Melb), MDSc (Melb), BDS (Otago), FRACDS (OMS), FRCS (Edin), FDSRCS (Eng)
Head, Oral & Maxillofacial Surgery Program
Department of Plastic & Maxillofacial Surgery
The Royal Children's Hospital of Melbourne
Melbourne, Victoria
Australia

Kaushik H. Sharma, BDS, DMD, MPA
Adjunct Clinical Assistant Professor
Department of Oral & Maxillofacial Pathology, Medicine and Surgery
Temple University Kornberg School of Dentistry, Philadelphia
Pennsylvania
United States;
Oral/Head & Neck Oncologic and Microvascular Reconstructive Surgeon
Department of Oral and Maxillofacial Surgery
St Luke's University Hospital
Bethlehem, Pennsylvania
United States

Brett Shirley, DDS, MD, FACS
Oral and Maxillofacial Surgery
Ochsner LSU Health Science Center
Shreveport Louisiana
United States;
Maxillofacial Oncology and Reconstructive Surgery
John Peter Smith Hospital
Fort Worth, Texas
United States;
Oral and Maxillofacial Surgery
Piney Woods Oral and Maxillofacial Surgery
Nacogdoches, Texas
United States

Paul Shivers, MD, DMD
Clinical Instructor
Oral and Maxillofacial Surgery
University of Michigan
Ann Arbor, Michigan
United States

Raymond P. Shupak, MD, DMD, MBE
Assistant Professor
Geisinger Commonwealth School of Medicine
Department of Oral Medicine and Maxillofacial Surgery
Geisinger Health System
Danville, Pennsylvania
United States

Joseph E. Van Sickels, DDS, FACD, FICD, FACS
Professor and Program Director
Oral and Maxillofacial Surgery
University of Kentucky
Lexington, Kentucky
United States;
Robert D. Marciani Professor for Oral and Maxillofacial Surgery

Douglas P. Sinn, DDS
Clinical Professor
Department of Surgery, Division of Oral and Maxillofacial Surgery
UT Southwestern Medical Center
Dallas, Texas
United States

Kevin Smith, DDS, FACS, FACD
Professor and Residency Program Director
Oral and Maxillofacial Surgery
The University of Oklahoma;
Co-Director
JW Keys Cleft and Craniofacial Clinic
The University of Oklahoma, Oklahoma
City Oklahoma
United States;
Co-Director
MK Chapman Cleft and Craniofacial Clinic
The University of Tulsa
Tulsa, Oklahoma
United States

Miller H. Smith, DDS, MD, FRCD(C), FACS, FRCS (Edin)
Clinical Assistant Professor
Department of Surgery, Division of Oral Maxillofacial Surgery
Cumming School of Medicine—University of Calgary;
Private Practice
South Calgary Oral Maxillofacial Surgery
Calgary Alberta
Canada;
Clinical Assistant Professor
Faculty of Medicine & Dentistry
University of Alberta
Edmonton, Alberta
Canada

Luke C. Soletic, DDS, MD
Oral and Maxillofacial Surgery
NYU-Langone/Bellevue Hospital Center
New York University
Bellevue Hospital Center
New York, New York
United States

Joel Stanek, MD
Staff Physician
Otolaryngology - Head and Neck Surgery
Hennepin County Medical Center
Minneapolis, Minnesota
United States

David Stanton, MD, DMD (Deceased)
Associate Professor
Oral & Maxillofacial Surgery
University of Pennsylvania Health System;
Attending Surgeon
Oral & Maxillofacial Surgery
Children's Hospital of Philadelphia
Philadelphia, Pennsylvania
United States

Martin B. Steed, DDS, FACS
Professor and James B. Edwards Chair
Department of Oral and Maxillofacial Surgery
Medical University of South Carolina
James B. Edwards College of Dental Medicine
Charleston, South Carolina
United States

Mark Stevens, DDS
Professor Emeritus (Retired)
Department of Oral and Maxillofacial Surgery
Augusta University
Augusta, Georgia
United States

Marissa Suchyta, PhD
Research Fellow
Division of Plastic Surgery
Mayo Clinic
Rochester, Minnesota
United States

Steven M. Sullivan, DDS, FACS, FACD
Professor and Chair
Department of Surgical Sciences/Oral and Maxillofacial Surgery
University of Oklahoma College of Dentistry
Oklahoma City, Oklahoma
United States

Omotara Sulyman, MD
Otolaryngology
University of Minnesota
Minneapolis, Minnesota
United States

Srinivas M. Susarla, DMD, MD, FACS, FAAP
Associate Professor
Oral and Maxillofacial Surgery
University of Washington School of Dentistry;
Associate Professor
Surgery (Plastic)
University of Washington School of Medicine
Seattle, Washington
United States

David Knight Sylvester II, DDS
Assistant Clinical Professor
Oral & Maxillofacial Surgery
OU Health Sciences Center, Oklahoma
City Oklahoma
United States;
Private Practice Oral & Maxillofacial Surgeon
ClearChoice Dental Implant Centers
St. Louis, Missouri
United States

Jean-Claude Talmant, MD
Plastic Surgeon Head
Cleft Palate Team
Clinique Jules Verne
Nantes, France

Rahul Tandon, DMD, MD
Oral and Maxillofacial Surgeon
Private Practice
Hinsdale Oral & Maxillofacial Surgery
Hinsdale, Illinois
United States

Jayini Thakker, DDS, MD, FACS
Associate Professor, Program Director
Oral and Maxillofacial Surgery
Loma Linda University
Loma Linda, California
United States

Stone Thayer, MD, DMD, FACS
Assistant Professor
Plastic Surgery
Univ of California San Diego, San Diego
United States

Paul S. Tiwana, DDS, MD, MS, FACS, FACD
Francis J. Reichmann Professor and Chair
Division of Oral & Maxillofacial Surgery
College of Dentistry;
Professor
Department of Surgery
College of Medicine
The University of Oklahoma Health Sciences Center
Oklahoma City, Oklahoma
United States

Pasquale G. Tolomeo, MD, DDS
Cosmetic Surgery
Private Practice
Advanced Body Sculpting
Fall River, Massachusetts;
Cosmetic Surgery
Private Practice
Tulsa Surgical Arts
Tulsa, Oklahoma;
Adjunctive Faculty
Bellevue Oral & Maxillofacial Surgery
New York University
New York, New York
United States

Dan Q. Tran, DDS
Assistant Professor of Surgery
Oral and Maxillofacial Surgery
VCU Medical Center
Richmond, Virginia
United States

Trevor E. Treasure, DDS, MD, MBA, FRCD(C)
Assistant Professor
Oral and Maxillofacial Surgery
University of Texas-School of Dentistry
Houston, Texas
United States

David C. Trent, DDS, MD
Clinical Assistant Professor
Department of Oral and Maxillofacial Surgery
University of California—San Francisco
San Francisco California
United States;
Private Practice
Sacramento, California
United States

R. Gilbert Triplett, DDS, PhD
Regents Professor
Oral & Maxillofacial Surgery
Texas A&M University College of Dentistry
Dallas, Texas
United States

Greg Tull, DMD (Deceased)
Assistant Professor and Associate Program Director
Oral and Maxillofacial Surgery
University of Oklahoma
Oklahoma City, Oklahoma
United States

Michael D. Turner, DDS, MD, MSc, FACS
Associate Professor
Division of Oral and Maxillofacial Surgery
Icahn School of Medical School at Mount Sinai;
Chief of Oral and Maxillofacial Surgery
Division of Oral and Maxillofacial Surgery
Mount Sinai Hospital
New York, New York
United States

Timothy A. Turvey, DDS, FACS
Professor
Oral and Maxillofacial Surgery
University of North Carolina
Chapel Hill, North Carolina
United States

Rachel Uppgaard, DDS
Associate Professor
Developmental and Surgical Sciences
University of Minnesota
Minneapolis, Minnesota
United States

Craig E. Vigliante, DMD, MD
Oral and Maxillofacial Surgeon/Cosmetic Facial Surgeon
Private Practice
Potomac Surgical Arts, PC
Leesburg, Virginia;
Reston Advanced Oral & Cosmetic Facial Surgery, PLLC
Reston, Virginia
United States

Christopher F. Viozzi, MD, DDS, FACS
Consultant and Assistant Professor
Oral and Maxillofacial Surgery and Pediatric Adolescent Medicine
Mayo Clinic
Rochester, Minnesota
United States

John Vorrasi, DDS
Associate Professor, Program Director
Oral and Maxillofacial Surgery and Hospital Dentistry
University of Rochester
Rochester, New York
United States

Peter D. Waite, MPH, DDS, MD, FACS
Professor Emeritus
Oral and Maxillofacial Surgery
University of Alabama
Birmingham, Alabama
United States

Kenneth Wan, MBBS (1st Hons), BDSc (Hons), FRACDS (OMS)
Consultant in Oral & Maxillofacial Surgery
Fiona Stanley Hospital
Murdoch Western Australia
Australia;
Consultant
Oral and Maxillofacial Surgery
West Perth Oral & Maxillofacial Surgery
West Perth, Western Australia
Australia

Brent B. Ward, DDS, MD, FACS, FACD
Professor, Chair and Fellowship Program Director
Oral and Maxillofacial Surgery
University of Michigan
Ann Arbor, Michigan
United States

Todd R. Wentland, DDS, MD
Oral and Maxillofacial Surgery
John Peter Smith Hospital
Forth Worth, Texas;
Piney Woods Oral and Maxillofacial Surgery
Nacogdoches, Texas
United States

Fayette C. Williams, DDS, MD, FACS
Director, Division of Maxillofacial Oncology & Reconstructive Surgery
Oral & Maxillofacial Surgery
John Peter Smith Hospital
Fort Worth, Texas
United States

Jennifer E. Woerner, DMD, MD
Associate Professor
Department of Oral and Maxillofacial Surgery
Louisiana State University Health Sciences Center;
Fellowship Director of Craniofacial and Cleft Surgery
Department of Oral and Maxillofacial Surgery
Louisiana State University Health Sciences Center;
Associate Dean of Academic Affairs
School of Medicine
Louisiana State University Health Sciences Center
Shreveport, Louisiana
United States

Larry M. Wolford, DMD
Clinical Professor
Department of Oral and Maxillofacial Surgery
Texas A&M University College of Dentistry;
Clinical Professor
Department of Orthodontics
Texas A&M University College of Dentistry
Dallas, Texas
United States

Patrick Wong, DDS, MD
Oral and Maxillofacial Surgery
Texas A&M College of Dentistry
Dallas, Texas
United States

Brian M. Woo, DDS, MD, FACS
UCSF-Fresno/Community Medical Centers
Department of Oral and Maxillofacial Surgery
Program Director
Director Head and Neck Oncologic Surgery, Microvascular Reconstruction
Assistant Director Cleft Craniofacial Surgery
Fresno, California
United States

Mariusz K. Wrzosek, DMD, MD, FACS
Associate Professor
Oral & Maxillofacial Surgery
Loyola University Medical Center
Maywood, Illinois
United States

Duke Yamashita, DDS
Attending Staff
Plastic and Maxillofacial Surgery
Children Hospital Los Angeles
Los Angeles, California
United States;
Attending Staff
Dentistry, OMS
Rancho Los Amigos National Rehabilitation Center
Downey, California
United States

David M. Yates, DMD, MD, FACS
Division Chief of Cleft & Craniofacial Surgery
El Paso Children's Hospital
El Paso, Texas
United States

Melvyn Yeoh, DMD, MD
Associate Professor
Oral and Maxillofacial Surgery
University of Kentucky
Lexington, Kentucky
United States

Yedeh Ying, MD, DMD, FACS
Associate Professor
Oral and Maxillofacial Surgery
University of Alabama at Birmingham
Birmingham, Alabama
United States

George Zakhary, DDS, MD, FACS
Assistant Clinical Professor
Oral & Maxillofacial Surgery
University of California San Francisco
Fresno, California
United States

John R. Zuniga, DMD, MS, PhD
Robert V. Walker DDS Chair in Oral and Maxillofacial Surgery
Professor, Departments of Surgery and Neurology
University of Texas Southwestern
Dallas, Texas
United States

Foreword

2016 marked the introduction of the first edition of this comprehensive atlas of Oral and Maxillofacial Surgery and it quickly became the authoritative atlas for this discipline. Six years later (2022), the second edition of this treatise goes to press. Like all other surgical specialties, oral and maxillofacial surgery continues to rapidly evolve, and the new edition reflects the changing nature of surgery, the technological advances and the therapeutic modalities that have developed over this short timeframe. Why this atlas is titled Oral and Maxillofacial Surgery and not Craniomaxillofacial Surgery is bewildering. The title does not reflect the encompassing scope of surgery included in this book. This authoritative atlas will have appeal to multiple specialties from the traditional fields interested in facial, head, neck and oral surgery.

Having edited several textbooks involving multiple authors, I have experienced the complexities involved with the ambitious undertaking of this atlas. Deepak and Paul are very well organized and disciplined and have achieved success with this challenging task. They have recruited almost 300 contributors to provide 116 chapters for the new edition of this atlas. The work is divided into 13 sections which provides a comprehensive overview of the topics of: head and neck anatomy, oral surgery, implants, orthognathic surgery, craniofacial surgery, cleft lip and palate surgery, craniomaxillofacial trauma surgery, benign facial pathology surgery, malignant pathology involving the skull base, face and neck including the thyroid and parathyroid glands, reconstructive surgery including soft tissue, bone, cartilage, nerve, and facial transplantation, facial cosmetic surgery, TMJ surgery and obstructive sleep apnea surgery. This inclusive scope of practice is beyond most but embodies the multiple pathways available to contemporary surgeons wanting to pursue craniomaxillofacial surgery. The latest edition includes a separate section on obstructive sleep apnea surgery, which adds to the comprehensiveness of this edition. As with the first edition, the chapters are well illustrated and are encyclopedic.

Most of the authors are representative of the contemporary training of oral and maxillofacial surgeons including both dental and medical degrees, general surgery experience, as well as fellowship training. The commonality of most of the authors is their dental and medical background and surgical expertise dedicated exclusively to the head, face, oral cavity, and neck. Most of the chapters are co-authored by well known and experienced clinicians teamed with more nascent surgeons who are the future leaders of the specialty. Deepak and Paul are known internationally and have networked with many current and future leaders of the specialty. The international representation of the contributors (numerous countries on 6 continents) has an appealing draw and reflects the global practice of craniomaxillofacial surgery.

Deepak and Paul have similar educational backgrounds, credentials, and career pathways as well as being fellowship trained providers of surgical care. They are both very experienced clinicians and educators. Both have research experience, and both are active administratively with their respective institutions and with service commitments to multiple national and international organizations. Fellowship training pursued by Deepak was oncology and microvascular reconstruction, while Paul pursued fellowship in cleft and craniofacial surgery. The 2 editors have a dynamic synergism which is reflected in this high-quality comprehensive work. Their energy and enthusiasm for what they do is apparent. This atlas mirrors their love and dedication to their work, their patients, their residents and fellows, and to the future of craniomaxillofacial surgery.

by, Timothy A. Turvey, DDS, FACS

Foreword

I am honored to provide comment on the second edition of what I consider to be the most complete, and masterfully illustrated, atlas of oral and maxillofacial surgery ever published. This encyclopedic overview will enable our trainees, and practicing surgeons, to make evidence-based surgical decisions and afford our patients better outcomes. It is a stunning display in text, photographs, and illustration of the breadth and complexity of contemporary oral and maxillofacial surgery. A fledgling discipline that began formally in 1918 as "oral surgery," was propelled, in the first fifty years, by advances in office-based surgery, anesthesia, pharmacology, surgical instrumentation, sterile technique, and experiential wisdom gained from trauma surgery in two World Wars. Starting in the late '60s, and early '70s, our training programs were formalized and broadened to include more exposure to general surgery and surgical subspecialties. An explosion of knowledge in surgical instrumentation, reconstructive and craniofacial techniques, microsurgery, biomaterials, implants, and imaging in the last fifty years has brought us to the current state of our specialty. This remarkable tome is not only the quintessential reference in oral and maxillofacial surgery, but a testimonial to that century of progress.

Dr. Ira Rutkow in *American Surgery: An Illustrated History* stated that "there is no way to separate present day surgery, and one's own practice routines, from the experiences of all the surgeons and all the years that have gone before." This exceptional text brings an organized, consistent, visual pedagogic methodology covering office-based minor procedures to the most complicated head and neck reconstructive surgeries. In the late 19th century, the English novelist Samuel Butler once said, "Diseases come of their own accord, but cures come difficult and hard." Drs. Kademani and Tiwana have created an exceptional single-source reference for our most current understanding of maxillofacial surgical procedures. Contemporary therapeutic decisions must be based on fact, evidence, and experience. Only scientific evidence can adjudicate those difficult decisions we all make daily as surgeons. I personally am indebted to Deepak and Paul for this Herculean effort to synthesize the past, present, and future of our specialty.

—Peter D. Quinn, DMD, MD
Chief Physician Executive [emeritus]
University of Pennsylvania Health System
Schoenleber Professor-Oral & Maxillofacial Surgery
University of Pennsylvania School of Dental Medicine

Preface

The first edition of *Atlas of Oral and Maxillofacial Surgery* was received positively. While many operations do not change significantly with the passage of time, the incorporation of refinements to technique and new technology begins the process of reshaping old into new. These modifications in technique, and the ever-broadening depth of our specialty, provided us the impetus to write this updated edition.

Although our foundations are based in dentistry, the specialty of Oral and Maxillofacial Surgery has evolved to include both a medical and a dental basis of training. While variations in the scope of practice still occur in the specialty across regions of the world, we have observed that these gaps have perceptibly narrowed with time. This change has been driven through the globalization of educational experiences, research, and clinical fellowships. The latter is the most important in this process of driving the specialty forward into a *Pangaea*. This Atlas was written to take advantage of the unifying strengths of our specialty as the premier surgical specialty caring for oral, craniomaxillofacial, and head & neck conditions that require operative intervention. It provides a navigational aid that can guide both experienced surgeons and surgeons in training through new operations and provide a basis for refinements of already established operations in their repertoire. Each chapter is organized in a similar fashion, guiding surgeons through the complex anatomy, instrumentation, technical operative surgery, and modifications. Besides updating chapters from the first edition, many new chapters and a new section on Obstructive Sleep Apnea have been added. Our aim is that this Atlas will define and capture the current global perspective of Oral and Maxillofacial Surgery.

This book is written to provide practicing surgeons, residents, and students the most up-to-date reference for the technical performance and reasoning behind the many types of operations used in our specialty. From the basic to the most complex, readers will find that each chapter is sequentially organized to provide a comprehensive, concise, and practical description of the operative details needed for the contemporary surgical delivery of oral and maxillofacial surgical care. A formal section on relevant surgical anatomy has been incorporated to further assist the reader. Each chapter has been written by an expert surgeon and author who has a specific area of expertise. We would like to express our gratitude to all the section editors and authors for lending their time and expertise to the development of this Atlas.

It is our hope that the information presented here will continue to define the scope of practice of Oral and Maxillofacial Surgery and will provide a basis for education and training for surgeons in the future, with the goal of improving the quality of patient care across the world.

Acknowledgments

We are deeply grateful to our many friends and colleagues who have supported us and contributed to this Atlas. We wish to thank our section editors, Gary F. Bouloux, Eric R. Carlson, Joseph E. Cillo Jr., Richard Allen Finn, Ghali Ghali, Alan S. Herford, Deepak G. Krishnan, Faisal A. Quereshy, Martin Steed, Steven M. Sullivan, and Brent B. Ward, who worked tirelessly to complete their editorial efforts. We thank them immensely for sharing their expertise and for their confidence and support in bringing this project to fruition.

We are also indebted to the many authors who gave their time and expertise in contributing to this book to make it a reality. We owe a particular debt of gratitude to our artist on this project, Joe Chovan. His artistic interpretation of anatomy and surgical procedures has set a new standard for the specialty and was simply breathtaking.

Contents

PART IX
Malignant Pathology

PART X
Reconstructive Surgery

Video Contents

CHAPTER 91

Biopsy Techniques

J. Michael McCoy

Armamentarium

#15 Scalpel blade and handle
2 × 2 and 4 × 4 gauze sponges
Appropriate sutures
Biopsy punch (sizes 3 to 6)
Bottles of 10% buffered formalin
Bottles of Michel's transport solution
Cytopathology request form
Fine tissue scissors
Local anesthetic with or without vasoconstrictor
Needle holders
Pick-ups with and without teeth
Several hemostats
Shave biopsy knife
Skin/oral disinfectant
Skin and oral retractors or hooks
Skin scribe
Surgical pathology request form

History of the Procedure

A biopsy is a surgical procedure in which a tissue sample is removed from a patient and submitted for laboratory examination. The word *biopsy* is of Greek derivation, originating from the words *bio* (life) and *opsia* (to see).[1] The first recorded biopsies were probably performed by the Arabs in the 12th century. During that time, fragments of neck masses were removed to "diagnose" a thyroid goiter.[2] The modern term *biopsy* was introduced into medical terminology by the French dermatologist Besnier in 1879,[3] whereas the first true diagnostic biopsy was performed by the Russian Rudnev in 1875.[4] Although surgical biopsies only came into generalized usage in the early 1900s, many types of biopsy procedures are currently available. Soft tissue biopsy procedures in use today include the shave (Fig. 91.1A), the ellipse (Fig. 91.1B), and the punch varieties (Fig. 91.1C). Each biopsy may also be categorized as incisional (Fig. 91.1D) or excisional (Fig. 91.1E), depending on the amount of tissue removed.

Indications for the Use of the Procedure

A biopsy is a diagnostic study often performed by an oral and maxillofacial surgeon. Fresh tissue, of either soft or hard character, is either partially or completely removed, allowing the oral and maxillofacial surgical pathologist to microscopically evaluate the cell morphology of this tissue. This biopsied tissue can also be evaluated chemically and occasionally radiographically. In oral and maxillofacial surgical patients, oral and sinus mucosa, bone, soft tissue, skin, and lymph nodes are the most commonly evaluated tissues in an office or hospital biopsy.

When the patent's clinical presentation, past history, or imaging studies do not allow a definitive diagnosis, the biopsy is the indicated procedure. In addition, occasionally the patient's health insurance company may require a biopsy prior to authorizing a definitive procedure. Prior to the biopsy, a differential diagnosis is of great importance for choosing the correct or most appropriate biopsy technique. Any mucosal, skin, or bone abnormality that persists despite either removal of the associated irritant or treatment with adjunctive indicates a biopsy. In addition, any lesions suspected to be of neoplastic origin are indicated for biopsy, as are vesiculobullous lesions and the majority of pigmented mucosal lesions.

Various biopsy techniques are available today. These include the elliptical biopsy, the core needle biopsy (CNB), the fine-needle aspiration (FNA) biopsy, and the bone trephine biopsy.[5] Incisional and excisional biopsies are also characterized as ellipse, punch, or shave types. In addition, cytologic smears are a tissue identification method available to the oral and maxillofacial surgeon.

Limitations and Contraindications

There are few absolute contraindications to a biopsy. In most instances, an area of infection has no need of a biopsy. Occasionally, an area of infection may also resemble neoplastic disease of bone or soft tissue. In such cases, a biopsy may be warranted. Patients with known allergies to local anesthetics or those who have a history of bleeding may require an alteration in the usual biopsy routine. Patients with deeply positioned lesions or lesions of bone may need computed tomography (CT) or ultrasound (US) to determine the exact type of biopsy needed. One must also carefully consider the use of a bone biopsy in patients undergoing treatment with intravenous or oral bisphosphonates as well as in patients who would require a bone biopsy in the area of prior irradiated bone.

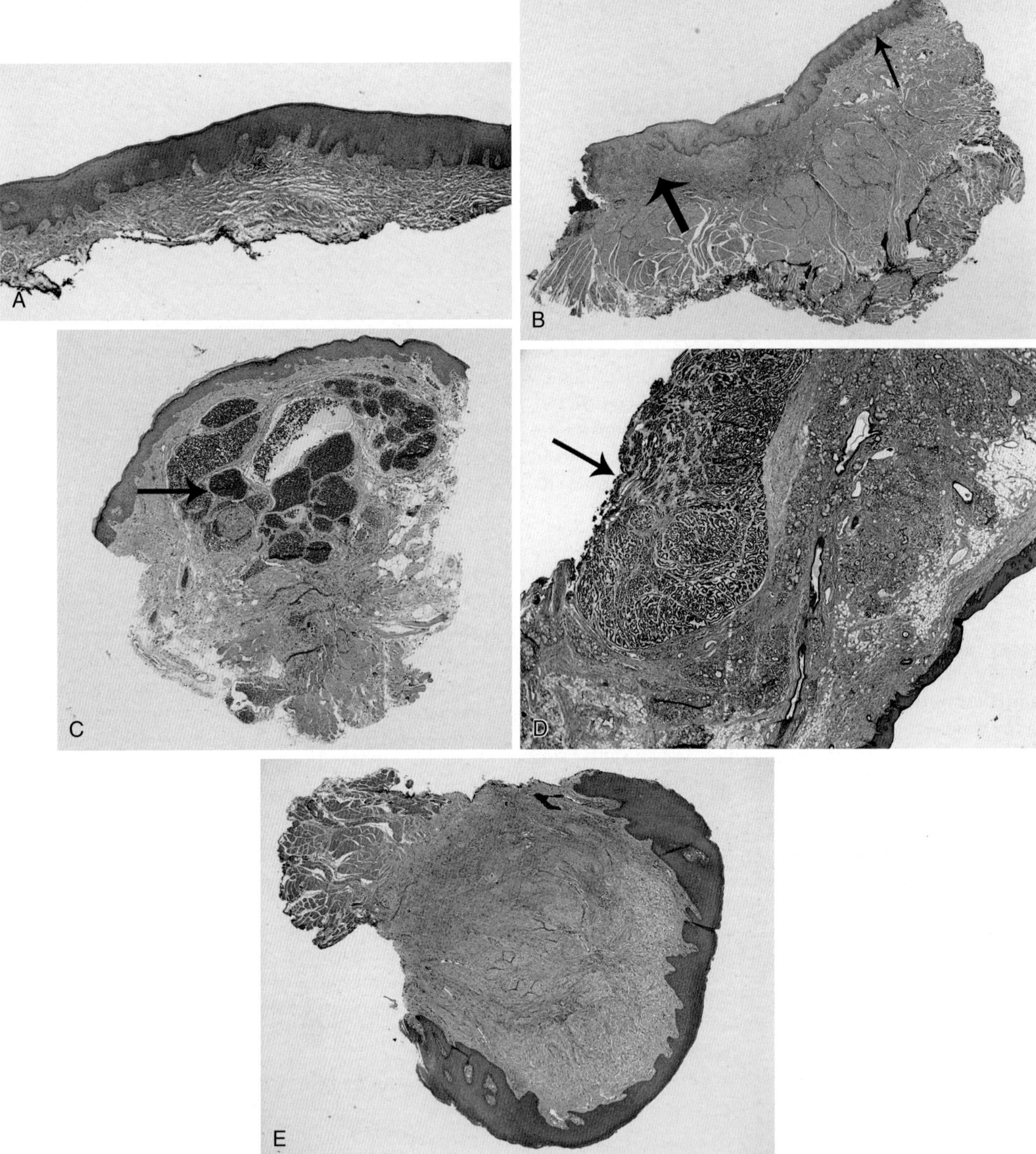

Figure 91.1 **A,** Histology of a shave biopsy. Note the scant amount of connective tissue below the epithelium. **B,** Histology of an ellipse biopsy. Note the normal epithelium at one end (*small arrow*) and dysplastic cells at the other (*large arrow*). **C,** Histology of a punch biopsy. Note the normal anatomic arrangement of the biopsy showing the hemangioma beneath the epithelium (*arrow*). **D,** Histology of an incisional biopsy. Note the salivary gland tumor deep in the biopsy, which has been incompletely removed (*arrow*). **E,** Histology of an excisional biopsy. Note that the biopsy contains the entire traumatic fibroma.

TECHNIQUE: Biopsy

Most skin and mucosal biopsies are of the elliptical type. Elliptical biopsies are often mandatory for the complete or partial removal of larger lesions. In addition, these biopsies are either incisional or excisional depending on the size of the lesion or its clinical characteristics. The larger amount of tissue removed with this biopsy technique will often provide enough tissue for multiple samples, and thus multiple tests, such as immunofluorescence or culture. Elliptical incisional or excisional biopsies always require sutures to close the wound, are more time-intensive, and scar more readily. In addition, they often require advanced surgical training prior to the procedure. This chapter describes an example of an incisional or excisional skin biopsy technique. The technique involving a mucosal biopsy is almost identical; thus, this skin biopsy procedure can easily be substituted for a mucosal biopsy.

STEP 1: Patient and Site Preparation

The patient is placed in a satisfactory pose with the proposed biopsy site positioned upward toward the surgeon. The biopsy site is then prepared with a skin antiseptic such as povidone-iodine or chlorhexidine. The area to be biopsied should then be outlined with a surgical marker/scribe so that the local anesthetic will not obliterate the actual biopsy outline.

STEP 2: Local Anesthesia

The area is next infiltrated with a local anesthetic, usually containing epinephrine to decrease the surgical bleeding, prolong the anesthetic, and limit the inherent toxicity of the anesthetic agent. The anesthetic may be injected directly into a smaller lesion or at the periphery of a larger one.

STEP 3: Surgical Outline

The position of the relaxed skin tension lines surrounding the biopsy site is established.[5] The surgeon aligns the long axis of the planned surgical procedure parallel to these lines (Fig. 91.2).

STEP 4: Incision

Using the prior diagramed ellipse lines, a #15 surgical blade is positioned almost perpendicular to the tissue and held like a pen. A 2- to 5-mm margin of normal-appearing tissue should surround the lesion to be excised. The length of the biopsy ellipse should be three times the width. As the incision continues, the blade's angle to the skin decreases but once again becomes perpendicular at the apex of the ellipse.

STEP 5: Removal and Handling of the Specimen

Carefully lift the biopsy ellipse with tissue forceps and undermine the ellipse parallel to the mucosal/skin surface. Then remove the biopsied material. If the biopsy procedure is excisional in nature, mark the specimen with a suture, thus allowing the oral and maxillofacial pathologist to accurately determine involved or uninvolved surgical margins. Once the biopsy tissue is removed and marked, immediately place it into the 10% buffered formalin fixation/carrying solution.

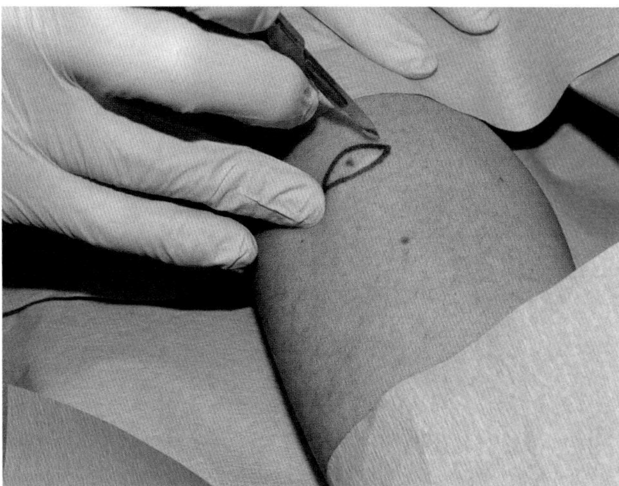

Figure 91.2 Clinical ellipse biopsy. Note the planned surgical incision lines and the angulation of the scalpel blade.

TECHNIQUE: Biopsy—*cont'd*

STEP 6: Specimen Labeling

Immediately complete the surgical pathology request form, including the differential diagnosis and other appropriate clinical information. Depict the biopsy as either incisional or excisional. This written form is necessary for the oral and maxillofacial pathologist to correctly identify the biopsied tissue.

STEP 7: Closure of Biopsy Site

If the biopsied area is small, it may be closed with surface sutures only. If larger, undermine the tissue edges either bluntly or sharply and close the wound in multiple layers. The deeper layers are then closed with resorbable suture, whereas the surface epithelium is closed with either resorbable or nonresorbable suture.

ALTERNATIVE TECHNIQUE 1: Punch Biopsy

Alternatives to the elliptical biopsy include punch biopsies. The punch biopsy is quick and accurate. It allows the oral and maxillofacial pathologist to view the entire biopsy in its natural anatomic arrangement. The punch can be utilized to remove small lesions or to incisionally biopsy larger ones. Three-millimeter or smaller diameter punches need no sutures but often provide inadequate tissue for pathologic analysis. Any larger diameter punch will require at least one suture. Punch biopsies rarely scar or become infected.

With the punch biopsy, the area to be studied is infiltrated with local anesthetic after careful cleansing. The surgeon then holds the tissue between the thumb and forefinger of the nondominant hand, stretching this tissue into a slightly ovoid appearance. The punch is placed perpendicular to the skin/mucosa and rotated in a twisting motion while applying pressure. Once the depth of the punch reaches the connective tissue below the epithelium, the surgeon removes the punch and elevates the biopsy cylinder with small pickups, taking great care not to distort the tissue. Either fine tissue scissors or a small scalpel blade is used to incise the biopsy cylinder base. The biopsied tissue is then placed into 10% buffered formalin and handled in a like manner to the previously discussed elliptical biopsy. The punch biopsy is usually closed with one or more sutures, depending on its diameter (Fig. 91.3).

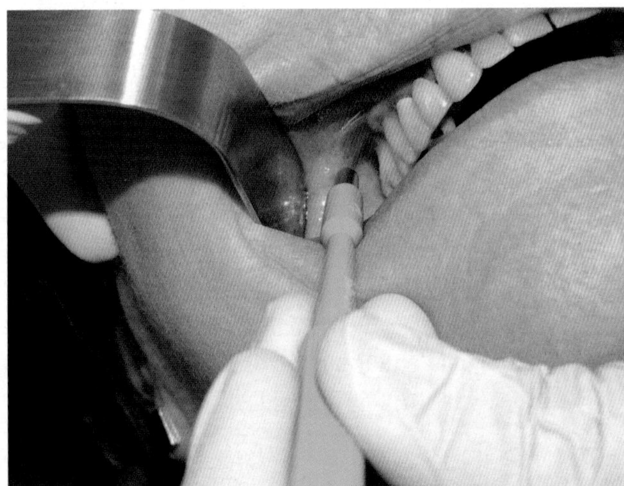

Figure 91.3 Clinical punch biopsy. Note the perpendicular position of the punch in relation to the mucosa.

ALTERNATIVE TECHNIQUE 2: Shave Biopsy

The shave biopsy is delegated to lesions that are either very thin or predominantly elevated. Examples are a skin nevus and leukoplakia from the floor of the mouth mucosa. The objective is to include the surface epithelium and a small amount of underlying connective tissue. The shave is quick and requires no sutures but again should only be used for either very thin or elevated lesions. This technique should never be used for pigmented lesions, infiltrative lesions, or lesions thought to be malignant.

The selected area is cleansed and then infiltrated with a local anesthetic. Once again, the area of the lesion is held between the thumb and forefinger, causing the soft tissue to become somewhat taut. Either a #15 surgical blade or a shave biopsy knife is held tangential to the tissue surface. With a sweeping motion, this sharp instrument is passed across and just beneath the lesion. No sutures are needed, as pressure alone should suffice to stop the oozing. As with the other biopsy techniques, the biopsied tissue is placed into 10% buffered formalin fixing/carrying solution. When completing the pathology request form, the surgeon should describe the submitted tissue as either a shave or a punch biopsy. This allows the histopathology laboratory to accurately orient the biopsy specimen (Fig. 91.4).

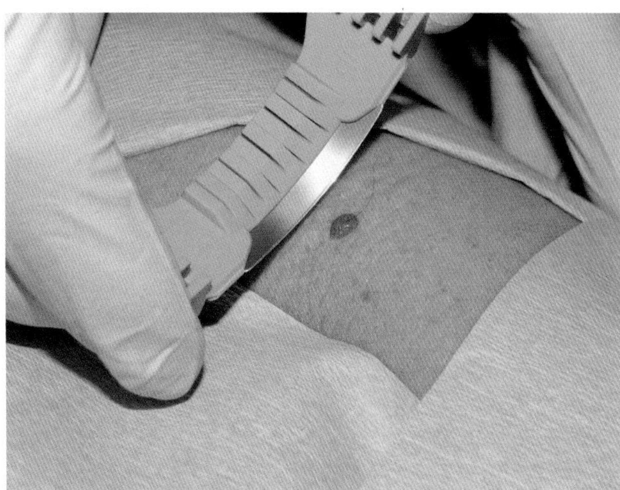

Figure 91.4 Clinical shave biopsy. Note the position of the shave knife in relation to the biopsy site.

ALTERNATIVE TECHNIQUE 3: Fine-Needle Aspiration Biopsy

The FNA biopsy is recognized as one of the most useful diagnostic procedures in the evaluation of head and neck masses. As with any type of biopsy procedure, the FNA biopsy is indicated for soft tissue or a bone mass that defies clinical or radiologic delineation and classification.[6] For cases in which the tumor type is known, the FNA biopsy is helpful in determining persistence or recurrence of the lesion after definitive treatment. If the lesion cannot be palpated or grossly identified, US or CT can be useful as a guidance tool for biopsy needle placement. The FNA biopsy is relatively safe, simple, easily learned, and cost-effective. Almost any head and neck mass that can be localized by palpation or imaged is suitable for FNA biopsy.

Place the patient in a comfortable position with the affected area upward. Cleanse the skin with an appropriate agent, and infiltrate a small amount of local anesthetic. Try not to distort the mass with the anesthetic agent. You may wish to mark the mass with a skin scribe prior to the administration of the local anesthetic. Grasp the mass between the fingers of the nonoperative hand and immobilize the area as much as possible. Attach the 23- or 25-gauge needle to the aspiration syringe barrel and advance the needle into the mass. Apply suction with the syringe only when the needle has entered the mass. Move the needle back and forth within the mass, making sure that the needle does not exit the skin or mucosa. After four or five short strokes, release the syringe suction completely. Then and only then can you remove the needle from the skin or mucosa. Please note that the biopsy material will most likely be only in the needle and the needle hub; thus, do not expect to visualize any cellular material in the syringe barrel itself. Carefully remove the needle from the hub and fill the syringe with air. Reattach the needle and place its tip on or just above the surface of a glass slide. Expel the contents of the needle on the slide, trying not to spray the contents elsewhere. Once again, remove the needle and repeat this air expulsion twice, each time keeping the needle on or near the slide. Take two more passes through the mass using the same needle and an identical technique, but each pass should be in a somewhat different angle or direction.[7]

The object of expelling the needle contents on a slide is to produce a thin layer of cells to be viewed microscopically. For this examination to be useful, a smear must be produced. To prepare this smear, hold the specimen slide in your right hand and then place a second non-specimen slide in the other. This second slide is parallel to and just above the specimen slide. In one fluid motion, pull the upper slide downward and across the specimen slide, thus producing a thin smear of cells. To microscopically examine the biopsied cells, the cells on each slide must be fixed. The two favored methods are air-dried fixation and alcohol or wet fixation. The wet fixation consists of placing each slide immediately into ethyl alcohol. Do not use formalin. The so-called dry technique is simply allowing each slide to air-dry. One can also dry the slide with a warm-air hair drier. In both instances, the air-dried slides or the alcohol-fixed slides are sent to a cytopathology laboratory. In addition to the microscope slides, a cytopathology request form must be filled out completely and sent with the slides. When filled out accurately, these forms aid the laboratory in determining the pathologic dilemma. Each laboratory is unique, and the clinician should question his or her own cytopathologist regarding the specific laboratory needs prior to performing a FNA biopsy (Fig. 91.5).

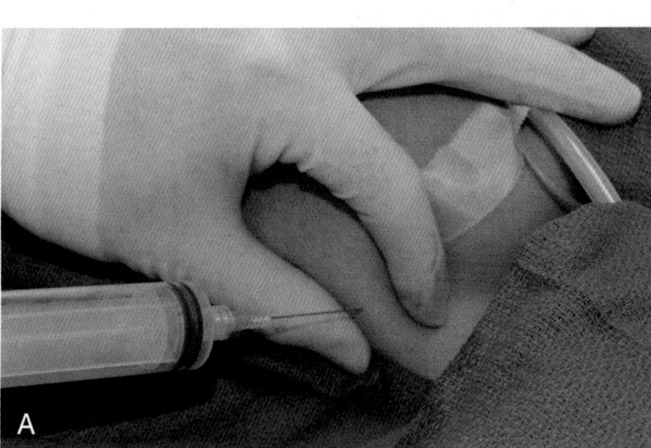

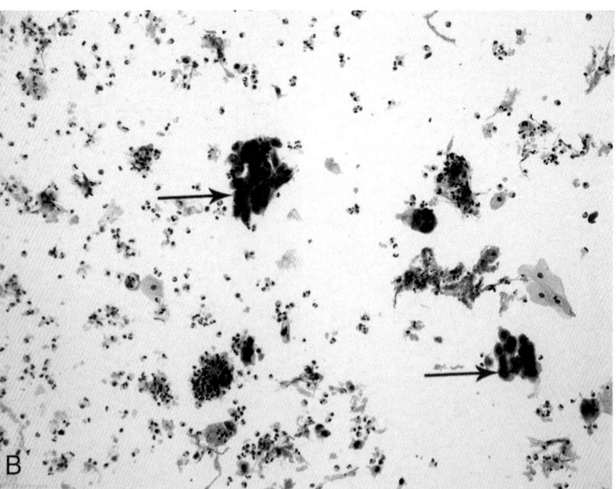

Figure 91.5 **A,** FNA biopsy of the neck. Note the small 25-gauge needle advancing into the neck mass. **B,** Cytology of an FNA biopsy of a neck mass. Note the malignant cells suggestive of metastatic squamous cell carcinoma (*arrows*).

ALTERNATIVE TECHNIQUE 4: Direct Immunofluorescent Biopsy

Vesiculobullous or blistering diseases of the oral and nasal mucosa are an important group of immunologic diseases caused by pathologic autoantibodies directed against antigens located within or just below the mucosal surface.[8] Direct immunofluorescence studies allow today's clinicians to diagnose, treat, and better understand problems such as erosive lichen planus, benign mucous membrane pemphigoid, pemphigus vulgaris, linear IgA disease, epidermolysis bullosa, and similar diseases that occur within the mucosa of the head and neck area[9] (Fig. 91.6).

The indicated soft tissue is removed as described previously and obtained as a shave, punch, or elliptical biopsy. Unlike routine biopsies, this tissue is immediately placed in Michel's[10] transport medium, which contains ammonium sulfate to help prevent tissue degradation. If Michel's is not available, one can wrap the biopsied tissue in saline-moistened gauze, but for no longer than 24 hours. If stored or transported in Michel's solution, the biopsy tissue will be acceptable for use by the histopathology laboratory for up to 2 weeks, although a shorter amount of time is more acceptable. As an alternative to Michel's medium, the biopsied tissue can also be preserved by snap-freezing in liquid nitrogen, although this procedure is extremely time-consuming and cost-prohibitive. Once again, it is imperative that a surgical pathology request form be accurately supplied with the biopsy material.

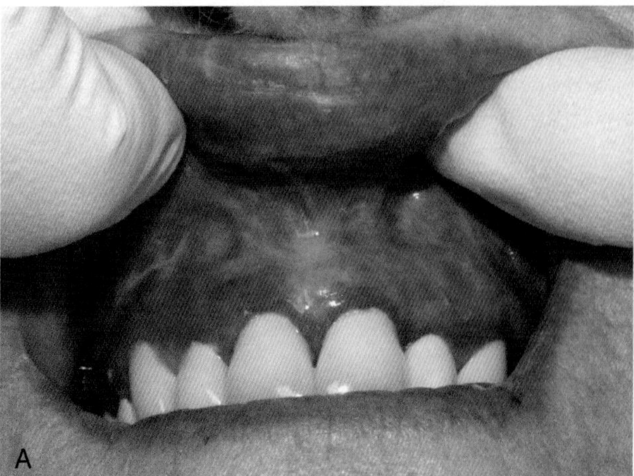

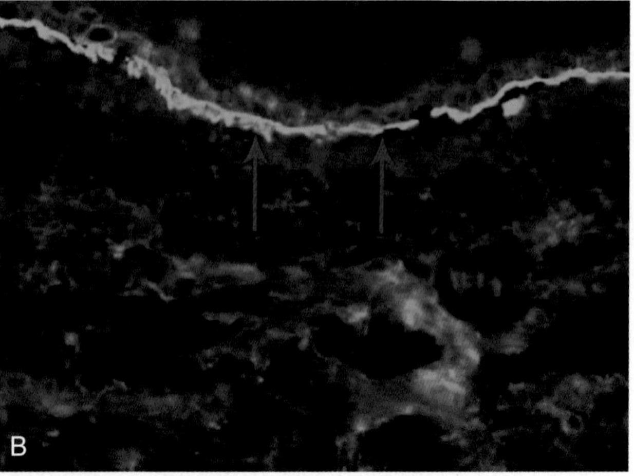

Figure 91.6 **A,** Clinical presentation of benign mucous membrane pemphigoid. Note the erythematous nature of practically all of the gingiva. **B,** Direct immunofluorescence histology of pemphigoid. Note the well-defined fluorescent line (*arrows*) at the junction of the epithelium and connective tissue.

ALTERNATIVE TECHNIQUE 5: Image-Guided Core Needle Biopsy

Even though this type of biopsy is rarely if ever performed by the oral and maxillofacial surgeon, the option of such a biopsy technique should always be a consideration in many neoplastic diseases of the head and neck. In various head/neck/oral diseases, particularly those that are neoplastic, the oral and maxillofacial surgeon only need consult the radiology group of local medical center or imaging center for their biopsy aid. Such imaging/biopsy procedures are often performed by a radiologist using either US or CT guidance and thus avoiding the complications of an open biopsy, as well as the problems associated with the FNA biopsy. In addition, these CNB studies are usually performed under local anesthesia, thus avoiding a general anesthetic. Currently US is the more commonly used imaging technique when performing both FNA biopsies and CNBs. The predominant reason for this is the absolute lack of patient radiation when using US guidance.

In recent years the needle biopsy, both FNA biopsy and CNB biopsy have changed the management and treatment strategies involving head and neck tumors.[11] Previously, the only way such lesions could be biopsied was either by an open incisional biopsy or by the much more involved and expensive surgical removal with frozen section aid while the patient is undergoing a general anesthetic. In fact, at present, the CNB has become the preferred diagnostic technique for lesions of the thyroid, salivary gland, and lymph nodes.[12]

CNBs are performed using larger cutting needles (usually 16 to 20 gauge) as opposed to the 23 to 25 gauge needle used for FNA biopsies. This allows larger tissue samples for the oral and maxillofacial pathologist, thus preserving a more accurate architectural and anatomic tissue alignment. As opposed to FNA biopsies, the diagnostic yield is much greater with the CNB, especially when examining salivary gland and cervical lymph nodes. The greatest disadvantage is the possible increase in significant complications. These include, but are not limited to, excessive bleeding, nerve damage, and possible tumor implantation along the needle tract. The experienced radiologist rarely experiences such complications.

Avoidance and Management of Intraoperative Complications

Careful incision design planning can obviate unsightly and unwanted scarring. One should attempt dissection away from major vessels to prevent post-biopsy hematomas. For biopsies of deeply positioned masses, CT or US guidance is often desirable (Figs. 91.7 and 91.8). Appropriate intraoperative specimen labeling with sutures and/or appropriate means will not only aid the surgical pathologist but also perhaps prevent a second unneeded biopsy procedure. Evaluation of the patient's past medical history can often decrease or prevent untoward allergic events, as well as avoiding periods of excessive bleeding. Careful consideration should be given to both the biopsy site and the selection of biopsy type so that tumor seeding can be avoided. In addition, during the biopsy, the clinician should consider definitive surgical needs so as not to disturb the anatomic design of the ultimate surgical procedure.

Postoperative Considerations

As a rule, the biopsy procedure has few complications as long as careful patient selection and consideration of biopsy type

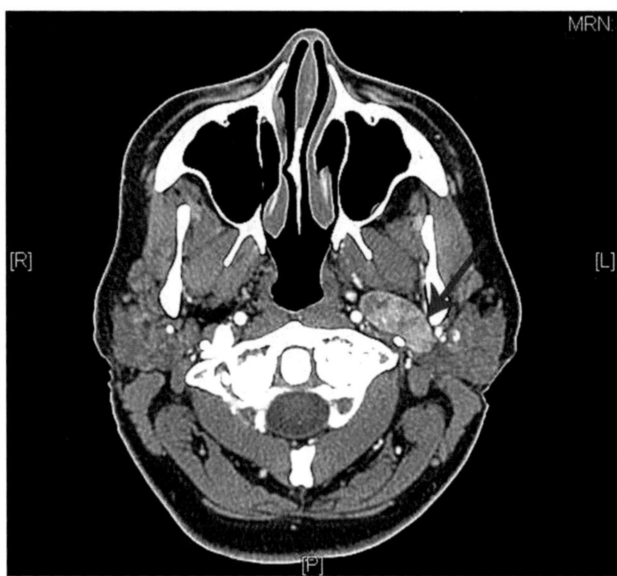

Figure 91.7 Contrast CT of the neck to aid in fine needle placement. Note the left neck mass (*arrow*) suggestive of a deep lobe parotid tumor.

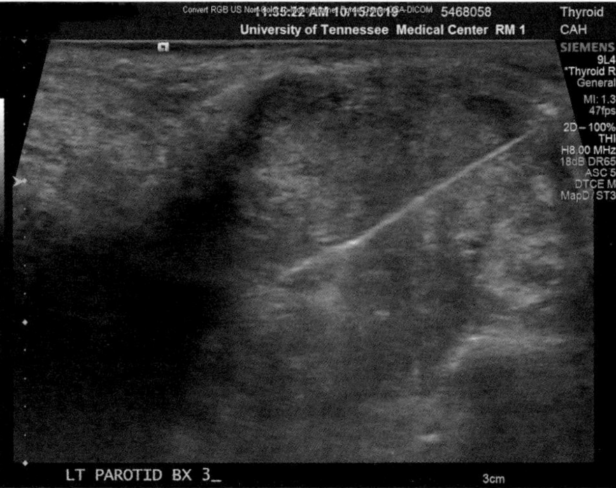

Figure 91.8 Ultrasound-guided core needle biopsy. Note the needle seen entering the hypoechoic parotid mass.

is followed both prior to and during the procedure. As with other invasive procedures, one should expect swelling and some mild postoperative pain. The swelling can be controlled with pressure and ice and the pain with mild analgesics. These medications will range from nonsteroidal anti-inflammatory drugs to narcotics, depending on both the specific patient and the tissue alteration caused by the biopsy procedure.[13] The oral and maxillofacial surgeon should carefully examine the area to be biopsied when designing the biopsy configuration so that as little scarring as possible is produced. Once again, careful pre-biopsy preparation is essential. Biopsies adjacent to major nerves and vessels should be avoided if at all possible. If these biopsy locations are unavoidable, intravenous sedation or general anesthetic to limit patient movement should be considered. The use of an operating microscope may also be a consideration. If a high-grade malignancy is suspected, one should carefully reflect on the design of the biopsy to avoid spreading tumor cells through the tract of the biopsy. If a lymphoid malignancy is suspected, one should ask the histopathology laboratory to furnish the additional fixative material needed for such lesions. When obtaining incisional biopsies, consideration should be given to the definitive surgical procedure needed to entirely remove the lesion. Two separate areas of scarring should be avoided.

Conclusion

In the diagnoses of pathologic tissue, the ultimate tools of greatest benefit unquestionably are an excellent clinical examination and sound medical judgment by the oral and maxillofacial surgeon. These human qualities may obviate the need for a tissue biopsy. At other times, a clinician will encounter entities of uncertain potential significance. In these instances, the biopsy could provide the simplest, most convenient, least morbid, and least costly avenue of access needed to make these determinations. At the time of biopsy, a bit of forward planning and prudence can vastly improve the procedure's outcome and thus allow the appropriate biopsy material to be collected. In addition, correct technique and handling of the biopsy material will greatly increase the chances of a correct histologic diagnosis. Inadequate care and consideration at any of the biopsy stages could conclude with the need for a further procedure or even an incorrect diagnosis.

References

1. Borroni G, Baldry A. The language of dermatology and dermatopathology from Robert Willan to A. Bernard Ackerman. *Am J Dermatopathol.* 1990;12(6):617–621.
2. Anderson JB, Webb AJ. Fine-needle aspiration biopsy and the diagnosis of thyroid cancer. *Br J Surg.* 1987;74(4):292–296.
3. Nezelof C, Guinebretiere JM. 1879, Ernest Besnier, inventor of the word "biopsy," (French). *Rev Prat.* 2006;56:2080.
4. Zerbino DD. [Biopsy: its history, current and future outlook]. *Lik Sprava.* 1994;(3–4):1–9.
5. Goldberg LH, Silapunt S, Alam M, Peterson SR, Jih MH, Kimyai-Asadi A. Surgical repair of temple defects after Mohs micrographic surgery. *J Am Acad Dermatol.* 2005;52(4):631–636.
6. Tryggvason G, Gailey MP, Hulstein SL, et al. Accuracy of fine-needle aspiration and imaging in the preoperative workup of salivary gland mass lesions treated surgically. *Laryngoscope.* 2013;123(1):158–163.
7. Irisawa A, Hikichi T, Bhutani MS, Ohira H. Basic technique of FNA. *Gastrointest Endosc.* 2009;69(2 suppl):S125–S129.
8. Lazarova Z, Yancey KB. Reactivity of autoantibodies from patients with defined subepidermal bullous diseases against 1 mol/L salt-split skin. Specificity, sensitivity, and practical considerations. *J Am Acad Dermatol.* 1996;35(3 Pt 1):398–403.
9. Schmidt E, Zillikens D. Pemphigoid diseases. *Lancet.* 2013;381(9863):320–332.
10. Vaughn Jones SA, Palmer I, Bhogal BS, Eady RA, Black MM. The use of Michel's transport medium for immunofluorescence and immunoelectron microscopy in autoimmune bullous diseases. *J Cutan Pathol.* 1995;22(4):365–370.
11. Warshavsky A, Rosen R, Perry C, et al. Core needle biopsy for diagnosing lymphoma in cervical lymphadenopathy: meta-analysis. *Head Neck.* 2020;42(10):3051–3060.
12. Monfore N, Jarmakani M, Wagner JM. The role of Core-Needle Biopsy in the evaluation of head and neck lesions. *J Am Osteopath Coll Radiol.* 2018;7(1):5–12.
13. Daniels SE, Desjardins PJ, Talwalker S, Recker DP, Verburg KM. The analgesic efficacy of valdecoxib vs. oxycodone/acetaminophen after oral surgery. *J Am Dent Assoc.* 2002;133(5):611–621.

CHAPTER 92

Temporal Artery Biopsy

Michael Awadallah

Armamentarium

Hand-held Doppler
Water-based lubricating jelly
#15 Blade
Double-ended skin hooks
Curved mosquito hemostat
Right-angle hemostat
3-0 Silk ties
Small-medium ligature clips
Electric hair shaver
Marking pen
Tenotomy scissors
Bipolar cautery
Bovie electrocautery
Frazier suction 8, 10, 12
Normal saline irrigation
Adson-Browns forceps
1% or 2% lidocaine without epinephrine
Small Weitlaner retractors
Specimen cup with formalin
4 × 4 gauze
3-0 Vicryl sutures
5-0 Monocryl sutures
Nerve integrity monitor
Kittners

History of the Procedure

We do know the procedure is historically linked with aiding in the diagnosis of giant cell arteritis (GCA). GCA is an immune-mediated granulomatous pan-vasculitis affecting small- to medium-sized arteries throughout the body and is the most common vasculitis in individuals 50 years old or greater. It affects women more than men in a 3:1 ratio and is associated with Scandinavian descent. The pathophysiology is believed to be a T-cell mediated inflammatory response in the arterial walls leading to obstruction and subsequent ischemia to the local and regional tissues.[1] Clinical manifestations depend on the site of obstruction and degree of collateral perfusion. Signs and symptoms most commonly occur in the head and neck area and include but are not limited to constitutional symptoms (fever, anemia, fatigue, malaise), jaw claudication, new onset headaches, and abrupt monocular vision loss. Other clinical manifestations include stroke, upper and/or lower extremity claudication, aortitis, aortic aneurysm, and peripheral neuropathy.[2,3] The American College of Rheumatology has published certain criteria that need to be met before the diagnosis of GCA can be made (Table 92.1). Three of the following criteria need to be met before establishing a diagnosis of GCA: a positive arterial biopsy showing granulomatous infiltration, erythrocyte sedimentation rate of at least 50 mm/h, age 50 years old or greater, new onset localized headache, and temporal artery tenderness or decreased temporal artery pulse pressure.[4,5]

Indications for the Procedure

The temporal artery biopsy is exclusively used in aiding the clinician in diagnosing cranial GCA. Historically, the literature has reported a sensitivity and specificity of 93.5% and 91.2%, respectively, for the temporal artery biopsy in diagnosing GCA.[2] However, other studies show a sensitivity range of 24%–90% and a specificity range of 81%–100%.[6] Pathognomic histopathology of the temporal artery specimen will show full thickness chronic granulomatous inflammation with infiltration of multinucleated giant cells, macrophages, and epithelioid histocytes in the tunica media and the breakdown of the internal elastic lamina.

Limitations and Contraindications

Diagnosis of GCA can be made clinically without the need of a biopsy. The biggest drawback of performing a biopsy aside from the complications of surgery and anesthesia is the false negative rate, which can range from 10% to 60%.[2,6,7] The false negative rate of biopsy is associated with skin lesions, inadequate length of specimen, inaccurate reading of histopathology, and glucocorticoid treatment.[2,8,9] A retrospective study by Narvaez et al. demonstrates that positive diagnostic accuracy decreases as time from provisional diagnosis increases. and this can be contributed to the expedient initiation of high-dose steroid therapy upon diagnosis.[10,11] Historically, a positive temporal artery biopsy

Table 92.1 American College of Rheumatology Criteria for Giant Cell Arteritis. Adapted from Hunder et al.

Criteria	Definition
Age of disease onset ≥ 50 years	Development of symptoms or findings at age 50 or older
New onset headache	New type of localized pain in the head
Abnormality of the temporal artery	Tenderness and/or decreased pulsations unrelated to arteriosclerosis of the cervical arteries
Elevated erythrocyte sedimentation rate	Erythrocyte sedimentation rate ≥ 50 mm/hour
Abnormal artery biopsy	Biopsy showing mononuclear cell infiltration, or granulomatous inflammation

is the gold standard for diagnosis for GCA; however, a negative biopsy does not rule out the diagnosis.[12] Upon suspicion or diagnosis of GCA based on the clinical criteria made by the American College of Rheumatology (ACR), treatment with a high-dose steroid is initiated and maintained for treatment, regardless of the biopsy result (see Table 92.1). According to Hunder et al., if at least three or more criteria are met by the patient, the diagnosis of GCA has a sensitivity and specificity of 93.5% and 91.2% respectively.[4] The temporal artery biopsy result does not change management and is used to confirm diagnosis of GCA; this is especially true for patients with a score of 3 or above on the ACR criteria for GCA.[13] High-resolution magnetic resonance angiography has also been used in the literature as an adjunctive aid in the diagnosis of GCA with a collective sensitivity of 73% and a specificity of 88%.[14]

SURGICAL TECHNIQUE AND STEPS

STEP 1: ANESTHESIA, PATIENT POSITIONING, AND DRAPING

This procedure can be performed under local or general anesthesia. The author of this chapter has performed it exclusively under general anesthesia; this allows for more patient comfort, surgeon comfort, free communication between the surgical team members, and better management of any intraoperative complications. A standard oral-tracheal intubation is performed by the anesthesia team, and the patient is placed in a supine position. An adequate strip of hair is removed from preauricular region to the lower temporal region of the scalp. Usually, a 2 × 5 cm area superior to the preauricular lesion will provide enough exposure to allow for a comfortable dissection, location, and harvesting of the superficial temporal artery (STA). The remaining hair is pinned down appropriately using silk or paper tape. The area is then scrubbed using standard sterile technique and squared off using blue towels.

STEP 2: MARKING OUT STA AND THE PARIETAL RAMUS

Using a hand-held Doppler the STA is initially located in the preauricular region, and then traced superiorly and posteriorly to locate the posterior ramus. This is mapped out using a marking pen during the process (Fig. 92.1). Local anesthesia is then injected at least 1.5 cm anterior and posterior from the markings to minimize distortion of the anatomy. Wait 5 minutes to allow for periincisional diffusion. Some literature advocates abundant use of local anesthesia to allow for hydrodissection, but this can work against the surgeon by distorting the delicate anatomy in this area.

STEP 3: INCISION

A 3–5 cm incision is then performed using a #15 blade in an oblique fashion parallel the direction of the hair follicles through skin and the subcutaneous layers to minimize incisional alopecia. This incision is then carried down to the level of the tempoparietal fascia. Adequate undermining with Bovie cautery is then performed to allow for further exposure and retraction of tissues. Any bleeding at this point can be readily controlled with bipolar cautery. At this point the surgical bed can be cleaned and bluntly dissected with Kittners.

STEP 4: LOCATING THE PARIETAL RAMUS OF THE STA

At this point, if the aforementioned steps were followed appropriately, the parietal ramus and accompanying vein(s) can be located with direct vision through the thin tempo-parietal fascia (Fig. 92.2). Direct palpation and/or hand-held Doppler can be used to confirm the nature of the vessel along with dissection down to the STA proper if necessary.

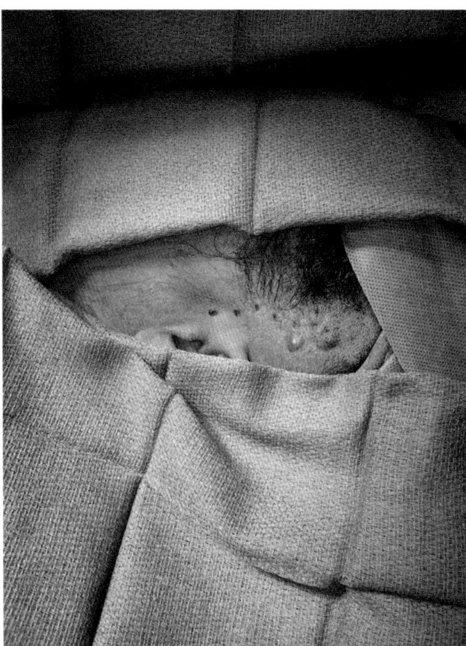

Figure 92.1 Mapping out the posterior rami of the superficial temporal artery (STA).

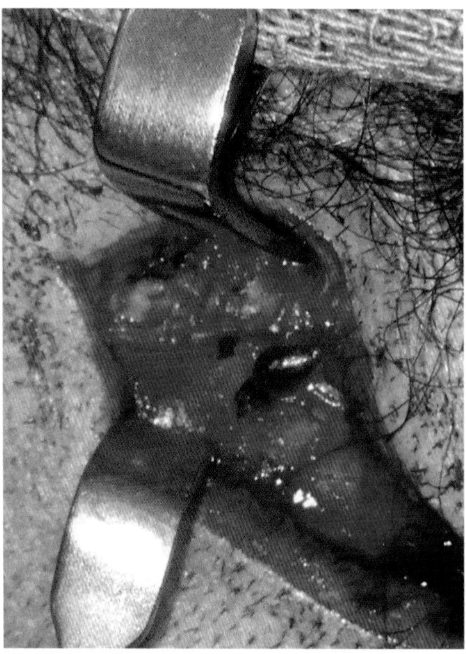

Figure 92.2 Visualization of the posterior rami of the superficial temporal artery (STA) through the tempo-parietal fascia.

SURGICAL TECHNIQUE AND STEPS—cont'd

STEP 5: STA HARVESTING AND CLOSURE

Once the artery has been located, proper isolation from the surrounding fascia and accompanying vein(s) should be performed using a combination of blunt and sharp dissection. Sharp dissection using tenotomy scissors and tissue pick-ups is utilized to incise the fascia over the artery along its exposed length and harvesting of the artery. The author prefers to use mosquito dissection to create separation between the artery and the vein. The literature indicates the length of the harvested artery contributes to false negative rates, with a minimal harvest threshold of 1.5 cm and preferably 2–3 cm for reduction of false negatives[15-17] (Fig. 92.3). After proper harvesting, the area is washed with copious amounts of normal saline and proper hemostasis is achieved. The area is then closed in layers, and the skin can be closed with staples or sutures.

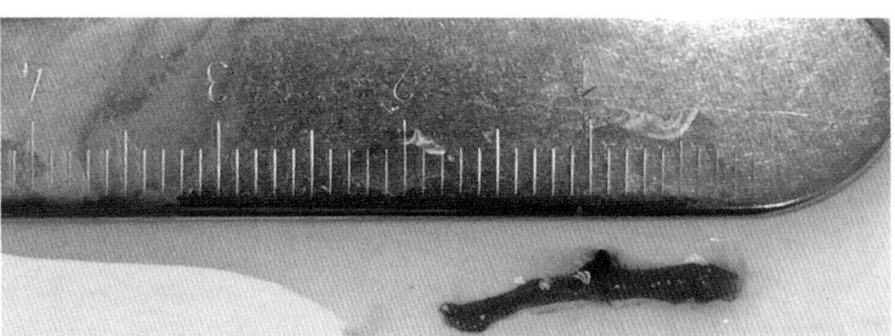

Figure 92.3 Harvested vessel (approximately 2 cm).

ALTERNATIVE TECHNIQUE 1: STA Biopsy in the Preauricular Region

The STA can be more readily mapped out in this area with only palpation because the vessel size and pulsations are more prominent. The multiple surrounding structures in this area include the cartilaginous canal and the parotid gland, and the auriculotemporal nerve located below the tragus can potentially lead to further complications if injured.[18] In the middle to low preauricular region, the STA lies within the superficial lobe of the parotid gland, and a deeper dissection is necessary to harvest it. This area also does fall into the "danger zone" and can lead to increased risk of inadvertent injury to the temporal/frontal branch of the facial nerve. In this area, there are multiple contributories from the STA that need to be identified and ligated prior to harvesting the artery. While the STA is more identifiable in this area, it comes at the cost of increased complications secondary to injury to adjacent structures and potentially more hemorrhage. The surgical steps and their order in this procedure are overall very similar to the standard technique described above. The main differences are centered around the local anatomy of the region and better need for vascular control. Meticulous takedown of the contributories from the STA should be performed prior to harvesting the artery. The fascial layers of dissection will be through the superficial musculoaponeurotic system, through the parotid-masseteric fascia, and finally through the superficial lobe of the parotid gland.

Avoidance and Management of Intraoperative Complications

Local and general anesthesia complications may arise during surgery and include cerebrovascular accident, myocardial infarction, death, and lidocaine toxicity. General surgical complications of this procedure include but are not limited to pain, bleeding, infection, swelling, local alopecia, and scarring. A site-specific surgical complication is limited to the injury of the temporal/frontal branch of the facial nerve leading to ipsilateral brow ptosis. A detailed understanding of the course of the STA and its bifurcations into a parietal and frontal ramus and the course of the temporal/frontal branch of the facial nerve is imperative to avoid injury and the sequela of brow ptosis.[19,20] The STA is a terminal branch of the external carotid artery, but more often than not it does bifurcate into a frontal and a parietal ramus as it travels superiorly. The STA and the temporal/frontal branch of the facial nerve are located between the tempo-parietal fascia and the temporalis fascia in the superior anterior preauricular region. Ideally, the biopsy should be taken from the parietal ramus of the STA as this falls out of the danger zone area described by Yoon et Al.[20] This zone is described as an area where the temporal/frontal branch of the facial nerve courses relatively superficially and immediately beneath the superficial temporal fascia and in intimate proximity with the frontal ramus of the STA. This area is bounded (A) the tragus of the ear, (B) the junction of the zygomatic arch and lateral orbital rim, (C) an area 2 cm superior to the superior orbital rim, and (D) the point superior to the tragus and in horizontal alignment with (C).[20] If a preauricular approach is used, further complications can occur, including damage to the cartilaginous external auditory canal (EAC) potentially leading to partial hearing loss, damage to the parotid capsule leading to potential salivary fistula, damage to the auriculotemporal nerve potentially leading to neuralgia, and/or Frey syndrome. If possible, any identified nerve injury or injury to the EAC should be directly repaired. The parotid capsule should be primarily closed if the preauricular approach is used along with a postoperative pressure dressing and an antisialagogue for 5 to 7 days.

Postoperative Considerations

Postoperative facial nerve assessment is crucial, especially the temporal/frontal branch. A standard pressure wound dressing is left on for 48 to 72 hours for both hemostasis and reduction in swelling. A gross hearing test can be performed postoperatively if the EAC has a confirmed or suspected injury. Postoperative wound infection is rare, and there is no need for routine postoperative antibiotics especially that this is a clean wound. If Frey syndrome occurs, then anticholinergics can be administered orally indefinitely, or periodic injections of botulism toxin A can also be administered. As stated previously, if the biopsy result is negative, it does not rule out disease, and a contralateral biopsy is not indicated, especially if the patient does meet ACR criteria for GCA. A postoperative arterial venous fistula can occur but is rare. Clinical manifestations include tinnitus, bruit, and a palpable thrill. The fistula can be excised and embolized, or local sclerotherapy can be utilized to eradicate the lesion.[13,21]

References

1. Jivraj I, Tamhankar M. The treatment of giant cell arteritis. *Curr Treat Options Neurol.* 2017;19(1):2.
2. Hussain O, McKay A, Fairburn K, Doyle P, Orr R. Diagnosis of giant cell arteritis: when should we biopsy the temporal artery? *Br J Oral Maxillofac Surg.* 2016;54(3):327–330.
3. Généreau T, Lortholary O, Pottier MA, et al. Temporal artery biopsy: a diagnostic tool for systemic necrotizing vasculitis. French Vasculitis Study Group [published correction appears in Arthritis Rheum 2000 Apr;43(4):929]. *Arthritis Rheum.* 1999;42(12):2674–2681.

4. Hunder GG, Bloch DA, Michel BA, et al. The American College of Rheumatology 1990 criteria for the classification of giant cell arteritis. *Arthritis Rheum*. 1990;33(8):1122–1128.
5. Meyers AD, Said S. Temporal artery biopsy: concise guidelines for otolaryngologists. *Laryngoscope*. 2004;114(11):2056–2059.
6. Bowling K, Rait J, Atkinson J, Srinivas G. Temporal artery biopsy in the diagnosis of giant cell arteritis: does the end justify the means? *Ann Med Surg (Lond)*. 2017;20(20): 1–5.
7. Ing EB, Wang DN, Kirubarajan A, et al. Systematic review of the yield of temporal artery biopsy for suspected giant cell arteritis. *Neuro Ophthalmol*. 2018;43(1):18–25.
8. Gonzalez-Gay MA, Garcia-Porrua C, Llorca J, Gonzalez-Louzao C, Rodriguez-Ledo P. Biopsy-negative giant cell arteritis: clinical spectrum and predictive factors for positive temporal artery biopsy. *Semin Arthritis Rheum*. 2001;30(4):249–256.
9. Banz Y, Stone JH. Why do temporal arteries go wrong? Principles and pearls from a clinician and a pathologist. *Rheumatology (Oxford)*. 2018;57(suppl 2):ii3–ii10.
10. Sait MR, Lepore M, Kwasnicki R, Allington J, Srinivasaiah N. Temporal artery biopsy: time matters!. *Intern Med J*. 2017;47(12):1465.
11. Narváez J, Bernad B, Roig-Vilaseca D, et al. Influence of previous corticosteroid therapy on temporal artery biopsy yield in giant cell arteritis. *Semin Arthritis Rheum*. 2007;37(1): 13–19.
12. Hall JK, Volpe NJ, Galetta SL, Liu GT, Syed NA, Balcer LJ. The role of unilateral temporal artery biopsy. *Ophthalmology*. 2003;110(3):543–548.
13. van Uden DJ, Truijers M, Schipper EE, Zeebregts CJ, Reijnen MM. Superficial temporal artery aneurysm: diagnosis and treatment options. *Head Neck*. 2013;35(4):608–614.
14. Aghdam KA, Sanjari MS, Manafi N, Khorramdel S, Alemzadeh SA, Navahi RAA. Temporal artery biopsy for diagnosing giant cell arteritis: a ten-year review. *J Ophthalmic Vis Res*. 2020;15(2):201–209.
15. Grossman C, Ben-Zvi I, Barshack I, Bornstein G. Association between specimen length and diagnostic yield of temporal artery biopsy. *Scand J Rheumatol*. 2017;46(3):222–225.
16. Papadakis M, Kaptanis S, Kokkori-Steinbrecher A, Floros N, Schuster F, Hübner G. Temporal artery biopsy in the diagnosis of giant cell arteritis: bigger is not always better. *Am J Surg*. 2018;215(4):647–650.
17. Oh LJ, Wong E, Gill AJ, McCluskey P, Smith JEH. Value of temporal artery biopsy length in diagnosing giant cell arteritis. *ANZ J Surg*. 2018;88(3):191–195.
18. Cahais J, Houdart R, Lupinacci RM, Valverde A. Operative technique: superficial temporal artery biopsy. *J Visc Surg*. 2017;154(3):203–207.
19. Murchison AP, Bilyk JR. Brow ptosis after temporal artery biopsy: incidence and associations. *Ophthalmology*. 2012;119(12):2637–2642.
20. Yoon MK, Horton JC, McCulley TJ. Facial nerve injury: a complication of superficial temporal artery biopsy. *Am J Ophthalmol*. 2011;152(2):251–255.e1.
21. Janssen M, Vaninbroukx J, Fourneau I. Arteriovenous fistula after superficial temporal artery biopsy. *Ann Vasc Surg*. 2013;27(4):500.e1–500.e5.

CHAPTER 93

Enucleation and Curettage of Benign Oral and Maxillofacial Pathology

Joseph E. Cillo Jr.

Armamentarium

#9 Periosteal elevator
#15 Scalpel blade
Allis or Addison clamps
Appropriate sutures
Carnoy's solution liquid nitrogen
Double-ended dental curette
Fissure or round carbide bur rongeurs
Local anesthetic with vasoconstrictor
Minnesota and Seldin retractors
Small round diamond bur

History of the Procedure

Surgical management of oral cysts was described as early as 1892 by Partsch and involved the intraoral exposure of the cyst lining (marsupialization), and was termed the *Partsch I procedure.*[1] Because the Partsch I procedure frequently led to inadequate cyst removal and complications in the preantibiotic era, Partsch described the Partsch II procedure (enucleation) in 1910.[2] Dowsett[3] and Wassmund[4] further developed the technique, thereby improving access for complete enucleation of the cyst through a wide intraoral osteotomy. Surgical techniques continued to improve over the decades, and the incidence of recurrence and infection subsequently declined. As the distinct benign pathologic processes of the oral and maxillofacial region became more clearly defined, it became more evident that the enucleation and curettage method was a primary choice for the initial definitive management of the majority of these lesions.[5] For example, the odontogenic keratocyst (OKC) has a high rate of recurrence, and the addition of chemical curettage, in addition to physical curettage, with enucleation has been shown to significantly decrease or eliminate the recurrence rate.[6] The development of chemical curettage also progressed with the utilization of Carnoy's solution[6] and liquid nitrogen,[7] as these methods have shown some success in decreasing the recurrence rates of some lesions.

Indications for the Use of the Procedure

Enucleation is the surgical treatment of benign pathology that involves the complete removal of the entity. It is the procedure of choice for removal of most cysts and other benign pathology of the oral and maxillofacial region that are anatomically distinct from the surrounding tissue and amenable to this type of therapy. Physical or chemical curettage may be added to the enucleation procedure in certain pathologies that require additional removal of surrounding bone to help ensure complete removal and to decrease the persistence of the lesion. Curettage may be completed with a sharp curette or a round diamond bur with copious cool irrigation to remove 1 to 2 mm of bone and any pathology remnants. Meticulous technique in the performance of the enucleation and curettage procedure is particularly important in the surgical management of lesions that tend to have high recurrence or persistence rates, such as the OKC. In this situation, the addition of Carnoy's solution to curettage or peripheral ostectomy has been shown to be more effective in decreasing the recurrence rate than the enucleation procedures alone.[6] Liquid nitrogen has also been used for chemical curettage with some success in the management of the luminal and intraluminal subtypes of ameloblastoma.[7] Enucleation and curettage may also be indicated as a second procedure in lesions that have persisted following the initial procedure of enucleation and curettage.

Simple enucleation and curettage may be indicated for unicystic ameloblastomas of the luminal and intraluminal subtype that have not shown evidence of extraosseous spread. However, if this option is utilized, routine radiographic follow-up is recommended, as the recurrence rate of unicystic ameloblastoma treated with enucleation and curettage has been shown to be unacceptably high.[8] Multicystic ameloblastomas are not amenable to enucleation and curettage, as this treatment results in an unacceptable recurrence rate and should be addressed with an extended surgical resection[9] (Table 93.1).

Table 93.1 Benign Oral and Maxillofacial Pathology Amenable to Enucleation and Curettage

Odontogenic Cysts	Dentigerous cyst
	Radicular cyst
	Odontogenic keratocyst (OKC)
	Calcifying odontogenic cyst
	Glandular odontogenic cyst
	Botryoid odontogenic cyst
	Buccal bifurcation cyst
Odontogenic Tumors	Odontoma
	Adenomatoid odontogenic tumor (AOT)
	Unicystic ameloblastoma
	Luminal subtype
	Intraluminal subtype
	Ameloblastic fibroma
	Ameloblastic fibroodontoma
	Cementoblastoma
	Central cementifying fibroma
	Cemento-ossifying fibroma
Fibroosseous Lesions	Central ossifying fibroma
	Central giant-cell granuloma
	Aneurysmal bone cyst
	Osteoma
	Osteoid osteoma
	Osteoblastoma
Other Lesions	Hemangioma
	Eosinophilic granuloma
	Neurilemmoma
	Neurofibroma
	Pigmented neuroectodermal tumor

Limitations and Contraindications

The enucleation and curettage procedure is limited in the treatment of multicystic lesions for which the treatment of choice might otherwise be the unicystic counterpart. Benign multicystic lesions of the oral and maxillofacial region may have numerous loculations and invaginations that would make access extremely difficult even using an extraoral approach and almost impossible if using an intraoral approach. In addition, the enucleation process may not remove the pathology in its entirety, and physical and chemical curettage may not be able to access or remove all remnants of the lesion. This will invariably lead to persistence of the lesion, particularly a high recurrence lesion such as OKC or in aggressive benign lesions such as the multicystic ameloblastoma.

The enucleation and curettage approach is contraindicated in solid locally aggressive benign and malignant lesions. Solid benign aggressive lesions such as ameloblastoma would have an extremely high recurrence rate with enucleation and curettage[8] and require resection with at least 1-cm margins in the mandible and partial maxillectomy.[7] Malignant lesions require a more aggressive composite resection, which is not possible with the enucleation and curettage approach.

TECHNIQUE: Enucleation and Curettage

STEP 1: Radiographic Evaluation

All available radiographic imaging results, such as panoramic radiographs and medical and cone beam computed tomography scans, must be thoroughly assessed. This will help determine the intrabony and soft tissue extent of the lesion and the anatomic structures such as tooth roots and nerves that may be involved (Fig. 93.1A).

STEP 2: Incision

An incision is marked to ensure that it is placed over an area of sound bone that allows for adequate tissue closure. This placement is vital, because it ensures the closure of the incision will not be placed over a bony defect. Placement of the incision over a bony defect may cause the wound to break down into the lesion cavity. This may cause defects in the surgical area that may result in functional and reconstructive difficulties (Fig. 93.1B).

STEP 3: Lateral Corticotomy

A small round or fissure bur is used to create a lateral corticotomy over the lesion. The lateral corticotomy should be made over an area of sound bone that will not be involved in closure of the incision line. This will allow for adequate access to the lesion that is not over the area of bony defect and maintain the integrity of the surrounding anatomy. The corticotomy should be of sufficient size to allow for adequate access to the lesion and to preserve surrounding tissue (Fig. 93.1C).

TECHNIQUE: Enucleation and Curettage—*cont'd*

STEP 4: Enucleation

Enucleation of the lesion is initiated at its most readily accessible point. A double-ended curette is used with the sharp edge placed against the bone. It may be necessary to decompress the cyst during the procedure to facilitate greater access and removal of the lesion. It is vital to use the sharp end of the curette between the lesion and against the bone so that the sharp edge of the curette is not against the lesion. This will allow for enucleation of the lesion and minimize the occurrence of tear of the pathologic entity. A cyst lining tear may occur if the sharp end of the curette is introduced against the lesion lining and may result in inadequate enucleation and eventual persistence of the lesion. This is particularly important in lesions such as the OKC, which has a significantly thin and friable cellular lining and is highly susceptible to tear. When careful enucleation is not performed, remnants of the pathology may result in the persistence of the lesion (Fig. 93.1D).

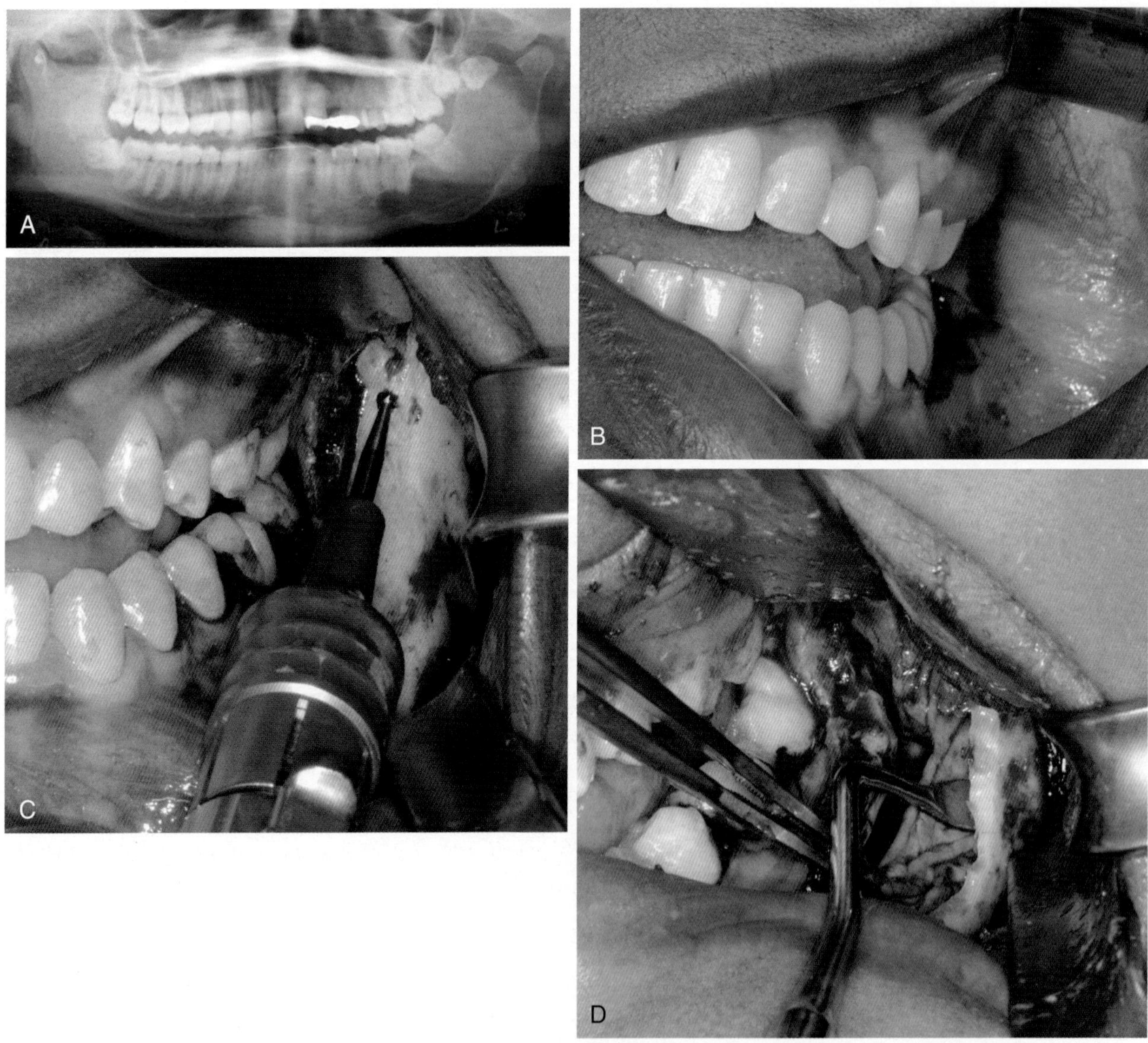

Figure 93.1 **A,** A panoramic radiograph revealing a well-circumscribed radiolucency associated with the crown of a completely impacted and grossly displaced lower left mandibular third molar that encompasses the entire left mandibular ramus and extends into the body of the mandible. **B,** An incision line is demarcated in the sagittal plane over an area of sound bone. **C,** Following subperiosteal dissection, an area of bone is revealed over which a round or fissure may be used to create a lateral osteotomy through which the lesion may be accessed. **D,** A sharp curved curette is used with the sharp edge against the bone to enucleate the cystlike lesion.

TECHNIQUE: Enucleation and Curettage—*cont'd*

STEP 5: Pathology Removal
Once the lesion has been successfully enucleated, it is removed intact from its cavity (Fig. 93.1E).

STEP 6: Curettage or Peripheral Ostectomy
The cavity that remains is examined thoroughly for any gross remnants of the lesion. At this time, a sharp curette may be used to ensure that the cavity is thoroughly curetted and that no gross pathology remains. A peripheral ostectomy may also be completed with a large round diamond bur with copious cool irrigation to remove 1 to 2 mm of surrounding bone until the cavity is clear of all visible pathology. In the case of the OKC, the addition of chemical curettage with Carnoy's solution may also be a consideration and has been shown to significantly decrease recurrence rates,[8] or liquid nitrogen may be used[9] (Fig. 93.1F and G, Box 93.1).

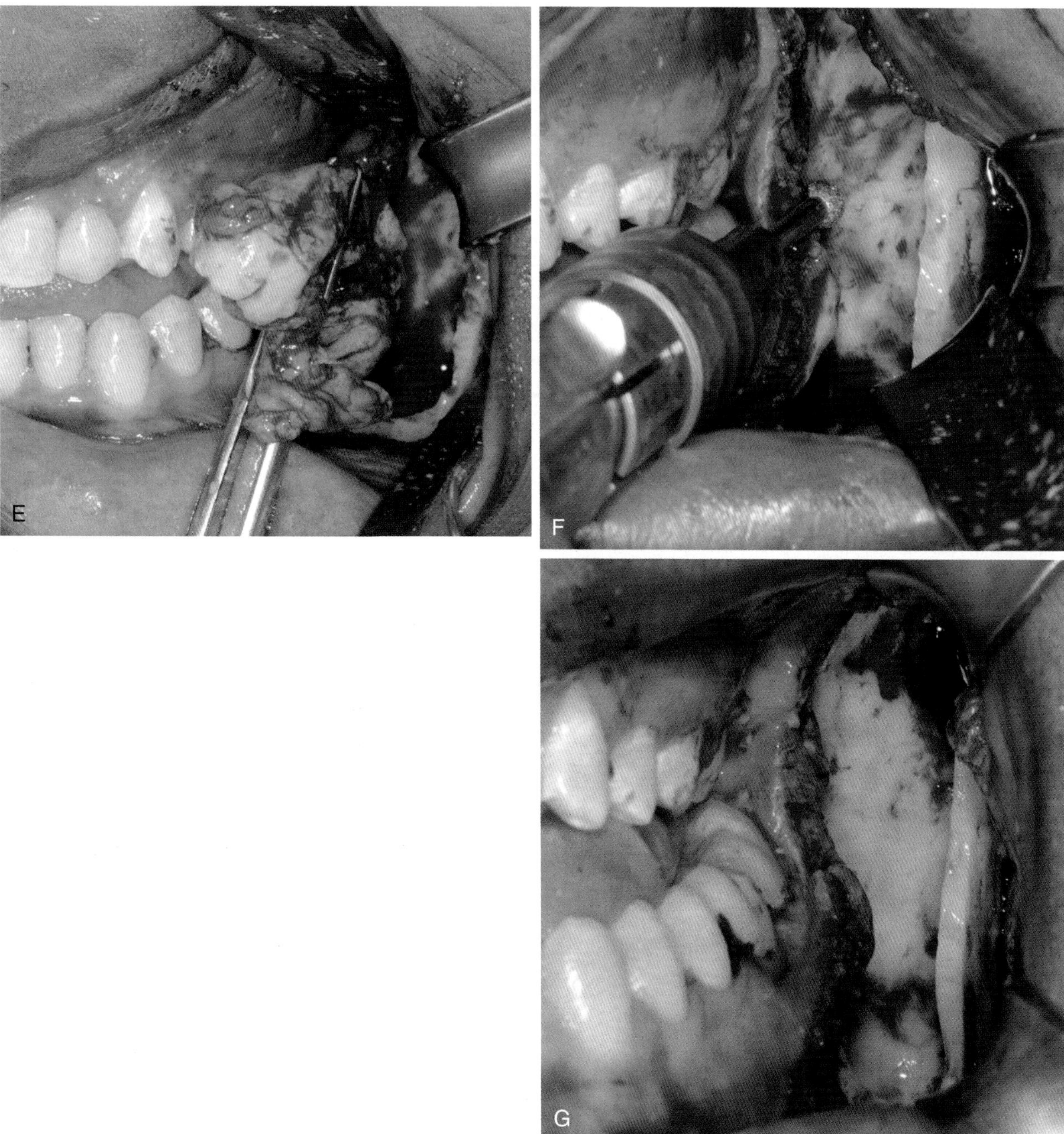

Figure 93.1, cont'd **E,** The lesion is removed in its entirety with the associated impacted mandibular third molar. **F,** A peripheral ostectomy is completed with either a sharp curette or a large round diamond bur to remove any potentially remaining lining of the lesion. **G,** Once the peripheral ostectomy is completed, the cavity that once contained the lesion should be free of all visible pathology.

Continued

BOX 93.1 Carnoy's Solution

Ferric Chloride	1 g
Absolute alcohol	60%
Chloroform	30%
Glacial acetic acid	10%

TECHNIQUE: Enucleation and Curettage—*cont'd*

STEP 7: Bone Grafting (Optional)

The option to immediately reconstruct the defect caused by the enucleation and curettage of benign pathology of the oral and maxillofacial region is controversial.[10] There are currently no known prospective randomized clinical trials comparing simple blood clot healing with different reconstructive techniques. The clinical studies that do exist advocate autogenous bone grafting, tissue-engineered bone substitutes,[11] or platelet-rich plasma.[12] Some studies have recommended that benign lesions that have undergone enucleation and curettage have immediate bone graft reconstruction to maintain mandibular integrity, reduce the risk of pathologic fracture, and permit restoration of function with implant-supported prostheses.[13] The option to bone graft the bony void left by the enucleation of pathology may be determined on a case-by-case basis. As it has been shown that there is spontaneous bone regeneration in osseous defects from enucleation and curettage,[14] the decision to bone graft is generally based on several factors such as the size, extent, and location of the lesion; the age of the patient; and the patient's physiologic capacity to undergo the procedure. Larger lesions will leave a void that may weaken the mandible and thereby make it more susceptible to fracture. These defects may benefit from an autogenous bone graft that may decrease the amount of time required to allow for bony fill and improve the structural integrity of the mandible. The age of the patient is also a consideration, as younger patients are able to regenerate bone into the defect faster and more effectively than older patients, thereby returning the mandible to structural integrity sooner. Also, elderly patients may not have the physiologic reserve to undergo a prolonged procedure to facilitate the harvesting and placement of an autogenous bone graft or the ability to recover from it.

STEP 8: Closure

The incision site is then closed in layers with resorbable sutures. A watertight closure is recommended with interrupted horizontal mattress sutures (Fig. 93.1H).

STEP 9: Post Removal Examination of the Lesion

The lesion should be examined to ensure that it has been removed in its entirety. It is advisable to open the lesion prior to processing for histologic microscopic evaluation to determine if any hidden pathologic entity, such as squamous cell carcinoma or another solid tumor, is present[15] (Fig. 93.1I).

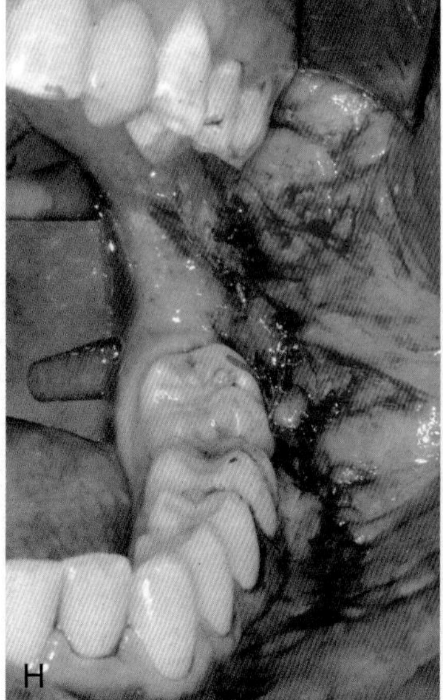

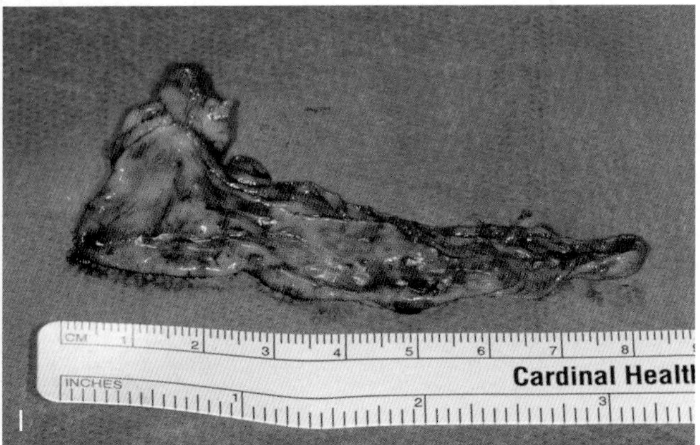

Figure 93.1, cont'd **H,** Primary closure is then achieved with resorbable sutures over an area of sound bone to prevent breakdown of the incision. **I,** The lesion is then inspected to ensure that it has been removed in its entirety, or for the presence of any solid masses within it.

TECHNIQUE: Enucleation and Curettage—*cont'd*

STEP 10: Postoperative Panoramic Radiograph

Postoperative and follow-up radiographs are obtained to assess the extent of the procedure, to ensure that the lesion has been successfully removed, to determine if there have been any pathologic or surgical fractures of the affected area, and to evaluate any reconstructive procedures that may have been performed. Aggressive benign lesions, such as the unicystic ameloblastoma or OKC, should be radiographically evaluated for an extended period of time following removal of the lesion (Fig. 93.1J).

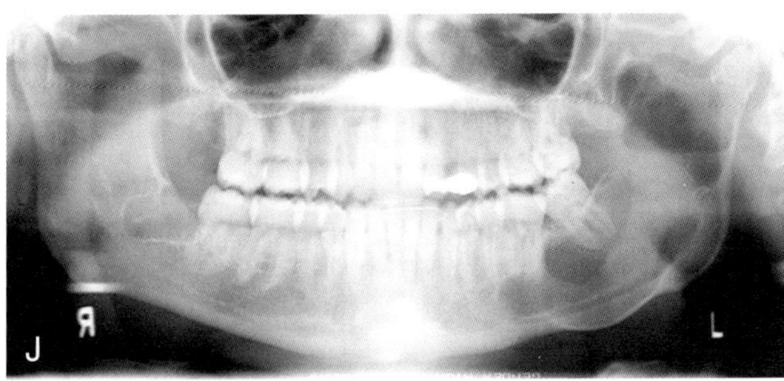

Figure 93.1, cont'd **J,** A postoperative panoramic radiograph is obtained to evaluate the surgical site for possible persistent or recurrent pathology and pathologic fractures.

ALTERNATIVE TECHNIQUE 1: Extraoral Approach

The extraoral approach to enucleation and curettage of benign pathology of the mandible may at times be warranted due to the greatly improved surgical access provided to the lesion. This may be particularly important when vital structures, such as the inferior alveolar nerve, are involved[16–18] or when placement of a rigid fixation plate is required to prevent a mandibular fracture that may result from the loss of structural integrity as a combined result of the enucleation and curettage of the lesion.[19] This approach may improve visibility to the lesion to prevent damage to these structures. The major disadvantages of the extraoral approach are scar formation and potential facial nerve injury. The benefits and risks should be weighed on a per-patient basis to determine if this approach is warranted (Fig. 93.2).

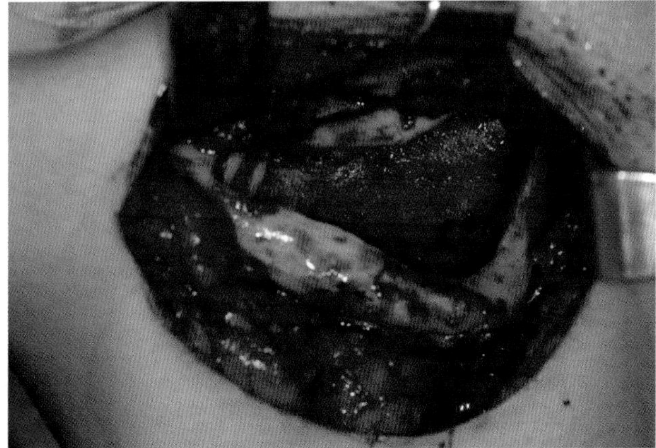

Figure 93.2 The mandible is accessed via an extraoral approach with combined retromandibular and submandibular approaches. This allows for superior access to the mandibular lesion when warranted.

ALTERNATIVE TECHNIQUE 2: Endoscopic Approach

The endoscopic approach to the enucleation and curettage of benign oral and maxillofacial pathology can be applied for both maxillary[20] and mandibular lesions.[21–23] Endoscopic transnasal surgery for maxillary odontogenic pathology is less invasive than the conventional approach, as the access incision is significantly smaller. It may also be advantageous for preserving the affected teeth and surgically managing odontogenic cysts that extend to the maxillary sinus.[20] The endoscopic enucleation and curettage method of mandibular pathology has been used successfully to manage lesions that are large[23] or difficult to access (such as the condyle)[21,22] without an extraoral approach. The endoscopically assisted enucleation and curettage procedure may decrease the risk of scar formation and facial nerve injury, reduce hospitalization time, and improve functional recovery[22] (Fig. 93.3).

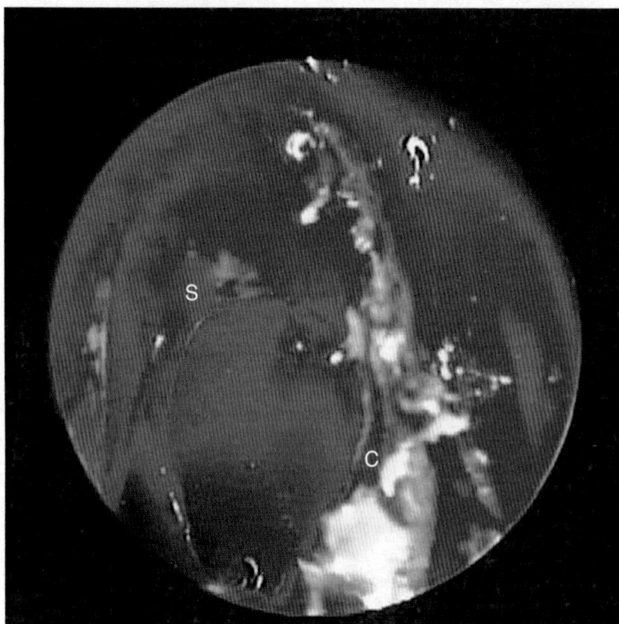

Figure 93.3 The view through an endoscope during an endoscopic approach for intraoral enucleation of a solitary cyst of the mandibular condyle. (From Kretzschmar DP, Postma GN, Inman JL. Intraoral endoscopic enucleation of a central mandibular condylar lesion. *J Oral Maxillofac Surg*. 2005;63(6):865-869.)

Avoidance and Management of Intraoperative Complications

Damage to adjacent structures is the most common intraoperative complication of this technique, which may include damage to adjacent teeth and nerves. Because most oral and maxillofacial pathology that is amenable to enucleation and curettage in this region is intimately involved with structures such as teeth and nerves, careful attention to surgical technique is vital. For example, the enucleation and curettage of lesions such as a OKC may be heavily interdigitated around teeth and into interproximal areas, so these may be difficult areas in which to perform curettage. The best way to avoid this complication is to attain the best possible intraoperative access by securing visibility, which is an important part of the surgical approach. In these situations, the utilization of chemical curettage with Carnoy's solution[6] or liquid nitrogen[7] may be warranted, based on the surgeon's preference and familiarity with their use. Good visibility may prevent iatrogenic damage to structures such as tooth roots or the inferior alveolar neurovascular bundle.

Tearing of the lesion is another intraoperative complication that is avoidable with careful attention to meticulous technique. Tearing of the lesion lining may result in remnants that persist. The surgeon can avoid this complication by carefully handling the curette gently between the lesion and bone, always with the sharp edge against the bone. The temptation to use the sharp edge of the curette against the lining of the lesion may cause tearing and inadequate enucleation.

Enucleation and curettage in the mandible, particularly large lesions that have resorbed a significant amount of bone, may lead to intraoperative results.[24] Large mandibular pathology may have already significantly weakened the mandible, and after enucleation of the lesion, curettage may reduce the structural integrity of the mandible further, resulting in fracture. Even without curettage, the mandible may have been weakened to the degree that any amount of manipulation would result in fracture. The preoperative radiographic assessment of the lesion is extremely important in this situation. If the lesion has resorbed the mandible so much that the chance of mandibular fracture following enucleation and curettage has increased, precautions should be taken to manage or prevent this situation. This may involve a simple procedure such as placing the patient on a soft nonchew diet until it can be radiographically confirmed that the regenerative process has begun in the mandible and there has been some bone fill in the area of potential fracture. Additional preventive treatment may involve the application of maxillomandibular fixation with arch bars for a period of time to help prevent fracture due to mandibular movement or mastication. Also, a rigid titanium plate may be placed, either intraorally or extraorally, whichever is more accessible, to stabilize and strengthen the mandible while it regenerates enough bone, either spontaneously or through a bone graft, to restore the structural integrity necessary for normal mandibular function.

Postoperative Considerations

The most common potential postoperative complication of enucleation and curettage of benign oral and maxillofacial pathology is infection. Because most procedures can be performed intraorally, contamination with oral bacteria into the blood-filled cavity of the pathology is always a possibility. Antibiotics, such as amoxicillin and metronidazole, have been shown to be present in measurable quantities in cyst walls, fluid, and surrounding tissues and to reduce the number of bacteria in the cystic fluid.[25] It is therefore recommended that patients receive antibiotics before and after surgery to help prevent infections.

Another consideration is the need for postoperative root canal therapy on teeth that have intimate root involvement with the pathology. The enucleation and curettage of lesions such as the OKC that is heavily interdigitated around tooth roots may be performed without the need for root canal therapy.[26] Apical curettage of tooth roots may lead to denervated but not devitalized results, as there is an extensive vascular architecture that provides vascularity through the periodontal ligament.[27]

Enucleation and curettage of maxillary pathology may extend into the maxillary and nasal sinuses and result in perforation and possible oroantral communication and fistula. Oroantral communications, when less than 2 mm in diameter, may heal spontaneously. However, when spontaneous healing does not occur, intervention may be required. A plethora of surgical[28,29] and nonsurgical[30] techniques have been developed to close oroantral fistulas. The most common and simple techniques are the buccal advancement flap and the buccal fat pad advancement. Location of the communication is important in the method of closure. Posteriorly, such as in the third molar area, or palatally located oroantral, communications are less amenable to the use of the buccal advancement flap, as the tension on the flap increases due to the need for excessive mobilization to cover the defect. This also obliterates the vestibule in this area, making potential reconstruction, such as with a denture or obturator, more difficult. In these situations, the buccal fat pad advancement technique may be more advantageous because it may extend a pedicle of vascularized fat to an area of almost 6 cm in diameter and not require primary coverage as it will heal by secondary intention and eventually completely undergo epithelialization.[31]

Late fracture of the mandible is a postoperative complication that may also occur from the combination of the enucleation of the pathologic lesion (which may have already significantly decreased the structural integrity of the mandible) and the curettage, which may further weaken the mandible following removal of a few millimeters of bone. A surgically induced fracture may ensue, which would require definitive treatment. Postoperative fracture of the mandible may occur at any time until the mandible has regenerated enough bone to reach its prepathologic structural state. Depending on the displacement and location of the fracture, treatment options for this complication range from a period of maxillomandibular fixation to extraoral open reduction and rigid internal fixation.

References

1. Partsch C. Uber kiefercysten. *Dtsch Monatsschr Zahnheilkd.* 1892;10:271.
2. Partsch C. Zur behandlung der kieferzysten. *Dtsch Monatsschr Zahnheilkd.* 1910;28:252.
3. Dowsett EB. Unique dental cyst. *Proc R Soc Med.* 1933;26(12):1562.
4. Wassmund M. *Textbook of the Practical Surgery of the Mouth and the Pine [Lehrbuch der praktischen Chirurgie des Mundes und der Kiefer].* Vol. 1. Leipzig, Germany: Hermann Meusser; 1935.
5. Stoelinga PJ. The management of aggressive cysts of the jaws. *J Maxillofac Oral Surg.* 2012;11(1):2–12.
6. Kaczmarzyk T, Mojsa I, Stypulkowska J. A systematic review of the recurrence rate for keratocystic odontogenic tumour in relation to treatment modalities. *Int J Oral Maxillofac Implants.* 2012;41(6):756–767.
7. Pogrel MA, Montes DM. Is there a role for enucleation in the management of ameloblastoma? *Int J Oral Maxillofac Implants.* 2009;38(8):807–812.
8. Ghandhi D, Ayoub AF, Pogrel MA, MacDonald G, Brocklebank LM, Moos KF. Ameloblastoma: a surgeon's dilemma. *J Oral Maxillofac Surg.* 2006;64(7): 1010–1014.
9. D'Agostino A, Fior A, Pacino GA, Bedogni A, Santis D, Nocini PF. Retrospective evaluation on the surgical treatment of jaw bones ameloblastic lesions. Experience with 20 clinical cases. *Minerva Stomatol.* 2001;50(1–2):1–7.
10. Ettl T, Gosau M, Sader R, Reichert TE. Jaw cysts—filling or no filling after enucleation? A review. *J Craniomaxillofac Surg.* 2012;40(6):485–493.
11. Pradel W, Eckelt U, Lauer G. Bone regeneration after enucleation of mandibular cysts: comparing autogenous grafts from tissue-engineered bone and iliac bone. *Oral Surg Oral Med Oral Pathol Oral Radiol Endod.* 2006;101(3):285–290.
12. Nagaveni NB, Praveen RB, Umashankar KV, Pranav B, Sreedevi R, Radhika NB. Efficacy of platelet-rich-plasma (PRP) in bone regeneration after cyst enucleation in pediatric patients—a clinical study. *J Clin Pediatr Dent.* 2010;35(1):81–87.
13. Barry CP, Kearns GJ. Case report—odontogenic keratocysts: enucleation, bone grafting and implant placement: an early return to function. *J Ir Dent Assoc.* 2003;49(3):83–88.
14. Ihan Hren N, Miljavec M. Spontaneous bone healing of the large bone defects in the mandible. *Int J Oral Maxillofac Surg.* 2008;37(12):1111–1116.
15. Jain M, Mittal S, Gupta DK. Primary intraosseous squamous cell carcinoma arising in odontogenic cysts: an insight in pathogenesis. *J Oral Maxillofac Surg.* 2013;71(1):e7–e14.
16. Bali A, Bali D, Sharma A, Iyer N. Extraoral enucleation of dentigerous cyst: a case report of rare treatment option and review of literatures. *Indian J Oral Sci.* 2012;3:53.
17. Yüzügüllü B, Araz K. Validity of conventional surgical treatment methods for mandibular dentigerous cysts. Two case reports. *N Y State Dent J.* 2011;77(2):36–39.
18. Savitha K, Cariappa KM. An effective extraoral approach to the mandible. A technical note. *Int J Oral Maxillofac Surg.* 1998;27(1):61–62.
19. Mintz S, Allard M, Nour R. Extraoral removal of mandibular odontogenic dentigerous cysts: a report of 2 cases. *J Oral Maxillofac Surg.* 2001;59(9):1094–1096.
20. Seno S, Ogawa T, Shibayama M, et al. Endoscopic sinus surgery for the odontogenic maxillary cysts. *Rhinology.* 2009;47(3):305–309.
21. Giovannetti F, Cassoni A, Battisti A, Gennaro P, Della Monaca M, Valentini V. Endoscopic approach to benign lesion involving the mandibular condyle. *J Craniofac Surg.* 2010;21(4):1234–1237.
22. Saia G, Fusetti S, Emanuelli E, Ferronato G, Procopio O. Intraoral endoscopic enucleation of a solitary bone cyst of the mandibular condyle. *Int J Oral Maxillofac Implants.* 2012;41(3):317–320.
23. Sembronio S, Albiero AM, Zerman N, Costa F, Politi M. Endoscopically assisted enucleation and curettage of large mandibular odontogenic keratocyst. *Oral Surg Oral Med Oral Pathol Oral Radiol Endod.* 2009;107(2):193–196.
24. Tieghi R, Consorti G, Clauser LC. Pathologic fracture of the mandible after removal of follicular cyst. *J Craniofac Surg.* 2011;22(5):1779–1780.
25. Traina AA, Deboni MC, Naclério-Homem MdaG, Cai S. Action of antimicrobial agents on infected odontogenic cysts. *Quintessence Int.* 2005;36(10):805–811.
26. Marx RE, Stern D. *Oral and Maxillofacial Pathology: A Rationale for Diagnosis and Treatment.* Carol Stream, Illinois: Quintessence Publishing; 2003.
27. Kramer IR. The vascular architecture of the human dental pulp. *Arch Oral Biol.* 1960;2:177–189.
28. Nezafati S, Vafaii A, Ghojazadeh M. Comparison of pedicled buccal fat pad flap with buccal flap for closure of oro-antral communication. *Int J Oral Maxillofac Implants.* 2012;41(5):624–628.
29. Batra H, Jindal G, Kaur S. Evaluation of different treatment modalities for closure of oro-antral communications and formulation of a rational approach. *J Maxillofac Oral Surg.* 2010;9(1):13–18.
30. Burić N, Jovanović G, Krasić D, et al. The use of absorbable polyglactin/polydioxanon implant (Ethisorb®) in non-surgical closure of oro-antral communication. *J Craniomaxillofac Surg.* 2012;40(1):71–77.
31. Baumann A, Ewers R. Application of the buccal fat pad in oral reconstruction. *J Oral Maxillofac Surg.* 2000;58(4):389–392.

Marsupialization

Mehran Hossaini-Zadeh

Armamentarium

#15 Blade
Adson or DeBakey forceps
Appropriate sutures
Drill with round bur
Local anesthetic with vasoconstrictor
Minnesota retractor
Round dental curette
Weider retractor

History of the Procedure

The *American Heritage Medical Dictionary* defines marsupialization as a surgical alteration of a cyst or similar enclosed cavity by making an incision and suturing the flaps to the adjacent tissue, creating a pouch.[1] Various authors have described marsupialization, including Jacobson, who provided the first description in 1950 for management of the Bartholin duct cyst.[2,3] He constructed a mucocutaneous junction by suturing the cyst lining to the skin, thus creating a continuous decompression of the lesion. This was in contrast to drainage of the cystic lesion and packing the cavity with iodoform gauze, where failure occurred due to the retraction of wound edges and stenosis. With the introduction of various types of catheters, the use of marsupialization seems to have declined. In oral and maxillofacial surgery, the use of marsupialization has been reported in the management of various odontogenic and nonodontogenic lesions such as the odontogenic keratocyst and ranula.[4,5]

Indications for the Use of the Procedure

One indication for marsupialization is to create a new accessory tract for drainage of a gland.[2] Various authors have reported this technique for the management of oral ranula, particularly in the pediatric population.[6–8] However, the reported recurrence rate associated with simple marsupialization can range from 14% to 67%.[9] Due to this recurrence rate, a modification of the technique, including packing the marsupialized cavity, has been described.[5,8] Based on a literature review by Patel, the average rate of recurrence for oral ranula after simple or modified marsupialization is 20%.[10] Excision of the ipsilateral sublingual gland along with the ranula has been demonstrated to be the most definitive treatment with the lowest rate of recurrence. However, despite its higher recurrence rate, marsupialization of the oral ranula may be considered a first-line treatment.[7,10,11]

Another indication for marsupialization is when continuous decompression of a lesion is desired, such as in the management of an odontogenic cyst.[4] Marsupialization has been described as an effective treatment modality for the management of an odontogenic keratocyst (OKC)[4,12] Upon marsupialization and decompression, substantial histologic changes have been reported in the epithelium of an OKC.[13–15] Based on cytokeratin-10 immunohistochemical staining, a treatment time of at least 9 months is required to demonstrate these histologic changes.[15] These findings indicate that marsupialization can be an effective technique for managing a keratocystic odontogenic tumor. However, a recurrence rate of 12% has been reported with this technique.[16] Despite these reports, marsupialization is an effective treatment modality for managing an OKC.

Marsupialization has been reported in the management of benign odontogenic tumors such as ameloblastoma. However, the rate of recurrence continues to be concerning.[17]

Limitations and Contraindications

Use of marsupialization is limited to cystic lesions that require continuous drainage. As a result, it cannot be used to manage solid lesions. The utility of marsupialization is debatable when the lesion is not composed of an epithelial lining that can be sutured to the surrounding mucosa or skin. Marsupialization is contraindicated when previous attempts at conservative treatment have failed and when complete or marginal resection is indicated.

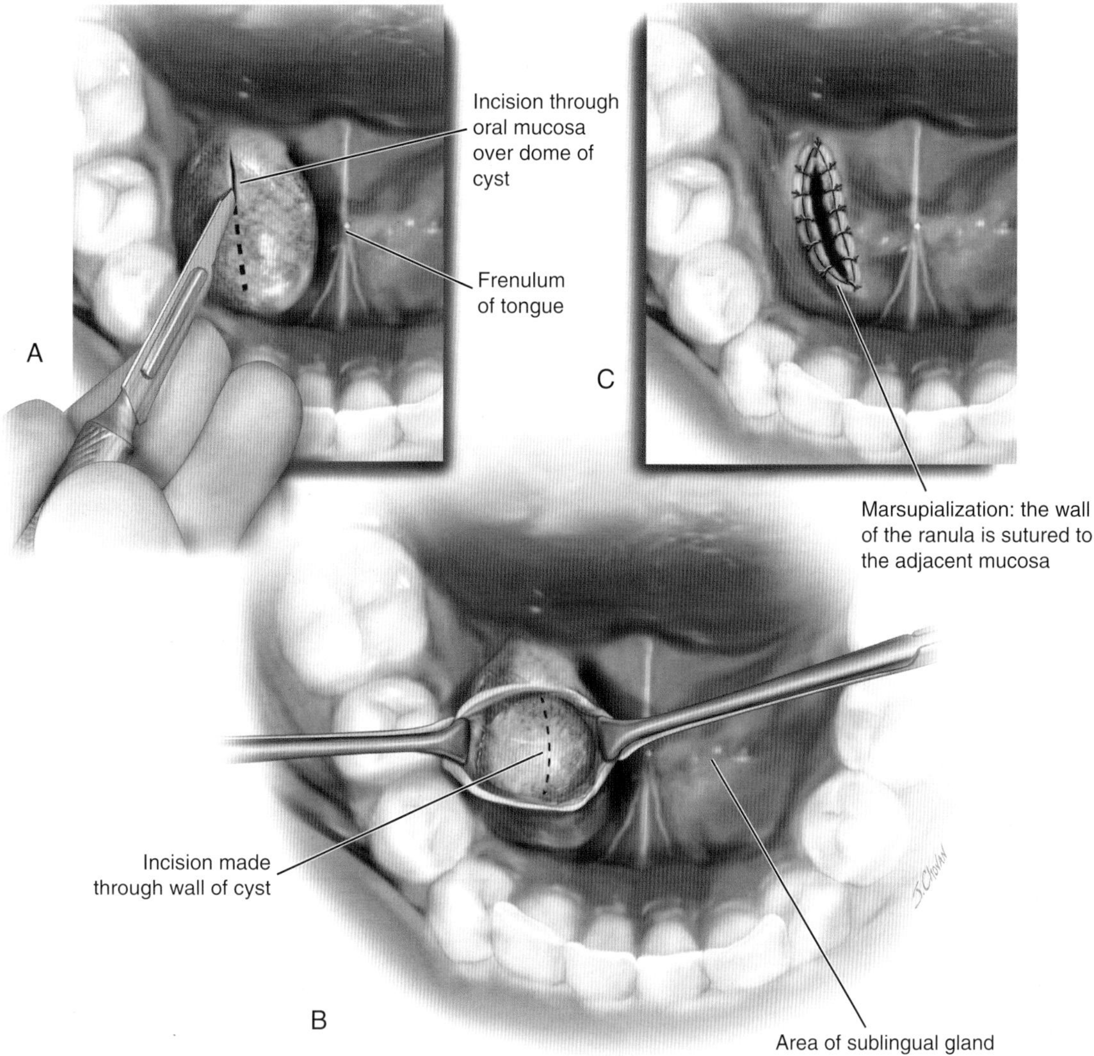

Figure 94.1 Marsupialization of a floor-of-the-mouth ranula.

TECHNIQUE: Marsupialization

STEP 1: Anesthesia and Patient Positioning

Marsupialization can be carried out under local anesthesia in an office setting. However, factors such as access to the lesion, the patient's level of anxiety or cooperation, and the ability to achieve adequate anesthesia to carry out the procedure should be considered. Therefore, performing the procedure under general anesthesia in the operating room setting may be considered as an alternative. The management of lesions in the posterior mandible, maxilla, or floor of the mouth is often most predictable in the operating room setting. General anesthesia is administered in conjunction with nasotracheal or oral Ring-Adair-Elwyn endotracheal intubation.

In addition to a local anesthesia block or general anesthesia, the incision site is infiltrated with 2% lidocaine and 1/100,000 epinephrine, or a similar alternative, for hemostasis and postoperative pain control. For soft tissue cystic lesions, such as ranula, Peterson described the simplest marsupialization technique.[18,19] In this technique, a ring of interrupted sutures is placed around the base of the intact cyst.

Patients can be positioned supine on the operating table or in a semireclined position on the operating chair.

STEP 2: Cyst Entry

In case of a ranula, it is advisable to cannulate the associated duct with a lacrimal probe to protect it from injury. A fine noncutting (round) needle with 4-0 Vicryl suture is passed into the cystic cavity, penetrating the mucosa and the cyst lining, and brought out approximately 3 mm from the point of entry.

Continued

TECHNIQUE: Marsupialization—cont'd

STEP 3: Suturing Cyst Lining to Oral Mucosa

The suture is tied, and the procedure is repeated until sutures 6 to 10 mm apart encircle the cyst (Figs. 94.1 and 94.2). With careful passing of the needle and suture, little to no cystic content should escape during this procedure. Once all the sutures are placed, an incision is made into the cystic cavity and the superior portion of the lesion is removed above the suture line. The remainder of the cyst is left undisturbed. At this point the surgical site is irrigated, and surgery is deemed to be complete. When the site has healed, the cystic lesion will be contiguous with the oral mucosa.

STEP 4: Osteotomy

For bony cystic lesions, the technique is slightly modified. For this technique, a mucosal incision is made in the standard fashion and will include the mucosa directly over the cystic lesion. If the lesion has not perforated the cortical plate, subperiosteal dissection is performed to expose the overlying bone.

STEP 5: Marsupialization

Using a round bur, the surgeon de-roofs the cystic lesion by removing the cortical bone overlying the lesion, being careful not to remove the cystic lining. A round dental curette or the broad end of a Woodson elevator is used to carefully dissect the cystic lining from the bony edges. The most superior portion of the cystic lesion is grasped with Adson or DeBakey forceps and excised. At this point, the free margins of the cystic lining are sutured to the free gingival margins, using a fine noncutting (round) needle with 4-0 Vicryl suture. The remainder of the mucosal incision is closed primarily, ensuring the cystic access remains open.

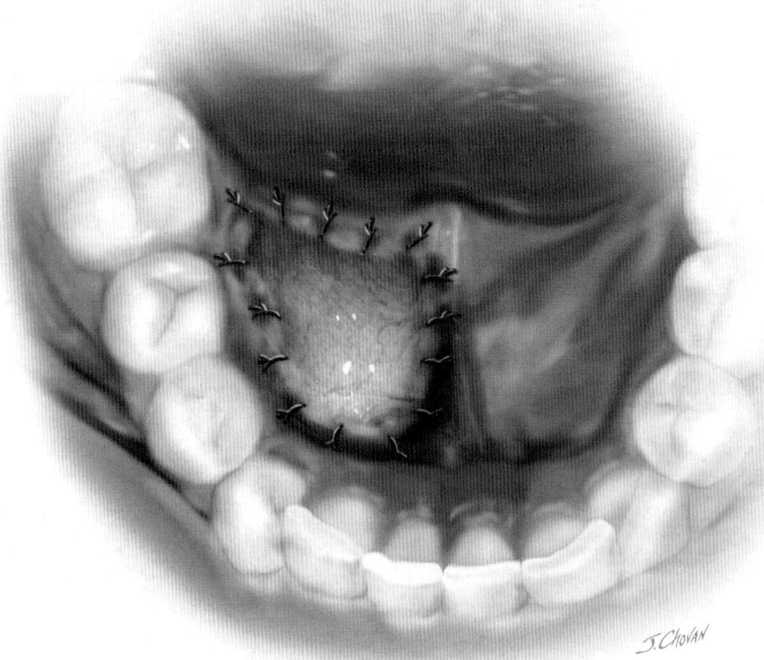

Figure 94.2 Sutures around the periphery of the marsupialized lesion.

ALTERNATIVE TECHNIQUE: Catheter Utilization

The alternative technique is to utilize a catheter to create an opening into the cystic cavity; this is technically a method of decompression. However, the terms *marsupialization* and *decompression* are often used interchangeably. As it has been described, marsupialization in the true sense indicates conversion of a cyst into a pouch contiguous with skin or mucosa. In contrast, decompression implies creating an access into a cystic lesion to reduce its internal pressure. For this technique, an incision is made through the overlying mucosa, and an opening of at least 1 cm in diameter is created into the cystic lesion. Once the cystic content is drained and irrigated, a catheter is inserted into the cystic cavity. The catheter can be fashioned from items such as a nasopharyngeal airway, 16 French rubber catheter, or similar items. The catheter can be secured in place with a nonresorbable suture to the adjacent mucosa. Alternatively, the catheter can be secured to the adjacent teeth using a circumdental ligature wire. The catheter is often left in place until evidence of resolution of the lesion is observed. For mandibular lesions, the catheter requires daily irrigation by the patient for as long as 6 to 9 months (Fig. 94.3).

Avoidance and Management of Intraoperative Complications

A number of intraoperative events may occur that will require a decision-making algorithm. Despite the working diagnosis of a cyst, the lesion may consist of a solid mass. If this is encountered during the surgery, marsupialization or decompression is no longer the appropriate treatment. The lesion may be devoid of content and epithelial lining; this can confirm the diagnosis of entities such as a simple bone cyst or aneurysmal bone cyst. This type of lesion resolves predictably without further treatment; therefore, marsupialization or decompression is not indicated. When dealing with cystic lesions in the soft tissue, the loss of the cystic content and collapse of the lesion will render the dissection and identification of the cystic lining quite challenging. Therefore, the intact cystic lining and contents are critical to the successful completion of the marsupialization technique. When performing marsupialization for the management of a ranula, there is a risk of damage to the corresponding salivary gland duct. Therefore, care should be exercised to identify and protect this and other adjacent ducts and anatomic structures.

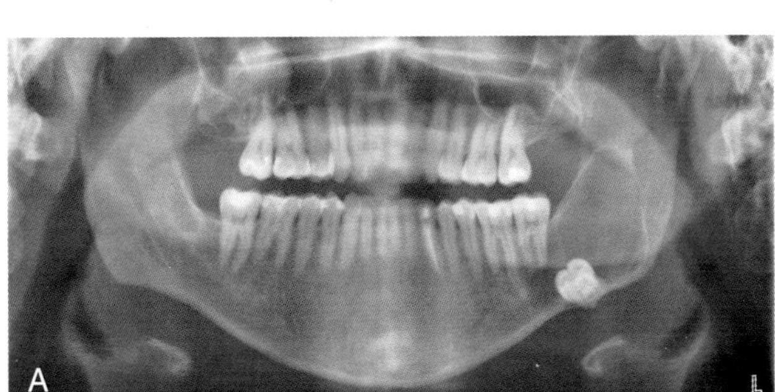

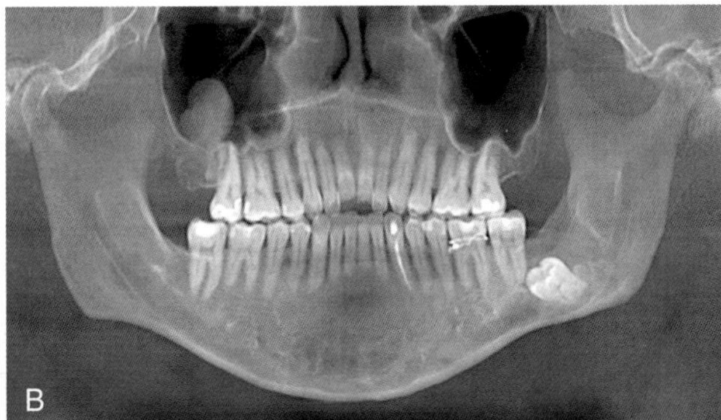

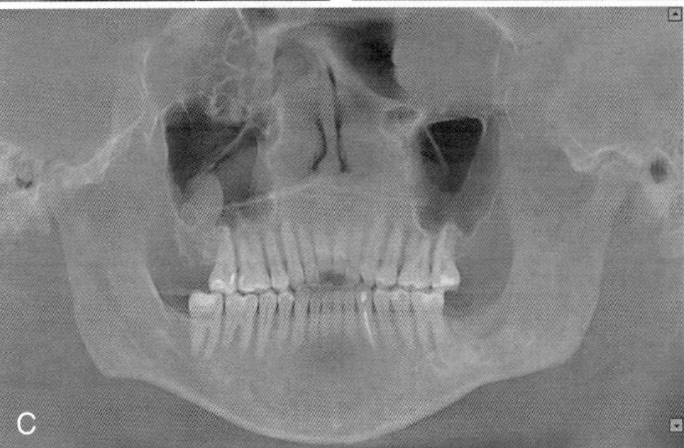

Figure 94.3 **A** Marsupialization of an odontogenic keratocyst. **B** A catheter was utilized to decompress the cyst and permit partial resolution. **C** Thereafter, the remaining cyst was subjected to an enucleation and curettage surgery as definitive management with curative intent.

Postoperative Considerations

The main postoperative complication associated with marsupialization is stenosis of the pouch, thereby reestablishing the cystic cavity. Other complications include infection, an inability to maintain adequate wound hygiene, dislodgement, or blockage of the catheters.

References

1. *The American Heritage Medical Dictionary.* Boston, MA: Houghton Mifflin Company; 2004, 2007.
2. Jacobson P. Vulvovaginal (Bartholin) cyst treatment by marsupialization. *West J Surg Obstet Gynecol.* 1950;58(12):704–708.
3. Omole F, Simmons BJ, Hacker Y. Management of Bartholin's duct cyst and gland abscess. *Am Fam Physician.* 2003;68(1):135–140.
4. Blanas N, Freund B, Schwartz M, Furst IM. Systematic review of the treatment and prognosis of the odontogenic keratocyst. *Oral Surg Oral Med Oral Pathol Oral Radiol Endod.* 2000;90(5):553–558.
5. Baurmash HD. Marsupialization for treatment of oral ranula: a second look at the procedure. *J Oral Maxillofac Surg.* 1992;50(12):1274–1279.
6. Haberal I, Göçmen H, Samim E. Surgical management of pediatric ranula. *Int J Pediatr Otorhinolaryngol.* 2004;68(2):161–163.
7. Yuca K, Bayram I, Cankaya H, Caksen H, Kiroğlu AF, Kiriş M. Pediatric intraoral ranulas: an analysis of nine cases. *Tohoku J Exp Med.* 2005;205(2):151–155.
8. Sandrini FA, Sant'ana-Filho M, Rados PV. Ranula management: suggested modifications in the micro-marsupialization technique. *J Oral Maxillofac Surg.* 2007;65(7):1436–1438.
9. Zhao YF, Jia Y, Chen XM, Zhang WF. Clinical review of 580 ranulas. *Oral Surg Oral Med Oral Pathol Oral Radiol Endod.* 2004;98(3):281–287.
10. Patel MR, Deal AM, Shockley WW. Oral and plunging ranulas: what is the most effective treatment? *Laryngoscope.* 2009;119(8):1501–1509.
11. Mortellaro C, Dall'Oca S, Lucchina AG, et al. Sublingual ranula: a closer look to its surgical management. *J Craniofac Surg.* 2008;19(1):286–290.
12. Pogrel MA, Jordan RC. Marsupialization as a definitive treatment for the odontogenic keratocyst. *J Oral Maxillofac Surg.* 2004;62(6):651–655.
13. Marker P, Brøndum N, Clausen PP, Bastian HL. Treatment of large odontogenic keratocysts by decompression and later cystectomy: a long-term follow-up and a histologic study of 23 cases. *Oral Surg Oral Med Oral Pathol Oral Radiol Endod.* 1996;82(2):122–131.
14. Rodu B, Tate AL, Martinez MG Jr. The implications of inflammation in odontogenic keratocysts. *J Oral Pathol.* 1987;16(10):518–521.
15. August M, Faquin WC, Troulis MJ, Kaban LB. Dedifferentiation of odontogenic keratocyst epithelium after cyst decompression. *J Oral Maxillofac Surg.* 2003;61(6):678–683.
16. Pogrel MA. Decompression and marsupialization as definitive treatment for keratocysts—a partial retraction. *J Oral Maxillofac Surg.* 2007;65(2):362–363.
17. Hong J, Yun PY, Chung IH, et al. Long-term follow up on recurrence of 305 ameloblastoma cases. *Int J Oral Maxillofac Surg.* 2007;36(4):283–288.
18. Peterson LW. In: Kruger GO, ed. *Textbook of Oral Surgery.* 2nd ed. St Louis, MO: Mosby; 1964.
19. Topazian RG. A marsupialization technique for treatment of ranulae. *Aust Dent J.* 1966;11(1):9–12.

CHAPTER 95

Marginal Mandibulectomy

Jasjit K. Dillon, Karl Pennau, and Li Han Lai

Armamentarium

#1, #2, #3 Dierks dissectors
#9 Periosteal elevators
#15 Scalpel blades
Appropriate sutures
Bipolar electrocautery
Bite block
Bone pencil
Cheek retractors (optional)
CO_2 laser (optional)
Dental elevators
Dental forceps
Dermis allograft (optional)
Langenbach retractors
Local anesthetic with vasoconstrictor
Malleable retractors
Mallet
Mayo scissors
Metzenbaum scissors
Minnesota retractors
Molt mouth prop
Monopolar electrocautery
Osteotomes
Peanut/Kittner sponges
Pineapple bur
Reciprocating saw
Ruler
Vascular clips
Weider retractor

History of the Procedure

In 1923, Crile described the marginal mandibulectomy as an incision that is "carried down to the bone and thence into the bone by a sharp chisel or saw, so that a slice of bone can be split off in one piece, bearing the undisturbed cancer off as on a bone platter."[1] Even today, surgery remains the primary treatment for malignant disease of the mandible and its surrounding soft tissues due to the risk of osteoradionecrosis and oral cavity squamous cell carcinoma's relative radio-insensitivity. In the mid-20th century, a segmental resection was the only treatment option for larger gingival and floor of the mouth lesions, or any bony lesions, as it was thought that malignant spread could occur through the periosteal lymphatics of the mandible.[2] In the 1970s, Marchetta et al. refuted this theory and showed that metastasis occurred through local lymphatics and not through the periosteum.[2,3] This discovery allowed for the possibility of marginal (rim or sagittal) mandibulectomy over a segmental resection. The marginal resections have had excellent early oncologic success and have remained a sound surgical treatment for perimandibular carcinomas.[4] In 1993, Barttelbort and Ariyan published a benchmark paper that showed a significant decrease in mandibular strength when the remaining basilar bone height was shortened below 10 mm.[5] He also compared rim resection to sagittal resection, and rim resection showed both greater strength and better oncologic treatment of affected bone.[5] Controversy still exists as to how carcinoma invades the bone. Brown reported that bony invasion is via direct infiltration of the bone, not preferentially to a certain bone location or through the inferior alveolar canal. This allows the inferior alveolar nerve (IAN) to be spared if not clinically or radiographically involved.[6]

This was a significant change for patients, especially in the prereconstruction plate and vascular graft era, who had to suffer significant cosmetic and functional deficits with segmental resections. As technology and imaging have improved, there are now more accurate ways to determine the extent of lesions in and around the mandible, giving us better reconstructive options and diagnostic planning tools to aid in surgical planning for resection. Use of marginal mandibulectomy over segmental resection does remain somewhat controversial, but several studies have shown its efficacy as a treatment for oral carcinoma with minimal invasion into the cortical bone.[7–11]

Indications for the Use of the Procedure

Marginal mandibulectomy is a useful surgical procedure for treating a few malignant and benign processes. It is useful for malignant lesions that affect the soft tissues of the alveolus, buccal sulcus, or floor of the mouth that abut the mandibular periosteum but have not invaded into the marrow space of the mandible. Marginal resection is also indicated when advanced imaging or an intraoperative examination of bone using periosteal stripping shows changes in cortical bone.[9,12,13] Tei and colleagues determined that if there is radiographic erosion, not a "moth-eaten" defect, of the mandible above the inferior alveolar canal secondary to squamous cell carcinoma of the alveolus or gingiva, the inferior border of the mandible can be preserved; if the defect is a moth-eaten defect that is confined to the alveolus, only marginal resection is acceptable.[11] Marginal mandibulectomy is also an excellent alternative to segmental resection for nononcologic processes such as osteonecrosis,[14] osteomyelitis, or benign tumors that leave at least 10 mm of basilar bone.[4]

Limitations and Contraindications

There are several circumstances that preclude marginal mandibulectomy. Patients who have previously undergone radiation therapy are poor candidates for marginal resection.[7,8] Irradiated bone is more susceptible to osteoradionecrosis, and there is an increased likelihood of bony invasion of the disease process and fracture of the residual mandible. Primary bone carcinomas or gross invasion of the medullary space require segmental resection, not marginal resection.[7,8,11] Edentulous patients with an affected atrophic mandible should not have a marginal mandibulectomy because there could be insufficient remaining basilar bone to withstand the forces of mastication and it could potentially lead to pathologic fracture.[10] Preoperative imaging, such as a panoramic radiograph, is helpful for assessing the superior-inferior height of the mandible along with oncologic imaging, such as computed tomography or magnetic resonance imaging scans, according to preference (Fig. 95.1). When there is extensive bone invasion or a thin atrophic mandible, a segmental resection is the resection of choice.

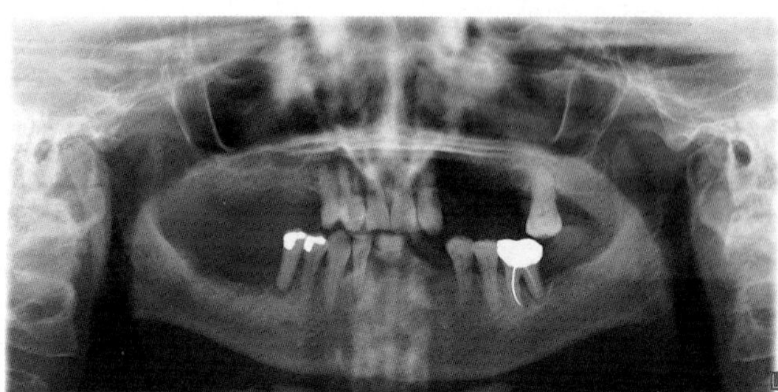

Figure 95.1 Height of mandible.

TECHNIQUE: Marginal Mandibulectomy

STEP 1: Intubation

Nasoendotracheal intubation with the tube secured to the forehead using tape and sutured to the membranous septum and columella, or a tracheostomy secured with appropriate taping or sutures is the preferred airway, depending on the extent of soft tissue resection planned with the procedure. For smaller lateral sulcus lesions that do not include the floor of mouth, oral Ring-Adair-Elwyn intubation could be considered. If using a carbon dioxide (CO_2) laser, the surgeon must consider the use of an armored endotracheal tube depending on the location of the lesion and the type of intubation (Fig. 95.2A and B).

STEP 2: Identify and Isolate

Place the bite block or Molt mouth prop on the contralateral side. Insert a moistened throat pack. Use Weider, Langenbeck, and Minnesota retractors to visualize the lesion. Identify teeth at the margins that need to be extracted, if any. These teeth will be in the line of the osteotomy. Use a marking pen or monopolar cautery to mark an outline of the planned surgical margin, if appropriate. Infiltrate the planned incision with 1% lidocaine with 1:100,000 epinephrine for additional hemostasis (Fig. 95.2C and D).

STEP 3: Dental Extractions and Incision

Use a #15 scalpel to make a sulcular incision around the teeth to be extracted. Release the periodontal ligament with a #9 periosteal elevator. Luxate the teeth with a dental elevator and extract with dental forceps. Using monopolar cautery, make an incision along the previously outlined margin through the mucosa. This could also be done with a CO_2 laser if so desired. If using a CO_2 laser, be sure to use appropriate eye protection for the patient and operating room personnel (Fig. 95.2E).

STEP 4: Dissection

Dissect deeper soft tissues with #1, #2, or #3 dissectors or scissors as desired, and divide subcutaneous tissues and muscle using an electrocautery/laser or Metzenbaum scissors down to the bone. Care should be taken of the surrounding anatomy, such as the lingual nerve, submandibular duct, mental nerve, and facial artery, all of which may or may not be sacrificed. Peanut/Kittner sponges often aid in their visualization and blunt dissection. Cauterize, or ligate, and divide any vessels that inhibit dissection.

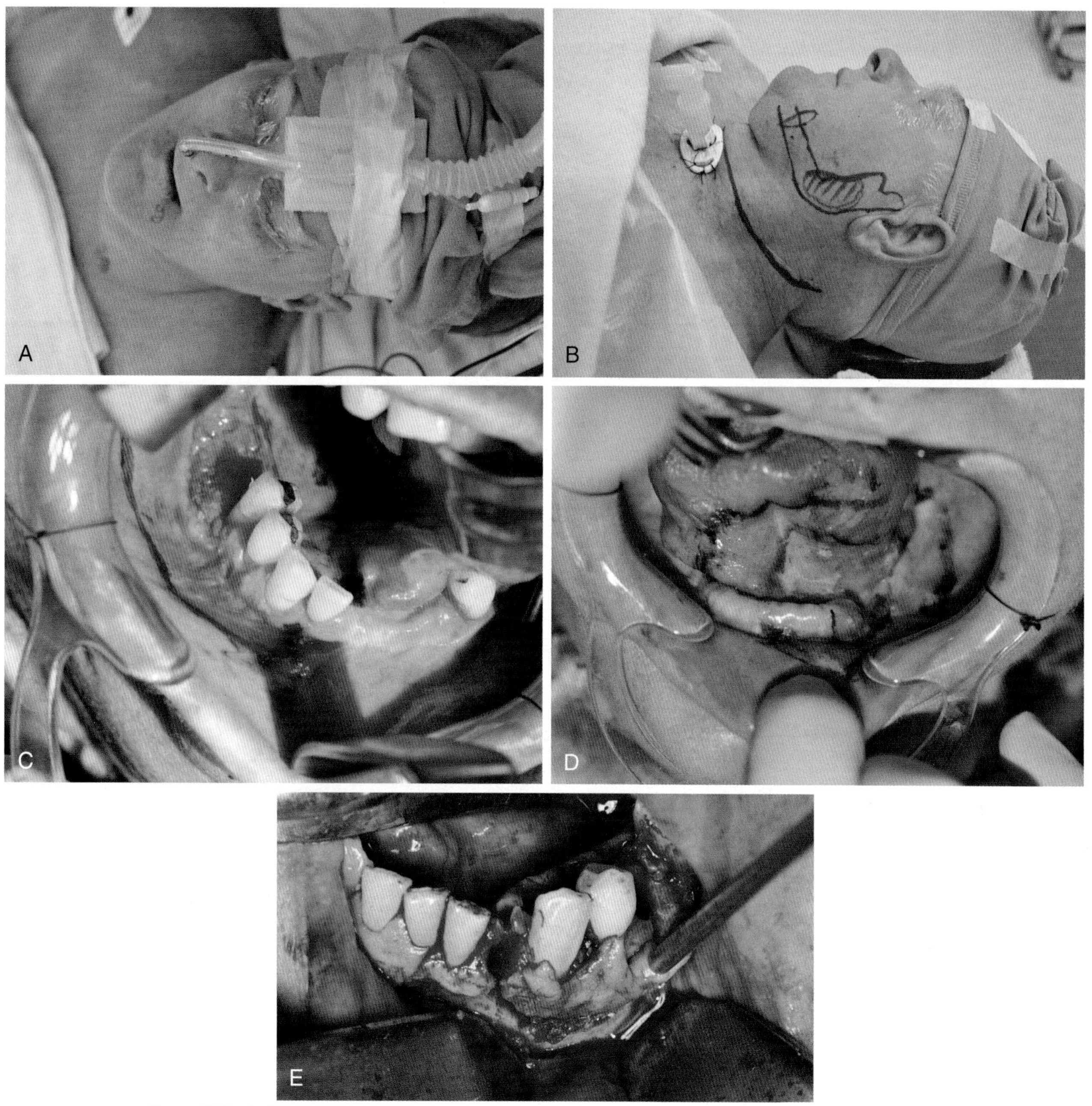

Figure 95.2 **A,** Nasoendotracheal intubation. **B,** Tracheostomy. **C** and **D,** Resection area demarcated. **E,** Extracted teeth around osteotomy sites.

Continued

TECHNIQUE: Marginal Mandibulectomy—*cont'd*

STEP 5: Bone Margins

Raise soft tissue off the bone in a subperiosteal plane with #9 periosteal elevators at the site of the osteotomy to visualize bone beneath the lesion. Note any cortical changes to aid in guiding bone margins. Also preserve pathologic soft tissue and bone continuity to avoid tumor spillage and erroneous final pathologic margins. Mark an outline of the planned surgical margin, using standard oncologic margins if appropriate, with a bone pencil. Plan for the osteotomy to be in a curvilinear fashion, not right angled, for added strength of the remaining mandible.[4] Also consider the height of the remaining bone (at least 10 mm) and the location of the inferior alveolar neurovascular bundle. If possible, preserve the IAN. If the remaining mandible will be left thin, consider removing the coronoid process separately or with a specimen to decrease the proximal pull of the temporalis (Fig. 95.2F).

STEP 6: Osteotomy

With good retraction and protection of surrounding soft tissues, insert the reciprocating saw and try to maintain 90-degree angulation to the bone. Using copious irrigation, make the osteotomy in curvilinear fashion along the predetermined line. Depending on the location of the lesion, this may be technically challenging via a purely intraoral approach. If in conjunction with neck access such as a neck dissection, the transcervical approach can be used for part or all of the osteotomy. If there is no neck dissection, a curved osteotome and mallet may be used to complete a portion of the osteotomy not reachable with the reciprocating saw (Fig. 95.2G).

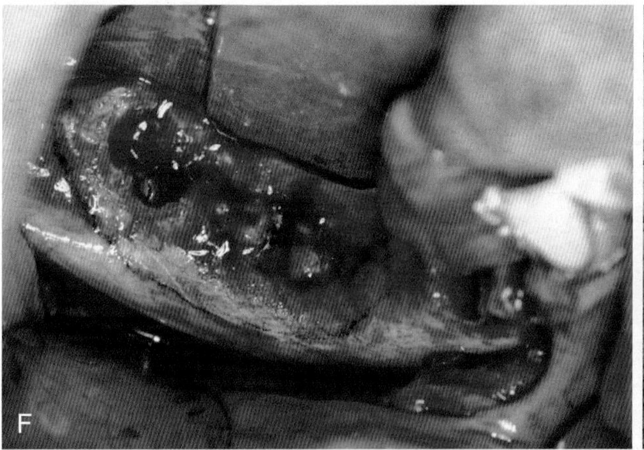

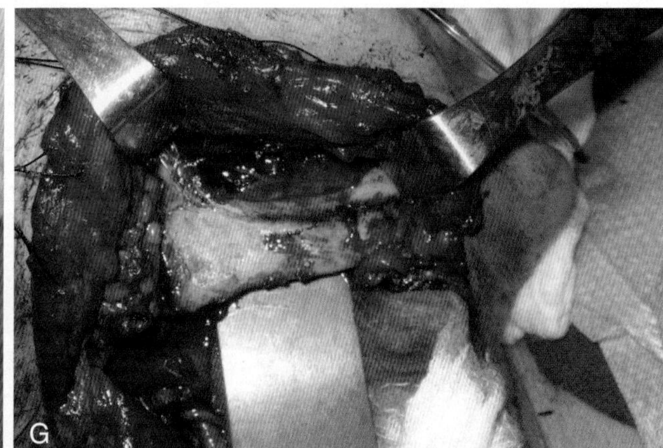

Figure 95.2, cont'd F and G, Bone markings with pencil.

TECHNIQUE: Marginal Mandibulectomy—*cont'd*

STEP 7: Specimen Removal

Remove the bone and soft tissue specimen from the mouth. Control any bleeders within the surgical site. Place 3-0 silk orientation sutures into the specimen, place it in formalin, and send it to pathology. If so desired, take frozen sections or a touch preparation evaluation of the cancellous bone at the margins of the surgical site with Metzenbaum scissors and curettes (Fig. 95.2H–J).

STEP 8: Bone Contouring

Remove sharp edges of the remaining mandible with a pineapple bur and irrigation. Ensure the osteotomy is curved and any straight-line angles are converted to smooth round surfaces to decrease the likelihood of a pathologic fracture. Again, use appropriate retraction of soft tissues and protect vital anatomy (Fig. 95.2K and L1).

STEP 9: Internal Fixation (Optional)

If the IAN has been sacrificed and a minimal height of basilar bone remains in the mandible, consider placement of a load-bearing reconstruction plate. Adapt a plate to the lateral border of the mandible, extending at least two screws proximal and distal to the affected bone. Secure the plate with appropriate locking or nonlocking screws, whichever is preferred (Fig. 95.2M).

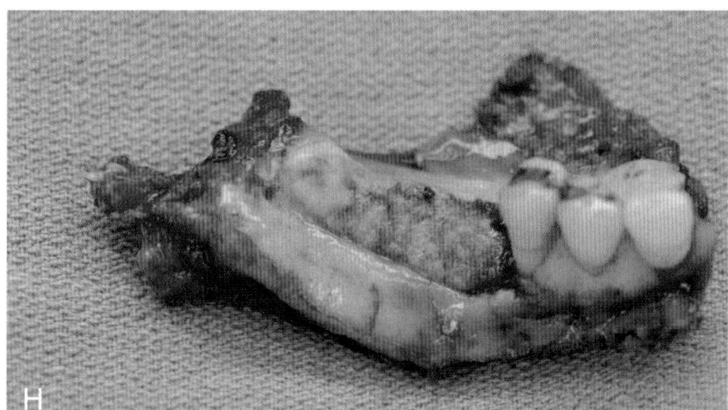

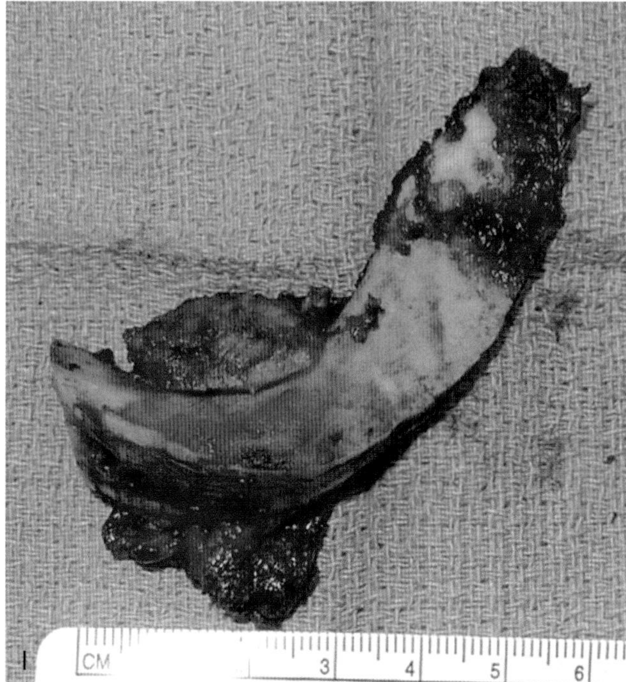

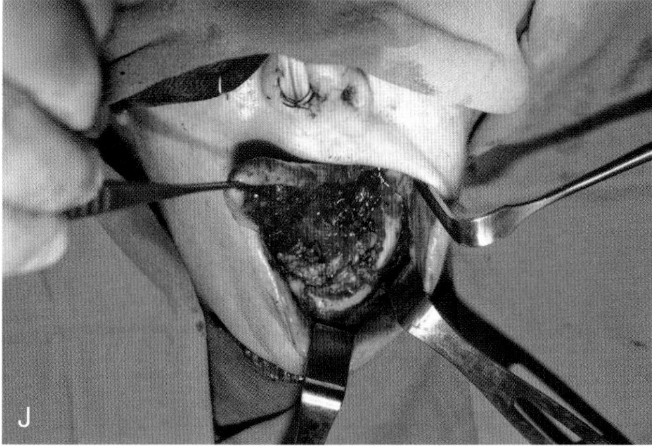

Figure 95.2, cont'd **H,** Specimen. **I,** Undersurface of specimen. **J,** Anterior marginal resection with floor of mouth.

Continued

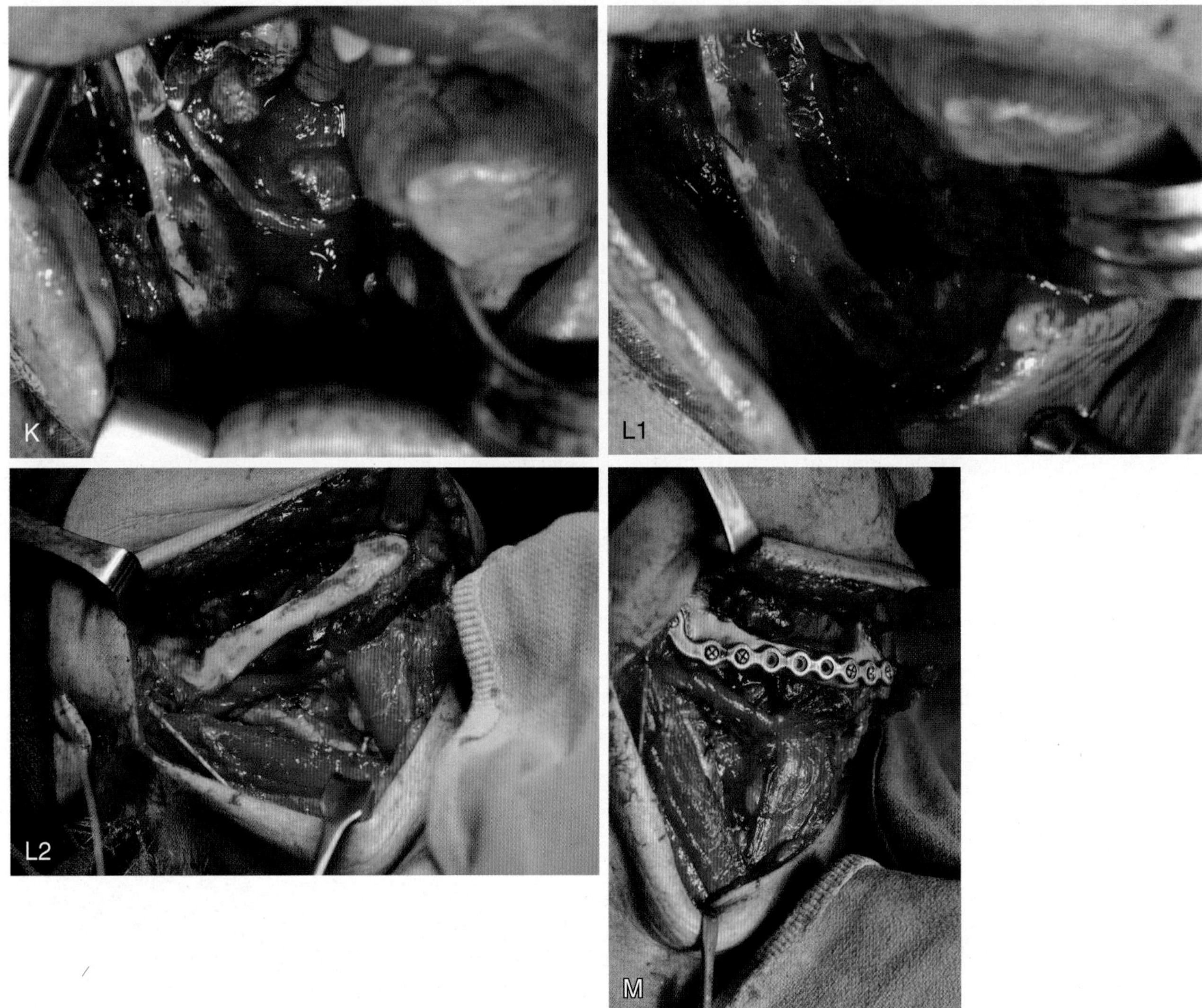

Figure 95.2, cont'd **K,** Osteotomy with lingual nerve preserved. **L1,** Osteotomy with lingual nerve retracted. **L2,** Osteotomy showing curved edges. **M,** Reconstruction plate.

TECHNIQUE: Marginal Mandibulectomy—*cont'd*

STEP 10: Closure

There are several options. Primary closure after undermining of surrounding soft tissue, buccal fat pad (BFP) advancement, split-thickness skin graft (STSG), allograft, and free/pedicled vascularized graft, depending on the size of the existing defect as well as giving consideration to possible postoperative radiation.[15,16] In each case, thoroughly irrigate the site and confirm hemostasis. Aim for a tension-free closure when insetting a graft or primary closure. Close with 3-0 Vicryl sutures. Consider suturing in petroleum-impregnated gauze bolster for nonvascularized grafts with 3-0 silk sutures. Irrigate and suction the oral cavity (Fig. 95.2N and O).

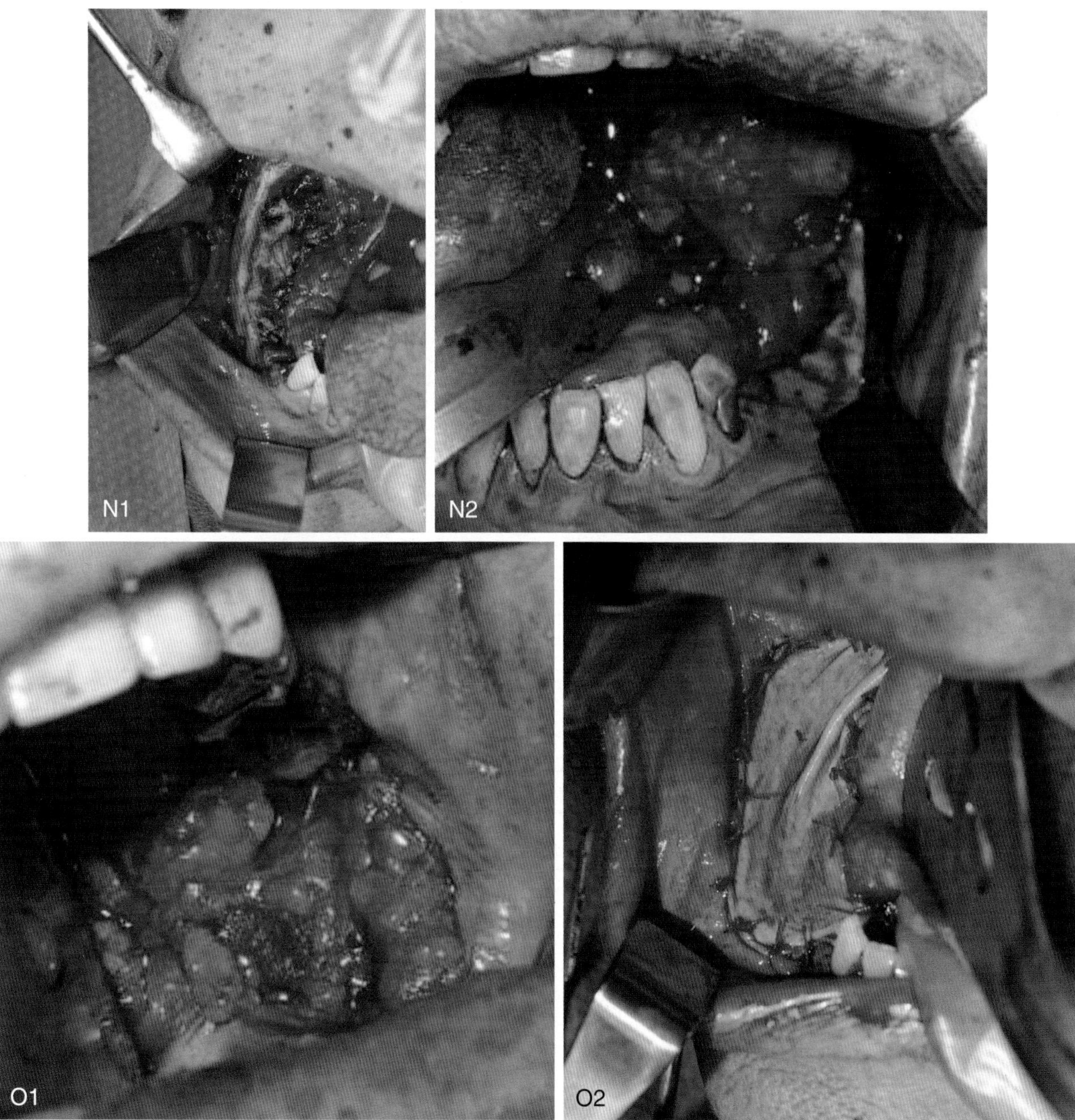

Figure 95.2, cont'd **N1** and **N2,** Buccal fat pad flap being inset. **O1,** Buccal fat pad inset. **O2,** Split-thickness skin graft for mucosal closure.

ALTERNATIVE TECHNIQUE 1: Transbuccal Technique

A modification of the standard marginal mandibulectomy has been described by Hirsch and Dierks.[17] They described using standard intraoral retraction and incisions around the lesion. However, to make the osteotomies, a percutaneous stab incision is made within the relaxed skin tension lines at a point midway in the course of the osseous cut, utilizing techniques of transbuccal instrumentation. The shank of a reciprocating saw blade is passed through the transbuccal wound from inside to outside. The shank is then loaded in a drill guide to protect the soft tissues during the osteotomy. The hand piece is then attached to the blade extraorally. The osteotomy is then created.[16] Standard irrigation is performed, and care is taken to protect surrounding soft tissues. This modification is also useful for the placement of screw fixation if needed. The skin is closed with a single horizontal mattress suture (Fig. 95.3).

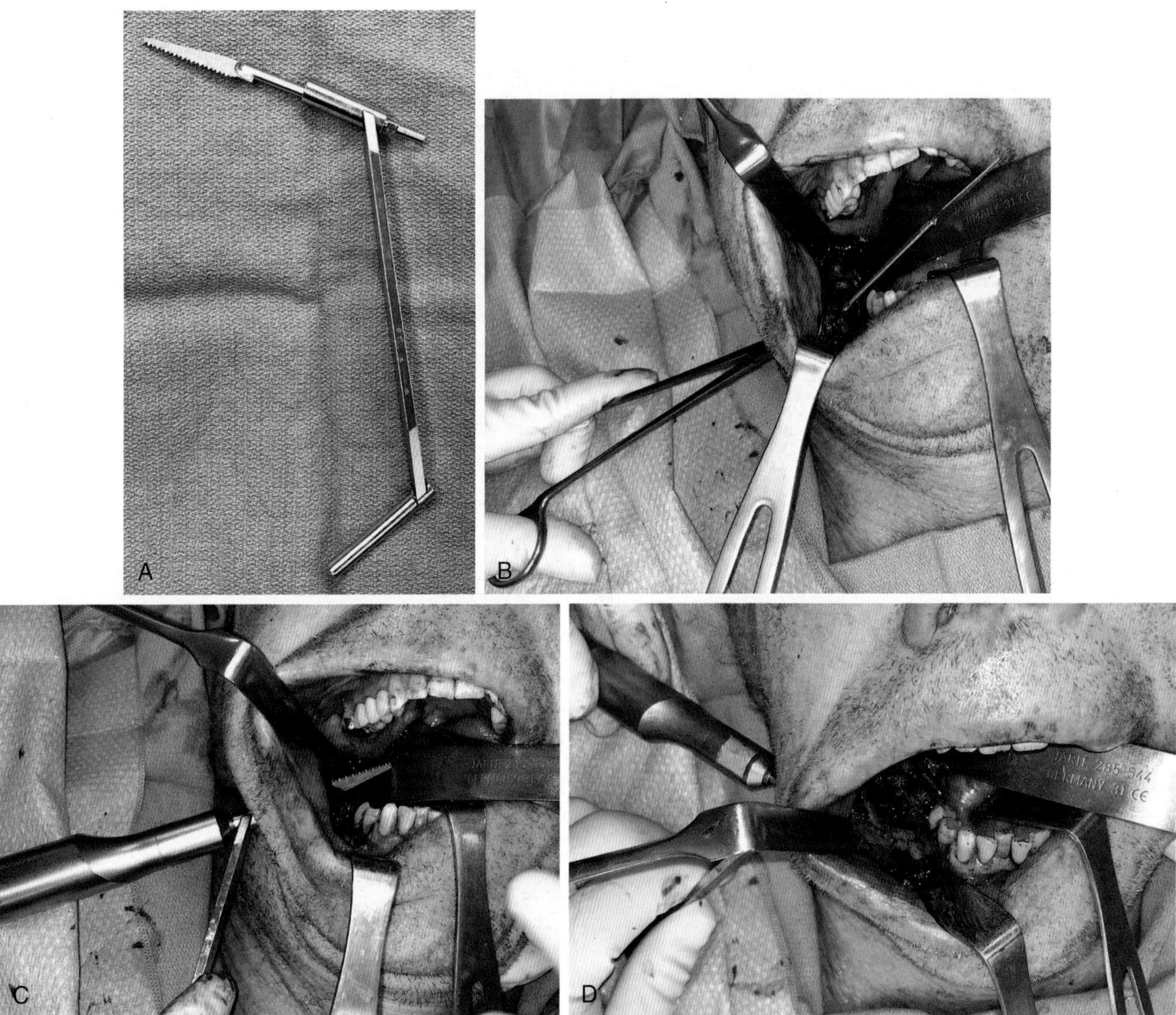

Figure 95.3 Transbuccal approach. A, The shank of the reciprocating saw in the protective drill guide. **B,** Passing the shank of the saw from inside to outside through the transbuccal incision. **C,** Attaching the handpiece to the shank of reciprocating saw extraorally. **D,** Making the osteotomy with drill guide intact to protect the surrounding soft tissues.

ALTERNATIVE TECHNIQUE 2: Cheek-Splitting Transbuccal Approach

Again, access to the posterior mandibular osteotomy via an intraoral approach alone is challenging, if not impossible, in some cases. In the absence of transcervical access due to either patient comorbidities or desires, Ohba and colleagues described a modification to the intraoral-only approach. They added a "combination archwise and serriform incision from the lower lip to the cheek skin," explaining "few critical anatomical structures exist around this area unless the incision is made too posteriorly. This incision allows marginal resection at the posterior mandible under direct vision via a transbuccal approach, resulting in a shorter operative duration and less surgical invasion"[18] (Fig. 95.4).

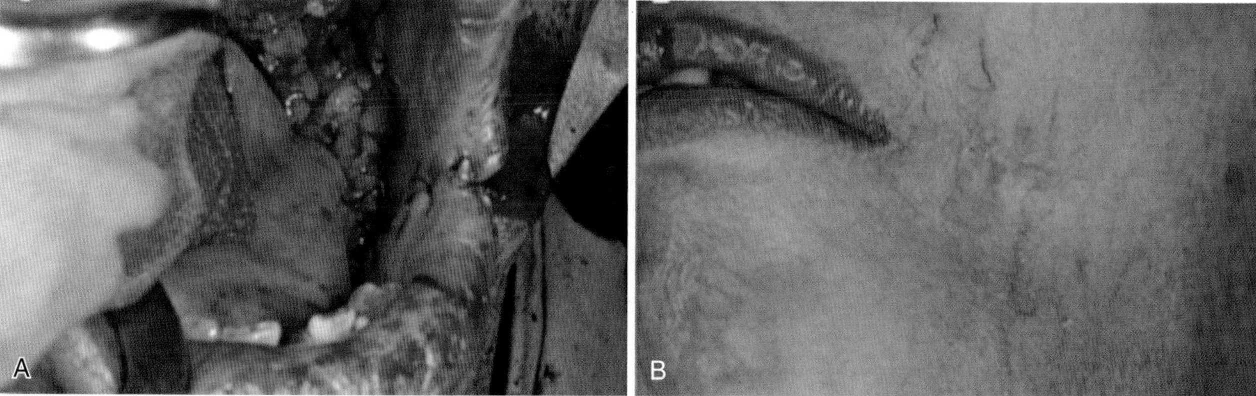

Figure 95.4 **A,** The incision line on the cheek. **B,** The marginal mandibulectomy with the cheek splitting. (From Ohba S, Yamashita H, Takashi I, et al. Marginal mandibulectomy for lower gingival carcinoma with a cheek-splitting transbuccal approach and reconstruction by buccal fat pad flap: a case report. *J Oral Maxillofac Surg.* 2013;71:e143.)

Avoidance and Management of Intraoperative Complications

Obtaining surgical access for a marginal mandibulectomy is one of the greatest challenges the surgeon will face. Direct visualization of the osteotomy and protected soft tissues is paramount to success. It is easy to misalign the reciprocating saw and damage vital structures. The saw tip will naturally want to point posteriorly on the posterior cut due to interference from the cheek. This puts the IAN and lingual nerve at risk for transection. To avoid this complication, there are several options: (1) do not make the posterior cut purely through a transoral approach; (2) use either of the modifications listed previously; (3) use a transcervical approach if in conjunction with a neck dissection; or (4) perform the marginal mandibulectomy separately from the coronoidectomy if the lesion is far enough anteriorly to obtain good oncologic margins posteriorly.

Another common complication is violation of the submandibular duct. If transection of the duct is required, or inadvertently occurs, and the submandibular gland is not planned for removal, then the proximal end of the duct should be identified, dissected free, and sutured to the floor of the mouth mucosa in a formal sialodochoplasty.

Bleeding is expected with surgery; however, the floor of the mouth and lateral buccal regions have several potential sources for unwanted additional bleeding. Care must be taken to avoid transection of the lingual, buccal, and facial vessels. Depending on the size of the lesion and its location, the surgeon must be aware of the surrounding anatomy and be prepared to identify and control bleeds from these areas. If resection is performed in conjunction with a neck dissection, more proximal identification of these vessels should have already occurred, providing an excellent opportunity for their control. If care is taken, it is rarely necessary to enter the neck solely to control bleeding from this procedure.

Postoperative Considerations

The patient will likely be admitted postoperatively to the floor or intensive care unit (ICU), depending on the extent of surgery for pain control and monitoring. Occasionally, the procedure can be considered outpatient surgery if the lesion is small and the primary closure was obtained at the time of surgery. A 48-hour course of steroids is reasonable to reduce edema.

If the patient had a BFP closure, fairly aggressive mouth-opening exercises will be required to decrease trismus starting on postoperative day 5 to 7, depending on the healing of the graft. Occasionally, the trismus will be severe enough to warrant release of scar tissue from the BFP graft. If an STSG has been taken or a dermis allograft used, the bolster must be removed 1 week postoperatively with appropriate antibiotic coverage while the bolster is in situ. Standard donor site care should be taken if the STSG was harvested from the thigh. If a vascular graft was used for reconstruction, then assume typical vascular monitoring in the ICU and floor per the vascular surgeon's recommendations. Patients may fracture the mandible, so pre/postoperative instructions should be given, notably regarding the care that should be taken when chewing hard foods. Dental rehabilitation can also be a challenge with these cases, and patients should be informed of this possibility prior to the surgery. Obtain a postoperative radiograph (Fig. 95.5) to assess the osteotomy and for baseline documentation. The patient should return for standard oncologic follow-up visits per guidelines for patient disease.

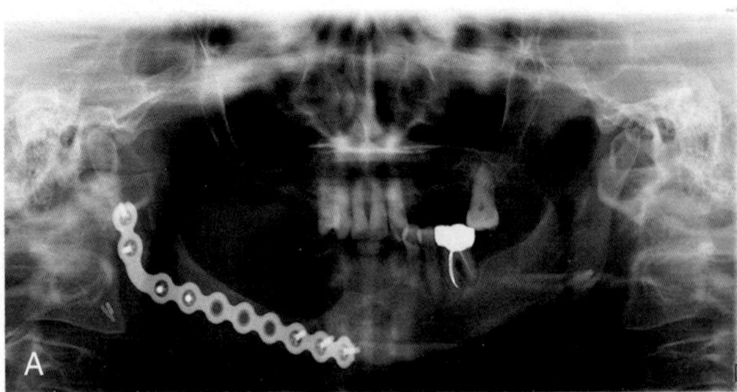

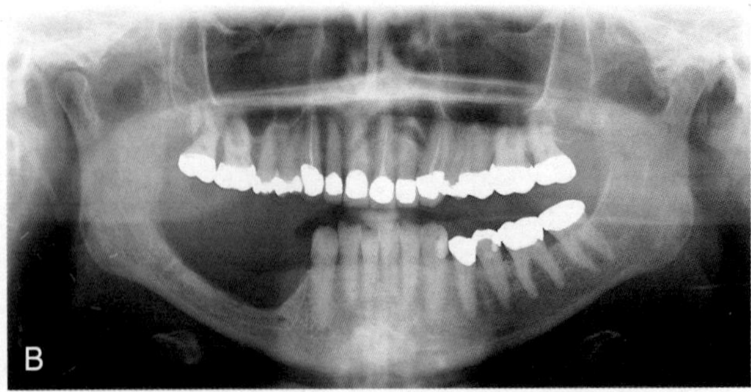

Figure 95.5 Postoperative Panorex with reconstruction plate **(A)** and without **(B)**.

References

1. Crile GW. Carcinoma of the jaws, tongue, cheek and lips. *Surg Gyn Obs*. 1923;36:132.
2. Marchetta FC, Sako K, Badillo J. Periosteal lymphatics of the mandible and intraoral carcinoma. *Am J Surg*. 1964;108:505–507.
3. Marchetta FC, Sako K, Murphy JB. The periosteum of the mandible and intraoral carcinoma. *Am J Surg*. 1971;122(6):711–713.
4. Pogrel MA. The marginal mandibulectomy for the treatment of mandibular tumours. *Br J Oral Maxillofac Surg*. 1989;27(2):132–138.
5. Barttelbort SW, Ariyan S. Mandible preservation with oral cavity carcinoma: rim mandibulectomy versus sagittal mandibulectomy. *Am J Surg*. 1993;166(4):411–415.
6. Brown J. Mechanisms of cancer invasion of the mandible. *Curr Opin Otolaryngol Head Neck Surg*. 2003;11(2):96–102.
7. Genden EM, Rinaldo A, Jacobson A, et al. Management of mandibular invasion: when is a marginal mandibulectomy appropriate? *Oral Oncol*. 2005;41(8):776–782.
8. Wax MK, Bascom DA, Myers LL. Marginal mandibulectomy vs segmental mandibulectomy: indications and controversies. *Arch Otolaryngol Head Neck Surg*. 2002;128(5):600–603.
9. Patel RS, Dirven R, Clark JR, Swinson BD, Gao K, O'Brien CJ. The prognostic impact of extent of bone invasion and extent of bone resection in oral carcinoma. *Laryngoscope*. 2008;118(5):780–785.
10. Politi M, Costa F, Robiony M, Rinaldo A, Ferlito A. Review of segmental and marginal resection of the mandible in patients with oral cancer. *Acta Otolaryngol*. 2000;120(5):569–579.
11. Tei K, Totsuka Y, Iizuka T, Ohmori K. Marginal resection for carcinoma of the mandibular alveolus and gingiva where radiologically detected bone defects do not extend beyond the mandibular canal. *J Oral Maxillofac Surg*. 2004;62(7):834–839.
12. Chen YL, Kuo SW, Fang KH, Hao SP. Prognostic impact of marginal mandibulectomy in the presence of superficial bone invasion and the nononcologic outcome. *Head Neck*. 2011;33(5):708–713.
13. Pandey M, Rao LP, Das SR. Predictors of mandibular involvement in cancers of the oromandibular region. *J Oral Maxillofac Surg*. 2009;67(5):1069–1073.
14. Notani K, Yamazaki Y, Kitada H, et al. Management of mandibular osteoradionecrosis corresponding to the severity of osteoradionecrosis and the method of radiotherapy. *Head Neck*. 2003;25(3):181–186.
15. Ertem SY, Uckan S, Ozden UA. The comparison of angular and curvilinear marginal mandibulectomy on force distribution with three dimensional finite element analysis. *J Craniomaxillofac Surg*. 2013;41(3):e54–e58.
16. Deleyiannis FW, Dunklebarger J, Lee E, et al. Reconstruction of the marginal mandibulectomy defect: an update. *Am J Otolaryngol*. 2007;28(6):363–366.
17. Hirsch DL, Dierks EJ. Use of a transbuccal technique for marginal mandibulectomy: a novel approach. *J Oral Maxillofac Surg*. 2007;65(9):1849–1851.
18. Ohba S, Yamashita H, Takashi I, et al. Marginal mandibulectomy for lower gingival carcinoma with a cheek-splitting transbuccal approach and reconstruction by buccal fat pad flap: a case report. *J Oral Maxillofac Surg*. 2013;71(2):e143–e146.

CHAPTER 96

Maxillectomy for Benign Tumors

Jonathan Bailey, Craig Norbutt, and Baxter Jones

Armamentarium

#9 Periosteal elevator
Freer elevator
#15 Bard-Parker scalpels and handle
Colorado tip Bovie/bipolar cautery
26-Gauge wire with wire cutters
Adson tissue forceps, delicate (fine teeth)
Gerald tissue forceps
3 3/4 in DeBakey thoracic tissue forceps
Appropriate sutures
Halsey needle holders
Army-Navy retractor
Obwegeser retractors
Senn double-ended retractors
Sewall orbital retractor set
Malleable retractors
Weider tongue depressor
Mouth prop
Single and double skin hooks
Extraction elevators and forceps
Rongeurs
Bone file
Bone hook, 9 × 1 inches
Dean suture scissors
Tenotomy scissors
5 1/2 in Metzenbaum dissecting scissors, curved
Lacrimal probes
Drill
Straight reciprocating saw
Right-angled fan reciprocating saw
Frazier suction tip
Local anesthetic with vasoconstrictor
Small and medium hemoclip applicator
Weider tongue depressor

History of the Procedure

The maxillectomy was designed for the surgical treatment of tumors involving the maxilla, the maxillary sinus, and associated structures of the midface including the nasal cavity and periorbita, which is more commonly involved in malignant neoplasms. Lazars first described the procedure in 1826 and attempted the first maxillectomy in 1827, but the procedure was aborted because of excessive blood loss.[1] Later that year, Joseph Gonsoul successfully completed this operation but credited Lazars for his initial description of the procedure.[2,3] In 1829, Syme performed the first successful maxillectomy with orbital exenteration.

The initial attempts to remove maxillary tumors resulted in high patient morbidity, including disfigurement and facial scarring. In 1927, Portmann and Rotrouvey described a transoral approach for a maxillectomy.[4] This method provided an additional approach to the maxilla and reduced the need for surgical incisions on the face. This notwithstanding, the greatest risks associated with a maxillectomy included postoperative wound infection and extensive blood loss. In the 1950s, significant advancements in anesthetic techniques helped to reduce intraoperative blood loss, thus decreasing the patient morbidity and mortality often seen with this procedure. During this time, the Weber-Ferguson approach to the maxillectomy was described, which eliminated a deforming scar while still providing excellent access to the midfacial skeleton.

Advancements in surgical techniques and improved instrumentation have allowed for a less invasive approach to some maxillary tumors. In 1977, Sessions and Larson described the medial maxillectomy for lesions of the lateral nasal wall.[5–7] Later on, with the development of the nasal endoscope, smaller lesions extending from the lateral nasal wall could be removed with improved visualization. The maxillectomy procedure has continued to evolve, while both improving patient outcomes and decreasing complications.

In 2000, Brown proposed a classification system of maxillary defects (Fig. 96.1). He developed his classification system as a tool for planning maxillary osteotomies, predicting complications, and postoperative needs based on anatomy affected during the maxillectomy, and to aid in defining appropriate reconstruction options. The classification system is based on both the vertical (class 1–4) dimension and horizontal (a–c) dimensions. For lesions confined to the alveolus, a Brown class 1 maxillectomy defect would be anticipated. This type of maxillectomy does not result in an oral-antral or oral-nasal communication. For neoplasms that extend into the maxillary sinus, a higher-level resection, including the maxillary sinus walls, would be indicated, resulting in a Brown class 2 defect. Class 1 and 2 defects are most common with benign odontogenic disease (Fig. 96.2). A Brown class 3 defect involves vertical extension including the floor of the orbit with or without peri-orbita and with or without skull base resection. Within the Brown classification, horizontal margins of the resection are described. The letter "a" is

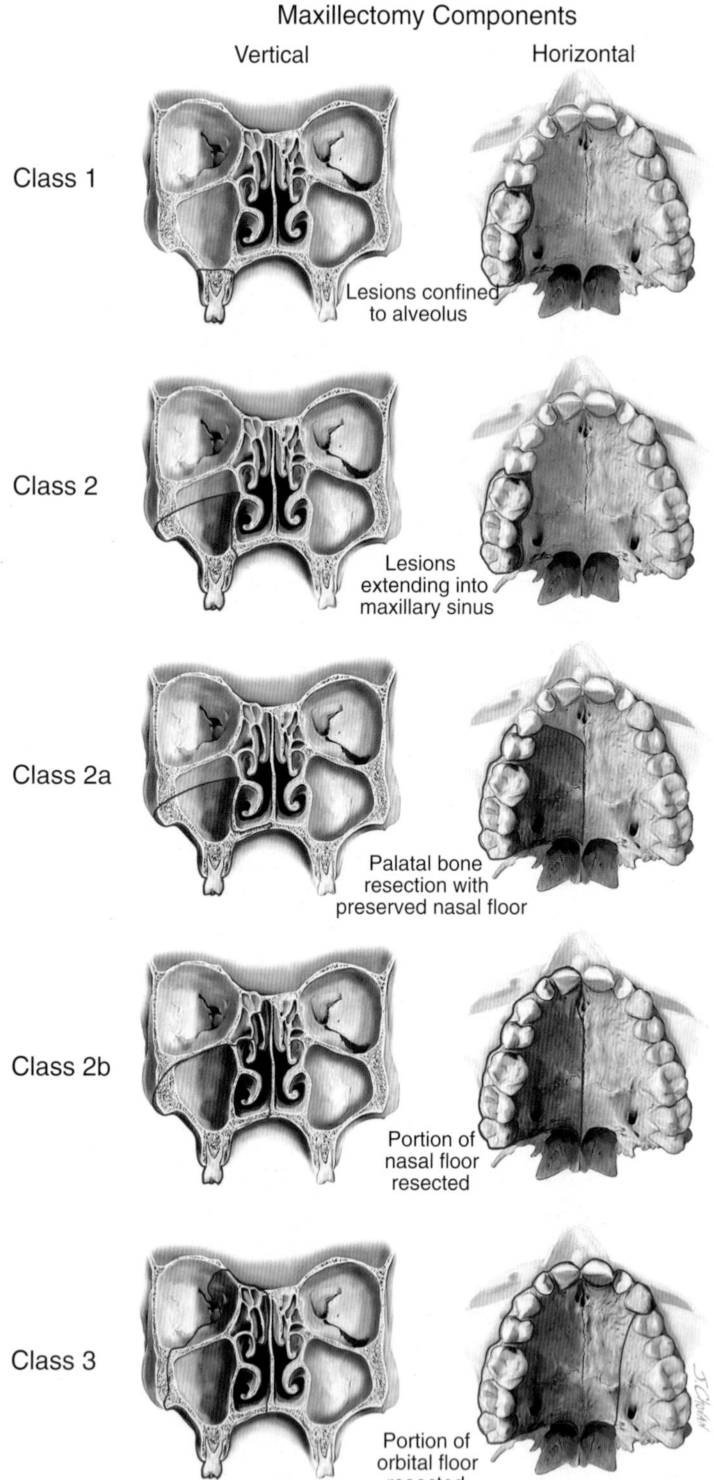

Figure 96.1 The Brown classification system.

designated for lesions requiring resection of the alveolar maxilla and hard palate with less than or equal to half the alveolar and hard palate resection not involving the nasal septum or crossing midline. More extensive or anterior lesions may require sacrifice of the bilateral maxillary alveolus and hard palate including the nasal septum. These would be designated with the letter "b." Letter "c" is reserved for removal of the entire alveolar maxilla and hard palate.[8–10]

Indications for the Use of the Procedure

The primary indication for maxillectomy is ablation of malignant and specific benign pathology, inflammatory processes, and trauma. The treatment of invasive carcinoma and sarcomas involves resection of tumor and tissue beyond the tumor that can leave a significant defect. Often, due to the extent

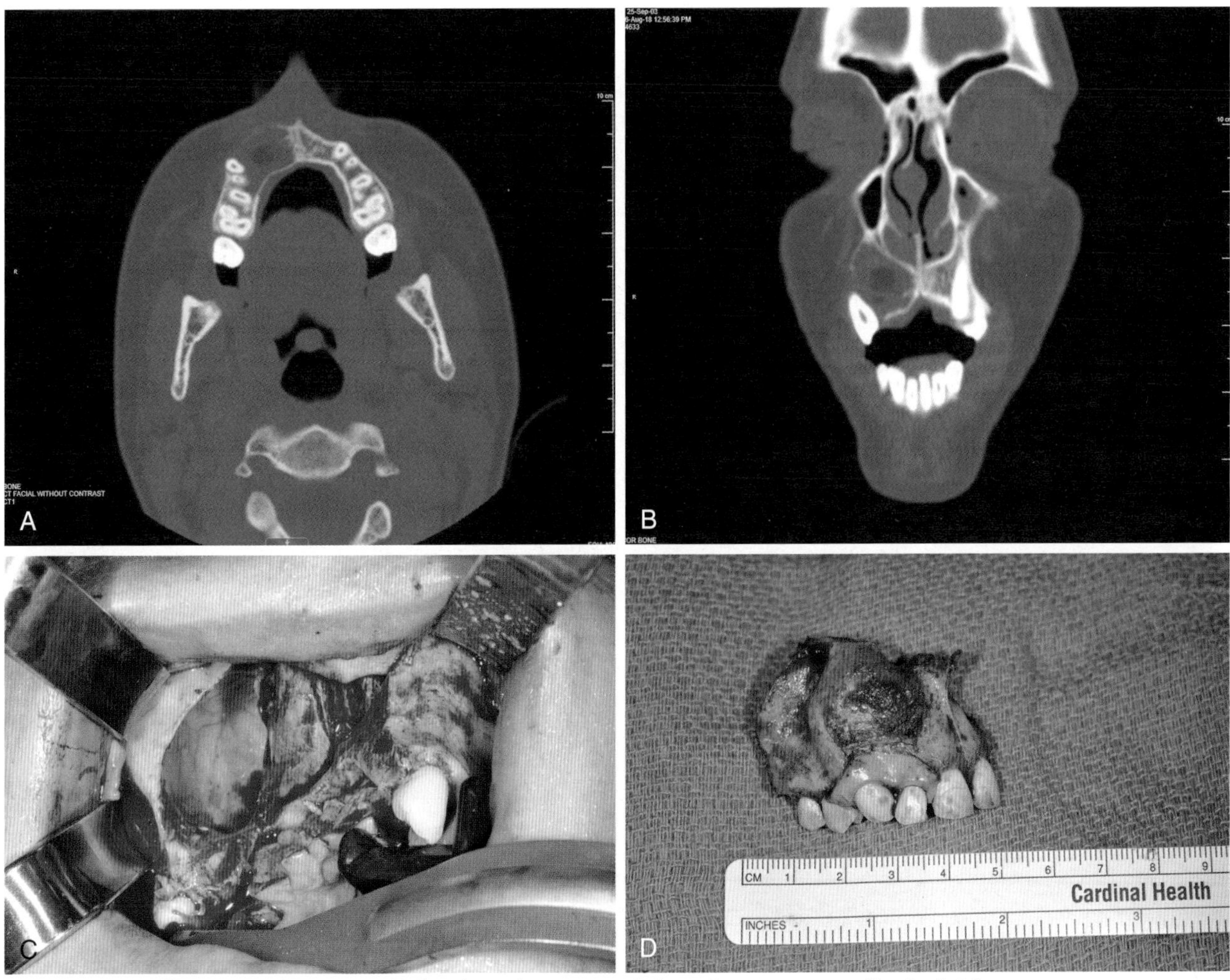

Figure 96.2 A 14-year-old female with myxoma of the right anterior maxilla. A, Axial computer tomography (CT) scan showing cortical perforation. **B,** Coronal CT scan showing extension up to the lateral nasal wall. **C,** Postablative picture of Brown class 2b defect. **D,** Specimen with gingiva remaining in areas 6/7.

of malignant tumors, the incision must be extended beyond that used in an intraoral approach to the maxilla for removal of benign disease. Some of the more commonly encountered benign processes of the maxilla that require maxillectomy include ameloblastoma, calcifying epithelial odontogenic tumor, myxoma, medication related osteonecrosis, osteoradionecrosis, and osteomyelitis. Additional indications for maxillectomy include advanced fungal disease such as mucormycosis and aspergillosis.[11] Here, we address the intraoral approach to the maxilla, or Keen approach, a variation of which includes the midfacial degloving approach. The Weber-Ferguson approach, and its many variations, is more commonly used when wide exposure of the midface, including the periorbita, is required. It is the purpose of this chapter to describe the indications, limitations, and technique for maxillectomy for benign disease via an intraoral approach.

Resection margins for locally aggressive benign odontogenic lesions such as ameloblastoma or myxoma traditionally include 1 cm of bone and one intact anatomic barrier.[11,12] The periosteum and the overlying mucosa may be preserved if the lesion is contained within the maxilla and has not extended beyond the confines of the bone. However, tumors that have perforated the maxilla require sacrifice of the adjacent overlying periosteum. The extent of the resection is dependent on the histologic diagnosis as well as the size and location of the neoplasm.

Limitations and Contraindications

Limitations of the maxillectomy technique are primarily due to anatomic features of the individual lesion, as indicated previously. Careful preoperative radiographic evaluation in all three planes is required, with particular attention to possible extension beyond the confines of the maxilla in the region of the nasal floor, orbital floor, and posterior maxilla (Fig. 96.3). Surgical limitations may also be affected by the available reconstructive options, including the skill set of the reconstructive surgeon. It is important to mention that all patients undergoing maxillectomy should be evaluated by a dentist and have preoperative impressions to facilitate reconstruction and dental rehabilitation postoperatively. There are no specific contraindications to maxillectomy.

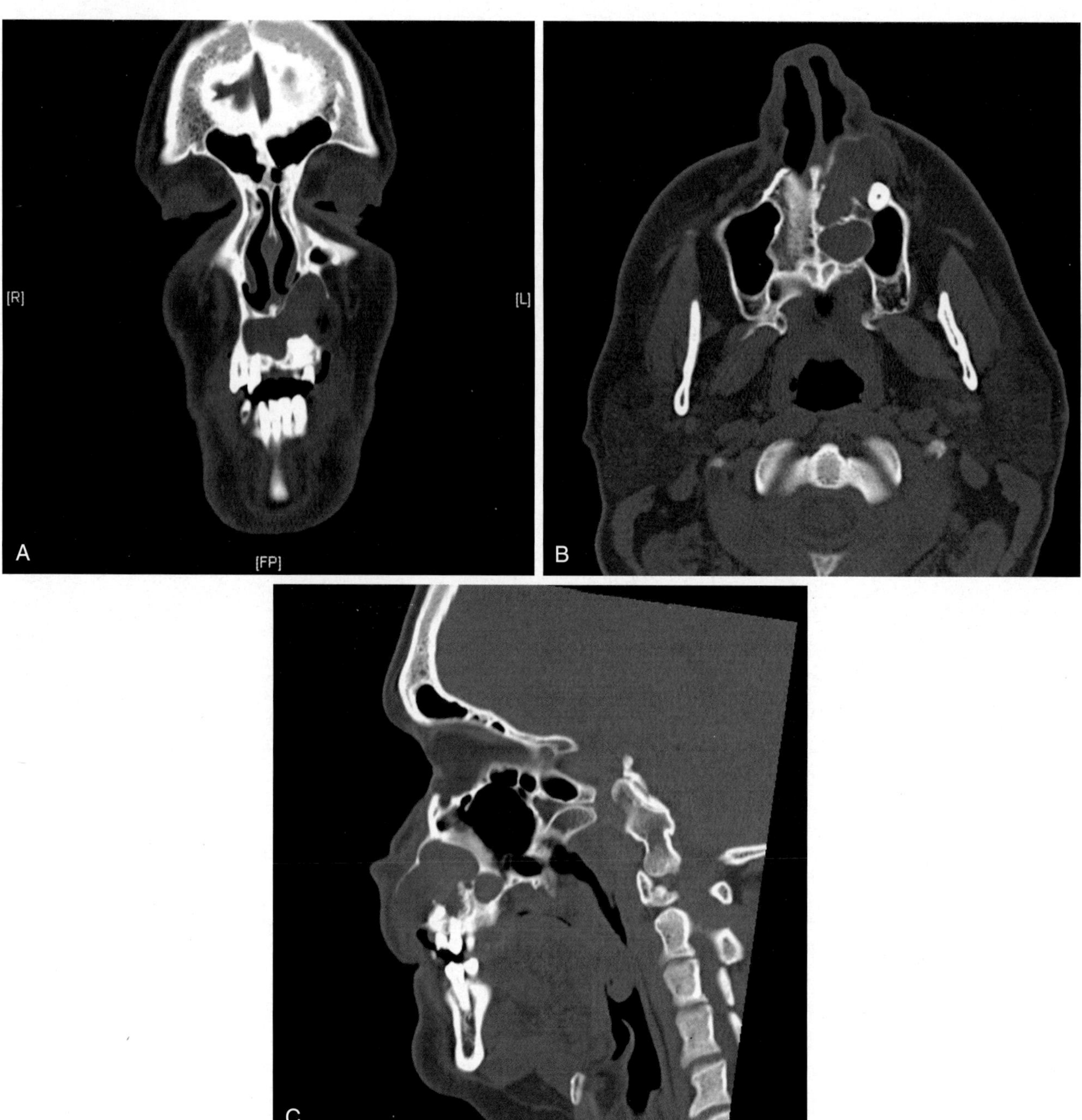

Figure 96.3 CT of facial bones of a 33-year-old male with ameloblastoma of the left maxilla showing anticipated Brown class 2b defect. A, Coronal view: In this view, the bony erosion through the anterior maxilla can be seen. **B,** Axial view: The left maxillary lesion is eroding into the anterior maxilla and displacing the septum, deviating the nose to the right. **C,** Sagittal view.

TECHNIQUE: Maxillectomy for Benign Tumors

STEP 1: Patient Preparation

For this procedure, oral endotracheal intubation, nasal intubation, or submental intubation may be utilized depending on the location of the tumor. For nasal and oral intubation, the endotracheal tube should be passed contralateral to the surgical site. Weight-specific steroids and antibiotics are given within 30 minutes of the incision and are redosed appropriately throughout the procedure.[13–15] The patient is turned 180 degrees and prepped and draped for an oral and maxillofacial surgery procedure. The oral cavity is suctioned, and a bite block and throat pack are placed. Two percent lidocaine with 1:100,000 epinephrine is injected into the maxillary vestibule and palate (Fig. 96.4A). Hypotensive anesthesia may be utilized as indicated and if tolerated to reduce intraoperative bleeding.

TECHNIQUE: Maxillectomy for Benign Tumors—*cont'd*

STEP 2: Incision

A #15 blade is used to make a sulcular incision on the buccal and palatal aspect of the maxillary teeth with proximal and distal releases if required. If the lesion has perforated the bone and at the site of prior biopsy, a layer of periosteum must be left over this area, and the initial incision design must take this into account.

STEP 3: Surgical Dissection and Exposure

A buccal full-thickness mucoperiosteal flap is reflected superiorly to the infraorbital nerve, medially to the piriform rim, and posteriorly to the maxillary tuberosity. The palate is similarly exposed, and the greater palatine neurovascular bundle is isolated and ligated. The muscular attachments of the soft palate to the bony hard palate are released.

For resections that include the nasal floor, a Freer elevator is used to dissect the nasal mucosal off the lateral and inferior nasal walls. The nasal septum is released with a double-guarded osteotome. A thin malleable retractor is placed to protect the nasal mucosa (Fig. 96.4B and C).

Continued

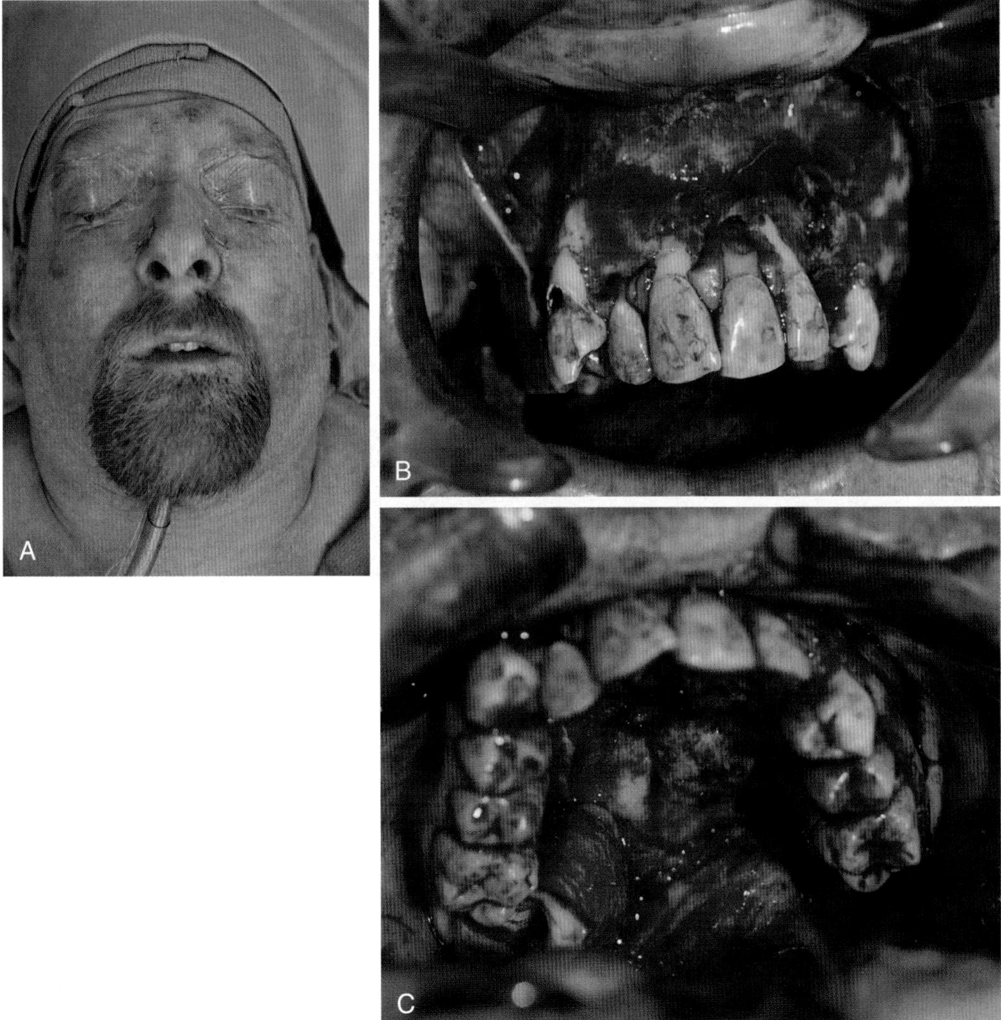

Figure 96.4 A 33-year-old male with ameloblastoma of left maxilla. A, Patient prepped for surgery with submental intubation. **B,** The anterior maxilla exposed with a full-thickness mucoperiosteal flap from a sulcular incision to preserve the keratinized tissue. **C,** The palate was exposed in a similar fashion with a full-thickness mucoperiosteal flap. Preserving the keratinized tissue will aid in a watertight closure.

TECHNIQUE: Maxillectomy for Benign Tumors—*cont'd*

STEP 4: Osteotomies

With the soft tissue dissection completed, the planned bone margins are identified. A reciprocating saw is used to create vertical anterior and posterior osteotomies across the alveolus. In the dentate patient, teeth may be extracted at the site of the osteotomies. Preoperative imaging determines the superior extent of the osteotomies. A buccal horizontal osteotomy is then completed to connect the anterior and posterior vertical osteotomies. Next, a sagittal palatal osteotomy is completed to connect the vertical osteotomies on the medial resection margin. For lesions extending anteriorly or to the midline, an osteotomy of the lateral nasal wall is performed with a guarded osteotome. The junctions of the osteotomies are then connected with an osteotome or saw.

If the resection includes the tuberosity, the osteotomy at the pterygoid plates is performed last. A broad curved osteotome is placed below the pterygomaxillary fissure and directed in an inferomedial direction. Palpation with the opposite hand in the hamular notch assists in correctly placing and orienting the osteotome.

STEP 5: Mobilization

The specimen is then sequentially mobilized and delivered using a broad osteotome. The specimen should then be inspected to ensure appropriate gross margins were obtained (Fig. 96.4D and E).

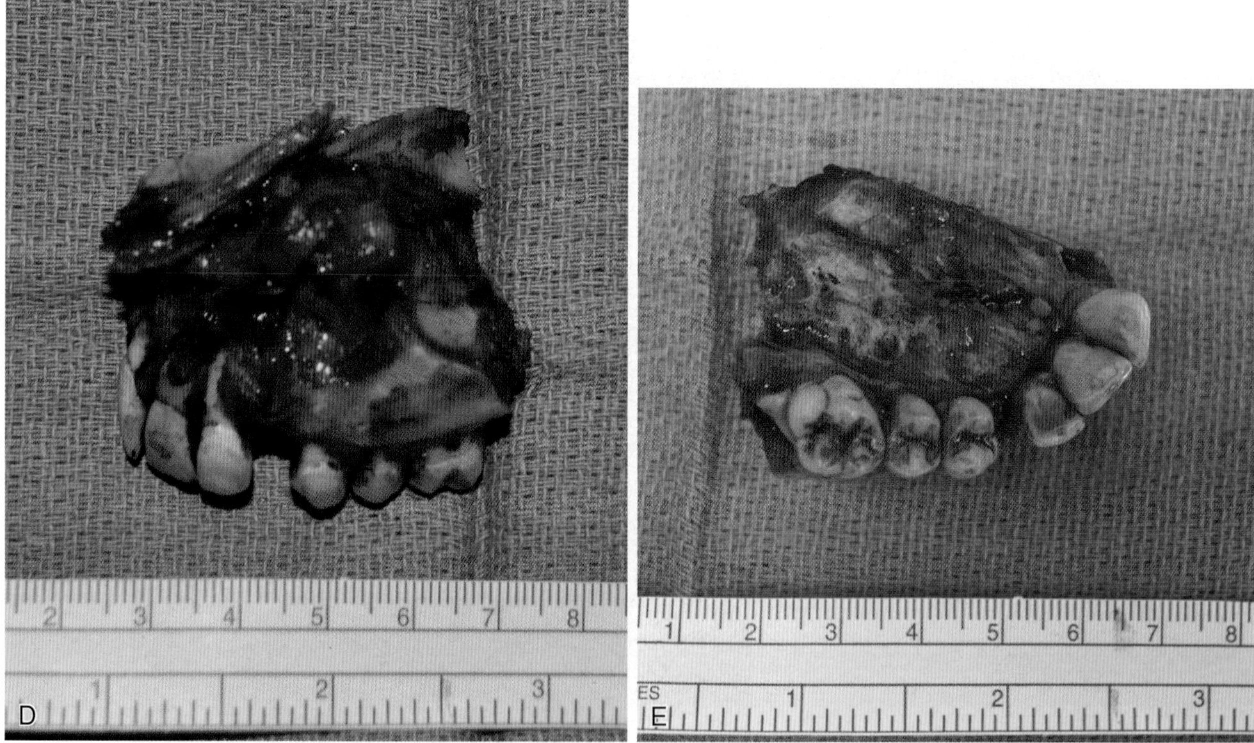

Figure 96.4, cont'd D and E, Resected partial maxillectomy specimen.

TECHNIQUE: Maxillectomy for Benign Tumors—*cont'd*

STEP 6: Closure

The defect should then be inspected to evaluate the gross adequacy of the resection, hemostasis, and the sinus communication and integrity of the nasal mucosa. A buccal fat flap may be mobilized through the defect to assist in closure (Fig. 96.4F and G). For Brown class 1, 2a, and 2b maxillectomy defects, the mucosal flaps are closed primarily with 3-0 Vicryl sutures (Fig. 96.4H).

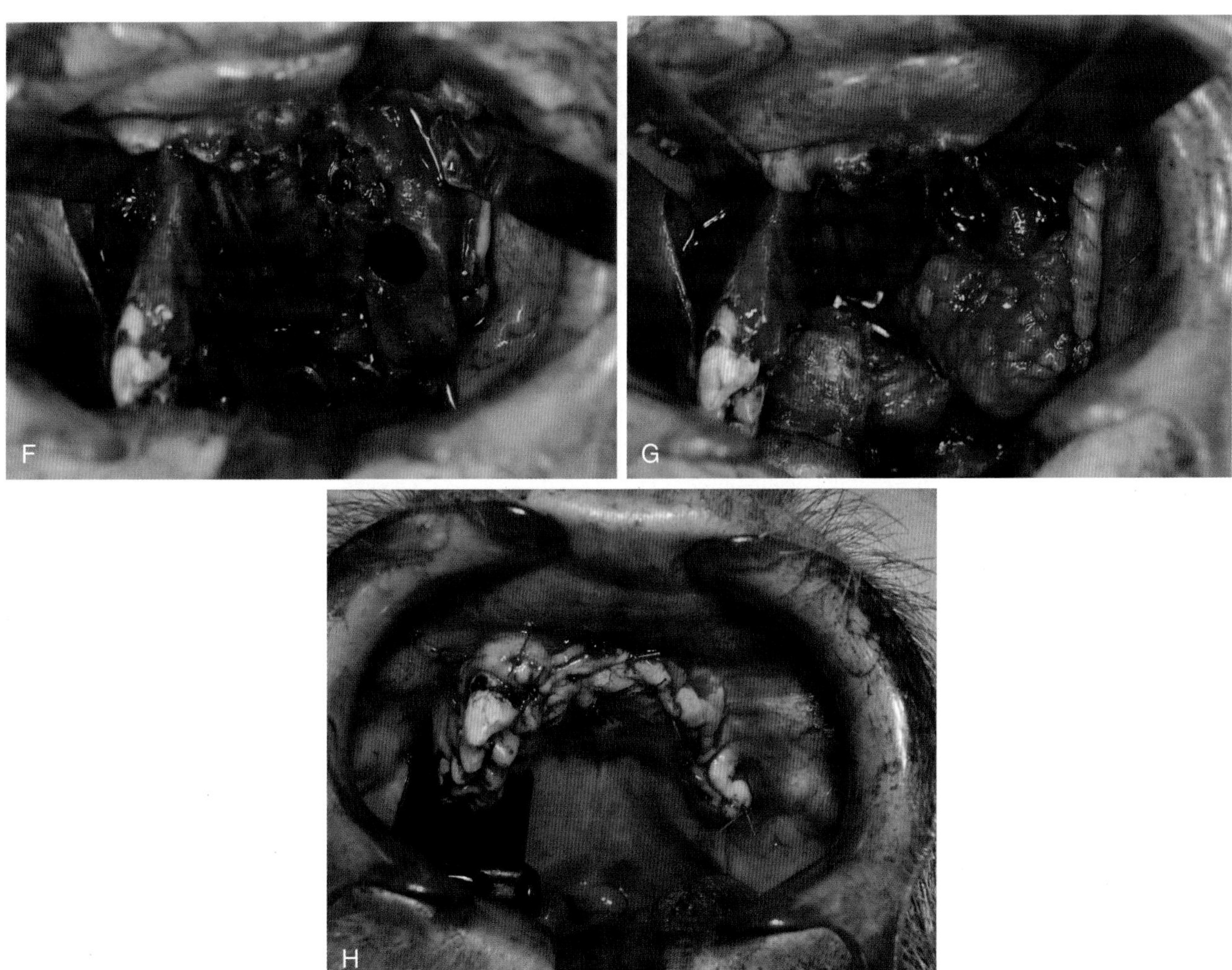

Figure 96.4, cont'd **F,** Brown class 2b maxillectomy defect with the nasal mucosa preserved and osteotomy into the left maxillary sinus. **G,** A left pedicled buccal fat pad graft is dissected and placed over the defect to help with preventing a communication to the oral cavity. **H,** Watertight layered closure over the left maxillary defect.

ALTERNATIVE TECHNIQUE: Maxillectomy With Weber-Ferguson Incision

For more extensive lesions that involve the orbital floor, a Weber-Ferguson incision is indicated. This surgical technique is described elsewhere in this atlas (Fig. 96.5A and B).

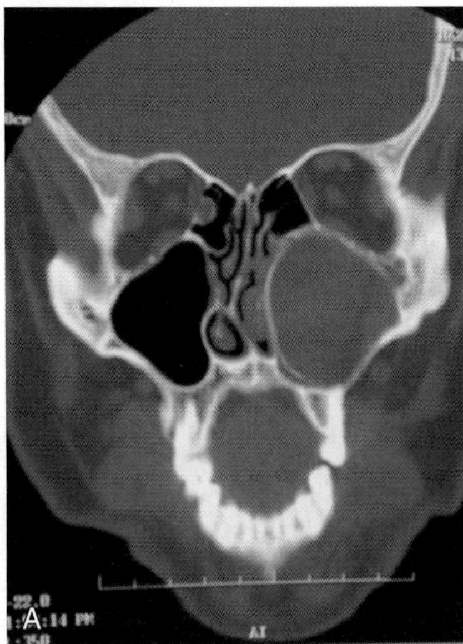
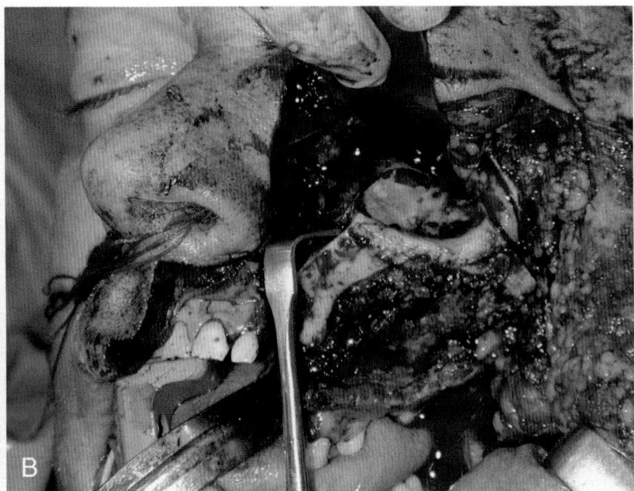

Figure 96.5 A 43-year-old male with ameloblastoma of the left maxilla with extension into orbital floor with anticipated Brown class 3 defect. **A,** CT of facial bones showing extension of the lesion to the orbital floor. **B,** Weber-Ferguson approach providing transfacial access for maxillectomy.

Avoidance and Management of Intraoperative Complications

The primary intraoperative complication in maxillary surgery is bleeding. Hypotensive anesthesia technique may be warranted, if tolerated by the patient. The most likely source of venous bleeding is the pterygoid plexus, which may be controlled with packing and topical hemostatic agents. The most common sources of arterial bleeding are the posterior superior alveolar artery and the greater palatine artery. The descending palatine artery is typically injured while completing the lateral nasal wall osteotomy and can be preserved by extending the osteotomy no more than 30 mm (35 mm in males) posteriorly. The descending palatine artery can be identified and controlled while down-fracturing the maxillectomy specimen, as in orthognathic surgery. If the osteotomy crosses the midline, bleeding may be encountered from the nasopalatine artery. The internal maxillary artery can also be injured while the surgeon is completing the pterygoid plate disjunction for a posteriorly located tumor.[16–18] When completing this osteotomy, the surgeon should orient the osteotome in an inferior, anterior, and medial direction. Bleeding that cannot be controlled with direct packing or ligation may require embolization by an interventional radiologist.

Oral-antral or oral-nasal fistula formation may occur after maxillectomy. The palatal and alveolar mucosa typically may be preserved during resection for benign disease that has not perforated the surrounding bone.[18–21] However, communication with the maxillary sinus and nasal cavity commonly occur. Smokers or diabetics may have delayed soft tissue healing, which may result in fistula formation. Careful closure of any violation of the nasal mucosa, as well as the oral mucosa, is required. Additional local flap techniques such as the buccal fat flap, at the time of resection, may decrease fistula formation.

With higher-level resections, ectropion or increased scleral show may result from the lower lid extension of the Weber-Ferguson incision. Diplopia and enophthalmos are potential complications after orbital floor resection, and therefore immediate reconstruction is indicated.[21–25] Alloplastic or autogenous reconstruction of the orbital floor and rim is completed at the time of resection.[25–28]

Epiphora may result from disruption of the nasolacrimal duct. Placement of lacrimal stents is indicated if the drainage system is violated during the resection. Atrophic rhinitis may result from disruption of the nasal and/or sinus membrane. This is a chronic condition that may be treated with regular irrigation and/or antibiotics as indicated. Gustatory rhinorrhea has also been described as a potential complication following maxillectomy, presumably due to aberrant regeneration of parasympathetic nerves, similar to Frey syndrome.[29] Other potential complications include corneal abrasion, traumatic optic neuropathy, and retrobulbar hematoma. All of these potential complications should be reviewed with the patient and family prior to surgery.

Postoperative Considerations

At the conclusion of the procedure, patients are admitted to the surgical floor for 24 to 72 hours for postoperative pain control with intravenous and oral analgesics and for observation of postoperative hemostasis. Postoperative antibiotics are prescribed for 48 hours, then discontinued, while oral care is completed with a chlorhexidine mouth rinse twice a day for 7 days.

Patients are placed on sinus precautions for the first 2 weeks to allow the soft tissues to heal. This includes no nose blowing, forceful sucking, valsalva, or any devices delivering positive pressure such as a continuous positive airway pressure machine. Diet is restricted to clear liquids for the initial 48 hours, followed by a soft, nonchewing diet with protein-supplemented shakes until soft tissue healing matures. For at least 2 to 3 days postoperatively, the head should be elevated to decrease swelling. On discharge, the patient should practice meticulous oral hygiene, and may be allowed gentle saltwater rinses for debris clearance and comfort.

References

1. McGuirt WF. Maxillectomy. *Otolaryngol Clin North Am*. 1995;28(6):1175–1189.
2. Benmoussa N, Kerner J, Josset P, Conan P, Charlier P. A 1842 skull from Dupuytren's museum of Paris: an original artifact of Joseph Gensoul first maxillectomy technique. *Eur Arch Otorhinolaryngol*. 2017;274(1):175–179.
3. Tsoucalas G, Gentimi F, Kousoulis AA, Karamanou M, Androutsos G. Joseph Gensoul and the earliest illustrated operations for maxillary sinus carcinoma. *Eur Arch Otorhinolaryngol*. 2013;270(1):359–362.
4. Portmann G, Rotrouvey H. *Le cancer du nex*. Paris: Gaston Dein et Cie; 1927.
5. Sessions RB, Larson DL. En bloc ethmoidectomy and medial maxillectomy. *Arch Otolaryngol*. 1977;103(4):195–202.
6. Sadeghi N, Al-Dhahri S, Manoukian JJ. Transnasal endoscopic medial maxillectomy for inverting papilloma. *Laryngoscope*. 2003;113(4):749–753.
7. Dierks EJ, Holmes JD. The Le Fort island approach: an alternative access for partial maxillectomy. *J Oral Maxillofac Surg*. 2002;60(11):1377–1379.
8. Brown JS, Rogers SN, McNally DN, Boyle M. A modified classification for the maxillectomy defect. *Head Neck*. 2000;22(1):17–26.
9. Brown JS, Shaw RJ. Reconstruction of the maxilla and midface: introducing a new classification. *Lancet Oncol*. 2010;11(10):1001–1008.
10. Spiro RH, Strong EW, Shah JP. Maxillectomy and its classification. *Head Neck*. 1997;19(4):309–314.
11. Ghali G, Lustig JH. Treatment of benign lesions of the maxillary sinus. *Oral Maxillofac Surg*. 1999;1:101.
12. Diecidue R, Streck P, Spera J, et al. Diagnosis of benign lesions of the maxillary sinus. *Oral Maxillofac Surg Clin North Am*. 1999;11:83.
13. Bratzler DW, Houck PM. Surgical infection prevention guidelines writers workgroup; American Academy of Orthopaedic Surgeons; American Association of Critical Care Nurses; American Association of Nurse Anesthetists; American College of Surgeons; American College of Osteopathic Surgeons; American Geriatrics Society; American Society of Anesthesiologists; American Society of Colon and Rectal Surgeons; American Society of Health-System Pharmacists; American Society of PeriAnesthesia Nurses; Ascension Health; Association of periOperative Registered Nurses; Association for Professionals in Infection Control and Epidemiology; Infectious Diseases Society of America; medical letter; premier; Society for Healthcare Epidemiology of America; Society of Thoracic Surgeons; Surgical Infection Society. Antimicrobial prophylaxis for surgery: an advisory statement from the National Surgical Infection Prevention Project. *Clin Infect Dis*. 2004;38(12):1706–1715.
14. Lotfi CJ, Cavalcanti RC, Costa e Silva AM, et al. Risk factors for surgical-site infections in head and neck cancer surgery. *Otolaryngol Head Neck Surg*. 2008;138(1):74–80.
15. Simo R, French G. The use of prophylactic antibiotics in head and neck oncological surgery. *Curr Opin Otolaryngol Head Neck Surg*. 2006;14(2):55–61.
16. Kaban LB, Pogrel AM, Perrott DH. *Complications in Oral and Maxillofacial Surgery*. Philadelphia: Saunders; 1997.
17. Cocke EW Jr, Robertson JH, Robertson JT, Crook JP Jr. The extended maxillotomy and subtotal maxillectomy for excision of skull base tumors. *Arch Otolaryngol Head Neck Surg*. 1990;116(1):92–104.
18. Eisele DW, Smith RW. *Complications in Head and Neck Surgery*. 2nd ed. Philadelphia, Pennsylvania: Mosby/Elseiver; 2009.
19. Acero J, García E. Reoperative midface reconstruction. *Oral Maxillofac Surg Clin North Am*. 2011;23(1):133–151, vii.
20. Andrades P, Militsakh O, Hanasono MM, Rieger J, Rosenthal EL. Current strategies in reconstruction of maxillectomy defects. *Arch Otolaryngol Head Neck Surg*. 2011;137(8):806–812.
21. Okay DJ, Genden E, Buchbinder D, Urken M. Prosthodontic guidelines for surgical reconstruction of the maxilla: a classification system of defects. *J Prosthet Dent*. 2001;86(4):352–363.
22. Pollice PA, Frodel JL Jr. Secondary reconstruction of upper midface and orbit after total maxillectomy. *Arch Otolaryngol Head Neck Surg*. 1998;124(7):802–808.
23. Smolka W, Iizuka T. Surgical reconstruction of maxilla and midface: clinical outcome and factors relating to postoperative complications. *J Craniomaxillofac Surg*. 2005;33(1):1–7.
24. Lethaus B, Lie N, de Beer F, Kessler P, de Baat C, Verdonck HW. Surgical and prosthetic reconsiderations in patients with maxillectomy. *J Oral Rehabil*. 2010;37(2):138–142.
25. Futran ND. Primary reconstruction of the maxilla following maxillectomy with or without sacrifice of the orbit. *J Oral Maxillofac Surg*. 2005;63(12):1765–1769.
26. Kessler P, Thorwarth M, Bloch-Birkholz A, Nkenke E, Neukam FW. Harvesting of bone from the iliac crest—comparison of the anterior and posterior sites. *Br J Oral Maxillofac Surg*. 2005;43(1):51–56.
27. Nkenke E, Weisbach V, Winckler E, et al. Morbidity of harvesting of bone grafts from the iliac crest for preprosthetic augmentation procedures: a prospective study. *Int J Oral Maxillofac Surg*. 2004;33(2):157–163.
28. Stern SJ, Goepfert H, Clayman G, Byers R, Wolf P. Orbital preservation in maxillectomy. *Otolaryngol Head Neck Surg*. 1993;109(1):111–115.
29. Zubair U, Salam O, Haque R. A case report of gustatory rhinorrhea after maxillectomy performed for squamous cell carcinoma. *Int J Health Sci (Qassim)*. 2018;12(1):83–84.

CHAPTER 97

Segmental Resection of the Mandible

Ricardo Lugo, George Zakhary, and D. David Kim

Armamentarium

#9 Periosteal elevator
#15 Scalpel blade
Appropriate sutures
Crile and Hallstatt mosquito hemostats
DeBakey forceps
Electrocautery unit
Freer elevator
Gerald forceps with teeth
Local anesthetic with vasoconstrictor
Malleable retractor
Mayo scissors
Metzenbaum scissors
Needle holder
Obwegeser turned-in and turned-out retractors
Plating system
Reciprocating sagittal saw
Senn retractors
Weider retractor

History of the Procedure

Prior to Crile's description of a marginal mandibular resection in 1923[1] and his description of the marginal resection as oncologically safe,[2–4] the segmental resection was the primary procedure for extirpation of benign and malignant pathology of the mandible. Given that a composite resection results in a continuity defect of the mandible with loss of soft tissue structures, reconstruction of the mandible has led to an improvement of quality of life for patients undergoing a segmental mandibulectomy.[5–8]

Mandibular resections in the first half of the 20th century were rarely reconstructed, leading to obvious facial deformities. The term *Andy Gump deformity* was used to describe the appearance of patients who underwent anterior mandibular resection without reconstruction. The character Andy Gump was portrayed as an antihero in US comic strips from 1917 to 1959 and is characteristically drawn with a large nose and mustache, but completely lacking a mandible.[9] Early descriptions of mandibular resection, reconstruction, or fixation in the literature used similar techniques for the resection but differed in immediate reconstruction. In 1942, Brown and McDowell described the use of Kirschner wires to fixate the mandible after resection.[10] In 1945, Winter and colleagues described the use of a cobalt chrome implant fixated with screws, with the implant lasting 1 year.[11] This was followed by several other surgeons using cobalt chrome or alloys, which lasted from 1 to 5 years. Additional reconstructive methods included the use of maxillomandibular fixation for several months followed by stainless steel wiring of blocs of iliac crest in the defect.[12] The more recent development of rigid internal fixation has increased the success and ability to reconstruct large segmental defects of the mandible.

Indications for the Use of the Procedure

Segmental resection is indicated in the treatment of benign or malignant mandibular pathology requiring bony margins involving the entire vertical height of the mandible or when a marginal resection would compromise the structural integrity of the mandible.

Limitations and Contraindications

The method is contraindicated in cases of cysts or small tumors that can be adequately treated by marsupialization, enucleation, or marginal resection, thereby preserving the structural integrity of the mandible.

TECHNIQUE: Lateral Mandibular Resection

STEP 1: Preparation

The sterile field should include both sides of the face and neck as well as landmarks for the orientation and monitoring of facial nerve function, including the earlobe, the oral commissure, and chin. Including a wide area in the sterile field allows for ease in extending the resection if clinically indicated without the need to reprep and drape. If the oral cavity is to be entered (typically resections involving tooth-bearing areas), this should be anticipated and the necessary extractions and arch bar placement performed prior to prepping. The anesthesia provider should be made aware that muscle relaxant use during induction should be short-acting in nature, as monitoring of facial nerve function intraoperatively could be rendered impossible. Injection of a local anesthetic with a vasoconstrictor should be completed in a superficial subcutaneous plane. Inadvertent injection of local anesthetic with a vasoconstrictor deep to the level of the platysma can affect conduction of the facial nerve (Fig. 97.1A).

Technique: Lateral Mandibular Resection—*cont'd*

STEP 2: Incision

A submandibular incision is made through subcutaneous tissue to the level of the platysma, at least 1.5 cm below the inferior border of the mandible, preferably in a neck skin crease, which is typically found lower. Placing the incision in a neck crease allows for a well-hidden scar but increases the amount of dissection and retraction necessary. The length of the incision must be extended beyond the planned resection to allow sufficient retraction of the wound for plate application. This can be done using a gentle curve anteriorly as the midline is approached or continued along the neck crease to the contralateral neck for a less perceptible scar (Fig. 97.1B).

STEP 3: Approach

Undermining the subcutaneous tissue from the platysma 1 to 2 cm along the wound increases the amount of retraction possible and allows for easy closure of the wound layers with a good approximation of the skin margins. With the skin retracted, the platysma is undermined and divided. This division should be continued across the full length of the skin incision to maximize the amount of exposure. The superficial layer of the deep cervical fascia is divided, noting that deep to this layer are the facial vessels and submandibular gland. Using the inferior portion of the gland as a landmark will generally guide the dissection deep to the level of the facial nerve and orient the surgeon to the facial vein lying superficial or just posterior to the gland. The facial vein once encountered can be divided and retracted superiorly to protect the marginal mandibular branch of the facial nerve. As long as dissection is carried out deep to this plane, along the submandibular gland, the nerve is safe from harm. The facial artery typically accompanies the vein but many times passes through the gland itself. When necessary, the artery may be divided for access. The dissection described above is appropriate for approaching the mandible in benign pathology. In approaching a mandible for malignant pathology with an associated neck dissection, special attention must be directed to the identification of perifacial lymph nodes, which should be taken with the neck dissection specimen if possible.

When dissection is intended to access the ramus and angle regions, the abovementioned landmarks may not be encountered and care must be taken to remain at the level of the skin incision or at least 1.5 cm below the inferior border of the mandible to prevent injury to the facial nerve. The anterior border of the sternocleidomastoid and the posterior belly of the digastric may be followed superiorly to locate the angle of the mandible. The external jugular vein and one of its tributaries, the retromandibular vein, may be encountered in this approach[13] (Fig. 97.1C and D).

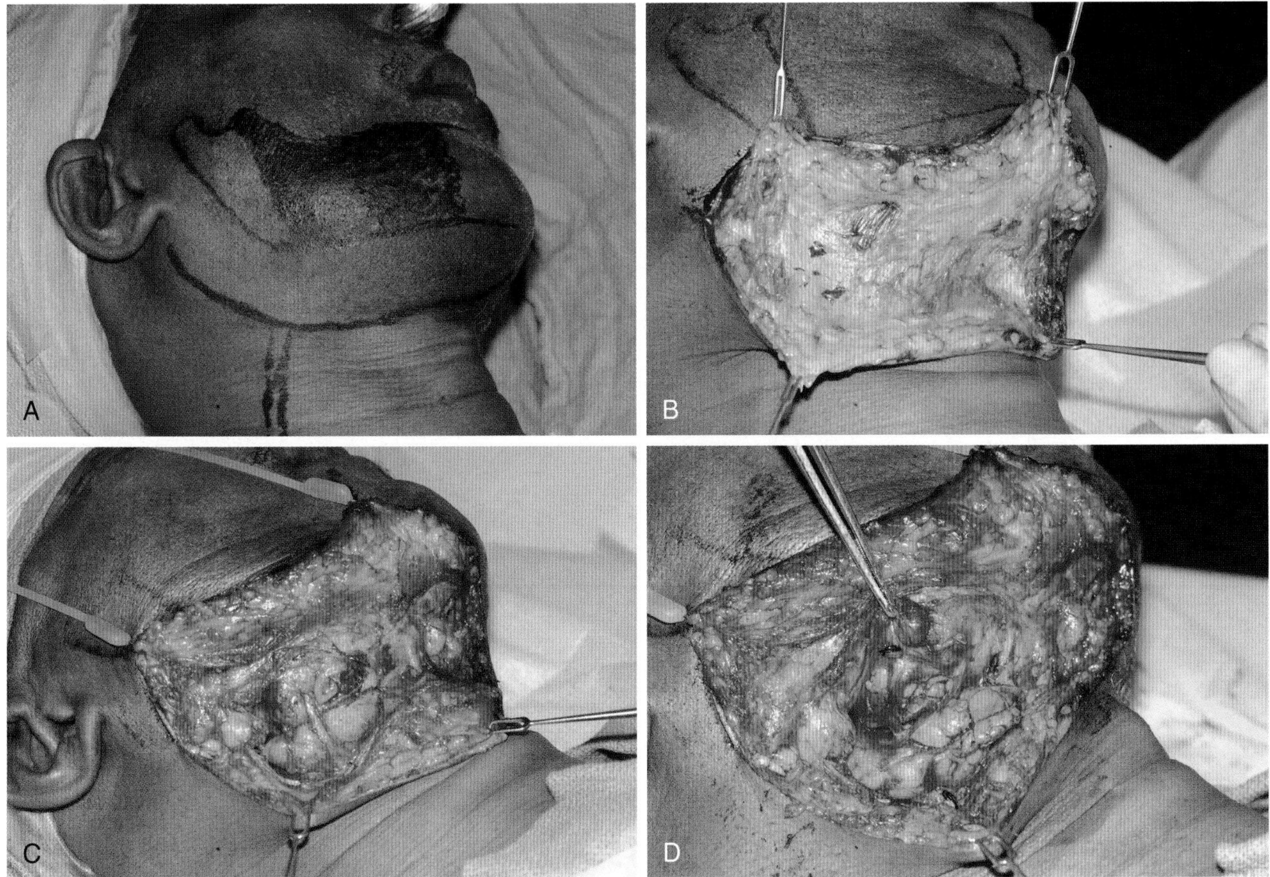

Figure 97.1 **A,** Preoperative markings for proposed resection and incision placement. **B,** Skin and subcutaneous tissue reflected to expose the platysma. **C,** Submandibular gland and facial vein exposed. **D,** Lymph node of Starr retracted superiorly with the facial artery visible.

Continued

Technique: Lateral Mandibular Resection—*cont'd*

STEP 4: Mandibular Exposure

The periosteum of the mandible is encountered in the body region after the submandibular gland is dissected and the gland is retracted inferiorly. In the ramus and angle regions, the pterygomasseteric sling surrounds the mandible. Depending on the anatomic barrier needed for adequate margins, a supraperiosteal or subperiosteal dissection is then performed. Unless the tumor or cyst has eroded through the inferior border of the mandible into the masseteric space, the pterygomasseteric sling may be sharply divided along the inferior border of the mandible. Once the subperiosteal, supraperiosteal, or muscular plane dissection of the lateral border of the mandible is complete, the lingual dissection can be performed in the appropriate anatomic plane, with care taken not to injure the lingual nerve. Many times the lingual dissection will not be completed until the osteotomies have been performed, allowing additional access to the medial surface of the mandible (Fig. 97.1E).

STEP 5: Mandibular Resection

Teeth involved in the proposed resection should be included in the specimen. One tooth on either side of the proposed osteotomy is typically removed to allow for adequate margins and to facilitate the osteotomy. If the attached gingiva can be reflected from the teeth along the planned resection, this should be performed, but many times the attached gingiva is included in the specimen. If the dissection is subperiosteal or only a thin layer of tissue is to be included with the resection, the reconstruction plate can be preadapted to the mandible with holes for fixation screws drilled. At this point the plate is removed, and the lingual tissues are dissected subperiosteally at the sites of the proposed osteotomy and protected using a broad malleable retractor. The osteotomy is performed using a reciprocating sagittal saw with normal saline irrigation (Fig. 97.1F).

STEP 6: Plate Application

Immediate reconstruction with free bone grafting, microvascular free tissue transfer, or bone morphogenetic proteins is generally ideal for the patient; however, this is not always possible due to intraoral communication or the nature of the pathology (to demonstrate adequate resection prior to reconstruction). With maxillomandibular fixation in place, a reconstruction plate that is adapted either prior to or after resection is fixated with a minimum of three bicortical locking screws on either side of the defect. In some cases, a trochar can be used for transcutaneous screw placement when exposure is limited (Fig. 97.1G and H).

STEP 7: Closure

Any intraoral communication should be closed to a watertight approximation. The pterygomasseteric sling should be reapproximated around the inferior border of the mandible or the reconstruction plate with resorbable sutures. Following this step, the platysma layer is reapproximated with resorbable suture and the skin is then closed with skin sutures or staples.

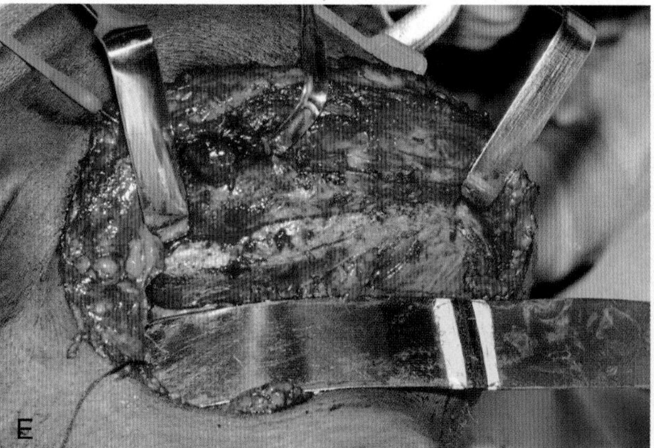

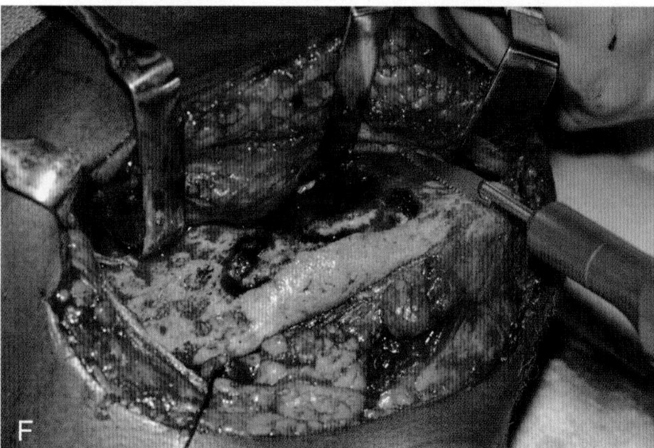

Figure 97.1, cont'd **E,** Inferior border of the mandible exposed, anterior belly of the digastric origin visible. **F,** Reciprocating saw used for a traditional osteotomy.

Technique: Lateral Mandibular Resection—*cont'd*

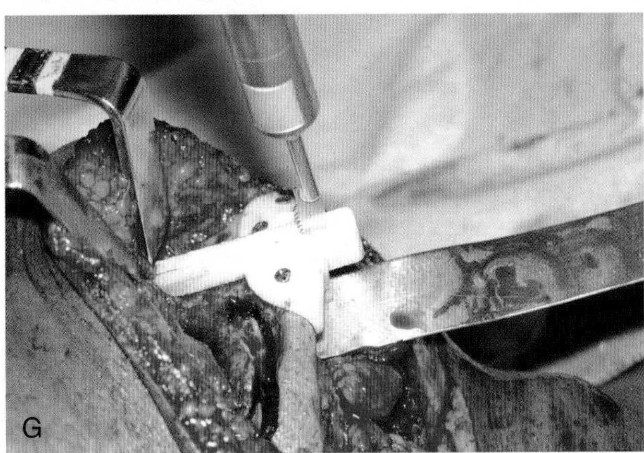

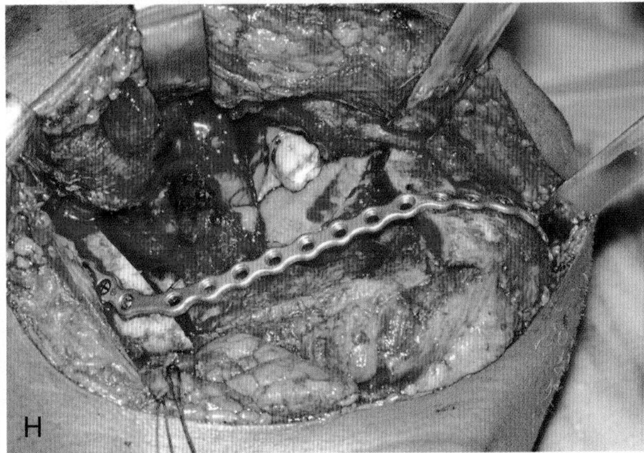

Figure 97.1, cont'd **G,** Use of cutting guides as part of the virtual surgical planning for immediate fibula free flap reconstruction. Note the protection of lingual tissues with a broad malleable retractor. **H,** Plate fixated with bicortical screws measured to length. Note the superiorly located position of the anterior plate in anticipation of fibula free flap reconstruction.

ALTERNATIVE TECHNIQUE 1: Crossing the Midline

When crossing the midline, the incision should be extended to the contralateral neck. The remainder of the procedure continues as previously described with the suprahyoid muscles freed from the inferior border of the mandible and then resuspended to the reconstruction plate during closure. The mental nerve on one side should be preserved when possible, if the resection does not necessitate its removal. A supraperiosteal dissection that crosses midline is shown. Virtual surgical planning allows for precise cutting guides, as well as improved accuracy and efficiency in plate adaptation (Fig. 97.2A and B).

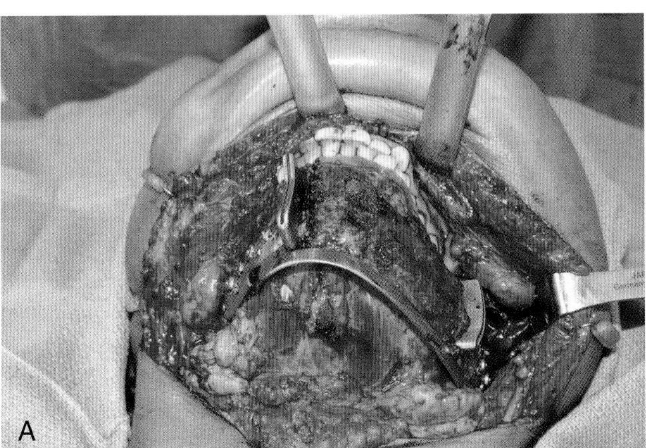

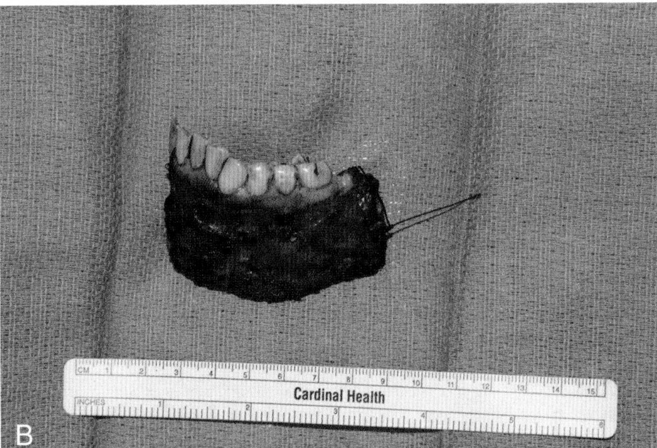

Figure 97.2 **A,** Segmental resection crossing the midline with custom cutting guides. **B,** Supraperiosteal segmental resection of the mandible.

ALTERNATIVE TECHNIQUE 2: Condylar Resections

For resections involving the mandibular condyle, care must be taken when approaching the area medial to the condyle. The anatomy in proximity to the condyle and ramus includes the inferior alveolar nerve, lingual nerve, facial nerve, external carotid artery, internal maxillary artery, middle meningeal artery, masseteric artery, and pterygoid venous plexus. Care must be exercised when resecting the ramus and condylar portions of the mandible in order to protect the structures deep and posterior to this region. Bleeding can be difficult to control due to limited access and visibility near the skull base. A reconstruction plate with a condylar prosthesis may be used in preparation for a later temporomandibular joint prosthesis, costochondral graft, or microvascular fibula reconstruction (Fig. 97.3A–D).

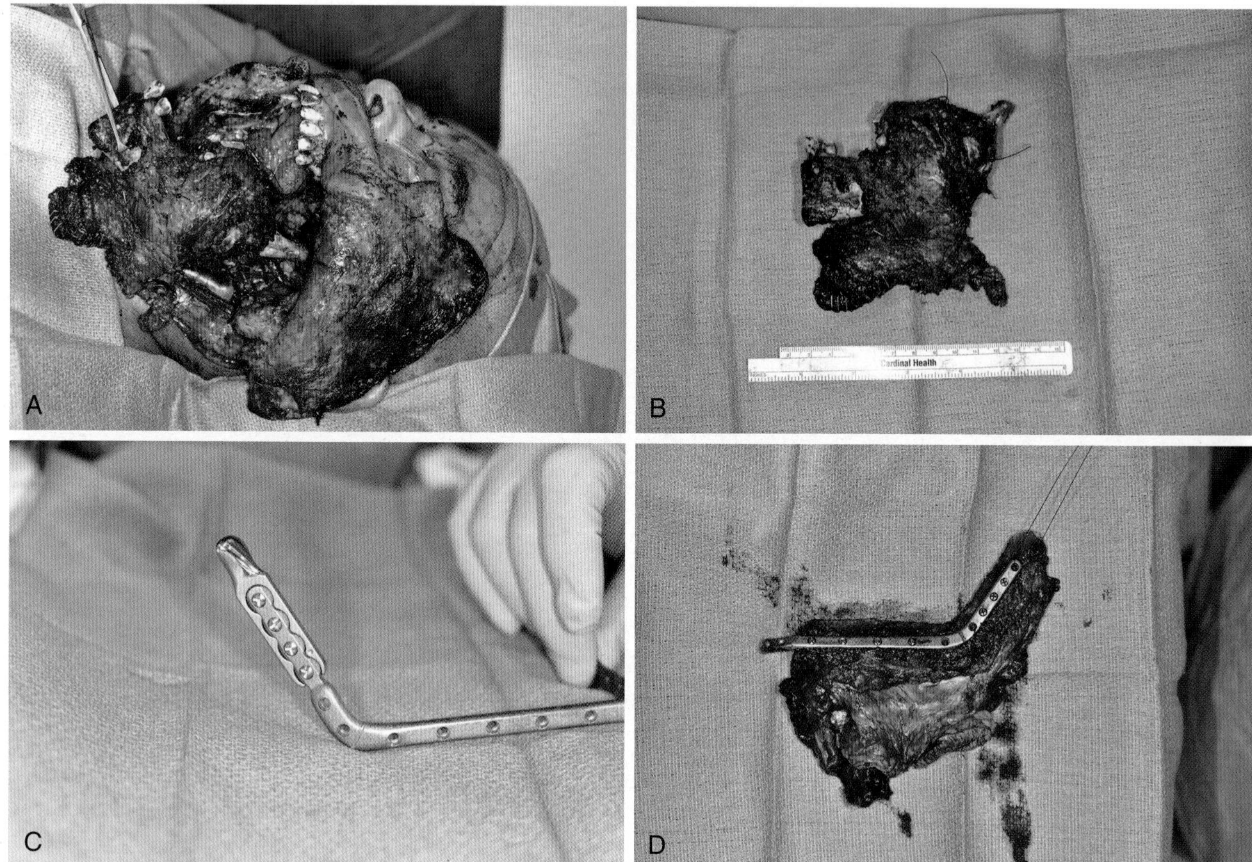

Figure 97.3 **A,** Segmental resection with a condylar disarticulation. **B,** Segmental resection. Note the supraperiosteal dissection over the malignant tumor and subperiosteal dissection proximal and distal to the proposed margins. **C,** Custom reconstruction plate with a stock condylar prosthesis. **D,** Fibula free flap with condylar reconstruction.

Avoidance and Management of Intraoperative Complications

Injury to the marginal mandibular branch of the facial nerve can be avoided by incising 1.5 cm below the inferior border of the mandible in the area posterior to the facial artery.[14] As described earlier, dissecting in a plane deep to the superficial layer of the deep cervical fascia will protect the marginal mandibular branch of the facial nerve by elevating the fascia along with the nerve. Alternatively, the nerve can also be protected by locating and dividing the facial vein and dissecting along the anterior border of the sternocleidomastoid muscle or deep to the submandibular gland capsule.

Injury to the lingual nerve can occur during the medial dissection, particularly in a supraperiosteal approach. Blunt dissection into the lingual soft tissues will allow the lingual nerve to come into view. If the lingual dissection is delayed until after the mandibular osteotomies, access will be improved thereby facilitating a safer dissection of the lingual nerve. Estimating bony margins prior to surgery can be misleading due to distortion or lack of detail of the region of the mandible in question on panoramic radiograph. A medical-grade computed tomography scan can improve accuracy in predicting intraoperative bony margins. Intraoperative plain films of the specimen can help the surgeon to visualize clinical margins.

Accuracy in reconstruction can be improved using virtual surgical planning with cutting guides for resection. In the case where a patient elects to pursue dental implants, virtual surgical planning allows for precise fibular osteotomies as well as simultaneous placement of dental implants into the fibula at the time of harvesting. This virtual planning allows for improved accuracy in the placement of the fibula for alveolar continuity as well as accuracy of dental implant placement into the fibula for eventual reconstruction.

Postoperative Considerations

Meticulous control of bleeding and drain placement when indicated can minimize postoperative hematoma, which in itself can compromise bone graft or free tissue transfer success. Avoidance of over- or underadaptation of the reconstruction plate can prevent asymmetry in facial form, especially in defects crossing the midline of the mandible.

Underadaptation of the reconstruction plate can also place excessive pressure on the overlying skin. This is especially problematic in patients with a history of radiation to the neck as it increases the risk of skin breakdown and plate exposure in the future. Symmetry and appropriate soft tissue draping can be achieved through preadaptation prior to resection and redraping of tissues intraoperatively to assess anterior and lateral projection of the plate. Alternatively, with virtual surgical planning, the reconstruction plate can be planned to mirror the pre-resection mandibular archform.

References

1. Crile GW. Carcinoma of the jaws, tongue, cheek and lips. *Surg Gyn Obs*. 1923;36:159–162.
2. Marchetta FC, Sako K, Badillo J. Periosteal lymphatics of the mandible and intraoral carcinoma. *Am J Surg*. 1964;108:505–507.
3. Marchetta FC, Sako K, Murphy JB. The periosteum of the mandible and intraoral carcinoma. *Am J Surg*. 1971;122:711–713.
4. Pogrel MA. The marginal mandibulectomy for the treatment of mandibular tumours. *Br J Oral Maxillofac Surg*. 1989;27:132–138.
5. Zavalishina L, Karra N, Zaid W, El-Hakim M. Quality of life assessment in patients after mandibular resection and free fibula flap reconstruction. *J Oral Maxillofac Surg*. 2014;72:1616–1626.
6. Zhu J, Xiao Y, Liu F, Wang J, Yang W, Xie W. Measures of health-related quality of life and socio-cultural aspects in young patients who after mandible primary reconstruction with free fibula flap. *World J Surg Oncol*. 2013;11:250–255.
7. Young CW, Pogrel MA, Schmidt BL. Quality of life in patients undergoing segmental mandibular resection and staged reconstruction with nonvascularized bone grafts. *J Oral Maxillofac Surg*. 2007;65:706–712.
8. Warshavsky A, Fliss D, Frenkel G, et al. Long-term health-related quality of life after mandibular resection and reconstruction. *Eur Arch Otorhinolaryngol*. 2019;276:1501–1508.
9. Pogrel MA. Who was Andy Gump? *J Oral Maxillofac Surg*. 2010;68:654–657.
10. Brown JB, McDowell F. Internal wire pin fixation for fractures of the jaw. *Surg Gynecol Obstet*. 1942;74:227–230.
11. Winter L, Lifton JC, McQuillan AS. Embedment of a Vitallium mandibular prosthesis as an integral part of the operation for removal of an adamantinoma. *Am J Surg*. 1945;69:318–324.
12. Kazanjian VH. Resection of tumor of the mandible and repair of the deformity: report of case. *J Oral Surg*. 1951;9:59–64.
13. Ellis E, Zide MF. *Surgical Approaches to the Facial Skeleton*. 2nd ed. Philadelphia, PA: Lippincott Williams & Wilkins; 2005:153–184.
14. Dingman RO, Grabb WC. Surgical anatomy of the mandibular ramus of the facial nerve based on the dissection of 100 facial halves. *Plast Reconstr Surg Transplant Bull*. 1962;29:266–272.

CHAPTER 98

Sublingual Gland Excision and Ductal Surgery

Brian M. Woo

Armamentarium

#11 and #15 scalpel blades
Allis clamp
Appropriate Sutures
Bipolar electrocautery
Bite block or Molt mouth prop
Blunt tenotomy scissors
Bowman lacrimal probes
DeBakey forceps
Gerald serrated and toothed forceps
Headlight
Kelly hemostats (curved and straight)
Local anesthetic with vasoconstrictor
Loupe magnification (2.5×)
Mayo scissors
Mosquito hemostats
Needle electrocautery
Schnidt right-angle tonsil forceps (Sawtell or Mixter)
Schnidt tonsil forceps (Boettcher)
Single skin hook
Skin staples (used if a cervical incision is made)
Surgical peanut sponges or Kittner sponges
Weider tongue retractor

History of the Procedure

It is difficult to find a report of the very first sublingual gland excision in the literature; however, early descriptions of the procedure can be found that are mainly related to the treatment of oral and plunging ranulas. Therefore, it is necessary to discuss the etiology, pathogenesis, and treatment of oral and plunging ranulas. Ranulas have been described for centuries, but there has always been controversy over their etiology. Hippocrates and Celsius believed that they were inflammatory in origin.[1] In 1585, Banister wrote that a "ranula is a tumor in that laxe and saufte parte of the mouth, which is under the tongue." He tried to cure ranulas first with the application of medicaments, and if that was unsuccessful, he opened them with cautery and applied the medicaments to the opened cavity.[2] In 1676, Wiseman observed that ranulas caused a croaking speech, and he described the oral ranula's blue-domed, cystic appearance as resembling the bulging underbelly or air sac of a frog—hence the term *ranula* (*rana* is the Latin word for frog) (Fig. 98.1A).[2] Early theories about the origin of the ranula included the existence of a submucosal bursa, possibly branchial in origin, or possibly originating from remnants of the external paralingual groove, or from remnants of the thyroglossal duct and chronic myxangitis of a salivary gland or chronic inflammation (Fig. 98.1B–E).[2] It was not until 1887 that Suzanne, followed by von Hipple in 1897, associated the sublingual gland with the origin of the ranula and recommended removal of the sublingual gland and ranula. In 1957, Crile performed sublingual gland excisions for recurrent plunging ranulas after attempts to remove the plunging ranulas through a cervical approach without removal of the sublingual gland and after removal of the submandibular gland failed. He concluded that the excision of the ranula without the removal of the sublingual gland resulted in recurrence.[3,4] In 1965, Cohen and Tiecke equated ranulas pathologically with mucoceles of minor salivary glands and, as for mucoceles, recommended excision of the lesion and the associated gland, the sublingual gland.[3] In 1969, Catone et al.[3] published nine cases of nonplunging ranulas successfully treated with excision of the sublingual gland and proposed that the sublingual gland and its excretory system were the origin of the ranula. In 1973, Roediger et al.[4] confirmed that the sublingual gland was the source of plunging ranulas by comparing the fluid contained within the plunging ranulas to the secretions of the different major salivary glands. They found that the cyst fluid and sublingual gland secretions had a higher amylase content than that of serum, but a lower amylase and higher protein content than that of the submandibular and parotid glands because of its more mucinous than serous production.

It is currently believed that there are two varieties of ranulas. The less common variety is the result of a mucus retention phenomenon; the other variety is the result of mucous extravasation or the mucous escape phenomenon. In 1685, Diemerbrock theorized that ranulas resulted from obstruction and retention of saliva in the excretory duct of a salivary gland.[3] This theory, that ranulas developed after complete or partial obstruction of an excretory duct and, therefore, led to

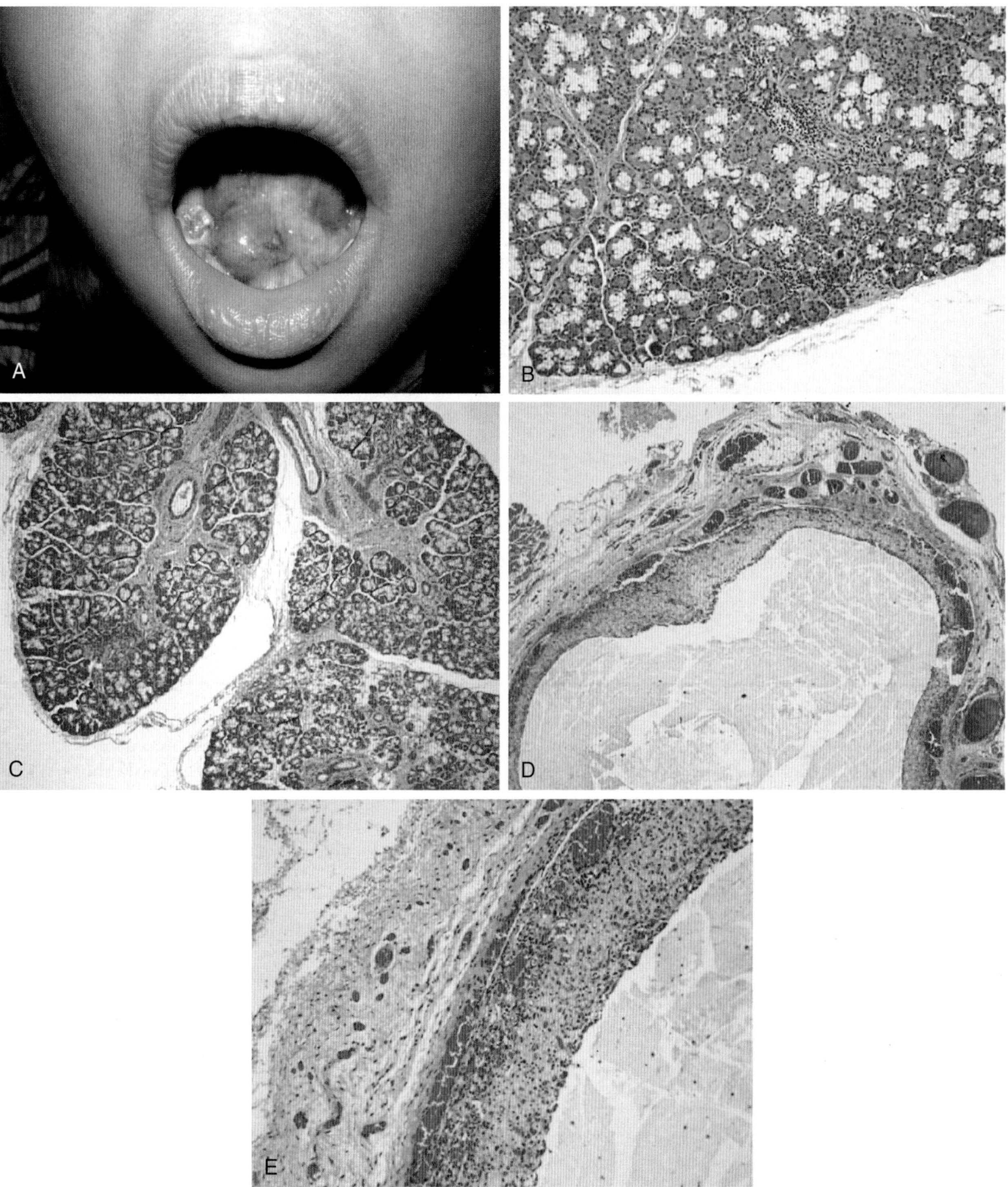

Figure 98.1 **A,** Photograph of a recurrent oral ranula in a 5-year-old female initially treated with marsupialization. She was subsequently treated with sublingual gland excision. **B** and **C,** Histologic sections of the patient's sublingual gland show a mild, patchy, chronic inflammatory infiltrate of lymphocytes. The sublingual gland also shows either no capsule or an incomplete capsule compared to the other major salivary glands; no capsule is observed in these sections. **D** and **E,** Histologic sections of the plunging ranula seen in the patient show a large pseudocyst with a thin, fibrous wall. Mucous contents are present. The pseudocyst wall varies from a dense fibrous layer with no evident epithelial lining to a more inflamed and congested wall with possible residual mucous epithelium. Some areas show intramural macrophages with probable mucinous contents.

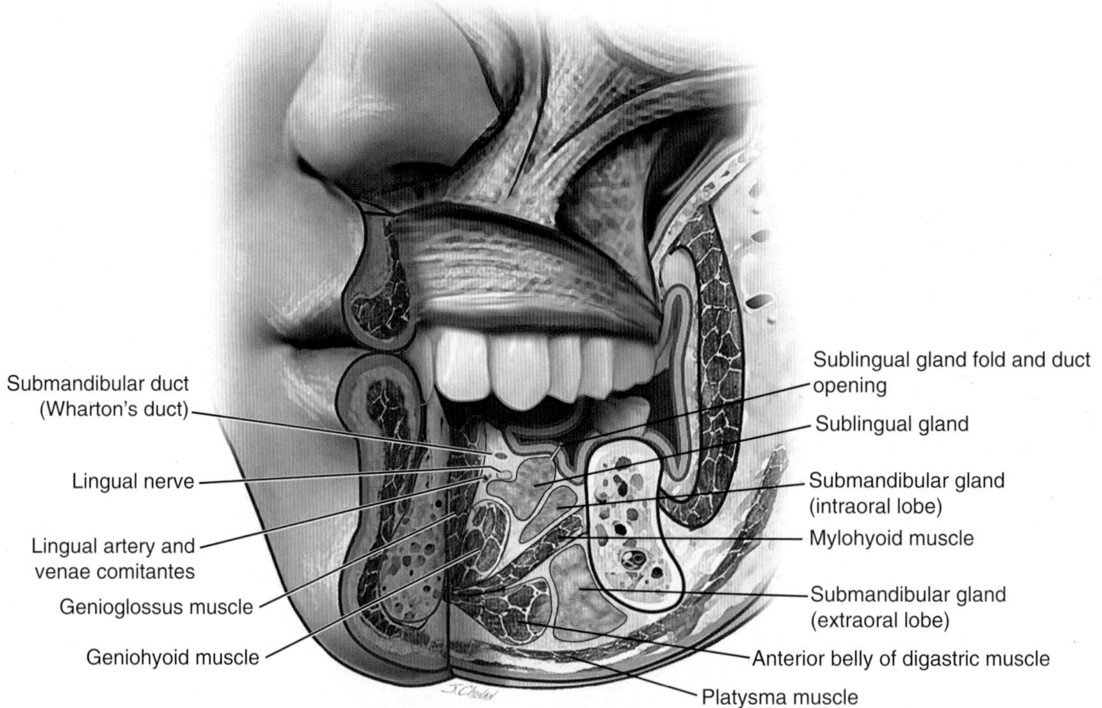

Figure 98.2 Frontal section through the tongue and sublingual and submandibular regions.

ductal dilation and the eventual formation of an epithelial-lined retention cyst, persisted for many years. However, in 1956, Bhaskur et al. reviewed 19 of their surgical specimens of ranulas and found that they were lined only by connective tissue.[5] In 1959, Standish and Shafer reviewed 97 cases of ranulas. They found that in 91 cases, the lesions were composed of a dense connective tissue capsule and that only six contained a partial or complete epithelial lining.[5] In 1964, Robinson and Hjorting-Hansen reviewed 125 ranulas and found that only 22 contained a partial or complete epithelial lining. Crile and others were also able to show that mucous extravasation and pseudocyst formation were the etiology of plunging ranulas (Figs. 98.2 and 98.3).[6]

Indications for the Use of the Procedure

Indications reported in the literature for sublingual gland excision include conditions, such as chronic sialadenitis, sialolithiasis, a floor of the mouth ranula arising from the sublingual gland, a plunging ranula, benign sublingual gland pathology (e.g., a pleomorphic adenoma), chronic and excessive drooling/sialorrhea, and enlargement of the sublingual gland that impeded prosthetic reconstruction.[3,2,7–13] An additional indication for sublingual gland excision is the recurrence of a ranula arising from the sublingual gland after marsupialization or other conservative treatment. The failure rate for marsupialization alone has been reported to be 61% to 89%, with recurrence occurring between 6 weeks and 12 months.[14] Bridger found that 44% of plunging ranulas were iatrogenic and usually occurred after single or multiple treatments of an oral ranula with marsupialization or simple drainage.[14] He believed that failed procedures could result in surface fibrosis that diverted the salivary leakage inferiorly, either through defects in the mylohyoid muscle or around the posterior edge of the mylohyoid muscle, leading to the formation of a plunging ranula (Fig. 98.4).

Limitations and Contraindications

In the author's opinion, there are no absolute contraindications for the excision of the sublingual gland for the previously listed indications; however, in some cases the surgeon should consider not performing a sublingual gland excision as the initial treatment. For example, with congenital ranulas, excision of the sublingual gland should not be considered the first-line therapy because some of these ranulas have been reported to resolve spontaneously. Some ranulas result in airway compromise at delivery or feeding difficulties; these require initial treatment with more conservative therapies, such as aspiration, unroofing, and marsupialization. Other types of ranulas have been shown to be epithelium-lined cysts or retention cysts instead of pseudocysts and require only marsupialization (with or without sialodochoplasty) or spontaneous rupture for cure.[15–17] Congenital ranulas are thought to arise from atresic, imperforate, or duplicated sublingual or submandibular ducts. Because congenital ranulas could also arise from the submandibular ducts, excision of the sublingual gland should

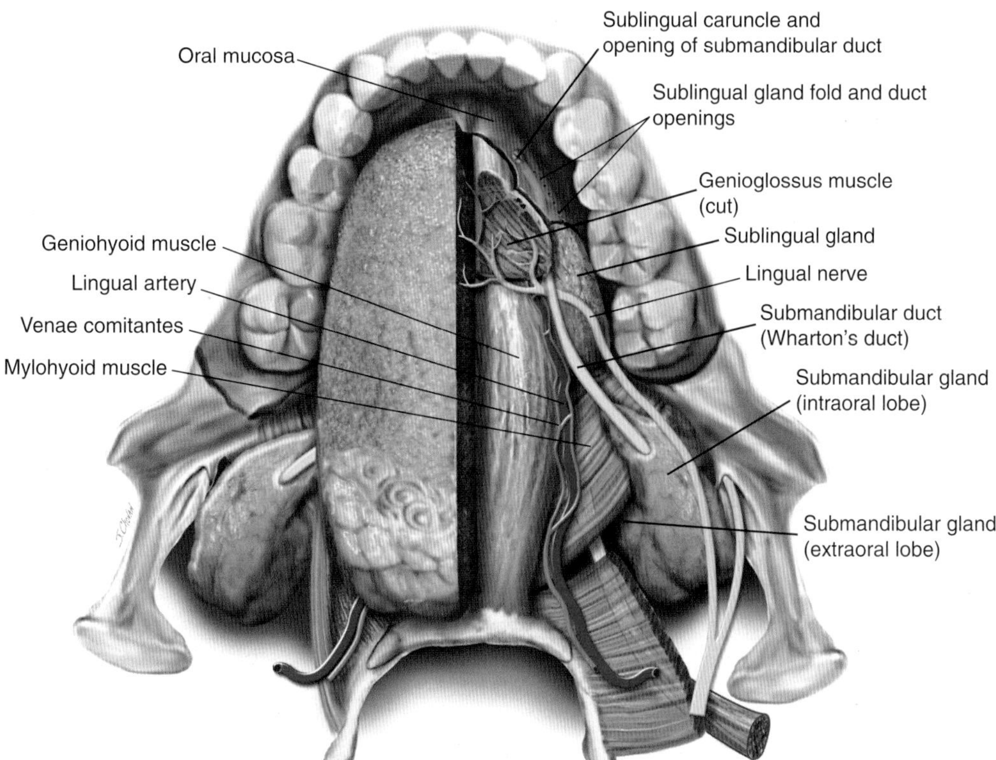

Figure 98.3 Submandibular and sublingual glands. Note the following: (1) With the tongue removed and the genioglossus and geniohyoid muscles cut, the submandibular and sublingual glands are exposed and their relationship to the inner aspect of the mandible is shown; (2) The submandibular duct measures about 5 cm and courses anteriorly between the sublingual gland and genioglossus muscle (cut). It opens in the floor of the mouth at the sublingular caruncle.

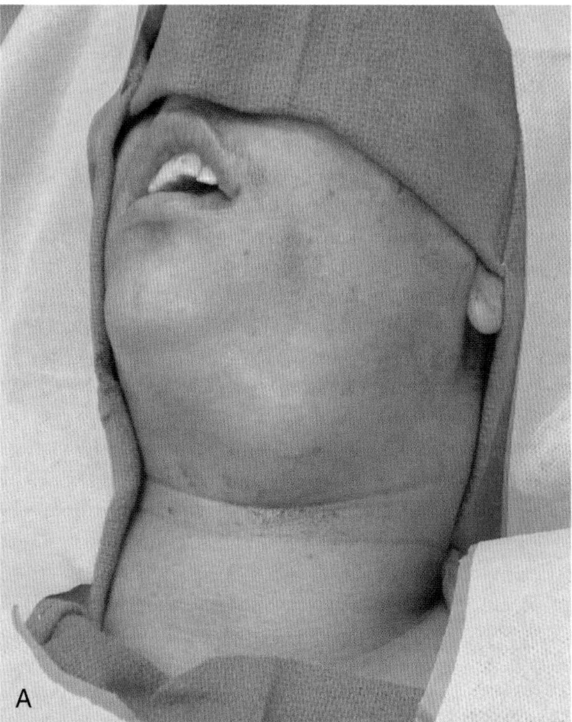

Figure 98.4 **A,** Note the bulge of the plunging ranula in the patient's left submandibular region, along with the previous incision for the incision and drainage.

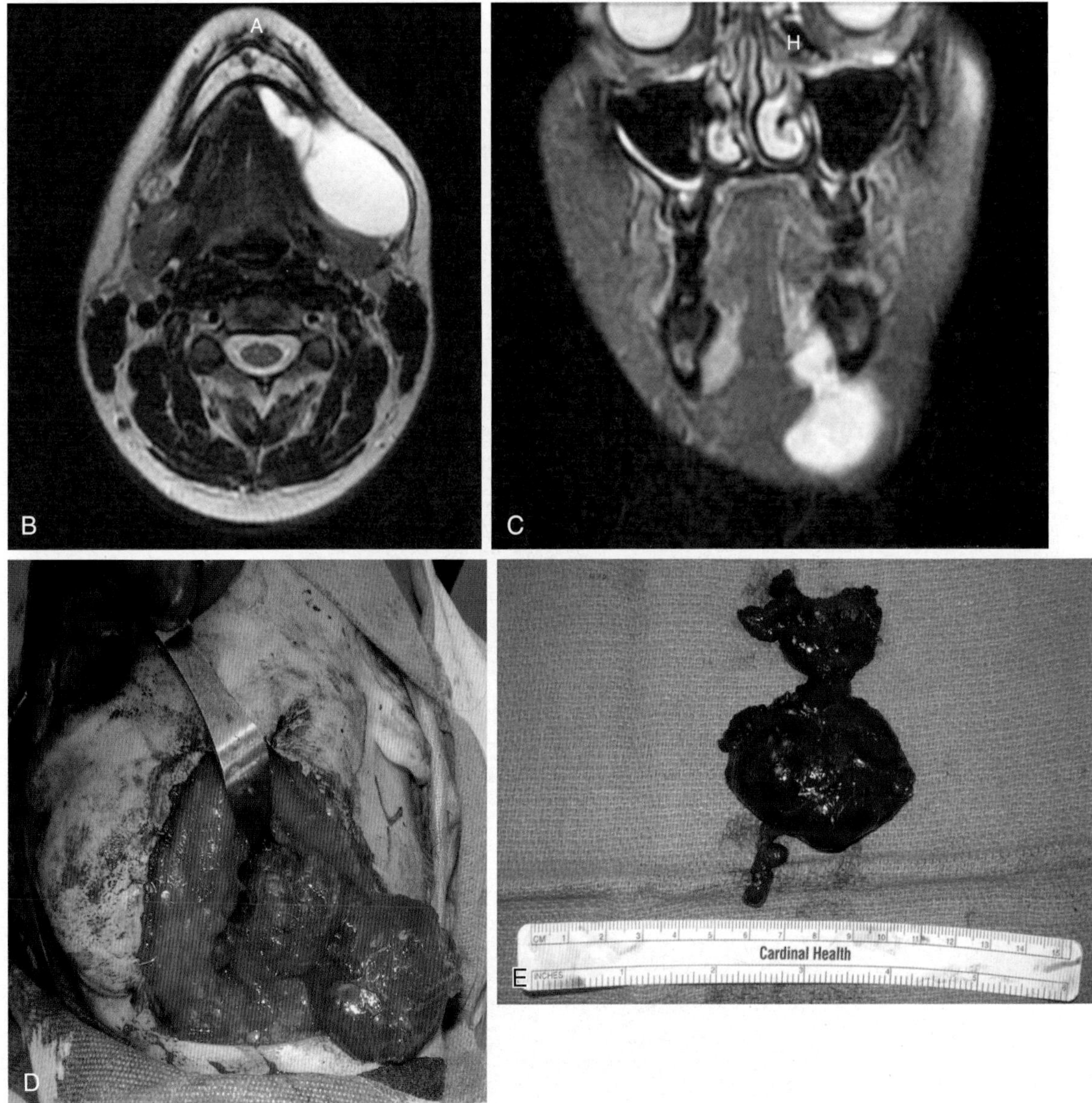

Figure 98.4, cont'd **B** and **C,** A T2-weighted magnetic resonance imaging scan with axial and coronal cuts shows the communication between the plunging ranula and the left sublingual gland through a defect in the mylohyoid muscle. **D,** The cervical approach is shown, with the plunging ranula and sublingual gland removed in continuity via a combined intraoral and cervical approach. A defect was found in the mylohyoid muscle at the time of surgery. **E,** The specimen alone with the plunging ranula and the sublingual gland attached superiorly.

not be considered the first-line therapy. Increasingly, reports in the literature are demonstrating an association between patients who are positive for the human immunodeficiency virus (HIV) and ranulas.[18,19] Benign lymphoepithelial cysts of the parotid glands in HIV-positive patients have been shown to respond to highly active antiretroviral drug therapy (HAART).[19] Some recent publications have shown possible regression of HIV-related ranulas with HAART; however, in a recent prospective study, Syebele and Bütow found that HIV-related ranulas did not respond, as well or as rapidly as, benign lymphoepithelial cysts.[18,19] Nevertheless, because HAART offers the possibility of regression, this approach should be considered before surgical excision of the sublingual gland.

TECHNIQUE: Sublingual Gland Excision

STEP 1: Anesthesia and Patient Positioning

The author prefers to perform the procedure under general anesthesia, because it allows greater patient comfort and greater retraction and visualization. In addition, it frees the surgeon from having to manage the airway and anesthesia (if an intravenous anesthetic is used); this allows the surgeon to focus on meticulous dissection and hemostasis. A nasal endotracheal tube is used instead of an oral endotracheal tube to keep the tube out of the surgical field. The procedure is performed with the patient in the supine position and in slight reverse Trendelenburg position. A shoulder roll can be placed if a cervical incision is needed. However, as mentioned previously, studies have shown that a plunging ranula is a pseudocyst and can be treated entirely through an intraoral approach; there is no need for dissection and complete removal of the plunging ranula. After the sublingual gland has been excised, a portion of the pseudocyst can be biopsied to confirm the diagnosis, and its contents can be evacuated using an intraoral approach. The pseudocyst usually resolves 2 to 3 months after excision of the sublingual gland. Betadine or an equivalent surgical preparation is painted on the lower face, around the oral cavity, and on the upper neck. The surgeon should don a headlight before beginning the procedure to improve visualization.

STEP 2: Retraction

A bite block or Molt mouth prop is placed in the mouth on the side opposite the sublingual gland to be excised. The Weider tongue retractor then is placed to retract the tongue and expose the floor of the mouth on the affected side. Retraction of the tongue with the Weider retractor should expose the lesion or ranula (if applicable), the plica sublingualis, and the orifice of the submandibular duct. The author finds it helpful to use loupe magnification to cannulate the Wharton duct on the affected side. This is performed with lacrimal probes, starting with the smallest probe (usually a 00 or 000) and progressing to a larger probe; this later facilitates identification and dissection of the sublingual gland away from the submandibular duct. When the lacrimal probe is inserted into the submandibular orifice and duct, care must be taken not to create a false passage. After the submandibular duct has been cannulated, local anesthetic with epinephrine can be injected around the margin of the ranula, using a multiple injection technique, to hydrodissect the mucosa off the ranula. After an initial plane between the ranula and the mucosa has been created at the periphery of the ranula, additional injections can be given in the newly hydrodissected plane, working toward the center. For these injections, the surgeon should use a small needle (30 gauge), and the bevel of the needle should face the ranula. If there is no ranula or lesion, a local anesthetic can be injected to hydrodissect the mucosa away from the sublingual gland. The epinephrine in the local anesthetic aids in hemostasis.

STEP 3: Incision

Multiple incision designs have been described in the literature. Surgeons have described linear incisions over the ranula or sublingual gland, 1 cm from the inner cortex of the mandible and parallel to the mandible, between the submandibular duct and the plica sublingualis, over the submandibular duct, and between the submandibular duct and the tongue. Others have described an elliptical incision over the ranula and the sublingual gland, and even a trapdoor incision incorporating the submandibular duct and its orifice.[3,11,20,21] The author prefers to make a linear incision with a #15 blade over the ranula or the gland, taking care to use light pressure and to incise only through the mucosa (Fig. 98.5A).

STEP 4: Dissection

The dissection is begun by grabbing the edges of the mucosa along the incision with a Gerald forceps. As the mucosal edge is lifted with the forceps, a mosquito hemostat or blunt tenotomy scissors is used to dissect the mucosa away from the ranula or sublingual gland by spreading the tips of the hemostat or scissors. If the incision needs to be extended, the mosquito hemostat can be used to dissect and tunnel under the mucosa through the existing incision, and a #15 blade or needle electrocautery can then be used to incise the mucosa over the closed mosquito hemostat.

After the mucosal flaps have been elevated, silk retraction sutures can be placed in the flaps and Kelly hemostats placed on the silk sutures to aid retraction. It is satisfying to be able to remove the ranula intact, but this is not essential. Some authors recommend deflating larger ranulas to gain better access to the floor of the mouth. Takimoto et al. recommend aspirating the ranula contents and then filling it with fibrin glue to make it firm and rubbery and easier to dissect.[22] The mucosa is dissected off the ranula until it can easily be moved side to side, allowing access to the sublingual gland and the contents of the floor of the mouth. If the ranula ruptures before this and the surgeon is unable to dissect it free in its entirety, a portion of it should be sent for permanent histologic examination to confirm the diagnosis, and further dissection should focus on the sublingual gland.

The author prefers to start with the lateral dissection, first separating the sublingual gland from the periosteum of the mandible, down to the level of the mylohyoid muscle. The author uses a combination of sharp and blunt dissection, but predominantly blunt dissection with surgical peanut sponges loaded on straight Kelly hemostats, especially posteriorly, to avoid injury to the lingual nerve as it crosses underneath the submandibular duct. The use of blunt dissection with peanut sponges is a must and is invaluable in identifying and preserving key structures. During the dissection, hemostasis is achieved with judicious use of needle and bipolar electrocautery.

Continued

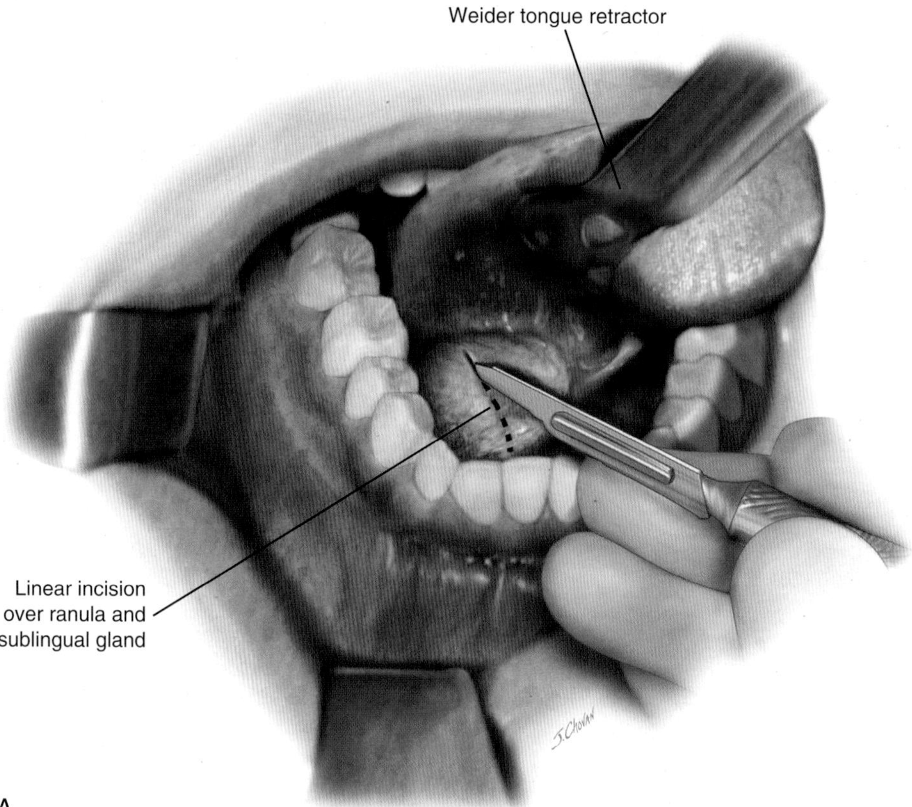

Figure 98.5 **A,** Excision of the sublingual gland using a linear incision and a medial approach through the mucosa of the floor of the mouth. A Weider tongue retractor is used to retract the tongue and expose the floor of the mouth on the affected side. A linear incision is preferred by the author.

TECHNIQUE: Sublingual Gland Excision—*cont'd*

Next, with the lacrimal probe in the submandibular duct, the medial dissection is started. A combination of blunt dissection with the peanut sponges or mosquito hemostats, and sharp dissection with tenotomy scissors is used to separate the sublingual gland from the submandibular duct anteriorly. In some instances, anterior sharp dissection with either tenotomy scissors or bipolar electrocautery is needed to separate the anterior portion of the sublingual gland from the periosteum lining the inner cortex of the anterior mandible. After the sublingual gland has been separated from the periosteum of the mandible and the submandibular duct anteriorly dissected, the portion of the sublingual gland that has been dissected free laterally and anteriorly can be grasped initially with a DeBakey or Gerald forceps, and later an Allis clamp, and retracted laterally. While lateral traction is applied, the medial dissection is carried out from anterior to posterior, using mainly blunt dissection with the peanut sponges. Some sharp dissection with the mosquito hemostat or blunted tenotomy scissors is used to separate the sublingual gland off the submandibular duct and then the lingual nerve, as the dissection proceeds posteriorly and the lingual nerve is identified. Posteriorly, the lingual nerve crosses from lateral to medial underneath the submandibular duct, and the posterior sublingual gland usually is continuous with the uncinate process of the submandibular gland that lies superior to the mylohyoid muscle. Therefore, the posterior sublingual gland is divided from the uncinate process of the submandibular gland by passing a mosquito hemostat or a Schnidt right-angle tonsil forceps underneath the posterior edge of the sublingual gland; then, needle electrocautery or bipolar electrocautery is used to cauterize through the gland onto the hemostat or forceps. While performing this step, the surgeon must identify and protect the lingual nerve and the Wharton duct. Some authors also recommend ligating the glandular tissue left behind before dividing the two glands. The sublingual gland now can be removed (Fig. 98.5B–E).

STEP 5: Hemostasis and Closure

During dissection of the sublingual gland and after the gland has been removed, hemostasis is achieved with judicious use of the needle electrocautery and bipolar electrocautery. After hemostasis has been obtained, the mucosal flaps can be loosely reapproximated with chromic gut suture, or they can be left open to heal secondarily.

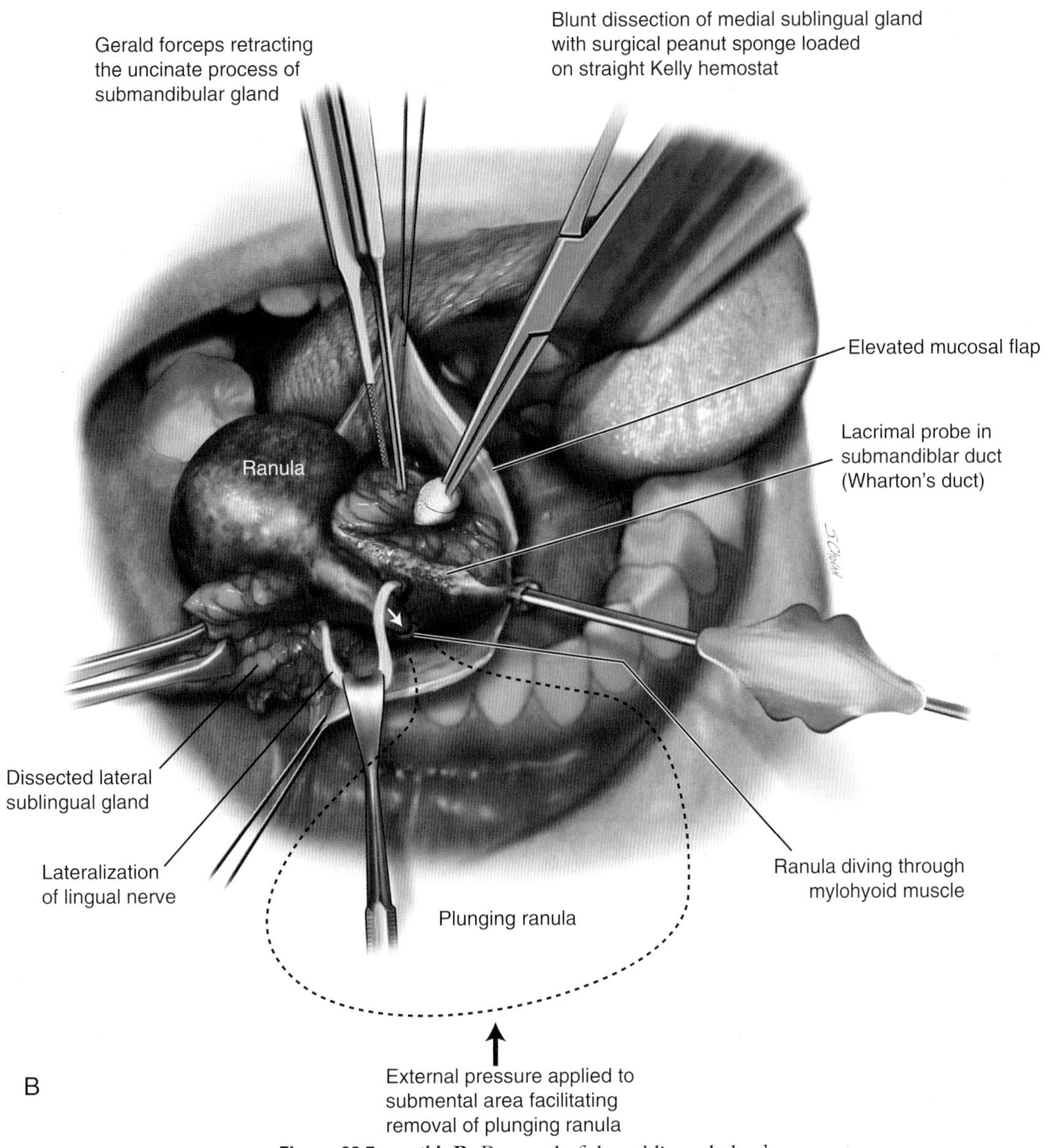

Figure 98.5, cont'd **B,** Removal of the sublingual gland.

Continued

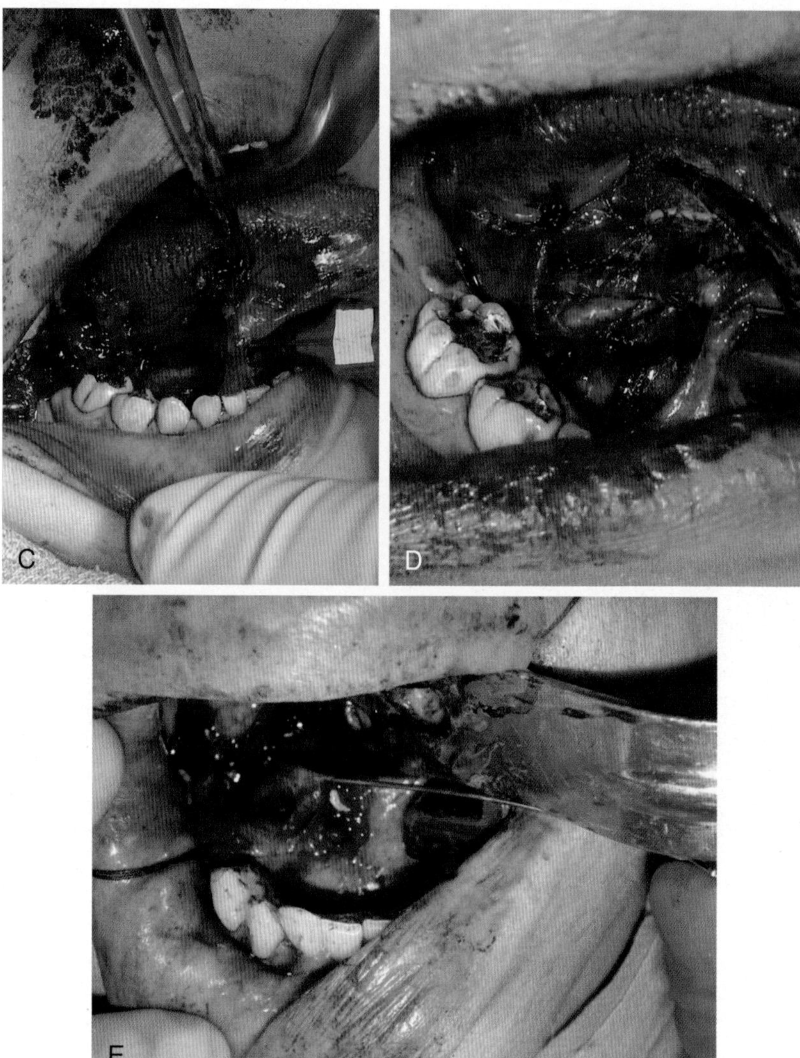

Figure 98.5, cont'd **C,** Medial dissection of the sublingual gland off the submandibular duct and lingual nerve. The sublingual gland can be seen posterior to the primary first molar. **D,** Use of a peanut sponge for blunt dissection, with the lingual nerve running underneath the submandibular duct. **E,** Overlying mucosa and submandibular duct incised over a lacrimal probe to expose a sialolith in the submandibular duct. A retraction suture in the mucosal flap also can be seen.

ALTERNATIVE TECHNIQUE 1: Lateral Approach to the Sublingual Gland

Galloway et al.[23] describe a lateral approach to the sublingual gland. An incision is made in the lingual gingival sulcus, starting in the first molar region and extending across the midline. A full-thickness mucoperiosteal flap is elevated off the medial surface of the mandible to the level of the floor of the mouth. The subperiosteal flap is retracted medially and posteriorly, and the sublingual gland can be seen bulging against the opposite side of the periosteum. An incision is made through the periosteum, and the sublingual gland is allowed to herniate through the incision. The gland then is separated and removed from the surrounding connective tissue with sharp and blunt dissection. Around the lingual nerve and submandibular duct, only blunt dissection is used. After adequate hemostasis has been achieved, the incision in the lingual gingival sulcus is closed (Fig. 98.6).

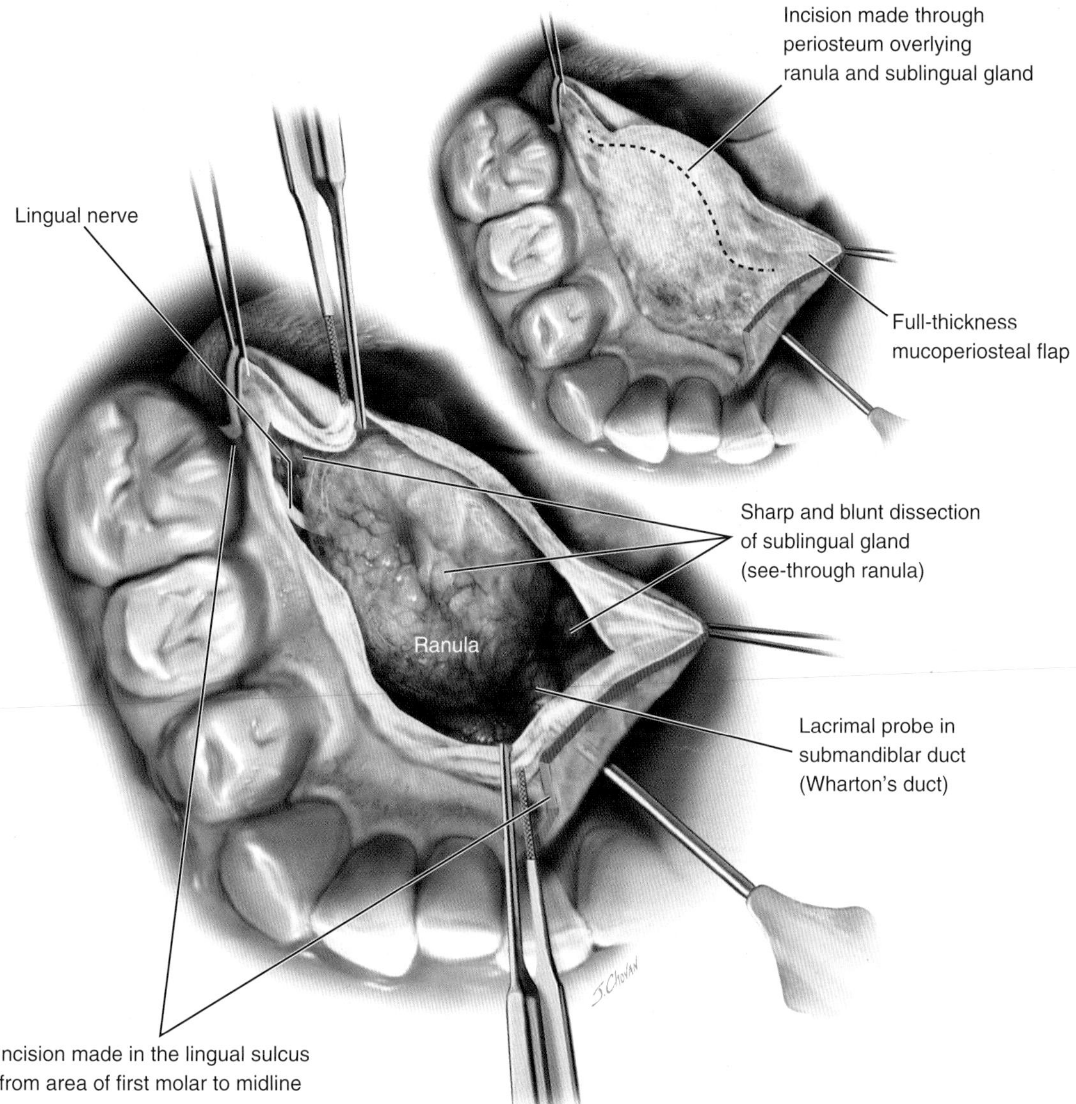

Figure 98.6 An alternate technique for removal of the sublingual gland using a lateral approach through the lingual periosteum of the mandible.

ALTERNATIVE TECHNIQUE 2: Sialodochoplasty

Obstruction of the submandibular duct usually is due to sialolithiasis or stricture. If the obstruction is anterior to the first and second molar region or the posterior edge of the mylohyoid muscle, it often can be treated with a sialodochoplasty via an intraoral approach. If the obstruction is at the posterior edge of the mylohyoid muscle, it is best treated by excision of the submandibular gland. The position of the sialolith or stricture is noted on imaging. If the sialodochoplasty is performed for a sialolith, a suture is thrown around the submandibular duct posterior to the sialolith and used as a traction suture to occlude the duct and prevent the sialolith from being displaced posteriorly. Next, the duct is cannulated with lacrimal probes, proceeding from smaller to larger and stopping in the region of the stone or stricture. The probe is then used to tent up the duct and its overlying mucosa. A #15 blade is used to incise longitudinally over the stone and the lacrimal probe to open the duct. If the duct needs to be opened more posteriorly, the lacrimal probe sometimes can be depressed and the tip of a fine scissors can be introduced into the duct lumen and used to extend the opening farther down the duct. After the duct has been opened, the sialolith can be milked forward and expressed. Afterward, the duct is irrigated to remove microliths, and the edges of the duct wall are sutured to the mucosa of the floor of mouth.

ALTERNATIVE TECHNIQUE 3: Repositioning/Transposition of the Submandibular Duct

Chronic excessive drooling/sialorrhea leads to maceration of the chin and neck, can lead to fluid depletion requiring parenteral replacement, and increases the risk of aspiration pneumonia. It is seen in patients with neurologic injury, cerebral palsy, myasthenia gravis, muscular dystrophy, mental retardation, and other conditions that result in poor neuromuscular coordination. These disorders cause incoordination of the oral phase of swallowing, resulting in pooling of saliva in the anterior mouth and subsequent spillage.[10–12] Sialorrhea usually is not caused by increased production of saliva. Repositioning/transposition of the submandibular duct has been shown to be an effective treatment for sialorrhea and is often accompanied by sublingual gland excision.[10,11,21] It is also performed if a portion of the submandibular duct has been resected or transected or damaged.

For drooling, repositioning of the submandibular duct is performed by using a #11 blade or a pair of fine sharp scissors to circumscribe and harvest a cuff of mucosa around the submandibular papilla. A submucosal tract or tunnel is then formed by blind dissection under the mucosa to a point behind the palatoglossal fold, and an incision is made through the mucosa at this point. The papilla with a small cuff of mucosa is then lifted in continuity with the duct, and a Gerald forceps or skin hook is used to gently grab the cuff of mucosa around the papilla and apply anterior traction on the duct as it is dissected circumferentially under the mucosa with a tenotomy scissors or mosquito forceps. A 4-0 or 5-0 Vicryl suture can then be passed through the mucosal cuff around the papilla and is used to help pull the papilla and duct submucosally through the tunnel and out the incision made behind the palatoglossal fold, using a mosquito forceps to pass the suture through the tunnel and out the incision at the palatoglossal fold. Care should be taken not to twist the duct as it is pulled through. Some surgeons pass a few sutures through the cuff of mucosa, leave the needles on, and pass the papilla and duct with the sutures and needles so that they can be used to suture the mucosal cuff to the mucosal opening behind the palatoglossal fold. The author prefers just to use a suture without a needle to pass the papilla and duct, and then to suture the cuff of mucosa around the papilla to the mucosal opening behind the palatoglossal fold with new sutures. If transposition of the submandibular duct is performed simultaneously with sublingual gland excision, a tunnel is not needed, and the transposition can be performed through the same incision as the sublingual gland excision. If a portion of the submandibular duct is resected or if the duct is damaged or transected, the proximal portion of the duct can be repositioned posteriorly to avoid tension and sutured to a hole in the floor of the mouth. If there is enough duct length remaining, the author prefers to incise the end of the remaining proximal duct and suture the edges of the duct to the mucosal hole in the same fashion as a sialodochoplasty. Reanastomosis of the proximal and distal duct ends after a transection is not recommended, because the circumferential suture line leads to stricture.

Additional Alternative Techniques

Many alternative techniques have been published in the literature. McGurk et al.[24] described a technique in which the oral ranula is approached through a longitudinal incision, dissected free from adjacent tissues, and then aspirated, allowing better identification of that portion of the sublingual gland to which the ranula is attached. The ranula and the portion of the sublingual gland to which it is attached are then excised using cutting diathermy. Baurmash[14,25,26] as mentioned previously, argued against blanket removal of the sublingual gland and provided examples of floor of the mouth lesions less than 1.5 cm that can be treated with a simple unroofing procedure with or without a sialodochoplasty. His examples included: (1) a mucocele of the incisal gland, which is treated with unroofing and removal of all glandular tissue, with or without peripheral margin suturing; (2) a retention cyst of the Wharton duct, which is treated with unroofing and sialodochoplasty; (3) a submandibular duct injury with salivary fluid leakage, which is treated with removal of the overlying mucosa, identification of the damaged area of the duct, and a sialodochoplasty posterior to the area of damage; and (4) a retention cyst of the sublingual gland, which is treated with simple unroofing. Baurmash also described a superficial dissecting ranula that crosses the midline and clinically appears bilaterally, which he marsupializes and explores to determine from which sublingual gland it arose. He then packs it with a positive pressure gauze packing. He does this for lesions greater than 1.5 cm, because these lesions are from the body of the sublingual gland and are pseudocysts from mucus extravasation. Baurmash recommends unroofing the pseudocyst, allowing complete evacuation of the mucus, and insertion of positive pressure gauze packing into the cavity for 7 to 10 days; this initially seals the leak and evokes an inflammatory response to initiate sufficient fibrosis to permanently seal the leak, leading to acinar atrophy and healing. He also reports having used this technique to successfully manage a plunging ranula.

Other techniques that have been reported to evoke an inflammatory response leading to fibrosis, or that promote fibrosis alone include the use of OK-432, a sclerosing agent (a lyophilized streptococcal preparation contraindicated in patients allergic to penicillin), carbon dioxide laser, ER,CR:YSGG laser, and cryotherapy.[2,27] Micromarsupialization of oral ranulas by seton, in which sutures are inserted into the roof of the ranula, has been used to theoretically allow mucosal epithelium to grow along the sutures into the ranula. This establishes epithelium-lined tracts and allows the flow of saliva from the ranula to persist,

Continued

ALTERNATIVE TECHNIQUE 3: Repositioning/Transposition of the Submandibular Duct—*cont'd*

relieving pressure on the wall of the pseudocyst. As a result, the walls of granulation tissue collapse and reduce the lumen until the epithelially lined tracts fuse with the torn glandular end of a duct of Rivinus to create a regenerated duct.[2]

Injection of botulinum toxin into the ranula and sublingual gland has been used to inhibit parasympathetic secretory stimulation, which shifts the balance away from secretory activity toward the opposing effects of macrophages, which absorb mucus, and the extensive connective tissue response leading to fibrosis.[2]

Transoral robotic surgery (TORS) is becoming more widely used for the treatment of oncologic disease of the tonsil and base of tongue, and for surgical treatment of tumors of the oropharynx, hypopharynx, larynx, and parapharyngeal spaces. TORS is also being used in the surgical treatment of obstructive sleep apnea. Advantages of robotic surgery utilizing a video-endoscope includes improved visualization with an illuminated high-resolution, magnified, three-dimensional view of the surgical field, direct line of sight, hand tremor elimination with similar or improved surgical dexterity, and improved ergonomics for the surgeon. The first robotic-assisted transoral removal of bilateral floor of the mouth ranulas and sublingual glands was described in 2011 by Walvekar et al.[28] Since then, TORS with and without sialendoscopy has been increasingly utilized for the treatment of floor of the mouth ranulas and plunging ranulas with sublingual gland excision, for the treatment of salivary stones, and for the treatment of minor salivary gland tumors.[29–32] Sialendoscopy through the submandibular papilla is used with TORS to help better visualize and localize the sublingual duct of Bartholin, the submandibular duct, stenosis/obstructions, and salivary calculi. After TORS sublingual gland excision and after TORS salivary calculi removal, sialendoscopy is also used to look for residual calculi or obstructions, and to visualize ligation of the sublingual duct of Bartholin and repairs of the submandibular duct if done. Extraoral and transoral submandibular gland excision using the robot has also been reported.[31,32]

Avoidance and Management of Intraoperative Complications

The most common intraoperative complications of sublingual gland excision are lingual nerve injury and submandibular duct injury. The surgeon can best prevent these complications by having a thorough understanding of the anatomy, achieving adequate retraction and hemostasis during surgery (thus improving visualization), using a lacrimal probe when possible to help identify the submandibular duct during surgery, and performing careful dissection. If transection of the lingual nerve is observed, immediate nerve repair should be performed. If the submandibular duct is transected or damaged, the proximal portion of the submandibular duct should be repositioned, with or without a sialodochoplasty, as described previously. If the remaining proximal portion of the submandibular duct is too short to be repositioned, the duct should be ligated. Subsequent symptoms are minimal and subside with atrophy of the submandibular gland. In their review of 571 patients treated for ranulas, Zhao et al.[33] found the complication of lingual nerve deficit in 4.89% of the patients and submandibular duct damage in 1.82% of the patients.[33] In their review, numbness of the tongue resulting from lingual nerve damage was more common after excision of both the sublingual gland and the ranula than after excision of the sublingual gland alone. Fortunately, all the patients who had numbness of the tongue regained sensation within 6 months of sublingual gland excision.

Postoperative Considerations and Complications

Overnight observation generally is not required. The patient is placed on a liquid diet for a few days, then advanced to a soft diet, and then to a regular diet as tolerated. The patient is given a prescription for pain medication and a short course of antibiotics. Recurrence of a ranula is the most common postoperative complication and is due to either conservative treatment that did not initially require removal of the sublingual gland or to sublingual gland tissue that was left behind. Both of these complications are treated by removing the remaining sublingual gland. In a review of 580 treated ranulas, Zhao et al.[34] reported a 66.75% recurrence rate after marsupialization alone, a 57.69% recurrence rate after excision of the ranula alone, and a 1.2% recurrence rate after excision of the sublingual gland alone or of the gland and the ranula.[34] A floor of the mouth hematoma, which may lead to airway obstruction in severe cases, can result if meticulous hemostasis is not achieved before closure. This complication is managed by securing the airway, evacuating the hematoma, and identifying and stopping any sources of bleeding. Zhao et al. have also reported postoperative infections managed by incision and drainage and administration of antibiotics.[33]

References

1. Black RJ, Croft CB. Ranula: pathogenesis and management. *Clin Otolaryngol Allied Sci*. 1982;7(5):299–303.
2. Harrison JD. Modern management and pathophysiology of ranula: literature review. *Head Neck*. 2010;32(10):1310–1320.
3. Catone GA, Merrill RG, Henny FA. Sublingual gland mucus-escape phenomenon—treatment by excision of sublingual gland. *J Oral Surg*. 1969;27(10):774–786.
4. Roediger WE, Lloyd P, Lawson HH. Mucous extravasation theory as a cause of plunging ranulas. *Br J Surg*. 1973;60(9):720–722.
5. Quick CA, Lowell SH. Ranula and the sublingual salivary glands. *Arch Otolaryngol*. 1977;103(7):397–400.
6. van den Akker HP, Bays RA, Becker AE. Plunging or cervical ranula. Review of the literature and report of 4 cases. *J Maxillofac Surg*. 1978;6(4):286–293.
7. Flaitz CM. Chronic sclerosing sialadenitis of the sublingual gland. *Am J Dent*. 2001;14(5):335–336.
8. Hong KH, Yang YS. Sialolithiasis in the sublingual gland. *J Laryngol Otol*. 2003;117(11):905–907.
9. Okura M, Hiranuma T, Shirasuna K, Matsuya T. Pleomorphic adenoma of the sublingual gland: report of a case. *J Oral Maxillofac Surg*. 1996;54(3):363–366.
10. Lal D, Hotaling AJ. Drooling. *Curr Opin Otolaryngol Head Neck Surg*. 2006;14(6):381–386.
11. McGurk M. The surgical management of salivary gland disease of the sublingual gland and floor of mouth. *Atlas Oral Maxillofac Surg Clin North Am*. 1998;6(1):51–74.
12. Ethunandan M, Macpherson DW. Persistent drooling: treatment by bilateral submandibular duct transposition and simultaneous sublingual gland excision. *Ann R Coll Surg Engl*. 1998;80(4):279–282.
13. Domaneschi C, Maurício AR, Modolo F, Migliari DA. Idiopathic hyperplasia of the sublingual glands in totally or partially edentulous individuals. *Oral Surg Oral Med Oral Pathol Oral Radiol Endod*. 2007;103(3):374–377.
14. Baurmash HD. Marsupialization for treatment of oral ranula: a second look at the procedure. *J Oral Maxillofac Surg*. 1992;50(12):1274–1279.
15. Steelman R, Weisse M, Ramadan H. Congenital ranula. *Clin Pediatr (Phila)*. 1998;37(3):205–206.
16. Cavalcante AS, Rosa LE, Costa NC, Hatakeyama M, Anbinder AL. Congenital ranula: a case report. *J Dent Child (Chic)*. 2009;76(1):78–81.
17. Akyol MU, Orhan D. Lingual tumors in infants: a case report and review of the literature. *Int J Pediatr Otorhinolaryngol*. 2004;68(1):111–115.
18. Syebele K. Regression of both oral mucocele and parotid swellings, following antiretroviral therapy. *Int J Pediatr Otorhinolaryngol*. 2010;74(1):89–92.
19. Syebele K, Bütow KW. Comparative study of the effect of antiretroviral therapy on benign lymphoepithelial cyst of parotid glands and ranulas in HIV-positive patients. *Oral Surg Oral Med Oral Pathol Oral Radiol Endod*. 2011;111(2):205–210.
20. Yates C. A surgical approach to the sublingual salivary gland. *Ann R Coll Surg Engl*. 1994;76(2):108–109.
21. Nadershah M, Salama A. Removal of parotid, submandibular, and sublingual glands. *Oral Maxillofac Surg Clin North Am*. 2012;24(2):295–305.
22. Takimoto T, Ishikawa S, Nishimura T, et al. Fibrin glue in the surgical treatment of ranulas. *Clin Otolaryngol Allied Sci*. 1989;14(5):429–431.
23. Galloway RH, Gross PD, Thompson SH, Patterson AL. Pathogenesis and treatment of ranula: report of three cases. *J Oral Maxillofac Surg*. 1989;47(3):299–302.
24. McGurk M, Eyeson J, Thomas B, Harrison JD. Conservative treatment of oral ranula by excision with minimal excision of the sublingual gland: histological support for a traumatic etiology. *J Oral Maxillofac Surg*. 2008;66(10):2050–2057.
25. Baurmash HD. Mucoceles and ranulas. *J Oral Maxillofac Surg*. 2003;61(3):369–378.
26. Baurmash HD. Treating oral ranula: another case against blanket removal of the sublingual gland. *Br J Oral Maxillofac Surg*. 2001;39(3):217–220.
27. Bodner L, Tal H. Salivary gland cysts of the oral cavity: clinical observation and surgical management. *Compendium*. 1991;12(3):150, 152, 154-156.
28. Walvekar RR, Peters G, Hardy E, et al. Robotic-assisted transoral removal of a bilateral floor of mouth ranulas. *World J Surg Oncol*. 2011;9:78.
29. Carey RM, Hodnett BL, Rassekh CH, Weinstein GS. Transoral robotic surgery with sialendoscopy for a plunging ranula. *ORL J Otorhinolaryngol Relat Spec*. 2017;79(6):306–313.
30. Capaccio P, Montevecchi F, Meccariello G, et al. Transoral robotic surgery for hilo-parenchymal submandibular stones: step-by-step description and reasoned approach. *Int J Oral Maxillofac Implants*. 2019;48(12):1520–1524.
31. Kane A, et al. Robotic surgery for salivary gland disease. *Curr Otorhinolaryngol Rep*. 2014;2:97.
32. Marzouk MF. Robot-assisted glandular surgery. *Atlas Oral Maxillofac Surg Clin North Am*. 2018;26(2):153–157.
33. Zhao YF, Jia J, Jia Y. Complications associated with surgical management of ranulas. *J Oral Maxillofac Surg*. 2005;63(1):51–54.
34. Zhao YF, Jia Y, Chen XM, Zhang WF. Clinical review of 580 ranulas. *Oral Surg Oral Med Oral Pathol Oral Radiol Endod*. 2004;98(3):281–287.

Submandibular Gland Excision

Eric R. Carlson and Andrew W. C. Lee

Armamentarium

#15 Bard Parker scalpel blade
2-0 Silk suture
3-0 Vicryl suture
5-0 Nylon suture
5-0 Vicryl suture
Electrocautery unit
Fine curved hemostats
Gerald forceps
Mayo scissors
Metzenbaum scissors
Penrose drain
Skin hooks

History of the Procedure

The history of submandibular gland excision demonstrates two chronologic reflections and scientific reporting. First reflection literature (1950s to 1970s) provided general comments related to submandibular gland tumors and nonneoplastic processes, and second reflection literature (1980s to present) reviewed morbidity associated with excision of the submandibular gland. A description of pathologic processes of the major salivary glands was initially provided by McFarland in 1926 and later by the same author in 1933.[1] This author's observations and reflections focused exclusively on parotid gland neoplasms due to their much higher incidence with no mention of the very rare submandibular gland tumors. In these two initial reports, 135 tumors of the parotid gland formed the basis for comments on the outcomes of surgical and nonsurgical therapy as a function of the size of the parotid tumor. The specific microscopic diagnosis was not discussed by the author in his review of these cases. Rather, McFarland described the outcomes of tumors smaller than a walnut (a bean, hazel nut, grape, marble, or almond), those of ordinary size between a walnut and a lemon (walnut, plum, egg, Seckel pear, or lemon), and tumors larger than a lemon (apple, goose egg, orange, grapefruit, two fists, or a human head). Moreover, the author did not comment on the techniques of surgical treatment for the tumors of the parotid gland. Finally, McFarland indicated that it was not advisable to operate on small parotid tumors and that the complications of facial nerve palsy, salivary fistula, and recurrence should be carefully considered for fear that more harm than good could occur.

In 1936 McFarland reported on 301 tumors of the major salivary glands, including 278 parotid gland tumors, 22 submandibular gland tumors, and one sublingual gland tumor.[2] This paper represents the first discussion of submandibular gland tumors. As in the author's 1933 publication, no specific comments were made regarding surgical technique, including those for the 22 submandibular gland tumors in the report. Nonetheless, the author indicated that 8 of the 22 submandibular gland tumors recurred.[2] It was not until the 1953 review by Foote and Frazell that a specific assessment of the histologic diagnosis of major salivary gland tumors was presented in the international scientific literature.[3] Eight hundred seventy-seven major salivary gland tumors were analyzed, of which 107 were in the submandibular gland. These included 47 benign mixed tumors, 11 malignant mixed tumors, 17 adenoid cystic carcinomas, and 8 mucoepidermoid carcinomas, among others. In fact, this paper served as a clinicopathologic review of tumors of the major salivary glands, again without specific mention of the technical aspects of the surgery performed for the removal of these tumors.

It was not until 1966 that Work introduced comments regarding the surgical excision of major salivary glands associated with benign and malignant neoplastic diagnoses.[4] In the case of parotid tumors, the author advised against enucleation procedures and reported that parotidectomy was infrequently combined with elective prophylactic neck dissection in cases of primary parotid malignant disease. Nonetheless, he astutely recommended prophylactic neck dissection in the case of a primary submandibular gland malignancy. In 1966 Work and Gates reviewed treatment of nonneoplastic diseases of the major salivary glands.[5] Transcutaneous excision of the submandibular gland was recommended in the case of a sialolith located within or near to the submandibular gland. In addition, the authors recommended submandibular gland excision in the case of severe injury to the gland and duct.

In 1967, Work recapitulated comments regarding surgery for neoplastic and nonneoplastic disorders of the major salivary glands.[6] A facial nerve preserving parotidectomy was recommended in the case of neoplastic disease of the parotid gland. An excision of the tumor and gland was recommended when encountering neoplastic disease of the submandibular gland. Also in 1967, the largest series of submandibular gland tumors was published by Eneroth and Hjertman who reviewed 187 cases of tumors of the submandibular gland, of which 125 were benign and 62 were malignant.[7] Of the benign tumors, 95 were diagnosed as mixed tumors. Treatment for these benign mixed tumors consisted of excision of the tumor in 50 cases, and evacuation of the submandibular region in 45 cases including 4 of which underwent radical neck dissection. Forty-one of these 95 patients also underwent preoperative or postoperative radiation therapy. Five of these patients accounted for 18 recurrences related to surgery/radiation therapy for these benign mixed tumors. In 1968 Seward published three papers on the topic of anatomic surgery for nonneoplastic processes of the major salivary glands. These included salivary calculi that addressed the symptoms, signs, and differential diagnosis[8]; calculi in the anterior part of the submandibular duct[9]; and calculi in the posterior part of the submandibular duct.[10] These papers emphasized surgical principles, specifically related to the salivary ducts rather than to the surgical excision of the submandibular gland. Finally, Rafla[11] reported on 35 submandibular gland tumors in 1970. This report commented on 13 benign tumors and 22 malignant tumors, of which 3 were metastatic tumors. Enucleation of benign submandibular gland tumors was performed in three cases, and the author was not critical of this technique.

Second reflection literature related to the submandibular gland pathology first appeared in the 1980s and has largely centered on clinical outcomes associated with submandibular gland excision.[12–17] Complications specifically related to the submandibular gland excision for benign disease are discussed in the avoidance and management of intraoperative complications section of this chapter.

Indications for the Use of the Procedure

Sialolithiasis of the Submandibular Gland

Submandibular sialolithiasis is a common diagnosis with post-mortem studies suggesting the prevalence of salivary calculi between 1% and 2%.[18] Sialolithiasis is the most common cause of salivary gland obstruction and occurs primarily in the submandibular gland (80% to 90%), with only 5% to 10% of sialoliths occurring in the parotid gland.[18,19] Submandibular sialolithiasis represents more than 50% of major salivary gland diseases and is the most common cause of acute and chronic salivary gland infections.[20] Some authors consider sialolithiasis to be a consequence as well as a cause of sialadenitis.[21] For example, the presence of a sialolith may result in the obstruction of salivary flow, thereby predisposing the submandibular gland to retrograde infection. In addition, the presence of sialadenitis may change the characteristics of the saliva, thereby favoring the deposition of calcium with the development of a sialolith. A series of 245 patients with sialolithiasis showed that 94.3% of stones were present in the submandibular gland system with the remaining stones located primarily in the parotid gland. A discussion of sialolithiasis, therefore, centers nearly exclusively on the submandibular gland. Distribution between right and left submandibular gland stones was nearly equal, and only about 1% of submandibular stones were present bilaterally.[22] Swelling was present in 94% of patients, pain in 65.2%, pus secretion in 15.5%, and fever in 6%, and 2.4% of patients in this series were asymptomatic.[22] Radiographically, approximately 80% of submandibular sialoliths are radiopaque, compared with 60% of parotid sialoliths that are radiopaque.[23] Most submandibular sialoliths are single in nature compared to parotid sialoliths, which more commonly occur as multiple stones.

Pathophysiologically, it has been suggested that the bend or genu in the submandibular duct may be an etiological factor in the formation of salivary stones since this bend may encourage stagnation of saliva. The submandibular duct emerges from the superficial aspect of the gland and passes over the free posterior margin of the mylohyoid muscle. It courses forward and slightly superiorly on the mylohyoid muscle before opening at the sublingual papilla. Drage et al.[24] investigated the genu of the submandibular duct in terms of whether its angle was of significance in the development of submandibular sialadenitis and sialolithiasis. One hundred and two sialograms were analyzed from three groups of patients including 18 normal patients, 61 patients with salivary calculi, and 23 patients with sialadenitis. Their study concluded that there is a wide variation in the angle of the genu of the submandibular duct in the sagittal plane in normal glands and in disease that does not appear to be associated with either sialadenitis or sialolithiasis. The length of the submandibular duct, the dependent anatomic position of the submandibular gland, and the alkaline nature of saliva along with its relatively high viscosity and high content of calcium salts probably account for the higher incidence of sialolithiasis of the submandibular gland compared with the other salivary glands.[25] The components of salivary stones were once believed to include desquamated epithelial cells, foreign bodies, mucous plugs, and microorganisms.[25,26] In 2004 Kasaboglu et al.[27] studied the chemical composition and micromorphology of sialoliths using X-ray diffraction analysis and scanning electron microscopy. In six examples of sialoliths, only hydroxyapatite crystals were identified, with no signs of foreign bodies or microorganisms identified at the core of the sialolith.

The involvement of a biofilm in the pathophysiology of sialolithiasis remains very controversial. Kao et al.[28] evaluated five salivary stones retrieved by sialoendoscopy with the hypothesis that bacteria form a core biofilm around which layers of calcium phosphate and hydroxyapatite are deposited. They proposed that biofilm formation within a single salivary gland or duct promotes local ductal injury. The biofilm induced ductal injury results in the activation of the host immune response that interacts with the biofilm and calcium nanoparticles, thereby creating a scaffold upon which further calcium deposition occurs. The development of infection of salivary stones related to biofilm formation has been studied by Perez-Tanoira et al.[29] These authors prospectively studied 55 salivary stones and assessed for biofilm formation using fluorescence microscopy and sonication. Biofilm formation was confirmed on the surface of 39 (71%) stones. A total of 96 microorganisms were isolated from 45 (81.8%) salivary stones. Two or more organisms were isolated in 33 (73.3%) cases. The primary isolates were *Streptococcus mitis/oralis* (*n* = 27; 28.1%), *Streptococcus anginosus* (*n* = 10; 9.6%), *Rothia* species (*n* = 8; 8.3%), *Streptococcus constellatus* (*n* = 7; 7.3%), and *Streptococcus gordonii* (*n* = 6; 6.2%). All patients who demonstrated the presence of a biofilm showed preoperative (12 cases) or perioperative (3 cases) drainage of pus. The authors concluded their study by stating that bacterial biofilm was related to more severe cases of sialadenitis.

The association of sialolithiasis and systemic lithiasis has been studied extensively. Patients with nephrolithiasis and sialolithiasis are not routinely examined for stones in other organs. Due to the composition of salivary and kidney stones being primarily calcium carbonates and calcium phosphates, intuition suggests there could be concordance in patients with both kidney and salivary stones. Choi et al.[30] studied nephrolithiasis as a risk factor for sialolithiasis by using data from the national cohort study from the Korean Health Insurance Review and Assessment Service. In doing so they selected 24,038 patients with nephrolithiasis and a control group of 96,152 patients without nephrolithiasis. The incidence of sialolithiasis in the two groups was compared over a 12-year follow-up period. The overall incidence of sialolithiasis among the nephrolithiasis patients was 0.08% (19/24,038) and 0.1% (92/96,152) in the control group. The adjusted hazard ratios (HR) of nephrolithiasis for sialolithiasis were not statistically significant. The adjusted HR of nephrolithiasis for sialolithiasis was 0.81. This study found no evidence that nephrolithiasis is associated with an increased risk of sialolithiasis after adjusting for age, gender, income, region of residence, hypertension, diabetes, and dyslipidemia.

Kim et al.[31] evaluated the association between cholelithiasis and sialolithiasis using a national sample cohort of the Korean population and two study designs. In their first study, the authors examined 21,170 cholelithiasis patients and 84,680 control patients without cholelithiasis and measured the occurrence of sialolithiasis. In their second study, 761 sialolithiasis patients were matched with 3044 control patients with sialolithiasis and the occurrence of cholelithiasis was measured. The HR for sialolithiasis was 1.49 (95% CI = 0.88 to 2.52) in the cholelithiasis group, and the HR for cholelithiasis was 1.18 (95% CI = 0.53 to 2.59) in the sialolithiasis group. These results are perhaps intuitive since the stone composition is very different between gallstones and salivary stones, and the risk factors for respective stone development are also different. The authors concluded that there is no association between sialolithiasis and cholelithiasis.

Stack and Norman[32] performed a retrospective analysis of 3000 primary hyperparathyroidism patients and identified 18 patients (0.6%) with documented sialolithiasis prior to parathyroid surgery. Sialolithiasis was the first presenting symptom in six patients that led to the diagnosis of primary hyperparathyroidism. The remaining 12 patients had kidney stones as their first presenting symptom (*n* = 5) or hypercalcemia (*n* = 7). Based on a reported incidence of sialolithiasis, of 0.45% in the United Kingdom, the authors interpreted their 0.6% incidence of sialolithiasis in their primary hyperparathyroidism cohort as significantly different and therefore relevant. Nonetheless, these authors are from the United States where the incidence of sialolithiasis is approximately 1% to 2%. It is unclear why the authors selected the incidence of sialolithiasis in the United Kingdom to compare their United States cohort of patients in whom sialolithiasis was diagnosed. The authors offered conclusions that parathyroid surgeons should be aware of the possible existence of sialolithiasis in their patients and salivary gland surgeons should be aware of the possible existence of primary hyperparathyroidism in their patients.

Kraaij et al.[33] performed a retrospective case-control study of 208 patients (112 males, 96 females) with salivary gland stones and a control group of 208 patients (112 males, 96 females). The submandibular gland was affected in 85.6% of patients, the parotid gland in 9.6%, and the sublingual gland in 2.4%. When evaluating for the presence of cholelithiasis, nephrolithiasis, and gout, no relationship was identified between sialolithiasis and the presence of systemic disease. Interestingly, there was a higher incidence of cholelithiasis in the control group than in the sialolithiasis group. The incidence of nephrolithiasis and gout was equal in both groups.

Regardless of the suspected etiology and the patient's medical comorbidity, the treatment of submandibular sialolithiasis is a function of the size and location of the sialolith. Transoral sialolithotomy is the preferred procedure for submandibular sialolithiasis when the sialolith is palpated on transoral examination.[34] This is particularly apparent since increasing evidence shows that the submandibular gland regains function after stone removal.[18] As such, submandibular gland excision is generally reserved for cases of submandibular sialolithiasis when the stone is noted radiographically to exist within the gland or its hilum where transoral retrieval of the stone is not possible. Preoperative imaging is therefore indicated to provide precise localization of the stone or stones (Fig. 99.1).

Sialadenitis of the Submandibular Gland

Sialadenitis, a generic term referring to salivary gland inflammation and infection, is a common affliction of the submandibular gland. Numerous etiologies exist for acute and chronic submandibular sialadenitis, including bacterial, viral, fungal, mycobacterial, parasitic, and immunologic causes. The diagnosis of sialadenitis is based on a thorough medical history, physical examination, and imaging studies. Numerous modifiable, nonmodifiable, or relatively nonmodifiable predisposing factors can result in sialadenitis.[35] Specifically, dehydration with or without recent surgery and anesthesia, the presence of a sialolith in the intraglandular or extraglandular ducts of the

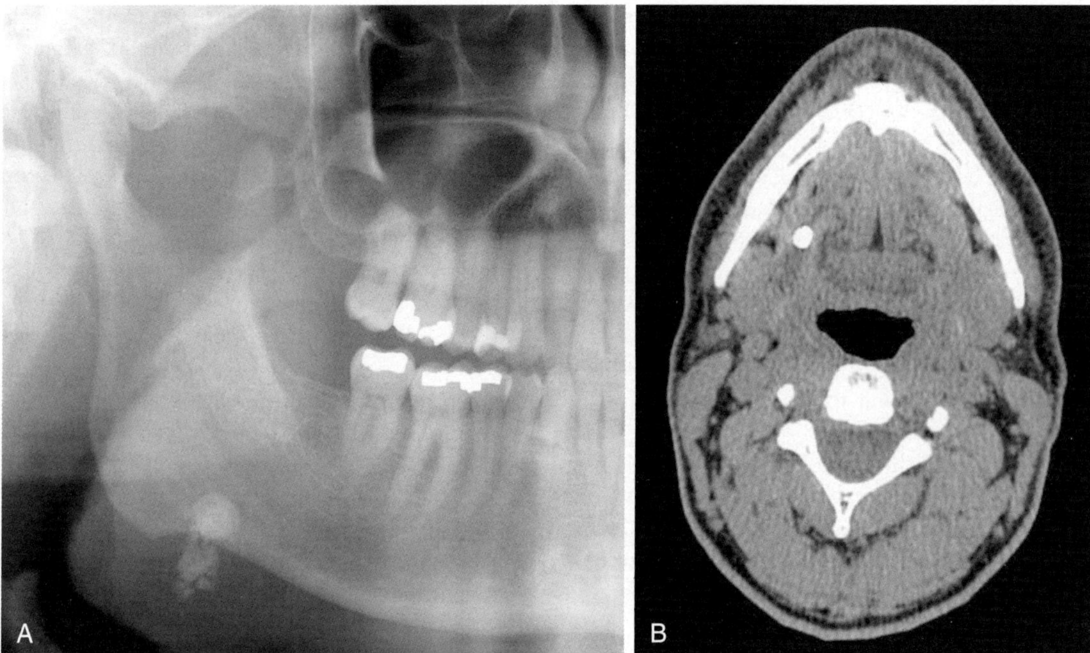

Figure 99.1 **A,** Panoramic radiograph that identifies several sialoliths within the right submandibular gland. The panoramic radiograph represents the minimum radiographic study to be obtained in all patients with a diagnosis of sialadenitis of the submandibular gland to rule out sialolithiasis as the cause of the sialadenitis. This patient underwent submandibular gland excision. **B,** This computed tomography (CT) scan identifies an extraglandular stone within the right Wharton duct. Ductal ectasia is noted proximal to the stone. This patient underwent submandibular gland excision with removal of the extraglandular stone.

submandibular gland, and medications with known anticholinergic properties are of significance in the development of submandibular sialadenitis.

Acute bacterial submandibular sialadenitis (ABSS) is a community-acquired disease most commonly diagnosed in association with a sialolith. The diagnosis of ABSS is less frequently associated with dehydration and an in-patient admission to the hospital than with acute bacterial parotitis. The history and clinical presentation of ABSS include submandibular swelling and pain that commonly occur related to eating. The presence of an enlarged submandibular gland should primarily suggest sialadenitis with a neoplasm ruled out as a remote, second diagnosis.[36] The presence of pus may be noted at the opening of the Wharton duct in the floor of mouth, under which circumstances the diagnosis of ABSS is made rapidly. The most common cause of ABSS is obstruction of the Wharton duct, typically from a sialolith, such that obtaining a panoramic radiograph is of paramount importance in the initial workup of a patient with a clinical diagnosis of submandibular sialadenitis. The use of computed tomography (CT) scans in patients with ABSS is indicated when complicated sialadenitis is diagnosed as noted by a febrile and toxic patient, when an abscess requiring drainage is suspected or when initial management does not resolve the infection (Fig. 99.2). The management of ABSS is initially medical, including the use of empiric antistaphylococcal/antistreptococcal antibiotics, hydration, massage of the affected submandibular gland, heat, and tart sour ball candies (sialogogues) to stimulate obstructed salivary flow. A sialolith located in the distal extraglandular duct should be promptly removed if possible when it is identified. More aggressive therapy is rarely required, and the compliant patient only rarely requires submandibular gland excision for a diagnosis of ABSS.

Chronic recurrent submandibular sialadenitis is usually the result of ineffective treatment of ABSS due to a noncompliant patient, the presence of a previously undiagnosed sialolith, or the presence of unrecognized or untreated chronic sialadenitis at the time of the initial evaluation of the patient. Chronic recurrent submandibular sialadenitis occurs more frequently than chronic bacterial parotitis. Under such circumstances, patients usually report symptoms of submandibular postprandial pain and swelling lasting longer than 1 month. Physical examination typically demonstrates an indurated gland that may be smaller than the unaffected contralateral submandibular gland due to scar contracture. Initial recommended medical management is like that for ABSS, but most patients with chronic sialadenitis ultimately require submandibular gland excision.

A firm swelling of the submandibular gland that is clinically diagnosed as sialadenitis may be indicative of chronic inflammation that should produce a differential diagnosis including a Kuttner tumor or IgG4-related disease. IgG4-related disease primarily affects middle-aged to elderly men and typically presents as single organ disease. A complete workup, however, commonly divulges widespread disease. IgG4-related disease can affect almost every organ but

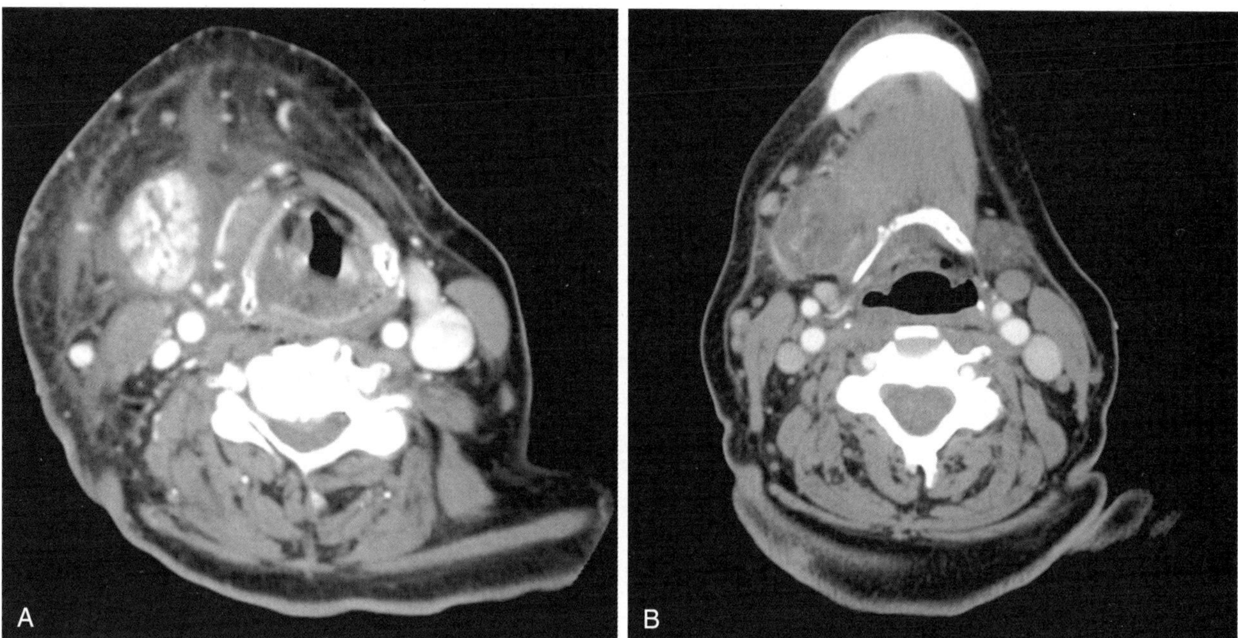

Figure 99.2 **A,** An axial computed tomography (CT) with intravenous contrast from a patient with right acute bacterial submandibular sialadenitis whose clinical presentation included significant swelling of the right neck. The CT scan demonstrates signs consistent with acute bacterial submandibular sialadenitis (ABSS), including fat stranding in the right neck, an enlarged right submandibular gland, and diffuse uptake of the intravenous contrast in the submandibular gland. This patient was admitted to the hospital for the administration of intravenous antibiotics. Incision and drainage were not required. The sialadenitis resolved without the need for submandibular gland excision. **B,** An axial CT scan image of ABSS with an abscess of the right submandibular gland. The right submandibular gland is significantly larger than the left gland. This patient required incision and drainage of the right submandibular gland. Subsequent excision of this submandibular gland was not required.

preferentially involves the pancreas and the salivary glands followed by the lacrimal glands, lymph nodes, biliary tract and gallbladder, retroperitoneum, thyroid gland, kidney, lung, periorbital tissues, aorta, and liver.[37]

Benign Tumor of the Submandibular Gland

Tumors of the submandibular gland are very rare, accounting for approximately 10% of all salivary gland tumors, whereas 80% of all salivary gland tumors occur in the parotid gland.[38] The fact that approximately 50% of submandibular gland tumors are benign translates to a paucity of available information regarding surgery and follow-up for benign submandibular gland tumors. Of the 13,749 primary epithelial salivary gland tumors reported by the Armed Forces Institute of Pathology in 1991, a total of 1235 (9%) submandibular tumors were identified, of which 725 (58.7%) were benign and 510 (41.3%) were malignant.[39] Of the 725 benign submandibular tumors, 657 (90.6%) were diagnosed as pleomorphic adenomas and 16 (2.2%) were diagnosed as Warthin tumors. Most experiences regarding benign submandibular gland tumors, therefore, are related to the pleomorphic adenoma. Two types of pleomorphic adenomas of the submandibular gland exist anatomically, including those frequently small tumors that are completely contained

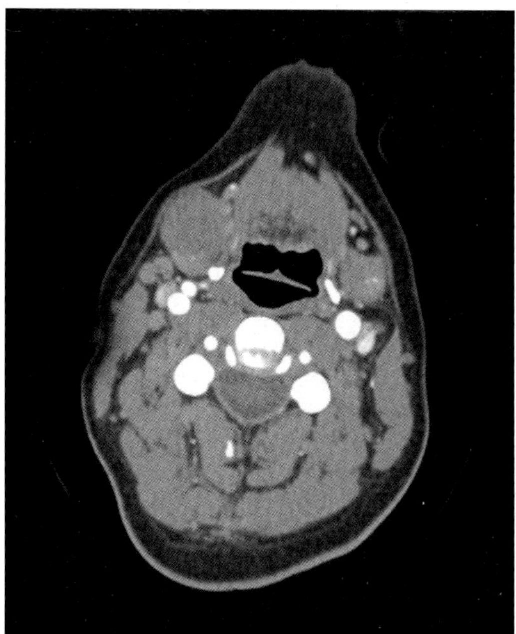

Figure 99.3 This large pleomorphic adenoma of the right submandibular gland has exited the parenchyma/capsule of the gland. As such, a meticulous dissection of the tumor's pseudocapsule was required during submandibular gland/tumor excision to ensure complete tumor removal with the avoidance of tumor spillage.

within the gland and those larger tumors that tend to extend beyond the gland capsule (Fig. 99.3). The former type of tumor is surgically approached in a manner identical to that for nonneoplastic submandibular gland lesions with a subfascial dissection. The pleomorphic adenoma that extends beyond the gland, however, requires a meticulous approach to the dissection of the pseudocapsule of the tumor, identical to extracapsular dissections of pleomorphic adenomas of the parotid gland.[40,41] In these cases, it is important to dissect the pseudocapsule of the tumor without inadvertently spilling the tumor that would predispose the patient to recurrence of the tumor. With careful surgical technique, excision of the submandibular gland and tumor results in a very low incidence of recurrence.[14] Preoperative fine-needle aspiration of a tumor of the submandibular gland is indicated to perform proper surgery for the tumor.[13] Specifically, benign cytologic findings will permit the surgeon to perform submandibular gland and tumor removal, while malignant cytologic findings will likely require the performance of a neck dissection, inclusive of the submandibular gland and tumor for proper management.

Penetrating Trauma of the Submandibular Gland

Injury to the submandibular gland is rare due to the protective nature of the mandible[42] (Fig. 99.4). This notwithstanding, when injuries do occur they may result in salivary extravasation into soft tissue or the development of a cutaneous salivary fistula. As such, complications of parenchymal submandibular gland injury typically involve these issues such that excision of the submandibular gland may be required. Removal of the submandibular gland is indicated if significant damage to the gland exists or if conservative therapy fails for salivary extravasation.[43]

Limitations and Contraindications

Excision of the acutely inflamed submandibular gland has historically been the subject of great controversy. Excision of the “hot” submandibular gland affected by acute sialadenitis or acute on chronic sialadenitis is relatively contraindicated for two reasons. The first reason is that most cases of ABSS are effectively managed with nonsurgical therapy as outlined previously. Acute sialadenitis of the submandibular gland can be resolved and reversed with maintenance of function of the gland. As such, excision of the gland in the acute setting is likely not necessary and therefore cannot be justified. The second reason for deferring excision of the “hot” submandibular gland is that the acute inflammatory response can complicate the dissection involved in the surgical procedure. The loss of surgical planes in the acutely inflamed submandibular region will increase the possibility of inadvertent injury to sensory and motor nerves in the surgical bed during the dissection. For these reasons, it is appropriate to defer excision of the submandibular gland that is acutely inflamed.

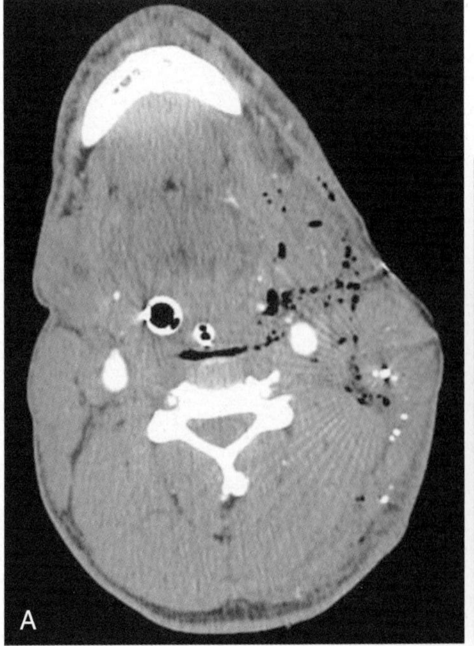

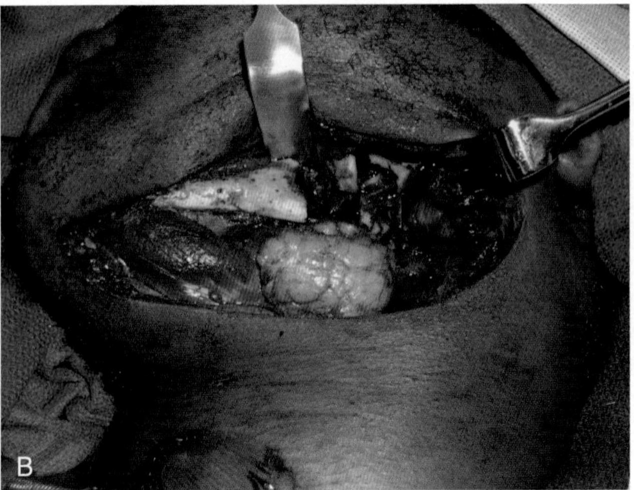

Figure 99.4 **A,** A gunshot to the left neck shows obvious trauma to the left submandibular region. **B,** The mandible received significant energy resulting in comminuted fracture from the gunshot wound, yet the submandibular gland was pristine upon exploration of the neck and repair of the hard- and soft-tissue injury.

TECHNIQUE: Submandibular Gland Excision for Sialolithiasis

STEP 1: Preoperative Imaging
The panoramic radiograph (Fig. 99.5A) serves the purpose of identifying a sialolith, while the CT scan (Fig. 99.5B) confirms the anatomic presence of a sialolith in the submandibular gland system that guides the surgery as well as providing an exact count in the case of a patient with multiple sialoliths. This count is essential to duplicate clinically at the time of excision of the gland and stone(s).

STEP 2: Intubation
Most patients undergoing submandibular gland excision for sialolithiasis confined to the gland and proximal duct can undergo orotracheal intubation. Under such circumstances the endotracheal tube is secured to the side of the face opposite the side of the planned neck incision. A nasoendotracheal intubation is preferred when sialoliths are located in the gland and distal duct requiring neck and oral dissection. Surgeon preference will dictate whether the operating room table is turned to isolate the side of the neck to be operated.

STEP 3: Incision
The skin incision for submandibular gland excision is centered over the submandibular gland and typically extends 2 to 3 cm anterior and posterior to the anatomic extent of the palpable gland and parallel to the inferior border of the mandible (Fig. 99.5C). This incision is commonly placed approximately two fingerbreadths below the inferior border of the mandible.

STEP 4: Dissection of the Musculature and Fascia of the Neck
Surgical excision of the submandibular gland involves surgical dissection of the platysma muscle and underlying investing layer of the deep cervical fascia (Fig. 99.5D). Most commonly, the muscle and fascia are divided with the electrocautery unit. The facial vein is isolated as it courses vertically in the neck within the investing layer of the deep cervical fascia. The vein is ligated, commonly with 2-0 silk suture. The dissection proceeds in a surgical plane deep to the ligated facial vein to avoid trauma to the marginal mandibular branch of the facial nerve that is predictably located superficial to the facial vein. The investing fascia is elevated off the submandibular gland's superficial, deep, anterior, and posterior surfaces and the dissection proceeds superiorly. Care is taken to avoid excessive superior retraction of soft tissues at the inferior border of the mandible to avoid trauma to the marginal mandibular branch of the facial nerve. The placement of a retraction suture in the submandibular gland permits its inferior retraction with resultant ease in the superior dissection at the inferior border of the mandible. The facial vein and artery are ligated with 2-0 silk suture as they enter the superior surface of the submandibular gland.

STEP 5: Separation of the Submandibular Gland From the Lingual Nerve
The mylohyoid muscle is retracted anteriorly, and the lingual nerve/submandibular ganglion are visualized (Fig. 99.5E). The submandibular ganglion and accompanying vein are ligated with 2-0 silk suture. The Wharton duct will be located inferior to the nerve as the duct exits the anterior aspect of the gland (Fig. 99.5F). The duct is ligated as far distally as possible without traumatizing the lingual nerve.

STEP 6: Delivery of the Submandibular Gland and Inspection of the Wound bed
The submandibular gland is delivered (Fig. 99.5G) following complete dissection of the investing fascia, ligation of the facial artery and vein, and ligation of the submandibular ganglion and duct. Thereafter, one should inspect the wound for verification of the integrity of ligated blood vessels (Fig. 99.5H). Often, the hypoglossal nerve is identified within the fascia medial to the mylohyoid muscle. The removal of the sialolith(s) is confirmed on inspection of the gland (Fig. 99.5I), which is very important when sialoliths in the extraglandular system are noted by CT scans and could be retained in the tissue bed if not properly accounted.

Continued

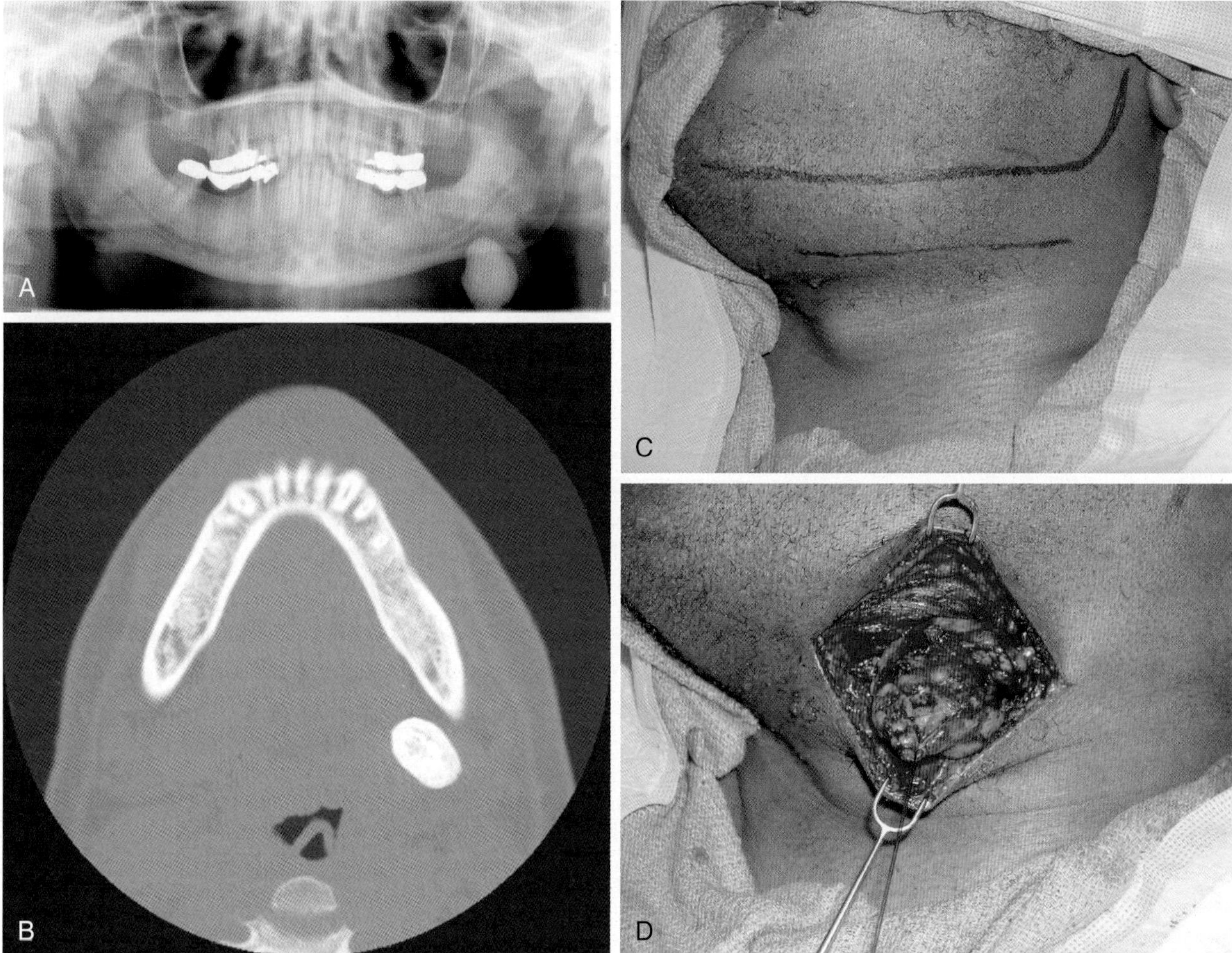

Figure 99.5 **A,** This panoramic radiograph identifies a sialolith likely located in the left submandibular gland. **B,** A review of computed tomography (CT) scans demonstrate that the submandibular sialolith in (A) is solitary and located in this patient's intraglandular duct. **C,** The incision measures approximately 6 to 8 cm in length and is centered over the palpable submandibular gland and parallel to the inferior border of the mandible. **D,** The soft-tissue dissection proceeds sharply through the skin, subcutaneous tissues, platysma muscle, and investing layer of the deep cervical fascia.

TECHNIQUE: Submandibular Gland Excision for Sialolithiasis—cont'd

STEP 7: Placement of a Drain

The removal of a submandibular gland inherently creates dead space within the neck, thereby requiring the placement of a drain. Two options exist for drain placement including a suction drain or a passive Penrose drain. If a Penrose drain is placed, a pressure dressing should be placed around the neck that also serves the purpose of collecting drainage from the drain. The removal of the submandibular gland for a diagnosis of sialolithiasis is a surgical procedure with little morbidity and predictable healing.

STEP 8: Transoral Removal of Distal Wharton Duct Stones if they are Present

It is important to identify the exact number of extraglandular stones by preoperative CT scans, with concordant intraoperative recovery during the surgical procedure. This is essential when multiple sialoliths are identified on preoperative CT scans. Therein, preoperative imaging of the patient with submandibular sialolithiasis serves not only to establish the precise location of the sialolith(s) but also serves to quantify the number of stones that must be accounted for at the time of surgery.

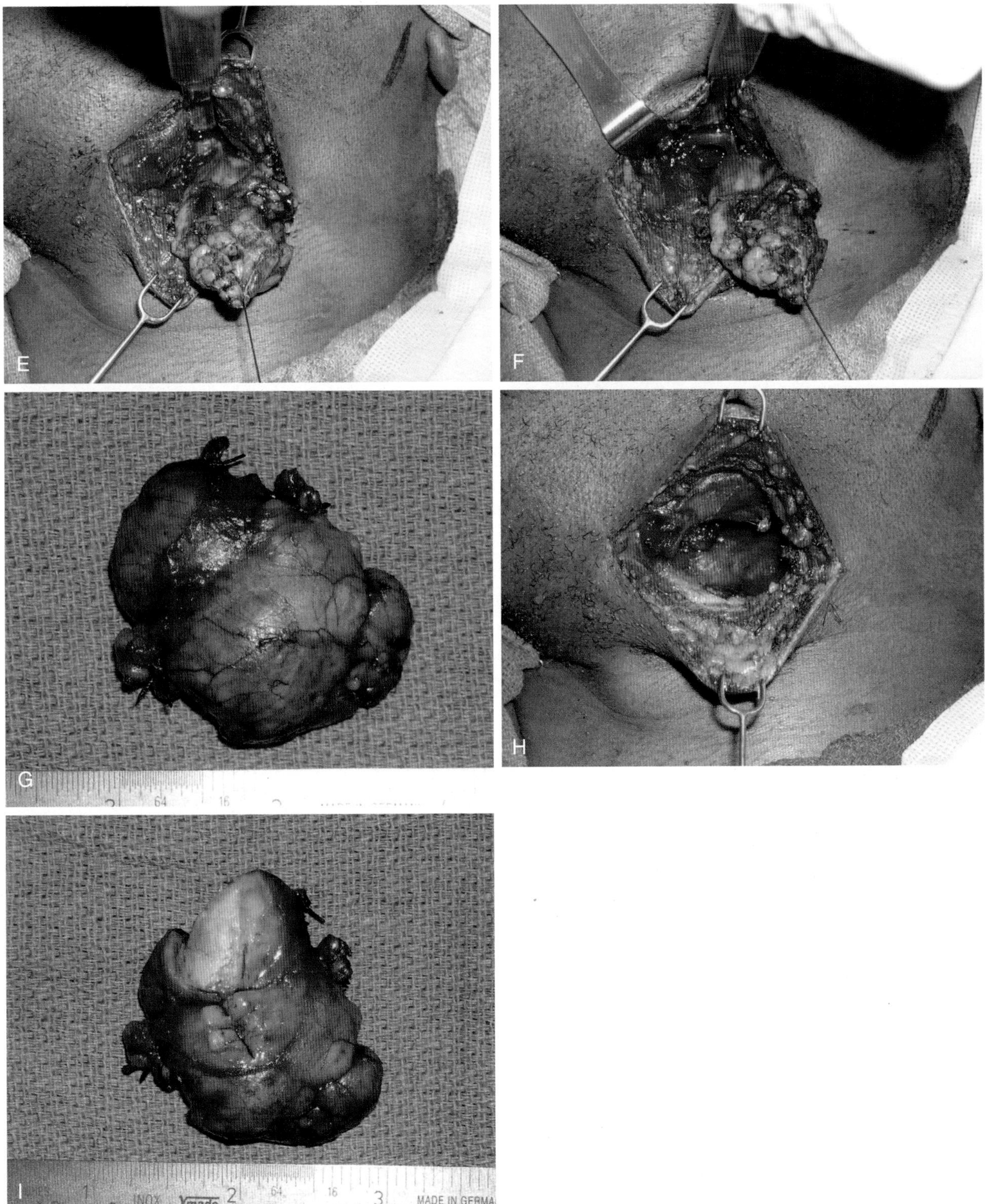

Figure 99.5,cont'd **E,** Continued superior dissection deep to the ligated facial vein permits anterior retraction of the mylohyoid muscle and initial identification of the lingual nerve. **F,** Additional dissection and inferior retraction of the gland permit full identification of the lingual nerve, the submandibular ganglion, and the inferiorly located Wharton duct. The submandibular ganglion and Wharton duct are ligated separately. **G,** The submandibular gland and intraglandular stone are delivered. **H,** The tissue bed is inspected for effective ligation of vessels. **I,** The large submandibular sialolith is exposed by incising the gland.

ALTERNATE OR MODIFIED TECHNIQUE # 1: Submandibular Gland Excision for Sialadenitis

The principles of excision of the submandibular gland for sialadenitis (Fig. 99.6) are nearly identical to those for a diagnosis of sialolithiasis. When chronic in nature, sialadenitis produces periglandular scarring that obscures the surgical planes between the submandibular gland, lingual nerve, and Wharton duct. Careful dissection is required to prevent injury to the lingual nerve under these circumstances.

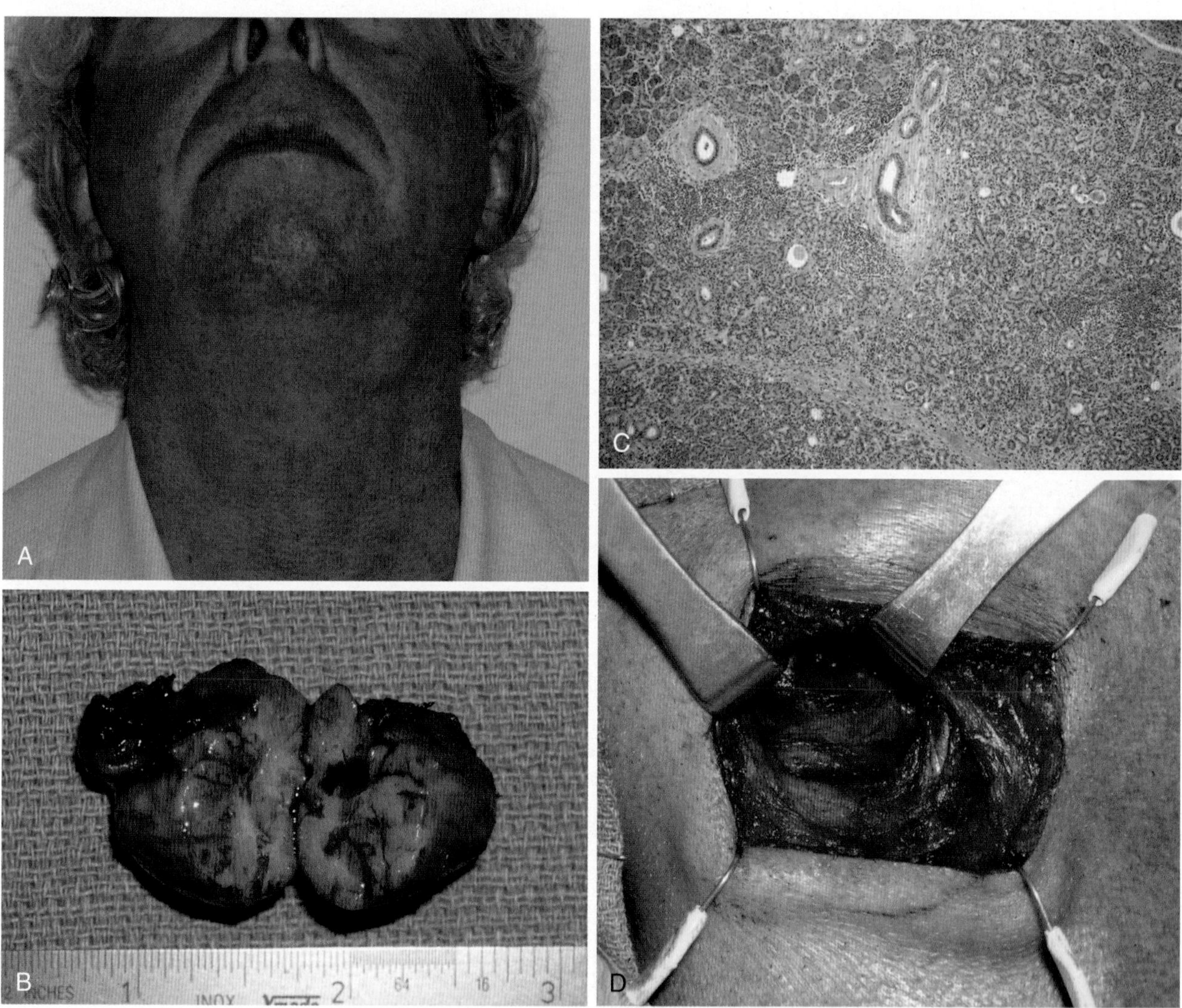

Figure 99.6 **A,** A patient with a visibly enlarged and palpably indurated left submandibular gland, who had been conservatively managed for acute sialadenitis for 12 months. A diagnosis of chronic sialadenitis was made, and he was advised to undergo submandibular gland excision. **B,** The bivalved submandibular gland specimen demonstrates scarred parenchyma of the gland, indicative of the chronic inflammatory state. **C,** The microscopic sections of the specimen identify a chronic sclerosing sialadenitis (hematoxylin and eosin, original magnification ×10). **D,** The remaining tissue bed will often permit visualization of the hypoglossal nerve.

ALTERNATE OR MODIFIED TECHNIQUE 2: Submandibular Gland Excision for Benign Tumor

The excision of a benign submandibular gland tumor is an en bloc procedure that requires strict attention to the location of the tumor. Preoperative imaging with CT scans will precisely locate the tumor and guide the dissection of the pseudocapsule of the tumor. Those benign tumors that are located within the submandibular gland are surgically excised by a traditional submandibular gland excision with little concern for tumor spillage (Fig. 99.7). However, the benign tumor that perforates through the gland parenchyma must be managed with a precise dissection of the tumor's pseudocapsule to prevent violation of the pseudocapsule with tumor spillage (Fig. 99.8). Tumor spillage is to be avoided to decrease the incidence of persistence of a benign tumor that might otherwise occur.

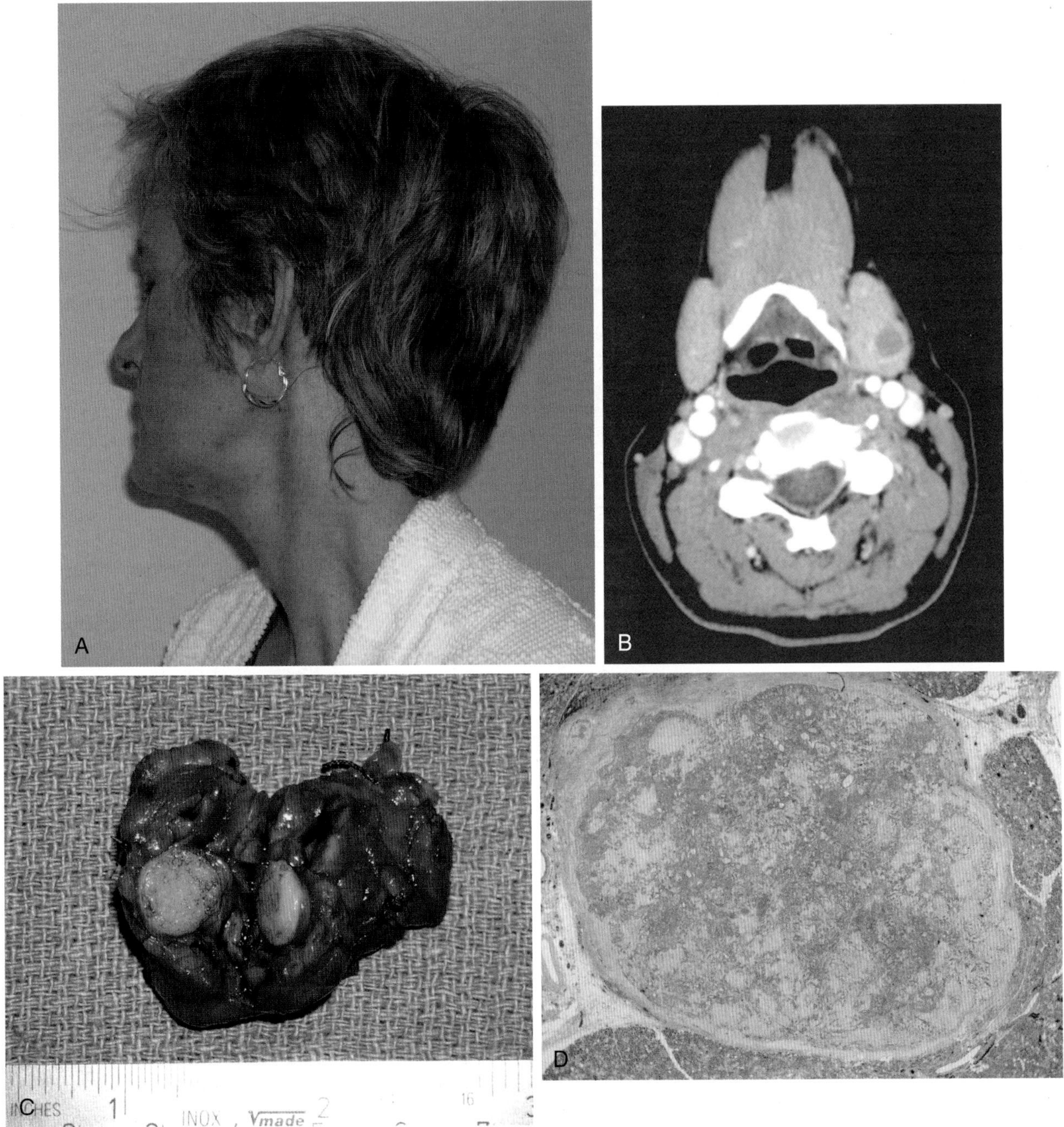

Figure 99.7 **A,** A patient with a visibly and palpably enlarged left submandibular gland. A discrete mass within the submandibular gland was observed on physical examination that led to the acquisition of computed tomography (CT) scans. **B,** The axial CT scans identified the presence of an intraglandular tumor without violation of the surface of the gland. A preoperative fine-needle aspiration biopsy was performed that identified benign disease, suggestive of a pleomorphic adenoma. **C,** A submandibular gland excision was performed without encountering the pseudocapsule of the tumor. Bivalving the specimen demonstrated the presence of the intraglandular tumor. **D,** The microscopic sections of the specimen identified a well-circumscribed pleomorphic adenoma completely encased within unremarkable salivary gland tissue (hematoxylin and eosin, original magnification ×2).

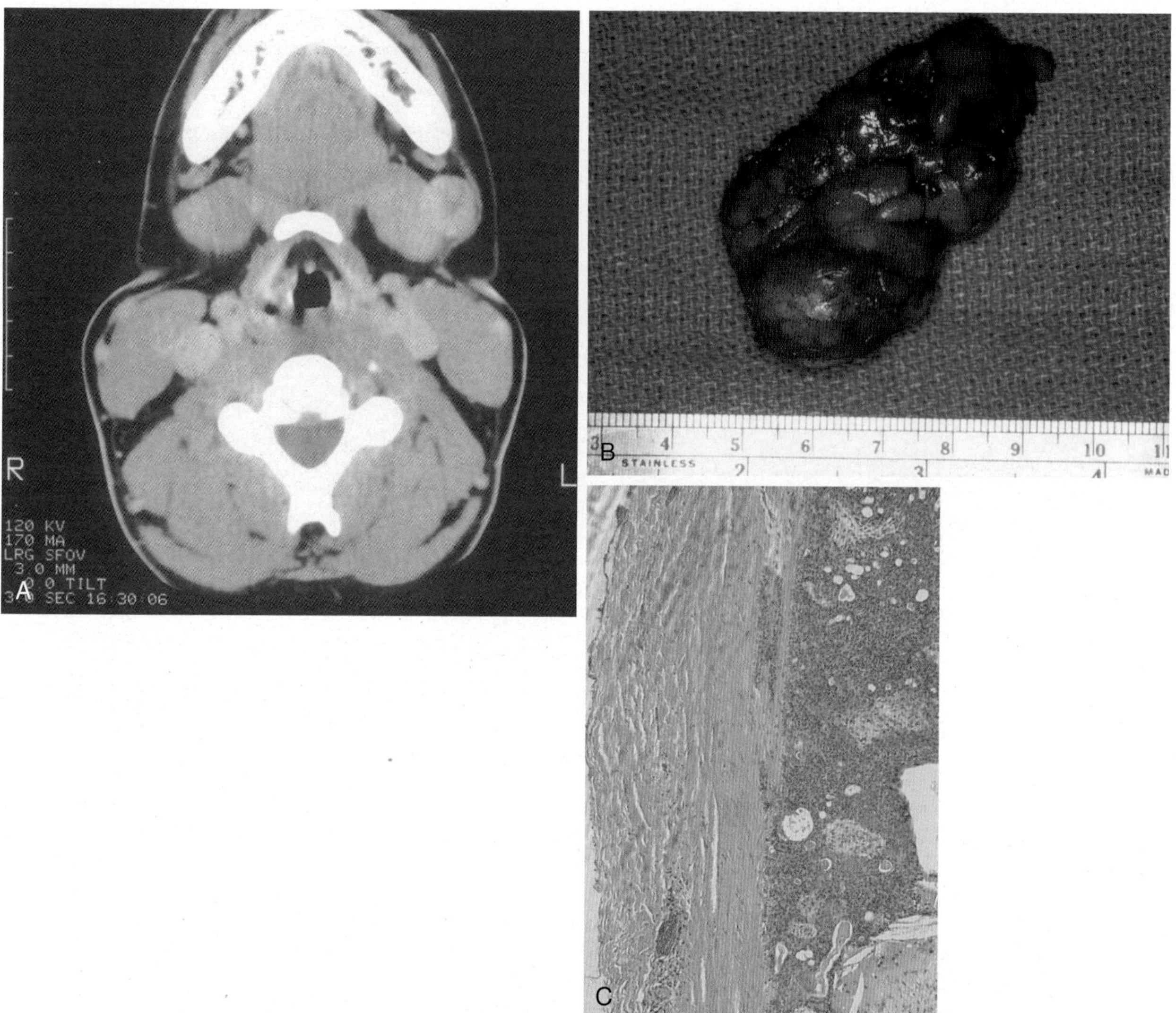

Figure 99.8 **A,** A left submandibular gland tumor exiting the gland as noted on axial computed tomography (CT) scan. Preoperative fine-needle aspiration biopsy suggested pleomorphic adenoma such that the patient underwent excision of the gland/tumor. **B,** Due to the extraglandular presence of the tumor, intraoperative dissection of the pseudocapsule of the tumor was required that permitted the delivery of the tumor/gland in an en bloc fashion. **C,** The microscopic sections of the specimen identified pleomorphic adenoma with an intact pseudocapsule (hematoxylin and eosin, original magnification ×10).

ALTERNATE OR MODIFIED TECHNIQUE 3: Transoral Excision of the Submandibular Gland

The unavoidable presence of a scar of the neck and possible nerve injury associated with traditional transcutaneous excision of the submandibular gland has led investigators to perform transoral excision of the submandibular gland. One such study compared the results of eight transoral submandibular gland excisions to eight transcutaneous submandibular gland excisions.[44] The mean operating time was significantly longer in the transoral approach compared with the transcervical approach. No transoral approach required conversion to a transcutaneous approach. As expected, temporary and permanent marginal mandibular palsy was more frequent in the transcutaneous approach, but temporary lingual nerve injury was more frequent in the transoral approach. There were no hypoglossal nerve injuries in either group.

ALTERNATE OR MODIFIED TECHNIQUE 4: Endoscopic Excision of the Submandibular Gland

Minimally invasive endoscopic surgery was developed to be a frequently performed, if not the standard procedure in many surgical disciplines. Such operations are not yet a standard procedure in the head and neck region due to the anatomic complexity in this region.[45] This notwithstanding, reviews exist of endoscopic submandibular gland excision that avoids a prominent scar in the neck and reduces the incidence of marginal mandibular nerve palsy. Chen et al.[45] performed 12 endoscopic submandibular gland excisions through a 2.0 to 2.5 cm incision at the hyoid midline. Three of the submandibular gland excisions were performed for benign tumors, six for sialolithiasis, and three for chronic sialadenitis. The mean duration of the procedures was 70 minutes (range 50 to 125 minutes), and no complications, including nerve injury or tumor recurrence, were reported. The authors pointed to superior visualization, magnification of key anatomic structures, and concealment of the scar in a cosmetic area to represent advantages of the endoscopic approach over the traditional transcervical approach for submandibular gland excision.

Avoidance and Management of Intraoperative Complications

Intraoperative complications related to submandibular gland excision for benign diagnoses are rare. Excessive bleeding can occur but is typically uncommon. The presence of the marginal mandibular branch of the facial nerve and the lingual nerve in the field of dissection can lead to temporary or permanent damage to these nerves. Numerous assessments have been reported regarding these and other morbidities associated with the submandibular gland excision. Preuss et al.[15] evaluated 258 submandibular gland excisions for a variety of diagnoses including sialolithiasis (n = 119), sialadenitis (n = 88), benign tumors (n = 27), and malignant tumors (n = 24). Overall, 38 (15%) complications were noted, including 22 cases (9%) of transient palsy of the marginal mandibular branch of the facial nerve, 4 cases (2%) of transient lingual nerve injury, 6 cases (2%) of wound infection, 4 cases (2%) of hematoma, and 2 cases (1%) of salivary fistula. The incidence of complications was higher in the group of malignant patients (25%) compared with the remaining benign conditions (13.7%), although this difference was statistically insignificant (p = .484). Only 1 of the 22 cases of transient palsy of the marginal mandibular branch of the facial nerve proved to be permanent, and this occurred in a patient undergoing excision of the submandibular gland for malignant disease. The authors pointed out that the performance of a neck dissection in patients with malignant tumors did not influence the rate of complications. Springborg and Moller[17] identified 302 patients who underwent excision of the submandibular gland during a 10-year period and reported long-term clinical outcomes in 139 of these patients, all of whom had benign diagnoses. Paresis of the marginal mandibular branch of the facial nerve was noted in 26 patients (18.7%), and 3 of these cases were permanent. Postoperative hematoma was noted in 14 patients, 3 of whom required reoperation. Thirteen cases of wound infection were identified, and 3 of these patients required surgical drainage. No cases of hypoglossal nerve injury were identified in this study, although five patients displayed permanent lingual nerve injuries on long-term follow-up examinations. Hypesthesia of the neck skin was the most common complication noted in 26 patients on long-term follow-up examination. This finding should probably be considered the norm rather than a complication. Chua et al.[16] reported on 13 of 101 patients undergoing submandibular gland excision for a variety of benign and malignant diagnoses. Complications were noted in 13 of 101 patients (12.9%), with temporary marginal mandibular branch injury being the most common, occurring in 5 of 13 patients. Lingual nerve injury occurred in three patients, and one patient experienced a temporary injury of the marginal mandibular branch of the facial nerve and a lingual nerve injury.

Postoperative Considerations

Considerations following submandibular gland excision for benign diagnoses depend on the specific diagnosis, the observation of early and late complications, and the removal of sutures and the drain. One issue to consider is whether patients require an overnight stay following excision of the submandibular gland for a benign diagnosis.[46] Experience demonstrates that patients can be operated on an ambulatory basis when a skilled surgeon proceeds with the surgery in a meticulous fashion to minimize the chance for postoperative bleeding. In general terms, patients may undergo drain removal within a few days following their surgery and suture removal between 7 and 10 days postoperatively. A review of the final histopathology of the excised specimen is important, particularly in the case of the excision of the submandibular gland for a suspected benign neoplasm. Additional postoperative considerations surround the surveillance of morbidity, including following the progress of a nerve injury if one is diagnosed postoperatively.

References

1. McFarland J. Tumors of the parotid region. Studies of one hundred and thirty-five cases. *Surg Gynecol Obstet.* 1933;57:104–114.
2. McFarland J. Three hundred mixed tumors of the salivary glands, of which sixty-nine recurred. *Surg Gynecol Obstet.* 1936;63:457–468.
3. Foote FW Jr, Frazell EL. Tumors of the major salivary glands. *Cancer.* 1953;6(6):1065–1133.
4. Work WP. Therapy of salivary gland tumors. *Arch Otolaryngol.* 1966;83(2):89–91.
5. Work WP, Gates GA. Non-neoplastic diseases of the major salivary glands. *J La State Med Soc.* 1966;118(5):190–195.
6. Work WP. Disease of the major salivary glands: classification, diagnosis and treatment. *Minn Med.* 1967;50(6):937–940.
7. Eneroth CM, Hjertman L. Benign tumours of the submandibular gland. *Pract Otorhinolaryngol (Basel)* . 1967;29(3):166–181.
8. Seward GR. Anatomic surgery for salivary calculi. Part I. Symptoms, signs, and differential diagnosis. *Oral Surg Oral Med Oral Pathol.* 1968;25:150–157.
9. Seward GR. Anatomic surgery for salivary calculi. II. Calculi in the anterior part of the submandibular duct. *Oral Surg Oral Med Oral Pathol.* 1968;25(3):287–293.
10. Seward GR. Anatomic surgery for salivary calculi. 3. Calculi in the posterior part of the submandibular duct. *Oral Surg Oral Med Oral Pathol.* 1968;25(4):525–531.
11. Rafla S. Submaxillary gland tumors. *Cancer.* 1970;26(4):821–826.
12. Gallina E, Gallo O, Boccuzzi S, Paradiso P. Analysis of 185 submandibular gland excisions. *Acta Otorhinolaryngologica Belg.* 1990;44(1):7–10.
13. Weber RS, Byers RM, Petit B, Wolf P, Ang K, Luna M. Submandibular gland tumors. Adverse histologic factors and therapeutic implications. *Arch Otolaryngol Head Neck Surg.* 1990;116(9):1055–1060.
14. Laskawi R, Ellies M, Arglebe C, Schott A. Surgical management of benign tumors of the submandibular gland: a follow-up study. *J Oral Maxillofac Surg.* 1995;53(5):506–508.
15. Preuss SF, Klussmann JP, Wittekindt C, Drebber U, Beutner D, Guntinas-Lichius O. Submandibular gland excision: 15 years of experience. *J Oral Maxillofac Surg.* 2007;65(5):953–957.
16. Chua DYK, Ko C, Lu KS. Submandibular mass excision in an Asian population: a 10-year review. *Ann Acad Med Singap.* 2010;39(1):33–37.
17. Springborg LK, Moller MN. Submandibular gland excision: long-term clinical outcome in 139 patients operated in a single institution. *Eur Arch Otorhinolaryngol.* 2013;270(4):1441–1446.
18. McGurk M, Escudier MP, Brown JE. Modern management of salivary calculi. *Br J Surg.* 2005;92(1):107–112.
19. McGurk M, Makdissi J, Brown JE. Intra-oral removal of stones from the hilum of the submandibular gland: report of technique and morbidity. *Int J Oral Maxillofac Surg.* 2004;33(7):683–686.
20. Escudier MP. The current status and possible future for lithotripsy of salivary calculi. *Atlas Oral Maxillofac Surg Clin North Am.* 1998;6(1):117–132.
21. Berry RL. Sialadenitis and sialolithiasis: diagnosis and management. *Oral Maxillofac Surg Clin North Am.* 1995;7:749. 503.
22. Lustmann J, Regev E, Melamed Y, Sialolithiasis. A survey on 245 patients and a review of the literature. *Int J Oral Maxillofac Surg.* 1990;19(3):135–138.
23. Miloro M. The surgical management of submandibular gland disease. *Atlas Oral Maxillofac Surg Clin North Am.* 1998;6(1):29–50.
24. Drage NA, Wilson RF, McGurk M. The genu of the submandibular duct—is the angle significant in salivary gland disease? *Dentomaxillofac Radiol.* 2002;31(1):15–18.
25. Carlson ER, Ord RA, eds. *Textbook and Color Atlas of Salivary Gland Pathology. Diagnosis and Management.* 2nd ed. Hoboken, New Jersey: Wiley-Blackwell; 2015:109–129.
26. Bodner L. Salivary gland calculi: diagnostic imaging and surgical management. *Compendium.* 1993;14(5):572–584.
27. Kasaboğlu O, Er N, Tümer C, Akkocaoğlu M. Micromorphology of sialoliths in submandibular salivary gland: a scanning electron microscope and X-ray diffraction analysis. *J Oral Maxillofac Surg.* 2004;62(10):1253–1258.
28. Kao WK, Chole RA, Ogden MA. Evidence of a microbial etiology for sialoliths. *Laryngoscope.* 2020;130(1):69–74.
29. Perez-Tanoira R, Aarnisalo A, Haapaniemi A, Saarinen R, Kuusela P, Kinnari TJ. Bacterial biofilm in salivary stones. *Eur Arch Otorhinolaryngol.* 2019;276(6):1815–1822.
30. Choi HG, Bang W, Park B, Sim S, Tae K, Song CM. Lack of evidence that nephrolithiasis increases the risk of sialolithiasis: a longitudinal follow-up study using a national sample cohort. *PLoS One.* 2018;13(4):e0196659.
31. Kim SY, Kim HJ, Lim H, et al. Association between cholelithiasis and sialolithiasis: two longitudinal follow-up studies. *Medicine (Baltim).* 2019;98(25):e16153.
32. Stack BC Jr, Norman JG. Sialolithiasis and primary hyperparathyroidism. *ORL J Otorhinolaryngol Relat Spec.* 2008;70(5):331–334.
33. Kraaij S, Karagozoglu KH, Kenter YAG, Pijpe J, Gilijamse M, Brand HS. Systemic diseases and the risk of developing salivary stones: a case control study. *Oral Surg Oral Med Oral Pathol Oral Radiol.* 2015;119(5):539–543.
34. Park JS, Sohn JH, Kim JK. Factors influencing intraoral removal of submandibular calculi. *Otolaryngol Head Neck Surg.* 2006;135(5):704–709.
35. Carlson ER. Diagnosis and management of salivary gland infections. *Oral Maxillofac Surg Clin North Am.* 2009;21(3):293–312.
36. Gallia LJ, Johnson JT. The incidence of neoplastic versus inflammatory disease in major salivary gland masses diagnosed by surgery. *Laryngoscope.* 1981;91(4):512–516.
37. Puxeddu H, Capecchi R, Carta F, Tavoni AG, Migliorini P, Puxeddu R. Salivary gland pathology in IgG4 related disease: a comprehensive review. *J Immunol Res.* 2018;2018:6936727.
38. Pogrel MA. The diagnosis and management of tumors of the submandibular and sublingual salivary glands. *Oral Maxillofac Surg Clin North Am.* 1995;7:565–571.
39. Auclair PL, Ellis GL, Gnepp DR, et al. Salivary gland neoplasms: general considerations. In: Ellis GL, Auclair PL, Gnepp DR, eds. *Surgical Pathology of the Salivary Glands.* Philadelphia, PA: WB Saunders Co; 1991:135–164.
40. Carlson ER, Webb DE. The diagnosis and management of parotid disease. *Oral Maxillofac Surg Clin North Am.* 2013;25(1):31–48, v.
41. Carlson ER, McCoy JM. Margins for benign salivary gland neoplasms of the head and neck. *Oral Maxillofac Surg Clin North Am.* 2017;29(3):325–340.
42. Betts NJ, Cottrell KR. Diagnosis and management of traumatic salivary gland injuries. In: Fonseca R, Walker, eds. *Oral and Maxillofacial Trauma.* 3rd ed. St. Louis, Missouri: Elsevier Saunders.
43. Singh B, Shaha A. Traumatic submandibular salivary gland fistula. *J Oral Maxillofac Surg.* 1995;53(3):338–339.
44. Chang YN, Kao CH, Lin YS, Lee JC. Comparison of the intraoral and transcervical approach in submandibular gland excision. *Eur Arch Otorhinolaryngol.* 2013;270(2):669–674.
45. Chen MK, Su CC, Tsai YL, Chang CC. Minimally invasive endoscopic resection of the submandibular gland: a new approach. *Head Neck.* 2006;28(11):1014–1017.
46. Laverick S, Chandramohan J, McLoughlin PM. Excision of a submandibular gland: a safe day case procedure? *Br J Oral Maxillofac Surg.* 2012;50(6):567–568.

CHAPTER 100

Superficial Parotidectomy

Daniel Oreadi

Armamentarium

#15 Scalpel
1/4-inch Penrose drain
Ace elastic wrap
Adson pickup with and without teeth
Allis clamp
Appropriate sutures
Army-Navy retractors
Babcock forceps
Baby Mixter forceps
Bipolar electrocautery
Cotton ball
Curved hemostats
DeBakey forceps
Gerald pickup with and without teeth
Iris scissors, straight and curved
Jacobson hemostat
Kerlix gauze roll
Kittner sponge
Kocher clamps
Local anesthetic with vasoconstrictor
Lone Star self-retractors
Loupe magnification (preference)
Metzenbaum scissors
Needle electrocautery
Neuro suction tip
NIM-Response nerve stimulator (optional)
Right-angle dissector
Senn retractors
Skin hooks (10-mm double prong)
Tenotomy scissors
Vari-Stim nerve locator
Webster needle holder

History of the Procedure

Salivary gland surgery dates back to the 16th century. The anatomy of the parotid gland and the role of the main ducts were described in the mid-17th century. The earliest references to "para-auricular swellings," as the Greeks called them, described the findings associated with calculi and inflammation.

Between 1650 and 1750, salivary gland surgery was limited to the treatment of ranulas and oral calculi. The concept of surgical excision of a parotid tumor has been attributed to Bertrandi in 1802. The initial applications of this surgery involved an extensive approach, which caused serious disfiguration and disability.

In about the 1850s, the focus shifted toward dissection and the intimate relationship between the facial nerve and the parotid gland. Attempts were made to perform the surgery with nerve preservation. John C. Warren, a physician, was the first to use ether inhalation anesthesia during resection of a parotid tumor in Boston in 1846. In 1892, Codreanu (a Romanian native) performed the first total parotidectomy with facial nerve preservation.

Before the 1950s, enucleation of benign neoplastic processes (e.g., pleomorphic adenoma) was the most common extirpative procedure; however, it was associated with elevated recurrence rates. The reason enucleation should be performed rather than removal of the gland was because of concern regarding injury to the facial nerve.

In 1958, Beahrs and Adson[1] eloquently described the relevant anatomy and surgical technique of current parotid gland surgery. They stressed the importance of surgical landmarks for avoiding injury to the facial nerve and advocated complete removal of the superficial portion of the parotid gland for noninvasive lesions confined to that location.

Indications for the Use of the Procedure

An estimated 75% to 80% of parotid neoplasms are benign. Pleomorphic adenoma and Warthin tumors account for most of the neoplasms encountered. When malignancy is encountered, adenoid cystic carcinoma and mucoepidermoid carcinoma are approximately equally represented. Adenocarcinoma, acinic cell carcinoma, carcinoma ex-pleomorphic adenoma, squamous cell carcinoma, and malignant mixed tumor may occasionally be encountered. Lymphoma may arise in the intraparotid or paraparotid lymph nodes. The lymph nodes may also be sites of metastases from cutaneous squamous cell carcinoma and melanoma of the face and scalp. In rare cases, tumors may metastasize to parotid lymph nodes from distant sites.[2]

Superficial parotidectomy is indicated for most benign and malignant tumors limited to the superficial lobe, for chronic sialadenitis, and as part of a lymphadenectomy for skin cancer of the scalp. Although some evidence suggests that certain lesions of the parotid gland can be treated or investigated with enucleation, it is the author's opinion that this is an unsafe practice and should not be encouraged because of the risk of tumor spillage and recurrence, in addition to the increased risk of facial nerve injury during revision surgery. In certain situations, such as for the treatment of pleomorphic adenoma, the presence of a pseudocapsule allows the surgeon to remove less parotid parenchyma relative to tumor size, making partial superficial parotidectomy the procedure of choice. Tumors that extend into the deep lobe may require total parotidectomy.[3]

Although the incisional parotid biopsy is the diagnostic procedure of choice for systemic disease involving the parotid, the superficial parotidectomy remains the minimal biopsy of choice for a mass suspected to be a neoplasm in the parotid.[4]

Limitations and Contraindications

In about 20% of patients, the parotid gland is really one lobe with an accessory lobe along the Stensen duct. The delineation of two lobes (the superficial lobe and the deep lobe), based on cranial nerve (CN) VII, is not so much anatomic as surgical.[5]

The contents of the triangular space anterior and inferior to the auricle include, among others, numerous sensory and autonomic nerves, the external carotid artery and its branches, and the retromandibular vein.

The integrity of the facial nerve is among the most important considerations during treatment of parotid gland diseases (Fig. 100.1).

Davis et al.[6] described six different facial nerve branching patterns, with no predominant pattern. In all types, the temporal and zygomatic branches arise from the upper division, and the cervical and marginal mandibular branches arise from the lower division. The major variations are in the origin of the buccal branch and the degree of cross-innervation

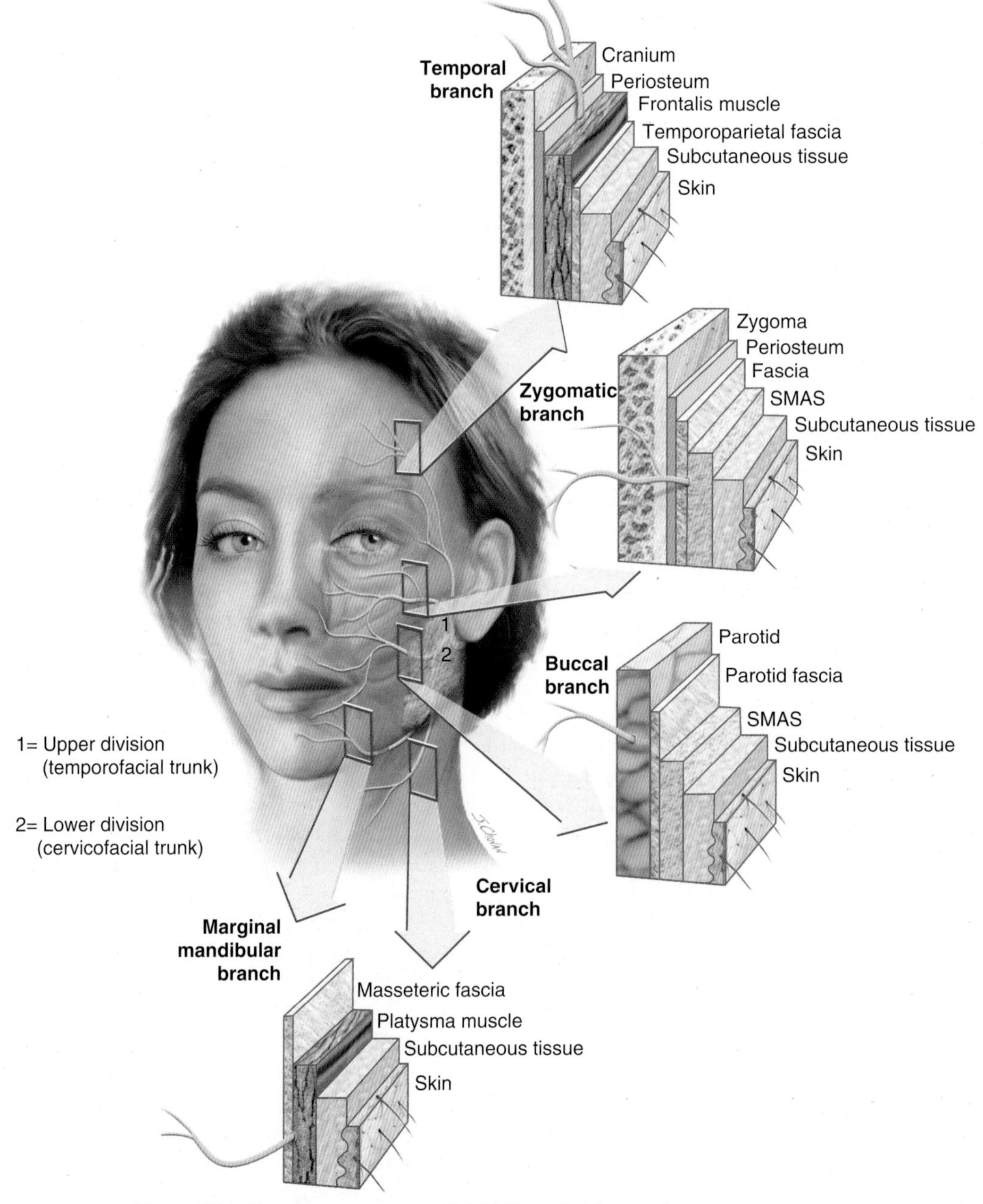

Figure 100.1 Facial nerve anatomy. *SMAS*, Superficial musculoaponeurotic system.

between adjacent terminal branches. Such branching patterns have no particular significance during the surgical procedure, mainly because of the constancy of the main trunk as it enters the parotid gland.

Because of the benign nature of most parotid tumors, patients commonly expect intact motor function of the face after surgery. However, in addition to variations in nerve anatomy, the surgery may be further complicated by other factors, including previous surgery, infection, and a history of radiation therapy. The tumor's size and type and its relation to the facial nerve may also increase the complexity of parotid surgery.[7]

Poor general health is the only relative contraindication to parotid surgery. In general, the superficial parotidectomy procedure is well tolerated by patients, even those medically optimized to undergo general anesthesia.[8]

TECHNIQUE: Superficial Parotidectomy

STEP 1: Intubation

Oral endotracheal intubation with either a conventional tube or a right-angle endotracheal tube is preferred. The tube is secured with skin adhesive and tape. Wiring the tube to the existing dentition, if present, is another option in cases when tube security is at risk. Avoidance of neuromuscular paralysis is important during the procedure to better identify the facial nerve.

STEP 2: Patient Positioning

Patient positioning is an important aspect of the surgical procedure. Proper positioning guarantees the surgeon's comfort and helps avoid limitations in access. The patient is placed in the supine position on the operating room table; the head is extended and turned to the contralateral side. The table is then rotated 90 degrees, with the operative side of the patient away from the anesthesia machine.

STEP 3: Prepping and Draping

A sterile cotton ball is used to block the external auditory canal; this prevents tympanic membrane irritation in the event of Betadine accumulation after prepping. A corneal protector is then placed over the ipsilateral globe, and the face and neck are prepped with Betadine scrub. The entire operative field is then draped in a sterile fashion, exposing the patient's ipsilateral eye, commissure, and chin to allow for visualization of facial movements during stimulation of the facial nerve (Fig. 100.2A).

Continued

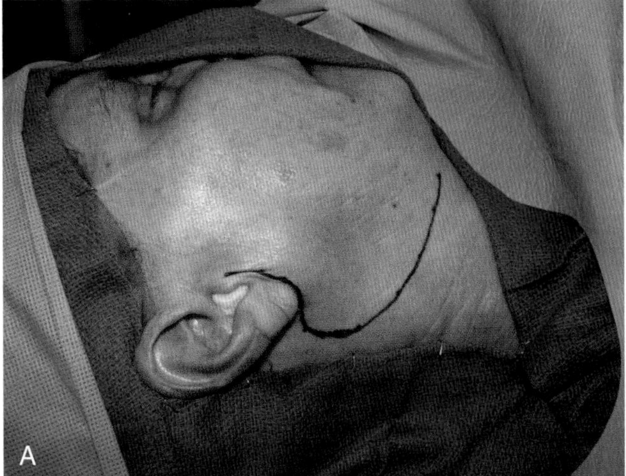

Figure 100.2 **A,** The patient is draped in a way that allows facial nerve stimulation to be assessed.

Technique: Superficial Parotidectomy—*cont'd*

STEP 4: Incision and Superficial Dissection

A marking pen is used to delineate a modified Blair incision, beginning in the preauricular region and extending into the upper aspect of the neck in a curvilinear fashion at the level of the hyoid bone, about two fingerbreadths below the angle of the mandible. Infiltration of 1% lidocaine with 1:100,000 epinephrine is then performed along the entire proposed incision only at the subcutaneous level; avoiding deep injection is important to prevent facial nerve impairment. A 2-0 silk suture is used to retract the ear lobule away from the incision site. With a #15 Bard-Parker blade, an incision is made through the skin and subcutaneous tissues. Dermal bleeding points are controlled using monopolar electrocoagulation. The author prefers to address the neck portion of the incision first. After the platysma muscle is exposed, its transection allows for exposure of the investing layer of the deep cervical fascia. Dissection is continued bluntly to expose the external jugular vein (EJV), greater auricular nerve (GAN), and sternocleidomastoid muscle (SCM). If the surgeon is able to avoid sacrificing the EJV, this will reduce later bleeding in the gland to some degree. The GAN can be preserved, if possible, although sacrificing it does not have long-term implications postoperatively.[9] On occasion, the anterior branches of the GAN can be divided to limit postoperative morbidity. In the preauricular region, dissection to the parotid capsule is performed. Metzenbaum scissors are used to undermine the skin flap superficial to the parotid capsule up to the anterior edge of the parotid gland, with special care taken not to enter the substance of the gland or the tumor. The posterior skin is elevated off the tail of the gland and the superior aspect of the SCM (Fig. 100.2B and C).

STEP 5: Deeper Dissection and Removal of the Gland

Once the inferior aspect of the parotid has been separated from the SCM, proper retraction anteriorly is necessary to continue bluntly dissecting the parotid gland from the surface of the cartilaginous ear canal toward the level of the cartilaginous (tragal) pointer. At this point, a couple of Babcock or Kocher clamps are placed in the posterior edge of the gland and retracted anteriorly. Palpation with a finger can be performed to assess for the cartilaginous prominence. Continuous exposure of the anterior border of the SCM and the cartilaginous ear canal must have been obtained at the end of this part of the procedure. Careful dissection of the soft tissue in this area is performed using a right-angle dissector or fine Jacobson hemostat. Several veins in this area may require suture ligation. At this point, only bipolar electrocautery (not monopolar) should be used to dissect through vessels and control bleeding.

Dissection then continues in a deeper direction to identify the posterior belly of the digastric muscle. A common mistake is to look for this muscle too low in the surgical field, risking the integrity of the accessory nerve and the jugular vein. Palpation of the mastoid tip allows for appreciation of the muscle entering the digastric groove; careful dissection of the tissues with a right-angle dissector allows exposure of the muscle. The gland is then freed from the superior and anterior edge of the digastric muscle, and the search for the main trunk of the facial nerve begins.

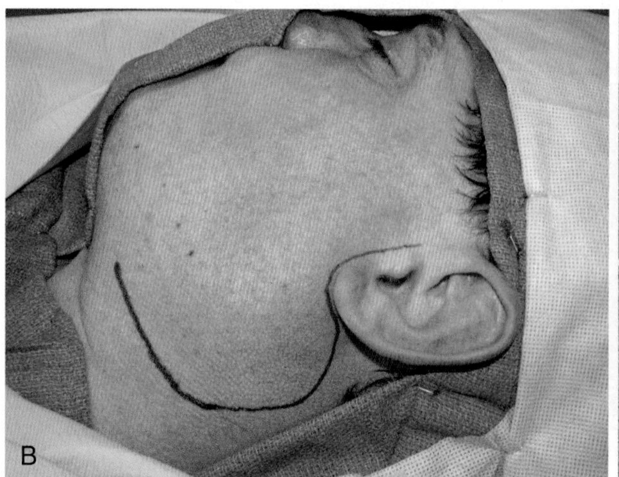

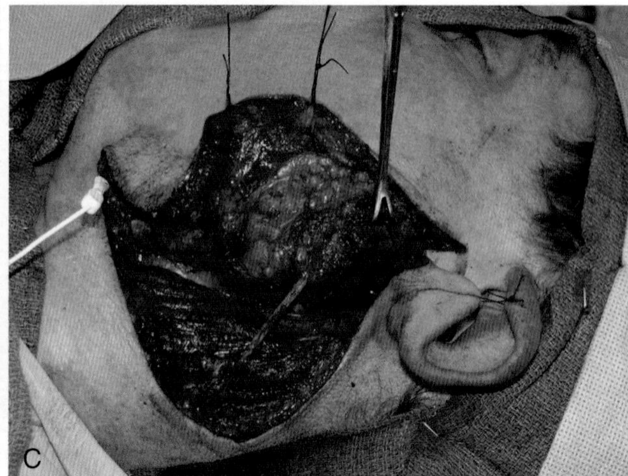

Figure 100.2, cont'd **B,** The modified Blair incision (also known as a lazy S incision) is designed along a preauricular and a cervical crease. **C,** Complete initial dissection to identify superficial landmarks in the cervical region.

Technique: Superficial Parotidectomy—*cont'd*

The posterior belly of the digastric muscle is not always a reliable landmark. Studies have shown that the main trunk of the facial nerve was found, on average, to be 4 to 5 mm anterocranial to its superior border.[10,11] The "pointers" cartilage should be identified; approximately 10 to 15 mm below it, the main trunk of the facial nerve can be found. Another reliable landmark is the tympanomastoid suture. The facial nerve is medial to this palpable landmark. Nerve stimulation is performed with a Vari-Stim III nerve locator or the checkpoint nerve stimulator and locator during the entire dissection of the nerve and its branches. Alternatively, some surgeons prefer to use nerve integrity monitoring (NIM) systems during the procedure. The author believes that either method provides a safe way to identify the facial nerve and its associated branches.

Careful dissection is then carried distally to the pes anserinus (Fig. 100.2D), following the upper and lower divisions of the nerve by dividing the parenchyma that lies superficial to the branches. At this point, as the dissection progresses, the anatomy of the nerve is variable; therefore, the surgeon must take care not to injure small branches. During dissection of the buccal nerve branches, the parotid duct may be encountered. The duct may resemble the nerve; therefore, the surgeon should not attempt to isolate it in order to avoid the unnecessary risks of injuring the small braches that run along its course. The gland eventually becomes pedicled to the duct, at which point it can be safely suture-ligated.

After the gland has been removed, the specimen is oriented for the pathologist, and the surgical field is carefully inspected to assess for bleeding vessels. Hemostasis using multiple Valsalva maneuvers is essential to prevent postoperative hematoma. The integrity of the facial nerve is confirmed by stimulating each branch (Fig. 100.2E).

Continued

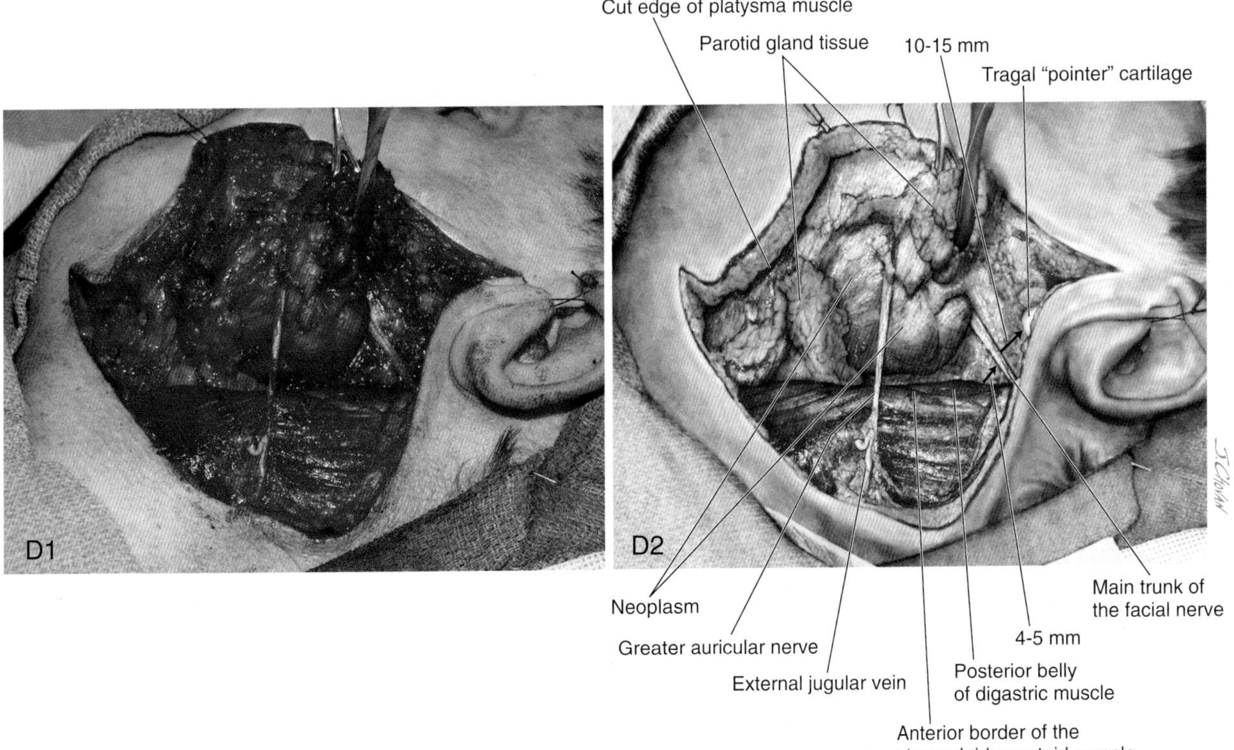

Figure 100.2, cont'd **D,** The main trunk of the facial nerve is identified.

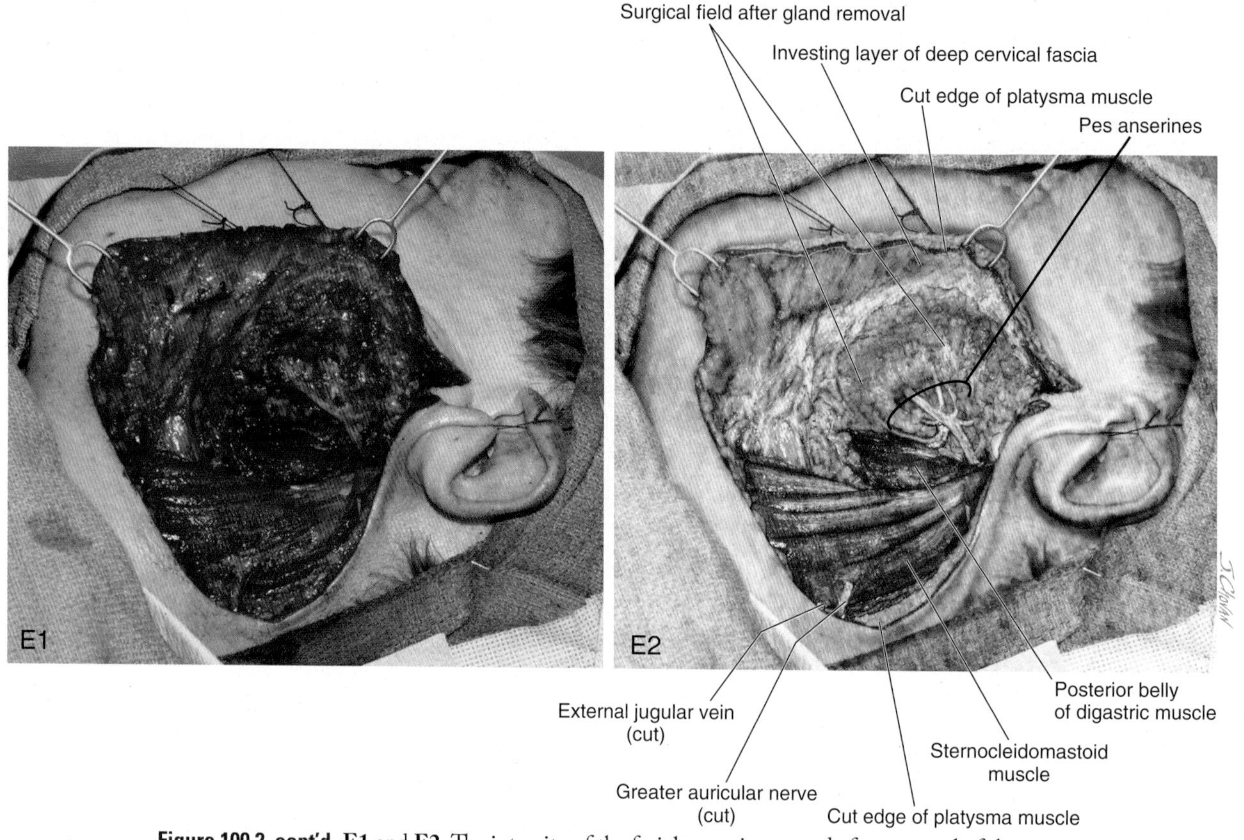

Figure 100.2, cont'd **E1** and **E2,** The integrity of the facial nerve is assessed after removal of the tumor.

Technique: Superficial Parotidectomy—*cont'd*

STEP 6: Irrigation, Drain Placement, Wound Closure, and Dressing

A 4 × 4 gauze pad is placed over the facial nerve (Fig. 100.2F), and then gentle irrigation with room-temperature saline can be performed safely, without negative effects on the nerve. A 1/4-inch Penrose drain is placed into the defect and away from the nerve. The drain is secured at the skin surface with 2-0 silk suture.

A three-layer closure is then carried out, beginning with the deep soft tissues. The platysma muscle is reapproximated using interrupted 3-0 Vicryl sutures. The subcuticular layer is closed with 5-0 Vicryl sutures, and the skin surface is closed with 5-0 nylon sutures in an interrupted fashion (Fig. 100.2G). The suture line is treated with Bacitracin ointment, and a pressure dressing consisting of Kerlix fluffs and a JawBra is placed.

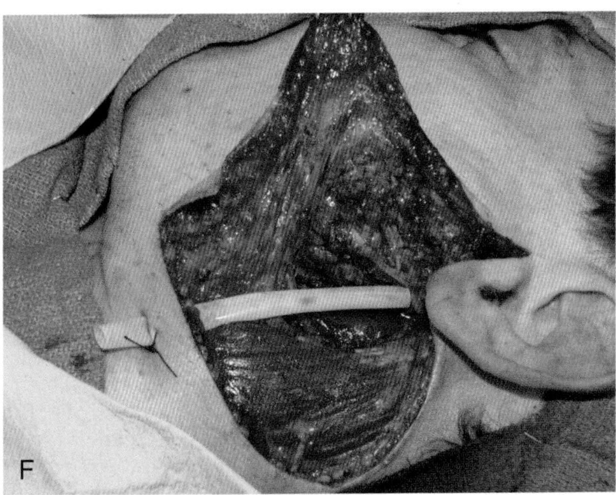

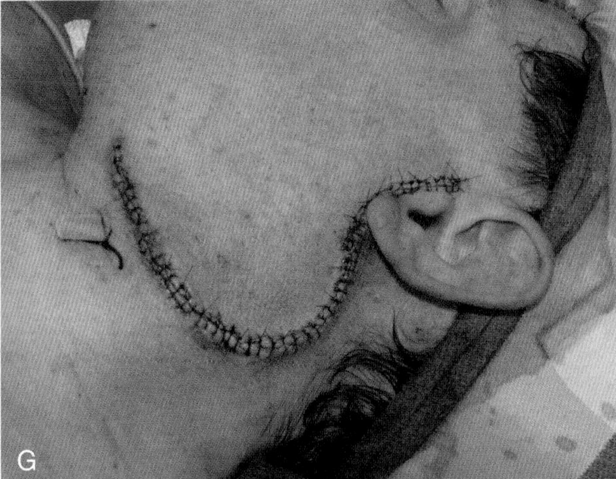

Figure 100.2, cont'd F, A nonsuction drain is placed along the sternocleidomastoid muscle and secured to the skin away from the wound edges. **G,** The wound is closed in layers, and the suture line is treated with antibiotic ointment.

ALTERNATIVE TECHNIQUE 1: Partial Superficial Parotidectomy

In certain situations, when tumors are confined to the parotid tail or a small area of the lateral aspect of the parotid gland, limited excision of the tumor, surrounded by a cuff of normal parotid, can be considered an acceptable treatment option. This type of procedure, known as a partial superficial parotidectomy, allows for identification and dissection of the facial nerve branches in the vicinity of the sacrificed normal parotid gland. The surgeon follows the same steps described for the superficial parotidectomy procedure until the main trunk of the facial nerve is identified; dissection of the facial nerve branches then continues based on the location of the tumor. For example, if the tumor is confined to the parotid tail, the cervicofacial division of the nerve must be dissected. Similarly, if the tumor lies above the level of the meatus, only the zygomaticofacial trunk should be dissected and the corresponding part of the gland removed.

The author believes that tumor size plays an important role in the decision of which surgical procedure should be performed. Small malignant tumors can be safely removed with a partial superficial parotidectomy procedure; however, when adequate margins are required and the tumor involves a considerable portion of the supraneural parotid gland, a superficial parotidectomy is recommended (Figs. 100.3–100.6A).

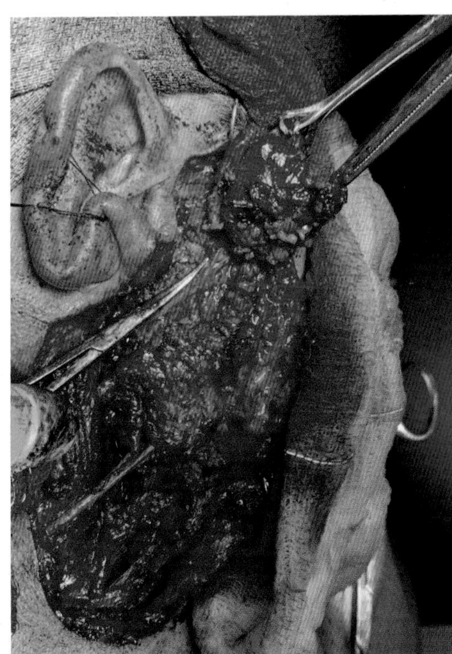

Figure 100.3 Partial superficial parotidectomy of a small lesion in the superior aspect.

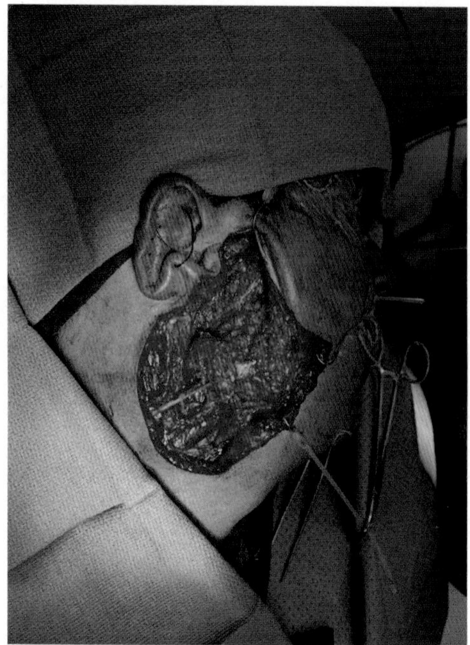

Figure 100.4 Residual defect after tumor removal.

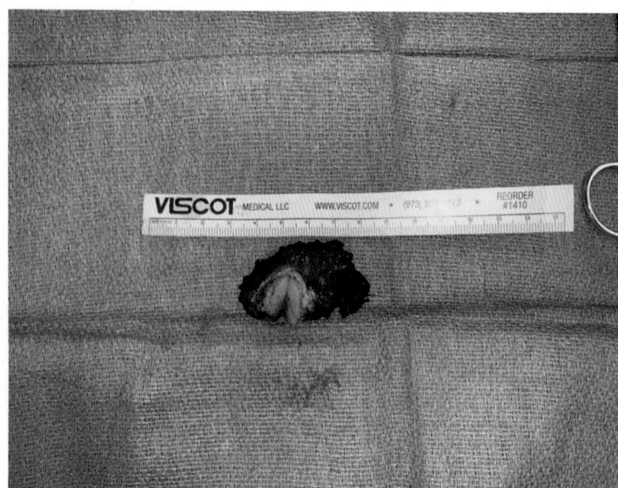

Figure 100.5 Bivalved specimen to be submitted for permanent section examination.

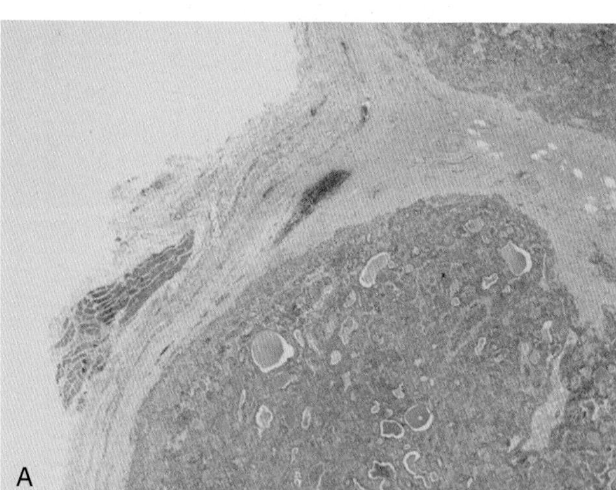

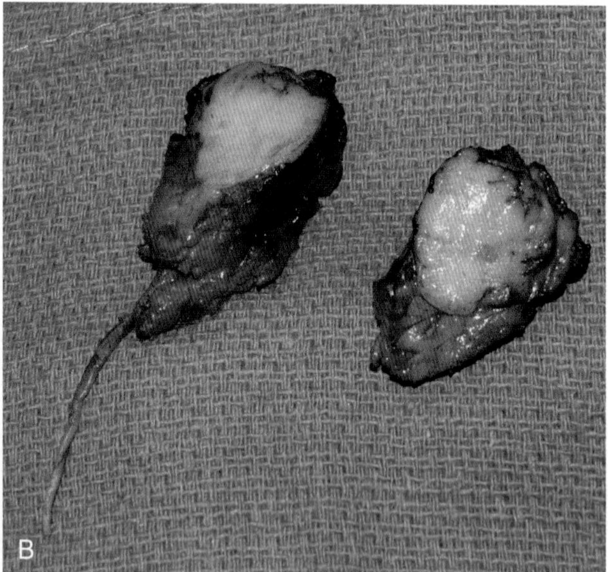

Figure 100.6 **A,** Medium-power microphotograph showing the pseudocapsule in a pleomorphic adenoma removed by superficial parotidectomy. **B,** Clinical photograph of a bilobed specimen showing the thin capsule surrounding the tumor.

ALTERNATIVE TECHNIQUE 2: Extracapsular Dissection

The traditional enucleation procedure for tumors involving the parotid gland led to frequent recurrences (20% to 45%)[12] and the need for revision surgery, thereby increasing the risk of injury to the facial nerve. Extracapsular dissection (ECD) is a more conservative approach to parotid tumors that limits the dissection immediately outside the tumor pseudocapsule.

ECD should be used only for benign pathologic entities. The need to identify the main trunk or branches of the facial nerve is avoided unless the pseudocapsule is in close proximity to any of the branches; ECD, therefore, is less invasive than the conventional superficial or the partial superficial parotidectomy. The standard approach for ECD is a preauricular incision with cervical extension. Certain modifications can be made, depending on the amount of parotid gland to be exposed. The skin is raised in a plane immediately superficial to the parotid fascia. Once the skin flap has been raised, the periphery of the tumor is marked in ink (Fig. 100.7A), and an incision is made with at least 1 cm of margin from the edges of the tumor to improve access. The key to ECD is finding a safe plane of dissection. The uninvolved parotid tissue is retracted away from the tumor (Fig. 100.7B and C), revealing loose tissue planes and 2 or 3 mm of tumor capsule. Avoiding tumor pulling reduces the likelihood of capsule rupture, allowing the surgeon to stay away from the capsule. As dissection continues to a deeper level, the proximity to branches of the facial nerve is evaluated by the use of a nerve stimulator. Slow dissection is recommended at this point. Once the tumor has been delivered (Fig. 100.7D), the parotid fascia is reapproximated and closed with 3-0 Vicryl sutures in an interrupted fashion. This restores the contour loss seen in conventional and sometimes partial superficial parotidectomy and eliminates any dead space; also, the closed fascia eliminates the possibility of Frey syndrome. The skin flap is closed in two layers over a Penrose drain, and a pressure dressing is applied.

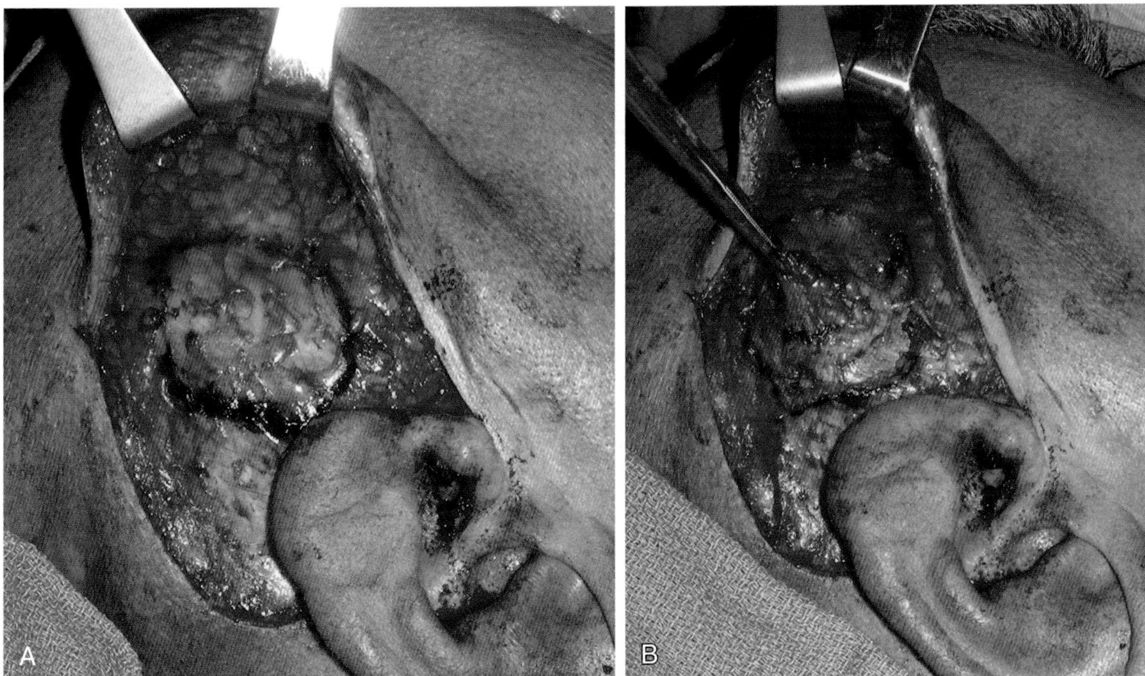

Figure 100.7 Extracapsular dissection (ECD) of a benign parotid gland tumor. **A,** Delineation of tumor limits. **B,** ECD procedure.

Continued

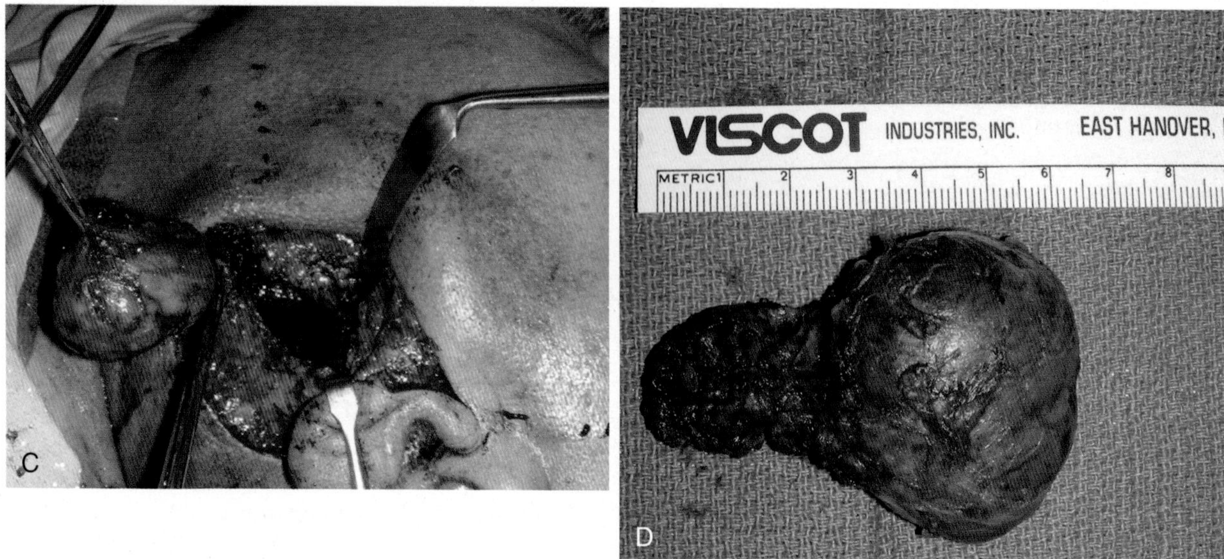

Figure 100.7, cont'd **C,** Dead space left behind after tumor removal. **D,** Tumor specimen with intact capsule and overlying parotid parenchyma. (Images provided by Eric Dierks, DMD, MD, FACS. In: Carlson ER, Webb DE. The diagnosis and management of Parotid disease. *Oral Maxillofac Surg Clin North Am*. 2013;25(1):31–48.)

Avoidance and Management of Intraoperative Complications

Every surgical procedure poses the risk of complications, as does resection of parotid tumors. Although damage to the facial nerve could be considered the most significant complication, there are others worth considering.

Thorough planning and a meticulous preoperative workup reduce the possibility of intraoperative complications. Adequate illumination and loupe magnification should be considered at all times; surgery of the parotid gland is one of the most challenging procedures in the head and neck region, requiring a high degree of expertise.

Inadvertent injury to the facial nerve occurs in 3% to 5% of cases.[13] This assumes that the facial nerve has been adequately identified and preserved during the course of the surgery. When the bulk of the tumor may obstruct direct access, which affects identification of the main trunk, anterograde identification of the branches toward the main trunk should be considered. If nerve injury occurs, primary immediate neurorrhaphy should be performed under magnification. When branches of the nerve are electively divided, the postoperative findings are predictable. On occasion, seemingly innocuous trauma to the facial nerve may be associated with neurapraxia and temporary paresis. More commonly, this paresis is due to excessive stimulation of the nerve intraoperatively; therefore, judicious stimulation is recommended. Stretching the nerve with excessive retraction could also negatively affect the status of the nerve postoperatively. Observation of postoperative movement, however slight, should be considered an indication of a good prognosis, and full recovery can be predicted. Steroid administration to reduce the incidence of neurapraxia associated with parotidectomy failed to demonstrate efficacy in a randomized trial.[14]

Careful consideration should also be given to blood vessels in the area near the facial nerve. The posterior auricular artery or its branch can cross the main trunk of the facial nerve and cause significant bleeding; therefore, proper identification and adequate ligation are paramount while the supraneural parotid is dissected to prevent loss of visualization, which could lead to nerve injury. When bleeding occurs, careful inspection should be performed, vessel ends should be tied or clipped, and bipolar electrocautery can be used, with extreme care taken to not transmit heat to nearby branches of the facial nerve.

In many cases, the recurrence of benign entities, such as pleomorphic adenomas, could be considered a preventable situation. Although rare, capsular rupture during surgery is a great concern for the surgeon. Reports suggest that tumor spillage need not be associated with an increased incidence of recurrence[15,16]; however, the oncologic surgeon invariably fears the chance for recurrence when safe oncologic planes are not obtained, regardless of the nature of the tumor. If tumor spillage is suspected, the author recommends that, at the completion of the procedure, the surgical wound be carefully irrigated with copious amounts of sterile, room-temperature saline solution, during which the facial nerve is protected with a 4 × 4 gauze pad.

Frey syndrome is a complication experienced in a small subset of patients after parotidectomy. This syndrome is thought to represent aberrant innervation between the severed postganglionic parasympathetic nerve branches of the auriculotemporal nerve that stimulate the parotid gland to secrete saliva, and the severed sympathetic innervation to the cutaneous eccrine sweat glands.[17] When the parasympathetic nerves are stimulated to increase salivary production during eating, gustatory flushing and sweating occur instead. Symptoms generally do not present for at least 6 to 12 months (which supports the reinnervation theory) and become more prevalent over time, presumably due to the time necessary for nerve regrowth (52% at 1 year, 83% after an average of 18 months).[18] Blocking the path of the cut parasympathetic nerve branches to the cutaneous sweat glands with allograft dermis has been one approach used to prevent Frey syndrome. Alternatively, the development of a thicker skin flap and the use of different flaps (e.g., sternocleidomastoid, platysma, temporalis fascia, and superficial muscular aponeurotic system), in addition to the use of adipose tissue, fascia lata, and lipolyzed dura, have been reported, with variable results.[19]

Rare complications, such as the development of a salivary fistula, sialocele, or seroma, occasionally occur after parotidectomy. Several studies have reported low rates of seroma/salivary fistula/sialocele, ranging from 2.7% to 6.6% without defining diagnostic criteria.[20,21]

Patients who had a superficial parotidectomy have a smaller chance of developing salivary fistula/sialocele compared to those who had partial superficial parotidectomy or ECD. When an ECD is performed, it is important to close the parotid fascia so that it is watertight; additionally, placement of a nonpressure drain reduces the possibility of a seroma developing.

Necrosis of skin flaps is rarely encountered. It occurs after the formation of a hematoma or due to the poor design of the incision and mishandling of the skin edges. Similarly, when the skin is elevated in a very superficial plane, compromise of the blood supply may ensue. The best management of skin necrosis is prevention, which includes proper planning of the skin incision, elevation of the flap in the correct plane, and prompt evacuation of a hematoma if encountered.

Unsightly scarring is rarely encountered in properly performed parotid surgery. Locating the facial scar in a preauricular skin crease and a cervical crease allows for uneventful healing. Wound closure should include approximation of subcutaneous tissues and careful reapproximation of the epithelium. This usually results in a highly acceptable and easily camouflaged scar.

Postoperative Considerations

The integrity of the facial nerve should be evaluated in the immediate postoperative period. Even with careful dissection, temporary postoperative facial nerve weakness may be present and should be transient. Systemic steroid therapy, as mentioned earlier, may not be of benefit; use of these drugs is guided by the surgeon's preference.

Transection of the GAN results in periauricular and earlobe numbness. Patients should be advised to protect the affected earlobe in cold weather. This condition is self-limiting, although recovery takes months and is usually incomplete.

Postoperative wound infection rarely occurs after parotidectomy. In a series of 175 parotidectomies performed without perioperative antibiotics, infection occurred in fewer than 5% of patients.[22] Routine administration of antibiotic prophylaxis is not indicated unless infection is present preoperatively. If infection is encountered, the wound should be drained and antibiotics administered based on the findings of Gram staining and culture and sensitivity data.

First bite syndrome, which refers to pain upon eating, is believed to be caused by local spasm and may resolve spontaneously.

The use of botulinum toxin for intracutaneous injections in the treatment of Frey syndrome has been found satisfactory.[23] Suture line care is just as important as closure; the use of antibiotic ointment during the initial postoperative care is helpful in preventing complications associated with skin wound healing.

The pressure dressing is left in place for 24 to 48 hours; the drain is removed based on fluid production (usually 5 to 7 days postoperatively). Sutures also can be removed 5 to 7 days after surgery, unless wound tension is present secondary to postoperative swelling. Steri-Strips are placed after suture removal as necessary.

References

1. Beahrs OH, Adson MA. The surgical anatomy and technic of parotidectomy. *Am J Surg*. 1958;95(6):885–896.
2. Johnson JT. Parotid. In: *Operative Otolaryngology: Head and Neck Surgery*. Philadelphia, Pennsylvania: Saunders; 1997.
3. Hsu AK, Kutler DI. Indications, techniques, and complications of major salivary gland extirpation. *Oral Maxillofac Surg Clin North Am*. 2009;21(3):313–321.
4. Marx RE. Incisional parotid biopsy for diagnosis of systemic disease. *Oral Maxillofac Surg Clin North Am*. 1995;7:505.
5. Lore JM, Medina JE. The parotid salivary gland and management of malignant salivary gland neoplasia. In: *An Atlas of Head and Neck Surgery*. 4th ed. Philadelphia, Pennsylvania: Saunders; 2005.
6. Davis RA, Anson BJ, Budinger JM, Kurth LR. Surgical anatomy of the facial nerve and parotid gland based upon a study of 350 cervicofacial halves. *Surg Gynecol Obstet*. 1956;102(4):385–412.
7. Nadershah M, Salama A. Removal of parotid, submandibular, and sublingual glands. *Oral Maxillofac Surg Clin North Am*. 2012;24(2):295–305, x.
8. Cawson RA, Gleeson MJ, Eveson JW. The surgery of salivary disease. In: *The Salivary Glands: Pathology and Surgery*. Oxford, UK: Isis Medical Media; 1997.
9. Min HJ, Lee HS, Lee YS, et al. Is it necessary to preserve the posterior branch of the great auricular nerve in parotidectomy? *Otolaryngol Head Neck Surg*. 2007;137(4):636–641.
10. de Ru JA, van Benthem PP, Bleys RL, Lubsen H, Hordijk GJ. Landmarks for parotid gland surgery. *J Laryngol Otol*. 2001;115(2):122–125.
11. Reid AP. Surgical approach to the parotid gland. *Ear Nose Throat J*. 1989;68(2):151–154.

12. Barzan L, Pin M. Extra-capsular dissection in benign parotid tumors. *Oral Oncol.* 2012;48(10):977–979.
13. Henry LR, Ridge JA. Parotidectomy. In: Souba WW, Mitchel P, Fink MD, et al., eds. *ACS Surgery: Principles and Practice.* 6th ed. Ontario, Canada: Decker; 2007.
14. Lee KJ, Fee WE Jr, Terris DJ. The efficacy of corticosteroids in postparotidectomy facial nerve paresis. *Laryngoscope.* 2002;112(11): 1958–1963.
15. Natvig K, Søberg R. Relationship of intraoperative rupture of pleomorphic adenomas to recurrence: an 11-25 year follow-up study. *Head Neck.* 1994;16(3):213–217.
16. Buchman C, Stringer SP, Mendenhall WM, Parsons JT, Jordan JR, Cassisi NJ. Pleomorphic adenoma: effect of tumor spill and inadequate resection on tumor recurrence. *Laryngoscope.* 1994;104(10):1231–1234.
17. Hoff SR, Mohyuddin N, Yao N. Complications of parotid surgery. *Oper Tech Otolaryngol.* 2009;20:123.
18. Dulguerov P, Quinodoz D, Cosendai G, Piletta P, Marchal F, Lehmann W. Prevention of Frey syndrome during parotidectomy. *Arch Otolaryngol Head Neck Surg.* 1999;125(8):833–839.
19. de Bree R, van der Waal I, Leemans CR. Management of Frey syndrome. *Head Neck.* 2007;29(8):773–778.
20. Upton DC, McNamar JP, Connor NP, Harari PM, Hartig GK. Parotidectomy: ten-year review of 237 cases at a single institution. *Otolaryngol Head Neck Surg.* 2007;136(5):788–792.
21. Al Salamah SM, Khalid K, Khan IA, Gul R. Outcome of surgery for parotid tumours: 5-year experience of a general surgical unit in a teaching hospital. *ANZ J Surg.* 2005;75(11):948–952.
22. Arriaga MA, Myers EN. The surgical management of chronic parotitis. *Laryngoscope.* 1990;100(12):1270–1275.
23. Arad A, Blitzer A. Botulinum toxin in the treatment of autonomic nervous system disorders. *Oper Tech Otolaryngol.* 2004;15:118.

CHAPTER 101

Sialendoscopy

Maryam Akbari and Michael D. Turner

Armamentarium

Balloon dilators
Blunt-tip tapered dilators
Imaging system (light source, video camera, and monitor)
Integrated sialendoscope
Irrigation system (20-mL saline syringe with extension tubing)
Lacrimal probes
Microburs (0.38 mm and 0.8 mm)
Microforceps (0.38 mm and 0.8 mm)
Off-angle-tip sialendoscope
Salivary duct bougies
Salivary duct introducer
Stents/drains
Stone retrieval baskets (stainless steel and nitinol)
Straight-tip sialendoscope

History of the Procedure

In 1990, Konigsberger and Gundlach independently reported the first application of sialendoscopy during intracorporeal lithotripsy of salivary gland stones.[1] In 1991, Katz described a diagnostic sialendoscopy using a 0.8-mm flexible endoscope.[2] Following this, there were multiple reports of the use of intracorporeal lithotripsy by various authors with mixed results. In 1997, Nahlieli reported his 3-year experience using a semirigid modular system for the treatment of sialoliths and strictures. Since then, the technology and techniques have evolved to make sialendoscopy a common procedure for the treatment of obstructive salivary gland disorders.[3,4]

Sialendoscopy is an excellent tool for the management of obstructive salivary gland disease, either on its own or in conjunction with an open procedure. Prior to its development, the only recourse for patients with these issues was removal of the offending gland. Appropriate imaging for the diagnosis of the etiology of the obstruction should be obtained. The most common causes of salivary gland obstructions are mucous plugs, sialoliths, and strictures. The first step in treatment is identification of the orifice of the gland. Once the orifice is visualized, dilation probes are then placed. If the orifice cannot be seen, a papillotomy is performed, and the duct is identified and skeletonized. Once the opening into the duct, either through the orifice or the duct wall incision, is dilated to an appropriate size, a sialoendoscope is then placed. If the sialoendoscope will be inserted and removed multiple times, salivary duct introducer should be placed. If a sialolith is present, a retrieval basket is deployed through the working port of the scope, and the basket is rotated to surround the stone. Light pressure is applied, and the sialolith is removed either through the orifice or through a small incision. If a stricture is present, attempt to dilate with hydrodissection, dilation balloons, and microforceps. The need for the placement of a cylindrical drain is considered on a case-by-case basis secondary to the concern of adhesion formation from trauma to the duct.

The leading complication is perforation of the duct wall, resulting in extravasation of the fluid into the surrounding tissue. If there is a perforation and the sialoendoscope cannot be placed into the proximal duct, the procedure should be discontinued. If the obstruction cannot be resolved, a sialadenectomy of the gland for definitive treatment or injection of botulinum toxin for palliative treatment should be performed.

Indications for the Use of the Procedure

Sialendoscopy is an effective and safe procedure for the treatment of obstructive salivary gland disorders, particularly for the management of sialolithiasis. Sialoliths make up 60% to 70% of all obstructions. Sialendoscopy is a minimally invasive technique that maintains glandular function as well as providing a means for removing the obstruction. A growing body of literature has highlighted the efficacy of sialendoscopy. For example, an observational study of 5525 consecutive patients treated with minimally invasive techniques, including sialendoscopy, reported that 80% of salivary calculi were removed, with only 2.9% of the patients having refractory symptoms that required removal of the salivary gland.[5]

Sialoliths are composed of calcium salts, desquamated epithelial cells, bacterial colonies, and mucus. The etiology of sialolithiasis is not exactly known. It is hypothesized that the initiating factor is salivary stasis from mucus, which causes a

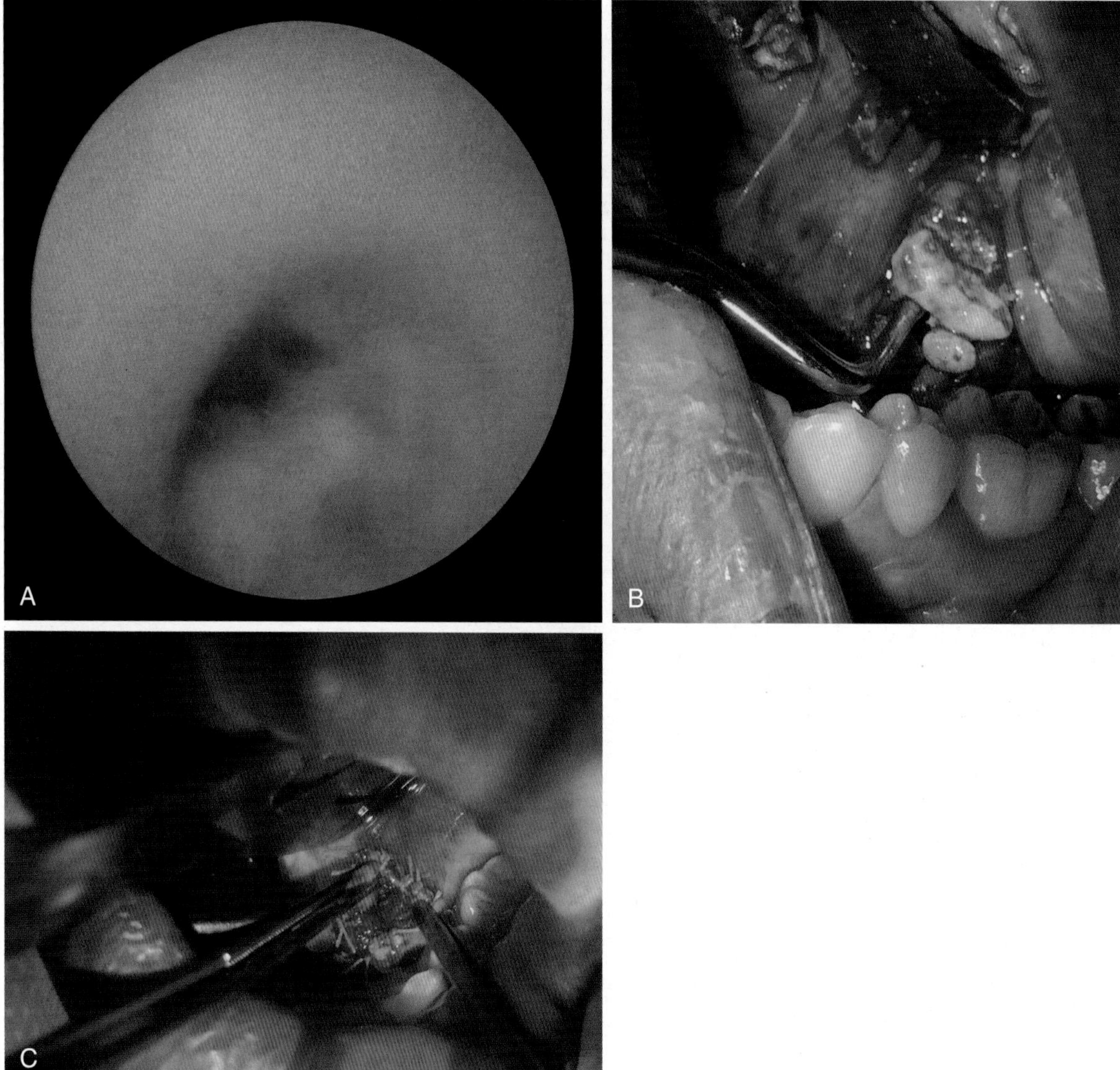

Figure 101.1 Left large submandibular obstructive and infected sialolith. **A,** Sialendoscopy view through a 1.1 sialendoscope confirming patency of the Wharton duct and removal of proximal fibrous adhesions. **B,** Removal of sialolith through a transoral incision. **C,** Creation of a complex sialodochoplasty. By having a patent duct and a sialodochoplasty, postoperative obstruction becomes unlikely because of the redundant drainage pathways.

concentration of saliva. A precipitation of the salivary minerals occurs, resulting in a calcification of the mucous plugs. Over time, these sialoliths, depending on their location, become large enough in size to cause a full or partial obstruction.

Sialoliths most often occur in the submandibular glands (90%) because of the high mucous content, and to a much lesser extent, in the parotid glands (10%) because the saliva is more serous in composition. There are a small number of cases where sialoliths have been found in sublingual glands. Submandibular gland stones are located in the hilum of the glands (57%), within the submandibular ducts (34%), and with much less frequency, in the gland parenchyma (9%). The areas with the highest amount of stasis are the puncta, where the orifice of the duct is narrowed or obliterated; at the junction of the lingual nerve and the duct; and proximal to the mylohyoid muscle, where the duct joins the hilum. Parotid gland sialoliths are mainly found in distal parotid ducts (64%), the smaller proximal ducts (23%), and in the hilum (13%).[6,7]

Interventional sialendoscopy is utilized to retrieve small mobile stone (<5 mm). Mobilization and fragmentation can be attempted for soft stones up to 7 mm. Extracorporeal shock-wave therapy can be utilized for sialoliths between 5 and 7 mm, or when a sialolith has an adherent fibrous capsule. The major reason it has not been adopted as an adjunctive modality is that it has a low target precision, and more importantly, there is a lack of approved devices globally. Because of this, it has fallen out of the treatment algorithm for most providers. Impacted stones and stones larger than 10 mm need to be removed with sialendoscopy combined approaches. In the submandibular gland, an intraoral incision is used for exposure and removal, and for the parotid gland, transfacial glandular access along with a transglandular dissection to the sialolith is used[7] (Figure 101.1).

Clinically, patients with an obstruction commonly present with prandial pain and swelling. It has been reported in the literature that swelling is present in 94% of cases, followed by pain in 65.2%, and purulent discharge in 15.5%. There are a small group of patients (2.4%) who are asymptomatic, although this number is not necessarily accurate because most asymptomatic stones are found incidentally.[7] With sialoliths, the magnitude of symptoms depends on their location and size and the mobility of the calculi. A concurrent infection can also be present, presenting with exudate drainage. Patients with obstructive salivary gland disease do not necessarily have a secondary infection, and patients with salivary gland infections do not necessarily have a salivary gland obstruction, although both can be present at the same time.

Nonsurgical treatment of patients with an obstructive gland condition includes hydration (up to 2 L of IV or PO intake of nonalcoholic fluid), glandular massage, and the use of moist heat. Most obstructive conditions are caused by mucous plugs that resolve spontaneously or can be quickly disrupted on examination. In managing salivary obstructions, sialagogues should be avoided, particularly in the presence of nonmobile sialoliths because of the pain and swelling from accumulation of saliva proximal to the obstruction.[6] Mucous plugs tend to resolve within 24 hours. The diagnosis of a sialolith or stricture should be considered in the presence of recurrent obstructions.

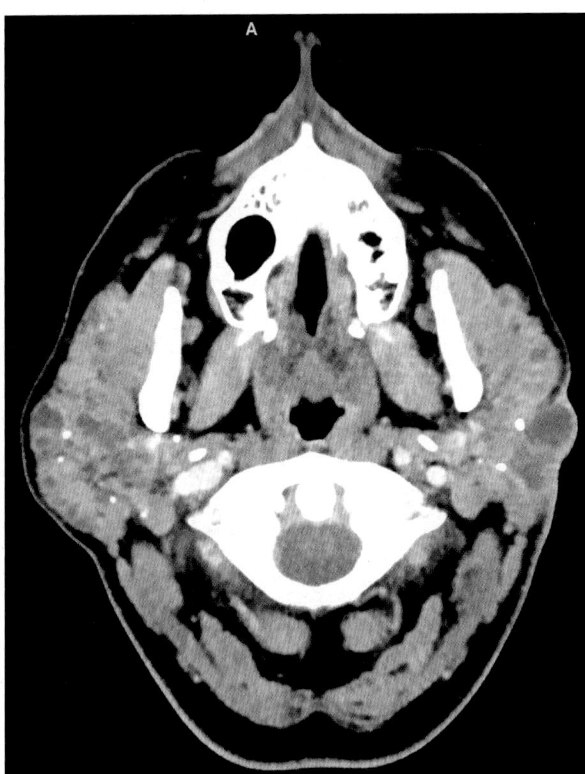

Figure 101.2 Patient CT with 15-year history of Sjögren syndrome with concurrent obstructive disease and infections. Visible sialectasias, calcifications, and abscesses.

Sialadenitis

Inflammation and edematous thickening of duct walls are characteristics of sialadenitis. Sialadenitis is most common in the parotid gland and often presents with recurrent salivary gland swelling and mucous plugs. Its management centers around irrigation, ductal dilation, and intraductal steroid administration via sialendoscopy.

Although the main obstructive etiologies are sialoliths (60% to 70%), stenosis and strictures (15% to 25%), and sialadenitis of unknown origin (5% to 10%). A small number of cases are due to anatomic variations of the duct system or retained foreign bodies.

Stenosis

There are two forms of stenosis of the duct. The first is a stricture, which is a localized narrowing stenosis of the duct by a scar band, and the second is a generalized stenotic duct, which is a fibrosis of the majority of the duct wall. The majority of strictures occur in the parotid duct. They are primarily located in the middle third of the duct, followed by the proximal third. A majority of stenosis cases are due to chronic sialadenitis of the glands or embedded sialoliths.[8]

Salivary duct stenosis is primarily idiopathic in nature, and they can be secondary to other disease processes. One of the most common causes of secondary stenosis are autoimmune diseases. The two most common autoimmune diseases are Sjögren syndrome and systematic lupus erythematosus. The pathophysiology of Sjögren syndrome was initially hypothesized as a direct auto-antibody destruction of saliva-secreting acinar cells. This model has become more complex due to advancements in genetics and molecule technology. The comorbidities posed by decreased saliva formation include increased incidences of dental caries, chronic periodontal disease, and oral *Candida*. Hyposalivation also leads to loss of pH buffering, mechanical cleansing, and the loss of function of the salivary immune system.[9]

In patients with Sjögren syndrome, 25% to 50% experience enlargement of one or both parotid glands. The etiology of the enlargement includes inflammation, stricture formation, mucous plugging, or a combination of all three. Sialography highlights the presence of multiple sialectasias and strictures of the salivary gland duct, which is a pathognomonic finding of the Sjögren syndrome diseased gland. Ultrasonography, computed tomography (CT), and sialograms can reveal multiple small hypoechogenic areas and punctate calcification[10] (Figure 101.2).

Management of the inflammation involves nonsteroidal antiinflammatory medications and conservative therapy. Disease progression results in the lysis of the acinar cells and an increase in the percentage of the salivary mucous content. This leads to the formation of mucous plugs, obstruction of the gland, and further sialadenitis.

Other etiologies of stenosis are changes secondary to radioactive iodine used in the management of thyroid cancer. The average radioiodine dose administered for therapy ranges

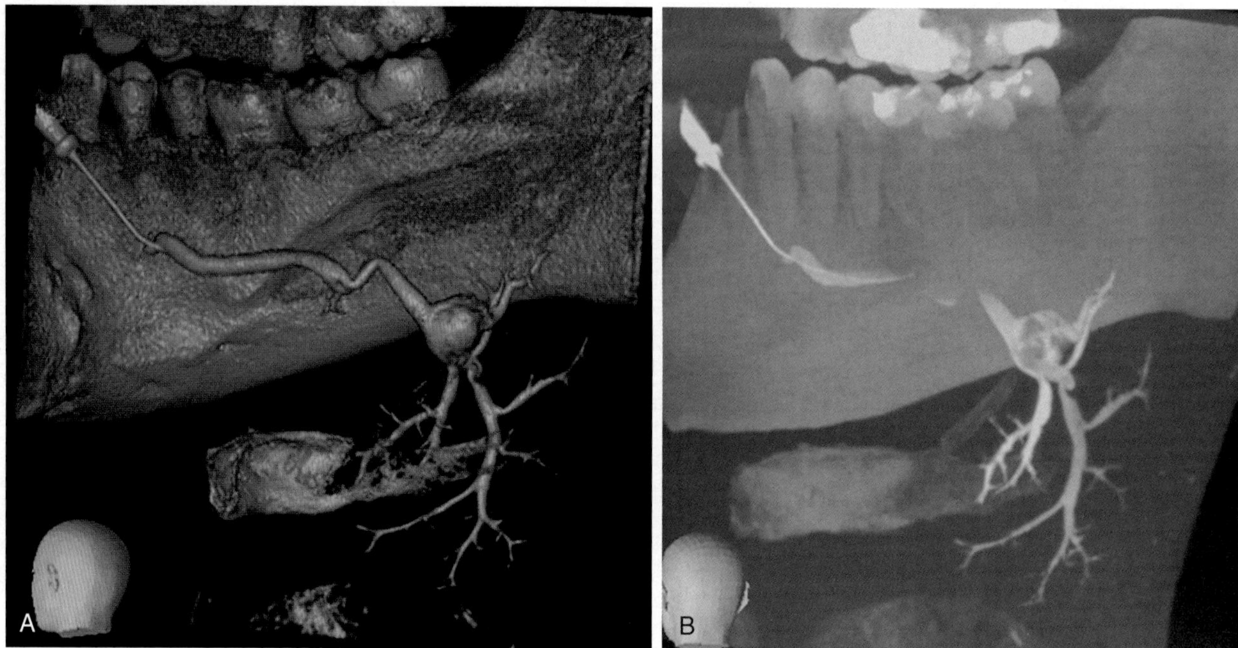

Figure 101.3 Imaging of a right submandibular gland sialolith. A, Cone-beam computed tomography sialogram three-dimensional reconstruction. B, Cone-beam computed tomography sialogram sagittal view. (Courtesy of Dr. Oded Nahlieli)

from 0.81 to 4.05 MBq. Serous salivary cells, like the thyroid, have cellular wall sodium-iodine symporters that bring radioactive iodine into the cells. Because the parotid gland is composed primarily of serous cells, it is the most commonly affected salivary gland. Clinical presentation of this disease entity consists of postprandial episodes of swelling and severe tenderness on palpation. Other etiological factors of stenosis are trauma and iatrogenic and congenital anomalies.

Imaging

The four commonly utilized imaging techniques in patients with salivary gland obstructions are ultrasound, CT, sialogram (or a combination CT/sialogram), and magnetic resonance imaging (MRI). Noncontrast CT remains the gold standard for diagnostic purposes, although a CT-sialogram better shows the etiology and location of the obstruction as well as the anatomy of the duct system (Figure 101.3).

Radiographically, the majority of salivary calculi are radiopaque (80% of submandibular calculi and 60% of parotid calculi). Ultrasound is also an accurate technique with no radiation and is significantly less expensive. It can be performed by the provider during their examination, although the procedure is technique sensitive and inaccurate in inexperienced hands. Ultrasound has the advantage of providing information about the condition of the gland in addition to size, location, and number of sialoliths. MRI is excellent for diagnosing masses and cysts but is expensive and no more accurate than a CT in diagnosing obstructions.[11]

Conventional and CT sialography, as well as ultrasonography, are useful for diagnosing these conditions. However, the only tool that can directly evaluate the extent and severity of the stenosis is sialendoscopy. The degree of stenosis is assessed by visualization of the duct lumen at the location of the stricture utilizing a 1.1-mm sialoendoscope for minor stenosis and 0.8-mm sialoendoscope for moderate to severe cases. The considerations for treatment of stenosis are location, degree of obstruction, and the length and type of tissue in the affected areas.

Limitations and Contraindications

Limited mouth opening, intraparenchymal stone, acute sialadenitis, and complete distal duct stenosis are contraindications for sialendoscopy.

STANDARD TECHNIQUE

Sialendoscopy is a clean-contaminated technique; therefore, prophylactic antibiotics are indicated prior to the procedure (ampicillin sodium/sulbactam sodium 3.0 g or clindamycin 600 mg). Intravenous corticoid steroid can also be administered to decrease postsurgical edema.

STANDARD TECHNIQUE:—*cont'd*

STEP 1: POSITIONING

If the procedure is being performed under general anesthesia, nasotracheal intubation is recommended to allow for unimpeded access to the oral cavity. Patients should be placed in a supine position with their back, with head and torso elevated between 15 degrees and 45 degrees. The surgeon stands contralateral to the operative site. For the office setting, sialagogues, such as lemon juice, can be placed on the tongue to stimulate salivary flow and dilation of the orifice. Regional local anesthesia with vasoconstrictors is used for regional nerve blocks for dilation and surgical incision sites. A mouth prop is placed contralateral to the operative site.

STEP 2: ACCESS AND DILATION

The next step is localization and visualization of the orifice to the duct, which can be challenging. The gland should first be palpated and pressure applied in a distal direction. Magnification is recommended for ideal results. If the orifice is seen, a pair of small-toothed forceps is used to pull the mucosa 2–3 mm anterior to the orifice. Grasping the papilla will cause bleeding, punctures into the papilla, and distortion of the local anatomy, and can lead to the creation of a false passage.

Dilation probes are placed sequentially. Circular movements at the orifice with the probe will stretch the lumen with light pressure. The smaller diameter probes can perforate the duct walls, creating a false passage. During dilation, the sialolith can be dislodged proximally, deeper into the gland where it can lodge in a smaller duct, so judicious use of force is recommended. The vector of insertion of the probes needs to be maintained uniformly at all times. If the sialendoscope will be inserted multiple times during the procedure, a salivary gland duct introducer should be inserted to prevent continued injury to the duct wall and papilla (Figure 101.4).

STEP 3: SIALENDOSCOPY

Once the duct is dilated, a sialoendoscope is introduced. If the cause of the obstruction is unknown, then a diagnostic sialendoscopy is performed with a 0.8- or 1.1-mm sialoendoscope. Irrigation tubing is attached to the irrigation port, and normal saline or lactated Ringer's solution is infiltrated to create an optical cavity. To identify a perforation of the duct, careful monitoring (of the floor of the mouth for the submandibular duct and the juncture of the masseter and buccinator muscles for the parotid duct) is necessary to identify signs of fluid extravasation.

The endoscope is then advanced down the center of the duct lumen, navigating the turns and major branches of the duct system. In the parotid gland, the most difficult area to traverse is between the masseter and buccinator muscles. This is the region where the duct turns from its deep position (closer to the oral cavity) to a more superficial location prior to the entrance into the parotid gland proper. Excessive force in this area can cause a perforation through the duct wall. If this occurs, it is difficult, although not impossible, to locate the proximal duct. Discontinuing the procedure can be considered at this time to prevent further injury or even transection of the duct. The area that is difficult to access in the submandibular duct is at the posterior border of mylohyoid muscle. Because the submandibular duct and the lingual nerve are in close proximity in this region, a perforation of the duct can result in a nerve injury (Figure 101.5).

The duct should be examined for vascularity and corrugation. In the absence of a sialolith, the scope should be advanced to the hilum and into the gland. If treating obstructive mucous plugs, this hydrodissection into the gland is, for the most part, curative. Within the gland, the ducts begin to branch into smaller ducts. The different ducts should each be explored, if possible (depending upon the diameter of the duct and the size of the sialendoscope being utilized).

For patients with duct stenosis, hydrostatic pressure is used to dilate the duct. The duct can also be expanded using microforceps and dilating balloons. A high-pressure dilation balloon can rupture the duct so deployment must be performed with endoscopic visualization when in the submandibular duct or with ultrasound guidance when in the parotid duct. Following dilation, the sialoendoscope should be inserted again, and loose scar tissue and debris should be removed.

Nonmobile sialoliths are usually associated with an overlying fibrous capsule. The sialendoscope should not be pushed past the sialolith since this can result in deflection and perforation of the duct, or displacement of the stone deeper into the gland, making it irretrievable, and further fracturing of the sialolith into multiple pieces. A fractured sialolith can be problematic since it will create multiple areas of deeper, inaccessible obstructions. To decrease the risk of this occurence, a microforceps is used to remove the fibrous tissue so that the sialolith can be visualized.

Continued

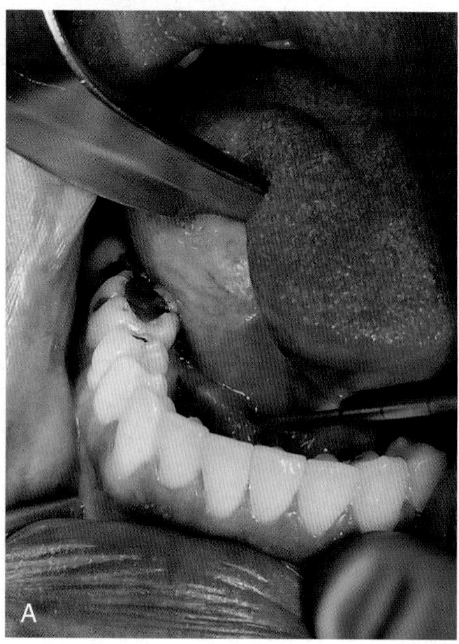

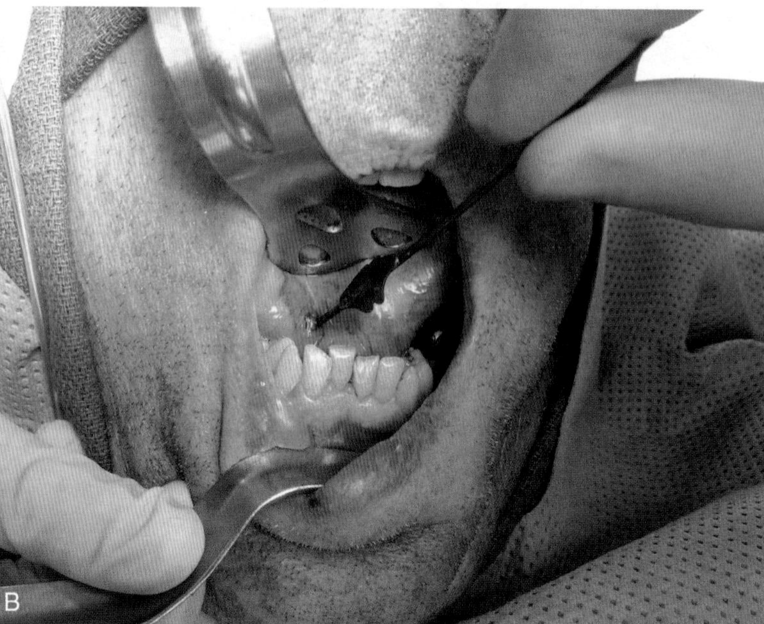

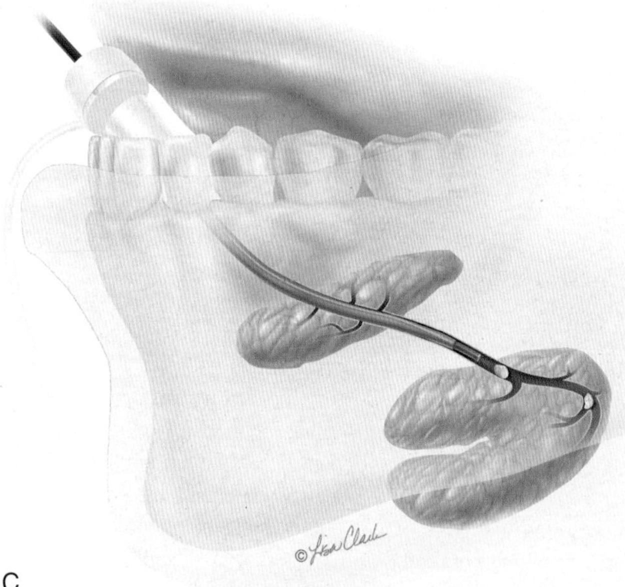

Figure 101.4 Dilation of the orifice of the duct can be performed with a variety of instrumentations. **A,** Dilation of right submandibular duct using a tapered Schaitkin probe (Karl Storz, Tuttlingen, Germany). **B,** Dilation utilizing a lacrimal probe. **C,** Insertion of Kolenda Salivary Duct Introducer. (© 2011 Lisa Clark.)

STANDARD TECHNIQUE:—*cont'd*

STEP 5: RETRIEVAL OF THE SIALOLITH

Once the sialolith is identified, a wire retrieval basket is inserted through the sialendoscope and extended into the duct. For sialoliths that have a regular contour and are parallel along the major axis, either a side-loading retrieval basket or front grasping basket can be used. To use a side-loading basket, the tip is placed proximal to the stone; it is then opened and pulled back until the basket strands are between the wall of duct and the stone. The basket is then rotated with a twirling motion until the stone is within the basket (Figure 101.6). Once the stone is acquired, the basket is fully closed. Constant pressure is applied with visualization while the sialendoscope and stone are removed. Excessive force should be avoided to prevent avulsion of the duct. The front grasping basket has the advantage of not having to pass between the lumen and the stone, although they are difficult to use in sialoliths that are embedded into the duct wall. If the sialolith is unable to pass through the duct orifice, a small incision using either a scalpel or electrocautery should be made overlying the palpable stone.

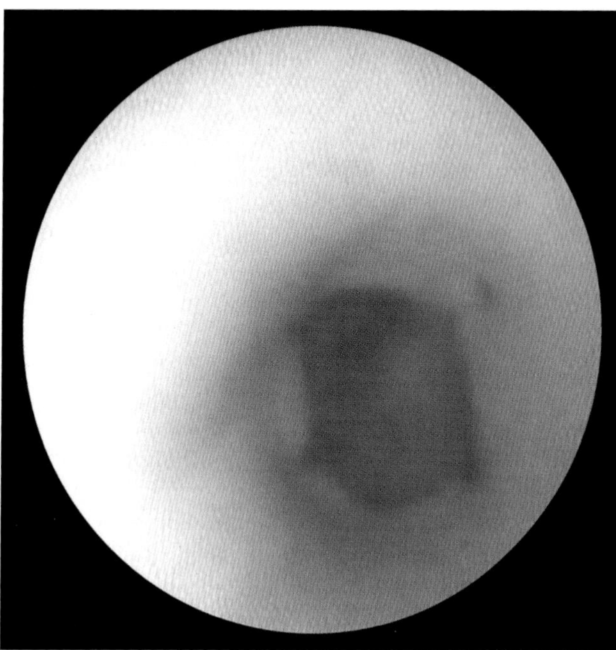

Figure 101.5 Perforation of the salivary duct with visualization of the interstitial tissue.

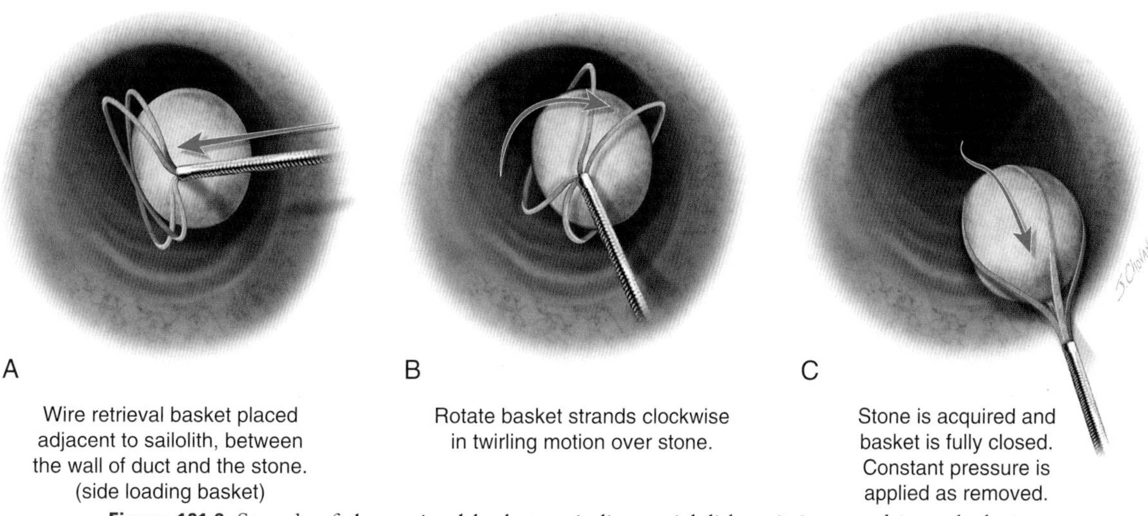
A
Wire retrieval basket placed adjacent to sailolith, between the wall of duct and the stone. (side loading basket)
B
Rotate basket strands clockwise in twirling motion over stone.
C
Stone is acquired and basket is fully closed. Constant pressure is applied as removed.

Figure 101.6 Strands of the retrieval basket encircling a sialolith as it is rotated in a clockwise direction.

STANDARD TECHNIQUE:—*cont'd*

STEP 6: REEXPLORATION AND DRAIN PLACEMENT

All branches of the salivary duct need to be retraced prior to exiting the lumen in order to detect and remove any residual calculi. Placement of the drain is necessary in the parotid gland because of the high rate of stenosis of the orifice failing manipulation. Submandibular ducts do not always need to have a drain placed if no incision were made or if the duct was not traumatized by the procedure. If a drain is placed (ideally under endoscopic visualization into the hilum), it should be secured into position with 4-0 Vicryl sutures. The drain should remain in place for 2 to 4 weeks, although it is not unusual for it to be dislodged out of the duct from the movement of the tongue and the cheek.

ALTERNATE OR MODIFIED TECHNIQUE

ALTERNATIVE TECHNIQUE FOR DILATION

Sialendoscopy can be utilized purely as a diagnostic tool in patients with unknown etiologies as well as a means of treatment, including adjunctive enhancement when used with open surgical procedures. Sialendoscopy via hydrodissection and microinstrumentation is utilized for disruption of mucous plugs and infiltration of an intraglandular corticoid steroid. A retrospective study of endoscopic management of 34 patients with Sjögren syndrome with obstructive salivary gland symptoms reported a significant symptomatic improvement following treatement.[9] Similar to other studies, strictures and mucous plugs were the common etiology of the obstruction. In this cohort, only three patients experienced relapse of their symptoms after one year of being symptomatic.

Dilation of the duct can also be performed by using a low-pressure dilation balloon within the distal portion of the duct. If a balloon dilator is not available, a size 3 or 4 Fogarty catheter can be used instead. Bougie dilators are another alternative instrument for dilation, either by themselves or in conjunction with a guidewire. If using a guidewire, care should be taken not to inadvertently perforate the duct wall. Sialendoscopy with insufflation, hydrodissection, and injection of 100 mg hydrocortisone has been used successfully to manage this condition. Studies have found that patients remained symptom free for 1 to 4 years after their initial sialendoscopy.[12]

Interventions based on clinical findings are as follows:

- Nonvisible duct orifice.
  - When the orifice in the papilla is not visible, a light coat of methylene blue can be painted over the region. The orifice can be dilated and visualized unless it is completely stenosed by either using pressure on the gland or a sialagogue if the patient is awake.
  - If the orifice of the duct is stenosed, a papillotomy should be performed. It is a U-shaped incision made around the papilla, avoiding transection of the duct. The duct is then located and skeletonized free from the surrounding tissues. A small incision is made into the duct wall using a #11 blade, and the sialoendoscope is advanced into the duct. Care should be taken not to place the tip of the blade too deep into the lumen or the opposite duct wall can be inadvertently incised as well.
  - If the parotid papilla cannot be identified, conversion to a transoral or extraoral combined approach can be considered. The description of these procedures goes beyond the scope of this chapter.
- Ductal stenosis in the distal parotid duct with a visible papilla is challenging if the adhesions or strictures are present within 2 cm of the orifice. A technique that can be used in this situation is placement of a guidewire through the working port of the sialoendoscope. If the wire can be passed through the stenosis, the scope can be removed and a dilation balloon is inserted over the guidewire and insufflated. If a focal stricture is encountered, a handheld microdrill can also be used, but once again, perforation of the duct wall can occur.
- Hilar and intraductal stenoses are difficult to correct. If the patient has persistent symptoms despite multiple dilation attempts, palliative relief can be achieved through injections of botulinum toxin or the definitive treatment of a sialadenectomy.

Avoidance and Management of Intraoperative Complications

- Airway compromise: The airway can be compromised because of extravasated fluid into the floor of the mouth from a perforated duct. If this occurs, the patient should remain intubated. The saline is absorbed into the surrounding tissue, and the edema will decrease within 24 hours.
- Perforation of the duct wall is a common occurrence and can be prevented (in most cases) by maintaining the vector insertion of dilators and using light pressure. Early recognition should allow for recannulation of the proximal duct. If the proximal duct cannot be located, the procedure should either be discontinued or converted to an open approach.
- Injury to the lingual nerve can occur if the duct is perforated or during the dissection in a combined approach. In a combined procedure, the duct should be identified and dissected until the lingual nerve is identified. The nerve should be skeletonized away from the duct to avoid it being injured.
- Small sialoliths may not be initially visualized. Care should be taken to not irrigate aggressively since this can displace the sialoliths proximally, making them irretrievable.
- A drain that is shorter than the duct can move deeper into the gland. The drain should ideally be radiopaque so it can be located on imaging and retrieved.

Postoperative Considerations

Postoperatively, glandular massage and maintaining daily hydration help maintain patency. If the drain is removed or dislodged earlier than expected, and obstructive symptoms return, both regular and frequent sequential dilation of the duct should be performed or the procedure repeated, as indicated.

References

1. Gundlach P, Scherer H, Hopf J, Leege N, Muller G, Hirst L, et al. Endoscopic-controlled laser lithotripsy of salivary calculi. In vitro studies and initial clinical use. *HNO*. 1990;38(7):247–250. PubMed PMID: 2394601. Epub 1990/07/01.
2. Katz P. New method of examination of the salivary glands: the fiberscope. *Inf Dent*. 1990;72(10):785–786. PubMed PMID: 2387611. Epub 1990/03/08.
3. Nahlieli O, Neder A, Baruchin AM. Salivary gland endoscopy: a new technique for diagnosis and treatment of sialolithiasis. *J Oral Maxillofac Surg*. 1994;52(12):1240–1242.
4. Zenk J, Hosemann WG, Iro H. Diameters of the main excretory ducts of the adult human submandibular and parotid gland: a histologic study. *Oral Surg Oral Med Oral Pathol Oral Radiol Endod*. 1998;85(5):576–580.
5. Iro H, Zenk J, Escudier MP, et al. Outcome of minimally invasive management of salivary calculi in 4,691 patients. *Laryngoscope*. 2009;119(2):263–268.
6. Koch M, Zenk J, Iro H. Algorithms for treatment of salivary gland obstructions. *Otolaryngol Clin North Am*. 2009;42(6):1173–1192 (Table of Contents).
7. Turner MD. Combined surgical approaches for the removal of submandibular gland sialoliths. *Atlas Oral Maxillofac Surg Clin North Am*. 2018;26(2):145–151.
8. Jackson EM, Walvekar RR. Surgical techniques for the management of parotid salivary duct strictures. *Atlas Oral Maxillofac Surg Clin North Am*. 2018;26(2):93–98.
9. Turner MD. Salivary gland disease in Sjögren's syndrome: sialoadenitis to lymphoma. *Oral Maxillofac Surg Clin North Am*. 2014;26(1):75–81.
10. Shacham R, Puterman MB, Ohana N, Nahlieli O. Endoscopic treatment of salivary glands affected by autoimmune diseases. *J Oral Maxillofac Surg*. 2011;69(2):476–481.
11. Hoffman HT, Pagedar NA. Ultrasound-guided salivary gland techniques and Interpretations. *Atlas Oral Maxillofac Surg Clin North Am*. 2018;26(2):119–132.
12. Nahlieli O, Nazarian Y. Sialadenitis following radioiodine therapy—a new diagnostic and treatment modality. *Oral Dis*. 2006;12(5):476–479.

CHAPTER 102

Thyroidectomy

Curtis Hanba, Brendan H. G. Pierce, Ashok R. Jethwa, and Maria Evasovich

Armamentarium

#15 Scalpel blade
Appropriate sutures
Army-Navy retractor
Bipolar cautery
Carmalt clamp
Fine-tipped dissector
Ligaclips
Local anesthetic with vasoconstrictor
Monopolar cautery
Nerve monitoring
Scalpel
Self-retractor
Senn retractors
Spoon

History of the Procedure

Accounts of thyroid pathology date back to 2700 BC. At the time, seaweed and iodine-rich sea sponges were used by the Chinese in an attempt to medically manage hypertrophic goiters. It was over a thousand years later that the Romans documented operative treatment for enlarged thyroid pathology. Leonardo da Vinci was one of the first artists to detail thyroid anatomy, doing so around 1500 AD, yet thyroid surgery continued to be a dangerous endeavor into the 1800s. In one account Samuel Gross warned "every stroke of the knife will be followed by a torrent of blood," and he further stated "no honest and sensible surgeon would ever engage in it."[1] It was not until later in the 19th century that Theodor Kocher revised thyroidectomy technique and lowered the procedure's mortality through increased antiseptic practices. In doing so, thyroidectomy would reach a mortality rate of less than 1%[2] by the middle of the 20th century.

The operative approach to thyroidectomy has evolved extensively with the advent of new surgical tools. In 1998, Miccoli and his group at the University of Pisa reported an endoscopic technique for thyroidectomy that has since become a widely used practice by minimal-access surgeons around the globe. Robotic-assisted thyroidectomy offers another minimal-access approach to the gland.

Despite the introduction of these novel techniques, conventional open thyroidectomy is still considered the surgical gold standard management of thyroid disease. This chapter details indications, workup, and technique for conventional open management of thyroid pathology.

Indications for Thyroidectomy

Thyroid disease is relatively common, and several medical associations have developed consensus guidelines for the medical and surgical management of thyroid pathology.[3–5] Surgery for benign thyroid pathology is primarily reserved for patients with symptomatic or compressive goiters. However, in some cases, benign, noncompressive thyroid nodules are removed based on patient requests as they may affect their quality of life.

Thyroidectomy remains a potentially definitive treatment for Graves disease. Indications for the procedure include moderate to severe associated ophthalmopathy, pregnancy or breastfeeding status, persistent hyperthyroidism after radioablation and/or maximal medical therapy, suspicion or diagnosed malignancy, or compressive symptoms.[6] Hyperactive multinodular goiters with thyroidal volume greater than 80 mL can also demonstrate a decreased ability for successful ablation using radioactive iodine, encouraging primary thyroidectomy as an appropriate management strategy.[7]

Concern for malignancy is often an indication for either partial or total thyroidectomy.

Thyroid nodules are clinically palpable in 4% to 7% of patients, with ultrasound identifying additional nodules in up to 50% of asymptomatic persons.[3,4,8,9] In concordance with National Comprehensive Cancer Network (NCCN) and American Thyroid Association (ATA) guidelines, the initial evaluation of a nodule should include measurement of serum thyrotropin levels, with ultrasound or radioiodine uptake scans utilized as appropriate.

Ultrasound-guided fine-needle aspiration remains the standard of care for cytologically assessing suspicious thyroid nodules. The utility of fine-needle aspiration is most commonly guided by nodule size and ultrasound characteristics as classified by the 2017 ACR Thyroid Imaging Reporting and Data System (TI-RADS).[10] Coincidentally, 2017 also introduced a revision to the Bethesda System for Reporting Thyroid Cytopathology (BSRTC), the most commonly implemented cytological classification system for reporting thyroid FNA cytology.[11] In agreement with the ATA and

NCCN recommendations, the 2017 BSRTC also introduced molecular testing as an option for patients with indeterminant cytology after fine-needle aspiration.[3,4] Currently, three clinically validated molecular tests are available for use in the United States (Table 102.1). Alternatively, one can consider observation, repeat fine-needle aspiration, or surgical lobectomy for managing indeterminant thyroid nodules, with the decision in part based on clinical assessment and patient preference.

Often, surgical lobectomy is the procedure of choice for managing differentiated thyroid malignancy. Indications for total thyroidectomy include known metastasis, extrathyroidal extension, a primary tumor >4 cm, cervical lymph node involvement, and poorly differentiated disease.[3] Consideration for total thyroidectomy is appropriate in the setting of known radiation exposure or bilateral thyroidal nodularity.[3]

Surgical Workup

Thyroidectomy is most commonly performed under general anesthesia. Prior to the operation, a general practitioner and anesthesia team should assess a patient's candidacy to safely undergo the operation. Additionally, it is the surgical team's responsibility to assess a patient's neck, remarking on prior surgical intervention, abnormally palpable vasculature, and surgical access limitations related to anticipated positioning challenges. A patient's voice should be assessed, and laryngoscopy should be performed in the setting of vocal abnormalities, history of prior neck or chest surgery, or suspected extralaryngeal spread of thyroid pathology.[12] Ideally, the vocal cords should be examined or evaluated prior to every thyroid surgery. Abnormal vocal fold movement can be observed in up to 60% of patients preoperatively, and if noted, should be documented in the patient's medical chart prior to performing the procedure.[13,14] Finally, a lateral and central compartment neck ultrasound should be performed to evaluate for lymphadenopathy, with lymph node biopsy suggested for nodules greater than 0.8 to 1.0 cm in size.[3,4] Thyroglobulin washout studies can increase the diagnostic yield of fine-needle aspiration, especially in cystic or hypervascular nodules.[15] Thyroglobulin levels >1 ng/mL support a diagnosis of metastatic disease in the context of indeterminant fine-needle aspiration.[15]

Postoperative Considerations and Management

Total thyroidectomy requires lifelong thyroid hormone replacement. A patient must reliably have access to this medication prior to offering surgery. For patients with uncontrolled hyperthyroidism, or autoimmune-related thyroid pathology, surgical manipulation can trigger an acute release of thyroid hormone requiring medical and anesthetic management to avoid devastating consequence related to thyroid storm. In this scenario, postoperative monitoring and hormone replacement should involve an endocrinology team when available. Pregnancy can be both an indication and contraindication to performing thyroidectomy. In cases of refractory hyperthyroidism, surgical treatment can be potentially curative, although anesthetic risks to the future child may outweigh the necessity of the operation.[16] A multidisciplinary approach to managing thyroid pathology in pregnancy should be utilized when available. Generally, differentiated thyroid malignancies are observed during pregnancy and treated surgically following delivery.

Table 102.1 Three Clinically Validated Molecular Tests

Assessment	NPV	PPV	SN	SP	Prevalence[a]
MPTX	95%	74%	93%	90%	30%
ThyroSeq v3	97%	66%	94%	82%	28%
Afirma GSC	96%	47%	91%	68%	24%

[a]Malignancy prevalence within tested cohort.
NPV, Negative predictive value; *PPV*, positive predictive value; *SN*, sensitivity; *SP*, specificity.

TECHNIQUE: Total Thyroidectomy

Open thyroidectomy remains the gold standard in thyroid surgery. Alternative techniques include robotic-assisted or endoscopic approaches. These procedures should be performed at specialized institutions familiar with the equipment and protocols necessary to offer a safe alternative to conventional thyroidectomy.

STEP 1: Incision Location

In the preoperative unit with the patient in an upright position, a midline 4-cm planned incision is marked in a natural skin crease below or at the level of the cricoid cartilage to best camouflage the scar. The incision can be lengthened for large goiters or complicated cases (Fig. 102.1A).

STEP 2: Intubation and Prep

It is important to discuss with your anesthesia colleagues the need to refrain from using long-term paralytics on induction and during the surgery, as this impedes the ability to stimulate the recurrent laryngeal nerves, which is necessary for an electromyographic (EMG) endotracheal tube (ET). A video laryngoscope is used for intubation so the surgeon and anesthesiologist can observe the correct placement of the surface electrode laryngeal EMG ET. By doing so, the surgeon can identify the correct depth of the intubation and ensure that the ET electrodes are in contact with the true vocal cords (Fig. 102.1B).

The skin of a premarked incision is (optionally) cleaned with alcohol and injected with 1% lidocaine and epinephrine at a 1:100,000 mixture. A shoulder roll is placed for mild neck extension, and the patient's head rests on a surgical foam donut. The patient is prepped from the chin to at least 4 cm below the clavicles and laterally to the trapezius, then draped for surgery (Fig. 102.1C and D).

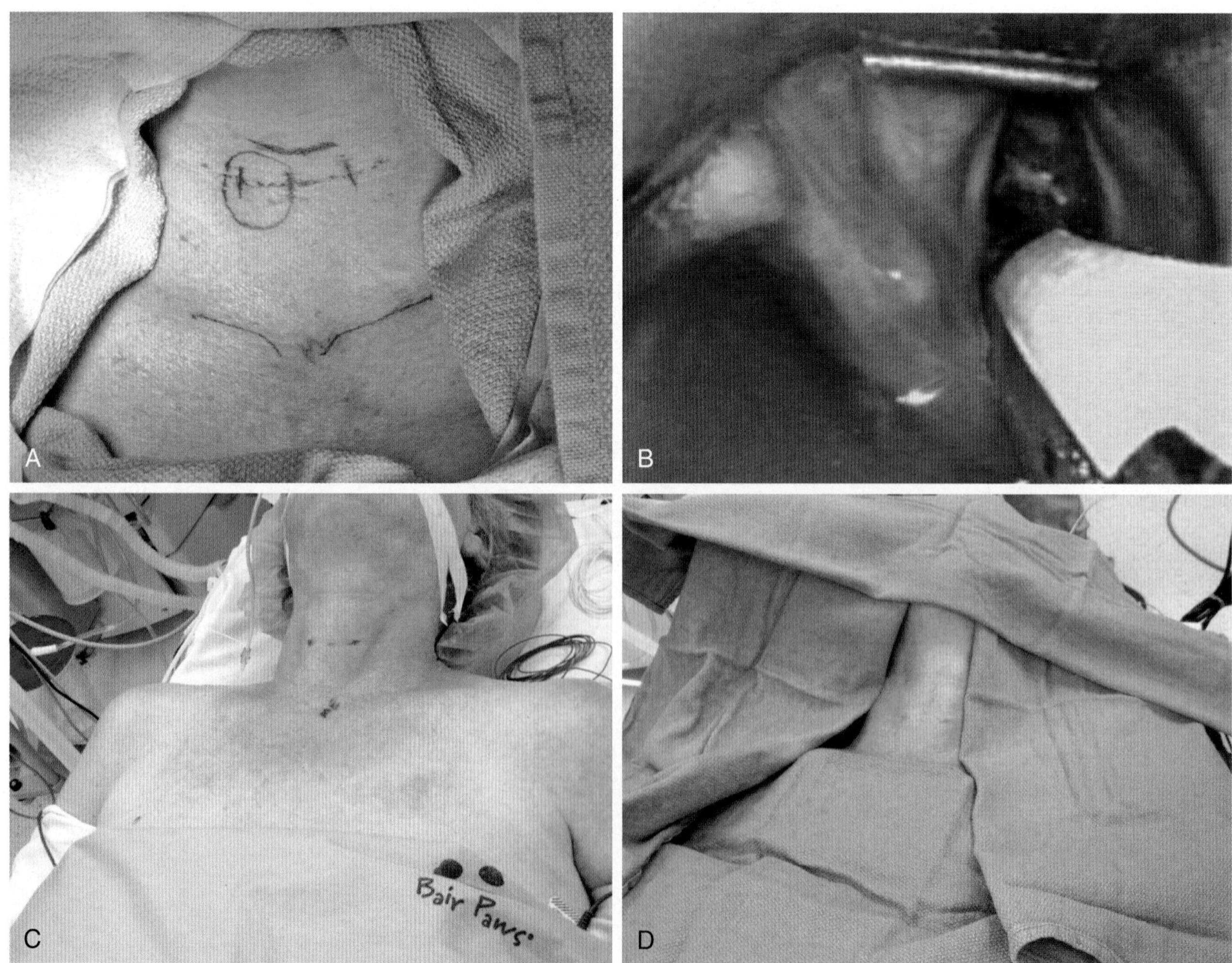

Figure 102.1 **A,** Cricoid cartilage marked, incision marked with the size of the nodule, and clavicles marked. **B,** Endotracheal tube as it is being placed; the white portion of the tube must be in contact with the true vocal cord. **C,** Patient with a marked incision, slightly extended with a shoulder roll in place. **D,** Patient prepped.

TECHNIQUE: Total Thyroidectomy—*cont'd*

STEP 3: Incision

Incision with a knife is made through the skin, dermis, superficial cervical fascia, and the platysma. Note that the platysma is absent at the midline. The anterior jugular veins will be deep to the superficial cervical fascia layer as the platysma and may need to be ligated with either suture or the harmonic scalpel (Ethicon Endosurgery, Cincinnati, Ohio) or LigaSure (Covidien, Dublin, Ireland) if they interfere with exposure. Smaller vessels may be cauterized, but minimal cautery is used at skin edges, as this may exacerbate scar formation.

STEP 4: Raising Subplatysmal Flaps

Senn retractors can be used to assist in raising the subplatysmal flap, extending from the thyroid cartilage to the level of the sternal notch. The correct plane should be avascular.

STEP 5: Divide the Midline Straps

The fatty tissue over the superficial layer of the deep cervical fascia is dissected midline down through the midline raphe. The assistant and surgeon retract the sternohyoid muscles. Dissection continues vertically in the avascular plane. Dissection is continued to the thyroid capsule. The strap muscles are retracted laterally and bluntly dissected inferiorly and superiorly to maximize visualization of the gland. If a lobectomy is to be performed, only elevate the ipsilateral strap muscles to decrease scar formation in the event that a completion thyroidectomy needs to be performed in the future. With larger goiters or invasive thyroid masses, it may be necessary to divide the strap muscles for greater exposure. When dividing the strap muscles, do so superiorly to preserve the ansa cervicalis innervation.

STEP 6: Ligating the Superior Pedicle

Use a Carmalt or a Kelly clamp to superficially grasp the capsule and a small amount of the gland; clamping a larger amount of thyroid gland increases the risk of bleeding from the thyroid. Manually retracting the gland is an alternate option. An assistant retracts the gland inferolaterally, the surgeon dissects between the trachea and gland to expose the Joll triangle. It is within this space that the external branch of the superior laryngeal nerve (ESLN) may be seen between the superior thyroid artery (STA), midline, and the cricothyroid muscle. The ESLN usually enters the larynx 1 cm superior to the thyroid gland.[17] Dissection of the ESLN need not be performed to minimize the risk of injury. Dissection is continued parallel to the superior thyroid vessels. The STA and vein are ligated individually as they enter the gland to minimize trauma to the ESLN. Ligation is performed as close to the gland as possible in a medial to lateral direction[18] to minimize the risk of injury to the SLN.[19] Ligations using suture, LigaSure,[20] a harmonic scalpel,[21] or clips are all acceptable methods. As you approach the dissection inferiorly and on the posterior portion of the gland, you should encounter the superior parathyroid glands, which present as a subtle caramel color. Once we identify the superior parathyroid gland, it is swept from the thyroid capsule, carefully maintaining its blood supply and viability (Fig. 102.1E–H). At this point, you can identify the recurrent laryngeal nerve slightly inferior and medial to the medial aspect of the superior parathyroid gland prior to or after addressing the middle thyroid vein.

STEP 7: Capsular Dissection and Ligation of Middle Thyroid Vein

Once the superior vessels have been ligated, the gland can be retracted inferiorly and medially to aid in dissection. The avascular tissue lateral and posterior to the thyroid is gently dissected, and any bleeding should be controlled with brief bipolar cautery. Dissection lateral to the capsule of the gland continues until the middle thyroid vein is encountered and ligated.

STEP 8: Identifying the Recurrent Laryngeal Nerve

Once the middle thyroid vein is divided, the gland can easily be retracted anteromedially, again with a Carmalt, Kelly clamp or manually. Visualization of the recurrent laryngeal nerve (RLN) is essential to good surgical outcomes, as demonstrated by lower incidence of vocal paresis with visualization.[22,23] Dissection to identify the RLN is done within the fatty tissue of the tracheoesophageal groove superior to the inferior thyroid artery (ITA). A Dietrich clamp is used to dissect parallel to the presumed course of the nerve due to its design, which offers a wide area to atraumatically dissect and visualize the structures between the tips. At this point, the NIM or similar nerve stimulator is beneficial to aid in mapping the course of the RLN. Especially in the area of the RLN, bipolar cautery and local pressure are used to control bleeding during dissection. As the nerve is traced superiorly, the branches can be identified at the level of or inferior to the cricothyroid membrane. The RLN is then dissected inferiorly to the ITA. It is paramount that all branches of the RLN are spared. The anterior branch supplies the motor fibers to the larynx, with the branching point commonly superior to the ITA. Do not use the ITA as a landmark to identify the nerve because of its variable course. The RLN is found running posterior to the artery 35% to 50% of the time in patients; it passes between the arterial branches in 24% to 30% of patients and is anterior to the artery in 21% to 32%.[24,25] The ligament of Berry is also not a reliable landmark, as a study of 143 cadavers found the RLN lateral to the ligament of Berry in 88.1%,[25] though

Continued

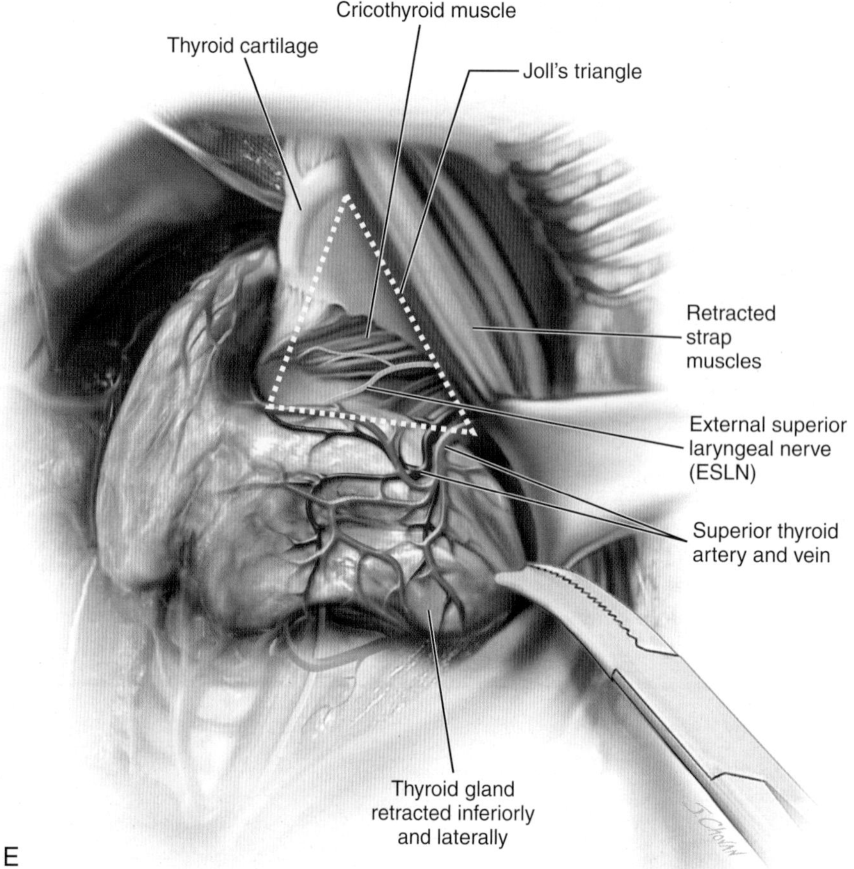

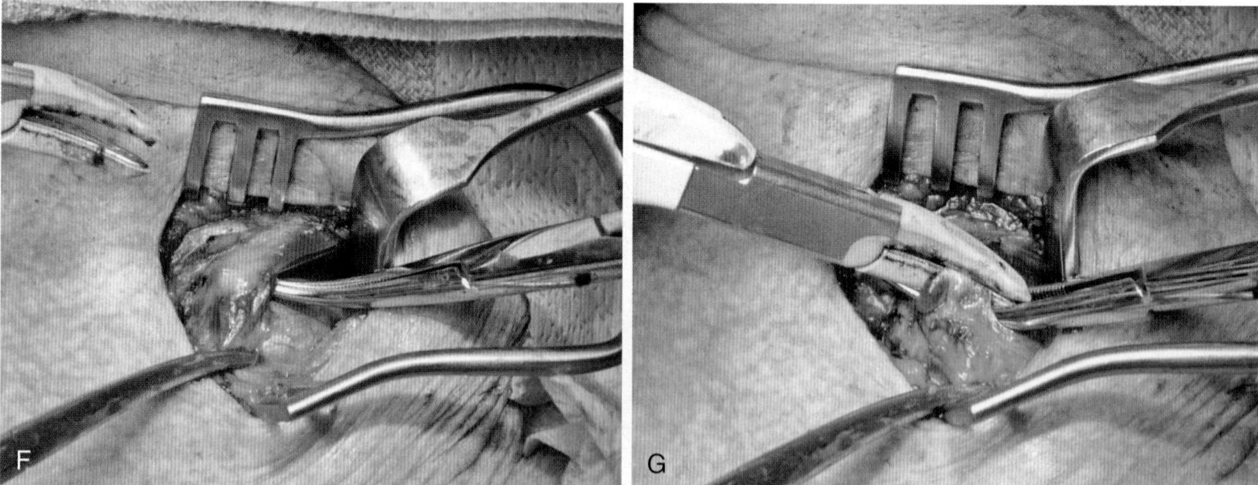

Figure 102.1,cont'd **E,** Surgical anatomy of the thyroid bed. **F,** Dissection of the superior vessels as they enter the gland. **G,** Superior vessel is ligated using the LigaSure device.

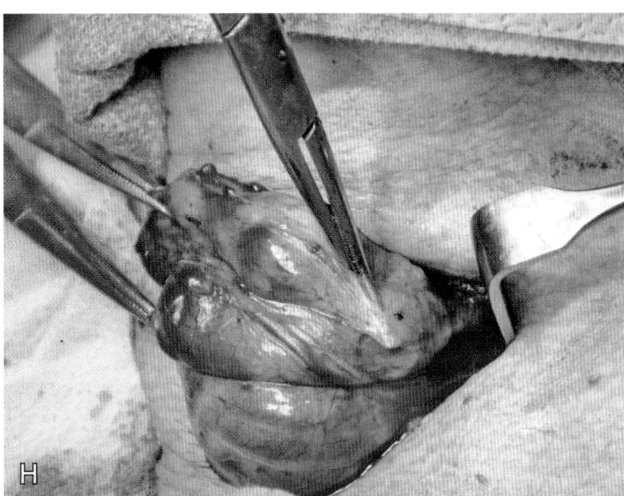

Figure 102.1,cont'd H, Dissection of the superior parathyroid gland off the thyroid, which is then gently swept off the thyroid.

TECHNIQUE: Total Thyroidectomy—*cont'd*

it can be found passing deep to it, through it, or even through the gland before it enters the larynx behind the cricothyroid articulation. Most publications comment on a right nonrecurrent laryngeal nerve, which is present in less than 1% of patients and often associated with an aberrant retroesophageal subclavian artery or other congenital malformation.[26,27] A left nonrecurrent laryngeal nerve is even more rare. Once the nerve has been found, dissection continues along the nerve inferiorly past the inferior parathyroid gland and vessel, before ligation of the inferior vessels. A reliable landmark where the RLN enters the larynx is the cricothyroid joint (Fig. 102.1I and J).

Continued

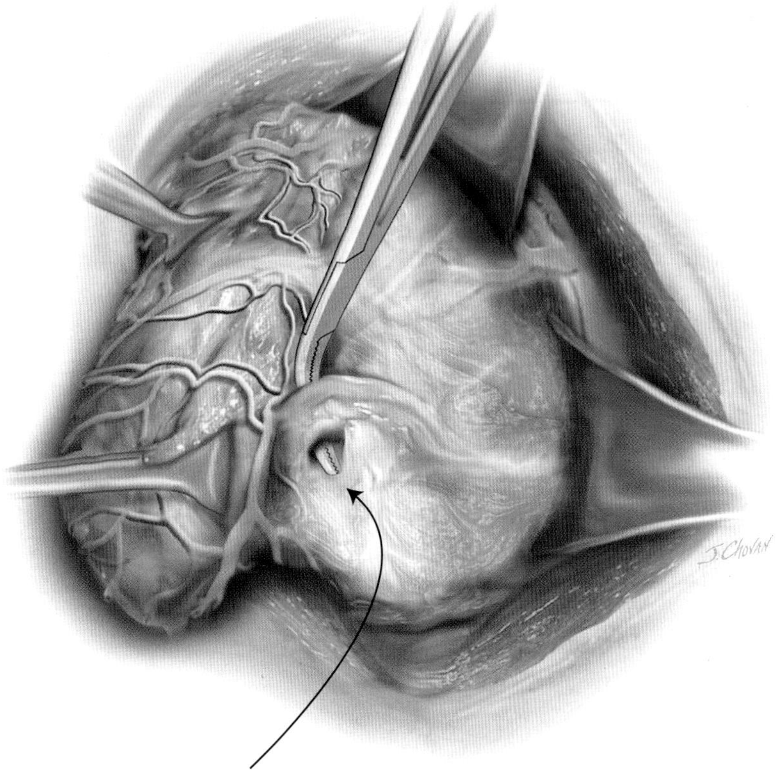

Figure 102.1,cont'd I, Dissection of the inferior thyroid artery.

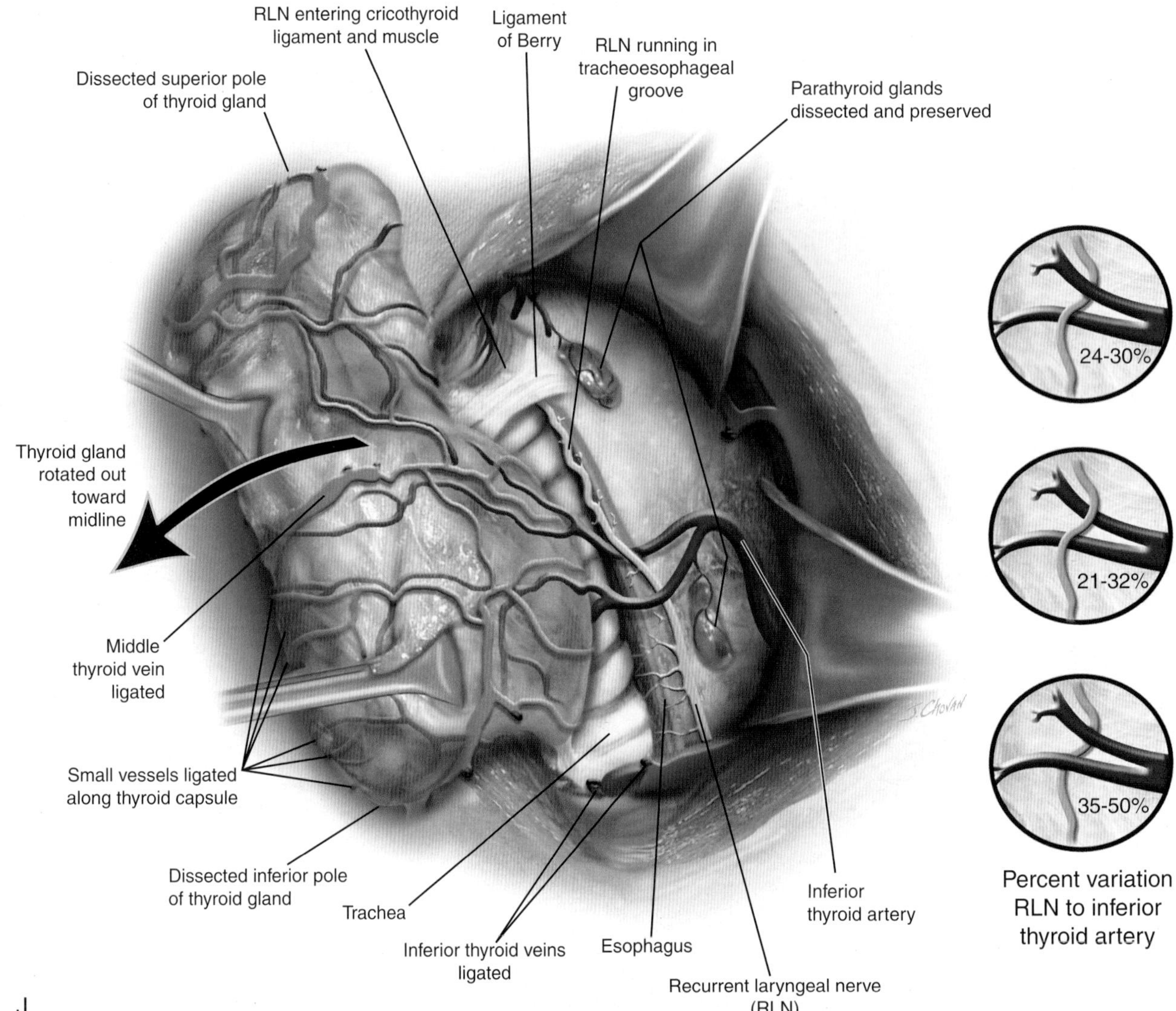

Figure 102.1,cont'd J, Thyroid gland is mobilized to identify the recurrent laryngeal nerve in the tracheoesophageal groove.

TECHNIQUE: Total Thyroidectomy—*cont'd*

STEP 9: Inferior Pole

Using a Carmalt or Kelly clamp, the gland continues to be retracted anteromedially along the trachea. The inferior vessels are skeletonized and then ligated as close to the gland as possible. Because the ITA supplies both the inferior and superior parathyroid glands, it is imperative that the ITA is ligated as it enters the thyroid as close to the capsule as possible. Remember, the parathyroid glands can be identified by their caramel color. The parathyroid gland is dissected off the undersurface of the thyroid gland and swept posteriorly and laterally.

If the surgeon is uncertain if there is a parathyroid gland present on the thyroid specimen or if there is concern that the gland has been devascularized, it can be placed in saline solution. Parathyroid gland tissue will sink, but fat will float. A small portion of the presumed parathyroid gland should be sent for pathology to ensure that it is not metastatic thyroid cancer. To minimize hypocalcemia, parathyroid autotransplantation is performed by sectioning the parathyroid into fine 2- to 3-mm pieces.[28] The sections are placed in small pockets within the strap or sternocleidomastoid muscles via blunt dissection and closed with several surgical clips. The parathyroid gland sections will revascularize in 4 to 6 weeks, and the clips will mark their position should they need to be removed in the future (Fig. 102.1K).

TECHNIQUE: Total Thyroidectomy—*cont'd*

STEP 10: Removing Thyroid off Trachea

The thyroid gland now remains attached to the trachea by the fascia (i.e., ligament of Berry). If the nerve has been identified and followed as it enters the larynx, then cautery can be used sparingly in the avascular plane between the thyroid and trachea. The RLN must be visualized as it enters the larynx at the cricothyroid joint before any cautery is used on the ligament of Berry (Fig. 102.1L).

STEP 11: Dividing the Thyroid

Division of the thyroid gland can be performed lateral to the isthmus with a harmonic scalpel, bipolar, monopolar, or LigaSure. This division during the total thyroidectomy procedure is optional and may allow additional space to operate, ensure a smaller incision, and aid the pathologist in clearly identifying the two different lobes (Fig. 102.1M).

Continued

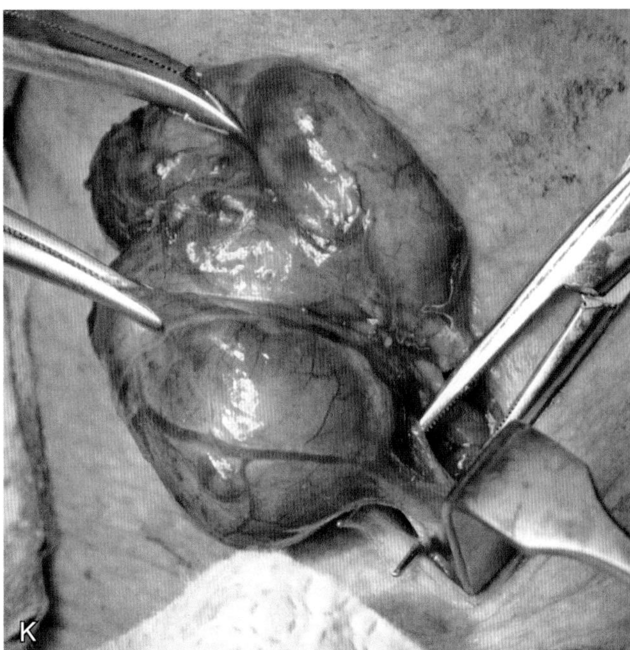

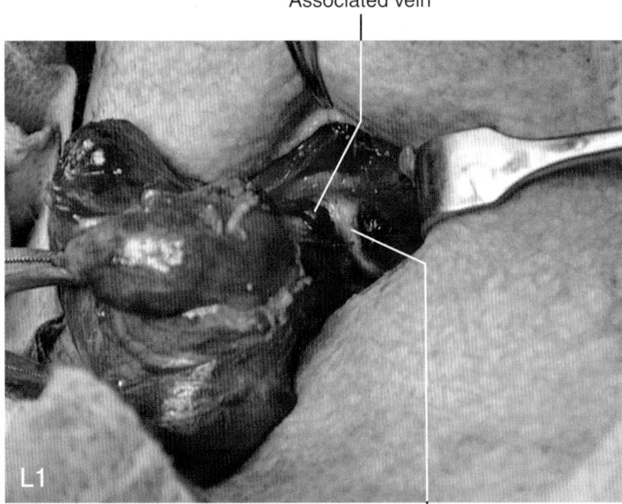

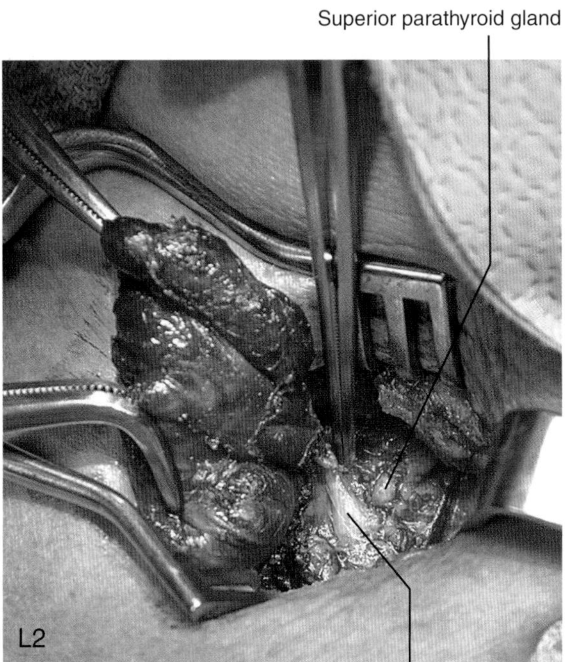

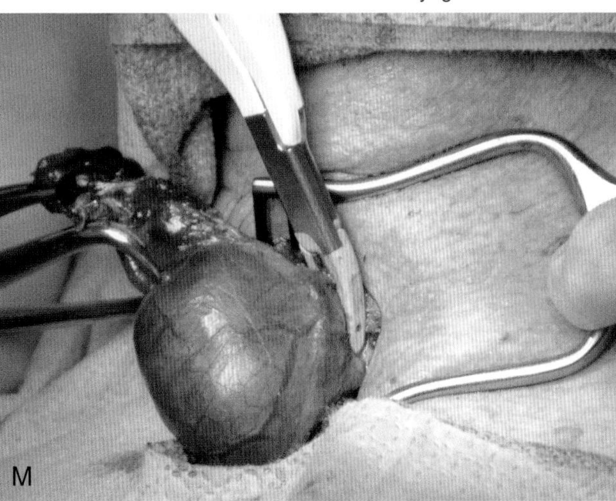

Figure 12.1,cont'd **K,** Dissection of inferior vessels. **L1** and **L2,** RLN as it enters the larynx, along with the small vein often next to the RLN; cautery can now be used to assist in removing the thyroid from the trachea. **M,** Right thyroid lobe is ligated at the isthmus with the LigaSure.

TECHNIQUE: Total Thyroidectomy—*cont'd*

STEP 12: Completing the Thyroidectomy

Repeat steps 5 through 9.

STEP 13: Prior to Closing

After the thyroid has been removed, irrigate the surgical bed. Using the suction over a gauze may help reduce trauma to the parathyroid glands or RLN. If a nerve monitoring ET is being used, the nerve stimulator can be used to stimulate the RLN proximally to ensure its integrity. One may also use this prior to beginning dissection on the contralateral lobe to ensure a signal is present. If the signal is lost, a staged operation may be considered.

STEP 14: Closure

Reapproximate the straps with interrupted dissolvable sutures, leaving an opening of 1 to 1.5 cm inferiorly to allow for blood or fluid to be evacuated to the subplatysmal plane, thereby minimizing the risk of tracheal compression should bleeding or seroma occur. The platysma is reapproximated with interrupted dissolvable sutures, and the skin is closed using a knotless subcutaneous running closure with a 5-0 Monocryl suture. The suture is cut, leaving a 5-mm untied tail. Dermabond (Ethicon Inc., Johnson & Johnson, Somerville, New Jersey) is placed over the closed incision. The surgeon may opt for alternative dressings, but we have found the described closure to have excellent cosmetic results and makes future suture removal unnecessary. A 2007 Cochrane review showed no benefit in placing surgical drains after thyroidectomy with regards to hematoma or seroma prevention. As a result, we do not routinely use drains.[29] A neck drain is indicated in a thyroidectomy with lateral neck dissection (Fig. 102.1N and O).

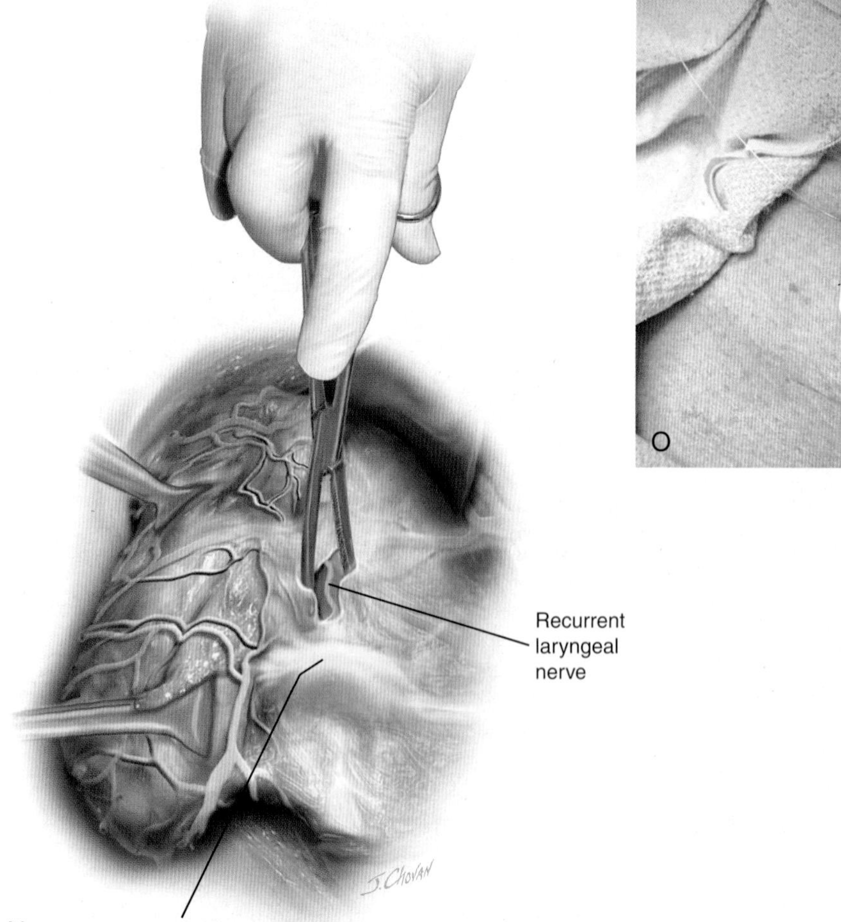

Figure 102.1,cont'd **N,** The recurrent laryngeal nerve is identified in the tissue bed. **O,** Skin closure before application of Dermabond, and cutting of loose suture ends.

Avoidance and Management of Intraoperative Complications

Recurrent Laryngeal Nerve Invaded by Tumor

The importance of preoperative laryngeal assessment is crucial for intraoperative decision making.[30] If the RLN is not functioning preoperatively, invasion of the nerve should be expected. If there is evidence that the nerve is invaded, the nerve should be resected en bloc with the tumor. Patients should be counseled that voice function may worsen and aspiration is possible. Even in patients with preoperative vocal cord paralysis, the RLN may be contributing to vocal tone. If the RLN is functioning preoperatively and found to be encased or invaded by tumor, every attempt should be made to dissect the nerve free of the tumor. All gross disease should be resected. The decision to resect a functioning nerve in the setting of a thyroid malignancy must be viewed in terms of the overall benefit to the patient. Two studies have found that papillary thyroid cancer invading or encasing the RLN can be left intact and treated with T_4 suppression and radioactive iodine, with no change in survival.[31,32] The discussion should be made with the patient preoperatively.

Management of a Severed Recurrent Laryngeal Nerve

If the nerve is severed during surgery without a significant loss of length, a primary neurorrhaphy should be performed in a tension-free closure using two to three 9-0 epineural sutures. After 6 to 12 months, the ipsilateral larynx should have some increased tone, and voice and swallowing should have improved. However, the vocal cord will not move in a coordinated fashion. In the interim, the patient can undergo a temporary vocal cord injection laryngoplasty to aid with voice performance.

If there is a segmental loss of the RLN and a tension-free anastomosis is not possible, an ansa cervicalis to distal RLN anastomosis is an option. The outcome will take 6 to 12 months, with the goal to maintain neural input to the ipsilateral larynx and maintain motor tone. The option of temporary injection medialization still exists and, if the patient is satisfied with this result, a permanent injection medialization. There is limited literature to suggest that medialization is favored in older patients with unilateral vocal cord paralysis.[33]

Postoperative Complications

Postoperative calcium management is standardized in our patients with a 2-week calcium/vitamin D protocol. Patients are prescribed 1 g of calcium three times a day for the first week, then twice a day for the second week. Patients are instructed to take an additional 1 g of calcium every hour and call the physician if they are experiencing symptoms of hypocalcemia, such as perioral or extremity numbness or tingling. This regimen has been shown to be safe and effective in the hands of an experienced thyroid surgeon.[34] Alternatively, parathyroid hormone monitoring has been demonstrated to predict postoperative hypocalcemia and can serve as an alternate strategy for initiating calcium replacement. Vescan et al. suggest a 1-hour postoperative parathyroid hormone draw, with aggressive calcium replacement suggested for laboratory values <10.4 pg/mL. Levels >15.1 pg/L were associated with normocalcemia postoperatively and helped to facilitate timely hospital discharge.[35]

Postoperative thyroid hormone replacement should start immediately after surgery to prevent surgery-induced hypothyroidism and suppress stimulated growth of persistent thyroid tissue. A general weight-based thyroid replacement of 1.4 to 2.2 μg/kg should be initiated, with further titration depending on a diagnosis of benign versus malignant disease.

References

1. Gross SD. 4th ed. *A System of Surgery*. Vol. II. Philadelphia, Pennsylvania: H.C. Lea; 1886.
2. Thompson NW, Olsen WR, Hoffman GL. The continuing development of the technique of thyroidectomy. *Surgery*. 1973;73(6):913–927.
3. Haddad RI, Nasr C, Bischoff L, et al. NCCN guidelines insights: thyroid carcinoma, version 2.2018. *J Natl Compr Canc Netw*. 2018;16(12):1429–1440.
4. Haugen BR, Alexander EK, Bible KC, et al. 2015 American Thyroid Association Management Guidelines for adult patients with thyroid nodules and differentiated thyroid cancer: the American Thyroid Association Guidelines Task Force on thyroid nodules and differentiated thyroid cancer. *Thyroid*. 2016;26(1):1–133.
5. Paschke R, Cantara S, Crescenzi A, Jarzab B, Musholt TJ, Sobrinho Simoes M. European thyroid association guidelines regarding thyroid nodule molecular fine-needle aspiration cytology diagnostics. *Eur Thyroid J*. 2017;6(3):115–129.
6. Smithson M, Asban A, Miller J, Chen H. Considerations for thyroidectomy as treatment for Graves disease. *Clin Med Insights Endocrinol Diabetes*. 2019;12:1179551419844523.
7. Bartsch DK, Luster M, Buhr HJ, Lorenz D, Germer CT, Goretzki PE, German Society for General and Visceral Surgery. Indications for the surgical management of benign goiter in adults. *Dtsch Arztebl Int*. 2018;115(1–02):1–7.
8. Lupo MA, Walts AE, Sistrunk JW, et al. Multiplatform molecular test performance in indeterminate thyroid nodules. *Diagn Cytopathol*. 2020;48(12):1254–1264.
9. Steward DL, Carty SE, Sippel RA, et al. Performance of a multigene genomic classifier in thyroid nodules with indeterminate cytology: a prospective blinded multicenter study. *JAMA Oncol*. 2019;5(2):204–212.
10. Tessler FN, Middleton WD, Grant EG, et al. ACR Thyroid Imaging, Reporting and Data System (TI-RADS): white paper of the ACR TI-RADS Committee. *J Am Coll Radiol*. 2017;14(5):587–595.
11. Cibas ES, Ali SZ. The 2017 Bethesda system for reporting thyroid cytopathology. *J Am Soc Cytopathol*. 2017;6(6):217–222.
12. Chandrasekhar SS, Randolph GW, Seidman MD, American Academy of Otolaryngology-Head and Neck Surgery, et al. Clinical practice

guideline: improving voice outcomes after thyroid surgery. *Otolaryngol Head Neck Surg*. 2013;148(suppl 6):S1–S37.
13. Farrag TY, Samlan RA, Lin FR, Tufano RP. The utility of evaluating true vocal fold motion before thyroid surgery. *Laryngoscope*. 2006;116(2):235–238.
14. Randolph GW, Kamani D. The importance of preoperative laryngoscopy in patients undergoing thyroidectomy: voice, vocal cord function, and the preoperative detection of invasive thyroid malignancy. *Surgery*. 2006;139(3):357–362.
15. Khadra H, Mohamed H, Al-Qurayshi Z, Sholl A, Killackey M, Kandil E. Superior detection of metastatic cystic lymphadenopathy in patients with papillary thyroid cancer by utilization of thyroglobulin washout. *Head Neck*. 2019;41(1):225–229.
16. Alexander EK, Pearce EN, Brent GA, et al. 2017 Guidelines of the American Thyroid Association for the diagnosis and management of thyroid disease during pregnancy and the postpartum. *Thyroid*. 2017;27(3):315–389.
17. Kierner AC, Aigner M, Burian M. The external branch of the superior laryngeal nerve: its topographical anatomy as related to surgery of the neck. *Arch Otolaryngol Head Neck Surg*. 1998;124:301.
18. Wiseman S, Tomljanovich P, Rigual N. Thyroid lobectomy: operative anatomy, technique, and morbidity. *Oper Tech Otolaryngol Head Neck Surg*. 2004;15:210.
19. Bellantone R, Boscherini M, Lombardi CP, et al. Is the identification of the external branch of the superior laryngeal nerve mandatory in thyroid operation? Results of a prospective randomized study. *Surgery*. 2001;130(6):1055–1059.
20. Pons Y, Gauthier J, Ukkola-Pons E, et al. Comparison of LigaSure vessel sealing system, harmonic scalpel, and conventional hemostasis in total thyroidectomy. *Otolaryngol Head Neck Surg*. 2009;141(4):496–501.
21. Ecker T, Carvalho AL, Choe JH, Walosek G, Preuss KJ. Hemostasis in thyroid surgery: harmonic scalpel versus other techniques—a meta-analysis. *Otolaryngol Head Neck Surg*. 2010;143(1):17–25.
22. Jatzko GR, Lisborg PH, Müller MG, Wette VM. Recurrent nerve palsy after thyroid operations—principal nerve identification and a literature review. *Surgery*. 1994;115(2):139–144.
23. Hvidegaard T, Vase P, Jørgensen K, Blichert-Toft M. Identification and functional recording of the recurrent nerve by electrical stimulation during neck surgery. *Laryngoscope*. 1983;93(3):370–373.
24. Skandalakis JE, Droulias C, Harlaftis N, Tzinas S, Gray SW, Akin JT Jr. The recurrent laryngeal nerve. *Am Surg*. 1976;42(9):629–634.
25. Asgharpour E, Maranillo E, Sañudo J, et al. Recurrent laryngeal nerve landmarks revisited. *Head Neck*. 2012;34(9):1240–1246.
26. Fancy T, Gallagher D III, Hornig JD. Surgical anatomy of the thyroid and parathyroid glands. *Otolaryngol Clin North Am*. 2010;43(2):221–227, vii.
27. Randolph GW. *Surgical Anatomy of the Recurrent Laryngeal Nerve. Surgery of the Thyroid and Parathyroid Glands*. Philadelphia, Pennsylvania: Saunders; 2003.
28. Adams M, Doherty G. Conventional thyroidectomy. *Oper Tech Otolaryngol Head Neck Surg*. 2009;20:2.
29. Samraj K, Gurusamy KS. Wound drains following thyroid surgery. *Cochrane Database Syst Rev*. 2007;17(4):CD006099.
30. Steurer M, Passler C, Denk DM, Schneider B, Niederle B, Bigenzahn W. Advantages of recurrent laryngeal nerve identification in thyroidectomy and parathyroidectomy and the importance of preoperative and postoperative laryngoscopic examination in more than 1000 nerves at risk. *Laryngoscope*. 2002;112(1):124–133.
31. Falk SA, McCaffrey TV. Management of the recurrent laryngeal nerve in suspected and proven thyroid cancer. *Otolaryngol Head Neck Surg*. 1995;113(1):42–48.
32. Nishida T, Nakao K, Hamaji M, Kamiike W, Kurozumi K, Matsuda H. Preservation of recurrent laryngeal nerve invaded by differentiated thyroid cancer. *Ann Surg*. 1997;226(1):85–91.
33. Paniello RC, Edgar JD, Kallogjeri D, Piccirillo JF. Medialization versus reinnervation for unilateral vocal fold paralysis: a multicenter randomized clinical trial. *Laryngoscope*. 2011;121(10):2172–2179.
34. Singer MC, Bhakta D, Seybt MW, Terris DJ. Calcium management after thyroidectomy: a simple and cost-effective method. *Otolaryngol Head Neck Surg*. 2012;146(3):362–365.
35. Vescan A, Witterick I, Freeman J. Parathyroid hormone as a predictor of hypocalcemia after thyroidectomy. *Laryngoscope*. 2005;115(12):2105–2108.

CHAPTER 103

Parathyroid Gland Surgery for Hyperparathyroidism

Brett A. Miles and Matthew R. Idle

Armamentarium

#15 Scalpel blade
Adson forceps, toothed
Appropriate sutures
Baby Metzenbaum, 14 cm, 5 ¼ in
Bipolar insulated, 4 in, 0.5-mm tip
DeBakey straight, 1.5-mm tip
Delicate Allis clamps, 7 ½ in
Frozen section analysis
Gerald forceps, 1 × 2 teeth
Intraoperative parathyroid hormone monitoring
Jamison scissors, curved, 7 in
Jamison-Metz scissors, curved, 6 in
Jarit flat-tip scissors, 5 in
Kittner dissector sponges
Local anesthetic with vasoconstrictor
Medium clip appliers
Monopolar cautery, insulated tip
Petit point Mixter forceps, 7 ¼ in
Petit point mosquito, 7 ⅛ in, curved
Polar Army-Navy retractors
Semken needle forceps, carbide, delicate, 6 in
Small clip appliers
Stevens tenotomy scissors, curved, 15 cm, 6 in

Optional

Endoscope/videoscopic assisted equipment
Gamma probe (for radioguided parathyroid gland identification)
Harmonic scalpel/vessel sealing device
Recurrent laryngeal nerve monitor, dissector

History of the Procedure

The relationship of the parathyroid gland and hyperparathyroidism was first recognized in 1903 by Askanazy, and the theory that parathyroid adenoma may be responsible for hyperparathyroidism was put forth by Schlagenhaufer in 1915.[1,2] The first operation to remove a parathyroid tumor was performed by Felix Mandl in Vienna, Austria, in 1925 with local anesthesia.[3] Subsequent work by Albright, Castleman, and Cope set the stage for our current understanding of the pathology of parathyroid glands and the surgical management of hyperparathyroidism.[4–6] In the 1950s and 1960s, an understanding of the activity of parathyroid hormone developed.[7] Continued understanding of the anatomy of the parathyroid region and gland physiology led to improved gland localization and improved accuracy of surgical technique.[8–14] The introduction of intraoperative parathyroid hormone (PTH) monitoring was revolutionary in the management of benign parathyroid disease.[15] However, despite more than 100 years of parathyroid surgery, the historical challenges, including gland localization, determining biologic cure, and reoperative surgery, remain relevant today.

Hyperparathyroidism is a disorder of bone and mineral metabolism caused by the hypersecretion of PTH. The majority of cases (80% to 90%) are due to solitary secretory parathyroid adenoma (Fig. 103.1). This is termed *primary hyperthyroidism,* the subject of this chapter. The prevalence of primary hyperparathyroidism is estimated to be 0.2% to 1%.[16] Between 5% and 15% of cases of primary parathyroid hyperplasia involve four-gland hyperplasia. Secondary and tertiary hyperparathyroidism are related to renal disease or other disruptions of calcium metabolism. Secondary hyperparathyroidism is a result of overactive parathyroid glands in the setting of renal osteodystrophy. Tertiary hyperparathyroidism typically occurs in patients with longstanding secondary hyperparathyroidism who undergo renal transplantation. Parathyroid carcinoma, although rare, may cause significant hyperparathyroidism and can be associated with debilitating symptoms. These types of hyperparathyroidism are beyond the scope of this chapter, although surgical treatment is often indicated in these disorders as well.

Surgical intervention is the single definitive treatment of primary hyperparathyroidism.[4] Traditionally, resection of the abnormal parathyroid glands was accomplished by a bilateral neck exploration (BNE) with evaluation of all four parathyroid glands. Intraoperative frozen section confirmation of parathyroid tissue was performed, and the offending gland was then resected. Current strategies have progressed toward minimally invasive parathyroidectomy (MIP), radioguided

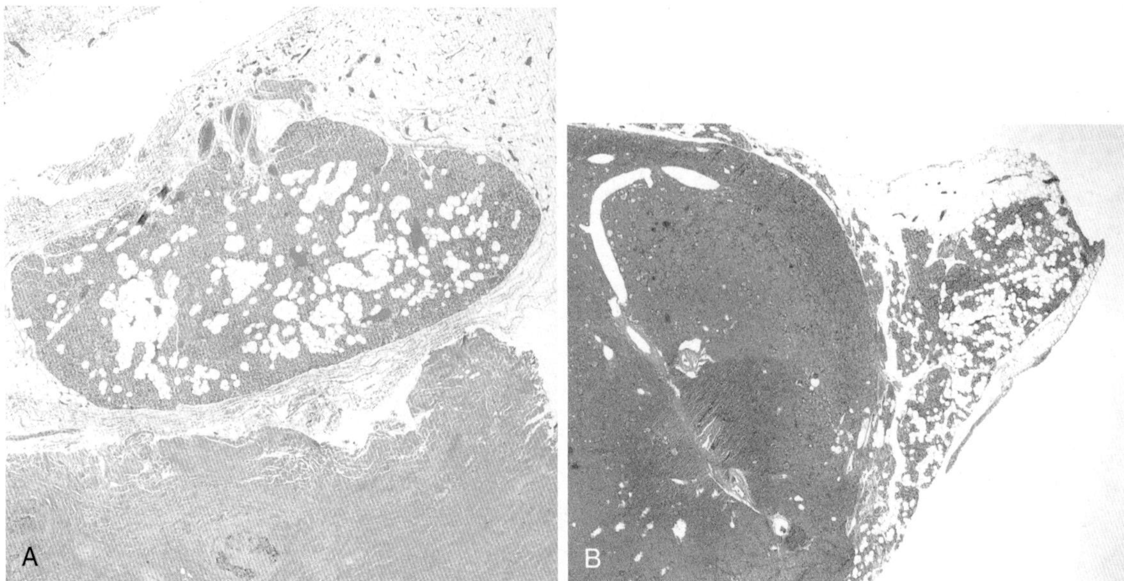

Fig. 103.1 **A,** Hematoxylin-eosin-stained, normal parathyroid gland, magnification 20×. **B,** Hematoxylin-eosin-stained, parathyroid adenoma, magnification 20×.

parathyroidectomy, video-assisted parathyroidectomy, and endoscopic parathyroidectomy.[17] Currently, 10% of surgeons practice BNE, 68% practice limited exploration, and 22% have a mixed practice. Most surgeons prefer a focal, single-gland examination under general anesthesia and 23-hour observation.[18] Interestingly, controversy related to long-term outcomes still exists among surgeons regarding routine versus minimally invasive approaches, despite advances in biochemical testing, imaging, and surgical techniques since the 1960s.[19,20] A Cochrane review showed that the success rates of MIP and BNE were similar. However, MIP demonstrated a lower risk of symptomatic perioperative hypocalcemia but a higher risk of vocal cord paralysis.[21]

Preoperative Parathyroid Localization

One of the most important steps in the preoperative evaluation of a patient with hyperparathyroidism, when primary hyperparathyroidism is suspected, is localization of the adenoma. Various imaging modalities are utilized to pinpoint the offending parathyroid gland or glands. These include ultrasound, 99mTc-sestamibi, computed tomography (CT), magnetic resonance imaging (MRI), and a variety of other imaging modalities. Most surgeons employ a combination of 99mTc-sestamibi and cervical ultrasound of the parathyroid glands. Nuclear imaging scanning uses a radiotracer that is preferentially taken up by the metabolically active parathyroid, thyroid, and cardiac tissue. The tracer washes out of the thyroid gland, revealing the location of the enlarged parathyroid glands. Because 99mTc-sestamibi scanning can be difficult to interpret and has issues with sensitivity, alternative imaging modalities are often utilized. Fusion with single-photon emission computed tomography (SPECT) or CT scanning improves anatomic information. Data suggest that the combination of CT-99mTc-sestamibi-SPECT is the best approach for preoperative localization for patients with one-gland disease.[22] The addition of ultrasound is likely more sensitive than 99mTc-sestamibi, but this decreases when thyroid nodules are present. Deep superior glands and other ectopic glands are also difficult to localize via ultrasound. Also, parathyroid adenomas in the mediastinum are generally seen by 99mTc-sestamibi scans but not by ultrasound. Additional modalities such as CT protocols, MRI, positron emission tomography (PET), and four-dimensional CT offer excellent promise to improve the localization of adenomas in the future and vary depending on the institution.[22,23] Four-dimensional CT may offer superior accuracy compared with that of ultrasonography and 99mTc-sestamibi scanning.[24] MRI with contrast has superior soft tissue imaging capabilities relative to CT and may be helpful in identifying ectopic parathyroid glands. Sensitivity is reported to be greater than 75% for localization of adenomas.[15] PET scanning may have a role in these situations as well.[25] ^{11}C-Choline PET/CT has demonstrated similar sensitivity to 99mTc-sestamibi imaging with reduced cost and radiation dose.[26]

Indications for the Use of the Procedure

With the use of routine blood screening tests, most patients who present with hyperparathyroidism are asymptomatic. Many patients express somewhat nonspecific symptoms such as fatigue, musculoskeletal pains and aches, depression, constipation and abdominal discomfort, and decreased memory. Symptoms related to the effects of PTH may occur, however, and some patients may present with renal calculi (10% to 20%) or rarely osteitis fibrosis. Parathyroidectomy has been shown to restore normocalciuria in 79% of patients with hypercalciuria.[27]

Current guidelines for the indications for parathyroidectomy are as follows[28]:

- All patients with symptomatic primary hyperparathyroidism
- Serum calcium greater than 1 mg/dL (0.25 mmol/L) above normal levels (generally >12 mg/dL)

- Creatinine clearance reduced to less than 60 mL/min
- Overt manifestations of hyperparathyroidism (such as nephrolithiasis, osteitis fibrosa cystica, or classic neuromuscular disease)
- Bone density T score <2.5 (>2.5 standard deviations below peak mass) standard deviation at any site or previous fragility fracture at the lumbar spine, hip, or distal radius
- Age <50 years in the absence of objective or subjective features
- Note that elevated 24-hour urine calcium is no longer an indication (previously >400 mg/day was a recommendation for parathyroidectomy)
- Neurocognitive and/or neuropsychiatric symptoms secondary to primary hyperparathyroidism

Patients with an elevated intact PTH level and a calcium concentration in the normal range often have secondary hyperparathyroidism. Secondary hyperparathyroidism can result from insufficient calcium or vitamin D intake, decreased intestinal calcium absorption, vitamin D malabsorption, or renal hypercalciuria. Parathyroidectomy in the setting of secondary hyperparathyroidism related to renal failure is a complex surgical issue. Supernumerary parathyroid tissue in ectopic locations is commonly encountered (discussed later). Thorough preoperative workup and surgical exploration with excision of the offending glandular tissue will ensure the best outcomes and should be performed by experienced clinicians. Cervical thymectomy may also be indicated due to intrathymic parathyroid glands.[29,30]

Limitations and Contraindications

Although there are several relative contraindications for parathyroidectomy depending on the clinical situation, an absolute contraindication is the presence of familial hypocalciuric hypercalcemia (FHH). Patients can present with elevated calcium and PTH levels, mimicking the serum biochemical characteristics of primary hyperparathyroidism. The differentiation of FHH from primary hyperparathyroidism may be revealed with the 24-hour urine calcium excretion. In FHH, the secretion of calcium is lower than expected in comparison with the serum calcium level. Calcium excretion over 24 hours is <100 mg in a majority of FHH patients but usually >200 mg in patients with primary hyperparathyroidism. In addition, PTH levels are generally mildly elevated or normal in FHH. FHH is not treated with parathyroidectomy, and referral to an endocrinologist is warranted.

Note also that thiazide diuretics and lithium administration may cause elevated PTH and serum calcium levels in some patients. The novel antidiabetic agent dapagliflozin (SGLT-2 inhibitor) has also been shown to cause raised PTH.[31] This fact is important to recognize prior to embarking on surgical exploration for patients with elevated PTH and calcium levels who are taking these medications, and appropriate preoperative investigation is warranted.

TECHNIQUE: Parathyroid Exploration and Gland Excision

The following surgical technique focuses on targeted parathyroid surgery for an identified parathyroid adenoma. Although there continues to be controversy regarding the risks and benefits of four-gland exploration, two-gland exploration, or targeted parathyroidectomy, a majority of surgeons perform minimally invasive, targeted surgery after preoperative localization of the gland. Quality-of-life data indicate that targeted parathyroidectomy offers a lasting advantage over traditional bilateral exploration, irrespective of surgical approach.[32] Despite the improving accuracy of localizing imaging technology, the surgeon should always be prepared to extend the surgical exploration, and patients should be appropriately informed, in the event of ectopic or multigland disease. Intraoperative PTH baseline levels prior to or after induction should be obtained prior to surgical manipulation of the glands.

STEP 1: Incision

The surgical incision is designed in a horizontal skin fold, generally below the level of the cricoid cartilage approximately 2 to 3 cm above the sternal notch, depending on the location of the suspected adenoma. The length of the incision may vary from 2 to 4 cm depending on the habitus of the patient and the required exposure. Incision design may vary widely with technique if video-assisted or endoscopic technology is utilized. The incision is carried through skin, subcutaneous tissue, platysma, and superficial cervical fascia, with subplatysmal dissection to increase the surgical access. The midline raphe of the infrahyoid strap musculature is identified (Fig. 103.2A and B).

STEP 2: Flap Elevation

The infrahyoid strap muscles are divided vertically at the midline raphe, and the cricoid cartilage is palpated. Inferior to the cricoid, the thyroid isthmus and ipsilateral thyroid lobe are identified. Blunt capsular dissection is then performed with Kittner dissectors to allow exposure and medial retraction of the thyroid lobe. Small perforating vessels of the capsule are carefully divided with bipolar electrocautery to avoid hemorrhage. The sternohyoid muscle may be divided at this point if additional access is required or an abnormally large thyroid lobe is present. At this point, initial identification of the carotid sheath is performed bluntly to avoid vascular injury (Fig. 103.2C).

Continued

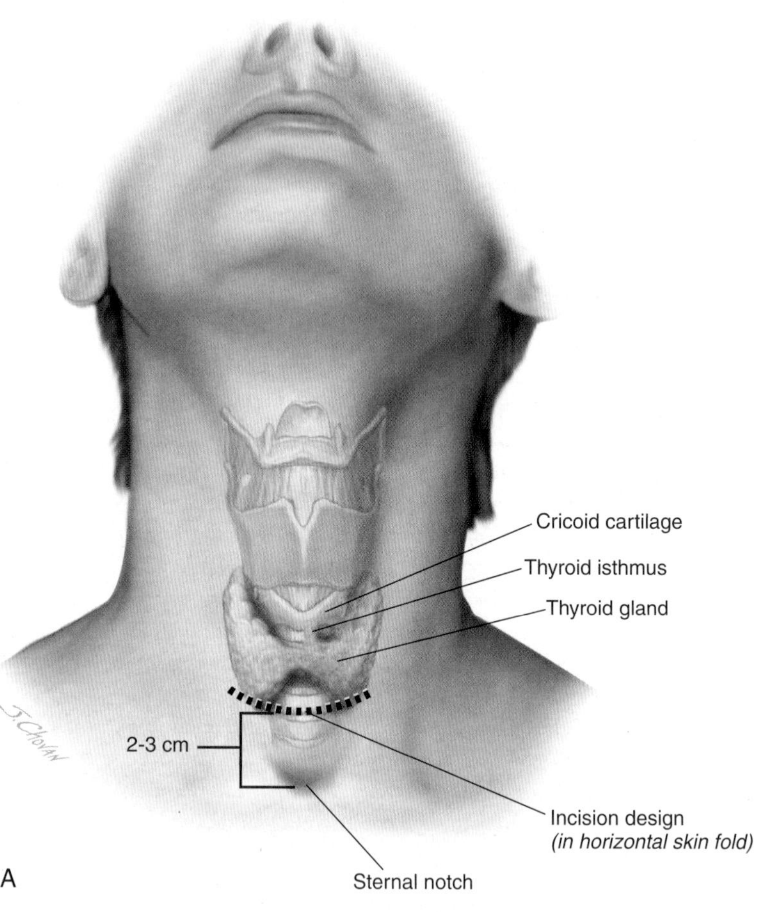

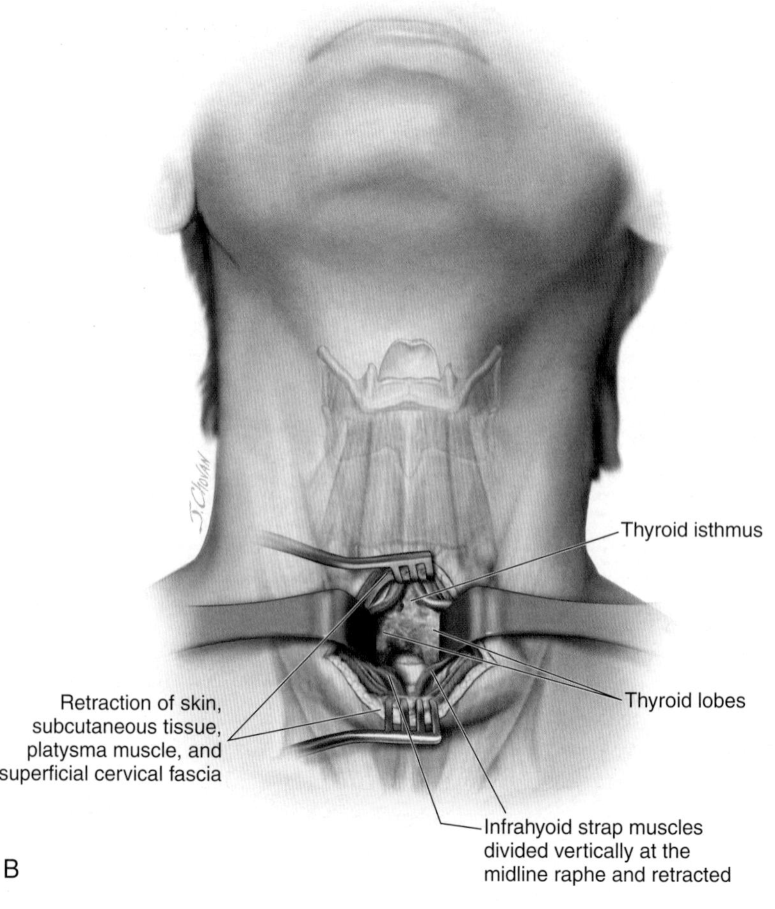

Fig. 103.2 A, Incision design: a 2- to 3-cm incision as shown will allow access to most parathyroid glands. **B,** Midline raphe of the infrahyoid strap musculature has been identified and retracted to reveal the thyroid isthmus.

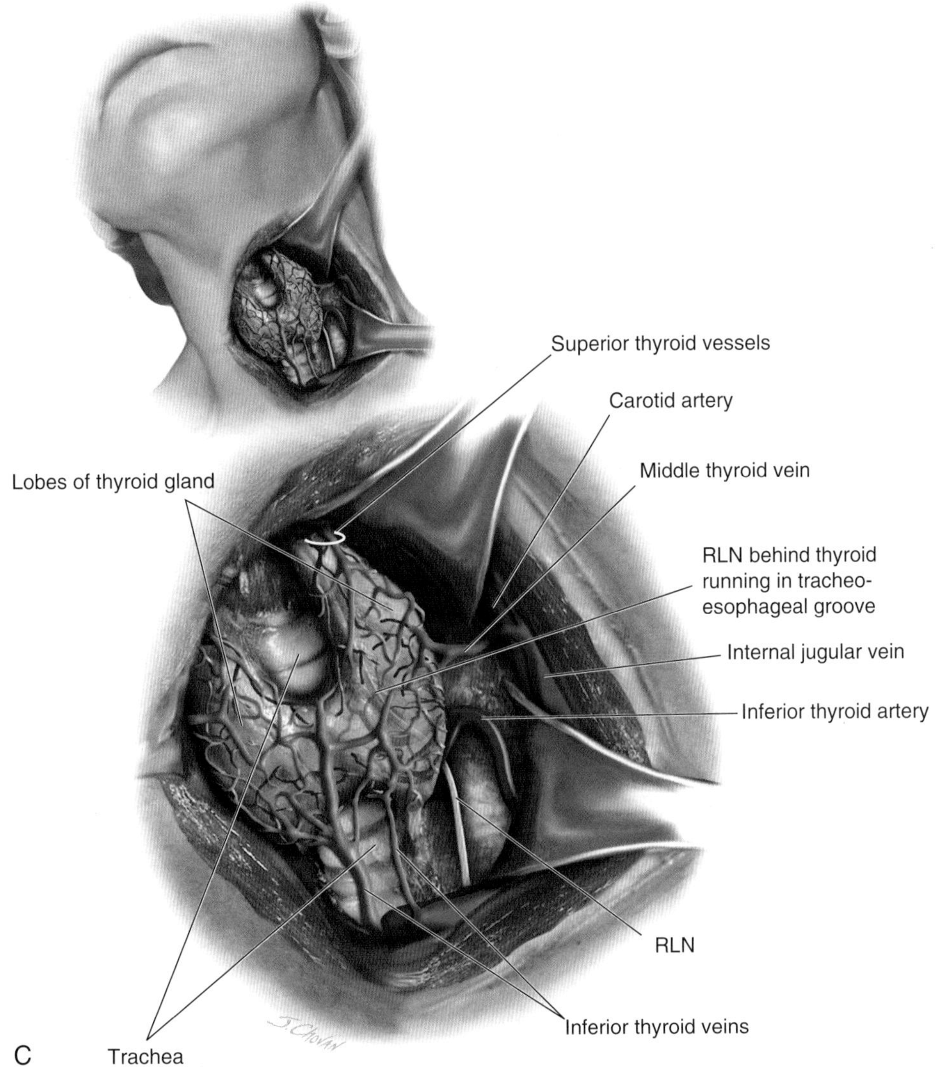

Fig. 103.2 cont'd C, Blunt capsular dissection has been performed to allow medial rotation of the gland, identifying the carotid sheath, parathyroid glands, and recurrent laryngeal nerve (*RLN*).

TECHNIQUE: Parathyroid Exploration and Gland Excision—cont'd

STEP 3: Dissection

Continued blunt capsular dissection of the thyroid lobe is performed, and the anterior/medial rotation of the gland improves surgical exposure. Often, the middle thyroid vein is identified and ligated to allow further medial retraction of the gland. Additionally, in some cases, ligation of the superior thyroid artery and vein may be required to allow further rotation of the gland to obtain adequate visualization of the paratracheal region. Initial identification of the tracheoesophageal groove, cricoid cartilage, and medial surface of the thyroid lobe with careful capsular dissection is performed (see Fig. 103.2C).

Continued

TECHNIQUE: Parathyroid Exploration and Gland Excision—cont'd

STEP 4: Parathyroid Localization

At this time, the paratracheal and tracheoesophageal region is explored to locate the suspected parathyroid adenoma or parathyroid gland. The carotid artery sheath, inferior thyroid artery, recurrent nerve, and glands are identified. Hemostasis is critical at this stage of the operation as hemorrhage within the fascial planes makes identifying the parathyroid glands difficult and may increase the risk of recurrent laryngeal nerve (RLN) injury. In general, bipolar electrocautery or other modalities such as harmonic technology are helpful to allow for a bloodless field. Ligating clips may be used; however, in certain cases they may affect postoperative surveillance imaging, and overuse of clips should be avoided.

Normal parathyroid glands are light brown in contrast to the surrounding fat, which is more yellow. Parathyroid adenomas are also brown but tend to appear darker than normal parathyroid tissue. Any tissue suspected of being parathyroid should be interrogated with frozen section analysis. Lymph nodes, thyroid nodules, and small fat globules may appear similar in size and color to parathyroid tissue, and frozen section analysis avoids unnecessary removal of normal parathyroid glands, as well as inadvertent removal of tissue with the assumption that the offending parathyroid has been removed. Rapid intraoperative measurement of parathyroid hormone via needle aspiration has been used as an alternative to frozen section analysis.[33] Many parathyroid adenomas can be palpated as soft nodules in the appropriate region to aid in identification. Continued careful dissection, hemostasis, and palpation are the hallmarks of successful parathyroid surgery.

The superior parathyroid gland is generally located at the posterior and lateral aspect of the thyroid gland. Careful dissection of the perithyroidal fat planes often reveals the superior parathyroid adherent to the gland in this region. The superior gland is most commonly located deep to the plane of the RLN and superior to the intersection of the RLN and the inferior thyroid artery, which provide anatomic landmarks. Note, however, that this relationship is variable, and careful dissection is required to avoid avulsion of the gland or recurrent nerve injury. Palpation of the cricotracheal groove and trachea can help with orientation during exploration. Careful, blunt dissection of the fibroareolar tissue in these regions facilitates the location of both normal and abnormal parathyroid glands and avoids nerve injury. Routine identification of the RLN is not required, but identification and dissection of the nerve often facilitate gland location and avoid nerve transection. The superior gland is posterior to the plane of the RLN and can often be found in the tracheoesophageal groove, in the posterior mediastinum, or adjacent or posterior to the esophagus. If additional exposure is needed, the superior thyroid artery can be ligated as it enters the superior aspect of the thyroid, and the thyroid gland can be further rotated anteromedially (Fig. 103.2D and E).

Exploration to locate the inferior gland begins at the inferior and posterior aspect of the thyroid lobe. The inferior gland is generally located anterior to the plane of the RLN and medial and anterior to the intersection of the RLN and the inferior thyroid artery. Inspection of the thyrothymic ligament and the superior aspect of the thymus is often required due to the variability of the inferior parathyroid gland location (Fig. 103.2C and F).

STEP 5: Intraoperative PTH Evaluation

Intraoperative PTH evaluation is then performed after excision and frozen section verification of the suspected adenoma. Although a variety of strategies exist, in general approximately 10 to 15 minutes after the abnormal gland is removed, the PTH sample should be within normal limits and should have decreased by more than 50% from the initial baseline value. In a majority of patients with primary hyperparathyroidism, this method provides biochemical confirmation of hyperfunctional gland removal and predicts both a eucalcemic state and a surgical cure. If the PTH level does not decrease by 50% and fall into the normal range, the surgeon should continue exploring until additional abnormal parathyroid glands are identified and removed.[34] The fact that targeted gland excision enhanced by intraoperative PTH monitoring does not result in a biologic cure for all patients (especially when monitored long term) has led some to advocate other techniques, such as handheld gamma probe localization and routine four-gland exploration.[20] However, utilization of intraoperative PTH monitoring has been shown to be 99% sensitive and results in curative surgery in approximately 90% of patients. It is also a critical technique for recognizing and resecting additional image-negative hyperfunctioning lesions.[35]

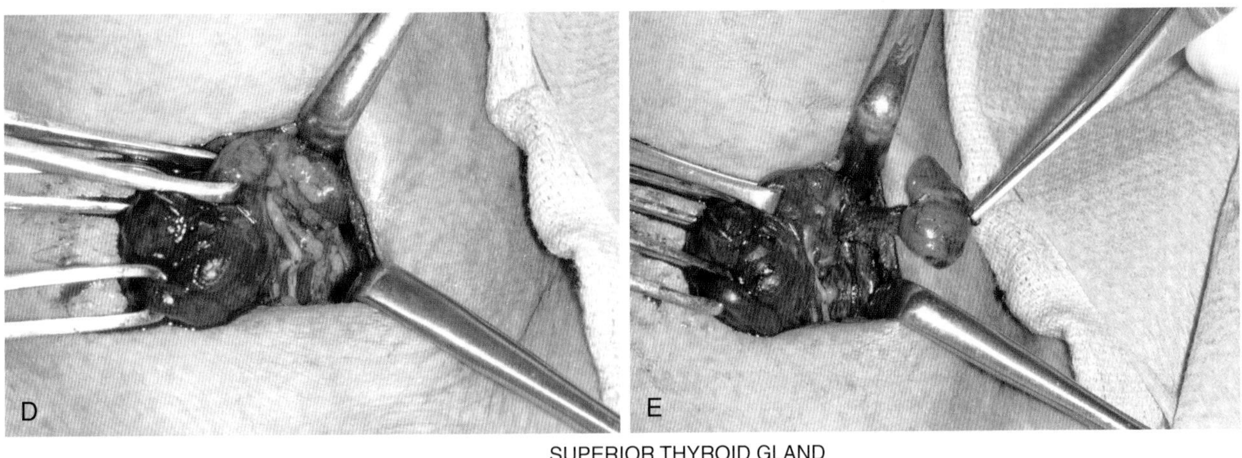

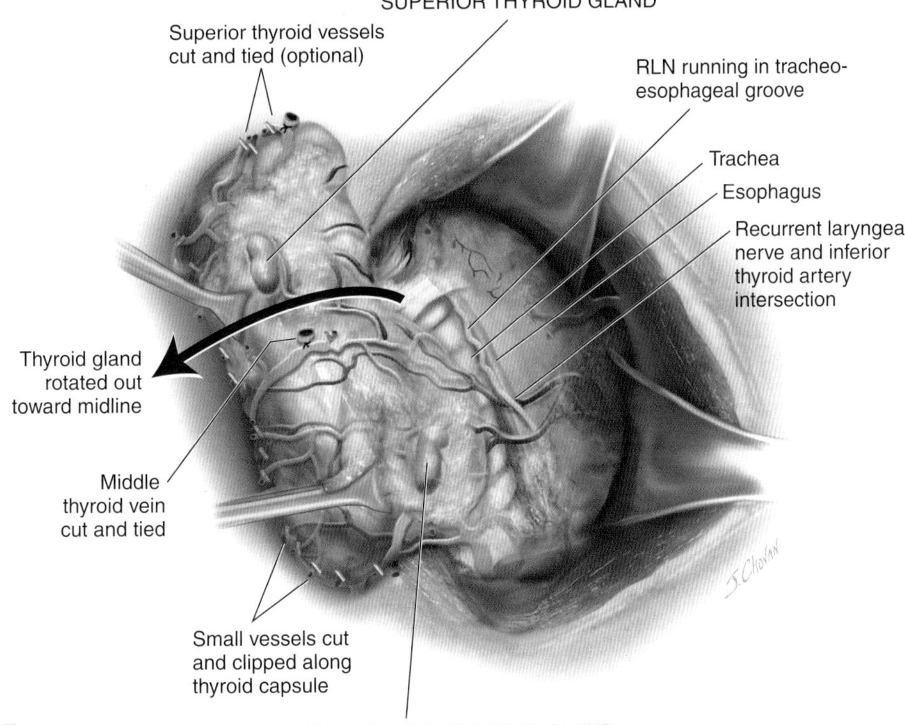

Fig. 103.2 cont'd D, With the left thyroid lobe retracted medially, the RLN is clearly visible with superior parathyroid adenoma lateral to the nerve with associated periglandular fat. **E,** Parathyroid adenoma, isolated on its blood supply prior to removal. **F,** Parathyroid glands are identified with careful dissection; the recurrent laryngeal nerve may be outlined if necessary. Occasionally, ligation of the superior vascular pedicle may be required for adequate visualization.

TECHNIQUE: Parathyroid Exploration and Gland Excision—cont'd

STEP 6: Closure

After verification of adequate surgical excision of the offending glands, the wound is irrigated and closure is performed. Hemostasis is achieved with judicious bipolar electrocautery. In general, no drains are required. Reapproximation of the infrahyoid strap musculature is important to avoid scarring of the overlying skin to the trachea and poor cosmetic results. This is performed with resorbable polyglactin sutures. The dermis is then closed with subcutaneous poliglecaprone sutures. The skin is sealed with cyanoacrylate skin adhesive, and no external sutures are placed to improve cosmesis (Fig. 103.2G).

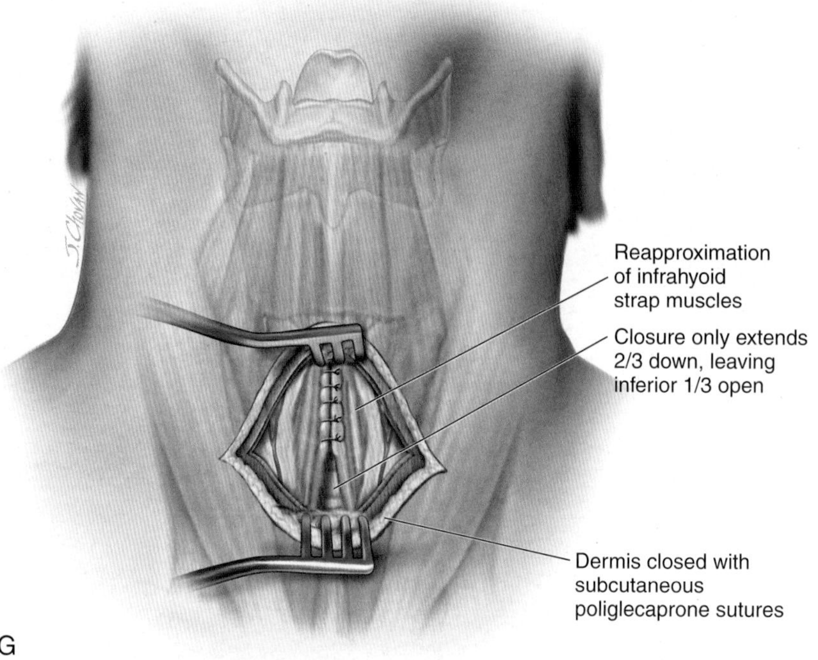

Fig. 103.2 cont'd G, Wound closure includes midline infrahyoid strap muscle approximation to prevent the overlying soft tissue from adhering to the trachea and resulting in poor cosmesis.

ALTERNATIVE TECHNIQUE 1: Four-Gland Exploration

Occasionally, in cases of four-gland parathyroid hyperplasia or ectopic parathyroid adenoma, a formal four-gland exploration is warranted. The surgical techniques are identical to the previously described technique; however, the procedure is performed bilaterally. Rarely, hemithyroidectomy is performed to facilitate exploration. When performing additional exploration for ectopic adenoma, the embryology of the parathyroids should be kept in mind, as there are implications on gland location. The superior parathyroid glands arise from the fourth branchial pouch, mirror the migration of the ultimobranchial bodies, and are usually located along the posterior part of the middle third of each thyroid lobe. The inferior parathyroid glands, which arise from the third branchial pouch, initially migrate with the thymus until they separate to take their final position, usually at the level of the inferior pole of each thyroid lobe. Note that the superior parathyroid glands show less anatomic variation than the inferior thyroid glands do, which can be especially important when attempting to locate ectopic parathyroid deposits.

When performing a four-gland exploration/three-and-a-half gland excision, intraoperative PTH levels should decrease further with each gland removal. After 3.5 glands have been removed, the PTH level should be in the normal range and at least 50% below the starting level. If the PTH level falls below the lower limit of normal autotransplantation (discussed later), the use of some previously removed parathyroid tissue should be considered.[36]

Surgical exploration for ectopic parathyroid glands can be an extensive undertaking, given the variety of locations known to harbor parathyroid tissue (Fig. 103.3). Formal thymectomy or resection of the hemithyroid lobe on the side of the missing parathyroid may be required and often reveals the offending gland on frozen section analysis. Surgical exploration of the carotid sheath regions bilaterally and the superior mediastinum may be required, as well as formal superior mediastinal dissection from the hyoid to the arch of the aorta, between the carotid sheaths. Conventional transcervical parathyroidectomy usually achieves satisfactory results, especially for upper mediastinal glands. Sternotomy approaches are effective but are seldom indicated and increase morbidity. In cases of deep and lower hyperfunctioning mediastinal parathyroids, video-assisted thoracoscopic approaches represent a less invasive alternative and may be the technique of choice.[37] If the offending gland is not located, surgical clips are placed near the known parathyroid glands in the event of future surgical interventions/imaging.

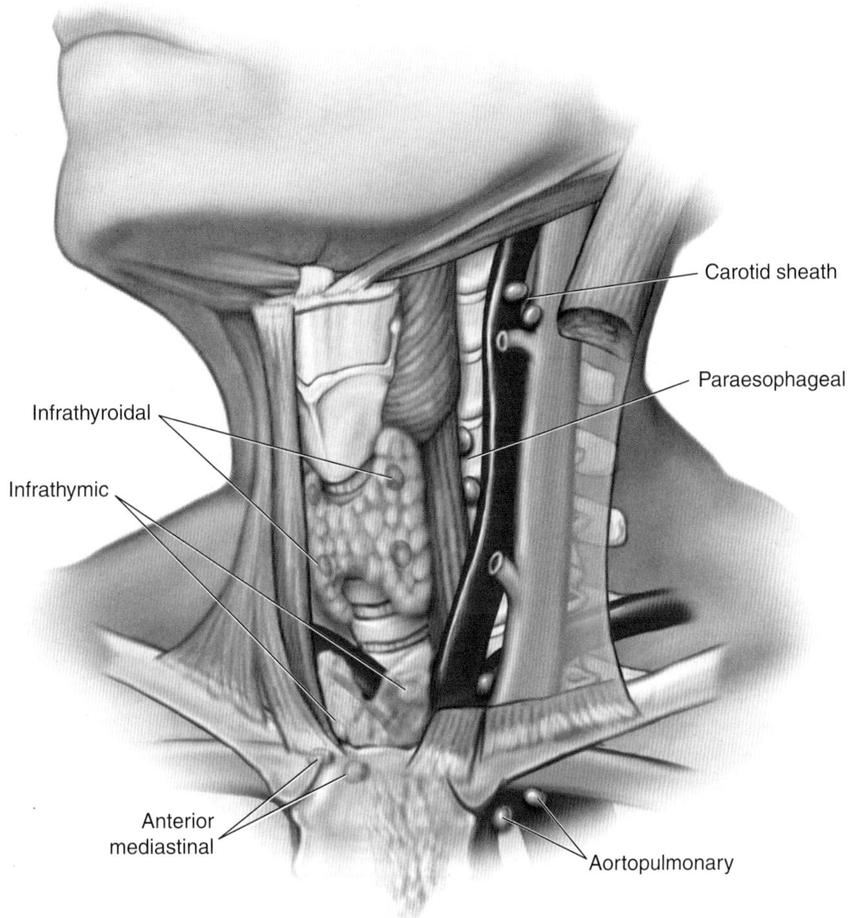

Fig. 103.3 Anatomic locations of ectopic parathyroid glands. Formal neck exploration and midline sternotomy may be required in rare cases of ectopic gland location.

ALTERNATIVE TECHNIQUE 2: Parathyroid Reimplantation

Occasionally, surgical hypoparathyroidism occurs (verified with intraoperative PTH) and this requires reimplantation of parathyroid tissue. In general, this tissue is reimplanted in the sternocleidomastoid muscle and the location marked with metallic clips to facilitate postsurgical imaging/localization. The tissue should be minced into small fragments and carefully placed in a pocket in the muscle. Frozen section verification of normal parathyroid tissue is a requirement of this technique. If a distant site is required, implantation into the brachioradialis muscle is readily achieved with a small incision. This allows for monitoring of the tissue at a site distant from the cervical region so there is no confusion related to ectopic parathyroid tissues/recurrence (Fig. 103.4). It may also be desirable to cryopreserve parathyroid tissue for later use if the risk of permanent hypoparathyroidism is recognized.

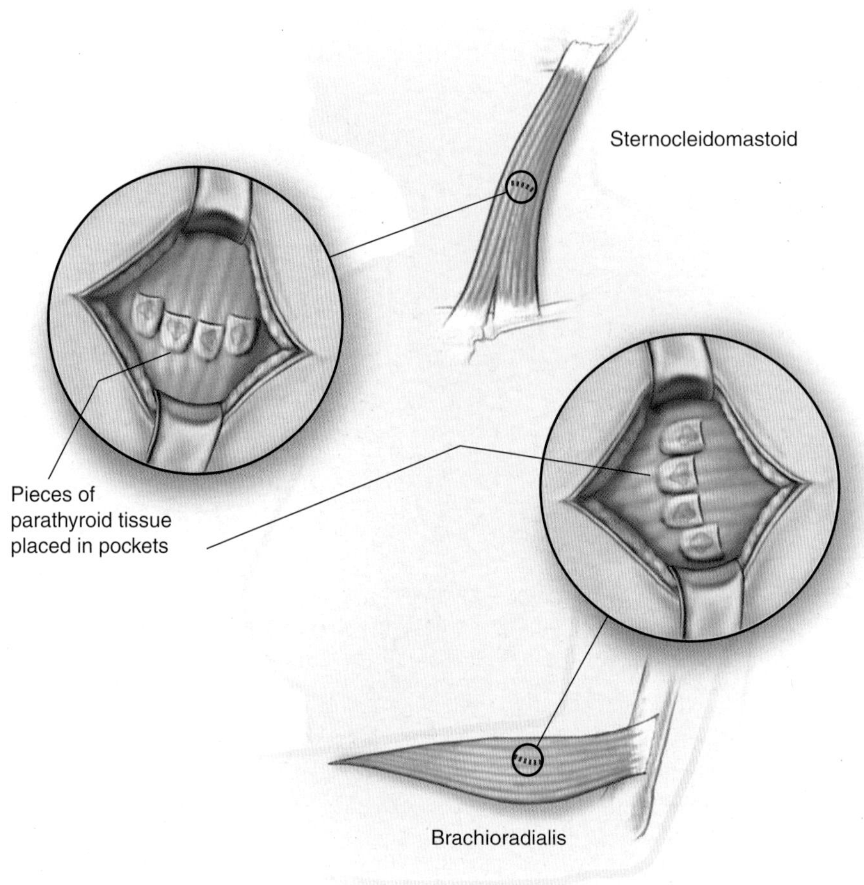

Fig. 103.4 Parathyroid reimplantation options include the sternocleidomastoid muscle or the brachioradialis muscle. The gland is morselized and placed into small muscle pockets to promote neovascularization.

Avoidance and Management of Intraoperative Complications

The risk of intraoperative RLN injury in routine parathyroid surgery is very low (1% to 2%) and increases with revision surgery.[17,32,36] Some surgeons perform intraoperative laryngeal nerve monitoring with special endotracheal tubes that have electromyographic capability. This technology cannot be used in operations performed with local anesthesia for obvious reasons. RLN monitoring has generated some controversy and is not used in many institutions due to increased cost, false signals related to electrode placement, and the lack of significantly improved outcomes in the scientific literature. Although the use of the intraoperative nerve monitor has not been shown to improve outcomes in thyroid/parathyroid surgery, the technology can provide valuable information to surgeons about the functioning of the RLN and external branch of the superior laryngeal nerve. This is especially true for revision parathyroidectomy and heavily scarred surgical beds. Surgeons should not overestimate the benefits of neuromonitoring when discussing the technology with patients, and there is no substitute for meticulous technique in the region of the RLN to prevent nerve injury.[38,39]

Postoperative Considerations

The most common postoperative concern for parathyroidectomy is transient hypocalcemia; this is of greater concern when four-gland exploration or total thyroidectomy is performed.[40] Vascular insult to the glands may result in hypocalcemia, which may require PO or intravenous calcium supplementation in the perioperative period. Intraoperative PTH monitoring has been shown to decrease the incidence of postoperative hypoparathyroidism (2% vs. 9%).[36] A 1-hour postoperative PTH level of

2.5 pmol/L or less can identify individuals at risk for developing symptomatic hypocalcemia. Early calcium supplementation for these patients is warranted.[41] Permanent hypocalcemia should be avoided at all costs, with autotransplantation of parathyroid tissue being effective when performed at the time of surgery.[40] Fortunately, other surgical complications such as infection, hematoma, vocal cord paralysis, and permanent hypocalcemia are relatively rare.[17,32,36]

References

1. Askanazy M. Ueber ostitis deformans ohne osteoides Gewebe. *Arb Path Inst Tubingen.* 1903;4:398.
2. Schlagenhaufer FS. Two cases of parathyroid tumour [German]. *Wien Klin Wochenschr.* 1915;28:1362.
3. Mandl FM. Therapeutic attempt in generalised osteitis fibrosa by extirpation of an epithelial gland tumour [in German]. *Wien Klin Wochenschr.* 1925;50:1343.
4. Cope O, Barnes BA, Castleman B, Mueller GC, Roth SI. Vicissitudes of parathyroid surgery: trials of diagnosis and management in 51 patients with a variety of disorders. *Ann Surg.* 1961;154(4):491–508.
5. Cope O, Keynes WM, Roth SI, Castleman B. Primary chief-cell hyperplasia of the parathyroid glands: a new entity in the surgery of hyperparathyroidism. *Ann Surg.* 1958;148(3):375–388.
6. Dunhill TP. Parathyroid glands in relation to surgery. *BMJ.* 1924;1(3288):5–7.
7. Egdahl RH, Canterbury JM, Reiss E. Measurement of circulating parathyroid hormone concentration before and after parathyroid surgery for adenoma or hyperplasia. *Ann Surg.* 1968;168(4):714–719.
8. Wang C. The anatomic basis of parathyroid surgery. *Ann Surg.* 1976;183(3):271–275.
9. Mason EE, Hoines J, Freeman JB. Hyperparathyroidism: evaluation of four decades of parathyroid surgery. *Can J Surg.* 1975;18(5):422–429.
10. Percival RC, Blake GM, Urwin GH, Williams JL, Kanis JA. Thallium-technetium subtraction scintigraphy as an aid to parathyroid surgery. *Br J Urol.* 1985;57(2):133–136.
11. Barraclough BH, Reeve TS, Duffy PJ, Picker RH. The localization of parathyroid tissue by ultrasound scanning prior to surgery in patients with hyperparathyroidism. *World J Surg.* 1981;5(1):91–95.
12. Cady B, Sedgwick CE. History of thyroid and parathyroid surgery. *Major Probl Clin Surg.* 1980;15:1–5.
13. Bröte L, Fagerberg G, Gillquist J, Larsson L. Parathyroid localization in patients with previous neck surgery. *Acta Chir Scand.* 1978;144(7–8):445–449.
14. Nussbaum SR, Thompson AR, Hutcheson KA, Gaz RD, Wang CA. Intraoperative measurement of parathyroid hormone in the surgical management of hyperparathyroidism. *Surgery.* 1988;104(6):1121–1127.
15. Robertson GS, Iqbal SJ, Bolia A, Bell PR, Veitch PS. Intraoperative parathyroid hormone estimation: a valuable adjunct to parathyroid surgery. *Ann R Coll Surg Engl.* 1992;74(1):19–22.
16. Coker LH, Rorie K, Cantley L, et al. Primary hyperparathyroidism, cognition, and health-related quality of life. *Ann Surg.* 2005;242(5):642–650.
17. Bellantone R, Raffaelli M, DE Crea C, Traini E, Lombardi CP. Minimally-invasive parathyroid surgery. *Acta Otorhinolaryngol Ital.* 2011;31(4):207–215.
18. Greene AB, Butler RS, McIntyre S, et al. National trends in parathyroid surgery from 1998 to 2008: a decade of change. *J Am Coll Surg.* 2009;209(3):332–343.
19. Hodin R, Angelos P, Carty S, et al. No need to abandon unilateral parathyroid surgery. *J Am Coll Surg.* 2012;215(2):297.
20. Norman J. Controversies in parathyroid surgery: the quest for a "mini" unilateral parathyroid operation seems to have gone too far. *J Surg Oncol.* 2012;105(1):1–3.
21. Ahmadieh H, Kreidieh O, Akl EA, El-Hajj Fuleihan G. Minimally invasive parathyroidectomy guided by intraoperative parathyroid hormone monitoring (IOPTH) and preoperative imaging versus bilateral neck exploration for primary hyperparathyroidism in adults. *Cochrane Database Syst Rev.* 2020;10:CD010787.
22. Mohebati A, Shaha AR. Imaging techniques in parathyroid surgery for primary hyperparathyroidism. *Am J Otolaryngol.* 2012;33(4):457–468.
23. Adler JT, Sippel RS, Chen H. New trends in parathyroid surgery. *Curr Probl Surg.* 2010;47(12):958–1017.
24. Hunter GJ, Schellingerhout D, Vu TH, Perrier ND, Hamberg LM. Accuracy of four-dimensional CT for the localization of abnormal parathyroid glands in patients with primary hyperparathyroidism. *Radiology.* 2012;264(3):789–795.
25. Wein RO, Weber RS. Parathyroid surgery: what the radiologists need to know. *Neuroimaging Clin N Am.* 2008;18(3):551–558 (ix. ix).
26. Ismail A, Christensen JW, Krakauer M, et al. 11C-Choline PET/CT vs. 99mTc-MIBI/123Iodide subtraction SPECT/CT for preoperative detection of abnormal parathyroid glands in primary hyperparathyroidism: a prospective, single-centre clinical trial in 60 patients. *Diagnostics.* 2020;10(11):E975.
27. Shariq OA, Strajina V, Lyden ML, et al. Parathyroidectomy improves hypercalciuria in patients with primary hyperparathyroidism. *Surgery.* 2020;168(4):594–600.
28. Wilhelm SM, Wang TS, Ruan DT, et al. The American association of endocrine surgeons guidelines for definitive management of primary hyperparathyroidism. *JAMA Surg.* 2016;151(10):959–968.
29. Bilezikian JP, Khan AA, Potts JT Jr. Third International Workshop on the Management of Asymptomatic Primary Hyperthyroidism. Guidelines for the management of asymptomatic primary hyperparathyroidism: summary statement from the third international workshop. *J Clin Endocrinol Metab.* 2009;94(2):335–339.
30. Dumasius V, Angelos P. Parathyroid surgery in renal failure patients. *Otolaryngol Clin North Am.* 2010;43(2):433–440 (x-xi).
31. Akhanlı P, Hepsen S, Ucan B, Saylam G, Cakal E. Hypercalcemic patient diagnosed with primary hyperparathyroidism after dapagliflozin treamtent. *AACE Clin Case Rep.* 2020;6(6):e319–e321.
32. Adler JT, Sippel RS, Chen H. The influence of surgical approach on quality of life after parathyroid surgery. *Ann Surg Oncol.* 2008;15(6):1559–1565.
33. Miccoli P. Intraoperative parathyroid hormone assay during surgery for secondary hyperparathyroidism: is it time to give up the chase at the hormone? *Endocrine.* 2012;42(3):459–460.
34. Pellitteri PK. The role of intraoperative measurement of parathyroid hormone in parathyroid surgery. *ORL J Otorhinolaryngol Relat Spec.* 2008;70(5):319–330.
35. Sugino K, Ito K, Nagahama M, et al. Minimally invasive surgery for primary hyperparathyroidism with or without intraoperative parathyroid hormone monitoring. *Endocr J.* 2010;57(11):953–958.
36. Richards ML, Thompson GB, Farley DR, Grant CS. Reoperative parathyroidectomy in 228 patients during the era of minimal-access surgery and intraoperative parathyroid hormone monitoring. *Am J Surg.* 2008;196(6):937–942.
37. Iacobone M, Mondi I, Viel G, et al. The results of surgery for mediastinal parathyroid tumors: a comparative study of 63 patients. *Langenbeck's Arch Surg.* 2010;395(7):947–953.
38. Angelos P. Ethical and medicolegal issues in neuromonitoring during thyroid and parathyroid surgery: a review of the recent literature. *Curr Opin Oncol.* 2012;24(1):16–21.
39. Randolph GW, Dralle H, Abdullah H, et al. International Intraoperative Monitoring Study Group. Electrophysiologic recurrent laryngeal nerve monitoring during thyroid and parathyroid surgery: international standards guideline statement. *Laryngoscope.* 2011;121(suppl 1):S1–S16.
40. Testini M, Rosato L, Avenia N, et al. The impact of single parathyroid gland autotransplantation during thyroid surgery on postoperative hypoparathyroidism: a multicenter study. *Transplant Proc.* 2007;39(1):225–230.
41. Lim JP, Irvine R, Bugis S, Holmes D, Wiseman SM. Intact parathyroid hormone measurement 1 hour after thyroid surgery identifies individuals at high risk for the development of symptomatic hypocalcemia. *Am J Surg.* 2009;197(5):648–653.

CHAPTER 104

Thyroglossal Duct Cyst

Omotara Sulyman, Tanisha Hutchinson, and David Hamlar

Armamentarium

Allis clamp
Bipolar and monopolar cautery
Blunt dissectors
Blunt retractors
Curved retractor
Lacrimal probes
Penrose or Jackson-Pratt drain
Small bone cutter/heavy scissors
Tenaculum forceps

History of the Procedure

Thyroglossal duct cysts (TGDC) are among the most common congenital neck masses. The thyroglossal duct is a remnant epithelial tract that forms as the thyroid gland migrates from its origin at the foramen cecum (between the junction of the anterior and posterior tongue) to its final position in the anterior neck.[1] The primitive thyroid usually descends anterior to the hyoid bone, but in 30% of cases, the thyroglossal duct is located posterior to the hyoid bone.[1–4] The thyroglossal duct typically involutes and atrophies between 7 and 10 weeks of gestation following migration of the primitive thyroid to its final pretracheal position in the inferior neck.[1,2] A remnant of the inferior thyroglossal duct commonly forms the pyramidal lobe of the thyroid gland. Persistence of other portions of the thyroglossal duct may give rise to cysts.[2] The locations of TGDC can be classified into four subdivisions: intralingual, suprahyoid and/or submental, thyrohyoid, and suprasternal.[5]

Simple excision of the thyroglossal duct without excision of the entire tract is associated with a high recurrence rate. In 1893, Schlange described excision of the thyroglossal duct en bloc with the central portion of the hyoid bone.[6] Schlange's approach was associated with a lower recurrence rate compared with simple excision. In 1920, Sistrunk explained that "the majority of operations for the cure of thyroglossal cysts are unsuccessful unless the epithelium-lined tract, running from the cyst to the foramen caecum, is completely removed".[7] Sistrunk extended Schlange's approach to include excision of a cuff of tissue between the hyoid bone and the foramen cecum.[7] Sistrunk's procedure reduced the recurrence rate from about 50% to 5%.[5,8] Today, the Sistrunk procedure is considered the standard management approach for thyroglossal duct cyst.

Indications for Use of the Procedure

TGDC commonly present as a midline neck mass, although 25% are found just lateral to the midline, with the majority on the left side.[9] In 2016, Thompson et al. found that of the 685 cases of TGDC, 520 (76%) were below the hyoid bone, and 165 (24%) were above the hyoid bone.[9] The diagnosis of TGDC is mostly based on history and physical examination. Ultrasonography should be performed to confirm the cystic lesion and the presence of a normal thyroid gland. Surgical excision of the TGDC is indicated in the setting of recurrent infection, recurrent drainage, and cosmesis, and to rule out the presence of malignancy. TGDCs occur in approximately 1% of TGDC.[10,11]

Thyroglossal Duct Cyst

In some cases, the TGDC may represent the only functioning thyroid tissue. If so, excision of the TGDC will result in permanent hypothyroidism requiring thyroid hormone replacement. Surgical excision is also contraindicated in the setting of active infection, as this is associated with a higher rate of recurrence. The infection should be treated and should have resolved prior to excision of the TGDC.[12]

TECHNIQUE: Sistrunk Procedure

This procedure is usually performed under general anesthesia with endotracheal intubation. Preoperative antibiotics may be given for perioperative prophylaxis. Decadron may be considered to decrease postoperative airway edema.

STEP 1: Position and Incision

The patient is placed in the supine position using a shoulder roll to provide neck extension. A transverse incision is marked in the midline through a skin crease in the upper neck slightly below the level of the hyoid bone. If there is a sinus tract or fistula, this should be encompassed within an elliptical incision.

Infiltrate the marked site with local anesthetic consisting of 1% lidocaine with 1:100,000 epinephrine.

The patient is sterilely draped in a manner that provides access to the oral cavity. Square off the surgical site from chin to clavicles and laterally from one sternocleidomastoid muscle to the other (Fig. 104.1).

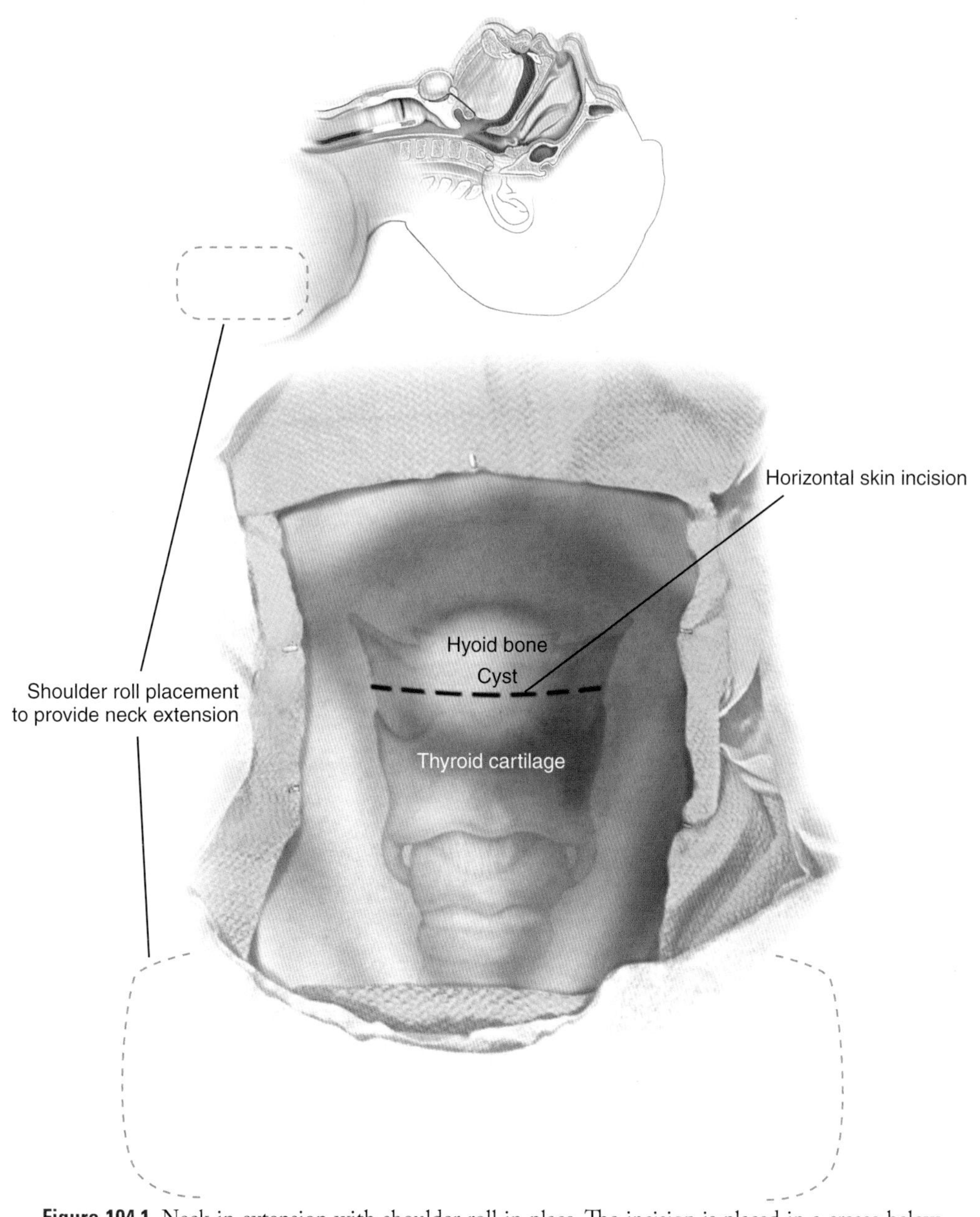

Figure 104.1 Neck in extension with shoulder roll in place. The incision is placed in a crease below the level of the hyoid bone.

TECHNIQUE: Sistrunk Procedure—*cont'd*

STEP 2: Identifying the Cyst

The incision is made in the skin and carried down through the subcutaneous tissue. The platysma muscle is divided. The strap muscles are identified and separated at the midline raphe. Extra care should be taken when separating the midline raphe as the cyst usually lies underneath the raphe. The strap muscles are retracted laterally exposing the cyst. The fascia overlying the cyst is divided (Fig. 104.2).

STEP 3: Dissecting the Cyst

The cyst is bluntly dissected free from the thyroid cartilage and the surrounding tissue, and left pedicled to the hyoid bone superiorly. A cuff of tissue should be taken with the cyst and tract to ensure complete excision. It is important to stay oriented to the midline to avoid injuring structures in close proximity. Straying from the midline risks injury to the superior laryngeal nerve (Fig. 104.3).

Continued

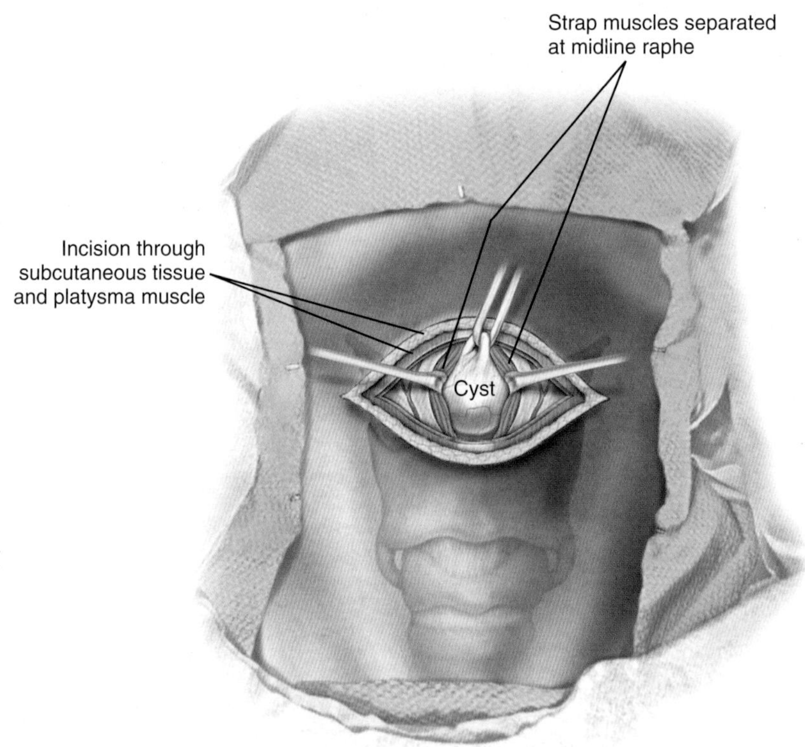

Figure 104.2 Incision carried through platysma with strap muscles separated exposing the cyst.

TECHNIQUE: Sistrunk Procedure—*cont'd*

STEP 4: Dissecting the Hyoid Bone

The hyoid bone is skeletonized sharply and grasped with tenaculum forceps. Avoid sharply dissecting directly on the superior and inferior aspect of the hyoid bone to prevent transecting the tract. Resect about 10 to 15 mm of the middle portion of the hyoid bone by making lateral bone cuts with a heavy scissors or a small bone cutter. The cuts should be medial to the lesser cornu of the hyoid bone to avoid injury to the hypoglossal nerves. The hypoglossal nerves are at risk for injury if the cuts are made too lateral (Fig. 104.4).

STEP 5: Dissecting the Superior Cuff

A cuff of tissue superior to the cut hyoid bone is dissected toward the foramen cecum. A curved retractor or finger can be inserted into the vallecula to displace the foramen cecum inferiorly to facilitate dissection (Fig. 104.5).

STEP 6: Excising the Specimen

At this point of the dissection, the specimen should be pedicled to the foramen cecum. With a finger or curved retractor pressing down the foramen cecum, the specimen is excised with a cuff of tissue still around the foramen cecum. The defect created may be closed with absorbable sutures (Fig. 104.6).

STEP 7: Closing the Wound

The wound should be irrigated and hemostasis should be confirmed. A drain is placed in the skin crease lateral to the incision. The wound is closed in a layered fashion by reapproximating the strap muscles loosely in the midline with absorbable suture (Fig. 104.7). The platysmal layer (if present) and deep dermal layer are reapproximated with dissolvable sutures. The skin is closed with absorbing or nonabsorbing sutures. Antibiotic ointment or Steri-Strips may be applied to the incision.

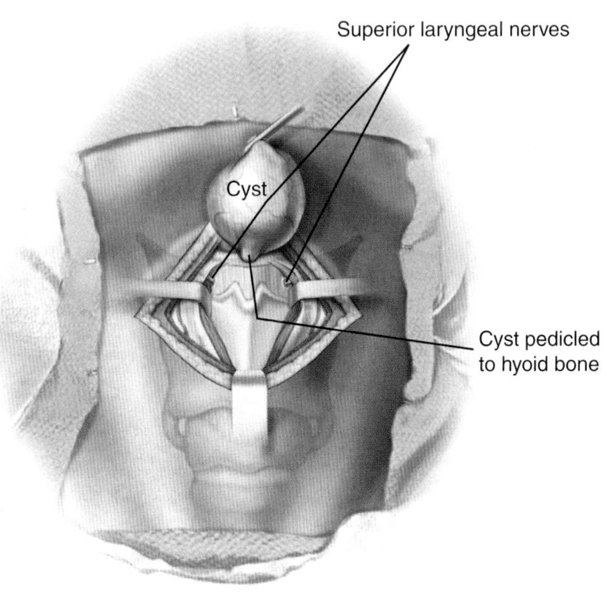

Figure 104.3 Cyst dissected from surrounding tissue and pedicled superiorly on the hyoid bone. Note the location of the superior laryngeal nerve.

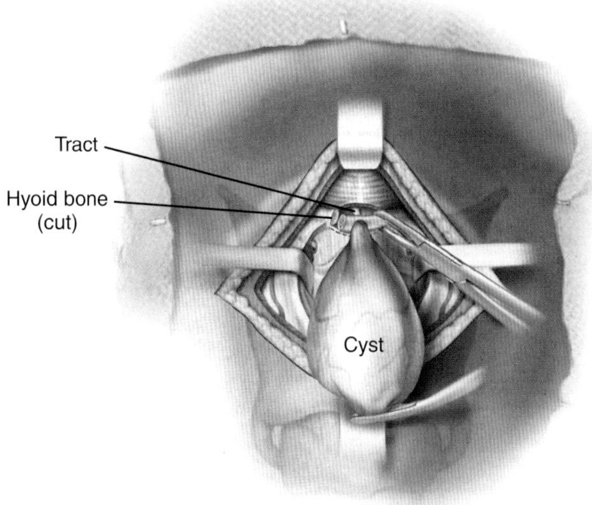

Figure 104.4 Middle portion of the hyoid bone is resected in continuity with the cyst.

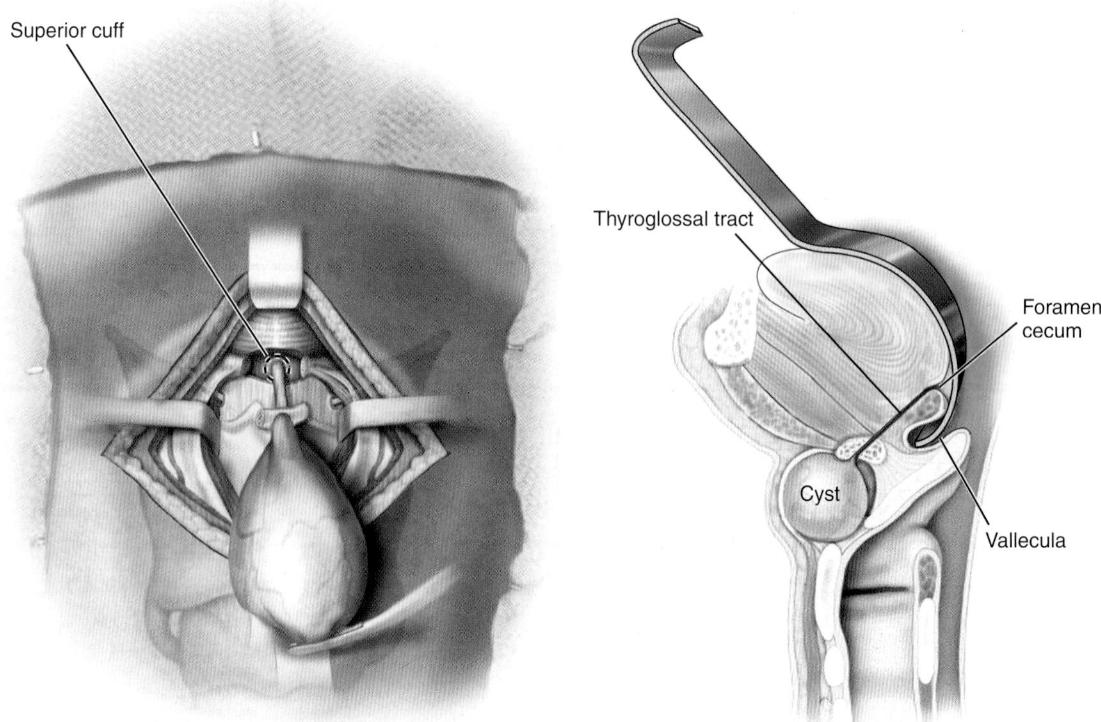

Figure 104.5 Suprahyoid portion of the tract is dissected. The cyst and tract are resected with a cuff of tissue at the tongue base. A retractor placed in the vallecula facilitates the resection.

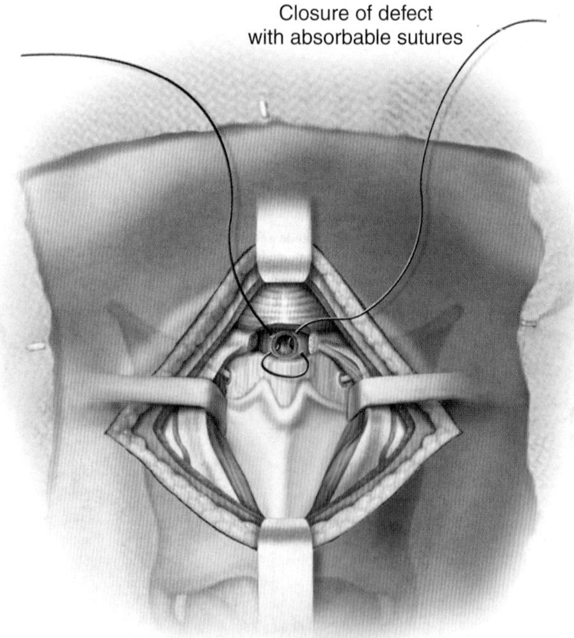

Figure 104.6 Closure of tongue base defect.

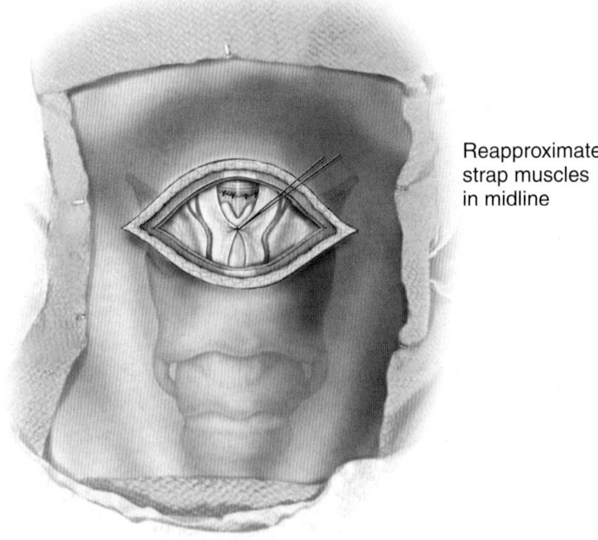

Figure 104.7 Strap muscles reapproximated.

ALTERNATE OR MODIFIED TECHNIQUE #1

During excision of the TGDC, if a draining sinus tract or previously infected cyst is present, an elliptical incision around the sinus opening or involved skin can be used to incorporate the involved skin into the incision. A lacrimal probe may also be introduced into the sinus tract to facilitate dissection (Fig. 104.8).

Avoidance and Management of Intraoperative Complications

Complications of the Sistrunk procedure are generally minor when anatomic landmarks are properly identified. Complications include wound infections, wound dehiscence, seroma, hematoma, recurrence, injury to the superior laryngeal nerve, injury to the hypoglossal nerve, inadvertent entry into the airway and pharynx, orocutaneous fistula, and hypothyroidism.[13,14] Major complications have been reported, including injury to the larynx requiring reconstruction with poor voice outcomes.[13]

If the pharynx is entered during the procedure, the defect should be repaired, a temporary nasogastric feeding tube should be considered to allow time for the defect to heal, and the patient should be given postoperative antibiotics. Inadvertent entry into the airway can be avoided by identifying the notch of the thyroid cartilage and the thyrohyoid membrane.[13] For unintentional airway injury, primary repair should be attempted, and tracheostomy should be considered. If the airway injury is just a puncture wound, then a drain should be placed to allow for egress of air as the wound heals by secondary intention.[13]

Staying oriented to the midline during the entire procedure and carefully identifying anatomic structures, especially in children, reduces the risk of major complications.

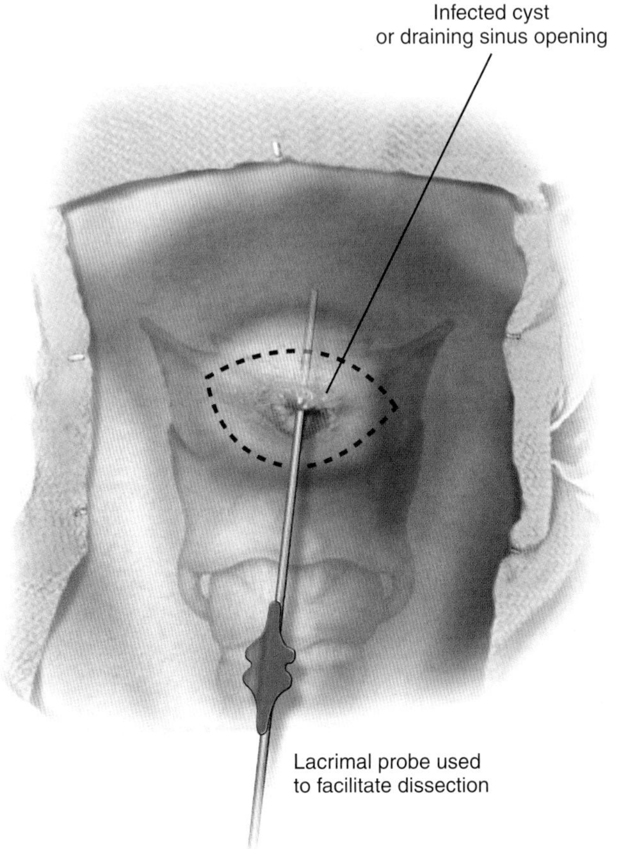

Infected cyst
or draining sinus opening

Lacrimal probe used
to facilitate dissection

Figure 104.8 Elliptical incision is used when the skin is involved. A lacrimal probe is placed into sinus to facilitate complete dissection of the tract.

Postoperative Considerations

Postoperatively, the patient is monitored for signs of hematoma. If a Penrose drain is used, the drain is removed when there is significant decrease in drainage. If a Jackson-Pratt drain is used, the drain is removed when the output is less than 30 mL in a 24-hour period. In most cases, the drain is removed on postoperative day 1. When limited dissection is performed, the wound may be closed without a drain. It is important to review the pathology of the resected specimen to ensure it is benign (Fig. 104.9).

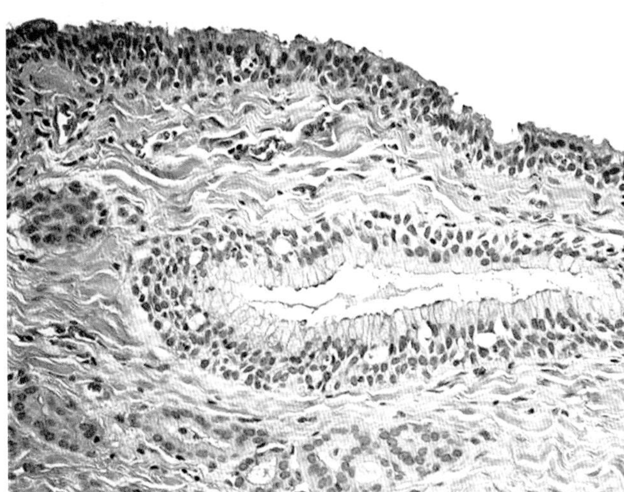

Figure 104.9 Histology of the thyroglossal duct cyst is shown here with a ciliated columnar-lined cyst.

References

1. Schoenwolf GC, Bleyl SB, Brauer PR, Francis-West PH. *Development of the Pharyngeal Apparatus and Face. Larsen's Human Embryology*. Elsevier; 2009.
2. Moore KL, Mark G, Torchia TVNP. *The Developing Human: Clinically Oriented Embryology*. Elsevier; 2019.
3. Ellis PDM, van Nostrand AWP. The applied anatomy of thyroglossal tract remnants. *Laryngoscope*. 1977;87(5 Pt 1):765–770.
4. Maddalozzo J, Alderfer J, Modi V. Posterior hyoid space as related to excision of the thyroglossal duct cyst. *Laryngoscope*. 2010;120(9):1773–1778.
5. Shah R, Gow K, Sobol SE. Outcome of thyroglossal duct cyst excision is independent of presenting age or symptomatology. *Int J Pediatr Otorhinolaryngol*. 2007;71(11):1731–1735.
6. Schlang H. Ueber die Fistulla colli congenita. *Arch Klin Chir*. 1893;46:390–2.
7. Sistrunk WE. The surgical treatment of cysts of the thyroglossal tract. *Ann Surg*. 1920;71(2):121, 2.
8. Ducic Y, Chou S, Drkulec J, Ouellette H, Lamothe A. Recurrent thyroglossal duct cysts: a clinical and pathologic analysis. *Int J Pediatr Otorhinolaryngol*. 1998;44(1):47–50.
9. Thompson LDR, Herrera HB, Lau SK. A clinicopathologic series of 685 thyroglossal duct remnant cysts. *Head Neck Pathol*. 2016;10(4):465–474.
10. Motamed M, McGlashan JA. Thyroglossal duct carcinoma. *Curr Opin Otolaryngol Head Neck Surg*. 2004;12(2):106–109.
11. Allard RHB. The thyroglossal cyst. *Head Neck Surg*. 1982;5(2):134–146.
12. Simon LM, Magit AE. Impact of incision and drainage of infected thyroglossal duct cyst on recurrence after Sistrunk procedure. *Arch Otolaryngol Head Neck Surg*. 2012;138(1):20–24.
13. Maddalozzo J, Venkatesan TK, Gupta P. Complications associated with the Sistrunk procedure. *Laryngoscope*. 2001;111(1):119–123.
14. Wootten CT, Goudy SL, Rutter MJ, Willging JP, Cotton RT. Airway injury complicating excision of thyroglossal duct cysts. *Int J Pediatr Otorhinolaryngol*. 2009;73(6):797–801.

CHAPTER 105

Management of Branchial Cleft Cysts, Sinuses, and Fistulae

Mehmet Ali Altay and Dale A. Baur

Armamentarium

#9 Molt periosteal elevator
#15 Blade
Adson forceps
Allis clamp
Appropriate sutures
Army-Navy retractors
Bipolar electrocautery
Bovie electrocautery
DeBakey forceps
Frazier suction
Freer elevator
Hemostats
Iris curved scissors
Lacrimal probes
Langenbeck retractors
Local anesthetic with vasoconstrictor
Methylene blue
Metzenbaum curved scissors
Minnesota retractor
Needle holders
Nerve stimulator
Senn retractors
Sweetheart retractor
Tenotomy scissors
Tissue forceps
Two-pronged skin hook
Weitlaner retractors

History of the Procedure

The development of the branchial anomalies, presenting as cysts, branchial sinuses, or branchial fistulas, is widely accepted to be the result of incomplete involution of the branchial apparatus.[1–3] In 1832, Ascherson first used the term *branchial cyst*.[2] In 1864, Housinger introduced the term *branchial fistula*.[4] Since then, many terms have been widely used in literature and practice. Many treatment modalities have been applied to branchial anomalies including incision and drainage, and sclerotherapy; however, complete surgical excision has proved to be the definitive treatment.[2,5–17] Historically, the cysts were only excised after becoming symptomatic, but recurrence rates as high as 20% were reported.[6,8,17] Current literature supports prophylactic excision in that these lesions are a significant source of morbidity from secondary infection, which can increase the difficulty of excision and the possibility of incomplete resection from postinflammatory fibrosis or scar.[7,11] To fully excise the tract of the sinus or fistula, an incision along the anterior border of the sternocleidomastoid muscle was once applied but later substituted with the classical and more cosmetic "stepladder" incision first described by Bailey in 1933.[5] Later, stripping techniques (or a combined approach) were successfully introduced for complete excision of the branchial sinus and fistula.[17,18] More recently, endoscopic and microscopic approaches have been applied.[14,15,17,18]

Etiology

Several theories have been proposed for the development of branchial anomalies, including branchial apparatus theory, cervical sinus theory, thymopharyngeal theory, and squamous epithelium inclusion theory. The branchial apparatus theory is the most commonly accepted.[1–3,19–21] Branchial anomalies are a consequence of abnormal development of the branchial apparatus during embryogenesis. Persistence of branchial apparatus remnants—due to incomplete closure or incomplete obliteration of the fetal branchial arches, pouches, or both—results in anomalies such as cysts, sinuses, fistulas, or an island of cartilage[20,22] (Fig. 105.1).

Presentation

Branchial anomalies are divided into first cleft, second cleft, and third and fourth pouch anomalies. Among these categories, second cleft anomalies account for 95%, and first cleft anomalies account for 1% to 4%. Third and fourth pouch anomalies, most of which are sinuses and similarly presented around the piriform sinus, are rare and are studied as case reports in the literature.[2,4,8,23–25] Most cases are diagnosed in the first and second decades but may present well into adulthood. Clinically, a branchial anomaly may present as a cyst, sinus, or fistula. A cyst is lined by epithelium but has no external opening. A sinus is a blind pocket that opens internally (persistence of a pouch) or externally (persistence of a cleft). A fistula is a tract that has both internal and external

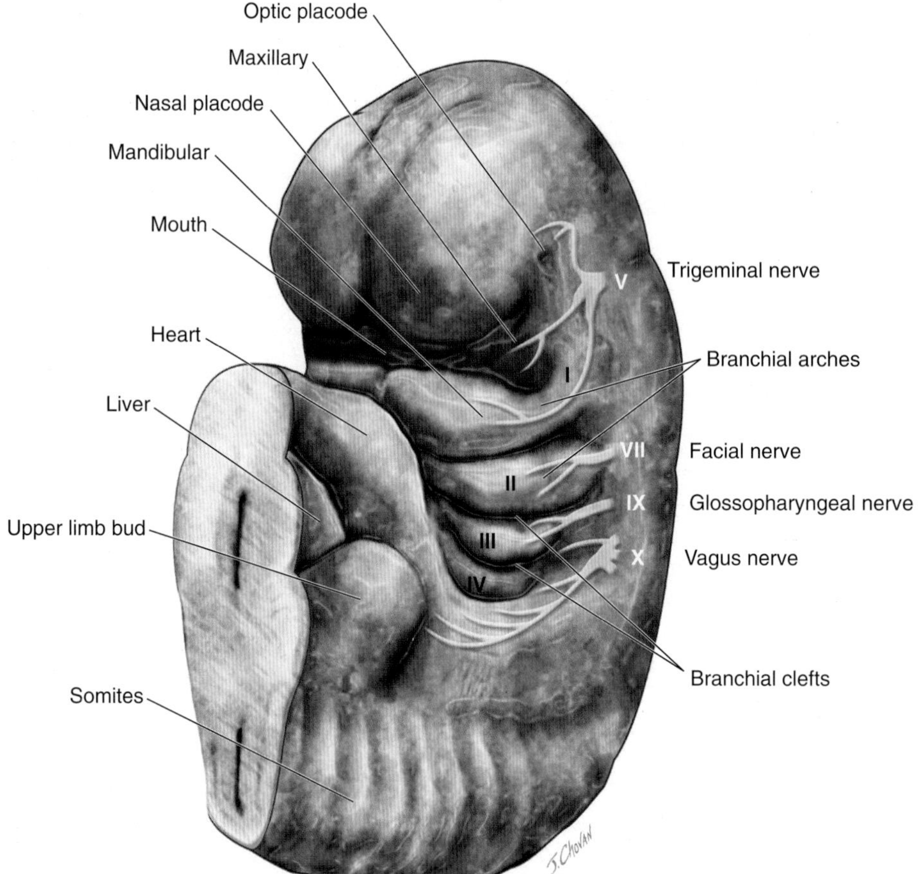

Figure 105.1 Embryology of branchial arches.

openings.[2,4,8,13,16–23,25–27] Branchial fistulas and sinuses seem to be diseases of childhood, whereas branchial cysts occur mainly in adulthood. Branchial cleft is a common congenital cervical anomaly in children,[28] and it can be accompanied by congenital developmental abnormalities of local tissues and organs, such as the first and second branchial arch syndrome, preauricular fistula, accessory auricles, auricle dysplasia, and atresia of the external auditory canal. A branchial anomaly may also be part of branchiootorenal syndrome[29] that was first described by Melnick et al.[30] and Fraser et al.[31] It is generally believed that the distribution of these diseases has no statistically significant difference in sex or side,[2,6,23,27,32–34] except that the fourth branchial pouch anomalies are predominantly left-sided (95% to 97%).[33] The branchial cleft cyst typically is a unilateral, painless, slow-growing, fluctuant, and smooth mass, sometimes with episodes of inflammation. Although rare, bilateral presentation of first branchial cleft anomalies has also been reported with a higher rate in familial cases.[34] It usually appears and enlarges after an upper respiratory infection. If infected, it can present as a firm, painful, immobile mass with or without systemic symptoms and signs of infection. The cyst may become abscessed, which can lead to rupture and cause a permanent sinus or recurrent cyst. It is reported that approximately 20% of lesions have been infected at least once by the time of surgery[35] (Fig. 105.2). Interim infection causes acute morbidity and increases the difficulty of complete excision. In the case of a branchial cleft sinus or fistula, about 80% of sinuses open to the skin and fewer open to the pharynx.[23] The presence of skin anomalies or swelling can be seen, sometimes with mucous or purulent discharge from the tract.

The location of branchial anomalies, usually parallel to a line from the tragus to the sternoclavicular joint,[8] differs according to their origin. First branchial remnants are relatively rare and are classified as type I or type II lesions.[36] Type I lesions present in the parotid or preauricular region as cysts or sinuses, whereas type II lesions present more posterior or inferior to the angle of the mandible. Either may extend into the external auditory canal (Fig. 105.3). The external opening is usually in the preauricular region or cervical region above the hyoid bone. Second branchial cleft remnants are located anterior to the sternocleidomastoid muscle, mostly in the junction between the upper one-third and lower two-thirds, and have been classified by Bailey[2] as type I (superficial cysts lying anterior to the sternocleidomastoid muscle and adjacent to it), type II (cysts lying on the great vessels and may be adherent to the internal jugular vein), type III (lesions extending between the internal and external carotid arteries), and type IV (lesions lying in the parapharyngeal space next to the pharyngeal wall) (Fig. 105.4).

If the cyst is large enough, it may cause mass effect and asymmetry of the neck as well as dyspnea, dysphagia, and dysphonia. Third and fourth cleft anomalies (Fig. 105.5) with

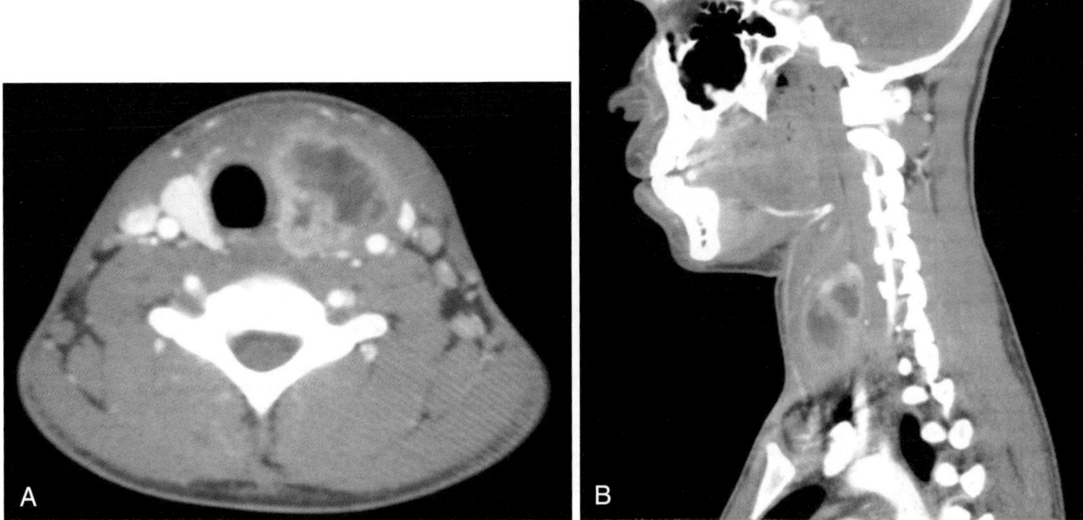

Figure 105.2 Contrast-enhanced axial (A) and sagittal (B) computed tomography scans showing a left-sided infected branchial cleft cyst with significant deviation of the airway. (Courtesy Joseph Carter, MD, Chair, Department of Otolaryngology, Metro Health Center, Cleveland, OH.)

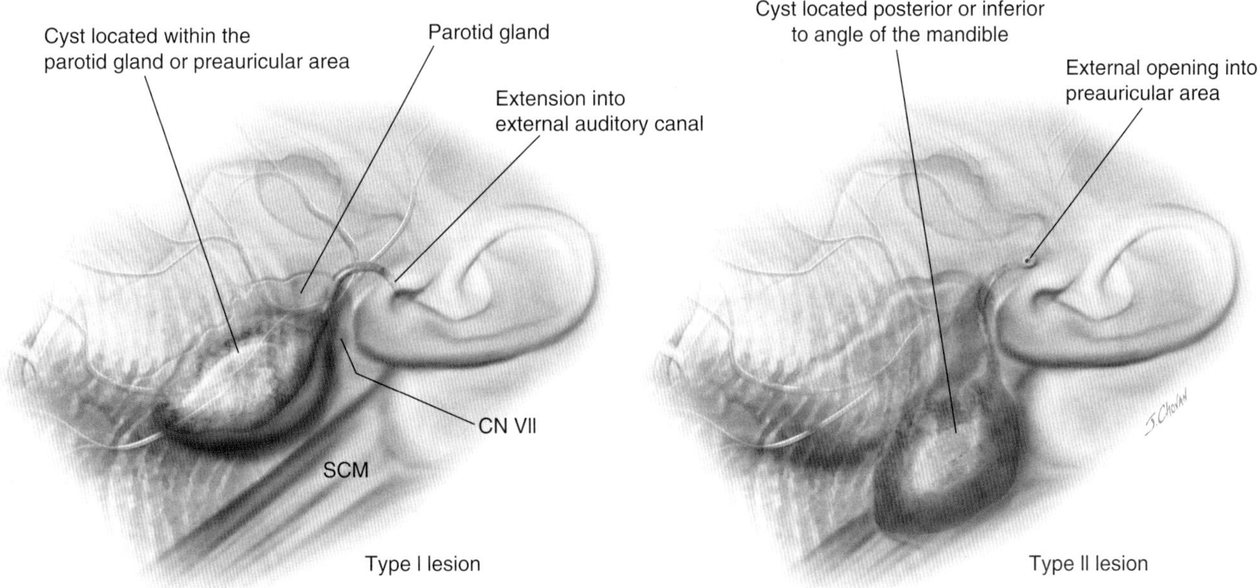

Figure 105.3 Type I and type II variants of the first branchial cleft cyst. *CN*, Cranial nerve.

noncommunicating or noninfected communicating cysts may initially present as cold thyroid nodules. When infected, there will be a recurrent upper respiratory tract infection, neck or thyroid pain and tenderness, and neck swelling. Other presentations include cellulitis, hoarseness, odynophagia, thyroiditis, abscess, and stridor. The third and fourth branchial pouch sinus connects to the piriform fossa (Fig. 105.6) or proximal esophagus (fourth), which can lead to tracheal compression and respiratory distress in infancy due to rapid enlargement as the infant swallows saliva, formula, or milk. An external opening to the skin is rarely present but can sometimes be found in the lower neck mostly secondary to recurrent infection and repeated surgery. The cephalic third pouch remnants, associated with thymic tissue, are described as passing superior to the superior laryngeal nerve and posterior to the common carotid artery, whereas the caudal fourth pouch remnants, associated with thyroid tissue, usually emerge caudal to the thyroid cartilage and cricothyroid muscle and pass between the superior and recurrent laryngeal nerves, looping under the aortic arch on the left side and subclavian artery on the right side.[2,24,27,33]

Histopathology

Histopathologically, there are differences between different anomalies.[2,16,23,24] The first cleft anomalies have squamous

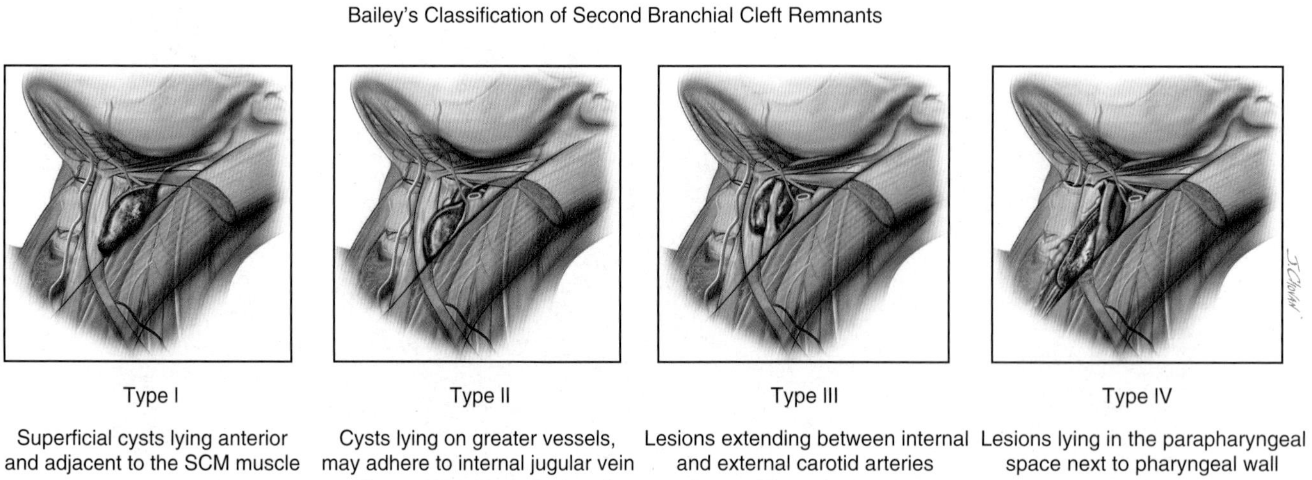

Bailey's Classification of Second Branchial Cleft Remnants

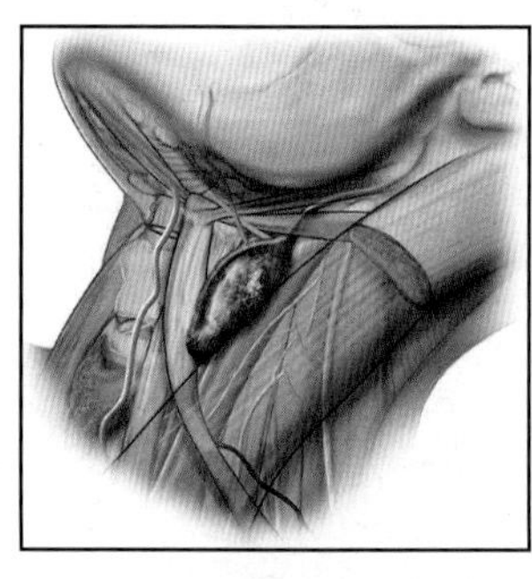
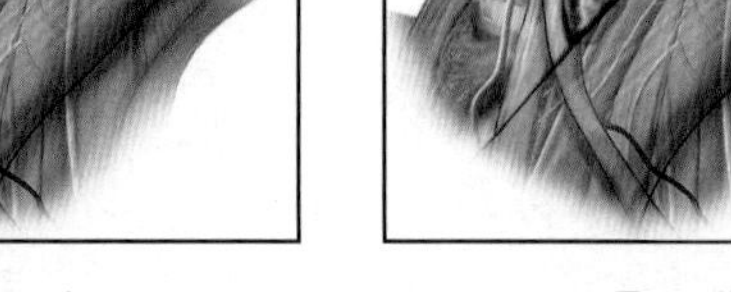
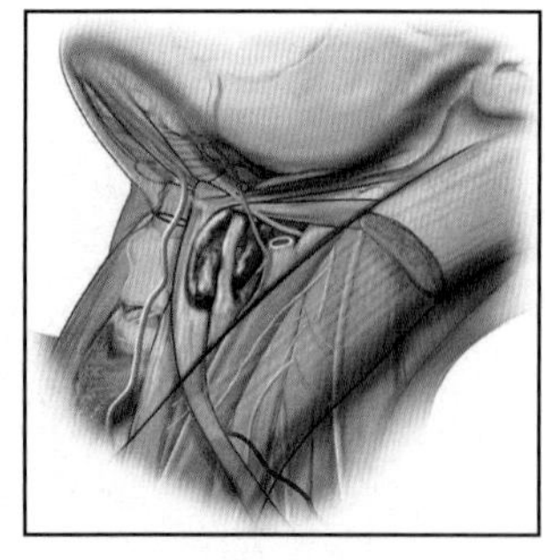
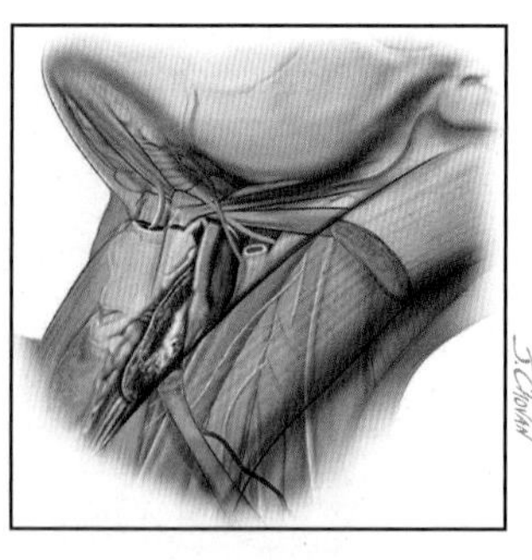

Figure 105.4 Bailey's classification of second branchial cleft cyst.

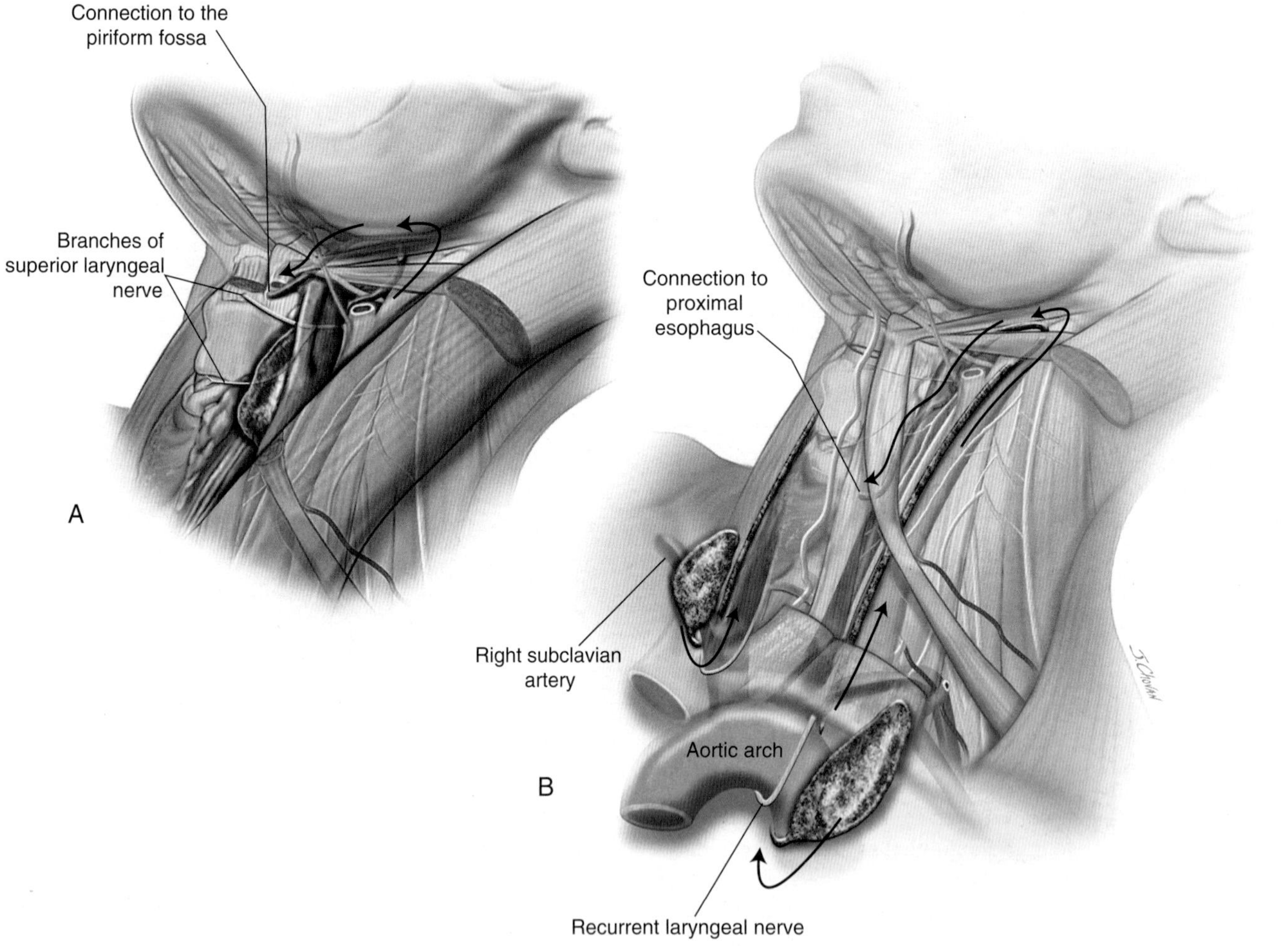

Figure 105.5 Third (A) and fourth (B) branchial cleft cysts, respectively.

epithelium (type I) or are mixed with skin adnexa or cartilage (type II). The second cleft anomalies are composed of a fibrocollagen wall surrounded by lymphoid tissue with follicle structures and a stratified squamous or columnar epithelium and occasionally respiratory epithelium (Fig. 105.7).

The sinus tracts of third and fourth cleft anomalies are lined by stratified squamous epithelium, which may be replaced in areas with respiratory epithelium. Squamous cell carcinoma has been reported to originate within branchial cleft lesions in adults, although it is extremely rare and controversial.[23,35]

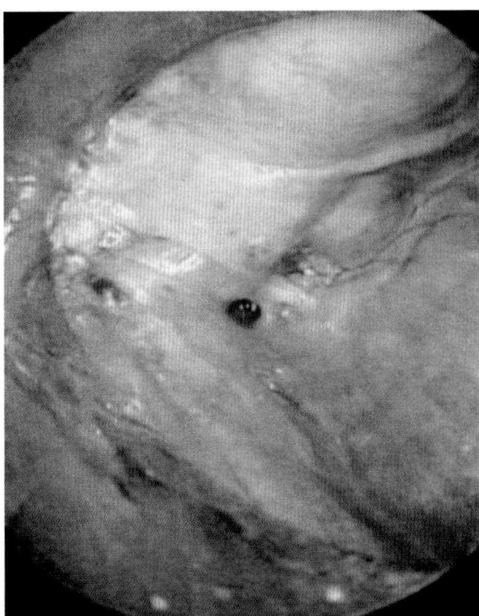

Figure 105.6 Direct laryngoscopic view of the right piriform sinus showing sinus tract opening from the third branchial cleft cyst. (Courtesy Joseph Carter, MD, Chair, Department of Otolaryngology, Metro Health Center, Cleveland, OH.)

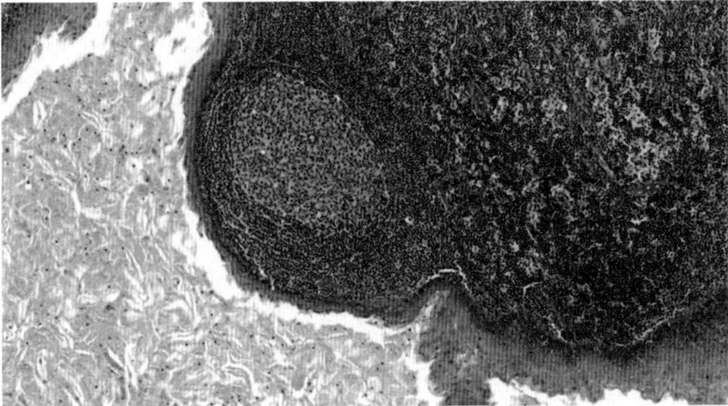

Figure 105.7 Stratified squamous epithelial lining of the cyst and germinal center in the wall of the branchial cyst. (Courtesy of Dr. Kelly Magliocca, Emory University, Atlanta, GA.)

Diagnosis

The diagnosis of a branchial cleft cyst is primarily based on medical history, clinical presentations, and exclusion. Branchial anomalies should be suspected for any unexplained lateral neck masses or recurrent neck space infections. Diagnostic procedures include ultrasonography, computed tomography (CT), CT fistulography, magnetic resonance imaging (MRI), and fine-needle aspiration (FNA), as well as sinogram or barium contrast study for third and fourth cleft anomalies.[2,16,19,23,37,25–27,32–40] Ultrasonography is a safe, inexpensive, and valuable exam that offers a reliable method to prove the cystic nature of the lesions. After the lesion has been proven cystic, CT and MRI can be performed to define the exact dimensions and the relationship with the neighboring anatomic structures. As an established diagnostic procedure in the diagnosis of a neck mass, FNA may not be diagnostic but aids in confirming the cystic and benign nature of a neck swelling. Cyst aspiration may appear as a turbid, yellowish fluid that microscopically may exhibit squamous cells, polymorphonuclear cells, lymphocytes, and cholesterol crystals. A barium esophagogram may reveal a sinus tract of third and fourth anomalies.

Differential Diagnosis

As cervical masses are common in clinical practice, branchial anomalies, although rare, should be included in the differential diagnosis. A differential diagnosis includes, toxoplasmosis, tuberculosis-scrofula, thyroglossal duct cyst, cervical abscess, dermoid cyst, hydatid cyst[32] cystic hygroma, paragangliomas, cystic metastasis of squamous cell carcinoma, and thyroid papillary carcinoma.[41] Guldfred et al.[32] reported a positive predictive value of 86% for the preoperative diagnosis of branchial cleft cysts and suggested considering every cystic lesion on the neck in the adult population as a potential cystic metastasis until proven otherwise. When left untreated, further enlargement or an extremely low risk of malignancy exist. Therefore, FNA is considered a mainstay in differential diagnosis.[42]

Treatment

Because the branchial cleft lesions will not resolve spontaneously, an early complete surgical excision of an asymptomatic lesion could preclude or minimize the chance of infection and is considered the definitive treatment, whereas other treatment modalities, such as sclerosing agents, chemocauterization, radiation therapy, and incision and drainage, are considered noncurative or controversial.[2,7–9,12–23,25–27,32–34,35] If there is no airway compromise or abscess formation, excision may be deferred beyond 3 to 6 months of age or after treatment of an acute infection. Recently, Ning et al.[43] proposed selective neck dissection to treat second, third, and fourth branchial cleft anomalies with recurrent or repeated neck infections, in an effort to reduce the difficulty of the surgery. In their study, the selective neck dissection technique was reported to be safe and effective in the treatment of branchial cleft anomalies with recurrent or repeated neck infection.

Robotic surgery is a recently defined technique that can be performed either through transoral route or by remote access retroauricular approaches for neck masses. It is reported to yield better functional and cosmetic outcomes compared with conventional open approaches in the management of oropharyngeal/laryngeal lesions. Widely considered a safe and effective technique, pediatric robotic surgery enables the surgeon to perform excision of branchial lesions without a visible neck scar.[44,45]

Limitations and Contraindications

Although a complete surgical excision of branchial anomalies is advocated, some limitations must be considered. Active infection must be controlled with antibiotics, with or without incision and drainage, before surgery can be performed. For these patients, surgery should be scheduled 4 to 6 weeks after symptoms resolve.[8,23,25,26] There is a general agreement in the literature that surgery of an inflamed cyst is associated with an increased risk of incomplete excision, recurrence, and complications. Schroeder et al.[46] have previously stated that 67% of branchial cleft sinuses/fistulae are infected before surgery. However, appropriate treatment of inflamed cysts is not clear. Kadhim et al.[47] recommends hospitalization of all patients for IV antibiotic application before surgery. In addition, the age of the child should be considered. An infant or a very young child with asymptomatic branchial anomalies can be followed for years to allow for a larger operative field and less potential damage to surrounding normal anatomic structures,[11] except in the case of aerodigestive tract compromise. Aspiration and decompression may be indicated if the patient is too young to undergo excision.[1,11,24]

TECHNIQUE: Excision of Branchial Cyst, Sinus, and Fistula

STEP 1: Anesthesia

This operation can be done under local anesthesia for superficial anomalies. However, general anesthesia is usually required due to the complexity of the dissection. Oral or nasal intubation can be applied for general anesthesia with the tube secured on the contralateral side of the lesion. The patient is positioned supine and routinely prepped and draped in sterile fashion.

STEP 2: Incision

The patient is positioned with the neck moderately extended and the face turned away from the surgeon for full exposure. For the sake of cosmetic outcomes, the course of the incision should be considered. Generally, horizontal or transverse incisions should be made along Langer lines or the crease of skin, and vertical incisions should be avoided. Incisions providing adequate exposure could be made directly over the surface of the cyst or elliptically, encompassing the sinus opening. Some surgeons even recommend a postauricular incision for the second cleft cyst with good cosmetic outcome. If a first cleft anomaly is deep to the skin, an additional standard S-shaped parotidectomy incision is recommended because of the close proximity to the facial nerve. When a submandibular incision is used, it should be at least two fingerbreadths below the mandible. A second parallel incision or "stepladder" incision may be required if the entirety of the cyst and sinus tract cannot be accessed with the initial incision (Fig. 105.8A).

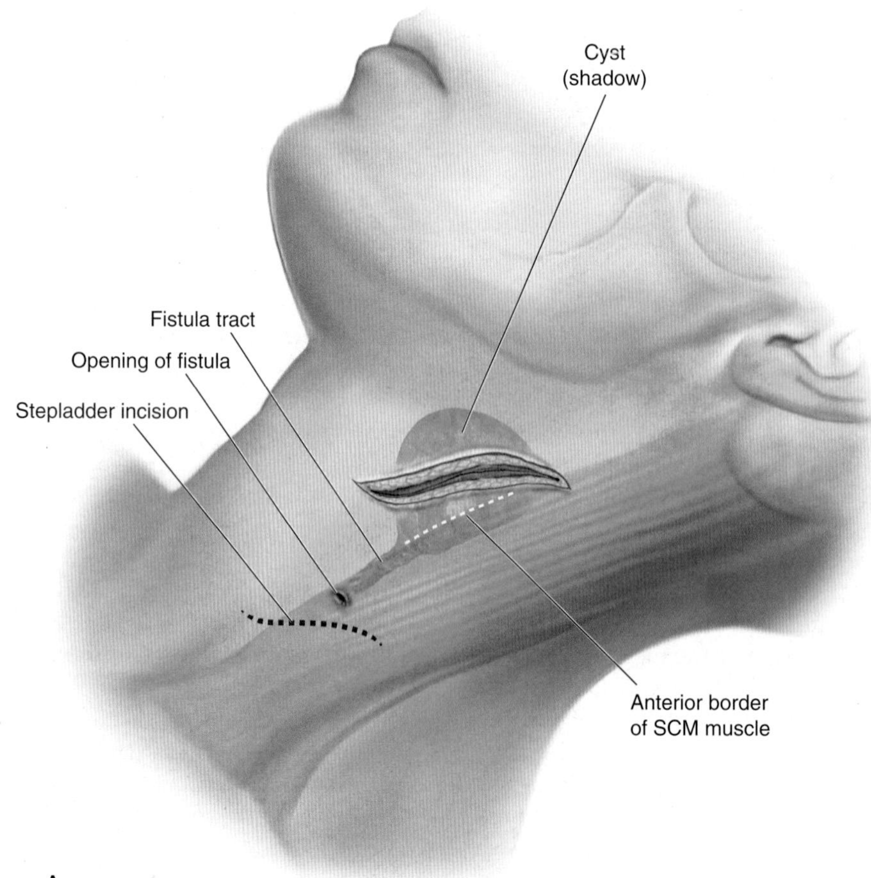

Figure 105.8 **A,** Standard incision for the second and third branchial cleft cyst with an additional stepladder incision, if indicated.

TECHNIQUE: Excision of Branchial Cyst, Sinus, and Fistula—cont'd

STEP 3: Dissection and Excision of Cyst, Sinus, and Fistula

After the incision is made, dissection proceeds through the subcutaneous tissues, platysma, and the superficial layer of the deep cervical fascia. If the cyst is large, partial aspiration may be helpful to facilitate dissection. Dissection of the cyst is relatively uncomplicated if it is intact. Cases with sinus or fistula are more challenging because of the complexity of the tracts. Injection of the tract with methylene blue or insertion of a malleable probe may help the surgeon to identify the tract. For third and fourth branchial anomalies, the internal opening of the sinus can be identified by rigid endoscopy near the piriform fossa. Nerve monitors may be used throughout the procedure due to the close proximity of the cranial nerves and their branches.

First branchial cleft anomalies may lie superficial or deep to the facial nerve. The facial nerve and its branches should be carefully identified and preserved first, and then the dissection proceeds in a manner similar to that used for a parotidectomy. Partial parotidectomy should be performed together with the cyst excision if necessary. When the fistula or sinus extends to the external auditory canal, adjacent canal skin and cartilage should be removed for complete excision. In rare cases, the tract may extend to the middle ear space or even extend along the eustachian tube. The associated tissue should be excised as far as possible. Second branchial cysts can be found along the upper third of the anterior border of the sternocleidomastoid muscle. The cyst is separated from the superficial layer of the deep cervical fascia. The sternocleidomastoid muscle is then retracted posteriorly to expose the posterior border of the cyst. If the cyst is deep, dissection continues to the carotid sheath to identify the internal jugular vein, the common carotid artery, and the vagus nerve. In this area, special care should be taken to avoid injury to vital structures. Posteriorly, second branchial cysts may cross cranial nerve XII and run deep to the posterior belly of the digastric and stylohyoid muscles, with or without a duct passing between the external and internal carotid arteries to the wall of the pharynx. At this point, a finger or a bougie placed in the oropharynx will be useful for complete excision.

For the second branchial fistula, the skin of the opening and surrounding tissues should be included in the excised margins. If the tract is too long, an additional stepladder incision is needed and the tract can be threaded through it for the convenience of complete excision. The third and fourth branchial anomalies can be found in the lower two-thirds of the neck. They perforate the thyrohyoid membrane and pass through the upper border of the left lobe of the thyroid, in close proximity to recurrent and superior laryngeal nerves. The current standard for surgical management of these lesions should include a partial or total thyroid lobectomy and complete dissection of the tract to the piriform sinus apex. Dissection should be carried out along the tracts. The laryngotracheal complex should be exposed. The ipsilateral thyroid lobe is mobilized and retracted medially to expose the cricothyroid joint. Recurrent and superior laryngeal nerves should be identified in this area and should be carefully preserved. Dissection then continues above the cricothyroid and runs to the piriform fossa through the thyroid cartilage. With sharp dissection the entire tract can then be excised along with surrounding thyroid tissue and part of the posterior thyroid cartilage if necessary. The superior parathyroid gland should be preserved in this procedure (Fig. 105.8B).

STEP 4: Closure

After copious irrigation, hemostasis should be achieved with electrocautery and ligation. The wound of the face and neck should be closed in a layered fashion. If there is a piriform or parapharyngeal wound, it should be closed with a pursestring suture or interrupted sutures of 3-0 to 4-0 Vicryl. An active or passive drain should be placed to prevent seroma or hematoma.

Continued

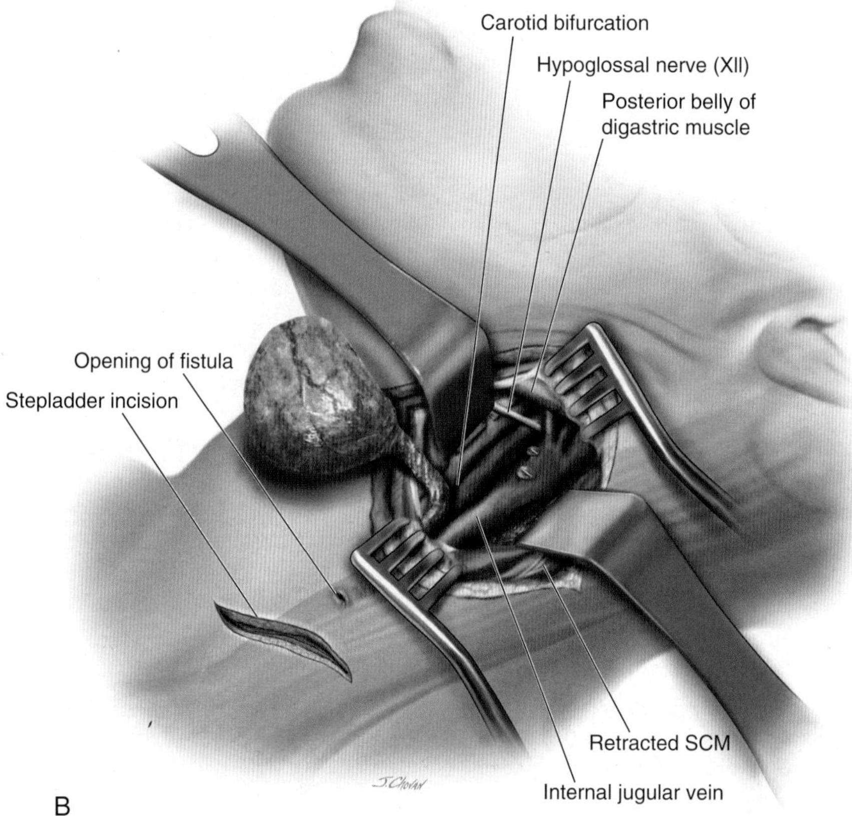

Figure 105.8 **B,** Dissection of the second branchial cyst inferior to the posterior belly of the digastric muscles.

ALTERNATIVE TECHNIQUE: Excision of Second Branchial Cleft Cysts via Retroauricular Approach

As the most common branchial cleft anomaly, the second cleft cyst is excised routinely by horizontal cervical incision. Some surgeons introduced the retroauricular incision for this procedure, with reported improved cosmetic outcome and patient satisfaction compared with conventional cervical incision.[10] The procedure is shown in Fig. 105.9. As an alternate method, transoral excision of second branchial anomalies has been described.[41] Ipsilateral tonsillectomy during the removal of second branchial anomalies has also been reported, but due to postoperative pain and risk of hemorrhage, it was found not to provide any outcome benefits.[48]

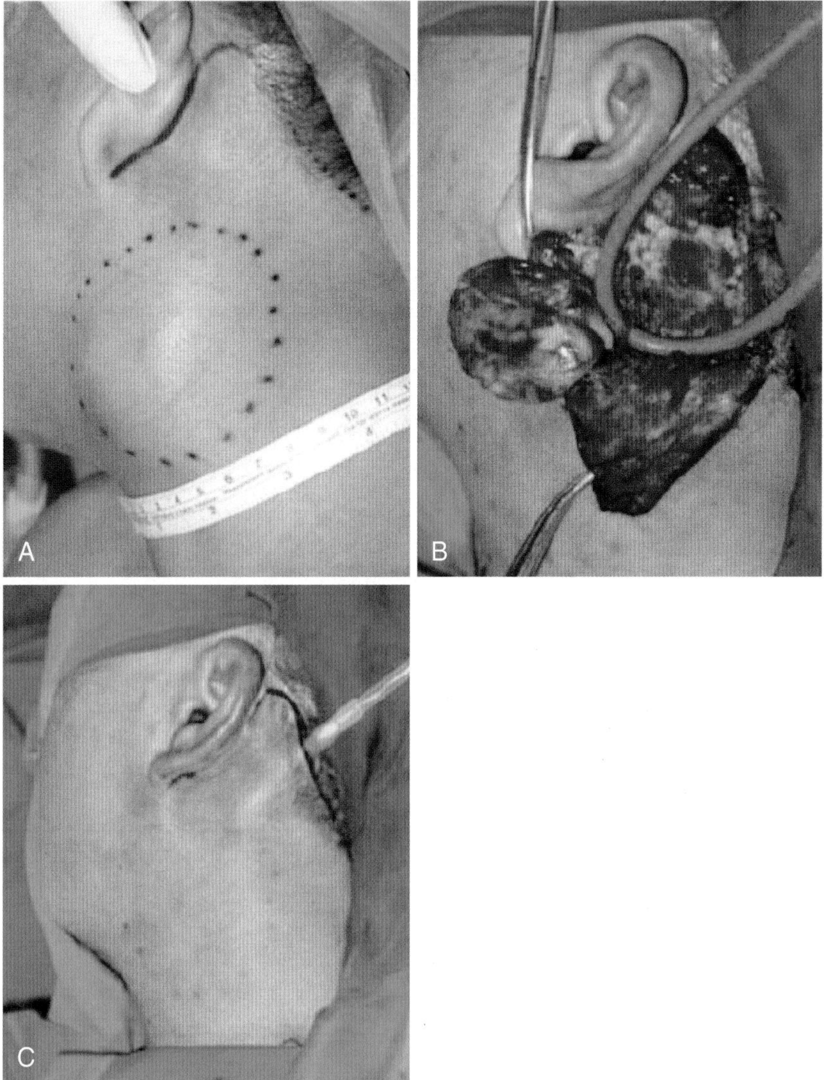

Figure 105.9 Retroauricular approach for removal of second branchial cleft cyst. **A,** Outline of the proposed incision for the removal of a second brachial cleft cyst using the retroauricular approach. **B,** Surgical removal of the cystic lesion. **C,** Closure of the wound with a drain in place. (From Chen WL, Fang SL. Removal of second branchial cleft cysts using a retroauricular approach. *Head Neck.* 2009;31:695.)

Avoidance and Management of Intraoperative Complications

The most common complication of branchial cleft anomalies is recurrence. Complete excision as a primary procedure offers the best results. Excision of the first branchial anomalies may pose specific surgical challenges. LaRiviere et al.[49] state that it is uncommon to successfully excise the first branchial arch anomalies in entirety at the first procedure. The average number of procedures to completely excise first cleft lesions is reported to be 2.4 per patient.[50] It should be kept in mind that repeated drainage procedures or failed attempts to remove the lesions carry an increased risk of injury to the facial nerve from scarring, which emphasizes the importance of a complete resection at the first attempt when possible. When the dissection is carried out, the cyst, sinus, or fistula must be excised together with adequate amounts of supporting connective tissue around the anomaly to ensure the entire removal of all epithelial remnants. Sometimes the wall of the cyst and tract may be thin and tenuous. Unexpected rupture can make the dissection difficult, so traction and dissection must be gentle and deliberate. To ensure complete excision, the tract may be injected with methylene blue. However, this can stain surrounding tissue and make the rest of the dissection more challenging.[3] In effort to simplify excision, Pitak-Arnnop et al.[51] have recently described the combination of fibrin sealant and methylene blue dye for surgery of branchial cleft cysts. These authors reported that sectioning of the lesion, with the proposed technique, proves a safer option in cases of high operative risk, such as injury to an important organ. Using a 2-0 or 3-0 monofilament suture or a lacrimal probe for the indication of the tract has also been documented.[52] For second cleft anomalies, bimanual palpation near the pharyngeal area will help confirm the attachment of the sinus tract to the tonsillar fossa, and direct laryngoscopy or endoscopy can be used for third and fourth cleft piriform sinuses. If there are suspected remnants, chemocauterization or electrocauterization may be applied to minimize the chance of recurrence after excision.

Other common complications include injury to adjacent important structures, including the previously mentioned cranial nerves, vessels, and parathyroid gland. Resection of these anomalies requires a specific and full understanding of anatomy. Excision of third and fourth anomalies should be performed in cooperation with the thoracic surgeon if the tracts run inferior to either the subclavian vein or the aortic arch.[3] A nerve monitor is useful for identifying the cranial nerves. Early excision is recommended due to the increased difficulty of excision following infection. Recently, Li et al.[53] proposed an algorithm (Fig. 105.10) for the management of branchial sinuses to avoid complications. In their approach, surgical options range from traditional open surgery to neck dissection and may also involve the use of carbon dioxide (CO_2) laser.

Postoperative Considerations

The airway should be evaluated if the surgery is conducted under general anesthesia. For cases with parapharyngeal or piriform incisions, systemic steroids should always be used to decrease postsurgical edema. For all cases, postoperative antibiotics are recommended due to the high risk of infection.

Patients should be followed up at 1 and 6 months after surgery. Wound healing, infection, recurrence, and cranial nerves should be examined. Endoscopic examination should be performed to evaluate the pharynx and piriform sinus.

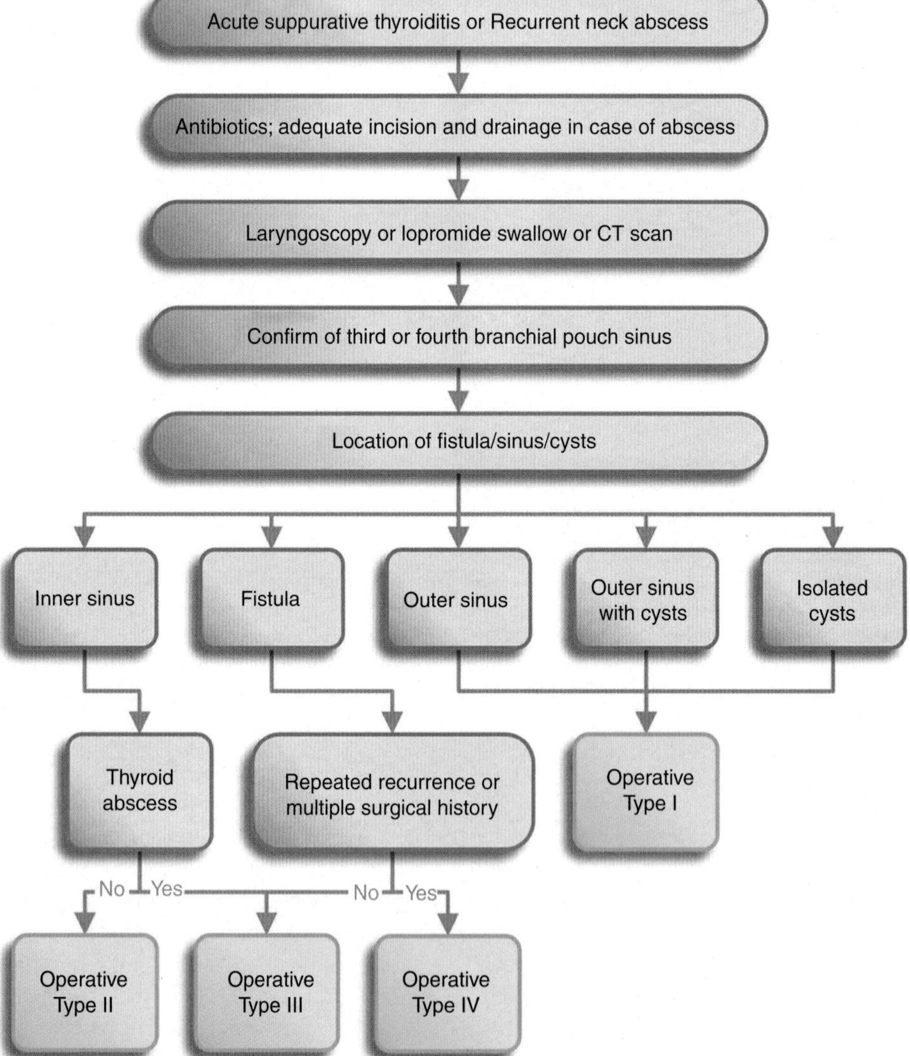

Figure 105.10 The algorithm proposed by Li et al.
Operative type I: Traditional open surgery
Operative type II: Internal fistula resection by carbon dioxide (CO_2) laser under a suspension laryngoscope and endoscope
Operative type III: Internal fistula resection by CO_2 laser combined with external fistula resection by small neck incision
Operative type IV: Complete resection of the fistula, assisted by the lumbar anesthesia tube as a metal probe combined with a pattern of neck dissection. (From Li Y, Lyu K, Wen Y, et al. Third or fourth branchial pouch sinus lesions: a case series and management algorithm. *J Otolaryngol Head Neck Surg.* 2019;48(1):61.)

References

1. Choi SS, Zalzal GH. Branchial anomalies: a review of 52 cases. *Laryngoscope*. 1995;105(9 Pt 1):909–913.
2. Bajaj Y, Ifeacho S, Tweedie D, et al. Branchial anomalies in children. *Int J Pediatr Otorhinolaryngol*. 2011;75(8):1020–1023.
3. Waldhausen JH. Branchial cleft and arch anomalies in children. *Semin Pediatr Surg*. 2006;15(2):64–69.
4. Amr M. Cervical cysts, sinuses, and fistulae of branchial, pharyngothymic duct, and thyroglossal duct origin. *Br J Plast Surg*. 1964;17:148–167.
5. Baumgartner CJ. Lateral cysts and fistulas of the neck. *Calif Med*. 1950;73(6):466–472.
6. Van de Mark TB, Weinberg S, Weizel HA, Gryfe JH, Zosky JG. Branchial cleft cysts. A review and case report. *Oral Surg Oral Med Oral Pathol*. 1969;28(2):149–156.
7. Deane SA, Telander RL. Surgery for thyroglossal duct and branchial cleft anomalies. *Am J Surg*. 1978;136(3):348–353.
8. Chandler JR, Mitchell B. Branchial cleft cysts, sinuses, and fistulas. *Otolaryngol Clin North Am*. 1981;14(1):175–186.
9. Neame JH. Stripping branchial fistulae. *Ann R Coll Surg Engl*. 1983;65(2):123.
10. Chen WL, Fang SL. Removal of second branchial cleft cysts using a retroauricular approach. *Head Neck*. 2009;31(5):695–698.
11. Cunningham MJ. The management of congenital neck masses. *Am J Otolaryngol*. 1992;13(2):78–92.
12. Kim MG, Lee NH, Ban JH, Lee KC, Jin SM, Lee SH. Sclerotherapy of branchial cleft cysts using OK-432. *Otolaryngol Head Neck Surg*. 2009;141(3):329–334.
13. Feldman JI, Kearns DB, Pransky SM, Seid AB. Catheterization of branchial sinus tracts. A new method. *Int J Pediatr Otorhinolaryngol*. 1990;20(1):1–5.
14. Chan KC, Chao WC, Wu CM. Surgical management of first branchial cleft anomaly presenting as infected retroauricular mass using a microscopic dissection technique. *Am J Otolaryngol*. 2012;33(1):20–25.
15. Chen EY, Inglis AF, Ou H, et al. Endoscopic electrocauterization of pyriform fossa sinus tracts as definitive treatment. *Int J Pediatr Otorhinolaryngol*. 2009;73(8):1151–1156.
16. Agaton-Bonilla FC, Gay-Escoda C. Diagnosis and treatment of branchial cleft cysts and fistulae. A retrospective study of 183 patients. *Int J Oral Maxillofac Surg*. 1996;25(6):449–452.
17. Olusesi AD. Combined approach branchial sinusectomy: a new technique for excision of second branchial cleft sinus. *J Laryngol Otol*. 2009;123(10):1166–1168.
18. De PR, Mikhail T. A combined approach excision of branchial fistula. *J Laryngol Otol*. 1995;109(10):999–1000.
19. Golledge J, Ellis H. The aetiology of lateral cervical (branchial) cysts: past and present theories. *J Laryngol Otol*. 1994;108(8):653–659.
20. Little JW, Rickles NH. The histogenesis of the branchial cyst. *Am J Pathol*. 1967;50(3):533–547.
21. McClure MJ, McKinstry CS, Stewart R, Madden M. Late presentation of branchial cyst. *Ulster Med J*. 1998;67(2):129–131.
22. Maran AGD, Buchanan DR. Branchial cysts, sinuses and fistulae. *Clin Otolaryngol Allied Sci*. 1978;3(1):77–92.
23. Glosser JW, Pires CA, Feinberg SE. Branchial cleft or cervical lymphoepithelial cysts: etiology and management. *J Am Dent Assoc*. 2003;134(1):81–86.
24. Liberman M, Kay S, Emil S, et al. Ten years of experience with third and fourth branchial remnants. *J Pediatr Surg*. 2002;37(5):685–690.
25. Houck J. Excision of branchial cysts. *Operat Tech Otolaryngol*. 2005;16:213.
26. Papadogeorgakis N, Petsinis V, Parara E, Papaspyrou K, Goutzanis L, Alexandridis C. Branchial cleft cysts in adults. Diagnostic procedures and treatment in a series of 18 cases. *Oral Maxillofac Surg*. 2009;13(2):79–85.
27. Telander RL, Deane SA. Thyroglossal and branchial cleft cysts and sinuses. *Surg Clin North Am*. 1977;57(4):779–791.
28. Teo NWY, Ibrahim SI, Tan KKH. Distribution of branchial anomalies in a paediatric Asian population. *Singapore Med J*. 2015;56(4):203–207.
29. Li HX, Zhou P, Tong M, Zheng Y. Branchial cleft fistula to branchio-oto-renal syndrome: a case report and literature review. *J Int Med Res*. 2020;48(7):300060520926363.
30. Melnick M, Bixler D, Silk K, Yune H, Nance WE. Autosomal dominant branchiootorenal dysplasia. *Birth Defects Orig Artic Ser*. 1975;11(5):121–128.
31. Fraser FC, Ling D, Clogg D, Nogrady B. Genetic aspects of the BOR syndrome—branchial fistulas, ear pits, hearing loss, and renal anomalies. *Am J Med Genet*. 1978;2(3):241–252.
32. Guldfred LA, Philipsen BB, Siim C. Branchial cleft anomalies: accuracy of pre-operative diagnosis, clinical presentation and management. *J Laryngol Otol*. 2012;126(6):598–604.
33. Godin MS, Kearns DB, Pransky SM, Seid AB, Wilson DB. Fourth branchial pouch sinus: principles of diagnosis and management. *Laryngoscope*. 1990;100(2 Pt 1):174–178.
34. Doshi J, Anari S. Branchial cyst side predilection: fact or fiction? *Ann Otol Rhinol Laryngol*. 2007;116(2):112–114.
35. Roback SA, Telander RL. Thyroglossal duct cysts and branchial cleft anomalies. *Semin Pediatr Surg*. 1994;3(3):142–146.
36. Work WP. Newer concepts of first branchial cleft defects. *Laryngoscope*. 1972;82(9):1581–1593.
37. Bhaskar SN, Bernier JL. Histogenesis of branchial cysts; a report of 468 cases. *Am J Pathol*. 1959;35(2):407–443.
38. Dutta A, Vallur S. An Unusual case of bilateral first branchial cleft anomaly: a case report with review of literature. *Indian J Otolaryngol Head Neck Surg*. 2020;72(3):381–384.
39. Blackwell KE, Calcaterra TC. Functional neck dissection for treatment of recurrent branchial remnants. *Arch Otolaryngol Head Neck Surg*. 1994;120(4):417–421.
40. Thorpe RK, Policeni B, Eigsti R, Zhan X, Hoffman HT. CT fistulography and histopathologic correlates for surgical treatment of branchial cleft sinuses. *Ear Nose Throat J*. 2020;145561320933015.
41. Zaifullah S, Yunus MR, See GB. Diagnosis and treatment of branchial cleft anomalies in UKMMC: a 10-year retrospective study. *Eur Arch Otorhinolaryngol*. 2013;270(4):1501–1506.
42. Coste AH, Lofgren DH, Shermetaro C. StatPearls Publishing; 2021 Dec. Branchial Cleft Cyst. [Updated 2021 Dec 15] In: StatPearls [Internet]. Treasure Island, FL. Available from: https://www.ncbi.nlm.nih.gov/books/NBK499914/.
43. Ning Y, Li C, Wang X, et al. Resection of second, third, and fourth branchial cleft anomalies with recurrent or repeated neck infection using the selective neck dissection technique. *ORL (Oto-Rhino-Laryngol) (Basel)*.2020;82(2):1–8.
44. Venkatakarthikeyan C, Nair S, Gowrishankar M, Rao S. Robotic surgery in head and neck in pediatric population: our experience. *Indian J Otolaryngol Head Neck Surg*. 2020;72(1):98–103.
45. Vidhyadharan S, Krishnan S, King G, Morley A. Transoral robotic surgery for removal of a second branchial arch cyst: a case report. *J Robot Surg*. 2012;6(4):349–353.
46. Schroeder JW Jr, Mohyuddin N, Maddalozzo J. Branchial anomalies in the pediatric population. *Otolaryngol Head Neck Surg*. 2007;137(2):289–295.
47. Kadhim AL, Sheahan P, Colreavy MP, Timon CV. Pearls and pitfalls in the management of branchial cyst. *J Laryngol Otol*. 2004;118(12):946–950.
48. Kajosaari L, Mäkitie A, Salminen P, Klockars T. Second branchial cleft fistulae: patient characteristics and surgical outcome. *Int J Pediatr Otorhinolaryngol*. 2014;78(9):1503–1507.
49. LaRiviere CA, Waldhausen JH. Congenital cervical cysts, sinuses, and fistulae in pediatric surgery. *Surg Clin North Am*. 2012;92(3):583–597 (viii).
50. Ford GR, Balakrishnan A, Evans JN, Bailey CM. Branchial cleft and pouch anomalies. *J Laryngol Otol*. 1992;106(2):137–143.
51. Pitak-Arnnop P, Subbalekha K, Sirintawat N, Auychai P, Klaisiri A, Neff A. Intraoperative injection of combined fibrin sealant and methylene blue dye for surgery of branchial cleft cysts: a case report. *J Stomatol Oral Maxillofac Surg*. 2019;120:378–382.
52. Acierno SP, Waldhausen JH. Congenital cervical cysts, sinuses and fistulae. *Otolaryngol Clin North Am*. 2007;40(1):161–176 (vii-viii).
53. Li Y, Lyu K, Wen Y, et al. Third or fourth branchial pouch sinus lesions: a case series and management algorithm. *J Otolaryngol Head Neck Surg*. 2019;48(1):61.

CHAPTER 106

Carotid Body Tumor

Julio Acero and Fernando Almeida

Armamentarium

#10 and #15 Scalpel blades
Appropriate sutures
Arterial graft instruments
Basic soft tissue room setup
Bipolar forceps (normal or irrigating)
Encircling tapes
Fogarty catheters
Hemoclip applicator
Magnifying loops
Major instrument head and neck tray (stringed instruments: Halstead mosquito, Kelly, and other forceps, Metzenbaum and Mayo dissecting scissors, retractors, brain spatula, skin and Joseph double hooks, Frazier or Yankauer suction tubes, others)
Mayfield headrest
Microsurgery tray
Nerve stimulator
Rubber shod clamps
Tracheotomy tray
Vascular 5-¬0 to 9-¬0 nylon sutures
Vascular grafts (vein graft or prothesis)
Vascular scissors
Vessel loops
Wound drain

History of the Procedure

The carotid body is the largest collection of paraganglia in the head and neck and is found in the carotid space. The term *paraganglia* was first described by Kohn in the early 20th century and is the most appropriate nomenclature from the embryologic aspect. The carotid body was first described by von Haller in 1743. Head and neck paragangliomas constitute less than 0.5% of all head and neck tumors and approximately 0.03% of all human tumors. Head and neck paragangliomas are named according to their site of origin (e.g., carotid body, jugular, vagal, tympanic). The carotid body tumor (CBT) is the most frequent head and neck paraganglioma, with a rate of 60% to 78%. Although mostly benign, their malignancy rate is 6% to 10%.[1] CBTs are also known as chemodectomas because of the physiological function of the carotid body as a chemoreceptor. CBTs were first reported by Von Luschka in 1862. In 1891 Marchand described the first removal attempted by Reigner in 1880, but the patient died. In 1886 Maydl reported a CBT resection, but the patient developed a stroke and became aphasic and hemiplegic. In 1891 Marchand reported the first description of the histologic appearance of CBTs. The first successful tumor resection of a carotid body in the American literature was reported by Scudder in 1903.[2,3] In 1953 James pointed out that the treatment of these tumors should be surgical resection except in those patients showing a potential risk of mortality or postoperative disabilities. In 1971 the Shamblin research group introduced a classification system for CBTs according to their relationship with the carotid arteries to determine the resectability of these tumors. Shambin type I tumors are small lesions at the carotid bifurcation and can generally be removed without difficulty. Shambin type II tumors are larger and significantly splay the carotid bifurcation but do not circumferentially encase the carotid arteries. Shamblin type III tumors are large and encase the vessels and are the most difficult when attempting resection. According to the Shamblin classification, type III tumors are associated with more perioperative neurovascular complications and complex surgical procedure.[4] In 2008 Hurtado-Lopez et al. were the first to successfully treat a theoretically inoperable case by combining traditional surgery with the preoperative insertion of two coated stents between the common and internal carotids beyond the base of the skull. This excluded the external carotid but maintained cerebral flow during the resection, which was performed 40 days later.[5]

Indications for the Use of the Procedure

There are three types of CBTs: sporadic, which is the most common (about 85% of CBTs); familiar, which is most common in younger patients; and hyperplastic. Familiar paragangliomas exhibit autosomal dominant transmission and are commonly seen in patients with von Hippel-Lindau disease, type I neurofibromatosis, and type II multiple endocrine neoplasia (MEN 2A, MEN 2B). The hyperplastic type is frequently associated with living at high elevation, as chronic hypoxic conditions including cyanotic heart

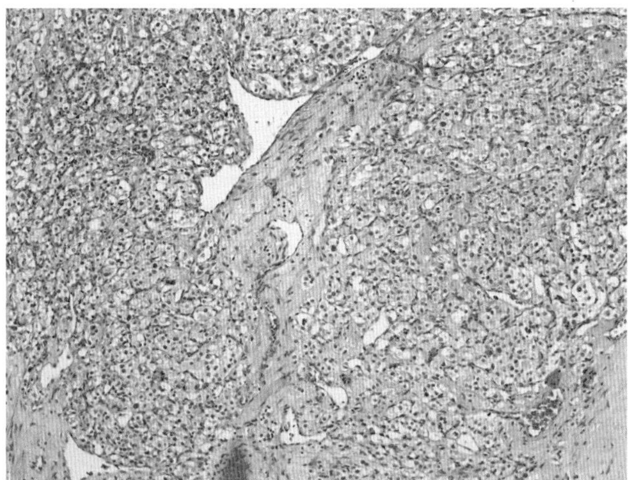

Figure 106.1 Carotid body tumor histology. Hematoxylin and eosin staining showing the nest of epithelioid cells with hyperchromatic nuclei surrounded by sustentacular cells.

disease and chronic obstructive pulmonary disease can lead to hypertrophy, hyperplasia, and then neoplasia of chief cells. There tends to be a higher female predominance, particularly in higher elevations. A molecular basis has been suggested. Mutation in six genes has been described, which has been shown to be related to the development of some paragangliomas.[6]

CBTs consist of a nest of epithelioid cells (type I cells), often with enlarged hyperchromatic nuclei arranged in groups called zellballen surrounded by a flattened layer of sustentacular cells (type II cells), and are positive for S-100 protein (Fig. 106.1). Although a minority of cases are described as histologically malignant, the pathological features cannot predict the biological behavior.[7]

Complete surgical resection is curative and is thus the mainstay of treatment, although tumor recurrence has been referred in 2.9% of cases after a presumed total resection. These tumors are particularly challenging to resect given their extensive vascularity arising from branches of the external carotid artery. The basic principles of the surgery involve locating and preserving the cranial nerves prior to dissecting the tumor. In large hypervascularized tumors with involvement of critical vascular and neural structures, total resection may be associated with bleeding and a high rate of morbidity and eventual mortality. Although single-stage resection is the gold standard, staged surgery has also been used, mainly in bilateral tumors and in cases with intracranial involvement. The surgical indication depends on the symptoms of the patient, size and location of the tumor, age and general condition of the patient, and risk of the surgical procedure concerning potential postoperative neurological impairment.[6]

Limitations and Contraindications

There are no absolute contraindications, except in elderly patients with associated morbidity and poor life expectancy. Although traditional therapy for CBTs is surgical resection, there are some limitations to its indication, such as the simultaneous treatment of bilateral CBTs, since blood pressure maintenance could be compromised by bilateral carotid body denervation. Other limitations are patients with high risk of stroke related to a potential carotid resection or ligation, and patients with malignant tumors with intracranial extension. Radiotherapy has been used in patients who cannot undergo surgery in order to control tumor growth, but complete regression of tumors with this modality is extremely rare.[4]

TECHNIQUE: Resection of Carotid Body Tumor

STEP 1: Patient Position

General anesthesia with orotracheal or nasotracheal intubation is administered with the patient in the supine position on the operating table with the neck extended and rotated to the contralateral side. In case of secretory tumors, premedication by the anesthesiologist with alpha and beta blockers is imperative. In cases where the resection of segments of the carotid artery with the tumor is expected, the lower extremity is prepared to obtain a vein graft (Fig. 106.2).

STEP 2: Incision

Incision should be based on tumor size. A longitudinal incision, parallel to the anterior edge of the sternocleidomastoid muscle, is the classic approach to carotid surgery. However, a curved horizontal incision along the cervical creases allows for a better approach to the surgical field and better aesthetic outcomes and can be expanded if necessary. Large tumors extended superiorly may need an extension of the incision including the preauricular area. Upper and lower skin flaps are elevated in the usual fashion. Careful dissection in a subplatysmal plane should be carried out to avoid injuries to the mandibular branch of the facial nerve or to the greater auricular nerve. Due to the high vascularity of this tumor, rough handling or dissection in an inappropriate plane will cause significant blood loss (Fig. 106.3).

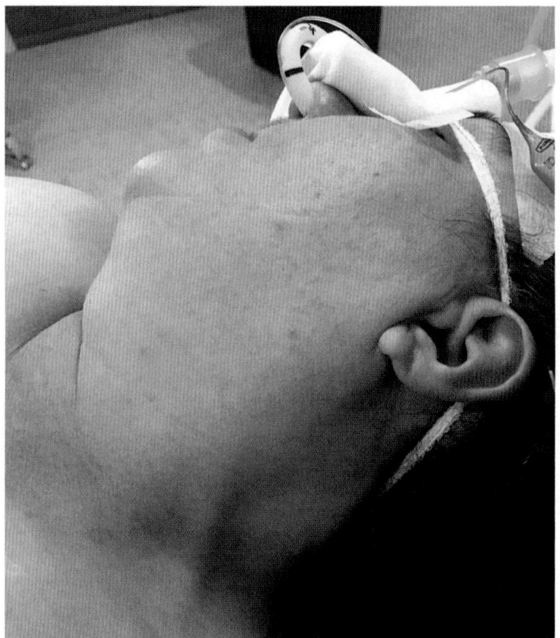

Figure 106.2 Patient position. Patient in the supine position on the operating table with the neck extended and rotated to the contralateral side.

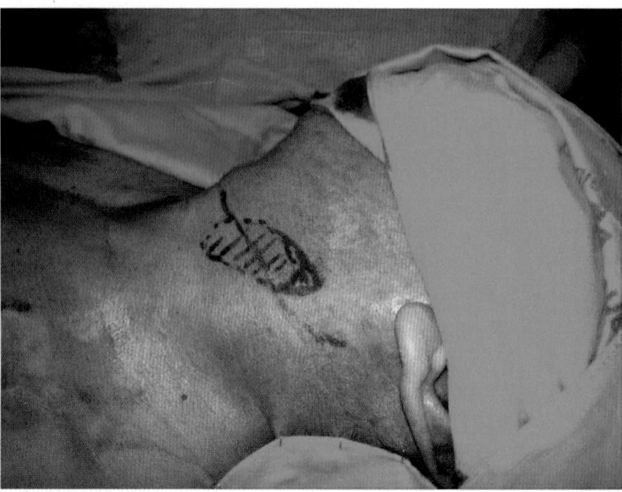

Figure 106.3 Incision along the cervical creases in the mid neck.

TECHNIQUE: Resection of Carotid Body Tumor—*cont'd*

STEP 3: Tumor Approach

Expose the anterior border of the sternocleidomastoid muscle. Retraction of the muscle allows for the identification and dissection of the internal jugular vein and the common, external, and internal carotid arteries. The approach to tumors showing superior extension can require the transection of the stylomandibular ligament.

Superior and inferior control of the blood vessels is an important step. Vessel loops are placed in the arteries and in the jugular vein allowing for retraction and potential occlusion in case of bleeding. The hypoglossal, ansa cervicalis, superior laryngeal, and vagus nerves should be identified and preserved (Fig. 106.4).

Continued

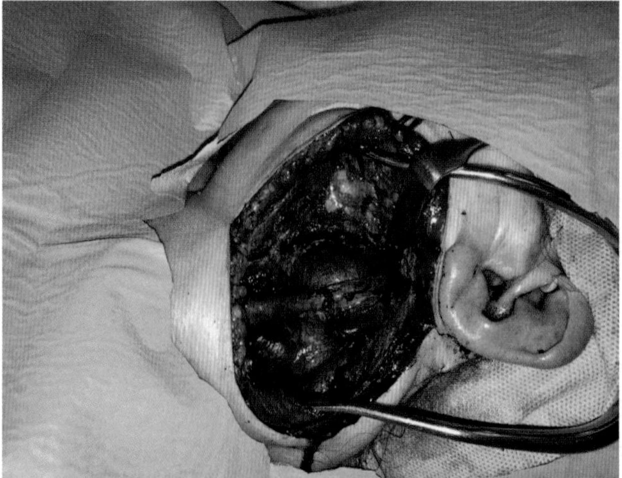

Figure 106.4 Tumor approach. Exposure of the anterior border of the sternocleidomastoid muscle and identification and dissection of the internal jugular vein.

TECHNIQUE: Resection of Carotid Body Tumor—*cont'd*

STEP 4: Tumor Dissection

Once proximal control of the common carotid artery is secured, dissection of the tumor begins. At this juncture, it is important that the vagus and hypoglossal nerves are identified and dissected to preserve their integrity. Dissection of the CBT should be performed in a subadventitial plane in order to reduce the risk of bleeding. This is usually a tedious, slow, and meticulous dissection because of the presence of multiple small feeder vessels. Cranio-caudal dissection of the tumor from the carotid vessels is performed into the carotid bifurcation. Careful hemostasis is obtained by means of bipolar coagulation and the use of clips. Crucial points at the dissection are the superior pole of the tumor, especially in cases of large tumors close to the skull base, and the posterior face of the bifurcation, where the majority of vascular injuries occur (Fig. 106.5A and B).

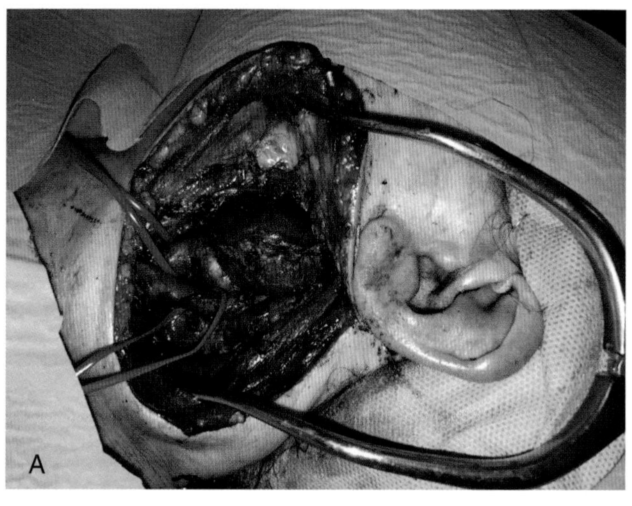

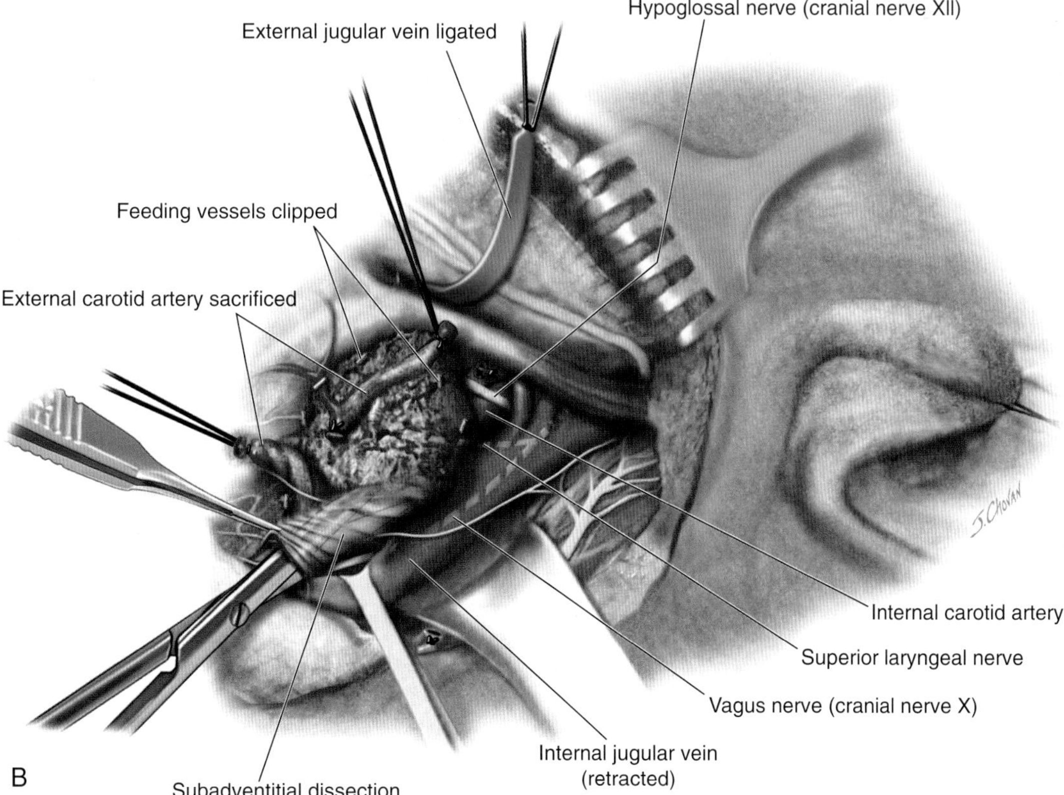

Figure 106.5 **A,** Dissection of the carotid body tumor. Subadventitial dissection with preservation of the cranial nerves. **B,** Dissection of the carotid body tumor (schematic resection). Subadventitial dissection with preservation of the cranial nerves.

TECHNIQUE: Resection of Carotid Body Tumor—*cont'd*

STEP 5: Removal of the Tumor

In complex cases, sacrifice of the internal jugular vein or the external carotid artery can provide better exposure and facilitate the tumor's excision. After complete exposure of the tumor has been achieved, it remains attached to the common and internal carotid arteries. Dissection of the tumor at this point, including ligation of the last feeding vessels, leads to its removal. Potential injuries of the vascular wall can occur and should be repaired using 5-0 vascular sutures. When the internal carotid artery is enveloped by the tumor or in case of malignant CBTs, internal carotid resection and vascular reconstruction either with a vascular prosthesis or a vein graft may be necessary (Fig. 106.6A and B).

STEP 6: Wound Closure

Once hemostasis and carotid permeability are assured, a Redon-type aspirative drain is placed. Two-layer closure of the wound is performed with 3-0 resorbable polyglactin suture at the subcutaneous layer while the skin is closed using staples or a 3-0 monofilament suture.

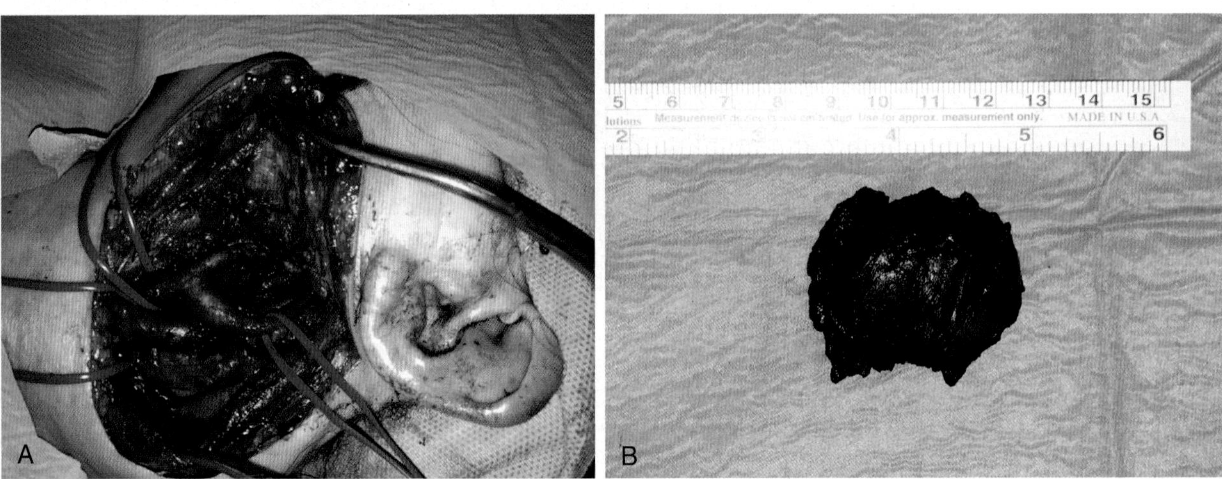

Figure 106.6 **A,** Removal of the tumor. Intraoperative aspect of the resection. **B,** Macroscopic aspect of a surgical specimen.

ALTERNATIVE OR MODIFIED TECHNIQUE

In cases of large tumors with cranial extension that require large exposed areas or exposure of the parapharyngeal space, a mandibular osteotomy at the ascending ramus can be performed (Fig. 106.7A–C).

In cases where resection of the internal carotid artery is necessary, reconstruction of the artery may be performed with an autogenous vein graft or a prosthetic graft (Fig. 106.7D1 and D2). Heparin solution should be injected proximally and distally. Proximal and distal anastomoses are performed using 5-0 vascular sutures. The patency of the graft is evaluated at the end of the procedure. Adequate repositioning of the mandible is ensured by previous positioning of the miniplates (Fig. 106.7E).

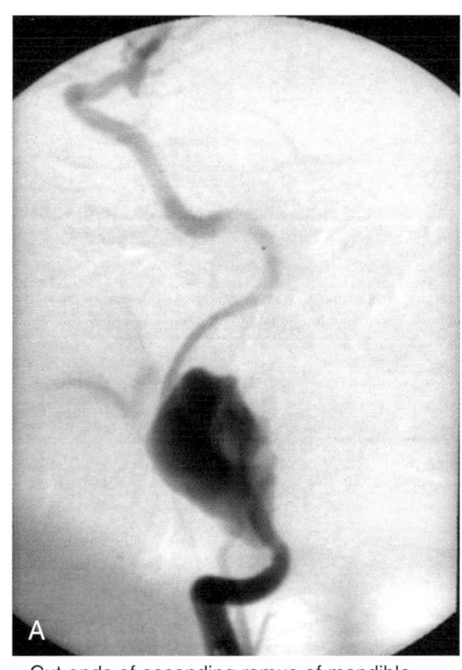

Figure 106.7 **A,** Internal carotid artery aneurysm. Preoperative angiography. **B,** Approach to the lesion through a mandibular osteotomy at the ascending ramus (schematic aspect). *SCM,* Sternocleidomastoid.

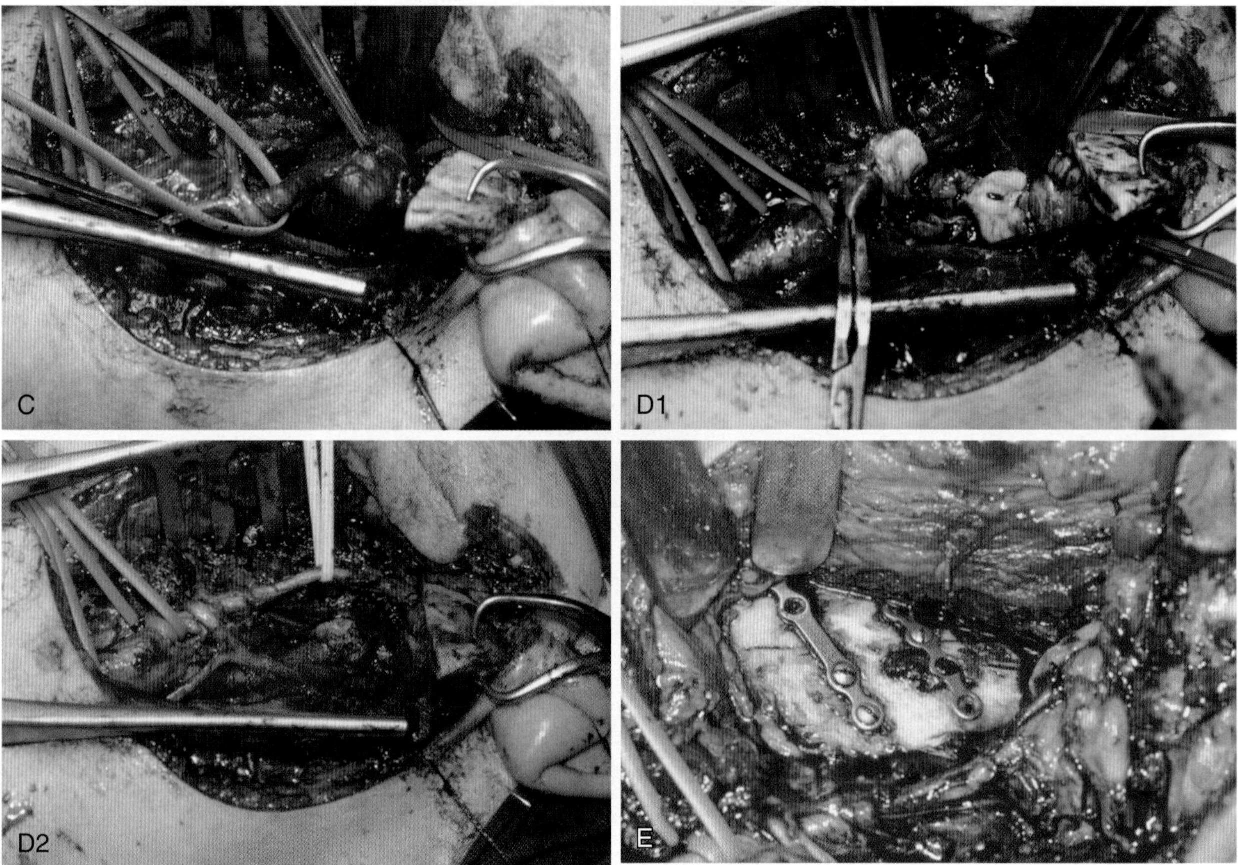

Figure 106.7, cont'd **C,** Approach to the lesion through a mandibular osteotomy at the ascending ramus (intraoperative aspect). **D1,** Internal carotid artery resected. **D2,** Reconstruction of the internal carotid artery with an autogenous vein graft. **E,** Adequate repositioning of the mandible is ensured by previous positioning of the miniplates.

Avoidance and Management of Intraoperative Complications

CBT surgery can result in significant morbidity. In experienced hands and with proper patient selection and counseling, morbidity can be significantly reduced. Meticulous preoperative evaluation, involving the measurement of catecholamines and alpha- and beta-adrenergic blockade, and soft intraoperative manipulation of the tissues are essential to avoid life-threatening complications. Patients with symptoms of a hyperfunctional tumor (headaches, excessive sweating, palpitations, etc.) should be evaluated with a 24-hour urine collection for norepinephrine and the metabolites metanephrine and vanillylmandelic acid. Serum catecholamines can also be measured.[8]

Preoperative imaging is required in order to evaluate the CBT. Doppler ultrasound, computed tomography (CT), magnetic resonance imaging, and angiography play important roles in the clinical diagnosis of CBTs. CBTs can be easily detected using CT or magnetic resonance angiography, showing a mass with enlarged feeding arteries in T2-weighted images that usually displaces the external carotid artery anteromedially and the internal carotid artery posteromedially, thus splaying the carotid bifurcation. The lesion has a "salt and pepper" appearance related to the low signal flow voids and the high signal foci of hemorrhage[4] (Fig. 106.8A–C). The most definitive method for determining vessel integrity is angiography. Angiography allows the opportunity to perform preoperative balloon occlusion studies and embolization if deemed appropriate. CBTs have classic features with angiography. The external and internal carotid arteries are splayed when a CBT is present. This is referred to as the lyre sign, which was named after the shape of the ancient stringed instrument. The presence of multiple paraganglioma can also be excluded at the imaging tests[8] (Fig. 106.9A and B).

Most of the neural tumors and paragangliomas, including CBTs, in the head and neck area are in close anatomical relation to adjacent arteries and cranial nerves; thus, the resection can result in neurovascular injury; stroke; cranial nerve dysfunction, potentially affecting the nerves IX, X, XI, and XII; and excessive blood loss. The incidence of intraoperative complications including vascular injury or cranial nerves lesions is in close relation to the tumor size. The highest risk is observed in tumors larger than 5 cm and grade 3 of Shamblin's classification.[9] Embolization of CBTs has been controversial. Although preoperative arterial embolization has been considered to

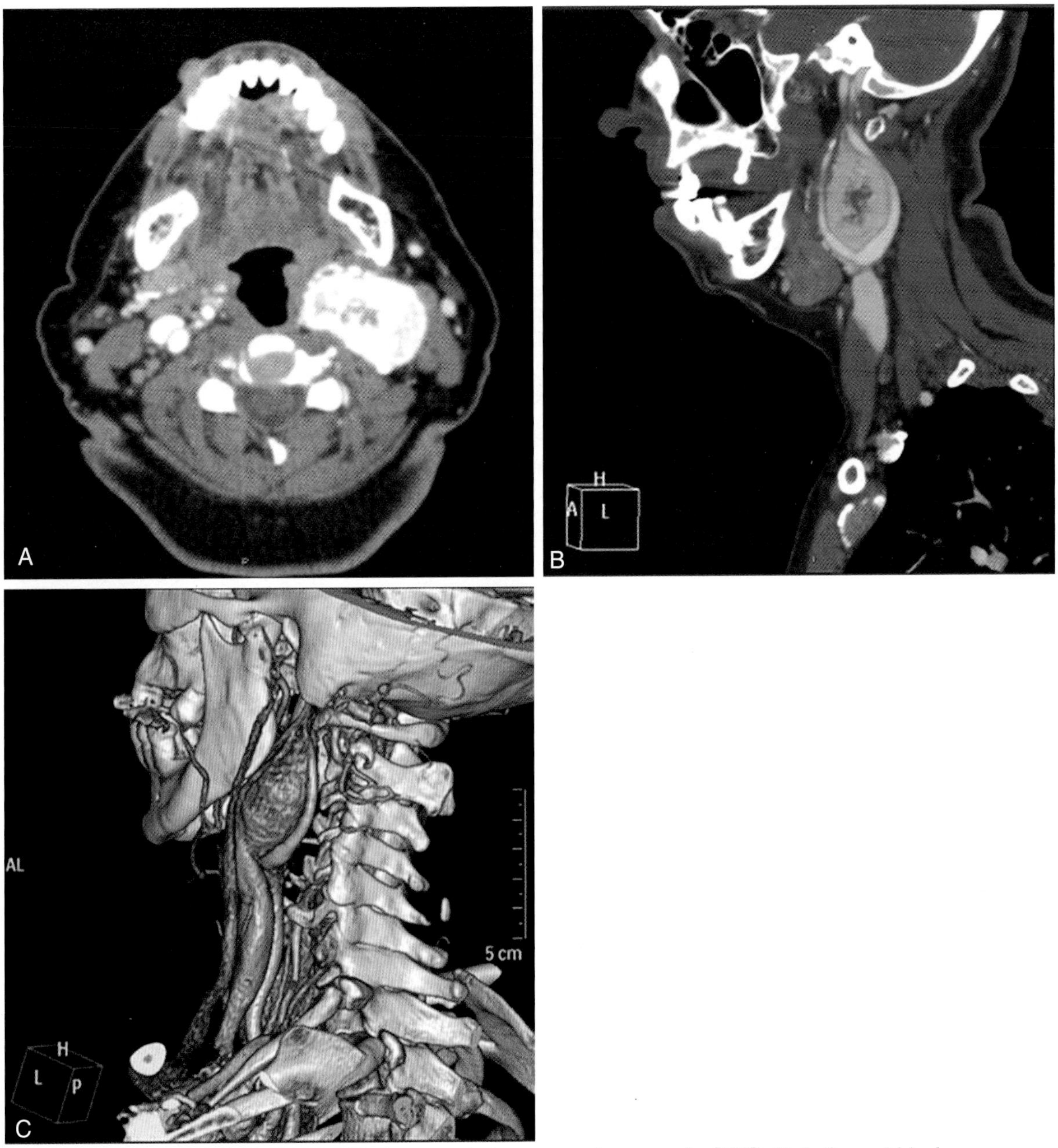

Figure 106.8 **A,** Left carotid body tumor (axial computed tomography [CT]). **B,** Left carotid body tumor (sagittal CT). **C,** Three-dimensional CT reconstruction showing a hypervascular mass within the left carotid bifurcation.

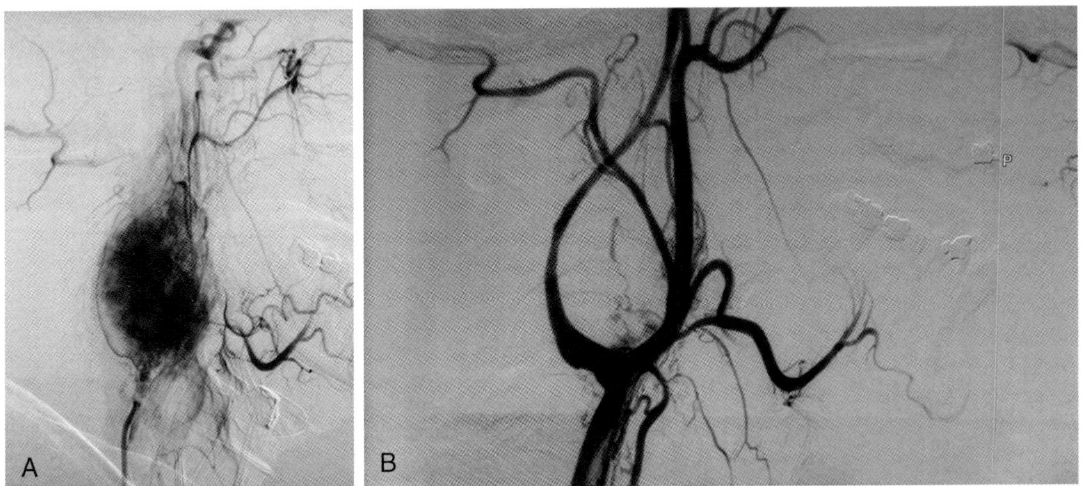

Figure 106.9 **A,** Preembolization angiography showing a carotid body tumor with splaying of the internal and external carotid arteries (lyre sign). **B,** Postembolization angiography.

attenuate the complication risk, presently it seems that there is no significant difference among the patient with or without embolization.[1,10] Internal carotid artery injury or manipulation including reconstruction or ligation significantly increases the incidence of stroke. A carotid balloon occlusion test should be carried out in case of high risk of carotid resection related to the tumor situation. A total of 65% of patients had a stroke after ligation of the internal carotid artery, while 25% of patients who passed a balloon occlusion test can have a delayed stroke. Intraoperative electroencephalographic and cerebral blood monitoring could be necessary. Adequate exposure of the distal internal carotid artery at the skull base in tumors extended superiorly through mobilization or resection of the parotid gland or temporary mandibular osteotomy can decrease the rate of severe intraoperative complications.[11]

Careful dissection of the tumor is also necessary to avoid the injury of the cranial nerves.[12] At the long-term follow-up, the rate of permanent nervous dysfunction is lower than 15%. The superior laryngeal nerve has been reported to be the most injured nerve during the posterior dissection of CBTs. Injury to the vagus nerve or the superior laryngeal branch results in vocal cord paralysis with hoarseness and increased aspiration risk.[4] Speech and swallowing problems result from hypoglossal nerve damage. Damage to the cervical sympathetic chain can lead to two different issues: Horner syndrome and first-bite syndrome. Horner syndrome leads to ptosis, miosis, and anhidrosis, and it is usually well tolerated. It usually resolves if the sympathetic chain has been preserved. First-bite syndrome consists of the development of pain in the parotid region after the first bite of each meal and can be seen after surgery of the parapharyngeal space and has been related to the loss of sympathetic nerve function to the parotid, causing a denervation. In case of surgical injury of the nerves, primary reanastomosis may be necessary. Greater auricular or sural nerve graft interposition can be indicated in case of failure.[8]

Postoperative Considerations

The patient should remain in the intensive care unit for a minimum of 24 hours for hemodynamic and respiratory control. The semi-Fowler position is recommended. Once the patient leaves the critical unit, drains can be removed, if applicable, and start progressive wandering. Patients should be heparinized after vascular reconstruction. Observation should include close monitoring of blood pressure and surveillance for postoperative bleeding or stroke.

Routine long-term follow-up is necessary in all paraganglioma patients because they may need rehabilitation. Rehabilitation of patients has improved over the years in the areas of voice and swallowing dysfunction, baroreflex failure, and first-bite syndrome. Most patients with postoperative deficits show good functional recovery with time and rehabilitation.[13,14]

References

1. Gözen ED, Tevetoğlu F, Kara S, Kızılkılıç O, Yener HM. Is preoperative embolization necessary for carotid paraganglioma resection: experience of a tertiary center. *Ear Nose Throat J.* 2020;145561320957236: 145561320957236. Epub ahead of print.
2. Scudder CL. *Am J Med Sci.* 1903:126–384.
3. Wilson H. Carotid body tumors surgical management. *Ann Surg.* 1964;159(6):959–966.
4. Mascia D, Esposito G, Ferrante A, Grandi A, Melissano G, Chiesa R. Carotid body tumor contemporary management in a high-volume center. *J Cardiovasc Surg (Torino).* 2020;61(4):459–466.
5. Hurtado-Lopez LM, Fink-Josephi G, Ramos-Méndez L, Dena-Espinoza E. Non-resectable carotid body tumor: hybrid surgical procedure to achieve complete and safe resection. *Head Neck.* 2008;30(12):1646–1649.
6. Wernick BD, Furlough CL, Patel U, et al. Contemporary management of carotid body tumors in a Midwestern academic center. *Surgery.* 2021;169(3):700–704.
7. Offergeld C, Brase C, Yaremchuk S, et al. Head and neck paragangliomas: clinical and molecular genetic classification. *Clinics (São Paulo).* 2012;67(suppl 1):19–28.
8. Head MO, Paragangliomas N. Multimodal management. In: *Head and Neck Cancer.* Springer; 2011.
9. Makeieff M, Raingeard I, Alric P, Bonafe A, Guerrier B, Ch M-A. Surgical management of carotid body tumors. *Ann Surg Oncol.* 2008;15(8):2180–2186.
10. Han T, Wang S, Wei X, et al. Outcome of surgical treatment for carotid body tumors in different shambling type without preoperative embolization: a single-center retrospective study. *Ann Vasc Surg.* 2020;63:325–331.
11. Hallett Jr JW, Nora JD, Hollier LH, Cherry Jr KJ, Pairolero PC. Trends in neurovascular complications of surgical management for carotid body and cervical paragangliomas: a fifty-year experience with 153 tumors. *J Vasc Surg.* 1988;7(2):284–291.
12. Cobb AN, Barkat A, Daungjaiboon W, et al. Carotid body tumor resection: just as safe without preoperative embolization. *Ann Vasc Surg.* 2020;64:163–168.
13. Sevil FC, Tort M, Kaygin MA. Carotid body tumor resection: long-term outcome of 67 cases without preoperative embolization. *Ann Vasc Surg.* 2020;67:200–207.
14. Suárez C, Rodrigo JP, Mendenhall WM, et al. Carotid body paragangliomas: a systematic study on management with surgery and radiotherapy. *Eur Arch otorhinolaryngol.* 2014;271(1):23–34.

CHAPTER 107

Excision of Facial Skin Malignancy

Thomas Schlieve, Pooja Gangwani, and Antonia Kolokythas

Armamentarium

#11 and #15 Blades
Adson forceps
Appropriate sutures
Curved Mayo scissors
DeBakey forceps
Dermatologic curettes
Electrocautery
Hemostats
Local anesthetic with and without vasoconstrictor
Metzenbaum scissors
Needle holder
Skin hook
Surgical marking pen
Surgical skin prep of choice (e.g., Betadine, ChloraPrep)
Suture scissors
Wood lamp

History of the Procedure

Skin cancer is the most common malignancy of humans, and its incidence continues to rise despite increased awareness of the disease among both practitioners and the general public.[1] Nonmelanoma skin cancer (NMSC), primarily squamous cell carcinoma (SCC) and basal cell carcinoma (BCC), is estimated to account for nearly 5.4 million[2] new cancer cases per year, representing 95% of all skin cancers (Figs. 107.1 and 107.2).[3] The incidence of NMSC has been rising at a rate of 5% per year, and it is estimated that 1 in 6 Americans develops skin cancer during their lifetime.[3,4] Although the incidence of NMSC is high, the 5-year survival remains above 95%, with most deaths occurring from metastatic SCC.[4,5] The overall incidence of metastatic disease in BCC is very low (0.0028% to 0.1%); favored sites include regional lymph nodes, the liver, lungs, bone, and skin.[6] SCC more frequently develops metastatic disease, with an overall rate of 2% to 6% for the primary lesion and 24% to 45% for recurrent SCC.[5,7,8] The presence of metastatic disease reduces the 5-year survival rate to only 34%; therefore, complete removal of disease at the time of initial surgery is essential.[7] Melanoma accounts for 75% of skin cancer-related deaths, but only 5% of all skin neoplasms (Fig. 107.3). Approximately 80,000 new cases of melanoma skin cancer are diagnosed per year in the United States, and the patient's age at diagnosis is younger than for most cancers. This makes melanoma the most common cancer diagnosis in women 20 to 29 years of age.[9,10]

Surgical excision of facial skin malignancy continues to be the gold standard treatment and is the procedure most often performed by oral and maxillofacial surgeons and other surgical specialists.[11,12] Other treatment modalities, such as cryotherapy, curettage and electrodessication, Mohs micrographic surgery (MMS), and laser treatment are available, and when used for specific indications by individuals well trained in the technique, they have similar rates of success. It should be noted that not every technique can be used for all lesions in all patients, and factors such as the histologic diagnosis, lesion size, patient comorbidities, and lesion site play a role in treatment planning. Although this chapter focuses on the standard surgical excision of lesions, the discussion of this procedure would not be complete without mentioning alternative treatment modalities.

Standard surgical excision is the most common treatment modality among plastic, ear, nose, and throat, and oral and maxillofacial surgeons, and the cure rate ranges from 93% to 95%. Surgical excision is advantageous because it allows for tissue diagnosis and assessment of completion of excision through frozen sections (if used) and final specimen histologic analysis. In addition, the cosmetic outcome often is superior, regardless of whether immediate or delayed closure is performed, especially for lesions amenable to primary closure. Excision is also the standard technique for removal of cutaneous melanomas as Mohs surgery remains a highly controversial treatment technique for this malignancy.[13–16] Disadvantages of standard surgical excision include the patient's perception of increased invasiveness, time, and potential increased expense.[17]

For BCC, it is important to distinguish between histologic subtypes. The morpheaform BCC is well known for its significant subclinical extension, and therefore a minimum 7-mm to 1-cm margin or consideration for Mohs surgery is advisable.[18] The National Cancer Care Network (NCCN) recommends surgical excision with 4 mm clinical margins and postoperative margin assessment for low-risk lesions.[19] For high-risk lesions, MMS or surgical excision with wider surgical margins and postoperative margin assessment is recommended.[19] However, the NCCN guidelines do not propose a

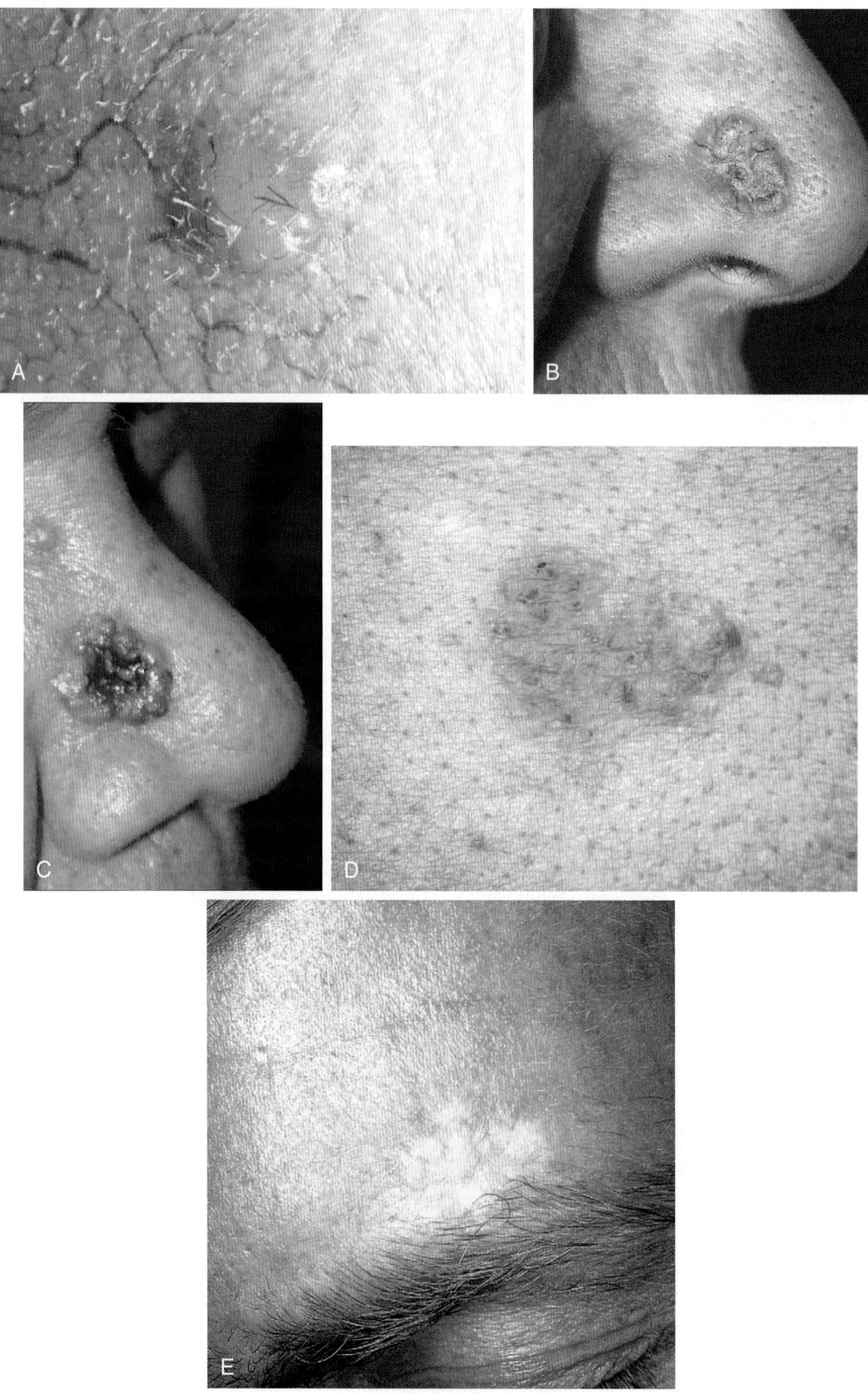

Figure 107.1 Types of basal cell carcinoma. **A,** Nodular, early. **B,** Nodular, ulcerated. **C,** Pigmented. **D,** Superficial. **E,** Morpheaform/sclerosing. (A and B courtesy of Habif T. Premalignant and malignant nonmelanoma skin tumors. In: Habif T, ed. *Clinical Dermatology.* 5th ed. St Louis, Missouri: Mosby; 2010; C and D courtesy of Rigel D, Cockerell C, Carucci J, Wharton J. Actinic keratosis, basal cell carcinoma, and squamous cell carcinoma. In: Bolognia J, Jorizzo J, Rapini R, eds. *Dermatology.* 2nd ed. St Louis, Missouri: Mosby; 2008.)

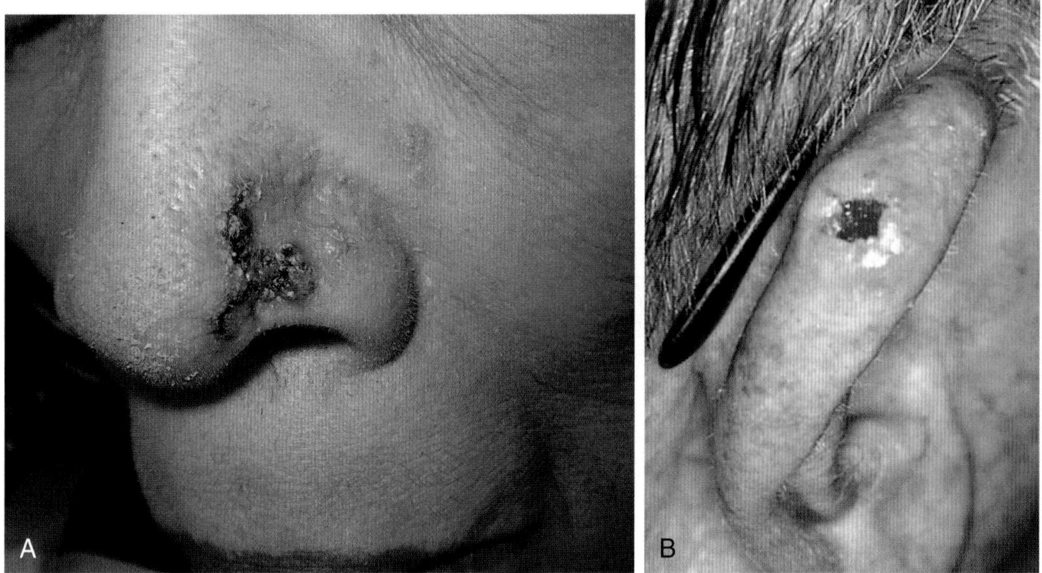

Figure 107.2 **A** and **B,** Squamous cell carcinoma. (Courtesty of Kenneaster DG. Introduction to skin cancer. *Oral Maxillofac Surg Clin North Am.* 2005;17:133.)

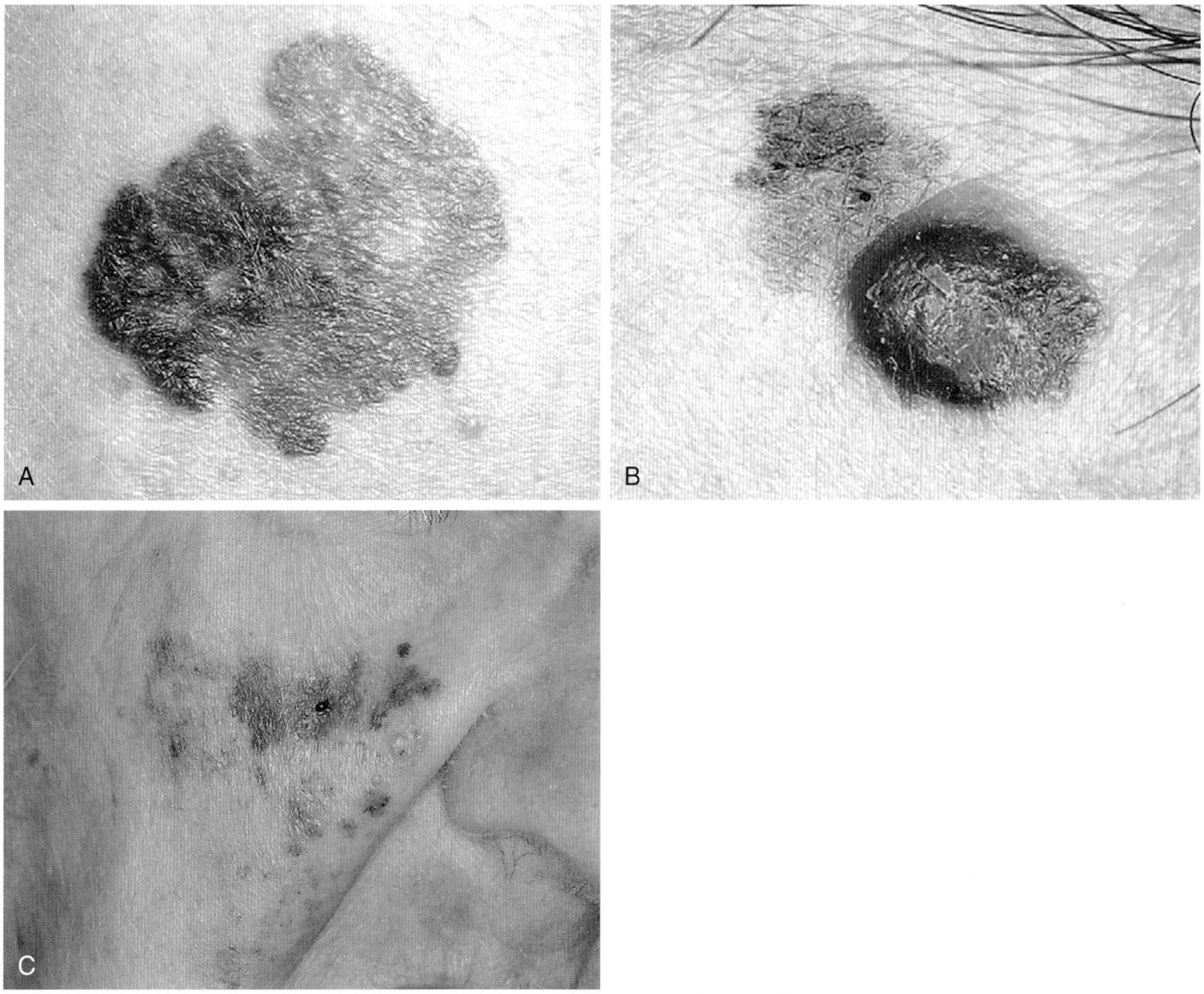

Figure 107.3 Type of melanoma. **A,** Superficial spreading. **B,** Nodular. **C,** Lentigo maligna melanoma. (A and B courtesy of Habif T. Nevi and malignant melanoma. In: Habif T, ed. *Clinical Dermatology.* 5th ed. St Louis, Missouri: Mosby; 2010; C courtesy of Nestle F, Halpern A. Melanoma. In: Bolognia J, Jorizzo J, Rapini R, eds. *Dermatology.* 2nd ed. St Louis, Missouri: Mosby; 2008.)

number for these wider margins.[19] Please see Table 107.1 for the description of low- and high-risk lesions.

In SCC, lesions of less than 1 cm can be excised with a 5-mm margin, provided there is no perineural invasion and the lesion is not poorly differentiated. These adverse histologic features are indications for Mohs surgery and/or consideration of wider margins (Table 107.2). Advanced SCC lesions with poor differentiation, invasion of adjacent structures, large size (greater than 2 cm), or recurrence often require 1- to 2-cm margins for tumor clearance. Finally, SCC originating in an area of radiation, chronic ulceration, or burn injury is a more aggressive tumor with an increased rate of metastatic disease and should be treated accordingly.[20] For in situ melanoma, a 5-mm margin should be included; lesions 0.5 to 1 mm thick

Table 107.1 Risk Factors for Recurrence[19]

H and P	Low Risk	High Risk
Location/Size	Trunk, extremities < 2 cm	Trunk, extremities ≥ 2 cm Cheeks, forehead, scalp, neck, and pretibia (any size) Head, neck, hands, feet, pretibia, and anogenital (any size)[3]
Borders	Well defined	Poorly defined
Primary vs. recurrent	Primary	Recurrent
Immunosuppression	(-)	(+)
Site of prior RT	(-)	(+)
Pathology[3]		
Subtype	Nodular, superficial[1]	Aggressive growth pattern[2]
Perineural involvement	(-)	(+)

[1]Low risk histologic subtypes
[2]This area constitutes high risk based on location, independent of size
Low-risk histologic subtypes include nodular, superficial, and other non-aggressive growth patterns such as keratotic, infundibulocystic, and fibroepithelioma of Pinkus
[3]Having (mixed) infiltrative, micronodular, morpheaform, basosquamous, sclerosing or carcinosarcomatous differentiation features in any portion of the tumor
Pathology: pathologic report noting the presence of any features that would increase the risk for local recurrence including invasion of tumor beyond reticular dermis and presence of perineural invasion
Adapted with permission from the NCCN Clinical Practice Guidelines in Oncology (NCCN Guidelines®) for Basal Cell Skin Cancer V.2.2022.

Table 107.2 Indications for Mohs Microscopic Surgery[37]

Tumor Characteristics
Large size of lesion measuring >2 cm anywhere on the body
Aggressive histological subtypes (morpheaform/fibrosing/sclerosing BCC, infiltrative BCC, micronodular BCC, sclerosing SCC, basosquamous, pagetoid, poorly differentiated SCC, spindle cell SCC)
Perineural invasion
Ill-defined margins
Incompletely excised or recurrent lesions

Anatomical Site
High-risk anatomical locations such as mask areas of the face (central face, eyebrows, eyelids, periorbital area, nose, lips, chin, mandible, preauricular and postauricular areas, temple, ears)
Areas in close proximity to embryonic fusion planes (periorbital, periauricular, perinasal, temporal)
Need for tissue preservation to achieve functional outcomes (hands, feet, genitals)
Skin cancers arising in scars, chronic wounds, or previously irradiated areas

Patient Factors
Immunocompromised patients (patients on immunosuppressive drugs, organ transplant recipients, patients with hematological malignancies or human immunodeficiency virus)
Genetic syndromes (basal cell nevus syndrome, xeroderma pigmentosum)
Environmental exposures (arsenic)

BCC, Basal cell carcinoma; *SCC,* squamous cell carcinoma.
Adapted from Chen ELA, Srivastava D, Nijhawan RI. Mohs micrographic surgery: development, technique, and applications in cutaneous malignancies. *Semin Plast Surg.* 2018;32:60–68.

require a 1-cm margin; and melanoma 1 to 2 mm thick necessitates a 1- to 2-cm margin. Lesions greater than 2 mm thick must be treated with 2-cm margins.[10] The necessary margin for lesions greater than 4 mm in depth (stage T4) has not been adequately studied, and early reports have failed to prove decreased local recurrence, disease-free results, or overall survival benefit to margins greater than 2 cm for these lesions.[21–23]

Skin Cancer in Organ Transplant Patients

Organ transplant recipients are on long-term immunosuppressant medications to prevent graft rejection. This in turn leads to reduced immune-mediated tumor surveillance and places them at an increased risk of developing skin cancers, particularly SCC, BCC, malignant melanoma, Merkel cell carcinoma, and Kaposi sarcoma.[24] Over 90% of the skin cancer seen in the transplant recipients are BCC and SCC, with SCC being four times more common than BCC, and the majority of them occurring in the head and neck region.[25]

Increase in the incidence of malignancy is directly proportional to the duration and intensity of immunosuppressive therapy.[25] Other risk factors include being Caucasian, advanced age at the time of transplantation, male sex, a history of pretransplant skin cancer treatment, and over-exposure to ultraviolet radiation.[26] The type of transplant also plays a role in determining the risk of posttransplant skin cancer. Due to the requirement of more intensive immunosuppressive therapy and older age at the time of transplant, thoracic organ (heart and lung) recipients have a higher risk of developing SCC than kidney transplant recipients.[26]

Furthermore, tumors in transplant recipients are more aggressive and are noted to respond poorly to the standard therapies.[24] Therefore, posttransplantation surveillance and the use of preventive strategies pertaining to sun protection, such as, use of sunscreen and wearing protective clothing are essential. The management of skin carcinomas in transplant recipients depends on the type and extent of the lesion.[24]

Management of Locally Advanced Head and Neck BCC and SCC

Locally advanced BCCs and SCCs of the head and neck region are typically large lesions that often infiltrate into structures such as the craniofacial bones and the surrounding tissues, and are challenging to treat.[27] These advanced lesions directly influence the metastatic potential, resulting in a negative impact on patient survival. Reconstructive options such as the use of pedicled flaps and free tissue transfer are driven by the size and the location of the resulting defect. Wide local excision with tumor-free margins, followed by immediate reconstruction and postoperative radiotherapy is the treatment of choice for locally advanced head and neck BCCs and SCCs.[27]

Indications for the Use of the Procedure

Before treatment of facial skin malignancy, a biopsy of the lesion in question should be performed. Several biopsy techniques are available, such as shave biopsy, punch biopsy, and incisional or excisional biopsy. The choice of biopsy technique depends on the lesion's size and appearance, the preliminary diagnosis, and the surgeon's preference. A shave biopsy is a simple, quick method of obtaining a specimen, but it may be too superficial to determine the depth of invasion and thus should be reserved for lesions that are clearly superficial in nature; it should never be used for melanoma. It is best used for papular or pedunculated lesions and blisters.[23] The punch biopsy specimen contains subcutaneous tissue and therefore characterizes lesion depth; however, seeding of deeper tissues in superficial SCC lesions is a concern. Punch biopsy sizes range from 2 to 8 mm, although 3- to 4-mm punches are used most often. By stretching the skin perpendicular to relaxed skin tension lines, the final shape of the biopsy site takes on an elliptical appearance and the site can be left to heal secondarily or closed primarily. The decision to use an excisional or incisional biopsy is based on the lesion's size and location and the clinical diagnosis. For suspected melanoma, excisional biopsy with a thin 2-mm margin is the preferred method. If the lesion is greater than 2 cm or involves anatomic subsites such as the ear or eyelid, incisional biopsy of the darkest or most abnormal-appearing zone of the lesion is acceptable.[21] It is important to note that no data suggest that incisional or punch biopsy of melanoma increases the likelihood of metastatic disease, and a lesion not amenable to excisional biopsy with a thin margin of normal tissue should be biopsied in this fashion.[28]

Surgical excision is indicated for all NMSCs and melanoma lesions that are considered resectable in a patient who will tolerate not only the excision but also the potential reconstruction. The goal of surgical excision is complete removal of the tumor with negative margins while maintaining acceptable cosmesis and function. Any lesion that cannot be resected with this goal in mind should be considered for palliative treatment and/or radiation treatment.

Limitations and Contraindications

Standard surgical excision is not appropriate for the treatment of patients who cannot withstand the surgery and reconstruction. Patients with multiple medical comorbidities may fall into this category, as may patients with advanced disease whose functional outcome after surgery would be unacceptable. When surgery is combined with radiation therapy, local disease control as high as 93% has been reported.[29] Standard surgical excision should be used with caution in the treatment of recurrent disease. Although recurrent disease can be cleared with reexcision using standard techniques in many cases, the possible role of Mohs surgery should be considered for any patient with recurrent BCC or SCC. This is especially true for patients reconstructed with flaps because these tumors are known to spread underneath flaps without clinical evidence of disease.

TECHNIQUE: Excision of Facial Skin Malignancy

STEP 1: Preparation

Using a surgical marking pen, the surgeon marks the intended margin of healthy-appearing tissue to be excised along with the lesion. The necessary margin will vary, as mentioned previously. A flexible ruler trimmed down to a few centimeters' length and held with a hemostat can be useful for marking a uniform margin. After it has been marked, the skin should be appropriately cleansed with the surgeon's preferred medium. Next, the surgical site should be appropriately draped and isolated. A local anesthetic with epinephrine can be infiltrated away from the lesion or used for nerve blockade to provide both anesthesia and assistance with hemostasis. If a local flap is planned, use of a local anesthetic without epinephrine should be considered to allow for assessment of vascularity (Fig. 107.4A).

STEP 2: Incision

The surgeon should make an incision along the previously marked margin using a #15 or #11 blade. An attempt should be made to create this incision with the blade angled outward at a 5- to 10-degree angle. This not only keeps the margin uniform as the incision is carried into deeper tissues, but also improves closure by creating a slight eversion of the wound margins. This incision should be initiated with a vertical stab, and then the blade angle is decreased to cut using the belly of the blade. Additionally, a minimum number of strokes should be performed to obtain a uniform depth. As the incision progresses toward the starting incision point, the blade should be returned to vertical to prevent cross-hatching. Excision to the next uninvolved anatomic barrier is completed. For most skin lesions, this includes skin and sub-cutaneous tissue down to fascia; however, muscle, periosteum, and/or bone should be included in the excision if direct tumor extension is present. Dissection with hemostats or scissors can be used after skin incision to access deeper tissues, as needed. The surgeon should make sure the depth of the incision around the lesion is uniform before proceeding to orientation and excision.

For BCC, curettage of the lesion with dermatologic curettes before excision, with remarking of the surgical margin, has been shown to increase the chance of tumor clearance by 25%.[30] To perform this procedure, the surgeon senses with the curette the "soft feel" of the BCC in relation to the adjacent normal tissue. Once it is thought that all tumor has been curetted, the lesion margin is confirmed, and excision is performed as described previously (see Fig. 107.4A).[30]

STEP 3: Orientation of the Specimen

Before it is removed from the surgical bed, the specimen should be marked in a standard fashion to provide orientation to the pathologist and to help determine the location of any positive margin should it be noted on final pathology. Markings should be placed in a clock face fashion and 90 degrees to each other for easy communication. For example, a short silk stitch can be placed at the superior margin and a long silk stitch at the left or lateral margin. Whichever means the surgeon chooses to orient the specimen, he or she should use it consistently so that there is no question, on final pathology, what each marking indicates (Fig. 107.4B).

STEP 4: Amputation of the Specimen

After orientation, the specimen is amputated from the patient. The surgeon should gently grasp the specimen with an Adson forceps, taking care not to crush the tissues, and undercut the specimen with a blade, Bovie, iris, or Mayo scissors at a uniform depth. Alternatively, skin hooks can be used to elevate the lesion to visualize the deep margin during removal (Fig. 107.4C).

STEP 5: Hemostasis and Wound Care

After the specimen has been placed in the proper medium, hemorrhage should be controlled using electrical or thermal cautery, pressure, or topical hemostatic aids as needed. For wounds left to heal by secondary intention or that are to be reassessed later, oxidized cellulose polymer can be placed at the base of the wound for additional hemostasis and left in place until the dressing is removed 24 to 72 hours later. The wound is then lined with an antimicrobial ointment and covered with a nonadhesive dressing (Fig. 107.4D).

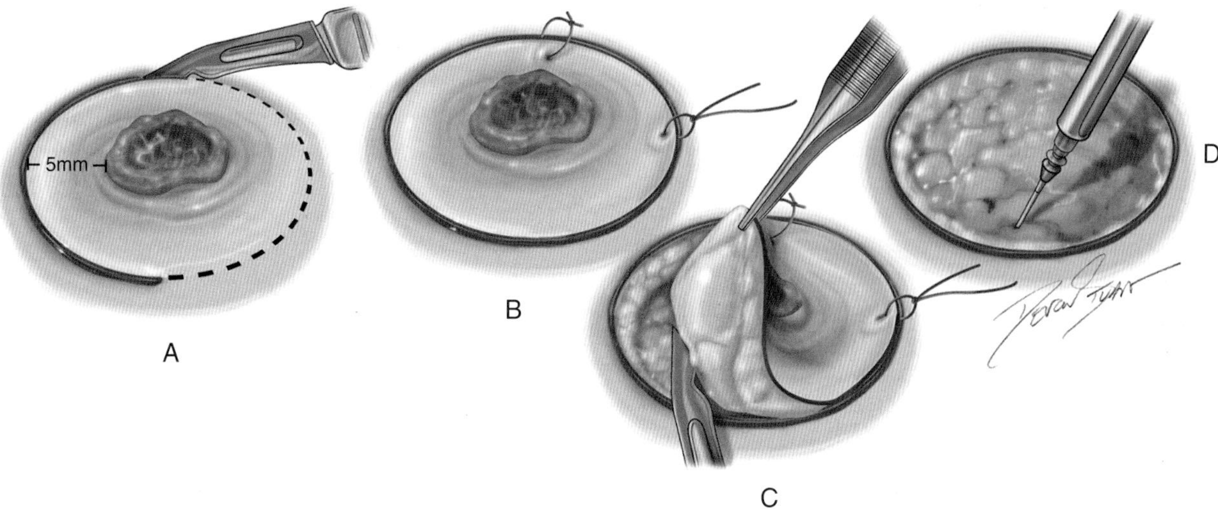

Figure 107.4 **A,** Basal cell carcinoma with marked 5-mm margin of normal-appearing skin. Initial incision, with #15 blade held at a 10-degree angle. **B,** Surgical specimen marked with a long stitch on the left margin and a short stitch on the superior margin. **C,** Completion of lesion excision at a uniform depth. **D,** Specimen removed and wound bed hemostatic.

ALTERNATIVE TECHNIQUE 1: Primary Closure of Excised Skin Malignancy

Primary wound closure is commonly planned before surgery. If a skin lesion is small and well demarcated, if frozen section margin analysis is to be used, if a sizeable margin of healthy tissue is to be removed, or if the patient refuses delayed closure, primary closure of the surgical site can be effectively performed. The lesion is excised in a fusiform or elliptical fashion, oriented parallel to the resting skin tension lines. The length should be three times the width with 30-degree angles at each corner. Alternatively, an M-plasty–type incision can be used to assist with closure and scar cosmesis. The adjacent tissue should be appropriately undermined with scalpel or scissor dissection to assist in achieving tension-free closure. After confirmation of a hemostatic wound, a layered closure is performed according to the surgeon's preference (Fig. 107.5).

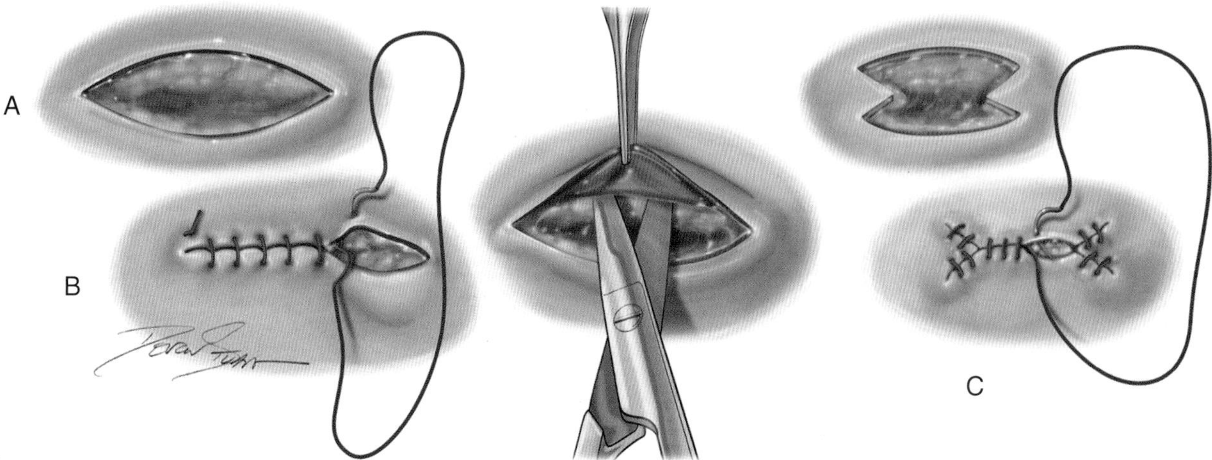

Figure 107.5 **A,** Fusiform incision for planned linear closure. **B,** Wound closure in a linear fashion with everted margins. **C,** M-plasty incision and final wound appearance after closure.

ALTERNATIVE TECHNIQUE 2: Special Considerations for Melanoma

When excising a melanoma, the surgeon might consider using a Wood lamp for improved visualization of tumor extent.[10] The Wood lamp (ultraviolet light with a wavelength of approximately 365 nanometers) is shone onto the skin, revealing varying fluorescence between the lesion pigmentation and normal skin; this shows possible extension not visible to the naked eye. Although not the standard of care, the Wood lamp may be a helpful adjunct in delineating tumor margins because frozen section identification of melanocytes is difficult. This is one reason Mohs surgery for melanoma remains controversial and, according to some, contraindicated.[10]

Sentinel lymph node biopsy (SLNB) currently is considered a staging tool for melanomas greater than 1 mm in thickness or for lesions less than 1 mm with ulceration, Clark level IV invasion, or a high mitotic count.[21] SLNB should not be performed in the setting of clinically positive nodes because these patients require formal lymphadenectomy. Patients who would otherwise not undergo completion lymphadenectomy should not undergo SLNB. Also, some surgeons do not perform SLNB in lesions greater than 4 mm in depth; instead, they perform elective lymphadenectomy for diagnostic purposes. SLNB can be completed at the time of primary lesion excision or after excision. The surgical scar then is used to guide injection of radioactive colloid and isosulfan blue dye.[10] (See Chapter 104 for more information on sentinel node biopsy.)

ALTERNATIVE TECHNIQUE 3: Cryotherapy

Cryotherapy is often used by dermatologists and general practitioners and has a cure rate of 94% to 99% for actinic keratosis, BCC, and superficial SCC. Small and well-demarcated lesions are often addressed in this manner because this technique provides no specimen for pathology, and healing occurs by secondary intention with a flat area of hypopigmentation. Many small lesions can be treated for a low cost in a single visit, often without the need for local anesthesia due to the anesthetic cooling effect of the procedure itself. The technique involves the application of liquid nitrogen (-50° to -60°C) in a spray or as a cryoprobe, through several freeze-thaw cycles, with resulting destruction of the lesion. A 4- to 6-mm margin of adjacent normal-appearing tissue should also be treated to ensure removal of the entire lesion.[17]

ALTERNATIVE TECHNIQUE 4: Curettage and Electrodesiccation

Curettage with electrodesiccation is a technique-sensitive treatment used mostly by dermatologists to treat small BCCs and the occasional well-differentiated SCC at specific anatomic subsites. Its advantages are the short surgical time and the ability to treat multiple lesions in a single visit. The lesion is aggressively curetted with multiple dermatologic curettes until normal tissue is palpated. Next, desiccation or fulguration with an electrosurgery device is performed. The resulting eschar is curetted to living tissue, and the process is repeated several times until the surgeon believes that a comfortable margin has been achieved. Due to the potential for a prolonged healing time, hypertrophic scarring, and hypopigmentation, this technique is not often chosen for facial malignancies.[17] The cure rate ranges from 91.5% for BCCs less than 5 mm to less than 74% for larger lesions.[31]

ALTERNATIVE TECHNIQUE 5: Mohs Micrographic Surgery

Mohs micrographic surgery (MMS) was pioneered by Frederic E. Mohs in the 1930s and 1940s.[32,33] The value of this technique lies in its ability to minimize removal of uninvolved tissue and to allow the surgeon to examine the status of the entire margin during surgery, whereas traditional pathologic analysis allows examination of only approximately 1% of the specimen margin.[33] Despite this apparent benefit, the time, cost, and lack of availability of a Mohs surgeon in all communities limit the application of the technique. The recommendations and indications for MMS are often debated; however, most oral and maxillofacial surgeons refer patients to a Mohs surgeon for treatment of lesions in locations where maximum tissue preservation is necessary, such as the eyelid. Additional relative indications include lesions with an increased risk of recurrence due to location in the H-zone of the face, recurrent disease, morpheaform BCC, tumors with ill-defined borders or aggressive histologic features, and NMSC lesions larger than 2 cm. Cure rates range from 99% for a BCC less than 2 cm to 94% to 99% for SCC.[32,33]

The technique is most often accomplished with local anesthetic due to the long duration of the procedure, possibly up to several hours for a small lesion. The tumor is first debulked with dermatologic curettes. The surgeon then performs a 45-degree, beveled excision, tapering off to horizontal at the depth of the lesion, thus creating a craterlike defect. Next, the specimen itself is oriented with a specimen map, and frozen sections are processed, with documentation of residual tumor on the specimen map. Successive layers are excised from the lesion until a clear margin is obtained on frozen sections. The surgeon then takes a final thin margin as a permanent specimen.[32,33] A detailed discussion of sectioning, mapping, and processing is beyond the scope of this chapter (Fig. 107.6).

Avoidance and Management of Intraoperative Complications

Intraoperative complications include bleeding, damage to adjacent structures, inability to obtain disease-free margins, and inability to reconstruct the surgical defect. Excessive bleeding can be caused by local or systemic factors. Proper surgical technique with ligation of vessels as they are encountered and judicious use of cautery can assist in controlling hemorrhage. Drains can be used to prevent hematoma formation when necessary, and pressure bandaging can be used. Systemic causes of bleeding can be anticipated by a thorough review of the patient's medical history. The inability to obtain clear margins, the inability to reconstruct a surgically created defect, or damage to adjacent structures can be avoided or anticipated by thorough preoperative planning and workup. Large lesions with extensive soft tissue involvement, long-standing scalp lesions, or lesions with increased likelihood of lymph node involvement should be imaged appropriately with magnetic resonance imaging or computed tomography. Patients with preoperative facial nerve palsy are unlikely to recover neurologic function after surgery and should be so

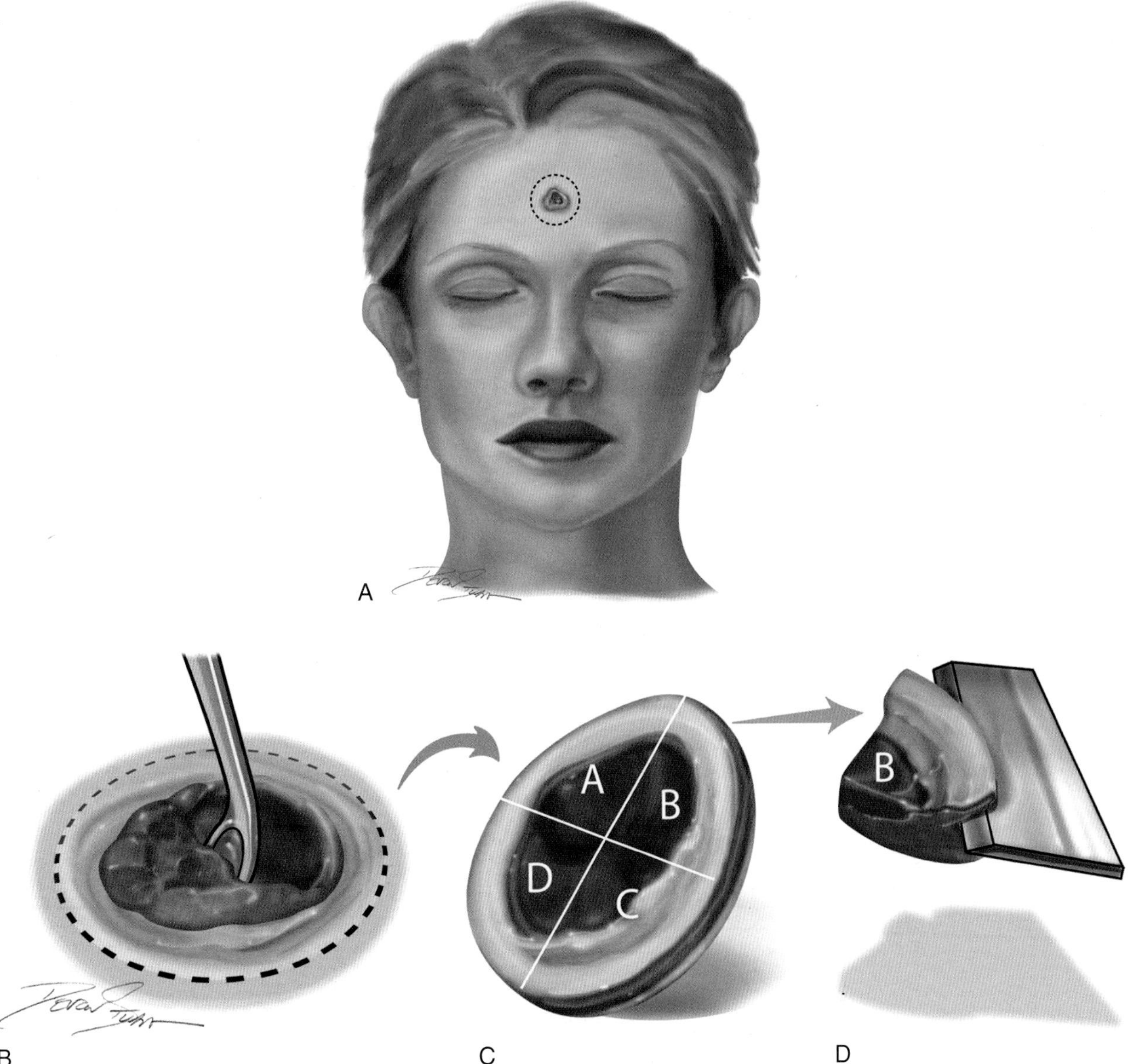

Figure 107.6 **A,** Basal cell carcinoma of the middle forehead. **B,** Dermatologic curette used to remove the bulk of the lesion. **C,** Excision of the entire lesion base and margin as a single specimen. **D,** Mapping of the surgical specimen followed by microscopic analysis.

advised. Involvement of the parotid requires appropriate parotidectomy and involvement of underlying bone requires ostectomy. Each of these findings can be anticipated based on preoperative imaging, and both excisional and reconstructive surgery can be planned with this in mind.

Postoperative Considerations

Positive margins on final pathology can be disheartening for both patient and surgeon. Positive margins may reflect aggressive biologic behavior, which may not be predictable preoperatively. If a positive margin is encountered, reexcision is generally appropriate, followed by a second pathologic evaluation of the margins. Consideration may be given to referral for Mohs surgery. If the lesion cannot be reexcised, adjuvant radiation therapy should be considered. An advantage of delayed repair of surgically excised lesions is the ability to return to the operating suite for reexcision of margins or to take down flaps used in reconstruction. Intraoperative frozen section margins can also be used in cases of large lesions, lesions planned for immediate reconstruction, or morpheaform BCC to confirm complete excision. The accuracy of frozen section margins is 85% to 98%; however, this requires additional time and expense and generally involves an operating room setting.[34] For smaller lesions, the surgeon can remove a slightly wider margin to increase the likelihood of tumor clearance. Historically, positive BCC margins were not always reexcised, and a "wait and watch" approach was used. The reason for this is the relatively low recurrence rate of 3.1% to 39% for BCC with positive margins. Further research has demonstrated the presence of tumor nests in 32% to 54% of patients who undergo further excision. The general consensus is that the surgeon should reexcise positive margins.[35]

Follow-up examination is very important for patients after a skin malignancy diagnosis due to a possible field cancerization effect and an increased risk for subsequent cancers. Patients with a prior SCC or BCC have a 3-year cumulative risk of developing a second lesion of 18% and 44%, respectively. A patient with a second BCC has a 50% chance of developing a third BCC.[36]

References

1. Housman TS, Feldman SR, Williford PM, et al. Skin cancer is among the most costly of all cancers to treat for the Medicare population. *J Am Acad Dermatol*. 2003;48(3):425–429.
2. Bander TS, Nehal KS, Lee EH. Cutaneous squamous cell carcinoma: updates in staging and management. *Dermatol Clin*. 2019;37(3):241–251.
3. National Cancer Institute at the National Institutes of Health: Skin Cancer. http://www.cancer.gov/.
4. Gloster HM Jr, Brodland DG. The epidemiology of skin cancer. *Dermatol Surg*. 1996;22(3):217–226.
5. Skidmore RA Jr, Flowers FP. Nonmelanoma skin cancer. *Med Clin North Am*. 1998;82(6):1309–1323 (vi).
6. Goldberg DP. Assessment and surgical treatment of basal cell skin cancer. *Clin Plast Surg*. 1997;24(4):673–686.
7. Padgett JK, Hendrix JD Jr. Cutaneous malignancies and their management. *Otolaryngol Clin N Am*. 2001;34(3):523–553.
8. Roth JJ, Granick MS. Squamous cell and adnexal carcinomas of the skin. *Clin Plast Surg*. 1997;24(4):687–703.
9. Rigel DS, Friedman RJ, Kopf AW. The incidence of malignant melanoma in the United States: issues as we approach the 21st century. *J Am Acad Dermatol*. 1996;34(5 Pt 1):839–847.
10. Wargo JA, Tanabe K. Surgical management of melanoma. *Hematol Oncol Clin North Am*. 2009;23(3):565–581.
11. Garner KL, Rodney WM. Basal and squamous cell carcinoma. *Prim Care*. 2000;27(2):447–458.
12. Bruce AJ, Brodland DG. Overview of skin cancer detection and prevention for the primary care physician. *Mayo Clin Proc*. 2000;75(5):491–500.
13. Zitelli JA, Brown C, Hanusa BH. Mohs micrographic surgery for the treatment of primary cutaneous melanoma. *J Am Acad Dermatol*. 1997;37(2 Pt 1):236–245.
14. Bhardwaj SS, Tope WD, Lee PK. Mohs micrographic surgery for lentigo maligna and lentigo maligna melanoma using Mel-5 immunostaining: University of Minnesota experience. *Dermatol Surg*. 2006;32(5):690–696.
15. Bienert TN, Trotter MJ, Arlette JP. Treatment of cutaneous melanoma of the face by Mohs micrographic surgery. *J Cutan Med Surg*. 2003;7(1):25–30.
16. Temple CL, Arlette JP. Mohs micrographic surgery in the treatment of lentigo maligna and melanoma. *J Surg Oncol*. 2006;94(4):287–292.
17. Stucker F, Nathan C, Lian T. Cutaneous malignancy. In: Bailey B, Johnson J, Newlands S, eds. *Head and Neck Surgery: Otolaryngology*. Philadelphia: Lippincott Williams & Wilkins; 2006.
18. Bailey JS, Goldwasser MS. Surgical management of facial skin cancer. *Oral Maxillofac Surg Clin North Am*. 2005;17(2):205–233 (vi).
19. NCCN Guidelines Version 1. Basal Cell Skin Cancer. https://www.nccn.org/professionals/physician_gls/pdf/nmsc.pdf. Accessed on 8/26/2020.
20. Brodland DG, Zitelli JA. Surgical margins for excision of primary cutaneous squamous cell carcinoma. *J Am Acad Dermatol*. 1992;27(2 Pt 1):241–248.
21. Tsao H, Atkins MB, Sober AJ. Management of cutaneous melanoma. *N Engl J Med*. 2004;351(10):998–1012.
22. Kanzler MH, Swetter SM. Malignant melanoma. *J Am Acad Dermatol*. 2003;48(5):780–783.
23. Neitzel CD. Biopsy techniques for skin disease and skin cancer. *Oral Maxillofac Surg Clin North Am*. 2005;17(2):143–146. v.
24. Mittal A, Colegio OR. Skin cancers in organ transplant recipients. *Am J Transplant*. 2017;17(10):2509–2530.
25. O'Reilly Zwald F, Brown M. Skin cancer in solid organ transplant recipients: advances in therapy and management: part I. Epidemiology of skin cancer in solid organ transplant recipients. *J Am Acad Dermatol*. 2011;65(2):253–261.
26. Garrett GL, Blanc PD, Boscardin J, et al. Incidence of and risk factors for skin cancer in organ transplant recipients in the United States. *JAMA Dermatol*. 2017;153(3):296–303.
27. Diamantopoulos P, Deskoulidi P, Dalianoudis I, et al. The management of locally advanced head and neck squamous and basal cell carcinomas. *J BUON*. 2018;23(4):1118–1124.
28. Bailey EC, Sober AJ, Tsao H, et al. Cutaneous melanoma. In: Goldsmith LA, Katz SI, Gilchrest BA, et al., eds. *Fitzpatrick's Dermatology in General Medicine*. ed 8. New York: McGraw-Hill; 2012. http://www.accessmedicine.com/content.aspx?aID=56062430.

29. Zablow AI, Eanelli TR, Sanfilippo LJ. Electron beam therapy for skin cancer of the head and neck. *Head Neck*. 1992;14(3):188–195.
30. Werlinger KD, Upton G, Moore AY. Recurrence rates of primary nonmelanoma skin cancers treated by surgical excision compared to electrodesiccation-curettage in a private dermatological practice. *Dermatol Surg*. 2002;28(12):1138–1142.
31. Spencer JM, Tannenbaum A, Sloan L, Amonette RA. Does inflammation contribute to the eradication of basal cell carcinoma following curettage and electrodesiccation? *Dermatol Surg*. 1997;23(8):625–630.
32. Snow SN, Madjar DD Jr. Mohs surgery in the management of cutaneous malignancies. *Clin Dermatol*. 2001;19(3):339–347.
33. Shriner DL, McCoy DK, Goldberg DJ, Wagner RF Jr. Mohs micrographic surgery. *J Am Acad Dermatol*. 1998;39(1):79–97.
34. DiNardo LJ, Lin J, Karageorge LS, Powers CN. Accuracy, utility, and cost of frozen section margins in head and neck cancer surgery. *Laryngoscope*. 2000;110(10 Pt 1):1773–1776.
35. Wilson AW, Howsam G, Santhanam V, et al. Surgical management of incompletely excised basal cell carcinomas of the head and neck. *Br J Oral Maxillofac Surg*. 2004;42(4):311–314.
36. Marcil I, Stern RS. Risk of developing a subsequent nonmelanoma skin cancer in patients with a history of nonmelanoma skin cancer: a critical review of the literature and meta-analysis. *Arch Dermatol*. 2000;136(12):1524–1530.
37. Chen ELA, Srivastava D, Nijhawan RI. Mohs micrographic surgery: development, technique, and applications in cutaneous malignancies. *Semin Plast Surg*. 2018;32(2):60–68.

CHAPTER 108

Local Flaps for Facial Reconstruction

Hans C. Brockhoff II and Felix Jose Amarista

Armamentarium

Adhesive wound closure strips (Steri-Strips)
Appropriate sutures
Liquid tissue adhesive
Local anesthetic
with bicarbonate (e.g., 1 mEq bicarbonate to 10 mL lidocaine)
with/without vasoconstrictor as indicated
Marking pen
Monopolar and bipolar electrocautery
Pickups
Adson and Adson-Brown
Ruler
Scalpel
#15, #10, #11 as indicated
Skin hooks
Single and double
Skin staples
Straight end curved, large and small
Suture and wound closure materials
Suture scissors
Tissue-cutting scissors

History of the Procedure

Soft tissue repair of the face originated around 600 BC, when Sushruta Samhita of India described nasal reconstruction with a cheek flap.[1] As surgery evolved, our reconstructive options multiplied into a prolific body of literature.

Facial defects can often cross facial subunits and be grossly disfiguring, resulting in negative social perception. Comprehensive assessment of the wound includes the location, size, depth, layers, function, and relationship to the surrounding facial subunits and tissues.[2]

The ideal reconstructive approach for any facial defect respects esthetic boundaries, closes under minimal tension, and provides a favorable cosmetic result with the least distortion of surrounding facial subunits.[2]

Reconstructive flaps are definitive procedures, which often benefit from adjustment or revision. They may compromise adjacent tissue with scars and may live or die depending on the (1) condition of the patient, (2) viability of adjacent skin, (3) choice of flap, and (4) timing of repair.

Patient-specific defect characteristics (size, subunit involved, nature of tissue involved) and patient clinical factors can alter the surgeon's choice for reconstruction.[3] For example, smoking (most common patient-related factor associated with increased risk for flap failure)[4] and diabetes may impact the viability of a flap. Other considerations include prior radiation therapy, previous surgery around the planned operative area, collagen-vascular disease, anticoagulants, and immunosuppression.

The viability of adjacent skin heavily influences choices. Traumatic wounds often have crushed borders, gunshots produce areas of hyperemia and stasis of the tissue, and prior scars and radiation often limit flap mobility and viability. Local flaps, when indicated, are considered ideal for reconstruction of facial defects due to excellent color and texture match from adjacent skin,[2] and should be preferred over free flaps whenever possible as far as the esthetic outcome is concerned.[5]

Other reconstructive options that might be considered include doing nothing, which allows healing via secondary intention, and split- or full-thickness skin grafting. These options may be superior for traumatic avulsion wounds.

Healing by secondary intention, rather than primary wound closure, may be a superior choice when shrinkage of the wound circumference would be beneficial. Certain areas can heal nearly imperceptibly and without distortion, such as the periauricular area, the posterior scalp, and small medial canthal defects. Secondary healing necessitates patient motivation and reliability, as well as a commitment to home care of the open wound. This is a relatively painless option, provided the wound is covered. Secondary healing can also be a useful temporary option for wound management. There is still opportunity at any time during the secondary epithelialization process to intervene with a flap or graft.

Advantages to grafting include the elimination of complex wound care, simplification of closure in compromised patients, reduction in future flap size, and observation for possible tumor recurrence.

Using skin grafts provides a less elegant wound closure, is patient- and surgeon-dependent, and relies primarily on a well-nourished bed of tissue for survival. Full-thickness skin grafts provide more volume, less contracture, and a better color match; however, split-thickness grafts achieve better survival rates with larger defects and do not require donor site closures.[2]

Indications for the Use of the Procedure

Correct timing of any wound repair influences success. Two concepts are noteworthy.

First, immediate flap coverage for either trauma or tumor resection is rarely emergently indicated. Exceptions to this standard are limited to unusual circumstances such as covering the brain or a major vessel. Open wounds may be left unrepaired for extended times, as long as debris and bacteria are removed, and the wound is covered. Appropriate coverage may consist of ointment or a simple bandage.

Second, delay of wound repair may offer opportunities to increase flap success. Delay maneuvers before final repair can enhance adjacent tissue viability, shrink defect size, and allow an augmented vascular base of granulation tissue. Delay allows the surgeon to carefully plan the approach. Surgical delays (e.g., limited flap lifting or tissue expansion) can precondition the flap and promote neovascularization and angiogenesis.

The surgeon should develop a schematic progression of reconstructive possibilities. This progression begins by mentally trying to close any wound by direct advancement of tissue in or near resting skin tension lines (RSTLs) if possible. Repositioning of end triangles and harnessing tissue creep modifications may be necessary. After the advancement flap has been considered, possible rotational flaps are evaluated. Finally, transposition and interpolation flaps are assessed. Obviously, there are locations on the face (e.g., the lips and nose) where a specific type of flap works optimally.

Flap Concepts

Early facial defect closures were directed toward "filling the hole," whereas more elegant and esthetic solutions now allow opportunities to create a natural harmonious result. The fundamental concepts of local flap reconstruction are listed in Box 108.1.

Anatomy

The most superficial layer of the skin is the epidermis. Beneath the epidermis, the dermis is subdivided into the superficial papillary and the deeper reticular layers.

BOX 108.1 Fundamental Concepts of Local Flap Reconstruction

1. Consider flap mobility blood supply
2. Consider tension forces within the flap and the effects on or of local anatomy
3. Consider where excess tissue may be ultimately positioned
4. Consider allowable wound tension at closure and where any technical maneuvers may be reasonable
5. Consider flap incisions near topographic borders within relaxed skin tension lines or hidden from obvious frontal views

Adapted from Zoumalan RA, Murakami CS. Facial flap complications. *Facial Plast Surg.* 2012;28(3):347–353.

There is both a superficial and deep intradermal vascular plexus, which typically runs parallel to the surface of the skin and provides nutrients to a large surface area. These vascular networks are extensive but by themselves cannot support tissue viability alone after significant tissue undermining is performed. The deeper, subdermal plexus lies beneath the dermis within the superficial subcutaneous tissue and plays a critical role in flap physiology. These vessels are often preserved in an advancing flap edge through the retention of a trace layer of fat on the undersurface of the tissue. A "random flap" depends upon this blood supply.[6]

Deep to the network of intradermal plexuses are the larger caliber axial "named" vessels (i.e., superficial temporal artery). Axial vessels lie deep to the subcutaneous fat on the surface of the superficial fascia, roughly parallel to the skin surface. These vessels within the flap dramatically enhance vascularity, thus offering options for lengthening the flap without compromising viability (e.g., forehead and Abbe flaps).

Musculocutaneous arteries, which are deeper interconnecting vessels, are perpendicular to the skin surface. These vessels exit the muscle and enter the subcutaneous tissue to supply a smaller region of the skin. Collectively, the septocutaneous and musculocutaneous arteries contribute to a diffuse interconnecting vascular network of dermal and subdermal arteries that create some vascular redundancy in the skin (Fig. 108.1).[7]

Flap Terminology

The Defect

A primary defect is any defect created by trauma or tumor. Direct advancement flaps close a primary defect by stretching the adjacent skin over the defect. When the elliptical advancement flap is ineffective, tissue must still be otherwise mobilized to fill the primary defect without undue tension. The use of additional incisions and maneuvers (e.g., backcuts) can allow tension-free closure.

A secondary defect is a defect that occurs as a result of movement of the flap and develops behind the advancing flap edge. Flap design compensates for the secondary defect by allowing the surgeon to close this defect as well. Sometimes the secondary defect is closed by dissipation of forces elsewhere or by grafting in an inconspicuous location.

Inherent Extensibility

Adequate skin mobility is partially attributable to skin extensibility (stretching of the elastic fibers). Low-tension closure minimizes scar widening, wound dehiscence, tissue ischemia, and anatomic distortion. On the face, tense closures can break down. This is less of a problem on the more forgiving forehead and scalp. There is generally more extensibility among older patients. A mid-cheek defect of only 1 cm may be the terminal limit of easy closure in an adolescent, 2.5 cm in a 40-year-old, and over 4 cm in a 75-year-old. On the face, no additional stretch/extensibility will be gained after 3 to 4 cm of undermining. Overstretching on the face will produce tears or striae, which can be permanent (Fig. 108.2).

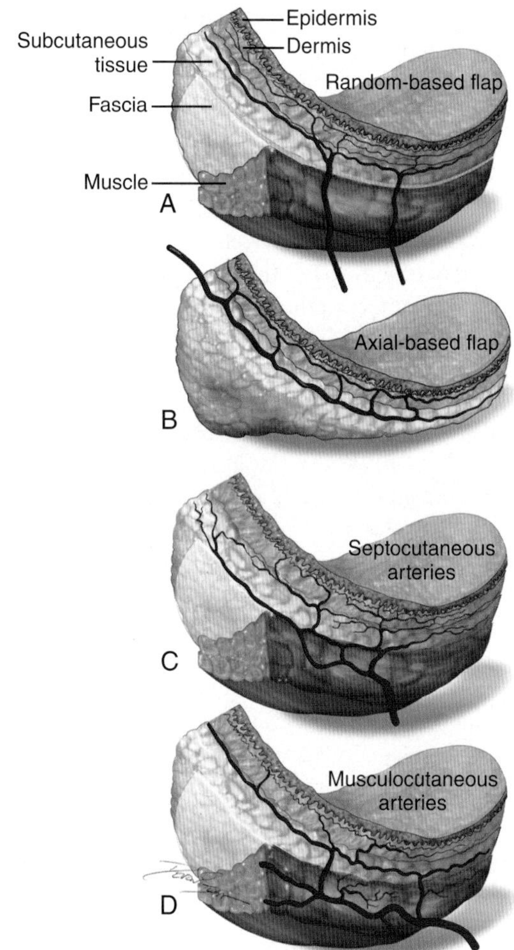

Figure 108.1 **A,** Vascularity is dependent upon diffuse subdermal plexus. Viability of long flaps is critically susceptible to local angiosomes, host conditions (e.g., scarring, diabetes), and social habits (e.g., smoking). **B,** Paramedian forehead flap. Vascularity is dependent upon named vessel allowing significant length. **C,** Septocutaneous flap. Vascularity is dependent upon perforating vessels (e.g., anterior lateral thigh free flap). This yields a pliable soft tissue flap since muscle is left at the donor site. **D,** Musculocutaneous flap. Vascularity dependent upon large vessels in muscle.

Mechanical Creep

Mechanical creep is the tendency for any solid material to move slowly or deform under the influence of stress, and skin is no exception. Skin held at a constant tension may require less tension over time. A common characteristic of mechanical creep can be observed following a tightly closed avulsive forehead wound. After a few days, the tissue relaxes.

Three principles of mechanical creep may be functionally garnered to help close tight flaps: presuturing, cyclic loading, and deep scoring of tense tissues:

- Presuturing pulls tissues together and can be employed from days to only minutes prior to attempting wound closure. This technique can gain millimeters to centimeters of additional length. Commercially available instrumentation is available, but the use of sutures can achieve the same result.
- Cyclic loading performs the same purpose at surgery. The surgeon cyclically loads the tissue with skin hooks or by inflating a catheter balloon to stretch it. Each cycle extracts additional stretch or creep from the tissue, yielding greater overall length.
- Deep tissue scoring, particularly of the galea, can also augment mechanical creep.

Biologic Creep

Biologic creep is the slow, methodic stretching of the skin, producing new skin. This physiologic property is reflected in severe obesity, pregnancy, and skin expansion.[7,8]

Surgical Flap Delay

Blood supply to the terminal portion of a random flap (flaps dependent on the subdermal plexus) is not as much a function of width, but rather one of length. Flap length can be limited by vascular compromising factors such as the small veins of diabetes or vasoconstriction from nicotine. The tissue perfusion pressure decreases as the length of the flap increases from its base. When this pressure falls below a critical closing pressure of the arterioles, flap necrosis occurs beyond that point. On the face, the original studies based the actual length on angiosomal units of vascularity (Fig. 108.3).

Augmenting the viable length of a flap may be critical to success. The delay technique for a local flap involves circumferential incision alone, subcutaneous undermining alone through small incisions, or circumferential and subcutaneous undermining without mobilization. Two weeks after the delay procedure, the flap may be transferred to the recipient site. This delay results in enhanced circulation to the flap through the closure of arteriovenous shunts and the realignment of the vasculature within the subdermal plexus.[9]

Angiosomal Unit

The angiosomal unit is the three-dimensional territory supplied by source arteries and veins. Identification of the anatomic territory of an individual perforator can help the surgeon define an area that may be safely lifted for a reconstructive effort with or without flap delay. The cutaneous perforator vessels at the flap base where the anastomotic connections usually occur can exhibit a reduced caliber, in which case they are named "choke arteries." These narrowed anastomoses can produce vascular insufficiency and ultimate necrosis at the flap edge.[10,11]

Facial Architecture

There is a wide variety of structural differences of the face depending on the location. These differences are often described and categorized as the *facial units,* examples of which are the eyelids, cheeks, nose, lips, mentum, and auricles. Some of these units can be further divided into *subunits* based on visible creases and differences in skin quality.[12]

Central units including the eyes, nose, and lips (central triangle of the face) usually draw more attention when viewing normal, novel faces, while peripheral facial units (cheeks, temple, and forehead) generally draw less attention allowing for more tolerable scar irregularity.

When designing an ideal flap for reconstruction, the most favorable result will be one that respects the facial subunits

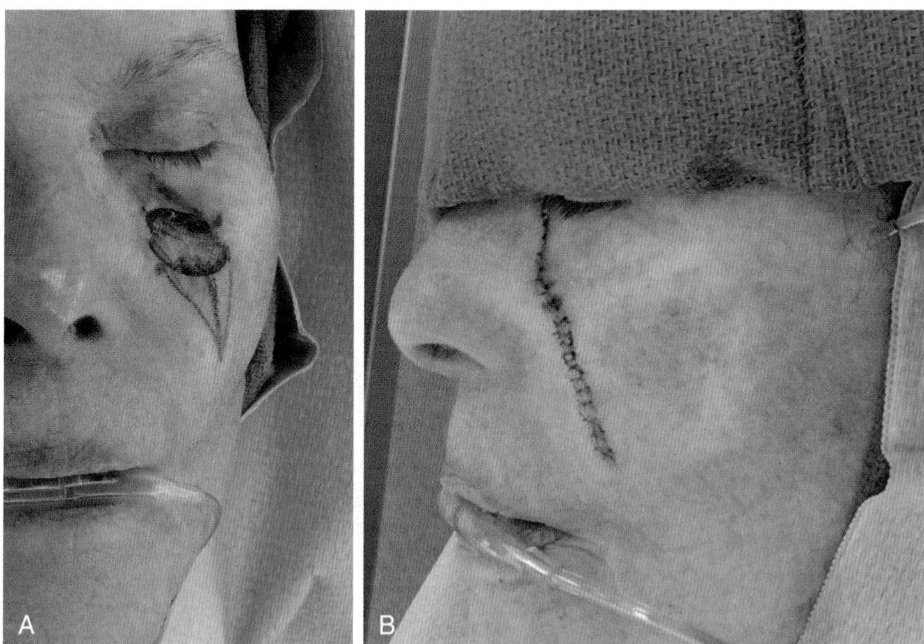

Figure 108.2 **A,** Advancement flap. The first choice to close a defect is in the resting skin tension lines. **B,** Undermining more than 3 to 4 cm on the face will usually not increase advancement distance. In older patients, more than 4 cm may be closed with direct advancement versus 1 cm in adolescents.

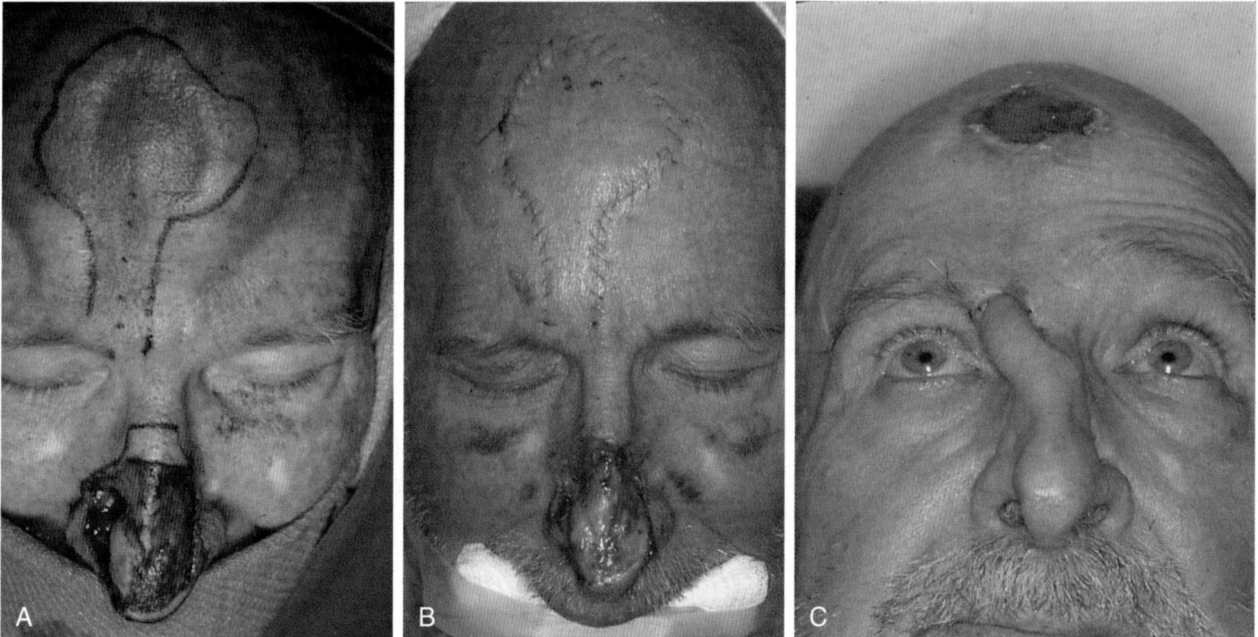

Figure 108.3 **A,** Flap delay. In compromised patients (e.g., smoking, diabetes, scarring), delayed maneuvers enhance flap viability and length. In the clinic, a template of the nasal defect was constructed. The pattern was unfolded, drawn on the forehead, and local anesthesia was injected. The dotted line, 17 to 22 mm from the midline, indicates the probable course of the artery. **B,** This flap was incised circumferentially, but an adequate delay also might have involved small incisions at the periphery and complete undermining. At 2 weeks, the flap can be mobilized with confidence. The open nasal tissues are kept covered and moist during the delay. **C,** Two or 3 weeks after the flap placement, the patient is ready for thinning or division and inset. The upper forehead, with an original defect more than 4 cm, is healing secondarily. The open forehead wound is covered with ointment and bandaged until wound tackiness is gone.

and their boundaries. Scars that lie directly along the borders of these units will be naturally camouflaged. Therefore, the surgeon who encounters a defect encompassing over half of a subunit such as the nasal tip or lip philtrum may consider removal of the entire subunit prior to reconstruction. The surgeon may consider independent repair of adjacent unit(s) so that large reconstructions do not flow nonanatomically from one unit to another (Fig. 108.4).

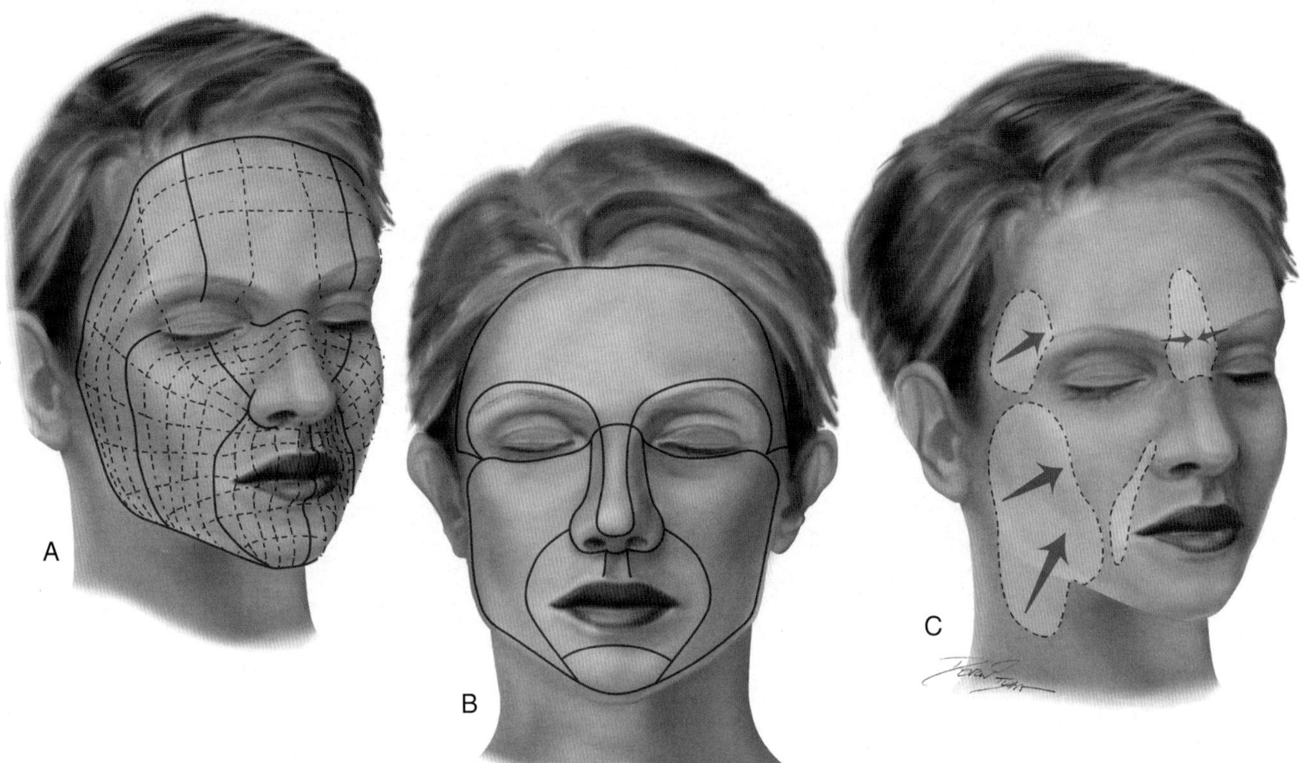

Figure 108.4 Flap choices hinge upon optimal esthetics and ease of mobilization. **A,** Flaps designed close to resting skin tension lines (RSTL) produce less obvious scars. The opposite directions to the RSTL are the lines of maximum extensibility. In most, but not all, situations, this direction allows greater flap mobility. **B,** Borders of topographical units of the face are also good places for scars because they are natural changes in visible planes. **C,** Mobility of tissue depends upon age, direction, location, and previous scars.

TECHNIQUE: Basic Concepts in Local Flap Design

Most flaps are somewhat ischemic to a certain extent initially, because the original tissue perfusion has been compromised by flap elevation (most tissue can survive on 10% of its average blood flow).[4]

The simplest flaps are elliptical advancement flaps, which are usually designed in a 3:1 or 4:1 length-to-width proportion. Elasticity of the dermis determines how easily the ellipse can be closed.

The three quandaries to flap control are as follows:

1. What to do with the triangular end of advancement excisions (Burow triangles)
2. What to do with the excess tissue or bunching (*dog ears,* which form as tissue moves into a defect) (Box 108.2)
3. How to handle flap tension (refer to specific flap sections)

BOX 108.2 Management of Dog Ears

1. Do nothing (works well on the scalp where bunched tissue lies down over time)
2. Close opposite lines of uneven lengths by spreading out the problem (halving)
3. Remove the excess to a hidden area (an end or middle triangle)
4. Lengthen the incision (to eliminate bunching)
5. Perform an M-plasty (which shortens the problem)
6. Reverse the S-loop (effectively hiding the excess elsewhere)
7. Advance the dog ear as a flap (subcutaneous "island")

Modified from Zide MF, Yan T. Head and neck skin cancer. In: Miloro M, Ghali GE, Larsen PE, Waite PD, eds. *Peterson's Principles of Oral and Maxillofacial Surgery.* 3rd ed. Shelton, CT: People's Medical Publishing House-USA; 2011.

TECHNIQUE: Basic Concepts in Local Flap Design—*cont'd*

TRIANGLES

There are two general options: remove the excess somewhere, throw it away, or use it as a free graft, or mobilize the excess on a subcutaneous pedicle (Fig. 108.5A–D).

ADVANCEMENT FLAPS[13,14]

Advancement flaps mobilize tissue in a single direction. They can be constructed with multiple modifications: simple, square, bilateral, Burow triangle repositioning, and A-to-T or O-to-T shaped designs.[8] The modifications of the advancement flap include those shown in Fig. 108.5E–J. These flaps are often useful in the repair of defects involving the forehead or eyebrow (Box 108.3).[15–18]

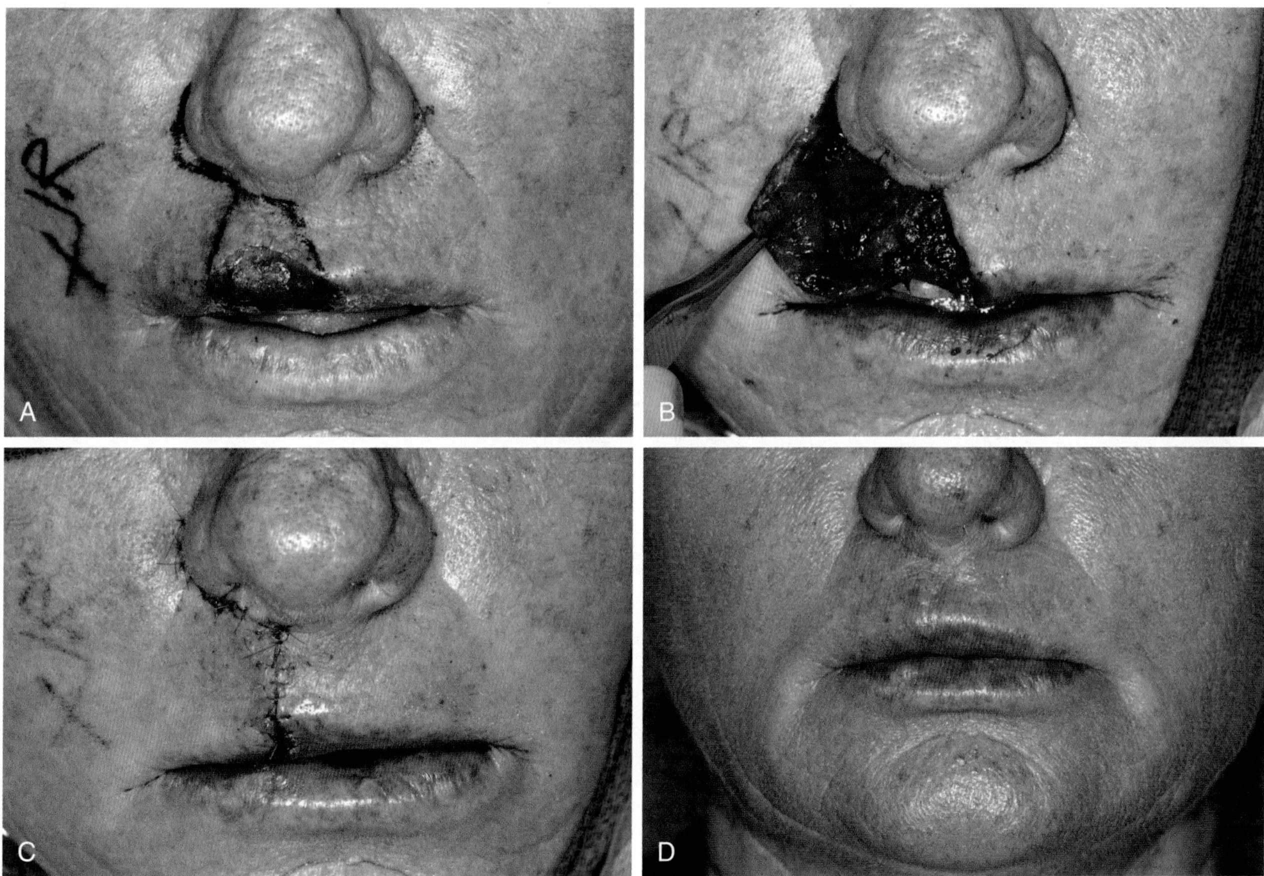

Figure 108.5 **A,** Medial lip defects less than 1.4 cm will produce minimal shifting of the philtral column. Visible shifts will occur above that size here. The more lateral the defect, the less obvious the philtral shift. Some surgeons close this defect with through-and-through excision without undermining. Regardless, the dog ears are removed in the alar area 1 mm out of the crease and include the oral mucosa above the muscle. **B,** Undermining above the muscle allows the flap to move over the defect. Tension on the flap may be reduced by excision of the small blue triangle of the orbicularis oris, which is rejoined before closure. **C,** At surgery, the critical factor is aligning the vermilion cutaneous border, since a 1-mm discrepancy is visible at conversational distance. **D,** After suture removal, there is a well-aligned lip, with minimal philtral shift.

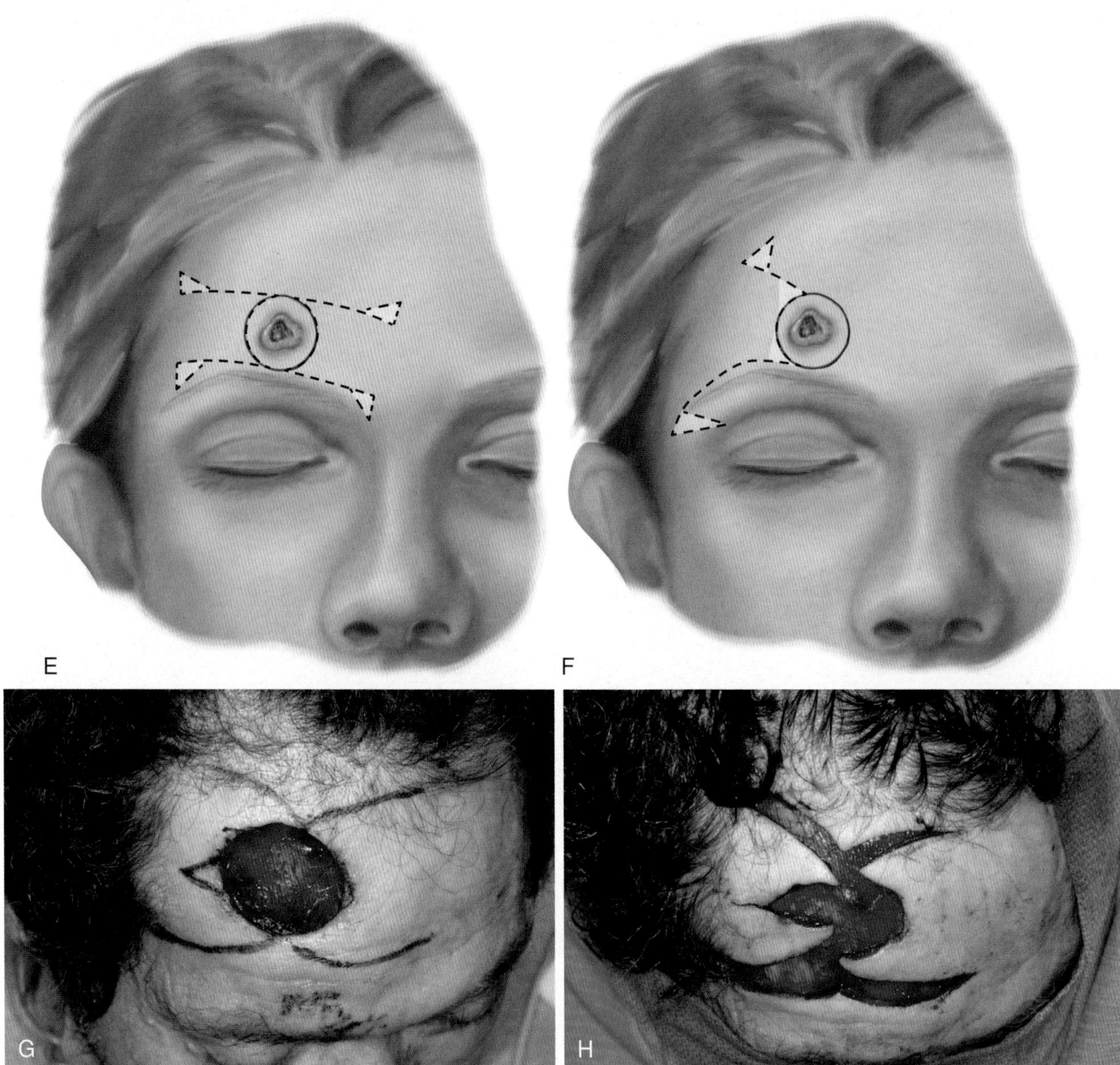

Figure 108.5, cont'd **E,** This often published "H" type of flap is a poor choice for three reasons. Long flaps get smaller as they advance, and they won't fit as drawn. Long random flaps like this should be subgaleal to survive, but that might injure motor or sensory nerves. Mobility of tissue here is mostly from the lateral direction, so the medial flap may not be indicated. **F,** A better option than the "H" flap. The direction of movement is mostly from the lateral. Dog ears are removed in topographic borders or other areas of tissue excess. **G,** Modifications of advancement flaps have reduced necessary movement in wide defects. In this case, a small triangle is removed from the advancing flap. The concave edge of the left flap will encircle the closing right flap. This wide defect, too large for the "classic H" closure, could also be closed with a scalp rotation flap. **H,** The flaps advance on each other half the distance of the classic "H" flap.

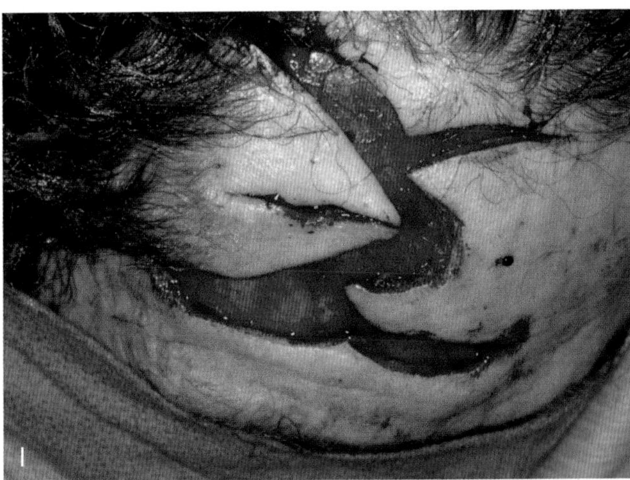

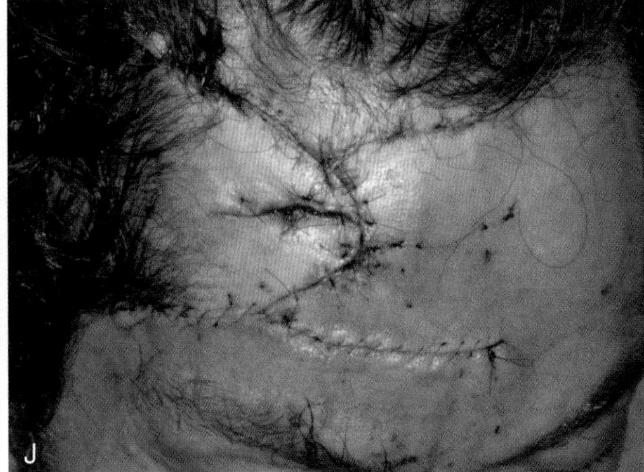

Figure 108.5, cont'd I, Closure ensuing. Flap elevated at subgaleal level provides vascularity to flaps at expense of sensory loss to high medial and lateral forehead. Critical eyebrow movement is maintained below the flap area. **J,** Flaps almost closed reveal more movement medially from the lateral flap. Minor dog ear removal behind hairline.

BOX 108.3 Advancement Flaps Pearls

Comments

1. Ideal to close the ends before middle
2. Undermining more than 3 to 4 cm on the face will not produce more laxity
3. Move end triangles to correct for local anatomy
4. Ideal for smaller defects
5. Advancement flaps work best in areas of skin with great elasticity
6. Provide very good aesthetic and functional results and a high level of patient satisfaction[19]

Concerns

1. Tension: If high, consider relief with mechanical creep enhancements (pexing, presuturing, scoring galea, intraoperative skin expansion)
2. If relief methods do not work, change plan or graft defect[13,14,20]

BOX 108.4 Rotational Flap Pearls

Comments

1. Redirects tension vectors
2. A backcut at the end of the rotational flap enhances mobility
3. Standing cutaneous deformities occur at the base of the flap; hence the 30-degree triangular excision; when the excision may compromise blood supply, it can be deferred until later

Concerns

1. Pivotal restraint
2. A backcut can compromise the flap's blood supply[21]

TECHNIQUE: Basic Concepts in Local Flap Design—*cont'd*

ROTATIONAL FLAPS

Rotational flaps are "pivotal flaps" that transfer tissue to an immediately adjacent defect through the utilization of an arc. Ultimately, the defects become triangular shaped.[22] Rotational flaps partially redistribute and redirect closure tension away from the primary defect; however, the curved incisions may not lie within the RSTLs. Rotational flaps can be random or axial if a named vessel is included. The random platform of blood supply is acceptable for large facial flaps but can be limited for large cervicofacial flaps, which extend low onto the neck or chest. In these cases, a deeper dissection plane and inclusion of the platysma muscle will augment the overall blood supply. An advantage to the rotational flap is that it may be rotated again at a future date should additional tissue need to be removed secondary to tumor presence (Box 108.4).[8]

TECHNIQUE: Basic Concepts in Local Flap Design—*cont'd*

KEY CONCEPTS IN ROTATIONAL FLAPS

1. The length of the arc of rotation is related to the restriction at the pivot point. On the face and nose, an arc of approximately four times the defect width is adequate. In the scalp, six times the defect width or more may be necessary.
2. The defect should ideally be in the configuration of an inverted 30-degree triangle. The shape of the legs of the triangle may conform to anatomic borders, such as the hairline.[17]
3. A shorter rotational flap produces a wider secondary defect, increasing the secondary defect closure tension.[9,23]
4. Pivot-point control will change depending on flap location (Fig. 108.5K–GG).[24–27]

Continued

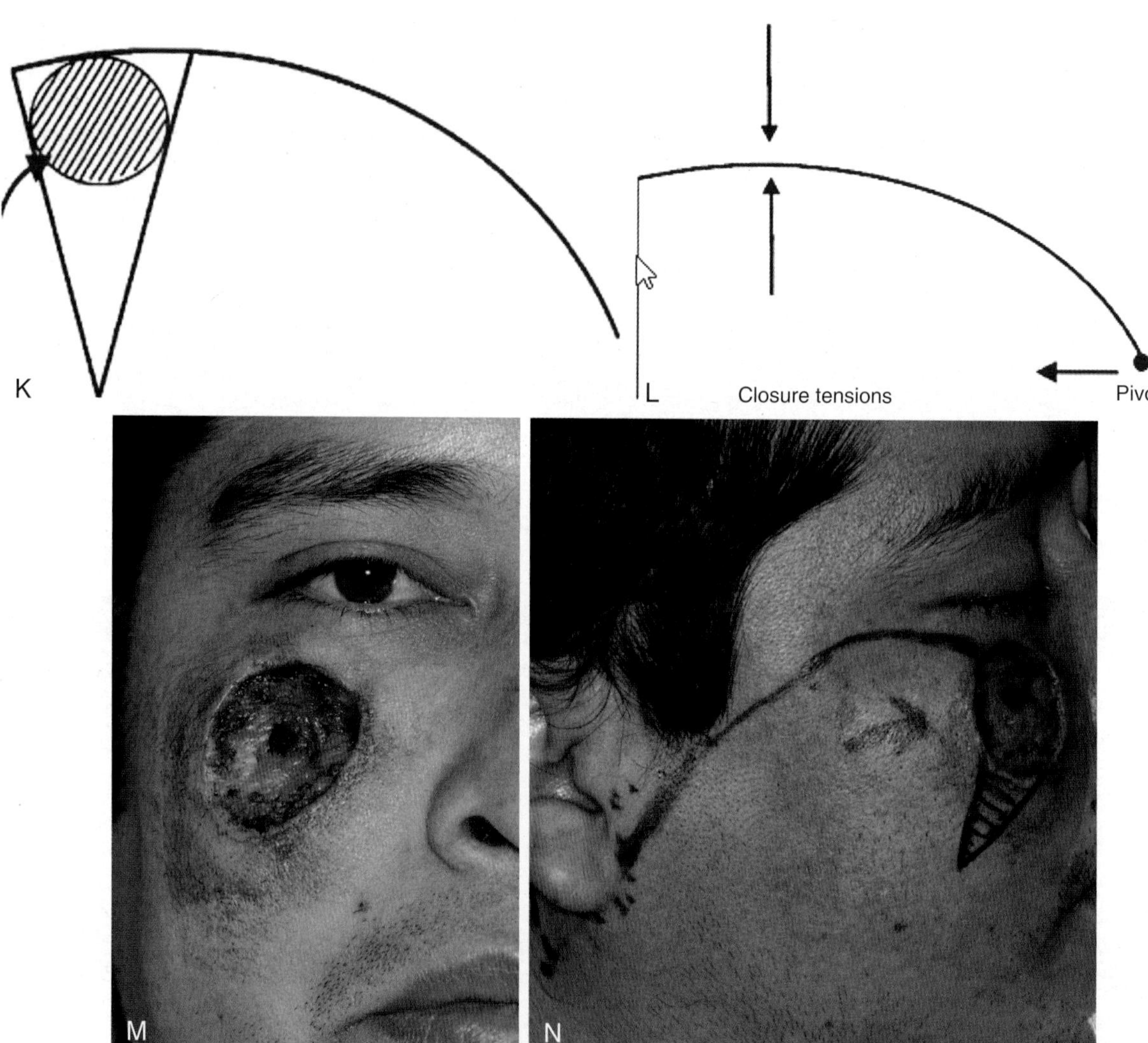

Figure 108.5, cont'd **K** and **L,** Closure forces of the rotation flap show that the pivot point moves toward the defect, and there is tension on the arc of closure. To design a rotation flap, these two aspects must be controlled. **M,** Central Mohs defect. **N,** Classic design with mobile pivot point at end of arc. The arc is barely three to four times the width of the defect because of tissue laxity.

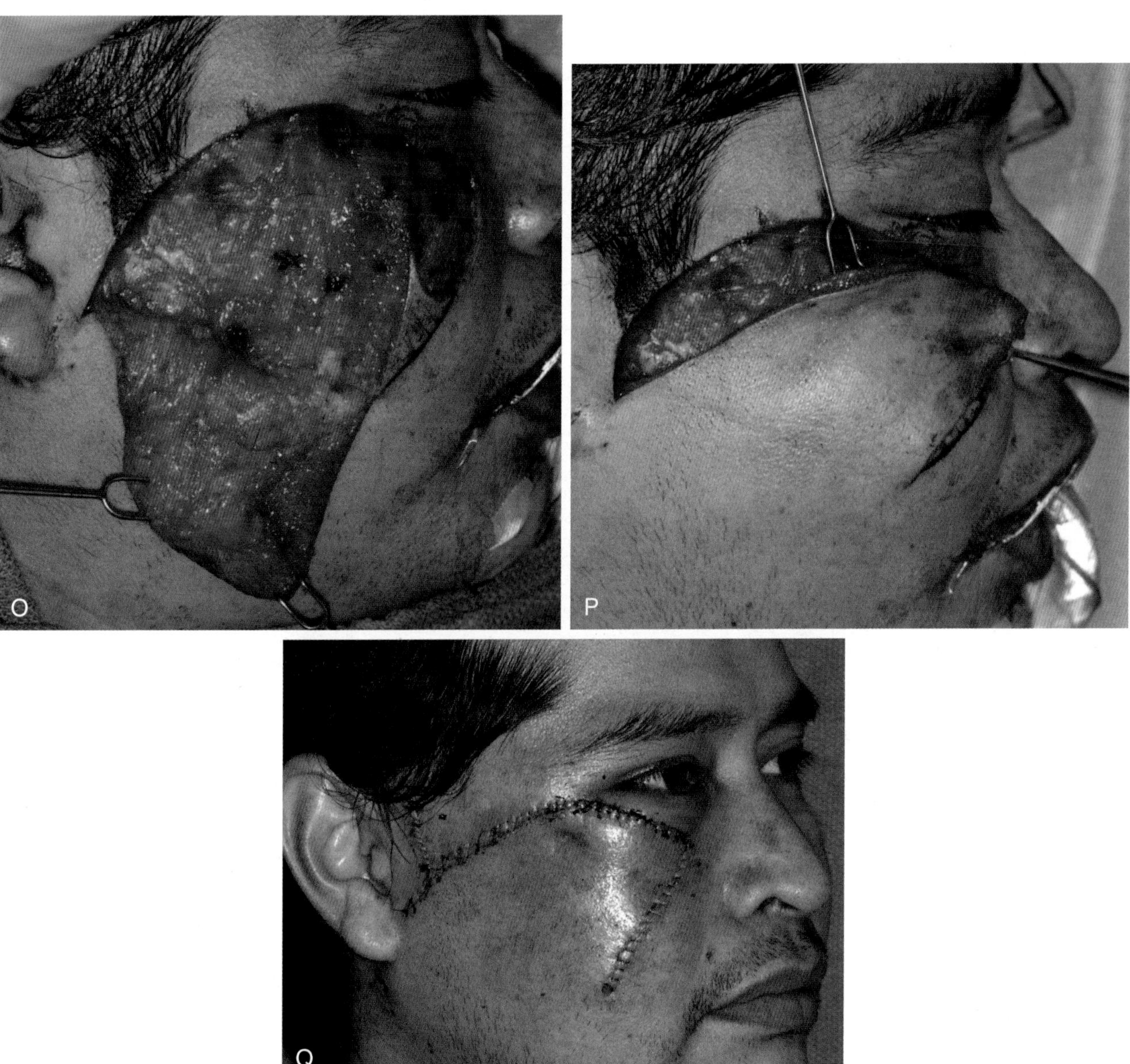

Figure 108.5, cont'd **O,** The random rotation flap. Only bipolar cautery controls bleeding beneath a flap. The 30-degree dog ear is removed last. More flap laxity may be obtained with the increase of the arc length or a back cut behind the ear. **P,** Easily mobilized flap exposes the secondary defect in the arc of the flap. A pexing suture to the orbital rim, at the point of the double skin hook, will prevent eyelid retraction. **Q,** Rotation flap with semi-permanent pexing suture at the lateral rim. This divot, from catching the dermis with the suture, will efface in 2 weeks.

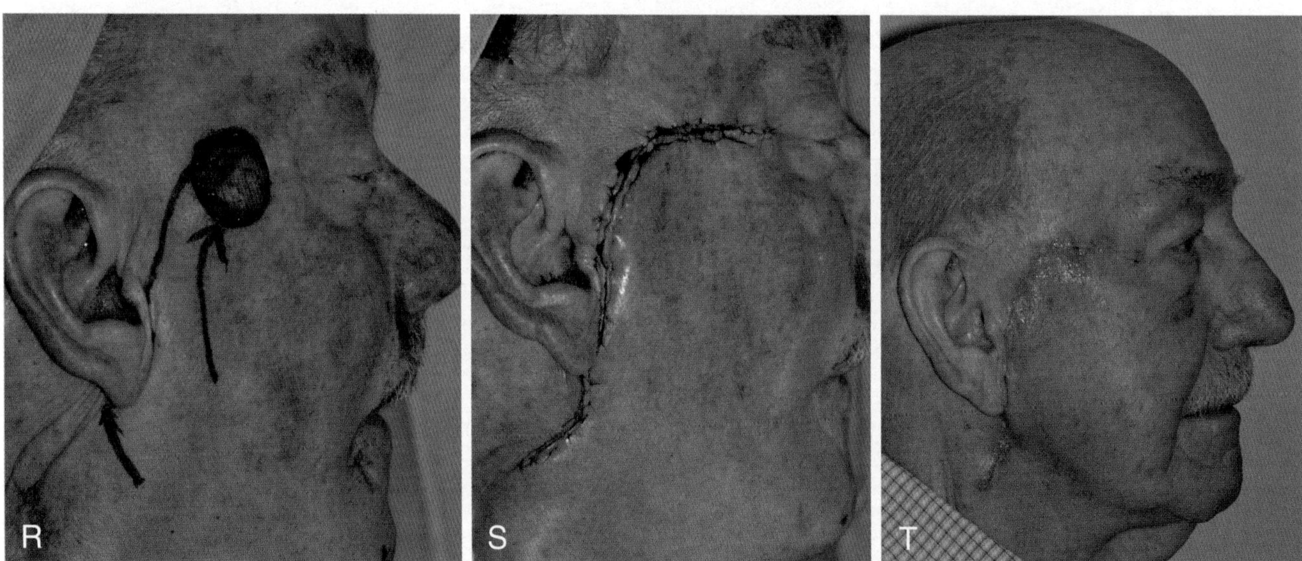

Figure 108.5, cont'd **R,** Right temporal resection defect and rotational flap design. **S,** Adequate rotation of flap and primary closure with nonresorbable suture. **T,** Two weeks postop. After suture removal, there is good healing and an adequate cosmetic result.

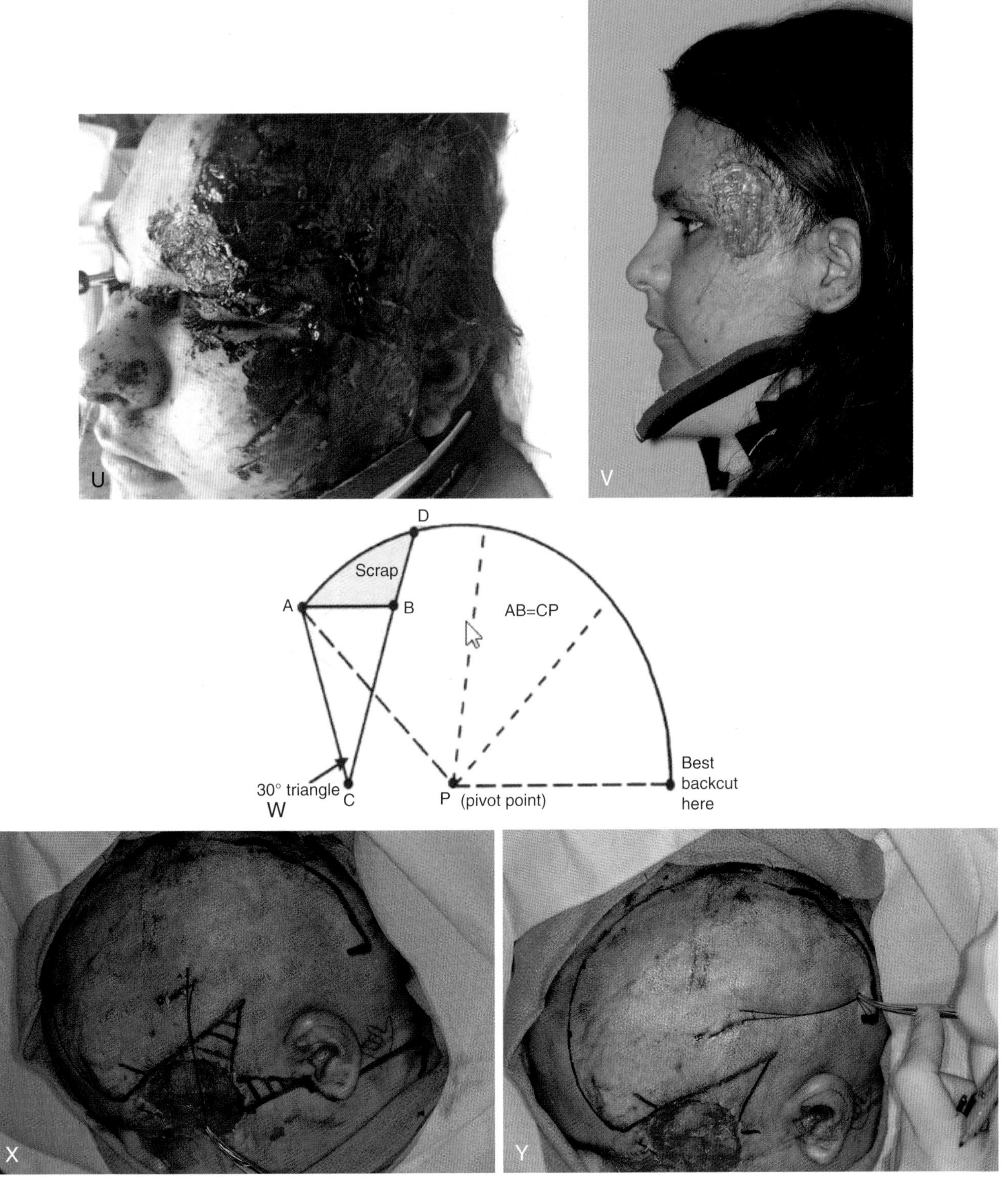

Figure 108.5, cont'd **U,** Necrotic tissue at left temporal area in emergency room photo. **V,** Residual temporal defect at 2 to 3 weeks after initial debridement and moist bandage coverage. The rounded edges and lack of peripheral inflammation manifest a clean wound ready for closure, surface scraping, and marginal excision. **W,** Design of a rotation flap in fixed scalp tissue demands modification. The pivot point must be moved from the end of the arc to the middle of a circle. If the pivot point is at the end of the arc, as in a classic rotation flap, the tip of the flap (*D*) will not cover the defect. Placing *D* in the higher position allows it to move to point *A*. The base length of the 30-degree triangle, *AB*, is moved to *CP*. *P* is the new pivot point. From here, the arc of the rotation is drawn (*dotted lines*). If enhanced rotation is indicated, a back cut may be included. **X,** Rotation flap. The pivot point has been sutured (*black suture*). The diameter of the arc has been selected, just as in the diagram for rotation flap with fixed scalp tissue. The smaller triangle, cross-hatched, will be removed to allow cheek advancement superiorly. **Y,** The scalp rotation has been designed by rotating the suture around the pivot point. At the back of the flap, a potential back cut has been drawn. The short lines are drawn to align the patient hair line.

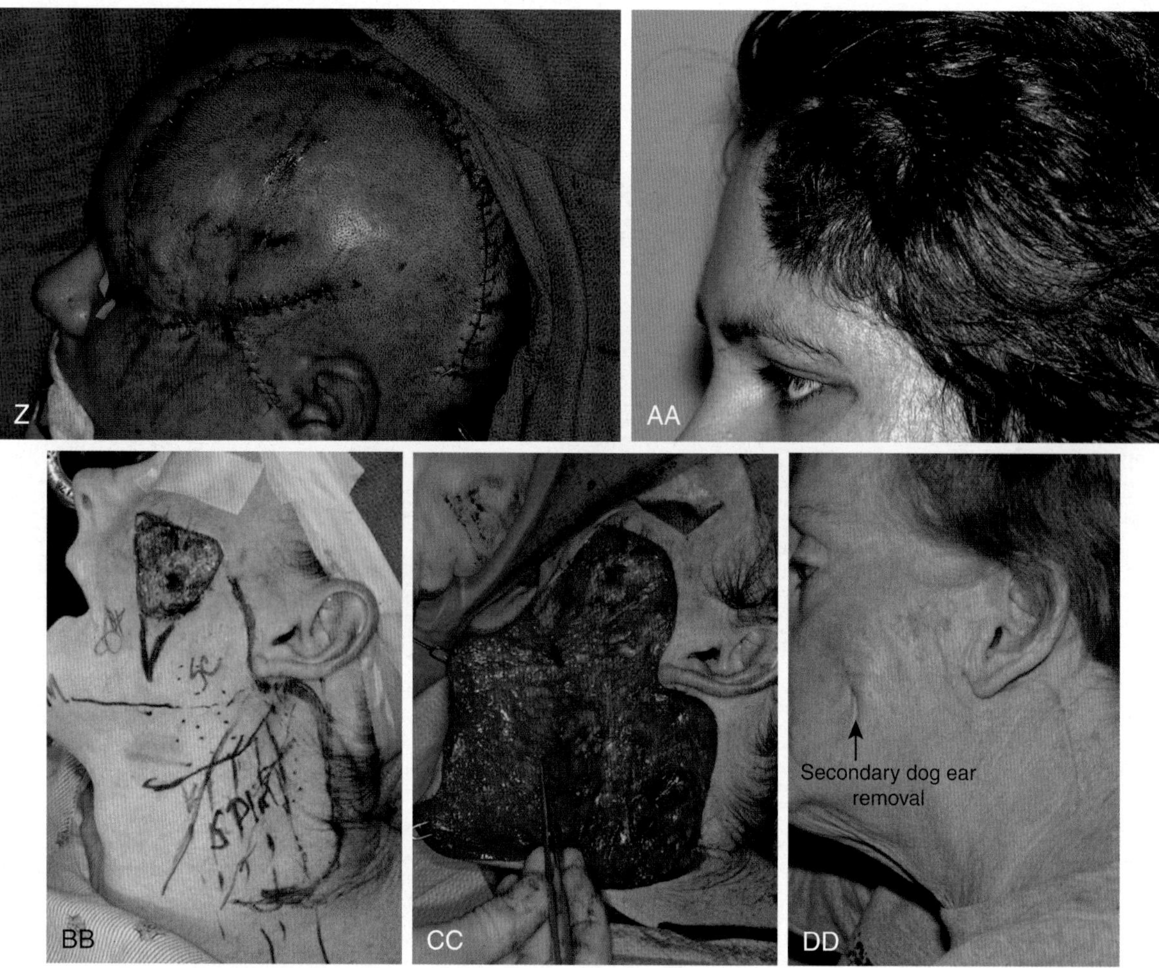

Figure 108.5, cont'd **Z,** Scalp rotation flap in place. A small amount of advancement was needed from the cheek. **AA,** Final result of scalp/temporal rotation flap at 2 months. Complex rotation flaps. **BB,** Cervicofacial rotation flap is subcutaneous (*SC*) on the face but under the platysma 2 cm below the mandible. The triangular dog ear will not be removed at the initial surgery. **CC,** Dissection accomplished with back cut in neck. **DD,** At 3 weeks, the residual dog ear may be removed easily in the office.

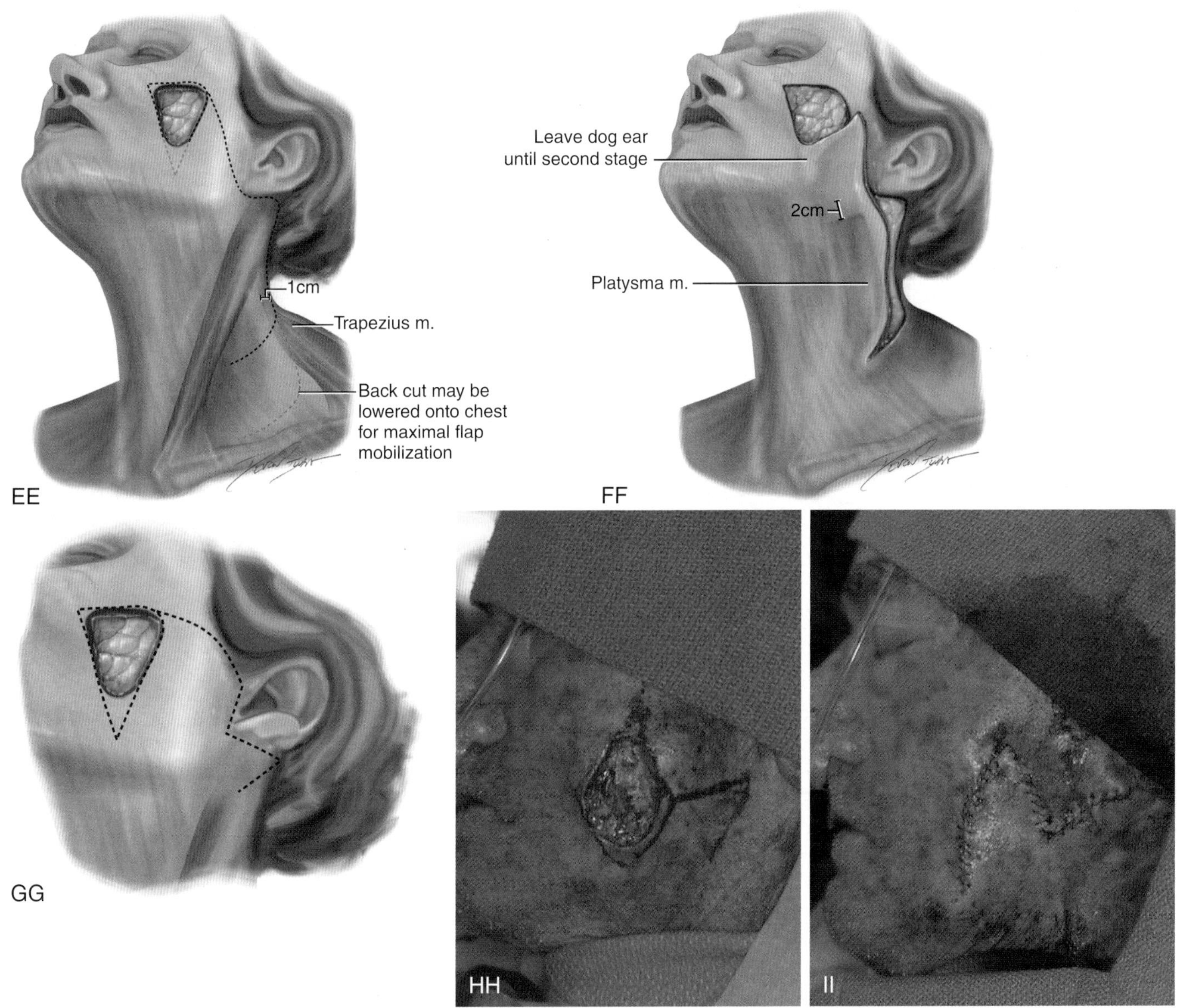

Figure 108.5, cont'd **EE,** Size of the cervicofacial flap is dependent upon the need for coverage. Therefore, the back cut may be on the neck or chest. The flap will not move adequately until the back cut is done. Scar contracture may be reduced by placing the arc of rotation 1 cm behind the border of the trapezius muscle. High behind the sternocleidomastoid, the flap is dissected superficially to avoid injury to the spinal accessory nerve. **FF,** In large cervicofacial flaps, which have "random flap" vascularity, the dog ear should be retained for at least 3 weeks. Vascularity is enhanced by dissection under the platysma in the neck from 2 cm below the border of the mandible, or under the superficial musculoaponeurotic system in the face. **GG,** An alternative to the long cervicofacial flap involves a back cut behind the ear, moving this tissue in front of the ear. **HH,** Rhomboid flap, designed so that the direction of the "short diagonal," from the obtuse angle origin of the rhomboid to the tip of the flap, is in the lines of maximum extensibility (LME). Easy transposition will be expected. **II,** The rhomboid flap was easily transposed. Unfortunately, some scars are not in the resting skin tension lines, and hair growth in men may be out of alignment.

TECHNIQUE: Basic Concepts in Local Flap Design—*cont'd*

TRANSPOSITION FLAPS

The transposition flap is a pivotal flap with a linear characteristic that combines advancement and rotation and moves adjacent tissue to an area that is under less tension. Similar to the rotational flap, a transposition flap creates a standing cutaneous deformity at the base of the flap.

Actual tissue movement may be rotational, linear, or both. Mechanically, the flap tends to be more confined than a rotational flap. Unfortunately, the transposition flap design violates RSTLs more than rotational or advancement flaps; therefore, some scars may be obtrusive. The design and placement of the flap's pivot point is a critical factor. Some flaps (e.g., nasal bilobed flaps) have both rotational and transpositional components.

One of the advantages for selecting a transposition flap include the ability to harvest the flap at a site that is not contiguous with the defect. This allows the surgeon the ability to choose areas of the face that possess greater skin elasticity as well as the option to place the donor scar in a more favorable location. (Fig. 108.5HH–RR).

Various configurations of transposition flaps exist and include but are not limited to bilobed, rectangular, parabola, Z-plasty, island, and rhombic. The classic transpositional design is the rhombic flap, which consists of an equilateral parallelogram with oblique angles. It was first described by Limberg with two angles of 120 degrees and two angles of 60 degrees.[28] Newer modifications of classic flaps remove less tissue and move easier (Box 108.5).[29]

Key Concepts in Transposition Flaps

As a pivotal flap, the length of the flap from its harvest position will shorten as the arc of pivotal movement increases. This length reduction must be factored into the design during planning.

A disadvantage in the use of this flap is the potential for the development of a "trapdoor" or "pincushion" deformity. Therefore, very small flaps should be avoided, and circumferential undermining is necessary to disperse forces of scarring. After a few weeks, steroid injection or silicone gel sheeting may speed effacement.

Continued

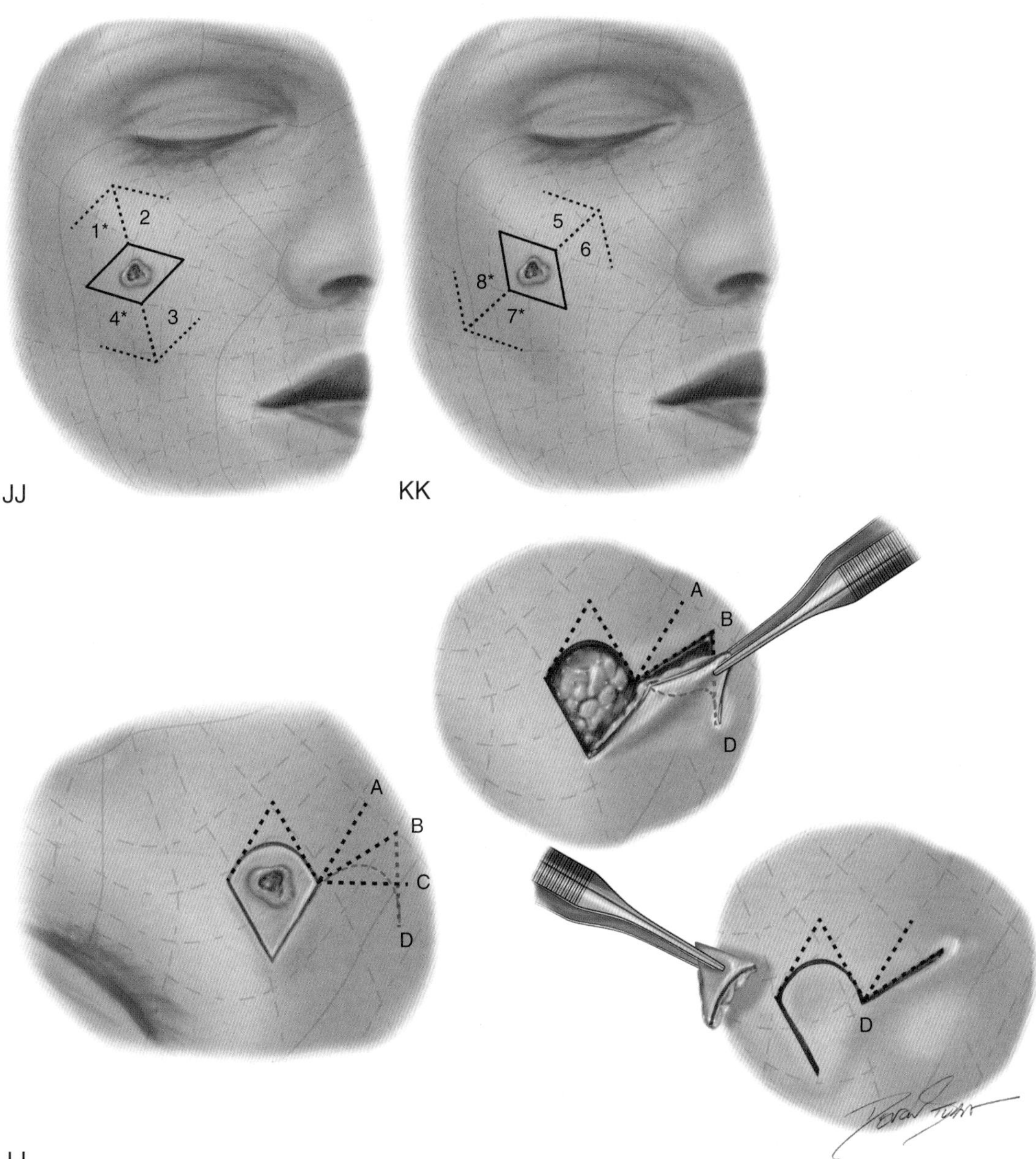

Figure 108.5, cont'd JJ, Rhomboid flaps are designed with two parallel lines in the LME. From these, parallelograms or rhomboids are designed. Out of the obtuse angles of the flaps, an umbrella is drawn, with sides equal to the sides of the rhomboid. The starred flaps show transposition option, which will not be hampered by fixed anatomy (e.g., a canthus) and will have a "short diagonal" (from the base of the flap to the tip) in the direction of the LME or mobile tissue. In this case, flaps #1 and #4 would be acceptable. **KK,** This second option produces four more flaps. Here, flaps #7 and #8 would be acceptable. **LL,** Newer modifications of classic flaps remove less tissue and move easier. (Courtesy of Tamborini F, Cherubino M, Scamoni S, Frigo C, Valdatta L. A modified rhomboid flap: the "diamond flap." *Dermatologic Surg*. 2012;38(11):1851–1855.)

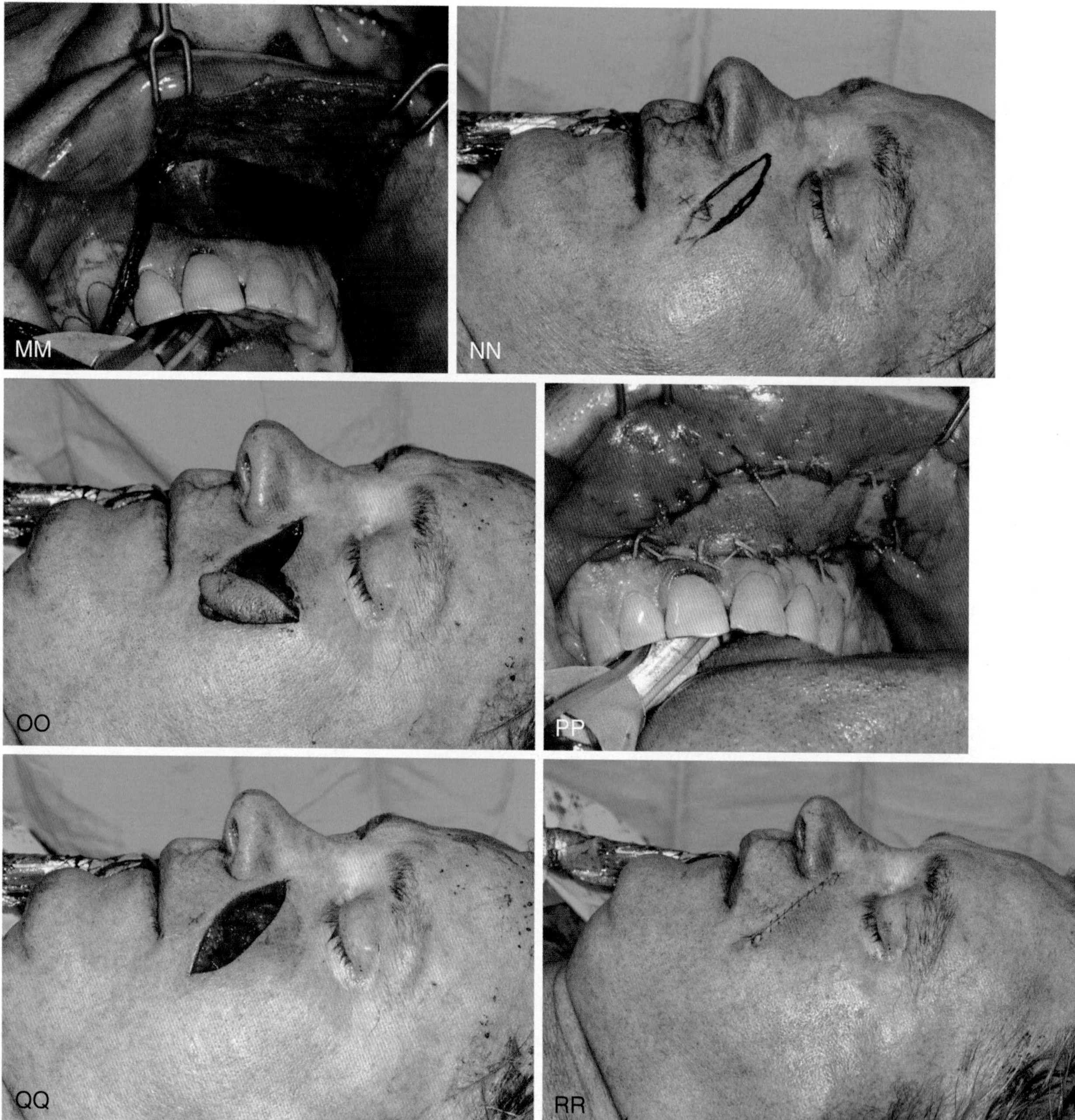

Figure 108.5, cont'd **MM,** Anterior maxillary defect that involved mucosa and part of the orbicularis oris. **NN,** Facial artery perforator flap was designed and marked according to the size of the defect centered on the perforator which was marked using Doppler identification. **OO,** The facial artery perforator flap was then raised completely on one visible facial artery perforator with a small cuff of surrounding fatty tissue to protect the small vessel from damage. **PP,** Flap was tunneled intraorally, rotated, and advanced medially. Inset of the flap was done with resorbable suture, and adequate coverage of anterior maxillary defect was obtained. **QQ,** Remaining left cheek defect produced after flap was tunneled intraorally. **RR,** Minor undermining of the subcutaneous layer along defect was performed and primary closure obtained with running nonresorbable suture.

BOX 108.5 Transposition Flap Pearls

Comments

1. The flap end does not have to be contiguous with the defect (only the base)
2. Blood supply is usually random

Concerns

1. The length of the flap shortens as the arc of pivotal movement increases
2. Propensity for development of trapdoor deformities (appearance of the flap is bulky like a pincushion)

TECHNIQUE: Basic Concepts in Local Flap Design—*cont'd*

INTERPOLATED FLAPS

The interpolated flap (e.g., the paramedian forehead flap, Abbe flap) is similar to the previously described transposition flap, but the flap base is not contiguous with the defect. The pedicle extends over a strip of intervening tissue. A secondary procedure will be required to divide and inset the pedicle and the flap (Fig. 108.5SS–FFF).

PARAMEDIAN FOREHEAD FLAP

The paramedian forehead flap is an ideal flap to reconstruct nasal defects greater than 1.5 cm. There is a similar color match to the recipient site and minimal donor site morbidity. The flap is axially based off the supratrochlear artery located approximately 17 to 24 mm lateral to the midline (Box 108.6).

Key Concepts for Paramedian Forehead Flaps

1. In nonsmokers with thick skin, the distal portion of the flap can be debulked of muscle and subcutaneous fat. A two-stage division and inset can then occur. To thin the skin to 2.5 mm over larger defects, a secondary intermediate procedure is advisable at 2 to 3 weeks.
2. A delay of 3 weeks is recommended prior to the separation of the pedicle to allow for adequate collateral blood supply to develop at the recipient site.
3. Flaps wider than 4.5 cm will be too wide to allow for complete closure of the secondary donor site.[30] In this case, secondary healing or skin expansion may be considered.

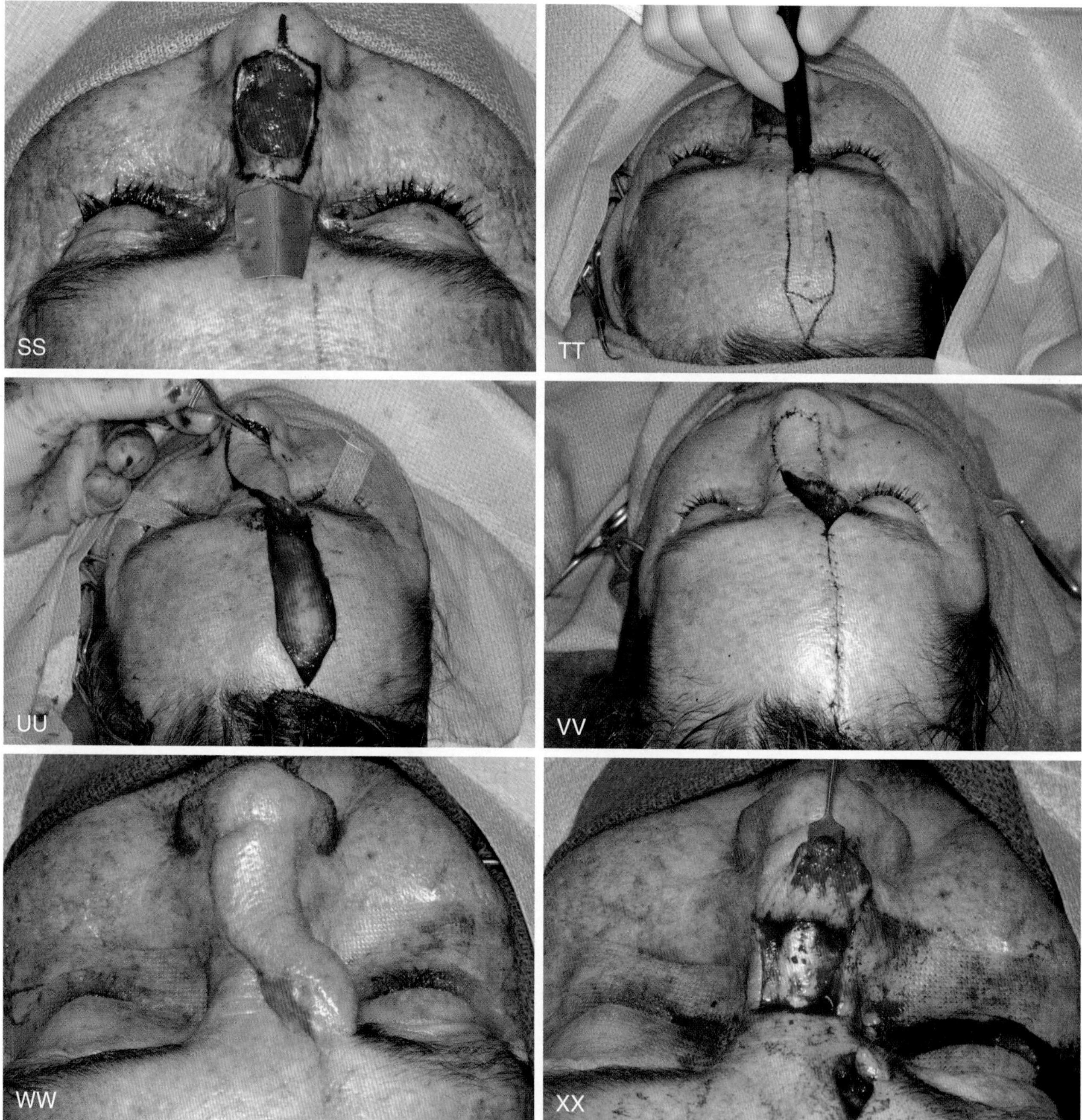

Figure 108.5, cont'd **SS,** Forehead flaps may be paramedian or median. Examples are shown. In all cases, a contoured template of the defect and the residual esthetic unit, or the contralateral unaffected nose, should be designed. The remainder of the topographic unit should be removed if more than two-thirds is involved. The flap should be ipsilateral to the defect if designed as a paramedian. **TT,** Paramedian forehead flap. Doppler may be used, but paramedian flaps will survive with a 12- to 13-mm base with the medial margin at the medial eyelid. The supratrochlear vessels are 17 to 22 mm from the midline. Since the flap can be extended more than 1 cm below the eyebrow, hair does not need to be included in the flap. Paramedian flaps, which will be thinned at the first surgery, should be mobilized without local anesthesia with epinephrine. **UU,** Paramedian flaps should be ipsilateral to the defect they cover. Donor defects of up to 4 cm may be closed by undermining the forehead subgaleally to the lateral eyebrow. **VV,** Paramedian flap in place. The exposed tissue will begin to round and tube but may be skin grafted. Simple wrapping with loose, nonadherent moist gauze is all that is necessary. **WW,** The paramedian flap is ready for thinning or division and inset. When indicated, cartilage may be placed under the flap at a primary or secondary thinning stage. **XX,** Division and inset at 3 weeks with thinning of residual flap.

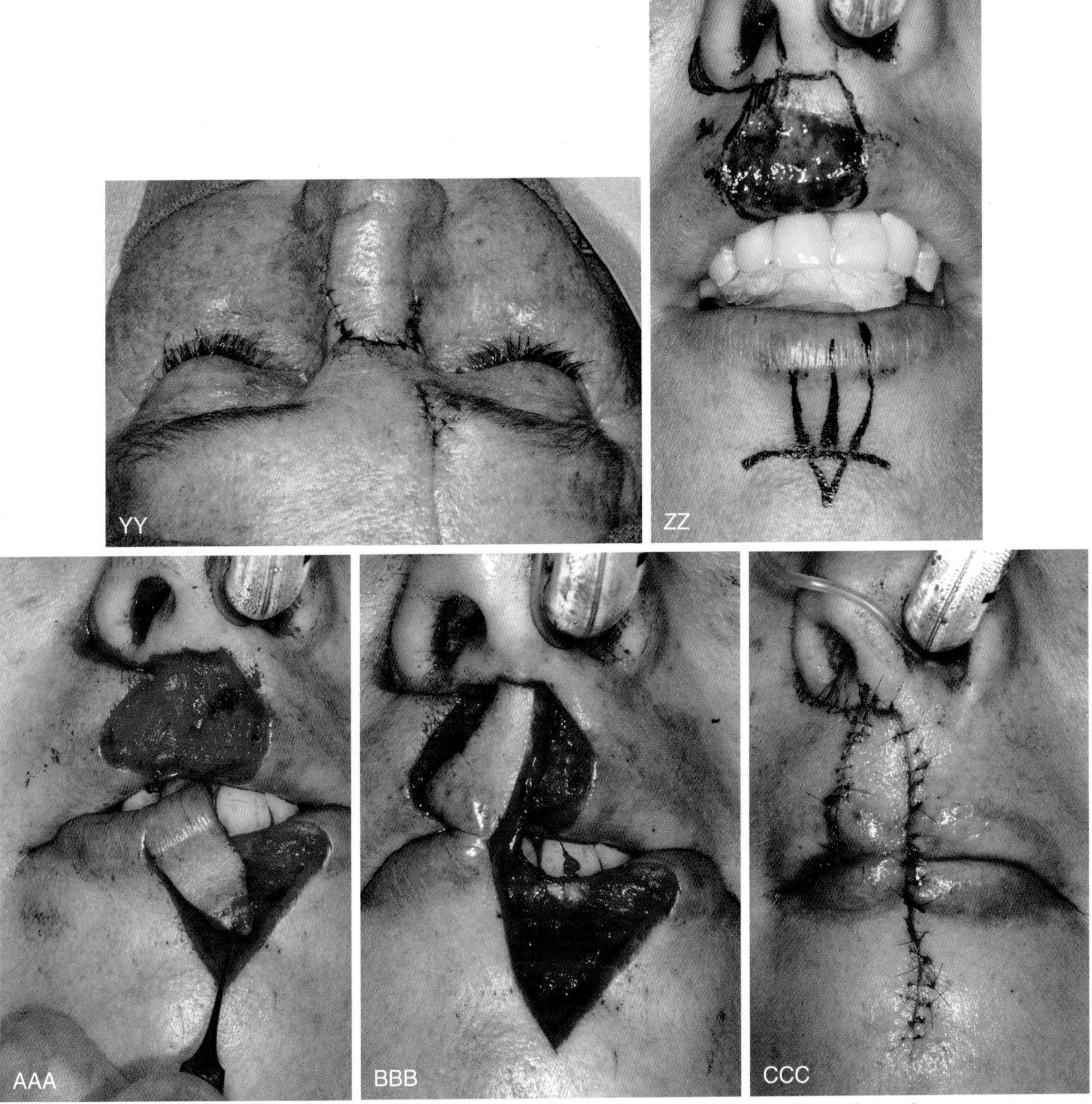

Figure 108.5, cont'd **YY,** After division and inset. **ZZ,** The lip Abbe flap may be designed to replace the entire defect (with extension into the nostril sill) or just the philtrum. In this case, the philtral area should be replaced. The vermilion cutaneous border has been tattooed with methylene blue in the upper and lower lips. In the lower lip donor site, when there is a significant concavity under the vermilion, a Z-plasty is optional to abrogate contracture. **AAA,** The Abbe flap is mobilized, leaving 12 to 13 mm of mucosa attached. The position of the labial vessel has been noted with the first cut through the lip. The edge of the Abbe flap should be de-epithelialized and pexed to the base of the nose or anterior nasal spine. The lateral advancement flap should move medially. **BBB,** The flap has been pexed into place, and the blue dots are ready for alignment. **CCC,** Abbe sutured into place.

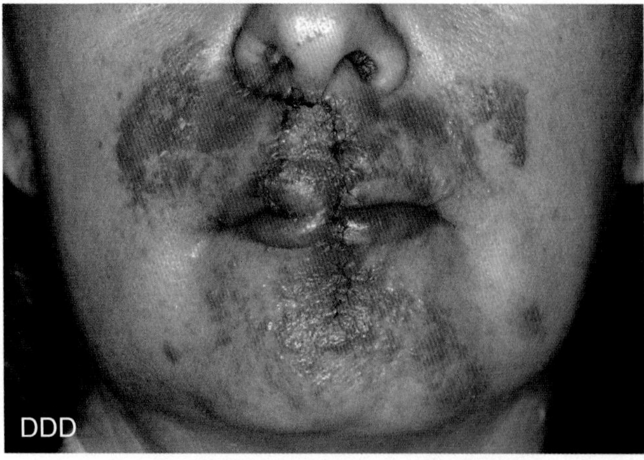

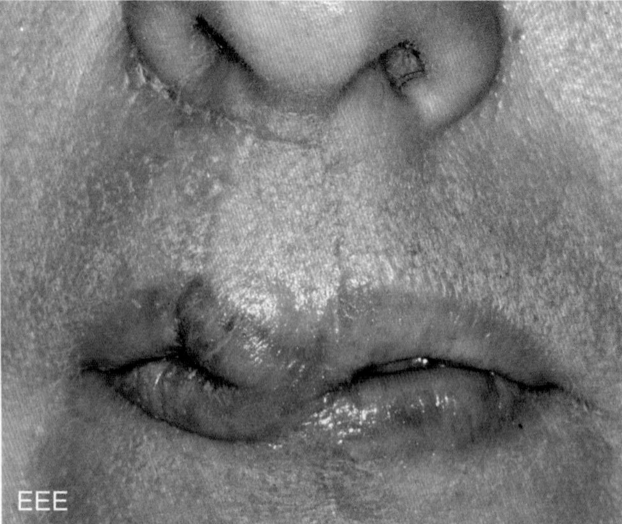

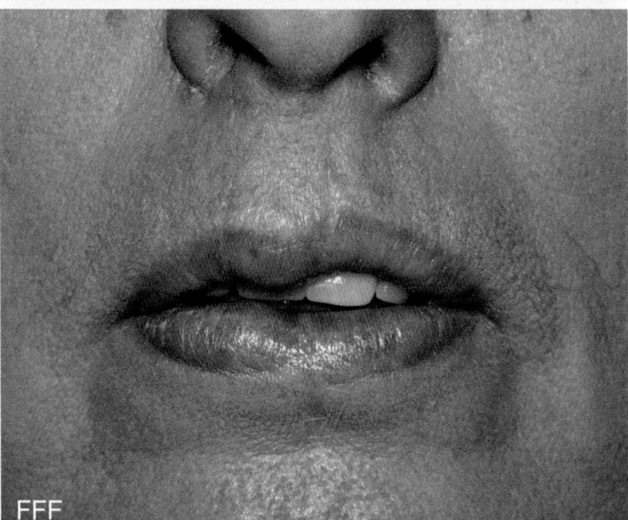

Figure 108.5, cont'd **DDD,** At 1 week, the antibiotic ointment produced an allergy. The patient stopped and applied over-the-counter hydrocortisone. **EEE,** At 3 weeks, division and inset occurred in the clinic under local anesthesia. There is never a need to wire teeth together, and diet restriction was textural only. **FFF,** When the tissue softens a few months after division and inset, minor revisions may be performed.

BOX 108.6 Paramedian Forehead Flap Pearls

Comments

1. Abundant blood supply (axial based)
2. Potential for two or three vertically oriented forehead flaps
3. Flap thinning at the end of the flap will not compromise blood supply; the supratrochlear artery runs superficial to the subcutaneous/subdermal tissue from a point approximately 1 cm superior to the level of the eyebrow[30]
4. Excellent skin match from the forehead to the nose

Concerns

1. A second surgery is required for separation of the pedicle at 3 weeks
2. Visible donor site scar[31,32]

Postoperative Complications

Preventing complications is especially true in facial reconstruction with local flaps because complications threaten not only the functional reconstruction but also the cosmetic appearance of the patient. A failed flap practically warrants another reconstruction attempt. The best suitable reconstructive modality usually is chosen and used at the first attempt.[4]

The most common complications include wound tension necrosis, hemorrhage, hematoma or seroma, and infection. Common causes of wound edge necrosis are ischemia from cigarette smoking (potentially prevented by cessation of smoking 2 days before and 2 weeks after)[4] and shortening of the flap base as a result of removal of a standing cone.[33]

A local flap may distort adjacent anatomy, especially in the perioral and periorbital regions. Local flaps for lip reconstruction have a lower rate of complications than other oral sub-sites; however, there are some potential complications associated like microstomia (5% to 25%), lip asymmetry (1% to 20%), paresthesia (15% to 20%), and oral competence (2% of cases).[3] Periorbital distortion produces scleral show or ectropion. With hair-bearing skin, there is a potential for abnormal hair distribution or direction. For example, non-hair-bearing skin of the cheek, ideally, should not be moved into the lip of a hirsute male. Either hair transplantation or laser removal of hair may correct some of these outcomes.

Pincushioning or trapdoor deformities can occur after local tissue transfer. Etiologies include lack of peripheral undermining to compensate for flap retraction, lymphatic obstruction, excessive subcutaneous tissue in the flap, asymmetric tissue contracture during scarring, and too small a flap. Options to mitigate these adverse effects include dermabrasion, flap revision or debulking, and intralesional corticosteroid injections.[33]

References

1. Kayser M. Surgical flaps. *Sel Read Plast Surg.* 1999;9(2).
2. Rabbani CC, Hwang MS, Byrne PJ, Desai SC. Management of large facial defects. *Facial Plast Surg.* 2020;36(2):148–157.
3. Comini LV, Spinelli G, Mannelli G. Algorithm for the treatment of oral and peri-oral defects through local flaps. *J Craniomaxillofac Surg.* 2018;46(12):2127–2137.
4. Vural E, Key JM. Complications, salvage, and enhancement of local flaps in facial reconstruction. *Otolaryngol Clin North Am.* 2001;34(4):739–751,vi.
5. Obermeier K, Smolka W. Comparison of aesthetic outcome of different facial reconstruction techniques after resection of cutaneous squamous cell carcinoma. *J Craniomaxillofac Surg.* 2020;48(1):117–121.
6. Patel KG, Sykes JM. Concepts in local flap design and classification. *Oper Tech Otolaryngol Head Neck Surg.* 2011;22(1):13–23.
7. Goding G, Hom D. Skin flap physiology. In: Baker SR, ed. *Local Flaps in Facial Reconstruction.* 3rd ed. Philadelphia, PA: Elsevier Saunders; 2017:14–29.
8. Zide MF, Yan T. Head and neck skin cancer. In: Miloro M, Ghali GE, Larsen PE, Waite PD, eds. *Peterson's Principles of Oral and Maxillofacial Surgery.* 3rd ed. Shelton, CT: People's Medical Publishing House-USA; 2011:743–771.
9. Baker SR. Flap classification and design. In: Baker SR, ed. *Local Flaps in Facial Reconstruction.* 3rd ed. Philadelphia, PA: Elsevier Saunders; 2017:71–107.
10. Taylor GI, Corlett RJ, Dhar SC, Ashton MW. The anatomical (angiosome) and clinical territories of cutaneous perforating arteries: development of the concept and designing safe flaps. *Plast Reconstr Surg.* 2011;127(4):1447–1459.
11. Saint-Cyr M, Wong C, Schaverien M, Mojallal A, Rohrich RJ. The perforasome theory: vascular anatomy and clinical implications. *Plast Reconstr Surg.* 2009;124(5):1529–1544.
12. Zoumalan RA, Murakami CS. Facial flap complications. *Facial Plast Surg.* 2012;28(3):347–353.
13. Dzubow LM. Advancement flaps. In: Dzubow LM, ed. *Facial Flaps: Biomechanics and Regional Application.* East Norwalk, CT: Appleton & Lange; 1990:166.
14. Krishnan R, Garman M, Nunez-Gussman J, Orengo I. Advancement flaps: a basic theme with many variations. *Dermatol Surg.* 2005;31(8 Pt 2):986–994.
15. Sugg KB, Cederna PS, Brown DL. The V-Y advancement flap is equivalent to the Mustardé flap for ectropion prevention in the reconstruction of moderate-size lid-cheek junction defects. *Plast Reconstr Surg.* 2013;131(1):28e–36e.
16. Salmon PJM, Klaassen MF. The rotating island pedicle flap: an aesthetic and functional improvement on the subcutaneous island pedicle flap. *Dermatol Surg.* 2004;30(9):1223–1228.
17. Braun M Jr, Cook J. The island pedicle flap. *Dermatol Surg.* 2005;31(8 Pt 2):995–1005.
18. Yoo SS, Miller SJ. The crescentic advancement flap revisited. *Dermatol Surg.* 2003;29(8):856–858.
19. Schnabl SM, Breuninger H, Iordanou E, et al. Patient satisfaction in 1,827 patients following various methods of facial reconstruction based on age, defect size and site. *J Dtsch Dermatol Ges.* 2018;16(4):426–433.
20. Harahap M. The modified bilateral advancement flap. *Dermatol Surg.* 2001;27(5):463–466.
21. Baker SR. Rotation flaps. In: Baker SR, ed. *Local Flaps in Facial Reconstruction.* 3rd ed. Philadelphia, PA: Elsevier Saunders; 2017:108–130.
22. Throckmorton GS, Williams FC, Potter JK, Finn R. The geometry of skin flap rotation. *J Oral Maxillofac Surg.* 2010;68(10):2545–2548.
23. Dzubow LM. Facial flaps biomechanics and regional application. In: Dzubow LM, ed. *Facial Flaps: Biomechanics and Regional Application.* East Norwalk, CT: Appleton & Lange; 1990:166.
24. Goldman GD. Rotation flaps. *Dermatol Surg.* 2005;31(8 Pt 2):1006–1013.
25. Zide MF, Topper D. Pivot point and secondary defect problems with rotation flaps. *J Oral Maxillofac Surg.* 2004;62(9):1069–1075.
26. Ahuja RB. Geometric considerations in the design of rotation flaps in the scalp and forehead region. *Plast Reconstr Surg.* 1988;81(6):900–906.
27. Ahuja RB. Mechanics of movement for rotation flaps and a local flap template. *Plast Reconstr Surg.* 1989;83(4):733–737.
28. Chasmar LR. The versatile rhomboid (Limberg) flap. *Can J Plast Surg.* 2007;15(2):67–71.
29. Tamborini F, Cherubino M, Scamoni S, Frigo C, Valdatta L. A modified rhomboid flap: the "diamond flap." *Dermatol Surg.* 2012;38(11):1851–1855.
30. Baker SR. Interpolated paramedian forehead flaps. In: Baker SR, ed. *Local Flaps in Facial Reconstruction.* 3rd ed. Philadelphia, PA: Elsevier Saunders; 2017:108–130.
31. Kishi K, Imanishi N, Shimizu Y, Shimizu R, Okabe K, Nakajima H. Alternative 1-step nasal reconstruction technique. *Arch Facial Plast Surg.* 2012;14(2):116–121.
32. Schreiber NTN, Mobley SR. Elegant solutions for complex paramedian forehead flap reconstruction. *Facial Plast Surg Clin North Am.* 2011;19(3):465–479.
33. Chu EA, Byrne PJ. Local flaps I: bilobed, rhombic, and cervicofacial. *Facial Plast Surg Clin North Am.* 2009;17(3):349–360.

CHAPTER 109

Panendoscopy

Michael R. Markiewicz and Tuan G. Bui

Armamentarium

Intubation tray (if using local anesthesia)
10-mL Syringe
Bag-valve ventilator with mask
Endotracheal tube (7-0 and 8-0)
Laryngoscope (with Macintosh and Miller blades)
Local anesthetic with vasoconstrictor
Lubrication (xylocaine jelly)
Oropharyngeal airway
Stethoscope
Stylet
Tape
Yankauer suction
Tracheostomy tray (for difficult airways)
#15 Blade
Adson forceps with teeth
Appropriate sutures
Army/navy retractors
Cricoid hook
Crilc forceps
Cuffed Shiley tracheostomy tube
Curved Mayo scissors
Electrocautery
Hemostatic clips
Trach collar
Tracheal dilator
Uncuffed Shiley tracheostomy tube
Direct laryngoscopy (Figs. 109.1 and 109.2)
45-cm Hopkins rod telescope
Anesthesia circuit adapter
Cotton pledget (if using local anesthesia)
Cup forceps (for biopsy)
Light source
Macintosh laryngoscope
Rigid bronchoscope
Rigid laryngoscope
Suction
Tetracaine or benzocaine spray (if using local anesthesia)
Tooth protector
Rigid Bronchoscopy
Forceps
Hopkins lens rigid telescope
Light source
Suction
Video equipment
Flexible Bronchoscopy (Fig. 109.3)
2.7-mm Flexible bronchoscope (2.0-, 3.5-, 4.0-mm endotracheal tubes)
3.5-mm Flexible bronchoscope (4.5-, 5.0-, 5.5-endotracheal tubes)
Antifog solution
Biopsy forceps
Silicone lubricant
Swivel adapter (Bodi connector)
Esophagoscopy (Fig. 109.4)
2% Viscous lidocaine
Air/water supplier
Biopsy forceps
Defogging agent
Flexible alligator forceps
Hopkins telescope
Light carriers
Light source
Metal suction
Neo-Synephrine
Round or oval esophagoscope
System monitors

History of the Procedure

Using a wax candle as a light source, in 1806, Bozzini used a combination of an angled speculum with a mirror insert to examine multiple cavities of the body, including the larynx.[1] In 1829, Babbington reported on the use of the glottiscope, a three-blade device consisting of a stainless steel mirror and tongue retractors.[1] In 1853, the "father of endoscopy," Desmoreaux, improved upon Bozzini's endoscope by attaching a gaslight and condenser to project a beam of light down the tube.

Around this time, Garcia developed a separate device consisting of a dental mirror, a hand mirror, and sunlight to visualize his own pharynx. Turck, Czermak, and then MacKenzie were all credited for refining techniques in endoscopy. Killian developed an apparatus for suspending the laryngoscope using a headlight.[2] In 1897, he used a rigid endoscope to examine the airways and reported the first incidence of removing a foreign body from the bronchial tree without performing tracheostomy.[3] Chevalier Jackson made major refinements to endoscopy in the early 1900s by inventing distal lighting for endoscopic equipment, developing a variety of endoscopic instruments and, along with Brunings of Germany, advocating the use of magnification in endoscopy.[4] The Zeiss operating microscope, developed in the 1950s along with laryngoscope development by Jako, led to increased quality of binocular magnification.[1]

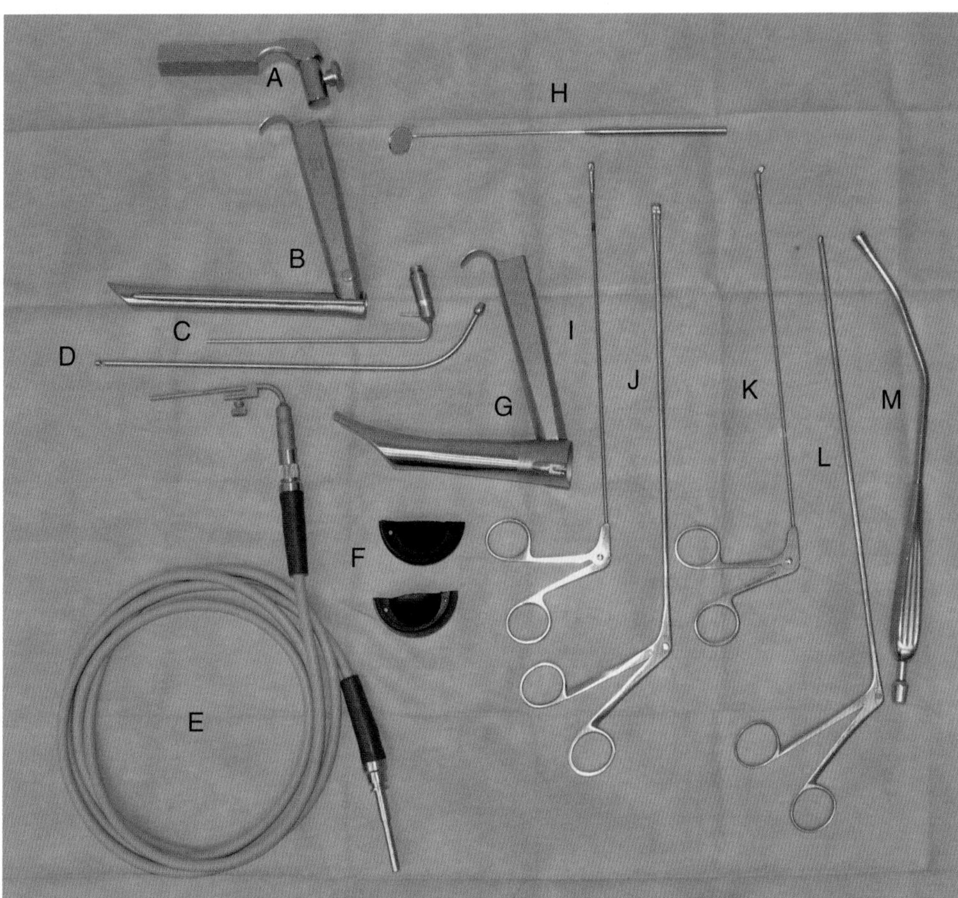

Figure 109.1 Direct laryngoscopy setup. **A,** Laryngoscope handle. **B,** Holinger anterior commissure laryngoscope. **C,** Fiberoptic light carrier. **D,** Jackson Velvet Eye aspirating suction. **E,** Fiberoptic light carrier and cord. **F,** Tooth guards. **G,** Lindholm operating laryngoscope. **H,** Laryngeal mirror. **I,** Small Jackson laryngeal forceps. **J,** Straight spoon forceps. **K,** Curved spoon forceps. **L,** Large Jackson laryngeal forceps. **M,** Yankauer suction.

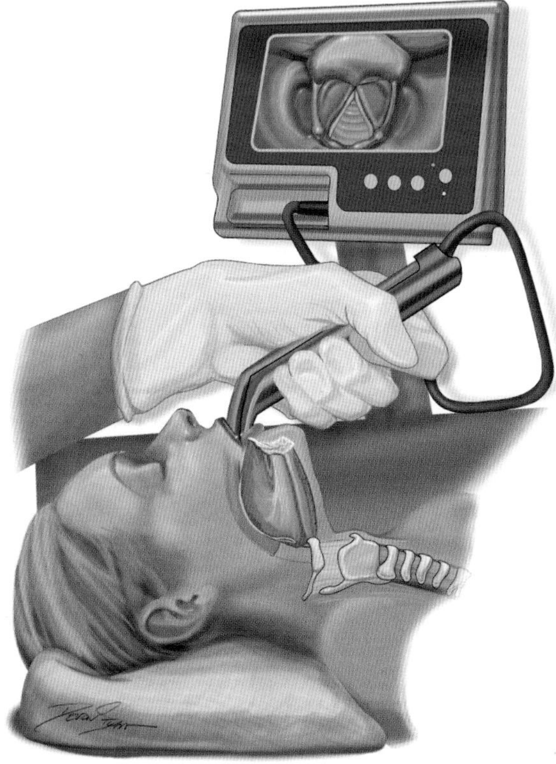

Figure 109.2 Use of the GlideScope in the airway.

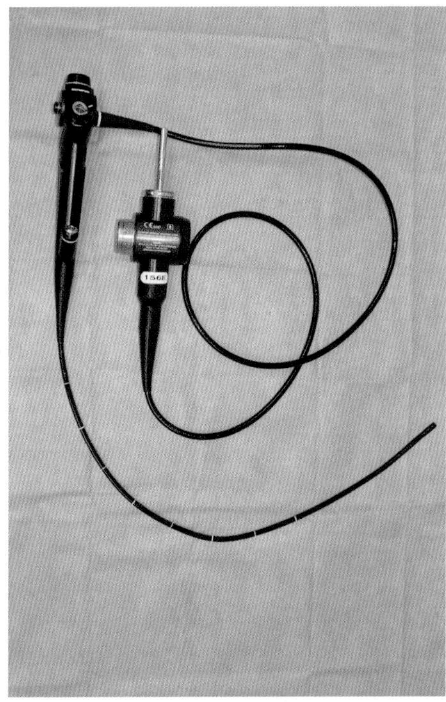

Figure 109.3 Flexible bronchoscope with side suction port and light source.

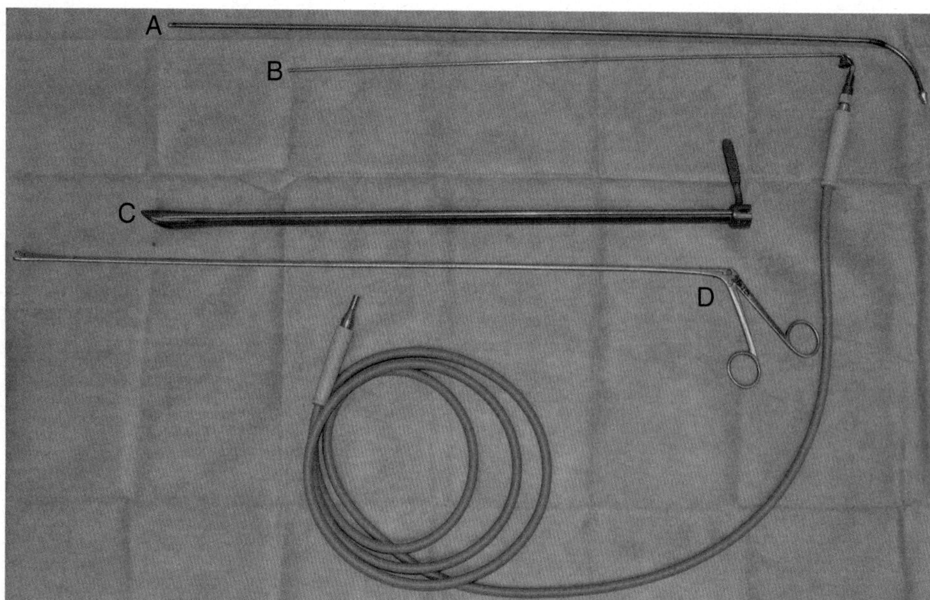

Figure 109.4 Esophagoscopy setup. **A,** Long suction. **B,** Light source. **C,** Esophagoscope. **D,** Alligator forceps.

Interestingly, optimal patient positioning in endoscopy was actually derived from physicians' work with sword swallowers. Desmoreaux, after assessing the technique of sword swallowers, was able to look into the stomach using a 47-cm tube; this technique, however, was never published.[5] Leiter, an instrument maker, in collaboration with Kussmaul and Johann von Mikulicz-Radecki, fabricated a light source for straight tube esophagoscopy. As von Mikulicz described it in his 1881 publication, *Zur Technik der Gastroskopie und Oesophagoskopie*, the two crucial moments during sword swallowing occur during passage of the sword through the upper and lower esophageal sphincters. Sword swallowers cannot change position (as is the case for patients undergoing esophagoscopy) and therefore must optimize the position of the proximal esophagus by displacing the lower jaw, hyoid bone, and tongue base anteriorly.[5]

The flexible fiberoptic bronchoscope was introduced by Shigeto Ikeda in the 1960s.[2] At approximately the same time, Hopkins developed a rod lens telescope that modified the ridged endoscope by adding angled and wide-angled lens.[6] More modern endoscopic instruments are able to capture pictures and video.

Indications for the Use of the Procedure

Panendoscopy for head and neck surgery, which includes direct laryngoscopy, esophagoscopy, and bronchoscopy, was classically considered an essential part of the workup for malignancies of the head and neck region.[7–10] The theory behind panendoscopy in the initial evaluation or follow-up for malignancies of the head and neck is that if a patient develops malignancy in those regions, they are at increased risk for lesions of other areas of the aerodigestive tract.[11,12] Lesions that are identified as a second malignancy, are distinct and geographically separated by normal nonneoplastic mucosa, and are not of metastatic origin are defined as synchronous tumors. These lesions must be identified at the time of initial tumor evaluation. Lesions discovered at some point in the future, after discovery of the primary lesion, are defined as metachronous tumors. The reported rate of synchronous cancers varies from 1.5% to 18%.[11,13,14] Although panendoscopy has been the gold standard,[10] some have questioned its economic and therapeutic effectiveness compared with contemporary techniques such as standard computed tomography (CT)[15–18] and 18F-fluoro-2-deoxy-d-glucose positron emission tomography/computed tomography (F-FDG PET/CT).[9–11,15,17,18] Davidson et al.[11] reported that the rate of synchronous tumors found in patients undergoing direct laryngoscopy, bronchoscopy, and esophagoscopy was 2.6% for pulmonary lesions, 1.3% for head and neck mucosal lesions, and 0% for esophageal lesions. Newer technologies, such as virtual three-dimensional F-FDG PET/CT[18], have been reported as an alternative to bronchoscopy for evaluating pharyngeal and laryngeal malignancies.[19] In a study comparing panendoscopy with ^{18}F-FDG PET/CT, the prevalence of tumors detected was 4.5% by panendoscopy versus 6.1% by ^{18}F-FDG PET/CT. However, given the lower specificity and the cost of ^{18}F-FDG PET/CT, panendoscopy is endorsed by many as a reliable method of investigation for secondary primary tumors and for follow-up screening.

Attempts at direct laryngoscopy should be made to obtain a general sense of the aerodigestive tract. If available, preoperative imaging should be reviewed to examine the precise location of any radiographically appreciable lesions. Consent for tracheostomy should be considered in patients with a tenuous airway. Although it may be performed under local anesthesia, endoscopy is usually performed under general anesthesia. Chevalier Jackson noted "Endoscopic ability cannot be bought with the instruments. As with all mechanical procedures, facility can be obtained only by educating the eye and the fingers in repeated exercise of a particular series of maneuvers. As with learning to play a musical instrument, a fundamental knowledge of technique, positions, and landmarks is necessary, after which only continued manual practice makes for proficiency."[4] Panendoscopy should be methodical, effective, and efficient, and all three skills are brought about by repetition.

Direct Laryngoscopy

In the patient with head and neck tumors, direct laryngoscopy may be used to identify and biopsy lesions of the pharynx and larynx. Suspicion of malignancy combined with symptoms such as chronic hoarseness, dyspnea, dysarthria, globus sensation, chronic dysphagia, pharyngitis, odynophagia, odynophonia, chronic choking episodes, chronic cough, and voice changes should be further investigated with direct laryngoscopy. (Other uses for direct laryngoscopy, such as drainage or removal of laryngeal scars, strictures, synechiae, or webs; procedures on the vocal cords; and exploration in patients with neurologic disease, are not discussed here.) Limited laryngoscopy can be performed in the office. For more accurate visualization of the airway and biopsy, the examination should be performed under general anesthesia in the operating room.

In the office, laryngoscopy can be performed using a 70- or 90-degree rigid telescope. Patient positioning is similar to that for indirect mirror laryngoscopy. However, this technique limits the speech sounds that can be elicited, especially in children. The stroboscope, initially developed by Oertel in 1878,[20] emits rapid pulses of light at a preset rate. This rate is usually synchronized with the vocal frequency of the patient during phonation. The stroboscope is usually used along with a rigid or fiberoptic endoscope and video recording device and a microphone, which is placed over the lateral neck to measure the acoustics of the patient's voice. The frequency of the light pulse is compared with the patient's vocal frequency; when they are synchronized, the image appears static. Deviations from this and changes in the true vocal cord vibratory pattern may reveal vocal cord pathology that could not otherwise be visualized. Another examination performed by speech pathologists is fiberoptic endoscopic evaluation of swallowing. This may be used along with videofluoroscopic examination for patients with dysphagia or aspiration.[21]

Bronchoscopy

In the patient with head and neck cancer, bronchoscopy is most commonly used for staging of malignancy and follow-up. Bronchoscopy can also be therapeutic, as in the case of obstruction by retained secretions (the details of this are not discussed here). The literature suggests an additional yield of bronchoscopy over chest radiography of less than 1% in identifying synchronous tumors.[7,22] However, the role of bronchoscopy in the presence of a normal thoracic CT scan has been questioned.[23,24] Bronchoscopes are either rigid or flexible. In general, the large, open lumen of a rigid bronchoscope is useful for retrieving foreign bodies or for performing therapeutic maneuvers such as electrocautery. Flexible bronchoscopes contain a fiberoptic lighting and viewing system that can display images on an attached eyepiece or external monitor. Flexible bronchoscopy also offers the advantage of digital photography. Fiberoptic bronchoscopes can be inserted farther toward the periphery of the bronchial tree than can rigid bronchoscopes, especially in the upper lobes. Davidson et al.[11] found no difference in the ability to find synchronous lesions between patients undergoing rigid bronchoscopy and those undergoing flexible bronchoscopy.[11]

Esophagoscopy

Indications for esophagoscopy include a history of organic disease of the esophagus, to assess caustic ingestion when a foreign body of the esophagus is suspected, when clinical or radiographic examination indicates esophageal disease, or in patients with squamous cell carcinoma of the hypopharynx.[11,25,26] The role of esophagoscopy in the head and neck cancer workup is controversial, with a less than 2% additional reported yield of finding synchronous tumors over barium swallow.[25,26]

For patients being evaluated for head and neck cancer, flexible esophagoscopy is routinely performed during percutaneous endoscopic gastrostomy tube placement and allows the surgeon to take digital photographs of any pathology that might be encountered. Imaging studies can guide the surgeon to any areas of concern. Esophagoscopy is usually performed under general anesthesia and may be carried out with either rigid or flexible instruments. Rigid esophagoscopy must be performed under general anesthesia; however, flexible esophagoscopy can be performed under sedation. The use of general anesthesia lessens the chance of trauma to the upper teeth and perforation of the esophagus and minimizes muscular resistance to passage of the endoscope. Rigid esophagoscopy is optimal for evaluation, biopsy, and management of the pharyngoesophageal segment and, like rigid bronchoscopy, can be performed with standard operating room instrumentation. Flexible endoscopy usually requires coordination with the endoscopy team.

Limitations and Contraindications

Contraindications to any element of panendoscopy include any local or systemic disease that limits the use of local or general anesthesia. A relative contraindication to direct laryngoscopy includes any condition that would result in either airway deterioration or crisis. Such patients should undergo awake tracheostomy, or the surgeon should be prepared to intervene to create a surgical airway. Other contraindications to direct laryngoscopy include patients with cervical spinal injury or stiff necks and patients with extremely obese necks. Severe retrognathia is considered a relative contraindication to laryngoscopy. Contraindications to bronchoscopy include a borderline pulmonary status, cachexia, and severe spondylosis or spondylarthrosis of the cervical or thoracic spine. Rigid esophagoscopy is relatively contraindicated in patients with deformities of the cervical and thoracic spine and those with maxillofacial or dental anatomy that limits passage of a rigid scope. In such cases, flexible scopes can be used. Additionally, fiberoptic bronchoscopy is contraindicated in patients with unstable arrhythmias, hemodynamic instability, increased intracranial pressure, severe hypoxia, hypercapnia, systemic coagulopathy, or thrombocytopenia.[27] Other factors include vasopressor use, a mean arterial pressure less than 65 mm Hg, positive end-expiratory pressure greater than or equal to 15 cm H_2O, and a partial pressure of arterial oxygen (PaO_2) of 70 mm Hg despite a fraction of inspired oxygen (FIO_2) greater than 70%.[28]

TECHNIQUE: Direct Laryngoscopy (Direct Laryngoscopy With Rigid Laryngoscope)

STEP 1: Anesthesia and Preparation

Local anesthesia is not required for direct laryngoscopy. However, a local anesthetic may be used and may be either sprayed into the pharynx or injected through the skin adjacent to the greater horn of the thyroid cartilage to block the superior laryngeal nerves. Alternatively, cotton pledgets soaked in cocaine solution may be placed in the piriform sinus to anesthetize the superior laryngeal nerve distribution.[29,30] The use of atropine or other antisialagogues is often helpful in limiting secretions.

STEP 2: Positioning

The endoscopist should be comfortably positioned at the head of the patient so that instruments can be passed over the right shoulder. The table should include a joint (Mayfield head holder) so that the patient's neck position can be adjusted. Before inserting the scope, the surgeon should digitally palpate the floor of the mouth, anterior tongue, retromolar trigone, buccal vestibule, soft palate, tonsils, vallecula, base of the tongue, pre-epiglottic space, palatoglossal folds, and piriform sinus. Although general anesthesia is preferred, forced inhalation of anesthetic gases and jet ventilation may also be used. Supraglottic jet ventilation still exposes the surgeon to anesthetics and aerosols from the airway, although to a lesser extent than insufflation techniques. Pharmacologic neuromuscular blockade is generally helpful. The assistant should guide the distal tip of instruments to the proximal opening of the laryngoscope. The patient is placed in a supine "sniffing position" or Boyce-Jackson position, which includes extension at the atlanto-occipital joint and flexion at the neck. This facilitates examination of the oropharynx and hypopharynx. A variety of laryngoscopes can be used, including those with an open or a side slit, scopes for suspension and those that view the anterior commissure. Side laryngoscopes can be used to deliver oxygen and anesthetic to the hypopharynx. The patient should be in a deep plane of anesthesia to prevent laryngospasm. A cuffed endotracheal tube is preferred to prevent contamination of the infraglottic airway with blood. Throughout direct laryngoscopy, a gentle touch should be used so as not to crush the tongue on the lower incisors or cause trauma to the larynx. When an anterior and superior vector of force is applied, the tongue base should be lifted, not pried, and the surgeon should be careful not to apply pressure to the anterior maxillary teeth (Fig. 109.5A).

STEP 3: Introduction of the Endoscope

The head position is based on the patient's anatomy. If the head of the operating table is adjustable, a shoulder roll is not required. While the neck is kept flexed, the atlanto-occipital joint is flexed by raising the head of the table to obtain a view of the anterior larynx. The hypopharynx and cervical esophagus can be examined best with the atlanto-occipital joint and neck extended. A plastic tooth guard is placed on the anterior maxillary teeth to prevent damage. While grasping the scope with the left hand, the surgeon uses the right hand to "scissor" open the mouth by placing the thumb on the mandibular incisors and index finger on the maxillary incisors and spreading.

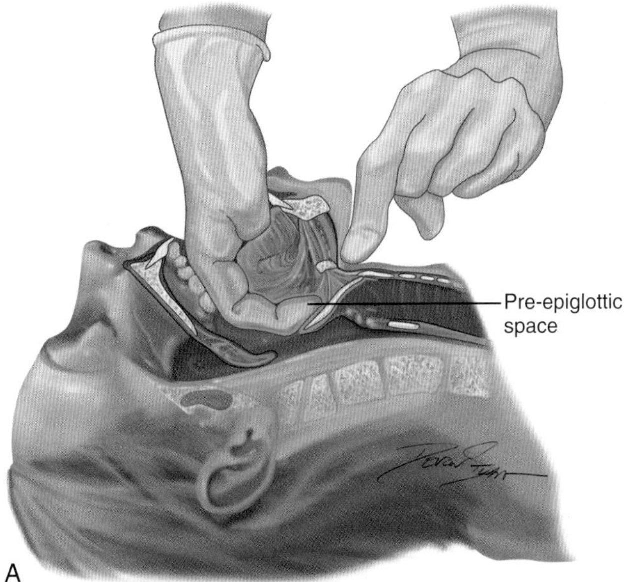

Figure 109.5 A, Before initiating direct laryngoscopy, bimanual palpation is performed on the floor of the mouth, anterior tongue, retromolar trigone, buccal vestibule, soft palate, tonsils, vallecula, base of the tongue, pre-epiglottic space, and palatoglossal folds. The anterior larynx is best evaluated by maintaining the neck and atlanto-occipital joint in a flexed position. The hypopharynx and cervical esophagus are best viewed with the atlanto-occipital joint and neck extended.

TECHNIQUE: Direct Laryngoscopy (Direct Laryngoscopy With Rigid Laryngoscope)—*cont'd*

STEP 4: Laryngoscopy

As the laryngoscope is advanced, the larynx comes into view. The tip of the laryngoscope is first placed into the vallecula, and the lingual tonsils, glossotonsillar sulci, right and left sides of the vallecula, and the epiglottic petiole are examined, as is the lingual surface of the epiglottis. Exposure of the larynx is performed by elevation of the epiglottis and its tissues attached to the hyoid bone. The surgeon then inserts the scope to the right of the tongue, thereby displacing it to the left. The larynx is then examined. With the glottis in view, the laryngeal surface of the epiglottis is seen and each aryepiglottic fold is inspected. If the anterior commissure of the vocal cords is not visualized, external digital pressure on the thyroid cartilage can improve visualization. The laryngoscope is advanced to view the anterior commissure of the glottis. Use of a small endotracheal tube facilitates this examination. If needed, brief removal and replacement of the endotracheal tube can facilitate evaluation of lesions of the edges of the true vocal cords. The tip of the laryngoscope is then positioned into the anterosuperior aspect of the right piriform recess, where it is lifted slightly to open the right piriform recess, allowing full inspection. Examination of the left piriform recess requires repositioning of the scope such that the tongue is deviated to the right. The false vocal cords are examined on either side, and although the laryngeal ventricle cannot be directly seen on direct laryngoscopy, tumors arising from this small area often can be identified. The tip of the laryngoscope is then placed beneath the endotracheal tube so as to lift the tube anteriorly. This allows inspection of the posterior commissure and arytenoids. The surgeon should note any interarytenoid fixation; to determine this, the arytenoids can be palpated with a long, slender instrument, such as the laryngeal suction tip. The lifting motion on the endotracheal tube also opens the esophageal introitus such that the postcricoid region can be viewed. In children, a posterior laryngeal cleft should be ruled out (Fig. 109.5B).

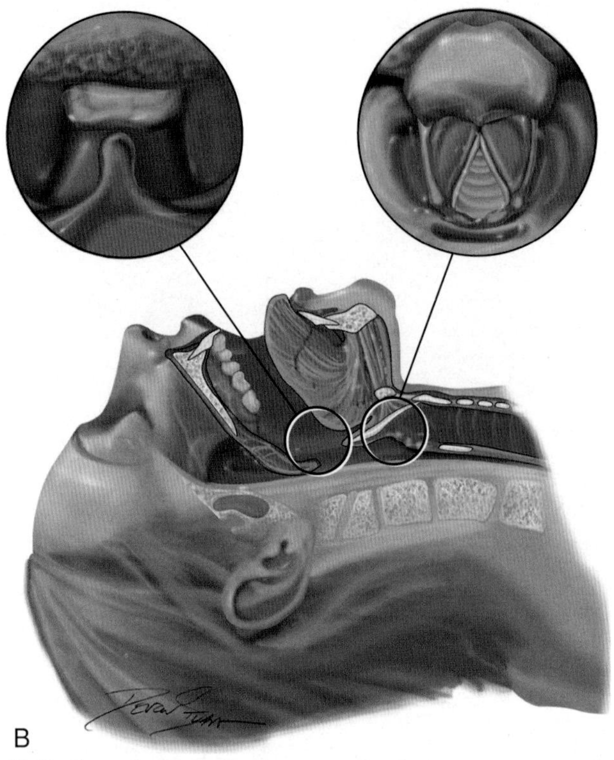

Figure 109.5, cont'd **B,** Once the larynx has been visualized, the examination of the larynx should note the appearance of the piriform sinus, interarytenoid space, false versus true vocal folds, aryepiglottic fold, vallecula, and epiglottic petiole.

ALTERNATIVE TECHNIQUE 1: Flexible Fiberoptic Nasopharyngoscopy/Laryngopharyngoscopy (Nasoendoscopy)

A mixture of topical anesthetic (e.g., benzocaine) and a decongestant (e.g., oxymetazoline) is sprayed twice into each naris, along the floor of the nose, so that it drips down into the posterior pharynx. When a typical nasopharyngoscope is inserted, the endoscopist's left hand rests lightly on the patient's nasal dorsum and the right thumb operates the angulation lever. The head of the scope is held between the third and fifth digits and the thenar eminence of the right hand. If a scope with a suction portal is used (e.g., a pediatric bronchoscope), the right index finger can control the suction. With the patient sitting upright or supine, three maneuvers may be used to guide the scope into the intended direction: (1) rolling the scope between the thumb and finger of the left hand, placing a C-loop in the scope to allow easy rotation of the scope; (2) advancing the scope by walking the scope between the thumb and finger with a finger rest on the nose; and (3) controlling the tip of the scope with flexion and extension.

The endoscope is then advanced through the nose just below the middle turbinate because the inferior meatus is generally too narrow to allow easy passage of the scope. The examination begins at the choana. To turn the corner from the nose to the nasopharynx, a slight inferior bend of the scope may aid its advancement. The pharynx may collapse upon entering. To improve visualization, the neck may be extended or the patient can protrude the tongue. The choana, eustachian tube orifice, fossa of Rosenmüller, and torus tubarius are examined bilaterally. The Passavant ridge and the adenoid pad should also be examined. Soft palate closure can be evaluated by having the patient say "cake." Any asymmetries should be noted because lesions of the nasopharynx are often submucosal.

Once the pharynx has been visualized, the base of the tongue, vallecula, glossoepiglottic fold, superior hypopharynx, posterior pharyngeal wall, epiglottis, aryepiglottic folds, arytenoids, false vocal folds, immediate subglottis, and true vocal folds are evaluated. The operator may ask the patient to protrude the tongue to visualize the vallecula and lingual surface of the epiglottis, turn the head to the right and left to visualize the contralateral piriform sinus, and insufflate the cheeks to open up the pharynx and hypopharynx. The glottis can be visualized during inspiration, or the true vocal folds and glottic closure can be visualized by phonating (Fig. 109.6).

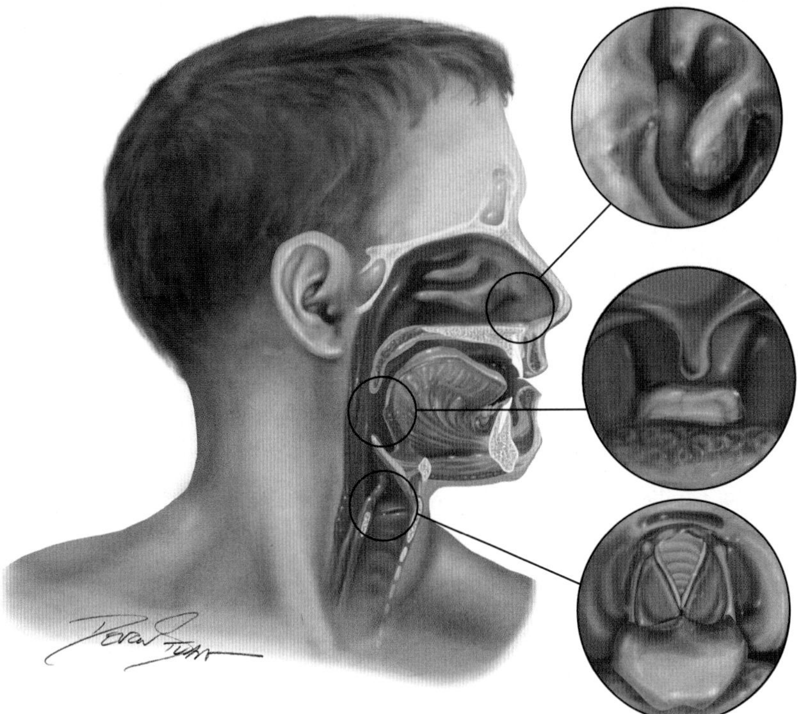

Figure 109.6 After the flexible nasopharyngoscope is passed into the nose, the pharynx, base of the tongue, vallecula, glossoepiglottic fold, superior hypopharynx, posterior pharyngeal wall, epiglottis, aryepiglottic folds, arytenoids, false vocal folds, true vocal cords, and subglottis should be evaluated. The rigid bronchoscope can be inserted into the oral cavity or through a Jackson laryngoscope. After the bronchoscope has been inserted through the laryngoscope, it is rotated 90 degrees to the left or right so that the leading edge of the scope is centered in the larynx by looking directly at the true vocal cord. This prevents trauma to the larynx. To access the right main bronchus, the head may be rotated to the left; to access the left bronchus, the head may be turned to the right.

ALTERNATIVE TECHNIQUE 1: Flexible Fiberoptic Nasopharyngoscopy/Laryngopharyngoscopy (Nasoendoscopy)—*cont'd*

Rigid Bronchoscopy

The rigid ventilating bronchoscope allows ventilation during the examination, although the blow-by of anesthetic gases can be considerable. Maintenance of general anesthesia using intravenous agents and avoidance of inhalation anesthesia during the procedure can be helpful. Insertion of the rigid bronchoscope can be performed after direct laryngoscopy, with intubation of the trachea with the bronchoscope. The patient can be adequately ventilated through the bronchoscope.[31]

When the bronchoscope is inserted at the level of the glottis, it should be rotated 90 degrees to the left or right so that the leading edge of the scope is centered within the larynx. The field of view should look directly at the true vocal cord. This maneuver helps avoid trauma to the larynx. Once in the trachea, the bronchoscope is stabilized between the thumb and index finger of the left hand with the longer fingers resting on the palate behind the incisors. Once past the larynx, the bronchoscope may be rotated back. The right hand is then used to pass instruments down the bronchoscope.

The examination of the subglottic airway can be performed under apnea or spontaneous ventilation with the insufflation technique, using the ventilation port of the bronchoscope. If a tracheostomy tube is in place, it can be removed and the tracheostomy stoma digitally occluded to allow inspection of the trach site.

Examination of the trachea ensues with attention to the width and shape of the subglottis and proximal trachea. The tracheal rings should be carefully examined for their shape. The trachea should be examined for any evidence of compression for external force, tracheomalacia, stenosis, or collapse. The examiner must keep in mind that an area of stenosis with loss of the tracheal rings can dilate somewhat under positive-pressure ventilation. Normal tracheal mucosa should be pink, with small vessels visualized over the underlying cartilage. The carina should be sharply delineated. Any lesions should be noted, as should any purulent or other discharge from either main stem bronchus. A widened carina may indicate an enlarged lymph node at the bifurcation.

The head may be rotated to the left to access the right main bronchus and to the right to access the left bronchus.

Continued

ALTERNATIVE TECHNIQUE 1: Flexible Fiberoptic Nasopharyngoscopy/Laryngopharyngoscopy (Nasoendoscopy)—*cont'd*

The lower lobe segmental bronchi are best seen with a 0-degree telescope. The anterior and posterior bronchi can be seen only with a 0- to 120-degree telescope. The lingular bronchus is best seen with a 30-degree telescope. Biopsies with a cup forceps may be taken as needed. If the operator wishes, a flexible scope can be advanced past the rigid scope to visualize past the segmental bronchi. Foreign bodies may be retrieved through the rigid bronchoscope, using a grasping or biopsy forceps. Removal of larger foreign bodies may necessitate simultaneous removal of the forceps, foreign body, and bronchoscope, followed by reintubation.

The bronchoscope itself can be used to tamponade any bleeding. Bronchoalveolar lavage and cytology could be considered in lieu of biopsy.

ALTERNATIVE TECHNIQUE 2: Bronchoscopy (Flexible Bronchoscopy)

The preparation and anesthesia for flexible bronchoscopy are similar to those for flexible direct laryngoscopy. Flexible bronchoscopy can be performed through the nose or mouth or through an endotracheal or tracheostomy tube. If the patient is intubated, a 2.7-mm flexible bronchoscope is used for 2.0-, 3.5-, and 4.0-mm endotracheal tubes; a 3.5-mm flexible bronchoscope will work for 4.5-, 5.0-, and 5.5-mm endotracheal tubes. A ventilating T-adapter is placed on the hub of the endotracheal or tracheostomy tube and connected to the ventilator tubing, which allows simultaneous ventilation during the examination. The flexible bronchoscope is inserted through the portal of the T-adapter, which provides an excellent seal and minimal leakage of anesthetic gases. A variety of flexible instruments can be advanced through the suction portal, but their size is limited. Foreign body retrieval baskets can be placed in this manner and deployed, but their removal with the foreign body requires complete removal of the bronchoscope. Just as with flexible esophagoscopy, flexible bronchoscopy offers the advantage of digital still and video photography. Flexible endoscopy currently is performed much more commonly than are rigid bronchoscopy and esophagoscopy (Fig. 109.7A).

Rigid Esophagoscopy

As in direct laryngoscopy, a shoulder roll may be used. General anesthesia with full pharmacologic neuromuscular blockage is most helpful. A surgical lubricant should be placed on the shaft of the esophagoscope. The presence of natural teeth and/or limited jaw opening makes rigid esophagoscopy much more challenging. The esophagoscope can be passed either with or without guidance though a laryngoscope; however, a laryngoscope generally does not need to be used in adults. With the endotracheal tube taped to the left, the esophagoscope and associated instruments can be passed to the right. The esophagus is approximately 23 to 25 cm long, extending from the hypopharynx to the stomach, and begins at approximately the lower border of the cricoid cartilage. The esophagus starts at the midline, curves gently to the left, and finally returns to the midline.

The neck is extended, bringing the esophagus in line with the mouth. The rigid esophagoscope is passed through the cervical esophagus and hypopharynx; then, while the examiner protects the maxilla with the thumb and forefinger, the scope is gently leveled off. The bevel of the esophagoscope should face down. If difficulty is encountered, an assistant can cradle the patient's head and slightly lift it off the headrest to facilitate passage (Fig. 109.7B and C).

The surgeon should be aware of the four narrowest portions of the esophagus. The first is the esophageal inlet at the cricopharyngeal muscle; the second is the crossing of the aorta approximately 25 to 30 cm from the teeth; the third is the crossing of the left bronchus; and the fourth is the diaphragmatic hiatus approximately 40 cm from the teeth (Fig. 109.7D). The cricopharyngeus muscle forms the upper esophageal sphincter, which begins approximately 20 cm from the teeth. Normally a collapsed lumen, the esophagus can be distended up to 2 cm. There is also a subtle fifth narrowing, just below the cricopharyngeus at the superior aperture of the thorax. In the "high-low" technique described by Jackson, the procedure is divided into four stages: entering the right piriform sinus, passing the cricopharyngeus muscle, passing through the thoracic esophagus, and passing the hiatus.

In a paralyzed patient, the cricopharyngeus should be entered with only light pressure. After the esophageal introitus and cricopharyngeus have been entered, the head of the operating table is lowered to a horizontal position. The esophagoscope then can be rotated so that it lies on the right side of the mouth, which facilitates passage of suction and instruments with the endoscopist's right hand. If the positioning is correct, the scope will "glide through" the thoracic esophagus. Pulsations are felt on the endoscope as it passes through the area of the aortic arch. To avoid perforations, the esophageal lumen should be visualized ahead of the esophagoscope as it is advanced.

As the esophagoscope is passed through the hiatus of the diaphragm, the head is lowered and positioned horizontally to the right axis so that the tube coincides with the lower

Continued

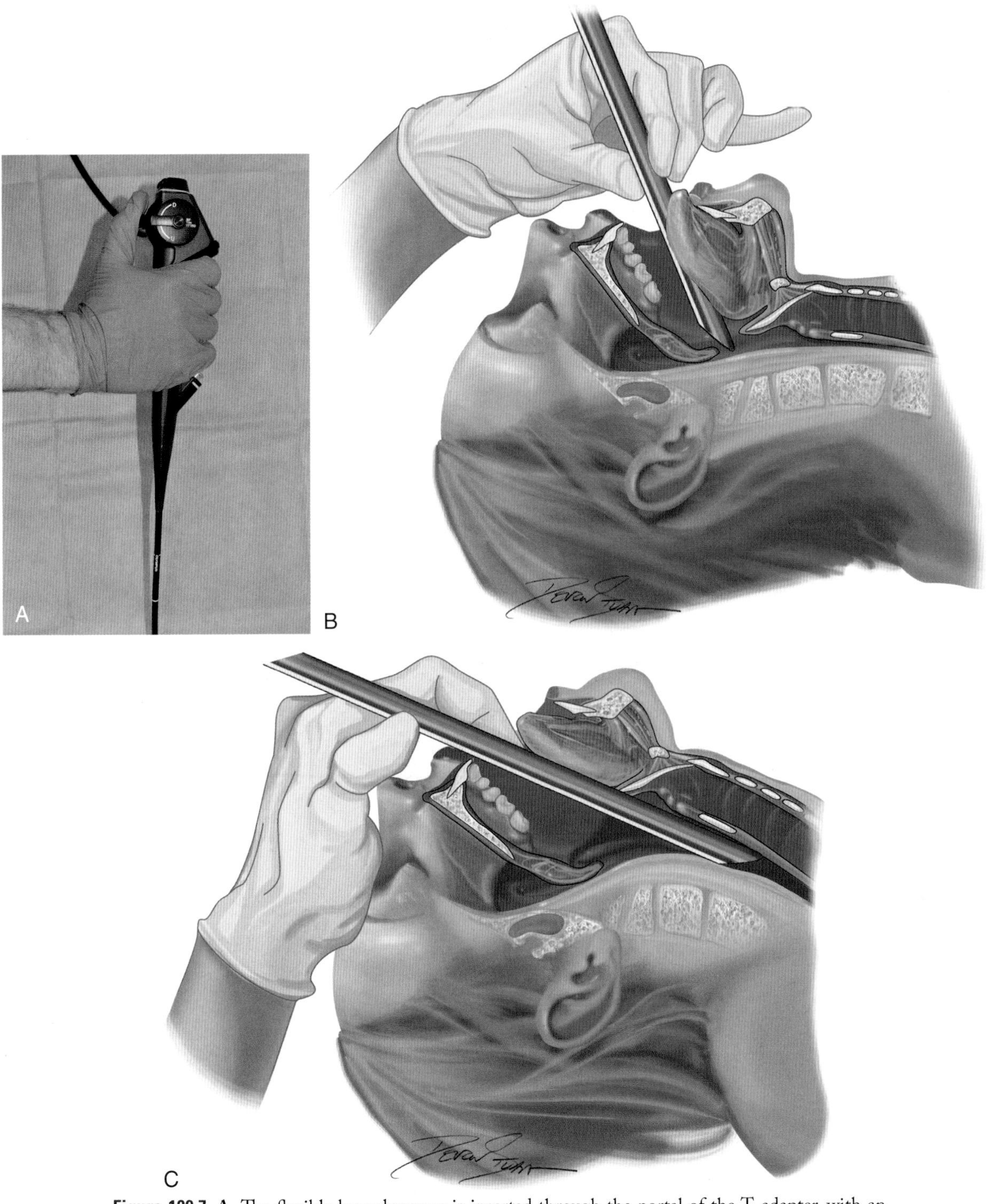

Figure 109.7 **A,** The flexible bronchoscope is inserted through the portal of the T-adapter, with an excellent seal and minimal leakage of anesthetic gases. **B,** Rigid esophagoscopy with side suction port and light source. **C,** Positioning of the patient, with the esophagus in line with the oral cavity. The tip of the esophagoscope is gently passed through the cervical esophagus. The neck is extended, bringing the esophagus in line with the mouth. The thumb serves as a fulcrum to maneuver the scope.

ALTERNATIVE TECHNIQUE 2: Bronchoscopy (Flexible Bronchoscopy)—*cont'd*

third of the esophagus. The scope is gently advanced, and the esophagus is examined for strictures, mucosal lesions, and tumors. The lumen of the esophagus is usually shiny and pink. Tumors can appear as ulcerations or submucosal obstructing spheres. Biopsies of the mucosal lining can be performed through the lumen of the rigid esophagoscope.[4] After rigid esophagoscopy or bronchoscopy, a postoperative chest radiograph can be helpful to rule out pneumothorax.

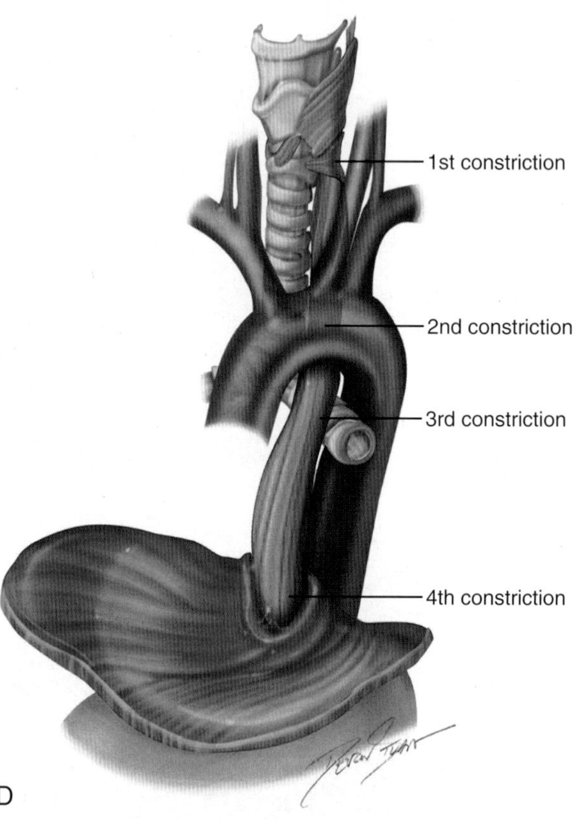

Figure 109.7,cont'd **D,** There are four areas of constriction in the esophagus: the first is the esophageal inlet at the cricopharyngeal muscle, the second is the crossing of the aorta approximately 25 to 30 cm from the teeth, the third is the crossing of the left bronchus, and the fourth is the diaphragmatic hiatus.

Avoidance and Management of Intraoperative Complications

Complications in esophagoscopy include cricoarytenoid joint dislocation, bleeding, perforation, and pneumothorax. Such complications usually can be prevented by careful instrumentation, proper instrument size choice, and minimizing attempts at passage of the scope.[32] Esophageal perforation can occur during manipulation of the esophagoscope, dilation, repair of a tracheoesophageal fistula, or biopsy; patients with ulceration, erosion from malignancy, and ectopic gastric mucosa may be at increased risk.[33] The complication rate for rigid esophagoscopy is reported to be higher than that for flexible esophagoscopy.[33] Perforations tend to occur at the weakest point in the esophagus (just below the cricopharyngeus), in the distal one fifth, or at the site of a lesion.

Postoperative Considerations

If there is concern about the airway, especially after biopsy of the aerodigestive tract, the patient should be admitted for observation and a postoperative chest radiograph should be taken. If the biopsy sites are hemostatic and there is no threat of airway compromise, the patient can be discharged. With extensive surgery of the larynx or insult from biopsy, systemic steroids and antibiotics should be considered. Humidified air, cough suppressants, and mucolytics should be considered.

After esophagoscopy the patient should be kept on nothing by mouth (NPO) status for 6 hours and monitored for any evidence of perforation. Fever, subcutaneous emphysema, or retrosternal pain often are signs and symptoms of perforation.[32] Barium swallow should not be used if perforation is suspected because extravasation of barium in the chest makes leaks more difficult to identify. A water-soluble contrast material should be used. Perforations can be managed by NPO status and antibiotics. Consideration can be given to open placement of a gastrostomy tube. Mortality is high with perforation and once this condition has been recognized, consultation with thoracic surgery should be arranged for assistance in managing the condition and for possible thoracic surgical intervention and drainage.

References

1. Karmody CS. Part I: historical perspectives, the history of laryngology. In: Fried MP, ed. *The Larynx: A Multidisciplinary Approach*. St. Louis: Mosby; 1996:3–11.
2. Prakash UB. Advances in bronchoscopic procedures. *Chest*. 1999;116(5):1403–1408.
3. Steiner W. Techniques of diagnostic and operative endoscopy of the head and neck (Part 2). Tracheoscopy, bronchoscopy, esophagoscopy, mediastinoscopy, interdisciplinary panendoscopy. *Endoscopy*. 1979;11(2):151–157.
4. Jackson C. *Bronchoscopy and Esophagoscopy: A Manual of Peroral Endoscopy and Laryngeal Surgery*. Philadelphia, London: W.B. Saunders Company; 1922.
5. Huizinga E. On esophagoscopy and sword-swallowing. *Ann Otol Rhinol Laryngol*. 1969;78(1):32–39.
6. Storz K. The world of endoscopy: extract from catalog endoscopes and instruments for ENT. In: *Karl Storz Endoscopy-America*. California: Culver City; 1997.
7. McGuirt WF. Panendoscopy as a screening examination for simultaneous primary tumors in head and neck cancer: a prospective sequential study and review of the literature. *Laryngoscope*. 1982;92(5):569–576.
8. McGuirt WF, Matthews B, Koufman JA. Multiple simultaneous tumors in patients with head and neck cancer: a prospective, sequential panendoscopic study. *Cancer*. 1982;50(6):1195–1199.
9. Priante AV, Castilho EC, Kowalski LP. Second primary tumors in patients with head and neck cancer. *Curr Oncol Rep*. 2011;13(2):132–137.
10. Shaha A, Hoover E, Marti J, Krespi Y. Is routine triple endoscopy cost-effective in head and neck cancer? *Am J Surg*. 1988;155(6):750–753.
11. Davidson J, Gilbert R, Irish J, et al. The role of panendoscopy in the management of mucosal head and neck malignancy-a prospective evaluation. *Head Neck*. 2000;22(5):449–454.
12. Dhooge IJ, De Vos M, Albers FW, Van Cauwenberge PB. Panendoscopy as a screening procedure for simultaneous primary tumors in head and neck cancer. *Eur Arch Oto-Rhino-Laryngol*. 1996;253(6):319–324.
13. Haerle SK, Strobel K, Hany TF, Sidler D, Stoeckli SJ. (18)F-FDG-PET/CT versus panendoscopy for the detection of synchronous second primary tumors in patients with head and neck squamous cell carcinoma. *Head Neck*. 2010;32(3):319–325.
14. Hujala K, Sipilä J, Grenman R. Panendoscopy and synchronous second primary tumors in head and neck cancer patients. *Eur Arch Oto-Rhino-Laryngol*. 2005;262(1):17–20.
15. Rodriguez-Bruno K, Ali MJ, Wang SJ. Role of panendoscopy to identify synchronous second primary malignancies in patients with oral cavity and oropharyngeal squamous cell carcinoma. *Head Neck*. 2011;33(7):949–953.
16. Guardiola E, Pivot X, Dassonville O, et al. Is routine triple endoscopy for head and neck carcinoma patients necessary in light of a negative chest computed tomography scan? *Cancer*. 2004;101(9):2028–2033.
17. Kerawala CJ, Bisase B, Lee J. Panendoscopy and simultaneous primary tumours in patients presenting with early carcinoma of the mobile tongue. *Br J Oral Maxillofac Surg*. 2009;47(5):363–365.
18. Pattani KM, Goodier M, Lilien D, Kupferman T, Caldito G, Nathan CO. Utility of panendoscopy for the detection of unknown primary head and neck cancer in patients with a negative PET/CT scan. *Ear Nose Throat J*. 2011;90(8):E16–E20.
19. Buchbender C, Treffert J, Lehnerdt G, et al. Virtual 3-D ^{18}F-FDG PET/CT panendoscopy for assessment of the upper airways of head and neck cancer patients: a feasibility study. *Eur J Nucl Med Mol Imaging*. 2012;39(9):1435–1440.
20. Bless DM, Swift E. Stroboscopy: new diagnostic techniques and applied physiology. In: Fried MP, ed. *The Larynx: A Multidisciplinary Approach*. St. Louis: CV Mosby; 1996:81–100.
21. Leder SB, Karas DE. Fiberoptic endoscopic evaluation of swallowing in the pediatric population. *Laryngoscope*. 2000;110(7):1132–1136.
22. Toyoshima M, Chida K, Enomoto N, Nakamura Y, Imokawa S, Suda T. A case of diffuse alveolar hemorrhage associated with interstitial pneumonia and systemic sclerosis. *Nihon Kokyuki Gakkai Zasshi*. 2005;43:437–441.
23. Guardiola E, Chaigneau L, Villanueva C, Pivot X. Is there still a role for triple endoscopy as part of staging for head and neck cancer? *Curr Opin Otolaryngol Head Neck Surg*. 2006;14(2):85–88.
24. Loh KS, Brown DH, Baker JT, Gilbert RW, Gullane PJ, Irish JC. A rational approach to pulmonary screening in newly diagnosed head and neck cancer. *Head Neck*. 2005;27(11):990–994.
25. Grossman TW, Toohill RJ, Lehman RH, Duncavage JA, Malin TC. Role of esophagoscopy in the evaluation of patients with head and neck carcinoma. *Ann Otol Rhinol Laryngol*. 1983;92(4 Pt 1):369–372.
26. Shapshay SM, Hong WK, Fried MP, Sismanis A, Vaughan CW, Strong MS. Simultaneous carcinomas of the esophagus and upper aerodigestive tract. *Otolaryngol Head Neck Surg*. 1980;88(4):373–377.
27. Cordasco EM Jr, Mehta AC, Ahmad M. Bronchoscopically induced bleeding. A summary of nine years' Cleveland clinic experience and review of the literature. *Chest*. 1991;100(4):1141–1147.
28. GU M, Chastre J. The standardization of bronchoscopic techniques for ventilator-associated pneumonia. *Chest*. 1992;102(5-suppl 1):557S–564S.
29. Gotta AW, Sullivan CA. Anaesthesia of the upper airway using topical anaesthetic and superior laryngeal nerve block. *Br J Anaesth*. 1981;53(10):1055–1058.
30. Gotta AW, Sullivan CA. Superior laryngeal nerve block: an aid to intubating the patient with fractured mandible. *J Trauma*. 1984;24(1):83–85.
31. Hunsaker DH. Anesthesia for microlaryngeal surgery: the case for subglottic jet ventilation. *Laryngoscope*. 1994;104(8 Pt 2 suppl 65):1–30.
32. Rabinovich S, Smith IM, McCabe BF. Rupture of the esophagus. *Arch Otolaryngol*. 1967;85(4):410–415.
33. Tsao GJ, Damrose EJ. Complications of esophagoscopy in an academic training program. *Otolaryngol Head Neck Surg*. 2010;142(4):500–504.

CHAPTER 110

Cricothyroidotomy and Tracheostomy

Raymond P. Shupak, Fayette C. Williams, and Roderick Y. Kim

Armamentarium

#15 and #11 Blades
Appropriate sutures
Army-Navy retractors
Cricoid hook
Kittner sponges
Local anesthetic with vasoconstrictor
Curved Mayo scissors
Senn retractors
Sterile 10-cc syringe
Trach ties or Velcro strap
Tracheal hook
Tracheostomy tube
Trousseau dilator
6-0 Armored tube

History of the Procedure

Surgical airways were once created only by a brave few who risked loss of their patients and their reputation. The procedure was frequently condemned, only to later be rediscovered. Although Egyptians likely performed the first tracheostomies around 3600 BCE as pictured on ancient tablets, the first "medical" reference noting a healed tracheostomy scar was described in 2000 BC in the sacred book of Hindu medicine, *Rig-Veda*. The first known written description of the tracheostomy technique came from Egypt around 1500 BC during the time of Imhotep. In 100 BC, Asclepiades further described the technique of the surgery, even though other experts of his time condemned the procedure. Whereas Hippocrates cited risks to the carotid arteries as the main reason to avoid a tracheostomy, Aretaeus of Cappadocia warned of infectious complications.[2] Asclepiades' enthusiasm for tracheostomy was later ridiculed by Caelius Aurelianus as a "senseless, frivolous, and even criminal invention of Asclepiades."

Much of our historical understanding of tracheostomy comes from legends passed down through time. Alexander the Great reportedly used his sword to open the trachea of a soldier suffocating on a bone. The Babylonian Talmud describes placing a reed into the newborn trachea to assist in ventilation.[3] Dante[1] proclaimed tracheostomy "a suitable punishment for a sinner in the depths of the Inferno." Perhaps the most interesting detailed report came from Antyllus in 100 AD. His description of a horizontal incision between the tracheal rings mirrors the technique most commonly used today. Further historical accounts were sparse until the Renaissance. During the 16th and 17th centuries, publications by Brasavola, Sanctorius, and Habicot reported on tracheostomies for airway obstruction due to infection and foreign bodies. In 1883, Trousseau reported on his lifesaving tracheostomies in 200 patients with diphtheria.[2]

Astonishingly, only since the 20th century has tracheostomy been considered a truly safe, predictable, and routine procedure. In 1921, Chevalier Jackson solidified modern tracheostomy indications and techniques, although he still advised against cricothyroidotomy. Tracheostomy is now routinely performed as an elective procedure and continues to serve as a lifesaving maneuver in both the hospital and the field.

Indications for the Use of the Procedure

Indications for a tracheostomy and a cricothyroidotomy have been debated for centuries; the indications are still debated but more rationalized.[4] Most indications can be summarized as upper airway obstruction or impending upper airway obstruction.[5] Although utilized interchangeably, *tracheotomy* refers to the procedure of creating an opening into the trachea, whereas *tracheostomy* refers to the actual opening resulting from the procedure.

Prolonged intubation with inability to wean from mechanical ventilation is a common indication for a tracheostomy. If a patient is expected to require mechanical ventilation for longer than 7 to 10 days, a tracheostomy is indicated. This improves patient comfort and has been shown to decrease the incidence of pneumonia, as well as shorten hospital stays.[6,7] Glottic injury due to prolonged intubation is also avoided with an early tracheostomy. Recent systematic reviews have shown decreases in the cost and duration of sedation in critically-ill patients who received an early tracheostomy.[8,9]

The inability to intubate and ventilate is an indication for placement of a tracheostomy or cricothyroidotomy depending on the urgency of the situation and armamentarium available. When considering a cricothyroidotomy, other airway maneuvers in the difficult airway algorithm should also be considered. The surgeon should become familiar with the American Society of Anesthesia difficult airway algorithm, in order to act expeditiously during an airway crisis.[10] Similarly, patients with upper airway obstruction and stridor, air hunger, retractions, or bilateral vocal cord paralysis are indicated for surgical airway.[11]

Head and neck trauma including facial fractures can also be an indication for a surgical airway, in addition to severe subcutaneous emphysema, airway edema, airway burns/eschar, and facial fractures compromising the airway. Patients with these findings progressing toward loss of the airway should be considered for a surgical airway.

Tracheostomy is the gold standard for treatment of obstructive sleep apnea and has a 100% cure rate. It bypasses the area of obstruction and can be used as a temporary or permanent (skin-lined tracheostomy) treatment depending on the severity of disease.[12]

Tracheostomy is useful in extensive head and neck surgical procedures for control of the airway during surgery and in the immediate postoperative period. The surgeon should consider a tracheostomy when a major head and neck operation may cause significant upper airway edema or otherwise compromise the patient's ability to maintain a safe airway. Further discussion of this topic can be found in the literature.[13]

Limitations and Contraindications

There are no true absolute contraindications, but there are instances when the surgical technique may need to be altered, such as the presence of a high-riding innominate artery, goiter, significant pulmonary disease, obesity, poor functional residual capacity, history of radiation, thyroid/laryngeal mass, and active communicable pulmonary disease. In the pediatric population, a cricothyroidotomy is contraindicated because of the unfavorable hourglass anatomy and the high risk for tracheal stenosis postoperatively.[14] Therefore, a formal tracheotomy should be performed on the pediatric population (Fig. 110.1).

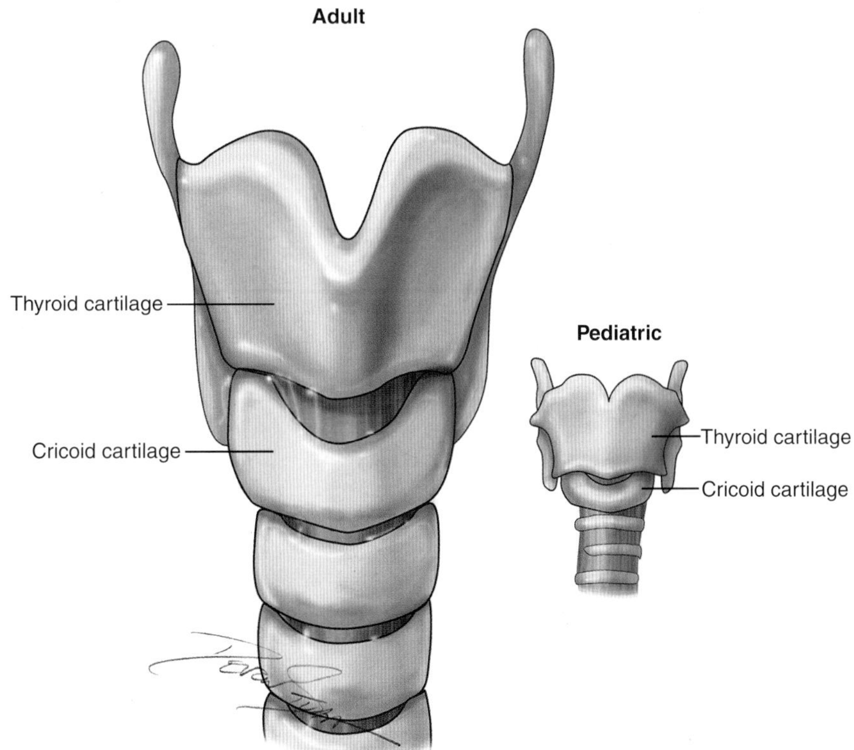

Figure 110.1 The thyroid cartilage covers the cricothyroid membrane in the pediatric airway.

TECHNIQUE: Tracheostomy

STEP 1: Positioning

The patient is positioned on a shoulder roll with the neck in extension to maximize the distance between the cricoid cartilage and the sternal notch. Draping is performed to include the upper chest region in continuity with the neck. Landmarks are palpated and marked. The sternal notch and the cricoid cartilage are the most important landmarks, as the dissection will be performed between these two structures. A 4-cm horizontal incision line should be drawn halfway between the sternal notch and the cricoid cartilage. Alternatively, the surgeon may simply mark the incision two fingerbreadths above the sternal notch. If the surgeon is to remove the endotracheal tube, it should be prepped into the field with enough slack to be reconnected to the tracheostomy tube. If the anesthetist is to remove the tube, the tube should be positioned for access under the drapes. Communication is key between the surgical team and the anesthetist throughout the whole procedure. When a tracheostomy is performed as part of a larger head and neck procedure, the endotracheal tube is managed most simply by prepping it into the field along with the entire head and neck (Fig. 110.2A and B).

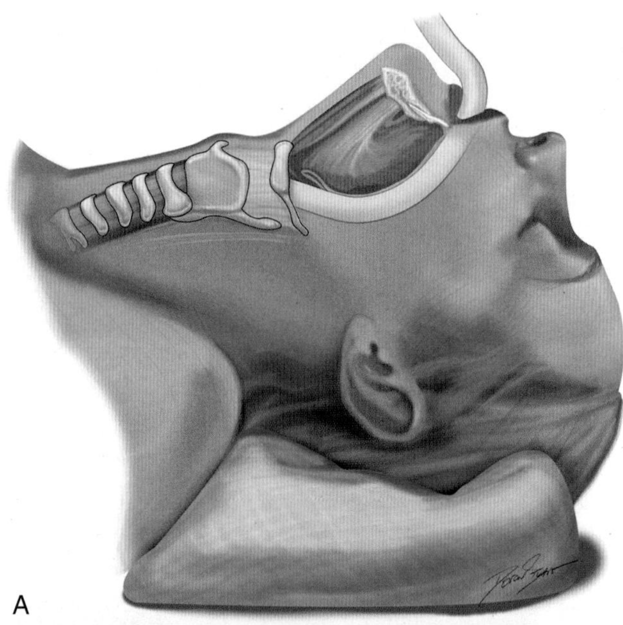

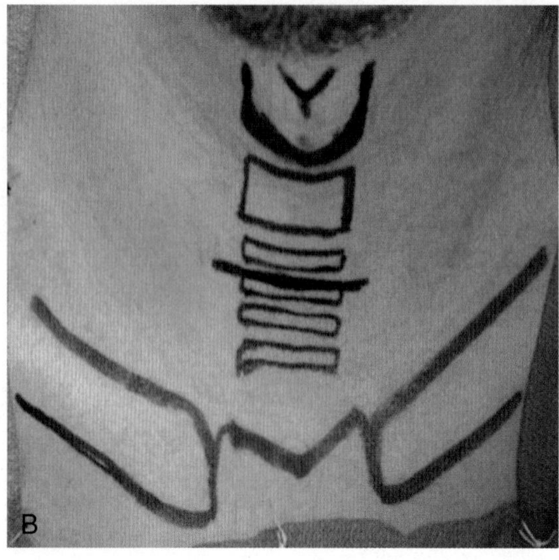

Figure 110.2 **A,** The neck is positioned in extension to allow access to the trachea. A shoulder roll often improves extension. **B,** Skin markings include the cricoid cartilage and the sternal notch. The incision is marked between these landmarks.

TECHNIQUE: Tracheostomy—cont'd

STEP 2: Skin Incision

The incision is performed with a scalpel or electrocautery down through skin into subcutaneous fat. Electrocautery maintains a more hemostatic incision and does not result in a worse scar, because the final wound heals secondarily after tracheostomy removal. Also, to decrease the chance of fire, the patient is placed on room air from 100% oxygen. The dissection is continued with electrocautery in a horizontal plane until the strap muscles are reached. Superficial anterior jugular veins are commonly encountered while reaching this plane. These veins are often sizable and should be suture-ligated or hemo-clipped if they cannot be retracted laterally. In the obese patient, a subcutaneous lipectomy can be performed down to the strap muscles to facilitate the deeper dissection. The fascia over the strap muscles is reached, and the avascular raphe is identified vertically in the midline between the strap muscles. A sponge wrapped tightly around the surgeon's finger can be used to vertically sweep this plane open to define the anatomy. Senn or Army-Navy retractors are used to pull the subcutaneous tissue superiorly and inferiorly. A Weitlaner retractor may also be used to retract vertically in a self-retaining fashion (Fig. 110.2C).

STEP 3: Division of Strap Muscles

Dissection continues with electrocautery, vertically in the midline raphe between the strap muscles. Once the fascia over the thyroid gland is reached, the strap muscles can be mobilized off the gland with blunt dissection. This allows the Army-Navy retractors to be horizontally positioned under the strap muscles to expose the thyroid isthmus. An alternative technique for lateral retraction of the strap muscles is to grasp the medial edge of the muscles with an Allis clamp and retract laterally. These clamps are allowed to hang off the side of the neck by their own weight to assist in lateral retraction of the strap muscles. The trachea and cricoid cartilage should be palpated again at this stage to ensure the dissection will proceed to the region of the second tracheal ring (Fig. 110.2D and E).

Continued

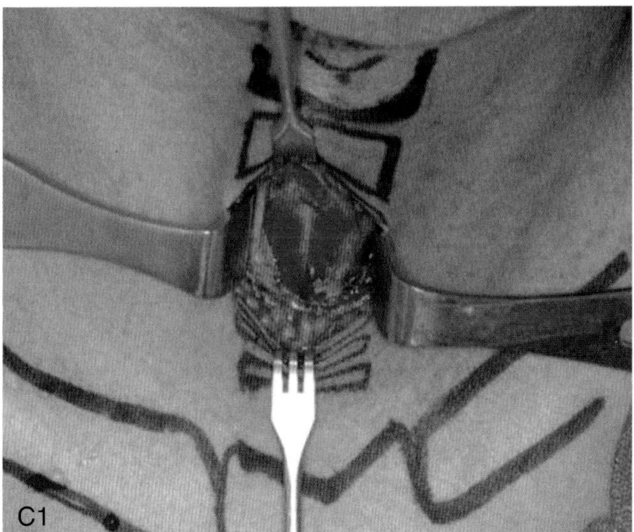

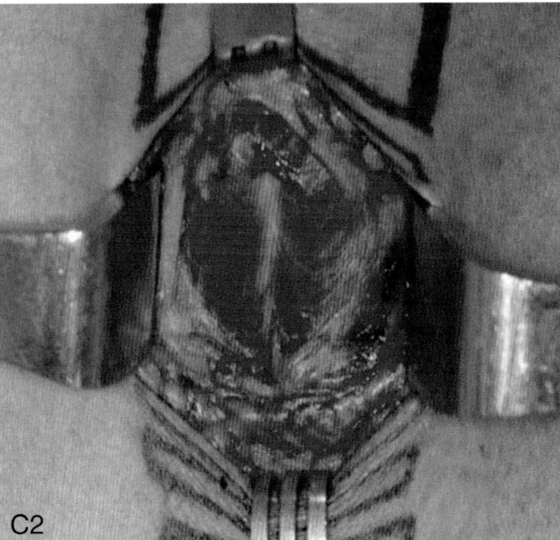

Figure 110.2,cont'd **C1** and **C2,** After dissection through the subcutaneous plane, the strap muscles and midline raphe are visualized.

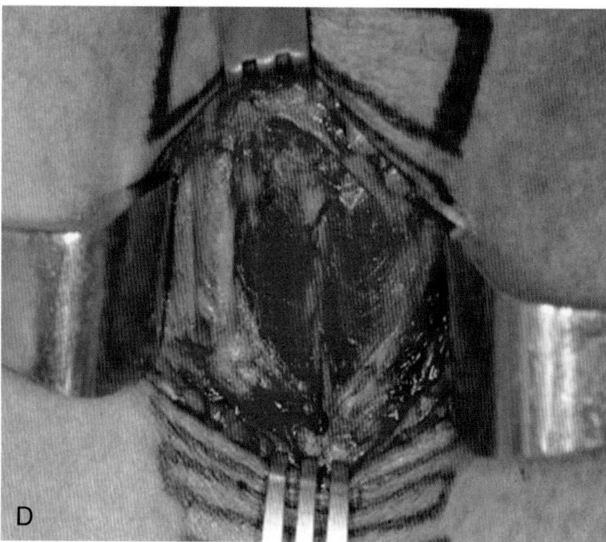

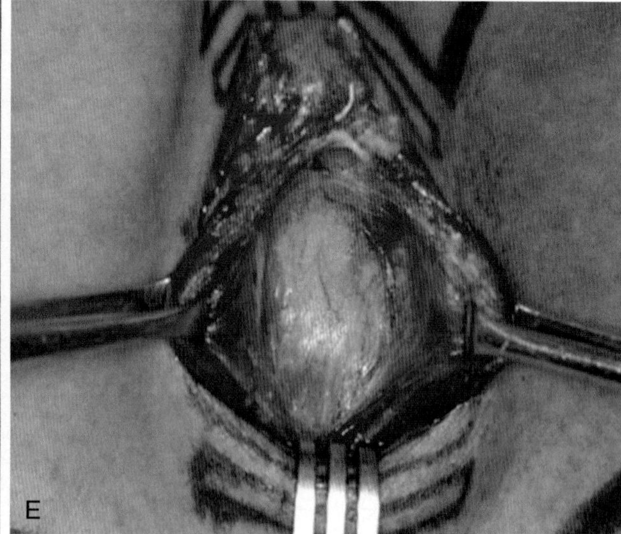

Figure 110.2,cont'd **D,** After mobilizing the strap muscles laterally, Army-Navy retractors are placed deep to the strap muscles. **E,** The strap muscles may also be retracted laterally using Allis clamps.

Continued

TECHNIQUE: Tracheostomy—cont'd

STEP 4: Division of Thyroid Gland

The isthmus of the thyroid gland must be managed after the strap muscles have been retracted. Although some surgeons recommend superior or inferior retraction of the gland, troublesome bleeding may ensue postoperatively, which is the most common complication of tracheotomy, as the tracheostomy tube rubs against the thyroid isthmus. Division of the isthmus moves the thyroid gland out of the field and decreases the chance for postoperative bleeding. The thyroid gland is easily divided vertically in the midline with cautery. Slow and thorough cautery through this highly vascular gland is recommended to ensure hemostasis. The surgeon should use caution because the trachea lies just deep to the thyroid isthmus. To avoid inadvertent entrance into the trachea with the cautery, the thyroid gland can be mobilized and lifted off the trachea bluntly with a tonsil or right angle hemostat. This maneuver allows cautery through the thyroid gland to proceed while safely protecting the underlying airway. Once the thyroid gland is divided, the tracheal rings are exposed and cleaned with Kittner sponges. Lateral pockets are developed immediately adjacent to the trachea and Army-Navy retractors are placed to retract the soft tissues laterally. This creates safe access directly onto the anterior wall of the trachea for entrance into the airway. These retractors should not be removed until the tracheostomy tube is in place and the anesthetist confirms that ventilation is adequate (Fig. 110.2F and G). At this time, the anesthetist may switch to 100% oxygen to preoxygenate before entrance of the airway, and the electrocautery is moved out of the field.

STEP 5: Entrance into the Trachea

Communication with the anesthesia team is especially critical during this step. Excellent hemostasis should be obtained prior to entering the airway, as cautery in an oxygen-enriched environment can lead to an airway fire. The tracheostomy tube cuff should be tested with a 10-cc syringe to verify no leaks are present. The cuff on the endotracheal tube is deflated and advanced 5 cm to avoid rupturing the cuff when entering the airway with a scalpel. A cricoid hook can be placed around the cricoid cartilage to stabilize the trachea. Tracheal incision design is a matter of personal preference. Multiple tracheal incision designs have been advocated, although no difference in outcomes has been demonstrated. Common incisions to enter the trachea include a vertical incision through rings 2 and 3, a horizontal incision between rings 2 and 3, a cruciate incision, and an H-shaped incision. For an inferiorly based flap of the anterior tracheal wall, a 1-cm horizontal incision is made with a #11 blade between the first and second tracheal rings.[12] Vertical releasing incisions are made inferiorly on each side through the second to third tracheal rings to develop an inferiorly based Bjork flap. Alternative tracheal incision designs may be utilized (Fig. 110.2H). The endotracheal tube is visualized within the trachea. A 3-0 Vicryl suture is used to fixate the tracheal flap to the dermis of the inferior skin incision with a horizontal mattress suture. This allows the stoma to remain patient if accidental decannulation occurs in the early postoperative period. If needed, the cuff may be reinflated to maintain ventilation until the endotracheal tube is ready to be withdrawn. Additional 2-0 Prolene temporary "stay" sutures may be placed through the tracheal rings lateral to the tracheal opening if desired (Fig. 110.2I and J).

Continued

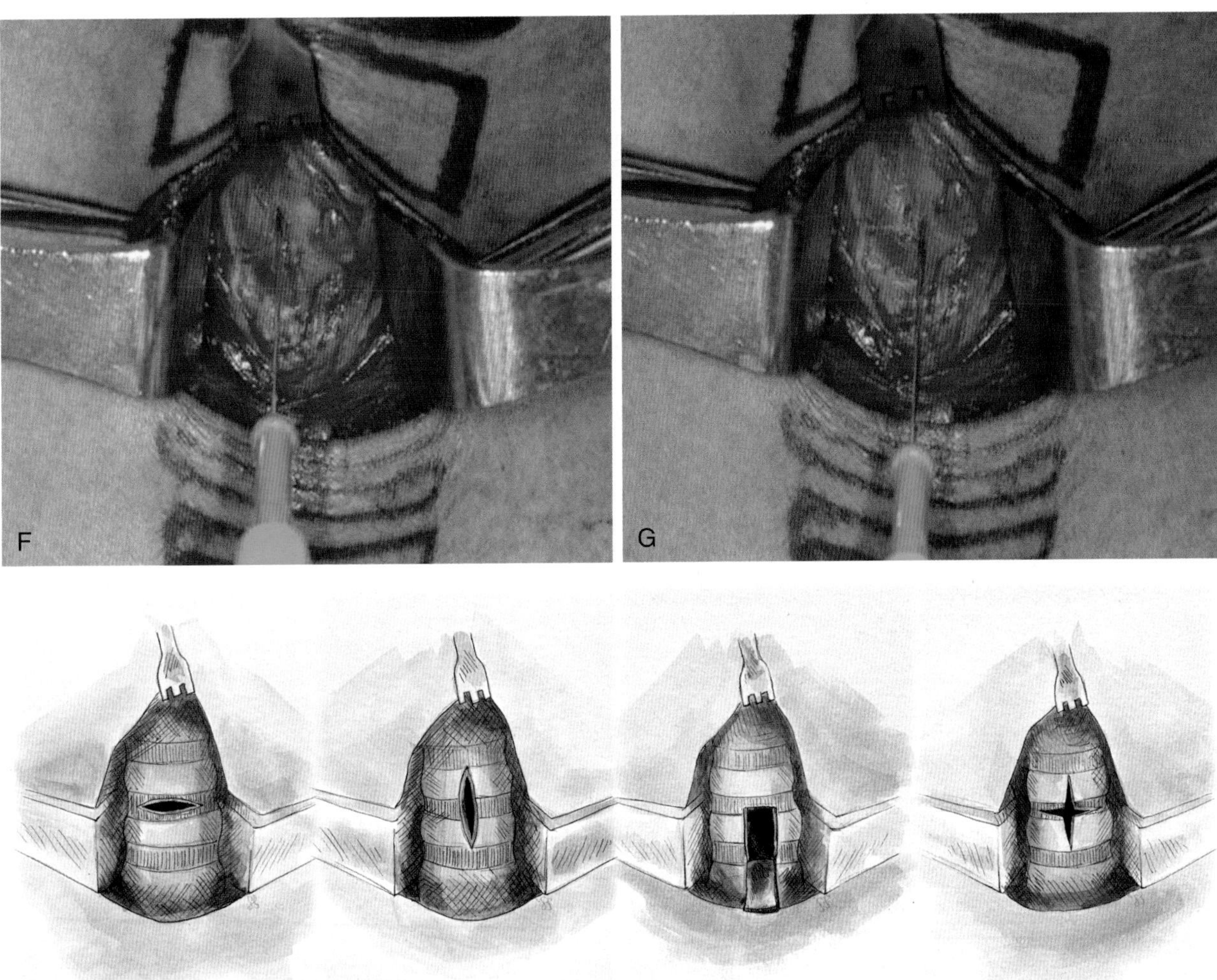

Figure 110.2,cont'd **F,** The isthmus of the thyroid gland is lifted off the trachea bluntly and divided with cautery. **G,** The Army-Navy retractors are positioned directly adjacent to the trachea. Hemostasis is confirmed prior to airway entry. **H,** Alternative tracheal incision designs.

TECHNIQUE: Tracheostomy—cont'd

STEP 6: Placement of Tracheostomy Tube

An appropriate size tracheostomy tube is selected, typically a size 6 or 8 depending on the adult patient's size. A special tracheostomy tube with increased proximal length is useful for obese patients with an increased distance from trachea to skin. The cuff on the endotracheal tube is deflated as the surgeon observes through the newly created tracheal window. Once the beveled edge of the endotracheal tube reaches the superior aspect of the opening, the tube is maintained in this position until the tracheostomy tube is secure. This allows advancement of the endotracheal tube back to its original position in the trachea should the surgeon have difficulty placing the tracheostomy tube. The airway is suctioned free of blood, and the tracheostomy tube is gently placed into the trachea with the obturator seated. Force should never be required, as this indicates either a stoma that is too small or a malpositioned tracheostomy tube outside the trachea. A Trousseau dilator can be useful to enlarge the tracheal opening if necessary. Once passively rotated into the trachea, the obturator is immediately removed from the outer cannula and replaced with the inner cannula, which is locked into place. The cuff is inflated with a 10-cc syringe, and the anesthesia circuit is attached to the tracheostomy tube. The anesthesia team verifies ventilation and return of end tidal carbon dioxide prior to removing the endotracheal tube and the Army-Navy retractors. Once confirmed, the flanges of the tracheostomy tube are sutured to the skin with 2-0 silk sutures. A trach tie around the neck may be used, but its use is discouraged in the setting of a head and neck operation with flap reconstruction (Fig. 110.2K and L).

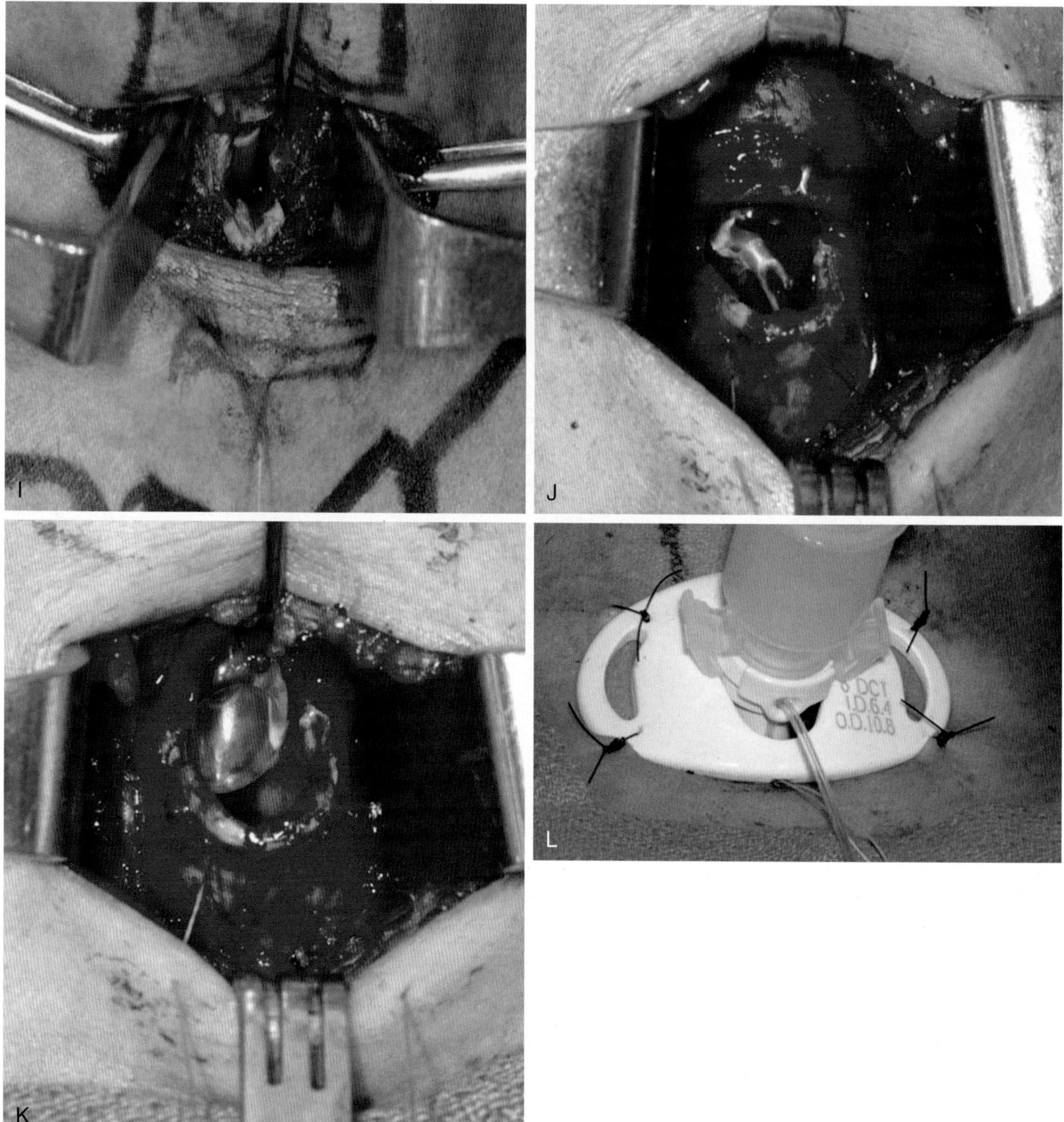

Figure 110.2,cont'd **I,** An inferiorly based flap is incised and reflected inferiorly to reveal the endotracheal tube within the trachea. **J,** The tracheal flap is sutured to the dermis with a 3-0 Vicryl. The endotracheal tube is still visualized within the lumen. **K,** The endotracheal tube is slowly pulled superiorly until the end of the tube is positioned at the top of the tracheal window. **L,** The tracheostomy tube is placed into the airway under direct visualization. (B–G and I–L, Courtesy of Dr. Edward Ellis III).

ALTERNATIVE TECHNIQUE: Cricothyroidotomy

A cricothyroidotomy is an alternative surgical airway used in emergent cases of airway loss. Most difficult airway algorithms place cricothyroidotomy as the final option in a "cannot intubate, cannot ventilate" scenario. Advantages of cricothyroidotomy include the minimal distance between the skin and the airway and the absence of major vascular structures.

The surgeon's nondominant hand should palpate the cricothyroid membrane with the index finger and stabilize the larynx with the thumb and middle finger. A vertical skin incision is recommended to allow for easy superior or inferior extension if necessary. The scalpel is used to cut down through skin and subcutaneous tissue to the cricothyroid membrane.

Palpation through the open incision confirms the position of the cricothyroid membrane. Troublesome bleeding may occur, but this is of secondary importance in an acute airway situation. The surgeon enters the cricothyroid membrane transversely with the scalpel. In a bloody field, this incision is made by palpation just above the cricoid cartilage. A hemostat is often needed to spread this space open large enough to accept a tracheostomy tube. Alternatively, a bloody endotracheal tube is usually immediately present in this unfortunate situation and may be inserted into the cricothyroidotomy. A small tube is advisable. The anesthesia circuit is connected to the tube and ventilation is verified. Consideration can be given to immediate conversion to a formal tracheotomy, in which case the cricothyroidotomy incision is left to close spontaneously (Fig. 110.3).

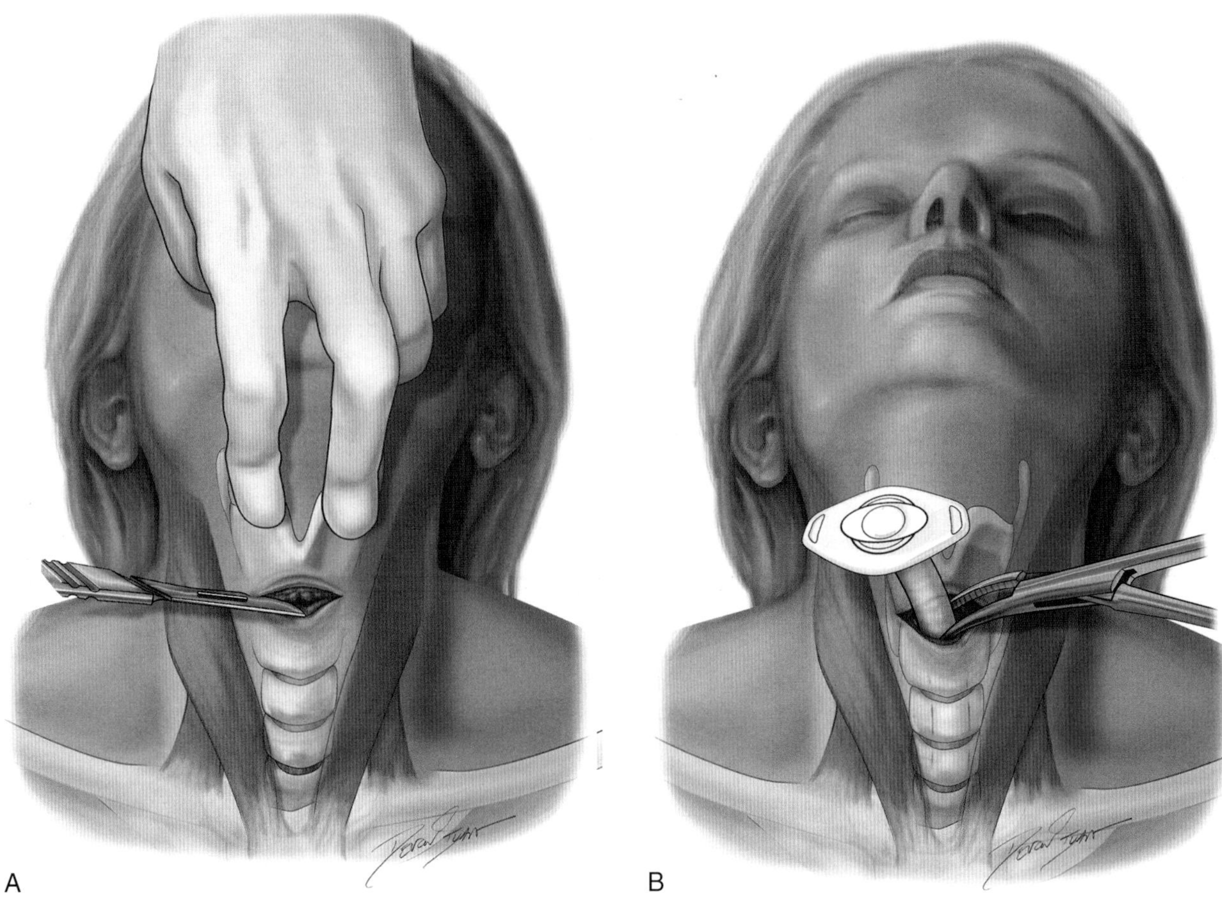

Figure 110.3 **A,** For an emergency surgical airway, the nondominant hand stabilizes the trachea while the other hand incises down to the trachea. **B,** Due to the limited opening of the cricothyroid membrane, a blunt hemostat is useful to widen the stoma while the tube is inserted.

ALTERNATIVE TECHNIQUE: Percutaneous Tracheostomy

Percutaneous tracheostomy is an alternative technique to the traditional operative tracheostomy. The procedure was initially described in the mid-20th century and draws inspiration from Seldinger's technique for vascular cannulation.[15,16] Since then, the procedure has undergone different modifications; however, the principal remains the same.[17] The indications for percutaneous tracheostomy parallel that of the operative technique. Potential advantages of percutaneous tracheostomy versus operative tracheostomy include decreased cost, operative time, bleeding, and wound infections.[18–21]

Percutaneous tracheostomy can be performed in multiple settings. The technique is often utilized bedside in the intensive care unit. Commercially available kits are available to aid in the performance of the procedure. The patient is placed in a supine position with a shoulder roll similar to a surgical tracheostomy. General anesthesia or intravenous sedation is used throughout the procedure. Standard landmarks (thyroid, cricoid cartilages, and sternal notch) are palpated and marked. The site is prepped and draped in normal fashion and local anesthesia is introduced by subcutaneous injection and administration of lidocaine through the endotracheal tube. A horizontal incision is carried out (approximately 2 cm) at the level of the first and second or second and third tracheal rings. A combination of blunt finger dissection and a curved hemostat are used to dissect down to the anterior tracheal wall. At this point a fiberoptic bronchoscope is inserted into the endotracheal tube for visualization within the airway. An introducer needle connected to a saline-filled syringe is inserted between tracheal rings. This can be observed under direct visualization via the bronchoscope. A guidewire is placed and the introducer needle is removed. A series of dilators are then used to increase aperture size. To finish, a tracheostomy tube is inserted over the guidewire and secured into position. The bronchoscope is used to confirm placement.

Although percutaneous tracheostomy is a relatively safe procedure, contraindications do exist. General considerations should be given to address coagulopathies and comorbidities prior to the procedure. Percutaneous tracheostomy should be avoided in the pediatric population, emergency situations, abnormal anatomical variations (high innominate artery), presence of tumor, and when unable to identify anatomic landmarks.[22] Complications coincide with that of surgical tracheostomy. Perforation of the posterior tracheal wall perforation has been reported with increased incidence utilizing this technique.[23] Finally, the procedure should be performed by those with advanced training in this technique to decrease complication rate.[24]

Avoidance and Management of Intraoperative Complications

Prevention of intraoperative complications for all surgical procedures begins with preoperative planning. Although a tracheostomy must sometimes be performed in an awake patient under local anesthesia, the ideal setting will have a protected airway with an endotracheal tube placed under general anesthesia. This is usually not possible when an emergent cricothyroidotomy is required, which results in a complication rate greater than elective tracheostomy.[25] Many complications of tracheostomy may be avoided by keeping the dissection in the midline of the neck.

Palpation and accurate landmark identification must be performed prior to incision. In the thick or obese neck, this task may be more difficult. After the incision is made into the subcutaneous fat, palpation should be performed again to verify proper orientation. The trachea should be palpated throughout the procedure to maintain the dissection safely in the midline. Furthermore, ample exposure and preventing a narrowing of the field as the dissection deepens can prevent deviation from the trachea.

Hemorrhage can occur from a variety of sources. Small veins traversing the surgical field are routinely encountered and should be ligated. The thyroid gland commonly bleeds during division of the isthmus and should be carefully controlled with cautery. Palpation above the sternal notch of a pulsatile mass should alert the surgeon to a high-riding innominate artery, which may result in catastrophic hemorrhage if injured. The common carotid arteries can also be placed at risk if the dissection wanders off the midline. The trachea is mobile in the horizontal plane and can be unknowingly retracted within the soft tissues held by Army-Navy retractors. This can allow movement of the common carotid artery into the surgical field, increasing the risk of injury. Therefore, the two retractors should work together to keep the trachea midline.

A tracheoesophageal fistula can be created by incision of the posterior wall of the trachea and anterior wall of the esophagus. More commonly, a tracheostomy tube can be placed forcibly into the trachea, producing laceration of the posterior wall of the trachea with the cannula. Prevention requires visualization of the tracheostomy tube as it enters the trachea and avoidance of force. Again, if the insertion requires force, the tracheostomy either needs to be widened with a blade, or dilated further. Small tears into the esophagus can be managed by placing a nasogastric tube under endoscopic guidance while positioning the tracheostomy tube distal to the site of injury on the posterior tracheal wall. Although this conservative treatment should allow small defects to close, larger defects require surgical exploration and repair. Passive drainage of the site of an esophageal tear is advisable.

One-third of all surgical fires occur in the airway with an oxygen-enriched environment. As mentioned briefly, if patient physiology allows, the anesthesia team should decrease the fraction of inspired oxygen below 25% because oxygen is ignitable at 26%.[26,27] In an oxygen-enriched environment, bipolar cautery is considered safer than monopolar cautery, although both should be avoided. Nitrous oxide is also flammable and should not be used. If an airway fire is encountered, the surgeon should immediately remove the burning endotracheal tube from the airway. The trachea should be intubated and the aerodigestive tract evaluated.[27] Again, communication with the anesthetist is key.

Postoperative Considerations

Various degrees of bleeding are common after tracheostomy. Up to 6% of patients can exhibit bleeding in the postoperative period.[28,29] Fortunately, most episodes in the early postoperative period are due to slow oozing, which is easily addressed with conservative measures. The thyroid gland and anterior jugular veins are the most common sources of bleeding due to irritation from the tracheostomy tube and inadequate hemostasis at the time of surgery. Local measures such as hemostatic packing around the tracheostomy tube are usually sufficient treatment. We prefer a single sheet of hemostatic packing around the tracheostomy tube, which is removed 24 hours postoperatively. If bleeding persists, exploration in the operating room should be considered. Consideration should also be given to a tracheo-innominate fistula for bleeding between the first and third weeks after surgery.[30] This devastating complication results from erosion of the end of the tracheostomy tube through the anterior wall of the trachea. Although a tracheostomy low in the trachea has been thought to be the greatest risk factor, the innominate artery has a highly variable course across the trachea, which places all patients at risk.[31] These patients sometimes present with a pulsatile tracheostomy tube or a significant "sentinel bleed," which should prompt a fiberoptic examination of the trachea for a source of bleeding. Profuse bleeding should be managed with retrosternal finger dissection and pressure to occlude the innominate artery (the Utley maneuver).[32] Although definitive management has historically consisted of innominate artery ligation, endovascular techniques may be considered in the stable patient.[33,34]

Mucous plugs and blood clots are common sources of obstruction within tracheostomy tubes, especially in the pediatric population.[35] Routine care by nursing staff should include cleaning of the inner cannula several times daily. Humidified air and regular suction may also minimize this problem. Early detection is important because an occluded airway can be catastrophic.

Accidental decannulation is of greatest concern during the first 3 to 7 days, when the tract between the trachea and skin has not matured and collapse of the wound edges is possible. Choosing a tracheostomy tube of proper size and length minimizes this complication, and when needed, with proximal extension. The flanges of the tracheostomy tube should be sutured to the skin. Tracheostomy ties around the neck, may also be used if a flap reconstruction has not been performed. The surgeon should anticipate swelling in the neck, which may increase the distance from the skin to the trachea. The flange of the tracheostomy tube will move with the skin and potentially decannulate the tube from the trachea, although the flanges are still seated flush against the skin (slow displacement phenomenon type 1).[36] If the tracheostomy tube is completely removed from the stoma, it should be replaced as quickly as possible. False passage into the peritracheal soft tissue is possible in this scenario. Lastly, endotracheal tube intubation of the stoma or even orotracheal intubation as a rescue maneuver may be considered if conditions necessitate.

Unintended movement of air into closed spaces occurs in several forms. Subcutaneous air emphysema is possible when air leaking out of the trachea is not allowed to escape past the skin edges. For this reason, the skin edges around a tracheostomy tube should be left open and not sutured. Pneumothorax and pneumomediastinum are possible after tracheostomy and can occur in up to 5% of cases.[37] A chest radiograph is recommended immediately after surgery. If a pneumothorax is detected, a chest tube should be placed.

Tracheal stenosis is a long-term complication of narrowing of the lumen of the trachea. The most likely etiology is ischemia of the tracheal wall due to pressure from an overinflated cuff. Cuff pressure should be monitored, and when clinically appropriate, the cuff should be deflated early in the postoperative period to minimize ischemia.

References

1. Dante Alighieri, 1265-1321. *The Divine Comedy of Dante Alighieri : Inferno, Purgatory, Paradise.* New York :The Union Library Association; 1935.
2. Frost EA. Tracing the tracheostomy. *Ann Otol Rhinol Laryngol.* 1976;85(5 Pt.1):618–624.
3. Szmuk P, Ezri T, Evron S, Roth Y, Katz J. A brief history of tracheostomy and tracheal intubation, from the Bronze Age to the Space Age. *Intensive Care Med.* 2008;34(2):222–228.
4. Booth JB. Tracheostomy and tracheal intubation in military history. *J R Soc Med.* 2000;93(7):380–383.
5. el-Kilany SM. Complications of tracheostomy. *Ear Nose Throat J.* 1980;59(3):123–129.
6. Durbin CG Jr. Indications for and timing of tracheostomy. *Respir Care.* 2005;50(4):483–487.
7. Cai SQ, Hu JW, Liu D, et al. The influence of tracheostomy timing on outcomes in trauma patients: a meta-analysis. *Injury.* 2017;48(4):866–873.
8. Meng L, Wang C, Li J, Zhang J. Early vs late tracheostomy in critically ill patients: a systematic review and meta-analysis. *Clin Respir J.* 2016;10(6):684–692.
9. Herritt B, Chaudhuri D, Thavorn K, Kubelik D, Kyeremanteng K. Early vs. late tracheostomy in intensive care settings: impact on ICU and hospital costs. *J Crit Care.* 2018;44:285–288.
10. Apfelbaum JL, Hagberg CA, Caplan RA, et al. American Society of Anesthesiologists Task Force on Management of the Difficult Airway. Practice guidelines for management of the difficult airway: an updated report by the American Society of Anesthesiologists Task Force on Management of the Difficult Airway. *Anesthesiology.* 2013;118(2):251–270.
11. Goldenberg D, Golz A, Netzer A, Joachims HZ. Tracheotomy: changing indications and a review of 1,130 cases. *J Otolaryngol.* 2002;31(4):211–215.
12. Bjork VO. Partial resection of the only remaining lung with the aid of respirator treatment. *J Thorac Cardiovasc Surg.* 1960;39:179–188.
13. Gigliotti J, Cheung G, Suhaym O, Agnihotram RV, El-Hakim M, Makhoul N. Nasotracheal intubation: the preferred airway in oral cavity microvascular reconstructive surgery? *J Oral Maxillofac Surg.* 2018;76(10):2231–2240.
14. Schroeder AA. Cricothyroidotomy: when, why, and why not? *Am J Otolaryngol.* 2000;21(3):195–201.
15. Shelden CH, Pudenz RH, Freshwater DB, Crue BL. A new method for tracheotomy. *J Neurosurg.* 1955;12(4):428–431.
16. Seldinger SI. Catheter replacement of the needle in percutaneous arteriography; a new technique. *Acta Radiol Suppl.* 1953;39(5):368–376.
17. Ciaglia P, Firsching R, Syniec C. Elective percutaneous dilatational tracheostomy. a new simple bedside procedure; preliminary report. *Chest.* 1985;87(6):715–719.
18. Freeman BD, Isabella K, Lin N, Buchman TG. A meta-analysis of prospective trials comparing percutaneous and surgical tracheostomy in critically ill patients. *Chest.* 2000;118(5):1412–1418.
19. Silvester W, Goldsmith D, Uchino S, et al. Percutaneous versus surgical tracheostomy: a randomized controlled study with long-term follow-up. *Crit Care Med.* 2006;34(8):2145–2152.
20. Dempsey GA, Morton B, Hammell C, Williams LT, Tudur Smith C, Jones T. Long-term outcome following tracheostomy in critical care: a systematic review. *Crit Care Med.* 2016;44(3):617–628.
21. Delaney A, Bagshaw SM, Nalos M. Percutaneous dilatational tracheostomy versus surgical tracheostomy in critically ill patients: a systematic review and meta-analysis. *Crit Care.* 2006;10(2):R55.

22. Warren WH. Percutaneous dilational tracheostomy: a note of caution. *Crit Care Med.* 2000;28(5):1664–1665.
23. Trottier SJ, Hazard PB, Sakabu SA, et al. Posterior tracheal wall perforation during percutaneous dilational tracheostomy: an investigation into its mechanism and prevention. *Chest.* 1999;115(5):1383–1389.
24. Seder DB, Lee K, Rahman C, et al. Safety and feasibility of percutaneous tracheostomy performed by neurointensivists. *Neurocrit Care.* 2009;10(3):264–268.
25. Chew JY, Cantrell RW. Tracheostomy. Complications and their management. *Arch Otolaryngol.* 1972;96(6):538–545.
26. Thompson JW, Colin W, Snowden T, Hengesteg A, Stocks RM, Watson SP. Fire in the operating room during tracheostomy. *South Med J.* 1998;91(3):243–247.
27. Tykocinski M, Thomson P, Hooper R. Airway fire during tracheotomy. *ANZ J Surg.* 2006;76(3):195–197.
28. Goldenberg D, Ari EG, Golz A, Danino J, Netzer A, Joachims HZ. Tracheotomy complications: a retrospective study of 1130 cases. *Otolaryngol Head Neck Surg.* 2000;123(4):495–500.
29. Smith DK, Grillone GA, Fuleihan N. Use of postoperative chest x-ray after elective adult tracheotomy. *Otolaryngol Head Neck Surg.* 1999;120(6):848–851.
30. Jones JW, Reynolds M, Hewitt RL, Drapanas T. Tracheo-innominate artery erosion: successful surgical management of a devastating complication. *Ann Surg.* 1976;184(2):194–204.
31. Oshinsky AE, Rubin JS, Gwozdz CS. The anatomical basis for post-tracheotomy innominate artery rupture. *Laryngoscope.* 1988;98(10):1061–1064.
32. Utley JR, Singer MM, Roe BB, Fraser DG, Dedo HH. Definitive management of innominate artery hemorrhage complicating tracheostomy. *J Am Med Assoc.* 1972;220(4):577–579.
33. Guimaraes M, Schönholz C, Phifer T, D'Agostino H. Endovascular repair of a tracheoinnominate fistula with a stent graft. *Vascular.* 2008;16(5):287–290.
34. Hafez A, Couraud L, Velly JF, Bruneteau A. Late cataclysmic hemorrhage from the innominate artery after tracheostomy. *Thorac Cardiovasc Surg.* 1984;32(5):315–319.
35. Carr MM, Poje CP, Kingston L, Kielma D, Heard C. Complications in pediatric tracheostomies. *Laryngoscope.* 2001;111(11 Pt 1):1925–1928.
36. Dierks EJ. Tracheotomy: elective and emergent. *Oral Maxillofac Surg Clin North Am.* 2008;20(3):513–520.
37. Barlow DW, Weymuller EA Jr, Wood DE. Tracheotomy and the role of postoperative chest radiography in adult patients. *Ann Otol Rhinol Laryngol.* 1994;103(9):665–668.

CHAPTER 111

Local Excision of Oral Malignancy

Brian Louis Ruggiero and Justine Moe

Armamentarium

#9 Molt periosteal elevator
#15 Scalpel blade
1% Lidocaine with 1:100,000 epinephrine
Adson-Beckman retractor
Appropriate sutures
Army-Navy retractor
Bipolar cautery
Cushing tissue forceps with teeth
Dingman mouth gag
Fibrillar collagen sheets
Fine curved hemostat
Flowable fibrin hemostatic matrix
Handheld Doppler probe
Local anesthetic with vasoconstrictor
McIndoe forceps
Malleable retractor
Marking pen
Molt mouth prop
Needle tip electrocautery
Reciprocating saw
Sagittal saw
Weider tongue retractor

History of the Procedure

Oral cavity cancers account for approximately 30% of all head and neck cancers, with squamous cell carcinoma as the most common histopathologic subtype. In 2020, oral and pharyngeal cancers represented 2.9% of new cancer cases and 1.8% of cancer deaths in the United States.[1,2] In 2018, oral cavity and lip cancers comprised 2.0% of new cancers and 1.9% of cancer deaths worldwide.[3]

While tobacco-related cancers including oral cavity squamous cell carcinoma (OSCC) have decreased in the last decade in the developed world,[4] human papilloma virus (HPV)-related oropharyngeal cancer has increased during the same timeframe.[5,6] Treatment principles for HPV-positive and HPV-negative oropharyngeal cancers are considered elsewhere.

The workup and treatment of OSCC follows the National Cancer Center Network (NCCN) guidelines.[7] Surgical extirpation to cancer-free margins is the mainstay of therapy, with primary radiation considered for early OSCC in select cases. Adjuvant radiation with or without systemic therapy is indicated for advanced stage disease and disease with adverse features.[7]

This chapter focuses primarily on the ablative surgical techniques for OSCC. While the extent of ablative surgery should be guided by oncologic principles rather than reconstructive considerations, the reconstructive plan needs to be considered prior to surgery such that the ablative surgery does not preclude a successful reconstruction. For example, target vessels should be preserved during neck dissection for planned free flap reconstruction, and incisions should be planned to incorporate planned local flap reconstruction.

Indications for the Use of the Procedure

OSCC can arise in the following subsites: tongue, floor of mouth, buccal mucosa, retromolar trigone, hard palate, gingiva/alveolar ridge, and lip (Fig. 111.1). In the ablation of the primary tumor, it is critical that a margin of healthy tissue is taken around all structures with tumor and may include mucosa, skin, muscle, bone, and nerve. A tumor-free pathologic margin is an independent predictor of decreased local and regional recurrence and increased overall survival.[5,6]

Clinically apparent neck disease (enlarged lymph nodes on clinical exam, or enlarged, morphologically abnormal, or necrotic lymph nodes on radiographic exam) warrants therapeutic neck dissection at the time of ablative surgery. The reported rate of occult nodal metastasis varies with the stage of disease and ranges from 20% to 44%.[8] Patients with T2 to T4a OSCC with a clinically negative neck should undergo elective neck dissection due to a high risk of occult nodal metastasis.[9] In T1N0 OSCC, elective neck dissection based on pathologic features (e.g., depth of invasion, perineural invasion) or sentinel lymph node biopsy can add a prognostic and therapeutic benefit for this subgroup of patients.[8,10]

Limitations and Contraindications

Postoperative complications in ablative surgery of OSCC vary per oral cavity subsite (Table 111.1). Very advanced OSCC including unresectable primary tumor (T4b), unresectable nodal disease, and distant metastasis (M1) at presentation should be considered for clinical trial enrollment and are treated with systemic therapy, radiation therapy, or supportive care. Additional relative contraindications to surgical treatment of OSCC include a high risk of surgical morbidity, and a patient systemically unfit for general anesthesia or surgery.

Margin Selection and Assessment

Surgical resection of oral cavity cancers is historically well studied with the overwhelming consensus amongst surgeons being that sufficient local control of the primary tumor is the single most important factor in long term survival.[11] Nevertheless, there is no universal agreement on what are considered adequate margins. Further complicating matters is the common use of vague terms like "close margin" and "near close margin," which only serve to create more ambiguity.[12]

For mucosal cancers, the lesion is often visible on gross examination, allowing for an adequate cuff of tumor-free tissue, or gross margins, to be excised. Unfortunately, there is no wealth of retrospective or prospective data analyzing these macroscopic margins, though a minimum 10 mm from the discernable tumor edge based on palpation and/or visual inspection is commonly practiced.

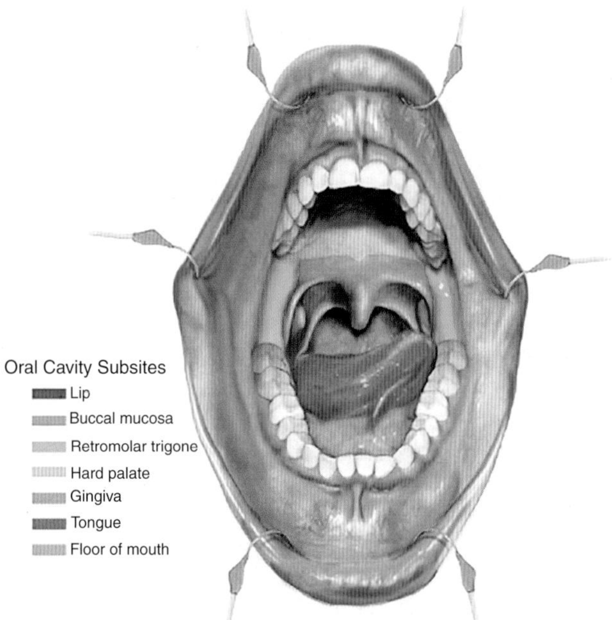

Figure 111.1 Oral cavity subsites.

Even with acceptable tumor visualization, this approach can be inconsistent. The surrounding mucosa may be easily stretched and distorted, leading to inadequate margins after resection.[13] Furthermore, the margin deep to the lesion is rarely measured but instead assessed by palpation and gross examination alone.[14]

There is, however, good data regarding pathologic/microscopic margins. It has been shown that negative pathologic margins >7.0 mm are associated with better local disease control, though most institutions/surgeons consider pathologic margins >5.0 mm to be adequate.[15,16] The degree of tissue shrinkage following excision and fixation can be quite significant and should always be considered by the surgeon. When excising the lesion, a gross margin of approximately 1 cm is therefore recommended to account for the tissue shrinking and has become a widely accepted standard of care.[16]

Intraoperative pathologic analysis allows for margin analysis at the time of surgery and immediate margin revision if necessary. Two methods of specimen sectioning for intraoperative analysis can be utilized, each with advantages and disadvantages. The radial method involves sectioning the specimen perpendicular to the margin such that both the tumor and tumor-free tissue can be analyzed in relationship to the margin. This allows for the distance between tumor and margin to be measured, providing the surgeon with an objective and measurable standard. In this method, however, only a small sample of the margin is examined. While multiple radial sections may be taken to assess a greater proportion of the margins, this can be burdensome and increase intraoperative time. The shave method involves sectioning the specimen parallel to the margin, allowing for a greater surface area of the margin to be assessed. However, this method does not provide a measurement from the tumor to the margin, nor does it distinguish between a close and a negative margin.[14,16]

Following excision, the surgeon can base margins on the specimen itself (specimen-driven margins) or on the resection bed from which the specimen was taken (patient/defect driven margins). At present, intraoperative margins are predominantly assessed from a specimen-driven approach; however, there are many circumstances where a combination of these techniques may be employed. These include complex resections, positive margins requiring revision, concern for perineural involvement, and others.[13]

Table 111.1 Commonly Encountered Structures and Postoperative Complications in Excision of an Oral Malignancy

Site	Commonly Encountered Structures	Postoperative Complications
Buccal mucosa	Stensen duct and buccal branch of facial nerve	Trismus, sialocele, facial palsy
Maxilla/palate	Maxillary sinus, greater palantine artery	Oral-antral fistula, hypernasal speech, velopharyngeal incompetence
Mandible/retromolar trigone	Lingual and inferior alveolar nerves	Trismus, neurosensory deficits
Tongue/floor of the mouth	Lingual nerve, Wharton duct	Neurosensory deficits, dysarthria, oral phase dysphagia
Lip/labial mucosa	Labial arteries	Sialorrhea, labial incompetence, microstomia, dysarthria

TECHNIQUE

Patients diagnosed with OSCC undergo workup per NCCN guidelines,[17] including history and physical examination, incisional biopsy, fiberoptic pharyngoscopy/laryngoscopy, contrast-enhanced computed tomography or magnetic resonance imaging of the head and neck, chest imaging, possible positron emission tomography, possible panendoscopy (see Chapter 96), dental evaluation, speech and swallow evaluation, and nutritional evaluation.

Resection of an OSCC is best performed under general anesthesia to allow for patient comfort, adequate access and retraction, and airway protection. Excision under local anesthesia in a clinic setting may be considered for small T1N0 lesions; however, the need for possible margin revision and possible neck dissection pending the final pathologic report and margin assessment must be strongly considered. Infiltration of local anesthetic with a vasoconstrictor can assist with hemostasis during the tumor resection, but it can distort tissue planes.

Site-Specific Surgical Management And Local Reconstruction Options: Buccal Mucosa

ALTERNATIVE TECHNIQUE

STEP 1: Marking

A marking pen or needle tip cautery is used to draw a planned mucosal incision with 1-cm circumferential margins from the visible and palpable tumor. If the planned resection involves the Stensen duct, a sialodochoplasty may be necessary in reconstruction. Cannulation with a lacrimal probe can assist with identification of the duct during resection (Fig. 111.2).

STEP 2: Mucosal Incision

Incision with a blade or needle tip electrocautery along the marked line is completed to underlying connective tissue. Care is taken not to handle the mucosal edge of the specimen aggressively because this may interfere with the histopathologic analysis of margins.

STEP 3: Circumferential Resection

Gentle opposite traction of the wound edges with a toothed forceps is used to visualize the deep margin. Needle tip electrocautery is used to deepen the incision through connective tissue and the buccinator muscle, remaining at least 1 cm from the tumor's edge. Using digital palpation to assess gross margins, the surgeon should frequently check that the incision is not deviating toward the tumor, both in circumference and depth.

STEP 4: Deep Resection

The depth of resection is planned based on preoperative imaging and bimanual palpation of gross tumor. If the overlying cheek skin is fixed to the tumor, or closer than 5 mm to the deep margin of the tumor, it should be excised en bloc with the intraoral buccal mucosal component. If a surgical plane exists between the tumor and cheek skin, a full-thickness resection may not be necessary. In such cases, it is important to be aware of the depth of the tumor so as to remove it successfully with oncologically sound margins. This often involves resection of the underlying buccinator muscle and may include subcutaneous fat with the specimen. Prior to removal from the field, the tumor is oriented with a suture (e.g., long suture anterior, short suture superior).

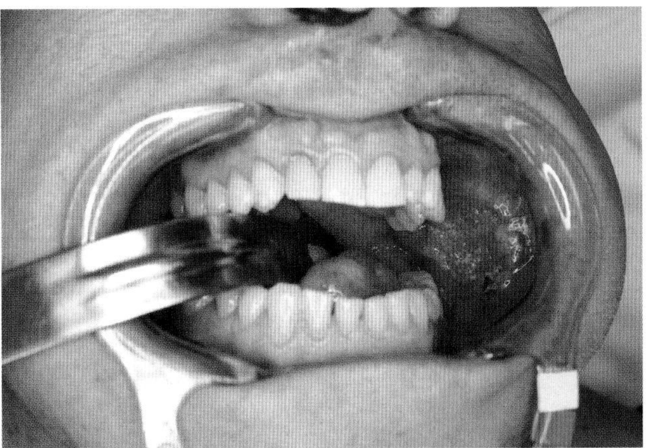

Figure 111.2 Squamous cell carcinoma of the left buccal mucosa involving the Stenson duct.

ALTERNATIVE TECHNIQUE-*cont'd*

STEP 5: Intraoperative Margin Evaluation
Intraoperative margin evaluation may be completed from the specimen or tumor bed as discussed above. Specimen-driven margins are taken after orientation by the surgeon to the pathologist and may be radial or shave margins. For tumor bed margins, Metzenbaum scissors are used to excise a thin circumferential mucosal margin, in addition to a deep margin to be evaluated by the pathologist. These should not be excised with electrocautery as cautery artifact reduces the accuracy of histologic analysis. If a margin returns "close" or positive for tumor, wider resection may be necessary.

STEP 6: Reconstruction
Small resection beds with viable underlying muscle may be amenable to healing by secondary intention or skin graft reconstruction. Larger, through-and-through, and composite defects may be reconstructed with local flap (e.g., buccal fat advancement flap), regional (e.g., pectoralis major myocutaneous flap), or free flaps (e.g., anterolateral thigh, radial forearm free flap). The buccal fat pad flap is an excellent local option for reconstructing small buccal mucosa defects, given its proximity to the defect, ease of harvest, hearty blood supply, and minimal donor site morbidity.[18]

ALTERNATIVE TECHNIQUE 1: Mandibular Gingiva/Retromolar Trigone

OSCC involving the mandibular gingival and retromolar trigone can invade the mandible secondarily. Patterns of mandibular invasion include through periosteum, foramina, attached mucosa, cortical bone defects in the edentulous mandible, and periodontal ligament in the dentate mandible.[19–21] Mandibular involvement should be suspected in gingival SCC even in the absence of gross bone involvement clinically or on imaging. For mandibular SCC with early bone involvement and in non-atrophic mandibles, a marginal mandibulectomy may be satisfactory to achieve negative margins while maintaining mandibular continuity. Segmental mandibulectomy is necessary for gross invasion of cancellous bone.[22]

STEP 1: Marking
A marking pen or needle tip cautery is used to draw a planned mucosal incision with 1-cm circumferential margins from the visible and palpable tumor.

STEP 2: Mucosal Incision
Needle tip electrocautery is used to create a mucosal incision along the planned circumferential resection.

STEP 3: Circumferential Soft Tissue Resection
The surgeon should leave an adequate cuff of uninvolved tissue around the tumor and, if possible, leave the periosteum over intact bone of the mandible. If a marginal mandibulectomy is indicated, a periosteal incision should be made on the buccal and lingual aspects of the mandible where the osteotomy is planned. From this incision, it is important not to reflect periosteum and soft tissue toward the tumor because this would violate the surgical margins.

STEP 4: Osteotomy
Determination of the extent of bony resection should be made based preoperatively on clinical and radiographic examination. For OSCC arising from the mandibular gingiva or retromolar trigone with no or minimal bone involvement where 1 cm or greater of mandibular height is anticipated to be preserved, a marginal mandibulectomy with preservation of the inferior border of the mandible can be planned (Fig. 111.3A–C). When 5 mm of mandibular height is anticipated to be preserved with the bony resection, a marginal mandibulectomy and placement of a reconstruction plate can be planned. Tumors with significant bone involvement or with less than 1 cm bone height between the affected bone and inferior border of the mandible should be planned for a segmental mandibulectomy (Fig. 111.4A–E). For example, OSCC of the mandibular gingiva or retromolar trigone overlying a severely atrophic mandible without bone involvement often require segmental mandibulectomy. If alveolus and teeth are present, the surgeon should plan to extract teeth in the line of osteotomy or plan to create an interdental osteotomy during the marginal or segmental resection.

Subperiosteal exposure of the buccal and lingual aspects of the mandible along the path of the planned osteotomy is completed with a periosteal elevator. Subperiosteal dissection is completed away from the tumor for adequate access. For a marginal mandibulectomy, a reciprocating or sagittal saw is used to create a full-thickness osteotomy from posterior to anterior, preserving the inferior border of the mandible. The marginal mandibulectomy

ALTERNATIVE TECHNIQUE 1: Mandibular Gingiva/Retromolar Trigone—*cont'd*

osteotomy is most commonly performed through a transoral approach; rarely, however, a small stab cheek incision can be made to facilitate the posterior aspect of the osteotomy.[23] It is crucial to create a rounded osteotomy, with no sharp line angles, to reduce areas of concentrated tensile stress during mandibular function, which can predispose to fracture. For a segmental mandibulectomy, the posterior and anterior osteotomies are completed from the lateral aspect.

The mobilized mandibular segment is lateralized, and the medial soft tissue dissection is completed, preserving a cuff of normal tissue around the tumor. If the lingual nerve can be preserved, it is dissected along its course and medialized.

In large retromolar trigone lesions, the ablative surgery may include the maxillary tuberosity and the adjacent buccal mucosa. In these cases, a marginal mandibulectomy and marginal maxillectomy may be necessary (Fig. 111.5).

STEP 5: Intraoperative Margin Evaluation

Circumferential mucosal margins can be analyzed as discussed previously. Bone margins should be evaluated via fresh-frozen or imprint cytologic analysis of curetted bone marrow from the native mandible.[24] The intraoperative identification of a positive bone invasion requires additional bone margins to be taken and may include the conversion of a marginal mandibulectomy to a segmental mandibulectomy.

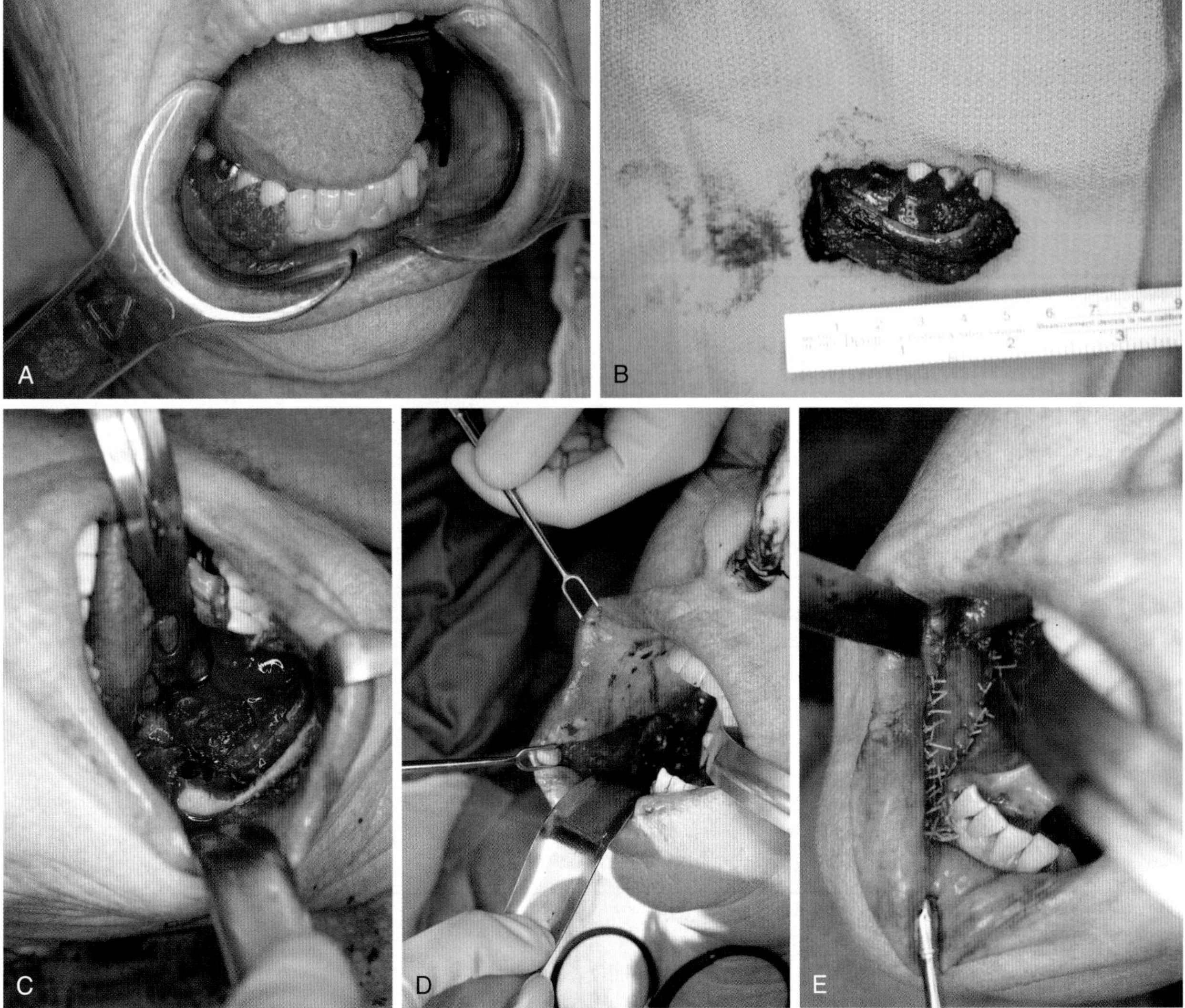

Figure 111.3 **A,** Squamous cell carcinoma of the right mandibular gingiva. **B,** Excised specimen. **C,** Marginal mandibulectomy. **D,** Planned soft tissue reconstruction with a facial artery myomucosal flap. **E,** Flap inset.

ALTERNATIVE TECHNIQUE 1: Mandibular Gingiva/Retromolar Trigone—*cont'd*

STEP 6: Reconstruction

Marginal mandibulectomy with a small soft tissue defect of the mandibular gingiva or retromolar trigone may be closed primarily. Larger soft tissue defects may require local flaps (e.g., buccal fat advancement flap, facial artery myomucosal flap) (Fig. 111.3D and E) or free flap (e.g., radial forearm fasciocutaneous flap). Split-thickness skin grafts or palatal gingival grafts can prevent the retraction of the mandibular vestibule and require immobilization with a wire-retained denture or surgical stent. If less than 1 cm of vertical bone height remains at the inferior border of the native mandible, prophylactic application of a reconstruction plate may be indicated to prevent fracture under function.

Segmental mandibulectomy necessitates regional or free flap reconstruction. Regional flaps (e.g., pectoralis major myocutaneous flap) allow for soft tissue reconstruction only, whereas free flap reconstruction allows for bony (e.g., fibula free flap) and/or soft tissue reconstruction (e.g., anterolateral thigh free flap) (Fig. 111.4F–I).

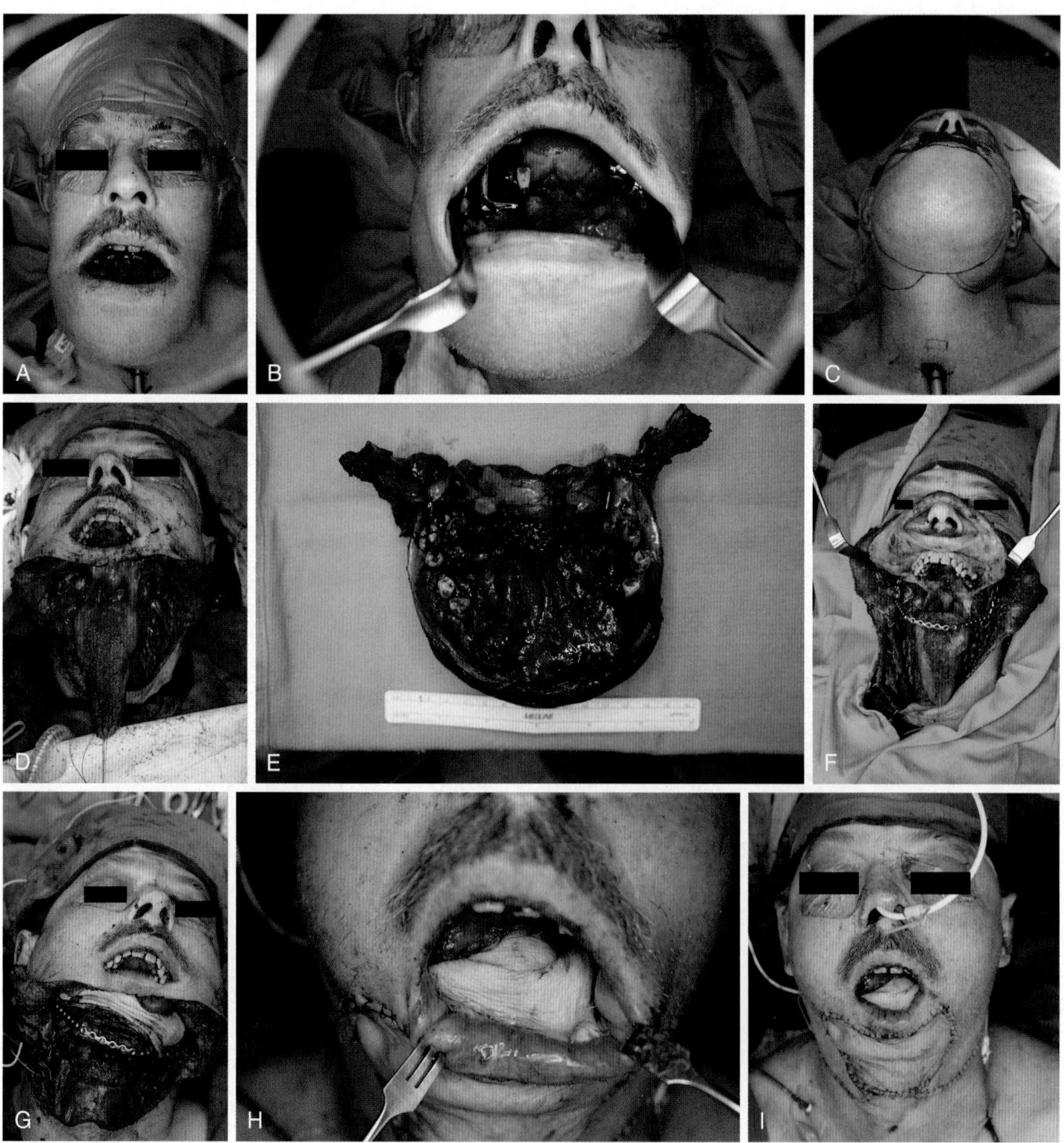

Figure 111.4 **A** and **B,** Squamous cell carcinoma of the bilateral mandible with involvement of the floor of mouth, ventral tongue, and chin. **C,** Planned resection with 1-cm skin margins. **D,** Composite resection including segmental mandibulectomy from mandibular ramus to ramus. **E,** Resection specimen. **F** and **G,** Mandibular reconstruction with a mandibular reconstruction plate and fibular free flap. **H,** Fibula skin paddle reconstruction of the intraoral mucosal defect. **I,** Reconstruction of the skin defect with a radial forearm free flap.

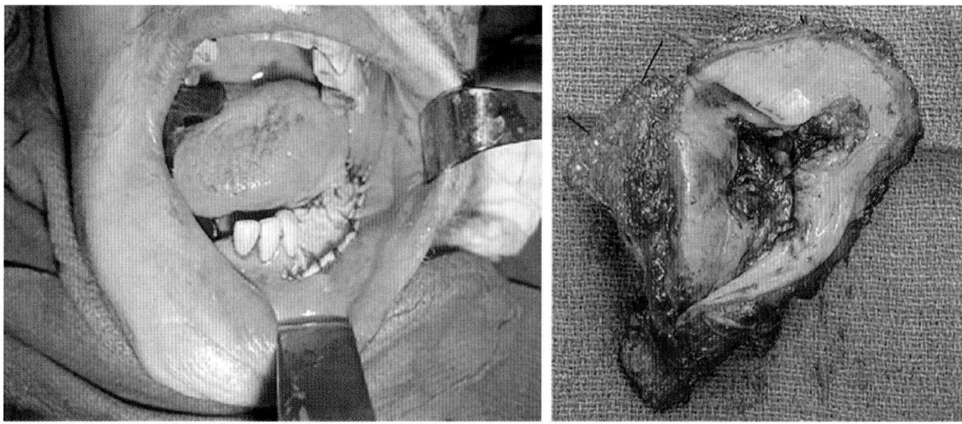

Figure 111.5 Composite resection of retromolar trigone, mandibular alveolus, maxillary alveolus, and buccal mucosa.

ALTERNATIVE TECHNIQUE 2: Maxillary Gingiva/Palate

OSCC involving the maxillary gingiva can invade the maxilla secondarily, and adequate resection of maxillary gingival cancers usually requires resection of a portion of the underlying alveolar bone. Depending on the extent of disease, OSCC of the maxilla can involve the maxillary alveolus, palate, maxillary sinus, nasal cavity, orbit, ethmoid and sphenoid sinuses, and base of skull. The anticipated resection should be characterized using the Brown and Okay classification systems (Fig. 111.6).[25]

Approaches to the maxilla vary based on disease extent. Most Brown class I or II defects can be approached transorally. The midfacial degloving incision including sublabial and rhinoplasty incisions improves access to the bilateral anterior maxilla and paranasal sinuses. The Weber-Ferguson incision allows wide access to the entire maxilla and orbital floor. A lip split mandibulotomy improves access to tumors of the posterior maxilla with extension into the pterygoid plates or infratemporal fossa.[22]

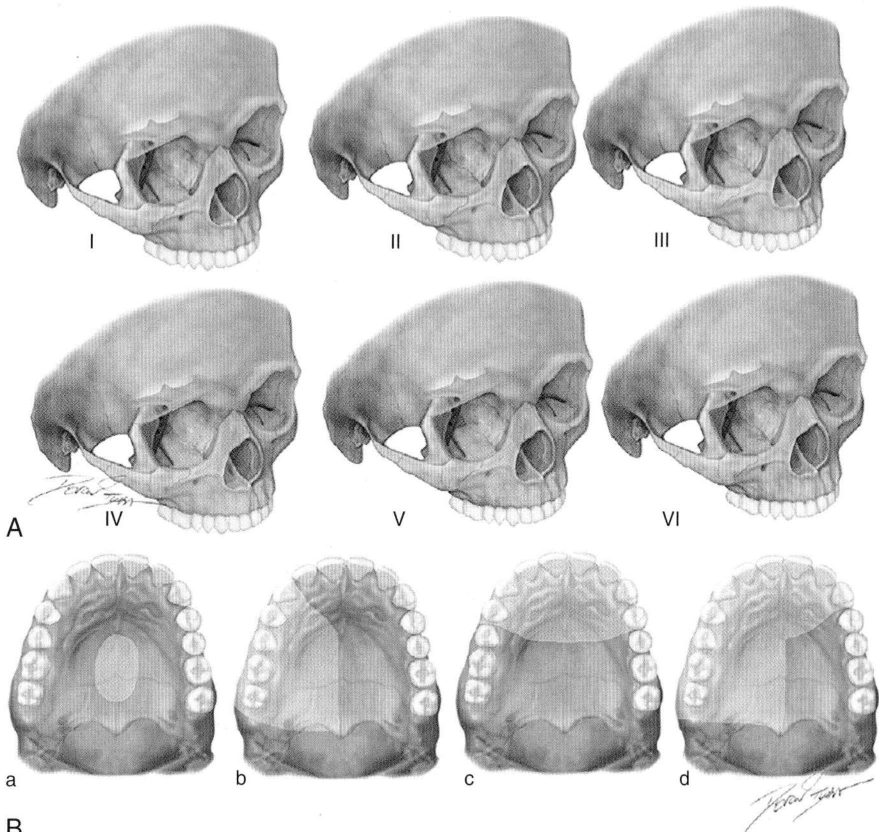

Figure 111.6 **A,** Vertical Component: Class I-VI; Class I- not involving oronasal/oroantral fistula; II- not involving orbital floor; III involving orbital floor without involving orbital contents; IV requiring orbital enucleation; V orbitomaxillary defects not involving alveolus; VI nasomaxillary defect. **B,** Horizontal component: a- palatal defect only; b-less than or equal to ½ unilateral; c- less than or equal to ½ bilateral; d- greater than ½ maxillectomy.

ALTERNATIVE TECHNIQUE 2: Maxillary Gingiva/Palate—*cont'd*

STEP 1: Marking

For lesions localized to the maxillary gingiva, a 1-cm circumferential margin is marked from visible and palpable tumor. Preoperative injection of an epinephrine-containing local anesthetic can assist in minimizing blood loss during the resective surgery (Fig. 111.7).

STEP 2: Mucosal Incision

Needle tip electrocautery is used to create a mucosal incision along the planned circumferential resection. This should be carried down through the periosteum to disease-free bone over the alveolus and palate. The buccal dissection may proceed superiorly in a supraperiosteal fashion until a safe distance from tumor has been achieved; then it is carried through the periosteum.

STEP 3: Circumferential Resection

On the buccal vestibular portions of the dissection, care should be taken to leave an adequate cuff of soft tissue around the tumor before approaching the maxilla. The alveolar and palatal incisions are carried to bone, and subperiosteal dissection is completed circumferentially to expose the planned osteotomy lines.

STEP 4: Osteotomy

With a reciprocating saw, osteotomies are created through the palate, alveolus, and lateral/anterior walls of the maxilla and lateral nasal wall. It is important to control the depth of saw penetration to protect the nasal mucosa and nasoendotracheal tube. If indicated, osteotomes are used along the pterygoid plates, lateral nasal wall, and nasal septum.

STEP 5: Intraoperative Margin Evaluation

Circumferential mucosal margins and bone margins can be analyzed as discussed previously.

STEP 6: Reconstruction

Reconstructive options for the maxilla vary, depending on the extent of the maxillary bony defect and soft tissue defect. Obturation has traditionally been the standard method of maxillary rehabilitation, with the primary goals of defect closure and separation of the oral cavity from the sinonasal cavities. Endosseous and zygomatic implants can facilitate retention and support of large obturators.

Smaller defects involving only soft tissue or small Brown class I defects are amenable to reconstruction with local flaps (e.g., buccal fat pad advancement, facial artery myomucosal flap). Brown class III, IV, and V defects often require free flap reconstruction and orbital reconstruction. Free tissue transfer allows for primary reconstruction, with fibula free flaps and deep circumflex iliac artery free flaps providing bone stock for dental rehabilitation with endosseous implants. Ablative defects involving the soft palate may also require free flap reconstruction (e.g., radial forearm free flap), as obturator reconstruction alone is not well tolerated.

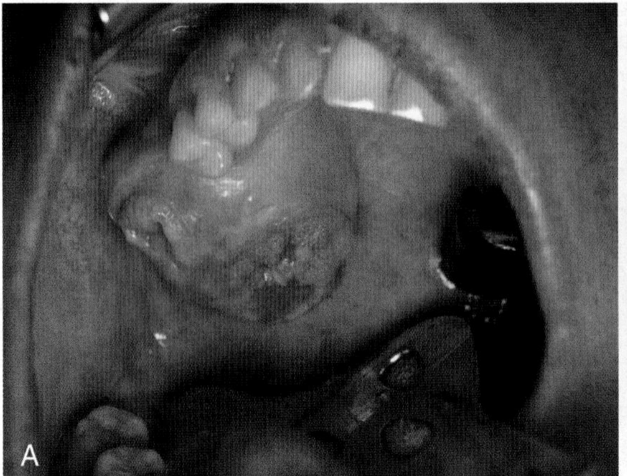

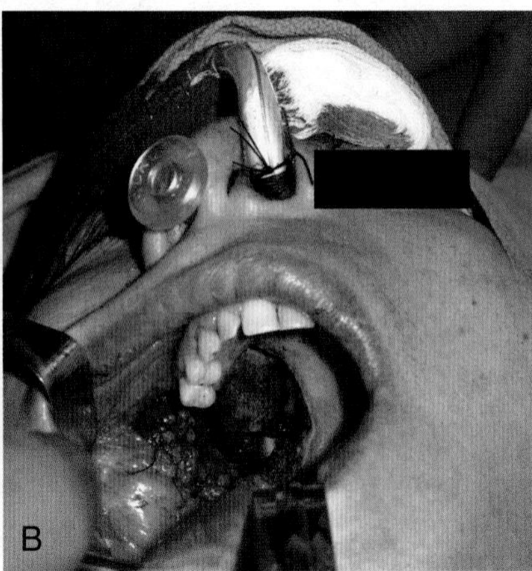

Figure 111.7 **A,** Carcinoma ex-pleomorphic adenoma of the hard palate. **B,** Ablative defect involving the hard palate and maxillary alveolus. The buccal fat pad was mobilized to provide bulk to the lateral soft palate and to improve the seal for the surgical obturator.

Option 1: Mandibulotomy Approach

The transoral approach can provide limited access for oncologic resection of tumors of the oropharynx, posterior maxilla, infratemporal and parapharyngeal spaces. In these cases, the midline or paramedian mandibulotomy can improve access for oncologic resection and reconstruction.

In the midline mandibulotomy, a full-thickness vertical incision through the midline lower lip is designed and carried along midline through the chin or laterally around the chin. Incisions are made in a full-thickness fashion, through periosteum and onto bone to expose the anterior mandible. The mandibulotomy is designed with a vertical osteotomy at or lateral to midline extending superiorly through the interproximal region between adjacent teeth or through an extraction site of an incisor. The osteotomy is planned anterior to the mental foramen in a stepped fashion. Prior to completing the osteotomy, one or two 4-hole miniplates are adapted to the anterior mandible at the site of the osteotomy and screw fixation holes are predrilled to allow ease of fixation and maintenance of dental occlusion. The mandibulotomy is then completed with a reciprocating saw (Fig. 111.8).

The mandibular segments are lateralized by separating the bony segments from the lingual mucoperiosteum and mylohyoid muscle, stripping attachments as necessary for adequate exposure.[26]

Option 2: Weber-Ferguson Approach

The Weber-Ferguson approach improves surgical access to tumors involving the maxilla, paranasal sinuses, orbit, and zygoma. The incision is designed with a vertical subnasal incision below the columella in the midline and extending inferiorly through the vermilion of the lip. Alternatively, this vertical incision can be made along ipsilateral philtral column with small steps at 90-degree angles in an effort to prevent future scar contracture.

At the superior extent of the subnasal incision, the incision extends 90 degrees laterally, 1 to 2 mm below the base of the nose, around the alar base, and then superiorly within the nasofacial sulcus to the level of the medial canthus. Depending on the involvement of the orbit or lateral maxilla, the incision may be extended laterally below the eyelid via a subciliary, subtarsal, or infraorbital incision or superiorly toward the ipsilateral brow. An upper eyelid extension is designed if orbital involvement is anticipated (Fig. 111.9A).

The cutaneous incision is carried in a full-thickness fashion through the upper lip and made continuous with an intraoral incision in the ipsilateral mucobuccal fold extending posteriorly to the maxillary tuberosity. The intraoral incision can be carried posteriorly within the gingival sulcus to preserve the

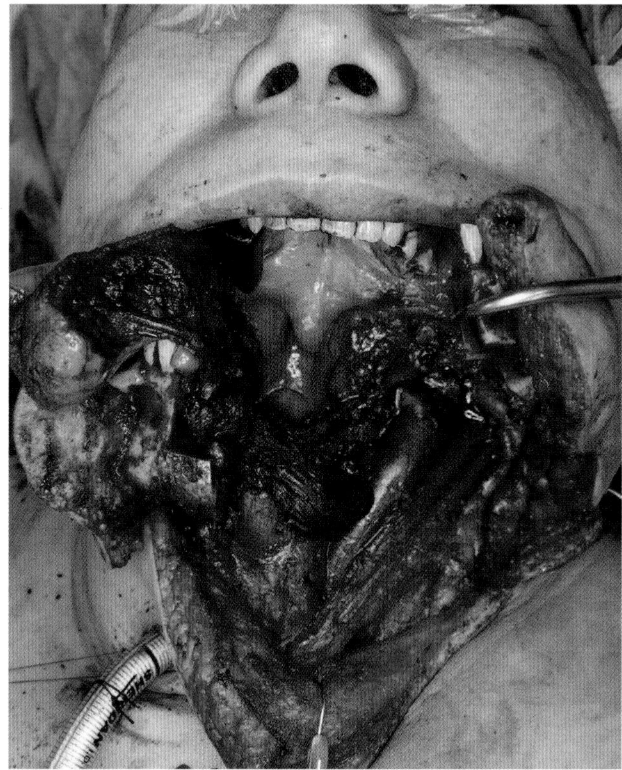

Figure 111.8 Mandibulotomy approach for base of tongue tumor.

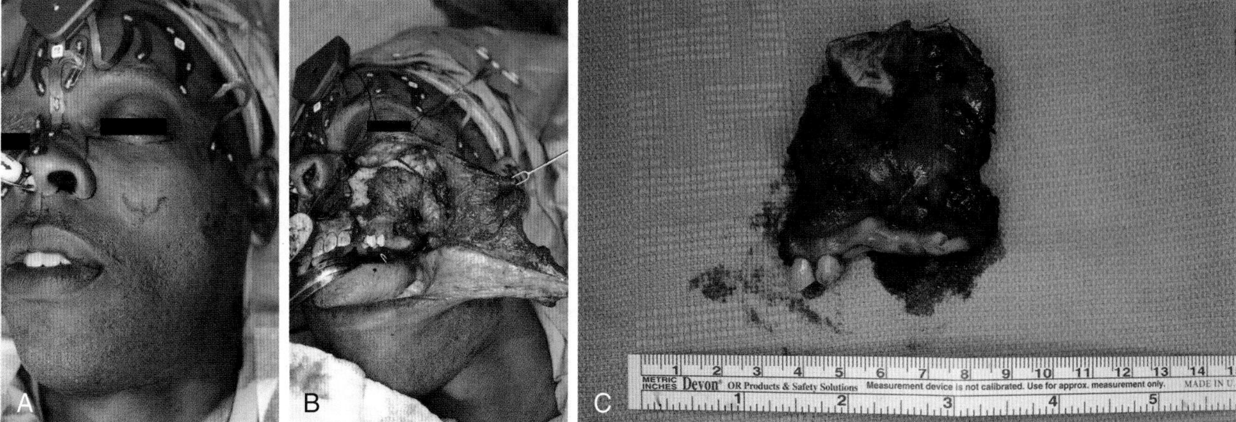

Figure 111.9 **A,** Weber-Ferguson incision design for excision of a maxillary ameloblastoma. **B,** Exposure of the inferior orbital rim, maxilla, and zygoma utilizing the Weber-Ferguson approach and osteotomies completed. **C,** Resected specimen.

keratinized gingiva if oncologically sound. Finally, the flap is then lateralized in a supra- or subperiosteal plane along the lateral maxilla, depending on the extent of the tumor involvement (Fig. 111.9B).

Option 3: Midface Degloving Approach

The midface degloving approach can provide greater access to tumors of the maxilla and paranasal sinuses below the level of the inferior orbital rim as compared with the transoral approach. The midface degloving approach utilizes endonasal and transoral incisions, circumventing the need for cutaneous incision, and therefore allowing a favorable aesthetic outcome.

Bilateral circumferential endonasal incisions are made including a complete transfixation incision, bilateral intercartilaginous incisions, and bilateral circumvestibular incisions along the piriform aperture. Dissection in a subperichondral plane is carried superiorly to elevate the soft tissues from the dorsum of the nose and then continued subperiosteally at the inferior edge of the nasal bone.

Transorally, a maxillary vestibular incision from the first molar to opposite first molar is made. In a subperiosteal plane, the soft tissues are elevated off the maxilla. At the level of the piriform aperture, the vestibular incision can be connected to the intranasal incisions bilaterally. This approach allows the midface to be elevated superiorly up to the level of the infraorbital rim.

ALTERNATIVE TECHNIQUE 3: Tongue/Floor of the Mouth

STEP 1: Marking

A marking pen or needle tip cautery is used to mark a 1-cm mucosal margin circumferentially from the visible and palpable tumor. Preoperative imaging and bimanual palpation are used to estimate tumor depth. Careful inspection and thorough palpation of the lesion is especially important in the resection of tongue lesions given their propensity for extension into deeper tissues. Lesions of the lateral tongue should be carefully evaluated for extension to the ventral tongue and floor of mouth. Depending on the location of the tumor, tongue retraction via silk traction sutures and/or a penetrating towel clip can facilitate surgical access.

STEP 2: Mucosal Incision

Needle tip electrocautery is used to create a mucosal incision along the planned circumferential resection. In floor of the mouth lesions, this may or may not include the lingual mandibular periosteum.

STEP 3: Circumferential Resection

Frequent digital palpation is helpful in determining the depth of resection through intrinsic tongue muscle. If margins allow, the lingual nerve should be identified and preserved. Resection of a portion of the submandibular duct can require sialodochoplasty. The tumor is delivered and immediately oriented with marking sutures.

STEP 4: Intraoperative Margin Evaluation

Circumferential and deep margins are taken as described previously.

STEP 5: Reconstruction

Extensive defects of the tongue and floor of the mouth generally require volume replacement with a fasciocutaneous or myocutaneous free flap; however, several local options exist for small to moderate tongue defects (more than two-thirds of native tongue remaining). Healing by secondary intention has proven to be effective in superficial tongue and floor of the mouth defects. Split-thickness skin grafting, particularly in the floor of the mouth, can be successful if adequate immobility with a bolster dressing can be achieved. Lateral tongue defects can also be primarily closed with vertical mattress sutures. Normal tongue movement can result in partial dehiscence of primary wound closure, but such defects heal dependably by secondary intention. Posterior oral tongue defects can be reconstructed with sliding tongue flaps.[27]

ALTERNATIVE TECHNIQUE 4: Lip/Labial Mucosa

STEP 1: Marking

SCC of the lip is less aggressive with less tendency to recur as than OSCC, behaving more similarly to SCC of the skin. T1N0 lesions of the lip fair remarkably well following surgical excision, with a local recurrence of 1.5% and 5-year survival of >90%.[28,29] As such, 5-mm margins are generally accepted as safe during resection of lip cancers. However, it is important to estimate the depth of the lesion as larger lesions (i.e., >2 cm). Tumors that invade the subcutaneous tissues have a higher rate of recurrence, and 1 cm margins may be required.[30]

Oncologically sound incisions should be designed in consideration of an aesthetic reconstruction. Bulky or thick cancers of the labial mucosa may require a full-thickness resection including skin and mucosal margins. It is especially important to note the position of the white roll as precise reapproximation of the vermilion border is essential for an aesthetic outcome. For wedge excisions, described in more detail below, the apices should fall in the labiomental crease for excisions of the lower lip and in the nasolabial fold for lesions of the upper lip.

STEP 2: Superficial Incision

The marked incision is completed with a #15 scalpel blade through the skin and lip vermilion. The remainder of the mucosal incision is completed with a blade or needle tip electrocautery. In patients with lip cancers secondary to chronic sun exposure, actinic cheilitis may diffusely involve the lip vermilion. In cases of diffuse vermilion involvement, a vermilionectomy or "lip shave" may be indicated, in which the plane of dissection should remain submucosal with a small cuff of underlying connective tissue. Alternatives to a vermilionectomy for actinic cheilitis include laser ablation and nonsurgical therapies such as 5-fluorouracil and imiquimod.

STEP 3: Circumferential Resection

Most often, resections of lip cancers are full thickness with removal of both the overlying skin and underlying oral mucosa in a single specimen. Larger and more invasive lesions may infiltrate deeper tissues and require a composite resection to include underlying bone and periosteum. Additionally, if there is numbness or paraesthesia, the mental nerve should be partially resected and sent for frozen histopathologic analysis.

STEP 4: Intraoperative Margin Evaluation

Circumferential and deep margins are taken as described previously.

STEP 5: Reconstruction

Reconstruction of the lips is complex and challenging because of the unique texture of the tissues, sphincter and salivary dam function, the effect on speech and mastication, and the lips' central location on the face. Depending on the size, depth, and location of the lesion and subsequent defect, several reconstructive approaches have been described. Two key points in any primary closure of lip and labial mucosal defects are (1) the reapproximation of the orbicularis oris muscle to restore oral sphincter function, and (2) the closure of the intraoral component with a Z-plasty to minimize scar contracture and resultant notching of the lip (Fig. 111.10).

Lower lip defects are generally more amenable to closure due to the lack of philtral columns and the presence of more redundant tissue. Primary closure may be achieved if the medio-lateral length of the defect is less than one-fourth in the upper lip and one-third in the lower lip.[31] Wedge excision with primary closure is used frequently for smaller lip lesion, and may be designed as a simple V-shaped, a W-shaped, or a shield-shaped resection. For the V excision, oncologically sound margins should be marked on either side of the lesion and then a V-shaped incision should be planed such that the apex lies in the labiomental crease (lower lip) or nasolabial fold (upper lip). The W excision is similar to the V-shaped incision but with two vertical components that can be closed into an inverted Y allowing for wider excision as compared to the V-shaped excision. In the shield excision, the vertical components meet each other in an angled or curvilinear fashion at the apex of the incision. In cases of a vermilionectomy, the labial mucosa can be advanced to achieve primary closure (Fig. 111.11A–D).[32]

Larger lesions are not amenable to primary closure and require more complex reconstruction. The Abbe-Estlander, or lip switch flap, is a feasible option for defects involving one-half to two-thirds of a single lip. This involves wedge resection of the lesion and mirrored incision on the opposite lip that is the same vertical height and approximately 50% the width of the anticipated defect. The flap is then rotated and inset into the defect and the harvest site is closed primarily (Fig. 111.12A–C). This is a pedicled rotational flap based on the labial artery and care must be taken to identify this vessel during harvest. This technique requires a second stage at 2 weeks to divide the pedicle after the flap has taken.[33,34]

Full-thickness ablative defects involving the oral commissure can be reconstructed using a Zisser commissuroplasty, a combination wedge excision, and mucosal advancement flap. Vertical Burrow's triangles with incisions hidden in the nasolabial and mentolabial folds and a horizontal triangle are designed. The vertical triangles are excised down to but not including oral mucosa, and the horizontal triangle is deepithelialized. The flaps are ad-

ALTERNATIVE TECHNIQUE 4: Lip/Labial Mucosa—*cont'd*

vanced medially to create a neo-commissure, undermining the buccal mucosa, which is inset into the horizontal triangles (Figs. 111.13 and 111.14).

The Karapandzic flap allows for closure of defects that are up to 80% of the lip.[35] These are designed as either unilateral or bilateral partial thickness flaps paralleling the lip margin and continuing superiorly in a curvilinear fashion to lie withing the nasolabial fold. Branches of the facial artery and nerve should be carefully identified and preserved during the dissection. The flaps can then be advanced and closed primarily. Gillies and McGregor flaps are also used for larger defects involving one-half to two-thirds of the lip; however, these procedures involve denervation of the lip and are therefore not the primary choice for reconstruction in these instances.[32]

Defects greater than two-thirds or those resulting in complete removal of the lip and underlying tissue can be reconstructed with free tissue transfer, including the radial forearm free flap with palmaris longus tendon sling, anterolateral thigh free flap, and osteocutaneous flaps such as the fibula and scapula free flaps for composite defects. Free flap reconstruction of larger defects is discussed at length elsewhere.

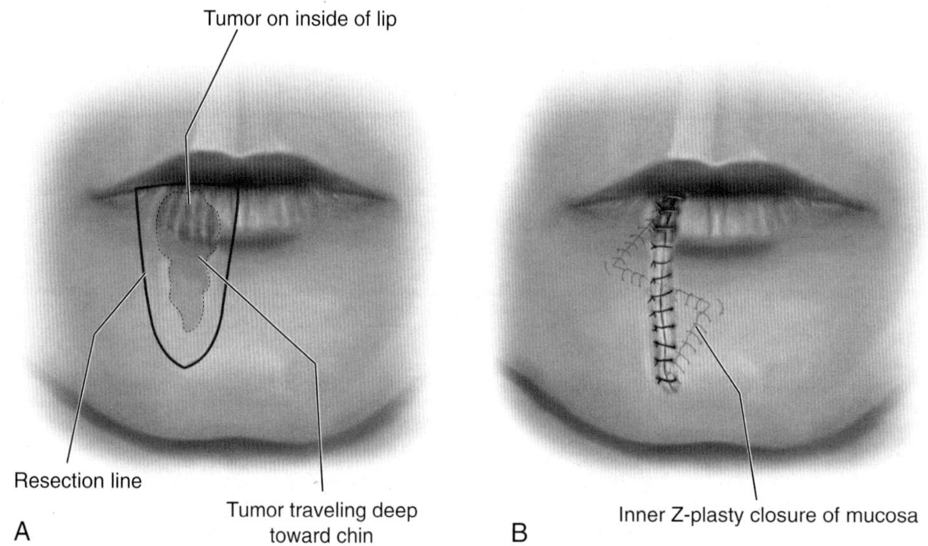

Figure 111.10 **A,** Wedge or V-type excision of a lower lip tumor. **B,** Primary lip closure with intraoral Z-plasty to minimize scar contracture.

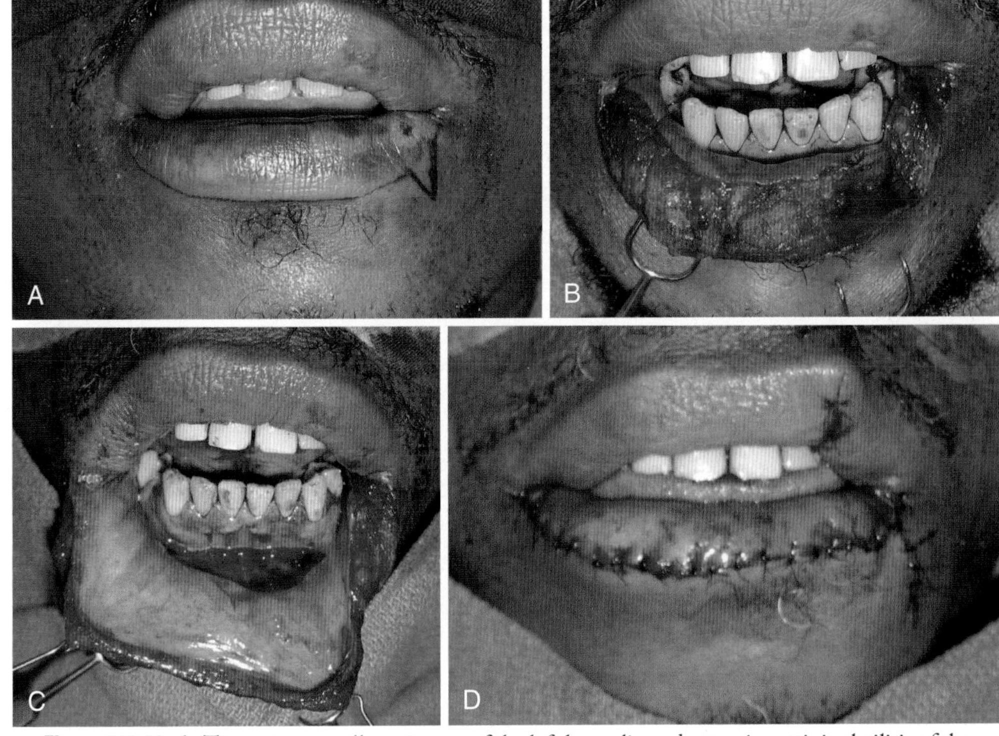

Figure 111.11 **A,** T1 squamous cell carcinoma of the left lower lip and extensive actinic cheilitis of the remaining lower lip, with markings for left lower lip wedge resection and total superficial lip shave. **B,** Ablative defect. **C,** Elevation of bipedicled labial mucosal flap. **D,** Flap inset with wedge closure of the left lateral lip defect.

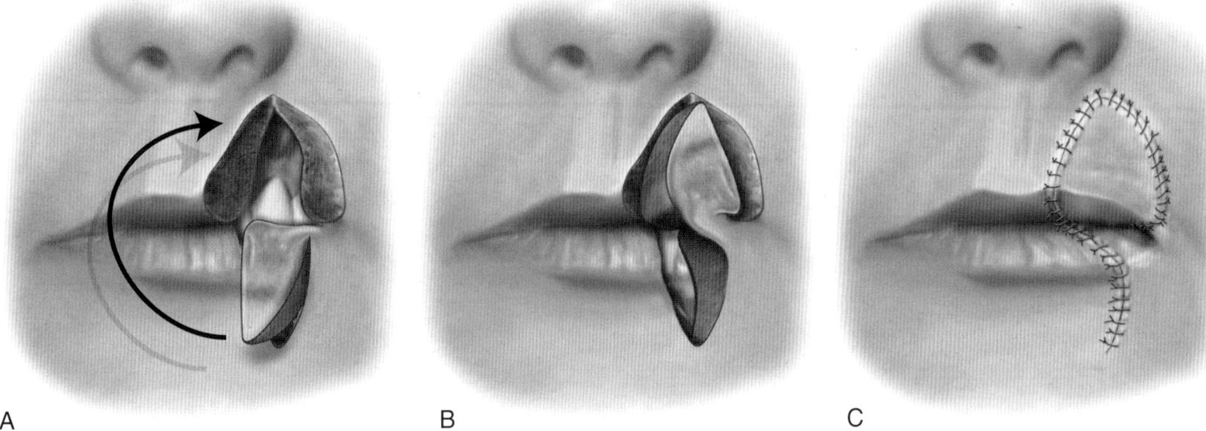

Figure 111.12 **A,** Elevation of an Estlander flap of the left lower lip. **B,** Flap inset into the defect of the left upper lip involving the commissure. **C,** Incision closure.

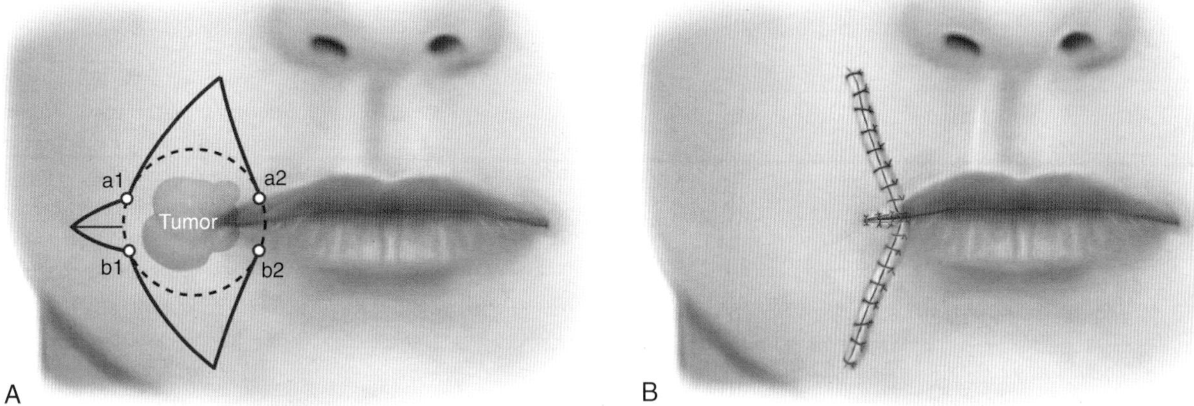

Figure 111.13 **A,** Zisser commissuroplasty design. **B,** Flap advancement and closure.

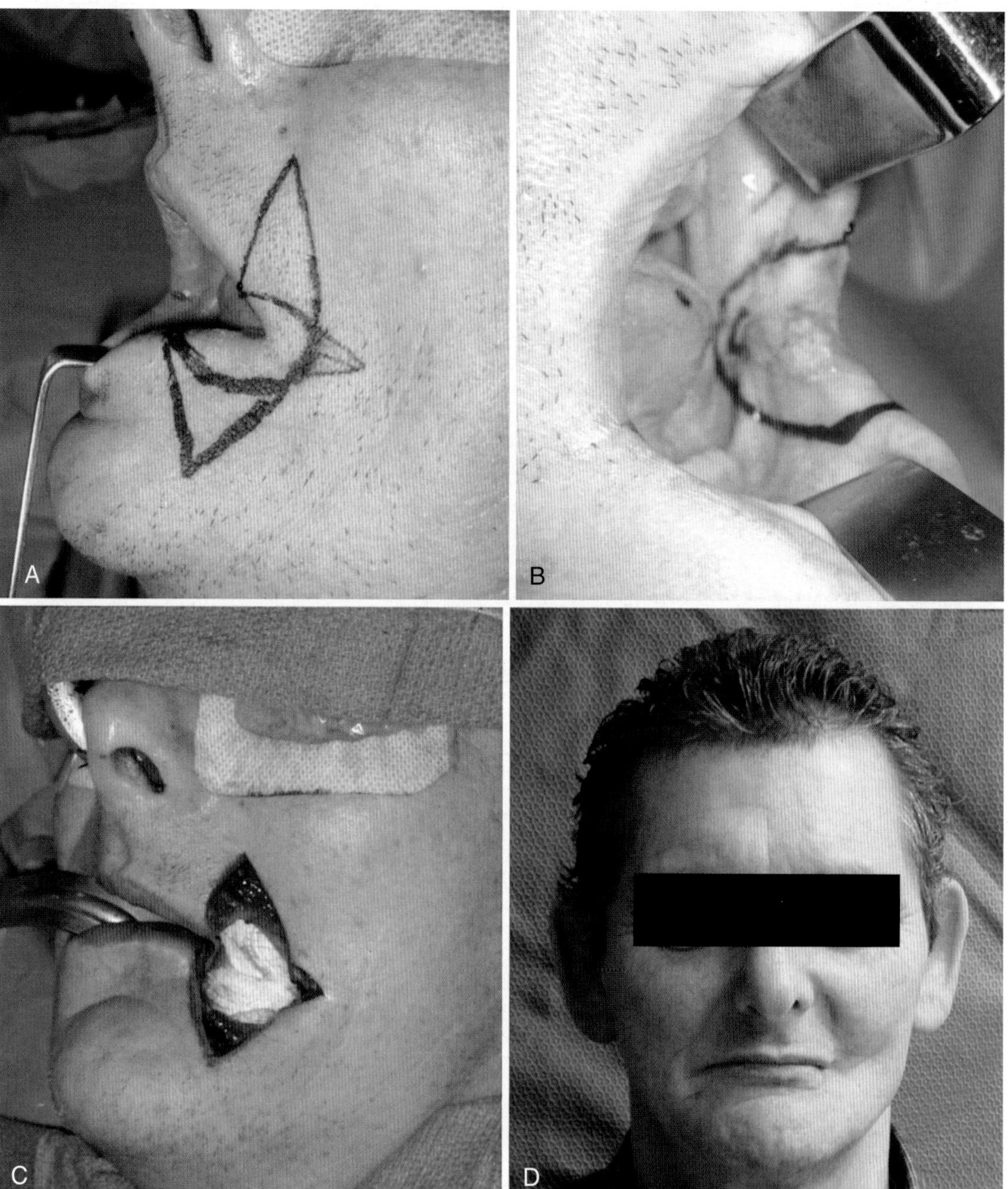

Figure 111.14 **A,** Zisser commissuroplasty design for a squamous cell carcinoma of the anterior buccal mucosa involving the oral commissure. **B,** Resection margins delineated along the buccal mucosa and lips. **C,** Ablative defect following creation of vertical and horizontal triangles. **D,** Flap advancement and closure.

Intraoperative Complications and Postoperative Considerations

Many complications in ablative surgery of OSCC can be prevented by thoughtful preoperative planning and careful surgical dissection; however, to obtain clear margins, sacrifice of functional structures may be necessary. Intraoperative and postoperative complications are specific to OSCC subsites and are mostly related to interruption of specific structures. Table 111.1 presents postoperative complications associated with commonly excised structures in the surgical treatment of OSCC.

The mainstay of surgical treatment for OSCC is sound oncologic margins without unnecessary resection of normal tissue. This concept is critically important as negative margins have consistently been associated with increased disease-free survival and increased overall survival in OSCC.[36] Negative margins on the first pass alone are paramount to successful treatment and are associated with a decreased local recurrence.[37]

References

1. Siegel RL, Miller KD, Jemal A. Cancer statistics, 2017. *CA Cancer J Clin.* 2017;67(1):7–30.
2. NIH. *Cancer Stat Facts Oral Cavity and Pharynx Cancer.* NIH; 2020. Available from: https://seer.cancer.gov/statfacts/html/oralcav.html.
3. Bray F, Ferlay J, Soerjomataram I, Siegel RL, Torre LA, Jemal A. Global cancer statistics 2018: GLOBOCAN estimates of incidence and mortality worldwide for 36 cancers in 185 countries. *CA Cancer J Clin.* 2018;68(6):394–424.
4. Chaturvedi AK, Anderson WF, Lortet-Tieulent J, et al. Worldwide trends in incidence rates for oral cavity and oropharyngeal cancers. *J Clin Oncol.* 2013;31(36):4550–4559.
5. Chaturvedi AK, Engels EA, Pfeiffer RM, et al. Human papillomavirus and rising oropharyngeal cancer incidence in the United States. *J Clin Oncol.* 2011;29(32):4294–4301.
6. Weatherspoon DJ, Chattopadhyay A, Boroumand S, Garcia I. Oral cavity and oropharyngeal cancer incidence trends and disparities in the United States: 2000-2010. *Cancer Epidemiol.* 2015;39(4):497–504.
7. NCCN. Head and Neck Cancers (Version 1.2021). Available from: https://www.nccn.org/professionals/physician_gls/pdf/head-and-neck.pdf.
8. Pentenero M, Gandolfo S, Carrozzo M. Importance of tumor thickness and depth of invasion in nodal involvement and prognosis of oral squamous cell carcinoma: a review of the literature. *Head Neck.* 2005;27(12):1080–1091.
9. D'Cruz AK, Vaish R, Kapre N, et al. Head and Neck Disease Management Group, Elective versus therapeutic neck dissection in node-negative oral cancer. *N Engl J Med.* 2015; 373(6):521–529.
10. Melchers LJ, Schuuring E, van Dijk BA, et al. Tumour infiltration depth ≥4 mm is an indication for an elective neck dissection in pT1cN0 oral squamous cell carcinoma. *Oral Oncol.* 2012;48(4):337–342.
11. Jesse RHSE, Sugarbaker EV. Squamous cell carcinoma of the oropharynx: why we fail. *Am J Surg.* 1976;132(4):435–438.
12. Hinni ML, Ferlito A, Brandwein-Gensler MS, et al. Surgical margins in head and neck cancer: a contemporary review. *Head Neck.* 2013;35(9):1362–1370.
13. Gooi ZAN. *Difficult Decisions in Head and Neck Oncologic Surgery*; 2019:23–39.
14. Shah AK, AK S. Postoperative pathologic assessment of surgical margins in oral cancer: a contemporary review. *J Oral Maxillofac Pathol.* 2018;22(1):78–85.
15. Liao CT, Chang JT, Wang HM, et al. Analysis of risk factors of predictive local tumor control in oral cavity cancer. *Ann Surg Oncol.* 2008;15(3):915–922.
16. Wenig BM. Intraoperative consultation (IOC) in mucosal lesions of the upper aerodigestive tract. *Head Neck Pathol.* 2008;2(2):131–144.
17. Network NCCN. *Head and Neck Cancers*; 2020:2.
18. Squaquara R, Kim Evans KF, Spanio di Spilimbergo S, Mardini S. Intraoral reconstruction using local and regional flaps. *Semin Plast Surg.* 2010;24(2):198–211.
19. McGregor AD, MacDonald DG. Patterns of spread of squamous cell carcinoma to the ramus of the mandible. *Head Neck.* 1993;15(5):440–444.
20. He Y, Zhang ZY, Zhu HG, Sader R, He J, Kovacs AF. Free fibula osteocutaneous flap for primary reconstruction of T3-T4 gingival carcinoma. *J Craniofac Surg.* 2010;21(2):301–305.
21. Pandey M, Rao LP, Das SR, Mathews A, Chacko EM, Naik BR. Patterns of mandibular invasion in oral squamous cell carcinoma of the mandibular region. *World J Surg Oncol.* 2007;5:12.
22. Moe JBA, Ward B. Surgical factors affecting outcomes in oral squamous cell carcinoma. In: Kademani D, ed. *Improving Outcomes in Oral Cancer.* Springer; 2020:43–63.
23. Hirsch DL, Dierks EJ. Use of a transbuccal technique for marginal mandibulectomy: a novel approach. *J Oral Maxillofac Surg.* 2007;65(9):1849–1851.
24. Yadav GS, Donoghue M, Tauro DP, Yadav A, Agarwal S. Intraoperative imprint evaluation of surgical margins in oral squamous cell carcinoma. *Acta Cytol.* 2013;57(1):75–83.
25. Brown JS, Shaw RJ. Reconstruction of the maxilla and midface: introducing a new classification. *Lancet Oncol.* 2010;11(10):1001–1008.
26. Spiro RHGF, Gerold FP, Strong EW. Mandibular "swing" approach for oral and oropharyngeal tumors. *Head Neck Surg.* 1981;3(5):371–378.
27. Lam DK, Cheng A, Berty KE, Schmidt BL. Sliding anterior hemitongue flap for posterior tongue defect reconstruction. *J Oral Maxillofac Surg.* 2012;70(10):2440–2444.
28. de Visscher JGAM, van den Elsaker K, Grond AJK, van der Wal JE, van der Waal I. Surgical treatment of squamous cell carcinoma of the lower lip: evaluation of long-term results and prognostic factors—a retrospective analysis of 184 patients. *J Oral Maxillofac Surg.* 1998;56(7):814–820.
29. Bhandari K, Wang DC, Li SC, et al. Primary cN0 lip squamous cell carcinoma and elective neck dissection: systematic review and meta-analysis. *Head Neck.* 2015;37(9):1392–1400.
30. Golubović M, Asanin B, Jelovac D, Petrović M, Antunović M. Correlation between disease progression and histopathologic criterions of the lip squamous cell carcinoma. *Vojnosanit Pregl.* 2010;67(1):19–24.
31. K C. Reconstruction of small- and medium-sized defects of the lower lip. *Am J Otolaryngol.* 1992;13:16–22.
32. Urbanek DBJ. In: Springer LC, ed. *Reconstruction Considerations Based on Size of Defect.* A K; 2014:59–78.
33. Abbe R. A new plastic operation for the relief of deformity due to double harelip. R A *Plast Reconstr Surg.* 1968;42(5):481–483.
34. J E. Eine Methode, aus der einen Lippe Substanzverluste der anderen zu Ersetzen. *Arch Klin Chir Arch Klin Chir.* 1872;14:622.
35. Closmann JJ, Pogrel MA, Schmidt BL. Reconstruction of perioral defects following resection for oral squamous cell carcinoma. *J Oral Maxillofac Surg.* 2006;64(3):367–374.
36. Kurita H, Nakanishi Y, Nishizawa R, et al. Impact of different surgical margin conditions on local recurrence of oral squamous cell carcinoma. *Oral Oncol.* 2010;46(11):814–817.
37. Ettl T, El-Gindi A, Hautmann M, et al. Positive frozen section margins predict local recurrence in R0-resected squamous cell carcinoma of the head and neck. *Oral Oncol.* 2016;55:17–23.

CHAPTER 112

Glossectomy

Allen C. Cheng and Jonathan James Jelmini

Armamentarium

2-0 Silk sutures
Shoulder roll or Mayfield adjustable horseshoe headrest
3-0 Polyglactin sutures
Allis clamps
Army-Navy retractors
Blake drains
Bite block or Molt mouth prop
Crile hemostats
Debakey or other tissue forceps
Electrocautery with spatula or needle tip
Harmonic scalpel
Gerald toothed forceps or other
Green retractors
Lahey clamps Langenbeck retractors
Mayo-Hegar needle drivers
Metzenbaum scissors
Nasal RAE tube or armored endotracheal tube and cuffed tracheostomy tube
Plastic cheek retractors
Skin staples
Surgical blades (#10 and 15 Bard-Parker)
Tenotomy scissors
Tissue dissectors (Dierks dissectors #1, 2, and 3 or other)
Tonsil clamp
Vein retractor
Vessel clips, small and medium
Yankauer suction
Hemostatic agents
Suction drains

History of the Procedure

Some of the earliest descriptions of tongue diseases and their remedies are found in the ancient Egyptian text, Papyrus Ebers, dating back to 1550 BC. The first surgical text describing tongue surgery was written by Indian surgeon Sushruta between 600 BC and 300 BC.[1] Hunerick, the king of the Vandals, removed the tongues of his enemies as early as 484 AD. Later, henchman of Ludwig IX improved upon the technique by using a hot iron to cauterize the tongue, thus reducing mortality. However, it was not until 1664 that Marchetti, Professor of Surgery in Padua, performed the first glossectomy for removal of tongue carcinoma.[2,3] Much later, D'Arcy Power, an English surgeon, described an alarming increase in "squamous" tongue cancer incidence in the late 19th century England. He astutely observed that its rise seemed to coincide with the increased prevalence of tobacco use, although the common thinking at that time linked tongue cancer to syphilis.[4]

By the 19th century, glossectomy became the procedure of choice when treating malignancies of the tongue. Bernhard von Langenbeck, Emil Theodor Kocher, Theodor Billroth, and their contemporaries utilized varying surgical approaches to remove tongue tumors.[3] George Crile and others incorporated Halstedian principles by combining glossectomy with radical neck dissection.[5] Although techniques for diagnosis, management of the neck, and reconstruction have evolved over the last 120 years, the primary treatment of malignancy of the tongue is still glossectomy.

Indications for the Glossectomy

Glossectomy is indicated for treatment of oral premalignant and malignant lesions of the tongue. The most common malignancy of the tongue is squamous cell carcinoma (SCC).

The treatment of premalignant tongue dysplasia is surgical. Several nonsurgical therapies have been studied, including topical agents and systemic medications. None of these have led to long-lasting resolution of oral dysplastic lesions.[6] Superficial partial glossectomy, taken just below mucosa with minimal 5 to 10-mm margins, decreases, but does not eliminate, the risk of dysplasia recurrence.[7] More importantly, it allows for pathologic review of the lesion and possible early identification of occult SCC.

SCC of the oral tongue is primarily treated by glossectomy. Radiotherapy as primary treatment has not been found to be as effective and has detrimental long-term side effects.[8,9]

Varied terminology has been used to describe glossectomy including partial glossectomy, hemiglossectomy, subtotal glossectomy, transoral glossectomy, total glossectomy, cuneiform glossectomy, and compartmental glossectomy. Some authors propose a more precise classification system for uniform and consistent documentation.[10] Regardless of classification, glossectomy to treat SCC usually includes removal of the tumor with a 1 to 1.5-cm margin of grossly normal tissue, with the ultimate goal of 5 mm of pathologically clear margins.

Compartmental glossectomy involves resection of the entire muscle compartment. Because it is more comprehensive, proponents of this approach argue that it leads to improved local control. However, it is a more invasive approach to glossectomy, and the data, albeit favorable, are limited to small patient cohorts at only a few institutions.[11,12] In larger tumors that invade deeply into the extrinsic tongue musculature, this method is practical and intuitive.

Radiotherapy with or without chemotherapy is used in the adjuvant setting when the tumor exhibits high risk pathologic features such as late stage (T4), bone invasion, lymph node metastasis, perineural invasion, lymphovascular invasion, close or positive margins, or extracapsular extension. .

For early-stage (T1 or T2) base of tongue (BOT) SCC, the advent of transoral robotic surgery (TORS) has allowed BOT partial glossectomy without open surgical approaches. TORS is indicated for BOT SCC tumors that do not extend into the vallecula, that are not deeply infiltrative, are well lateralized, and that the surgeon expects to be able to remove with negative margins. Review of outcomes from retrospective data from TORS for oropharynx SCC followed by adjuvant radiotherapy with or without chemotherapy has found comparable local and regional control of disease but with improved swallowing function after treatment.[13,14]

Other indications for glossectomy include the treatment of macroglossia secondary to various systemic illnesses and obstructive sleep apnea. The discussion of these techniques are beyond the scope of this chapter.

Limitations and Contraindications

The tongue is an enormously complex array of muscles essential to speech and swallowing, both of which are central aspects of daily living and social interaction. Consequently, the most challenging aspect and greatest limitation of treating SCC of the tongue with glossectomy is adequately restoring function. The current techniques available for tongue reconstruction are crude, relying on the functionality of the unresected, native tongue to maintain speech and swallowing.

The critical components of a functioning tongue, in order of importance, are mobility, anterior tip shape, size of the tongue, and sensation. Deficits following glossectomy vary based on the extent of the resection, the type of reconstruction, volume of reconstructed tongue, and postoperative tongue mobility.[15,16] Tumors requiring resection of less than 50% of its overall volume usually can preserve adequate speech and swallowing function.[17] Studies assessing quality of life after partial glossectomy have concluded short-term decline in speech and swallowing with an overall return to baseline by 1 year.[18] Tumors involving greater than 50% of the tongue and/or involve the floor of mouth benefit from microvascular free tissue transfer to preserve adequate tongue mobility.

BOT malignancy presents the surgeon with a difficult challenge in regards to access for both ablation and reconstruction. The development of TORS has afforded a less invasive approach to removal of smaller tumors (T1 and T2) of the BOT. Because disease control rates for TORS and chemoradiotherapy are similar to BOT SCC, the key factor in deciding between surgical and nonsurgical therapies as first-line treatment is the anticipated functional outcome.[19–21] BOT SCC that is likely to require adjuvant chemoradiotherapy should be considered for primary treatment with chemoradiotherapy, as the functional outcome is not likely to be improved with the addition of surgery, and disease control may be sufficient without surgery.

Larger tumors invading the BOT often require subtotal or total glossectomy where microvascular free tissue transfer is needed for reconstruction where more invasive access is required. Minimally invasive open techniques for access to the BOT through a floor of mouth window have been described in cadaveric studies. These, at least conceptionally, would allow for larger resections with reconstruction.[22]

Advances in reconstruction with microvascular free tissue transfer have led to improvements in reestablishing premorbid form and function. The radial forearm and anterior lateral thigh donor sites (discussed in other chapters) have become workhorses for reconstructing major defects providing adequate bulk to preserve swallowing and speech, even in patients requiring subtotal and total glossectomy.[23,24] Several studies have looked at which reconstructive option is superior with near equal efficacy.[23–25] Innervated free flaps that provide sensation have been described with high sensory fidelity. Although this should theoretically improve function, this has not been demonstrated and has largely been abandoned due to the risk of dysesthesias.[26,27]

Few contraindications exist for removal of invasive SCC via glossectomy, and they are limited to medical comorbidities that would place the patient at significant risk of death administered general anesthetic.

TECHNIQUE: Partial Glossectomy

STEP 1: Establishing a Secure Airway

Because of the risk of airway embarrassment from tongue swelling or hemorrhage, glossectomy is most often performed under general anesthesia. For T1 and smaller T2 oral tongue SCC, intubation with a nasal right-angle endotracheal (RAE) tube often suffices.

For larger SCC (T3 or T4) or when a free flap is planned, a tracheostomy is wise (see Chapter 110). Placement of an armored endotracheal tube in the tracheostomy during the procedure results in a lower profile than a tracheostomy tube and keeps the tubing away from the surgical field. The endotracheal tube is secured to the skin of the chest wall with 2-0 silk sutures in a mattress fashion (Fig.112.1A and B).

Continued

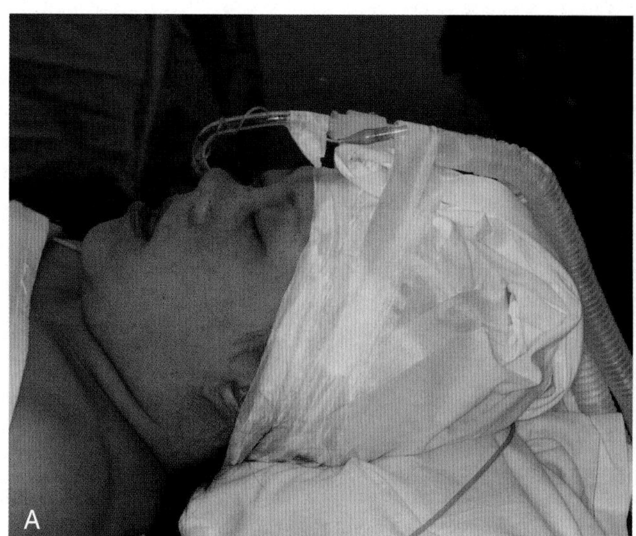

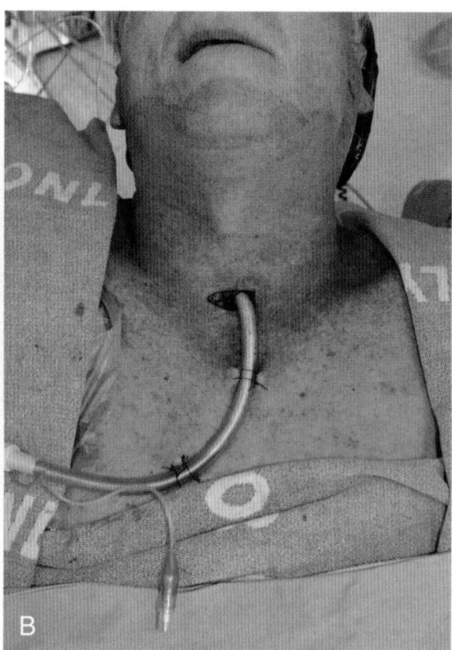

Figure 112.1 **A,** Secure the nasal right-angle endotracheal (RAE) tube to a head drape while taking pressure off the nasal ala. **B,** An armored endotracheal tube has a lower profile and keeps the circuit away from the surgical field during the operation.

TECHNIQUE: Partial Glossectomy—*cont'd*

STEP 2: Preparing the Patient

Position the patient supine with slight reverse Trendelenburg. Prepare and drape the patient in standard fashion.

We often use clear blue plastic cheek retractors to facilitate exposure of the oral cavity. These can be secured with 2-0 silk transbuccal sutures. We often forgo the use of these check retractors in tumors that are quite posterior as they may interfere with sufficient retraction of the ipsilateral cheek.

Place one or more 2-0 silk sutures passed through the tongue in a mattress fashion for tongue retraction. The retraction stitch should be well away from the planned resection margin. Place a bite block or Molt mouth prop on the contralateral side of the planned surgery (Fig. 112.2A–C).

STEP 3: Making the Mucosal Incision and Taking It to Depth

Carefully examine the tumor visually and with bimanual palpation to determine its extent. Next, use a guarded needle point electrocautery to mark out a 1 to 1.5-cm margin surrounding the lesion on the "cut" or "blend" setting. Adjust the power of the electrocautery to be just enough to allow for sufficient hemostasis without causing excessive char. Although excessive use of cautery can make the pathologic analysis of the margin much more difficult, in our experience, judicious use of electrocautery has not limited our pathologists ability to perform their assessment.

Extend the incision is down to the desired and uniform depth circumferentially, leaving the inferior portion of the incision for last. Alternate between "cut" and "coagulation" to maintain hemostasis. Avoid angling the incision toward the tumor center prematurely. Likewise, avoid moving away from the center and undermining the adjacent mucosa. Erring on the side of dissecting away from the tumor is preferred over taking the margin too close. The conceptual goal for this initial dissection is to create a cylindrical specimen down to the appropriate depth (Fig. 112.3A and B).

During sharp dissection, the assistant must maintain sufficient tension with forceps to allow for clean separation. This allows for early visualization of critical structures as they are approached. Also, the surgeon must continually examine the tumor visually and by palpation to ensure a sufficient margin is being maintained. Keep in mind that the incised tongue tissue will shrink toward the tumor up to 40%, so the surgeon must include a generous cuff to maintain an adequately clear margin.[28–30]

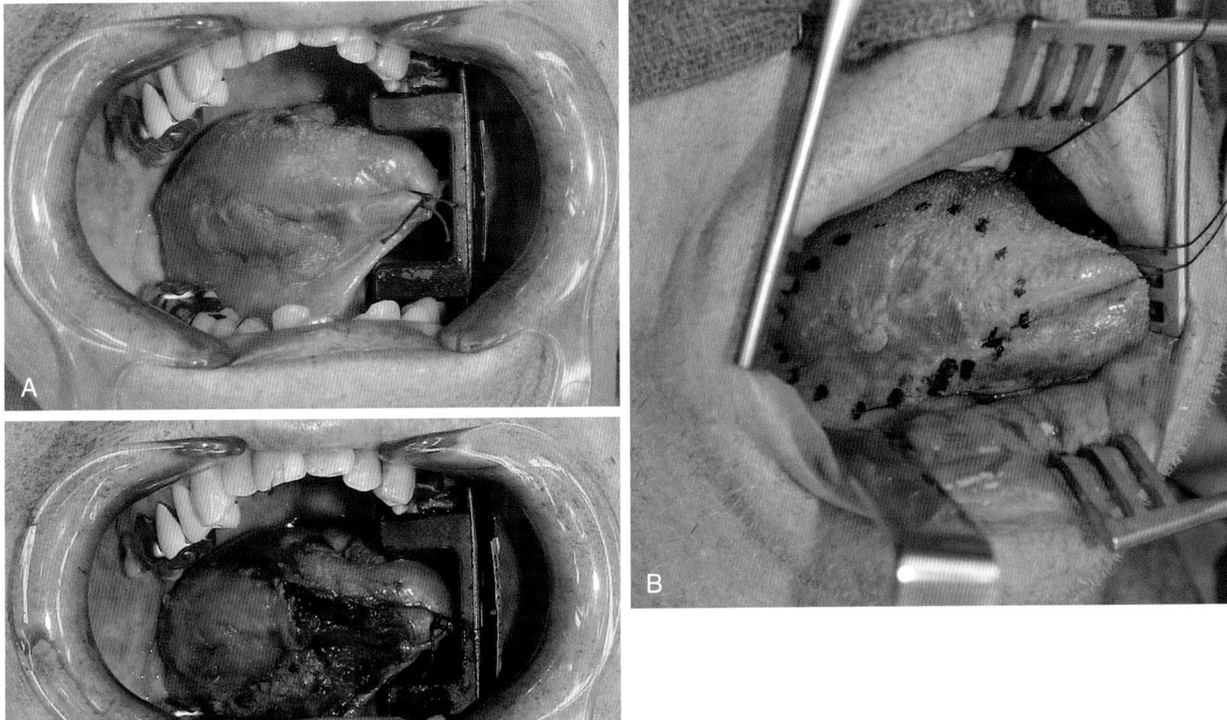

Figure 112.2 **A,** Use of plastic cheek retractors to expose the oral cavity. **B,** Use of articulating self-retaining Adson-Beckman retractors to expose the oral cavity. Note the marked-out resection margin and the retention sutures placed strategically to provide optimal retraction and tension. **C,** Mucosal incision is taken to depth circumferentially.

TECHNIQUE: Partial Glossectomy—*cont'd*

STEP 4: Completing the Inferior Incision and Control of the Lingual Artery and Its Branches

Before making the inferior portion of the incision, it is often necessary to identify and ligate the lingual artery and veins as they run medial to the hyoglossus muscle, particularly along the posterior and inferior margins of an anterolateral tongue tumor. Use a dissector to bluntly dissect through the hyoglossus muscle fibers. Blunt finger dissection with gauze can help tease the vessels into view. Timely identification of these vessels allows the surgeon to avoid brisk bleeding (Fig. 112.3C). If they are within or entering the tumor, ligate and divide them.

STEP 5: Identify and Protect the Lingual Nerve if Not Involved by Tumor

If the resection encroaches upon the location of the lingual nerve but does not require its sacrifice, blunt dissection is used to identify and preserve it after incising through mucosa, submucosa, and mylohyoid muscle. The tines of a tissue dissector are spread in small amplitudes along the direction of the nerve, as it passes posterior to anterior, biased obliquely towards the midline. The nerve runs parallel to the lingual plate of the mandible in the region of the retromolar pad and palatoglossal arch, before curving medially towards the tongue around the premolar region.[31–33] Once the nerve has been identified, it is dissected both proximally and distally to determine its proximity to the tumor. If the lingual nerve is safely away from the tumor, it is partially skeletonized and gently retracted away from the specimen. If the nerve is seen traveling into or out of the tumor specimen, it should be sacrificed.

Continued

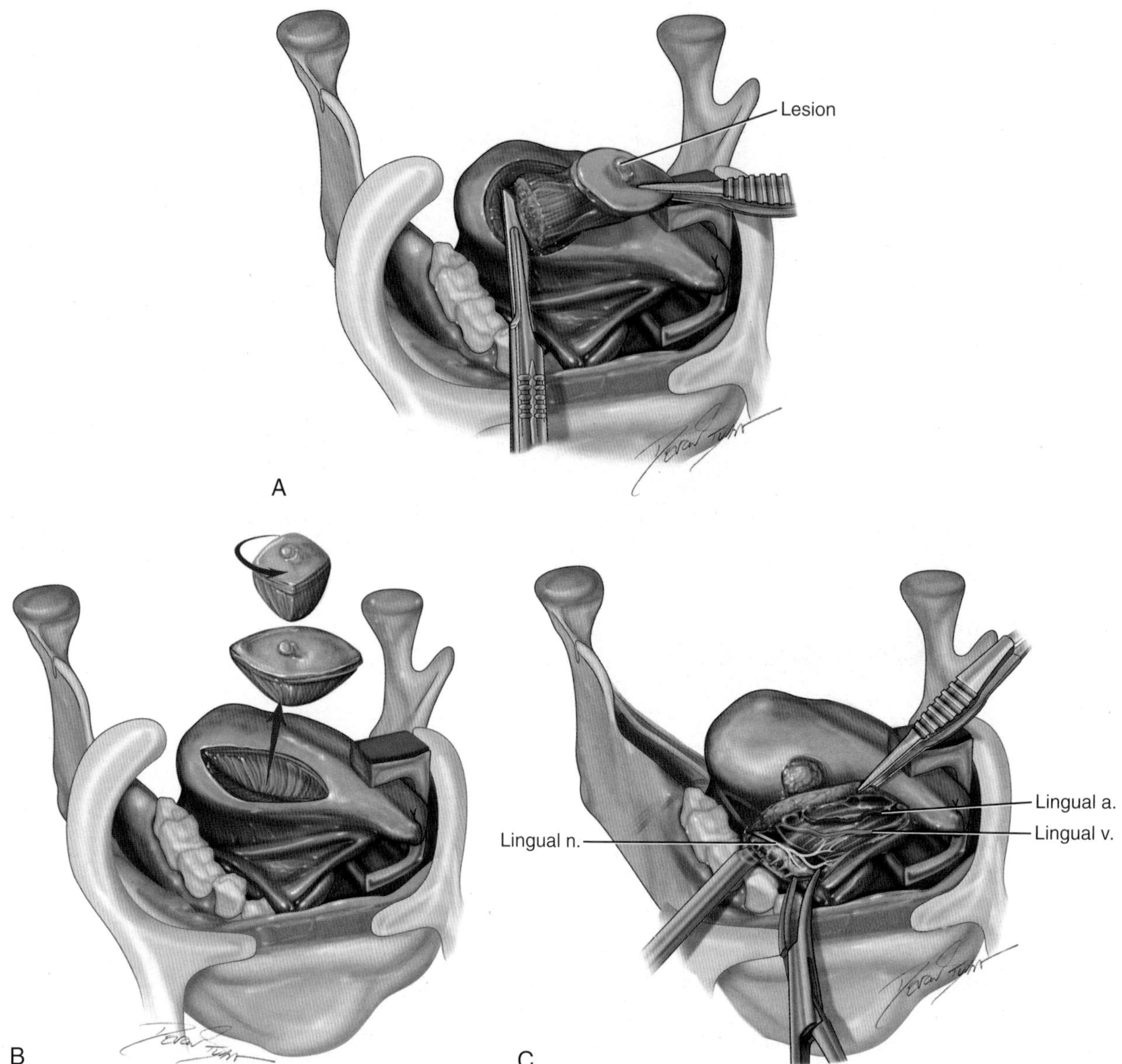

Figure 112.3 **A,** Taking the mucosal incision to depth 19 circumferentially; the goal is to create a cylinder. **B,** Making the deep margin the "keel of a boat." **C,** The lingual artery, its branches, and the lingual nerve are identified and protected.

TECHNIQUE: Partial Glossectomy—*cont'd*

STEP 6: Dissect Out and Protect or Ligate the Submandibular Duct

The Wharton duct is seen lateral to the hyoglossus and medial to the mylohyoid muscle, intimately related to the lingual nerve. If not involved with tumor, dissect it free and protect it. If either the duct or its opening along the lingual frenum is involved, dissect it out proximally, ligate and divide it. If the submandibular gland is not being removed as part of a neck dissection, consider reconstituting the duct by performing a sialodochoplasty.

TECHNIQUE: Partial Glossectomy—*cont'd*

STEP 7: Deep Portion of the Resection

Once these structures are dealt with, the dissection is then taken to the appropriate depth at the inferior incision. The dissection then proceeds centripetally with the deepest point of the dissection 1 to 1.5 cm deep to the body of the tumor. Visualize the specimen as having a shape similar to a keel of a boat or an upside-down glacier with 1.5 cm of native tissue surrounding the tumor in all dimensions. Keep the orientation of the specimen in mind as it is removed.

STEP 8: Intraoperative Margin Analysis

There are several ways to perform intraoperative margin analysis. The procedure can be simplified into two strategies, taking the margins from the resection bed or taking the margins from the specimen. We describe an approach that encompasses both.

After the specimen is logged, take the glossectomy specimen to the pathology laboratory. With the pathologist, orient and ink the margins of the specimen prior to fixation. Then, breadloaf the specimen so that the resection can be viewed in cross section (Fig. 112.4A–C). This allows for a more accurate view of areas where the tumor may be close to the resection margin. Sample these areas for frozen section analysis. In areas that are especially close, go back to the patient and take an additional margin from the resection bed.

Continued

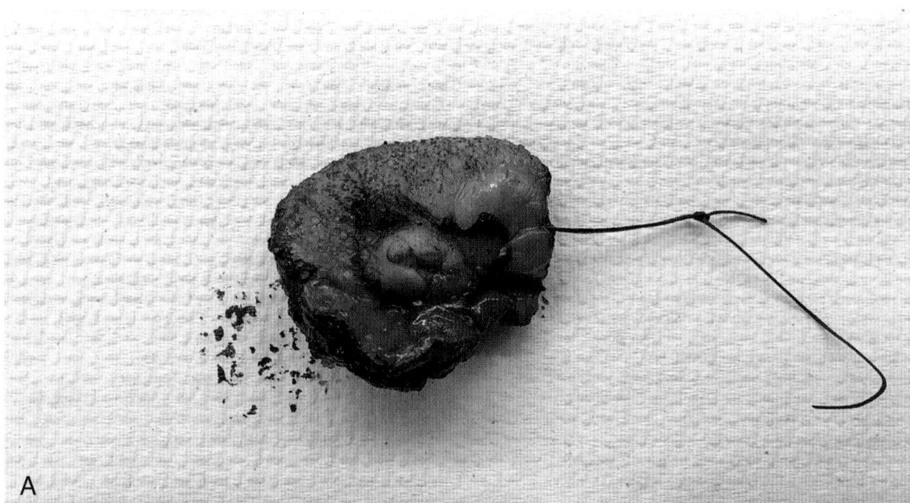

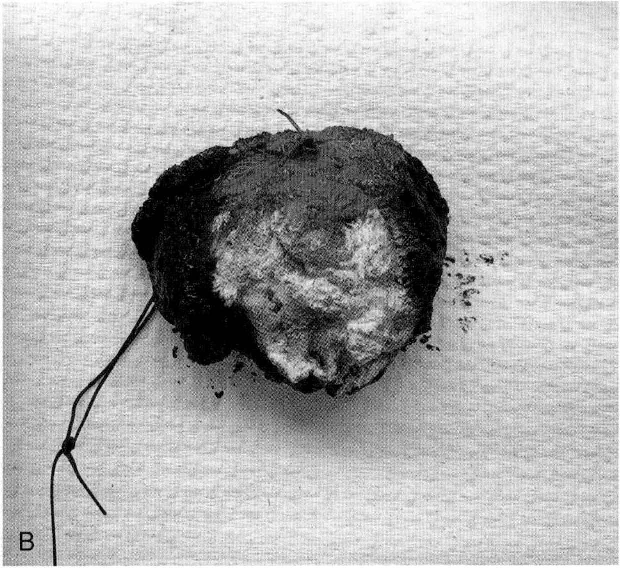

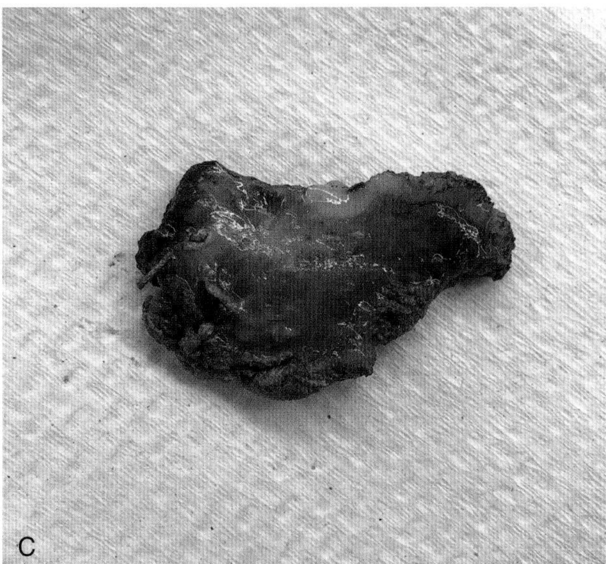

Figure 112.4 **A,** Glossectomy specimen oriented for pathologist prior to fixation. **B,** Margins of tumor inked. **C,** Tumor breadloafed for cross sectional review.

TECHNIQUE: Partial Glossectomy—*cont'd*

STEP 9: Modification that Includes En Bloc Resection with the Mandible

The tumor dictates the extent of the resection. If the tumor encroaches upon the lingual aspect of the mandible but is without frank periosteal invasion, the adjacent bone should be taken as an additional anatomic margin from the tumor. A composite resection with a marginal mandibulectomy should be considered (see Chapter 95).

When the mandibular bone is involved clinically or radiographically, one should consider a segmental mandibulectomy (see Chapter 97).

STEP 6: Closure or Reconstruction (in Order of Complexity)

HEALING BY SECONDARY INTENTION

Superficial partial glossectomies are amenable to healing by secondary intention. Healing by secondary intention will lead to scarring and contracture, as with any other site in the body, causing deviation towards the defect side. It should be avoided when the floor of mouth is involved in the resection because of the likelihood of tongue tethering.

PRIMARY CLOSURE

Primary closure should be reserved for partial glossectomy of superficial tumors without any floor of mouth involvement. When closing primarily, it is important to eliminate dead space from the defect, reducing the risk of postoperative hematoma. Deep mattress sutures are effective to approximate the intrinsic muscles of the tongue. The mucosal edges are best closed with 3-0 polyglactin sutures in horizontal mattress fashion for strength and wound edge eversion. For more longitudinal defects, incorporating a T incision can help reduce the shortening and flattening of the ipsilateral side by distributing the closure between two dimensions. This simple method of closure avoids additional donor site morbidity but does cause deviation of the contralateral tongue to the defect (Fig. 112.5A).

SPLIT-THICKNESS SKIN GRAFTING

Split-thickness skin grafting requires a donor site, usually from the patient's thigh, which adds minor postoperative morbidity. This method is best utilized when less than 50% of the tongue has been removed. It provides less tongue contracture than the two previous methods but does not recreate tongue bulk. A split-thickness skin graft is harvested with slightly more thickness (0.16 inch) when compared to reconstructing other areas of the body. The key to successful graft integration, just as in other parts of the body, relies on meticulous immobilization of the graft to the recipient site. This is inherently difficult in the highly mobile tongue. Pie crusting of the skin graft with numerous sutures is required. Adjuncts such as fibrin tissue adhesives (Tisseel) aid in obtaining a more stable graft to the wound bed interface. Use of a bolster made of petroleum impregnated gauze greatly facilitates immobilization of the graft but is uncomfortable for the patient (Fig. 112.5B).

LOCAL AND REGIONAL PEDICLED FLAPS

Local and regional flaps can be used for larger defects and offer the advantage of having their own blood supply. These contract less than the previous mentioned methods and restore the loss of tongue bulk. A variety of options are available and are described elsewhere but may include the hemi-tongue advancement flap, submental island flap, supraclavicular flap, and the pectoralis major flap. In patients without known or suspected metastatic lymphadenopathy and adequate submental tissue, the submental island flap is a reliable method that can be incorporated within the neck dissection incision (Fig. 112.5C and D).

FREE FLAPS

Microvascular free tissue transfer provides the most predictable restoration of form and function as previously discussed in this chapter.[23–27] The radial forearm and anterior lateral thigh are the workhorse flaps for tongue reconstruction. Techniques for these reconstructions are described elsewhere. While these options optimize tongue bulk and mobility, they are considerably more complex surgeries that require specialized postoperative care with extended hospital stays (Fig. 112.5E).

TECHNIQUE: Partial Glossectomy—*cont'd*

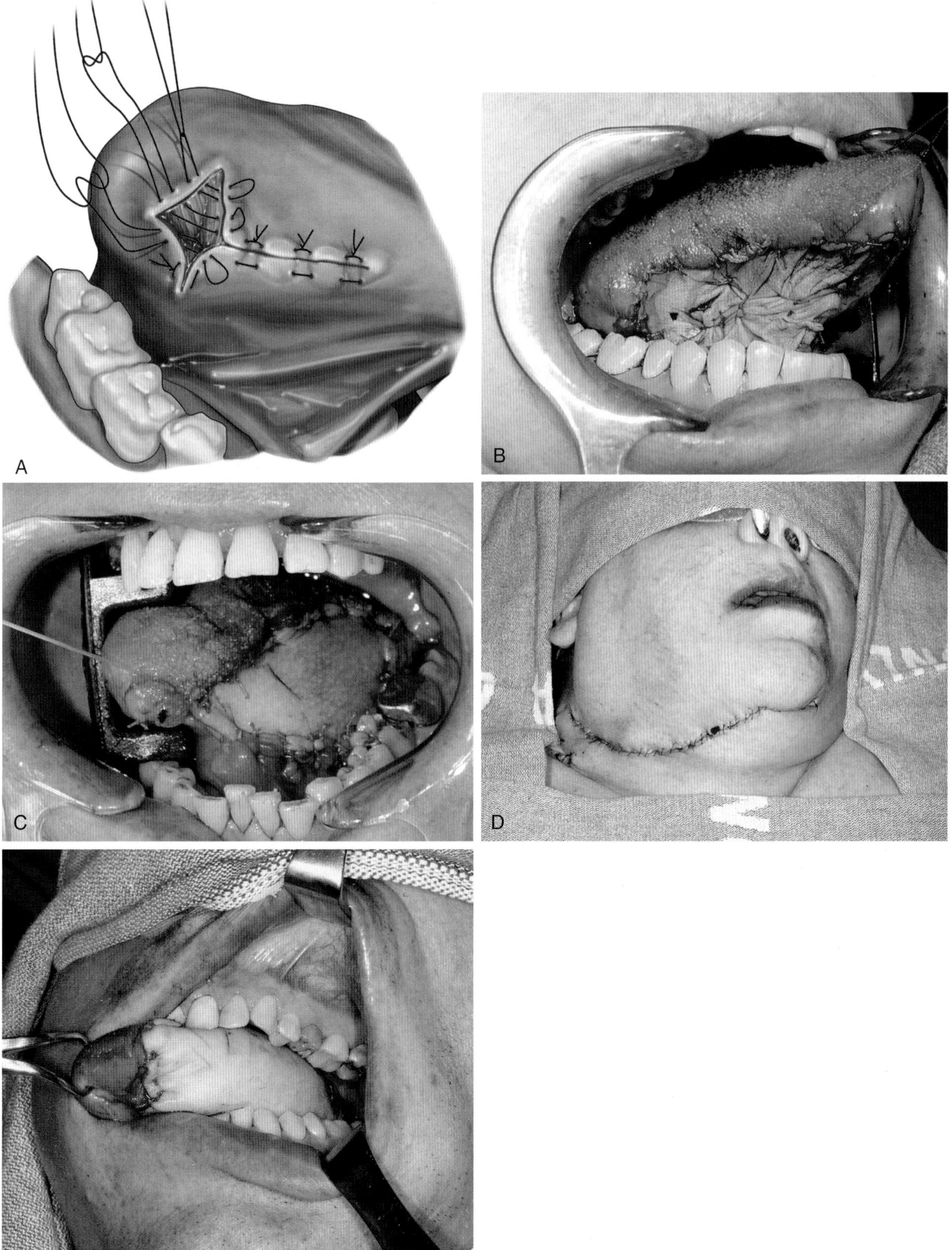

Figure 112.5 **A,** Closure of the defect into a T incision. **B,** Reconstruction of the defect with a split-thickness skin graft. **C,** Reconstruction of the defect with a submental island flap. **D,** Note the minimal local deformity from harvesting of the submental island. **E,** Reconstruction of the defect with a radial forearm free flap.

ALTERNATIVE TECHNIQUE 1: Access to the Base of Tongue

As mentioned previously, SCC of the BOT presents the surgeon with difficult access to obtain adequate margins and reconstructive inset. This requires augmented access for visualization and palpation of the tumor in three dimensions as well as the ability for free flap inset to the posterior aspect of the resection.

The lip-split mandibulotomy technique is described elsewhere and provides the greatest access, but is the most invasive (Fig. 112.6A–C).

There are two pharyngotomy approaches that can also be used: the suprahyoid and lateral pharyngotomy. A suprahyoid pharyngotomy is used for BOT tumors that do not involve the vallecula (Fig. 112.7A and B). It is performed as follows. The suprahyoid musculature is exposed via the same approach used for a neck dissection, and if a neck dissection is planned, this is done first. Otherwise, electrocautery is used to cut through the fibroadipose tissue down to the hyoid bone. An Allis clamp is placed on the hyoid bone and retracted

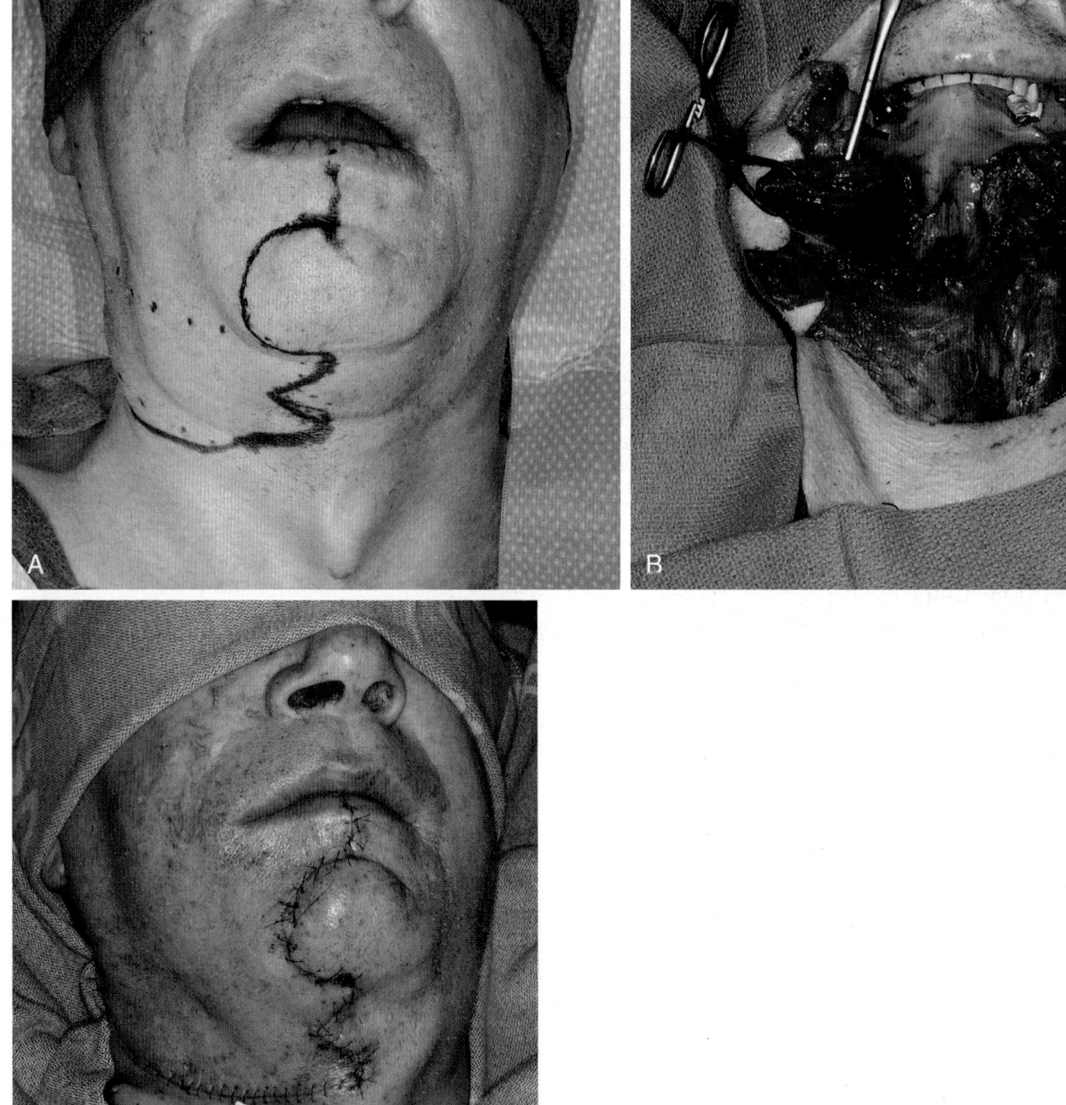

Figure 112.6 **A,** Preoperative, surgical access, and postoperative closure of lip-split with mandibulotomy. **B,** Preoperative, surgical access, and postoperative closure of lip-split with mandibulotomy. **C,** Preoperative, surgical access, and postoperative closure of lip-split with mandibulotomy.

ALTERNATIVE TECHNIQUE 1: Access to the Base of Tongue—*cont'd*

anteriorly for stabilization. The attachments of the suprahyoid musculature are divided, starting at the midline and working posteriorly towards the greater cornu on both sides. Stay close to bone to avoid injury to the lingual artery and hypoglossal nerve. As the dissection proceeds towards the greater cornu, the assistant surgeon presses on the contralateral hyoid to displace the working side outward, facilitating dissection.

A right-angle retractor, such as a Deaver or Langenbeck, is placed transorally with its tip in the vallecula. The instrument is used to displace the vallecula anteriorly into the wound so that it can be identified by palpation. The pharyngotomy is created by cutting down to the retractor, and the retractor is passed through this initial pharyngotomy. The tip of the epiglottis is grasped with an Allis clamp and brought into the neck. Metzenbaum scissors are used to extend the pharyngotomy laterally along the edge of the epiglottis toward the piriform recess. This maximizes the posterior mucosal margin away from the tumor.

Once the pharyngotomy is complete and open, the BOT is grasped with an Allis clamp positioned away from tumor, and the BOT is pulled through the pharyngotomy into the surgical field.

Once the resection is completed, repair of the pharyngotomy is performed in layers. The mucosal edges are closed with horizontal mattress sutures of 3-0 polyglactin, everting the closure into the pharyngeal lumen. The deep intrinsic muscles are then sutured to the hyoid bone with either 0 polyglactin or nonresorbable sutures.

Larger BOT SCC with extension into the vallecula, piriform recess, lateral pharyngeal wall, or larynx requires greater access than that provided by a suprahyoid pharyngotomy. A lateral pharyngotomy, with or without a mandibulotomy, provides reasonable access to the oropharynx (Fig. 112.7C and D).

A neck dissection is performed initially; otherwise, the sternocleidomastoid is skeletonized along its medial surface and is retracted posteriorly. The internal jugular vein is mobilized and retracted posteriorly. The hypoglossal (CN XII) nerve is identified and is generously skeletonized posteriorly and anteriorly. The descendens hypoglossi is divided to allow retraction of the hypoglossal nerve cephalad. The superior laryngeal nerve is identified medial to the carotid bifurcation, just superficial to the pharyngeal constrictors. It is skeletonized and superiorly retracted as well. In some instances, it may have to be divided to provide sufficient access although this should be avoided if possible.

The digastric and stylohyoid muscles are divided at their attachments to the hyoid bone. The ipsilateral hyoid is skeletonized as described for the suprahyoid pharyngotomy approach. A portion of the hyoid can be resected to aid in exposure.

The inferior constrictor attachments to the thyroid ala are divided along the posterior edge of the cartilage. The assistant facilitates by pressing on the contralateral side of the thyroid ala, displacing and rotating it into the surgical field. The mucosa of the piriform recess is reflected off the medial aspect of the thyroid ala for a short distance with a Freer elevator.

A Yankauer suction tip is placed transorally into the pharynx and is directed into the piriform recess so that it can be palpated through the cervical wound. The pharyngotomy is created by incising over the Yankauer suction into the hypopharynx. While retracting the hypoglossal nerve superiorly, the pharyngotomy is extended superiorly with scissors while simultaneously inspecting the pharyngeal side so that adequate exposure of the BOT is achieved. An Allis clamp is placed on the epiglottis to pull the BOT through the pharyngotomy and into view. Penetrating towel clips can also be placed medially and laterally to the tumor to pull the BOT into the cervical wound.

Once the tumor has been removed, closure of the pharyngotomy is performed with horizontal mattress 3-0 polyglactin sutures, everting into the pharyngeal lumen. Prolonged nasogastric tube feeding is to be anticipated.

Finally, TORS provides a minimally invasive approach to the BOT. This technique is outside of the scope of this chapter.

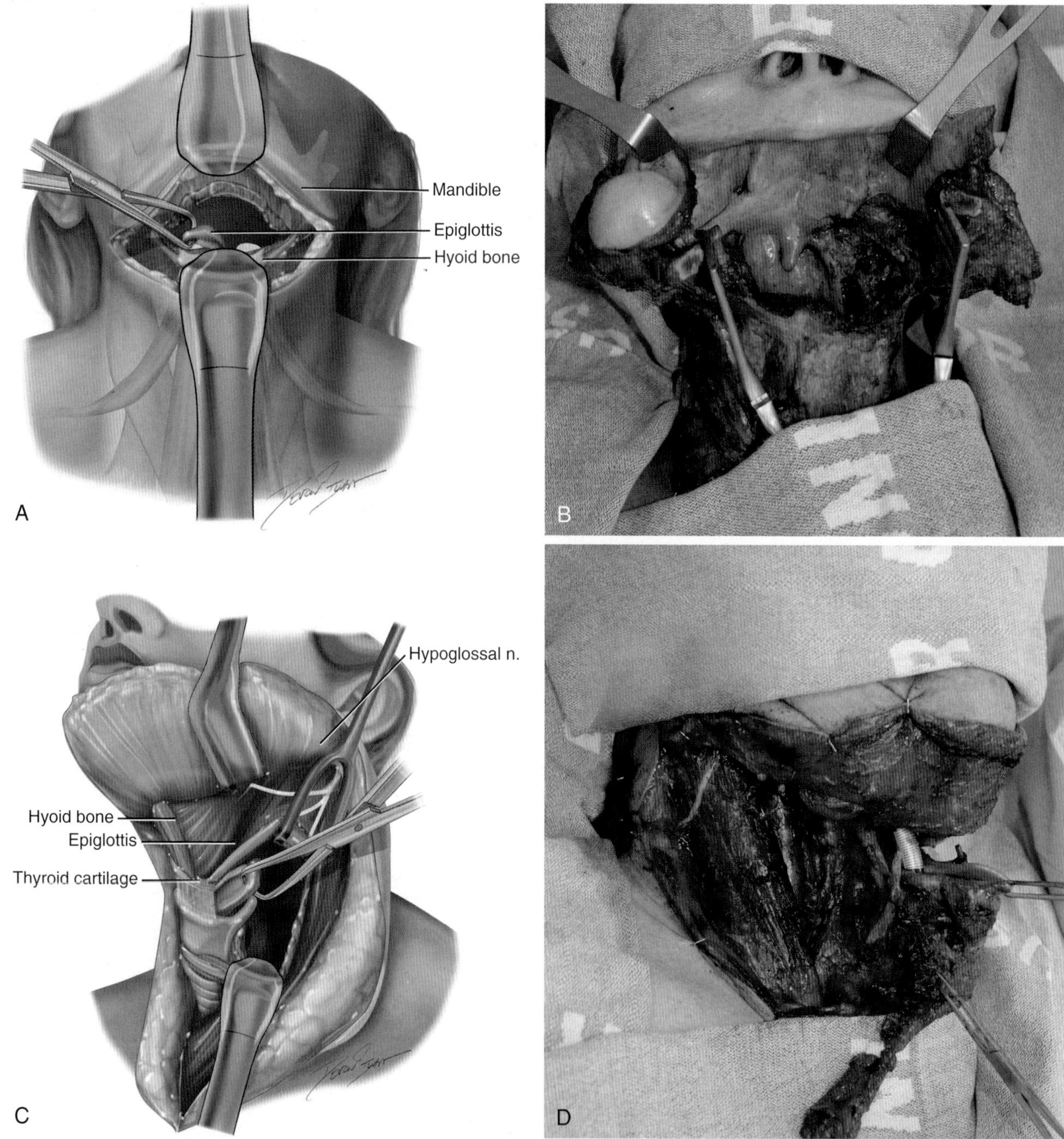

Figure 112.7 **A** and **B,** Midline mandibulotomy approach with suprahyoid pharyngotomy for total glossectomy. **C** and **D,** Suprahyoid pharyngotomy.

ALTERNATIVE TECHNIQUE 2: Compartmental Resection

The aim of compartmental resection is to remove the primary tumor with along with potential in transit metastases.[12] For advanced tumors of the tongue, compartmental resection can be done through a mandibular lingual release or lip split with mandibulotomy. The mandibular lingual release approach has been shown to be equally effective in tumor eradication with less postoperative risk of orocutaneous fistula formation when compared to the lip-split technique.[34,35]

A traditional skin incision for neck dissection is used and formal neck dissection is completed prior to tumor resection. Care is taken to leave the dissected contents of the neck in continuity with the primary lesion, which is approached through the submental triangle. Begin by using blunt and sharp dissection to detach the mylohyoid from the hyoid bone inferiorly and the contralateral mylohyoid anteriorly. With the mylohyoid reflected, the tumor can be palpated

ALTERNATIVE TECHNIQUE 2: Compartmental Resection—*cont'd*

through the geniohyoid and genioglossus muscles. This also allows for palpation of the septum of the tongue, an avascular plane useful to follow during the resection.

Next, detach the hyoglossus from the hyoid bone where the lingual artery and hypoglossal nerve should be encountered, ligated and divided. The mandibular attachment of the mylohyoid is now divided, and reflection will allow for visualization of the floor of mouth and lingual nerve. The lingual nerve and styloglossus muscle are traced as far proximally as possible and divided, and the genioglossus is detached from its tubercle attachment and separated from its contralateral counterpart. At this point, the fibrofatty node bearing tissue, submandibular glandular tissue, and suprahyoid musculature are pedicled to the tumor, and resection can be carried out from above and below the mandible. The hemiglossectomy is completed in an anterior to posterior direction and the specimen is removed en bloc (Fig. 112.8A and B).

Compartment resection results in a large defect and communication between the oral cavity and neck. This necessitates either a free flap or pedicled flap to fill and close.

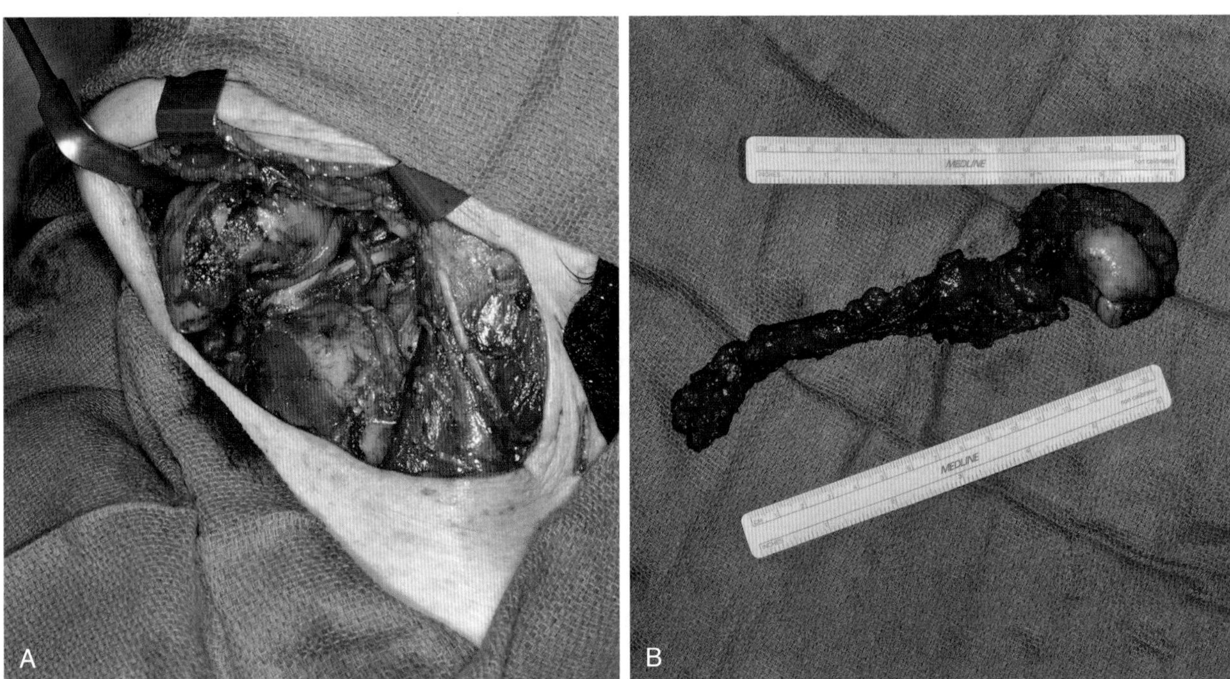

Figure 112.8 **A,** Suprahyoid pharyngotomy with exposure of the tongue base with the tumor being pulled through the neck incision. **B,** Compartmental resection hemiglossectomy.

Avoidance and Management of Intraoperative Complications

Hemorrhage

The tongue is a richly vasculature structure. Appropriate slow electrocautery dissection with tension across the incision line helps to minimize blood loss. Identification and ligation of the lingual artery and its branches and oversewing with mattress sutures are effective techniques to control bleeding.

Nerve Injury

If the lingual and hypoglossal nerves are not involved in the tumor, every effort should be made to preserve them. The lingual nerve follows a predictable course, as described above, and the hypoglossal nerve lies deeper within the musculature. If inadvertently injured, an attempt should be made to repair these nerves with microneurosurgical techniques.

Neuropraxia from retraction and skeletonization is common postoperatively and will typically show improvement over the course of 6 months to a year.

Postoperative Considerations

Postoperative Swelling and Airway Embarrassment

The tongue is highly vascular and prone to developing bleeding, swelling, and hematoma, all of which can lead to airway embarrassment. Signs of any of these should prompt a return to the operating room to secure the airway, evacuate hematoma, and obtaining hemostasis. Perioperative corticosteroids can help minimize edema leading to airway embarrassment. Because of this, we have a very low threshold to performing elective tracheostomy.

Communication with anesthesia colleagues intraoperatively and hospitalist and nursing colleagues postoperatively helps avoid unexpected problems. The surgeon and staff should be prepared to mobilize the equipment, resources, and providers to efficiently perform an emergent intubation or surgical airway, if necessary. Information that is important to communicate includes the airway anatomy, type of airway present, size of tube for reintubation, size of tracheostomy tube to be used, location of a tracheostomy surgical tray, and contact information for the surgical team.

Free flap reconstructions after glossectomy results in more significant postoperative edema, both within the flap and the native tongue. We routinely perform elective tracheostomy for patients after glossectomy that require free flap reconstruction.

Postoperative Infection

Given the contaminated nature of the oral cavity, postoperative infection is not an uncommon occurrence. However, there is a dearth of evidence to guide surgeons on what is the most optimal regimen for antibiotic prophylaxis.

Several studies looking at this question have demonstrated that the type of antibiotic is of utmost importance and that the duration should be at least 24 hours postoperatively.[36–38] It is common practice in free flap reconstructions to administer intravenous antibiotics 5 to 7 days postoperatively. In our practice, we typically use intravenous ampicillin/sulbactam, cefazolin with metronidazole, or clindamycin (in patients with penicillin allergy).

Enteral Nutrition

Placement of a nasogastric feeding tube such as a 12 French Dobhoff tube, serves as a temporary means for enteral nutrition. Postoperative swallowing difficulties lasting longer than 3 weeks should prompt consideration of gastrostomy tube placement. This is especially important in patients who had severe malnutrition preoperatively or patients who will undergo postoperative chemoradiation therapy.

Resumption of oral feeding is tailored to patient-specific factors. The risks and benefits of resumption of oral feeding should be weighed by the surgeon in collaboration with a speech language pathologist (SLP). The potential risk of surgical site infection from nutritional substrate must be considered as well as the potential for aspiration. Patients with free flap reconstructions demonstrating maintenance of watertight wound closure can generally begin oral intake around postoperative day 5 or 6[39] after SLP evaluation. Early oral intake has been demonstrated to lead to shorter hospital stays without adverse outcomes in select patients.[40]

Speech and Swallow Rehabilitation

Swallowing dysfunction after glossectomy represents a significant morbidity for patients. High body mass index, smaller resections, and absence of adjuvant therapy correlate with an increased return to total oral diet.[41] Early SLP consultation and treatment provide patients with exercises and coping skills to maximize their chances of effective swallowing and speech. In cases of severe dysarthria, they can assist in providing other mechanisms for effective communication.

Oral/Pharyngeal Cutaneous Fistulas

Combined approaches to glossectomy through the neck place the patient at risk for developing fistula formation between the aerodigestive tract and the skin. While meticulous layered closure with marginal edge eversion limits the occurrence, they are not always avoidable. If a fistula forms, the treatment is largely conservative and involves local wound care. The patient should be kept nulla per os and enteral nutrition provided. When infection is present, systemic antibiotics are employed, and wet to dry packing soaked in 0.25% acetic acid or 0.125% sodium hypochlorite (Dakins's solution) aids in antimicrobial colonization. When the wound bed is free from infection a negative pressure dressing such as a vacuum-assisted wound closure can aid in healing. Persistent fistulas may require surgical removal via fistulectomy and possibly additional locoregional flap or free flap reconstruction. Patients who demonstrate chronic wound healing problems should be investigated for malnutrition, hypothyroidism, and other causes for poor wound healing.

References

1. Ring ME. The treatment of macroglossia before the 20th century. *Am J Otolaryngol.* 1999;20(1):28–36.
2. Folz BJ, Silver CE, Rinaldo A, et al. An outline of the history of head and neck oncology. *Oral Oncol.* 2008;44(1):2–9.
3. Absolon KB, Rogers W, Aust JB. Some historical developments of the surgical therapy of tongue cancer from the seventeenth to the nineteenth century. *Am J Surg.* 1962;104:686–691.
4. Power D. Cancer of the tongue: abstract of the Bradshaw lecture delivered before the royal college of surgeons of England. *BMJ.* 1919;1(3028):37–38.
5. Crile G. Excision of cancer of the head and neck: with special reference to the plan of dissection based on one hundred and thirty-two operations. *J Am Med Assoc.* 1906;47:1780–1788.
6. Lodi G, Franchini R, Warnakulasuriya S, et al. Interventions for treating oral leukoplakia to prevent oral cancer. *Cochrane Database Syst Rev.* 2016;7:CD001829.
7. Mehanna HM, Rattay T, Smith J, McConkey CC. Treatment and follow-up of oral

dysplasia—a systematic review and meta-analysis. *Head Neck*. 2009;31(12):1600–1609.

8. Robertson AG, Soutar DS, Paul J, et al. Early closure of a randomized trial: surgery and postoperative radiotherapy versus radiotherapy in the management of intra-oral tumours. *Clin Oncol (R Coll Radiol)*. 1998;10:155–160.
9. Wolfensberger M, Zbaeren P, Dulguerov P, Müller W, Arnoux A, Schmid S. Surgical treatment of early oral carcinoma-results of a prospective controlled multicenter study. *Head Neck*. 2001;23(7):525–530.
10. Ansarin M, Bruschini R, Navach V, et al. Classification of GLOSSECTOMIES: proposal for tongue cancer resections. *Head Neck*. 2019;41(3):821–827.
11. Calabrese L, Bruschini R, Giugliano G, et al. Compartmental tongue surgery: long term oncologic results in the treatment of tongue cancer. *Oral Oncol*. 2011;47(3):174–179.
12. Calabrese L, Giugliano G, Bruschini R, et al. Compartmental surgery in tongue tumours: description of a new surgical technique. *Acta Otorhinolaryngol Ital*. 2009;29(5):259–264.
13. Weinstein GS, O'Malley BW Jr, Magnuson JS, et al. Transoral robotic surgery: a multicenter study to assess feasibility, safety, and surgical margins. *Laryngoscope*. 2012;122(8):1701–1707.
14. Weinstein GS, Quon H, Newman HJ, et al. Transoral robotic surgery alone for oropharyngeal cancer: an analysis of local control. *Arch Otolaryngol Head Neck Surg*. 2012;138(7):628–634.
15. Sun J, Weng Y, Li J, Wang G, Zhang Z. Analysis of determinants on speech function after glossectomy. *J Oral Maxillofac Surg*. 2007;65(10):1944–1950.
16. Takatsu J, Hanai N, Suzuki H, et al. Phonologic and acoustic analysis of speech following glossectomy and the effect of rehabilitation on speech outcomes. *J Oral Maxillofac Surg*. 2017;75(7):1530–1541.
17. Chuanjun C, Zhiyuan Z, Shaopu G, Xinquan J, Zhihong Z. Speech after partial glossectomy: a comparison between reconstruction and nonreconstruction patients. *J Oral Maxillofac Surg*. 2002;60(4):404–407.
18. Dzioba A, Aalto D, Papadopoulos-Nydam G, Head and Neck Research Network, et al. Functional and quality of life outcomes after partial glossectomy: a multi-institutional longitudinal study of the head and neck research network. *J Otolaryngol Head Neck Surg*. 2017;46(1):56.
19. Hamilton D, Paleri V. Role of transoral robotic surgery in current head & neck practice. *Surgeon*. 2017;15(3):147–154.
20. Golusiński W. Functional organ preservation surgery in head and neck cancer: transoral robotic surgery and beyond. *Front Oncol*. 2019;9:293.
21. Mercante G, Ruscito P, Pellini R, Cristalli G, Spriano G. Transoral robotic surgery (TORS) for tongue base tumours. *Acta Otorhinolaryngol Ital*. 2013;33(4):230–235.
22. Chung J, Bender-Heine A, Lambert HW. Improving exposure for transoral oropharyngeal surgery with the floor of mouth window: a cadaveric feasibility study. *J Otolaryngol Head Neck Surg*. 2019;48(1):62.
23. Han AY, Kuan EC, Mallen-St Clair J, et al. Total glossectomy with free flap reconstruction: twenty-year experience at a tertiary medical center. *Laryngoscope*. 2019;129(5):1087–1092.
24. Tarsitano A, Vietti MV, Cipriani R, Marchetti C. et al. Functional results of microvascular reconstruction after hemiglossectomy: free anterolateral thigh flap versus free forearm flap. *Acta Otorhinolaryngol Ital*. 2013;33:374–379.
25. de Vicente JC, de Villalaín L, Torre A, Peña I. Microvascular free tissue transfer for tongue reconstruction after hemiglossectomy: a functional assessment of radial forearm versus anterolateral thigh flap. *J Oral Maxillofac Surg*. 2008;66(11):2270–2275.
26. Namin AW, Varvares MA. Functional outcomes of sensate versus insensate free flap reconstruction in oral and oropharyngeal reconstruction: a systematic review. *Head Neck*. 2016;38(11):1717–1721.
27. Kuriakose MA, Loree TR, Spies A, Meyers S, Hicks Jr WL. Sensate radial forearm free flaps in tongue reconstruction. *Arch Otolaryngol Head Neck Surg*. 2001;127(12):1463–1466.
28. Johnson RE, Sigman JD, Funk GF, Robinson RA, Hoffman HT. Quantification of surgical margin shrinkage in the oral cavity. *Head Neck*. 1997;19(4):281–286.
29. Cheng A, Cox D, Schmidt BL. Oral squamous cell carcinoma margin discrepancy after resection and pathologic processing. *J Oral Maxillofac Surg*. 2008;66(3):523–529.
30. Mistry RC, Qureshi SS, Kumaran C. Post-resection mucosal margin shrinkage in oral cancer: quantification and significance. *J Surg Oncol*. 2005;91(2):131–133.
31. Pogrel MA, Renaut A, Schmidt B, Ammar A. The relationship of the lingual nerve to the mandibular third molar region: an anatomic study. *J Oral Maxillofac Surg*. 1995;53(10):1178–1181.
32. Kikuta S, Iwanaga J, Kusukawa J, Tubbs RS. An anatomical study of the lingual nerve in the lower third molar area. *Anat Cell Biol*. 2019;52(2):140–142.
33. Zur KB, Mu L, Sanders I. Distribution pattern of the human lingual nerve. *Clin Anat*. 2004;17(2):88–92.
34. Li H, Li J, Yang B, Su M, Xing R, Han Z. Mandibular lingual release versus mandibular lip-split approach for expanded resection of middle-late tongue cancer: a case-control study. *J Craniomaxillofac Surg*. 2015;43(7):1054–1058.
35. Cilento BW, Izzard M, Weymuller EA, Futran N. Comparison of approaches for oral cavity cancer resection: lip-split versus visor flap. *Otolaryngol Head Neck Surg*. 2007;137(3):428–432.
36. Oppelaar MC, Zijtveld C, Kuipers S, et al. Evaluation of prolonged vs short courses of antibiotic prophylaxis following ear, nose, throat, and oral and maxillofacial surgery: a systematic review and meta-analysis. *JAMA Otolaryngol Head Neck Surg*. 2019;145(7):610–616.
37. Mitchell RM, Mendez E, Schmitt NC, Bhrany AD, Futran ND. Antibiotic prophylaxis in patients undergoing head and neck free flap reconstruction. *JAMA Otolaryngol Head Neck Surg*. 2015;141(12):1096–1103.
38. Haidar YM, Tripathi PB, Tjoa T, et al. Antibiotic prophylaxis in clean-contaminated head and neck cases with microvascular free flap reconstruction: a systematic review and meta-analysis. *Head Neck*. 2018;40(2):417–427.
39. Guidera AK, Kelly BN, Rigby P, MacKinnon CA, Tan ST. Early oral intake after reconstruction with a free flap for cancer of the oral cavity. *Br J Oral Maxillofac Surg*. 2013;51(3):224–227.
40. McAuley D, Barry T, McConnell K, Smith J, Stenhouse J. Early feeding after free flap reconstruction for oral cancer. *Br J Oral Maxillofac Surg*. 2015;53(7):618–620.
41. Chen DW, Wang T, Shey-Sen Ni J, et al. Prognostic factors associated with achieving total oral diet after glossectomy with microvascular free tissue transfer reconstruction. *Oral Oncol*. 2019;92:59–66.

CHAPTER 113

Composite Resection

Robert Ord and Donita Dyalram

Armamentarium

#9 Molt periosteal elevator
#10 and #15 scalpels
Appropriate sutures
Army-Navy retractors
Banana blade for saw
Bipolar electrocautery
Burs (fissured and oval)
Langenbeck toe-out retractor
Local anesthetic with vasoconstrictor
Malleable retractors
Mandibular plating system
Needle electrocautery
Nerve stimulator
Reciprocating saw
Small and medium hemoclips

History of the Procedure

The management of cancer of the mandible has been primarily surgical over the past 60 years. The decision between segmental and marginal resection is based on the proximity of the cancer to the jaw and the pattern and extent of bone invasion. In the 1950s, segmental resection was advocated based on the premise that the lingual periosteal lymphatics of the mandible were responsible for drainage of the tongue and floor of the mouth.[1] In 1959, Panagopoulos[2] proposed that bony invasion of the mandible occurred by direct extension of the tumor through nutrient canals, based on his finding of tumor cells in Volkmann's canals in a few cases. Involvement of the inferior alveolar canal was another consideration in the planning of resection of the mandible.[3]

Various routes of tumor entry into the mandible have been described. Byars[4] suggested invasion could occur through the occlusal surface of the mandible or through the mental foramen from primary tumors in the lip or gingiva and through the inferior border of the mandible from cancer in the neck. Other studies have suggested invasion via the periodontal membrane in dentate patients or occlusal cortical defects in the edentulous mandible.[5,6]

There are two histologic patterns of invasion of the mandible.[7,8] In the erosive pattern of spread, the tumor spreads on a broad front with a connective tissue layer with osteoclasts, separating the tumor and the bone. In the invasive pattern of spread, islands of tumor advance independently, with little osteoclastic activity and no separation of the tumor from the bone.

Brown and Browne[6] studied patterns of invasion and how they can determine the type of mandibular resection. They studied 33 patients who required segmental or rim/marginal resection and found that, with more extensive bone involvement, the pattern was invasive. In areas where alveolar bone remained, the pattern was more likely to be erosive, and as the tumor extended into basal bone, its pattern became invasive. In areas where less alveolar bone is present (posterior mandible), the pattern is invasive, unlike the symphysis of the mandible. Brown and Browne proposed that in dentate patients, the site of entry is at the junction of the attached and reflected mucosa, which is usually 10 mm below the crest of the ridge. A surgeon considering a marginal resection should estimate from this area, rather than from the crest, to ensure clear margins. In a study of 100 mandibular resections, true bone invasion was seen in 8/35 (23%) of rim resections and 54/65 (83%) segmental resections.[9] Local control is not associated with bone invasion or the extent of mandibular resection but was significantly impacted by positive soft tissue margins.[10]

Indications for the Use of the Procedure

The term *composite mandibulectomy* can be defined as the excision of a portion of the mandible in continuity with the associated involved soft tissues, plus or minus a neck dissection. Although composite mandibulectomy may be indicated for benign disease (e.g., ameloblastoma), this chapter discusses the management of cancer. Cancers may arise primarily within the jaw (e.g., sarcoma, intraosseous carcinomas); however, most oral cancers are squamous cell carcinomas that arise in the oral mucosa and secondarily involve bone.

Marginal resection of the mandible is defined as resection of the superior (alveolar) portion of the mandible, leaving the lower border in continuity. Preserving the inferior border of the mandible during cancer resection, where possible, simplifies the reconstructive plan and spares the patient the morbidity associated with a free flap transfer. The decision to perform a marginal resection rather than a segmental resection is based on the extent of bony invasion and the proximity of the tumor to the mandible, such that 1-cm oncologic margins can be obtained. When bone is uninvolved by tumor clinically and radiologically and the periosteum can be easily stripped from intact cortical bone, and there is no oncologic indication for bone removal, bone still may be removed (e.g., gingival tumor) to ensure a 1-cm margin. When the tumor is stuck to the periosteum and/or there is limited invasion of only cortical bone, a marginal resection is indicated. For small lesions (T1 or T2) lying close to the gingivolingual gutter on the lingual aspect of the mandible, the local control rates for rim/marginal resection were comparable to those for other procedures.[11] Bartellbort et al.[12] recommended that when the rim/marginal mandibulectomy is performed, smooth, curved osteotomies without step-offs were simple, biomechanically sound, and resulted in a low complication rate. A panoramic radiograph can be used to assess the vertical height of the mandible, to ensure that at least 1 cm of bone can be maintained at the lower border.

Marginal mandibular resections, especially in the anterior region, may be approached intraorally. In a retrospective study of 46 patients, Ord et al.[13] found that clinical examination, panoramic radiographs, and computed tomography (CT) scans were 82.6% accurate in diagnosing mandibular invasion. They found that the mandible was involved in 65% of patients who underwent segmental resection and 7.6% of those who had marginal resection. They concluded that indications for marginal resection were cancer in close proximity to the bone, minimal cortical invasion, or an early erosive pattern of invasion.

If there is evidence of bony invasion through the cortex into medullary bone, a segmental resection is indicated. Most segmental resections require an in-continuity neck dissection and are approached through a cervical incision.

Using the Cawood and Howell[14] classification of the edentulous mandible, Brown et al.[15] suggested a guide for determining whether continuity of the mandible can be preserved with a safe oncologic margin. This was a retrospective case study based on 77 patient orthopantomograms, bone scintigraphy, and magnetic resonance imaging (MRI). They found that marginal resection was suitable in 58% of class I/ II (dentate or immediate extraction); 43% of class III /IV (greater than 20-mm well-rounded or knife-edge ridge); and 6% among class V /VI (less than 20-mm flat or depressed ridge form). Not surprisingly, the more resorbed mandible (i.e., class V/VI) required a segmental resection. CT and MRI are complementary in assessing bone invasion.[16]

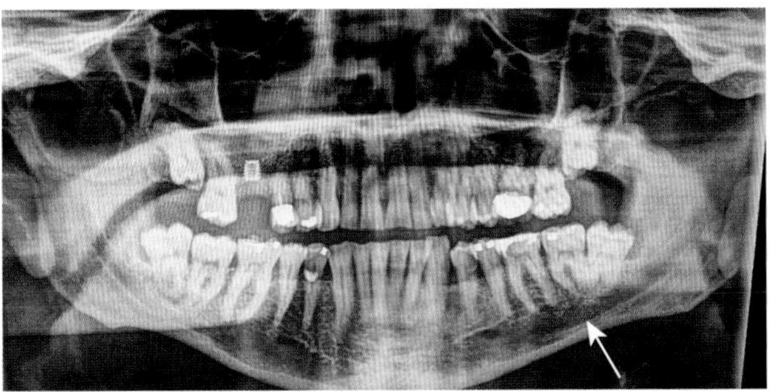

Figure 113.1 The Panorex film shows subtle loss of bone on the superior aspect of the ridge between teeth 20, 21, and 22. The patient complained of anesthesia of the lower lip, and clinically the T1 gingival cancer extended to the mental foramen. The radiograph also shows an expanded mental foramen. The white arrow indicates a widened inferior alveolar nerve (IAN) canal with loss of its cortical walls. At surgery, biopsy of the IAN at the lingula was positive for squamous carcinoma, and the nerve was traced cranially to the foramen ovale and skull base to obtain a clear margin.

When medullary bone invasion occurs in the body of the mandible, the entire nerve-bearing segment of bone is removed due to the potential for perineural spread by tumor along the inferior alveolar nerve[17,18] (Fig. 113.1). Posterior tumors (e.g., retromolar fossa) may require a lip-split/mandibulotomy approach. Bone invasion alone does not worsen the prognosis if resection margins are adequate.[19] Considerations in presurgical planning for mandibular resection include the type of incision to be used, the management of the neck, and the extent of the soft tissue and bone resection.

TECHNIQUE: Composite Marginal Mandibular Resection

STEP 1 Preparation of Patient for Composite Marginal Mandibular Resection

Composite marginal mandibular resection is usually undertaken for anterior floor of the mouth tumors, involving the lingual periosteum/lingual cortical bone (Fig. 113.2A). The patient is positioned on either a Mayfield headrest or on a doughnut with a shoulder roll. General anesthesia with nasal intubation is used, although tracheotomy may be required. When neck dissection is indicated, it is usually performed as a discontinuity procedure. In the case of a larger T3 or T4 tumor, an in-continuity marginal resection with neck dissection can be performed using a pull-through approach (discussion of that procedure is beyond the scope of this chapter).

STEP 2 Planning Incision for the Composite Marginal Mandibular Resection

An intraoral approach is used. The oral mucosa is dried with suction and a laparotomy sponge. A 1-cm margin is marked with a marking pen around the palpable margin of the tumor. This margin usually includes the attached gingival tissue on the buccal aspect, even when the tumor is lingual in the floor of the mouth. The mucosa on the buccal aspect is incised with needle tip electrocautery. Dissection is carried down to the mandibular bone through muscle, and the periosteum at the depth of the cut is elevated with a periosteal elevator. A sulcular incision is made along the teeth distal to the proposed bone cuts on both sides to prevent tearing of the mucosa, a precaution that facilitates closure of the defect.

Continued

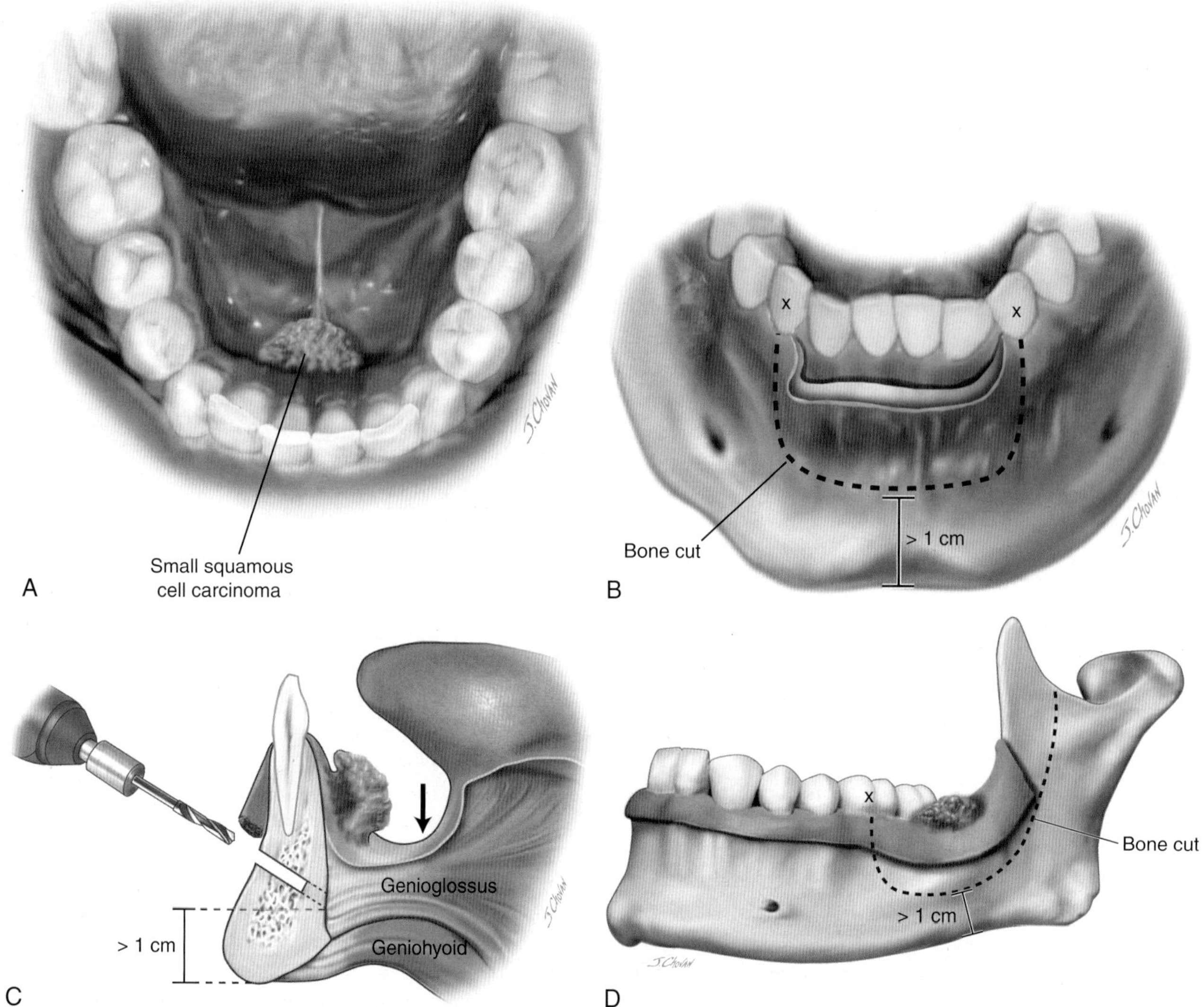

Figure 113.2 **A,** View from above shows a small squamous cell carcinoma of the anterior floor of the mouth stuck to the periosteum/cortical bone of the lingual aspect of the mandible. **B,** View from the buccal aspect: teeth 22 and 27 are to be extracted (marked with an X). The bone cut is below the apices of the teeth. A minimum height of 1 cm should be preserved at the inferior border of the mandible. **C,** Sagittal view of marginal resection. **D,** The dotted line indicates the proposed osteotomy for the marginal resection in the posterior mandible for a gingival/retromolar cancer. Maintaining a minimum height of 1 cm of bone at the inferior border of the mandible is preferred. If possible, the inferior alveolar nerve and vascular bundle are preserved. X marks the tooth to be extracted.

TECHNIQUE: Composite Marginal Mandibular Resection—*cont'd*

STEP 3 Soft Tissue Dissection

With a periosteal elevator, the soft tissue flaps defined by the sulcular incisions are raised in a subperiosteal plane, dissecting away from the tumor. Care is taken to identify the mental nerves, which can be preserved, if not within the oncologic margin. The flaps are extended to the midline bilaterally, passing inferior to the buccal gingival tissue previously outlined for resection. This exposes the buccal aspect of the anterior mandible to the chin (Fig. 113.2B).

STEP 4 Outline of the Osteotomies into the Mandible

Any teeth that were preplanned for extraction to allow a 1-cm bony margin are extracted. The bony osteotomy is marked with a #2 side-cutting bur, with a series of holes through the buccal cortex. The cut should be 3 to 4 mm beneath the apices of the teeth and leave at least 1 cm of bone height at the lower border. The corners of the cut where the vertical osteotomy meets the horizontal should be rounded to avoid a right angle, which could result in weakness, leading to stress fracture.

TECHNIQUE: Composite Marginal Mandibular Resection—*cont'd*

STEP 5 Performing Osteotomy

The osteotomy cut is made with either a #2 side-cutting bur or a banana blade reciprocating saw, depending on the surgeon's preference. The bony cut is made at an angle, sloping lingually for a tumor located on the lingual side (Fig. 113.2C). The cut is made through both cortices. It frequently is difficult to be sure that the entire lingual cortex has been cut, especially at the corners, and the osteotomy may require completion with gentle use of a mallet and thin osteotome to release the bony segment. Once the osteotomy is complete, the resected bone segment can be gently dislocated buccally, with care taken not to tear the lingual mucosa. The lingual gingiva and floor of the mouth can now be seen and the lingual soft tissue resection completed under direct visualization. This is especially helpful in dentate patients with retro-inclined incisors.

STEP 6 Preparation of the Site for Reconstruction

The specimen is now released, and frozen sections are harvested from the soft tissue margins. The osteotomized bone edges are smoothed with a large round bur or file. Reconstruction depends on the size of the defect and may involve primary closure, skin grafting, a local flap, or a microvascular free flap.

STEP 7 Management of the Retromolar or the Posterior Gingival Tumor

In the posterior mandible, for a retromolar or posterior gingival tumor, the osteotomy may include the anterior vertical ramus. The approach may be intraoral or cervical. The osteotomy is continued vertically through the sigmoid notch to include the coronoid process (Fig. 113.2D). A Langenbeck toe-out retractor is placed in the notch during the osteotomy. The temporalis muscle fibers are dissected off the coronoid with electrocautery. A right-angle clamp is useful for spreading the superior and lingual temporalis attachments, to facilitate resection with Bovie electrocautery.

TECHNIQUE: Composite Segmental Mandibular Resection

The most common mandibular resection is a hemi-mandibulectomy without sacrifice of the condyle (Fig. 113.3A).

STEP 1 Tumor Delineation

Neck dissection is nearly always performed via a subplatysmal horizontal cervical "apron" incision. The neck dissection remains pedicled to the lower border of the mandible. At this point, provided the primary tumor does not involve the buccal soft tissues or extend through the buccal cortex of the mandible, the periosteum at the lower border is incised with electrocautery. If still present, the facial artery and common facial vein are divided between ligatures.

STEP 2 Management of the Masseter Muscle and Mental Nerve

If the masticatory muscles at the angle of the mandible are not involved by the tumor, the pterygo-masseteric sling is sectioned at the lower border. The masseter muscle is then elevated off the mandible with electrocautery or a periosteal elevator, sweeping from superior to inferior. A Langenbeck toe-out retractor is placed in the sigmoid notch to expose the entire buccal surface of the vertical ramus. A saw is used to make a vertical subsigmoid osteotomy cut through the buccal cortex only (Fig. 113.3B). The periosteum is raised to a height of 1 cm along the lower border of the horizontal body, extending to the parasymphyseal region. The mental nerve is identified, and a vertical saw cut is made anterior to the nerve, through the buccal cortex only, as dictated by the position of the tumor.

STEP 3 Preplating the Mandible Before Resection

At this point, a reconstruction plate can be contoured to the mandible and temporarily screwed into position. A prebent plate from a three-dimensional stereolithographic model can also be used but is not advisable if the buccal soft tissues overlying the lower border of the mandible are infiltrated or if the mandible itself is expanded.

STEP 4 Management of the Intraoral Component of the Resection

If the tumor involves the buccal gingiva, sulcus, or cheek, a 1-cm margin is incised around the tumor with electrocautery and is carried through the deep tissues to bone, with the cut angled away from the tumor. With a periosteal elevator, the tissues inferior to the resection are raised off the mandible to communicate with the lower border dissection, creating a tunnel between the mouth and the neck. The cervical skin flap can now be retracted superiorly, allowing direct visualization of the buccal surface of the mandible with the attached tumor. At this point, the bone cuts are completed using a reciprocating saw through the buccal and lingual cortices of the mandible. Please refer to Step 5 of composite marginal mandibular resection on how to conduct the osteotomies.

Continued

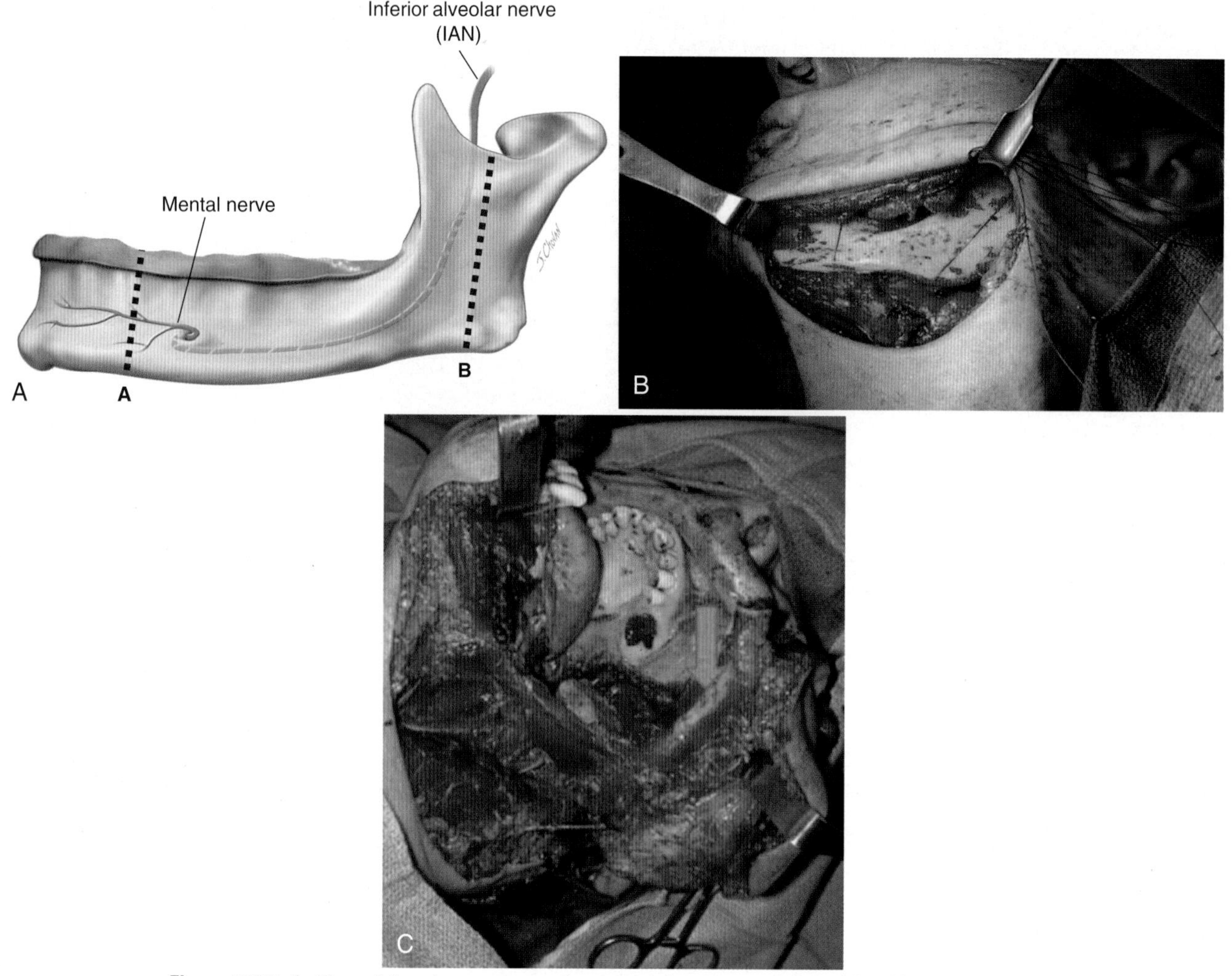

Figure 113.3 **A,** Dotted line A, anterior to the mental foramen, and dotted line B, proximal to the lingula, show the proposed segmental resection encompassing the nerve-bearing segment of the mandible. **B,** The subsigmoid cut has been outlined through the buccal cortex with a reciprocating saw. **C,** After lip-split and mandibular swing, the retromolar fossa and infratemporal contents are resected under direct vision (arrow points to the retracted mandible).

TECHNIQUE: Composite Segmental Mandibular Resection—*cont'd*

STEP 5 Modification of Technique for Tumors on the Lingual Aspect of the Mandible

If the tumor is located primarily on the lingual side of the mandible, the buccal tissues are elevated subperiosteally either by a sulcular or horizontal incision below the fixed gingiva, depending on the oncologic margin required. This allows the whole buccal surface of the mandible to be exposed. This is followed by elevation of the cervical flap, buccal osteotomy cuts, and plate placement, as previously described. Before the osteotomies are completed, a vertical cut is made with electrocautery from the lingual gingiva to the floor of the mouth 1 cm anterior to the tumor. This acts as a "stop" cut and prevents inadvertent tearing of the lingual mucosa toward the tumor during the mandibular osteotomy. The distal bone cut is made with a saw completely through the entire mandible. The proximal subsigmoid cut is made full thickness, beginning at the lower border. The cut is then carried cephalad. The subsigmoid portion is cut last in case of injury to a branch of the maxillary artery, which should be protected by the Langenbeck toe-out retractor. If arterial bleeding occurs, completing the osteotomy will allow access to the vessel.

TECHNIQUE: Composite Segmental Mandibular Resection—*cont'd*

STEP 6 Resection of the Tumor
Returning to the distal bone cut, the lingual periosteum is now sectioned with electrocautery, and the mandible is rotated toward the buccal side (gently so as not to tear the lingual mucosa) to allow complete access to the lingual side (Fig. 113.3C). The tumor of the floor of the mouth is palpated, and 1-cm margins around the tumor are marked with electrocautery. The dissection is deepened using electrocautery or scissors through the mylohyoid muscle, maintaining a 1-cm margin, until the tumor is pedicled to the mandible. The lingual nerve is preserved or sacrificed depending on its relationship to the tumor. As the mylohyoid muscle is divided, the mandible can be "swung" farther buccally, providing improved access to the posterior lingual region.

STEP 7 Completion of the Proximal Osteotomy
At this point, whether the tumor was primarily buccal or lingual, the horizontal body of the mandible is free of tissue attachments. The surgeon's attention now turns to the proximal osteotomy cut, which is distracted to divide residual lingual attachments of the medial pterygoid muscle to the vertical ramus. The inferior alveolar bundle is identified, and the artery is clipped as it emerges from the mandibular foramen. The inferior alveolar nerve can be clipped or followed to the skull base and foramen ovale if perineural invasion is suspected (Fig. 113.1). Frozen sections can be taken from the sectioned nerve.

STEP 8 Completion of the Tumor Resection
At this point, only the temporalis attachment to the coronoid process is holding the specimen. These fibers are divided close to the bone with electrocautery. The superior and lingual fibers can be difficult to access. In this case, the mandible is retracted inferiorly, and a right-angle clamp is used to spread and define the tendinous muscle attachments for division. The mandibular specimen is mobilized and removed in continuity with the neck dissection.

In some cases, the temporalis attachments can prevent the buccal swing of the mandible, for tumor resection. If this is the case, they can be detached as described in Step 7 of composite marginal mandibular resection.

ALTERNATIVE TECHNIQUE 1: Resection of the Overlying Skin

Involvement of facial skin is not common for intraoral tumors. It can occur laterally from buccogingival cancers (Fig. 113.4A and B) or anteriorly from extensive floor of the mouth cancers. In these cases, excision of the involved skin is incorporated into the neck dissection incision (Fig. 113.4B) to allow maximum access. The skin excision is done with a #15 scalpel blade or a needle tip electrocautery, allowing a 1-cm margin around the involved skin. The corresponding intraoral incision also is made through mucosa around the tumor with a 1-cm margin. The two incisions are joined to create a through-and-through defect using scissors or electrocautery. To facilitate dissection in a safe oncologic plane, repeated bimanual palpation is useful. In difficult cases, a needle can be inserted from the skin incision through to the mucosal incision to define the path of dissection to avoid cutting too close to the tumor. The skin resection is in continuity with the neck dissection and allows excellent access for the osteotomies. The mandibular resection proceeds as previously detailed. Careful planning of the skin incision can allow adjacent facial and cervical skin to be used to reconstruct the skin defect; this avoids a second flap or a different-color skin paddle (Fig. 113.4C and D).

ALTERNATIVE TECHNIQUE 2: Resection of the Condyle and Masticatory Muscles[20]

STEP 1 Exposure of the Condyle
The condyle rarely requires resection for oral tumors. In cases of extensive involvement of the vertical ramus and masticatory musculature, it is excised (Fig. 113.5A). Because the primary tumor is usually retromolar or oropharyngeal, a lip-split incision is combined with the cervical incision to allow posterior access. If the tumor extends into the infratemporal fossa, the mastoid portion of the cervical incision is carried anteriorly into a preauricular and hemicoronal incision (Fig. 113.5B).

STEP 2 Lip-Split Approach
The lip-split and cervical incisions are raised, dissecting through the buccal tissues overlying the horizontal body of the mandible, as dictated by any anterior/buccal involvement of the tumor. The dissection, with scissors, proceeds from anterior and inferior, passing superficial to the fascia of the masseter muscle. This isolates the masseter muscle on the specimen side and passes deep to the parotid and branches of the facial nerve, which are retracted and preserved. In some cases, a formal superficial parotidectomy is used to identify any involved branches of the facial nerve. In most cases, this is not necessary.

Continued

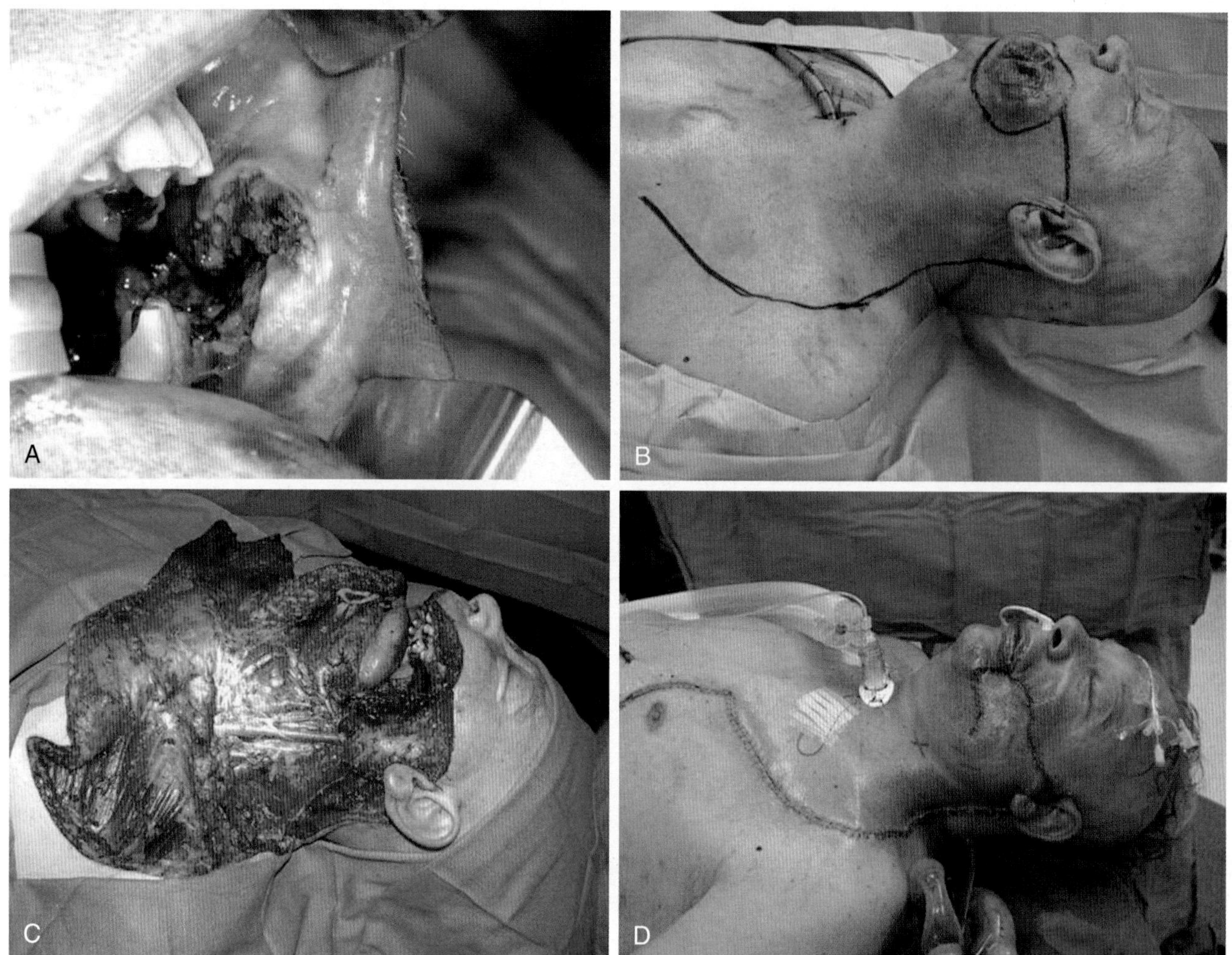

Figure 113.4 **A,** A T4 squamous cell carcinoma of the buccal mucosa involving the mandible. **B,** Obvious extension of oral cancer through the skin. The incision is designed to accommodate a neck dissection and a cervicofacial rotation flap for skin reconstruction and to allow resection of the involved facial skin with a 1.5-cm margin. **C,** Defect after resection of the cheek and mandible and elevation of the cervical rotation flap. Reconstruction of the mandible and mucosa will be accomplished with a fibular flap. **D,** Inset of the cervical rotation flap.

ALTERNATIVE TECHNIQUE 2: Resection of the Condyle and Masticatory Muscles[20]—*cont'd*

STEP 3 Complete Resection of the Masseter and Temporalis Muscles

The masseter is followed to its origin at the zygomatic arch by retraction of the parotid superficially to form a tunnel. The fibers of the masseter attachment to the zygomatic arch are cut close to the bone with electrocautery. The superior attachment of the masseter is reflected inferiorly, and the temporalis muscle insertion onto the coronoid and anterior vertical mandibular ramus is directly visualized deep to the masseter. The temporalis attachment to the coronoid is cut with electrocautery. This completes the buccal dissection. If the temporalis muscle is involved by tumor, the hemicoronal flap is raised to allow resection of the temporalis muscle (Fig. 113.5B).

STEP 4 Approach to the Lingual Aspect of the Tumor via an Anterior Mandibular Osteotomy

The anterior mandibular osteotomy through the horizontal body of the mandible with division of the lingual periosteum is carried out as previously described. The lingual tissues in the floor of the mouth and the mylohyoid muscle are dissected as dictated by the size and involvement of the tumor. This allows the mandible to be swung lingually, as previously described.

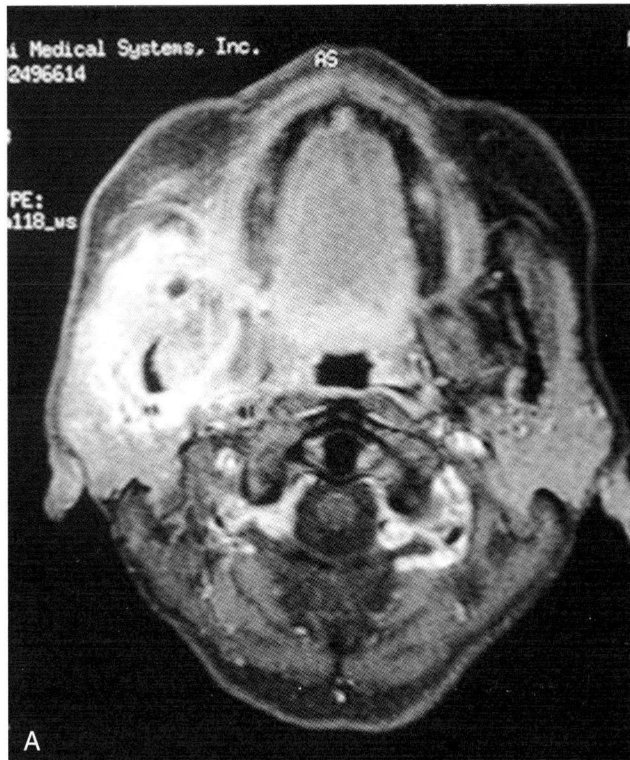

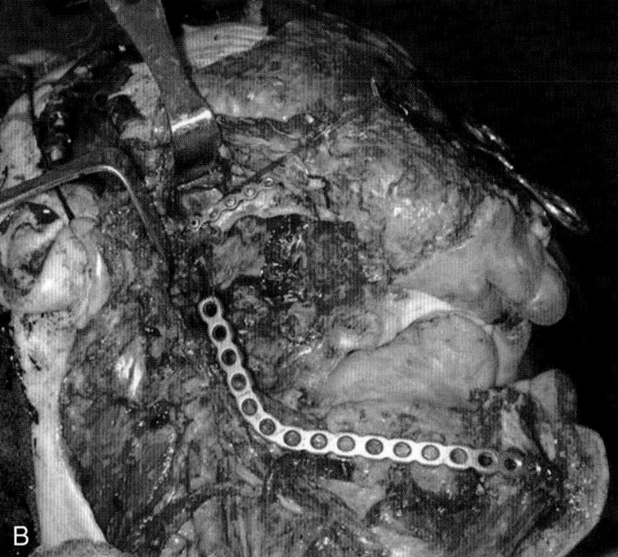

Figure 113.5 **A,** MRI shows extensive involvement of the masseter and pterygoid muscles with destruction of the mandible and extension into the infratemporal fossa by squamous cell carcinoma. **B,** Surgical approach demonstrating lower lip split extended into a hemicoronal flap. Army-Navy retractors are retracting the sectioned temporalis muscle. The malar arch was osteotomized for skull base access and has been plated back in place; the bone of the skull base is seen lateral to the malar arch.

ALTERNATIVE TECHNIQUE 2: Resection of the Condyle and Masticatory Muscles[20]—*cont'd*

STEP 5 Resection of the Medial Pterygoid Muscle

At this point, the mandibular swing allows visualization of the medial pterygoid muscle, which is followed to its insertion at the pterygoid plates. The muscle is cut close to the plate with electrocautery; the surgeon should take care to spread the muscle with a mosquito or right-angle clamp to identify and avoid the maxillary artery. Once the medial pterygoid has been resected, the lateral pterygoid fibers are visible.

STEP 6 Management of the Maxillary Artery and the Lateral Pterygoid Muscle

The maxillary artery can lie superficial or deep to the lateral pterygoid muscle. It should be identified and double-ligated. If it is accidentally cut, it can retract into muscle and cause problematic bleeding. If the lateral pterygoid muscle is to be resected, its insertions to the pterygoid plates and skull base are sectioned with needle point Bovie electrocautery.

STEP 7 Disarticulation of the Condylar Head

The surgeon's attention now turns to the condyle. It is approached from the buccal (lateral) side through the access gained by sectioning the masseter muscle from the zygomatic arch. The condylar neck is palpated buccally, and a subperiosteal dissection is made, reflecting the overlying soft tissues superiorly. This includes sectioning of the lateral capsule of the joint. The periosteal elevator is used to separate the disk from the head of the condyle so that it can be preserved. The attachments of the lateral pterygoid muscle to the condylar head and disk anteriorly are identified and carefully divided close to the bone with electrocautery. The mandible is rotated buccally and inferiorly to partially dislocate the condylar head from the fossa, exposing the lateral pterygoid attachments more lingually. These are divided, staying close to the bone with the needle tip electrocautery, directly or after spreading the muscle with a right-angle clamp. This is done cautiously because the internal maxillary artery lies close to the posterior and lingual surfaces of the neck of the condyle. The condyle is now dislocated from the fossa completely.

STEP 8 Management of the Inferior Alveolar Nerve

The inferior alveolar bundle is identified, clipped, and divided. Residual attachments that may interfere with release of the specimen (e.g., the stylomandibular and sphenomandibular ligaments) are divided, and the specimen is released.

ALTERNATIVE TECHNIQUE 3: Composite Resection of the Anterior Mandible

STEP 1 Planning Incisions for Composite Resection

Composite resection of the anterior mandible is usually performed for large floor of the mouth cancers. In the authors' experience, the skin of the chin is quite frequently invaded by cancer. The approach is usually cervical because bilateral neck dissections will have been performed. If the skin of the chin is to be resected, the skin paddle is incorporated into the cervical incision to allow access as described for composite resection of the lateral mandible (Fig. 113.6A).

STEP 2 Resection of the Tumor

The cervical flap is raised as a "visor" approach, and the mental nerves are preserved only if the bone resection allows (Fig. 113.6B). The buccal dissection and the mandibular osteotomies are carried out as previously described. On the lingual side, the geniohyoid and genioglossus muscles are divided as indicated by the depth and size of the tumor. The genial muscles that have not been resected are marked with polypropylene suture so that they can be identified and sutured to the mandibular reconstruction, to prevent tongue retro-position during the reconstruction.

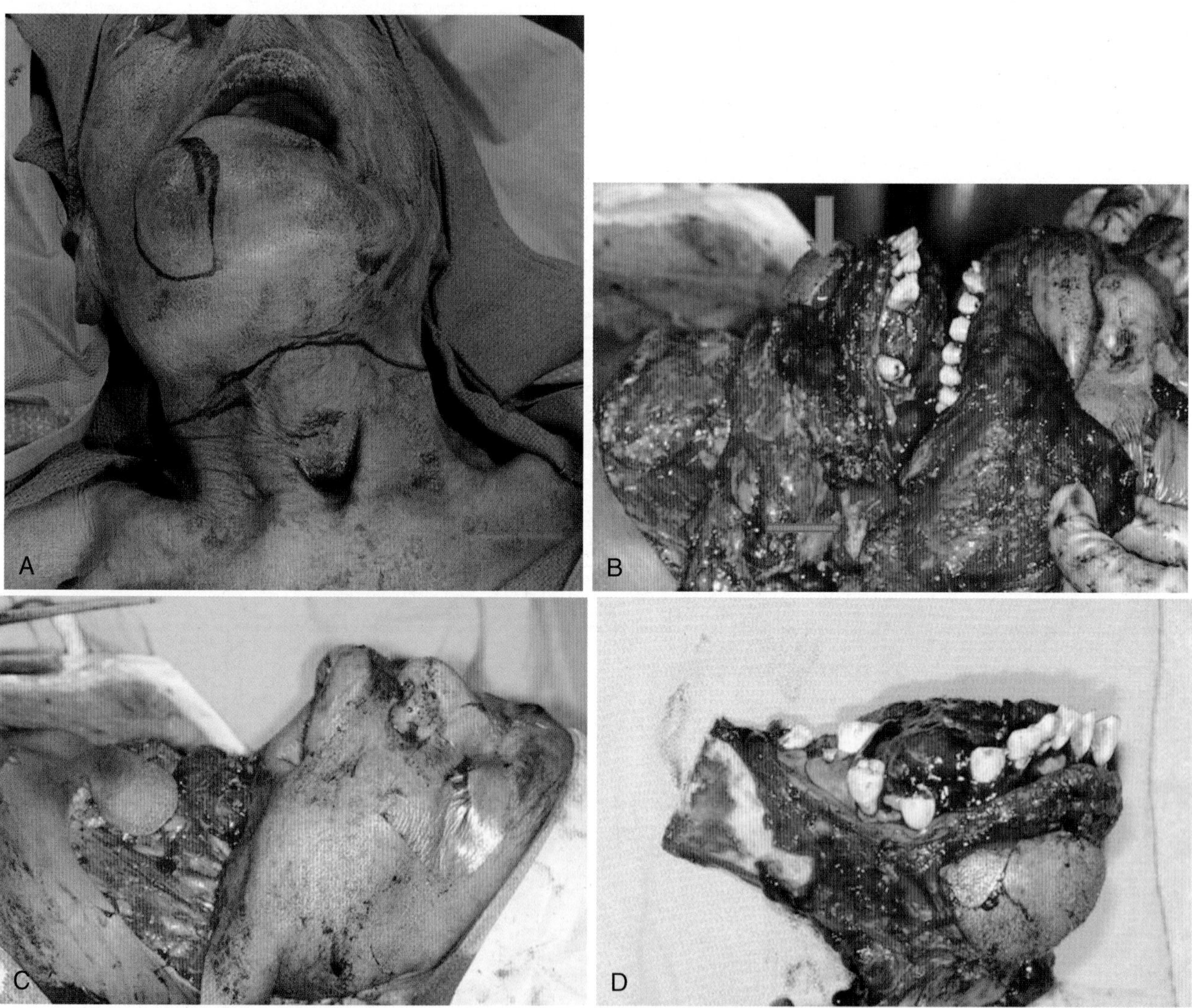

Figure 113.6 **A,** A T4 SCC of the mandible and involving the skin on the face. A visor incision is planned for the neck dissection, and the skin excision is outlined. **B,** In this patient, a central area of chin skin has been excised *(thick blue arrow)*. The cervical flaps are raised cephalad to the mandible retracted by the surgeon's fingers on the left. The bone at the angle of the mandible is exposed for resection *(thin blue arrow)*. **C,** Resection of from angle to angle of the mandible causes a gross "Andy Gump" deformity that mandates reconstruction. **D,** The resected specimen involves angle to angle of the mandible. Note the facial skin paddle and the displaced teeth secondary to bone invasion by the large floor of the mouth squamous cell carcinoma (SCC).

ALTERNATIVE TECHNIQUE 3: Composite Resection of the Anterior Mandible—*cont'd*

STEP 3 Consideration for Hyoid Bone Resuspension
After the resection and removal of the anterior mandible, the size of the defect is evaluated (Fig. 113.6C and D). Identification of the hyoid bone and suspension with 0 polypropylene sutures to the subsequent mandibular reconstruction will control laryngeal sag and help with future swallowing.

Avoidance and Management of Intraoperative Complications

A major intraoperative complication in any surgery is uncontrolled and/or persistent hemorrhage. In composite mandibular resection, this can be a problem in the pterygoid region with the maxillary artery or its branches. To avoid inaccessible bleeding from the masseteric artery, the subsigmoid osteotomy is completed from the lower border initially, leaving the superior cut through the sigmoid notch until last. This allows the mandible to be quickly separated if the artery is cut. Bleeding from the maxillary artery can be profuse and difficult to stop if the artery retracts into muscle. If the inferior alveolar bundle has been identified, the inferior alveolar artery can be followed cephalad until its junction with the maxillary artery trunk is identified. The maxillary artery crosses the inferior alveolar nerve laterally (superficially) as it emerges around the condylar neck and can be ligated at this point. Diffuse bleeding from the pterygoid venous plexus can also be challenging to control. When arterial or venous bleeders from the muscles cannot be identified, large silk sutures can be passed around blocks of muscle as hemostatic sutures, which frequently stop the hemorrhage.

Another intraoperative complication is tearing of the lingual tissues while "swinging" the mandible buccally. These mucosal tears can extend into the tumor, making it very difficult to maintain a proper oncologic margin. This can be prevented firstly by a vertical "stop cut" through the lingual mucosa, once the tooth at the site of the mandibular osteotomy has been extracted. Secondly, the osteotomy should be completed with the drill or saw through both cortices as a clean cut. If the cut is not complete and the surgeon attempts to complete the split of the mandible by twisting an osteotome, a fracture of the lingual plate that extends distal or proximal to the osteotomy site can tear the lingual tissues when the mandible is swung buccally. Finally, the lingual periosteum must be completely divided before the mandible is gently swung buccally. The lingual margin can then be cut under direct vision.

Postoperative Complications

In cases of buccal/gingival tumor with invasion into the cheek or chin region, excision with preservation of skin can leave the facial skin very thin. Unless a muscle flap or muscle tissue from an osteo-cutaneous free flap is placed over the reconstruction plate, the plate will erode through the skin. This usually occurs during or shortly after radiation therapy (Fig. 113.7A).

When radical composite resection requires a lip-split incision in combination with a cervical and extended hemicoronal incision, the blood supply of the skin flap can be compromised. This is especially true in heavy smokers and in patients who have had previous radiation therapy. The authors have seen loss of the lower lip and the cervical portion of the flap (Fig. 113.7B). Excision with skin grafting or flap repair is usually required.

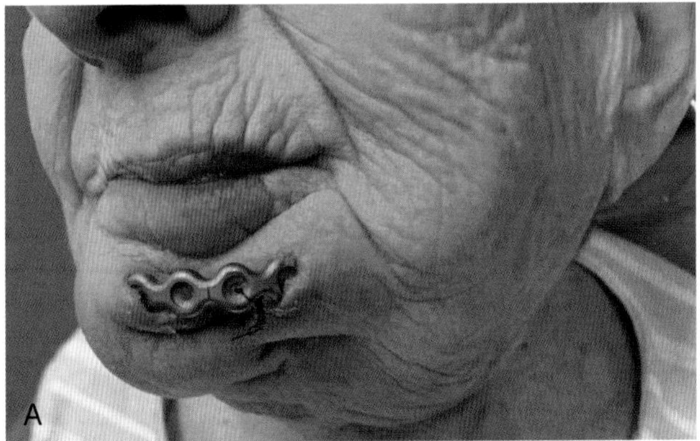

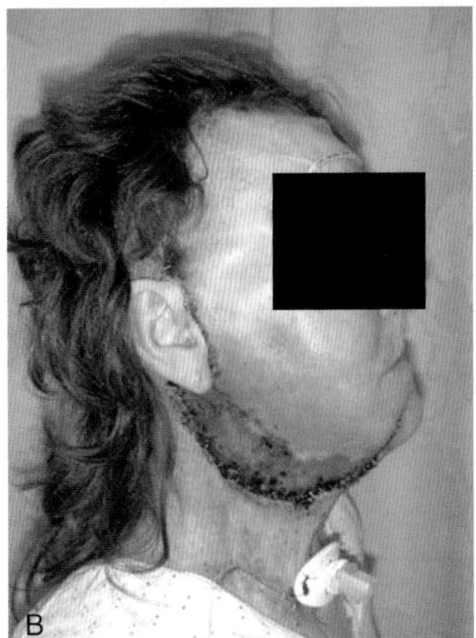

Figure 113.7 **A,** Plate exposure after radiation therapy. **B,** Patient in Fig. 113.4 is shown 10 days after surgery. The inferior portion of the cervical flap is ischemic and necrotic. The area of necrosis is well demarcated, the dead skin is debrided, and either skin grafting or flap reconstruction is performed.

References

1. Ward GE, Robben JO. A composite operation for radical neck dissection and removal of cancer of the mouth. *Cancer*. 1951;4(1):98–109.
2. Panagopoulous AP. Bone involvement in maxillofacial cancer. *Am J Surg*. 1959;98:898.
3. Southam JC. The extension of squamous carcinoma along the inferior dental neurovascular bundle. *Br J Oral Surg*. 1970;7(3):137–145.
4. Byars LT. Extent of manidbular resection required for treatment of oral cancer. *AMA Arch Surg*. 1955;70(6):914–922.
5. McGregor AD, MacDonald DG. Routes of entry of squamous cell carcinoma to the mandible. *Head Neck Surg*. 1988;10(5):294–301.
6. Brown JS, Browne RM. Factors influencing the patterns of invasion of the mandible by oral squamous cell carcinoma. *Int J Oral Maxillofac Surg*. 1995;24(6):417–426.
7. Carter RL, Tsao SW, Burman JF, Pittam MR, Clifford P, Shaw HJ. Patterns and mechanisms of bone invasion by squamous carcinomas of the head and neck. *Am J Surg*. 1983;146(4):451–455.
8. Totsuka Y, Usui Y, Tei K, et al. Mandibular involvement by squamous cell carcinoma of the lower alveolus: analysis and comparative study of histologic and radiologic features. *Head Neck*. 1991;13(1):40–50.
9. Brown JS, Kalavrezos N, D'Souza J, Lowe D, Magennis P, Woolgar JA. Factors that influence the method of mandibular resection in the management of oral squamous cell carcinoma. *Br J Oral Maxillofac Surg*. 2002;40(4):275–284.
10. O'Brien CJO, Adams JR, McNeil EB, et al. Influence of bone invasion and extent of mandibular resection on local control of cancers of the oral cavity and oropharynx. *Int J Oral Maxillofac Surg*. 2003;32(5):492–497.
11. Flynn MB, Moore C. Marginal resection of the mandible in the management of squamous cancer of the floor of the mouth. *Am J Surg*. 1974;128(4):490–493.
12. Barttelbort SW, Bahn SL, Ariyan SA. Rim mandibulectomy for cancer of the oral cavity. *Am J Surg*. 1987;154(4):423–428.
13. Ord RA, Sarmadi M, Papadimitrou J. A comparison of segmental and marginal bony resection for oral squamous cell carcinoma involving the mandible. *J Oral Maxillofac Surg*. 1997;55(5):470–477.
14. Cawood JI, Howell RA. A classification of the edentulous jaws. *Int J Oral Maxillofac Surg*. 1988;17(4):232–236.
15. Brown J, Chatterjee R, Lowe D, Lewis-Jones H, Rogers S, Vaughan D. A new guide to mandibular resection for oral squamous cell carcinoma based on the Cawood and Howell classification of the mandible. *Int J Oral Maxillofac Implants*. 2005;34(8):834–839.
16. Bouhir S, Mortuaire G, Dubrulle-Berthelot F, et al. Radiological assessment of mandibular invasion in squamous cell carcinoma of the oral cavity and oropharynx. *Eur Ann Otorhinolaryngol Head Neck Dis*. 2019;136(5):361–366.
17. Bilodeau EA, Chiosea S. Oral squamous cell carcinoma with mandibular bone invasion: intraoperative evaluation of bone margins by routine frozen section. *Head Neck Pathol*. 2011;5(3):216–220.
18. Wysluch A, Stricker I, Hölzle F, Wolff KD, Maurer P. Intraoperative evaluation of bony margins with frozen-section analysis and trephine drill extraction technique: a preliminary study. *Head Neck*. 2010;32(11):1473–1478.
19. Mücke T, Hölzle F, Wagenpfeil S, Wolff KD, Kesting M. The role of tumor invasion into the mandible of oral squamous cell carcinoma. *J Cancer Res Clin Oncol*. 2011;137(1):165–171.
20. Blanchaert RH, Ord RA. Vertical ramus compartment resection of the mandible for deeply invasive tumors. *J Oral Maxillofac Surg*. 1998;56(1):15–22.

CHAPTER 114

Maxillectomy

Brandyn Herman and Melvyn Yeoh

Armamentarium

#9 Periosteal elevators
#11 and #15 Scalpel blades
Appropriate sutures
Curved Mayo or other heavy scissors
Dermatome
Fixation devices
Freer elevators
Kerrison rongeurs
Local anesthetic with vasoconstrictor
Malleable retractors
Needle cautery tip
Obwegeser retractors
Osteotomes
Reciprocating saw
Seldin retractors
Topical decongestant nasal packing
Unipolar and bipolar electrocautery
Weider tongue depressor

History of the Procedure

For history and evolution of the maxillectomy procedure, please refer to the discussion of partial/infrastructure maxillectomy in Chapter 84.

Indications for the Use of the Procedure

Complete unilateral maxillectomy or one of its variants is commonly performed for surgical resection of benign or malignant tumors of the maxilla, whether they originate from bone, minor salivary glands, sinus tissue, or dental tissues. The comprehensive treatment of malignant diseases of the maxilla commonly entails a combined approach utilizing adjuvant radiotherapy or chemotherapy, especially when dealing with advanced stage disease. Surgical resection is the treatment of choice for the majority of these tumors, except for those that are highly responsive to radiotherapy or chemotherapy such as lymphoreticular malignancies.

Surgical resection of the maxilla and its contiguous structures can be divided into three main types: partial maxillary resection with the preservation of the roof and superior portions of the antrum, total maxillary resection with preservation of the globe, and total maxillary resection with orbital exenteration. The precise limit of surgical resection is determined by the extent of the tumor.

Determination of the extent of resection is especially challenging in the preoperative evaluation of maxillary tumors, as the bulk of the tumor is rarely visualized during physical examination. Preoperative evaluation should include a standard head and neck examination, focused on the oral cavity, nasal cavity, and orbital regions. Flexible nasopharyngoscopy can provide more thorough visualization of the nasal cavity, nasopharynx, and oropharynx and has become a standard adjunct to clinical head and neck examination. Imaging studies such as computed tomography (CT) scans and magnetic resonance imaging (MRI), when correlated with clinical examination, will help stage the tumors accurately.

Ohngren's line is an imaginary plane drawn from the medial canthus to the angle of the mandible[1] (Fig. 114.1). This plane roughly divides the maxillary sinus into an anteroinferior aspect and a posterosuperior aspect. Not surprisingly, tumors that are located within or have extended into the posterosuperior aspect of the maxillary sinus tend to be associated with a poor prognosis, as they are more likely to exhibit involvement of the orbit and infratemporal fossa. Obvious signs of invasion of orbital contents include proptosis and impairment of extraocular muscle function that will necessitate orbital exenteration for complete resection of the lesion. Ophthalmologic consultation is frequently helpful when trying to ascertain if orbital contents have been invaded, and it is especially valuable to assess the status of the opposite eye.

Total ipsilateral maxillary resection is not always required. Tumors originating from the inferior aspect of the maxilla or maxillary sinus (below Ohngren's line) can commonly be treated with a partial maxillectomy involving the inferior portion of the maxilla, thereby preserving the zygomatic complex, the orbital floor, and the inferior orbital rim (see Chapter 84). Likewise, tumors involving only the medial maxillary wall or lateral nasal wall, such as an inverted papilloma, can be treated with a medial maxillectomy. Bilateral, total maxillectomy is occasionally required and entails much greater complexity in reconstruction. A variety of vascularized bone flaps can be utilized, as can support of an obturator prosthesis on four zygomatic implants.[2] On occasion, the tumor will have extended

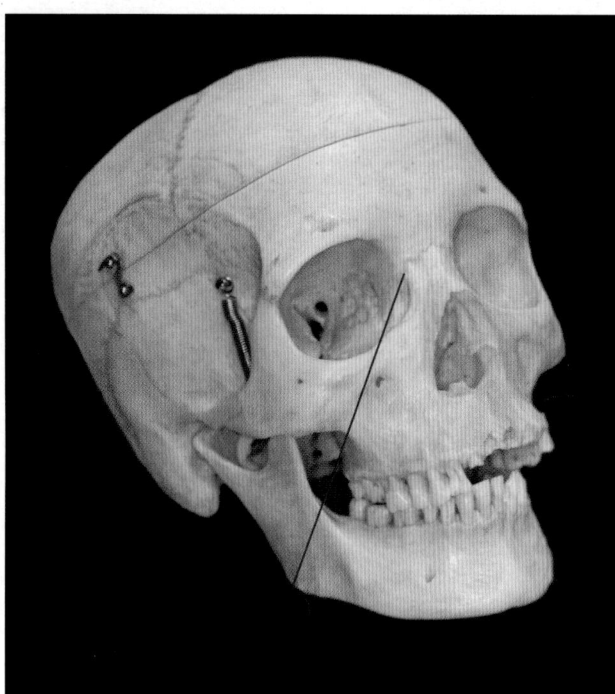

Figure 114.1 Ohngren's line.

beyond the confines of the maxillary antrum into adjacent structures such as the ethmoid sinus, sphenoid sinus, pterygomaxillary and infratemporal fossae, and the orbit. Extended maxillectomy or craniofacial resection may be required if the tumor is amendable to resection.

Benign and malignant tumors of the maxilla and maxillary sinuses are histologically diverse, as they arise from varied structures. They can arise from within the Schneiderian membrane, from the bone surrounding the maxillary sinus, or from odontogenic tissues within the alveolar process, or they can extend into the maxilla or maxillary sinus through contiguous spread from surrounding structures such as the oral cavity, orbit, nasopharynx, skull base, or overlying skin. Evaluation of patients with these tumors requires three-dimensional imaging, and both MRI and CT scans are helpful in discriminating the extent of tumor mass from backed-up secretions within the maxillary sinus lumen or within adjacent paranasal sinuses.

Ideally, a multidisciplinary team in conjunction with a hospital tumor board is required to provide comprehensive evaluation, treatment, and adjunctive therapy. A multidisciplinary team approach has been shown to provide improved patient quality of life, function, and survival for head and neck cancer patients.[3] Optimally, the team would include a head and neck ablative and reconstruction surgeon, dentist, oral-facial prosthodontist, specialist in radiation oncology, medical oncologist, clinical pathologist, pain and palliative care team, registered dietitian, speech language pathologist, physical and occupational therapists, and social worker. Tumor boards help to ensure access to the "best current thinking about cancer management" and provide a variety of ideas and perspectives and the use of cutting-edge technologies and treatments.[3]

Limitations and Contraindications

The decision to perform surgery is based on the type and extent of the tumor and the patient's general health, comorbidities, and wishes. Absolute contraindications for performing a maxillectomy include the patient's refusal to provide consent for surgery, diseases such as lymphoreticular tumors that are best treated by nonsurgical means, or a debilitated patient who is unable to tolerate surgery due to poor overall health. Relative contraindications center on situations where maxillectomy with curative intent may not be feasible and a palliative course of treatment may be preferable. Such situations may involve patients with untreatable distant metastases. A palliative treatment plan may be more appropriate for patients with large tumors that require bilateral orbital exenteration and for tumors with extensive intracranial invasion.

TECHNIQUE: Total Ipsilateral Maxillectomy With Orbital Preservation via the Weber-Ferguson Approach

The Weber-Ferguson surgical approach is indicated for access to maxillary tumors that either extend superiorly toward the orbital floor or involve the orbit or for tumors that extend posteriorly toward the posterior wall of the maxillary antrum. This approach provides a wide access to all areas of the maxilla and orbital floor.

STEP 1: Patient Preparation

Oral-endotracheal intubation with a reinforced tube is a standard airway for maxillectomy, although contralateral nasal endotracheal intubation can be used for unilateral maxillectomy. A tracheotomy is always appropriate and is recommended for extended maxillectomy and for maxillectomy along with a craniofacial resection. Hypotensive anesthesia to minimize blood loss is advisable. Preoperative packing of the nasal cavity with decongestant-soaked materials and regional injection of epinephrine-containing local anesthesia in a manner similar to that for a septorhinoplasty can reduce blood loss. The eye is protected with a temporary 5-0 silk tarsorrhaphy suture prior to incision if orbital preservation is planned.

STEP 2: Skin Incisions

An incision line is drawn along the crest of the ipsilateral philtral column of the lip from the nostril sill inferiorly to the white roll. The incision then turns medially 90 degrees and is extended within the white roll to the midline of cupid's bow. Here, the incision line turns inferiorly 90 degrees to extend through the vermilion of the lip, thereby creating a step-off, which will resist scar contracture and subsequent notching of the lip. Creation of a Z-plasty on the mucosal

TECHNIQUE: Total Ipsilateral Maxillectomy With Orbital Preservation via the Weber-Ferguson Approach—*cont'd*

inner surface of the lip at the time of closure also helps avoid notching. From the superior extent of the philtral column incision at the nostril sill, the incision line turns 90 degrees laterally to extend around the base of the nose, and superiorly along the nasofacial groove (at the border of the esthetic units) terminating just below the medial canthus. This incision will be adequate for most maxillectomies. If further lateral release is needed, the subciliary extension can be created. The incision line is drawn extending laterally within a skin crease approximately 3 to 4 mm below the ciliary line to just below the lateral canthus. This incision line can be modified to extend further laterally or superiorly, as required for tumor removal.

A #15 blade is then used to make the lateral rhinotomy portion of the incision. Skin and subcutaneous tissue is incised along the nasofacial groove, and the incision is brought inferiorly, transecting the full thickness of the upper lip through the vermilion. The superior labial artery is ligated or coagulated. The subciliary incision of the Weber-Ferguson approach is then begun laterally at the lateral canthus and is brought medially in the subciliary level, approximately 3 to 4 mm below the lower eyelid and extended slightly inferior to the medial canthus toward the superior end of the lateral rhinotomy incision. The underlying orbicularis oculi muscle is then incised in a tangential direction and directed inferiorly down to bone in a preseptal plane, utilizing electrocautery. This method of incision through the orbicularis oculi muscle will maintain the integrity of the orbital septum (Fig. 114.2A).

STEP 3: Oral Incisions

Utilizing electrocautery, an incision is made in the ipsilateral mucobuccal fold approximately 1 cm away from the free gingival junction. It extends from end of the lip-splitting incision to the third molar-tuberosity area. If oncologically safe, this incision can be made partially or completely within the gingival sulcus to preserve gingiva. A facial cheek flap is then elevated in a subperiosteal plane off the maxilla in a subperiosteal plane. In the event of tumor extension through the anterolateral maxillary wall, a supraperiosteal dissection of appropriate thickness will be necessary. The cheek flap is reflected superiorly toward the infraorbital rim. Care is taken to preserve the infraorbital nerve if possible; however, sacrifice of this nerve in conjunction with the subciliary extension significantly improves posterior access.

The facial flap is elevated not only to expose the anterior maxilla but to carry it laterally over the zygomatico-maxillary buttress. If possible and oncologically appropriate, identification and clipping the internal maxillary artery at the pterygomaxillary fissure at this juncture are ideal, as they will minimize the blood loss as the procedure proceeds.

Continued

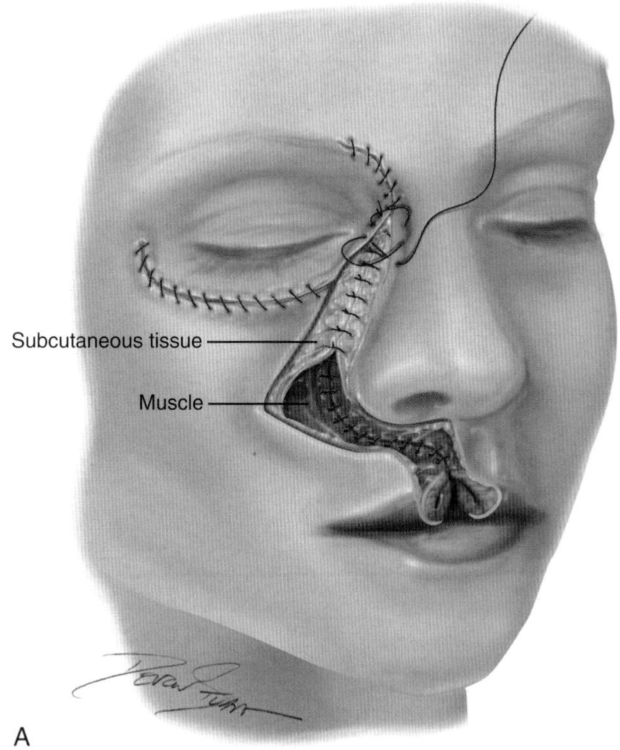

Figure 114.2 **A,** Traditional Weber-Ferguson approach in various stages of closure with subciliary extension and supraorbital extension.

TECHNIQUE: Total Ipsilateral Maxillectomy With Orbital Preservation via the Weber-Ferguson Approach—*cont'd*

After full exposure of the anterior and lateral walls of the maxilla, an incision in the soft palate is made, starting at the posterior portion of the ipsilateral maxillary buccal vestibule incision. This incision is made with electrocautery and extends medially along the hard-soft palate junction, posterior to the tumor. The muscles are transected from their hard palate bony attachments. This incision is brought medially toward the palatal midline or medial to the lesion. The exact placement of this incision is dictated by tumor position and adequacy of margins and may involve inclusion of the entire hemisoft palate with the specimen. The incision turns anteriorly through the mucoperiosteum of the hard palate. It follows a paramedian line medial to the lesion, thereby joining the anterior portion of the maxillary vestibular incision. The maxilla and tumor are then encircled by the oral component of the incision.

After elevation of the facial flaps, attention is directed to the orbital contents. If preoperative imaging has demonstrated that the tumor approaches the antral roof, the periorbita is elevated inferiorly and medially to expose the floor of the orbit, lacrimal fossa, and lamina papyracea. The lacrimal sac is then identified and retracted, which stretches and exposes the nasolacrimal duct. The nasolacrimal duct is then transected at the junction with the sac. Direct extension of the tumor through the periorbita is an indication for orbital exenteration (see Chapter 103). If the orbital contents are to be preserved, the lacrimal sac is marsupialized by dividing the sac and fixating each half to the surrounding periorbita allowing drainage into the nasal cavity (Fig. 114.2B and C).

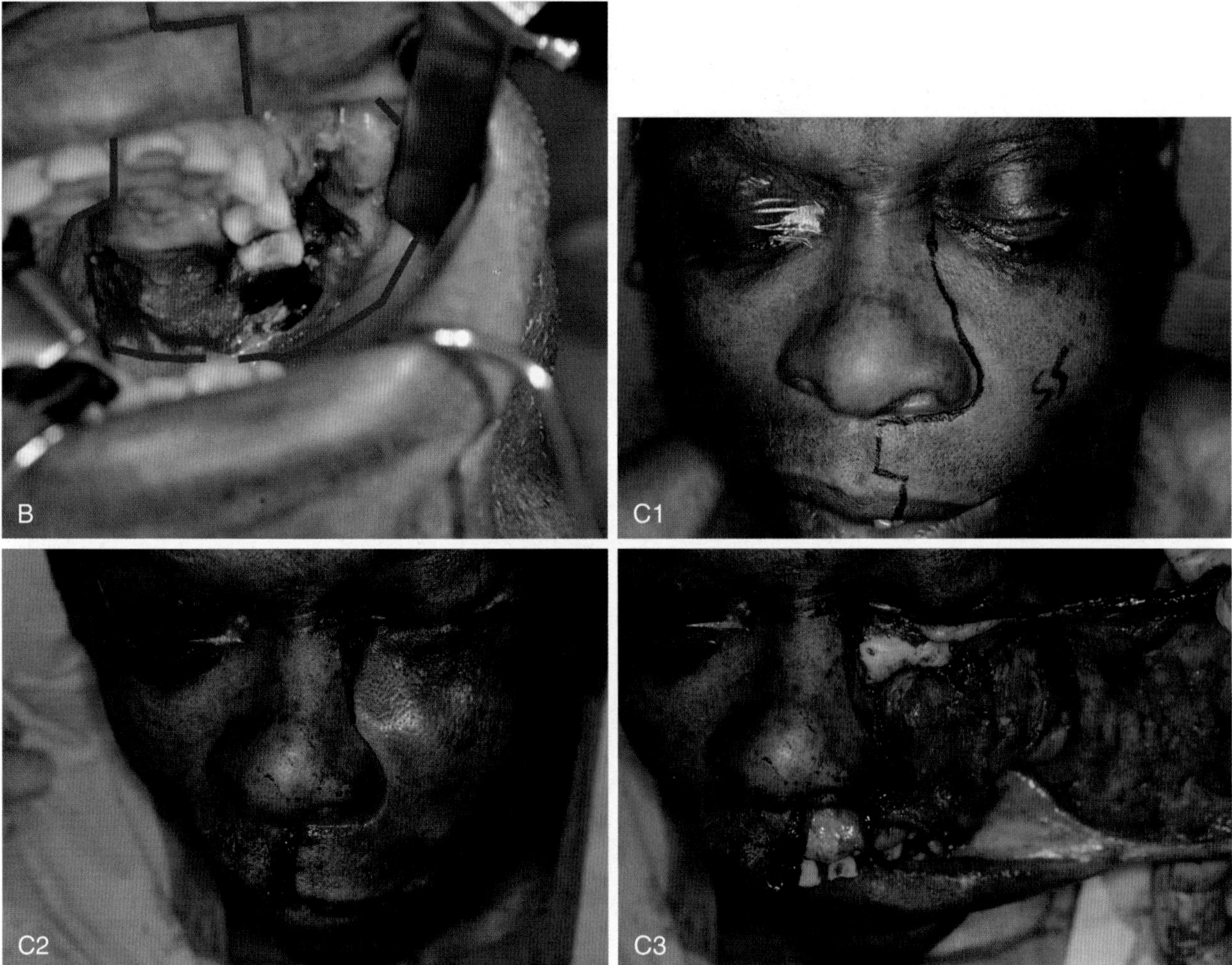

Figure 114.2, cont'd **B,** Intraoral view of the Weber-Ferguson approach illustrating the view of the hard and soft palate incisions joining with the maxillary buccal vestibular incision. **C1,** Marked Weber-Ferguson approach exposure for resection of a maxillary squamous cell carcinoma tumor. **C2,** Incised Weber-Ferguson approach for resection of a maxillary squamous cell carcinoma tumor. **C3,** Reflected Weber-Ferguson flap for resection of a maxillary squamous cell carcinoma tumor.

TECHNIQUE: Total Ipsilateral Maxillectomy With Orbital Preservation via the Weber-Ferguson Approach—*cont'd*

STEP 4: Osteotomies for Ipsilateral Maxillectomy With Orbital Floor Resection

(For osteotomy design for infrastructure maxillectomy, please refer to Chapter 84.)

The first osteotomy is made with a reciprocating saw at the junction of the frontal and body process of the zygoma. A vertical bone cut is then made, separating the maxilla from the nasal bones. This cut is extended superiorly to the frontoethmoidal suture line. From this point, the osteotomy is carried posteriorly, just inferior to the level of the anterior and posterior ethmoid arteries to a point 1 to 2 mm posterior to the posterior ethmoid foramen, avoiding the optic foramen.

An osteotomy is then made through the orbital floor passing laterally and connecting the medial orbital wall osteotomy to the lateral orbital wall by crossing the inferior orbital fissure. The lateral orbital wall is then osteotomized approximately 1 to 1.5 cm inferior to the frontozygomatic suture, and the osteotomy is connected to the first osteotomy at the junction of the frontal and body process of the zygoma.

Following removal of vasoconstrictive nasal packing, a reciprocating saw is then used to osteotomize the hard palate in a paramedian position, medial to the tumor. Careful control of the amount of "plunge" of the reciprocating saw helps avoid unnecessary laceration of the highly vascular turbinates.

A chisel is then placed in the pterygomaxillary fissure and directed in a posterior-superior direction to separate the maxilla from the skull. If the tumor involves the posterior maxillary wall, the pterygoid plates can be resected along with the maxilla by directing the chisels at the superior aspect of the pterygoid plates or by utilizing heavy curved scissors to sharply cut the plates along with the pterygoid musculature. The posterior and superior attachments of the inferior turbinate are sharply divided, and the specimen can then be removed with an anterior inferior rocking movement (Fig. 114.2D and E).

Continued

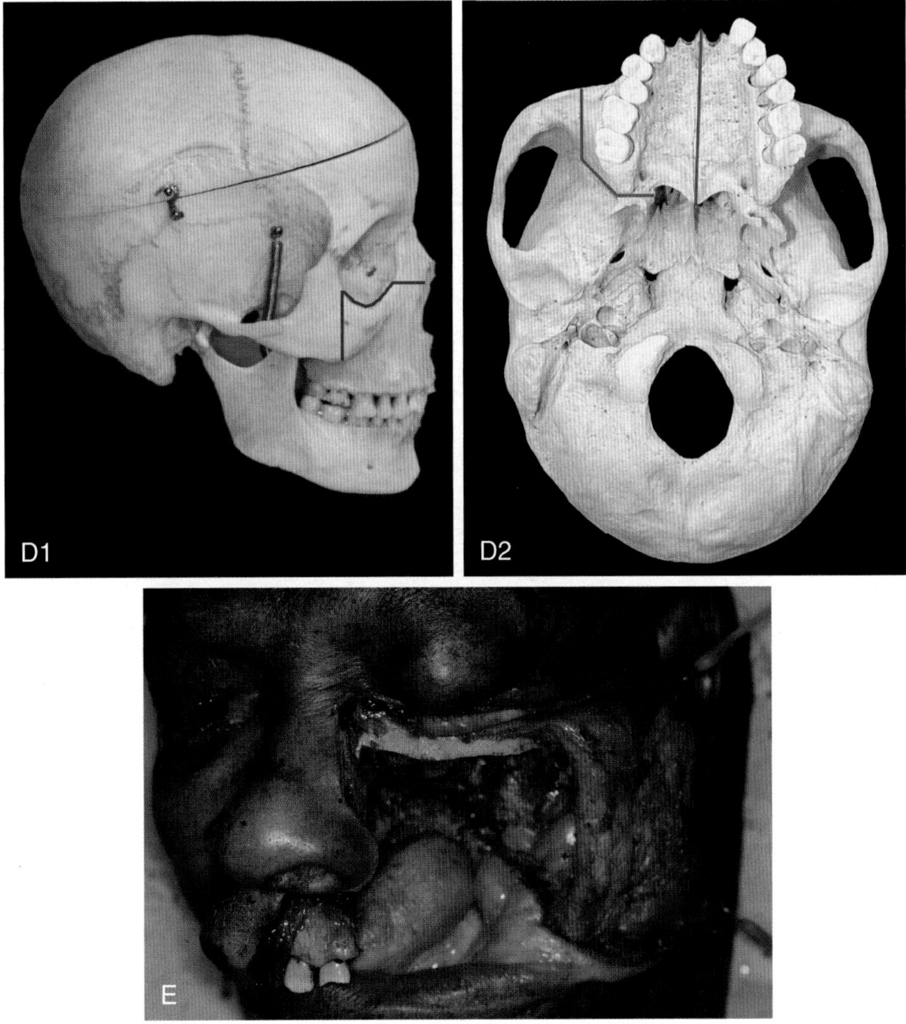

Figure 114.2, cont'd **D,** Outline of osteotomies illustrated on a skull for a total maxillectomy with orbital content preservation. **D1,** Profile view. **D2,** Inferior view. **E,** Maxillectomy defect.

TECHNIQUE: Total Ipsilateral Maxillectomy With Orbital Preservation via the Weber-Ferguson Approach—*cont'd*

STEP 5: Reconstruction

After the total ipsilateral maxillectomy specimen is removed and hemostasis achieved, attention should first be directed toward reconstruction of the missing inferior orbital floor and rim. Reconstruction of the orbital floor can be completed with either alloplasts such as a titanium mesh or a preformed custom implant or with autogenous tissues, such as free bone grafts from the hip, cranium, or osteocutaneous free microvascular flaps. The ipsilateral coronoid process pedicled to the temporalis can be rotated medially to support the orbital floor.[4] The type of reconstruction depends on the size of the defect as well as the experience and preference of the surgeon.

If the maxillary cavity is not to be reconstructed with a microvascular free flap, the defect should be lined with a split-thickness skin graft or acellular dermis. Lining the inner aspect of the cavity promotes rapid healing and helps to limit contraction of the surgical cavity, leading to subsequent collapse of the midface.

The ipsilateral temporalis muscle flap can be used to cover the orbital floor and, in some situations, is used to obliterate the cavity. Because of disuse atrophy of muscle, this flap will atrophy, and the result will be inferior to that of a microvascular free flap containing fat and fascia.

Ideally, a surgical obturator can be fabricated preoperatively and is placed immediately after the resection. If the dentition does not allow for clasp retention of the obturator, lag screws can be placed through to the remaining hard palate. The prefabricated obturator can support a skin or dermal graft. Alternatively, the prosthetic obturator can be fabricated in a delayed fashion once the incisions have healed. The maxillary defect can be initially packed with an antibiotic impregnated gauze or sponge to bolster the skin graft and to maintain facial shape. After 1 week, the skin graft has taken and the packing can be removed. The patient will have difficulty articulating and eating until the prosthetic obturator can be fitted (Fig. 114.2F and G).

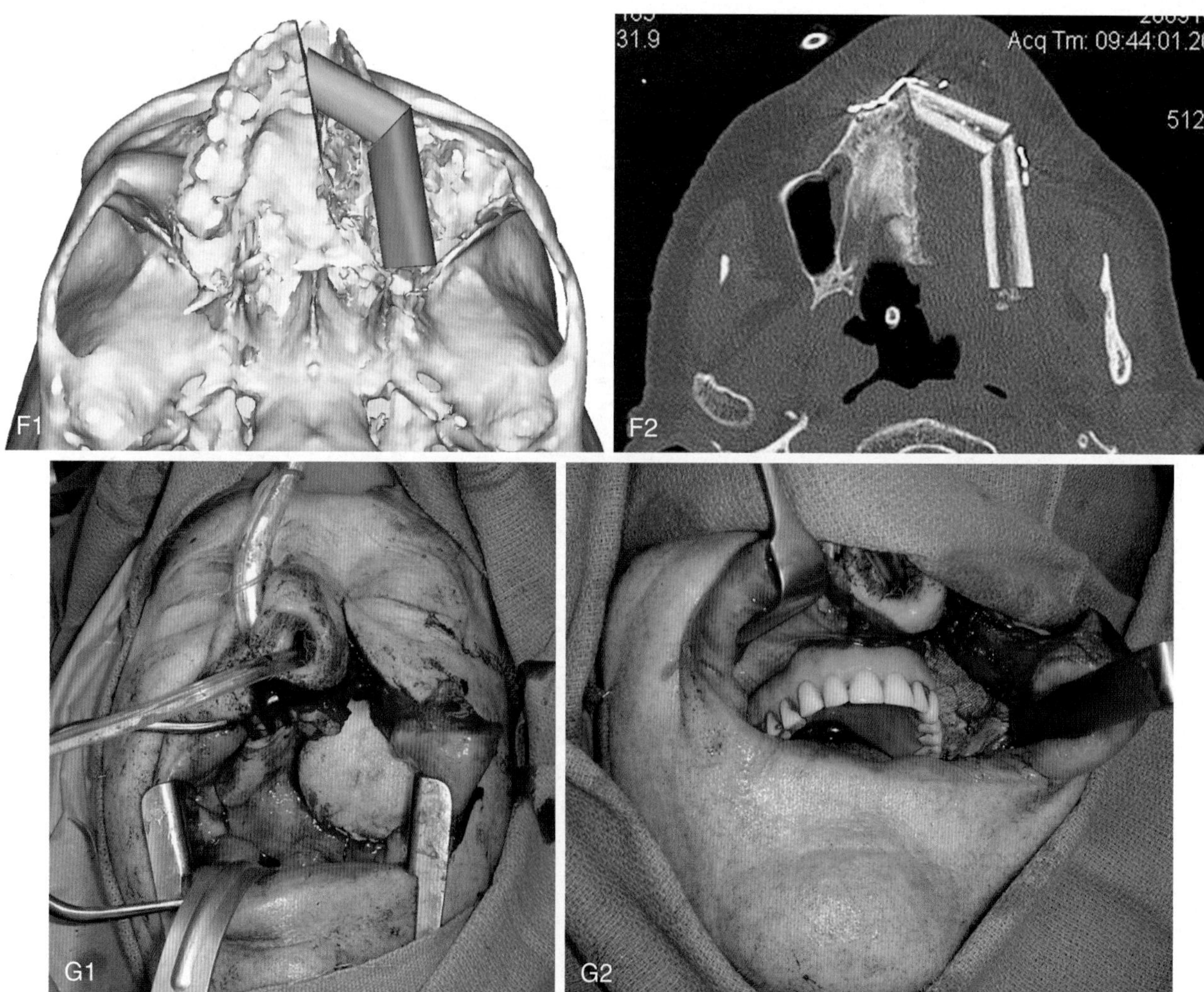

Figure 114.2, cont'd **F1,** Computer planning of microvascular fibula reconstruction of left ipsilateral maxillectomy defect. **F2,** Postoperative CT scan of fibular reconstruction. **G1,** Gauze-wrapped, antibiotic ointment-impregnated sponge obturator supports split-thickness skin graft that lines the defect. **G2,** Denture prosthesis is secured to maxilla with screws, supporting the sponge obturator.

ALTERNATIVE TECHNIQUE 1: Mandibulotomy Approach to Posterior Maxillectomy

Tumors situated in the posterior aspect of the maxilla with extensive involvement of the pterygoid plate area can be effectively approached and widely exposed via a lower lip-splitting incision and median or paramedian mandibulotomy.[5] When used for access to maxillary tumors, there is rarely need for any upper lip or midfacial incisions (Fig. 114.3).

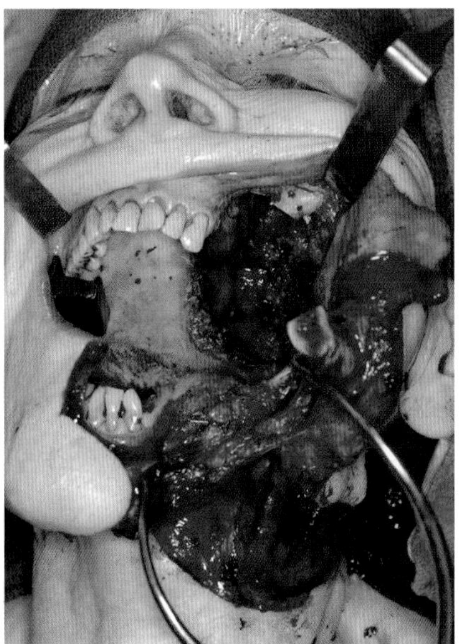

Figure 114.3 Maxillectomy via the mandibulotomy approach.

ALTERNATIVE TECHNIQUE 2: Transoral Approach

The transoral approach obviates the need for a facial incision but is primarily indicated for access when the maxillary tumor is isolated to the inferior aspect of the maxilla or maxillary antrum. Edentulism greatly facilitates the transoral approach in patients with adequate jaw opening (Fig. 114.4).

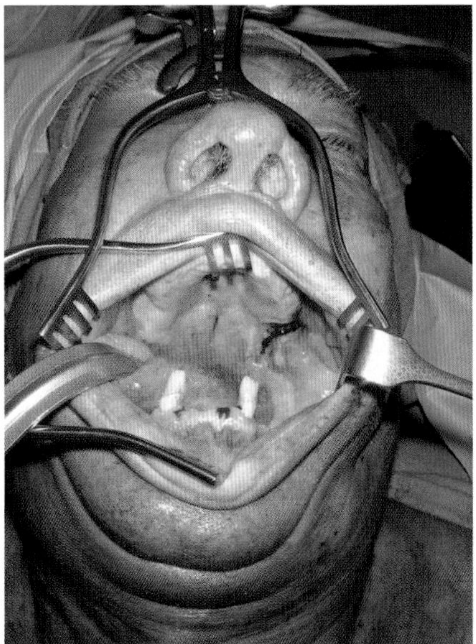

Figure 114.4 Transoral approach for maxillectomy.

ALTERNATIVE TECHNIQUE 3: Midfacial Degloving Approach

The midfacial degloving approach, like the transoral approach, obviates the need for a facial skin incision. This approach provides more exposure than the traditional transoral approach but is only indicated for maxillary tumors that are located anteroinferiorly and have minimal to no ethmoidal involvement.

The first step of this procedure is to create a circumferential endonasal incision of the nasal vestibules, bilaterally. This begins with a complete transfixion incision, which is connected to bilateral intercartilaginous incisions. The intercartilaginous incision is further extended laterally, then caudally and medially across the floor of the vestibule back to the transfixion incision. After this circumferential endonasal incision is made, elevation of soft tissues from the nasal dorsum is performed through the intercartilaginous incision, passing in a subcutaneous plane over the upper lateral cartilages, which remain in place. The elevation of the soft tissue is carried superiorly toward the medial canthal and glabella region and laterally over the anterior wall of the maxilla to the infraorbital foramina. A long maxillary vestibular incision is made from the maxillary first molar crossing the midline to its opposite counterpart. This incision can be carried posteriorly toward the third molar if more exposure is needed. In a subperiosteal plane, facial soft tissues are elevated over the anterior wall of the maxilla bilaterally. At the piriform aperture area, this intraoral circumvestibular incision is sharply connected to the intranasal incisions. Soft tissue attachments to the anterior margin of the septal cartilage are released. This allows the nasal tip, along with the lower lateral cartilages and adjacent midface soft tissues, to be elevated in a subperiosteal and subcutaneous plane up to the level of the infraorbital rim and taking care to preserve the infraorbital nerves. Judicious use of periosteal release incisions enhances retraction and access (Fig. 114.5).

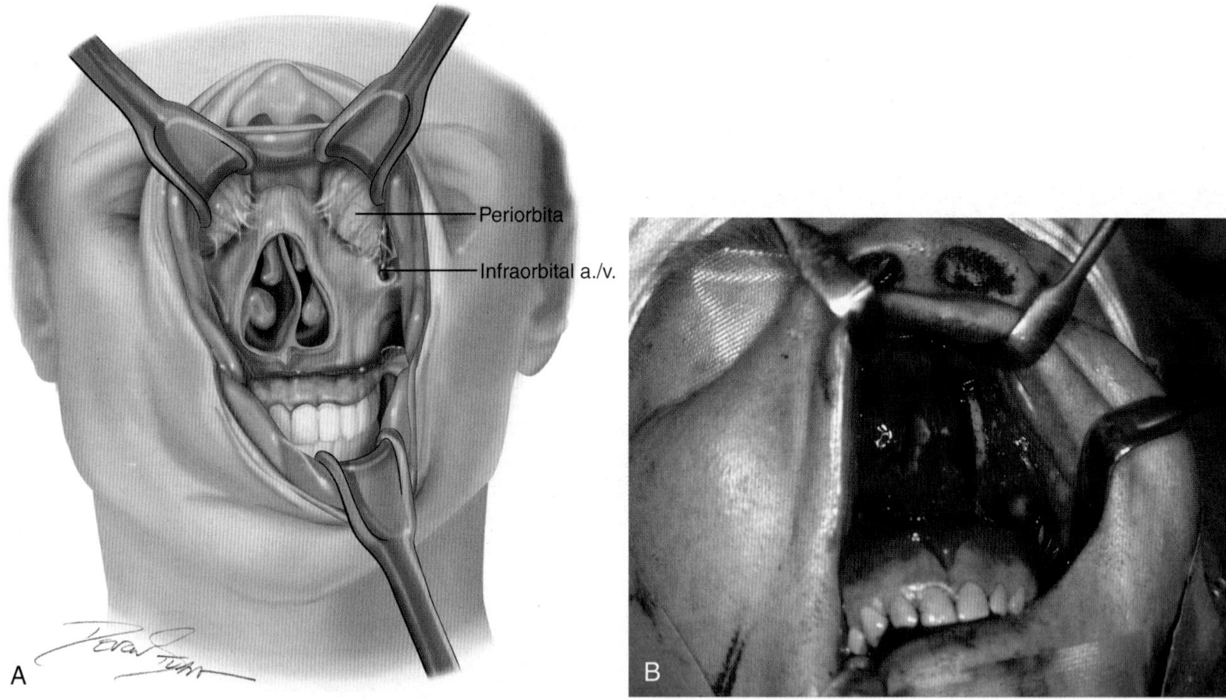

Figure 114.5 **A,** Facial degloving incision exposing the nose, nasal radix, and ethmoid region. **B,** Circumferential endonasal incisions (intercartilaginous incision and transfixion incisions).

ALTERNATIVE TECHNIQUE 4: Medial Maxillectomy

The medial maxillectomy is indicated for smaller tumors that involve the common wall separating the maxillary and nasal cavities or tumors of the inferior ethmoid region. Although medial maxillectomy can be performed via an endoscopic approach, an open approach may be preferable for malignant tumors. The lateral rhinotomy incision is begun just below the medial aspect of the eyebrow and extends inferiorly in the nasofacial groove curving laterally to fall within the alar sulcus and terminating within the nostril. The orbital contents are dissected from the medial and inferior walls of the orbital cavity in a subperiosteal plane exposing the lacrimal sac, as well as the anterior and posterior ethmoid arteries.

A window is created through the medial aspect of the anterior wall of the maxillary sinus using a 4-mm osteotome. This window is enlarged vertically with a Kerrison rongeur, extending inferiorly to the level of the nasal floor. If oncologically safe, consideration can be given to removing the piriform buttress and grafting it back into position at the conclusion of the operation. At the inferior extent of the resection, a reciprocating saw is used to cut horizontally at the level of the nasal floor, through the lateral nasal wall into the maxillary sinus, extending posteriorly to the posterior limit of the sinus. A vertical cut is then made from the anterior-medial orbital floor inferiorly through the orbital rim into the anterior ethmoid cells just behind the medial maxillary buttress, passing further inferiorly into the maxillary sinus. This passes lateral to the lacrimal fossa, which usually is included in the specimen. The inferior aspect of the lacrimal sac is transected. Orbital contents are then retracted laterally. A horizontal saw cut is made from the orbit into the anterior ethmoid labyrinth, extending from the previous vertical cut anteriorly to the anterior ethmoid artery. This artery is ligated and divided to allow further posterior extension of the cut. This superior horizontal cut is made at a level below the frontoethmoidal suture line as that marks the level of the cribriform plate. The final cut, which is the most difficult, is a posterior vertical osteotomy made with angled scissors such as Dean scissors from the posterior nasal floor to the posterior tip of the superior turbinate and posterior ethmoid cells. This osteotomy is usually between the palatine bone and pterygoid process of the sphenoid bone (Fig. 114.6).

Reconstruction of the medial maxillectomy defect is unnecessary. The bone defect is typically of no esthetic or functional consequence, especially if the piriform buttress is preserved. If the medial canthal tendon has been transected, reattachment is recommended, and if the lacrimal duct has been transected, the remaining portion is drained into the nasal cavity as described previously.

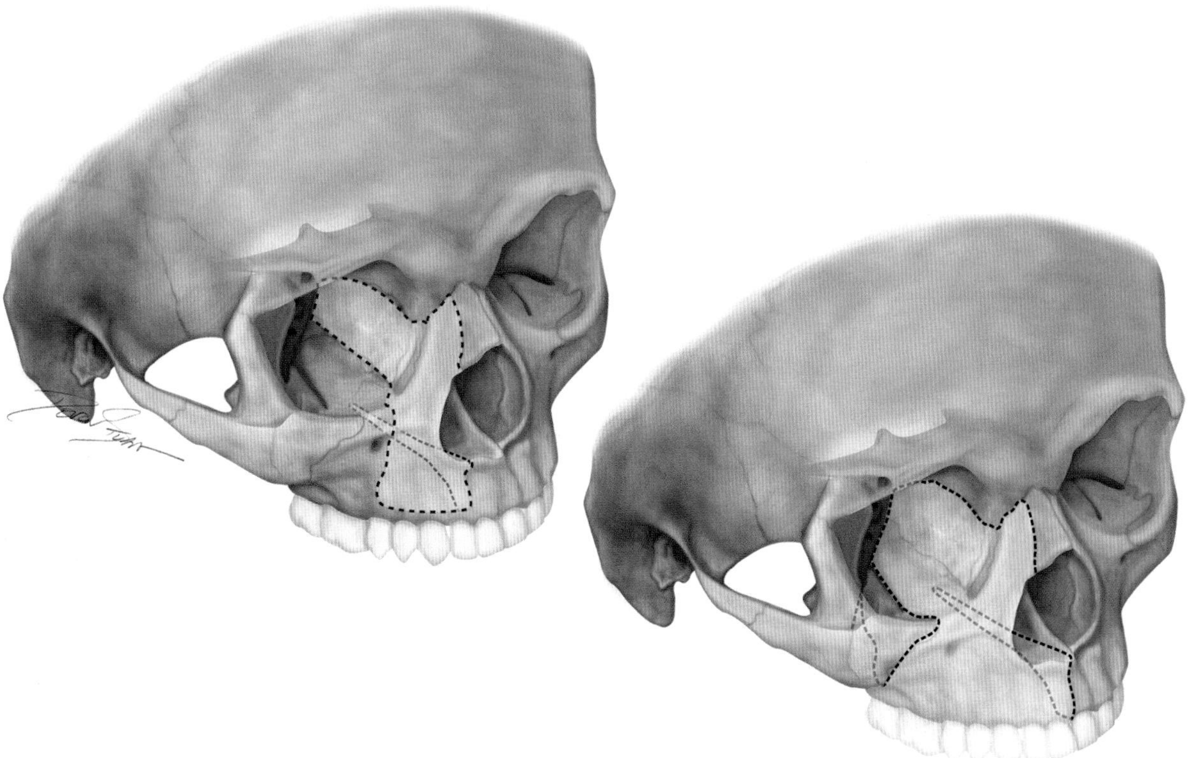

Figure 114.6 Osteotomy design for medial maxillectomy.

Avoidance and Management of Intraoperative Complications

Hemorrhage is the most frequent intraoperative and early postoperative complication of maxillectomy. The maxilla and the midfacial region are well-vascularized areas of the body, and the maxillary artery and its branches are located directly in the surgical field. A moderate amount of bleeding is expected during this procedure and can emanate from multiple obscure sites such as the soft palate, hard palate mucosa, pterygoid plexus, and skin flaps. The most common cause of brisk hemorrhage during the maxillectomy procedure is transection or laceration of the internal maxillary artery. Hemorrhage from this vessel can be life-threatening if not controlled. It is ideal to isolate and ligate this vessel during the exposure, prior to osteotomy. Because of aberrations in anatomy, tumor location, and patient body habitus, this is not always possible. If significant bleeding is encountered during the osteotomies, the maxillectomy should be completed expeditiously and direct pressure applied to the wound bed with a laparotomy sponge. With the aid of suction, the maxillary artery can then be identified and clipped or suture-ligated. Should the bleeding occur postoperatively or if the surgeons are unable to find the bleeding source, angiography and embolization can be utilized. If the patient's medical condition permits, intraoperative hypotensive anesthesia is recommended.

Other intraoperative complications include corneal injury from exposure or abrasion during surgery. This can usually be prevented by placement of a temporary tarsorrhaphy suture. The optic nerve can be directly injured during the procedure or it can be indirectly injured from overpacking the maxillary defect causing vascular compromise. If an acute decrease in visual acuity is identified, any packing or obturator should be removed and prompt ophthalmologic consultation should be obtained. Epiphora is also frequently noted in the immediate postoperative period. This can commonly be attributed to postsurgical edema surrounding the lacrimal sac and nasolacrimal duct remnant, and should resolve spontaneously.

Postoperative Considerations

Patients who have undergone total ipsilateral maxillectomy are generally admitted to the intensive care unit for close monitoring. Tracheotomy is usually performed on patients who have undergone concomitant neck dissection or a free flap reconstruction of the defect. Perioperative corticosteroid administration can be helpful for appropriate patients, as can a 30-degree elevation of the head of the bed to minimize edema. If orbital contents have been preserved, repeated visual checks are performed to look for signs of optic nerve compromise. If a microvascular free flap was performed, the usual flap surveillance protocol is followed to monitor flap survival. If a surgical obturator prosthesis is placed or the wound is packed, the patient can be progressed from a liquid to a soft-mechanical diet within a few days. Once the patient is tolerating an oral diet, ambulating, and showing signs of recovery, hospital discharge usually occurs from 2 to 7 days postsurgery. The packing or obturator prosthesis is removed approximately 1 week postoperatively and the wound inspected.

Intermediate complications such as infection, microvascular free flap failure, and failure of prosthesis can occur shortly after surgery to a few weeks postoperatively. Transient ipsilateral serous otitis media with hearing loss can result from edematous obstruction of the eustachian tube. Chronic complications and complaints from the patients such as reflux of contents into the nasal cavity, velopharyngeal insufficiency, trismus, chronic epiphora, and unacceptable cosmesis can occur and remain for years after the surgery.

References

1. Ohngren LG. Malignant tumors of the maxilla-ethmoid region. *Acta Otol.* 1933;19(suppl):101–106.
2. Schmidt BL, Pogrel MA, Young CW, Sharma A. Reconstruction of extensive maxillary defects using zygomaticus implants. *J Oral Maxillofac Surg.* 2004;62(9 suppl 2):82–89.
3. Varkey P, Liu YT, Tan NC. Multidisciplinary treatment of head and neck cancer. *Semin Plast Surg.* 2010;24(3):331–334.
4. Pryor SG, Moore EJ, Kasperbauer JL, Hayden RE, Strome SE. Coronoid-temporalis pedicled rotation flap for orbital floor reconstruction of the total maxillectomy defect. *Laryngoscope.* 2004;114(11):2051–2055.
5. Nair S, Sridhar KR, Shah A, Kumar B, Nayak K, Shetty P. Maxillectomy through mandibulotomy—a retrospective clinical review. *J Oral Maxillofac Surg.* 2011;69(7):2040–2047.

Orbital Resection

Beomjune Kim, Matthew Radant, and Deepak Kademani

Armamentarium

#9 Molt periosteal elevator
#10 and #15 scalpel blades
#701 Bur
Adson forceps with teeth
Adson forceps without teeth, serrated tips
Appropriate sutures
Austin retractor
Bipolar electrocautery
Channel retractor
Curved Mayo scissors
Dietrich or other right-angle hemostat
Double-guarded nasal septal osteotome
Fomon lower lateral alar scissors (14 cm)
Hair elastics
Local anesthetic with vasoconstrictor
Malleable retractors
Mayfield headrest
Needle electrocautery, including Colorado tip
Neurosurgical cottonoids (1/2 × 3 inches)
Obwegeser retractors
Osteotomes, sharp, curved (4 to 6 mm)
Osteotomes, sharp, straight (4 to 6 mm)
Oxymetazoline decongestant (0.05% solution)
Pterygoid osteotome
Raney clips
Reciprocating saw
Seldin elevator

History of the Procedure

The first mention of exenteration can be found in a German textbook of ophthalmology written by Bartisch in 1583.[1] The same surgical approach was proposed for certain cases of exophthalmos. Langenbeck in 1821 and Dupuytren in 1833 were the earliest to undertake this surgical technique. Collins in 1864 and von Arlt in 1874 provided detailed accounts of the surgical method of orbital exenteration as it is performed today. The operation was reserved for malignant tumors of the orbit and the periorbital tissues, and the exenteration socket was left to spontaneously epithelialize by granulation tissue. In 1872, Streatfeild introduced the conservative orbital exenteration with the lid-sparing technique, in which the eyelids were sutured together, thus hiding the empty orbital cavity. In 1909, Golovine[2] proposed the extended orbital exenteration, which included adjacent structures such as the maxillary sinuses.

Indications for the Use of the Procedure

The removal of the eye is one of the most morbid and dreaded procedures in head and neck surgery but is sometimes unavoidable. Enucleation is often due to the tumor invading the orbit or arising within the globe itself (Fig. 115.1). Its indications can be categorized into malignant tumor, benign but locally aggressive tumor, intractable infection, intractable orbital or ocular pain, penetrating orbital trauma, and disfigurement with meaningful vision (Table 115.1).[3]

The emotional effect that eye removal has on a patient should be taken into consideration. For many it is a life-changing event that can transform social relationships as well as their overall well-being. The decision to proceed to orbital exenteration is often made intraoperatively. Orbital exenteration is appropriate for patients with tumor invasion of periorbita. The risk of preserving the eye must be weighed against the benefit of oncologic control.

Preoperative Evaluation

A thorough history and physical examination and a complete ophthalmological examination of both eyes are paramount for any condition requiring orbital surgery. If possible, it is advisable to consult ophthalmology and a maxillofacial prosthodontist before the surgery. Otherwise, the preoperative evaluation for orbital surgery varies with different conditions and indications. For malignant tumors, presurgical cancer workups based on the National Comprehensive Cancer Network guidelines are indicated including a biopsy for histological diagnosis, computed tomography (CT), magnetic resonance imaging (MRI), or positron emission tomography (PET). Before committing to orbital resection, all the available therapeutic options should be discussed by the tumor board and exhausted. For infection, culture and sensitivity data are crucial for conservative medical therapy. Multidisciplinary care with infectious disease experts is crucial in achieving control of aggressive infections. Adequate antibiotic therapy, conservative incision, and drainage and/or debridement should be attempted until orbital exenteration

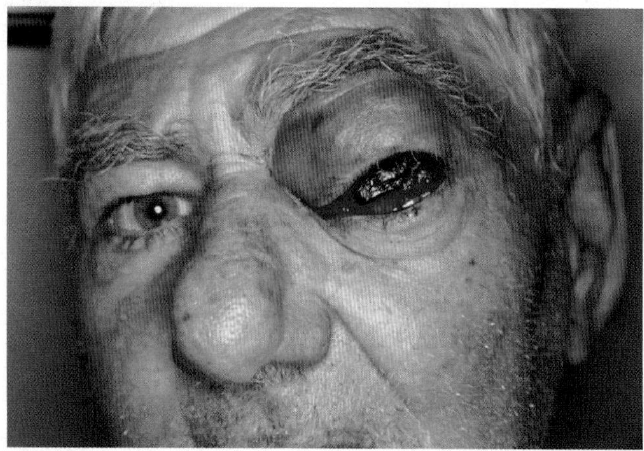

Figure 115.1 Patient with an orbital lymphoma. Note proptosis with marked congestion of the conjunctiva and chronic chemosis.

Table 115.1 Tumor Categories

Indication	Example
Malignant tumor	Squamous cell carcinoma, basal cell carcinoma, melanoma, sebaceous cell carcinoma[3] Orbital tumors can be categorized into primary orbital tumor; secondary extension from adjacent structures such as skin, oral/nasal cavity, and sinus tumors; and metastatic tumors
Benign but locally aggressive tumor	Lymphangioma, meningioma, Stevens-Johnson syndrome[1,4]
Infection	*Aspergillus*[5] rhino-orbital-cerebral mucormycosis[6] especially in immunocompromised patients[7]
Intractable ocular pain[8]	Stevens-Johnson syndrome or other inflammatory or autoimmune conditions
Trauma	Globe rupture, avulsion of periorbital tissue with insufficient remaining tissue for protection of the globe
Disfigurement of the eye without meaningful vision	Phthitis bulbi from trauma, pathology, infection, or surgery[9]

is deemed necessary to control the infection. Again, imaging studies are recommended to evaluate the extent of the infection and involved anatomic structures. Before the operation, a complete blood count with platelets, coagulation studies, and at least type and screen for potential transfusion should be performed.

During the informed consent process, the rationale behind removing an eye should be clearly discussed with the patient and family. The decision whether to exenterate the orbit is frequently made during surgery. It must be made very clear that every effort will be made to preserve the eye provided that it will not affect the prognosis of disease/survival of the patient. Moreover, the implications of losing an eye should be thoroughly discussed, including the reconstructive options. A formal psychiatric evaluation and counseling can be extremely beneficial and should be considered in every patient undergoing removal of their globe.

TECHNIQUE: Surgical Procedure—Orbital Exenteration

- A lid-sparing technique (subtotal exenteration) can be utilized for most cases of benign disease and for tumors involving the posterior portion of the orbit (Fig. 115.2). If possible, this technique provides an excellent color match to facial skin and is more esthetically desirable.[10]
- Total exenteration should be planned for tumors involving the anterior portion of the orbit and the skin, conjunctiva, or lacrimal gland (Fig. 115.3).
- Total exenteration

STEP 1: Positioning

The patient is placed in a reverse Trendelenburg position and the head in an extended position with a shoulder roll. A suture tarsorrhaphy is usually helpful.

STEP 2: Marking

A circumferential incision is made through the skin overlying the orbital rim and deepened through the orbicularis oculi, and blunt dissection in the pretarsal/preseptal plane is then carried out to the orbital rim. Periosteum/periorbita is incised a few millimeters outside the orbit along the orbital rim (Fig. 115.4A and B).[7,11]

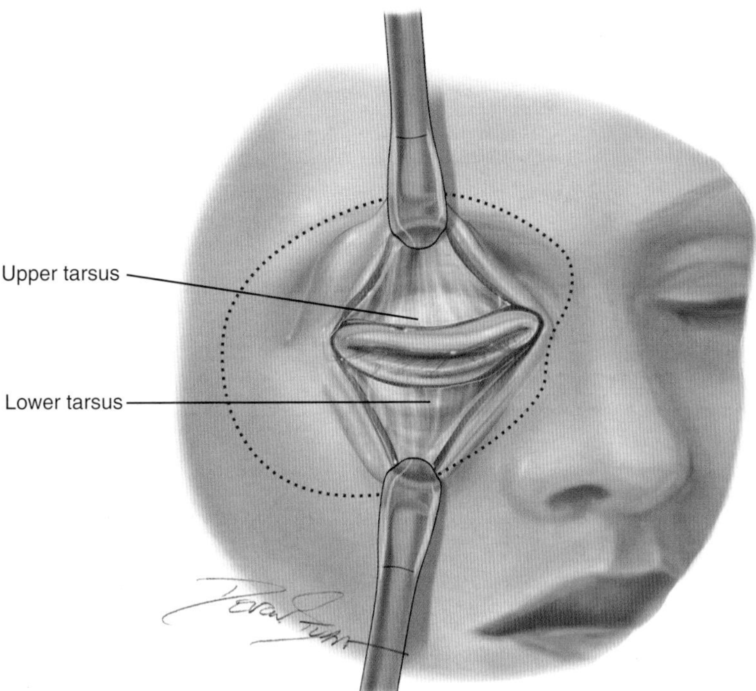

Figure 115.2 The skin incision is placed approximately 2 to 3 mm above and below the lash lines in the upper and lower eyelids, respectively.

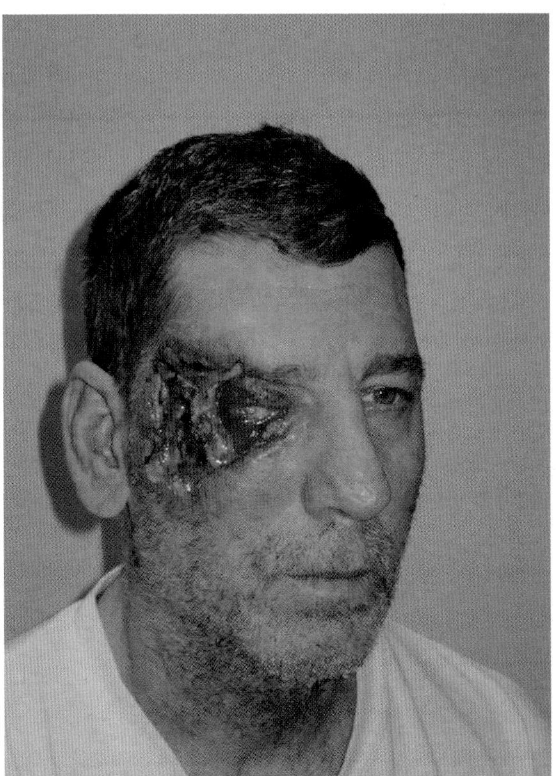

Figure 115.3 Total exenteration should be planned for tumors involving the anterior portion of the orbit and the skin, conjunctiva, or lacrimal gland.

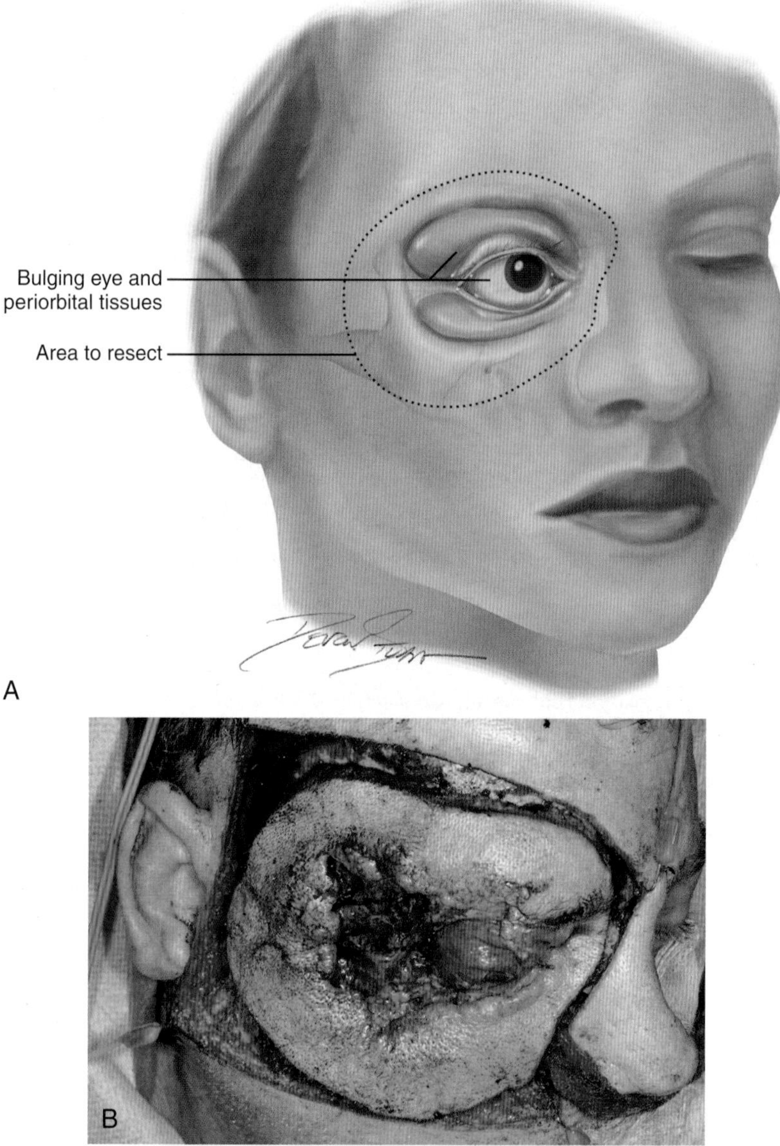

Figure 115.4 **A** and **B,** Positioning and marking.

TECHNIQUE: Surgical Procedure—Orbital Exenteration—*cont'd*

STEP 3: Dissection

The periorbita is then carefully elevated with a Molt #9 or Freer elevator. Dissection continues in this plane circumferentially and posteriorly reflecting the orbital contents. Dissection is usually started at the supero-temporal portion of the orbit where the bone is thickest. In the medial aspect of the orbit, care is taken to avoid fracturing the fragile orbital plate of the ethmoid. It should be kept in mind that sino-orbital or naso-orbital fistulas are most easily created over the lamina papyracea and result in chronic discharge. The lacrimal sac is reflected laterally to be included with the orbital resection and the nasolacrimal duct is ligated and cut. Sharp dissection is usually necessary at the trochlea and at the canthal ligaments. The anterior and posterior ethmoidal arteries should be identified on the superomedial wall and either clipped or cauterized to avoid bleeding (Fig. 115.5). The zygomaticofacial and zygomaticotemporal vessels on the lateral wall can be cauterized.

STEP 4: Posterior orbital dissection

As dissection proceeds posterior toward the orbital apex, careful elevation of the periorbita is recommended, particularly in the posteromedial aspect of the orbit where an iatrogenic cerebrospinal fluid leak can be created. Monopolar cautery should be avoided in the posterior orbit.

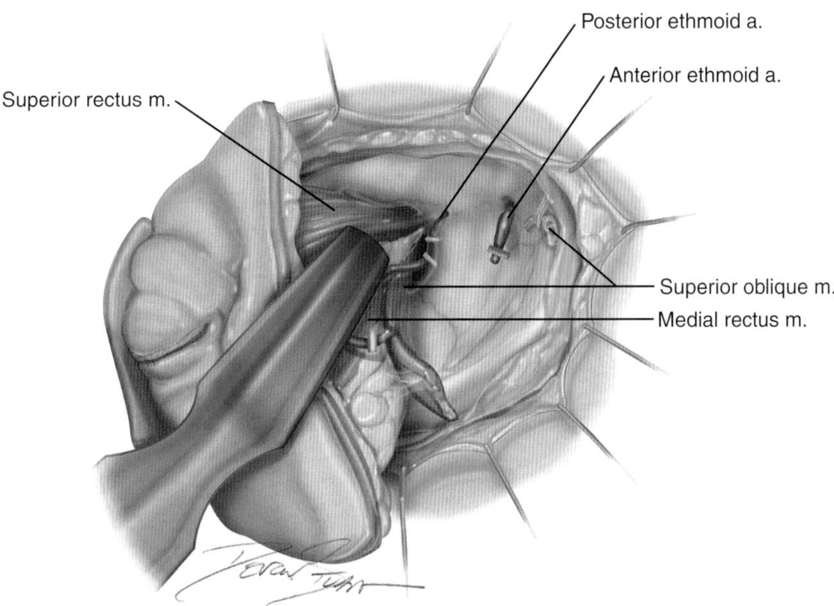

Figure 115.5 Elevation of the periorbita and clipping of the anterior and posterior ethmoid arteries.

TECHNIQUE: Surgical Procedure—Orbital Exenteration—*cont'd*

STEP 5: Tumor excision

At the orbital apex, the contents of the superior and inferior orbital fissures and the apical stump are now divided (Fig. 115.6). A right-angle hemostat is utilized to clamp the apical tissue avoiding any undue tension and monopolar cautery, which can cause injury to the optic chiasm. Any pressure in this region can cause an oculocardiac reflex with transient bradycardia or asystole so the anesthesiologist should be informed. The tissue above the hemostat is now cut with a curved pair of scissors or knife. Now the specimen is delivered (Fig. 115.7). The apical stump is tied off with 2-0 silk stitch. After removal of the orbital contents, identification of bleeding sources is now easier, and hemostasis is further achieved with bipolar cauterization.

Continued

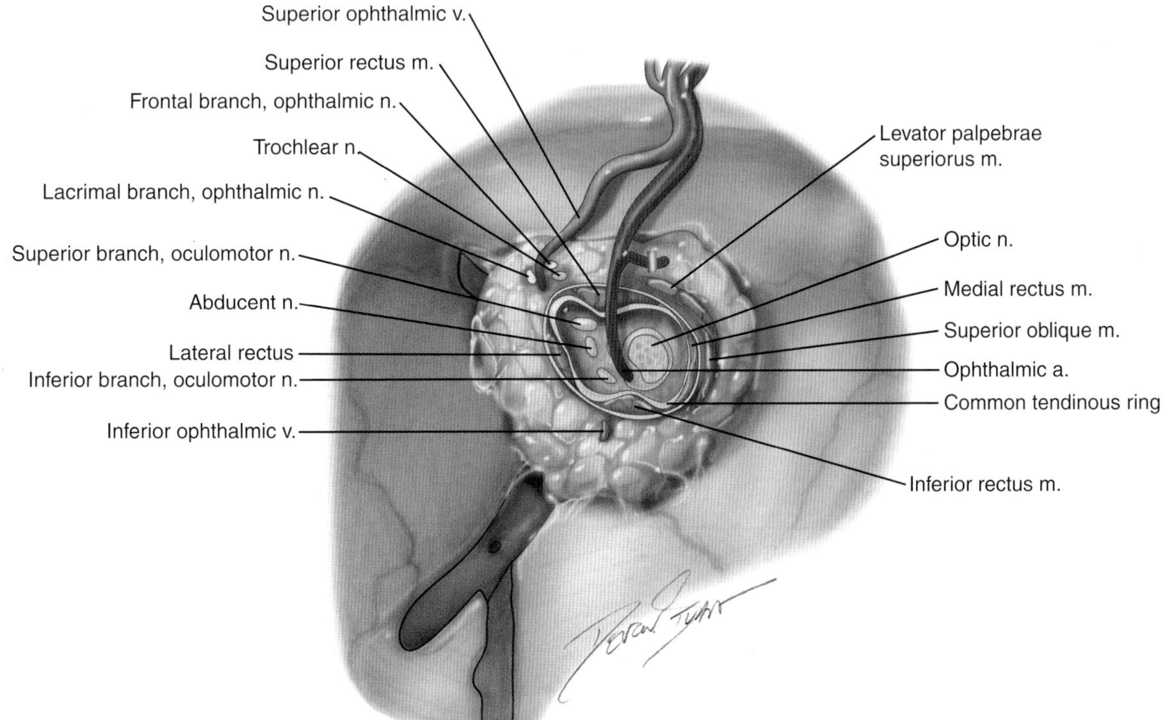

Figure 115.6 Transection of orbital apex tissues.

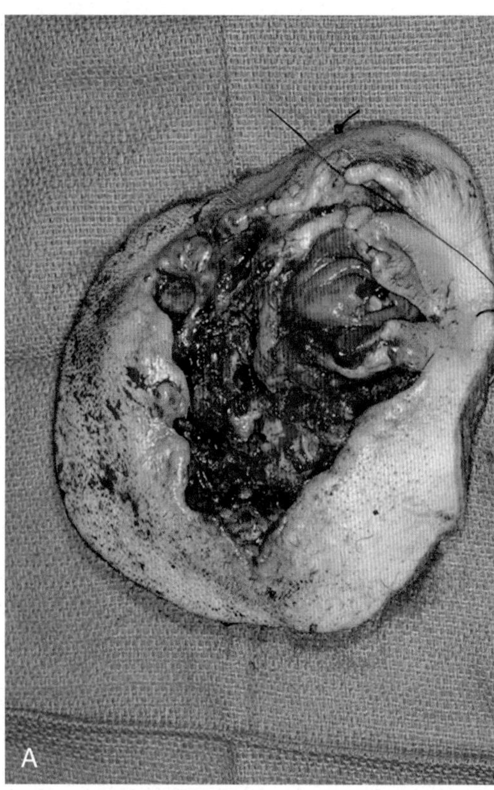

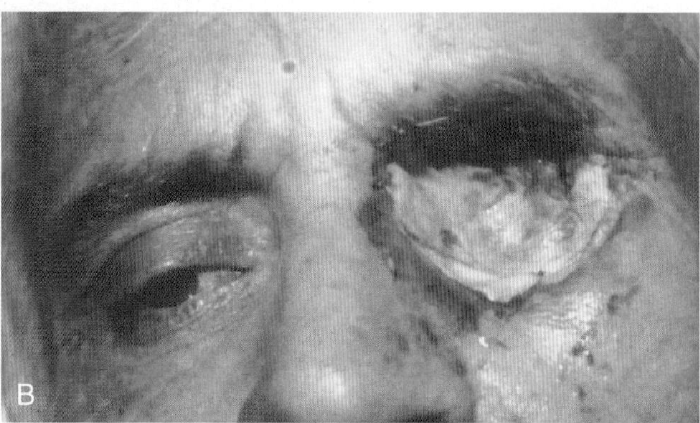

Figure 115.7 **A** and **B,** Initial phase of epithelialization with the skin graft lining the orbital cavity.

TECHNIQUE: Surgical Procedure – Orbital exenteration—*cont'd*

RECONSTRUCTIVE OPTIONS

- The orbit can heal by granulation (Fig. 115.8). Healing by granulation should be reserved for tumors without bony involvement of the orbit. Healing by granulation can take up to 2 months. The orbit should be lined with a nonadherent dressing such as Telfa or Xeroform gauze and packed with fluffed gauze with appropriate antibiotic coverage and bandaged tightly. The dressing must be changed regularly. If the eyelids have been preserved, the margins can be sewn together (Fig. 115.9), draped over the orbital rim, or used to retain a prosthesis depending on the restorative plan.[12]

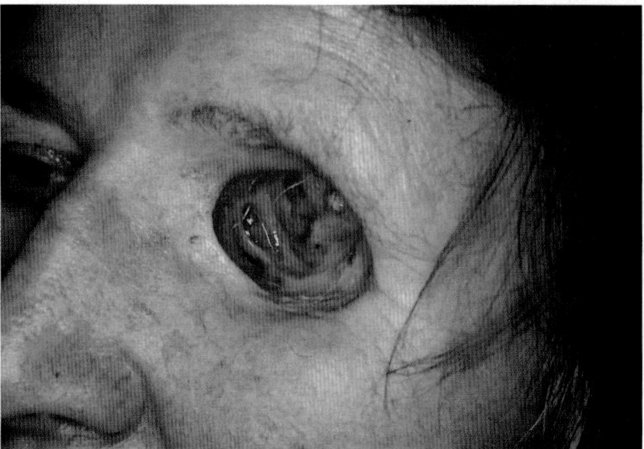

Figure 115.8 Clinical photograph of a patient after orbital exenteration. The cavity was left to granulate by secondary intention. There are signs of communication between the exenterated orbital cavity and the anterior ethmoids. This communication between the nasal cavity and the orbit creates several problems for the patient, mainly due to the inability to blow his nose because the air escapes through the communicating ethmoids.

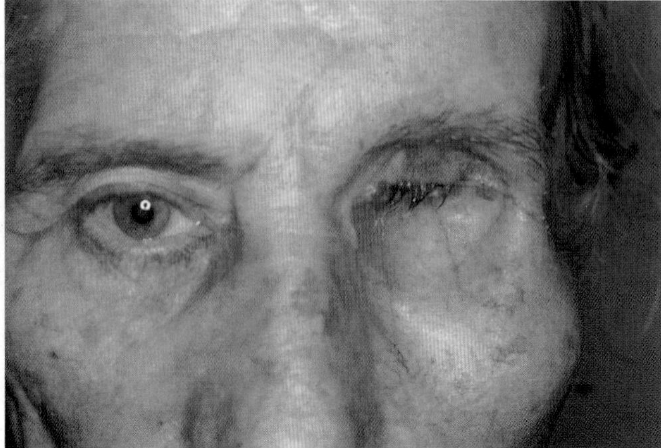

Figure 115.9 Patient after an orbital exenteration via a lid-sparing technique. Sewing the upper and lower lids together results in minimal functional and esthetic impairment.

TECHNIQUE: Surgical Procedure – Orbital exenteration—*cont'd*

- Split-thickness skin graft is frequently used for lining of the orbital cavity. Skin grafting aids in faster epithelialization and prevents respiratory epithelial migration from the sinuses. The respiratory epithelial lining is friable, produces mucus, and bleeds easily, and thus is not an ideal surface for a prosthesis. Skin graft is usually harvested from the thigh and placed and sutured to the edges of the remaining periorbital skin. Then the orbit is packed with antibiotic-impregnated gauze for apposition of the graft to the orbit.
- Various pedicled or free vascularized flap options are available for obliteration and reconstruction of the orbit. If only soft tissue reconstruction is desired, paramedian forehead (Fig. 115.10A and B),[13] temporalis (Fig. 115.11),[14,15] cervicofacial,[16] radial forearm,[17] anterolateral thigh, rectus abdominus and latissimus dorsi flaps[18] are commonly used. If bony reconstruction is desired, osteo-cutaneous fibula, deep circumflex iliac artery, and scapula flaps can be utilized (Fig. 115.12A and B).
- There are several advantages of leaving the orbital cavity open without sophisticated reconstructive surgery including the ease of tumor surveillance by direct visualization and better prosthetic retention and flexibility in options.[19] Obviously, an open orbital cavity can be examined daily by the patient, which is impossible with an orbital defect that has been obliterated with a flap, which requires an MRI, CT, or PET scan for tumor surveillance. An orbital defect obliterated with a flap may quire a secondary revision to accommodate a prosthetic eye.
- A spectacle-mounted or adhesive-secured prosthesis can be used for stability and retention of the prosthesis. If the volume and density of the surrounding bone allow, osseo-integrated implants are another armamentarium available to help with prosthetic support (Fig. 115.13A–C).[20,21]

Continued

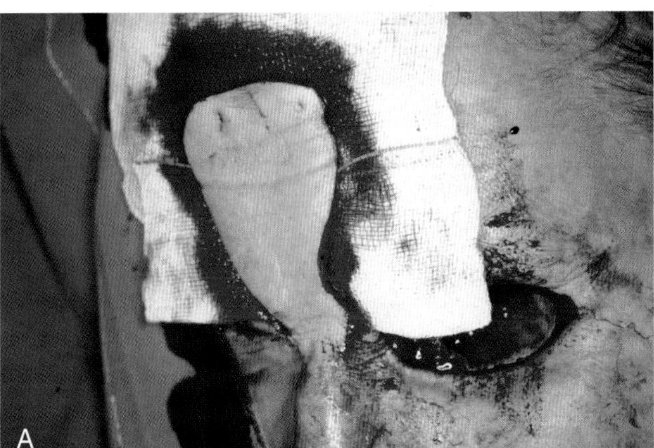

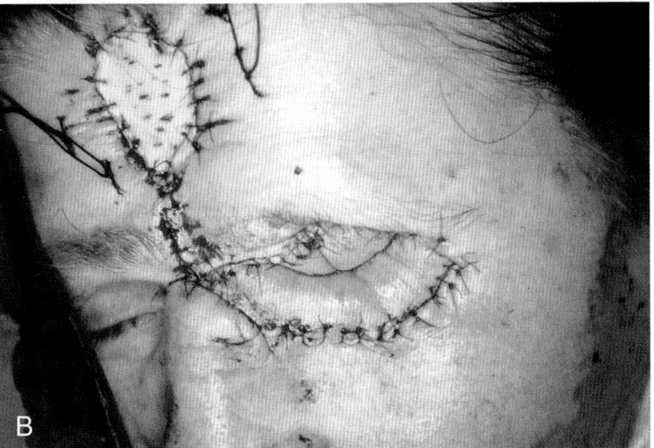

Figure 115.10 **A,** The flap is transposed 90 degrees from its axis and covers the orbital cavity. **B,** The forehead defect is lined with a full-thickness skin graft from the supraclavicular area.

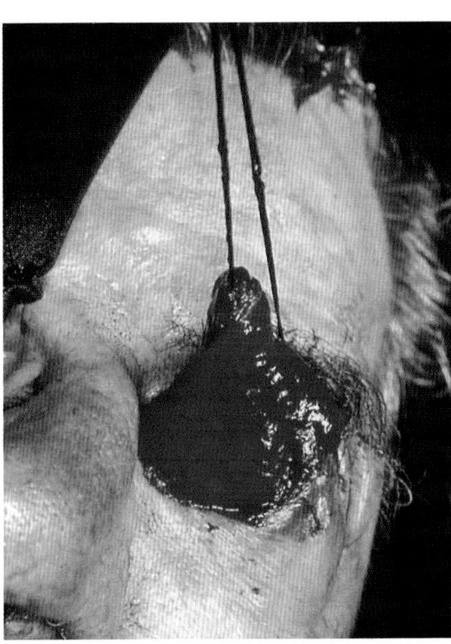

Figure 115.11 The transposed temporalis flap is shown retracted through the orbital cavity.

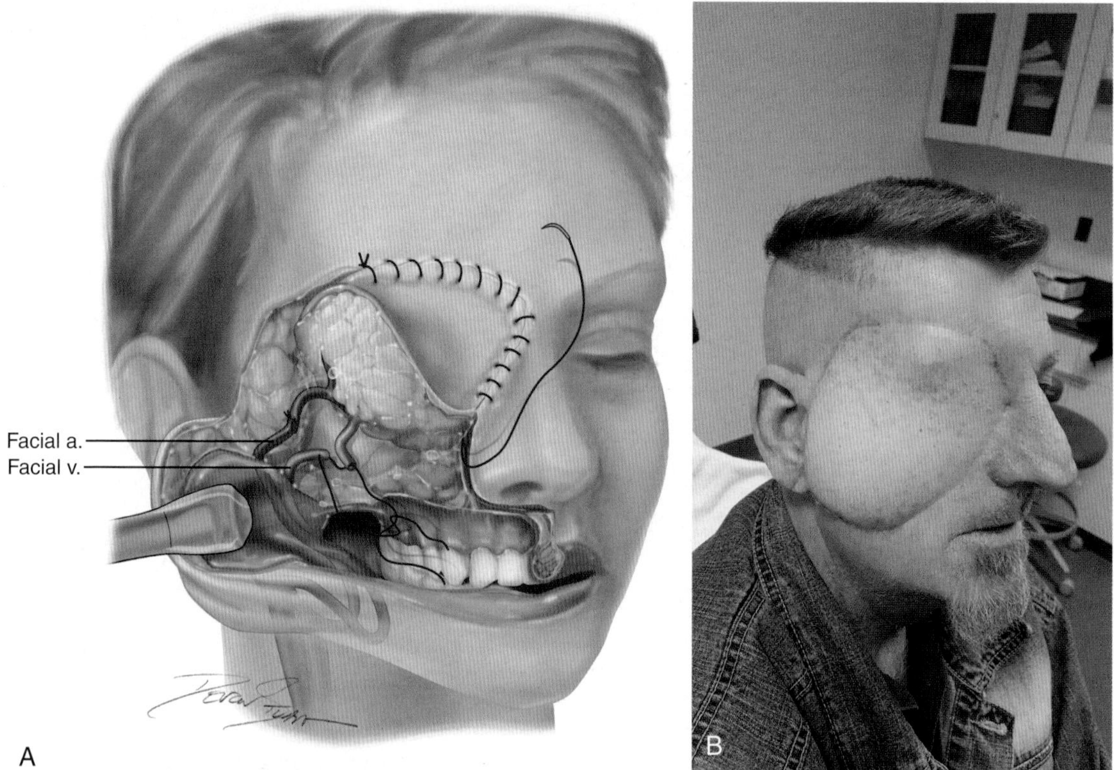

Figure 115.12 **A** and **B,** Inset of an anterolateral thigh free flap into an orbitomaxillectomy defect.

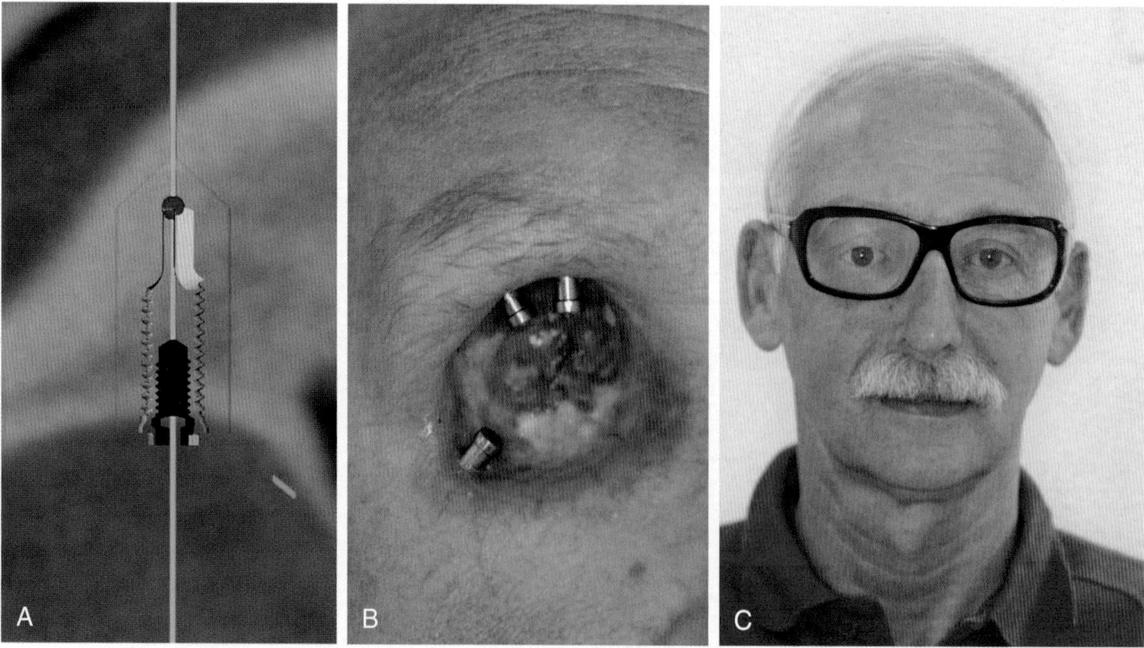

Figure 115.13 **A,** Placement of a dental implant into the orbital rim. **B,** Implant-supported magnets around orbital defect. **C,** Final prosthesis in place with eyeglasses. (Courtesy of Gert Meijer, Radboud UMC, Nijmegen, the Netherlands.)

TECHNIQUE: Surgical Procedure – Orbital exenteration—*cont'd*

Although orbital exenteration is the most common orbital ablative surgery utilized by head and neck surgeons, orbital enucleation and evisceration are also useful procedures in certain clinical situations. Evisceration involves removal of the contents of the eye itself, but preservation of the sclera and all of its attachments. Enucleation refers to the removal of the entire globe, as opposed to evisceration where only the contents of the eye are removed. As discussed previously, exenteration involves removal of the eye as well as the soft tissue contents of the orbit. The choice of procedure performed is guided by the nature of the disease.[22]

Enucleation and evisceration are indicated in clinical situations where removal of only the globe or intraocular contents does not compromise the prognosis or therapeutic outcome (e.g., glaucoma, phthisis bulbi, ocular trauma, endophthalmitis, or uveitis). For malignant tumor involving the orbit, these limited procedures are contraindicated. In suspected sympathetic ophthalmia, severe phthisis bulbi, clinically resistant bacterial endophthalmitis, and intraocular malignancy (e.g., melanoma or retinoblastoma), enucleation is preferred over evisceration.[22,23] If structural preservation of more intraorbital contents is desired, evisceration achieves a better cosmetic outcome that enucleation. In addition, the incidence of implant extrusion is lower with evisceration.[24]

- Preoperative Care
  - The physical and psychosocial implications of losing an eye must be thoroughly discussed with the patient and family. Prosthetic rehabilitation of the eye can mitigate negative psychosocial outcomes and should be thoroughly discussed as well. The total absence of light perception should be documented when relevant. Anticoagulants should be discontinued prior to the elective surgery.
- Evisceration

EVISCERATION

STEP 1: Patient Positioning

The patient is placed supine on the operating table, and it is elevated in a slight reverse Trendelenburg position. A small shoulder roll is used to extend the neck and allow for access to the surgical field. The patient is draped appropriately for the procedure, taking into account a wide field of sterility dependent on the adjunct procedures to be performed. The use of local anesthetic is entirely up to surgeon preference.

STEP 2: Incision

A 360-degree incision is made with a #15 blade through the conjunctiva close to the limbus. Once this is complete, Wescott scissors are used to undermine the conjunctiva as well as the Tennon capsule. This allows the conjunctiva to be recessed several millimeters to expose the insertions of the rectus muscles. A full-thickness circumferential incision is made around the limbus and the cornea is removed.

STEP 3: Removal of the Ocular Contents

The ocular contents are then removed with an evisceration spoon. Care must be taken to remove any residual pigment that is attached to the sclera. Tenotomy scissors are then used to make a cut posteriorly from the limbus between any two of the rectus muscles. A similar cut is then made 180 degrees from the original.

STEP 4: Removal of the Optic Disc

The optic disc can now be identified. It is found just nasal to the most posterior extent of the sclera. A circular cut is made around the disc to free it from the sclera. Once removed, two radial cuts can be made in the posterior sclera that extend back toward the equator of the globe. These should be made at right angles to the original anterior limbus cuts. The intraconal fat can now be accessed.

STEP 5: Implant Placement

An implant usually sized 20 to 22 mm is selected and inserted into the sclera, partially pushing it into the intraconal fat. The flaps in the anterior sclera are then overlapped and then closed with 6-0 resorbable suture. The Tenon capsule and conjunctiva are then closed in layers with 7-0 absorbable suture. A conformer is then placed over this and held in place by the eyelids. A temporary prosthesis can then be fitted in 2 to 3 weeks and a permanent prosthesis after 3 months of healing.

- Enucleation[25]

ENUCLEATION

STEP 1: Patient Positioning

Patient positioning and preparation are the same as those for evisceration.

STEP 2: Incision and Dissection

A 360-degree peritomy is carried out, where an incision is made at the limbus in order to reflect the conjunctiva and Tenon capsule of the eye. The conjunctiva and Tenon capsule are separated posteriorly to the insertion of extraocular muscles. Blunt and sharp dissection is used to eliminate all adhesions. Each muscle insertion is identified and isolated using a muscle hook. The muscles are cut with tenotomy scissors close to the sclera.

Continued

TECHNIQUE: Surgical Procedure – Orbital exenteration—*cont'd*

STEP 3: Separation at the Orbital Apex

The speculum is depressed and the globe relaxes. The globe is pulled medially and upward, which allows the curved hemostat to be placed inside the orbit from the lateral side. The optic nerve is clamped as far posteriorly as possible by sliding the hemostat towards the optic canal (at least 6 to 10 mm from the globe in case of intraocular malignancy). Enucleation scissors are introduced again from the lateral side and the nerve is sectioned. The optic nerve stump is cauterized and the hemostat is released.

STEP 4: Implant Placement

The chosen implant is placed inside the cavity, and the four rectus muscles are sutured to the implant. The Tenon capsule is attached to the implant using resorbable sutures. The conjunctiva is closed with a continuous suture. A conformer should be used to maintain the fornices.

- Postoperative Care
  - — Analgesics are given as indicated.
  - — Antibiotics are typically given for 5 to 7 days.
  - — Fitting of the prosthesis should begin 4 to 8 weeks after surgery.

Avoidance and Management of Intraoperative Complications

- Intraoperative bleeding can be controlled with packing/pressure and prothrombotic agents applied to the orbital apex, blood pressure control, and transfusion of packed red blood cells or platelets, as necessary. In some instances, completion of exenteration facilitates identification of bleeding sources and efficient control of hemorrhage.
- Postoperative hematoma can be prevented by meticulous hemostasis during surgery and avoidance of postoperative hypertension. It should be controlled aggressively if it occurs under a skin graft or a flap. The former may be drained by a simple incision and drainage and then replacing the pressure dressing, while the latter should be drained by opening the incision and thoroughly removing all the clots and rinsing. With significant hematoma, the flap viability can be compromised by venous congestion. Thus, it should be identified and addressed in an urgent fashion.
- Postoperative infection is rare but must be vigorously treated with antibiotics, incision and drainage, and surgical debridement of devitalized tissue.
- Sino-nasal or sino-orbital fistulas are quite common and cause a prolonged healing time, chronic mucus discharge, and hygiene problems. Dural exposure and cerebrospinal fluid leaks can result with the bony dehiscence and occur in the superior aspect of the orbit. If noted intraoperatively, a small flap of extraocular muscle and fat may be spared and used to repair either the bony dehiscence or dural tear.[26] Flap reconstruction of the orbital defects results in a lower rate of fistula formation.

Postoperative Considerations

Orbital resection is a complicated procedure that can lead to significant psycho-social issues. The patient should have a plan for postoperative psychologic support. Additionally, the patient will also need have considerations of type of orbital prosthesis post resection. A temporary spacer or orbital prosthesis can be placed at the time of initial resection with the final prosthesis fabricated once the surgical wounds have healed. It is also critical that the health of the remaining eye be optimized with frequent ophthalmologic evaluation.

References

1. Bartisch G II. Ophthalmic laboratorians. *Am J Ophthalmol*. 1952;35(9):1365–1367.
2. Golovine SS. Orbitosinus exenteration. *Ann Ocul*. 1909;141:413.
3. Levin PS, Dutton JJ. A 20-year series of orbital exenteration. *Am J Ophthalmol*. 1991;112(5):496–501.
4. Bartley GB, Garrity JA, Waller RR, Henderson JW, Ilstrup DM. Orbital exenteration at the mayo clinic. 1967–1986. *Ophthalmology*. 1989;96(4):468–473.
5. Dhiwakar M, Thakar A, Bahadur S. Invasive sino-orbital aspergillosis: surgical decisions and dilemmas. *J Laryngol Otol*. 2003;117(4):280–285.
6. Peterson KL, Wang M, Canalis RF, Abemayor E. Rhinocerebral mucormycosis: evolution of the disease and treatment options. *Laryngoscope*. 1997;107(7):855–862.
7. Kraus D, Bullock J. Orbital infections. In: Pepose JS, Holland GN, Wilhelmus KR, eds. *Ocular Infection & Immunity*. St Louis, MO: Mosby-Year Book; 1996.
8. Rose GE, Wright JE. Exenteration for benign orbital disease. *Br J Ophthalmol*. 1994;78(1):14–18.
9. Odugbo OP, Wade PD, Samuel OJ, Mpyet CD. Indications for destructive eye surgeries among adults in a tertiary eye care center in North Central Nigeria. *J West Afr Coll Surg*. 2015;5(2):134–153.
10. Looi A, Kazim M, Cortes M, Rootman J. Orbital reconstruction after eyelid- and conjunctiva-sparing orbital exenteration. *Ophthalmic Plast Reconstr Surg*. 2006;22(1):1–6.
11. Rapidis AD. Orbital resection and reconstruction. In: Langdon J, Patel M, Ord R, Brennan P, eds. *Operative Oral and Maxillofacial Surgery*. 2nd ed. London, UK: Hodder Arnold; 2011.
12. Coston TO, Small RG. Orbital exenteration—simplified. *Trans Am Ophthalmol Soc*. 1981;79:136–152.
13. Price DL, Sherris DA, Bartley GB, Garrity JA. Forehead flap periorbital reconstruction. *Arch Facial Plast Surg*. 2004;6(4):222–227.

14. Menon NG, Girotto JA, Goldberg NH, Silverman RP. Orbital reconstruction after exenteration: use of a transorbital temporal muscle flap. *Ann Plast Surg*. 2003;50(1):38–42.
15. Altindas M, Yucel A, Ozturk G, Sarac M, Kilic A. The prefabricated temporal island flap for eyelid and eye socket reconstruction in total orbital exenteration patients: a new method. *Ann Plast Surg*. 2010;65(2):177–182.
16. Cuesta-Gil M, Concejo C, Acero J, Navarro-Vila C, Ochandiano S. Repair of large orbito-cutaneous defects by combining two classical flaps. *J Craniomaxillofac Surg*. 2004;32(1):21–27.
17. Tahara S, Susuki T. Eye socket reconstruction with free radial forearm flap. *Ann Plast Surg*. 1989;23(2):112–116.
18. Beasley NJ, Gilbert RW, Gullane PJ, Brown DH, Irish JC, Neligan PC. Scalp and forehead reconstruction using free revascularized tissue transfer. *Arch Facial Plast Surg*. 2004;6(1):16–20.
19. Kuo CH, Gao K, Clifford A, Shannon K, Clark J. Orbital exenterations: an 18-year experience from a single head and neck unit. *ANZ J Surg*. 2011;81(5):326–330.
20. Nerad JA, Carter KD, LaVelle WE, Fyler A, Brånemark PI. The osseointegration technique for the rehabilitation of the exenterated orbit. *Arch Ophthalmol*. 1991;109(7):1032–1038.
21. Konstantinidis L, Scolozzi P, Hamedani M. Rehabilitation of orbital cavity after total orbital cavity after total orbital exenteration using oculofacial prostheses anchored by osseointegrated dental implants posed as a one-step surgical procedure. *Klin Monatsbl Augenheilkd*. 2006;223:400–404.
22. Tyers AG, Medel R, Vasquez LM (eds): Orbital Surgery. ESASO Couse Series. Basel, Karger, 2014(5);73–91.
23. Al-Dahmash SA, Bakry SS, Almadhi NH, Alashgar LM. Indications for enucleation and evisceration in a tertiary eye hospital in Riyadh over a 10-year period. *Ann Saudi Med*. 2017;37(4):313–316.
24. Timothy NH, Freilich DE, Linberg JV. Evisceration versus enucleation from the ocularist's perspective. *Ophthalmic Plast Reconstr Surg*. 2003;19(6):417–420.
25. Perman KI, Baylis HI. Evisceration, enucleation, and exenteration. *Otolaryngol Clin North Am*. 1988;21(1):171–182.
26. Bartley GB, Kasperbauer JL. Use of a flap of extraocular muscle and fat during subtotal exenteration to repair bony orbital defects. *Am J Ophthalmol*. 2002;134(5):787–788.

CHAPTER 116

Neck Dissection

Deepak Kademani, Scott T. Claiborne, and Kaushik H. Sharma

Armamentarium

Shoulder roll
#10, #15 Surgical blades
Bovie electrocautery
Bipolar cautery
Local anesthesia with vasoconstrictor
Tissue dissectors (McCabe, Dierks #1, 2, 3)
Army-Navy retractors
Green thyroid retractor
Surgical clips (small, medium, large)
Satinsky vascular clamps
Silk sutures 2-0
Mosquito clamps
Curved Mayo scissors
Babcock clamps
Flat Blake drains
3-0, 2-0 Polyglycolic sutures
Skin staples or 5-0 prolene sutures

History of the Procedure

Originally based on the Halstedian principles of en bloc removal of lymph nodes in the neck, neck dissection is a standard procedure for the management of patients with head and neck tumors. The term *neck dissection* has evolved to encompass several different operations that may be selected based on the nature of the patient's disease. The neck dissection was first described in the late 19th century surgery by von Langenbeck, Billroth, von Volkmann, and Kocher, who developed and reported the early cases of different types of neck dissection. However, it was George Crile, in 1906, who popularized neck dissection and reported the first significant series of radical neck dissection, bringing this procedure to the attention of the medical world as an effective operation with reproducible technique and results.[1] The greatest impetus to the status of this surgical procedure came from Martin, who published a report in 1951 of 1450 cases that established the place and technique of radical neck dissection in the modern treatment of head and neck cancer.[2] The traditional radical neck dissection now is reserved for patients with bulky metastatic neck disease or those who have a regional failure after first-line therapy. In 1967 Bocca described the concept of a functional neck dissection with limited surgical morbidity with equivalent oncologic safety as a radical neck dissection.[3]

Anatomic Classification of the Zones of the Neck

The lymph node basins within the neck have been described in various levels first by Memorial Sloan Kettering Cancer Center and then further subdivided by Suen and Goepfert (1987) at MD Anderson Cancer Center.[4,5] The anatomic basis of neck node level classifications is described and provides the basis for surgical extirpation of lymph node areas of the neck based on the site of the primary tumor and first echelon lymphatic drainage. Fig. 116.1 illustrates the different zones and levels of the neck.

LEVEL I: LYMPH NODE GROUPS: SUBMENTAL AND SUBMANDIBULAR

Level IA: Submental triangle

Boundaries: anterior bellies of the digastric muscle and hyoid bone

Level IB: Submandibular triangle

Boundaries: body of the mandible, anterior and posterior belly of the digastric muscle

LEVEL II: LYMPH NODE GROUPS: UPPER JUGULAR

Boundaries

1. Anterior: lateral border of the sternohyoid muscle
2. Posterior: posterior border of the sternocleidomastoid muscle
3. Superior: skull base
4. Inferior: level of the hyoid bone (clinical landmark) or carotid bifurcation (surgical landmark)

Levels IIA and **IIB** are arbitrarily designated anatomically by splitting level II with the spinal accessory nerve.

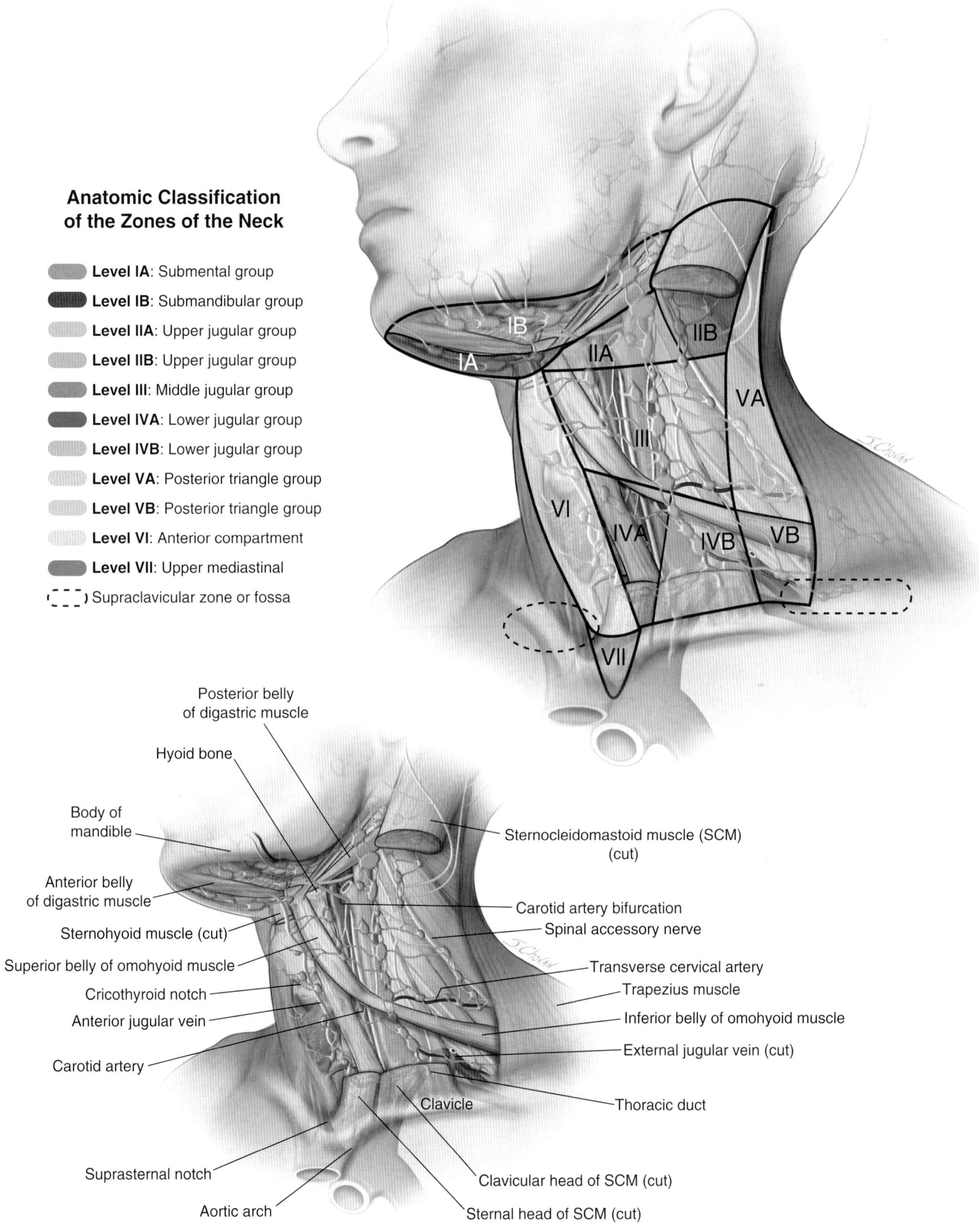

Figure 116.1 Anatomic depiction of all the lymphatic levels of the neck with their surrounding structures. *SCM*, Sternocleidomastoid.

LEVEL III: LYMPH NODE GROUPS: MIDDLE JUGULAR

Boundaries

1. Anterior: lateral border of the sternohyoid muscle
2. Posterior: posterior border of the sternocleidomastoid muscle
3. Superior: hyoid bone (clinical landmark) or carotid bifurcation (surgical landmark)
4. Inferior: cricothyroid notch (clinical landmark) or omohyoid muscle (surgical landmark)

LEVEL IV: LYMPH NODE GROUPS: LOWER JUGULAR

Boundaries

1. Anterior: lateral border of the sternohyoid muscle
2. Posterior: posterior border of the sternocleidomastoid muscle
3. Superior: cricothyroid notch (clinical landmark) or omohyoid muscle (surgical landmark)
4. Inferior: clavicle

Level IVA denotes the lymph nodes that lie along the IJV but immediately deep to the sternal head of the SCM. **Level IVB** denotes the lymph nodes that lie deep to the clavicular head of the SCM.

LEVEL V: LYMPH NODE GROUPS: POSTERIOR TRIANGLE

Boundaries

1. Anterior: posterior border of the sternocleidomastoid muscle
2. Posterior: anterior border of the trapezius muscle
3. Inferior: clavicle

Level VA denotes those lymphatic structures in the upper part of level V that follow the spinal accessory nerve. **Level VB** refers to those nodes that lie along the transverse cervical artery. Anatomically, the division between these and the subzones is the inferior belly of the omohyoid muscle.

LEVEL VI: LYMPH NODE GROUPS: PRELARYNGEAL (DELPHIAN), PRETRACHEAL, PARATRACHEAL, AND PRECRICOID (DELPHIAN) LYMPH NODES (ALSO KNOWN AS THE ANTERIOR COMPARTMENT)

Boundaries

1. Lateral: carotid sheath
2. Superior: hyoid bone
3. Inferior: suprasternal notch

LEVEL VII: LYMPH NODE GROUPS: UPPER MEDIASTINAL

Boundaries

1. Lateral: carotid arteries
2. Superior: suprasternal notch
3. Inferior: aortic arch

Supraclavicular zone or fossa: relevant to nasopharyngeal carcinoma

Boundaries

1. Superior margin of the sternal end of the clavicle
2. Superior margin of the lateral end of the clavicle
3. The point where the neck meets the shoulder

Classification of Neck Dissection

In 1991, the Committee for Head and Neck Surgery and Oncology of the American Academy of Otolaryngology/Head and Neck Surgery developed a system for the classification of neck dissections.[6] It is based on the following concepts:

1. Radical neck dissection (RND) is the standard basic procedure for cervical lymphadenectomy, with removal of lymph nodes in levels I–V with sacrifice of the sternocleidomastoid (SCM), internal jugular vein (IJV), and spinal accessory nerve (cranial nerve [CN] XI).
2. Modified radical neck dissection (MRND) includes the preservation of any nonlymphatic structures while maintaining nodal sampling in levels I–V.
3. Selective neck dissection (SND) is any procedure that preserves one or more groups or levels of lymph nodes.
   a. Supra-omohyoid type (levels I–III).
   b. Lateral type (II–IV)
   c. Posterolateral type (II–V)
   d. Anterior compartment type (VI)
4. An extended neck dissection (END) refers to the removal of additional lymph node groups or nonlymphatic structures relative to the RND.

In 1989 Medina[7] suggested that the term *comprehensive neck dissection* be used whenever all the lymph nodes contained in levels I through V have been removed and recommended three subtypes of MRND. Medina's classification for MRND is as follows:

1. Type I (XI preserved)
2. Type II (XI, IJV preserved)
3. Type III (XI, IJV, and SCM preserved)

Indications for the Use of the Procedure

Neck dissection is indicated in the majority of patients with head and neck cancer. The goal of neck dissection has two primary objectives: pathologic staging and therapeutic intervention. Pathologic staging of the neck further determines whether therapy is warranted in the case of a clinically staged N0 neck. This is strong evidence to suggest that neck dissection also has therapeutic benefits in all stages of head and neck cancer with improvement in patient survival. Radical neck dissections are typically reserved for patients with bulky neck disease with local invasion and extension of the tumor into nonlymphatic structures. RND is typically reserved in situations where oncologic safety cannot be obtained with preservation of the nonlymphatic structures of the SCM, IJV, or spinal accessory nerve and lymphatic contents in level I–V are interrogated. MRND is indicated in patients with clinical or radiographic evidence of nodal metastasis to the neck that does not directly infiltrate or adhere to the nonlymphatic structures which can be preserved, with dissection of levels I–V. The rationale for supraomohyoid neck dissection was developed for treatment of the N0 neck in patients with oral cavity carcinomas. This was established by Lindberg[8] in 1972 where the distribution of lymph node metastasis in head and neck squamous cell carcinomas was considered. He showed that the level II midjugular nodes were the most frequently metastasized node from primary tumors of the head and neck and the distribution pattern of lymphatics drainage from all sites within the head and neck. SND is indicated in patients with primary tumors arising from the oral cavity without clinical or radiologic evidence of cervical metastasis but who have a high probability of occult lymphatic disease. Kligerman et al.[9] established the basis of SND with a risk of occult metastasis of greater than 20% as a basis. The therapeutic implications are that all patients with T2 tumors and greater and any oral cavity tumors with a thickness greater than 3 to 4 mm exceed the relative risk of 20% of occult metastasis and should be given consideration for an SND.

Limitations and Contraindications

Neck dissection is an operation aimed at addressing the lymphatic basins at risk or those involved with metastatic disease. Although neck dissection is an important operation for control of neck disease, it is often augmented with postoperative radiotherapy or chemotherapy where there is pathologic evidence of extracapsular nodal extension of tumor or multiple or multilevel nodal disease. In situations of tumors approaching the midline, often bilateral nodal basins are at risk of metastatic disease and therefore bilateral neck dissections should be performed. Sacrifice of the IJV bilaterally should be avoided simultaneously due to the risk of severe cerebral and/or facial edema, and should this be required, it can be performed in a staged fashion to allow for revascularization. Neck dissection can be particularly challenging in patients who have received previous medical therapies such as chemoradiotherapy or radiotherapy as primary management of their head and neck tumors.

TECHNIQUE

The following procedure describes an SND with alterative techniques of an RND and an MRND.

STEP 1: Intubation

Oral intubation can be used when a neck dissection is being performed in isolation. However, either nasal intubation or a surgical airway is required for patients undergoing an extirpation of a primary head and neck tumor with neck dissection. A shoulder roll should be placed to allow mild neck extension. The endotracheal tube should be secured to allow manipulation of the neck. Typically, no paralytic agents should be used on induction to facilitate peripheral nerve monitoring.

STEP 2: Incisions

There are several variations of neck dissection incisions that have been historically used (Fig. 116.2A). For a straight-line neck dissection, the incision should be placed in a resting skin tension line midway between the angle of the mandible and clavicle extending just slightly anterior to the auricle to the midline. Prior to incision, the incision should be marked and infiltrated with local anesthetic with a vasoconstrictor.

STEP 3: Raising the Subplatysmal Flaps

A #10 blade knife can be used to create an incision through the skin and subcutaneous tissues. The underlying platysma is visualized. A Bovie electrocautery is then be used to transect the platysma muscle. Once the platysma is divided, subplatysmal flaps are then raised to the level of the inferior border of the mandible superiorly and the omohyoid muscle inferiorly. This can be extended to be superior to the clavicle should further dissection of level IV be required. Care should be exercised to preserve the greater auricular nerve. The external jugular vein should be skeletonized, ligated, and divided. Skin flaps can then be secured superiorly and inferiorly (Fig. 116.2B).

STEP 4: Dissection of Level 1 Lymph Nodes

The marginal mandibular branch of the facial nerve transverses the neck within the superficial layer of deep cervical fascia, and in most patients is within a distance of 1.5 cm inferior to the inferior border of mandible. The superficial layer of the deep cervical fascia is dissected and raised to the level of the inferior border of the mandible

Continued

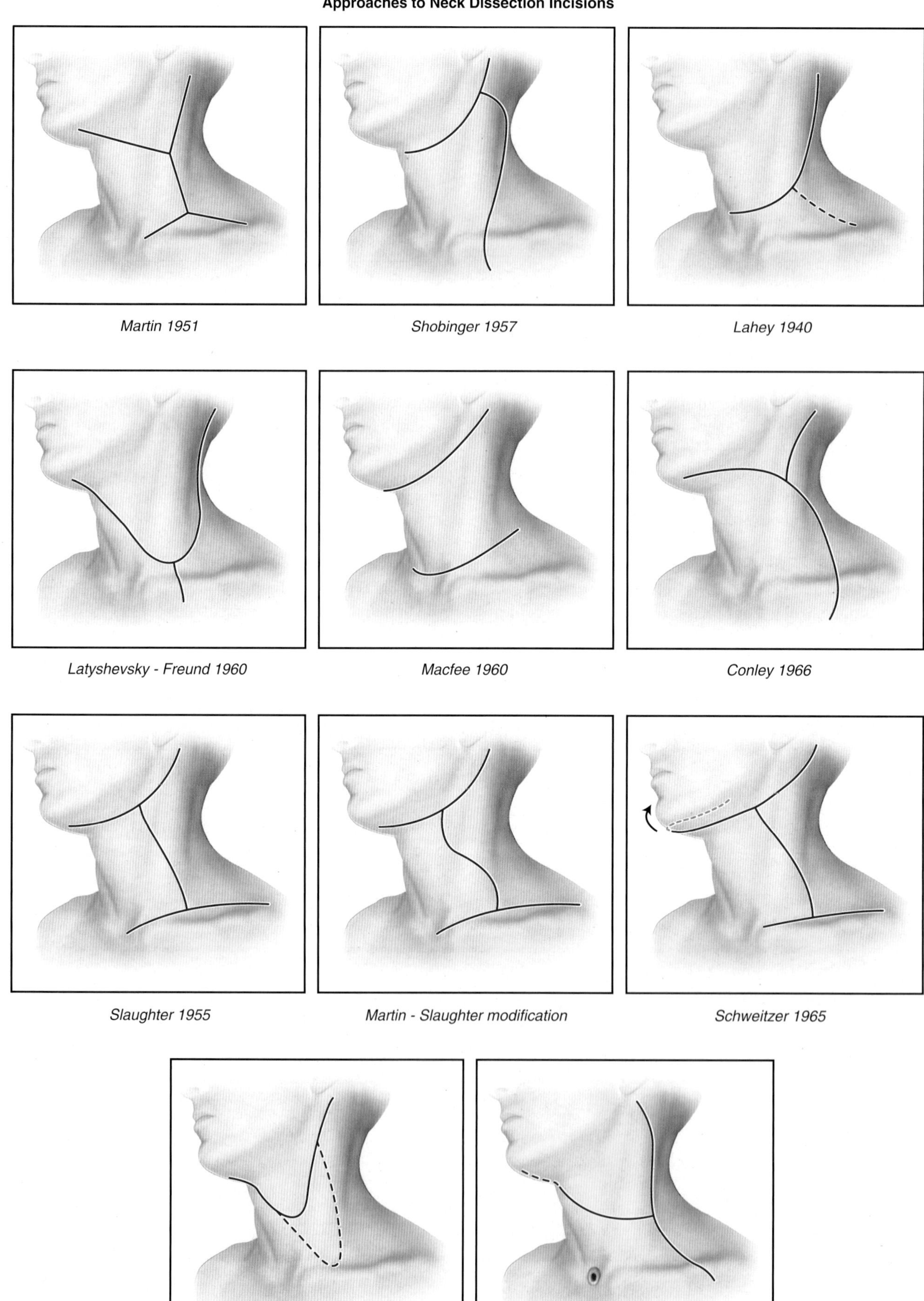

Figure 116.2 **A,** Variations of the neck incisions used historically.

Supraomohyoid Neck Dissection (Levels I-III)

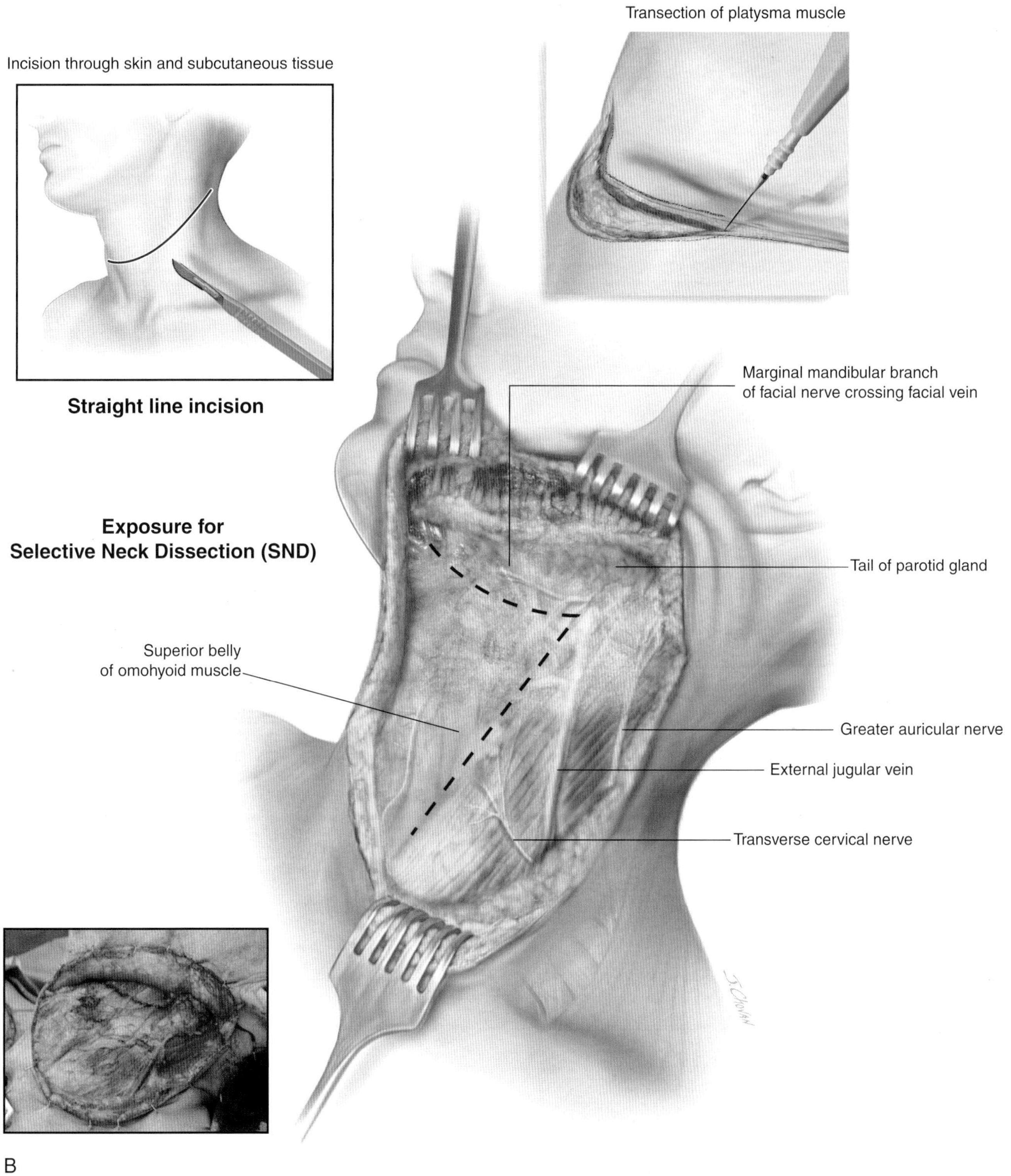

Figure 116.2, cont'd B, The subplatysmal flaps have been raised to the inferior border of the mandible superiorly and the clavicle inferiorly. Skin flaps are raised in a subplatysmal plane to expose the superficial layer of the deep cervical fascia.

TECHNIQUE—*cont'd*

to protect the marginal mandibular branch of the facial nerve. The capsule of the submandibular gland should now be exposed. Bovie electrocauterization is used to dissect the fascia from superficial to the anterior belly of the digastric muscle in the submental triangle; this is continued posteriorly to the submandibular gland. The lateral limit of the dissection is the midline diatheses or the contralateral anterior belly of the digastric muscle. The submandibular gland is then retracted inferiorly into the neck and is circumferentially dissected along the contents of level I. The common facial vein and artery are identified and ligated as they traverse the posterior aspects of the gland. Anteriorly, they are once again identified and ligated and are typically encountered on the medial side of the submandibular gland. Once this division has occurred, the gland is further retracted into the neck, and an Army-Navy retractor is placed beneath the mylohyoid muscle to retract it superiorly. The lingual nerve is typically visualized here with the parasympathetic rami to the submandibular gland. The rami are transected with care to protect the lingual nerve. The submandibular duct is then identified, skeletonized, and divided. The entire contents on level I should be pedicled inferiorly on the digastric muscle (Fig. 116.2C).

STEP 5: Identification of the Spinal Accessory Nerve

Mosquito clamps are now applied to the fascia overlying the anterior border of the SCM superiorly from the level of the digastric muscle inferiorly to the omohyoid muscle. The fascia is then separated from the muscle with Bovie electrocauterization. When the inferior surface of the SCM is reached, care should be taken, as the jugular sheath will be proximal to this area. The muscle continues to be retracted posteriorly as the fascial contents are dissected posteriorly. Approximately 1 cm above the Erb point (the point where the greater auricular nerve crosses the posterior border of the SCM) is the area where the spinal accessory nerve can be identified. The care should be exercised in dissecting the nerve in this location since it can be relatively superficial and easily injured (Fig. 116.2D).

STEP 6: Dissection of Level IIB

Once the spinal accessory nerve is identified, it can be skeletonized laterally from several centimeters, dissected free, and retracted from the underlying fascia. When a clearance of level IIb is desired, the fascia above the CN XI is dissected deep to the level of the levator scapulae and splenius capitis. This fascia packet is then brought inferiorly beneath the nerve. The retromandibular vein and tail of the parotid gland may be encountered in the superficial compartment of this dissection.

STEP 7: Dissection of Level IIA

Once level IIb is pedicled inferiorly beneath the CN XI, the fascia is sharply dissected posteriorly to the jugular sheath. The cervical roots form the posterior limit of the dissection, and fascia should be removed superficial to the nerve rootlets. Dissection deeper than the cervical roots should be avoided to avoid injury to the transverse cervical vessels and preserve the prevertebral fascia, which overlies the phrenic nerve and brachial plexus. Once the fascia is dissected anteriorly, the posterior border of the IJV and carotid sheath are encountered. The fascia should then be retracted over the jugular sheath (Fig. 116.2 E and F).

STEP 8: Dissection of Level III

Once the white roll of the IJV is identified on the anterior border of the IJV, a #15 blade can be used to skeletonize the fascia from the vein sharply. Care should be taken here to maintain tension on the fascia and IJV to facilitate separation and inadvertent injury to the IJV or carotid artery. The inferior thyroid vein is the first branch of the vein identified on the anterior border and is skeletonized, ligated, and divided. Once this is done, the fascia from the jugular sheath is advanced superficially from the posterior belly of the digastric and the omohyoid muscle inferiorly to the level of the level I dissection, which is pedicled on the digastric. As the dissection continues, the anterior jugular veins are identified and ligated. The specimens can now be removed from the patient and orientated by level (Fig. 116.2G).

STEP 9: Closure of the Neck

Once the surgical field is rendered hemostatic, the Valsalva maneuver can be performed to ensure there is no evidence of chyle leak or pneumothorax. A flat #10 Blake drain is placed and secured. Closure is then performed with a polyglactic suture for approximation of the platysma muscle along with skin closure and the application of antibiotic ointment.

STEP 10: Extubation

Extubation should be performed with minimal agitation while holding pressure to the surgical site to avoid postoperative hematoma formation.

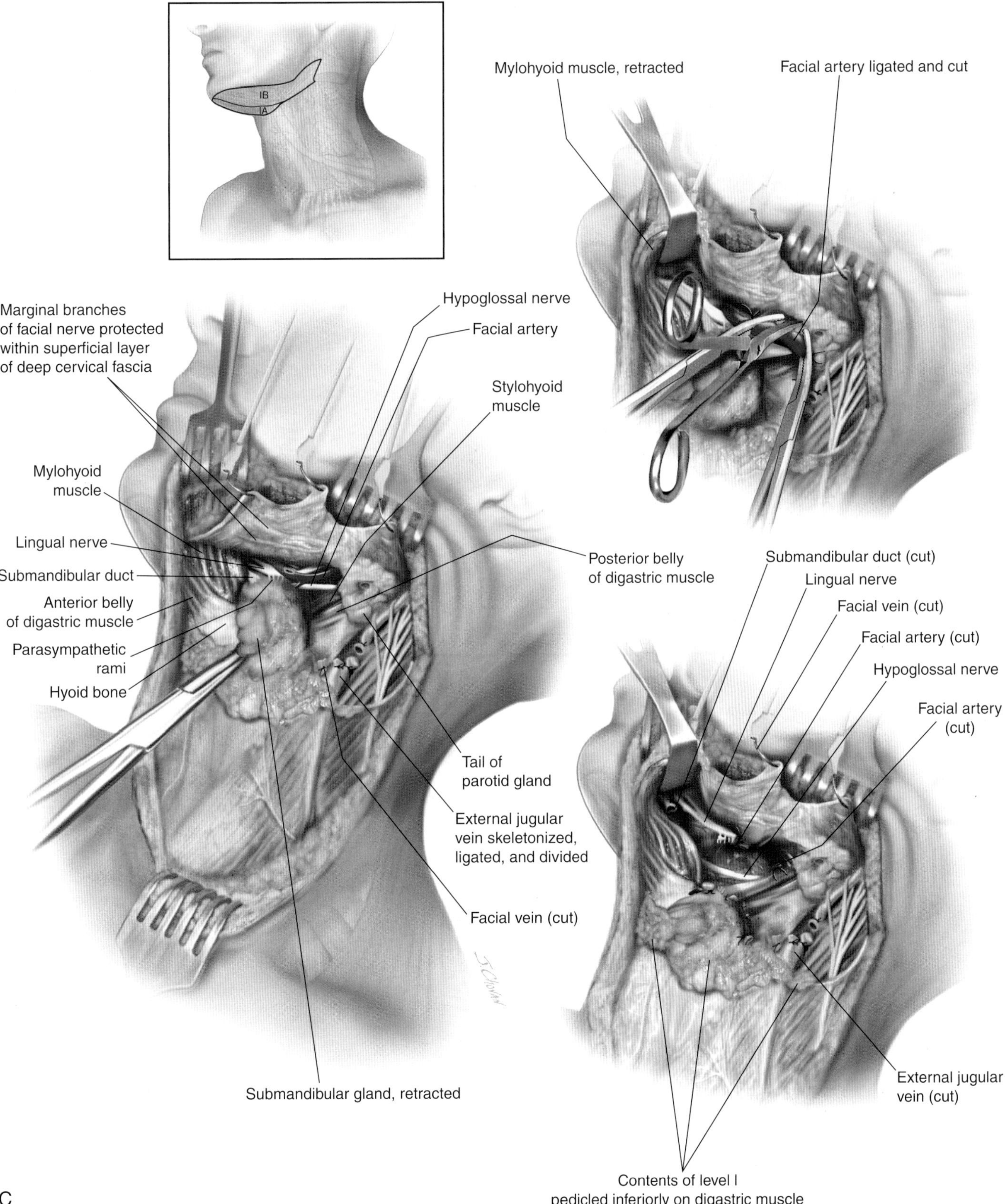

Figure 116.2, cont'd **C,** The anatomic location of the marginal mandibular nerve is shown. The nerve is protected by raising the superficial layer of the deep cervical fascia. The facial artery and vein are ligated to facilitate mobilization of the submandibular gland.

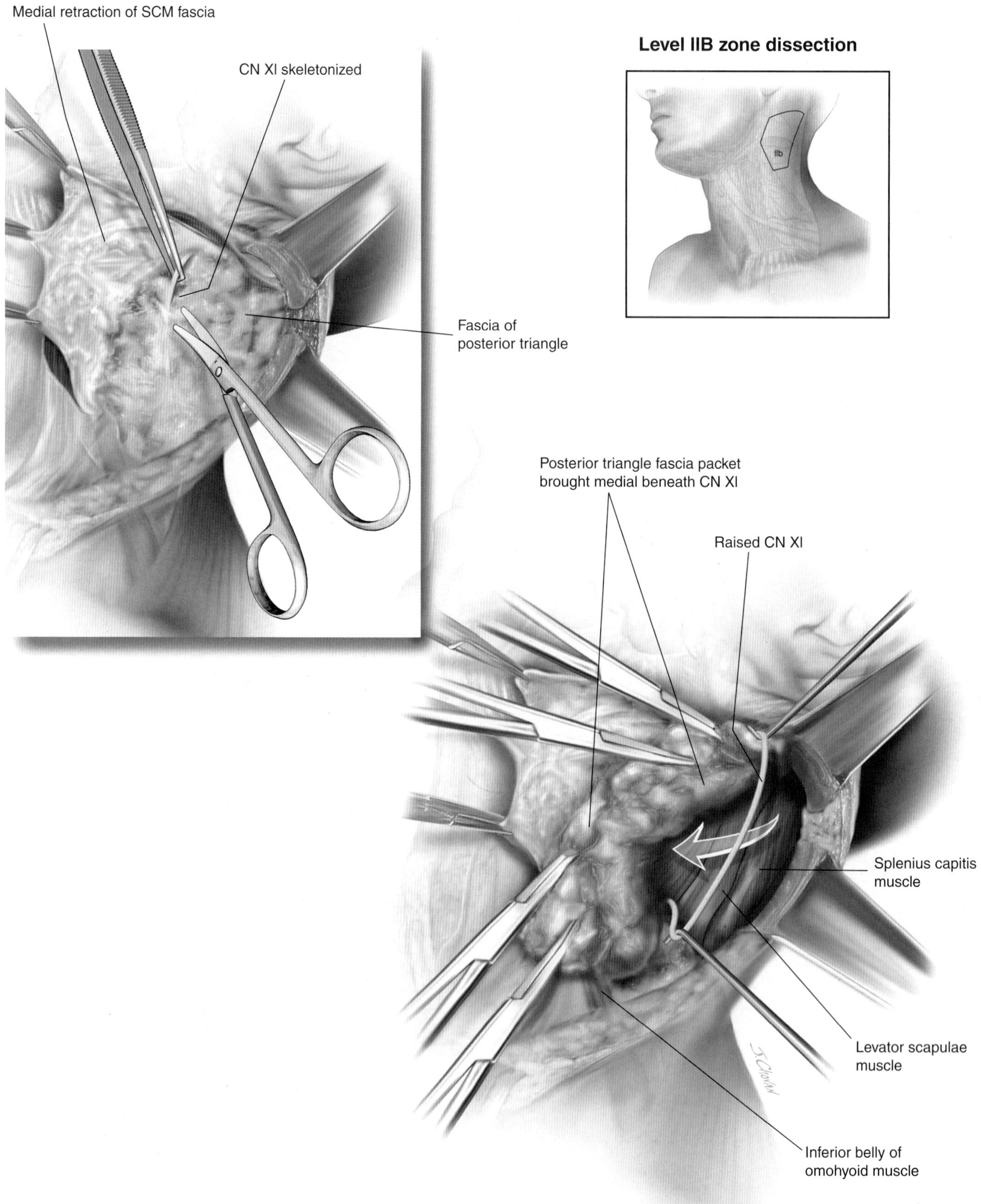

Figure 116.2, cont'd D, The spinal accessory nerve is identified approximately 1 cm above the Erb point. Once the nerve is identified, it can be skeletonized to facilitate dissection and mobilization of the lymphatic compartment in level IIB from the muscular floor of the splenius capitis and the levator scapulae. When level IIB is to be removed in continuity with the remainder of the neck dissection, the fascial compartment is brought beneath the spinal accessory nerve to maintain continuity with the remainder of the specimen.

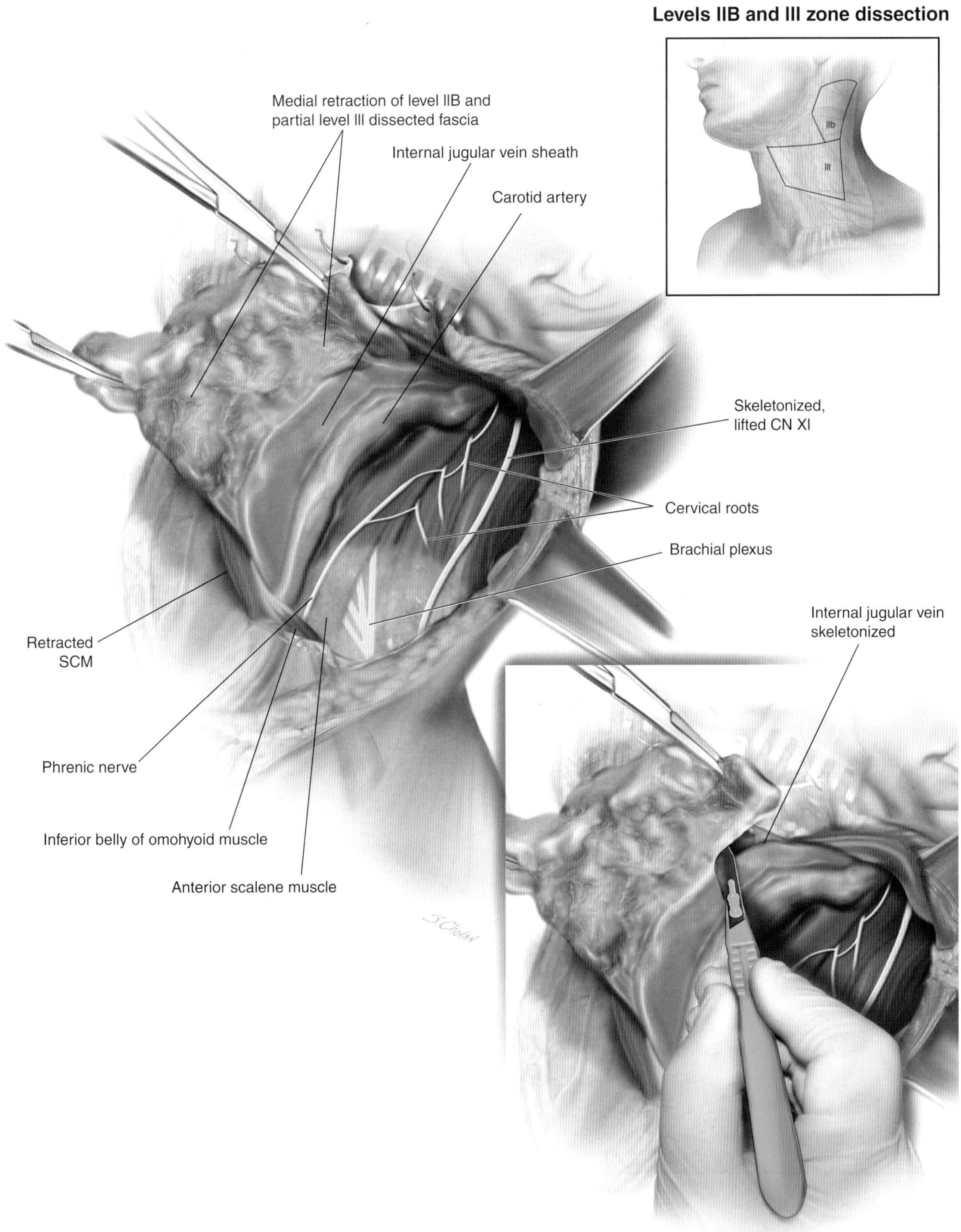

Figure 116.2, cont'd E, The cervical fascia is then mobilized anteriorly from the cervical roots. This establishes the posterior boundary of the neck dissection specimen. The IJV and carotid artery are then encountered, and the fascia is retracted medially and sharply and carefully separated from the IJV.

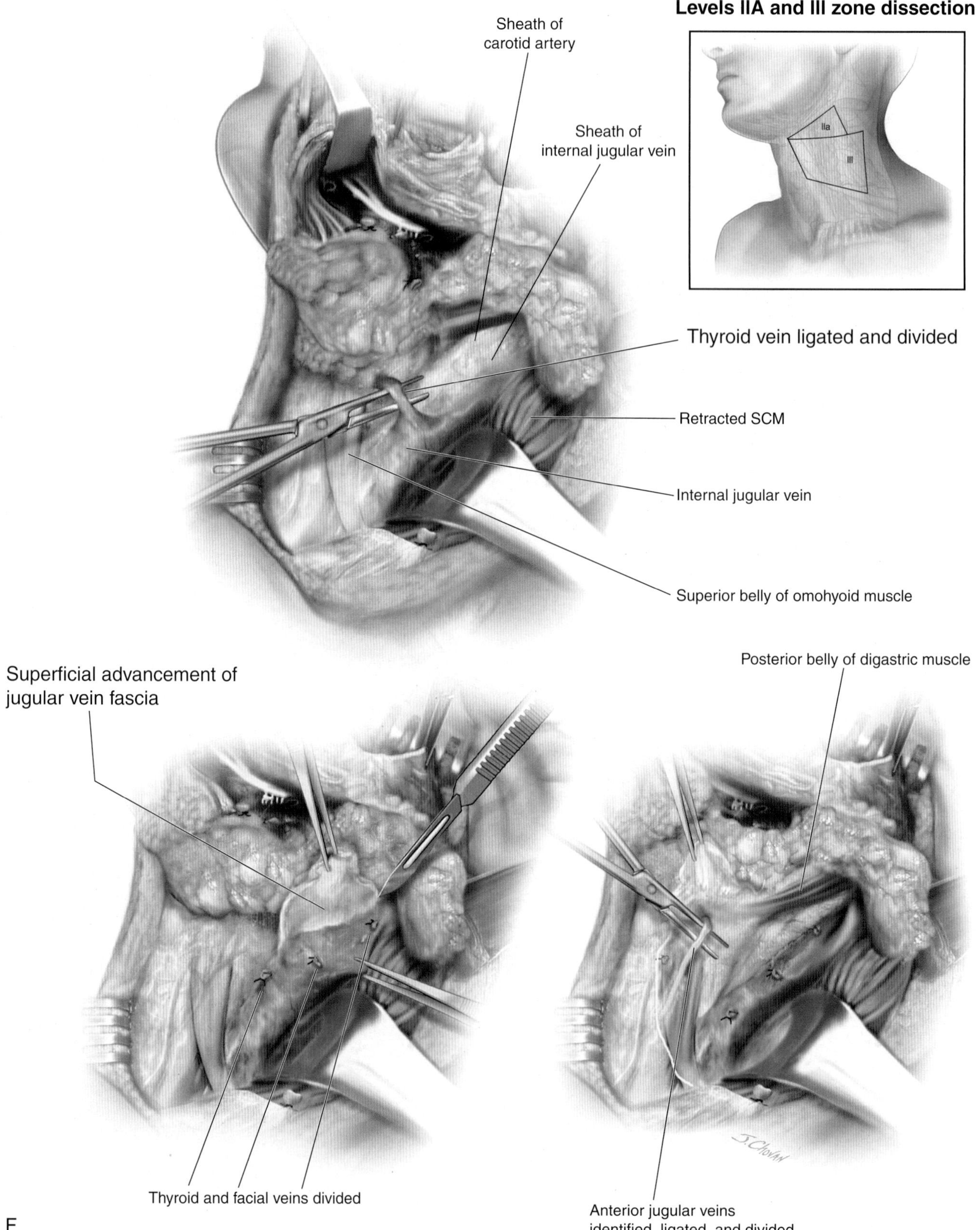

Figure 116.2, cont'd F, The thyroid veins are identified and divided. Once the lymphatic tissue is separated from the IJV and in the submandibular triangle, the fascia along the digastric and hyoid musculature can be skeletonized to remove the remaining attachments of the specimen.

Completion of the Supraomohyoid Neck Dissection (Levels I-III)

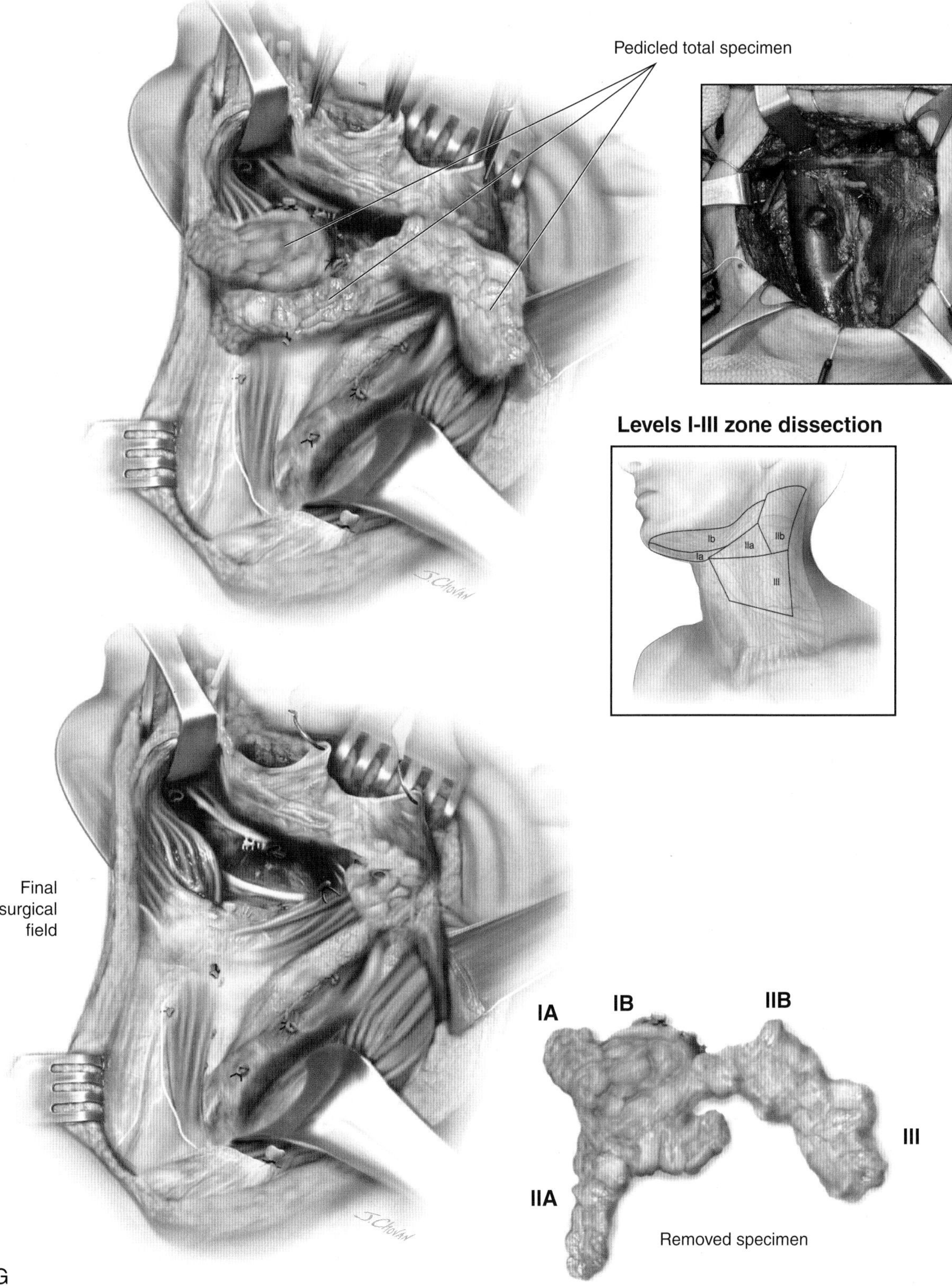

Figure 116.2, cont'd G, Complete removal of the fibrofatty tissue specimen containing all the lymph nodes and its orientation. Note that level IIB can be taken in continuity or separately. Surgical field after completed neck dissection. Note the relationship of the posterior belly of the digastric to the IJV and carotid artery. The spinal accessory nerve and the cervical roots can also be appreciated lateral to the IJV.

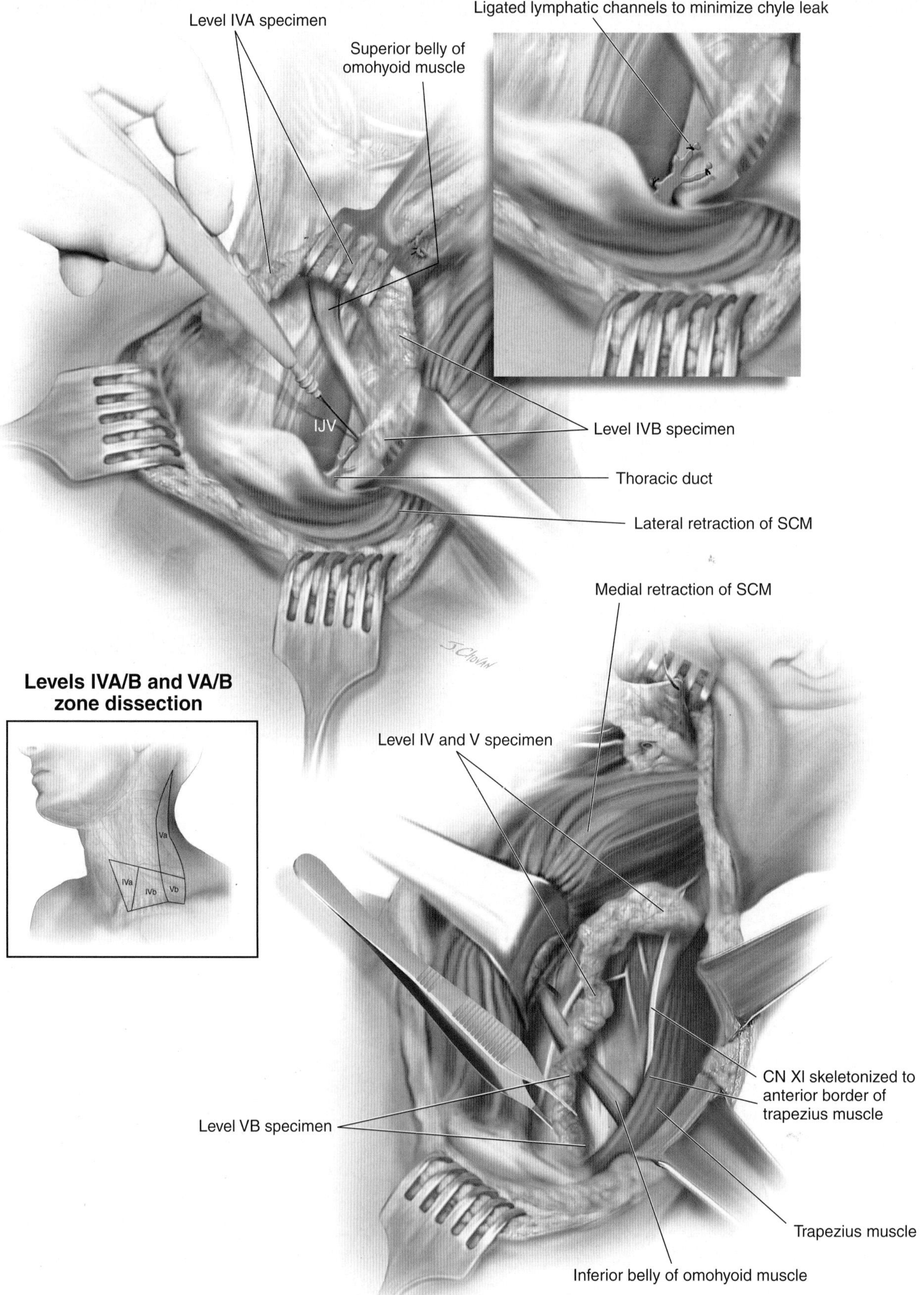

Figure 116.2, cont'd **H,** An MRND is defined by removing the lymphatic contents in levels I–V with preservation of the sternocleidomastoid muscle, IJV, and spinal accessory nerve. The extension of a supraomohyoid neck dissection into levels IV–V is performed with gentle retraction and skeletonization of the fascia from the surrounding musculature inferior to the omohyoid muscle. Care should be exercised to avoid injury to the thoracic duct and the transverse cervical vessels.

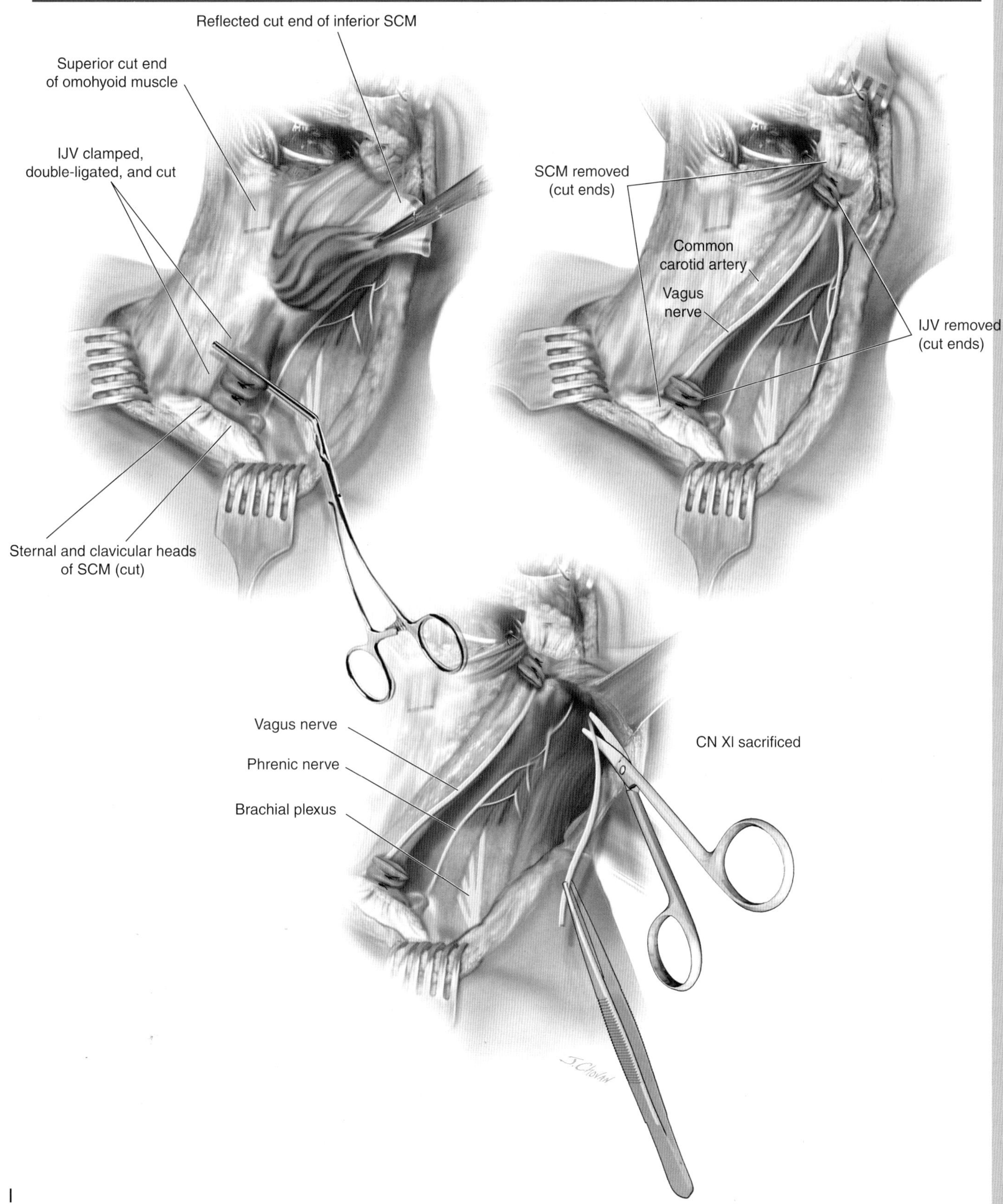

I

Figure 116.2, cont'd I, An RND involves dissection of the lymphatic contents in levels I–V with sacrifice of the sternocleidomastoid muscle, IJV, and spinal accessory nerve. The clavicular and sternal heads of the SCM are divided to expose the IJV. The IJV is then ligated and dissected from the carotid artery superiorly. Both the SCM and the IJV are then divided and ligated in a similar fashion at the superior limit of the neck dissection. Once the spinal accessory nerve is identified and skeletonized to the anterior boundary of the trapezius muscle, it may be divided to facilitate mobilization and removal of the neck dissection specimen in levels I–V.

ALTERNATIVE TECHNIQUE #1

MODIFIED RADICAL NECK DISSECTION

The MRND involves sampling of all five levels of the lateral neck. In addition to the supraomohyoid neck dissection, the removal of additional levels IV and V is facilitated in the following way. Level IV is dissected as an extension from level III inferior to the omohyoid muscle and superior to the clavicle. The fascial contents in this location are loosely adherent and can be retracted manually up into the surgical field and then sharply transected with cautery. The most inferior aspects of the dissection that bring fascia up from beneath the clavicle can place the thorax duct particularly on the left side of the neck at risk of injury.[10] This area should be carefully dissected and cauterized with bipolar cautery. The lymphatic channels can be ligated and divided to minimize the risk of chyle leak.

Level V is addressed by skeletonizing the CN XI further laterally in the neck than was previously described at the anterior border of the trapezius muscle. Care should be exercised during this dissection so as not to injure or inadvertently transect the nerve (Fig. 116.2H).

ALTERNATIVE TECHNIQUE #2

RADICAL NECK DISSECTION

In addition to levels I–V, the RND removes the SCM, IJV, and CN XI. The clavicular and sternal heads of the SCM are divided to reveal the IJV. Satinski vascular clamps are applied to the IJV, which is then divided and double ligated with 2-0 silk sutures. Care should be taken to protect the carotid artery inferior to the IJV. Superiorly, the SCM is divided to expose the IJV, which is once again ligated and double ligated. Once this is done, posterior dissection will reveal the CN XI as previously described, which can then be sacrificed to ensure complete removal of the lymph node basin to the muscular floor of level V and the anterior border of the trapezius muscle (Fig. 116.2I).

Avoidance and Management of Intraoperative Complications

The complication rate for neck dissection is relatively low if good surgical technique is used and the surgeon has an in-depth knowledge of the anatomy; however, some problems can arise from this surgery.[11] In all cases, prevention is the best course of action.

Incisions

A variety of approaches exist for the approach to neck dissections that usually simply rely on the surgeon's preference. The vascular supply of the cervical skin is derived from the external carotid artery superiorly and the subclavian artery inferiorly. Trifurcations or incisions parallel to the carotid artery should be avoided, particularly in salvage cases after radiotherapy. In the latter instances, some surgeons prefer the security of a McFee incision, which avoids some of the potential problems of three-point access. A straight-line incision that is placed in a resting skin tension line heals well postoperatively and is well camouflaged in a skin crease (Fig. 116.2J).

Flap Elevation and Closure

Flaps should be elevated in the subplatysmal plane to maximize their blood supply unless local disease dictates otherwise. Tissue should be incised in stages, particularly if bilateral flaps are employed as this limits blood loss. Skin flaps should not be allowed to dry out, and if necessary, 2 to 3 mm of the edges should be excised before closure. If a tracheostomy is to be performed, it should not be incorporated into the main surgical field to avoid contamination.

Cardiac Arrythmias

Perioperative cardiac complications due to manipulation of the carotid bulb can often be minimized using intraoperative lignocaine on the carotid sinus to counter potential arrhythmias caused by digital manipulation. Early hypertension

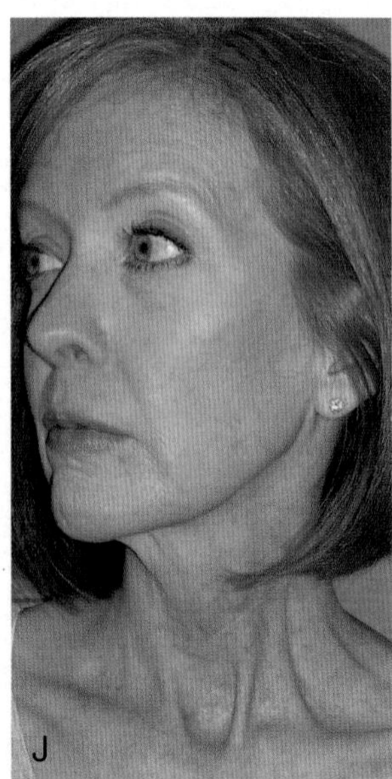

Figure 116.2, cont'd J, Neck incision within a skin crease has healed well within the resting lines of tension. *IJV*, internal carotid vein; *SCM*, sternocleidomastoid.

may follow RND possibly as a result of either carotid sinus denervation or a Cushing's reflex associated with intracranial hypertension.

Air Embolus

Air embolus, which can occur following injury to the IJV, is a rare event. Large emboli can produce sudden falls in end-tidal carbon dioxide and arterial blood pressure. A precordial Doppler probe may detect the characteristic murmur of venous embolus. Local pressure should be applied and the patient placed in the Trendelenburg position. In severe cases, attempts can be made to pass a catheter and aspirate air from the right side of the heart.

Pneumothorax

This may occur when working low in the neck, particularly if the lung apex is high as may occur in overinflation secondary to inadvertent one-lung intubation. Any tears in the pleura should be closed and their integrity tested by hyperinflation of the lung, placing the patient in the Trendelenburg position, and irrigating the area with clear fluid to observe bubbles. Chest tube placement is rarely needed after neck dissection.

Chyle Leak

The thoracic duct arises from the cisternal chyli at the level of the second lumbar vertebra and rises into the neck between the aorta and the azygos vein. In the thorax it crosses to the left, and after passing behind the aortic arch and left subclavian artery, it lies on the anterior scalene muscles and phrenic nerve. The duct terminates most commonly in the left IJV, although less commonly it may enter the left subclavian, left external jugular, left brachiocephalic (innominate) vein or right IJV. Up to 50% of patients exhibit more than one termination of the duct. The right lymphatic duct drain terminates at the junction of the right subclavian vein and IJV. The key to treatment of a chyle fistula is prevention, which demands knowledge of the relevant anatomy. Postoperative leaks are usually identified when feeding is commenced. Multiple approaches to the treatment of an established leak have emerged, including parenteral nutrition with surgical therapy reserved for high-output situations.

Neural Structures

Reparative processes of transected cervical nerves may lead to neuromas in the early or late postoperative period.

In limiting neural injury during neck dissection, the surgeon arguably focuses mainly on the spinal accessory nerve (SAN), which can be safely preserved without jeopardizing the integrity of tumor exenteration as long as it not grossly involved by disease. Care should be taken when elevating the skin flaps in the posterior triangle, as occasionally the SAN lies surprisingly superficially. Consistent and rapid identification of the SAN in the upper neck during dissection can be facilitated by a number of methods, many of which rely on the identification of the Erb point. The attachment of the SCM to the mastoid process is usually tendinous laterally, the inferior extent of this portion of the muscle often corresponding to the emergent point of the SAN from the medial muscle. A small vessel invariably lies immediately over the SAN in a relationship analogous to the artery that it often encountered while exposing the main trunk of the facial nerve. If significantly reduced shoulder pain and disability are apparent in the early postoperative phase, then progressive physical therapy should be instituted in an attempt to minimize its impact and improve quality of life.

Whereas the ansa cervicalis is frequently sacrificed, the vagus, lingual, hypoglossal, and marginal mandibular branch of the facial nerves should be identified and preserved. Identification of the latter should be attempted early on in the neck dissection following flap elevation. If the nerve cannot be identified by visual inspection through the layers of the deep cervical fascia, its integrity should be preserved by dividing the facial vessels approximately 1 cm below the lower border of the mandible and then retracting the divided ends upwards, thus lifting the marginal mandibular branch of the nerve away from the surgical field. The hypoglossal nerve can be identified crossing the external carotid artery and then emerging from underneath the posterior belly of digastric on the hyoglossus muscle. It is at risk of inadvertent damage at both sites. Transient neuropraxia to the phrenic nerve is often manifested subclinically in the postoperative period with changes on plain radiography, but if a severe pulmonary problem exists, especially with concurrent pectoris major flap harvest, respiration may be compromised. Bilateral phrenic nerve palsies may necessitate periods of prolonged mechanical ventilation. Although the carotid plexus of the sympathetic trunk is at risk of injury, the presence of Horner syndrome in the postoperative period is less than 1%. The brachial plexus lies between scalenus anterior and medius muscles as it crosses the posterior triangle. It is not usually encountered other than in the extended RND, but knowledge of its location is important in preventing further readily avoidable complications. Intentional transection of the vagus nerve can result in intraoperative cardiac problems, of which the anesthetist needs to be forewarned. Whenever possible, integrity of the cranial nerves should be maintained unless this compromises tumor resection.

Drains

Drainage is used following neck dissection to prevent the collection of fluid and to aid healing. The drain placement should be carried out separately from the incision to reduce the risk of infection.

Special Considerations

Bilateral Neck Dissection

Increased morbidity and mortality have been demonstrated in patients undergoing simultaneous bilateral neck dissections.[10] Higher rates of infections and fistulae occur and complications such as facial edema and swelling are commonplace, particularly if both IJVs are transected simultaneously. Raised intracranial pressure (ICP) occurs following bilateral IJV ligation with secondary systemic hypertension (Cushing's reflex). This rise in ICP commonly requires aggressive treatment with hyperventilation, fluid restriction, steroids, and mannitol. The ICP frequently returns to normal within 24 hours. There can be a significant rise in ICP in a staged second neck dissection even if the subsequent operation is undertaken many years after the initial surgery. Even in cases of bilateral neck dissections where one IJV is preserved, postoperative imagining demonstrates thrombosis in up to 30% of cases. Meticulous technique with prevention of drying of the preserved IJV and minimization of excess trauma likely reduces the incidence of this occurrence.

The Previously Treated Neck

Previous treatment of the neck, be it radiation, chemoradiation, or surgery, can have a significant impact, both in terms of practicalities and postoperative complications. Previous radiation encourages fibrosis between tissue planes such that subsequent dissection can be a laborious process. These problems are often compounded when previous neck surgery has taken place and is of particular issue if vascular access needs to be preserved to form the basis of recipient vessels for free tissue transfer. In such circumstances, some of the more commonly used vessels (e.g., facial or superior thyroid arteries) may well have been sacrificed. There is rarely a role for preoperative arterial imaging. Instead, the surgeon should be wary of preserving vessels in and around the surgical field. The transverse cervical artery and vein are useful recipient vessels since they are rarely irradiated, are of near constant caliber throughout their course, and are not commonly affected by atherosclerosis.

Carotid Blowout

Carotid blowout is associated with over 60% morbidity and 50% mortality. Neurological sequelae of emergency ligation include hemiplegia, hemi-anesthesia, aphasia, and dysarthria. The incidence is increased following radiation and salivary fistulae. Damage to the adventitial layer during surgery may be another contributory factor. If impending blowout is suspected (sentinel bleed), endovascular techniques with stent-grafts may be indicated rather than open ligation, although short-term complications still occur.

References

1. Crile G. Excision of cancer of the head and neck: with special reference to the plan of dissection based on 132 operations. *J Am Med Assoc.* 1906;47:1780–1785.
2. Martin H, Del Valle B, Ehrlich H, Cahan WG. Neck dissection. *Cancer.* 1951;4(3):441–499.
3. Bocca E, Pignataro O. A conservation technique in radical neck dissection. *Ann Otol Rhinol Laryngol.* 1967;76(5):975–987.
4. Suen JY, Goepfert H. Standardization of neck dissection nomenclature. *Head Neck Surg.* 1987;10(2):75–77.
5. Shah JP. Patterns of cervical lymph node metastasis from squamous carcinomas of the upper aerodigestive tract. *Am J Surg.* 1990;160(4):405–409.
6. Robbins KT, Medina JE, Wolfe GT, Levine PA, Sessions RB, Pruet CW. Standardizing neck dissection terminology: official report of the Academy's Committee for Head and Neck Surgery and Oncology. *Arch Otolaryngol Head Neck Surg.* 1991;117(6):601–605.
7. Medina JE. A rational classification of neck dissections. *Otolaryngol Head Neck Surg.* 1989;100(3):169–176.
8. Lindberg R. Distribution of cervical lymph node metastases from squamous cell carcinoma of the upper respiratory and digestive tracts. *Cancer.* 1972;29(6):1446–1449.
9. Kligerman J, Lima RA, Soares JR, et al. Supraomohyoid neck dissection in the treatment of T1/T2 squamous cell carcinoma of oral cavity. *Am J Surg.* 1994;168(5):391–394.
10. Kerawala CJ, Heliotos M. Prevention of complications in neck dissection. *Head Neck Oncol.* 2009;1:35.
11. Kerawala CJ. Complications of head and neck cancer surgery—prevention and management. *Oral Oncol.* 2010;46(6):433–435.

Sentinel Node Biopsy for Oral Squamous Cell Carcinoma

Marcus A. Couey, Andrew M. Baker, and R. Bryan Bell

Armamentarium

#15 Scalpel blades
1% Isosulfan blue dye (optional)
1% Lidocaine with 1:100,000 epinephrine
25-gauge Needle on a tuberculin syringe
Appropriate sutures
Bipolar electrocautery
Electrocautery
Fine curved hemostat or dissectors
Handheld gamma probe
Lahey clamps
Local anesthetic with vasoconstrictor
Lymphoscintigraphy (gamma camera; nuclear medicine suite)
MacIndoe forceps
Marking pen
Radiotracer—99mTc tilmanocept (lymphoseek) or 99mTc sulfur colloid
Weitlaner retractor

History of the Procedure

The most important factor affecting the outcome of patients with oral squamous cell carcinoma (OSCC) is the presence of cervical lymph node metastasis at diagnosis.[1] However, even in early-stage tumors with no clinical or radiographic evidence of regional disease, approximately 23% will in fact harbor occult cervical metastasis.[2] This has led most investigators to recommend that patients with OSCC undergo elective, selective neck dissection (SND) of the clinically N0 neck if they have primary tumors that demonstrate clinical prognostic indicators of metastasis, such as a size greater than 2 cm in diameter or a depth of invasion greater than 2 to 4 mm.[3] SND in the clinically N0 patient is beneficial when the tumor is found on pathologic evaluation of the specimen; this allows for early removal of metastatic disease and accurate staging information on which to base adjuvant therapy. Unfortunately, this approach has led to unnecessary surgery in 65% to 75% of patients with early-stage OSCC. Additionally, neck dissection is associated with neurogenic shoulder dysfunction and esthetic deformity in a significant number of individuals.

Sentinel lymph node biopsy (SLNB) is a minimally invasive technique that is currently under investigation for staging of OSCC and offers the potential of reducing the morbidity associated with SND.[4] The concept of the *sentinel node* is premised on the filtering mechanism of lymph nodes: metastatic tumor cells tend to deposit within the first echelon lymph nodes along the lymphatic drainage pathway of a primary tumor. The term was initially coined by Gould et al., when describing a level II cervical lymph node consistently identified during parotidectomy for malignant tumors, the status of which guided the surgeons to complete or forego neck dissection.[5] Following advancements in lymphatic mapping using injectable radiotracers and/or dyes in the late 20th century, the definition of *sentinel node* evolved to denote the lymph node(s) within the primary tumor-draining echelon being most likely to harbor metastatic disease. Since Morton et al.'s landmark study demonstrating intraoperative lymphatic mapping in 1992,[6] rigorous evaluation of SLNB has led to its broad acceptance as a less-invasive staging procedure for early primary tumors in cutaneous melanoma and breast cancer.[6] More recently, SLNB has shown promise as an alternative to observation as well as elective node dissection (END) in early-stage oral cancer.

SLNB has been shown to accurately predict nodal metastases in numerous clinical studies, wherein patients underwent SLNB followed by END.[7] These findings have been validated in several prospective multicenter studies over the last decade, with negative predictive values (NPV) ranging from 88.1% to 97.0%.[8–12] The SENT trial, the largest prospective study to date, surgically staged 415 patients with cT1-T2 N0 oral SCC using SLNB. Positive SLNs were found in 94 patients (23%), which led to a neck dissection within 3 weeks. Overall survival and disease-free survival rates were 92% and 94%, respectively, over 3 years. Contralateral drainage was identified in 12% of cases, and positive SLNs were found on the contralateral side in 6%, which would have been missed if ipsilateral END was performed. This suggests that SLNB may be a more accurate staging tool than END.

Most of the published studies on SLNB used 99mTc sulfur colloid or similar radiotracer (with or without injected dye). These agents loosely diffuse within injected tissues and have been associated with "shine-through" radioactivity from the primary site, which can confound SLN identification.[13] This is particularly relevant for floor-of-mouth cancers, which have a close proximity to the level I nodal basin. While some studies, including the SENT trial, reported no problems with shine-through, two multicenter studies reported substantially higher false-negative rates for floor-of-mouth tumors.[9,10] 99mTc Tilmanocept was developed to minimize shine-through and increase the specificity of SLNB through preferential accumulation of radiotracer within lymph nodes.[14] In 2015, Agrawal et al. reported results from a phase III trial of 99mTc tilmanocept in oral cancer, which enrolled patients from 13 institutions in the United States and Canada.[15] SLNB with 99mTc tilmanocept demonstrated a NPV of 97.8%, and a false-negative rate of only 2.6% (positive lymph node on neck dissection specimen in the presence of a negative SLN). Furthermore, they reported no problems with shine-through. In 100% of patients in floor-of-mouth tumors (*N* = 20), at least one SLN was identified, 12 of which were positive and none were false negatives. Injected dye was not used in this study.

Recently, abstracts from two controlled clinical trials of SLNB in cT1-T2 N0 oral cancer were presented to the American Society of Clinical Oncology, in which patients were randomized to receive either upfront END or SLNB followed by SND in cases of positive SLN. In 2019, Hasegawa et al. reported results from 265 patients enrolled at 16 institutions in Japan.[16] Three-year recurrence-free survival (RFS) and overall survival were 80% and 89%, respectively, in the SLNB group, with 81% and 86% in the upfront END group, respectively. In 2020, Garrel et al. reported results from the SentiMERORL trial, which enrolled 279 patients at 10 institutions in France.[17] Two-year and 5-year RFS were 90.7% and 89.4%, respectively, in the SLNB arm, with 89.6% and 89.6% in the END arm, respectively. Both trials reported improved functional outcomes within 3 to 6 months of surgery. While we are awaiting the final manuscripts with detailed methods and results for these two trials, the data published thus far suggest noninferior oncologic outcomes and decreased morbidity with SLNB compared with upfront END.

Indications

Current indications for SLNB include biopsy-confirmed T1 or T2 oral cavity squamous cell carcinoma of all subsites, including the tongue, floor of the mouth, retromolar trigone, buccal mucosa, alveolus/gingiva, hard palate, and lip, clinically negative for neck disease based on the physical examination and advanced imaging (e.g., contrast-enhanced CT or MRI). SLNB can be beneficial in staging ipsilateral or bilateral necks for unilateral or midline tumors, respectively.

Limitations and Contraindications

SLNB is a minimally invasive staging technique for early cancers of the oral cavity and oropharynx with clinically negative neck disease. Patients with clinical or radiographic evidence of neck metastasis should undergo formal therapeutic neck dissection and/or definitive radiotherapy. Current contraindications to SLNB include the following:

- Lack or unavailability of a nuclear medicine facility
- Clinically evident neck disease
- History of cancer or surgery in the neck
- History of radiation to the neck
- Recent neck trauma
- Advanced primary tumor that requires free tissue transfer and neck dissection for vascular access

SLNB for floor-of-mouth tumors is limited by the shine-through effect of a radiotracer and interference with evaluation of the nearby level I lymph nodes (Fig. 117.1).

TECHNIQUE: Sentinel Node Biopsy

STEP 1: Injection of Radiotracer

In the nuclear medicine suite, the area of the oral cavity tumor is anesthetized with local or topical anesthetic. 500 mCi of either 99mTc tilmanocept (lymphoseek) or 99mTc sulfur colloid is evenly injected submucosally around the tumor using a tuberculin syringe. A total of four injections, given in quadrants around the lesion, is generally sufficient. Typically, this is performed by the nuclear medicine suite staff but the assistance of a member of the surgical team may be required (Fig. 117.2A).

STEP 2: Lymphoscintigraphy

Approximately 30 minutes after injection of the radioactive tracer, the patient should undergo multiview planar lymphoscintigraphy with a gamma camera in the nuclear medicine suite. Anterior, lateral, and oblique views are obtained. When available, single-photon emission computed tomography is recommended, as it provides the surgeon with three-dimensional orientation of the sentinel node.[18] The images are reviewed to identify laterality and the site of the first echelon of lymph nodes draining the primary tumor (Fig. 117.2B).

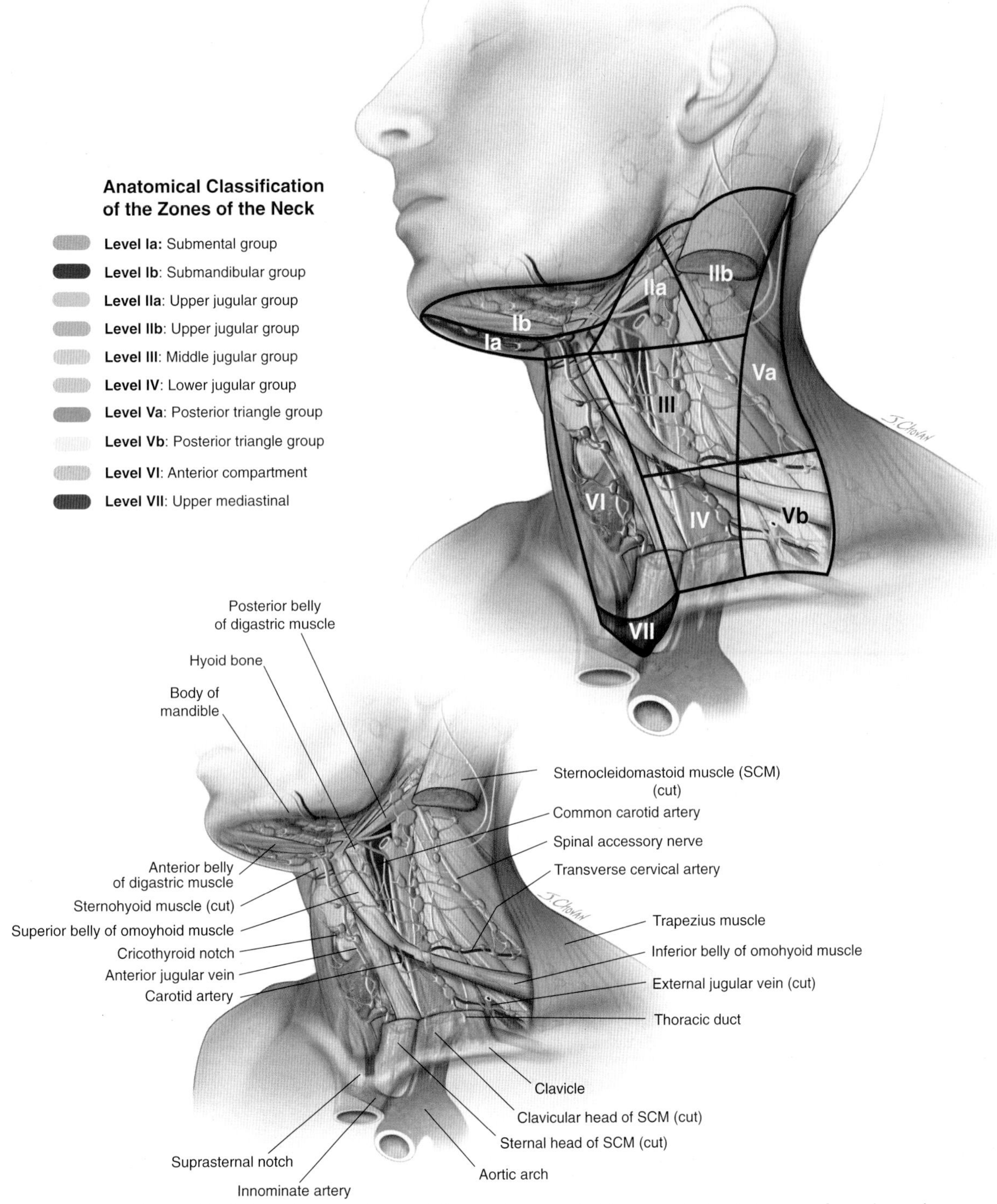

Figure 117.1 Lymphatic drainage of the head and neck. Note the chain of drainage from the oral cavity subsites to the cervical chain.

Continued

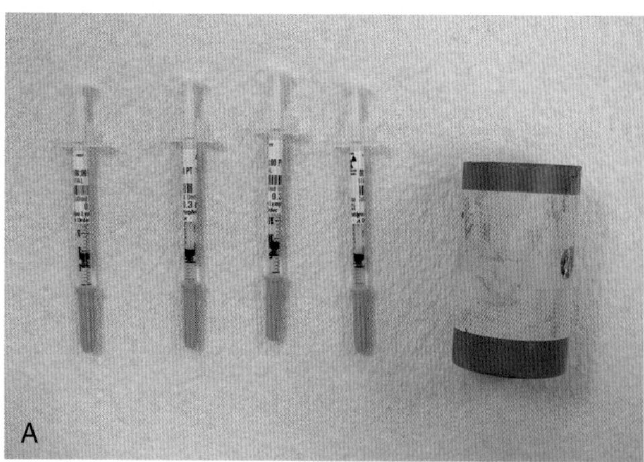

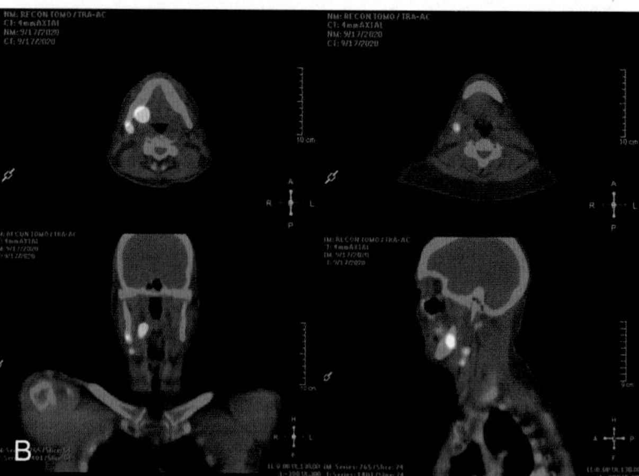

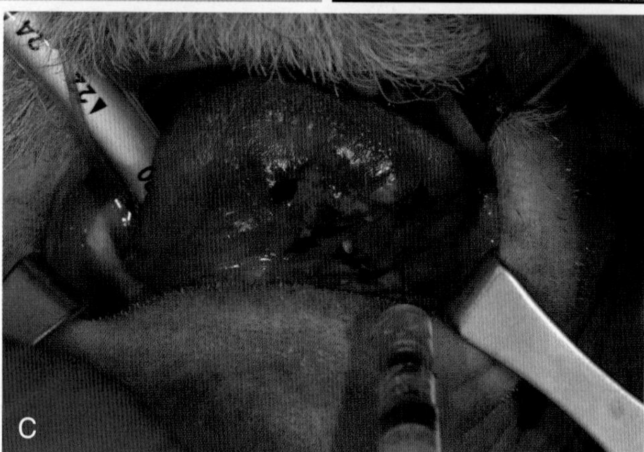

Figure 117.2 **A,** Radiotracer prepared in syringes for submucosal peritumor injection. The site is divided into quadrants and injected evenly. **B,** SPECT/CT revealing radiotracer at the site of injection around the right tongue tumor, as well as two foci of radiotracer uptake within the ipsilateral level II lymph node basin (sentinel nodes). **C,** Injection of blue dye into the peritumor submucosa. Note the flow of dye through the lymphatics that becomes "trapped" in the first echelon of lymph nodes.

TECHNIQUE: Sentinel Node Biopsy—cont'd

STEP 3: Dye Injection (Optional)

The patient is brought to the operating room within 24 hours of radioactive tracer injection and prepped and draped in the standard fashion for an oncologic operation. As an adjunct to the radiotracer, 0.5 to 1 cc of vital blue dye is injected submucosally around the periphery of the tumor 10 to 15 minutes prior to tumor resection. Isosulfan blue (1%) is traditionally used for its protein binding characteristics and propensity to accumulate in lymph nodes;[19] however, it carries a risk of allergic reactions, including anaphylaxis.[20] Methylene blue (1%) may be used as an alternative dye, with equal efficacy for visual identification of the sentinel node and less potential for allergic reaction (Fig. 117.2C).[21]

STEP 4: Resection of the Primary Tumor

The primary tumor is resected in accordance with basic oncologic principles (Fig. 117.2D). This is done to prevent shine-through when attempting to locate the sentinel nodes. Although the radiotracer injected around the tumor drains into the lymphatic channels and becomes lodged in the first echelon of nodes, some will remain in the tumor bed and surrounding tissues. This can interfere with lymphatic mapping of the neck because the primary tumor may emit a substantial amount of radiation, creating a false-positive or inaccurate reading on the gamma probe. This is a particularly troublesome technical limitation when the level I lymph node basins are interrogated for floor-of-mouth cancers; however, use of 99mTc tilmanocept may minimize this phenomenon compared with 99mTc sulfur colloid.[15,22]

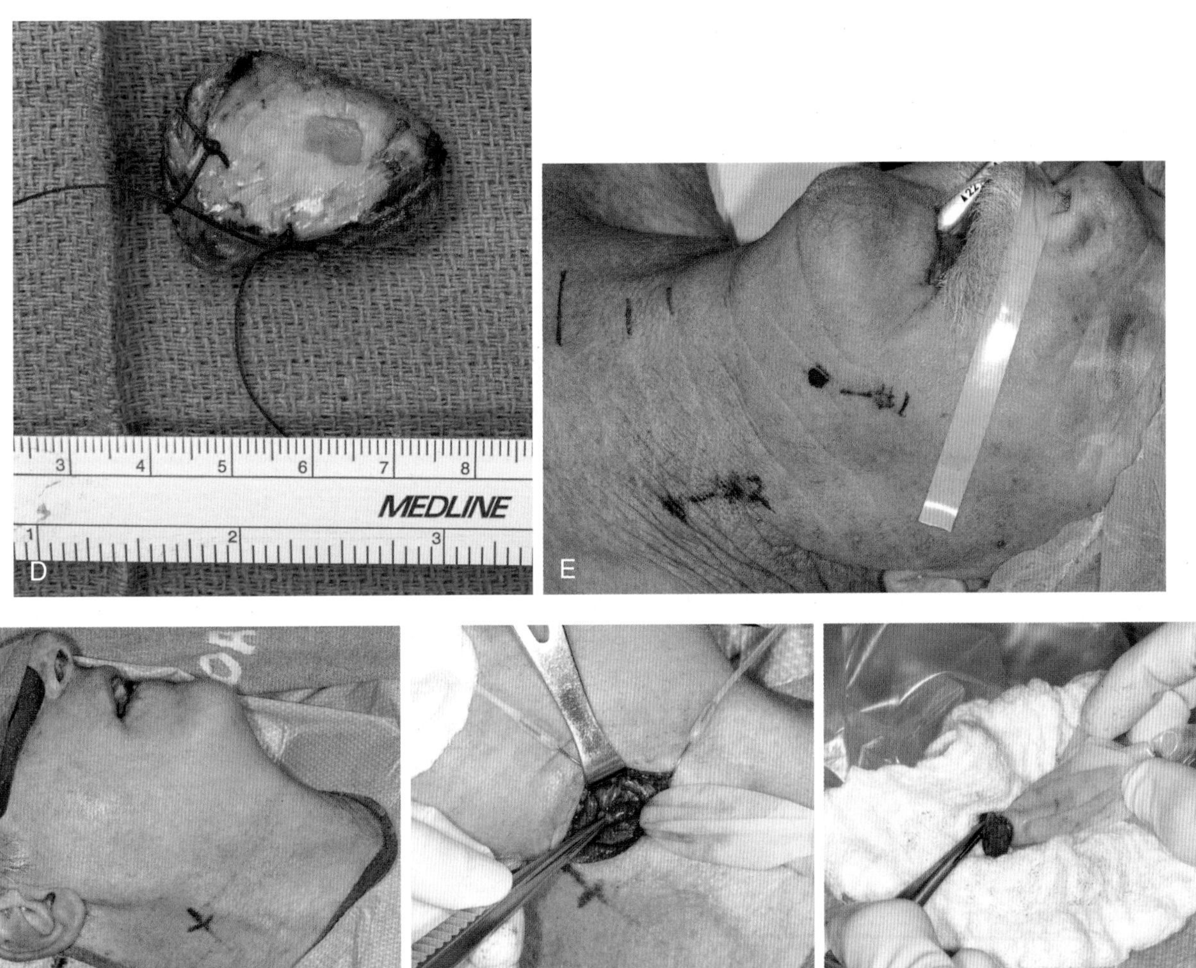

Figure 117.2, cont'd **D,** Resected primary tumor specimen. This is done before lymph node biopsy to prevent shine-through. Note the blue staining of the tumor from isosulfan blue dye. **E,** The gamma probe is placed on the skin of the neck using the lymphoscintigram as a guide. Once a hot spot is identified, a skin incision is marked to harvest that set of lymph nodes. **F,** When possible, the incision should be positioned so that it can be extended for a neck dissection. **G,** Identification of the sentinel node(s) with the gamma probe and removal with blunt dissection. **H,** The excised specimen is examined for radioactivity with the gamma probe ex vivo to confirm that it is the sentinel lymph node.

TECHNIQUE: Sentinel Node Biopsy—cont'd

STEP 5: Intraoperative Lymphatic Mapping

The handheld gamma probe is calibrated to detect the specific radiotracer injected and placed directly on the neck in the area of radiotracer uptake as revealed on lymphoscintigraphy. The probe is used to identify hot spots, or areas of increased gamma radiation. A gamma count of at least three times the measured in vivo background count is considered hot. This area is marked (Fig. 117.2E).

STEP 6: Harvesting the Sentinel Node

A skin incision is marked along lines of resting tension over the area of highest radioactivity, and a local anesthetic with vasoconstrictor is injected subcutaneously. When possible, the incision should be positioned so that it can be extended for a neck dissection, should this be required (Fig. 117.2F). A #15 blade is used to incise the skin, and sharp dissection with electrocautery to and through the platysma muscle is completed. Subplatysmal flaps are created superiorly and inferiorly with electrocautery. A self-retaining Weitlaner retractor is placed under the flaps to expose the superficial layer of the deep cervical fascia and fibroadipose tissue containing the cervical lymphatics.

Continued

TECHNIQUE: Sentinel Node Biopsy—cont'd

The gamma probe is reintroduced into the wound directly over the superficial layer of the deep cervical fascia to help locate the sentinel node. Pale blue staining from dye injection may also aid visual identification of the node. Blunt dissection in the hottest area with a fine curved clamp through the cervical fascia is completed, and the sentinel node is identified (Fig. 117.2G). This and any immediately adjacent nodes are sharply excised from the neck and placed on a sterile table away from the patient. A direct gamma count of the specimen is obtained ex vivo (Fig. 117.2H).

STEP 7: Examining the Neck

The gamma probe is reintroduced directly into the surgical bed and immediately surrounding areas. The gamma count should be 10% or less than that of the hottest node removed; if it is not, further harvesting of lymph nodes is completed until a 10:1 ratio of ex vivo node to surgical bed is obtained.

STEP 8: Histopathologic Examination

Perhaps the most important step of SLNB lies out of the surgeon's hands. An active working relationship with the pathologist examining the nodes is imperative in obtaining accurate results for staging purposes. The guidelines established by the Second International Conference on Sentinel Node Biopsy in Mucosal Head and Neck Cancer are most widely used by pathologists participating in SLNB.[23]

The node is fixed and cleared of surrounding adipose tissue, then bisected along its longest axis. If each hemisphere is thicker than 2.5 mm, the halves are sectioned into 2.5-mm slices. Step serial sectioning (SSS) of the segments is completed at 150 μm, and four adjacent slices are mounted at a time. One is stained with hematoxylin and eosin (H&E), and one is evaluated by immunohistochemistry (IHC) for cytokeratin. The remaining two sections are reserved for future analysis, if necessary. If all the sections are negative by H&E and IHC, the node is declared tumor-free. If a section stains positive for cytokeratin, the adjacent serial section stained with H&E is thoroughly reexamined for tumor cells. This detailed histopathologic examination can accurately identify macrometastasis, micrometastasis, and individual tumor cells in the first echelon nodes of the cervical lymphatics.

Intraoperative frozen section or touch preparation/imprint cytology may be used to assess the sentinel node(s) intraoperatively, allowing the surgeon to make decisions about further surgical interrogation of the neck. Although time constraints limit, thorough and detailed histopathologic analysis with thin SSS and IHC as described previously, identification of carcinoma in sentinel node biopsies with these techniques has been successful and on par with the techniques described previously.[24,25] However, some literature does not support the use of monoslice frozen section analysis and imprint cytology as an intraoperative tool because it may not be as sensitive as SSS and IHC in the identification of micrometastasis in SLNB.[26,27]

STEP 9: Completion of Neck Dissection

If intraoperative frozen sections were sent and returned positive for carcinoma, a formal neck dissection can be completed immediately to allow for more complete staging. If preoperative suspicion for occult neck disease is high, a neck dissection may also be completed, with the SLNB used as an adjunctive staging tool regardless of intraoperative pathologic analysis.

If no intraoperative frozen sections were sent and the final pathology is positive for carcinoma, the patient may benefit from returning to the operating room for a completion neck dissection. This can provide therapeutic benefit and allows for more comprehensive assessment of the need for postoperative adjunctive radiotherapy or chemotherapy.

Avoidance and Management of Intraoperative Complications

Lymphatic mapping with isosulfan blue and technetium-99m radiotracer is relatively safe, with an overall adverse drug reaction rate of 1.1% to 1.5%. Most reactions are limited to pruritus, rash, and blue hives. About 0.1% to 0.5% of patients have developed hypotensive or anaphylactic responses to lymphatic mapping agents, with isosulfan blue usually being the culprit.[20,28] Patients with sulfa allergy have not been shown to be at higher risk for these reactions. Caution in administering these drugs, as with any other drug, and vigilance for drug reactions, may avoid life-threatening injury. As described earlier, methylene blue may be used in place of isosulfan blue because it has a lower incidence of adverse effects.[21]

From a surgical standpoint, SLNB is similar to neck dissection, and care must be taken to avoid similar potential complications. Although the incision and access for SLNB are smaller than for formal neck dissection, injury to important structures can be problematic. Incision through the superficial layer of the deep cervical fascia must be 1.5 to 2 cm below the inferior mandibular border to prevent transection of the marginal mandibular branch of the facial nerve. Because the surgical access is small, it is important not to lose orientation in regard to the mandible. Posteriorly, the greater auricular nerve and external jugular veins lie superficial to the superficial layer of the deep cervical fascia. Deep to this, the spinal accessory nerve, hypoglossal nerve, and branches of the external carotid can be found. Careful dissection is necessary to avoid injury to these structures.

If gamma counts remain very high after excision of multiple lymph nodes, radiation shine-through may be culpable; this phenomenon mostly occurs in the level I lymph node basin in cases of floor-of-mouth cancer and can be problematic even when the primary tumor is excised first. However, data suggest that shine-through is greatly reduced when using 99mTc tilmanocept.[15,22] If the surgeon still experiences difficulty locating the sentinel lymph node in the absence of shine-through, this may be an indication to convert to a formal neck dissection.

As mentioned above, the current guidelines for pathologic processing of SLNB tissue incorporate both IHC and SSS at 150 μm intervals. The pathologist must be comfortable in following the protocol, particularly SSS, to limit false negatives and potentially down-stage a patient. While there is some evidence that standard sectioning at 2-mm intervals may be sufficient for the detection of micrometastasis,[25,29] this has yet to be tested against SSS in a large prospective trial.

Postoperative Considerations

From a surgical standpoint, the major postoperative considerations are bleeding and hematoma formation, marginal mandibular nerve palsy, and wound infection. Strict adherence to surgical and aseptic principles can limit these problems, making SLNB a minimally invasive and safe procedure.

The major postoperative considerations with SLNB stem from the final pathology. Because this is a pure staging procedure, the status of the sentinel node can direct the surgeon and patient in how to proceed. Although recent data report excellent sensitivity and specificity with SLNB, there is a possibility of missing occult neck disease with this procedure and potentially under-staging a patient.

Based on our experience and that of others, it is thought that SLNB currently has a role in the management of patients with OSCC, although that role has yet to be clearly defined. In the future, it likely will be used as an adjuvant to clinical and radiographic staging, either alone or in combination with SND, based on the size and location of the primary tumor. Because a significant number of patients undergoing surgery for N0 OSCC require microvascular free tissue transfer, performing a SND in this setting as a matter of routine seems reasonable. However, the SLNB concept may be advantageous for identifying aberrant or unexpected patterns of lymphatic drainage, such as in patients with contralateral drainage, "skip metastasis" to level IV of the neck, or "in transit" lymph nodes located above the inferior border of the mandible or within the parotid gland, even when a SND is planned. The so-called sentinel lymph node–assisted neck dissection may be particularly useful for midline tumors in an effort to limit the neck dissection to only one side.

Ample evidence already supports the use of the SLNB technique as an alternative to watch and wait for patients with T1N0 OSCC, regardless of primary tumor depth. In our opinion, there is little use for simply watching an N0 neck. Even in primary tumors less than 3 mm deep, the risk of occult metastasis is not 0, and SLNB may provide valuable staging and prognostic information in that select group of patients with small primary tumors and no clinical or radiographic evidence of nodal metastasis in whom microvascular reconstruction is not planned.

The question remains as to whether SLNB is a safe and efficacious option in patients who might otherwise undergo END. In addition to the clinical trials from Japan and France mentioned in the beginning of this chapter, this question may be answered by another very large phase II/III multicenter randomized clinical trial of SLNB using 99mTc tilmanocept, which opened to enrollment in the United States in mid-2020 (NRG HN-006 – NCT04333537). With a targeted accrual of 618 patients with cT1-T2 N0 oral cancer, this trial will evaluate neck and shoulder functional outcomes (phase II) and DFS (phase III), with secondary endpoints, including quality of life and costs comparisons. With the increasing focus on minimally invasive surgery and value in health care, these data are expected to be highly relevant to the treatment of patients with early-stage oral cancer moving forward.

References

1. Shah JP. Cervical lymph node metastases—diagnostic, therapeutic, and prognostic implications. *Oncology (Williston Park)*. 1990;4(10):61–69;discussion 72, 76.
2. Massey C, Dharmarajan A, Bannuru RR, Rebeiz E. Management of N0 neck in early oral squamous cell carcinoma: a systematic review and meta-analysis. *Laryngoscope*. 2019;129(8):E284–E298.
3. Spiro RH, Huvos AG, Wong GY, Spiro JD, Gnecco CA, Strong EW. Predictive value of tumor thickness in squamous carcinoma confined to the tongue and floor of the mouth. *Am J Surg*. 1986;152(4):345–350.
4. Crocetta F, Botti C, Pernice C, et al. Sentinel node biopsy versus elective neck dissection in early-stage oral cancer: a systematic review. *Eur Arch Oto-Rhino-Laryngol*. 2020.
5. Gould EA, Winship T, Philbin PH, Kerr HH. Observations on a "sentinel node" in cancer of the parotid. *Cancer*. 1960;13(1):77–78.
6. Sondak VK, Wong SL, Gershenwald JE, Thompson JF. Evidence-based clinical practice guidelines on the use of sentinel lymph node biopsy in melanoma. *Am Soc Clin Oncol Educ Book*. 2013;33(1):e320–e325.
7. Kim DH, Kim Y, Kim SW, Hwang SH. Usefulness of sentinel lymph node biopsy for oral cancer: a systematic review and meta-analysis. *Laryngoscope*. 2021;131(2):E459–E465.
8. Civantos FJ, Zitsch RP, Schuller DE, et al. Sentinel lymph node biopsy accurately stages

the regional lymph nodes for T1–T2 oral squamous cell carcinomas: results of a prospective multi-institutional trial. *J Clin Oncol.* 2010;28(8):1395–1400.

9. Alkureishi LW, Ross GL, Shoaib T, et al. Sentinel node biopsy in head and neck squamous cell cancer: 5-year follow-up of a European multicenter trial. *Ann Surg Oncol.* 2010;17(9):2459–2464.
10. Flach GB, Bloemena E, Klop WMC, et al. Sentinel lymph node biopsy in clinically N0 T1–T2 staged oral cancer: the Dutch multicenter trial. *Oral Oncol.* 2014;50(10):1020–1024.
11. Schilling C, Stoeckli SJ, Haerle SK, et al. Sentinel European Node Trial (SENT): 3-year results of sentinel node biopsy in oral cancer. *Eur J Cancer.* 2015;51(18):2777–2784.
12. Miura K, Hirakawa H, Uemura H, et al. Sentinel node biopsy for oral cancer: a prospective multicenter Phase II trial. *Auris Nasus Larynx.* 2017;44(3):319–326.
13. Hornstra MT, Alkureishi LW, Ross GL, Shoaib T, Soutar DS. Predictive factors for failure to identify sentinel nodes in head and neck squamous cell carcinoma. *Head Neck.* 2008;30(7):858–862.
14. Surasi DS, O'Malley J, Bhambhvani P. 99mTc-Tilmanocept: a novel molecular agent for lymphatic mapping and sentinel lymph node localization. *J Nucl Med Technol.* 2015;43(2):87–91.
15. Agrawal A, Civantos FJ, Brumund KT, et al. [99m Tc] Tilmanocept accurately detects sentinel lymph nodes and predicts node pathology status in patients with oral squamous cell carcinoma of the head and neck: results of a phase III multi-institutional trial. *Ann Surg Oncol.* 2015;22(11):3708–3715.
16. Hasegawa Y, Tsukahara K, Yoshimoto S, et al. Neck dissections based on sentinel lymph node navigation versus elective neck dissections in early oral cancers: a randomized, multicenter, non-inferiority trial. *Am Soc Clin Oncol.* 2019.
17. Garrel R, Perriard F, Favier V, Richard F, Daures JP, De Boutray M. Equivalence randomized trial comparing treatment based on sentinel node biopsy versus neck dissection in operable T1–T2n0 oral and oropharyngeal cancer. *Am Soc Clin Oncol.* 2020.
18. Giammarile F, Schilling C, Gnanasegaran G, et al. The EANM practical guidelines for sentinel lymph node localisation in oral cavity squamous cell carcinoma. *Eur J Nucl Med Mol Imaging.* 2019;46(3):623–637.
19. Tsopelas C, Sutton R. Why certain dyes are useful for localizing the sentinel lymph node. *J Nucl Med.* 2002;43(10):1377–1382.
20. Montgomery LL, Thorne AC, Van Zee KJ, et al. Isosulfan blue dye reactions during sentinel lymph node mapping for breast cancer. *Anesth Analg.* 2002;95(2):385–388.
21. Thevarajah S, Huston TL, Simmons RM. A comparison of the adverse reactions associated with isosulfan blue versus methylene blue dye in sentinel lymph node biopsy for breast cancer. *Am J Surg.* 2005;189(2):236–239.
22. Marcinow AM, Hall N, Byrum E, Teknos TN, Old MO, Agrawal A. Use of a novel receptor-targeted (CD206) radiotracer, 99mTc-tilmanocept, and SPECT/CT for sentinel lymph node detection in oral cavity squamous cell carcinoma: initial institutional report in an ongoing phase 3 study. *JAMA Otolaryngol Head Neck Surg.* 2013;139(9):895–902.
23. Stoeckli SJ, Pfaltz M, Ross GL, et al. The second international conference on sentinel node biopsy in mucosal head and neck cancer. *Ann Surg Oncol.* 2005;12(11):919–924.
24. Tschopp L, Nuyens M, Stauffer E, Krause T, Zbären P. The value of frozen section analysis of the sentinel lymph node in clinically N0 squamous cell carcinoma of the oral cavity and oropharynx. *Otolaryngol Head Neck Surg.* 2005;132(1):99–102.
25. Bell RB, Markiewicz MR, Dierks EJ, Gregoire CE, Rader A. Thin serial step sectioning of sentinel lymph node biopsy specimen may not be necessary to accurately stage the neck in oral squamous cell carcinoma. *J Oral Maxillofac Surg.* 2013;71(7):1268–1277.
26. Vorburger MS, Broglie MA, Soltermann A, et al. Validity of frozen section in sentinel lymph node biopsy for the staging in oral and oropharyngeal squamous cell carcinoma. *J Surg Oncol.* 2012;106(7):816–819.
27. Trivedi NP, Ravindran HK, Sundram S, et al. Pathologic evaluation of sentinel lymph nodes in oral squamous cell carcinoma. *Head Neck.* 2010;32(11):1437–1443.
28. Amr D, Broderick-Villa G, Haigh PI, Guenther JM, DiFronzo LA. Adverse drug reactions during lymphatic mapping and sentinel lymph node biopsy for solid neoplasms. *Am Surg.* 2005;71(9):720–724.
29. Jefferson G.D., Sollaccio D., Gomez-Fernandez C.R., Civantos F. Jr. Evaluation of immunohistochemical fine sectioning for sentinel lymph node biopsy in oral squamous cell carcinoma. *Otolaryngol Head Neck Surg.* 2011;144(2):216–219.

CHAPTER 118

Laryngectomy

Marcus A. Couey and Ashish A. Patel

Armamentarium

#9 Molt periosteal elevator
#10, #15 Surgical blades
2-0 Polypropylene suture
3-0 Polyglactin sutures
4-0 Chromic gut suture
Allis clamp
Army-Navy retractor
Babcock clamps
Bovie electrocautery
Crile hemostats
Cuffed tracheostomy tube
DeBakey or other tissue forceps
Dietrich right-angle clamp
Flat Blake drains
Lahey clamps
Langenbeck retractor (long, toe-in)
Local anesthetic with vasoconstrictor
Lone Star elastic stays
Metzenbaum scissors
Nasogastric tube (14-French)
Shoulder roll or Mayfield horseshoe head holder
Skin staples
Standard Neck Dissection Instrumentation
Tissue dissectors (Dierks #1, #2, #3, or other)
Vessel clips (small and medium)
Weitlaner retractor
Wire-reinforced endotracheal tube (standard, or anatomically shaped laryngectomy tube)

History of the Procedure

Total laryngectomy (TL) entails the complete removal of the larynx with separation of the digestive tract from the lower respiratory tract and establishment of a permanent tracheal stoma. A patient who has undergone TL is known as a *laryngectomee*.

The first TL was performed by Theodor Billroth in 1873, on a 36-year-old patient with carcinoma of the larynx that had recurred after narrow excision. To conclude the operation, the trachea was secured to the skin, the pharyngeal fistula was narrowed with sutures, and the wound was packed open. Remarkably, less than 3 weeks later the patient was eating by mouth and his feeding tube was removed.[1] He lived for 7 months before dying of recurrent disease.[2] Multiple other reports from throughout Europe soon followed, but the operation was fraught with complications and carried a high mortality rate. TL did not achieve a level of acceptable safety until the early 20th century.

An assortment of open partial laryngectomy procedures evolved in the mid-20th century. These operations were often able to preserve some form of lung-powered speech; however, they shared a high prevalence of chronic aspiration and recurrent pneumonias. While partial laryngectomy procedures continue to be used effectively in carefully selected patients with smaller tumors, their utilization has been largely supplanted by radiotherapy and newer surgical techniques such as transoral laser microsurgery and transoral robotic surgery.[3,4]

Between 1997 and 2008, new cases of laryngeal cancer in the United States decreased by 33%, while the number of TLs performed decreased by 48%.[5] The trend toward nonsurgical management followed the landmark Veterans Affairs Laryngeal Cancer Trial in 1991[6] and multiple subsequent studies that supported chemoradiotherapy (CRT) in the primary management of most laryngeal cancers (RTOG 91-11, 2013).[7] This shifted the role of TL toward salvage treatment in cases of recurrent or persistent disease after chemoradiation, and for primary management of very advanced cancers.

Indications

Advanced laryngeal cancer is usually treated with CRT in an effort to preserve the larynx.[8,9] However, primary TL is indicated for very advanced laryngeal tumors associated with major cartilage destruction or extralaryngeal spread (i.e., T4a tumors).[10,11] TL may rarely be indicated in cases of extensive tongue cancer requiring total glossectomy.

TL is often used as salvage treatment for recurrent laryngeal cancer following failure of radiotherapy alone or CRT. Radionecrosis of the larynx after CRT is an uncommon complication that may be difficult to differentiate from cancer recurrence, but it usually is an indication for TL.[12] TL may also be indicated for tumor-free patients who have undergone prior partial laryngectomy or major glossectomy and/or radiotherapy and who have developed intractable aspiration with recurrent pneumonia or other irreversible laryngeal dysfunction after cancer therapy.[13]

Preoperative Considerations

Obtaining cross-sectional imaging, either computed tomography (CT) or magnetic resonance imaging (MRI), is essential for assessing the primary tumor and lymph nodes. For previously untreated laryngeal tumors with suspected cartilage involvement, it is important to differentiate between erosion of the inner cortex of the thyroid cartilage (indicating a T3 lesion, which can be treated with CRT) and erosion of the outer cortex (defining a T4a tumor, requiring surgical management).[14] If the imaging findings are equivocal, dual-energy CT or diffusion-weighted MRI may be helpful in determining the extent of cartilage involvement.[15,16] Chest imaging and/or positron emission tomography/CT should also be performed, and the case should be discussed at a multidisciplinary tumor board.

Patients should be evaluated by flexible laryngoscopy to assess tumor extent and vocal cord mobility; it is rare that a patient with mobile vocal cords will require TL. Direct laryngoscopy is also essential to map the extent of the tumor and to collect tissue for histologic diagnosis if not already obtained. Tumors with extensive involvement of the pharyngeal walls or invasion of the base of tongue should be planned for an interpositional regional or free flap reconstruction. For patients with a history of radiation, we always perform flap reconstruction, either interpositional for pharyngeal reconstruction, or onlay to bolster the pharyngeal closure and reduce the risk of fistula formation. Subglottic and tracheal extension of carcinoma may require significant tracheal resection; however, the trachea can almost always be mobilized cephalad out of the chest and pexed to the sternal periosteum, allowing for construction of an adequate stoma. Sometimes, a vascularized skin flap is required to line the cephalad portion of the stoma when extensive tracheal resection is required. Rarely, the tracheal stump can be rerouted under the innominate artery with the aid of manubrial resection to create an anterior mediastinal tracheostomy as initially described by Sisson.[17,18]

Before surgery, the patient must be fully prepared for the permanent loss of lung-powered speech, and the patient should have a preoperative consultation with a speech-language pathologist. Plans must be made for the patient to be able to communicate with the medical and nursing staff after surgery, using writing equipment, word boards, or other devices. The medical and nursing staff should be aware that the patient's only airway is the tracheal stoma; if the need for bag mask ventilation arises, it must be performed using a pediatric mask over the tracheostoma or through a cuffed tube through the stoma; ventilation through the nose and mouth will not be possible. The patient should also be prepared for the impaired ability to smell after laryngectomy, which results from a lack of airflow through the nose.

Concurrent Neck Dissection

For patients with previously untreated T4a laryngeal cancer undergoing TL, management of the regional lymph nodes is indicated, with a selective neck dissection (jugular lymph node chain levels II–IV) for N_0 disease being the minimum operation.[19,20] In cases of clinically evident cervical lymphadenopathy, all additional involved levels should be cleared. For well-lateralized glottic tumors, ipsilateral neck dissection could be considered; however, tumors requiring primary TL are generally advanced and often encroach upon or cross the midline. We generally perform bilateral neck dissection for patients undergoing primary TL, and we have found this to be a minimal source of morbidity in this setting.

Neck dissection for N_0 disease in the salvage setting is controversial. Several studies have found no survival advantage with elective neck dissection, and in fact concurrent neck dissection may confer a higher rate of complications including pharyngocutaneous fistula.[21,22] In our practice, patients undergoing TL for salvage after radiation will be reconstructed with a free flap, either as an interpositional flap for pharyngeal reconstruction or as an onlay over the pharyngeal closure. In these cases, at least one side of the neck will be dissected to facilitate vascular anastomosis and minimize the risk of recurrence at the vascular pedicle.

TECHNIQUE: Total Laryngectomy

The patient is positioned on the operating table with the head extended, using either a Mayfield horseshoe head holder or a shoulder roll. The arms are tucked, and the elbows are padded, as for any major head and neck operation. Placement of an arterial line frequently is performed before laryngectomy, and adequate venous access is ensured. The patient is intubated orally unless a prior tracheostomy has been performed. A GlideScope (Verathon, MA) is useful for intubation to visualize the extent of the tumor. We also perform direct laryngoscopy following intubation to again visualize the extent of the tumor involvement for planning the point of entry for pharyngotomy during TL.

STEP 1: Cervical Incision and Elevation of Skin Flaps

An apron-type (Gluck-Sorenson) incision is made with a horizontal limb that lies just below the level of the cricoid cartilage, and the incision follows a curvilinear path along the posterior border of the sternocleidomastoid muscle to the mastoid process bilaterally. If a tracheostomy has not been performed prior to TL, a V-shaped appendage can be designed into the midline of the flap (Fig. 118.1A1), which will facilitate creation of a wider stoma as described in Step 11. If a tracheostomy has been performed prior to TL, it will need to be excised as part of the TL specimen (Fig. 118.1A2).

The incision is extended through the platysma with a scalpel or electrocautery, and a subplatysmal flap is raised to a level above the hyoid. Care should be taken to maintain the appropriate depth of the skin flap, particularly in the midline where the platysma may be absent. A moist lap sponge can be secured over the skin flap with Lone Star elastic retractor hooks to prevent tissue desiccation.

TECHNIQUE: Total Laryngectomy—*cont'd*

STEP 2: Exposing the Hyoid

Electrocautery is used to separate the suprahyoid musculature from the superior aspect of the hyoid bone (Fig. 118.1B1). Working from medial to lateral facilitates protection of the hypoglossal nerve. Care should be taken to stay superficial to the preepiglottic space to avoid premature entry into the pharynx. Each greater horn of the hyoid is exposed circumferentially using the finger ring of a mosquito hemostat toward the midline (Fig. 118.1B2).

Continued

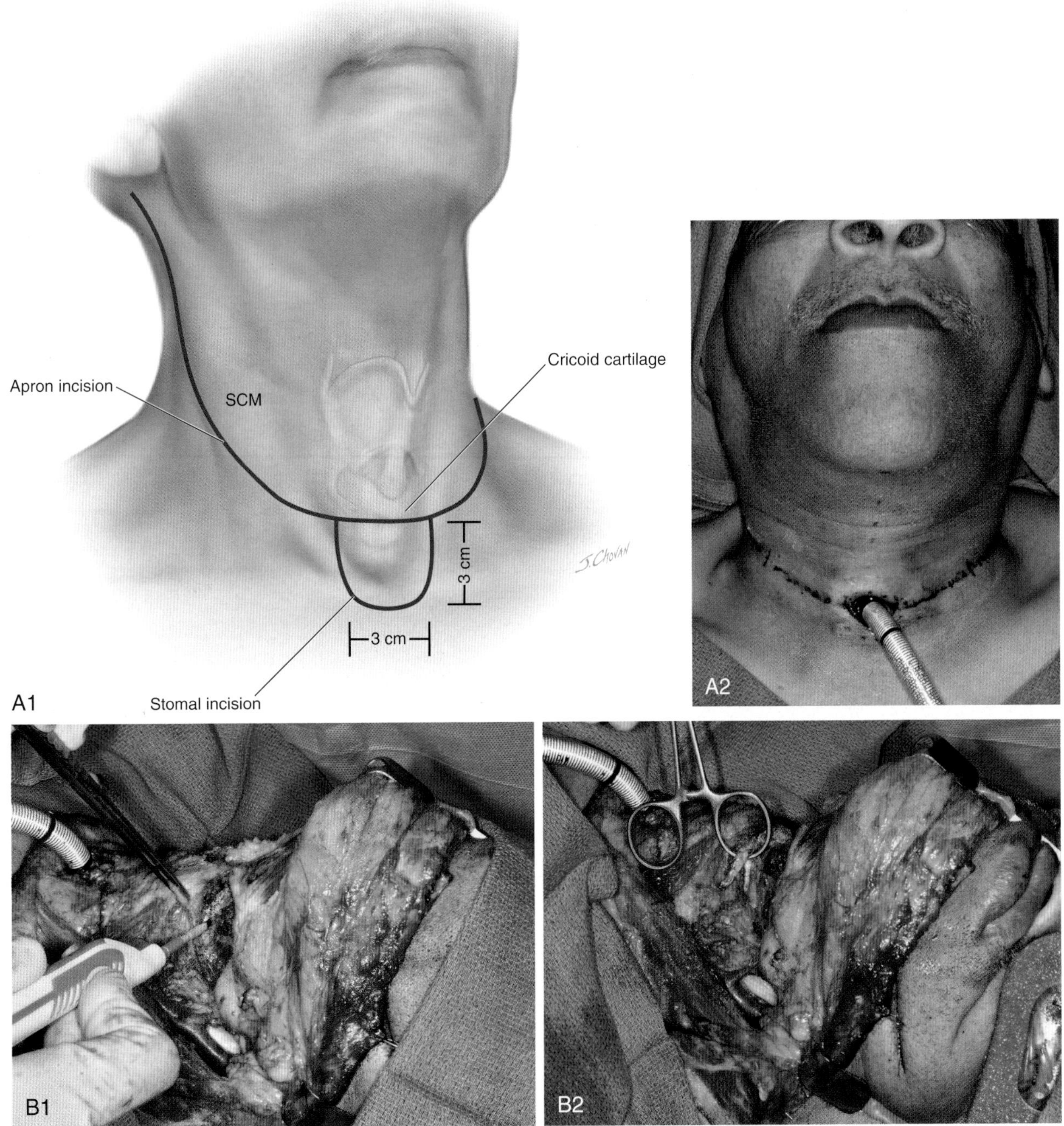

Figure 118.1 **A1,** Cervical incision without preexisting tracheostomy. **A2,** Cervical incision with preexisting tracheostomy. **B1** and **B2,** Each greater horn of the hyoid is exposed circumferentially. *SCM*, sternocleidomastoid.

TECHNIQUE: Total Laryngectomy—*cont'd*

STEP 3: Skeletonizing the Lateral Aspect of the Thyroid Cartilage

The entire length of the inferior pharyngeal constrictor musculature is then incised with electrocautery vertically, just anterior to the palpable posterior border of the thyroid cartilage. This incision is extended through the perichondrium (Fig. 118.1C1). A #9 Molt periosteal elevator is then used to reflect the perichondrium posteriorly around the posterior border of the thyroid cartilage (Fig. 118.1C2). This allows for preservation of as much piriform recess sinus mucosa as possible, facilitating eventual pharyngeal closure; however, tumor extension into the piriform recess can preclude this maneuver on the involved side. The lateral aspect of the thyroid cartilage is skeletonized and exposed bilaterally.

The thyroid lobe ipsilateral to the tumor is usually included in the specimen and remains attached to the thyroid cartilage and proximal trachea. Both superior and inferior thyroid arteries and veins are ligated and divided on that side. The contralateral thyroid lobe and inferior thyroid vessels are preserved, and the superior thyroid artery can be preserved by dividing the superior laryngeal vessels distally.

STEP 4: Creating the Inner Tunnel

If ipsilateral or bilateral neck dissections are performed prior to TL, the sternocleidomastoid muscle can be retracted laterally, creating the so-called outer tunnel. This is not an absolute requirement, but it can facilitate skeletonization of the internal jugular vein and medial dissection along the carotid artery to create the required inner tunnel. Neck dissection specimens can be either pedicled to the lateral aspect of the thyroid cartilage or can be divided, oriented, and sent separately to pathology. In this chapter, we consider any neck dissections to have been removed from the larynx specimen.

The carotid is dissected free on its medial extent, and the hypoglossal nerve and superior thyroid artery are identified on each side. The strap muscles are divided inferiorly above the level of the manubrium and included with the surgical specimen. The anterior jugular veins are divided inferiorly (Fig. 118.1D).

STEP 5: Performing the Initial Pharyngotomy

At this point, the larynx and hyoid complex should be circumferentially mobilized from its superior and lateral attachments (Fig. 118.1C1–C2). A long toe-in Langenbeck retractor is placed transorally into the vallecula, which is used as a guide for entry through the mucosa. With electrocautery, a transverse incision is made into the vallecula through the preepiglottic space with care to avoid the hypoglossal nerve. When cancer involves the vallecula, the pharynx is entered through the piriform recess area contralateral to the tumor. Once the pharyngotomy has been performed, the epiglottis can be grasped with an Allis clamp to provide gentle forward traction and displace it into the neck wound (Fig. 118.1E).

STEP 6: Vertical Incision Lateral to Each Aryepiglottic Fold

Metzenbaum scissors are inserted such that the inner tine of the scissors lies on the mucosal surface of the medial aspect of the piriform recess, hugging the lateral edge of the aryepiglottic (AE) fold while maintaining at least a 1-cm margin around the tumor. The outer tine lies on the underside of the mucosa beneath the previously skeletonized greater horns of the hyoid bone and thyroid cartilage (Fig. 118.1F1). A vertical incision is then made through the pharyngeal wall, terminating at the level of the base of the piriform recess, adjacent to the posterior aspect of the cricoid (Fig. 118.1F2). In cases of tumor involvement of the piriform recess, the vertical incision may have to be placed more posteriorly on the lateral pharyngeal wall. It is important to perform this maneuver first on the side contralateral to the tumor to allow for safe oncologic margins and better visualization of the pharyngeal mucosa.

STEP 7: Postcricoid Transverse Incision

Using Metzenbaum scissors, the postcricoid transverse incision connects the inferior limbs of the incisions made in Step 8 (Fig. 118.1G). If there is significant post cricoid hypopharyngeal involvement of tumor, this dissection should proceed caudally to the cervical esophagus to generate oncologically sound margins.

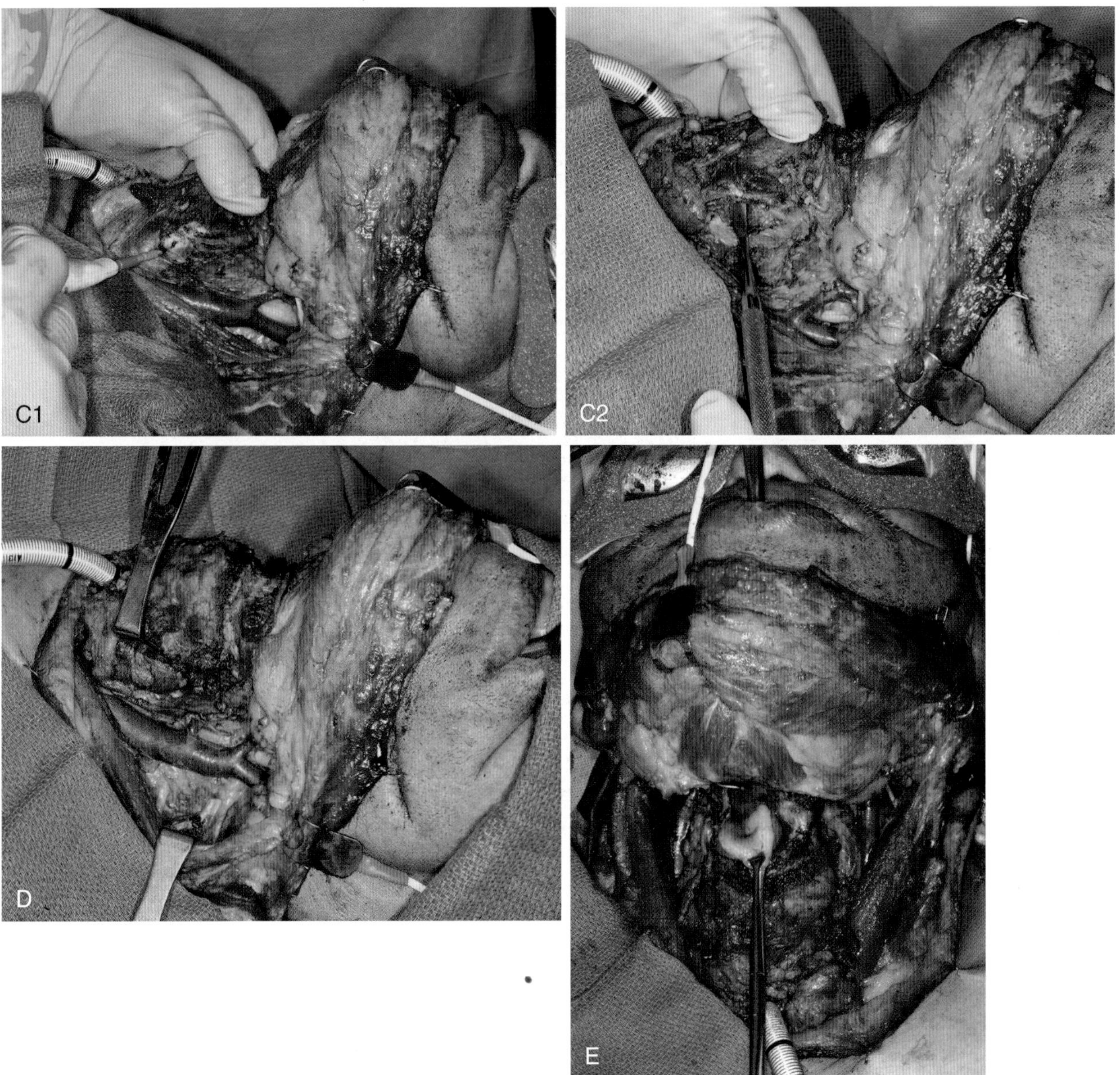

Figure 118.1, cont'd **C1** and **C2,** Skeletonizing the lateral aspect of the thyroid cartilage. **D,** Developing the inner tunnel. **E,** Pharyngotomy completed with epiglottis retracted ventrally.

Continued

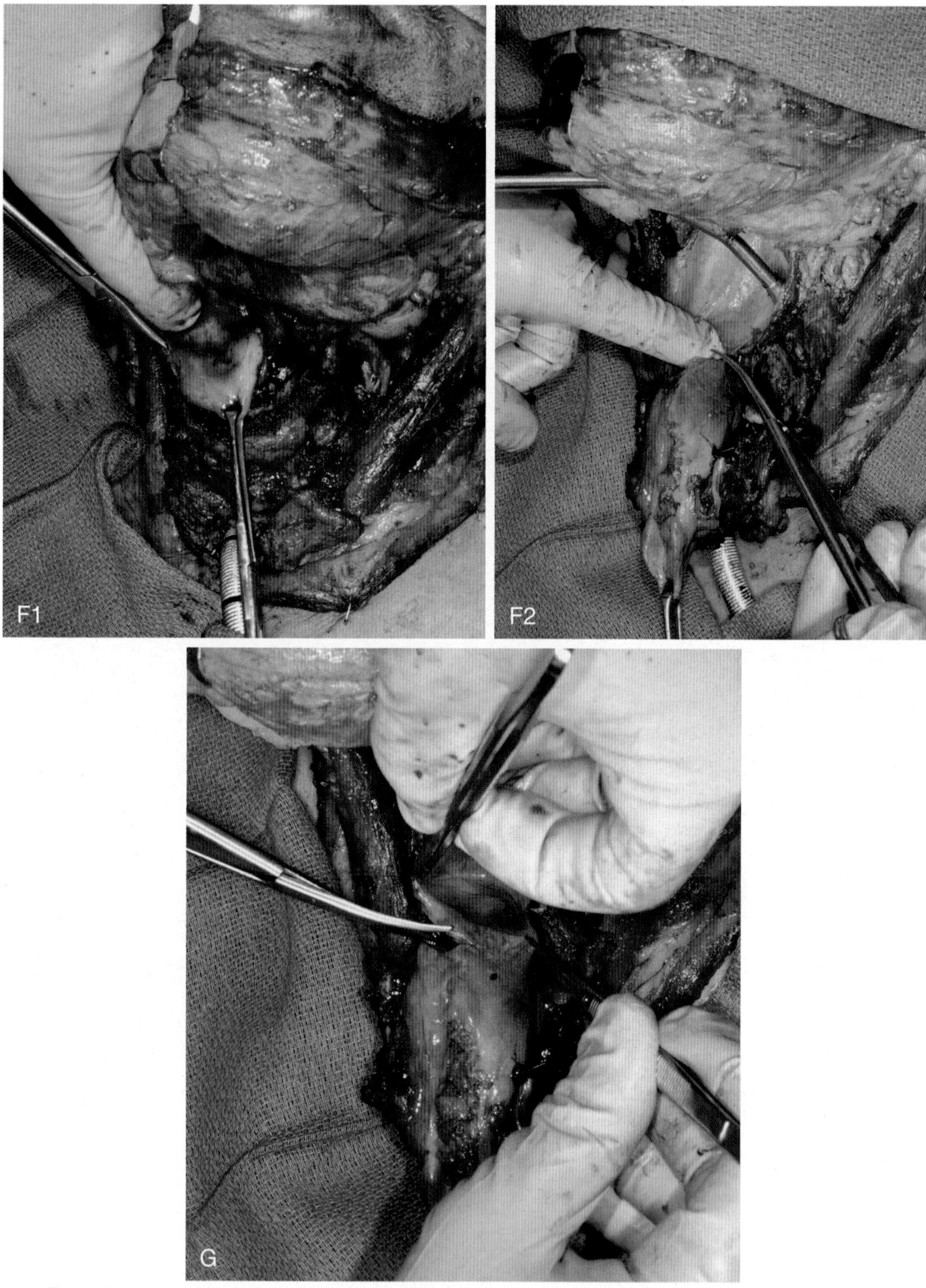

Figure 118.1, cont'd **F1** and **F2,** Vertical incision lateral to each aryepiglottic fold. **G,** Postcricoid incision.

TECHNIQUE: Total Laryngectomy—*cont'd*

STEP 8: Exposing the Trachea

The thyroid isthmus is divided. The thyroid on the side opposite of the tumor is reflected off the trachea from medial to lateral with sharp and blunt dissection. The preserved hemithyroid remains pedicled to the superior and inferior thyroid vessels.

STEP 9: Developing the Tracheoesophageal Plane and Transecting the Trachea

The tracheoesophageal groove is identified bilaterally, and the recurrent laryngeal nerves are severed. The trachea is sharply dissected from the esophagus with scissors (Fig. 118.1H1). The trachea is then divided horizontally to deliver the specimen (Fig. 118.1H2). Typically, the tracheotomy is between the second and third ring; however, it may need be placed more caudal to include a previous tracheotomy within the resection or if there is subglottic extension of the tumor. The distal trachea is grasped with a Babcock clamp, and a wire-reinforced "armored" endotracheal tube and ventilation circuit is then inserted and secured to the chest skin with 2-0 silk sutures. It is important to avoid the tube "popping out" of the stoma for the remainder of the case, which can lead to aspiration of blood and resultant pneumonitis or pneumonia; an anatomically shaped preformed tube such as the Rusch Laryngoflex (Willy Rusch GMBH) can be helpful in this regard.

The specimen is then oriented to the pathologist, and appropriate frozen sections are obtained (Fig. 118.1H3).

Continued

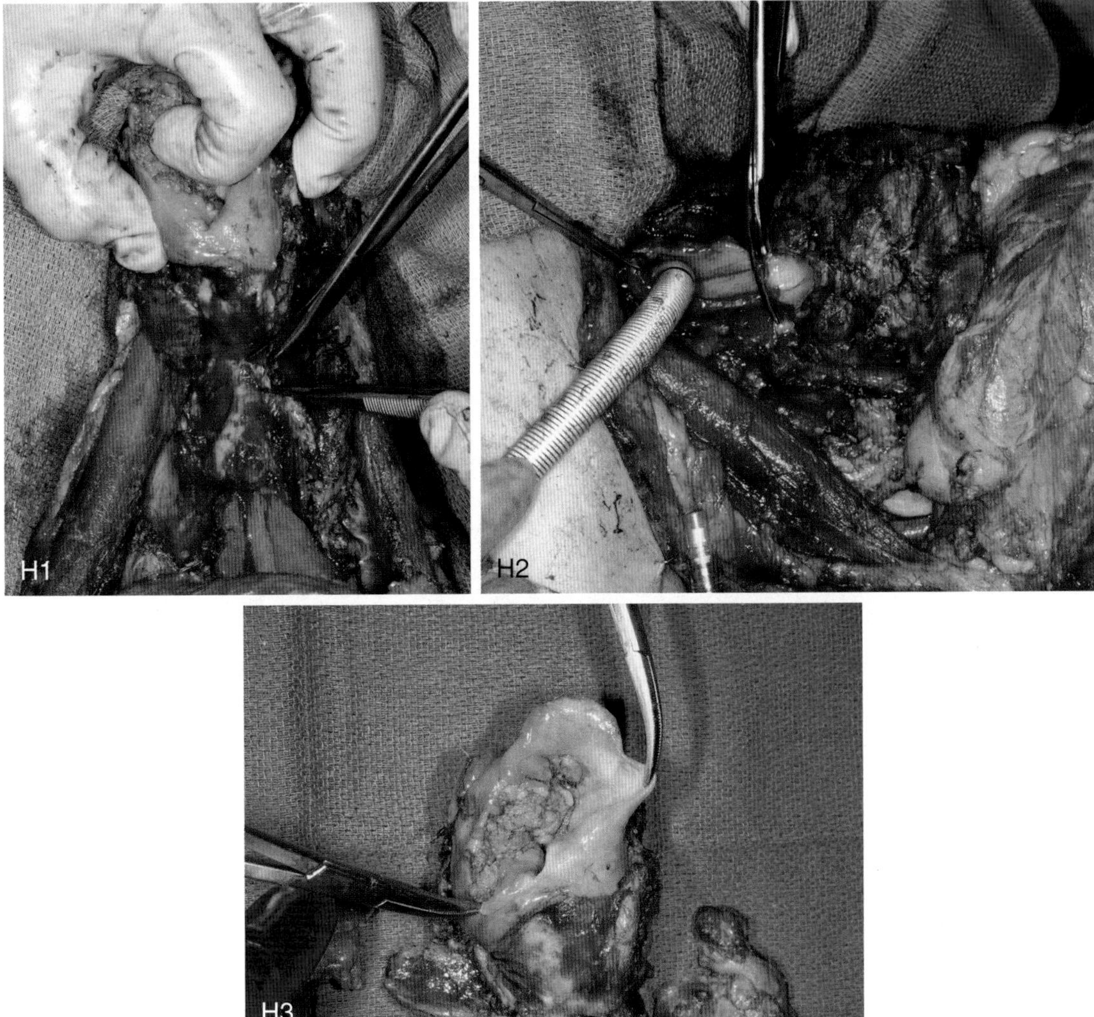

Figure 118.1, cont'd H1, Exposing the trachea and developing the tracheoesophageal plane. **H2,** Transecting the membranous trachea. **H3,** Removed specimen.

TECHNIQUE: Total Laryngectomy—*cont'd*

STEP 10: Cricopharyngeal Myotomy

Division of the cricopharyngeus muscle (upper esophageal sphincter) is helpful for facilitating swallowing and optimizing esophageal speech. The surgeon's nondominant index finger is placed into the distal esophagus, dilating the esophagus and tensing the circular fibers of the cricopharyngeus. A gauze sponge is then placed beneath the surgeon's nondominant thumb to provide traction. A scalpel is used to meticulously divide the muscle fibers vertically, down to the level of the underlying esophageal mucosa (Fig. 118.1I1 and I2). Care must be taken to avoid overzealous myotomy and esophageal perforation.

STEP 11: Pharyngeal Closure

This is also an opportune time to place a nasogastric feeding tube, if the patient does not already have a gastrostomy tube. The feeding tube can be inserted through the nose and into the esophagus under direct visualization and secured with a nasal bridle. Closure of defect is performed over the nasogastric tube or salivary bypass tube using inverting, interrupted Connell sutures of 3-0 polyglactin (Fig. 118.1J1–J3). It is critical to invert all mucosal edges into the lumen of the pharynx to reduce the risk of pharyngeal leak and fistula formation. An attempt is made to preserve as much circumferential pharyngeal mucosa as possible; therefore, smaller tissue bites are appropriate, as long as a water-tight closure can be obtained. The closure begins on the inferior aspect, and as it proceeds superiorly, the typical T-formation of the closure is seen. The horizontal limbs of the T are each closed from lateral to medial. The three limbs of the closure meet in the midline with a three-point inverting suture (Fig. 118.1J1–J3). The integrity of the pharyngeal closure can be tested by insufflating the pharynx with dilute povidone iodine solution (1:1 with saline) through the mouth using an Asepto syringe. Leakage of fluid is easily detected given the dark color of the iodine solution. The esophagus should be occluded manually during this test to prevent insufflation of the stomach, and the residual solution should subsequently be suctioned. Any sites of leakage should be identified and buttressed with additional interrupted sutures. Pharyngeal closure may also be performed over a salivary bypass tube, which may reduce the risk of fistula formation.[23]

At this point, regional or free flap inset can proceed if being utilized in an onlay fashion to bolster the closure. The flap is laid over the pharyngeal closure and secured to the suprahyoid musculature, sternocleidomastoids, and mandibular periosteum prior to microvascular anastomosis.

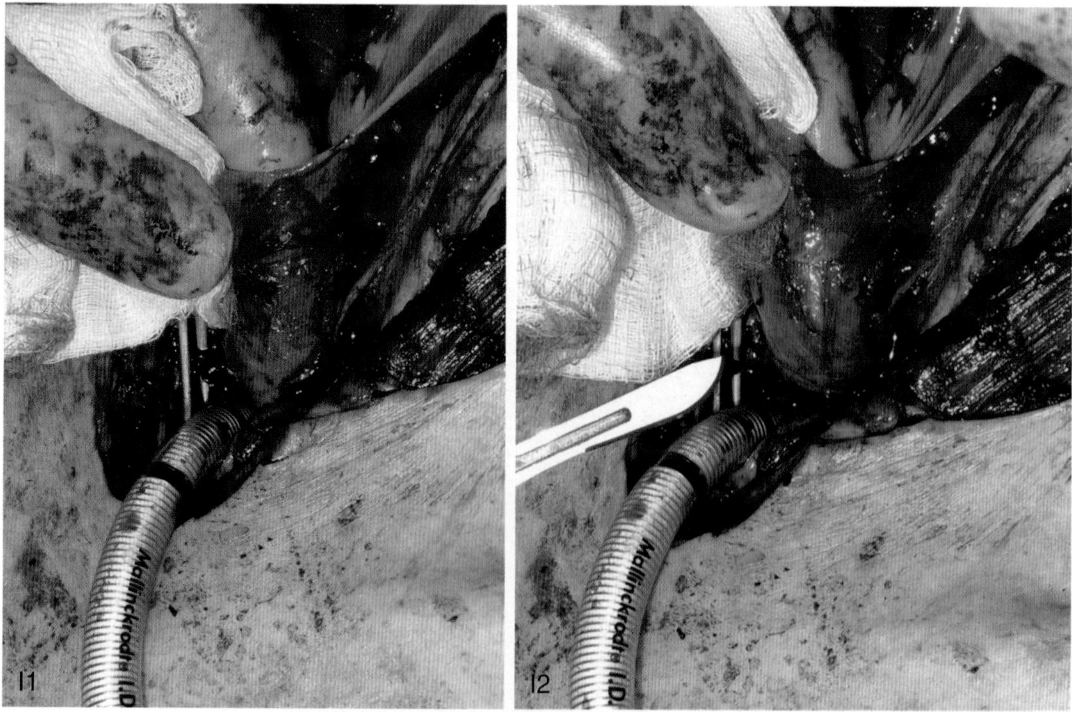

Figure 118.1, cont'd **I1** and **I2,** Cricopharyngeal myotomy.

TECHNIQUE: Total Laryngectomy—*cont'd*

STEP 12: Maturing the Stoma and Wound Closure

A U-shaped skin excision centered over the suprasternal notch is then performed to allow for maturing of the stoma. The position and size of the excision will depend on the size of the tracheal stoma, and whether there had been a previous tracheostomy performed as the surrounding skin should be included in the excision in such cases. The anterior wall of the trachea is secured to the periosteum of the manubrium with three interrupted, nonresorbable 2-0 polypropylene sutures starting in the midline. These sutures support the trachea and should result in the most superior tracheal ring lying just beneath the level of the subcutaneous tissue of the skin surrounding the stoma. It is important to pass these sutures around a stable tracheal ring, usually one or two rings below the terminal ring of the stump, in a submucosal fashion to prevent granulation tissue and crusting in the tracheal lumen.

A Crile hemostat is then placed in the lumen of the tracheal stoma and is spread laterally, tensing the posterior tracheal wall. Metzenbaum scissors are used to create a full-thickness vertical incision through the midline membranous trachea, at a distance of approximately 1.5 cm. This allows the stoma to widen transversely during closure. Spatulating the trachea in this fashion creates a V-shaped defect that is best closed by creating a corresponding V in the midline of the superior skin flap, which is sutured to the posterior tracheal wall during the final skin flap closure.

Starting in the midline and working laterally on each side, skin-to-tracheal closure is begun with interrupted, buried 3-0 polyglactin sutures, which are placed to approximate the dermis of the skin to the perichondrium of the highest tracheal cartilage. An effort is made to pass the sutures around the tracheal cartilage without penetrating the tracheal mucosa. This closure draws in the adjacent skin and helps open the tracheal stoma.

After irrigation and drain placement, closure of the neck begins with the midline advancement of the superior skin flap inferiorly into the V-shaped defect created in the posterior tracheal wall, using submucosal-to-subcutaneous 3-0 polyglactin sutures. Skin-to-mucosal closure around the stoma is performed with interrupted 4-0 chromic gut suture. The remainder of the neck platysmal closure and skin stapling are performed in a routine fashion (Fig. 118.1K1–K3).

At the conclusion of the operation, the wire-reinforced endotracheal tube is replaced with a cuffed tracheostomy tube for postoperative ventilatory support.

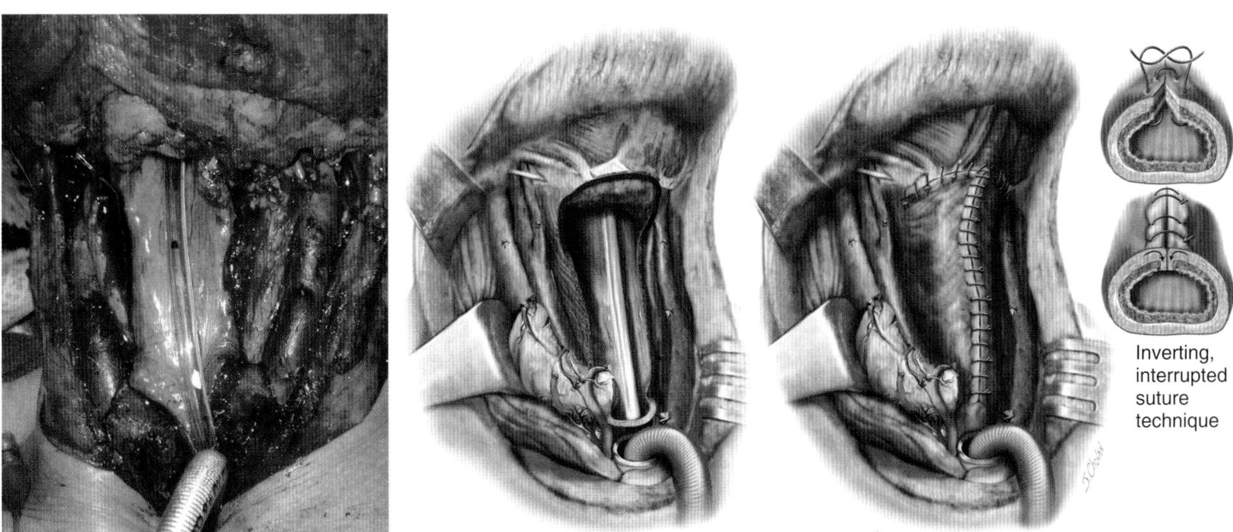

Figure 118.1, cont'd **J1** and **J2,** Specimen removed and nasogastric tube placed. **J3,** T-shaped pharyngeal closure with 3-0 polyglactin sutures.

Continued

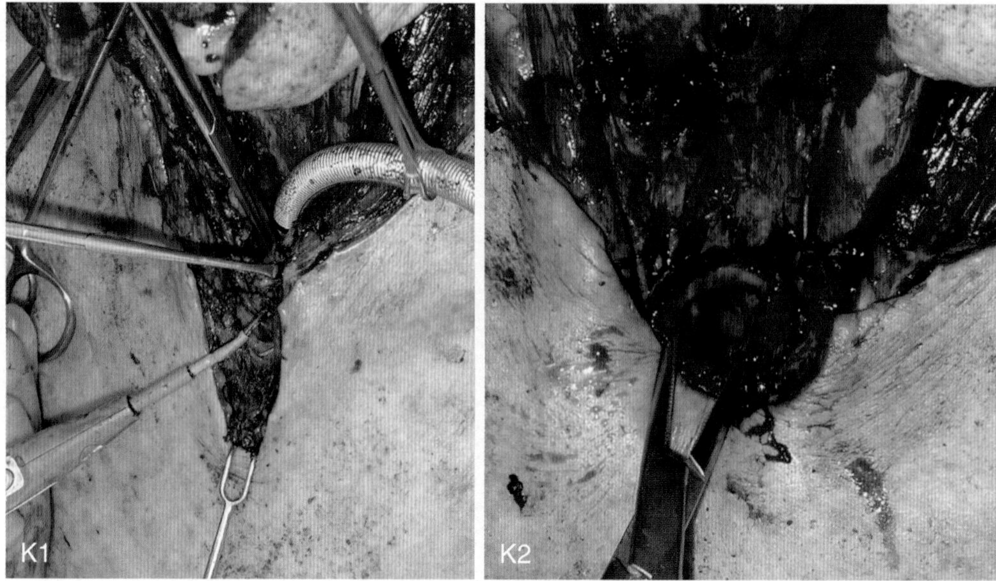

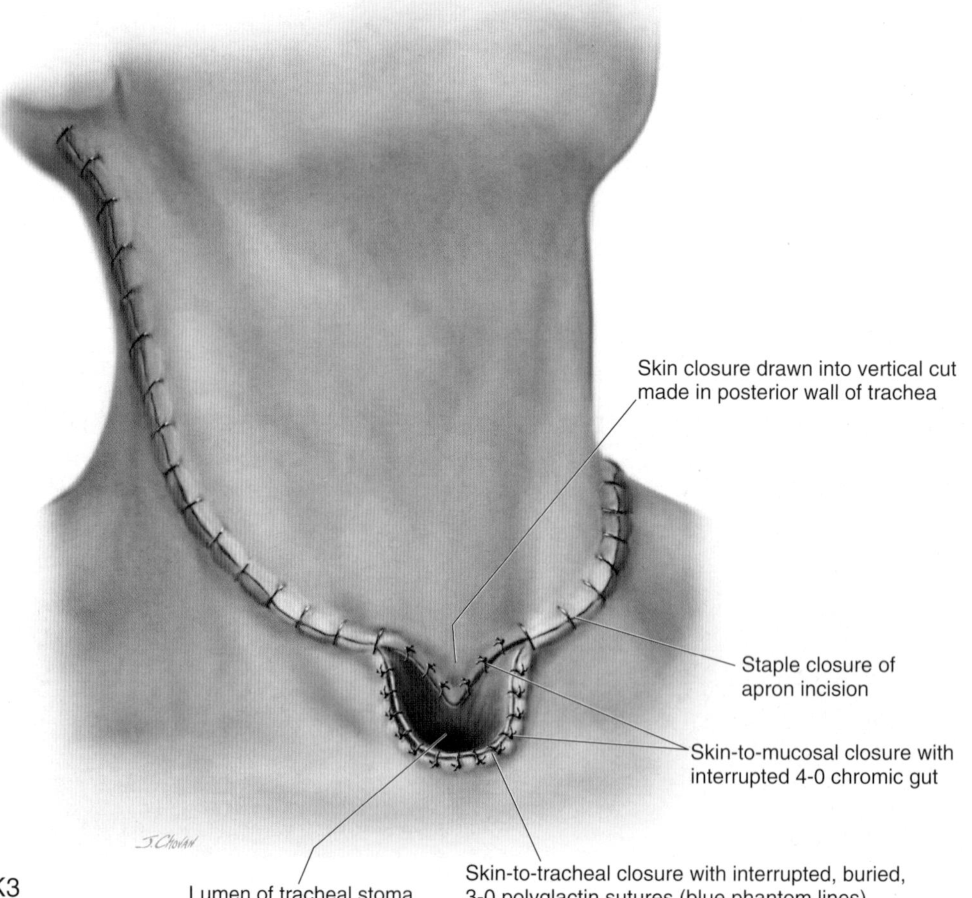

Figure 118.1, cont'd **K1,** U-shaped skin excision. **K2,** Spatulating the posterior trachea. **K3,** Matured stoma and neck closure.

ALTERNATIVE TECHNIQUE 1: Laryngopharyngectomy With Interpositional Free Flap Reconstruction

In some situations, extension of the cancer onto the adjacent pharyngeal wall or walls is such that none or only a thin vertical strip of posterior pharyngeal wall mucosa remains connecting the oropharynx to the esophagus. Even if only a small strip exists, this should be preserved, if at all possible, to avoid stenosis. The inset of a vascularized flap can be performed to allow pharyngoesophageal reconstruction of a sufficient diameter to avoid stenosis. Inset of the flap is performed with 3-0 polyglactin horizontal mattress sutures using standard techniques. In total laryngopharyngectomy with cervical esophagectomy, creating a tubed fasciocutaneous free flap requires approximately 9 cm of width to support an adequate luminal diameter. Suspension of the flap to the prevertebral fascia with multiple pexing sutures is very helpful for resisting inferior displacement, particularly with a pedicled pectoralis major flap (Fig. 118.2).

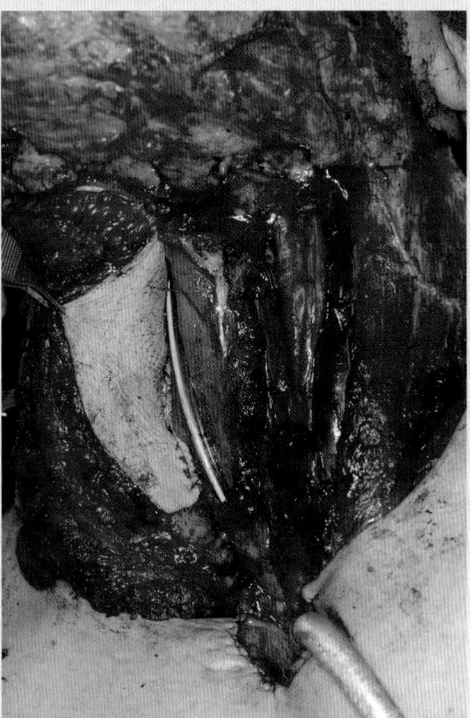

Figure 118.2 Inset of free flap into the pharyngeal closure.

ALTERNATIVE TECHNIQUE 2: Total Laryngectomy With Base of Tongue Resection and Free Flap Reconstruction

In cases of laryngeal cancer with base of tongue involvement, or extensive tumor originating in the oral cavity or oropharynx and invading the supraglottic larynx, the TL procedure must be approached differently. Often, the superior margin can be initially delineated through a transoral approach to resect the base of tongue toward the hyoid. Then, a cuff of suprahyoid muscles is resected transcervically to join the base of tongue incision. After these steps, the TL can proceed as described in the main text. Occasionally, alternative approaches will be required, such as the lingual pull-through or lip split with mandibulotomy in cases requiring total or subtotal glossectomy, respectively (Fig. 118.3A–F). Extensive tongue cancer involving the mandible and supraglottic larynx may require total glossectomy, mandibulectomy, and TL (Fig. 118.4A–F).

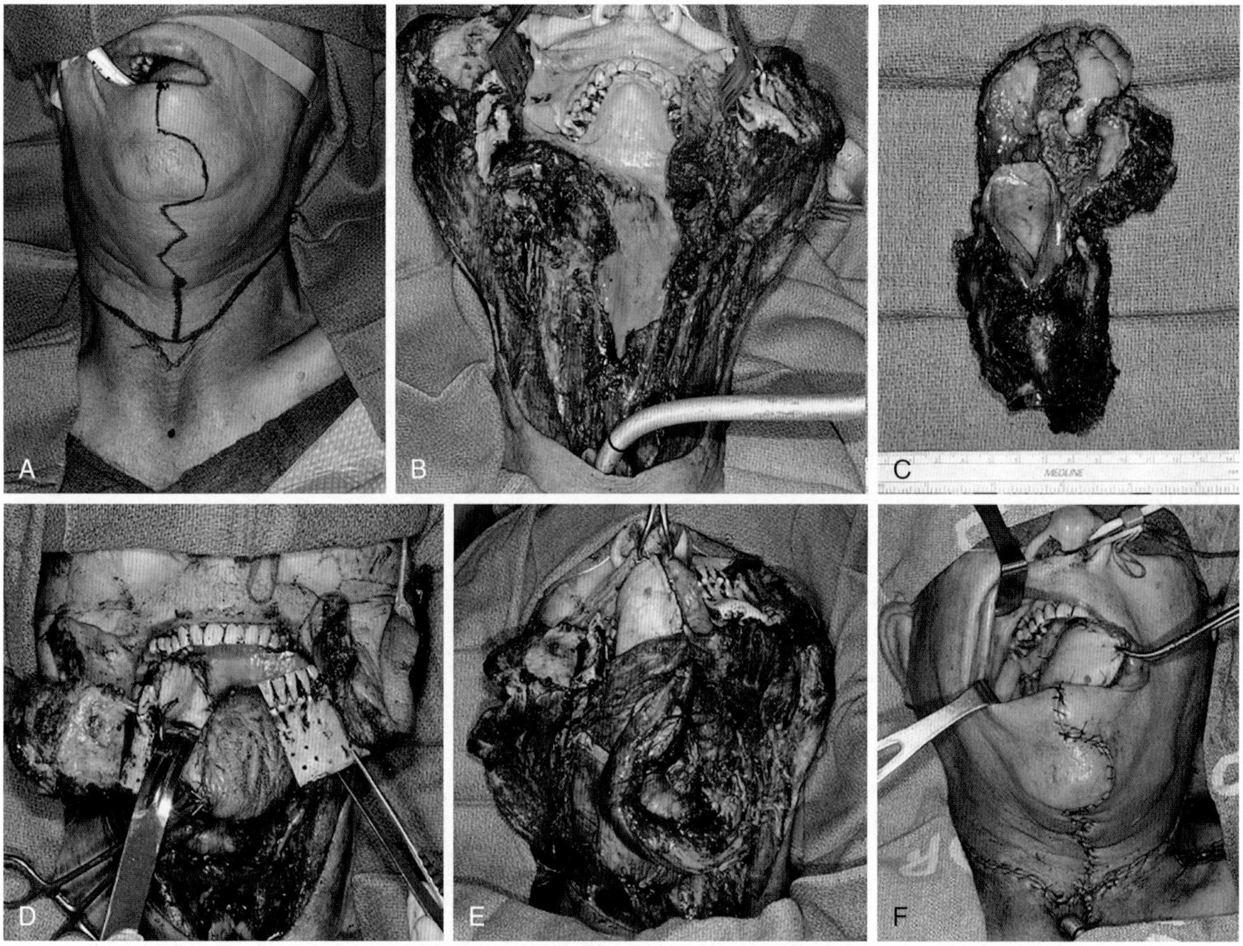

Figure 118.3 **A–F,** Extensive base of tongue cancer involving the epiglottis, requiring subtotal glossectomy through lip split mandibulotomy approach, total laryngectomy, and free flap reconstruction.

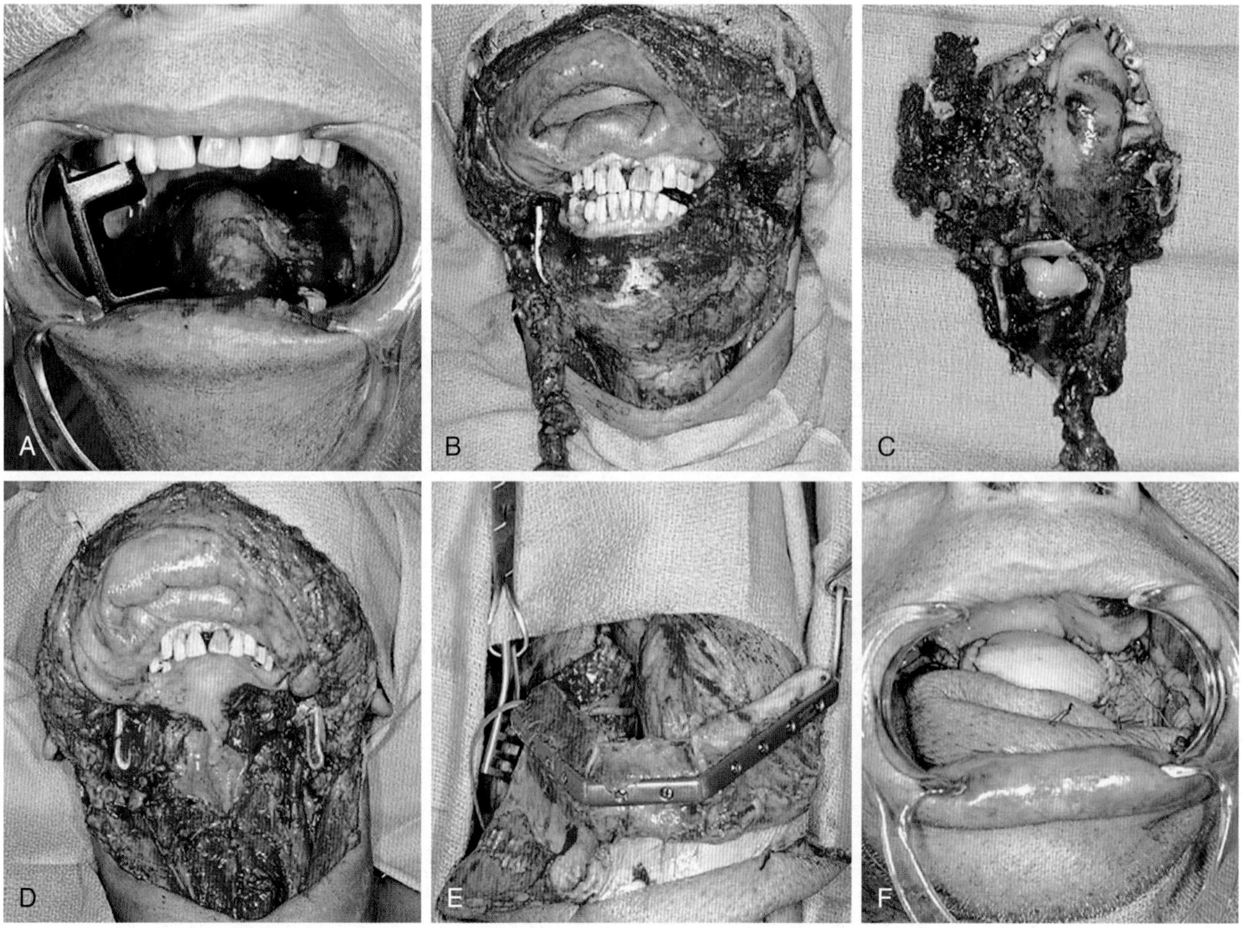

Figure 118.4 **A–F,** Extensive tumor involving the mandible and entire tongue, requiring subtotal mandibulectomy, total glossectomy, total laryngectomy, and free flap reconstruction.

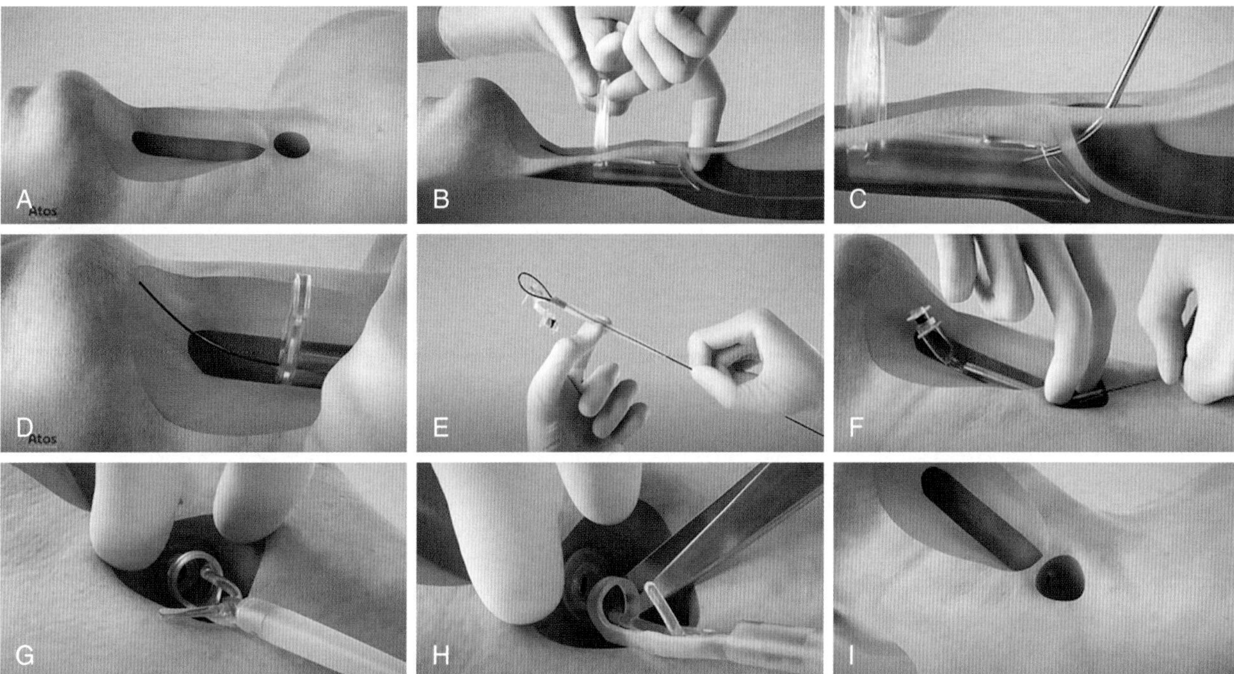

Figure 118.5 **A–I,** Tracheoesophageal puncture at the time of total laryngectomy. (Courtesy of Atos Medical.)

ALTERNATIVE TECHNIQUE 3: Tracheoesophageal Puncture at the Time of Laryngectomy

Historically, most laryngectomees were trained to produce classic esophageal speech by swallowing air and controlling eructation, which allows a staccato series of short phrases that results in guttural but understandable speech. Significantly better speech is produced after tracheoesophageal puncture (TEP), the patency of which is maintained by a one-way speech prosthesis.[24,25] TEP entails insertion of the speech prosthesis, a puncture through the "party wall" between the superior aspect of the tracheal stoma and the lumen of the cervical esophagus. When the tracheal stoma is occluded by the laryngectomee, pulmonary air is diverted through the grommet into the cervical esophagus, which allows phonation by reverberations of the walls of the reconstructed pharynx.

The TEP can be performed as a secondary procedure, after the laryngectomy and reconstruction are well healed. TEP can also be performed primarily, at the time of TL. Primary TEP should not be performed in patients with pulmonary compromise or impaired manual dexterity. Although there is evidence that primary TEP is safe in patients with a history of radiation, we generally prefer to wait in these patients, and perform secondary TEP in 4 to 6 months. When performing primary TEP, the posterior tracheal wall at the site of the stoma should not be split to enhance stomal size, and the party wall between the trachea and esophagus must not have been separated during the resection.

Several methods for TEP have been described. We prefer to use the Provox Vega puncture set, which streamlines prosthesis placement into a single-stage procedure. First, ensure the patient's head and neck are in a neutral position. After removal of the larynx and maturation of the stoma are performed (Fig. 118.5A), the pharyngeal protector is placed into the esophagus at the party wall (Fig. 118.5B). The tip of the pharyngeal protector is palpated through the trachea and the planned puncture site is identified. The puncture site should be sufficiently low on the posterior wall of the membranous trachea, as placement too close to the superior margin of the residual trachea will result in a prosthesis that is angled downward and difficult for the patient to see and clean. The puncture needle is inserted through the party wall until the needle enters the lumen of the pharyngeal protector (Fig. 118.5C). The guidewire is pushed through the needle until it extends out of the lumen of the pharyngeal protector for approximately 20 cm (Fig. 118.5D). The puncture needle is removed first, followed by the pharyngeal protector. The guidewire is inserted into the puncture dilator and pushed until it extends through the dilator exit hole (Fig. 118.5E). The tip of the guidewire is inserted into the hole next to the exit hole, and the guidewire is tightened to secure it to the puncture dilator (Fig. 118.5E). Dilate the puncture site by carefully pulling the guidewire until the dilator has passed the puncture site, while using finger pressure from the nondominant hand to support the tracheoesophageal wall (Fig. 118.5F). Carefully pull the guidewire until the prosthesis exits the puncture site and unfolds in the trachea (Fig. 118.5G). The prosthesis is then turned in the correct position and the safety strap is cut (Fig. 118.5H). The patient can begin using the prosthesis for speech under the guidance of the speech-language pathologist at any time postoperatively.

Avoidance and Management of Intraoperative Complications

Excessive Resection of the Piriform Recess and Pharyngeal Wall Mucosa

During the creation of the vertically oriented incisions along the AE fold coursing through the piriform recess area (Step 8), overzealous anterior retraction can result in a vertical tear of the mucosa before the Metzenbaum scissors can create the properly oriented incision. This mucosal tear tends to track horizontally and may result in the need for excessive resection of the lateral pharyngeal wall. Such a situation requires importation of a vascularized flap to restore an adequate circumference to the pharyngeal reconstruction. Complete circumferential resection of the pharyngeal wall results in a laryngopharyngectomy, which becomes much more difficult to reconstruct.[26]

Avoiding the Creation of a Too-Small Stoma

Stomal problems are best avoided rather than treated later. The vertical incision in the posterior tracheal wall does not devascularize the trachea because it receives its blood supply from lateral vascular arcades. An effort should be made to preserve the lateral blood supply to the trachea whenever possible. Excision of an adequate skin window for the tracheostomy position, excision of a small triangle of the medial edge of the sternocleidomastoid adjacent to the stoma, and advancement of the skin flap into the created V all help create a large stoma that will resist scarification and secondary stomal stenosis (Fig. 118.6). Occasionally, additional room must be created for the stoma by excising triangular wedges from the medial aspect of the sternocleidomastoid muscles bilaterally. This can be performed by grasping the medial aspect of the sternal head of the muscle with an Allis clamp just lateral to the stomal site and excising a wedge of muscle at the position where the sternal head of the muscle lies closest to the lateral border of the stoma.

Postoperative Considerations

As soon as ventilatory support is no longer needed, the tracheostomy tube is exchanged for a soft silicone laryngectomy tube, and humidified air is directed to the airway with an external humidifier (tracheostomy mask) or heat-moisture exchanger (HME). Use of an HME in the immediate postoperative period has been shown to have multiple benefits over external humidifiers, including increased compliance, fewer pulmonary complaints, and better sleep.[27] Anecdotally, we have also found in our practice that HME use results in less soaking of the incision with humidity and less propensity for wound dehiscence. A speech-language pathologist should be consulted immediately postoperatively for communication including use of an electrolarynx,

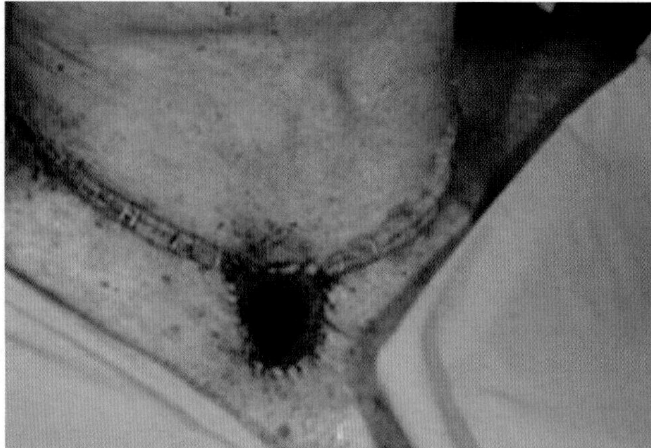

Figure 118.6 Creation of a large stoma that will resist scarification and secondary stomal stenosis.

or TEP if placed primarily. Patients are kept nil per os with enteral feeds for 2 weeks, at which time we perform a modified barium swallow exam to assess for leak from the pharyngeal closure. If no leak is identified, the patient can start per os trials. Secondary TEP can be offered at 4 to 6 months postoperatively, after completion of wound healing and adjuvant therapy, if applicable.

Complications

Pharyngocutaneous Fistula Formation

The complication of pharyngocutaneous fistula (PCF) formation adds to patient morbidity and prolongs recovery after TL. A meta-analysis of 26 papers identified a published incidence of PCF ranging from 2.3% to 65.4%. Variables associated with PCF included a hemoglobin lower than 12.5 g/dL, previous tracheotomy, preoperative radiotherapy, and concurrent neck dissection in patients with prior radiation.[28]

Fistulas usually occur within the first 1 to 2 weeks after TL and are heralded by erythema over the cervical skin, followed by what appears to be a localized infection. The fistula develops along the path of least resistance and tends to drain through the cervical closure line. Unfortunately, this often occurs just above the tracheal stoma. Treatment generally requires opening the wound, frequent packing, antibiotics, nil per os, and enteral nutritional support until closure is obtained. Maintenance of a euthyroid state is critical for wound healing. In cases of chronic PCF, flap closure may be required.

Tracheal Crusting and Mucous Plug Occlusion of the Trachea

Maintenance of humidified air intake to the tracheal stoma assists the patient in transitioning from inspiration of air that has been warmed and humidified by the nasopharynx to relatively dry and cool room air. Some patients, especially smokers, create copious tracheobronchial secretions during this transition phase, and appropriate suctioning requires adequate humidification of inspired air. Patients should use external humidified trach mist or an HME at all times following TL, and the benefits of HME in particular are mentioned above under the section Postoperative Considerations. After hospital discharge, it is helpful for patients to use a home humidifier in their bedroom, particularly during the winter months, in addition to using the HME. Intratracheal crust formation can result in respiratory compromise, and direct transstomal removal may be necessary. Most patients eventually master this process themselves.

Premature Dislodgement or Removal of the Nasogastric Tube

The nasogastric tube should be securely fixed by suturing to the membranous portion of the nasal septum or by placement of a nasal bridle to avoid inadvertent loss of this tube. The duration of nasogastric feeding varies, depending on the nature of the pharyngeal closure (e.g., primary closure or inset of a vascularized flap), whether the patient has a history of preoperative radiotherapy, and the surgeon's preference.[29] If the tube is lost or removed prematurely, the tube should be replaced under direct visualization (e.g., using a video laryngoscope under sedation). If this is not possible, consideration may be given to performance of an open gastrostomy.

Hypothyroidism

Laryngectomees usually have sustained dual insults to their thyroids: initial radiotherapy, followed by ipsilateral hemithyroidectomy performed at the time of TL. As a result, the remaining hemithyroid often undergoes a progressive decrease in function. One study with a follow-up longer than 10 years showed an overall incidence of hypothyroidism of 49%.[30] We routinely assess thyroid function prior to surgery in patients with a history of radiation, and also within 2 to 3 weeks after laryngectomy in most patients. Long-term serial monitoring of thyroid function tests is advisable, as for all patients with a history of radiation to the head and neck.

References

1. Schwartz AW, Devine KD. Some historical notes about the first laryngectomies. *Laryngoscope*. 1959;69(2):194–201.
2. Gussenbauer C. Uber die erste durch Th. Billroth am Menschen ausgefuhrte Kehlkopf-Extirpation und die Anwendung eines Kunstlichen Kehlkopfes. *Arch Klin Chir*. 1874;17:343–356.
3. Thomas L, Drinnan M, Natesh B, Mehanna H, Jones T, Paleri V. Open conservation partial laryngectomy for laryngeal cancer: a systematic review of English language literature. *Cancer Treat Rev*. 2012;38(3):203–211.
4. Weinstein GS, O'Malley BW Jr, Snyder W, Hockstein NG. Transoral robotic surgery: supraglottic partial laryngectomy. *Ann Otol Rhinol Laryngol*. 2007;116(1):19–23.
5. Maddox PT, Davies L. Trends in total laryngectomy in the era of organ preservation: a population-based study. *Otolaryngol Head Neck Surg*. 2012;147(1):85–90.
6. Wolf GT, Fisher SG, Hong WK, et al. Department of Veterans Affairs Laryngeal Cancer Study Group. Induction chemotherapy plus radiation compared with surgery plus radiation in patients with advanced laryngeal cancer. *N Engl J Med*. 1991;324(24):1685–1690.
7. Forastiere AA, Zhang Q, Weber RS, et al. Long-term results of RTOG 91-11: a comparison of three nonsurgical treatment strategies to preserve the larynx in patients with locally advanced larynx cancer. *J Clin Oncol*. 2013;31(7):845–852. https://doi.org/10.1200/JCO.2012.43.6097.
8. Strojan P, Haigentz M Jr, Bradford CR, et al. Chemoradiotherapy vs. total laryngectomy for primary treatment of advanced laryngeal squamous cell carcinoma. *Oral Oncol*. 2013;49(4):283–286.
9. American Society of Clinical Oncology; Pfister DG, Laurie SA, Weinstein GS, et al. American Society of Clinical Oncology clinical practice guideline for the use of larynx-preservation strategies in the treatment of laryngeal cancer. *J Clin Oncol*. 2006;24(22):3693–3704.
10. van der Putten L, de Bree R, Kuik DJ, et al. Salvage laryngectomy: oncological and functional outcome. *Oral Oncol*. 2011;47(4):296–301.
11. Hartl DM, Ferlito A, Brasnu DF, et al. Evidence-based review of treatment options for patients with glottic cancer. *Head Neck*. 2011;33(11):1638–1648.
12. Cukurova I, Cetinkaya EA. Radionecrosis of the larynx: case report and review of the literature. *Acta Otorhinolaryngol Ital*. 2010;30(4):205.
13. Theunissen EA, Timmermans AJ, Zuur CL, et al. Total laryngectomy for a dysfunctional larynx after (chemo)radiotherapy. *Arch Otolaryngol Head Neck Surg*. 2012;138(6):548–555.
14. Edge SB, Edge SB. *AJCC Cancer Staging*. Manual. 8th ed. Springer; 2017.
15. Kuno H, Onaya H, Iwata R, et al. Evaluation of cartilage invasion by laryngeal and hypopharyngeal squamous cell carcinoma with dual-energy CT. *Radiology*. 2012;265(2):488–496.
16. Taha MS, Hassan O, Amir M, Taha T, Riad MA. Diffusion-weighted MRI in diagnosing thyroid cartilage invasion in laryngeal carcinoma. *Eur Arch Oto-Rhino-Laryngol*. 2014;271(9):2511–2516.
17. Sisson GA, Straehley CJ Jr, Johnson NE. Mediastinal dissection for recurrent cancer after laryngectomy. *Laryngoscope*. 1962;72:1064–1077.
18. Gomes MN, Kroll S, Spear SL. Mediastinal tracheostomy. *Ann Thorac Surg*. 1987;43(5):539–543.
19. Brazilian Head and Neck Cancer Study Group. End results of a prospective trial on elective lateral neck dissection vs type III modified radical neck dissection in the management of supraglottic and transglottic carcinomas. *Head Neck*. 1999;21(8):694–702.
20. Spiro RH, Gallo O, Shah JP. Selective jugular node dissection in patients with squamous carcinoma of the larynx or pharynx. *Am J Surg*. 1993;166(4):399–402.
21. Bohannon IA, Desmond RA, Clemons L, Magnuson JS, Carroll WR, Rosenthal EL. Management of the N_0 neck in recurrent laryngeal squamous cell carcinoma. *Laryngoscope*. 2010;120(1):58–61.
22. Dagan R, Morris CG, Kirwan JM, et al. Elective neck dissection during salvage surgery for locally recurrent head and neck squamous cell carcinoma after radiotherapy with elective nodal irradiation. *Laryngoscope*. 2010;120(5):945–952.
23. Punthakee X, Zaghi S, Nabili V, Knott PD, Blackwell KE. Effects of salivary bypass tubes on fistula and stricture formation. *JAMA Facial Plast Surg*. 2013;15(3):219–225.

24. Blom ED, Singer MI, Hamaker RC. Tracheostoma valve for postlaryngectomy voice rehabilitation. *Ann Otol Rhinol Laryngol.* 1982;91(6 Pt 1):576–578.
25. Deschler DG, Emerick KS, Lin DT, Bunting GW. Simplified technique of tracheoesophageal prosthesis placement at the time of secondary tracheoesophageal puncture (TEP). *Laryngoscope.* 2011;121(9):1855–1859.
26. Piazza C, Taglietti V, Nicolai P. Reconstructive options after total laryngectomy with subtotal or circumferential hypopharyngectomy and cervical esophagectomy. *Curr Opin Otolaryngol Head Neck Surg.* 2012;20(2):77–88.
27. Mérol JC, Charpiot A, Langagne T, Hémar P, Ackerstaff AH, Hilgers FJ. Randomized controlled trial on postoperative pulmonary humidification after total laryngectomy: external humidifier versus heat and moisture exchanger. *Laryngoscope.* 2012;122(2):275–281.
28. Paydarfar JA, Birkmeyer NJ. Complications in head and neck surgery: a meta-analysis of postlaryngectomy pharyngocutaneous fistula. *Arch Otolaryngol Head Neck Surg.* 2006;132(1):67–72.
29. Prasad KC, Sreedharan S, Dannana NK, Prasad SC, Chandra S. Early oral feeds in laryngectomized patients. *Ann Otol Rhinol Laryngol.* 2006;115(6):433–438.
30. Ho ACW, Ho WK, Lam PKY, Yuen APW, Wei WI. Thyroid dysfunction in laryngectomees—10 years after treatment. *Head Neck.* 2008;30(3):336–340.

CHAPTER 119

Pharyngectomy

Moni A. Kuriakose and Swagnik Chakrabarti

Armamentarium

#15 Scalpel
Allis forceps
Appropriate sutures
Cat paw retractors
Dissecting forceps
Dissecting scissors
Freer elevator
Langenbeck retractors
Local anesthetic with vasoconstrictor
Monopolar and bipolar electrocautery
Nasogastric tube
Needle holder
Skin hooks
Suction drains of choice
Tooth and nontooth Adson forceps

History of the Procedure

The history of pharyngectomy dates back to 1878, when Cheever described lateral pharyngectomy with mandibulectomy and lymph node dissection for a large tonsil tumor.[1] Unfortunately, the patient developed local and regional recurrence. Various techniques for resection of hypopharyngeal cancer have evolved since then. Sebileau, in 1904,[2] described partial pharyngectomy via a lateral retrothyroid approach. This was followed by Trotter's development of the lateral pharyngectomy in 1913.[2] Supracricoid-hemilaryngopharyngectomy was subsequently described by Andre, Pinel, and Laccourreye (1962).[2] Ogura, in 1965,[2] developed extended supraglottic-laryngopharyngectomy. All of these procedures were suitable for T1 and T2 hypopharyngeal cancers. Following the refinement of radiation therapy techniques that evolved during the 20th century, these tumors could be treated with radical radiotherapy with similar oncologic outcomes and lower morbidity. Furthermore, owing to the high incidence of neck nodal metastasis even among T1 and T2 hypopharyngeal cancers, patients treated with partial pharyngectomy and neck dissection would often require adjuvant radiotherapy anyway. Thus, single modality radiotherapy or chemoradiotherapy was recommended to treat these patients, with surgery being reserved as a salvage procedure. Finally, hypopharyngeal cancers, because of their aggressive nature and tendency of submucosal spread (especially postcricoid cancers), require resection using wide surgical margins, which cannot be generally obtained by partial pharyngectomy. Today, the indication for conservative pharyngeal surgery is limited to endoscopic laser resection or transoral robotic surgery in a selected group of patients with early tumors (T1, T2, and rarely T3 tumors) performed by specially trained surgeons. Open surgery such as total laryngectomy with partial pharyngectomy, total laryngopharyngectomy, or total laryngopharyngoesophagectomy with appropriate reconstruction is indicated for T4a cancers and recurrent/residual cancers after radiotherapy or chemoradiotherapy. Table 119.1 lists various treatment options for hypopharyngeal cancers.

Indications for the Use of the Procedure

Patients who are candidates for this procedure include those with T4a cancers of the piriform sinus with the tumor not extending to the postcricoid region and not crossing the midline along the posterior pharyngeal wall.

Patients with T3 lateralized cancers of the piriform sinus with a nonfunctional larynx should also be considered,[3] such as patients with airway obstruction requiring tracheostomy or a feeding tube. These patients are less likely to regain a functional larynx even after cancer cure following organ-preservation radiotherapy or chemoradiotherapy, and therefore are considered as a relative indication for surgery.

Patients with lateralized piriform sinus cancers treated initially with organ-preservation therapy who present with recurrent/residual tumor may also benefit from the procedure.

Limitations and Contraindications

Some conditions do warrant limitations to this procedure, such as the presence of T4b hypopharyngeal cancer (tumor invasion of the prevertebral fascia, encasing the carotid artery by 270 degrees or greater or involving the mediastinal

Table 119.1 Pharyngectomy Reconstructive Options

Pectoralis Major Myocutaneous (PMMC) Flap (see Chapter 111)	**Introduced by Ariyian in 1979[3]** **First used by Whiters and colleagues[4] in the same year for reconstruction of circumferential hypopharyngeal defects in a tubed form**
Indications	Partial defects in the pharyngeal mucosa (the width of the flap is decided by the width of the remnant pharyngeal mucosa) Circumferential defects in the pharyngeal mucosa (the width of the flap required is 8–10 cm)
Contraindications	Resection margin reaching beyond the thoracic inlet Defects longer than 11–12 cm
Advantages	Operating time is reduced, which is especially important among emaciated and fragile hypopharyngeal cancer patients Fan-shaped muscular portion of the flap is helpful for protecting the carotid artery, especially in postradiotherapy patients No microsurgical training is required The flap donor site can be closed primarily with minimal morbidity
Disadvantages	This flap provides a suboptimal reconstructive choice when a significant part of the base of tongue or the lateral oropharyngeal wall has been resected; the weight and the downward traction of the flap significantly impair the mobility of the tongue, resulting in degradation of augmented speech and poorer swallowing function The bulkiness of the flap makes it difficult to be sutured at the relatively narrow cervical esophageal stump, resulting in circumferential stenosis; this can be partially overcome by performing interdigitations to provide a zigzag configuration at the distal anastomosis The bulkiness and rigidity of the PMMC flap reduce its vibratory properties, resulting in poor phonatory outcomes The flap can result in distortion and blocking of the tracheostoma in obese patients and patients with a short neck For circumferential defects, the three-point closure sites are prone to fistula formation and subsequent stenosis Complication rates in relation to stenosis and pharyngocutaneous fistula are higher than those of free flaps May result in significant breast deformity in female patients
Remarks	As the muscle bulk sometimes prevents complete tubulization, Fabian[5] and Spriano and colleagues[6] modified the technique by using a U-shaped reconstruction of the circumferential hypopharyngeal defect by suturing the flap edges to the prevertebral fascia, either covering the fascia by a skin graft[5] or leaving it bare[6] The PMMC flap can be considered a reconstructive option for thin male patients with partial hypopharyngeal defects and significant comorbidity where a prolonged operative time is to be avoided
Radial Forearm Free Flap (RFFF) (see Chapter 114)	**Introduced by Yang and colleagues[7] in 1981** **Used for hypopharyngeal reconstruction for the first time in 1985 by Harii and colleagues[8]**
Indications	Partial defects in the pharyngeal mucosa Circumferential defects in the pharyngeal mucosa
Contraindications	Resection margin reaching beyond the thoracic inlet
Advantages	The pharyngocutaneous fistula rates are lower than those with the PMMC flap and comparable with other free flaps Its long vascular pedicle, low donor site morbidity, good caliber vessels, tolerance to long ischemia times, and relative ease in harvesting make it a good option for pharyngeal reconstruction The radial artery and the cephalic vein have a certain degree of independence from each other, which makes microvascular anastomosis possible on recipient vessels located at considerable distance from each other, even on opposite sides of the neck A skin island of up to 12–14 cm^2 can easily be harvested without donor site problems The good pliability of the flap has a definite advantage over PMMC and anterolateral thigh (ALT) flaps, especially among obese patients, resulting in superior voice and swallowing outcome The low volume of the flap does not hamper primary closure of the neck Hair growth even in men is exceedingly low on the volar aspect of the forearm as compared with the thigh and the chest
Disadvantages	Potential donor site morbidities including tendon exposure, partial loss of skin graft, hypovascularization with cold intolerance, and transient or permanent numbness of the first two fingers and dorsum of hand The flap does not provide muscle for covering the carotids or reinforcing the pharyngeal closure Three-point closure is required for circumferential defects

Table 119.1 Pharyngectomy Reconstructive Options—cont'd

Anterolateral Thigh Flap (ALT) (see Chapter 119)	Introduced by Song and colleagues[9] in 1984
Indications	Partial defects in the pharyngeal mucosa Circumferential defects in the pharyngeal mucosa
Contraindications	Resection margin reaching beyond the thoracic inlet obvious severe peripheral vascular disease (preoperative angiography is warranted in these circumstances)
Advantages	The pharyngocutaneous fistula rate of the ALT flap is lower than that observed in the RFFF flap; this may be related to the generous amount of vascularized fascia lata that can be harvested with the flap, which can be used as a second layer closure; a lower fistula rate is associated with a lower rate of stenosis formation In selected patients, an extensive portion of the vastus lateralis muscle can be harvested with the skin or independently, and it can be used for a second layer closure over the suture line or for protecting the great vessels of the neck Large skin paddles or two separate skin paddles can be harvested with minimal donor site morbidity Remoteness of the thigh from the head and neck makes the two-surgical-team approach possible, thus reducing the operating time As hypopharyngeal cancer patients are frequently emaciated, they have decreased thigh bulk, which facilitates tubing the flap for circumferential defects The diameter of the tubed flap corresponds well with the diameter of the remnant oropharyngeal mucosa in circumferential defects
Disadvantages	In obese patients, the bulk of the flap impairs the vibratory property of the neopharynx, resulting in poor speech Mismatch in lumen diameter between the tubed flap and the cervical esophagus in circumferential defects Three-point closure is required for circumferential defects
Remarks	As a general rule, the ALT free flap is the first-line reconstructive option for pharyngeal defects; the only limiting factors are the requirement for microvascular expertise and prolonged operating time
Jejunal Free Flaps	**Introduced by Seidenberg and colleagues[10] in 1959**
Indications	Circumferential pharyngeal defects
Contraindications	Resection margin reaching beyond the thoracic inlet
Advantages	Diameter of the jejunum matches with the esophageal stump mucosa For circumferential defects, there is no three-point closure, as required in tubed fasciocutaneous or PMMC flaps Mucosa is replaced by mucosa Intrinsic peristaltic activity of the jejunum helps in bolus propulsion; however, the initial peristaltic movements are not coordinated, and patients usually complain of dysphagia in the early postoperative period
Disadvantages	Perioperative donor site complications are high; mortality ranges from 0% to 17% (mean, 2.5%), which is four times higher than that for fasciocutaneous free flaps; morbidities of an abdominal surgery include bowel obstruction, abdominal bleeding, acute gastric dilatation, superior mesenteric syndrome, laparocele, wound infection or dehiscence, abdominal wall hematoma, and prolonged ileus Limited ischemic tolerance of the jejunal flap commonly results in partial necrosis, pharyngocutaneous fistula, and subsequent stenosis The length of the vascular pedicle (10–15 cm) is roughly half that usually observed in RFFF and ALT free flaps Voice (in patients with a tracheoesophageal puncture) is usually "wet and gurgly" Tolerance of the jejunum to radiotherapy is only 50 Gy, which is lower than the recommended dose of postoperative adjuvant radiotherapy in head and neck cancer patients Three intestinal and two microvascular anastomoses are required The flimsy and friable nature of vessels (particularly the vein) as compared to fasciocutaneous flaps There is a frequent mismatch in diameter at the pharyngeal end External skin defect, if present, requires another flap

Continued

Table 119.1 Pharyngectomy Reconstructive Options—cont'd

Gastroomental Flap	Introduced by Baudet[11] in 1979
Indications	Circumferential pharyngeal defects
Contraindications	Resection margin reaching beyond the thoracic inlet
Advantages	The main advantage over a jejunal free flap is the provision of a generous amount of highly vascularized greater omentum to be draped around the neopharyngeal conduit, covering the great vessels and filling dead space Length of gut that can be obtained is about 30 cm Good caliber vessels and superb independent mobility of the gastroepiploic vascular pedicle
Disadvantages	High perioperative donor site complications (similar to jejunal flap)
Remarks	Gastroomental free flap is currently recommended in the management of select, complicated high-risk conditions in which a generally healthy patient (able to withstand the potential complications of an abdominal procedure) is associated with a serious local wound problem owing to infection, hypovascularization, or necrosis
Gastric Pull-Up	Introduced by Ong and Lee[12] and popularized by Le Quesne and Ranger in 1966[13]
Indications	Only reconstructive option when the tumor extends to the thoracic esophagus or the resection margin reaches beyond the thoracic inlet
Contraindications	High upper limit of resection of pharynx (oropharynx or above) where reach of mobilized stomach is difficult
Advantages	One-stage procedure and a single intestinal anastomosis required No microvascular expertise required
Disadvantages	Complications of abdominal surgery as previously mentioned Gastric reflux and early satiety

structures), cancer originating from or involving the postcricoid region, and primary posterior pharyngeal wall tumors or piriform sinus tumors involving the posterior pharyngeal wall.

Careful consideration must also be given to patients who have extensive tumor involvement of the base of tongue. These patients require total glossectomy along with laryngopharyngectomy and exhibit significant morbidity in speech and swallowing function following surgery. Although this condition is not a contraindication for surgery, these patients may initially be treated with induction chemotherapy. Further management can be planned depending on the response assessment. If there is no response or progressive disease, surgery may be performed or consideration can be given to palliative care. In patients with complete or partial response, concurrent chemoradiotherapy may be a treatment option.

This procedure is contraindicated for patients who are medically unfit for surgery or who are unwilling to consent to surgery.

TECHNIQUE: Total Laryngectomy With Partial Pharyngectomy

STEP 1: Patient Preparation

Pulmonary and nutritional status should be optimized prior to this extensive surgery. Most patients with hypopharyngeal cancers are nutritionally deprived due to chronic dysphagia, and nutritional supplementation should be provided before the surgical procedure.

STEP 2: Patient Positioning

Patient is positioned supine, with the neck extended with a shoulder bag and the head stabilized with a head ring.

STEP 3: Maintenance of Airway

If the patient has already undergone a tracheotomy, a flexible endotracheal tube is inserted through the existing stoma. If the patient has not undergone a previous tracheotomy, nasal or oral tracheal intubation is usually performed and maintained in situ until tracheal transection is performed at the end of the laryngopharyngectomy. Patients with bulky tumors or borderline obstruction should undergo preliminary tracheotomy under local anesthesia. In this setting, it should be performed at a higher level between the first and second tracheal rings to allow incorporation of the tracheostomy within the surgical resection.

TECHNIQUE: Total Laryngectomy With Partial Pharyngectomy—*cont'd*

STEP 4: Incision and Exposure

Neck incision, exposure, neck dissection, and the initial steps of laryngectomy are completed as in Steps 1 through 4 in Chapter 105 (Fig. 119.1A).

STEP 5: Skeletonization of the Larynx

This part is similar to the description provided in Chapter 105, with few salient differences.

The suprahyoid muscles are divided, staying close to the superior aspect of the hyoid bone. It is unlikely that hypopharyngeal cancer will have extension to the vallecula region, which is likely to occur in a supraglottic carcinoma of larynx. During this part of the dissection, care should be taken to preserve the lingual artery, which lies just superior to the greater cornu of the hyoid bone. The muscles divided from the medial to lateral direction include mylohyoid, geniohyoid, pulley of digastric, and hyoglossus. Cautery is best avoided lateral to the lesser cornu of the hyoid bone to prevent injury to the lingual artery and the hypoglossal nerve. As an alternative, one may consider dividing the greater cornu of the hyoid bone with a bone cutter and leaving it in situ.

The constrictor muscles are divided along the lateral aspect of the thyroid ala to expose the piriform fossa mucosa on the unaffected side. The decision of whether the apparent normal mucosa can be preserved has to be determined by intraoperative frozen-section examination. This is essential in hypopharynx cancer with a high incidence of submucous spread of the tumor event up to 2 cm away from the clinical tumor borders, which is rare in laryngeal cancers.

The contralateral thyroid lobe to be preserved is dissected away from the tracheal-esophageal groove along with the parathyroid glands. Bipolar electrocautery facilitates this dissection. Both the superior thyroid vascular pedicle and the inferior thyroid artery need to be preserved to provide adequate blood supply to the thyroid gland and the parathyroid glands.

With the use of a Freer elevator, the contralateral uninvolved piriform sinus along with the internal perichondrium of thyroid cartilage along the lateral wall of the piriform sinus is mobilized from the thyroid cartilage. Superior dissection is followed along the hyoepiglottic ligament up to the epiglottis and the vallecula to avoid entry into the preepiglottic space (Fig. 119.1B–F).

Continued

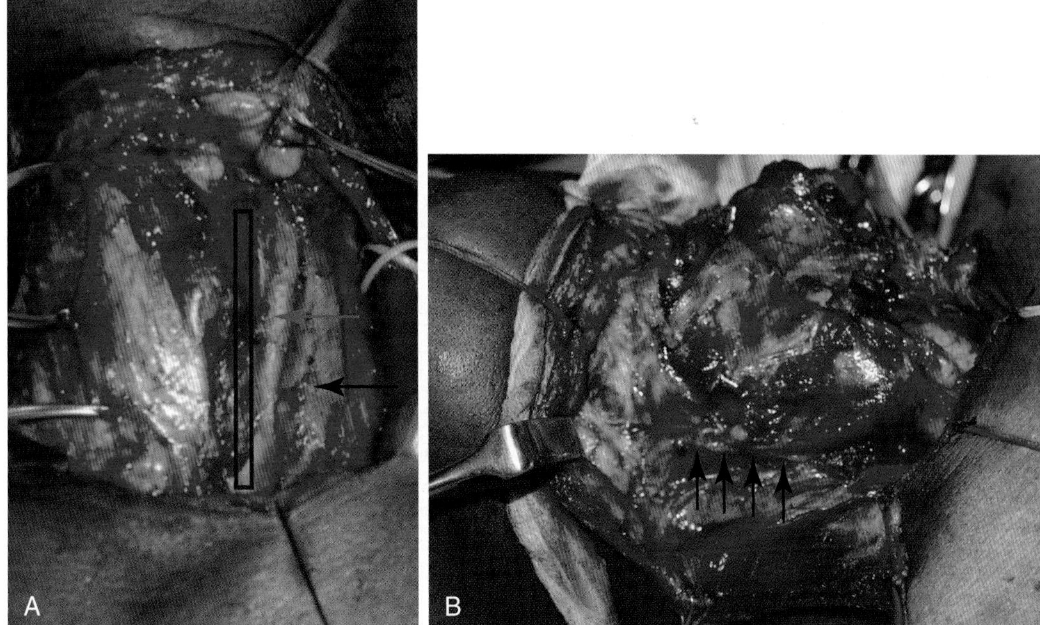

Figure 119.1 **A,** After the skin flap has been elevated and neck dissection completed as outlined in Chapter 105, the laryngopharynx complex is separated from the carotid fascia. To undertake this step, a plane (rectangle) between the carotid artery *(blue arrow)* and the constrictor muscles is developed. The internal jugular vein *(black arrow)* is seen lateral to the carotid artery. **B,** The superior thyroid vessels *(black arrows)* are preserved on the side of the thyroid lobe being preserved.

TECHNIQUE: Total Laryngectomy With Partial Pharyngectomy—*cont'd*

STEP 6: Entry Into the Upper Aerodigestive Tract

In patients with hypopharyngeal (rather than laryngeal) cancers, it is best to enter the pharynx in the vallecula, contralateral to the tumor (see Chapter 105). The tumor can then be visualized from the end of the table. Under direct vision of the pharyngeal mucosa and tumor, the mucosal incision could be extended along the thyrohyoid membrane to the laryngoepiglottic fold, preserving as much normal pharyngeal mucosa as possible. This may allow primary reconstruction of the pharynx or a patch flap pharyngoplasty, avoiding the need for tubed flap reconstruction. If there is suspicion about the involvement of the vallecula, entry is made through the uninvolved piriform sinus.

The trachea is transected anteriorly between the second and third tracheal rings with a #15 blade. To avoid perforation of the endotracheal tube balloon, one may request the anesthesiologist to deflate the cuff prior to making this incision.

Curved heavy scissors can be used to complete the tracheal transection to the lower border of the cricoid cartilage. The endotracheal tube is then withdrawn and a new tube is inserted through the tracheostomy incision. A 2-0 polypropylene suture is used to stabilize the trachea to the anterior neck skin flap.

The membranous trachea is then separated from the esophagus up to the level of the posterior cricoarytenoid musculature. If there is suspicion about significant subglottic extension of the tumor, this step is delayed until the tumor can be visualized directly. This is rare in hypopharyngeal cancer, as opposed to laryngeal cancer, where a transglottic tumor can have subglottic extension, necessitating removal of more than one tracheal ring (Fig. 119.1G–I).

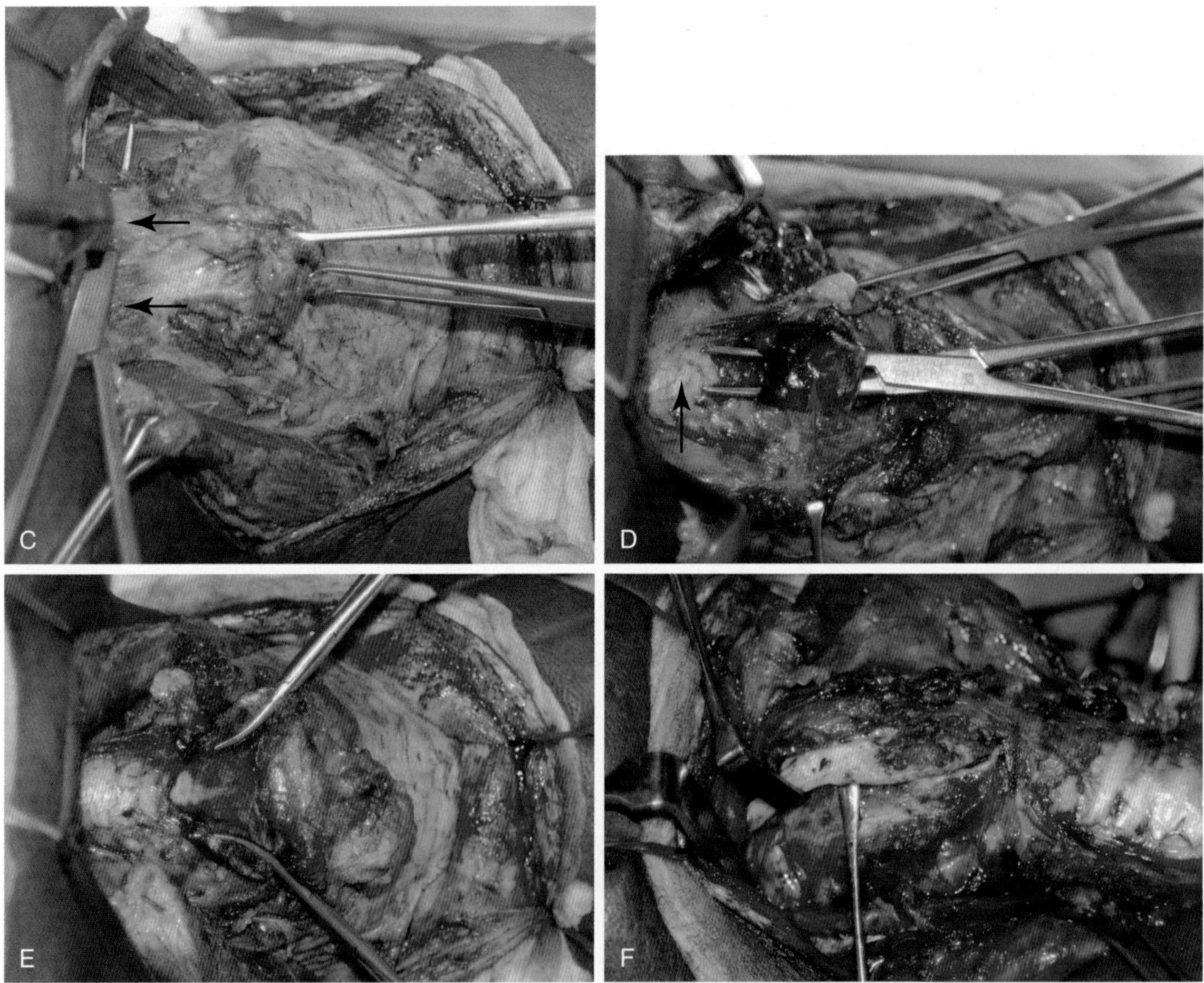

Figure 119.1, cont'd **C,** The strap muscles *(black arrows)* are divided inferiorly above the suprasternal notch. The right sternothyroid muscle has been lifted with an artery forceps. **D,** The trachea *(black arrow)* and the thyroid isthmus *(blue arrow)* are exposed after dividing the strap muscles. **E,** The thyroid lobe is divided (the two ends are held by artery forceps) and ligated, and the lobe to be preserved is dissected off the tracheal wall up to the tracheal-esophageal groove using bipolar cautery. Care should be taken to preserve the parathyroid glands and their blood supply. **F,** The constrictor muscles are divided at the lateral aspect of the thyroid. The uninvolved piriform mucosa is mobilized from the thyroid cartilage using a Freer elevator.

TECHNIQUE: Total Laryngectomy With Partial Pharyngectomy—*cont'd*

STEP 7: Removal of the Tumor

If entry is made through the vallecula, the epiglottis is grasped with an Allis clamp. While standing at the head end of the table and under direct vision, the operator can assess the margins and make the mucosal cuts. This requires at least 2 cm of unstretched normal mucosa, usually 3 cm inferiorly and 2 cm both superiorly and laterally due to the high risk of submucous spread of hypopharyngeal tumors.[14] If the uninvolved piriform sinus is entered first, the laryngopharynx is opened up like a book and the pharyngeal wall is resected with adequate margins (Fig. 119J and K).

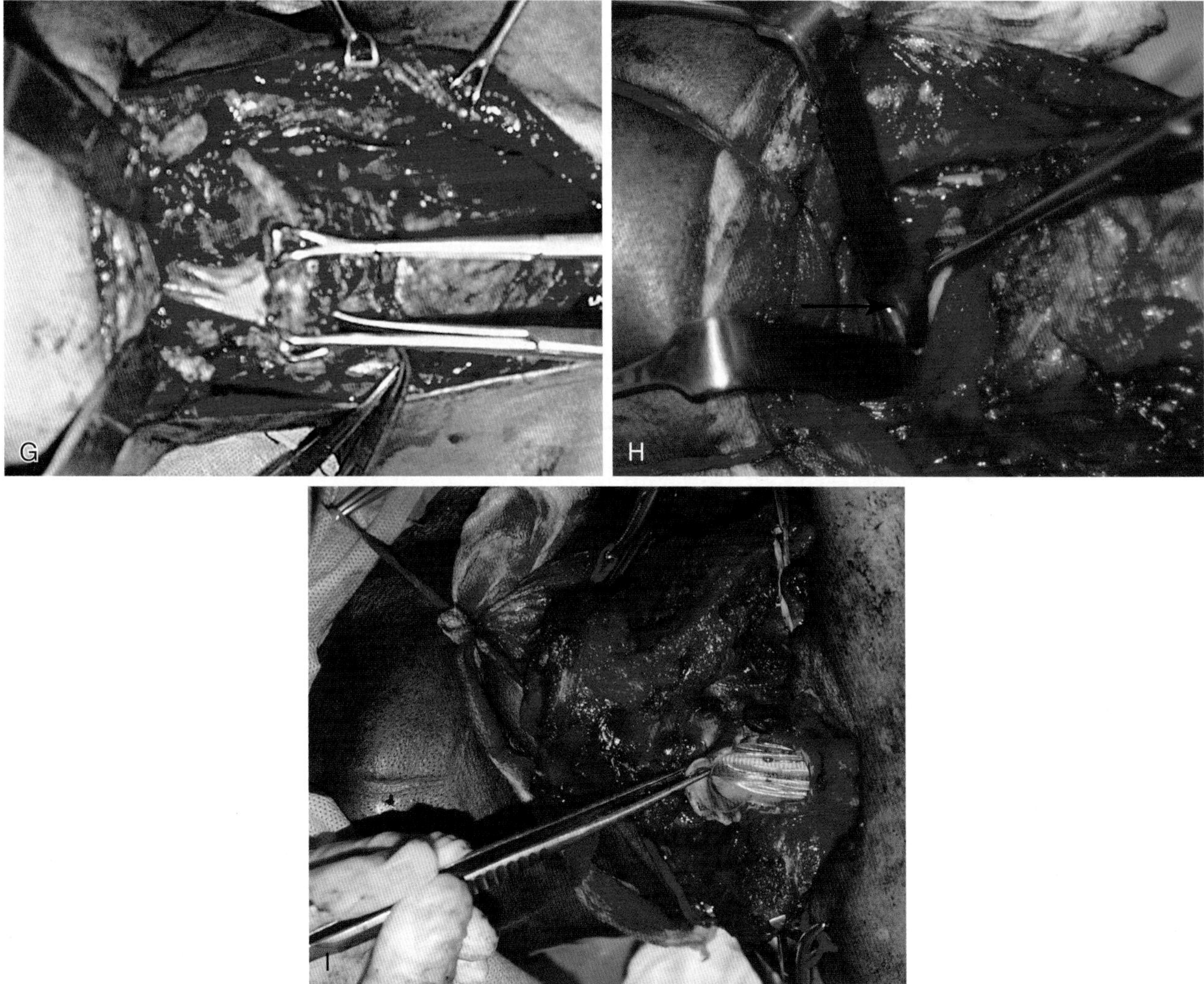

Figure 119.1, cont'd **G,** The hyoid bone being skeletonized. Arrows depict the position of the hyoid bone. **H,** The upper aero digestive tract is entered through the vallecula of the noninvolved side. The tip of the epiglottis is held with Babcock forceps and the base of tongue mucosa *(black arrow)* is retracted superiorly. **I,** The anterior tracheal wall is transected at a desired level with adequate margin from the tumor. It is held with forceps and retracted; the endotracheal tube is seen inside the trachea.

Continued

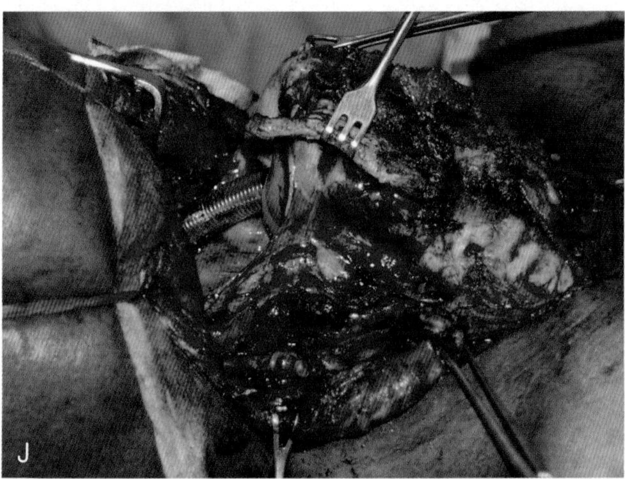

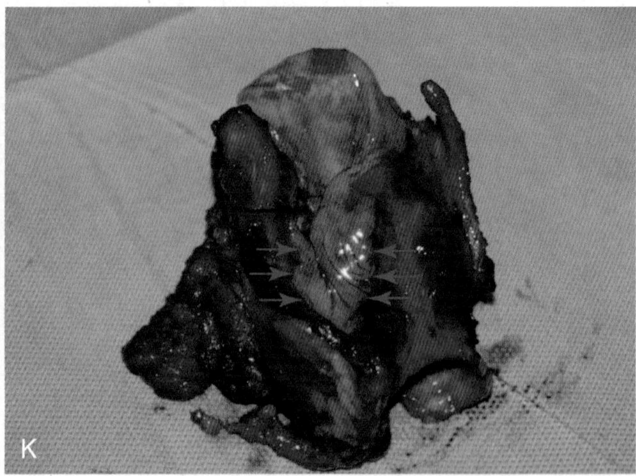

Figure 119.1, cont'd **J,** The hypopharynx is exposed by extending the pharyngotomy along the uninvolved pharyngeal mucosa. **K,** Specimen of total laryngectomy with partial pharyngectomy. The tumor is present in the left aryepiglottic fold *(black arrow)*. The pharyngeal mucosal cut margins are shown with *blue arrows*.

INDICATIONS FOR THE USE OF THE PROCEDURE

Several situations may warrant the use of a pharyngectomy, such as the presence of T4a piriform sinus cancer crossing the midline or involving the postcricoid region or the presence of T3/T4a postcricoid or posterior pharyngeal wall cancer. As for T1/T2 postcricoid or posterior pharyngeal wall cancer presenting with obstruction, such lesions are better managed by total laryngopharyngectomy, as they are likely to develop permanent stricture of the cervical esophagus following radiotherapy.

Another indication is a postcricoid, posterior pharyngeal wall or upper cervical esophageal cancer previously treated with organ-preservation therapy presenting with recurrent/residual disease.

LIMITATIONS AND CONTRAINDICATIONS

There are some limitations to the use of a pharyngectomy, including the presence of T4b hypopharyngeal cancer involving tumors that have invaded the prevertebral fascia, encasing the carotid artery by 270 degrees or greater or involving the mediastinum, as well as tumors involving the membranous trachea and extending below the clavicle. This procedure is contraindicated for patients who are medically unfit for surgery or who are unwilling to consent to surgery.

TECHNIQUE: Total Laryngopharyngectomy

Steps from incision to exposure are essentially the same as that of total laryngectomy with partial pharyngectomy (see Chapter 105).

STEP 1: Assessment of Resectability

Once the carotid sheath is identified, it is retracted laterally and the prevertebral fascia is identified by blunt dissection. Finger palpation is then used to determine whether the cancer has infiltrated into the retropharyngeal or retroesophageal space or into the prevertebral fascia. If cancer is adherent to the prevertebral fascia, the fascia should be included in the resection. However, if there is gross prevertebral fascia involvement, the surgery may serve only as a palliative procedure to temporarily improve oral feeding. Abandoning the procedure at this point may be considered, as would a palliative feeding gastrostomy or tracheostomy to alleviate symptoms.

STEP 2: Entry Into the Pharynx

A transhyoid circumferential pharyngotomy is carried out, and the retropharyngeal fascia is separated from the prevertebral fascia in the retropharyngeal space up into the level of the transhyoid incision. The epiglottis is grasped with an Allis forceps, and the entire larynx and hypopharynx are elevated anteriorly from the alar layer of the prevertebral fascia. If there is no tracheal involvement, the usual transection of the trachea between the second and third tracheal rings is appropriate. However, if cancer has extended into the trachea, more of the distal trachea may need to be resected.

Assessment of the distal extent of the resection is essential to plan whether the patient will require a total laryngopharyngectomy with tubed flap reconstruction or a total laryngopharyngoesophagectomy with gastric pull-up. To make this decision, it is advisable to expose, incise, and biopsy the cervical esophagus with frozen section to determine the need for esophagectomy.

TECHNIQUE: Total Laryngopharyngectomy—*cont'd*

STEP 3: Mobilization of the Laryngopharynx and Cervical Esophagus

If a laryngopharyngectomy is planned, a circumferential incision is made at the desired level (2 cm away from the tumor) of the hypopharynx and the cervical esophagus, and the specimen is delivered. Most tumors of the postcricoid region require total laryngopharyngoesophagectomy and a gastric pull-up reconstruction.

After the tracheal resection is carried out and the distal trachea is stabilized to the anterior neck skin, the specimen containing the larynx, pharynx, and cervical esophagus is then separated from the membranous tracheal wall. Care should be taken not to damage the membranous trachea by leaving a rim of esophageal serosa and muscle on the tracheal side. This should be followed by dissection along the avascular retroesophageal plane into the mediastinum. The segmental blood supply to the esophagus that enters it laterally is cauterized with a bipolar cautery and divided. This should be done close to the esophageal wall to avoid damage to the pleura. Gentle traction of the specimen allows superior mobilization of the specimen. The specimen remains attached to the distal esophagus until the stomach is mobilized (Fig. 119.2A).

STEP 4: Mobilization of Stomach

The abdomen is opened and the stomach is mobilized by the general surgical team, either through midline laparotomy incision or laparoscopically. The stomach is drawn into a tube, and kocherization of the duodenum is often required to obtain adequate mobilization of the stomach up to the oropharynx.

Blunt dissection in the mediastinum from the abdomen below and from the neck above allows the specimen to be mobilized and the stomach to be delivered into the neck by applying gentle traction. The esophagus is then transected at the gastroesophageal junction and the total laryngopharyngoesophagectomy specimen is delivered en bloc.

STEP 5: Reconstruction

After surgical removal of the tumor, a neopharynx is created to reestablish the conduit of the digestive tract. Various surgical options are available, each with its advantages and disadvantages (Fig. 119.2B).

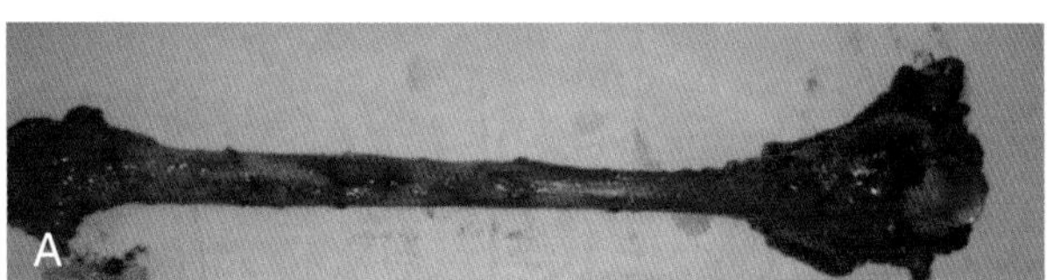

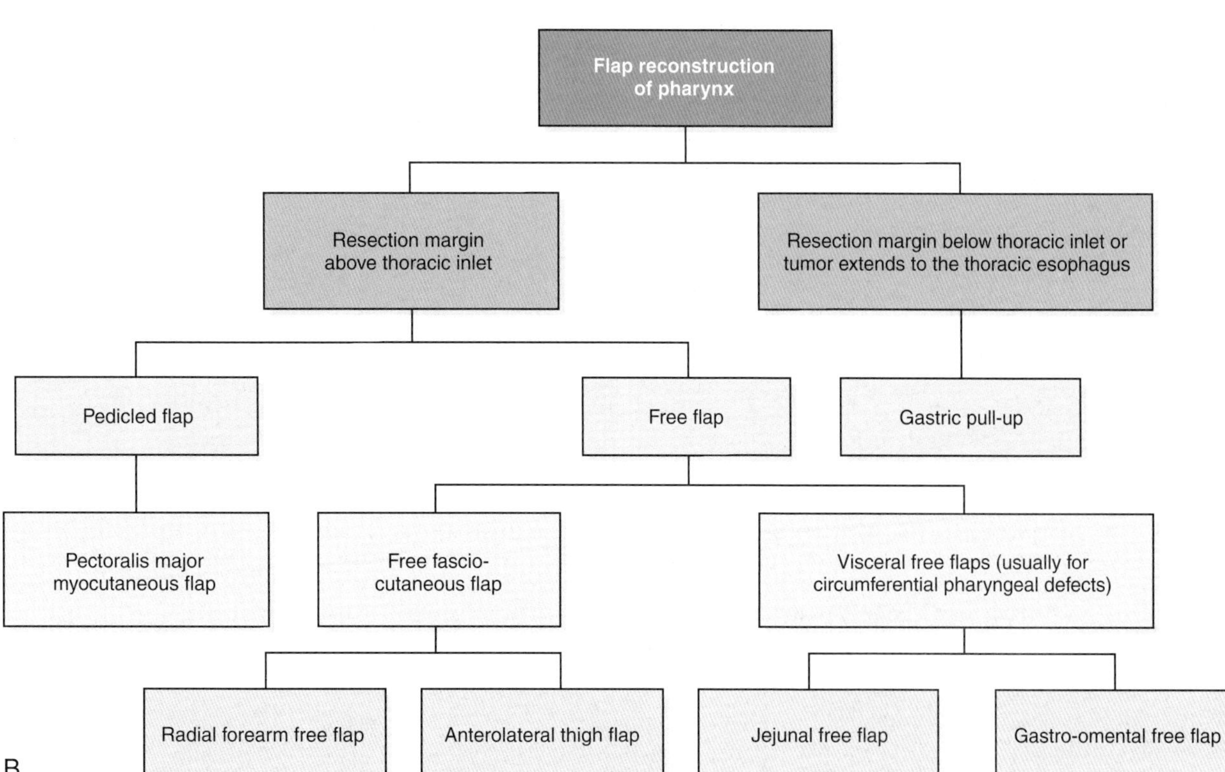

Figure 119.2 **A,** The specimen containing the larynx, pharynx, and cervical esophagus. **B,** Surgical options algorithm.

TECHNIQUE: Total Laryngopharyngectomy—*cont'd*

STEP 6: Primary Closure

As reported by Hui and colleagues,[15] in a group of 52 patients who underwent total laryngectomy with or without partial pharyngectomy, the minimum width of unstretched and stretched remnant pharyngeal mucosa for primary closure without excessive risk of pharyngocutaneous fistula or stenosis was 1.5 cm and 2.5 cm, respectively, and the mean width of mucosa was 3.24 cm of unstretched and 4.83 cm of stretched mucosa. As safe resection of hypopharyngeal cancer requires a margin of 2 to 3 cm, a remnant mucosa adequate for primary closure is usually not available except for small tumors confined to the medial wall of the piriform sinus or the postcricoid region. Moreover, as most early tumors are treated with organ-preservation strategies with surgery reserved for salvage, the possibility of primary closure is further reduced, owing to the devascularized and heavily radiated nature of the residual pharyngeal mucosa. An overview of flap reconstruction of pharyngeal defects is depicted in Fig. 119.2D–E (note Fig. 119.2C–F).

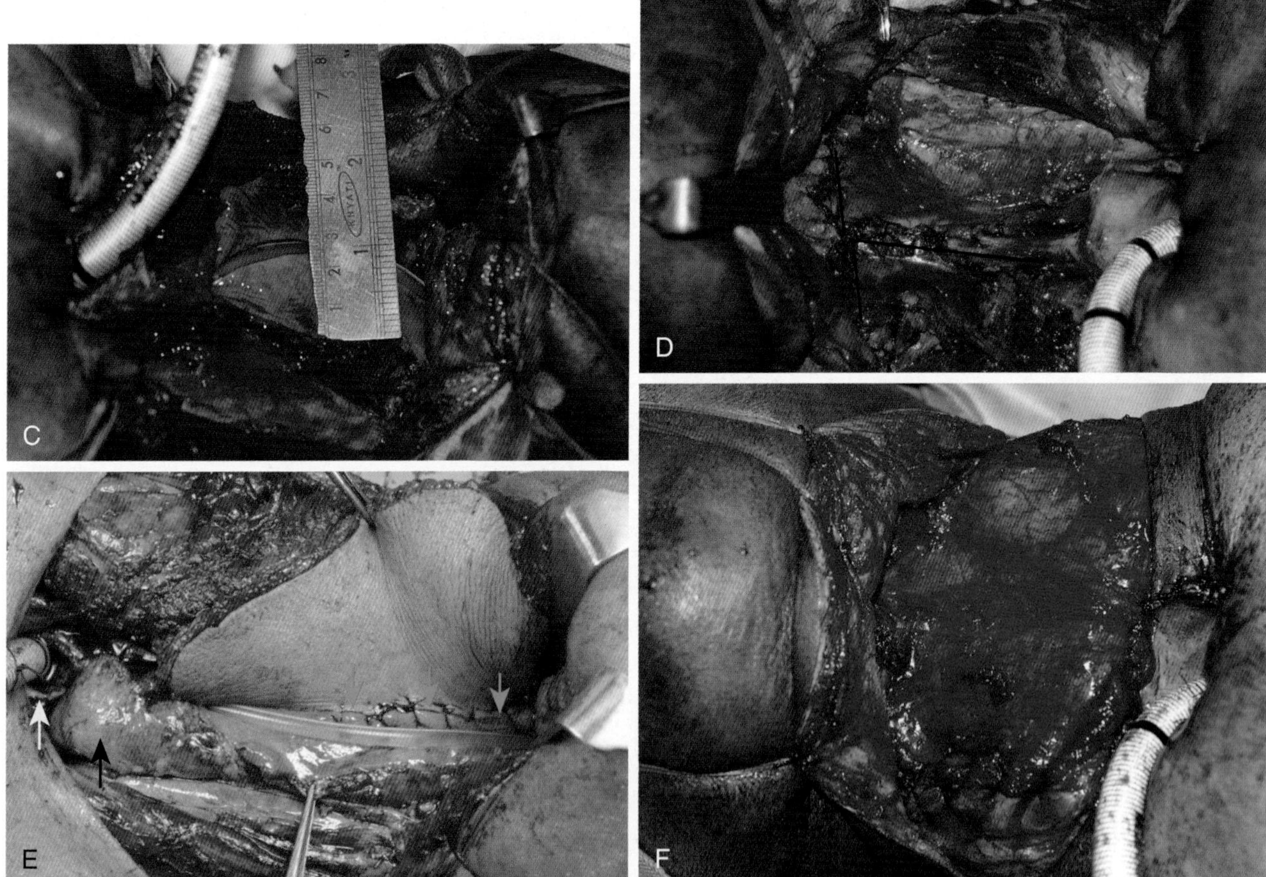

Figure 119.2 cont'd C and **D,** Remnant pharyngeal mucosa (unstretched) with 3.5 cm width is present after resection of a squamous cell carcinoma of the left aryepiglottic fold. This defect can be closed primarily. **E,** The skin of the pectoralis major myocutaneous flap is used as patch pharyngoplasty. It is sutured to the remnant pharyngeal mucosa *(green arrows)*. Also shown are the preserved left lobe of the thyroid gland *(black arrow)* and the tracheal cut end *(yellow arrow)*. **F,** Pectoralis major muscle used to reinforce a primary pharyngeal closure in a postradiotherapy patient to minimize pharyngocutaneous fistula.

Avoidance and Management of Intraoperative Complications

Drain Failure

Failure of the drains to hold vacuum represents a serious threat, as it may cause patients to develop a hematoma and interfere with wound healing. This condition results from a leak in the pharynx, skin, or the stoma closure, and it leads to dead space within the wound with increased chances of hematoma, infection, and, most important, carotid or internal jugular vein blowout. The leak needs to be promptly detected and corrected.

Hematoma

Although rare, hematoma can be caused by inappropriate hemostasis or ligature failure. This can lead to pressure separation of the pharyngeal repair and wound infection. Hematoma can be avoided by meticulous hemostasis and a Valsalva maneuver performed at the end of the surgery to look for any bleeding points.

A hematoma detected in the postoperative period needs to be evacuated after taking the patient back to the operating room and opening up the wound. Any detectable bleeder is ligated and new drains inserted, as the previous drains are likely to be blocked by clots.

Pharyngocutaneous Fistula

Typically, pharyngocutaneous fistula develops on the first postoperative week in nonradiated patients and the second postoperative week in previously radiated patients. Predisposing factors include inappropriate closure of the neopharynx, poor nutritional status, and previous radiotherapy. Clinical signs include erythema and edema around the suture line and an increasingly turbid drain output. When the skin sutures are opened, purulent material and saliva drain out of the wound.

Pharyngocutaneous fistula can be avoided by meticulous closure of the neopharynx. Tight closure is avoided. Three-point closures are reinforced with additional sutures. At sites with luminal mismatch, multiple Z-plasties can be carried out. In previously irradiated patients, fresh nonradiated tissue (usually pectoralis muscle) can be used to cover the pharyngeal closure. When feasible, the nutritional status of the patient should be optimized in the preoperative period and maintained postoperatively. Patients should be kept on a high-protein diet unless contraindicated. Skin and stoma closure should be meticulous so that the skin flap sticks well to the underlying tissue, thus eliminating the dead space.

Management of an established fistula is usually conservative. The patient is given nothing by mouth. Regular wound dressing changes are performed with packing of defects as needed. A proper antibiotic based on culture and sensitivity of the pus from the wound is started. A pressure dressing is sometimes useful, and the suction drain is kept for a prolonged period. If the conservative measures fail and the fistula persists for more than 2 weeks in a nonradiated patient or 3 weeks in a radiated patient, surgical closure using a pedicled or a free flap can be considered.

Hypocalcemia

Transient hypocalcemia (serum calcium <8 mg/dL [4.24 mmol/L] or ionized calcium <4 mg/dL [1.12 mmol/L]) is a fairly common complication following laryngopharyngectomy. It occurs as a result of vascular shock to the parathyroids, variations in serum protein binding due to alterations in postoperative acid-base status, or hypoalbuminemia.

Symptoms of mild hypocalcemia include perioral and upper and lower extremity tingling and numbness and a feeling of anxiety. Severe hypocalcemia presents with mental status changes, muscle cramps, tetany, hypotension, seizures, laryngospasm, and stridor. An electrocardiogram will show a prolonged QT interval. Chvostek and Trousseau signs may become positive with increasing neuromuscular irritability.

Hypocalcemia can be prevented in the intraoperative period by meticulously preserving the parathyroids when separating the preserved thyroid lobe from the tracheal surface and by preserving the inferior thyroid artery on the side of the preserved thyroid lobe.

Mild asymptomatic hypocalcemias are managed with an oral supplementation of calcium with vitamin D_3 (15 mg/kg/day of elemental calcium with 0.25 to 0.5 μg/day of vitamin D_3), gradually tapered as the serum calcium rises. Symptomatic or severe hypocalcemia (ionized calcium <1 mmol/L) is treated with 10 mL of 10% intravenous calcium gluconate in 50 to 100 mL of 5% dextrose in water over a period of 10 minutes, titrated according to the patient's symptoms or serum calcium levels.

Carotid Blowout

Carotid blowout is a dreaded complication that carries a high mortality and morbidity and usually occurs within the first postoperative week. Predisposing factors include wound infection, pharyngocutaneous fistula, and previous radiation. Careful handling of the carotids during the surgery by keeping the vessels moist and preserving the adventitia, which contains the vaso vasorum, is important for preventing blowout. In postradiated patients, covering the vessel with a vascularized flap is warranted. Preventing a salivary fistula by meticulous closure of the pharynx helps to protect the carotid from salivary contamination and later blowout.

Pharyngoesophageal Stricture

Stricture of the neopharynx can be a late sequel of a pharyngoesophageal fistula. Patients with benign stricture usually complain of a progressive dysphagia; however, a malignant stricture should always be ruled out in patients presenting with an acute onset of dysphagia. Intraoperatively, cricopharyngeal myotomy and proper closure of the neopharynx with inlay of a vascularized flap when necessary to enhance the luminal diameter of the neopharynx will help to reduce the chances of stricture. Benign strictures are managed by repeated dilation, but persistent strictures require secondary flap reconstruction.

Hypothyroidism

The combination of pre- or postoperative radiotherapy plus hemithyroidectomy usually conspires to produce eventual hypothyroidism.[16,17] Appropriately titrated thyroid hormone replacement is then required.

Postoperative Considerations

Apart from the routine postsurgical care, laryngopharyngectomy patients need specific care in the immediate postoperative period. This includes fluid balance, oxygenation, wound drain vacuum retention, and output measurement and skin flap monitoring. Tracheostoma care includes steam inhalation and humidification. Appropriate tracheobronchial suction helps prevent pulmonary complications, and early ambulation reduces the risk of deep vein thrombosis. Appropriate pain management is done. Nasogastric feeding for laryngectomy/partial pharyngectomy or jejunal feeding for total laryngopharyngoesophagectomy is initiated once the bowel sounds appear, usually in the first postoperative day. Oral feeding is usually started on 7th postoperative day in nonradiated patients and 12th to 14th postoperative day in previously radiated patients. In patients with a pharyngeal leak, oral feeds are withheld until the leak subsides. Neck drains are removed once the output is <20 mL on two consecutive days and is serous in nature, usually by the fifth to seventh postoperative day. Barring complications, patients are generally discharged by the 7th to 10th postoperative day.

References

1. Cheever DW. Cancer of the tonsil: removal of the tumor by external incision (a second case). *Boston Med Surg J*. 1878;99:133.
2. Uppaluri R, Sunwoo JB. Neoplasms of the hypopharynx and cervical esophagus. In: Cummings CW, Flint PW, eds. *Otolaryngology Nead and Neck Surgery*. 4th ed. Philadelphia, Pennsylvania: Elsevier; 2005.
3. Ariyan S. The pectoralis major myocutaneous flap. A versatile flap for reconstruction in the head and neck. *Plast Reconstr Surg*. 1979;63(1):73–81.
4. Withers EH, Franklin JD, Madden Jr JJ, Lynch JB. Pectoralis major musculocutaneous flap: a new flap in head and neck reconstruction. *Am J Surg*. 1979;138(4):537–543.
5. Fabian RL. Reconstruction of the laryngopharynx and cervical esophagus. *Laryngoscope*. 1984;94(10):1334–1350.
6. Spriano G, Piantanida R, Pellini R. Hypopharyngeal reconstruction using pectoralis major myocutaneous flap and pre-vertebral fascia. *Laryngoscope*. 2001;111(3):544–547.
7. Yang G, Chen B, Gao Y, et al. Forearm free skin flap transplantation. *Zhonghua Yixue Zazhi*. 1981;61:139.
8. Harii K, Ebihara S, Ono I, Saito H, Terui S, Takato T. Pharyngoesophageal reconstruction using a fabricated forearm free flap. *Plast Reconstr Surg*. 1985;75(4):463–476.
9. Song YG, Chen GZ, Song YL. The free thigh flap: a new free flap concept based on the septocutaneous artery. *Br J Plast Surg*. 1984;37(2):149–159.
10. Seidenberg B, Rosenak SS, Hurwitt ES, Som ML. Immediate reconstruction of the cervical esophagus by a revascularized isolated jejunal segment. *Ann Surg*. 1959;149(2):162–171.
11. Baudet J. Reconstruction of the pharyngeal wall by free transfer of the greater omentum and stomach. *Int J Microsurg*. 1979;1:53.
12. Ong GB, Lee TC. Pharyngogastric anastomosis after oesophago-pharyngectomy for carcinoma of the hypopharynx and cervical oesophagus. *Br J Surg*. 1960;48:193–200.
13. Le Quesne LP, Ranger D. Pharyngolaryngectomy, with immediate pharyngogastric anastomosis. *Br J Surg*. 1966;53(2):105–109.
14. Ho CM, Ng WF, Lam KH, Wei WJ, Yuen AP. Submucosal tumor extension in hypopharyngeal cancer. *Arch Otolaryngol Head Neck Surg*. 1997;123(9):959–965.
15. Hui Y, Wei WI, Yuen PW, Lam LK, Ho WK. Primary closure of pharyngeal remnant after total laryngectomy and partial pharyngectomy: how much residual mucosa is sufficient? *Laryngoscope*. 1996;106(4):490–494.
16. Sinard RJ, Tobin EJ, Mazzaferri EL, et al. Hypothyroidism after treatment for nonthyroid head and neck cancer. *Arch Otolaryngol Head Neck Surg*. 2000;126(5):652–657.
17. Tell R, Sjödin H, Lundell G, Lewin F, Lewensohn R. Hypothyroidism after external radiotherapy for head and neck cancer. *Int J Radiat Oncol Biol Phys*. 1997;39(2):303–308.

CHAPTER 120

Buccal Fat Pad Flap

Adam P. Fagin and Peter B. Franco

Armamentarium

#15 Scalpel blades
Appropriate sutures
Bipolar electrocautery
Dissecting forceps
Ligature forceps, hemostat
Lip and cheek retractor
Local anesthetic with vasoconstrictor
Metzenbaum scissors
Mouth gag
Needle electrocautery
Periosteal elevator
Soft tissue retractor

History of the Procedure

Lorenz Heister first identified the buccal fat pad (BFP) in 1727. He thought it was glandular in nature and identified it as the "glandula molaris" in his *Compendium Anatomicum.* In 1801, Marie-Francois-Xavier Bichat was the first to provide the anatomic description of the BFP as a fatty tissue.[1] Since then, it has been referred to in the medical literature by different names, including the boule de Bichat, masticatory fat pad, sucking pad, and sucking cushion.

The BFP had limited clinical use for many years. It was considered a surgical nuisance because it could be accidentally encountered during various surgical procedures in the oral cavity and pterygomaxillary space.[2,3] Its use increased after Egyedi[4] described methods of using the BFP for closing oronasal and oroantral communications and as a versatile pedicle graft for closing postsurgical maxillary defects. Tideman et al.[5] described its detailed anatomy and vascular supply and the appropriate operative technique. Rapidis et al.,[6] Hao,[7] Dean et al.,[8] and Toshihiro et al.[9] used the pedicle BFP for reconstruction of small- and medium-sized postsurgical oral defects of malignant lesions.

Indications for the Use of the Procedure

Within the past decade, many reports have described the use of the BFP as a flap for oral reconstruction after tumor removal or for other oral lesions. The BFP has also been successfully used as an unlined pedicle graft for maxillary defects, such as defects in the alveolar crest, maxilla, hard and soft palate, cleft, retromolar region of the mandible, and vestibular sulcus.[10] In addition, the BFP has often been used to repair palatal defects.[11]

Surgery involving the hard palate frequently can leave oroantral or oronasal defects, resulting in considerable difficulty in speech and deglutition. Because of its close proximity to oral defects, the BFP can be used for reconstruction. It can also be used to effectively reconstruct small- to medium-sized posterior maxillary alveolar defects.[12] Thus, the BFP can be used to cover defects resulting from traumatic injury or malignant tumors of the soft tissue of the oral cavity. Pedicle fat pad grafts are advantageous because they reduce the invasiveness and duration of the operation, and BFPs used to reconstruct defects have been shown to reduce pain and operative trauma. In addition, the rich blood circulation to the soft tissue promotes the healing of nearby structures. The grafted fat pad also functions as a site for granulation (thus limiting scar contraction) and can physically close dead space of a defective area.[13] Furthermore, the BFP has strong antiinfection and reconstruction advantages, with little necrosis or reabsorption (Fig. 120.1).[11]

Clinical Uses of the Buccal Fat Pad Flap (Fig. 120.2)

1. Closure of oral antral communication/oral antral fistula (OAF)[4]
2. Closure of oral nasal communication[8]
3. Closure of mucosal defects[5–9,12]
4. Treatment of oral submucosal fibrosis[14,15]
5. Repair of primary cleft[16]
6. Reconstruction of the temporomandibular joint[17–19]
7. Membrane in sinus floor augmentation[20]
8. Coverage of severe gingival recession defect[21,22]
9. Closure of anterior and middle skull base defects[23,24]
10. Treatment in osteonecrosis and medication-related osteonecrosis of the jaws[25–29]
11. Coverage of zygomatic implants (extrasinus technique)[30]

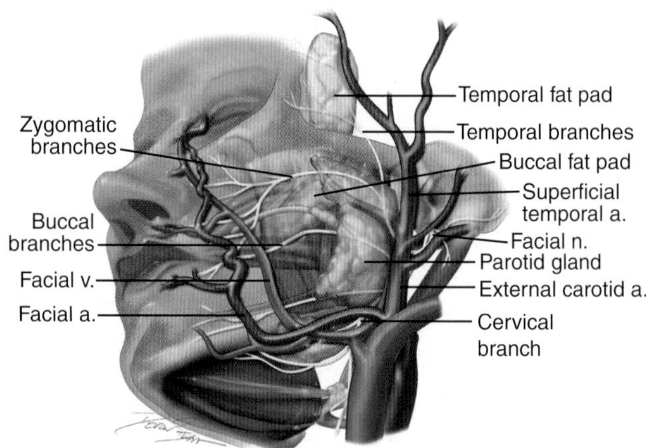

Figure 120.1 Schematic representation of the buccal fat pad (BFP) with important landmarks in the face.

12. Prevention of Frey syndrome[31,32]
13. Augmentation of facial contour deformity[33]
14. Treatment of peri-implantitis[34]

Limitations and Contraindications

The BFP is versatile in terms of its location and application. It can be used as far anteriorly as the superior alveolar ridge canine tooth region and up to, but not beyond, the midline of the palate extending laterally to the superior buccal sulcus and buccal mucosa. Posteriorly, it can be used in the hard palate, the tuberosity region, the retromolar area, the soft palate (up to the midline), and the anterior tonsillar pillar.[35] The critical factor in successful use of the BFP seems to be the size of the defect treated; although the literature reports that defects 7 × 5 × 2 cm have healed successfully, most authors recommend 5 × 4 cm defects (medium-sized) for reconstruction with the BFP.

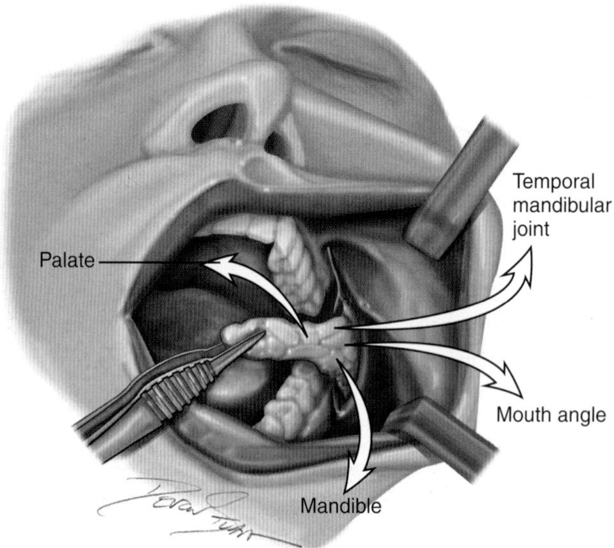

Figure 120.2 Applicability of the buccal fat pad (BFP).

Limitations of the pedicle BFP include the following:

- Only small to medium defects can be covered.
- The pedicle BFP can be used only for coverage of defects, not for adding bulk.
- The procedure may result in a small depression.[8]

TECHNIQUE: Buccal Fat Pad Flap

STEP 1: Incision

Under either local or general anesthesia, an upper mucosal incision posterior to the area of the zygomatic buttress is made, followed by a simple incision through the periosteum and fascial envelope of the BFP. At times the surgical exposure for the excision or additional reconstruction techniques has already exposed this area in which case only the fascial envelope of the BFP needs to be bluntly entered with a forceps (Fig. 120.3C).

STEP 2: Exposure and Mobilization of Buccal Fat

Once the fascial capsule has been entered the surgeon works with a curved forceps or Metzenbaum scissors to spread around the buccal fat. Spreading around the fat and widening the fascial opening under gentle traction will serve to gently coax the buccal fat from its anatomic environment and into the oral cavity where it can be utilized. This technique is important because the buccal fat itself is friable. Pulling on the exposed fat will thin the pedicle and disrupt its vascular plexus, which can compromise its eventual regenerative potential. Direct mechanical suction should also be avoided as this too can damage and thin the pedicle of the fat pad.

STEP 3: Inset

Continue progressive teasing and spreading around the buccal fat until an adequate reconstructive volume and pedicle length to reach and cover the target defect are achieved. Verify that tension-free coverage of the defect can be obtained, and continue the dissection process above if additional pedicle length is required, but do not pull on the fat pad. Now, spread the distal portion of the fat pad over the defect to obtain the desired reconstruction (Fig. 120.3D). Secure the graft into place with interrupted, circumferential, resorbable tacking sutures such as 3-0 polygalactin.

STEP 4: Closure

If the buccal fat is to be used as a deep layer of a layered closure, then the superficial layer can now be mobilized and closed over the fat pad (Fig. 120.3E). However, direct closure of the opening used to access the BFP is not needed and typically should be avoided as not to strangulate the graft's pedicle.

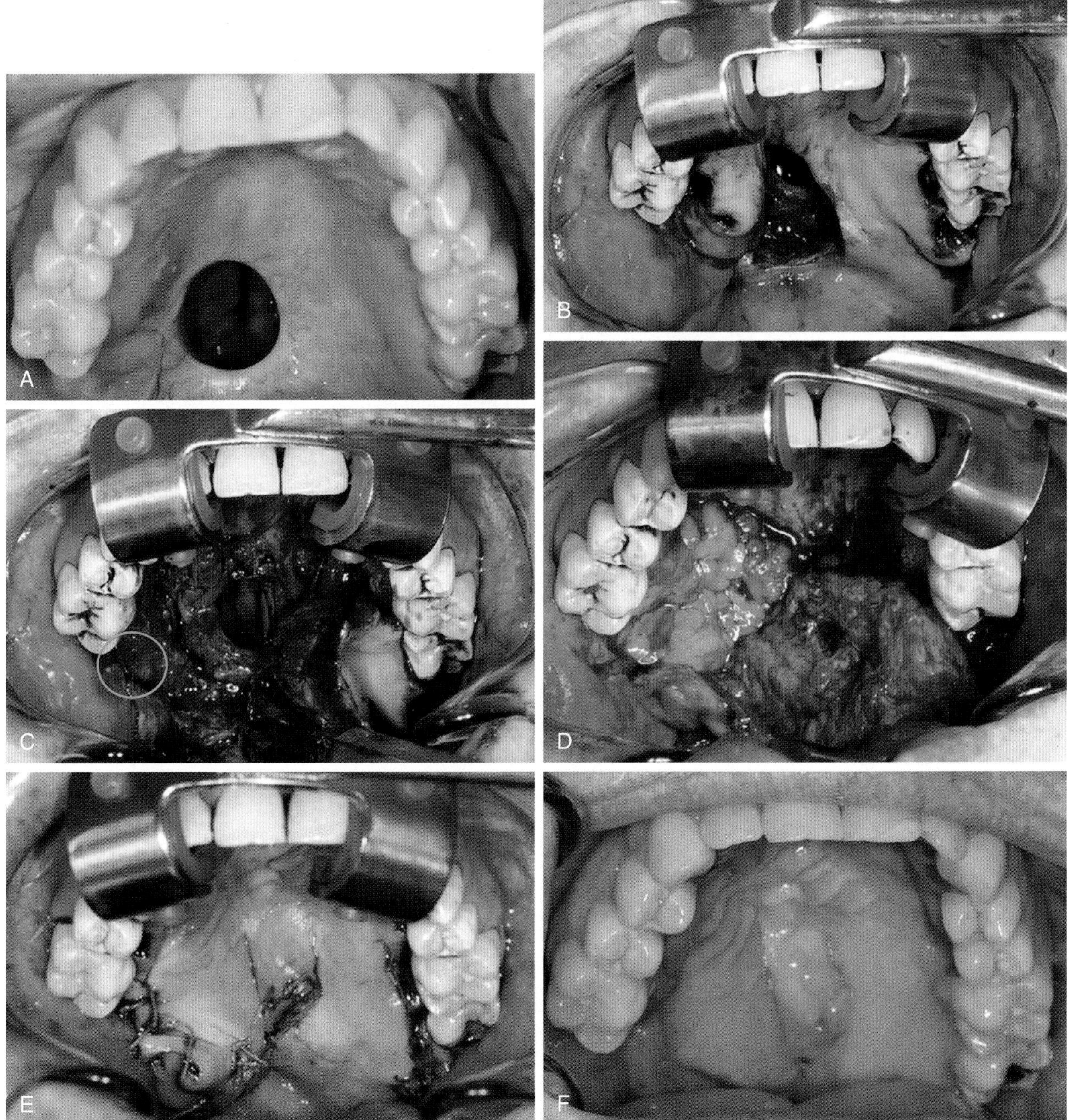

Figure 120.3 **A,** A 3 × 2 cm oronasal fistula defect. **B,** Sulcular, palatal incision from molar to molar and excision of fistula tissue. **C,** Reflection of the palatal flap demonstrating fistula defect and displaying easy access to the buccal fat pad (BFP), just behind the zygomatic buttress and first molar, indicated with a circle. **D,** Inset of the BFP over the defect creating the nasal layer of the planned two-layered closure. **E,** Oral layer, creating the second layer of closure, with advancement of the palatal flap medially on all sides leaving the sulcular aspect of the palate to granulate. **F,** Two weeks postoperative with complete closure of the oronasal fistula. (Photos courtesy of Daniel Petrisor, DMD, MD, FACS, FICD)

ALTERNATIVE TECHNIQUE 1: Temporomandibular Joint Reconstruction

The BFP is approached through the same preauricular incision as is used for temporomandibular joint (TMJ) ankylosis exposure. The main body of the BFP and its temporal extension lie in close proximity to the coronoid process and temporalis muscle tendon. Blunt dissection is performed with a curved hemostat anterior and medial to the coronoid process to breach the periosteum. External pressure is applied over the cheek area by an assistant. The BFP can be easily manipulated and brought to the TMJ region. Depending on the amount of fat required, the temporal or buccal process (or both) are used. The BFP is sutured to the adjacent tissue with one or two absorbable sutures using a curved, round-body needle.[17–19]

ALTERNATIVE TECHNIQUE 2: Skull Base Reconstruction

With an orbitozygomatic bone flap or supraorbital or lateral orbital flap, the superior margin of the BFP bulges over the site of the osteotomy, and its dissection is performed by mobilization of its body and temporal and buccal processes on the vascularized pedicle, which is presented by the pterygopalatine process. The latter is long enough to translocate the BFP to the skull base defect.[23] A fenestrated or gripping forceps is used to grab the temporal process and body, which are gently pulled out together with the buccal process.[24]

Avoidance and Management of Complications

Among the few complications associated with use of the BFP are recurrence of OAF and partial loss of the flap, which have mostly been seen with large defects.[36–39] A rare visible change in facial contour has been reported in patients only when the BFP is used for reconstruction of a large defect. The surgeon might consider a contralateral buccal lipectomy to correct this alteration. Cheek deformity has also been reported.[16,40] Trismus from scarring has been reported, mainly when the BFP is used for reconstruction of retromolar trigone or buccal mucosa defects. Occasional hematoma and hemorrhage also have been reported; these were found to be caused by problems with one of the pedicles of the flap,[35] and they responded to conservative treatment. Mild obliteration of the vestibule, which corrects in due course of time, has also been reported.

Postoperative Considerations

For the intraoral use of a BFP reconstruction, the surgeon should consider several additional considerations. The patient should adhere to a soft diet for 2 weeks to avoid trauma associated with mastication on the reconstruction. In addition, the patient should be instructed to refrain from smoking for at least 2 weeks. Finally, if the reconstruction involves the antrum or nasal cavity, the patient should be placed on standard sinus precautions and avoid any forceful nose blowing or intentional change in the pressure of their sinus cavity for 4 weeks. Additionally, a short postoperative course of antibiotics that provides coverage for sinus flora should be considered for 3 to 7 days (e.g., amoxicillin clavulanic acid). Optionally, a chlorhexidine gluconate 0.12% mouth rinse may be prescribed.

References

1. Marzano UG. Lorenz Heister's "molar gland". *Plast Reconstr Surg*. 2005; *115*(5), 1389–1393. https://doi.org/10.1097/01.prs.0000157014.77871.8d.
2. Wolford DG, Stapleford RG, Forte RA, Heath M. Traumatic herniation of the buccal fat pad: report of case. *J Am Dent Assoc*. 1981;103(4):593–594.
3. Messenger KL, Cloyd W. Traumatic herniation of the buccal fat pad. Report of a case. *Oral Surg Oral Med Oral Pathol*. 1977;43(1):41–43.
4. Egyedi P. Utilization of the buccal fat pad for closure of oro-antral and/or oro-nasal communications. *J Maxillofac Surg*. 1977;5(4):241–244.
5. Tideman H, Bosanquet A, Scott J. Use of the buccal fat pad as a pedicled graft. *J Oral Maxillofac Surg*. 1986;44(6):435–440.
6. Rapidis AD, Alexandridis CA, Eleftheriadis E, Angelopoulos AP. The use of the buccal fat pad for reconstruction of oral defects: review of the literature and report of 15 cases. *J Oral Maxillofac Surg*. 2000;58(2):158–163.
7. Hao SP. Reconstruction of oral defects with the pedicled buccal fat pad flap. *Otolaryngol Head Neck Surg*. 2000;122(6):863–867.
8. Dean A, Alamillos F, García-López A, Sánchez J, Peñalba M. The buccal fat pad flap in oral reconstruction. *Head Neck*. 2001;23(5):383–388.
9. Toshihiro Y, Nariai Y, Takamura Y, et al. Applicability of buccal fat pad grafting for oral reconstruction. *Int J Oral Maxillofac Implants*. 2013;42(5):604–610.
10. Baumann A, Ewers R. Application of the buccal fat pad in oral reconstruction. *J Oral Maxillofac Surg*. 2000;58(4):389–392.
11. Hai HK. Repair of palatal defects with unlined buccal fat pad grafts. *Oral Surg Oral Med Oral Pathol*. 1988;65(5):523–525.
12. Amin MA, Bailey BMW, Swinson B, Witherow H. Use of the buccal fat pad in the reconstruction and prosthetic rehabilitation of oncological maxillary defects. *Br J Oral Maxillofac Surg*. 2005;43(2):148–154.
13. Shibahara T, Watanabe Y, Yamaguchi S, et al. Use of the buccal fat pad as a pedicle graft. *Bull Tokyo Dent Coll*. 1996;37(4):161–165.
14. Lai DR, Chen HR, Lin LM, Huang YL, Tsai CC. Clinical evaluation of different treatment methods for oral submucous fibrosis. A 10-year experience with 150 cases. *J Oral Pathol Med*. 1995;24(9):402–406.
15. Mehta AK, Panwar SS, Verma RK, Pal AK. Buccal fat pad reconstruction in oral submucosal fibrosis. *Med J Armed Forces India*. 2003;59(4):340–341.
16. Levi B, Kasten SJ, Buchman SR. Utilization of the buccal fat pad flap for congenital cleft palate repair. *Plast Reconstr Surg*. 2009;123(3):1018–1021.
17. Singh V, Dhingra R, Sharma B, Bhagol A, Kumar P. Retrospective analysis of use of buccal fat pad as an interpositional graft in temporomandibular joint ankylosis: preliminary study. *J Oral Maxillofac Surg*. 2011;69(10):2530–2536.
18. Singh V, Dhingra R, Bhagol A. Prospective analysis of temporomandibular joint reconstruction in ankylosis with sternoclavicular graft and buccal fat pad lining. *J Oral Maxillofac Surg*. 2012;70(4):997–1006.
19. Rattan V. A simple technique for use of buccal pad of fat in temporomandibular joint reconstruction. *J Oral Maxillofac Surg*. 2006;64(9):1447–1451.

20. Hassani A, Khojasteh A, Alikhasi M, Vaziri H. Measurement of volume changes of sinus floor augmentation covered with buccal fat pad: a case series study. *Oral Surg Oral Med Oral Pathol Oral Radiol Endod*. 2009;107(3):369–374.
21. Panda S, Del Fabbro M, Satpathy A, Das AC. Pedicled buccal fat pad graft for root coverage in severe gingival recession defect. *J Indian Soc Periodontol*. 2016;20(2):216–219.
22. Deepa D, Arun Kumar KV. Clinical evaluation of class II and class III gingival recession defects of maxillary posterior teeth treated with pedicled buccal fat pad: a pilot study. *Dent Res J*. 2018;15(1):11–16.
23. Jackson IT. Anatomy of the buccal fat pad and its clinical significance. *Plast Reconstr Surg*. 1999;103(7):2059–2060.
24. Cherekaev VA, Golbin DA, Belov AI. Translocated pedicled buccal fat pad: closure of anterior and middle skull base defects after tumor resection. *J Craniofac Surg*. 2012;23(1):98–104.
25. Nabil S, Ramli R. The use of buccal fat pad flap in the treatment of osteoradionecrosis. *Int J Oral Maxillofac Implants*. 2012;41(11):1422–1426.
26. Rotaru H, Kim MK, Kim SG, Park YW. Pedicled buccal fat pad flap as a reliable surgical strategy for the treatment of medication-related osteonecrosis of the jaw. *J Oral Maxillofac Surg*. 2015;73(3):437–442.
27. Duarte LFM, Alonso K, Basso EC, Dib LL. Surgical treatment of bisphosphonate-related osteonecrosis of the jaws with the use of buccal fat pad: case report. *Braz Dent J*. 2015;26(3):317–320.
28. Berrone M, Florindi FU, Carbone V, Aldiano C, Pentenero M. Stage 3 medication-related osteonecrosis of the posterior maxilla: surgical treatment using a pedicled buccal fat pad flap: case reports. *J Oral Maxillofac Surg*. 2015;73(11):2082–2086.
29. Gallego L, Junquera L, Pelaz A, Hernando J, Megías J. The use of pedicled buccal fat pad combined with sequestrectomy in bisphosphonate-related osteonecrosis of the maxilla. *Med Oral Patol Oral Cir Bucal*. 2012;17(2):e236–e241.
30. de Moraes EJ. The buccal fat pad flap: an option to prevent and treat complications regarding complex zygomatic implant surgery. Preliminary report. *Int J Oral Maxillofac Implants*. 2012;27(4):905–910.
31. Kim JT, Naidu S, Kim YH. The buccal fat: a convenient and effective autologous option to prevent Frey syndrome and for facial contouring following parotidectomy. *Plast Reconstr Surg*. 2010;125(6):1706–1709.
32. Torretta S, Pignataro L, Capaccio P, Brevi A, Mazzola R. The buccal fat: a convenient and effective autologous option to prevent Frey syndrome and for facial contouring following parotidectomy. *Plast Reconstr Surg*. 2011;127(2):998.
33. Komatsu S, Ikemura K, Kimata Y. Pedicled buccal fat pad for the augmentation of facial depression deformity: a case report. *Medicine (Baltim)*. 2017;96(30):e7599.
34. Kablan F. The use of buccal fat pad free graft in regenerative treatment of peri-implantitis: a new and predictable technique. *Ann Maxillofac Surg*. 2015;5(2):179–184.
35. Chakrabarti J, Tekriwal R, Ganguli A, Ghosh S, Mishra PK. Pedicled buccal fat pad flap for intraoral malignant defects: a series of 29 cases. *Indian J Plast Surg*. 2009;42(1):36–42.
36. Poeschl PW, Baumann A, Russmueller G, Poeschl E, Klug C, Ewers R. Closure of oroantral communications with Bichat's buccal fat pad. *J Oral Maxillofac Surg*. 2009;67(7):1460–1466.
37. Colella G, Tartaro G, Giudice A. The buccal fat pad in oral reconstruction. *Br J Plast Surg*. 2004;57(4):326–329.
38. Zhong LP, Chen GF, Fan LJ, Zhao SF. Immediate reconstruction of maxilla with bone grafts supported by pedicled buccal fat pad graft. *Oral Surg Oral Med Oral Pathol Oral Radiol Endod*. 2004;97(2):147–154.
39. Martín-Granizo R, Naval L, Costas A, et al. Use of buccal fat pad to repair intraoral defects: review of 30 cases. *Br J Oral Maxillofac Surg*. 1997;35(2):81–84.
40. Dubin B, Jackson IT, Halim A, Triplett WW, Ferreira M. Anatomy of the buccal fat pad and its clinical significance. *Plast Reconstr Surg*. 1989;83(2):257–264.

CHAPTER 121

Tongue Flap

Daniel J. Meara

Armamentarium

#15 Scalpel blade
2-0 silk suture
3-0 Vicryl suture
Adson pickups
DeBakey pickups
Dingman mouth gag
Hemostats
Intermaxillary fixation screws or Erich arch bars
Local anesthetic with vasoconstrictor
Mayo suture scissors
Molt or Denhart mouth gag
Needle electrocautery
Needle driver
Stainless steel wires or elastic bands
Tenotomy tissue scissors

History of the Procedure

The tongue flap is a specialized pedicled flap for reconstruction of the oral cavity and is frequently utilized for the correction of congenital or acquired defects. The tongue has a robust vasculature supply, making the flap durable and readily utilized as a primary method of reconstruction or as a salvage procedure when other reconstruction efforts have failed. Inherent flap effects on oral function limit its clinical application and tolerance by patients. However, the technique has been documented since the early 1900s. Eiselsberg, in 1901, described a pedicled tongue flap for the reconstruction of intraoral defects and Lexer reported the use of a tongue flap for retromolar and tonsillar defects in 1909.[1] In 1956 Klopp and Schurter reintroduced the technique in the reconstruction of soft palate defects and in 1966 Guerrero-Santos and Altamirano discussed the technique for the closure of hard palatal fistulas.[2] Jackson, in 1972, suggested the utility of tongue flaps for the closure of palatal fistulae in children.[3] Subsequent articles have reviewed the use of tongue flaps for the correction of floor-of-mouth defects, lip defects, cleft-related fistulas, and tongue defects.[4] Specifically, Lam et al. describe a sliding anterior hemitongue flap for hemitongue glossectomy defects after a squamous cell carcinoma resection and Buchbinder and St-Hilaire describe a sliding posterior tongue flap for lateral defects up to 6 cm.[4,1] Comini et al. suggested an algorithm for the treatment of oral and perioral defects through local flaps, with the tongue flap being a key contributor (Fig. 121.1).[5]

Indications for the Use of the Procedure

The tongue flap is indicated in the treatment of congenital and acquired defects of the oral cavity, such as residual fistulas in cleft palate patients or for reconstruction status post tumor resection or traumatic injury repair. General categories to consider for the use of a pedicled tongue flap include[1,3,4]:

- oronasal communications,
- oroantral communications,
- floor-of-mouth or buccal mucosal defects,
- lip defects, and
- tongue defects.

Limitations and Contraindications

Patient tolerance is likely to be the main limitation of the use of a tongue flap in reconstructive surgery. No absolute contraindications exist, but relative contraindications include: (1) prior tongue flap, (2) tobacco use, due to its effects on wound healing, and (3) significant medical comorbidities, such as anxiety disorders, diabetes, seizures, and severe malnutrition, which may be affected by tongue flap surgery and associated maxillomandibular fixation (MMF), if utilized.

TECHNIQUE

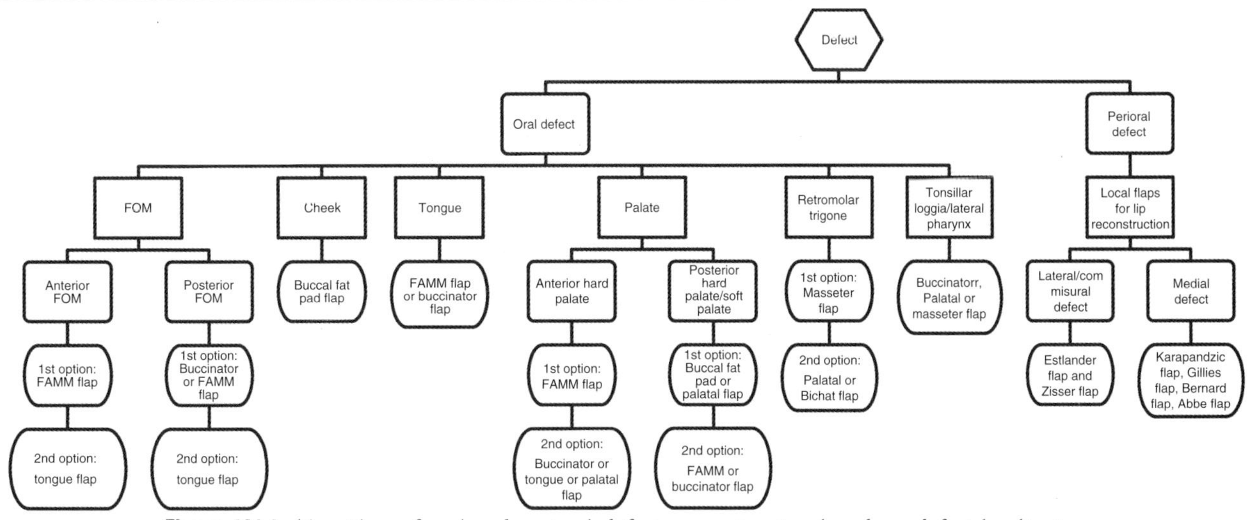

Figure 121.1 Algorithm of oral and perioral defects reconstruction based on defect localization. (From Comini L, Spinelli G, Mannelli G. Algorithm for the treatment of oral and peri-oral defects through local flaps. *J Cranio Maxillofac Surg*. 2018;46:2127–2137.)

TECHNIQUE: Tongue Flap

The surgical design of a tongue flap is dictated by the defect, but two main flap types exist: (1) anterior based and (2) posterior based (Fig. 121.2).[2] Posterior-based flaps are typically utilized for defects of the soft palate, retromolar area, and posterior buccal mucosa.[2] Anterior-based flaps are more ideal for defects of the hard palate, upper

Continued

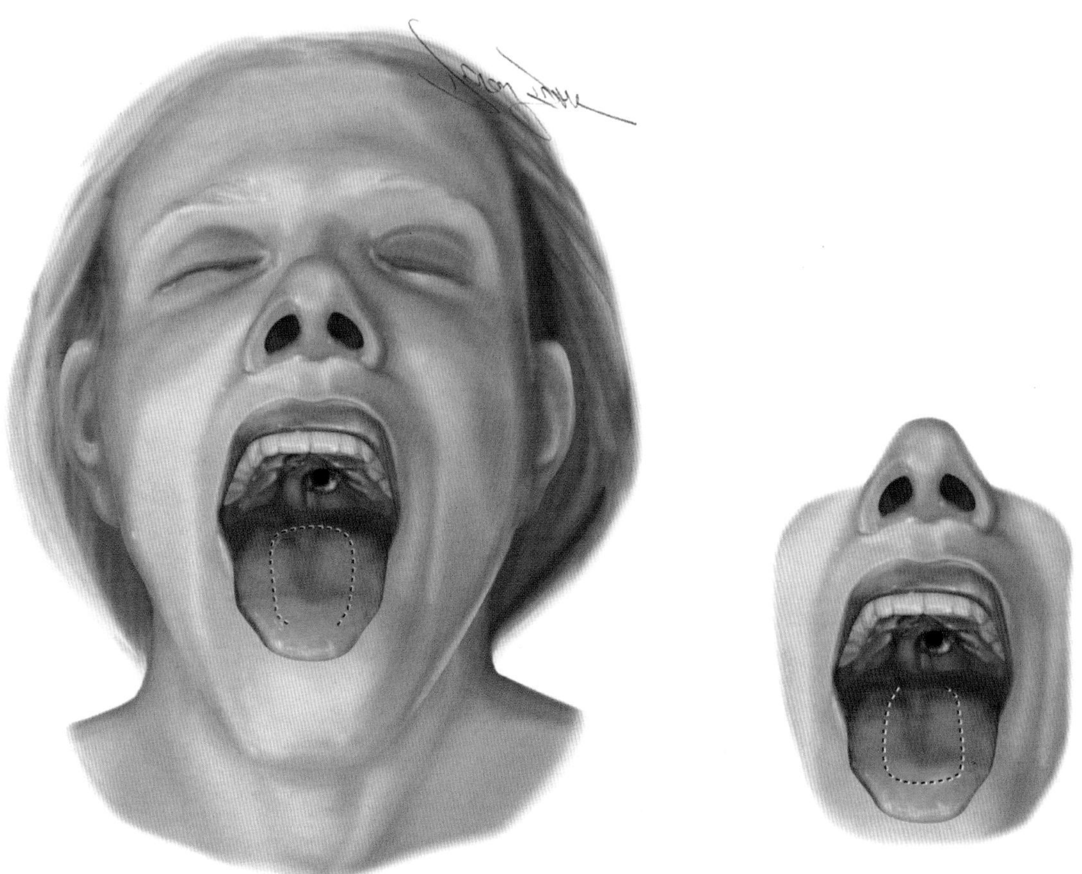

Figure 121.2 Left, posterior-based tongue flap. Right, anterior-based tongue flap. (From Steinhauser E. Experience with dorsal tongue flaps for closure of defects of the hard palate. *J Oral Maxillofac Surg*. 1982;40:787–789.)

TECHNIQUE: Tongue Flap—*cont'd*

and lower lips, and anterior buccal mucosa.[2] The central or paramedial tongue flap, either anterior or posterior dorsal, is a random pattern flap with robust vascularity from branches of the lingual artery.[6] The lateral tongue flap, however, may be an axial pattern flap, if the dorsal lingual artery is included.[1]

STEP 1: Intubation

To facilitate access and visibility and possible MMF, a nasoendotracheal intubation is preferred. The tube is secured after proper placement is confirmed.

STEP 2: Surgical Field Exposure

The Molt or Denhart mouth gag is placed and the tongue and the defect requiring reconstruction are exposed. A 2-0 silk stay suture is placed through the tongue, approximately 1 cm posterior to the tip, for retraction and additional exposure. A throat pack is placed after the oral cavity is suctioned free and the tail of the pack is left visible as a reminder for removal at the end of the case, especially before placement into MMF. Then, 2% lidocaine with 1:100,000 epinephrine is infiltrated into the surgical sites for local anesthesia and vasoconstriction. The application of Erich arch bars, intermaxillary fixation screws, or ivy loops is completed if MMF is part of the treatment plan. MMF is recommended as a means to limit tongue movement and minimize tension on the flap during the initial healing phase. Failure to do so for any tongue flap, depending on patient compliance, increases the risk of incomplete flap incorporation or even frank detachment.

STEP 3: Flap Design, Anterior-Based Flap

The flap design is delineated with a marking pen. Electrocautery is then utilized to develop the flap with attention to key anatomical design elements (Figs. 121.3A and B). Specifically, flap thickness should be approximately 3 mm, with a gradual increase to 5 mm at the base.[7] Length is dictated by the location and extent of the defect but may extend, posteriorly, to within 1 cm of the circumvallate papilla and anteriorly to within 1 cm of the tip of the tongue (Fig. 121.4).[7] The flap width should be slightly greater than the defect size and the length should facilitate passive positioning of the flap at the reconstruction site.[7] Deepithelialization is performed, as needed. Hemostasis is obtained at the donor site with electrocautery and pressure to minimize blood loss. The throat pack is removed.

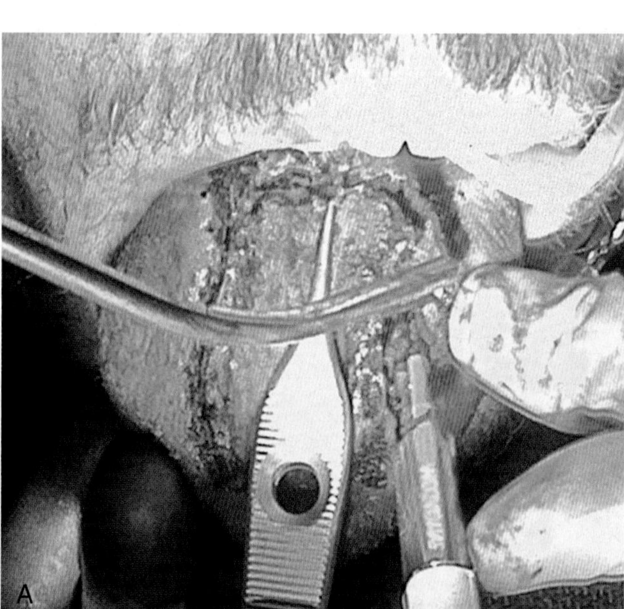

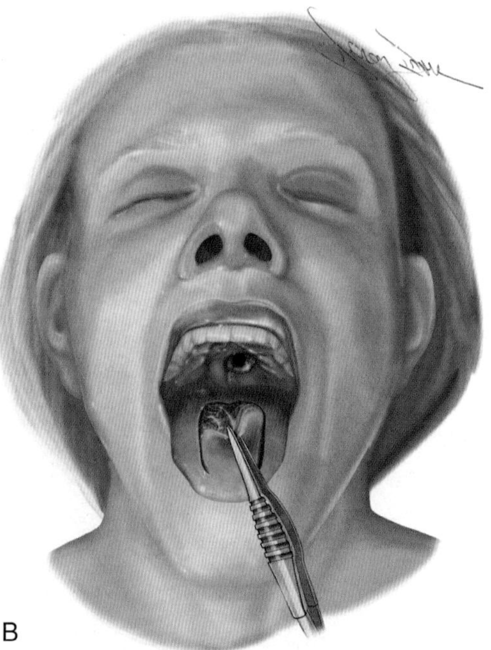

Figure 121.3 **A,** Marking pen outline and initial incision and elevation of posteriorly based tongue flap for the reconstruction of oronasal communication status post gunshot wound. **B,** Surgical site marked on the dorsal surface of the tongue. Elevation of a median tongue flap. (Courtesy Dr. Daniel J. Meara; from Elyassi A, Helling E, Closmann J. Closure of difficult palatal fistulas using a "parachuting and anchoring" technique with the tongue flap. *Oral Surg Oral Med Oral Pathol Oral Radiol.* 2011;112:711–714)

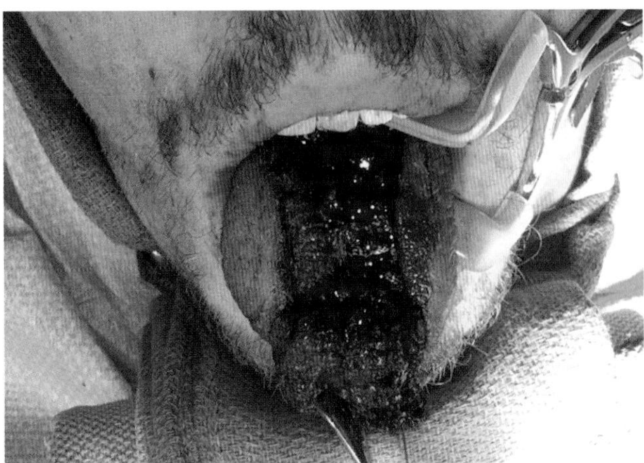

Figure 121.4 Clinical example of the elevated median, anterior-based tongue flap, demonstrating thickness and preservation of key landmarks. (Courtesy of Dr. Daniel J. Meara.)

TECHNIQUE: Tongue Flap—*cont'd*

STEP 4: Flap Inset

The tongue flap is positioned within the defect and all horizontal mattress sutures are placed before any of the knots are tied, so as to maximize visibility and to facilitate a secure and stable flap inset, especially in palatal defects where access is limited and worsens with each tied knot. 3-0 Vicryl is the suture of choice for inset due to its strength and adsorption properties. The anterior aspect of the defect and both lateral margins are the key stitches to secure the flap, as the posterior aspect will be addressed at the flap division and contouring stage, in approximately 2 to 3 weeks.[7] The donor site is then primarily closed, via a running stitch, with 3-0 Vicryl (Figs. 121.5A–C). Avoidance of overclosure at the pedicle base is critical to flap perfusion and, ultimately, flap success. MMF is then applied, if desired.

Continued

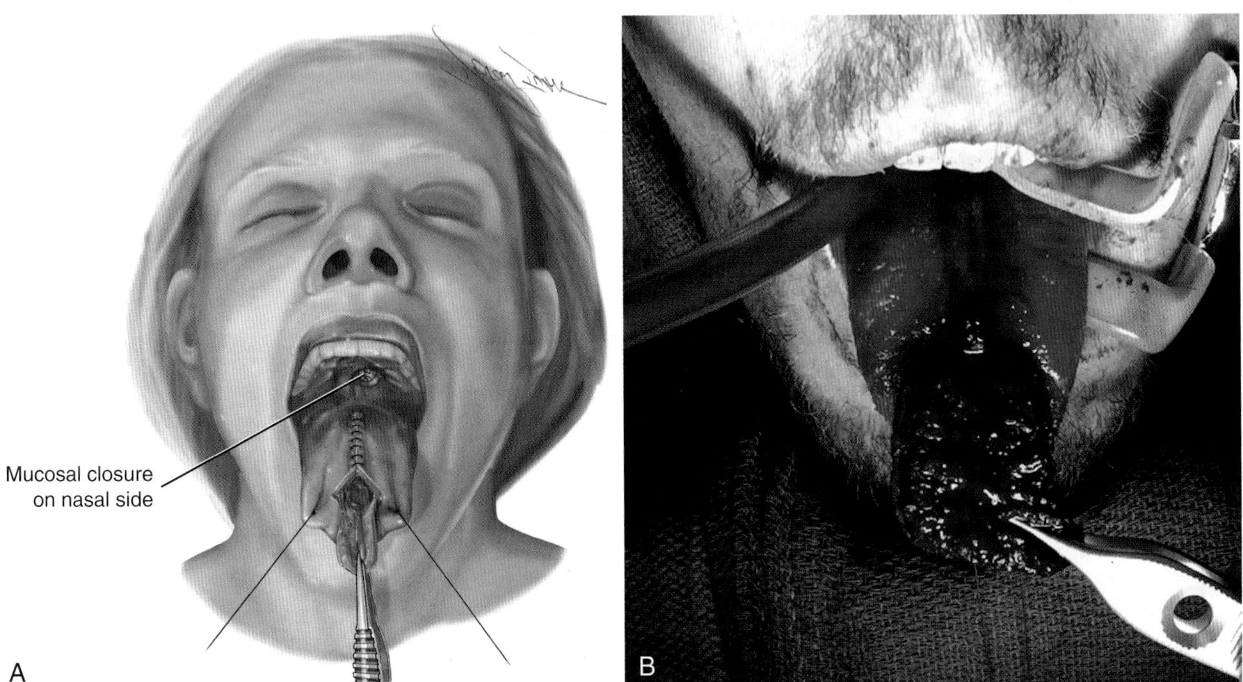

Figure 121.5 **A,** Top, median tongue flap with donor site closed and flap deepithelialized, ready for inset. **B,** Clinical example of medial tongue flap with donor site closed and ready for inset.

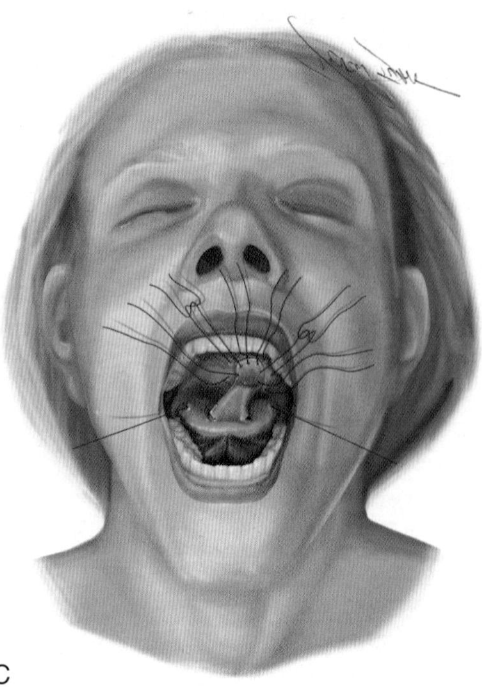

Figure 121.5, cont'd **C,** Top, tongue flap with donor site closed and flap deepithelialized, ready to be secured to catheter and inset into defect. (From Elyassi A, Helling E, Closmann J. Closure of difficult palatal fistulas using a "parachuting and anchoring" technique with the tongue flap. *Oral Surg Oral Med Oral Pathol Oral Radiol.* 2011;112:711–714. Courtesy of Dr. Daniel J. Meara.)

TECHNIQUE: Tongue Flap—*cont'd*

STEP 5: Flap Division and Contouring

Flap division occurs 2 to 3 weeks postoperatively, under general anesthesia. A nasoendotracheal tube is secured, MMF is released, and the flap is divided. The division site, within the pedicle, is determined by the tissue required to reconstruct the remaining defect. A Dingman mouth gag is placed for ideal exposure, contouring, and inset of the residual defect. 3-0 Vicryl suture, via horizontal mattress sutures, is utilized to evert the margins. Judicious debulking can occur, so as to create ideal contours; however, excessive debulking can compromise tissue viability and should be avoided. The Dingman mouth gag is removed and the tongue donor site is contoured, with a #15 blade and local tissue rearrangement, to recreate an esthetic and functional tongue (Fig. 121.6).

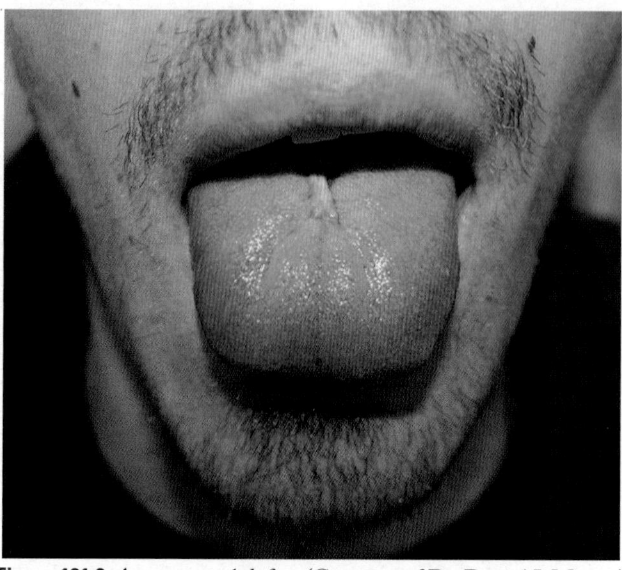

Figure 121.6 An oro-nasal defect (Courtesy of Dr. Daniel J. Meara.)

ALTERNATE OF MODIFIED TECHNIQUE 1: Posterior-Based Flap

The core tongue flap design principles are unchanged. However, the posterior-based flap hinges at the posterior aspect of the tongue, anterior to the circumvallate papilla (Fig. 121.7). This modification is desired in the oral reconstruction of soft palate, retromolar, and posterior buccal mucosal defects.[2]

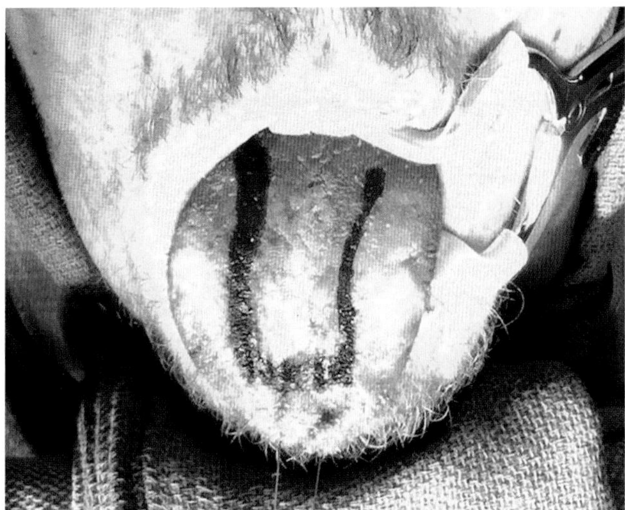

Figure 121.7 Marking pen incision outline for posteriorly based tongue flap, to address posterior hard palate and soft palate defects. (Courtesy of Dr. Daniel J. Meara.)

ALTERNATE OF MODIFIED TECHNIQUE 2: Transit Flap

Fischinger and Zargi suggest a slight modification of the central or paramedian tongue flap for floor-of-mouth defects. The dorsal flap is developed and then tunneled through the ventral tongue to the FOM defect. Critical to this modification is the avoidance of flap constriction by inadequate tunnel dimensions.[8]

ALTERNATE OF MODIFIED TECHNIQUE 3: Lateral-Based Flap

The lateral tongue flap is indicated for the reconstruction of lip commissure, buccal mucosa, floor-of-mouth, alveolar, and lateral palatal defects. This flap is particularly useful for oroantral defects and maintains the principles previously outlined for the central or paramedian tongue flaps. However, to facilitate tongue donor site primary closure, the lateral tongue flap is designed with a V-shape or wedge design.[9,1]

ALTERNATE OF MODIFIED TECHNIQUE 4: Parachute and Anchoring

Primarily an option for the closure of difficult palatal fistulas. The dorsal tongue flap is developed and a red rubber catheter is passed through the nose and palatal fistula into the oral cavity. The catheter is then secured to the distal end of the tongue flap with 3-0 Vicryl suture.[10] Next, the catheter is pulled back out of the nose, resulting in elevation or "parachuting" of the tongue flap into the defect.[10] The tongue flap is anchored to the nasal septum with 3-0 Vicryl, minimizing early detachment (Fig. 121.8). The prepassed horizontal mattress sutures are tied to coapt the deepithelialized margins of the tongue flap to the deepithelialized tissues of the fistula site.[10]

Continued

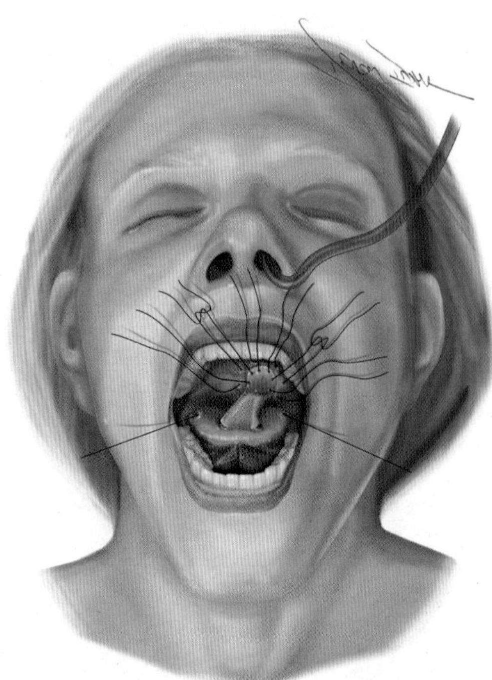

Figure 121.8 Catheter, while secured to tongue flap, is pulled through nose "parachuting" the flap and previously passed sutures into the palatal defect. (From Elyassi A, Helling E, Closmann J. Closure of difficult palatal fistulas using a "parachuting and anchoring" technique with the tongue flap. *Oral Surg Oral Med Oral Pathol Oral Radiol.* 2011;112:711–714.)

ALTERNATE OF MODIFIED TECHNIQUE 5: Double Tongue Flaps

The double tongue flap technique is best suited for large palatal defects or salvage cases, especially for cases in which the defect is actually divided into two fistulas, such as in cleft palate patients, by the caudal end of the nasoseptum. In this technique, the dorsal tongue is divided into two separate tongue flaps, with a preserved island of tissue between the flaps. Flap dimensions are roughly 20 mm width × 50 mm length × 3 mm thickness and are inset into the nasal floor, with 4-0 Vicryl suture (Fig. 121.9).[11] Specifically, the nasal layer is first reconstructed by suturing palatal mucosa tissue, from the defect margins, to the midline vomer flaps. Next, the double tongue flaps are sutured to the recipient sites with a large permanent suture. In this technique, closure of the donor site is often challenging and thus, in an attempt to avoid a secondary tongue deformity, the donor sites are allowed to heal by secondary intention, though "tacking" sutures, to partially close the donor sites, can be placed at the distal aspect of the wounds.

Avoidance and Management of Intraoperative Complications

The correct choice of tongue flap, adequate mobilization, and appropriate flap thickness are the three main intraoperative steps that must be accurately executed, so as to minimize the complications associated with the procedure. The choice of a central, posteriorly based tongue flap for an anterior, hard palate defect will likely result in a pedicled flap that is unable to reach the desired defect site. Such a miscalculation would require inset of the flap back to its original position and the creation of a new, lateral, anterior-based flap or cessation of the procedure and rescheduling for a later date. Similarly, if the correct flap is developed but is not adequately mobilized, difficulty will ensue with inset due to tension. Flap extension should be maximized and a back-cut may be employed to gain additional flap length, so as to reduce tension. This will also reduce the likelihood of postoperative flap detachment.

According to the anatomic study by Shangkuan et al., the body of the tongue is nourished by approximately 25 arterial branches from the deep lingual artery (Figs. 121.10A and B).[6] The robust perfusion facilitates the success of a pedicled tongue flap. However, the creation of a narrow or a thin flap may predispose to flap necrosis, especially if the flap is under tension. Attention to the core principles of flap development, as discussed above, reduces the incidence of intraoperative or postoperative complications. This particular issue can be minimized by maintaining a thick base and minimizing flap tension.

Lastly, restriction of tongue movement during the initial healing period is advantageous. Controversy exists regarding the need for MMF, though intuitively, limitation of tongue flap movement is likely to minimize flap failure by reducing flap detachment and facilitating vascular in-growth at the site of inset.

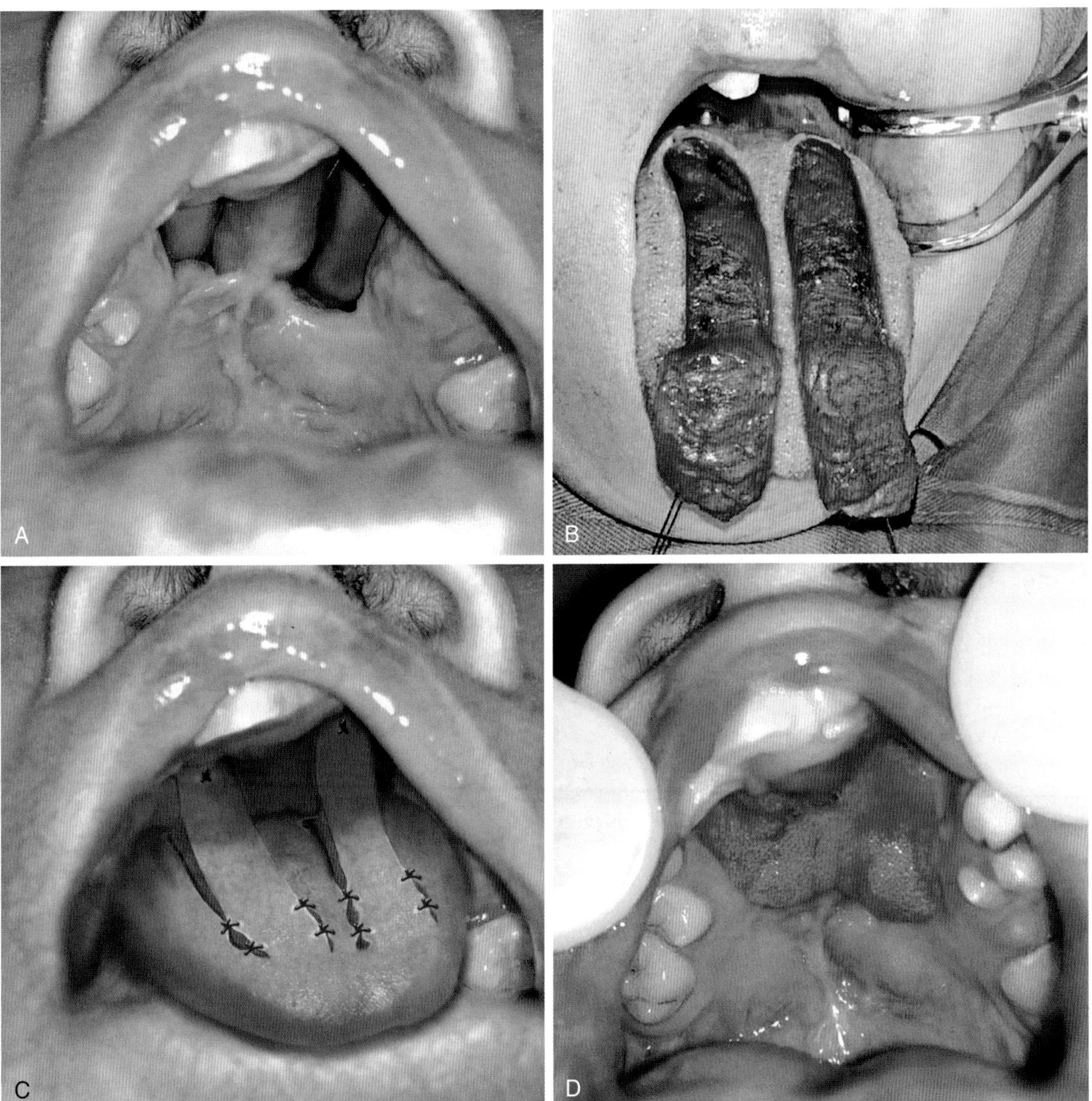

Figure 121.9 Double tongue flap technique best suited for large palatal defects or salvage cases, especially for cases in which the defect is actually divided into two fistulas. **A,** The fistula on anterior hard palate with deviated mobile premaxilla; **B,** double tongue flaps (dimensions around 2 cm width × around 5 cm length) were lifted up with about 3-mm thickness; **C,** picture of tongue dorsal view taken 1 month after the division of tongue flap pedicles. (From Zhou X, Ma L. Double tongue flaps for anterior huge palatal fistula closure. *Plast Reconstr Surg Glob Open*. 2019;7:e2246.)

Postoperative Considerations

Immediate postoperative tongue edema is expected and the patient should be monitored for any airway compromise. Perioperative steroids, such as Decadron, can blunt the edematous response and should be considered in patients without contraindications. Also, if MMF is employed, wire cutters should be with the patient at all times and appropriate patient education and anticipatory guidance is mandatory.

Bleeding from the raw surface of the flap is rare if attended to during the surgery with judicious use of electrocautery and dressing with oxidized cellulose strips. However, if significant bleeding does occur, adequate visibility is critical and requires the release of any forms of mandibular restriction. Hemostatic agents, electrocautery, and gentle pressure can be applied. Ultimately, the patient may require return to the operating room and even flap takedown to address any persistent or significant hemorrhage.

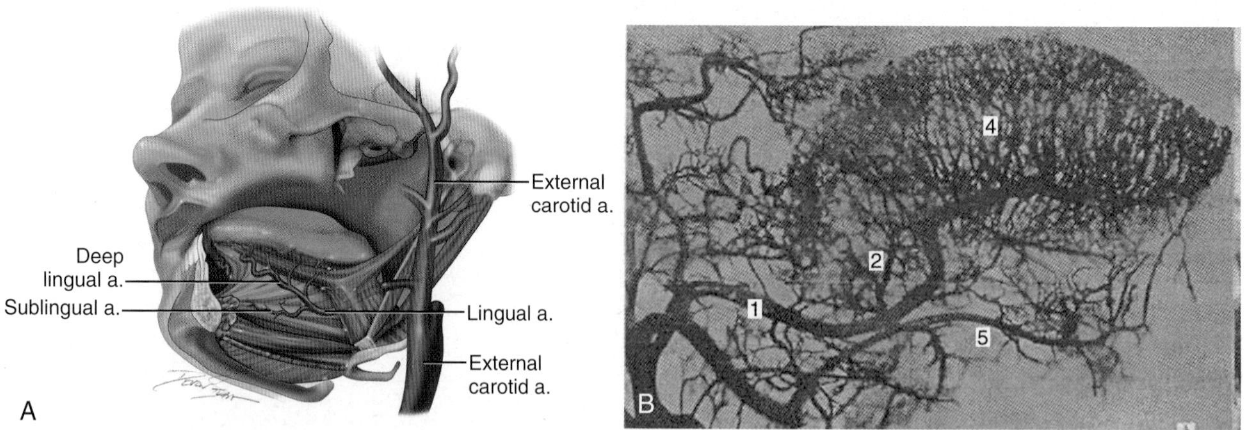

Figure 121.10 **A,** Diagram showing segmentation of the lingual artery. **B,** Branches of the lingual artery. View of the lingual artery. 1, Lingual artery; 2, lingual root artery; 3, lingual body artery; 4, submental branch of the facial artery; 5, lingual frenal artery. (From Shangkuan H, Xinghai W, Zengxing W, et al. Anatomic bases of tongue flaps. *Sug Radiol Anat*. 1998;20:83–88.)

Salvage

Detachment of the tongue flap during the postoperative period is a significant and unfortunate complication. Consequently, Agrawal and Panda detailed an innovative means to salvage a detached flap during the postoperative period in palatal reconstruction cases.[12] Specifically, they advocate the insertion of a contoured silicone block into the anterior palatal region via stainless steel wires to adjacent teeth.[11] The tongue flap is then transfixed to the block, to support and stabilize the flap during healing to the defect site (Fig. 121.11).[12]

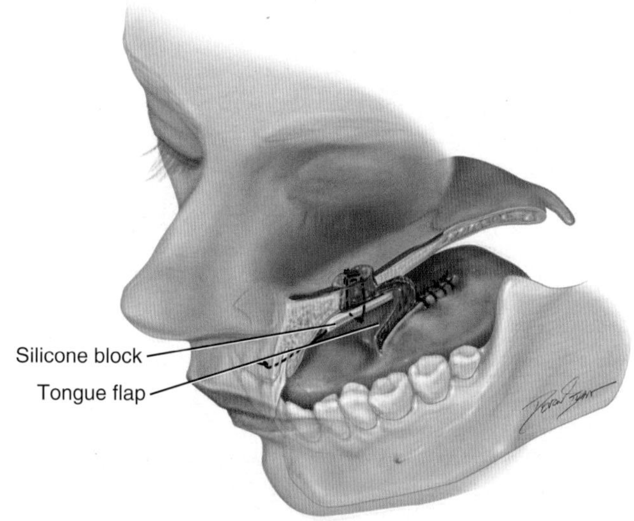

Figure 121.11 Sagittal view showing fixation of the silicone block under the tongue flap. The block has been fixed to the teeth with stainless steel wire. A transfixation suture passes through the sutured nasal mucosa, tongue flap, and silicone block. (From Agrawal K, Panda K. Management of a detached tongue flap. *Plast Reconstr Surg*. 2007;120(1):151–156.)

Patient Education

Patient education is critical so as to demystify the procedure and the postoperative concerns, such as effects on feeding, speech, taste, and sensation. Kinnebrew suggests that defects of the anterior one-third of the tongue can induce sibilance or "lisping."[13] However, speech, taste, and sensation alterations are typically limited. As for feeding, a liquid diet will be required until flap division. Thus, nutritional education is critical and should include discussion regarding supplements, such as protein drinks. Lastly, wound care should include gentle chlorhexidine rinses and perioperative intravenous antibiotics are sufficient.

References

1. Comini L, Spinelli G, Mannelli G. Algorithm for the treatment of oral and peri-oral defects through local flaps. *J Craniomaxillofac Surg*. 2018;46:2127–2137.
2. Buchbinder D, St-Hilaire H. Tongue flaps in maxillofacial surgery. *Oral Maxillofac Surg Clin N Am*. 2003;15:475–486.
3. Steinhauser E. Experience with dorsal tongue flaps for closure of defects of the hard palate. *J Oral Maxillofac Surg*. 1982;40:787–789.
4. Posnick J, Getz S. Surgical closure of end-stage palatal fistulas using anteriorly-based dorsal tongue flaps. *J Oral Maxillofac Surg*. 1987;45:907–912.
5. Lam D, Cheng A, Berty K, et al. Sliding anterior hemitongue flap for posterior tongue defect reconstruction. *J Oral Maxillofac Surg*. 2012;70:2440–2444.
6. Shangkuan H, Xinghai W, Zengxing W, et al. Anatomic bases of tongue flaps. *Surg Radiol Anat*. 1998;20:83–88.
7. Guzel M, Altintas F. Repair of large, anterior palatal fistulas using thin tongue flaps: long-term follow-up of 10 patients. *Ann Plast Surg*. 2000;45:109–117.
8. Fischinger J, Zargi M. Repair of anterior floor of mouth defects by a central or paramedian island tongue flap. *J Laryngol Otol*. 2003;117:391–395.
9. Johnson P, Banks P, Brown A. Use of the posteriorly based lateral tongue flap in the repair of palatal fistulae. *Int J Oral Maxillofac Surg*. 1992;21:6–9.

10. Elyassi A, Helling E, Closmann J. Closure of difficult palatal fistulas using a "parachuting and anchoring" technique with the tongue flap. *Oral Surg Oral Med Oral Pathol Oral Radiol.* 2011;112: 711–714.
11. Zhou X, Ma L. Double tongue flaps for anterior huge palatal fistula closure. *Plast Reconstr Surg Glob Open*. 2019;7:e2246.
12. Agrawal K, Panda K. Management of a detached tongue flap. *Plast Reconstr Surg*. 2007;120(1):151–156.
13. Kinnebrew M. Use of the tongue flap for intraoral reconstruction: a report of 16 cases. *J Oral Maxillofac Surg*. 1998;56:720–721.

CHAPTER 122

The Palatal Flap

Sharon Aronovich and Paul Shivers

Armamentarium

#9 Periosteal elevator
#15 and #12 Scalpel blades
4-0 Polyglycolic acid suture on RB-1 and TF needles
#7 Scalpel handle (long)
Bipolar electrocautery
Blair "hockey stick" elevator
Cottle osteotome, 7-inch curved
DeBakey forceps
Gauze—estimate length of flap by simulating expected rotation
Gerald toothed forceps
Kilner-Dott mouth gag
Local anesthetic with vasoconstrictor
Mallet
Needle electrocautery
Pencil Doppler probe
Shoulder roll
Woodson elevator

History of the Procedure

The palatal flap is an axial flap based on the greater palatine artery. It can be used as a rotational flap or an interpolated flap with an intervening bridge of oral epithelium. Its first reported description was credited to Ashley in 1939.[1] Since then, several authors have demonstrated the use of this flap and its modifications in closure of oroantral fistulas, oronasal fistulas, and a variety of small to medium-sized ablative defects.[2–8] In 1967, Moore and Chong described the use of the "sandwich" palatal island flap for palatal lengthening in the treatment of hypernasal speech.[9] Henderson expanded on the use of the palatal island flap based entirely on the greater palatine artery in the closure of oroantral fistulae.[10]

In 1977, Gullane and Arena used the total palatal island flap based unilaterally on one single greater palatine artery with 180 degrees rotation for large ablative oral defects.[11] This was supported by Maher's anatomic studies in 1977, which demonstrated a "macronet" of submucosal vessels forming anastomoses between the right and left palatal arteries (Fig. 122.1).[12] This technique was reevaluated by Genden and colleagues in 2001 with 100% success in five cases.[13] Alternatively, the flap may be deepithelialized and inverted posteriorly. Reports on this technique have noted complete donor site reepithelialization by 4 weeks in all cases.

In 2003, Anavi and colleagues reported good outcomes in a series of 63 patients with oroantral fistulas treated with a palatal rotation-advancement flap. They reported on the use of this axial flap for defects as large as 2 × 4 cm.[14]

Advantages include location adjacent to defect site, similar or "like" tissue, good vascularity, maintenance of sensory innervation, adequate thickness, minimal donor site morbidity, simple anatomy, and short procedure time.

Indications for the Use of the Procedure

Although many authors advocate the primary use of a Rehrman's buccal advancement flap for the closure of oroantral fistula, an axial palatal rotation flap is reserved as an option for failed repairs and large communications. As noted previously, the palatal flap carries its own blood supply from the greater palatine artery and is a reliable, locally available source of highly bound oral mucosa. Use of this flap prevents obliteration of the buccal vestibule where future denture use is planned.

The palatal flap has been successfully used for reconstruction of sizable ablative oral defects of the maxillary alveolus and tuberosity, hard palate, anterior soft palate, retromolar trigone, and tonsillar fossa. Salins and Benjamin emphasized the benefits of the palatal flap compared with alternative options in overcoming challenges specific to the retromolar trigone region.[15] The rotation of this "like tissue" is sufficiently stout to recreate the pterygomandibular raphe as well as support the tongue base. If the neurovascular pedicle is maintained during elevation, the sensate flap also offers proprioceptive advantage with regard to swallowing.

In pediatric patients with oronasal fistulas secondary to failed cleft palate repair, anterior defects of the hard palate may be repaired with a palatal rotation flap and nasal side closure. This approach is an option provided that one of the greater palatine arteries is intact and that adequate adjacent hard palate tissue is available. Children over the age of 5 are eligible for this repair; earlier palatal flap elevation can compromise maxillary growth in a manner analogous to a primary cleft repair.[13] Other options include the anteriorly based tongue flap and the facial artery myomucosal flap.

Lastly, the palatal rotation flap may be considered in the management of acquired oronasal fistulas, which may be

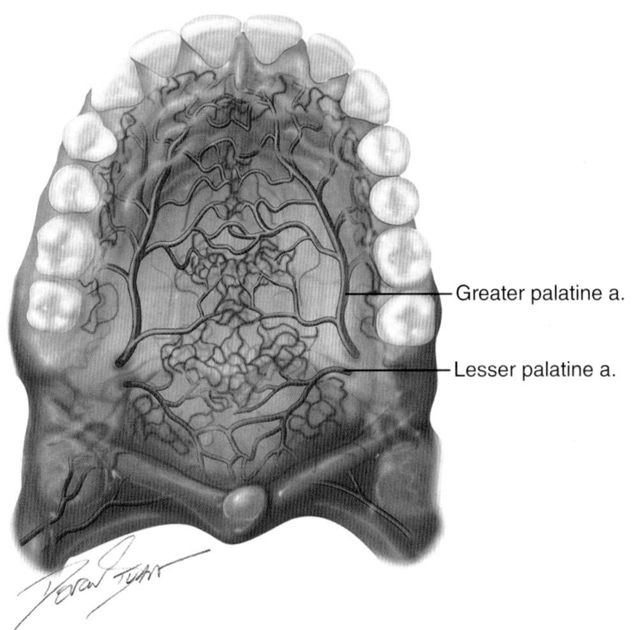

Figure 122.1 Vascular supply of the palatal flap. The right-sided palatal finger flap is elevated based on the greater palatine artery. There are anastomosing connections with the sphenopalatine artery and the submucosal vascular plexus crossing the midline.

secondary to ablative defects, trauma, infection (i.e., tertiary syphilis), autoimmune vasculitis (i.e., Wegener granulomatosis), or the use of illicit substances such as cocaine.

Limitations and Contraindications

In some of the abovementioned indications, compromise of the descending or greater palatine artery secondary to prior palatoplasty or traumatic injuries is a distinct possibility and may be a contraindication. The availability of a patent greater palatine artery must be confirmed prior to raising a palatal flap. Otherwise the flap is raised as a random pattern flap limiting the possible length-to-width ratio.

As with any surgical procedure, careful patient selection requires good clinical judgment and an appreciation for the social, medical, and surgical components that make each case unique. Concerns for a patient's ability to tolerate a secondary flap inset procedure or follow home care instructions may be relative contraindications. Medical comorbidities that may compromise healing include tobacco smoking, use of continuous positive airway pressure or bilevel positive airway pressure, or coagulopathies.

Prior to considering oroantral fistula repair, clinical and radiographic evaluation should assess for signs of maxillary sinus infection as well as foreign bodies. The authors favor three-dimensional radiographic studies over orthopantogram as they are more sensitive in the detection of these issues. Any active infection or sinusitis should be managed preoperatively to prevent failure of the reconstruction effort.[16] Antibiotic coverage for acute bacterial sinusitis is typically 5 to 7 days of amoxicillin/clavulanate in uncomplicated cases.[17] Chronic sinusitis can be managed medically, though details are beyond the scope of this chapter.

In the setting of resistant chronic maxillary sinusitis, the prognosis of oroantral fistula repair may be improved with treatment of the affected sinus via functional endoscopic sinus surgery (FESS).[18] FESS is a minimally invasive approach for renewal of normal sinus drainage patterns and has largely supplanted the traditional Caldwell-Luc procedure.[19] In a case series by Andric et al.,[18] a palatal flap and FESS were performed simultaneously for 14 patients suffering from an oroantral fistula in the setting of chronic maxillary sinusitis. Ten of the 14 patients were followed for greater than 6 months, and there were no reports of flap failure. While these results are captivating, evidence for concurrent treatment remains limited.

Large defects of the palate or maxilla (>1.5 to 2 cm) may require a prosthetic reconstruction or other local, regional, or distant flaps. Examples include the anteriorly based tongue flap, the temporoparietal fascia flap, and radial free forearm flap, respectively.

Excessive rotation of the flap >90 degrees, such as to the molar areas, may be a relative contraindication and depends on the surgeon's comfort level with the technique. The concern is that kinking of the greater palatine artery pedicle may compromise the blood supply.

TECHNIQUE: Palatal Rotation Flap

STEP 1: Positioning and Access

The patient may be intubated nasally or orally with a Ring-Adair-Elwyn (RAE) tube. A shoulder roll is placed extending the neck just enough for adequate exposure to the palate. A Kilner-Dott mouth gag depresses the tongue and oral RAE while anchoring the maxillary dentition superiorly. This gives excellent access for palatoplasty. For oroantral fistulas, a bite block may be used with a nasal RAE tube.

STEP 2: Ablation or Recipient Site Preparation

The defect to be reconstructed is first established. This may include a wide local excision of a neoplasm with frozen sections to confirm negative margins or excision of marginal mucosa during a secondary reconstruction.

A critical distinction must be made between an oroantral communication and an oroantral fistula. Communications are less amenable to two-layer closure as they have not yet developed an epithelial-lined tract. Nasal side closure of such a defect would require modification to the palatal flap, such as a double overlapping

Continued

TECHNIQUE: Palatal Rotation Flap—*cont'd*

hinge flap, or the utilization of a secondary flap. Fistulae develop as a sequela of communications that fail to close spontaneously, for any of the aforementioned reasons.

When closing an oroantral or oronasal fistula, the authors prefer to identify the bony margins of the defect by sounding down with a 25-gauge needle on a syringe. A circumferential incision is carried down to sound bone and includes a small cuff of nasal or antral mucosa. A subperiosteal dissection is carried out to mobilize the nasal or antral mucosa with a Woodson elevator or a Blair "hockey stick" elevator. This layer is then closed with a resorbable suture on a TF or M-1 (Ethicon) half-round needle to facilitate closure in a confined space. The defect size can now be accurately measured. If the defect is too large to close this inner layer, the marginal epithelium may be simply excised, exposing the underlying bony defect (Fig. 122.2A).

STEP 3: Palatal Flap Anatomy and Surgical Markings

The greater palatine artery is a terminal branch of the descending palatine artery and arises within the hard palate at the greater palatine foramen, which is situated medial to the second or third maxillary molar where the maxillary alveolus meets the horizontal plate of the palatine bone and the palatine process of the maxilla. The greater palatine artery has anastomosing branches anteriorly with the terminal posterior septal branch of the sphenopalatine artery, arising from the incisive foramen (see Fig. 122.1). The greater palatine foramen can usually be identified by manual palpation. If the location or viability of the greater palatine artery is uncertain, a pencil Doppler probe may be used for confirmation. Once the origin is marked, the flap is outlined. The length and shape are estimated by using a template. This will slightly underestimate the total length necessary given the kinking of tissue at the base of the flap. As the flap is rotated around a fixed pivot point of the greater palatine artery, the available length of the flap is shortened. After the flap has been outlined with a marking pen, local anesthetic with vasoconstrictor may be injected in the distal two-thirds of the flap and peripherally, avoiding accidental damage to the artery at the origin.

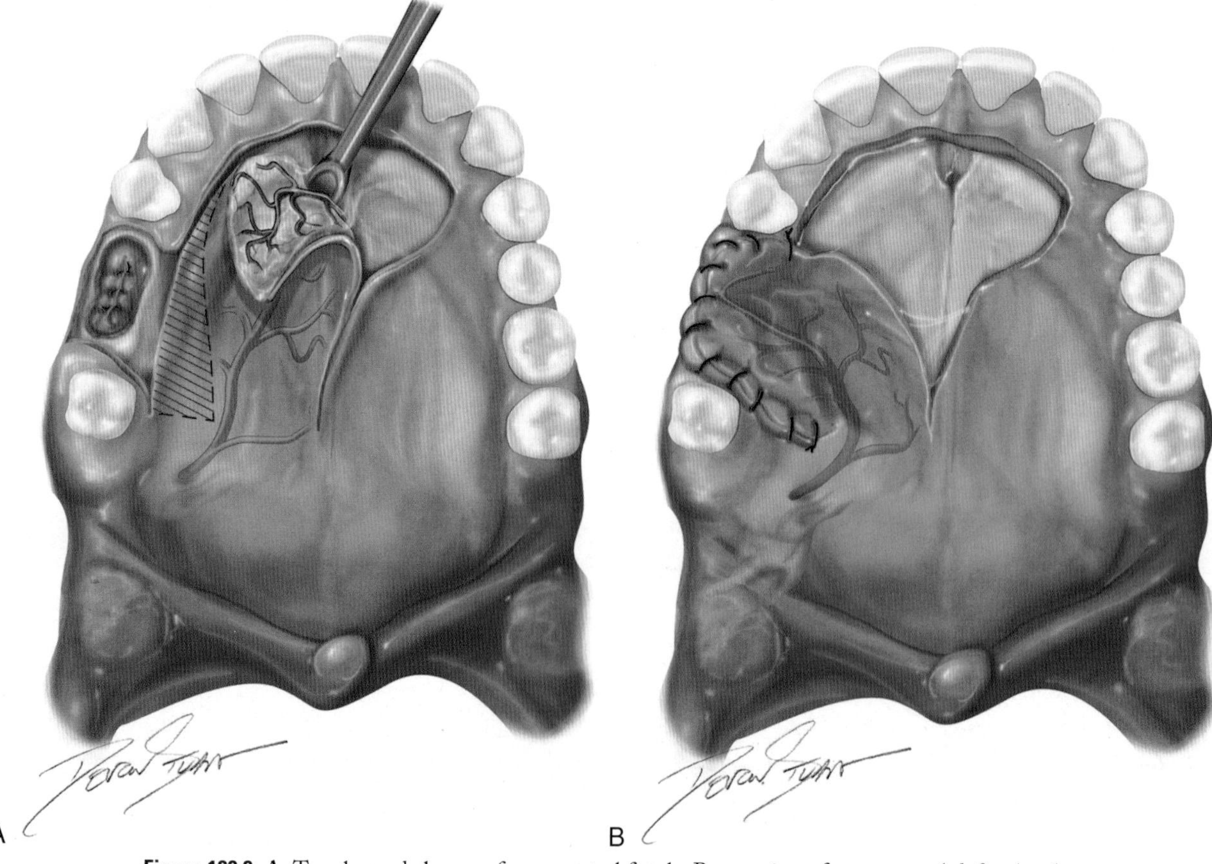

Figure 122.2 **A,** Two-layered closure of an oroantral fistula. Preparation of an oroantral defect by elevating the marginal mucosa off the bony margins of the defect in a subperiosteal plane and repair of the antral mucosa with inverted mattress sutures. The bony defect is measured and appropriate palatal rotation flap designed. **B,** Palatal flap rotated and sutured over sound bone for defect reconstruction.

TECHNIQUE: Palatal Rotation Flap—*cont'd*

STEP 4: Incision and Reconstruction

An incision is made starting anteriorly, outlining a flap design based on the shape of the defect. On the alveolar side, a 3- to 5-mm margin of palatal gingiva may be maintained to preserve the periodontal support of adjacent teeth. The incision is carried posteriorly leaving adequate tissue on either side of the greater palatine artery at the base. Preferably, a full-thickness mucoperiosteal palatal flap is elevated, and subperiosteal dissection is carried out posteriorly until the artery is identified. The flap contains oral mucosa, fibrofatty connective tissue, minor palatine salivary glands, and periosteum.

Alternatively, a supraperiosteal dissection may be started distally to avoid leaving denuded bone. The latter dissection must include an adequate thickness of fibrofatty palatal tissue converting to a subperiosteal dissection at the proximal one-half to one-third to ensure preservation of the artery. The flap is rotated and should reach the defect in a tension-free manner. This may be accomplished with conservative triangular back cuts on the inner aspect of the flap's rotational base. Care should be taken to avoid compromising vascular supply. The flap should cover the defect allowing closure over sound bone using resorbable 3-0 or 4-0 polyglycolic acid sutures or nonresorbable sutures. Hemostasis at the donor site may be achieved with a palatal stent, bone wax, or local hemostatic material such as gelatin sponges or oxidized regenerated cellulose with stay sutures (Fig. 122.2B).

Large midline defects often generated from oncologic resection can employ bilateral palatal flaps for closure in a VY pushback fashion. As described by Dings et al., this technique distributes the amount of tissue mobilization amongst the two flaps.[20] Thus, tissue redundancy and pedicle kinking are reduced.

STEP 5: Insetting Procedure

If used as an interpolation flap, a second surgical procedure for dividing and insetting the flap must be planned 3 weeks after the primary operation. Prior to proceeding with the second operation, collateral blood supply to the flap is assessed by occluding the pedicle with a suture while assessing the vascularity of the flap distally.

ALTERNATIVE TECHNIQUE 1: Modification of the Palatal Rotation Flap Using an Extended Palatal Incision

When using a palatal flap for coverage of an oroantral communication of the posterior maxillary alveolus, the flap may be designed with a wide base. Laterally, the incision extends in a sulcular fashion posterior to the defect location, and the incision is carried on the maxillary tuberosity with a slight lateral curve posteriorly into mobile or unattached tissue. Posterior dissection into the soft palate within the subglandular plane provides the good mobility necessary for rotation and ensures good vascularity to the flap while avoiding the need for a back cut near the artery. If posterior molars are present, high-riding tissue may be conservatively excised (Fig. 122.3).[5]

ALTERNATIVE TECHNIQUE 2: Nasal Mucosal Closure With Vomerine Flaps in Combination With a Palatal Rotation Flap

Whenever possible, oronasal fistulas are repaired using a two-layered tension-free closure. If the nasal septum is accessible through the defect, a midseptal incision is performed with anterior and posterior lateral releasing incisions. A subperiosteal and subperichondrial dissection is performed to elevate cranially based septo-vomerine flaps unilaterally or bilaterally. This is sutured to the mobilized nasal mucosa for tension-free closure of the nasal layer. A palatal rotation flap is then elevated and mobilized for oral-side closure (Fig. 122.4).

ALTERNATIVE TECHNIQUE 3: Layered Closure of Oroantral Communication With a Buccal Flat Pad Flap and a Palatal Rotation Flap

After elevation of a buccal mucoperiosteal flap, the periosteum at the base is incised revealing the underlying buccal flap pad. This vascularized buccal fat pad is gently teased out and advanced into the oroantral defect as an additional layer. The palatal flap is then rotated and sutured to the elevated buccal flap (Fig. 122.5).

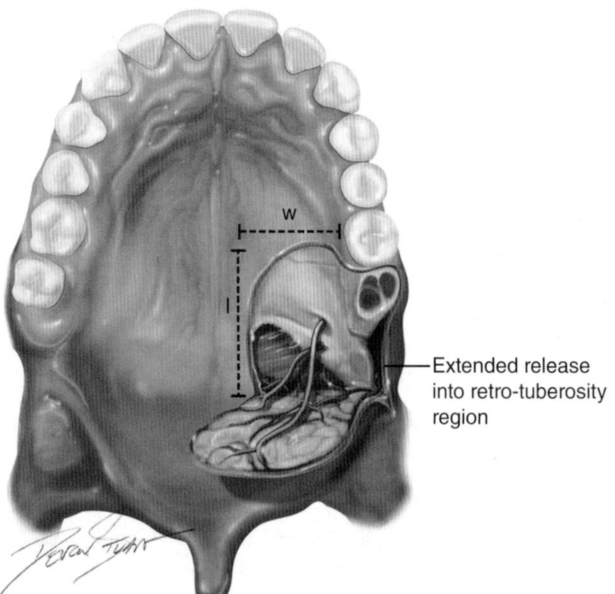

Figure 122.3 Wide-based palatal rotation flap with a length-to-width ratio of 2. Incision carried into the soft palate and retrotuberosity region for increased mobility and rotation of the flap for closure of a maxillary tuberosity defect.

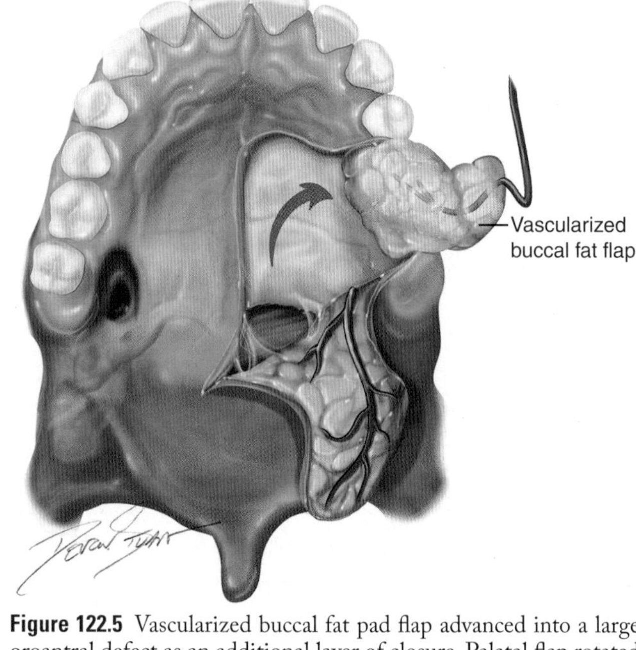

Figure 122.5 Vascularized buccal fat pad flap advanced into a large oroantral defect as an additional layer of closure. Palatal flap rotated and sutured to the elevated buccal flap.

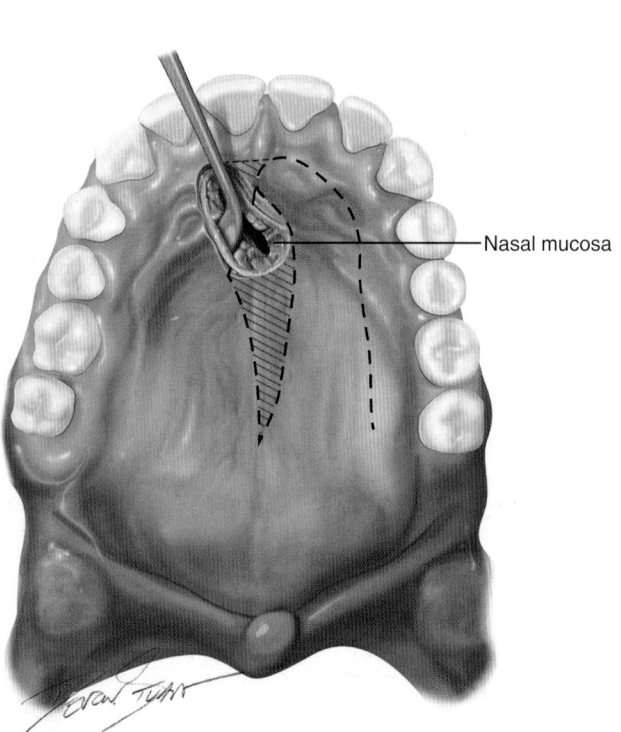

Figure 122.4 Two-layered closure of a midline oronasal fistula of the anterior hard palate. Identification of sound underlying bone. Incision of the marginal mucosa and subperiosteal dissection to mobilize the nasal flaps with a Blair "hockey stick" elevator. Bilateral vomerine flaps mobilized to aid in repair of the nasal layer first. Closure of the oral defect with a palatal flap with wedge excision of medial mucosa to avoid an epithelial bridge.

Avoidance and Management of Intraoperative Complications

Laceration or transection of the greater palatine artery must be avoided by designing a large base that includes the artery at its exit from the foramen. If the artery is accidentally damaged, hemostasis is achieved, and the blood supply is that of a random pattern flap from the submucosal vascular plexus. As evidenced by sacrifice of the descending palatine arteries during Le Fort I osteotomies, the palatal tissue can survive based on the robust collateral circulation from branches of the facial and ascending pharyngeal arteries. There are, however, limitations to the palatal tissue tolerance of random pattern flap design.

In 2002, Lee and colleagues treated 21 patients with oroantral fistulas in the maxillary third molar area using a random palatal flap with ligation of the greater palatine artery. They reported a success rate of 76.2% with necrosis and breakdown of the repair in five patients. The mean length-to-width ratio was 2.23 and 2.40 for the success and failure groups, respectively. No flap necrosis was encountered with a ratio below 2.15, whereas a ratio above 2.49 was always associated with distal necrosis and flap failure. Their results support the use of the palatal rotation flap as a random flap, in the event the arterial supply is damaged, as long as the design of the flap includes a wide base with an optimal length-to-width ratio.[21]

Insufficient flap length to cover the defect or closure with tension can be prevented by ensuring that the anterior extent of the flap exceeds the diameter needed to reach the end of the bony defect after rotating the flap.

Difficulty rotating the palatal flap into the defect can be encountered at molar sites and defects of the posterior hard palate. Triangular wedge excisions may be performed conservatively to rotate the flap, but this option carries the risk of vascular compromise. Extension of the incision to the soft palate, in a layer between minor salivary glands and tensor aponeurosis, may be another option to facilitate rotation but may require coagulation of the lesser palatine artery if bleeding is encountered. Lastly, osteotomies at the hamulus or at the posterior aspect of the descending palatine canal may help the patient to gain some mobility but must be accomplished with care.

Vascular insufficiency of the flap evidenced by pallor or inadequate capillary refill should signal that the greater palatine artery is kinked. Increased mobility must be achieved as discussed previously or postoperative flap necrosis may ensue. Venous congestion of the flap can be avoided by developing a full-thickness mucoperiosteal flap for its entire length and careful tissue handling with serrated nontoothed tissue forceps such as DeBakey forceps.

Postoperative Considerations

Use of the palatal rotation flap usually leaves areas of exposed palatal bone, which are a source of postoperative pain and undergo secondary epithelialization. A soft plastic or acrylic palatal stent may be used for hemostasis and patient comfort. This stent must not compress the palatal flap or its vascular origin. It may be removed during the second postoperative week. Patients should begin with a liquid or nonchew blenderized diet for the first week and advance to a soft mechanical diet thereafter. Antibiotic coverage can be based on the surgeon's preference for minor maxillofacial procedures; the authors prescribe a course according to the unique requirements of an individual case and have no set regimen. Pain is typically controlled with the use of nonsteroidal antiinflammatory medications and opioids. Patients are to avoid strenuous physical activity throughout the first week in order to avoid bleeding at the donor site. Complete reepithelialization of the exposed donor site defect can be expected in 3 to 4 weeks postoperatively.

References

1. Ashley REA. A method of closing antroalveolar fistulae. *Ann Otol Rhinol Laryngol.* 1939;24:433.
2. Chonkas NC. Modified palatal flap technique for closure of oroantral fistula. *J Oral Surg.* 1974;32:12.
3. Quayle AA. A double flap technique for the closure of oro-nasal and oro-antral fistulae. *Br J Oral Surg.* 1981;19(2):132–137.
4. Sokler, Klara, Vanja Vuksan, and Tomislav Lauc. "Treatment of oroantral fistula." *Acta stomatologica Croatica: International journal of oral sciences and dental medicine.* 2002;36(1): 129–134.
5. Kale TP, Urolagin S, Khurana V, et al. Treatment of oroantral fistula using palatal flap: a case report and technical note. *J Int Oral Health.* 2010;2:77.
6. Borgonovo AE, Berardinelli FV, Favale M, Maiorana C. Surgical options in oroantral fistula treatment. *Open Dent J.* 2012;6:94–98.
7. Rintala A. A double, overlapping hinge flap to close palatal fistula. *Scand J Plast Reconstr Surg.* 1971;5(2):91–95.
8. Salins PC, Kishore SK. Anteriorly based palatal flap for closure of large oroantral fistula. *Oral Surg Oral Med Oral Pathol Oral Radiol Endod.* 1996;82(3):253–256.
9. Moore FT, Chong JK. The "Sandwich" technique to lengthen the soft palate. *Br J Oral Surg.* 1967;4(3):183–188.
10. Henderson D. The palatal island flap in the closure of oro-antral fistulae. *Br J Oral Surg.* 1974;12(2):141–146.
11. Gullane PJ, Arena S. Palatal island flap for reconstruction of oral defects. *Arch Otolaryngol.* 1977;103(10):598–599.
12. Maher WP. Distribution of palatal and other arteries in cleft and non-cleft human palates. *Cleft Palate J.* 1977;14(1):1–12.
13. Genden EM, Lee BB, Urken ML. The palatal island flap for reconstruction of palatal and retromolar trigone defects revisited. *Arch Otolaryngol Head Neck Surg.* 2001;127(7):837–841.
14. Anavi Y, Gal G, Silfen R, Calderon S. Palatal rotation-advancement flap for delayed repair of oroantral fistula: a retrospective evaluation of 63 cases. *Oral Surg Oral Med Oral Pathol Oral Radiol Endod.* 2003;96(5):527–534.
15. Salins PC, Benjamin P. Anatomic basis for reconstitution of retromolar region: significance of palatal flap. *J Oral Maxillofac Surg.* 2009;67(5):1141–1148.
16. Yih WY, Merrill RG, Howerton DW. Secondary closure of oroantral and oronasal fistulas. *J Oral Maxillofac Surg.* 1988;46:359.
17. Chow AW, Benninger MS, Brook I, et al, Infectious Diseases Society of America; IDSA clinical practice guideline for acute bacterial rhinosinusitis in children and adults. *Clin Infect Dis.* 2012;54(8):e72–e112.
18. Andric M, Saranovic V, Drazic R, Brkovic B, Todorovic L. Functional endoscopic sinus surgery as an adjunctive treatment for closure of oroantral fistulae: a retrospective analysis. *Oral Surg Oral Med Oral Pathol Oral Radiol Endod.* 2010;109(4):510–516.
19. Lal D, Stankiewicz JA. Primary sinus surgery. In: Flint PW, ed. *Cummings Otolaryngology: Head and Neck Surgery.* 7th ed. Philadelphia, PA; 2021.
20. Dings JP, Mizbah K, Bergé SJ, Meijer GJ, Merkx MA, Borstlap WA. Secondary closure of small- to medium-size palatal defects after ablative surgery: reappraisal of reconstructive techniques. *J Oral Maxillofac Surg.* 2014;72(10):2066–2076.
21. Lee JJ, Kok SH, Chang HH, Yang PJ, Hahn LJ, Kuo YS. Repair of oroantral communications in the third molar region by random palatal flap. *Int J Oral Maxillofac Surg.* 2002;31(6):677–680.

CHAPTER 123

Temporalis Axial Flap

Jeffrey S. Dean and Rahul Tandon

Armamentarium

#9 Periosteal elevator
#10 and #15 Scalpel blades
#701 Bur
Adson forceps with teeth
Allis clamps
Appropriate sutures
Bipolar electrocautery
Channel retractor
Curved Mayo scissors
DeBakey forceps
Doppler ultrasound
Hair elastics
Local anesthetic with vasoconstrictor
Malleable retractors
Mayfield headrest
Midfacial plating system
Needle electrocautery
Obwegeser retractors
Raney clips
Reciprocating saw
Seldin retractor
Sinn rakes
Skin staples

History of the Procedure

Correction of soft tissue and bony defects has some of the most challenging tasks for the reconstructive surgeon. The use of tissue flaps has become a common technique in reconstructive surgery due to their demonstrated success. Flaps have been documented as far back as 600 BC, when an Indian hermit, Sushrutha, reconstructed the nose with a forehead flap, a technique that continues to be used to this day.[1] However, it was not until the late 19th century, when Golovine and Lentz performed reconstructions on an eviscerated orbital defect and a resected condylar neck, respectively, that the first descriptions of the temporalis flap were documented.[2,3] This type of flap also was used in early reconstructive efforts on the temporomandibular joint (TMJ), as a portion of the temporalis muscle was attached to the temporalis fascia.[4,5] In 1948, Campbell described the use of the temporalis flap in the reconstruction of a left maxillary defect,[6] and nearly 10 years later, the same flap was used in middle ear and mastoid cavities.[7]

Later years saw the anatomic boundaries expanded by Bakamjian[8] and Horton,[9] who used the flap to reconstruct the palate and maxilla after tumor resection. Nevertheless, reconstruction of exenterated orbital defects remained the primary use for most surgeons, as demonstrated by a study by Tessier and Krastinova.[10] They described 14 cases in which the flap was transposed through the lateral orbital wall, preserving the eyelids. Further developments, combined with a better understanding of the anatomic site, allowed surgeons to carry the flap to defects that once seemed too far to reconstruct.

Over the past few decades, the temporalis flap has been used in a myriad of reconstructive efforts for the orbit, eyelids, cranial base, maxilla and palate, and mandible.[11–15] This flap even found a use in the treatment of craniofacial deformities, such as Treacher Collins syndrome, after van der Meulen et al.[16] modified the technique proposed by McCarthy and Zide.[17] The temple region is an appropriate donor site because it has a copious vascular supply and several layers of tissue, which provide it with the versatility seen surgically. The advantages of this flap have been demonstrated in previous studies, and its popularity continues to increase, along with its evolution. With its robust blood supply and proven versatility, the temporalis flap has shown staying power as a treatment for more than 2000 years, which can be attributed to its reliability and its ability to cover many areas in the maxillofacial region.

Indications for the Use of the Procedure

The goals of maxillofacial reconstruction should focus on accurately reproducing the original form, providing the patient with appropriate esthetics, and restoring functional needs.

The vascular supply of the temporalis muscle is from the temporal artery, one of two terminal branches of the external carotid artery. The temporal artery divides into three primary arteries: the anterior deep temporal artery, the posterior deep temporal artery, and the middle temporal artery. Each primary artery branches into secondary arterioles and then into the terminal arterioles. In the coronal plane, the vessels are located mainly on the lateral and medial aspects of the muscle, with a significantly lower vascular density in the midline (Fig. 123.1). The versatility of the temporalis

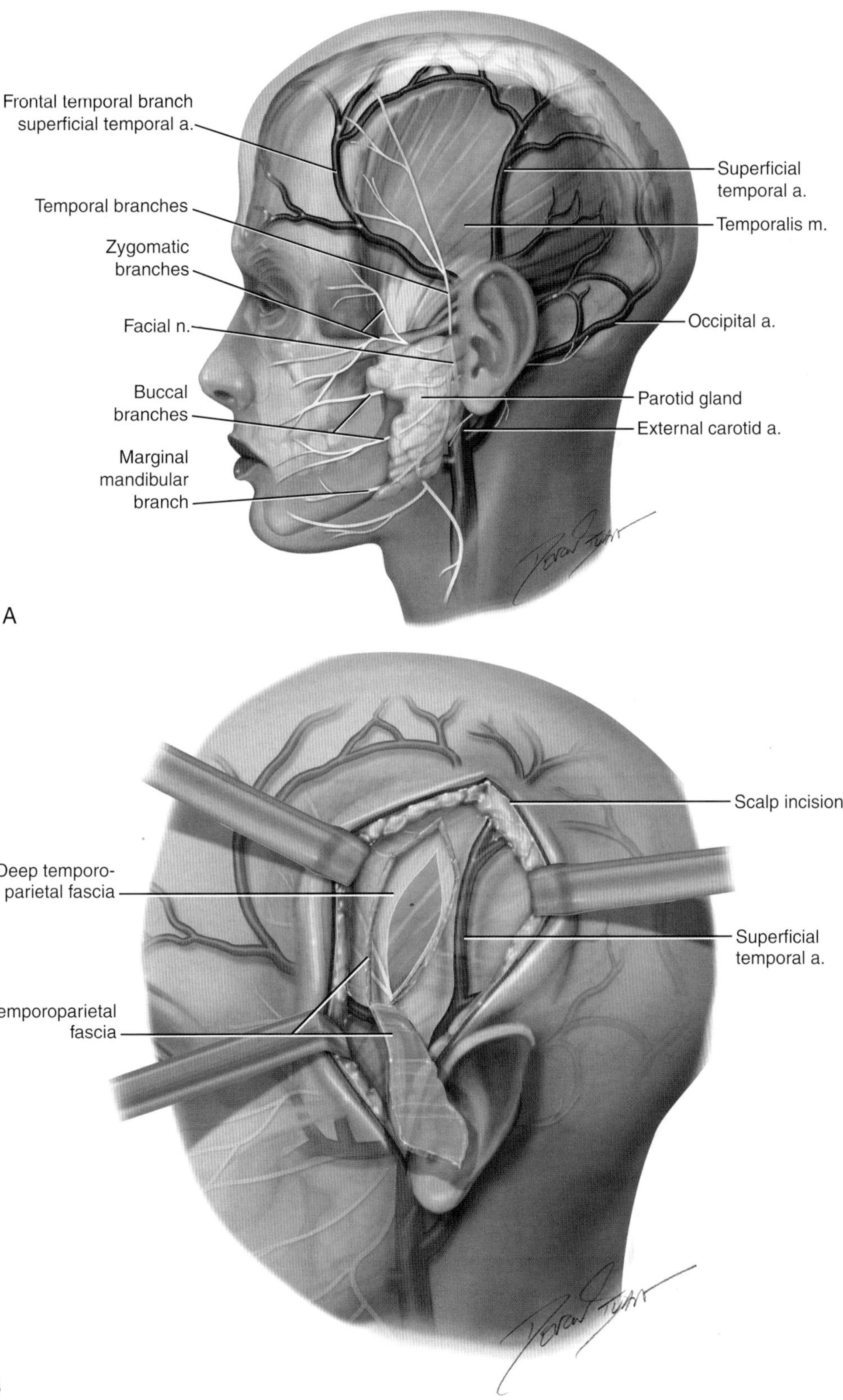

Figure 123.1 **A,** The delicate regional anatomy requires meticulous surgical technique when planning a temporalis axis flap. **B,** The diversity of tissue layers allows for flap versatility in reconstruction.

muscle flap enables surgeons to accomplish multiple tasks, whether the defect is traumatic, pathologic, or developmental in origin.

In cases of extensive en bloc resection of the maxilla, orbits, and cranial base, in which communication with the anterior skull base occurs, the temporalis muscle flap can provide appropriate coverage and a watertight seal. The flap is also used in the reconstruction of oral-mandibular defects and TMJ ankylosis, the reconstruction of palatal defects in cleft patients, and even in reanimation of total unilateral facial paralysis.[4] The temporalis flap also is ideal for other maxillofacial defects of the cheek and palate caused by pathologic lesions, such as ameloblastoma, myxoma, and giant cell tumor.[18] In the field of dentistry, it can be used as a soft tissue bed for later placement of bone grafts and implants,[19] with epithelialization taking approximately 4 to 6 weeks to complete.[20–22] Nevertheless, its popularity is largely due to its ability to resurface enormous defects of the orbital region, particularly the orbit. Donor site esthetics often are acceptable to patients, and they also provide great flexibility and versatility. Additionally, compared with other flaps, the temporalis flap is less bulky, more malleable, originates in a relatively hairless region, and is in close proximity to the oral cavity and other potential donor areas.

Limitations and Contraindications

One of the most important limitations to note with the use of the temporalis muscle flap is donor defect, which could result in temporal hollowing. This hollowing may result from temporalis fat pad wasting and/or lack of muscular support. However, meticulous attention to surgical detail can prevent such an occurrence. If temporal hollowing does occur, a secondary surgical procedure involving one of three grafts can be undertaken: a sliced autogenous rib cartilage graft, a dermal fat graft, or a deepithelialized lateral arm free flap.[12] Implants also can be used to correct such defects. In addition, following the use of the anterior portion of the temporalis flap, advancement of the posterior portion into the defect can mitigate this effect.[19] The bulkiness of the flap can has certain disadvantages, such as possible TMJ limitation and pain due to loss of temporalis function.[15] Although many of these disturbances can be debilitating, they can be mitigated, and possibly eliminated, through physiotherapy for the patient. Reconstruction of the hypopharynx/mandibular region may cause dysphagia, resulting in food emanating from the nose. Following reconstruction after a maxillectomy, some patients have demonstrated continued hypernasality[4] caused by retraction of the soft palate in the course of flap healing, which reduces the posterior soft palate/pharyngeal seal.

TECHNIQUE: Temporalis Flap for Intraoral Defects

The versatility of the temporalis muscle flap provides the surgeon with several options, yet the technique may differ for each option, depending on which flap is needed. Nevertheless, common approaches in every variation of the flap must be considered.

STEP 1: Assessment of Anatomic Structures

It is important to first define the margins, establish the branches of the superficial temporal artery, and determine and mark the pivot point. A Doppler ultrasound can be used if palpation is insufficient. The distance from the pivot point to the nearest border of the defect helps define the length of the pedicle.

STEP 2: Incision

A coronal incision using a #15 blade is carried through the skin, with dissection beneath the galea to the supraorbital ridge. In some cases a hemicoronal incision also can be made, extending inferiorly to the preauricular region at the level of the tragus. This initial incision should be made to the level of the temporal fascia and hidden within the hairy temporoparietal region. The dissection eventually becomes periosteal, extending in the plane toward the lateral orbital rim to the zygomatic arch. The dissection is then continued through to the superficial fascia of the temporalis muscle; it is important for the surgeon to avoid injury to the frontal branch of the facial nerve. The dissection is carried over the muscle to its posterior border (Fig. 123.2A and B).

STEP 3: Dissection and Mobilization of the Temporalis Flap

Once the posterior portion of the temporalis muscle has been detached, leaving a strip attached at the anterior border, the entire muscle is elevated with a periosteal elevator. Dissection is continued from under the zygomatic arch, mobilizing everything except for the portion attached to the coronoid process. If necessary, the muscle can be split in the coronal plane because the blood supply is still maintained.

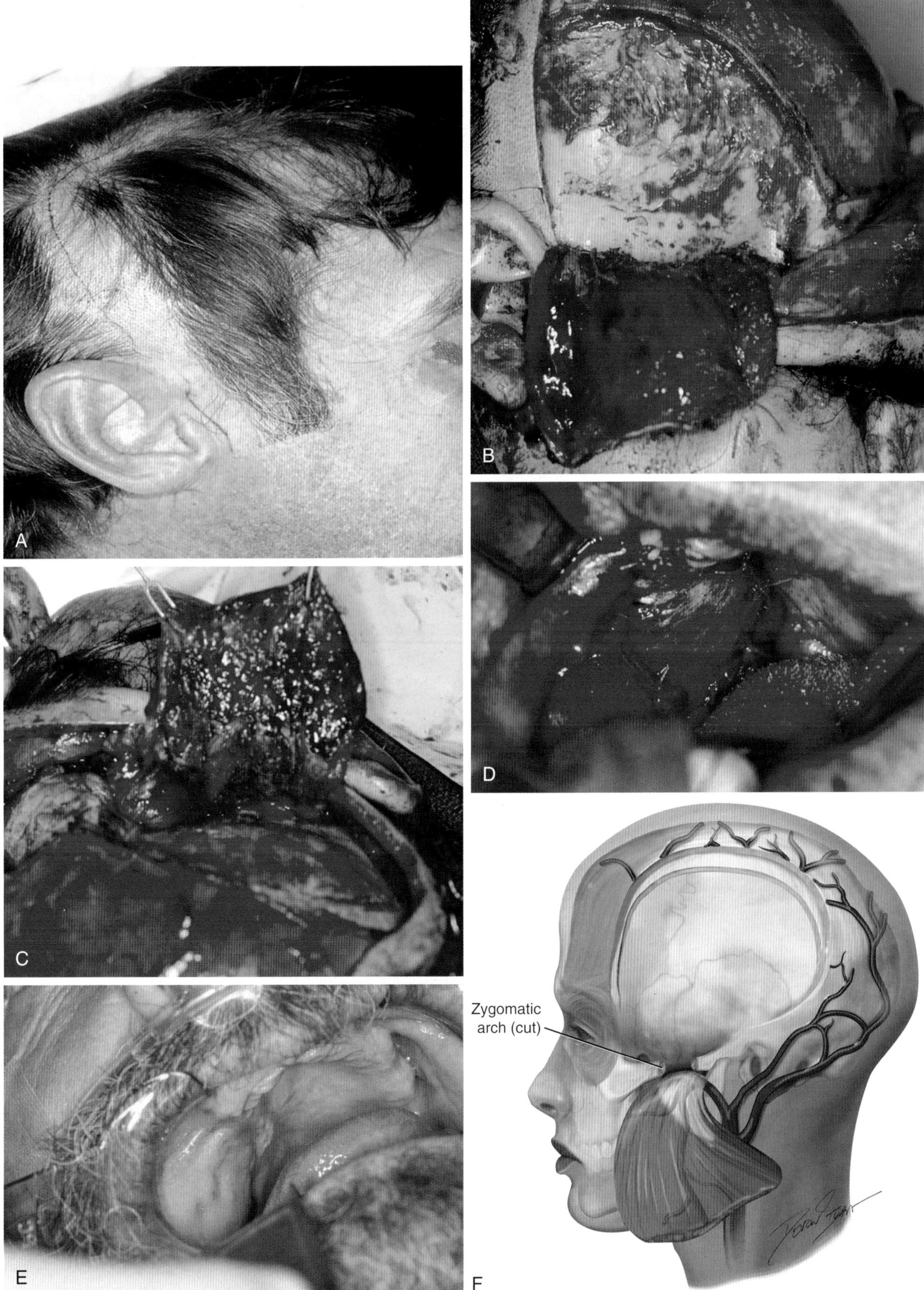

Figure 123.2 **A,** Outline of the hemicoronal incision, which extends inferiorly to the preauricular region at the level of the tragus. **B,** Detachment of the posterior portion of the temporalis muscle. **C,** Isolation of the flap. **D,** Positioning of the flap. **E,** Intraoral defect requiring reconstruction. **F,** Division of the zygomatic arch allows for mobilization of the flap into the lower third of the face.

TECHNIQUE: Temporalis Flap for Intraoral Defects—*cont'd*

STEP 4: Positioning of the Flap

It may be advantageous at this point to resect the zygomatic arch so as to avoid compression of the pedicle. This allows for increased rotation of the flap, which is needed for reconstruction of intraoral defects and to avoid compression or strangulation of the pedicle. A subperiosteal tunnel is created with a rongeur to help transpose the muscle to the recipient site; it may be useful to guide the flap into the oral cavity with two silk sutures. Once the muscle has been approximated, it is sutured into position (Fig. 123.2C–F).

STEP 5: Closure of the Flap

A suction drain is placed in the subgaleal plane, and the coronal flap is closed in layers at the donor site. Prophylactic antibiotics are administered intravenously four times a day for the first 24 hours after surgery.

ALTERNATIVE TECHNIQUE 1: Temporalis Flap for Temporomandibular Joint (TMJ) Reconstruction

In addition to reconstruction of intraoral defects, the temporalis flap is useful for the treatment of TMJ ankylosis. In this case, a gap arthroplasty is performed with a condylectomy. In some cases, a costochondral graft is used as a substitute for the condylar head. A temporalis flap approximately 1.5 to 2 fingerbreadths thick is then isolated and mobilized over the zygomatic arch and reflected inferiorly over it. This portion is then sandwiched between the remnant of the condylar process (or chondral end of the costochondral graft) and the temporal bone. Once appropriate positioning has been established, the muscle is sutured in both the anterior and posterior directions.[23]

ALTERNATIVE TECHNIQUE 2: Temporalis Flap for Orbital Reconstruction

The temporalis flap can also be used to reconstruct orbital floor defects caused by resection of maxillofacial tumors or for reconstruction of the orbital cavity after exenteration. The muscle is exposed and isolated as previously described. It is then split coronally, and if the orbital floor is reconstructed, the anterior portion of the muscle or a portion pedicled to the coronoid process is used.[4] If the lateral wall is resected or obliterated due to trauma, the muscle is mobilized through a subcutaneous tunnel into the orbit; if the lateral wall is present, a tunnel can be created. It is important to avoid compromising the blood supply as it is placed within the defect. The flap is then sutured in place and covered with a local skin flap.[24] The coronal incision is closed in layers as previously described (Fig. 123.3).

Avoidance and Management of Intraoperative Complications

As with any large reconstructive procedure, several complications can occur with temporalis flap procedures. Complications that occur during the reconstructive effort include unilateral frontal palsy, partial ossification of the flap, and complete loss of the distal portion of the flap.[12] During exposure of the muscle, the surgeon can avoid injury to the temporal branch of the facial nerve by using the modified preauricular approach.[25] Injury to the underlying arteries, particularly the superficial temporal artery, should be judiciously avoided. Doppler ultrasound can be used to determine the length of the flap and its location, but some have advocated the use of digital palpation for this purpose.[26] The frontal branch of the superficial temporal artery serves as a demarcation that should not be crossed.[27] Although a wide pedicle is sometimes needed, a pedicle that is too bulky may limit the arc of rotation, leading to possible disfigurement of the skin.[26] Studies have also shown that symptoms from the donor site can be minimized if care is taken during the raising of the flap not to incise through the inner epimysium and pericranium, leaving a few millimeters of muscle fibers.[13] Fluid collection at the donor site can also occur but is alleviated by evacuation pressure followed by a dressing.[4]

Postoperative Considerations

The temporalis flap should be evaluated and assessed for the color of the flap, suture dehiscence, the presence of infection, and necrosis of the flap.[11] Prevention of infection can be accomplished by administering antibiotic prophylaxis; dexamethasone can also be administered three times a day during this time. Depending on the site reconstructed, postoperative rehabilitation is crucial to the success of the procedure.

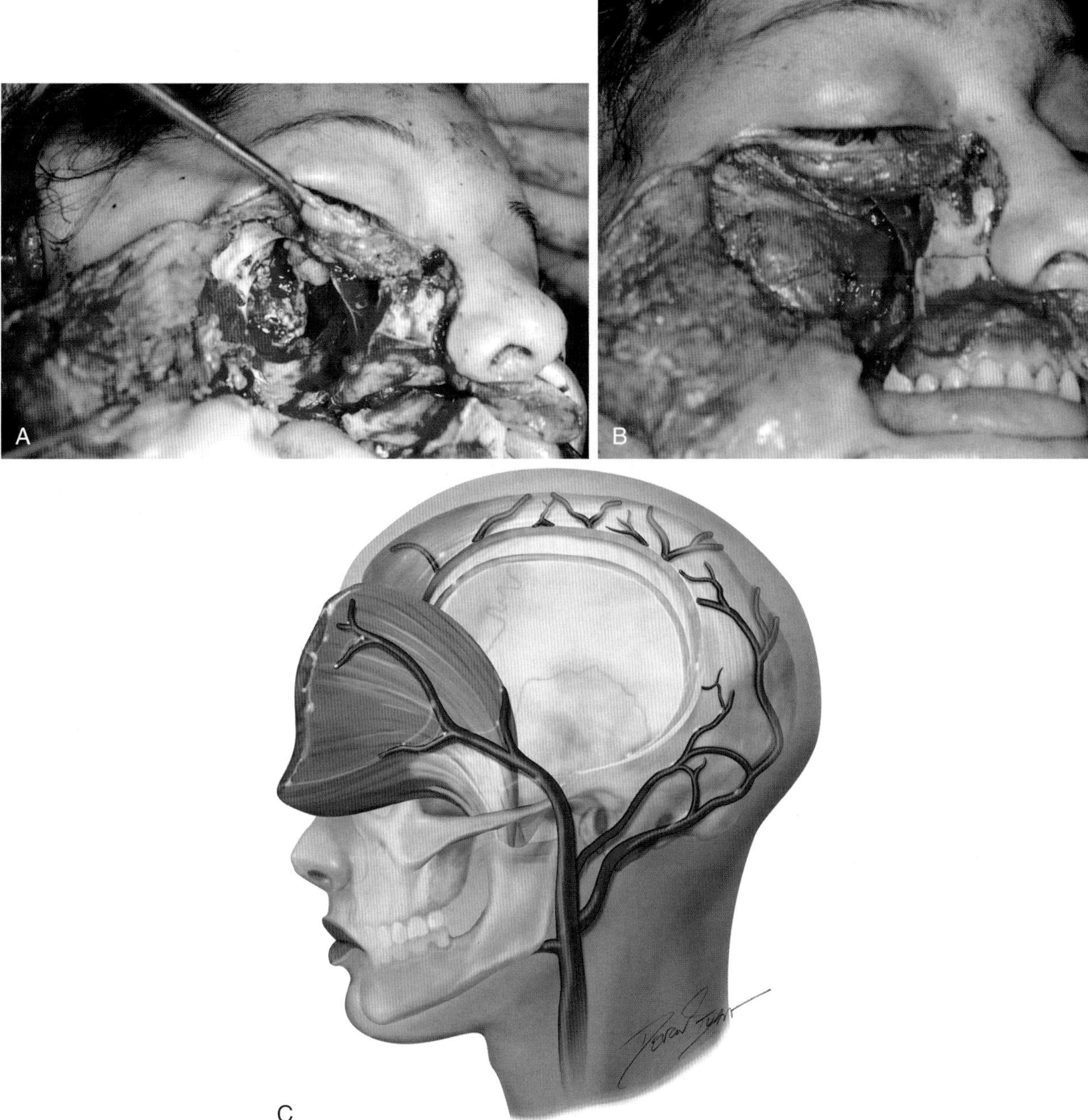

Figure 123.3 **A,** Orbital floor defect in a young patient. **B,** Reconstruction of the floor defect with a temporalis flap. **C,** The temporalis flap is an excellent choice for orbital defects and is facilitated by being above the zygomatic arch.

Parameters such as improvements in mastication, speech, and appropriate facial contours should be assessed at weekly, monthly, and yearly follow-ups. Neurosensory disturbances may lead to panic in both the patient and clinician; however, they often do not constitute an irreversible complication. The transposed muscle eventually reepithelializes and becomes covered with superficial sensory receptors, restoring the normal sensory functions.[28]

References

1. Bajpai H, Saikrishna D. The versatility of temporalis myofascial flap in maxillo-facial reconstruction: a clinical study. *J Maxillofac Oral Surg*. 2011;10(1):25–31.
2. Golovine SS. Procede de cloture plastique de l'orbite après l'exenteration. *Arch Ophthalmol.* 1898;18:679.
3. Lentz J. Ankylose osseuse de la machoire inferieure, resection du col condyle avec interposition du muscle temporal entre les surfaces de resection. *Congress Franc De Chir*. 1895;113.
4. Clauser L, Curioni C, Spanio S. The use of the temporalis muscle flap in facial and craniofacial reconstructive surgery. A review of 182 cases. *J Cranio-Maxillo-Fac Surg.* 1995;23(4):203–214.
5. Speculand B. The origin of the temporalis muscle flap. *Br J Oral Maxillofac Surg.* 1992;30(6):390–392.
6. Campbell HH. Reconstruction of the left maxilla. *Plast Reconstr Surg*. 1948;3(1):66–72.

7. Rambo JHT. Musculoplasty: a new operation for suppurative middle ear deafness. *Trans Am Acad Ophthalmol Otolaryngol*. 1958;62(2):166–177.
8. Bakamjian V. A technique for primary reconstruction of the palate after radical maxillectomy for cancer. *Plast Reconstr Surg*. 1963;31:103–117.
9. Horton CE. Tumors of the maxilla and orbit. In: Gaisford JC, ed. *Symposium on Cancer of the Head and Neck*. St Louis, Missouri: Mosby; 1969.
10. Tessier P, Krastinova D. La transposition du muscle temporal dans l'orbite anophtalme. *Ann Chir Plast*. 1982;27:213.
11. Yadav S, Dhupar V, Dhupar A, Akkara F. Temporalis muscle flap in midfacial region defects. *Internet J Plast Surg*. 2011;7(1).
12. Cordeiro PG, Wolfe SA. The temporalis muscle flap revisited on its centennial: advantages, newer uses, and disadvantages. *Plast Reconstr Surg*. 1996;98(6):980–987.
13. Holmlund A, Lund B, Weiner CK. Mandibular condylectomy with osteoarthrectomy with and without transfer of the temporalis muscle. *Br J Oral Maxillofac Surg*. 2012.
14. Bradley P, Brockbank J. The temporalis muscle flap in oral reconstruction. A cadaveric, animal and clinical study. *J Maxillofac Surg*. 1981;9(3):139–145.
15. Habel G, Hensher R. The versatility of the temporalis muscle flap in reconstructive surgery. *Br J Oral Maxillofac Surg*. 1986;24(2):96–101.
16. van der Meulen JC, Hauben DJ, Vaandrager JM, Birgenhager-Frenkel DH. The use of a temporal osteoperiosteal flap for the reconstruction of malar hypoplasia in Treacher Collins syndrome. *Plast Reconstr Surg*. 1984;74(5):687–693.
17. McCarthy JG, Zide BM. The spectrum of calvarial bone grafting: introduction of the vascularized calvarial bone flap. *Plast Reconstr Surg*. 1984;74(1):10–18.
18. El-Sheikh M, Zeitoun I, El-Massry MAK. The temporalis muscle flap in maxillofacial reconstruction. *Saudi Dent J*. 1991;3:13.
19. Abubaker AO, Abouzgia MB. The temporalis muscle flap in reconstruction of intraoral defects: an appraisal of the technique. *Oral Surg Oral Med Oral Pathol Oral Radiol Endod*. 2002;94(1):24–30.
20. Alonso del Hoyo J, Fernandez Sanroman J, Gil-Diez JL, Diaz Gonzalez FJ. The temporalis muscle flap: an evaluation and review of 38 cases. *J Oral Maxillofac Surg*. 1994;52(2):143–147.
21. Colmenero C, Martorell V, Colmenero B, Sierra L. Temporalis myofascial flap for maxillofacial reconstruction. *J Oral Maxillofac Surg*. 1989;47:197.
22. Wolff KD, Dienemann D, Hoffmeister B. Intraoral defect coverage with muscle flaps. *J Oral Maxillofac Surg*. 1995;53(6):680–685.
23. Mani V, Panda AK. Versatility of temporalis myofascial flap in maxillofacial reconstruction—analysis of 30 cases. *Int J Oral Maxillofac Surg*. 2003;32(4):368–372.
24. Kummoona R. Periorbital and orbital malignancies: methods of management and reconstruction in Iraq. *J Craniofac Surg*. 2007;18(6):1370–1375.
25. Al-Kayat A, Bramley P, AI-Kayat A. A modified pre-auricular approach to the temporomandibular joint and malar arch. *Br J Oral Surg*. 1979;17(2):91–103.
26. Tan O, Atik B, Ergen D. Temporal flap variations for craniofacial reconstruction. *Plast Reconstr Surg*. 2007;119(7):152e–163e.
27. Lopez R, Dekeister C, Sleiman Z, Paoli JR. The temporal fasciocutaneous island flap for oncologic oral and facial reconstruction. *J Oral Maxillofac Surg*. 2003;61(10):1150–1155.
28. Caldana L, Marenzi R, Pennello B. Riabilitazione dopo riscontruzione del palate con limbo di muscolo temporale. *Chirs Testa E Collo*. 1989;6:1.

CHAPTER 124

Pectoralis Major Myocutaneous Flap

Kaushik H. Sharma, Scott T. Claiborne, and Deepak Kademani

Armamentarium

#10 and #15 Surgical blades
Appropriate sutures
Army-Navy retractors
Babcock clamps
Bipolar cautery
Blake drains
Bovie electrocautery
Curved Mayo scissors
Doppler probe
Local anesthetic with vasoconstrictor
Mosquito clamps
Ridge retractor
Satinsky vascular clamps
Shoulder roll
Surgical clips (small, medium, and large)
Tissue dissectors (McCabe, Dierks #1, #2, and #3)

History of the Procedure

The pectoralis major myocutaneous (PMMC) flap has always been considered the workhorse flap for oral, head, and neck reconstruction. In 1979, Ariyan was the first to describe the use of the PMMC flap in head and neck reconstruction.[1] Before Ariyan described its use for head and neck defect reconstruction, Pickrell and colleagues used the PMMC flap to reconstruct chest wall defects as a turnover flap to close sternal wounds.[2] Ariyan described the use of the flap for reconstruction in 11 patients with oropharyngeal, cervicofacial, orofacial complex, orbit, and temporal defects.[3] This work led to a lot of head and neck surgeons using this flap for primary reconstruction of head and neck defects. The current advancements with the successful use of vascularized free flaps, the use of the PMMC pedicled flap has decreased significantly. Currently, for head and neck reconstruction, the PMMC flap has been typically used as a salvage flap after failure of a free vascularized flap or in patients who are poor candidates for free flaps; alternatively, they are used for reconstruction of large head and neck defects as a chimeric flap with a free vascularized flap.[4] Despite this limited use, the flap remains a versatile and reliable option for head and neck reconstruction.

The main advantages of this flap are that it offers one-stage reconstruction, the patient's position need not be changed during the procedure, and multiple skin paddles can be harvested to close complex defects.[5,6]

Disadvantages of the flap are that one can lose muscle function due to weakness in arm adduction/rotation. Poor contour defects can be noted after the flap has been harvested over the chest wall, and a bulge is usually visible over the supraclavicular region due to the arc of the pedicle. This supraclavicular bulge can be prevented by dissecting the pedicle. In cases where the flap has been used to close a defect caused by a cancer ablation, the pectoralis muscle prevents visualization of any recurrences, making follow-up complicated.[7,8] Serial computed tomography scans are used to rule out any tumor recurrences in these patients. In women, harvest of the flap can lead to asymmetry of the breast tissue, whereas in males, hair can grow over the skin paddle when placed intraorally. In males, the flap can be harvested without a skin paddle to avoid the problem of hair and bulkiness in the oral cavity.

Anatomy

The pectoralis is a large, fan-shaped muscle that covers the anterior chest wall, lying over the pectoralis minor, subclavius, serratus anterior, and the intercostal muscles on the anterior thoracic wall. Its origins are divided into a cephalic (clavicular) portion that attaches to the medial one-third of the clavicle, a central (sternal) portion that arises from the sternum and the first six ribs, and a caudal (abdominal) portion that arises from the aponeurosis of the external oblique muscle portion. The muscle converges to form a tendon that attaches to the greater tubercle of the humerus and forms the axillary fold.[9]

Laterally, the pectoralis major is closely associated with the medial aspect of the deltoid muscle, forming the deltopectoral groove, which consistently contains the cephalic vein. The superior surface of the pectoralis major is surrounded by a layer of deep cervical fascia. The inferior surface is separated from the pectoralis minor by the clavipectoral fascia. The clavipectoral fascia extends cephalad to insert into the inferior aspect of the clavicle, splitting just before its insertion to surround the subclavian muscle.

The blood supply to this muscle includes the pectoral branch of the thoracoacromial artery, the lateral thoracic artery, the superior thoracic artery, and the intercostal

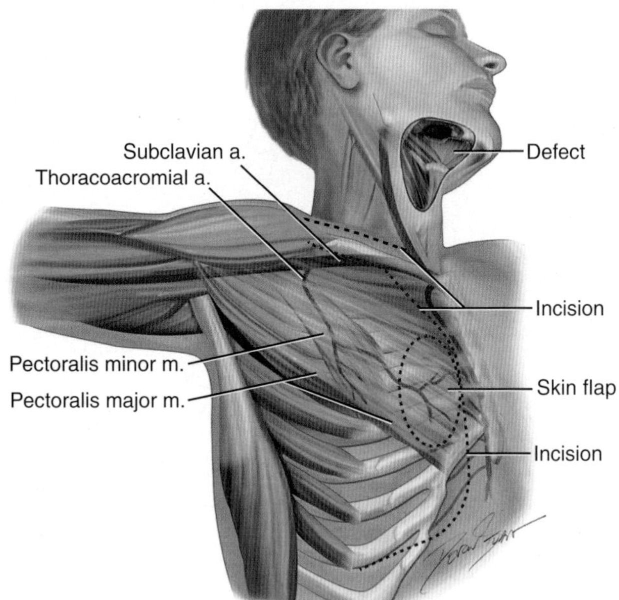

Figure 124.1 Pectoralis muscle delineated with the vascular supply.

artery.[10] The pectoralis artery supplies the pectoralis major and arises from the thoracoacromial artery, which in turn originates from the second portion of the axillary artery. The lateral pectoral artery is also contained within the neurovascular bundle, although it is not believed to contribute significantly to the blood supply of the muscle and often is sacrificed to improve the arc of rotation of the muscle. Both arteries are accompanied by their respective venae comitantes (Fig. 124.1).[11]

The tendinous insertion of the pectoralis major on the greater tubercle of the humerus is sacrificed completely to improve the arc of rotation and to increase the effective length of the pedicle. The pectoralis major and overlying skin are supplied by the internal mammary perforators, which anastomose with the thoracoacromial artery branches. Thus, the medial aspect of the muscle is the most reliable area on which to design a skin paddle.[12] Inferiorly, the skin overlying the muscle adjacent to the rectus abdominis is supplied by the superior epigastric artery and is the least reliable for skin transfer. The total skin territory of the pectoralis major is almost 400 cm^2, although it is rare to require such a large skin paddle for a head and neck reconstruction.[9]

The medial (C5–C7) and lateral (C8–T1) pectoral nerves supply motor innervation to the muscle. The neurovascular bundles pass through the clavicular pectoral fascia en route to the deep surface of the muscle. The function of the pectoralis major is to adduct and medially rotate the arm. Motor branches from C5 and C6 supply the clavicular head while fibers from C7, C8, and T1 supply the sternocostal head of the pectoralis muscle. Sensory innervation is from the same spinal nerves through C5, C6, C8, and T1.[13]

Indications for the Use of the Procedure

The PMMC flap can be used to reconstruct a variety of defects of the head and neck, defects that affect the oral cavity, and oropharyngeal, pharyngoesophageal, and skull base defects. In the oral cavity, the flap can be used to reconstruct the tongue, palate, floor of mouth, buccal mucosa, and segmental defects of the mandible.

For oral, head, and neck reconstruction, this pedicle flap may be used to close an orocutaneous fistula, cover an exposed carotid artery, add bulk to a radical neck dissection site, or restore complex defects with inner and outer epithelial linings.[14] If the muscle flap is used to cover intraoral defects, the muscular surface mucosalizes without the use of a skin paddle. In patients with severe comorbidities, the PMMC can be used as an alternative to free vascularized flaps to close head and neck defects. The upper limit of this flap is usually cephalad to the level of the zygomatic arch.

Many authors have described the use of this flap as a myofascial, myocutaneous, or a myo-osseous flap. Myofascial and myocutaneous uses were described earlier. The use of the PMMC as a myo-osseous flap has also been described in the literature, although its utility is questionable. The flap is usually taken with a rib and used to reconstruct segmental defects of the mandible in addition to providing soft tissue coverage for intraoral or extraoral defects simultaneously. Its advantage is that the curvature of the rib resembles the curvature of the mandible. Combining a rib graft with a PMMC flap, however, does have limitations, including resorption of the graft, pain at the donor site, an increased length of hospital stay, and an increased failure rate.[15] The PMMC flap may also be used to close chest/sternal wounds after cardiothoracic surgery.

Limitations and Contraindications

PMMC flaps are predominantly used as salvage flaps in head and neck reconstruction and therefore have relatively few contraindications. Some patients may have a congenital absence of the pectoralis muscle, as in the case of Poland syndrome, which is also accompanied by cutaneous syndactyly. Previous trauma to the chest wall or surgery (e.g., mastectomy, subclavian lines, cardiac pacemaker, breast implants) to the chest wall could compromise blood supply to the muscle, leading to a poorly vascularized muscle.[14] Shah and colleagues described a possible contraindication in morbidly obese patients, as they may have a nonviable skin paddle and increased bulk, limiting functional reconstruction.[16] Additionally, some patients have vocations that require full range of movement of their shoulders and arms, therefore raising a pectoralis flap could lead to functional restrictions in adduction/abduction of the shoulders.

TECHNIQUE: Pectoralis Major Myocutaneous Flap

STEP 1: Patient Positioning and Preparation

Oral intubation can be used when a PMMC flap is being considered and will be performed in isolation. However, either nasal intubation or a surgical airway is required for patients undergoing an extirpation of a primary head and neck tumor with neck dissection with a PMMC reconstruction. A shoulder roll should be placed to allow mild neck extension. The endotracheal tube should be secured to allow manipulation of the neck. Paralytic agents can usually be used when performing a PMMC flap. The use of a tracheostomy should be strongly considered when performing this flap due to edema that could be experienced in the postoperative setting.

STEP 2: Incisions

The incision site should be delineated with a surgical marker, and the skin paddle length and width should correlate to the size of the defect in the head and neck region. The site prior to incision should be marked and infiltrated with local anesthetic with vasoconstrictor. The skin paddles marked are based on the perforators and usually the goal is to capture the perforating vessels during the harvest. Adjunctive measures to localize the perforators could include a Doppler or SPY Intraoperative Imaging System for Graft Assessment by Lifecell. The SPY system can also be used at the end of the procedure to ensure good vascularity to the skin paddle.

The clavicle and the lateral border of the sternum are outlined. The vascular pedicle runs vertically along a line drawn from the acromion to the xiphoid process. The skin paddle should be marked on the inferomedial portion of the flap corresponding to the size of the defect. A curving C-shaped incision is made to encompass the skin paddle and allow the breast and skin to be elevated off the chest wall. This incision allows for preservation of vessels (internal mammary perforators) for a deltopectoral flap in case there is vascular compromise of the pedicle or when the deltopectoral flap is needed as an adjunctive measure (Fig. 124.2A).

Continued

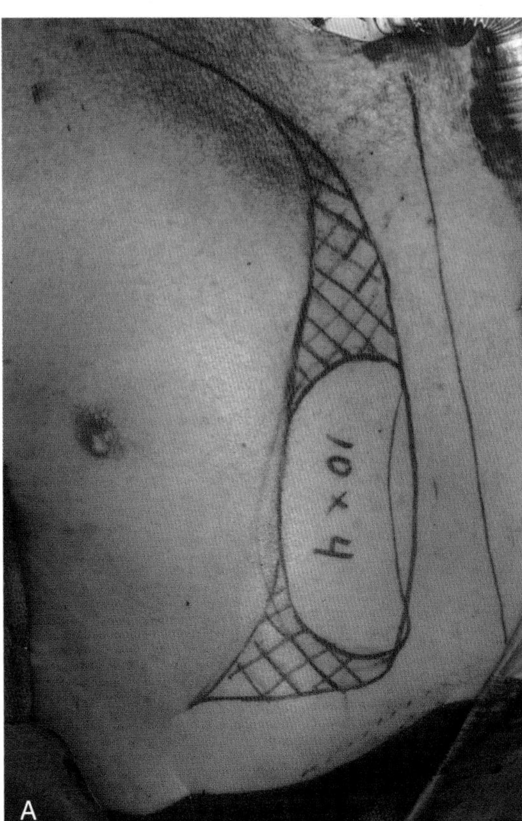

Figure 124.2 A, The skin paddle is delineated with a surgical marker. The size of the skin paddle corresponds to the size of the defect to be closed.

TECHNIQUE: Pectoralis Major Myocutaneous Flap—*cont'd*

STEP 3: Pectoralis Muscle Dissection

A #10 blade knife can be used to create an incision through the skin and subcutaneous tissue down to the pectoralis fascia encircling the skin paddle. Once the muscle is identified, the inferolateral aspect of the muscle flap is identified and the plane between the pectoralis major and the minor is entered and bluntly dissected. To prevent shearing of the perforators, the skin paddle can be sutured to the pectoralis muscle flap. A broad-based flap is usually harvested to ensure good capture of the perforating vessels to the pectoralis muscle flap.

Dissection is then performed medially on the lateral aspect of the sternum, maintaining a submuscular plane of dissection to the clavicle. Internal mammary perforators are usually encountered between the second and fourth intercostal spaces and need to be identified and clipped to prevent bleeding. This plane should be carefully dissected to prevent inadvertent entry or bleeding into the chest cavity (Fig. 124.2B).

STEP 4: Vascular Pedicle Identification

As the pectoralis flap is advanced cephalad, the plane of dissection between the major and minor is encountered along the clavipectoral fascia. The plane is relatively avascular and can be opened easily with blunt dissection.

The vascular pedicle is located on the upper lateral portion of the flap. The pectoral branch of the thoracoacromial artery can be seen on the deep surface of the pectoralis major and medial to the pectoralis minor (Fig. 124.2C).

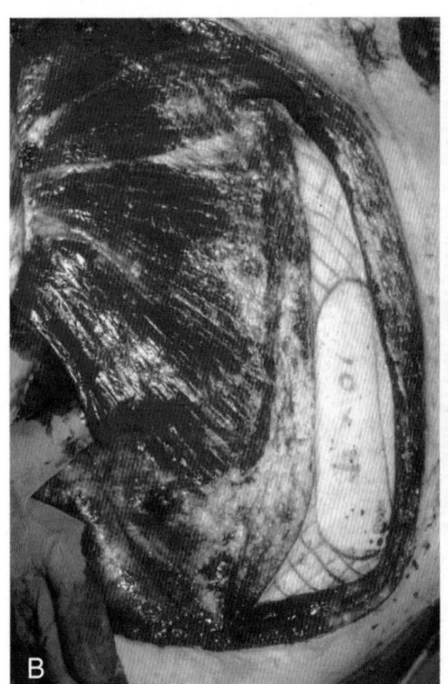

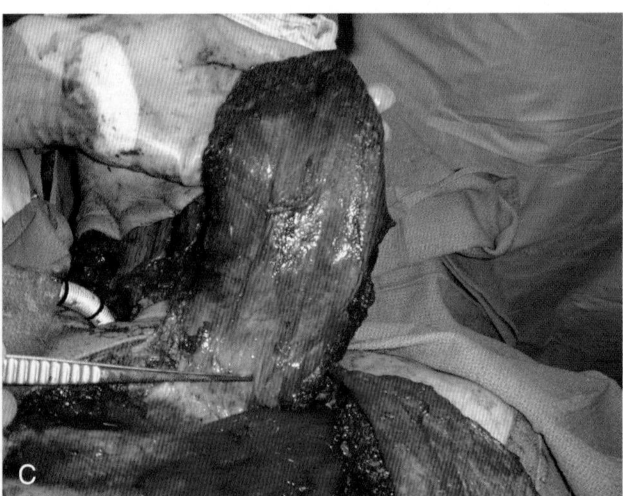

Figure 124.2, cont'd B, The skin paddle is shown with the pectoralis muscle and a broad cuff of subcutaneous tissue to capture perforators. The lateral border of the pectoralis muscle is also shown to illustrate the deep aspect of the dissection. **C,** The vascular pedicle can be seen on the deep surface of the pectoralis major muscle with the lateral thoracic and the thoracoacromial vessels.

TECHNIQUE: Pectoralis Major Myocutaneous Flap—*cont'd*

STEP 5: Humeral Release

The muscle divides laterally as it courses toward the humeral insertion. The lateral and medial pectoral nerves, along with the lateral vascular pedicle, are sacrificed to allow for a greater arc of rotation and to avoid flap contraction with subsequent arm movement. The transection of the pectoral nerves leads to atrophy of the flap, which is beneficial in head and neck defects, especially if gross contour defects are visible extraorally, and to minimize the torsion/head pull of the flap (Fig. 124.2D).

STEP 6: Tunneling in the Head and Neck

Once the flap is elevated, a broad tunnel is created in the subcutaneous plane to allow the flap to be passed through into the neck. Typically, three to four fingerbreadths of space are needed to ensure that the pedicle is not compressed or compromised. The flap is subsequently tunneled through the subcutaneous plane created with the skin paddle oriented to prevent torquing of the pedicle (Fig. 124.2E and F).

Continued

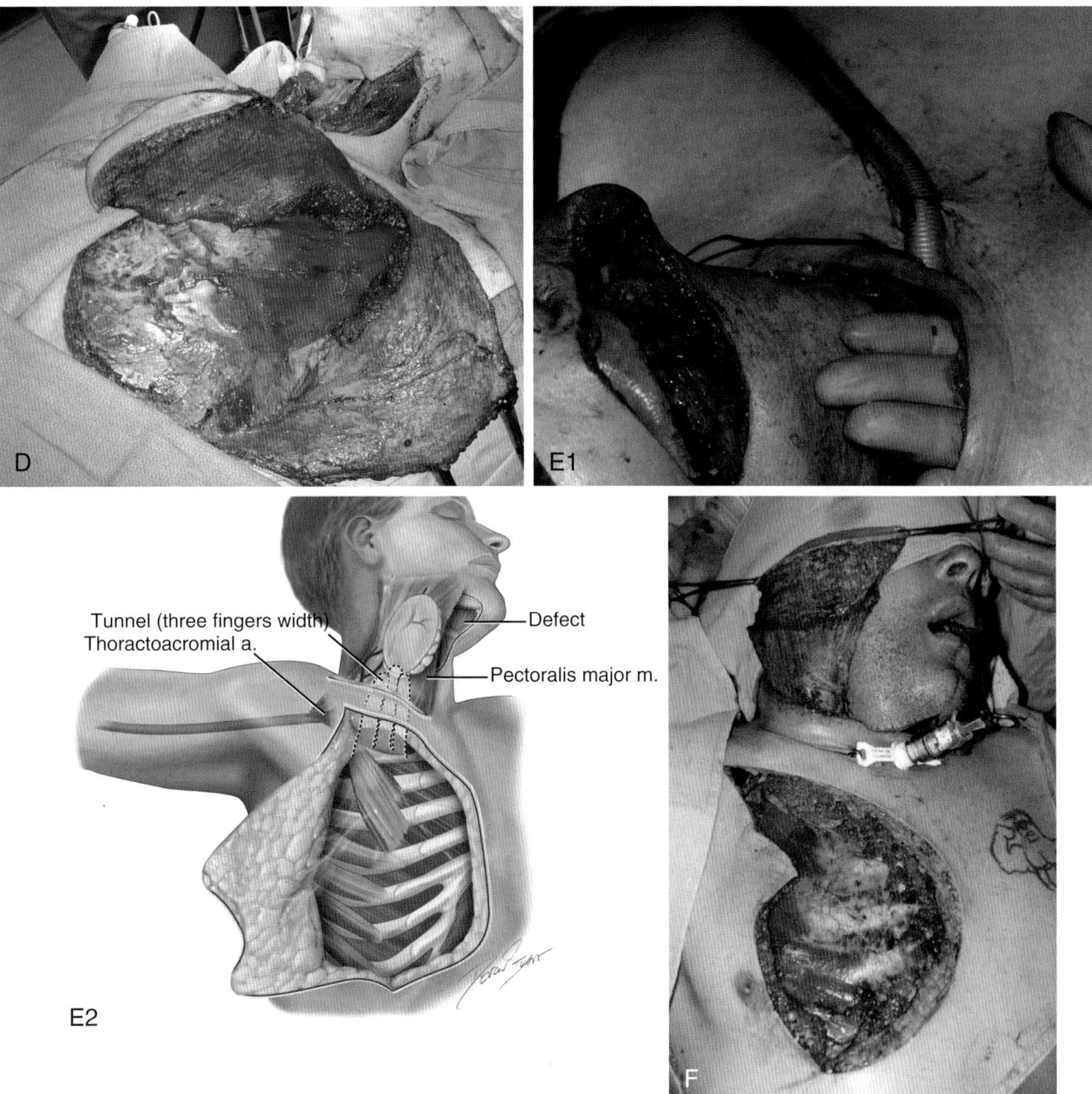

Figure 124.2, cont'd D, The pectoralis muscle is released off the humeral head to increase the arc of rotation with careful preservation of the vascular pedicle. Sometimes the lateral thoracic artery is sacrificed to increase the arc of rotation. **E1** and **E2,** A tunnel three to four fingerbreadths wide is made in the subcutaneous plane to prevent compression/compromise of the vascular pedicle. **F,** The entire flap with the skin paddle is tunneled through the subcutaneous tunnel to be inset in place.

TECHNIQUE: Pectoralis Major Myocutaneous Flap—*cont'd*

STEP 7: Closure

Once the flap skin paddle is sutured in place, drains are placed into the donor site in a dependent fashion. The donor site is closed primarily; however, if a large skin paddle is used, then a skin graft needs to be placed over the exposed muscle. The site is closed in a layer fashion with 3-0 Vicryl sutures after the dependent drains are placed and secured with 2-0 nylon sutures. Staples or nylon sutures can be used to close the skin (Fig. 124.2G and H).

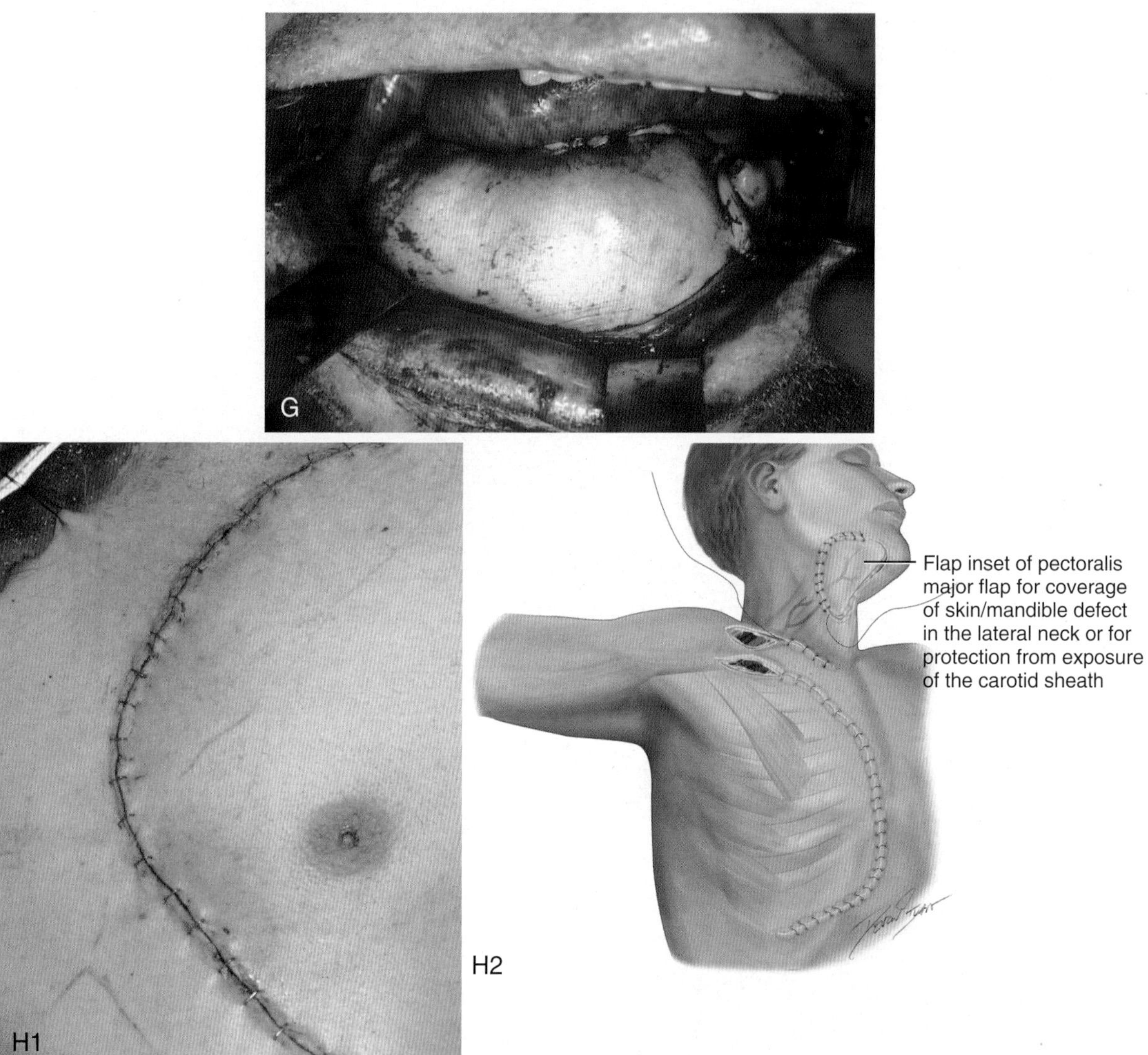
G
H1
H2
Flap inset of pectoralis major flap for coverage of skin/mandible defect in the lateral neck or for protection from exposure of the carotid sheath

Figure 124.2, cont'd **G,** The flap is inset in place and sutured with 3-0 Vicryl sutures. **H1** and **H2,** The donor site is closed in a layered fashion with drains. Staples can be used to close the skin, or alternatively the skin could be closed with nylon sutures.

Alternative Technique: Deltopectoral Flap

In the mid-1960s, Bakamjian used the deltopectoral flap for head and neck reconstruction.[21] The deltopectoral flap is an axial fasciocutaneous flap based on the second and third perforators of the internal mammary artery. The superior incision is made parallel to the clavicle inferiorly and made through skin, subcutaneous, and pectoral fascia. The distolateral extent of the flap is determined by the location of the defect relative to the rotational length of the flap. The flap is elevated in a subfascial plane from lateral to medial and is transposed to the recipient site. The donor site can be closed primarily or a split-thickness skin graft can be used to cover the muscle over the donor site.

The deltopectoral flap is mainly used to reconstruct cutaneous defects of the neck. Due to the advent of microvascular surgery, this flap has limited use in orofacial or pharyngeal reconstruction. The limitations associated with the deltopectoral flap are the lack of bulk, the need for a skin graft for closure of the donor defect, and sometimes the unreliability of the flap's distal random perforators.

Avoidance and Management of Intraoperative Complications

The most common complication associated with this flap is partial or total flap necrosis during the development of the PMMC flap. Several authors have studied the complications of the PMMC flap. The largest study was conducted by Vartanian and colleagues from Brazil, who studied 437 patients who underwent head and neck reconstruction with a PMMC flap.[17] They concluded that there was an overall complication rate of 36.1%, with only 2.4% of the cases involving total flap necrosis. The flap-related complications noted were fistula formation in 11.8%, partial necrosis in 9.7%, infection in 8.3%, dehiscence in 2.8%, and total necrosis in 2.4% of all the patients. When the complication rate of the PMMC flap was compared with other pedicled flaps, there was a significantly lower complication rate with this flap ($p < 0.004$).[17]

Shah and colleagues studied their complication rates and noted a variety of issues that were highly correlated to the failure of the pectoralis muscle flap. These authors found that several factors were associated with poor flap outcomes, including age >70 years, female gender, nomographic overweight, albumin levels less than 4 g/dL, use of the flap for oral cavity reconstruction after a major glossectomy, and the presence of systemic diseases such as diabetes mellitus, hypertension, atherosclerotic heart disease, peripheral vascular disease, renal failure, and collagen vascular disease.[16] The main complications noted were wound infection, fistula formation, and wound dehiscence, and these were increased in irradiated patients. Larger skin paddles led to the greater capture of vessel perforators, leading to a decreased loss of the skin paddle compared with smaller skin paddles that led to vascular insufficiency.[12] Electrocautery should be used judiciously; overzealous use can lead to coagulation of the vessels and compromising the pedicle through retrograde thrombosis. Incorporation of the lateral thoracic artery is important for flap viability.

Metha and colleagues also studied their complication rates in PMMC flaps in 220 patients.[18] They noted similar complication rates. Their flap necrosis rate was 27.3% (2.7% total and 24.6% partial loss), fistula formation (12.7%), infection (20.5%), dehiscence (14.5%), and hematoma formation (4.5%). They further described the high risk factors for flap necrosis with odds ratios of 10.83 when using bipedicled flaps and 10.32 in diabetic patients. Other high factors also described included female gender, defect size, primary site (tongue had the highest risk), and prior chemotherapy.[18]

Direct comparisons between the myocutaneous flap and microvascular free flaps have been highlighted in two studies. The first, conducted by Nayak and Swain, found that in the microvascular group there was a 13% difference between the cosmesis and functional differences between the two groups.[19] Patients from the microvascular free flaps group had an average operating time that was 4 hours greater and a hospitalization stay that was 3 days longer, and the average cost of treatment was doubled when compared to the myocutaneous flap. Of note, there were greater flap failure rates and reexploration rates in the microvascular group. Another matched control study conducted by Smeele and colleagues looked at the morbidity and cost differences between free flap reconstruction and pedicled flap reconstruction in oral and oropharyngeal cancer treatment.[20] The outcome variables that were analyzed included operative time, blood loss, admission length (including intensive care unit and coronary care unit stay), complications, secondary interventions, readmissions, and feeding status. The study showed there was no difference between the two groups in all the variables except for a difference noted in operative time ($p < 0.0001$).[20]

Postoperative Considerations

Once a pectoralis flap is used for head and neck reconstruction there may be a need for postoperative physical therapy to ensure the arm as adequate function. Also in the irradiated patient there may be contracture of the neck which may be need to released or have the pedicled taken down to improve range of motion. In the female patient there will likely be a contour deformity of the breast which may need to be addressed secondarily if this of concern to the patient.

References

1. Ariyan S. The pectoralis major myocutaneous flap. A versatile flap for reconstruction in the head and neck. *Plast Reconstr Surg.* 1979;63(1):73–81.
2. Pickrell KL, Baker HM, Collins JP. Reconstructive surgery of the chest wall. *Surg Gynecol Obstet.* 1947;84(4):465–476.
3. Ariyan S. Further experiences with the pectoralis major myocutaneous flap for the immediate repair of defects from excisions of head and neck cancers. *Plast Reconstr Surg.* 1979;64(5):605–612.
4. Righi PD, Weisberger EC, Slakes SR, Wilson JL, Kesler KA, Yaw PB. The pectoralis major myofascial flap: clinical applications in head and neck reconstruction. *Am J Otolaryngol.* 1998;19(2):96–101.
5. Ord RA, Avery BS. Side-by-side double paddle pectoralis major flap for cheek defects. *Br J Oral Maxillofac Surg.* 1989;27(3):177–185.
6. Wilson JS, Yiacoumettis AM, O'Neill T. Some observations on 112 pectoralis major myocutaneous flaps. *Am J Surg.* 1984;147(2): 273–279.
7. Ossoff RH, Wurster CF, Berktold RE, Krespi YP, Sisson GA. Complications after pectoralis major myocutaneous flap reconstruction of head and neck defects. *Arch Otolaryngol.* 1983;109(12):812–814.
8. Schuller DE. Limitations of the pectoralis major myocutaneous flap in head and neck cancer reconstruction. *Arch Otolaryngol.* 1980;106(11):709–714.
9. Kademani D, Dierks E. *Reconstruction of Ablative Maxillofacial Defects.* Vol. 4. OMS Knowledge Updates; 2006:153–171.

10. Freeman JL, Walker EP, Wilson JS, Shaw HJ. The vascular anatomy of the pectoralis major myocutaneous flap. *Br J Plast Surg*. 1981;34(1):3–10.
11. Saraceno CA, Santini H, Endicott JN, Martinez C, Shah C. The pectoralis major myocutaneous flap: an angiographic study. *Laryngoscope*. 1983;93(6):756–759.
12. Teo KG, Rozen WM, Acosta R. The pectoralis major myocutaneous flap. *J Reconstr Microsurg*. 2013;29(7):449–456.
13. Carlson ER, Layne JM. The pectoralis major myocutaneous flap for reconstruction of soft-tissue oncologic defects. *Atlas Oral Maxillofac Surg Clin North Am*. 1997;5(2):15–35.
14. Carlson ER. Pectoralis major myocutaneous flap. *Oral Maxillofac Surg Clin North Am*. 2003;15(4):565–575 (vi).
15. Ord RA. The pectoralis major myocutaneous flap in oral and maxillofacial reconstruction: a retrospective analysis of 50 cases. *J Oral Maxillofac Surg*. 1996;54(11):1292–1295.
16. Shah JP, Haribhakti V, Loree TR, Sutaria P. Complications of the pectoralis major myocutaneous flap in head and neck reconstruction. *Am J Surg*. 1990;160(4):352–355.
17. Vartanian JG, Carvalho AL, Carvalho SM, Mizobe L, Magrin J, Kowalski LP. Pectoralis major and other myofascial/myocutaneous flaps in head and neck cancer reconstruction: experience with 437 cases at a single institution. *Head Neck*. 2004;26(12):1018–1023.
18. Metha S, Sarkar S, Kavarana N, Bhathena H, Metha A. Complications of the pectoralis major myocutaneous flap in oral cavity reconstruction: a prospective evaluation of 220 cases. *Plast Reconstr Surg*. 1997;98:31–37.
19. Nayak UK, Swain B. Myocutaneous v/s micro vascular free flaps in oral cavity reconstruction—a comparative study. *Indian J Otolaryngol Head Neck Surg*. 2004;56(2):96–98.
20. Smeele LE, Goldstein D, Tsai V, et al. Morbidity and cost differences between free flap reconstruction and pedicled flap reconstruction in oral and oropharyngeal cancer: matched control study. *J Otolaryngol*. 2006;35(2):102–107.
21. Bakamjian VY. Total reconstruction of pharynx with medially based deltopectoral skin flap. *N Y State J Med*. 1968;68(21):2771–2778.

CHAPTER 125

Submental Island Flap for Reconstruction of Head and Neck Defects

Dale A. Baur, David Collette, and Petra Olivieri

Armamentarium

#9 Molt periosteal elevator
#15 Blade
Adson forceps
Allis clamp
Appropriate sutures
Army-Navy retractors
Bipolar electrocautery
Bovie electrocautery
DeBakey forceps
Doppler and lube
Frazier suction
Hemostats
Iris curved scissors
Langenbeck retractors
Local anesthetic with vasoconstrictor
Metzenbaum curved scissors
Mosquito hemostats
Needle holders
Nerve stimulator
Senn retractors
Skin marking pen
Tenotomy scissors
Two-pronged skin hook

History of the Procedure

Surgeons often must treat head and neck defects caused by ablative surgery or injury. Reconstruction of complex head and neck defects with functional and morphologic restoration has long been a highly challenging and complex surgical undertaking. Many techniques have been developed to treat these defects, including skin grafts, local or regional flaps, free vascularized tissue transfer, and tissue expansion for reconstruction. Although skin grafting is technically simple and can provide good esthetic results with low morbidity, it cannot be used for complex defects. Tissue expansion is another option for cutaneous coverage, but this technique requires multiple operative procedures and a significant commitment by the patient. Random pattern flaps (advancement flap, rotation flap) and platysma myocutaneous flaps[1,2] can provide a good color match for the face; however, they are often unreliable,[3] and mobility and the amount of tissue that can be used are limited. Also, in many cases the scars at the donor site are unacceptable. A pedicled flap, such as a trapezius or pectoralis myocutaneous flap, can provide sufficient transplant tissue and is suitable for reconstructing large head and neck defects.[4] However, this flap is too bulky to be suitable for reconstructing small or medium-sized defects in the head and neck region.

Advances in microsurgery have allowed many complex facial defects to be reconstructed with free flaps, such as radial forearm or other free fasciocutaneous flaps; however, the color and texture of these flaps show a definite demarcation with the neighboring facial skin. In addition, these flaps are more surgically complex and have the potential for flap failure associated with microsurgical techniques.[5,6] For reconstruction of head and neck defects, the flap should be reliable, pliable, and functionally and cosmetically acceptable; it also should have minimum donor site morbidity and should match the recipient site in color, texture, and thickness.[7]

In 1993, Martin et al.[5] first described a new axial-patterned island flap based on the submental artery. This new flap, the submental island flap, enhanced the reliability and mobility of the random cervical platysma myocutaneous flap and was also free of the limitations of the latter, described previously. The submental island flap consists of thin, pliable tissues with a perfect color match and is similar to facial skin. It also has a robust blood supply and a good arc of rotation. This procedure can also reduce the submental fullness and jowling associated with the aging face and has positive esthetic results.[8] Significant research on its anatomy and applications has shown that the submental island flap is ideal for head and neck reconstruction. This flap also has been described as a free flap.[5] All these advantages make the submental island flap easy to work with, and it is widely used by numerous oral and maxillofacial surgeons.[9–11]

Anatomy

The basis for the submental island flap is the submental artery, which is reported to be a well-defined, consistent branch of the facial artery with a diameter of 1 to 2 mm.[5,9,10] It arises

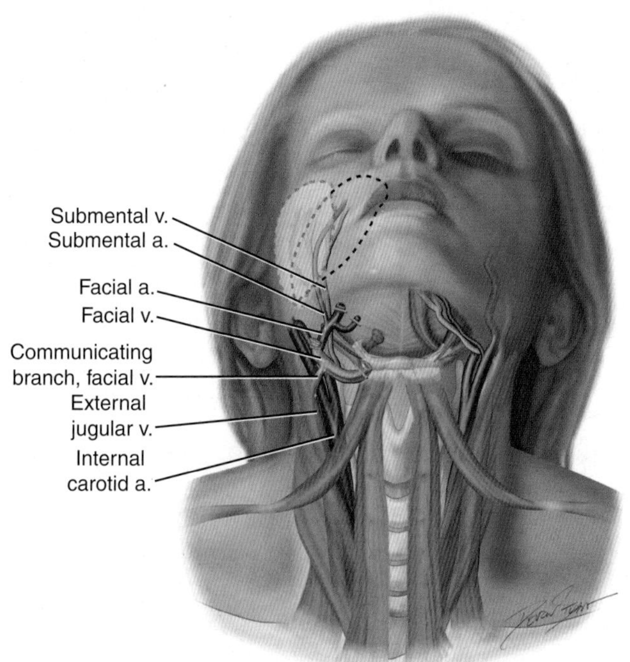

Figure 125.1 Anatomy of the submental artery.

from the facial artery, deep or superficial to the submandibular gland, approximately 1.5 to 2 cm below the inferior border of the mandible, and passes forward and medially on the mylohyoid muscle below the mandibular border, ending behind the mandibular symphysis just lateral to the midline.[5,12] Most commonly, it runs deep to the anterior belly of the digastric muscle and sends off some branches to the submental skin, lower lip, and sublingual gland (Fig. 125.1).[5,10–12,14]

Along its course, one to four cutaneous perforators are found piercing the overlying platysma, forming a subdermal plexus that anastomoses extensively with the contralateral branches, providing a possible large random extension on the other side. Venous drainage of this flap is through the submental vein into the facial vein. There are one to three anastomoses between these vessels and the external jugular vein, which plays a major role in the surgical procedure and, in some cases, may be used for the venous drainage of the flap.[5,14] Because of its reliable blood supply, this flap can be harvested from mandibular angle to mandibular angle, with the width determined by the flaccidity of the neck skin; this allows direct closure with a well-hidden donor scar of up to 18 × 7 cm in size. The pedicle may be up to 8 cm long, and the arc of the pedicle is such that the flap easily reaches defects of the face.[5–7,15]

Indications for the Use of the Procedure

For reconstruction of head and neck defects, the ideal is to achieve both functional and esthetic outcomes. Additional donor site morbidity should be avoided, especially with benign diseases.[5,7] The proximity of the donor site and its characteristics of reliability, excellent skin match, minimal donor site morbidity, and a long pedicle make the submental island flap an ideal method for reconstruction of head and neck defects caused by trauma, burns, or surgical defects. Furthermore, the relative simplicity of raising this flap gives the additional benefit of a shorter operative time. In direct comparison to radial forearm free flap reconstruction, submental island flap reconstruction was associated with shorter operative times, shorter length of hospital stay, and overall cost savings.[16] When appropriate, these advantages make the submental island flap especially important to consider in patients with head and neck cancer, who are elderly and with a poor comorbidity profile.

Since its introduction, the submental flap has achieved great success in the intraoral reconstruction of floor of the mouth, gingival, palate, cheek, oropharynx, and esophageal defects, in addition to cutaneous reconstruction of the lip, nose, preauricular region, and temporal region; some surgeons have even reported its use for forehead defects.[5–7,9,10,18–27] With a rich vascular network between the ipsilateral and contralateral facial arteries and veins, the submental flap can be used for contralateral defects, in which case a Y–V technique or other procedure is required to increase the length of the pedicle.[22,27] This flap can also be designed as a free flap, if required, or as an axial-pattern osteocutaneous flap in the reconstruction of facial bony defects through the use of a segment of the mandibular rim.[5,11] As an island flap, it can also be used safely for patients who received prior radiation treatment in a therapeutic dose.[7,28] However, in those cases, direct closure of the donor site may be incomplete and may require skin grafts. This flap is particularly suited for reconstruction of hair-bearing areas in men.[11,17,20,24]

Limitations and Contraindications

Use of the submental island flap in head and neck reconstruction has some specific limitations and contraindications. For example, metastatic disease in either the submental (level Ia) or submandibular (level Ib) lymph node basins, is a contraindication.[14,17] Another contraindication is injury or ligation of the submental or facial vascular system during previous neck surgery.[27,29] Although the pedicle of the flap is reliable and constant as reported, anatomic anomalies of the vessels are a contraindication; the authors recommend preoperative examination of these vessels to exclude anatomic anomalies. Preoperative identification of the facial and submental arteries with three-dimensional computed tomography angiography has been reported to be helpful in evaluating the vessels and avoiding injury.[30] Relative limitations and contraindications include an obese neck[17] and reconstruction of hairless facial regions in men.[27]

TECHNIQUE: Reconstruction With a Submental Island Flap

A submental island flap can be harvested by two methods: in an anterograde fashion from the facial vessels and in a retrograde manner from the submental vessels. The techniques applied are the same, but the sequence of flap dissection is different. However, no significant differences are seen in the outcomes. The authors prefer the retrograde manner, which is described below.

STEP 1: Anesthesia, Positioning, and Armamentarium

The submental flap procedure is performed under general anesthesia. The method of intubation is based on the site of the defect and must take into account surgical convenience. The patient is placed in the supine position, with the neck moderately extended before harvesting of the flap begins. If tolerated by the patient, a shoulder roll may be placed to aid in extension of the neck. The armamentarium consists of a standard soft tissue tray, nerve stimulator, and vascular clips or ties. Doppler ultrasound may be useful for locating the vessels.

STEP 2: Flap Design

Depending on the defect created by excision of the lesions, the flap is horizontally designed in the area served by the submental artery. It should be a little bigger in size than the defect, although the maximum dimension that can be reliably harvested is 15 × 7 cm.[5] The flap should be spindle-shaped or elliptical to facilitate primary closure. Its superior limit should be at least 1 cm below the inferior border of the mandible to prevent inferior lip eversion and to hide the donor site scar as much as possible. The lower limit, defined above the cervicomental angle, depends on the laxity of the skin and could be determined by a simple pinch test. To perform this test, the surgeon pinches the skin of the submental area between two fingers before outlining the flap; this helps evaluate skin laxity and the likelihood of performing direct closure. The length of the skin paddle can be determined by the distance from the pivot point below the ipsilateral antegonial notch to the most distal point of the defect. This length should equal the distance from the ipsilateral antegonial notch to the most distal extent of the designed flap along the course of the ipsilateral submental artery. It is important to note that the flap design may cross the midline and will be based on the excellent collateral flow of the vessels in this region. The borders of the flap can be marked, and relevant vessels are identified preoperatively (Fig. 125.2A–C).

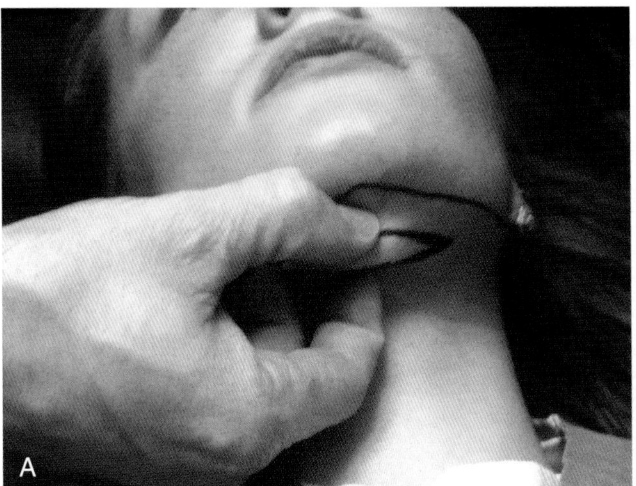

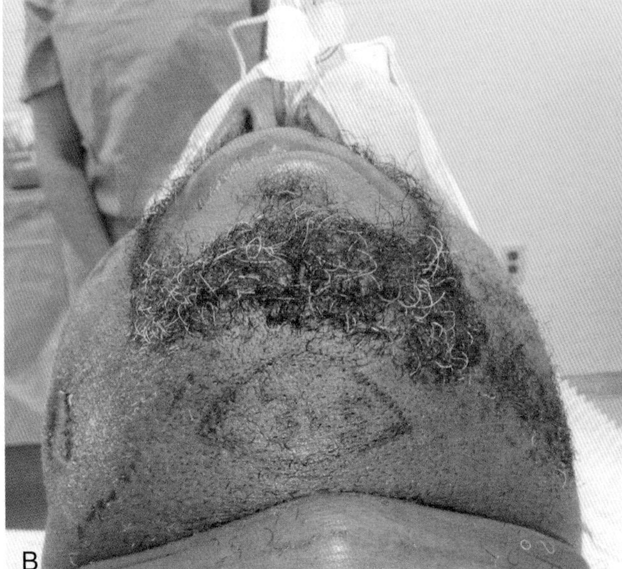

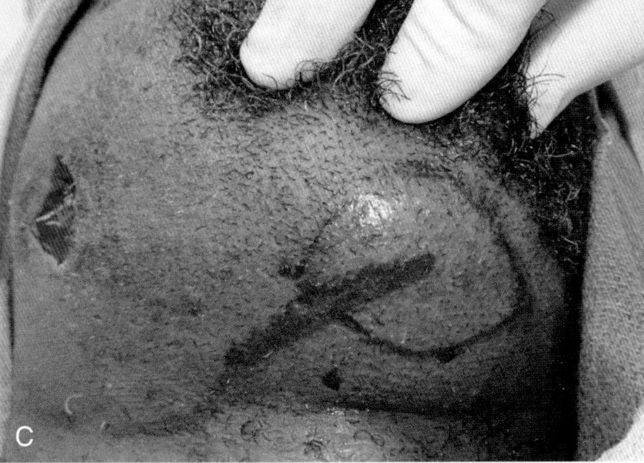

Figure 125.2 **A,** Skin pinch test. **B,** Flap design. The dimensions of this flap are 3 × 5 cm. **C,** Flap design and course of the submental artery based on Doppler imaging.

TECHNIQUE: Reconstruction with a Submental Island Flap—*cont'd*

STEP 3: Incisions and Dissection of the Flap

After the elliptical portions of the flap have been marked, an incision is made through skin, subcutaneous tissue, and platysma. The dissection starts on the contralateral side. After incision of the upper border of the flap, the marginal mandibular branch of the facial nerve is identified near the lateral edge of the flap within the superficial layer of the deep cervical fascia, just deep to the platysmal plane. Dissection continues to the submandibular gland. The facial and submental vessels of the contralateral side are dissected. After ligation of the vessels and their perforators to the submandibular gland and deep tissues, the flap is detached from the underlying muscles in the subplatysmal plane above the digastric muscle. Dissection is carried out continuously toward the origin of the pedicle. When the midline is reached, dissection proceeds carefully to identify the ipsilateral submental vessels. Dissection is carried deeper into level Ia down to the mylohyoid muscle. The ipsilateral anterior belly of the digastric muscle is then raised by dissection off the mandible and hyoid bone; the mylohyoid muscle remains intact. A modified technique for resident training has been described, which advocates including the mylohyoid muscle in the flap.[31] Although this is probably not necessary, it provides an additional margin of safety in preserving the submental artery and perforating vessels and makes the dissection easier.[11,15] Although this may provide additional pedicle bulk, in some cases this helps with reconstruction. If the mylohyoid muscle is included in the flap, it should be released from its attachments. The submental artery and vein then are dissected from the deep fascia connections. Care must be taken to identify and protect the ipsilateral marginal mandibular branch of the facial nerve during the dissection. When the dissection reaches the origin of the submental vessels, all branches to the submandibular gland are ligated and the submental artery island is created with a wide arc of rotation. If this flap is designed as a free flap, it may be harvested according to the required pedicle length. It is crucial that, in malignant cases, the submandibular nodes are always checked during flap elevation, followed by selective dissection.[6,9] Also, the pedicle should be skeletonized to minimize the possibility of metastasis (Fig. 125.2D–E).

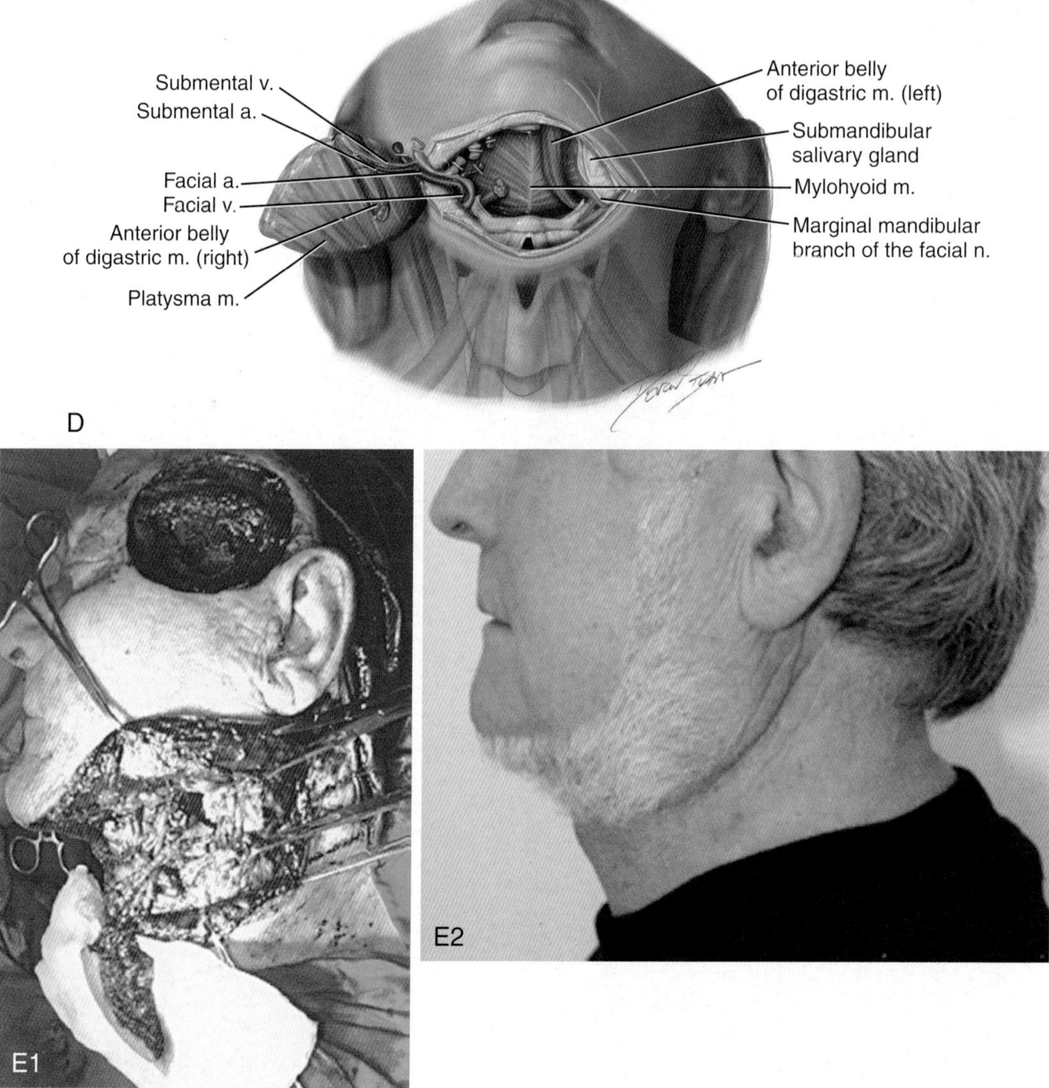

Figure 125.2, cont'd **D,** Flap design and incision. **E1–E2,** Submental island flap elevated, post surgery.

TECHNIQUE: Reconstruction with a Submental Island Flap—*cont'd*

STEP 4: Elongation of the Pedicle

A pedicle length of approximately 5 cm is easily obtained when the dissection is completed with the entire facial artery retained; this is usually sufficient.[5,27] A longer pedicle may be achieved by dividing the facial vessels distal to the origin of the submental artery or by dividing and anastomosing the taut submental or common facial vein to a suitable vein close to the recipient site[14]; this provides an additional 1 to 2 cm of pedicle length. Another procedure that increases the length of the pedicle is the Y–V procedure. By ligating the facial vessels proximal to the origin of the submental artery with the corresponding vein, the surgeon can design the flap as a reverse-flow flap, which is supplied by the distal facial artery pedicle; in this way, extra length can be obtained, and the flap will reach up to the infraorbital region. A Y–V procedure can also be accomplished using the external jugular vein. This is done by locating a communicating branch between the facial and external jugular veins. The trunk of the facial vein is divided proximal to this communicating branch. Consequently, the Y-vascular pattern turns into a V-vascular pattern that allows up to 5 cm of additional distal mobilization of the flap.[32]

STEP 5: Tunnel Preparation and Flap Transfer

After the flap has been created, a tunnel may be made from the origin of the pedicle to the defect, if needed. This tunnel can be submucosal, subcutaneous, or a combination of these. The tunnel should be broad enough so as not to compress the flap. The skin paddle is carefully passed through the tunnel or primarily existing incision to the defect. Excessive stretching of the flap should be avoided. For further pedicle advancement and a greater arc of rotation, the marginal mandibular branch of the facial nerve can be dissected off the facial pedicle and the elevated submental artery island flap passed under the marginal mandibular nerve (Fig. 125.2F).[6]

STEP 6: Closure and Drainage

When the flap is transferred to the site of the defect, it is trimmed to a shape suitable for the defect. After complete hemostasis and copious irrigation, the flap is sutured layer by layer to the margins of the defect without excessive tension. Usually the donor site can be closed directly without additional dissection, especially in elderly patients. The cervical skin can be sutured to the hyoid bone to maintain the cervicomental angle. In cases that pose difficulty with direct closure, skin on the cervical side, rather than the mandible side, should be mobilized to prevent eversion of the lower lip. Flexion of the neck to facilitate closure should be avoided, because it causes subsequent hypertrophic scars. Passive drains should be placed in the donor site and the subcutaneous tunnel to prevent a compressive hematoma (Fig. 125.2G).

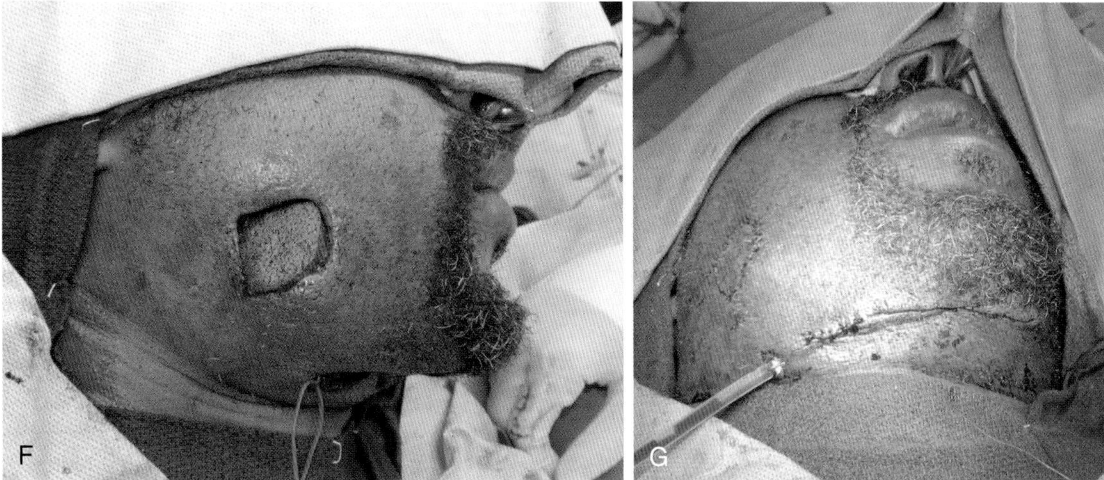

Figure 125.2, cont'd **F,** Tunnel created and flap inset through tunnel. **G,** Inset of flap and closure of donor site.

Avoidance and Management of Intraoperative Complications

A sufficient blood supply to the submental island flap is crucial for successful reconstruction. When the flap is designed, the surgeon must make sure that its size and the length of the pedicle are adequate for reconstruction. Submental vessels must be carefully protected during flap harvesting. A flap that includes the ipsilateral anterior belly of the digastric muscle provides better venous drainage and prevents failure. The authors recommend the use of loupes for dissecting submental vessels. Care should be taken, in the creation of the tunnel, to ensure that it is broad enough to allow transfer of the flap to the recipient site without excessive tension on or trauma to the skin paddle. Also, the surgeon should avoid distorting or over manipulating the pedicle. Vascular anomalies should be excluded before surgery by ultrasound or computed tomography angiography, although only a few cases of such anomalies have been reported.[5,12] Care should be taken to avoid injury to the marginal mandibular nerve when the flap is raised. The surgeon can prevent this type of injury by identifying and preserving the marginal mandibular nerve either before raising the flap or when dissection reaches this site.

A visible scar or eversion of the lower lip can be avoided if the flap is created and sutured according to the techniques described in this chapter.

Postoperative Considerations

Airway management is paramount for any case involving the head and neck region. Although airway swelling with submental flaps is minimal in the author's experience, it warrants consideration. Also, the patient should avoid wearing neckties during the initial postoperative period to avoid compromising the vascular pedicle. Although the success rate of the submental island flap is very high, partial or total loss of the flap cannot be entirely avoided. After surgery, moderate immobilization of the head is suggested, along with a perioperative course of steroids and antibiotics.

Intensive observation of the flap after surgery is important, including its color, texture, temperature, and capillary refill.[33] Almost all failures of submental flaps are caused by venous congestion. In most cases, this development resolves gradually; however, the surgeon should evaluate the cause to determine whether surgical intervention, decompression, or puncture of the flap is needed.

For cases involving oral reconstruction, the patient should be fed through a nasogastric tube or should have liquid food without chewing for 7 to 14 days. Oral care should be carefully performed three or four times every day. Drains may be removed when the drainage has decreased to less than 30 mL in a 24-hour period. If the flap needs to be debulked for cosmetic purposes, this should be done 6 months after surgery.

References

1. Futrell JW, Johns ME, Edgerton MT, Cantrell RW, Fitz-Hugh GS. Platysma myocutaneous flap for intraoral reconstruction. *Am J Surg*. 1978;136(4):504–507.
2. Hurwitz DJ, Rabson JA, Futrell JW. The anatomic basis for the platysma skin flap. *Plast Reconstr Surg*. 1983;72(3):302–314.
3. Céruse P, Disant F, Cote I, Dessenon C, Morgon AH. [Submental myocutaneous island flaps: anatomical study and prospective use]. *Rev Laryngol Otol Rhinol*. 1996;117(5):389–392.
4. Chen WL, Deng YF, Peng GG, et al. Extended vertical lower trapezius island myocutaneous flap for reconstruction of cranio-maxillofacial defects. *Int J Oral Maxillofac Surg*. 2007;36(2):165–170.
5. Martin D, Pascal JF, Baudet J, et al. The submental island flap: a new donor site. Anatomy and clinical applications as a free or pedicled flap. *Plast Reconstr Surg*. 1993;92(5):867–873.
6. Chen WL, Li JS, Yang ZH, Huang ZQ, Wang JU, Zhang B. Two submental island flaps for reconstructing oral and maxillofacial defects following cancer ablation. *J Oral Maxillofac Surg*. 2008;66(6):1145–1156.
7. Vural E, Suen JY. The submental island flap in head and neck reconstruction. *Head Neck*. 2000;22(6):572–578.
8. Pelissier P, Casoli V, Martin D, Demiri E, Baudet J. [Submental island flaps. Surgical technique and possible variations in facial reconstruction]. *Rev Laryngol Otol Rhinol*. 1997;118(1):39–42.
9. Curran AJ, Neligan P, Gullane PJ. Submental artery island flap. *Laryngoscope*. 1997;107(11 Pt 1):1545–1549.
10. Yilmaz M, Menderes A, Barutçu A. Submental artery island flap for reconstruction of the lower and mid face. *Ann Plast Surg*. 1997;39(1):30–35.
11. Faltaous AA, Yetman RJ. The submental artery flap: an anatomic study. *Plast Reconstr Surg*. 1996;97(1):56–60.
12. Magden O, Edizer M, Tayfur V, Atabey A. Anatomic study of the vasculature of the submental artery flap. *Plast Reconstr Surg*. 2004;114(7):1719–1723.
13. Moubayed SP, Rahal A, Ayad T. The submental island flap for soft-tissue head and neck reconstruction: step-by-step video description and long-term results. *Plast Reconstr Surg*. 2014;133(3):684–686.
14. Sterne GD, Januszkiewicz JS, Hall PN, Bardsley AF. The submental island flap. *Br J Plast Surg*. 1996;49(2):85–89.
15. Uysal AC, Alagöz MS, Unlü RE, Sensöz O. An anatomic study and clinical applications of the reversed submental perforator-based island flap. *Plast Reconstr Surg*. 2003;112(2):690–691.
16. Forner D, Phillips T, Rigby M, Hart R, Taylor M, Trites J. Submental island flap reconstruction reduces cost in oral cancer reconstruction compared to radial forearm free flap reconstruction: a case series and cost analysis. *J Otolaryngol Head Neck Surg*. 2016;45:11.
17. Merten SL, Jiang RP, Caminer D. The submental artery island flap for head and neck reconstruction. *ANZ J Surg*. 2002;72(2):121–124.
18. Demir Z, Kurtay A, Sahin U, Velidedeoğlu H, Celebioğlu S. Hair-bearing submental artery island flap for reconstruction of mustache and beard. *Plast Reconstr Surg*. 2003;112(2):423–429.
19. You YH, Chen WL, Wang YP, Liang J. The feasibility of facial-submental artery island myocutaneous flaps for reconstructing defects of the oral floor following cancer ablation. *Oral Surg Oral Med Oral Pathol Oral Radiol Endod*. 2010;109(6):e12–e16.
20. Multinu A, Ferrari S, Bianchi B, et al. The submental island flap in head and neck reconstruction. *Int J Oral Maxillofac Surg*. 2007;36(8):716–720.
21. Genden EM, Buchbinder D, Urken ML. The submental island flap for palatal

reconstruction: a novel technique. *J Oral Maxillofac Surg*. 2004;62(3):387–390.

22. Janssen DA, Thimsen DA. The extended submental island lip flap: an alternative for esophageal repair. *Plast Reconstr Surg*. 1998;102(3):835–838.
23. Kummoona R. Use of lateral cervical flap in reconstructive surgery of the orofacial region. *Int J Oral Maxillofac Surg*. 1994;23(2):85–89.
24. Kitazawa T, Harashina T, Taira H, Takamatsu A. Bipedicled submental island flap for upper lip reconstruction. *Ann Plast Surg*. 1999;42(1):83–86.
25. Koshima I, Inagawa K, Urushibara K, Moriguchi T. Combined submental flap with toe web for reconstruction of the lip with oral commissure. *Br J Plast Surg*. 2000;53(7):616–619.
26. Sebastian P, Thomas S, Varghese BT, Iype EM, Balagopal PG, Mathew PC. The submental island flap for reconstruction of intraoral defects in oral cancer patients. *Oral Oncol*. 2008;44(11):1014–1018.
27. Abouchadi A, Capon-Degardin N, Patenôtre P, Martinot-Duquennoy V, Pellerin P. The submental flap in facial reconstruction: advantages and limitations. *J Oral Maxillofac Surg*. 2007;65(5):863–869.
28. Wu Y, Tang P, Qi Y, Xu Z. Submental island flap for head and neck reconstruction: a review of 20 cases. *Asian J Surg*. 1998;21:247.
29. Higgins KM, Backstein R. The submental island flap: a regional and free flap with a myriad of reconstructive applications. *J Otolaryngol*. 2007;36(2):88–92.
30. Zhang DM, Chen WL, Lin ZY, Yang ZH. Use of a folded reverse facial-submental artery submental island flap to reconstruct soft palate defects following cancer ablation. *J Cranio-Maxillo-Fac Surg*. 2014;42(6):910–914.
31. Patel UA, Bayles SW, Hayden RE. The submental flap: a modified technique for resident training. *Laryngoscope*. 2007;117(1):186–189.
32. Pistre V, Pelissier P, Martin D, Lim A, Baudet J. Ten years of experience with the submental flap. *Plast Reconstr Surg*. 2001;108(6):1576–1581.
33. Haskins N. Intensive nursing care of patients with a microvascular free flap after maxillofacial surgery. *Intensive Crit Care Nurs*. 1998;14(5):225–230.

Latissimus Dorsi Flap

Genevieve C. Bonin and Nicholas M. Makhoul

Armamentarium

#15 and #10 Scalpel blades
Appropriate sutures
Bipolar electrocautery
Curved Mayo scissors
Gerald forceps
Jackson-Pratt drains with bulb suction
Kelly retractors (24.1 cm; blade, 3.8 × 6.3 cm)
Kelly retractors (26.6 cm; blade, 8.8 × 7.6 cm)
Local anesthetic with vasoconstrictor
Malleable flexible ribbon retractors
Metzenbaum dissecting scissors
Needle electrocautery
Skin staples
Tenotomy dissecting scissors
Vascular clips
Vessel loops

History of the Procedure

The latissimus dorsi myocutaneous flap was the first musculocutaneous flap described in the medical literature. Initially, it was reported by Tansini in 1896 as a modality for reconstruction after a mastectomy.[1] He advocated excision of the skin in the mammary region to reduce the risk of cutaneous recurrences after breast cancer, and he detailed the transfer of the adjacent latissimus dorsi flap to reconstruct the defect. He further described his anatomic findings on the importance of axial circulation to such flaps, including the presence of perforators in myocutaneous flaps and the latissimus dorsi myocutaneous unit. In 1912, D'Este[2] further developed this technique for breast reconstruction. It was not until decades later, however, that the use of the latissimus dorsi flap was expanded, due to its numerous advantages, to encompass indications for shoulder and upper extremity defects.[3,4] The first documented use of this flap for head and neck reconstruction was described by Quillen and colleagues in 1978.[5,6] The pedicled latissimus dorsi flap, based on the thoracodorsal vasculature, was tunneled under the subcutaneous tissue and superficial to the pectoralis major, serving as an island rotational flap to reconstruct lateral neck and cheek defects resulting from the resection of a mandibular carcinoma with skin involvement.

The use of the latissimus dorsi flap as a free flap in the head and neck region was first reported by Watson et al.[7] in 1979. The free flap was used to reconstruct a deep posterior neck dehiscence after the excision of a large mass and also to correct a large defect subsequent to hemifacial microsomia with partial absence of the mandible and malar and temporal bones. Further modification of the latissimus dorsi flap technique introduced motor innervation of a reconstructed tongue by anastomosis of the thoracodorsal nerve to the hypoglossal nerve,[8] in addition to the reanimation of hemifacial paralysis with anastomosis to the facial nerve.[9–12] Osseous reconstruction of the mandible and scalp with the inclusion of a rib for an osteomyocutaneous flap was reported by Maruyama et al.[13] and Hirase et al.,[14] respectively; however, this technique has not gained favor because of the advent of more suitable osteomyocutaneous free flaps, particularly for the reconstruction of the maxillofacial region.

Indications for the Use of the Procedure

The substantial versatility and safety of the latissimus dorsi flap are due partly to the ease of flap raising, the high-caliber and excellent length of the vessels, a consistent vascular anatomy, ample available donor tissue, minimal donor site morbidity, and the high density of myocutaneous perforators to the skin paddle.[15–17] The total area covered by each latissimus dorsi muscle is 25 to 40 cm, which provides a large source of robust tissue for defect closure (Fig. 126.1). The neurovascular anatomy has been well established; the thoracodorsal artery and vein arise off the subscapular vessels, which are located in the third part of the axillary artery. The thoracodorsal artery has major branches to the serratus anterior, teres major, latissimus dorsi, and tip of the scapula (Fig. 126.2). The ability of this flap to function as either a pedicled flap or a free microvascular tissue transfer adds to its versatility as a major musculocutaneous flap.

As a pedicled flap, the latissimus dorsi flap can be used in a number of reconstructions of the head and neck by passing it through the axilla and between the pectoralis minor and major muscles. Possible applications include mucosal defects of the pharynx and oral cavity; resurfacing of large defects of the face and neck, scalp, and temporal or occipital regions; and also orbital, maxillary, palatal, and midface cutaneous defects. Augmenting the arc of rotation of the

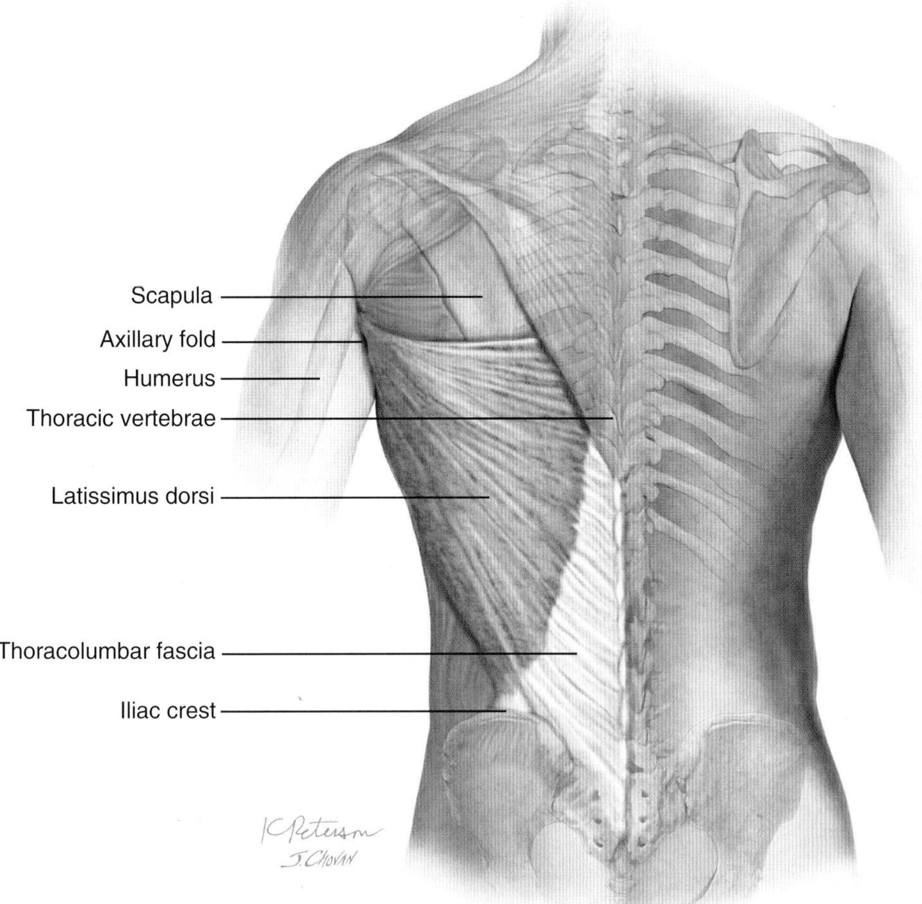

Figure 126.1 The latissimus dorsi muscle originates from the thoracic vertebrae, the thoracolumbar fascia, and the middle to the posterior iliac crest. It overlaps the scapular tip and forms the posterior axillary fold before inserting on the medial surface of the humerus.

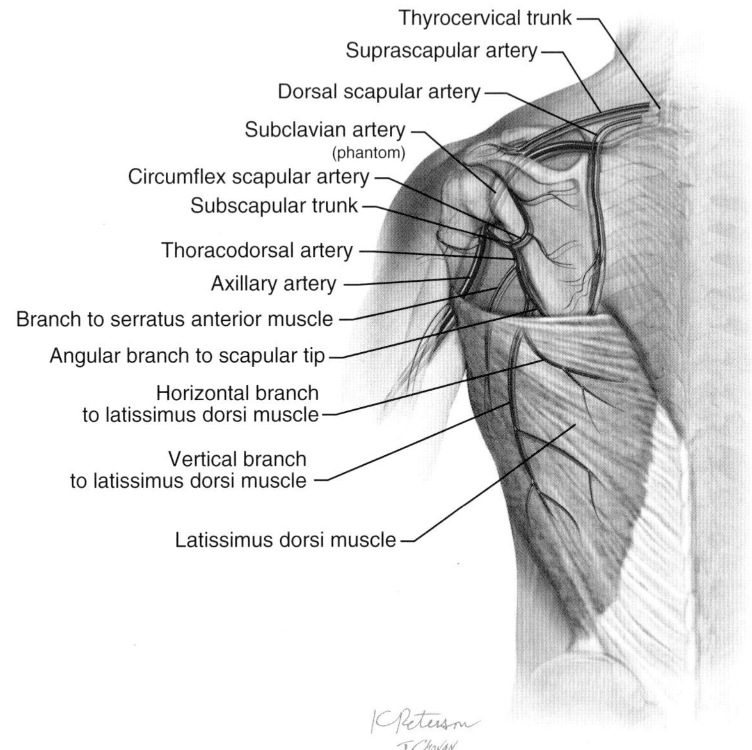

Figure 126.2 The thoracodorsal artery and vein arise from the bifurcation of the subscapular trunk, along with the circumflex scapular artery (CSA). The main branches of the thoracodorsal artery are to the serratus anterior muscle and the scapular tip (via the angular branch); its vertical and horizontal branches are to the latissimus dorsi muscle. The thoracodorsal vascular pedicle is approximately 10 cm long and has a diameter of 1 to 4 mm.

pedicled flap facilitates its use in some of the more distant sites. Limitations of the arc of rotation are due to the attachment of the thoracodorsal pedicle to major branches, such as the serratus anterior branches, which cause tethering of the inferior thoracodorsal pedicle. A greater arc of rotation can be gained by mobilizing the thoracodorsal pedicle off the circumflex scapular artery (CSA); however, caution must be used with this maneuver because this superior tethering to the CSA keeps the thoracodorsal pedicle from kinking when used as a pedicled flap.[18] Fashioning the skin paddle over the most distal angiosome can permit reach of the flap for scalp and forehead reconstruction; however, the density of perforators in this area is much reduced, leading to a potential for loss of distal skin viability. Nevertheless, the advent of microvascular tissue transfer has enabled the use of this robust flap throughout the head and neck without major concern.

Through-and-through soft tissue defects of the oral and maxillofacial region involving both skin and mucosa can be reconstructed with the latissimus dorsi flap by folding over the skin paddle and deepithelializing the intervening skin bridge (Fig. 126.3). Another technique for reconstructing

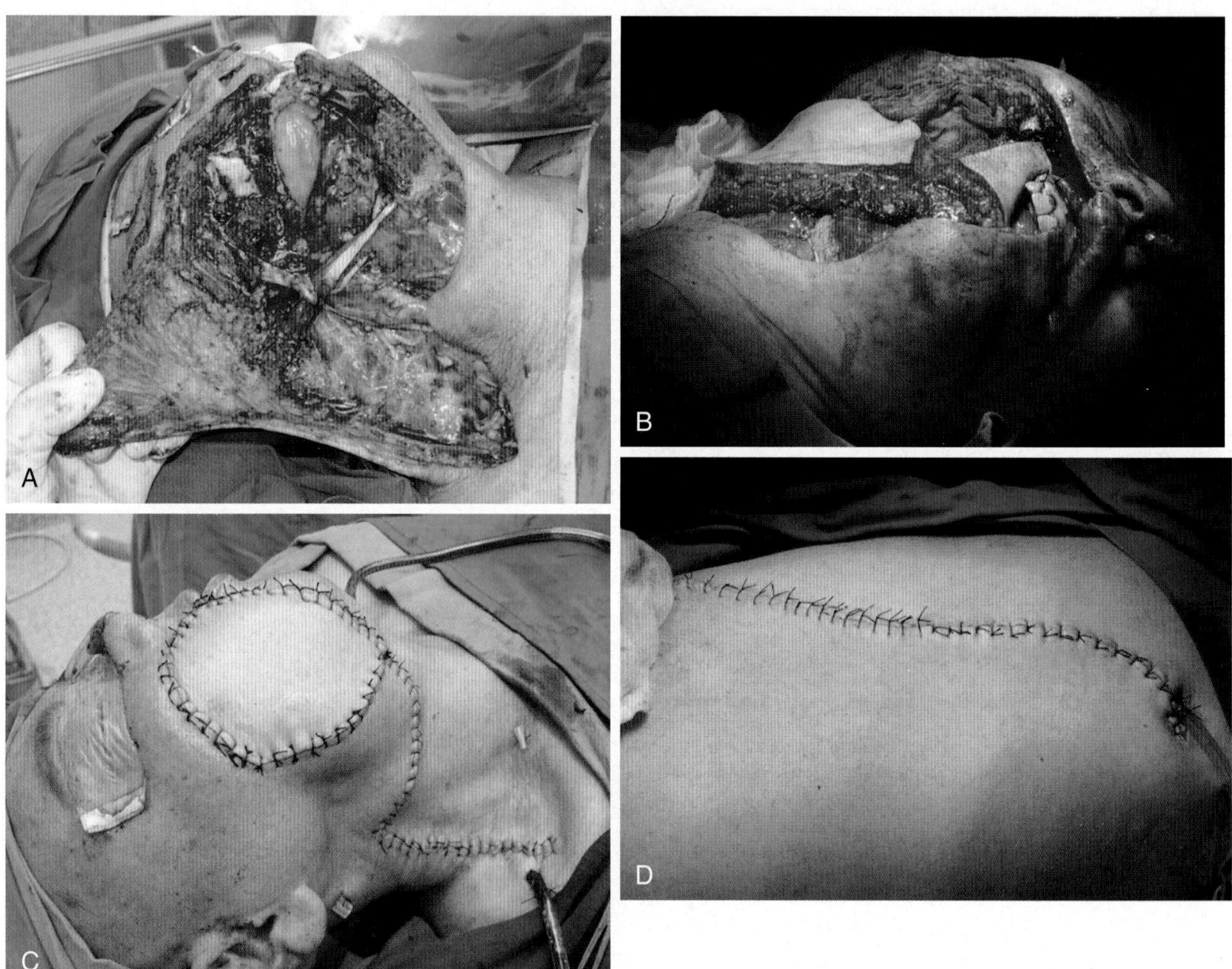

Figure 126.3 **A,** A 54-year-old male with T4aN2b squamous cell carcinoma of the right mandible. Surgical treatment involved composite resection of the right mandible, buccal mucosa, right floor of the mouth, and right cheek skin, with right modified neck dissection. **B,** Separation of the large skin paddle taken from the latissimus dorsi into two separate skin paddles for closure of both the intraoral defect and the cutaneous defect. A scalpel is used to separate the skin just into the subcutaneous fat; care is taken to preserve the muscle layer continuity to ensure perfusion of both skin paddles. Further deepithelialization of the skin paddle can be done to fit both defects. The two skin paddles are used in the composite defect of the cheek and mouth. A separate flap is created for bony reconstruction of the region. **C,** Use of the two-skin paddle latissimus dorsi flap facilitates closure of the oral cavity; the deepithelialized bridge allows separation of the cheek flap while maintaining the commissure and chin subunit. The bulk of muscle harvested is used to augment the right cheek area. **D,** Closure of the donor skin. Mobilization of the skin toward the midline allows harvesting of a 10 cm skin flap and primary closure with no difficulties.

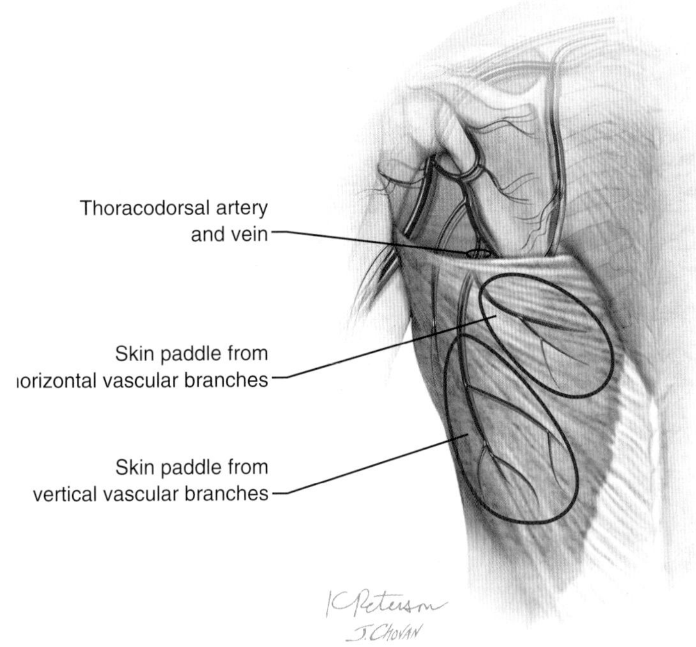

Figure 126.4 Two separate skin paddles can be harvested based on the horizontal and vertical branches of the thoracodorsal artery and vein.

these multiunit defects involves the creation of two skin paddles on the vertical and descending branches of the thoracodorsal pedicle, as described by Tobin et al.[19] (Fig. 126.4). However, caution must be exercised when this flap is used due to its bulkiness, particularly when folded; the need for a secondary debulking procedure is not uncommon.

The free-flap form of the latissimus dorsi flap has many applications in the maxillofacial region. Its use for the closure of large orbitomaxillary defects has been advocated, especially when significant bulk is needed to obliterate a defect after orbital exenteration. Two-pedicle techniques similar to those described previously have been used to close palatal and midface defects.[20] Defects of the temporal and occipital scalp region can be reconstructed with either a pedicled or a free flap; however, if the defect is very large or includes the vertex of the scalp, a free flap typically is required. A common technique for large scalp defects involves the harvesting of muscle only, with primary skin grafting over the muscle flap (Fig. 126.5). This technique eliminates the need for primary closure of the donor site, allows the muscle to be stretched easily over the convex skull, and achieves closure to all points over the cranium.[21]

The latissimus dorsi flap has also been proposed for use as a composite flap that includes rib bone. This technique has not gained much popularity due to the relatively poor bone stock available and because better alternative flaps can be made for reconstructing bone in the maxillofacial region. However, when the latissimus dorsi flap is harvested with the subscapular system, it can be used in large defects as a composite "mega flap" with scapular bone for complex multisubunit defects of the maxillofacial region (Fig. 126.6).

The latissimus dorsi flap has also been used as a sensate flap in the maxillofacial region, using the dorsal rami and posterior branches of the lateral cutaneous branch of the intercostal nerve.[22,23] Different techniques for dynamic facial reanimation have also been successfully described, involving the use of the thoracodorsal nerve and the neurotization of the myocutaneous flap using branches of the facial nerve.[9,24] Although the use of the latissimus dorsi flap as a neurotized myocutaneous free flap for facial reanimation has been well documented, application of this technique for tongue reconstruction has produced poorer results due to the complexity of muscular movement in the tongue.[8,25]

The latissimus dorsi flap has been used extensively for pharyngeal reconstruction as a tubed musculocutaneous flap for circumferential pharyngoesophageal reconstructions.[26] An advantage of this technique, as advocated by its authors, is the ability to achieve a well-sealed pharyngeal reconstruction by suturing the harvested muscle to the surrounding tissues and the skin to remaining mucosa. Other well-established applications in the lower aerodigestive tract include a large tissue transfer in the case of stomal recurrences and the use of a large amount of tissue to cover an extensive neck defect.[21]

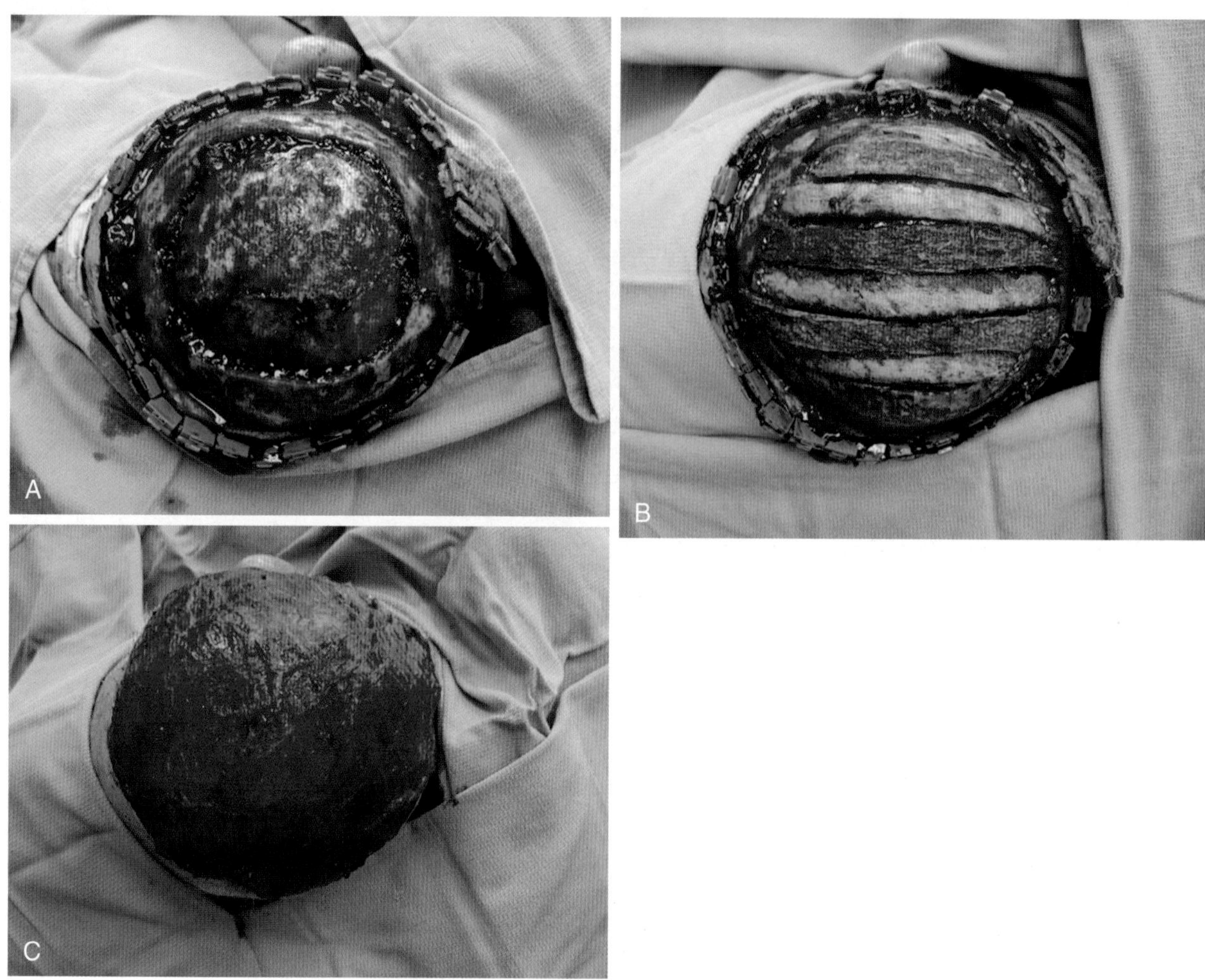

Figure 126.5 **A,** T4aN0 squamous cell carcinoma of the scalp that perforates the outer cortex of the skull. Composite resection of the scalp and skull to the dura was performed. **B,** Use of split rib grafts to restore coverage over the dura. **C,** Use of the free latissimus dorsi flap. Placement of muscle only facilitates the closure of the vertex and provides adequate coverage of split rib grafts. A large amount of muscle was harvested with primary closure of the donor site, which did not require grafting. Split-thickness skin grafts are used to cover the muscle on the neoscalp.

Limitations and Contraindications

Although the latissimus dorsi flap is a popular procedure in head and neck reconstruction, certain limitations and disadvantages must be noted. These include the need to place the patient in a lateral decubitus position for harvesting. This position does not allow for a simultaneous, two-team approach for tumor resection in the head and neck region. In addition, care must be taken to avoid injury to the contralateral shoulder by stabilizing it appropriately during patient positioning. Some studies have reported injuries to the ipsilateral brachial plexus and radial nerve, with subsequent permanent loss of sensation or complete motor function of the upper extremity.[27–29] Generalized muscle weakness surrounding the operated shoulder has been detailed, which puts limits on certain sports and some basic daily activities.

If a large skin paddle is harvested (i.e., greater than 10 cm in width), a skin graft may be required because the donor site may not be amenable to primary closure; this often produces a poor esthetic result.

The myocutaneous latissimus dorsi flap may be too bulky for certain oral cavity defects because the regional anatomy of the donor site can include a significant amount of adipose tissue between the muscle and the skin. In contrast, subsequent atrophy of the muscle layer can transform a favorably bulky flap, in the setting of facial contour augmentation, into an unfavorable outcome due to volume loss over time.

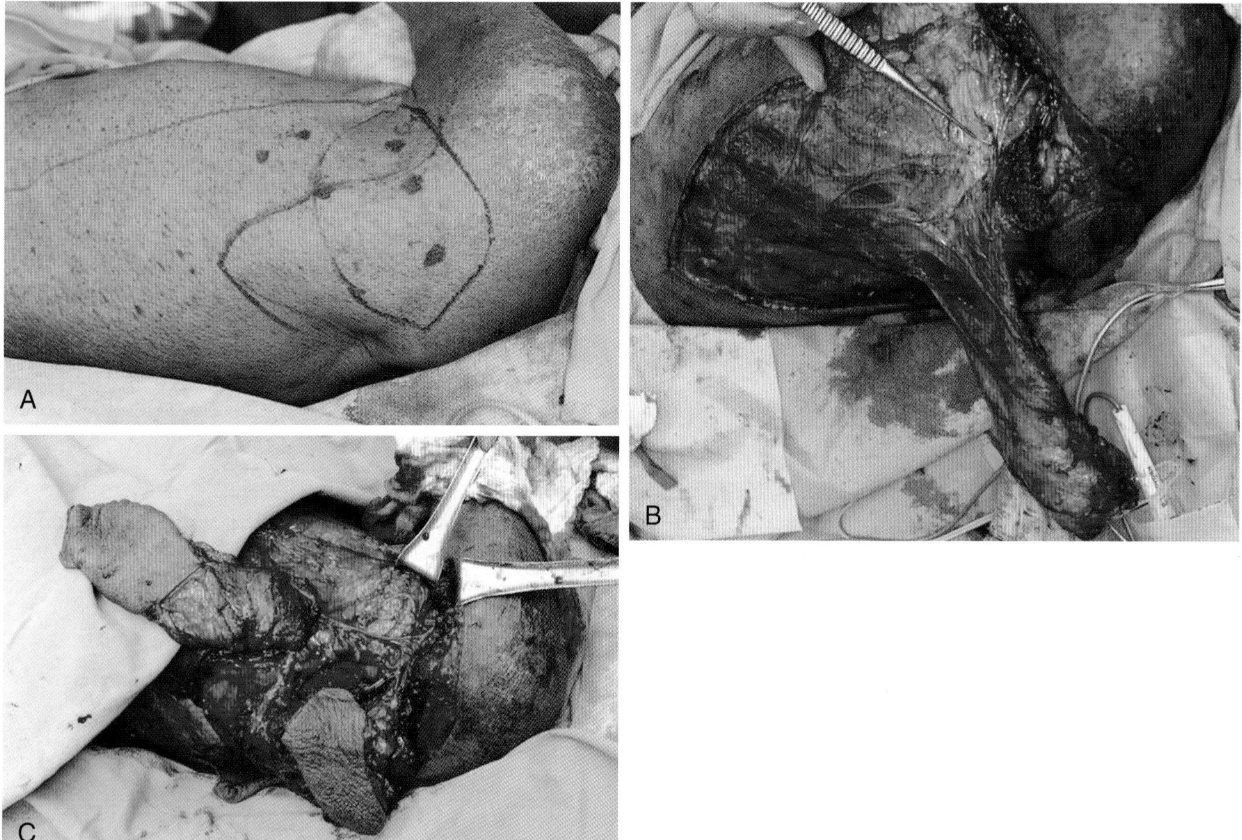

Figure 126.6 A, Markings for the harvest of a chimeric flap based on the subscapular system. A midaxillary line is drawn to represent the anterior border of the latissimus dorsi muscle. The patient is positioned in the lateral decubitus position on a bean bag, and the ipsilateral arm is stabilized by an orthopedic hydraulic arm device. Care is always taken to reduce compression on the contralateral arm and neck. The flap harvested was used to reconstruct a composite defect of the floor of the mouth, tongue, base of the tongue, lower lip, chin, and bony mandible from the left angle to the right body. The muscle bulk of the latissimus dorsi is used to support the neofloor of the mouth and separate the scapula skin flap. The skin of the latissimus is then used to close the cutaneous defect. **B,** The latissimus flap is raised, and the thoracodorsal vessels under the muscle are identified. The vessels are dissected up to the previously dissected CSA; then, careful dissection of the subscapular artery allows the transfer of the latissimus dorsi musculocutaneous flap, scapular tip, lateral scapular bone, and skin flap. **C,** Latissimus flap with thoracodorsal pedicle leading up to the subscapular artery.

TECHNIQUE: Free Vascularized Latissimus Dorsi Flap

STEP 1: Patient Positioning

The patient is placed in the lateral decubitus position. Care must be taken to avoid nerve compression injuries; therefore the head should be supported by placing a pad between the shoulder and the neck. The ipsilateral arm can be allowed to move freely and can be included in the surgical field, along with the lateral thorax, shoulder, axilla, and back. To obtain primary closure without tension, the ipsilateral arm can be draped and excluded from the operative field. If the latissimus dorsi is to be harvested with the scapula as a chimeric flap, a Spider Arm Positioner (Smith & Nephew, Memphis, TN) can be helpful for manipulating the arm intraoperatively. If bilateral harvesting of the latissimus dorsi is necessary, it is best to place the patient in the prone position.

TECHNIQUE: Free Vascularized Latissimus Dorsi Flap—*cont'd*

STEP 2: Flap Design and Markings

Other than in patients who have undergone previous surgery or radiation therapy in the area, the vascular anatomy is consistent, and multiple perforator vessels supply the overlying skin in this region. Therefore no preoperative studies are necessary for the evaluation of the anatomy (Fig. 126.7A).

When the latissimus dorsi flap is to be harvested as a free flap for distant reconstruction, the typical skin paddle design is oriented in an oblique direction to the muscle to facilitate the largest skin paddle dimension. However, this creates a less esthetic scar with primary closure compared to the transverse skin paddle orientation typically used in breast reconstruction, in which esthetics are a significant concern. In most instances the skin flap is based on the vertical branch of the thoracodorsal artery and is drawn in a fusiform shape to assist in closure.

The most important landmarks to be determined before incision are the midpoint of the axilla, the iliac crest, and the scapular tip. The anterior margin of the latissimus dorsi muscle can be marked at the posterior axillary line while the patient is standing or sitting. Alternatively, a line can be drawn between the midpoint of the axilla and a point that lies approximately between the anterior superior iliac spine and the posterior superior iliac spine, which represents the anterior border of the muscle. The superior margin of the muscle lies 3 to 4 cm above the scapular tip and overlies the attachment of the teres major to the scapular bone. The posterior margin of the muscle is represented by the vertebral column, and the inferior margin of the muscle is marked at the level of the posterior superior iliac crest. The skin island is marked 4 to 5 cm posterior to the anterior edge of the latissimus dorsi muscle, and it should be less than 10 cm wide to allow for primary closure unless skin grafting of the donor site is planned. The inferior edge of the skin island should be placed at least 8 cm superior to the posterior superior iliac crest. If two skin paddles are required, each island can be based separately off the vertical and transverse branches of the thoracodorsal artery.

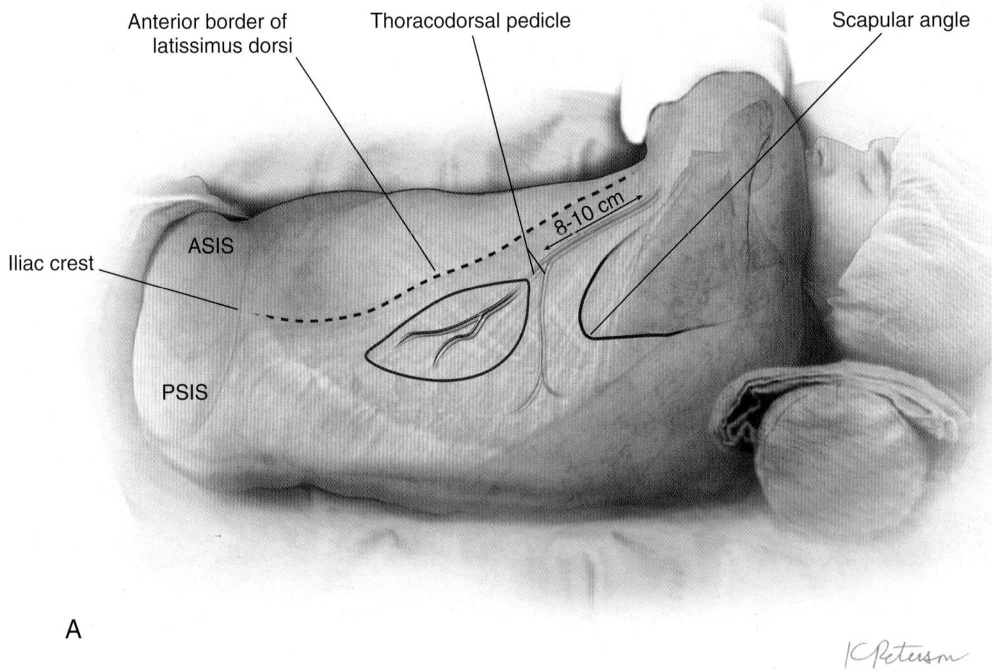

Figure 126.7 **A,** Anatomic landmarks to be identified include the scapular tip, iliac crest, and a line drawn from the midaxilla to the midpoint between the anterior superior iliac spine (ASIS) and posterior superior iliac spine (PSIS). The dashed line represents the anterior border of the latissimus dorsi muscle; the skin paddle is drawn to follow the vertical branch of the thoracodorsal artery and vein. The vascular pedicle bifurcates 8 to 10 cm below the axilla and runs underneath the muscle. The donor site can be closed primarily when less than 10 cm in widest diameter.

TECHNIQUE: Free Vascularized Latissimus Dorsi Flap—*cont'd*

STEP 3: Incision and Anterior Flap Dissection

The incision through the skin and subcutaneous tissue is performed along the anterior margin of the skin island and is continued toward the axilla. Variability in the amount of subcutaneous tissue can be observed based on the patient's body habitus. The dissection is pursued along the anterior margin down to the underlying muscle fibers. The anterior aspect of the latissimus dorsi muscle can be identified by anteriorly retracting the serratus muscle, which comes into view after dissection through the fibrofatty tissue. Differentiation superiorly between the teres major muscle and the latissimus dorsi is made by identifying the attachment of the teres major to the scapular bone; the latissimus dorsi overlies the scapula. Care must be taken to avoid dissecting the fatty tissue under the region of the skin paddle from the underlying latissimus dorsi muscle (Fig. 126.7B).

STEP 4: Visualization of the Thoracodorsal Artery and Its Branches

Once the latissimus dorsi muscle is in view, the vascular pedicle should be identified. The vascular pedicle enters the undersurface of the muscle 8 to 10 cm below the midpoint of the axilla. The first branch typically encountered is the branch to the serratus anterior. This branch supplies the anterior serratus muscle and can be found at the anterior margin of the latissimus dorsi muscle. The branch to the serratus muscle is carefully dissected proximally toward its bifurcation with the trunk of the thoracodorsal artery. Typically, 1 to 2 cm below the scapular tip, the thoracodorsal artery bifurcates into vertical and horizontal branches, which are the basis of the two skin island flaps.

The latissimus dorsi muscle is dissected and raised along its anterior border; this allows the vascular pedicle to be traced proximally and gently dissected toward the axilla. The angular branch of the thoracodorsal artery running off toward the scapular tip can be observed during this proximal dissection; this typically is clipped unless a chimeric flap is harvested that includes the scapular tip. The vascular pedicle is dissected to a suitable length for the flap inset and microvascular anastomosis. The proximal vascular pedicle can be taken at the subscapular trunk or distal to the bifurcation with the CSA.

The surgeon must take care to avoid injury to the pedicle while continuing the elevation of the latissimus dorsi muscle by blunt dissection. Segmental vessels to this muscle that originate from the intercostal arteries can be encountered at the medial and distal aspects of the muscle (Fig. 126.7C).

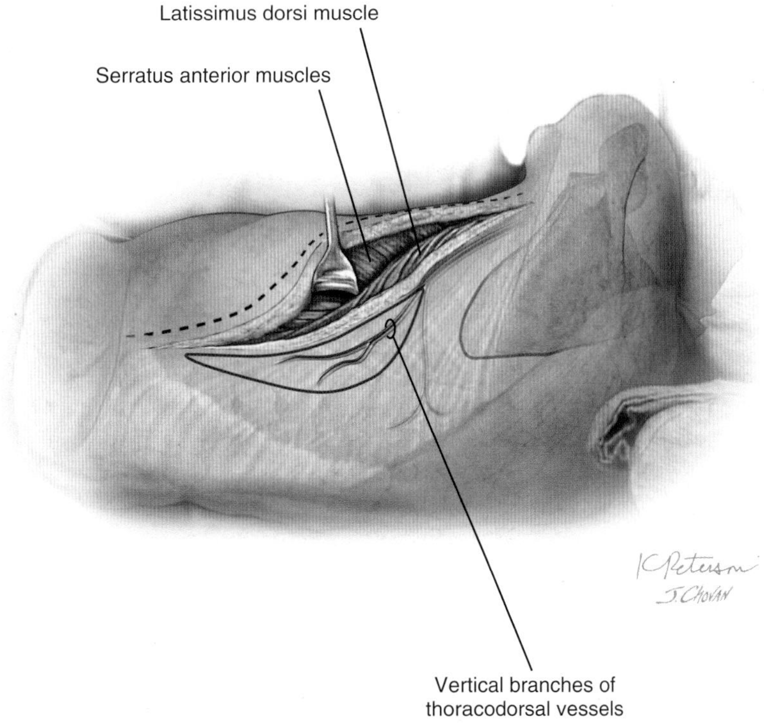

Figure 126.7 cont'd B, The anterior incision is performed first along the anterior border of the latissimus dorsi. The serratus anterior muscle and latissimus dorsi muscle are identified once the subcutaneous fat has been dissected. The anterior border of the latissimus should be separated from the serratus anterior by gentle retraction of the anterior muscles. Care should be taken to maintain skin attachment to the underlying muscle.

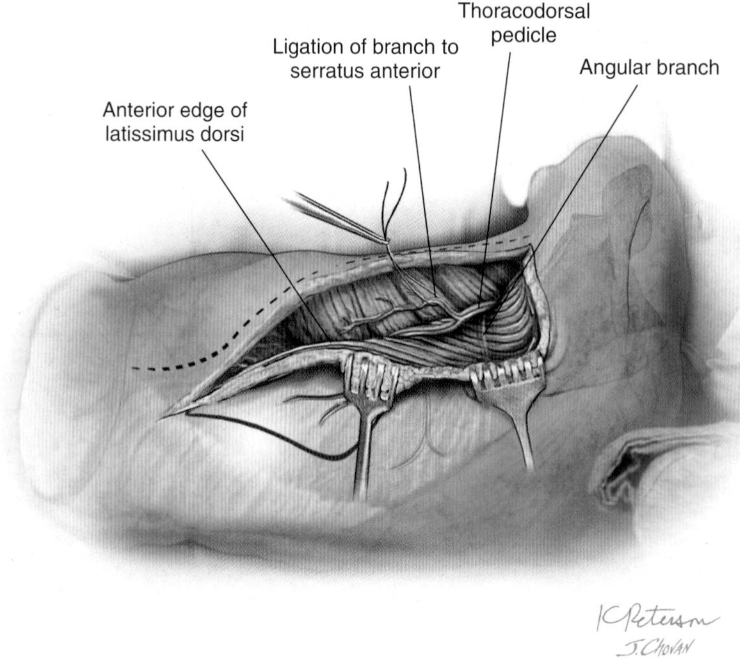

Figure 126.7 cont'd **C,** Careful retraction on the latissimus dorsi exposes the branch to the serratus anterior muscle. Proximal dissection of the main vascular pedicle can then be accomplished by tracing the thoracodorsal artery and vein. Careful ligation of the serratus anterior branch is done to free the inferior pedicle.

TECHNIQUE: Free Vascularized Latissimus Dorsi Flap—*cont'd*

STEP 5: Posterior Flap Dissection

The skin and subcutaneous tissue along the posterior edge of the skin paddle are incised, and dissection is continued down to the muscular fascia. The posterior edge of the latissimus dorsi muscle is elevated along the same plane as performed anteriorly. Because the inferior and posterior aspects of the skin paddle most likely do not correspond to the inferior and posterior edge of the latissimus dorsi muscle, the muscle fibers must be transected before the elevation of the inferior and posterior poles of the skin paddle (Fig. 126.7D).

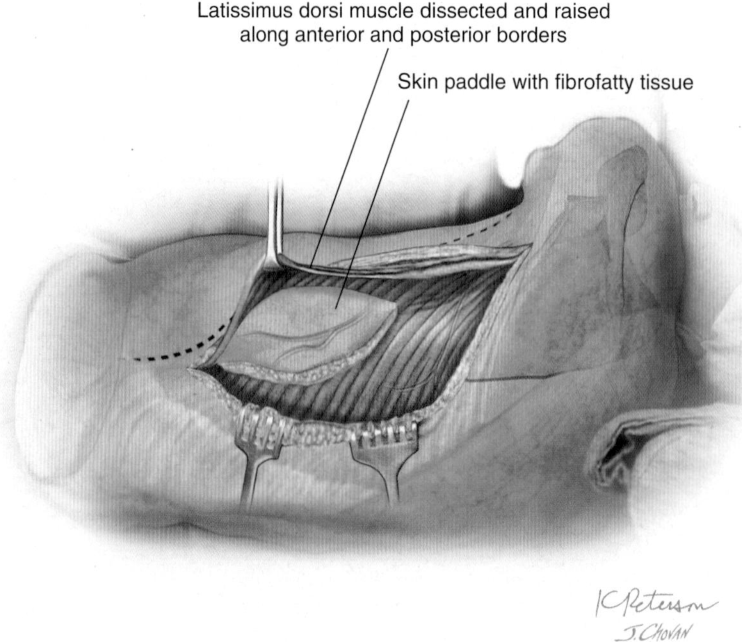

Figure 126.7 cont'd **D,** Posterior skin incision is completed down to the level of the muscle. Dissection of the muscle toward the midline allows for mobilization of the skin for donor site closure. Additional muscle can be harvested, if desired, along with the skin paddle. The muscle is then divided inferiorly, laterally, and toward the midline, with care taken to avoid damage to the underlying pedicle.

TECHNIQUE: Free Vascularized Latissimus Dorsi Flap—*cont'd*

STEP 6: Elevation of the Flap

An attachment remains between the cranial aspect of the skin paddle and the vascular hilum containing the important vertical branch of the thoracodorsal artery. Retraction of the neurovascular bundle allows better visualization of the remaining muscle fibers that need to be transected.

STEP 7: Harvesting of the Flap and Closure

Once the recipient vessels have been prepared for microvascular anastomosis, perfusion of the flap is assessed before its vascular supply is disconnected. After the flap has been transferred, hemostasis is achieved, and two drains are positioned, sutured to the overlying skin, and placed on bulb suction. Primary closure can be achieved if the skin island is less than 10 cm wide and if the patient's skin laxity permits. Otherwise, a split-thickness skin graft can be sutured in place overlying the exposed muscle, and a pressure dressing can be placed.

Avoidance and Management of Intraoperative Complications

It may be difficult to assess the anterior border of the latissimus dorsi muscle in certain patients (e.g., obese individuals). Typically the anterior edge of the muscle runs along a straight line from the dorsal axillary fold to the midline of the iliac crest. In slim patients, adduction of the arm should allow for proper palpation of the anterior muscle edge.

As previously mentioned, the serratus branch of the thoracodorsal artery is the first branch visualized during the dissection. Care must be taken to avoid mistaking this branch for the actual main trunk of the thoracodorsal artery; to aid with this, the division of the serratus branch can be performed once the myocutaneous flap has been completely elevated and the proximal pedicle dissected. Trauma, including complete transection, to the vertical branch of the thoracodorsal artery can occur if the muscle flap is too narrow. Care should be taken to ensure that the muscle flap is as wide as, if not even slightly wider than, the overlying skin paddle and that no oblique dissection from the superficial aspect of the skin paddle deep toward the muscle layer has been performed (Fig. 126.8).

The bulky aspect of the skin paddle can allow for shearing forces that injure the perforator vessels, leading to

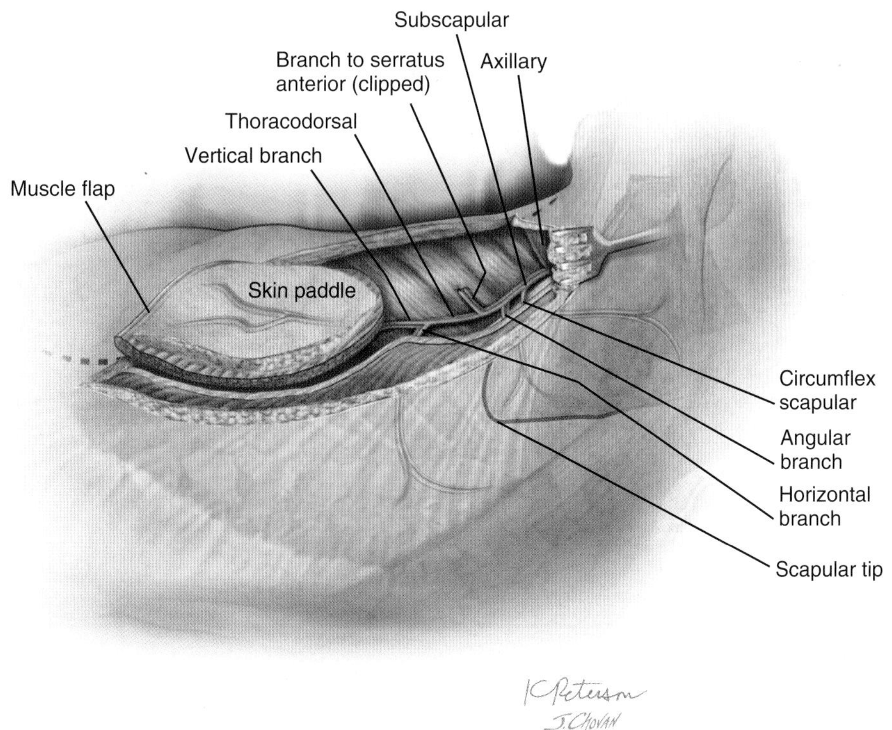

Figure 126.8 Complete dissection of the thoracodorsal pedicle and release of the muscle attachments allows the surgeon to visualize the circumflex scapular artery (CSA), angular branch, and subscapular artery. The surgeon can take the vascular pedicle from whatever area provides the appropriate length and vascular width.

compromised perfusion to the skin island. To avoid trauma of this nature, stay sutures should be placed to fix the skin paddle to the underlying muscle; these can remain in place until careful inset of the flap.

Postoperative Considerations

Complications from the development of a hematoma or seroma at the donor site are minimized by proper intraoperative hemostasis and the placement of two drains on bulb suction. These drains are monitored for daily output and may be kept in place for up to 5 to 7 days after surgery. Large donor site defects have been treated effectively with negative-pressure wound therapy.[30] Normal movement of the arm can be performed on the first postoperative day; however, strenuous physical activity (e.g., heavy lifting) should be avoided for the first 6 weeks after surgery. Gentle physiotherapy to regain adequate range of motion in the arm can be performed within a few days after surgery.

References

1. Maxwell GP. Iginio Tansini and the origin of the latissimus dorsi musculocutaneous flap. *Plast Reconstr Surg*. 1980;65:686.
2. D'Este S. La technique de l'amputation de la mamelle pour carcinome mammaire. *Rev Chir*. 1912;18:62.
3. Mendelson BC, Masson JK. Treatment of chronic radiation injury over the shoulder with a latissimus dorsi myocutaneous flap. *Plast Reconstr Surg*. 1977;60:681.
4. Silverton JS, Nahai F, Jurkiewicz MJ. The latissimus dorsi myocutaneous flap to replace a defect on the upper arm. *Br J Plast Surg*. 1978;31:29.
5. Quillen CG. Latissimus dorsi myocutaneous flaps in head and neck reconstruction. *Plast Reconstr Surg*. 1979;63:664.
6. Quillen CG, Shearin JC, Giorgiade NG. Use of the latissimus dorsi myocutaneous island flap for reconstruction in the head and neck area. *Plast Reconstr Surg*. 1978;62:113.
7. Watson JS, Craig P, Orton CI. The free latissimus dorsi myocutaneous flap. *Plast Reconstr Surg*. 1979;64:299.
8. Haughey BH. Tongue reconstruction: concepts and practice. *Laryngoscope*. 1993;103:1132.
9. Mackinnon SE, Dellon AL. Technical considerations of the latissimus dorsi muscle flap: a segmentally innervated muscle transfer for facial reanimation. *Microsurgery*. 1988;9:36.
10. Wei W, Zuoliang Q, Xiaoxi L, et al. Free split and segmental latissimus dorsi muscle transfer in one stage for facial reanimation. *Plast Reconstr Surg*. 1999;103:473.
11. Takushima A, Harii K, Asato H, et al. Fifteen-year survey of one-stage latissimus dorsi muscle transfer for treatment of longstanding facial paralysis. *J Plast Reconstr Aesthet Surg*. 2013;66:29.
12. Biglioli F, Colombo V, Pedrazzoli M, et al. Thoracodorsal nerve graft for reconstruction of facial nerve branching. *J Craniomaxillofac Surg*. 2014;42(1):e8–e14. doi:10.1016/j.jcms.2013.03.001.
13. Maruyama Y, Urita Y, Ohnishi K. Rib–latissimus dorsi osteomyocutaneous flap in reconstruction of a mandibular defect. *Br J Plast Surg*. 1985;38:234.
14. Hirase Y, Kojima T, Kinoshita Y, Bang HH, Sakaguchi T, Kijima M. Composite reconstruction for chest wall and scalp using multiple ribs–latissimus dorsi osteomyocutaneous flaps as pedicles and free flaps. *Plast Reconstr Surg*. 1991;87(3):555–561. doi:10.1097/00006534-199103000-00027.
15. Pirgousis P, Fernandes R. Contemporary methods in tongue reconstruction. In: Bagheri SC, Bell B, Khan HA, eds. *Current Therapy in Oral and Maxillofacial Surgery*. St. Louis: Saunders; 2012.
16. Wolff KD, Holzle F. *Raising of Microvascular Flaps: A Systematic Approach*. 2nd ed. Berlin: Springer; 2011.
17. Slavin SA, Fox S. Latissimus dorsi myocutaneous flap. In: Guyuron B, Eriksson E, Persing JA, eds. *Plastic Surgery: Indications and Practice*. Philadelphia: Saunders; 2009.
18. Friedrich W, Berbenhold C, Lierse W. Vascularization of the myocutaneous latissimus dorsi flap. *Acta Anal (Basel)*. 1988;131:97.
19. Tobin G, Moberg A, DuBou R, et al. The split latissimus dorsi myocutaneous flap. *Ann Plast Surg*. 1981;7:272.
20. Baker S. Closure of large orbital-maxillary defects with free latissimus dorsi myocutaneous flaps. *Head Neck Surg*. 1984;6:828.
21. Pennington D, Stern H, Lee K. Free flap reconstruction of large defects of the scalp and calvarium. *Plast Reconstr Surg*. 1989;83:655.
22. Dabb R, Conklin W. A sensory innervated latissimus dorsi musculocutaneous free flap: case report. *J Microsurg*. 1981;2:289.
23. Gordon L, Bunche H, Alpert B. Free latissimus dorsi muscle flap with split-thickness skin graft cover: a report of 16 cases. *Plast Reconstr Surg*. 1982;70:173.
24. Maruyama Y, Nakajima H, Fossati E, Fujino T. Free latissimus dorsi myocutaneous flaps in the dynamic reconstruction of cheek defects: a preliminary report. *J Microsurg*. 1979;1:231.
25. Haughey B, Fredrickson J. The latissimus dorsi donor site: current use in head and neck reconstruction. *Arch Otolaryngol Head Neck Surg*. 1991;117:1129.
26. Watson JS, Roberston GA, Endrum J, et al. Pharyngeal reconstruction using the latissimus dorsi myocutaneous flap. *Br J Plast Surg*. 1982;35:401.
27. Logan AM, Black MJ. Injury to the brachial plexus resulting from shoulder positioning during latissimus dorsi flap pedicle dissection. *Br J Plast Surg*. 1985;38:380.
28. Freedlander E. Brachial plexus cord compression by the tendon of a pedicled latissimus dorsi flap. *Br J Plast Surg*. 1986;39:514.
29. Siegmund CJ, Tighe JV. Sensory and motor function impairment after brachial plexus cord compression by a pedicled latissimus dorsi flap. *Br J Plast Surg*. 2001;54:449.
30. Schmedes GW, Banks CA, Malin BT, Srinivas PB, Skoner JM. Massive flap donor sites and the role of negative pressure wound therapy. *Otolaryngol Head Neck Surg*. 2012;147(6):1049–1053. doi:10.1177/0194599812459015.

CHAPTER 127

Radial Forearm Flap

Joshua E. Lubek

Armamentarium

#15 Scalpel blades
Allis clamps
Appropriate sutures
Bipolar electrocautery
Dermatome
Hemostats
Heparinized saline flushes
Local anesthetic with vasoconstrictor
Microvascular forceps (jeweler forceps)
Microvascular vessel clamps (Acland clamps)
Monopolar needle tip electrocautery
Needle drivers
Papaverine irrigation
Senn retractors
Skin hooks
Surgical loupes
Suture scissors
Tenotomy scissors
Tourniquet/Esmarch bandage
Vascular forceps (Jerrold)
Vascular hemostatic titanium clips
Vessel loops
Warm saline irrigation

History of the Procedure

The radial forearm flap was first reported by Yang et al.[1] in 1981 for resurfacing the neck secondary to burn contractures. Use of the flap became popular shortly after Soutar and McGregor[2] in 1986 published a report on a series of 60 consecutive cases in which the radial forearm flap was used for intraoral reconstruction. Since then, numerous articles and book chapters have been written describing both the technique and applications for use of the radial or ulnar artery-based forearm flap for reconstruction in the oral and maxillofacial regions.

This chapter focuses on the radial forearm flap technique and discusses the ulnar forearm flap as an alternate technique for forearm flap reconstruction.

Indications for the Use of the Procedure

The radial forearm flap is a reliable, versatile flap, based on the radial artery, that can be applied to the reconstruction of many anatomic structures in the head and neck. Passing under the bicipital aponeurosis, the brachial artery divides into the radial and ulnar arteries. The radial artery courses deep to the brachioradialis muscle and the pronator teres in the upper third of the forearm and between the tendons of the brachioradialis and flexor carpi radialis in the lower two-thirds of the forearm. From this point it travels into the hand, passing through the anatomic "snuff box" and contributing to the dual blood supply of the hand. The skin paddle of the radial forearm flap is supplied by approximately 7 to 10 fasciocutaneous branches (average diameter, 0.5 mm) that originate directly from the radial artery (Fig. 127.1). Venous drainage is via two independent systems (the superficial [cephalic] vein or the deep venae comitantes traveling with the radial artery), either of which can adequately drain the flap. The pedicle length averages 10 to 12 cm, with good vessel diameter (2.5 mm). Sensory innervation is derived from the lateral antebrachial cutaneous nerves traveling with the cephalic vein or, in the case of an ulnar forearm flap, the median antebrachial cutaneous nerves coursing with the basilic vein. These sensory nerves can be harvested with the flap to provide sensory reinnervation to structures such as the tongue.[3–6] Most commonly the lingual nerve or inferior alveolar nerve is the selected recipient nerve. Since Urken and colleagues[7,8] produced the initial reports on sensory radial forearm flap reconstruction for oral and oropharyngeal defects, numerous retrospective cohort series have been detailed.[9–14] Most series use the contralateral hemitongue as a control. The results have shown significant differences in neurosensory recovery, with statistical improvements in light touch, temperature sensation, and two-point discrimination. These results have also been confirmed on histologic evaluation, with larger, better-arranged, and more numerous nerve fibers identified.[9]

Controversy does exist as to the validity of sensory forearm flap reinnervation with regard to true functional outcomes (speech and swallowing) compared with nonsensate flaps. Many studies are marked by a lack of randomization; poor description of the method of speech and swallow evaluation; and poor reporting of the location and size of the defect and of confounding variables (e.g., adjuvant radiotherapy). Biglioli et al.[10] reported improved oral function and quality of life with innervated flaps, but Mah et al.[11] found no significant difference between innervated and noninnervated

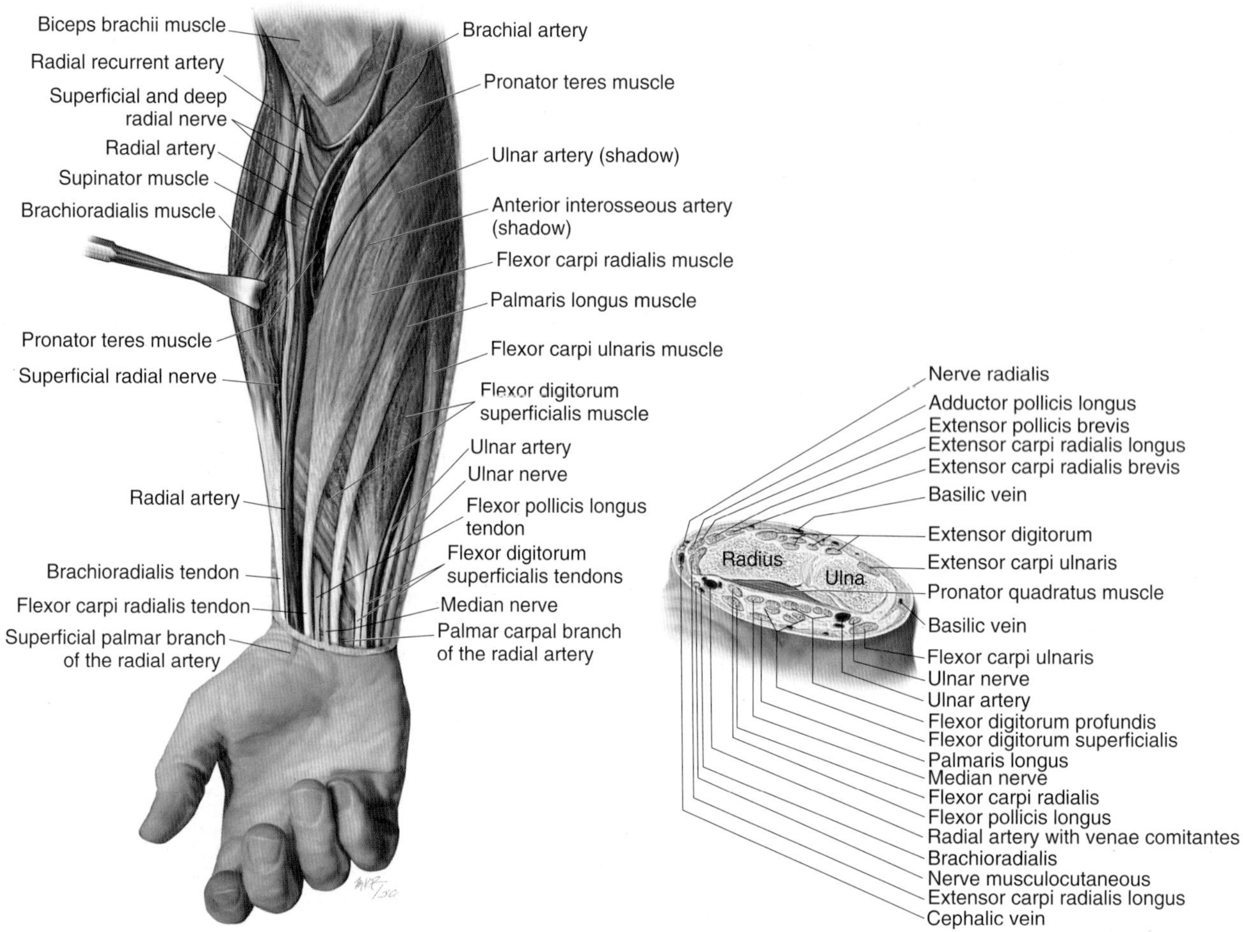

Figure 127.1 Course of the radial artery within the forearm.

free flaps in terms of speech, swallowing function, or quality of life. Sabesan et al.[12] even demonstrated some level of neurosensory recovery in their series of 40 noninnervated radial forearm flaps.

The superficial branch of the radial nerve supplies sensation to the dorsal aspect of the thumb and index finger. It is located in close proximity to the radial artery and its vena comitans and should be preserved during flap harvest. The flap can be harvested as a fasciocutaneous flap or, if required, bone or tendon also can be transferred. Although many elaborate shapes and designs have been devised, the author routinely uses a rectangular shape and has not found any issue with matching a specific defect. Any redundant tissue can be deepithelialized or removed during flap inset. The radial artery supplies blood to the bone via fascioperiosteal branches through the intermuscular septum and musculoperiosteal branches through the flexor pollicis longus and pronator quadratus muscles. Up to 10 cm of length and 40% of the cross section of the radius may be safely harvested.[5,15–17]

The ulnar forearm flap has similar properties to the radial forearm flap in terms of tissue pliability and thickness. The ulnar artery courses deep to the antebrachial flexor muscles of the upper forearm. In the middle and distal third of the forearm, it travels deep to the muscle and tendons of the flexor carpi ulnaris and flexor digitorum superficialis along an imaginary line from the medial epicondyle of the humerus to the lateral edge of the pisiform bone. The ulnar artery gives off perforating branches to the skin, mostly located in the distal third of the vessel just before traveling into the wrist superficial to the flexor retinaculum. The ulnar nerve is a mixed sensorimotor nerve that travels medially and in close proximity to the ulnar vessels. Preservation of the ulnar nerve is essential for the proper function of the hand.[4,6,18,19]

The ulnar artery pedicle generally is shorter than the radial artery pedicle; however, donor site morbidity for the ulnar flap is considered comparable or even superior to the radial flap. Some authors have reported decreased donor site morbidity in terms of neurosensory effects, function, and skin graft loss rates compared with the radial forearm donor site. Other suggested advantages of the ulnar flap, compared with the radial forearm flap, include a skin paddle with less hair and a more aesthetic, hidden donor site scar (Fig. 127.2).[19]

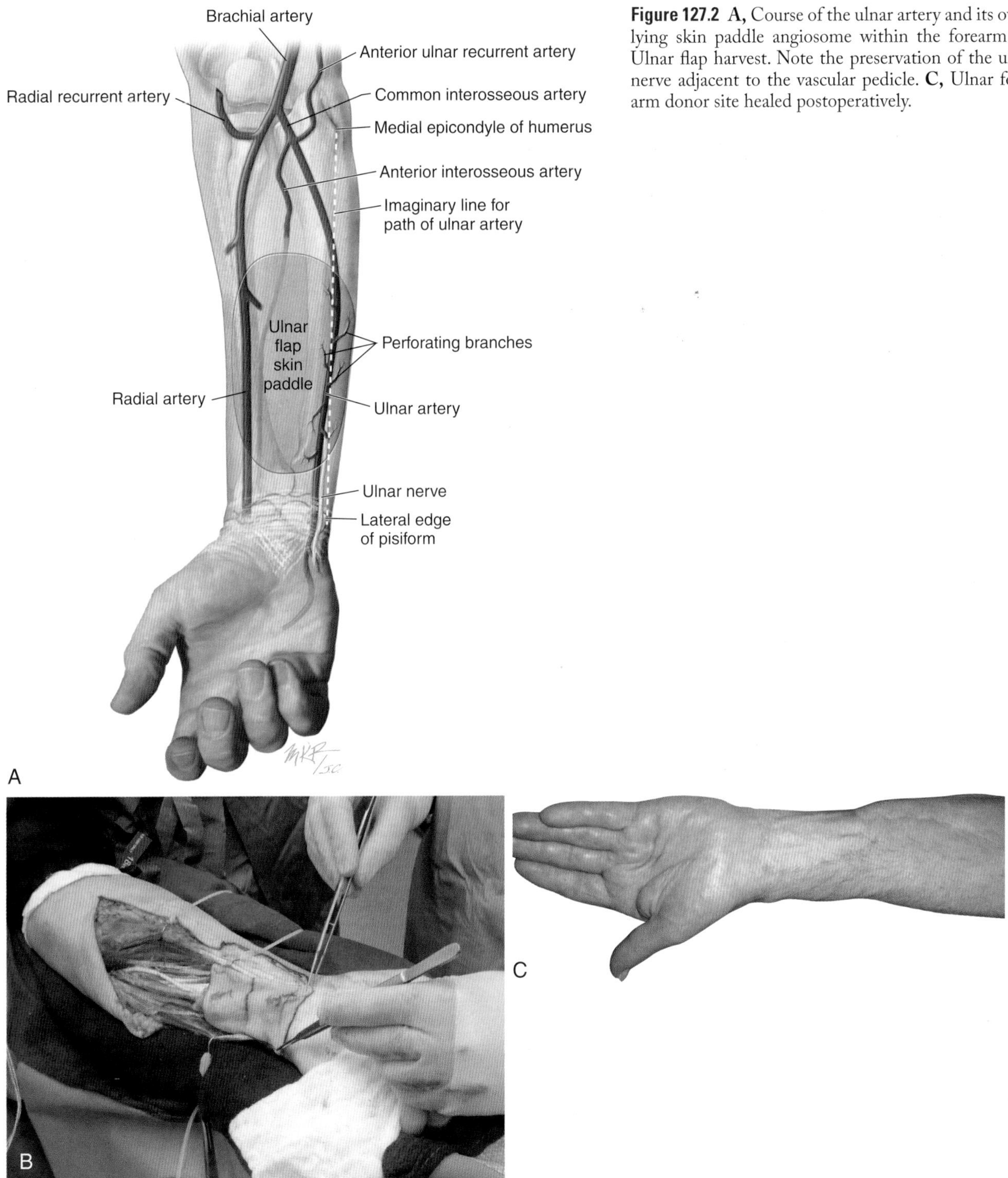

Figure 127.2 **A,** Course of the ulnar artery and its overlying skin paddle angiosome within the forearm. **B,** Ulnar flap harvest. Note the preservation of the ulnar nerve adjacent to the vascular pedicle. **C,** Ulnar forearm donor site healed postoperatively.

Huang et al.[6] reported on both the anatomy and donor site morbidity in a series of 50 successful ulnar flaps used for reconstruction in the head and neck. The mean diameters of the ulnar artery and vein were 2.3 mm (± 0.6) and 1.7 mm (± 0.6), respectively. The mean number of sizable perforators was 4.3 (± 1.2), and most of the first perforators were located within 5 cm of the proximal wrist crease. There were no long-term complications reported concerning the ulnar nerve.

The forearm flap is ideally suited to reconstruct defects of the oral cavity (floor of the mouth, tongue, buccal mucosa, and posterior maxillectomy defects) and oropharynx and also laryngopharyngectomy defects (Fig. 127.3).[2,5,7,8,15,16,20,21]

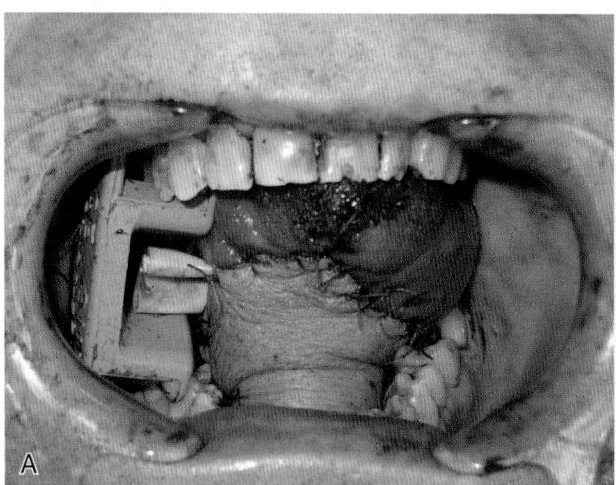

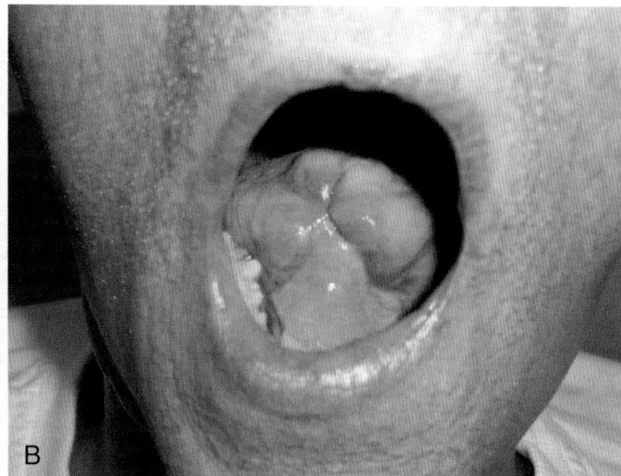

Figure 127.3 **A,** Forearm flap used to reconstruct a floor of the mouth defect. **B,** Forearm flap for a floor of the mouth defect after completion of adjuvant radiotherapy.

Limitations and Contraindications

Limitations on the use of the forearm flap are based on two main considerations: adequate blood supply to the donor site hand and the type of defect in the head and neck to be reconstructed. The blood supply to the hand is based on the deep and superficial palmar arches. In general terms, the two palmar arches of the hand communicate with each other and form a complete dual loop that communicates with itself to create a dual redundant blood supply to the digits. Blood flow to the deep palmar arch is predominantly supplied by the radial artery, and the superficial arch is predominantly supplied by the ulnar artery. The Allen test should be performed before surgery to verify an adequate dual blood supply to the hand. In a series of 650 anatomic forearm dissections by Coleman and Anson,[4] 10% of the cases had no branches of the superficial palmar arch to the thumb and index finger, and in 50% of the cases, the deep arch did not connect to the ulnar artery. Approximately 5% of the time, both variations are present; in such cases, the blood supply to the thumb and index finger is derived entirely from the radial artery. If there is any question about the integrity of the palmar arches, whether from anatomic variation, previous trauma, or atherosclerotic disease, color flow Doppler ultrasound can be used to assess the adequacy of the palmar arch blood flow. If the forearm donor site is determined to be the best tissue choice for reconstruction and the radial artery is the dominant supply to the hand, the author uses the ulnar forearm flap in the reconstruction of the head and neck defect.

Defects of the head and neck that require large amounts of bulky soft tissue (e.g., subtotal glossectomy, maxillectomy with orbital exenteration, and large skull base defects) are often better suited to reconstruction using donor sites such as the thigh, latissimus dorsi, or rectus abdominis. These donor sites provide more adequate tissue bulk, and their use often avoids the need for donor site skin grafts (as are required with the forearm flap).

The amount of bone available for harvest in the radial forearm osteofasciocutaneous flap is quite limited for reconstruction of the maxillofacial region. Although the use of this flap has been described for short mandibular, maxillary, and orbital rim defects, better donor sites are available, such as the fibula, vascularized iliac crest, and scapula. The latter donor sites provide better bone quality and quantity, allowing for reconstruction of larger bony defects and possibly dental implant rehabilitation as well. Preplating of the osteofasciocutaneous radial forearm donor site has dramatically reduced donor site morbidity; complaints of donor site stiffness and mild wrist weakness are common but do not limit daily activities.[5,15,17]

TECHNIQUE: Radial Forearm Flap Harvest

STEP 1: Allen Test to Confirm Adequate Redundant Blood Supply to the Hand

The nondominant hand usually is selected. The radial artery and the ulnar artery are palpated at the wrist. The patient is asked to make a fist, and the arteries are occluded with the surgeon's fingers. The palm of the hand will appear white. The finger pressure over the ulnar pulse is released, and the hand and digits (including the thumb and index finger) should reperfuse to a healthy color within 15 seconds.

TECHNIQUE: Radial Forearm Flap Harvest—*cont'd*

STEP 2: Flap Design and Tourniquet Insufflation

The skin paddle is designed based on the radial artery. The distal end of the skin paddle should be at least 1 cm from the flexor crease of the wrist. Superficial veins (e.g., the cephalic vein) also can be easily identified and marked out on the skin. The forearm is exsanguinated with an Esmarch bandage, and a sterile tourniquet is applied and insufflated to 250 mm Hg (Fig. 127.4A).

STEP 3: Identification of the Brachioradialis Muscle With Preservation and Dissection of the Cephalic Vein

An incision is made through the skin and into the subcutaneous tissue, outlining the skin paddle. The incision along the proximal aspect of the skin paddle toward the antecubital fossa is made in a linear or "lazy S" fashion at the same depth. The surgeon performs the dissection on the radial side of the flap, identifying the cephalic vein in the proximal forearm and ligating vessels branching lateral to it. The fascia over the brachioradialis muscle is identified and exposed. At this time, the lateral cutaneous nerve can be identified in close proximity to the cephalic vein and can be preserved for possible use with a sensate flap, if so desired. Dissection continues along the cephalic vein distally, along its lateral aspect, toward the most distal aspect of the skin paddle. The distal end of the cephalic vein can be ligated, and subfascial dissection over the brachioradialis muscle and tendon must be performed. Care must be taken to preserve the paratenon of the brachioradialis tendon. The superficial branches of the radial nerve should be identified at the distal aspect and preserved to maintain sensation to the dorsum of the hand. The communicating veins medial to the main trunk of the cephalic vein must be preserved the full length of the flap because these will provide the drainage route from the flap to the cephalic vein proximally. The cephalic vein can be circumferentially skeletonized at its proximal extent near the antecubital fossa.

STEP 4: Identification of the Flexor Carpi Radialis Muscle, Palmaris Longus, and Vascular Pedicle

On the ulnar aspect of the forearm, dissection is carried down to the flexor carpi radialis muscle and palmaris longus tendon. A subfascial dissection is performed, with care taken to preserve the paratenon of the flexor carpi radialis tendon. The vascular pedicle can now be easily identified in the intermuscular septum between the muscle bellies of the flexor carpi radialis and brachioradialis (Fig. 127.4B).

STEP 5: Identification and Ligation of the Vascular Pedicle Distally

Superficial vessels encountered during the distal dissection near the flexor crease of the wrist can be ligated with hemoclips or bipolar cautery. The distal aspect of the radial artery and the vena comitans pedicle can now be identified and ligated with 2-0 silk suture and vascular clips between the brachioradialis and flexor carpi radialis tendons (Fig. 127.4C).

Continued

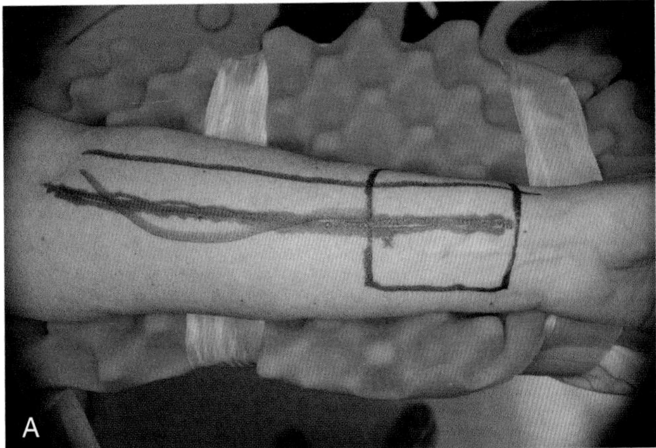

Figure 127.4 **A,** Radial forearm flap is marked out before exsanguination and tourniquet insufflation. The *red line* outlines the course of the radial artery; the *green line* is the skin incision; and the lateral *blue line* marks the course of the cephalic vein.

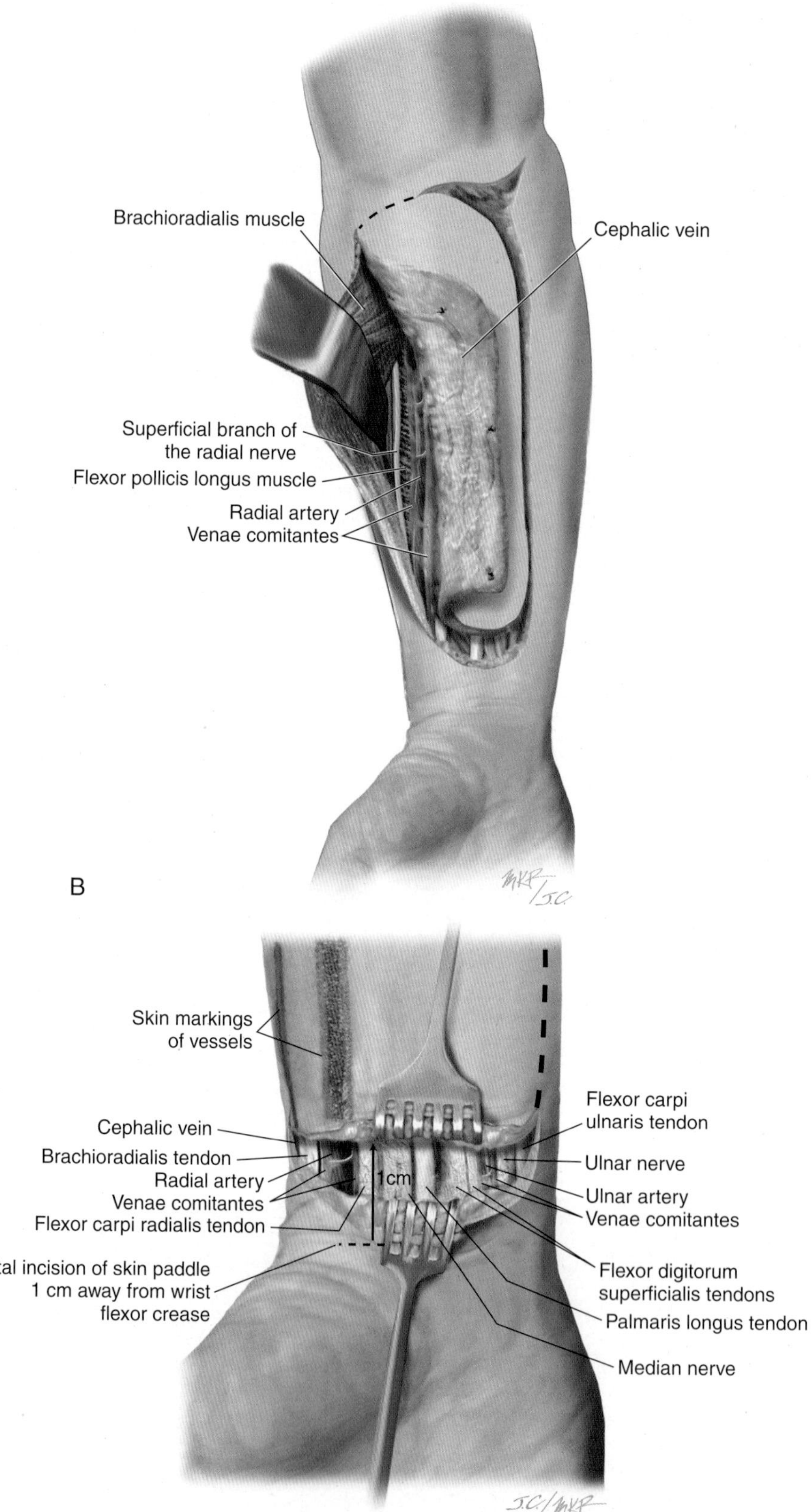

Figure 127.4, cont'd **B,** Identification of the radial artery vascular pedicle between the muscle bellies of the brachioradialis and flexor carpi radialis. **C,** Identification of the pedicle distally within the flexor crease of the wrist.

TECHNIQUE: Radial Forearm Flap Harvest—*cont'd*

STEP 6: Elevation of the Radial Forearm Flap

The flap can now be elevated off the flexor digitorum superficialis and flexor pollicis longus muscle in a surgical plane deep to the vascular pedicle. Dissection proceeds in a distal to proximal direction toward the antecubital fossa between the muscle bellies of the flexor carpi radialis and brachioradialis. Small branching blood vessels are either clipped with vascular clips or cauterized with bipolar cautery (Fig. 127.4D).

STEP 7: Release of the Tourniquet and Division of the Pedicle

Once the flap harvest is complete, the tourniquet can be released. Meticulous attention should be paid to hemostasis of the flap and forearm donor site using hemoclips and bipolar cautery. Heparinized saline, papaverine, and warm saline irrigation should be used at this point. Hand perfusion should be verified with identification of adequate capillary refill to all of the digits. The flap should be allowed to reperfuse for at least 20 minutes before division of the pedicle. The vascular pedicle then can be divided with 2-0 silk suture proximally.

STEP 8: Closure of the Forearm and Skin Grafting of the Donor Site Defect

The proximal portion of the forearm can be closed in a layered fashion with 3-0 Vicryl suture for the subcutaneous tissue and staples for the skin. In rare cases the skin paddle defect can be closed primarily or with a VY advancement flap. A skin graft can be harvested in a full-thickness or split-thickness fashion and secured with gut suture. A suction drain should be placed proximally, and a medication-impregnated, nonstick dressing and gauze wrap should be placed over the skin graft. A volar splint should be used to immobilize the hand for 5 to 7 days in a neutral position and to protect the graft (Fig. 127.4E).

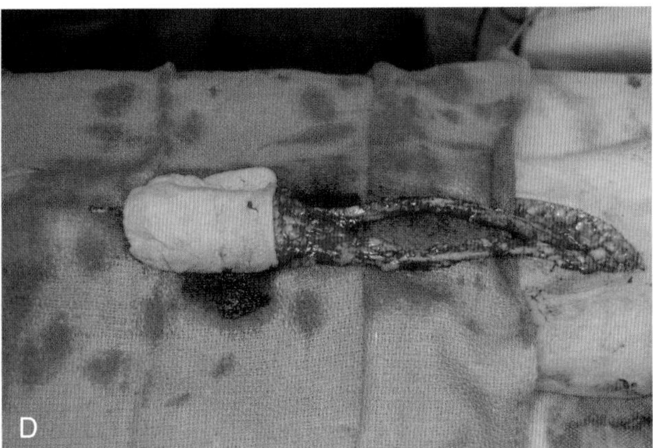

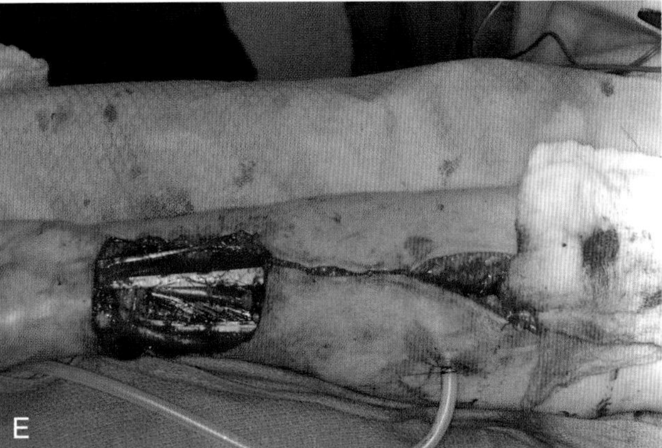

Figure 127.4, cont'd **D,** Elevation of the flap in a distal to proximal direction. The flap remains pedicled proximally. Note both the preservation of the vascular pedicle and the cephalic vein laterally. **E,** Closure of the radial forearm flap donor site. A suction drain has been placed. A skin graft has not yet been secured over the skin paddle defect.

ALTERNATIVE TECHNIQUE 1: Harvesting With the Palmaris Longus Tendon

For harvesting with the palmaris longus tendon, dissection is carried out in a manner similar to that described in steps 1 through 3. On the ulnar aspect of the forearm, dissection is carried down to the flexor carpi radialis muscle and palmaris longus tendon. The entire length of the tendon and muscle should be exposed. A subfascial dissection should be performed deep to the tendon selected for reconstruction (i.e., the palmaris longus), keeping it attached to the forearm flap skin paddle. The vascular pedicle can be identified distally and ligated. The remainder of the flap can be elevated in a fashion similar to that previously described (Fig. 127.5).

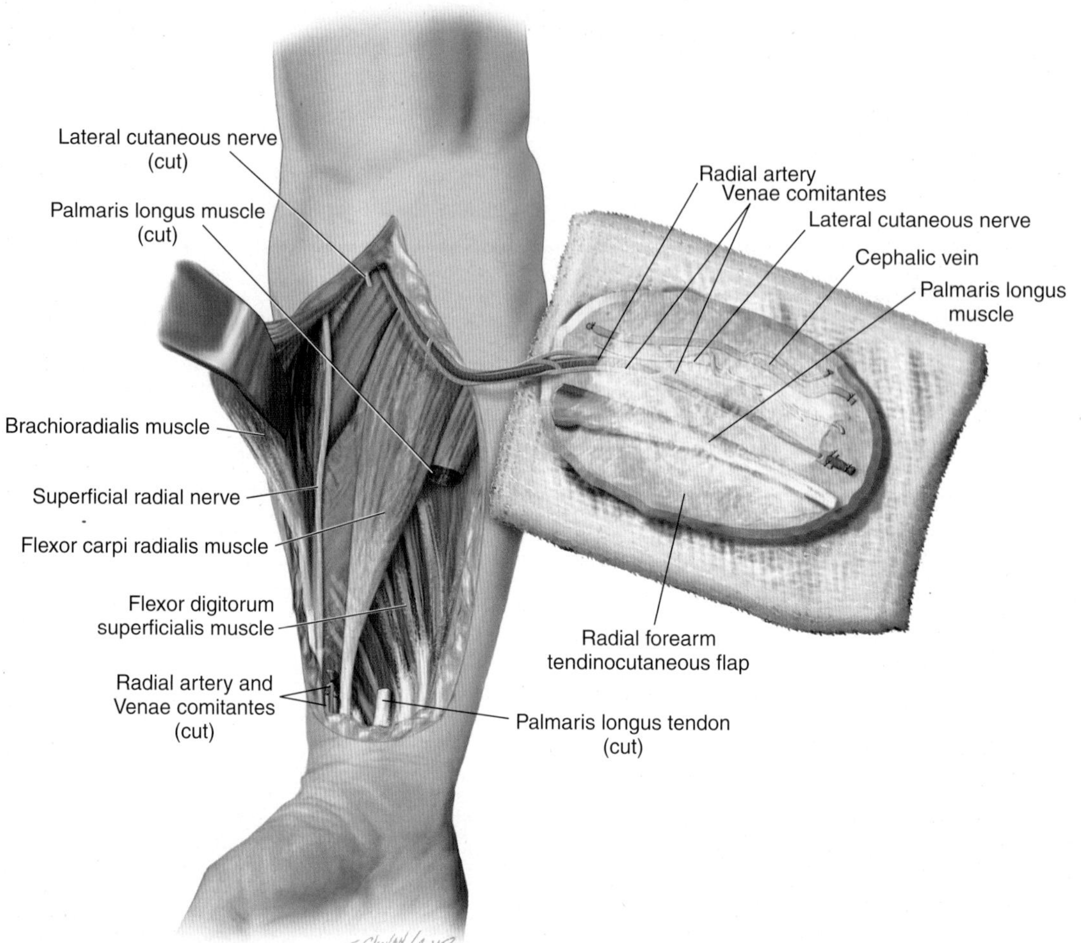

Figure 127.5 Radial forearm flap elevated with the palmaris longus tendon.

ALTERNATIVE TECHNIQUE 2: Radial Forearm Osteocutaneous Flap

For a radial forearm osteocutaneous flap, dissection is carried out in a fashion similar to that described in steps 1 through 4. The vascular pedicle is identified in the intermuscular septum from the ulnar aspect. The brachioradialis muscle is retracted laterally. While the superficial branch of the radial nerve is protected, the periosteum is incised lateral to the intermuscular septal perforators for the desired length of the radius bone to be harvested.

The vascular pedicle is tied off distally, and the flexor carpi radialis muscle is retracted medially. The muscle bellies of the flexor pollicis longus and pronator quadratus are incised, exposing the periosteum over the radius bone from the ulnar aspect. The radius bone segment is osteotomized, preserving the intermuscular septum bounded by both the flexor digitorum superficialis and flexor pollicus longus medially and both the brachioradialis and extensor pollicus muscles laterally while remaining attached to the flap's fasciocutaneous component superficially. The remainder of the flap is elevated in a standard fashion as previously described (Fig. 127.6).

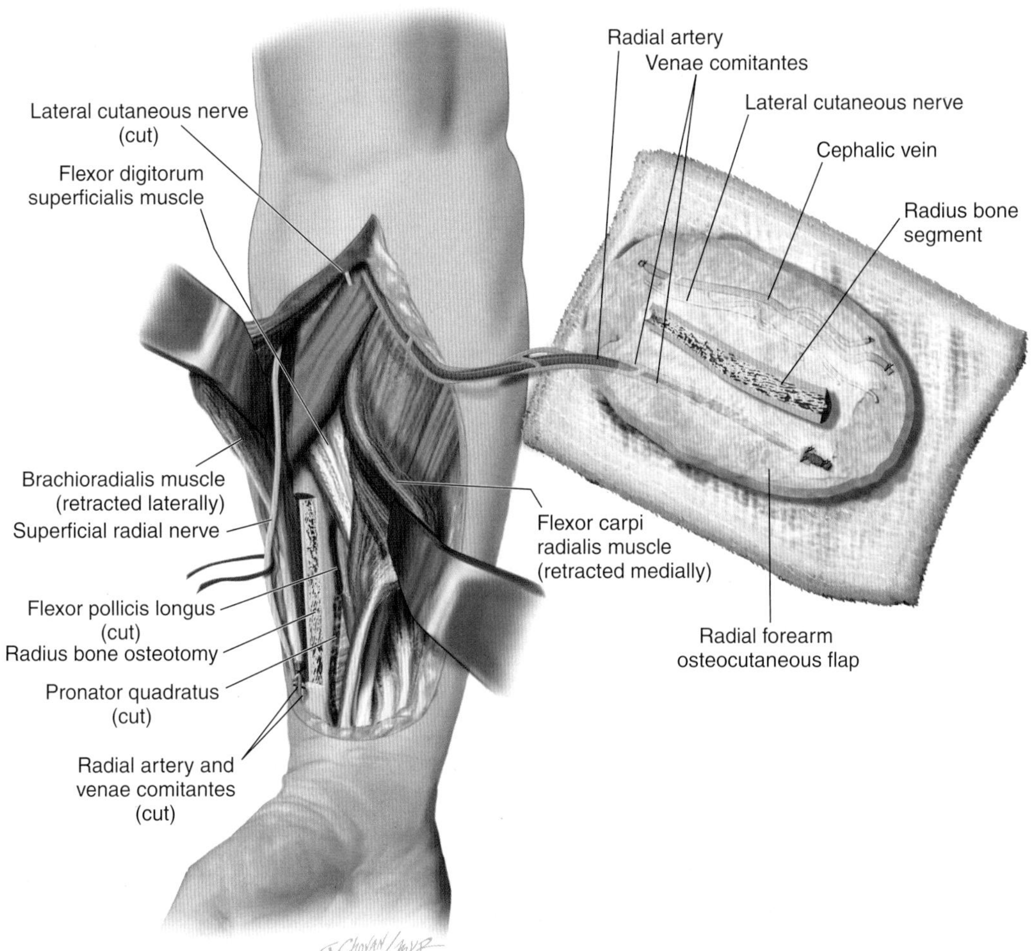

Figure 127.6 Radial forearm flap harvested with a section of radius bone from the distal third.

ALTERNATIVE TECHNIQUE 3: Harvesting the Ulnar Flap

PRESERVATION OF THE BASILIC VEIN AND IDENTIFICATION OF THE VASCULAR PEDICLE

The ulnar flap can be harvested under sterile tourniquet technique after exsanguination. The skin paddle is based on the ulnar artery along the medial aspect of the forearm. The initial incision is made through subcutaneous tissue, and the flexor carpi ulnaris, flexor carpi radialis, palmaris longus, and flexor digitorum superficialis muscle bellies are identified. The basilic vein can be encountered medially and ligated distally. Lateral branching vessels from the basilic vein into the skin paddle must be preserved if this vein is to be used. The ulnar vascular pedicle can be identified in the fascia between the muscle bellies of the flexor carpi ulnaris and flexor digitorum superficialis.

PRESERVATION OF THE ULNAR NERVE AND ELEVATION OF THE FASCIOCUTANEOUS FLAP

The flexor carpi ulnaris is retracted medially, and the ulnar nerve is gently dissected and mobilized from the vascular pedicle. The lateral aspect of the skin flap is elevated in a subfascial plane above the flexor digitorum superficialis tendon. The ulnar vascular pedicle is now ligated distally, with elevation of the skin paddle and pedicle in a distal to proximal direction superficial to the flexor digitorum profundus. Any branching vessels to the muscle are ligated with suture or hemostatic clips. The pedicle can be dissected proximally to the takeoff of the common interosseous artery (Fig. 127.7).

Continued

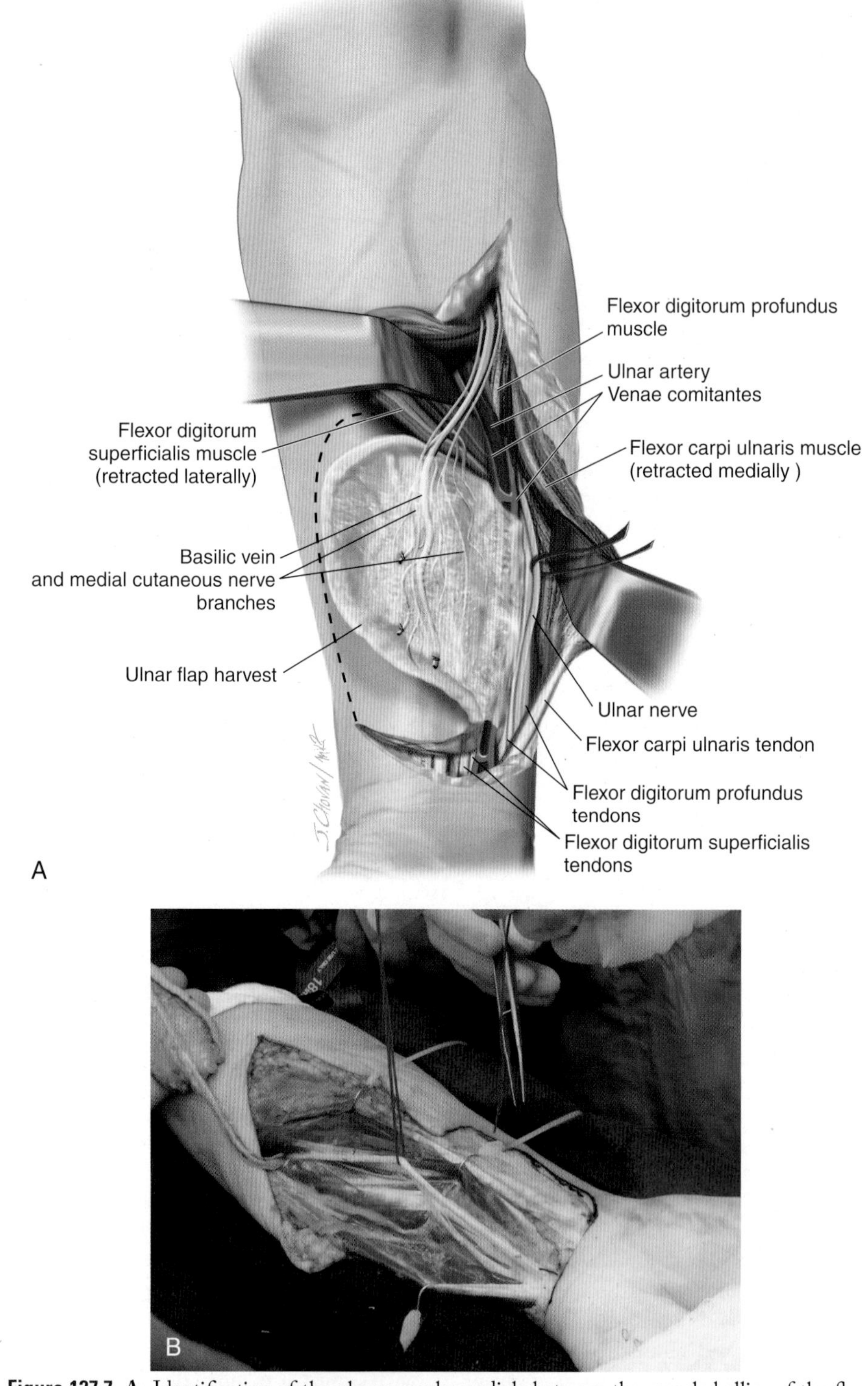

Figure 127.7 **A,** Identification of the ulnar vascular pedicle between the muscle bellies of the flexor digitorum superficialis and the flexor carpi ulnaris. **B,** Ulnar forearm flap elevated. The vessel loop isolates the ulnar nerve, which must be preserved during the harvest.

Avoidance and Management of Intraoperative Complications

As previously described, a preoperative Allen test is essential to confirm the adequacy of redundant blood supply to the hand based on either the radial or ulnar artery. Clear marking of the selected donor site forearm should be performed in the preoperative staging area. This should include communication with the anesthesia team to ensure avoidance of unnecessary blood draws and placement of intravenous or intraarterial lines that may damage vessels selected for use in microvascular anastomosis.

Although only a single venous anastomosis is required from either system to adequately drain the flap, many surgeons are more comfortable with multiple venous anastomoses for redundancy against possible venous thrombosis.[3,5,18] Other advantages of including the cephalic vein for anastomosis comprise the larger-caliber vessel (2 to 4 mm) versus the small-diameter (1 to 2 mm), thin-walled vena comitans. Theoretical disadvantages of using the superficial system include increased flap harvest time and increased flap tissue bulkiness. Some authors advocate preservation of the communicating vein between the venae comitantes and the cephalic vein at the antecubital fossa to allow both systems to drain off a single vessel. However, studies have shown numerous communicating branches between the two systems throughout the forearm, with adequate drainage via either system.[3,5] The surgeon must also be aware that the cephalic vein could be heavily scarred, resulting in poor flow and inadequate flap drainage, because of previous trauma (e.g., iatrogenic from multiple intravenous lines or blood draws or from self-abuse, such as intravenous drug use). The ulnar flap also can be drained off either its superficial venous system (basilic vein) or the ulnar vena comitans, allowing for a single venous anastomosis.[6,19,20]

To minimize flap ischemia time, pedicle division and flap transfer should be performed once the recipient vessels have been prepared and hemostasis is noted at the head and neck defect site. The cephalic vein can be divided first to assess the adequacy of venous outflow. If added venous length is needed, the cephalic vein may be dissected proximally beyond the antecubital fossa into the upper arm before vascular pedicle division.

Aberrant anatomy of the radial artery can result in a higher takeoff in the axilla or upper arm off the brachial artery (12% to 15% of cases). This does not affect flap harvest or flap success. A low takeoff also has been described (5 to 7 cm distal to the antecubital fossa). This does not affect flap harvest, but a short pedicle results, and vein grafting may be required if added length is needed for a successful reconstruction.[5]

A superficial ulnar artery is reported in 0.7% to 9% of cases. The artery is usually identified superficial to the bicipital aponeurosis, and the incidence is reportedly higher with the absence of the palmaris longus tendon. When the radial forearm flap is raised, any arteries that cross the forearm in a superficial layer should be identified before dividing. The radial artery also should be identified before division of the superficial artery as it may be the ulnar artery. Division of both the radial artery and ulnar artery will result in a disastrous loss of blood supply to the hand. One of the transected arteries will require reanastomosis and restoration of blood supply to the hand. The tourniquet can be released before division of the vessels to confirm the superficial artery and to recheck an Allen test. If the ulnar artery is inadvertently divided, the flap can be converted to an ulnar artery-based flap (obviously, with preservation of the radial artery).[19]

The size and shape of the head and neck defect to be reconstructed should be evaluated before flap harvest to ensure that an adequate amount of tissue is harvested for reconstruction.

An adequate amount of thin, pliable tissue is required during tongue and floor of the mouth reconstruction, both to seal off the oral cavity from the neck to prevent salivary leaks and to provide unrestricted movement for the native tongue tissue. If more bulk is required, a larger flap can be harvested, with a portion deepithelialized and rolled on itself. Sensory nerves, such as the antebrachial cutaneous nerve, can be harvested with the flap and reanastomosed to nerves in the head and neck for partial flap sensation.[2,5–12]

Tendinocutaneous forearm flaps can be used to reconstruct total or subtotal lower lip defects; this is especially true in cases involving previous irradiation or local flap reconstruction. Although oral muscular competence will be altered, because there is no replacement of the orbicularis oris sphincter, the flap will help prevent microstomia and provide partial competence, with generally good results. Most commonly, the palmaris longus tendon can be harvested with the flap and attached to the end fibers of the orbicularis oris or the periosteum of the malar region for added suspension. The flap is folded over the tendon to reline both the oral mucosa and skin of the chin and lip. It is important to overcompensate when the flap is suspended to account for postoperative flap drooping in the future. The brachioradialis tendon or flexor carpi radialis tendon may also be selected in cases of an absent palmaris longus (10%) or if a thicker tendon band is required (Fig. 127.8).[5,6,16]

Defects involving the retromolar fossa or tonsillar fossa are easily reconstructed with the forearm flap. The flap can easily be extended to provide coverage onto the soft palate or extension into the glossotonsillar sulcus. Flap inset is usually performed under direct visualization via a lip-split mandibulotomy; however, newer techniques using robotic inset have been described in cases of minimal access resection surgery. Parachuting sutures placed before flap inset, rather than individual thrown sutures, help with flap inset. The surgeon must pay careful attention to closure of the most inferior portion to help prevent a salivary leak.

The goals of soft palate reconstruction should focus on minimizing velopharyngeal dysfunction and insufficiency, and the resultant hypernasality of speech and nasal regurgitation. The forearm flap can be folded upon itself to reline both the palatal mucosal and nasal mucosal surfaces if the surgeon wants to avoid a raw fascial flap nasal mucosal surface. There is no difference in outcomes, and the nasal side can be left to granulate without any adverse effects in flap healing. The surgeon must remember that the forearm flap becomes an adynamic sling that contracts secondarily due to scarring. To help avoid hypernasality and velopharyngeal insufficiency, the flap should be sutured to a portion of the posterior pharyngeal wall, or a superiorly based pharyngeal flap should be used in conjunction with the forearm flap (Fig. 127.9).[5,22]

Forearm flap reconstruction can be applied to defects of the buccal mucosa to help limit postoperative trismus.

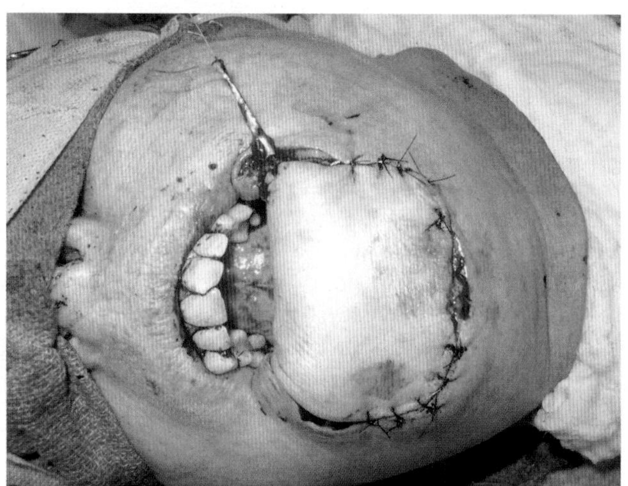

Figure 127.8 Total lower lip reconstruction with a radial forearm flap. The palmaris longus tendon is used for lip support.

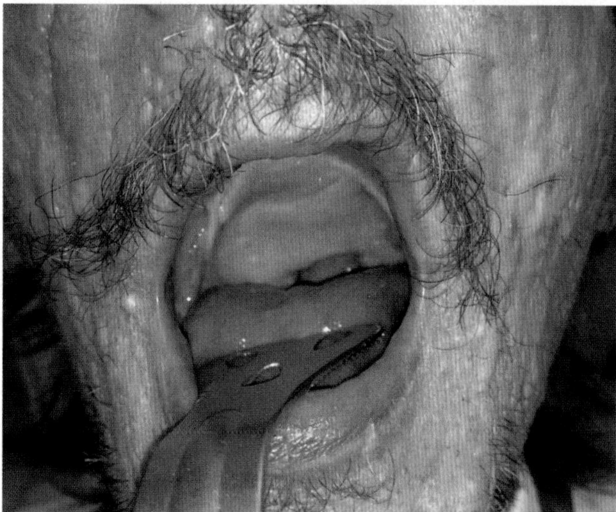

Figure 127.9 Radial forearm flap used for a total soft palate reconstruction. Note the narrowed nasopharyngeal port, which reduces speech hypernasality.

Full-thickness defects involving the cheek and buccal mucosa can be reconstructed with the folded forearm flap technique.

Pharyngoesophageal reconstruction after laryngopharyngectomy can also be performed using a tubed forearm flap. The flap can be prefabricated before division of the pedicle or tubed during inset in the neck. The flap can be sutured around a large-caliber nasogastric tube or salivary bypass tube. Some redundancy of tissue should be accounted for to allow for postoperative flap contracture, minimizing the risk of neopharyngeal stricture. A two-layered closure can be performed at the anastomotic suture line (excess tissue to be deepithelialized is harvested, and vascularized fascia is used for a second layer of closure). This technique can help reduce the risk of postoperative leakage or fistula formation, especially in previously irradiated tissue. An external skin paddle can be incorporated into the flap design and used to assist in monitoring of otherwise buried free flaps (Fig. 127.10).[5,23]

The radius bone should be preplated after harvesting of the osteocutaneous flap, regardless of whether an actual radius fracture occurred. This is due to a 20% risk of radius fracture if preplating is not performed after radius bone harvest.[5,15,17]

During flap inset, the surgeon must ensure the adequacy of any subcutaneous tunnels created from the defect to the recipient vessels to avoid compression of the pedicle and vascular compromise. Vessel geometry is also of great importance; the surgeon must pay careful attention to obtaining a tension-free anastomosis without too much vessel redundancy resulting in kinking of the pedicle. Soft drains (e.g., Penrose drains) should be placed to help prevent hematoma formation and to reduce the risk of flap compromise after flap inset.

Postoperative Considerations

Postoperative monitoring of free flap viability should be performed per unit protocol. As with all free flaps, the risk of vascular compromise is highest in the first 48 hours. Many microsurgical services monitor flaps every hour for the first 24 hours and every 2 hours for the subsequent 48 hours. Standard monitoring includes assessment of color, turgor, temperature, capillary refill, and Doppler signal. The use of various antiplatelet and antithrombotic medications is highly controversial; no clear benefit has ever been demonstrated in randomized controlled trials. Regardless, successful flap salvage depends on early recognition of problems and prompt reexploration in the operative setting.[18,24]

Most often the forearm donor site requires skin grafting (allogeneic or autogenous) to close the donor site defect. No significant difference in functional or esthetic outcomes has been seen between full-thickness skin grafts and split-thickness skin grafts.[5,21,25] The author prefers split-thickness skin grafts from the lateral thigh and full-thickness skin grafts from the groin or medial upper arm (Fig. 127.11). Davis et al.[21] performed a retrospective review of the donor site skin graft in 47 patients who underwent radial forearm free flap reconstruction. They concluded that there was no statistically significant difference between the split-thickness skin graft and the full-thickness skin graft in the number of postoperative dressings, incidence of tendon exposure, time to healing at the skin graft donor site, and time to healing at the skin graft recipient site. Some trends indicated improved subjective patient esthetics in the full-thickness skin graft group.

The skin graft should be well adherent with a bolster dressing, and the forearm should be immobilized with the hand in a neutral position for 5 to 7 days to allow adequate time for graft neovascularization. A volar splint should be fabricated to immobilize and protect the skin graft. Physical therapy for the forearm and hand should begin on postoperative day 7 and should be continued until range of motion and strength return to preoperative baseline levels.

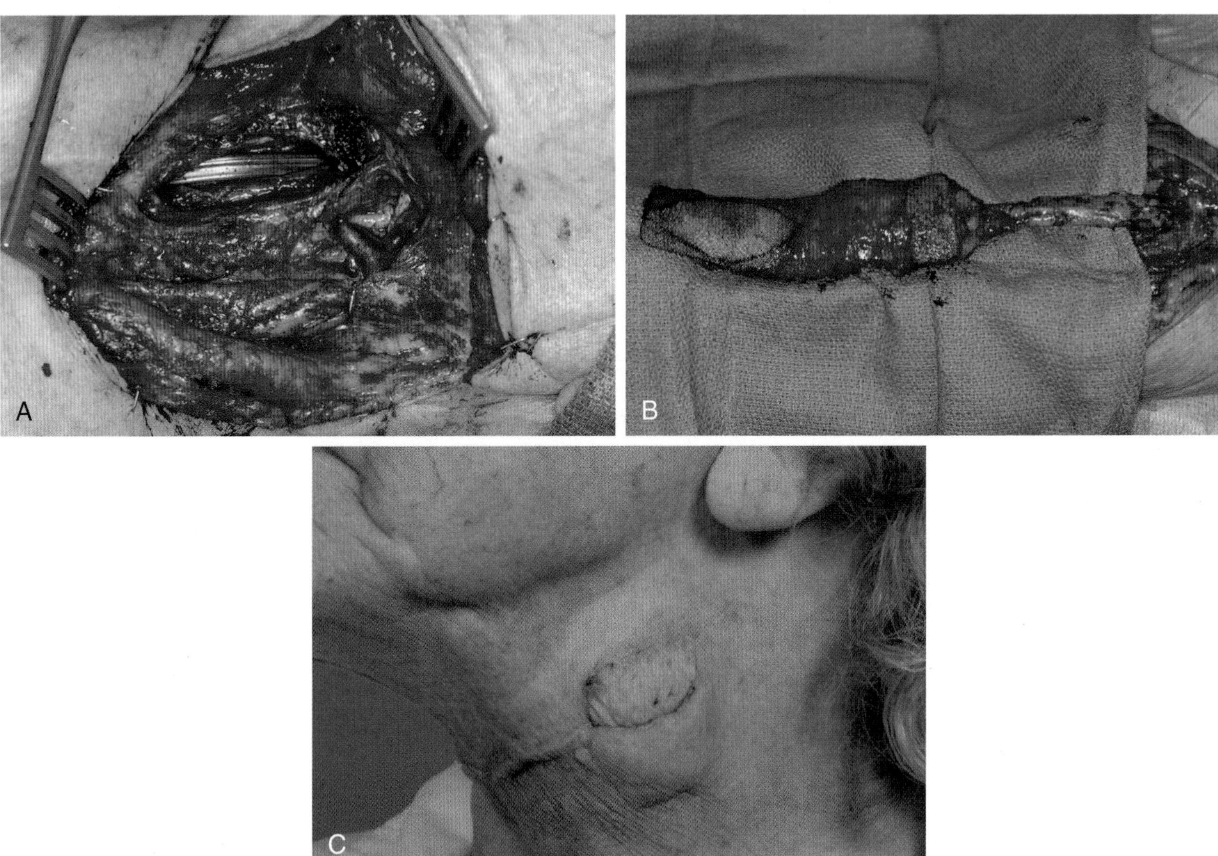

Figure 127.10 **A,** Pharyngeal stricture excision after a failed attempt at esophageal dilation. The patient had undergone previous laryngectomy and radiotherapy. **B,** Radial forearm flap harvest for pharyngeal wall reconstruction. An external skin paddle for flap monitoring has been designed. **C,** Healed forearm flap for pharyngeal stricture reconstruction. Note the healed external skin monitor within the neck incision. The patient regained normal swallowing function after reconstruction.

A temporary feeding tube should be considered for lip, oral cavity, and oropharyngeal reconstructions during the initial postoperative period to allow for early nutrition during the acute healing phase. Flap hair growth also can be a concern to patients; however, this is usually not an issue in patients who require postoperative adjuvant radiotherapy. Options for hair removal include laser removal or skin paddle deepithelialization.

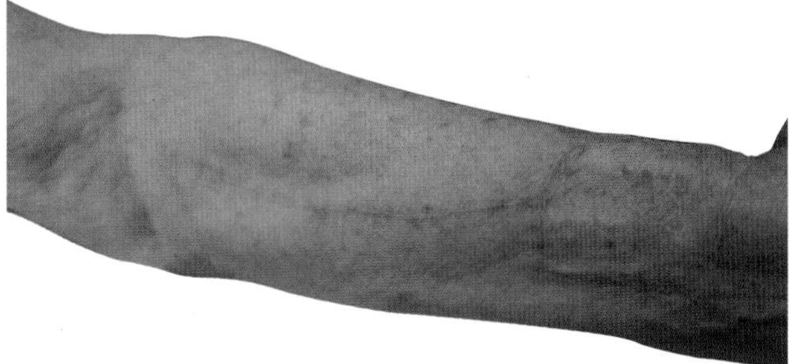

Figure 127.11 Healed forearm donor site after skin grafting, with overall good aesthetics.

References

1. Yang G, Chen B, Gao Y, et al. Forearm free skin flap transplantation. *Zhonghua Yixue Zazhi.* 1981;61:139.
2. Soutar DS, McGregor IA. The radial forearm flap in intraoral reconstruction: the experience of 60 consecutive cases. *Plast Reconstr Surg.* 1986;78(1):1–8.
3. Thoma A, Archibald S, Jackson S, Young JE. Surgical patterns of venous drainage of the free forearm flap in head and neck reconstruction. *Plast Reconstr Surg.* 1994;93(1):54–59.
4. Coleman SS, Anson BJ. Arterial patterns in the hand based upon a study of 650 specimens. *Surg Gynecol Obstet.* 1961;113:409–424.
5. Futran ND, Gal TJ, Farwell DG. Radial forearm free flap. *Oral Maxillofac Surg Clin North Am.* 2003;15(4):577–591. vi-vii.
6. Huang JJ, Wu CW, Lam WL, et al. Anatomical basis and clinical application of the ulnar forearm free flap for head and neck reconstruction. *Laryngoscope.* 2012;122(12):2670–2676.
7. Urken ML, Weinberg H, Vickery C, Biller HF. The neurofasciocutaneous radial forearm flap in head and neck reconstruction: a preliminary report. *Laryngoscope.* 1990;100(2 Pt 1):161–173.
8. Urken ML, Biller HF. A new bilobed design for the sensate radial forearm flap to preserve tongue mobility following significant glossectomy. *Arch Otolaryngol Head Neck Surg.* 1994;120(1):26–31.
9. Kim JH, Rho YS, Ahn HY, Chung CH. Comparison of sensory recovery and morphologic change between sensate and nonsensate flaps in oral cavity and oropharyngeal reconstruction. *Head Neck.* 2008;30(8):1099–1104.
10. Biglioli F, Liviero F, Frigerio A, Rezzonico A, Brusati R. Function of the sensate free forearm flap after partial glossectomy. *J Cranio-Maxillo-Fac Surg.* 2006;34(6):332–339.
11. Mah SM, Durham JS, Anderson DW, et al. Functional results in oral cavity reconstruction using reinnervated versus nonreinnervated free fasciocutaneous grafts. *J Otolaryngol.* 1996;25(2):75–81.
12. Sabesan T, Ramchandani PL, Ilankovan V. Sensory recovery of noninnervated free flap in oral and oropharyngeal reconstruction. *Int J Oral Maxillofac Surg.* 2008;37(9):819–823.
13. Santamaria E, Wei FC, Chen IH, Chuang DC. Sensation recovery on innervated radial forearm flap for hemiglossectomy reconstruction by using different recipient nerves. *Plast Reconstr Surg.* 1999;103(2):450–457.
14. Kuriakose MA, Loree TR, Spies A, Meyers S, Hicks WL Jr. Sensate radial forearm free flaps in tongue reconstruction. *Arch Otolaryngol Head Neck Surg.* 2001;127(12):1463–1466.
15. Villaret DB, Futran NA. The indications and outcomes in the use of osteocutaneous radial forearm free flap. *Head Neck.* 2003;25(6):475–481.
16. Sadove RC, Luce EA, McGrath PC. Reconstruction of the lower lip and chin with the composite radial forearm-palmaris longus free flap. *Plast Reconstr Surg.* 1991;88(2):209–214.
17. Sinclair CF, Gleysteen JP, Zimmermann TM, et al. Assessment of donor site morbidity for free radial forearm osteocutaneous flaps. *Microsurgery.* 2012;32(4):255–260.
18. Evans BCD, Evans GRD. Microvascular surgery. *Plast Reconstr Surg.* 2007;119(2):18e–30e.
19. Sieg P, Jacobsen HC, Hakim SG, Hermes D. Superficial ulnar artery: curse or blessing in harvesting fasciocutaneous forearm flaps. *Head Neck.* 2006;28(5):447–452.
20. Hekner DD, Abbink JH, van Es RJ, Rosenberg A, Koole R, Van Cann EM. Donor-site morbidity of the radial forearm free flap versus the ulnar forearm free flap. *Plast Reconstr Surg.* 2013;132(2):387–393.
21. Davis WJ III, Wu C, Sieber D, Vandevender DK. A comparison of full and split thickness skin grafts in radial forearm donor sites. *J Hand Microsurg.* 2011;3(1):18–24.
22. Brown JS, Zuydam AC, Jones DC, Rogers SN, Vaughan ED. Functional outcome in soft palate reconstruction using a radial forearm free flap in conjunction with a superiorly based pharyngeal flap. *Head Neck.* 1997;19(6):524–534.
23. Anthony JP, Singer MI, Deschler DG, Dougherty ET, Reed CG, Kaplan MJ. Long-term functional results after pharyngoesophageal reconstruction with the radial forearm free flap. *Am J Surg.* 1994;168(5):441–445.
24. Chen KT, Mardini S, Chuang DCC, et al. Timing of presentation of the first signs of vascular compromise dictates the salvage outcome of free flap transfers. *Plast Reconstr Surg.* 2007;120(1):187–195.
25. Sidebottom AJ, Stevens L, Moore M, et al. Repair of the radial free flap donor site with full or partial thickness skin grafts. A prospective randomised controlled trial. *Int J Oral Maxillofac Surg.* 2000;29(3):194–197.

CHAPTER 128

Fibula

David R. Kang and Brent B. Ward

Armamentarium

#9 Periosteal elevator
#15 and #10 blades
Appropriate sutures
Bipolar electrocautery
Broad periosteal elevator
Cutting guides or sterile tongue blades or sterile foam blocks
Dermatome (if skin graft required)
Dingman bone clamps
Full guard or two periosteal elevators for osteotomies
Heel support
Hip bump
Jackson-Pratt drain, size 10 flat
Knee support
Metzenbaum scissors
Pen Doppler
Reciprocating or oscillating saw can be substituted with a Gigli saw
Richardson retractor
Ruler
Tenotomy scissors
Tourniquet inflated to 350 mm Hg

History of the Procedure

The restoration of form and function to the maxillofacial complex has always been a challenge. This region is the most complex regarding function in the human body, with the airway and gastrointestinal system traversing its structures, and the skeleton providing the framework for the dentition and oral cavity; this area is critical for esthetics, speech, breathing, and nutritional intake. Failure to reconstruct maxillofacial defects after trauma or oncologic resection results in unopposed muscle action leading to collapse to the ipsilateral side, cosmetic asymmetry, loss of function, and decreased quality of life.

The need for immediate reconstruction of head and neck defects results in the development of the deltopectoral flap and pectoralis major flap, but immediate bony reconstruction for complex oncologic defects was not performed in the head and neck.[1,2] The reconstruction of complex head and neck oncologic defects was revolutionized with microvascular free tissue transfer and the ability to immediately reconstruct mandibular defects.

In 1971, Strauch and coworkers were isolating a rib on a vascular pedicle and transposing this to the mandible in dogs as an island flap, and in 1974 Östrup and Fredrickson described microvascular rib transfer to the mandible in dogs.[3,4] In 1973, Daniel and Taylor introduced the clinical reality of a free flap with an iliofemoral island flap transposed to the distal extremity.[5,6] Taylor, in 1975, described the first free fibula flap transfer in humans, explaining the repair of traumatic injuries to the tibia in two patients.[7] In 1977, the first free flap reconstruction of the mandible using a vascularized rib occurred,[8,9] and Chen and Yan, in 1979, described the first osteocutaneous free fibula flap transferred to treat the traumatic loss of the radius.[10] In the same year, Gilbert introduced the lateral approach to the fibula, which was more efficient compared with Taylor's posterior approach, which required the patient to be in a prone position.[11] Ten years would pass until Hidalgo, in 1989, introduced the osteocutaneous fibula free flap for use in mandibular reconstruction when he presented 12 cases of segmental mandibular defects averaging 13.5 cm.[12]

Since then, the fibula free flap has become the gold standard for reconstruction of a large variety of mandibular defects due to its consistency in size, vascular pedicle length, vessel diameter, and the ability to incorporate a reliable skin paddle with the bone flap. Wei and colleagues, in 1986, published an anatomic and clinical study showing the reliability of the osteocutaneous fibula free flap.[13] The perforator anatomy has been revisited numerous times, confirming four to eight perforators along the fibula, most commonly located along the junction of the middle third and distal third of the fibula. These are more commonly septocutaneous, with the proximal perforators more likely to be musculocutaneous, traversing through the soleus or flexor hallucis longus muscle.[14,15] The diameter of the peroneal artery ranges from 1 to 2.5 mm and the width of the venae comitantes ranges from 2 to 4 mm with a total pedicle length of up to 15 cm. The bone dimensions may range from a width of 1 to 3 cm, averaging 2 cm, with a length up to 26 cm. The skin paddle can be made up to a length of 32 cm and a width of 14 cm.[16,17]

Many authors have described the reliability and viability of the fibula free flap with a success rate greater than 95%.[18,19] Hidalgo showed the reliability more than a decade after surgery with 70% of patients tolerating a regular diet with maintenance of good esthetic outcomes.[20]

Alternatives to the fibula free flap are also available, including nonvascularized corticocancellous bone grafts, vascularized scapula free flaps, osteocutaneous radial forearm free flaps, and the vascularized iliac crest free flap. Many contend that nonvascularized bone grafts offer better anatomic reconstructions with superior alveolar bone height, symmetric arch form, and graft width, whereas others state that the risk of infection, failure rates approaching 50%, and overall complication rates nearing 70% with nonvascularized corticocancellous bone grafts all make the approach too risky.[21–23]

Frodel and coworkers and Moscoso and coworkers both compared the bone thickness and stock from four free flap donor sites—the iliac crest, scapula, fibula, and radius—and found that the iliac crest proved to be the most reliable implant donor site followed by the scapula, fibula, and radius; however, the difference between the iliac crest and scapula and between the scapula and fibula did not achieve statistical significance.[24,25] The iliac crest has several disadvantages, such as having a bulky soft tissue cuff, difficult to inset, short vascular pedicle, the risk of postoperative hernia, and an inherent shape that sometimes makes contouring to the anterior mandible difficult.[26] The disadvantages of the scapula include the lack of segmental blood supply, which does not tolerate osteotomies, the inability to use a two-team approach, and the risk of weakness and loss of range of motion associated with harvesting this flap. The radius provides a thin monocortical bone segment that does not tolerate osteotomies well, and the radius bone at the donor site is at risk for postoperative fractures.[26]

In many cases, the fibula free flap provides the best option for mandibular reconstruction. Its long bicortical bone, which is consistently uniform in terms of width and length, allowing reconstruction of extensive mandibular defects including the condyle; its consistent pedicle length and diameter with dual medullary and periosteal blood supply; the ability to incorporate a skin and muscular component; and the ability to use a two-team approach all make this the free flap of choice for most extensive mandibular reconstructions.[26–28]

Indications for the Use of the Procedure

The goal of maxillofacial reconstruction using the fibula free flap is not only to restore continuity to the mandible or maxilla but also to restore form and function, allowing a return to normal speech, chewing, and swallowing. There are several indications for fibula reconstruction, such as oncologic surgery, allowing for aggressive resection and reliable reconstruction of previously unreconstructable defects. In these cases, the fibula or other free tissue transfer has the significant advantage of withstanding postsurgical radiotherapy. Other indications include posttraumatic defects, osteoradionecrosis, osteomyelitis, and congenital deformities.[29–31] Mandibular defects larger than 4 to 6 cm are typically used for a fibula flap, and this osseous flap surpasses all others when the anterior mandibular segment is involved, or for those requiring condylar reconstruction.[26,32,33]

Preoperative Assessment

Preoperative assessment prior to harvesting a fibula free flap begins with the attainment of a thorough medical history and physical examination that may reveal poor reliability of the peroneal artery and venae comitantes to include prior trauma, deep vein thrombosis, or peripheral vascular disease as well as diabetes and hypertension. Signs of previous trauma or surgery or atypical skin temperature, skin lesions, and hair growth should be examined for evidence of peripheral vascular disease.

Vascular studies have become extremely useful in preoperative preparation for free fibula harvest. Some groups have advocated that thorough physical examination and noninvasive Doppler examination are sufficient,[17,34] whereas others have concluded that preoperative angiography with its high positive predictive value and sensitivity can improve the chances of a successful outcome.[35,36] Kim and colleagues reviewed the variations in 1000 femoral arteriograms, and normal branching of the popliteal artery was present in 92.2%. Of the 7.8% with variations, most had a high origin of the anterior tibial artery or a trifurcation pattern. Of the variant patterns to the foot, the most common (5.6%) reflected the supply to the distal posterior tibial artery from the peroneal artery.[37] In 0.2% to 8% of the population, the peroneal artery is the dominant blood supplier to the foot, also known as peroneal artery magna, secondary to the absence or hypoplasia of the anterior and posterior tibial arteries.[16,27,37]

Conventional angiography evaluation of the lower extremity for the fibula free flap has been associated with risks of hemorrhage and thrombosis from the arterial catheterization and has now evolved into less invasive studies such as computed tomography angiography (CTA), magnetic resonance angiography (MRA), and color Doppler flow examinations. CTA and MRA are comparable except that a CTA is faster than an MRA and exposes the patient to radiation. Both are able to image the trifurcation of vessels and are able to image perforators. On the other hand, Doppler ultrasound is operator-dependent and unable to image the trifurcation of vessels.[38] MRA also cannot be used for patient-specific modeling during virtual surgical planning.

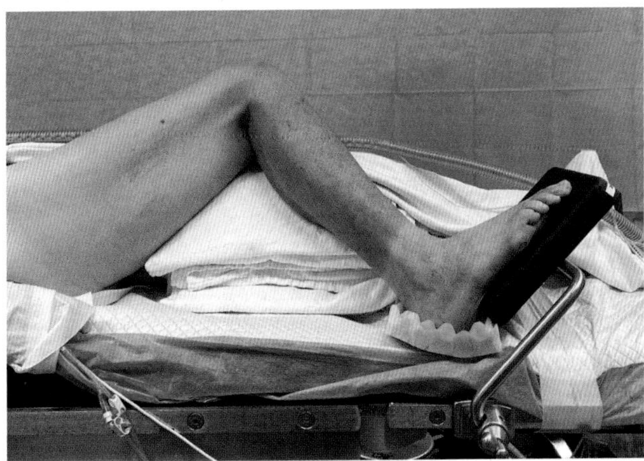

Figure 128.1 Orthopedic footrest to better support the 90-degree bent leg.

TECHNIQUE: Osteocutaneous Fibula Harvest

STEP 1: Patient Positioning and Preparation

The patient's leg is positioned so that it is supported by a hip bump internally rotating the leg and pelvis with knee and foot support, which positions the leg with a 90-degree bend at the knee, giving better access to the lateral and posterior portions of the leg (Fig. 128.1). The entire lower extremity is prepped, and the toes may be prepped or covered, but exposure of the foot for Doppler assessment of the posterior tibial artery and dorsalis pedis pulses allows for confirmation of vascular flow to the foot throughout the procedure. The topographic anatomy is marked with a line along the posterior border of the fibula, from the fibular head superiorly and the lateral epicondyle of the ankle inferiorly. This line approximates the intermuscular septum. The fibula is marked 6 to 8 cm distal to the fibular head and proximal to the lateral malleolus, denoting the bone that will be spared to preserve knee and ankle stability.

The peroneal nerve is indicated on the illustration with a line 1 to 2 cm below the fibular head. A Doppler may be utilized to mark potential perforators for inclusion in the skin paddle; however, for efficiency the perforators can be identified after the initial anterior skin incision and dissection of the intermuscular septum. The skin paddle can then be fabricated around the identified septocutaneous perforators. It should be noted that harvest of the fibula and skin more distally generates a longer vascular pedicle, which may be of importance particularly when the contralateral neck vessels are to be utilized for anastomosis. Generally, the dominant septocutaneous perforators are located more distally, allowing the centering of the flap in the region of the distal and middle thirds of the leg. The design of the skin paddle must take into account the fixed length of the skin perforators and intermuscular septum. The orientation of the left or right fibula into the right or left mandible or maxilla will dictate the location of the perforators and skin paddle as demonstrated by the orientation of the left fibula into the right mandible. If the peroneal vessels come off of the mandible anteriorly, the perforators and skin paddle will be along the inferior aspect of the neo-mandible, making intraoral rotation of the skin paddle more difficult but facilitating reconstruction of a cervical defect. Therefore, if intraoral reconstruction is needed with this orientation, the skin paddle can be made much larger to accommodate this lack of rotation. Alternatively, the fibula can be flipped and the vessels can come off posteriorly (Fig. 128.2A–C).

STEP 2: Incision

The leg is exsanguinated and the thigh tourniquet inflated to 350 mm Hg (however, a tourniquet is not mandatory for this procedure). A curvilinear incision is made anterior to the marking of the intermuscular septum along the peroneus longus and carried down to the fascia over the peroneus longus and brevis muscles. Dissection proceeds anteriorly in a suprafascial plane in order to incorporate additional fascia as needed. The fascia is then incised anterior to the intermuscular septum, revealing the peroneus longus and brevis muscles. Blunt subfascial dissection is carried posteriorly in this plane separating the fascia from the underlying muscle; this leads to the identification of the septocutaneous perforators at the posterior crural septum, which must be carefully protected. In cases where perforators are not identified in this region, musculocutaneous perforators are likely, necessitating a cuff of flexor hallucis longus and soleus later in the dissection. In approximately 6% of cases, no septocutaneous or musculocutaneous perforators are evident, in which case harvest of both the crural septum and anticipated site of musculocutaneous perforators is indicated, and a guarded prognosis but not absolute failure for the skin paddle should be assumed (Fig. 128.2D and F).

Continued

TECHNIQUE: Osteocutaneous Fibula Harvest—*cont'd*

STEP 3: Muscle and Vascular Pedicle Dissection

Once the perforators are identified, the peroneal muscles are retracted laterally and the lateral aspect of the fibula is palpated. The intermuscular septum is divided proximal to the perforators to facilitate retraction of the peroneal muscles anteriorly and the soleus posteriorly. Sharp or electrocautery dissection of the peroneus longus and brevis is continued along the lateral and anterior aspect of the fibula, leaving a generous 3-mm cuff of muscle on the bone to preserve the periosteal circulation. Dissection continues along the anterior aspect of the fibula until the intermuscular septum of the anterior compartment is reached. This is then incised, revealing the extensor digitorum and extensor hallucis muscles, which are swept medially using a broad periosteal elevator, revealing the interosseous membrane. The anterior tibial artery

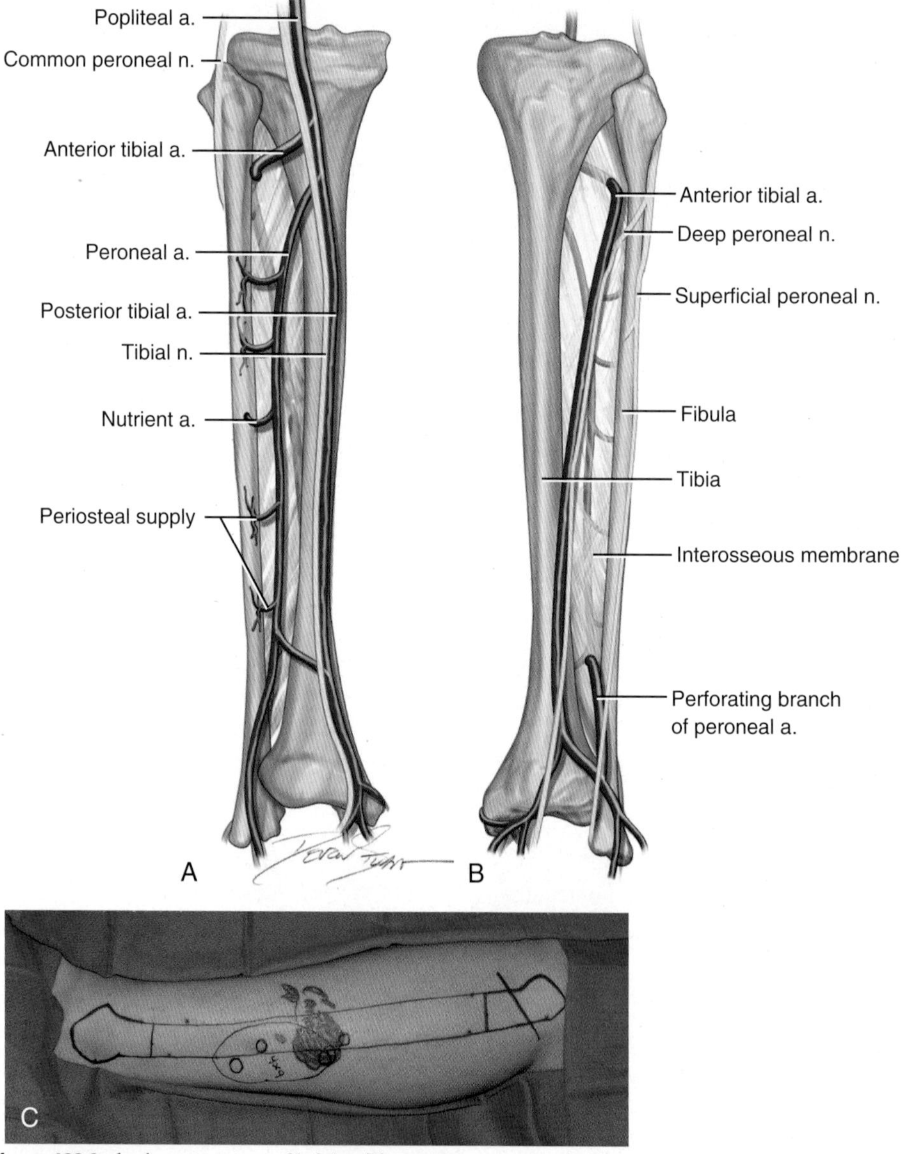

Figure 128.2 **A,** Anterior view of left leg. The common peroneal nerve crosses the fibular neck, dividing into the superficial and deep peroneal nerves. The anterior tibial vessel descends with the deep peroneal nerve along the anterior medial aspect of the interosseous membrane. The distal aspect of the peroneal artery passes through the interosseous membrane into the anterior compartment. **B,** Posterior view of left leg. The popliteal artery branches into the anterior tibial artery and the posterior tibial artery, which branches into the peroneal artery, provides the blood supply to the fibula through a nutrient artery and numerous periosteal vessels. **C,** Fibula illustrated with 6 cm marked from fibular head and lateral malleolus. Peroneal nerve illustrated inferior to fibular head. Perforators marked in circles and a 4 × 9 cm skin paddle is drawn out.

TECHNIQUE: Osteocutaneous Fibula Harvest—*cont'd*

and vein as well as the deep peroneal nerve are identified and retracted medially. The interosseous membrane is then divided, often with a Metzenbaum scissor proximal to distal with the right hand on the left leg, or distal to proximal on the right leg for a right hand dominant surgeon. Attention is turned to the proximal and distal portions of the fibula 6 to 8 cm from the fibular head and lateral malleolus, where circumferential dissection in a subperiosteal plane is completed to protect the vascular pedicle. A full guard or two #9 periosteal elevators can then be passed in a subperiosteal fashion around the fibula to protect the vascular pedicle. The osteotomies can then be completed with a reciprocating saw. The fibula is retracted laterally with Dingman bone clamps for increased visualization of the remaining dissection. If difficulty is encountered retracting the fibula bone laterally after the osteotomies are complete, the interosseous membrane is likely still attached and needs to be released. The tibialis posterior muscle is identified deep to the interosseous membrane, and the peroneal vessels are found deep to this muscle between the tibialis posterior and flexor hallucis muscles. The tibialis posterior muscle is divided distally first, leaving a 3-mm cuff of muscle on the fibula, unroofing the peroneal vasculature. The peroneal vessels are then identified and ligated distally, facilitating lateral retraction of the flap. The flexor hallucis muscle is then divided medial to the peroneal artery and vein. Additional flexor hallucis muscle can be harvested here for increased muscle bulk for coverage of defects without a skin paddle, such as in the maxilla. The posterior incision for a skin paddle is then outlined based upon the location of the perforators and previously made anterior incision. If additional skin paddle coverage is needed, this can be made up here. Incision is made through the skin and fascia, and blunt dissection is carried anteriorly in a subfascial plane to join the anterior dissection and the intermuscular septum and perforators.

The entire flap can now be easily retracted laterally, and the pedicle can be dissected proximally to its takeoff point from the posterior tibial vessels, taking care to prevent shearing of the pedicle from the fibular bone during lateral retraction. A large vein will often be branching medially along the proximal aspect of the pedicle and give the appearance of the posterior tibial bifurcation; however, this is usually not the posterior tibial trunk and the vein can be divided and dissected more proximally to give several centimeters of length to the overall pedicle. The tourniquet may then be released and bleeding controlled. Prior to the ligation of vessels, the flap may be assessed for vascular supply as well as verification of pulses to the foot (Fig. 128.2G–L).

Continued

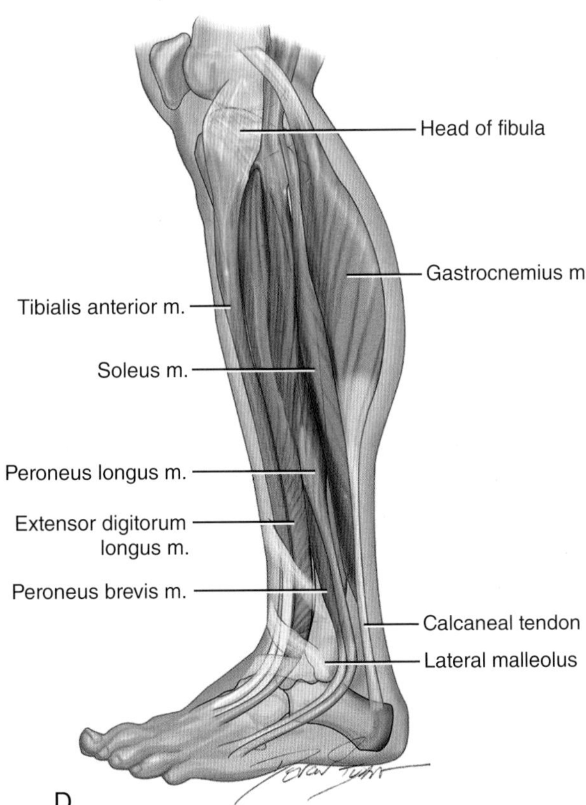

Figure 128.2, cont'd D, The posterior crural septum is located between the peroneus longus and brevis muscles and the soleus and gastrocnemius muscles. The position of the posterior crural septum can be approximated with a line drawn from the head of the fibula to the lateral malleolus.

TECHNIQUE: Osteocutaneous Fibula Harvest—*cont'd*

STEP 4: Osteotomy

The fibula may be shaped at the leg with the vascular pedicle attached or at the head following proximal ligation of the vessels based on anticipated complexity and desire for brevity in the total ischemic time of the flap. Shaping is completed based on the anatomic requirements of the defect with planning for the segments required. Closing wedge osteotomies are utilized for contouring the fibular bone. Cutting guides from virtual planning, sterile tongue blades, or sterile foam blocks can be used to guide the closing wedge osteotomies when complex reconstruction is required. The vascular pedicle should be carefully protected during the completion of osteotomies by using subperiosteal dissection and placement of the #9 periosteal between the vascular pedicle and saw blade. The periosteum can be extended at the most proximal and distal ends of the fibula osteotomy sites so that this periosteum can overlap with the butt joint of the recipient

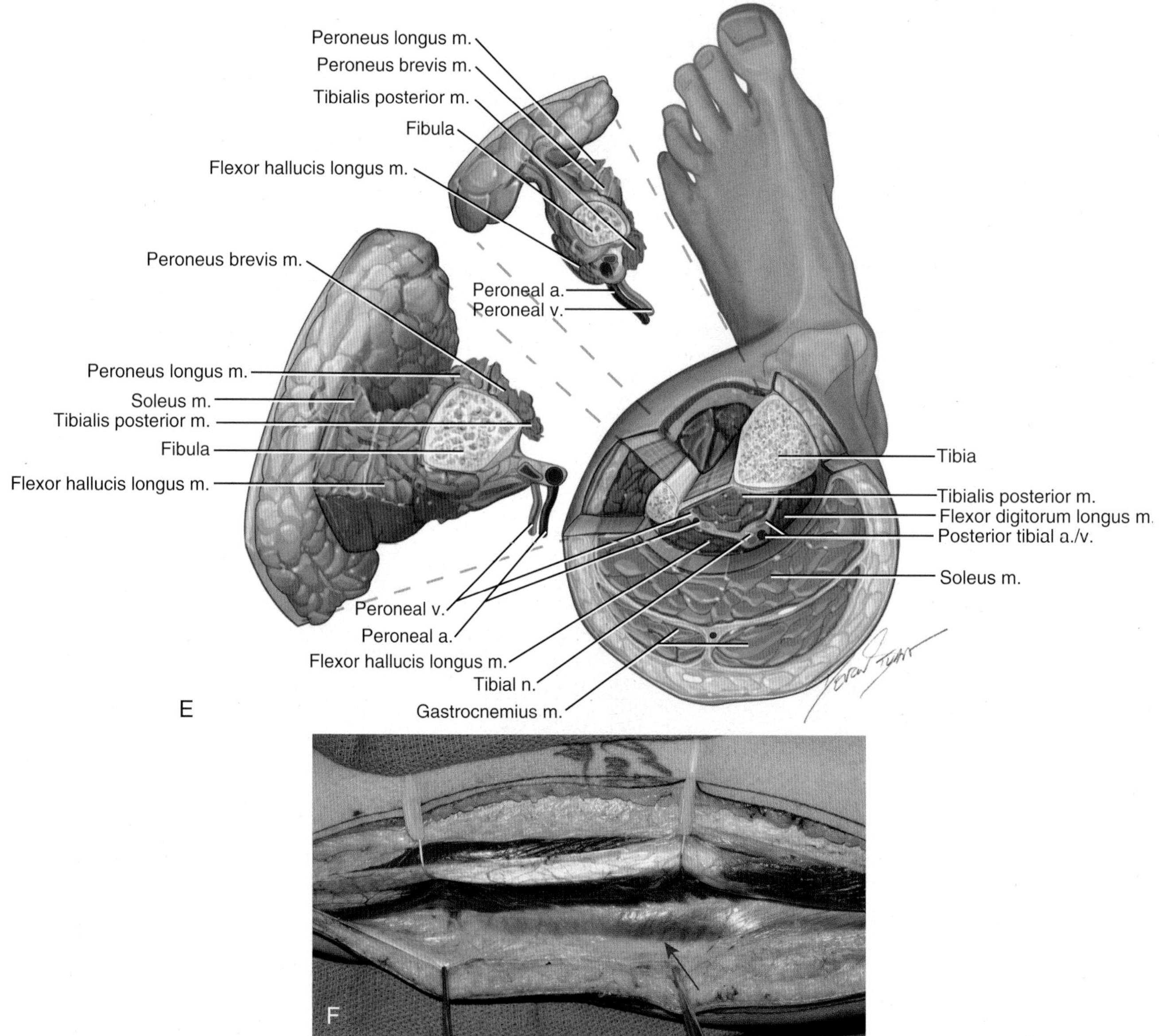

Figure 128.2, cont'd **E,** Cross-sectional anatomy of the leg depicting the path of the septocutaneous perforators, which may run purely through the septum or partially through the flexor hallucis longus (FHL) muscle, requiring harvest of a cuff of FHL to protect these perforators. Musculocutaneous perforators run their course entirely through FHL and soleus muscle, requiring a cuff of both muscles to protect the vascular pedicle. **F,** Peroneus longus and brevis retracted medially, revealing the posterior crural septum. A septocutaneous perforator is visualized at the distal blue arrow, and a small musculocutaneous perforator is visualized at the proximal red arrow.

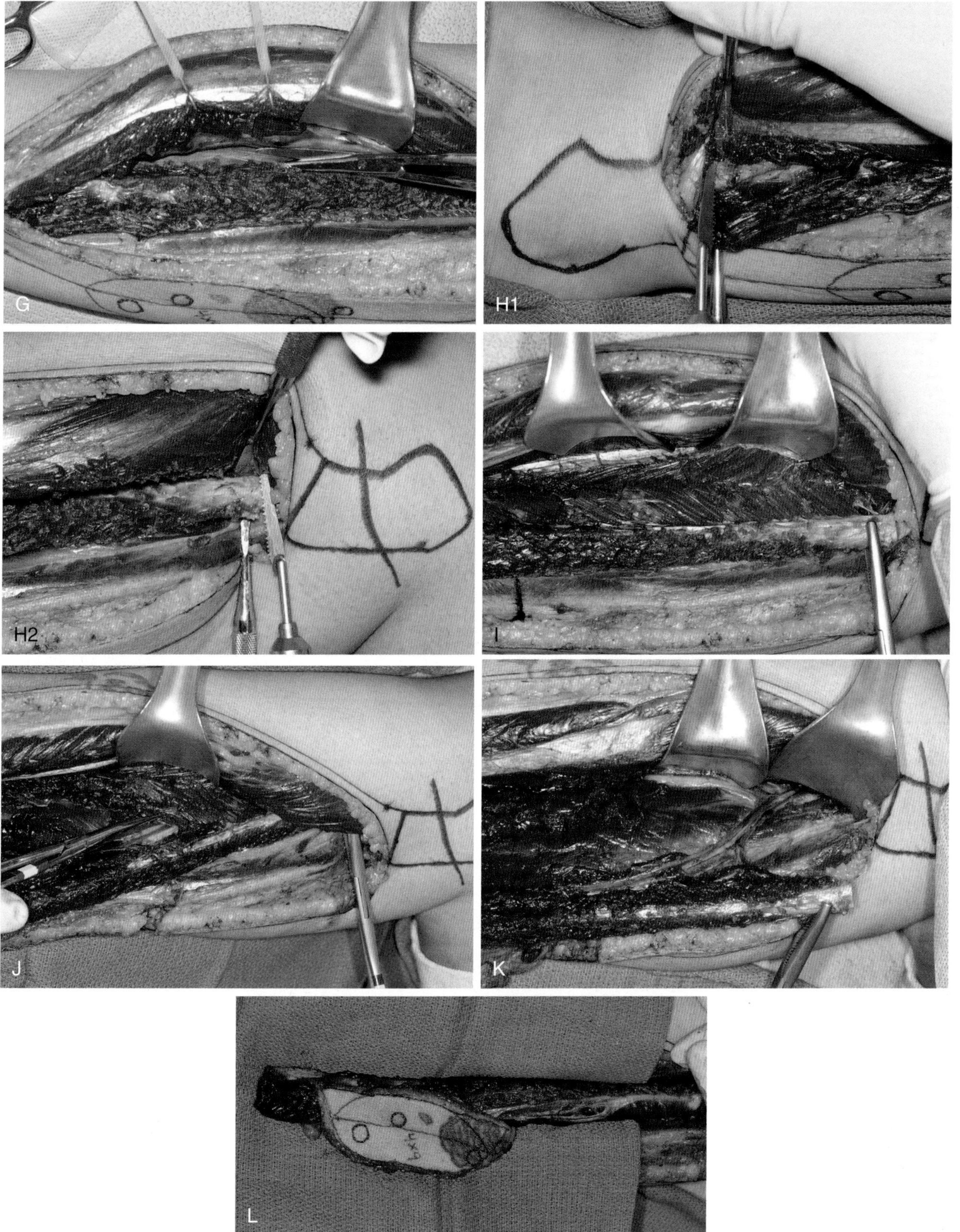

Figure 128.2, cont'd **G,** Peroneus longus and brevis muscles dissected off the fibula, leaving a 3-mm cuff of muscle, and retracted medially revealing the underlying anterior tibial vessels and deep peroneal nerve. Medially, the interosseous membrane is visualized and divided with scissors. **H1** and **H2,** Two periosteal elevators placed around the proximal and distal fibula in a subperiosteal plane to protect the underlying pedicle during osteotomy. **I,** After completion of the proximal and distal fibular osteotomies and division of the interosseous membrane, the extensor digitorum and extensor hallucis are retracted medially revealing the characteristic chevron-shaped fibers of the tibialis posterior muscle. **J,** The tibialis posterior muscle is divided with fine scissors unroofing the underlying peroneal vessels. **K,** Dissection completed with the peroneal vessels branching off the posterior tibial artery and veins. **L,** Fibula flap raised with skin paddle and ready for osteotomies either at the leg with pedicle attached or at the head and neck with pedicle detached.

Continued

TECHNIQUE: Osteocutaneous Fibula Harvest—*cont'd*

site. Where preoperative assessment allows for harvest of either fibula, planning for osteotomies and fixation should include consideration for the desired final location of the cutaneous paddle and the pedicle, as preferences of right versus left do exist based on these desired final positions. The number of osteotomies and size of segments should be carefully evaluated. Shorter segments and multiple osteotomies increase the chance for total or partial failure. A cadaver study indicated that segments shorter than 1 cm are unlikely to possess adequate vascularity and should not be utilized unless the recipient bed can support a nonvascularized graft. The vascular supply of the fibular bone is via two routes: the periosteal blood supply as well as a nutrient vessel to the fibula medullary bone. This nutrient artery is a branch off the peroneal artery, which takes off posteriorly to the interosseous membrane and enters midfibula through the nutrient foramen. This vessel is frequently divided during reconstruction of maxillofacial defects, but the periosteal blood supply is adequate for survival of the bone flap (Fig. 128.2M–O).

STEP 5: Inset

The fibula is brought to the recipient site and fixated to its final position. Depending on the needs of the location to be reconstructed, this may be accomplished with a variety of plating techniques including miniplates, reconstruction plates, and custom printed or milled plates. Fibular segments should be adequately stabilized with multiple monocortical screws or single screws if bony contacts provide adequate additional stability. The skin paddle is sutured in place and a small suture can be placed onto the skin paddle to facilitate pen Doppler evaluation of the skin perforators. Several modalities can be utilized for monitoring the integrity of the flap, including internal veinous or arterial Doppler, external Doppler, or with a tissue oximeter such as Vioptix (Fig. 128.2P).

STEP 6: Microvascular Anastomosis

Anastomosis of vessels is completed in the standard fashion (Figs. 128.2Q–T). In some patients, severe atherosclerosis of the entire length of the peroneal artery is encountered. These calcifications are often found in the tunica intima and innermost media. Try and identify portions that are not calcified and divide the pedicle at this location for anastomosis. If the entire length of the pedicle is calcified, a larger 7-0 tapered needle may be attempted. What the authors prefer for severe calcifications of the peroneal artery is to carefully circumferentially remove the calcifications, which will include the tunica intima and innermost media. With the remaining outermost media and tunica externa, the vessels can be carefully anastomosed. The suturing technique will need to be modified by suturing the compromised vessel inside out to prevent inward collapse of the calcified intima.

STEP 7: Closure

The donor and recipient sites are closed. The donor site of the leg can frequently be closed primarily depending on the size of the cutaneous paddle, typically 4 cm or less in width. Some advocate the approximation of the flexor hallucis longus muscle loosely to the interosseous membrane with the foot placed in a neutral 90-degree angle and with the great toe extended to prevent weakness in dorsiflexion, whereas others advocate leaving the muscle unattached to prevent contracture or "claw toe."[16,39] When necessary, the site can be prepared for skin grafting to avoid excess tension of skin and possible constriction of vessels to the foot. A suction drain is utilized and maintained based on standard protocols. (Fig. 128.2U).

ALTERNATIVE TECHNIQUES

Minimal technique variations exist in the harvest of the fibula, with the most prominent being the harvest of a fibula without a skin paddle. In these cases, a linear incision in the skin may be utilized to complete a circumferential dissection around the fibula, similar to the dissection completed for the osteocutaneous fibula but without maintenance of a skin paddle. The incision in these cases is closed primarily.

Although harvesting is fairly standard, a wide variety of modifications exist for flap inset based on location, and these variations deserve discussion.

Condylar Reconstruction

The length of the harvested fibula is adequate for angle-to-angle reconstruction of the mandible. Where single or multiple condylar reconstruction will be completed, some surgeons have opted for a combination of fibula with harvested rib in cases where an associated free graft is acceptable. Where the fibula alone is utilized, it may be shaped to adapt to the glenoid fossa. Maintenance of the fibula in the fossa has on occasion been problematic, prompting some surgeons to advocate wire

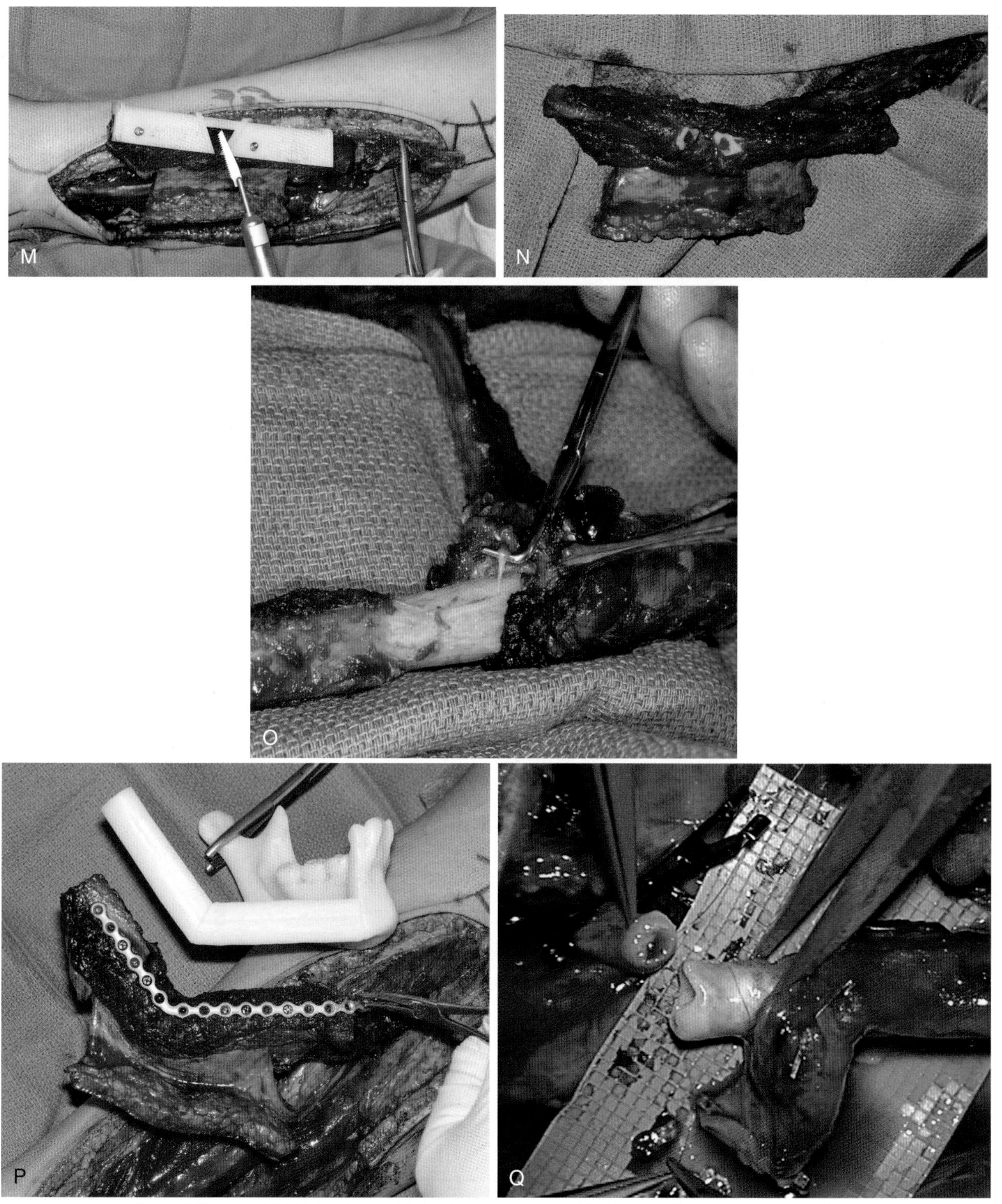

Figure 128.2, cont'd **M,** Cutting guide in place screwed in with intermaxillary fixation screws, closing wedge osteotomies about to be completed using a reciprocating saw. **N,** Osteotomies completed; note bleeding medullary bone and skin paddle edges. **O,** Nutrient artery found near the midpoint of the fibula, often divided for head and neck applications. **P,** Fibula plated using a 2.5 mm thick plate and compared to adjacent model for symmetry. **Q,** Complete calcification of the entire length of the peroneal artery.

Continued

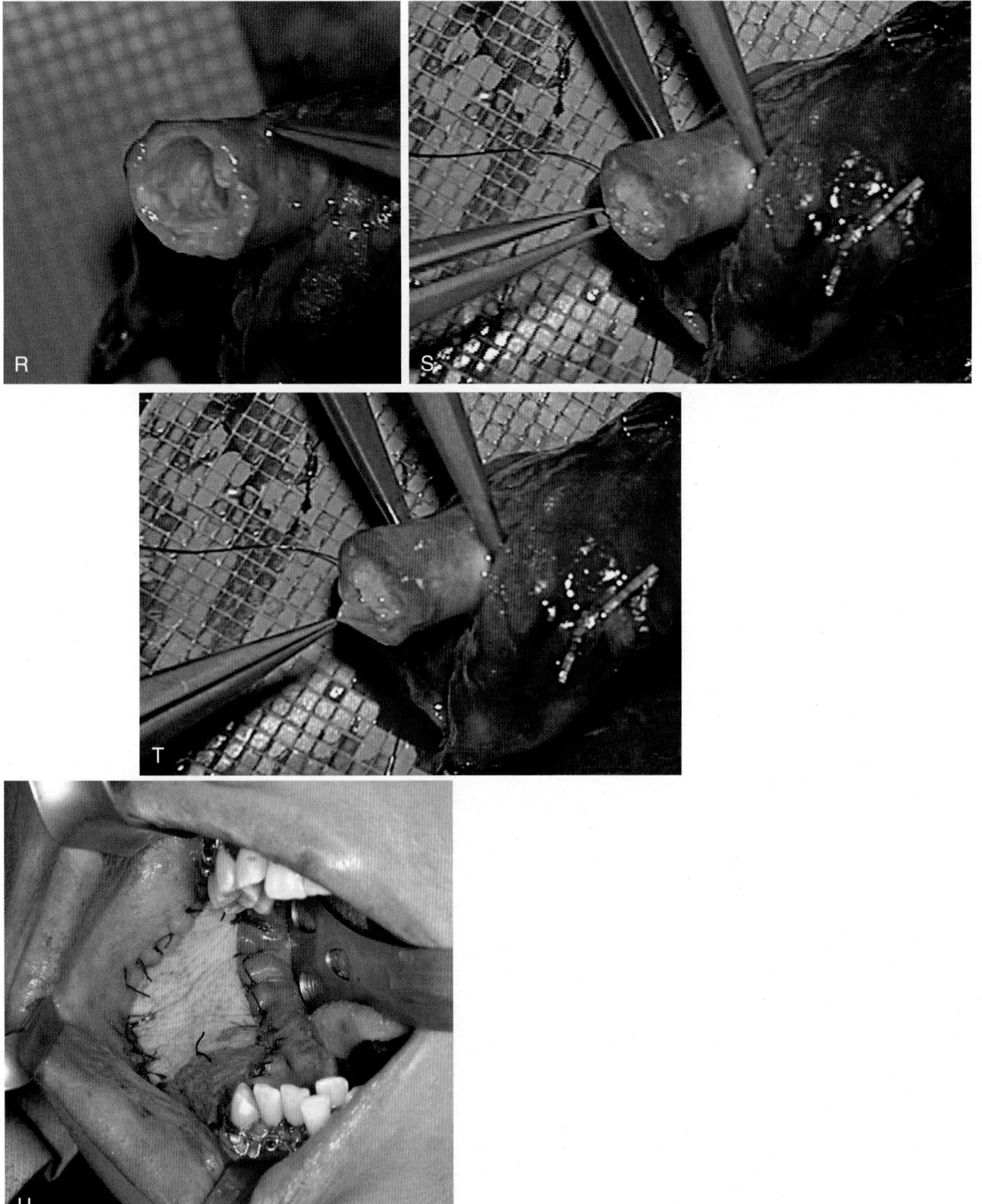

Figure 128.2, cont'd **R,** Lumen of the calcified peroneal artery. **S,** Calcifications, tunica intima, and innermost media of the peroneal artery being removed. **T,** New edge of calcified vessel with remaining outermost media and tunica externa/adventitia. **U,** Skin paddle inset into oral cavity with a 4-0 silk suture marking perforator location for pen Doppler placement.

ALTERNATIVE TECHNIQUE—*cont'd*

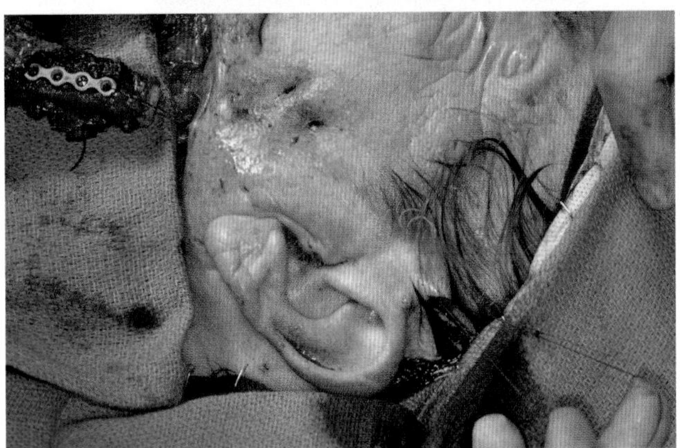

Figure 128.3 Fibula suspended superiorly with a nylon suture passed through a small incision in the temporal region through a spinal needle, passed through a hole in the plate and passed back through the spinal needle, which has been reset into a new position. This suture is then passed through the temporalis fascia and tied down after the mandible has been inset to help suspend the new condyle.

or suture suspension superiorly. As an alternative, some have utilized a protocol with postoperative intermaxillary fixation followed by guiding elastics to assist in maintaining condylar position. The location of the vascular pedicle in condylar reconstruction is an important consideration. Reconstructing the condyle with the vessels oriented distally along the neomandible allows the pedicle to exit anteriorly to the contralateral neck or with a gentle 180-degree turn back to the ipsilateral side. Alternatively, reconstructing the condyle with the pedicle oriented proximally generally requires a somewhat acute turn in the pedicle and removal of some of the vascular supply to the most superior extent of the proximal fibula with an anticipated small segment of free graft fibula (Fig. 128.3).

Reconstruction of the Mandible With Anticipated Placement of Implants

The width of the fibula is adequate for placement of endosseous implants but certainly does not match a removed dentate mandible. Fibulas placed at the inferior border can be successfully reconstructed with implants using standard prosthodontics, which obviates the need for alternative reconstructive techniques. Additionally, a number of technical modifications have been proposed to optimize the vertical implant position, each with some limitations. Placement of the fibula superior to the inferior border offers a more optimal implant position but poor facial esthetics. This can be mitigated with placement of the reconstruction plate along the inferior border of the mandible and fixation of the fibula bone superiorly with miniplates. Some have advocated a midway position so as to not overly compromise facial esthetics while utilizing this approach. In cases where free grafting is feasible, additional segments of free grafted fibula may be utilized in the inferior border for facial form. As an alternative where free grafting is not advised, the double-barreled fibula has been proposed where a segment of bone is removed such that the vascular pedicle and remaining bone can make a 180-degree turn for vascularized fibular bone-to-bone contact with fixation. The limitation of this technique is the increased technical demands and increased failure rate given the necessary pedicle position. Finally, some have advocated the use of vertical distraction osteogenesis of the fibula segment to increase the vertical height following placement at the inferior border.[40]

Maxillary Reconstruction

Maxillary reconstruction with the fibula flap is the preferred technique for many surgeons, yet replacement of three-dimensional form and function of both the infrastructure and superstructure of the maxilla presents a significant challenge for the reconstructive surgeon. A number of modified techniques have been described utilizing the fibula to address this challenge, which mirror those utilized in the mandible. The use of free graft segments and double/triple barrel techniques has each been described. The final prosthetic plan is crucial in decision making given that optimal bone placement for endosseous implants becomes a driving force when this is the final reconstructive plan. Computer-guided modeling may be of significant benefit in complex cases to simulate the final desired position of the vascularized fibula. Where a skin paddle is expected to close an oral defect, care must be taken to protect the vascular pedicle, given possible exposure through the superior surface to the residual maxillary sinus and nasal cavity. To address this issue, some have advocated the use of a second fascial free flap for nasal closure. In the author's experience, a generous cuff of fascia for vessel protection as well as positioning the vessels laterally toward the cheek offers adequate coverage of vessels during the postoperative healing period.

Avoidance and Management of Intraoperative Complications

Intraoperative complications may occur during osteotomies and inset of the fibula flap. The pedicle can be injured during fibula osteotomies; to prevent this occurrence, a subperiosteal dissection and protection of the pedicle with a #9 elevator are essential. Additionally, monocortical screws are recommended to protect the vascular pedicle. Poor periosteal blood supply to the fibular segments can be avoided by ensuring that there is a generous 3-mm cuff of muscle around the periosteum and by having adequate fibular segment lengths (Fig. 128.4). Intraoperative loss of the skin paddle can occur if the delicate perforators are injured.

With virtual planning, osteotomies can be planned with precision using prefabricated cutting guides and a

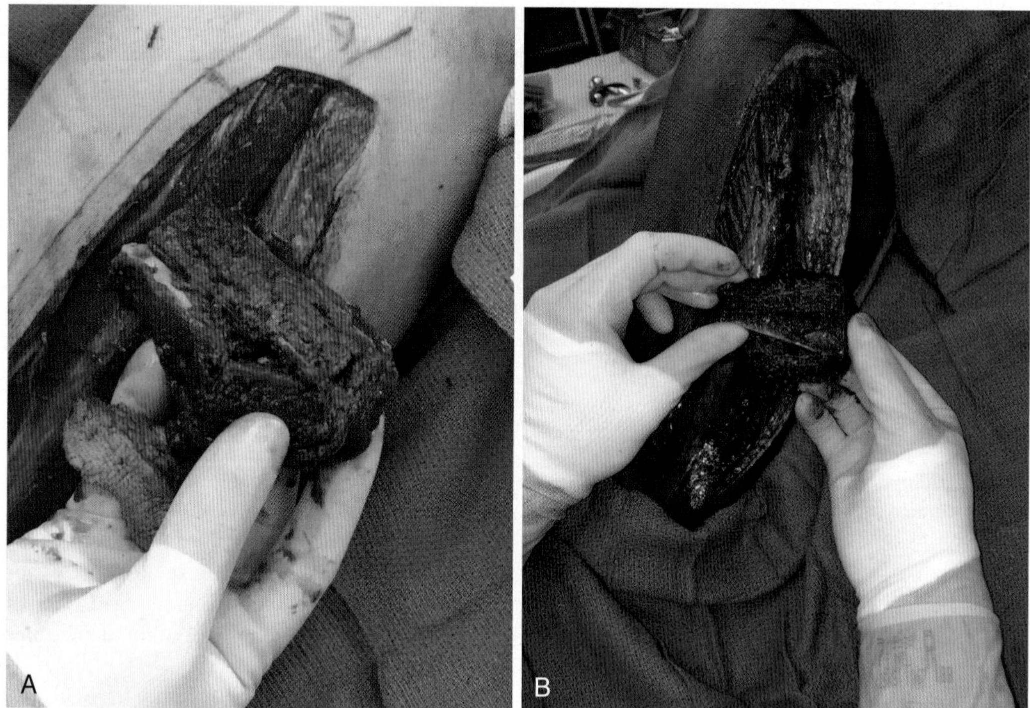

Figure 128.4 **A,** Double barrel two-piece fibula with angled inferior edge to better contour the inferior border. **B,** Double barrel four-piece fibula, note shortened vascular pedicle.

prefabricated plate that fits perfectly. However, osteotomies are still difficult, with soft tissue and protection of the pedicle obscuring vision. Do not hesitate to change saw blades if there is difficulty cutting or stop and reposition as needed. Do not take the cutting guide off after completion of only a portion of the osteotomy, as the guide may be placed back into the incorrect position, eliminating the precision the guides provide. Sterile tongue blades or foam cutting blocks can be used as templates to make closing wedge osteotomies when virtual planning has not been utilized.

Posterior open bite may result after condylar disarticulation due to condylar sag after reconstruction using a fibular segment. This can be prevented by a short 1- to 2-week course of intermaxillary fixation. Suspension of the condyle can be completed using suture suspension to the temporal bone or the temporalis fascia to assist in the prevention of condylar sag; however, this technique may result in mild lateral displacement of the neocondyle.

The pedicle may also be in danger of kinking due to unfavorable geometry in relation to the takeoff from the anterior or posterior fibula and the location of the recipient vessels. If the pedicle comes off the fibula to the ipsilateral neck too anteriorly, the pedicle may be required to be released from the fibula a few centimeters to prevent kinking of the vessels. After anastomosis is completed, the patient's head should be rotated to the left and right to observe pedicle orientation. If there is any kinking or unfavorable compression of the vessels, the pedicle may need to be redraped across the neck, and tacking sutures may need to be applied.

Postoperative Considerations

Postoperative monitoring of the fibula free flap involves physical examination as well as the use of adjunctive methods such as the external Doppler, implantable Doppler, and tissue oximetry. Physical examination changes may at times be subtle with minimal physical signs of pending flap failure. Capillary refill, temperature, turgor, and color are monitored every hour for the first 48 hours. Two obvious late findings include a pale flap, which is suffering from arterial thrombosis, and a blue flap, which indicates venous congestion secondary to a venous thrombosis or compression of the pedicle due to anatomy or hematoma.

The external pen Doppler is commonly used to evaluate the vascular pedicle and the skin perforators, but the clinician may inadvertently pick up adjacent vessels, and the venous signal may be difficult to find. The implantable Doppler is a 20-MHz ultrasound probe mounted on a silicone cuff that can be placed around an arterial or venous pedicle, which is then plugged into a portable monitor.[41] Bui and colleagues reviewed 1193 cases and found that venous thrombosis (which occurred in 74% of the cases) was more common than arterial thrombosis (which occurred in 40%)[42]; therefore the internal Doppler should be placed on the vein distal to the anastomosis. However, the external and internal Doppler share a common problem in that it is difficult to define what signal quality changes necessitate exploration.

Tissue oximetry with a near-infrared monitor uses an emission of near-infrared light to measure local tissue oxygen saturation with a probe that is either taped to the external skin paddle or sutured to the intraoral skin paddle. Lin and colleagues were able to increase their flap salvage rate from 57.7% to 93.75%, which they attributed to the earlier detection and earlier intervention before significant thrombosis occurred.[43,44]

Lohman and colleagues found that physical changes in the flap lagged behind the adjunctive methods of flap monitoring, ranging from 30 to 60 minutes. Their conclusion was that if veteran personnel were not available, physical examination is insufficient for flap monitoring.[44]

Flap monitoring of the buried flap presents additional challenges given that no visual cues are present. A higher reliance on internal or external Doppler is key in these cases. Recognizing the limitations of these adjunctive devices is critical so as to appropriately explore flaps that may be compromised.

Several reports describe interruption of the vascular pedicle in free flaps as early as 6 days with survival of the flap. Burns and colleagues described three radial forearm free flaps surviving after interruption of either the venous drainage or the arterial connection at 6 to 19 days.[45] Godden and Thomas reported the survival of a radial forearm free flap after loss of venous and arterial flow at 9 days.[46] These cases describe thin radial forearm flaps but may not be indicative of when the fibula osteocutaneous flap becomes independent in its own blood supply. Mücke and colleagues, in a prospective clinical study, evaluated the hemoglobin oxygenation and capillary flow in 50 free flaps, of which 15 were osteocutaneous fibula free flaps, during occlusion of the vascular pedicle after 4 weeks and 3 months. They found that flap autonomization rates were higher in the mandible and nonirradiated sites, with fasciocutaneous flaps to be autonomized faster than osseomyocutaneous flaps. On the other hand, myocutaneous flaps were never autonomized after 4 weeks. Approximately 40% of the osseomyocutaneous flaps were autonomized at 4 weeks.[47]

Because the fibula free flap has become the workhorse flap for mandibular reconstruction as well as extremity reconstruction, several groups have looked at the morbidity and function of the donor site after harvest of this flap.[48,49]

As described by Gilbert in 1979, the lateral approach to the fibula is now standard, creating an incision approximately 6 cm distal to the head of the fibula to just 6 cm proximal to the lateral malleolus. A skin graft is commonly placed if the wound cannot be closed primarily, usually if the skin paddle is greater than 4 cm wide.[11,16] In 2011, Momoh and colleagues evaluated 157 consecutive patients who underwent fibula free flap reconstruction for head and neck defects and found that the overall perioperative complications after fibula harvest totaled 31%, including partial skin graft loss, total skin graft loss, cellulitis, wound dehiscence, and abscess, but only 3% of these patients required operative intervention. They noted that 33% of their skin-grafted patients had complications versus 29% of their patients who had primary closure. This group also evaluated the timing of ambulation following harvest of the fibula and found that there was no significant association between the timing of ambulation postsurgery and the incidence of complications.[50]

Ling and colleagues performed a systematic search of the English and Chinese literature from 1966 to 2011, retrieving 42 relevant articles. They separated the postoperative complications into early donor site morbidity and late donor site morbidity. The weighted mean incidence of early donor site morbidity was wound infection, 1.07%; wound dehiscence, 7%; partial skin graft loss, 8.1%; and total skin graft loss, 4.7%. Where wounds were closed primarily, the complication rate was 9.9% versus those closed with skin graft at 19%. The weighted mean incidence of late donor site morbidity was chronic pain, 6.5%; considerable gait abnormality, 3.9%; ankle instability, 5.8%; limited range of motion in the ankle, 11.5%; reduced muscle strength, 4.0%; claw toe, 6.1%; dorsiflexion of the great toe, 3.6%; and sensory deficit, 6.95%.[51]

Lin and coworkers described, in 2009, the donor site morbidity of bilateral fibula free flap transfer in seven patients, where the second fibula was used due to previous fibula flap failure, development of osteoradionecrosis after postoperative radiation, or in one patient with an extensive mandibular defect, the need for an additional bone segment to match the length of the defect. The patients were evaluated using a subjective questionnaire and an objective balance and gait test, and the researchers found that the long-term functional deficits were minimal and evident only when subjected to unfavorable sensory feedback conditions.[52]

Compartment syndrome is rare and there are only a handful of reports in the literature.[54–57] These cases of compartment syndrome were discovered several days or weeks after surgery in a delayed fashion, due to masking of symptoms by narcotics, expected postoperative pain, and splint or cast in place preventing complete examination. Compartment syndrome occurs within a closed anatomic space, when the tissue perfusion pressure is lower than tissue pressure, leading to hypoperfusion resulting in tissue necrosis. This can be the result of externally applied compressive forces or internally expanding structures such as a hematoma.[57,58]

Clinical assessment is the examination of choice for compartment syndrome. The signs are pain disproportionate to the severity of injury, increase in pain on passive stretch, progressive paresthesia, paralysis, and loss of pulses. Diagnosis is difficult, especially for head and neck cancer patients who may have difficulty communicating and giving a clear history, or participating in a complete examination. Pressure measurements can be taken using the needle manometer, wick catheter, slit catheter, or the Stryker intracompartmental pressure monitor system.[60–63] Biomarkers can also be evaluated for compartment syndrome. In a study by Valdez and colleagues, the researchers identified 39 out of 97 patients with compartment syndrome. Using the model of creatinine kinase greater than 4000 U/L, chloride level greater than 104 mg/dL, and blood urea nitrogen level less than 10 mg/dL, 0 of 6 patients had compartment syndrome when all three variables were absent; however, when one, two, or three variables were present, the percentage of patients with compartment syndrome was 36%, 80%, and 100%, respectively.[63] Ulmer assessed, through an English literature search from 1966 to 2001, whether the diagnosis of compartment syndrome could be based on clinical findings. Using the clinical findings of pain, paresthesia, pain on passive stretching, and paresis, Ulmer described the odds of compartment syndrome in relation to the number of clinical findings present. With the presence of one clinical finding, the odds were 25%; with the presence of two clinical findings (pain, pain on passive flexion), 68%; with the presence of three clinical findings (pain, pain on passive flexion, paresthesia), 93%; and with the presence of four clinical findings, there was a 98% chance that the patient would have a diagnosis of compartment syndrome.[64]

Most patients begin weight-bearing ambulation with an Aircast boot (which is easier to examine the leg for wound complications) or cast on postoperative day 1 or 2 and maintain this boot for approximately 4 weeks. If a skin graft is placed, the bolster dressing is taken down after 5 to 7 days and redressed with a nonadherent petroleum-based gauze. To avoid complications, care should be taken to prevent shearing of the skin graft by keeping the foot in a 90-degree position, which also assists in preventing contracture of the toes and claw deformity. Adequate drainage of the wound with a Jackson-Pratt drain and dressing the wound gently with care to avoid compression of the lower leg. A wound vacuum-assisted closure (VAC) device can also be applied to the skin graft in place of a bolster dressing and taken down at 5 to 7 days with Mepitel or Adaptic gauze placed in between the VAC sponge and skin graft. If the skin graft does not appear to have taken completely, the VAC may be reapplied for another 5 to 7 days. During this time, the patient's foot should be immobilized in a neutral position with an Aircast boot or cast when ambulating and a L'nard Multi-Podus boot while in bed to prevent shearing of the skin graft. If no skin graft is placed, the dressing is taken down on postoperative day 2 to evaluate the lower extremity clearly. The Jackson-Pratt drain is removed once the drainage is less than 30 cc in a 24-hour period for 2 consecutive days.

References

1. Bakamjian VY. A two stage method for pharyngoesophageal reconstruction with a primary pectoral skin flap. *Plast Reconstr Surg.* 1965;36:173–184.
2. Ariyan S. The pectoralis major myocutaneous flap. A versatile flap for reconstruction in the head and neck. *Plast Reconstr Surg.* 1979;63(1):73–81.
3. Strauch B, Bloomberg AE, Lewin ML. An experimental approach to mandibular replacement: island vascular composite rib grafts. *Br J Plast Surg.* 1971;24(4):334–341.
4. Östrup LT, Fredrickson JM. Distant transfer of a free, living bone graft by microvascular anastomoses. An experimental study. *Plast Reconstr Surg.* 1974;54(3):274–285.
5. Taylor GI, Daniel RK. The free flap: composite tissue transfer by vascular anastomosis. *Aust N Z J Surg.* 1973;43(1):1–3.
6. Daniel RK, Taylor GI. Distant transfer of an island flap by microvascular anastomoses. A clinical technique. *Plast Reconstr Surg.* 1973;52(2):111–117.
7. Taylor GI, Miller GD, Ham FJ. The free vascularized bone graft. A clinical extension of microvascular techniques. *Plast Reconstr Surg.* 1975;55(5):533–544.
8. Buncke HJ, Furnas DW, Gordon L, Achauer BM. Free osteocutaneous flap from a rib to the tibia. *Plast Reconstr Surg.* 1977;59(6):799–804.
9. Serafin D, Villarreal-Rios A, Georgiade NG. A rib-containing free flap to reconstruct mandibular defects. *Br J Plast Surg.* 1977;30(4):263–266.
10. Chen ZW, Yan W. The study and clinical application of the osteocutaneous flap of fibula. *Microsurgery.* 1983;4(1):11–16.
11. Gilbert A. Surgical technique: vascularized transfer of the fibular shaft. *Int J Microsurg.* 1979;1:100.
12. Hidalgo DA. Fibula free flap: a new method of mandible reconstruction. *Plast Reconstr Surg.* 1989;84(1):71–79.
13. Wei FC, Chen HC, Chuang CC, Noordhoff MS. Fibular osteoseptocutaneous flap: anatomic study and clinical application. *Plast Reconstr Surg.* 1986;78(2):191–200.
14. Iorio ML, Cheerharan M, Olding M. A systematic review and pooled analysis of peroneal artery perforators for fibula osteocutaneous and perforator flaps. *Plast Reconstr Surg.* 2012;130(3):600–607.
15. Yu P, Chang EI, Hanasono MM. Design of a reliable skin paddle for the fibula osteocutaneous flap: perforator anatomy revisited. *Plast Reconstr Surg.* 2011;128(2):440–446.
16. Wei FL, Mardini S. *Flaps and Reconstructive Surgery.* Saunders Elsevier; 2009:443–445.
17. Wallace CG, Chang YM, Tsai CY, Wei FC. Harnessing the potential of the free fibula osteoseptocutaneous flap in mandible reconstruction. *Plast Reconstr Surg.* 2010;125(1):305–314.
18. Wei FC, Seah CS, Tsai YC, Liu SJ, Tsai MS. Fibula osteoseptocutaneous flap for reconstruction of composite mandibular defects. *Plast Reconstr Surg.* 1994;93(2):294–304.
19. Urken ML, Buchbinder D, Costantino PD, et al. Oromandibular reconstruction using microvascular composite flaps: report of 210 cases. *Arch Otolaryngol Head Neck Surg.* 1998;124(1):46–55.
20. Hidalgo DA, Pusic AL. Free-flap mandibular reconstruction: a 10-year follow-up study. *Plast Reconstr Surg.* 2002;110(2):438–449.
21. Carlson ER, Marx RE. Part II. Mandibular reconstruction using cancellous cellular bone grafts. *J Oral Maxillofac Surg.* 1996;54(7):889–897.
22. Adamo AK, Szal RL. Timing, results, and complications of mandibular reconstructive surgery: report of 32 cases. *J Oral Surg.* 1979;37(10):755–763.
23. Foster RD, Anthony JP, Sharma A, Pogrel MA. Vascularized bone flaps versus nonvascularized bone grafts for mandibular reconstruction: an outcome analysis of primary bony union and endosseous implant success. *Head Neck.* 1999;21(1):66–71.
24. Moscoso JF, Keller J, Genden E, et al. Vascularized bone flaps in oromandibular reconstruction. A comparative anatomic study of bone stock from various donor sites to assess suitability for enosseous dental implants. *Arch Otolaryngol Head Neck Surg.* 1994;120(1):36–43.
25. Frodel JL Jr, Funk GF, Capper DT, et al. Osseointegrated implants: a comparative study of bone thickness in four vascularized bone flaps. *Plast Reconstr Surg.* 1993;92(3):449–455.
26. Chim H, Salgado CJ, Mardini S, Chen HC. Reconstruction of mandibular defects. *Semin Plast Surg.* 2010;24(2):188–197.
27. Fernandes R. Fibula free flap in mandibular reconstruction. *Atlas Oral Maxillofac Surg Clin North Am.* 2006;14(2):143–150.
28. Yim KK, Wei FC. Fibula osteoseptocutaneous flap for mandible reconstruction. *Microsurgery.* 1994;15(4):245–249.
29. Wong CH, Wei FC. Microsurgical free flap in head and neck reconstruction. *Head Neck.* 2010;32(9):1236–1245.

30. Wei FL, Mardini S. General principles and analysis of defects in head and neck reconstructions. *Semin Plast Surg*. 2003.
31. Sun GH, Patil YJ, Harmych BM, Hom DB. Inpatients with gunshot wounds to the face. *J Craniofac Surg*. 2012;23(1):e62–e65.
32. Kademani D, Keller E. Iliac crest grafting for mandibular reconstruction. *Atlas Oral Maxillofac Surg Clin North Am*. 2006;14(2):161–170.
33. Jewer DD, Boyd JB, Manktelow RT, et al. Orofacial and mandibular reconstruction with the iliac crest free flap: a review of 60 cases and a new method of classification. *Plast Reconstr Surg*. 1989;84(3):391–403.
34. Ahmad N, Kordestani R, Panchal J, Lyles J. The role of donor site angiography before mandibular reconstruction utilizing free flap. *J Reconstr Microsurg*. 2007;23(4):199–204.
35. Kelly AM, Cronin P, Hussain HK, Londy FJ, Chepeha DB, Carlos RC. Preoperative MR angiography in free fibula flap transfer for head and neck cancer: clinical application and influence on surgical decision making. *AJR Am J Roentgenol*. 2007;188(1):268–274.
36. Urken ML, Cheney ML, Blackwell KE, et al. *Atlas of Regional and Free Flaps for Head and Neck Reconstruction*. 2nd ed. Lippincott Willaims & Wilkins; 2011:412.
37. Kim D, Orron DE, Skillman JJ. Surgical significance of popliteal arterial variants. A unified angiographic classification. *Ann Surg*. 1989;210(6):776–781.
38. Rozen WM, Ashton MW, Stella DL, Phillips TJ, Taylor GI. Magnetic resonance angiography and computed tomographic angiography for free fibular flap transfer. *J Reconstr Microsurg*. 2008;24(6):457–458.
39. Sassu P, Acland RD, Salgado CJ, Mardini S, Ozyurekoglu T. Anatomy and vascularization of the flexor hallucis longus muscle and its implication in free fibula flap transfer: an anatomical study. *Ann Plast Surg*. 2010;64(2):233–237.
40. Wong CH, Wei FC. Microsurgical free flap in head and neck reconstruction. *Head Neck*. 2010;32(9):1236–1245.
41. Poder TG, Fortier PH. Implantable Doppler in monitoring free flaps: a cost-effectiveness analysis based on a systematic review of the literature. *Eur Ann Otorhinolaryngol Head Neck Dis*. 2013;130(2):79–85.
42. Bui DT, Cordeiro PG, Hu QY, Disa JJ, Pusic A, Mehrara BJ. Free flap reexploration: indications, treatment, and outcomes in 1193 free flaps. *Plast Reconstr Surg*. 2007;119(7):2092–2100.
43. Lin SJ, Nguyen MD, Chen C, et al. Tissue oximetry monitoring in microsurgical breast reconstruction decreases flap loss and improves rate of flap salvage. *Plast Reconstr Surg*. 2011;127(3):1080–1085.
44. Lohman RF, Langevin CJ, Bozkurt M, Kundu N, Djohan R. A prospective analysis of free flap monitoring techniques: physical examination, external Doppler, implantable Doppler, and tissue oximetry. *J Reconstr Microsurg*. 2013;29(1):51–56.
45. Burns A, Avery BS, Edge CJ. Survival of microvascular free flaps in head and neck surgery after early interruption of the vascular pedicle. *Br J Oral Maxillofac Surg*. 2005;43(5):426–427.
46. Godden DR, Thomas SJ. Survival of a free flap after vascular disconnection at 9 days. *Br J Oral Maxillofac Surg*. 2002;40(5):446–447.
47. Mücke T, Wolff KD, Rau A, Kehl V, Mitchell DA, Steiner T. Autonomization of free flaps in the oral cavity: a prospective clinical study. *Microsurgery*. 2012;32(3):201–206.
48. Shpitzer T, Neligan P, Boyd B, Gullane P, Gur E, Freeman J. Leg morbidity and function following fibular free flap harvest. *Ann Plast Surg*. 1997;38(5):460–464.
49. Shindo M, Fong BP, Funk GF, Karnell LH. The fibula osteocutaneous flap in head and neck reconstruction: a critical evaluation of donor site morbidity. *Arch Otolaryngol Head Neck Surg*. 2000;126(12):1467–1472.
50. Momoh AO, Yu P, Skoracki RJ, Liu S, Feng L, Hanasono MM. A prospective cohort study of fibula free flap donor-site morbidity in 157 consecutive patients. *Plast Reconstr Surg*. 2011;128(3):714–720.
51. Ling XF, Peng X. What is the price to pay for a free fibula flap? A systematic review of donor-site morbidity following free fibula flap surgery. *Plast Reconstr Surg*. 2012;129(3):657–674.
52. Lin JY, Djohan R, Dobryansky M, et al. Assessment of donor-site morbidity using balance and gait tests after bilateral fibula osteoseptocutaneous free flap transfer. *Ann Plast Surg*. 2009;62(3):246–251.
53. Berzofsky C, Shin E, Mashkevich G. Leg compartment syndrome after fibula free flap. *Otolaryngol Head Neck Surg*. 2013;148(1):172–173.
54. Fodor L, Dinu C, Fodor M, Ciuce C. Severe compartment syndrome following fibula harvesting for mandible reconstruction. *Int J Oral Maxillofac Implants*. 2011;40(4):443–445.
55. Kerrary S, Schouman T, Cox A, Bertolus C, Febrer G, Bertrand JC. Acute compartment syndrome following fibula flap harvest for mandibular reconstruction. *J Craniomaxillofac Surg*. 2011;39(3):206–208.
56. Sun G, Yang X, Wen J, Wang A, Hu Q, Tang E. Treatment of compartment syndrome in donor site of free fibula flap after mandibular reconstruction surgery. *Oral Surg Oral Med Oral Pathol Oral Radiol Endod*. 2009;108(5):e15–e18.
57. Mabee JR, Bostwick TL. Pathophysiology and mechanisms of compartment syndrome. *Orthop Rev*. 1993;22(2):175–181.
58. Matsen FA III, Winquist RA, Krugmire RB Jr. Diagnosis and management of compartmental syndromes. *J Bone Joint Surg Am*. 1980;62(2):286–291.
59. Rorabeck CH, Castle GS, Hardie R, Logan J. Compartmental pressure measurements: an experimental investigation using the slit catheter. *J Trauma*. 1981;21(6):446–449.
60. Mubarak SJ, Hargens AR, Owen CA, Garetto LP, Akeson WH. The wick catheter technique for measurement of intramuscular pressure. A new research and clinical tool. *J Bone Joint Surg Am*. 1976;58(7):1016–1020.
61. Boody AR, Wongworawat MD. Accuracy in the measurement of compartment pressures: a comparison of three commonly used devices. *J Bone Joint Surg Am*. 2005;87(11):2415–2422.
62. Hammerberg EM, Whitesides TE Jr, Seiler JG III. The reliability of measurement of tissue pressure in compartment syndrome. *J Orthop Trauma*. 2012;26(1):24–31.
63. Valdez C, Schroeder E, Amdur R, Pascual J, Sarani B. Serum creatine kinase levels are associated with extremity compartment syndrome. *J Trauma Acute Care Surg*. 2013;74(2):441–445.
64. Ulmer T. The clinical diagnosis of compartment syndrome of the lower leg: are clinical findings predictive of the disorder? *J Orthop Trauma*. 2002;16(8):572–577.

CHAPTER 129

Scapular Free Flap

Marina Morante Silva and Rui P. Fernandes

Armamentarium

Flap Harvest
#9 Periosteal elevator
Appropriate sutures
Army/Navy retractors
Colorado-tip monopolar electrocautery
DeBakey forceps
Fine-tipped bipolar electrocautery
Local anesthetic with vasoconstrictor
Reciprocating saw (for bone flap harvest)
Richardson retractors
Senn retractors
Skin hooks
Straight osteotomes
Tonsil clamps
Microvascular Instruments
Appropriate sutures
Coupler instrument
Heparinized saline
Jeweler's forceps ×3
Microneedle holders
Microscissors
Papaverine
Single and double microvascular clamps
Venous coupler
Vessel dilators
Donor Site Closure
19-French Jackson-Pratt suction drain
Appropriate sutures
Flap Insetting
Appropriate sutures
Bone plating system

History of the Procedure

First described by dos Santos in 1980,[1] the scapular flap, along with the subscapular artery system upon which it is based, is recognized as the most dynamic donor region available for free tissue transfer to the head and neck.[2] The subscapular artery system gives rise to a variety of flaps: fasciocutaneous (scapular/parascapular/thoracodorsal artery perforator), osteofasciocutaneous (scapular/parascapular with lateral scapular border or tip), musculocutaneous (latissimus dorsi/serratus anterior), and musculo-osteocutaneous (latissimus dorsi/serratus anterior + rib). Vascularized bone, muscle, fat, skin, and fascia may be transferred as discrete components or combined as a chimeric flap on a single pedicle for composite reconstruction involving disparate axes.[3]

The first clinical application of the scapular free flap was reported by Gilbert and Teot in four cases of lower extremity reconstruction.[4] This was followed by a number of successful cases of fasciocutaneous transfer, citing a substantial improvement in postoperative morbidity compared with the latissimus dorsi myocutaneous flap.[5–7] These studies were possible following earlier dye injection cadaver studies by Saijo, which elucidated the angiosomes of the circumflex scapular, thoracodorsal, and posterior intercostal arteries. He predicted that a fasciocutaneous flap based on the circumflex scapular artery could supply up to 15 × 20 cm of thin, pliable skin supplied by a consistent pedicle of sufficient caliber for microvascular anastomosis.[8] Teot and coworkers first identified the potential for vascularized bone transfer in their report describing the pedicled lateral scapular border as part of an osteocutaneous flap.[9] Further anatomic studies outlined the neurovascular and musculoskeletal anatomy of the subscapular system, providing microsurgeons with parameters to optimize flap perfusion and bone volume.[1,10–13] Novel modifications soon followed and multiple combinations have been proposed in relation to the flaps of the subscapular system. Nassif described the vertically oriented parascapular flap as a fasciocutaneous flap based on a vertical branch of the circumflex scapular artery, with the potential to include a portion of latissimus dorsi muscle inferiorly.[14] Batchelor and Bardsley introduced a biscapular fasciocutaneous flap, anastomosing bilateral circumflex scapular arteries in the upper and lower leg for a 40-cm soft tissue defect.[15] Suitability of the superficial temporal artery for anastomosis to the circumflex scapular artery was initially reported in 1984 in several cases of scalp reconstruction.[16,17] In 1985 Koshima first discussed the possibility of combining a scapular and parascapular flap to reconstruct a leg defect.[18] More recently, in 2015, Shaw et al.[19] described the TDAP-Scap flap, which involved combining the scapular flap (utilizing the circumflex scapular artery) with the thoracodorsal artery perforator flap that Agrigiani described in 1995. Pau et al. modified this flap to a chimeric thoracodorsal perforator-scapular flap based on the angular artery (TDAP-Scap-aa) that has longer pedicle (up to 20 cm).[20]

Mandibular and maxillary reconstruction using scapular bone has been cited extensively with laudable results. Swartz and colleagues first employed lateral borders and lateral border/scapular tip bones for reconstruction in 26 cases of maxillectomy and composite mandibular defects.[21] The course of the angular artery and its periosteal perforators supplying the scapular tip was later described by Deraemaecker and colleagues,[22] leading to its popularization as a source of bone stock. Coleman and Sultan initially described using the scapular tip for mandibular and midface reconstruction as a bipedicled osteocutaneous flap, with a separate skin paddle based on the circumflex scapular artery.[23] The medial border may be harvested for improved pedicle length, but this bone is of poorer stock than the lateral border and must remain attached to the overlying skin.[24,25] Baker and Sullivan noted the advantage of separate pedicles for soft tissue and bone segments in their report on one-stage mandibular reconstruction. Large cutaneous or mucosal defects up to 12 × 10 cm with corresponding segmental bone gaps of up to 14.5 cm were restored simultaneously.[26] Suitability for dental implants was reported by Moscoso and colleagues in their study of 28 cadavers. Serial cross sections of the lateral border of the scapula showed greater implantability distal from the glenohumeral joint, where bone stock is thickest. Overall, 78% of harvested scapular bone segments were deemed fit for implant placement, defined as those with a neomandibular height of 10 mm and a width of 5 mm or more. This was significantly more consistent than the fibula free flap.[27] Likewise, the possibility of implants in the scapular tip flap has been evaluated.[28–31] In their study of scapular flaps, Lanzer et al. observed an increase in bone density after one year, which allows implant placement.[32] Numerous studies have upheld the importance of dental rehabilitation and mastication in functional outcomes,[28–33] along with labial competence, deglutition, facial cosmesis, and speech. Since its introduction, the scapular free flap has maintained its role as a readily harvested flap with negligible donor site morbidity and wide reconstructive applications.

Indications for the Use of the Procedure

Scapular and parascapular osteocutaneous flaps are probably the most versatile flaps, associated with acceptable donor site features, including the potential for primary closure without a skin graft, a well-hidden scar, and limited functional impairment. The circumflex scapular artery provides up to 4 cm of length, with a caliber of 2.5 to 4 mm before dividing into transverse and descending scapular branches, which supply the scapular and parascapular skin paddles, respectively.[34] In patients with peripheral vascular disease affecting the lower extremities and precluding the use of the fibular or deep circumflex iliac artery osteocutaneous flaps, the scapular system provides reliable vessels and good bone stock for reconstruction and is rarely affected by atherosclerosis,[35,36] making it a good alternative for elderly patients. Also, because of the possibility of a chimeric flap, it is the best option for complex defects avoiding the use of two free flaps.[37]

Head and Neck Reconstruction

Total Hard Palate Reconstruction

The scapular tip conforms well to defects resulting from subtotal or total maxillectomy without orbital exenteration.[2,38] Although not always amenable to dental implant rehabilitation, the scapular tip in horizontal orientation adapts well to hard palate defects, effectively separating the oral and nasal cavities. Mertens et al. described the possibility of implant rehabilitation in the scapular tip.[39] In their series of 46 patients, Brown and associates cited successful use of the scapular flap in head and neck reconstruction, including midfacial reconstruction with the latissimus dorsi–scapular tip.[40]

Mandible

Mandibular continuity defects may be reconstructed using a scapular tip for anterior defects[41] or a lateral or medial border for posterior defects. Boahene et al. have successfully applied the scapular tip to temporomandibular reconstruction as a novel condylar head replacement[41] (Fig. 129.1A–G).

Orbitomaxillary

In their 2007 retrospective review of 21 patients, Kosutic and associates evaluated latissimus dorsi–scapular free flap reconstruction of orbitomaxillary defects. They cited the necessity of using muscle and bone flaps, each with separate arcs of rotation, for restoring complex three-dimensional defects of the orbit and midface. Decreased flap morbidity was attributed to the use of a single anastomosis for multiple tissue types, as opposed to a combination of multiple flaps.[42]

Calvarian. In 2013 Hasan et al. described a series of five patients reconstructed with the angle of scapula combined with latissimus dorsi and long pedicle using the thoracodorsal vessels, with good results.[43]

Soft Tissue Contour Deformities

Buried, deepithelialized scapular or parascapular flaps or adipofascial flaps may be used for facial soft tissue augmentation. These flaps have been described extensively for the treatment of hemifacial microsomia and Romberg disease.[44] Tanna and colleagues compared inframammary extended scapular flaps with serial multistage fat grafting in hemifacial microsomia patients with similar orbit, mandible, ear, nerve, soft tissue (OMENS) system scores, noting similar postoperative symmetry scores between the two techniques.[45] The burn sequelae of the neck have also been described in Angrigiani et al.[46] Outside the head and neck, the subscapular artery system has long provided reliable tissue for axial and extremity reconstruction.[47,48] The free fasciocutaneous thoracodorsal artery perforator flap combined with the vascularized scapula has been reported successfully for covering traumatic Gustilo IIIb lower extremity wounds.[49] Pedicled reconstruction of the axilla, shoulder, back, and upper extremity has also been widely reported with unquestionable success.

Limitations and Contraindications

Potential donor site risks involved in the harvest of subscapular artery system flaps include shoulder dysfunction resulting from detachment of the teres major muscle. Brachial plexopathy has been noted as a complication from patient positioning. When harvesting bone, maintaining 1 cm of bone inferior to the glenoid fossa is recommended to avoid inadvertent entry into the joint capsule.[2] Axillary node dissection for breast malignancy and previous trauma to the donor site represent significant risks of vascular compromise and should be carefully evaluated prior to initiating flap harvest.

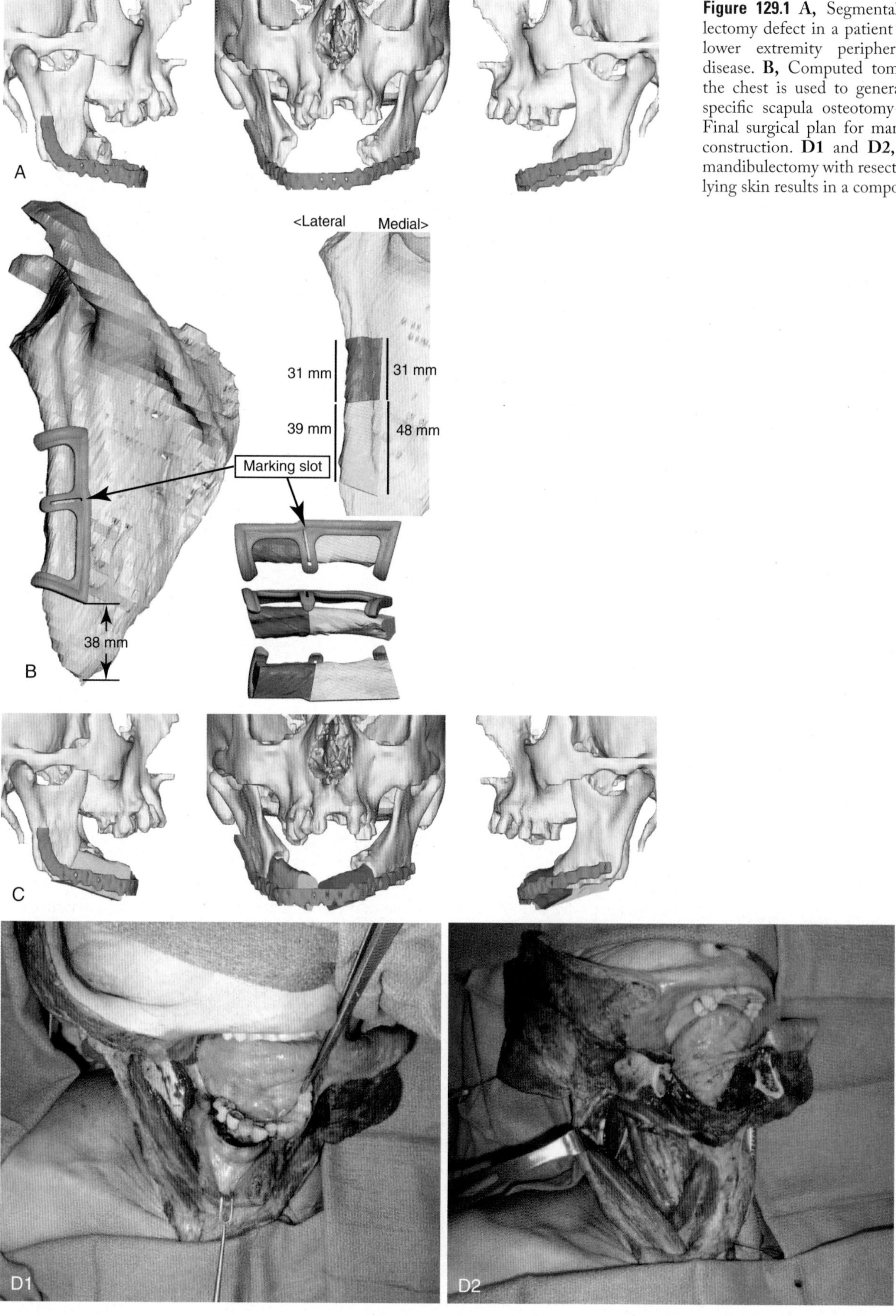

Figure 129.1 **A,** Segmental mandibulectomy defect in a patient with severe lower extremity peripheral vascular disease. **B,** Computed tomography of the chest is used to generate patient-specific scapula osteotomy guides. **C,** Final surgical plan for mandibular reconstruction. **D1** and **D2,** Segmental mandibulectomy with resection of overlying skin results in a composite defect.

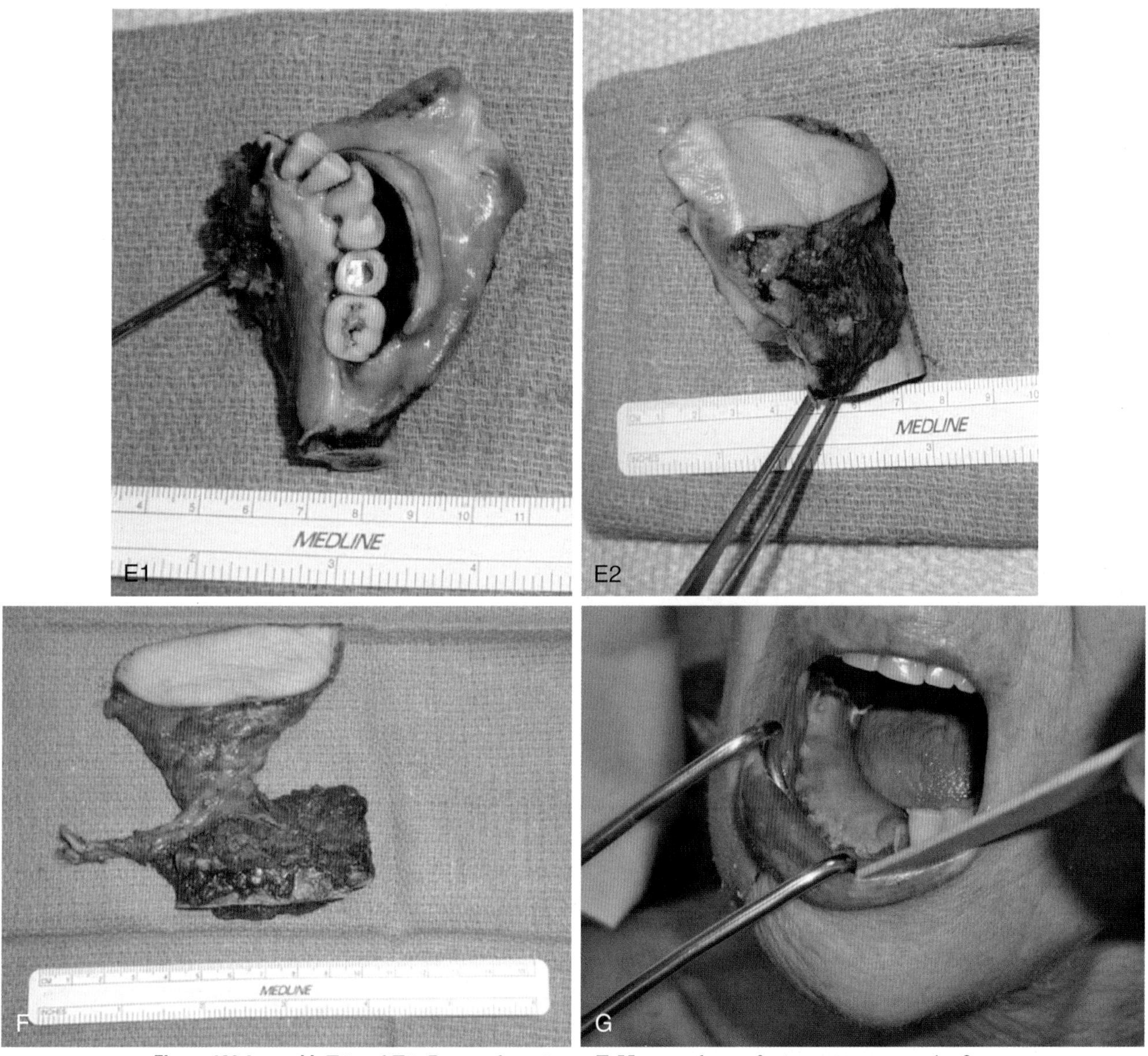

Figure 129.1, cont'd **E1** and **E2,** Resected specimen. **F,** Harvested osteofasciocutaneous scapular flap. **G,** Well-healed reconstructed composite defect. Lower lip defect was repaired primarily.

TECHNIQUE: Scapular Flap Harvest (Fig. 129.2A)

STEP 1: Positioning

When harvesting a scapular flap, patient positioning is determined by its intended use. If a resection is also being performed, a two-team approach should be employed. Thus, the lateral decubitus position is preferred because it allows the recipient site to be prepared simultaneously. If the flap is to be used in a pedicled fashion, having the arm prepped and in the field in lateral decubitus will allow for simulation of arc of rotation. Ultimately, it is the surgeon's preference in terms of positioning in lateral decubitus or prone. The prone position requires that the patient be turned supine after the harvest and closure of the donor site. This can also add operative time to the procedure (Fig. 129.2B).

STEP 2: Doppler and Anatomic Markings

Palpate and mark the tip, as well as the medial and lateral borders of the scapula. The triangular fossa is then identified; it is bounded superiorly by the teres minor, inferiorly by the teres major, and laterally by the long head of the triceps brachii muscle. This is where the circumflex scapular vessels emerge from the subscapular artery. The vessel location can be confirmed with Doppler at this time. The circumflex scapular artery divides into a descending branch, a transverse branch, and ascending branches as it courses through the triangular space (Fig. 129.2C).

Continued

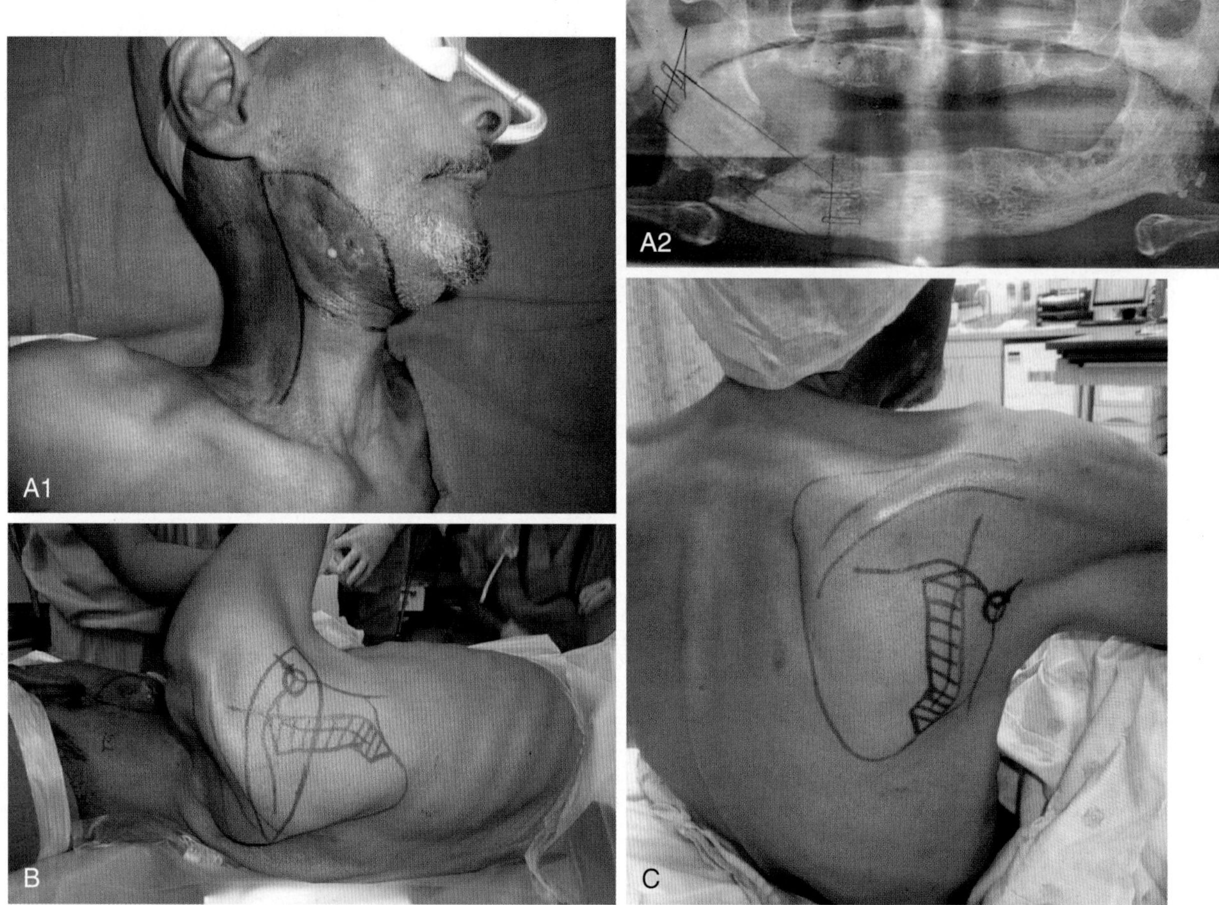

Figure 129.2 **A1** and **A2,** Osteoradionecrosis with planned segmental mandibulectomy. **B,** Left lateral decubitus position for flap harvest and recipient site preparation obviates the need for intraoperative repositioning. **C,** Landmarks for scapular free flap harvest.

TECHNIQUE: Scapular Flap Harvest—*cont'd*

STEP 3: Skin Paddle Design

Incorporation of the triangular space ensures vascularity of the skin paddle. The skin paddle is designed according to the soft tissue requirements of the defect. A horizontal design incorporating the transverse branch is termed a scapular flap, whereas a longitudinal design incorporating the descending branch is termed a parascapular flap. Two further designs may be superior: the first based on the ascending branch, and the second, inferior-lateral using the inframammary extended circumflex scapular artery (ascending branch of the descending artery), which is called the IMECC flap. A skin paddle width of about 10 cm or less can be closed primarily. Paddle lengths of up to 25 cm can be obtained without skin grafting. Skin paddle sizes as large as 25 × 35 cm can be obtained with skin grafting to the donor site. If bone is being harvested from either the medial or lateral scapula, it can be accessed through the existing skin incisions (Fig. 129.2D).

STEP 4: Skin Paddle Elevation and Vessel Identification

Two approaches to vessel identification can be used. In the first, the superior- and lateral-most incisions are made, and the dissection proceeds directly to the triangular space. The fascia overlying the teres major and deltoid muscles is removed to allow a safe dissection to the circumflex scapular artery and its venae comitantes. Once the vessels are isolated, dissection can quickly proceed medially. In the second method, the pedicle is approached from the medial position in a subfascial plane until the lateral edge of the scapula is approached; the fasciae overlying the teres muscles are included at this point until the pedicle is isolated. Branches to the teres muscles are divided, and the dissection proceeds to the subscapular system (Fig. 129.2E).

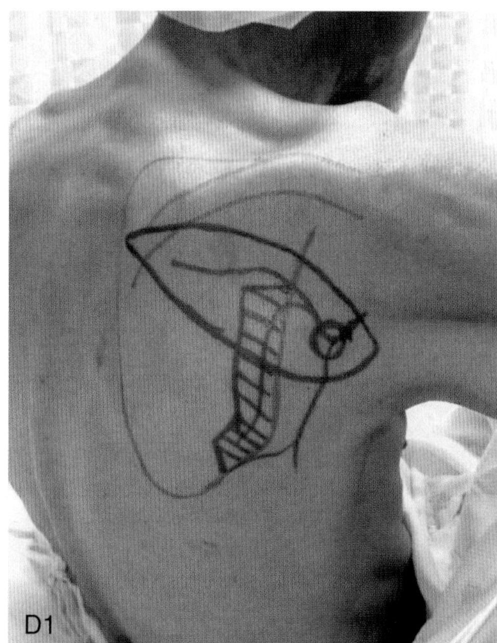

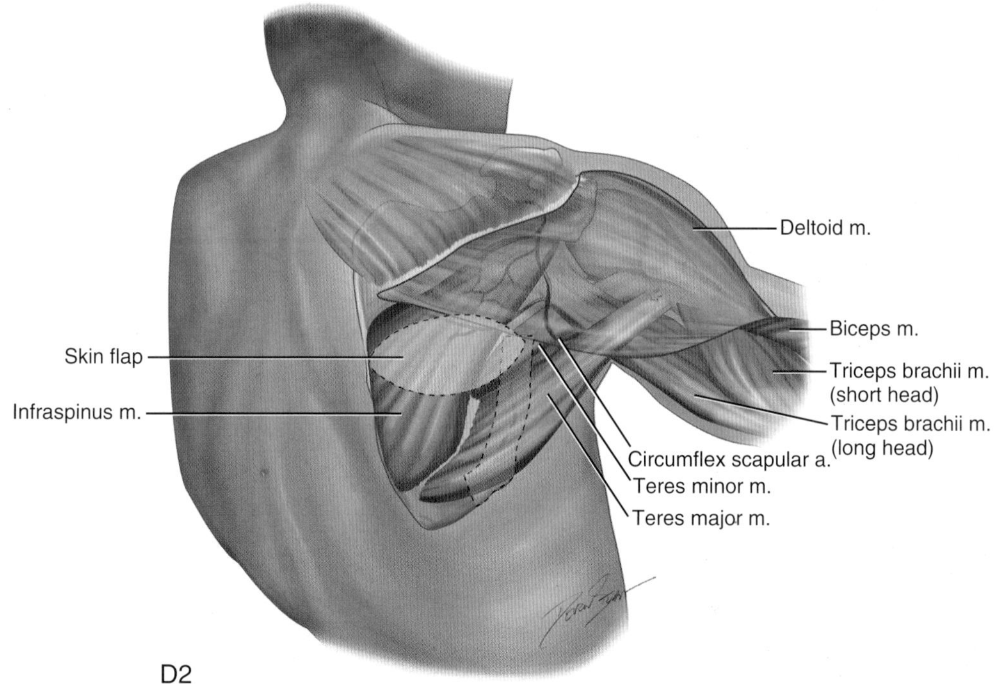

Figure 129.2, cont'd **D1** and **D2,** Transverse (scapular) skin paddle design centered over the triangular fossa.

TECHNIQUE: Scapular Flap Harvest—*cont'd*

STEP 5: Muscular Dissection and Osteotomy

When bone is required in addition to soft tissue, the lateral border of the scapula is favored over the medial border given its greater thickness (3 cm vs. 1.5 cm). A bone length of 10 to 14 cm can be harvested. The latissimus dorsi muscle is reflected to expose the muscle overlying the bone. The teres minor and major are directly incised, exposing the periosteum of the dorsal surface of the scapula. The osteotomies are performed once the periosteum has been incised and reflected. The attachment of the serratus muscle to the inferior angle of the scapula is maintained. Having completed the osteotomies, the surgeon can continue the dissection to the subscapular system. Of note, the inferior angle of the scapula should be preserved to ensure shoulder stability.

If the medial part of the scapula is to be harvested, the distal portion of the flap is left attached. A bone segment 2-cm thick and 10- to 12-cm long can be harvested. An incision is made through the infraspinatus muscle, exposing the periosteum on the dorsal surface of the scapula. The rhomboid major muscle is released from its medial attachment. The serratus and subscapularis muscles are also released from the anterior surface of the

Continued

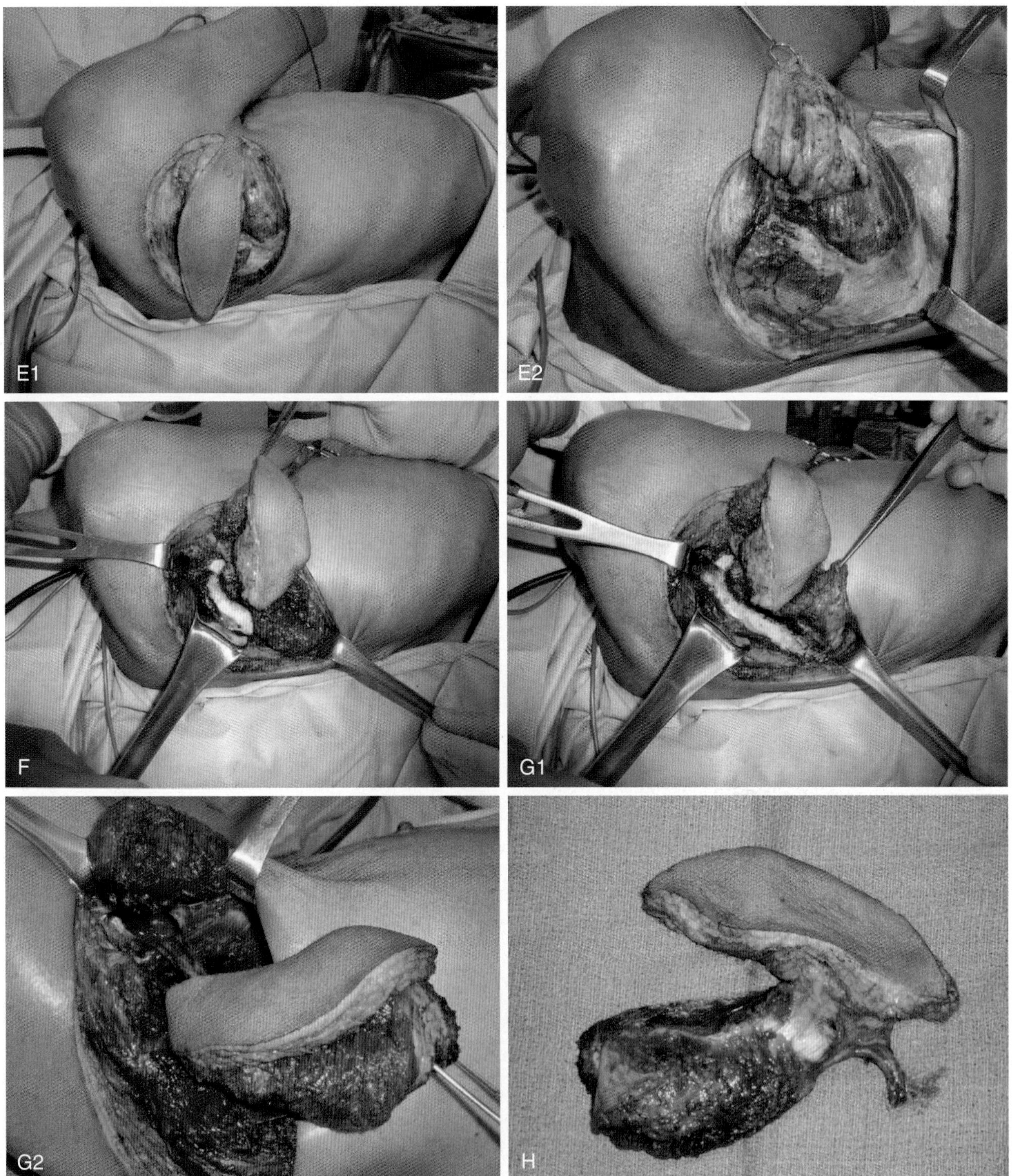

Figure 129.2, cont'd **E1,** Skin paddle elevation. **E2,** Elevation proceeds in a subfascial plane. **F,** Muscular dissection exposing the bone before osteotomy. **G1,** Complete exposure of the bone before osteotomy. **G2,** Completed osteotomy before pedicle division. **H,** Harvested flap before transfer.

TECHNIQUE: Scapular Flap Harvest—*cont'd*

osseous segment but must be reattached to the medial portion of the scapula. If the scapula tip is harvested, the teres major and the rhomboid muscles are released and the infraspinatus is elevated from the scapula. The pedicle is identified by retracting the latissimus dorsi inferiorly and lateral, so the angular artery is seen emerging from the thoracodorsal artery. After the osteotomy, the subscapularis muscle is divided. To have a longer pedicle, the direction of the thoracodorsal artery is performed[50] (Fig. 129.2F–H).

TECHNIQUE: Scapular Flap Harvest—*cont'd*

STEP 6: Closure

Primary closure should be the goal; however, if soft tissue flap widths greater than 10 cm are harvested, skin grafts may be needed. Significant undermining in a suprafascial layer is performed until tension-free closure can be achieved. The serratus, latissimus, and teres major muscles should be reinserted through drill holes or anchor sutures in the remaining scapula. Deep fascia should be closed with 2-0 Vicryl sutures. Deep subcutaneous layers should also be closed with 2-0 Vicryl sutures. The skin can be closed with 3-0 Prolene/nylon sutures. A suction drain should be placed because seroma formation can occur with early mobilization of the arm. The arm is placed in a shoulder immobilizer for 5 to 7 days. Physical therapy is initiated at that point (Fig. 129.2I–K).

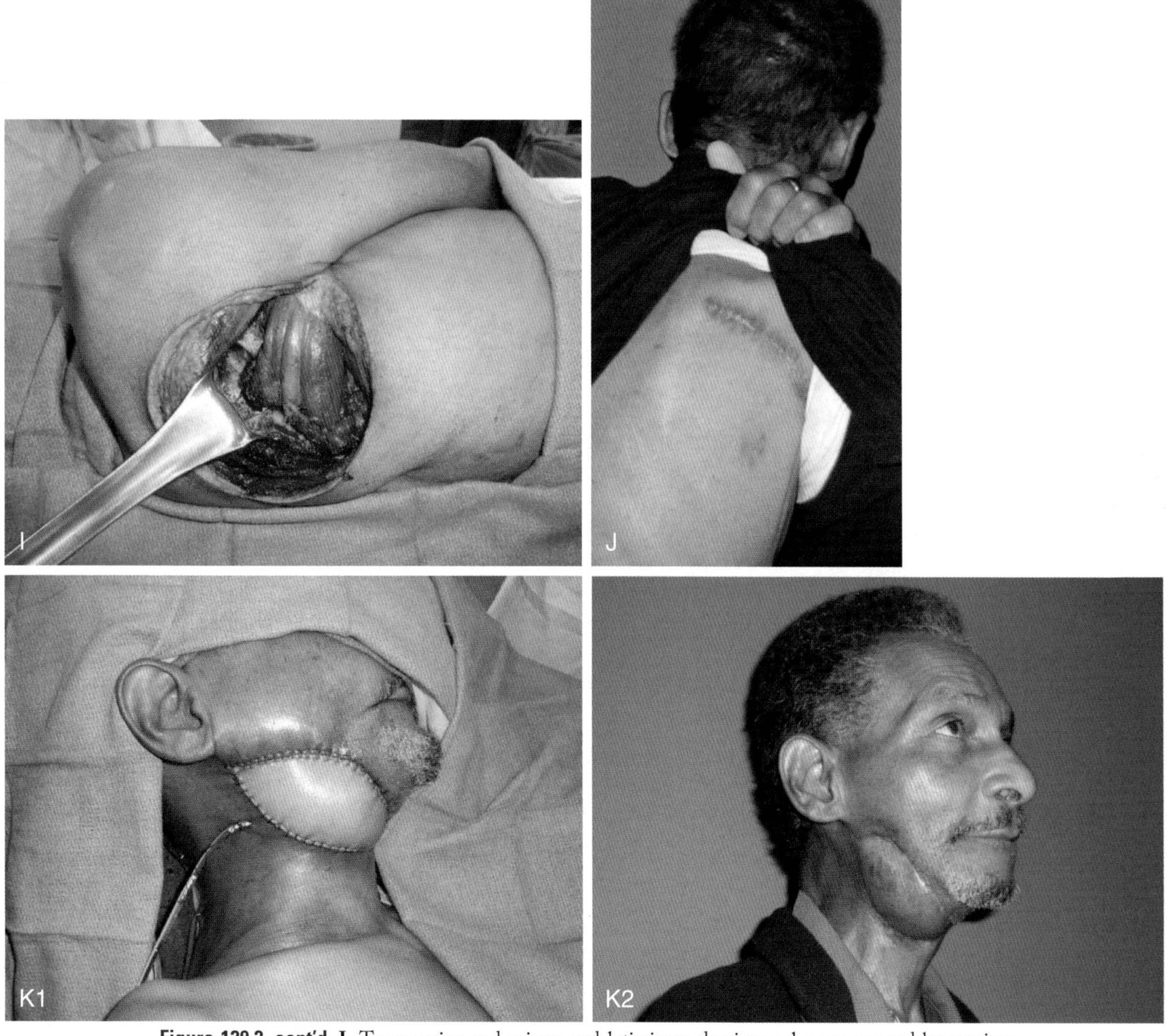

Figure 129.2, cont'd **I,** Teres major and minor and latissimus dorsi muscles are secured by passing heavy suture through holes drilled in the osteotomized scapular border. **J,** Healed donor site incision. **K1** and **K2,** Osteofasciocutaneous scapular free flap in situ.

Avoidance and Management of Intraoperative Complications

For secondary reconstructions or benign disease, where time allows, tissue expanders can be placed to preexpand the skin so as to avoid skin grafting to close the harvest site. Intraoperatively, care must be taken during dissection of the main pedicle, as numerous large caliber vessels must be ligated and nerves must be preserved. Potential injury to the long thoracic nerve can result in a "winged scapula" appearance. The two most common postoperative complications are excessive scar formation and shoulder weakness/stiffness. Patel et al. demonstrated that the range of motion is decreased in the operated arm compared with the contralateral arm, but there were no subjectives disabilities perceived by the patients.[51] In the immediate postoperative period, there will be significant limitations to shoulder movement, but with physical therapy initiated within the first week, patients can regain full function by 2 to 4 weeks. Excessive scar formation is secondary to wound separation as a result of early mobility. Patient counseling regarding the formation of a scar and the need for arm immobility for 5 to 7 days is critical.

Postoperative Considerations

The major concern following subscapular system free flap harvest is the development of an unesthetic scar, which is exacerbated by early, excessive arm movement. Otherwise, donor sites closed primarily demonstrate few postoperative complications. Chest radiograph abnormalities may occasionally present concerns to radiologists unfamiliar with this harvest site. In their review of 82 patients who underwent scapular bone harvest, 29 radiologists reviewed 884 postoperative chest radiographs. Only one radiologist correctly identified the scapular surgical defect, which is concerning because of the lack of awareness among radiologists regarding this increasingly utilized flap source.[52]

References

1. dos Santos LF. Retalho escapular: um novo retalho liver microcirurgico. *Rev Bras Cir.* 1980:70.
2. Urken M. Scapular and parascapular fasciocutaneous and osteofasciocutaneous and subscapular mega flap. In: *Regional and Free Flaps for Head and Neck Reconstruction.* Baltimore, Maryland: Lippincott Williams & Wilkins; 2012.
3. Fairbanks GA, Hallock GG. Facial reconstruction using a combined flap of the subscapular axis simultaneously including separate medial and lateral scapular vascularized bone grafts. *Ann Plast Surg.* 2002;49(1):104–108.
4. Gilbert A, Teot L. The free scapular flap. *Plast Reconstr Surg.* 1982;69(4):601–604.
5. Barwick WJ, Goodkind DJ, Serafin D. The free scapular flap. *Plast Reconstr Surg.* 1982;69(5):779–787.
6. Urbaniak JR, Koman LA, Goldner RD, Armstrong NB, Nunley JA. The vascularized cutaneous scapular flap. *Plast Reconstr Surg.* 1982;69(5):772–778.
7. Hamilton SG, Morrison WA. The scapular free flap. *Br J Plast Surg.* 1982;35(1):2–7.
8. Saijo M. The vascular territories of the dorsal trunk: a reappraisal for potential flap donor sites. *Br J Plast Surg.* 1978;31(3):200–204.
9. Teot L, Bosse JP, Moufarrege R, et al. The scapular crest pedicled bone graft. *Int J Microsurg.* 1981;3:257.
10. Cormack GC, Lamberty BG. The anatomical vascular basis of the axillary fascio-cutaneous pedicled flap. *Br J Plast Surg.* 1983;36(4):425–427.
11. Mayou BJ, Whitby D, Jones BM. The scapular flap—an anatomical and clinical study. *Br J Plast Surg.* 1982;35(1):8–13.
12. dos Santos LF. The vascular anatomy and dissection of the free scapular flap. *Plast Reconstr Surg.* 1984;73(4):599–604.
13. Rowsell AR, Davies DM, Eisenberg N, Taylor GI. The anatomy of the subscapular-thoracodorsal arterial system: study of 100 cadaver dissections. *Br J Plast Surg.* 1984;37(4):574–576.
14. Nassif TM, Vidal L, Bovet JL, Baudet J. The parascapular flap: a new cutaneous microsurgical free flap. *Plast Reconstr Surg.* 1982;69(4):591–600.
15. Batchelor AG, Bardsley AF. The bi-scapular flap. *Br J Plast Surg.* 1987;40(5):510–512.
16. Chiu DT, Sherman JE, Edgerton BW. Coverage of the calvarium with a free parascapular flap. *Ann Plast Surg.* 1984;12(1):60–66.
17. Batchelor AG, Sully L. A multiple territory free tissue transfer for reconstruction of a large scalp defect. *Br J Plast Surg.* 1984;37(1):76–79.
18. Koshima I, Soeda S. Repair of a wide defect of the lower leg with the combined scapular and parascapular flap. *Br J Plast Surg.* 1985;38(4):518–521.
19. Shaw R, Ho M, Brown J. Thoracodorsal artery perforator-scapular flap in oromandibular reconstruction with associated large facial skin defects. *Br J Oral Maxilofac Surg.* 2015;53(6):569–571.
20. Pau M, Wallner J, Feichtinger M, et al. Free thoracodorsal, perforator-scapularflap based on the angular artery (TDAP-scap-aa): clinical experiences and description on a novel technique for single flap reconstruction of extensive oromandibular defects. *J Cranio-Maxillo-Fac Surg.* 2019;47(10):1617–1625.
21. Swartz WM, Banis JC, Newton ED, Ramasastry SS, Jones NF, Acland R. The osteocutaneous scapular flap for mandibular and maxillary reconstruction. *Plast Reconstr Surg.* 1986;77(4):530–545.
22. Deraemaecker R. *The Serratus Anterior-Scapular Free Flap: A New Osteomuscular Unit for Reconstruction after Radical Head and Neck Surgery (Abstract).* Proceedings of the Second International Conference on Head and Neck Cancer; 1988.
23. Coleman JJ III, Sultan MR. The bipedicled osteocutaneous scapula flap: a new subscapular system free flap. *Plast Reconstr Surg.* 1991;87(4):682–692.
24. Thoma A, Archibald S, Payk I, Young JE. The free medial scapular osteofasciocutaneous flap for head and neck reconstruction. *Br J Plast Surg.* 1991;44(7):477–482.
25. Nkenke E, Vairaktaris E, Stelzle F, Neukam FW, Stockmann P, Linke R. Osteocutaneous free flap including medial and lateral scapular crests: technical aspects, viability, and donor site morbidity. *J Reconstr Microsurg.* 2009;25(9):545–553.
26. Baker SR, Sullivan MJ. Osteocutaneous free scapular flap for one-stage mandibular reconstruction. *Arch Otolaryngol Head Neck Surg.* 1988;114(3):267–277.
27. Moscoso JF, Keller J, Genden E, et al. Vascularized bone flaps in oromandibular reconstruction. A comparative anatomic study of bone stock from various donor sites to assess suitability for enosseous dental implants. *Arch Otolaryngol Head Neck Surg.* 1994;120(1):36–43.
28. Urken ML, Buchbinder D, Weinberg H, et al. Functional evaluation following microvascular oromandibular reconstruction of the oral cancer patient: a comparative study of reconstructed and nonreconstructed patients. *Laryngoscope.* 1991;101(9):935–950.
29. Tang JA, Rieger JM, Wolfaardt JF. A review of functional outcomes related to prosthetic

treatment after maxillary and mandibular reconstruction in patients with head and neck cancer. *Int J Prosthodont (IJP)*. 2008;21(4):337–354.

30. Cuesta-Gil M, Ochandiano Caicoya S, Riba-García F, Duarte Ruiz B, Navarro Cuéllar C, Navarro Vila C. Oral rehabilitation with osseointegrated implants in oncologic patients. *J Oral Maxillofac Surg*. 2009;67(11):2485–2496.
31. Solís R, Mahaney J, Mohhebali R, et al. Digital imaging evaluation of the scapula for prediction of endosteal implant placement in reconstruction of oromandibular defects with scapular free flaps. *Case Reports: Microsurgery*. 2019;39(8):730–736.
32. Lanzer M, Gander T, Grätz K, Rostetter C, Zweifel D, Bredell M. Scapular free vascularised bone flaps for mandibular reconstruction: are dental implants possible? *J Oral Maxillofac Res*. 2015;6(3):e4.
33. Lukash FN, Sachs SA. Functional mandibular reconstruction: prevention of the oral invalid. *Plast Reconstr Surg*. 1989;84(2):227–233.
34. Zenn MJ. Scapular/parascapular flap. In: *Reconstructive Surgery: Anatomy, Technique, and Clinical Applications*. St. Louis, Missouri: Quality Medical Publishing; 2012.
35. Hanasono MM, Skoracki RJ. The scapular tip osseous free flap as an alternative for anterior mandibular reconstruction. *Plast Reconstr Surg*. 2010;125(4):164e–166e.
36. Smith RB, Henstrom DK, Karnell LH, Chang KC, Goldstein DP, Funk GF. Scapula osteocutaneous free flap reconstruction of the head and neck: impact of flap choice on surgical and medical complications. *Head Neck*. 2007;29(5):446–452.
37. Wolfer S, Wohlrath R, Kunzler A, Foos T, Ernst C, Schultze-Mosgau S. *Br J Oral Maxillofac Surg*. 2020;58(4):451–457.
38. Vaienti L, Soresina M, Menozzi A. Parascapular free flap and fat grafts: combined surgical methods in morphological restoration of hemifacial progressive atrophy. *Plast Reconstr Surg*. 2005;116(3):699–711.
39. Mertens C, Freudlsperger C, Bodem J, Engel M, Hoffmann J, Freier K. Reconstruction of the maxilla following hemimaxillectomy defects with scapular tip grafts and dental implants. *J Cranio-Maxillo-Fac Surg*. 2016;44(11):1806–1811.
40. Brown J, Bekiroglu F, Shaw R. Indications for the scapular flap in reconstructions of the head and neck. *Br J Oral Maxillofac Surg*. 2010;48(5):331–337.
41. Boahene KD, Owusu JA, Collar R, Byrne P, Ishii L. Vascularized scapular tip flap in the reconstruction of the mandibular joint following ablative surgery. *Arch Facial Plast Surg*. 2012;14(3):211–214.
42. Kosutic D, Uglesic V, Knezevic P, Milenovic A, Virag M. Latissimus dorsi-scapula free flap for reconstruction of defects following radical maxillectomy with orbital exenteration. *J Plast Reconstr Aesthet Surg*. 2008;61(6):620–627.
43. Hasan Z, Gore SM, Ch'ng S, Ashford B, Clark JR. Options for configuring the scapular free flap in maxillary, mandibular, and calvarial reconstruction. *Plast Reconstr Surg*. 2013;132(3):645–655.
44. Iñigo F, Jimenez-Murat Y, Arroyo O, Fernandez M, Ysunza A. Restoration of facial contour in Romberg's disease and hemifacial microsomia: experience with 118 cases. *Microsurgery*. 2000;20(4):167–172.
45. Tanna N, Wan DC, Kawamoto HK, Bradley JP. Craniofacial microsomia soft-tissue reconstruction comparison: inframammary extended circumflex scapular flap versus serial fat grafting. *Plast Reconstr Surg*. 2011;127(2):802–811.
46. Angrigiani C, Neligan P, Thrikutam N. Anterior neck resurfacing using a single free flap. Comparison of flap descent in patients with burn sequalae of the neck/chest and patients with burn sequelae of only the neck. *Ann Plast Surg*. 2019;83(6):642–646.
47. Izadi D, Paget JT, Haj-Basheer M, Khan UM. Fasciocutaneous flaps of the subscapular artery axis to reconstruct large extremity defects. *J Plast Reconstr Aesthet Surg*. 2012;65(10):1357–1362.
48. Germann G, Bickert B, Steinau HU, Wagner H, Sauerbier M. Versatility and reliability of combined flaps of the subscapular system. *Plast Reconstr Surg*. 1999;103(5):1386–1399.
49. Momeni A, Krischak S, Bannasch H. The thoracodorsal artery perforator flap with a vascularized scapular segment for reconstruction of a composite lower extremity defect. *Microsurgery*. 2006;26(7):515–518.
50. Choi N, Cho J-K, Jang JY, Cho JK, Cho YS, Baek CH. Scapular tip free flap for head and neck reconstruction. *Clin Exp Otorhinolaryngol*. 2015;8(4):422–429.
51. Patel K, Tsu-Hui H, Partridge A, et al. Assessment of shoulder function following scapular free flap. *Head Neck*. 2020;42(2):224–229.
52. Powell DK, Nwoke F, Urken ML, et al. Scapular free flap harvest site: recognising the spectrum of radiographic post-operative appearance. *Br J Radiol*. 2013;86(1023):20120574.

CHAPTER 130

Rectus Abdominis Free Flap

Andrew Salama and Rushil R. Dang

Armamentarium

Appropriate sutures
Army-Navy retractors
Curved forceps, hemostat or Halsted mosquito
Curved Jameson dissection scissors
Curved Metzenbaum dissection scissors
Deaver retractors
DeBakey forceps ×2
Double skin hook retractors ×2
Irrigating bipolar forceps
Local anesthetic with vasoconstrictor
Lone star retraction hooks
Medium and small vascular clips
Protected Bovie tip
Scalpel handle and blades (#10, #15)
Surgical tissue pouches ×3
Surgical tissue stapler
Suture scissors
Vessel loops

History of the Procedure

The reconstructive utility of the rectus abdominis flap was first described in cardiothoracic surgery literature as a modality to reconstruct chest wall defects following sternotomy complications. A regional rotational epigastric island skin flap based on the deep inferior epigastric vessels was used to reconstruct chest wall defects.[1] Taylor et al. elegantly clarified the cutaneous perfusion of the abdominal skin based on the deep inferior epigastric artery and vein through ink injection studies. Pennington and Pelly subsequently reported some of the first clinical applications of the free rectus abdominis musculocutaneous flap.[2–4] The rectus abdominis free flap (RAFF) has been used to reconstruct a multitude of surgical defects crossing multiple anatomic regions and surgical disciplines. The reliable anatomy, ease of harvest, and availability for a two-team approach have made it a first-tier choice for complex reconstructions including sternal wounds, lower extremity defects (especially those in the distal one-third of the leg), perineal defects, and breast reconstruction following mastectomy.[4–9]

Indications for the Use of the Procedure

Although advances in radiotherapy and chemoradiotherapy have vastly altered the practice of head and neck oncology since the late 1980s, surgery remains a mainstay in advanced-stage disease as a component of multimodality therapy. Evidence from the Veterans Affairs larynx trial is often credited for initiating a paradigm shift that focused on organ preservation and quality of life. Thereafter, many patients with index tumors in areas other than the larynx were subjected to radiation therapy with curative intent rather than surgery.[10] A primary tenet of oncologic surgery is complete surgical extirpation of a tumor including a margin of histologically uninvolved tissue to achieve negative surgical margins. Surgical margins are influenced by the underlying clinical behavior of the tumor as well as proximity to vital structures; however, the intent of surgery remains improved local-regional control translating into improved disease-specific survival. Among all head and neck subsites, squamous cell carcinoma to the oral cavity continues to be managed primarily with surgery based on superior response rates evidenced by improved locoregional control.[11] Moreover, surgical salvage is commonly employed in the setting of local-regional failure among many cancer subsites within the head and neck. The advent of reliable reconstructive options in head and neck surgery gave birth to a new category of surgical defects, creating an ongoing process of discovery.

The introduction of vascularized free flaps revolutionized the extirpative approach to surgical therapy for head and neck cancer and expanded the envelope of surgical feasibility for advanced disease that would not have been otherwise treated with surgery. Reliable regional flaps and free tissue transfer to a greater degree have also improved or maintained form, function, and quality of life for head and neck oncology patients.[12] Nakatsuka and colleagues reported some of the initial favorable results of head and neck reconstruction utilizing the RAFF.[4] Following widespread acceptance in the surgical community, the RAFF continues to serve as a workhorse flap in head and neck reconstruction because of its consistent anatomic landmarks, long vascular pedicle, ease of harvest, and reproducible results.[4,13,14] The RAFF filled a void left by the available reconstructive options prior to its development, in particular the broadly celebrated pectoralis major myocutaneous flap. Some of the head and neck indications of this flap include the following advantages.

Advantages

1. Reliable soft tissue donor.[15,16]
2. Long pedicle that allows for anastomosis to the contralateral side of the defect.
3. Favorable vessel diameter for microvascular anastomosis.
4. The flap can be harvested with multiple skin islands, which allows for reconstruction of large through-and-through defects. This can be a great advantage compared with the use of two flaps (free flap and a regional flap or two free flaps); the latter option has a significantly increased operating time, increased donor site morbidity, and increased risk of flap loss as well as the increased need for anatomizing vessels in the neck, which might be decreased by irradiation or previous neck dissection.[14]
5. Easily located landmarks.
6. Possibility of motor nerve harvest by including the segmental nerve.
7. Allows two simultaneously working surgical teams.[13,16–18]
8. Primary closure of the donor site, avoiding the morbidity of a second donor site.
9. Minimum volume changes to the RAFF after radiation therapy.[19]
10. Can be used as a single flap to reconstruct radical composite through-and-through defects.

Total and Subtotal Glossectomy Defects

The goal of total and subtotal glossectomy reconstruction is to provide ample, durable tissue bulk to provide glossopalatal contact, which is a key component for bolus transport in the swallowing sequence. Dynamic glossopalatal closure preserves swallowing, creates a narrow oropharyngeal space, and relies on the creation of height and roundness in the neotongue.[6] The RAFF is ideally suited for tongue reconstruction in part because of the inherent bulk imparted by variable degrees of muscle and adipose tissue. Design modifications, including surgical overbulking, functionally improve speech and swallowing and prevent aspiration.[6,15,18] Larger defects commonly include portions of the tongue and floor of mouth. The RAFF has the advantage of structurally creating a new mylohyoid muscle through suspension of the anterior rectus sheath to the anterior and posterior mandible to form a hammock-like configuration. From a reconstruction perspective, this maneuver maintains flap bulk while counteracting flap ptosis and thereby preserving necessary glossopalatal contact.

Maxillary and Midface Reconstruction

The incidence of maxillary and midface malignancies is comparatively lower than that in other head and neck subsites; however, the functional and cosmetic implications often require free tissue transfer as a component of the surgical treatment plan.[1,20] Several classifications have been described, commonly sharing the goal of providing a reconstructive scaffold to guide clinical decision making.[3,4,21–23] The Brown classification is a defect-based algorithm that includes vertical and horizontal dimensions and opines broad recommendations according to defect characteristics. A subsequent expanded classification by the same authors included orbital and nasomaxillary defects (Fig. 130.1).[4–9,24] An ideal maxillary reconstruction should aim not only to isolate the mouth from the sinus and nasal cavity but also to provide bone for potential dental rehabilitation with endosseous implants. The RAFF has been used extensively for maxillary defects, predominantly for class III defects involving the orbital contents.

The advantages of primary midface and maxillary reconstruction include immediate functional restoration and isolation of the nasal cavity and maxillary sinus from the oral cavity, preventing hypernasal speech and alimentary regurgitation. Immediate reconstruction decreases the time frame to begin radiation therapy.[11,25] Yetzer and Fernandes demonstrated improved quality of life in patients who underwent soft tissue maxillary reconstruction compared with patients who elected obturators as their reconstructive modality.[12,26] Composite reconstruction of radical midface defects has included the use of non vascularized bone graft and titanium mesh to reconstruct the osseous orbital walls in conjunction with the RAFF.[4,24,25,27] The use of the RAFF has been advocated for reconstructing through-and-through defects of the cheek. The available bulk, design versatility, and pedicle length make the RAFF a viable choice for midface and maxillary reconstruction when bone is not required.

Mandibular Reconstruction

The gold standard for composite segmental mandibular reconstruction is free tissue transfer such as the fibula free flap, deep circumflex iliac artery free flap, and scapula free flap.[12,28] Altered vascular anatomy, venous insufficiency, and functionally significant atherosclerosis of the peroneal vascular system, for instance, may preclude the use of the fibula free flap.[6,15,17,29,30] Pure soft tissue reconstruction of lateral defects is also used when patients have significant medical comorbidities, lack available donor sites, or are unwilling to undergo composite free tissue transfer. Soft tissue reconstruction of lateral mandibular segmental defects can be used in selected cases, and the RAFF has been used to reconstruct such defects with and without mandibular hardware.[6,31,32] The RAFF can be easily modified to accommodate through-and-through defects, particularly of the cheek through the creation of multiple skin islands or partial segmental deepithelialization.[13,27] In an effort to decrease plate exposure in soft tissue lateral defects, Yokoo and colleagues

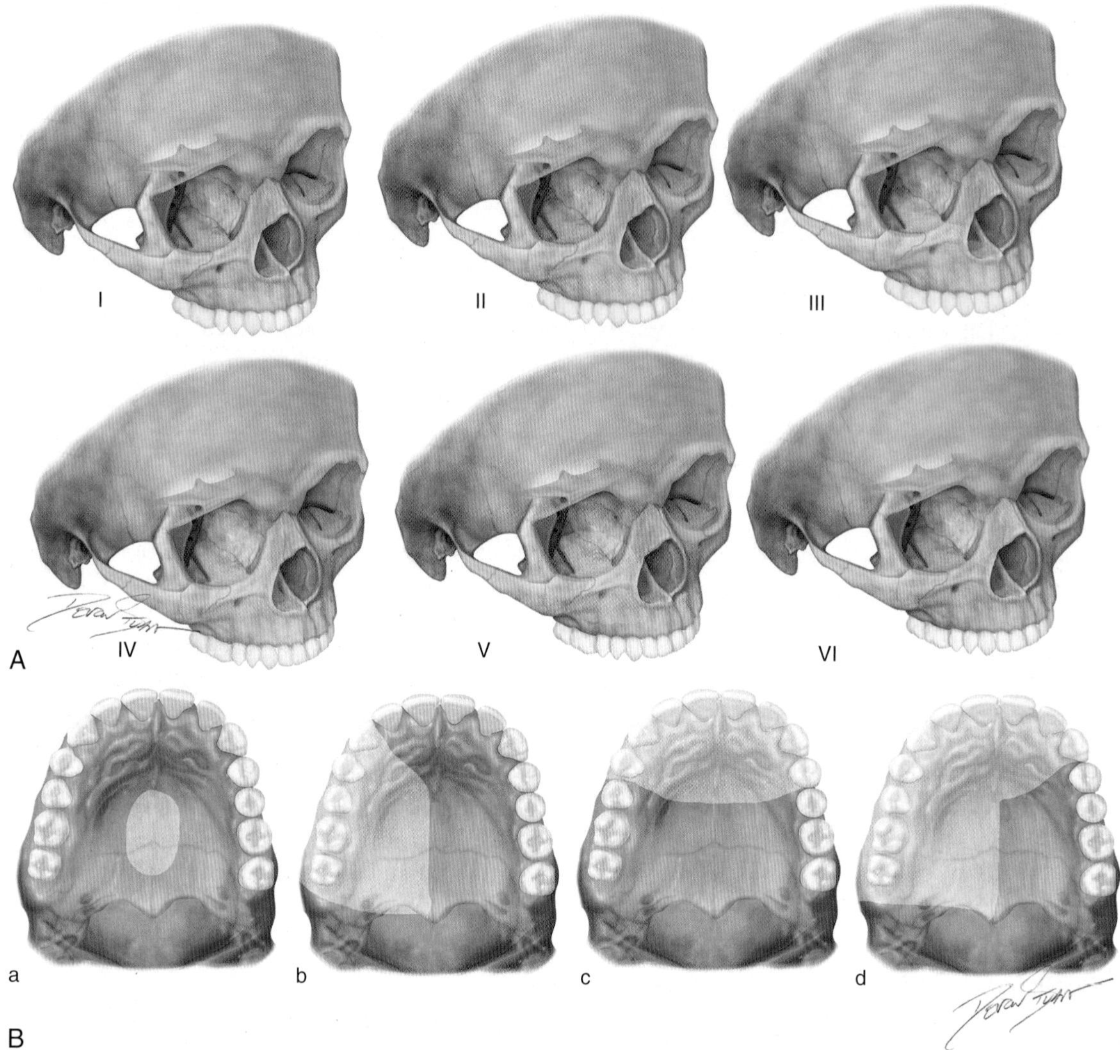

Figure 130.1 **Classification of vertical and horizontal maxillectomy and midface defects.** **A,** Vertical classification: **I,** maxillectomy not causing an oronasal fistula; **II,** not involving the orbit; **III,** involving the orbital adnexa with orbital retention; **IV:** with orbital enucleation or exenteration; **V,** orbitomaxillary defect; **VI,** nasomaxillary defect. **B,** Horizontal classification: **a,** palatal defect only, not involving the dental alveolus; **b,** less than or equal to half unilateral; **c,** less than or equal to half bilateral or transverse anterior; **d,** greater than half maxillectomy. Letters refer to the increasing complexity of the dentoalveolar and palatal defect, and qualify the vertical dimension. (Redrawn from Brown JS, Shaw RJ. Reconstruction of the maxilla and midface: introducing a new classification, *Lancet Oncol.* 2010;11:1002.)

espoused a wrapping technique in which the hardware is circumferentially wrapped with muscle, and a portion is deepithelialized to facilitate closure. The anterior rectus sheath fascia is placed in proximity to the hardware, and the cutaneous element is used for intraoral closure. Wound complications including plate exposure and extrusion are less frequent with this approach.[6]

Dynamic Facial Reanimation

Adynamic reconstruction for patients with Bell's palsy and facial paralyses provides good resting symmetry and shorter operating time; however, the use of free tissue transfer has allowed dynamic facial reanimation, which adds the emotional component to the reconstruction. The innervated RAFF has been utilized in dynamic facial reanimation by harvesting the segmental nerve.[6,15,18,33]

Craniofacial Defects/Skull Base

The RAFF is widely used in skull base reconstruction following radical resection of skull base tumors. The muscle bulk is ideally suited for obliteration of paranasal sinus and frontal lobe defects. Moreover, the rectus may be used for dural reconstruction in instances of persistent cerebrospinal fluid leaks where the site may not be identifiable. It is important to understand the concept of the "three-cavity defect" when addressing craniofacial defect reconstruction. This distinction helps to address the reconstructive needs of the nasal, oral, and intracranial cavities.[15,34]

Limitations and Contraindications

The varieties of clinical applications that soft tissue free flap afford are nearly limitless. However, the use of the RAFF in head and neck surgery is generally reserved for larger, complex anatomic defects. From a flap design perspective, the RAFF is among the most versatile and modifiable, yet it is often harvested as a myocutaneous free flap containing skin, subcutaneous fat, fascia, and muscle. Variations including muscle only, and segmental flaps are also employed depending on case-specific reconstructive demands.[27] One limitation of a skin-bearing RAFF in the head and neck is the quantity of subcutaneous adipose tissue. In this regard, obesity and the increased volume of abdominal fat may complicate the flap inset. Furthermore, skin perforators, which traverse the fat layer, are prone to shearing forces, increasing the risk for full/partial skin and fat necrosis.

The rectus muscle originates from the anterior aspect of the costal cartilages (sixth, seventh, and eighth) and the xiphoid process and inserts on the pubic symphysis. The average muscle dimensions are 30 cm in length and 6 cm in width. The entire muscle can be harvested; however, there appears to be an anecdotal relationship between the amount of muscle harvested and the development of abdominal wall hernias. Flap bulk plays a critical role in the postoperative functional capacity of RAFF, particularly for total and subtotal glossectomy defects. Flap atrophy and the resultant loss of volume affects long-term function in some patients. Although loss of bulk is likely multifactorial, muscle and fat atrophy as well as scarring contribute to this phenomenon. Volumetric changes in flap dimensions have been described and are most notable in the first 6 months. Yamaguchi and colleagues[19] quantitatively analyzed volumetric changes and found a 30% loss of flap volume, which mostly occurred in the first few postoperative years. Initial flap volume is artificially elevated from the combination of postoperative surgical edema and the absence of lymphatic drainage. Denervation of the rectus muscle is largely unavoidable and leads to long-term muscle atrophy. Technical modifications have been suggested to avoid flap atrophy and include dynamic reinnervation and intentional flap overbulking to counteract flap atrophy.[15,17]

Contraindications to RAFF include previous surgical procedures that disrupted the vascular pedicle or skin perforators including but not limited to previous abdominal surgery, laparotomy, and hernia repair.[31] The reconstructive surgeon should inspect the abdominal wall for transverse scars, including the Kocher subcostal incision that commonly divides the rectus muscle. Previous abdominoplasty is a relative contraindication, although the procedure is technically feasible based on case reports described in the breast reconstruction literature. A superiorly based RAFF is contraindicated in patients with a history of cardiac revascularization utilizing the internal mammary artery despite the presence of distal anastomosis between the superior epigastric artery and the costomarginal artery.[27]

TECHNIQUE: The Myocutaneous Rectus Abdominis Free Flap Harvest

RELATIVE SURFACE ANATOMY

The rectus abdominis is a long, longitudinally oriented, broad skeletal muscle measuring 30 cm in length and 6 cm in width that spans the full length of the anterior abdominal wall. The flap has two dominant vascular pedicles, making it type III according to the Mathes and Nahai flap classification. The RAFF has dual blood supply, the deep superior epigastric artery (DSEA) proximally, and the deep inferior epigastric artery (DIEA) distally. Anastomotic communication between the DSEA and DIEA coalesces at the umbilicus and form small-caliber vessels known as choke vessels. The importance of the choke vessels rises in staged reconstructions where the ligation of the DSEA causes dilatation of these choke vessels. This maneuver is rarely needed in head and neck reconstruction procedures. Taylor's study in the mid-1980s is considered a landmark study because it introduced the concept of angiosomes and choke vessels. The other important observation was the ability to harvest a lower abdominal flap solely on large periumbilical perforator vessels of the DIEA; this observation opened the door for the deep inferior epigastric artery perforator (DIEAP) flap, which gained popularity for use during breast reconstruction.[2,27] In their study, Kang et al. showed a 93% success rate for DIEAP in head and neck defects with three key advantages, including a long pedicle, moldable fat, and reconstruction of defects within contained spaces.[35]

The average length of the nutrient vessel is 13 cm. The diameters of the DIEA and vein average between 3.4 mm and 2.5 to 4.4 mm, respectively. The abdominal wall has been divided into four anatomic zones to facilitate flap design. More than 90% of the major perforators are located within a 6-cm radius lateral and inferior to the umbilicus, which corresponds to the middle and medial thirds of the muscle.[2,4,14,27] The RAFF is commonly raised based on the DIEA and vein in a musculocutaneous fashion, which allows an increased diameter for skin harvest.[15,16,18] The DIEA branch of the external iliac ascends superficial to the inguinal ligament where it courses superomedially to run along the deep lateral aspect of the muscle. Various skin paddle designs have been implemented to serve various reconstructive purposes; they include vertical, oblique, and transverse skin paddles.[4] The pedicle enters the muscle 1 to 2 cm away from the arcuate line (4 to 6 cm above the pubic bone). A thorough understanding

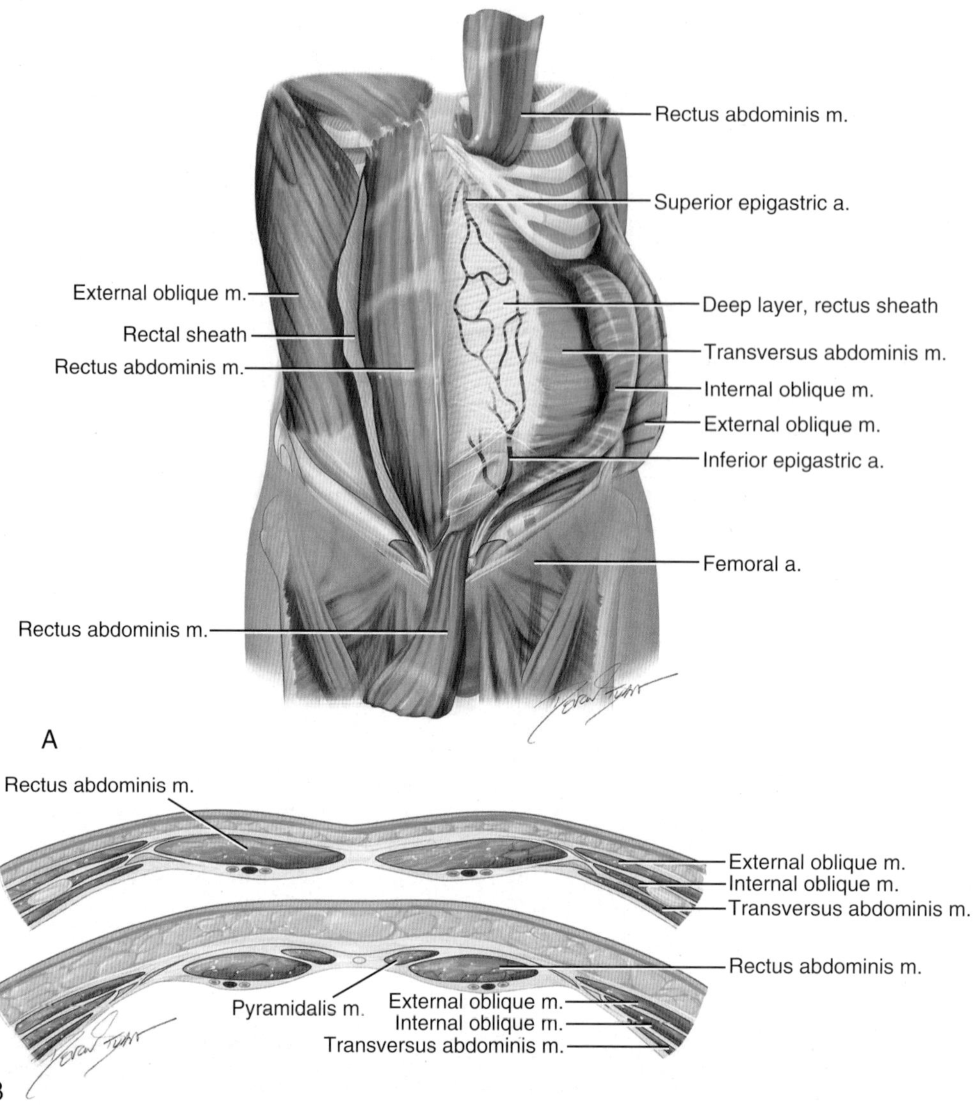

Figure 130.2 **A,** Regional anatomy of the rectus abdominis muscle. **B,** The variation of the posterior abdominal rectus sheath. **a,** Superior to the arcuate line. **b,** Inferior to the arcuate line. Harvesting the rectus sheath inferior to the arcuate line will likely lead to an abdominal hernia.

TECHNIQUE: The Myocutaneous Rectus Abdominis Free Flap Harvest—*cont'd*

of the rectus sheath is critical for flap harvest, which is formed by aponeurotic extensions of three abdominal muscles (internal oblique, transversus abdominis, and external oblique). The composition of the rectus sheath is not consistent along its course. The likelihood of weakening the abdominal wall if the flap is harvested below the arcuate line corresponding to the superior iliac spine is very high due to a weak posterior rectus sheath at that level, which is composed mainly of tranversus abdominis fascia (Fig. 130.2A and B).

STEP 1: Positioning, Exposure, and Anatomic Landmarks

The patient is placed in a supine position; this allows for the participation of two simultaneous working surgical teams. The surgeon needs to make sure to include the lower rib arch, posterior axillary line, and upper thigh in the prepping and draping. It is also important to mark the linea alba, linea semilunaris, inguinal ligament, symphysis, costal margin, and arcuate line at the level of the anterior iliac spine.

STEP 2: Initial Skin Incision and Sheath Exposure

The skin is incised with a #10 blade, and electrocautery is used to carefully dissect through the fat, while trying to capture and not violate the large-caliber musculocutaneous perforators. The depth of cephalic dissection is carried down to the rectus abdominis sheath.

TECHNIQUE: The Myocutaneous Rectus Abdominis Free Flap Harvest—*cont'd*

STEP 3: Sheath Incision and Rectus Muscle Exposure

The anterior sheath is then incised sharply to reveal the rectus abdominis muscle, which is exposed along its full length. The remaining skin incision is completed by the caudal incision that is performed in the same fashion down to the rectus abdominis sheath. Some have advocated tacking sutures from the skin to the anterior rectus sheath to preserve these perforators and prevent shearing (Fig. 130.2C and D).

STEP 4: Elevation of the Rectus Muscle

The skin paddle along with the underlying rectus muscle is elevated off the posterior sheath from inferior to superior directions. After the rectus muscle is freed from the posterior rectus sheath, blunt dissection is recommended because the vascular pedicle will be encountered and should be identified at the arcuate line where it is dissected free from the inferior rectus muscle. The pedicle dissection should continue until the external iliac vessels where the pedicle is divided after ligation has been reached (Fig. 130.2E–G).

STEP 5: Donor Site Closure

The fascia at the donor defect is closed with special attention to include the internal oblique muscle in the closure. Failure to pay attention to this step increases the risk that the patient will develop an abdominal bulge.

Continued

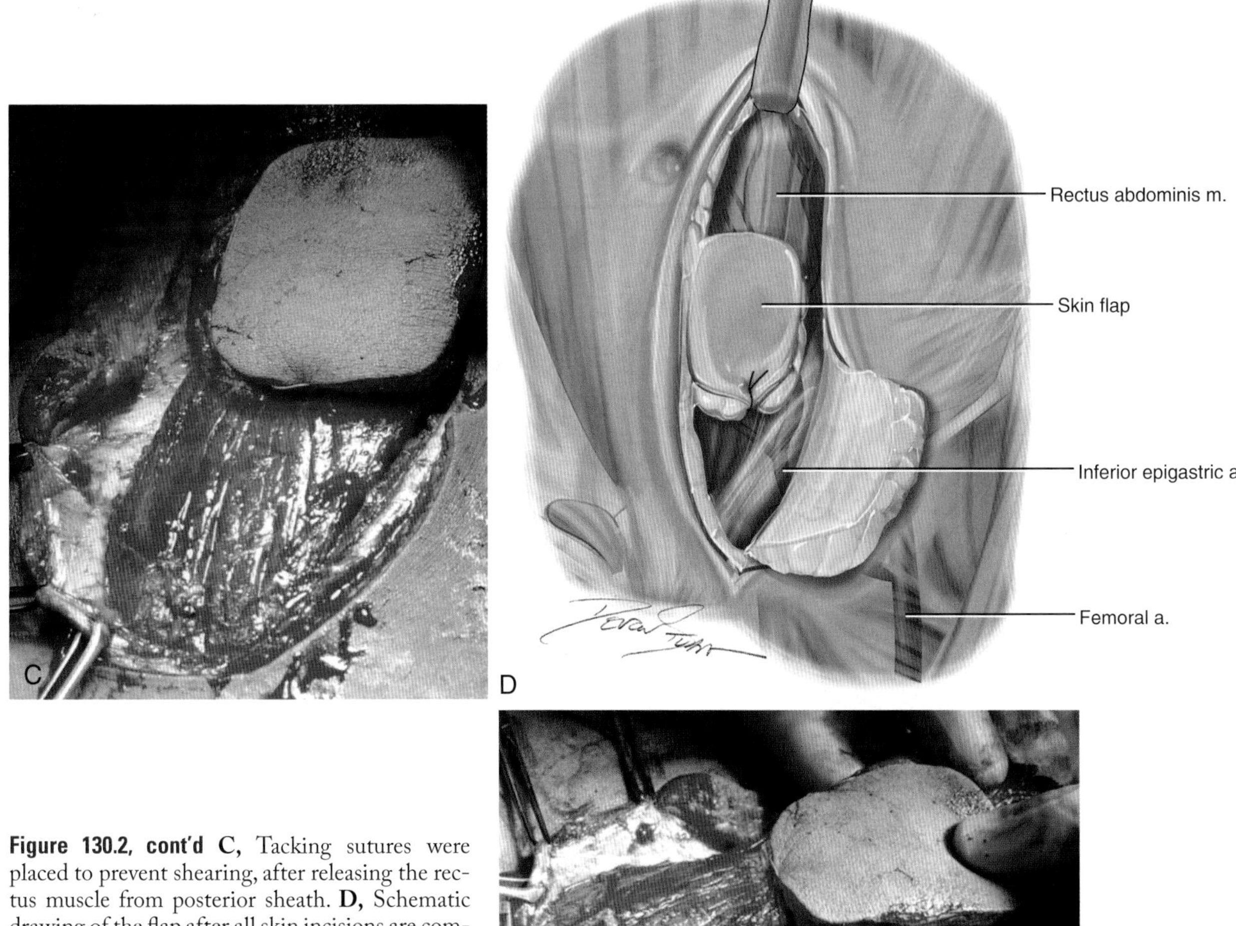

Figure 130.2, cont'd C, Tacking sutures were placed to prevent shearing, after releasing the rectus muscle from posterior sheath. **D,** Schematic drawing of the flap after all skin incisions are completed, showing the vascular pedicle in the inferior portion of the rectus muscle. Skin island after skin incisions are made and dissection of the vascular pedicle. **E,** RAFF after dissection completion and freeing it from the posterior rectus sheath.

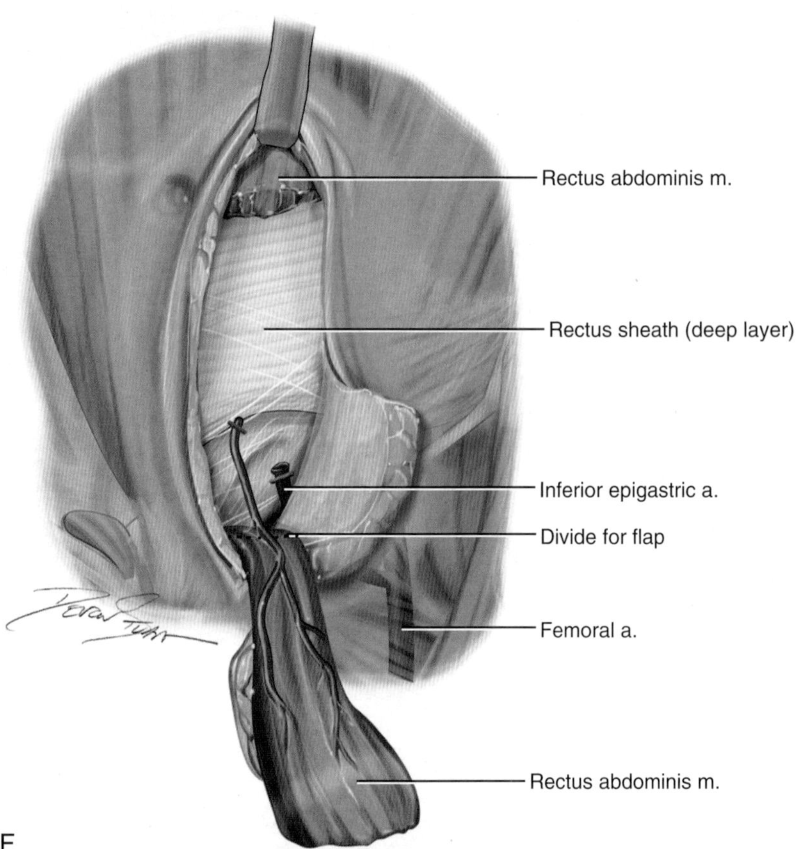

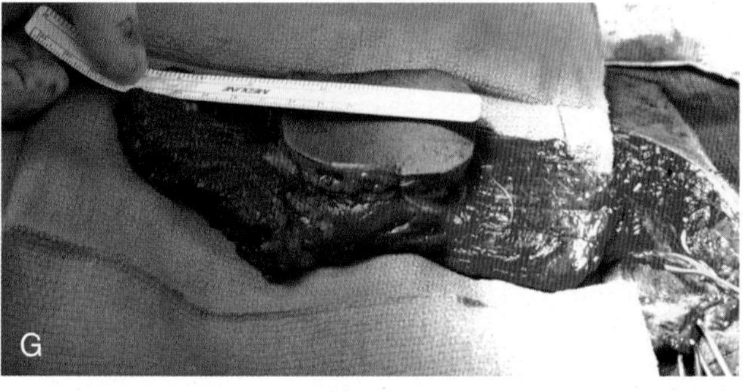

Figure 130.2, cont'd **F,** Schematic drawing demonstrating the RAFF released from the posterior rectus sheath and vascular pedicle dissected, ready to be divided and transferred; note maintaining of the rectus abdominis muscle below the arcuate line. **G,** The RAFF has been fully dissected and the DIEA isolated from the external iliac artery.

Avoidance and Management of Intraoperative Complications

Depending on the reconstructive goal, a desired thin pliable flap is sometimes needed and primary thinning of the flap by dissecting the musculocutaneus perforators through the muscle may be performed. A disadvantage of this technique is that there is an increased risk of damaging small perforator vessels due to their unpredictable course. An advantage of the technique of flap harvest, however, is the ability to maintain abdominal wall integrity.[15,27]

The RAFF is a heavy, bulky flap, and proper suspension of the flap is necessary to help prevent flap ptosis. Prolene or polydioxanone sutures may be used to suspend the flap to adjacent bone. This common practice is very useful, especially in maxillary reconstructions.

To overcome the limitations associated with thick skin and subcutaneous tissues, particularly in overweight patients, some authors have advocated harvesting the flap in a muscular fashion with fascia and augmenting the flap with a split-thickness skin graft.[15] This approach may decrease the risk of skin necrosis in these patients.

Thin patients with a limited quantity of abdominal tissue restricting the harvest of the flap, or in cases where more flap tissue is needed from areas that are less well vascularized, the concept of "super charging" the flap becomes helpful to improve the blood supply to the additional volume of tissue included in the flap. This is done by harvesting additional vascular pedicles and anastomosing them to recipient vessels in the neck.

The incidence of abdominal bulging (1.7% to 4%) can be decreased by maintaining the rectus fascia below the arcuate line. Herniation occurs if the internal abdominal pressure does not match that in the abdominal wall muscles.[15,16,29,33] Preserving at least 1 cm on each side of the anterior rectus muscle sheath has also been advocated to facilitate closure.[14]

Placing sutures to tug the undermined skin flap to the rectus aponeurosis reduces "dead space," decreasing the incidence of hematomas and seromas at the donor site. Extra plication of the aponeurosis of the rectus muscle achieves a better body contour for the patient.

During the closure of the anterior rectus sheath, the surgeon should pay attention to both the internal and external oblique muscles.

The abdominal binder application for the donor site is determined according to the surgeon's preference; some authors have recommended its use for a month postoperatively.[27]

It is important to avoid extensive undermining of the skin flaps, which may lead to necrosis of the abdominal flap. This donor site complication is usually treated with minor local debridement and dressing changes.

The incidence of seroma is low due to the routine use of suction drains, but if they occur, needle aspiration and pressure dressing should be the first line of management. Persistence of the problem requires surgical evacuation.

Postoperative Considerations

Flap-related considerations include the following:

- Standard flap monitoring for early signs of flap failure related to venous or arterial thrombosis
- Partial or total flap necrosis
- Infection
- Bleeding

Suspending the flap to the adjacent bone might counteract anticipated flap ptosis due to increased flap bulk. Another technique to overcome this problem is to perform a secondary debulking procedure or liposuction.

Donor site complications (8.5% to 14.3%) include the following:

- Hematoma
- Seroma
- Ileus
- Pain
- Hernia
- Abdominal bulging and back pain
- Adhesions
- Scar

The reconstructive surgeon needs to be aware of the relevant anatomy and technique to harvest the RAFF flap as a workhorse flap in head and neck reconstruction, and this may be the first choice for selected patients. Proper closure of the anterior sheath is important to prevent hernia. Mesh can also be used to reinforce the abdominal wall.

References

1. Drever JM, Hodson-Walker N. Closure of the donor defect for breast reconstruction with rectus abdominis myocutaneous flaps. *Plast Reconstr Surg*. 1985;76(4):558–565.
2. Taylor GI, Corlett RJ, Boyd JB. The versatile deep inferior epigastric (inferior rectus abdominis) flap. *Br J Plast Surg*. 1984;37(3):330–350.
3. Pennington DG, Pelly AD. The rectus abdominis myocutaneous free flap. *Br J Plast Surg*. 1980;33(2):277–282.
4. Nakatsuka T, Harii K, Yamada A, Asato H, Ebihara S. Versatility of a Free Inferior Rectus Abdominis Flap for Head and Neck Reconstruction. *Plastic and Reconstructive Surg*. 1994;93(4):762–769.
5. Jacobsen WM, Meland NB, Woods JE. Autologous breast reconstruction with use of transverse rectus abdominis musculocutaneous flap: mayo clinic experience with 147 cases. *Mayo Clin Proc*. 1994;69(7):635–640.
6. Yokoo S, Komori T, Furudoi S, et al. Indications for vascularized free rectus abdominis musculocutaneous flap in oromandibular region in terms of efficiency of anterior rectus sheath. *Microsurgery*. 2003;23(2):96–102.
7. Georgiade GS, Riefkohl R, Levin LS. *Georgiade Plastic, Maxillofacial, and Reconstructive Surgery*. 3rd ed. New York, New York: Lippincott Williams & Wilkins; 1997.
8. Nagarjuna M, Patil BR, Nagraj N, Gopalkrishnan K. Use of superiorly based vertical rectus abdominis myocutaneous flap for the correction of costal osteomyelitis at the pectoralis major myocutaneous flap donor site. *J Oral Maxillofac Surg*. 2013;71(2):e132–e136.
9. Greer SE. *Handbook of Plastic Surgery*. CRC Press; 2004.
10. Fung K, Lyden THT, Lee J, et al. Voice and swallowing outcomes of an organ-preservation trial for advanced laryngeal cancer. *Int J Radiat Oncol Biol Phys*. 2005;63(5):1395–1399.
11. Lubek JE, Clayman L. An update on squamous carcinoma of the oral cavity, oropharynx, and maxillary sinus. *Oral Maxillofac Surg Clin North Am*. 2012;24(2):307–316 (x).
12. Bak M, Jacobson AS, Buchbinder D, Urken ML. Contemporary reconstruction of the mandible. *Oral Oncol*. 2010;46(2):71–76.
13. Mosahebi A, Chaudhry A, McCarthy CM, et al. Reconstruction of extensive composite posterolateral mandibular defects using nonosseous free tissue transfer. *Plast Reconstr Surg*. 2009;124(5):1571–1577.
14. Patel NP, Matros E, Cordeiro PG. The use of the multi-island vertical rectus abdominis myocutaneous flap in head and neck reconstruction. *Ann Plast Surg*. 2012;69(4):403–407.
15. Urken ML, Cheney ML, Blackwell KE, et al. *Atlas of Regional and Free Flaps for Head and Neck Reconstruction*. 2nd ed. New York, New York: Lippincott Williams & Wilkins; 2012.
16. Grabb WC. *Grabb and Smith's Plastic Surgery*. 6th ed. New York, New York: Lippincott Williams & Wilkins; 2007.
17. Matsui Y, Ohno K, Shirota T, Imai S, Yamashita Y, Michi K. Speech function following maxillectomy reconstructed by rectus abdominis myocutaneous flap. *J Cranio-Maxillo-Fac Surg*. 1995;23(3):160–164.
18. Langdon J, Patel M, Ord R, Brennan P. *Operative Oral and Maxillofacial Surgery*. 2nd ed. London: CRC Press; Hodder Arnold Publication; 2010.
19. Yamaguchi K, Kimata Y, Onoda S, Mizukawa N, Onoda T. Quantitative analysis of free flap volume changes in head and neck reconstruction. *Head Neck*. 2012;34(10):1403–1407.
20. Futran ND, Mendez E. Developments in reconstruction of midface and maxilla. *Lancet Oncol*. 2006;7(3):249–258.
21. Cordeiro PGP, Chen CMC. A 15-year review of midface reconstruction after total and subtotal maxillectomy: part I. Algorithm and outcomes. *Plast Reconstr Surg*. 2012;129(1):124–136.
22. Spiro RH, Strong EW, Shah JP. Maxillectomy and its classification. *Head Neck*. 1997;19(4):309–314.

23. Andrades P, Militsakh O, Hanasono MM, Rieger J, Rosenthal EL. Current strategies in reconstruction of maxillectomy defects. *Arch Otolaryngol Head Neck Surg.* 2011;137(8):806–812.
24. Brown JS, Shaw RJ. Reconstruction of the maxilla and midface: introducing a new classification. *Lancet Oncol.* 2010;11(10):1001–1008.
25. Bianchi B, Bertolini F, Ferrari S, Sesenna E. Maxillary reconstruction using rectus abdominis free flap and bone grafts. *Br J Oral Maxillofac Surg.* 2006;44(6):526–530.
26. Yetzer J, Fernandes R. Reconstruction of orbitomaxillary defects. *J Oral Maxillofac Surg.* 2013;71(2):398–409.
27. Bianchi B, Bertolini F, Ferrari S, Tullio A. The rectus abdominis myocutaneous flap combined with vascularized costal cartilages for orbito-malar facial reconstruction. *J Oral Maxillofac Surg.* 2005;63(7):1026–1029.
28. Wei F-C, Mardini S. *Flaps and Reconstructive Surgery*. Saunders; 2009.
29. Kekatpure VD, Manjula BV, Mathias S, Trivedi NP, Selvam S, Kuriakose MA. Reconstruction of large composite buccal defects using single soft tissue flap—analysis of functional outcome. *Microsurgery.* 2013;33(3):184–190.
30. Butler CE, Lewin JS. Reconstruction of large composite oromandibulomaxillary defects with free vertical rectus abdominis myocutaneous flaps. *Plast Reconstr Surg.* 2004;113(2):499–507.
31. Cappiello J, Piazza C, Taglietti V, Nicolai P. Deep inferior epigastric artery perforated rectus abdominis free flap for head and neck reconstruction. *Eur Arch Oto-Rhino-Laryngol.* 2012;269(4):1219–1224.
32. Kroll SS, Robb GL, Miller MJ, Reese GP, Evans GR. Reconstruction of posterior mandibular defects with soft tissue using the rectus abdominis free flap. *Br J Plast Surg.* 1998;51(7):503–507.
33. Spector M, Kim K. The latissimus dorsi, pectoralis minor, and rectus abdominus free flaps for dynamic reconstruction of the paralyzed face. *Operative Techniques in Otolaryngology-Head and Neck Surgery.* 2012;23(4):268.
34. Tokoro K, Fujii S, Kubota A, et al. Successful closure of recurrent traumatic csf rhinorrhea using the free rectus abdominis muscle flap. *Surg Neurol.* 2000;53(3):275–280.
35. Kang SY, Spector ME, Chepeha DB. Perforator based rectus free tissue transfer for head and neck reconstruction: new reconstructive advantages from an old friend. *Oral Oncol.* 2017;74:163–170.

CHAPTER 131

Deep Circumflex Iliac Artery Free Flap

Daniel A. Hammer, Brett Shirley, and Fayette C. Williams

Armamentarium

#10 Blade
#10 Jackson-Pratt drain
#15 Blade
Appropriate sutures
Bone wax
Heavy osteotomes
Large Weitlaner retractors
Local anesthetic with vasoconstrictor
Malleable retractors
Obwegeser retractors
Prolene mesh
Reciprocating saw
Vessel clips

History of the Procedure

Early attempts of vascularized iliac crest harvest were based on the superficial iliac vessels supplying the groin. Success rates were limited before surgeons gained an accurate understanding of the blood supply to the ilium. In 1979, Taylor et al. and Sanders and Mayou recognized the superiority of the deep circumflex iliac artery (DCIA) as the dominant blood supply to the bone.[1,2] Only a year later, reports of mandible reconstruction emerged using this new flap.[3] Surgeons quickly realized that the skin paddle associated with this flap was often bulky due to "obligatory muscle cuff" and the tethering of the skin to the bone, which renders soft tissue placement problematic in complex oromandibular reconstructions.[4] These limitations often required secondary revision procedures when used in oral cavity reconstruction.

To avoid these limitations, surgeons investigated other soft tissues associated with the anatomical region that could be used for composite oral defects. They quickly adapted the harvest of the internal oblique free muscle flap, based on the ascending branch of the DCIA, with their traditional DCIA harvest. The internal oblique free flap was first described in 1984 for lower extremity reconstruction.[5] This flap modification quickly began to replace the skin paddle as the soft tissue component of choice when harvesting the DCIA free flap. In 1989, Urken and colleagues described the iliac crest bone flap with the internal oblique muscle to resurface oral and pharyngeal defects when combined with mandible reconstruction.[6,7] The DCIA flap with internal oblique was eventually used for maxillary reconstruction as popularized by Brown almost a decade later.[8–10] Further refinements of the internal oblique muscle technique were soon published.[11,12]

Recently, perforator flaps have gained significant attention due to their ability to limit the size of the soft tissue bulk harvested and donor site morbidity. In addition, anatomic studies of the macroscopic vascular anatomy of the DCIA and its contribution to the skin overlying the iliac crest have determined a perforator-based skin paddle was feasible and predictable for the DCIA flap.[13] This technique was first described by Kimata in 2003 for the reconstruction of composite oromandibular defects.[14,15] With further refinement and study, the DCIA perforator flap has become more predictable.[16,17]

Continued innovation has led to the development of a chimeric flap including the lateral iliac crest, based on the ascending branch of the lateral femoral circumflex artery with components of the anterolateral thigh, and fascia lata flaps were used to reconstruct a composite defect of the oral cavity.[18] In addition, a medial approach to the flap using a minimally invasive approach has been described that does not require a lateral dissection and maintains the iliac crest integrity. This technique combined with virtual surgical planning and CAD/CAM technology has led to decreased patient morbidity and successful reconstruction of complex oromandibular defects.[19]

Indications for the Use of the Procedure

The DCIA free flap is an excellent source of bone and soft tissue for composite defects of the head and neck. Of the major sources of vascularized bone, the iliac crest provides the most anatomic reconstruction of the mandible due to the natural contours corresponding to the curvature of the mandible. In addition, no other vascularized bone source can replace both the height and width of the native mandible.

This large quantity of available bone makes the DCIA free flap especially appealing when planning for osseointegrated

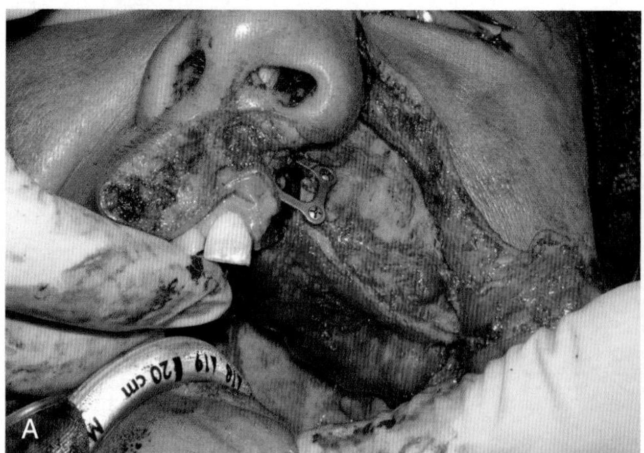

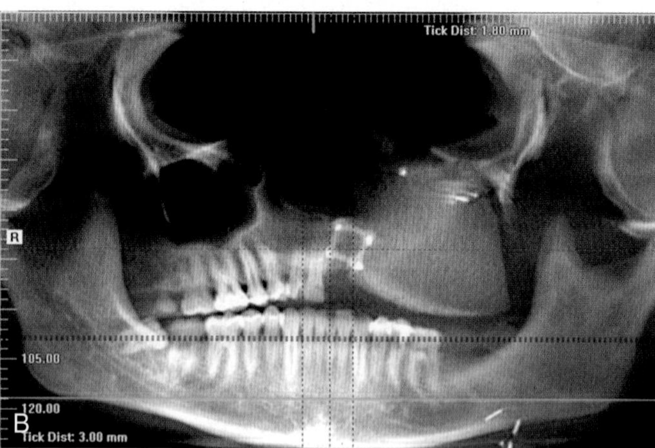

Figure 131.1 A and B, Vertical positioning of a deep circumflex iliac artery (DCIA) bone flap into the maxilla. The internal oblique muscle is sutured to the palate.

dental implant placement.[20] Long-term dental implant success is optimized with minimal bone resorption, and outcomes data can be inconsistent when comparing various osteocutaneous flaps used in head and neck reconstruction. When comparing the volume reduction of the bone flap over 2 years immediately after mandibular reconstruction, the volume loss was least in the fibula free flap, most significant in the scapula free flap, with the DCIA flap in between.[21] When studying periimplant bone resorption over time, no significant difference was noted in the periimplant bone resorption 3 years after placement in a fibula free flap versus a DCIA flap.[22] Last, for patients who will undergo radiation therapy after reconstruction, there is no significant difference in the rates of osteoradionecrosis between the free fibula and DCIA flaps.[23]

For intraoral reconstruction, the internal oblique muscle or a perforator-based skin paddle is often used as the soft tissue component to avoid the unnecessary bulk of the traditional cutaneous skin paddle. If the muscle flap is chosen, the muscle layer drapes easily in the oral cavity and can be trimmed as needed. Within a month the muscle is mucosalized and conforms nicely to the contours of the bone. Advantages of perforator dissection techniques are that they allow thinning and customization of the skin paddle. However, as previously discussed, the skin perforator may be unreliable and should be confirmed to be present preoperatively.

For through-and-through defects of the oral cavity requiring both mucosal and skin replacement, the internal oblique may be used to resurface the oral cavity, while a cutaneous skin paddle simultaneously replaces the external skin defect.[24]

For maxillary reconstruction, the iliac crest may be positioned vertically (Fig. 131.1) or horizontally as dictated by the defect. The internal oblique muscle is draped across the palate to separate the sinonasal cavity from the oral cavity.[8] This muscle eventually atrophies and becomes a taut band of vascularized tissue resembling the native hard palate.

Limitations and Contraindications

Although the DCIA free flap has great versatility, certain disadvantages exist. The skin paddle has limited mobility in relation to the bone, making accurate reconstruction of complex defects more challenging. Superior chimeric properties exist within the subscapular system, which allows for easier three-dimensional insetting. However, as previously discussed, chimeric options for the DCIA do exist with the fascia lata and anterolateral thigh free flaps based off of the ascending branch of the lateral femoral circumflex artery.[18]

The bone stock of the vascularized iliac crest is generally limited to 16 cm, which is not sufficient for total mandibular reconstruction. Osteotomies are performed on the lateral surface of the ilium the majority of the time to protect the vascular supply on the medial surface. This produces open segments at the osteotomy sites, which may need to be grafted with corticocancellous bone. Recently, Dumonta et al. described the Pararectus approach to the DCIA flap harvest to increase the quantity of bone harvested while maintaining the integrity of the lateral femoral cutaneous and genitofemoral nerves.[25] Lastly, the vascular pedicle is relatively short. With an average pedicle length of 5 to 7 cm, vein grafting should be anticipated in vessel-depleted necks or with maxillary reconstruction.

Contraindications to harvest of the DCIA free flap include prior surgery in the region of the flap harvest, existing hernias, and obesity. Preoperative physical exam should focus on the presence of scars or hernias. Obesity is a relative contraindication, as the bulky skin paddle is less reliable and often too large to be useful.

TECHNIQUE: DCIA With Internal Oblique Muscle

STEP 1: Positioning and Skin Marking

The patient is placed supine with the iliac crest exposed. Draping should include the midline of the abdomen medially, the costal margin superiorly, the groin crease inferiorly, and down to the operating room bed laterally. For larger bone flaps, a cushioned beanbag under the hip provides additional exposure to the gluteal region. The anterior superior iliac spine is palpated and marked along with the remainder of the iliac crest posteriorly. An incision line is drawn along the superior aspect of the iliac crest. The incision extends from the palpable femoral pulse in the groin crease to the midaxillary line posteriorly (Fig. 131.2A).

STEP 2: Incision and Muscle Exposure

The incision is performed with a #15 blade down into subcutaneous tissue. Electrocautery continues the dissection through subcutaneous fat down to the external oblique muscle. This muscle has thick fibers superiorly but becomes a tendinous sheath more inferiorly. The external oblique muscle is divided from the iliac crest to expose the internal oblique muscle. The plane between these two muscles is easily identified by recognizing the muscle fibers that travel in opposite directions. Additionally, a loose areolar plane separates the two muscles. A simple technique to identify this plane is to make an incision (parallel to the skin incision) inferiorly through the aponeurosis of the external oblique. Fat and loose areolar tissue immediately become apparent. Blunt finger dissection can be performed in this plane to lift the external oblique muscle off the internal oblique. This incision through the external oblique is extended along the superior aspect of the iliac crest until the appropriate length of bone is exposed. Further blunt dissection superiorly and medially will lift the external oblique from the internal oblique. This plane should be developed to visualize the rectus sheath and the costal margin to gain full exposure of the internal oblique muscle (Fig. 131.2B).

STEP 3: Incorporating the Internal Oblique

The dimensions of bone to be harvested should be decided at this point. When reconstructing smaller bone defects, consideration should be given to harvesting a portion of iliac crest a few centimeters posterior to the anterior superior iliac spine. This effectively lengthens the vascular pedicle and decreases morbidity by keeping the anterior superior iliac spine intact. The portion of the internal oblique muscle to be harvested is marked and centered over the anticipated bone segment. The internal oblique is divided sharply with a #10 blade down to the transversus abdominis muscle. Unlike the loose plane superficial to the internal oblique, this plane must be developed sharply. The safest region to begin transecting the internal oblique is at the superior extent (below the costal margin) because the muscle is thickest in this region. The plane between the internal oblique and transversus abdominis is marked by a thin avascular fascial layer. This layer must be included on the deep surface of the internal oblique muscle, as this plane contains the ascending branch of the DCIA, which supplies the muscle. Therefore the dissection should proceed directly onto the bare muscle fibers of the transversus abdominis. The internal oblique muscle is elevated inferiorly and laterally toward the iliac crest in this plane with further sharp dissection. Caution is advised when approaching within 2 cm of the iliac crest to avoid injury to the DCIA and the ascending branch. A 2- to 3-cm cuff of muscle should be left undisturbed on the medial aspect of the iliac crest to protect this vascular pedicle. Once the internal oblique muscle flap is isolated on the iliac crest, the inferior portion of the remaining internal oblique is divided medial to the inguinal ligament down into the groin region (Fig. 131.2C and D).

Continued

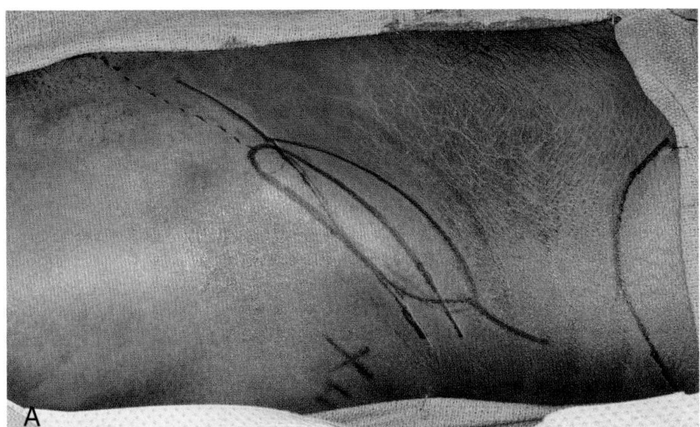

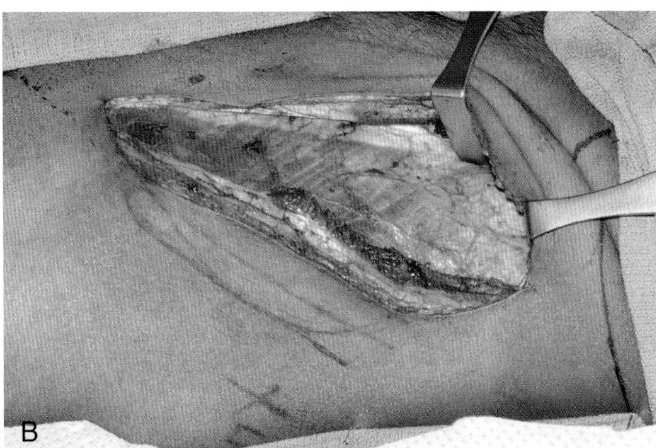

Figure 131.2 **A,** The left iliac crest is outlined. The dotted line marks the inguinal ligament and the costal margin is included superiorly. A skin paddle is outlined over the superior aspect of the iliac crest if desired. **B,** The external oblique muscle is divided and retracted to expose the internal oblique muscle up to the costal margin. The rectus sheath is seen medially.

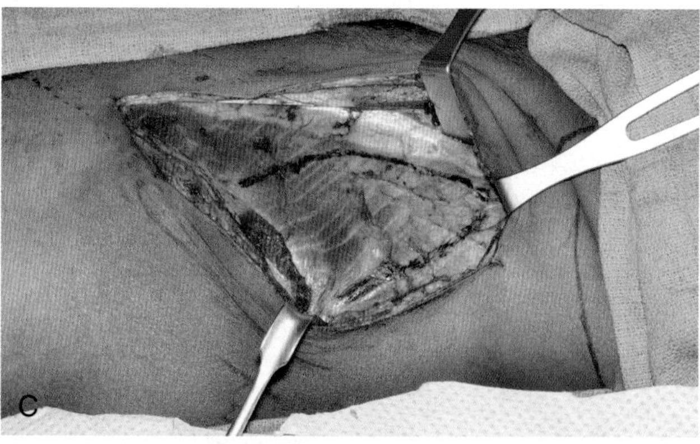

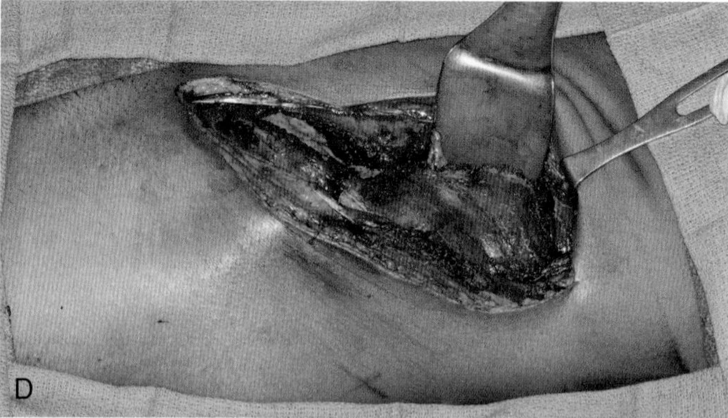

Figure 131.2, cont'd **C,** A segment of internal oblique muscle is marked for incision. The rectus sheath noted medially should remain undisturbed. **D,** The internal oblique muscle is harvested and pedicled on the iliac crest. The remainder of the internal oblique inferiorly is divided parallel to the previous division of the external oblique.

TECHNIQUE: DCIA With Internal Oblique Muscle—*cont'd*

STEP 4: Completing the Abdominal Muscle Dissection

The transversus abdominis attachment is divided from the medial surface of the ilium while leaving a 2-cm cuff of muscle on the bone. Similar to the internal oblique, the transversus abdominis is further divided down to the iliac vessels, which are easily palpated through the soft tissue. This is easiest to accomplish if the internal oblique muscle flap attached to the iliac crest is reflected laterally out of the wound. Deep to the transversus abdominis muscle is where the deep circumflex iliac vessels lie. As the transversus abdominis muscle is divided, the preperitoneal fat bulges into the surgical field. The only remaining muscle attachment on the medial aspect of the ilium is the iliacus muscle. The vascular pedicle runs in the groove between the insertion of the iliacus and transversus abdominis muscles on the medial aspect of the ilium and has a palpable pulse. The iliacus muscle should be divided below the bone attachment, leaving a small cuff to avoid the vicinity of the pedicle. The preperitoneal fat is retracted medially with large malleable retractors to visualize the iliacus muscle during division. An incision is made down to bone on the lateral aspect of the iliac crest. The attachments of the tensor fascia lata and gluteal muscles are stripped inferiorly in a subperiosteal plane. The segment of bone to be harvested is fully exposed in preparation for the osteotomies (Fig. 131.2E).

STEP 5: Osteotomies

Bone cuts can be made from either the medial or lateral aspect of the ilium. Access is usually better from the lateral aspect after full exposure of the outer cortex. Osteotomies are performed with either a reciprocating or an oscillating saw under copious irrigation. The vertical cuts are performed first from the iliac crest down to the planned horizontal osteotomy. The abdominal contents are retracted medially and protected during the bone cuts. During the vertical osteotomies, extra care should be taken to avoid inadvertent transection of the DCIA pedicle running on the medial surface of the ilium. The horizontal osteotomy should be performed inferior to the vascular pedicle at the same level of the iliacus transection performed on the medial surface. Heavy osteotomes can be used to complete the osteotomies if necessary. All three osteotomies should be beveled in such a manner that the bone segment can be fractured inward toward the abdominal cavity where the vascular pedicle lies (Fig. 131.2F).

STEP 6: Dissection of the Vascular Pedicle

Once the bone cuts are completed, the flap is isolated on the pedicle. There are usually some soft tissue attachments remaining around the anterior superior iliac spine. When these attachments are released, the vascular pedicle lies medial to the bone and must not be injured.

The ascending branch of the DCIA emerges from the main pedicle at variable distances from the external iliac artery. In rare cases, the ascending branch may have a separate takeoff and not be connected to the DCIA. The pedicle is dissected out circumferentially toward the external iliac artery, which is palpated in the soft tissue. The lateral femoral cutaneous nerve commonly runs close to the pedicle and should be preserved when possible. As the pedicle is traced more proximally, the artery and vein separate as the external iliac vessels are approached. Whereas the paired venae comitantes travel with the arterial pedicle, these veins usually merge into a single vein within 1 to 2 cm of the external iliac vein (Fig. 131.2G).

STEP 7: Layered Closure With Mesh

Closure of the iliac crest donor site begins with hemostasis. The cut edges of bone are a common source of slow but persistent bleeding. Bone wax may be burnished into the marrow spaces for tamponade. The iliacus muscle is closed to the transversus abdominis muscle with deep sutures without violating the peritoneal cavity. Reinforcement of these muscles may be improved by attaching these sutures to drill holes in the immediately adjacent iliac bone.

TECHNIQUE: DCIA With Internal Oblique Muscle—*cont'd*

A suction drain is now placed into the wound and should rest in the deepest layer of the dissection near the bone. The missing internal oblique muscle is reconstructed using mesh to establish continuity with the ilium. Various materials have been advocated, including polyester fiber mesh, polypropylene mesh, and AlloDerm (Allergan, US).[26] This mesh is sutured into place with heavy prolene sutures. The lateral aspect of the mesh should be fixated to the iliac crest and the lateral muscle attachments. Proper insetting of the mesh is accomplished by overlapping the muscle 1 to 2 cm. The external oblique muscle is closed to itself and to the lateral muscle attachments superficial to the mesh. Remaining skin and subcutaneous planes are closed in layers (Fig. 131.2H and I).

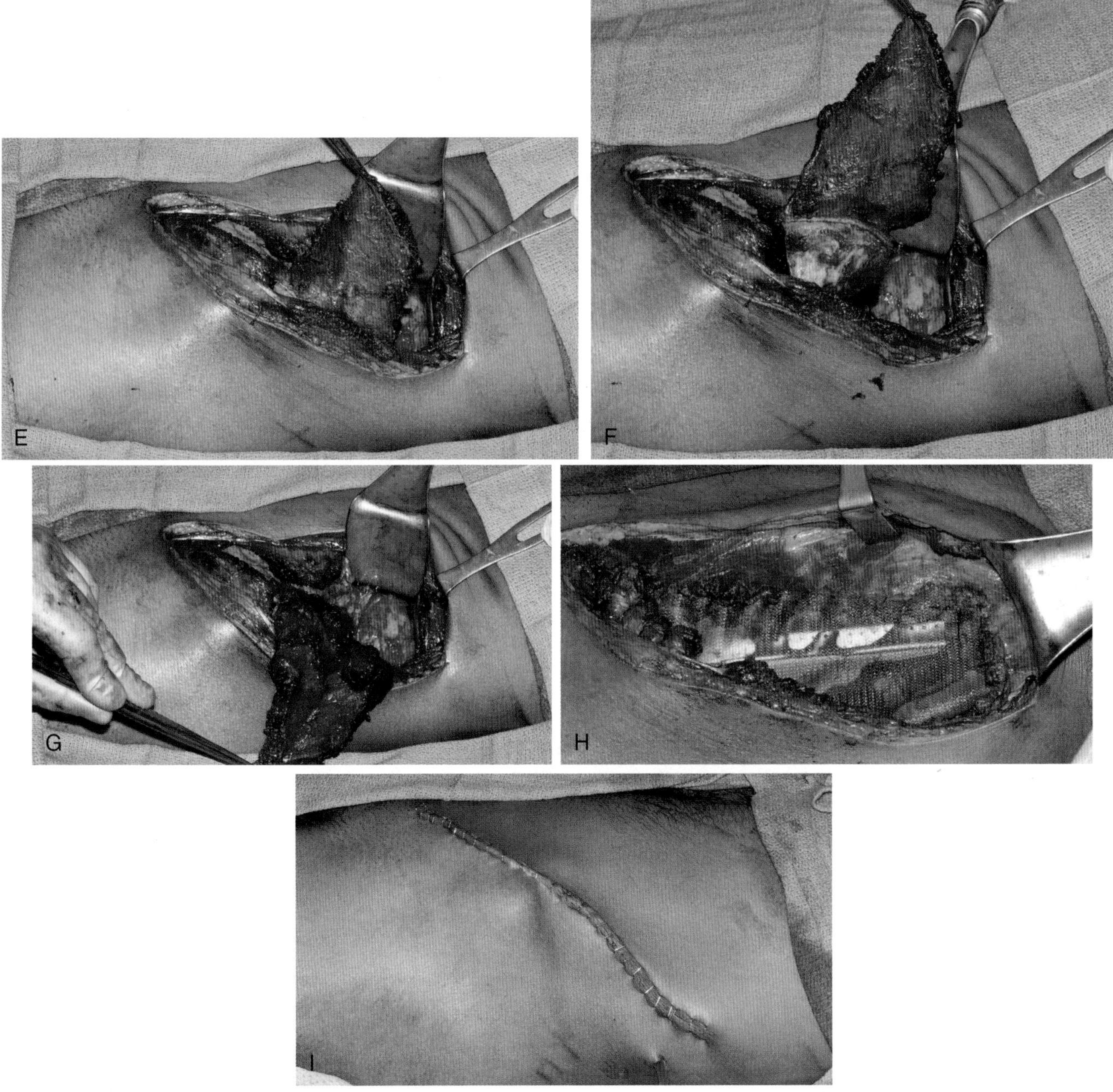

Figure 131.2, cont'd **E,** The harvested portion of the internal oblique muscle is lifted to expose the underlying transversus abdominis for division. **F,** Completion of bone osteotomies allows the harvested bone and internal oblique muscle to be mobilized. **G,** The composite flap is positioned laterally while the abdominal contents are retracted medially to allow dissection of the pedicle. **H** and **I,** After closing the transversus abdominis to the iliacus muscles, a mesh is used to replace the missing segment of internal oblique muscle. A closed suction drain is placed deep to this layer. The external oblique muscle is then repaired, followed by the final skin closure.

ALTERNATIVE TECHNIQUE: DCIA With Skin Paddle

STEP 1: Skin Marking

Although the skin paddle based on perforators from the DCIA was initially considered unreliable, more recent investigations have improved our understanding of the vascular basis for this flap.[17,27] Musculocutaneous perforators are most numerous 2 cm superior and 5 to 10 cm posterior to the anterior superior iliac spine.[17] A handheld Doppler device may be useful to locate these perforators.[28] The skin paddle should include this area and extend parallel to the iliac crest. Releasing incisions on either side should be extended along the inguinal ligament anteriorly and the iliac crest posteriorly. Skin paddles may be as large as 10 × 15 cm (Fig. 131.3A).[28]

STEP 2: Incision and Muscle Exposure

The superior aspect of the skin paddle is incised first along with the releasing incisions. The dissection proceeds through subcutaneous tissue down to the external oblique muscle and aponeurosis. The superior aspect of the skin paddle may be reflected off the external oblique toward the iliac crest, but the surgeon should take care to stay 3 cm away from the iliac crest. This is a critical region to leave undisturbed in order to preserve the skin perforators arising through the external oblique within 2 cm of the iliac crest. Alternatively, the skin paddle may be harvested with perforator dissection techniques to reduce the bulk and improve the mobility of the skin relative to the bone.[16,17,27] The inferior aspect of the skin paddle is incised down to the muscle layer and elevated superiorly to the iliac crest (Fig. 131.3B).

STEP 3: Muscular Dissection

The external oblique muscle is transected 3 cm superior to the iliac crest. A 3-cm muscle cuff must be preserved to protect the musculocutaneous perforators originating from the DCIA. The internal oblique muscle is divided similarly to expose the transversus abdominis. The ascending branch of the DCIA is located deep to the internal oblique and must be ligated. Alternatively, a sheet of the internal oblique muscle may be harvested in addition to the skin paddle by incorporating this muscle layer with the ascending branch. The transversus abdominis is transected with a 3-cm cuff of muscle left on the ilium to expose the underlying preperitoneal fat. Dissection at this point continues as described previously.

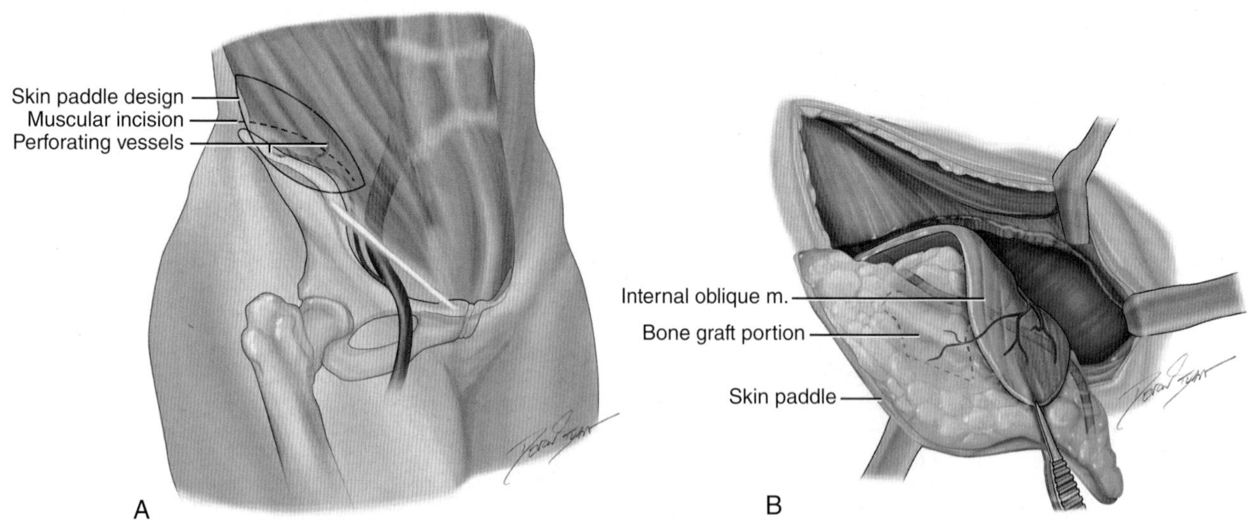

Figure 131.3 **A,** A skin paddle must include the region directly over the iliac crest and extend superiorly to capture skin perforators. **B,** Skin perforators are identified superficial to the external oblique muscle.

Avoidance and Management of Intraoperative Complications

Careful attention to detail is required during both the harvest and donor site closure. Accurate palpation of the iliac crest is often difficult in obese patients when marking skin incisions. After the skin incision is extended down to the external oblique muscle, the iliac crest and anterior superior iliac spine should again be palpated to confirm the location. During dissection of the vascular pedicle, the lateral femoral cutaneous nerve must be identified and protected. Less commonly, the ilioinguinal nerve can also be injured. Numbness and occasional pain in the thigh may result.

Removal of the iliac crest results in contour abnormalities in up to 38% of patients.[29] This may be prevented by using only the inner aspect of the ilium instead of a complete bicortical harvest. Postoperative ambulation is also improved with this technique by preserving the gluteal attachments to the lateral iliac crest. The abdominal contents should be retracted and protected during osteotomies. Injury to abdominal contents is avoided by identifying the preperitoneal fat as the transversus abdominis muscle is divided. This layer should not be dissected, as the thin peritoneum lies just beneath this plane. The anesthesia team may paralyze the patient to minimize protrusion of the abdominal contents into the surgical field.

Postoperative Considerations

A reputation for high donor site morbidity has limited the use of the DCIA free flap in many institutions. Reports on the incidence of donor site complications are varied. Difficulty in ambulation during the early postoperative period is common. Initial weakness produces a limp, which usually resolves after 3 to 6 months.[30] When compared with other commonly employed osteocutaneous flaps for head and neck reconstruction (forearm, fibula, and scapula), the DCIA flap had the lowest rate of delayed healing of the donor site with 5%, compared with 20% for the forearm and fibula and 10% for scapula free flaps.[31] When DCIA was directly compared with the fibula free flap regarding donor site morbidity and quality of life, no significant superiority of either flap was determined.[32]

Postoperative incisional hernias are a risk, especially if inadequate abdominal wall reconstruction is performed during closure. Hernias may develop in 3% to 9% of patients.[33] The risk of herniation increases with denervation of the rectus muscle. These nerves lie in the plane between the internal oblique and transversus abdominis muscles. Careful preservation of these nerves may preserve innervation to the rectus muscles.[34] An abdominal binder may be useful during the first postoperative month to allow adequate healing of the abdominal wall while avoiding herniation and wound dehiscence. If a hernia develops, surgical repair with mesh is often necessary.

Hematomas and postoperative bleeding are rare, but they most commonly develop from the oozing surface of the medullary bone. The cut edges of muscle are another common source. The surgeon should also maintain surveillance for a bleeding vessel in the region of the pedicle dissection. Blood collections are typically retroperitoneal and can hide a large amount of blood before becoming clinically obvious. Excellent hemostasis should be verified prior to closure, as the presence of a drain will not prevent bleeding complications. If a hematoma is suspected, ultrasound or computed tomography may be helpful.[35]

Bowel sounds should be confirmed prior to feeding the patient after surgery. Abdominal examination should also search for acute signs such as guarding, rebound tenderness, or rigidity. Although the abdominal cavity is not entered, manipulation and retraction of the bowels may lead to the development of an ileus.

References

1. Taylor GI, Townsend P, Corlett R. Superiority of the deep circumflex iliac vessels as the supply for free groin flaps. *PRS*. 1979;64:595.
2. Sanders R, Mayou BJ. A new vascularized bone graft transferred by microvascular anastomosis as a free flap. *Br J Surg*. 1979;66:787.
3. Franklin JD, Shack RB, Stone JD, et al. Single-stage reconstruction of mandibular and soft tissue defects using a free osteocutaneous groin flap. *Am J Surg*. 1980;140:492.
4. Safak T, Klebuc MJ, Mavili E, et al. A new design of the iliac crest microsurgical free flap without including the "obligatory" muscle cuff. *PRS*. 1997;100:1703.
5. Ramasastry Tucker J, Swartz W, Hurwitz D. The internal oblique muscle flap: an anatomic and clinical study. *PRS*. 1984;73(5):721–733.
6. Urken ML, Vickery C, Weinberg H, et al. The internal oblique-iliac crest osseomyocutaneous microvascular free flap in head and neck reconstruction. *JRM*. 1989;5:203–215.
7. Urken ML, Vickery C, Weinberg H, et al. The internal oblique-iliac crest osseomyocutaneous free flap in oromandibular reconstruction: report of 20 cases. *Arch Otolaryngol Head Neck Surg*. 1989;115:339.
8. Brown JS. Deep circumflex iliac artery free flap with internal oblique muscle as a new method of immediate reconstruction of maxillectomy defect. *Head Neck*. 1996; 18:412.
9. Brown JS, Jones DC, Summerwill A, et al. Vascularized iliac crest with internal oblique muscle for immediate reconstruction after maxillectomy. *BJOMS*. 2002;40:183.
10. Bianchi B, Ferri A, Ferrari S, et al. Iliac crest free flap for maxillary reconstruction. *JOMS*. 2010;68:2706.
11. Maranzano M, Freschi G, Atzei A, Miotti AM. Use of vascularized iliac crest with internal oblique muscle flap for mandible reconstruction. *Microsurgery*. 2005;25:299.
12. Maranzano M, Atzei A. The versatility of vascularized iliac crest with internal oblique muscle flap for composite upper maxillary reconstruction. *Microsurgery*. 2007;27:37.
13. Taylor GI. The angiosomes of the body and their supply to perforator flaps. *Clin Plast Surg*. 2003;30:331.
14. Kimata Y. Deep circumflex iliac perforator flap. *Clin Plast Surg*. 2003;30:433.
15. Kimata Y, Uchiyama K, Sakuraba M, et al. Deep circumflex iliac perforator flap with iliac crest for mandibular reconstruction. *Br J Plast Surg*. 2001;54:87.
16. Wechselberger G, Schwaiger K, Hachleitner J, et al. Facial reconstruction with a unique osteomyocutaneous DCIA perforator flap variant: a case report. *Eur Surg*. 2016;48:129–133.
17. Bergeron L, Tang M, Morris S. The anatomical basis of the deep circumflex iliac artery perforator flap with iliac crest. *PRS*. 2007;120:252.

18. Dorafshar A, Seitz I, DeWolfe M, et al. Split lateral iliac crest Chimera flap: utility of the ascending branch of the lateral femoral circumflex vessels. *PRS*. 2010;125:574.
19. Modabber N, Ayoub A, Bock SC, et al. Medial approach for minimally invasive harvesting of a deep circumflex iliac artery flap for reconstruction of the jaw using virtual surgical planning and CAD/CAM technology. *BJOMS*. 2017;55:946–951.
20. Shimizu T, Ohno K, Matsuura M, et al. An anatomical study of vascularized iliac bone grafts for dental implantation. *J Craniomaxillofac Surg*. 2002;30:184.
21. Wilkman T, Apajalahti S, Wilkman E, et al. A comparison of bone resorption over time: an analysis of the free scapular, iliac crest, and fibular microvascular flaps in mandibular reconstruction. *JOMS*. 2017.
22. Kniha K, Mohlhenrich SC, Foldenauer AC, et al. Evaluation of bone resorption in fibula and deep circumflex iliac artery flaps following dental implantation: a three-year follow-up study. *J Cranio-Maxillo-Fac Surg*. 2017;45:474–478.
23. Lia H, Tana M, Grinsell D, et al. Comparative osteoradionecrosis rates in bony reconstructions for head and neck malignancy. *JPRAS*. 2019.
24. Shaw RJ, Brown JS. Osteomyocutaneous deep circumflex iliac artery perforator flap in the reconstruction of midface defect with facial skin loss: a case report. *Microsurgery*. 2009;29:299.
25. Dumonta CE, Keela MJ, Djonovb V, et al. The Pararectus approach provides secure access to the deep circumflex iliac vessel for harvest of a large sized and vascularized segment of the iliac crest. *Injury*. 2017;48:2169–2173.
26. Iqbal M, Lloyd CJ, Paley MD, Penfold CN. Repair of the deep circumflex iliac artery free flap donor site with Protack (titanium spiral tacks) and Prolene (polypropylene) mesh. *BJOMS*. 2007;45:96.
27. Ting JW, Rozen WM, Chubb D, et al. Improving the utility and reliability of the deep circumflex iliac artery perforator flap: the use of preoperative planning with CT angiography. *Microsurgery*. 2011;31:603.
28. Ting JW, Rozen WM, Grinsell D, et al. The in vivo anatomy of the deep circumflex iliac artery perforators: defining the role for the DCIA perforator flap. *Microsurgery*. 2009;29:326.
29. Valentini V, Gennaro P, Aboh IV, et al. Iliac crest flap: donor site morbidity. *J Craniofac Surg*. 2009;20:1052.
30. Shavlokhova V, Mertens C, Engel M, et al. Do Functional Scores of flap donor sites Recover after reconstruction of segmental jaw defects? *JOMS*. 2019;1:e1–e7.
31. Kearns M, Ermogenous P, Myers S, Ghanem A. Osteocutaneous flaps for head and neck reconstruction: a focused evaluation of donor site morbidity and patient reported outcome measures in different reconstruction options. *APS*. 2018;45:495–503.
32. Schardt C, Schmid A, Bodem J, et al. Donor site morbidity and quality of life after microvascular head and neck reconstruction with free fibula and deep-circumflex iliac artery flaps. *J Cranio-Maxillo-Fac Surg*. 2017;45:e304–e311.
33. Duncan MJ, Manktelow RT, Zuker RM, Rosen IB. Mandibular reconstruction in the radiated patient: the role of osteocutaneous free tissue transfers. *PRS*. 1985;76:829.
34. Hartman EH, Spauwen PH, Jansen JA. Donor-site complications in vascularized bone flap surgery. *J Invest Surg*. 2002;15:185.
35. Arrington ED, Smith WJ, Chambers HG, et al. Complications of iliac crest bone graft harvesting. *Clin Orthop Relat Res*. 1996;329:300.

CHAPTER 132

Anterolateral Thigh (ALT) Free Flap

Omar Breik, Prav Praveen, and Sat Parmar

Armamentarium

Addison tooth tissue forceps
Allis tissue forceps (2)
Appropriate sutures
Bipolar electrocautery
Bonney blue ink
Czerny retractors (2)
DeBakey tissue forceps
Gillies toothed dissecting forceps
Jameson tenotomy scissors
Langenbeck retractors (2)
Ligaclips
Local anesthetic with vasoconstrictor
Morris retractor
Mosquito artery forceps
Needle holders
Portable nondirectional handheld 10 MHz Doppler probe (e.g., Super Dopplex D900)
Rake retractors (2)
Rampley's swab-holding forceps
Scalpel handle and #12 and #15 scalpel blades
Skin clips
Sommerlad pen
Suture scissors
Travers self-retaining retractor

History of the Procedure

The anterolateral thigh (ALT) flap is a soft tissue perforator free flap normally pedicled on the descending branch of the lateral circumflex femoral artery (LCFA). It was first described by Song et al. as a septocutaneous flap in 1984.[1] It did not initially gain widespread popularity because it was found that in most cases, the ALT skin was supplied only by musculocutaneous perforators, and septocutaneous vessels were seldom present. However, as surgeons gained experience with perforator flaps and the skills for intramuscular perforator dissection improved, use of the flap became increasingly popular. Wei et al.,[2] in particular, have enthusiastically endorsed its versatility and reliability for head and neck reconstruction, pioneering the concept of the "free-style flap."[3]

The flap may be raised as a fasciocutaneous or myocutaneous flap. It also can be raised with multiple skin paddles or as a chimeric flap with separate skin and muscle components.[4] In this way, the flap can be custom-designed to fit almost any soft tissue defect in the head and neck. The perforators are reliably positioned,[5] and the pedicle is long and wide. Two-team surgery is easily performed without the need for patient repositioning. Long-term donor site morbidity is low, and in all but the largest diameter skin harvest, the donor site may be closed primarily. In their study, Brown et al.[6] reported that patients preferred the thigh donor site, which may be easily concealed, over the more visually apparent forearm donor site.

Indications for the Use of the Procedure

Intraoral Defects

The ALT has replaced the radial forearm as the flap of choice for intraoral reconstruction in many centers, particularly in Asia.[7] Caucasian patients have a greater amount of subcutaneous fat in the thigh, resulting in a thicker flap suitable for hemiglossectomy (Fig. 132.1), subtotal or total glossectomy, and other large oral cavity defects.[8,9] However, it is probably too bulky for reconstruction of smaller oral cavity defects, especially defects affecting the ventral tongue, anterior floor of the mouth, and buccal mucosa, where the thinner, more pliable tissue of the radial forearm flap is often more appropriate. For large orofacial defects involving significant facial and intraoral soft tissue loss, the versatility of the ALT makes it an ideal soft tissue option to consider either independently or in combination with other flaps such as a fibula.[10] Where perforators permit, multi-paddled chimeric ALT can also be used to reconstruct multiple subunits more anatomically using a single flap.[11]

Facial, Scalp, and Skull Base Defects

A large skin area may be harvested to reconstruct extensive defects resulting from cancer ablation or trauma. The skin is more pliable and may achieve a better contour compared with alternative donor sites, such as the latissimus dorsi and rectus abdominis. Flap thickness may be an advantage in

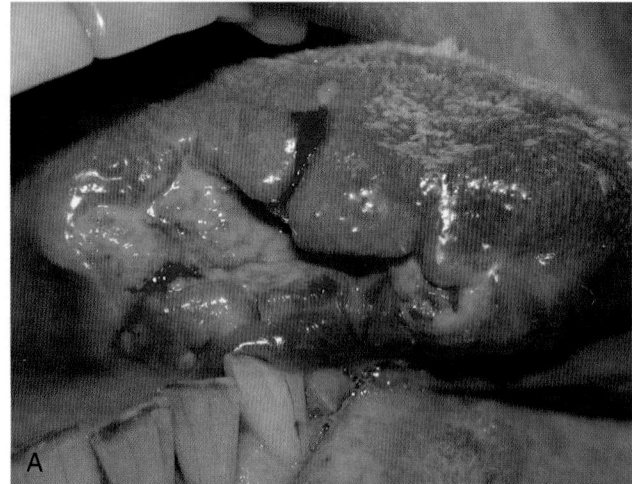

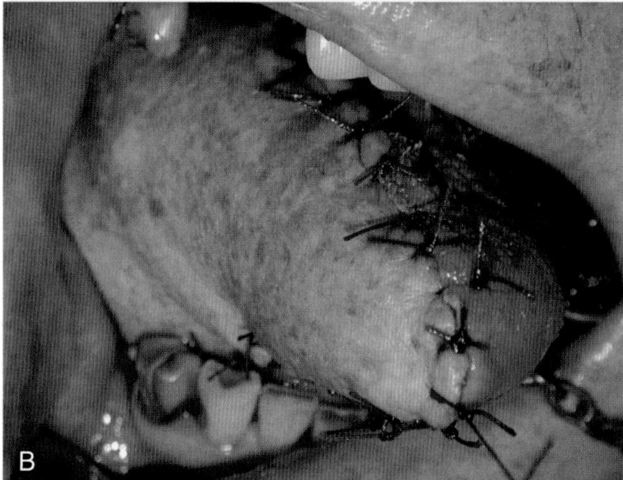

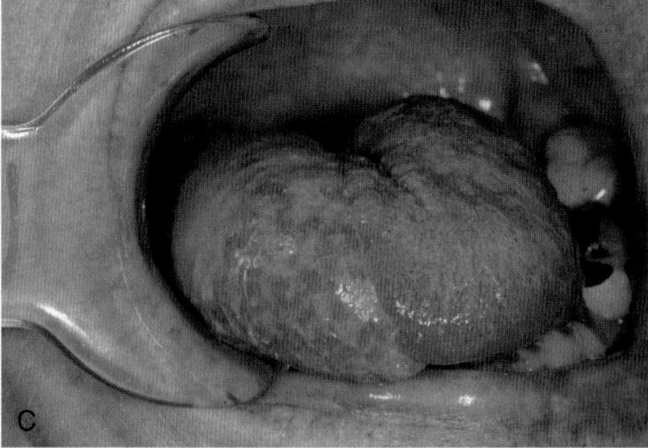

Figure 132.1 **A,** Patient with cT3 squamous cell carcinoma of the right lateral tongue. **B,** Tumor resected and reconstructed with anterolateral thigh flap. **C,** Six months after surgery, showing excellent integration of the flap to the tongue. (Courtesy RJ Shaw/JS Brown, Liverpool, UK.)

reconstruction of defects of the skull base and those resulting from radical composite parotid resection (Fig. 132.2). The flap bulk may be further augmented in these cases, if desired, by harvesting a segment of vastus lateralis muscle with the flap.

Pharyngolaryngectomy Defects

Partial pharyngeal reconstruction with an ALT or a radial forearm flap have been proven reliable. The advantage of the ALT over the radial forearm is the reduced donor site morbidity, more robust fascia for second layer coverage, larger possible skin paddle and the option of vascularized muscle flap for coverage of exposed great vessels. For circumferential pharyngeal reconstruction, the tubed ALT has gained in popularity over the jejunum for pharyngolaryngectomy reconstruction in recent years. The skin provides increased rigidity compared with the jejunum, and the ability to harvest a fascial flange surrounding the cutaneous aspect of the flap allows for two-layered, watertight closure. Some evidence suggests that the ALT is superior to jejunal flaps with regard to tracheoesophageal speech and swallowing and avoids the risks associated with a laparotomy.[12] However, the enthusiasm to abandon the jejunal flap in favor of the ALT is not universal, and these authors have reported an increased stricture rate for ALT reconstruction of circumferential defects.[13] This experience is consistent with the findings of a recent systematic review that also found fistula and stricture rates are higher in fasciocutaneous pharyngeal reconstructions than jejunum flaps.[14]

Surgical Anatomy

The ALT flap is pedicled on the descending branch of the LCFA, which is the largest branch of the profunda femoris system (Fig. 132.3). The pedicle is made up of one artery and usually two veins and runs in the intermuscular septum between the rectus femoris and vastus lateralis muscles, along with the motor nerve supply to the vastus lateralis. The pedicle length ranges from 8 to 16 cm. If harvested at its takeoff from the profunda femoral vessels, it has a vessel diameter of at least 2 mm,[15] and typically 4 mm for the artery and 6 mm for the veins. The pedicle gives off perforating branches to the rectus femoris and vastus lateralis and septocutaneous branches to the skin of the ALT (although, as already mentioned, these are not reliably present). Some of the vastus perforators terminate by piercing the deep fascia to supply the skin of the ALT. These perforating branches are dissected to harvest the flap.

Limitations and Contraindications

The anatomy of the ALT flap is less predictable than that of other soft tissue alternatives. Although perforators are rarely absent, their numbers and position can vary considerably. The variations are summarized well in a paper by Shieh et al., 2000.[16] This limits the surgeon's control over flap thickness and pedicle length. If the only suitable perforators are in a proximal position in the thigh (possibly originating from the transverse rather than the descending branch of the LCFA), the flap tends to be bulkier and to

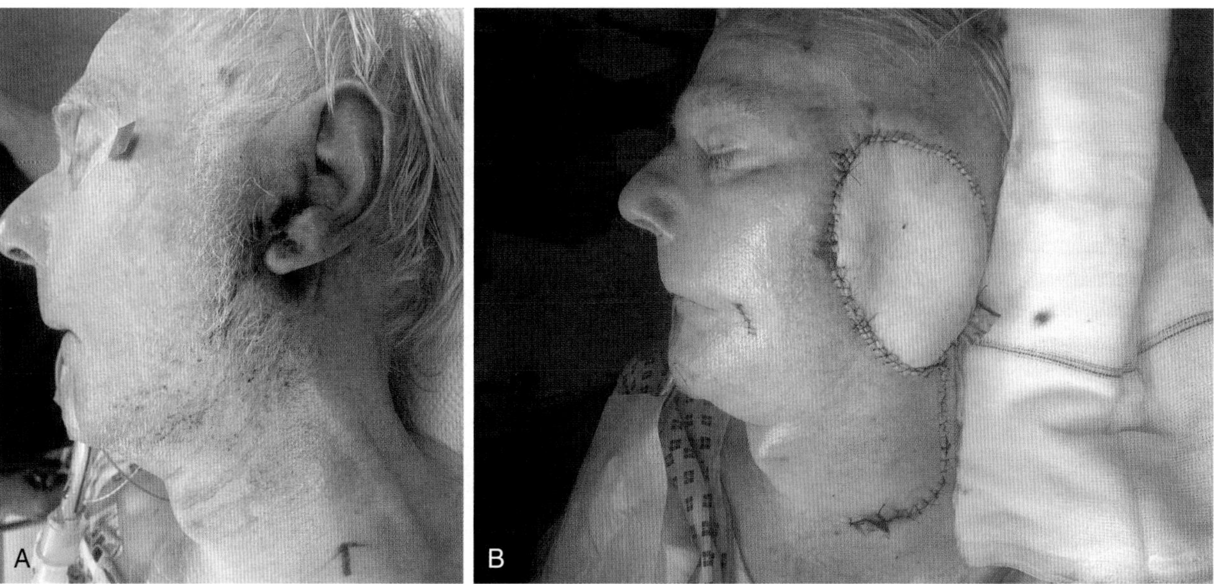

Figure 132.2 **A,** Squamous cell carcinoma of the right parotid fungating onto the cheek involving the pinna. **B,** After radical resection and reconstruction with an anterolateral thigh flap.

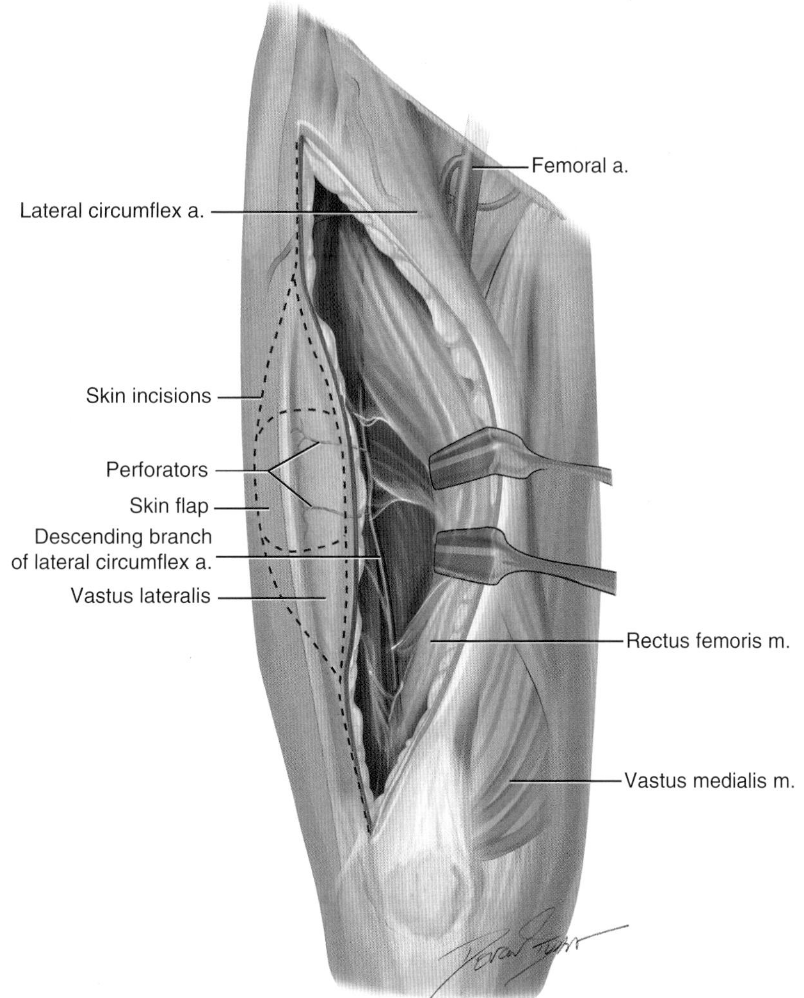

Figure 132.3 Surgical anatomy: The intermuscular septum between the vastus lateralis and the rectus femoris has been opened, and the rectus muscle has been retracted medially. The descending branch of the lateral circumflex femoral artery pedicle can be seen in the gutter between the muscles. Two perforators are seen coming off the pedicle to traverse the vastus muscle before piercing the fascia to supply the skin of the anterolateral thigh.

have a shorter pedicle. The harvest time is also very difficult to predict. Early identification of a large septocutaneous perforator can significantly reduce the harvest time to less than an hour. However, musculocutaneous dissection of multiple small, tortuous perforators can be a slow process, and raising of the flap should commence at the same time as the neck dissection.

Because of the increased bulkiness of the flap seen in overweight patients (particularly Caucasian females, who have increased subcutaneous fat in the thigh), the ALT probably should be avoided in such patients when thin, pliable tissue is required (e.g., for small intraoral defects or for a tubed reconstruction of a pharyngolaryngectomy defect). A simple pinch test (between thumb and index finger) is a good estimation of the suitability of the ALT. Some authors advocate aggressive flap thinning or suprafascial harvesting, but this is not recommended for those new to the technique, and an alternative reconstruction should be considered.

Donor site morbidity is low, and the site can nearly always be closed primarily (up to a maximum width of 8 to 10 cm, depending on the size of the thigh and the laxity of the skin). However, if a large flap has been harvested, the need for skin grafting of the donor site increases the morbidity and may result in a long, slow, healing process.

TECHNIQUE: ALT Harvest Technique

STEP 1: Setup and Marking

The flap may be harvested at the same time as tumor resection or neck vessel access. A right-handed surgeon will find the right leg easiest to dissect. With the foot in the neutral position, a line is marked from the anterior superior iliac spine (ASIS) to the superolateral margin of the patella (SLP). This line corresponds to the intermuscular septum between the rectus femoris and vastus lateralis muscles. The midpoint of the line is marked, and a circle with a 4-cm radius is drawn around this point. This circle is the most likely position of skin perforators from the LCFA. The position of the perforators is then mapped with a handheld Doppler probe and marked on the skin. These marks are used only as a guide because they do not always correlate reliably with the position or presence of the perforators on surgical exploration. The false-negative rate for Doppler mapping is higher in patients with a high body mass index, and the false-positive rate is higher in lean patients.[17] The apparent absence of audible perforators on Doppler mapping should not necessarily dissuade the surgeon from attempting the flap. After Doppler mapping, the line from ASIS to SLP is redrawn, bowing medially in the midpoint to avoid the marked perforators by about 4 cm (or more if a very wide flap is to be raised). This line is the incision line and forms the medial aspect of the skin paddle.

STEP 2: Prepping and Draping

The lower abdomen, ASIS, ipsilateral groin, and leg circumferentially to below the knee should be prepared with povidone-iodine solution. The foot and lower leg are covered with a sterile booty drape; a cuffed extremity drape is then passed over the foot and lower leg, advanced to the proximal limit of the limb, and fixed to skin, exposing the ASIS (Fig. 132.4A).

STEP 3: Incision

The incision follows the predrawn line from the ASIS to the SLP, bowing medially in the middle to avoid damage to the perforators. The incision is deepened through subcutaneous fat and deep fascia to expose the underlying muscle (see Fig. 132.4B).

STEP 4: Identification of Perforators

The cut fascial edge on the lateral side is sutured to the lateral skin edge with 2-0 suture, which is cut long to allow a heavy clip or Allis forceps to be suspended from its length to apply gentle lateral traction. More forceful lateral traction is not necessary and risks avulsion of the smaller perforators. The dissection proceeds laterally on the deep aspect of the fascia on a broad front; the surgeon must take care to avoid damage to the perforators, which are readily identified as small vessels piercing the deep aspect of the fascia from the muscle. This dissection may be performed carefully with a #15 blade or by inserting the tips of the dissection scissors just under the free edge of the fascia and opening the tips to open the plane between fascia and muscle. Once identified, the perforators are marked by drawing a semicircle in Bonney's blue ink on the fascia around the perforator. This helps prevent inadvertent damage to the perforator later on, when the field has become bloodied and the perforator has spasmed (see Fig. 132.4C). The authors also create a small V-shaped notch in the skin edge at the level of the perforators. This ensures the surgeon is always aware of the approximate position of the perforators even during inset.

STEP 5: Identification of the Pedicle

The rectus muscle is retracted superolaterally with skin hooks or rake retractors. The intermuscular septum between the rectus femoris and vastus lateralis is opened with a combination of sharp dissection along the lateral border of the rectus and blunt dissection by sweeping the thumb of the left hand into the plane to separate the muscles. Vessels supplying the rectus muscle will be encountered and must be ligated or coagulated. The rectus muscle is retracted medially with Langenbeck retractors to expose the descending branch of the LCFA, which runs in the gutter between the muscles (see Fig. 132.4D).

TECHNIQUE: ALT Harvest Technique—*cont'd*

STEP 6: Perforator Dissection

Magnification with loupes (×2.5) is recommended. If a septocutaneous perforator is identified, this can be quickly mobilized. In most cases, however, musculocutaneous perforators must be dissected. Dissection begins with deroofing of the muscle covering the perforator using fine tenotomy scissors (e.g., Jameson scissors). The scissor tips are inserted into the perivascular plane between the perforator and the overlying muscle to a depth of 0.5 to 1 cm. The muscle is then gently tented up and incised. Many tiny branches usually arise from the lateral aspects of the perforator to supply the adjacent muscle, but much less so from the top of the vessel. This allows incision of the overlying muscle normally without excess bleeding. The dissection proceeds in a similar way to the dissection of the facial nerve in a parotidectomy. The assistant should gently retract the cut edge of the muscle on either side of the perforator with Allis forceps to improve visibility. It is safest to stay right on the perforator to avoid inadvertently cutting it. Once the perforator has been deroofed, it must be mobilized from the muscular bed by lateral dissection. The tiny lateral branches must be managed with microvascular Ligaclips or low-power bipolar microdiathermy forceps. Placement of the tips of the bipolar forceps on or directly adjacent to the perforator should be avoided to prevent thermal damage to these vessels. Instead, the tips should be placed a few millimeters away from the vessels; in this way, a small cuff of muscle is raised with the perforator, affording it extra protection. The perforators often take a very tortuous route through the vastus muscle to reach the pedicle. This stage of the procedure should not be rushed, and adequate time must be

Continued

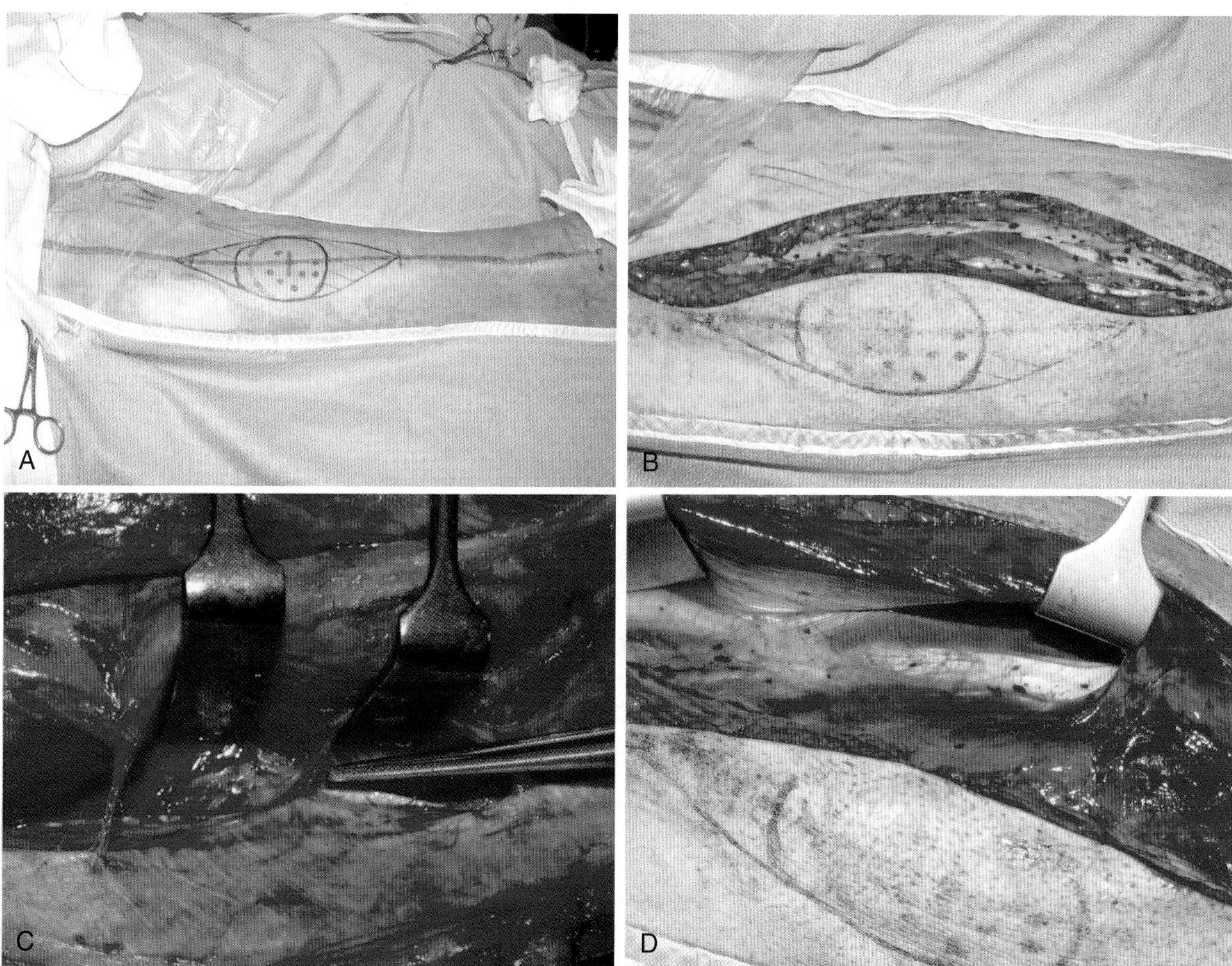

Figure 132.4 **A,** Right leg mapped for perforators using Doppler ultrasound. The leg has also been prepared and draped for surgery. **B,** Initial incision along a line from the anterior superior iliac spine to the superolateral patella. An incision is made through the skin, subcutaneous fat, and fascia to expose the underlying rectus femoris muscle. **C,** Careful dissection is performed on the deep aspect of the fascia to expose the perforators. **D,** Medial retraction of the rectus muscle exposes the pedicle (descending branch of lateral circumflex femoral artery).

TECHNIQUE: ALT Harvest Technique—*cont'd*

allowed for completion of the dissection without pressure. Starting from the most distal perforator, all identified perforators should be dissected before any decisions are made about the design of the flap paddle (see Fig. 132.4E and F). In the authors' experience, once the distal perforator is dissected to the pedicle, ligate the distal limb of the descending branch of the lateral circumflex artery. This improves flow through the perforators, making further perforator dissections easier.

STEP 7: Dissection of the Pedicle

The artery and its venae comitantes are dissected from the takeoff point of the most distal perforator proximally to the takeoff point of the pedicle from the LCFA. Dissection is aided by superomedial retraction of the rectus femoris muscle using a Czerny retractor or self-retaining retractor. Multiple branching vessels will be identified along the course of the pedicle and should be ligated unless, of course, a chimeric flap with a muscular paddle is planned. Mobilize the pedicle completely before completing the skin paddle dissection.

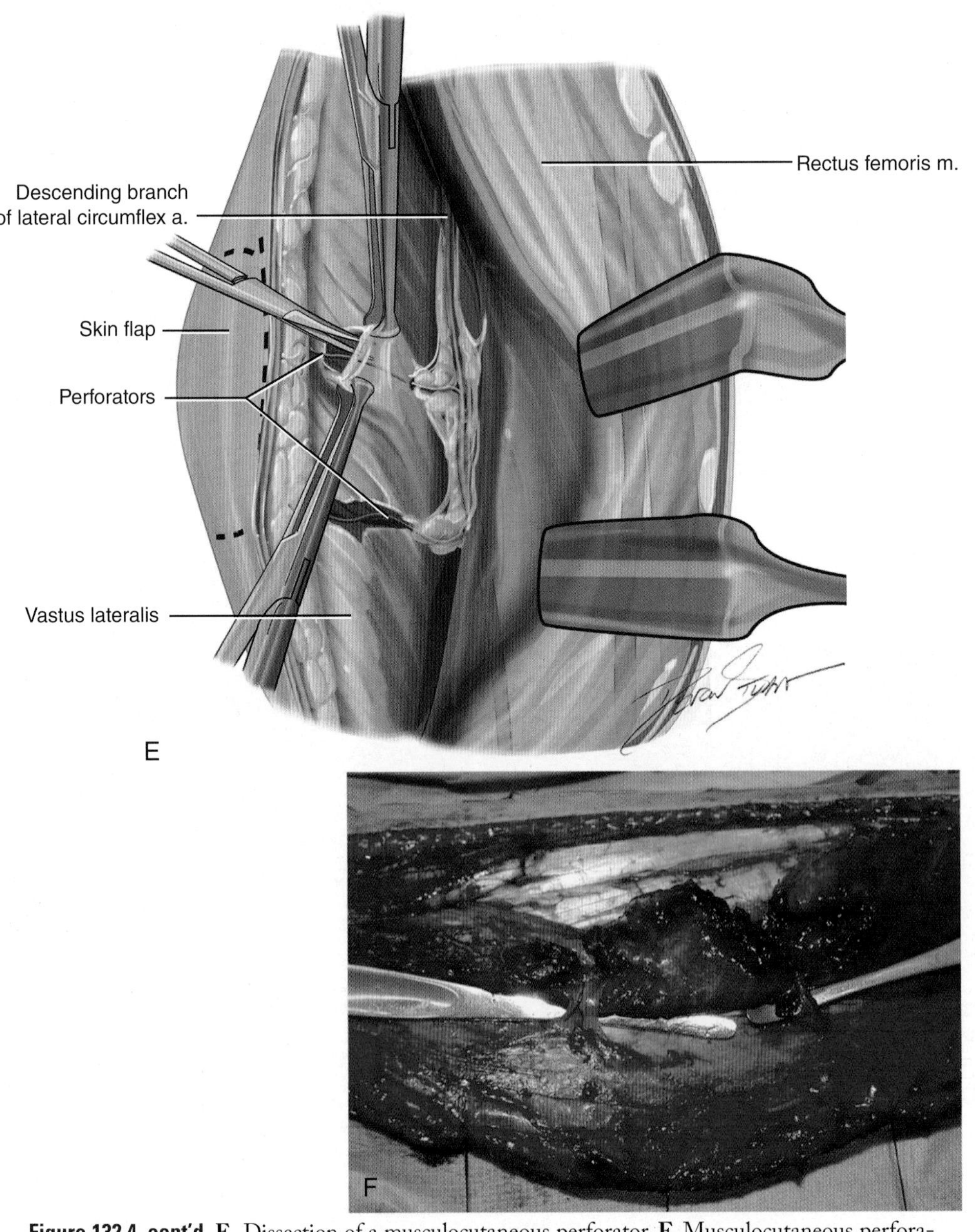

Figure 132.4, cont'd **E,** Dissection of a musculocutaneous perforator. **F,** Musculocutaneous perforators dissected.

TECHNIQUE: ALT Harvest Technique—*cont'd*

STEP 8: Considerations Before Final Flap Harvest and Detachment

The final skin incision and detachment of the flap should be delayed until the neck dissection and tumor ablation are complete. There are several benefits to this. First, it allows the final dimensions of the flap to be revised based on the size of the completed resection defect. Second, there is some scope for altering the diameter of the donor vessels, depending on what vessels are available in the neck after the neck dissection. The pedicle may be detached at the LCFA itself (i.e., above the trifurcation of the descending, oblique, and transverse branches), providing larger vessels for anastomosis, or, more commonly, below the trifurcation at the descending branch, providing a slightly smaller vessel that is often suitable for end-to-end anastomosis with the facial artery. Finally, in some cases in which there is a choice of potential perforators, the position of the flap in the thigh may be selected, depending on the desired thickness and pliability of the flap. The skin and subcutaneous fat are bulkiest in the proximal thigh and become progressively thinner distally. Some sources have suggested a flap thickness in Caucasians of 4 cm in the upper thigh, 3 cm in the midthigh, and 2 cm in the lower thigh. The desire for extra bulk must be offset by the reduced pedicle length that comes with a more proximal flap harvest.

Continued

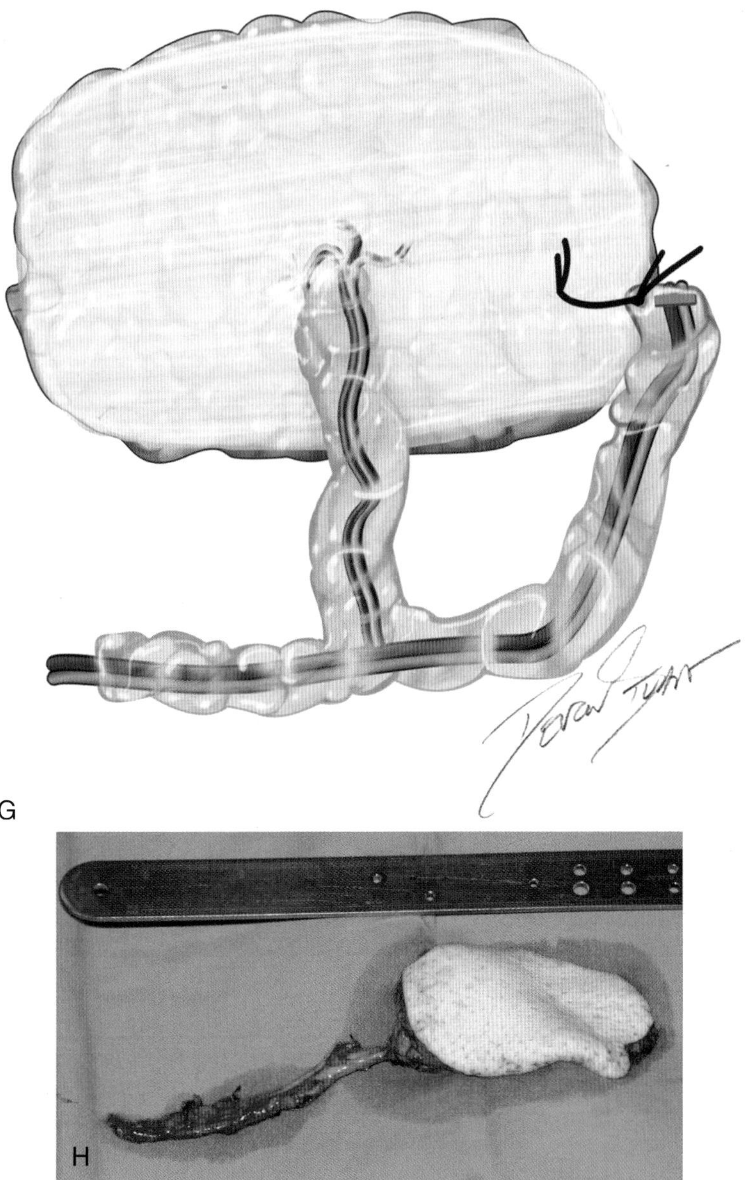

Figure 132.4, cont'd **G,** Detached flap with distal pedicle sutured to the edge of the fascia; this is done to help prevent twisting of the perforator/pedicle. **H,** Detached flap awaiting inset and anastomosis.

TECHNIQUE: ALT Harvest Technique—*cont'd*

This flap can be harvested based on a single perforator; however, this creates the possibility of inadvertent twisting of the perforator, resulting in flap compromise. Obviously, the best way to avoid this is to harvest the flap based on two or more perforators, but that is not always possible. The risk of twisting may be minimized by marking the top of the perforator and distal pedicle with Bonney's blue ink before detachment of the skin paddle from the leg. Another useful technique is to dissect out the pedicle distal to the perforator, section it, and suture this free end to the fascia at the edge of the flap. This provides the antitwisting benefits of a second perforator[8] (although obviously not the vascular perfusion benefits!) (see Fig. 132.4G).

STEP 9: Completion of the Skin Paddle Harvest

The surgeon draws the back-cut to outline the desired paddle size, making sure to include the perforators. The position of the perforators may be marked either with ink or, more accurately, by passing a suture through the skin from medial to lateral 1 cm below the perforator. The surgeon makes the incision through skin, fat, and fascia while holding the skin paddle in the nondominant hand with the ring and little fingers below the perforators, offering further protection. It is important to be mindful of the fact that once the skin incision is complete, the sometimes bulky skin paddle is attached to the leg only by the often flimsy perforator, which can easily become avulsed. The skin paddle is cradled in the nondominant hand and elevated so that any final dissection of the perforators and pedicle may be completed. Depending on the type of reconstruction, modification and shaping of the skin paddle can be performed after detachment during inset, or while the tissue is still vascularized before detachment. For a total glossectomy defect, an elliptical skin paddle can be inset and folded, de-epithelializing excess skin (and burying the de-epithelialized segments), to create a protruding tongue segment with a central anterior suture line within the skin paddle itself. If using this technique, then modification of the skin paddle can only be made intraorally once inset is commenced. However, if a specific design of skin paddle is being followed, then modification of the skin paddle can be made before detachment. For total and subtotal glossectomy reconstruction, various designs have been described in the recent literature, including the cathedral triptych,[18] mushroom-shaped,[19] or five-point eight-line segment design.[20] It remains unclear whether these designs lead to better functional outcomes.

STEP 10: Detachment

The vessels are clamped proximally, and the flap is passed to the top end for inset. The clamped vessels are ligated with a 3-0 transfixion suture (see Fig. 132.4H).

STEP 11: Donor Site Closure

Any bleeding points are coagulated with bipolar diathermy. A suction drain is inserted and fixed to the skin with a 2-0 silk suture. Defects of up to 10 cm usually can be closed primarily with 2-0 braided resorbable subcutaneous suture and 3-0 monofilament skin suture or skin staples for the skin. Very large defects may require closure with a split-thickness skin graft, necessitating an additional donor site. Tissue expansion to allow primary closure of the donor site has been reported but may not be practical for cancer surgery.

STEP 12: Monitoring

Flaps used for reconstruction of a cutaneous defect are easily monitored with handheld Doppler ultrasound probe positioned over the perforator. This may not be possible with an intraoral defect, for which reliance on the appearance of the flap and the ability to demonstrate a blanch and subsequent capillary refill on pressure are often necessary. Alternatively, the pedicle can be monitored with an implantable Cook-Swartz Doppler probe, which may provide reassurance with buried flaps (e.g., after ALT pharyngolaryngectomy reconstruction).

ALTERNATIVE TECHNIQUE: Pharyngeal Reconstruction

Pharyngeal reconstruction after laryngopharyngectomy requires a few unique techniques to optimize outcomes which are worthy of mention here. The shape of the skin paddle needs to be considered early.

Partial Pharyngectomy

Often a slightly wider part of the flap is needed for the proximal pharynx than the distal pharynx. A coffin-shaped skin paddle design provides extra width and skin proximally to ensure tension-free closure (Fig. 132.5A). Additionally, taking a cuff of fascia that is wider than the skin paddle provides a vascularized second layer over the mucosal anastomosis. When insetting this flap shape, the tip of the coffin is oriented anteriorly. The mucosal layer is closed first with a continuous Cushing suture or interrupted inverted double mattress sutures. The second layer of fascia is then sutured to surrounding muscle to further reinforce the mucosal repair (see Fig. 132.5B). These

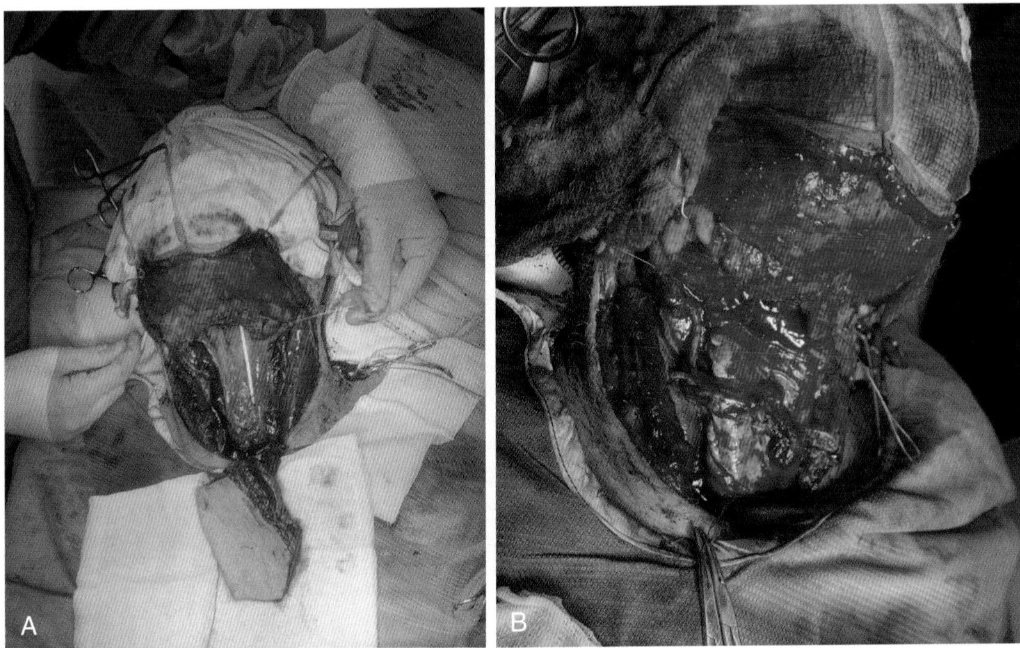

Figure 132.5 **A,** Partial pharyngectomy defect. Coffin-shaped anterolateral thigh laid out on the drapes prior to inset. The point on the coffin will be inset anteriorly to the proximal pharynx. **B,** Flap inset performed with double layer inset. Vascular anastomoses in the right neck.

closures are performed prior to anastomosis especially on the side of anastomosis as access is better.

Circumferential Pharyngectomy

The tubed ALT is designed in a rectangular or slightly trapezoidal shape, with the slightly wider end used for the proximal pharynx for the same reasons as described above (Fig. 132.6A). A cuff of fascia wider than the skin paddle is also valuable for a second layer closure, especially when the patient has a thick subcutaneous fat layer. The ALT is then fashioned into a tube shape around a salivary bypass tube (see Fig. 132.6B), and the skin closure can be performed while still vascularized in the leg with continuous Cushing sutures or interrupted inverted double mattress sutures (see Fig. 132.6C). If possible, a second layer of closure over the skin closure is performed with the fascia. Once inset into the pharynx, this anastomosed surface can be facing anteriorly or posteriorly depending on what seems preferable for the lie of the pedicle vessels. Where possible, having this surface facing the prevertebral fascia will be ideal. If the fascial layer is not wide enough for a second layer closure, then it could be sutured to the prevertebral fascia as close to the skin closure/anastomosis as possible. The proximal mucosal anastomosis is then performed, followed by the distal anastomosis. The salivary bypass tube is ideally kept in situ for 4 to 6 weeks.

Avoidance and Management of Intraoperative Complications

- Absence of perforators: Although this complication is rare (occurring in about 1% to 6% of cases),[21,22] it nevertheless is prudent to obtain the patient's prior consent for an alternative flap in case it becomes necessary.
- Perforator damage during the initial incision: The initial incision may result in irreparable damage to the largest or only perforator. This risk is minimized by ensuring that the marked incision line bows medially by 4 cm in the region of the marked perforator/midline, as suggested in the technique section.
- Perforator damage during dissection: A learning curve is associated with perforator flap harvesting, but damage to the delicate perforators may occur even in experienced hands. It is important to perform perforator dissection slowly and meticulously, without the pressure of time constraints.
- Perforator or pedicle twisting: This is one of the main causes of flap failure, and great care must be taken at the time of flap inset. The risk may be minimized by following the tips outlined in the technique section.

Postoperative Considerations

Regular flap observations and clinical assessment are required to ensure adequate perfusion to the ALT flap. Even if an implantable Doppler is used and it demonstrates good flow in the pedicle, it does not necessarily mean adequate perfusion through the perforators to the skin. Although as a rule, clinical assessment is more important than Doppler signal for monitoring all free flaps, it is especially relevant in perforator flaps such as the ALT.

Drain output is monitored postoperatively and is removed once the drain output is <30 mL per day. The main

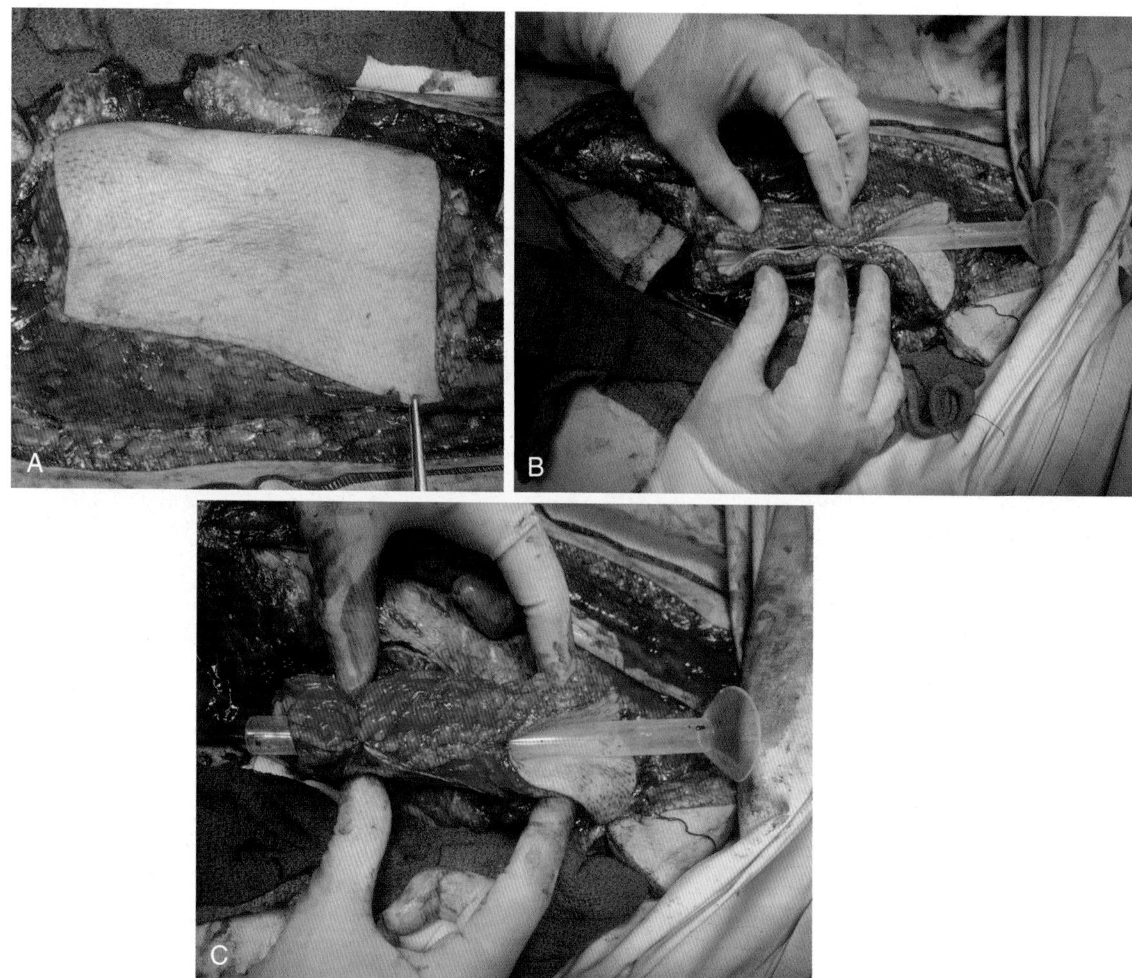

Figure 132.6 **A,** Trapezoidal-shaped skin paddle 12 cm width proximally and 10 cm width distally. **B,** Rolling the spin paddle around a salivary bypass tube. **C,** Skin closure is performed first. Note that thickness of the ALT in this case did not allow the fascia to be adequately wrapped around for a second layer over the repair. More fasciae should have been harvested.

postoperative risk is seroma formation likely secondary to the muscle disruption required in the perforator dissection. A simple dressing is applied unless a split-thickness skin graft is needed for closure. In this case, then a pressure dressing is applied for 10 days before inspection. There are no limitations to mobilization postoperatively. Overall, the incidence of short-term donor site morbidity is low, with lower rates of wound dehiscence and tendon exposure than the radial forearm free flap.[23] Minimal long-term donor site morbidity is associated with ALT flaps. Although the scar frequently runs the length of the thigh, patients generally prefer this to the alternative on the forearm. If the nerve supply to the vastus is sacrificed, which is not infrequent during dissection of the pedicle, a measurable but minimal thigh weakness results. Any gait disturbance normally resolves in the following weeks or months. Sensory alteration in the thigh may also occur.

References

1. Song YG, Chen GZ, Song YL. The free thigh flap: a new free flap concept based on the septocutaneous artery. *Br J Plast Surg.* 1984;37(2):149–159.
2. Wei FC, Jain V, Celik N, Chen HC, Chuang DC-C., Lin CH. Have we found an ideal soft-tissue flap? An experience with 672 anterolateral thigh flaps. *Plast Reconstr Surg.* 2002;109(7):2219–2226.
3. Wei F-C., Mardini S. Free-style free flaps. *Plast Reconstr Surg.* 2004;114(4):910–916.
4. Adler N, Dorafshar AH, Agarwal JP, Gottlieb LJ. Harvesting the lateral femoral circumflex chimera free flap: guidelines for elevation. *Plast Reconstr Surg.* 2009;123(3):918–925.
5. Yu P, Youssef A. Efficacy of the handheld Doppler in preoperative identification of the cutaneous perforators in the anterolateral thigh flap. *Plast Reconstr Surg.* 2006;118(4):928–933.
6. Katre C, Brown JS, Rogers SN, et al. Patient preference in placement of donor site scar in head and neck cancer free flap reconstruction. *Int J Oral Maxillofac Surg.* 2007;36(11):1059.
7. Wong C-H., Wei F-C.. Microsurgical free flap in head and neck reconstruction. *Head Neck.* 2010;32(9):1236–1245.
8. Shaw RJ, Batstone MD, Blackburn TK, Brown JS. The anterolateral thigh flap in head and neck reconstruction: "pearls and pitfalls". *Br J Oral Maxillofac Surg.* 2010;48(1):5–10.

9. Yu P, Robb GL. Reconstruction for total and near-total glossectomy defects. *Clin Plast Surg*. 2005;32(3):411–419. vii.
10. Brinkman J, Kambiz S, de Jong T, Mureau M. Long-term outcomes after double free flap reconstruction for locally advanced head and neck cancer. *J Reconstr Microsur*. 2019;35(1): 66–73.
11. Jiang C, Guo F, Li N, et al. Multipaddled anterolateral thigh chimeric flap for reconstruction of complex defects in head and neck. *PLoS One*. 2014;9(9):e106326.
12. Yu P, Hanasono MM, Skoracki RJ, et al. Pharyngoesophageal reconstruction with the anterolateral thigh flap after total laryngopharyngectomy. *Cancer*. 2010;116(7):1718–1724.
13. Parmar S, Al Asaadi Z, Martin T, Jennings C, Pracy P. The anterolateral fasciocutaneous thigh flap for circumferential pharyngeal defects—can it really replace the jejunum? *Br J Oral Maxillofac Surg*. 2014;52(3): 247–250.
14. Koh HK, Tan NC, Tan BK, Ooi ASH. Comparison of outcomes of fasciocutaneous free flaps and jejunal free flaps in pharyngolaryngoesophageal reconstruction: a systematic review and meta-analysis. *Ann Plast Surg*. 2019;82(6):646–652.
15. Chana JS, Wei FC. A review of the advantages of the anterolateral thigh flap in head and neck reconstruction. *Br J Plast Surg*. 2004;57(7):603–609.
16. Shieh SJ, Chiu HY, Yu JC, Pan SC, Tsai ST, Shen CL. Free anterolateral thigh flap for reconstruction of head and neck defects following cancer ablation. *Plast Reconstr Surg*. 2000;105(7):2349–2357.
17. Shaw RJ, Batstone MD, Blackburn TK, Brown JS. Preoperative Doppler assessment of perforator anatomy in the anterolateral thigh flap. *Br J Oral Maxillofac Surg*. 2010;48(6):419–422.
18. Leymarie N, Karsenti G, Sarfati B, Rimareix F, Kolb F. Modification of flap design for total mobile tongue reconstruction using a sensitive antero-lateral thigh flap. *J Plast Reconstr Aesthet Surg*. 2012;65(7):e169–e174.
19. Longo B, Pagnoni M, Ferri G, Morello R, Santanelli F. The mushroom-shaped anterolateral thigh perforator flap for subtotal tongue reconstruction. *Plast Reconstr Surg*. 2013;132(3):656–665.
20. Fan S, Zhang H, Li Q, et al. A novel anatomy-based five-points eight-line-segments technique for precision subtotal tongue reconstruction: a pilot study. *Oral Oncol*. 2019;89:1–7.
21. Wong C-H., Wei F-C., Fu B, Chen Y-A., Lin J-Y.. Alternative vascular pedicle of the anterolateral thigh flap: the oblique branch of the lateral circumflex femoral artery. *Plast Reconstr Surg*. 2009;123(2):571–577.
22. Yu P. Characteristics of the anterolateral thigh flap in a Western population and its application in head and neck reconstruction. *Head Neck*. 2004;26(9):759–769.
23. Knott PD, Seth R, Waters HH. Short-term donor site morbidity: a comparison of the anterolateral thigh and radial forearm fasciocutaneous free flaps. *Head Neck*. 2016;38(1):E945–E948.

CHAPTER 133

Skin Grafting

Miller H. Smith and Colin MacIver

Armamentarium

Appropriate sutures
Cotton balls
Dermabond/Indermil
Dermatome knife
Dermatome, motorized
Dilute epinephrine–soaked gauze (ampule of 1:1000 mixed in 500 mL normal saline 0.9%)
Local anesthetic with vasoconstrictor
Mepitel silicone dressing
Metzenbaum scissors
Mineral oil
Monocryl or Prolene/nylon suture
Scalpel, #15 blade
Silk suture
Tegaderm/OpSite dressing
Thermoplastic beads
Topical thrombin spray
Xeroform gauze or Alginate dressing

History of the Procedure

Reverdin first noted the success of skin grafting in a human patient in 1869, when he removed multiple small pieces of epidermis and autotransplanted them onto a bed of granulation tissue. Due to techniques with "pinch" grafting, Lawson demonstrated success with larger full-thickness grafts in 1870. Ollier thereafter reported improved success with grafts when the donor site was prepared and débrided to healthy fresh tissue. Thiersch evolved the principles of proper debridement and was the first to demonstrate success using thinner grafts with improved survival and allowing the donor site to heal by reepithelialization without an open wound. Blair and Brown's paper published in 1929 highlighted the benefits and disadvantages of split-thickness grafts and explained how to achieve reliable success and survival. The current focus is on tissue preparation, innovative dressings to improve and accelerate healing, and tissue engineering techniques that will expand cell populations for vastly reduced donor site size.[1,2]

Indications for the Use of the Procedure

Within the scope of oral maxillofacial surgery, there are several indications for split-thickness and full-thickness grafting. Grafts are frequently required to repair defects to the head and neck region related to trauma, pathologic/oncologic resection, facial burns, contracture release, and congenital or developmental conditions. In addition, the reconstructive maxillofacial surgeon also utilizes grafts to repair donor site defects following microvascular free flap surgery harvest (Fig. 133.1).

Skin grafts inherently differ based on the amount of dermis harvested. The epidermal layer is quite thin (0.075 to 0.15 mm) compared with the dermis (1 to 4 mm) and is completely harvested in all types of skin grafts. The dermal layer has much more variability in thickness based on location and patient age. Thinner dermis is located on the eyelids; it increases in thickness over the temples and scalp and is thickest over the back. The dermis thickens as children mature to adulthood and then thins out after the fifth decade.[1]

Full-thickness grafts harvest the entirety of both the epidermis and dermis, thereby requiring the donor site to be closed primarily over top of the underlying subcutaneous tissue to allow for proper healing. Split-thickness grafts split the dermal layer to leave the residual dermis overlying the subcutaneous tissue to heal with secondary reepithelialization. A split-thickness graft can be harvested at a variety of selected thicknesses (0.3 to 0.45 mm/0.012 to 0.018 inch). As thinner grafts are believed to be more reliable for success, often the 0.012-inch setting is used. A handheld purpose-made knife can be used for harvest, but some irregularity and variable thickness can result. Air-driven or electric dermatomes have adjustable thickness controls and interchangeable footplates for the preselected width of the harvest. These dermatomes can allow for uniform harvest at a reliable thickness (Fig. 133.2). The donor site often heals within a period of 7 to 21 days, and a variety of dressings are advocated to minimize delays in healing.[3]

Grafting can be considered as a primary treatment strategy or can be delayed if necessary, depending on the wound. When evaluating the recipient site, the surgeon addresses several requirements to optimize graft healing and minimize failures. These include good regional vascularity, the absence of local infection, and a lack of residual tumor. Certain tissue types may afford decreased success rates during healing due to complicating factors. An actively bleeding wound bed will not allow good contact with the graft due to fluid tension

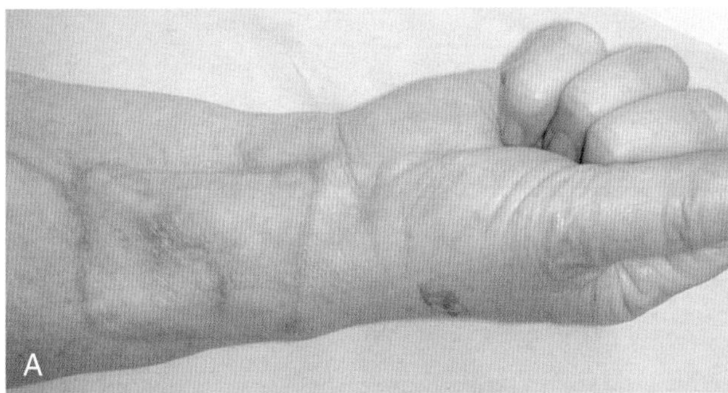

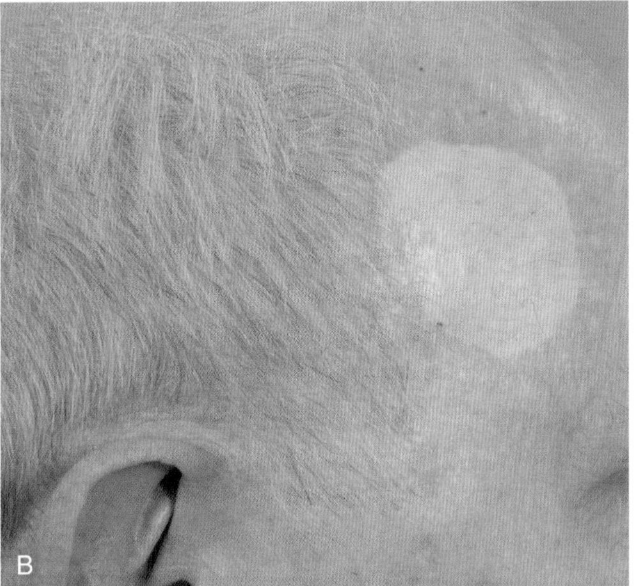

Figure 133.1 Healed skin graft to radial forearm defect (**A**) and to temple defect (**B**).

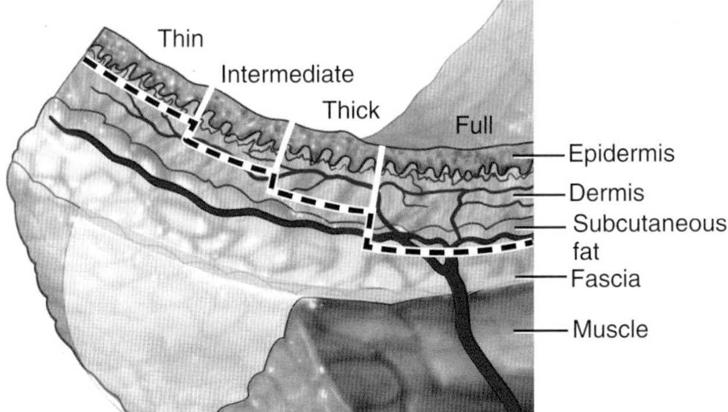

Figure 133.2 Depth of split-thickness and full-thickness skin grafts.

and ballooning. Exposed cortical bone, cartilage, and tendons pose difficulties for complete graft take.[4,5] Maintaining a small layer of periosteum, perichondrium, and paratenon is helpful but not if it sacrifices marginal clearance during tumor excision. Hypovascular tissues can be problematic due to fibrosis of the adjacent arterial and venous supply caused by prior irradiation or underlying scar tissue from burns or repeated surgeries. In these challenging cases it is usually necessary to employ additional graft and wound bed preparation along with the use of specialty dressings.

Many wounds demonstrate a bed of granulation tissue, and it is imperative that this tissue is healthy and has minimal bacterial colonization. Sampling tissue for approximate bacterial counts from the recipient bed in delayed procedures can help guide treatment to avoid untoward difficulties with graft healing. It is well accepted that bacterial counts less than 10^5/g tissue can successfully take a graft, with lower counts affording better results in ideal situations. Local and systemic antibiotics and dressing management can help surgeons to disinfect and decontaminate the wound. In an open wound, frequent dressing changes (two to three times a day) may be necessary to optimize healing and decrease contamination. In addition, the graft should be immobilized during healing to ensure optimal contact between the graft and the recipient site while minimizing shear forces. Immobilization can include the use of bolsters or figure-eight quilting sutures. Although it is ideal to replace tissue defects with identical tissue, skin grafts can be used in multiple applications and offer significant benefits compared with local or regional flaps within the head and neck region.

During the first 24 hours of healing, there is plasma, or more appropriately serum imbibition, which allows nutrients to transfer from the recipient bed to the graft. In addition, fibrinogen release by the capillary system allows for anchorage of the graft. This matures to form vascular inosculation channels primarily at the base and periphery with the adjoining subdermal plexus. Vascular flow is reestablished thereafter, often starting by postoperative day 3 or 4 (Table 133.1). It is imperative to maintain stabilization of the graft during this early healing phase.

Split-Thickness Donor Sites

Despite the inherent capacity for the donor site to heal, it is subject to discoloration (hypo- or hyperpigmentation as well as erythema), irregularity, and scarring. Therefore, it is preferable to locate donor sites in inconspicuous areas that clothing can easily hide. Considerations in choosing a site include ease of access during surgery, ease of managing wounds, and postoperative discomfort. Many areas on the proximal extremities and trunk are used, including the upper anterior thigh, lateral thigh, lower abdomen, buttocks, and infrequently the flank of the back. Many other sites are referenced in the literature but are used infrequently for maxillofacial surgical procedures.

Split-Thickness Recipient Site Applications

Although this is by no means a comprehensive listing of all sites, it affords several examples of applications given a multitude of clinical scenarios.

Soft Tissue Defect

Large Open Wounds to the Scalp and External Cheek. Despite the unappealing properties of poor color match and contracture, split-thickness grafts are frequently used to obtain initial healing of the defect. They may also be applied

Table 133.1 Key Differences Between the Two Grafting Techniques

Split-Thickness Grafts	Full-Thickness Grafts
Increased survivability	Improved tissue color and consistency
Increased contracture	Decreased contracture
Can be placed on mobile tissues if bolstering or quilting used	Require complete stabilization
Tolerate less vascularity (periosteum, paratenon, perineurium, prepared bone)	Require healthy vascularized bed of soft tissue

in medically compromised patients to decrease the morbidity associated with larger pedicled flap procedures or microvascular free tissue transfer.

Buccal Mucosa, Partial Tongue, Limited Floor of Mouth Reconstruction. Due to the lack of esthetic concerns intraorally, split-thickness grafts are often used in an attempt to resurface defects.[6,7] Contracture is expected, and therefore grafting is undertaken for smaller defects of the aforementioned sites. For larger defects, flaps would be ideally recommended to improve the function and bulk of the resected areas[8] (Fig. 133.3).

Exposed Muscle From a Pedicled or Microvascular Flap in the Head and Neck Region. Pedicled flaps or even microvascular tissue transfer can create areas of exposed muscle that cannot be closed over, primarily due to soft tissue swelling and tension or concerns over pedicle blood supply. Some grafts may be considered temporary measures to be excised at a later date if necessary.[9]

Covering Exposed Paratenon or Muscle in Microvascular Free Flap Harvest (Common Areas Include Radial Forearm and Fibula Donor Sites). Donor tissue sites may frequently create a defect in areas that possess minimal esthetic needs. Controversy continues to exist over the use of full-thickness versus split-thickness grafts to cover these defects.[10] Many accept that split-thickness grafts offer a greater chance of graft success, especially when placed over paratenon (radial forearm defect) due to decreased vascularity.

Oral Rehabilitation

Maxillectomy With Use of Obturator. Several authors believe that a split-thickness skin graft within the buccal or labial defect of a maxillectomy can be used to provide a scar band that can stabilize an obturator. The contraction that occurs with the healing of a skin graft is used advantageously by the maxillofacial prosthodontist for additional retention of the prosthesis.[11–13]

Oral Rehabilitation

Vestibuloplasty With Floor of Mouth Lowering. Preprosthetic site preparation has been utilized to improve tissue attachment and subsequent denture retention. With the increasing use of microvascular free tissue transfer for managing ablative defects, there is an increased need for flap revision, debulking, and skin grafting.[14] Minimizing the soft tissue thickness allows for more successful oral rehabilitation with dental implants.

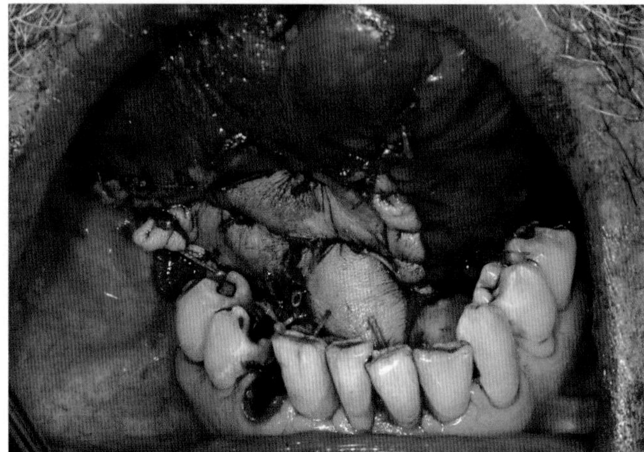

Figure 133.3 Split-thickness skin graft to a floor of mouth defect following cancer resection.

Full-Thickness Donor Sites

To satisfy cosmetic requirements of the face, full-thickness grafts can offer optimized color match, consistency, and texture. A multitude of harvest sites can allow for inconspicuous residual scars, including the upper lid, preauricular, postauricular, nasolabial, supraclavicular, and upper neck (Fig. 133.4).[3] When esthetic demands are not paramount, any body site can be utilized, including the abdomen, thigh, upper arm, and even skin from an avulsive injury or from resection of soft tissue flaps. As these sites require primary closure, elliptical incisions are used. The elliptical incisions parallel the relaxed or resting skin tension lines of the face or neck and are oriented perpendicular to the lines of maximum extensibility. Often, excess tissue is harvested to allow for tension-free closure while avoiding the creation of standing cutaneous (cone) deformities ("dog ears") at the edges of the harvest site. The pinch test is an easy tool that can be used to ensure optimal harvest with minimal tension closure.

Full-Thickness Recipient Site Applications

Given the improved success rates of healing with split-thickness skin grafts, the full-thickness skin graft is targeted primarily to higher esthetic needs of the head and neck. A full-thickness graft can replace a shallow defect with like tissue that allows minimal to no discernible depression to the surgical defect area. Use of a bolster dressing is imperative to adapt the graft to the defect and avoid untoward shear stresses. After placement and healing of the graft, subtle

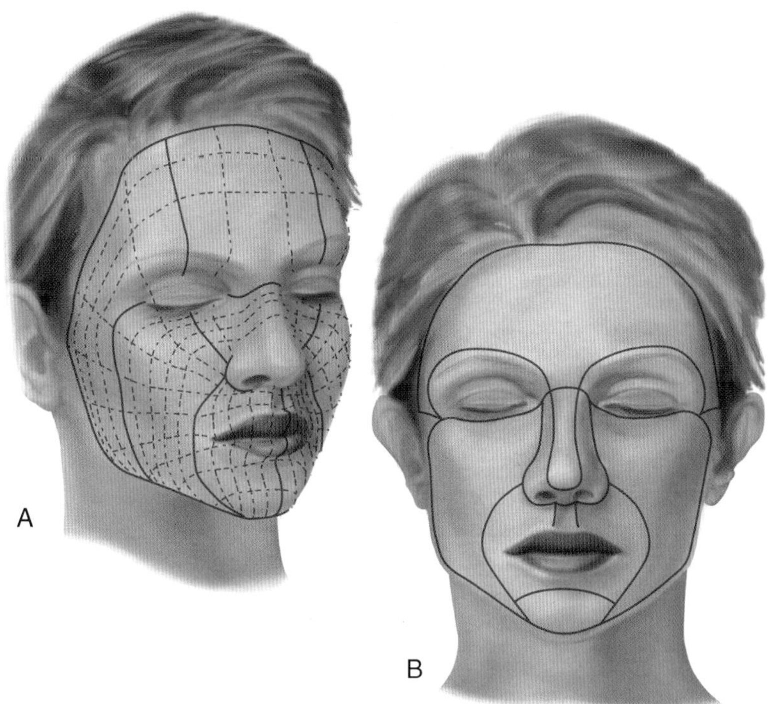

Figure 133.4 **A,** Resting skin tension lines. **B,** Full-thickness skin graft head and neck esthetic donor sites.

irregularities in color and texture can often be managed with selective dermabrasion.

Soft Tissue Defect

Small Defects in High Esthetic Areas. Resection of cutaneous neoplasms is a common occurrence. Based on the esthetic subunits of the face, grafts may be preferred over local-regional flaps. A small full-thickness graft can be used for reconstruction in areas with thin skin or thin defect depth. These include the eyelids and medial canthus, cheek, nose (especially over the lateral alar lobule and dorsum), and auricle. These grafts are tailored to the defect by matching size and shape (Fig. 133.5).

Oral Cavity. Oral cavity defects rarely require full-thickness grafts, as there is a tolerance for less ideal esthetics and increased scarring without impeding function. In addition, the moist oral environment can reduce graft success. The operator will often preferentially choose a split-thickness graft of thin or moderate thickness due to improved success in healing and graft take.

Composite Full-Thickness Donor Sites

Epidermis, dermis, and underlying tissues can all be harvested as a single graft. Additional tissues may include fat, hair follicles, or cartilage.[15] As more tissue is harvested, the success rates decrease because these other tissues lack reliable immediate blood flow. Therefore, only small grafts are indicated, and immobilization overlying a healthy well-vascularized tissue bed is paramount.

Composite Full-Thickness Recipient Site Applications

Hair Transplantation

Although newer techniques of follicular cell transfer or micrografting have become commonplace,[16] composite skin and hair follicle grafts have been used in the eyebrow region. Ensuring proper follicular hair orientation from the harvest site can allow for a proper pattern for new brow hair growth.[3]

Nasal Alar and Auricular Cartilage Reconstruction

Most grafts harvested are free cartilaginous grafts from the ear with a local flap repair; however, some may include auricular or alar cartilage and skin for small (<1 cm) full-thickness alar defects. In these instances it is important to harvest a slightly larger graft to compensate for inevitable graft contracture.[3]

Limitations and Contraindications

Due to the limitations of donor site morbidity and slightly reduced survival, full-thickness grafts are limited to smaller defects.

Esthetic subunits must be considered during repair to avoid poor cosmesis following healing. In some instances a combination of local flap repair and a skin graft is necessary. Often, a skin graft may be used to offer initial healing of the wound and then is more formally excised and repaired in a secondary fashion. Such instances are common following burns, large traumatic defects, or malignancy monitoring. The

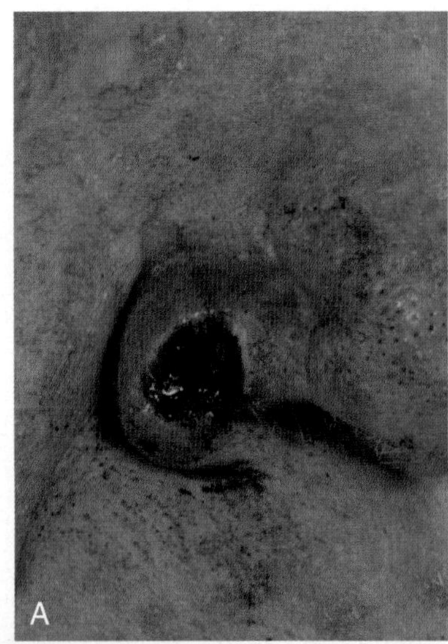

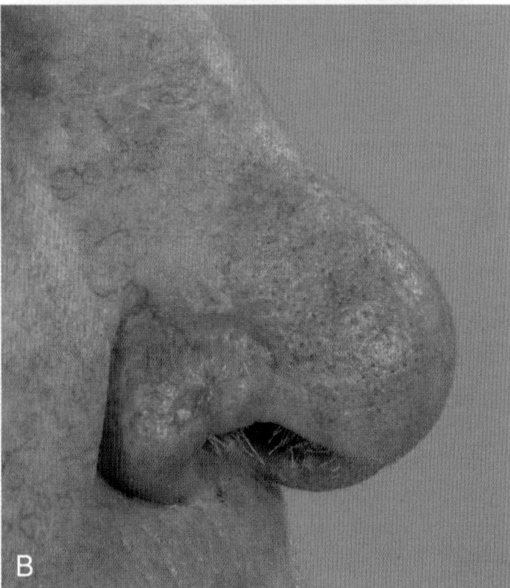

Figure 133.5 **A,** Nasal alar rim defect following cancer resection. **B,** Early postoperative healing from full-thickness skin graft.

grafted areas can thereafter be replaced with local-regional flaps with or without the use of tissue expanders or, in some instances, microvascular free tissue transfer. In addition, some advocate dermal fat grafting or dermabrasion to improve tissue texture and color to camouflage inconsistencies.

Skin grafts are contraindicated in infected wound beds, over avascular tissues, or with incomplete clearance of malignant disease. Although there are improved tolerances for success even in debilitated patient populations as compared to flaps, some situations may not be appropriate for grafting. These include irradiated tissue beds, areas of severe vasculitis or arterial insufficiency, and patients with severe malnutrition or inflammatory disease. Patients with high cosmetic needs may not be suitable candidates.

TECHNIQUE: Split-Thickness Skin Grafting

STEP 1: Recipient Site/Defect Preparation

Analysis of the wound is paramount. Ideally the tissue bed should have uniform depth and be beveled at the edges in esthetic areas to allow blending of the margins into the adjacent native tissues. Hemostasis should be achieved with monopolar or bipolar electrocautery. A template can be used to measure the defect size and shape and can factor up to a 10% to 20% larger size necessary to allow for contracture. The template should not be fabricated from an intraoral site and transferred to a separate sterile area. If necessary, the template can be sandwiched between an OpSite (Smith & Nephew, London, UK) dressing to ensure sterility with transfer.[17]

TECHNIQUE: Split-Thickness Skin Grafting—*cont'd*

STEP 2: Split-Thickness Skin Graft Harvest

The donor site is identified, and the hair is trimmed with clippers. The site is then sterilized with Betadine or chlorhexidine prep and draped in a sterile fashion. Mineral oil is then used to moisten the skin in the desired area. A dermatome blade and appropriately sized footplate (1 to 4 inches wide) are secured to the motorized dermatome. The desired thickness (commonly 0.012 inch) is selected with the control lever, and a #15 scalpel blade is inserted between the blade edge and the dermatome drum to ensure no warping or malpositioning of the dermatome blade. The scalpel should slide freely with no impingement. An assistant uses gauze to help flatten and retract the tissues, while the operator similarly uses counter-retraction. The dermatome should make initial contact at a 45-degree angle at full speed, then flatten during skin contact and harvest. After harvesting the desired length, the dermatome is angled away from the skin at a 45-degree angle and the motor is stopped. If necessary, the distal edge is cut free from the donor site. Saline-soaked gauze is placed directly onto the wound (Fig. 133.6A and B).

STEP 3: Graft Inspection and Preparation

The graft will have a dull side (epidermis) and a shiny side (dermis), and this can be unrolled onto a plastic tray (or kidney basin). Depending on the site, small incisions (1- to 2-mm "pie-crusting") can be made into the skin graft using a #15 scalpel blade to help with egress of fluid and better adaptation into the defect. Conversely, meshing (using a custom lattice pattern: 1.5:1, 2:1, 3:1) can expand the graft to a larger surface area and adapt to a convoluted wound. This step decreases cosmesis and increases contracture due to secondary wound healing with a checkerboard pattern. If the graft is not to be used for a period of time, it should be covered and protected with saline-soaked gauze to avoid desiccation. The harvest site is then inspected, and a variety of dressings can be used (Fig. 133.6C).

STEP 4: Donor Site Management

Hemostasis can be achieved at the donor site with the use of direct pressure, dilute epinephrine spray, or topical thrombin spray. Commonly, a large occlusive adhesive dressing OpSite (Smith & Nephew, London, UK) or Tegaderm (3M, Saint Paul, MN, USA) or an antibacterial petrolatum gauze dressing (Xeroform, Covidien, Mansfield, MA, USA) is used to protect the donor site wound. Blood may collect under the dressing and can be aspirated in the postoperative period using a sterile needle with a syringe (Fig. 133.6D). Alternatively, an alginate dressing (which will promote haemostasis and healing in a moist wound environment) can be placed on the wound and covered with a dry dressing. The overlying dry dressing can be replaced every 3 to 5 days and the underlying alginate left in place to allow for absorbance of excess fluid until complete wound healing been completed, usually after 2 to 3 weeks.

STEP 5: Recipient Site Grafting

Hemostasis is once again confirmed within the recipient site. The graft is positioned with tacking sutures to help orient and optimize positioning within the wound. Excess can be trimmed freehand, allowing for some redundancy. A variety of sutures are used based on the site (for the face, polypropylene/nylon, chromic gut, or polyglactin sutures can be applied; for intraoral applications, chromic gut, Vicryl/polyglactin or Monocryl/poliglecaprone sutures can be used). The graft edges are secured with suture in a continuous or interrupted fashion to allow primary closure. Once inset, the graft can be immobilized using quilting sutures (Fig. 133.6E). Skin glue can also be used as an alternative to suturing the graft at the peripheral margins; however, it is still advisable to use quilting sutures to maintain graft contact with the underlying wound and to reduce shear and potential serum/haematoma formation between graft and wound.

STEP 6: Bolster Dressing or Stent

BOLSTER

Silk sutures are positioned around the periphery of the wound (either at the margin or a small distance from the margin). Four stitches are minimum, but often eight or more are used in pairs to secure the dressing, depending on size. A silicone dressing, Mepitel (Molnlycke, Gothenburg, Sweden) or Adaptic (3M-KCI, Saint Paul, MN, USA) is often trimmed to fit within the wound to allow fluid egress and avoid adherence. A sheet of Xeroform (Covidien, Mansfield, MA, USA) is opened over the wound and mineral oil–soaked cotton balls are equally distributed over the Xeroform. The Xeroform is folded over the top, and the silk sutures are then tied opposing one another to secure the bolster in place. For larger defects, foam sponge can be cut to the defect size and secured with staples overlying the silicone and Xeroform dressing (Fig. 133.6F and G).

Stent

Acrylic stents fabricated preoperatively from impressions or dentures/obturators are used to help the graft adapt to the wound. In some instances a stent can be fabricated intraoperatively using thermoplastic beads molded to the defect shape after heating with a water bath. The stent can then be secured to the underlying bone by way of two positional screws or circummandibular wires (Fig. 133.6H).

Continued

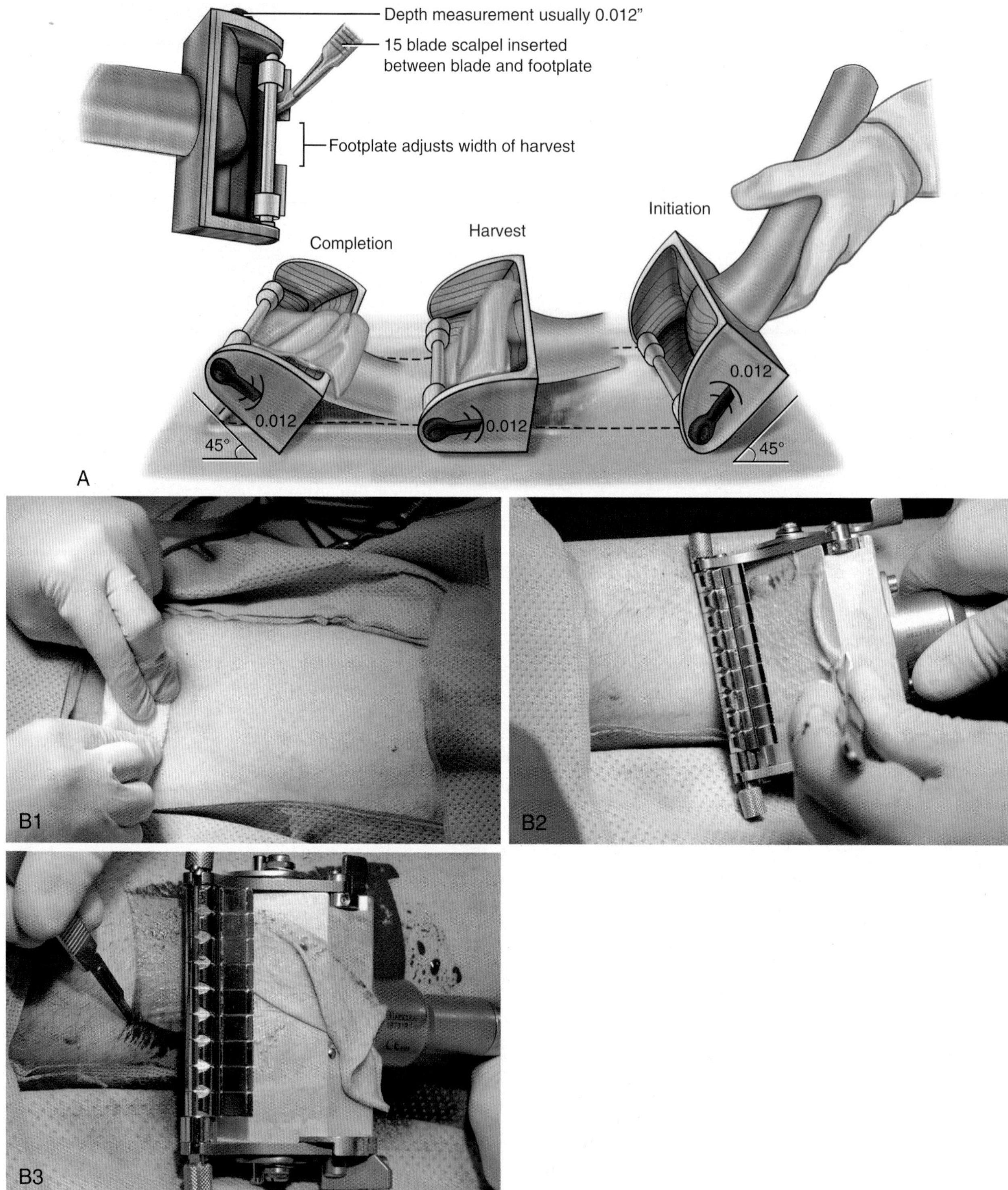

Figure 133.6 **A,** Motorized dermatome harvest technique. **B,** Initial harvest of split-thickness skin graft with counter-retraction **(B1)**, harvest **(B2)**, and sectioning of graft from donor site **(B3)**.

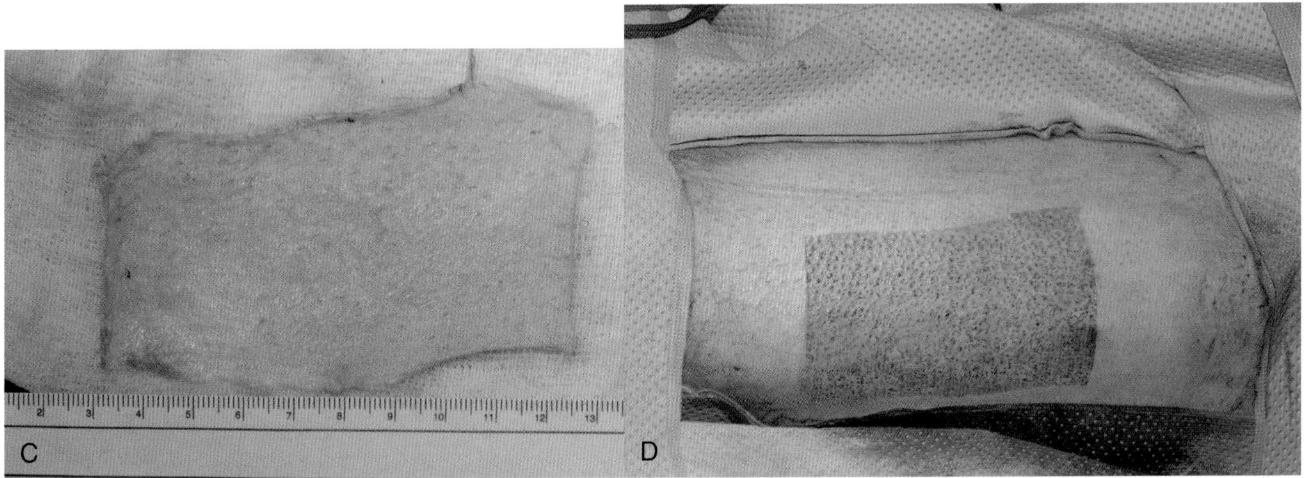

Figure 133.6, cont'd **C,** Inspection of graft to reveal epidermal (dull) and dermal (shiny) surfaces and preservation with saline-soaked gauze. **D,** Topical thrombin applied to donor site for hemostasis and OpSite, Xeroform, or Alginate dressing subsequently placed.

ALTERNATIVE TECHNIQUE 1: Full-Thickness Skin Graft Harvest

The appropriate donor site is prepped in a sterile fashion and a pinch test is used to demonstrate appropriate elasticity for wound closure. A template can be used to outline a slightly larger graft size and shape, allowing for contracture, and local anesthetic is infiltrated after tracing. An elliptical incision is outlined parallel to the resting skin tension lines to allow for primary closure of the wound. The scar may end up two to three times the length of the desired graft width to minimize standing cone deformities at the edges of the wound. The skin incision is made with a scalpel, and this or scissors can be used to undermine in a subdermal plane at one corner of the wound. Some may roll the graft over a finger with a skin hook or gauze to evaluate the thickness of the graft and to minimize fat. Hemostasis is achieved with bipolar electrocautery. The wound edges are undermined to allow for tension-free closure. The wound is closed in a layered fashion with deep dermal sutures followed by subcuticular or skin closure. All subcutaneous tissue is removed from the deep surface of the harvested graft to reveal the shiny dermis, using scissors with the graft stretched over an index finger. Similar to split-thickness grafts, small (1- to 2-mm) incisions can be used to help adapt the graft (pie-crusting). If the graft is not used immediately, it can be covered with saline-soaked gauze (Fig. 133.7).

ALTERNATIVE TECHNIQUE 2: Recipient Site Preparation and Skin Substitutes

In some circumstances of exposed bone or poor vascularity, attempts can be made to optimize success by providing a granulation tissue bed prior to grafting.[18] Although some authors have advocated skin grafting directly onto bone, more reliable results can be achieved by grafting onto a bed of vascularized tissue. With large scalp defects this can be particularly challenging. A more reliable method is removal of the outer table of calvarial bone and exposure of the underlying well vascularized cancellous bone. This will granulate over a period of 2 to 4 weeks and provide an improved vascularized soft tissue base for grafting. Application of a negative pressure dressing after bone removal will increase the rate of granulation tissue formation. This technique requires replacement of the negative pressure dressing every 3 to 5 days, thereby avoiding daily dressing changes. Once a well-vascularized base has been established, a skin graft can be placed directly over the wound bed and secured with sutures or skin glue to the margins. The application of the negative pressure dressing for a further period of 5 days allows the graft to be immobilized and compressed to the wound bed reducing shear and minimizing detrimental haematoma and seroma formation (Fig 133.8).

Many products are available on the market to promote the formation of a healthy layer of granulation tissue. Some additionally provide antibacterial properties with impregnated silver. Based on the wound type, different components can be used to promote wound health, including collagen, alginate, and cellulose with or without impregnated silver. In addition, skin substitutes can be used to provide a temporary bed of soft tissue to allow for future grafting or regional flaps. Such substitutes may include cadaveric allografts and engineered synthetic and cultured bilaminar grafts.

As a quick overview, wound preparation products can include Promogran (3M-KCI, Saint Paul, MN, USA), a combination of collagen and cellulose that helps to reduce proteases and

Continued

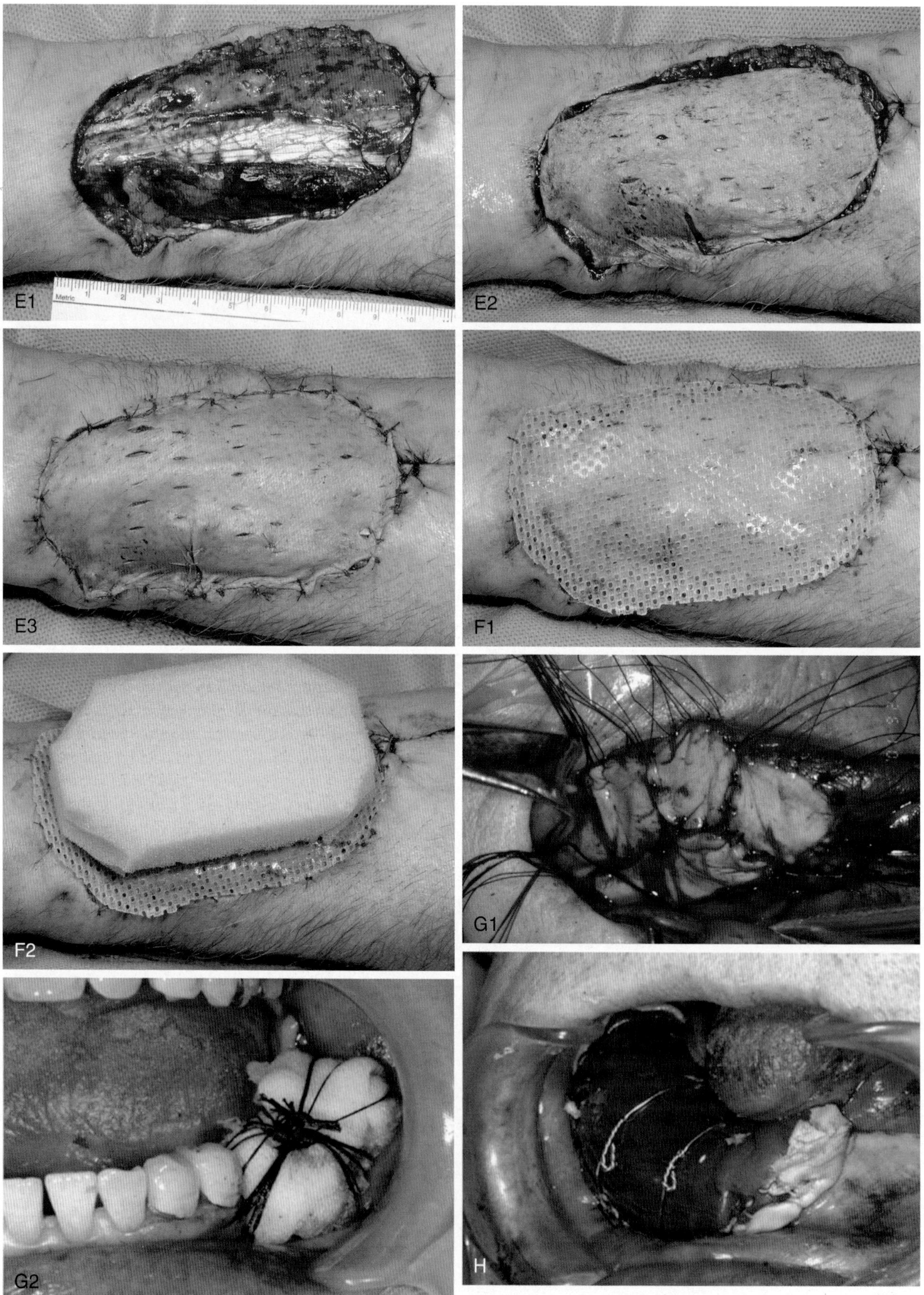

Figure 133.6, cont'd **E1,** Skin graft pie-crusted to allow fluid egress and better adaptation to wound. **E2,** Tacked into place using several sutures and subsequently trimmed to site. **E3,** Remainder of graft sutured in place. **F1,** Silicone dressing placed onto recipient site. **F2,** Sterile sponge adapted to defect. **G1,** Silk sutures placed into wound to adapt bolster. **G2,** Xeroform and cotton balls bolster in place. **H,** Surgical stent adapted and secured with circummandibular wires.

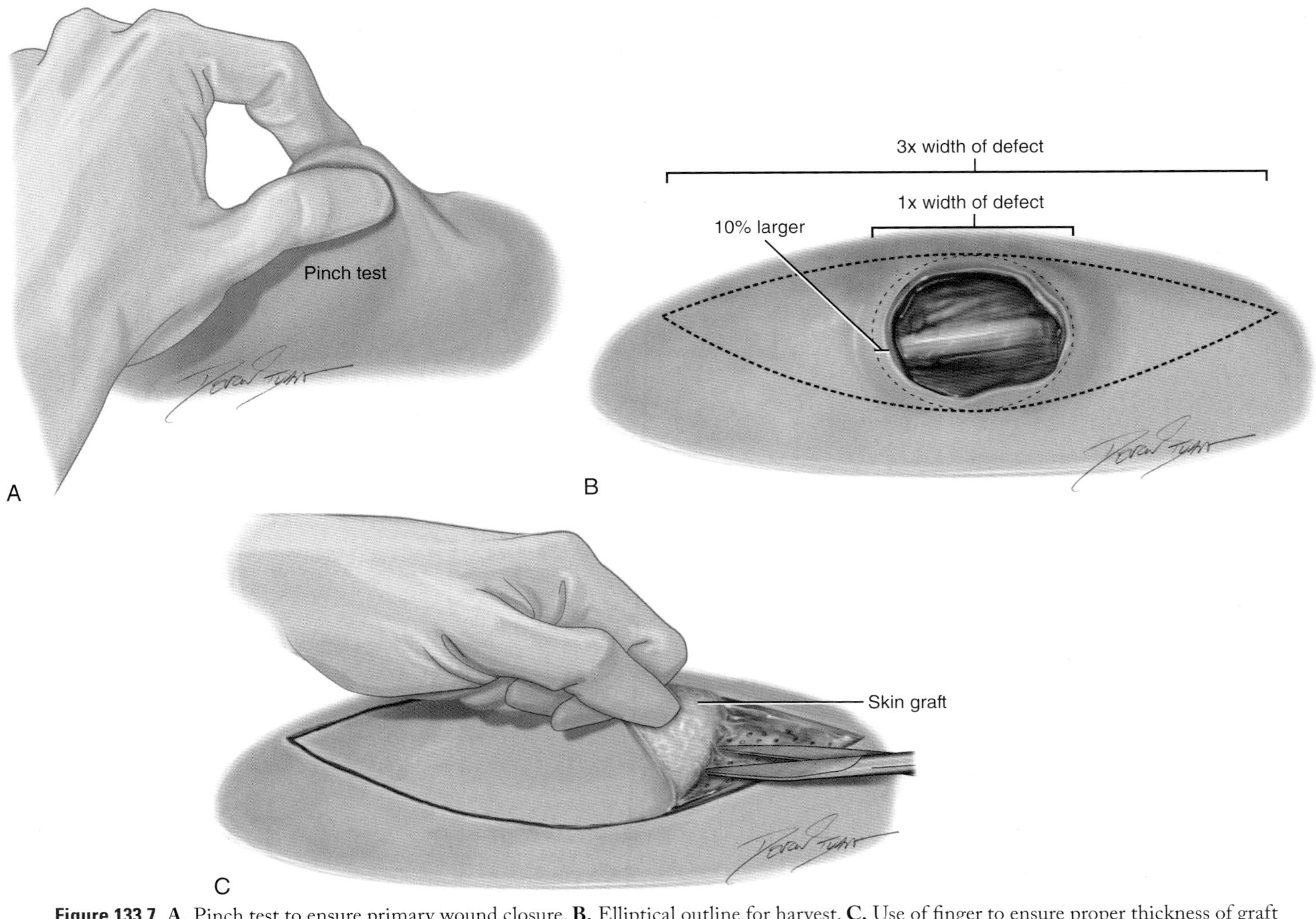

Figure 133.7 **A,** Pinch test to ensure primary wound closure. **B,** Elliptical outline for harvest. **C,** Use of finger to ensure proper thickness of graft harvest.

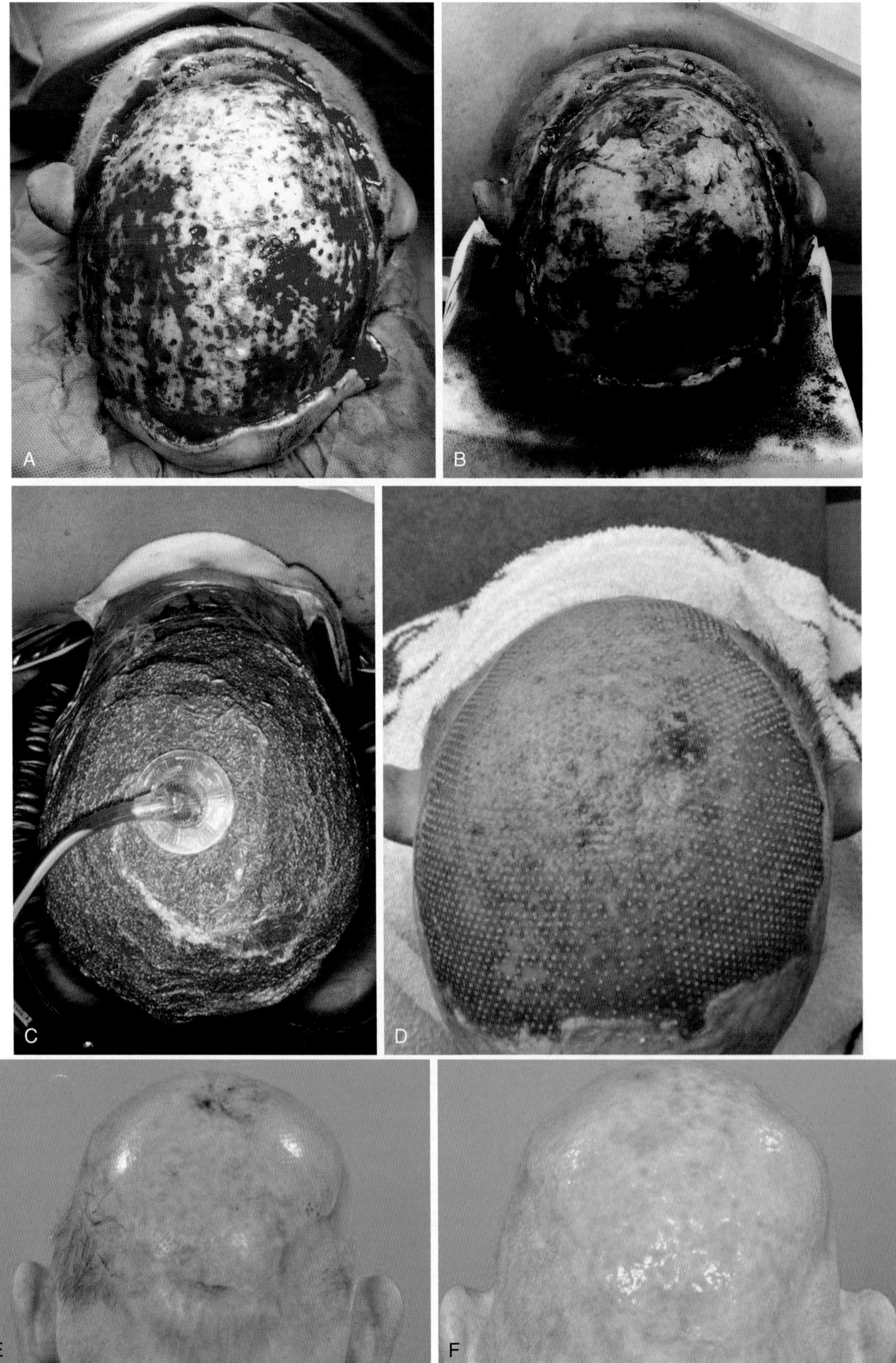

Figure 133.8 **A,** Large scalp defect. **B,** Bone prepared to remove outer table. **C,** Application of wound vac for negative pressure dressing. **D,** Removal of vac with underlying bed of granulation tissue. **E,** Skin graft at 1 month. **F,** Skin graft well healed at 6 months.

ALTERNATIVE TECHNIQUE 2: Recipient Site Preparation and Skin Substitutes—*cont'd*

resultant wound degradation with or without silver; Melgisorb (Molnlycke, Gothenburg, Sweden), an alginate-based product that absorbs exudate from the wound) with or without silver; and Allevyn (Smith & Nephew, London, UK), a hydrocellular product used to help absorb fluid and wick away from wound. A variety of similar and unique products are also offered by Covidien (Mansfield, MA, USA), 3M (St. Paul, MN, USA), Integra Life Sciences (Princeton, NJ, USA), and Covalon (Mississauga, Ontario, Canada). These can be used for several weeks to prepare the wound site for appropriate skin grafting or skin substitutes.

Skin substitutes can be placed onto a wound bed to help mitigate the need for a donor site. They often provide a temporary solution to help delay the need for grafting, although some more permanent solutions do exist. Cadaveric allografts and xenografts are on the market for temporary wound closure to provide a barrier during healing. Their uses are limited due to epidermal sloughing, disease transmission, and antigenic properties. Engineered single layer and bilaminates are useful to avoid these problems for temporary wound management. These include Biobrane (Smith & Nephew, London, UK), Integra (Integra Lifesciences, Princeton, NJ, USA), Apligraf (Organogenesis Holdings., Canton, MA, USA), and Theraskin (LifeNet Health, Virginia Beach, VA, USA) (Fig. 133.9).[19–21] Please note that many other wound care products are available.

ALTERNATIVE TECHNIQUE 4: Cultured Autologous Epidermal Replacements

Tissue engineering has also offered the promise of providing cultured keratinocytes harvested from the patient and expanded onto manufactured scaffolds/constructs. This allows for small, well-tolerated donor sites. Epicel (Vericel Corp, Cambridge, MA, USA) has been used as an expanded epidermal autograft. It is produced by taking two biopsies from the patient and expanding the keratinocytes over 15 to 21 days onto mouse-derived fibroblasts. Due to the lack of clinical trials and its application as a humanitarian use device, approval by the US Food and Drug Administration is limited to its use on patients with burns over greater than 30% of the body surface area.[19] Ex vivo produced oral mucosa equivalents (cultured epithelial cells onto Alloderm acellular dermis constructs; LifeCell, Bridgewater, NJ, USA) are also under clinical trials as a means to improve healing and avoid donor site morbidity for oral reconstruction.[22–24]

A more conservative and rapid approach has introduced onsite preparation and processing to allow delivery of autologous keratinocytes in a spray-on technique. ReCell (Avita Medical, Valencia, CA, USA) utilizes a small split-thickness biopsy (1 × 1 cm) harvested from the patient.[25–28] A sterile single-use kit is used intraoperatively for graft processing, keratinocyte segregation, and suspension in a mere 30 minutes. The spray can thereafter be used to resurface a variety of wounds for improved healing and color match. For the head and neck region, a useful application can be to improve the color match of distant flaps or skin grafts with hypopigmentation. Dermabrasion is used to create a healthy wound surface, and the ReCell spray can cover up to 80 times the surface area of the harvested skin graft. Due to transfer of melanocytes and keratinocytes, improved pigmentation matching is noted, and the wounds heal better than with dermabrasion alone. In addition, the keratinocyte spray can be used to accelerate wound healing at a donor site and thereby minimize scarring[28] (Fig. 133.10A and B).

Avoidance and Management of Intraoperative Complications

Few major complications result during grafting procedures for maxillofacial purposes. Commonly, an intraoperative concern may be related to a smaller graft harvest than necessary. The harvested grafts and recipient sites should be managed in a gentle manner. A graft harvested over an underlying bone protuberance may not allow for uniform harvest and create a jagged edge. This can be unsightly for patients, and this is a reason to advocate two-person harvest with counter-retraction and flattening of the tissues.

Postoperative Considerations

Dressings are frequently left in place for 5 to 7 days to avoid any untoward shear forces on the graft during the critical early healing phase. Extreme care should be taken during the first dressing change to prevent disruption of the healing tissues. If the bandages adhere to the underlying tissues, a small amount of sterile saline can be used to moisten the dressing during removal. Upon removal, the wound bed should be evaluated for evidence of graft take.

Despite optimal grafting techniques, partial or even complete graft failure can occur.[29] Treatment of partial graft loss often requires dressing management (every 1 to 3 days or longer depending on the product used) and allowing the graft to granulate secondarily. Careful management of the wound can avoid delayed infections. On occasion, a secondary grafting procedure may be necessary. Once a defect has healed and the graft has become integrated, unsightly tissues and scars can be revised with future surgeries. This can include serial excision, scar revision, dermabrasion, and tissue expansion with local flap reconstruction.[30,31]

Continued

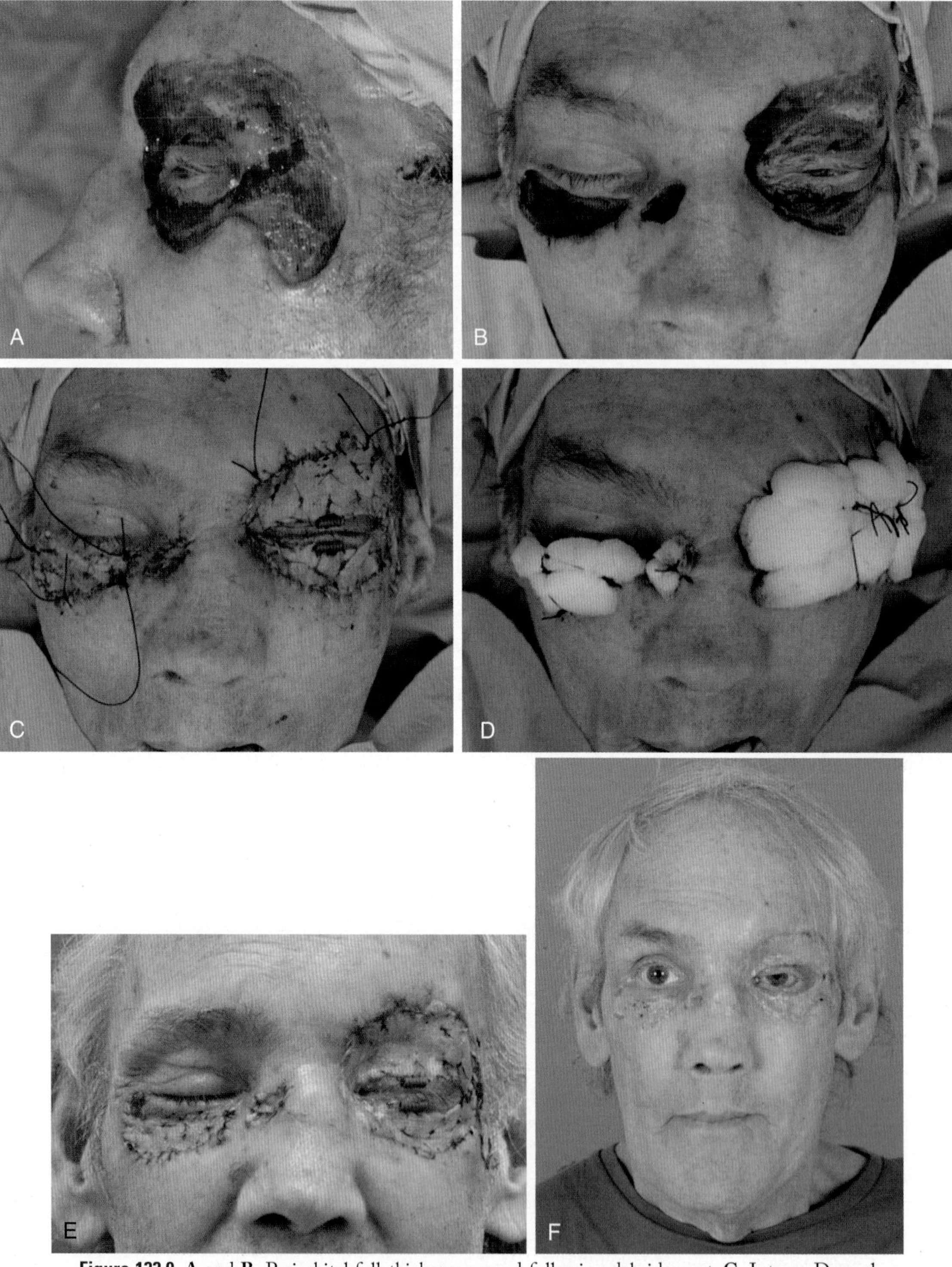

Figure 133.9 **A** and **B,** Periorbital full-thickness wound following debridement. **C,** Integra Dermal Regeneration Template Single Layer Thin applied to the wound with overlying split-thickness skin grafting. **D,** Application of bolster. **E,** Early healing and graft take at 2 weeks. **F,** Six weeks postop result. (From Wounds International, with permission,)

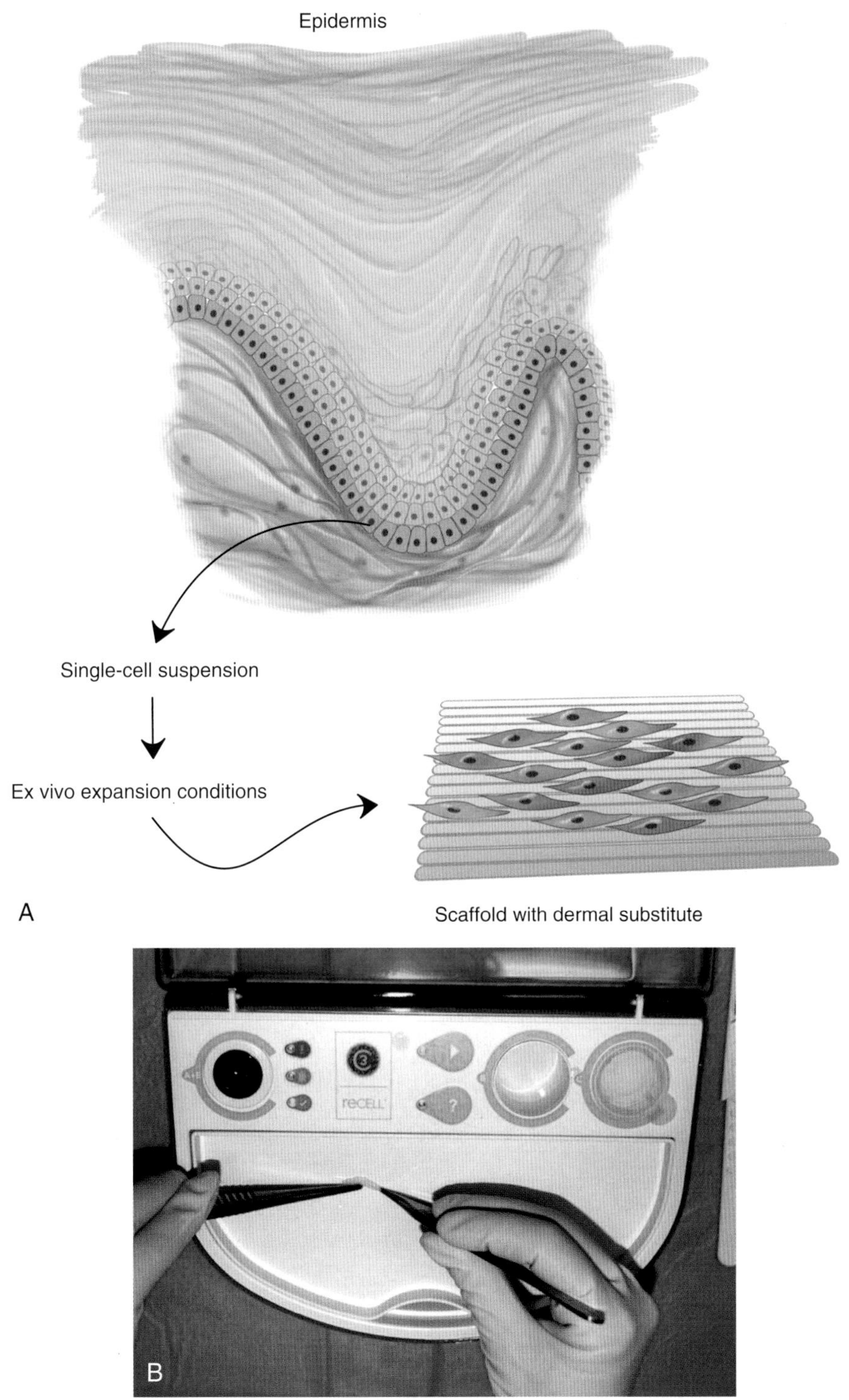

Figure 133.10 **A,** Cultured keratinocytes harvested from the patient and expanded onto manufactured scaffolds/constructs. **B,** Sterile single-use ReCell keratinocyte spray kit.

ALTERNATIVE TECHNIQUE 4: Cultured Autologous Epidermal Replacements—*cont'd*

Donor sites for split-thickness grafts may form excessive granulation tissue and may require debridement or further dressing management to help control exudate and allow the wound bed to heal over. Removal of the initial dressing at 5 to 7 days postharvest can help avoid this occurrence. The scar will appear red and erythematous for 6 to 12 months postoperatively and on occasion become either hypo- or hyperpigmented.

Full-thickness donor sites infrequently develop infection, wound dehiscence, or visible scars. Many of these problems can be mitigated by sterile preparation and adhering to principles of resting skin tension lines and proper closure techniques.

References

1. Hentz VR, Mathes SJ. *Plastic Surgery*. 2nd ed. Philadelphia, PA: WB Saunders; 2006.
2. Santoni-Rugiu P, Sykes PJ. *A History of Plastic Surgery*. Heidelberg, Germany: Springer; 2007.
3. Baker SR. *Local Flaps in Facial Reconstruction*. 2nd ed. St. Louis, MO: Mosby; 2007.
4. Stallings JO, Huffman WC, Bernstein L. Skin grafts on bare bone. *Plast Reconstr Surg*. 1969;43(2):152–156.
5. Tran LE, Berry GJ, Fee WE Jr. Split-thickness skin graft attachment to bone lacking periosteum. *Arch Otolaryngol Head Neck Surg*. 2005;131(2):124–128.
6. Alvi A, Myers EN. Skin graft reconstruction of the composite resection defect. *Head Neck*. 1996;18(6):538–543.
7. Girod DA, Sykes K, Jorgensen J, Tawfik O, Tsue T. Acellular dermis compared to skin grafts in oral cavity reconstruction. *Laryngoscope*. 2009;119(11):2141–2149.
8. Hansen SL, Leon P. Reconstruction of the oral cavity. *Semin Plast Surg*. 2003;17:387.
9. Lutz BS. Beauty of skin-grafted free muscle flaps in head and neck reconstruction. *Microsurgery*. 2006;26(3):177–181.
10. Sidebottom AJ, Stevens L, Moore M, et al. Repair of the radial free flap donor site with full or partial thickness skin grafts. A prospective randomised controlled trial. *Int J Oral Maxillofac Surg*. 2000;29(3):194–197.
11. Brown KE. Peripheral consideration in improving obturator retention. *J Prosthet Dent*. 1968;20(2):176–181.
12. Okay DJ, Genden E, Buchbinder D, Urken M. Prosthodontic guidelines for surgical reconstruction of the maxilla: a classification system of defects. *J Prosthet Dent*. 2001;86(4):352–363.
13. Aramany MA. Basic principles of obturator design for partially edentulous patients. Part II: design principles. *J Prosthet Dent*. 1978;40(6):656–662.
14. Moy PK. Alveolar ridge reconstruction with preprosthetic surgery: a precursor to site preservation following extraction of natural dentition. *Oral Maxillofac Surg Clin North Am*. 2004;16(1):1–7.
15. Holt DS. Should all skin grafts be low fat? Composite skin and fat grafts in facial reconstruction. *Br J Oral Maxillofac Surg*. 2012;50(2):137–140.
16. Bunagan MJK, Banka N, Shapiro J. Hair transplantation update: procedural techniques, innovations, and applications. *Dermatol Clin*. 2013;31(1):141–153.
17. Sood V, Misra A, Brown I, Devine J. Technique for transfer of a template in free flap design. *Br J Oral Maxillofac Surg*. 2010;48(7):557.
18. Tausche A-K, Sebastian G. Wound conditioning of a deep tissue defect including exposed bone after tumour excision using PROMOGRAN* Matrix, a protease-modulating matrix. *Int Wound J*. 2005;2(3):253–257.
19. Ehrenreich M, Ruszczak Z. Update on tissue-engineered biological dressings. *Tissue Eng*. 2006;12(9):2407–2424.
20. Snyder D., Sullivan N., Margolis D., Schoelles K. Skin Substitutes for Treating Chronic Wounds, AHRQ Technology Assessment Program—Technical Brief. Project ID: WNDT0818. www.ahrq.gov
21. Dantzer E, MacIver C, Moiemen N, Schiavon M, Schiestl CM, Thomas C. Using Integra dermal Regeneration template single layer thin in practice. *Wounds International*. 2018;9:71.
22. Izumi K, Terashi H, Marcelo CL, Feinberg SE. Development and characterization of a tissue-engineered human oral mucosa equivalent produced in a serum-free culture system. *J Dent Res*. 2000;79(3):798–805.
23. Izumi K, Takacs G, Terashi H, Feinberg SE. Ex vivo development of a composite human oral mucosal equivalent. *J Oral Maxillofac Surg*. 1999;57(5):571–577.
24. Izumi K, Tobita T, Feinberg SE. Isolation of human oral keratinocyte progenitor/stem cells. *J Dent Res*. 2007;86(4):341–346.
25. Currie LJ, Martin R, Sharpe JR, James SE. A comparison of keratinocyte cell sprays with and without fibrin glue. *Burns*. 2003;29(7):677–685.
26. Wood FM, Giles N, Stevenson A, Rea S, Fear M. Characterisation of the cell suspension harvested from the dermal epidermal junction using a ReCell® kit. *Burns*. 2012;38(1):44–51.
27. Tenenhaus M, Rennekampff HO. Surgical advances in burn and reconstructive plastic surgery: new and emerging technologies. *Clin Plast Surg*. 2012;39(4):435–443.
28. Cervelli V, De Angelis B, Spallone D, Lucarini L, Arpino A, Balzani A. Use of a novel autologous cell-harvesting device to promote epithelialization and enhance appropriate pigmentation in scar reconstruction. *Clin Exp Dermatol*. 2010;35(7):776–780.
29. Salama AR, McClure SA, Ord RA, Pazoki AE. Free-flap failures and complications in an American oral and maxillofacial surgery unit. *Int J Oral Maxillofac Implants*. 2009;38(10):1048–1051.
30. Hoffmann JF. Tissue expansion in the head and neck. *Facial Plast Surg Clin North Am*. 2005;13(2):315–324, vii.
31. Kim EK, Hovsepian RV, Mathew P, Paul MD. Dermabrasion. *Clin Plast Surg*. 2011;38(3):391–395, v-vi.

CHAPTER 134

Anterior Iliac Crest Bone Grafting (AICBG)

Ravi Agarwal and George Obeid

Armamentarium

#10 Scalpel blades
Appropriate sutures
Bone gouges
Cobb elevators
Curved osteotomes
Electrocautery
Gluteal bump
Key (periosteal) elevators
Liston bone cutters
Local anesthetic with vasoconstrictor
Mallet
Microfibrillar collagen
Obwegeser iliac crest retractor
Oscillating saw
Putti bone rasp
Reciprocating saw
Rongeurs
Straight and angled bone curettes
Straight spatula
Taylor retractor
Weitlaner retractors

History of the Procedure

Anterior iliac crest bone grafting (AICBG) has been part of oral and maxillofacial surgery reconstruction for close to a hundred years. Its use was initially noted during the First World War by German surgeons, Lindemann of Dusseldorf and Klapp of Berlin.[1] By 1917, the use of iliac crest bone grafts for mandibular reconstruction had become widespread practice. The ilium was firmly established as a source of bone for defects of the jaw in July 1920, when Gilbert Chubb[2] reported on 60 cases of bone grafting in the mandible. Original reconstructive methods for the facial bones relied on free bone graft blocks, which often are dense and have little cellularity.

In 1944, Rainsford Mowlem[3] used cancellous chip grafts for reconstruction, noting increased cellularity and satisfactory healing within weeks. With further refinement of fixation techniques, corticocancellous blocks or particulate bone chips from the ilium were used for mandibular reconstruction, with good success. The technique for harvesting bone from the anterior ilium has largely gone unchanged. The soft tissue surgical approach is universally accepted by patients. Minor modifications in the bone harvesting techniques are mostly attempts to reduce postoperative pain and gait disturbances. Minimally invasive outpatient techniques also are available for harvesting cancellous bone from the anterior ilium with trephines and reamers.[4]

Indications for the Use of the Procedure

The anterior ilium can be a source for bone grafting in most facial reconstruction cases that can be managed by a free nonvascularized autograft. The ilium, once considered the gold standard as a donor site, allows transplantation of a large concentration of osteocompetent cells. However, with free tissue transfer and advancements in tissue engineering, the use of the ilium is changing. A discussion of the indications for free tissue transfer versus nonvascularized bone grafts is beyond the scope of this chapter.

The anterior ilium, unlike other sites such as the calvaria or tibia, can provide both corticocancellous blocks and just cancellous marrow for use in grafting. Most reconstructive cases that require 50 cc or less of bone can be managed with a single anterior ilium.[5] This amount of bone can reconstruct a 5-cm defect, assuming each centimeter of defect requires 10 cc of bone. Another indication is based on the ability to harvest the anterior ilium in a two-team approach for a free bone graft; this can shorten operating room and anesthesia time.[6]

The most common procedures that use the anterior ilium include correction of posttraumatic deformities (malunion, nonunion), postablative reconstruction of the jaws (odontogenic cysts, small benign tumors), orthognathic procedures, alveolar cleft grafts, and reconstruction of atrophic jaws for future dental implants (sinus augmentation, ridge augmentation) (Fig. 134.1).

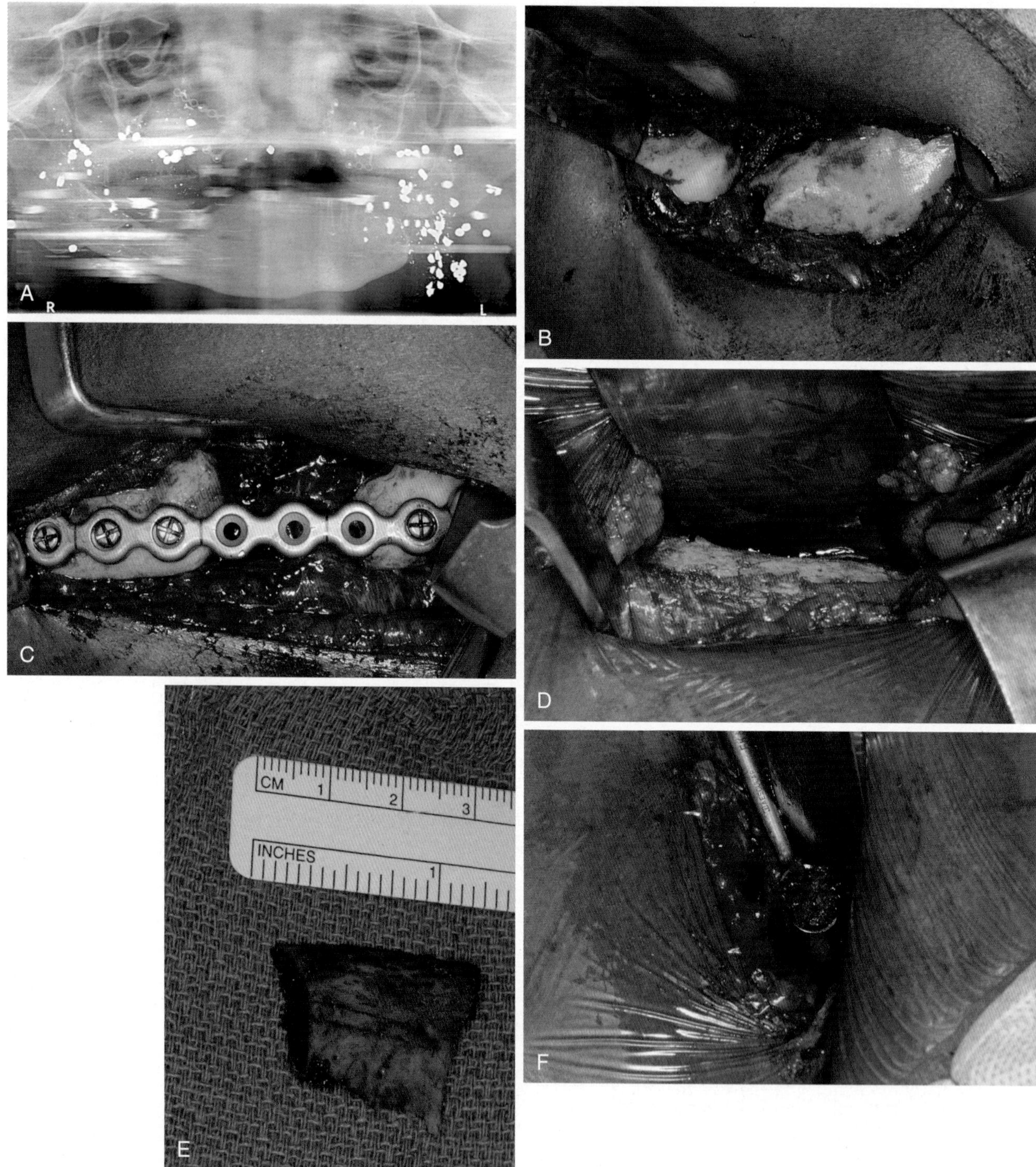

Figure 134.1 **A,** Preoperative radiograph of patient with a history of left mandibular nonunion after sustaining a gunshot injury. **B,** Exposure of the left mandibular nonunion through a submandibular approach without violating the oral mucosa. **C,** Reconstruction plate adapted; note that defect is approximately 3 cm in size. **D,** Exposure of the anterior iliac crest with medial wall exposure. **E,** Corticocancellous block obtained from the medial wall. **F,** Harvesting of cancellous bone using a bone curette.

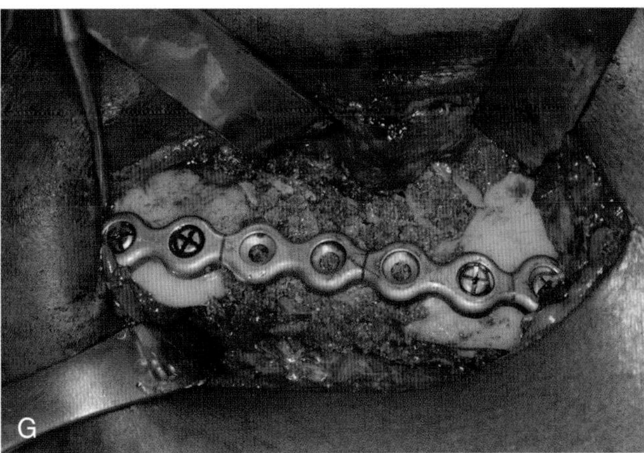

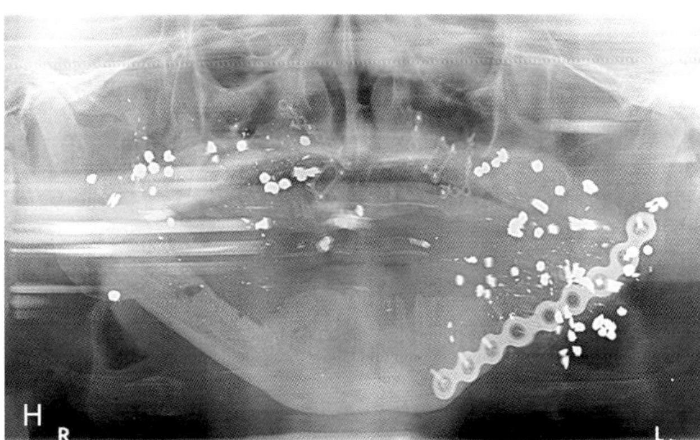

Figure 134.1, cont'd **G,** The block was particulated, mixed with cancellous bone, and then grafted into the mandibular defect. **H,** A 3-month postoperative radiograph of the reconstruction.

Limitations and Contraindications

Use of the anterior ilium requires strict sterile technique, often necessitating general anesthesia in the operating room. On average, the region of bone harvest in the anterior ilium yields 15 to 20 cc of noncompressed bone, with a maximum of 50 cc in some individuals.[7,8] Consequently, defects larger than 4 to 5 cm cannot be reconstructed from a single harvest site. Another limitation is obesity, which can distort the anatomy and make the surgical approach more difficult. Patients with a history of hernia repairs can be at risk for inadvertent abdominal penetration. In patients with hip prostheses, the anterior ilium should not be harvested on the affected side to avoid any confusion of symptoms and to reduce the risks of hardware failure and infection.

Contraindications to anterior ilium harvest include previous trauma or infection of the surgical site. Systemic factors, such as metabolic bone diseases, should also be taken into consideration. Relative contraindications include bisphosphonate use, chemotherapy, irradiation of the site, and/or long-term steroid use.[5]

TECHNIQUE: Medial Approach

STEP 1: Patient Preparation and Positioning

General anesthesia is obtained using endotracheal intubation, and the patient is placed in the standard supine position. A soft roll or saline bag wrapped in a towel is used as a bump under the gluteal region on the side of harvest to elevate and rotate the hip, making it more accessible. More often, the bone harvest involves a two-team approach, and the second surgical site should be separately draped in anticipation. In prolonged procedures, the bump should be removed from underneath the gluteal region once the bone graft has been obtained. Keeping the lower spine rotated for an extended period may add to the postoperative discomfort of the patient (Fig. 134.2A).

STEP 2: Landmark Identification

The surgeon should palpate and mark the location of the anterior superior iliac spine (ASIS). Marking is continued along the anterior iliac crest until the widest portion is encountered; this is the iliac tubercle. The incision marking is made 2 cm lateral to the iliac crest to create an inconspicuous scar, to prevent injury by a belt or low waistband, and to reduce the incidence of nerve injury.[9] This incision marking can be made 4 to 8 cm in length, depending on the amount of harvest needed. This marking should be 1.5 to 2 cm short of the ASIS to reduce injury in the 2.5% of the population whose lateral femoral cutaneous nerve runs over the anterior superior spine.[10] Posteriorly, the iliohypogastric nerve and subcostal nerves course laterally over the region of the iliac crest and tubercle; these nerves sometimes can be unavoidable because they can cross the iliac crest approximately 5 to 6 cm posterior to the ASIS.[9,11,12] Once marked, the subcutaneous tissue can be injected with a local anesthetic containing a vasoconstrictor. The subperiosteal plane over the crest can also be infiltrated. The field is then prepped and appropriately draped. An antimicrobial incise drape can be used to prevent contamination from the pubic area (Fig. 134.2B).

Continued

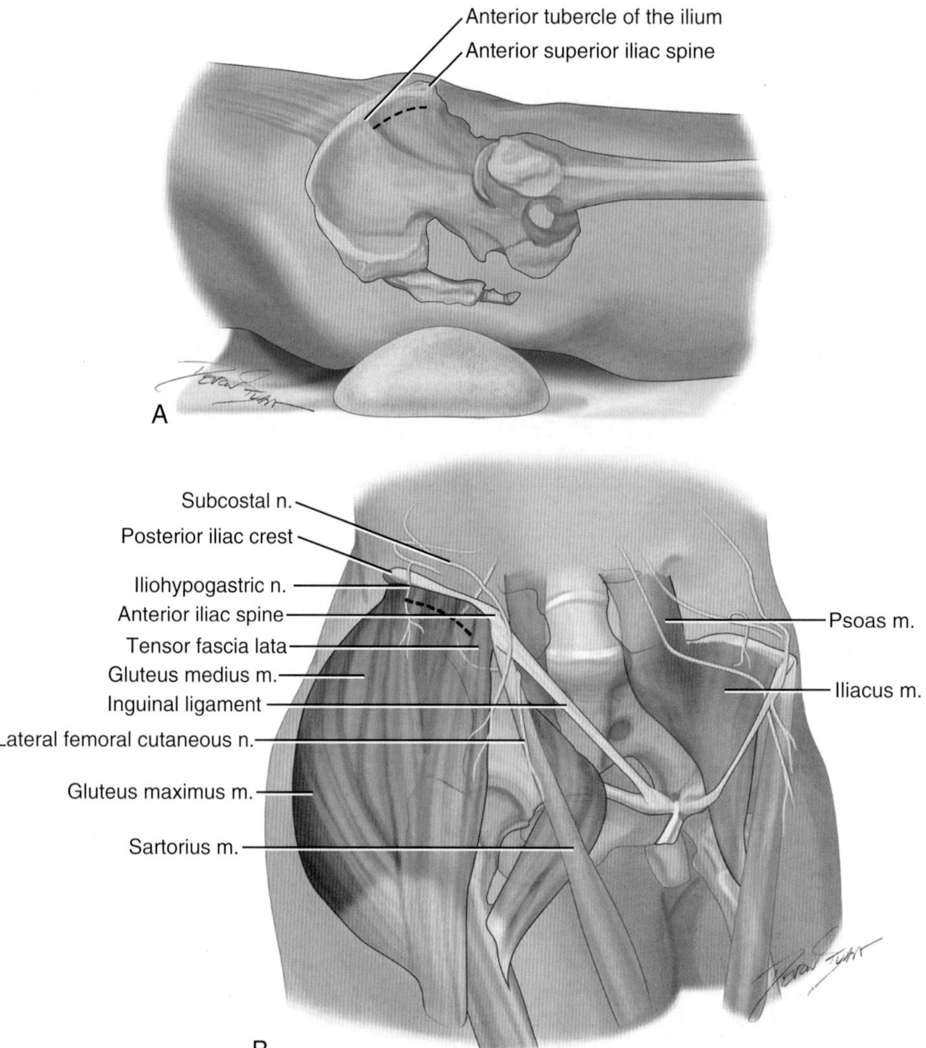

Figure 134.2 **A,** Lateral view demonstrating placement of a soft roll to elevate the anterior iliac crest. The incision *(dashed line)* is placed lateral to the crest and posterior to the anterior iliac spine. **B,** Anterior view of the anterior iliac crest shows the relationships of the muscular and neural structures as they relate to the proposed incision *(dashed line)*. Although not typically visualized during harvest, the iliohypogastric nerve may be encountered with posterior extension of the incision.

TECHNIQUE: Medial Approach—*cont'd*

STEP 3: Incision

Gentle pressure is placed against the abdomen superior and medial to the incision line, which slides the incision over the iliac crest. A #10 blade is then used to sharply incise the skin along the marked incision. The subcutaneous tissues are sharply incised with a blade or electrocautery to the level of the overlying superficial abdominal fascia, the layers of which are known as the Camper fascia and Scarpa fascia. This fascia can be sharply incised with a blade or electrocautery. Once below the abdominal fascia, the crest should be palpated. Using a sponge or pledget, the surgeon should bluntly dissect any remaining fat or layers over the crest and identify muscular fibers medially from the external oblique muscle and laterally from the tensor fascia lata muscle. A periosteal incision then can be made sharply onto the crest of the ridge, staying in between the two muscles.

TECHNIQUE: Medial Approach—*cont'd*

STEP 4: Dissection

Once on the crest, a subperiosteal dissection is performed along the crest using the Key elevator, staying at least 1.5 to 2 cm posterior to the anterior iliac spine. If only cancellous bone is to be harvested, no further dissection is required, and osteotomies can be performed for access. However, if a corticocancellous block is needed, the Key elevator then is turned onto the medial cortex to reflect the iliacus muscle off the medial wall. Safe dissection can be performed to a depth of 5 to 7 cm using a Cobb elevator and medial retractor (Fig. 134.2C).

STEP 5: Osteotomies and Bone Harvest

If only cancellous bone is to be harvested, a variety of options for harvest are available. A narrow, 5 × 20 mm cortical window can be made on the crest with an osteotome, a saw, or a fissure bur. This cortical window can then be removed, allowing access to the marrow. The cancellous bone can be harvested using a combination of bone gouges and bone curettes.

The preferred method for obtaining corticocancellous blocks is to take them from the medial wall of the anterior ilium.[13] This approach also maximizes the bone available in the least morbid fashion, whereas the lateral approach produces more discomfort and gait disturbance due to disturbance of the tensor fascia lata.[11] With a medial retractor in place, protecting the soft tissue, osteotomies should be outlined along the midcrest and vertically through the crest onto the medial wall. The anterior vertical cut should be at least 2 cm posterior to the ASIS. The posterior cut can be variable, depending on the amount of bone required; it usually is made 4 to 5 cm posterior to the anterior cut. A template previously fashioned to the desired shape of the bone graft can also be used to mark the osteotomies. The cuts are then made with spatula osteotomes or a reciprocating saw. The medial cut is made with a curved osteotome or an oscillating saw. If a medial osteotomy is not adequate, levering the bone block may propagate a fracture at an incorrect level, compromising the size and shape of the desired graft. When making the osteotomies, the surgeon must keep in mind that the cortical plate in these regions is generally thin, 1 to 2 mm. Once the block has been removed, the remaining cancellous bone and adjacent marrow sites are harvested with bone gouges and bone curettes. Typically, cancellous bone is harvested to the depth of the confluence of the cortical plates (Fig. 134.2D).

Continued

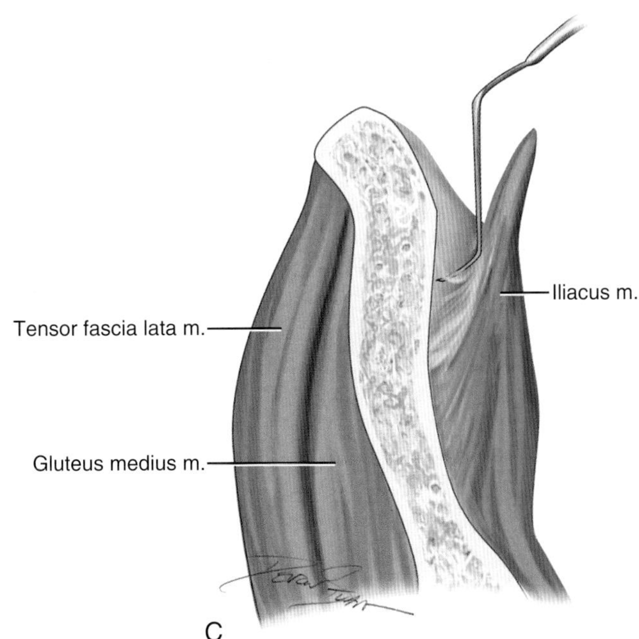

Figure 134.2, cont'd **C,** Typical donor site of the anterior iliac crest after medial wall exposure. Note the position of the medial retractor placed in a subperiosteal plane to retract the iliacus muscle and protect the intraabdominal contents. With a medial wall approach, there is the preservation of the lateral cortex, which limits trauma to the insertion of the tensor fascia lata.

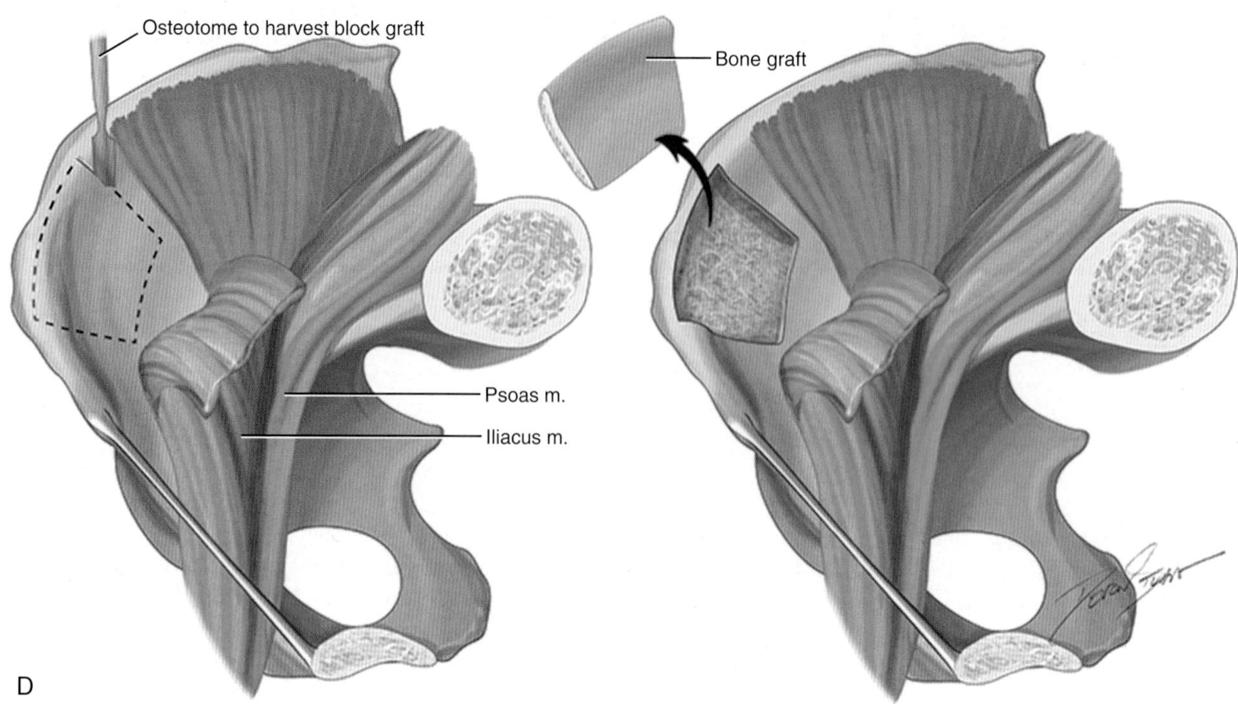

Figure 134.2, cont'd **D,** Harvesting of a corticocancellous block from the medial aspect of the anterior ilium after reflection of the iliacus muscle. An osteotome or saw can be used for the corticotomies in the suggested design. After retrieval of the block, the exposed underlying cancellous bone can be harvested utilizing bone curettes and gouges.

TECHNIQUE: Medial Approach—*cont'd*

STEP 6: Closure

All sharp bony edges should be smoothed with rongeurs or bone files. Any bleeding points considered to be more than general marrow oozing can be managed with electrocautery. General hemostasis is obtained by fluffing 1 g of microfibrillar collagen (e.g., Avitene) into the defect. The use of suction drains after bone harvesting is not necessary; however, if they are used, the authors prefer not to place them within the bony cavity.

The periosteum and muscular fascia should be closed with a strong, resorbable suture, such as 2-0 Vicryl. The subcutaneous tissues are then closed with 3-0 resorbable Vicryl suture. The skin can be closed with 4-0 transdermal sutures, skin staples, or a subcuticular suture.

The surgical site is then dressed with a transparent, permeable dressing for 48 hours. A pressure dressing using gauze and elastic tape is optional.

ALTERNATIVE TECHNIQUE 1: Pediatric Anterior Iliac Crest Bone Harvest

Harvesting of anterior iliac crest bone in a pediatric patient is essentially the same as in the adult, with one exception. In pediatric patients, the crest of the ilium has a cartilaginous cap that serves as an ossification center; therefore, harvesting bone below the cap does not affect growth. To harvest particulate marrow, the cartilaginous cap, including the perichondrium/periosteum complex, must be divided midcrestal and reflected to one side, typically medially. Occasionally, an H-incision may be required on either side to facilitate reflection of the cap. Once the cap has been reflected, the marrow space is exposed, allowing harvesting with bone gouges and curettes. When harvesting is complete, the cartilaginous cap is reapproximated with wires or strong sutures (Fig. 134.3).

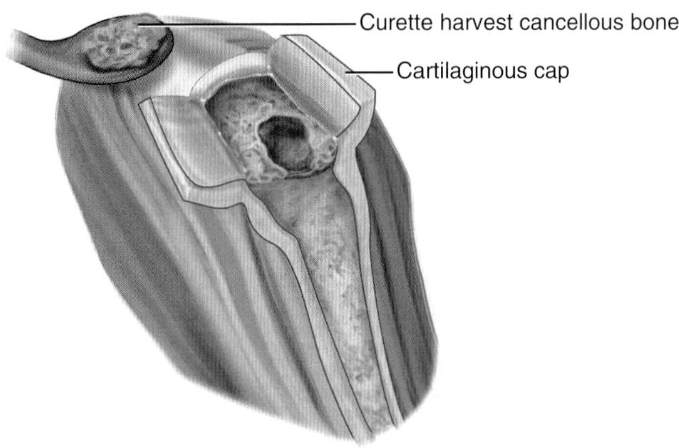

Figure 134.3 Pediatric anterior ilium with cartilaginous cap incised to expose the underlying cancellous marrow. A bone curette can be used to harvest cancellous chips.

ALTERNATIVE TECHNIQUE 2: Optional Crest Preservation

An alternative approach to harvesting bone involves preserving the integrity and muscular attachments to the crest, as described by Grillon et al.[14] By leaving the muscular attachments and periosteum attached to the crest, an osteoperiosteal cap can be created to allow access to the marrow and medial wall. Harvesting then can be completed in a fashion similar to that described previously. At the end of the procedure, the osteoperiosteal cap can be fixated in place. This procedure is thought to avoid crest deformities; eliminate dead space, making the use of postoperative drains unnecessary; and reduce gait disturbance by good fixation of the cap with its musculature.[14]

This procedure is accomplished by marking the same surgical incision described previously and dissection down to the periosteum without disrupting any of the muscular fascia. A horizontal incision is made through the periosteum just lateral to the crest. The length of this incision is determined by the length of the desired cap. On each end of this horizontal incision, a 1-cm vertical incision is made laterally to medially across the crest. With a saw or osteotomes, a rectangular bony cap is cut free and reflected medially, hinging on the periosteum and musculature. The side cuts can be made at a 45-degree angle to allow better reseating of the cap. Once the cap has been reflected, the medial dissection can proceed as described previously for graft harvest. The cap is then repositioned and secured with strong, nonabsorbable suture or wires by creating drill holes to rigidly secure the bone. Soft tissue closure is the same as previously described (Fig. 134.4).

ALTERNATIVE TECHNIQUE 3: Bone Marrow Aspirate

With recent advancements in tissue engineering and processing of blood products in tissue engineering, the use of bone marrow aspirate concentrates has significantly increased. The anterior iliac crest serves as a source for aspiration of mesenchymal stem cells, other osteoprogenitor cells, and growth factors.[15] The preparation for this procedure is similar to traditional harvesting techniques with the addition of a bone marrow aspirate kit which contains trocars, hollow-aspiration needle, syringe, and anticoagulant solution. The puncture sites for the anterior ilium should be safely placed 2–6 cm posterior to the anterior superior spine to access wider region of the anterior ilium. Once the puncture sites have been marked, local anesthesia can be deposited into the skin and outer cortex. A small (2–4 mm) stab incision in the skin is all that is needed. Hemostats are then used to create a blunt path to the outer cortex. The sharp trocar is placed within the aspiration

Continued

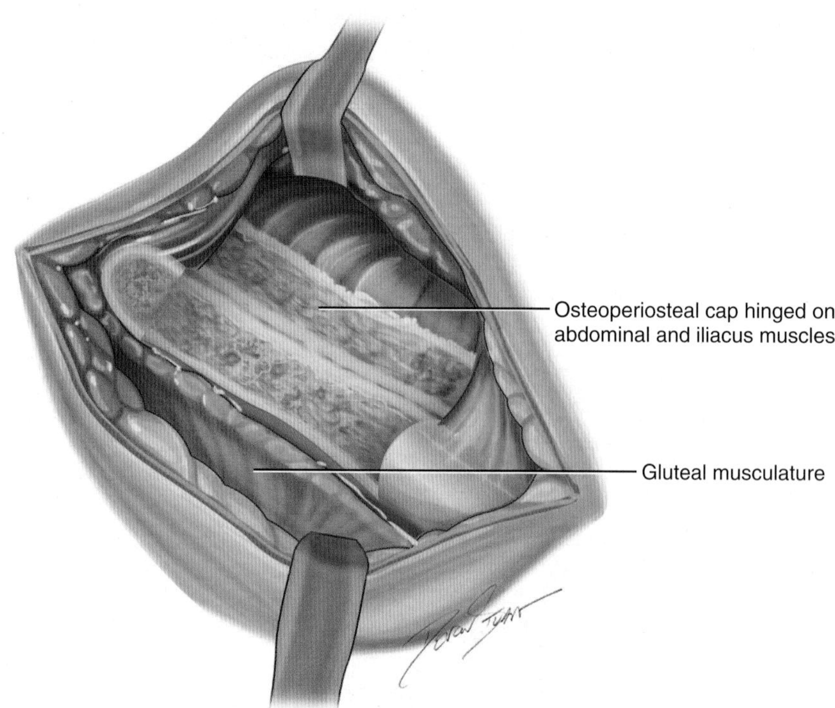

Figure 134.4 With a crestal preservation technique, an osteoperiosteal cap is created to hinge on the periosteum and iliac musculature. This exposes the marrow for harvesting of cancellous chips. If there is a need for a corticocancellous block, further medial dissection would be required below the cap.

ALTERNATIVE TECHNIQUE 3: Bone Marrow Aspirate—*cont'd*

needle and is then advanced through outer cortex while rotating the wrists back and forth. Palpation of the ilium is important to direct the trocar between the medial and lateral cortices, attempting to stay centered within the marrow to avoid inadvertent cortical perforations. Once advanced into the marrow, the sharp trocar is removed and a syringe with anticoagulant is used to aspirate bone marrow. Rotation of the needle can be done to reach marrow circumferentially. If further marrow aspirate is needed, the trocar can be reintroduced to reposition the needle into adjacent marrow spaces or a second puncture site may be used. On completion of aspiration, the syringe can then be handed off the field for processing (Fig. 134.5). The skin incision is closed with appropriate sutures and a simple sterile dressing is applied.

Avoidance and Management of Intraoperative Complications

Complications from AICBG include bleeding problems, nerve injuries, hernia development, gait disturbances, wound breakdown, cosmetic defects, chronic pain, and pathologic fractures.[16] Inadequate landmark identification, excessive soft tissue dissection, and overzealous bone harvesting are common causes of intraoperative complications.

The ASIS should be palpated and marked. Incision and bone harvesting should be kept at least 1 cm posterior to the ASIS to prevent pathologic avulsion fracture and to avoid damage to the lateral femoral cutaneous nerve, which can aberrantly travel over the ASIS.[16] Posteriorly, the incision can course through the path of the iliohypogastric nerve, which travels near the iliac tubercle, causing some numbness of that nerve's small distribution.

Minimizing soft tissue dissection to the crest and medial aspect of the anterior ilium (if needed) has been shown to reduce pain and gait disturbance because the outer (lateral) table muscles remain undisturbed.[16] This, in fact, tends to be the most recommended technique for anterior ilium bone harvesting. If the medial table and musculature are stripped, it is important to maintain a subperiosteal dissection with gentle retraction. Excessive retraction on the medial ilium can increase postoperative pain and risks traction injury to the lateral femoral cutaneous nerve, in addition to the ilioinguinal nerve. Similarly, this dissection and excessive retraction of the inner table musculature/abdominal wall can increase the risk of adynamic ileus and hernia.[17] Closure and reconstruction of the soft tissue musculature and fascia can also minimize gait disturbance and pain.

The techniques described often provide a unicortical block and some particulate marrow for reconstruction.

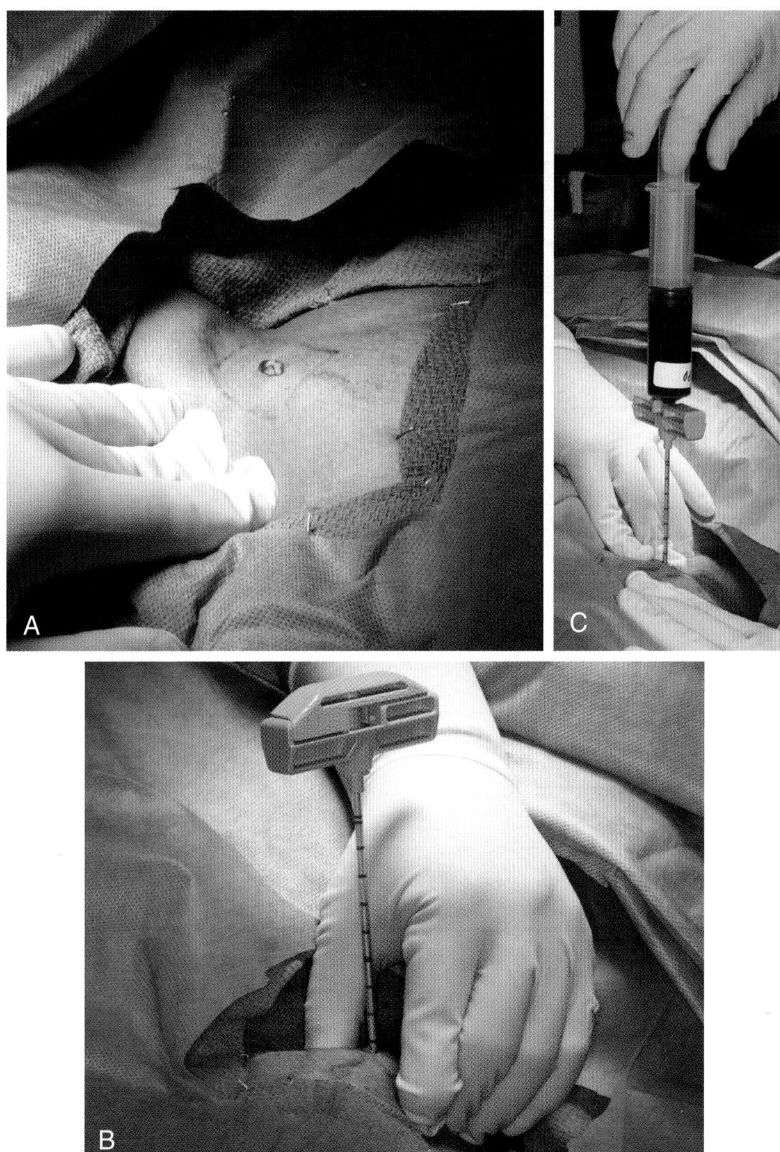

Figure 134.5 **A,** Small skin incision with blunt dissection to the iliac crest. **B,** Trocar positioned within the anterior ilium; note the manual palpation of the cortices serving as a guide to position the needle. **C,** Aspiration syringe with bone marrow aspirate; note the appearance is similar to blood.

Techniques for obtaining bicortical or tricortical blocks, which involve full-thickness defects inside the ilium, account for most of the complications reported in the literature.[17] Harvesting bone from beyond the limits described can undermine the ASIS, leading to avulsion fracture, bleeding from adjacent vasculature, and increased pain and gait disturbance.[18] To prevent contour deformities, a portion of the crest should be left intact if a crest preservation technique is not used.[19] Bleeding from the marrow is often managed with a hemostatic agent, such as gelatin sponges or microfibrillar collagen. Brisk bleeding can be managed with electrocautery, whereas a bleeding vessel in the soft tissues requires dissection and ligation. Suction drains can also be used, but this may not affect the likelihood of wound complications.[19]

Postoperative Considerations

Pain control is important in the postoperative phase.[20] Appropriate nonsteroidal antiinflammatory drugs and narcotics often provide adequate control. Postoperative continuous local anesthetic infusions can help reduce acute narcotic needs.[19] Most postoperative pain resolves within 2 weeks after surgery; however, chronic pain lasting longer than 3 months is the most common minor complication noted in the literature.[19]

Gait disturbance associated with the anterior ilium is common postoperatively. The patient can begin ambulation on postoperative day 1 but should use caution. Most gait disturbances are self-limiting, typically lasting less than 2 weeks.[16] During those 2 weeks, the patient should be advised to avoid climbing more than one flight of stairs and to refrain from extensive physical activities. Patients may use a cane for ambulation assistance in the immediate postoperative phase, although this is rarely necessary.

Suction drains, if used, can be removed once output is less than 25 mL over 24 hours; typically this is seen on postoperative day 2. Pressure dressings can be transitioned to a surgical dressing after 24 to 48 hours. After inspection of the wound and suture line, a simple dressing can be placed and changed as necessary. Skin sutures or staples usually are removed 10 to 14 days after surgery.

References

1. Rowe NL, Killey HC. *Fractures of the Facial Skeleton*. 2nd ed. London, UK: Churchill Livingstone; 1969.
2. Chubb G. Bone-grafting of the fractured mandible. *Lancet*. 1920;196:9.
3. Mowlem R. Cancellous chip bone grafts: report on 75 cases. *Lancet*. 1944;244:7467.
4. Freilich MM, Sándor GK. Ambulatory in-office anterior iliac crest bone harvesting. *Oral Surg Oral Med Oral Pathol Oral Radiol Endod*. 2006;101(3):291–298.
5. Marx RE, Stevens MR. Anterior ilium. In: Marx RE, Stevens MR, eds. *Atlas of Oral and Extraoral Bone Harvesting*. Chicago, Illinois: Quintessence; 2010.
6. Kessler P, Thorwarth M, Bloch-Birkholz A, Nkenke E, Neukam FW. Harvesting of bone from the iliac crest—comparison of the anterior and posterior sites. *Br J Oral Maxillofac Surg*. 2005;43(1):51–56.
7. Hall MB, Vallerand WP, Thompson D, Hartley G. Comparative anatomic study of anterior and posterior iliac crests as donor sites. *J Oral Maxillofac Surg*. 1991;49(6):560–563.
8. Ahlmann E, Patzakis M, Roidis N, Shepherd L, Holtom P. Comparison of anterior and posterior iliac crest bone grafts in terms of harvest-site morbidity and functional outcomes. *J Bone Joint Surg Am*. 2002;84(5):716–720.
9. Hwang K, Nam YS, Kim DJ, Han SH, Hwang SH. Could skin retraction incision minimize nerve injury over the iliac crest? *J Craniofac Surg*. 2007;18(6):1447–1450.
10. Mischkowski RA, Selbach I, Neugebauer J, Koebke J, Zöller JE. Lateral femoral cutaneous nerve and iliac crest bone grafts—anatomical and clinical considerations. *Int J Oral Maxillofac Surg*. 2006;35(4):366–372.
11. Kademani D, Keller E. Iliac crest grafting for mandibular reconstruction. *Atlas Oral Maxillofac Surg Clin North Am*. 2006;14(2):161–170.
12. Chou D, Storm PB, Campbell JN. Vulnerability of the subcostal nerve to injury during bone graft harvesting from the iliac crest. *J Neurosurg Spine*. 2004;1(1):87–89.
13. Nkenke E, Weisbach V, Winckler E, et al. Morbidity of harvesting of bone grafts from the iliac crest for preprosthetic augmentation procedures: a prospective study. *Int J Oral Maxillofac Surg*. 2004;33(2):157–163.
14. Grillon GL, Gunther SF, Connole PW. A new technique for obtaining iliac bone grafts. *J Oral Maxillofac Surg*. 1984;42(3):172–176.
15. Chahla J, Mannava S, Cinque ME, Geeslin AG, Codina D, LaPrade RF. Bone marrow aspirate concentrate harvesting and processing technique. *Arthrosc Tech*. 2017;6(2):e441–e445.
16. Fasolis M, Boffano P, Ramieri G. Morbidity associated with anterior iliac crest bone graft. *Oral Surg Oral Med Oral Pathol Oral Radiol*. 2012;114(5):586–591.
17. Kurz LT. Techniques and complications of bone graft harvesting. In: Herkowitz HN, Garfin SR, Eismont FJ, Bell GR, eds. *Rothman-Simeone the Spine*. 6th ed. Philadelphia, Pennsylvania: Elsevier; 2011.
18. Ebraheim NA, Yang H, Lu J, Biyani A, Yeasting RA. Anterior iliac crest bone graft. Anatomic considerations. *Spine*. 1997;22(8):847–849.
19. Myeroff C, Archdeacon M. Autogenous bone graft: donor sites and techniques. *J Bone Joint Surg Am*. 2011;93(23):2227–2236.
20. Becker ST, Warnke PH, Behrens E, Wiltfang J. Morbidity after iliac crest bone graft harvesting over an anterior versus posterior approach. *J Oral Maxillofac Surg*. 2011;69(1):48–53.

CHAPTER 135

Posterior Iliac Crest Bone Grafting

Shahid R. Aziz

Armamentarium

#15 Blade scalpel
#703 Bur
Appropriate sutures
Army-Navy retractors
Banana-shaped reciprocating saw blade
Bennett retractor
Caliper
Hohman retractor
Local anesthetic with vasoconstrictor
Mallet
Metzenbaum scissors
Needle driver
Needle electrocautery
Osteotomes (straight, curved; wide, narrow; large, medium, small)
Periosteal elevators
Rasp
Reciprocating saw
Rongeur
Small, medium, and long curettes
Smith spreaders
Vertical ramus osteotomy saw
Vertical ramus osteotomy saw blade
Exparel
Weitlaner self-retaining retractors

History of the Procedure

The first documented use of the posterior ilium as a site for bone graft harvest was in 1946 in the orthopedic surgery literature.[1] In 1950, Dingman advocated using the posterior ilium for craniomaxillofacial defects.[2] Since the 1980s, oral and maxillofacial surgeons have used the posterior ilium as a source of corticocancellous bone.[3,4]

Indications for the Use of the Procedure

The posterior iliac crest bone graft (PICBG) is indicated for maxillofacial reconstruction of skeletal defects requiring a significant volume of cortical, cancellous, or corticocancellous bone. Typically, defects requiring more than 40 mL of cancellous bone marrow or defects requiring large corticocancellous blocks are appropriate for PICBG. The PICBG can provide greater than 100 mL of cancellous bone marrow or maximum 5 × 5 cm cortical block.[5]

Limitations and Contraindications

The most significant limitation of the PICBG harvest is the prone positioning required. Placing the patient prone and then switching to the supine position following harvest can add 1 to 2 hours of surgical time. In addition, unlike the anterior iliac crest bone harvest, only one surgical team is able to operate during PICBG harvest, adding further operating time and, in turn, increased anesthesia time and hospital cost. Absolute contraindications are few but include previous fracture, radiation to site, infection at site, and any type of systemic metabolic bone disease such as osteoporosis. In addition, because this harvest is completed under general anesthesia, any contraindication to general anesthesia is a contraindication to the PICBG harvest. Relative contraindications include current use of oral or intravenous bisphosphonates or chronic steroid use.[6]

TECHNIQUE: Posterior Iliac Crest Bone Graft Harvest

Prior to any surgery, a review of pertinent surgical anatomy is critical. The largest amount of bone reservoir in the ilium is in the area of the posterior tubercle, or the area that the ilium posteriorly articulates with the sacrum. The PICBG provides up to 100 cc of uncompressed bone. Muscular attachments in this area include the gluteus maximus muscle and the gluteus minimus muscle. Most of the bone is located beneath the insertion of the gluteus maximus and is defined by the presence of a well-defined palpable triangular fossa. The gluteus medius attaches to the posterior ilium inferior to the gluteus maximus insertion. Superiorly, the thoracodorsal fascia of the latissimus dorsi attaches to the posterior ilium. Blood supply to this area is via the deep circumflex iliac artery. Pertinent neural anatomy includes the superior and medial cluneal nerves. The superior cluneal nerves are dorsal rami from L1, L2, and L3, which pierce the lumbodorsal fascia superior to the posterior iliac crest and innervate the skin over the posterior medial buttocks. While the medial cluneal nerves arise from S1, S2, and S3 and arise from the sacral foramina and course laterally to innervate the medial buttocks, the insertion of the gluteus maximus is between the superior and medial cluneal nerves. The sciatic notch and nerve, which supply the motor innervation to the lower extremity, are 6 to 8 cm inferior to the posterior iliac crest and should not be encountered during routine dissection. An incision placed between these nerves will prevent sensory loss postoperatively (Fig. 135.1A).

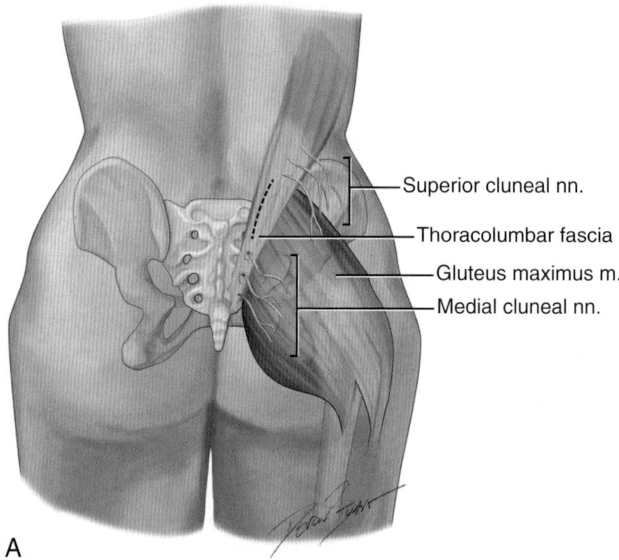

Figure 135.1 **A,** Outline demonstrating incision design in relation to the superior cluneal and medial cluneal nerves.

STEP 1: Patient Preparation

Patient positioning for the harvest of the PICBG is important to provide maximal access and because this positioning is unique among procedures performed by the maxillofacial surgeon. The patient is placed in a prone jackknife position with the table flexed at 210 degrees. Note that the patient is first nasally intubated supine and then carefully rolled to a prone position. Care must be given to appropriate padding as well as the position of extremities and genitalia in a male patient to avoid pressure-related injury. Typically the upper extremities are extended superiorly with shoulders abducted a maximum of 90 degrees. A roll is placed along the midsection/pelvis to enhance the jackknife position. Sandbags are placed as well along the anterior ilium for support[7] (Fig. 135.1B).

STEP 2: Incision

Prior to incision, intravenous antibiotics that cover dermal flora should be administered as well as perioperative steroids. Once properly positioned and prepped, the posterior ilium is palpated, located, and identified using the local anesthetic needle. Local anesthetic is infiltrated, typically 1% lidocaine with 1:100,000 epinephrine. A curvilinear incision is made starting 1 cm from the posterior superior iliac spine and extending 5 to 6 cm along the crest superolaterally. The initial incision is through skin and subcutaneous tissue. As noted previously, this incision design will minimize risk to associated sensory nerves (Fig. 135.1C).

TECHNIQUE: Posterior Iliac Crest Bone Graft Harvest—*cont'd*

STEP 3: Dissection and Iliac Crest Exposure

Blunt dissection with a periosteal elevator is completed through the fascia down to the periosteum; dissection may be facilitated by the use of an electrocautery with a needle tip. Care should be taken to dissect along the peak of the crest to avoid incising the gluteal muscles, thus minimizing postoperative gait issues. Subperiosteal dissection is essential as well to avoid disrupting associated musculature. Dissection should stay 1 cm away from the posterior superior iliac spine to avoid disturbing the sacroiliac ligament. Subperiosteal dissection then occurs along the lateral aspect of the posterior ilium to a maximum depth of 6 cm. Weitlaner self-retaining retractors as well as a Bennett retractor are used to facilitate dissection. At this point, 5 to 6 cm of the posterior iliac crest as well as 5 to 6 cm of the lateral aspect of the ilium should be exposed (Fig. 135.1D).

STEP 4: Osteotomy and Bone Harvest

Prior to surgery, a determination of the size and type of graft should be made (cancellous, cortical block, etc.). Based on this conclusion, the harvest osteotomies can be determined. Note that obtaining a graft larger than 5 × 5 cm increases risk of fracture and therefore should not be attempted.[6] With a marking pen or electrocautery, the dimensions of the harvest osteotomies can be outlined. Note that the superior aspect of the harvest osteotomy is just inferior to the crest of the posterior iliac ridge to minimize fracture risk. In this author's experience, a banana-shaped reciprocating saw blade as well as a vertical ramus osteotomy saw (90-degree, fan-shaped oscillating saw) can be used.

Continued

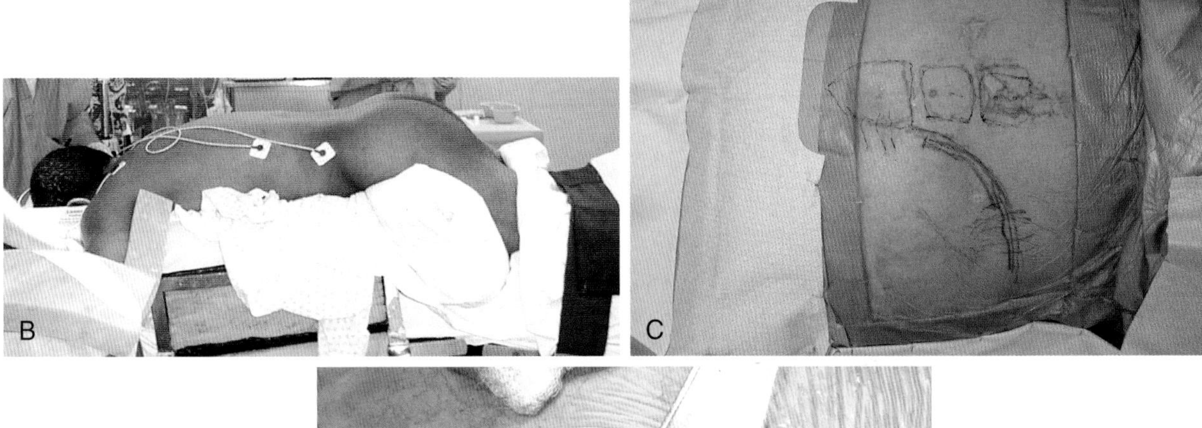

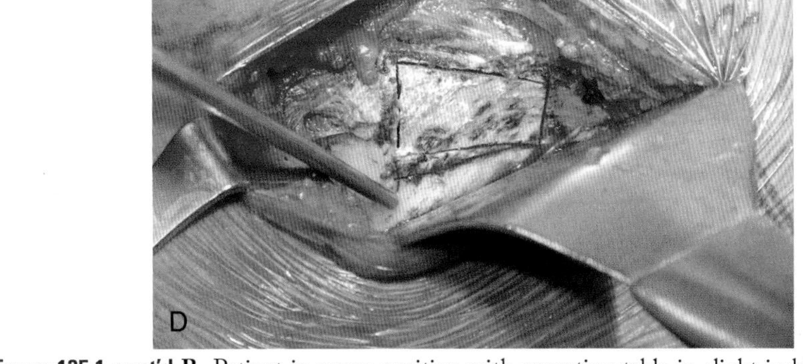

Figure 135.1 cont'd B, Patient in prone position with operating table in slight jackknife. Note importance of pressure point padding. **C,** Curvilinear incision design with patient prepped/draped. **D,** Dissection down to expose crest and lateral aspect of posterior ilium.

TECHNIQUE: Posterior Iliac Crest Bone Graft Harvest—*cont'd*

With copious saline irrigation, the banana blade can be used to score the vertical and crestal osteotomies. The vertical ramus saw can be used to score the inferior osteotomy. Once the surgeon is satisfied with the score marks, the osteotomies can be deepened through cortical bone to a depth of no greater than 3 mm, just penetrating the lateral cortex. Straight and curved osteotomes can then be utilized to complete the osteotomies into cortical bone. A Smith spreader can be then used along with osteotomies to remove the cortical block, exposing the underlying cancellous bone. With curettes, >100 mL of cancellous bone can be harvested. Once the required amount of PICBG is harvested, the edges of the donor site can be smoothed with a rasp and the site irrigated with saline. Further, hemostasis can be hastened utilizing fibrinous collagen (Fig. 135.1E and F).

STEP 5: Closure

Closure is typically completed using 3-0 Vicryl for deeper layers, 3-0 chromic for subdermal layers, and 5-0 Monocryl for the dermal layer. A Jackson-Pratt drain may or may not be needed depending on the level of hemostasis achieved, and this decision is usually left to the surgeon's discretion. A pressure dressing is applied with care not to disturb closure, and a 0.25% bupivacaine plain may be infiltrated into the incision to assist in postoperative analgesia.

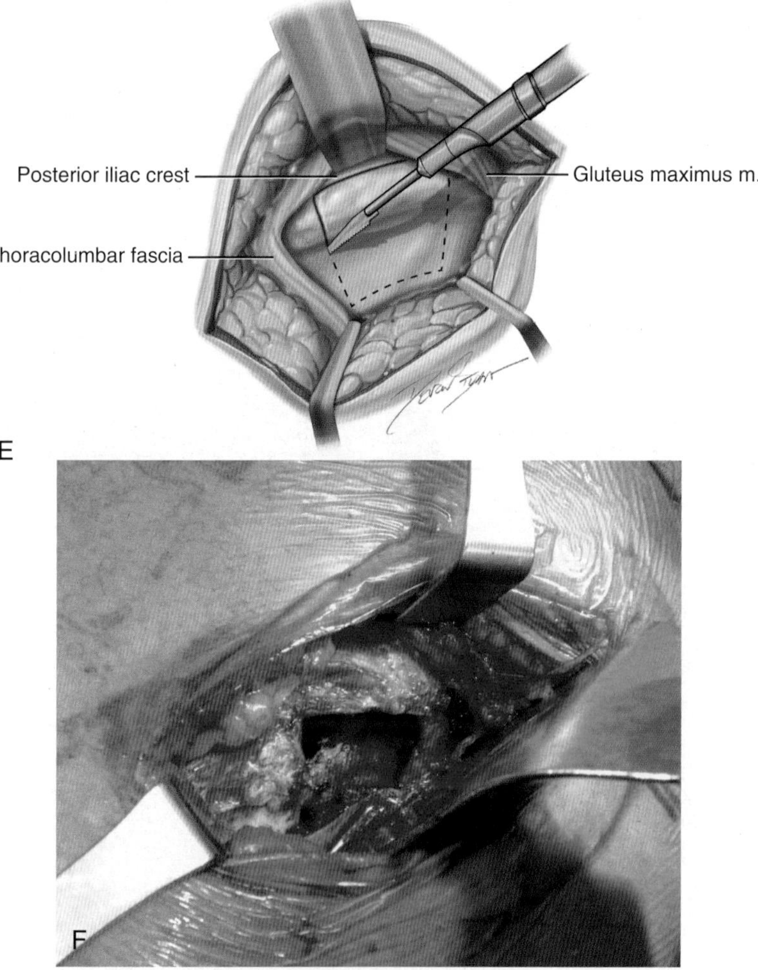

Figure 135.1 cont'd E, Outline of osteotomies. **F,** Donor site postharvest.

Avoidance and Management of Intraoperative Complications[6]

The following complications may arise.

Seroma

This is the most common complication following PICBG. Typically, seromas occur secondary to the failure to utilize a drain, premature removal of a drain, or premature exercise postoperatively. Treatment includes needle aspiration and pressure dressing.

Hematoma

This complication occurs due to poor hemostasis or failure to place a drain. Stable nonexpansile hematomas can be treated with a pressure dressing and observation. Expanding hematomas are typically associated with a significant bleed from the surgical site. This may require reexploration of the surgical site with appropriate hemostatic measures.

Fracture

This is a rare complication, usually associated with overaggressive osteotomies. This complication can be prevented with a combination of appropriate surgical technique and proper patient selection. Patients with osteoporosis or other bony morbidities are at increased risk for fracture; therefore, they are not ideal candidates for PICBG. Nondisplaced or greenstick fractures are treated with bed rest and pain management. Displaced/significant fractures may require open reduction/internal fixation and as such may need orthopedic surgical consultation/intervention.

Gait Disturbance

Gait disturbance is also a rare complication and is often secondary to disruption of the gluteal muscle attachments. Physical therapy typically will reestablish gait to normal function.

Postoperative Considerations

Pain management is essential. Postoperative use of bupivacaine as well as acceptable oral and intravenous analgesia is indicated. Because the maxillofacial reconstruction may require maxillomandibular fixation, intravenous analgesia is required until oral intake can be achieved. Patient-controlled analgesia is an excellent option. Consultation with the institution's pain management service may be indicated. The extent of postoperative antibiotic use is an area of debate. This author advocates a week of antibiotics postoperatively, which covers postoral and skin flora. Finally, consultation with a physical therapist is indicated to provide initial ambulation assistance.

References

1. Dick IL. Iliac-bone transplantation. *J Bone Joint Surg Am*. 1946;28:1–14.
2. Dingman RO. The use of iliac bone in the repair of facial and cranial defects. *Plast Reconstr Surg*. 1950;6(3):179–195.
3. Mrazik J, Amato C, Leban S, Mashberg A. The ilium as a source of autogenous bone for grafting: clinical considerations. *J Oral Surg*. 1980;38(1):29–32.
4. Bloomquist DS, Feldman GR. The posterior ilium as a donor site for maxillo-facial bone grafting. *J Maxillofac Surg*. 1980;8(1):60–64.
5. Zouhary KJ. Bone graft harvesting from distant sites: concepts and techniques. *Oral Maxillofac Surg Clin North Am*. 2010;22(3):301–316.
6. Marx R, Stevens M. *Atlas of Oral and Extraoral Bone Harvesting, (Chapter 3): Posterior Ileum.* Hanover Park, Illinois: Quintessence Publishing; 2010.
7. Mazock JB, Schow SR, Triplett RG. Posterior iliac crest bone harvest: review of technique, complications, and use of an epidural catheter for postoperative pain control. *J Oral Maxillofac Surg*. 2003;61(12):1497–1503.

CHAPTER 136

Tibial Bone Graft

George M. Kushner and Brian Alpert

Armamentarium

Appropriate sutures
Hall drill with tapered fissure bur
Local anesthetic with vasoconstrictor
Lower extremity tourniquet/thigh blood pressure cuff
Needle driver
Orthopedic bone harvesting curettes
Osteotome and mallet
Periosteal elevator
Russian forceps
Scalpel
Seldin retractors
Stainless steel bowl to hold bone graft
Sterile dressing supplies
Suture scissors
Syringe with local anesthesia 0.5% Marcaine with epinephrine 1:200,000
Weitlaner self-retaining retractor

History of the Procedure

Autogenous bone grafts have a long and well-documented history in maxillofacial reconstruction. The first report of autogenous tibial bone graft for use in the maxillofacial region was by Catone in 1992.[1] Since that time, multiple citations in both the orthopedic and maxillofacial literature have demonstrated the effectiveness of the autogenous tibia bone graft harvest.[2–5] The tibia bone graft harvest provides an adequate quantity and quality of bone, is technically easy to perform, and has a low complication rate.

Indications for the Use of the Procedure

The autogenous tibia graft harvest provides cancellous bone that has multiple uses in the maxillofacial region. Essentially, any indication for cancellous bone grafting in the maxillofacial region can be accomplished using the autogenous tibia graft. Traditionally, these autogenous bone grafts were harvested from the iliac crest. Alternatively, surgeons have the option of using banked bone, artificial bone, and now bone morphogenetic protein. The autogenous tibia graft harvest has given surgeons and patients another treatment option for maxillofacial reconstruction. The risks and benefits of each bone grafting technique must be evaluated and individualized for each patient.

Dental implantology, trauma, and reconstruction are the primary uses of autogenous bone grafting in the maxillofacial region.[6] Tibia bone grafts have been used for maxillary sinus lift procedures and to augment existing bone for placement of dental implants.[7] In trauma, tibia bone grafts have been used to treat difficult clinical situations such as defect fractures and atrophic edentulous fractures of the mandible. There is a wide range of reconstructive needs that can be fulfilled by the autogenous tibia bone graft, such as treatment of pathology defects, alveolar cleft grafting in skeletally mature patients, and restoring continuity defects of the jaws.

Limitations and Contraindications

Any surgical procedure has limitations and contraindications, and this certainly applies to the tibia bone graft harvest technique. This procedure is generally performed on skeletally mature patients. There is a growth plate in the tibial plateau region, which can be damaged during the harvest technique. Therefore, we do not perform this procedure on growing patients. However, several authors have successfully reported the safe use of autogenous tibia bone grafts for alveolar cleft grafting procedures in children.[8,9] The skin over the harvest site should be free of infection or pathology and be in good general condition. It is recommended to avoid sites that have had prior surgery such as fractures with orthopedic hardware or total joint replacements. Careful evaluation of the patient's activity level should be considered. We have avoided tibia graft harvest on distance runners who place large amounts of force on the tibial plateau on a repetitive basis. Lastly, the surgeon must consider the volume of bone required for the procedure. One can predictably harvest 25 cc of bone from the proximal tibia.[10] Reports have revealed that one may obtain 40 cc of bone from the proximal tibia, which is generally equivalent to an anterior iliac crest bone graft harvest. If larger amounts of bone are required, the surgeon must consider the addition of fillers or an additional autogenous bone graft harvest site. Simultaneous bilateral tibia bone graft harvests have been performed.

TECHNIQUE: Tibial Bone Graft

STEP 1: Preparation

The patient should have a sterile surgical preparation of the operative field, which extends 12 inches above and below the planned incision site. The patient is given a broad-spectrum antibiotic prophylaxis such as a cephalosporin within 30 minutes of incision time. Once the incision site has been marked, local anesthesia is infiltrated into the subcutaneous tissues to bone. We have used Marcaine with epinephrine for its vasoconstriction properties and long half-life for patient comfort. A lower extremity tourniquet is applied to the upper thigh and inflated to 50 mm Hg above the patient's systolic blood pressure. If a formal tourniquet is not available, a thigh blood pressure cuff can be used. Time with the tourniquet inflated should be monitored and not exceed 2 hours.

The surgical procedure is generally done in the operating room under general anesthesia as an adjunct to the main maxillofacial procedure. However, the procedure can easily be adapted to the office and performed under intravenous sedation and local anesthesia. The tibia graft harvest techniques can also be done under local anesthesia alone in cooperative patients[11] (Fig. 136.1A).

STEP 2: Incision

The key to the lateral approach to proximal tibia graft harvest is to locate Gerdy's tubercle. Gerdy's tubercle is a bony protuberance located between the patellar tendon and the head of the fibula. When palpating the proximal tibia, the patellar tendon is identified as the midline structure. Palpating 90 degrees laterally, one can easily identify the head of the fibula. Gerdy's tubercle is a bony protuberance between these two structures and is easily palpated. The incision will be placed over Gerdy's tubercle and approximately 3 to 4 cm in length. There are no major anatomic structures overlying Gerdy's tubercle.

The surgical dissection is minimal. The incision is carried through the skin and subcutaneous tissues. The iliotibial tract, which is a dense fascial band running from the lateral ilium to the lateral surface of the tibia, is encountered. The iliotibial tract is incised sharply. The iliotibial tract is identified and will be important as a layer in the closure. The incision is carried through periosteum to bone. The periosteum is elevated and Gerdy's tubercle is fully exposed[2] (Fig. 136.1B–E).

STEP 3: Bony Window

A bony window must be made in the proximal lateral tibia to gain access to the cancellous bone to be harvested. The surgeon has two choices for this osteotomy: a drill with a cutting bur or an osteotome with a mallet. We have favored a drill and bur to make the oval window, as it is easy, quick, and atraumatic. We favor an oval or round window with no sharp corners, which can be stress risers. Alternatively, the surgeon can use osteotomes and a mallet to cut the cortical bone and gain access to the cancellous bone. The cortical window is removed and not replaced. This cortical window can be used as a cortical graft, morselized and used with the cancellous graft, or discarded. Removing the cortical window essentially eliminates Gerdy's tubercle[2] (Fig. 136.1F and G).

STEP 4: Bone Harvest

Cancellous bone is accessed and harvested with orthopedic bone curettes. The surgeon scoops out the cancellous bone by going across the proximal tibia and down the shaft of the tibia. Great care must be taken harvesting bone in a superior direction, as you can enter the joint space or significantly undermine the tibial plateau. Trephines have also been used to harvest cancellous bone from the proximal tibia.[12] One can predictably obtain 25 cc of cancellous bone from the proximal tibia. The surgeon should be able to adequately predict the amount of bone needed and harvest that amount. The surgeon should only take the amount of bone needed and not waste the patient's autogenous bone. The autogenous bone graft should be placed in the patient's own blood or saline until it is needed for the reconstructive procedure. The total time for harvesting the graft is generally 30 minutes or less[2] (Fig. 136.1H–J).

STEP 5: Closure

The incision is closed in layers. The iliotibial tract is easily identified and closed with a 2-0 resorbable suture such as Vicryl. Subcuticular sutures are placed with a 4-0 resorbable suture such as Vicryl. The thigh tourniquet or blood pressure cuff is deflated and hemostasis is checked. The skin suture is generally a 4-0 nonresorbable suture such as Prolene.

A sterile dressing is placed. We prefer a compressive dressing such as an Ace wrap or Coban dressing over the site[2] (Fig. 136.1K).

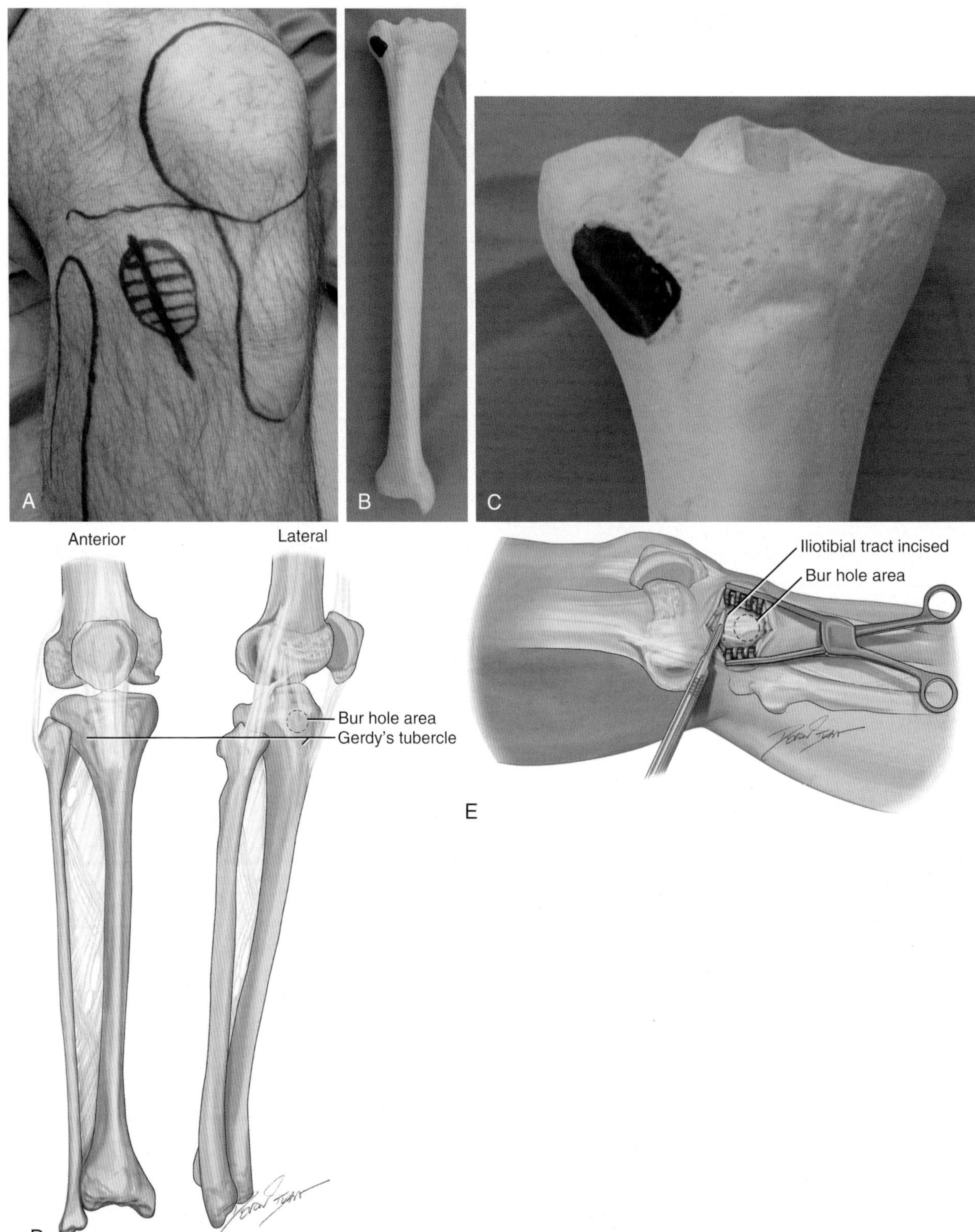

Figure 136.1 **A,** Incision marked over Gerdy's tubercle. **B,** Right tibia with Gerdy's tubercle marked. **C,** Close-up of right proximal tibia with Gerdy's tubercle marked. **D,** Anterior and lateral views of bur hole over Gerdy's tubercle. **E,** Bur hole outlined over Gerdy's tubercle after soft tissue retracted.

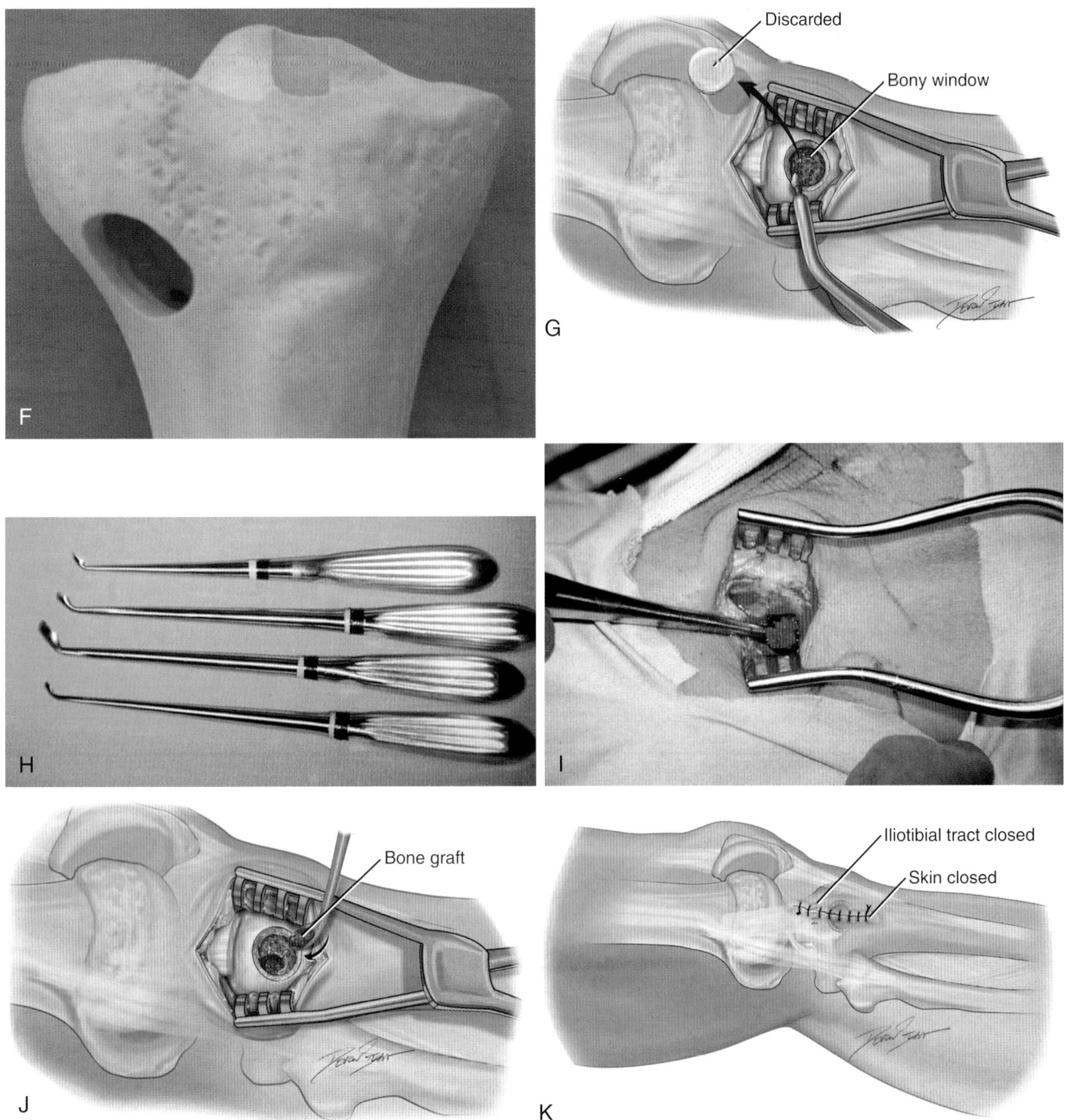

Figure 136.1, cont'd F, Oval window into proximal tibia over Gerdy's tubercle. **G,** Cortical window removed exposing cancellous bone at Gerdy's tubercle. **H,** Orthopedic bone harvest curettes. **I,** Bone graft harvest from proximal tibia. **J,** Cancellous bone being removed using orthopedic curette. **K,** Incision over Gerdy's tubercle closed in layers.

ALTERNATIVE TECHNIQUE: Proximal Tibial Bone Graft

As an alternative technique, the proximal tibia graft harvest can be approached from the medial surface. The anterior medial region of the proximal tibia can easily be used to access cancellous bone graft. The dissection is minimal, and the harvest technique is similar to the lateral approach. A 3- to 4-cm skin incision is made in the anterior medial tibia region of the proximal tibia. A bony window is made with the drill and cutting bur. The cortical window is removed and not replaced. The cancellous bone is harvested with orthopedic curettes or trephines. The layered closure is similar to the lateral approach. However, the iliotibial tract is not present on the medial approach to provide soft tissue coverage over the bony window. There is a potential disadvantage of having an incision over a bony window, which may lead to wound breakdown[9,10,12] (Fig. 136.2).

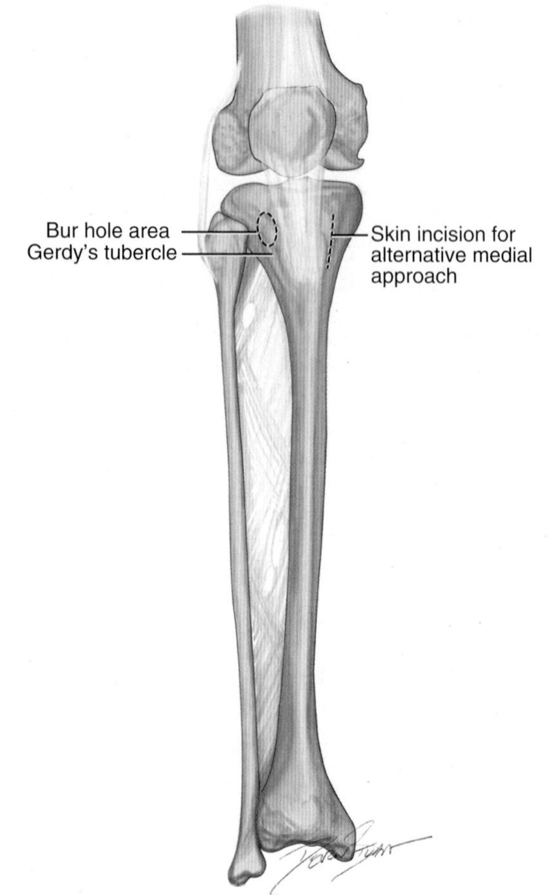

Figure 136.2 Surface anatomic landmarks for tibial bone graft harvest site.

Avoidance and Management of Intraoperative Complications

The area overlying Gerdy's tubercle is devoid of any major anatomic structures, so damage to associated structures such as blood vessels and nerves should be extremely low. Round or oval access osteotomy cuts prevent sharp angles in the cortical bone and negate the possibility of stress risers. Using a drill and cutting bur is precise and is less traumatic to the cortical bone when compared with using an osteotome and mallet to perform the cortical osteotomy. When harvesting the cancellous graft, the surgeon should extend across the proximal tibia and down the shaft of the tibia. Great care should be taken, or the surgeon should possibly avoid altogether the urge to harvest bone in a superior direction. Harvesting bone in a superior direction could lead to undermining (and weakening) the tibial plateau or surgical misadventure into the joint space. If this occurs, consultation with an orthopedic surgeon is advised. Lastly, the final closure of the skin is performed with the tourniquet deflated to check hemostasis and decrease the chance of hematoma formation.

POSTOPERATIVE CONSIDERATIONS

Immediately postoperatively, the patient is instructed to allow weight bearing as tolerated. Patients are not generally given crutches, canes, or walkers. However, some patients may occasionally require some assistance with ambulation. If possible, rest with the harvest site elevated is recommended. The surgical site is kept dry for 48 hours. The sutures are removed in 10 to 14 days. No contact sports or vigorous physical activity is recommended for 6 weeks postoperatively. Analgesics that are sufficient for the primary procedure are generally adequate for the tibia bone graft harvest. Hydrocodone or the equivalent will generally suffice for most patients.

The postoperative course for the tibial bone graft harvest is usually uneventful. The postoperative pain is less than a corresponding iliac crest bone graft harvest. Possible complications include hematoma at the site, wound breakdown, and wound infection. There is obviously an external scar, which has the potential to be unsightly for the patient. Fracture at the graft harvest site is a possibility, as removing bone temporarily weakens the region. Fracture of the proximal tibia has been reported after an autogenous bone graft harvest.[13–17] Clinicians should be vigilant in monitoring the tibia harvest site postoperatively. Continued pain or a new onset of significant pain should prompt the surgeon to obtain a radiograph of the area to evaluate the harvest site for possible fracture. If a fracture is confirmed, consultation with an orthopedic surgeon is recommended (Figs. 136.3-136.5).

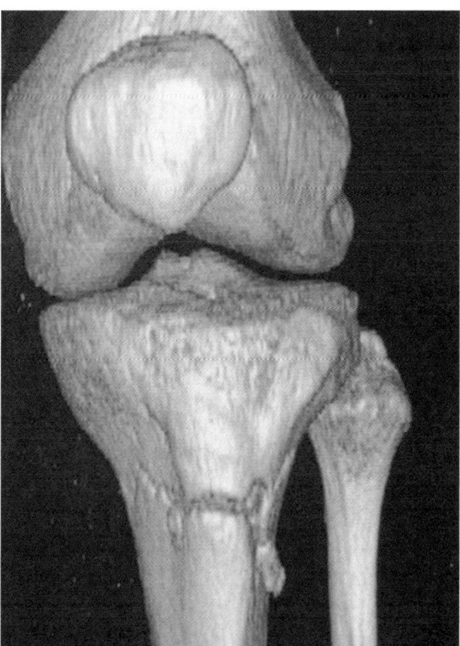

Figure 136.3 Fracture of proximal tibia after bone graft harvest.

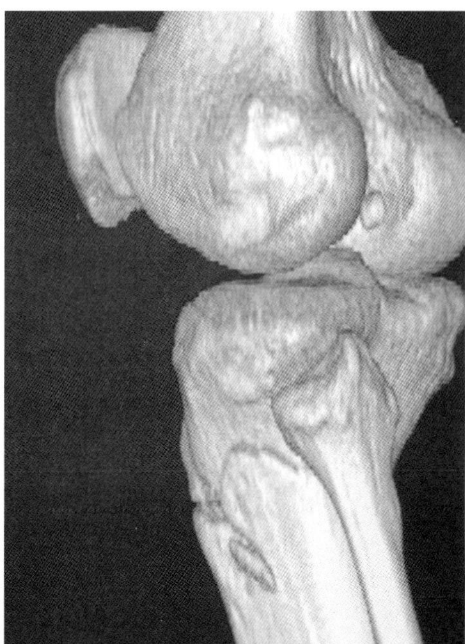

Figure 136.4 Fracture of proximal tibia after bone graft harvest.

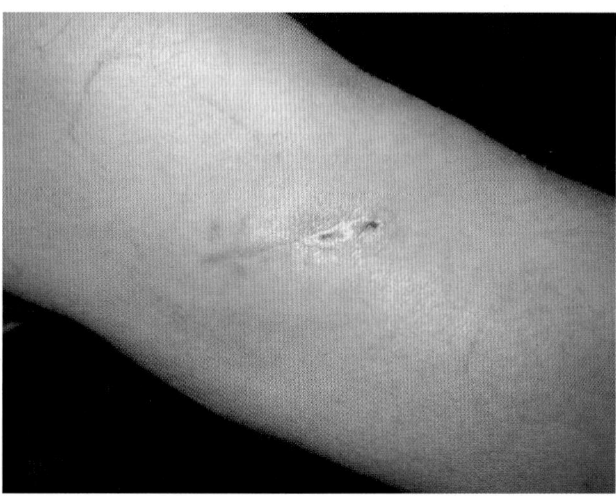

Figure 136.5 Minor incision breakdown with superficial infection.

References

1. Catone GA, Reimer BL, McNeir D, Ray R. Tibial autogenous cancellous bone as an alternative donor site in maxillofacial surgery: a preliminary report. *J Oral Maxillofac Surg*. 1992;50(12):1258–1263.
2. Kushner GM. Tibia bone graft harvest technique. *Atlas Oral Maxillofac Surg Clin North Am*. 2005;13(2):119–126.
3. Myeroff C, Archdeacon M. Autogenous bone graft: donor sites and techniques. *J Bone Joint Surg Am*. 2011;93(23):2227–2236.
4. Mauffrey C, Madsen M, Bowles RJ, Seligson D. Bone graft harvest site options in orthopaedic trauma: a prospective in vivo quantification study. *Injury*. 2012;43(3):323–326.
5. Whitehouse MR, Lankester BJ, Winson IG, Hepple S. Bone graft harvest from the proximal tibia in foot and ankle arthrodesis surgery. *Foot Ankle Int*. 2006;27(11):913–916.
6. Mazock JB, Schow SR, Triplett RG. Proximal tibia bone harvest: review of technique, complications, and use in maxillofacial surgery. *Int J Oral Maxillofac Implants*. 2004;19(4):586–593.
7. Peysakhov D, Ferneini EM, Bevilacqua RG. Maxillary sinus augmentation with autogenous tibial bone graft as an in-office procedure. *J Oral Implantol*. 2012;38(1):43–50.
8. Al Harbi H, Al Yamani A. Long-term follow-up of tibial bone graft for correction of alveolar cleft. *Ann Maxillofac Surg*. 2012;2(2):146–152.
9. Walker TW, Modayil PC, Cascarini L, Williams L, Duncan SM, Ward-Booth P. Ret-

rospective review of donor site complications after harvest of cancellous bone from the anteriomedial tibia. *Br J Oral Maxillofac Surg.* 2009;47(1):20–22.

10. Herford AS, King BJ, Audia F, Becktor J. Medial approach for tibial bone graft: anatomic study and clinical technique. *J Oral Maxillofac Surg.* 2003;61(3):358–363.
11. Kirmeier R, Payer M, Lorenzoni M, Wegscheider WA, Seibert FJ, Jakse N. Harvesting of cancellous bone from the proximal tibia under local anesthesia: donor site morbidity and patient experience. *J Oral Maxillofac Surg.* 2007;65(11):2235–2241.
12. Lezcano FJ, Cagigal BP, Cantera JM, de la Peña Varela G, Blanco RF, Hernández AV. Technical note: medial approach for proximal tibia bone graft using a manual trephine. *Oral Surg Oral Med Oral Pathol Oral Radiol Endod.* 2007;104(1):e11–e17.
13. Herford AS, Dean JS. Complications in bone grafting. *Oral Maxillofac Surg Clin North Am.* 2011;23(3):433–442.
14. Chen YC, Chen CH, Chen PL, Huang IY, Shen YS, Chen CM. Donor site morbidity after harvesting of proximal tibia bone. *Head Neck.* 2006;28(6):496–500.
15. Michael RJ, Ellis SJ, Roberts MM. Tibial plateau fracture following proximal tibia autograft harvest: case report. *Foot Ankle Int.* 2012;33(11):1001–1005.
16. Van Damme P. Fracture of the tibia: complication of bone grafting to the anterior maxilla. *J Craniomaxillofac Surg.* 1998;26(suppl 1):197.
17. Galano GJ, Greisberg JK. Tibial plateau fracture with proximal tibia autograft harvest for foot surgery. *Am J Orthop.* 2009;38(12):621–623.

CHAPTER 137

Costochondral Graft

Deepak G. Krishnan

Armamentarium

#10 and #15 Scalpel blades and blade handles
#701 Bur/reciprocating saw blade
Adson tissue forceps fine with teeth
Appropriate sutures
Army-Navy retractors
Bipolar electrocautery
Doyen retractor
Fixation devices (P&S or internal/external DO devices)
Frazier suction
Giertz rib-cutting shears
Kocher Ochsner clamp (straight/curved)
Local anesthetic with vasoconstrictor
Mayo Hager needle holders
Mayo scissors
Needle electrocautery
Periosteal elevators
Weitlaner self-retaining retractors (6 1/2 blunt)

History of the Procedure

The current technique for mandibular ramus/condyle/temporomandibular joint (TMJ) reconstruction using an autogenous rib graft was popularized by Poswillo.[1,2] However, much credit goes to Sir Harold Gillies, who, in the 1920s, was the first to describe the use of the costochondral graft (CCG).[3] Although other techniques have been tried and tested, the CCG still remains a workhorse in the reconstruction of the ramus-condyle unit (RCU) in a growing child and often enough in an adult. The main advantage of the CCG is that it is a biologically compatible autograft that has some growth potential.[4,5] One of the disadvantages of the use of CCG for reconstruction of the RCU is the unpredictable growth pattern of the graft itself. From their experience, Kaban and Perrott[6] hypothesized that the transfer of a large cartilaginous cap may be the cause of this overgrowth; these authors advocate the use of a 1- to 2-mm cartilaginous cap to avoid this problem. CCGs also tend to be flexible and almost elastic, which often can lead to deformation of these grafts in function. In addition, this predisposes them to intraoperative problems with fixation and the possibility of resorption or failure. Several authors have assessed the long-term fate of CCGs and reaffirmed the challenge of the unpredictability of its growth pattern. In addition to overgrowth, undergrowth and ankylosis have been reported. Reviews by Mulliken et al.[7] suggested that most of the growth of the CCG occurs in the first 2 months after placement and that the graft often does not have a linear pattern of growth, but rather follows a slow, irregular pattern, although there are many variations of this general rule.

A better understanding of CCG growth patterns and rigid fixation techniques, in addition to the ability to simulate and perform virtual treatment planning of the graft, has led to a more predictable technique.

Indications for the Use of the Procedure

1. Reconstruction of the RCU in growing children
2. Reconstruction of the RCU in disarticulation resections of the mandible in adults
3. Reconstruction of other continuity defects or articulation defects in the adult mandible and maxilla
4. Costal cartilage grafts for reconstruction of cartilaginous defects in the ear and nose
5. Additional bone graft strut to complement another autogenous cancellous marrow graft harvested from elsewhere, often as a crib or a sandwich

Limitations and Contraindications

Limitations

Although the CCG provides form and function, it often does not provide bulk and is not an ideal source for osteogenic regeneration. The flimsy rib does not reconstruct the horizontal and vertical height of the ramus or the body of the mandible. Muscular attachments of the latissimus dorsi restrict the access and limit the length of the rib that can be harvested.

Contraindications

1. Metabolic bone diseases (e.g., osteogenesis imperfecta, osteopetrosis)
2. Infective conditions affecting the ribs (e.g., osteomyelitis)
3. A history of irradiation of the chest
4. A recent history of trauma to the chest or pneumothorax
5. Severe restrictive pulmonary disease (e.g., cystic fibrosis, sarcoidosis)

TECHNIQUE: Costochondral Graft Harvesting

STEP 1: Patient Positioning and Preparation

The fifth, sixth, or seventh rib is chosen, ideally from the side contralateral to the defect to match the curvature of the rib. The patient is placed in a standard supine position for most harvests. Occasionally, if a longer harvesting procedure is needed, a lateral approach or a lateral decubitus position is used. Chlorhexidine or Betadine is used to prep the chest widely over the area of the proposed incision, which is marked before the prep. The prep must cross the midline superiorly and must be above the nipple line and extend laterally beyond the midaxillary line. Standard draping is then completed. The surgeon's choice of local anesthetic with epinephrine is injected into the subcutaneous layer, to the depth of the rib, along the planned incision.

STEP 2: Incision and Flap Elevation

Ideally, the proposed incision is placed in the inframammary crease in both males and females for the best cosmetic outcome. This incision is placed as close as possible to the rib to be harvested. If more than one rib is to be obtained, alternate ribs are best chosen to minimize postoperative morbidity. A skin incision of approximately 4 to 5 cm is made with a #15 blade on a handle through the skin. Thereafter, a blade or needle tip electrocautery is used to obtain further exposure through subcutaneous tissue and fascia and between the pectoralis major and rectus abdominis muscles over the rib to be harvested (Fig. 137.1). As this incision is developed, the surgeon should place one finger in the intercostal space above the desired rib and another finger below that rib, thus straddling it. This precaution prevents inadvertent slippage of the blade into the intercostal spaces, causing a pleural puncture. A flap is reflected above and below to provide adequate tension-free exposure of the desired length of the rib and its adjoining cartilaginous junction.

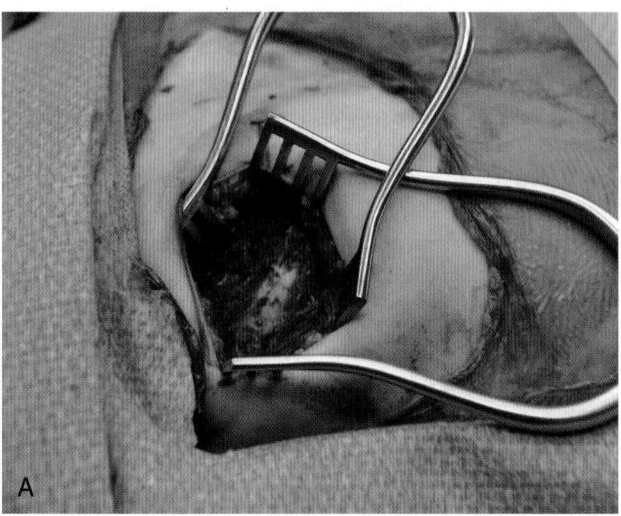

Figure 137.1 **A,** Incision made through the skin, fascia, and muscle, exposing the periosteum over the rib.

TECHNIQUE: Costochondral Graft Harvesting—*cont'd*

STEP 3: Graft Harvest

The surgeon now uses the same #15 blade to make an incision through the periosteum over the midline of the rib horizontally, taking care not to score through the cartilaginous cap. Standard #9 Molt periosteal elevators can be used to dissect in a subperiosteal plane all around the rib to be harvested. Longacre described the importance of maintaining this periosteum and closing it after removal of the rib, which allows regeneration of a new rib.[8] Similar to the precaution taken while making the incision over the rib, it helps to move the two fingers straddling the rib back and forth as this periosteal flap is elevated, thus preventing the dissection from slipping into the intercostal space and accidentally creating a pneumothorax or lacerating the intercostal vessels. A Doyen retractor or similar curved retractor is inserted underneath the periosteal sheath to detach it from the undersurface of the rib. The retractor is moved medially to gain subperiosteal dissection along the cartilaginous cap area also and is left there for protection while an incision is made through the cap. A fresh #15 blade is used to incise through the full depth of the desired thickness of the cartilage. The surgeon now swings the rib outward and laterally, peeling off any further periosteal attachments from beneath, and a protected rib cutter is inserted to cut and completely separate the rib at its desired length. The graft is then removed (Fig. 137.1B–D).

STEP 4: Wound Management

The wound is checked for hemostasis. Once hemostasis has been obtained, it is imperative to check for any pleural punctures. This is best done by filling the defect with normal saline, having the anesthesiologist introduce positive pressure, and then performing a Valsalva maneuver. Absence of bubbling air in the saline-filled defect suggests the absence of a pneumothorax. Once this has been confirmed, wound closure is initiated. The periosteal sleeve is closed first with interrupted 3-0 Vicryl sutures. As mentioned before, some suggest that this promotes de novo regeneration of the missing rib, especially in younger individuals. The deep and superficial fascial and muscular layers are closed with interrupted 3-0 Vicryl sutures. Once a subdermal closure has been achieved with the same suture, either a subcuticular running stitch with 4-0 Monocryl suture or proper skin suturing with nonresorbable sutures can be used (Fig. 137.1E).

Continued

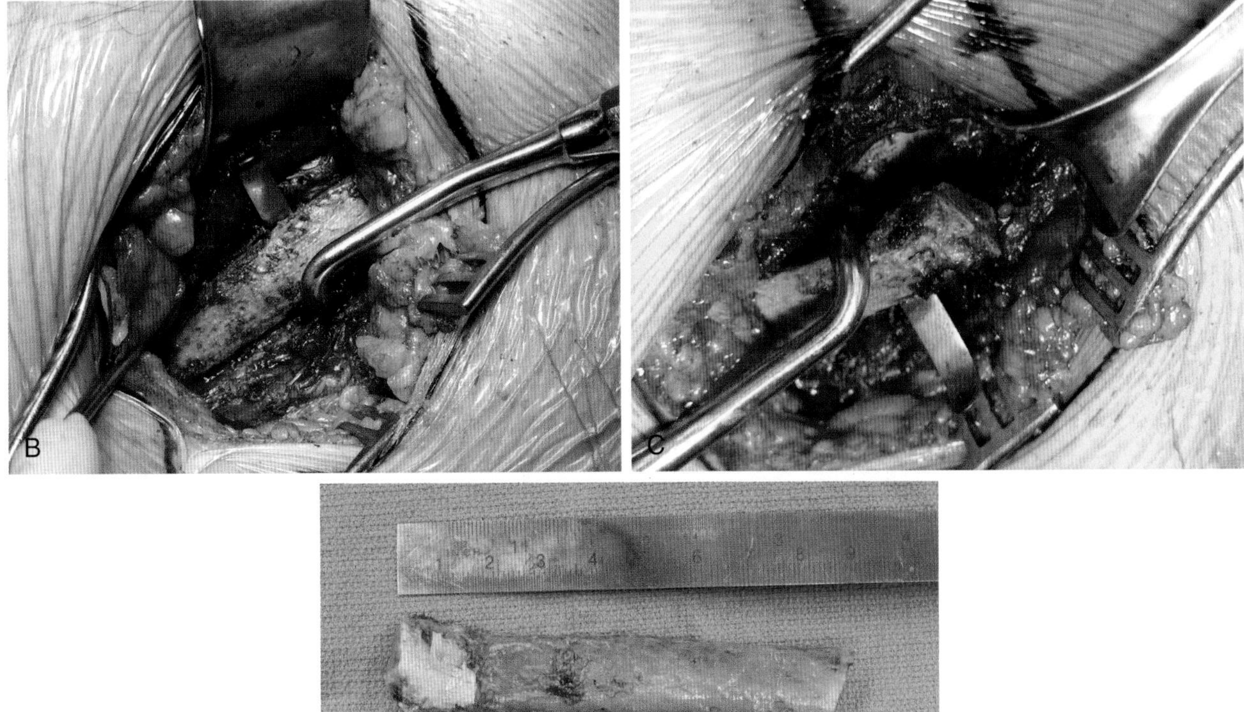

Figure 137.1 cont'd B, Medial elevation of the pleura and periosteum with a Doyen rib stripper. **C,** Careful elevation of the rib graft. **D,** Costochondral graft harvested. Note the presence of a cartilaginous cap.

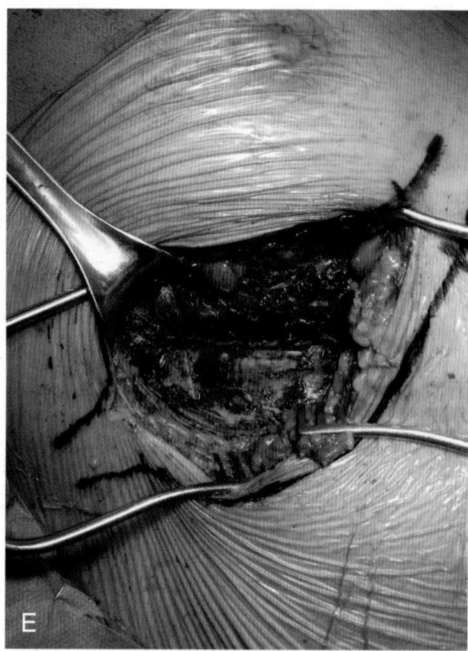

Figure 137.1 cont'd E, Intact pleura after removal of the rib.

TECHNIQUE: Costochondral Graft Harvesting—*cont'd*

STEP 5: Dressing

The skin surface is cleaned and dried. Steri-Strips are placed perpendicular to the incision directly over the wound. A small piece of cut gauze is placed over the Steri-Strips, and an occlusive dressing (e.g., Tegaderm) or an adhesive bandage may be placed. The wound is best left untouched before this dressing is removed in 5 to 7 days.

ALTERNATIVE TECHNIQUE 1: Pediatric Patients

When a rib is harvested in children, the costochondral junction must be managed slightly differently because of the risk of the cartilage separating from the rib. The surgeon can avoid this by taking no more than the necessary 3 mm of cartilage and by first sharply cutting through the perichondrium with a #15 blade and carefully separating it along with the graft. Also, care must be taken in young female patients to avoid placing the incision in a manner that could cause a breast deformity.

ALTERNATIVE TECHNIQUE 2: Virtual Surgical Planning

As a result of the availability of virtual surgical planning, CCGs now can be procured and trimmed to precision with cutting guides and splints. The technique involves preoperative computed tomography scanning of the desired rib and custom fabrication of a cutting guide for the surgeon for harvesting of the rib. This eliminates the guesswork regarding the required length of the graft, and it also aids in the adaptation of the grafted rib precisely to the native mandible, enabling good mandible-rib interface (Fig. 137.2).

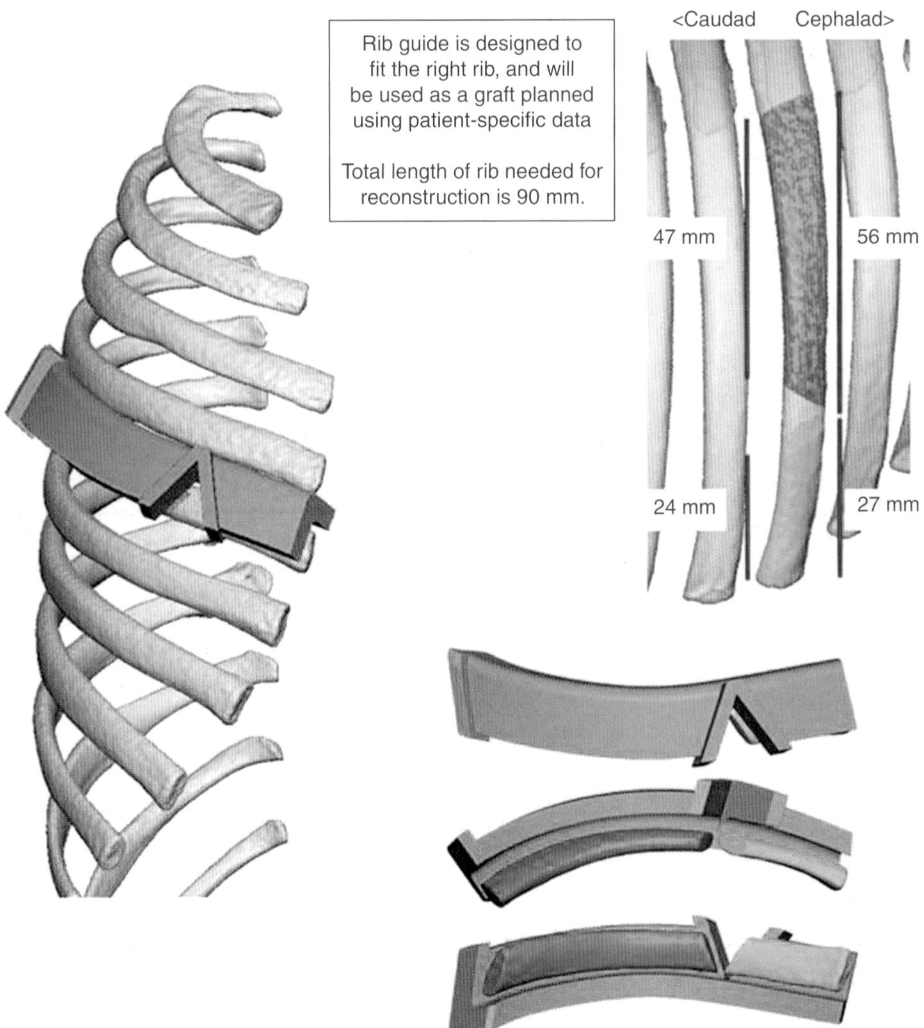
Rib guide is designed to fit the right rib, and will be used as a graft planned using patient-specific data
Total length of rib needed for reconstruction is 90 mm.
<Caudad
Cephalad>
47 mm
56 mm
24 mm
27 mm

Figure 137.2 A and B, Virtual surgical planning and surgical guide for rib grafting.

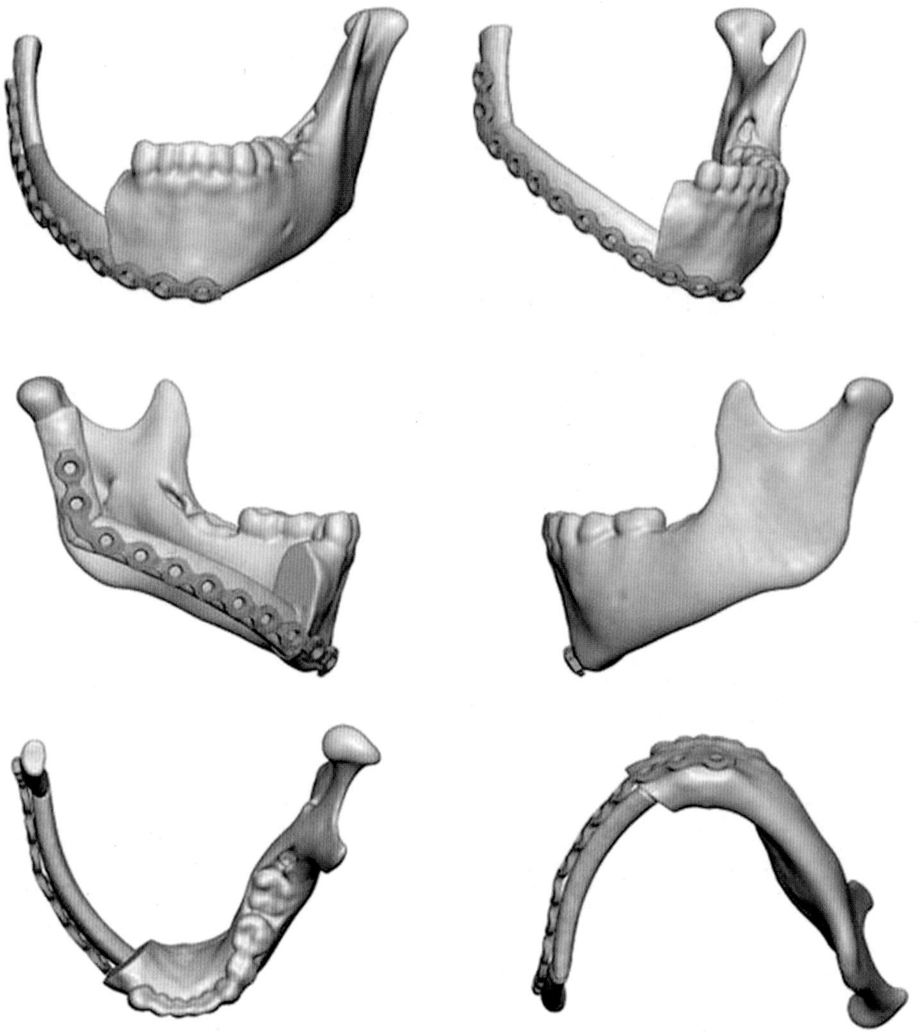

Figure 137.2 cont'd

Avoidance and Management of Intraoperative Complications

The dreaded complication of creating a pneumothorax can be easily avoided or recognized intraoperatively and managed effectively. These pneumothoraxes are generally small and are caused by a relatively small tear in the pleura. The underside of ribs often has small bony projections that are points of adherence of the parietal pleura. Rapidly stripping the pleural attachment from these can cause multiple small pleural punctures. Careful use of a curved elevator and stripping off the pleura before introducing a Doyen rib stripper are helpful in preventing pneumothoraxes. If a small pneumothorax is identified intraoperatively, it can be managed by placing a small suction drain catheter, around which a horizontal mattress suture is placed. The catheter is withdrawn under suction as the suture is tightened.

Bleeding from the blood vessels adjoining the rib may occur during harvesting of the graft. This is best avoided by neat subperiosteal dissection and careful local measures.

Postoperative Considerations

A postoperative chest radiograph is useful for identifying a pneumothorax. A small pneumothorax identified on a postoperative chest radiograph is managed conservatively. Most conservative management involves observation for at least 6 hours, after which reliable patients with ready access to emergency medical services theoretically can be discharged home if a repeat chest radiograph excludes progression of the pneumothorax. While the patient is hospitalized, supplemental oxygen should be administered to facilitate resorption of the pleural air. Air in the pleural space is reabsorbed when the communication between the alveoli and the pleural space collapses. The rate of resorption can be markedly increased if supplemental oxygen is administered.[9] In animal models, the rate of resorption increased six-fold when humidified 100% oxygen was administered.[10]

Unresolved pneumothoraxes or large pneumothoraxes must be managed by standard chest tube placement.

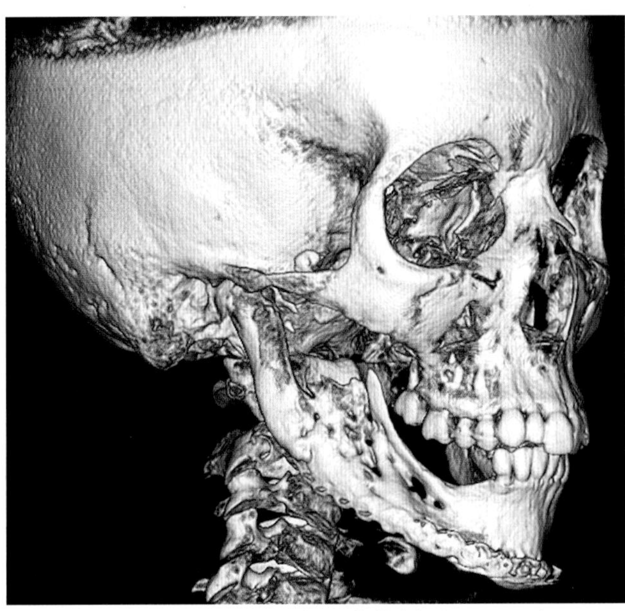

Figure 137.3 Seven-year follow-up imaging on rib graft. Rib has integrated into native mandible and formed a functional temporomandibular joint (TMJ), and there is de novo bone formation in the coronoid region.

When more than one rib is harvested, postoperative pain or pleuritis may occur. A local anesthetic depot device could be considered for the patient's comfort and can be placed at the time of the procedure.

Wound dehiscence or local infection of the incision site is managed by debridement and culture-based antibiotic therapy; it also may require wound packing to allow healing by secondary intention.

CCGs can potentially have some unpredicted growth patterns. When the periosteum of the native mandible is left behind (especially in children), it tends to encourage de novo bone formation eventually (Fig. 137.3).

References

1. Poswillo D. Experimental reconstruction of the mandibular joint. *Int J Oral Surg.* 1974;3(6):400–411.
2. Poswillo DE. Biological reconstruction of the mandibular condyle. *Br J Oral Maxillofac Surg.* 1987;25(2):100–104.
3. Gillies HL. *Plastic Surgery of the Face.* London, UK: Oxford University Press; 1920.
4. Ko EW, Huang CS, Chen YR. Temporomandibular joint reconstruction in children using costochondral grafts. *J Oral Maxillofac Surg.* 1999;57(7):789–798.
5. Kaban LB, Bouchard C, Troulis MJ. A protocol for management of temporomandibular joint ankylosis in children. *J Oral Maxillofac Surg.* 2009;67(9):1966–1978.
6. Kaban LB, Perrott DH. Discussion: unpredictable growth pattern of costochondral graft. *Plast Reconstr Surg.* 1992;90:887.
7. Mulliken JB, Ferraro NF, Vento AR. A retrospective analysis of growth of the constructed condyle-ramus in children with hemifacial microsomia. *Cleft Palate J.* 1989;26(4):312–317.
8. Longacre JJ, Destefano GA. Reconstruction of extensive defects of the skull with split rib grafts. *Plast Reconstr Surg.* 1957;19(3):186–200.
9. Northfield TC. Oxygen therapy for spontaneous pneumothorax. *BMJ.* 1971;4(5779):86–88.
10. Chernick V, Avery ME. Spontaneous alveolar rupture at birth. *Pediatrics.* 1963;32:816–824.

CHAPTER 138

Calvarial Bone Graft

William J. Curtis, Brent Golden, and Michael Jaskolka

Armamentarium

Appropriate sutures
Bone contouring/bending forceps
Bone mill
Bone shaving harvester
Bone wax
Cool saline-moistened sponge/lap
Egg-shaped bur
Gelfoam soaked in thrombin
Kocher bone clamp
Large Steiger bur
Local anesthetic with vasoconstrictor
Mallet
Midface plate and screw system
Needle electrocautery
Obwegeser retractors
Periosteal elevator
Raney clips
Reciprocating saw
Saline irrigation
Scalpel
Self-retaining retractor
Skin hooks (2)
Small Steiger bur
Small straight and curved osteotomes
Sterile secondary table

History of the Procedure

The current gold standard in reconstruction focuses on the use of recombinant hormones, stem cells, and scaffolds, with the goal of tissue regeneration. Although these technologies and techniques are surely the way of the future, autogenous bone grafting continues to play a primary role in the field of oral and craniomaxillofacial surgery.

The character of bone grafts harvested from different donor sites or derived from different germ cell layers and the behavior of these grafts when placed in different recipient sites have been a topic of much debate. Researchers and surgeons such as Wolff, Moss, Enlow, Whitaker, Axhausen, Boyne, Longaker, and Marx have all helped elucidate the details of bone graft healing; the importance of the interaction between bone and recipient soft tissue throughout the bone grafting process also has been highlighted.[1]

The ideal bone graft is difficult to identify due to the number of clinical scenarios that may require various combinations of onlay, inlay, block, and particulate grafts. A donor site that is readily available with ample volume, easily harvested without significant morbidity, and able to satisfy many different indications is as close to ideal as can be achieved. The calvarial bone graft applied through different techniques can fulfill most bone grafting requirements in the craniomaxillofacial skeleton.

In 1890, both Mueller and Koenig published on the use of the calvaria as a pedicled osteocutaneous flap for cranial defect reconstruction.[2] This technique was popular until 1903, when von Hacker simplified the technique by taking the outer table pedicled on only pericranium. The use of cranial bone as a free graft subsequently was described by Keen, Sohr, and Axhausen. This began a shift from allogeneic to autogenous cranial reconstruction, as described by Cushing in 1908. Further experience was gained from treatment of the many ballistic injuries that occurred during World War I and World War II. These injuries were increasingly reconstructed using calvarial grafts, as reported by Delageniere and Virenque, respectively. Calvarial grafts were applied to craniofacial reconstruction and widely championed by Paul Tessier through the 1960s and 1970s. Since his landmark publication in 1982, the cranial bone graft has become a staple in the armamentarium of maxillofacial surgeons around the world.[3–6]

Indications for the Use of the Procedure

The cranium provides a versatile stock of bone that can be used for autogenous grafting, and it has a number of advantages over other common harvest sites, such as the ilium, rib, or tibia. The skull is readily included in the primary surgical field, and access is quickly and easily achieved through the scalp. With proper positioning and technique, the risk of visible scarring is negligible. A large volume and surface area of bone with variable contour are available. The high proportion of cortical bone makes the outer cortex an ideal bone graft for onlay purposes. Through wide exposure, significant diploë can also be harvested and combined with morselized cortical bone for particulate grafting. Full-thickness harvest with immediate site reconstruction provides a source of thick bone for significant augmentation or reconstruction. There is limited postoperative donor site morbidity from all of these techniques. The following sections discuss specific indications for the cranial bone graft.

Cranial Vault Reconstruction

Patients who have undergone craniectomy for decompression, tumor (Fig. 138.1), trauma, or infection may present with full-thickness defects that require reconstruction. Autogenous cranium is an excellent option as compared with alloplastic materials, which have a high cost of fabrication and increased risk of complete loss as a result of exposure or infection.

In the pediatric patient, consideration must be given to the regenerative nature of the cranium owing to the osteogenic properties of the dura and to a lesser extent the pericranium. As the patient ages, the cranium is more prone to incomplete regeneration after surgical insult.

Depending on the age of the patient and the size of the defect, cranial reconstruction can be completed with resorbable mesh and cortical shavings, in situ split-thickness harvest and transposition, and full-thickness harvest with splitting and reconstruction of both the donor site and affected area.

Stabilizing Craniomaxillofacial Osteotomies

Wassmund, Axhausen, Schuchardt, Gillies, Trauner, Schmid, and others have reported cases of mobilization and advancement of the craniofacial skeleton for pathologic, congenital, and posttraumatic deformities; Obwegeser and Tessier refined and popularized many of the craniomaxillofacial procedures that are used contemporarily. Stabilization of osteotomy sites with bone grafts is recommended for significant advancements to aid in both healing and minimization of postoperative relapse. Grafts are commonly placed in an interpositional fashion at the zygomaticofrontal, nasofrontal, pterygomaxillary, and nasomaxillary buttresses (Fig. 138.2). Their use is also advised for significant advancement of the mandible with inverted L procedures and sliding step genioplasties.

Onlay Bone Augmentation

Conventional orthognathic surgical procedures (i.e., bilateral sagittal split and Le Fort I osteotomies) are primarily used to correct dentofacial relationships. However, patients with abnormal facial proportions often benefit from further hard tissue augmentation in addition to corrective surgery. Split-thickness calvarial onlay bone grafts can significantly improve the aesthetic outcome when appropriately applied (Fig. 138.3).

Cleft Bone Grafting

Patients born with cleft lip and/or palate often have an associated cleft involving the maxilla, alveolar ridge, and nasal floor. Although the anterior iliac crest is the gold standard for secondary bone grafting, the calvaria is a convenient and effective source of bone for all aspects of cleft reconstruction

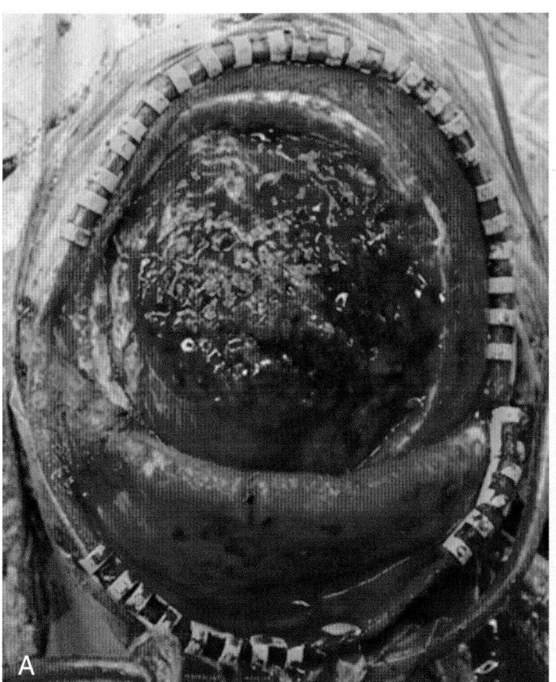

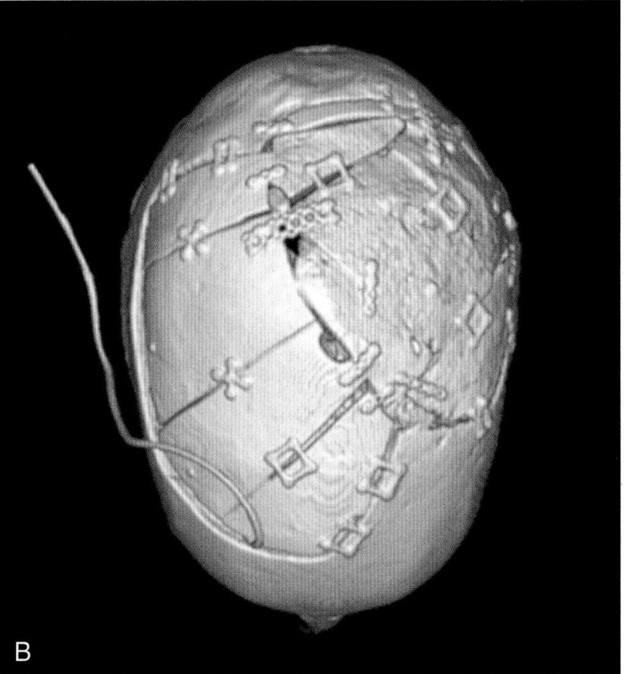

Figure 138.1 **A** and **B,** Reconstruction using split full-thickness graft after resection for adenocarcinoma metastasis.

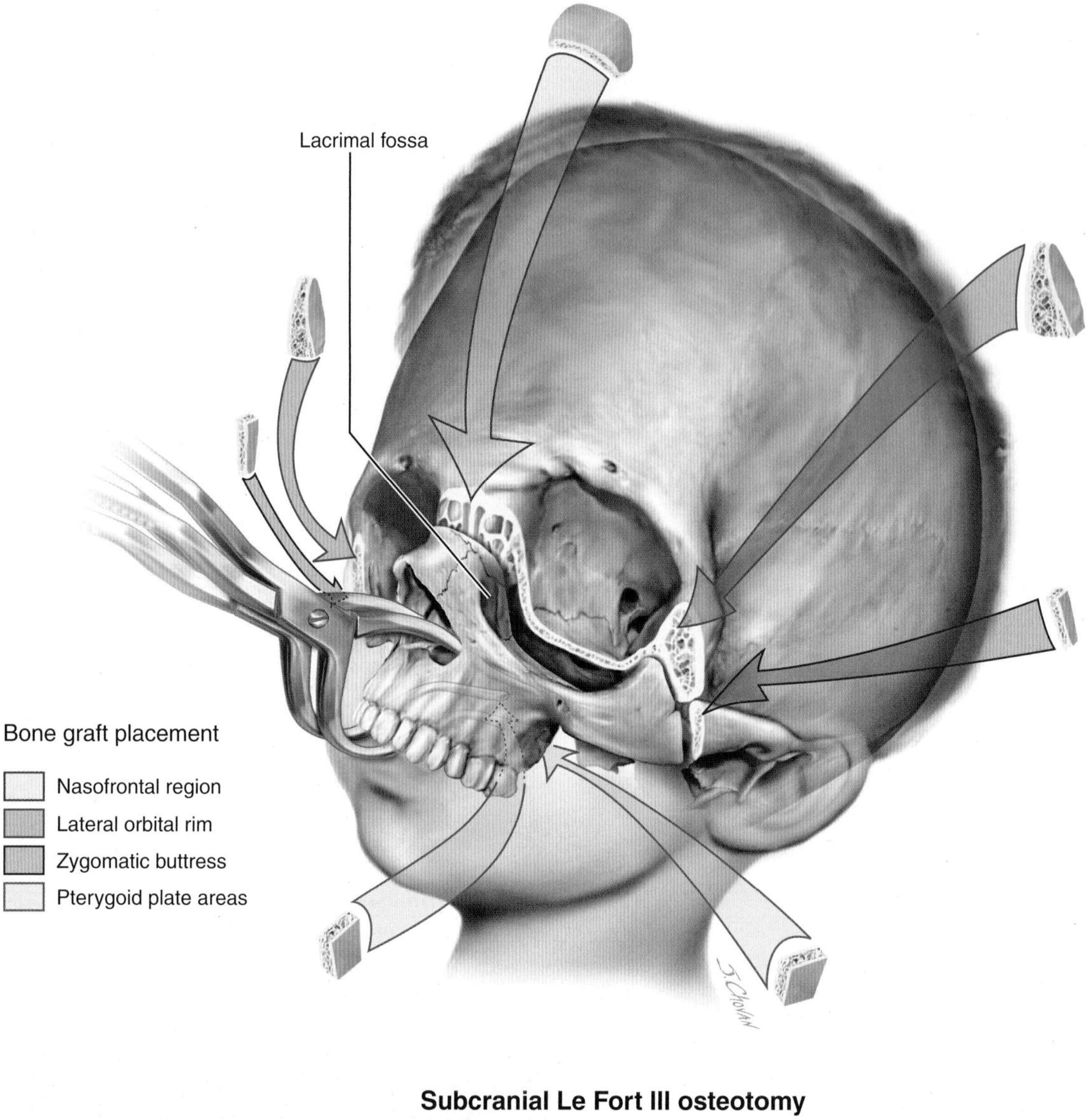

Lacrimal fossa

Bone graft placement

- Nasofrontal region
- Lateral orbital rim
- Zygomatic buttress
- Pterygoid plate areas

Subcranial Le Fort III osteotomy

Figure 138.2 Modified Le Fort III osteotomy stabilized with interpositional bone grafts.

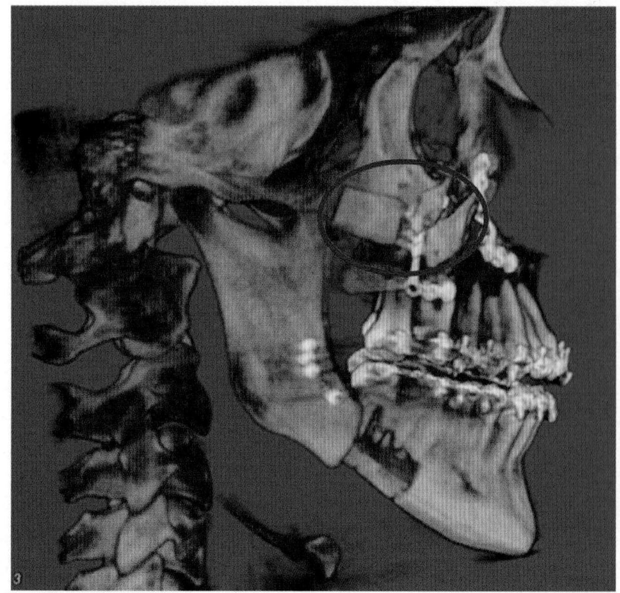

Figure 138.3 Augmentation of midface with split-thickness onlay grafting.

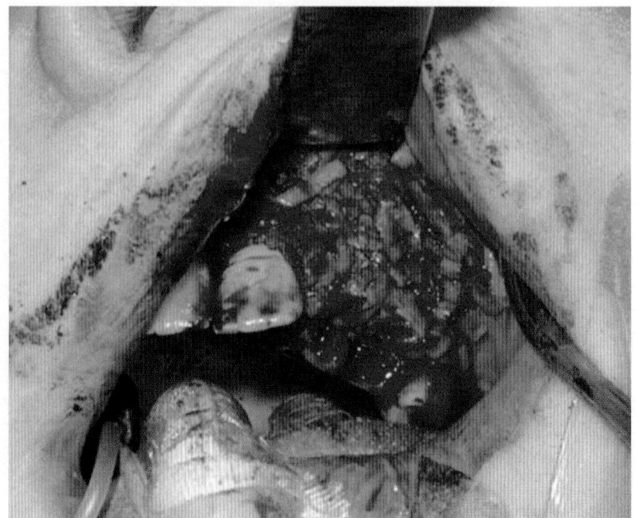

Figure 138.4 Cleft alveolar bone graft using cranial bone shavings.

(Fig. 138.4) or augmentation for prosthetic or orthodontic indications. Orthognathic surgery is also regularly indicated in the patient with a cleft to correct midface deficiency and may require a combination of alveolar grafting, grafting for osteotomy stabilization, and onlay augmentation.

Trauma

Trauma often results in damage to the craniomaxillofacial region. Of particular relevance are high-energy mechanisms (e.g., motor vehicle crashes, all-terrain vehicle accidents, gunshot injuries), which often lead to comminuted or avulsive injuries of the facial skeleton. Although microplate fixation techniques are helpful, primary split-thickness calvarial reconstruction of the frontal, nasal (Fig. 138.5), orbital, and zygomatic regions is often indicated to prevent posttraumatic deformity.

Pathology

Hard tissue defects resulting from pathologic extirpation may require significant bone stock for reconstruction. Depending on the volume and condition of the soft tissue recipient site, a free or pedicled full-thickness cranial bone graft may be a viable option for maxillary and mandibular reconstruction.

Congenital Conditions

Multiple congenital conditions are associated with deformity of the craniofacial skeleton. In the patient with craniosynostosis, split-thickness cranial grafts are regularly employed in primary reconstruction to stabilize expansion and prevent incomplete ossification (Fig. 138.6).

Treacher Collins syndrome and hemifacial microsomia are two other craniofacial conditions that benefit from a reconstructive approach. Full-thickness cranial bone is often used for orbitozygomatic reconstruction after the age of 7 once regional facial growth is complete.[7,8] Depending on the anatomic and functional status of the ramus and condyle unit, as most clearly described by Kaban et al.,[9] full-thickness calvaria may also be used for reconstruction and augmentation of the mandible and of the glenoid fossa in combination with cartilage or fascial lining.

Limitations and Contraindications

Every patient and clinical scenario must be evaluated individually. The status and health of the recipient tissue bed should

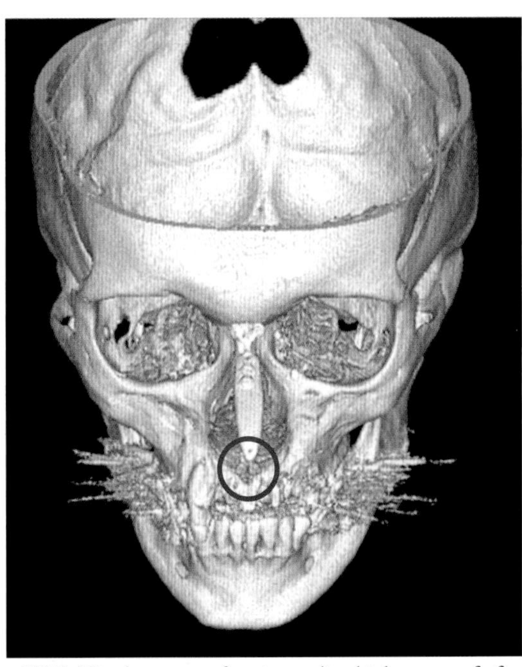

Figure 138.5 Nasal strut graft using split-thickness graft for nasal reconstruction.

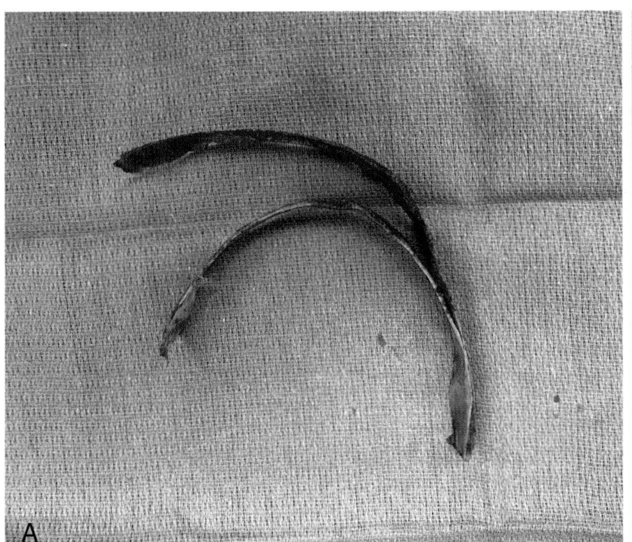

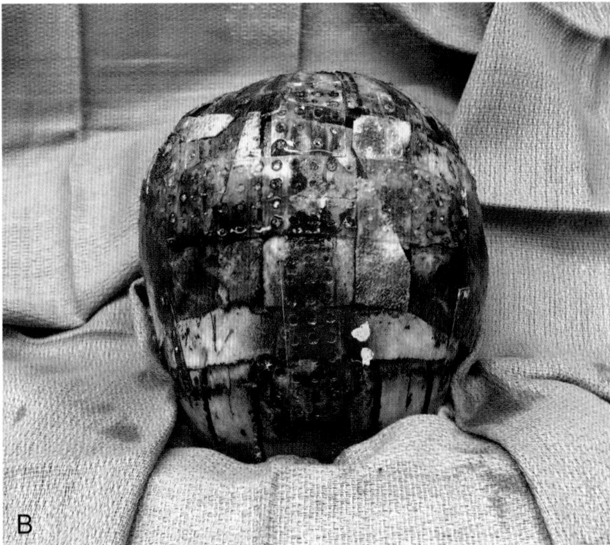

Figure 138.6 A, Splitting of the inner and outer table of the calvarium in a 9-month-old patient undergoing posterior cranial vault expansion for sagittal craniosynostosis. **B,** Completed posterior cranial vault reconstruction using split-thickness cranial bone grafts in a 9-month-old patient with sagittal craniosynostosis.

be specifically evaluated before the use of nonvascularized bone grafts. Consideration must be given to the type and volume of bone graft required because variation in the thickness of the skull and the absence of a diploic layer may limit the type of bone available or complicate split-thickness harvesting. Otherwise, there are few limitations and contraindications to harvesting bone from the cranium. Caution should be used when considering patients with the following conditions[10]:

- History of head trauma, ventricular shunt, implanted brain stimulator
- History of irradiation of the cranium
- History of osteomyelitis
- Metabolic or malignant bone disease (i.e., osteogenesis imperfecta, Paget disease of the skull, osteopetrosis, multiple myeloma, and metastatic tumor)

TECHNIQUE: Split-Thickness Cranial Bone Graft

STEP 1: Preoperative Evaluation

A thorough history and physical examination are key to preoperative evaluation. If there are no concerning findings, imaging may be deferred depending upon the comfort of the surgeon. Plain skull radiographs or cone beam computed tomography may be useful to ensure adequate thickness or the presence of a diploic space if desired. If the patient has undergone previous surgery or has a history of pathology or trauma, computed tomography of the head is warranted.

STEP 2: Site Selection

The preferred site for cranial bone harvesting is the parietal bone of the nondominant side; remaining posterior to the coronal suture protects the motor strip. The middle to posterior region is generally the thickest part of the cranium with the most developed diploic space.[11] At the superior aspect of the skull beneath the sagittal suture lies the sagittal sinus. The middle meningeal artery runs just deep to the squamous portion of the temporal bones near the squamoparietal suture. By remaining at least 1 cm from these two suture lines and in the "center" of the parietal bone during harvesting, the surgeon can avoid these important vascular structures (Fig. 138.7A).

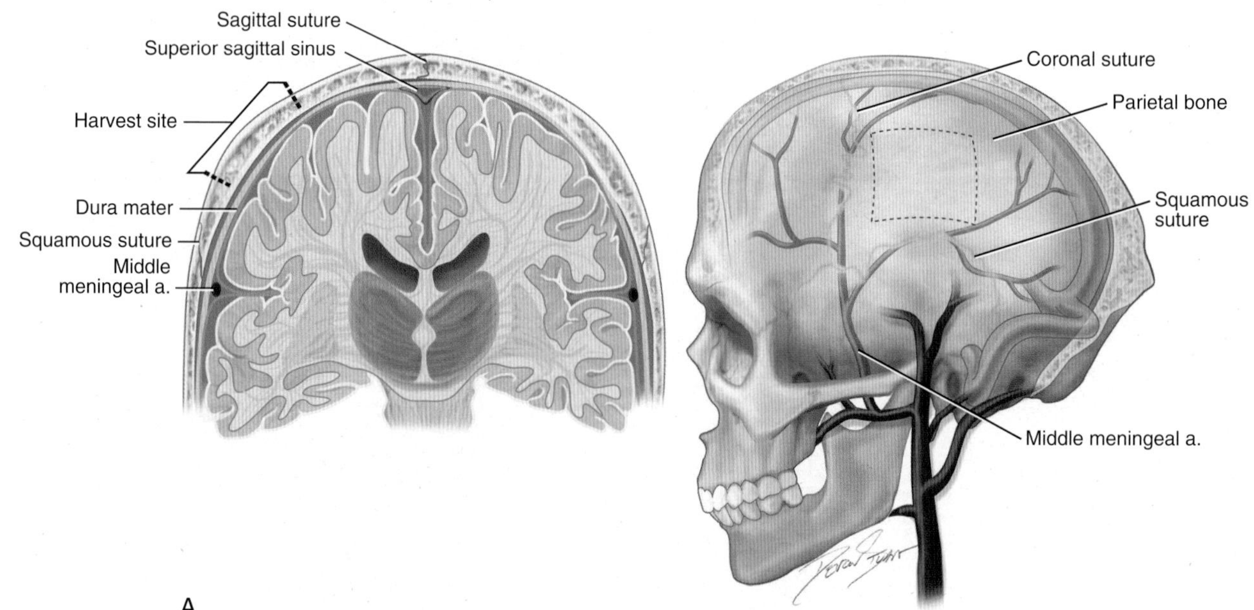

Figure 138.7 **A,** Ideal area for split-thickness cranial bone harvest.

TECHNIQUE: Split-Thickness Cranial Bone Graft—*cont'd*

STEP 3: Site Preparation

If the primary surgical procedure requires access through a coronal flap, cranial bone grafts can be easily harvested after dissection of the posterior flap. If a more remote site is being grafted, a local incision through the scalp directly over the harvest site is used. The scalp may be trimmed with clippers in the area of the planned incision if desired, but shaving the scalp is contraindicated. In general, for local graft harvesting the hair is first parted with surgical lubricant. The head is wrapped in a pillowcase; access through the pillowcase is cut over the incision site, and the edges are stapled to the scalp. This helps keep the hair contained out of the surgical field. Alternatively, the hair can be bound into small tufts with small elastics. The area is prepped sterilely and then toweled off, keeping important landmarks in the surgical field (e.g., the upper aspect of the ear) to aid orientation (Fig. 138.7B–D).

Continued

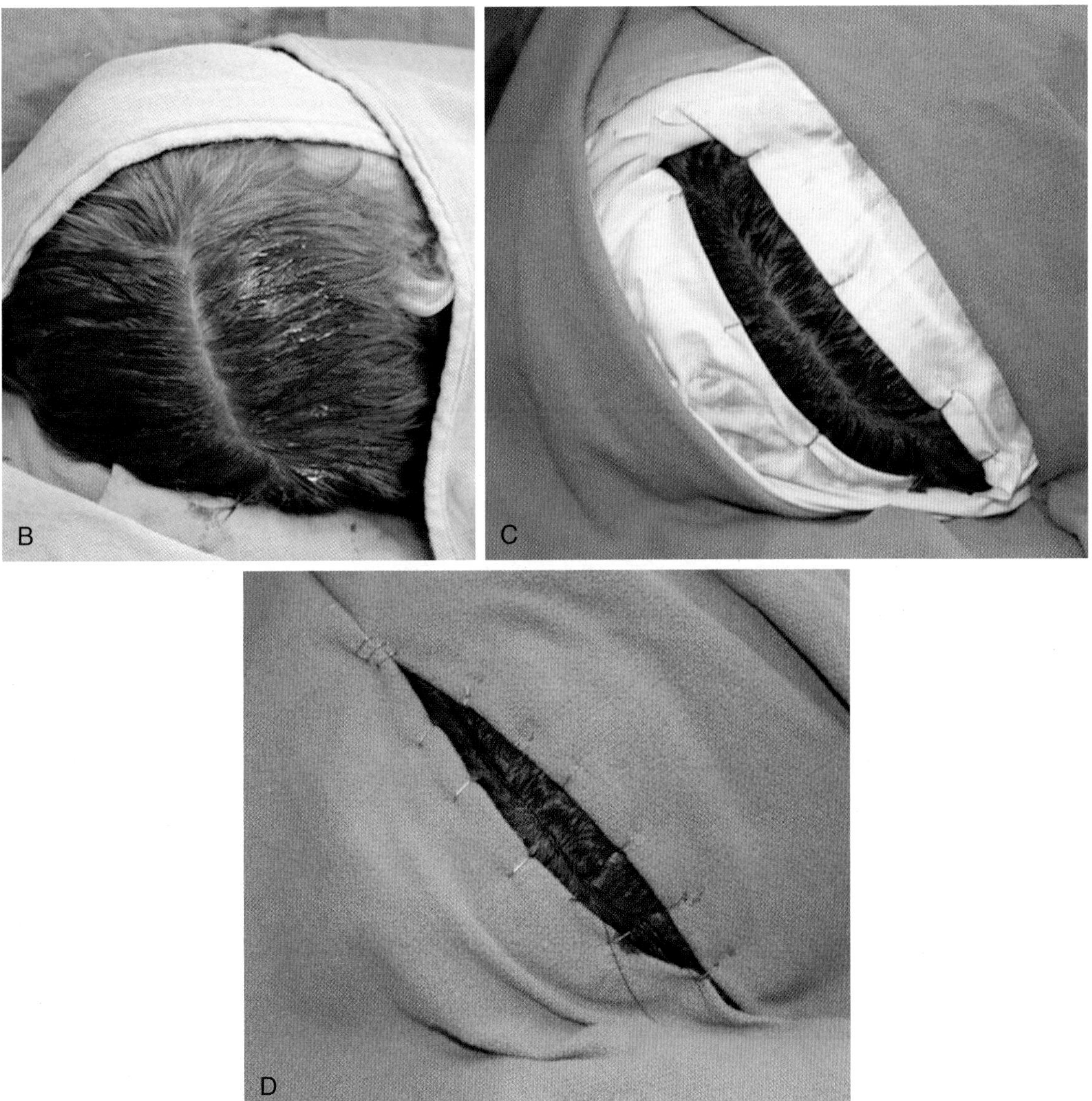

Figure 138.7, cont'd **B,** Hair parted and surgical lubricant applied. **C,** Pillowcase stapled in place for hair retraction. **D,** Area prepped over pillowcase and sterile drapes stapled in place.

Continued

TECHNIQUE: Split-Thickness Cranial Bone Graft—*cont'd*

STEP 4: Incision

The incision line is marked, and a local anesthetic with vasoconstrictor is injected along the planned incision site. A sufficient amount is injected to cause hydrodissection of the tissues. Sufficient time (5 to 7 minutes) is allotted to allow for vasoconstriction. A full-thickness incision is made with a #15 scalpel blade and any scalp bleeding is controlled. Electrocautery can be used deep to the hair follicles to prevent alopecia and Raney clips can be placed if necessary. Subperiosteal dissection is performed with a periosteal elevator. Skull bleeding can be controlled with Gelfoam soaked in thrombin or bone wax. When large incisions are used, it is beneficial to proceed in small increments to minimize blood loss, especially in the pediatric patient. Ruiz et al.[12] have provided a detailed description of the recommended technique for a coronal flap.

STEP 5: Outline Osteotomies

After exposure is complete and hemostasis has been achieved, the planned osteotomies are marked with a surgical marking pen or electrocautery. If strips are planned, the ideal dimensions are 1 to 1.5 × 3 to 4 cm for ease of harvesting and flexibility of application. If a larger contoured graft is desired, it may be beneficial to create a template of the area to be reconstructed and transfer it to the harvest area. A small Steiger bur is used to perform the initial osteotomy through the outer cortex to the underlying diploë. Copious irrigation should be used to flood and cool the bone at all times while power instruments are used. Care must be taken to avoid perforations through the inner cortex that could injure the underlying dura or brain. Irrigation, lighting, and suction are important to enable the surgeon to visualize the depth of the cut being performed (Fig. 138.7E).

STEP 6: Beveling Osteotomies

With the osteotomies outlined, additional contouring must be performed to allow visualization and direct access to the diploic space with osteotomes. A larger Steiger or egg-shaped bur is used to bevel the outer border of the initial osteotomies. Depending on the size and shape of the planned bone graft or struts, this may need to be completed in a circumferential fashion (Fig. 138.7F).

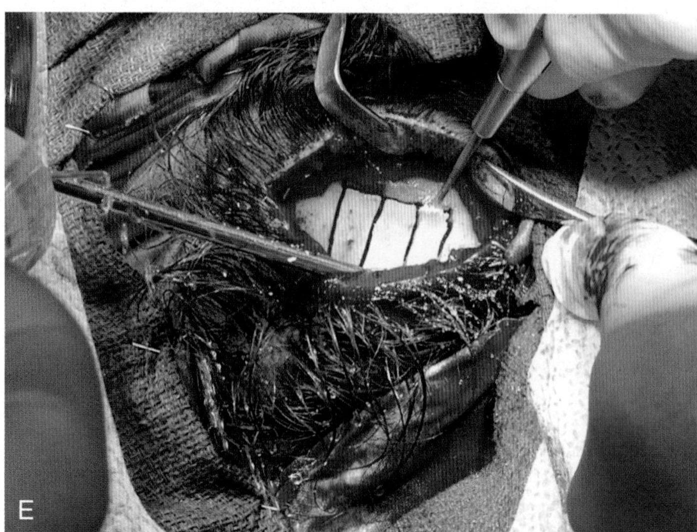

Figure 138.7, cont'd E, Outlining osteotomies.

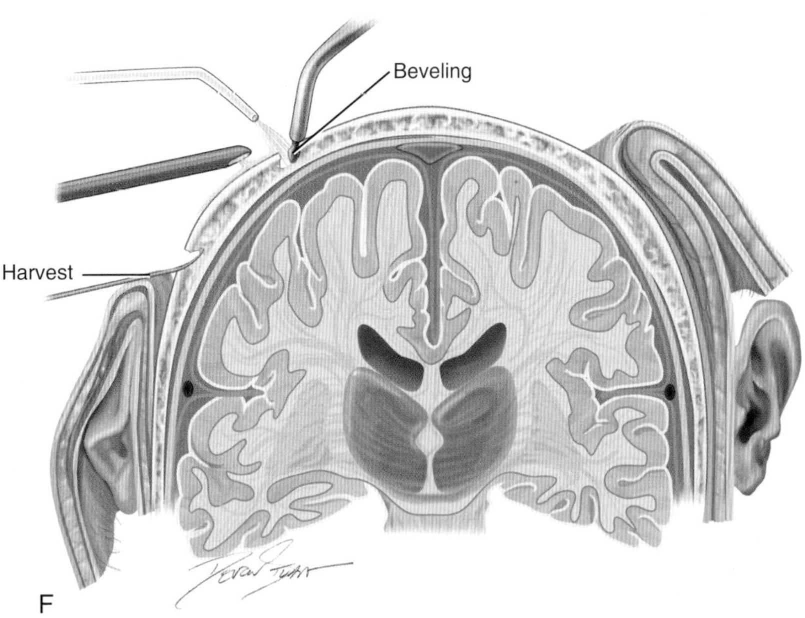

Figure 138.7, cont'd F, Beveling osteotomies.

TECHNIQUE: Split-Thickness Cranial Bone Graft—*cont'd*

STEP 7: Graft Harvest

If possible, the small Steiger bur is used again to develop the plane between the inner and outer cortices. A slightly curved osteotome then is malleted in 2- to 3-mm increments. Once entry into the appropriate plane has been confirmed, more aggressive use of wider curved or straight osteotomes can begin. Maintaining proper angulation at this point is of utmost importance to avoid violation of the inner cortex. This process needs to be completed in a controlled circumferential manner until the graft has been elevated. The graft should be stabilized with a bone clamp before removal, and it is then transferred to a basin with cool saline or moistened sponges. If strips are being harvested, once the first strip has been removed, access to the remainder of the outlined grafts is simplified. Overly aggressive use of the osteotome risks fracturing of the graft or causing full-thickness harvest and should be avoided.

Additional cancellous bone can be harvested at this time by using a curette in the marrow space. The amount harvested in this manner varies greatly depending on the thickness of the diploic space and the area of exposure.

STEP 8: Hemostasis

Once the grafts have been removed, hemostasis is achieved. Gelfoam soaked in thrombin can be placed in the defect, and this is usually sufficient to stop most bleeding. Areas that continue to bleed should be closely inspected to ensure that the inner cortex is intact and that there are no underlying vascular injuries. Bone wax should be used judiciously because it can prevent bone healing and regeneration. Historically, many different types of bone substitutes and putties were used to fill the donor site defect, but this approach is not recommended. Patients rarely have any complaints about contour or asymmetry if the harvest site is appropriately located.

STEP 9: Closure

The scalp is closed in layers. Use of 2-0 or 3-0 Vicryl suture on a CT-2 or SH needle is recommended to close the periosteum and galea, with the goal of slight eversion of the edges of the scalp. The skin is closed with 3-0 or 4-0 chromic gut suture in a running locking fashion. If meticulous hemostasis and underlying closure are performed, drains are not necessary. The incision is covered with antibiotic ointment, and a pressure dressing of Telfa, gauze fluff, Kerlix, and Coban can be placed for 24 hours to aid in hemostasis if desired.

Continued

ALTERNATIVE TECHNIQUE 1: Full-Thickness Cranial Bone Graft

Full-thickness cranial bone grafts can be used for calvarial reconstruction and for block grafting (e.g., zygoma reconstruction for Treacher Collins syndrome). A template is made of the area to be reconstructed and traced on adjacent bone. The neurosurgeon performs a full-thickness craniotomy, and the bone graft is removed to the back table. The bone block is then split in half with a reciprocating saw. One half is split again into inner and outer tables and is used to reconstruct the donor site with microplate fixation; the other half is used for the desired grafting indication (Fig. 138.8). Biodegradable hardware is preferred for pediatric patients.

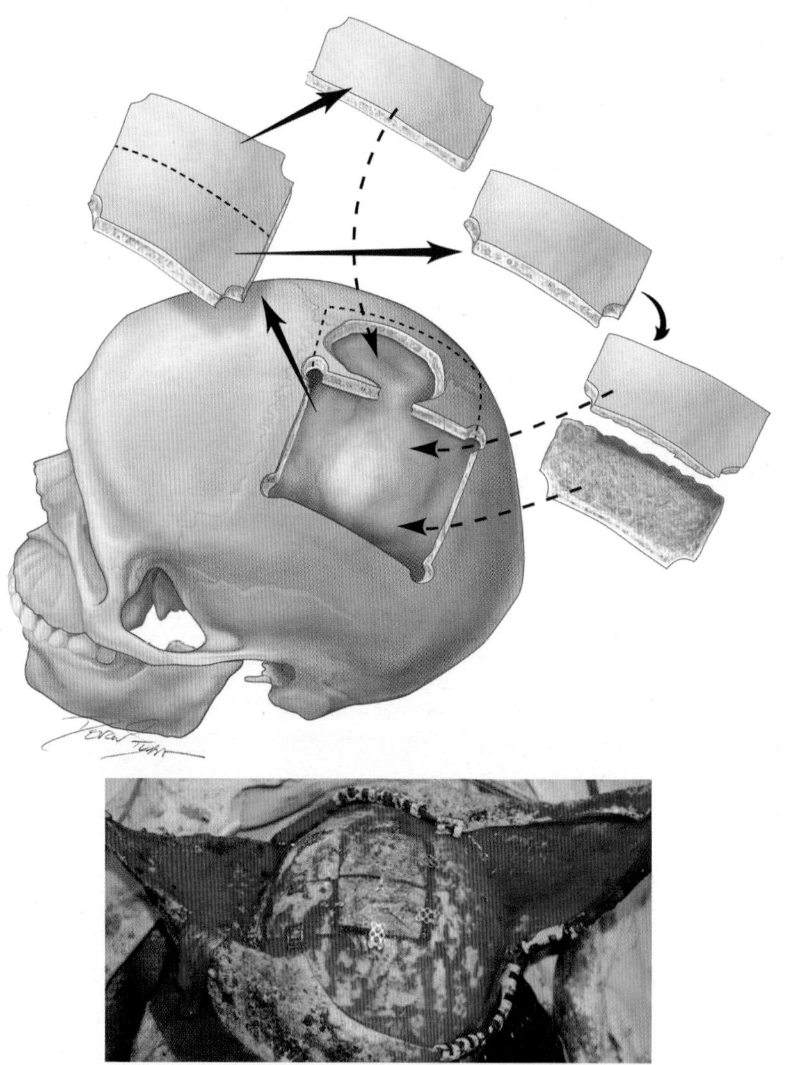

Figure 138.8 Reconstruction of a full-thickness defect with adjacent split full-thickness graft.

ALTERNATIVE TECHNIQUE 2: Myoosseous Pedicled Cranial Bone Graft

Myoosseous pedicled cranial bone grafting is similar to the full-thickness technique. The temporalis muscle can be left attached to the area of parietal bone being used for reconstruction. The neurosurgeon performs the craniotomy around the outlined graft. Tunneling under the periosteum at the inferior craniotomy site may be performed to allow access for the neurosurgeon, or this area may be out-fractured carefully. The pedicled graft can then be rotated into position for maxillary/zygoma reconstruction. Often this requires removal and replacement of the zygomatic arch or segmentation of the pedicled graft (Fig. 138.9). The donor site then is reconstructed using the full-thickness technique described previously.

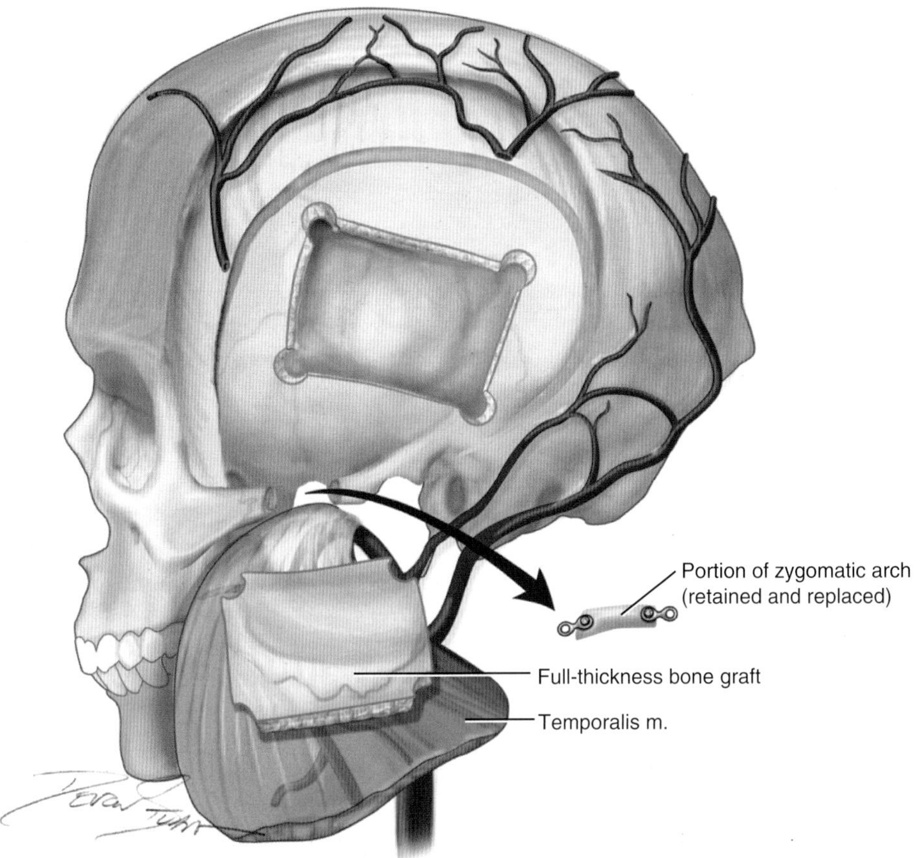

Figure 138.9 Pedicled full-thickness graft.

ALTERNATIVE TECHNIQUE 3: Cranial Bone Shavings

Large amounts of particulate bone can be harvested from the cranium using a shaving harvester (Fig. 138.10). A smaller local incision can be used, or the skull can be approached through a coronal flap. Care must be taken in the pediatric skull to avoid a full-thickness perforation, which can occur with overzealous use of the scraper.

A bone mill can be used in combination with any of the above techniques to morselize the harvested graft if desired.

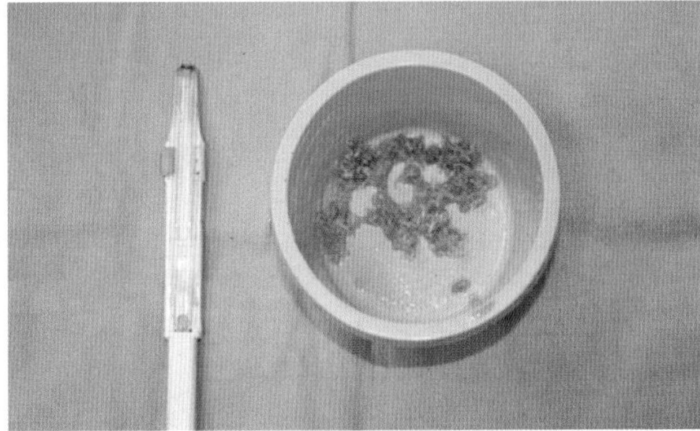

Figure 138.10 Shaving harvester and cortical shavings.

Avoidance and Management of Intraoperative Complications

Full-Thickness Perforation

Full-thickness defects should be inspected for underlying dural injuries and managed appropriately. If the skull defect is small, bone shavings can be placed and covered with a small piece of resorbable mesh and screws. If the defect is larger, a split-thickness graft should be harvested and fixated appropriately. Small defects (less than 1 cm) typically do not need grafting in the young pediatric patient (under 2 years of age).

Dural Injury

Dural injury may occur during the harvest of cranial bone. A partial thickness tear can be reinforced with a piece of Gelfoam. Full-thickness laceration is usually evident due to leakage of cerebrospinal fluid. A clean laceration may be directly sutured with braided nylon. Larger or irregular injuries may require a craniotomy to facilitate access to the brain, bleeding vasculature, or edges of the dura. After management of any underlying brain injury and hemostasis, the dura may need to be patched with autogenous pericranium or other regenerative materials (e.g., Duragen). Areas of the cranium that overly an area of dural injury must be completely reconstructed, especially in the pediatric patient, to prevent further complications, such as a leptomeningocele.

Fracture/Crazing of Bone Graft During Harvest

Advancing the osteotomes gradually in a controlled fashion during split-thickness harvesting is necessary to avoid fracture of the graft.

Postoperative Considerations

Patients are commonly monitored overnight, but the overall duration of admission and perioperative management is dictated by the primary surgical procedure. If used, the pressure dressing can be removed on the first or second postoperative day. Patients undergoing significant reconstruction may require a protective helmet in the postoperative period.

Postoperative antibiotics are dictated by the surgeon's preference and the primary surgical procedure. The incision should be cleaned with a mix of half-strength peroxide and water twice daily and lightly coated with antibiotic ointment. On the third postoperative day, the patient may begin showering and washing the hair with plain baby shampoo, but he or she should be instructed not to soak the wounds or aggressively scrub or dry the hair for 2 weeks.

Postoperative complications are rare but may involve the formation of hematomas, seromas, or surgical site infection.[13] These complications typically are easily managed with local wound care, antibiotics, and aspiration or incision and drainage if necessary. Neurologic injury, cerebrospinal fluid leakage, and leptomeningocele should be referred to and managed by a neurosurgeon.

References

1. Oppenheimer AJ, Tong L, Buchman SR. Craniofacial bone grafting: Wolff's law revisited. *Craniomaxillofac Trauma Reconstr.* 2008;1(1):49–61.
2. Jackson IT, Helden G, Marx R. Skull bone grafts in maxillofacial and craniofacial surgery. *J Oral Maxillofac Surg.* 1986;44(12):949–955.
3. Tessier P. Autogenous bone grafts taken from the calvarium for facial and cranial applications. *Clin Plast Surg.* 1982;9(4):531–538.
4. Tessier P, Kawamoto H, Matthews D, et al. Autogenous bone grafts and bone substitutes—tools and techniques: I. A 20,000-case experience in maxillofacial and craniofacial surgery. *Plast Reconstr Surg.* 2005;11(5 suppl):6S–24S.
5. Tessier P, Kawamoto H, Posnick J, Raulo Y, Tulasne JF, Wolfe SA. Taking calvarial grafts, either split in situ or splitting of the parietal bone flap ex vivo—tools and techniques: V. A 9650-case experience in craniofacial and maxillofacial surgery. *Plast Reconstr Surg.* 2005;116(suppl 5):54S–71S.
6. Tessier P, Kawamoto H, Posnick J, Raulo Y, Tulasne JF, Wolfe SA. Taking calvarial grafts—tools and techniques: VI. The splitting of a parietal bone "flap". *Plast Reconstr Surg.* 2005;116(suppl 5):74S–88S.
7. Waitzman AA, Posnick JC, Armstrong DC, Pron GE. Craniofacial skeletal measurements based on computed tomography: part II. Normal values and growth trends. *Cleft Palate Craniofac J.* 1992;29(2):118–128.
8. Posnick JC, Goldstein JA, Waitzman AA. Surgical correction of the Treacher Collins malar deficiency: quantitative CT scan analysis of long-term results. *Plast Reconstr Surg.* 1993;92(1):12–22.
9. Kaban LB, Moses MH, Mulliken JB. Surgical correction of hemifacial microsomia in the growing child. *Plast Reconstr Surg.* 1988;82(1):9–19.
10. Marx RE, Stevens MR. Cranial bone. In: Marx RE, Stevens MR, eds. *Atlas of Oral and Extraoral Bone Harvesting.* Chicago, Illinois: Quintessence; 2009.
11. Moreira-Gonzalez A, Papay FE, Zins JE. Calvarial thickness and its relation to cranial bone harvest. *Plast Reconstr Surg.* 2006;117(6):1964–1971.
12. Ruiz RL, Pattisapu JV, Costello BJ, Golden B. The coronal scalp flap: surgical technique. *Atlas Oral Maxillofac Surg Clin North Am.* 2010;18(2):69–75.
13. Tessier P, Kawamoto H, Posnick J, Raulo Y, Tulasne JF, Wolfe SA. Complications of harvesting autogenous bone grafts: a group experience of 20,000 cases. *Plast Reconstr Surg.* 2005;116(suppl 5):72S–73S.

CHAPTER 139

Intraoral Bone Harvesting Techniques

Hans C. Brockhoff II, David M. Yates, and Richard Allen Finn

Symphysis Armamentarium

Local anesthetic with epinephrine
Periosteal elevator
Needle electrocautery
703 Surgical bur
Piezosurgery device (optional)
Osteotomes and mallet
Obwegeser retractors
3-0 Vicryl suture
4-0 Vicryl suture
3-0 Chromic gut suture
Bone curette
Caliper
Double skin hooks
Mentalis dressing (Tensoplast, Benzoin, Tegaderm)

Body Ramus Armamentarium

Local anesthetic with epinephrine
Periosteal elevator
Needle electrocautery
703 Surgical bur
Piezosurgery device (optional)
Osteotomes and mallet
Obwegeser retractors
Mayo scissors
3-0 Chromic gut suture
Caliper
Sweetheart retractor
Bite block

History of the Procedure

Bone grafting in the maxillofacial region has experienced significant growth over the past two decades.[1–4] The options continue to expand as new products become available. Categorically speaking, current materials include autografts, allografts, xenografts, and alloplasts. Within these subcategories, there is a wealth of information to be explored that falls beyond the scope of this chapter. However, the gold standard for bone grafting has been and has continued to be autogenous bone. This bone offers three desirable biologic properties, namely, osteogenic, osteoinductive, and osteoconductive properties. The osteogenic property provides progenitor cells, which are contained within the graft and have the ability of self-renewal and proliferation. The osteoinductive potential aids in recruitment and induction of mesenchymal cells to differentiate into bone-forming osteoblasts, and lastly, the presence of a physical osteoconductive scaffolding facilitates tissue ingrowth (Fig. 139.1).

Simply put, the most obvious goal for bone augmentation is to facilitate new bone formation. Historically speaking, this was achieved with the mindset that a bone graft requirement only needed to serve as a biocompatible construct to allow for the ingrowth of new bone. However, with a better understanding of bone biology, it is understandable that the unique properties offered by autogenous bone are most desired. Despite this fact, it is noted that only 15% of augmentation procedures utilize autogenous bone.[3] It is likely that the ongoing pursuit of suitable substitute materials has been fueled by some of the shortcomings of autographs, including donor site morbidity and limited bone availability.

Regardless of the excitement for alternative grafting substitutes, which was a $2.58 billion industry in 2018,[5] autogenous bone grafting continues to play a pivotal role in the

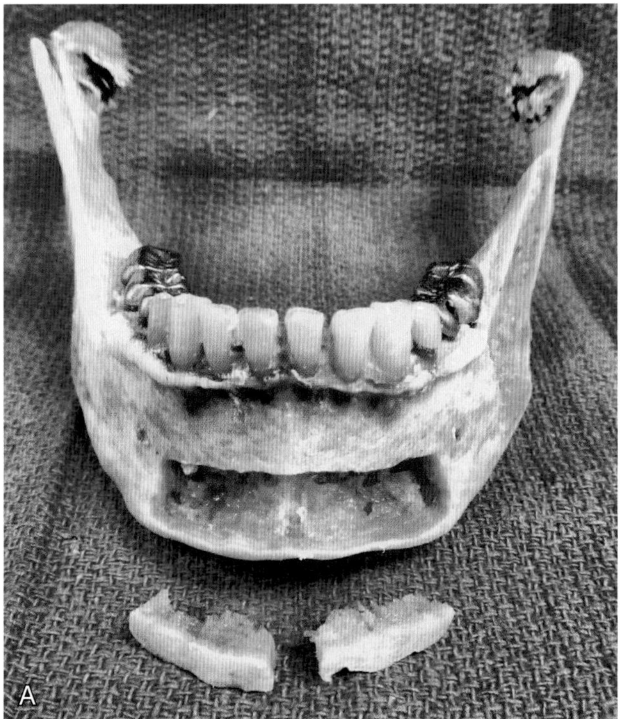

Figure 139.1 A, Symphysis bone graft.

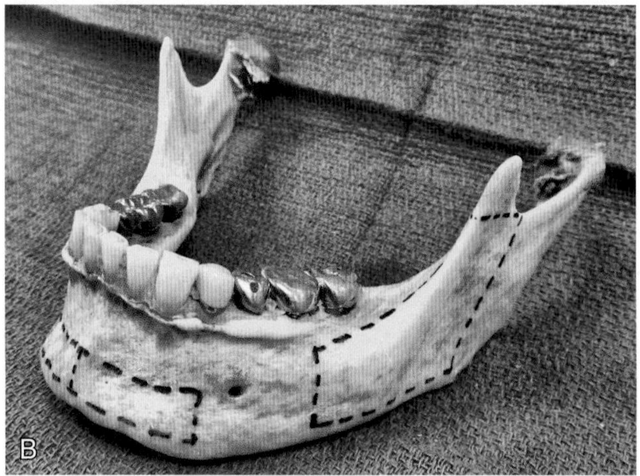

Figure 139.1, cont'd B, Body/ramus graft and symphysis grafts are marked.

hands of the maxillofacial surgeon. Intraoral bone graft techniques have been commonly used for the repair of maxillofacial bony defects. Applications have included dorsal nasal struts to repair orbital floor defects, augment alveolar ridges, cleft repair, and even for cosmetic augmentation in the paranasal region.[6–15] The body/ramus and symphysis grafts are composed of autogenous intramembranous bone, which is easily accessible while leaving no cutaneous scar. There is very minimal morbidity associated with these grafts, and they can easily be performed as in-office procedures thereby decreasing overall cost.

Table 139.1 Surface Area and Volume Harvestable from Various Intraoral Sites

Donor Sites	Surface Area of Corticocancellous Graft (mm^2)	Volume of Corticocancellous graft (mL)
Symphysis	358.9	1.15
Body/Ramus	855.6	2.02

Reference 16

Indications for the Use of the Procedure

Harvest site selection is dependent on a thorough understanding of the quality and quantity of bone needed for the intended reconstruction. One graft may be selected over another, for example, if a higher amount of cortical bone is desired. Symphysis grafts offer a robust quantity of cancellous bone in addition to cortical bone. In contrast, a body/ramus graft provides a large quantity of bone and is an excellent source of dense cortical bone; however, only minimal cancellous bone is available.[16]

The reported amounts of bone harvestable from intraoral sites are variable throughout the literature especially regarding total volume. The largest study to date performed on 59 cadavers looked at the surface area and volume harvestable from various intraoral sites (Table 139.1).[16]

SYMPHYSIS TECHNIQUE

STEP 1: Anesthetic

Inject local anesthesia with vasoconstrictor from second premolar to second premolar 7 minutes prior to incision.

STEP 2: Incision

Two incision designs are acceptable, sulcular and vestibular. The vestibular incision has a higher incidence of postoperative pain, scarification, dehiscence, decrease in vestibular length, and possible chin ptosis if the mentalis muscle is inadequately repaired.[17] However, it is a viable option if the periodontal health of the mandibular incisors is poor. This is because of increased gingival recession that can occur with a sulcular incision in this patient population.[17]

Sulcular Incision Technique

Double skin hooks are placed on the lower lip to provide gentle retraction and allow adequate visualization of the anterior symphysis. Using a #15 blade, a sulcular incision is made from first premolar to first premolar with distal releasing incisions bilaterally from the distal line angle of the first premolar.[17]

Vestibular Incision Technique

Double skin hooks are placed on the lower lip to provide gentle retraction and allow adequate visualization of the anterior symphysis. Using a #15 blade or Bovie electrocautery, a curvilinear incision is made extending from first premolar to first premolar. Anterior to the canine region, the vestibular incision should be 10 to 15 mm from the mucogingival junction; however, when in the premolar region, the incision should be only 5 to 10 mm from the mucogingival junction to avoid the mental nerve branches.

The incision is carried through mucosa only to avoid the mental nerve branches. Avoiding the mental nerve branches, incise the mentalis muscle using curved Mayo scissors at a 45-degree angle to the mandible, thereby simultaneously avoiding perforation through the skin and allowing myomucosal cuff preservation. Once to periosteum, incise using a #15 blade or Bovie electrocautery.

SYMPHYSIS TECHNIQUE—*cont'd*

STEP 3: Dissection

A full-thickness mucoperiosteal flap is developed using a periosteal elevator in all directions until the mental nerve foramen is identified bilaterally and the inferior border of the mandible is exposed.

STEP 4: Osteotomy

Using a sterile pencil, mark out the following osteotomy sites:

- Superior Osteotomy: In the dentate mandible, if the root bulge is visible, plan the osteotomy 5 mm inferior to the root of the canine teeth bilaterally. If the roots are fully encased in bone and no root bulge is noted, place the osteotomy 14 mm below the cemento-enamel junction of the canine teeth bilaterally.
- Inferior Osteotomy: 4 mm superior to the inferior border of the mandible
- Lateral Osteotomy: 5 mm anterior to the mental nerve foramen

Using a 703 bur (or Piezosurgery device) and extensive irrigation, remove cortical bone until bleeding from cancellous bone beneath is visualized at all locations. Additionally, transect the graft in the sagittal dimension at midline. Dependent on the size of the desired corticocancellous block, extend the corticotomies toward the lingual, taking care to avoid perforating the lingual cortical plate. Once the desired depth is achieved, curved osteotomes are placed and walked along the corticotomies. Upon delivery of the graft, additional bone curettage may be performed only in the lingual direction to harvest additional remaining cancellous bone. The graft is then preserved in normal saline until its use is required.

STEP 5: Closure

Extensively irrigate the defect to remove any residual debris. Use bone wax as needed for hemostasis. The donor site may have particulate allograft placed with the addition of a platelet concentrate (platelet-rich plasma/leukocyte platelet-rich fibrin). This is possible through the use of a centrifuge. When closing a vestibular approach, resuspend the mentalis muscle with three interrupted stitches utilizing 3-0 Vicryl. The mucosa can then be closed with a 3-0 chromic gut suture in a continuous fashion. If a sulcular incision was selected, place interdental papilla sutures with 4-0 Vicryl suture for closure.

STEP 6: Dressing

If a vestibular approach was selected and the bellies of the mentalis muscle were incised, it is necessary to place a mentalis dressing for 5 days.

BODY/RAMUS HARVEST TECHNIQUE

Many variations for a body/ramus graft have been described. The following is a description of the maximal quantity that can be achieved. Less bone can be harvested based on the reconstructive needs (Fig. 139.2).

STEP 1: Anesthetic

Inject local anesthesia with vasoconstrictor from second premolar to the lateral border of the mandible in addition to an inferior alveolar nerve (IAN) block 7 minutes prior to incision.

STEP 2: Incision and dissection

Begin with placement of a bite block and sweetheart retractor. Obwegeser right-angle retractors are positioned in the upper and lower vestibules and pulled taught to expose and stretch the mucosa overlying the ramus/body. Using Bovie electrocautery, a mucosal incision is made along the vestibule beginning 5 mm away from the mucogingival junction adjacent to the first molar. The incision extends 3 cm posteriorly paralleling the anatomy of the mandibular ramus. Continue the dissection through the buccinator muscle. The right-angle retractors are then moved inwardly and placed within the edges of the mucosal incision to retract and protect the remaining buccal tissue. The length of the bone along the incision is then sounded out with the Colorado tip of the Bovie electrocautery, and the dissection is then continued directly to bone. A #9 periosteal elevator is used to create a subperiosteal dissection beginning at the anterior edge of the ascending ramus. Begin by first exposing the lateral aspect of the body down toward the inferior border and sweep laterally to expose the angle. Return to the anterior ramus and concentrate on exposing some of the lingual side of the ascending ramus. A notched right-

Continued

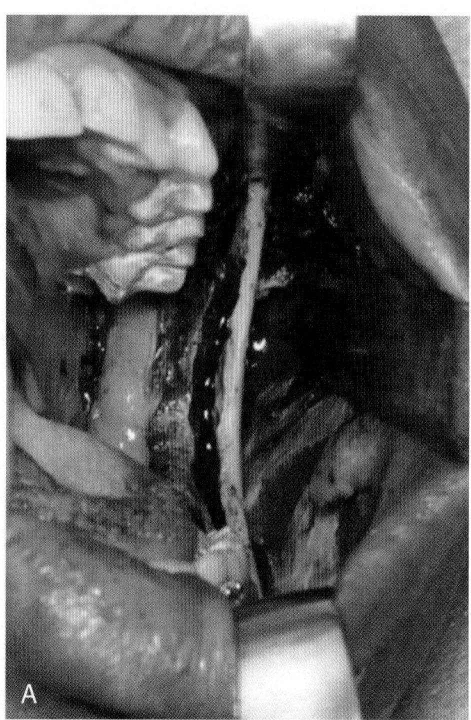

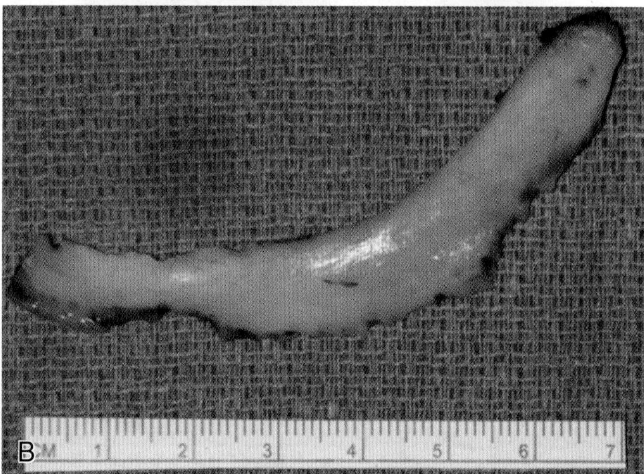

Figure 139.2 **A,** Intraoral harvest of a left body/ramus graft. The superior osteotomy is visualized. **B,** Completed harvest of a left body/ramus graft.

BODY/RAMUS HARVEST TECHNIQUE—*cont'd*

angle retractor can now be placed along the ascending ramus. The temporalis muscle fibers will now be encountered and often resist the upward retraction. The fibers can be stripped with the pointed edge of the periosteal elevator in the superior to inferior direction. Lastly, expose the most lateral aspect of the ramus to assist in complete visualization of the bony mandible. A second incision decision may alternatively be utilized for the harvesting this graft as well. Rather than a sagittal split incision, the incision design begins on the most distal aspect of the posterior mandibular tooth. The incision is then continued through the retromolar pad and up along the ascending ramus. This is carried toward the buccal side to allow for avoidance of injury to the lingual nerve. Anteriorly, the incision is carried in a sulcular fashion on the buccal side, and a releasing incision can be made at the level of the first premolar. The full-thickness mucoperiosteal flap may then be elevated in a similar fashion as previously described.

BODY/RAMUS HARVEST TECHNIQUE—*cont'd*

STEP 3: Osteotomy

Using a sterile pencil, mark out the following osteotomy sites:

- Superior Osteotomy: The external oblique cut is made along the anterior border of the ramus approximately one-third the width of the mandible (4 to 6 mm medial to the lateral surface). The osteotomy extends superior to the base of the coronoid and anteriorly to the distal half of the first molar area.
- Inferior Osteotomy: A partial thickness cut is made 4 mm superior to the inferior border of the mandible.
- Anterior Osteotomy: Extends to the distal half of the first molar area
- Posterior Osteotomy: Extends to the antilingula

A 703 bur (or Piezosurgery device) under copious amounts of irrigation is used to initiate the cuts on both the ascending ramus and anteriorly on the body of the mandible. This is carried through the cortical bone until bleeding cancellous bone is encountered. A round bur is then utilized for the inferior and posterior cuts but should only be used to score the cortex due to the close proximity of the IAN. A curved osteotome and mallet are then used via the superior cut to complete separation of the graft from the body of the mandible. It is critical to angle the curved osteotome toward the graft due to the close proximity of the IAN to the cortex in this area of the mandible.[18]

Once the graft is delivered, the remaining cut bone edges should be smoothed using a bone file. The defect is then extensively irrigated prior to closure.

STEP 4: Closure

Use bone wax as needed for hemostasis. The donor site may benefit from placement of platelet concentrate (platelet-rich plasma/leukocyte platelet-rich fibrin). This is possible through the use of a centrifuge but is not a requisite. The mucosa can then be closed with a 3-0 chromic gut suture in a continuous fashion for the sagittal incision approach versus 4-0 Vicryl for the extended distal hockey stick incision.

Avoidance and Management of Intraoperative Complications

Symphysis Harvest

One may prevent potential chin ptosis by appropriately resuspending the mentalis muscle and placing a postoperative mentalis dressing.

To avoid lip/chin paresthesia, visualization and protection of the mental nerve at the foramen bilaterally must be achieved. The osteotomy must be at least 5 mm anterior to the mental nerve foramen to ensure that there is no damage to the mental branches of the IAN. It has been well documented that the IAN will often progress anterior to the mental foramen prior to its exit from the osseous structure of the mandible. For this reason, the use of bone curettes to harvest additional cancellous bone is not recommended lateral to the created osteotomies.[19–23]

It is difficult to avoid potential damage to the incisive branch of the IAN, which is likely to be affected when harvesting from this area. As expected, the canal is highly varied, but in general it decreases in diameter from lateral to medial as it gives off branches to individual teeth. In general, it maintains a distance of 10 to 14 mm above the inferior border and nearly disappears toward the midline. This is thought to be due to the formation of a plexus-like network with small tributaries. This results in a loss of sensation to the mandibular anterior teeth and a sensation of "wooden" teeth.[19–24] However, this should not overly deter the harvesting of the graft. Even with complete disruption of the incisive canal, Hutchinson and MacGregor demonstrated revascularization and restoration of full vitality and function of almost all teeth after 6 to 12 months. The few patients who remained insensate were indifferent to their symptoms.[25]

Table 139.2 Complication of Symphysis Harvest

Symphysis Harvest Complications	Early Complications (%)	Continued Complications >1 year (%)
Altered sensation to mandibular anterior teeth	25	7
Altered sensation to chin	17–76	0–52
Subjective change in chin contour		34
Clinically detectable change in chin contour		0

References: 19–23

Body/Ramus Harvest

The incidence of complication is much less with body/ramus harvest as compared with symphysis harvest (Tables 139.2 and 139.3) However, injury to the IAN is still very possible when performing a body/ramus harvest. Two techniques are essential to avoid injury to the IAN. The cortex for the posterior and inferior osteotomies must only be scored using a

Table 139.3 Complications of Body/Ramus Harvest

Body/Ramus Harvest Complications	Early Complications (%)	Continued Complications >1 year (%)
Terminal branch of buccal nerve paresthesia	21	4
Altered sensation in IAN distribution	4.4–16	0–11.6

References: 19,20,23
IAN, Inferior alveolar nerve.

round bur. It is not advised to perforate through the cortex due to the close proximity of the IAN.[18] Additionally, when using osteotomes to free the graft, the osteotomes must be angled laterally toward the cortex, not into the substance of the mandible. Rajchel et al. demonstrated that the IAN may even directly come into contact with the lateral mandibular cortex in this region.[18–20,23]

Postoperative Considerations

Ramus/body and symphysis harvests are valuable sources of autogenous intramembranous bone that can be easily harvested with low morbidity, high patient satisfaction, and excellent clinical results. When selecting between the mandibular body/ramus or symphysis grafts, it is important to consider the reconstruction needs that must be met. The mandibular body/ramus offers a large area of cortical bone, whereas the symphysis offers mostly cancellous bone with a small cortical component. These techniques continue to be reliable and affordable methods in maxillofacial reconstruction.

References

1. Miron RJ, Hedbom E, Saulacic N, et al. Osteogenic potential of autogenous bone grafts harvested with four different surgical techniques. *J Dent Res*. 2011;90(12):1428–1433.
2. Giannoudis PV, Dinopoulos H, Tsiridis E. Bone substitutes: an update. *Injury*. 2005;36(suppl 3):S20–S27.
3. Pikos M, Miron R. *Bone Augmentation in Implant Dentistry*. Quintessence Publishing; 2019.
4. Pikos MA. Mandibular block autografts for alveolar ridge augmentation. *Atlas Oral Maxillofac Surg Clin North Am*. 2005;13(2):91–107.
5. Bone Grafts and Substitutes Market Size, Share & Trends Analysis Report by Material Type, by Application Type, by Region and Segment Forecasts 2019–2026. https://www.grandviewresearch.com/.
6. Montazem A, Valauri DV, St-Hilaire H, Buchbinder D. The mandibular symphysis as a donor site in maxillofacial bone grafting: a quantitative anatomic study. *J Oral Maxillofac Surg*. 2000;58(12):1368–1371.
7. Gellrich NC, Held U, Schoen R, Pailing T, Schramm A, Bormann KH. Alveolar zygomatic buttress: a new donor site for limited preimplant augmentation procedures. *J Oral Maxillofac Surg*. 2007;65(2):275–280.
8. Güngörmüş M, Yavuz MS. The ascending ramus of the mandible as a donor site in maxillofacial bone grafting. *J Oral Maxillofac Surg*. 2002;60(11):1316–1318.
9. Choung PH, Kim SG. The coronoid process for paranasal augmentation in the correction of midfacial concavity. *Oral Surg Oral Med Oral Pathol Oral Radiol Endod*. 2001;91(1):28–33.
10. Amrani S, Anastassov GE, Montazem AH. Mandibular ramus/coronoid process grafts in maxillofacial reconstructive surgery. *J Oral Maxillofac Surg*. 2010;68(3):641–646.
11. Herford AS. Dorsal nasal reconstruction using bone harvested from the mandible. *J Oral Maxillofac Surg*. 2004;62(9):1082–1087.
12. Mintz SM, Ettinger A, Schmakel T, Gleason MJ. Contralateral coronoid process bone grafts for orbital floor reconstruction: an anatomic and clinical study. *J Oral Maxillofac Surg*. 1998;56(10):1140–1144.
13. Güngörmüş M, Yilmaz AB, Ertaş U, Akgül HM, Yavuz MS, Harorli A. Evaluation of the mandible as an alternative autogenous bone source for oral and maxillofacial reconstruction. *J Int Med Res*. 2002;30(3):260–264.
14. Bähr W, Coulon JP. Limits of the mandibular symphysis as a donor site for bone grafts in early secondary cleft palate osteoplasty. *Int J Oral Maxillofac Surg*. 1996;25(5):389–393.
15. Li KK, Schwartz HC. Mandibular body bone in facial plastic and reconstructive surgery. *Laryngoscope*. 1996;106(4):504–506.
16. Yates DM, Brockhoff II HC, Finn R, Phillips C. Comparison of intraoral harvest sites for corticocancellous bone grafts. *J Oral Maxillofac Surg*. 2013;71(3):497–504.
17. Alfaro FH, ed. *Bone Grafting in Oral Implantology: Techniques and Clinical Applications*. Quintessence Publishing; 2006:1–234.
18. Rajchel J, Ellis III E, Fonseca RJ. The anatomical location of the mandibular canal: its relationship to the sagittal ramus osteotomy. *Int J Adult Orthodon Orthognath Surg*. 1986;1(1):37–47.
19. Weibull L, Widmark G, Ivanoff CJ, Borg E, Rasmusson L. Morbidity after chin bone harvesting—a retrospective long-term follow-up study. *Clin Implant Dent Relat Res*. 2009;11(2):149–157.
20. Clavero J, Lundgren S. Ramus or chin grafts for maxillary sinus inlay and local onlay augmentation: comparison of donor site morbidity and complications. *Clin Implant Dent Relat Res*. 2003;5(3):154–160.
21. Rabelo GD, de Paula PM, Rocha FS, Jordão Silva C, Zanetta-Barbosa D. Retrospective study of bone grafting procedures before implant placement. *Implant Dent*. 2010;19(4):342–350.
22. Nóia CF, Ortega-Lopes R, Olate S, Duque TM, de Moraes M, Mazzonetto R. Prospective clinical assessment of morbidity after chin bone harvest. *J Craniofac Surg*. 2011;22(6):2195–2198.
23. Cordaro L, Torsello F, Miuccio MT, di Torresanto VM, Eliopoulos D. Mandibular bone harvesting for alveolar reconstruction and implant placement: subjective and objective cross-sectional evaluation of donor and recipient site up to 4 years. *Clin Oral Implants Res*. 2011;22(11):1320–1326.
24. Vu DD, Brockhoff II HC, Yates DM, Finn R, Phillips C. Course of the mandibular incisive canal and its impact on harvesting symphysis bone grafts. *J Oral Maxillofac Surg*. 2015;73(2):258.e1–258.e12.
25. Hutchinson D, MacGregor AJ. Tooth survival following various methods of sub-apical osteotomy. *Int J Oral Surg*. 1972;1(2):81–86.

CHAPTER 140

Auricular Cartilage Graft Harvest

Joli Chou

Armamentarium

- #15 Scalpel blades
- 3-0 and 4-0 Nylon suture
- 4-0 Plain gut suture, 4-0 Vicryl suture
- 25- or 30-gauge needle with methylene blue
- Bipolar electrocautery
- Dental cotton roll or petroleum gauzes
- Double prong or single prong skin hooks
- Fine tissue forceps
- Local anesthetic with vasoconstrictor
- Tenotomy scissors or baby Metzenbaum scissors

History of the Procedure

The use of autologous cartilage graft in reconstruction surgery has been described as early as 1896 in the German literature by Konig.[1] Subsequently, in 1907, Sushruta Samhita in India performed cartilage grafting in the form of a composite graft.[2] In 1946, Brown and Cannon reported the use of auricular skin and cartilage composite grafts for reconstruction of the nose.[3] Since that time, multiple harvesting techniques for auricular cartilage have been described with variations in the location of skin incision, location of cartilage removal, and maximal amount of cartilage that can be removed without causing donor site deformity.[4]

Indication for the Use of the Procedure

Because of its elastic nature, pliability, and multiple contours, the auricular cartilage is one of the most versatile cartilage grafts. Indications for its use are many and are briefly reviewed. A detailed discussion of each indication is, however, beyond the scope of this chapter.

Nasal Reconstruction

In the esthetic and functional reconstruction of intrinsic, traumatic, or post-oncologic surgery defect of the nose, cartilage grafting is often required. Choices of donor cartilage include the nasal septal cartilage, costal cartilage, and auricular cartilage. The use of auricular cartilage is indicated: (1) in pediatric patients older than 4 years of age, (2) when the nasal defect encompasses the nasal septal cartilage, (3) when the amount of cartilage required exceeds the amount that the nasal septum can provide, and (4) when a skin/cartilage composite graft is required.[5] In addition, the ease of harvest and its ability to substitute for all the cartilaginous structures of the nose has made the auricular cartilage an ideal donor site for nasal reconstruction. The types of graft and areas of nose that can be reconstructed using the auricular cartilage are listed in Table 140.1.[4]

Orbital Floor/Wall Blowout Fracture Reconstruction

Various indications for treatment, surgical access for treatment, and reconstruction techniques of the orbital floor/wall blowout fractures have been described in the literature. Insufficient treatment may result in diplopia, entrapment of extraocular muscle, and enophthalmos due to an increase in orbital volume. Both autologous and alloplastic material can be used to repair the fractured orbital floor/wall. Castellani and colleagues reported that for relative small (up to 2 × 2 cm) orbital floor defects the use of auricular cartilage graft is comparable to other graft material reported in the literature.[6] Similarly, Kruschewsky et al. concluded in a prospective, randomized study of 20 patients that there is no significant esthetic or functional difference in orbital blowout fractures repaired with auricular cartilage or polyacid copolymer material.[7]

Tracheal Reconstruction

Reconstruction of tracheal window defects as result of tumor resection or repair of tracheoesophageal fistula requires the use of graft material that would allow for maintenance of the tracheal skeletal framework to preserve the tracheal lumen. The relative thin and pliable elastic cartilage of the auricle allows for easier attachment to the native tracheal wall when compared with costal cartilage.[8] In addition, the natural contour of the conchal cartilage prevents prolapse of the graft into the tracheal lumen and creates a skeletal support for the tracheal wall.[9]

Table 140.1 Auricular Cartilage and Nasal Reconstruction

Type of Graft	Region of Nose
Lateral crural strut graft	Ala
Spreader grafts	Dorsum
Columellar strut graft	Tip
Septal perforation repair	Septum
Dorsal onlay graft	Dorsum
Alar rim graft	Ala
Butterfly graft/shield graft	Tip

Tympanoplasty

Middle ear pathology, including tympanic membrane perforation, cholesteatoma, and atelectatic ear, may require reconstruction of the tympanic membrane after removal of the pathology. Conchal and tragal cartilage have been used with fair results in the reconstruction of the tympanic membrane.[10]

Eyelid Reconstruction

Partial-thickness lower eyelid defects with the loss of tarsal plate may result in entropion and retraction. Cartilage grafts can be used to lengthen or replace the tarsal plate loss. Full-thickness eyelid defects should be reconstructed to prevent injury to the cornea. The auricular cartilage can be used in conjunction with a vascularized cutaneous or musculocutaneous flap for reconstruction of full-thickness eyelid loss. Composite skin/cartilage grafts can also be used but are less reliable as they are more prone to ischemia.[11]

Interpositional Graft in Temporomandibular Joint Arthroplasty

Degenerative disease of the temporomandibular joint (TMJ) and TMJ ankylosis are often treated with TMJ arthroplasty after failure of nonsurgical therapy and minimally invasive therapy. Studies have suggested the effectiveness of TMJ arthroplasties without reconstruction.[12–14] However, the use of either allograft or autografts in TMJ arthroplasty may decrease occlusal disturbances and further degenerative changes of the joint surfaces.[15] Autogenous auricular cartilage has been used as an interpositional graft after TMJ discectomy and at TMJ ankylosis surgery to prevent re-ankylosis.[16–18] The harvested auricular cartilage may be fixed to the condylar head or the underside of the glenoid fossa or not fixated at all.[16–19]

Contralateral Ear Reconstruction

Finally, auricular cartilage can be used to establish the framework for reconstruction of the contralateral ear.[20]

Limitations and Contraindications

The contraindications for auricular cartilage graft harvesting include systemic diseases or conditions such as collagen vascular disease, rheumatic disease, lupus, polychondritis, sarcoid, Wegener granulomatosis, predilection to keloid formation, prior extensive auricular cartilage harvesting, and microtia. There might be impaired wound healing or poor quality/quantity of the donor cartilage in patient with these conditions or systemic diseases. In addition, auricular cartilage harvesting should be avoided in children under the age of 4 years to prevent growth restriction of the external ear.[5]

TECHNIQUE

STEP 1: Local Anesthesia

Harvesting of auricular cartilage may be performed with local anesthetic, under general anesthesia, or a combination of both. The greater auricular nerve, the lesser occipital nerve, and the auriculotemporal nerve, which provide sensation to the external ear, can be anesthetized by an infiltration of lidocaine with vasoconstrictor both medial and posterior to the auricle.[21] A 27-gauge or 30-gauge needle may be inserted in the subperichondrial plane either anteriorly or posteriorly over the conchal area to inject local anesthetics and create hydrodissection and facilitate later subperichondrial dissection.[4]

STEP 2: Marking

The boundary of the planned harvest should be determined from the anterior surface of the auricle.[21] Large portions of the concha may be removed without any postharvest ear deformity, making it the most common site of harvest. However, multiple different studies have shown that certain key auricular structures should not be violated during auricular concha cartilage harvest to preserve auricular morphology postoperatively.[4,22] These key structures include the antihelix, the root of the helix, and the boundary between the concha cavum and the posterior inferior margin of the external auditory canal.[4] Rarely, if only small strips of cartilage are to be harvested, they could also be harvested from the area between the helix and antihelix or the helical rim[21] (Fig. 140.1). A short, 25- to 30-gauge needle dipped in methylene blue is used to tattoo the planned field of cartilaginous resection. This is done by introducing the needle dipped in methylene blue into the skin of the anterior ear, and it is then pushed completely through the posterior surface of the ear (Fig. 140.2).

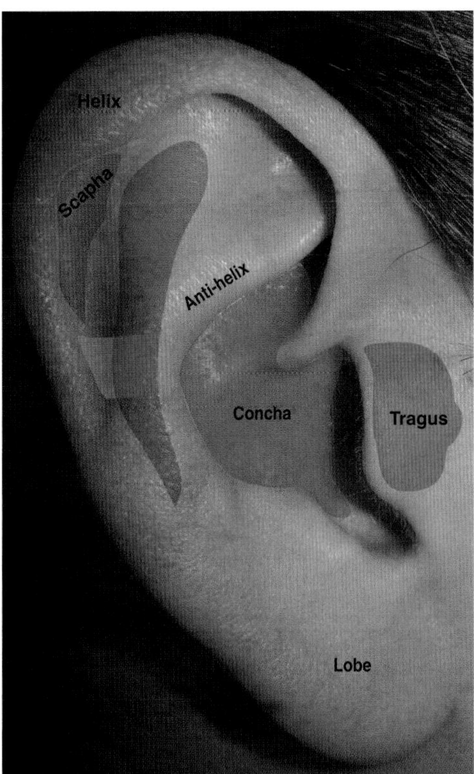

Figure 140.1 Potential sites of auricular cartilage harvest.

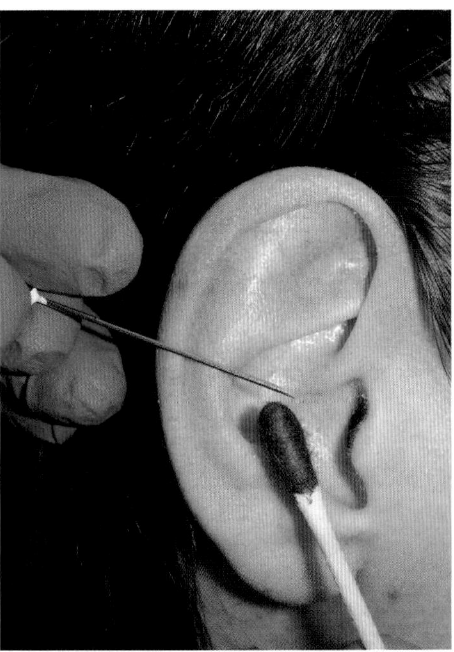

Figure 140.2 A needle with methylene blue used to tattoo the boundary of cartilage removal.

TECHNIQUE—*cont'd*

STEP 3: Cartilage Harvesting

Auricular concha cartilage could be harvested either via an anterior or a posterior approach. Non-conchal cartilage is harvested via the posterior approach.[21] The tragal cartilage is harvested via the tragal rim.[23] The anterior auricular incision is placed on the lateral edge of the concha on the inner aspect of the common and inferior crura of the antihelix.[5] A skin or skin/perichondrium flap is then raised. If a subperichondrial dissection is to be carried out, previous hydrodissection with local anesthetic would aid in this maneuver. Initial incision in the conchal cartilage is made parallel and slightly medial to the skin incision. Dissection is then continued posteriorly on the deep surface either in the subcutaneous or subperichondrial plane.[5,24] The cartilage is then liberated at its premarked medial boarder after the deep surface dissection is completed (Fig. 140.3). It is recommended that the perichondrium is left attached on one surface of the harvested cartilage to prevent fracture of the cartilage.[4]

Conchal cartilage harvest can also be accomplished via a posterior or retroauricular incision. A vertical incision is placed on the posterior surface of the auricular concha medially.[25] Dissection is then carried down to the perichondrium leaving the perichondrium attached to the cartilage posteriorly. This dissection is continued medially to the premastoid area. The conchal cartilage with its perichondrium is then separated from the mastoid fascia. Next, an incision into the cartilage is made in the medial boundary of the planed harvest. Another incision in cartilage is made in the lateral boundary of the graft after the anterior surface of the conchal bowl is elevated in the subperichondrial plane (Fig. 140.4).

Harvest of the cartilage in the scaphoid fossa of the ear is achieved by making an incision along the posterior rim of the helix once the posterior aspect of the ear is exposed with anterior retraction of the helix. Dissection is carried down to the subperichondrial plane. This plane is then extended until the desired amount of cartilage is exposed. Incision into the cartilage is then made carefully so as not to perforate the anterior skin. The cartilage incision should not be made directly beneath the skin incision but rather slightly medial to allow for additional 2 mm of cartilage to support the helix. Once the incision in the cartilage is complete, the cartilage is elevated away from the skin and perichondrium of the anterior auricular surface by a combination of blunt and sharp dissection with scissors.[26]

To harvest the tragal cartilage, an incision is made in the tragal rim. Then subperichondrial dissection is completed both anterior and posterior to the tragal cartilage. The facial nerve is located approximately 10 to 12 mm anterior to the lower end of the tragal cartilage, and care should be taken during dissection to avoid injury. The whole tragal cartilage could be removed except for a small rim at the site of the skin incision.[23]

Continued

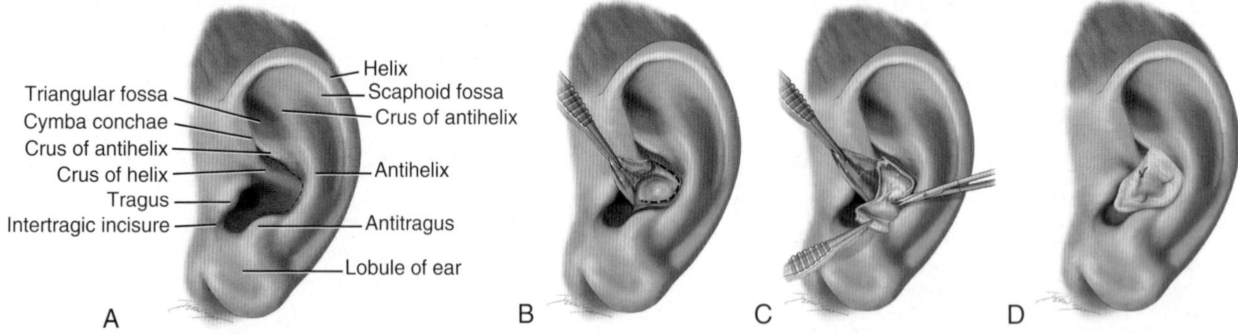

Figure 140.3 **A,** Anterior incision to harvest the conchal cartilage. The skin can be elevated with or without the underlying perichondrium. **B,** Dotted line showing incision through the cartilage or cartilage/perichondrium. **C,** Cartilage then separated from the posteromedial perichondrium on the deep surface. **D,** Closure.

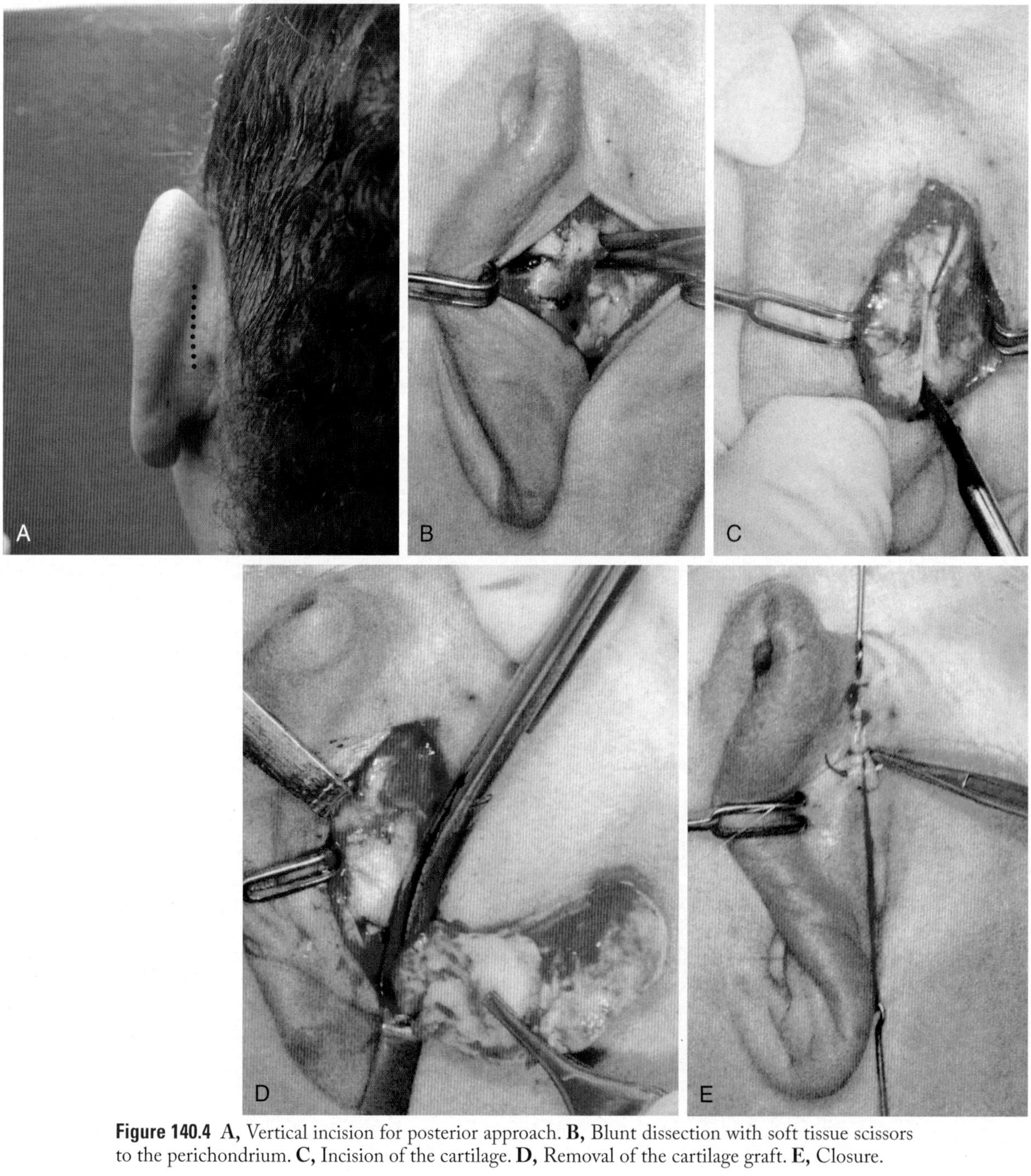

A B C D E

Figure 140.4 **A,** Vertical incision for posterior approach. **B,** Blunt dissection with soft tissue scissors to the perichondrium. **C,** Incision of the cartilage. **D,** Removal of the cartilage graft. **E,** Closure.

TECHNIQUE—*cont'd*

STEP 4: Closure and Dressing

Once the cartilage graft is removed, hemostasis should be obtained via bipolar cautery, as the skin envelops of the donor site are thin. The wound is then irrigated and closed with a few interrupted 4-0 Vicryl sutures in the subcutaneous layer. The skin is then approximated either with 4-0 plain gut suture or nylon suture in a continuous fashion.[4,22]

In a posterior approach harvest, a bolster dressing using cotton roll or folded petroleum gauze can be secured in the concha fossa in the following fashion. Prior to the skin closure, a horizontal suture using 4-0 Vicryl suture is placed through the anterior superior portion of the concha fossa. This stitch is taken through the mastoid fascia, and then brought out through the posterior superior portion of the concha fossa. A second similar suture is placed in the inferior portion of the concha fossa. The dressing material is placed in the concha fossa, and then the sutures are crisscrossed over the dressing and tied to press the skin of the conchal fossa against the mastoid fascia to eliminate the dead space[27] (Fig. 140.5A).

In an anterior approach harvest, the bolster dressing can be secured in the concha fossa using a through-and-through 3-0 or 4-0 nylon suture (Fig. 140.5B). This suture should hold the dressing in position and eliminate the dead space between the anterior and posterior skin but not strangulate the tissue. Antibiotic ointment could be applied to the conchal bowl prior to the placement of the dressing.[5]

No additional bolster dressing is applied when the cartilage is harvested for the tragus or scapha; however, a U-shaped 5-0 suture may be placed through the anterior and posterior surface of the tragus or scapha to avoid hematoma formation.[23]

Avoidance and Management of Intraoperative Complications

Perforation of the auricular skin flaps could occur during dissection. Injection of local anesthetic into the appropriate plane to create hydrodissection would allow for easier dissection and prevent perforation of the skin flaps. Injection of local anesthetic with vasoconstrictor prior to incision could assist in hemostasis during the procedure to minimize the use of cautery, which could also cause skin perforation. The inappropriate amount of cartilage harvest can be avoided by preoperative marking or tattooing of the cartilage to be harvested. If not premarked, the area of cartilage to be removed is difficult to assess once the dissection has begun and the preoperative morphology of the ear has been disturbed.[5]

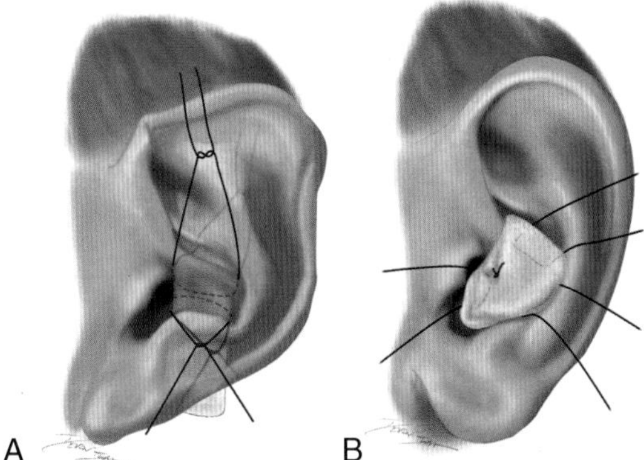

Figure 140.5 **A,** Superior and inferior horizontal suture for bolster dressing in posterior approach. **B,** Through-and-through sutures for bolster dressing in anterior approach.

Postoperative Considerations

Immediately after surgery, patients should avoid additional pressure on the donor site. For example, the patient should sleep on the contralateral side for the first two days after surgery to prevent distortion of the concha.[28] In addition, avoid excessive harvesting of the concha cartilage to prevent postoperative concha distortion.[4,5,22] Postoperative antibiotic is not indicated for the donor site but may be indicated for the graft site. The patient usually only requires mild analgesic for the donor site; however, they may require additional analgesic for the graft site.[21] The bolster dressing is left in place for 3 to 5 days postoperatively to prevent hematoma formation.[29]

References

1. Konig F. Reconstruction of the anterior tracheal wall. *Berl Klin Worchenschr.* 1896;33:1129.
2. Sushruta S, Bhishagratna KK, translator. *The Sushruta Samhita.* Calcutta, India: Kaviraj Kunja Lal Bhishagratna; 1907.
3. Brown JB, Cannon B. Composite free grafts of skin and cartilage from the ear. *Surg Gynecol Obstet.* 1946;82:253–255.
4. Lee M, Callahan S, Cochran CS. Auricular cartilage: harvest technique and versatility in rhinoplasty. *Am J Otolaryngol.* 2011;32(6):547–552.
5. Murrell GL. Auricular cartilage grafts and nasal surgery. *Laryngoscope.* 2004;114(12):2092–2102.
6. Castellani A, Negrini S, Zanetti U. Treatment of orbital floor blowout fractures with conchal auricular cartilage graft: a report on 14 cases. *J Oral Maxillofac Surg.* 2002;60(12):1413–1417.
7. Kruschewsky LS, Novais T, Daltro C, et al. Fractured orbital wall reconstruction with an auricular cartilage graft or absorbable polyacid copolymer. *J Craniofac Surg.* 2011;22(4):1256–1259.
8. Sugiyama A, Urushihara N, Fukumoto K, et al. Combined free autologous auricular cartilage and fascia lata graft repair for a re-

current tracheoesophageal fistula. *Pediatr Surg Int*. 2013;29(5):519–523.
9. Kaneko K, Sakaguchi K, Takano A, Jinnouchi S, Ishimaru K, Takahashi H. Tracheal reconstruction using S-shaped skin flaps and a conchal cartilage graft. *Ann Thorac Surg*. 2011;92(5):e111–e112.
10. Dornhoffer JL. Cartilage tympanoplasty. *Otolaryngol Clin North Am*. 2006;39(6):1161–1176.
11. Otley CC, Sherris DA. Spectrum of cartilage grafting in cutaneous reconstructive surgery. *J Am Acad Dermatol*. 1998;39(6):982–992.
12. Eriksson L, Westesson PL. Long-term evaluation of meniscectomy of the temporomandibular joint. *J Oral Maxillofac Surg*. 1985;43(4):263–269.
13. Holmlund AB, Gynther G, Axelsson S. Diskectomy in treatment of internal derangement of the temporomandibular joint. Follow up at 1, 3, 5 years. *Oral Surg Oral Med Oral Pathol*. 1993;76:266.
14. Takaku S, Toyoda T. Long-term evaluation of discectomy of the temporomandibular joint. *J Oral Maxillofac Surg*. 1994;52(7):722–726.
15. Merrill RG. Historical perspectives and comparisons of TMJ surgery for internal disk derangements and arthropathy. *Cranio*. 1986;4(1):74–85.
16. Tucker MR, Kennady MC, Jacoway JR. Autogenous auricular cartilage implantation following discectomy in the primate temporomandibular joint. *J Oral Maxillofac Surg*. 1990;48(1):38–44.
17. Hall HD, Link JL. Diskectomy alone and with ear cartilage interposition grafts in joint reconstruction. *Oral Maxillofac Clin North Am*. 1989;1:329.
18. Lei Z. Auricular cartilage graft interposition after temporomandibular joint ankylosis surgery in children. *J Oral Maxillofac Surg*. 2002;60(9):985–987.
19. Witsenburg B, Freihofer HP. Replacement of the pathological temporomandibular articular disc using autogenous cartilage of the external ear. *Int J Oral Surg*. 1984;13(5):401–405.
20. Firmin F, Sanger C, O'Toole G. Ear reconstruction following severe complications of otoplasty. *J Plast Reconstr Aesthet Surg*. 2008;61(suppl 1):S13–S20.
21. Hutchison I. Reconstructive surgery-bone and cartilage harvesting. In: Langdon JD, Patel MF, eds. *Operative Maxillofacial Surgery*. London, UK: Chapman & Hall; 1998.
22. Han K, Kim J, Son D, Park B. How to harvest the maximal amount of conchal cartilage grafts. *J Plast Reconstr Aesthet Surg*. 2008;61(12):1465–1471.
23. Kotzur A, Gubisch W. Tragal cartilage grafts in aesthetic rhinoplasty. *Aesthetic Plast Surg*. 2003;27(3):232–236.
24. Sclafani AP, Pearson JM. Nasal grafts and implants. In: Thomas JR, ed. *Advanced Therapy in Facial Plastic and Reconstructive Surgery*. Shelton, CT: People's Medical Publishing House-USA; 2010.
25. Boccieri A, Marano A. The conchal cartilage graft in nasal reconstruction. *J Plast Reconstr Aesthet Surg*. 2007;60(2):188–194.
26. Baylis HI, Rosen N, Neuhaus RW. Obtaining auricular cartilage for reconstructive surgery. *Am J Ophthalmol*. 1982;93(6):709–712.
27. Guyuron B. Simplified harvesting of the ear cartilage graft. *Aesthetic Plast Surg*. 1986;10(1):37–39.
28. Nicolle FV, Grobbelaar AO. Technique for harvesting of conchal cartilage grafts. *Aesthetic Plast Surg*. 1997;21(4):243–244.
29. Sherris DA, Larrabee WF Jr. Graft harvest techniques. In: Sherris DA, Larrabee WF Jr, eds. *Principles of Facial Reconstruction: A Subunit Approach to Cutaneous Repair*. 2nd ed. New York, NY: Thieme Medical Publishers; 2010.

CHAPTER 141

Facial Nerve Repair and Reanimation

David Hamlar, Kenneth Wan, Joel Stanek, and Sofia Lyford-Pike

Armamentarium

#10 and #15 blades
9-0 Suture
Army-Navy retractor
Appropriate suture
Castroviejo needle holder
DeBakey forceps
External eyelid weights and double-sided tape
Facial nerve monitor
Fibrin tissue glue
Gerald forceps
Heparinized saline
Implants
Jeweler forceps
Metzenbaum scissors
Microvascular instrumentation
Microscissors
Minnesota retractor
Microneedle holder
Nerve conduit or vein graft
Papaverine
Periosteal elevator
Reciprocating saw
Senn retractor
Soft tissue instrumentation
Venous coupler
Vessel dilators

History of the Procedure

The facial nerve serves myriad functions in the head and neck, including efferent motor function to the facial musculature; afferent gustatory sensation via chorda tympani; and parasympathetic function to the lacrimal, sublingual, and submandibular glands (Fig. 141.1). Facial nerve dysfunction results in marked esthetic and functional deficits, impacting the quality of life profoundly.[1] Reconstructive surgeons in the late 19th and early 20th centuries described some of the first facial reanimation techniques, many of which are still used to this day. Drobnick is credited with the first nerve transposition in 1879, utilizing the spinal accessory nerve as a donor nerve.[2] Manasse and Korte built upon this work by utilizing the hypoglossal nerve.[3,4] Functional muscle transfers using masseter and temporalis were pioneered by Lexer and Eden in 1911.[5] In 1970, Scaramella described the first report of a cross-face nerve graft (CFNG) from the normal to the affected side.[6] With the advent of improved microvascular equipment and techniques in subsequent decades, numerous authors described various neurotized free muscle transfers for restoration of spontaneous smile including pectoralis minor,[7] extensor digitorum brevis,[8] and gracilis,[9] which in combination with cross-face nerve grafting revolutionized the management of flaccid paralysis.

Indications for Use of the Procedure

Facial reanimation procedures can be separated broadly into static and dynamic procedures, based on the potential for volitional muscle movement. The decision to pursue various reconstructive options takes into account numerous variables including a patient's age, comorbid conditions, duration of paralysis, anatomic status of the proximal and distal facial nerve, need for adjuvant radiotherapy in cases of malignancy, and the patient's goals for therapy.

Whenever possible, primary repair or interposition grafting of the facial nerve is the reconstructive option of choice. In instances of malignancy (i.e., parotid neoplasms), facial nerve sacrifice can be anticipated and reconstructed at the time of extirpation. Penetrating facial nerve injuries should be explored and repaired within 72 hours of injury while distal nerve excitability remains intact. If repair is not possible at the time of exploration, distal branches should be identified and tagged for future reconstruction.

Static procedures are often recommended in patients who are too frail to undergo extensive, lengthy operations. As the name implies, these operations do not provide movement but rather suspend facial soft tissues. Static sling procedures can restore oral and nasal valve competence by elevating the commissure and the nasal valve tissues. Wedge excision and cheiloplasty can address the adynamic lower lip. Upper eyelid loading is indicated in any patient with exposure keratopathy symptoms from paralytic lagophthalmos and has the benefit of easy reversibility should nerve recovery occur. The use of static procedures does not impede future dynamic reconstruction should the patient desire, and in fact, they are useful adjuncts while axonal regeneration occurs.

Dynamic reconstructive options depend greatly on the duration of paralysis and the status of nerve donor candidates. Nerve transposition and cross-face nerve grafting rely on intact motor end plates and therefore must be completed

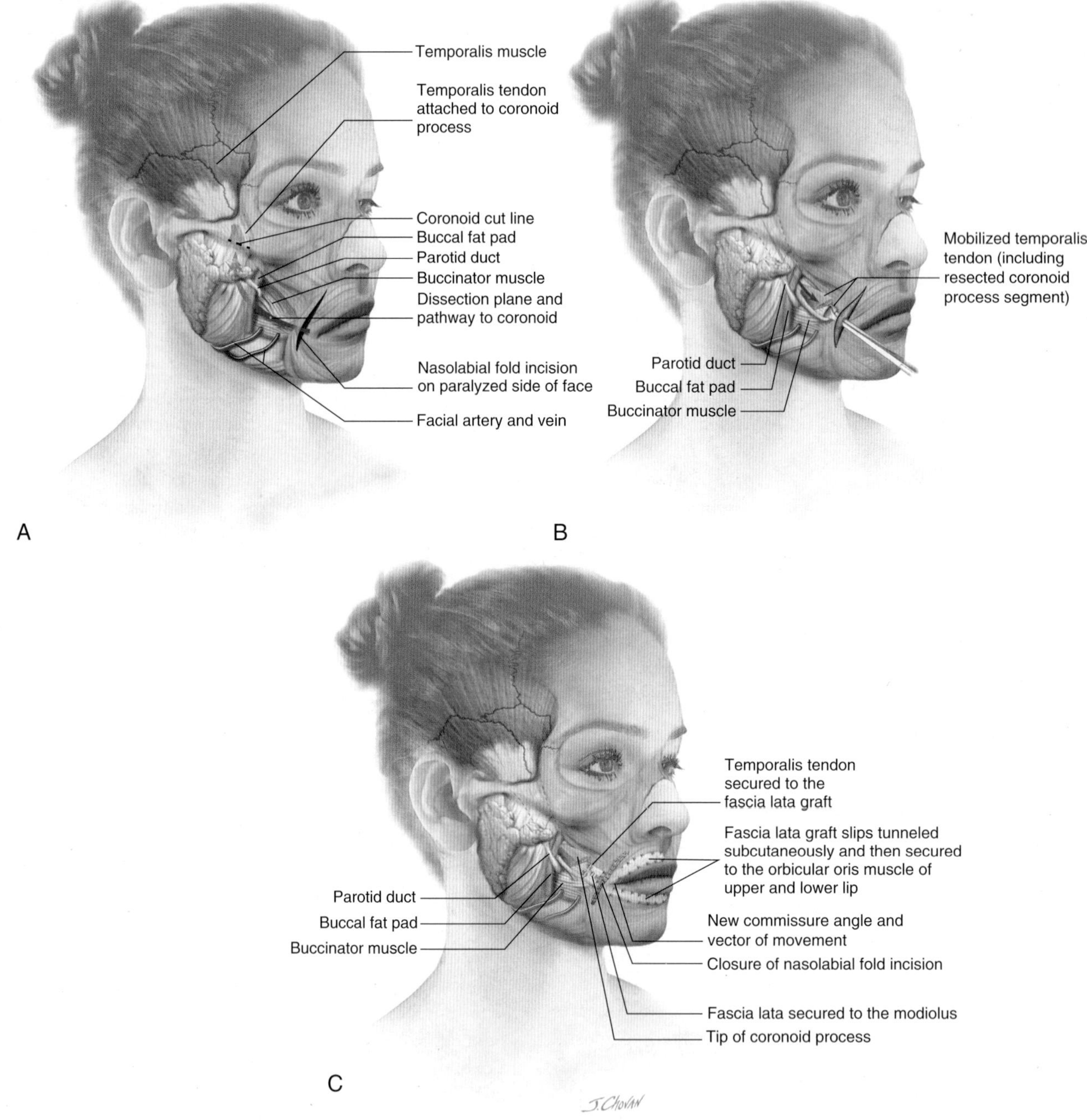

Figure 141.1 Orthodromic temporalis tendon transfer. **A** The coronoid process can be approached via an external incision at the nasolabial fold or a combined external/intraoral approach. The planned horizontal osteotomy is marked. **B** After completion of the osteotomy, the coronoid process and temporalis tendon are mobilized towards the modiolus. **C** A fascia lata graft is frequently incorporated. An upper and lower slip of the fascia are tunneled subcutaneously and secured to the orbicularis oris near the midline. The fascia proximal to the slips is secured to the modiolus.

within 12 to 18 months of paralysis onset before irreversible muscle atrophy has occurred.[10] These techniques are utilized when a proximal nerve stump is not available or viable such as injury at the skull base. If paralysis has been present for longer than 18 months, temporalis tendon or free muscle transfer must be considered for dynamic motion. Electromyography (EMG) can be used to determine if muscle is denervated, reinnervating, or electrically silent, indicating muscle atrophy. Temporary transposition of the hypoglossal nerve is another useful context to provide motor input to facial musculature to minimize atrophy while a CFNG is prepared, a so-called "babysitter" procedure.[11]

Limitations and Contraindications

Managing facial paralysis requires a holistic understanding of an individual patient's pathophysiology, anatomic constraints, functional deficits, and goals for treatment. As such, patients often require multiple procedures and a multidisciplinary approach to provide the most satisfactory outcomes.

Static reconstructions have relatively few limitations or contraindications. Static slings may require revisions over time as soft tissues become ptotic. Eyelid weights may become infected or extrude, requiring removal. A weight that is too heavy or too light may need to be exchanged. The adynamic lower lip can be difficult to manage surgically and is often best treated with botulinum toxin to the contralateral depressor labii inferioris for improved symmetry.

Patients undergoing neural-based dynamic reconstructions should be counseled regarding variability in results and timeline for recovery of function. This is usually 6 months or longer depending on the distance of required neural regeneration. Cross-face nerve grafting, while returning the ability for spontaneous facial expression, carries the highest variability in results, likely due to the lower number of recruited motor neurons.[12] As such, it is best utilized to power a single nerve division or free muscle graft. This technique also places the intact facial nerve at risk for injury. Nerves to masseter and hypoglossal transposition provide excellent motor power; however, both are limited by nonspontaneity of smile (requiring jaw clenching or tongue movement for muscle activation). Hypoglossal transposition is contraindicated in patients at risk for developing other cranial neuropathies or those with baseline dysphagia, as tongue dysfunction may exacerbate this problem. All nerve reconstructions carry a risk of developing synkinesis from misrouting of motor axons. This can be managed with botulinum toxin or selective neurectomy. Free muscle transfer carries a risk of flap failure, excessive muscle bulk, and change in position of the nasolabial fold.

TECHNIQUE: Static Procedures

STATIC SLING

Step 1: A standard preauricular rhytidectomy incision is made with a #10 or #15 scalpel blade and a skin flap is raised with rhytidectomy scissors to allow the exposure of the zygomatic arch, which will later serve to secure the proximal end of the static sling.

Step 2: We then turn our attention to making a small 1 cm vermillion border or nasolabial fold subcutaneous incision to expose the orbicularis muscle and modiolus. The addition of a subciliary incision can provide exposure to the inferior orbital rim that can provide additional anchor points that helps in finessing the vector of the static sling.

Step 3: A soft tissue tunnel is created with rhytidectomy scissors from the zygomatic arch area to the modiolus in a subcutaneous or subsuperficial musculoaponeurotic system (SMAS) plane.

Step 4: Select a static sling graft material according to the surgeon's preference: tensor fascia lata, palmaris longus tendon, expanded polytetrafluorethylene (Gore-Tex), or acellular human dermis (AlloDerm) can be used.

Step 5: Mattress-suture one end of the sling to the modiolus with nonresorbable polyethylene or nylon 3-0 suture, or alternatively, the sling can be split into two tongues and each individually sutured to the lateral aspect of the upper and lower orbicularis oris muscle.

Step 6: The sling is pulled through the soft tissue tunnel to exit in the zygomatic area.

Step 7: A posterior superior vector is desired. Determine the ideal vector and trim the length of the sling to create the correction tension and position of the commissure. Some overcorrection should be incorporated as all types of sling material stretch under tension over time.

Step 8: Fixate the proximal end of the sling to the zygomatic arch with Mitek anchors, miniplate or a nonresorbable nylon or polyethylene suture.

Step 9: The surgical wound is washed with copious normal saline and the surgical wound closed in layers according to the surgeon's preference.

Continued

TECHNIQUE: Static Procedures—*cont'd*

UPPER EYELID WEIGHT

Step 1: Mark supratarsal crease. The incision is centered over the midpupillary line and medial limbus and should measure about 2 cm.

Step 2: Incise through the skin and orbicularis oculi muscle. After infiltrating with local anesthetic with vasoconstrictor, the skin is incised sharply. Dissection through the muscle can be accomplished sharply with scissors or with high-temp loop cautery.

Step 3: Identify the orbital septum and expose the tarsal plate. Take care not to violate the orbital septum. Follow it inferiorly to identify the tarsal plate. A precise pocket should be created to avoid migration of the implant. The ideal placement of the implant is about 2 mm above the lash line to avoid extrusion at the lid margin.

Step 4: Place weight in the pocket and secure to the tarsal plate with partial-thickness sutures (5-0 or 6-0 polydioxanone). Avoid manipulating the implant excessively. Two sutures are placed to secure the implant to the tarsus. The lid can be everted after the placement of these sutures to ensure a full-thickness bite though the conjunctiva has not been taken.

Step 5: Reapproximate muscle (5-0 polyglactin) and close skin (5-0 fast-absorbing gut). Closing the muscle over the implant provides an extra barrier to extrusion or infection. The skin is closed per surgeon preference with either fine absorbable or nonabsorbable suture.

TECHNIQUE: Wedge Excision and Cheiloplasty

WEDGE EXCISION

Step 1: The planned wedge excision is marked. The lateral aspect of the incision is marked approximately 5 to 7 mm lateral to the oral commissure. The width of the excision is 2 to 2.5 cm. The superior cuts are perpendicular to the vermillion and the inferior aspect is triangular shaped to close without a standing cutaneous deformity.

Step 2: Full-thickness excision of the lower lip is performed. The lateral incision is made first to determine whether the extent of the planned excision is appropriate or will place the closure under undue tension. The medial incision can then be made.

Step 3: The lip is reapproximated in layers. Muscles are reapproximated with 3-0 polyglactin. The mucosa is closed with 4-0 chromic. The medial edge of the vermillion is intentionally placed lower than the vermillion laterally to allow for the eversion of the red lip.

CHEILOPLASTY

Step 1: A fusiform of skin is marked along the vermillion border. Only skin will be excised. This allows the red lip to evert more effectively and improve symmetry.

Step 2: Skin incisions are made with a #15 blade. Skin is excised and discarded.

Step 3: The wound is closed in layers.

TECHNIQUE: Dynamic Procedures

PRIMARY NEURORRHAPHY AND CABLE GRAFTING

Primary Neurorrhaphy

Step 1: A modified Blair or rhytidectomy incision is made with a #15 or #10 scalpel blade and a skin flap raised.

TECHNIQUE—Dynamic Procedures *cont'd*

Step 2: Anatomical landmarks such as the tympanomastoid suture and posterior belly of digastric or tragal pointer are used to identify the facial nerve trunk as it exits the stylomastoid foramen. The facial nerve is dissected distally to the area in need of primary neurorrhaphy and the proximal nerve stump is identified and mobilized. A mastoidectomy is necessary if the infratemporal portion of the facial nerve is the area of concern.

Step 3: The nerve ends are examined under magnification with an operating microscope and a colored background utilized to facilitate better visual delineation of the nerve. Microsurgical jeweler forceps are used to meticulously handle the nerve.

Step 4: Perform neurolysis and removal of scar tissue/epineurium from the site of injury if necessary.

Step 5: Coaptation of the nerve is carried out and the nerve ends are to meet tension-free. Blood on the nerve ends is irrigated away to prevent scar formation.

Step 6: Using 8-0 to 10-0 polypropylene sutures, two to three interrupted sutures are placed 180 or 120 degrees apart in the epineurium under magnification with microneedle holders and jeweler forceps.

Step 7: Nerve diameter mismatch can be corrected by beveling the smaller nerve to create better coaptation.

CABLE GRAFTING

Cable nerve grafting is a viable option if the length of the remaining facial nerve is insufficient for tension-free primary coaptation. The basic general microsurgery principles previously described in the primary neurorrhaphy section apply in cable grafting. It is important to obtain enough grafted nerve length with some redundancy such that upon completion of neurorrhaphy, the final coaptated nerve lies in a tension-free lazy S or C configuration. Sural, greater auricular, medial, and lateral antebrachial nerves are common autologous nerve graft donor options. Other options include decellularized cadaveric nerve allograft (Avance, Axogen), entubilization with autologous vein graft, or alloplastic biodegradable polymer nerve conduits (polylactide-caprolactone such as Neurotube, Neurolac, or type 1 collagen such as NeuraGen).

SURAL NERVE HARVESTING

Step 1: Mark the surgical incision: surgical access is made with an oblique incision with a #10 or #21 scalpel blade posterior to the lateral malleolus and anterior to the Achilles tendon (the nerve enters the foot at this landmark) down to the subcutaneous plane where the nerve lies. Once identified, aided by gentle traction and palpation of the nerve, additional 6 to 8 cm oblique incisions following its course proximally are made until the desired length of the nerve is achieved.

Step 2: Up to 40 cm of the sural nerve can be harvested if the skin incision is extended proximally all the way up to the popliteal fossa, whereby the number of fascicles increases proximally. As the nerve runs posteriorly up the posterior dorsal aspect of the lower leg in the subcutaneous plane, it descends deep between the two heads of the gastrocnemius muscle toward its origin in the popliteal fossa, where it is formed by the union of the branches of common fibular and tibial nerves.

Step 3: Small saphenous veins accompany the nerve and primary hemostasis can be achieved by bipolar cautery, vessel ties, or ligating clips.

Step 4: Once the desired length is dissected, the proximal and distal ends are cut and the proximal and distal nerve ends of the harvest sites should be tied or Liga-clipped.

Step 5: The surgical wound is closed in layers according to the surgeon's preference and surgical drain is not required.

Continued

TECHNIQUE—Dynamic Procedures *cont'd*

GREATER AURICULAR NERVE HARVESTING

Step 1: Mark the position of the greater auricular nerve: a line is drawn from the angle of the mandible to the mastoid tip. A second line is drawn that bisects the aforementioned line at a right angle. The second line corresponds to the path of the nerve from Erb's point of the neck to the area below the auricle.

Step 2: A modified Blair or rhytidectomy incision is made and a skin flap is raised.

Step 3: The nerve is dissected off the lateral aspect of the sternocleidomastoid muscle and traced to the auricle. Its path is posterior to the external jugular vein. Usually, 10 cm of nerve length can be harvested and the caliber of the nerve is constant throughout its course.

Step 4: Once the desired length is dissected, the proximal and distal ends are cut and the proximal and distal nerve ends of the harvest sites should be ligated or Liga-clipped.

Step 5: Surgical wound is closed in layers according to the surgeon's preference.

MEDIAN AND LATERAL ANTEBRACHIAL NERVE HARVESTING

Step 1: These nerves pose a good alternative if a radial forearm free flap is harvested at the same time for reconstruction; hence mark and make the incision per radial forearm free flap with the extension of the proximal incision to the antebrachial fossa.

Step 2: The lateral antebrachial cutaneous nerve is a terminal branch of the musculocutaneous nerve. Locate it as it emerges from the lateral aspect of the bicep tendon and follow it distally as it runs superficially to the brachialis muscle. Up to 12 cm can be harvested.

Step 3: For the median antebrachial nerve, locate it by marking a point two fingers' breadth distal to the medial epicondyle while the elbow is extended. Then draw a line two fingers' breadth medial to the first point, and this will be the approximate location of the nerve. Raise the skin flap in a subcutaneous plane and the nerve will be seen running close to the branchial vein. Up to 20 cm of graft can be obtained if the nerve is chased proximally up to the mid–upper arm, whether it divides into the anterior and posterior cutaneous divisions.

ORTHODROMIC TEMPORALIS TENDON TRANSFER

Step 1: The nasolabial fold is marked preoperatively on the paralyzed side of the face.

Step 2: The nasolabial fold incision is made sharply and carried into the subcutaneous fat.

Step 3: Dissection proceeds toward the mandibular ramus. The appropriate plane of dissection is between the buccal fat pad laterally and the buccinator muscle medially. Take care to avoid injuring the parotid duct that traverses this space. Once the ramus is reached, a limited portion of the masseter muscle may need to be elevated.

Step 4: Identify the coronoid and perform coronoidectomy. The coronoidectomy can be made with a reciprocating saw. Prior to the complete release of the coronoid, grasp the temporalis tendon with an Allis clamp, as it can retract into the infratemporal fossa and be difficult to retrieve.

TECHNIQUE—Dynamic Procedures *cont'd*

Step 5: Secure the temporalis tendon to the fascia lata graft. The graft should be harvested with a separate setup or prior to performing the approach for the temporalis tendon transfer to avoid contamination. A graft measuring at least 5 × 10 cm should be harvested. The graft is secured to the tendon with 3-0 polydioxanone mattress sutures.

Step 6: Secure the fascia lata graft to the upper/lower lip. Subcutaneous tunnels are made from the nasolabial incision medially toward the midline upper and lower lip along the vermillion border. A small incision is then made at the midline and the fascia, which has been divided into two slips for approximately half its length, is separately tunneled and secured to the orbicular oris muscle.

Step 7: The fascia lata graft is secured to the modiolus. The graft immediately proximal to the divided slips of fascia is secured to the modiolus with 3-0 polydioxanone mattress sutures. This step ensures the excursion of the oral commissure with the activation of the temporalis muscle. The vector of movement and excursion of the commissure can be assessed with transcutaneous stimulation of the temporalis muscle, and any adjustments can be made prior to closure.

Step 8: Incisions are closed in a layered fashion with resorbable deep sutures and fine cutaneous sutures per surgeon preference.

TWO-STAGE CROSS-FACE NERVE GRAFT

Step 1: A rhytidectomy or modified Blair incision is designed on the paralyzed side of the face. The incision is made down to the parotidomasseteric fascia and a SMAS flap is elevated with facelift scissors to the anterior border of the parotid gland. Facial nerve branches are identified.

Step 2: Facial nerve branches resulting in greatest oral commissure excursion are mapped with a nerve stimulator. Due to extensive anastomoses of the midface branches, one or two redundant branches are often available for transfer without impairing the nonparalyzed side. Ensure redundancy when selecting the donor nerve.

Step 3: A subcutaneous tunnel is fashioned to the contralateral canine fossa. The previously harvested nerve graft (sural, lateral antebrachial cutaneous, etc.) is tunneled from the midface dissection to the canine fossa.

Step 4: Perform anastomosis of the nerve graft to the donor facial nerve branch.

Step 5: The distal nerve graft is marked with clips or colored suture in the canine fossa. Incisions are closed per surgeon preference.

Step 6: Growth of axons along the nerve graft is followed with a Tinel sign. Tapping the skin along the course of the nerve graft will elicit a tingling sensation, which can be used to monitor the progress of axonal regrowth. When the Tinel sign is present at the canine fossa, the CFNG is ready for anastomosis.

NERVE TO MASSETER TRANSPOSITION

Step 1: A rhytidectomy or modified Blair incision is designed on the paralyzed side of the face as described under CFNG.

Continued

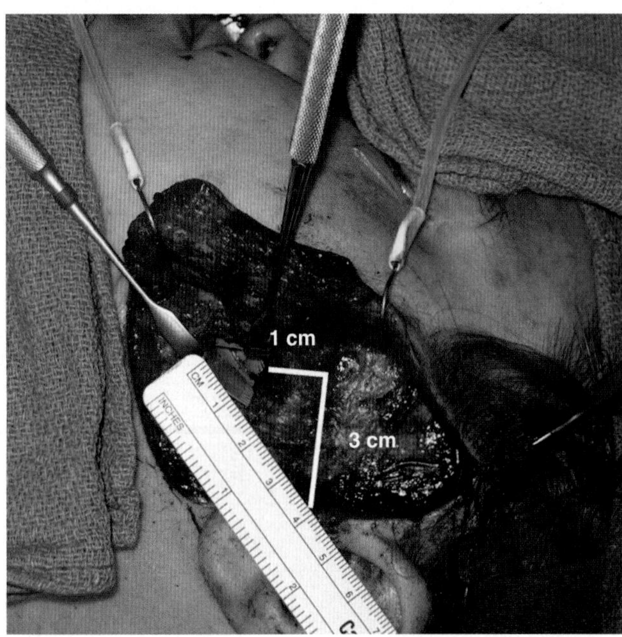

Figure 141.2 Dissection demonstrating the location of the nerve to masseter. The nerve to masseter is reliably identified approximately 1 cm inferior to the zygomatic arch and 3 cm anterior to the tragus as it passes through the sigmoid notch to innervate the muscle from the deep aspect.

TECHNIQUE—Dynamic Procedures *cont'd*

Step 2: A suitable nerve recipient is identified and selected.

As nerve excitability is no longer present, a robust branch to the zygomaticus is most often selected.

Step 3: The nerve to masseter is identified (Fig. 141.2).

The nerve is reliably found approximately 3 cm anterior to the tragus, 1 cm inferior to the zygoma, and 1.5 cm deep to the SMAS. The subzygomatic triangle approach is reliable beyond the use of surface landmarks. The nerve travels between the sigmoid notch of the mandible to innervate the masseter on the deep side. Dissection is performed bluntly through the muscle fibers. Muscle stimulation may be noted as dissection approaches the nerve. Once the nerve is identified, it is traced medially, where it begins to branch. The nerve is divided sharply proximal to any branching and reflected laterally.

Step 4: Perform anastomosis of the nerve to masseter to the distal midface nerve branch.

Step 5: Wound closure is done.

HYPOGLOSSAL NERVE TRANSPOSITION, END-TO-SIDE WITH JUMP GRAFT

Step 1: A rhytidectomy or modified Blair incision is designed on the paralyzed side of the face as described under CFNG.

Step 2: The main trunk of the facial nerve is identified (Fig. 141.3). Traditional landmarks include the tragal pointer, tympanomastoid suture, and posterior belly of digastric. The nerve can be dissected retrograde to the stylomastoid foramen. If desired, additional length of the facial nerve can be attained by completing a cortical mastoidectomy, dividing the nerve at the second genu, and reflecting it inferiorly into the neck. Some sternocleidomastoid muscle release may also help.

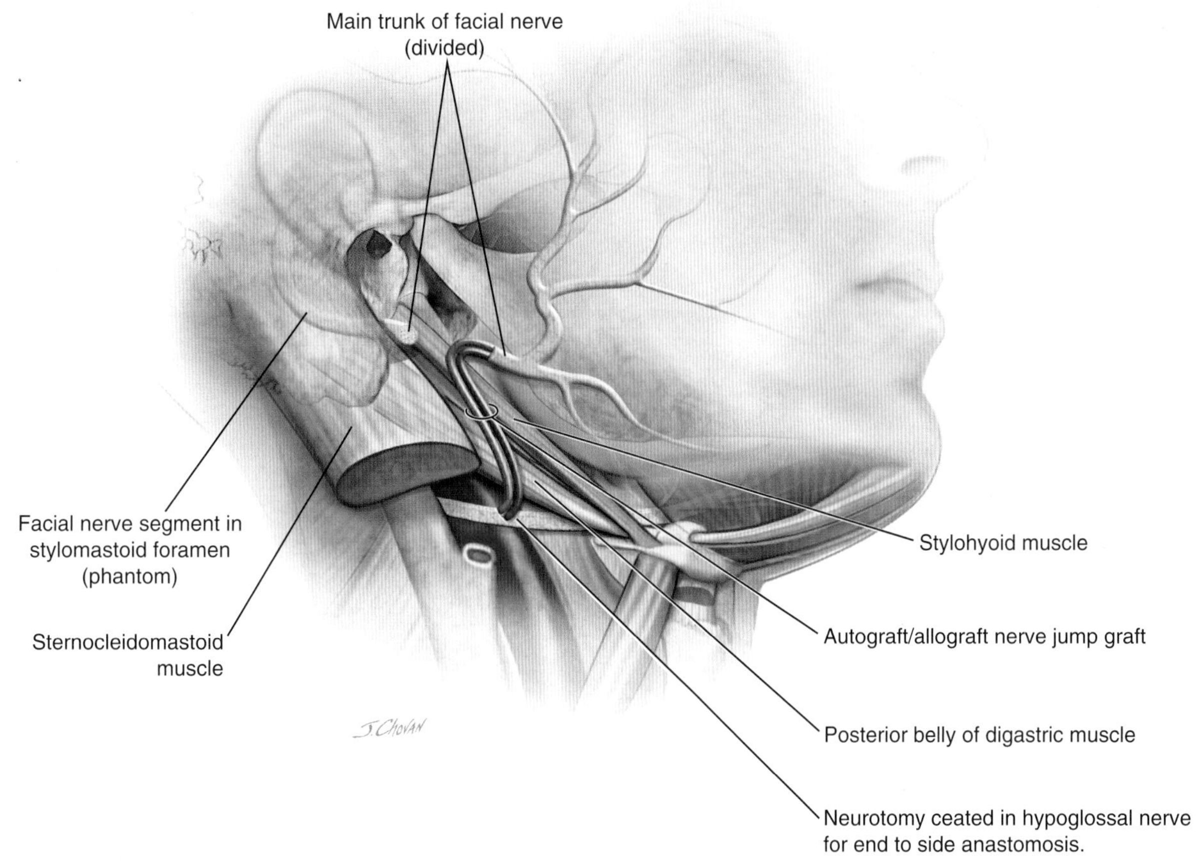

Figure 141.3 Schematic of end-to-side technique for facial-hypoglossal anastomosis. A jump graft is interposed between a neurotomy created in the hypoglossal nerve and the distal trunk of the facial nerve.

TECHNIQUE—Dynamic Procedures *cont'd*

Step 3: The hypoglossal nerve is identified medial to the posterior belly of digastric. The posterior belly of digastric can be followed anterior and inferior to the digastric tendon. The nerve lies just deep to the muscle and tendon. There are typically one or more large veins overlying the nerve, which must be ligated to improve exposure.

Step 4: A neurotomy is created in the hypoglossal nerve and an allograft/autograft nerve is anastomosed in an end-to-side fashion as a jump graft. Several variations in technique exist. Traditionally, the hypoglossal nerve was completely transected and anastomosed to the facial nerve. Partial nerve transfers have also been described. We prefer the end-to-side technique with jump graft to minimize morbidity associated with hypoglossal nerve palsy. Some surgeons prefer to perform the neurotomy distal to the ansa cervicalis.

Step 5: The jump graft is anastomosed to the main trunk of the facial nerve. The sacrifice of some facial nerve branches (e.g., cervical branches) may be performed to minimize synkinetic motion.

Step 6: Wound closure is performed per surgeon preference.

Continued

TECHNIQUE—Dynamic Procedures *cont'd*

GRACILIS FREE TISSUE TRANSFER

STEP 1: Preparation of Recipient Site

The paralyzed side of the face is approached through a rhytidectomy incision. Dissection is taken down to the parotidomasseteric fascia and carried anteriorly in a sub-SMAS plane. The modiolus is identified and can be found by following the zygomaticus major muscle medially. 4-0 or 5-0 polyglactin sutures are placed in the modiolus, checking placement by pulling on the sutures and noting the position relative to the commissure.

The facial artery and vein are next identified and prepared for microvascular anastomosis by dissecting an adequate length and assessing vessel diameter. The superficial temporal vessels can also be used if the facial vessels are not present.

Next, the motor input to the free muscle transfer is prepared. If a CFNG was performed previously, the distal end is identified and freshened sharply. If a nerve to masseter transfer is planned, this is performed as previously described.

STEP 2: Harvest of Gracilis Muscle (FIG. 141.4)

The thigh is abducted and flexed at the knee. Landmarks include the insertion of the adductor tendons on the superior pubic ramus superiorly and the medial condyle of the tibia inferiorly. An incision is designed 2 cm medially to a line drawn between these landmarks and measures 12 to 15 cm.

The skin is incised sharply with a #15 blade and carried through the subcutaneous tissues. The muscle belly is identified and exposed near its midpoint. The neurovascular pedicle is then identified. The artery and its venae comitantes are reliably identified 8 to 10 cm inferior to the pubic tubercle, passing between adductor longus anteriorly and adductor magnus posteriorly. The adductor artery, a branch of the deep femoral artery, gives off a branch to the gracilis, which enters on the deep surface of the muscle. The anterior obturator nerve enters the muscle at a more oblique course about 1 to 2 cm superior to the entry point of the artery. The necessary length of the muscle is marked. The muscle is then divided superiorly and inferiorly to approximately 50% of its width taking care not to injure the pedicle. A longitudinal incision is then made. The obturator nerve is divided. The artery and venae comitantes can be dissected to a length of about 6 cm where they are clipped.

STEP 3: Thinning of Muscle and Vessel Preparation

Muscle thinning can be performed in situ or on the back table. This is important to avoid excessive bulk transfer to the face. The ideal weight of the muscle is 15 to 25 g. The adventitia is cleaned from the vessels in preparation for anastomosis.

STEP 4: Muscle Inset

The muscle is oriented such that the pedicle exits inferiorly. The obturator nerve is tunneled toward the mouth if using a CFNG. The muscle is inset into the modiolus with the previously placed 4-0 or 5-0 polyglactin sutures in a figure-of-8 fashion. This is most easily accomplished after running a 3-0 polyglactin suture along the proximal and distal end of the muscle to prevent the insetting sutures from pulling through the muscle fibers. Three to four sutures are placed on the proximal portion of the muscle to the superficial layer of deep temporal fascia. The oral commissure should be set at about 50% of the anticipated smile excursion.

STEP 5: Arterial and Venous Anastomosis

The adductor artery is anastomosed to the facial artery with a 9-0 or 10-0 nylon suture. One vena comitans is anastomosed to the facial vein with an appropriately sized venous coupler.

STEP 6: Nerve Anastomosis

The obturator nerve is anastomosed to either the CFNG (with the neurorrhaphy completed intraorally) or the nerve to masseter with two to three interrupted 9-0 nylon sutures in the epineurium.

STEP 7: Closure of Neck and Leg

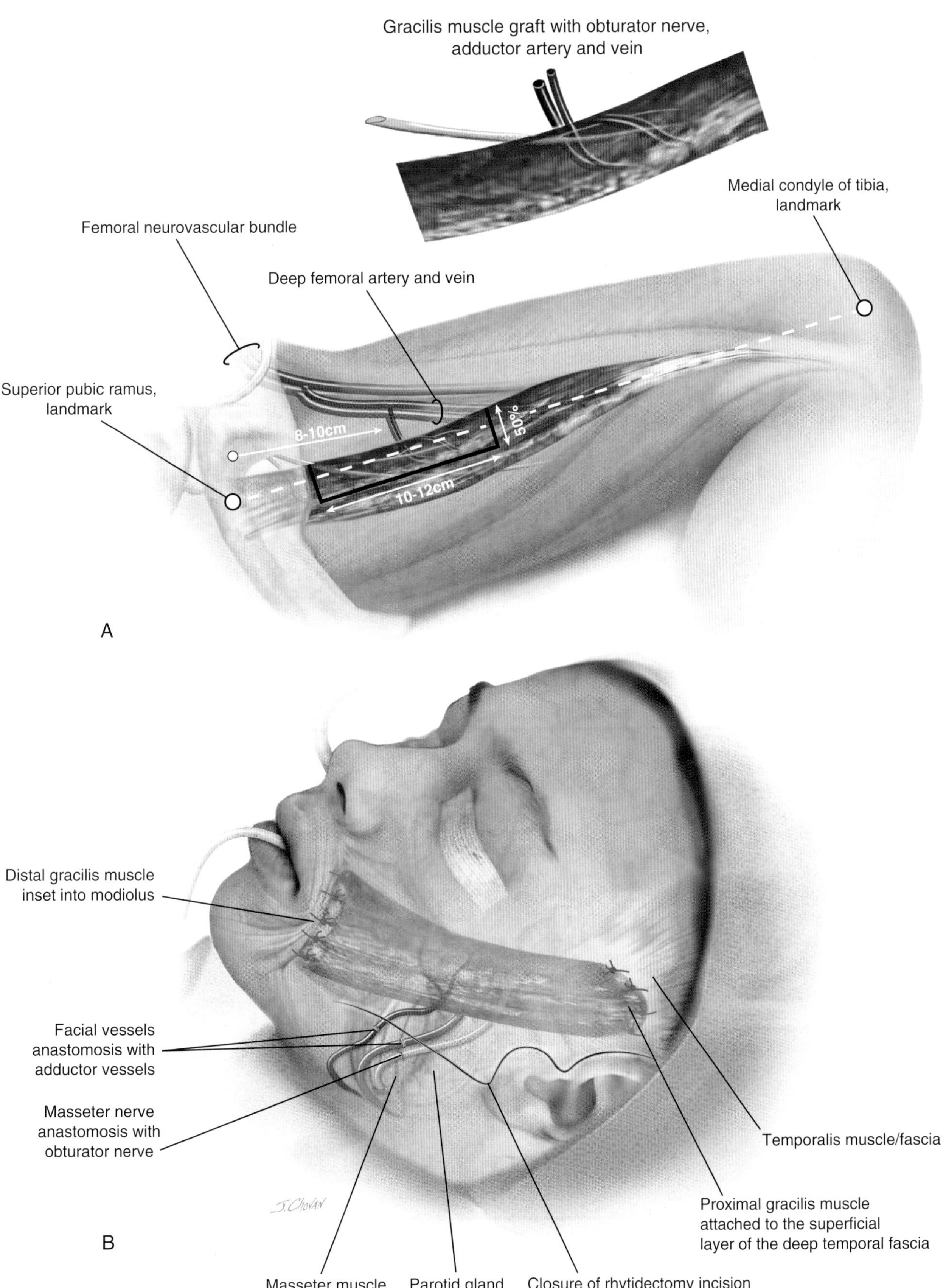

Figure 141.4 **A** Harvest of gracilis muscle with neurovascular bundle. Approximately 50% of the width of the muscle is harvested to avoid excessive bulk in the face. **B** The gracilis is inset into the modiolous distallly and to the temporalis fascia proximally. The adductor vessels are anastomosed to the facial vessels and the obturator nerve to the nerve to masseter.

Avoidance and Management of Intraoperative Complications

Upper Eyelid Weight

Care should be taken to avoid full-thickness passage of the suture through the tarsus and conjunctiva, which could result in corneal irritation. Excessive manipulation of the weight prior to implantation should be avoided and consideration should be given to soaking the implant in antibiotic-impregnated solution to minimize risk of infection.

Static Sling

Every attempt should be made to avoid violating the oral mucosa. Infection of the fascia graft is rare but can significantly impact the results of the procedure if infection compromises the viability of the free fascia graft.

Neurorrhaphy

Tension-free nerve repair is of utmost importance. An interposition nerve graft should be employed if there is any question of excessive tension.

Temporalis Tendon Transfer

The parotid duct runs in the vicinity of the dissection. If injured, the duct should be ligated to avoid postoperative salivary fistula. A pressure dressing and intraparenchymal botulinum toxin injection can be considered.

Gracilis Free Muscle Transfer

Careful thinning of gracilis muscle to avoid devascularizing muscle.

Postoperative Considerations

All patients should be monitored for infection in the immediate postoperative period. Antimicrobial prophylaxis is indicated for cases involving intraoral manipulation. With the exception of free tissue transfer, most patients are discharged home on the same operative day unless observation is otherwise indicated. Free tissue transfers are monitored per institution protocol, most commonly with Doppler stethoscope checks, as no skin paddle is available for monitoring. Aspirin is administered to avoid thrombosis at the anastomosis. The thigh should be monitored for any signs of a hematoma.

References

1. Nellis JC, Ishii M, Byrne PJ, Boahene KDO, Dey JK, Ishii LE. Association among facial paralysis, depression, and quality of life in facial plastic surgery patients. *JAMA Facial Plast Surg*. 2017;19(3):190–196.
2. Sawicki B. In: Chepault. The *Status of Neurosurgery*. JReuff, Paris, 1902. p. 189.
3. Manasse P. Uber vereinigung des N. facialis mit dem N. accesorius durch die Nervenpfropfung (Greffe nerveuse). *Arch Klin Chir*. 1900;62:805.
4. Korte W. Ein Fall von Nervenpfropfung: des Nervus facialis auf den Nervus hypoglossus. *Deutsche med Wihnschr*. 1903;17:293–295.
5. Lexer E, Eden R. Uber die chirurgische Behandlung der peripheren Facialislahmung. *Beitr Klin Chir*. 1911;73:116.
6. Scaramella LF. *Preliminary Report on Facial Nerve Anastomosis*. Osaka, Japan: Second International Symposium on Facial Nerve Surgery; 1970.
7. Terzis JK., Manktelow RT. Pectoralis minor: a new concept in facial reanimation. *Plast Surg Forum*. 1982;69:760–769.
8. Thompson N, Gustavson EH. The use of neuromuscular free autografts with microneural anastomosis to restore elevation to the paralysed angle of the mouth in cases of unilateral facial paralysis. *Chir Plast*. 1976;3(3):165–174.
9. Harii K, Ohmori K, Torii S. Free gracilis muscle transplantation, with microneurovascular anastomoses for the treatment of facial paralysis. a preliminary report. *Plast Reconstr Surg*. 1976;57(2):133–143.
10. May M. Nerve substitution techniques. In: May M, Schaitkin B, eds. *The Facial Nerve*. New York: Thieme Publishers; 1999:611–633.
11. Terzis JK, Tzafetta K. "Babysitter" procedure with concomitant muscle transfer in facial paralysis. *Plast Reconstr Surg*. 2009;124(4):1142–1156.
12. Chuang DC, Wei FC, Noordhoff MS. "Smile" reconstruction in facial paralysis. *Ann Plast Surg*. 1989;23(1):56–65.

CHAPTER 142

Face Transplant

Marissa Suchyta, Waleed Gibreel, Karim Bakri, Carrie E. Robertson, Thomas J. Salinas, Sebastian Cotofana, Hatem Amer, and Samir Mardini

Armamentarium

Face transplantation is an innovative procedure for patients with facial deformities who have exhausted traditional reconstructive options. Over 40 facial transplants have been performed worldwide for defects caused by a variety of etiologies, including ballistic injuries, animal attacks, severe burns, and advanced neurofibromatosis type 1.[1] Face transplants have included both soft tissue and underlying bones, including the maxilla and mandible, leading to immense functional and esthetic improvement for patients[2] (Fig. 142.1). This is a highly patient-specific procedure, as evidenced by the wide variety of facial defects that recipients have presented with. Face transplant thus adds to the armamentarium of reconstructive surgeons and is highly dependent on a multidisciplinary team that brings together the broad areas of expertise that are needed.

History of the Procedure

The first successful face transplant was performed in 2005 in Amiens, France, restoring both esthetic and function of the mid and lower-face in a 38-year-old woman following a dog bite.[3] This initial transplant demonstrated the success of both the surgical technique as well as long-term maintenance of the facial transplant with immunosuppression therapy. Since this initial paradigm-shifting success, there have been over 40 face transplants performed around the world. These included the first partial face transplant in the United States in 2008,[4] as well as the first full face transplant, which included all soft tissue of the face and underlying bone structure, in Barcelona in 2010.[5]

Indications for the Procedure

Candidates for face transplant usually have complex soft tissue with or without bone defects. The soft tissue deformity must involve more than one esthetic subunit of the face as well as a large percent of the total facial surface area.[6] In patients where it is deemed that multiple conventional reconstructive procedures would yield suboptimal function and esthetics, facial transplantation could be indicated as the primary procedure for that patient. The ideal candidate has improved function as a primary driver and motivation for the transplant; this may include blinking, oral continence, chewing, and breathing, among other essential functions.

Face transplants have been performed on patients whose disfigurements were caused by trauma, including animal attacks.[7] Individuals with severe ballistic injuries, which generally affect both the soft tissue and underlying skeletal structure, are also potential face transplant candidates. Advances in burn care have led to the survival of patients with extensive esthetic and functional deficits caused by facial burn contractures and scarring. Face transplant can lead to immense improvement in the quality of life for these patients.[8] Transplants have also been performed on patients with deformities from neurofibromatosis.[9,10] Concerns in these patients are the risk of transformation to neurofibrosarcoma once the immune system is compromised; also of concern is the risk related to sensory and motor involvement with tumors in these patients requiring nerve regeneration to innervate the transplanted face. Each individual case presents a unique circumstance that necessitates an individualized approach based upon the tissue defect and missing functional units.

Limitations and Contraindications

Perhaps one of the most important preoperative aspects of face transplantation is that of patient selection. The patient with a facial disfigurement that can be reconstructed with adequate function and esthetics using conventional techniques should not be considered for facial transplantation as the risk-benefit ratio would not weigh in favor of this procedure. Furthermore, the patient should be in good physical health, assessed through both physical exam and laboratory testing to exclude chronic conditions that increase risk from immunosuppression. Magnetic resonance imaging and computed tomography (CT) should be performed to assess any anatomical limitations to face transplant, including the absence of recipient vessels. The presence of a facial nerve is also crucial to the functional recovery aspect of face transplant and should be evaluated by electromyography and/or imaging studies. Careful assessment of the risk-benefit of face transplant must be discussed with potential recipients and compared with all other potential reconstructive options. The lifelong commitment to follow-up and the side effects of required immunosuppression must be stressed.

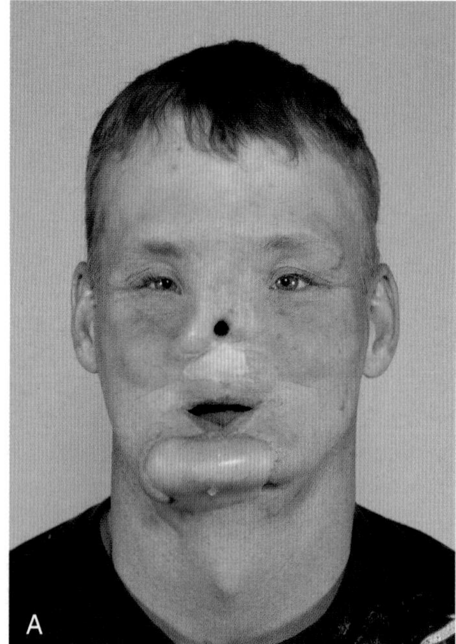

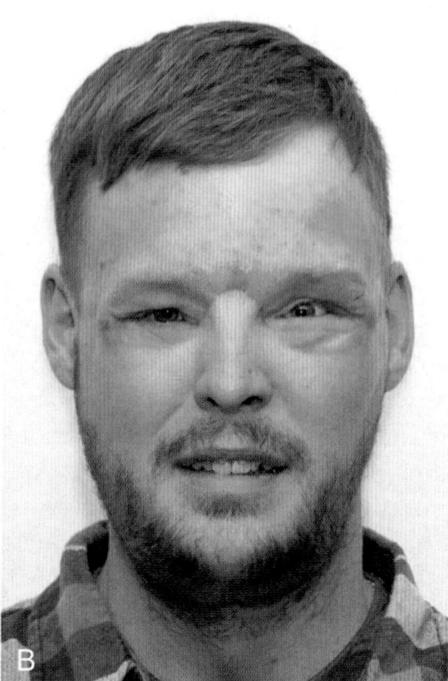

Figure 142.1 Face transplant can lead to an immense increase in quality of life for patients with facial defects who have exhausted the armamentarium of traditional reconstructive options. This patient, who was transplanted at our institution, is pictured preoperatively (A) with facial disfigurement due to a gunshot injury. He is shown in the postoperative period (B), demonstrating the large improvement that a face transplant can have in a patient in restoring both function and esthetic appearance. (Used with permission of Mayo Foundation for Medical Education and Research, all rights reserved.)

The social support and mental health of the potential recipient is equally as important as the recipient's physical health.[11] It is crucial that a psychiatrist well versed in evaluating and working with transplant patients is a member of the face transplant team. Psychiatric and psychological evaluation of potential recipients is an essential aspect of patient selection and, ultimately, is a major contributor to lifelong success of a procedure and adherence to immunosuppression protocols. This was demonstrated in the second face transplant performed in the world, 2 years after which the patient's nonadherence to immunosuppression led to immune rejection of the transplanted face and the patient's death.[12] As in all transplant surgeries, social support has been demonstrated to be critical to long-term positive outcomes in all composite allotransplant surgeries, and a clinical social worker should also be a vital member of the face transplant team.

Ethical Considerations

Certain groups of patients may require detailed ethical consideration due to their altered risk-benefit ratio, psychosocial condition, and support or their ability to provide a truly informed decision related consent to the procedure. This includes concerns regarding patients with prior malignancies, such as those who seek reconstruction after disfiguring head and neck oncologic resection.[13] The esthetic and functional potential benefits of face transplant to these patients are clear. However, the requirement of lifelong immunosuppression and the increased risk of recurrence and de novo malignancy due to these agents make the choice to proceed with facial transplantation less reasonable. There are conflicting opinions regarding whether traditional cancer remission times accepted in solid organ transplant recipients should also be applied to face transplant recipients. Current research on immune tolerance induction may further alter this risk-benefit ratio as immunosuppressive options are expanded.

Other questions of recipient selection include whether blind patients should be considered for face transplant.[14] Early arguments against blind individuals receiving face transplants largely questioned whether the benefits of the face transplant to a nonseeing individual would still outweigh the risks of immunosuppression and extensive surgical reconstruction. However, successful transplantation of blind patients has demonstrated a large increase in quality of life, particularly due to increased function and the ability to interact in society.[15,16]

Another ethical issue that has arisen in face transplants is that of the permissibility of performing a transplant on a child who does not yet have full autonomy to give informed consent nor the full capacity to perform a risk-benefit analysis of a lifelong commitment to immunosuppression.[17] Bilateral hand transplant was performed in a young child who was already a solid organ transplant recipient. It was argued that there was no increased risk due to immunosuppressive therapy since the

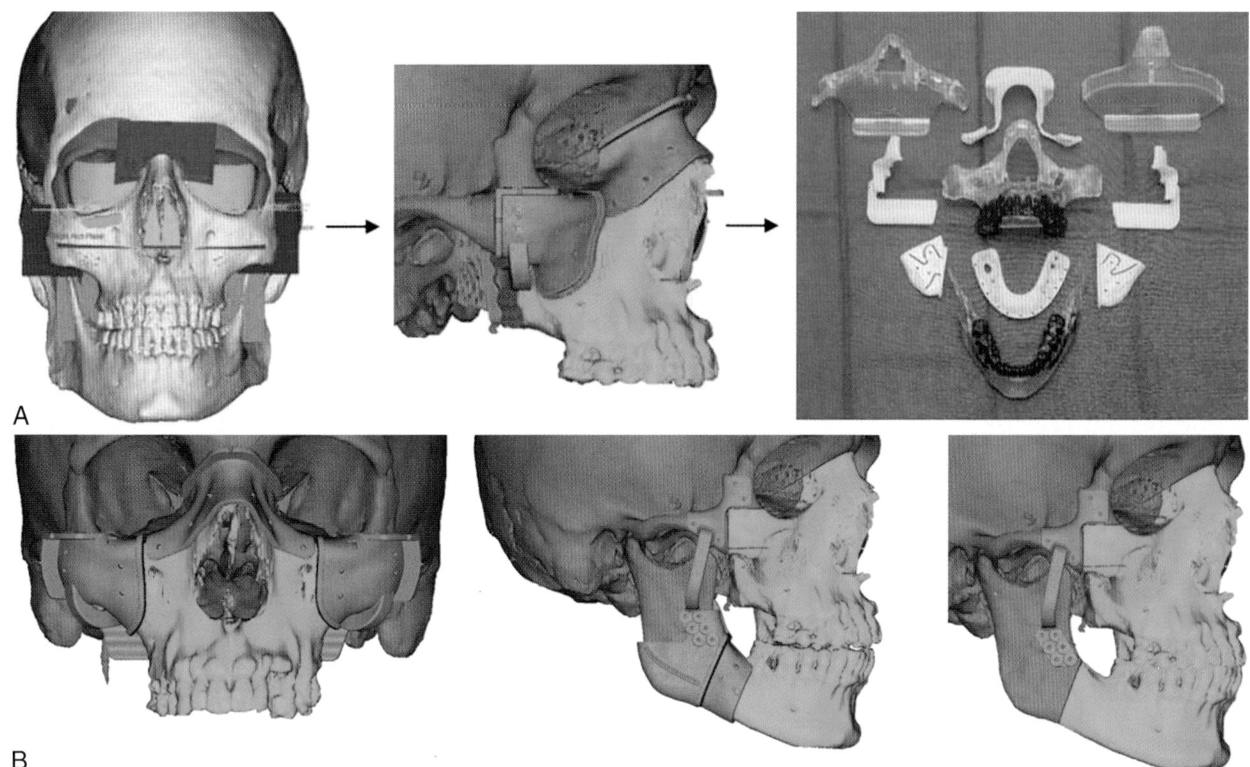

Figure 142.2 **A** and **B**, Preoperative virtual surgical planning demonstrating maxilla, zygoma, and mandible guides. (Used with permission of Mayo Foundation for Medical Education and Research, all rights reserved.)

patient was already committed to such drugs due to a lifesaving transplant. To get a sense of an ethicist view on the topic of face transplant in a child, a survey of clinical ethicists demonstrated that 61% of ethicists agreed or strongly agreed that it is permissible to perform a face transplant on a child.[18]

Another issue unique to face transplant is that of donor suitability. Donor-recipient human leukocyte antigen (HLA) screening is performed to avoid unacceptable antigens if anti-HLA antibodies are present in the recipient, as in solid organ transplant.[19] In addition, the viral serology status of both donor and recipient is identified for common latent infections, including cytomegalovirus and Epstein-Barr virus, which can then be prophylactically managed in the case of donor-recipient mismatch for cytomegalovirus or avoided for Epstein-Barr.[20] Unique to face transplants are donor-recipient esthetic match considerations. A suitable donor should have the same Fitzpatrick skin type if possible and not to exceed one grade difference. Studies have demonstrated that the donor should be within 10 years above and 20 years below the recipient.[21]

TECHNIQUE:

Face transplant surgery is an extremely individualized, highly complex procedure. Extensive preoperative assessment of the recipient's original facial defect, as well as prior reconstructive efforts, is crucial.

VIRTUAL SURGICAL PLANNING/3D GUIDE CREATION

Virtual surgical planning and three-dimensional (3D)-printed osteotomy and positioning guides are critical to obtaining optimal outcomes in face transplant. A high-resolution CT scan is taken of the recipient and donor. Utilizing a computer-aided design and manufacturing (CAD/CAM) environment, 3D reconstructed images are created. Additionally, the head and neck vasculature is assessed through these scans to ensure adequacy and patency of the recipient vessels and to plan the inset. A 3D reconstructed image of the ideal skeleton is created for the recipient. In the virtual planning sessions, the donor skeleton is superimposed on the recipient 3D reconstructions using a chosen anatomical point as reference points for aligning the facial skeletons dependent on the defect (such as the inferior orbital rims). The surgery is planned in the virtual environment, enabling crucial decision making regarding osteotomy placement allowing for more focus, less stress and less waisted time in the operating room. Utilizing this virtual plan, 3D-printed guides are created to guide osteotomies (Fig. 142.2A). In collaboration with 3D Systems, we have developed novel clear "fit guide" to aid in determining bony protuberances that would prevent ideal placement of the donor tissue on the recipient defect. Positioning guides are used to aid in inset of the bone to achieve the plan outlined in the virtual surgical planning session. Close collaboration with biomedical engineers in creation of these 3D guides is crucial.

VASCULATURE

Recipient and donor vessel selection in face transplant is dependent upon the tissues transplanted and the defect to be reconstructed. For most parts of the face, the facial vessels (facial artery and vein) are used for the donor face, as these are sufficient in supplying and draining both the maxilla and mandible[22] and most soft tissue of the face except the occipital scalp and some of the parietal scalp. Alternatively, the external carotid can be used for the donor tissue if the internal maxillary vessels, superficial temporal, or posterior occipital vessels are needed to supply a larger portion of the facial soft tissue or bony skeleton. To include the entire scalp, the posterior auricular or superficial temporal arteries should also be considered. Venous outflow is established via the common facial vein, which is sufficient to drain the face. Theoretically, including the internal maxillary artery would provide better blood supply, although no reports have demonstrated a lack of blood supply to the maxilla supplied only through periosteal blood supply coming from the facial vessels. In our anatomic dissections we found it feasible to dissect the internal maxillary artery to the point where it supplies the maxilla; however, the site of osteotomy often precludes inclusion of the vessel branches.

NERVE RECONSTRUCTION

Face transplant success is highly dependent upon regeneration of the facial nerve, leading to restoration of facial movement and function.[23,24] Coaptation location of the donor and recipient facial nerves is a subject of debate in the field. Some groups coapt the facial trunk proximally, advocating simplifying the neurorrhaphy technique and decreasing operative time. However, to avoid synkinesis, we advocate that nerve branches be coapted close to target muscles to prevent aberrant regeneration and the development of synkinesis. This requires mapping of facial nerve function using an intraoperative nerve stimulator, which we suggest performing while the face is videorecorded so that muscle movement can be analyzed more carefully (Fig. 142.2B). In this manner, careful notation of movement patterns elicited by stimulation of individual nerve branches can be performed, and the ideal nerve branches in donor and recipient can be matched. Neurorrhaphies of sensory nerves of the donor and recipient should also be performed if possible, including of the infraorbital nerve, mental nerve, and supraorbital nerve if the forehead is transplanted. Sensory recovery has been reported among patients for whom sensory nerve coaptation was not performed, most likely from regeneration of nerve fibers originating in the recipient bed and allograft margins.[25] However, coaptation of sensory nerves leads to more predictable reinnervation and protection of donor tissue and thus should be performed whenever possible.

SURGICAL STEPS

STEP 1: Donor Procurement

Our preference is that total intravenous anesthesia rather than inhalational anesthesia is used throughout the donor and recipient surgery until all nerve branches have been identified and stimulated. Planning of incisions in face transplant should be placed in locations that provide the most inconspicuous scarring. The amount of tissue transplanted should factor in the parts of the recipient's face that are missing function and whether the entire structure should be replaced. Each individualized defect requires specific planning. For midfacial defects the incisions are pretragal in the temple and are designed the way a cervicofacial flap is with the rest of the incision in the lower eyelid skin and across the radix of the nose. Corresponding incisions are made in the donor and recipient. Subcutaneous skin flaps are raised past the parotid gland. Then, a high superficial musculoaponeurotic system (SMAS) flap is elevated with a design similar to a high SMAS facelift, enabling identification of the facial nerve branches distal to the parotid gland (site of final nerve anastomosis). Attention is then drawn to the tragus where a plane is dissected down to the tragal pointer where the trunk of the facial nerve is located inferior and posterior to that point. The facial nerve is dissected proximally to the stylomastoid foramen. A superficial parotidectomy along with dissection of the nerve branches from proximal to distal is performed. This enables identification of the facial nerve branches and allows for less bulk in the cheek following inset. The facial nerves are then functionally identified using an intraoperative nerve stimulator and tagged with sutures. The main trunk of the facial nerve is transected as it exists the stylomastoid foramen and reflected anteriorly with the skin flap. Any desired sensory nerves are also identified (infraorbital, supraorbital, supratrochlear, mental) and transected as proximal as possible to provide enough redundancy to be able to perform coaptation with the recipient sensory nerves following bony inset. All necessary soft tissue to restore the recipient defect should be included in the graft. The decision whether to include the masseter with the flap is dependent on whether the recipient's pterygomasseteric sling is intact. Following careful dissection, the osteotomy guides are then placed on the facial bones in the planned locations and secured in place. Osteotomy guides with a metal insert with the exact width of the planned bone saw are used to guide the angle of the planned osteotomy. A sagittal bone saw or piezoelectric saw (DePuy Synthes, Raynham, MA) is preferred for the bony cuts. When upper and lower jaws are included in the transplant, the inner cheek mucosa, hard palate, and some soft palate, along with all the oral mucosa, are included in the donor procurement. The neck vessels are then explored to identify the external carotid, facial artery, superficial temporal, internal maxillary, and occipital vessels. The artery is transected at the takeoff of the external carotid artery. The common facial vein is identified and dissected proximally and included along with a segment of the internal jugular vein. Timing of transection of the vessels is coordinated closely with the recipient's preparation.

TECHNIQUE: Surgical Steps—*cont'd*

STEP 2: Recipient Preparation and Reconstruction

Donors for face transplants will most likely be donors for other solid organs; therefore, close coordination by the organ procurement organization with the solid organ teams is critical. Incisions are planned on the recipient to enable donor procurement to be aborted should the donor become unstable and the solid organ teams need to interrupt facial procurement to begin solid organ procurement. For midfacial reconstructions including upper and lower jaw and overlying soft tissues, the incisions are planned in the nasolabial folds and the skin flaps are dissected from medial to lateral in the subcutaneous plan. This exposure allows for exposure and dissection of the facial nerve branches distal to the parotid gland and identification of the function of each branch through stimulation. In case procurement is aborted due to donor instability, the skin flaps can be repositioned and closed. Of note, identification of facial nerve function in the recipient may be more difficult due to the initial defect, leading to the absence of facial mimetic muscles. The recipient facial nerves should then be transected as distally as possible to maximize donor-recipient nerve overlap and minimize any possible nerve tension at the coaptation site. Next, recipient vessels are also identified in the neck. Depending on the units that are procured with the donor tissue to provide optimal function and esthetics, the donor dissection and resection is performed to accommodate the donor tissue. Beyond the point of nerve exposure and identification and recipient vessel exposure, the rest of the recipient preparation will cause extensive irreversible damage and should be performed only if the donor is stable. Once it is deemed that the donor is stable and solid organ teams can wait to procure their organs, the sites of bone cuts are identified and 3D-printed surgical guides are then affixed at the location of planned bony osteotomies. The osteotomies are performed, and the recipient tissue is then disimpacted and removed to complete creation of the planned recipient defect. Areas of bony prominence on the recipient defect are then assessed and rongeured to correct the contour needed to best fit the donor graft. Our group again utilizes novel clear, 3D-printed fit guides that aid in determining whether there are bony prominences in the recipient defect. The donor segment is also placed against the reciprocal clear fit assessment guide of the planned recipient defect and burred as needed. The donor graft is then brought into the field and bony fixation is performed. On each side of the face, the donor and recipient vessels are approximated, and end-to-end anastomoses are performed using standard microsurgical technique. Following revascularization of the donor tissue, facial nerve branches are matched between donor and recipient utilizing the prior functional assessment of each branch's motor function. Tension-free neurorrhaphies between branches with identical function are performed. Sensory nerve coaptations between the infraorbital, supraorbital, and inferior alveolar nerves of the donor and recipient are performed. Because of the redundancy left from proximal dissection of the donor nerve and distal dissection of the recipient nerve, the sensory nerve coaptation can be performed following bony fixation in the orbit for the infraorbital nerve and below the mandible border for the inferior alveolar nerve.

Finally, all soft tissue is approximated and closed. This includes the intraoral soft tissue, suturing the donor to recipient palate and buccal mucosa. The skin is tailored and closed. The recipient is then placed in mandibulomaxillary fixation with rubber bands.

A sentinel flap can also be transplanted from the donor to recipient to monitor for immune rejection and provide a secondary site for skin biopsies.[26] We suggest procuring a posterior tibial artery free flap from the donor (on the posterior tibial artery and vein), which places the operating surgeon far from the solid organ transplant teams during organ procurement. This flap can then be inset into the groin region of the recipient.

ALTERNATIVE OR MODIFIED TECHNIQUE

Prior to committing to a face transplant, a plan for continued conventional reconstruction is clearly outlined and discussed with the patient. For midfacial defect patients, we outline three phases of reconstruction: (1) upper and lower jaw reconstruction with bone flaps, osteointegrated implants, and prosthesis; (2) nasal reconstruction with a free flap for inner nasal lining, cartilage grafts for structural support, and a forehead flap for outer nasal lining; and (3) lip reconstruction with a gracilis functional flap along with other cheek flaps.

Avoidance and Management of Intraoperative Complications

The ideal means to avoid intraoperative complications in face transplant is to be well versed as an operative team in the steps of the procedure and operative plan. Preoperative rehearsals with full cadaver surgeries are invaluable prior to the procedure to come up with a protocol for the particular patient, to prepare the team, to build confidence, and to familiarize all other team members in addition to the surgeons on the steps of the procedure, including nurses and scrub techs. Engineers are invited to the rehearsals to help develop and refine the cutting and positioning guides.

Blood Transfusion

The extensive nature of face transplant surgeries may lead to high rates of blood loss, with reported volume loss of 0.5 to 12.5 L.[27] Thus, it is important to have blood products readily available for transfusion both intraoperatively as well as postoperatively.

Complications

As in free flap surgery, intraoperative issues come up routinely and postoperative complications need to be dealt with in a timely fashion. Vessel kinking, spasm, or thrombosis can occur intraoperatively. Postoperatively, hematomas, thrombosis, skin loss, and partial or total flap loss can occur.

Postoperative Considerations

Acute Postoperative Concerns

Immediately after face transplant, postoperative concerns mirror those of complex free flap surgeries. These include anesthesia recovery after the extended operative time of these procedures. Adequate arterial inflow and venous outflow into the grafted tissue are essential, and Doppler monitoring is necessary to ensure pedicle vessel patency. Venous congestion is also an important concern. Additionally, as in free flap surgeries, acute postoperative concerns include wound healing complications, infection, and hematomas.

Donor Restoration

One unique postoperative consideration in face transplant is restoration of the donor face following procurement, which is an essential aspect of most face transplant protocols and, in many countries, required by law.[28] Collaboration with skilled anaplastologists is necessary in order to create handmade masks from silicone or resin. Alternatively, 3D printing of a donor mask is also another option.

Immunosuppression Considerations

Unlike in traditional free flap surgeries, additional concerns exist regarding immune suppression and acceptance of the transplanted tissue. Induction therapy is initiated during surgery and is usually a combination of antithymocyte globulin (a T-cell depleting agent) and methylprednisolone.[29] Some centers use alemtuzumab, while a few have used nondepleting induction with basiliximab. Maintenance therapy is usually a triple therapy consisting of a calcineurin inhibitor (commonly tacrolimus), antiproliferative agent (commonly mycophenolate mofetil), and corticosteroids.

Acute cellular rejection can occur, frequently within the first year posttransplant. Antibody-mediated rejections can occur in sensitized recipients due to preformed donor-specific antibodies (DSA) or due to de novo DSA in the setting of reduction in immunosuppression or nonadherence.[30] Almost all face transplant recipients reported in the literature have experienced an episode of acute rejection within a year postsurgery. Cutaneous signs of rejection include erythema, edema, mucosal lesions, and exanthema. Skin biopsies taken during postoperative follow-up are crucial in the evaluation of acute rejection. These biopsies should be read according to the Banff CTA criteria by a trained dermatopathologist, who can attempt to separate common dermatologic conditions.[31] Acute rejection is typically treated with oral or intravenous steroids, T-cell depleting agents, and in some programs, with topical corticosteroids or tacrolimus.

Chronic rejection has been observed in follow-up of face transplant recipients. Chronic rejection leads to fibrosis and excess collagen deposition, leading to changes in both the graft and its vasculature.

Graft versus host disease (GVHD) is also an immunological complication that is of concern in all transplant surgeries, including face transplant, due to its high mortality rate. Reassuringly, GVHD is a rare complication in both solid organ transplant and has not yet been reported in face transplant. In this condition, donor lymphocytes attack recipient tissue.

The required immune suppression increases the risk of certain malignancies and opportunistic infections in face transplant recipients. There are also metabolic complications attributed to some of the agents used. These include post-transplant diabetes, hyperlipidemia, and nephrotoxicity.[32,33]

Since face transplants are nonvital transplants, strategies to decrease the toxicity of immunosuppression protocols as well as induction of tolerance would benefit the wider applicability of these transplants.

Nerve Regeneration Considerations

The success of face transplant is largely dependent on the restoration of spontaneous, symmetric facial movement, smile, and emotional expression. Nerve regeneration into the donor tissue is thus a crucial outcome following face transplant, which is integral to functional recovery. A mask-like appearance is to be expected in face transplant patients for several months until facial nerve regeneration occurs, which is estimated at a speed of 1 mm of nerve regeneration to the distal target daily. Our group's preference is to perform neurorrhaphies of distal facial nerve branches rather than at the facial nerve root to minimize the risk of aberrant regeneration and subsequent synkinesis. It is also crucial to initiate physical, biofeedback-driven facial reanimation therapy and neuromuscular rehabilitation early in the postoperative period, as this can improve facial reanimation outcomes and enable early identification and treatment of synkinesis through mirror feedback and retraining therapy. Recovery of clinically appreciable facial movement has been reported as early as 2 to 3 months, with an average of 6 to 8 months.[34–36] Sensation of thermal stimuli has been reported within 2 weeks of face transplant, with normal pressure sensation at 6 months postoperative.[25] Research regarding the effect of electrical stimulation and immune protocols (particularly the effect of tacrolimus on facial nerve regeneration) has demonstrated promising therapeutic options that may improve face transplant reanimation outcomes in the future.[37]

Dental Considerations

Dental health and rehabilitation are critical to achieve optimal functional and esthetic outcomes.[38] Dental restoration in face transplant recipients is important to overall health and optimization of occlusion. Postoperative occlusion correction can include orthodontic treatment, dental prosthetics, and orthognathic surgery. We also advocate the inclusion of a speech and language pathologist on the face transplant team to guide speech therapy following transplant.

References

1. Siemionow M. The decade of face transplant outcomes. *J Mater Sci Mater Med.* 2017;28(5):64.
2. Lantieri L. Face transplant: a paradigm change in facial reconstruction. *J Craniofac Surg.* 2012;23(1):250–253.
3. Dubernard J-M, Lengelé B, Morelon E, et al. Outcomes 18 months after the first human partial face transplantation. *N Engl J Med.* 2007;357(24):2451–2460.
4. Siemionow MZ, Papay F, Djohan R, et al. First U.S. near-total human face transplantation: a paradigm shift for massive complex injuries. *Plast Reconstr Surg.* 2010;125(1):111–122.
5. Barret JP, Gavaldà J, Bueno J, et al. Full face transplant: the first case report. *Ann Surg.* 2011;254(2):252–256.
6. Pomahac B, Diaz-Siso JR, Bueno EM. Evolution of indications for facial transplantation. *J Plast Reconstr Aesthet Surg.* 2011;64(11):1410–1416.
7. Siemionow M, Ozturk C. An update on facial transplantation cases performed between 2005 and 2010. *Plast Reconstr Surg.* 2011;128(6):707e–720e.
8. Sosin M, Ceradini DJ, Levine JP, et al. Total face, eyelids, ears, scalp, and skeletal subunit transplant: a reconstructive solution for the full face and total scalp burn. *Plast Reconstr Surg.* 2016;138(1):205–219.
9. Krakowczyk Ł., Maciejewski A, Szymczyk C, Oleś K, Półtorak S. Face transplant in an advanced neurofibromatosis type 1 patient. *Ann Transplant.* 2017;22:53–57.
10. Sicilia-Castro D, Gomez-Cia T, Infante-Cossio P, et al. Reconstruction of a severe facial defect by allotransplantation in neurofibromatosis type 1: a case report. *Trans Pro.* 2011 Sep;43(7):2831–2837.
11. Soni CV, Barker JH, Pushpakumar SB, et al. Psychosocial considerations in facial transplantation. *Burns.* 2010;36(7):959–964.
12. Murphy BD, Zuker RM, Borschel GH. Vascularized composite allotransplantation: an update on medical and surgical progress and remaining challenges. *J Plast Reconstr Aesthet Surg.* 2013;66(11):1449–1455.
13. Diaz-Siso JR, Sosin M, Plana NM, Rodriguez ED. Face transplantation: complications, implications, and an update for the oncologic surgeon. *J Surg Oncol.* 2016;113(8):971–975.
14. Bramstedt KA, Plock JA. Looking the world in the face: the benefits and challenges of facial transplantation for blind patients. *Prog Transplant.* 2017;27(1):79–83.
15. Carty MJ, Bueno EM, Lehmann LS, Pomahac B. A position paper in support of face transplantation in the blind. *Plast Reconstr Surg.* 2012;130(2):319–324.
16. Hendrickx H, Blondeel PN, Van Parys H, et al. Facing a new face: an interpretative phenomenological analysis of the experiences of a blind face transplant patient and his partner. *J Craniofac Surg.* 2018;29(4):826–831.
17. Marchac A, Kuschner T, Paris J, Picard A, Vazquez MP, Lantieri L. Ethical issues in pediatric face transplantation: should we perform face transplantation in children. *Plast Reconstr Surg.* 2016;138(2):449–454.
18. Suchyta MA, Sharp R, Amer H, Bradley E, Mardini S. Ethicists' opinions regarding the permissibility of face transplant. *Plast Reconstr Surg.* 2019;144(1):212–224.
19. Siemionow MZ, Gordon CR. Institutional review board-based recommendations for medical institutions pursuing protocol approval for facial transplantation. *Plast Reconstr Surg.* 2010;126(4):1232–1239.
20. Razonable RR, Amer H, Mardini S. Application of a new paradigm for Cytomegalovirus disease prevention in Mayo Clinic's first face transplant. In: Mayo Clinic Proceedings. 2019.
21. Aflaki P, Nelson C, Balas B, Pomahac B. Simulated central face transplantation: age consideration in matching donors and recipients. *J Plast Reconstr Aesthet Surg.* 2010;63(3):e283–e285.
22. Pomahac B, Gobble RM, Schneeberger S. Facial and hand allotransplantation. *Cold Spring Harb Perspect Med.* 2014;4(3):a015651.
23. Arun A, Abt NB, Tuffaha S, Brandacher G, Barone AAL. Nerve regeneration in vascularized composite allotransplantation: current strategies and future directions. *Plast Aesthet Res.* 2015;2:226–235.
24. Suchyta MA, Sabbagh MD, Morsy M, Mardini S, Moran SL. Advances in peripheral nerve regeneration as it relates to VCA. *Vascularized Composite Allotransplant.* 2016;3(1–2):75–88.
25. Siemionow M, Gharb BB, Rampazzo A. Pathways of sensory recovery after face transplantation. *Plast Reconstr Surg.* 2011;127(5):1875–1889.
26. Kueckelhaus M, Fischer S, Lian CG, et al. Utility of sentinel flaps in assessing facial allograft rejection. *Plast Reconstr Surg.* 2015;135(1):250–258.
27. Ricci JA, Pomahac B. Face transplantation. In: Wei F-C, Mardini S, eds. *Flaps and Reconstructive Surgery E-Book.* Elsevier Health Sciences; 2016.
28. Quilichini J, Hivelin M, Benjoar MD, Bosc R, Meningaud JP, Lantieri L. Restoration of the donor after face graft procurement for allotransplantation: report on the technique and outcomes of seven cases. *Plast Reconstr Surg.* 2012;129(5):1105–1111.
29. Siemionow M, Ozturk C. Face transplantation: outcomes, concerns, controversies, and future directions. *J Craniofac Surg.* 2012;23(1):254–259.
30. Haug V, Kollar B, Obed D, et al. The evolving clinical presentation of acute rejection in facial transplantation. *JAMA Facial Plast Surg.* 2019;21(4):278–285.
31. Cendales LC, Kanitakis J, Schneeberger S, et al. The Banff 2007 working classification of skin-containing composite tissue allograft pathology. *Am J Transplant.* 2008;8(7):1396–1400.
32. Lantieri L, Grimbert P, Ortonne N, et al. Face transplant: long-term follow-up and results of a prospective open study. *Lancet.* 2016;388(10052):1398–1407.
33. Lellouch AG, Ng ZY, Kurtz JM, Cetrulo CL. Mixed chimerism-based regimens in VCA. *Curr Transplant Rep.* 2016;3(4):390–394.
34. Aycart MA, Perry B, Alhefzi M, et al. Surgical optimization of motor recovery in face transplantation. *J Craniofac Surg.* 2016;27(2):286–292.
35. Khalifian S, Brazio PS, Mohan R, et al. Facial transplantation: the first 9 years. *Lancet.* 2014;384(9960):2153–2163.
36. Lantieri L, Hivelin M, Audard V, et al. Feasibility, reproducibility, risks and benefits of face transplantation: a prospective study of outcomes. *Am J Transplant.* 2011;11(2):367–378.
37. Saffari TM, Bedar M, Zuidam JM, et al. Exploring the neuroregenerative potential of tacrolimus. *Expert Rev Clin Pharmacol.* 2019;12(11):1047–1057.
38. Brooks JK, Lubek JE. Face transplantation: general review and long-term management of the dental patient. *Quintessence Int.* 2020;51(4):334–342.

CHAPTER 143

Autogenous Auricular Reconstruction

Omotara Sulyman, Tsung-yen Hsieh, and David Hamlar

Armamentarium

#15 Scalpel
Blunt dissectors
Blunt retractors
Cautery—bipolar and monopolar
Doyen rib raspatory
Freer elevator
Penrose or Jackson-Pratt drain
Self-retaining retractors
Xeroform fashioned into a bolster dressing

Introduction

Auricular reconstruction is one of the most complex and intricate surgeries performed by facial plastic surgeons. The ear is a three-dimensional structure and for optimal esthetic outcomes, auricular size, location, orientation, and anatomic landmarks are characteristics that need to be maintained during reconstructive endeavors.[1] Throughout the history of auricular reconstruction, there are two major challenges that have plagued reconstructive surgeons: construction of an appropriate, biologically safe auricular framework, and completely draping the framework with skin.

History of Procedure

The early history of auricular reconstruction was associated with the repair of oncologic and traumatic defects.[2] Through their work, Berghaus and Toplak found that partial auricular reconstructions were performed as early as 600 BC.[3] Celsus, Susruta, the Sicilian Branca family, Italian surgeon Gaspare Tagliacozzi, and the famous Berlin surgeon Dieffenbach were all credited for their early documentation of partial auricular defect reconstructions.[2] However, even as late as the 19th century, reconstruction for the complete replacement of an ear was considered impossible.[2] Until the end of the 19th century, attempts at total auricular reconstruction were frowned upon and famous surgeons, such as Dieffenbach, Nelaton, Ombredanne, Fritze, and Reich, considered total reconstruction of an auricle to be impractical.[2–4]

As documented by Berghaus and Toplak, the early pioneers of total reconstruction of an auricle were Kuhnt, and his assistant, Schanz (1890 in Germany), who used the ipsilateral auricular cartilage rudiment; Randall (1893 in Philadelphia), who used a frame of fresh rabbit cartilage; and Körte (1905 in Berlin), who used a composite graft from the normal ear with the mastoid skin of the affected side and a free skin transplant for the reconstruction.[3] As one can imagine, early attempts were fraught with high complication rates and less-than-ideal esthetic results.

In the early 1930s, a new era in auricular reconstruction was ushered in based on the clinical use of autogenous cartilage reported by Pierce and others.[5] Starting from approximately the mid-20th century, detailed publications on total auricular reconstruction based on the innovative works of Tanzer, Converse, Brent, Nagata, and Weerda began to appear in the literature.[4,6–9]

To date, most ear reconstructive techniques have been derived from the principle that uses a framework placed beneath the skin to create an ear form. Numerous materials have been used to fabricate the ear framework, including allogenous cartilage, xenogenous cartilage, autogenous bone, alloplastic materials, metals, and other synthetic materials. However, autologous cartilage has long been considered the standard material.[2,3] Autologous costal cartilage has been revered for its biocompatibility, durability, and stability over time but is not without shortcomings.

Ear Embryology

Auricular development begins between 21 and 22 days after conception.[6] By day 38 postconception, six mesenchymal hillocks evolve, arranged around the first branchial cleft. Three hillocks are derived from the first (mandibular) and three from the second (hyoid) branchial arches. The first three cranial ventral hillocks of the first branchial arch form the anterior part of the external ear: tragus, helical crus, and helix. The caudal and dorsal three hillocks of the second branchial arch form the posterior part of the ear: antihelix, antitragus, and lobule.[2] The concha and the external auditory canal develop from the first branchial cleft. As the ear develops, it moves from an initially anterocaudal position into a dorsocranial position.[2] The last portion of the pinna to develop is the concha and by week 20 and the auricle is nearly anatomically complete.[10]

Anatomy and Esthetic Units

The external ear includes the pinna and the external auditory canal. The framework of the auricle is formed by elastic cartilage, which has a thickness of 1 to 3 mm.[6,11,12] The overlying anterior skin is about 0.8 to 1.2 mm thick and adherent to the perichondrium without any underlying subcutaneous tissue. In contrast, the posterior auricular skin has a subcutaneous layer of 1.2 to 3 mm and increased mobility over the cartilage.[12]

The blood supply of the auricle is variable and dominated by branches of the superficial temporal and posterior auricular vessel. Cervical nerves (the great auricular nerve—C2, C3) and the lesser occipital nerve (C2) innervate the posterior aspect of the auricle and lobule. These nerves are variable in size and distribution, but the majority of the time, the lesser occipital nerves have been found to innervate the superior ear and the mastoid region. On the other hand, the inferior ear and a portion of the preauricular area are supplied by the great auricular nerve.[13] The anterior surface of the ear and the tragus are supplied by the trigeminal nerve (auriculotemporal nerve V3). The auricular branch of the vagus nerve (Arnold nerve) supplies the external auditory meatus, and the concha is innervated by a branch of the facial nerve.[13]

The length and width of the auricle depend on body stature and age. On average, the auricle reaches 85% of its final length by the age of 6 and 90% by age 9.[2] The width of the auricle reaches 95% of its final width by the age of 6.[2] Auricular projection remains almost constant throughout life. On average, the ear projection is 20.6 ± 4 mm, with a range between 12 and 28 mm.[2] The auricular rim is positioned 10 to 12 mm from the mastoid at the superior helix, 16 to 18 mm from the mastoid at midear, and 20 to 22 mm from the mastoid in the lower third (Fig. 143.1).[13]

Indications for the Procedure

Microtia occurs as a broad and variable range of deformities involving the first and second branchial arches. Adverse events that occur during the sixth through eighth weeks of gestation can lead to the clinical spectrum of microtia.[13] The cause of microtia is thought to be heterogeneous, including genetic anomalies, teratogens, and vascular abnormalities. Large multinational registries of congenital malformations suggest that the prevalence of microtia is from 0.76 to 2.35 per 10,000 births.[14–19] There is a lower incidence of microtia among Whites and Blacks than in Hispanics and Asians. In unilateral cases, the right side appears to be more frequently affected than the left side. Microtia, especially in isolated forms, is more prevalent in males than females.[2]

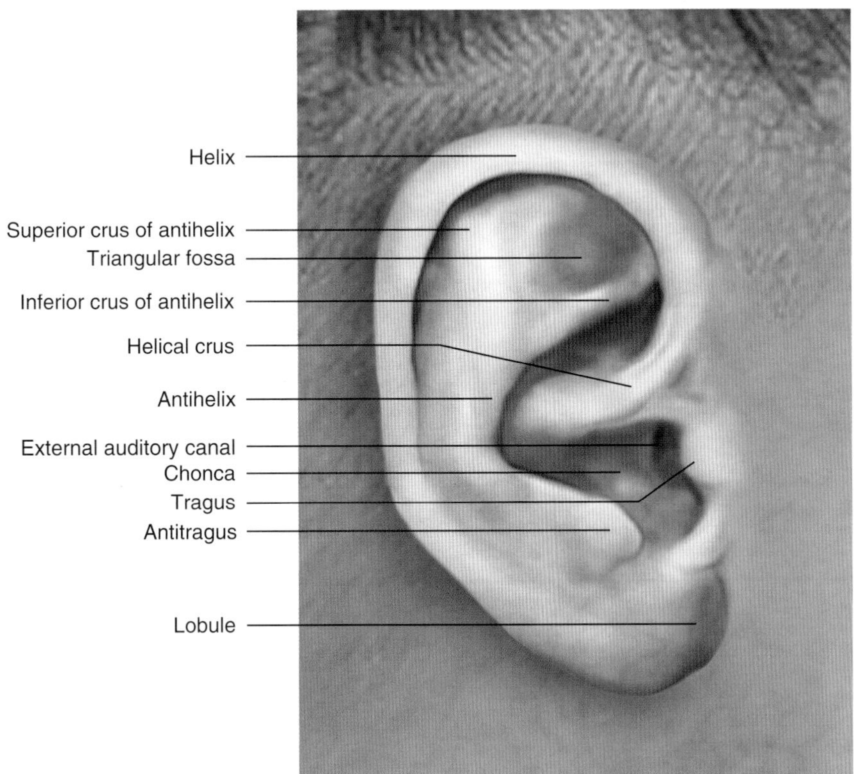

Figure 143.1 Esthetic units of ear.

Microtia is usually classified according to the vestigial structures present. Nagata proposed a classification of this disorder, relevant to the surgical correction of each deformity. He classifies microtia into the lobule type, concha type, and small concha type. Anotia is the most severe of microtia, which represents the complete absence of the external ear.[9,20–22]

Marx and Meurman also graded microtia based on the vestigial remnant.[23,24] In grade I microtia, all of the auricular structures are present but with variable degrees of hypoplasia of the auricle and variable external auditory stenosis. In grade II, there is variable hypoplasia of the concha along with by absence of the external auditory canal. In grade III, the auricle is absent and the lobule has an abnormal shape and position. Grade IV (also called anotia) is the most severe form of microtia, which is characterized by the complete absence of the external ear.[23,24]

Limitations and Contraindications

Initial assessment of patients with microtia should include a thorough physical examination, including the evaluation of the face, facial symmetry, facial animation, ear structure, ear symmetry, and dental occlusal relationships. Physical examination along with family history and genetic counseling or testing will help address any syndromic issues.[2]

The severity of the external deformity appears to correlate with the severity of the temporal bone abnormalities but no association between the severity of the dysmorphic features and the degree of hearing loss has been found.[14] The middle ear deformity may range from minor ossicular chain disruption (the stapes is usually normal) to the complete absence of the tympanic cavity.[25] Sensorineural, conductive, and mixed (sensorineural and conductive) hearing loss may be present in the affected ear, with the most predominant hearing deficit in microtia being conductive hearing loss (80% to 90%).[2,25] Given the risk of otologic issues, complete audiologic evaluation and radiographic study of the temporal bones is critical in all patients with microtia.[2]

The most important factors to consider when determining the most appropriate timing for auricular reconstruction include the age of the patient, external ear maturity, the availability of adequate rib cartilage, and risk of peer ridicule.[26] The ear reaches 95% of its final length and 85% of its final width by age 6.[2] The ear reaches its adult width at about age 10.[27,28] Rib cartilage becomes sufficient at about age 5 to 6 years, which coincides with the beginning of schooling.[8,29] It has been documented that autologous cartilage framework usually grows at a similar rate to the normal ear and sometimes may become slightly larger than the native ear. Based on the above, many surgeons like Brent begin microtia ear reconstruction at around 6 years of age.[8,30] However, some surgeons may delay the surgery until a later age.[13,30] Surgeons like Nagata prefer to begin microtia reconstruction when the patient is 10 years old or older and with a chest circumference of at least 60 cm at the level of the xiphoid process.[31]

Hearing Restoration

Consideration is given to the possibility of hearing restoration if the canal atresia and middle ear ossicular disruption is favorable. Jahrsdoerfer formulated the original criteria for middle ear reconstruction.[32] Based on his findings, attempted canaloplasty and middle ear surgery were considered therapy. There is a myriad of options available today and not indicated for this text.

TECHNIQUE: Surgical Technique

The procedure is performed under general anesthesia in an operating room. The patient should be positioned supine on the operating table. The table should be rotated 180 degrees from the anesthesia machine. The ipsilateral chest wall and entire face are left exposed and sterilely prepped. The following description is based on the technique described by Nagata,[9] with some modifications.

STEP 1: Skin Marking and Auricular Site Preparation

Mark the external ear position with the help of a transparent template using the dimensions of the normal-looking contralateral ear. The distances of the helical root to the orbit and lobule to oral commissure along with the axis of the ear–nasal dorsum serve as landmarks to place the future ear. These landmarks from the normal contralateral side are drawn on the abnormal side and should remain visible during surgery.[33] In craniofacial microsomia due to the asymmetry of the face, these distances cannot always be respected; therefore the surgeon will need to be creative in achieving the best esthetic outcome.[33]

A Z-plasty on the caudal aspect of the rudiment is planned on an individual basis. The goal of the planned incision is to optimally use the skin of the lower rudiment for the reconstruction and prepare the remaining skin for the coverage of the upper two-thirds of the pinna.[2] Attempts should be made to preserve cartilaginous structures of the rudiment and if esthetically favorable, the tragus should be left intact. Other unfavorable cartilaginous rudiment in the area of the pedicle should be removed. The skin flap is then prepared by creating thin subcutaneous flaps.[2] It is critical that the subcutaneous pedicle in the region of the future concha is left intact in order to maintain full vascularization of the skin flap.[2] The surrounding skin is then undermined and mobilized beyond the planned ear position except for the skin of the lower one-third and the skin overlying the mastoid area.[2]

TECHNIQUE: Surgical Technique—*cont'd*

STEP 2: Cartilage Graft Harvesting

The cartilage framework is usually harvested from the synchondrosis of the sixth, seventh, and eighth ribs, and the ninth rib. It was initially thought that the preservation of perichondrium on the surface of the cartilage may help with construct adherence to the recipient site and promote graft viability; however, due to problems with anterior chest wall deformity, many surgeons now recommend leaving at least some remnant of the perichondrium in situ to support cartilage regeneration at the harvest site and decrease chest wall depression.[26,30,34–36]

The ipsilateral anterior chest wall is prepped and draped for harvesting. The skin incision outline for the harvesting of the costal cartilage is determined by placing a mark at the xiphoid process of the sternum and the inferior margin of the rib cage. A 9-cm horizontal line is drawn between the two markings from the medial margin of the rib cage laterally to the seventh rib.[31]

A #15 scalpel is used to incise the skin and subdermal tissue. Using blunt dissection, the muscular fascia of the rectus abdominis muscle and external oblique muscle are exposed. The muscle layers are bluntly dissected until the perichondrium of the sixth to ninth ribs is exposed and the intercostal muscle is visible. Dissection should be gently performed so as not to puncture the intrathoracic cavity. Self-retaining retractors or Army-Navy retractors can be used to expose the surgical site. Using a scalpel, the perichondrium is incised at the center of the cartilage. It is important that the incision is made superficially to maintain an appropriate subperichondrial plane for elevation and to avoid cutting the costal cartilage. A freer elevator is used to undermine the perichondrium from the costal cartilage. Difficulty with undermining may suggest that the elevation is being done in the wrong plane.

The posterior surface of the costal cartilage is then carefully undermined, ensuring that the tip of the elevator remains in contact with the costal cartilage to prevent accidental entry of the intrathoracic cavity. Extreme caution should be taken at this point because entry into the thoracic cavity can lead to pneumothorax. The Doyen rib raspatory is used to elevate the posterior cartilage off the posterior periosteum and to serve as a cutting board to avoid penetration of the intrathoracic cavity. Using a scalpel, an incision is made medial to the costochondral junction. The sixth and seventh costal cartilages are harvested *en bloc* the eighth and ninth costal cartilages are undermined starting from the free edge and then harvested. The costal cartilages are harvested while leaving the perichondrium intact.

After the cartilage has been harvested, a leak test is performed by infiltrating the surgical site with saline. A Valsalva maneuver is then performed to increase the intrathoracic pressure to about 30 cm H_2O. The presence of bubbles at the surgical site will indicate violation of the thoracic wall. If no evidence of a leak, then closure of the surgical site can ensue after the harvested cartilage is successfully fabricated into the auricular framework (Fig. 143.2).

If there are unused pieces of cartilage after the framework fabrication, these pieces are cut into small 2-mm blocks and placed back into the perichondrial pocket.[31] The perichondrium is reapproximated using 4-0 Polydioxanone (PDS, Ethicon) sutures, ensuring that the returned pieces of cartilage remain in the pocket. Before layered closure of the surgical site, Marcaine 0.25% is used for intercostal nerve block to decrease postoperative pain.[33] For older patients, an ON-Q ropivacaine pain pump can be placed in the wound bed to be removed 24 hours postsurgery. A Penrose drain is placed beneath the muscle layer and then the wound is closed in layers. The muscle, muscular fascia, and subdermal layers are sutured with 4-0 Vicryl sutures. The dermis is sutured with 5-0 nylon and a clean gauze dressing is taped over the wound.[31]

STEP 3: Auricular Framework

An auricular framework is constructed from the harvested costal cartilage. The framework should include a base plate, antihelix, tragus–antitragus complex, and helix.[2] A spare piece of cartilage is then stored under the thoracic skin to reconstruct the posterior wall of the concha during the second stage.[33] The base plate is formed from the synchondrotic parts of the seventh and eighth ribs.[2] If needed, it can be thinned to a maximum thickness of 8 mm.[2] Using carving knives, the typical contour of the scapha and triangular fossa are created, as well as the base frame. The antihelix and its crura are carved from the rest of the eighth rib and the tragus–antitragus complex is carved from the rest of the seventh rib cartilage. The helix is carved from the ninth rib cartilage. All components are then combined and held together with sutures (Fig. 143.3).

The auricular framework is inserted into the previously prepared skin pocket and positioned appropriately, utilizing the normal contralateral ear as a reference. Two flat suction drains are placed and help hold the framework in its desired position. The drains are left in for 3 or 4 days.[2] After the implantation and positioning of the auricular framework, excess skin at the upper skin flap is carefully excised. The skin edges are then closed in a tension-free manner. The surgical site is closed with 5-0 Prolene. Bolsters are then sutured over the skin flaps and left in the place for 2 weeks.[37]

Continued

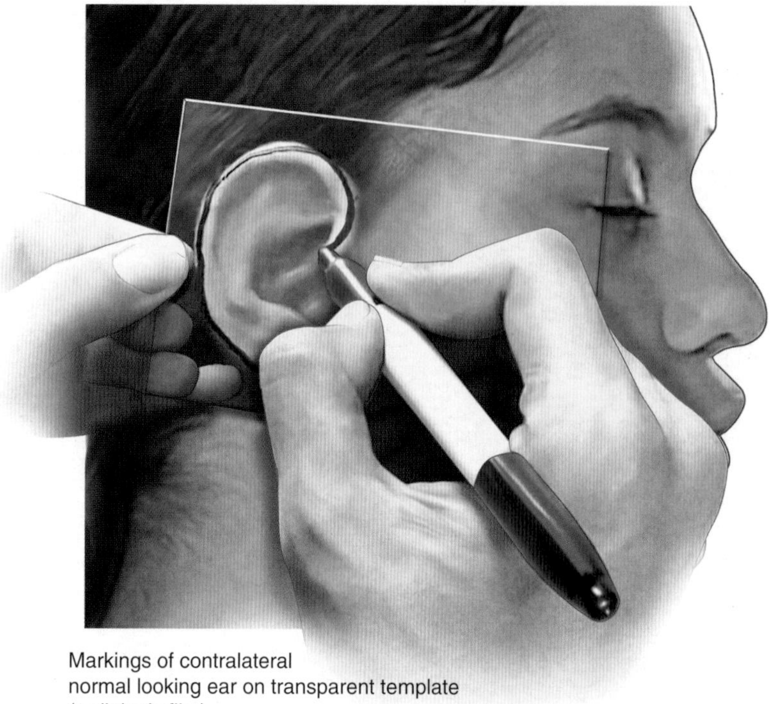

Markings of contralateral
normal looking ear on transparent template
(radiologic film)

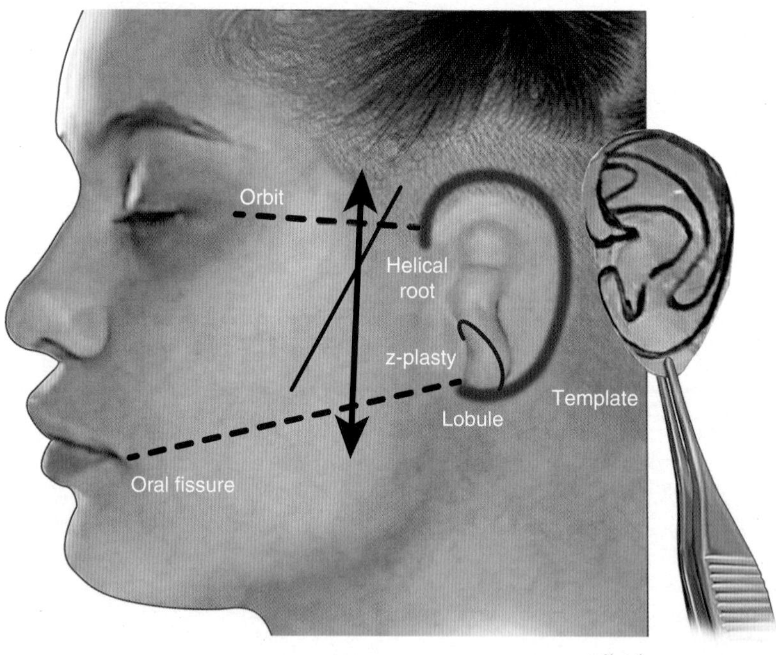

Figure 143.2 Cartilage graft harvesting.

TECHNIQUE: Surgical Technique—*cont'd*

STEP 4: Elevation of the Auricle and Construction of the Retroauricular Sulcus

The retroauricular sulcus is an important esthetic element of the pinna.[2] The creation of the retroauricular sulcus occurs about 6 months after the first operation. A semicircular incision is made approximately 1 cm from the helix of the constructed ear, from the inferior crus to the front of the lobule. The framework is then released from the underlying tissue while preserving the vascularized connective tissue overlying the framework. A fascia layer becomes visible medially. This fascia is a continuation of the temporoparietal fascia (TPF) and superficial musculoaponeurotic system (SMAS). This fascia layer is incised in the direction of the antihelix and released from the deep temporal fascia and the periosteum of the mastoid plane.[2] This provides a well-vascularized flap that would cover the cartilage wedge and revascularize the skin graft that would be used during this operation. From one remaining piece of costal cartilage (sixth rib), which was previously stored in a subcutaneous pocket of the chest wound, a cartilage wedge is carved. The height of the wedge is based on the desired auricular projection. The cartilage wedge is then secured with Vicryl sutures and covered with the previously elevated SMAS flap. The retroauricular wound is then covered with a split-thickness skin graft from the head or a full-thickness skin graft from the abdomen.[2] A bolster is placed over the skin graft and then removed in 1 week (Fig. 143.4).

Continued

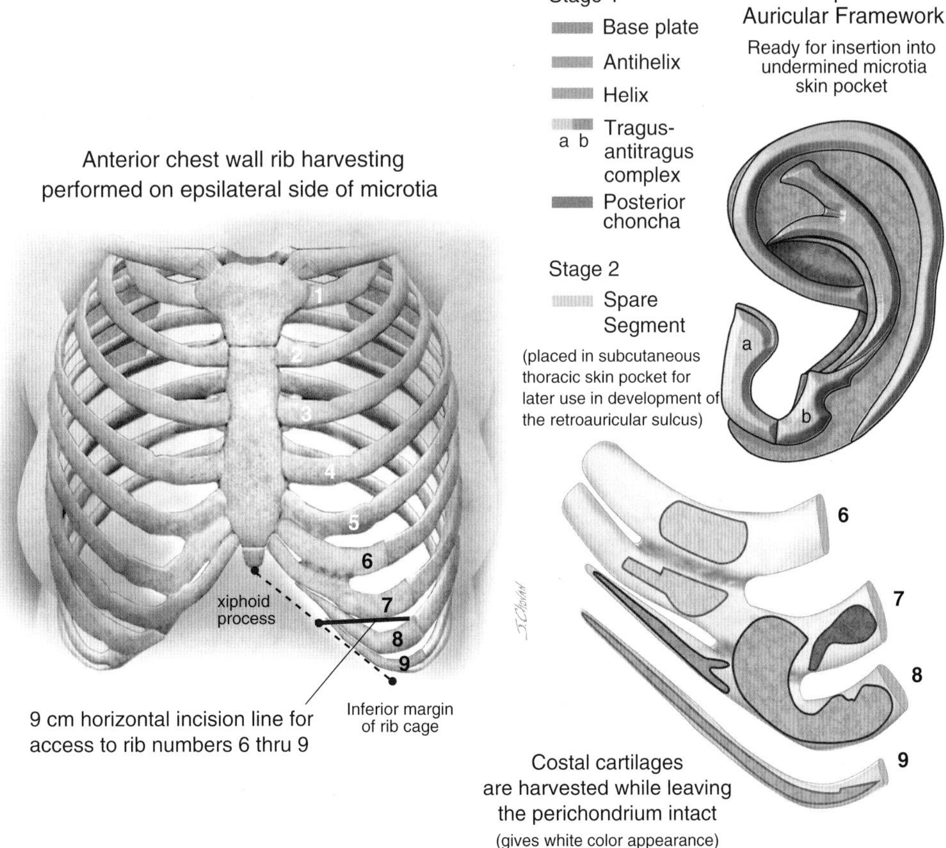

Figure 143.3 Auricular framework.

Stage 2 - Creation of Retroauricular Sulcus

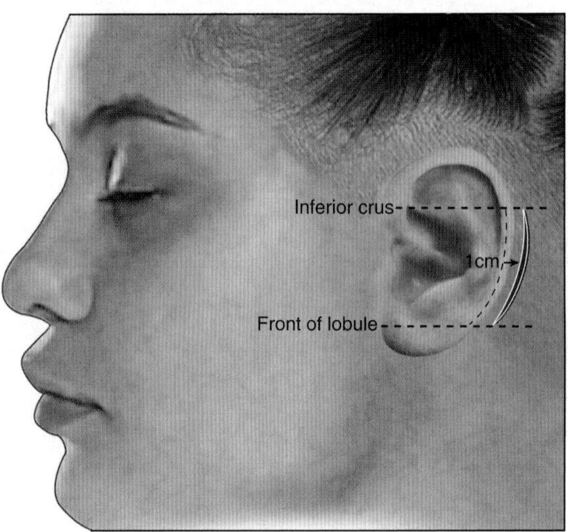

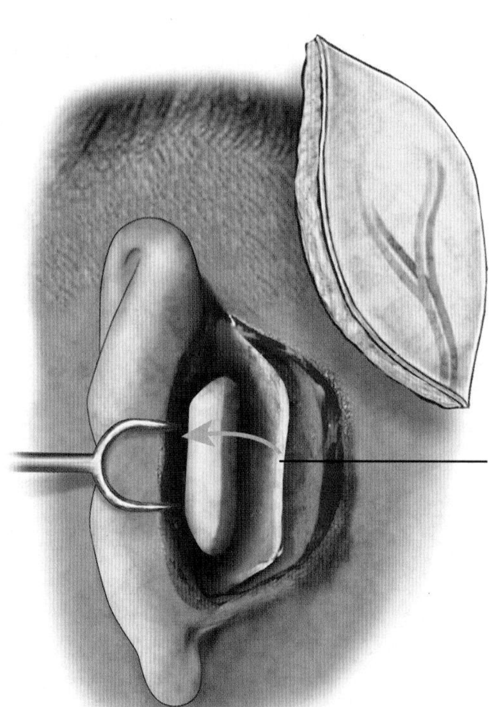

Figure 143.4 Retroauricular sulcus.

Postoperative Considerations and Avoidance of Complications

The complications of this surgery are rarely major. However, even minor complications can progress to the loss of the graft if not addressed appropriately. Some early complications include hematoma formation, skin flap or skin graft necrosis, infection, and pneumothorax. If, as a result of skin flap/skin graft necrosis, the cartilage framework becomes exposed, the patient is placed on antibiotics with *Staphylococcus* and *Pseudomonas* coverage. In addition, the exposed area should be covered with moist dressing. If the area is small with some perichondral covering, the wound may heal secondarily. If there is bare cartilage that is exposed, early coverage of the area with a vascularized local flap or TPF flap with a skin graft may be used to prevent desiccation, devitalization, or infection of the framework. The patient may then need to be on a long-term course of antibiotics to prevent infection of the cartilage and subsequent resorption of the graft. Pneumothorax, while rare, can occur from violation of the pleura during costal cartilage harvest. A leak test should be performed after cartilage harvest and before closure to rule out pneumothorax. In addition, a chest X-ray should be performed postoperatively to ensure pneumothorax has not occurred.

Other minor complications may include scarring and poor esthetic outcome. Minor scar revisions can be addressed surgically but care must be taken not to expose the cartilage framework. Poor esthetic outcomes secondary to malpositioning are usually related to existing asymmetry or poor preoperative planning. Meticulous preoperative evaluation, recognition of preexisting ear or facial asymmetries, and careful surgical planning are crucial in order to ameliorate the risk of poor positioning.

Postoperative Considerations

Autogenous auricular reconstruction is a challenging and humbling procedure. A thorough understanding of the embryology and anatomy is crucial. Proper training, comprehensive preoperative evaluation, and meticulous surgical planning are essential for a successful reconstruction. Each patient, each ear deformity is unique and challenges the surgeon to continually strive for improved esthetic and functional outcomes. The management of these patients can be an incredibly rewarding experience.

References

1. Wang T. Auricular reconstruction. In: Papel I, Frodek J, Holt R, et al., eds. *Facial Plastic and Reconstructive Surgery*. 4th ed. Thieme Publishers; 2016:708–717.
2. Siegert R, Magritz R. Congenital auricular deformities. In: Papel I, Frodel J, Holt R, et al., eds. *Facial Plastic and Reconstructive Surgery*. 4th ed. Thieme Publishers; 2016:861–874.
3. Berghaus A, Toplak F. Surgical concepts for reconstruction of the auricle: history and current state of the art. *Arch Otolaryngol Neck Surg*. 1986.
4. Converse JM. Reconstruction of the auricle–part 1. *Plast Reconstr Surg*. 1958.
5. Pierce GW, Klabunde EH, Bergeron VL. Useful procedures in plastic surgery. *Plast Reconstr Surg*. 1947.
6. Weerda H. *Chirurgie Der Ohrmuschel. Verletzungen, Defekte, Anomalien*. Thieme; 2004.
7. Tanzer RC. Total reconstruction of the external ear. *Plast Reconstr Surg*. 1959.
8. Brent B. Ear reconstruction with an expansile framework of autogenous rib cartilage. *Plast Reconstr Surg*. 1974.
9. Nagata S. A new method of total reconstruction of the auricle for microtia. *Plast Reconstr Surg*. 1993.
10. Karmody CS, Annino DJ. Embryology and anomalies of the external ear. *Facial Plast Surg*. 1995.
11. Danter J, Siegert R, Weerda H. Ultrasonographische Haut- und Knorpeldickenmessungen an gesunden und rekonstruierten Ohren mit einem 20-MHz-Ultra-schallgerät [Ultrasound measurement of skin and cartilage thickness in healthy and reconstructed ears with a 20-MHz ultrasound device]. *Laryngorhinootologie*. 1996;75(2):91–94.
12. Siegert R, Krappen S, Kaesemann L, Weerda H. Computer-assisted anthropometry of the auricle. *Face*. 1998;6:1–6.
13. Beahm EK, Walton RL. Auricular reconstruction for microtia: part I. Anatomy, embryology, and clinical evaluation. *Plast Reconstr Surg*. 2002.
14. Llano-Rivas I, Ariadna, Del Castillo V, Reyes R, Carnevale A. Microtia: a clinical and genetic study at the National Institute of Pediatrics in Mexico City. *Arch Med Res*. 1999.
15. Figueroa AA, Friede H. Craniovertebral malformations in hemifacial microsomia. *J Craniofac Genet Dev Biol*. 1985.
16. Bennun RD, Mulliken JB, Kaban LB, Murray JE. Microtia: a microform of hemifacial microsomia. *Plast Reconstr Surg*. 1985.
17. Rahbar R, Robson CD, Mulliken JB, et al. Craniofacial, temporal bone, and audiologic abnormalities in the spectrum of hemifacial microsomia. *Arch Otolaryngol Head Neck Surg*. 2001. https://doi.org/10.1001/archotol.127.3.265.
18. Shibazaki-Yorozuya R, Nagata S. Preferential associated malformation in patients with anotia and microtia. *J Craniofac Surg*. 2019.
19. Rogers BO. Microtic, lop, cup and protruding ears: four directly inheritable deformities? *Plast Reconstr Surg*. 1968.
20. Nagata S. Modification of the stages in total reconstruction of the auricle: part III. Grafting the three-dimensional costal cartilage framework for small concha-type microtia. *Plast Reconstr Surg*. 1994.
21. Nagata S. Modification of the stages in total reconstruction of the auricle: part I. Grafting the three-dimensional costal cartilage framework for lobule-type microtia. *Plast Reconstr Surg*. 1994.
22. Nagata S. Modification of the stages in total reconstruction of the auricle: part IV. Ear elevation for the constructed auricle. *Plast Reconstr Surg*. 1994.
23. Marx H. Die Mißbildungen des Ohres. In: *Die Krankheiten Des Gehörorgans*.; 1926.
24. Meurman Y. Congenital microtia and meatal atresia: observations and aspects of treatment. *AMA Arch Otolaryngol*. 1957.
25. Yeakley JW, Jahrsdoerfer RA. CT evaluation of congenital aural atresia: what the radiologist and surgeon need to know. *J Comput Assist Tomogr*. 1996.

26. Tanzer RC. Total reconstruction of the auricle: the evolution of a plan of treatment. *Plast Reconstr Surg*. 1971.
27. Adamson JE, Hortox CE, Crawford HH. The growth pattern of the external ear. *Plast Reconstr Surg*. 1965.
28. Farkas LG. Anthropometry of normal and anomalous ears. *Clin Plast Surg*. 1978.
29. Nagata S. Modification of the stages in total reconstruction of the auricle: part II. Grafting the three-dimensional costal cartilage framework for concha-type microtia. *Plast Reconstr Surg*. 1994.
30. Brent B. Technical advances in ear reconstruction with autogenous rib cartilage grafts: personal experience with 1200 cases. *Plast Reconstr Surg*. 1999.
31. Kawanabe Y, Nagata S. A new method of costal cartilage harvest for total auricular reconstruction: part I. Avoidance and prevention of intraoperative and postoperative complications and problems. *Plast Reconstr Surg*. 2006.
32. Jahrsdoerfer RA, Yeakley JW, Aguilar EA, Cole RRGL. Grading system for selection of aural atresia. *Am J Otol (NY)*. 1992;13(1):6–12. https://doi.org/10.1016/j.fsc.2017.09.005.
33. Firmin F, Marchac A. A novel algorithm for autologous ear reconstruction. *Semin Plast Surg*. 2011.
34. Tanzer RC. Microtia—a long-term follow-up of 44 reconstructed auricles. *Plast Reconstr Surg*. 1978.
35. Ohara K, Nakamura K, Ohta E. Chest wall deformities and thoracic scoliosis after costal cartilage graft harvesting. *Plast Reconstr Surg*. 1997.
36. Kirkham HLD. The use of preserved cartilage in ear reconstruction. *Ann Surg*. 1940.
37. Nagata S. Total auricular reconstruction with a three-dimensional costal cartilage framework. *Ann Chir Plast Esthet*. 1995.

CHAPTER 144

TMJ Arthrocentesis

Gary F. Bouloux

Armamentarium

60-cc syringe
22-gauge 1.5-inch hypodermic needle (2)
Iodine swab (2)
Intravenous tubing (12 inch)
Lactated Ringer's solution
Local anesthetic such as 2% lidocaine with 1:100,000 epinephrine (dental cartridge) with 27-gauge hypodermic needle
Small round adhesive bandage (2)

History of the Procedure

Arthrocentesis of the temporomandibular joint (TMJ) was developed in the late 1980s following some initial success with the use of intraarticular pumping of the superior joint space as well as arthroscopic lysis and lavage.[1,2] The procedure has been shown to improve pain and range of motion in patients with arthralgia, internal derangement, closed lock and inflammatory arthropathy.[3–13] Arthrocentesis of the TMJ is typically performed in the superior joint space using 60 to 200 cc of lactated Ringer's (LR) solution as an irrigant. A volume of 60 cc is sufficient to remove more than 95% of inflammatory mediators.[14,15] It is also sufficient to distend the joint, potentially resulting in the disruption of immature adhesions and/or a "stuck" disk. Performing arthrocentesis or injection within the inferior joint space, in addition to the superior joint space, has been reported, but it is difficult to perform and the supporting evidence is weak.[16]

The use of adjunct medication following arthrocentesis remains controversial. Various medications have been used, including corticosteroids, hyaluronic acid, morphine and most recently platelet concentrates. The latter consists of platelet-rich plasma, platelet-rich fibrin, and platelet-rich growth factors. Comparing the efficacy of these medications is challenging, given the heterogeneity between studies. Although some studies report additional benefit from the use of adjunct medication, the majority of well-controlled randomized clinical trials, systematic reviews, and meta-analyses suggest that arthrocentesis alone is sufficient to reduce pain and improve range of motion.[5,6,17–20]

The pain reduction following superior joint space arthrocentesis varies considerably between studies. This is likely the result of heterogeneity in the diagnosis and procedures between studies. A pain reduction of 33% to 86% has reported following arthrocentesis with a mean pain reduction of 47%.[5,12,21–32] Several factors are thought to adversely influence the efficacy of the procedure, including more severe baseline pain, advanced osteoarthritis (Wilkes stage IV and V) and maladaptive psychosocial comorbid diagnoses.

The increase in maximum incisal opening following arthrocentesis also varies between studies, with a mean increase of 13%.[6,12,16,29–32] Patient-reported outcome measures following arthrocentesis have infrequently been used, although improvement in the Jaw Function Limitation Scale has been reported.[6]

Indications

As with all surgical procedures for the management of TMJ pain, it remains critical to identify an intraarticular source prior to performing a surgical procedure. However, orofacial pain may have multiple causes, and it is important to consider a broad differential diagnosis in all patients. The most robust and validated approach to correctly identifying temporomandibular dysfunction (TMD), including intraarticular pathology, is with the use of the diagnostic criteria for temporomandibular disorders (DC/TMD).[33] The DC/TMD guides a structured history taking and physical examination that facilitates the formation of an axis I and II diagnoses. Axis I diagnoses include pain-related temporomandibular disorders such as myalgia, local myalgia, myofascial pain, myofascial pain with referral, arthralgia and headache attributed to TMD. Axis I also includes intraarticular temporomandibular disorders such as disk displacement with reduction, disk displacement with reduction and intermittent locking, disk displacement without reduction with limited opening, disk displacement without reduction without limited opening, degenerative joint disease and subluxation. The axis I intraarticular diagnoses are all appropriate candidates for arthrocentesis. Although not included in the DC/TMD axis I diagnoses, stuck disk phenomenon, inflammatory arthropathy, metabolic disease (gout and pseudogout), and suppurative arthritis are also appropriate diagnoses for arthrocentesis. The use of the DC/TMD guidelines will enable many of the listed diagnoses to be made with a high sensitivity and specificity. This remains a key element in making the correct diagnosis and therefore selecting a treatment that is appropriate to the diagnosis. Patients who also have non intraarticular TMJ sources of pain may still be candidates for arthrocentesis as long as the other sources of pain are actively being treated. In addition, patients with multiple pain sources should have realistic expectations for the outcome following arthrocentesis in the setting of other pain sources.

Contraindications and Limitations

Arthrocentesis requires a joint space in which to place needles and irrigate. It should not be performed in patients with bony or fibrous ankylosis, suspected malignant TMJ pathology, or a known middle cranial fossa perforation. The presence of any skin infection overlying the proposed injection sites is also a contraindication to the procedure. Although arthrocentesis has been shown to significantly reduce pain, its efficacy for improving range of motion is more limited. When pain reduction and a modest increase in range of motion are desired, arthroscopy remains a better choice for most patients.

TECHNIQUE

Arthrocentesis can be performed under local anesthesia either with or without deep sedation/general anesthesia. The consent should include the potential for temporary weakness of the facial nerve. There are many technical variations for performing the procedure but all revolve around the same basic steps. The use of the Holmlund-Hellsing (HH) line has traditionally been advocated to identify the posterior and anterior needle puncture sites. A line is drawn from the lateral canthus of the eye to the mid-tragus. The posterior puncture site is located 10 mm anterior to the posterior edge of the tragus and 2 mm inferior to the HH line. The anterior puncture site is an additional 10 mm anteriorly along the HH line and 10 mm inferior. These puncture sites correspond to the posterior recess and apex of the articular eminence but are much more suited for arthroscopy. A relatively simple technique for double puncture arthroscopy includes the following steps:

1. Place a disposable surgical head cap on the patient to hold the hair out of the surgical field. The additional use of surgical tape to secure the edge of the cap to the skin at a level near the pinna of the ear is very helpful (Fig. 144.1).

2. Use the nail of the index finger to identify the lip of the glenoid fossa and posterior slope of the articular eminence by pressing moderately firmly against the skin. Mark the outline carefully with a skin marker ensuring accuracy (Fig. 144.2).

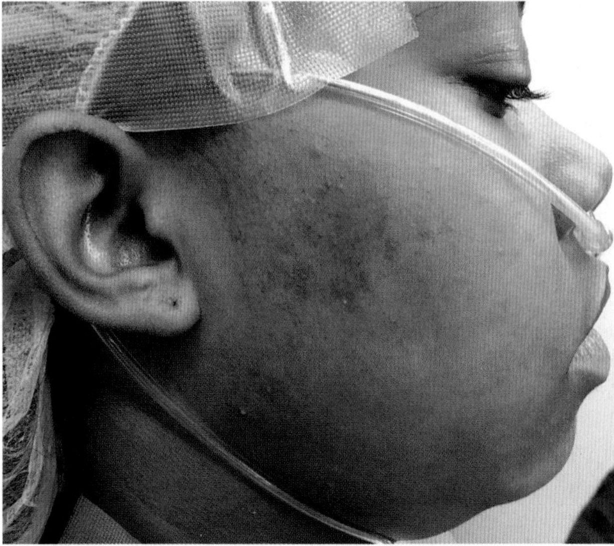

Figure 144.1 The surgical head cap is secured to the patient's head with surgical tape.

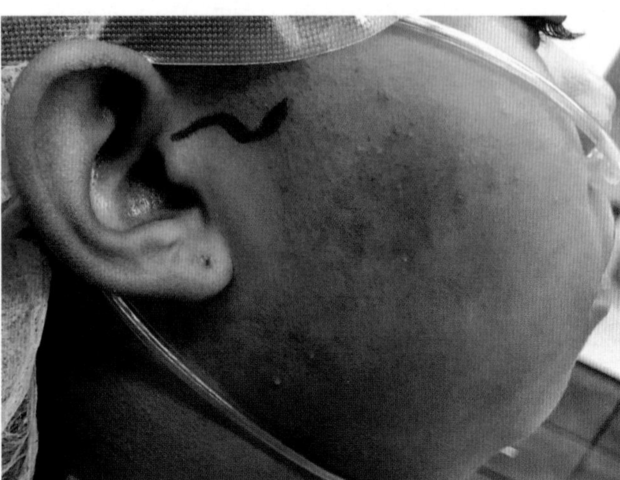

Figure 144.2 Mark the lip of the glenoid fossa and posterior slope of the articular eminence with a skin marker.

TECHNIQUE—*cont'd*

3. Place a mark at the junction of the midpoint of the tragus and outlined lip of the glenoid fossa. This is the initial puncture site for the posterior needle.

4. Paint the skin with iodine (Fig. 144.3).

5. Place the tip of the local anesthetic needle over the posterior puncture site. Angle the needle approximately 15 degrees anteriorly and superiorly. Gently puncture the skin and begin to inject 2% lidocaine with 1:100,000 epinephrine (1 dental cartridge) immediately under the skin to form a weal. Allow the anesthetic to diffuse, and then gently advance the needle while depositing local anesthesia. Resistance will be felt when the joint capsule is encountered. Gently puncture the capsule and advance the needle gently until the glenoid fossa roof is encountered. Be gentle to avoid scuffing the fossa. A 1.5-inch needle should be at a minimal depth of approximately 3/4 to 1 inch to ensure correct positioning. The remaining half of the dental cartridge should be injected into the superior joint space before removing the needle (Fig. 144.4).

6. If the local anesthetic needle encounters bone too prematurely based on the depth of the needle, the most likely cause is an excessive superior angle striking the lip of the glenoid fossa or an excessive inferior angle striking the lateral pole of the condyle. Adjust the needle accordingly.

7. Wait several minutes to allow adequate anesthesia.

8. Insert a 22-gauge needle using the same puncture site and trajectory that was used for the local anesthesia. This needle has a larger diameter but should also pass through the capsule and gently strike the roof of the glenoid fossa (Figs. 144.5 and 144.6).

Continued

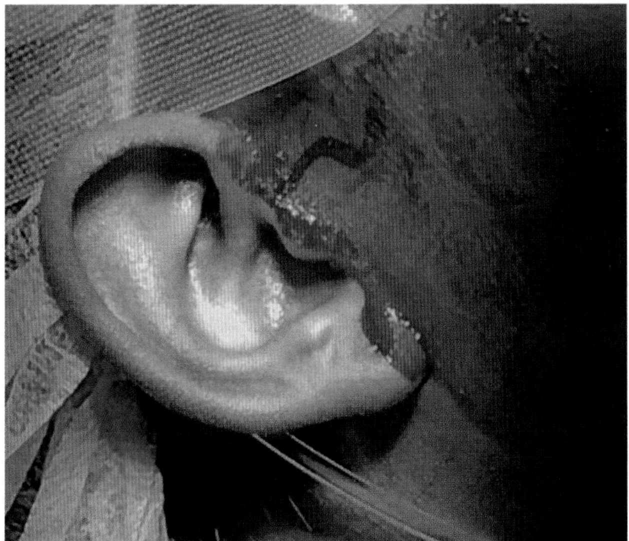

Figure 144.3 The patient's skin is painted with iodine.

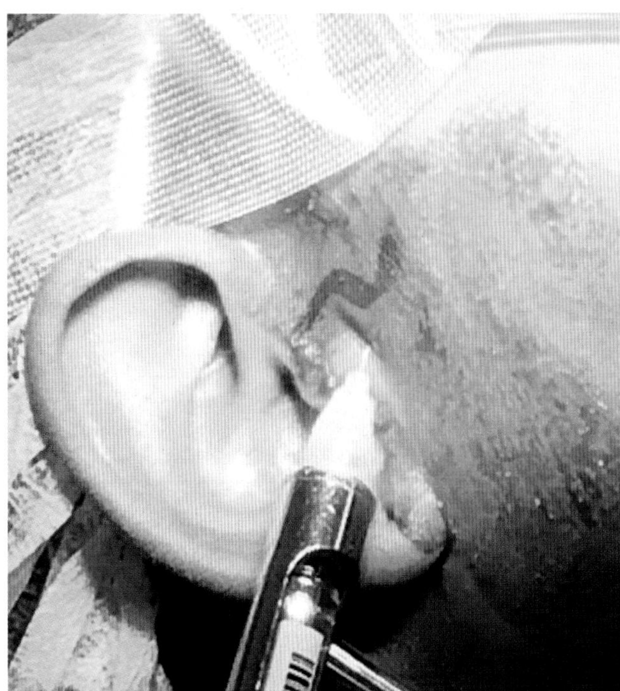

Figure 144.4 Inject the local anesthetic.

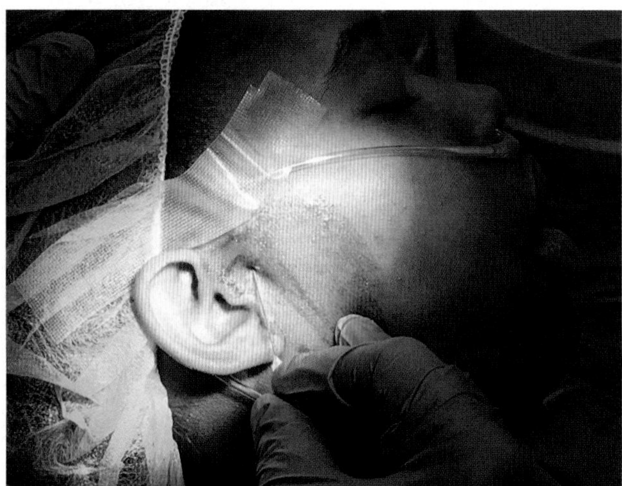

Figure 144.5 The 22-gauge needle is inserted in the same puncture site and trajectory that was used for the local anesthesia.

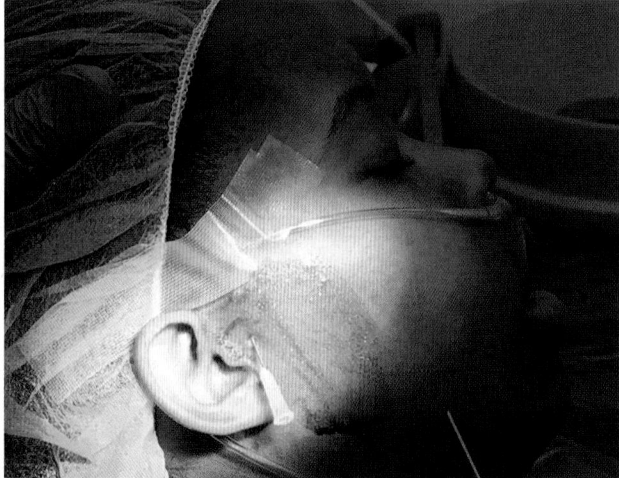

Figure 144.6 The 22-gauge needle has a larger diameter but should also pass through the capsule.

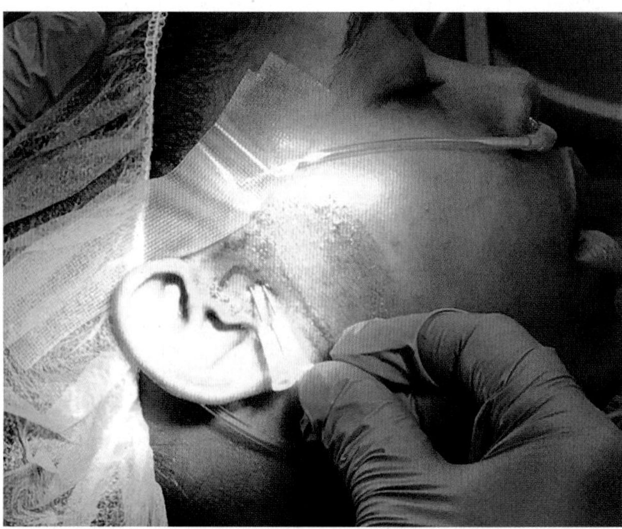

Figure 144.7 A second 22-gauge needle is inserted 3 to 4 mm anterior to the posterior needle (keeping parallel to the first needle at all times).

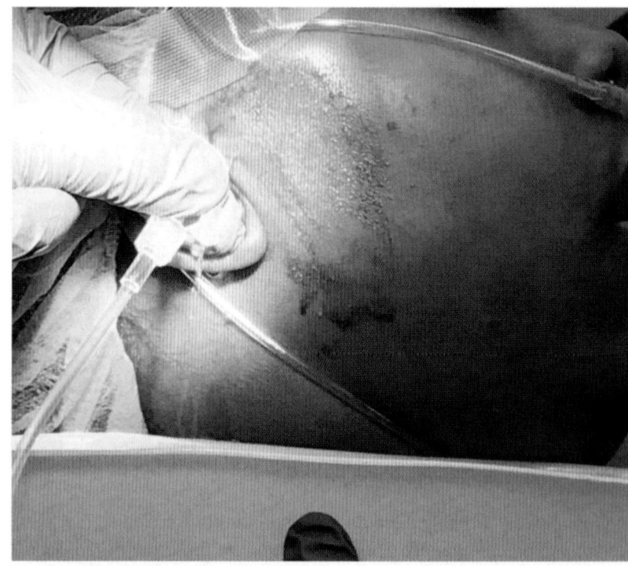

Figure 144.8 Irrigate the full 60 cc of lactated Ringer's (LR) solution while ensuring the outflow from the other needle.

TECHNIQUE—*cont'd*

9. Take a second 22-gauge needle and insert it 3 to 4 mm anterior to the posterior needle, being sure to keep the needle parallel to the first needle at all times. The needle will also encounter resistance as it passes through the capsule before gently striking the roof of the glenoid fossa (Fig. 144.7).

10. Take a 60-cc syringe/12-inch tubing filled with LR solution and connect it to the hub of the one needle. Hold the hub firmly to prevent undue movement which can scuff the fossa.

11. Irrigate the full 60 cc of LR while ensuring the outflow from the other needle. If irrigation is difficult, take a moment to advance both needles to ensure they are resting on bone. Additionally, gently rotate one needle at a time to ensure the bevel is not pressed against intraarticular tissue. It is sometimes helpful to move the irrigating tubing between needles if irrigation is difficult (Figs. 144.8 and 144.9).

TECHNIQUE—*cont'd*

12. Irrigation should be with intermittent pressure to ensure a variation in intraarticular pressure which can disrupt a stuck disk and immature fibrous adhesions.

13. Manipulate the jaw to obtain maximum incisal opening and translation toward the end of the procedure prior to the last 10 cc of irrigation.

14. If unable to irrigate the majority of the 60 cc despite adjusting needles and manipulating the jaw, remove the anterior needle and instill 0.5 cc of corticosteroid through the posterior needle before removing.

15. Manipulate the jaw again to ensure maximal mouth opening and joint translation.

16. Place a small adhesive bandage over the puncture sites.

17. Ensure patients receive a written program of jaw exercises to be performed several times per day over several weeks.

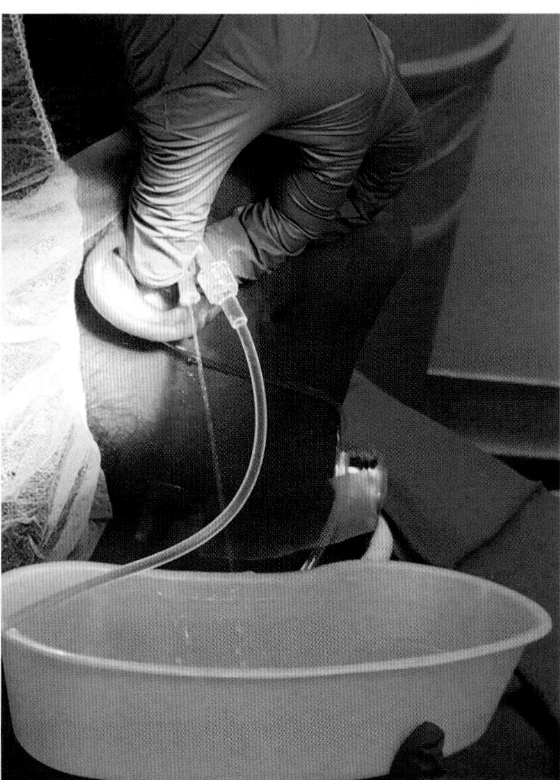

Figure 144.9 If irrigation is difficult, gently rotate one needle at a time to ensure the bevel is not pressed against intraarticular tissue.

Avoidance and Management of Intraoperative Complications

Arthrocentesis is a relatively simple procedure. Intraoperative complications can be avoided if attention to detail is maintained during the procedure. Identify landmarks accurately, particularly the lip of the glenoid fossa, postglenoid tubercle, and articular eminence. Use a soft and gentle touch when inserting needles so that the capsular resistance to needle penetration is appreciated. Use a soft and gentle touch when the roof of the glenoid fossa is sounded to avoid iatrogenic scuffing or perforation of the middle cranial fossa.

Ensure that the irrigation fluid is exiting the outflow needle at all times to prevent extravasation within the soft tissues or capsular rupture. Reposition and rotate the bevel of the needles as needed to ensure good flow. The use of a handheld syringe for irrigation and the tactile feel of the pressure needed to obtain flow is the most ideal technique to prevent barotrauma. The use of insufflation bags for irrigation is discouraged as they often result in soft tissue swelling when the outflow is obstructed for even short periods of time.

On occasion, it is difficult or impossible to obtain outflow despite multiple attempts to reposition or rotate needles. This may be the result of chondromalacia, fibrosis, degenerative joint disease, or stuck disk. The inability to lavage the joint will prevent the elution of inflammatory mediators or degraded proteins. In these situations, it is best to simply inject 0.5 to 1 cc of a corticosteroid within the joint. The use of coricosteroid should also be coinsidered when performing arthrocentesis in patients with known inflammatory arthropathy (e.g., rheumatoid arthritis, etc.).

On occasion, insertion of the needle through the soft tissue results in the outflow of blood that can be brisk. This suggests that the needle is within the lumen of a blood vessel, most likely the superficial temporal artery or vein. It is recommended that the needle be immediatley removed and not advanced through the capsule to avoid the introduction of blood within the superior joint space which can result in fibrosis. Bleeding may occur at the skin puncture site, which can be easily managed with digital pressure. Once bleeding has stopped, reinsert a new needle in a different location to avoid the blood vessels.

Postoperative Considerations

Pain following arthrocentesis is generally very mild and responds to several days of over-the-counter nonsteroidal antiinflammatory drugs (NSAIDs). Prescription NSAIDs and opioids are not required.

Postoperative exercises are crucial following any TMJ procedure including arthrocentesis. They are important to prevent disk adhesion and promote synchronous movement of the condyle and disk. Exercises should begin the same day as the procedure. The four basic movements include maximal opening without deviation, protrusion without deviation, and left/right lateral excursions. Each of the 4 movements require 10 repetitions. The exercises should be performed hourly at least 10 times per day.

Dietary modification is typically unnecessary, although patients may feel less discomfort with a softer diet.

References

1. Murakami KI, Iizuka T, Matsuki M, Ono T. Recapturing the persistent anteriorly displaced disk by mandibular manipulation after pumping and hydraulic pressure to the upper joint cavity of the temporomandibular joint. *Cranio*. 1987;5(1):17–24.
2. Nitzan DW, Dolwick MF, Heft MW. Arthroscopic lavage and lysis of the temporomandibular joint: a change in perspective. *J Oral Maxillofac Surg*. 1990;48(8):798–801.
3. Al-Belasy FA, Dolwick MF. Arthrocentesis for the treatment of temporomandibular joint closed lock: a review article. *Int J Oral Maxillofac Surg*. 2007;36(9):773–782.
4. Alpaslan C, Dolwick MF, Heft MW. Five-year retrospective evaluation of temporomandibular joint arthrocentesis. *Int J Oral Maxillofac Surg*. 2003;32(3):263–267.
5. Bouloux GF, Chou J, Krishnan D, et al. Is hyaluronic acid or corticosteroid superior to lactated ringer solution in the short-term reduction of temporomandibular joint pain after arthrocentesis? Part 1. *J Oral Maxillofac Surg*. 2017;75(1):52–62.
6. Bouloux GF, Chou J, Krishnan D, et al. Is hyaluronic acid or corticosteroid superior to lactated ringer solution in the short term for improving function and quality of life after arthrocentesis? Part 2. *J Oral Maxillofac Surg*. 2017;75(1):63–72.
7. Brennan PA, Ilankovan V. Arthrocentesis for temporomandibular joint pain dysfunction syndrome. *J Oral Maxillofac Surg*. 2006;64(6):949–951.
8. Carvajal WA, Laskin DM. Long-term evaluation of arthrocentesis for the treatment of internal derangements of the temporomandibular joint. *J Oral Maxillofac Surg*. 2000;58(8):852–855.
9. Emshoff R. Clinical factors affecting the outcome of arthrocentesis and hydraulic distension of the temporomandibular joint. *Oral Surg Oral Med Oral Pathol Oral Radiol Endod*. 2005;100(4):409–414.
10. Emshoff R, Rudisch A. Determining predictor variables for treatment outcomes of arthrocentesis and hydraulic distention of the temporomandibular joint. *J Oral Maxillofac Surg*. 2004;62(7):816–823.
11. Emshoff R, Rudisch A, Bösch R, Strobl H. Prognostic indicators of the outcome of arthrocentesis: a short-term follow-up study. *Oral Surg Oral Med Oral Pathol Oral Radiol Endod*. 2003;96(1):12–18.
12. Onder ME, Tüz HH, Koçyiğit D, Kişnişci RS. Long-term results of arthrocentesis in degenerative temporomandibular disorders. *Oral Surg Oral Med Oral Pathol Oral Radiol Endod*. 2009;107(1):e1–e5.
13. Spallaccia F, Rivaroli A, Cascone P. Temporomandibular joint arthrocentesis: long-term results. *Bull Group Int Rech Sci Stomatol Odontol*. 2000;42(1):31–37.
14. Emshoff R, Puffer P, Strobl H, Gassner R. Effect of temporomandibular joint arthrocentesis on synovial fluid mediator level of tumor necrosis factor-alpha: implications for treatment outcome. *Int J Oral Maxillofac Surg*. 2000;29(3):176–182.
15. Kaneyama K, Segami N, Nishimura M, Sato J, Fujimura K, Yoshimura H. The ideal lavage volume for removing bradykinin, interleukin-6, and protein from the temporomandibular joint by arthrocentesis. *J Oral Maxillofac Surg*. 2004;62(6):657–661.
16. Long X, Chen G, Cheng AH, et al. A randomized controlled trial of superior and inferior temporomandibular joint space injection with hyaluronic acid in treatment of anterior disc displacement without reduction. *J Oral Maxillofac Surg*. 2009;67(2):357–361.
17. Davoudi A, Khaki H, Mohammadi I, et al. Is arthrocentesis of temporomandibular joint with corticosteroids beneficial? A systematic review. *Med Oral Patol Oral Cir Bucal*. 2018;23(3):e367–e375.
18. Bergstrand S, Ingstad HK, Møystad A, Bjørnland T. Long-term effectiveness of arthrocentesis with and without hyaluronic acid injection for treatment of temporomandibular joint osteoarthritis. *J Oral Sci*. 2019;61(1):82–88.
19. Cömert Kiliç S, Güngörmüş M, Sümbüllü MA. Is arthrocentesis plus platelet-rich plasma superior to arthrocentesis alone in the treatment of temporomandibular joint osteoarthritis? A randomized clinical trial. *J Oral Maxillofac Surg*. 2015;73(8):1473–1483.
20. Zotti F, Albanese M, Rodella LF, Nocini PF. Platelet-rich plasma in treatment of temporomandibular joint dysfunctions: narrative review. *Int J Mol Sci*. 2019;20(2):20.
21. Manfredini D, Rancitelli D, Ferronato G, Guarda-Nardini L. Arthrocentesis with or without additional drugs in temporomandibular joint inflammatory-degenerative disease: comparison of six treatment protocols. *J Oral Rehabil*. 2012;39(4):245–251.
22. Giraddi GB, Siddaraju A, Kumar A, Jain T. Comparison between Betamethasone and sodium hyaluronate combination with Betamethasone alone after arthrocentesis in the treatment of internal derangement of TMJ-using single puncture technique: a preliminary study. *J Maxillofac Oral Surg*. 2015;14(2):403–409.
23. Giraddi GB, Siddaraju A, Kumar B, Singh C. Internal derangement of temporomandibular joint: an evaluation of effect of corticosteroid injection compared with injection of sodium hyaluronate after arthrocentesis. *J Maxillofac Oral Surg*. 2012;11(3):258–263.
24. Tabrizi R, Karagah T, Arabion H, Soleimanpour MR, Soleimanpour M. Outcomes of arthrocentesis for the treatment of internal derangement pain: with or without corticosteroids? *J Craniofac Surg*. 2014;25(6):e571–e575.
25. Malik AH, Shah AA. Efficacy of temporomandibular joint arthrocentesis on mouth opening and pain in the treatment of internal derangement of TMJ-A clinical study. *J Maxillofac Oral Surg*. 2014;13(3):244–248.
26. Monje-Gil F, Nitzan D, González-Garcia R. Temporomandibular joint arthrocentesis. Review of the literature. *Med Oral Patol Oral Cir Bucal*. 2012;17(4):e575–e581.
27. Vos LM, Huddleston Slater JJ, Stegenga B. Arthrocentesis as initial treatment for temporomandibular joint arthropathy: a randomized controlled trial. *J Craniomaxillofac Surg*. 2014;42(5):e134–e139.
28. Nitzan DW, Samson B, Better H. Long-term outcome of arthrocentesis for sudden-onset, persistent, severe closed lock of the temporomandibular joint. *J Oral Maxillofac Surg*. 1997;55(2):151–157.

29. Basterzi Y, Sari A, Demirkan F, Unal S, Arslan E. Intraarticular hyaluronic acid injection for the treatment of reducing and nonreducing disc displacement of the temporomandibular joint. *Ann Plast Surg*. 2009;62(3):265–267.
30. Manfredini D, Bonnini S, Arboretti R, Guarda-Nardini L. Temporomandibular joint osteoarthritis: an open label trial of 76 patients treated with arthrocentesis plus hyaluronic acid injections. *Int J Oral Maxillofac Implants*. 2009;38(8):827–834.
31. Guarda-Nardini L, Masiero S, Marioni G. Conservative treatment of temporomandibular joint osteoarthrosis: intra-articular injection of sodium hyaluronate. *J Oral Rehabil*. 2005;32(10):729–734.
32. Guarda-Nardini L, Stifano M, Brombin C, Salmaso L, Manfredini D. A one-year case series of arthrocentesis with hyaluronic acid injections for temporomandibular joint osteoarthritis. *Oral Surg Oral Med Oral Pathol Oral Radiol Endod*. 2007;103(6):e14–e22.
33. Schiffman E, Ohrbach R, Truelove E, et al. International RDC/TMD Consortium Network, International association for Dental Research; Orofacial Pain Special Interest Group, International Association for the Study of Pain; Diagnostic Criteria for Temporomandibular Disorders (DC/TMD) for clinical and research applications: recommendations of the International RDC/TMD Consortium Network and orofacial pain special interest group. *J Oral Facial Pain Headache*. 2014;28(1):6–27.

CHAPTER 145

Temporomandibular Joint Arthroscopy

Joseph P. McCain, Reem H. Hossameldin, and Christopher A. Fanelli

Armamentarium

Basic Armamentarium
1.9-mm TMJ arthroscope, 30-degree angle
Arthroscopy tower: light source, HD camera, monitors
Two similar 2-mm scored cannulas
Sharp trocar
Blunt obturator
Straight probe
French #3 myringotomy suction tip
IV Line, stop cock
Lactated Ringer/1:300,000 epinephrine irrigation fluid
Lavage needle, 22 gauge × 1.5 inch
Local anesthetic with vasoconstrictor
Appropriate sutures

Advanced Armamentarium
Basic armamentarium plus the following:
2.4-mm suction punch
Biopsy forceps and needles
Meniscus mender set, with appropriate suture/wire, button
Other hand instruments: bone rasps and bone curettes
Radiofrequency coblation micro debridement
Holmium YAG laser
Monopolar and bipolar electrocautery probes
Motorized instruments: full radius shaver

History of the Procedure

The first report of diagnostic arthroscopy of the temporomandibular joint (TMJ) was given by Ohnishi,[1] who utilized the no. 24 arthroscope first developed by Watanabe.[2] The puncture technique was further refined by Holmlund and Hellsing, who identified puncture sites that correlated with the tragal-lateral canthus line.[3–7] This was supported by Johnson who further reported on the diagnostic arthroscopy of the joint,[8] and Murakami who described a safe and effective method for joint puncture as well as normal anatomy and histology.[9–12] A succinct summary and appropriate nomenclature were subsequently published by Murakami and Hoshino.[10] The results of the first TMJ arthroscopy in the US were presented and published by McCain in 1985.[13] The initial report detailed his experience with puncture techniques, irrigation systems, diagnostic observations, and complications. Shortly thereafter, Sanders published articles describing the therapeutic benefits of arthroscopy in patients with acute painful hypomobility of the joint.[14,15] McCain followed with an article describing normal anatomy, a refined technique for joint arthroscopy, the appearance of joint pathology, and the complications associated with the procedure.[16]

Diagnostic and operative arthroscopy of the TMJ provides a minimally invasive procedure that can facilitate diagnosis, reduce pain, and improve jaw function. The majority of the literature supporting arthroscopy are case series and cohort studies, all with some degree of confounding and bias.[17] It is generally accepted that in patients with pain and limited function due to TMJ internal derangement, natural progression without nonsurgical or surgical intervention usually results in resolution of symptoms in 67% to 75% of patients.[18] Arthrocentesis, arthroscopy, and open surgical techniques have all been shown to produce varying degrees of reduction in signs and symptoms in 80% to 90% of patients.[19] Long-term follow-up following diagnostic and surgical arthroscopy in multiple studies has shown the efficacy and safety of the procedure.[20–23]

When comparing outcomes following arthroscopy with outcomes following arthrocentesis and open surgical techniques, arthroscopy has been shown to be superior.[24,25] Comparison between arthroscopy and arthrocentesis also shows an improved reduction of pain with variable rates among different studies ranging from 38% to 67% with a mean of 55.7%, with increased range of motion ranging from 22% to 58% with mean of 41.08%, and comparable complication rates.[26,27] The long-term benefit of arthroscopy over arthrocentesis and open procedures is clear when managing patients with internal derangement, particularly those with Wilkes stage I, II, and III disease.[28–30]

The success rate of diagnostic arthroscopy in relation to Wilkes classification was reported to be 70.5% for Wilkes stage II, 64.0% for Wilkes stage III, 70.0% for Wilkes stage IV, and 63.5% for Wilkes stage V.[31] In addition, a study shows that performing operative arthroscopic discopexy in 42 joints resulted in a 69% success rate: 86.7% for the Wilkes II and III group versus 25% for the Wilkes IV and V group.[32] Factors that may adversely affect the outcome of TMJ arthroscopy include the lack of required surgical skills that allow for iatrogenic complications, improper selection criteria in relation to the performed surgical technique, number of surgeries performed on the same patient, and lack of postoperative rehabilitation. Given the ability of arthroscopy to facilitate visualization and ultimately diagnosis, it remains a robust workhorse in the diagnosis and management of intraarticular pathology.[33–36]

Indications for the Use of the Procedure

Arthroscopic surgery is well suited to the patient with intraarticular pain and dysfunction. Reducing joint inflammation, chondromalacia, synovitis, and eliminating fibrous adhesions, pseudowalls, and synovial plica are all possible with arthroscopy and often result in long-term benefits.[32]

As with all procedures that are considered, the correct diagnosis is critical. A thorough history and clinical examination with the required diagnostic aids that follow the Diagnostic Criteria for Temporomandibular Disorders with both axes I and II diagnoses remains paramount.[37] Diagnostic arthroscopy should be considered in patients who present with unexplained persistent joint pain that is unresponsive to medical forms of therapy. This is particularly beneficial when there is also an absence of positive findings on imaging studies. Finally, it is also useful for the biopsy of suspected lesions or diseases.

Operative arthroscopy has distinct indications. It provides an opportunity to manage synovitis, which is often present within the TMJ in patients with inflammatory arthropathy, including rheumatoid arthritis and juvenile idiopathic arthritis.[38] Operative arthroscopy also allows for treatment of various stages of internal derangements as classified according to Wilkes criteria.[39] In either situation, arthroscopy is used to wash out and remove the inflammatory mediators, degraded proteins, or any mechanical barrier to reduce pain and improve maximal incisal opening. Hypomobility secondary to intra-joint adhesions can be effectively managed during operative arthroscopy by releasing adhesions. Operative TMJ arthroscopy is also used for patients with degenerative joint disease and for the management of hypermobility resulting in painful subluxation or dislocation. Hypermobility and TMJ dislocation are common and are generally treated with conservative therapy. In some patients, they can become a chronic recurrent condition. Recurrent temporomandibular joint dislocation (RTD) can significantly decrease the patient's quality of life and require some form of surgical intervention for correction. The incidence has been described as acute, chronic, recurrent, and longstanding.[40] Operative TMJ arthroscopy presents a minimally invasive alternative treatment for RTD.[41]

Limitations and Contraindications

Arthroscopy, although a versatile procedure, does have some limitations in its application. Patients with bony ankylosis of the TMJ require an open procedure for management. Other circumstances that may prevent the use of TMJ arthroscopy include patients with significant overlying skin infections and situations in which the surgeon is concerned that tumor seeding may occur from surgical instrumentation. Like all surgical procedures, the surgeon must consider the medical circumstances unique to each patient. The effective and safe use of arthroscopy also requires significant operator skill and experience.

TECHNIQUE 1: Basic TMJ Arthroscopy (Single-Puncture Arthroscopy)

STEP 1: Patient Preparation

Primary arthroscopy is performed under local anesthesia, local anesthesia and intravenous sedation, or monitored anesthesia care (MAC). The patient is brought to the operating suite, placed in the dorsal supine position, and brought to the proper anesthesia plane for MAC. Examination under anesthesia should be performed to confirm or modify the preoperative diagnosis. The patient's head should be turned to the contralateral side to ensure the operative field is horizontal. The hair is placed in a bouffant cap and secured by silk tape. After digital localization of the greatest concavity of the glenoid fossa, the preauricular skin is prepped with Betadine and draped in the usual manner for TMJ arthroscopy, and an ear wick is placed for protection (Fig. 145.1A).

STEP 2: Local Anesthesia

After standard landmarks have been marked, local anesthesia is deposited using 2% lidocaine with 1:100,000 epinephrine using a 30-gauge needle in the preauricular area (Fig. 145.1B).

STEP 3: Insufflation

The superior joint space is then insufflated via an inferior and lateral approach utilizing a 30-gauge needle and insufflated with 2.5 cc of the local anesthesia to ensure good plunger rebound (Fig. 145.1C).

Continued

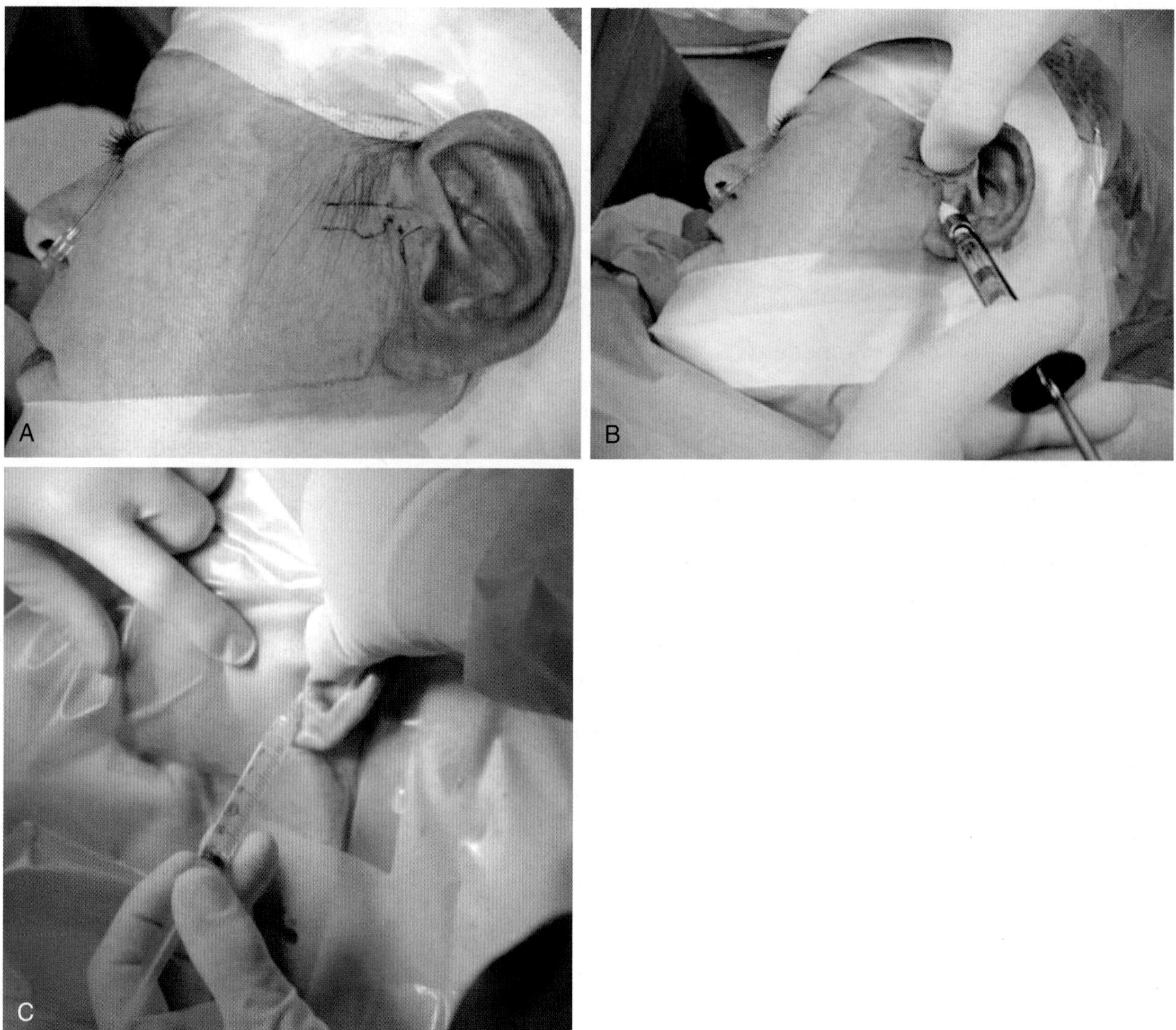

Figure 145.1 **A,** Patient preparation and draping. **B,** Instillation of local anesthesia. **C,** Insufflation of superior joint space.

TECHNIQUE 1: Basic TMJ Arthroscopy (Single-Puncture Arthroscopy)—*cont'd*

STEP 4: Fossa Portal Puncture

The first puncture is always placed at the maximum concavity of the glenoid fossa while the mandible is in protruded position. Hold the cannula/trocar in the dominant hand and grip the cannula with an index finger, controlling the tip and the base of the cannula in the palm of the hand. Experienced TMJ arthroscopists may hold the trocar and puncture with the nondominant hand. Using the trocar, penetrate the skin at the fossa puncture site with a slow rotational motion. The fossa puncture should be made deliberately and carefully in an attempt to pass one time through the lateral capsule and into the joint space to avoid extravasation problems. Advance the trocar until contact is felt with the lip of the glenoid fossa. Always sound this bony landmark; never pass the instrument straight through the capsule without locating the bone. Allow the trocar to feel the junction of the lateral lip of the glenoid fossa and the superior aspect of the capsule. Advance the cannula completely into the joint space. At this point, the cannula should be inserted approximately 20 to 25 mm as measured from the skin to the center of the joint, which is known as the safety zone. Then remove the trocar and attach the scope (Fig. 145.1D).

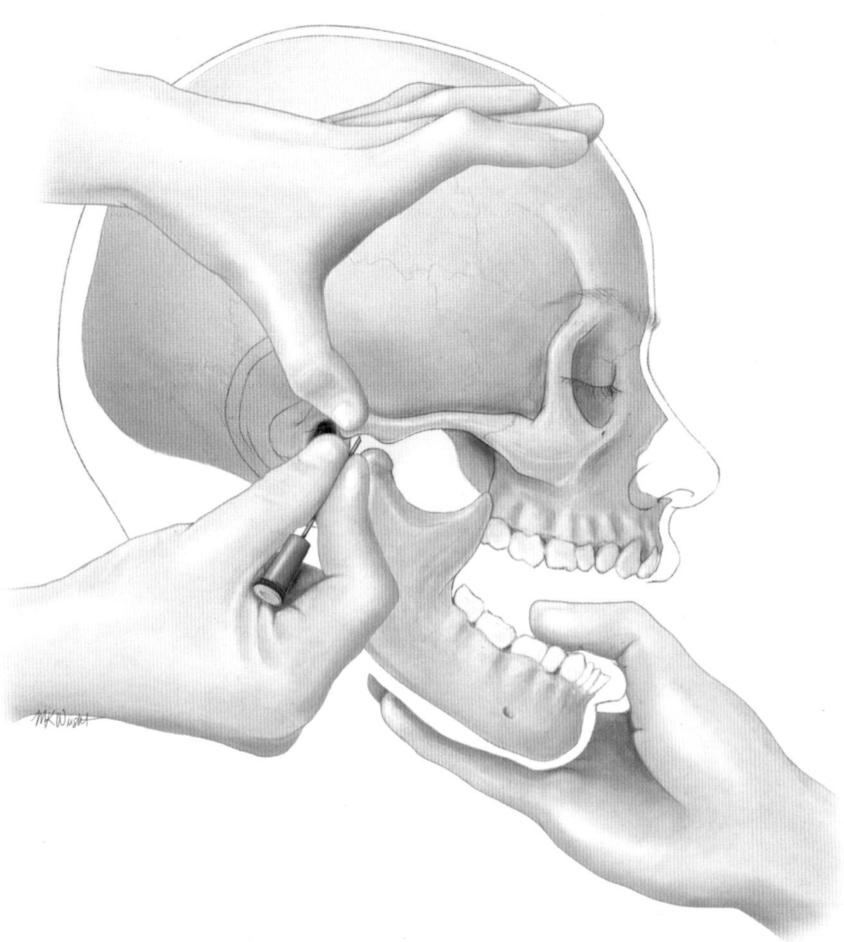

D

Figure 145.1, cont'd **D,** Fossa portal puncture.

TECHNIQUE: Basic TMJ Arthroscopy (Single-Puncture Arthroscopy)—*cont'd*

STEP 5: Insertion of Outflow Needle

With the mandible maintained in a protrusive position, instruct the surgical assistant to insufflate the joint with approximately 2 to 3 mL of fluid using the direct irrigation syringe and to maintain pressure on the plunger to retain distention of the joint. Then insert a 22-gauge, 1.5-inch needle approximately 5 mm anterior and 5 mm inferior to the fossa puncture site while observing the flow of irrigation fluid through the needle consisting of lactated Ringer's solution with 1:300,000 epinephrine (Fig. 145.1E).

STEP 6: First Level of Treatment

The first level of treatment begins with an arthroscopic arthrocentesis, which is done with a minimum of 120 cc of irrigation fluid with turbulent flow in order to remove inflammatory substrates as well as lysis of any small adhesions present.

This is followed by the diagnostic sweep that provides an accurate diagnosis of normal and pathologic states in the superior joint space by describing the seven points of interest as well as joint motion (Fig. 145.1F).

Continued

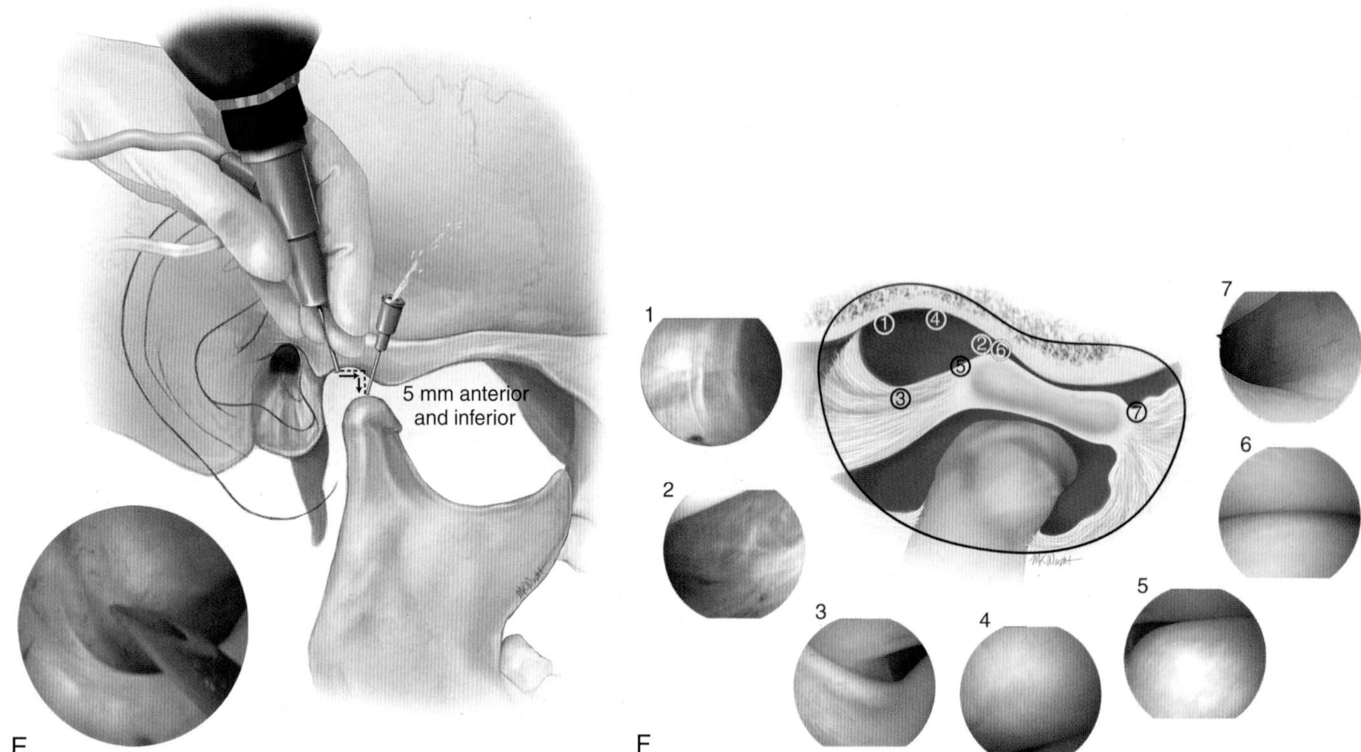

Figure 145.1, cont'd **E,** Insertion of outflow needle. **F,** Diagnostic sweep.

TECHNIQUE: Basic TMJ Arthroscopy (Single-Puncture Arthroscopy)—*cont'd*

STEP 7: Second Level of Treatment

The second level of treatment involves the instillation of intraarticular medications, as indicated in certain cases, including the following:

- Injection of sclerosing agents into the retrodiskal tissue crease in cases of dislocated disks, using the lavage needle
- Injection of steroid agents into a severely inflamed retrodiskal tissue (Fig. 145.1G)
- Intraarticular injection of hyaluronic acid acting as an adhesive bandage for microbleeders and synovial fluid replenishing agent as well as lubricant
- Intraarticular injection of regenerative medicine agents (platelet-rich plasma, stem cells, etc.)

STEP 8: Closure

Once the procedure is complete, all instruments are removed while maintaining direct pressure over the puncture sites, and then the patient's head is elevated slightly to aid in hemostasis. The fossa puncture site is closed using single suture of 6-0 nylon and then covered with bacitracin ointment and a spot adhesive bandage. Finally, the ear wick is removed.

STEP 9: Jaw Manipulation

With the patient's head facing upwards, the surgeon manipulates and stretches the mandible, and the range of motion is recorded afterward.

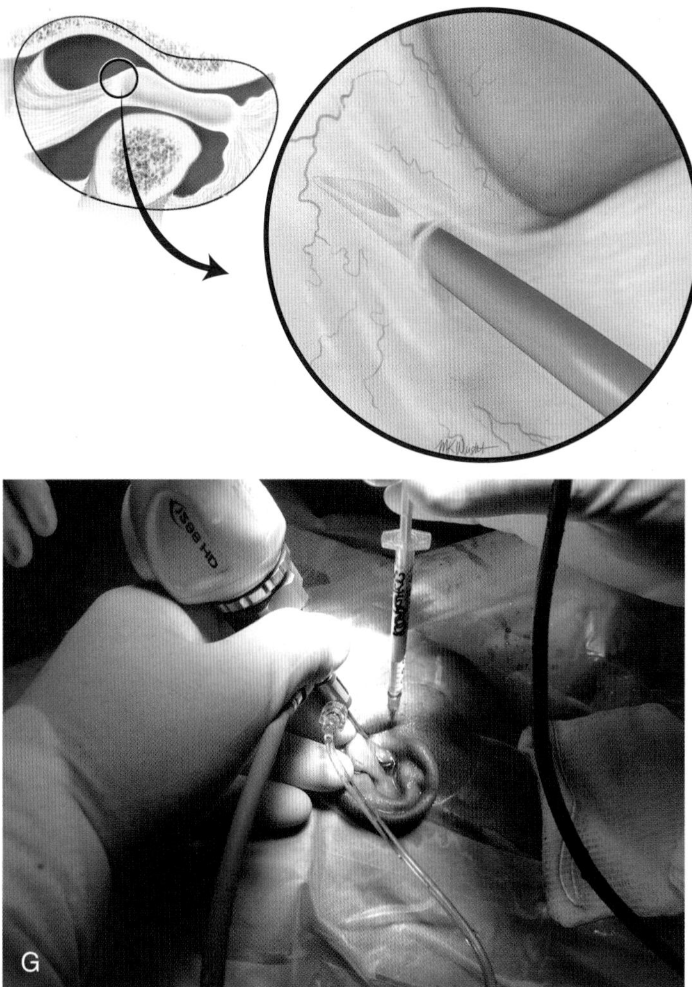

Figure 145.1, cont'd G, Direct intraarticular injection and instillation of medications.

TECHNIQUE 2: Operative TMJ Arthroscopy (Double-Puncture Arthroscopy)

STEP 1: Intubation

The patient is placed in a dorsal supine position and brought to the proper plane of general anesthesia via nasotracheal intubation.

STEP 2: Patient Examination and Preparation

The patient is examined under anesthesia. Then the patient is positioned, prepped, and draped in the usual manner for TMJ arthroscopy. A sterile ear wick is placed in the ear for protection.

STEP 3: Fossa Portal Puncture with Lysis and Lavage

Steps 2 through 6 of the primary arthroscopy technique are repeated.

STEP 4: Second Cannula Puncture

After completion of the diagnostic sweep, the second puncture needs to be placed exactly in the most anterior and lateral corner of the superior joint space to ensure maximum flexibility of the operative cannula. While the condyle is being seated in the fossa, the irrigation needle is removed and then the puncture site is located according to triangulation principles, creating an equilateral triangle in the following manner:

- A second measuring cannula is positioned flat against the tegument with the tip (0-mm marking) contiguous with the scope at the point of entry (skin) and continuous (in a straight line) with the plane of the arthroscope. The depth of the scope penetration is now translated to the cannula.
- The site for the second puncture has now been established. In a fashion similar to that used for the fossa puncture, the assistant insufflates the joint with 2 mL of irrigation fluid. The

Continued

TECHNIQUE 2: Operative TMJ Arthroscopy (Double-Puncture Arthroscopy)—*cont'd*

sounding 22-gauge needle followed by the trocar/cannula penetrate perpendicular to the tegument and then continue in the same direction. The trocar is rotated through the skin and advanced until encountering bone at the junction between the anterior aspect of the anterior slope of the articular eminence and the continuation of the zygomatic arch. Next, the trocar/cannula is rotated through the capsule and synovium.

- The trocar is observed on the monitor entering the joint space. Once intraarticular, the trocar is removed and drainage of the irrigating fluid is noted through the cannula (Fig. 145.2A).

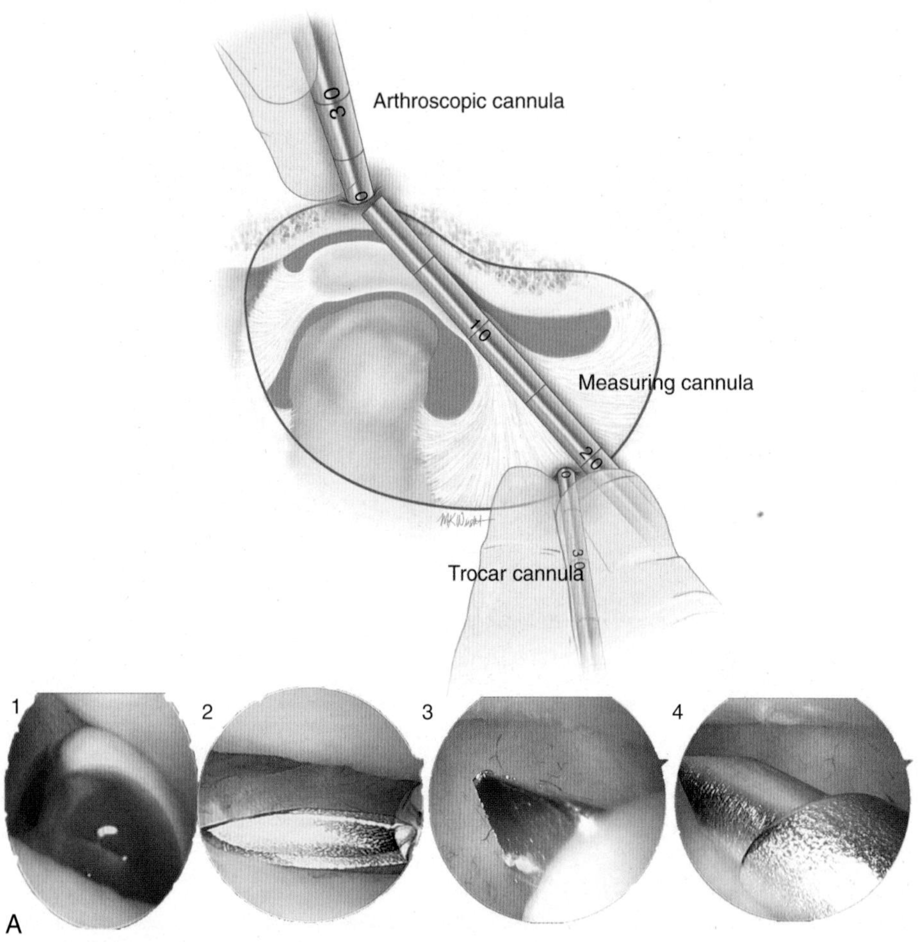

Figure 145.2 **A,** Double-puncture technique with vector measuring system.

TECHNIQUE: Operative TMJ Arthroscopy (Double-Puncture Arthroscopy)—*cont'd*

STEP 5: Advanced Arthroscopic Procedure

At this stage of the operation, different additional procedures can be performed as needed, including the following:

1. Synovial biopsy: either using cup forceps punch full-thickness biopsy or soft-tissue biopsy needles (Fig. 145.2B).
2. Arthroscopic debridement: performed in cases of arthrofibrosis, synovial hyperplasia, chondromalacia stages III and IV, synovial plica, and ankylosing osteoarthritis. It is advisable to start debridement in the anterior recess and do as much of the debridement as efficiently as you can in the anterior recess, then work your way to the intermediate zone and then finally the posterior pouch. An effective joint debridement is one where the instruments can pass freely from the front to the back of the joint. You have increased joint space once the debridement has been completed. Debridement is performed using different instruments and motorized devices that can be inserted through the second working cannula to ablate or coagulate any adhesions or redundant tissue, including the following:
   - Hand instruments such as a straight probe, curved probe, cup biopsy forceps, bone curettes, bone files, and banana blade
   - Holmium laser fiber tip
   - Motorized mini shaver with full radius or barrel tips
   - Coblation therapy
   - Bipolar and monopolar electrocautery
   - Ultrasonic aspirator
3. Arthroscopic discopexy: This technique is used for both the reducing and the nonreducing disk. It consists of the following steps:
   a. Anterior release (pterygoid myotomy): The incision is made with electrocautery, coblation, or a laser through the synovial membrane extending laterally to the vascular hump, penetrating the synovial membrane, and slicing the capsule. The pterygoid muscle is identified and then cut; the intention is to release the superior belly of the pterygoid muscle from its insertion into the articular disk.
   b. Disk reduction: Once the anterior release has been completed, the operative cannula and the scope are then walked back in the lateral sulcus to the posterior pouch. Once these two instruments reach the peak of the articular eminence, the condyle is pulled forward, and then both instruments can drop into the posterior pouch. The disk is reduced by compressing the retrodiskal tissue laterally with a straight probe while the condyle is in a forward or forward and contralateral position. Occasionally, the disk will hold its position but most of the time it will slip back forward, which will require deepening of the anterior release (Fig. 145.2C).
   c. Retrodiskal scarification or contracture: The target area of the retrodiskal contracture is generally the boggy and redundant synovium found lateral to the oblique protuberance. Low-voltage laser, bipolar cautery, or coblation is used to weld that tissue, accomplishing synovectomy superficially and then penetrating deeper into the bilaminar zone, causing scar contracture.
   d. Disk fixation: A disk fixation can be accomplished in one of two ways. The first and more traditional way is the suture or wire/button discopexy. A second way is by rigid fixation with either resorbable or titanium screws. Regardless of the methodology of fixation, the disk is held in reduction during the course of the fixation. The target area of fixation is the posterior lateral corner of the disk-condyle assembly, the area of the lateral pole where the disk attaches to the condyle (Fig. 145.2D).
   e. Arthroscopic contracture: This procedure is indicated in cases of recurrent TMJ dislocation cases. Once the second puncture is established, then the scope and the working cannula are moved to the posterior pouch. Utilizing a Holmium laser on weld mode, coblation, electrocautery, or chemical sclerosing agent injection, multiple lesional burns or scars are created in the oblique protuberance. The posterior synovectomy is completed to enact scar contracture and then penetrate the retrodiskal tissue into the bilaminar zone with laser, coblation, or electrocautery and again enact multiple regional burns to contract that retrodiskal tissue of the posterior capsule. Then the patient is taken through jaw function to check the existence of any dislocation; if no dislocation is present, then the procedure is done (Fig. 145.2 C and D).

Continued

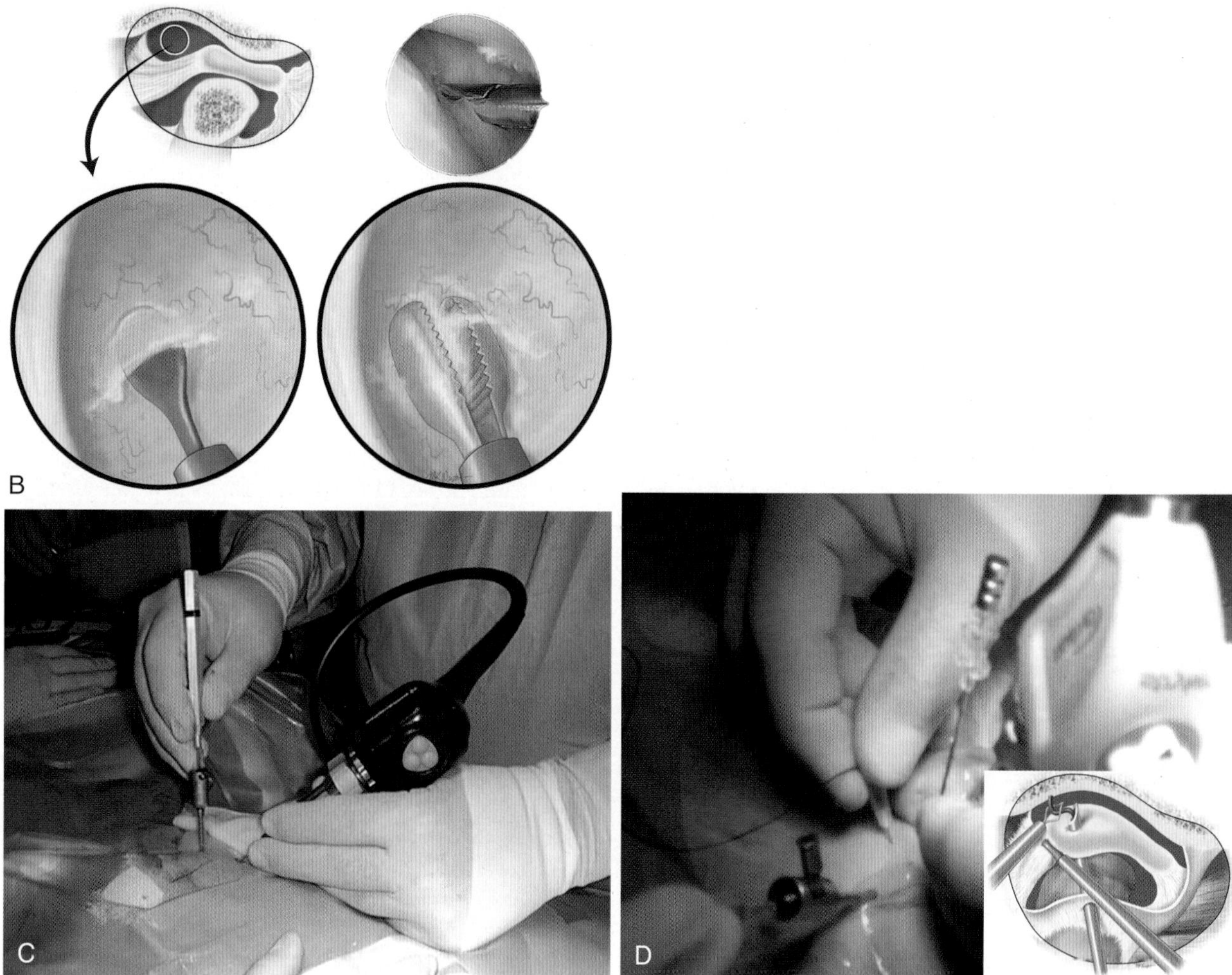

Figure 145.2, cont'd **B,** Synovial biopsy technique in the anterior recess. **C,** Lysis of adhesions using straight probe. **D,** Discopexy technique for disk repositioning.

Avoidance and Management of Intraoperative Complications

The potential intraoperative complications are numerous but should be reduced through the use of careful and meticulous surgical technique. Injury to the facial nerve remains a significant potential complication. Prevention of this injury requires proper placement of cannulas and care in joint lavage to avoid extravasation. Injury to other significant trigeminal nerve branches can also occur. These include the auriculotemporal nerve, the lingual nerve, and the inferior alveolar nerve. Prevention requires exact puncture measurement, anterior to the tragus. The surgeon must also avoid medial drape perforation that can occur by overextending the cannula by more than 35 mm. Care must also be taken to avoid medial extravasation by careful puncture technique, observation of surgical site, gentle pressure to irrigation, patent inflow/outflow system, and routine postoperative parapharyngeal space examination using laryngoscope. Fortunately, these injuries are rare, and most patients regain nerve function within 6 months postoperatively.

Injury to the vestibulocochlear nerve and dysfunction of the auditory system can also occur during arthroscopy. Attention should be paid to angulate the trocars anteriorly, with the same angulation of the tragus to avoid any perforation into the middle ear. Not advancing the arthroscope past 25 mm is also prudent. If the tympanic membrane is punctured, the surgeon should immediately stop the procedure, avoid irrigation, and obtain an intraoperative otolaryngology consultation. Usually, if the tympanic membrane injury is less than 30% of the drum surface, healing should occur with no sequela. Any minor ear hemorrhage is controlled by bipolar cautery, while the external auditory meatus is treated with hydrocortisone drops for up to 2 weeks.

Scuffing of the fibrocartilage lining can also occur intraoperatively. This is mitigated by avoiding repeated attempts of irrigation needle insertion. During glenoid fossa puncture, attention to the direction of trocar insertion as well as intraarticular manipulation should be taken into account. If scuffing is minor, fibrocartilage regenerates with little consequence. Injury to major vascular structures can also occur during arthroscopy. The vertical distance of the maxillary artery from the usual arthroscopic approaches 20 mm. Although a rare complication, it may result in an arteriovenous (AV) fistula with a pathognomonic patient complaint of a persistent hissing sound, which requires medical attention and treatment. Injury to the overlying superficial temporal vessels may also occur. This is managed by applying controlled pressure without sequela. On rare occasions, injury to these vessels results in an AV fistula or pseudoaneurysm, which should be managed surgically.

Perforation of the glenoid fossa during arthroscopy is a severe complication of the procedure. Prevention focuses primarily on controlling the direction of instruments toward the tubercle and away from the fossa. Extreme caution during attempting triangulation must also be observed. If the skull base is perforated, an intraoperative neurosurgical consultation and the use of prophylactic antibiotics are recommended. Postoperative computed tomography with intravenous contrast must be obtained to help identify any extradural or subdural hematoma. Most cerebrospinal fluid leaks will heal spontaneously. If a cerebrospinal fluid leak persists, a pressure dressing should be applied with patient hospitalization and head elevation. A leak that has persisted for longer than 48 hours is an indication for lumbar subarachnoid drain placement. Surgical repair of the middle cranial fossa dura, although an option, is rarely necessary.

Injuries to the disk may also occur during the procedure. The surgeon should avoid any deviation from standard technique of capsular puncture to prevent this complication. If disk perforation occurs, small perforations should be sutured using a 20-gauge needle. The avascular area of the meniscus shows a fibrous tissue healing response 4 to 6 weeks postoperatively. Hemarthrosis can be a difficult intraoperative problem to manage, so it should be prevented by not tearing the superficial temporal artery. It may also be caused by excessive bleeding from severely inflamed synovium/retrodiskal tissue upon joint entrance and by bleeding from the pterygoid artery when the surgeon is performing a myotomy for an anterior release procedure. Minor hemorrhage can be tamponaded by pressure irrigation. Excessive hemorrhage can be difficult to manage. Initially, increasing pressure in the irrigation bag can be attempted. Other initial maneuvers may include injecting a small amount of hyaluronic acid intraarticularly, using cautery or a laser on the bleeding area, or injecting local anesthetic with a vasoconstrictor into the bleeding site via spinal needle or as insufflation. Additional methods to apply pressure to stop the bleeding include insufflating the entire joint under pressure while all cannulas are obturated for 5 minutes or removing all instruments while direct palmar external pressure is applied for 5 minutes. For added pressure, the condyle is seated in the fossa if the source of the bleeding is located posteriorly, and it protrudes if bleeding anteriorly. It is also possible to apply pressure through the use of a #4 catheter balloon inserted through a working portal and inflated with normal saline, which is left in place for 5 minutes as well. If all measures are not successful, the joint is approached via open technique.

Like all surgical procedures, infection remains a risk with TMJ arthroscopy. Adherence to a proper sterile operating environment and technique, proper perioperative antibiotic prophylaxis, high-volume irrigation, and the absence of any adjacent skin infections are all important considerations. If an infection occurs, administration of cephalosporin for 7 days is prudent. If the infection persists, exploration of the area under local anesthesia with removal of any residual suture and further cephalosporin administration for 7 days may be helpful. In the presence of frank purulence, arthrocentesis or incision and drainage are necessary with copious antibiotic solution lavage, debridement with placement drain (to be removed in 3 days), and intravenous antibiotic coverage. Noninfectious effusions of the joint may also occur. Prevention of this complication is aimed at instructing patients to avoid overzealous use of the jaw or bruxing habits. If it does occur, initial management is directed at joint rest and a soft diet with heat application and nonsteroidal antiinflammatory drugs for pain management. If the effusion persists after 6 weeks, aspiration can be performed and, if this fails, a steroid injection will help to settle underlying inflammation. If the effusions develop some months after surgery, the surgeon should view this as an indication of degenerative disease progression.

Any minimally invasive procedure in a tight space carries with it the risk of instrument breakage and loose bodies. TMJ arthroscopy is no exception. Avoid instruments with manufacturing defects. Care must be exercised to not misuse any instruments, and if an instrument has worn out, it should be replaced. All instruments with flexible parts should be tested prior to the insertion into the joint. One must never apply excessive force or bending during the procedure. The use of ferromagnetic instruments is also recommended. If an instrument fracture occurs, immediately stop the procedure and maintain the position of arthroscope and cannulas. Keep the broken instrument in view and ensure the joint space is distended for optimal visibility. Next, measure the depth of the instrument with a scored cannula. Consider using fluoroscopic assistance to localize the piece if it cannot be visualized. Finally, remove the fragment. It may be desirable if this particular complication occurs to switch systems to a larger, 3 mm working cannula with a switch stick technique and retrieve the broken fragments with a golden retriever.

Postoperative Considerations

Postoperatively, patients are placed in a self-regime of physical therapy that includes stage II exercises as outlined by Wilk and McCain,[41] or jaw motion rehabilitation device exercises at 20 repetitions, four times a day. The goal of management is to achieve a normal range of motion. Immediately postoperatively, patients will present with decreased range of motion, probably secondary to pain. However, patients need to be mobilized if an adhesive phenomenon is to be prevented. Later, the physical therapy is modified to prevent excessive range of motion.

Patients are maintained on a soft consistency diet for 3 to 6 months before being advanced to a regular diet. Analgesics are provided as required. They are also instructed to wear the flat occlusal orthotic. Follow-up is maintained at 1 week, 1 month, 3 months, 6 months, and then every 6 months thereafter. Preoperative and postoperative assessment parameters include the improvement index measured with a visual analog scale, range of motion measured vertically in millimeters, and diet consistency. The patient should maintain the immediate postoperative opening, and pain should be limited to the first postoperative week.

In cases of mandibular dislocation, four brackets should be applied to the cuspids, on which medium elastics are applied to each side, holding jaws in a fixed position.

References

1. Ohnishi M. Arthroscopy of the temporomandibular joint. *1 Stomatal Soc Jpn*. 1975;42:207.
2. Ohnishi M. Clinical application of arthroscopy in the temporomandibular joint diseases. *Bull Tokyo Med Dent Univ*. 1980;27(3):141–150.
3. Hellsing G. Experiences from dissectional and arthroscopic studies of the TMJ. *Aust Prosthodont Soc Bull*. 1986;16:59.
4. Hellsing G, Holmlund A, Nordenram A, Wredmark T. Arthroscopy of the temporomandibular joint. Examination of 2 patients with suspected disk derangement. *Int J Oral Surg*. 1984;13(1):69–74.
5. Hellsing G, L'Estrange P, Holmlund A. Temporomandibular joint disorders: a diagnostic challenge. *J Prosthet Dent*. 1986;56(5):600–606.
6. Holmlund A, Hellsing G. Arthroscopy of the temporomandibular joint. An autopsy study. *Int J Oral Surg*. 1985;14(2):169–175.
7. Holmlund A, Hellsing G, Wredmark T. Arthroscopy of the temporomandibular joint. A clinical study. *Int J Oral Maxillofac Surg*. 1986;15(6):715–721.
8. Johnson L. *Arthroscopic Surgery: Principles and Practice*. 3rd ed. St. Louis: Mosby; 1986:1297–1300.
9. Murakami K, Hoshino K. Histological studies on the inner surfaces of the articular cavities of human temporomandibular joints with special reference to arthroscopic observations. *Anat Anz*. 1985;160(3):167–177.
10. Murakami K, Hoshino K. Regional anatomical nomenclature and arthroscopic terminology in human temporomandibular joints. *Okajimas Folia Anat Jpn*. 1982;58(4–6):745–760.
11. Murakami K, Ito K. Arthroscopy of the temporomandibular joint: arthroscopic anatomy and arthroscopic approaches in the human cadaver (in Japanese; abstract in English). *Arthroscopy*. 1981;6:1.
12. Murakami K, Ono T. TMJ arthroscopy by inferolateral approach. *Int J Oral Maxillofac Surg*. 1986;15:410.
13. McCain I.P.. Arthroscopy of the human temporomandibular joint. In: *Proceedings From the AAOMS Meeting*. Washington, DC; 1985.
14. Sanders B. Arthroscopic surgery of the TMJ: treatment of internal derangement with persistent lock. *Oral Surg*. 1986;62:361.
15. Sanders B, Buoncristiani R. Diagnostic and surgical arthroscopy of the temporomandibular joint: clinical experience with 137 procedures over a 2-year period. *J Craniomandib Disord*. 1987;1(3):202–213.
16. McCain JP. Arthroscopy of the human temporomandibular joint. *J Oral Maxillofac Surg*. 1988;46(8):648–655.
17. Chung KC, Swanson JA, Schmitz D, Sullivan D, Rohrich RJ. Introducing evidence-based medicine to plastic and reconstructive surgery. *Plast Reconstr Surg*. 2009;123(4):1385–1389.
18. Kurita K, Westesson PL, Yuasa H, Toyama M, Machida J, Ogi N. Natural course of untreated symptomatic temporomandibular joint disc displacement without reduction. *J Dent Res*. 1998;77(2):361–365.
19. Laskin D. Surgical management of internal derangements. In: Laskin DM, Greene CS, Hylander WL, eds. *Temporomandibular Disorders: An Evidenced-Based Approach to Diagnosis & Treatment*. Quintessence Publishing; 2006:469–481.
20. McCain JP, Sanders B, Koslin MG, Quinn JH, Peters PB, Indresano AT. Temporomandibular joint arthroscopy: a 6-year multicenter retrospective study of 4,831 joints. *J Oral Maxillofac Surg*. 1992;50(9):926–930.
21. Dimitroulis G. A review of 56 cases of chronic closed lock treated with temporomandibular joint arthroscopy. *J Oral Maxillofac Surg*. 2002;60(5):519–524.
22. Sanders B, Buonchristiani RD. A 5-year experience with arthroscopic lysis and lavage for the treatment of painful temporomandibular joint hypomobility. In: Clark GT, Sanders B, Bertolami CN, et al., eds. *Advances in Diagnostic and Surgical Arthroscopy of the Temporomandibular Joint*. Philadelphia: Saunders; 1993:51.
23. Murakami K, Segami N, Okamoto M, Yamamura I, Takahashi K, Tsuboi Y. Outcome of arthroscopic surgery for internal derangement of the temporomandibular joint: long-term results covering 10 years. *J Cranio-Maxillo-Fac Surg*. 2000;28(5):264–271.
24. Reston JT, Turkelson CM. Meta-analysis of surgical treatments for temporomandibular articular disorders. *J Oral Maxillofac Surg*. 2003;61(1):3–10.
25. Undt G, Murakami K, Rasse M, Ewers R. Open versus arthroscopic surgery for internal derangement of the temporomandibular joint: a retrospective study comparing two centres' results using the Jaw Pain and Function Questionnaire. *J Cranio-Maxillo-Fac Surg*. 2006;34(4):234–241.
26. De Souza, Raphael F, da Silva L, et al. Interventions for managing temporomandibular joint osteoarthritis. *Cochrane Database Syst Rev*. 2018;6.
27. Insel O, Glickman A, Reeve G, et al. New Criteria demonstrate successful outcomes following temporomandibular joint (TMJ) arthroscopy. *Oral Surg Oral Med Oral Pathol Oral Radiol*. 2020;130(1):e20–e21.
28. White RD. Arthroscopic lysis and lavage as the preferred treatment for internal derangement of the temporomandibular joint. *J Oral Maxillofac Surg*. 2001;59(3):313–316.
29. Indresano AT. Surgical arthroscopy as the preferred treatment for internal derangements of the temporomandibular joint. *J Oral Maxillofac Surg*. 2001;59(3):308–312.
30. Al-Moraissi EA. Arthroscopy versus arthrocentesis in the management of internal derangement of the temporomandibular joint: a systematic review and meta-analysis. *Int J Oral Maxillofac Implants*. 2015;44(1):104–112.
31. Hossameldin RH, McCain JP. Outcomes of office-based temporomandibular joint arthroscopy: a 5-year retrospective study. *Int J Oral Maxillofac Implants*. 2018;47(1):90–97.
32. McCain JP, Hossameldin RH, Srouji S, Maher A. Arthroscopic discopexy is effective in managing temporomandibular joint internal derangement in patients with Wilkes stage II and III. *J Oral Maxillofac Surg*. 2015;73(3):391–401.
33. McCain JP, Podrasky AE, Zabiegalski NA. Arthroscopic disc repositioning and suturing: a preliminary report. *J Oral Maxillofac Surg*. 1992;50(6):568–579.
34. Tarro AW. A fully visualized arthroscopic disc suturing technique. *J Oral Maxillofac Surg*. 1994;52(4):362–369.
35. Kaneyama K, Segami N, Sato J, Murakami K, Iizuka T. Outcomes of 152 temporomandibular joints following arthroscopic anterolateral capsular release by holmium: YAG laser or electrocautery. *Oral Surg Oral Med Oral Pathol Oral Radiol Endod*. 2004;97(5):546–551.
36. Nickerson JW, Boering G. Natural course of osteoarthritis as it relates to internal derangement of the temporomandibular joint. *Oral Maxillofac Surg Clin North Am*. 1989;1:27.
37. Schiffman E, Ohrbach R, Truelove E, et al. Diagnostic Criteria for Temporomandibular Disorders (DC/Tmd) for Clinical and Research Applications: recommendations of the International RDC/TMD Consortium Network* and

Orofacial pain Special Interest Group. *J Oral Facial Pain Headache.* 2014;28(1):6–27.

38. Angeles-Han S, Prahalad S. The genetics of juvenile idiopathic arthritis: what is new in 2010? *Curr Rheumatol Rep.* 2010;12(2):87–93.
39. Wilkes CH. Internal derangements of the temporomandibular joint. Pathological variations. *Arch Otolaryngol Head Neck Surg.* 1989;115(4):469–477.
40. Torres DE, McCain JP. Arthroscopic electrothermal capsulorrhaphy for the treatment of recurrent temporomandibular joint dislocation. *Int J Oral Maxillofac Surg.* 2012;41(6):681–689.
41. Wilk BR, McCain JP. Rehabilitation of the TMJ after arthroscopic surgery. *Oral Surg Oral Med Oral Pathol.* 1992;73:531.

CHAPTER 146

Arthroplasty and Eminectomy

Shyam Sunder Indrakanti, Helaman Erickson, and John R. Zuniga

Armamentarium

#15 Scalpel blade
#9 Periosteal elevator
0.02-inch Silastic sheet
702 Carbide bur
4-0 Vicryl, 4-0 Monocryl, 5-0 Prolene, or 5-0 fast-absorbing suture
Bone clamp
Bone file or reciprocating rasp
Cotton pellet or Merocel ear packing
Freer elevator
Headlight for operating surgeon
Kitner retractors
Local anesthetic with vasoconstrictor
Needle electrocautery/PEAK PlasmaBlade
Nerve stimulator/Checkpoint 9394 stimulator
Osteotomes
Right angle vascular clamp
Round bur
Senn retractor
TMJ retractors

History of the Procedure

Thomas Annandale is the first surgeon credited with describing temporomandibular joint (TMJ) surgery in 1887; however, both Humphrey's approach to condylectomy (1856) and Riedel's meniscectomy (1883) precede this time period. Annandale's curved incision over the lateral ligament, which was carried down to the capsule, was succeeded by Stimson's T-shaped incision (1897) and Murphy's L-shaped incision (1914).[1–3] The horizontal arm lies over the zygoma with both modifications, although the vertical portion was placed more posteriorly by Murphy and incorporated the use of temporal fat and fascia as an interpositional flap. In 1939, Professor Wakely of King's College published his arthroplasty technique utilizing a pedicled temporalis flap tunneled under the zygoma.[4] Eminectomy was first described in 1951 with Myrhaug's articular eminence reduction.[5] In 1967, Dautrey described moving a proximal segment of the zygoma downward and forward to mechanically prevent dislocation.[6]

The standard preauricular incision with a hockey stick extension superiorly has been preferred by practitioners since the mid-20th century. Since then, modifications such as incising posterior to the tragus while remaining endaural as well as the post auricular, intraoral, rhytidectomal, Blair, and submandibular approaches have been described and utilized by surgeons.

Indications

Surgery is indicated to either promote healing by replacing missing tissue with grafts, restore damaged tissue, or remove unsalvageable tissue. In 1994, Dolwick and Dimitroulis described absolute and relative indications for arthrotomy. Absolute indications include fibrous and osseous ankylosis, neoplasia, recurrent or chronic dislocation, and developmental disorders including condylar hyperplasia. The relative indications include internal derangement, osteoarthrosis, and trauma.[7] Dolwick further divided the need for TMJ surgery into general and specific indications. Surgery is indicated in patients who are unresponsive to nonsurgical therapy assuming the patient is compliant and any myofascial pain has been managed. Physical exam should localize pain to the TMJ, especially upon functional loading and movement; mechanical interference may also be appreciated. More specific indications include disorders not responding to TMJ arthrocentesis, chronic severe limited mouth opening, degenerative joint disease with intolerable pain and dysfunction, and severe joint disease identified on computed tomography (CT) or magnetic resonance imaging (MRI). Generally, the more localized the pain is to the TMJ area, the better the surgical prognosis.[8] Orbach and Dworkin's 2019 AAPT diagnostic criteria consider the clinical presence of pain to be vital to the diagnosis of temporomandibular dysfunction (TMD) and broadly categorizes it into myalgia, arthralgia, and secondary headaches, which can be verified via provocation testing of the muscles, TMJ, and masticatory system, respectively. The fourth category of TMD is titled "painful DJD," which can be simplified into the presence of the above three categories with imaging showing joint changes.[9]

Eminectomy is indicated for recurrent TMJ dislocation. A study conducted by Boering found a relatively low incidence of 1.8% in a population of 400 symptomatic TMJ patients.[10] Recurrent dislocations are often found in those with joint laxity, internal derangement of the TMJ, and with neurologic disorders who experience seizure or extra pyramidal symptoms from neuroleptic therapy. Recurrent dislocation causes injury to the disk, capsule, and ligaments, leading to internal derangement.[11]

Arthrocentesis, arthroscopy, and open surgery (arthrotomy/arthroplasty) remain the most common surgical procedures for patients when nonsurgical treatment has failed to reduce pain or improve function. A meta-analysis comparing open and arthroscopic surgery with respect to pain, maximum incisal opening (MIO), mandibular impairment, and clinical signs showed that pain reduction, increased MIO, and a reduction in mandibular impairment all favored open surgery.[12] Improvement in clinical signs (clicking, crepitus, joint pain) favored arthroscopic procedures (Fig. 146.1A–D).

Contraindication and Limitations

Patient selection is of vital importance, requiring compliance with treatment regimens, good understanding of the disorder, and having realistic expectations. Older individuals with multiple comorbidities who are not suitable candidates for general anesthesia can still be treated with conservative measures like injectables (autologous blood, sclerosing agents) with or without maxillomandibular fixation or local anesthesia based eminectomy technique described by Segami.[13,14] Patients with significant psychosocial and behavioral components contributing to their perceived or actual TMD based on the Axis II DC/TMD questionnaire should be considered more carefully for operative intervention.[15]

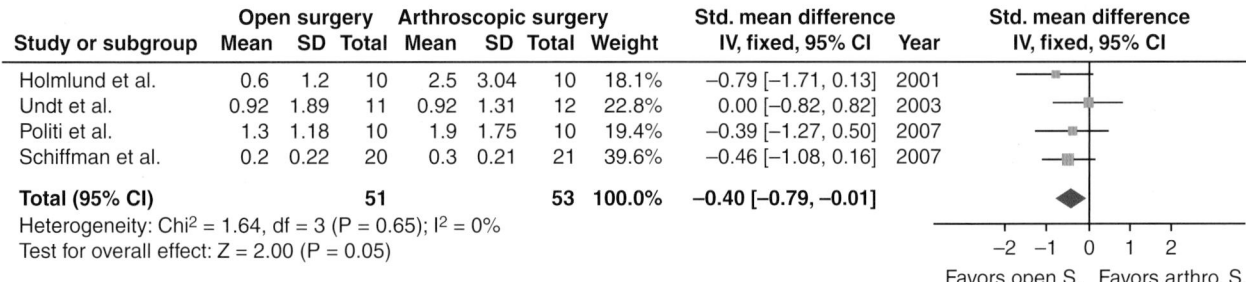

Study or subgroup	Open surgery Mean	SD	Total	Arthroscopic surgery Mean	SD	Total	Weight	Std. mean difference IV, fixed, 95% CI	Year
Holmlund et al.	0.6	1.2	10	2.5	3.04	10	18.1%	−0.79 [−1.71, 0.13]	2001
Undt et al.	0.92	1.89	11	0.92	1.31	12	22.8%	0.00 [−0.82, 0.82]	2003
Politi et al.	1.3	1.18	10	1.9	1.75	10	19.4%	−0.39 [−1.27, 0.50]	2007
Schiffman et al.	0.2	0.22	20	0.3	0.21	21	39.6%	−0.46 [−1.08, 0.16]	2007
Total (95% CI)			**51**			**53**	**100.0%**	**−0.40 [−0.79, −0.01]**	

Heterogeneity: Chi² = 1.64, df = 3 (P = 0.65); I² = 0%
Test for overall effect: Z = 2.00 (P = 0.05)

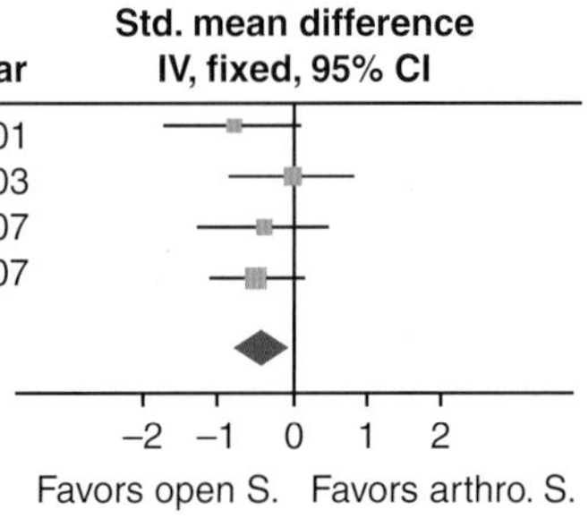

A

Study or subgroup	Open S. Events	Total	Arthro. S. Events	Total	Weight	Odds ratio M-H, fixed, 95% CI	Year
Holmlund et al.	8	10	8	10	18.2%	1.00 [0.11, 8.95]	2001
Politi et al.	8	10	7	10	15.9%	1.71 [0.22, 13.41]	2007
Hobeichi et al.	10	28	10	34	65.9%	1.33 [0.46, 3.88]	2008
Total (95% CI)		**48**		**54**	**100.0%**	**1.33 [0.56, 3.18]**	
Total events	26		25				

Heterogeneity: Chi² = 0.12, df = 2 (P = 0.94); I² = 0%
Test for overall effect: Z = 0.65 (P = 0.52)

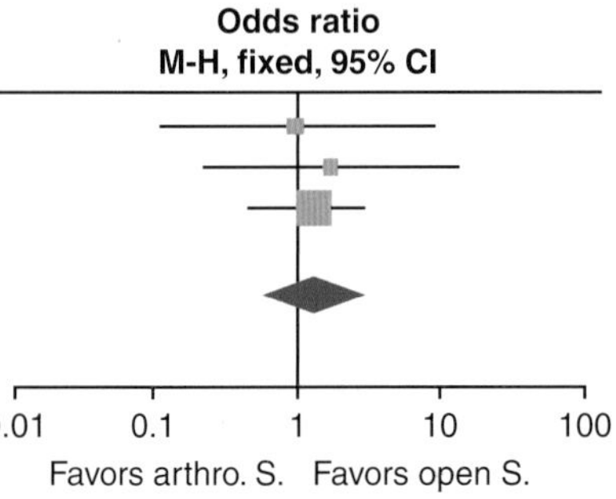

B

Study or subgroup	Open S. Mean	SD	Total	Arthro. S Mean	SD	Total	Weight	Mean difference IV, fixed, 95% CI	Year
Holmlund et al.	4.9	3.51	10	6.2	6.09	10	10.7%	−1.30 [−5.66, 3.06]	2001
Undt et al.	2.1	2.3	14	2.3	2.3	12	64.3%	−0.20 [−1.97, 1.57]	2003
Politi et al.	4.6	3.41	10	6.3	3.06	10	25.1%	−1.70 [−4.54, 1.14]	2007
Total (95% CI)			**34**			**32**	**100.0%**	**−0.69 [−2.12, 0.73]**	

Heterogeneity: Chi² = 0.85, df = 2 (P = 0.65); I² = 0%
Test for overall effect: Z = 0.96 (P = 0.34)

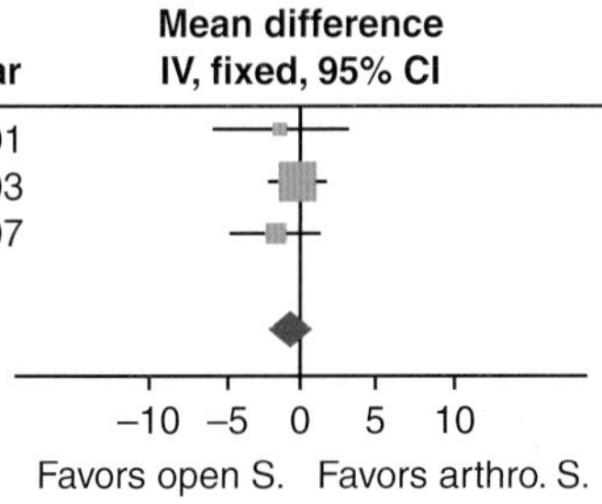

C

Study or subgroup	O. S Events	Total	A. S Events	Total	Weight	Odds ratio M-H, fixed, 95% CI	Year
Holmlund et al.	6	10	6	10	28.2%	1.00 [0.17, 5.98]	2001
Politi et al.	2	10	2	10	18.8%	1.00 [0.11, 8.95]	2007
Hobeichi et al.	14	28	10	34	53.0%	2.40 [0.84, 6.83]	2008
Total (95% CI)		**48**		**54**	**100.0%**	**1.74 [0.76, 3.98]**	
Total events	22		18				

Heterogeneity: Chi² = 0.98, df = 2 (P = 0.61); I² = 0%
Test for overall effect: Z = 1.32 (P = 0.19)

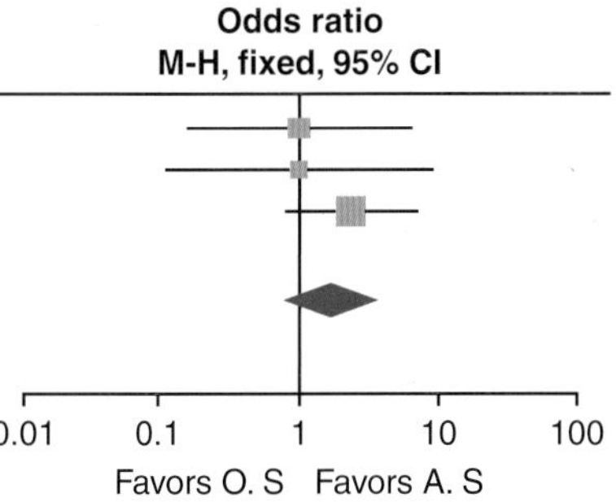

D

Figure 146.1 **A,** Forest plot for pain open surgery versus arthroscopy. **B,** Forest plot for MIO open versus arthroscopy. **C,** Forest plot for mandibular impairment open versus arthroscopy. **D,** Forest plot for postoperative clinical findings open versus arthroscopy. Figure 145.1A–D (Adapted from Al-Moraissi EA. Open versus arthroscopic surgery for the management of internal derangement of the temporomandibular joint: a meta-analysis of the literature. *Int J Oral Maxillofac Surg*. 2015;44(6):763–770).

TECHNIQUE 1: Arthroplasty

STEP 1: Prepping and Draping Patient

Open TMJ surgery is performed under general anesthesia. The patient is placed supine on the operating table with the head turned to expose the operative side. It is usually unnecessary to remove hair unless it will enter the wound during surgery and increase the likelihood of infections.[16] Prior to prepping the skin, an antibiotic ointment-impregnated cotton pellet, petroleum gauze, or an impregnated Merocel (Medtronic Merocel—Dublin, Ireland) ear packing is placed into the external auditory canal. This minimizes the entry of fluid into the ear during surgery, which could lead to postoperative irritation and pain of the canal or tympanic membrane. The skin is then prepped and draped to include the external ear, in case of the need for cartilage harvest, preauricular skin including the zygomatic arch to the lateral canthus, and inferiorly to the mandibular border. A sterile adhesive border is then applied with the ear exposed and sterile drapes are placed.

STEP 2: Incision

The endaural approach, a modification of the preauricular incision placed on the tragus instead of the pretragal crease, is described herein. If further access is required, Al-Kayat and Bramley describe an extension into the temporal area about 1 cm above the superior margin of the palpable zygomatic arch.[17] After marking out the incision, care must be taken to avoid injecting local anesthetic too deep or it may anesthetize the facial nerve. If a nerve stimulator is used, it is also crucial to communicate this to the anesthesia team and avoid the use of neuromuscular blockade. Newer and more sophisticated instruments such as Checkpoint (Checkpoint Surgical—Cleaveland, OH) have been studied and found to be equally reliable to electromyography in thyroid surgery.[18]

An incision is made from the uppermost point of the auricle inferior to the attachment of the ear lobule with the middle portion of the incision hidden in the posterior tragus. Care is taken to avoid tragal cartilage and minimize the risk of perichondritis, although some surgeons transect through the tragal cartilage (Fig. 146.2A). The incision is through the skin and subcutaneous tissue down to superficial temporalis fascia. A blunt instrument is then used to open a pocket anterior to the external auditory canal. The superficial temporal artery and vein are located deep to the subcutaneous tissue and may be encountered and ligated or retracted forward. Dissection is bluntly continued toward the superficial temporal fascia until the smooth, white, and well-defined surface of the superficial surface of the temporalis fascia is encountered (Fig. 146.2B). When a small pocket has been developed, a Senn retractor is placed into the wound down to this layer. Another Senn is placed in the pretragal incision. The soft tissue in the depth of the wound has clearly defined landmarks that can then be sharply released using scissors.

STEP 3: Dissection to the Temporomandibular Joint Capsule

The superficial layer of the deep temporal fascia is now visible the entire length of the wound. A scalpel is used to incise this layer just anterior to the plane of dissection and parallel to the skin incision. A Molt periosteal elevator is then utilized to dissect over the periosteum anteriorly. Dissecting in this layer protects and allows retraction of branches of the facial nerve (Fig. 146.2C). This plane is superior to the lateral capsule of the TMJ and the posterior attachment of the parotidomasseteric fascia. This attachment is cut just anterior to the auditory canal and the fascia retracted anteriorly to expose the lateral capsule to view (Fig. 146.2D). Kitner retractors are particularly useful and cause minimal soft tissue injury during this process, and if performed in the correct layer, bleeding is minimized.

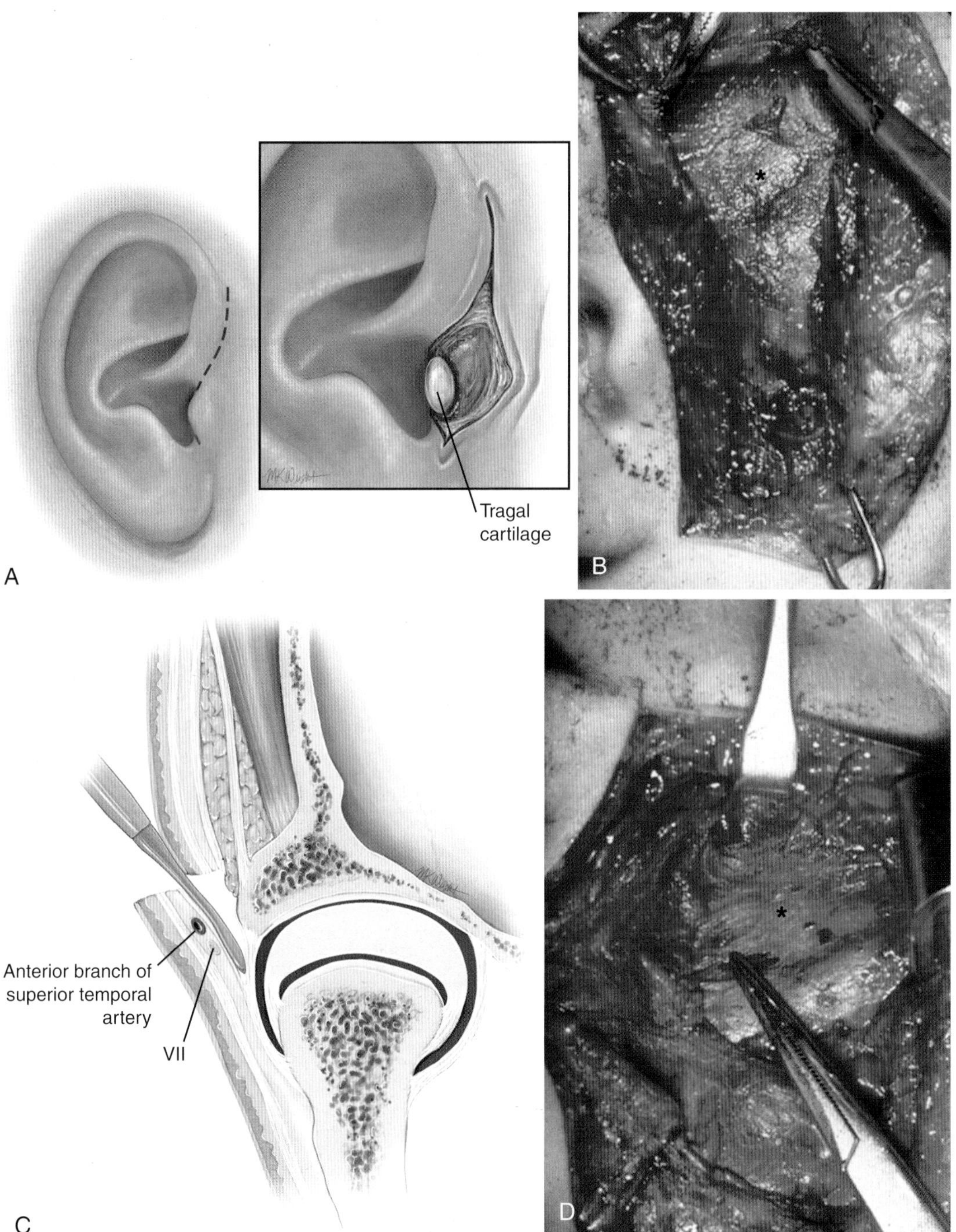

Figure 146.2 **A,** Incision. **B,** Temporalis fascia. **C,** Incision and reflection of superficial layer of deep temporal fascia. **D,** Incision and reflection of superficial layer of deep temporal fascia.

TECHNIQUE 1: Arthroplasty—*cont'd*

STEP 4: Exposing the Intraarticular Spaces

The lateral capsule is now well exposed and entry into the joint may be accomplished by making a 4 to 5 mm incision through the capsule parallel to the zygomatic arch and 2 to 3 mm below it (Fig. 146.2E). A Freer elevator is then used to enter the superior joint space and break up adhesions between retrodiscal tissues, disk, glenoid fossa, and articular eminence. The Freer elevator is then turned vertically into the lateral recess. At this point, the first decision for surgical management is made: if the superior surface of the disk is intact without perforations or evidence of condyle exposure, or cartilaginous degeneration, an additional "disk sparing" incision is performed instead of a "disk replacement" incision. A disk sparing incision is parallel to the incision described above but is placed below (about 1 cm) and through capsule, disk, and ligament down to the lateral bone of the condylar head. A subperiosteal dissection is performed, and a retractor is placed onto the lateral cortex of the condyle and a subperiosteal dissection is directed superiorly. Simultaneously, the mandible is retracted inferiorly by a surgical assistant so that the head of the condyle is exposed and inspected. This also allows examination of the articular disk through both the upper and lower TMJ compartments without cutting through the disk. A disk replacement incision is placed vertically from the middle of the superior joint access incision described above in a descending direction onto the lateral cortex of the condylar head and neck completing a T-shaped incision over the lateral capsule. This incision transects the lateral and superior portions of the articular disk and allows excellent access to the internal components (condylar neck, head, articular cartilage, and retrodiscal tissue) with the intent to resect/remove the articular disk (or condylar neck, etc.).

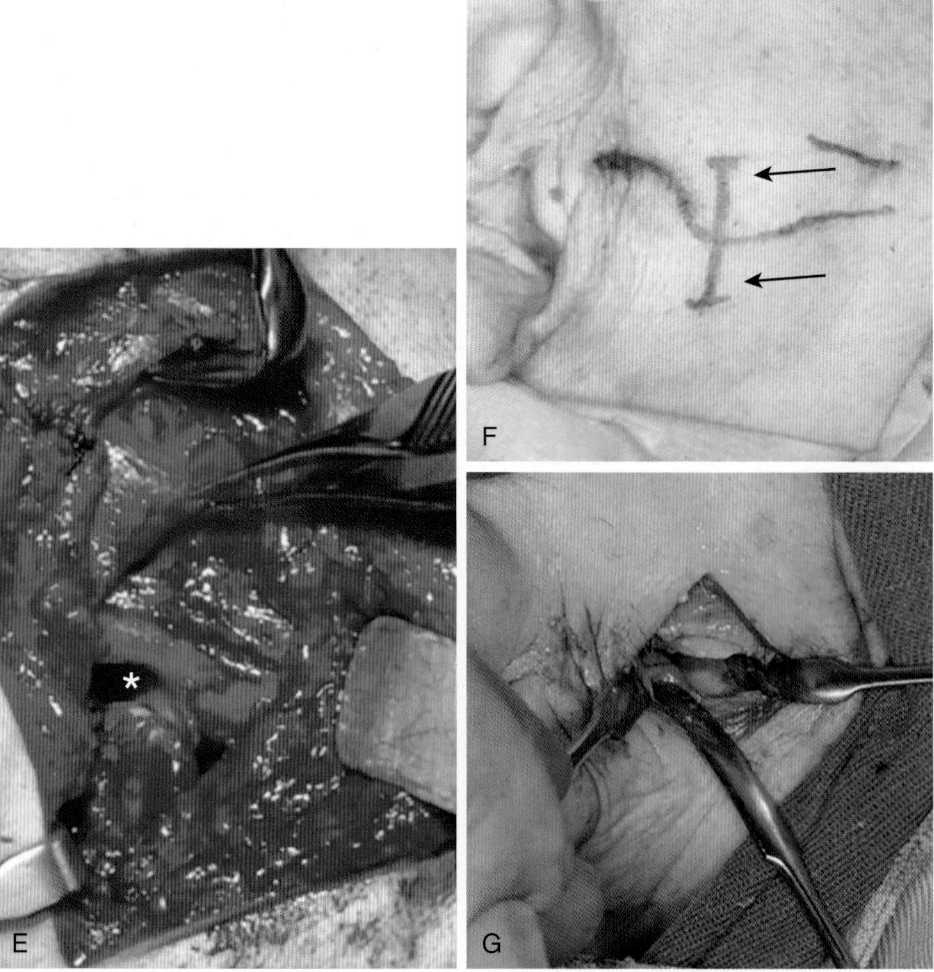

Figure 146.2, cont'd **E,** Entry into the joint. **F,** Eminectomy incision described by Segami. **G,** Eminectomy approach described by Segami.

TECHNIQUE 2: Eminectomy

The authors prefer to perform an eminectomy in addition to meniscoplasty. Ideally, the eminectomy is done prior since it significantly enhances the access to the disk during meniscoplasty. If surgical management requires meniscectomy, eminectomy is avoided to allow the autograft of choice to adapt and fixate to the unaltered fossa and eminence. Meniscectomy eliminates the possibility of disk recapture that may occur when the disk is repositioned with meniscoplasty. The eminence determines the movement of the disk during translation and rotation but does not affect the condylar head movement.[19] Thus, the eminectomy has a positive outcome on disk movement postoperatively without effecting condylar movement. Posteminectomy patients demonstrate normal opening and excursive movements and do not deviate on opening or protrusion since condylar pathways are not affected.

STEP 1: Exposure

After access to the TMJ is accomplished, eminectomy is performed with the aid of chisels, rotating burs, reciprocating rasps, or Piezosurgery device. Reducing the eminence as far medially as possible is important to a successful surgical outcome. An alternative exposure is described by Segami as a 2-cm vertical incision anterior to the pretragal crease for more direct access under local anesthesia[12] (Fig. 146.2F and G).

STEP 2: Reduction of the Eminence

Once the joint is exposed and the articular eminence is identified, a 1-mm fissure bur is utilized to make a horizontal cut into the lateral tubercle of the eminence that will allow for an unobstructed path of condylar translation (Fig. 146.3A). Complete bone removal is continued, with the surgeon ensuring at all times that the plane of the bur is directed inferiorly approximately 10 degrees as it proceeds medially, to follow the natural slope of the eminence toward its medial base. Approximately 90% of the cut in the eminence is made utilizing the 1-mm fissure bur.[20] An osteotome positioned with an inferior angulation is then used to complete the cut and avoid the skull base. A large round bur or reciprocating rasp smooths the eminence and completes the eminectomy as far medial as possible (Fig. 146.3B). During the cuts, a broad retractor is used to depress and protect the meniscus and condyle. At the end of the procedure, the bony surfaces should be well rounded and smooth.

STEP 3: Closure

After completion of the eminectomy, it has been recommended to reattach the lateral joint capsule by drilling holes into the lateral rim of the zygomatic arch and reinserting the joint capsule with resorbable sutures.[11] Arthroscopic eminoplasty has also been described.[21] The amount and location of bone removed from the eminence are subject to debate. Some advocate reducing the height and contouring the eminence, whereas others recommend complete resection.[22,23]

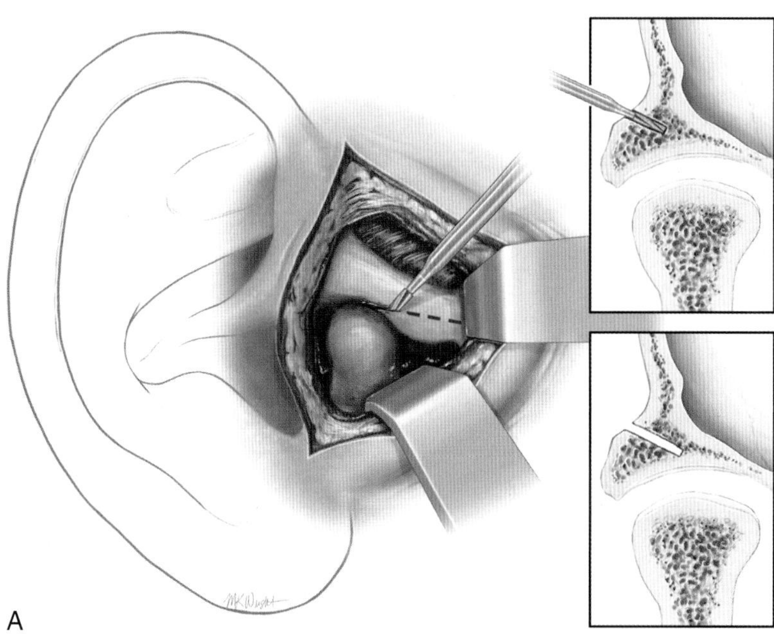

Figure 146.3 A, Lateral aspect eminectomy.

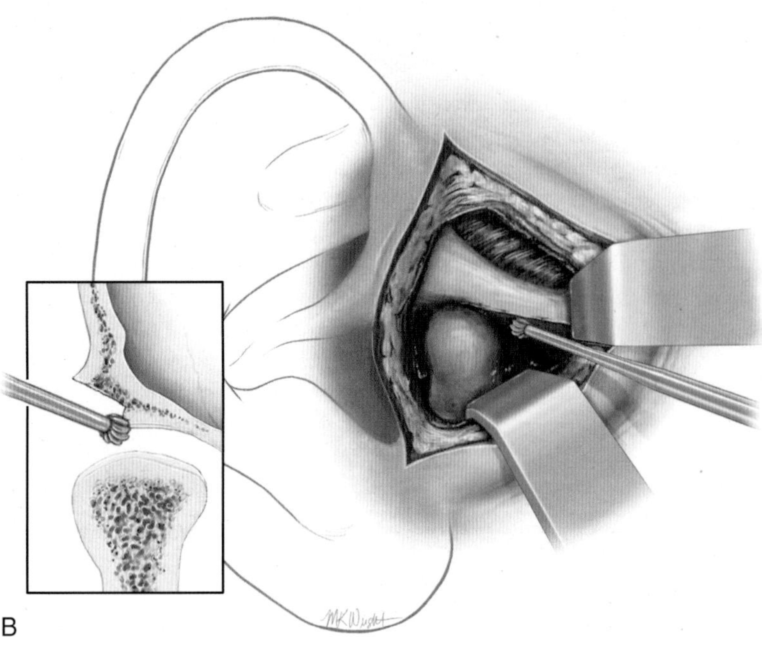

Figure 146.3, cont'd B, Medial aspect of eminectomy.

TECHNIQUE 3: Disk Imbrication, Plication, Mitek Implant, Meniscectomy

Reestablishment of the anatomic disk-condyle relationship has been described by utilizing plication, imbrication, and the use of implants. Typically, disks are displaced anteromedially; therefore, a posterior lateral vector will return the disk to a normal position. The directional relocation of the disk is the primary objective in these procedures.[20]

Meniscocondylar imbrication, also known as discopexy, is suturing of the disk to the lateral condyle, thus preventing the classic anteromedial displacement while attaining an appropriate vector to reduce the disk to its anatomic location. Utilizing a 701 fissure bur, a hole is drilled in the lateral condyle in a sagittal plane from posterior to anterior. The meniscus is freed up from adhesions so that it can passively lay over the height of the condyle. A 4-0 nonresorbable (Mersilene) (J&J Ethicon—Sommerville, NJ) suture is first passed through the hole in the lateral condylar neck from posterior to anterior. The suture is then placed through the meniscus from inferior to superior and as far medial as possible through the intermediate band and posterior attachment. The knot is tied in the posterior lateral aspect. The lateral border of the disk is then secured to the lateral capsular attachment utilizing four to six 4-0 Vicryl (J&J Ethicon—Sommerville, NJ) sutures. Adequacy of the sutures is then assessed by opening and closing the mandible.[20]

Disk plication is the partial or complete removal of retrodiscal tissue and suturing the remaining tissue to the posterior ligament. A partial meniscoplasty is performed by removing a wedge and repositioning the disc posterior and lateral.[24] Utilizing right angle vascular clamps, the anterior and posterior portion of the disc may be clamped for better control of wound edges and hemostasis (Fig. 146.4A). The disk is then sutured together utilizing 4-0 resorbable suture to recreate the natural position of the disk. A wedge plication can be tailored to control different vectors to return the disk to the appropriate position. After plication, range of motion exercises are performed in the operating room to evaluate for locking, catching, or obstruction. Often eminectomy is performed in conjunction with this procedure.

The use of Mitek (DePuy Mitek—Raynham, MA) mini anchors is commonly used to reposition the disk in its anatomical position. This implant is a bone anchoring system that is placed into the most posterior, superior, lateral condylar neck. The implant secures itself in bone with a cleat system that is activated upon insertion. The anchor has an eyelet where a nonresorbable suture is then passed through the posterior band of the disk. This allows the disk to be securely sutured in place preventing relapse.[25] The lateral capsule is the closed with 4-0 Vicryl.

When the disk is perforated, deformed, or irreparable and causing pain or inhibiting smooth pain free function, a meniscectomy may be required. Meniscectomy removes the central avascular portion as well as the posterior attachment that may be perforated. Care must be taken to minimize injury to the retrodiskal tissue, which is usually hyperemic; if it begins oozing, it is difficult to achieve hemostasis without extensive cauterization. Some literature suggests that the PEAK PlasmaBlade (Medtronic PEAK—Dublin, Ireland) facilitates better postoperative healing than traditional electrocautery.[26] The medial attachment of the disk is generally the most challenging to remove. The condyle must be retracted anterior and inferior to allow access to the medial attachment, which can then be incised using a curved TMJ scissor or a #15 blade. It is important to remove the entire meniscus and to trim any

TECHNIQUE 3: DISK IMBRICATION, PLICATION, MITEK IMPLANT, MENISCECTOMY—*cont'd*

loose or ragged edges to prevent adhesion or fibrosis. Care must be taken to avoid perforating the medial capsule, which may result in bleeding due to injury of the middle meningeal or internal maxillary artery, or the pterygoid venous plexus. Depending on disk and joint morphology, it may be prudent to remove the disk in pieces starting with the easily accessible lateral portion and proceeding deeper into the joint with improved vision and access.[16]

Post meniscectomy imaging shows flattening of the anterior-superior slope of the condyle while the anterior lip of the condyle might show sclerosis or some beaking.[27,28] Other potential postoperative changes include crepitus and fibrosis. Wilkes advocated a temporary silicone sheet placed into the joint space with a pullout tab so the sheet could be removed after a fibrous capsule is able to form 6 to 12 weeks later[28] (Fig. 146.4B).

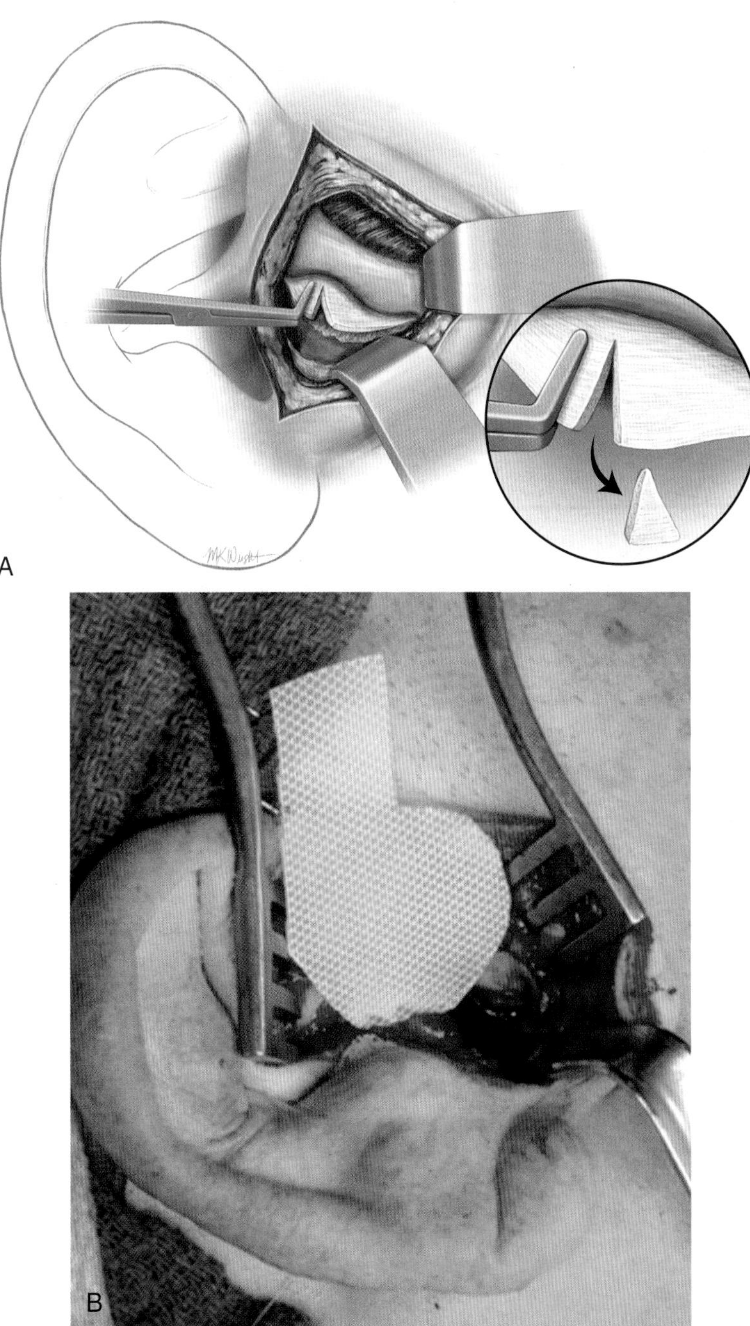

Figure 146.4 **A,** Wedge excision of retrodiscal tissue. **B,** Silastic pullout.

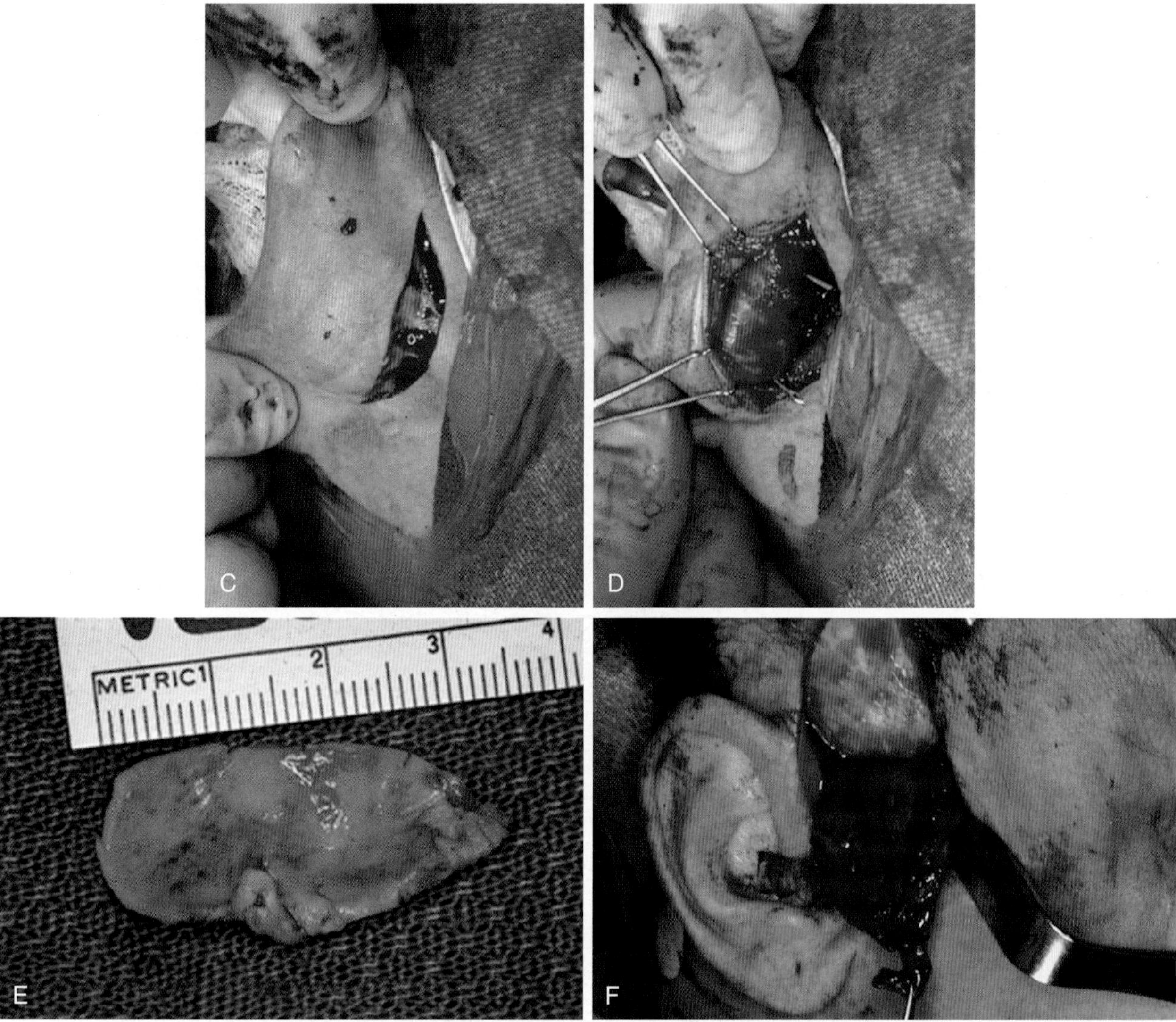

Figure 146.4, cont'd **C,** Incision placed in the posterior ear crease. **D,** Conchal bowl exposure in the posterior ear. **E,** Auricular cartilage graft after harvest. **F,** Temporalis flap.

TECHNIQUE 4: Interpositional Grafting

Following meniscectomy, some advocate temporary silicone implants while others recommend autogenous reconstructive options, including auricular cartilage, dermis, temporalis muscle flap, and fat. Matrix-associated chondrocytes have also been transplanted as a means of tissue regeneration with promising results.[29] Studies are equivocal, and most patients do well without reconstruction, but there is still concern about crepitus and regressive remodeling[30,31] (Table 146.1).

Table 146.1 Limitations of Existing Temporomandibular Joint (TMJ) Disk Replacement Material

Material	Limitations
Silastic, Proplast/Teflon	Foreign body reactions
Ear cartilage	Fragmentation and ankylosis
Fat	Fragmentation and poor handling
Full-thickness skin	Epidermoid cyst formation
Fascia and dermis	Insufficient bulk and difficult to anchor
Allogenic grafts	Potential cross-infection and unpredictable resorption
Temporalis muscle	Fibrosis and trismus
Dermis-fat graft, full-thickness skin, dermis	Visible scar in donor site
Tissue engineering	Untested in vivo

1. Medtronic PEAK—Dublin, Ireland
2. Medtronic Merocel—Dublin, Ireland
3. J&J Ethicon—Sommerville, NJ.
4. Checkpoint Surgical—Cleaveland, OH.
5. DePuy Mitek—Raynham, MA.
6. Avanos Medical On-Q—Alpharetta, GA.
7. Pacira Biosciences Inc. Exparel—Parsippany-Troy Hills, NJ.

Reproduced from Dimitroulis G. A critical review of interpositional grafts following temporomandibular joint discectomy with an overview of the dermis-fat graft. *Int J Oral Maxillofac Surg.* 2011;40:561.

TECHNIQUE 4: Interpositional Grafting—*cont'd*

EAR CARTILAGE HARVEST

Auricular cartilage is commonly used during arthroplasty to replace the disk. This is accomplished through an incision in the posterior ear. It is placed in the posterior ear crease so that it is well hidden and placed over intact cartilage. The graft is best harvested from the part of the conchal bowl that exhibits a curvilinear pattern that will readily adapt to the glenoid fossa[32] (Fig. 146.4C–E). The dissection is supraperichondrial to preserve the perichondrium on the convex "perichondral side" while it is subperichondral on the concave "cartilage side." Harvesting the graft in this fashion facilitates stable fibrous attachment to the fossa on the perichondral side and movement over the condylar head on the cartilage side without fibrous attachments. Additionally, should the subperichondral dissection on the concave surface lead to fracture of the elastic cartilage, the perichondral tissue will maintain the form of the graft. Once harvested, the graft is preserved in sterile saline until ready for insertion. The postauricular incision is closed with three deep sutures, each attaching the perichondral tissue retained on the concave side to the retromastoid fascia to close the dead space. Avoid using a compression dressing, as it has been associated with chondritis and skin necrosis. The incision is then closed with fast-absorbing suture.

The harvested graft is then inserted into the joint space so the lateral edge of the cartilage matches the lateral edge of the articular fossa and extends medially over the entire articular fossa and eminence such that when the condyle is seated and then translated, and there is contact with the graft during these movements. The graft is fixated to the articular fossa using two 1-0 or 2-0 Vicryl sutures anchored to the lateral edge of the articular fossa prepared by passing a wire-passing bur or 702 carbide bur from the lateral to the medial surfaces of the fossa to fixate the graft and prevent rotation during condylar movement. Finally, to prevent fragmentation, a 0.02 inch reinforced silastic sheet with a pullout tab is placed between the articulating condyle and the graft. The silastic sheet is removed in 12 weeks.

DERMIS GRAFT

The dermal graft is taken from the abdomen or lateral thigh. A #15 blade is used to make a 3 cm by 3 cm full-thickness elliptical incision accounting for contraction of the graft during handling. Using a dermatome to excise a split-thickness skin graft that is not detached is an acceptable alternative. The donor site skin is repositioned and sutured at the periphery. The dermal graft is then placed into the joint space and sutured to the anterior and posterior attachment with 4-0 resorbable suture.[33]

TEMPORALIS MUSCLE FLAP

Temporalis fascia is an inadequate graft; however, the temporalis myofascial flap is the most commonly used interpositional material because of minimal donor site cosmetic and functional morbidity.[34] This flap is harvested by extending the endaural incision into the temporal region about 3 cm. The superficial temporalis fascia is then identified. Utilizing a #15 blade, a full-thickness inferiorly based, pedicled flap including superficial fascia, temporalis muscle, and deep temporalis fascia is harvested. The distal edge of the flap needs to be wider than the joint space it is going to fill to account for contraction. In general, the length of the flap from the superior edge to the zygomatic arch is 5 to 6 cm and approximately 3 cm in width (Fig. 146.4F). The flap is then rotated laterally over the zygomatic arch and positioned in the joint space so that the temporalis periosteum is against the glenoid fossa. One issue with this rotation is the asymmetry of the ipsilateral face caused by the bulk of muscle that is lateral to the zygomatic arch. Alternatively, the posterior zygomatic arch may be osteotomized in two places to allow for the flap to rotate into the joint space. The segments of the arch are then returned and secured in place with rigid fixation.[35] The flap is held in position with two nonresorbable sutures that are passed through holes drilled in the posterior fossa and anterior eminence.[36] The flap may also be raised in the same manner as described above but passed through the infratemporal space passing it from the articular eminence posteriorly into the joint space. It is sutured in place as above.

TECHNIQUE 4: Interpositional Grafting—*cont'd*

MATRIX-ASSOCIATED CHONDROCYTE TRANSPLANTATION

While tissue regeneration has been employed in other joints, there are limited studies of its application in TMJ arthroplasty. The technique described by Undt et al. discussed the use of collagen scaffold combined with a suspension made from harvested rib chondrocytes and autologous blood.[29] It is secured with a 1-mm thick silicone sheet that was retrieved 4 to 5 months later and the graft could be analyzed for differentiation.

Avoidance and Management of Intraoperative Complications

The major associated intraoperative complications with TMJ surgery include damage to cranial nerve VII, bleeding associated with terminal branches of the external carotid artery and retromandibular vein, and damage to the parotid gland. Facial nerve injury of the temporal branch (occasionally the zygomatic branch) is the most significant complication associated with open surgery. Although total facial nerve paralysis is possible, it is rare. The inability to raise the eyebrow is the most commonly observed finding, occurring in 5% of the cases, and usually resolves in 3 months; it is permanent in <1% of cases. Other complications are limited opening and minor occlusal changes.[37] Avoidance of the facial nerve as well as anatomic variation and location has been well described. Al-Kayat described the distance utilizing many landmarks. The distance from the lowest point of the external bony auditory canal to the bifurcation of the facial nerve was 1.5 to 2.8 cm (mean: 2.3 cm), and the distance from the postglenoid tubercle to the bifurcation was 2.4 to 3.5 cm (mean: 3.0 cm). The most variable measurement was the point at which the upper trunk crosses the zygomatic arch. It ranged from 8 to 35 mm anterior to the most anterior portion of the bony external auditory canal (mean: 2.0 cm)[17] (Fig. 146.5).

Prior to eminectomy, imaging of the articular eminence is extremely important to prevent possible perforation into the middle cranial fossa, exposure of the temporal lobe, and possible cerebrospinal fluid leak.[36] It is important to identify the lateral tubercle of the temporal bone on CT or MRI and to estimate the thickness both laterally and medially to prevent penetration into the middle cranial fossa. Hall conducted an anatomic study of 38 cadaver heads to establish a guideline for eminectomy and found that the average distance from the lateral tubercle to the temporal bone is 9 mm with a range of 5 to 14 mm. The antero-posterior length of the eminence averaged 11 mm ranging from 9 to 18 mm, while the width was 21 mm ranging from 16 to 25 mm.[38] After eminectomy is completed, the mandible is manipulated to ensure unobstructed condylar motion during normal range of motion.

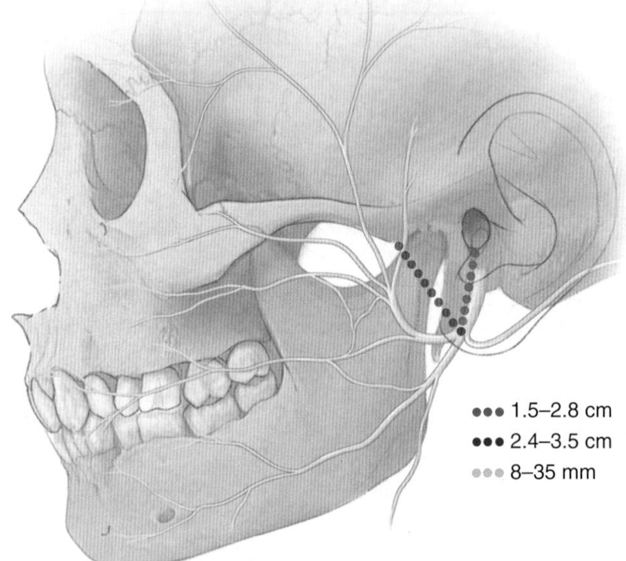

Figure 146.5 Facial nerve relationship.

Postoperative Considerations

Before closure of the capsule, an angiocath is placed in the surgical site, which is connected to an On-Q (Avanos Medical On-Q—Alpharetta, GA) pain pump after closure. The pump delivers a continuous infusion of anesthetic intraarticularly and has been shown to be effective in controlling postoperative pain.[39,40] This is usually left in place for 3 days postoperatively. A pressure dressing is also placed and is usually removed 24 hours later. Routine wound care is performed for the incision with application of antibiotic ointment twice per day until the sutures are removed 5 days later. A no-chew diet is prescribed for 3 weeks, and the patient is slowly advanced. Aggressive and early joint mobilization is required for any intraarticular joint surgery to succeed. Range of motion exercises begin on postoperative day 4 with the goal of improving range of motion and mobilizing postsurgical edema. Liposomal bupivacaine (Exparel; Pacira Biosciences Inc. Exparel— Parsippany-Troy Hills, NJ) may also be used as an alternative to the use of the On-Q pump.[41]

References

1. Annandale T. Displacement of the inter-articular cartilages of the lower jaws and its treatment by operation. *Lancet*. 1887;(8):411.
2. Stimson LA. *Manuel of Operative Surgery*. 3rd ed. Philadelphia: Lea Bross & Co; 1895.
3. Murphy JB. Arhthroplasty for intra-articular bony and fibrous ankylosis of temporomandibular articulation. *JAMA*. 1914;(62):1783–1794.
4. Wakely C. The surgery of the temporomandibular joint. *Surgery*. 1939;5:697–706.
5. Myrhaug H. A new method of operation for habitual dislocation of the mandible; review of former methods of treatment. *Acta Odontol Scand*. 1951;9(3–4):247–260.
6. Gosserez M, Dautrey J. Osteoplastic bearing for treatment of temporomandibular luxation. Transaction of Second Congress of the International Association of Oral surgeons Copenhagen, Munksgaard. *Int J Oral Surg*. 1967;IV:261.
7. Dolwick MF, Dimitroulis G. Is there a role for temporomandibular joint surgery? *Br J Oral Maxillofac Surg*. 1994;32(5):307–313.
8. Walters PJ, Geist ET. Correction of temporomandibular joint internal derangements via the posterior auricular approach. *J Oral Maxillofac Surg*. 1983;41(9):616–618.
9. Ohrbach R, Dworkin SF. AAPT diagnostic criteria for chronic painful temporomandibular disorders. *J Pain*. 2019;20(11):1276–1292.
10. de Leeuw R, Boering G, Stegenga B, de Bont LG. Temporomandibular joint osteoarthrosis: clinical and radiographic characteristics 30 years after nonsurgical treatment: a preliminary report. *Cranio*. 1993;11(1):15–24.
11. Undt G. Temporomandibular joint eminectomy for recurrent dislocation. *Atlas Oral Maxillofac Surg Clin North Am*. 2011;19(2):189–206.
12. Al-Moraissi EA. Open versus arthroscopic surgery for the management of internal derangement of the temporomandibular joint: a meta-analysis of the literature. *Int J Oral Maxillofac Implants*. 2015;44(6):763–770.
13. Renapurkar SK, Laskin DM. Injectable Agents versus surgery for recurrent temporomandibular joint dislocation. *Oral Maxillofac Surg Clin North Am*. 2018;30(3):343–349.
14. Segami N. A modified approach for eminectomy for temporomandibular joint dislocation under local anaesthesia: report on a series of 50 patients. *Int J Oral Maxillofac Implants*. 2018;47(11):1439–1444.
15. Schiffman E, Ohrbach R. Executive summary of the diagnostic criteria for temporomandibular disorders for clinical and research applications. *J Am Dent Assoc (1939)*. 2016;47(6):438–445.
16. Ness GM. Arthroplasty and discectomy of the temporomandibular joint. *Atlas Oral Maxillofac Surg Clin North Am*. 2011;19(2):177–187.
17. Al-Kayat A, Bramley P. A modified pre-auricular approach to the temporomandibular joint and malar arch. *Br J Oral Surg*. 1979;17(2):91–103.
18. Lawson BR, Kamani D, Shama M, Kyriazidis N, Randolph GW. Safety and reliability of a handheld stimulator for neural monitoring during thyroid surgery. *Laryngoscope*. 2020;130(2):561–565.
19. Isberg A, Westesson PL. Steepness of articular eminence and movement of the condyle and disk in asymptomatic temporomandibular joints. *Oral Surg Oral Med Oral Pathol Oral Radiol Endod*. 1998;86(2):152–157.
20. Weinberg S, Cousens G. Meniscocondylar plication: a modified operation for surgical repositioning of the ectopic temporomandibular joint meniscus. Rationale and operative technique. *Oral Surg Oral Med Oral Pathol*. 1987;63(4):393–402.
21. Segami N, Kaneyama K, Tsurusako S, Suzuki T. Arthroscopic eminoplasty for habitual dislocation of the temporomandibular joint: preliminary study. *J Craniomaxillofac*. 1999;27(6):390–397.
22. Cascone P, Ungari C, Paparo F, Marianetti TM, Ramieri V, Fatone M. A new surgical approach for the treatment of chronic recurrent temporomandibular joint dislocation. *J Craniofac Surg*. 2008;19(2):510–512.
23. Helman J, Laufer D, Minkov B, Gutman D. Eminectomy as surgical treatment for chronic mandibular dislocations. *Int J Oral Surg*. 1984;13(6):486–489.
24. Hall MB. Meniscoplasty of the displaced temporomandibular joint meniscus without violating the inferior joint space. *J Oral Maxillofac Surg*. 1984;42(12):788–792.
25. Ruiz Valero CA, Marroquin Morales CA, Jimenez Alvarez JA, Gomez Sarmiento JE, Vallejo A. Temporomandibular joint meniscopexy with Mitek mini anchors. *J Oral Maxillofac Surg*. 2011;69(11):2739–2745.
26. Peprah K, Spry C. *Pulsed Electron Avalanche Knife (PEAK) PlasmaBlade versus Traditional Electrocautery for Surgery: A Review of Clinical Effectiveness and Cost-Effectiveness*. Ottawa, ON: CA Agency for Drugs and Technologies in Health; 2019.
27. Agerberg G, Lundberg M. Changes in the temporomandibular joint after surgical treatment. A radiologic follow-up study. *Oral Surg Oral Med Oral Pathol*. 1971;32(6):865–875.
28. Wilkes CH. Surgical treatment of internal derangements of the temporomandibular joint. A long-term study. *Arch Otolaryngol Head Neck Surg*. 1991;117(1):64–72.
29. Undt G, Jahl M, Pohl S, et al. Matrix-associated chondrocyte transplantation for reconstruction of articulating surfaces in the temporomandibular joint: a pilot study covering medium- and long-term outcomes of 6 patients. *Oral Surg Oral Med Oral Pathol Oral Radiol*. 2018;126(2):117–128.
30. Holmlund AB. Surgery for TMJ internal derangement. Evaluation of treatment outcome and criteria for success. *Int J Oral Maxillofac Surg*. 1993;22(2):75–77.
31. Dimitroulis G. The role of surgery in the management of disorders of the temporomandibular joint: a critical review of the literature. Part 2. *Int J Oral Maxillofac Surg*. 2005;34(3):231–237.
32. Svensson B, Wennerblom K, Adell R. Auricular cartilage grafting in arthroplasty of the temporomandibular joint: a retrospective clinical follow-up. *Oral Surg Oral Med Oral Pathol Oral Radiol Endod*. 2010;109(3):e1–e7.
33. Dimitroulis G. A critical review of interpositional grafts following temporomandibular joint discectomy with an overview of the dermis-fat graft. *Int J Oral Maxillofac Implants*. 2011;40(6):561–568.
34. Herbosa EG, Rotskoff KS. Composite temporalis pedicle flap as an interpositional graft in temporomandibular joint arthroplasty: a preliminary report. *J Oral Maxillofac Surg*. 1990;48(10):1049–1056.
35. Bergey DA, Braun TW. The posterior zygomatic arch osteotomy to facilitate temporalis flap placement. *J Oral Maxillofac Surg*. 1994;52(4):426–427.
36. Quinn P. *Color Atlas of Temporomandibular Joint Surgery*. St. Louis, MO: Mosby; 1998.
37. Dolwick MF. Temporomandibular joint surgery for internal derangement. *Dent Clin North Am*. 2007;51(1):195–208.
38. Hall MB, Brown RW, Sclar AG. Anatomy of the TMJ articular eminence before and after surgical reduction. *J Cranio-Mandibular Pract*. 1984;2(2):135–140.
39. Zuniga JR, Ibanez C, Kozacko M. The analgesic efficacy and safety of intra-articular morphine and mepivicaine following temporomandibular joint arthroplasty. *J Oral Maxillofac Surg*. 2007;65(8):1477–1485.
40. Charous S. Use of the ON-Q pain pump management system in the head and neck: preliminary report. *Otolaryngol Head Neck Surg*. 2008;138(1):110–112.
41. Kenes MT, Leonard MC, Bauer SR, Wyman MJ. Liposomal bupivacaine versus continuous infusion bupivacaine via an elastomeric pump for the treatment of postoperative pain. *Am J Health Syst Pharm*. 2015;72(23 suppl 3):S127–S132.

CHAPTER 147

Custom Total Temporomandibular Joint Replacement

Louis G. Mercuri

Armamentarium

Appropriate sutures
Barton head dressing materials
Basic oral and maxillofacial surgery instruments
Change of gown and gloves
Custom temporomandibular joint screw and instrument kit
Eye lubricant and eye protection devices
Hair cutting shears and elastic adhesive tape
Jaw-exercising device
Local anesthetic with vasoconstrictor
Marking pen, bipolar cautery
Maxillomandibular fixation kit
Otic speculum, drops, and cotton pledgets
Otoscope, cotton pledgets, and mineral oil
Penfield elevator to place fat graft
Plastic adhesive and surgical isolation drapes
Power equipment, burs, saws, and Jacob's chuck
Soft-tissue surgical instruments
Temporomandibular joint surgical instruments
Vancomycin solution to soak implants

History of the Procedure

In 1992, the US Food and Drug Administration (FDA) banned the implantation of all temporomandibular joint (TMJ) devices due to the significant failure of TMJ devices containing Proplast-Teflon (Vitek, Houston, TX).[1] Thereafter, surgeons were forced into utilizing autogenous bone and/or temporalis flaps to manage these failed devices and end-stage TMJ cases. Many of these autogenous tissue reconstructions ultimately were doomed to fail because of the persistence of the toxic effects of fragmented Proplast-Teflon particles in and around the joint.[2]

Prior to the 1992 FDA ban because of the extent of the bony architectural damage caused by the local reaction to Proplast-Teflon, surgeons found it difficult, if not impossible, to adequately fit and stabilize the available stock TMJ replacement (TMJR) device components. In 1989, utilizing the computer-assisted design/computer-assisted manufacturing (CAD/CAM) developed for orthopedic hip and knee revision devices by Techmedica (Camarillo, CA), a custom TMJR device was designed to be manufactured from the same biocompatible materials successfully used in orthopedic joint replacement devices for over 50 years.[3] In 1990, Techmedica received FDA clearance to conduct clinical trials as an investigational patient-fitted TMJR device.

In 1995, the FDA reclassified all implantable TMJ devices into its most stringent category, class III. Class III devices are defined as those that support or sustain human life, are of substantial importance in preventing impairment of human health, or which present a potential, unreasonable risk of illness or injury.[4] Due to the perceived level of risk associated with class III devices, the FDA determined that general and special controls alone were insufficient to ensure the safety and effectiveness of class III devices. Therefore, the FDA's strictest scientific and regulatory review process, a Pre-Market Approval (PMA) application, was required for approval of any new implantable TMJ-related device.

In 1996, TMJ Concepts (Ventura, CA) assumed the Techmedica brand and developed the PMA application for FDA approval that included the investigational device prospective multicenter study data to satisfy the PMA clinical requirement[5]. In 1999, based on laboratory mechanical testing and the aforementioned prospective multicenter clinical study, the FDA deemed the TMJ Concepts patient-fitted system as safe and effective for the management of end-stage TMJ disorders.[6]

Clinical outcomes following TMJR with the Techmedica/TMJ Concepts custom prostheses have previously been reported. Clinical and statistically significant improvements in pain, mandibular function, and diet have been seen at 10, 14, and 20+ years after implantation, respectively. Patients also reported an average 85% to 87% improvement in their quality of life at all study periods. Furthermore, there were no instances of Techmedica\TMJ Concepts TMJR material-related failures in any of these reviews.[7–10]

Indications for the Use of the Procedure

Salvage of end-stage pathologic conditions that significantly alter temporal glenoid fossa and mandibular condyle/ramus bony architecture are considered indications for a custom TMJR device. The primary goal of TMJR is the long-term, safe, and effective restoration of mandibular function and form. The fundamental everyday activities of mastication, speech, deglutition, and airway support are supported by TMJ function and form. Therefore, over a lifetime, these tasks expose the TMJ complex to more cyclical loading and unloading than any other joint. Therefore, to provide successful long-term function and form, any TMJR device must be capable of managing the anatomic, functional, and esthetic discrepancies presented to it.[11]

Inflammatory Arthritis Involving the TMJ Not Responsive to Other Modalities of Treatment

Inflammatory arthritis involves a local synovial tissue-mediated, destructive local, or systemic disease process. Therefore, orthopedic surgeons opt for total joint replacement (TJR) because the long-term results are predictable.[12] When the mandibular condyle is extensively damaged, degenerated, or absent as the result of an inflammatory arthritic condition, TMJR provides a predictable approach to achieving optimal functional, esthetic, and symptomatic improvement.[13] TMJR is advocated, as opposed to autogenous tissues, because the composite materials are not affected by either the systemic or local pathology associated with any inflammatory arthritic disease process, it avoids the need for a second autogenous tissue donor site with potential associated morbidity, it decreases operating room time, and it allows for simultaneous mandibular advancement with predictable long-term stable results.[12]

Recurrent Fibrosis or Bony Ankylosis Not Responsive to Other Modalities of Treatment

In patients with bony or fibrous TMJ ankylosis, or reankylosis, autogenous reconstruction makes little sense. No recently published orthopedic literature discusses the use of autogenous bone for the reconstruction of any axial joint affected by bony or fibrous ankylosis. Alloplastic joint replacement is the recommended orthopedic procedure for such cases.[14,15] Traditional management of TMJ bony ankylosis, has been gap arthroplasty with autogenous tissue grafting or alloplastic hemiarthroplasty. Regardless of the technique, the ability to create acceptable form, secure fixation, and stabilization of any autogenous bone or soft-tissue graft at surgery necessarily delays early mandibular functional rehabilitation. Further, the consequences of autogenous bone graft mobility during the initial stages of healing or early physical therapy will severely compromise the free graft's incorporation into the host bone by impeding or hindering angioneogenesis.[16,17] Alloplastic TMJ hemiarthroplasty devices are no longer available. Therefore, in light of the orthopedic experience and other biophysiological considerations, TMJR should be considered the best management option for patients with TMJ fibrous and bony ankylosis.[18]

Failed Tissue Grafts (Bone and Soft Tissue)

Successful outcome of free autogenous bone and soft tissue grafting requires that the recipient site provide a rich vascular bed. Unfortunately, the scar or pathologically damaged tissue encountered in end-stage disease TMJ cases does not provide a vascular environment conducive to the predictable success of free autogenous hard- and soft-tissue grafts. Marx reported that capillaries can penetrate a maximum tissue thickness of 180 to 220 μm, whereas the thickness of scar tissue surrounding previously operated bone averages 440 μm.[19] This may account for the clinical observation that free autogenous tissue grafts, such as cartilage, costochondral, and sternoclavicular grafts, often fail in cases with extreme anatomic bony architectural discrepancies resulting from end-stage pathology.

A survey of experienced TMJ surgeons reported that 95.5% preferred TMJR over autogenous bone grafting for TMJ replacement. This preference was based on fewer postoperative complications and more predictable outcomes using TMJR. In cases where autogenous bone graft revision was indicated, a TMJR was preferred. Based on these responses it was concluded that surgeons should consider TMJR as the primary salvage option for reconstruction in the management of most end-stage TMJ pathology.[20]

Failed and Failing TMJR devices

Failed and failing TMJR devices require either revision or replacement. Revision means maintaining the same device in place, whereas replacement means the complete removal of the TMJR and implanting a new one.[21] Revision should be considered for cases with acute infections, dislocation, some malpositioned implants, malocclusion, and early heterotopic ossification. On the other hand, replacement should be considered for TMJR failures due to device component fracture, an adverse local tissue response, component loosening, late/chronic infections, or documented material hypersensitivity. However, patient selection and surgeon experience play a critical role in successful patient revision and replacement outcomes.[22]

Due to the osteolysis that occurs around failed TMJR components, substantial host bone anatomic architectural discrepancies occur. Therefore, it is difficult to adapt and stably fixate autogenous tissues or stock TMJR components to the host bone. Further, the adverse local tissue responses associated with failed or failing devices provide an unfavorable environment for the introduction of an autogenous graft. Therefore, custom TMJR components provide more predictable outcomes than autogenous tissue or stock TMJR devices.[23]

Loss of Vertical Mandibular Height or Occlusal Relationship Due to Bony Resorption, Trauma, Developmental Abnormalities, or Pathologic Lesions

Loss of posterior mandibular vertical dimension due to developmental abnormalities, end-stage TMJ pathology, neoplasia, or traumatic injury results in a discrepancy in mandibular function, facial esthetics, and the dental occlusion. In cases where the pathology directly involves the bone and associated soft tissues of the TMJ itself, TMJR rather than osteotomy or autogenous tissue reconstruction should be considered.[24] Custom TMJR has also been successfully utilized in the management of patients with congenital abnormalities[25–29] as well as end-stage TMJ pathology, neoplasia, or traumatic injury.[30,31]

Relative Limitations and Contraindications

Age of the Patient

Since TMJR devices have no intrinsic growth capability, the benefits of their utilization in growing patients over autogenous tissue led to the assumption that their use in skeletally immature patients was contraindicated. However, recent literature suggests that further investigation into TMJR use in skeletally immature patients may be warranted.[32–38] For more than 30 years, the orthopedic literature has reported improvement in function and quality of life for skeletally immature arthritic and tumor patients with the utilization of alloplastic joint replacement devices.[39–61]

One of the major arguments against the use of TMJR devices in skeletally immature patients has been that future revision surgery will be required. Most, if not all, autogenous tissue or orthognathic reconstruction options in this population require future revision surgery. Potential revision solutions for TMJR might include (1) replacement of the entire device or just the ramus/condyle component with one of more appropriate dimensions to correct any mandibular growth related deficiency; (2) performing a ramus orthognathic procedure, such as sagittal split osteotomy or intraoral vertical ramus osteotomy, since the ramus/condyle components screw fixation for custom TMJR devices is all posterior to the mandibular foramen; or (3) hybrid osseodistraction utilizing the TMJR ramus/condyle component as one unit of a custom-designed distraction apparatus.[62]

Based on the ankylosis and overgrowth complications reported with costochondral grafting for TMJ reconstruction in skeletally immature patients, the orthopedic experience with alloplastic joint replacement in growing patients, and preliminary pediatric TMJR studies, TMJR in skeletally immature patients may be an appropriate treatment modality for the following conditions: (1) high inflammatory TMJ arthritis unresponsive to other modalities of treatment, (2) recurrent fibrosis and/or bony ankylosis unresponsive to other modalities of treatment, (3) failed tissue grafts (bone and soft tissue), and (4) loss of vertical mandibular height and/or occlusal relationship due to bony resorption, trauma, or developmental abnormalities where there is a muscular matrix, benign neoplasia, or other pathological lesions.[63,64]

Physical and Mental Status of the Patient

Is the patient physically and psychologically prepared to cope with the permanent loss of a body part? Does the patient have realistic expectations for both subjective and objective outcomes? Do they understand that revision or replacement surgery may be required in the future? Is the patient willing or able to perform the post-TMJR physical therapy required to obtain maximum functional benefit from the procedure? In orthopedic joint replacement, the strongest predictors of outcome are reported to be preoperative pain/function (patients with less severe preoperative disease obtained the best outcome), diagnosis (patients with rheumatoid arthritis did better than those with osteoarthritis), deprivation (patients from poorer areas had worse outcomes), and anxiety/depression (patients with anxiety/depression were associated with less pain relief); older patients and women had poorer outcomes.[65–67] Further, the orthopedic literature also reveals that the greater number of preoperative comorbidities, the poorer the outcomes.[68–71]

These reports are consistent with TMJ patient data demonstrating that the presence of comorbid conditions explain why 50% of patients seeking care for TMJ pain, some of whom are multiply operated and/or were exposed to failed materials or devices, still report experiencing pain 5 years later and that 20% of chronic pain patients experience long-term disability from their pain.[72–76]

Therefore, it is absolutely essential that both surgeon and patient understand that the primary goal of TMJR is restoration of mandibular function and form, not complete pain relief. Any notable decrease in pain will only be a secondary benefit that may occur in some cases. When surgeons promise 100% pain relief, this only intensifies any unreasonable, unrealistic, and unattainable outcome expectations patients may already have developed.[77] Other variables that the clinician must consider are any pending litigation related to the onset of TMJ symptoms, drug or alcohol abuse resulting from chronic pain, and the patient's willingness to comply with the total TMJR management plan. Knowledge of those issues and the effects that prior management failures, comorbid conditions, genetics, and chronic centrally mediated pain have on patients allows clinicians to manage more appropriately any functional or end-stage disease process.

Uncontrolled Systemic Disease

As with any alloplastic implant, dental, orthopedic or TMJ, patients with potentially compromising medical comorbid conditions must have the condition brought under control and a risk/benefit ratio determined by the surgeon in discussions with the patient before plans proceed for TMJR surgery. Patients with significant comorbid conditions, when implanted, should be monitored closely postoperatively for complications.

Active Infection at the Implantation Site

As with any alloplast material, implantation into an infected or contaminated area can result in failure of the components of the device to stabilize, leading to micromotion and catastrophic failure under functional loading. *Cutibacterium acnes* (formerly *Propionibacterium acnes*) has increasingly become recognized as a causative agent of periarticular TMJR infection. *C. acnes* is a Gram-positive bacterium that forms part of the normal flora of the skin, oral cavity, large intestine, the conjunctiva, and the external auditory canal. Although primarily recognized for its role in acne, *C. acnes* is an opportunistic pathogen, causing a range of postoperative and device-related infections. Surgeons should consider *C. acnes* as a risk for infection in patients, especially those with a history of chronic acne or acne vulgaris.[78]

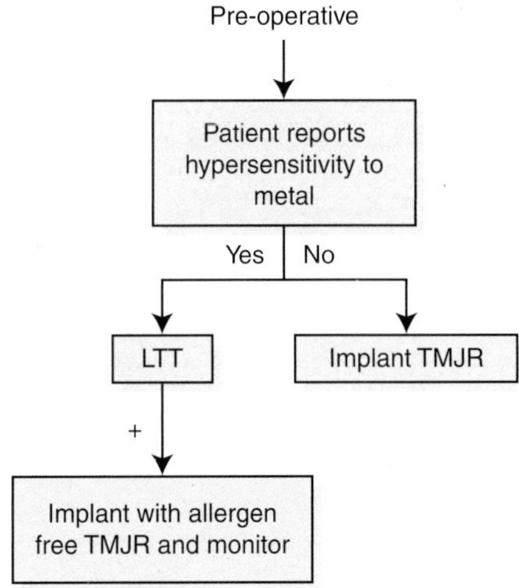

Figure 147.1 Pre-TMJR hypersensitivity testing algorithm. *LTT*, Lymphocyte transformation test; *TMJR*, temporomandibular joint replacement. (Modified from Christensen TJ, Samant SA, Shin AY. Making sense of metal allergy and hypersensitivity to metallic implants in relation to hand surgery. *J Hand Surg Am*. 2017;42:737 and Mercuri and Caicedo. Material Hypersensitivity and TMJ Replacement. *J Oral Maxillofac Surg*. 2019;77:1371–1376.)

Documented Hypersensitivity to TMJR Materials

Documented hypersensitivity to the materials typically used in the production of TMJR device components, commercially pure titanium (cpTi), titanium alloy (Ti6V4Al ELI), cobalt-chrome-molybdenum alloy (CoCrMo), and ultra-high molecular weight polyethylene (UHMWPE), is rare. Although approximately 10% of the population can be sensitive to the nickel (<1%) in the CoCrMo alloy, far fewer reports of such allergic reactions have been reported in the orthopedic literature.[79] Historically, there have been two testing modalities that have been used to diagnose hypersensitivity to implanted metals: skin patch testing (SPT) and the lymphocyte transformation test (LTT). SPT tests for hypersensitivity utilize macrophages (Langerhans cells) within the dermis, which are much different than the lymphocytic response cells found in deeper tissues (T lymphocytes) where joint implants are located. In addition, the interpretation of SPT results is purely subjective as there is no verified standard scoring system.[80,81] Skin testing using intradermal metal disks has been determined to be unreliable and is not recommended.[82]

The limitations of SPT led researchers to find another test to confirm preimplantation metal allergy. It has been demonstrated that the LTT measures the ability of lymphocytes to proliferate in the presence and the absence of a metal ion stimulus cultured with a patient's peripheral blood lymphocytes. Investigators have also used the LTT to evaluate orthopedic implant patients with symptoms indicating potential hypersensitivity to their implants to identify patients who might benefit from implant removal and replacement with components composed of nonreactive materials.[83] Currently, the diagnosis of alloplastic joint replacement material hypersensitivity appears to be one of exclusion, and there are no available validated management algorithms for the management of such cases. However, based on a review of the available orthopedic literature, a practical workup and management approach for hypersensitivity algorithm for TMJR were developed[84] (Fig. 147.1). Hypersensitivity testing prior to primary TMJR can be helpful when a patient reports a history of intolerance to jewelry or an allergic reaction to a prior metal implant. However, to date, routine testing is not supported by the literature.[84,85]

TECHNIQUE KEY POINTS: Custom TMJR

Patient and Operating Room Preparation

- After the proper diagnosis has been made indicating the need for TMJR and the patient's informed consent is obtained, the process of designing and manufacturing custom TMJR components can begin. The patient undergoes a protocol computed tomography (CT) scan from which a stereolithographic acrylic (SLA) model is developed. This model serves as the template for the design and manufacture of the patient-fitted custom TMJR components (Fig. 147.2).
- The surgeon and design engineer use the SLA model for planning the design for the TMJR device and any applicable host bone modifications (Fig. 147.3).
- In some cases, especially those involving combined TMJR and orthognathic procedures, a virtual surgical planning conference can be scheduled to coordinate the case planning.[86,87] The surgeon approves the surgical plan and implant design, and the custom TMJR components are manufactured, sterilized, and forwarded to the hospital.

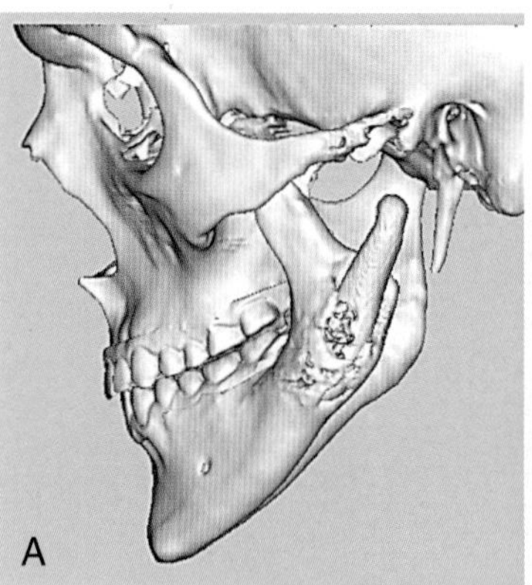

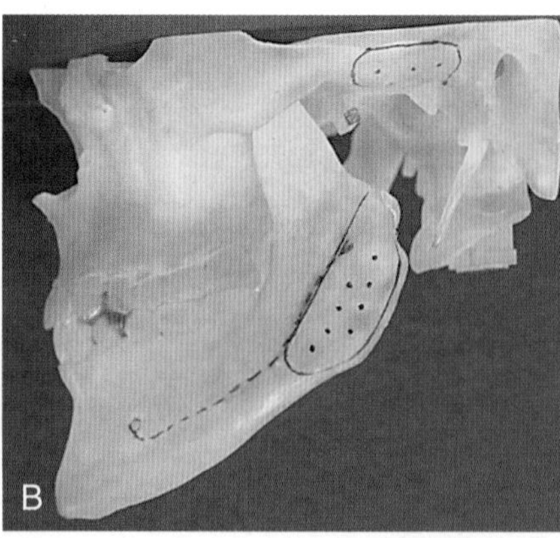

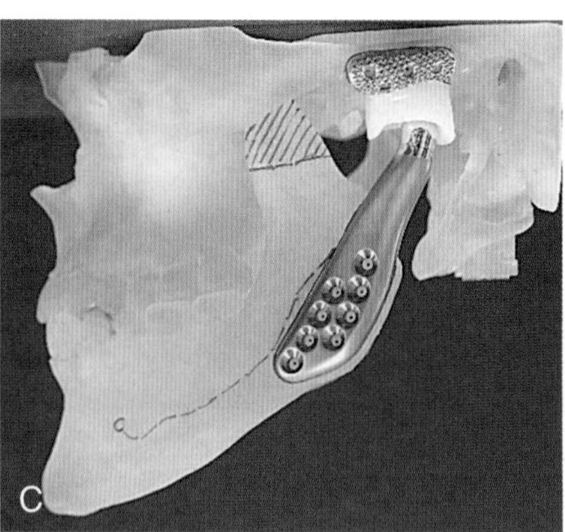

Figure 147.2 **A,** Failed autogenous graft stereolithographic acrylic (SLA) model. **B,** Component design. **C,** Completed custom temporomandibular joint replacement (TMJR).

TECHNIQUE KEY POINTS: Custom TMJR—*cont'd*

- While a CT arteriogram (CTA) is not necessary for every TMJ ankylosis case, it should be considered when the preoperative CT demonstrates possible involvement of the internal maxillary artery itself or any of its major branches in the planned surgical procedure.[88,89]
- Patients should be advised to wash their hair with mild shampoo before surgery and not use any hair sprays, gels, or facial makeup.
- The use of prophylactic antibiotics is the most important factor in preventing a periprosthetic joint infection. To reach the minimum inhibitory concentration in the end organs during surgery, the optimum time for weight-adjusted prophylactic antibiotic administration is 1 hour prior to the surgery.[90–92] A first- or second-generation cephalosporin is suggested. The timing can be extended up to 2 hours for vancomycin and fluoroquinolones.[93]
- Hair in the area of the preauricular incision should be sheared, not razored. Any remaining hair, the eyes, the auditory canal(s), and mouth should be appropriately isolated from the surgical field using adhesive iodine-impregnated drapes.
- Any maxillomandibular fixation (MMF) system can be positioned after general anesthesia induction and before the patient is prepped and draped for the sterile implantation procedure. The patient should not be placed into MMF at this stage of the procedure to allow for free movement of the mandible during the implantation procedure.
- All instruments and rotatory equipment used intraorally to apply MMF appliances, remove teeth, or to harvest autogenous abdominal fat must be strictly isolated from those used to implant the TMJR device components.[93]
- After removal from their sterile packaging under sterile conditions, it is the author's recommendation that the TMJR components be placed in a 1 g vancomycin/500 cc saline solution to soak during the procedure. After implantation of the TMJR components, the vancomycin solution should be used to irrigate the preauricular and retromandibular incisions thoroughly before closure.[94]

Custom TMJR Implantation

- The standard preauricular and retromandibular incisions, dissections, and steps for the implantation of the temporal fossa and ramus/condyle components of the TMJ Concepts custom TMJR system have been well documented and described.[95]
- To determine the anterior extent of the preauricular dissection, refer to the SLA model that should be available in the operating room. Sterilizing the anatomic bone model and handling during surgery in the sterile field is not recommended.
- Custom TMJR ramus/condyle and fossa components are patient fitted. Therefore, to avoid implantation errors, it is essential that the surgeon prepare the fossa and ramus host bone properly so that each component interfaces with the host bone as planned (Fig. 147.4). This is especially important at the medial aspect of the fossa; otherwise, the medial aspect of the fossa will lie away from the bone, resulting in an inappropriate or more lateral bearing relationship of the ramus/condyle component condylar head to the fossa. Using the fossa seating tool is important during fossa seating to ensure it is fully seated against the bone and does not "rock" (Fig. 147.5).
- The retromandibular incision provides not only good access to the mandibular ramus for implanting the TMJR ramus/condyle component but also access to the external carotid artery should uncontrollable hemorrhage arise from the internal maxillary artery or any of its branches.[96] Therefore, this incision and dissection to bone should be completed before condyle resection, especially in ankylosis cases.
- A subparotid rather than a transparotid dissection should be used to prevent contamination of the ramus/condyle component implant site by saliva and prevent potential postoperative sialocele formation.[97,98]
- There must be a minimum of 15 mm gap between the mandibular condylar resection and the height of the articular eminence area to accommodate the anterior flange of the TMJ Concepts fossa component (Fig. 147.6).

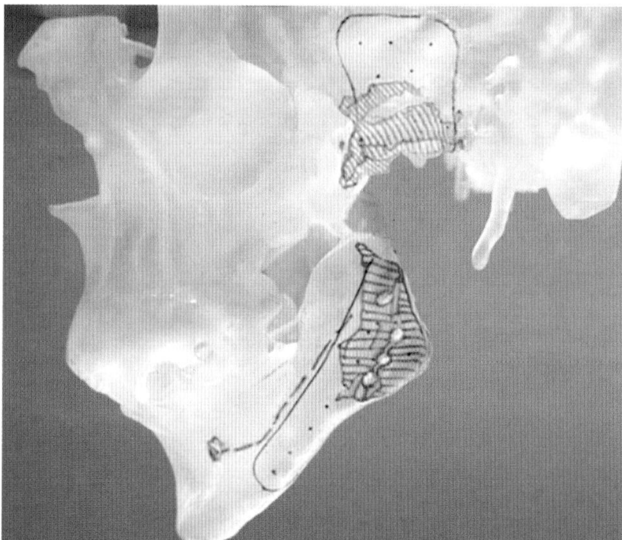

Figure 147.3 Areas marked in red on the preplanned stereolithographic acrylic (SLA) model showing where lateral mandibular ramus and fossa recontouring are required at implantation to obtain "best fit" for each component.

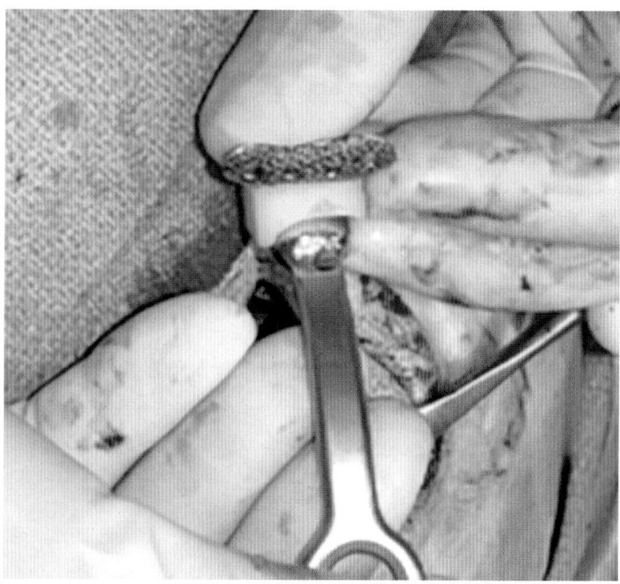

Figure 147.5 The fossa tool seating used to seat and confirm the passive positioning of this component without any movement and stabilizing the implant during fixation.

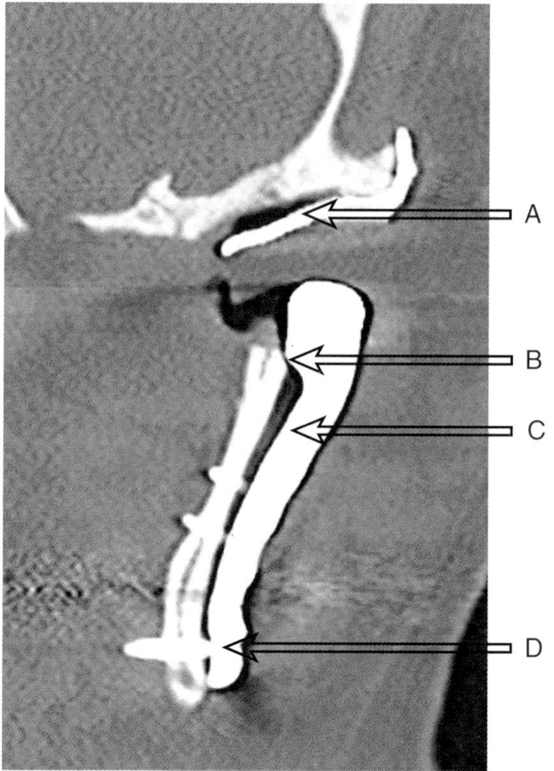

Figure 147.4 Errors to be avoided during implantation of custom temporomandibular joint replacement (TMJR) components. **A,** Incomplete removal of soft tissue from the medial aspect of the fossa preventing the fossa component from seating properly. **B,** Inadequate removal of bone at the superior aspect of the mandibular ramus preventing the ramus/condyle component from seating properly. **C,** The most superior screw is not placed. **D,** Improper screw length.

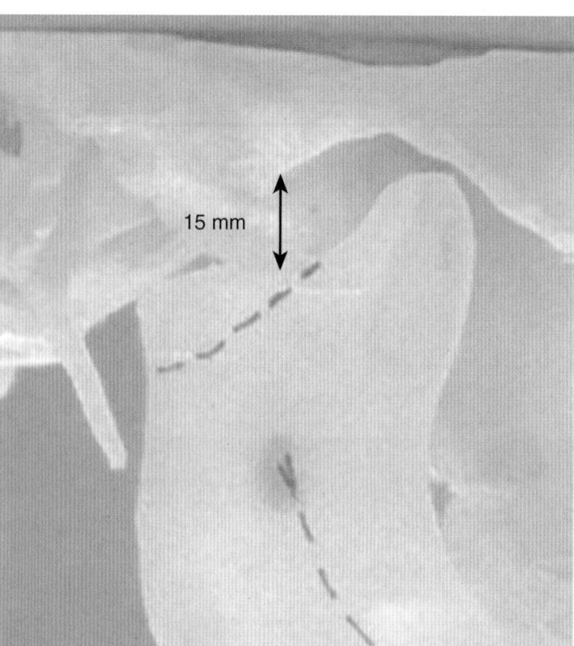

Figure 147.6 There must be a minimum of 15 mm gap between the mandibular condylar resection and the height of the articular eminence area to accommodate the anterior flange of the patient-fitted fossa component.

TECHNIQUE KEY POINTS: Custom TMJR—*cont'd*

- Custom TMJR ramus/condyle and fossa components are designed and manufactured to have a precise articulation. Therefore, the surgeon must be sure to fixate the components with the patient in the proper planned occlusion.
- Finite element analysis has confirmed that the maximum functional forces placed on a TMJR condyle/ramus component during function is concentrated at the most superior screw hole.[99] Therefore, the most superior screw is important for stabilization during function.
- The screw lengths are recommended for bicortical fixation and to avoid functional irritation of the medial pterygoid muscle or temporalis muscle by overextended screw tips. If a screw hole should happen to strip out or the quality of the host bone is poor, rescue screws provided in the instrumentation kit should be used. Loose screws should never be left in place. All screws should be placed and retightened before closure (Fig. 147.7).
- When drilling the pilot holes for the self-tapping fixation screws, the drill guide must be used to ensure that each drill hole is centered properly; otherwise, there is the possibility that the shoulder of the screw will prematurely contact the ramus condyle plate causing the screw to fracture at its collar as the screw is hand tightened into its recessed position in the plate. Slow speed and copious irrigation are essential as these holes are drilled to ensure that the bone retaining the screws remains viable (Fig. 147.8).
- If an autogenous fat graft is utilized, it must be packed all around the articulation (Fig. 147.9). A Penfield neurosurgical elevator works well to maneuver the fat medially.
- All wounds should be copiously irrigated with the remaining vancomycin solution and closed carefully in layers. Drains are typically not required.
- An intraoperative anterior-posterior skull image is advised to document proper component articulation, screw orientation, and placement (Fig. 147.10).
- While the patient is still under anesthesia, the auditory canal(s) and tympanic membrane(s) should be inspected with an ear speculum to ensure there was no intraoperative accumulation of irrigation fluid, blood, or inadvertent communication created between the TMJ area and these structures. This inspection should be documented in the operative notes. Blood clots should be removed with gentle, warm irrigation and careful suction. Instillation of antibiotic/steroid otic drops and occlusion of the external auditory canal with a cotton pledget are recommended to decrease the potential for the development of infection or inflammatory pain.
- Due to obscure involvement of the pathology with the auditory canal, perforation, tearing of the cartilaginous auditory canal or the tympanic membrane can occur. Should any of these occur or be discovered on inspection, consultation with an otolaryngologist is advised to determine the best management option.
- In cases where bilateral hyperplastic coronoid processes are removed (rheumatoid, ankylosis, condylar resorption, etc.), light training elastics maintained for 1 week will prevent potential TMJR dislocation.
- A pressure dressing should be applied and kept in place for 24 hours. When the pressure dressing is removed, the wounds should be cleansed at least twice daily with a 50:50 mixture of H_2O:H_2O_2 using a sterile cotton swab followed by a light coating of antiseptic ointment until the sutures are removed.

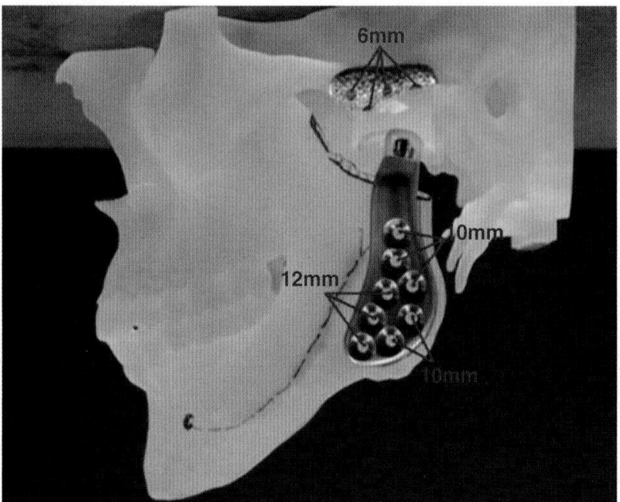

Figure 147.7 Patient-fitted temporomandibular joint replacement (TMJR) device on SLA model with exact fixation screw lengths indicated.

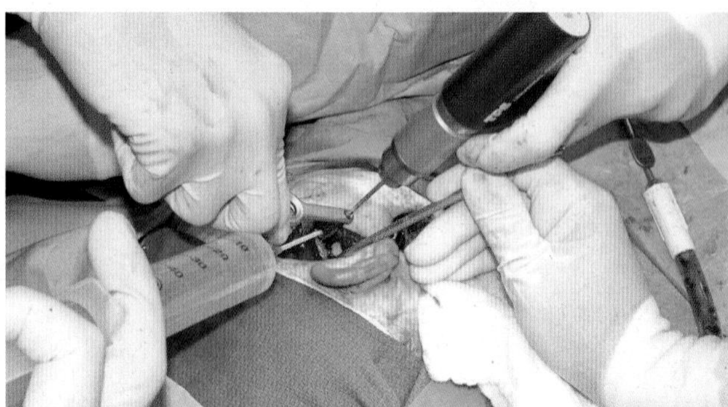

Figure 147.8 A slow-speed drill and drill guide used to prepare a screw hole into the host temporal and mandibular bones. Copious irrigation is essential as these holes are drilled to ensure that the bone retaining the screws remains viable.

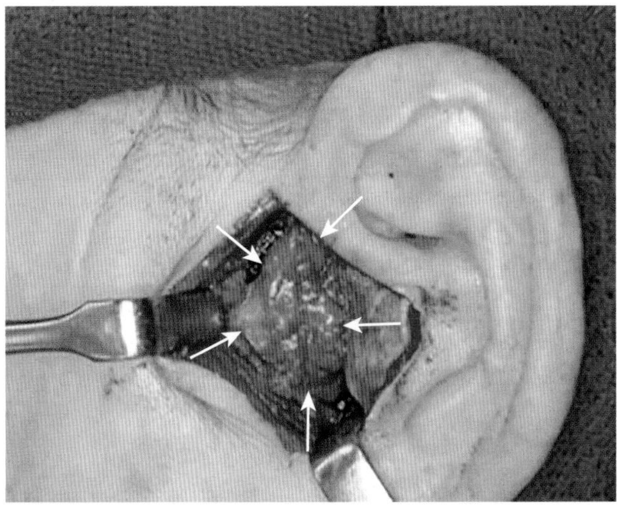

Figure 147.9 Packing autogenous fat around the articulation of a temporomandibular joint replacement (TMJR) to decrease the potential for development of heterotopic bone formation. (Wolford LM, Karras SC. Autologous fat transplantation around TMJ total joint prostheses: preliminary treatment outcomes. *J Oral Maxillofac Surg.* 1997;55:245.)

Management of Common Complications

Infection

The infection rate for TMJR devices has been reported to be 1.86%.[100]

Three types of TMJR postoperative infections can occur:

1. Superficial infections. It is recommended that "stitch abscesses" and seromas be aggressively managed before the organisms involved affect the deeper tissues and TMJR components.
2. Early deep infections. The earlier the diagnosis is made after TMJR surgery (2 to 5 days) and managed, following an aggressive early management protocol (Fig. 147.11), the greater the chance of salvaging the TMJR device.
3. Late deep infections. When signs and symptoms of infection appear weeks to months after TMJR implantation, a biofilm infection is the most likely culprit.[101] Management using the modified late management protocol (Fig. 147.12) is recommended.

Heterotopic Ossification

The incidence of heterotopic ossification associated with a TMJR is reported to be 0.58%.[102] Heterotopic bone formation is the presence of bone in the soft tissue surrounding a joint replacement device where bone normally does not exist, leading to decreased joint mobility and pain. History and imaging are used to distinguish it from other diagnostic possibilities. As prophylaxis, a nonsteroidal antiinflammatory drug (such as indomethacin), a diphosphonate (such as ethane-1-hydroxy-1,1-diphosphate), and local radiation therapy have all been recommended.[102] Surgical removal of

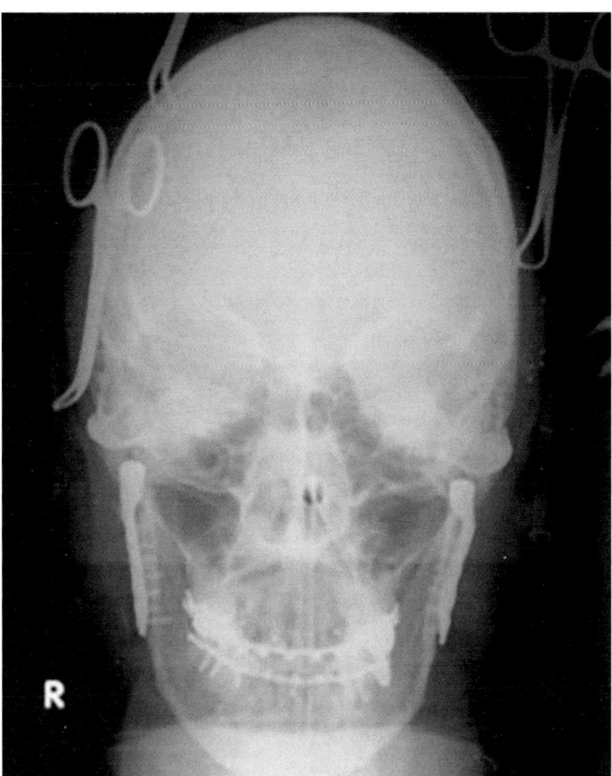

Figure 147.10 Intraoperative anterior-posterior skull imaging confirmation of component alignment, position, and fixation.

Early protocol
1. Infection identified
2. Broad-spectrum antibiotics started
3. Infectious disease consult
4. Surgery a. I/D, C&S, debridement b. Prosthesis scrubbed with toothbrush and betadine solution c. Placement of irrigating catheters/drains for 4–5 days
5. Irrigation of catheters Q4h with DAB for 4–5 days, then catheters/drains removed
6. PICC line placed
7. IV antibiotic therapy based on C&S
8. Outpatient IV antibiotics for 4–6 weeks

Key: I/D, incision and drainage; C&S, culture and sensitivity; DAB, double antibiotic solution (neomycin and polymyxin B).

Figure 147.11 Early temporomandibular joint (TMJ) total joint replacement (TJR) infection protocol. (Mercuri LG. Avoiding and managing temporomandibular joint total joint replacement surgical site infections. *J Oral Maxillofac Surg.* 2012;70:2280–2289.)

the heterotopic bone has been endorsed to preserve joint mobility, but heterotopic bone formation is likely to recur and possibly progress. Therefore, for prophylaxis in TMJR, it is recommended that an autogenous fat graft be packed around the TMJR articulation to decrease potential recurrence[103,104] (Fig. 147.9).

Late protocol
1. Infection identified
2. Broad-spectrum antibiotics started
3. Infectious disease consult
4. Surgery stage I a. I/D, C&S, debridement, device removed b. Placement of PMMA/tobramycin spacer
5. PICC line placed
6. IV antibiotic therapy based on C&S
7. Outpatient IV antibiotics for 6–8 weeks
8. Surgery stage II Replacement with new device at 8–10 weeks
9. IV antibiotics until discharge

Key: I/D, incision and drainage; C&S, culture and sensitivity; DAB, double antibiotic solution (neomycin and polymyxin B).

Figure 147.12 Late infection temporomandibular joint (TMJ) total joint replacement (TJR) protocol. (Mercuri LG. Avoiding and managing temporomandibular joint total joint replacement surgical site infections. *J Oral Maxillofac Surg*. 2012;70:2280–2289.)

Material Hypersensitivity

Long-term TMJR follow-up data reveal a reported postoperative material sensitivity of 0.14%.[84] Should a post-TMJR patient be documented by LTT as sensitive to any nickel containing alloy metal (CoCr alloy) used in the manufacture of a TMJR device (Fig. 147.13), the metal components of a replacement TMJR should be manufactured from a nonreactive material.

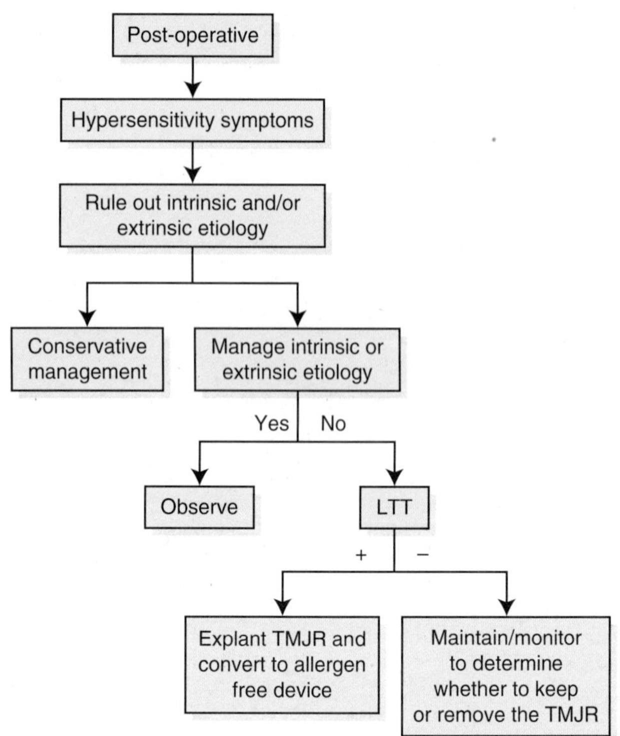

Key: LTT – lymphocyte transformation test.

Figure 147.13 Post-TMJR hypersensitivity testing algorithm. *LTT*, Lymphocyte transformation test; *TMJR*, temporomandibular joint replacement. (Mercuri LG, Caicedo MS. Material hypersensitivity and TMJ replacement. *J Oral Maxillofac Surg*. 2019; 77:1371–1376. Modified from Christensen TJ, Samant SA, Shin AY. Making sense of metal allergy and hypersensitivity to metallic implants in relation to hand surgery. *J Hand Surg Am*. 2017;42:737–746.)

Post-TMJR Chronic Pain

Persistent or chronic postsurgical pain can become both a significant clinical and economic issue. While the estimated mean incidence varies between 10% and 50% relative to a variety of surgical procedures, to date it has been rarely reported post-TMJR (0.43%).[105]

Acute pain almost always originates from nociception in somatic or visceral tissues (intrinsic pain); however, not every pain sensation originates from nociception (extrinsic pain).[106] After TMJR, there may be both intrinsic and extrinsic causes for pain. The surgeon must rule each out in a systematic manner to manage the etiology appropriately (Fig. 147.14).

Intrinsic Causes for Post-TMJR Pain

The Biologic Response to Metal Implants report states that when working up a patient with a painful total joint, hypersensitivity should be the last item on the list, since the literature clearly demonstrates that 1% or less of joint replacement device failures are causally related to material hypersensitivity.[107] Therefore, the most common causes for post-TMJR pain, infection, heterotopic ossification, micromotion, and loose hardware must be ruled out first. However, there are two other potential intrinsic causes of post-TMJR chronic pain: synovial impingement and an adverse local tissue response to material wear, both of which mimic hypersensitivity and should be ruled out before TMJR removal and replacement.

Synovial impingement syndrome has been reported as a cause of pain and dysfunction after orthopedic joint replacement.[108–111] After any joint replacement, a pseudosynovium develops. Westermark et al. and Monje et al. demonstrated this in TMJR patients.[112,113] Further, Murakami et al. demonstrated synovial plicae as invaginations of synovial tissue in the TMJ similar to those found in the hip and knee.[114] Davis et al. presented arthroscopic images of inflamed synovial plicae entrapped between the bearing surface of TMJR devices in patients with post-TMJR pain and dysfunction and demonstrated that the early clinical outcomes of arthroscopic management are with decreasing pain and increasing the MIO.[115] Larger studies with longer follow-up are needed to further classify the different causes of prosthetic failure and advance the approaches to management. TMJR arthroscopy should be reserved only for surgeons with level 3 arthroscopy skills.

Although rare in TMJR due to minimal functional TMJ loading compared with hips and knees, material wear results in the release of material wear particles and ions leading to synovial and periarticular soft-tissue inflammation.[116] Therefore, this local tissue response may act as another source

Intrinsic etiology	Extrinsic etiology
Infection	Prior misdiagnosis
Heterotopic bone formation	Chronic centrally mediated pain
Dislocation	Persistent myofascial/muscular pain
Material sensitivity	Complex regional pain syndrome I
Aseptic component or screw loosening	Neurologic injury (CPRS II)
Component or screw fracture	Temporalis tendonitis
Osteolysis	Coronoid impingement
Neuroma formation	Frey's neuralgia
Synovial entrapment syndrome	Integrin formation

Figure 147.14 Intrinsic and extrinsic causes for post-TMJ TJR pain. (*Mercuri LG. Complications associated with TMJ TJR: management and prevention. In: Mercuri LG (ed). Temporomandibular Joint Total Joint Replacement—TMJ TJR: A Comprehensive Reference for Researchers, Material Scientists and Surgeons. New York, NY: Springer, 2016.*)

of post-TMJR pain and dysfunction. Diagnostic local anesthesia infiltration may be diagnostic and careful debridement can be therapeutic.

Extrinsic Causes for Post-TMJR Pain

It is noteworthy that many of these painful and dysfunctional post-TMJR patients have been multiply operated and/or misdiagnosed as muscular TMD patients with multiple comorbidities and persistent centrally mediated muscle pain. A multicenter cross-sectional study to identify preoperative risk factors for pain at rest and with activity after total hip and knee replacement stated that moderate to severe pain was reported by 20% at rest and 33% with activity. Among the significant predictors for postoperative pain at rest were female sex, increased severity of preoperative pain in the hip or knee area, and preoperative use of opioids. Predictors for postoperative pain with activity were severity of the preoperative hip and/or knee pain, preoperative use of anticonvulsants and antidepressants, and prior previous hip/knee surgery.[117]

A prospective study of knee replacement patients identified possible predictors of outcome 6 months postoperatively. The strongest predictors of outcome were preoperative pain with function: those with less severe preoperative disease obtained the best outcome; diagnosis: those with rheumatoid arthritis did better than those with osteoarthritis; social status: economically needier patients had worse outcomes; and mental status: anxiety/depression were associated with poorer pain symptom relief.[118]

The orthopedic literature also reveals that the greater number of preoperative comorbidities, the poorer the outcomes.[119–122] These data are consistent with TMJ disorder data that demonstrated that the presence of comorbid conditions may perhaps explain why 50% of patients seeking care for TMJ pain, some of whom were multiply operated and/or exposed to failed materials or devices, still report experiencing pain 5 years later, and 20% of chronic TMJ pain patients experience long-term disability from their pain.[123–125]

The appropriate overall management of patients requiring TMJR requires the surgeon make the correct diagnosis and understand the patient's associated predictors of outcomes, especially any comorbid conditions. Then the surgeon must perform the surgery at the right time, correctly and aseptically, utilizing the appropriate TMJR system. This assures the results will be professionally satisfying for the surgeon and, most importantly, provide the best outcome for the patient.

Postoperative Considerations

Early active physical therapy, either with commercially available jaw-exercising devices or other methods, is essential to successful future function, especially in ankylosis cases.

While the American College of Surgeons stated there was no evidence that postoperative antibiotic decreased surgical site infections, an exception was made for orthopedic joint replacement.[90] Therefore, an antibiotic (first- or second-generation cephalosporin) that covers the spectrum of potential skin, ear, and saliva contaminants is recommended for 7 to 10 days postoperatively.[93]

Surgeons should educate the patient and relatives regarding proper wound care, personal hygiene, the early signs of a surgical site infection, and the importance of reporting symptoms to the surgeons as soon as they arise. Preprinted post-TMJR instructional and FAQs encompassing these issues should be provided on discharge.

References

1. Mercuri LG. History of TMJ TJR. In: Mercuri LG, ed. *Temporomandibular Joint Total Joint Replacement—TMJ TJR—A Comprehensive Reference for Researchers, Material Scientists and Surgeons*. New York: Springer; 2016:44–52.
2. Henry CH, Wolford LM. Treatment outcomes for temporomandibular joint reconstruction after Proplast-Teflon implant failure. *J Oral Maxillofac Surg*. 1993;51(4):352–358.
3. Mercuri LG. The TMJ Concepts patient fitted total temporomandibular joint reconstruction prosthesis. In: Donlon WC, ed. *Oral and Maxillofacial Surgery Clinics of North America*. 2000;12:73–91.
4. https://www.fda.gov/medical-devices/overview-device-regulation/classify-your-medical-device.
5. Mercuri LG, Wolford LM, Sanders B, White RD, Hurder A, Henderson W. Custom CAD/CAM total temporomandibular joint reconstruction system: preliminary multicenter report. *J Oral Maxillofac Surg*. 1995;53(2):106–115.
6. https://www.accessdata.fda.gov/cdrh_docs/pdf/P980052A.pdf.
7. Mercuri LG, Wolford LM, Sanders B, White RD, Giobbie-Hurder A. Long-term follow-up of the CAD/CAM patient fitted total temporomandibular joint reconstruction system. *J Oral Maxillofac Surg*. 2002;60(12):1440–1448.
8. Mercuri LG, Giobbe-Hurder A. Long term outcomes after total alloplastic TMJ reconstruction following exposure to failed materials. *J Oral Maxillofac Surg*. 2004;62:1088–1096.
9. Mercuri LG, Edibam NR, Giobbie-Hurder A. Fourteen-year follow-up of a patient-fitted total temporomandibular joint reconstruction system. *J Oral Maxillofac Surg*. 2007;65(6):1140–1148.
10. Wolford LM, Mercuri LG, Schneiderman ED, Movahed R, Allen W. Twenty-year follow-up study on a patient-fitted temporomandibular joint prosthesis: the Techmedica/TMJ Concepts device. *J Oral Maxillofac Surg*. 2015;73(5):952–960.
11. Mercuri LG. Custom TMJ TJR devices. In: Mercuri LG, ed. *Temporomandibular Joint Total Joint Replacement—TMJ TJR—A Comprehensive Reference for Researchers, Material Scientists and Surgeons*. New York: Springer; 2016:91–132.
12. Mercuri LG, Abramowicz S. Temporomandibular joint arthritic disease. In: Farah C, Balasubramaniam R, McCullough M, eds. *Contemporary Oral Medicine*. New York: Springer; 2018:1919–1954.
13. Mercuri LG. Surgical management of TMJ arthritis. In: Laskin DM, Greene CS, Hylander WL, eds. *Temporomandibular Joint Disorders: An Evidence-Based Approach to Diagnosis and Treatment*. Chicago: Quintessence; 2006:455–468.
14. Chapman MW, James MA. *Chapman's Comprehensive Orthopedic Surgery*. 4th ed. London: JP Medical Ltd; 2019.
15. Canale ST, Beaty JH. *Campbell's Operative Orthopaedics*. 12th ed. St. Louis: Mosby; 2012.
16. Matsuura H, Miyamoto H, Ishimaru J, Kurita K, Goss AN. Effect of partial immobilization on reconstruction of ankylosis of the temporomandibular joint with an autogenous costochondral graft: an experimental study in sheep. *Br J Oral Maxillofac Surg*. 2001;39(3):196–203.
17. Mercuri LG. Costochondral graft versus total alloplastic joint for TMJ reconstruction. In: Laskin DM, Renapukar SK, eds. *Current Controversies in the Management of Temporomandibular Disorders*. Philadelphia, Pennsylvania: Elsevier; 2018.
18. Movahed R, Mercuri LG. Management of temporomandibular joint ankylosis. *Oral Maxillofac Surg Clin North Am*. 2015;27(1):27–35.
19. Mercuri LG. Alloplastic temporomandibular joint reconstruction. *Oral Surg Oral Med Oral Pathol Oral Radiol Endod*. 1998;85(6):631–637.
20. Hawkins A, Mercuri LG, Miloro M. Are Rib grafts still used for temporomandibular joint reconstruction? *J Oral Maxillofac Surg*. 2020;78(2):195–202.
21. Mercuri LG, Anspach WE 3rd. Principles for the revision of total alloplastic TMJ prostheses. *Int J Oral Maxillofac Surg*. 2003;32(4):353–359.
22. Amarista F, Mercuri L, Perez D. TMJR revision and replacement: a survey and review of the literature. *J Oral Maxillofac Surg*. 2020.
23. Mercuri LG. Temporomandibular joint reconstruction. In: Fonseca R, ed. *Oral and Maxillofacial Surgery*. Philadelphia: Elsevier; 2008:945–960.
24. Mercuri LG. Alloplastic temporomandibular joint reconstruction. In: Bagheri SC, Bell RB, Kahn HA, eds. *Current Therapy in Oral and Maxillofacial Surgery*. Philadelphia: Elsevier; 2011:875–880.
25. Zanakis NS, Gavakos K, Faippea M, Karamanos A, Zotalis N. Application of custom-made TMJ prosthesis in hemifacial microsomia. *Int J Oral Maxillofac Implants*. 2009;38(9):988–992.
26. Schlieve T, Almusa M, Miloro M, Kolokythas A. Temporomandibular joint replacement for ankylosis correction in Nager syndrome: case report and review of the literature. *J Oral Maxillofac Surg*. 2012;70(3):616–625.
27. Wolford LM, Perez DE. Surgical management of congenital deformities with temporomandibular joint malformation. *Oral Maxillofac Surg Clin North Am*. 2015;27(1):137–154.
28. Cascone P, Vellone V, Ramieri V, Basile E, Tarsitano A, Marchetti C. Reconstruction of the adult hemifacial microsomia patient with temporomandibular joint total joint prosthesis and orthognathic surgery. *Case Rep Surg*. 2018;2018:2968983.
29. Polley JW, Girotto JA, Fahrenkopf MP, et al. Salvage or solution: alloplastic reconstruction in hemifacial microsomia. *Cleft Palate Craniofac J*. 2019;56(7):896–901.
30. Vega L, Meara D. Mandibular replacement utilizing TMJ TJR devices. In: Mercuri LG, ed. *Temporomandibular Joint Total Joint Replacement—TMJ TJR—A Comprehensive Reference for Researchers, Material Scientists and Surgeons*. New York: Springer; 2016:165–185.
31. Westermark A, Hedén P, Aagaard E, Cornelius CP. The use of TMJ Concepts prostheses to reconstruct patients with major temporomandibular joint and mandibular defects. *Int J Oral Maxillofac Implants*. 2011;40(5):487–496.
32. Mercuri LG, Swift JQ. Considerations for the use of alloplastic temporomandibular joint replacement in the growing patient. *J Oral Maxillofac Surg*. 2009;67(9):1979–1990.
33. Keyser BR, Banda AK, Mercuri LG, Warburton G, Sullivan SM. Alloplastic total temporomandibular joint replacement in skeletally immature patients: a pilot survey. *Int J Oral Maxillofac Surg*. 2020;S0901-S5027(20):30050–30053.
34. Sinn DP, Tandon R, Tiwana PS. Can alloplastic temporomandibular joint reconstruction be used in the growing patient?. A preliminary report. *J Oral Maxillofac Surg*. 2021;79:2267e1-2267.e16.
35. Granquist EJ. Treatment of the temporomandibular joint in a child with juvenile idiopathic arthritis. *Oral Maxillofac Surg Clin North Am*. 2018;30(1):97–107.
36. Resnick CM. Temporomandibular joint reconstruction in the growing child. *Oral Maxillofac Surg Clin North Am*. 2018;30(1):109–121.
37. Frid P, Resnick C, Abramowicz S, Stoustrup P, Nørholt SE. Temporomandibular Joint Juvenile Arthritis Work Group TMJaw. Surgical correction of dentofacial deformities in juvenile idiopathic arthritis: a systematic literature review. *Int J Oral Maxillofac Implants*. 2019;48(8):1032–1042.
38. Sekhoto MG, Rikhotso RE, Rajendran S. Management of unpredictable outcomes of costochondral grafts. *Int J Surg Case Rep*. 2019;62:144–149.
39. Arden GP, Ansell BM, Hunter MJ. Total hip replacement in juvenile chronic polyarthritis and ankylosing spondylitis. *Clin Orthop Relat Res*. 1972;84(84):130–136.
40. Aufranc OE. Surgery of the hip in rheumatoid arthritis and osteoarthritis. *Bull Rheum Dis*. 1964;14:335–338.
41. Bosquet M, Burssens A, Mulier JC. Long term follow-up results of a femoral megaprosthesis. A review of thirteen patients. *Arch Orthop Trauma Surg*. 1980;97(4):299–304.
42. Bsila RS, Inglis AE, Ranawat CS. Joint replacement surgery in patients under thirty. *J Bone Joint Surg Am*. 1976;58(8):1098–1104.

43. Carpenter EB. Resection of the proximal third of the femur for chondrosarcoma in a child: replacement with a metallic prosthesis. Case report. *J Bone Joint Surg Am.* 1979;61(4):628–630.
44. Halley DK, Charnley J. Results of low friction arthroplasty in patients thirty years of age or younger. *Clin Orthop Relat Res.* 1975;112:180–191.
45. Kitsoulis PB, Stafilas KS, Siamopoulou A, Soucacos PN, Xenakis TA. Total hip arthroplasty in children with juvenile chronic arthritis: long-term results. *J Pediatr Orthop.* 2006;26(1):8–12.
46. Manfrini M, Innocenti M, Ceruso M, Mercuri M. Original biological reconstruction of the hip in a 4-year-old girl. *Lancet.* 2003;361(9352):140–142.
47. Manoso MW, Boland PJ, Healey JH, Tyler W, Morris CD. Acetabular development after bipolar hemiarthroplasty for osteosarcoma in children. *J Bone Joint Surg Br.* 2005;87(12):1658–1662.
48. Ruddlesdin C, Ansell BM, Arden GP, Swann M. Total hip replacement in children with juvenile chronic arthritis. *J Bone Joint Surg Br.* 1986;68(2):218–222.
49. Salvati EA, Wilson PD Jr. Long-term results of femoral-head replacement. *J Bone Joint Surg Am.* 1973;55(3):516–524.
50. Sim FH, Chao EY. Hip salvage by proximal femoral replacement. *J Bone Joint Surg Am.* 1981;63(8):1228–1239.
51. Singsen BH, Isaacson AS, Bernstein BH, et al. Total hip replacement in children with arthritis. *Arthritis Rheum.* 1978;21(4):401–406.
52. van Kampen M, Grimer RJ, Carter SR, Tillman RM, Abudu A. Replacement of the hip in children with a tumor in the proximal part of the femur. *J Bone Joint Surg Am.* 2008;90(4):785–795.
53. Winkelmann WW. Type-B-IIIa hip rotationplasty: an alternative operation for the treatment of malignant tumors of the femur in early childhood. *J Bone Joint Surg Am.* 2000;82(6):814–828.
54. Witt JD, Swann M, Ansell BM. Total hip replacement for juvenile chronic arthritis. *J Bone Joint Surg Br.* 1991;73(5):770–773.
55. Donati D, Zavatta M, Gozzi E, Giacomini S, Campanacci L, Mercuri M. Modular prosthetic replacement of the proximal femur after resection of a bone tumour a long-term follow-up. *J Bone Joint Surg Br.* 2001;83(8):1156–1160.
56. Cage DJ, Granberry WM, Tullos HS. Long-term results of total arthroplasty in adolescents with debilitating polyarthropathy. *Clin Orthop Relat Res.* 1992;283:156–162.
57. Bessette BJ, Fassier F, Tanzer M, Brooks CE. Total hip arthroplasty in patients younger than 21 years: a minimum, 10-year follow-up. *Can J Surg.* 2003;46(4):257–262.
58. Wroblewski BM, Purbach B, Siney PD, Fleming PA. Charnley low-friction arthroplasty in teenage patients: the ultimate challenge. *J Bone Joint Surg Br.* 2010;92(4):486–488.
59. Tsukanaka M, Halvorsen V, Nordsletten L, et al. Implant survival and radiographic outcome of total hip replacement in patients less than 20 years old. *Acta Orthop.* 2016;87(5):479–484.
60. Levin AS, Arkader A, Morris CD. Reconstruction following tumor resections in skeletally immature patients. *J Am Acad Orthop Surg.* 2017;25(3):204–213.
61. Tsuda Y, Tsoi K, Stevenson JD, Fujiwara T, Tillman R, Abudu A. Extendable endoprostheses in skeletally immature patients: a study of 124 children surviving more than 10 years after resection of bone sarcomas. *J Bone Joint Surg Am.* 2020;102(2):151–162.
62. Cascone P, Basile E, Angeletti D, Vellone V, Ramieri V, PECRAM Study Group. TMJ replacement utilizing patient-fitted TMJ TJR devices in a re-ankylosis child. *J Craniomaxillofac Surg.* 2016;44(4):493–499.
63. Movahed R, Mercuri LG. Management of temporomandibular joint ankylosis. *Oral Maxillofac Surg Clin North Am.* 2015;27(1):27–35.
64. Wolford L, Movahed R, Teschke M, Fimmers R, Havard D, Schneiderman E. Temporomandibular joint ankylosis can be successfully treated with TMJ Concepts patient-fitted total joint prosthesis and autogenous fat grafts. *J Oral Maxillofac Surg.* 2016;74(6):1215–1227.
65. Judge A, Arden NK, Cooper C, et al. Predictors of outcomes of total knee replacement surgery. *Rheumatology (Oxford).* 2012;51(10):1804–1813.
66. Mehta SP, Perruccio AV, Palaganas M, Davis AM. Do women have poorer outcomes following total knee replacement? *Osteoarthritis Cartilage.* 2015;23(9):1476–1482.
67. Brummett CM, Urquhart AG, Hassett AL, et al. Characteristics of fibromyalgia independently predict poorer long-term analgesic outcomes following total knee and hip arthroplasty. *Arthritis Rheumatol.* 2015;67(5):1386–1394.
68. Jones CA, Voaklander DC, Suarez-Alma ME. Determinants of function after total knee arthroplasty. *Phys Ther.* 2003;83(8):696–706.
69. Lingard EA, Katz JN, Wright EA, Sledge CB, Kinemax Outcomes Group. Predicting the outcome of total knee arthroplasty. *J Bone Joint Surg Am.* 2004;86(10):2179–2186.
70. Escobar A, Quintana JM, Bilbao A, et al. Effect of patient characteristics on reported outcomes after total knee replacement. *Rheumatology (Oxford).* 2007;46(1):112–119.
71. Arendt-Nielsen L, Nie H, Laursen MB, et al. Sensitization in patients with painful knee osteoarthritis. *Pain.* 2010;149(3):573–581.
72. Drangsholt M, LeResche L. Temporomandibular disorder pain. In: Crombie IK, Croft PR, Linton SJ, LeResche L, Von Korff M, eds. *Epidemiology of Pain: A Report of the Task Force on Epidemiology of the International Association for the Study of Pain.* Seattle: IASP; 1999:203–233.
73. Fernández-de-las-Peñas C, Galán-del-Río F, Fernández-Carnero J, Pesquera J, Arendt-Nielsen L, Svensson P. Bilateral widespread mechanical pain sensitivity in women with myofascial temporomandibular disorder: evidence of impairment in central nociceptive processing. *J Pain.* 2009;10(11):1170–1178.
74. Popescu A, LeResche L, Truelove EL, Drangsholt MT. Gender differences in pain modulation by diffuse noxious inhibitory controls: a systematic review. *Pain.* 2010;150(2):309–318.
75. Velly AM, Look JO, Carlson C, et al. The effect of catastrophizing and depression on chronic pain—a prospective cohort study of temporomandibular muscle and joint pain disorders. *Pain.* 2011;152(10):2377–2383.
76. Lim PF, Maixner W, Khan AA. Temporomandibular disorder and comorbid pain conditions. *J Am Dent Assoc.* 2011;142(12):1365–1367.
77. Mercuri LG. Temporomandibular joint disorder management in oral and maxillofacial surgery. *J Oral Maxillofac Surg.* 2017;75(5):927–930.
78. Khader R, Tingey J, Sewall S. Temporomandibular prosthetic joint infections associated with Propionibacterium acnes: a case Series, and a review of the literature. *J Oral Maxillofac Surg.* 2017;75(12):2512–2520.
79. Hallab NJ. Material hypersensitivity. In: Mercuri LG, ed. *Temporomandibular Joint Total Joint Replacement—TMJ TJR—A Comprehensive Reference for Researchers, Material Scientists and Surgeons.* New York: Springer; 2016:227–249.
80. Gallo J, Goodman SB, Konttinen YT, Raska M. Particle disease: biologic mechanisms of periprosthetic osteolysis in total hip arthroplasty. *Innate Immun.* 2013;19(2):213–224.
81. Münch HJ, Jacobsen SS, Olesen JT, et al. The association between metal allergy, total knee arthroplasty, and revision: study based on the Danish Knee Arthroplasty Register. *Acta Orthop.* 2015;86(3):378–383.
82. Thomas P, Geier J, Dickel H, et al. DKG Statement on the use of metal alloy discs for patch testing in suspected intolerance to metal implants. *J Dtsch Dermatol Ges.* 2015;13:1001–1004.
83. Hallab NJ, Anderson S, Stafford T, Glant T, Jacobs JJ. Lymphocyte responses in patients with total hip arthroplasty. *J Orthop Res.* 2005;23(2):384–391.
84. Mercuri LG, Caicedo MS. Material hypersensitivity and TMJ replacement. *J Oral Maxillofac Surg.* 2019;77:1371–1376.
85. Jacobs JJ. Clinical manifestations of metal allergy. Adverse reactions to byproducts of joint replacements (AAOS/ORSI). Presented at: Annual Meeting of the American Academy of Orthopaedic Surgery. San Francisco, CA; 2012:7–11.

86. Movahed R, Teschke M, Wolford LM. Protocol for concomitant temporomandibular joint custom-fitted total joint reconstruction and orthognathic surgery utilizing computer-assisted surgical simulation. *J Oral Maxillofac Surg*. 2013;71(12):2123–2129.
87. Wolford LM. Computer-assisted surgical simulation for concomitant temporomandibular joint custom-fitted total joint reconstruction and orthognathic surgery. *Atlas Oral Maxillofac Surg Clin North Am*. 2016;24(1):55–66.
88. Susarla SM, Peacock ZS, Williams WB, Rabinov JD, Keith DA, Kaban LB. Role of computed tomographic angiography in treatment of patients with temporomandibular joint ankylosis. *J Oral Maxillofac Surg*. 2014;72(2):267–276.
89. Hossameldin RH, McCain JP, Dabus G. Prophylactic embolisation of the internal maxillary artery in patients with ankylosis of the temporomandibular joint. *Br J Oral Maxillofac Surg*. 2017;55(6):584–588.
90. Ban KA, Minei JP, Laronga C, et al. American College of Surgeons and Surgical Infection Society: surgical site infection guidelines, 2016 update. *J Am Coll Surg*. 2017;224(1):59–74.
91. Berríos-Torres SI, Umscheid CA, Bratzler DW, et al. Centers for disease control and prevention guidelines for the prevention of surgical site infection. *JAMA Surg*. 2017;152(8):784–791.
92. O'Hara LM, Thom KA, Preas MA. Update to the Centers for disease control and prevention and the Healthcare infection control Practices advisory Committee guideline for the prevention of surgical site infection (2017): a summary, review, and strategies for implementation. *Am J Infect Control*. 2018;46(6):602–609.
93. Mercuri LG. Prevention and Detection of TMJ prosthetic joint infections update. *Int J Oral Maxillofac Surg*. 2019;48:217–224.
94. Mercuri LG. Avoiding and managing temporomandibular joint total joint replacement surgical site infections. *J Oral Maxillofac Surg*. 2012;70(10):2280–2289.
95. Mercuri LG. Total reconstruction of the temporomandibular joint with a custom system. In: Ness G, ed. *Atlas of Oral and Maxillofacial Clinics of North America*. Philadelphia, PA: Elsevier; 2011.
96. Quinn PD, Granquist EJ. *Atlas of Temporomandibular Joint Surgery*. 2nd ed. Ames, IA: Wiley Blackwell; 2015:41–49.
97. Parihar VS, Bandyopadhyay TK, Chattopadhyay PK, Jacob SM. Retromandibular transparotid approach compared with transmasseteric anterior parotid approach for the management of fractures of the mandibular condylar process: a prospective randomised study. *Br J Oral Maxillofac Surg*. 2019;57(9):880–885.
98. Scolozzi P, Foletti JM. A closer examination of the retromandibular subparotid approach: surgical technique and anatomical considerations with a special focus on the angular tract. A cadaveric study and a technical note. *J Stomatol Oral Maxillofac Surg*. 2020;S2468-7855(20):30082–30083.
99. Kashi A, Chowdhury AR, Saha S. Finite element analysis of a TMJ implant. *J Dent Res*. 2010;89(3):241–245.
100. Mercuri LG. Avoiding and managing temporomandibular joint total joint replacement surgical site infections. *J Oral Maxillofac Surg*. 2012;70(10):2280–2289.
101. Mercuri LG. Microbial biofilms: a potential source for alloplastic device failure. *J Oral Maxillofac Surg*. 2006;64(8):1303–1309.
102. Mercuri LG, Saltzman BM. Acquired heterotopic ossification in alloplastic joint replacement. *Int J Oral Maxillofac Surg*. 2017;46:1562–1568.
103. Wolford LM, Karras SC. Autologous fat transplantation around temporomandibular joint total joint prostheses: preliminary treatment outcomes. *J Oral Maxillofac Surg*. 1997;55(3):245–251.
104. Mercuri LG, Ali FA, Woolson R. Outcomes of total alloplastic replacement with periarticular autogenous fat grafting for management of reankylosis of the temporomandibular joint. *J Oral Maxillofac Surg*. 2008;66(9):1794–1803.
105. Mercuri LG. Complications associated with TMJ TJR: management and prevention. In: Mercuri LG, ed. *Temporomandibular Joint Total Joint Replacement—TMJ TJR: A Comprehensive Reference for Researchers, Material Scientists and Surgeons*. New York: Springer; 2016:187–226.
106. Merskey H, Bogduk N. *Classification of Chronic Pain. Descriptions of Chronic Pain Syndromes and Definitions of Pain Terms*. 2nd ed. Seattle: IASP; 1994.
107. Biological Responses to Metal Implants. *U.S. Food and Drug Administration. Center for Devices and Radiological Health*; 2019. www.fda.gov.
108. Dupont JY. Synovial plicae of the knee. Controversies and review. *Clin Sports Med*. 1997;16(1):87–122.
109. Kent M, Khanduja V. Synovial plicae around the knee. *Knee*. 2010;17(2):97–102.
110. Funk L, Levy O, Even T, Copeland SA. Subacromial plica as a cause of impingement in the shoulder. *J Shoulder Elbow Surg*. 2006;15(6):697–700.
111. Ruiz de Luzuriaga BC, Helms CA, Kosinski AS, Vinson EN. Elbow MR imaging findings in patients with synovial fringe syndrome. *Skeletal Radiol*. 2013;42(5):675–680.
112. Westermark A, Leiggener C, Aagaard E, Lindskog S. Histological findings in soft tissues around temporomandibular joint prostheses after up to eight years of function. *Int J Oral Maxillofac Implants*. 2011;40(1):18–25.
113. Monje F, Mercuri L, Villanueva-Alcojol L, de Mera JJ. Synovial metaplasia found in tissue encapsulating a silicone spacer during 2-staged temporomandibular joint replacement for ankylosis. *J Oral Maxillofac Surg*. 2012;70(10):2290–2298.
114. Murakami K, Hori S, Yamaguchi Y, et al. Synovial plicae and temporomandibular joint disorders: surgical findings. *J Oral Maxillofac Surg*. 2015;73(5):827–833.
115. Davis CM, Hakim M, Choi DD, Behrman DA, Israel H, McCain JP. Early clinical outcomes of arthroscopic management of the failing alloplastic temporomandibular joint prosthesis. *J Oral Maxillofac Surg*. 2020;78(6):903–907.
116. Mercuri LG, Urban RM, Hall DJ, Mathew MT. Adverse local tissue responses to failed temporomandibular joint implants. *J Oral Maxillofac Surg*. 2017;75(10):2076–2084.
117. Liu SS, Buvanendran A, Rathmell JP, et al. Predictors for moderate to severe acute postoperative pain after total hip and knee replacement. *Int Orthop*. 2012;36(11):2261–2267.
118. Judge A, Arden NK, Cooper C, et al. Predictors of outcomes of total knee replacement surgery. *Rheumatology (Oxford)*. 2012;51(10):1804–1813.
119. Jones CA, Voaklander DC, Suarez-Alma ME. Determinants of function after total knee arthroplasty. *Phys Ther*. 2003;83(8):696–706.
120. Lingard EA, Katz JN, Wright EA, Sledge CB, Kinemax Outcomes Group. Predicting the outcome of total knee arthroplasty. *J Bone Joint Surg Am*. 2004;86(10):2179–2186.
121. Escobar A, Quintana JM, Bilbao A, et al. Effect of patient characteristics on reported outcomes after total knee replacement. *Rheumatology (Oxford)*. 2007;46(1):112–119.
122. Arendt-Nielsen L, Nie H, Laursen MB, et al. Sensitization in patients with painful knee osteoarthritis. *Pain*. 2010;149(3):573–581.
123. Drangsholt M, LeResche L. Temporomandibular disorder pain. In: Crombie IK, Croft PR, Linton SJ, LeResche L, Von Korff M, eds. *Epidemiology of Pain: A Report of the Task Force on Epidemiology of the International Association for the Study of Pain*. Seattle: IASP; 1999:203–233.
124. Velly AM, Look JO, Carlson C, et al. The effect of catastrophizing and depression on chronic pain—a prospective cohort study of temporomandibular muscle and joint pain disorders. *Pain*. 2011;152(10):2377–2383.
125. Lim PF, Maixner W, Khan AA. Temporomandibular disorder and comorbid pain conditions. *J Am Dent Assoc*. 2011;142(12):1365–1367.

Stock Alloplastic Temporomandibular Joint Reconstruction

Eric J. Granquist and Peter D. Quinn

Armamentarium

Antibiotic irrigation
Army-Navy retractors
Basic soft tissue set
Dingman bone-holding forceps
Dunn-Dautrey retractors
Flat diamond rasp
24-Gauge surgical wire
Malleable retractors
Molt curette
1-mm Side cutting fissure bur
Nasal freer
Needle-tip Bovie
Nerve stimulator
Obwegeser periosteal elevator
Oscillating saw
PDQ Zygoma retractors
Surgairtome
Sutures: 3-0, 4-0 Vicryl, 5-0 fast gut
T-bar osteotome

History of the Procedure

The history of alloplastic temporomandibular joint (TMJ) reconstruction has been marred by failures secondary to inappropriate design, poor preclinical trials, and a failure to appreciate outcomes in the orthopedic literature. Initially, alloplastic materials were used almost exclusively for recurrent ankylosis.[1] Eggers used tantalum foil in 1946 as an interpositional implant.[1] In 1960, Robinson used a stainless-steel fossa prosthesis, and Christensen used an array of cast vitallium fossae that were secured to the zygomatic arch.[1] Currently in the United States, there are two Food and Drug Administration (FDA)-approved TMJ replacement systems that both utilize metal-on-polyethylene designs. A complete understanding of the biomechanics, biomaterials, and occlusal considerations of the patient requiring total alloplastic joint reconstruction is essential to ensure good outcomes. An increasing number of patients with advanced degenerative joint disease (Wilkes IV and V) are now progressing directly to alloplastic reconstruction. Stock alloplastic joint reconstruction is a cost-effective solution in these patients.

In 2005, the FDA approved the Biomet TMJ prosthesis following a 10-year prospective investigational device exemption study on 224 patients.[2] At 3 years, patients had a significant improvement in pain, with postoperative scores decreasing from a mean of 8.5 (prior to total joint replacement [TJR]) to 2.8. Mouth opening also improved from 20.1 to 29.3 mm. Most importantly, patient satisfaction scores were high, with 99% of patients stating that they would have the surgery again. A 3.2% revision rate was seen, with no device-related mechanical failures. Westermark also reported on his experience with this prosthesis in 12 patients who were followed for up to 8 years. At 1-year follow-up, mean jaw opening increased from 3.8 to 30.2 mm.[3] Joint-related pain was eliminated in all but two patients. These two patients reported persistent muscle pain. No postoperative infections or device failures were seen. More recently, a post-market surveillance order to all manufacturers of TMJ implants in the United States was issued in order to evaluate outcomes of TMJ devices.[4] A prospective observational study involving 498 devices in 319 subjects with a mean follow-up of 8.6 years was completed. In this study, the overall device explantation rate was 4.2% with a reoperation rate of 7%. This translated into a Kaplan-Meir survivorship rate of 98% at 3 years, 96% at 5 years, and 94% at 10 years. The most common causes of either removal or reoperation included adhesion removal (2.6%, 13/498), heterotopic bone/ankylosis (2.0%, 10/498), and infection (1.6%, 8/498). The overall device failure rate was 1%, suggesting that the use of stock alloplastic joint replacement of the TMJ is safe and effective.

Indications for the Use of the Procedure

Indications for TMJ reconstruction include bony ankylosis, failed previous alloplastic reconstruction, failed autogenous joint reconstruction, posttraumatic condylar injury, avascular necrosis, posttumor reconstruction, developmental abnormalities, functional deformity, and severe inflammatory conditions that have failed conservative treatments[5–7] (Table 148.1).

Current reconstructive options for the surgeon include the use of either autogenous or alloplastic materials. In the skeletally mature population, alloplastic joint replacement offers the advantage of immediate function, lack of donor site morbidity, reduced operative time and most importantly, more predictable outcomes. In the pediatric population, autogenous reconstruction has the additional advantage of growth potential, particularly with costochondral grafts. It should be

Table 148.1 Indications for Stock total joint replacement (TJR)
Arthritic conditions: osteoarthritis, inflammatory arthritis
Ankylosis, reankylosis, and heterotopic bone formation
Failed autogenous reconstruction
Avascular necrosis
Multiple operated open joint procedures
Fracture
Functional deformity
Benign neoplasm/cysts
Malignancy
Degenerated and resorbed joints
Developmental abnormality

noted that in pediatric patients with ankylosis, growth has ceased, and alloplastic total joint reconstruction may be considered. The ability to achieve predictable, safe, long-lasting, and cost-effective reconstruction should be considered when deciding the method of joint reconstruction. Device longevity is unknown, although devices continue to function well after more than 15 years.

Careful preoperative planning and setting reasonable patient expectations are required for successful joint reconstruction. Maximal opening between 30 and 35 mm can be expected with a total joint prosthesis. Patients with prolonged preoperative decreased range of motion often have muscle and soft tissue contracture and scarring that requires attention during surgery. This may require coronoidectomy or muscle stripping. Patients should be aware that unilateral replacement causes deviation to the side of the prosthesis on terminal opening. Pain reduction for patients who have undergone multiple operations is often difficult to achieve. A direct correlation exists between the number of previous surgical procedures and the likelihood that presurgical symptoms will be reduced (Table 148.1).[8–10]

Limitations and Contraindications

Absolute contraindications for TJR include the presence of infection in the operative field, allergy to the prosthetic components, and systemic conditions rendering the patient unable to tolerate the operative procedure (Table 148.2). Nickel is the most common cause of allergy following TJR. Devices can be manufactured using only titanium alloy to avoid this issue. Skeletal immaturity is also considered a contraindication to alloplastic joint reconstruction. Mercuri and Swift have argued for consideration of alloplastic TMJ reconstruction in the pediatric population with previously failed autogenous grafts, high inflammatory arthritis unresponsive to other modalities, and loss of vertical height due to bony resoprtion.[11] Alloplastic reconstruction can avoid the complications associated with autogenous grafting such as ankylosis or graft resorption that may render subsequent revision surgeries more complicated. The lifespan of alloplastic prostheses is a concern in the younger patient population. It is unknown how long one can reasonably expect a TMJ prosthesis to function. In the young patient population, it is important to educate these patients that revision arthroplasty is expected, and the surgeon should plan their osteotomies accordingly. The use of a custom implant system is usually necessary in cases where there is a severe craniofacial deformity present with an anatomical discrepancy that precludes the use of a stock device.

Table 148.2 Contraindications
Active acute or chronic infections
Inadequate quantity or quality of bone
Allergy to implant components
Skeletally immature patients

Unacceptable failure rates in previous iterations of alloplastic TMJ implant systems provided valuable input for development of newer FDA-approved implants. Appreciation of biomechanical and orthopedic principals, along with appropriate clinical trials, has helped in the development of safe and effective devices.[1,12–14] It is important to recognize that these devices still have limitations. This includes a finite life expectancy, limited translation, the development of wear debris, and the potential for infection.[15–19]

TECHNIQUE: Alloplastic Temporomandibular Joint Reconstruction

STEP 1: Prep and Positioning

The patient should be intubated with a nasal RAE tube with the endotracheal tube either sutured in placed or secured to the head wrap to allow for head and mandible manipulation. A preoperative antibiotic should be given during this time to ensure adequate tissue levels prior to incision. Hair should first be removed from the proposed incision site, typically to the superior portion of the helix. A head wrap is then applied and secured with skin staples. The skin is prepped. The patient is then draped, and a urologic drape is then adapted and used as a sterile barrier to manipulate the mandible during the operation. Minimizing contamination from the oral cavity is critical for reducing postoperative infections. Attention to sterile technique, especially when alternating between the surgical site and the oral cavity, is the most important step in preventing prosthetic infection (Fig. 148.1). Finally, the surgeon should address the external auditory canal to minimize potential contamination of the surgical filed. This can be accomplished by irrigating the canal with antibiotic saline or isolating the canal through the use of mineral oil-impregnated cotton or suturing.

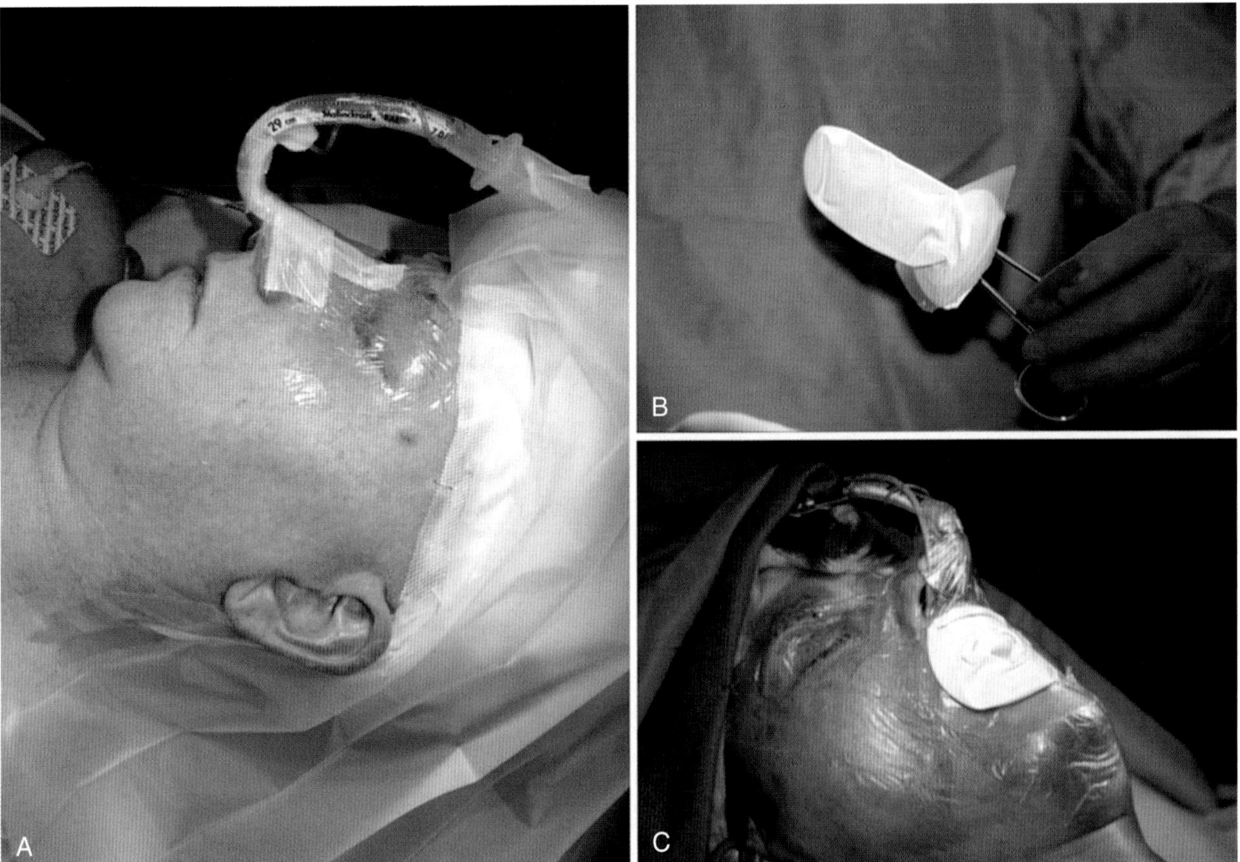

Figure 148.1 **A,** Patient positioned prior to face prep. Noted nasotracheal tube is secured to the nasal bridge and foam is used to support the tube and minimized pressure on the nasal tip. **B,** A urological drape is modified to allow for sterile manipulation of the mandible. **C,** Urologic drape in place and secured with Tegaderm.

TECHNIQUE: Alloplastic Temporomandibular Joint Reconstruction—*cont'd*

STEP 2: Endaural Incision

An endaural incision is the preferred approach to the mandibular condyle in alloplastic joint reconstruction. This approach provides an excellent cosmetic outcome. In addition, it allows for a stepped approach to the joint, which improves tissue coverage and increases the distance of the prosthetic device from the incision (Fig. 148.2).

STEP 3: Retromandibular Incision

The retromandibular incision is marked by placing a gloved finger from the lobule of the ear to the angle of the mandible. The incision is marked approximately 1 cm below the lobule of the ear to the premasseteric notch (Fig. 148.3). A nerve stimulator is used during this dissection to identify and avoid the marginal mandibular nerve. Once dissection through the superficial layer of the deep cervical fascia is completed, the angulation of the dissection changes to parallel the sternocleidomastoid muscle. A Kelly hemostat is used to define the plane between the submandibular gland and sternocleidomastoid muscle. This will expose the posterior belly of the digastric muscle, marking the deepest point of the dissection. An Army-Navy retractor is used to retract the facial artery anteriorly exposing the inferior border of the mandible and anterior portion of the pterygomasseteric sling. The sling is incised with a #15 blade along the avascular aponeurosis. A Molt curette can be used to strip any remaining periosteal attachment. This allows a clean dissection of the masseter from the lateral aspect of the mandible with the aid of an Obwegeser periosteal elevator. Once this dissection is complete, communication between the endaural and retromandibular incisions exists in a safe subperiosteal plane (Fig. 148.4). Care should be taken to minimize trauma between the small cuff of tissue between the two incisions, as the facial nerve travels in this plane.

Continued

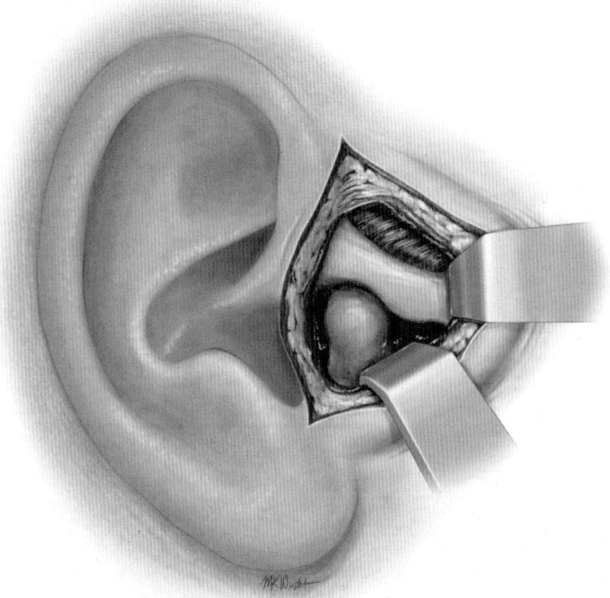

Figure 148.2 Diagram showing exposed temporomandibular capsule. Note the zygomatic retractor used to protect the facial nerve.

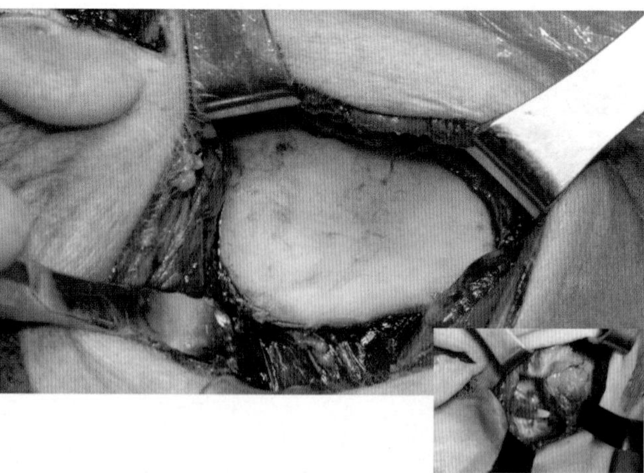

Figure 148.4 Exposed lateral aspect of the mandibular ramus to the condylar neck. Army-Navy retractors are used to retract and protect the facial artery *(right)* and trunk of the facial nerve *(top)*. Insert: Retromandibular approach before with pterygomasseteric sling intact. The posterior belly of the digastric and submandibular gland is visualized.

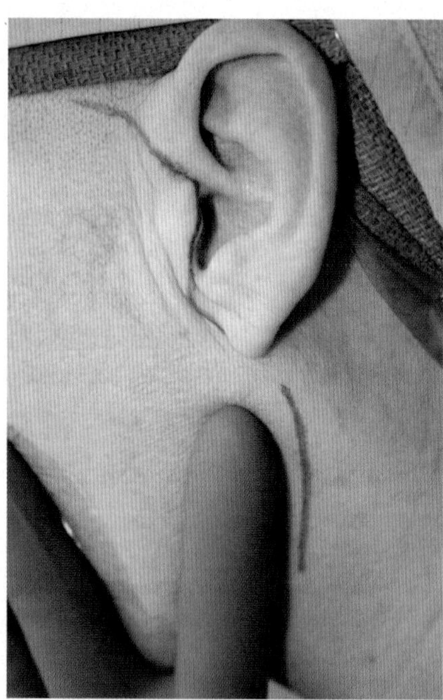

Figure 148.3 Endaural and retromandibular incisions marked. Note the gloved finger is used as a reference to palpate the angle of the mandible to aid in incision design.

TECHNIQUE: Alloplastic Temporomandibular Joint Reconstruction—*cont'd*

STEP 4: Condylectomy

It is essential to complete the retromandibular incision prior to the condylar osteotomy to ensure rapid access to the underlying vasculature, in case difficult-to-control bleeding is encountered. In cases of ankylosis or previous surgeries where altered anatomy may be encountered, thrombin-soaked sponges, collagen, or Floseal matrix should be available to control bleeding following removal of the condylar segment. A two-step osteotomy has been developed to minimize risk to the internal maxillary artery and ensure adequate bone removal for the fossa component. Two Dunn-Dautrey retractors and a condylar neck retractor should be placed in the subperiosteal plane at the level of the neck of the condyle. This allows improved visualization and protects adjacent soft tissue structures. Once the neck of the condyle is fully exposed, a 1-mm fissure bur is used to perform the condylectomy (Fig. 148.5). An osteotomy is performed by first starting at the midpoint of the condylar neck sparing the medial cortex. The cut is then extended both anteriorly and posteriorly toward the Dunn-Dautrey retractors. A T-bar osteotome is then used to complete the osteotomy (Fig. 148.6). Alternatively, a piezoelectric saw may be used. The condyle is then grasped with a bone-holding forceps, and the lateral pterygoid muscle is then carefully dissected free. Significant bleeding may occur during this portion of the procedure due to the rich vascularity in the region (Fig. 148.7). With the condyle removed, the mandible is superiorly repositioned by grasping the inferior border through the retromandibular incision with a bone-holding forceps. This allows for the second osteotomy, at the level of the inferior portion of the sigmoid notch, to occur at a safer distance from the internal maxillary artery.

STEP 5: Fossa Placement

Once adequate bone is removed from the mandible, attention is then directed to the articular eminence. The eminence is reduced to allow for tripod stability of the fossa component. This is best accomplished with a diamond rasp. While reducing the eminence, it is important that the rasp parallels the superior aspect of the zygomatic arch. This ensures correct angulation of the fossa and minimizes potential dislocation. Once the eminence is modified, fossa sizers should be placed to determine the correct implant size. If the fossa flange does not sit flush with the eminence, the rasp can be used to reduce any irregularities along the lateral aspect of the zygomatic arch (Fig. 148.8). It is important to note, the system utilizes trial sizers, which can be placed multiple times until satisfactory position and seating is obtained. Once satisfactory seating and angulation of the fossa has been accomplished with the trial sizer, the fossa implant is soaked in antibiotic-impregnated saline and then inserted into the modified glenoid fossa. This minimizes the potential for contamination. The fossa can then be initially secured with two screws until the adequacy of the fossa position can be confirmed, although five screws are typically used once this is verified (Fig. 148.9). An assistant should then place the mandible into occlusion, and the clearance between the mandible and fossa is checked. A nasal freer should easily pass between the fossa and the stump of the condylar neck. If resistance is met, a handheld rasp or fissure bur should be used to further reduce the mandible.

STEP 6: Intermaxillary Fixation

The patient is placed in intermaxillary fixation. This is best accomplished, in a stable and efficient manner, with the use of Ivy loops placed on the premolars. Alternatively, Erich arch bars, intermaxillary fixation screws or pigtail wires can be used. (Fig. 148.10). A separate intraoral instrument set should be utilized to minimize contamination of the joint. Reprepping and draping of the patient, as well as glove changes before returning into the surgical wounds, should also occur.

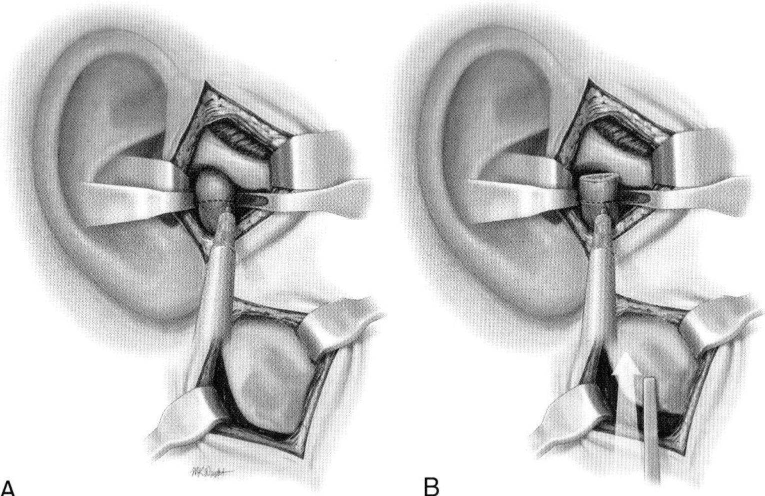

Figure 148.5 **A,** Fissure bur used to make osteotomy just below the condylar head. **B,** Second osteotomy at the level of the sigmoid notch, with the mandible superiorly repositioned.

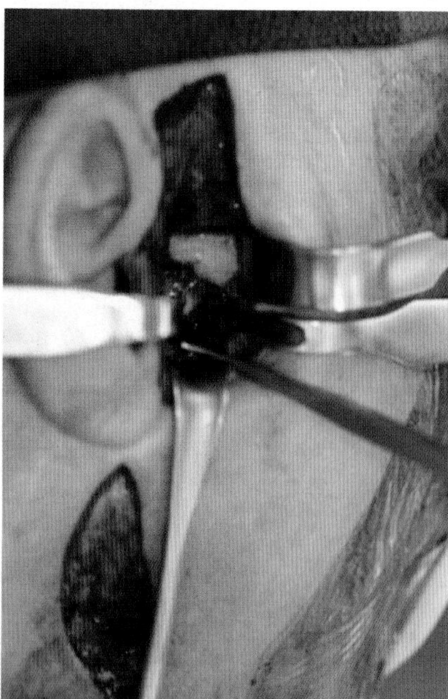

Figure 148.6 T-bar osteotome used to complete osteotomy.

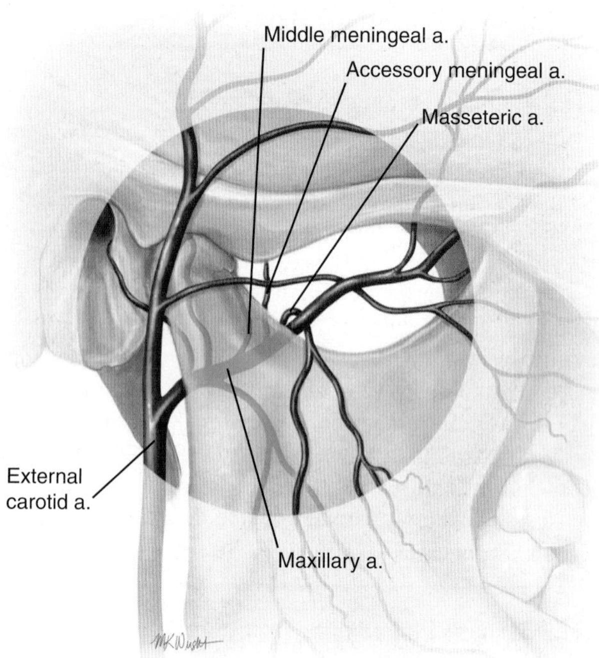

Figure 148.7 Medial view of the mandible. Note the proximity of the maxillary artery, masseteric artery, and middle meningeal artery to the temporomandibular joint (TMJ).

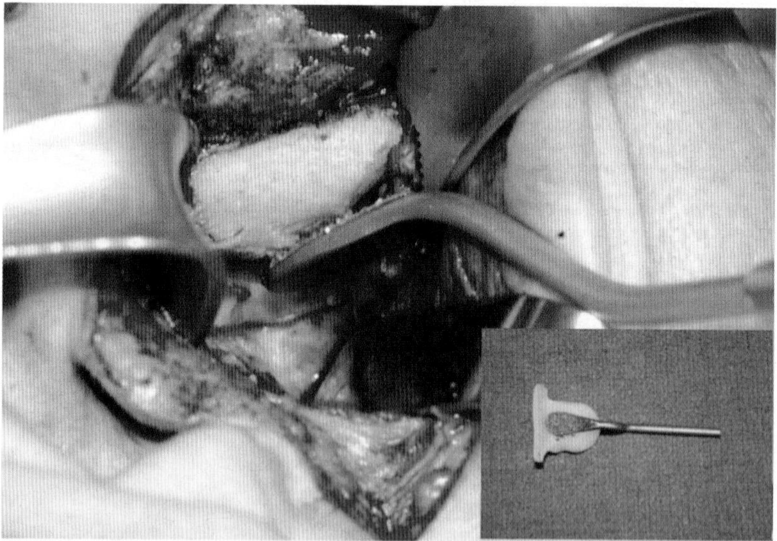

Figure 148.8 Diamond rasp used to reduce the articular eminence. Insert: Size of rasp in reference to the fossa component.

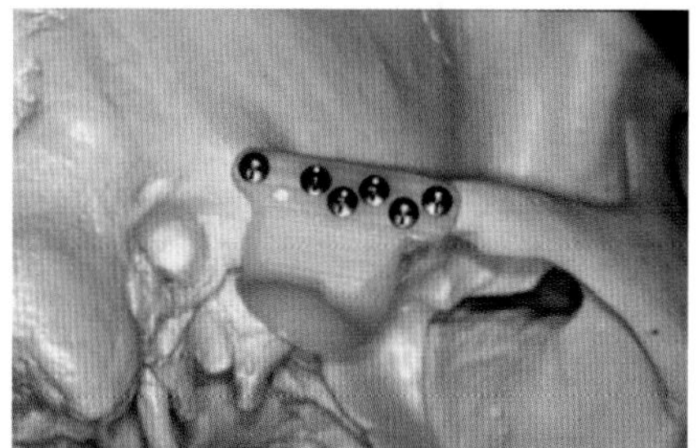

Figure 148.9 Mandibular fossa secured to model skull.

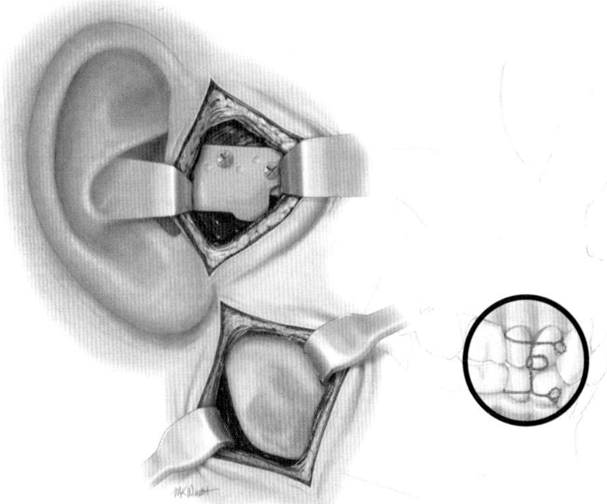

Figure 148.10 Diagram showing patient in internal maxillary fixation and fossa in place.

TECHNIQUE: Alloplastic Temporomandibular Joint Reconstruction—*cont'd*

STEP 7: Condylar Placement

The condylar component is placed through the retromandibular incision. Sizers are available to determine the correct size mandibular component. The condyle head should sit in a slight posterior direction and at the midpoint of the fossa in the medial-lateral dimension (Fig. 148.11). This will ensure good matching and function of the prosthesis. In order to achieve optimal placement, any irregularities in the lateral aspect of the mandible interfering with seating can be reduced with the reciprocating diamond rasp. Once satisfactory placement of the mandibular component is achieved, it should be secured with two screws.

STEP 8: Range of Motion

With the mandibular and fossa components in place, the intermaxillary fixation should be released and the range of motion and function should be checked. It is important to ensure that the prosthesis does not dislocate. Finally, the maximal opening should be measured. If a passive opening of less than 30 mm is found, a coronoidectomy should be considered. The osteotomy should occur through the endaural incision.

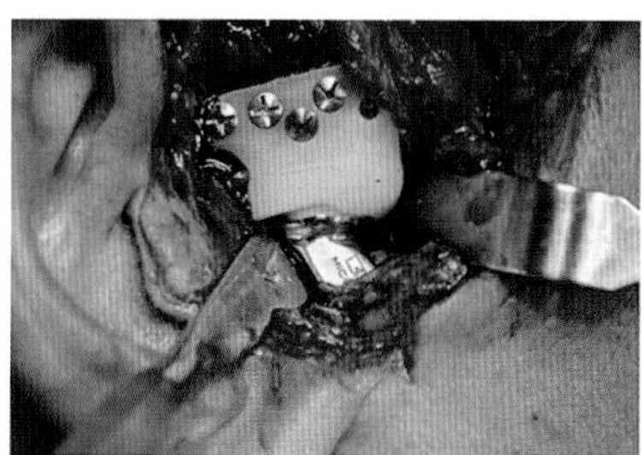

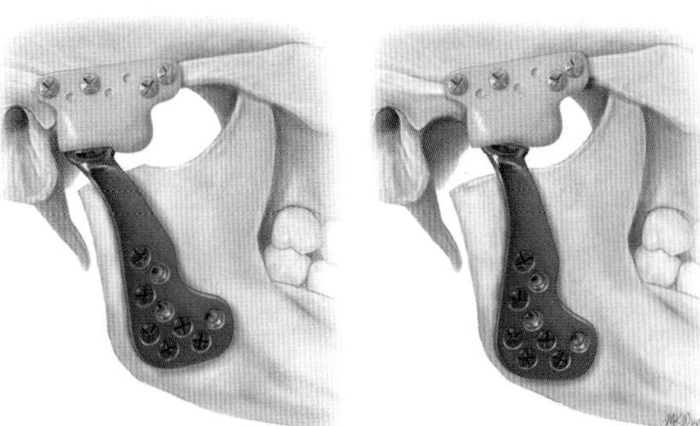

Figure 148.11 Photo of correct fossa-condyle orientation. Diagram *(below)* showing correct *(left)* and incorrect *(right)* fossa-condyle orientation.

TECHNIQUE: Alloplastic Temporomandibular Joint Reconstruction—*cont'd*

STEP 9: Final Screw Placement

Once optimal range of motion and position of the prosthesis have been achieved, final screw placement can occur. Care should be taken to ensure that the screw holes do not encroach on the inferior alveolar nerve when placing the mandibular screws. This is easily accomplished with the aid of standard radiographs.

STEP 10: Closure

Closure begins once all wounds have been thoroughly irrigated with antibiotic-impregnated saline. Hemostasis is confirmed and the endaural incision is closed in layers. The retromandibular incision is then irrigated and closed in layers beginning with the superficial layer of the deep cervical fascia after hemostasis is confirmed. The pterygomasseteric sling is left to passively reattach. The skin is then closed, and dressings are placed. Once the wounds are dressed, the intermaxillary fixation wires or screws are removed.

ALTERNATE OR MODIFIED TECHNIQUE

ANKYLOSIS

Ankylosis of the TMJ presents several additional challenges to reconstruction and restoration of TMJ function. Patients with massive ankylosis should have a computed tomography angiogram to identify any potential vasculature that may result in bleeding. If the internal maxillary artery is found to be adjacent to the bony mass, selective preoperative embolization can be utilized to minimize the potential for massive hemorrhage.

Intubation can be problematic with minimal mouth opening and may necessitate fiberoptic intubation. Close communication and planning with the anesthesia team are essential for the safe induction of anesthesia in these patients. Additional measures including awake intubation, or tracheostomy, may also be considered. The ankylotic bony mass often extends beyond the boundaries of the joint capsule. This presents three unique problems. First, the alteration of local anatomy and proximity to adjacent vasculature increases the risk of bleeding. Second, the bony mass renders the separation of the mandible from the skull base more difficult and increases the risk of middle cranial fossa exposure or perforation. Finally, limited movement of the mandible may cause fibrosis of musculature or elongation of the mandibular coronoid process, resulting in a secondary cause of trismus. In order to minimize or avoid the first two potential problems, the osteotomy for the condylectomy should be modified. The initial osteotomy is then placed at the most inferior aspect of the ankylosis to be removed. Once this lower osteotomy is completed and the mandible separated from the skull base, attention should be directed to removing the ankylotic mass. Often, a pseudoarthrosis, or evidence of previous meniscal anatomy is present. A 1-mm fissure bur should be used to initiate the osteotomy, with a slight inferior angulation. A curved T-bar osteotome can then be used to separate the remaining bony mass from the skull base (Fig. 148.12). The remaining bone can be carefully and judiciously removed with the aid of a diamond rasp or pineapple bur. Alternatively, the osteotomies may be aided by the use of virtual surgical planning and custom cutting guide fabrication (Fig. 148.13A–E). In this scenario, a saw may be considered for the osteotomy. The use of computed tomography-guidance may also be considered during this aspect of the procedure to minimize iatrogenic entry into the middle cranial fossa. Once bone removal is complete, jaw function should be evaluated. If opening is less than 30 mm, a coronoidectomy should be considered. It is also helpful to actively stretch the mandible with the aide of two Molt mouth props or a Bell retractor. Once the prosthesis is placed to prevent reankylosis, fat grafting should be utilized to minimize dead space and prevent adhesions and heterotopic bone formation.

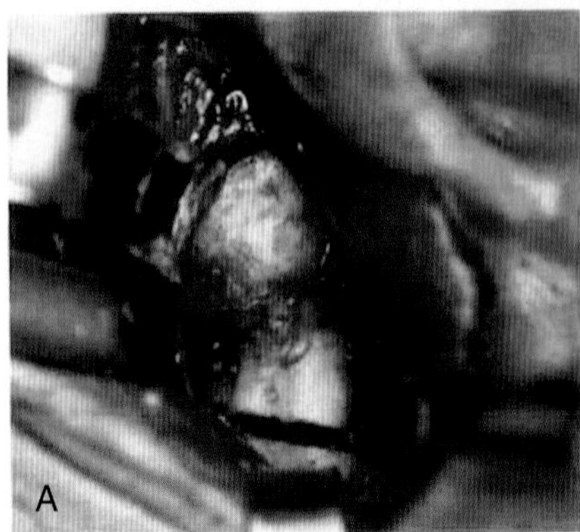

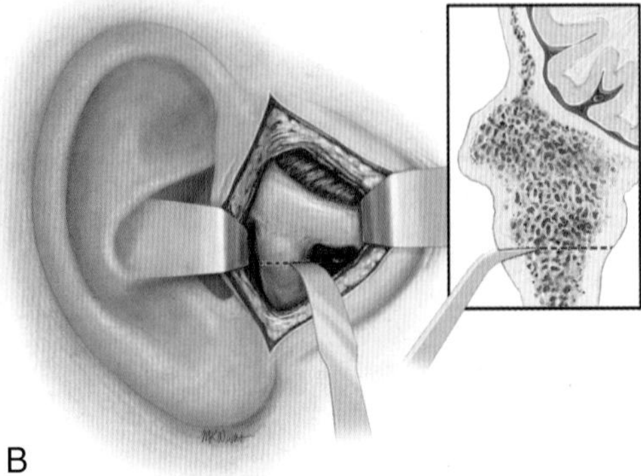

Figure 148.12 **A,** Image showing initial osteotomy in a patient with ankylosis. Note the osteotomy is placed lower, along the neck of the condyle where normal anatomy is present. **B,** Diagram showing separation of the ankylotic mass from the skull base. It is important this occurs after the mandible has been separated from the skull base to minimize middle cranial base perforation or skull base fracture.

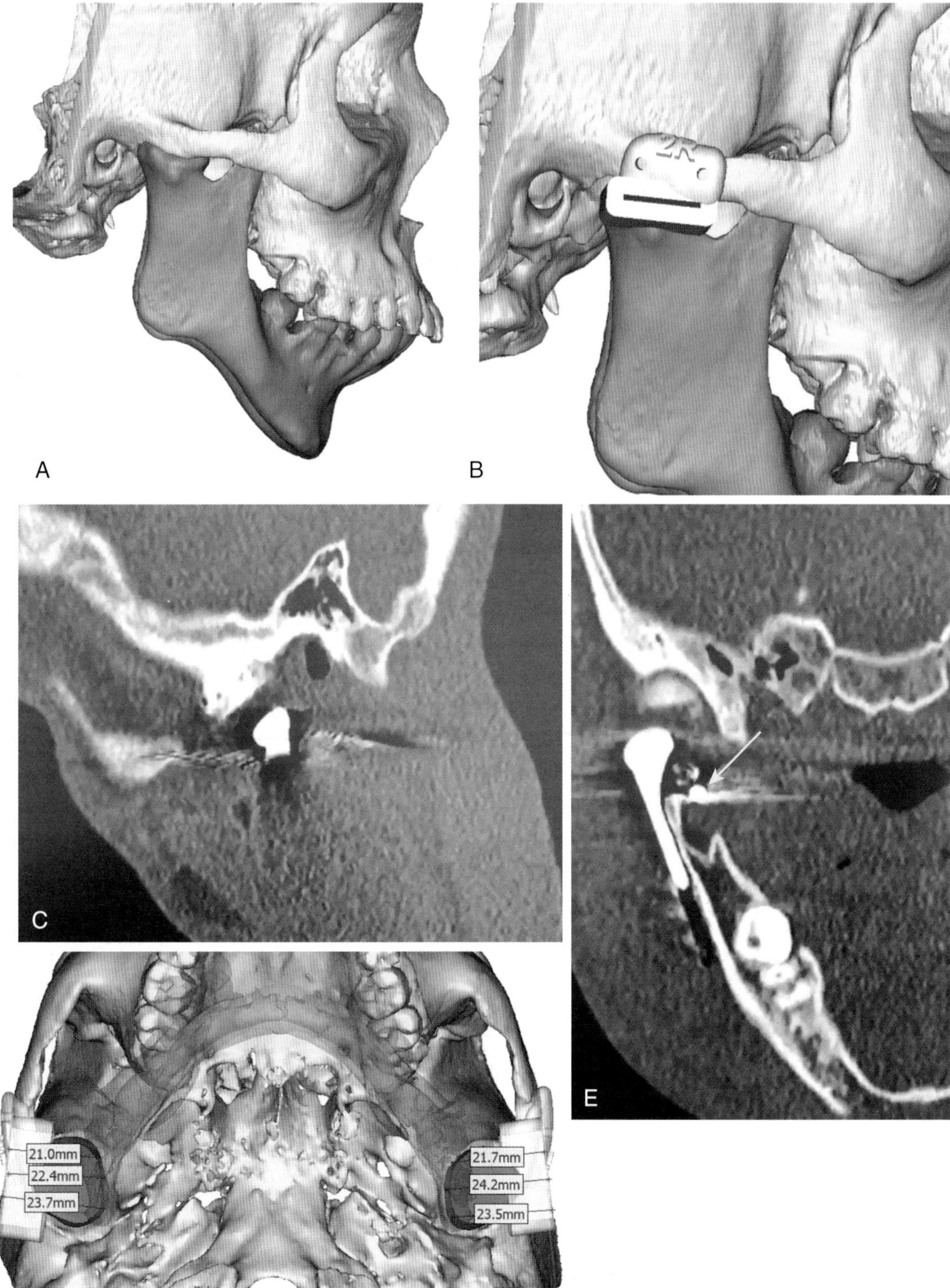

Figure 148.13 **A,** Preoperative computed tomography (CT) reconstruction demonstration temporomandibular joint (TMJ) ankylosis with loss of anatomic landmarks between the middle ear and intracranial fossa. **B,** Custom-designed cutting guide in predetermined position; note the flange design allows for placement of the saw, creating an ideal surface for the stock fossa prosthesis. **C,** Postoperative CT demonstrating flat osteotomy created with the aid of the custom cutting guide. **D,** Cutting guides in place with demonstration of depths from cutting surface. **E,** Postoperative CT with stock mandibular TMJ prosthesis in place. *Yellow arrow* notes position of preoperative selective embolization of the internal maxillary artery.

ALTERNATE OR MODIFIED TECHNIQUE—*cont'd*

CORRECTION OF FACIAL ASYMMETRY

Growing patients with TMJ disease will often have secondary facial asymmetry. In cases where the disease process results in loss or destruction of the native mandibular condyle, alloplastic joint reconstruction can serve to replace the nonfunctioning joint and be used to correct the preexisting dentofacial discrepancy in the skeletally mature patient. In conjunction with a LeFort I osteotomy, the skeletal asymmetry can be corrected in a single-stage surgery. (Fig. 148.14A and B). The use of an alloplastic joint further provides a stable platform for orthognathic reconstruction. The protocol for the reconstruction of facial asymmetry secondary to TMJ disease begins with a standard LeFort I osteotomy with repositioning of the maxilla utilizing an intermediate splint based on the position of the native mandible. Once the maxilla is secured in its new position, the total joint reconstruction proceeds with the condylectomy as described above. The mandible is then placed into its new position utilizing a final splint and the prosthesis is placed. If a midline correction or yaw correction is needed, a contralateral sagittal split osteotomy can be performed prior to placing the patient in intermaxillary fiction. The prosthetic device is the placed, and function checked. Once complete, a genioplasty may also be performed at the same time, if necessary.

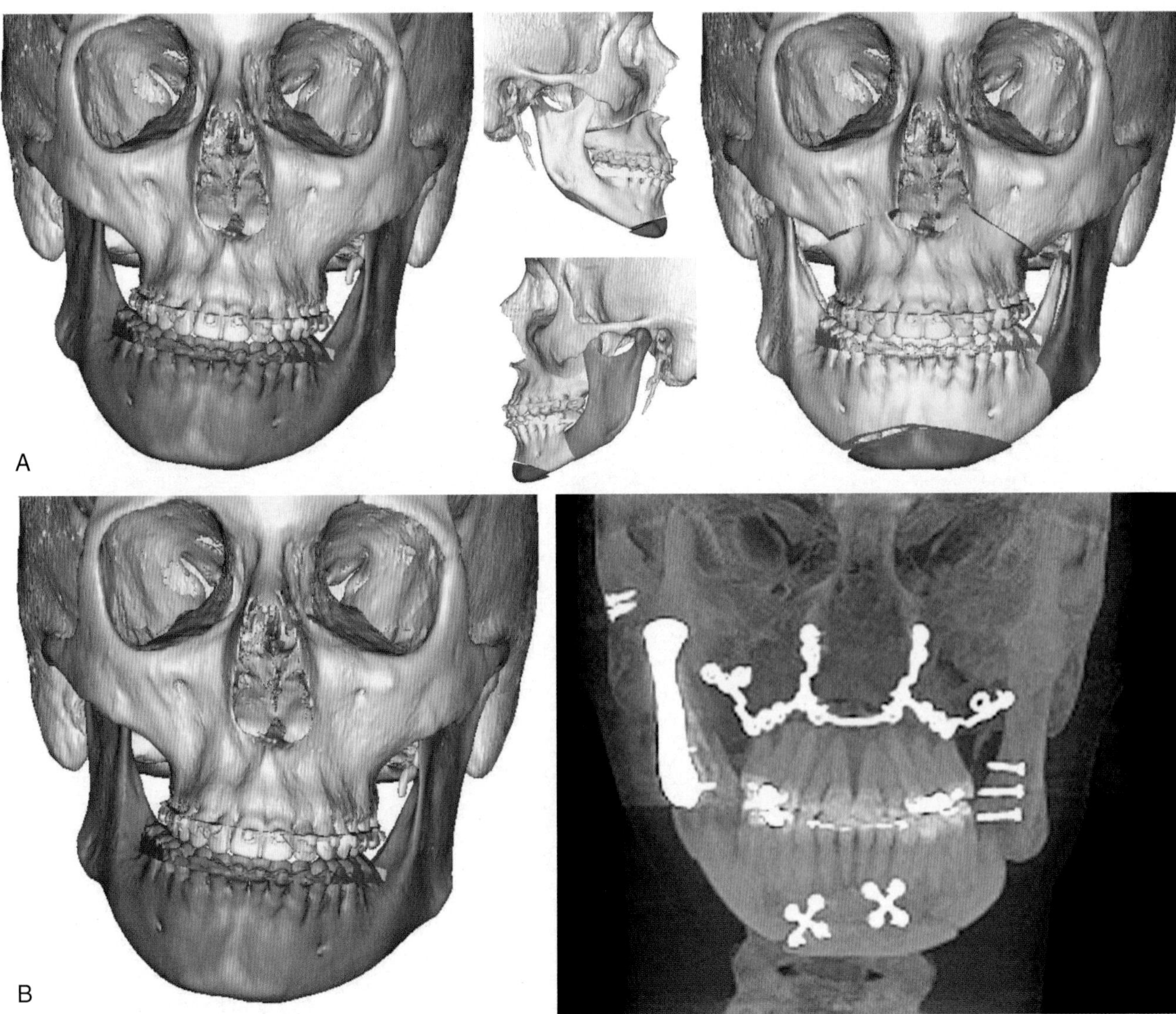

Figure 148.14 **A,** Preoperative computed tomography (CT) of patient with a history of left condylar hyperplasia and secondary right temporomandibular joint (TMJ) degeneration along with the virtual surgical planned Lefort I osteotomy, contralateral sagittal split osteotomy, genioplasty, and condylectomy planned. **B,** Preoperative CT and postoperative imaging with hardware in place.

Avoidance and Management of Intraoperative Complications

Surgical complications can be divided into failure of technique, failure of diagnosis, failure of device, failure secondary to patient disease, and relative failure secondary to patient expectation. Fortunately, TMJ prosthetic infection is rare, with an infection rate of 1.6%. Prosthetic joint infection can be difficult to treat and is often secondary to the formation of biofilms. The microbiology of TMJ device infection is often polymicrobial and typically consists of skin flora. Early infections (<3 months) may be treated with antibiotics, but intermediate or late infections often require device removal, prolonged intravenous antibiotics and a new prosthesis. In 2010, Wolford et al. published the results of his protocol for treating infections. Early prosthetic joint infections were treated by a periprosthetic antibiotic washout and debridement and placement of irrigation catheters, followed by 4 to 6 weeks of intravenous antibiotics. Patients with chronic infections were treated with a similar protocol, except the prosthesis was removed and replaced 8 to 10 weeks later. Wolford was able to salvage four of the five infected prostheses in the acute protocol and achieve resolution of all infections in the chronic protocol.[19] Strict attention to aseptic technique, the use of perioperative antibiotics, and minimizing cross-contamination from any intraoral procedure is key to decreasing prosthetic joint infection. Additional measures utilized include external auditory ear irrigation with antibiotic-impregnated saline and soaking components in antibiotic saline prior to implantation.

Heterotopic bone formation and reankylosis can be difficult problems, particularly in the multioperated patient. In addition to excessive bone formation, there is often extensive scarring, which renders achieving acceptable maximal incisal opening difficult. Several methods to combat heterotopic bone formation have been addressed in the orthopedic literature. This includes nonsteroidal antiinflammatory medication (indomethacin) and the use of low dose postsurgical radiation.[20] Reported regimens include 10 Gy in five fractionated daily doses in the immediate postoperative period.[21,22] Wolford and Karras reported the use of autogenous fat grafting around the prosthetic joint to prevent bone formation and scarring. In a case series of 37 joints, no patient grafted with fat formed heterotopic bone compared with 35% of the controls.[23]

Bleeding is most often encountered from the middle meningeal artery, internal maxillary artery, masseteric artery, or the lateral pterygoid muscles. Identification and ligation of the severed vessel are clearly preferred but often difficult. Several hemostatic agents should be available to help with bleeding, particularly since many of these vessels can be difficult to identify through the standard approaches. It is essential to achieve hemostasis prior to closure to prevent hematoma formation. Thrombin, collagen, or Floseal (Ethicon, Summerville NJ, USA) may be utilized to decrease bleeding. For more brisk bleeding, which is difficult to control, access to the external carotid artery is possible through the retromandibular incision. It is important to identify at least three branches to ensure proper identification of the external carotid artery before it is ligated. Collateral circulation can limit the effectiveness of ligation. Lastly, interventional radiology may be considered to identify and occlude a bleeding vessel.

Malocclusion following placement of the prosthesis is ideally identified prior to final screw placement. If only two screws were placed, the mandibular component can easily be repositioned without compromising stabilization. Prior to the release of the intermaxillary fixation, occlusion should be checked to ensure correct alignment and to confirm that there was no failure of the intermaxillary wires. The clearance between the fossa and mandible should also be checked for interference, and if present, must be addressed to obtain acceptable occlusion and function. The surgeon should not hesitate to reposition the components to ensure proper occlusion.

Finally, patients with chronic or centralized pain can be difficult to manage in the acute postoperative period. Unfortunately, many patients with TMJ disease have undergone multiple operations and subsequently developed centralized pain.[24] Consultation with a pain specialist is important in the care of these individuals. Several studies have shown that patients with fewer open TMJ procedures report significantly lower pain scores following total joint surgery compared to those with multiple operations.[8–10] This information suggests that following a failed open arthroplasty, patients may benefit from TJR instead of further revision procedures. Prior to the consideration of TMJ replacement surgery, the clinician should consider a diagnostic block to determine the percentage of pain resolution. For patients with minimal pain reduction, additional surgery should be avoided if possible.

Postoperative Considerations

Postoperative radiographs should be obtained prior to patient discharge in order to confirm correct angulation, screw position, and condylar seating. Patients are seen 10 days following discharge for suture removal, and passive jaw motion is encouraged. Active jaw physical therapy may be indicated for patients and is typically initiated for 4 to 6 weeks following surgery, beginning on postoperative day 1. Postoperative pain management should primarily consist of antiinflammatory medication and acetaminophen with narcotic medications for rescue. The patient should be quickly titrated off narcotic medication during the immediate postoperative period. For patients taking narcotic medication prior to surgery or a requiring narcotic pain medication for longer than 1 month, referral to a pain specialist should be considered.

References

1. Quinn PD. Alloplastic reconstruction of the temporomandibular joint. *Selected readings on oral and maxillofacial surgery*. 1996;7(5):1–20.
2. Giannakopoulos HE, Sinn DP, Quinn PD. Biomet Microfixation temporomandibular joint replacement system: a 3-year follow-up study of patients treated during 1995 to 2005. *J Oral Maxillofac Surg*. 2012;70:787–794.
3. Westermark A. Total reconstruction of the temporomandibular joint. Up to 8 years follow-up of patients with Biomet total joint prostheses. *Int J Oral Maxillofac Surg*. 2010;39:951–955.
4. Granquist EJ, Bouloux G, Dattilo D, et al. Outcomes and survivorship of Biomet Microfixation total joint replacement system: results from an FDA postmarket study. *J Oral Maxillofacial Surg*. 2020;78(9):1499–1508.
5. Guarda-Nardini L, Manfredini D, Ferronato G. Temporomandibular joint total replacement prosthesis: current knowledge and considerations for the future. *Int J Oral Maxillofac Surg*. 2008;37:103–110.
6. Quinn PD, Prosthesis L. *Oral Maxillofac Surg Clin North Am*. 2000;12:93–299.
7. Sidebottom AJ. Guidelines for the replacement of temporomandibular joints in the United Kingdom. *B J Oral Maxillofac Surg*. 2008;46:146–147.
8. Bradrick JP, Indresano AT. Failure rates of repetitive temporomandibular surgical procedures. *J Oral Maxillofac Surg*. 1992;50(suppl 3):145.
9. Henry CH, Wolford LM. Treatment outcomes for temporomandibular joint reconstruction after failed proplast-teflon implant failed. *J Oral Maxillofac Surg*. 1993;51:352.
10. Mercuri LG. Subjective and objective outcomes in patients reconstructed with a custom-fitted alloplastic temporomandibular joint prosthesis. *J Oral Maxillofac Surg*. 1999;57:1427–1430.
11. Mercuri LG, Swift JQ. Considerations for the use of alloplastic temporomandibular joint replacement in the growing patient. *J Oral Maxillofac Surg*. 2009;67:19709. 1990.
12. Driemel O, Braum S, Muller-Richter UDA, et al. Historical development of alloplastic temporomandibular joint replacement after 1945 and state of the art. *Int J Oral Maxillofac Surg*. 2009;38:909–920.
13. Quinn PD. Autogenous and alloplastic reconstruction of the temporomandibular joint. In: *Color Atlas of Temporomandibular Joint Surgery*. St. Louis, Missouri: Mosby; 1998.
14. Guarda-Nardini L, Manfredini D, Ferronato G. Temporomandibular joint total replacement prosthesis: current knowledge and considerations for the future. *Int J Oral Maxillofac Surg*. 2008;37:103–110.
15. Bhatt H, Goswami T. Implant wear mechanism—basic approach. *Biomed Mater*. 2008;3:042001.
16. Ingham E, Fisher J. Biological reactions to wear debris in total joint replacement. *Proc Inst Mech Engrs*. 2000;214:21–37.
17. McGloughlin TM, Kavanagh AG. Wear of ultra-high molecular weight polyethylene (UHMWPE) in total knee prostheses: a review of key influences. *Proc Inst Mech Eng H*. 2000;214:349–359.
18. Riegel R, Sweeney K, Inverso G, Quinn PD, Granquist EJ. Microbiology alloplastic total joint infections: a 20-year retrospective study. *J Oral Maxillofac Surg*. 2018;76:288–293.
19. Wolford LM, Rodrigues DB, McPhillips A. Management of the infected temporomandibular joint total joint prosthesis. *J Oral Maxillofac Surg*. 2010;68:2810–2823.
20. Kienapfel H, et al. Prevention of heterotopic bone formation after total hip arthroplasty. *Arch Orthop Trauma Surg*. 1999;119:292–302.
21. Durr ED, et al. Radiation treatment of heterotopic bone formation in the temporomandibular articulation. *Int J Radiat Oncol Bio Phys*. 1993;27:863–869.
22. Reid R, Cooke H. Postoperative ionizing radiation in the management of heterotopic bone formation in the temporomandibular joint. *J Oral Maxillofac Surg*. 1999;57:900–905.
23. Wolford LM, Karras SC. Autologous fat transplantation around temporomandibular joint total joint prostheses: preliminary treatment outcomes. *J Oral Maxillofac Surg*. 1997;55:245–251.
24. Milam SB. Failed implants and multiple operations. *Oral Surg Oral Med Oral Pathol Oral Radiol Endod*. 1997;83:156–162.

CHAPTER 149

Temporomandibular Joint (TMJ) Ankylosis

Nigel Shaun Matthews and Matthew H. Pham

Armamentarium

#9 Periosteal elevator
#15 Blade
Arch bars
Adson forceps
Bipolar forceps
Channel retractor
DeBakey tissue forceps
Double skin hooks
Dunn-Dautrey condyle retractor
Freer elevator
Hemostats
Kittner dissector sponges
Metzenbaum curved scissors
Microdrill
Needle tip microdissection needle
Nerve stimulator
Obwegeser-Freer curved and J-shaped elevators
Obwegeser right angled curved up and down retractors
Ruler
Rongeur
Sagittal saw
Scissors
Senn retractor
Seldin elevator
Ultrasonic handpiece (Piezo)
Tessier straight and curved osteotome
Virtual surgical planning cutting guides

History of the Procedure

Ankylosis, or the immobility of a joint secondary to fusion of bones, was one of the first temporomandibular joint (TMJ) disease processes to be treated surgically. The earliest report of the surgical treatment of TMJ ankylosis describes gap arthroplasty and the use of wood to mobilize the jaw in 1840.[1] A subsequent report by Murphy in 1914 also described a gap arthroplasty to treat ankylosis.[2] Ankylosis can be classified by location, type of tissue (fibrous or bony), and the extent of fusion (complete or partial).[3] Ankylosis is most commonly caused by trauma, but can also be due to infection, systemic arthropathy (ankylosing spondylitis, rheumatoid arthritis), osteoarthritis, irradiation, previous surgery, internal derangements, and perinatal events.[4]

Patients with a fibrous or bony ankylosis may commonly have facial asymmetry, restricted range of motion, and malocclusion. They may also present with an anterior open bite from a shortened ramus or midface abnormalities involving the piriform rim and orbits. Treatment for ankylosis depends on patient-specific factors but is almost invariably surgical. The three broad methods of treatment are gap arthroplasty, reconstruction or total joint replacement (TJR). Gap arthroplasty can be with or without the use of interpositional tissue. Interpositional tissue is thought to reduce the chance of ankylosis recurrence by eliminating dead space. Tissues commonly used include temporalis muscle, dermis-fat, fat, and auricular cartilage.[5] Reconstruction typically utilizes autogenous tissue while TJR utilizes alloplastic material.[6–10] Autogenous reconstruction typically involves the use of costochondral, sternoclavicular, fibular, iliac crest, or metatarsophalangeal grafts. The costochondral graft is the most widely used graft, particularly in children, and was first described by Harold Gillies in the 1920s.[11] Several authors have supported the use of costochondral graft for the reconstruction of the TMJ due to the graft's growth potential in juveniles.[12–14] Unfortunately, the costochondral graft has been shown to have an unpredictable growth pattern, which can lead to complications such as facial asymmetry and malocclusion.[15,16] Despite unpredictable growth, the costochondral graft is still considered by many to be the operative management of choice in children and adults who have not had prior surgery.[17,18]

TMJ reconstruction with alloplastic material should be considered in patients with ankylosis, reankylosis, failed tissue grafts, inflammatory arthritis not responsive to other treatment modalities, and failed previous alloplastic reconstruction.[19] Two devices are currently approved by the US Food and Drug Administration (FDA): the TMJ Concepts (TMJ Concepts, Ventura, CA, USA) custom joint (FDA approved in 1999) and the Zimmer Biomet (Zimmer Biomet Warsaw, IN, USA) total joint stock device (FDA approved in 2006). Stock joints require recontouring of the patient's bone prior to placement, which can lead to material fatigue or overload if not properly fitted. This creates micromotion and can lead to fibrous connective tissue surrounding the implant. A custom implant prosthesis is designed and contoured based on preoperative computed tomography (CT) to ensure superior adaptation to bony structures making it more appropriate for complex cases.[20] Long-term stability and function have been demonstrated with the TMJ Concepts custom prostheses.[21]

Outcomes following the treatment of TMJ ankylosis with various surgical approaches have been reported. A meta-analysis by De Roo reported that autogenous reconstruction had the highest average postoperative maximal opening at 30.6 mm.[22] Gap arthroplasty and gap arthroplasty with interpositional grafting reported openings of 26.2 mm and 26.7 mm, respectively.[10] A systematic review by Al-Moraissi et al. compared pain and reankylosis rates. Gap arthroplasty with interpositional graft (temporalis flap) was found to decrease reankylosis by 215% in comparison to gap arthroplasty alone.[23] Maximum incisal opening was also greater in the costochondral graft group compared with the alloplastic TJR. However, the alloplastic group had a substantial reduction in pain compared with that of the costochondral group[23] (Fig. 149.1A–D).

Indications

The broad goals of treatment for ankylosis are restoration of jaw form and function, prevention of reankylosis, and symmetrical growth of the mandible in a growing patient. More specific goals include establishing adequate oral opening, a satisfactory occlusion, appropriate facial form, ability to masticate, satisfactory speech, and an adequate airway.

A more conservative arthroplasty may be performed if the patient has minimal fibrous tissue causing fibrous ankylosis. However, gap arthroplasty (with or without interpositional tissue), autogenous reconstruction, or alloplastic TJR is needed if there is extensive fibrosis or bony ankylosis. Costochondral grafts are most useful in children who may benefit from continued growth of the cartilage cap. Alloplastic TJR has been shown to have excellent results in the setting of inflammatory arthritis involving the TMJ, recurrent ankylosis, failed reconstruction, and loss of vertical mandibular height.[24]

Making the correct diagnosis of ankylosis prior to treatment is imperative. The Diagnostic Criteria for Temporomandibular Disorders (DC/TMD) remains a robust tool to enable the correct diagnosis of both arthrogenous and muscle-related pain and limited function (Axis I).[25] Although TMJ ankylosis is not generally considered within the spectrum of TMD, it is included within the DC/TMD taxonomic description of TMJ diseases.[25] Masticatory muscle disorders may coexist with ankylosis and should be recognized and treated in addition to the ankylosis. It is also important to recognize any psychosocial diagnoses (Axis II) including anxiety, depression, and somatization that can adversely affect outcomes following the treatment of ankylosis.

Limitations and Contraindications

Gap arthroplasty with or without interpositional graft may reestablish jaw opening but it is unable to reposition the mandible. This prevents the ability to correct facial form, modify the occlusion, or increase the airway. The potential for reankylosis also remains high. Autogenous reconstruction with a costochondral graft is limited by overgrowth, undergrowth, resorption, and then potential for reankylosis. This graft should be used with caution in patients who have had prior attempts at TMJ reconstruction as the soft tissue vascularity is compromised, which may result in resorption of the graft. TJR provides the ability to accomplish all of the treatment goals but is not without limitations. Hardware failure, prosthesis infection, dislocation, and material hypersensitivity can all occur. The latter is typically related to nickel, cobalt, or chromium within the condylar head. The use of all titanium prostheses in patients with known allergy to these metals remains a better choice. Patients with any infection at the planned surgical site and those with severe acne are not good candidates for TJR given the risk of early and late periprosthetic infection.

TECHNIQUE

VIRTUAL SURGERY PLANNING

The management of individuals with TMJ ankylosis can be very challenging and requires coordination of care with radiology and anesthesiology. Essential radiology includes CT with axial, coronal, and sagittal images. Consideration should be given to the use of CT angiography if concern exists for the presence of blood vessels within the ankylotic mass. Measurements can be taken from the CT scan using identifiable landmarks to determine the superior and inferior boundaries of resection. Virtual surgical planning (VSP) can be an extremely helpful adjunct when doing this and allows for the development of a precise surgical plan. VSP can also provide splints to guide occlusal relationships and cutting guides for precise resection. If the patient has sufficient opening, dental models or intraoral scans can be incorporated into the CT to aid the accuracy of occlusal planning. The combination of VSP, stereolithographic models, and CT-based navigation has enhanced the safety, accuracy, and efficiency of ankylosis surgery. This approach reduces the need for intraoperative improvisation due to the accuracy of the planning and precision of surgical guides and navigation. In addition to enhancing the resection of the ankylosis, the use of VSP and models also enhances the design of the alloplastic joint replacement. Orthognathic occlusal splints are also used to facilitate functional occlusal relationships (Fig. 149.2A–F).

A plan for providing a safe airway should be coordinated with the anesthesiologist before surgery. Fiberoptic nasoendotracheal intubation is frequently required due to limited opening. The patient should be informed that a tracheostomy may be performed if fiberoptic intubation is unsuccessful.

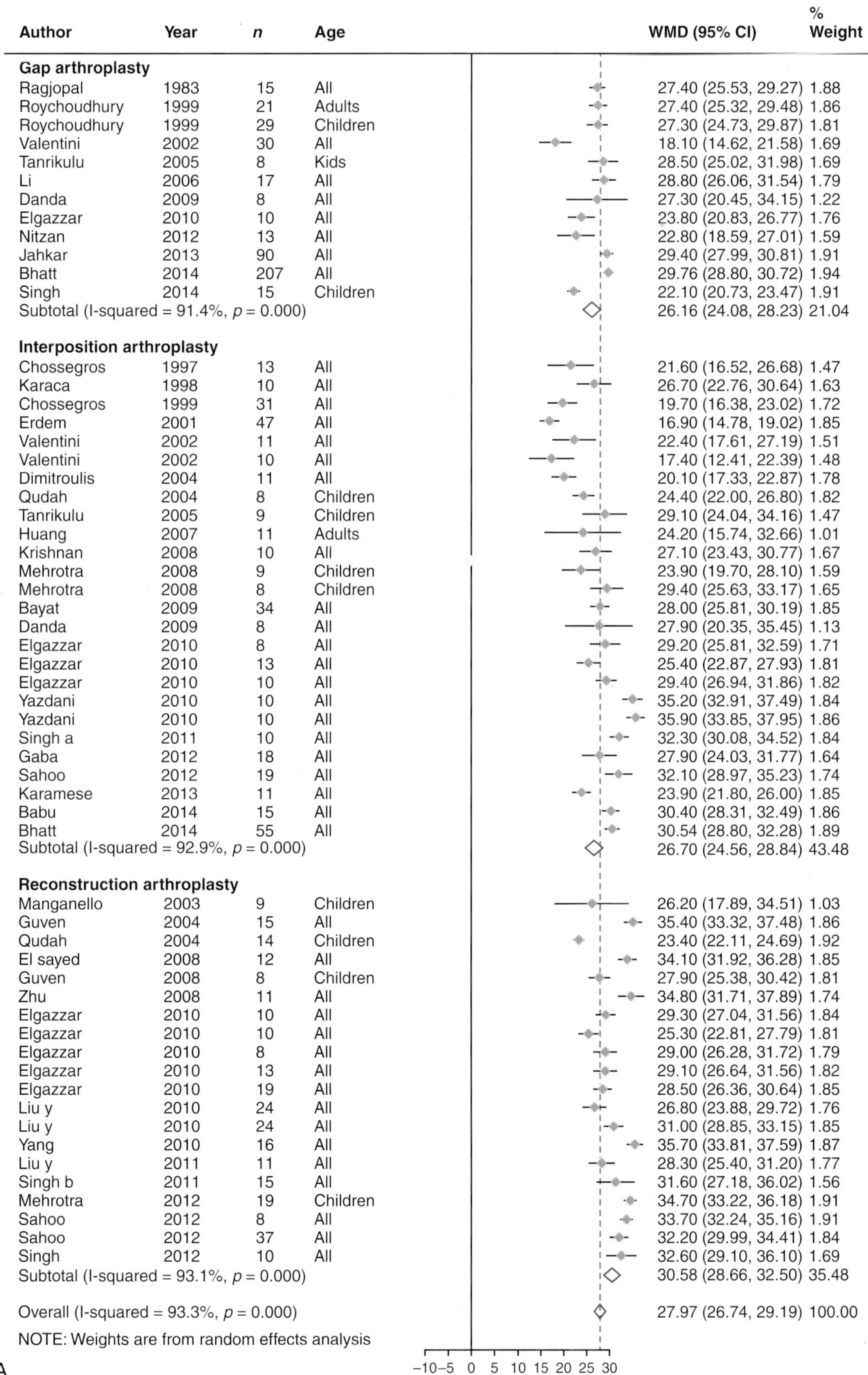

Author	Year	*n*	Age	WMD (95% CI)	% Weight
Gap arthroplasty					
Ragjopal	1983	15	All	27.40 (25.53, 29.27)	1.88
Roychoudhury	1999	21	Adults	27.40 (25.32, 29.48)	1.86
Roychoudhury	1999	29	Children	27.30 (24.73, 29.87)	1.81
Valentini	2002	30	All	18.10 (14.62, 21.58)	1.69
Tanrikulu	2005	8	Kids	28.50 (25.02, 31.98)	1.69
Li	2006	17	All	28.80 (26.06, 31.54)	1.79
Danda	2009	8	All	27.30 (20.45, 34.15)	1.22
Elgazzar	2010	10	All	23.80 (20.83, 26.77)	1.76
Nitzan	2012	13	All	22.80 (18.59, 27.01)	1.59
Jahkar	2013	90	All	29.40 (27.99, 30.81)	1.91
Bhatt	2014	207	All	29.76 (28.80, 30.72)	1.94
Singh	2014	15	Children	22.10 (20.73, 23.47)	1.91
Subtotal (I-squared = 91.4%, *p* = 0.000)				26.16 (24.08, 28.23)	21.04
Interposition arthroplasty					
Chossegros	1997	13	All	21.60 (16.52, 26.68)	1.47
Karaca	1998	10	All	26.70 (22.76, 30.64)	1.63
Chossegros	1999	31	All	19.70 (16.38, 23.02)	1.72
Erdem	2001	47	All	16.90 (14.78, 19.02)	1.85
Valentini	2002	11	All	22.40 (17.61, 27.19)	1.51
Valentini	2002	10	All	17.40 (12.41, 22.39)	1.48
Dimitroulis	2004	11	All	20.10 (17.33, 22.87)	1.78
Qudah	2004	8	Children	24.40 (22.00, 26.80)	1.82
Tanrikulu	2005	9	Children	29.10 (24.04, 34.16)	1.47
Huang	2007	11	Adults	24.20 (15.74, 32.66)	1.01
Krishnan	2008	10	All	27.10 (23.43, 30.77)	1.67
Mehrotra	2008	9	Children	23.90 (19.70, 28.10)	1.59
Mehrotra	2008	8	Children	29.40 (25.63, 33.17)	1.65
Bayat	2009	34	All	28.00 (25.81, 30.19)	1.85
Danda	2009	8	All	27.90 (20.35, 35.45)	1.13
Elgazzar	2010	8	All	29.20 (25.81, 32.59)	1.71
Elgazzar	2010	13	All	25.40 (22.87, 27.93)	1.81
Elgazzar	2010	10	All	29.40 (26.94, 31.86)	1.82
Yazdani	2010	10	All	35.20 (32.91, 37.49)	1.84
Yazdani	2010	10	All	35.90 (33.85, 37.95)	1.86
Singh a	2011	10	All	32.30 (30.08, 34.52)	1.84
Gaba	2012	18	All	27.90 (24.03, 31.77)	1.64
Sahoo	2012	19	All	32.10 (28.97, 35.23)	1.74
Karamese	2013	11	All	23.90 (21.80, 26.00)	1.85
Babu	2014	15	All	30.40 (28.31, 32.49)	1.86
Bhatt	2014	55	All	30.54 (28.80, 32.28)	1.89
Subtotal (I-squared = 92.9%, *p* = 0.000)				26.70 (24.56, 28.84)	43.48
Reconstruction arthroplasty					
Manganello	2003	9	Children	26.20 (17.89, 34.51)	1.03
Guven	2004	15	All	35.40 (33.32, 37.48)	1.86
Qudah	2004	14	Children	23.40 (22.11, 24.69)	1.92
El sayed	2008	12	All	34.10 (31.92, 36.28)	1.85
Guven	2008	8	Children	27.90 (25.38, 30.42)	1.81
Zhu	2008	11	All	34.80 (31.71, 37.89)	1.74
Elgazzar	2010	10	All	29.30 (27.04, 31.56)	1.84
Elgazzar	2010	10	All	25.30 (22.81, 27.79)	1.81
Elgazzar	2010	8	All	29.00 (26.28, 31.72)	1.79
Elgazzar	2010	13	All	29.10 (26.64, 31.56)	1.82
Elgazzar	2010	19	All	28.50 (26.36, 30.64)	1.85
Liu y	2010	24	All	26.80 (23.88, 29.72)	1.76
Liu y	2010	24	All	31.00 (28.85, 33.15)	1.85
Yang	2010	16	All	35.70 (33.81, 37.59)	1.87
Liu y	2011	11	All	28.30 (25.40, 31.20)	1.77
Singh b	2011	15	All	31.60 (27.18, 36.02)	1.56
Mehrotra	2012	19	Children	34.70 (33.22, 36.18)	1.91
Sahoo	2012	8	All	33.70 (32.24, 35.16)	1.91
Sahoo	2012	37	All	32.20 (29.99, 34.41)	1.84
Singh	2012	10	All	32.60 (29.10, 36.10)	1.69
Subtotal (I-squared = 93.1%, *p* = 0.000)				30.58 (28.66, 32.50)	35.48
Overall (I-squared = 93.3%, *p* = 0.000)				27.97 (26.74, 29.19)	100.00

NOTE: Weights are from random effects analysis

Figure 149.1 **A,** Forest plot showing weighted mean differences in postoperative maximal incisal opening after gap arthroplasty, interposition arthroplasty, and reconstruction arthroplasty.

Continued

Study or subgroup	GA Events	GA Total	IPG Events	IPG Total	Weight	Odds ratio M-H, fixed, 95% CI	Year
Tanrikulu et al.	0	8	1	9	27.6%	0.33 [0.01, 9.40]	2005
Ramezanian et al.	7	22	0	26	6.4%	25.65 [1.37, 480.52]	2006
Danda et al.	1	8	1	8	18.0%	1.00 [0.05, 19.36]	2009
Zhi et al.	3	24	0	17	10.3%	5.70 [0.28, 117.88]	2009
Elgazzar et al.	2	11	0	14	7.2%	7.63 [0.33, 177.14]	2010
Holmlund et al.	0	14	0	22		Not estimable	2013
Shaikh et al.	0	10	0	10		Not estimable	2013
Mansoor et al.	0	30	1	30	30.4%	0.32 [0.01, 8.24]	2013
Total (95% CI)		**127**		**136**	**100.0%**	**3.15 [1.17, 8.46]**	
Total events	13		3				

Heterogeneity: Chi² = 6.63, df = 5 (P = 0.25); I² = 25%
Test for overall effect: Z = 2.27 (P = 0.02)

B

Study or subgroup	AJR Mean	AJR SD	AJR Total	CCJ Mean	CCJ SD	CCJ Total	Weight	Mean difference IV, fixed, 95% CI	Year
Saeed et al.	21.15	11.39	50	23.9	13.02	49	46.3%	−2.75 [−7.57, 2.07]	2002
Tang et al.	23.95	11.07	23	23.6	11.34	28	28.2%	0.35 [−5.82, 6.52]	2009
Loveless et al.	9.4	9.7	14	18	9.7	22	25.5%	−8.60 [−15.10, −2.10]	2010
Total (95% CI)			**87**			**99**	**100.0%**	**−3.36 [−6.65, −0.08]**	

Heterogeneity: Chi² = 3.95, df = 2 (P = 0.14); I² = 49%
Test for overall effect: Z = 2.01 (P = 0.04)

C

Study or subgroup	AJR Mean	AJR SD	AJR Total	CCJ Mean	CCJ SD	CCJ Total	Weight	Mean difference IV, fixed, 95% CI	Year
Saeed et al.	4.55	3.72	50	5.7	3.38	49	37.5%	−1.15 [−2.55, 0.25]	2002
Tang et al.	3.6	1.7	23	4.4	2.4	28	57.7%	−0.80 [−1.93, 0.33]	2009
Loveless et al.	2.25	4.25	7	3.75	3.66	10	4.9%	−1.50 [−5.38, 2.38]	2010
Total (95% CI)			**80**			**87**	**100.0%**	**−0.97 [−1.82, −0.11]**	

Heterogeneity: Chi² = 0.22, df = 2 (P = 0.89); I² = 0%
Test for overall effect: Z = 2.21 (P = 0.03)

D

Figure 149.1, cont'd **B,** Forest plot showing gap arthroplasty (*GA*) versus interpositional gap arthroplasty (*IPG*) with regard to recurrence rate of ankylosis. **C,** Forest plot showing alloplastic joint reconstruction (*AJR*) versus costochondral joint (*CCJ*) with regard to maximal incisal opening. **D,** Forest plot showing alloplastic joint reconstruction (*AJR*) versus costochondral joint (*CCJ*) with regard to pain. (Part A adapted from Su-Gwan K. Treatment of temporomandibular joint ankylosis with temporalis muscle and fascia flap. *Int J Oral Maxillofac Surg.* 2001;30(3):189–193. Parts B–D adapted from Al-Moraissi EA, El-Sharkawy TM, Mounair RM, El-Ghareeb TI. A systematic review and meta-analysis of the clinical outcomes for various surgical modalities in the management of temporomandibular joint ankylosis. *Int. J. Oral Maxillofac.* Surg. 2015;44:470–482.)

TECHNIQUE—*cont'd*

SURGICAL PROCEDURE: STEP 1

After the induction of anesthesia and verification of endotracheal intubation, the endotracheal tube should be stabilized in a manner that prevents pressure necrosis of the nasal tip and forehead. Endotracheal tube stabilization should allow the head to be moved from right to left without dislodgement of the tube. The eyes should be lubricated and sealed shut with individual adhesive dressings. If adequate opening exists to place arch bars, this can be completed at this point. Complete a thorough sterile preparation of the face and neck with Betadine solution, chlorhexidine, or both. Place a sterile towel under the head, and seal the mouth and nose with a rectangular adhesive dressing. Isolate the surgical field with towels, a split sheet, and a head sheet (Fig. 149.3A).

STEP 2

Outline the preauricular incision within the skin crease closest to the tragus, making sure it is within 8 mm of the external auditory meatus. A question mark-shaped extension (Al Kayat and Bramley modification) into the temporal region can be utilized for better visualization of the temporalis fascia and muscle. Outline a retromandibular incision centered on the angle of the mandible between the antegonial notch and tragus in a natural fold approximately

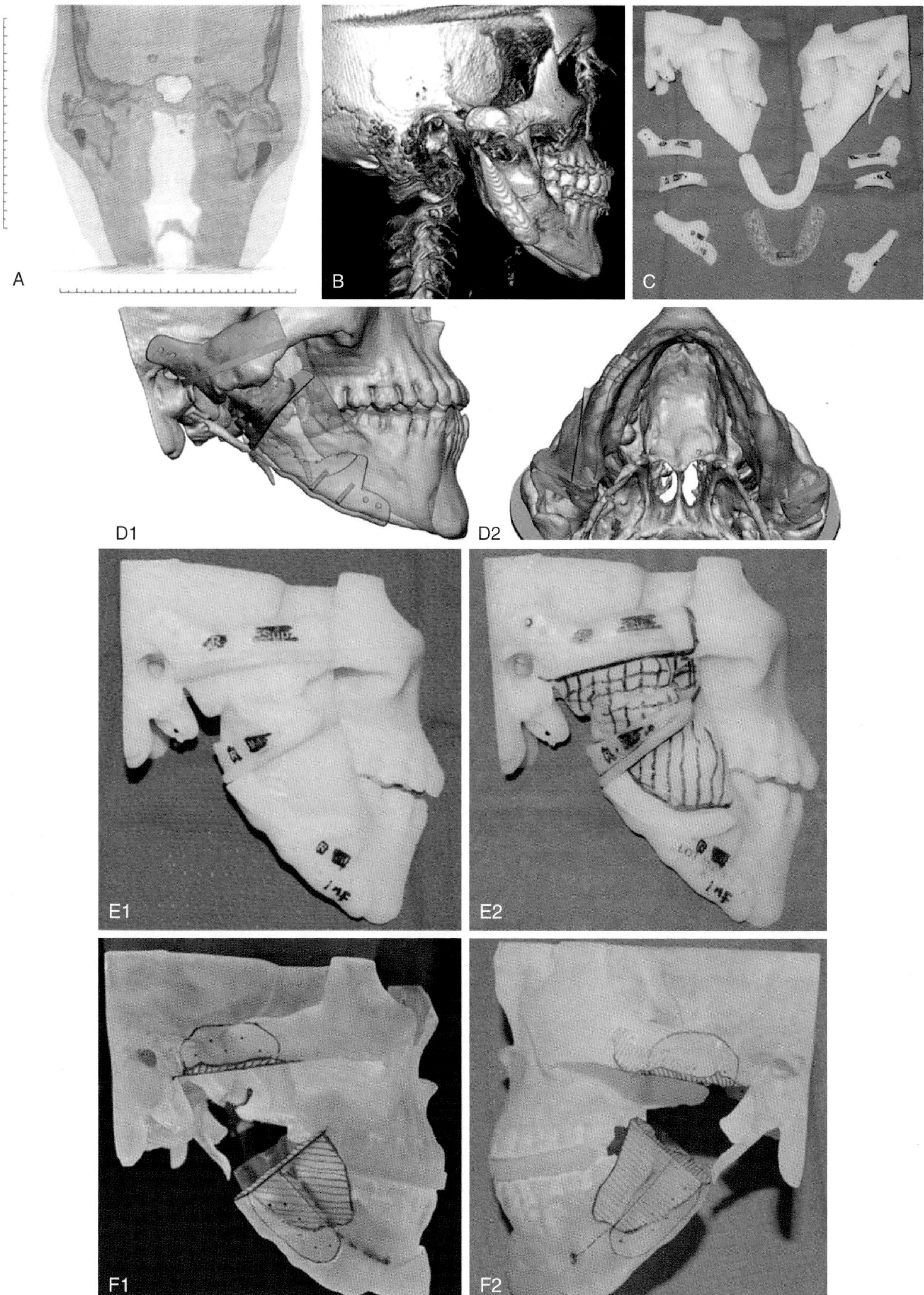

Figure 149.2 **A,** Computed tomography (CT) bone window of a coronal section through the temporomandibular condyles showing severe recurrent bony ankylosis of bilateral temporomandibular joints (TMJs). **B,** Three-dimensional CT image to correlate with navigation images. **C,** Stereolithographic model of the right and left side of the patient, cutting guides, and the repositioning guides. **D1** and **D2,** Surgical guides overlaid on CT scan. **E1** and **E2,** Ankylosis and planned resection and recontouring. **F1** and **F2,** Resected ankylosis, recontoured ramus/fossa, repositioned mandible, and prosthesis design.

TECHNIQUE—*cont'd*

1 cm inferior and posterior to the mandibular ramus angle inferior border outline. Preemptive analgesia and hemostasis are established by providing a subcuticular injection of local anesthetic along both incision outlines and by an auriculotemporal nerve block along the avascular pretragal plane. If surgical navigation is planned, the fiduciary system is placed and point-to-point indexing is completed. The availability of intraoperative navigation has significantly enhanced the accuracy of reconstruction cases. This technology is well-suited to the complex nature of recurrent TMJ cases. It allows safety in all aspects of the surgery, with particular attention to the superior and medial aspects of the surgery, where the anatomy can be particularly altered in patients with recurrent ankylosis (Fig. 149.3B).

STEP 3

The dissection is initiated in the pretragal fold with continuous, curvilinear skin incisions. The pretragal avascular plane is established with a mosquito hemostat. The plane of dissection is posterior to the superficial temporal artery and vein and the auriculotemporal nerve. The neurovascular structures are moved anteriorly during the dissection, using hemostats and Kittner dissectors, to avoid unnecessary neurovascular trauma. The superficial layer of the deep temporal fascia is identified, and an incision is made through it with the needle tip microdissector. The dissection is followed to the zygomatic arch, and the root of the zygoma is identified. A periosteal or Obwegeser elevator is used to expose the lateral aspect of the joint; great care is taken to remain subperiosteal to avoid trauma to the temporal branch of the facial nerve. The elevator should be lifted in a tenting motion as the tissue overlaying the zygomatic arch is dissected. If the joint capsule is present, insufflate with a local anesthetic, make an incision below the zygomatic arch, and open the capsule to inspect the ankylosis. At this point, the preauricular dissection is packed with moist gauze (Fig. 149.3C and D).

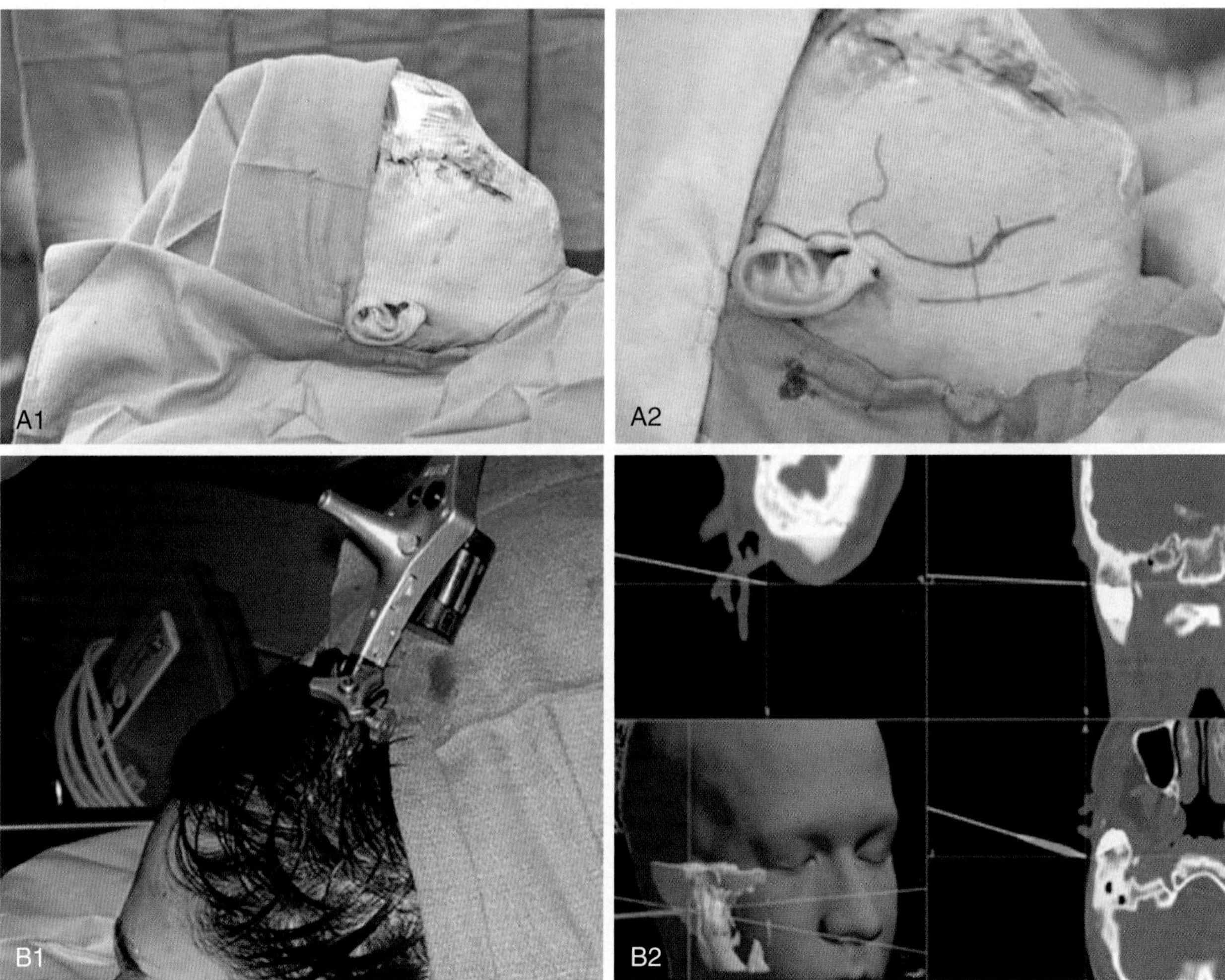

Figure 149.3 **A1** and **A2,** Patient prep and draping. **B1** and **B2,** Fiduciary marker and registration.

TECHNIQUE—*cont'd*

STEP 4

A layered retromandibular dissection is then completed with positive identification of the platysma, marginal mandibular branch of the facial nerve, and parotidomasseteric fascia. The pterygomasseteric sling is then divided, and the mandible is exposed (Fig. 149.3E).

The entire lateral surface of the mandible is exposed with careful protection of the retromandibular vein posteriorly. The entire posterior and anterior borders, condylar neck, sigmoid notch, and coronoid process should be visible. One toe-out retractor is placed on the anterior border at the base of the coronoid process, one into the sigmoid notch, and one above the coronoid process. If cutting guides were made during VSP, they should be applied at this time with two to three screws. The coronoidectomy is completed with a sagittal saw or Piezosurgery (Mectron, Carasco, GE, Italy) handpiece. The coronoid process is held with a Kelly clamp and dissected free with elevators and electrocautery. Of note, it can be helpful to ask anesthesia for brief paralysis during this time to decrease the pull of the temporalis. It is otherwise much more likely for the coronoid to be lost into the infratemporal space.

Continued

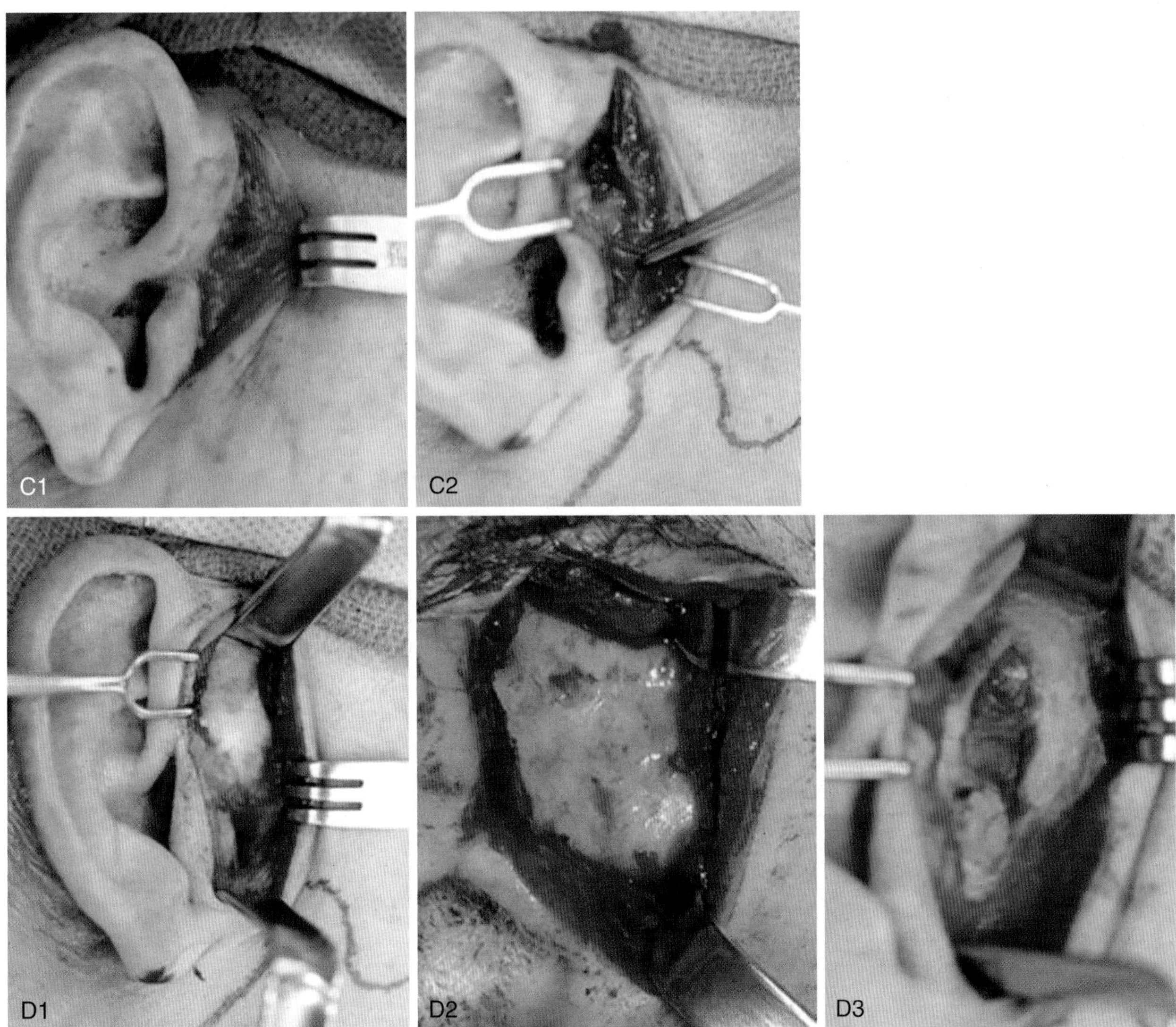

Figure 149.3, cont'd **C1** and **C2,** Preauricular approach through temporoparietal fascia. **D1** and **D3,** Identification and division of the temporalis fascia.

TECHNIQUE—*cont'd*

STEP 5

Once the ankylosis is well exposed, a caliper is used to score the superior line of resection based off the measurements from the CT scan in relation to an identifiable landmark, such as the superior border of the zygomatic arch. A second score line is marked approximately 1 cm inferior to the original line. Again, if VSP was used, the cutting guide can be placed and secured at this time. The initial resection is completed with a microsagittal saw, fissure bur, or Piezosurgery handpiece to a depth a few millimeters short of the dimension determined by CT measurements or to the depth determined by the cutting guides. Surgical navigation can also be used to guide the depth of resection. The resection is completed as necessary with judicious use of osteotomies. The surgeon should look for remnants of a joint space and follow that plane during final resection of bone from the fossa. The surgeon must be very careful during removal of bone from the posterior wall of the joint to avoid fracture of the bony external auditory canal. The resected bone must be carefully dissected from soft tissue with elevators and electrocautery. If bleeding is encountered, hemostasis can be achieved with bipolar cautery, needle tip electrocautery, vascular clips, and Surgicel (Johnson & Johnson, New Brunswick, NJ, USA). Once the resection is complete, it can be verified by inspection from the preauricular and retromandibular view and, if needed, by intraoperative CT (Fig. 149.4A and B).

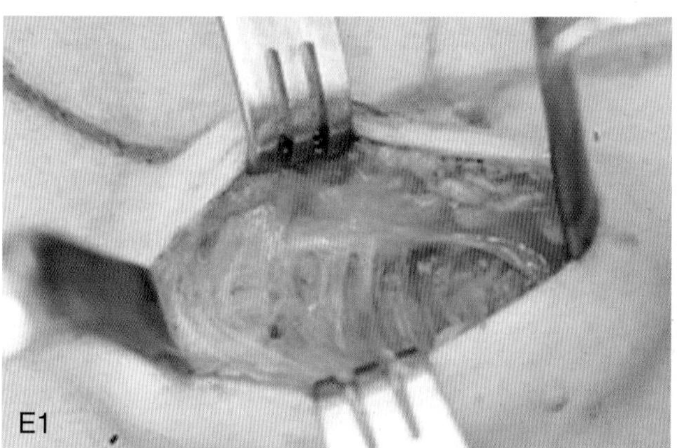

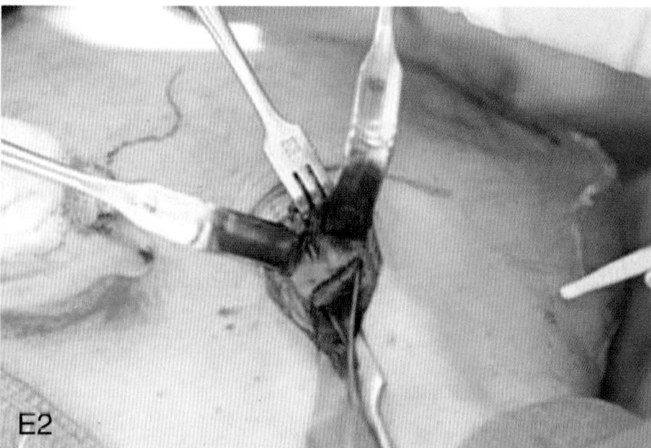

Figure 149.3, cont'd **E1** and **E2,** Retromandibular approach.

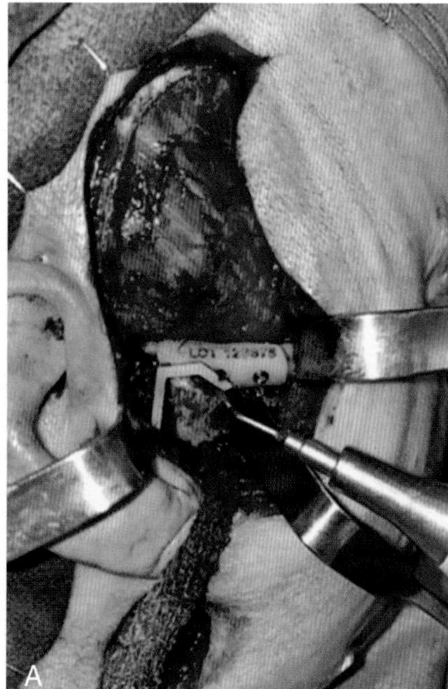

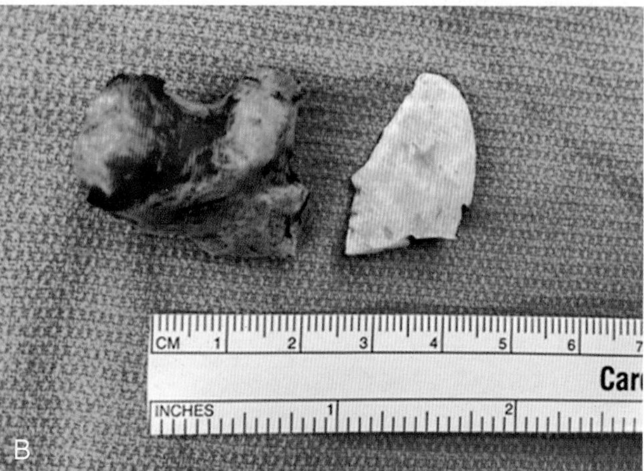

Figure 149.4 Resection of ankylosis and coronoid process. **A,** Cutting guide for resection of ankylosis. **B,** Resected ankylosed condyle coronoid.

TECHNIQUE—*cont'd*

STEP 6

Once the resection is complete, the reconstruction of choice is completed to maintain the gap. In adults without contraindications, the method of choice is a patient-specific joint replacement. The patient is placed into maxillomandibular fixation (MMF) prior to placement of the implant. The entire surgical team should change gloves and gowns, and the patient's oral cavity needs to be re-covered with adhesive dressings prior to turning attention back to the surgical site. At this point, a standard approach is used to complete a TJR (Fig. 149.5A–C).

The patient is released from MMF and function of the autogenous or alloplastic joint is verified. Intraoral guiding elastics are placed. Adhesive dressings are then replaced over the oral cavity prior to skin closure.

STEP 7

A 2 to 3 cm inferior curvilinear periumbilical incision is made after subcutaneous injection of local anesthesia. Dissection is carried out with hemostats until adipose tissue is encountered. Approximately 2 to 4 cc of fat graft is harvested and placed in saline. The site is irrigated and closed with deep Vicryl (Ethicon Inc, J & J Company, J494G) sutures and subcuticular or interrupted skin sutures. The fat graft is then placed around the condylar head of the TJR implant. It is important to tuck the graft into the medial and inferior space surrounding the implant to minimize the risk of ankylosis recurrence (Fig. 149.6A–C).

Continued

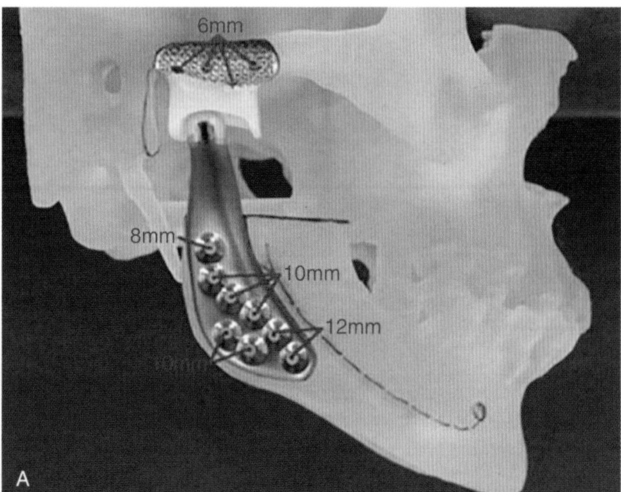

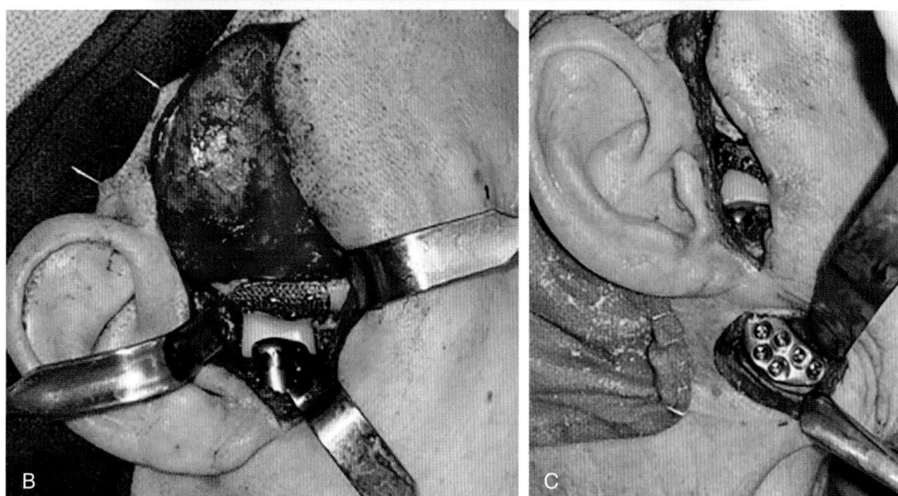

Figure 149.5 Insertion of total joint replacement. Patient-specific joint replacement, revealing the fossa and mandibular components in an appropriate relationship.

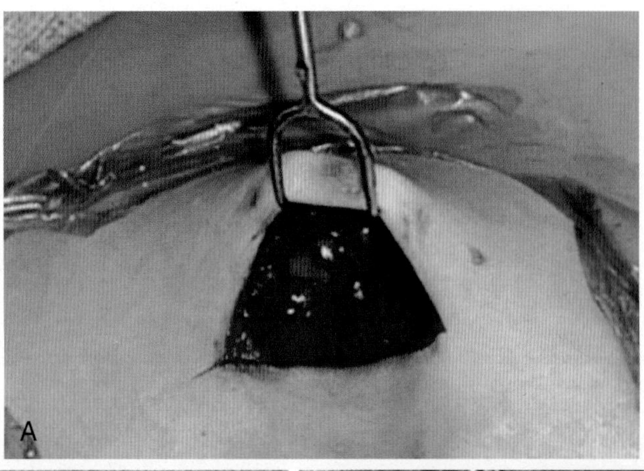

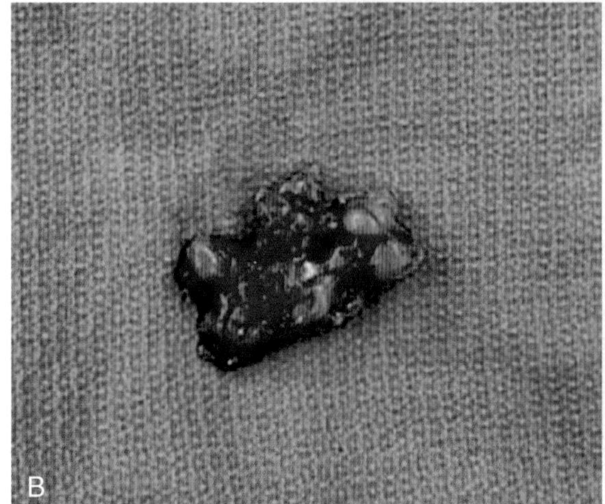

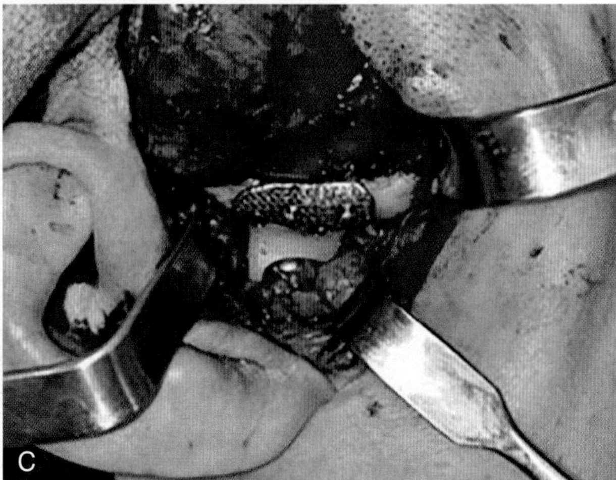

Figure 149.6 Fat graft harvest and placement around the total joint replacement (TJR). **A,** Incision for access to harvest abdominal fat. **B,** Harvested abdominal fat. **C,** Fat graft placed around condylar component.

TECHNIQUE—*cont'd*

STEP 8

Perioperative pain control can be enhanced by placing an On-Q pain pump (Avanos, Alpharetta, GA, USA) to deliver ropivacaine 0.2%. The On-Q set PM003 with a standard catheter delivers 2 cc/hour for 5 days. The total volume in the elastomeric pump is 270 cc. The catheter is introduced from inferior to the retromandibular incision in a subcuticular plane using the needle and plastic cannula contained in the set. It is advanced to the preauricular incision; the catheter is placed adjacent to the auriculotemporal nerve, not in the joint. It is secured with a Vicryl suture looped around the catheter. Where it exits the neck, the catheter is secured with Steri-Strips, and the full length of the tubing is covered with Opsite dressings. Closure is then carried out in a layered fashion, first closing the joint space with 3-0 Vicryl suture. Fascia and subcutaneous tissue are then reapproximated with 4-0 Vicryl suture followed by 5-0 nylon running suture to close the skin. The incisions are covered with Steri-Strips and an adhesive island dressing that is removed on the second postoperative day (Fig. 149.7A).

An alternative pain control modality is injection of 10 to 20 cc of liposomal bupivacaine (Exparel) (Pacira, Troy-Hills, NJ, USA) at each surgical incision site. This has been shown to decrease opioid requirements in other oral and maxillofacial procedures and helps to provide extended anesthesia postsurgery[25] (Fig. 149.7B).

Avoidance and Management of Intraoperative Complications

Correction of TMJ ankylosis is one of the most challenging procedures in oral and maxillofacial surgery. The medial aspect of the ankylosis is in close proximity to the middle meningeal artery, internal jugular vein, and internal carotid artery. VSP and the use of a Piezosurgery device can assist in avoidance of these structures. Access to the internal maxillary artery through the retromandibular incision is mandatory to control acute hemorrhage during resection. Temporary facial nerve weakness is not uncommon after TJR. Facial mimetic exercises, as well as adequate lubrication and taping of the eye, are imperative until the patient regains function. Parotid injury with sialocele or fistula formation are also possible, and they can be treated conservatively with pressure dressings,

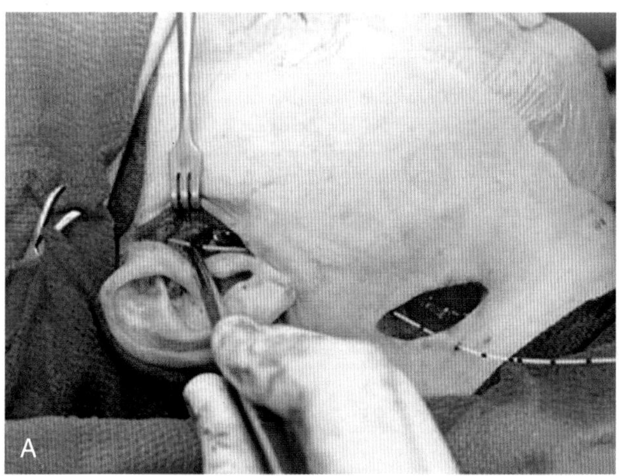
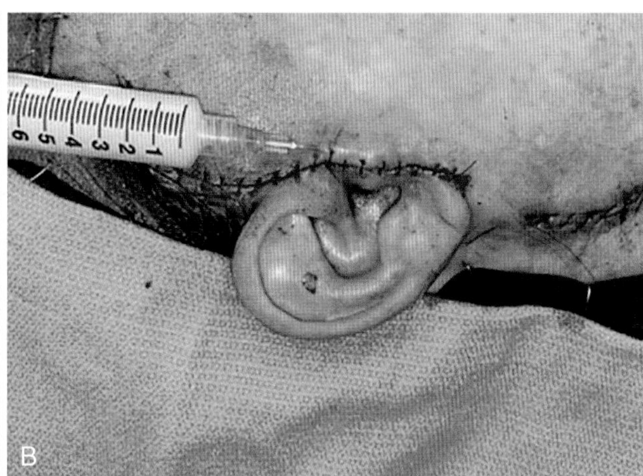

Figure 149.7 **A,** On-Q pain pump placement. **B,** Liposomal Bupivacaine injection.

antisialagogues, and botulinum toxin. Patients may experience decreased hearing due to edema surrounding the external auditory canal. Perforation of the tympanic membrane can also occur and can be treated with antibiotic drops, placement of an occlusive ear wick, and close follow-up.

Postoperative Considerations

Rehabilitation is the most significant concern in the postoperative period. Physical therapy should continue after the maximal incisal opening is established to prevent relapse.[26] The greatest advantage of alloplastic material over autogenous grafts is the ability to start physical therapy immediately following surgery. Returning the jaw to normal function reduces scar tissue formation, allowing for optimal range of motion.[27] An oral orthotic appliance is necessary for patients with parafunctional habits to reduce wear and increase the functional life of the prosthesis.

References

1. Carnochan JM. Mobilizing a patient's ankylosed jaw by placing a block of wood between the raw bony surfaces after resection. *Arch Med (Oviedo)*. 1860;2:284.
2. Murphy JB. Arthroplasty for intra-articular bony and fibrous ankylosis of temporomandibular articulation. *JAMA*. 1914;62:1783–1794.
3. Rowe NL. Ankylosis of the temporomandibular joint. *J R Coll Surg Edinb*. 1982;27(2):67–79.
4. Topazian RG. Etiology of ankylosis of the TMJ: analysis of 44 cases. *J Oral Surg Anesth Hosp Dent Serv*. 1964;22:227.
5. MacIntosh RB. The use of autogenous tissues for temporomandibular joint reconstruction. *J Oral Maxillofac Surg*. 2000;58(1):63–69.
6. Vasconcelos BC, Porto GG, Bessa-Nogueira RV, Nascimento MM. Surgical treatment of temporomandibular joint ankylosis: follow-up of 15 cases and literature review. *Med Oral Patol Oral Cir Bucal*. 2009;14(1):E34–E38.
7. Huang IY, Lai ST, Shen YH, Worthington P. Interpositional arthroplasty using autogenous costal cartilage graft for temporomandibular joint ankylosis in adults. *Int J Oral Maxillofac Surg*. 2007;36(10):909–915.
8. Loveless TP, Bjornland T, Dodson TB, Keith DA. Efficacy of temporomandibular joint ankylosis surgical treatment. *J Oral Maxillofac Surg*. 2010;68(6):1276–1282.
9. Mercuri LG, Ali FA, Woolson R. Outcomes of total alloplastic replacement with periarticular autogenous fat grafting for management of reankylosis of the temporomandibular joint. *J Oral Maxillofac Surg*. 2008;66(9):1794–1803.
10. Su-Gwan K. Treatment of temporomandibular joint ankylosis with temporalis muscle and fascia flap. *Int J Oral Maxillofac Surg*. 2001;30(3):189–193.
11. Gillies HD. *Plastic Surgery of the Face*. London, UK: Oxford University Press; 1920.
12. Kaban LB, Perrott DH, Fisher K. A protocol for management of temporomandibular joint ankylosis. *J Oral Maxillofac Surg*. 1990;48(11):1145–1151.
13. Ware WH, Brown SL. Growth centre transplantation to replace mandibular condyles. *J Maxillofac Surg*. 1981;9(1):50–58.
14. Poswillo DE. Biological reconstruction of the mandibular condyle. *Br J Oral Maxillofac Surg*. 1987;25(2):100–104.
15. Guyuron B, Lasa CI Jr. Unpredictable growth pattern of costochondral graft. *Plast Reconstr Surg*. 1992;90(5):880–886.
16. Peltomäki T, Rönning O. Interrelationship between size and tissue-separating potential of costochondral transplants. *Eur J Orthod*. 1991;13(6):459–465.
17. Kaban LB, Bouchard C, Troulis MJ. A protocol for management of temporomandibular joint ankylosis in children. *J Oral Maxillofac Surg*. 2009;67(9):1966–1978.
18. Saeed NR, Kent JN. A retrospective study of the costochondral graft in TMJ reconstruction. *Int J Oral Maxillofac Surg*. 2003;32(6):606–609.
19. Saeed N, Hensher R, McLeod N, Kent J. Reconstruction of the temporomandibular joint autogenous compared with alloplastic. *Br J Oral Maxillofac Surg*. 2002;40(4):296–299.
20. Mercuri LG, Giobbie-Hurder A. Long-term outcomes after total alloplastic temporomandibular joint reconstruction following exposure to failed materials. *J Oral Maxillofac Surg*. 2004;62(9):1088–1096.
21. Mercuri LG, Wolford LM, Sanders B, et al. Custom CAD/CAM total joint reconstruction system: preliminary multicenter report. *J Oral Maxillofac Surg*. 1995;53:106.
22. De Roo N, Van Doorne L, Troch A, Vermeersch H, Brusselaers N. Quantifying the outcome of surgical treatment of temporomandibular joint ankylosis: a systematic review and meta-analysis. *J Craniomaxillofac Surg*. 2016;44(1):6–15.
23. Al-Moraissi EA, El-Sharkawy TM, Mounair RM, El-Ghareeb TI. A systematic review and meta-analysis of the clinical outcomes for

various surgical modalities in the management of temporomandibular joint ankylosis. *Int J Oral Maxillofac Implants.* 2015;44(4):470–482.

24. Schiffman E, Ohrbach R, Truelove E, et al. International RDC/TMD Consortium Network, International association for Dental Research, Orofacial Pain Special Interest Group, International Association for the Study of Pain; Diagnostic Criteria for Temporomandibular Disorders (DC/TMD) for clinical and research applications: recommendations of the International RDC/TMD Consortium Network and orofacial pain special interest group. *J Oral Facial Pain Headache.* 2014;28(1):6–27.
25. Magraw C, Pham M, Neal T, et al. A multimodal analgesic protocol may reduce opioid use after third molar surgery: a pilot study. *Oral Surg Oral Med Oral Pathol Oral Radiol.* 2018;126(3):214–217.
26. Friedman MH, Weisberg J, Weber FL. Postsurgical temporomandibular joint hypomobility. Rehabilitation technique. *Oral Surg Oral Med Oral Pathol.* 1993;75(1):24–28.
27. Salter RB. *Continuous Passive Motion.* Baltimore, Maryland: Williams & Wilkins; 1993.

CHAPTER 150

Brow Lifting

Tirbod Fattahi and Sepideh Sabooree

Armamentarium

#9 Periosteal elevator
30" Pediatric sinus endoscope
Endoscope guard
Endoscopic muscle dissector
Endoscopic nerve hook
Endoscopic periosteal elevator
Endoscopic scissors
Endoscopic tower with monitor
Face lift "Bear Claw" retractor
Face lift scissors
Freer elevator
Long metzenbaum scissors

History of the Procedure

The history of brow lifting goes back nearly 100 years. Passot, in 1919, was credited with the first description of forehead lifting using several transverse skin excision of upper forehead skin.[1] In 1926, Hunt described coronal and hairline excision.[2] Others described undermining of the pericranium and resection of corrugator muscles in the following years.[3] In the 1960s, other modifications such as the pretrichial incision were introduced.[4] The first description of a "bi-planar" approach to the temporal region was described in the early 1970s.[5] Flowers has been given credit for emphasizing the importance of proper brow positioning *prior* to upper eye lid surgery.[6] In 1992, Isse introduced the concept of minimally invasive brow lifting via the endoscopic approach.[7] Since then, there have been a number of modifications to both the "open" and "endoscopic" approaches for forehead lifting.[8–13]

Indications for the Use of the Procedure

The main indication for brow lifting is to create a more youthful position for brows. There are certainly other secondary advantages of brow lifting such as improvement in the appearance of forehead rhytids, relaxation of glabellar muscles (corrugator, procerus, and depressor supercilia), improvement in the appearance of crow's feet, and enhancing the appearance of upper eye lids (by improving dermatochalasia of upper lids). An open, bright, and youthful appearance of the eyes and brows, especially in a female, is one of the first features of the face noticed in public (Fig. 150.1). It is important to note, as will be discussed later, that patients who have upper eye lid dermatochalasia should have their brows examined first before eye lid surgery. Many times, the real culprit of upper eye lid dermatochalasia is brow ptosis.

Limitations and Contraindications

There are several limitations and contraindications to consider when discussing brow lifting. Many of the limitations depend on the particular type of brow lifting. Open brow lifting can include coronal, pretrichial, mid-forehead, direct, and browpexy. The only other type of brow lifting is the endoscopic approach. Coronal brow lifting can lengthen the forehead; therefore, it should not be used in patients with high hairlines (long forehead). Direct brow lifting and browpexy can only lift the brows a few millimeters; they are not indicated for severe brow ptosis. Pretrichial brow lift is done in a subgaleal (preferred) or subcutaneous plane; this approach will limit correction/transection of procerous and corrugator muscles unless additional incisions are made. Endoscopic technique has an inherent learning curve and requires endoscopic instruments and monitors, which can be expensive. Endoscopic brow lifting is rather difficult to perform in patients with severe curvature of the forehead (sloping of the forehead in profile view).

Other limitations of brow lifting include the dilemma of performing a forehead lift on a bald patient or one with a receding hairline. Some have advocated performing a pretrichial lift and actually lowering the hair-bearing scalp (inferiorly). Others recommend endoscopic brow lifting as the best choice for a bald patient (multiple small incisions versus a coronal incision). Of note, it is important to place brows in the ideal position prior to performing upper eye lid blepharoplasty.

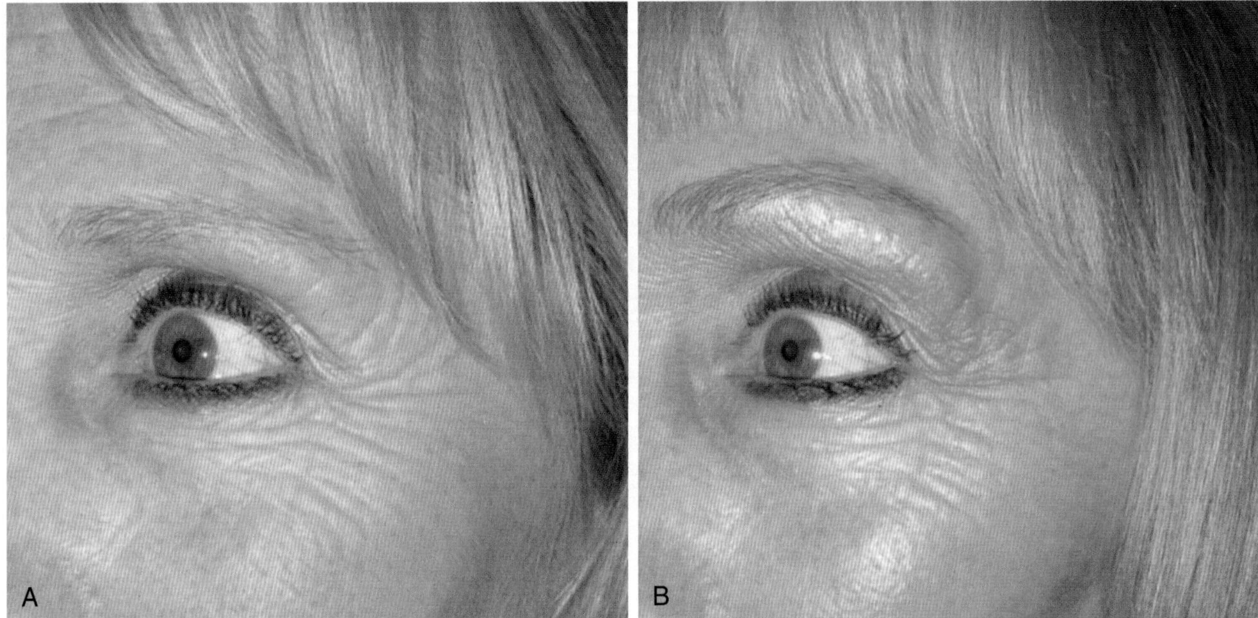

Figure 150.1 **A,** Preop image following brow lift. **B,** Postop image following brow lift.

TECHNIQUE: Endoscopic Brow Lift

Techniques for both endoscopic and pretrichial approaches will be described in a step-wise fashion.

STEP 1: Preparation

- Patient is placed in supine position in the surgical suite with head in a small "holder" such as a Mayfield head device or a "donut" head device to minimize movement. Protective eye shields (contact lenses) are placed in. Supra-orbital foramina/notches are marked. Standard prep solution is then used over the entire face and head. Local anesthesia with a vasoconstrictor is also given.

STEP 2: Incision

- A mid-line incision is made along the sagittal (median) plane, approximately 2 cm in length within (1.0 cm) the hairline. Incision is taken all the way down through the pericranium to bone. Two similar incisions are made (paramedian) in a line parallel to the lateral limbus/canthus areas, again deep to bone. Next two temporal incisions are made. These are slightly longer (2 to 3 cm) and are obliquely fashioned over the mid-temple area within the hair-bearing scalp perpendicular to a line from the nasal ala to the lateral canthus. These two incisions are deepened to the level of the deep temporal fascia. This creates a bi-planar level of dissection (subperiosteal and supra-fascial) (Figs. 150.2 and 150.3)

STEP 3: Dissection

- Using a #9 periosteal elevator, the entire forehead is dissected in a subperiosteal plane up to the supraorbital rims. An endoscopic guard can be used during the dissection to prevent the scalp flap from collapsing and diminishing the view of the surgical field (Fig. 150.4). This dissection is limited laterally by the temporal fusion lines and is performed through the 3 forehead ports (median and paramedian). Some advocate using the endoscope during the subperiosteal elevation near the supraorbital rims for direct visualization of the neurovascular bundles. Endoscopic elevators can also be used during this dissection.
- Using the temporal ports, dissection is carried medially toward the temporal fusion line staying on top of the deep temporal fascia. Once the temporal fusion line is reached, under direction visualization through one of the scalp ports, the fusion line is transected, creating a smooth transition from the skull (subperiosteal) to the suprafascial dissection over the deep temporal fascia (Figs. 150.5 and 150.6).

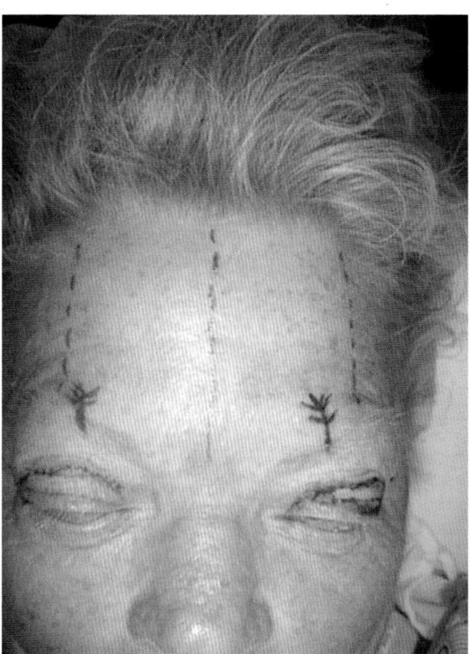

Figure 150.2 Location of three scalp ports for endoscopic brow lift.

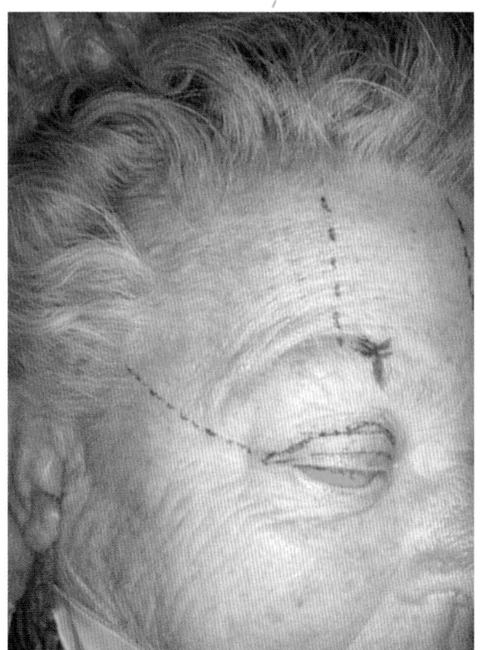

Figure 150.3 Location of temporal port for endoscopic brow lift.

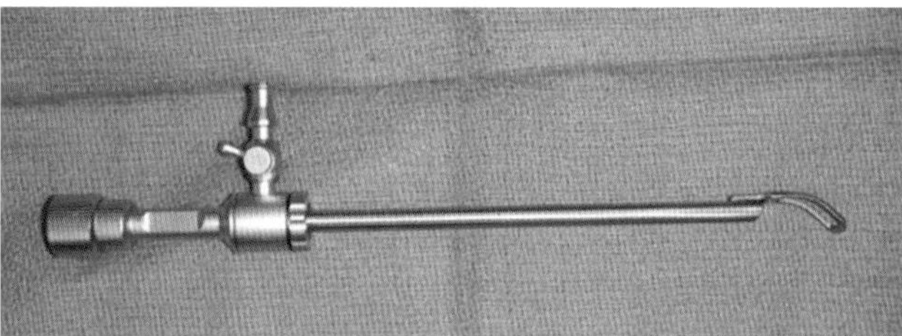

Figure 150.4 Endoscopic guard; note curvature of the tip, which aids in keeping the scalp elevated.

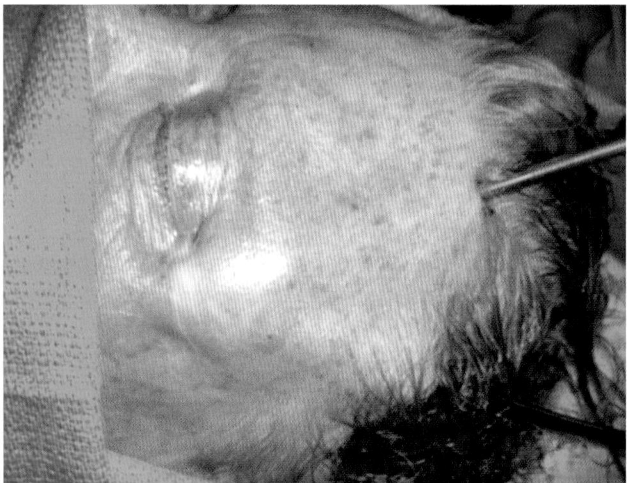

Figure 150.5 Dissection along the lateral orbital wall.

TECHNIQUE: Endoscopic Brow Lift—*cont'd*

STEP 4: Release and Scoring of Arcus Marginalis

- Once the entire subperiosteal dissection and temporal dissection are completed, under direct visualization, the released arcus marginalis is scored in a transverse direction from one side all the way to the other side. This is a critical step to allow mobilization of the forehead flap in a cephalad direction. The use of endoscopic elevators and nerve hook is helpful in this step.

Continued

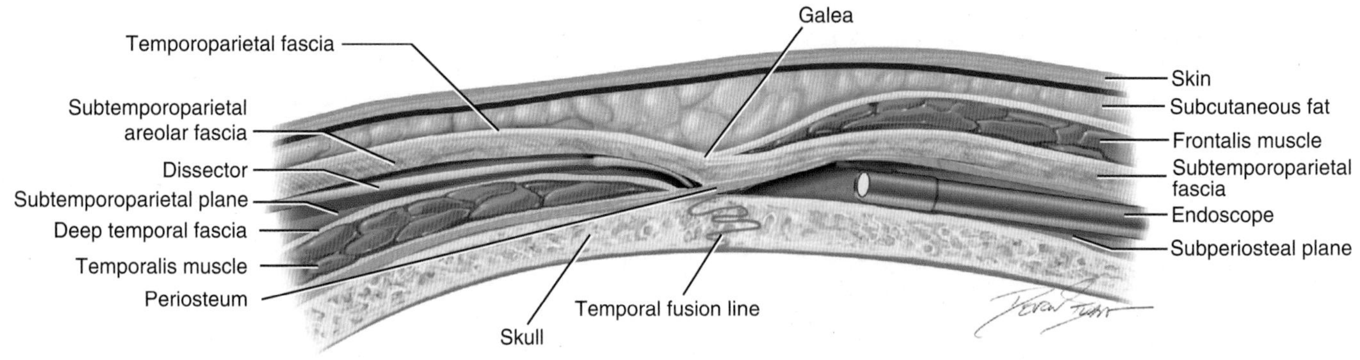

Figure 150.6 Bi-planar relationship between the pericranium and deep temporal fascia.

TECHNIQUE: Endoscopic Brow Lift—*cont'd*

STEP 5: Fixation

- Once satisfied with the amount of brow elevation, attention is directed to flap fixation. There are several techniques available to secure the elevated forehead flap. These include bone tunnels, resorbable anchor devices, and titanium plates and screws. Fixation devices are typically only used at the two paramedian ports; the temporal incisions are closed so that the elevated temporal flap (inferior flap) is secured to the deep temporal fascia on the intact temple (superior flap) in a cephalad direction. This closure aids significantly in elevating the tail of the brows. Fibrin sealants are also quite helpful in maintaining the forehead flap in an elevated state.

STEP 6: Dressing

- After the closure of scalp and temple incisions, the hair is washed in the operating room. A pressure dressing is placed circumferentially to minimize swelling and bruising. All brow lift patients should be seen within 24 hours in order to rule out a hematoma. Transient paresis of the temporal branch of the facial nerve may be present for a few days. Scalp and forehead numbness is much more common and may last for several months.

ALTERNATE TECHNIQUE: Pretrichial/Trichophytic Forehead Lift

STEP 1: Preparation

- Patient preparation for a pretrichial forehead lift is identical to an endoscopic technique. The patient is placed in supine position in the surgical suite with the head in a small "holder" such as a Mayfield head device or a "donut" head device to minimize movement. Protective eye shields (contact lenses) are placed in. Supra-orbital foramina/notches are marked. Standard prep solution is then used over the entire face and head. Local anesthesia with a vasoconstrictor is also given.

STEP 2: Incision

- An overly beveled incision is made just inside the villus hairs of the forehead. It is also critical to make the incision in a very "irregular" fashion. This incision extends from one temporal area to the other side (Fig. 150.7).

STEP 3: Dissection and Elevation

- The author only elevates the flap in a subgaleal plane (Fig. 150.8). Others have advocated elevating a subcutaneous forehead flap. Forehead skin flaps can become quite thin in the subcutaneous plane and chances of vascular compromise or creation of a "button-hole" exist. Elevation in a subgaleal plane should continue inferiorly until proper mobilization of the forehead and brows are obtained. Typically, dissection lateral to the temporal fusion lines can be performed if the elevation of the tail of the brow is necessary. Also, since the dissection is subgaleal, the arcus marginalis is not seen and does not require release.

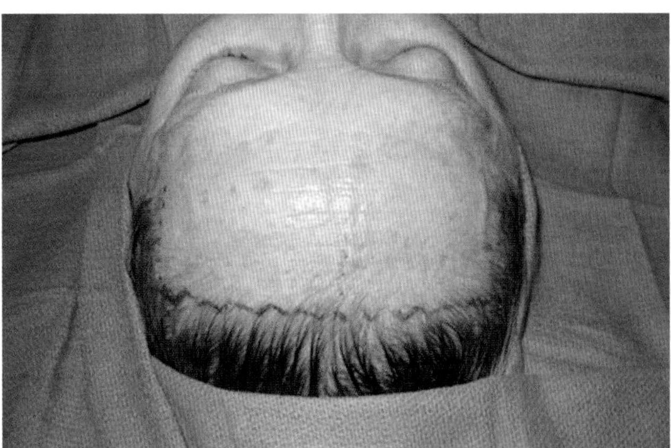

Figure 150.7 Irregular incision for trichophytic brow lift.

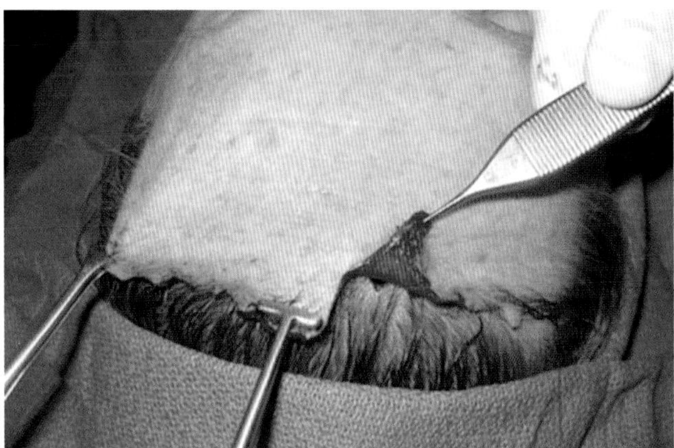

Figure 150.9 Separation of forehead flap into two sections; note amount of flap elevation and overlap.

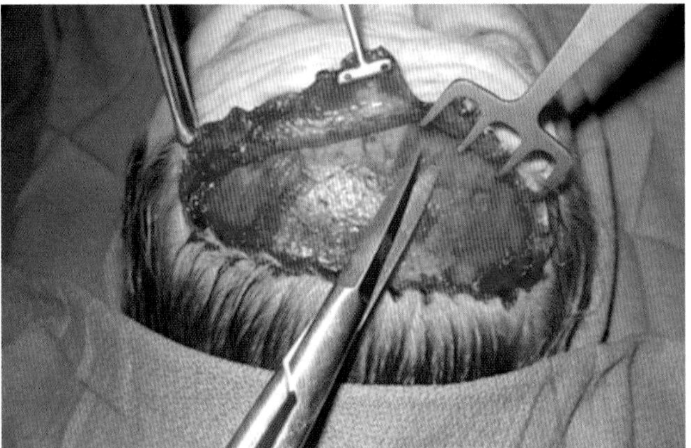

Figure 150.8 Elevation in a subgaleal plane.

ALTERNATE TECHNIQUE: Pretrichial/Trichophytic Forehead Lift—*cont'd*

STEP 4: Trimming and Inset of Forehead Flap

- Once the proper elevation has been made, a vertical midline incision can be made (approximately 1 to 2 cm in length) to create two separate forehead flaps (Fig. 150.9). This allows an easier manipulation of the right and left forehead flaps. Appropriate excision of the forehead flap is then done, after which an irregular incision design is created on the superior aspect of the forehead flap to match the irregular incision along the hear bearing scalp.

STEP 5: Closure

- Fibrin sealant is used in the subgaleal plane prior to closure. A deep closure and skin closure is then performed. No drains are necessary.

STEP 6: Dressing

- A pressure dressing is applied to the head circumferentially and maintained until the first postoperative visit, 24 hours later.

Avoidance and Management of Intraoperative Complications

Intraoperative complications from brow lifting typically stem from several areas. Technical issues during endoscopic brow lifting can be encountered during the elevation of the forehead flap. It is imperative to stay in a subperiosteal layer throughout the dissection of the central area of the forehead. Constant endoscopic visualization of the field is critical since dissection in a more superficial plane can jeopardize the frontal branch of the facial nerve. Another critical step is the complete release of the arcus marginalis; failure to do so will significantly hinder the elevation of the forehead and brows. Dissection along the medial aspect of the brows should be kept to a minimum since overzealous manipulation or aggressive resection of the glabellar muscles can lead to severe and unsightly separation and lateralization of the medial aspects of the brows.

During a pretrichial brow lift, complications can arise during the elevation of the flap. Elevation of a subcutaneous flap, as opposed to a subgaleal flap, must be done judiciously or avoided altogether; subcutaneous flaps can be quite thin, thereby compromising the subdermal plexus. As mentioned previously, it is the opinion of the author that pretrichial brow lifts should only be performed in a subgaleal plane. It is also critical not to excise too much skin from the forehead; excision of too much skin might require lowering of the hair-bearing scalp, which may or may not be a good aesthetic option for the patient (depending on the position of the hair and length of the forehead).

Postoperative Considerations

All brow lift patients should have a pressure dressing applied to their face/head at the completion of surgery. Drains can be avoided if hemostatic agents such as fibrin sealants are used during surgery. Patients should be seen within 24 hours following brow lifting. The main purpose of this appointment is to examine the patient for the possibility of a hematoma. Any hematoma should be drained in order to prevent flap necrosis. Pressure dressing can be maintained for a few more days if necessary. Patients are allowed to wash their hair gently with mild shampoo (such as baby shampoo) within 48 hours of surgery, although the application of antibiotic ointment along the incision sites should continue until complete epithelialization has occurred. Patients are reminded that anesthesia and hypesthesia of the scalp and forehead are common and can last weeks to months.

Hair growth should begin along the incision sites within weeks of surgery, although mild alopecia may be experienced. Final photographs are typically obtained around 3 to 4 months following surgery.

References

1. Passot R. Chirurgie Esthetique des rides du visage. *Presse Med.* 1919;27:258.
2. Hunt HL. *Plastic Surgery of the Head, Face and Neck.* Philadelphia: Lea and Febiger; 1926.
3. Fomon S. *Surgery of Injury and Plastic Repair.* Baltimore: Williams and Wilkins; 1939.
4. Marino H, Gandolfo E. Treatment of forehead wrinkles. *Prensa Med Argent.* 1964;34:406.
5. Regnault P. Complete face and forehead lifting, with double traction on crow's feet. *Plast Reconstr Surg.* 1972;49:123.
6. Flowers RS. Periorbital aesthetic surgery for men: eyelids and related structures. *Clin Plast Surg.* 1991;18:689.
7. Isse NG. Endoscopic facial rejuvenation: endoforehead, the functional lift. Case Reports. *Aesth Plast Surg.* 1994;18:21–29.
8. Vinas J, Caviglia C, Cortinas JL. Forehead rhytidoplasty and brow lifting. *Plast Reconsts Surg.* 1976;57:445.
9. Ramirez OM. Anchor subperiosteal forehead lift: from open to endoscopic. *Plast Reconstr Surg.* 2001;107:868.
10. Niamtu J. Endoscopic brow and forehead lift: a case for new technology. *J Oral Maxillofac Surg.* 2006;64:1464.
11. Rowe DJ, Guyuron B. Optimizing results in endoscopic forehead rejuvenation. *Clin Plast Surg.* 2008;35:355.
12. Nahai FR. The varied options in brow lifting. *Clin Plast Surg.* 2013;40:101.
13. Javidnia H, Sykes J. Endoscopic brow lifts: have they replaced coronal lifts? *Facial Plast Surg Clin N Am.* 2013;21:191.

CHAPTER 151

Facelift

Jon D. Perenack

Armamentarium

#11 and #15 scalpel blades
1.5-, 2-, 3-mm Single-hole liposuction cannulas
6-mm Spatula liposuction cannula
10-mm Malleable retractor
22-gauge spinal needle
Aerosolized fibrin sealant
Appropriate sutures
Brown-Adson pickups
Deaver retractor (small)
DeBakey forceps
Infusion device or 60-cc syringe
Iris scissors
Local anesthetic with vasoconstrictor
Marking pen
Metzenbaum scissors
Multipronged skin hook retractor
Needle electrocautery (short and extended tip)
Round-tip facelift scissors
Sharp-tip facelift scissors
Stapler
Suction capable of creating -20 mm Hg pressure
Tumescent solution (500 cc normal saline, 50 cc 1% lidocaine, 1 cc 1:1000 epinephrine, 1 g tranexamic acid)

History of the Procedure

The term facelift in current popular culture has come to describe any number of procedures that help rejuvenate the appearance of the lower face and neck and that may or may not involve an invasive surgical procedure. Early scientific descriptions of facelift surgery from the 19th century primarily dealt with single-plane elevation of the skin of the lower face and neck, posterior/superior pulling of excess tissue with excision of redundant skin, and closure. Skoog[1] first described a deeper plane approach to tightening the neck by undermining the posterior platysma and repositioning in a posterior/superior location. Mitz and Peyronie[2] described the superficial musculoaponeurotic system (SMAS) in 1976, which allowed for a better understanding of how to safely proceed with deeper dissections in the midface without injuring the facial nerve.[3–9] Biplanar lifts involving undermining of the skin and also the SMAS subsequently were advocated on grounds that a longer-lasting, more natural result could be obtained.[5] Authors noted that the SMAS could be repositioned in one vector and the skin in a slightly different vector to sculpt the face. Liposuction typically was advocated as an adjunct to the procedure. With the advent of aggressive resurfacing techniques, such as the carbon dioxide (CO_2) laser and phenol peels, deep plane lifts were described in which subcutaneous skin dissection was minimized to allow simultaneous resurfacing.[10] Lift was achieved solely through the undermining and repositioning of the SMAS layer. Hamra and others described modifications to allow elevation of the midface simultaneously with the facelift. Other authors described a simultaneous subperiosteal elevation[11] in the midface and mandible to release the true retaining ligaments of the face and allow more passive repositioning. As techniques became more aggressive, recovery periods and the potential for serious complications increased.

Over the past 10 to 15 years, the trend in facelifts has been toward less invasive lifts. In many ways, these facelifts resemble the lifts described in the 1970s, with less reliance on extensive subcutaneous dissection and some form of minimal modification of the SMAS. Adjunctive techniques involving additive volumizing, resurfacing, and selective liposuction are routinely performed along with the facelift so that one technique is no longer responsible for achieving the entire goal of the operation. Innovations in liposuction technique, utilizing radiofrequency, ultrasound, or laser technology to augment fat melting and skin tightening have also reduced the need for more aggressive lifts or midline platysmaplasty.[12–15]

Indications for the Use of the Procedure

As the history of the facelift suggests, the goal is to rejuvenate the lower face and neck through tightening of skin and adjacent superficial and deeper structures, with modification of fat planes as necessary.

Skin Laxity

General "looseness" of the skin of the face and neck is often the primary reason given by patients for seeking a facelift. It is important to evaluate the general thickness of the skin, its apparent elasticity and glandularity, and the presence of fine and coarse rhytids. The procedure is generally not successful at "pulling out" fine lines; these are best addressed with a resurfacing procedure, and the patient should be informed accordingly. Exceptionally thick or thin skin may be prone to relapse. Male patients classically have thicker skin that relapses in the neck region early (1 to 2 years) and may require a touch-up neck lift. Patients with thin, inelastic skin also tend to relapse early and form "sweeps" in unnaturally oriented resting skin tension lines along the jawline.[16] These patients benefit from adjunctive skin procedures that thicken and revitalize the dermis, such as resurfacing or radiofrequency tightening.

Muscle/SMAS Laxity

Often muscle/SMAS laxity is most notable in the formation of single or double (multiple) platysmal bands in the submental region. In the facial region, this laxity may manifest as jowling, deep nasolabial folds, and marionette lines. Invariably, there is also some component of skin laxity associated with these findings. The facelift procedure should be designed to allow adequate access to tighten the SMAS/platysmal layer and allow passive redraping of the skin as the facial musculature is repositioned.

Modification of Fat Planes

Fat is distributed in the face and neck in a superficial plane and in a deep plane. The superficial subcutaneous plane is contiguous throughout the face and neck, with fibrous attachments traversing it, between the deeper SMAS layer and the overlying dermis. The deeper fat planes are found in discrete anatomic pockets and are not as fibrous. In the aging face, the superficial plane often becomes more hypertrophied, whereas the deeper plane atrophies. One goal of the facelift is to sculpturally reduce excess superficial fat. This is typically accomplished with liposuction, direct excision, or suture repositioning. Patients who display fat atrophy, either local to one area or globally throughout the face, may benefit from facial volumizing. This may be accomplished through fat transfer, alloplastic implants, or injectable fillers.[12,13]

Limitations and Contraindications

Medical Clearance

The facelift is a completely elective procedure. As such, it should be performed only on patients who have an American Society of Anesthesiologists (ASA) 1 or 2 status, since this procedure is typically performed in an outpatient setting.

Anticoagulants

Patients who are unable to halt aspirin or other anticoagulant therapy during the perioperative period should be deferred or offered a limited surgical plan.

Smoking

The effects of tobacco use, particularly nicotine load, on wound healing have been well documented.[17] Some surgeons may refuse to operate on a patient until all smoking has ceased for several months preoperatively. As self-reporting of smoking cessation is unreliable, a urine cotinine test (a major metabolite of nicotine) is useful to determine if a patient has smoked or been exposed to nicotine in the previous 5 days. As a matter of practicality, most patients can safely undergo a facelift if they have limited themselves to two or three cigarettes per day.

Beyond these limitations, the main contraindications to the procedure are relative and are often a function of the patient's perception of the problem and the surgeon's accurate diagnosis.

Expectations

Most patients have a reasonable expectation of the likely result from facelift surgery. Some studies have suggested that a patient will appear approximately 7 to 10 years younger in the area of the lower face and neck after facelift surgery. Occasionally a patient demands a result that is unobtainable, such as complete elimination of all rhytids in a 75-year-old smoker. An attempt should be made to educate the patient as to the achievable results; however, if a consensus cannot be reached, surgery should be deferred.

Body Dysmorphic Disorder or Mental Illness

Patients with documented body dysmorphic disorder or mental illness are poor surgical candidates and should not be operated on for an elective facelift procedure. Unfortunately, not all patients arrive at the surgeon's office with documented history of these medical issues. Many surgeons rely on a prescreening mental health questionnaire along with observational documentation by the staff and surgeon to avoid operating on these "red flag" patients.

Relative Contraindications

Relative contraindications include recognition of adjunctive cosmetic problems and the need for additional procedures to create the patient's desired correction, as discussed in the following sections.

Skin. Fine rhytids, dyschromias, and other actinic-related changes of the skin are not a contraindication to the procedure, but the patient should be educated that the facelift will not improve these issues. Often, the patient may remark that dyspigmented patches actually become more apparent after a facelift, as folded and redundant skin is stretched flat. Appropriate skin care, adjunctive resurfacing, and the use of nonablative lasers may be indicated.

Bone. Patients may have underlying bony deficiencies in the area of the chin, piriform aperture, and/or mandibular angles that may not be favorable to achieving an outstanding cervicomental line angle and overall result. It has been well described that bone loss occurs in these anatomic regions with aging; in other cases, such deficiencies may have been present from a young age. Whenever possible, the surgeon should offer options to augment these areas to a more desirable contour.

Hyoid. The outstanding facelift result is more likely to be obtained in a patient with a hyoid that is superiorly positioned relative to the mandibular plane and is positioned posterior to the mandibular angle with a long mandibular body. This delineates the inferior aspect of the creation of a sharp cervicomental line angle. When this relationship is not present and a low hyoid is palpated with an anteroposterior short chin, the facelift result is somewhat compromised. Often an obtuse cervicomental line angle is obtained. The facelift may still be performed, but the patient should be shown the results obtained in patients with a similar hyoid configuration to avoid unreasonable expectations and disappointment.

Previous Liposuction/Facelift Surgery/Scarring. Patients should be made aware that the complication rate often is higher in individuals with a history of previous face/neck surgery. Such complications include scarring, skin compromise, and contour irregularity. These problems also may be seen in patients with a history of severe nodular cystic acne in the areas to be dissected or a history of subcutaneous volumizing with injectable filler. Patients who preoperatively display fat plane irregularity and dermal tethering are especially at risk for these complications. The surgeon should manually palpate the tethered areas to assess for restriction of movement, vascularity and vitality of skin, and the presence of fat plane irregularity and deep scar tissue formation.

TECHNIQUE: Facelift

STEP 1: Marking

The patient is marked in an upright, sitting position preoperatively. Permanent marker is used to outline the jawline and the level of the hyoid. A topographical style is used to mark fat deposits and deficiencies. The extent of subcutaneous dissection should be marked and the design and placement of the incision determined (Table 151.1).

STEP 2: Intubation or Intravenous Sedation

Oral intubation is recommended for patients to be treated under general anesthesia. General anesthesia is considered for any procedure that may last longer than 3 hours because a Foley catheter should be placed. IV sedation may be adequate for shorter procedures. The endotracheal tube should be secured midline to the chest and the patient prepped with a chlorhexidine solution and draped sterilely.

STEP 3: Tumescent Anesthesia

A tumescent solution is infiltrated subcutaneously throughout the face and neck with a 22-gauge spinal needle to create hydrodissection of the tissue plane. An infusion device hastens this step along nicely, but a 60-cc syringe is also effective. The tumescent solution may typically be 500 cc of normal saline or lactate Ringer's solution, containing 50 cc 1% lidocaine (for pain control), 1 cc of 1:1000 epinephrine (for blood vessel constriction to decrease bleeding during surgery), and 1 g tranexamic acid (TXA) (to decrease fibrinolysis of platelet plugs, decreasing delayed bleeding). The infusion should be extended 1 to 2 cm past the marking for the expected surgical dissection.

STEP 4: Lipodissection

A #11 blade is used to make a stab incision above each helix, the inferior earlobes, and at the midline submental incision. A 1.5- or 2-mm lipocannula set to no suction is used to gently create tunnels in the subcutaneous plane (lipodissection) in the area of planned elevation. The surgeon's hand holding the cannula creates a reciprocating action while the other hand palpates the subcutaneous placement of the cannula to ensure a proper plane of dissection. This is carried out preauricular, submental, and anterior to the sternocleidomastoid (SCM). The auricular ligament and tight mastoid attachments usually preclude lipodissection posterior to the SCM.

STEP 5: Closed Liposuction

In the neck/submentum region, areas of lipohypertrophy are treated with closed liposuction using the 1.5-, 2-, and 3-mm cannulas, in a sequential fashion, at −20 mm Hg suction. The edges of the area liposuctioned should be feathered so that a ridge or gouge is not created in the fat plane. A 3-mm cannula is usually required only in the central portion of a fatty deposit and should be used judiciously. Facial region lipohypertrophy, when present, is often in the jowl and nasolabial fold areas. Facial liposuction should be carried out only with a 1.5-mm, or at most a 2-mm, cannula. It is often useful to create an additional stab access with a #11 blade at the nasoalar junction to allow top-down liposuction in the nasolabial fold and jowl. The skin should be palpated for evenness of fat removal. In general, it is better to underresect than to overresect. Touch-up liposuction may be performed at 6 months after the surgery, if needed, and typically is an office procedure. Correcting fat plane unevenness, or dermal tethering, from excess removal of a fatty tissue is a far more difficult problem.

Continued

Table 151.1 Facelift Incision Options by Region

Incision Region	Incision Type	Advantages	Disadvantages
Temporal	Pretemporal tuft Vertical or stair-stepped	No displacement of temporal tuft Good scar camouflage	Visible scar May reduce or displace temporal tuft
Preauricular	Pretragal	No tragal blunting No beard hair displacement in males	Visible scar
	Endaural/post-tragal	Good scar camouflage	Tragal blunting Beard displacement into ear canal
Earlobe	Extension onto neck skin Skin advancement under earlobe	Decreased chance of pixie ear Good scar camouflage	Visible scar Secondary-intention healing of lobe undersurface
Postauricular	Conchal-mastoid crease	No beard hair displacement onto posterior ear Good scar camouflage	Possible scar migration onto neck skin
	On conchal bowl	Good scar camouflage	Beard hair displacement onto posterior ear Possible posterior ear tethering
Posterior hairline	Standard within hairline	Good scar camouflage	Less direct neck lift Requires excision of hair-bearing scalp
	Trichophytic	Excellent direct neck lift Minimal hair loss	Visible scar Inability of patient to wear hair "up"

TECHNIQUE: Facelift—*cont'd*

STEP 6: Open Liposuction and Platysmaplasty

A #15 blade is used to open the submental incision 10 to 12 mm and to undermine circumferentially 5 mm subcutaneously. The facelift scissors are opened 2 to 3 mm with the tips angled away from the dermis. A pushing motion is used to open the subcutaneous plane by slicing the scissors through the fibrous attachments between the dermis and platysma. During this portion of the operation, it is imperative that the assistant provide an adequate "jaw thrust" from the vertical ramus, to create a smooth platysmal plane for dissection. If the jaw thrust is inadequate, the platysma may roll upon itself, causing the surgeon to dissect out of plane.

Once the area of the submentum from angle to angle has been opened subcutaneously, a malleable retractor is inserted, and any bleeding points are cauterized with a long needle-point Bovie. If residual fat is seen adhering to the surface of the platysma, the 6-mm spatula cannula is used to "vacuum" it off directly with open liposuction. At this point, the anterior/medial edges of the platysma muscles should be visible. If the patient has minimal platysmal banding, the surgeon can merely advance and secure the edges together with interrupted 3-0 polyglycolate suture. With more profound banding, the medial 5 to 10 mm of each platysma should be excised, tapering to the level of the hyoid. Metzenbaum scissors are used to resect the bands. The cut ends are then sutured together to the level of the hyoid in an interrupted fashion (with 3-0 polyglycolate suture) and then oversewn in a running fashion back up to the submental incision. A horizontal backcut is created in the platysma for 2 to 3 cm at the level of the hyoid to prevent the sutured midline from forming a tight obtuse band after surgery. The underside of the skin flap is inspected for bleeding vessels, and any found are cauterized.

STEP 7: Lateral Face and Neck Dissection

A #15 blade is used to create the desired skin incision, coursing from the temple, around the ear, and into the posterior hairline. A number of variations can be used for each anatomic portion of the incision, and the desired path should be chosen preoperatively. Needle electrocautery is used to develop a subcutaneous plane preauricularly. The facelift scissors are used in the same fashion as for the submentum to open the subcutaneous plane to the desired extent. This is usually carried inferiorly and posteriorly to the auricular ligament. A multipronged skin hook retractor is used to pull the ear anterior while a skin flap is developed with the electrocautery just superficial to the mastoid fascia. This dissection is subsequently carried inferiorly into the neck, and the auricular ligament is released, connecting the two pockets. Any bleeding points are cauterized. Care is taken not to injure the great auricular nerve as it courses over the SCM. Dissection over the posterior border of the platysma proceeds carefully so as not to disrupt the external jugular vein.

TECHNIQUE: Facelift—*cont'd*

STEP 8: SMAS Modification

A 2-0 horizontal mattress polyglycolate suture is used to grasp the SMAS layer along the jawline approximately 3 cm from the angle of the mandible. The suture is pulled posteriorly to ensure that the SMAS moves passively with the pull. A posterior/superior vector is used to secure the suture to the fascia overlying the SCM. A similar mattress suture is passed through the preauricular SMAS, 1 cm below the zygomatic arch and 2 cm anterior to the incision. This portion of the SMAS is elevated in a 45-degree posterior/superior vector and secured. Intervening mattress sutures are placed to create a posterior displacement of the platysma in the neck coursing to a mostly superior vector just below the zygomatic arch. A running 2-0 polyglycolate suture oversews the interrupted mattress sutures to stabilize and smooth the plicated SMAS layer. Care is taken to ensure that the SMAS forms a smooth layer, without waviness or distortion.

STEP 9: Final Check of Subcutaneous Elevation and Submental Closure

After the SMAS plication has been deemed adequate, the patient's head is placed in a neutral position and the skin is redraped. The surgeon should evaluate for any points of rotation where inadequate subcutaneous elevation does not allow for passive redraping. Further subcutaneous undermining is accomplished with the facelift scissors until no pivot points or dermal tethering is noted. The underside of the skin flap should be inspected for bleeding points, which are cauterized.

The submental dissection is once again inspected to ensure that no bleeding has resumed. Normal saline is used to flush any extraneous blood from the field. The forehead is used to create the effect of a jaw thrust and a malleable retractor is inserted. Using a nitrogen tank and aerosolized sprayer, the surgeon applies fibrin sealant to the raw surfaces of the submental skin flap and platysma. Fibrin sealant has been shown to reduce postoperative ecchymosis and swelling and to reduce recovery time.[18] The skin then is placed manually against the platysma in the desired location. The submental incision is closed with three subcutaneous 4-0 poliglecaprone interrupted sutures. The skin is closed with a running 6-0 plain gut suture. A lap sponge is used to apply gentle pressure to prevent any shear or bleeding under the flap.

STEP 10: Excision of Skin and Closure of the Lateral Face and Neck Incision

Excision of excess skin is directed to obtaining a smooth and unpleated adaptation from the incision around the ear to the skin flap. This is accomplished by excising "dog ears" of excess skin at the temple and posterior hairline. The posterior flap is pulled superiorly and slightly anterior-posterior to the ear. A 0-0 polyglycolate suture is mattressed through a thick portion of the flap to the mastoid fascia behind the ear. Just before the mastoid suture is secured, aerosolized fibrin sealant is again sprayed onto the exposed surfaces, and the mastoid suture is pulled taut and tied. Sharp facelift scissors are used to excise the excess posterior skin, and the edges are stapled closed. The posterior hairline is matched across the incision as it is closed. At the temple, the flap is pulled posteriorly and superiorly, and excess is sharply excised. Closure in the hairline is again performed with staples. The remainder of the flap is passively draped and sharply excised. A subcutaneous closure is performed with 4-0 poliglecaprone interrupted sutures. Skin edges should be closely adapted after the deep closure. The incision in front of the ear is then closed with 6-0 plain gut running suture. No drains are placed with this technique.

Antibiotic ointment is applied to all incisions. Nonadherent pads are placed over the submental and preauricular incisions. A thick cotton pad is cut to extend from temple to temple around the submentum. Additional cotton is placed postauricularly. A tight Kerlix bandage is then used to wrap the face and neck, extending around the vertex. It is secured with silk tape.

ALTERNATIVE TECHNIQUE 1: Deep Plane Facelift

The anatomic plane of the SMAS has been well described as it relates to the region inferior to the zygomatic arch, superior to the mandibular plane, and anterior to the auricle extending to the oral commissure. Numerous facelift dissection techniques have been described that rely on elevation of the SMAS, superficial to the parotid capsule, and anteriorly, superficial to the branches of the facial nerve. The deep plane facelift technique is especially useful if the surgeon plans to perform medium or deep full face laser or chemical resurfacing simultaneously with the facelift procedure. The SMAS/skin flap provides a sturdy flap for lifting, and its robust blood supply allows adequate recovery from the resurfacing procedure.[19]

Continued

ALTERNATIVE TECHNIQUE 1: Deep Plane Facelift—*cont'd*

STEPS 1 TO 6:

Steps 1 through 6 are performed as described previously, except that lipodissection is performed only 2 to 3 cm in front of the ear.

STEP 7: Subcutaneous Undermining

The surgeon undermines the subcutaneous plane anterior to the auricular crease to the extent that skin excision is planned, typically 2 cm. Subcutaneous dissection below the mandibular plane is carried out approximately 2 cm anterior to the posterior border of the platysma. Additional undermining in this region may be necessary so that the neck skin may be repositioned posterior/superior passively without creating tether points or rippling. Subcutaneous undermining in the posterior neck is performed as previously described.

STEP 8: SMAS Elevation and Modification

The SMAS layer is incised from a point 1 cm below the zygomatic arch and 1 cm in front of the preauricular incision. The incision is carried inferiorly until the posterior border of the platysma is released over the SCM about 4 cm below the mandibular plane. Horizontal back-cuts are made in the SMAS 1 cm below the zygomatic arch for 2 to 3 cm and at the inferior aspect of the platysma incision for 3 cm. The SMAS layer is elevated anteriorly off the parotid capsule with Metzenbaum scissors using a vertical spreading technique. Once the parotid-cutaneous ligaments have been released, the dissection is carried anteriorly until the lateral face can be passively moved posteriorly by pulling on the SMAS flap. The branches of the facial nerve are often seen in the loose fascial tissue just below the plane of dissection. Sub-SMAS dissection is then carried inferior to the mandibular plane until the inferior backcut is reached. The facial SMAS flap is then repositioned posterior-superior with horizontal mattress 2-0 polyglactin sutures. Occasionally, a strip of SMAS, 1 to 2 cm wide may need to be excised to prevent excess tissue bulk anterior to the ear. The platysma is repositioned over the SCM posteriorly and superiorly and fixed with 2-0 polyglactin mattress sutures.

STEPS 9 AND 10:

Steps 9 and 10 are performed as previously described.

ALTERNATIVE TECHNIQUE 2: Neck Lift

A subset of patients present with negligible facial laxity and minor jowling, yet have moderate submental/neck laxity/lipohypertrophy and platysmal banding. These patients typically may be 40 to 50 years of age, previous facelift patients 5 to 10 years after the initial lift, or a male patient who wants to avoid preauricular incisions. A bariatric patient in his or her 30s may also qualify for neck lift surgery combined with facial fat augmentation. The neck lift is essentially the facelift procedure minus the incision and dissection superior to the earlobe, anterior to the ear.[20] Often it is necessary to carry the incision 5 to 10 mm up the anterior earlobe to reduce bunching of the preauricular skin as the skin of the neck is redraped posteriorly and superiorly. The postauricular and posterior hairline incisions are similar to those for the facelift. The submental dissection is required only if platysmal banding is present or if significant lipohypertrophy requires subcutaneous release of the skin from underlying attachments and open liposuction. Posterior neck SMAS modification is limited to posterior/superior plication of the posterior border of the platysma over the SCM fascia. Deep plane subplatysmal elevation may be performed if desired. Two 0-0 polyglycolate sutures are passed through the thick skin flap over the mastoid and drawn superiorly and anteriorly. Fibrin sealant may be applied as an aerosol before closure, as described previously.

ALTERNATIVE TECHNIQUE 3: Mini-tuck

The mini-tuck represents the subcutaneous facelift techniques described in the early surgical literature, before the more invasive SMAS techniques evolved. Mini-tucks involve subcutaneous dissection only, in an arc of 4 cm of skin anterior to the auricle and extending 2 to 4 cm below the mandibular plane. The SMAS may be plicated with three to five mattress sutures (2-0 polyglycolate) over and/or slightly anterior to the parotid and slightly below the mandibular plane. The incision usually does not extend posterior to the auricle except for the inferior 1 to 2 cm of the lobe. This lift represents many of the "named" or "trademarked" lifts that are heavily marketed to the public as revolutionary, requiring minimal recovery and performed under local anesthesia. Although this lift can be readily performed under local anesthesia (or with light sedation) and patients often can return to work the next day, it should be used only for patients requiring minimal lift in the facial and immediate submental regions. A good predictor of success is for the surgeon to simulate the lift by placing both hands in the preauricular region and pulling posteriorly/superiorly. If resolution of unwanted laxity is accomplished, this lift will likely succeed. If pull is required both preauricularly and inferiorly through the lateral neck, a more extensive postauricular and hairline dissection is needed to unwind dog ears and remove the excess skin.

ALTERNATIVE TECHNIQUE 4: No Midline Platysmaplasty and Use of Augmented Liposuction Technique

The open liposuction/midline platysmaplasty is considered by many surgeons to be necessary to correct submental banding and/or excessive submental lipomatosis. Corset techniques with or without a platysmal backcut at the level of the hyoid bone are mainstay techniques. Complications associated with this approach include increased chance of seroma/hematoma, and late findings of cosmetic deformity involving a "surgical" looking anterior neck, with unusual platysma V banding, "cobra neck" deformity, and subcutaneous volume deficiency in the area below the platysma backcut in the thin-skinned patient. One option to avoid these complications is to not perform an open procedure to the anterior neck at all. Instead, platysmal redundancy is resolved with an aggressive lateral approach with lateral platysmal undermining and posterolateral repositioning. Submental and jowl lipomatosis is corrected utilizing augmented liposuction techniques. Augmented liposuction techniques typically involve completing Steps 1 to 4. After completing lipodissection, the midline and jowl areas are treated with a device that causes lipodisruption of fat and heats skin using energy derived from either a radiofrequency, ultrasonic, or laser device. Upon completion of this step, "cold" liposuction can be carried out as per Step 5 with omission of Step 6 entirely. Steps 7 to 10 may be completed either as a SMAS imbrication technique or as the deep plane alternative technique previously described. Long-term results with this technique appear to be equivalent or superior to those obtained with classic midline platysmaplasty/open liposuction in most patient types, with less complications.[21,22] Patients with heavy midline platysmal redundancy or those requiring subplatysmal fat resection, typically still require midline platysmal plication with or without a hyoid-level backcut.

Avoidance and Management of Intraoperative Complications

Hematoma is the most common preventable intraoperative and immediate postoperative complication in facelift surgery. The reported incidence typically is 3% to 5%, although it may be as high as 20% in male patients.[23–25] Common patient risk factors for hematoma include smoking, dietary supplements, blood thinning medications, hypertension, and unrecognized clotting disorders. Intraoperative controllable factors include avoiding hypotension (normotensive status is best), use of tumescent solution containing TXA, lidocaine, and epinephrine, meticulous control of bleeding, and smooth extubation without straining against the tube or closed glottis. Postoperative pressure dressing may also be helpful in reducing seroma/hematoma and swelling.

Facial nerve injury is rare and is best avoided by maintaining dissection in the appropriate planes. SMAS sutures should be placed superficially so as to not lasso and strangulate a facial nerve branch.[26]

Errors in skin excision include creating ripples, creases, or folds in the skin flap or the removal of too much skin, requiring closure under tension. The systematic approach of removing the temporal and postauricular dog ears first minimizes these complications. Passive positioning of the skin flap helps prevent rippling.[23–25] If tethering is noted, the underside of the flap should be released subcutaneously until the dimple is relieved. Until the surgeon is comfortable with the excision component, guide cuts may be made in the flap to help locate the appropriate removal. If excessive skin is inadvertently removed, an attempt should be made to undermine and advance more skin. This typically occurs in the postauricular region. Deep 3-0 polyglycolate sutures may be placed 1 to 2 cm from the incision to relieve tension on the skin edge.

Irregular or excessive fat removal is best avoided by remembering that it is better to underresect than overresect. The flap should be manipulated during liposuction to palpate for even removal. The liposuction cannula should not be passed repetitively in the same location to prevent gouging. The surgeon should be aware that due to "handedness," a right-handed surgeon naturally has difficulty suctioning the right submentum compared with the left.

Postoperative Considerations

The patient's heavy support dressing is removed on postoperative day 1, and he or she is instructed to wear a light-support, removable wrap for 7 days, day and night, and then 7 days while sleeping only. Antibiotic ointment is applied to all skin incisions for 2 days; thereafter, the patient switches to a moist, occlusive, petroleum-based ointment, which is applied for 5 days. All staples are removed at 7 days. Oral antibiotics are prescribed for 5 days. If the patient presents on postoperative day 2 or 3 with profound edema, a short, tapering oral steroid course is prescribed. Patients typically see the final results in 3 to 4 months.

Hematomas

Hematoma formation typically occurs in the first 24 hours after surgery but may be seen as late as 7 days. Large hematomas are considered an emergency, and the patient must be taken back to surgery for evacuation, cauterization/tie-off of bleeding vessels, and reclosure.[23–25] If left untreated, large hematomas cause overlying skin pressure necrosis. Small, nonexpansile hematomas may be observed and aspirated with a needle around postoperative day 5 to 7 after they liquefy. Most hematomas progress to seroma formation.

Seromas

Seromas typically are treated with daily needle aspiration and gentle compression until they resolve.

Abnormalities or Loss of Sensation

Most patients report some sensory disturbance in the distribution of the greater auricular and transverse cervical nerves.[26] In most cases this is self-resolving over many months, and patient reassurance is recommended. For symptomatic dysesthesias, the author recommends a short, tapering course of an oral steroid and low dose oral amitriptyline.

Facial Nerve Weakness

Most injuries to the facial nerve are self-resolving in 3 to 6 months.[26] Because unilateral weakness in the marginal mandibular branch distribution is the most common presentation, low-dose botulinum toxin treatment to the contralateral depressor anguli oris transiently causes weakness and thus makes the facial expression more symmetric as the injury resolves.

Wound Dehiscence, Flap Necrosis, and Widened Scars

In most cases, wound dehiscence, flap necrosis, and widened scars are related to excess tension across the wound closure, an excessively thin flap, or aggressive cauterization of the flap. A widened, atrophic, hypopigmented scar is the typical result. Local wound care and a moist occlusive dressing should be applied until the site reepithelializes. After the scar matures (minimum 6 months), the site may be assessed for adjacent skin laxity that may allow scar excision and passive closure. If this is not possible, resurfacing with ablative laser energy improves the esthetic outcome.[23–25] A pulsed dye laser may be used to shrink adjacent telangiectasia and vascularity. Local steroid injection may be useful to reduce hypertrophic scarring or keloiding.

Cases

Case 1

A 57-year-old female with moderate jowling, facial/neck laxity, and platysmal bands. Preoperative and 4 months postoperative after lateral SMAS/platysma imbrication, midline corset platysmaplasty with hyoid backcut, and lipocontouring utilizing standard liposuction technique. Upper blepharoplasty also performed (Fig. 151.1).

Case 2

A 63-year-old female with moderate jowling, severe facial/neck laxity with lipomatosis, and moderate platysmal bands. Preoperative and 4 months postoperative after deep plane facelift, midline corset platysmaplasty with hyoid backcut, and lipocontouring utilizing standard liposuction technique (Fig. 151.2).

Case 3

A 53-year-old female with minimal jowling, minimal facial laxity, moderate midline submental laxity with platysmal band, and associated lipomatosis. Preoperative and 4 months postoperative after neck lift with lateral platysmal undermining and repositioning, midline corset platysmaplasty with hyoid backcut, and lipocontouring utilizing standard liposuction technique (Fig. 151.3).

Case 4

A 50-year-old female with mild jowling, facial and submental laxity, minimal platysmal band and moderate submental lipomatosis. Preoperative and 6 months postoperative after mini-tuck with lateral SMAS imbrication, and lipocontouring performed utilizing radiofrequency augmented liposuction technique. Endoscopic browlift also performed (Fig. 151.4).

Case 5

A 58-year-old female with moderate jowling, severe facial/neck laxity with lipomatosis, and moderate platysmal bands. Preoperative and 6 months postoperative after deep plane facelift, no midline platysmaplasty, and lipocontouring performed utilizing radiofrequency augmented liposuction technique. Lower blepharoplasty with lateral canthopexy and facial CO_2 laser resurfacing also performed (Fig. 151.5).

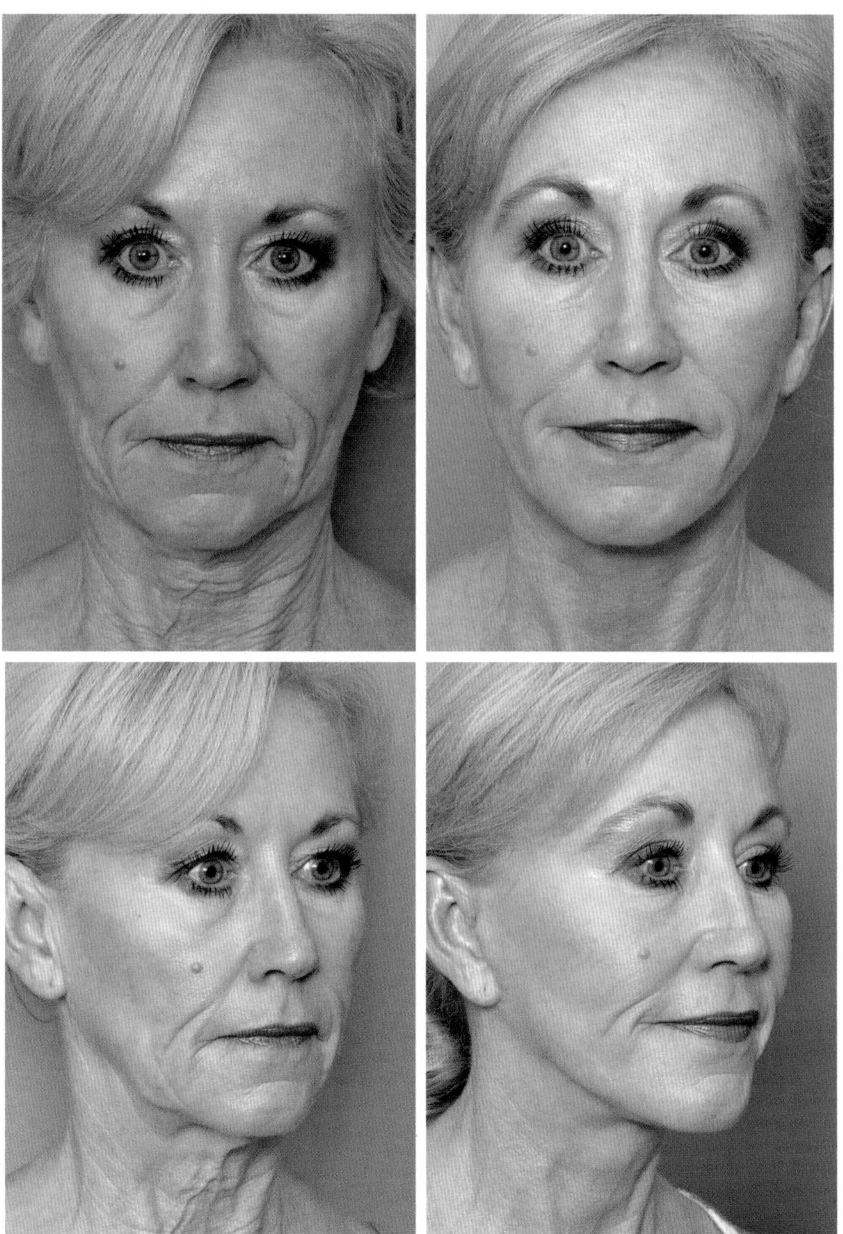

Fig. 151.1 Preoperative and postoperative photos of a 57-year-old female with moderate jowling, facial/neck laxity, and platysmal bands.

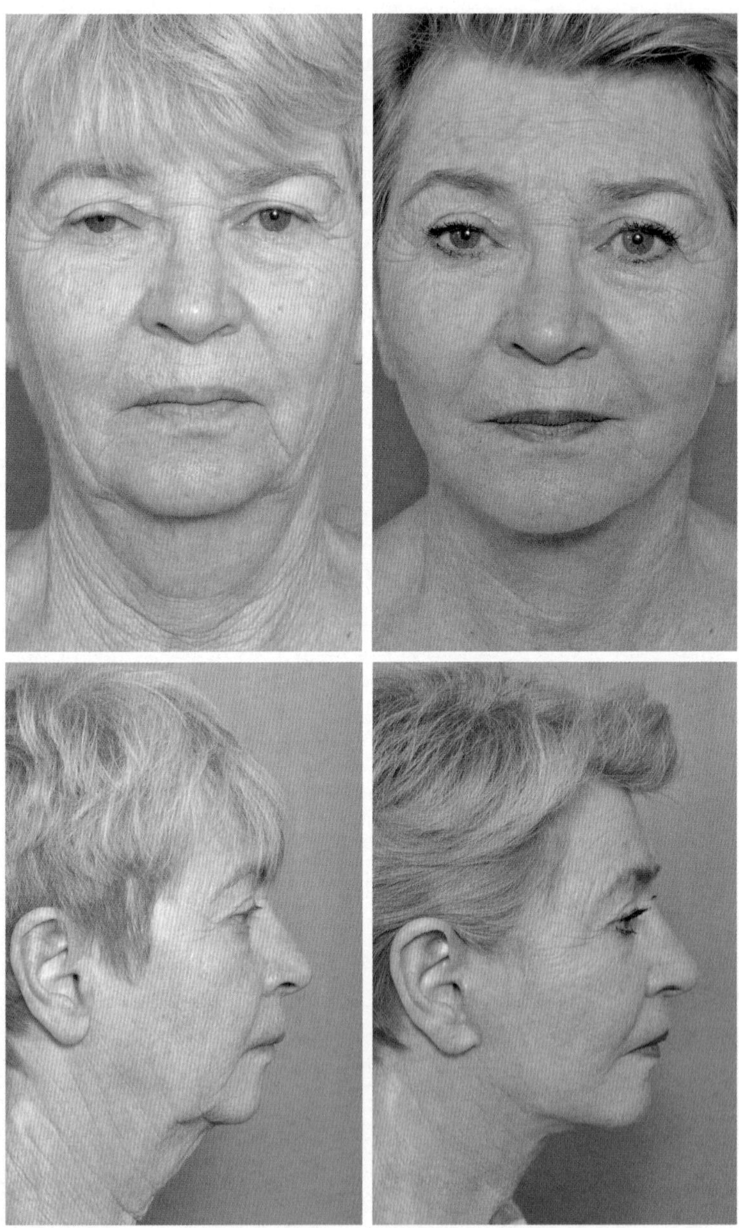

Fig. 151.2 Preoperative and postoperative photos of a 63-year-old female with moderate jowling, severe facial/neck laxity with lipomatosis, and moderate platysmal bands.

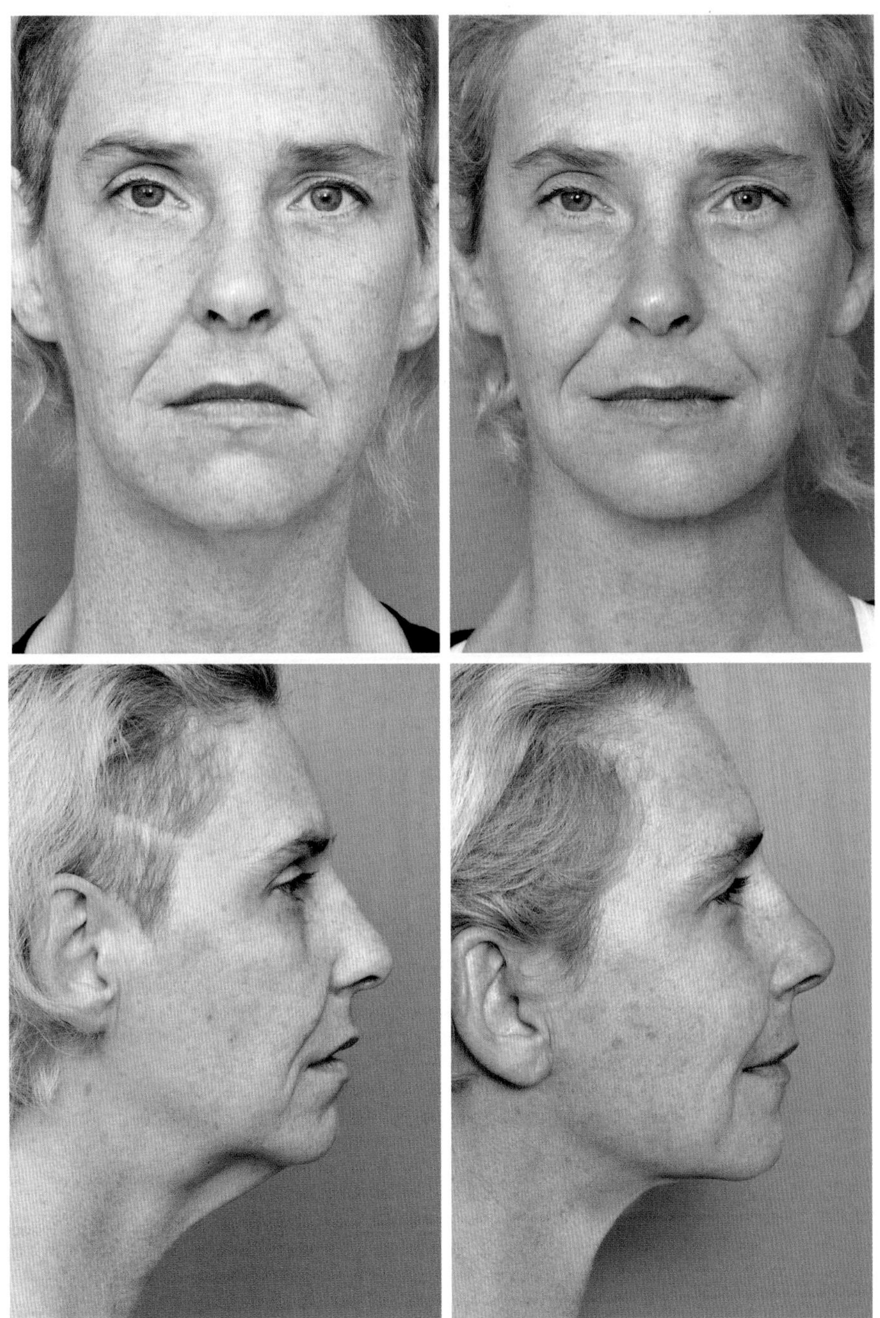

Fig. 151.3 Preoperative and postoperative photos of a 53-year-old female with minimal jowling, minimal facial laxity, moderate midline submental laxity with platysmal band, and associated lipomatosis.

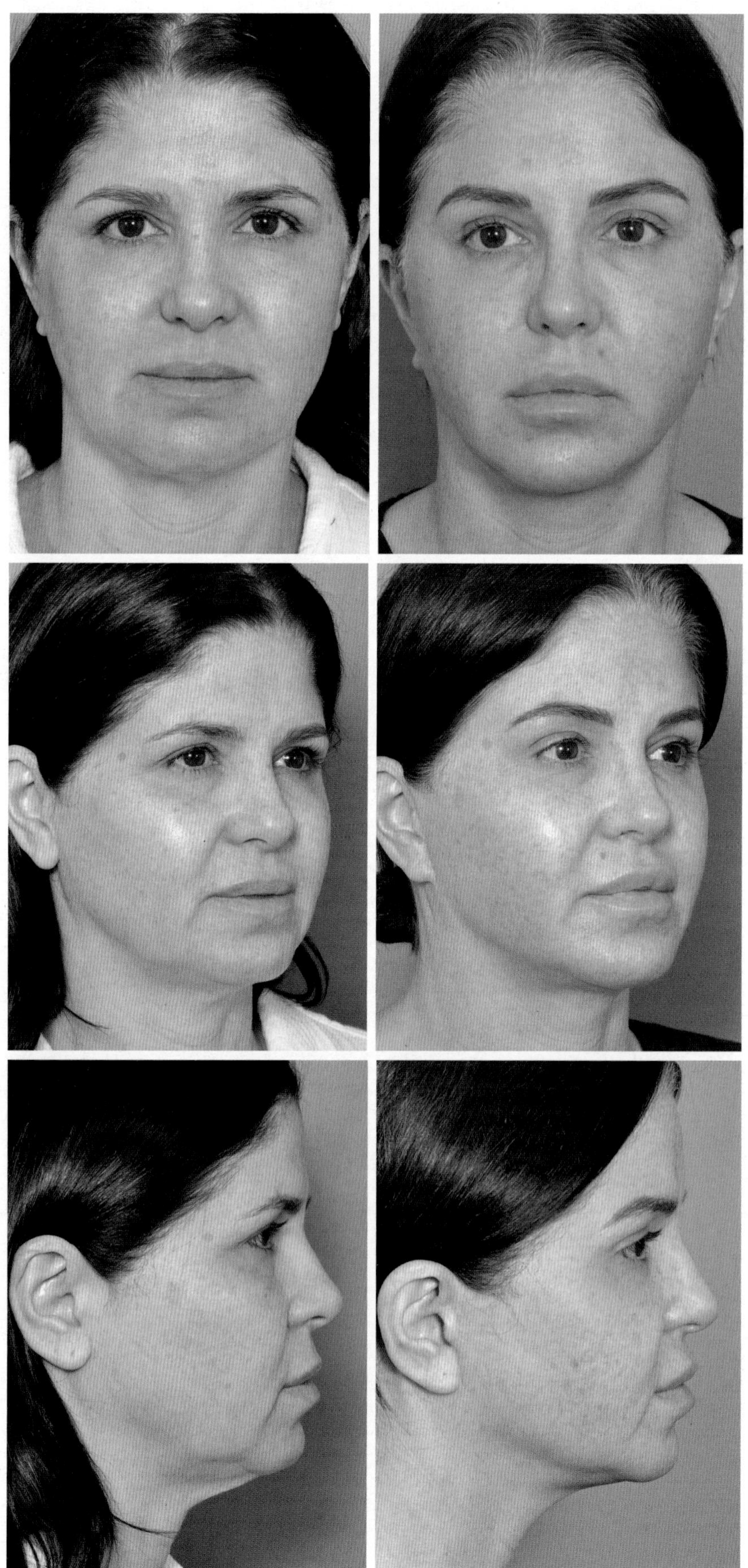

Fig. 151.4 Preoperative and postoperative photos of a 50-year-old female with mild jowling, facial and submental laxity, minimal platysmal band, and moderate submental lipomatosis.

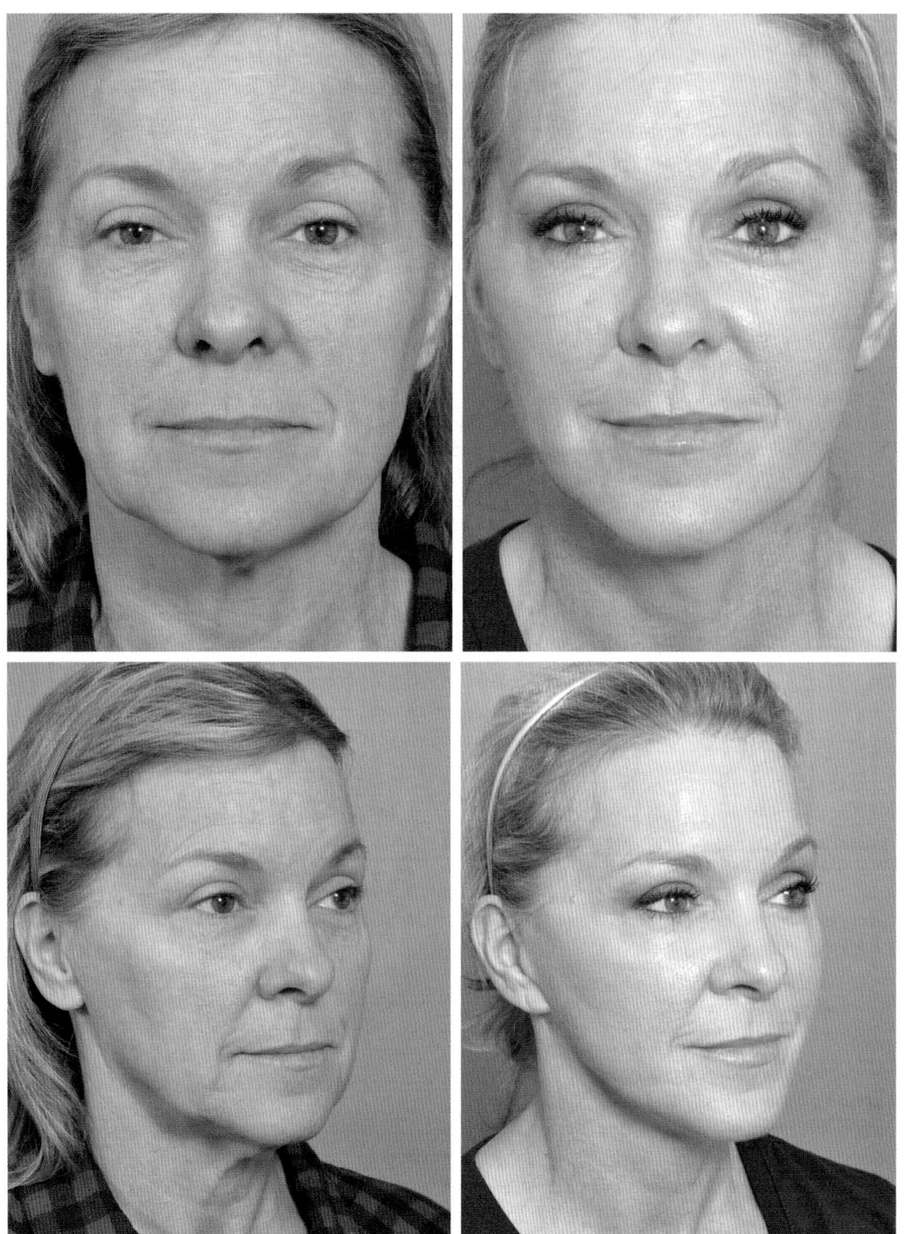

Fig. 151.5 Preoperative and postoperative photos of a 58-year-old female with moderate jowling, severe facial/neck laxity with lipomatosis, and moderate platysmal bands.

References

1. Skoog T. *Plastic Surgery: New Methods and Refinements*. Philadelphia, Pennsylvania: Saunders; 1974.
2. Mitz V, Peyronie M. The superficial musculo-aponeurotic system (SMAS) in the parotid and cheek area. *Plast Reconstr Surg*. 1976;58(1):80–88.
3. Adamson PA, Litner JA. Evolution of rhytidectomy techniques. *Facial Plast Surg Clin North Am*. 2005;13(3):383–391.
4. Lemmon ML, Hamra ST. Skoog rhytidectomy: a five-year experience with 577 patients. *Plast Reconstr Surg*. 1980;65(3):283–297.
5. Owsley JQ Jr. SMAS-platysma facelift. A bidirectional cervicofacial rhytidectomy. *Clin Plast Surg*. 1983;10(3):429–440.
6. Jost G, Levet Y. Parotid fascia and face lifting: a critical evaluation of the SMAS concept. *Plast Reconstr Surg*. 1984;74(1):42–51.
7. Bosse JP, Pappillon J. Surgical anatomy of the SMAS at the malar region. In: *Transactions of the Ninth International Congress of Plastic and Reconstructive Surgery*. New York: McGraw-Hill; 1987.
8. Thaller SR, Kim S, Patterson H, Wildman M, Daniller A. The submuscular aponeurotic system (SMAS): a histologic and comparative anatomy evaluation. *Plast Reconstr Surg*. 1990;86(4):690–696.
9. Stuzin JM, Baker TJ, Gordon HL. The relationship of the superficial and deep facial fascias: relevance to rhytidectomy and aging. *Plast Reconstr Surg*. 1992;89(3):441–449.
10. Hamra ST. The deep-plane rhytidectomy. *Plast Reconstr Surg*. 1990;86(1):53–61.
11. Ramirez OM. The subperiosteal approach for the correction of the deep nasolabial fold and the central third of the face. *Clin Plast Surg*. 1995;22(2):341–356.
12. Stuzin JM. Restoring facial shape in face lifting: the role of skeletal support in facial

analysis and midface soft-tissue repositioning. *Plast Reconstr Surg*. 2007;119(1):362–376.
13. Lambros V. Fat contouring in the face and neck. *Clin Plast Surg*. 1992;19(2):401–414.
14. Marcus BC. Rhytidectomy: current concepts, controversies and the state of the art. *Curr Opin Otolaryngol Head Neck Surg*. 2012;20(4):262–266.
15. Dulguerov N, D'Souza A. Update on treatment rationale and options for the ageing face. *Curr Opin Otolaryngol Head Neck Surg*. 2011;19(4):269–275.
16. Lambros V, Stuzin JM. The cross-cheek depression: surgical cause and effect in the development of the "joker line" and its treatment. *Plast Reconstr Surg*. 2008;122(5):1543–1552.
17. Rees TD, Liverett DM, Guy CL. The effect of cigarette smoking on skin-flap survival in the face lift patient. *Plast Reconstr Surg*. 1984;73(6):911–915.
18. Farrior E, Ladner K. Platelet gels and hemostasis in facial plastic surgery. *Facial Plast Surg*. 2011;27(4):308–314.
19. Sykes JM, Liang J, Kim JE. Contemporary deep plane rhytidectomy. *Facial Plast Surg*. 2011;27(1):124–132.
20. Rohrich RJ, Rios JL, Smith PD, Gutowski KA. Neck rejuvenation revisited. *Plast Reconstr Surg*. 2006;118(5):1251–1263.
21. Jacono AA, Malone MH. The effect of midline corset platysmaplasty on degree of face-lift flap elevation during concomitant deep-plane face-lift A cadaveric study. *JAMA Facial Plast Surg*. 2016:183–187.
22. Mustoe TA, Rawlani V, Zimmerman H. Modified deep plane rhytidectomy with a lateral approach to the neck: an alternative to submental incision and dissection. *Plast Reconstr Surg*. 2011;127(1):357–370.
23. Bloom JD, Immerman SB, Rosenberg DB. Face-lift complications. *Facial Plast Surg*. 2012;28(3):260–272.
24. Rodriguez-Bruno K, Papel ID. Rhytidectomy: principles and practice emphasizing safety. *Facial Plast Surg*. 2011;27(1):98–111.
25. Chang S, Pusic A, Rohrich RJ. A systematic review of comparison of efficacy and complication rates among face-lift techniques. *Plast Reconstr Surg*. 2011;127(1):423–433.
26. Baker DC, Conley J. Avoiding facial nerve injuries in rhytidectomy. Anatomical variations and pitfalls. *Plast Reconstr Surg*. 1979;64(6):781–795.
27. PD 1McKinney P, Katrana DJ. Prevention of injury to the great auricular nerve during rhytidectomy. *Plast Reconstr Surg*. 1980;66(5):675–679.

CHAPTER 152

Rhinoplasty and Septoplasty

Tirbod Fattahi

Armamentarium

Adson-Brown forceps
Adson forceps
Aufricht retractor
Ballenger Swivel septal knife
Bayonet forceps
Cartilage grid
Cottle elevator
Curved guarded osteotomes
Double ball retractor
Freer elevator
Joseph scissors
Joseph skin hooks
Nasal speculum
Nasal tip graft cookie-cutters
Rubin osteotome
Septal morselizer
Septal rasps
Serrated amalgam plugger

History of the Procedure

The origin of rhinoplasty involves nasal reconstruction more than the contemporary definition of rhinoplasty. It is believed that as early as 1600 BC, Egyptians were performing various types of nasal surgery and manipulations.[1] Indian physician, Sushruta Samhita, who lived around 1000 to 800 BC, is also recognized as one of the pioneers of rhinoplasty.[2] In 1818, German surgeon Carl van Graefe used the term "rhinoplasty" for the first time in his textbook. Other prominent surgeons, such as Johann Dieffenbach, John Roe, and Robert Weir, made significant contributions to the art of rhinoplasty in the mid- to late- 19th century. However, the father of modern rhinoplasty is considered to be Dr. Jacques Joseph (1865 to 1934), an orthopedic surgeon from Berlin who performed a rhinoplasty using "external incisions" in 1898. Three particular surgeons, Drs. Joseph Safian, Gustave Aufricht, and Samuel Fomon, traveled to Europe to learn Joseph's techniques. These three physicians were instrumental in bringing rhinoplasty to the United States in the 1940s. Two of Fomon's students, Drs. Irving Goldman and Maurice Cottle, became leaders in the field of rhinoplasty in the second half of the 20th century. These two individuals were also instrumental in developing various surgical and rhinoplastic societies in the United States. Other notable people involved in enhancing the art of rhinoplasty in this country include Drs. Jack Anderson, Richard Webster, Gaylon McCullough, and Jack Gunter. Jack Anderson is considered the first person to perform an "open rhinoplasty" in the early 1980s.

Indications for the Use of the Procedure

Septoplasty and rhinoplasty are indicated in the management of functional and cosmetic deformities of the nasal complex. Often combined together, these procedures are aimed at correcting various nasal air flow obstructions along the nasal complex and improving the appearance of the external nose (Fig. 152.1). An isolated septoplasty will address nasal deviation as well as breathing difficulties. Rhinoplasty can improve the appearance of the nose. When performed together, graft material can be obtained through septoplasty, which can then be used during the rhinoplasty portion of the operation. Essentially, all aspects of the nose or septum can be approached and modified through two main techniques: "open" and "closed or endonasal." Minor modifications of the nose can be approached through the "closed" technique, while the "open" technique is reserved for a more comprehensive and direct approach to the nose. The term "open structure rhinoplasty" was created to describe an open rhinoplasty procedure where procured grafts (from septoplasty or other sites) are used to "structure" or "build" a nose. Essentially, all aspects of the nose or septum can be approached and modified through two main techniques: "open" and "closed or endonasal."

Limitations and Contraindications

Limitations of septorhinoplasty are few; patients who suffer from radiographic-proven maxillary sinus disease (polyps,

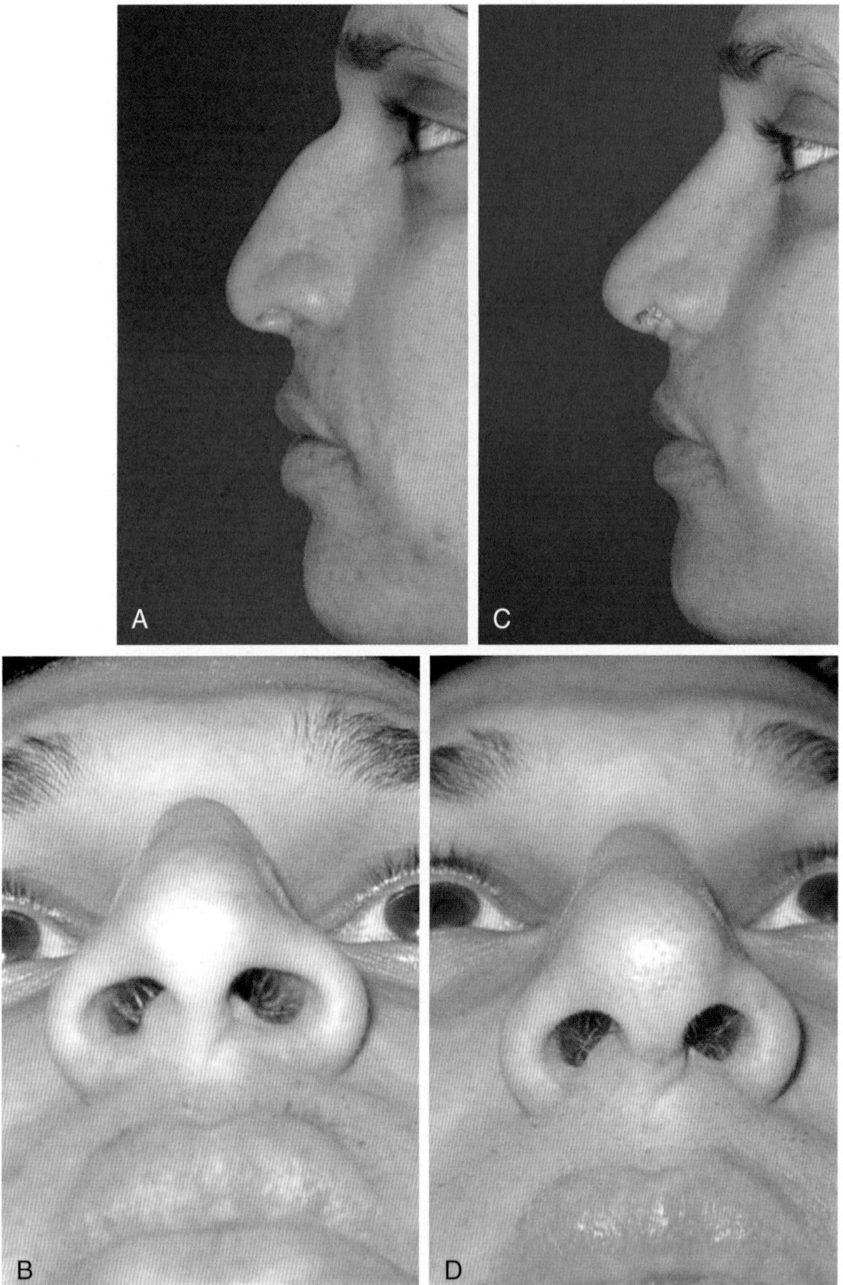

Figure 152.1 **A** and **B,** Preoperative photos. **C** and **D,** Postoperative photos.

etc.) may not benefit from an isolated septoplasty or rhinoplasty. It is prudent to differentiate between patients who have difficulty breathing because of sinus disease and those who have difficulty breathing because of a deviated nasal complex or those with allergy-mediated processes such as allergic rhinitis. Contraindication to a cosmetic rhinoplasty would be any psychiatric disorder, such as body dysmorphic disorder, where the patient has unrealistic expectations.[3]

TECHNIQUE: Open Rhinoplasty Including Septoplasty

STEP 1: Preparation of Nose

- All cases are done under general anesthesia. After securing the oral endotracheal tube, a throat pack is placed. Local anesthesia with a vasoconstrictor is injected into the nose, specifically along the caudal edge of lateral crus, columella, dome, and lateral nasal walls. The septum should also be injected

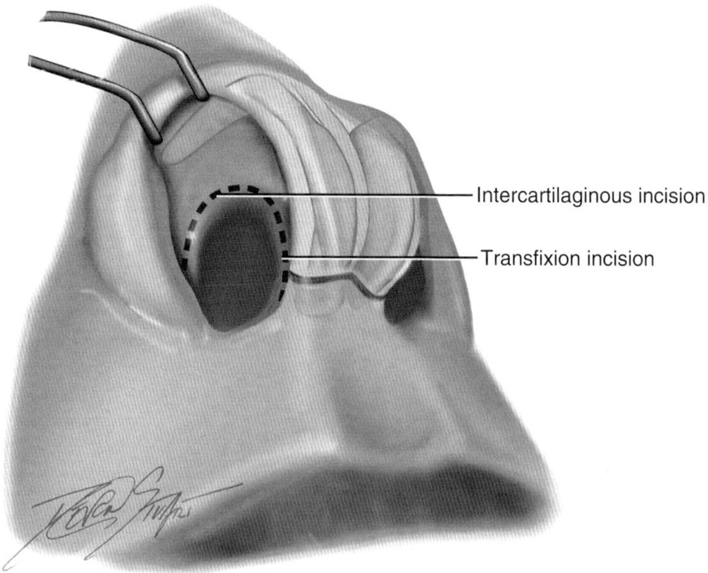

Figure 152.2 Marginal incision.

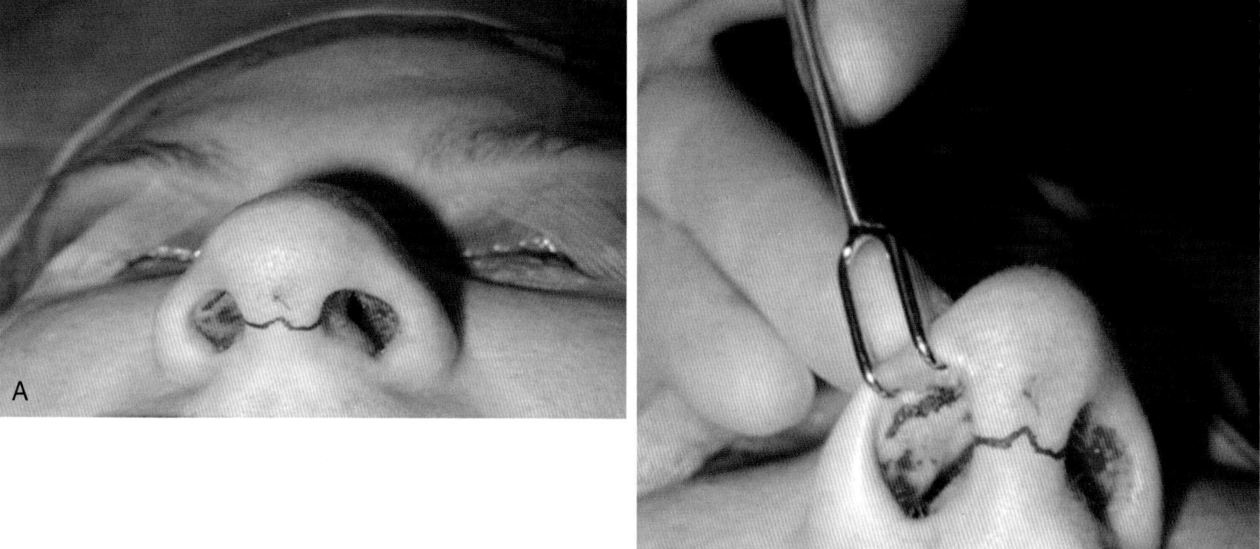

Figure 152.3 **A** and **B,** Placement of marginal and transcolumellar incisions.

TECHNIQUE: Open Rhinoplasty Including Septoplasty—*cont'd*

between the cartilage and nasal mucosa on both sides. After administration of local anesthesia, the nose is packed with cottonoid soaked in oxymetazoline. The nose is then prepped and draped for surgery. This sequence will allow ample time for the vasoconstriction of the nose prior to making an incision.

STEP 2: Incision

- Marginal (infracartilaginous) incision along the caudal edge of lower lateral cartilages, connected to a transcolumellar incision (Figs. 152.2 and 152.3). The vertical component (columellar side wall) of the marginal incision should be about 4 to 5 mm posterior to the cutaneous edge of the columellar skin. This incision is then connected to the transcolumellar incision. Care must be taken not to transect the medial crura while making

Continued

TECHNIQUE: Open Rhinoplasty Including Septoplasty—*cont'd*

the transcolumellar incision. There are multiple variations for the type of incision across the columella but the most common is an inverted "V" placed along the narrowest portion of the columella. Placing the incision too high can make it conspicuous.

STEP 3: Flap Elevation

- With the aid of skin hooks and finger traction and countertraction, elevate the skin-muscle flap in a subperichondrial fashion over the domal cartilages; it is easier to reflect the soft tissue from the columella upward (cephalad) since it will allow direct visualization of the caudal edges of the lateral crus, which should minimize inadvertent incision into the cartilage. Continue cephalad until nasal bones are seen and convert the dissection to a subperiosteal method (Fig. 152.4). Use double prong skin hooks to retract the dome inferiorly as you elevate the soft tissue envelope in a cephalad direction. Once a proper soft tissue envelope is formed, an Aufricht retractor is placed for retraction.

STEP 4: Dorsal Hump Reduction

- Using a double-guarded osteotome, remove the cartilaginous/bony hump in a fashion parallel to the ideal dorsal lines (Fig. 152.5); the cartilaginous component of the hump can be excised with a blade and the osteotome completes the bony component removal. Save all excised cartilage (in case needed later) (Fig. 152.6). The typical shape of the resected hump is that of a "canoe" with cartilage caudal and bone cephalad. A large hump resection will produce an open-roof deformity, which will necessitate lateral osteotomies (will be discussed later in the manuscript).

STEP 5: Septum Exposure

- Separate the medial crura, take down the transdomal ligaments (connecting the right and left medial crura), and find the caudal edge of the septum. Elevate a subperichondrial flap on both sides from a dorsal to ventral direction. A serrated amalgam plugger works well in elevating the perichondrium off of septal cartilage (Figs. 152.7 and 152.8). Elevation of the mucoperichondrial flaps must extend posteriorly toward the ethmoid and vomer bones. Exposure of the septum in the manner (dorsal approach) obviates the need for a transfixion incision.

STEP 6: Harvest of Septum

- Leaving at least 10 mm of cartilage dorsally and caudally, remove the remaining portion of the septum using a swivel knife. If a dorsal hump removal is anticipated, either perform the hump reduction first and then harvest the septum, or leave more than 10 mm of remaining cartilage since the removal of the cartilaginous hump will obviously decrease the 10 mm height. Right-angle swivel knives are preferred to straight swivel knives due to their ergonomic shape. After retrieval of the septum, check for perforations along the mucoperichondrium. Next, using a Keith needle, close the mucoperichondrial flaps in a quilting fashion in order to close the dead space

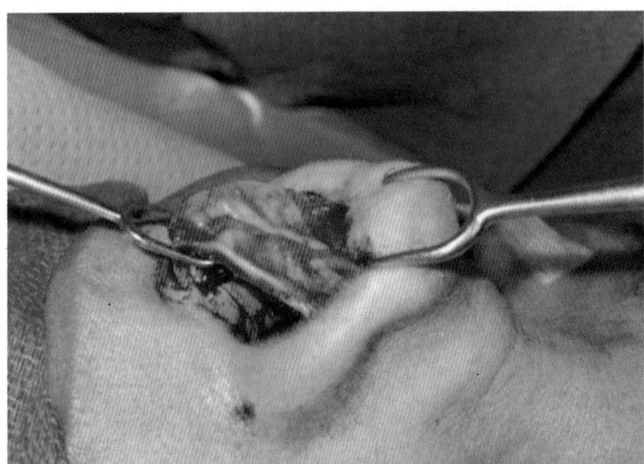

Figure 152.4 Degloving of the nose in a subperichondrial fashion.

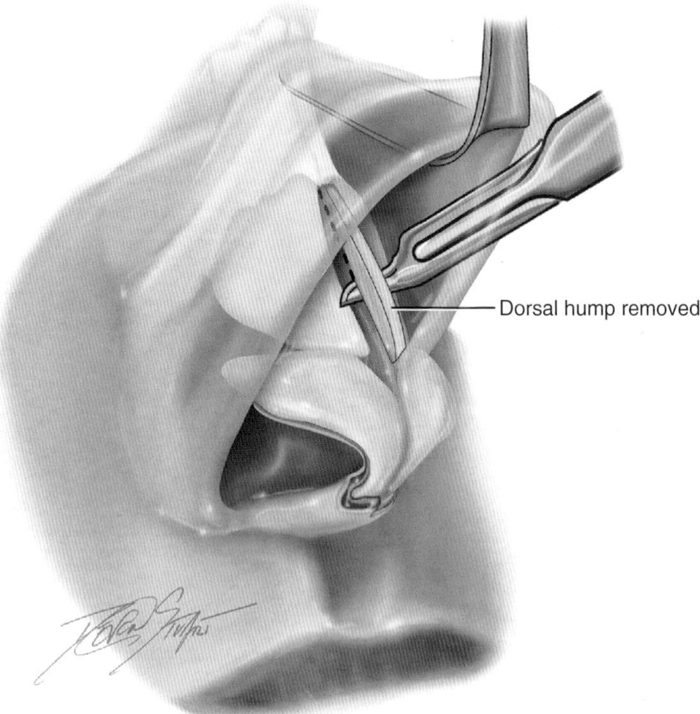

Figure 152.5 Hump reduction.

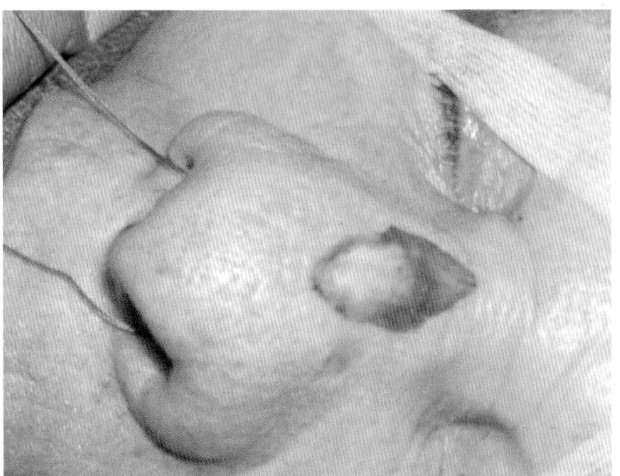

Figure 152.6 Typical appearance of the resected hump (note cartilaginous and bony components).

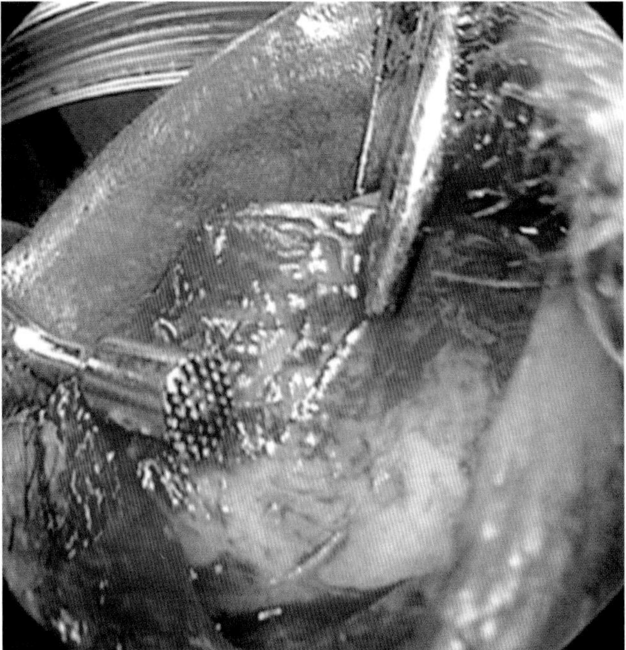

Figure 152.7 Serrated amalgam plugger used in elevating mucoperichondrium.

Continued

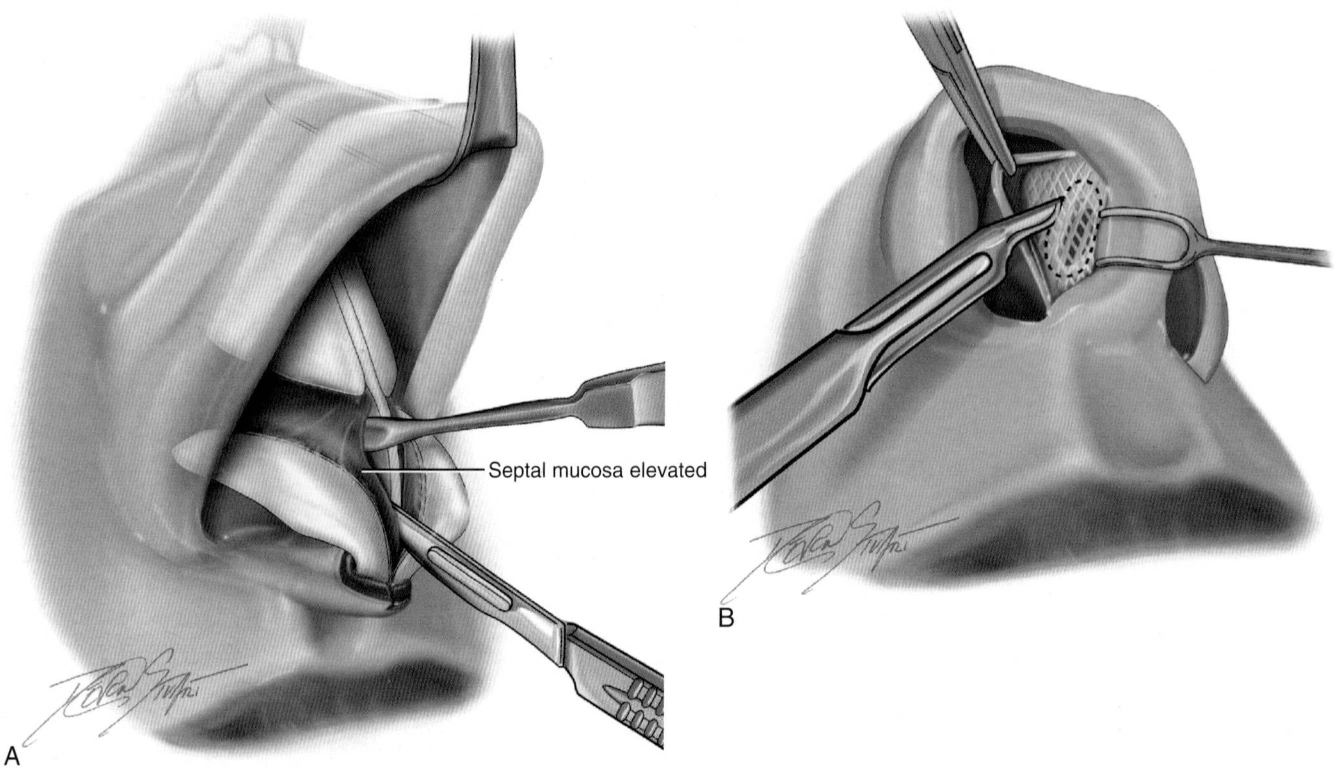

Figure 152.8 A and B, Elevation of mucoperichondrium in a dorsal to caudal direction.

TECHNIQUE: Open Rhinoplasty Including Septoplasty—*cont'd*

created after harvesting the septum. Note: if one has harvested more septum than needed, the unused portion of the septum can be placed back into the nose within the mucoperichondrial flaps for future use.

STEP 7: Lateral Osteotomy

- After hump reduction, it will be necessary to close an open roof deformity using lateral osteotomies. This can be done endonasally or externally through a percutaneous approach. When performing an endonasal lateral osteotomy, it is important not to include the inferior turbinate head in the osteotomy; this will cause medicalization of the inferior turbinate and air flow obstruction. Osteotomy should begin just cephalad to the head of the inferior turbinate, thereby preserving a triangular area commonly known as the Webster's triangle (head of the inferior turbinate, nasal floor, and lateral nasal sidewall) (Fig. 152.9). Percutaneous lateral osteotomies are favored by some in difficult cases where in-fracturing of the lateral side wall is incomplete.

STEP 8: Tip Plasty

- According to the indicated needs of the patient, tip plasty can be accomplished by performing cephalic trim, transdomal suturing, and dome division. Cephalic trim will cause a natural rotation of the tip of the nose (Fig. 152.10). Various suturing techniques exist in order to shape or narrow the domal cartilages (Figs. 152.11 and 152.12).

STEP 9: Grafting

- Harvested septum can be fashioned to be used as a columellar strut graft, spreader grafts, and tip/shield grafts. Spreader grafts are placed between the dorsal septum and upper lateral cartilages along the internal nasal valve area. Typical sizes are 20 × 5 mm. Spreader grafts are useful in "pinched" nasal midvaults or patients with collapse of the internal nasal valves (positive Cottle's test). They are secured using horizontal mattress sutures. Columellar strut grafts should be placed in all open rhinoplasty cases in order to restore support to the nasal tip (Fig. 152.13). The strut graft should be placed just above the anterior nasal spine and secured to the medial crura. The placement of the strut graft directly on the anterior nasal spine may cause "clicking sounds" when the patient moves the tip of his/her nose (Fig. 152.14). Shield grafts are also quite useful for creating a harmonious dome and tip. They can be

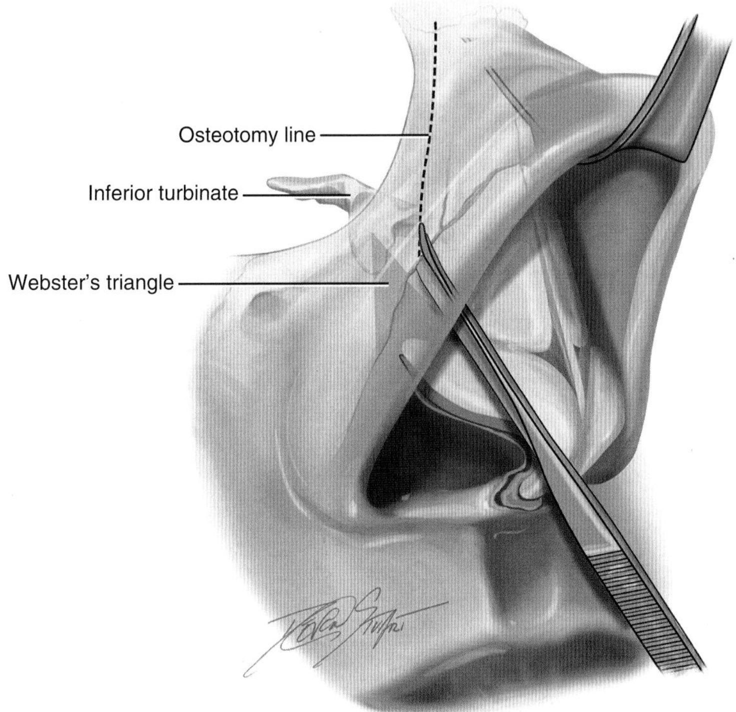

Figure 152.9 Orientation of lateral osteotomy with preservation of the Webster's triangle.

TECHNIQUE: Open Rhinoplasty Including Septoplasty—*cont'd*

hand-carved or one can use "cookie cutters" to procure them. Care should be taken to ensure that the edges of the graft are beveled to prevent palpation through a thin soft tissue envelope (Figs. 152.15 and 152.16).

STEP 10: Closure

- The transcolumellar incision is closed using multiple 6-0 nonresorbable sutures. Marginal incisions along the caudal edges of the lateral crus are closed using fast-absorbing sutures. Care should be exercised in not including cartilage in the closure (mucosa to mucosa only) to prevent warping or bossae formation.

STEP 11: Dressing

- External taping and splint should always be used in order to redrape the soft tissue envelope over the underlying skeleton. Internal splints can be useful to prevent septal hematoma or postoperative nose bleeds. All dressings and sutures are removed within the first 4 to 5 days following surgery and a new dressing is applied for another 5 to 7 days.

ALTERNATIVE TECHNIQUE

Rhinoplasty can also be performed through an endonasal approach, obviating the need for a transcolumellar incision.[4] This approach is ideal for isolated tip deformities; it does have a shorter recovery period and postoperative edema; however, visualization is greatly limited. This is the major difference between endonasal and open rhinoplasty. Most experts believe that the open technique offers a significantly wider surgical access and visualization, can allow for precise placement of grafting material, and is the technique of choice in post-traumatic rhinoplasty and revision surgery.[5–8] Endonasal approach is accomplished by performing a marginal incision as well as an intercartilaginous incision between upper and lower lateral cartilages. The lateral crus is then dissected off the overlying skin but maintained on its underside mucosal surface. The cartilage can then be "delivered" out of the nose while attached in a bipedicled fashion medially and laterally.

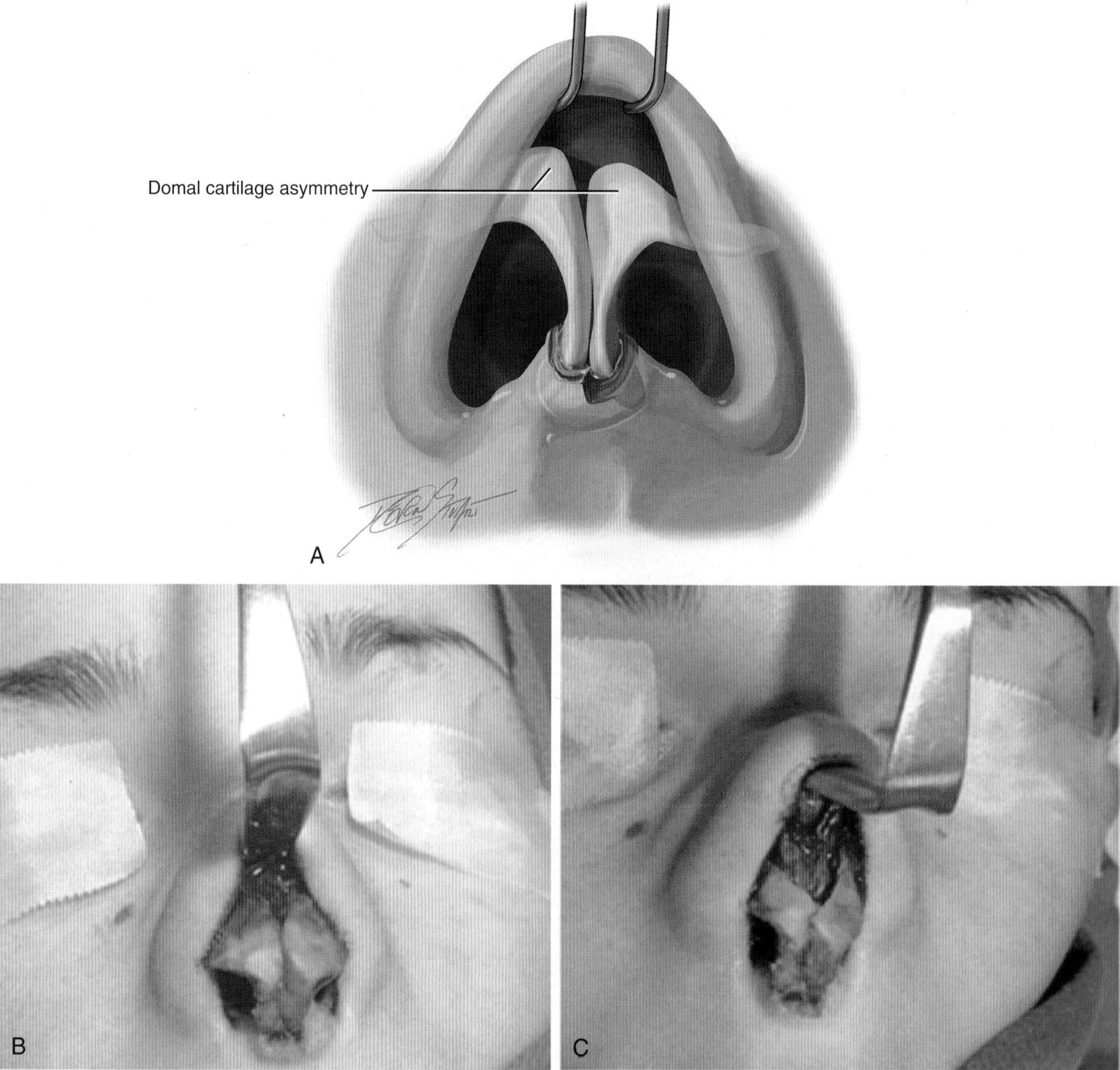

Figure 152.10 A–C, Cephalic trim.

Avoidance and Management of Intraoperative Complications

Intraoperative complications from rhinoplasty stem from technical issues. Technical issues can be encountered during the elevation of soft tissue envelope (not elevating in a subperichondrial fashion), leading to nasal tip flap necrosis, during the elevation of perichondrium off of septum, causing a "button-hole" within the septum that can then lead to a septal perforation and a saddle nose deformity, and failure to completely remove a dorsal hump, leading to a residual dorsal convexity.[9,10]

Postoperative Considerations

Patients are seen within 5 to 7 days following surgery to remove dressing/splints and sutures. Postoperative antibiotics and steroids should be used in most patients to reduce the risk of infection (especially with internal packs) and reduce bruising. Patients should be counseled appropriately about prolonged edema around the nasal tip due to the transcolumellar incision in open rhinoplasty. Revision surgery should be delayed for about a year to allow for edema and swelling to resolve; however, if the nose is grossly deviated following surgery, waiting an entire year is not warranted and revision surgery should be planned sooner.

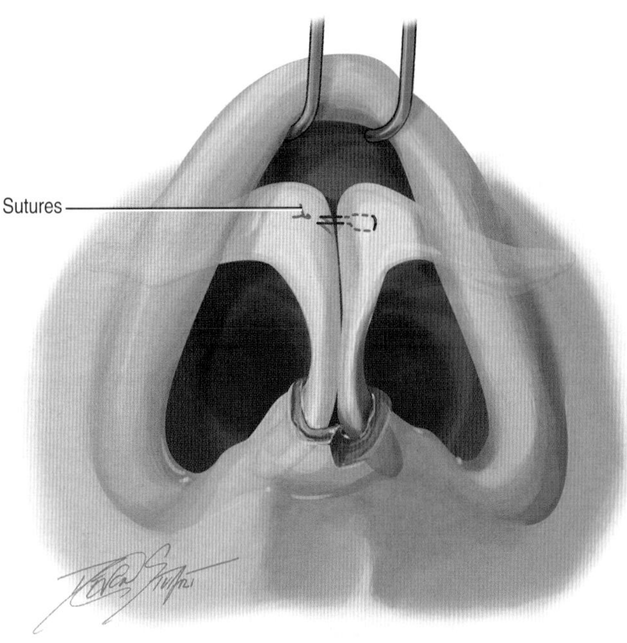

Figure 152.11 Transdomal suture placed within right dome.

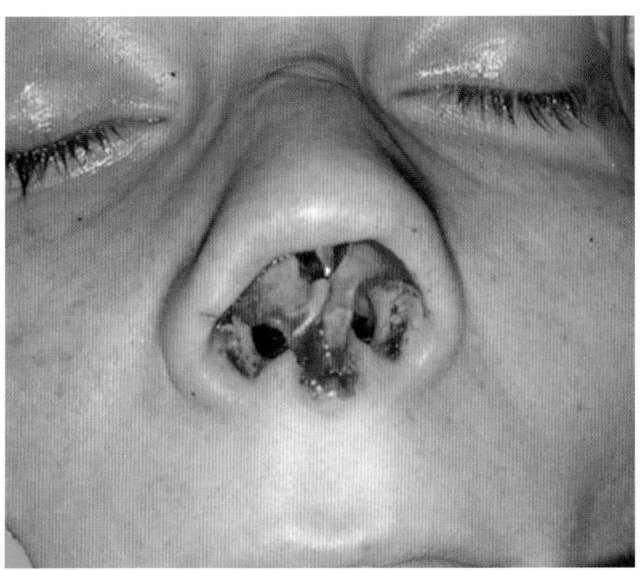

Figure 152.12 Right dome appearance following placement of transdomal suture.

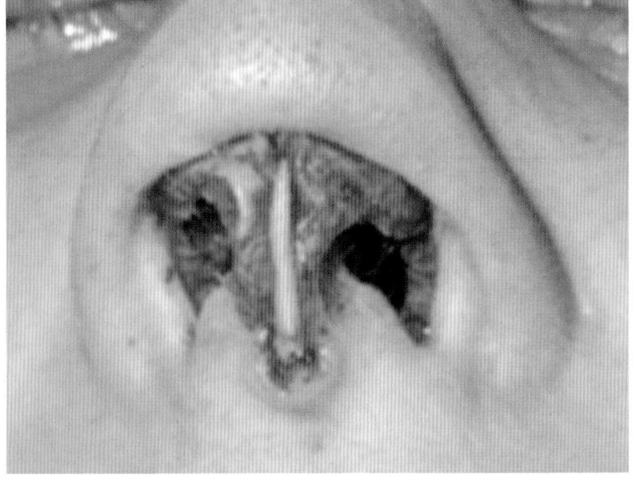

Figure 152.14 Columellar strut graft in place.

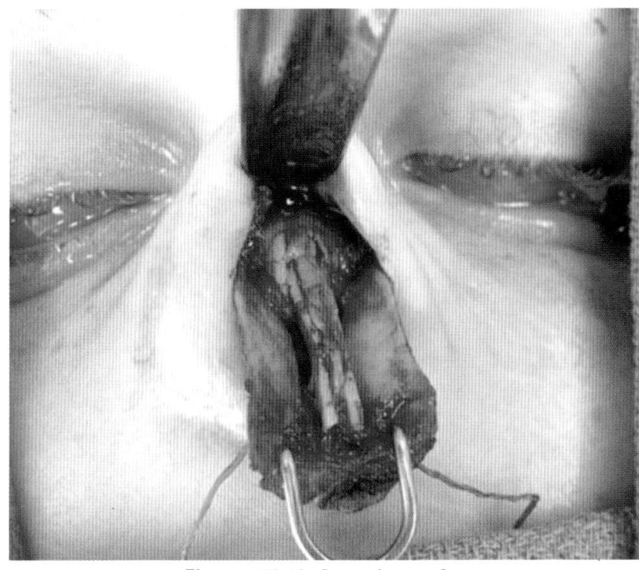

Figure 152.13 Spreader grafts.

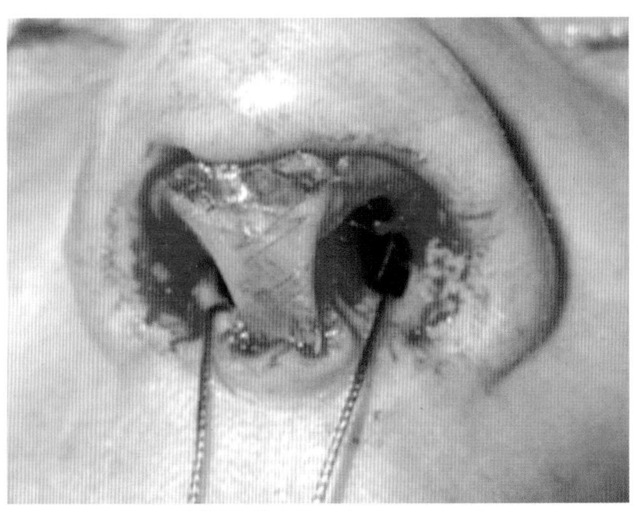

Figure 152.15 Shield graft sutured in place.

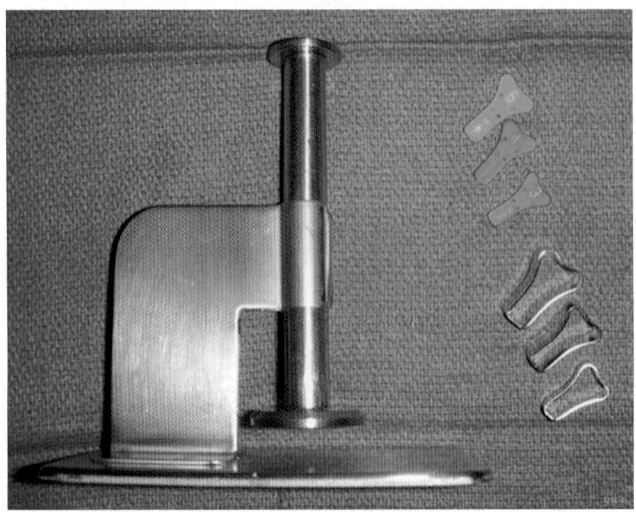

Figure 152.16 Cookie cutters used in shaping shield grafts.

References

1. Snell GED. A history of rhinoplasty. *Can J Otolaryngol.* 1973;2:224–230.
2. Simons RL. *Aligning the Stars: The History of Modern Rhinoplasty.* Video presentation at the American Academy of Facial Plastic and Reconstructive Surgery meeting. Washington, DC; 2007.
3. Adamson PA, Chen T. The dangerous dozen: avoiding potential problem patients in cosmetic surgery. *Facial Plast Surg Clin North Am.* 2008;16:195–202.
4. McCollough EG, English JL. A new twist in nasal tip surgery: an alternative to the Goldmand tip for the wide or bulbous lobule. *Arch Otolaryngol.* 1985;111:524–529.
5. Toriumi DM. Structural approach to primary rhinoplasty. *Aesthet Surg J.* 2002;22(1):72–84.
6. Toriumi DM. Structure approach in rhinoplasty. *Facial Plast Surg Clin North Am.* 2005;13(1):93–113.
7. Fattahi T. Internal nasal valve: significance in nasal air flow. *J Oral Maxillofac Surg.* 2008;66(9):1921–1926.
8. Fattahi T. Considerations in revision rhinoplasty: lessons learned. *Oral Maxillofac Surg Clin North Am.* 2011;23:101–108.
9. Tardy ME, Schwartz MS, Parras G. Saddle nose deformity: autogenous graft repair. *Facial Plast Surg.* 1989;6:121.
10. Tebbetts JB. Open vs. closed rhinoplasty: analyzing processes. *Aesthet Surg J.* 2006;26:456–459.

CHAPTER 153

Otoplasty

Faisal A. Quereshy and Ashley E. Manlove

Armamentarium

#15 Scalpel blade
30- and 27-Gauge needles
Adson and Adson-Brown forceps
Appropriate sutures
Colorado tip electrocautery
Curved iris scissors
Double skin hook
Frazier tip suction (7-French)
Local anesthetic with vasoconstrictor
Long-tipped cotton applicators
Marking pen
Methylene blue
Raytec sponges
Saline irrigation
Senn retractor
Smooth Crile-Wood needle holder
Smooth Webster needle holder
Straight iris scissors
Straight Mayo scissors
Straight Metzenbaum scissors

History of the Procedure

The prominent ear is a common aesthetic problem, affecting approximately 5% of the population.[1] Ears are considered protruded when they protrude more than 20 mm and greater than 35 degrees from the occipital scalp.[2] Common causes of a protruding ear include the following:

- Effacement of the antihelical fold
- Deep concha bowl
- Excessive helical root
- Cup ear deformity
- Excess fold of cartilage causing Stahl's ear, or a pointed ear
- Macrotia
- Overprojected lobule
- Prominent Darwin tubercle[2]

Otoplasty, or surgical correction of the protruded ear, is reported in the literature as far back as 1845. The first ear surgery performed is credited to Dieffenbach and involved the excision of the retroauricular skin with conchomastoid fixation (posttraumatic). This approach corrected only the cephaloauricular angle and not the underlying cartilage; therefore, relapse was high. Since 1845, more than 100 techniques have been described.[3] Surgical techniques can be broadly described at cartilage sparing, cartilage cutting, or a combination of both (Table 153.1).

The Mustarde technique was described in 1963 and continues to be one of the most popular cartilage-sparing approaches. The Mustarde otoplasty creates an antihelix with permanent conchoscaphal mattress sutures. Furnas described another cartilage-sparing approach with simple correction of the prominent ear with a well-formed antihelical fold but protruding conchal bowl using a conchal bowl-to-mastoid periosteum suture. Mustarde and Furnas techniques are often used together since a prominent ear is often the result of a lack of an antihelical fold and the presence of a large conchal bowl.

Otoplasty with cartilage cutting or scoring is also popular as this allows the surgeon to shape the cartilage and avoid using permanent suture material. Surgeons weaken the anterior cartilage with abrasion, rasping, cutting, or needle scoring so that the cartilage becomes more malleable.[3] With cartilage-cutting techniques, care must be taken not to disrupt the blood supply to the cartilage which would result in necrosis. Studies comparing cartilage-sparing with cartilage-cutting techniques do not show an improved outcome or increased complication rate for one method over the other.

Nonsurgical treatment of otoplasty is a great treatment modality if the ear formation is present and diagnosed immediately after birth. At birth, the ear cartilage is pliant and responsive to splinting or ear molding. Within 3 to 4 days of birth, the ear cartilage starts to stiffen and can no longer be managed nonsurgically. Unfortunately, many infants are born with normal appearing ear projection, but the ears become more prominent after one year of age.

Indications for the Use of the Procedure

Otoplasty is most commonly used for surgical correction of prominent ears that may involve an underdeveloped antihelix or an enlarged conchal bowl. Surgical correction may be indicated for grade I (mild) deformities, grade II (moderate) deformities, and grade III (severe auricular) deformities.

Table 153.1 Otoplasty Techniques

Cartilage Cutting	Cartilage Sparing	Combination
Stenstrom	Furnas	Converse
Weerda	Mustarde	Cihandide
Walter	Spira	Ersen
Pitanguy	Scaphomastoid	
Luckett		
Davis		

Understanding the normal auricular anatomy is important to determine the best surgical approach of the prominent ear. Protruding ears are the most common grade I deformity; however, a careful examination must be performed to distinguish deformity from a misshapen auricle. Proposed criteria to describe the normal ear include the following:[4–8]

- The helical rim should be 6 to 20 mm from the head.
- The angle between the mastoid and the helix should be less than 30 degrees.
- The axis of the ear should be parallel to the bridge of the nose.
- The auricle should be 55 to 70 mm posterior to the lateral orbital margin.
- The width of the auricle should be 50% to 60% of the length.
- The lobule should be parallel to the antihelical fold in the same plane.

McDowell[9] has proposed the following goals for otoplasty:

- All upper third ear protrusion must be corrected.
- The helix of both ears should be seen beyond the antihelix from the frontal view.
- The helix should have a smooth and regular line throughout.
- The postauricular sulcus should not be markedly decreased or distorted.
- The helix-to-mastoid distance should fall in the normal range of 10 to 12 mm in the upper third, 16 to 18 mm in the middle third, and 20 to 22 mm in the lower third.
- The position of the lateral ear border to the head should match within 3 mm at any point between the two ears.

Planning for otoplasty requires a thorough evaluation of the patient and his or her expectations, along with the goals of the parents. The surgeon should discuss with the patient the risks, benefits, and postoperative recovery before any surgery is planned. During the evaluation, take preoperative photographs and develop the surgical plan. A complete evaluation of prominent ears involves assessment of (1) the degree of antihelical fold; (2) the depth of the conchal bowl (if the bowl is greater than 2.5 cm, cartilage must be excised); (3) the plane of the lobule; (4) the angle between the helical rim and mastoid; and (5) the quality of the cartilage, which has more spring and pliability in a child than in an adolescent or adult.[10]

Limitations and Contraindications

There are very few contraindications to otoplasty. The best timing for otoplasty continues to be a topic of debate. Typically, surgical correction is performed around 6 to 7 years of age for two reasons. At this age, ear growth is nearly complete, and the cartilage has not completely stiffened and that patient is socially and emotionally better prepared for surgery.[11] The ears grow rapidly in the first decade with 95% to 97% of the total growth completed by age 10. However, at age 5 the child begins primary school, and the psychosocial implications of ear malformation must be taken into consideration when planning for surgery. For this reason, most surgical ear corrections are done around 5 to 7 years of age. Gosain et al.[10] along with Balogh and Millesi[12] have demonstrated that early surgical intervention does not negatively affect the growth of the ear.

Relative contraindications include young patients whose parents are pushing for surgery before the child is cooperative or patients who have unrealistic expectations for the outcome.

TECHNIQUE: Cartilage-Sparing Otoplasty

The cartilage-sparing technique combines the Furnas technique to address conchal bowl hypertrophy with the Mustarde technique for creating an antihelical fold.

STEP 1: Planning

Furnas concha markings: Apply gentle pressure, rotating the cavum posteriorly toward the mastoid. Mark the excess skin on the dorsal aspect of the cavum to be excised. As mentioned previously, if the conchal bowl is greater than 2.5 cm, the technique must be modified to a cartilage-cutting method (see Modified Technique 1 later in the chapter).

Mustarde antihelical fold markings: Apply gentle pressure to the superior helical rim and mark the crest of the projected antihelical fold. Through-and-through markings with methylene blue are placed at least 7 mm apart, parallel to the crest, to ensure that the fold is not too narrow (Fig. 153.1A–D).

Continued

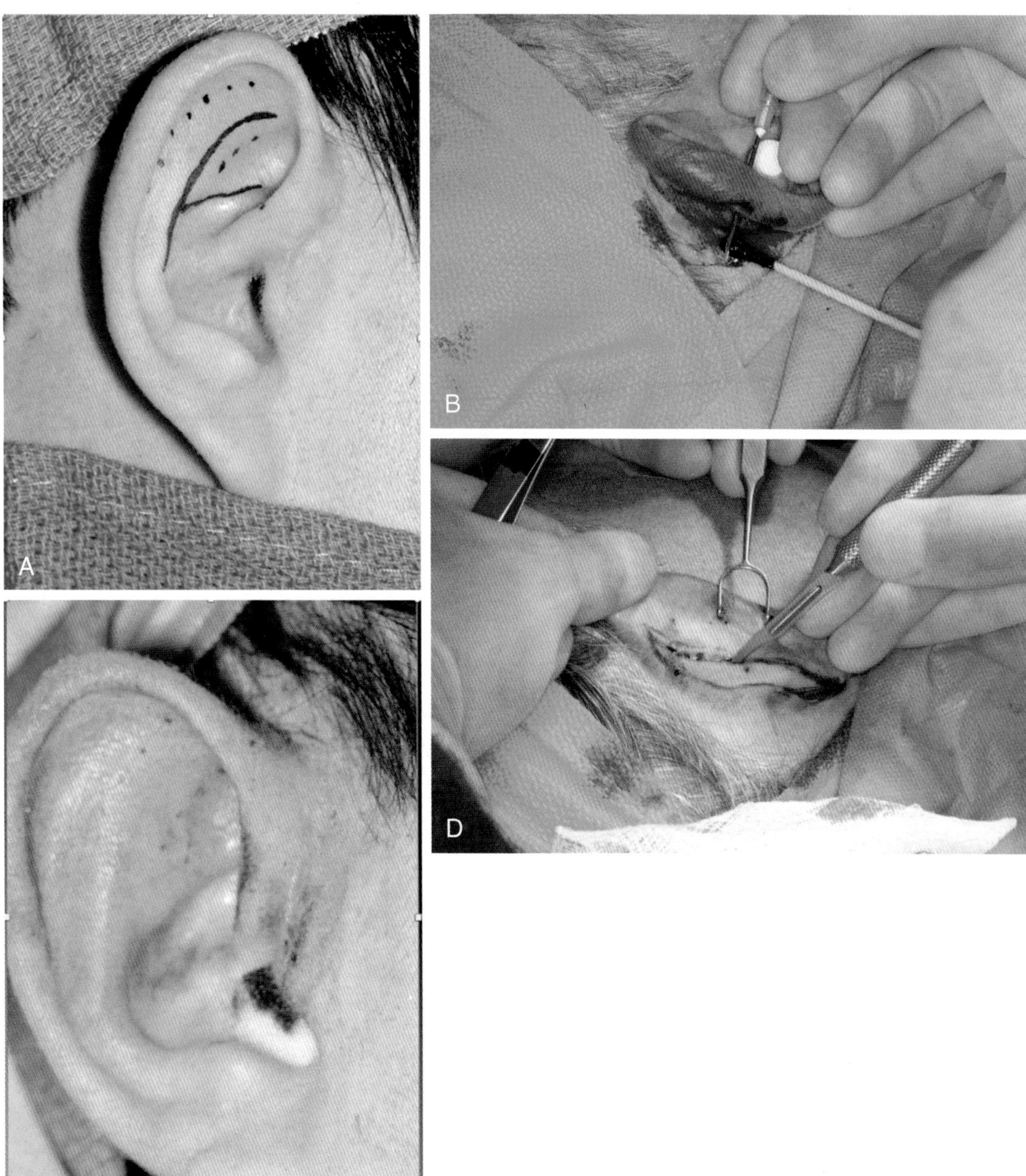

Figure 153.1 **A–C,** Presurgical marking of the conchal bulb and antihelical fold. **D,** Incision.

TECHNIQUE: Cartilage-Sparing Otoplasty—*cont'd*

STEP 2: Anesthesia

Inject a local anesthetic (1% lidocaine with epinephrine) to obtain anesthesia and to hydrodissect the anterior skin off the auricular cartilage and conchal bowl.

STEP 3: Incision

Furnas method: Expose the conchal cartilage through an elliptical incision on the posterior aspect of the auricle. The ellipse should be only wide enough to allow removal of excess retroauricular connective tissue, fatty tissue, and muscle tissue.

Mustarde method: Using the same retroauricular incision, make a small horizontal incision at the inferior aspect of the new antihelical fold and pass a Freer elevator through. Release the anterior auricular skin over the new antihelical fold. Weaken the anterior aspect of the anterior cartilage with Adson forceps or a rasp to create a subtle appearance for the new antihelical fold (Fig. 153.1E).

STEP 4: Suturing

Furnas method: Using 3-0 silk, place three or four conchomastoid horizontal mattress sutures in the lateral third of the concha parallel to the auricular curve, pinning the conchal bowl posteriorly. Be careful not to puncture the anterior skin of the ear and not to place the sutures too close to the external auditory canal. If excess cartilage is present, part of the conchal bowl must be excised to avoid constriction of the external auditory canal.

Mustarde method: Using nonresorbable horizontal mattress sutures (e.g., 4-0 Mersilene), secure the antihelical fold with permanent horizontal mattress sutures through the perichondrium and cartilage, medial to lateral, so that the knot is along the medial surface. Place the sutures perpendicular to the marked antihelical fold so that when they are tightened, they produce a well-rounded fold (Fig. 153.1F).

STEP 5: Dressing

In all surgical correction of the prominent ear, a pressure dressing is used to eliminate dead space and to help prevent hematoma formation. The dressing should be left in place for 2 weeks.

Furnas method: Tie the mattress sutures over a ball of Xeroform or a cotton ball soaked in triple antibiotic ointment placed in the caval fossa. The medicated cotton roll keeps the skin flat and stretched over the cartilage and maintains the depth of the caval fossa. This reduces dead space and helps prevent hematoma formation.

Mustarde method: Place petroleum gauze over the anterior and posterior aspect of the antihelix and scaphoid fossa. Cover the petroleum gauze with fluffs and place a tight head wrap to hold the dressing in place.

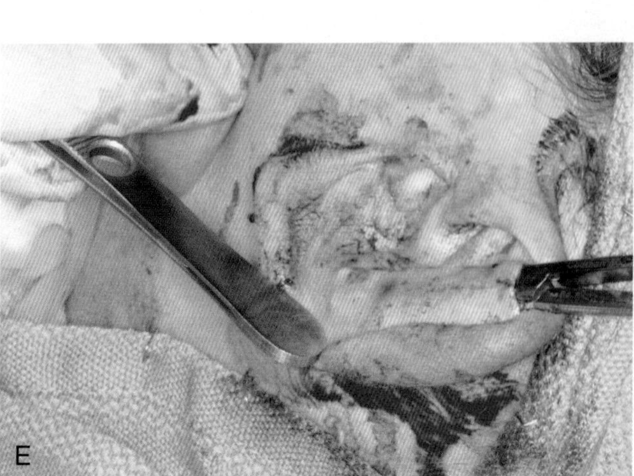

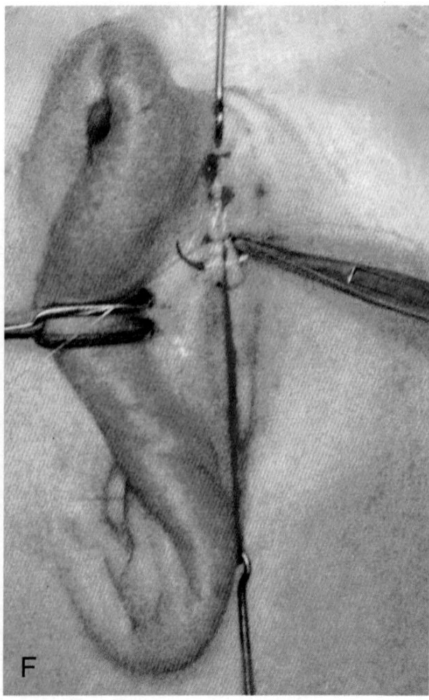

Figure 153.1, cont'd **E,** Conchal bulb exposure. **F,** Suturing.

ALTERNATIVE TECHNIQUE 1: Cartilage-Cutting Otoplasty for Hypertrophic Conchal Bowl

The Davis technique is an alternative to the Furnas method of treating conchal hypertrophy, which involves excising the cartilage.[13]

STEP 1: Planning

Mark the skin of the anterior surface of the conchal bowl with a marking pen, ensuring at least 8 mm of conchal wall height from the conchal scaphal junction. Use methylene blue transfixion tattoos to mark the posterior cartilage. Starting just inferior to the lower crus border with the marking pen, move anteriorly into the cymbal fossa and then curve around and inferior again, forming the top half of a kidney-bean shape. Continue anteriorly again and curve inferiorly along the posterior aspect of the external auditory canal; continue posteriorly into the cavum concha and then into the posterior conchal wall.

STEP 2: Anesthesia

Obtain local anesthesia and hydrodissection by infiltrating 2% lidocaine/1 : 100,000 epinephrine into the anterior skin of the conchal bowl.

STEP 3: Excision of Skin and Cartilage

Using a #15 blade, make an elliptical incision along the posterior aspect of the auricle. Do not make the ellipse any larger than the amount of skin to be excised because the skin must be tension-free at closure. The methylene blue tattoo marks should be visualized once the skin has been removed. Using a #15 blade, carefully cut full thickness through the cartilage, taking care not to damage the anterior conchal skin. Using a sharp Freer elevator, release the cartilage from the perichondrium. Position the ear posteriorly against the mastoid surface and evaluate for sharp cartilage edges or prominences. Remove postauricular muscle and connective tissue so that the skin closure is passive (Fig. 153.2A and B).

STEP 4: Conchal Bowl Fixation

Using 3-0 silk suture, place three or four sutures to fixate the ear, passing the suture through the anterior skin of the conchal bowl, deep through the postauricular muscle, and then back through the anterior skin of the conchal bowl. Tie the sutures over Xeroform gauze or a cotton ball coated with triple antibiotic ointment. Suture the postauricular skin with resorbable suture, such as 5-0 fast-absorbing gut. The silk sutures and Xeroform or cotton ball should be left in place for a minimum of 2 weeks (Fig. 153.2C).

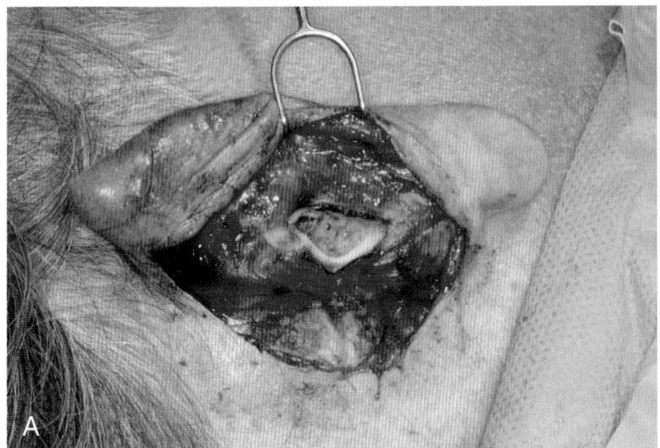

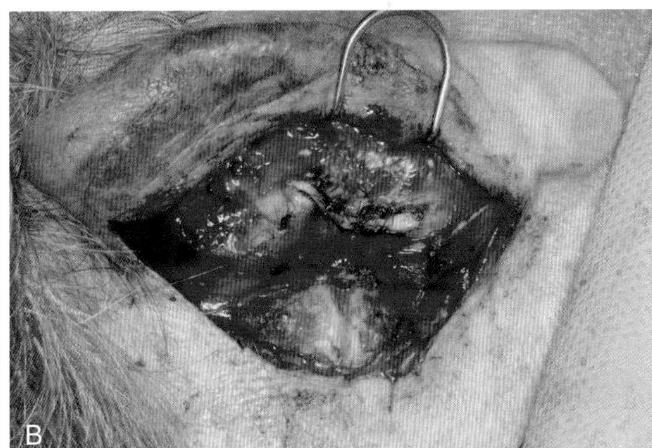

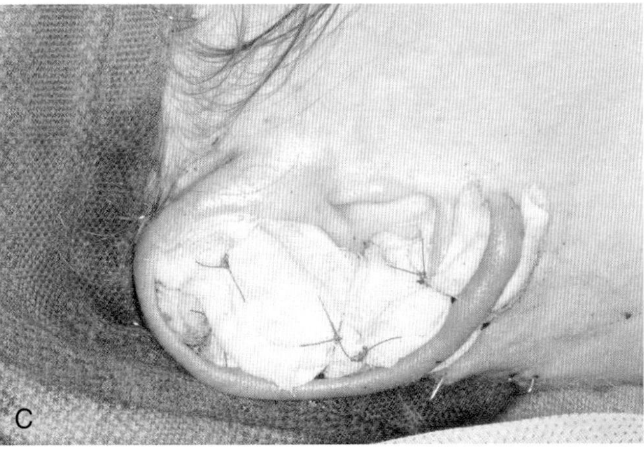

Figure 153.2 **A** and **B,** Cartilage scoring and harvest. **C,** Bolster packing in place to minimize the risk of postoperative hematoma.

ALTERNATIVE TECHNIQUE 2: Cartilage-Scoring Otoplasty for Prominent Helix

Mustarde's cartilage-sparing approach is popular to avoid unaesthetic sharp cartilage edges. In young patients who have pliable cartilage, this technique works very well. Patients who are older than 10 years of age often have more rigid cartilage and require a different approach. Scoring of the cartilage can weaken its structure and make it more compliant. Scoring can be done from the anterior or posterior aspect. Gibson and Davis[14] demonstrated that cartilage warps away from the scored surface. In older patients or patients with stiff cartilage, the surgeon should score the anterior aspect of the auricle, such as those described by Stenstrom[15] and Chongchet,[16] to achieve the appropriate shape.

STEP 1: Planning

Apply pressure to the superior helical rim and mark the crest of the antihelix with a marking pen. The marks are then transferred to the cartilage with methylene blue through transfixion.

STEP 2: Anesthesia

Local anesthesia and hydrodissection are achieved by injecting 2% lidocaine/1:100,000 epinephrine.

STEP 3: Incision and Scoring

Make an incision along the posterior aspect of the scaphoid fossa and expose the cartilage. A combination of scoring and cutting can accomplish the goal of creating the antihelical fold. Under direct visualization, a #15 blade can be used to score the anterior aspect of the cartilage along the methylene blue marks parallel to the scapha, weakening the cartilage so that it becomes pliable and folds to create the antihelix. Another option is to blindly rasp the anterior aspect of the cartilage in the subperichondrial plane. All scoring and rasping must be at least 4 mm from the helical edge. Temporary nonabsorbable mattress sutures are placed to hold the newly formed antihelix in the correct position. Occasionally the posterior skin is excised, but the surgeon must be mindful of passive closure to avoid keloid formation. The skin is closed with an absorbable suture.

STEP 4: Dressing

Place Xeroform or triple antibiotic cotton dressing against the anterior aspect of the helix, along with fluffs and a head wrap. Shape and dress the anterior aspect of the ear with a slightly compressive dressing to fill concavities and dead space. The dressing should remain dry and should be kept in place for approximately 2 weeks.

TECHNIQUE: Surgical Correction of the Protruding Earlobe

Patients with prominent ears often have prominent earlobes that need to be addressed in addition to the helix, antihelix, and conchal bowl. At the time of surgical planning and marking of the posterior auricular incision, the incision should be extended inferiorly. Numerous designs have been described, including a Z-plasty, a V shape, an ellipse, and a fishtail. Once the skin has been excised and hemostasis achieved, the skin edges are brought together and sutured with 4-0 plain gut.

Avoidance and Management of Intraoperative Complications

Intraoperative complications of otoplasty are rare. Blood loss with otoplasty should be minimal; however, occasionally excessive bleeding occurs that may require intraoperative treatment. Intraoperative bleeding can be minimized with the use of local anesthesia with epinephrine and use of bipolar electrocautery.

The great auricular nerve provides sensation to most of the external ear. Injury to the nerve or any of its branches may result in numbness or tingling of the skin covering the ear or the site of scar formation. The numbness commonly resolves, but there is a chance of permanent loss of sensation in the area of the surgery.

Postoperative Considerations and Complications

Complications of otoplasty are typically described as early and late complications. Early complications include hematoma formation, infection, pain, bleeding, pruritus, chondritis, and necrosis. Late complications include unaesthetic results, including hypertrophic scars, residual deformity, problems with sutures holding, granuloma formation, and dysesthesias.[5]

Hematoma formation and infection are the most dreaded complications of otoplasty surgery. Hematoma formation occurs in approximately 2% to 4% of patients and manifests as acute, severe pain that usually is unilateral.[17] Causes of hematoma include failure to control hemostasis during surgery, overly tight suturing without appropriate dependent drainage at the inferior aspect of the incision, trauma after surgery, hypertension, and bleeding disorders. If a hematoma is suspected, the head dressing should be removed immediately and the sutures released to drain the hematoma. Occasionally, exploratory surgery is necessary to identify the source. A pressure dressing must be reapplied to prevent another hematoma from forming. Fibrosis or cauliflower ear deformity can result if the hematoma goes untreated.

Infection from otoplasty manifests with redness, swelling, fever, and sometimes drainage from the incision site. It can be caused by dehiscence of the wound, poorly managed hematoma evacuation, or breach of sterile technique. Treatment of infection includes intravenous antibiotics and topical mafenide acetate cream. All sutures must be removed, including those placed in the cartilaginous reconstruction, and the cosmetic deformity must be dealt with once the infection completely clears. Infection can lead to chondritis and residual deformity of the ear. Chondritis is a surgical emergency and must be treated immediately with removal of all suture material, irrigation and drainage of infection, and antibiotics. The cosmetic deformity is addressed once the infection clears.

Hypertrophic scarring in otoplasty is most common in the posterior auricular region, especially when the incision is closed under tension. Patients prone to keloid formation must be treated aggressively with intraincisional steroid injection. The best treatment for hypertrophic scar formation is prevention with passive closure of the skin.

Narrowing or stricture of the external auditory canal can occur if the conchal bowl is rotated anteriorly while the ear is set back. This can be avoided by using the Davis technique and by excising redundant cartilage to avoid pressure on the canal.

Patient dissatisfaction with an unsightly appearance is apparent by postoperative month 6. A sharply ridged antihelical fold, irregular contours, lack of regular contour of the superior crus, a misshapen antihelical fold, and a narrow ear are some unaesthetic postoperative complications. These residual deformities are usually the result of poor surgical planning and execution.

Many studies have been performed on the success rates of cartilage-sparing versus cartilage-cutting techniques with regard to patient satisfaction and reoperation; however, these studies have shown conflicting results. Ultimately, the choice of technique is determined by the surgeon's preference.

References

1. Bardach J. Congenital ear deformities. Surgery for congenital and acquired malformation of the auricle. In: Cummings CW, ed. *Otolaryngology: Head and Neck Surgery*. St Louis, Missouri: Mosby; 1986.
2. Kelley P, Hollier L, Stal S. Otoplasty: evaluation, technique, and review. *J Craniofac Surg*. 2003;14(5):643–653.
3. Nazarian R, Eshraghi AA. Otoplasty for the protruded ear. *Semin Plast Surg*. 2011;25(4):288–294.
4. Naumann A. Otoplasty—techniques, characteristics and risks. *GMS Curr Top Otorhinolaryngol, Head Neck Surg*. 2007;6:Doc04.
5. Farkas LG. *Anthropometry of the Head and Face*. 2nd ed. New York, New York: Raven Press; 1994.
6. Siegert R, Krappen S, Kaesemann L, Weerda H. Computer assisted anthropometry of the auricle. *Face*. 1998;6:1.
7. Tolleth H. Artistic anatomy, dimensions, and proportions of the external ear. *Clin Plast Surg*. 1978;5(3):337–345.
8. Bozkir MG, Karakaş P, Yavuz M, Dere F. Morphometry of the external ear in our adult population. *Aesthetic Plast Surg*. 2006;30(1):81–85.
9. McDowell AJ. Goals in otoplasty for protruding ears. *Plast Reconstr Surg*. 1968;41(1):17–27.
10. Gosain AK, Kumar A, Huang G. Prominent ears in children younger than 4 years of age: what is the appropriate timing for otoplasty? *Plast Reconstr Surg*. 2004;114(5):1042–1054.
11. Janis JE, Rohrich RJ, Gutowski KA. *Otoplasty*. *Plast Reconstr Surg*. 2005;115(4):60e–72e.
12. Balogh B, Millesi H. Are growth alterations a consequence of surgery for prominent ears? *Plast Reconstr Surg*. 1992;89(4):623–630.
13. Davis JE. *Aesthetics and Reconstructive Otoplasty*. New York, New York: Springer-Verlag; 1987.
14. Gibson T, Davis W. The distortion of autogenous cartilage grafts: its cause and prevention. *Br J Plast Surg*. 1958;10:257.
15. Stenstrom SJ. A natural technique for correction of congenitally prominent ears. *Plast Reconstr Surg*. 1963;32:509–518.
16. Chongchet V. A method of antihelix reconstruction. *Br J Plast Surg*. 1963;16:268–272.
17. Adamson PA, Strecker HD. Otoplasty techniques. *Facial Plast Surg*. 1995;11(4):284–300.

Laser Skin Resurfacing

Craig E. Vigliante and Carrie E. Cera Hill

Armamentarium

Alcohol wipes or acetone
Appropriate sutures
Internal or external metal eye shields
Lacrilube
Laser equipment (CO_2 or erbium or combination)
"Laser in Use" sign for door
Laser-protective small particle masks for surgeon and staff
Laser safety equipment
Laser smoke evacuator
Laser-specific lens cleaning protocol
Laser-specific protective eye wear for surgeon and staff
Local anesthetic with vasoconstrictor
Makeup remover
Postoperative laser ice face mask
Postoperative laser ointment (Vaseline, CU3 Cream, Aquaphor, Vanicream ointment)
Proper staff and surgeon laser training
Saline eye wash
Tetracaine eye drops
Tongue blad

History of the Procedure

The acronym LASER stands for light amplification by stimulated emission of radiation, and describes the process by which light is produced. All laser systems contain four components: 1) gas, liquid or solid medium which is stimulated to generate laser light, 2) a source of energy to excite the medium, 3) mirrors to form an optical cavity surrounding the medium, and amplifies the radiation emission, 4) a delivery system. Light from a laser interacts with skin in four ways: reflection, scattering, transmission, and absorption. The following parameters control the effects of laser on tissue: wavelength, fluence, irradiance, spot size, and pulse duration. In ~1960, Dr. Leon Goldman became the first physician to use a laser to treat human skin.[1] Conditions which may be treated with lasers include Ablative Skin Resurfacing (to treat photoaging, scars, epidermal lesions), Non-ablative Skin Rejuvenation, Fractional Photothermolysis, Vascular lesions, Pigmented lesions and Tattoo Removal / Reduction, Laser Hair Reduction. In addition to lasers, Non-laser light sources include intense pulsed light (IPL) which emits polychromatic, non-coherent light for treatment of vascular lesions, pigmented lesions, hair removal / reduction, and non-ablative rejuvenation.

Ablative lasers include CO2 (10,600 nm) and Er:YAG (2940 nm) with a target chromophore of water. Light may be pulsed or scanned to ablate superficial tissue, causing a 'plume' of vaporized skin. Heat is removed via vaporization, with some residual heat remaining within skin surface. Indications including treatment of photoaging including rhytides and loss of elasticity, scars, and epidermal skin lesions. The result is resurfacing of the epidermis and contraction of the dermis. Downtime is 5-7 days and post-operative skin care is important to avoid complications.[1]

The carbon dioxide (CO_2) laser was invented by Kumar Patel in 1964. This was the first gas laser to produce high-power radiation continuously.[2] The CO_2 laser has more practical applications today than any other type of laser. The chromophore (light-absorbing compound) of the CO_2 laser is water. Because more than 80% of the epidermis is composed of water, the CO_2 laser is particularly useful in the treatment of the skin. This ablative laser allows surgeons to perform CO_2 laser skin resurfacing (LSR) accurately, safely, and effectively with precise depth control.

The first CO_2 lasers were continuous wave (CW) lasers. These CW lasers increased in popularity in the 1980s but had little thermal control. Treatments of the skin took a very long time because the spot sizes were small and optical scanners did not exist. In addition, these treatments were very technique-sensitive. Thermal relaxation times were often violated, resulting in prolonged healing times and scarring.[3] These clinical results were unacceptable, and short-pulse CO_2 laser energy was developed. These superpulsed CO_2 lasers were introduced in the 1990s. This dramatically reduced the incidence of scarring and the prolonged healing times seen with CW modalities.[3] The superpulsed lasers were a major advantage over the CW lasers because they decreased the size of the thermal zone, with shorter pulse widths resulting in greater safety, less discomfort, and less downtime.

The first high-energy CO_2 pulsed laser, operating at a wavelength of 10,600 nm, was developed by Lumenis (Yokneam, Israel) and named the UltraPulse Laser.[4] The advent of the Lumenis Ultrapulse Encore carbon dioxide ($LUPCO_2$) laser in the late 1990s changed everything for

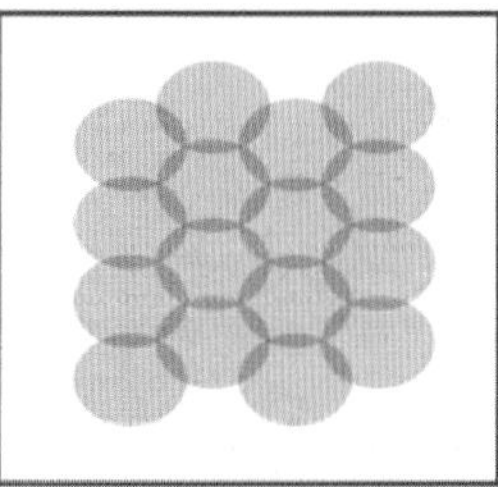

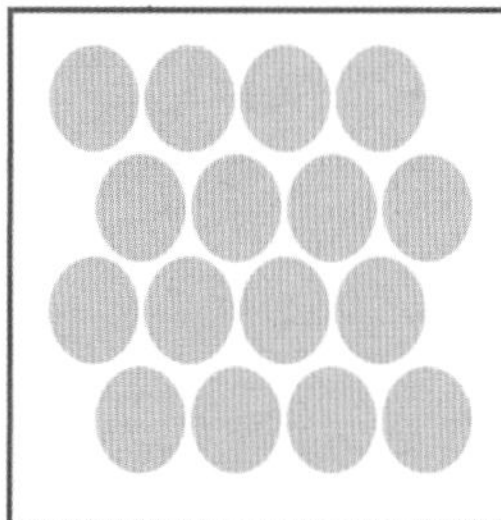

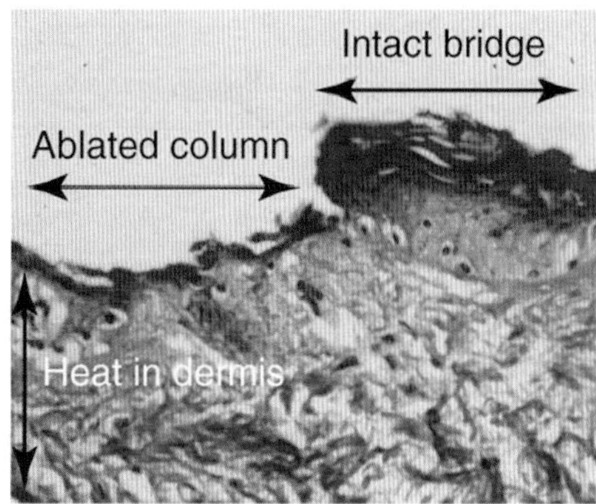

Figure 154.1 Histology showing fractional laser "microthermal zones" between bridges of unaffected tissue. (Courtesy Lumenis, Yokneam, Israel).

LSR. This laser provided the most safety with the shortest pulse width and narrowest thermal zone, resulting in less discomfort and less downtime. Erbium:YAG (yttrium-aluminum-garnet) lasers gained popularity in the 1990s and are still used today. The erbium:YAG laser emits a wavelength of 2940 nm, which is absorbed by water 10 times more efficiently than with the CO_2 laser.[3] Unfortunately, it does not remove wrinkles the way a CO_2 laser can, so clinical results are compromised. Heat generation is insufficient to promote clinically significant collagen shrinkage. The thermal energy zone is smaller and water absorption is greater, so the collagen in the skin is undertreated compared to a CO_2 laser. The yttrium, scandium, gallium garnet (YSGG) erbium laser (Cutera; Brisbane, California), with a 2790 nm wavelength, fills the gap between CO_2 and erbium:YAG lasers in terms of clinical use and effectiveness.

In 2004, Manstein et al.[5] introduced the concept of fractional photothermolysis. This concept was a major advance in laser skin rejuvenation. Instead of treating 100% of the skin surface, as does traditional CO_2 LSR, this method treats a fraction of the skin on each pass.[6] The computer coordinates drilling of multiple, small, vertically oriented holes, shaped like cylinders, of thermally damaged tissue called "microthermal zones." The surrounding areas of unaffected tissue act as reservoirs for healing by providing structural and nutritional support and a reservoir for keratinocyte migration (Fig. 154.1). The thermomechanical destruction that occurs when the microthermal zones are made is followed by a predictable and beneficial skin-tightening phase through a process of heat-induced shrinkage of collagen and the initiation of neocollagenesis. Clinically, this concept of focal damage with adjacent tissue sparing has led to improved patient comfort and recovery in the postprocedural period.[7]

Although the erbium laser wavelengths are very effective for resurfacing, the CO_2 laser has been found to be more effective for neocollagenesis because of its thermal damage, leading to dermal heating.[8] All skin resurfacing lasers continue to be compared to the CO_2 laser, both in terms of downtime and results. The CO_2 laser has the longest track record and is considered by many to be the gold standard for laser skin rejuvenation.

Indications for the Use of the Procedure

Laser skin rejuvenation (LSR) or Laser Resurfacing provides a very effective way to safely treat problematic areas of facial aging. Not many skin treatments can consistently give such dramatic results as laser skin treatment. The final results of many facial cosmetic surgical treatments, including facelifts and blepharoplasties, are greatly enhanced by the addition of LSR (Fig. 154.2). The addition of a laser to these procedures is considered "the icing on the cake," so to speak. It is no longer acceptable to rejuvenate the underlying structures and leave the damaged skin untreated.[9] The laser treatment can be done in conjunction with these surgical procedures or performed as an "a la carte" protocol. This depends on the surgeon's experience level and on variables such as the patient's level of compliance, healing capacity, medical history, and accepted recovery time. In fact, it is widely known that it is difficult to achieve the best facial cosmetic surgical results without the addition of some form of facial laser treatment.[10]

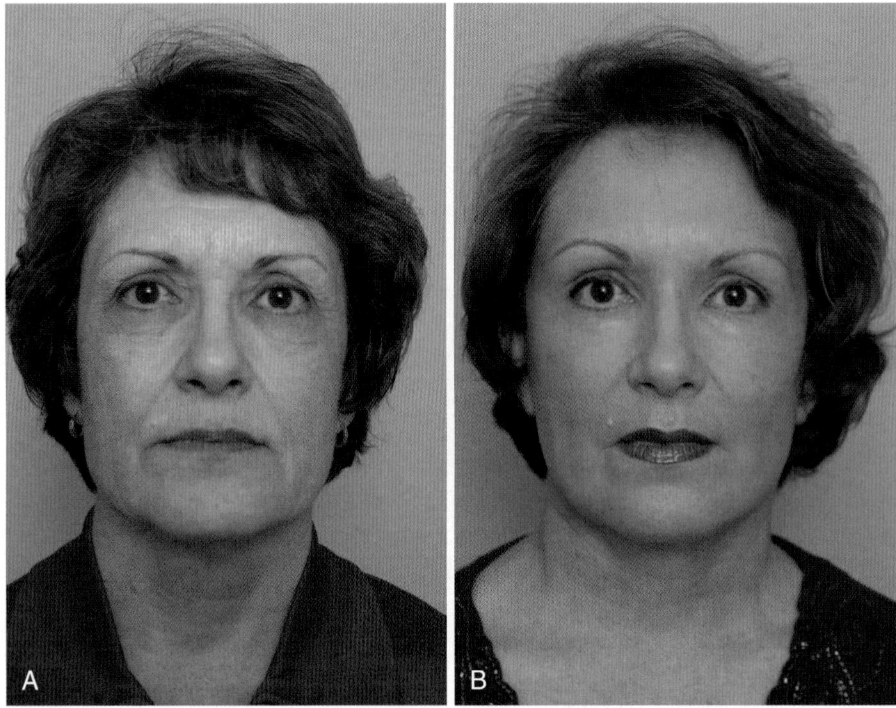

Figure 154.2 Before (**A**) and after (**B**) photographs for a facelift performed with the addition of CO_2 laser treatment.

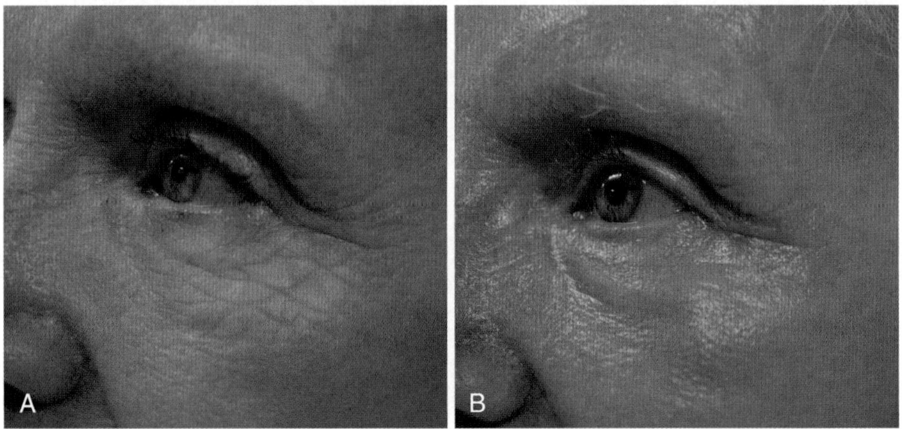

Figure 154.3 Before (**A**) and after (**B**) photographs for CO_2 laser treatment of the upper and lower eyelids.

Age certainly comes into play, but this is true for most facial cosmetic surgery. Many experienced surgeons do not consider a facelift complete without the addition of LSR.

The problem areas of facial skin aging include varying degrees of skin laxity (dermatochalasis), wrinkles, skin quality, pore size, texture, and sun damage (dyschromia). Laser treatment can address all of these issues simultaneously, resulting in significant improvements. Ablative lasers do a very good job of targeting specific areas of the face that need it the most, such as fine lines and wrinkles around the eyes and mouth. "Smoker's lines" around the lips can be identified and focused on appropriately. Dermatochalasis of the upper and lower eyelids can be treated with significant tightening and disappearance of wrinkles (Fig. 154.3). Pigment dyschromias confined to the epidermis are adequately treated with ablative lasers (Fig. 154.4). Vascular dyschromias are better treated with nonablative diode lasers or intense pulsed light treatments in the 515 to 560 nm wavelength spectrum with specific targets for hemoglobin.

Many practitioners agree that the laser must get down to the papillary dermis to really tighten the skin and treat the signs of facial aging.[10] Patients need to be sedated for work in the papillary dermis. The latest-generation $LUPCO_2$ is a high-energy, short-pulsed, scanned CO_2 laser with the added benefit of CoolScan technology (Fig. 154.5). This allows for safe and very effective treatment of a full face within 30 to 45 minutes. There are essentially no disposables. The laser has multiple treatment settings, ranging from fractional CO_2

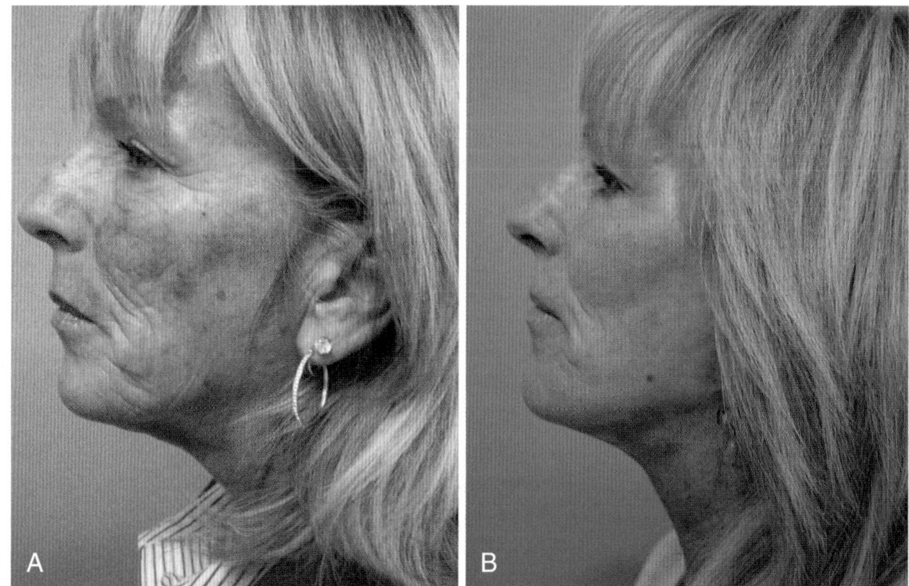

Figure 154.4 Before (**A**) and after (**B**) photographs for CO_2 laser treatment for severe sun damage.

Non-sequential Pattern Scan

Heat does not dissipate from adjacent pulses within the scan

1	2	3	4	5
10	9	8	7	6
11	12	13	14	15
20	19	18	17	16

Traditional CO_2
Uses **Sequential**
Scan Sequence

1	9	3	19	8
20	5	15	12	16
17	11	2	6	4
7	13	18	10	14

CoolScan™
Non-sequential,
non-adjacent
Scan Sequence

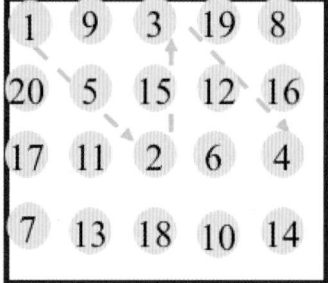

Figure 154.5 Traditional CO_2 laser and Lumenis CoolScan technology system. (Courtesy Lumenis, Yokneam, Israel).

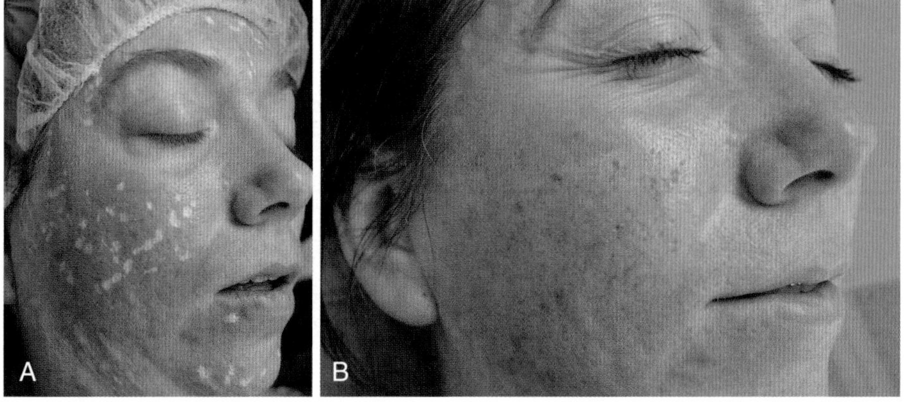

Figure 154.6 Trichloroacetic acid chemical reconstruction of skin scars (TCA CROSS) treatment of acne scarring with 60% TCA spot treatment and fractional CO_2 laser treatment.

(CO_2 Lite, ActiveFx, DeepFx) to full ablative CO_2 (MaxFx). This system is customizable by the surgeon for each patient, depending on the cosmetic facial subunits to be treated. The patient's age and degree of facial aging, the amount of acceptable patient downtime, acne scarring, and other factors all can be taken into account with the CO_2 laser settings. In general, fractional settings result in decreased healing time compared with totally ablative settings. In the author's experience, Active Fx alone requires approximately 5 days of patient recovery time. Adding Deep Fx to this treatment regimen requires approximately 7 to 10 days of patient recovery time. MaxFx also requires approximately 7 to 10 days of recovery time.

Shallow, dish-shaped acne scars can be improved with LSR, although the results are not as impressive as for wrinkle removal.[11] Usually, a combined treatment is necessary. Deep ice pack scars require dermal punch grafts, trichloroacetic acid chemical reconstruction of skin scars (TCA CROSS), subcision, other filling agents, or a combination of these (Fig. 154.6).[12]

Dermatologic problems in the epidermis, papillary dermis, or midreticular dermis are also improved or removed with LSR. These problems include epidermal nevi, actinic keratoses, seborrheic keratosis, lentigines, syringomas, xanthelasmas, and superficial basal cell carcinomas. Traumatic or surgical scars can be improved with LSR as well. The resurfacing is performed 6 to 8 weeks after injury, while collagen remodeling is still occurring. Irregularities in scar height respond best. Actinic cheilitis also responds well to laser treatment. Rhinophyma can be reshaped with the laser with minimal bleeding, better accuracy, and a quicker healing time.[11]

Limitations and Contraindications

Ablative skin resurfacing has its limitations, and the most important of these is patient selection by skin type. Human skin's reaction to direct sunlight has been clinically quantified by Fitzpatrick.[13] The Fitzpatrick classification (Table 154.1) gives us a barometer to follow when selecting patients for this procedure. In general, the best candidates are Fitzpatrick skin types I, II, or III. These patients can be treated very effectively, with less risk of postinflammatory hyperpigmentation, the most common treatable complication of LSR. Special care is advisable when treating patients who have skin that is darker than Fitzpatrick type III. Patients with darker skin phenotypes are at risk for permanent hypopigmentation with procedures that reach the depth of the reticular dermis.[14] Asian skin falls into the category of Fitzpatrick skin type IV. These patients can also be treated with minimal risk, as long as milder laser settings are used. Fitzpatrick skin types V and VI generally are not candidates for LSR due to the risk for permanent pigmentation changes.

Recent or current use of Accutane for acne is considered an absolute contraindication to LSR. The reepithelialization of the laser-treated skin is accomplished from the epithelium of the shafts of the hair follicles. Because Accutane shuts down the hair follicles and sebaceous glands on the face, adverse results can occur when patients are taking this medication. In addition, the risk of scarring is increased with Accutane use; therefore, it is generally recommended that patients refrain from using Accutane for 18 months to 2 years before any type of LSR. These patients have marked sebaceous gland destruction, so their ability to reepithelialize is markedly diminished.[15]

Table 154.1 Fitzpatrick Skin Classification

Skin Type	Skin Color	Characteristics
I	Ivory white	Always burns; never tans
II	White	Usually burns; tans minimally
III	White	Burns moderately; tans moderately
IV	Beige/light brown	Burns minimally; tans easily
V	Moderate brown	Rarely burns; tans profusely
VI	Dark brown/black	Never burns; tans profusely

From Obagi S, Bridenstine JB. Skin resurfacing. *OMS Knowledge Update 2001*. Rosemont, IL, AAOMS Publications.

Rules that apply to the face cannot be applied to other regions of the body.[3] It is important to note that the regenerative capacity of the neck and chest skin is much less than that of the facial skin. Because there are fewer pilosebaceous units in the thinner skin on the neck, a longer healing time and an increased risk of complications can be expected. Hypertrophic scarring and alteration in pigmentation occurs readily. However, the decreased thermal radiation of the erbium:YAG laser permits skin resurfacing of the neck without the scarring or pigmentary changes seen with the CO_2 laser.[3] Care must be taken when lasering the neck to turn down the laser fluence and density. Patients should be warned that LSR of the neck doubles the recovery time.

A relative contraindication to LSR is lasering of the facial skin right after a facelift. It is always considered safest to laser the face and perform a facelift at two separate operative visits. Sometimes this is not practical for the patient, but it is difficult to argue against this being the safest technique. Many experienced cosmetic facial surgeons perform facelifts and LSR at the same time. Although waiting 3 months for resurfacing traditionally has been recommended, Alster et al.[16] described 34 patients who underwent combination CO_2 or erbium:YAG LSR and surgical lifting procedures (S-lift rhytidectomy, blepharoplasty, and brow lift). The effects were found to be no different from those in patients undergoing the laser-only procedure. Performance of a facelift and simultaneous LSR requires a conservative preauricular undermining.[9] To reduce the risk of skin sloughing, the laser must be "turned down" over the raised portion of the facelift flap (Fig. 154.7). Only experienced facelift surgeons should

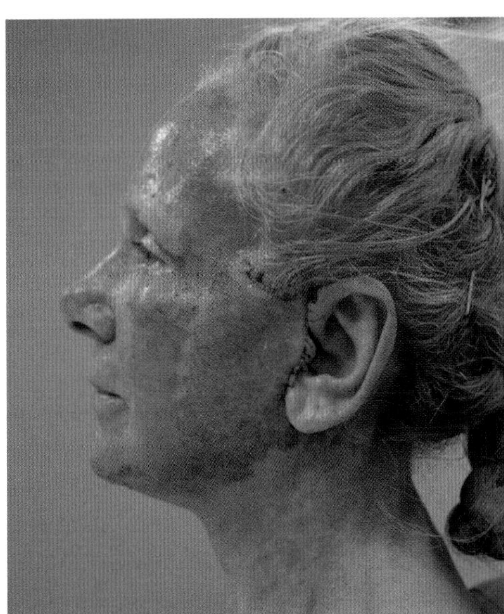

Figure 154.7 Patient who underwent a facelift and CO_2 laser treatment, 4 days after surgery. Laser fluence (J/cm^2) decreased over the facelift flap.

perform simultaneous LSR. Because the neck skin is much thinner and more vulnerable than the facial skin, the neck skin should never be laser-resurfaced concurrently with a neck lift/neck liposuction. The risks involved would most certainly outweigh the benefits.

Other limitations include a history of keloid scarring, connective tissue disease, poor diet, active cystic acne, excessive tanning, and current tretinoin (Retin-A) use. All of these inhibit skin regeneration postoperatively.

Laser safety and guidelines are outlined by the American National Standards Institute (ANSI) in the USA. Blindness in patients and practitioners are prevented with laser eye protection including protective eye wear and eye shields. Abalative lasers have a fire hazard risk of cloth materials, plastic or hair. Placing the laser in standby when not in use, moistening of hair nearby area of treatment reduce fire risk. Biohazardous plume inhalation, in particular during ablative laser use, should be minimized with use of a smoke evacuator, appropriate room ventilation, and high particulate face mask, ie N95, use.[1]

TECHNIQUE: Facial Laser Skin Resurfacing

STEP 1: Removal of Residual Makeup

The patient should be wearing no skincare products including makeup for this procedure. Preoperatively the skin should be clean and dry, as the target chromophore is water. Hair should also be pulled back, away from the face, with use of a disposable headband or similar.

STEP 2: Marking of the Face

Working with the patient, the surgeon uses a marking pen to mark the areas of concern. This allows for open communication and discussion so that these areas can be adequately treated. The inferior border of the mandible is marked with the patient in a sitting position to allow for irregular feathering of the laser into the neck; in this way, the mandible/neck transition is not overtreated (Fig. 154.8A).

STEP 3: Use of General Anesthesia

A state of comfort for the patient and the surgeon is necessary for effective LSR. As discussed, general anesthesia may be used, with the addition of local anesthesia nerve blocks to make the patient comfortable during the LSR procedure. Adequate anesthesia training is required. After the patient has been sedated, he or she is draped with blue operating room towels. In addition, local anesthesia with nerve blocks, tumescent anesthesia or compound topical numbing for 30 to 60 minutes prior to resurfacing are all used.

STEP 4: Use of Nonreflective Metal Internal Eye Shields

The surgeon should choose the size of nonreflective metal internal eye shields that best fits the patient. The medium size fits well in most patients. Two drops of 0.5% tetracaine eye drops are placed in each eye. Then a small amount of Lacrilube is placed on both sides of each metal eye shield while connected to a suction cup. The eyelids are gently opened and the metal shields are placed into each eye individually, with care taken to protect the cornea (Fig. 154.8B).

STEP 5: Achieving Adequate Anesthesia for the Face

V1, V2, and V3 blocks are routinely performed, along with tumescent anesthesia as necessary. A 27-gauge needle and aspirating syringe with 2% Lidocaine with 1:100,000 epinephrine is used for the nerve blocks. A 27-gauge needle and 20-cc syringe with 1% Lidocaine with 1:100,000 epinephrine is used to obtain the tumescent anesthesia in the subdermal plane of the face. Tumescent anesthesia can be very helpful for anesthetizing the dermal plexus of nerves to keep the patient comfortable. Local infiltration of the upper and lower eyelids is performed with a short 30-gauge needle and 5-cc syringe and 1% lidocaine with 1:100,000 epinephrine (Fig. 154.8C).

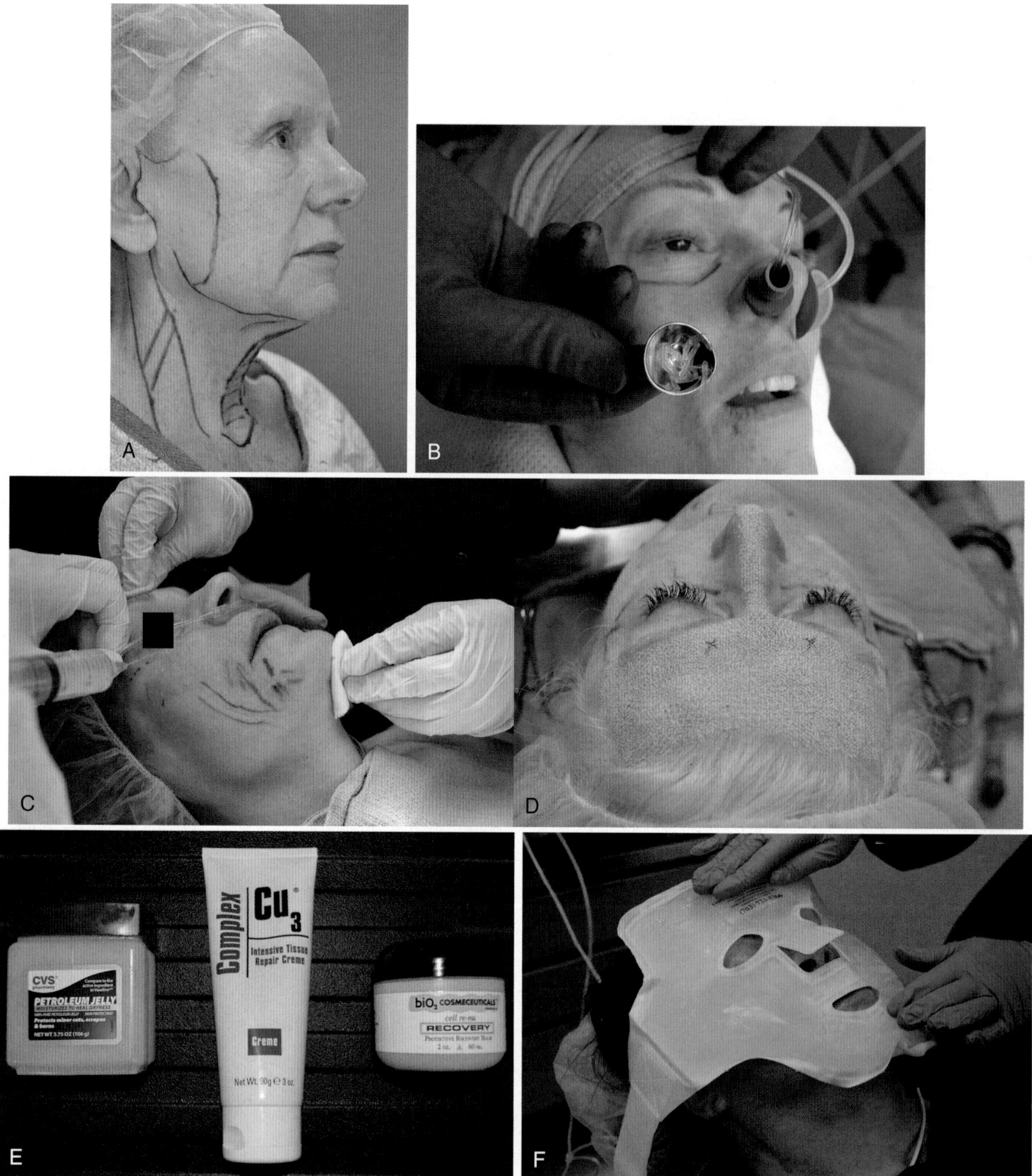

Figure 154.8 **A,** Preoperative facial markings before CO_2 laser treatment and facelift. **B,** Placement of internal metal eye shields. **C,** Adequate anesthesia is obtained with V1, V2, and V3 blocks and infiltration of a local anesthetic. **D,** The start of the CO_2 laser procedure; note the difference between the treated and the untreated skin. **E,** Various postoperative moisturizing ointments. **F,** Custom full face and eyelid postoperative laser ice pack.

TECHNIQUE: Facial Laser Skin Resurfacing—*cont'd*

STEP 6: Laser Skin Resurfacing

The surgeon must have a working knowledge of the laser and its effects to achieve good treatment outcomes. Many lasers have customizable settings, depending on the patient's needs. It is always better to err on the more conservative side to avoid complications. The laser is used with the optical Computer Pattern Generator (CPG) scanner to treat the face. The treatments can range from a light fractional setting to full ablative LSR. In addition, skin treatment can involve a single laser pass or a second laser pass. When performing LSR, the surgeon must follow a system so that some areas of the skin are not missed and others are not overtreated. It works well to start at the tip of the nose and follow the bridge of the nose back to the forehead. The forehead is divided in two, and each side is treated. Then, traveling down, the right temple, the right malar, and the right preauricular regions are treated. This is repeated down the left side of the face. The perioral and chin regions are treated next. The lip vermilion border is treated more aggressively to help eliminate vertical lip lines. After the full face has been treated, the upper and lower eyelids are treated. It is important to remember that the laser pattern size must be adjusted around the eyes, including the laser fluence. In addition, the lower eyelashes must be protected from the laser beam; this can be done with a wooden tongue blade. Last, the laser fluence is turned down and the transition zone is "feathered" from the face into the neck at the mandibular border. It is very important that each surgeon have a checklist for performing this procedure (Fig. 154.8D).

STEP 7: Application of Moisturizing Ointment

After the LSR is complete, it is very important to place a thin layer of protective ointment on the facial areas treated. The ointment can be cooled in the refrigerator ahead of time for patient comfort. Examples of such ointments include Vaseline petrolatum, Vanicream ointment, Aquaphor, CU3 Skin Repair Crème (Photomedex; Montgomeryville, Pennsylvania), and Bio2 Cosmeceuticals Protective Recovery Balm (Bio2 Cosmeceuticals; Harbor City, California) (Fig. 154.8E).

STEP 8: Removal of Metal Eye Shields

The eyelids are opened individually and the small suction cups are used to gently remove the metal eye shields. Care must be taken to avoid corneal trauma. Then the eyes are rinsed with copious amounts of saline eyewash to remove any residual Lacrilube.

STEP 9: Use of Facial Ice Pack

Custom ice packs can be used for immediate postoperative facial LSR. They include ice packs made specifically for the eyelids and ice packs made for the full face. These gel packs have a protective white layer on the side applied to the facial skin that protects it from frostbite. The patient will appreciate this in the immediate postoperative period because the face will feel very warm, equivalent to a sunburn (Fig. 154.8F).

STEP 10: Postprocedural Care Instructions

Postcare patient compliance is very important after LSR to minimize complications and optimize results. The patient should be instructed to soak the face with a white vinegar solution (1 teaspoon of white vinegar mixed into 2 cups of water) five or six times a day until the skin reepithelializes (in approximately 7 days). A soft cotton cloth is used to perform the soaks. No rubbing is necessary because this will make the skin very raw. After each soak, a thin layer of ointment should be applied to protect the skin from dryness and crusting. Strict sun avoidance is essential for 7-14 days, followed thereafter with daily mineral sunscreen SPF 30+.

Extended post procedural skin care, days 7 to 21, may involve prescription topicals such as topical steroids to treat post inflammatory erythema and prescription hydroquinone to treat and/or avoid post inflammatory hyperpigmentation.

Avoidance and Management of Intraoperative Complications

Intraoperative complications can be avoided by following the "rules" of LSR. Perhaps the most important rule is knowing when to stop.[16] In the beginning, it is prudent for the surgeon to be conservative with patients until he or she develops a good feel for the laser. The laser settings of energy and density are most important and vary, depending on the age of the patient, the degree of dermatochalasis, the amount of sun damage, the thickness of the dermal-epidermal unit, the duration of downtime acceptable to the patient, and Fitzpatrick skin type. There is no set formula or magic number of passes. Each case is unique and must be treated as such. Visually determining whether a wrinkle has been removed is relatively straightforward. The ability to evaluate the wound depth, however, is a part of laser education best gained by observation and mentoring.[16]

With a LUPCO$_2$ laser, most maxillofacial laser candidates (Fitzpatrick skin types I, II, and III) have a "good" result with a single pass set at 70 millijoules (mj) and a density of 5. Depending on the skin, the most aggressive the surgeon should get is setting the machine at 80 mj with a density of 6.[17] For lighter fractional ActiveFx treatments, setting the

CO_2 laser at 100 mj or less and a density of 3 or less would be appropriate. DeepFx treatments, if necessary, are usually performed right before ActiveFx treatments. The laser settings for an average DeepFx treatment over deep creases and wrinkles would be 15 mj with a density of 15 with a single pulse. Following these guidelines helps prevent poor outcomes and patient dissatisfaction. Scarring can be avoided in high-risk areas, such as the inferior border of the mandible, by decreasing the laser energy, gently feathering the laser treatment into the neck, avoiding multiple passes, and stretching the skin upwards towards the lower face, or downwards towards the neck for a flat uniform treatment surface. Feathering the treatment area. This also helps avoid an obvious face/neck delineation of treated and untreated skin in patients who have severe sun damage (Fig. 154.9).

There is no defense for laser ocular damage from this procedure. Preferably, internal nonreflective metal eye shields should be placed before any laser treatment on or near the upper or lower eyelids begins. The eyes of the surgeon and assistants also must be covered with protective laser goggles. When the laser is not being used, it should be placed in standby mode to avoid inadvertent laser firing. Mirrors and windows in the laser treatment room should be covered. Any supplemental oxygen source, such as a nasal cannula, must be turned off and removed from the patient during laser treatment to prevent intraoperative fires. Water should be quickly available to put out a laser fire, should one occur.

Contrary to popular belief in the past, it is advisable to leave the laser char in place as a biologic dressing to protect the skin and promote wound healing (Fig. 154.10). The skin should not be débrided between passes because this takes off the skin "Band-Aid" and leaves the skin raw and weepy.[10]

It is also very important to focus on the treatment at hand. If the goal of the procedure is one laser pass without overlap, care should be taken to accomplish this. Too much laser overlap and missed areas can easily be avoided with attention to detail. The surgeon must keep in mind that more than one pass on the skin with a fractional laser is not fractional treatment anymore. This can lead to overtreatment, longer downtime, increased complications, and unhappy patients. Again, when combining LSR with a facelift, the surgeon must take care to turn down the laser over skin that has undergone a facelift. This helps prevent the most dreaded complication, skin necrosis, which is very difficult to treat and explain.

Postoperative Considerations

Postoperative management of laser-treated skin can significantly influence treatment outcomes and patient satisfaction. Detailed oral and written preoperative instructions and postoperative instructions are given. Preoperative and postoperative medications also are given. Patient compliance with the postoperative skin care regimen is the single most important factor in achieving successful outcomes. Procedure complications include scarring, hyperpigmentation, hypoigmentation, prolonged erythema, and bacterial, viral, or fungal skin infections.

Practically speaking, the more downtime the patient can accept, the better results the patient can expect. From clinical observation, fractional lasers, such as the ActiveFx, have less downtime and quick recovery times but also less significant results. This must be discussed preoperatively with the patient to clarify his or her needs and wants. Use of a fully ablative laser, such as the MaxFx, increases the recovery time but can deliver dramatic postoperative results (Fig. 154.11). It all depends on what the patient wants and expects.

Patients can expect erythema after LSR. Erythema can last 2 weeks to 3 months. Prolonged erythema is considered any redness that lasts longer than 1 month. Topical steroids (e.g., clobetasol cream) are used to treat prolonged erythema. Recall phenomenon (facial redness) during showering is self-limiting. DeepFx treatments increase the risk of prolonged erythema because the laser energy treats deeper into the dermis (Fig. 154.12). Other contributing factors for prolonged erythema include attending hot yoga classes and spending time in steam rooms during the postoperative period. Such practices should be avoided for a few months because they prolong facial erythema.

Infections after LSR can be serious, especially if diagnosis is delayed. Normally, the patient has minimal pain after the skin is treated. For the first few hours, the skin will feel warm similar to a sunburn. Any severe pain after this time must be investigated. Possible infections include herpes simplex virus (HSV), impetigo, and fungus. Each is treated differently but aggressively. In patients with a history of herpes labialis, LSR can trigger an outbreak that can spread to involve the entire denuded skin surface, with resulting increased pain, prolonged healing, and an increased risk of scarring. Surgeons should keep in mind that HSV does not make vesicles on laser-treated skin because the epidermis has been removed. Many practitioners have encountered several instances in which patients denied any history of herpes labialis, yet developed severe herpes outbreaks after laser resurfacing. Therefore, all patients are given valacyclovir 500 mg by mouth twice a day starting up to 2 days before and continuing for at least 10 days after the procedure.[4] HSV outbreaks are treated with high doses of antiviral medications orally (e.g., valacyclovir) and topically with acyclovir. Bacterial infections are initially treated with oral antibiotics and with IV antibiotics, as needed, if there is no improvement. Fungal infection with *Candida albicans* can manifest as painful, burning, erythematous ulcerations. There may be pustules within the wound and beyond the wound margin where there is intact skin. Fungal infection may be the result of postoperative occlusive ointments. Semipermeable dressings can reduce this risk, as does frequent postoperative facial washing.[18] Fungal infections are treated with oral and topical antifungals, such as fluconazole and Nizoral cream, respectively. A few laser surgeons recommend a dose of fluconazole on the day of resurfacing to reduce the risk of candidal infection in the treated area. Some prescribe a short course (3 to 4 days) of oral corticosteroids

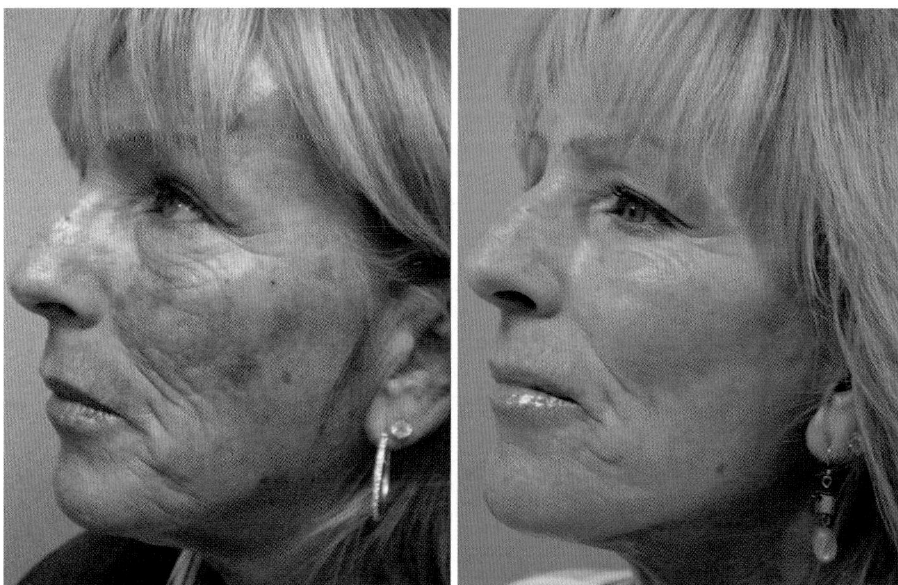

Figure 154.9 Obvious face and neck contrast between laser-treated skin and untreated skin.

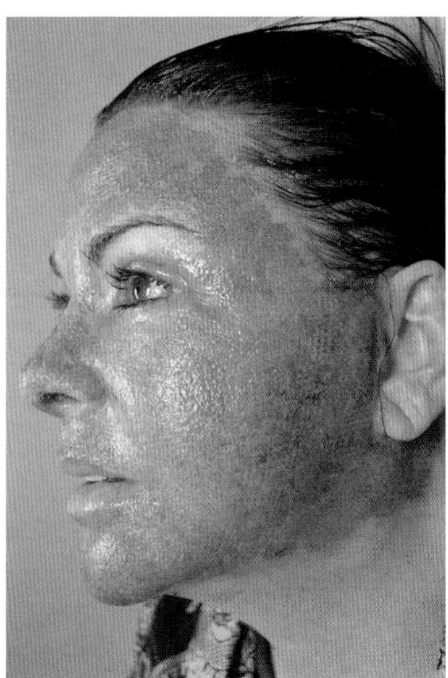

Figure 154.10 Patient immediately after laser treatment; laser char is left on the skin as a biologic wound dressing.

for the patient perioperatively to reduce the very significant edema that usually occurs during the first 72 hours after the procedure.[4] Persistent or severe bacterial infections must be cultured. Fungal infections can be diagnosed with potassium hydroxide preps, which reveal pseudohyphae. Herpes infections can be confirmed with Tzanck smears, which reveal multinucleated giant cells.

Postinflammatory hyperpigmentation (PIH) is a common postoperative sequela of LSR. This is especially true with darker skin types (Fitzpatrick skin types III to V).[3] Presurgical and postsurgical skin care regimens to suppress melanin activity may be useful in darker skin types.[11] PIH usually becomes clinically apparent 3 to 4 weeks after wounding (depending on the depth of injury) (Fig. 154.13). Therefore, it can be anticipated and treated prophylactically rather than after the fact. When PIH is present, its treatment becomes difficult and detracts from the patient's satisfaction with the overall surgery.[15] The condition is reversible with time and some medical treatment, including topical steroids (clobetasol cream) and bleaching agents (e.g., 4%+ hydroquinone).

Hypopigmentation presents with a delayed onset and is more serious because it is not reversible. Permanent hypopigmentation that develops up to 12 months after resurfacing, has been reported in up to 16% of patients, although it seems to be less frequent than after dermabrasion or deep chemical peels.[18] Permanent hypopigmentation is far easier to camouflage when the entire face is treated rather than regional resurfacing of cosmetic subunits.[4]

Patients often develop pruritus during the first few weeks after resurfacing, but this is usually self-limited.[4] The skin can get very itchy and dry during the normal healing process. This can be helped by applying topical steroid cream and using oral diphenhydramine. Patients need to trim their nails and wear gloves during sleep to protect their fragile new skin from scratching (Fig. 154.14). Patients can experience pruritus and skin tightness for 1 to 4 months after LSR.[4]

Milia and acne are very common after laser treatments. Milia are keratin-retention cysts, usually caused by plugged hair follicles, that develop 3 to 8 weeks after the treatment. They may be isolated or occur in dense clusters. Milia can be very upsetting to patients,[18] but they are usually self-limiting. Persistent milia can be treated with manual extraction and glycolic peels as needed (after reepithelialization has occurred). The etiology is comedogenic effects of many post-care ointments (e.g., CU3 cream, Vaseline) required in the immediate postoperative period. Acne is a frequent postoperative event, especially in patients with a past history of acne. It usually develops in the first few weeks after resurfacing.[3]

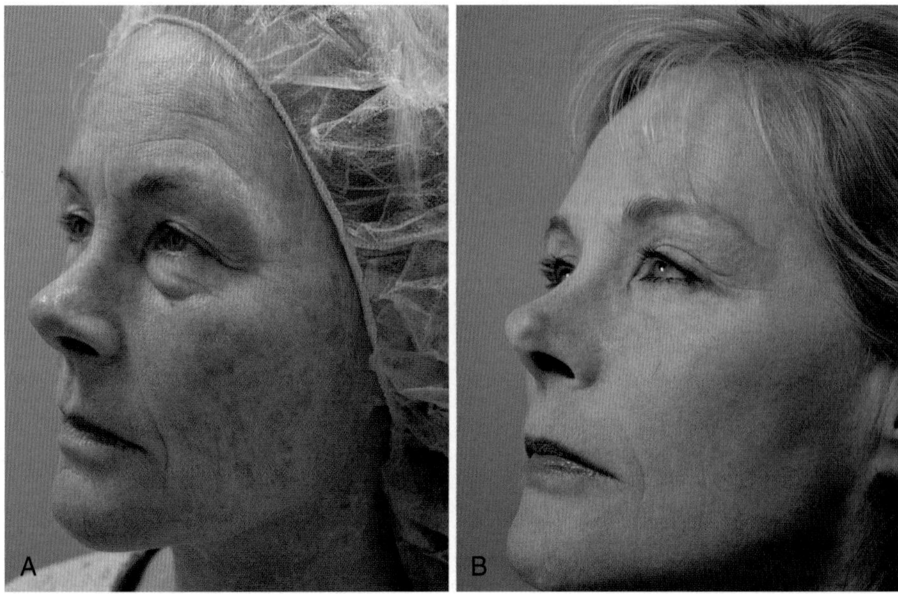

Figure 154.11 Full face before (**A**) and after (**B**) photographs of a patient who had a CO_2 laser treatment and upper and lower eyelid blepharoplasty.

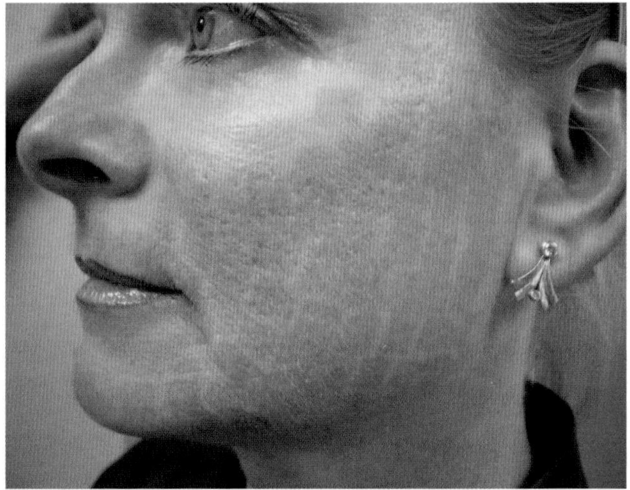

Figure 154.12 Patient with prolonged erythema after full face CO_2 laser treatment (ActiveFx + DeepFx).

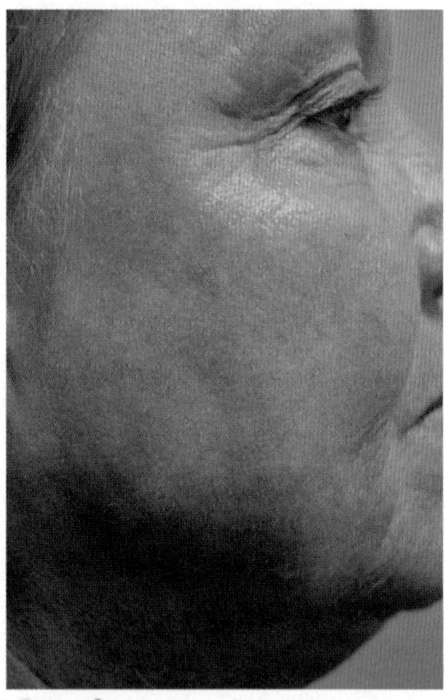

Figure 154.13 Postinflammatory hyperpigmentation (PIH) after CO_2 laser treatment.

Acne flares can be treated with topical and systemic treatments as necessary. Milia and acne can be minimized by use of less comedogenic ointments, such as Vanicream ointment, and transitioning to water based emollients including as gel-based emollients, ie EltaMD Laser Enzyme Gel, once reepithelization occurs.

Lower eyelid ectropion or scleral show, can occur after LSR therapy. A preoperative clinical examination for lid laxity and preexisting scleral show is imperative.[19] This complication can be limited by obtaining a thorough cosmetic history, including any history of lower eyelid blepharoplasty. Patients with previous skin-muscle lower lid blepharoplasties are at risk of ectropion, and conservative treatment should be used in these areas. Elderly patients also may have existing senile ectropion, which can be worsened by laser resurfacing.[20] The pull test and snap test of the lower eyelids should be done preoperatively and documented during the evaluation phase to help guard against this. Immediately after laser treatment of the lower lids, the skin can be stretched a bit to help avoid lower lid malposition.[10] Temporary ectropion may occur immediately after lid resurfacing and typically resolves in a few days or weeks.[21] Massage of the lower lids or lower lid taping in the postoperative period helps improve the ectropion with the hope of avoiding a lateral canthopexy.

Post–fractional laser dermatitis is rare and in most cases represents an irritant contact dermatitis variant.[21] This usually

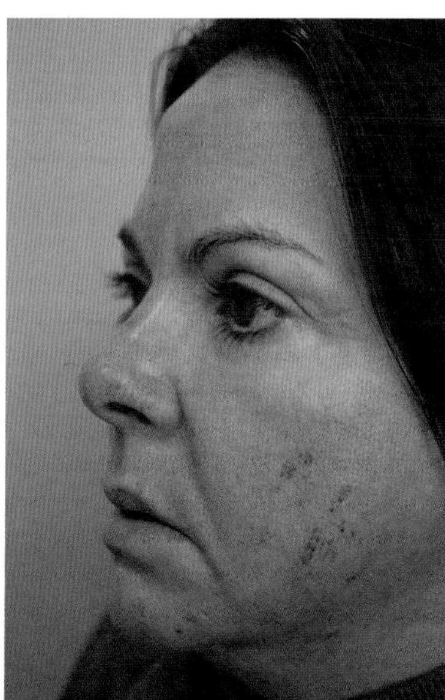

Figure 154.14 Facial scratching during sleep after CO_2 laser treatment.

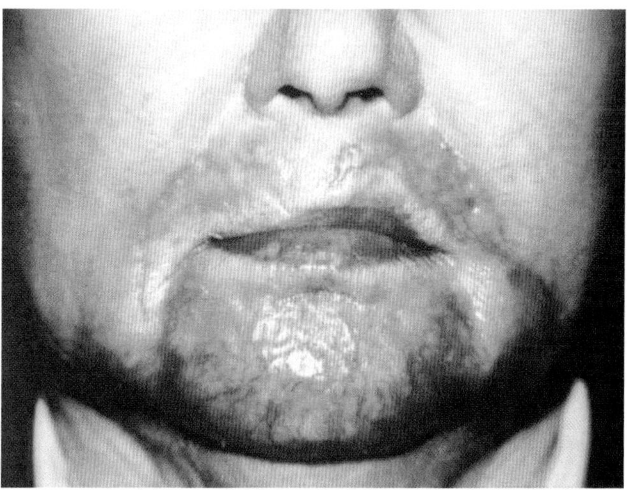

Figure 154.15 Severe perioral scarring resulting from older laser treatment protocol with a low-fluence, continuous wave CO_2 laser. (From Watson SW, Sawisch TJ. Cosmetic ablative skin resurfacing. *Oral Maxillofacial Surg Clin North Am*. 2004;16:225).

occurs when the patient deviates from the prescribed postoperative skin care regimen. Unfortunately, many products have ingredients that can irritate the healing skin. Frequent use of postoperative double and triple antibiotic ointments leads to contact dermatitis after LSR and thus should be avoided.[22] Because the cutaneous surface is without an epidermal barrier for up to 7 days postoperatively, any potential sensitizer, such as a fragrance, a preservative, or an antibiotic, has a greater opportunity to interact with the cutaneous immune system to produce a type IV allergic contact dermatitis.[23] Systemic steroids (e.g., Medrol Dose Pack or prednisone) may be necessary to treat this condition, which presents with itchiness, redness, a rash, and possibly hives. After the skin has fully healed (usually in 5 to 10 days, depending on the extent of the treatment), hypoallergenic mineral products with sun protection factor can be used.

Keratoacanthomas (KAs) may develop in areas of skin trauma including postoperative wounds. These are low-grade malignant skin tumors that are known to arise over sites of trauma. It is difficult to determine which KA will resolve spontaneously and which will continue to grow and destroy surrounding tissue. Multiple eruptive KAs have been reported after CO_2 laser resurfacing.[24] Trauma to the skin seems to act as a trigger for the development of a KA. Surgical excision is the standard treatment for a solitary KA. Multiple KAs have been treated successfully with oral retinoids.

Hypertrophic scarring is the most feared and serious of all LSR complications (Fig. 154.15). It is usually the result of overtreatment and damage to the deep dermal layers.[25] It may result from a large number of passes, use of excessive energy, or pulse stacking when a CO_2 laser is used (overlap of laser irradiated sites, especially after the first pass), resulting in excessive thermal damage.[26] It is better to do a touch-up procedure down the road than to go too deeply the first time in an attempt to totally eradicate the offending rhytids.[4] Hypertrophic scarring usually occurs around the lips or in the skin overlying bone, such as the chin, mandibular border, and malar region. An upper lip that has had previous extensive electrolysis or hair removal (which destroys dermal hair follicles) also can be at increased risk for scarring.[19] Focal areas of erythema and in duration 2 to 4 weeks after treatment are the first signs of potential scar formation.[21] In general, the highest risk of scarring is seen in patients with a prior history of irradiation or surgical procedures, involving the neck or eyelids and those who have experienced postoperative wound infection, contact dermatitis, or keloid scarring. Early treatment of hypertrophic scarring in such patients often involves the use of topical corticosteroids or silicone gel products, intralesional corticosteroid injections, 5-fluorouracil, and pulsed dye laser therapy.[27,28] High-potency fluorinated steroid creams (e.g., Temovate; 0.5% clobetasol propionate twice daily for 2 to 3 weeks) can be used on incipient scarring. Silicone sheets can be used. Silicone topical gel is more useful on the face (Kelocare Laser Gel, applied once daily).[19] Intralesional steroid injections are necessary if the topical therapy is ineffective. Triamcinolone acetonide (Kenalog, 10 mg/mL or 0.1 to 0.3 cc [0.1 to 0.3 mg]) is injected from a tuberculin syringe into the scar once a month. Surgeons who are not experienced in treating this complication should refer these patients to more experienced practitioners, as early as possible.[20] The injection must be placed in the center of the thickened scarred area to avoid adjacent dermal fat atrophy.[19]

References

1. Bolognia JL, Jorizzo JL, Rapini RP: Dermatology, Second Edition. 2008;136:2089.
2. Massachusetts Institute of Technology. *Inventors of the Week—Kumar Patel*; 2000. Inventors.about.com.
3. Watson SW, Sawisch TJ. Cosmetic ablative skin resurfacing. *Oral Maxillofac Surg Clin North Am*. 2004;16(2):215–230.
4. Airan LE, Hruza G. Current lasers in skin resurfacing. *Facial Plast Surg Clin North Am*. 2002;10(1):87–101.
5. Manstein D, Herron GS, Sink RK, Tanner H, Anderson RR. Fractional photothermolysis: a new concept for cutaneous remodeling using microscopic patterns of thermal injury. *Lasers Surg Med*. 2004;34(5):426–438.
6. Gardner VW, Nease CJ. The no-incision, dual-technique, laser facelift: a prospective series of 16 patients. *Am J Cosmet Surg*. 2013;30:28.
7. Saedi N, Petelin A, Zachary C. Fractionation: a new era in laser resurfacing. *Clin Plast Surg*. 2011;38(3):449–461. vii.
8. Alexiades-Armenakas M, Sarnoff D, Gotkin R, Sadick N. Multi-center clinical study and review of fractional ablative CO2 laser resurfacing for the treatment of rhytides, photoaging, scars and striae. *J Drugs Dermatol*. 2011;10(4):352–362.
9. Chisholm BB. Surgical facial rhytidectomy: the evolution of an esthetic concept. *Oral Maxillofac Surg Clin North Am*. 2000;12:719.
10. American Academy of Cosmetic Surgery. Twenty-Ninth Annual Scientific Meeting. *Las Vegas*. 2013:16–19.
11. Harsha BC. Preoperative considerations for laser skin resurfacing. *Oral Maxillofac Surg Clin North Am*. 2000;12:555.
12. Rullan P. Dermatology Institute, Chula Vista, CA. Personal communication.
13. Fitzpatrick TB. The validity and practicality of sun-reactive skin types I through VI. *Arch Dermatol*. 1988;124(6):869–871.
14. Obagi S. Pre- and postlaser skin care. *Oral Maxillofac Surg Clin North Am*. 2004;16(2):181–187.
15. Guttenberg SA, Emery III RW. Laser cosmetic skin resurfacing: superpulsed perspective. *Oral Maxillofac Surg Clin North Am*. 2004;16(2):197–213.
16. Alster TS, Doshi SN, Hopping SB. Combination surgical lifting with ablative laser skin resurfacing of facial skin: a retrospective analysis. *Dermatol Surg*. 2004;30(9):1191–1195.
17. Niamtu J. Virginia oral and facial surgery. Personal communication.
18. Bernstein LJ, Kauvar ANB, Grossman MC, Geronemus RG. The short- and long-term side effects of carbon dioxide laser resurfacing. *Dermatol Surg*. 1997;23(7):519–525.
19. Demas PN, Bridenstine JB. Diagnosis and treatment of postoperative complications after skin resurfacing. *J Oral Maxillofac Surg*. 1999;57(7):837–841.
20. Niamtu J. Common complications of laser resurfacing and their treatment. *Oral Maxillofac Surg Clin North Am*. 2000;12:579.
21. Metelitsa AI, Alster TS. Fractionated laser skin resurfacing treatment complications: a review. *Dermatol Surg*. 2010;36(3):299–306.
22. Fisher AA. Lasers and allergic contact dermatitis to topical antibiotics, with particular reference to bacitracin. *Cutis*. 1996;58(4):252–254.
23. Nanni CA, Alster TS. Complications of carbon dioxide laser resurfacing. An evaluation of 500 patients. *Dermatol Surg*. 1998;24(3):315–320.
24. Gewirtzman A, Meirson DH, Rabinovitz H. Eruptive keratoacanthomas following carbon dioxide laser resurfacing. *Dermatol Surg*. 1999;25(8):666–668.
25. Grover S, Apfelberg DB, Smoller B. Effects of varying density patterns and passes on depth of penetration in facial skin utilizing the carbon dioxide laser with automated scanner. *Plast Reconstr Surg*. 1999;104(7):2247–2252.
26. Fitzpatrick RE, Smith SR, Sriprachya-anunt S. Depth of vaporization and the effect of pulse stacking with a high-energy, pulsed carbon dioxide laser. *J Am Acad Dermatol*. 1999;40(4):615–622.
27. Alster T, Zaulyanov L. Laser scar revision: a review. *Dermatol Surg*. 2007;33(2):131–140.
28. Alster TS, Tanzi EL. Hypertrophic scars and keloids: etiology and management. *Am J Clin Dermatol*. 2003;4(4):235–243.

CHAPTER 155

Liposuction of the Face and Neck

Angelo L. Cuzalina and Pasquale G. Tolomeo

Armamentarium

Marking pen #11
Scalpel 1-,1.5-, or 2-mm liposuction cannulas
Gauge spinal needle 10 mL
1% lidocaine with 1:100,000 epinephrine
Wall suction
Tumescent solution (500 cc normal saline, 50 mL 1% lidocaine, 1 mL 1:1000 epinephrine)

History of the Procedure

The first reported use of suction to remove fat was performed by Dr. Charles Dujarier in the 1920s.[1] However, Italian gynecologists Arpad and Giorgio Fischer were recognized as the developers of modern liposuction. In 1974, the father and son pair created a blunt, hollow instrument that allowed them to suction fat while avoiding major blood vessels.[2] Around 1978, French physicians Yves-Gerard Illouz and Pierre Fournier sought to improve the armamentarium of liposuction. Illouz developed the "wetting technique" with the use of saline and hyaluronidase to minimize intraoperative bleeding. Furthermore, Illouz developed blunted cannulas with a decreased diameter to avoid damage to underlying structures.[3] Fournier introduced the use of local anesthesia as well as utilization of a crisscross method via multiple incision sites to improve contouring. Fournier is additionally credited with the recommendation of taped compression to aid in support and contour of the suctioned tissue.[4]

Liposuction gained popularity in the Unites States in the 1980s but met considerable adversity due to reports of excess bleeding and severe irregularities. It was not until 1985 when Dr. Jeffrey A. Klein, a dermatologist, improved the tumescent technique with the combination of saline, lidocaine, and epinephrine.[5] The advent of the perfected tumescent greatly decreased postoperative pain and bleeding.

Indications for the Use of the Procedure

As human life expectancy has improved over the years, the desire to maintain a youthful appearance or even reversal of the aging process has been a pivotal focus of society and surgeons. Facial aging is a dynamic process that involves ongoing changes to the skin, subcutaneous tissue, and underlying bony structures. The clinical findings that constitute aging are skin laxity, skin excess, rhytids, lipomatosis, alteration in skin tone, muscle atrophy, and volume loss.[6] The dynamic process is greatly influenced by intrinsic and extrinsic factors (Table 155.1).

The extracellular matrix plays a pivotal role in tissue function and is the foundation of all tissue. Collagen is one of the major proteins of the extracellular matrix and functions to maintain homeostasis of the tissue.[7] Type I and III collagens are the most abundant proteins of the soft tissue and are vital in the maintenance of the tissue. The peak of collagen formation occurs between the ages of 20 and 24 in both males and females. Type I collagen production significantly decreases at the age of 45 in men and age of 30 to 35 in women. Type III collagen significantly increases between the ages of 45 and 59 in men, and 55 and 59 in women; the presence of increased type III collagen causes excess fibrosis within the soft tissue. With this significant change in cell turnover, collagen formation and skin rejuvenation are greatly affected.[7] Type 1 collagen provides the infrastructure for healthy skin and plays a key part in skin elasticity and firmness. With a decrease in the production of Type 1 collagen, the formation of facial rhytids and skin laxity begin to develop.

As an individual ages, significant changes in metabolic function and hormonal regulation occur. Basal metabolic rates decrease in both females and males, leading to weight fluctuations with the distribution of fatty tissue in various body areas.[8] Women who have undergone menopause have decreased levels of estrogen with elevated levels of androgen. These hormonal changes lead to a decreased amount of soluble collagen, cell turnover rate and collagen synthesis, thus causing decreased skin resistance and pliability. The overlying skin is thin due to a 2.1% decrease in collagen content every postmenopausal year.[9] Estrogen affects normal bone remodeling via inhibition of osteoclasts and bone resorption. As estrogen levels decrease, osteoclast activity increases while osteoblast activity decreases, thus leading to bone resorption.[10] As men age, testosterone levels decrease approximately 1.6% per year after the age of 30 to 40 years.[11] Testosterone directly plays a role in the prevention of bone resorption via androgen receptors in osteocytes, while indirectly inhibiting osteoclast activity and activating osteoblasts following

Table 155.1 Aging Factors

Intrinsic Aging Factors	Extrinsic Aging Factors
Loss of cellular function	UV radiation
Decreased proliferative and repair capacity	Tobacco use
Chromosomal abnormalities	Alcohol use
Hormonal changes	Environmental factors
Gene mutation	Gravitational forces
Facial bone atrophy	Loss of elasticity
	Emotional stress

From Niamtu, J. *Cosmetic Facial Surgery.* 2nd ed. Edinburgh: Elsevier; 2018.

conversion to estrogen.[12] With low levels of testosterone, bone loss is accelerated. With the decrease in bone remodeling due to osteopenia/osteoporosis, the facial skeleton and dental structures undergo resorption. As facial resorption occurs, the support to the overlying soft tissue diminishes and leads to ptosis. The most common areas of the face that experience resorption are the maxilla, pyriform rims, orbital rims, and the mandible. Another aspect that adds to facial aging is the ligamentous attachments of the face. As bony resorption occurs, the facial ligaments suspend the soft tissue and accentuate hollowing in the areas where bony projection has been lost.[13]

The greatest factors that affect facial aging are substance/alcohol abuse, sun exposure, and emotional stress.[8] Lifestyle is another factor that affects facial structure. With the onset of obesity, fat is distributed to various parts of the body, most specifically in the areas of the submalar and submental region of the face. The deposition of fat in these areas gives a more jovial appearance with a rounded mid-face, yet significant fullness along the submental region gives an unaesthetic appearance. The presence of fat along the submental region may involve a genetic component as well.

Jowls

Jowl formation begins to develop around the fifth and sixth decades of life. The fat of the jowls is composed of subcutaneous fat compartments that are supported by the mandibular septum and is separate from the buccal fat. As the face ages, the mandibular and masseteric ligaments develop increased laxity, causing the descent of fat beyond the mandibular border and into the submandibular plane. In addition to laxity, photodamage, buccal fat pad descent, and weight gain contribute to loss of mandibular border definition[8] (Fig. 155.1).

When performing liposuction to this area, the surgeon must be conservative to avoid worsening of skin laxity. Furthermore, the surgeon should proceed with caution in the jowl region due to the presence of the marginal mandibular nerve and subsequent risk of paralysis should one cause damage to it.

Submental

The submental region is of primary concern for individuals around the third and fourth decades of life. The deposition

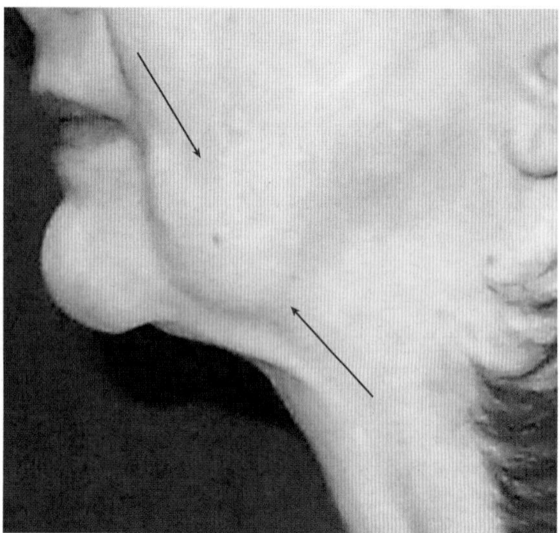

Figure 155.1 Presence of severe jowling. Jowling is due to the descent of fat beyond the mandibular border extending into the submandibular region.

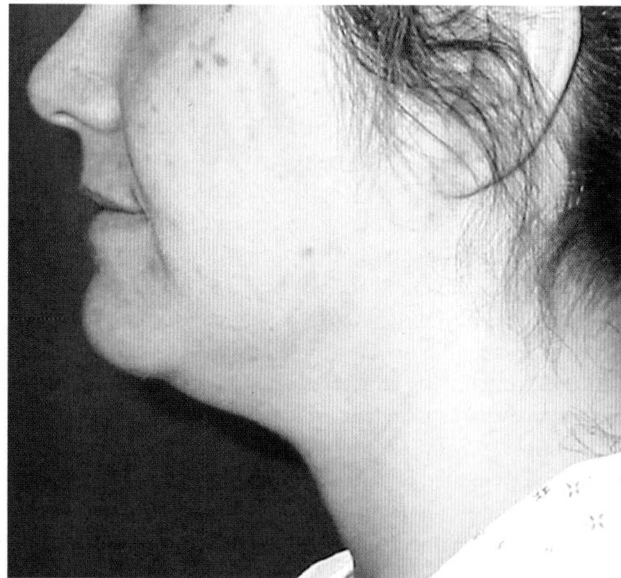

Figure 155.2 Presence of submental fat. Submental fat gives the appearance of a bulging neck.

of submental fat may be linked to genetic or environmental causes, skeletal deformities that highlight minute changes, or anatomical changes. As a patient's weight increases, fat is deposited along the preplatysma layer in the submental region, giving the appearance of a bulging neck (Fig. 155.2). For patients with a skeletal deformity such as microgenia or a retrognathic mandible, fat deposition in this area tends to have a more dramatic presentation due to an already decreased thyromental distance.

As the patient continues to age, so does the face. The hyoid bone begins to descend, creating an obtuse neck and loss of definition of the cervicomental angle. Fat deposition occurs along the submental region and leads to loss of chin definition (Fig. 155.3). The goal of submental liposuction is to restore the

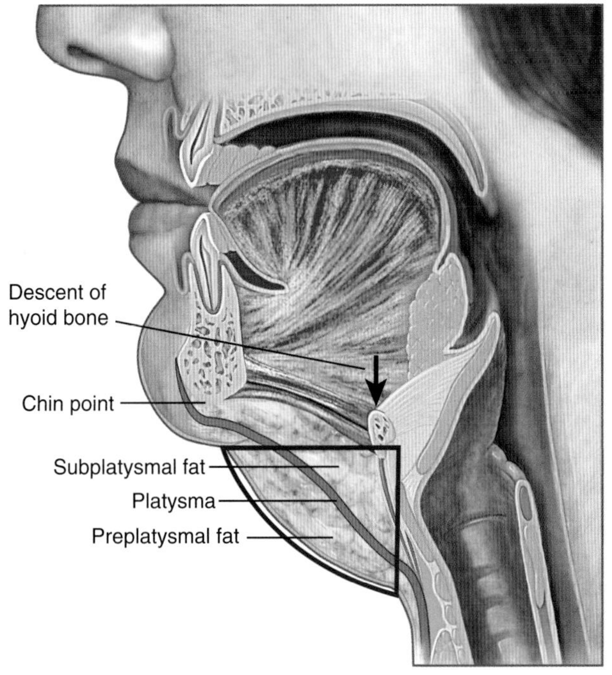

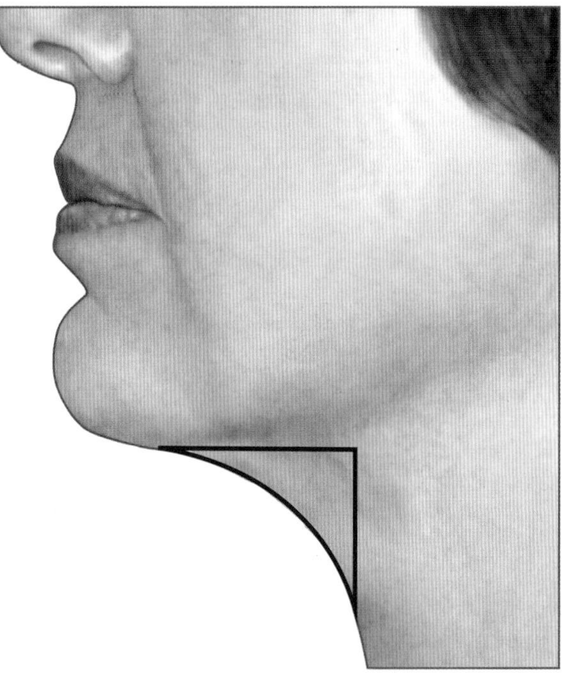

Figure 155.3 Hyoid descent and the obtuse neck. The cervicomental angle is formed by the intersection of the submental and cervical planes. This patient is considered a "difficult neck" due to the presence of an obtuse neck shape, subplatysmal fat, and low positioned hyoid.

contour between the neck and inferior border of the mandible, while reestablishing the ideal cervicomental angle.

The surgeon should assess the amount of supraplatysmal/submental fat to determine if liposuction alone is a viable treatment option. The area is evaluated by having the patient press their tongue against the roof of the hard palate, thus activating the suprahyoid and platysma muscles. Evaluation of the submental area is then performed with a digital pinch using the thumb and index fingers to approximate the volume of supraplatysmal fat versus subplatysmal fat.

Neck

The aesthetic neck is defined as having a superiorly distinct mandibular border, smooth and prominent mandibular angle, visible anterior border of the sternocleidomastoid muscle, visible thyroid bulge, cervicomental angle of 90 to 100 degrees, and healthy skin tone.[6] Changes that develop over time include muscular atrophy, inferior descent of the hyoid, atrophy of the chin and inferior border of the mandible, deposition of supra- and subplatysmal fat, and ptotic glands. These changes present a severe challenge to the surgeon. A majority of the time, liposuction alone is not sufficient to treat these conditions, and excision of facial tissue is required.

To aid surgeons in treatment planning, Angelo Cuzalina and Colin Bailey developed a classification of the cosmetic neck with recommended procedures for treatment (Fig. 155.4 and Table 155.2).

Patient Evaluation

Preoperative assessment of a patient is pivotal prior to any surgical procedure. First and foremost, it is critical to obtain the patient's medical history and chief complaint. The chief complaint should be in the patient's own words and should be the primary area of discussion. The provider should allow the patient to describe their concerns and assist the patient with open-ended questions. The provider should obtain a complete list of medical diagnoses, medications with proper dosages and frequencies, allergies, and past surgical history. The patient's social history should also be reviewed, and the discussion must focus on the use of tobacco or nicotine-containing products due to their effects on vasculature and wound healing. Additionally, social history should include the patient's profession, as surgery may affect work-related duties.

Physical examination involves a thorough assessment of the face including symmetry, facial animation, skin quality, areas of bony and soft tissue prominence, rhytids, areas of ptosis, and soft tissue volumes. Following the clinical examination, facial photographs should be obtained to demonstrate findings to the patient and establish a comparison for future evaluation. The pictures should include frontal, lateral, and oblique views in a neutral position.

Patient Discussion

After completion of the examination, it is pivotal to discuss the clinical findings and the proposed treatments with the patient. The first step is to address the patient's chief complaint and

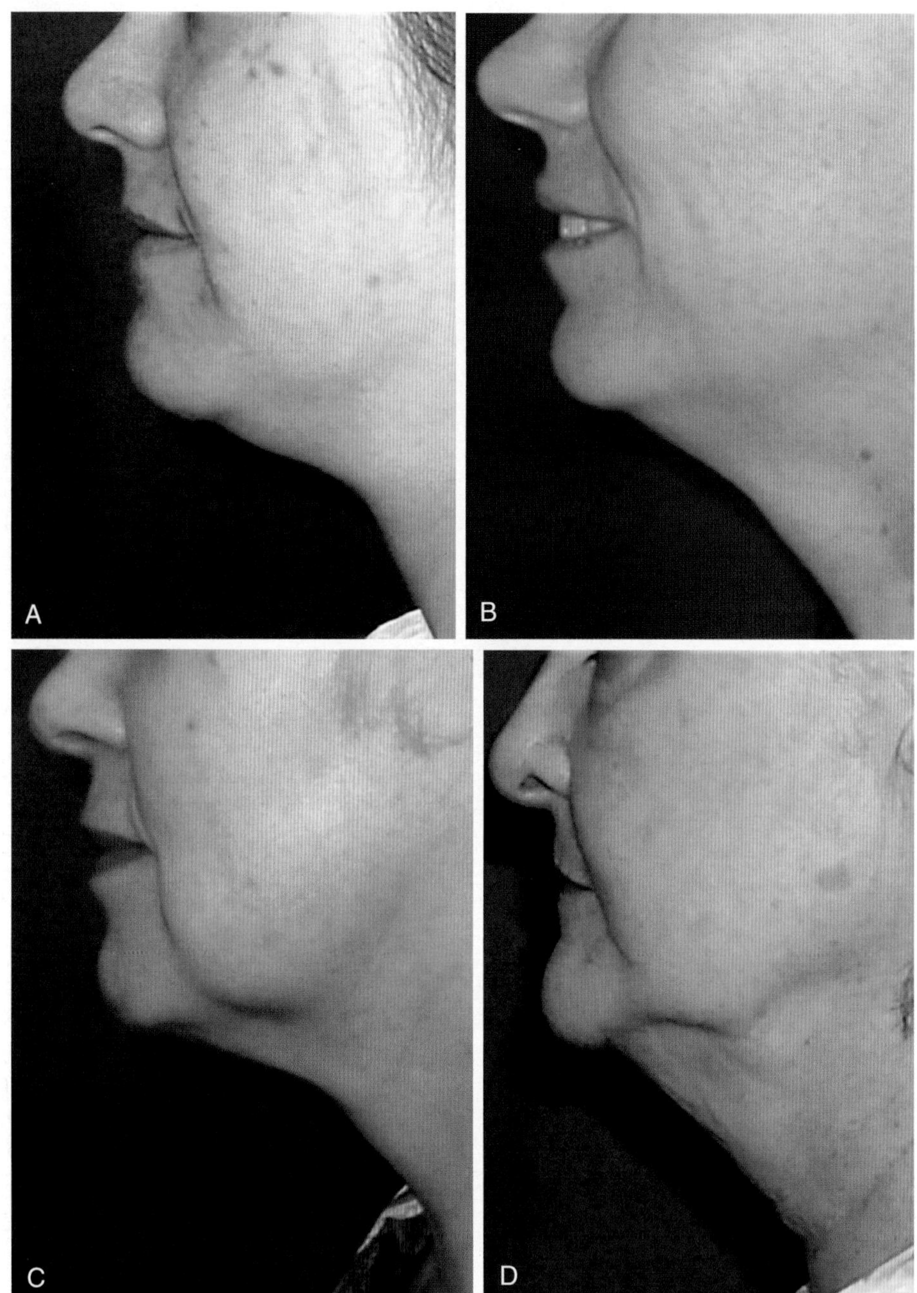

Figure 155.4 Cuzalina and Bailey cosmetic neck classification.[6] **A,** Type I. **B,** Type II. **C,** Type III. **D,** Type IV.

demonstrate the discoveries. The clinical findings should be presented in a manner that ensures the patient understands what is being described. To assist with this aspect of consultation, the use of photography and anatomic models is highly recommended. Once the patient is informed of the clinical problems, treatment options should be proposed along with the associated risks, benefits, and complications and if any alternative therapies are available. Never assume that the patient has a complete appreciation of the discussion and encourage the patient to ask questions or for clarifications.

The surgeon must focus on the patient's desires while maintaining sound surgical parameters. The patient should play an active role in the consultation by providing chief concerns as well as being an active participant in the clinical exam. An educated patient is one who understands the indications for various facial procedures and is aware of any limitations or possible complications. This assures a great provider-patient experience with an aesthetic outcome.

At the conclusion of the consult, the patient is be presented with a list of the proposed treatments and the associated costs. The surgical coordinator and the patient meet to review the cost of treatment, discuss finances, and set up the next steps in the surgical process.

Limitations and Contraindications

The ideal surgical candidate for liposuction of the face and neck presents with minimal jowling, platysmal banding, subplatysmal fat, and skin laxity as well as excellent skin tone and favorable hyoid position. The surgeon must be aware of the downfalls and limitations of liposuction. Excessive treatment of the affected areas may result in contour irregularities and damage to the underlying structures. While treating the jowls, the surgeon must remember that the presence of jowls is multifactorial, including ptotic fat compartments, buccal fat pad descent, and skin changes. Liposuction alone will reduce the presence of fat along the mid-face; however, it does not address the laxity of the facial suspensory system or the increase skin laxity. If the other components of the jowl are not rectified, liposuction as a sole treatment may lead to facial hollowing.

Table 155.2 Cuzalina and Bailey Cosmetic Neck Classification and Proposed Treatment

Cosmetic Neck Type	Proposed Treatment
Type I: Good skin tone, minimal subplatysmal fat, no platysmal banding, normal submandibular gland, minimal or no jowling	Liposuction only
Type II: Fair skin tone, subplatysmal fat bulging, platysmal banding with minimal or no jowling	Submentoplasty with or without liposuction
Type III: Jowling and neck laxity, with or without preplatysmal fat and minimal platysmal laxity	Rhytidectomy only
Type IV: Significant jowling, facial cutis laxity, major platysmal banding, heavy subplatysmal fat	Rhytidectomy with submentoplasty with or without liposuction
Subclassifications:	
A: Chin weakness	Genioplasty vs. chin implant
B: Submandibular gland fullness	Excision of submandibular gland
C: Low hyoid bone	Limited improvement capability

From, Cuzalina LA, Bailey CE. Cosmetic surgical rejuvenation of the neck. In: Erian A., Shiffman M, eds. *Advanced Surgical Facial Rejuvenation.* Berlin, Heidelberg: Springer; 2012.

Treatment of the submental and neck region may involve liposuction, platysmaplasty, submentoplasty, facelift, and chin implants. If the surgeon does not properly evaluate the submental and neck region, the postoperative outcome may appear worse than the preoperative situation. Submental lipohypertrophy may camouflage platysmal banding and render it difficult to assess its presence. The presence of platysmal banding requires a platysmaplasty only if there is minimal skin excess. The authors address this situation by creating a 2 cm submental incision followed by dissection until the platysma muscle is encountered. At this time, the platysma is cut back approximately 5 to 7 cm at the level of the hyoid bone, taking care to remain parallel to the mandibular border.

For patients with a moderate amount of subplatysmal fat and platysmal banding, a submentoplasty is required. A submentoplasty includes submental liposuction, platysmaplasty, and excision of subplatysmal fat. These patients are not ideal candidates for liposuction alone due to the persistent submental fullness and unaesthetic cervicomental angle. The submental region is accessed similarly to the platysmaplasty and dissection is continued down to the platysma, where the platysma back cuts and excision are performed. Once through the platysma, subplatysmal fat is encountered between the anterior bellies of the digastric muscles. This fat is then excised thus flattening the obtuse neck (Figs. 155.5 and 155.6). A platysmaplasty and a submentoplasty do

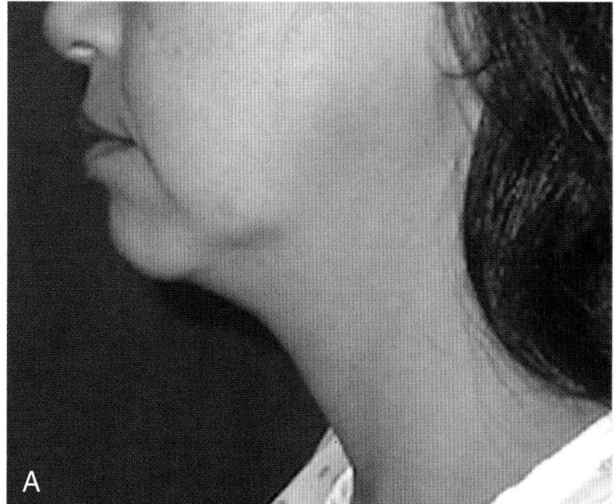

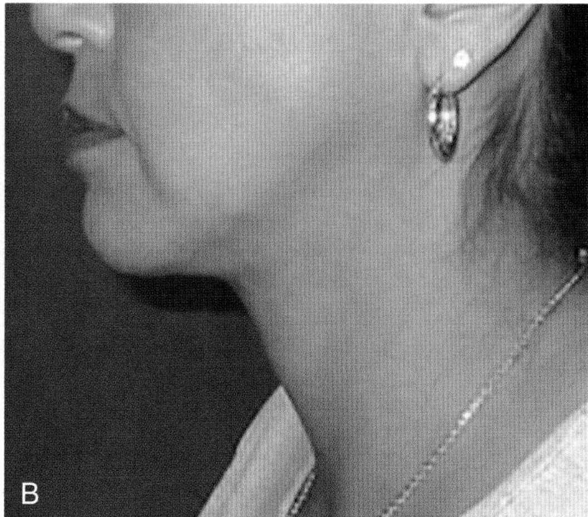

Figure 155.5 Submentoplasty. **A,** Preoperative. **B,** Postoperative submentoplasty with submental liposuction and chin implant.

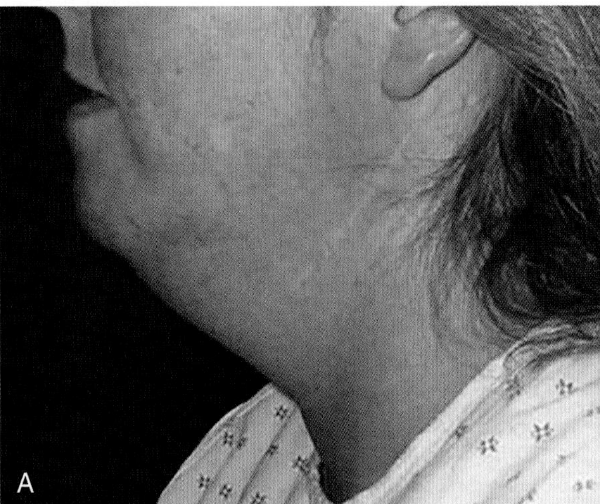

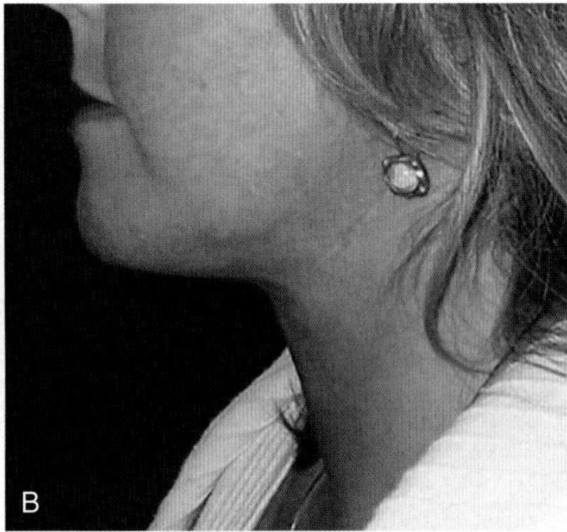

Figure 155.6 Submentoplasty. **A,** Preoperative. **B,** Postoperative submentoplasty with subplatysmal fat resection, submental liposuction, and chin implant.

TECHNIQUE: Face and Neck Liposuction

1. Marking

On the day of surgery, a final discussion is held with the patient, and all planned surgical procedures are reviewed and confirmed. It is important to allow patients to ask questions during this time and to ensure complete understanding of the surgical process. The patient is marked in the preoperative area while sitting in an upright position, therefore ensuring proper identification of facial landmarks and boundaries (Figs. 155.7 and 155.8).

Preoperative markings include the mandibular border, thyroid cartilage, sternocleidomastoid muscles, planned areas of treatment, and puncture sites.

2. Intubation and General Anesthesia

Patients for facial procedures are placed under general anesthesia and are intubated. This ensures the safety of the patient while maintaining the airway and avoiding extraneous movements from the patient.

3. Tumescent Anesthesia

The tumescent solution consists of 500 cc of 0.9% sodium chloride (normal saline), 50 cc of 1% lidocaine, and 1 cc of epinephrine.

Prior to infiltration of the tumescent anesthesia, the surgical site is preprepped with diluted Betadine.

The puncture sites are located posterior to each earlobe (2) and at the midline of the submental region (Fig. 155.9). The planned puncture sites are infiltrated with a total of 10 mL of 1% lidocaine with 1:100,000 epinephrine to assist with hemostasis and pain control. The tumescent solution is then injected via the puncture sites that are created through the use of a #11 blade. The tumescent is introduced into the face and neck with the use of a 22-gauge spinal needle; this allows for hydrodissection along the subcutaneous plane. While injecting the solution, the nondominant hand is applying gentle pressure to ensure proper placement and location of the needle. A total of 500 cc of tumescent is injected, with the end goal of skin blanching to signify adequate anesthesia.

The tumescent solution is infiltrated along the mandibular border from the submental region to the anterior border of the sternocleidomastoid muscles bilaterally and then inferiorly to the clavicles. Additional anesthesia is applied to the jowl region.

4. Closed Liposuction

While performing liposuction, the cannula opening must face away from the skin to avoid contour deformities and minimize injury to the subdermal plexus. The nondominant hand applies gentle pressure to allow for the localization of the cannula tip and identification of remaining tissue density. This technique assists with the prevention of overtreatment of an area and indentations. Liposuction is performed from a cranial to caudal direction with uniform radial strokes, creating a smooth contour. The surgeon must observe the consistency of the aspirated content; the presence of blood notifies the surgeon to avoid continued treatment in this area.

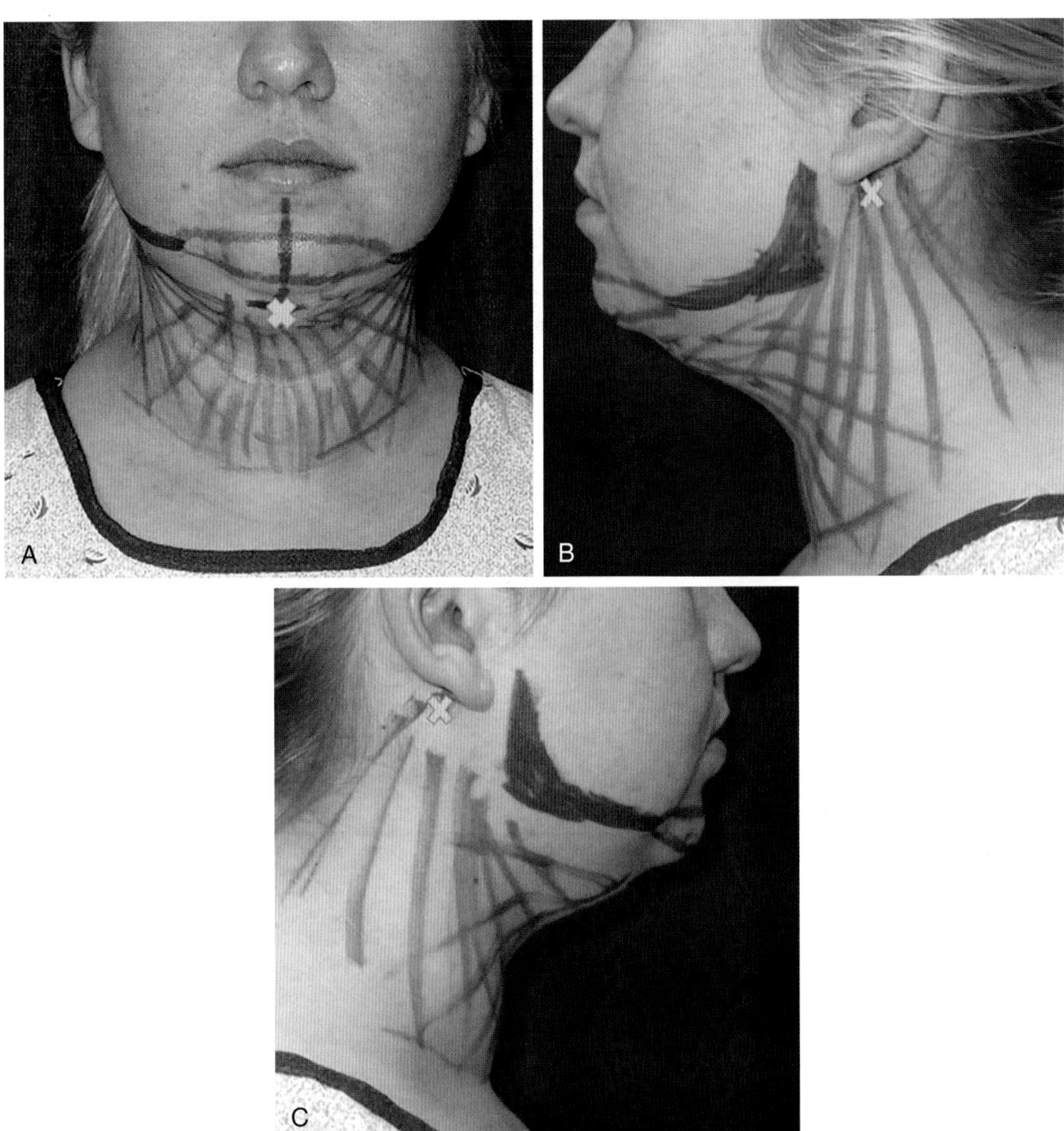

Figure 155.7 Preoperative markings. **A,** Frontal view. **B,** Left lateral view. **C,** Right lateral view. *Red:* outline of the mandible; *blue:* planned areas of liposuction; *green:* position of chin implant; *yellow:* puncture sites.

TECHNIQUE: Face and Neck Liposuction—*cont'd*

In the submental region, areas of lipohypertrophy are treated with the use of 1.5- and 2-mm cannulas connected to wall suction (Fig. 155.10). The cannula is advanced to the submental region, and liposuction is performed along the subcutaneous plane with the cannula opening facing toward the platysma. Liposuction is performed in short, radial strokes while maintaining pressure with the opposite hand. A digit is placed along the mandibular border, and liposuction is performed below the digit, thus extenuating the chin.

In the jowl region, areas of lipohypertrophy are treated with the use of 1-, 1.5- and 2-mm cannulas connected to wall suction. The cannula is advanced to the jowl area, and liposuction is performed along the subcutaneous plane with the cannula opening facing away from the skin. Liposuction is performed in short, radial strokes while maintaining pressure with the opposite hand. When addressing the mandibular border, liposuction should be performed above and below the inferior border of the mandible and should never be performed directly over the border (Fig. 155.11). To assist with defining the inferior border of the mandible, a digit is placed along the inferior border and liposuction is performed above

Continued

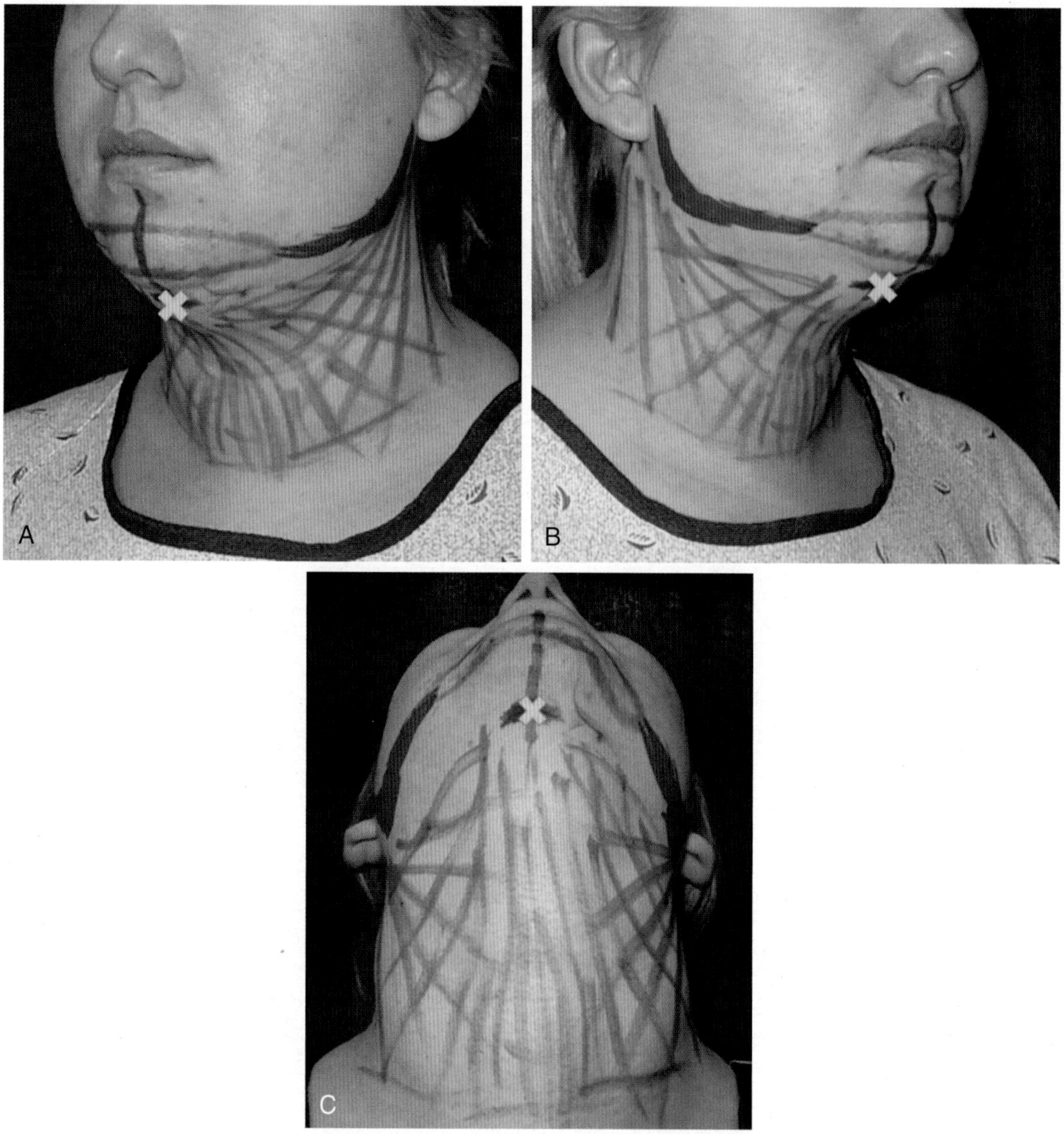

Figure 155.8 Preoperative markings. **A,** Left oblique view. **B,** Right oblique view. **C,** Worm's-eye view. *Red:* outline of the mandible; *blue:* planned areas of liposuction; *green:* position of chin implant; *yellow:* puncture sites.

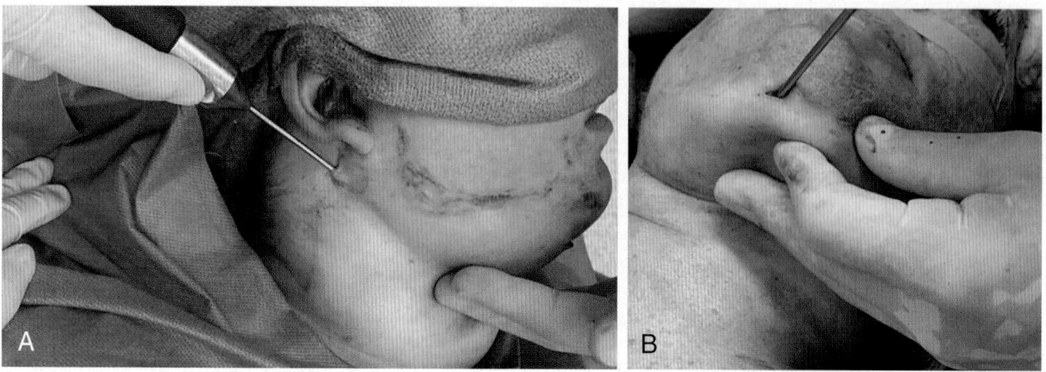

Figure 155.9 Puncture sites. **A,** Postauricular. **B,** Submental incision.

TECHNIQUE: Face and Neck Liposuction—*cont'd*

and below the digit. It is recommended that the superior aspect of the jowl be treated from the post-auricular puncture site while the inferior aspect of the jowl is treated from the submental site.

Areas of lipohypertrophy in the neck are treated in an identical fashion to areas of lipohypertrophy in the jowl, utilizing 1.5- and 2-mm cannulas (see Fig. 155.11). The inferior extent of the liposuction encroaches just superior to the clavicle, while the posterior extent is limited by the auricular and mastoid ligaments.

Near the end of the procedure, a pinch test is performed to assess the removal of fat and identify any discrepancies between the two sides. The surgeon must evaluate each side of the face and aim to create a mirror image with aesthetic results. A well-defined mandibular border signifies youth and reverses the effects of aging (Figs. 155.12 and 155.13).

5. Closure

Surgical puncture sites are allowed to spontaneously drain. A pressure dressing and head wrap are applied, and the patient is directed to remove the dressing after 24 hours.

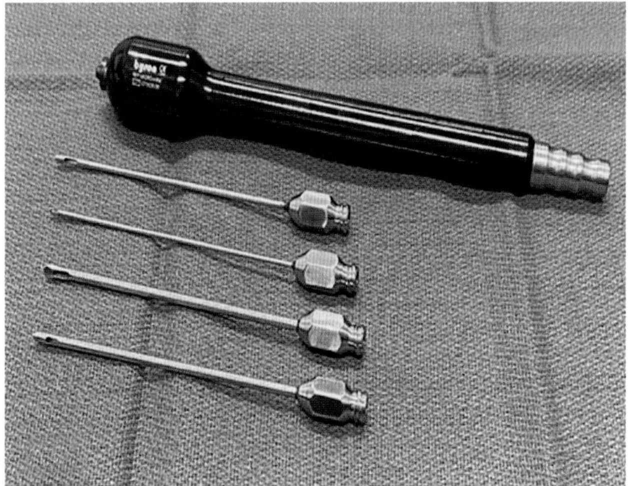

Figure 155.10 Microcannulas. Microcannula sizes range from 1 to 3 mm. An adaptor must be equipped to allow for attachment to wall suction.

not address the overlying skin laxity, and these patients will require a formal cervical rhytidectomy.

Submentoplasty offers patients an aesthetic neck with long-term stability in patients with supraplatysmal fat, subplatysmal fat, and platysmal banding. Of utmost importance is the need for a surgeon to recognize patient populations that require a formal cervical rhytidectomy when a platysmaplasty and submentoplasty would not be aesthetically appropriate.

Avoidance and Management of Intraoperative and Postoperative Complications

The most common complications following face and neck liposuction are contour irregularities, bleeding, hematoma, infection, hypesthesia, skin necrosis, hyperpigmentation, prolonged induration, marginal mandibular injury, and perforation into surrounding structures, with hematoma being the most common.

To minimize intraoperative bleeding, the surgeon must ensure the use of epinephrine in the tumescent anesthesia. The presence of epinephrine causes vasoconstriction of the facial vessels, thus decreasing the likelihood of bleeding as well as hematoma formation. To avoid significant contour irregularities, multiple steps must be taken. Liposuction should be performed from multiple directions to decrease the likelihood of overtreating an area. Further, a minimum of 5 mm of fat must remain along the dermis. If an excess amount of fat is removed, the dermal layer will be in close contact with the platysma and may lead to scarring and retraction (Fig. 155.14). To avoid injury to the marginal mandibular nerve and facial vessels, a micro cannula is utilized along the mandibular border and jowls while remaining in the subcutaneous plane.[6]

Postoperative Considerations

The patient must be made aware of clinical signs of infection, including fever, erythema, incremental increase in pain, and warmth at the surgical sites. Following the procedure, the patients are discharged on antibiotics to reduce the risk of infection. In order to reduce the risk of a hematoma/seroma, a compressive dressing is placed at the conclusion of the case. The patient is directed to maintain the dressing for 7 days; it may only be removed to shower and it must be immediately replaced. Patients are evaluated 7 days following the surgical procedure. At this time, the compressive dressing is removed, and the neck is evaluated for possible hematoma or seroma formation. Any areas that are concerning for fluid collection are aspirated and immediate pressure is reapplied. The patient is reevaluated in 1 to 2 days to assess for recollection.

The patient is given a new compressive dressing and directed to perform lymphatic massages with warm compresses to

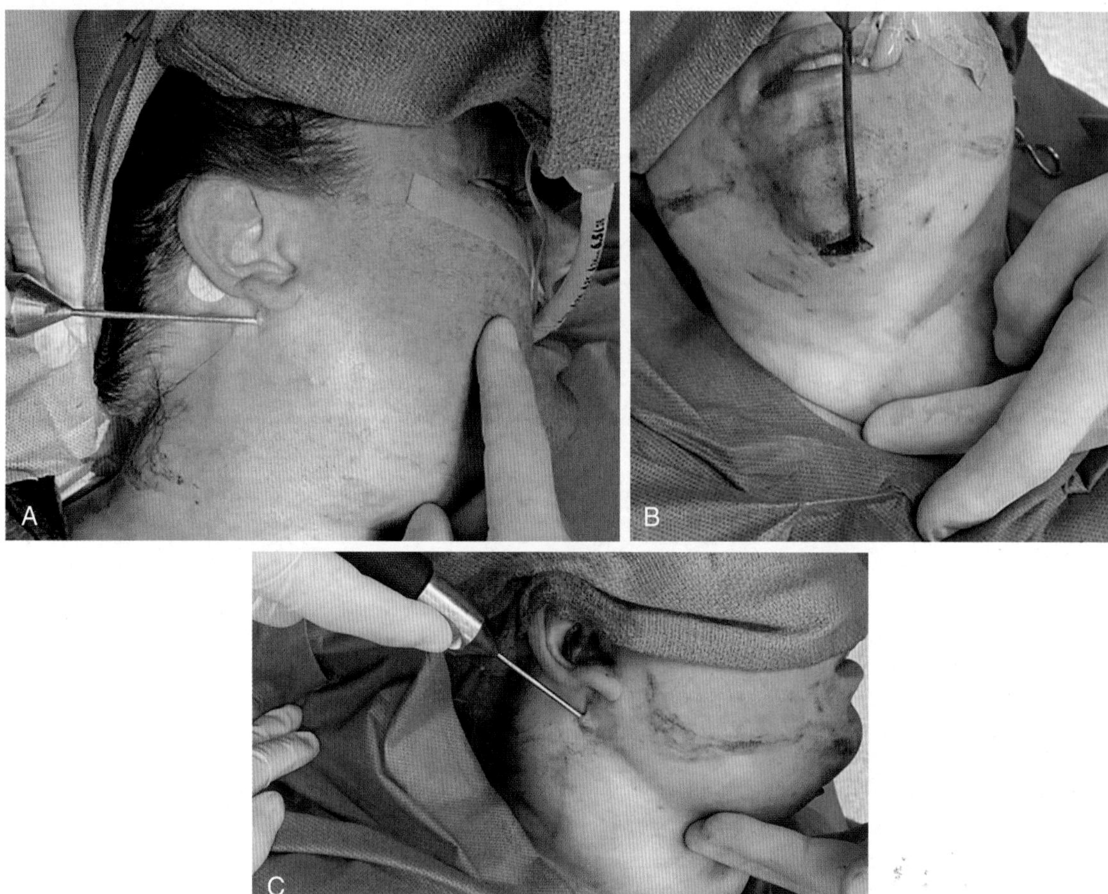

Figure 155.11 Treatment sites. **A,** Jowl region. **B,** Submental region. **C,** Neck.

assist the recovery process. The patient is directed to follow-up in 2 weeks or sooner if any acute changes occur. The patient is informed that 6 months of healing is required prior to complete assessment of aesthetic success. For those patients who develop contour deformities, fat grafting is a viable option to address these areas.

Other Treatment Modalities

Injection Lipolysis

Kybella (deoxycholic acid) has been approved by the Food and Drug Administration for the treatment of submental fullness due to an excess of submental fat. Kybella offers patients a minimally invasive option when compared to liposuction; however, multiple treatment sessions are required. Deoxycholic acid is a cytolytic solution that induces cell membrane lysis in protein poor tissue. As the acid is introduced into the subcutaneous plane, fat cells undergo apoptosis and induce an inflammatory response in the area. The inflammation induces stimulation of fibroblasts and collagen deposition leading to skin tightening. The results of treatment include reduction of submental fat and improved contour of the mandibular border and chin, thus restoring a youthful look.

Ultrasonic-Assisted Liposuction

Ultrasonic liposuction involves the use of mechanical and thermal energy via ultrasonic waves to liquify fat cells followed by traditional liposuction to remove these disrupted adipocytes. The ultrasonic liposuction generates heat that causes volumetric contraction of the overlying skin via induction of collagen formation. This allows for improved contour of the surgical area with decreased skin laxity. Extreme caution must be taken when utilizing this instrument due to increased risk of thermal injury to the overlying skin.

Laser-Assisted Liposuction

Laser-assisted liposuction is another adjuvant therapy to treat lipohypertrophy. This instrument utilized laser energy via a cannula to distribute light to the adipocytes. The transfer of light energy causes cell lysis and liquification of the fat cell. Just as in the ultrasonic-assisted liposuction technique, traditional liposuction is required to remove the content. Additional benefits of the instrument are coagulation of vessels, contraction of adipose and dermal collagen and reorganization of the reticular dermis due to the generation of new collagen fibrils. The clinical benefits of the above stated benefits are decreased blood loss and postoperative edema, improved skin contour, and laxity.[14]

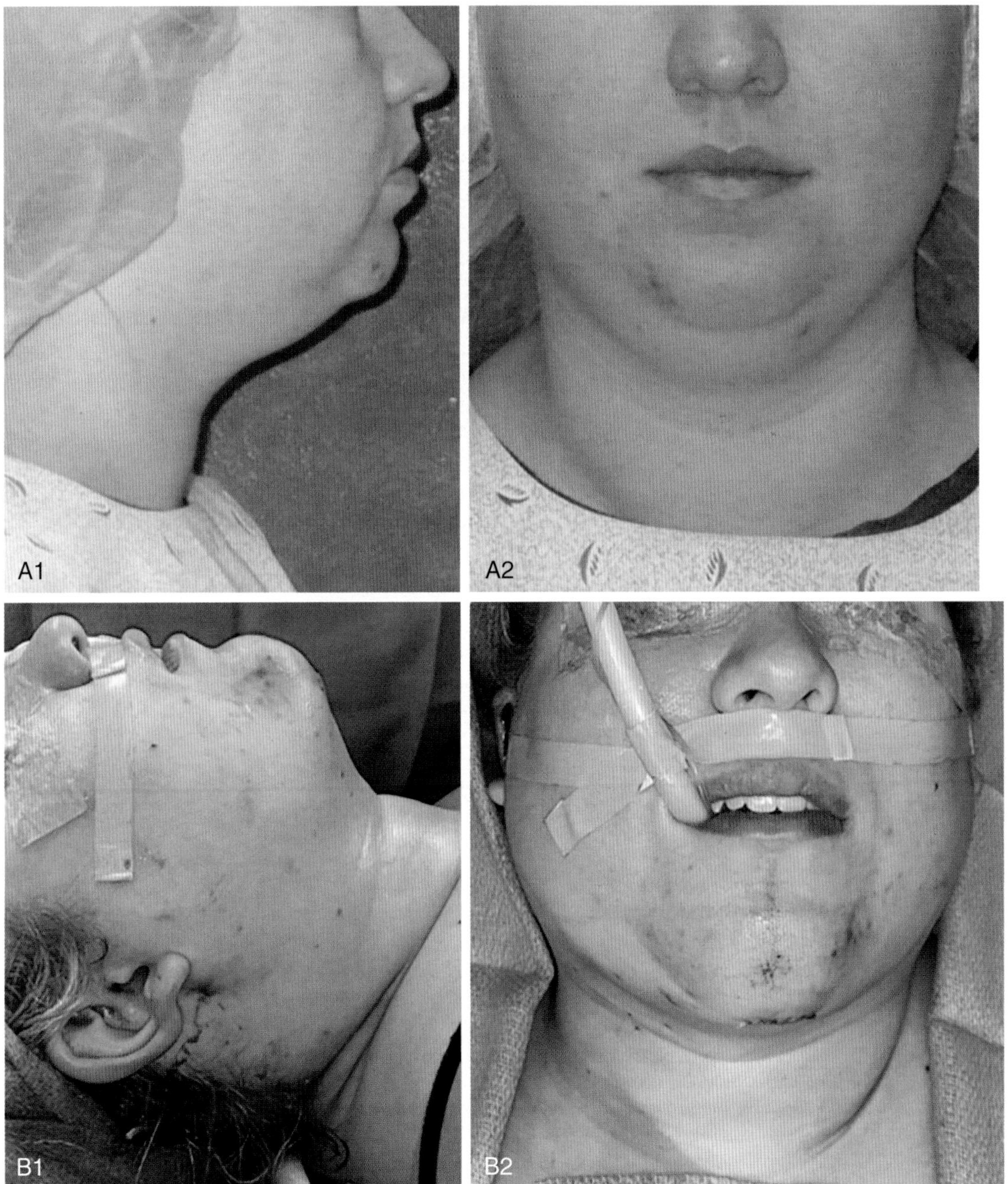

Figure 155.12 Liposuction and chin implant. **A,** Preoperative (**A1,** Right lateral view; **A2,** Frontal view). **B,** Postoperative (**B1,** Right lateral view; **B2,** Frontal view).

Plasma Energy for Treatment of Skin Laxity

For patients with lipohypertrophy and mild to moderate skin laxity, liposuction alone may not yield aesthetic results. Plasma energy and liposuction have demonstrated enhanced and noticeable outcomes in these patients. Plasma energy in conjunction with radiofrequency has been shown to effect specific proteins found in blood vessels, as well as collagen. With increasing temperatures due to the plasma energy, the bonds between protein molecules are disrupted, leading to denaturation. This process is reversed upon tissue cooling and leads to the development of a coagulum, aiding in blood vessel occlusion and hemostasis. Collagen is a key protein in the development and maintenance of connective tissue and skin. When exposed to temperatures greater than 66.8 °C, contraction of the collagen fibrils occur to approximately one-third of its original length.[15] The combination of protein denaturation and collagen contraction leads to a reduction of surface area and volume of the treated area. For patients with mild skin laxity, plasma energy with radiofrequency may be utilized to rejuvenate, tighten the skin of the neck and submental region, while contouring the mandibular jawline.[16,17]

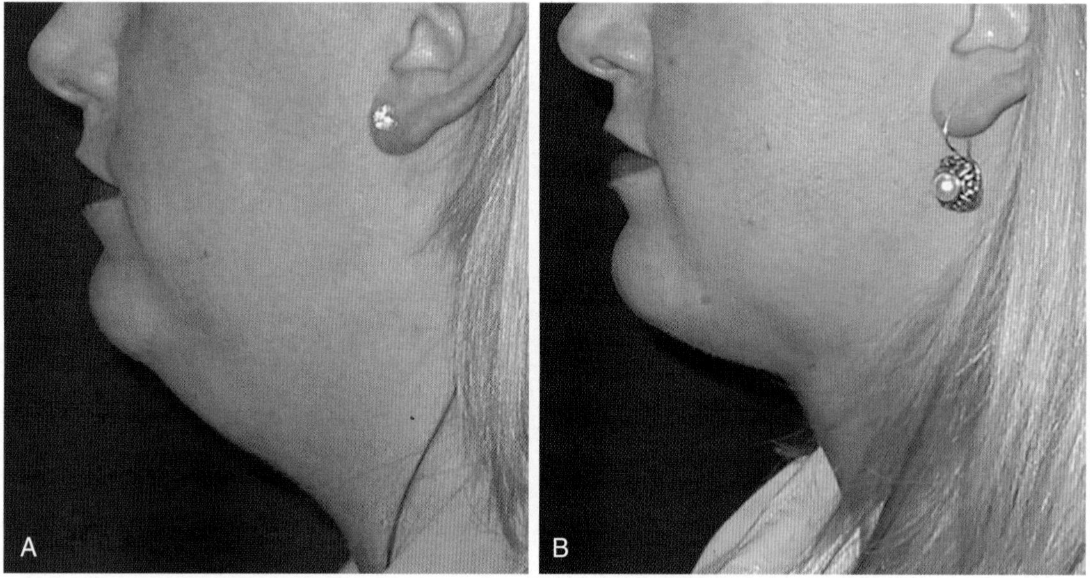

Figure 155.13 Submental liposuction. **A,** Preoperative. **B,** 1-month postoperative.

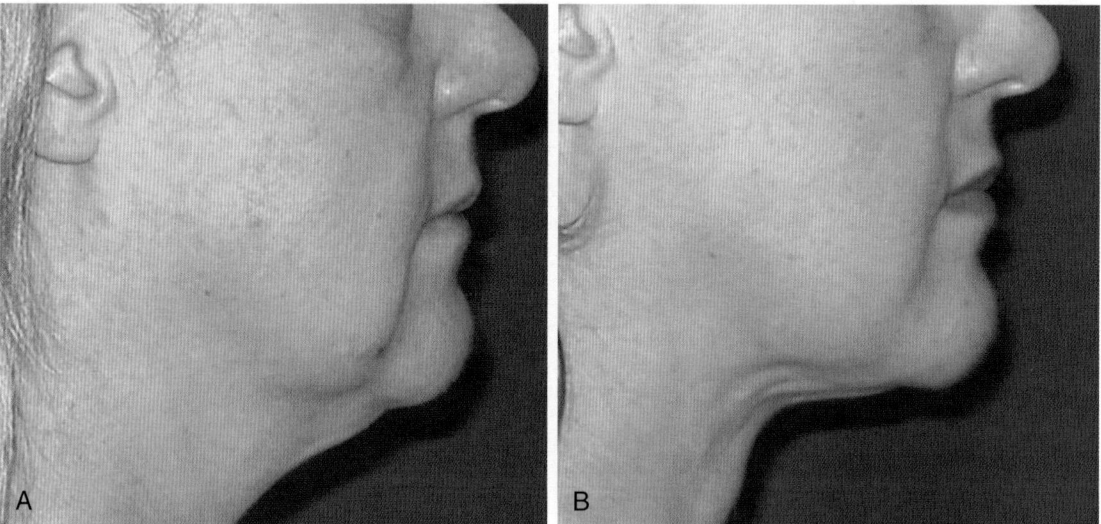

Figure 155.14 Contour irregularities. **A,** Preoperative. **B,** Postoperative. Presence of contour irregularities due to excess fat removal and underlying platysma banding.

References

1. Flynn TC, Coleman II WP, Field LM, Klein JA, Hanke CW. History of liposuction. *Dermatol Surg*. 2000;26(6):515–520.
2. Fischer A, Fischer G. First surgical treatment for molding body's cellulite with three 5 mm incisions. *Bull Int Acad Cosmet Surg*. 1976;3:35.
3. Illouz YG. Body contouring by lipolysis: a 5-year experience with over 3000 cases. *Plast Reconstr Surg*. 1983;72(5):591–597.
4. Bellini E, Grieco MP, Raposio E. A journey through liposuction and liposculture: review. *Ann Med Surg (Lond)*. 2017;24:53–60. Published 2017.
5. Klein JA. The tumescent technique for liposuction surgery. *Am J Cosmet Surg*. 1987;4:263–267.
6. Cuzalina LA, Bailey CE. Cosmetic surgical rejuvenation of the neck. In: Erian A, Shiffman M, eds. *Advanced Surgical Facial Rejuvenation*. Berlin, Heidelberg: Springer; 2012.
7. Kehlet SN, Willumsen N, Armbrecht G, et al. Age-related collagen turnover of the interstitial matrix and basement membrane: implications of age- and sex-dependent remodeling of the extracellular matrix. *PLoS One*. 2018;13(3):e0194458.
8. Niamtu J. In: *Cosmetic Facial Surgery*. 2nd ed. Edinburgh: Elsevier; 2018.
9. Lund KJ. Menopause and the menopausal transition. *Med Clin North Am*. 2008;92(5):1253–1271, xii.
10. Ji MX, Yu Q. Primary osteoporosis in postmenopausal women. *Chronic Dis Transl Med*. 2015;1(1):9–13. Published.
11. Stanworth RD, Jones TH. Testosterone for the aging male; current evidence and recommended practice. *Clin Interv Aging*. 2008;3(1):25–44. https://doi.org/10.2147/cia.s190.
12. Golds G, Houdek D, Arnason T. Male hypogonadism and osteoporosis: the effects, clinical consequences, and treatment of testosterone deficiency in bone health. *Int J Endocrinol*. 2017;2017:4602129.
13. Kahn DM, Shaw RB. Overview of current thoughts on facial volume and aging. *Facial Plast Surg*. 2010;26(5):350–355.
14. Low M. Submental liposuction. In: Erian A, Shiffman M, eds. *Advanced Surgical Facial Rejuvenation*. Berlin, Heidelberg: Springer; 2012.
15. Gardner ES, Reinisch L, Stricklin GP, et al. In vitro changes in non-facial human skin following CO_2 laser resurfacing: a comparison study. *Lasers Surg Med*. 1996;19(4):379–387.
16. Gentile DR. Cool atmospheric plasma (J-Plasma) and new options for facial contouring and skin rejuvenation of the heavy face and neck. *Facial Plast Surg*. 2018;34(1):66–74.
17. Zamora J, Roman S. Subcutaneous neck skin tightening. *Adv Cosmet Surg*. 2019:89–95.

CHAPTER 156

Scar Revision

Erik Jon Nuveen

Armamentarium

#15 Bard Parker blade
7 to 9 Inch facelift scissors
4-5 or 5-0 Monocryl suture
5-6 or 6-0 Prolene suture
Iris scissors
Local anesthetic
Method of cauterization
Surgical marking pen
Skin hooks

History of Scar Revision

Although the presence of scars undoubtedly preceded the written word, the origin of the word "scar" can be found in the Greek word "eskhara" and was first published in the 14th century in French literature as "escharre."[1] The current common definition of a scar includes any visual tissue marking the location where healing has occurred after injury or disease to the skin.[2] The skin is the largest organ of the body and functions to cover and seal the internal from the external in order to reduce evaporative body fluid loss and resist infection. Descriptive terms associated with scaring include redness, elevation, pigmentation (hypo or hyper), fibroproliferative, hypertrophic, or keloid. All may be the result of either normal or excessive healing during the evolution of repair of a wound. The cosmetic appearance of a scar is the most important criteria to judge the surgical outcome of a scar revision.

Normal Wound Healing

Wound healing is a physiological process consisting of of four phases: hemostasis, inflammation, proliferation, and remodeling.[2] Injury to skin, elective or otherwise, may result in tattered tear, a clean cut, or avulsive wound. Wounds with unopposed margins do not benefit from cellular communication and suffer a prolonged course of healing and increased risk of infection. Wounds that heal as a result of direct cellular contact of the wound edges heal with a lower likelihood of visible scaring. The physiological response to injury includes a diverse cellular response. Hemostasis is soon followed by platelet activation and clot formation. Angiogenesis involves endothelial cell proliferation, migration, and branching to form new blood vessels. Resident fibroblasts proliferate and invade the clot to form contractile granulation tissue. Reepithelialization simultaneously occurs and involves the proliferation and differentiation of stem cells. Growth factors and cytokines are released that are critical to cellular repair. Unopposed wounds heal through a process of granulation followed by reepithelialization.[3] Collagen remodeling takes place throughout a 12 to 18-month period and continues to gain tensile strength of 70% to 80% of uninjured skin.[4,5]

Abnormal Scar Formation

The International Advisory Panel on Scar Management classifies scarring into six categories: mature scar, immature scar, linear hypertrophic, widespread hypertrophic, and minor and major keloids.[6–8] Hypertrophic scars remain within the boundaries of the original incision. Redness, itching, or burning often accompanies these rope-like elevated scars. Keloid scars are a focally raised lesion extending beyond the borders of the original incision. These lesions extend and continue to grow over years and do not regress on their own. Minor keloids may begin to develop up to a year after the injury. Major keloids continue to spread into normal tissue over years and are raised greater than 0.5 cm from their origins. The Vancouver scar scale[9] for the timing of scar revision is important to improved outcomes. Immature scars are prone to hypertrophy and give poor results after scar revision. Adjunct treatments such as the use of silicone sheet and intralesional steroid injections can be given during this period. However, if early intervention is needed, it is wiser to do it only after 8 to 12 weeks in adults and 6 months in children smaller than 7 years of age[10] (Fig. 156.1).

Non-Surgical Treatment for Scars

A. Noninvasive treatment options: compression garments,[11] silicone gel sheeting,[12] massage and ultrasound therapy,[13] Micropore tape,[14] topical vitamin E,[15] radiation therapy,[16] retinoic acid,[17] cryotherapy,[18,19] and laser.[20]
B. Invasive treatment options: intralesional injections with 5-flourouracil,[21] triamcinolone,[22] interferon gamma,[23,24] botulinum toxin (Botox; Allegan Corp),[25] bleomycin,[26] and TGF modulators.[27] Surgical excision and closure are the mainstays of treatment. Recent suggested and

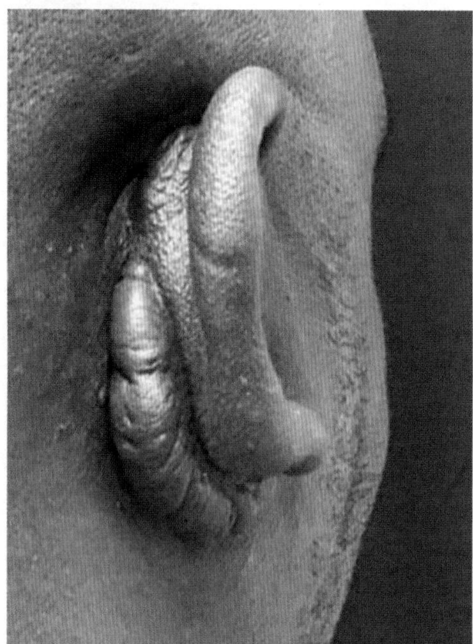
Figure 156.1 Keloid formation after cartilage harvest.

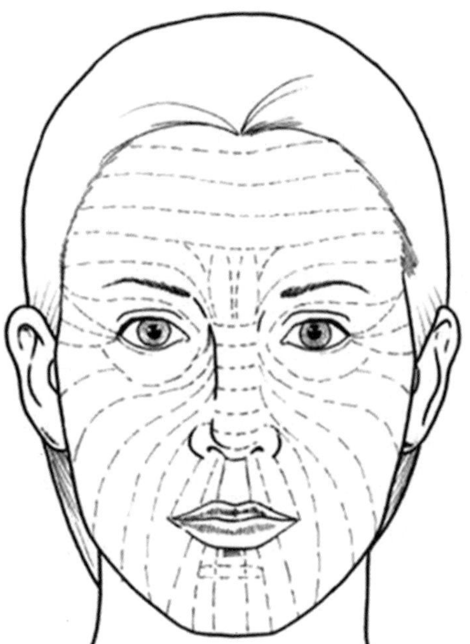
Figure 156.2 Relaxed skin tension lines.[39]

researched interventions for wound healing and scar formation include autologous fat grafting,[28] oral minocycline given in high doses,[29,30] angiotensin converting enzyme inhibitors,[31,32] angiotensin receptor blockers,[33] topical 1% prolyl 4-hydroxylase inhibitor,[34] procollagen C-proteinase inhibitor,[35] tamoxifin,[36] topical anti-TGF-β1 and 2 antibody, exogenous TGF-β3,[37] and topical celecoxib (a selective cyclooxygenase-2 inhibitor).[38]

Indications for the Procedure

A surgical scar revision should be considered when the benefits outweigh the risks. The principles of ideal scar revision technique include the following. Meticulous care of wound edges and handling of tissue, a tension free approximation, layered closure, wound margin eversion, and hemostasis.

An ideal scar revision procedure should leave the most imperceptible scar with minimal discoloration, distortion of adjacent tissue without depression or elevation of surrounding tissues. Utilization of facial esthetic subunit principles is also critical.

The general principles of scar revision are applied to all techniques of scar modification for improvement (Figs. 156.2 and 156.3).

The characteristics of ideal scar revision outcomes include the following:

1. The most imperceptible scar.
   a. Achieved by paralleling relaxed skin tension lines (RSTL)
   b. No discoloration (redness, pigmented, or amelanotic)
   c. No distortion of surrounding tissues
   d. No depression or elevation of levels
   e. Utilize facial esthetic unit principles if possible[40,41]

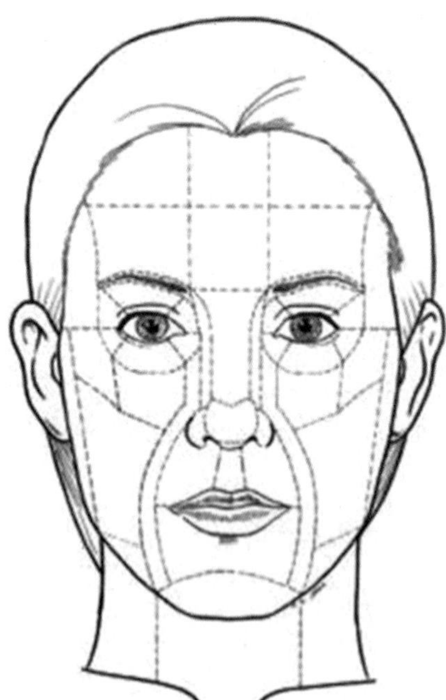
Figure 156.3 Facial esthetic subunits.

Limitations and Contraindications

Factors that may decrease patient satisfaction and esthetic outcome from scar revision surgery include unrealistic expectations, medical comorbidities that affect soft tissue healing, and the use of tobacco products.

1. Unrealistic expectations
2. Timing of scar/injury
3. Medical condition/medications of the patient
4. Use of tobacco products[42,43]

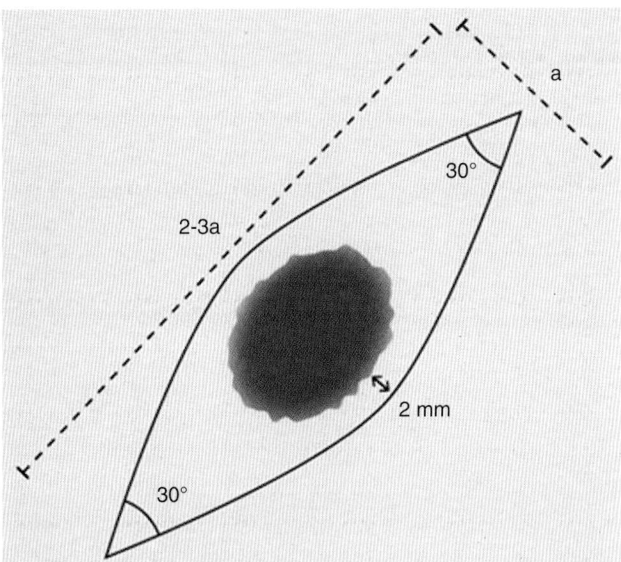

Figure 156.4 Diagrammatic of fusiform elliptical excision. (Illustration: Øystein Horgmo, University of Oslo.)[44]

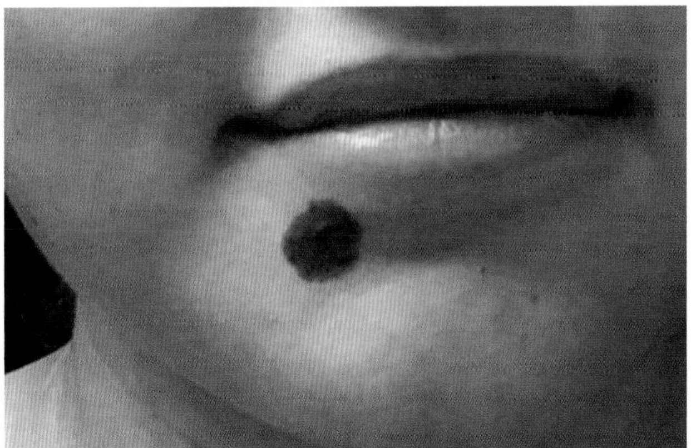

Figure 156.5 Pigmented lesion of the face.

TECHNIQUE: Fusiform Elliptical Excision

STEP 1: Planning

This technique is best utilized when the scar is mature, depressed, or widened and present along RSTLs and does not violate the esthetic facial subunits. The ratio of length to width is 3:1, and the ends of the excision do not exceed 30 degrees to prevent "dog ear" redundancy of tissue (Figs. 156.4 and 156.5).

Analysis of the lesion discloses it has been present since birth. No changes have been noticed in coloration, borders, redness, size or sensation. Anatomically, the lesion falls either immediately within the lines of skin tension or immediately adjacent and parallel to the RSTL. The options for treatment included elliptical fusiform excision, but the potential exists for distortion of the lip in this highly functional region. Alternatives include wide undermining and serial fusiform excision and local advancement reconstruction. This latter option would result in larger areas of excision with increased scar length. In this case, we chose serial excision using a fusiform pattern and wide undermining.

STEP 2: Anesthesia

A total of 5.0 cc of 2% lidocaine with 1:100,000 epinephrine is introduced in the local region with a 27-gauge needle and syringe. This was allowed to infiltrate for 10 minutes to achieve hemostasis and anesthesia.

STEP 3: Incision

Using a #15C Bard Parker blade, the skin is incised to the level of subcutaneous fat along the lines drawn preoperatively. Wide undermining is performed with iris scissors to approximately 2 to 3 cm distal to the incision placement. Electrocautery was used throughout for hemostasis; remaining in the subcutaneous plane minimized interruption of the more robust deeper blood supply.

STEP 4: Suturing

The skin edges are advanced with 4-0 Monocryl suture using vertical everting interrupted sutures. The subcutaneous layer is reapproximated with 6-0 nylon in a running fashion and externalized proximally and distally. Skin glue is applied. The nylon running suture is removed at postoperative day 6.

Of note, the geometry of this excision exceeded ideal parameters as indicated above in diagram with the width exceeding ideal versus the length and the proximal and distal angles of divergence exceeding ideal. As a result, this patient underwent a serial excision in order to minimize wound tension and dog ear formation (Figs. 156.6–156.8).

TECHNIQUE: Z-Plasty

STEP 1: Planning

a. This common technique allows for a change in direction of a linear scar to better reapproximate RSTLs.
b. A 60-degree angle formed between the common diagonal and the arm results in a gain of 75% in length and a change in direction of 90 degrees.
c. The scar is excised directly. The wound edges are widely undermined.
d. Full thickness rotation is achieved (Fig. 156.9).

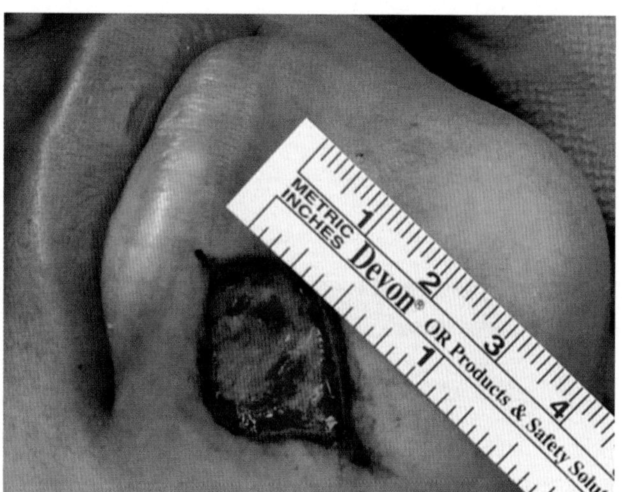

Figure 156.6 Fusiform excision and wide undermining.

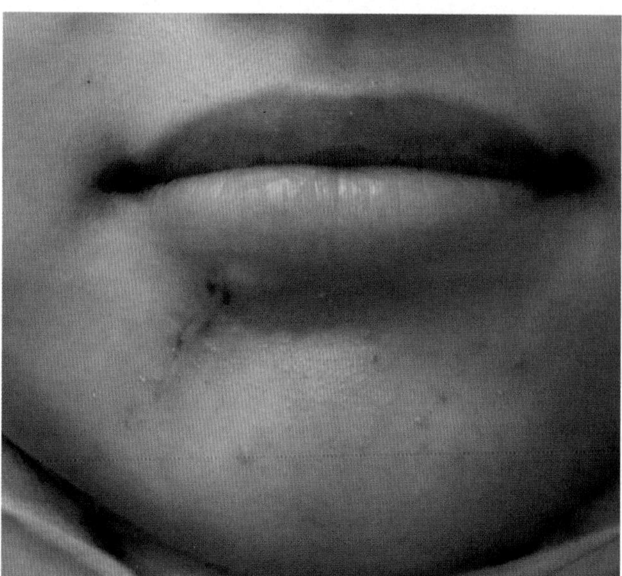

Figure 156.8 Three months postoperative.

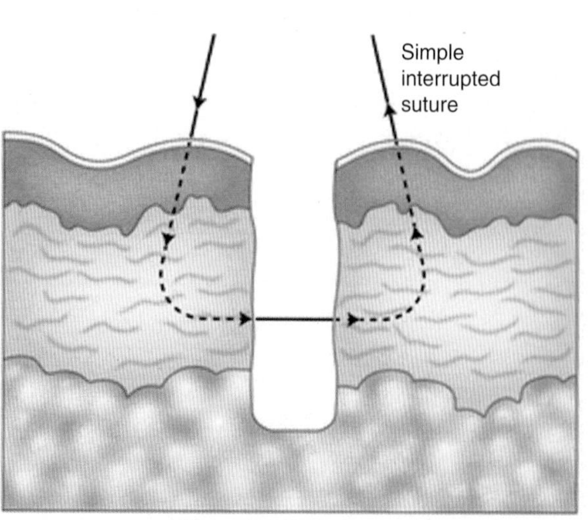

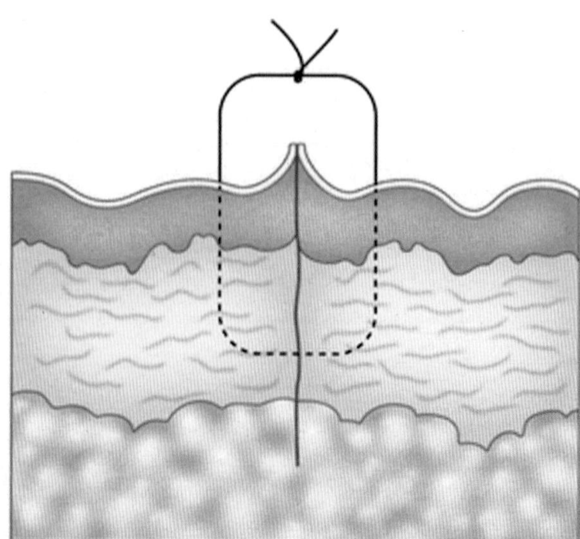

Figure 156.7 Cross sectional view of eversion suture technique with interrupted suture.[45]

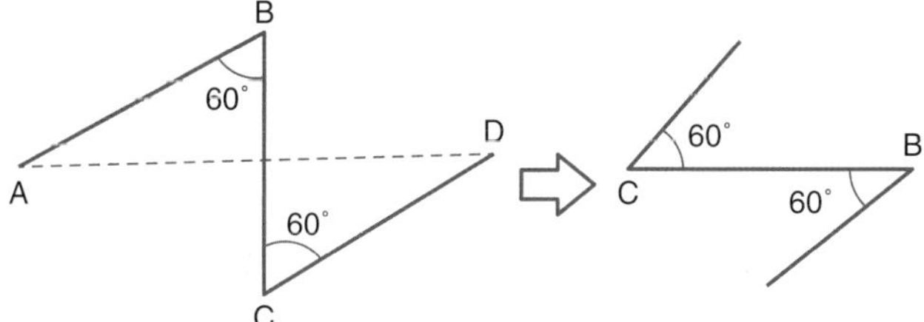

Figure 156.9 Basic Z-plasty scar revision.

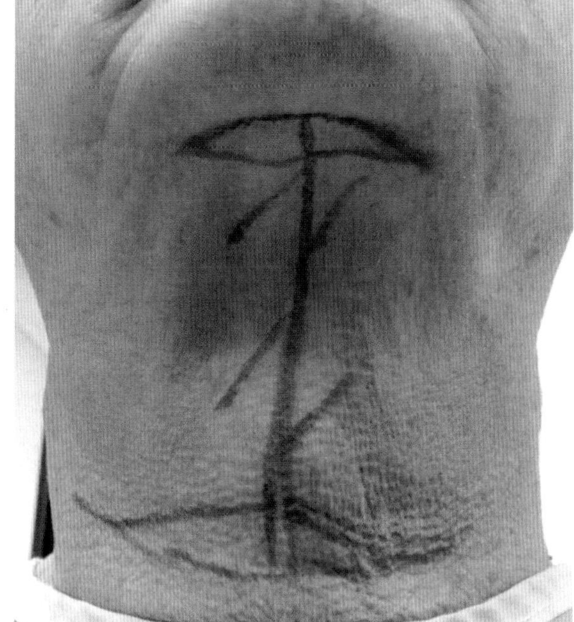
Figure 156.10 Proposed double goblet Z-plasty for neck laxity.

TECHNIQUE: Complex Z-Plasty

The goblet Z-plasty is commonly used for elective neck resection and combines a single or multiple Z-plasties and a goblet resection for a maximum gain in length and also irregularizes a linear scar.

STEP 1: Planning

This patient presented with a focused goal of improvement of his cervicomental laxity. He was resistant to consider a post auricular incision of the traditional neck lift surgery and alternatively underwent isolated anterior midline neck Z-plasty with platysmal corset. This procedure can safely and efficiently be performed under local anesthesia alone, but most choose intravenous sedation for psychological reduction of anxiety. Preoperative photographs were taken and recorded. The anticipated and optional single and double Z-plasty were diagrammed along with the goblet midline excision.

STEP 2: Anesthesia

A total of 10.0 cc of 2% lidocaine with 1:100,000 epinephrine was introduced in the area of planned incisions using a 27-gauge needle and syringe. A total of 300 cc of tumescent solution (1.0 cc of 1:1000 epinephrine, 500 mg lidocaine, 10 cc of $NaHCO_3$ in 500 cc normal saline IV infusion bag) was infused using a 22-gauge spinal needle into the subcutaneous tissues of the submental region, waiting a total of 15 minutes for hemostasis and anesthesia to be achieved.

STEP 3: Incision

Using a #10 Bard Parker blade, the skin was incised to the level of subcutaneous fat along the lines drawn preoperatively. Wide undermining was performed with iris scissors to approximately 5.0 cm distal to the incision placement. Electrocautery was used throughout for hemostasis, while remaining in the subcutaneous plane minimized interruption of the more robust deeper blood supply.

STEP 4: Suturing

The subcutaneous fat may be removed with lipoaspiration either directly (spatulated cannula 5.0 mm) or indirectly using a closed technique (2.5 mm Mercedes cannula). Midline 1.0 to 3.0 cm can be resected and midline plication with 4-0 PDS suture with inferior cutback of the platysma performed. The overlying skin is realigned with traditional rotational advancement of the flaps while maintaining a 60-degree angle for maximum perfusing of the most distal extent of the flap. Inset is performed at the dermis with 4-0 Monocryl. At the conclusion of deep closure, there should be no tension on the epidermal reapproximation. This can then be closed with either subcutaneous 5-0 or 6-0 Monocryl or a running external 5-0 fast-absorbing suture. Skin glue is a consideration for all skin closures. The fast-absorbing suture must be kept moist with an occlusive dressing ideally containing petroleum jelly for 6 days for ideal resorption and to minimize delayed resorption of the suture (Figs. 156.10–156.12).

Continued

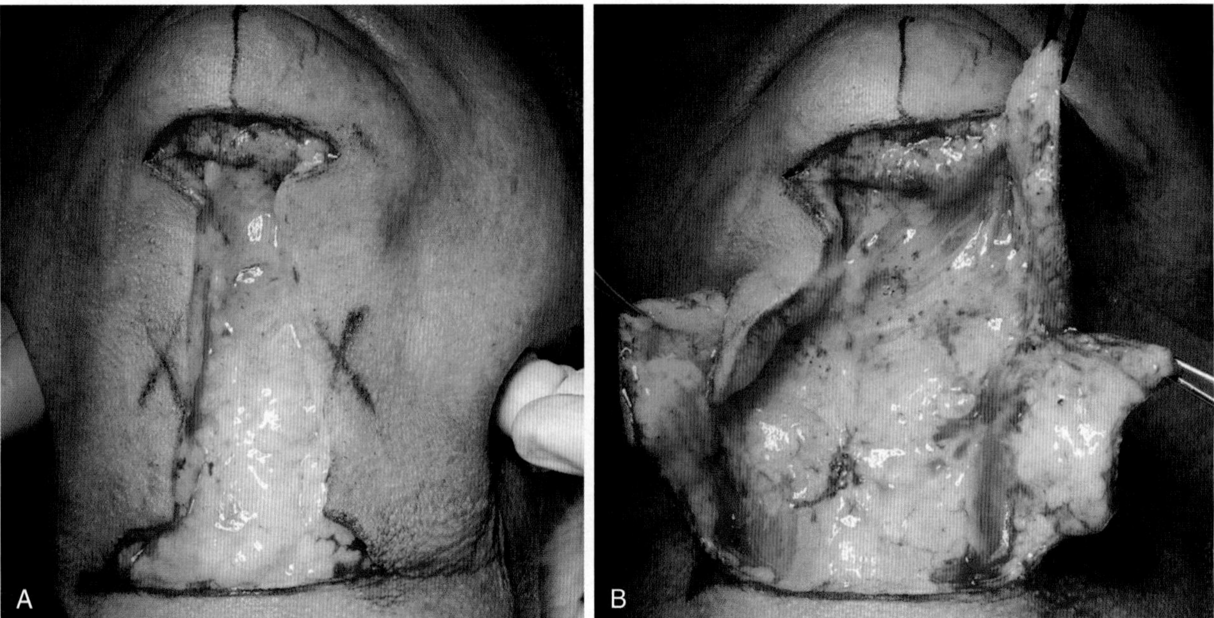

Figure 156.11 Wide undermining and advancement-rotation of flaps.

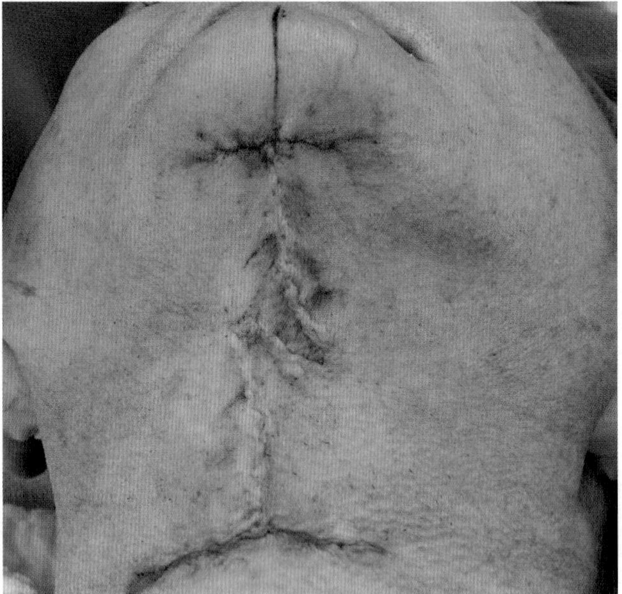

Figure 156.12 Single midline Z-plasty closure.

TECHNIQUE: Complex Z-Plasty—*cont'd*

STEP 5: Dressing

The head is wrapped with Coflex over one-half foam padding for 16 to 24 hours. This is followed by 4 days of near-continuous wear of a facial compression garment.

TECHNIQUE: W-Plasty

STEP 1: Planning

The concept of the W-plasty[46,47] is to break up the linear scar with irregularities[48] by applying a series of consecutive triangles, matched on the opposite side. The limb of each triangle should not be greater than 5.0 mm and not less than 3.0 mm. The triangular apex should not be less than 60 degrees to preserve viability. The interdigitation forms a single zig-zag line, effectively camouflaging the undesirable incision.

This scar resulted from excoriation after a routine facelift procedure. The wound was allowed to heal secondarily but resulted in the scar as seen at 1 year after initial presentation. Consent was obtained for W-plasty scar excision and serial dermabrasion or carbon dioxide laser treatment post operatively. Photos were taken and recorded. Diagrams were made to include a geometric opposing W-plasty incision for complete excision of the scar. This method was chosen primarily due to the scar crossing multiple aesthetic units of the face and it falls perpendicular to the RSTL. The W-plasty technique will allow the best randomization of the linear scar through careful interdigitation of fresh peripheral skin to reduce noticeability of the scar.

STEP 2: Anesthesia

A total of 10.0 cc of 2% lidocaine with 1:100,000 epinephrine is introduced in the area of planned incisions using a 27-gauge needle and syringe. A total of 100 cc of tumescent solution (1.0 cc of 1:1000 epinephrine, 500 mg lidocaine, 10 cc of $NaHCO_3$ in 500 cc normal saline IV infusion bag) was infused using a 22-gauge spinal needle into the subcutaneous tissues of the lateral cheek and jaw region, waiting a total of 15 minutes for hemostasis and anesthesia to be achieved.

STEP 3: Incision

Using a #11 blade, the skin is incised at full thickness along the lines diagrammed. The lateral tissue is undermined with facelift scissors to minimize tension upon closure.

STEP 4: Suturing

Closure is achieved with 4-0 Monocryl suture at the level of the dermis using a everting interrupted suture technique. Skin was reapproximated with 5-0 fast-absorbing suture.

STEP 5: Dressing

Petroleum jelly is applied as a postoperative dressing to assure proper resorption.

STEP 6: Postsurgical Scar Management

Dermabrasion with a fine diamond drum was performed at 6 weeks and two treatments with ScarFx (Luminis Ultrapulse carbon dioxide laser) using recommended parameters from the manufacturer (Figs. 156.13–156.16).

1. Advancement and rotational advancements of local and regional skin may be an ideal choice when local plasty techniques are insufficient for ideal reduction in scar appearance.
2. Skin graft or free flap reconstructive options exist for large defects that cannot otherwise be improved without distortion.

Avoidance and Management of Intraoperative Complications

The most important aspect of scar revision surgery is to ensure the patient is fully informed on the variety reconstructive options available including a discussion of donor site morbidity should a local, regional, or distant flap be used for reconstruction. The general principles of scar revision should be to minimize potential morbidity while providing the patient the greatest esthetic benefit.

Postoperative Considerations

Intraoperative injection may be appropriate with Botox or triamcinolone. All patients that undergo scar revision must be compliant with a rigid postoperative schedule of evaluation over the course of scar maturation, often extending beyond a year. The first visit should be at 24 hours to ensure no evidence of hematoma and excellence of viability and vascular return. Consideration should be made for intralesional injection at 2 weeks postoperatively. Topical silicone scar gel, silicone gel sheeting or compressive garments, and external ultrasound should be considered throughout the healing phases. Dermabrasion should be ideally considered at 6 to 8 weeks postoperatively to disrupt the later proliferative and early remodeling phase of the scar healing process. Often, these postoperative procedures are a challenge to monetize and are very consuming of staff and physician time and attention. Scheduled examination should take place every 6 to 8 weeks to ensure immediate intervention should pain, redness, itching, or elevation be identified.

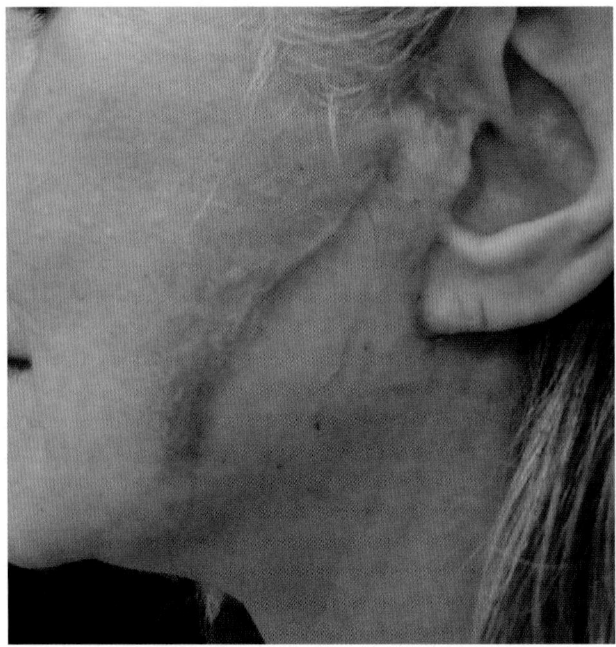

Figure 156.13 Scar prior to removal.

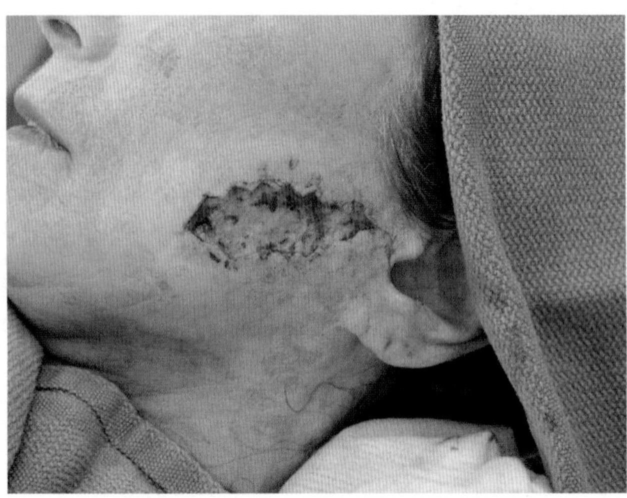

Figure 156.15 Excised region of W-plasty.

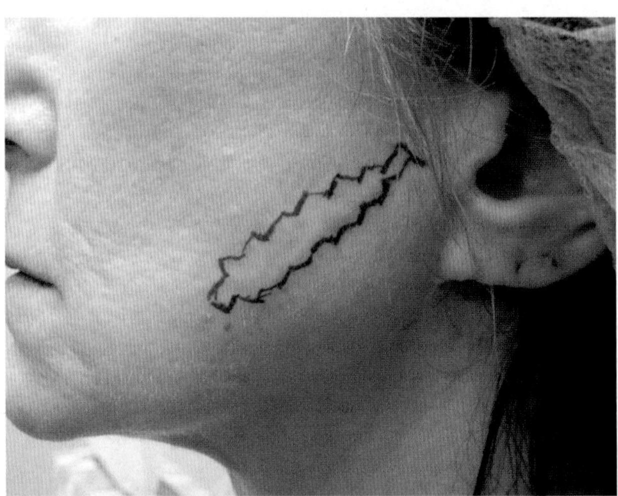

Figure 156.14 W-plasty design.

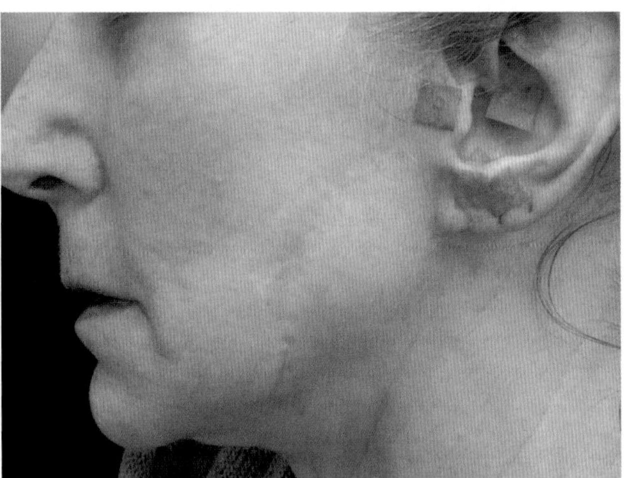

Figure 156.16 Results at 6 months.

References

1. Garg S, Dahiya N, Gupta S. Surgical scar revision: an overview. *J Cutan Aesthet Surg.* 2014;7(1):3–13.
2. Wallace HA, Basehore BM, Zito PM. Wound healing phases. In: *StatPearls.* StatPearls Publishing; 2020.
3. Rodrigues M, Kosaric N, Bonham CA, Gurtner GC. Wound healing: a cellular perspective. *Physiol Rev.* 2019;99(1):665–706.
4. Levenson SM, Geever EF, Crowley LV, Oates JF III, Berard CW, Rosen H. The healing of rat skin wounds. *Ann Surg.* 1965;161:293–308.
5. Ireton JE, Unger JG, Rohrich RJ. The role of wound healing and its everyday application in plastic surgery: a practical perspective and systematic review. *Plast Reconstr Surg Glob Open.* 2013;1(1):e10–e19. Published 2013.
6. Bayat A, McGrouther DA, Ferguson MW. Skin scarring. *BMJ.* 2003;326(7380):88–92.
7. Mustoe TA, Cooter RD, Gold MH, et al. International advisory panel on scar management. International clinical recommendations on scar management. *Plast Reconstr Surg.* 2002;110(2):560–571.
8. Gold MH, Berman B, Clementoni MT, Gauglitz GG, Nahai F, Murcia C. Updated international clinical recommendations on scar management: part 1—evaluating the evidence. *Dermatol Surg.* 2014;40(8):817–824.
9. Gold MH, McGuire M, Mustoe TA, et al. International advisory panel on scar management. Updated international clinical recommendations on scar management: part 2—algorithms for scar prevention and treatment. *Dermatol Surg.* 2014;40(8):825–831.
10. Powers PS, Sarkar S, Goldgof DB, Cruse CW, Tsap LV. Scar assessment: current problems and future solutions. *J Burn Care Rehabil.* 1999;20(1 Pt 1):54–60.
11. Schweinfurth JM, Fedok F. Avoiding pitfalls and unfavorable outcomes in scar revision. *Facial Plast Surg.* 2001;17(4):273–278.
12. Staley MJ, Richard RL. Use of pressure to treat hypertrophic burn scars. *Adv Wound Care.* 1997;10(3):44–46.
13. Hsu KC, Luan CW, Tsai YW. Review of silicone gel sheeting and silicone gel for the prevention of hypertrophic scars and keloids. *Wounds.* 2017;29(5):154–158.

14. Walker JJ. Ultrasound therapy for keloids. *S Afr Med J.* 1983;64(8):270.
15. Reiffel RS. Prevention of hypertrophic scars by long-term paper tape application. *Plast Reconstr Surg.* 1995;96(7):1715–1718.
16. Havlik RJ. Vitamin E and wound healing: safety and efficacy reports. *Plast Reconstruct Surg.* 1997;100(7):1901–1902.
17. Kovalic JJ, Perez CA. Radiation therapy following keloidectomy: a 20-year experience. *Int J Radiat Oncol Biol Phys.* 1989;17(1):77–80.
18. Janssen de Limpens AM. The local treatment of hypertrophic scars and keloids with topical retinoic acid. *Br J Dermatol.* 1980;103(3):319–323.
19. Rusciani L, Rossi G, Bono R. Use of cryotherapy in the treatment of keloids. *J Dermatol Surg Oncol.* 1993;19(6):529–534.
20. van Leeuwen MCE, van der Wal MBA, Bulstra AJ, et al. Intralesional cryotherapy for treatment of keloid scars: a prospective study. *Plast Reconstr Surg.* 2015;135(2):580–589.
21. Bailin P. Use of the CO_2 laser for non-PWS cutaneous lesions. In: Arndt KA, Noe JM, Rosen S, eds. *Cutaneous Laser Therapy: Principles and Methods.* John Wiley; 1983:187–200.
22. Bijlard E, Steltenpool S, Niessen FB. Intralesional 5-fluorouracil in keloid treatment: a systematic review. *Acta Derm Venereol.* 2015;95(7):778–782.
23. Morelli Coppola M, Salzillo R, Segreto F, Persichetti P. Triamcinolone acetonide intralesional injection for the treatment of keloid scars: patient selection and perspectives. *Clin Cosmet Investig Dermatol.* 2018;11:387–396. Published 2018.
24. Pittet B, Rubbia-Brandt L, Desmoulière A, et al. Effect of gamma-interferon on the clinical and biologic evolution of hypertrophic scars and Dupuytren's disease: an open pilot study. *Plast Reconstr Surg.* 1994;93(6):1224–1235.
25. Larrabee WF Jr, East CA, Jaffe HS, Stephenson C, Peterson KE. Intralesional interferon gamma treatment for keloids and hypertrophic scars. *Arch Otolaryngol Head Neck Surg.* 1990;116(10):1159–1162.
26. Bi M, Sun P, Li D, Dong Z, Chen Z. Intralesional injection of botulinum toxin type A compared with intralesional injection of corticosteroid for the treatment of hypertrophic scar and keloid: a systematic review and meta-analysis. *Med Sci Monit.* 2019;25:2950–2958.
27. España A, Solano T, Quintanilla E. Bleomycin in the treatment of keloids and hypertrophic scars by multiple needle punctures. *Dermatol Surg.* 2001;27(1):23–27.
28. O'Kane S, Ferguson MW. Transforming growth factor beta s and wound healing. *Int J Biochem Cell Biol.* 1997;29(1):63–78.
29. Klinger M, Caviggioli F, Klinger FM, et al. Autologous fat graft in scar treatment. *J Craniofac Surg.* 2013;24(5):1610–1615.
30. Henry SL, Concannon MJ, Kaplan PA, Diaz-Arias AA. The inhibitory effect of minocycline on hypertrophic scarring. *Plast Reconstr Surg.* 2007;120(1):80–88.
31. Yrjänheikki J, Tikka T, Keinänen R, Goldsteins G, Chan PH, Koistinaho J. A tetracycline derivative, minocycline, reduces inflammation and protects against focal cerebral ischemia with a wide therapeutic window. *Proc Natl Acad Sci USA.* 1999;96(23):13496–13500.
32. Schnee JM, Hsueh WA. Angiotensin II, adhesion, and cardiac fibrosis. *Cardiovasc Res.* 2000;46(2):264–268.
33. Steckelings UM, Wollschläger T, Peters J, Henz BM, Hermes B, Artuc M. Human skin: source of and target organ for angiotensin II. *Exp Dermatol.* 2004;13(3):148–154.
34. Reish RG, Eriksson E. Scars: a review of emerging and currently available therapies. *Plast Reconstr Surg.* 2008;122(4):1068–1078.
35. Kim I, Mogford JE, Witschi C, Nafissi M, Mustoe TA. Inhibition of prolyl 4-hydroxylase reduces scar hypertrophy in a rabbit model of cutaneous scarring. *Wound Repair Regen.* 2003;11(5):368–372. PubMed: 12950641.
36. Reid RR, Mogford JE, Butt R, deGiorgio-Miller A, Mustoe TA. Inhibition of procollagen C-proteinase reduces scar hypertrophy in a rabbit model of cutaneous scarring. *Wound Repair Regen.* 2006;14(2):138–141. PubMed: 16630102.
37. Mancoll JS, Macauley RL, Phillips LG. The inhibitory effect of tamoxifen on keloid fibroblasts. *Surg Forum.* 1996;47:718–720.
38. Brahmatewari J, Serafini A, Serralta V, Mertz PM, Eaglstein WH. The effects of topical transforming growth factor-beta2 and anti-transforming growth factor-beta2,3 on scarring in pigs. *J Cutan Med Surg.* 2000;4(3):126–131. PubMed: 11003716.
39. Wilgus TA, Vodovotz Y, Vittadini E, Clubbs EA, Oberyszyn TM. Reduction of scar formation in full-thickness wounds with topical celecoxib treatment. *Wound Repair Regen.* 2003;11(1):25–34. PubMed: 12581424.
40. Moran ML. Scar revision. *Otolaryngol Clin North Am.* 2001;34(4):767–780, vi.
41. Fattahi TT. An overview of facial aesthetic units. *J Oral Maxillofac Surg.* 2003;61(10):1207–1211.
42. Borges AF. Relaxed skin tension lines. *Dermatol Clin.* 1989;7(1):169–177.
43. Rees TD, Liverett DM, Guy CL. The effect of cigarette smoking on skin-flap survival in the face lift patient. *Plast Reconstr Surg.* 1984;73(6):911–915.
44. Riefkohl R, Wolfe JA, Cox EB, McCarty KS Jr. Association between cutaneous occlusive vascular disease, cigarette smoking, and skin slough after rhytidectomy. *Plast Reconstr Surg.* 1986;77(4):592–595.
45. Berg-Knudsen T, Ingvaldsen C, Mørk G, Tønseth K. Tidsskriftet. 29 June 2020 Tidsskr Nor Legeforen. https://aneskey.com/post-excisional-wound-closure-chapter-for-rural-surgeons/
46. Penn J. Zigzag modification of the tubed-pedicle flap. *Br J Plast Surg.* 1948;1(2):110.
47. Rodgers BJ, Williams EF, Hove CR. W-plasty and geometric broken line closure. *Facial Plast Surg.* 2001;17(4):239–244.
48. Goutos I, Yousif AH, Ogawa R. W-plasty in scar revision: geometrical considerations and suggestions for site-specific design modifications. *Plast Reconstr Surg Glob Open.* 2019;7(4):e2179.

CHAPTER 157

Neuromodulators and Injectable Fillers

Courtney Caplin

Neuromodulators

Armamentarium

Topical anesthetic of choice: BLT, EMLA	Botulinum toxin of choice: Botox, Dysport, Xeomin, Jeuveau	1-mL syringe with 25-gauge, 1-inch needle: used to draw up toxin. The longer needle allows the operator to reach the bottom of a bottle
Alcohol wipes to cleanse skin	0.9% Sodium chloride (normal saline): although many brands recommend normal saline without preservative, using bacteriostatic saline is less painful upon injection and often preferred by the injector	32-gauge, 1/2-inch needle: the 25-gauge needle is removed from the 1-mL syringe and replaced with the 32-gauge needle for injection
Gauze	3-mL syringe with 18-gauge, 1-inch needle: used to draw up saline to reconstitute the toxin	Alternatively, the rubber stopper can be removed from the bottle and 1-mL insulin syrgine can be used to draw up toxin and deliver

History of the Procedure

Botulism is derived from the Latin word for sausage, "betulus," after a food poisoning outbreak that occurred in Germany in the late 1700s. In the late 1800s, Van Ermengem concluded that botulism was not an infection but rather intoxication from a toxin produced by *Clostridium botulinum*, a spore-forming obligate anaerobic bacterium. Later in the 1900s, after another outbreak of food poisoning from canned white beans, doctors observed that their patients experienced xerostomia and xeropthalmia, which gave forth the idea of therapeutic use by modulating the neurotransmitter acetylcholine.[1]

The *Clostridium* bacterium was studied, and botulinum toxin A was isolated and purified. In the 1940s, the US government allowed academic investigations, and in 1977, the FDA approved clinical trials for strabismus. In the 1980s, while studying botulinum toxin A (Oculinum) for the treatment of blepharospasm, Dr. Jean Carruthers, an oculoplastics surgeon, noted that her patient's glabella rhytids were gone. Her husband, Dr. Alastair Carruthers, a dermatologist, investigated cosmetic treatment, which led to the first publication for cosmetic use in 1992.[1-3]

Although approved for alternative uses prior, Allergan Inc. received FDA approval for Botox for glabellar rhytids in 2002. Ipsen Pharmaceuticals introduced Dysport for cosmetic use in 2009. Merz followed shortly with Xeomin in 2010, and Jeuvau, the newest botulinum toxin for cosmetic use was introduced by Evolus in 2019 (Table 157.1).[4]

Indications for the Use of the Procedure

Botulinum toxin A has numerous indications, from migraines to bladder dysfunction; however, with regard to facial aesthetics, the toxin is used to weaken the muscles of facial expression, thereby softening or eliminating facial rhytids caused by muscular contraction. The most commonly treated areas include the horizontal lines of the forehead (caused by frontalis contraction), the vertical and horizontal lines of the glabellar region (caused by the paired corrugator supercilii muscles and procerus contraction), and crow's feet (caused by the orbicularis oculi contraction).[5]

For the mechanism of action, the botulinum toxin blocks neuromuscular transmission by irreversibly binding to the presynaptic terminal and inhibiting the release of acetylcholine. This inhibition occurs as the neurotoxin cleaves the Synaptosomal-Associated Protein, 25kDA (SNAP-25) SNAP-25, a protein necessary for exocytosis of acetylcholine from vesicles situated within nerve endings, inhibiting the communication of the neurotransmitter with the muscle.[5]

Table 157.1 Comparison of Neuromodulators[6,8,17]

Trademark Name	Generic Name	Manufacturer	Units per Standard Vial	Relative Units for Glabella
Botox	Onabotulinumtoxin A	Allergan	50, 100 unit vials	20 units
Dysport	Abobotulinumtoxin A	Galderma	300, 500 unit vials	50 units
Xeomin	IncobotulinumtoxinA	Merz	50, 100 unit vials	20 units
Jeuveau (Newtox)	PrabotulinumtoxinA	Evolus	100 units	20 units

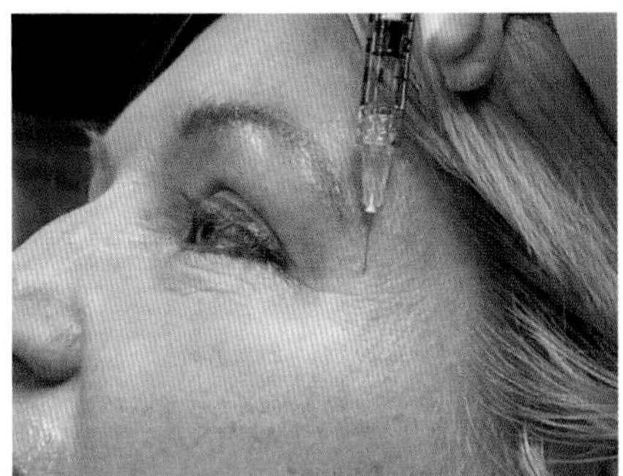
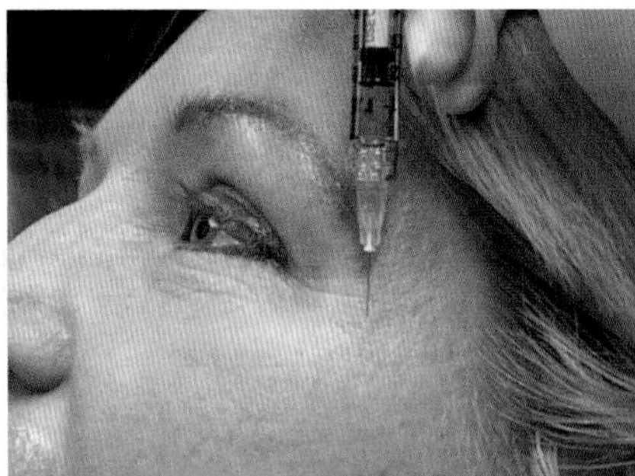
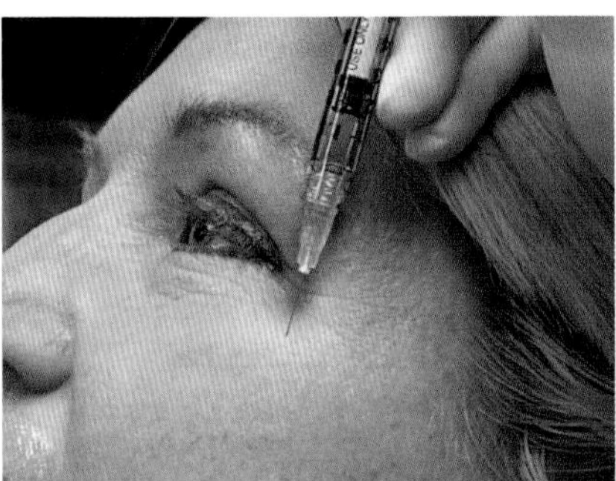

Figure 157.1 Injection sites for the orbicularis oculi.

Limitations

With any cosmetic procedure, expectations should always be set. The amount of correction may be limited with a single dosage. However, with time and serial neurotoxin injection, atrophy of the muscle can occur to further soften long-standing lines.

With regard to neurotoxins, one of the biggest limitations is the amount of weakening of the frontalis a patient can tolerate when brow ptosis is already present. As the frontalis is the only muscle of facial expression to raise the eyebrow, if neurotoxin is injected to weaken its action further, the brow will sit in its lowest position. The ideal brow position for a male sits 0 to 2 mm above the supraorbital rim. The ideal brow position for a female also starts at 0 to 2 mm above the supraorbital rim and then up arches 8 to 10 mm from the rim, and the tail can vary from 10 to 15 mm above the rim.

The desire to correct forehead wrinkles can be problematic for patients whose brows have descended and are chronically using their frontalis to keep their brows lifted. These patients are also the same ones who typically have the deepest rhytids from the hyperactivity of this muscle, and often present complaining of these lines. These patients must be cautioned that if the muscle is overly weakened, then the brow will sit lower and their eyelids will feel heavy. These patients are often best suited for a brow lift surgery.

General dosages are recommended by product manufactures; however, one must evaluate each individual as muscle strength and size vary. For example, 20 units of onabotulinum toxinA may be an average for the glabella; however, a 24-year-old, petite female with dynamic rhytids may need only 12 units, and a muscular, 53-year-old male with resting rhytids may need 50. Each patient and each area of injection should be assessed and dosed accordingly (Figs. 157.1 and 157.2).

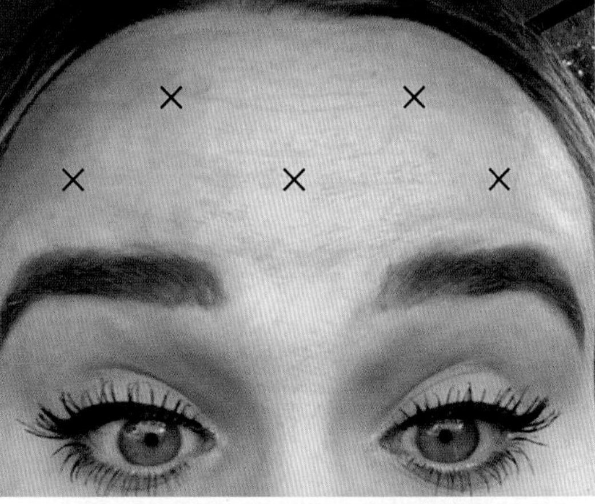
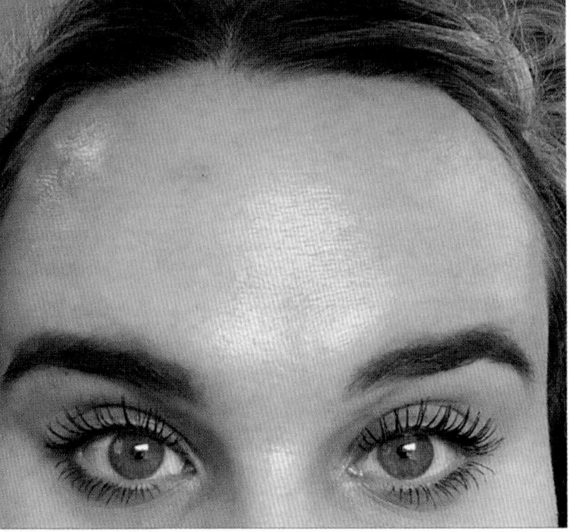

Figure 157.2 Frontalis injection sites.

Contraindication to Neurotoxins

- Known hypersensitivity or allergy to botulinum toxin (or any component including human albumin)
- Infection at injection site[5-8]

Relative Contraindications to Neurotoxin

- Known neuromuscular disease such as amyotrophic lateral sclerosis, myasthenia gravis, or Lambert–Eaton syndrome
- Use of aminoglycoside or spectinomycin antibiotics, which are known to affect neuromuscular transmission and potentiate the effects of botulinum toxin
- Pregnancy
- Lactation[5-8]

Table 157.2 Dilution Calculations

Vial	Saline
50 units	1.25 mL
100 units	2.5 mL

Table 157.3 Recommended Units of Botox per Location[7]

Location	Botox
Glabella	20 units
Frontalis	20 units
Orbicularis Oculi	24 units

TECHNIQUE: Toxin

STEP 1: Reconstitution Of Product

The injector can control how dilute the product is by the amount of saline added to the vial. The most common dilution is 4 units of Botox/Xeomin/Jeuveau /0.1 mL or 12 units of Dysport/0.1 mL (Table 157.2).

STEP 2: Preoperative Photos

Standard preoperative photos are taken at rest and with dynamic expression using the muscle to be injected with toxin.

STEP 3: Topical Anesthetic

Topical anesthetic is applied to the area of injection.

STEP 4: Injection

After the skin is properly cleansed, the patient may be asked to animate, and the needle is injected through skin to the level of the muscle. The injection should be aimed at the belly of muscle, not the rhytid itself. The desired amount of toxin is then injected (Table 157.3).

Postoperative Considerations and Complications

- After neurotoxin injection, patients should be instructed to avoid lying supine for four hours to help limit the potential migration of product.
- Headache: Care is taken not to hit the periosteum as this has an increased incidence of postoperative pain. Should headache occur, typical over the counter medication, such as acetaminophen, should be ample treatment.
- Eyelid edema: Edema can be a result of the trauma of injection. The patient should be instructed to keep head elevated and use ice as needed.
- Asymmetry: Symmetry of the face and muscular activity should be assessed prior to injection. If otherwise symmetric, uniform and consistent dosage of injection should be performed to keep muscular activity and the resulting facial expressions symmetric.
- Brow ptosis: Appropriate preoperative evaluation must be performed to avoid injecting an already ptotic brow as discussed previously. Additionally, treating the glabella simultaneously should be considered to help counteract the depressor muscles contributing to brow ptosis. Injection of the frontalis should also be kept at a minimum of 2 cm above the eyebrow.
- Eyelid ptosis: Care must be taken to avoid injecting too closely to the levator palpebrae superioris. As a rule of thumb, injection should be a minimum of 1 cm from the supraorbital rim and central eyebrow. Should eyelid ptosis occur, ipraclomide drops can be prescribed to help open the eye during social occasions. Although time for reinnervation of the levator muscle is the ultimate cure, alpha agonist drops work on Mueller's muscle for temporary relief.
- Injection site infection.[5]

Injectable Fillers

Armamentarium

Topical anesthetic of choice: BLT, EMLA
Alcohol wipes to cleanse skin
Injectable filler of choice
Gauze
Cold compress

Table 157.4 Comparison of Injectable Fillers[18-31]

Manufacturer	Product	Description	Duration of Action
Allergan	Juvederm Ultra	Hyaluronic acid	Up to 1 year
	Juvederm Ultra Plus	Hyaluronic acid	Up to 1 year
	Juvederm Volbella	Hyaluronic acid	Up to 1 year
	Juvederm Vollure	Hyaluronic acid	Up to 1.5 years
	Juvederm Voluma	Hyaluronic acid	Up to 2 years
Galderma	Restylane	Hyaluronic acid	Up to 1.5 years
	Restylane Silk	Hyaluronic acid	Up to 6 months
	Restylane Kysse	Hyaluronic acid	Up to 1 year
	Restylane Defyne	Hyaluronic acid	Up to 1 year
	Restylane Refyne	Hyaluronic acid	Up to 1 year
	Restylane Lyft	Hyaluronic acid	Up to 1.5 years
	Sculptra	Poly-L lactic acid	Up to 2 years
Suneva	Bellafill	Polymethylmethacylate (PMMA) and bovine collagen	Up to 5 years
Merz	Radiesse	Calcium hydroxylapatite	Up to 1 year
	Belotero	Hyaluronic acid	Up to 6 months
Alcon	Sikilon 1000	Silicone	Permanent

History of the Procedure

The most popular fillers are hyaluronic acid-based products that are hydrophilic in nature, absorbing water to plump, and then dissolve with isovolumetric degradation back into water and carbon dioxide. Galderma introduced Restalyne as the first FDA-approved cosmetic hyaluronic acid filler in 2003. Allergan followed shortly with Juvederm in 2005. Since then, many others have entered the cosmetic market. The various hyaluronic acid fillers differ by particle size, G prime, cross-linking, and duration of effect. Many also have the option to be premixed with lidocaine. Other types of fillers such as Bellafill and Sculptra are biostimulants, which promote the patient's own collagen production. These are considered longer lasting because even though the product itself has a finite duration, the collagen that the body produces remains.[9,10]

Indications and Limitations

As we age, we lose volume from the face, and as volume loss occurs, gravity takes effect and pulls on the skin creating lines and folds. By restoring volume, facial rejuvenation can be achieved. However, the degree of skin laxity must be assessed. Most fillers are purchased in syringes between 0.5 mL and 1.0 mL. Evaluation of the patient and assessment of the degree of skin laxity must be made in order to discuss options with the patient and when a surgical procedure will provide a greater benefit.

The intended site, depth, and frequency of the various fillers depend on the individual product's composition and properties, and the manufacturer's recommendations should be considered. Hyaluronic acid fillers are one of the most user friendly and versatile products. They are commonly used to augment the cheeks, nasolabial folds, lips, tear troughs, temples, and chin. Alternatively, polymethylmethacrylate should be avoided in and around the orbicularis oculi and orbicularis oris as the sphincter-like contraction of the muscle has been correlated with granuloma formation. Silicone is both permanent itself and a biostimulant and not suggested for the novice injector. It can be used in select cases for postsurgical corrections but is otherwise focused on lip augmentation (Table 157.4).[11-13]

Contraindications

- Known allergy or hypersensitivity to the filler or any of its components
- Infection at injection site

TECHNIQUE: For Cheeks

STEP 1: Preoperative Photos

Standard preoperative photos are taken in frontal, 3/4 quarter, and profile views at rest.

STEP 2: Topical Anesthetic

Topical anesthetic is applied to the area of injection.

STEP 3: Markings

After the area is cleansed, markings are made with one line running from the lateral canthus to oral commissure and a second line from lateral nasal sill to root of helix forming four quadrants in order to help symmetric analysis and augmentation with filler.

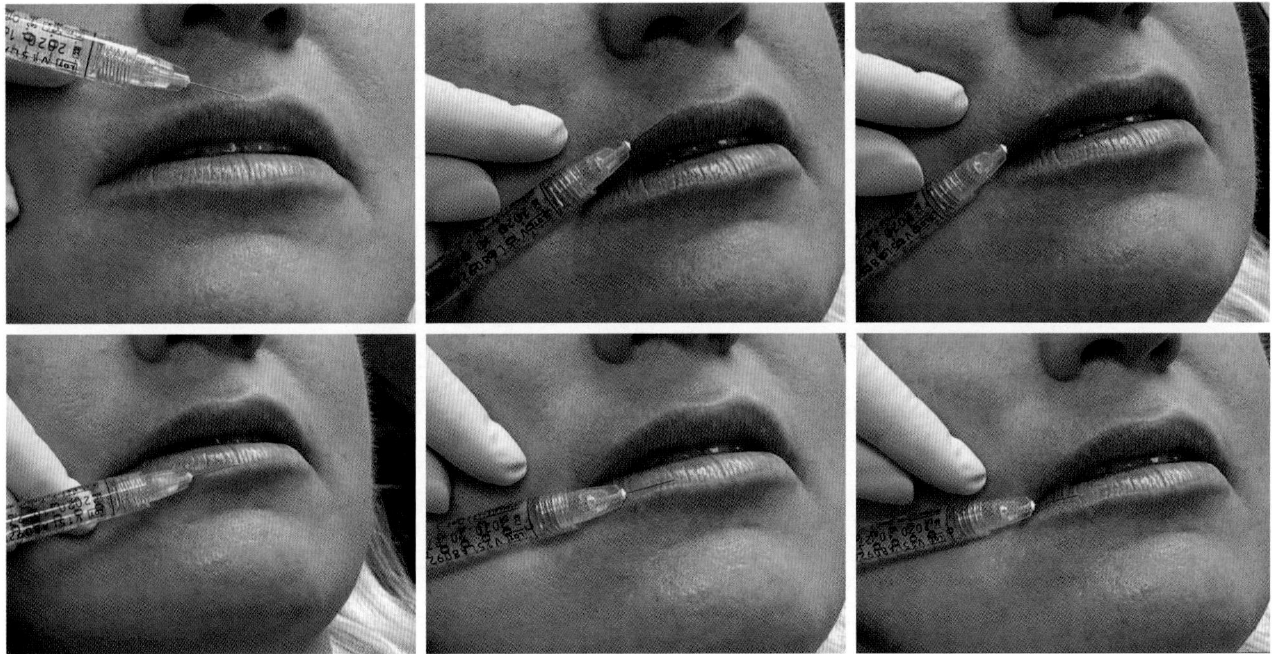

Figure 157.3 Step 3.

STEP 4: Injection Of Malar Eminence

The needle is inserted and aspiration attempted. Filler is then injected in small boluses in a deep plane above periosteum augmenting the zygoma in the superior lateral quadrant formed by the intersecting lines. The largest bolus should focus over the malar eminence approximately 1 cm lateral and 1.5 cm inferior to the lateral canthus.

STEP 5: Subsequent Injections

Sequential boluses are then injected at various depths for a smooth contour of the cheek.[14]

STEP 6: Aftercare

Massage as needed to smooth any lumpiness and apply cold compress.

TECHNIQUE: Nasolabial Folds

STEP 1: Preoperative Photos

Standard preoperative photos are taken in frontal, 3/4 quarter, and profile views at rest.

STEP 2: Topical Anesthetic

Topical anesthetic is applied to the area of injection.

STEP 3: Injection Of Pyriform Rim

After the area is cleansed, the needle is inserted, and aspiration attempted. Filler is then bloused deep along the pyriform rim, medial to the fold.

STEP 4: Subsequent Injections

Filler is then injected at varying depths (deeper for folds/more superficial for wrinkles) filling in the deficit medial to the fold in a retrograde fashion.[15]

STEP 5: Aftercare

Massage as needed to smooth any lumpiness and apply cold compress.

TECHNIQUE: For Lips

STEP 1: Preoperative Photos

Standard preoperative photos are taken in frontal, 3/4 quarter, and profile views at rest and smiling.

STEP 2: Topical Anesthetic

Topical anesthetic is applied to the lips and intraorally in the maxillary and mandibular vestibule.

STEP 3: Injection Of Vermillion Border

After the area is cleansed, the needle is inserted, an attempt is made to aspirate, and then filler is then injected along the white roll for lip definition followed by massage (Fig. 157.3).

STEP 4: Injection Of Lip

For added fullness and volume, the injector should attempt to aspirate, and then filler is injected into the body of the lip with care to avoid the labial artery (Fig. 157.4).

STEP 5: Aftercare

Massage as needed to smooth any lumpiness and apply cold compress (Fig. 157.5).

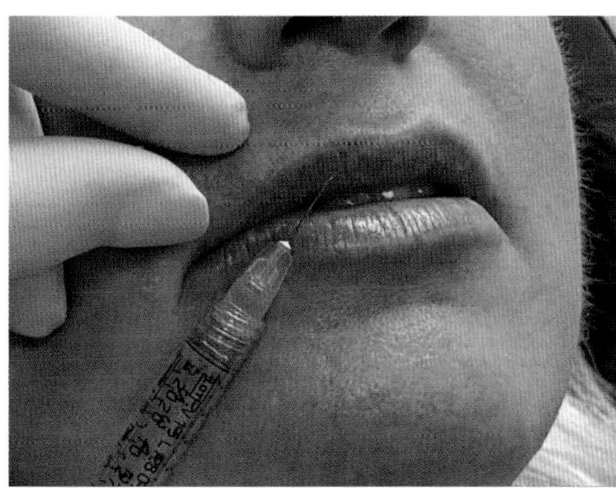
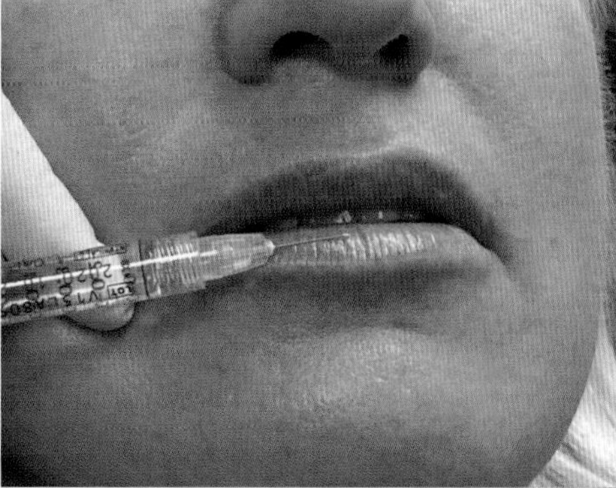

Figure 157.4 Step 4. Allergan Aesthetics.

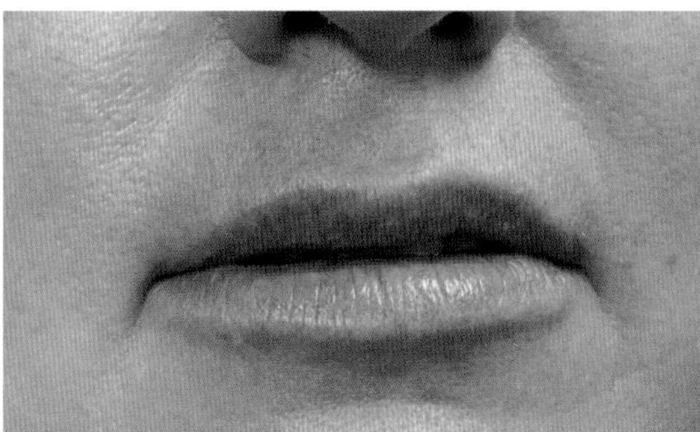
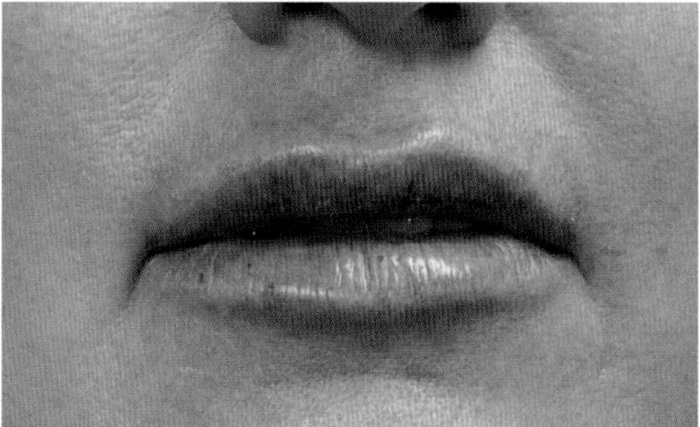

Figure 157.5 Before and after one syringe of hyaluronic acid filler.

Postoperative Considerations/Complications

- Edema and ecchymosis: These are the most common post injection reactions. As these are expected to an extent, it would be difficult to even consider them to be a complication. However, since most patients desire injectables as a noninvasive option, they must be prepared for the expected recovery process. If immediate bleeding occurs, pressure should be applied, and a cold compress should be provided post care. Patients should be instructed to keep their head elevated and consider sleeping with an additional pillow. Patients should be warned that after lying supine overnight, that edema can appear most alarming when they wake.
- Intravascular injection and necrosis: Should an intravascular injection occur, the injection site should immediately be injected with hyaluronidase and massaged. Additionally, a warm compress and nitroglycerin paste can be applied to region of decreased perfusion. A course of aspirin therapy should also be considered. Hyaluronidase is an emergency drug and should be readily available whenever a hyaluronic acid filler is being injected. A skin test can be considered to check for hypersensitivity depending on the emergency and severity of compromise. Knowledge of anatomy along with slow and deliberate aspiration and injection technique should be performed by the injector in order to minimize and avoid the possibility of vascular injection.
- Tyndall effect: Superficial injection can result in a blue hue and noticeable lump of filler. Should this occur, the area of injection can either be expressed after puncture of the site, or hyaluronidase can be used to dissolve it.
- Asymmetry: Symmetry of the face and volume should be assessed prior to injection. If the face is otherwise symmetric, uniform and consistent injection should be performed.
- Injection site infection[16]

References

1. Niamtu J. Neuromodulators (neurotoxins). In: *Cosmetic Facial Surgery*. Elsevier; 2018.
2. Carruthers A, Carruthers J. Practical botulinum toxin anatomy. In: *Botulinum Toxin*. 2nd ed. Saunders; 2008:31–42.
3. Carruthers J, Carruthers A. The use of botulinum toxin type A in the upper face. *Facial Plast Surg Clin North Am*. 2006;14(3):253–260.
4. Kontis TC, Lacombe VG. Neurotoxins overview. In: *Cosmetic Injection Techniques: A Text and Video Guide to Neurotoxins and Fillers*. Thieme; 2019:6–7.
5. Haggerty CJ, Laughlin RM, Panossian AJ. Botulinum toxin type A (botox). In: *Atlas of Operative Oral and Maxillofacial Surgery*. Wiley Blackwell; 2015.
6. Galderma Laboratories LP. *Dysport. Material safety data sheet*; 2019. galderma.com/dysport.
7. Allergan Aesthetics. *BOTOX Cosmetic. Material safety data sheet*; 2020. media.allergan.com.
8. Evolus Inc. *Jeuveau. Material safety data sheet*; 2019. jeuveau.evolus.com.
9. Niamtu J. Neuromodulators (neurotoxins). In: *Injectable Fillers, Lip Augmentations, Lip Reduction, Lip Lift*. Elsevier; 2018.

10. Allergan Aesthetics. *Juvéderm Ultra Plus. Material safety data sheet*; 2016. hcp.Juvederm.com.
11. Kontis TC, Lacombe VG. Fillers overview. In: *Cosmetic Injection Techniques: A Text and Video Guide to Neurotoxins and Fillers*. Thieme; 2019:92–94.
12. Kontis TC, Lacombe VG. Filler injection methods. In: *Cosmetic Injection Techniques: A Text and Video Guide to Neurotoxins and Fillers*. Thieme; 2019:98–99.
13. Kontis TC, Lacombe VG. Choosing the right filler. In: *Cosmetic Injection Techniques: A Text and Video Guide to Neurotoxins and Fillers*. Thieme; 2019:101–103.
14. Kontis TC, Lacombe VG. Filler injection for cheekbone augmentation. In: *Cosmetic Injection Techniques: A Text and Video Guide to Neurotoxins and Fillers*. Thieme; 2019:155–157.
15. Kontis TC, Lacombe VG. Filler injection for nasolabial folds. In: *Cosmetic Injection Techniques: A Text and Video Guide to Neurotoxins and Fillers*. Thieme; 2019:107–110.
16. Haggerty CJ, Laughlin RM, Panossian AJ. Soft tissue augmentation. In: *Atlas of Operative Oral and Maxillofacial Surgery*. Wiley Blackwell; 2015.
17. Allergan Aesthetics. *BOTOX Cosmetic. Material safety data sheet*; 2020.
18. Suneva Medical. *Bellafill. Material safety data sheet*; 2020. www.bellafill.com.
19. Galderma Labratories LP. *Sculptra. Material safety data sheet*; 2016. galderma.com/sculptra.
20. M. North America, Inc. *Belotero Balance. Material safety data sheet*; 2020. www.belotero.com.
21. Galderma Labratories LP. *Restylane Silk. Material safety data sheet*; 2017. galderma.com/restylane.
22. Galderma Labratories LP. *Restylane Kysse. Material safety data sheet*; 2020. galderma.com/restylane.
23. Galderma Labratories LP. *Restylane Defyne. Material safety data sheet*; 2016. galderma.com/restylane.
24. Galderma Labratories LP. *Restylane Lyft. Material safety data sheet*; 2018. galderma.com/restylane.
25. Galderma Labratories LP. *Restylane. Material safety data sheet*; 2016. galderma.com/restylane.
26. Galderma Labratories LP. *Restylane Refyne. Material safety data sheet*; 2016. galderma.com/restylane.
27. M. North America, Inc. *Radiesse. Material safety data sheet*; 2016. radiesse.com.
28. Allergan Aesthetics, Juvéderm Voluma VC. *Material safety data sheet*; 2020. Hcp.Juvederm.com.
29. Allergan Aesthetics. *Juvéderm Ultra. Material safety data sheet*; 2019. Hcp.Juvederm.com.
30. Allergan Aesthetics, Juvéderm Vollure XC. *Material safety data sheet*; 2019. Hcp.Juvederm.com.
31. Allergan Aesthetics, Juvéderm Volbella XC. *Material safety data sheet*; 2019. Hcp.Juvederm.com.

CHAPTER 158

Augmentation of the Midface and Mandible With Alloplastic Implants

Ron Caloss

Armamentarium

#10 Blade
Bone screws
Local anesthetic with epinephrine
Mayo scissors
Obwegeser retractors
Periosteal elevators
Tape/dressing material

History of the Procedure

Facial onlay implants have been used as standalone or with other esthetic procedures to rejuvenate and enhance facial contours for quite some time. Over the past three decades, onlay implants have been used as an adjunct to orthognathic surgery. Robiony was the first to report a case series on the simultaneous use of malar implants with a Le Fort osteotomy to correct malar hypoplasia.[1] Yaremchuk has described the use of implants as an adjunctive to orthognathic surgery by correcting contour irregularities or disharmonies after skeletal movements.[2,3] More recently, computer-assisted design (CAD)/computer-aided manufacturing (CAM) technology has allowed correction of facial asymmetries and residual deformities that exist in patients undergoing orthognathic surgery. In these situations, implants can be placed simultaneously or secondarily to improve facial balance and symmetry.[4]

Various polymers have been developed over time. These include silicone, high density porous polyethylene, polytetrafluoroethylene (Gore-Tex), methyl methacrylate, and polyether ether ketone. For the most part, these materials have been shown to be reliable with a relatively low complication profile and have several favorable characteristics, including structural stability. They are also easy to shape and are noncarcinogenic and bioinert to minimize inflammation and foreign body reaction.[5,6]

Indications for Use of the Procedure

Alloplastic onlay implants are used to improve the shape, definition, and balance of the face. They can be used alone or as an adjunct to other soft-tissue cosmetic procedures such as rhytidectomy.[7] They can be used in the setting of orthognathic surgery as an adjunct to improve facial balance in the infraorbital, malar, chin, and angle regions. Implants have also been used in the management of posttraumatic skeletal deformities. They offer a variety of advantages over autogenous grafts, including ease of shaping, the lack of resorption, and donor site morbidity.

Facial aging is characterized by ptosis of soft tissues and a loss of soft-tissue volume. The facial skeleton has itself been shown to change as one ages. If one has deficient skeletal support to begin with, the stigma of facial aging becomes even more pronounced over time.[8-10] Rejuvenation has come to focus on volume enhancement and not just repositioning of soft tissues with traditional rhytidectomy procedures. Fillers are commonly used to efface folds and contour irregularities. But when there is larger volume deficiency, implants can offer a more robust augmentation. Improving skeletal or hard tissue support enhances the suspension and drape of overlying soft tissue.[11,12]

Esthetic malar augmentation is indicated in individuals who frontally exhibit poor lateral cheek projection (bizygomatic width) in relation to the bigonial and bitemporal widths. Similarly, augmentation is indicated in those who exhibit poor cheek projection in the three-quarter oblique view.[13] A malar or submalar implant can be used to correct flattening that occurs secondary to ptosis and atrophy of the malar fat pad and create a smoother contour to the cheek. Infraorbital implants, such as a tear trough implant is indicated to correct a negative vector defect in which the globe is projecting anterior to the infraorbital rim. This implant may also efface a tear trough deformity.[14] If a patient presents with significant deficiency in both the infraorbital and malar region, stacked implants or custom implant may be indicated.

Table 158.1 Implantech and Medpor Implant Choices for Augmenting Various Regions of the Face.

Deficiency	Implantech	Medpor
Infraorbital	Flowers Tear Trough	———
Malar	Conform Terino Malar Shell	Extended Malar Shell
Infraorbital and malar	Flowers Tear Trough Extended Size	Design RZ Malar
Chin +/- jowling	Conform Extended Anatomical Chin	———
Jowling	Mittleman Prejowl	———
Angle lateral	Lateral Mandibular Angle	———
Angle vertical	Posterior Mandibular Angle	———
Angle lateral and inferior	———	Angle of the Mandible
Facial asymmetry	Stacked Stock or 3D Accuscan Patient-Specific (custom)	———

Esthetic chin augmentation is indicated when there is lack of adequate anterior projection of the chin relative to the midface and compromise of an esthetic cervicomental angle in profile view. In general, the chin should be 4 mm or so behind a line perpendicular to subnasally for females and less so for males. A well-defined smooth inferior border of the mandible separates the lower third of the face from the neck and enhances chin-neck esthetics.[13] An alloplastic extended chin implant is indicated if a patient is undergoing a rhytidectomy procedure and presents with microgenia and jowling. The implant will enhance support of the soft tissue, efface the jowls, and create a smoother contour to the inferior border.[7] A sliding osteotomy in this instance can accentuate jowling.

Mandibular angle augmentation is indicated when there is inadequate bigonial width or separation of the face and neck. In the esthetically pleasing face, the mandibular angle area is medial to the zygomatic area so that the face tapers slightly from the zygomatic area. The posterior body and angle can be augmented laterally and/or inferiorly to improve bigonial width and create a distinct separation of the face from the neck.[13]

The author utilizes implants as an adjunct to orthognathic procedures to manage skeletal deficiency or asymmetry that will not be corrected by the skeletal movements. Implants can bring balance to the entire face and counter the effects of aging. For instance, when a class III patient presents with significant midface hypoplasia that extends into the malar and infraorbital region, augmenting the midface above the Le Fort osteotomy will provide harmony to the entire midface, especially when a large advancement is indicated. When both the infraorbital and malar areas are deficient, the author likes to use an Implantech Flowers Tear Trough Extended implant (Table 158.1). This implant augments the infraorbital rim and extends laterally to also augment the malar area (Figs. 158.1 and 158.2). Additionally, patients that present with a prominent chin (class III) and deficient posterior facial height/high angle can benefit from augmentation of the angle. An implant in this situation will improve lower third harmony, angle definition, and separation of the face from the neck (Fig. 158.3).

Complex facial asymmetries can be difficult to manage with orthognathic procedures alone. After cant, yaw, and midline asymmetries are addressed, asymmetries sometimes persist. This is especially so with unilateral condylar hyperplasia and congenital deformities such as hemifacial microsomia. Facial implants, especially custom implants, are a great adjunct in these situations (Figs. 158.4 and 158.5).

Limitations and Contraindications

Implants should not be placed if there is active infection in surrounding areas. If skin, odontogenic, or sinus infections contaminate an adjacent implant, a biofilm may form on the implant surface. Chronic infections associated with bacteria living in biofilms are resistant to treatment with conventional antibiotics.[15] Therefore, the likelihood of needing to remove the implant is high.

The patient must have a recipient site that has adequate healing potential. A scarred or irradiated tissue bed should raise concern. Inadequate soft-tissue bulk and quality tissue overlying an implant increase the chance for implant extrusion. Any condition that leads to a patient being immunocompromised is a relative contraindication. This includes patients with uncontrolled diabetes and patients who smoke.[16]

Patients with a body dysmorphic disorder or similar psychiatric illness are not good candidates for cosmetic procedures. It is important to have a good understanding of a patient's motive and expectations when seeking cosmetic surgery. If the patient's perception or expectation appears unrealistic, consider not offering him/her treatment.

Implants can enhance orthognathic surgical procedures, but they should not be a substitute for managing skeletal hypoplasia associated with dentofacial deformities. One must recognize both the functional and esthetic benefits of moving the maxilla and/or mandible for someone that has an underlying skeletal malocclusion.

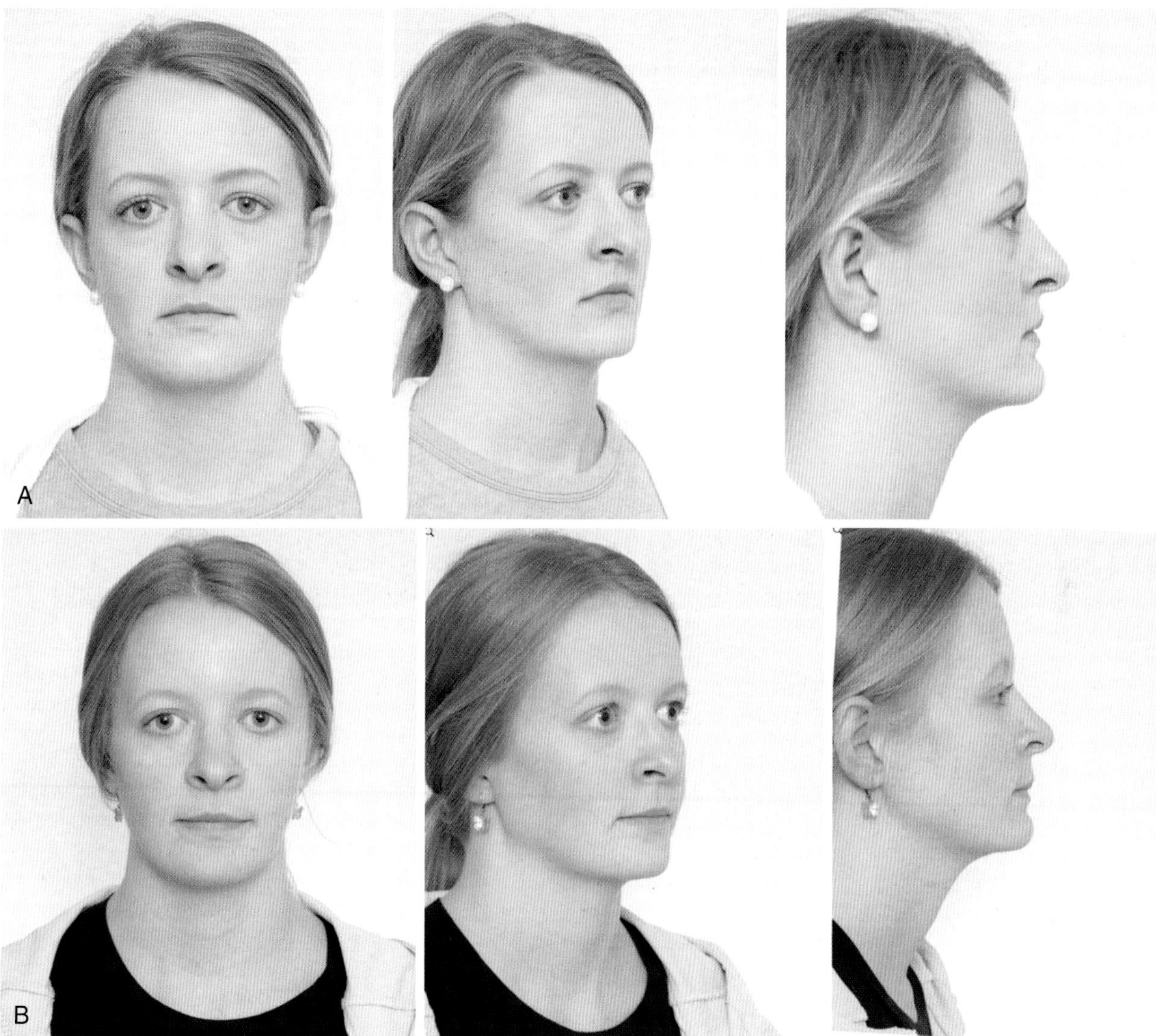

Figure 158.1 **A,** Preoperative. **B,** Twelve months postoperative. This patient underwent a Le Fort 1 advancement (7 mm) and down graft (3 mm) as well as a mandibular setback. She had simultaneous placement of an extended Implantech Flowers Tear Trough implant. This implant extends laterally over the body of the zygoma to also augment the malar area.

TECHNIQUE: Malar, Genial and Angle Augmentation

STEP 1: Selection of Appropriate Implant

The author will focus on the use of solid silicone (Implantech) and high density porous polyethylene (Medpor) implants. They come in a variety of stock designs and sizes to augment the midface and mandible as well as other areas such as the paranasal region and nasal bridge. Silicone implants eventually become encapsulated.[17] High density porous polyethylene allows soft-tissue and bone ingrowth over time.[18] This is thought to improve implant stability. A multitude of designs are available and can be found in both manufactures' catalogs.[19,20] Some of the various implants that the author uses are listed in Table 158.1.

Selection of the appropriate design and size of an implant is critical. Adding proper volume in the right location must be carefully considered. Incorrect choice can lead to patient and surgeon dissatisfaction. In most situations, a stock implant (as opposed to a custom one) will be used. Stock implants come in various shapes and styles. Sizes are typically small, medium and large, varying in width, height, and projection at the apex. Sizer sets are available to aid in the selection.

Continued

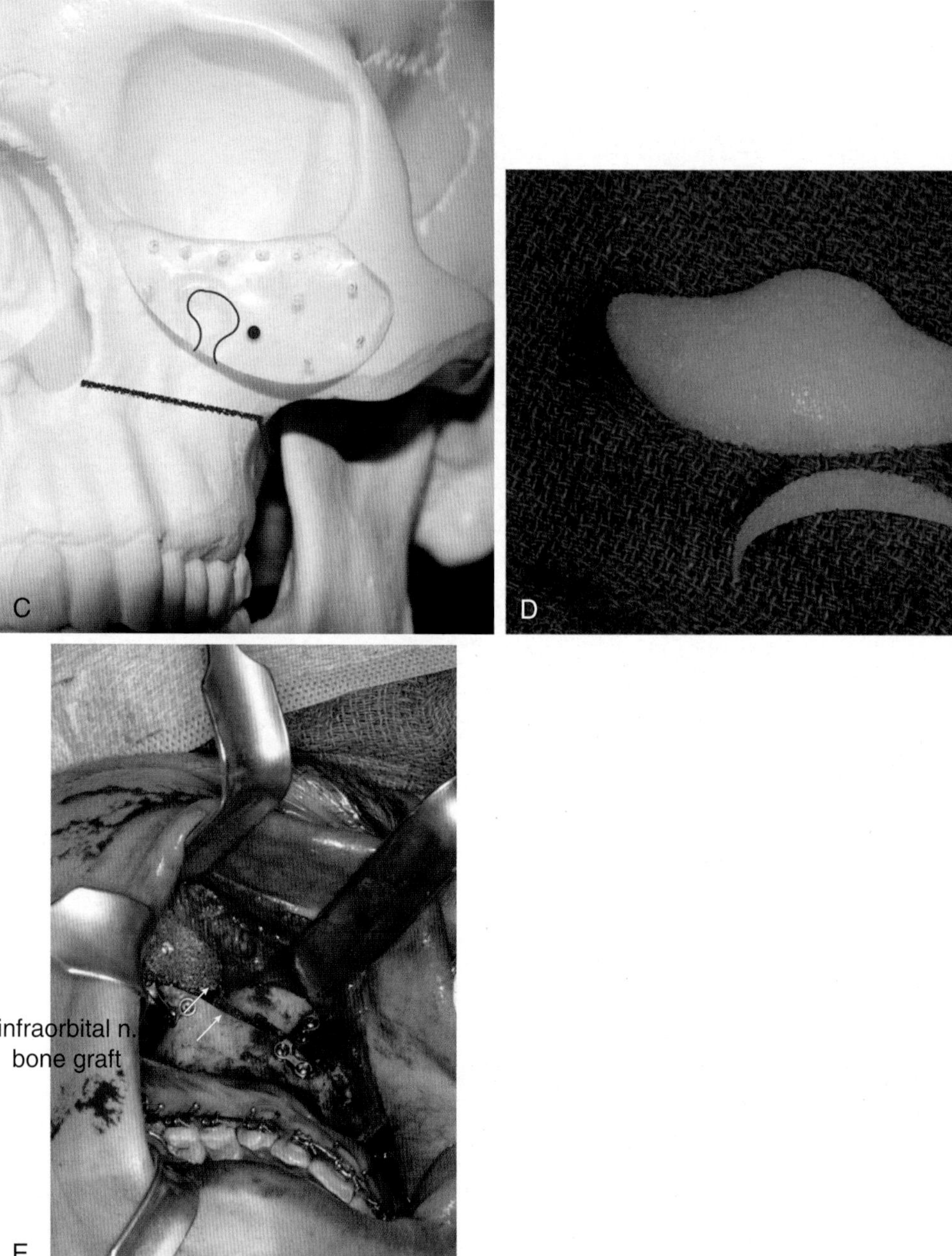

Figure 158.1, cont'd **C,** The Tear Trough implant is overlaid to the maxilla to show the relationship to the Le Fort osteotomy and infraorbital nerve. The red dot indicates the implant projection at the apex, which is 5 mm for this particular implant. Note that an extended Tear Trough implant extends laterally over the body of the zygoma to simultaneously augment the malar region. **D** and **E,** If a malar implant such as the Medpor one pictured here is placed when a Le Fort 1 advancement is being performed, the inferior aspect of the implant should be trimmed so that the implant sits above the osteotomy. The osteotomy gap can be bone grafted as shown here.

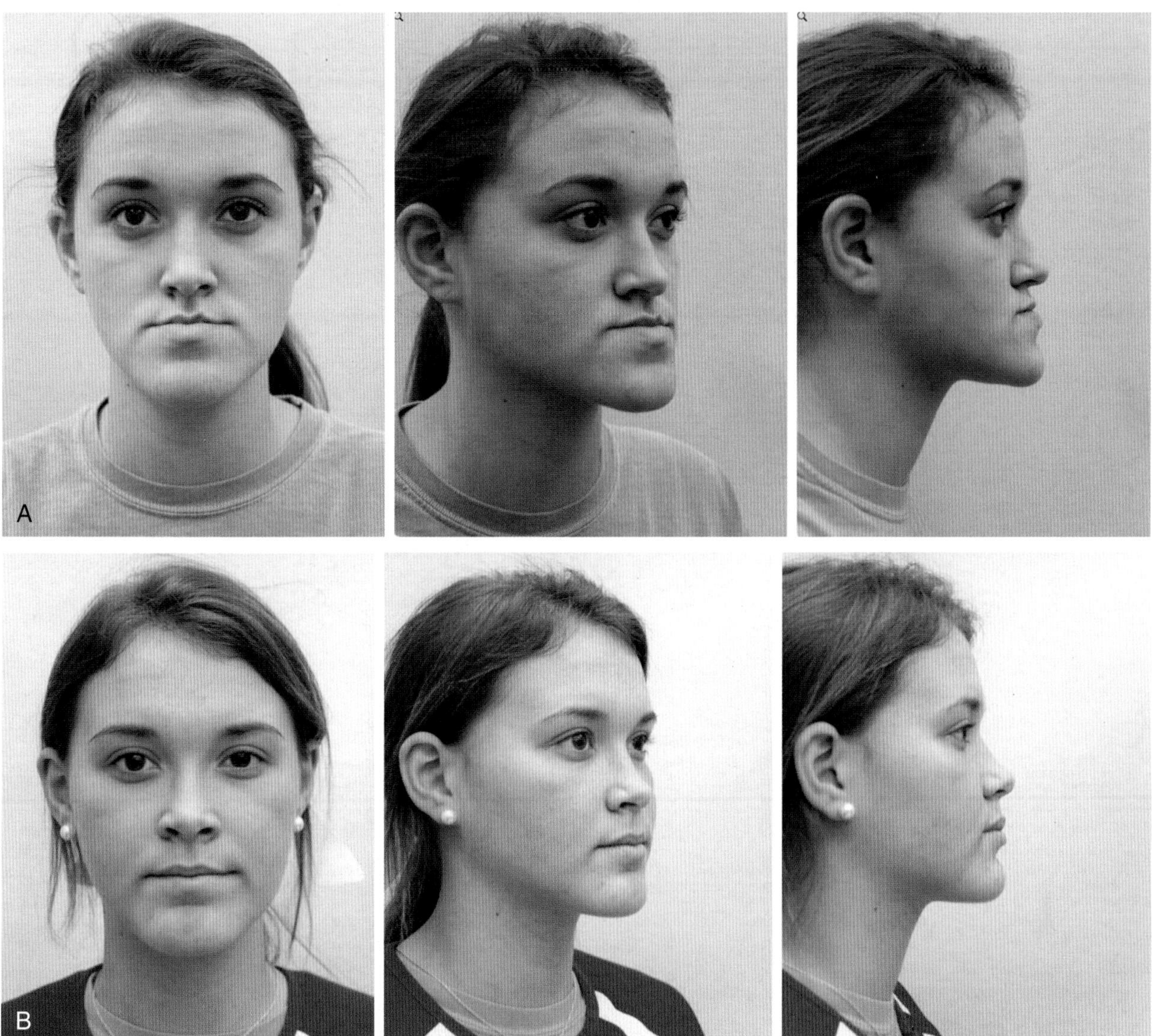

Figure 158.2 **A,** Preoperative. **B,** Two months postoperative. This patient underwent a Le Fort 1 advancement (10 mm), mandibular setback, and simultaneous placement of an Implantech custom midface implant.

TECHNIQUE—*cont'd*

Anthropometric measures can be helpful in selecting the most appropriate implant design. For instance, the malar prominence is around 10 mm lateral and 15 to 20 mm inferior to the lateral canthus. Cephalometric analyses can be used to assess proper chin projection relative to the skeletal base or soft tissue of the midface. Epker described a method of determining the amount of ideal vertical angle augmentation using a lateral cephalogram. The vertical linear distance between the patient's existing and constructed normal inferior border at the gonial angle is measured. This distance is the amount of vertical change in the angle that is indicated to create ideal skeletal support.[13]

Ultimately, an artistic feel is needed in determining the best implant design and size to achieve a favorable result. One needs to keep in mind the specific areas that are deficient in the midface (infraorbital, malar, paranasal) or mandible (chin, angle) and then select the appropriate implant(s) to address the deficient area(s). At times, it may be necessary to stack implants. For instance, if someone has both infraorbital and malar deficiency, one can simultaneously use both a tear trough and malar shell implant. Likewise, stacked implants may be indicated in cases of facial asymmetry (Fig. 158.4).

Continued

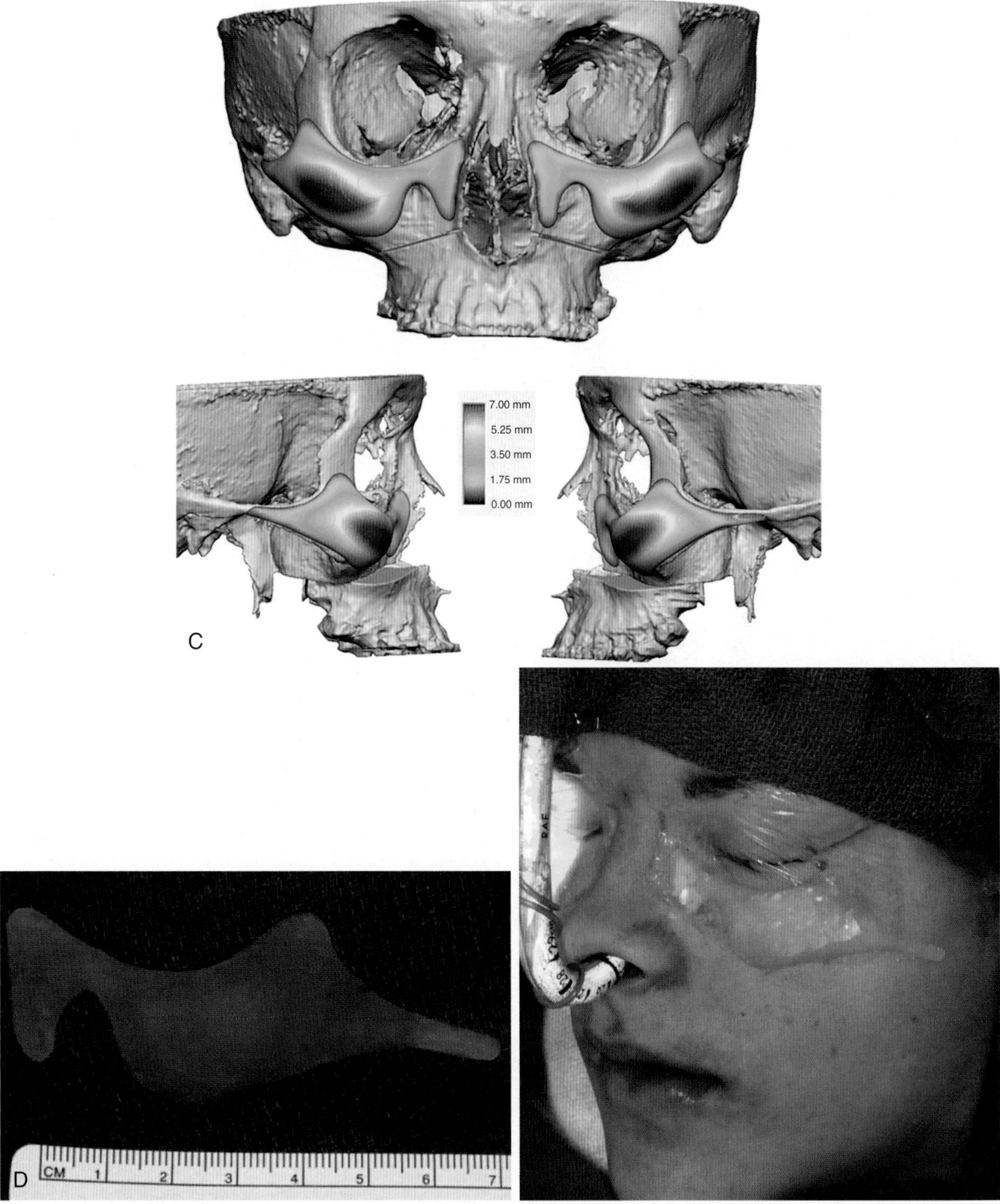

Figure 158.2, cont'd **C,** Computer-assisted design of the custom implant that was planned after virtual osteotomies to maintain balanced augmentation in the upper midface. The colormap shows the millimeter projection throughout the implant. **D,** Picture of the actual custom implant and its overlay to the face.

TECHNIQUE—*cont'd*

In most situations, the author prefers silicone implants over porous polyethylene. Silicone is softer and may feel more natural in areas where there is a thin soft-tissue drape. The harder feel of porous polyethylene is not an issue if there is a thicker soft-tissue drape such as the angle. Silicone is more flexible and has a smoother surface. It is easier to place through a smaller incision. A longer incision and more aggressive dissection are required for a porous polyethylene implant because it is less flexible and it has a rough textured surface. Silicone is more easily explanted due to the fact that it is encapsulated. Porous polyethylene is much more difficult to remove because of tissue ingrowth. This should be considered when placing implants in a younger patient, such as one undergoing concomitant orthognathic surgery. For various reasons, there may be a need to remove the implant later in life.

Continued

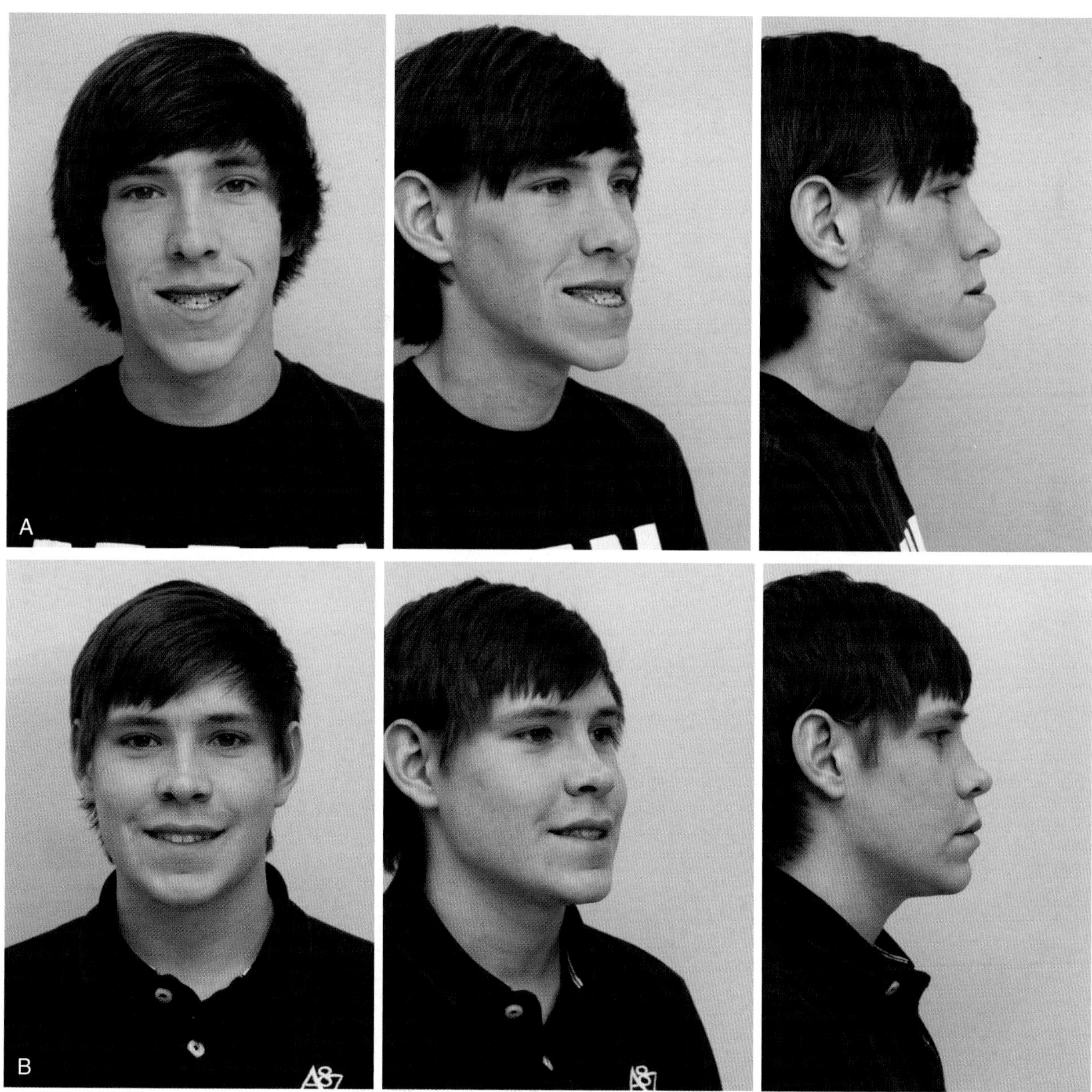

Figure 158.3 **A,** Preoperative. **B,** Twenty months postoperative. This patient underwent Le Fort 1 advancement (8 mm), mandibular setback, and (C) placement of Medpor Angle of the Mandible implants with a 7 mm lateral and 5 mm inferior projection at the angle. It provided balance of the posterior body and angle with his strong chin projection. This implant is bulky and often needs to be trimmed along its edges. He also had Medpor super petite Design RZ Malar implants placed.

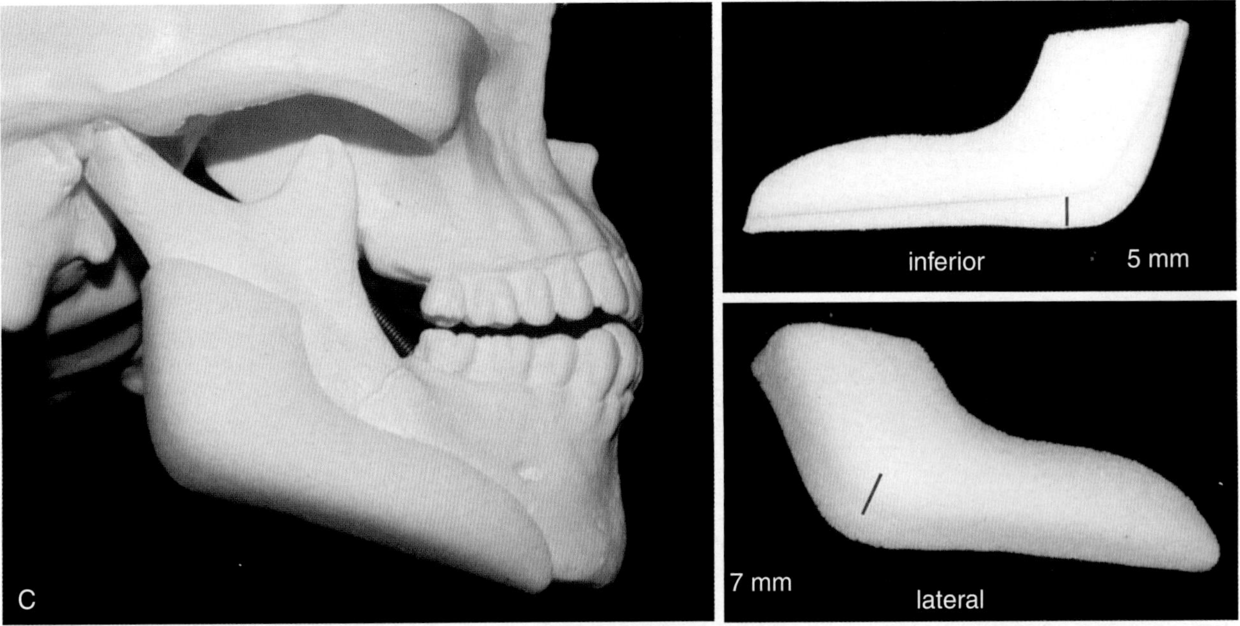

Figure 158.3, cont'd

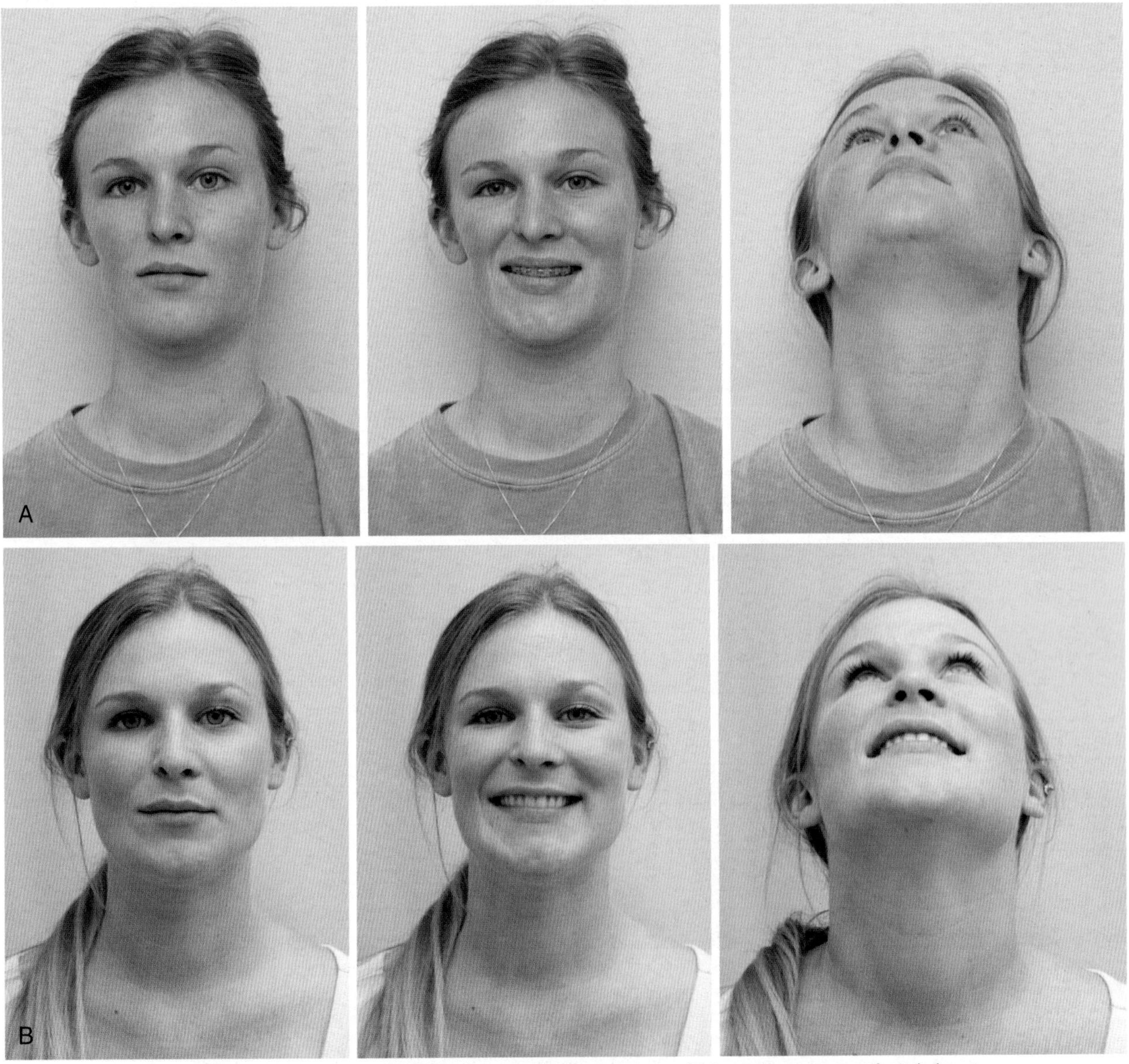

Figure 158.4 **A,** Preoperative. **B,** Twelve months postoperative. This patient presented with hemifacial atrophy (Parry–Romberg syndrome). She underwent a maxillary and mandibular osteotomy to correct her occlusal cant. She simultaneously had stacked malar and mandibular angle implants placed on her right side to improve the residual facial asymmetry.

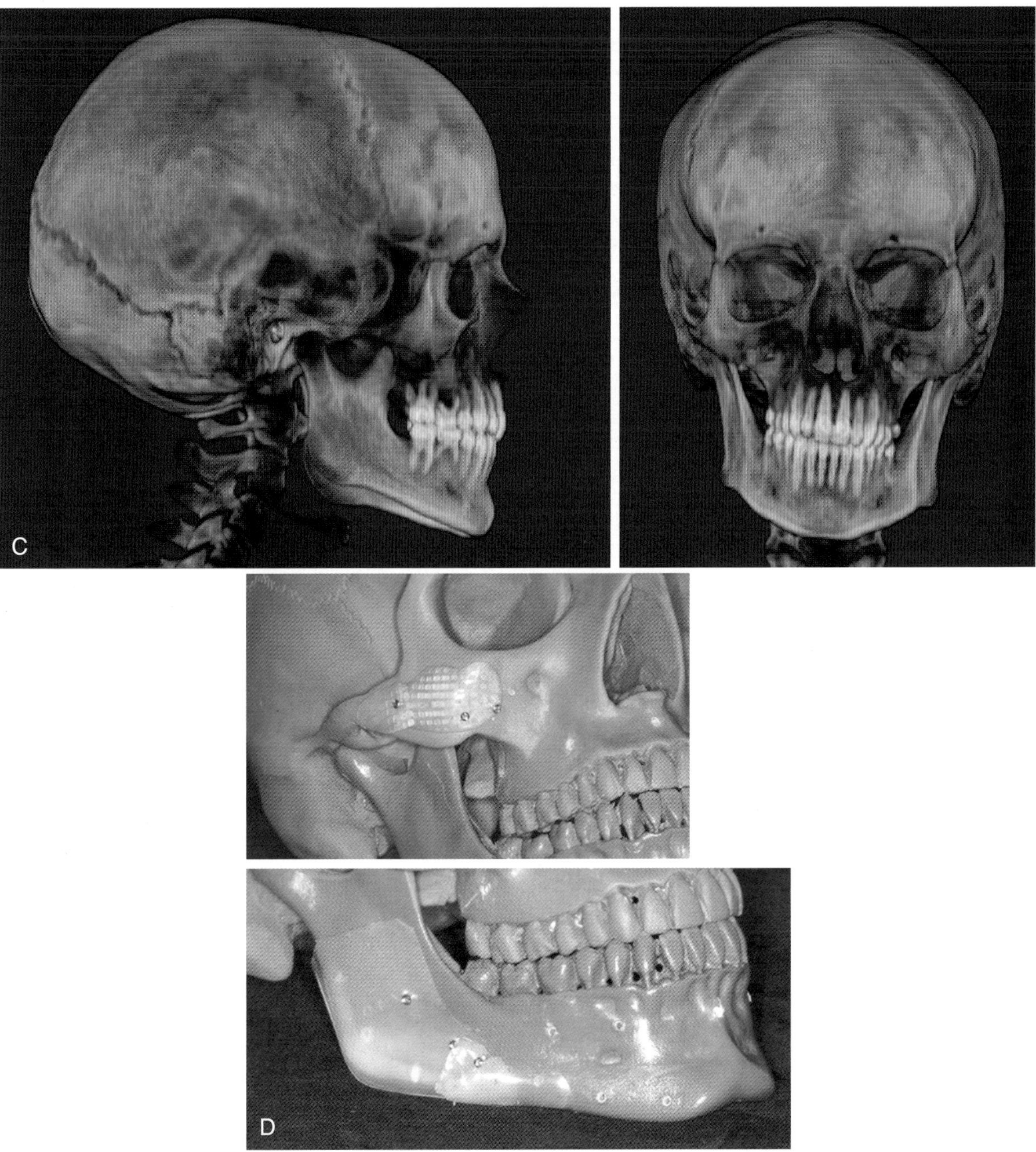

Figure 158.4, cont'd **C,** The cone beam computed tomography scan demonstrates the underlying skeletal atrophy throughout the midface and mandible. Soft tissues also exhibit atrophy with this syndrome. **D,** Implantech Conform Binder Submalar implants and Lateral Mandibular Angle implants were stacked in the fashion shown.

TECHNIQUE—*cont'd*

STEP 2: Anesthesia

Implants are generally placed in the operating room setting under general anesthesia, especially, if other procedures are being performed at the same time that warrant a general anesthetic. In certain situations, intravenous sedation with regional nerve blocks can be considered. Isolated placement of malar or chin implants would be an example. Regardless of the anesthetic technique, it is best to use sterile technique to minimize risk of infection. This would include extra- and intraoral prep with chlorhexidine or Betadine and sterile gowning and draping.

The incision line and areas of tissue dissection should be infiltrated with lidocaine with epinephrine. One should wait 7 to 10 minutes to allow for the hemostatic effect of epinephrine to occur. Marcaine with epinephrine blocks can be administered at the conclusion of surgery for preemptive analgesia.

STEP 3: Approach and Exposure

An intraoral approach may be used for placement of any implant in the midface and mandible. The author uses an intraoral approach with the exception of placing genial implants, in which case a submental crease incision is preferred. A transconjunctival approach can be used to place an infraorbital implant, but the author finds that an intraoral approach provides better access. Interestingly, placement of alloplastic implants with exposure to the oral cavity is generally not a concern for subsequent implant infection.

Bovie electrocautery with a needle tip is be used to incise through the mucosa and periosteum. A sharp periosteal elevator is used to carry out subperiosteal dissection to expose the area over which the onlay implant will lie. Implants are always placed beneath the periosteum directly onto bone.

For placement of malar implants, a standard maxillary vestibular incision is carried from first molar to first molar. Subperiosteal dissection is carried over the body of the zygoma, anterior extent of the zygomatic arch and lateral and infraorbital rims. If an infraorbital implant is going to be placed, the infraorbital nerve should be completely dissected around so that the implant lies passively on the rim above the nerve. The author finds that attempting to limit dissection in order to provide a tight pocket for implant stability hinders passive and accurate positioning. The lateral and infraorbital rim and infraorbital nerve can serve as landmarks for symmetric placement of the implant on each side. Screw fixation of the implant should provide initial stability to avoid implant migration. An in-turned Obwegeser retractor that extends the full length of dissection is used to retract the soft-tissue envelope.

A chin implant can be placed intraorally through a standard genioplasty incision but, as stated, the author prefers a submental crease incision. This approach offers better visualization and alignment of the implant along the inferior border. In addition, it provides access for submental lipectomy or platysmal plication at the same time if these procedures are planned. A 1.5 to 2 cm incision is made just posterior to the submental crease. This prevents deepening of the crease and keeps the incision well hidden underneath the chin when skin is advanced forward by the implant. A #15 blade is used to incise skin. Bovie electrocautery is used to incise through subcutaneous tissue above the platysma. The soft tissue is retracted forward to expose the inferior border. The Bovie needle tip is used to incise through the periosteum just anterior to the platysmal insertion on the inferior border. Subperiosteal dissection is carried out superiorly and laterally along the lateral aspect of the mandible. Liberal dissection is performed so that the implant will sit passively. Sinn retractors and a small in-turned Obwegeser retractors are used to retract the soft-tissue envelop.

Angle implants are placed via a standard sagittal split osteotomy incision in the posterior vestibule. The periosteum and overlying soft-tissue envelope should be aggressively stripped from the lateral ramus, angle, anterior, posterior, and inferior borders so that the implant can be passively placed. The anterior aspect of the ascending ramus can be used as a landmark for symmetric placement on both sides. An out-turned Obwegeser retractor can aid in visualization along the posterior border and angle. A Bauer retractor placed in the sigmoid notch can aid in retraction of the soft tissues superiorly. If porous polyethylene implants will be placed the incision and dissection will need to be extended because the material's stiffness and textured surface makes it more difficult to place as compared to silicone.

STEP 4: Placement and Securing Implants

Both silicone and porous polyethylene implants can be carved with Mayo scissors or a #10 blade to provide a more custom fit. Medpor Angle of the Mandible implants are fairly bulky and usually require trimming on the lateral aspects. The author usually does not modify Implantech implants if the appropriate design and size are chosen beforehand except when placing midface implants simultaneously with a Le Fort advancement. In this situation, the infraorbital or malar implant should be trimmed on the inferior aspect so that it lies above the osteotomy. The osteotomy gap can then be grafted with autogenous or allogenic bone.

As described in the previous step, use of surrounding anatomy is helpful in placing bilateral implants symmetrically. For instance, a malar implant can be referenced to its position relative to the lateral and infraorbital rims and the infraorbital nerve. When an Implantech Flowers Tear Trough implant is used, the surgeon must carve a notch on the inferior aspect of the implant to accommodate the nerve. The implant comes with an imprint of the area to be removed. This implant has to be inserted by pulling the medial portion above the nerve as it positioned. This is best accomplished by placing a mosquito hemostat above and medial to the nerve, grabbing the medial aspect, and pulling it through to seat the

TECHNIQUE—*cont'd*

notched portion over the nerve. The implant may extend slightly above the infraorbital rim. This can provide rejuvenation to the lower lid, or it may counter soft-tissue dissent that will occur with aging. However, overextension can lead to lower lid malposition and limit vision on downward gaze.

Genial implants should provide symmetry with the midline of the face. Skin overlying the midline of the chin is marked prior to the dissection to aid in proper placement. The Implantech extended chin implant has a midline mark that can be aligned with the skin reference mark.

Angle implants can be more challenging to place symmetrically because of limited visualization at the angle and posterior border. Care should be taken to ensure that the posterior and inferior shelf of the implant lie along the posterior and inferior borders of the mandible. Referencing the implant's position relative to the anterior ramus and mental nerve is helpful. If an angle implant is being placed after a sagittal split osteotomy, the technique for performing the osteotomy and fixation does not have to be altered. The implant can overlay lateral border plates without issue. Angle implants are not as suitable for placing simultaneous to an intraoral vertical ramus osteotomy if segments are overlapping laterally and not fixated.

Implants should be secured in place with two fixation screws to prevent rotation and migration. Rarely more than two are necessary. The author uses 1.5-mm screws that are long enough to traverse the implant and engage the outer cortex of bone. Self-tapping screws are preferred over self-drilling to minimize implant displacement as the screw is placed. Fixation screws are usually placed through the access incision. Angle implants require use of a transbuccal trochar in order to place a fixation screw in the mid ramus.

When placing a high density porous polyethylene implant, it should be vacuum impregnated with an antibiotic solution to minimize the risk of infection. Vancomycin is typically used. This is achieved by placing the implant into a 60- or 90-cc syringe with the antibiotic solution. The plunger is forcefully withdrawn while holding a finger over the end of the syringe. This will need to be done repeatedly in order to remove air from the porous implant and replace it with the antibiotic solution. When this process reaches its end point, the implant sinks in the solution. To bend the implant, it is placed in sterile hot saline; this removes its original memory and allows it to be readily molded to the underlying bone.[13]

STEP 5: Closure

The wounds should be thoroughly irrigated with antibiotic solution. Again, vancomycin is typically used. For maxillary vestibular incisions, the mucosa is closed in a single layer with a running chromic gut suture. For mandibular vestibular incisions, the wound is closed in two layers. The periosteum and buccinator muscle are closed with interrupted chromic gut. The mucosa is then closed with a running horizontal mattress chromic gut suture to ensure water-tight closure. This will prevent the saliva that pools in the lower vestibule from entering the wound.

STEP 6: Dressing

A pressure dressing is placed for 5 to 7 days to stabilize the implant and prevent hematoma formation. The author prefers using Mastisol and three layers of crisscrossed quarter inch brown paper tape dressing. The dressing should extend beyond the borders of the implant to include the surrounding tissue that was undermined. Dressings are covered with Tegaderm to minimize soiling of the tape.

ALTERNATIVE OR MODIFIED TECHNIQUE: Custom Implants

CAD/CAM technology makes custom implants a readily available option. For more complex cases, it is a good alternative to stock implants. In the case of a severe class III patient that has malar and infraorbital hypoplasia, a custom implant can be designed so that it augments the upper midface to balance the effects of the maxillary advancement. Because of the precise fit to underlying bone, the implant is likely to be more stable long term (Fig. 158.2).

Another use is in the management of facial asymmetries resulting from congenital, developmental, or posttraumatic deformities. Implants can be used in conjunction with orthognathic surgery in the management of unilateral condylar hyperplasia, hemifacial microsomia, Parry–Romberg syndrome (hemifacial atrophy), and hemifacial hyperplasia (Fig. 158.5).

A third-party planning company, such as 3D Systems, provides software support to design the implant with the surgeon. The CAD file is sent to the implant manufacturer, such as Implantech, for production of the custom implant. If orthognathic surgery is being performed simultaneously, virtual planning for this is carried out in the usual fashion.

The technique for placement of custom implants is essentially analogous to that of placing stock implants. More planning is obviously required beforehand. The turnaround time for production is typically 6 to 8 weeks. The expense is significantly higher when compared with stock implants.

Avoidance and Management of Intraoperative Complications

Any number of complications can occur and should be considered both before, during, and after performing surgery. These include improper implant selection or placement, asymmetry, neuropraxia, persistent edema, hematoma, seroma, infection, migration, soft-tissue contour changes surrounding the implant, palpability, extrusion, bone resorption, and need for revision.[16]

Time must be taken before surgery to properly choose the proper implant design and size. Attention to detail is essential when placing bilateral implants to make sure they are evenly placed using anatomic landmarks as previously discussed. Proper handling of soft tissue and maintaining a subperiosteal plane of dissection will minimize postoperative edema and hematoma formation. Careful dissection around the infraorbital and mental nerves will minimize injury and long-term paraesthesia.

Because infection and biofilm formation will likely result in the need for implant removal, using aseptic technique is important. Minimize handling of the implants prior to inserting them. Irrigate wounds with saline containing antibiotics prior to closure. Interestingly, the results of a recent systematic review indicated that some porous materials were associated with higher rates of infection than nonporous implant types.[6] Porous polyethylene allows for tissue ingrowth, and this is thought to decrease the chance for ingress of bacteria and subsequent implant infection. Porous polyethylene implants should be vacuum-impregnated with an antibiotic solution, as previously described. Mandibular vestibule incisions should be closed in two layers. Mucosa should be closed with a water-tight horizontal mattress suture to avoid ingress of bacteria into the wound from saliva pulling in the vestibule.

Two-point fixation of the implant is important for a number of reasons. Movement of the implant may cause continued tissue injury with resultant local inflammation and edema. Migration of the implant may also leave space between the

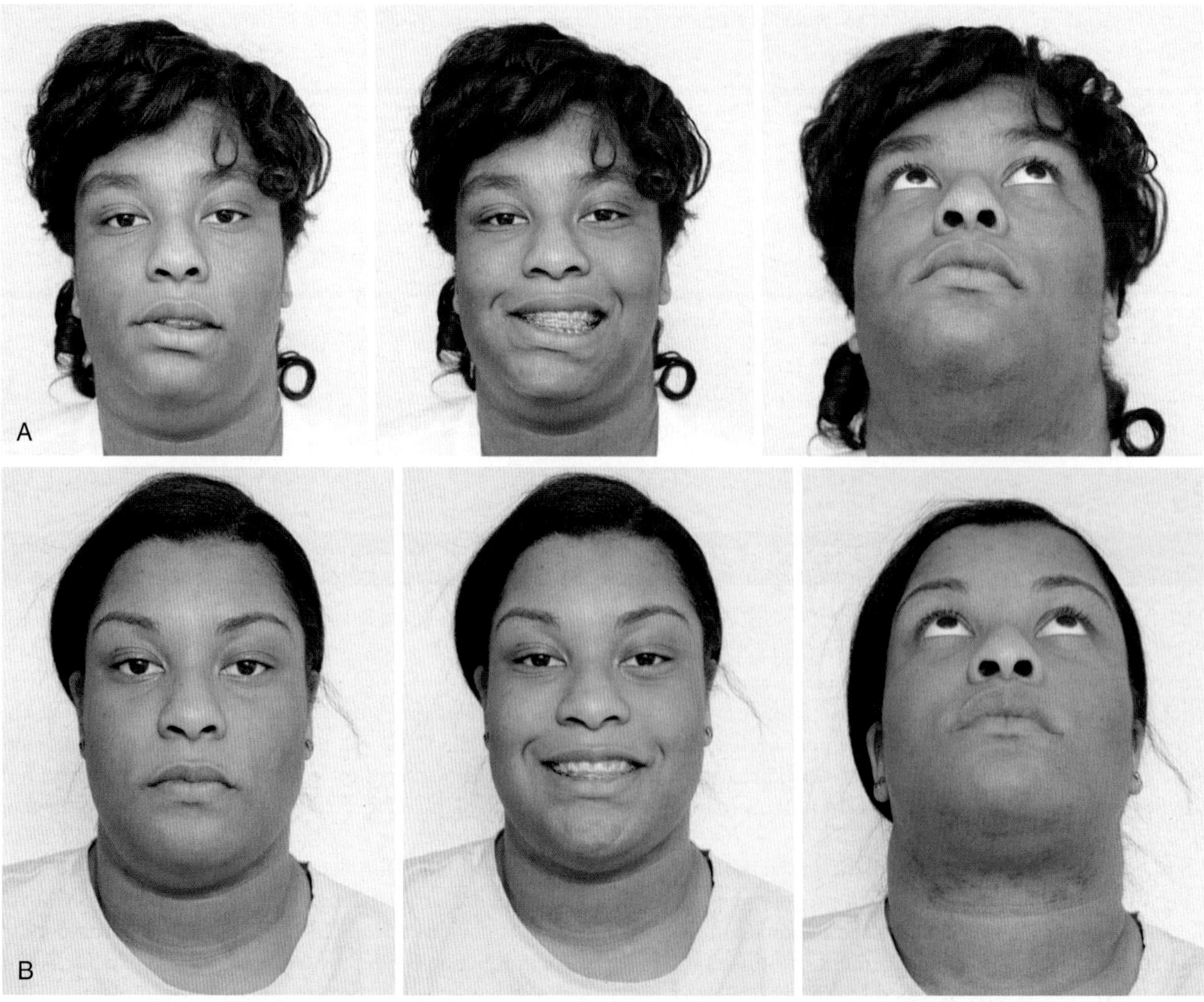

Figure 158.5 **A,** Preoperative. **B,** Fourteen months postoperative. This patient presented with hemifacial microsomia.

implant and surrounding tissue that may serve as a space for hematoma, seroma, or microbial invasion and infection. An implant is more likely salvageable if an early postoperative infection occurs if it is well fixated and nonmobile.[6,16]

Postoperative Considerations

The author places patients on antibiotics for a week. Amoxicillin and chlorhexidine rinse are routinely used if implants are placed through an intraoral incision. Cephalexin and a topical antibiotic ointment are used if an extraoral approach is used for placing chin implants. Patients should maintain a liquid diet for 1 day and a full liquid/pureed diet for approximately 1 week. Subsequently, they can advance to a soft, mechanical diet for the next 2 weeks, until the incisions are well healed. By 6 weeks, the implants should be stable enough to resume normal physical activity. Dressings can be removed as early as 48 hours, once edema and risk of hematoma formation subside. The author typically leaves the dressing in place until the first postoperative visit at 5 to 7 days.

Hematomas and seromas are best prevented with gentle handling of the tissues, maintaining a subperiosteal plane of dissection, placement of a pressure dressing, and control of blood pressure during and after the procedure. Smaller hematomas will likely resolve without treatment. Large hematomas need to be recognized and evacuated. A liquefied hematoma or seroma that occurs 2 to 4 weeks after surgery may be drained percutaneously.[16]

Patients should be informed that edema can last several weeks due to the body's inflammatory response to the implant. Persistent edema up to a year is uncommon but can occur due to the host immune reaction to the implant material. After cheek implants are placed, the patient is instructed to begin vigorous lip exercises after the incisions are healed to expedite resolution of residual edema and to improve natural lip motion. After placement of angle implants, patients will likely experience hypomobility due to trismus. At 2 weeks, they can be placed on range of motion exercises four times a day until full range of motion returns.

If a wound infection occurs, a broad-spectrum antibiotic should be used for at least 2 weeks. An infection does not

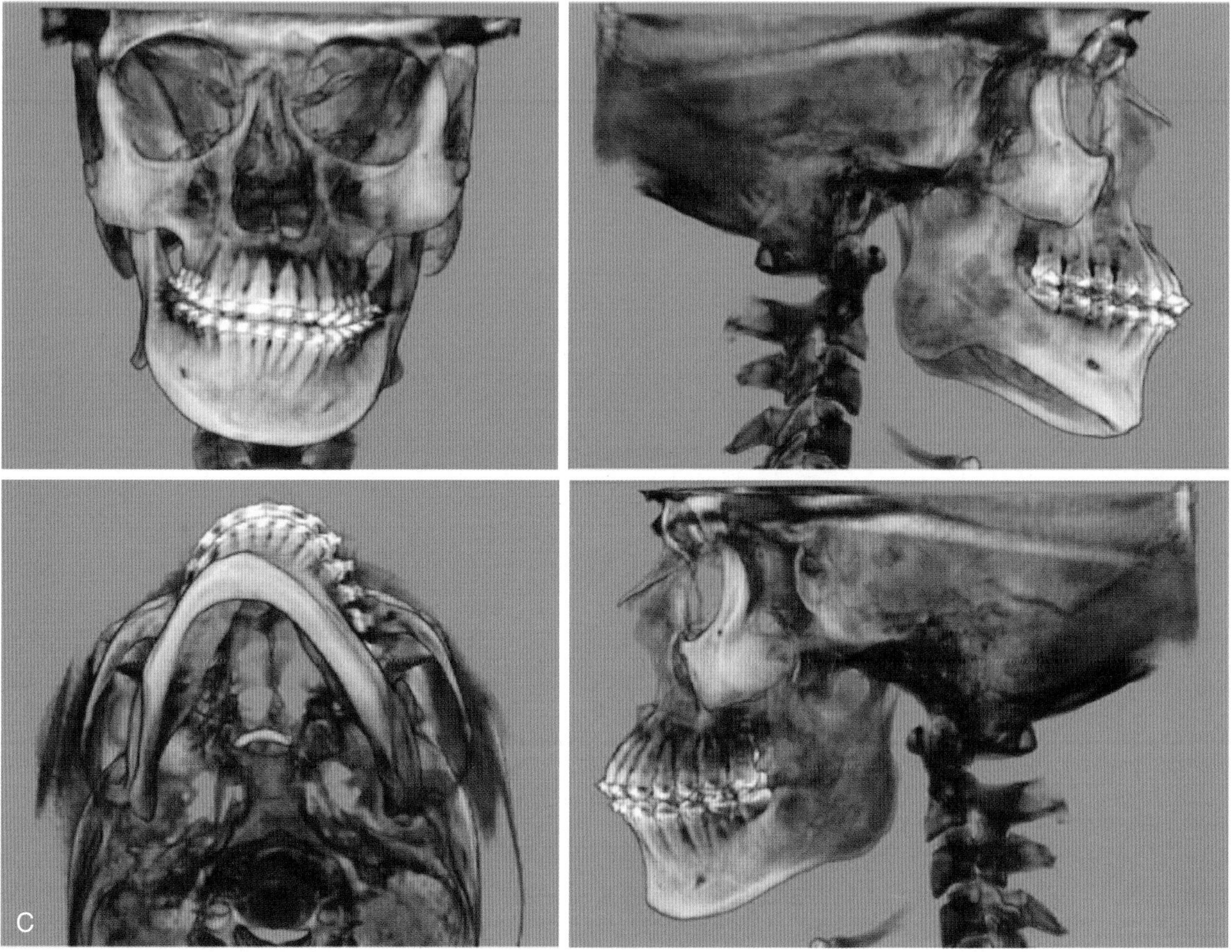

Figure 158.5, cont'd **C,** Her cone beam computed tomography scan demonstrates significant skeletal asymmetry.

Continued

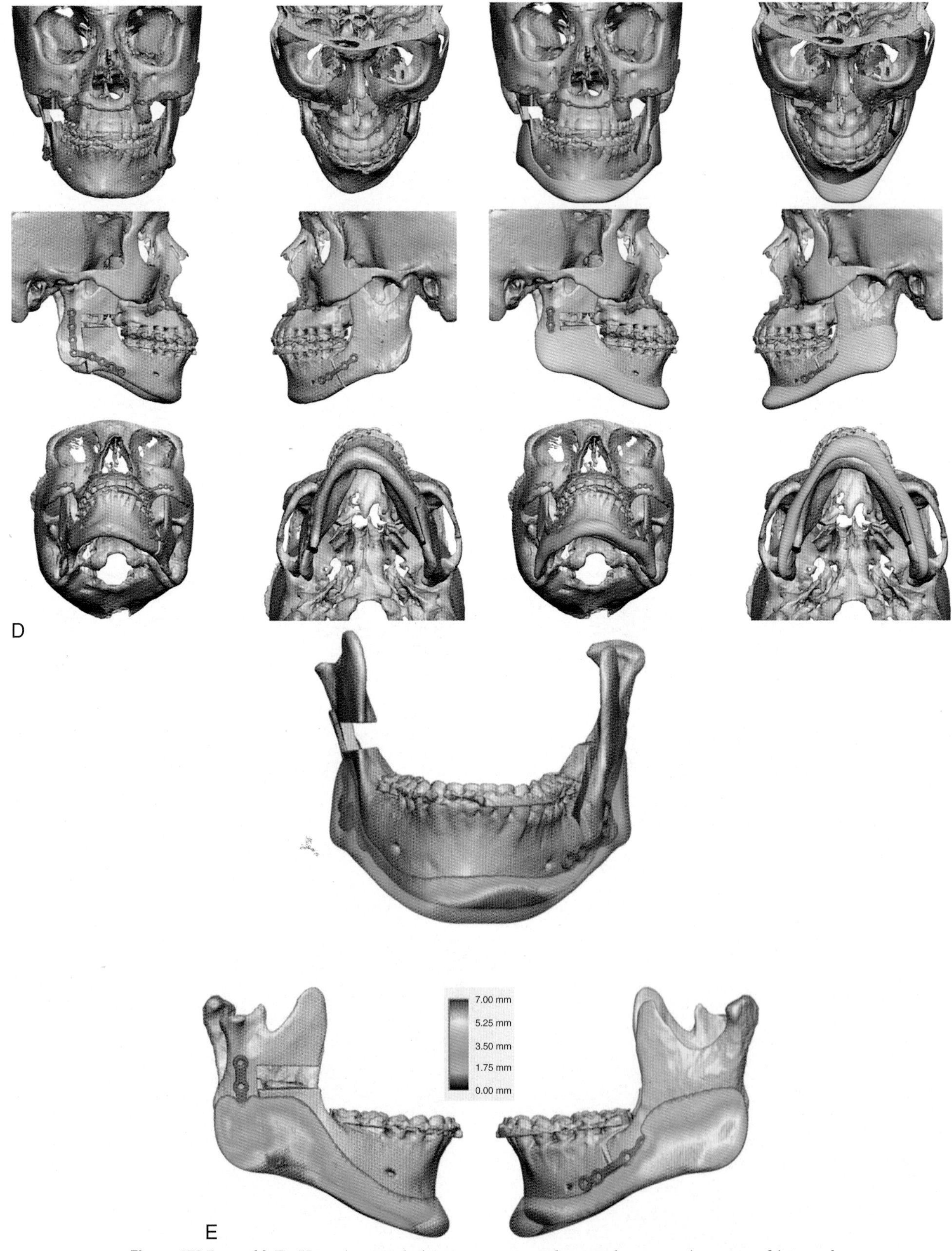

Figure 158.5, cont'd **D,** Virtual surgical planning was carried out and custom plates were fabricated as shown. There was residual skeletal asymmetry after her occlusal cant and yaw were corrected in addition to soft-tissue hypoplasia on the effected side seen with this disorder. **E,** Computer-assisted design of a custom mandibular implant was planned after virtual osteotomies to correct the residual chin and inferior border asymmetry. The colormap shows the millimeter projection throughout the implant.

necessary condemn the implant. However, if frank purulence is noted, the implant likely needs to be removed and infection cleared for several weeks before replacing the implant.

If the patient expresses concern about the esthetic appearance of the implant, they should be encouraged to wait several weeks to let edema resolve. If after that time there is still concern, explantation should be considered. When the surgeon sees the problem being a matter of improper implant selection or placement, or implant migration has occurred, it is reasonable to discuss a revision procedure with the patient. If there is concern that the patient has a body dysmorphic disorder, it may be best to remove and not replace the implant. Good patient communication is important regardless.[16]

The implant may have to be explanted in the future for any number of reasons. When placing implants in young patients, the need to explant later in life should be discussed. While they improve support of the soft-tissue envelope and thus would be expected to decrease the stigmata of aging, the longevity of esthetic enhancement is unknown. How overlying soft tissue responds with aging cannot be fully predicted. Implant visibility may occur with time. If the patient were to undergo a soft-tissue procedure such as rhytidectomy later in life, the presence of the implant may need to be taken into consideration.

Bone resorption underneath an implant is a rare occurrence. Chin button implants and mentalis muscle hyperactivity with implant displacement superiorly over thinner cortical bone are risk factors for resorption. Contemporary extended anatomic chin implants do not typically have this problem, likely due to distribution of the pressure forces over a broader anatomic area. Significant bone resorption associated with malar implants is rare. This is likely due to the large surface contact with underlying bone and the laxity of the overlying soft tissue with minimal muscle pull against the bone.[16]

References

1. Robiony M, Costa F, Demitri V, Politi M. Simultaneous malaroplasty with porous polyethylene implants and orthognathic surgery for correction of malar deficiency. *J Oral Maxillofacial Surg*. 1998;56:734–741.
2. Yaremchuk MJ, Doumit G, Thomas MA. Alloplastic augmentation of the facial skeleton: an occasional adjunct or alternative to orthognathic surgery. *Plast Reconstr Surg*. 2011;127(5):2021–2030.
3. Lee JH, Kaban LB, Yaremchuk MJ. Refining post-orthognathic surgery facial contour with computer-designed/computer-manufactured alloplastic implants. *Plast Reconstr Surg*. 2018;142(3):747–755.
4. Lutz JC, Assouline Vitale LS, Graillon N, Foletti JM, Schouman T. Standard and customized alloplastic facial implants refining orthognathic surgery: outcome evaluation. *J Maxillofacial Surg*. 2020;78:1832.e1831–1832.e1812.
5. Rubin JP, Yaremchuk MJ, JP R. Complications and toxicities of implantable biomaterials used in facial reconstructive and aesthetic surgery: a comprehensive review of the literature. *Plast Reconstr Surg*. 1997;100(5):1336–1353.
6. Oliver JD, Eells AC, Saba ES, et al. Alloplastic facial implants: a systematic review and meta-analysis on outcomes and uses in aesthetic and reconstructive plastic surgery. *Aesthetic Plast Surg*. 2019;43(3):625–636.
7. Schwartz D, Quereshy FA. Combined rhytidectomy and alloplastic facial implants. *Atlas Oral Maxillofac Surg Clin North Am*. 2014;22(1):69–73.
8. Matros E, Momoh A, Yaremchuk MJ. The aging midfacial skeleton: implications for rejuvenation and reconstruction using implants. *Facial Plast Surg*. 2009;25(4):252–259.
9. Shaw RB Jr, Katzel EB, Koltz PF, Kahn DM, Girotto JA, Langstein HN. Aging of the mandible and its aesthetic implications. *Plast Reconstr Surg*. 2010;125(1):332–342.
10. Mendelson B, Wong CH. Changes in the facial skeleton with aging: implications and clinical applications in facial rejuvenation. *Aesthetic Plast Surg*. 2012;36(4):753–760.
11. Binder WJ. Facial rejuvenation and volumization using implants. *Facial Plast Surg*. 2011;27(1):86–97.
12. Binder WJ, Dhir K, Joseph J. The role of fillers in facial implant surgery. *Facial Plast Surg Clin North Am*. 2013;21(2):201–211.
13. Epker BN. *Alloplastic Esthetic Facial Augmentation*. BC Becker Inc; 2004.
14. Yaremchuk MJ. Infraorbital rim augmentation. *Plast Reconstr Surg*. 2001;107(6):1585–1592.
15. Fux CA, Costerton JW, Stewart PS, Stoodley P. Survival strategies of infectious biofilms. *Trends Microbiol*. 2005;13(1):34–40.
16. Cuzalina LA, Hlavacek MR. Complications of facial implants. *Oral Maxillofac Surg Clin North Am*. 2009;21(1):91–104, vi-vii. vi-vii.
17. Vistnes LM, Ksander GA, Kosek J. Study of encapsulation of silicone rubber implants in animals. A foreign-body reaction. *Plast Reconstr Surg*. 1978;62(4):580–588.
18. Klawitter JJ, Bagwell JG, Weinstein AM, Sauer BW. An evaluation of bone growth into porous high density polyethylene. *J Biomed Mater Res*. 1976;10(2):311–323.
19. https://www.implantech.com/product-category/products/facial-implants/silicone-facial-implants/.
20. https://cmf.stryker.com/assets/files/5n/cmf_br_93-rev.-none_13908-medpor-oral-brochure.pdf.

CHAPTER 159

Micrografting and Hair Transplantation Surgery

David Stanton, Deepak Kademani, and Paul S. Tiwana

Armamentarium

Surgical marking pen
Wax pencil
Local anesthetic with vasoconstrictor
#10 Scalpel blades
#11 Scalpel blades
Multibladed scalpel handle
18-Gauge solid needle
19-Gauge solid needle
Jeweler's tissue forceps
Fine tissue forceps
3-0 Vicryl suture
Normal saline solution for injection
Telfa dressing
ABD dressing
#5 Tube gauze

History of the Procedure

In 1959, Norman Orentreich authored a paper on male pattern baldness (MPB) in which his most important observation was that grafts from the hair-bearing rim of the scalp were "donor dominant" and continued to grow hair when implanted into thinning or bald areas.[1] Thus, the concept of multiple scalp grafts for the treatment of baldness evolved. This movement of hair grafts from genetically preprogrammed, permanently growing sites to balding areas is the foundation of hair transplantation and micrografting as we know it today. This procedure, though used primarily for androgenetic alopecia or MPB, can also be used to cover scars secondary to scalp trauma or previous surgical procedures, radiation and thermal burns, and inactive phases of disease such as scleroderma and other cicatricial processes, as well as for some types of female alopecia.[2] Because MPB is a genetically determined phenomenon, transplantation procedures move permanently growing scalp hair from the sides and back of the head (donor area) to appropriate recipient sites in the frontal, mid-scalp, and vertex regions.[3]

During the initial years of hair restoration surgery, the most common type of graft was a cylindrical plug (punch graft) measuring approximately 4 mm and containing 10 to 20 hairs removed from the hair-bearing area and placed in a somewhat smaller cylindrical hole in the balding region of the scalp. Depending on the degree of baldness, one to three sessions of transplantation were required per area, with the placement of 50 to 100 grafts at each session. If previous grafts had been done, the later transplants were placed between the previous grafts to create a confluent pattern.

The newest and most recent refinement in hair transplant surgery is follicular unit (FU) transplantation. Studies of horizontal sections of the scalp have revealed that human scalp hairs grow in small compartments or FUs.[4] The FU was first described by Headington in 1984 and was shown to include one to four terminal follicles, one or two vellus follicles, and perifollicular vascular and neural plexuses, all surrounded by concentric layers of collagen fibers.[5] Seager demonstrated that single-hair micrografts, when created by sectioning larger FUs, had less growth than when the FUs were kept intact. This supports the concept of the FU as a physiologic entity rather than just an anatomic one.[6] Consequently, the concept of FU transplantation has developed, with intact FU groupings being dissected under microscopic magnification. Single-FU or multi-FU (two to three FUs) grafts are transplanted.

Micrografts consisting of one to three hairs are implanted along the anterior hairline to eliminate the doll's hair look that cylindrical plugs could cause and give the most natural appearance to the hairline.[7] Multi-FUs, which consist of four to six hairs, are placed behind the hairline grafts for added density. These grafts are cut from donor strips taken by ellipse or multibladed knives (Fig. 159.1). Loupe or microscope magnification is used to allow precise visualization of hair direction and permit careful creation of properly sized grafts.

The tiny full-thickness grafts are then implanted into wounds made with a small (1 to 2 mm) blade (slits) or into puncture receptor sites created by 18-, 19-, or 20-gauge solid needles (Fig. 159.2). In fact, hair replacement surgery is now performed with large quantities (800 to 2500) of micrografts and multi-FUs.

Indications for the Use of the Procedure

Male Pattern Baldness

MPB is the change from terminal hair to vellus hair. The true dimensions and complexity of this process have only recently

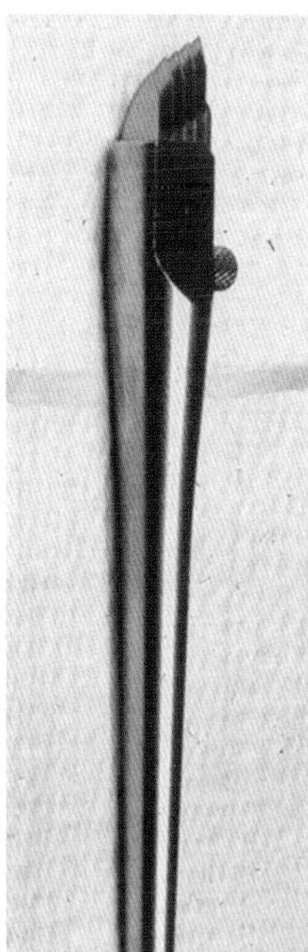

Figure 159.1 Multibladed knife with spacers to define donor strip width.

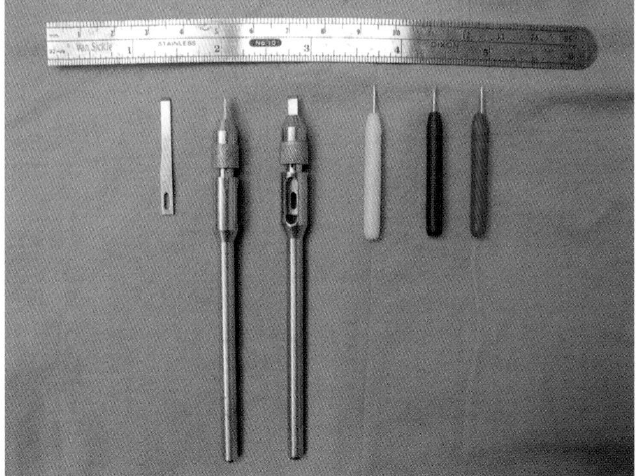

Figure 159.2 Instruments for recipient site preparation. Slit blade on left. Solid needles on right.

been appreciated. The progress of MPB is not linear; the condition develops in fits and starts. Terminal hair progresses to vellus hair far past the age at which it was thought that one could delineate the extent of MPB. Surgeons performing hair transplant surgery today realize that it is not the dramatic changes in MPB that occur between the ages of 20 and 35 years, but what can take place from 40 to 50 years and beyond.[2]

In Caucasians, normal male pattern hair loss is noticeable in about 30% of men by the age of 30 years and in 50% of men by 50 years. Certain racial groups, including the Japanese, Chinese, American Indians, and some tribes of Africans, are relatively immune to the condition, which in Caucasians follows a dominant trait with incomplete penetrance. Expression of this sex-limited gene depends on the level of circulating androgen. This hereditary incidence is noticeable not only in men but also in women who have a strong familial history of baldness.[8]

In men, hair loss can begin as early as the age of 20 years. With normal hair loss, one to several hundred hairs fall each day and are replaced by new hair. In the evolution of MPB, the new hair is fine and thin. Eventually, nothing is left on the scalp but the almost imperceptible fuzz of vellus hair. Simultaneously, hypertrophy of the sebaceous glands and hypersecretion of sebum usually occur and are provoked by androgenetic stimulation of the pilosebaceous follicles, which causes complete loss. MPB usually progresses in a definite pattern. First, the frontal hair regresses, and then loss of the more temporal hair becomes apparent with simultaneous thinning of the vertex. Ultimately, the most severe balding consists of total loss of the frontal and vertex hair. Norwood classified approximately seven different types of MPB.[9] Identification of these types is key to an understanding of proper planning of hair transplantation surgery (Fig. 159.3).[2]

Female Pattern Hair Loss

Like MPB, female pattern hair loss is most often due to heredity and aging. Hormonal influences in hereditary hair loss in women may be different from those in men, but researchers are continuing to study it. Unlike men, most women retain some of their natural hairline, which can be thickened to a delicate, yet fuller appearance.

Female pattern hair loss is not as obvious as MPB, but like men, it can be treated effectively. Frequently, women's patterns are more diffuse or spread out over the entire scalp (Fig. 159.4). Whether a female is a candidate for transplantation is determined at the initial consultation. A trained physician can also diagnose whether a woman is experiencing permanent female pattern hair loss and not temporary hair loss related to medical conditions such as pregnancy, disease, or stress.[2] Significant improvements in hairline definition, hair density, and facial aesthetics can be achieved.

Eyebrow Reconstruction

The periorbital region has an important role in the perception of facial esthetics and proportion, and it also imparts volumes to facial expression and nonverbal communication. The causes of eyebrow loss can be mechanical, such as overzealous plucking, electrolysis, or laser hair removal; trauma; or medical conditions such as hormonal imbalance or alopecia universalis.[10]

Hair loss patterns of the eyebrows include decreased density, short overall length of the eyebrow, a size or shape that is too narrow, or a hairless scar. With proper design and surgical technique, it is possible to reconstruct eyebrows with transplanted hairs growing at a natural angle and direction. The surgeon should keep in mind that a female eyebrow generally has a natural peak at the junction of the middle and lateral thirds, approximately at a line tangent to the lateral

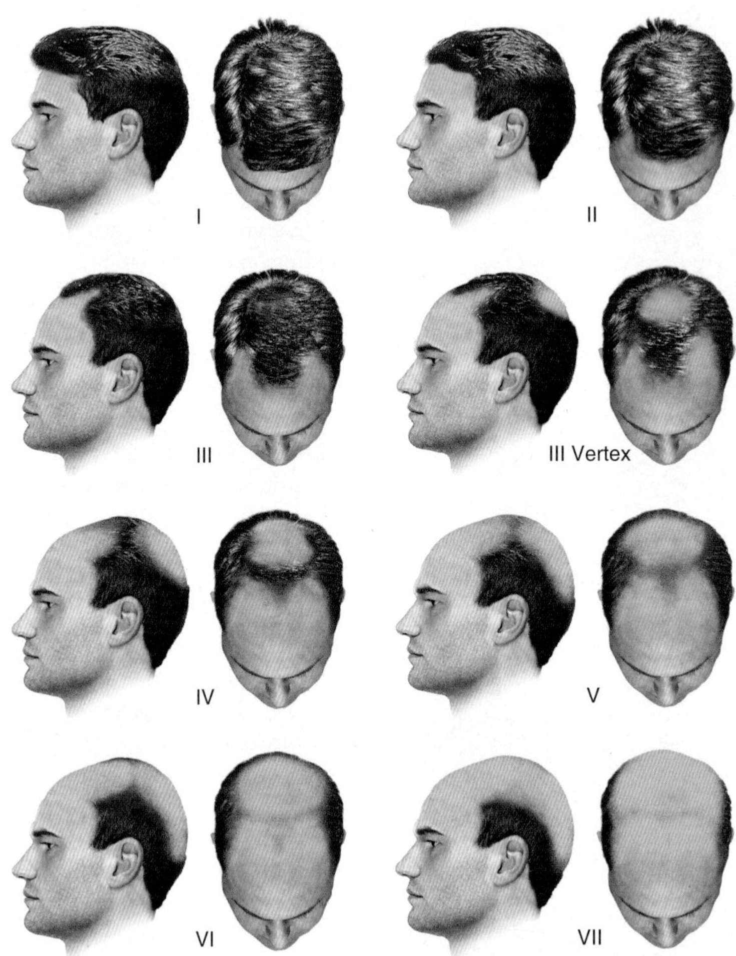

Figure 159.3 Norwood classification of male pattern baldness. (From Konior RJ, Nadimi S. Hair Restoration: Medical and Surgical Techniques. In: Flint PW. *Cummings Otolaryngology: Head and Neck Surgery*. 7th ed. Elsevier; 2021.)

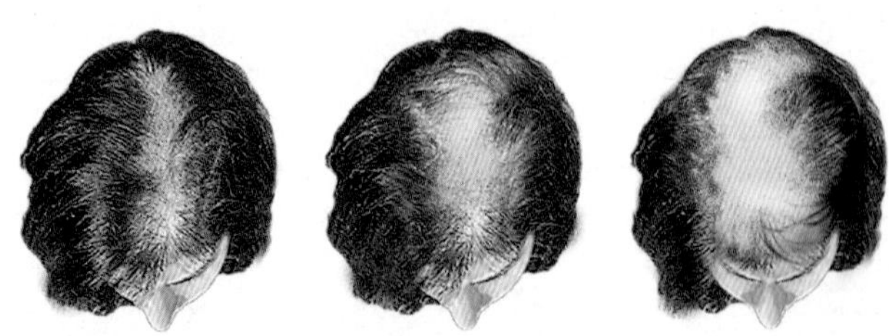

Figure 159.4 Female pattern hair loss. (From Konior RJ, Nadimi S. Hair Restoration: Medical and Surgical Techniques. In: Flint PW. *Cummings Otolaryngology: Head and Neck Surgery*. 7th ed. Elsevier; 2021.)

limbus of the eye. A male eyebrow is generally found to lie over the supraorbital ridge. Patients should participate in the eyebrow design and approve the size, shape, and location preoperatively.[2]

Recipient sites are created with 19- or 20-gauge solid needles and can be placed between existing eyebrow hairs with minimal risk of damage. It is not uncommon for 200 to 350 individual grafts to be placed into one eyebrow. The majority of these grafts will be single-hair grafts, but two-hair grafts can be used in the central portion of the eyebrow, particularly if the donor hair is fine. The "stick and place" technique seems to work well for eyebrow reconstruction (Fig. 159.5A and B).[2]

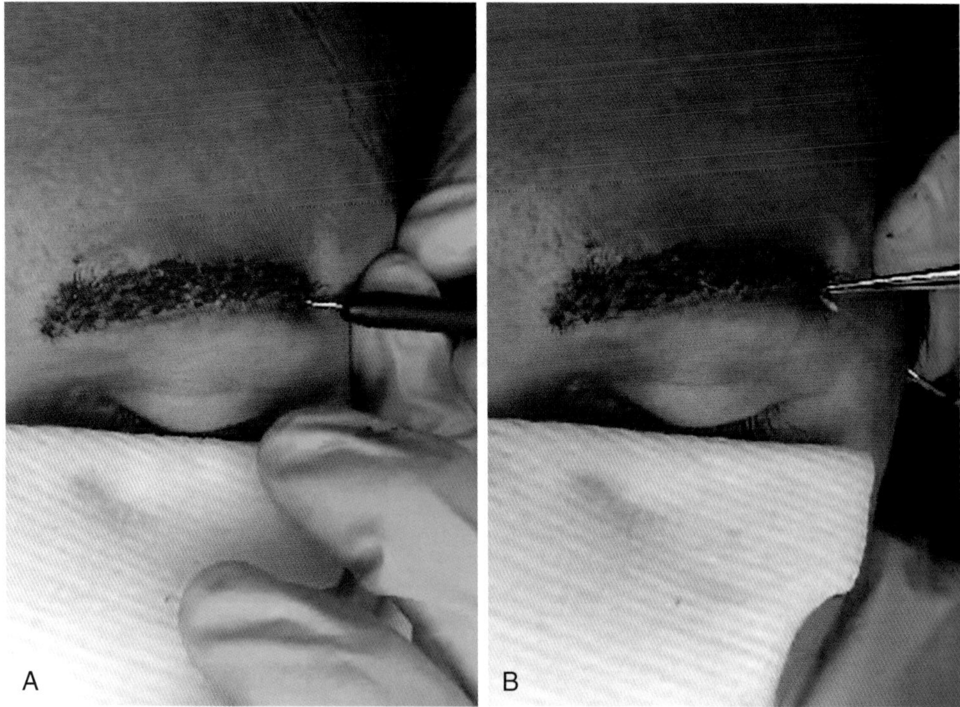

Figure 159.5 **A,** Solid needle for site prep. **B,** Placement of a graft into a brow site.

The donor area for eyebrow reconstruction is the lateral occipital scalp because this area has tremendous density and often has finer hair. The harvesting technique is as described later, and the donor hairs are dissected under magnification to select hardy single-hair or, occasionally, two-hair grafts.[10] Patients should be informed that the transplanted occipital hair will grow not to a finite length but as though it were still residing on the occipital scalp. Consequently, these transplanted hairs will require trimming.

Ninety percent of the transplanted hairs will grow. Despite proper placement, some of these hairs will grow in a less than optimal direction, such as too vertical or at an obtuse emergence angle from the skin. These hairs can be trained to grow in the proper direction with gels and combing. If these "wild" hairs are unresponsive to training, they can be trimmed short or plucked out.[2]

In the immediate postoperative period, the recipient sites can be gently cleansed with mild soap on postoperative day 1. Application of antibiotic ointment keeps the recipient site moist and can help minimize scabbing.

Scars in Hair-Bearing Skin

Grafting into scars generally requires the placement of single FU grafts, mimicking the angulation and growth pattern of the surrounding facial hair. The "stick and place" technique described for eyebrow reconstruction would be utilized. Grafting into scalp scars or temporal scars could utilize the grafts of single or multiple FUs, but the surgeon should always attempt to mimic the existing growth pattern of the surrounding hair.

Limitations and Contraindications

The contraindications for hair transplant include conditions with inadequate donor hair with an advanced Norwood type VII pattern, very thin donor region density, or a systemic condition such as alopecia areata. Systemic diseases or conditions that might result in poor wound healing, such as collagen vascular disease, lupus etc. or a predilection to keloid formation, would also be relative contraindications.

TECHNIQUE

HAIRLINE DESIGN AND PLACEMENT[2]

Positioning of the anterior frontal hairline is the most critical factor in a successful hair transplantation procedure. Successful placement begins with one's understanding of the concept of facial thirds. The somewhat rounded and tapered frontal hairline is placed with the apex approximately 2 cm above the perceived frontal hairline as defined by dividing the face into thirds. The lateral points of the hairline are made perpendicular to a line drawn to the outer canthus of the eyes. This somewhat posterior placement of the transplanted surgical hairline is a representation of a mature man's hairline through the normal aging process. In anticipating future hair loss, hair transplantation should provide an esthetic result throughout the decades of life.[11] A successfully placed hairline at 30 years of age must also retain the same esthetically pleasing look at age 60 years and beyond. Hairlines placed too low will, in most cases, be esthetically unacceptable as the patient reaches the fifth and sixth decades of life. In addition, the retropositioning of the surgically transplanted hairline will limit the number of grafts required for complete fullness and therefore help conserve the amount of donor hair used, especially in individuals with more advanced patterns of balding.

The anticipated hairline is drawn initially with a wax pencil, which can easily be removed with an alcohol wipe if revisions to hairline design are necessary. The final outline of the hairline design is then reinforced with an indelible fine-point marking pen. It must be symmetric and properly placed (Fig. 159.6). Some practitioners will then mark the anticipated recipient sites. Others will proceed to anesthesia and recipient site preparation without marking the recipient site. Either method is acceptable as long as the recipient sites are behind and confluent with the marked hairline in a staggered fashion.

ANESTHESIA[2]

With the patient in a sitting position, the donor site is anesthetized with 2% lidocaine with 1:100,000 epinephrine. Use of a vasoconstrictor is usually necessary to aid in hemostasis. A 30-gauge needle is used not only for subcutaneous infiltration for the donor sites but also to achieve a ring block for the recipient sites.[3] Oral anxiolytics, inhalational nitrous oxide and oxygen, or intravenous sedation can also be used during the injection of local anesthetic, which lasts approximately 1 to 2 minutes. Approximately 10 to 15 minutes is required for full vasoconstriction to take place before the procedure is begun.

RECIPIENT SITE PREPARATION[2]

Complete preparation of the recipient site involves the use of recipient slit blades and solid needles for micrografts and multi-FUs (i.e., stab wounds or needle punctures at each planned graft position) (Fig. 159.7). These wounds are created prior to the dissection for harvesting the grafts so that bleeding will have ceased before one attempt to insert the grafts. The recipient site must be accurately angled to match the angle at which the original hair emerged from the scalp. Usually, there is some terminal or lanugo hair to help determine this angle, but essentially all hair is placed in a forward direction. Exceptions to the forward placement of hair would be recipient sites in the temporal/sideburn regions, eyebrows, moustache, and beard regions. An additional requirement is that the blade or recipient punch passes deep to the skin into subcutaneous tissue.

Continued

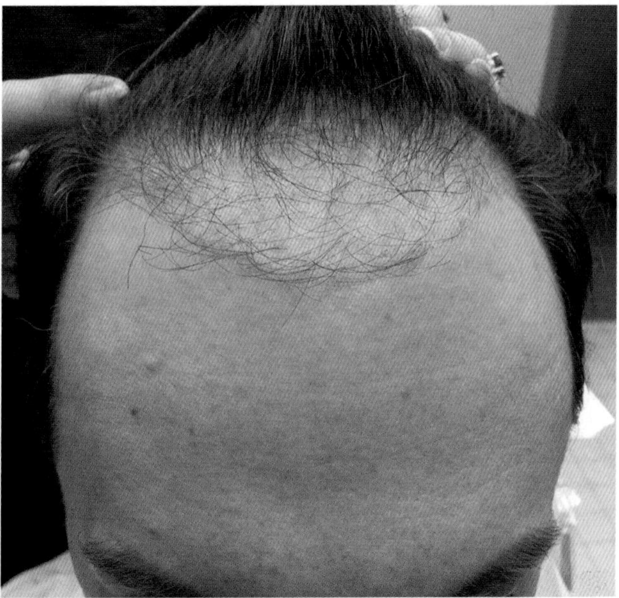

Figure 159.6 The anticipated hairline—symmetrical and rounded. This line acts as a guide for the placement of micro- and multifollicular grafts in needle punctures and slits.

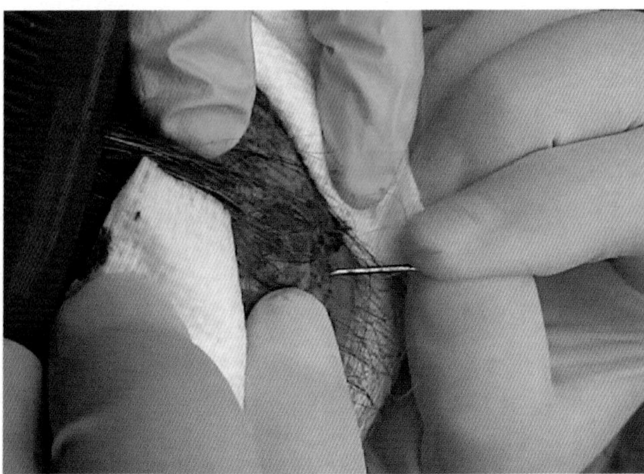

Figure 159.7 Preparation of a recipient site. The needle is oriented to mimic the growth direction of the surrounding hair and angled anteriorly.

TECHNIQUE—*cont'd*

DONOR SITE SELECTION AND PREPARATION[2]

After marking the recipient sites, appropriate donor areas are chosen that will match, as closely as possible, the texture and density of the recipient area. In essence, the donor site is hair that would typically exist in a type 6 or 7 pattern.[12] Thus, by visualizing the patient's head from behind, an arbitrary line drawn from the top of the ears would denote an area below which all hair would be genetically programmed to grow indefinitely when transplanted. Similarly, the hair remaining just above and behind the ears would appear to have that same potential.

An area that will provide the needed number of grafts is clipped to a length of approximately 2 mm with either scissors or clippers. One should be able to see the angled direction of the hair growth as it emerges from the scalp to achieve proper orientation in the recipient area. These hair follicles must also be visualized when using an ellipse or multibladed knife to take a long strip required for micrograft and multifollicular preparation. The area is prepared with an adequate antiseptic solution, either iodophor or alcohol-soaked sponges, to clean and remove any spicules of hair remaining on the surface (Fig. 159.8).

HARVESTING DONOR STRIPS[2]

In the patient, in a sitting position with the head firmly fixed, the donor site is injected with physiologic saline until maximum turgor is achieved to minimize skin distortion during the procedure. This tumescence is similar to that performed during liposuction procedures. Similar skin turgor is desired. The "fountain sign," when the tumescent solution squirts from the puncture site from adequate turgor, is also frequently noted.

Because hair transplantation involving micrografts and multifollicular grafting has now evolved into a procedure that generates and moves hundreds or thousands of much smaller grafts, the process adds significant time and complexity to the transplant procedure. To simplify and accelerate the production of grafts, the donor scalp is often harvested as long narrow strips with the aid of a multibladed knife. Grafts of single FUs, two to three FUs, or four to six FUs can easily be visualized and quickly cut from narrow donor strips.

Obtaining donor tissue as long narrow strips with a multibladed knife has become a mainstay of the transplant procedure for many surgeons, with the ideal strip being defined as one with a full complement of viable intact hairs along the entire length and a minimal number of transected hairs. The two key elements for cutting perfect strips are tumescence and proper angling of the cutting instrument. After maximal tumescence is obtained by injecting normal saline both subcutaneously and intradermally, #10 blades are placed on the multibladed knife. It is held by the fingers, and the angle of the knife is constantly changed while maintaining consistent alignment with the hair direction and checking for both parallel alignment of the knife blades and donor hairs. Depths greater than 6 mm should be avoided in an effort to remain in a dissection plane superficial to the galea, which minimizes the chance of excessive bleeding. After a single pass with the multibladed knife, removal of the strip is accomplished by sharp dissection with super sharp scissors or a scalpel, which is used to cut along a precise plane approximately 1 to 2 mm below the level of the hair follicles. Spacers of 2 to 3 mm define the width of strips, which again are best cut only into the subcutaneous fat layer to avoid the galea aponeurotica (Fig. 159.9). When the harvesting of micrografts and multifollicular grafts is complete, the donor site is generally closed in one layer with a 3-0 Vicryl suture to provide a thin scar completely covered by existing hair and actually preserving the amount of donor hair available for subsequent transplant procedures.[13,14] Occasionally, some tension is noted, and the superior and inferior scalp flaps are undermined. A two-layered closure is then performed.

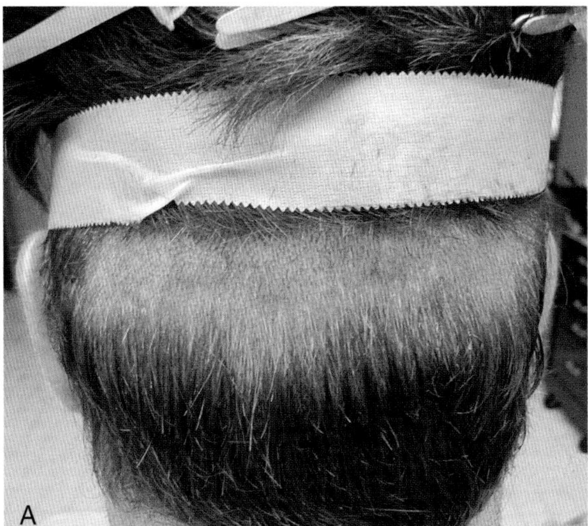

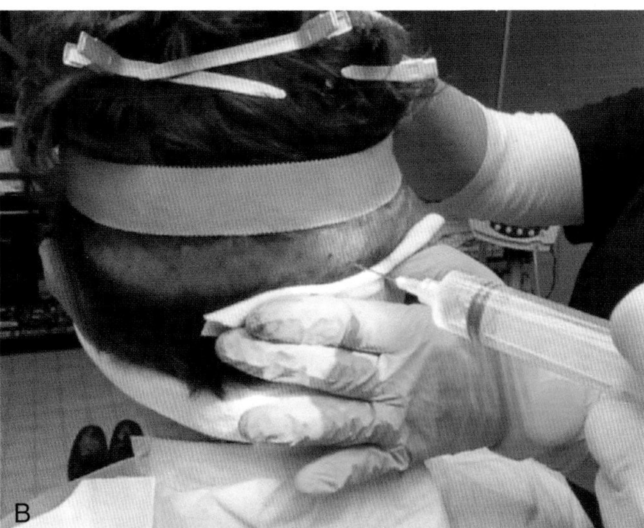

Figure 159.8 **A,** Prepared donor site. **B,** Tumescent injection of normal saline.

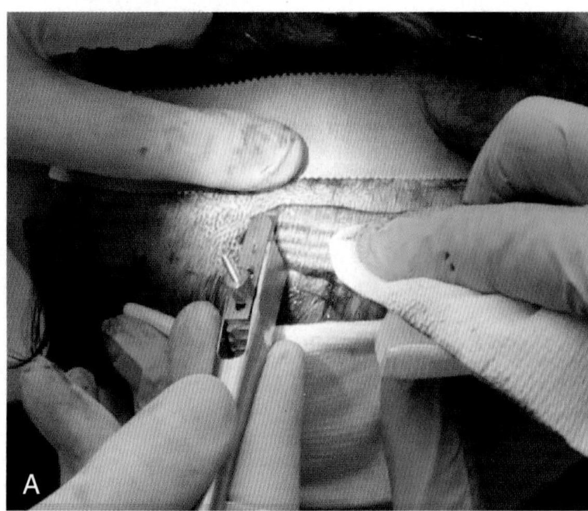

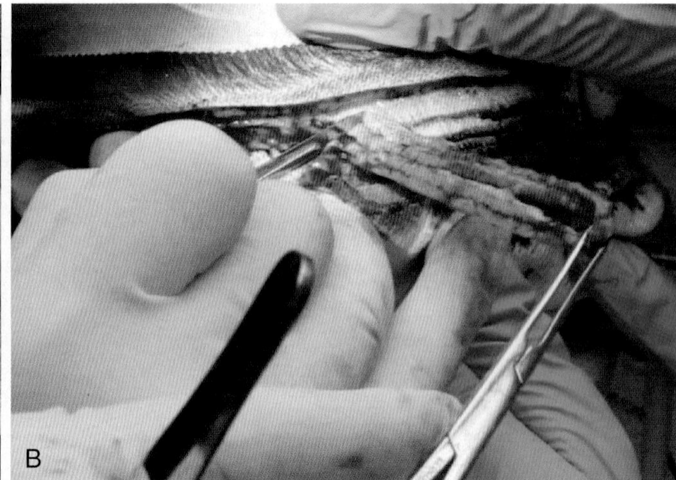

Figure 159.9 **A,** Harvest of the donor scalp strips with the multibladed knife. The blades should parallel the hair follicle in the subcutaneous tissue. **B,** Removal of the donor strips: dissection in the subcutaneous fat, deep to the hair follicles and superficial to the galea.

TECHNIQUE—*cont'd*

GRAFT PREPARATION

The harvested donor scalp should be kept moist in a normal saline solution at all times. If a prolonged ex-vivo time is anticipated, chilled normal saline solution can extend graft viability. Under loupe or microscopic magnification, excess subcutaneous fat should be trimmed from the harvested strips of scalp. Then under similar magnification, a #11 blade is used to dissect FU groupings from the donor scalp strip. Grafts containing one or two FUs are prepared for placement into the hairline. Multifollicular unit grafts containing four to six hairs are prepared for placement posterior to the rows of hairline grafts. These slightly larger grafts add density to the hair restoration (Fig. 159.10).

GRAFTING THE RECIPIENT AREA[2]

The recipient hole is approximately 0.25 mm smaller than the donor graft, and the graft is inserted to test for snugness of fit. A snug fit is essential because revascularization of the graft depends on blood vessels growing from the dermis of the recipient scalp into the dermis of the graft.

Angling of the recipient site improves the direction of hair growth and lengthens the recipient site, resulting in better accommodation of the graft from the thicker donor skin and preventing elevation of the graft.[7] Micrografts and multifollicular grafts are implanted with a small jeweler's forceps into 1- to 2-mm slits or needle puncture sites (Fig. 159.11).

Inexperienced operators will encounter considerable difficulty at first, and it is important for the recipient sites to have reached the sticky stage of coagulation before implantation is attempted, usually in 5 to 10 minutes. It should be remembered that for micrografts or multifollicular grafts, gentle pressure is applied with a swab or a finger to adjacent grafts while the grafts are inserted. Unquestionably, these procedures cannot be performed with consummate expertise and in a timely fashion without using a well-trained transplant team consisting of at least one surgeon who prepares and marks the operative sites and obtains the donor strip and two to three technicians who cut the grafts and place them just as rapidly as they are dissected (Fig. 159.12).

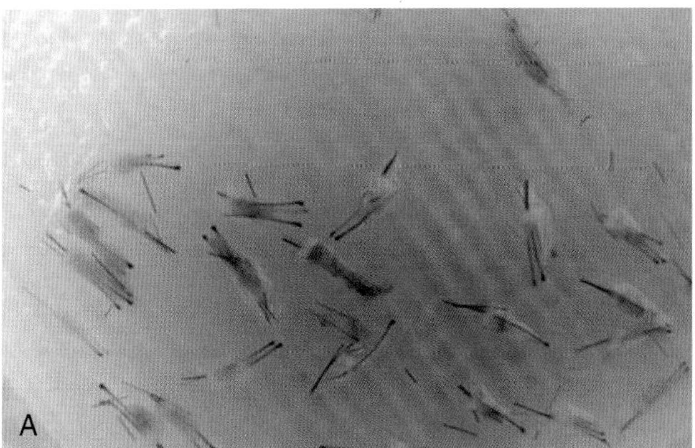

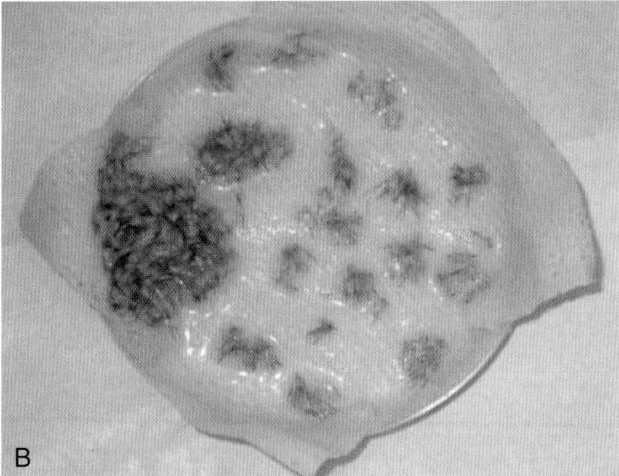

Figure 159.10 **A,** Micrografts. **B,** Multifollicular grafts cut in preparation for implantation.

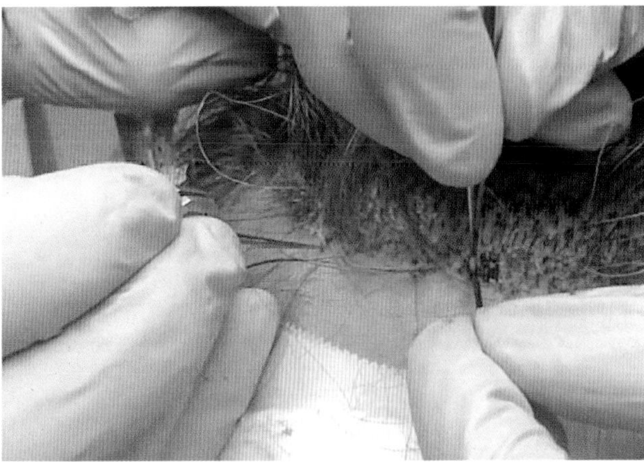

Figure 159.11 On left, placement of a graft with fine jeweler's forceps. On the right, placement facilitated with the use of the jeweler's forceps and slit blade.

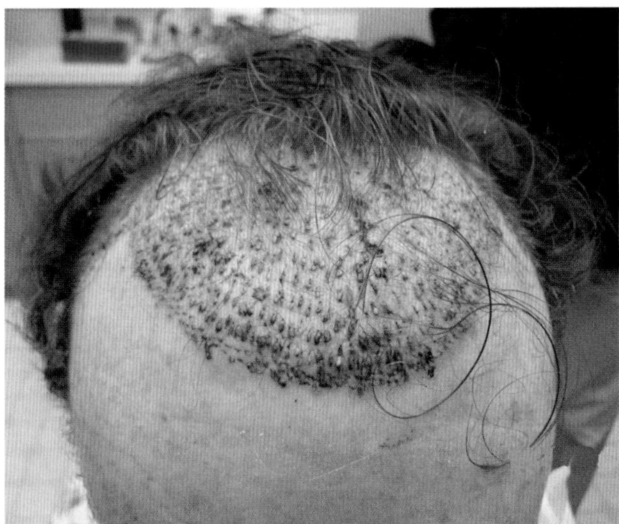

Figure 159.12 Recipient sites with grafts in place to correct a frontal hair loss pattern.

ALTERNATE TECHNIQUE

FOLLICULAR UNIT EXTRACTION

FU extraction is an alternate technique for harvesting donor grafts, one FU at a time with tiny skin punches. Some practitioners utilize machines to aid in the harvesting of donor grafts and/or placement of the grafts. One of these devices harvests with a motorized drill pneumatic system,[15,16] and another utilizes a robot.[15,16] Grafts containing one to three hairs are obtained. The donor site is a very large area of occipital scalp. This technique requires the trimming of this very large region of donor scalp and is almost impossible to camouflage in the immediate postoperative period. Hundreds to thousands of tiny punch holes remain after harvesting (Fig. 159.13). These do not require closure, but heal with very tiny circular scars; even though the technique is touted to be "scarless." Because only very tiny grafts are used, the resulting hair growth often does not provide the density achieved with multi-FU grafts, frequently necessitating additional procedures. It is not the preferred technique of the author.

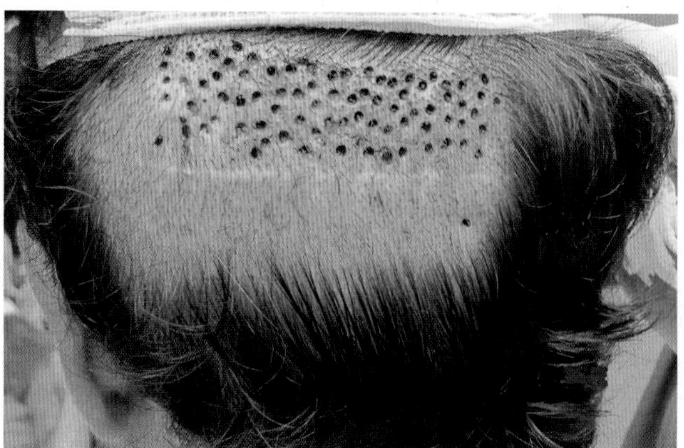

Figure 159.13 Follicular unit extraction technique. Note the large donor area and tiny punch harvests.

Avoidance and Management of Intraoperative Complications

Bleeding, both during and after the operation, is the most common complication. It usually occurs in patients who have taken aspirin or blood-thinning medications or supplements immediately before surgery. Thus, all patients are asked to abstain from aspirin or aspirin-containing products for at least 10 to 14 days before each transplant procedure. Other blood-thinning medications are adjusted accordingly. Operative bleeding is controlled by pressure, injection of additional epinephrine-containing anesthetic and saline into the bleeding site, or suturing. If adequate control takes place during the procedure, postoperative bleeding is rare.

Edema of the forehead may occur starting on the third or fourth postoperative day. It probably results from excessive anesthetic volume or surgical trauma, and it is particularly disturbing in the frontal area because most patients consider it to be cosmetically annoying. This swelling requires no treatment; however, systemic corticosteroids seem to help eliminate this problem. The corticosteroid regimen includes 10 mg of dexamethasone intramuscularly at the time surgery, followed by a 5-day postoperative course of decreasing dexamethasone dosage orally (Decadron 5-13 Pak, Merck, West Point, PA).

Infection is a possible complication, although the use of postoperative antibiotics and the requirement that patients wash their hair twice a day for the first 3 days following each surgical procedure virtually eliminates this potential. Patients are given 500 mg of tetracycline or 250 mg of cefuroxime (Ceftin) for 7 days postoperatively twice a day.

Cobblestoning, or irregular elevation of the grafts, is prevented by proper graft placement and by adequate cleansing postoperatively the morning after each surgical procedure.

Hypertrophic scarring occasionally occurs in patients with a history of poor scar formation. In this case a trial transplant is undertaken with a limited number of different-sized grafts placed in an unobtrusive area while making certain that they fit snugly in the recipient sites. If scarring and poor growth occur, further grafting on that patient should not be done.[3]

With proper patient selection, hairline design and placement, and meticulous surgical technique, an excellent result can be achieved in most patients.[2]

Postoperative Considerations

The donor and recipient sites may or may not be bandaged. If bandaging is preferred, a nonadhering Telfa (Kendall Company, Boston, MA) pad coated with antibiotic ointment is placed over the operative sites. Several layers of flattened gauze sponges (4 × 3 inches) and a layer of ABD dressings are then used to hold the Telfa in place. These dressings are then secured into position with #5 tube gauze. The dressing is removed the following morning, and the scalp and each graft are cleansed meticulously with a cotton swab and hydrogen peroxide. The hair is washed and styled to cover the operative sites. The patient is mandated to wash the hair twice a day for the first 3 days following each transplant procedure. Suture removal, when necessary, is accomplished 1 to 2 weeks after each procedure. The patient must, of course, be made aware that a lag phase exists before hair growth is initiated. After approximately 3 months, the telogen phase of the transplanted grafts ends and anagen begins.[2]

References

1. Orentreich N. Autografts in alopecias and other selected dermatological condition. *Ann N Y Acad Sci.* 1959;83:463–479.
2. Hendler BH, Stanton DC. Micrografting and hair transplantation surgery. In: Bagheri B, Khan, eds. *Current Therapy in Oral and Maxillofacial Surgery.* St Louis, Missouri: Elsevier; 2012.
3. Hendler BH. Hair transplantation. In: *OMS Knowledge Update, Vol I, Pt. II. Esthetic Surgery Section.* Rosemont, Illinois: American Association of Oral and Maxillofacial Surgeons (AAOMS); 1995.
4. Reed M. Hair transplantation. In: *Grabb and Smith's Plastic Surgery.* 6th ed. Philadelphia, Pennsylvania: Lippincott Williams & Wilkins; 2006.
5. Headington JT. Transverse microscopic anatomy of the human scalp—a basis for a morphometric approach to disorders of the hair follicle. *Arch Dermatol.* 1984;120:449–456.
6. Bernstein RM, Rassman WR. The logic of follicular unit transplantation. *Dermatol Clin.* 1999;17:277–295.
7. Nordstrom REA. "Micrografts" for improvement of the frontal hairline after hair transplantation. *Aesthetic Plast Surg.* 1981;5:97–101.
8. Stegman SJ, Tromovitch TA. *Cosmetic Dermatologic Surgery.* Chicago, Illiniois: Year Book Publishers; 1984.
9. Norwood OT. Classification and incidence of male pattern baldness. In: Norwood OT, Shiell RC, eds. *Hair Transplant Surgery.* 2nd ed. Springfield, Illinois: Charles C Thomas; 1984.
10. Gandleman M, Epstein JS. Hair transplantation to the eyebrow, eyelash, and other parts of the body. *Facial Plast Surg Clin North Am.* 2004;12:253–261.
11. Nordstrom REA. The initial interview. *Facial Plast Surg.* 1985;2:179–187.
12. Alt TH. Evaluation of donor harvesting techniques in hair transplantation. *J Dermatol Surg Oncol.* 1984;10:799–806.
13. Morrison ID. An improved method of suturing the donor site in hair transplantation surgery. *Plast Reconstr Surg.* 1981;67:378–381.
14. Pierce HE. Improved method of closure of donor sites in hair transplantation. *J Dermatol Surg Oncol.* 1979;6:475–476.
15. Shiell RC. A review of modern surgical hair restoration techniques. *J Cutan Aesthet Surg.* 2008;1(1):12–16.
16. Rose PT. The latest innovations in hair transplantation. *Facial Plast Surg.* 2011;27(4):366–377.

CHAPTER 160

Genioglossus Advancement/Hyoid Suspension for Obstructive Sleep Apnea (OSA)

David J. Dattilo

Armamentarium—Genioglossus Advancement

1.5 Low-profile fixation plates
Armamentarium—Hyoid Suspension
Calipers
Kelly forceps
Medium to small malleable retractors
Small tracheostomy hooks
Mini anchor system/with attached non-resorbable suture
Metzenbaum dissection scissors
Rake retractors
Reciprocating saw large bone bur, 1.5 drill
Small right-angle retractors

History of the Procedure

The genioglossus advancement (GA) procedure was first described by Riley and coworkers as a surgical treatment for obstructive sleep apnea (OSA) in 1984.[1] Following multiple clinical trials, it eventually became a reliable initial procedure in the two-staged surgical protocol put forth by the Stanford University team.[2] The procedure relies on the advancement of the genioglossus muscle in an anterior vector and, in doing so, relieves obstruction at the base of the tongue during sleep in patients suffering from hypopharyngeal OSA. This advancement is accomplished by advancing the genial tubercle, and thus the fan-shaped fibers of the genioglossus muscle throughout the tongue creating tension at the base and expanding the airway. The initial GA procedure reported by Riley and colleagues was simply an advancement genioplasty with the superior border rising high enough to capture the genial tubercles. Subsequent procedures where changes in the lower facial profile were not indicated or desired revolved around an osteotomized full thickness "window" in the anterior mandible.[3,4] This osteotomy would capture the entirety of the muscle attachment, pull it through the width of the mandible, a distance of approximately 13 mm and stabilize it in some way so as to create the desired tension but not distort the patient's profile. This initial blind window approach gave birth to multiple studies evaluating the variations in the position and dimensions of the tubercle to be captured, its distance to the apices of the mandibular teeth, and the inferior border of the mandible.[5,6] Based on this information, new designs were developed over the next 30 years that would safely capture the entire musculature, preserve the vitality of the teeth and prevent any long-term deformity of the mandible.[7–9]

The hyoid suspension procedure became popular based on two studies early on in the anatomic basis of OSA. The first study by Riley and coworkers involved the systematic comparison of cephalometric films of OSA patients to a controlled group. This study demonstrated a consistent trend of OSA patients having a more inferiorly displaced hyoid bone.[3] A second study by Van de Graff and coworkers while studying airway resistance in dogs demonstrated a significant reduction in airway resistance with anterior displacement of the hyoid bone concluding that in patients with OSA obstruction at the level of the hypopharynx/base of the tongue may be the result of decreased activity of the genioglossus and hyoid musculature.[10] The suspension procedure has since been added to the GA to help further enlarge the pharyngeal space.

The initial procedure relied upon wire or fascia latta wrapped around the hyoid bone and suspended anteriorly to the symphysis region of the mandible. This procedure was later modified by Riley et al. and again by Hormann and Baisch[11] to an inferior suspension to the thyroid cartilage. The techniques appear to be equally effective in assisting the GA in expansion of the airway and can be used at the discretion of the surgeon.

Indications for the Use of Procedure

The ideal candidate for this procedure is the patient with mild to moderate OSA with diagnostic evidence of decreased posterior airway space with hypopharyngeal collapse (Fugita II,III). From an objective standpoint, past studies have shown that patients with a respiratory disturbance index (RDI) of less than 40 have an 86% to 100% success rate based on accepted criteria of a RDI less than 20 or a 50% reduction over the preoperative study.[9,12,13] It should be mentioned that in these studies the procedure was accompanied by a palatal reduction procedure. As the RDI increased in the 44 to 60 range, the success rate fell to 57%, and beyond this level it was suggested that a maxillomandibular advancement would provide better and more predictable results. With class 2 retrognathic mandibles, the sliding advancement genioplasty is preferred and in such cases the hyoid suspension may not be necessary due to the additional attachment of the digastric and the geniohyoid musculature to the distal segment.

Limitations and Contraindications

Patients with clinically severe OSA with a high body mass index and radiographic evidence of obstruction at multiple levels of the upper airways cannot be expected to respond well to this procedure and should be considered for an Maxillo-Mandibular Advancement (MMA). Also, patients with micrognathia and edentulism are risks for fracture by not providing enough bone mass to support the muscle advancement. Patients with osteoporotic disease will always run the risk of fracture and should be avoided as candidates.

TECHNIQUE

The evolution of this surgical procedure arose from multiple attempts of different techniques that would preserve as much of the native bone tissue as possible while still obtaining the optimum advancement of the genioglossus muscle and the required anterior tension of the hyoid bone. These two procedures are described below as being done together through one extraoral incision that provides access to both surgical sites decreasing surgical time and sites of possible postsurgical morbidity. However, these procedures can be done separately and incisions can be placed intraorally or extraorally at the surgeon's discretion. The author prefers extraoral incisions to preserve the soft tissue cover over the anterior osteotomies, which prevents breakdown and provides functional molding of the underlying bone to more natural contours.

STEP 1: A 5-cm incision is made in or just posterior to the submental fold, providing adequate access for the hyoid procedure and the GA through the same incision. Dissection is first carried down through the platysma until the anterior bellies of the digastric muscles are located. Using these two muscle bellies as guides, blunt and sharp dissection is taken posteriorly, staying in the midline, until the hyoid bone can be palpated. Digital palpation is useful in this dissection to differentiate between the hyoid and thyroid bone, especially in large individuals. The hyoid is then isolated by placing a wide malleable retractor on the superior and inferior aspects. A small tracheostomy hook is placed on the inferior border of the hyoid to stabilize it for further dissection and placement of suspension sutures. Following stabilization of the hyoid, subperiosteal exposure of the anterior body with the midline spine is performed.

STEP 2: Minimal stripping of soft tissue of the anterior hyoid ensures that all muscle attachments remain intact maximizing the effect of the advancement on the airway and minimizing complications. Two types of suspension can be carried out at this point. The author prefers the Mitek mini anchor procedure, which does not require any disruption or dissection of the musculature.[14] With counter pressure being applied, two Mitek mini anchors are placed, one on each side of the central spine in the thicker bone comprising the inferior border of the hyoid by drilling a 2.1 mm hole and placing quick anchor with a preattached #0 Ethibond suture (Ethicon, Inc. Bridgewater, New Jersey) (Fig. 160.1). Once placement of the Mitek sutures is complete, hemostasis is obtained, and the sutures are laid aside until the remainder of the GA procedure is completed.

If a circumferential wire or suture procedure is desired an orthopedic rotator cuff suture passer (Linvatec, Largo, FL) is best used to facilitate the safe passing of the suture.[15] Because of the posterior inclination of the superior portion of the body of the hyoid, passing these sutures can be exceedingly difficult. Care must be taken to avoid the posterior portion of the midline of the hyoid in order to avoid damage to the hyo-epiglottic ligament, which stabilizes the hyoid to the epiglottis. Just lateral to the midline but still on the thicker bone of the body is where the sutures should be placed. Once the suture passer is placed around the hyoid from inferior to superior and is visualized, the sutures are passed through it from superior to inferior as the passer is withdrawn. This is carried out on both sides. Hemostasis is checked and the sutures are laid aside until the completion of the GA.

The hyoid portion of the operation is always done first so that the dissection is not complicated by alteration in anatomy or bleeding from the more superior GA operative site.

Continued

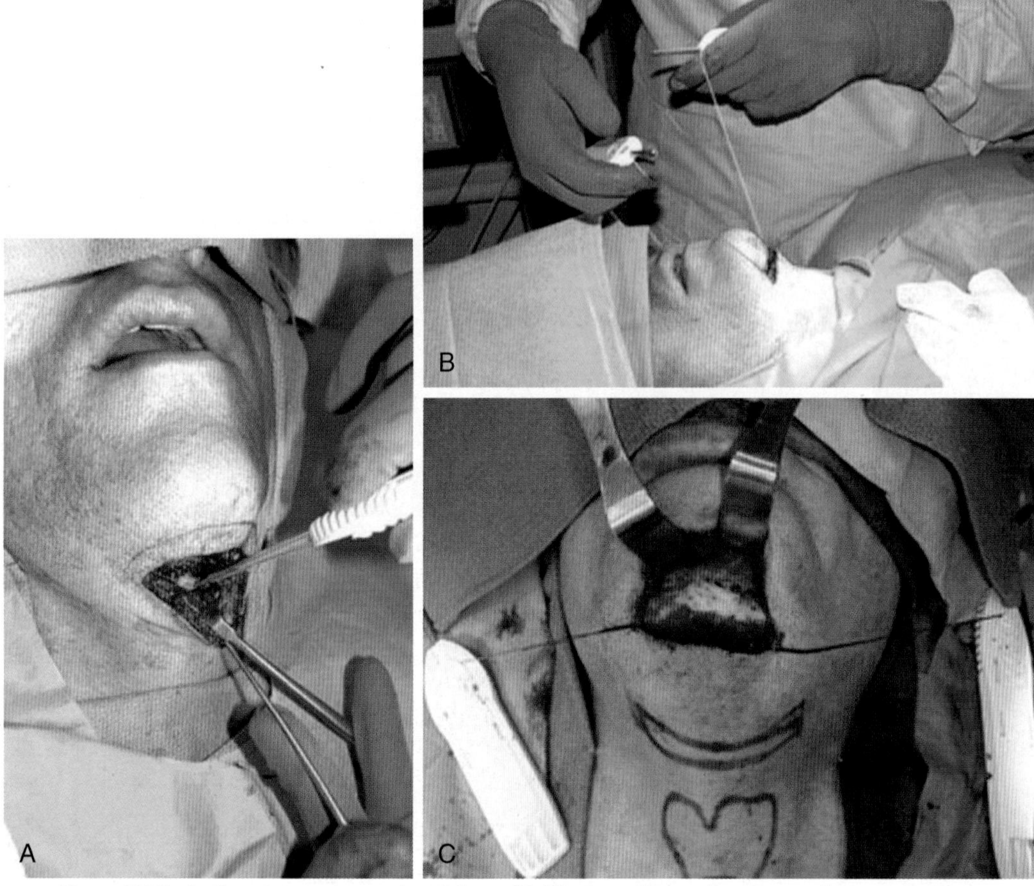

Figure 160.1 **A,** Securing anchor to hyoid bone. **B,** Placing additional anchor and testing stability. **C,** Placing sutures aside and exposing anterior mandible for GSA procedure.

TECHNIQUE—*cont'd*

STEP 3: Attention is then turned to the superior portion of the incision. The digastric muscles are followed again to the inferior border of the mandible. Subperiosteal dissection is carried out to lift the skin flap up exposing the anterior portion of the mandible out to the mental foramen and superior to a point where the canine prominence and, in some cases, the roots of the anterior teeth. Consideration of known distances between the genial tubercles and the roots of the mandibular teeth and the inferior border as well as the width of the muscle itself are all important at this point in order to design your bone incision. Average measurements indicate the tubercles are 14.2 mm from the inferior border and 11.8 mm from the root apices. Calipers are used to measure the most superior extent of your bone incision, which in a normal sized individual is approximately 15 mm from the inferior border of the mandible. This initial marking is important, and from it all other markings for the final design are taken. It can be altered depending on the size of the mandible and the presence of tooth roots and also can be assisted by the fabrication of a CT-generated surgical guide. The superior osteotomy should be a minimum of 5 mm inferior to the root apices to avoid denervation and devascularization of the individual teeth. The inferior incision is made approximately 5 to 6 mm above the inferior border so as to catch as much of the genial tubercle as possible but still preserve the strong cortical inferior border and prevent weakening of the mandible. The design is then tapered laterally on both sides to form an elliptical pattern that will avoid the roots of the teeth as well as provide a strong strut on the inferior mandible to provide support. The total horizontal length should be taken out to approximately one and a half to two times the vertical heights to ensure enough bone to overlap when the muscle is pulled forward and rotated 90 degrees taking into account the shorter lingual cortex due to the curvature of the mandible. This overlap should have enough bone to accommodate a 2.0 screw. Before the osteotomy is completed, a screw is placed in the center cortex to assist in pulling out and rotating the tethered segment.

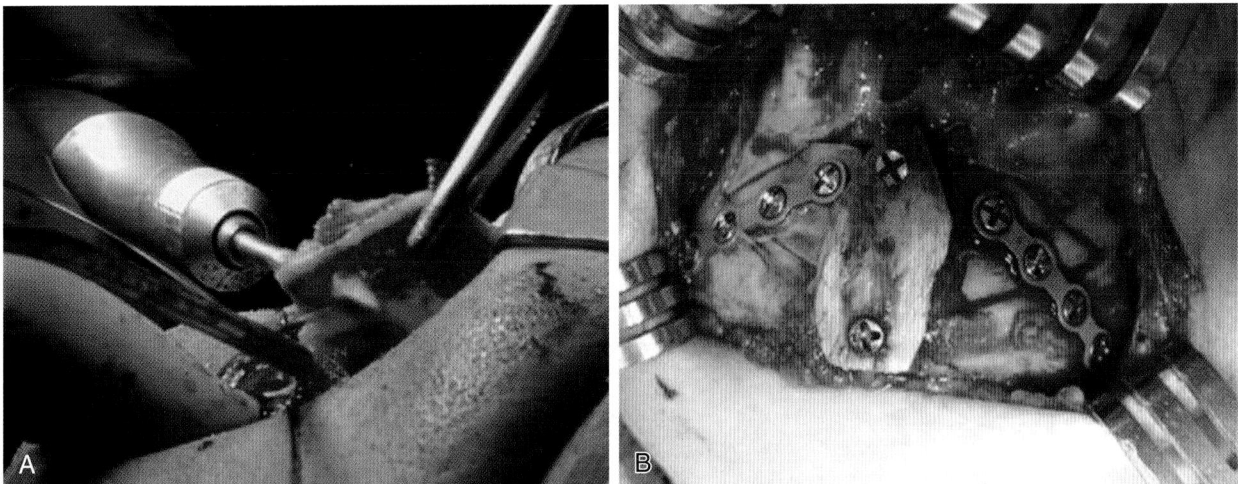

Figure 160.2 **A,** Removing cortical-cancellous portion of advanced segment. **B,** Grafting segment to lateral defects.

TECHNIQUE—*cont'd*

The osteotomy of the genioglossus attached bone segment is then completed, released, advanced, and rotated 90 degrees. With the lingual cortex now resting on the facial cortex of the outer mandible, the screw is removed, and the cortico-cancellous outer layer is removed with a reciprocating saw down to the lingual cortex. The remaining lingual cortex is taken down and recontoured with a barrel bur and a 2-mm screw is placed on the inferior and superior portion of the advanced segment. The free facial cortex that was removed is then split, the center portion is removed, and it is regrafted back into the surgical defect and secured with low-profile 2.0 miniplates (Fig. 160.2). These free bone grafts may have to be contoured on the medial side so as to not impinge upon the advanced belly of the genioglossus muscle.

STEP 4: Finally, the Mitek sutures anchored to the hyoid or the free circa mandibular sutures are passed underneath the belly of the digastric on each side and anchored to the inferior border of the mandible in line with the most lateral point of the osteotomy. Two holes are drilled into the inferior border of the mandible in these areas with a wire passing bur, and the suture needle of one arm is passed and tied with the other with mild tension maintaining the hyoid in an anterior vector but not significantly changing its anatomic position (Fig. 160.3). The purpose of the sutures is to suspend the hyoid, not to significantly advance it, which could cause fracture of this very fragile bone or a breakage of the suture. A suction drain is placed within the depth of the wound and the wound is closed in layers.

Avoidance and Management of Complications

Genioglossus Advancement

Intraoperative complications for the GA procedure can best be avoided through careful bony incision design measurements that keep away from structures that can cause long-term morbidity if damaged. If the superior margin of the incision is closer than 5 mm to the roots of the mandibular teeth, necrosis of the pulp chambers and desensitization can occur. If these symptoms persist postoperatively, an endodontic consult should be obtained. The horizontal dimension of the osteotomy needs to be sufficiently long enough to span the vertical defect when turned 90 degrees, considering the shorter curvature of the lingual cortex, in order to support the tension caused by the advanced musculature. If insufficient length of bone occurs, then the cortex can be rigidly fixed to either the upper or lower margin of the osteotomy with a single bone screw. Alternatively, a spanning plate can be placed across the defect to suspend the tethered boney segment in its desired anterior position. This procedure can also be used in the event of the muscular attachment being inadvertently stripped from the tubercles by too aggressive advancement of the tethered segment.

All attempts should be made to reconstruct any through and through defect of the mandible caused by the procedure through free bone grafting. Earlier descriptions of the pull-through "window" procedures left large defects on each side of the advancement, weakening the mandible, and causing

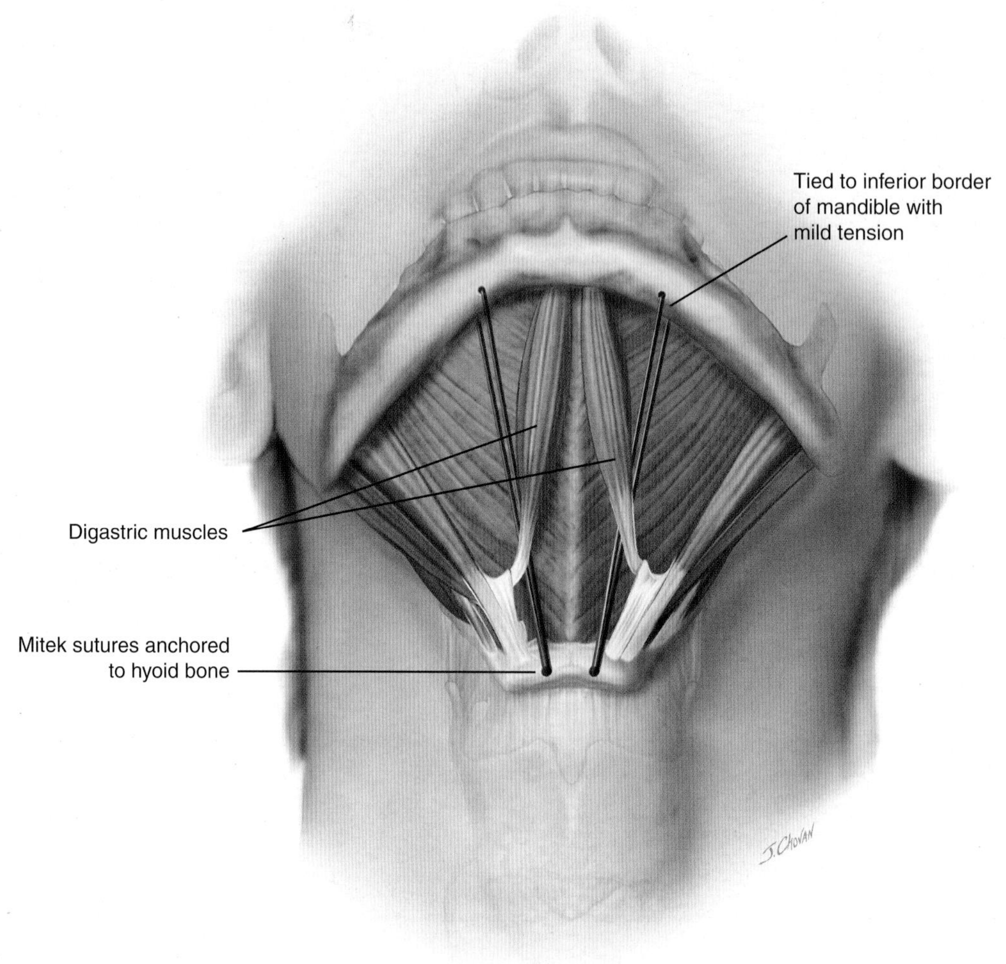

Figure 160.3 Osteotomy sites on mandible and hyoid for suture passage.

major difficulty in future dental reconstructive efforts as tooth loss and alveolar resorption occurred.

Hyoid Suspension

The surgical complications of this procedure mostly arise from the difficulties in exposing and manipulating this free-floating bone with multiple muscle attachments. If the surgeon does not correctly identify the midline of the hyoid, then stabilization, wire passing, and anchor placement can all result in fracture of this very fragile bone. If fracture occurs, reduction is necessary with a small low-profile plate. The hyo-epiglottic ligament attaches to the superior portion of the posterior hyoid in the midline. Therefore if a small tracheostomy hook is placed under the inferior border in the midline, it will avoid the ligament, stabilize the hyoid, and help the surgeon with a reference as to where the suspension suture anchors or the circum-hyoid sutures should be placed. Overaggressive advancement of the hyoid is to be avoided. Not only can it result in breakage of one or both of the suspension sutures, but fracture and postoperative difficulty in swallowing can also occur.[16] Over advancement can also result in the base of the tongue folding back over the hyoid, eliminating some of the airway expansion accomplished through the GA.

Postoperative Considerations

It is expected that all patients will have a floor-of-the-mouth ecchymosis and elevation of the tongue that can be quite prominent for the first week following surgery. The temporary changes in speech and difficulty swallowing may just require reassurance of the patient. The surgical drain can be removed the following day assuming minimal blood is present in the collection bulb over one full shift. Due to the multiple procedures close to the airway, it is recommended the patient spends 24 hours either in a monitored unit or at least in an area where multiple checks can be carried out by nursing staff. The patient should be advised to bring their CPAP/BIPAP with them for possible use during the postoperative period.

ALTERNATIVE TECHNIQUE 1: Hyoid–Thyroid Suspension (Hyoidthyroidpexia)

As a singular procedure for isolated hypopharyngeal airway collapse or in conjunction with a GA that is performed through an intraoral approach, this technique has also been found to be effective. The movement of the hyoid bone, however, is not in a forward anterior vector but limited to an inferior and slightly anterior position.[17] A horizontal incision is made in the midline of the neck at or just above the hyoid bone. Dissection is taken down to the level of the supra hyoid musculature isolating a portion of the body of the hyoid at the midline. The musculature attached to the inferior of the hyoid is stripped from its attachments and dissected clean. The styloid hyoid ligament is resected from the lesser cornu with the remaining suprahyoid musculature remaining intact. The thyroid notch and the thyroid lamina are exposed through a subcutaneous vertical incision.

A suture or surgical wire is then passed around the hyoid bone on both sides of the midline using a suture passer as mentioned above avoiding the midline and the hyo-epiglottic ligament. The thyroid notch and the superior lamina are then identified. The fixation sutures or wires are then placed through the thyroid cartilage lateral to the notch on each side, pulling the hyoid and its musculature down and forward over the thyroid. Because of the perichondral blood supply to the superior portion of the thyroid minimal dissection is warranted to prevent necrosis. The suspension material is made fast with the knot tucked away so as to not irritate the overlying skin. The wound is then closed in layers and a passive drain is placed.

Maintaining good anatomic landmarks throughout the dissection will keep the surgeon oriented and in the midline while identifying the hyoid and the thyroid cartilages. Staying lateral to the midline of these two structures while passing the suspension sutures will prevent any damage to the hyo-epiglottic ligament or the vocal cords.

ALTERNATIVE TECHNIQUE 2: Advancement Genioplasty (With Genial Tubercle Capture)

For the patient with a class ll profile and moderate obstructive airway disease, this technique offers excellent possibilities for correcting the airway obstruction and the retrusive lower facial profile with a single procedure. The technique can be accomplished either intra- or extraorally and usually does not require an accompanying hyoid suspension due to the advancement of the hyoglossus and genioglossus muscle.

After exposing the anterior mandible through either an intraoral or extraoral approach, similar measurements are made in the midline from the lower border of the mandible superior approximately 15 mm. Careful attention to the position of the anterior teeth keeping the planned osteotomy cut at least 5 mm from the roots of the teeth. The cut is then extended to the inferior border of the mandible on each side at a level just below the mental foramen. The distal segment of the osteotomy is separated and advanced, along with the genioglossus attachment forward to the desired position. A rigid stepped plate is first placed in the midline to maintain the anterior position of the advanced segment and then additional plates can be placed on the lateral wings to maintain stabilization and prevent movement of the segment while healing.

The more superior placement of the osteotomy cut as compared with the routine advancement genioplasty does come with it the risk of fracture through the narrowed basal bone beneath the anterior alveolus. Placement of an arch bar on the mandibular teeth can help avoid this complication. Endodontic consultation maybe necessary if the patient suffers from prolonged symptoms of desensitization of the anterior teeth. Due to the sometimes large advancement of the distal segment and the subsequent formation of a step between the two segments, a bone graft may be utilized to soften the contour of the vestibule. If this is anticipated, serious thought should be given to an extraoral approach to allow better healing of the surgical site.

References

1. Riley R, Guilleminault C, Powell N, Derman S. Mandibular osteotomy and hyoid bone advancement for obstructive sleep apnea: a case report. *Sleep*. 1984;7(1):79–82.
2. Riley RW, Powell NB, Guilleminault C. Obstructive sleep apnea syndrome: a surgical protocol for dynamic upper airway reconstruction. *J Oral Maxillofac Surg*. 1993;51(7):742–747.
3. Riley RW, Powell NB, Guilleminault C. Inferior mandibular osteotomy and hyoid myotomy suspension for obstructive sleep apnea: a review of 55 patients. *J Oral Maxillofac Surg*. 1989;47(2):159–164.

4. Li KK, Riley RW, Powell NB, Troell RJ. Obstructive sleep apnea surgery: genioglossus advancement revisited. *J Oral Maxillofac Surg*. 2001;59(10):1181–1184.
5. Mintz SM, Ettinger AC, Geist JR, Geist RY. Anatomic relationship of the genial tubercles to the dentition as determined by cross-sectional tomography. *J Oral Maxillofac Surg*. 1995;53(11):1324–1326.
6. Silverstein K, Costello BJ, Giannakpoulos H, Hendler B. Genioglossus muscle attachments: an anatomic analysis and the implications for genioglossus advancement. *Oral Surg Oral Med Oral Pathol Oral Radiol Endod*. 2000;90(6):686–688.
7. Dattilo DJ, Aynechi M. Modification of the anterior mandibular osteotomy for genioglossus advancement with hyoid suspension for obstructive sleep apnea. *J Oral Maxillofac Surg*. 2007;65(9):1876–1879.
8. Dattilo DJ. The mandibular trapezoid osteotomy for the treatment of obstructive sleep apnea: report of a case. *J Oral Maxillofac Surg*. 1998;56(12):1442–1446.
9. Emara TA, Omara TA, Shouman WM. Modified genioglossus advancement and uvulopalatopharyngoplasty in patients with obstructive sleep apnea. *Otolaryngol Head Neck Surg*. 2011;145(5):865–871.
10. Van de Graaff WB, Gottfried SB, Mitra J, van Lunteren E, Cherniack NS, Strohl KP. Respiratory function of hyoid muscles and hyoid arch. *J Appl Physiol*. 1984;57(1):197–204.
11. Hörmann K, Baisch A. The hyoid suspension. *Laryngoscope*. 2004;114(9):1677–1679.
12. Vilaseca I, Morelló A, Montserrat JM, Santamaría J, Iranzo A. Usefulness of uvulopalatopharyngoplasty with genioglossus and hyoid advancement in the treatment of obstructive sleep apnea. *Arch Otolaryngol Head Neck Surg*. 2002;128(4):435–440.
13. Dattilo DJ, Drooger SA. Outcome assessment of patients undergoing maxillofacial procedures for the treatment of sleep apnea: comparison of subjective and objective results. *J Oral Maxillofac Surg*. 2004;62(2):164–168.
14. Dattilo DJ, Kolodychak MT. The use of the Mitek mini anchor system in the hyoid suspension technique for the treatment of obstructive sleep apnea syndrome. *J Oral Maxillofac Surg*. 2000;58(8):919–920.
15. Schmitz JP, Bitonti DA, Lemke RR. Hyoid myotomy and suspension for obstructive sleep apnea syndrome. *J Oral Maxillofac Surg*. 1996;54(11):1339–1345.
16. Richard W, Timmer F, van Tinteren H, de Vries N. Complications of hyoid suspension in the treatment of obstructive sleep apnea syndrome. *Eur Arch Otorhinolaryngol*. 2011;268(4):631–635.
17. Riley RW, Powell NB, Guilleminault C. Obstructive sleep apnea and the hyoid: a revised surgical procedure. *Otolaryngol Head Neck Surg*. 1994;111(6):717–721.

CHAPTER 161

UPPP, LAUP, and RAUP Procedures for Obstructive Sleep Apnea

Joseph E. Cillo Jr.

Armamentarium

Oral RAE endotracheal intubation
Dingman or Crowe-Davis mouth retractor
Coblation device
Suction coagulator, 10-Fr
Tonsil sponges
Ear bulb syringe
10 cc Control top syringe
Needle: 27-gauge
Bipolar cautery
Handheld CO_2 laser with backstop (for LAUP)
Radiofrequency electrode (for RAUP)

History of the Procedures

Several surgical palatal procedures have been developed to help alleviate nocturnal obstruction in the upper airway for management of snoring obstructive sleep apnea (OSA). Uvulopalatopharyngoplasty (UPPP) was introduced by Fujita et al.[1] in 1981 as the first surgical procedure intended to address OSA. Its primary purpose was to alleviate obstruction of the retropalatal airway through the reduction and rearrangement of the contributing and surrounding soft tissues. These generally included removal of the tonsils and uvula with repositioning of the surrounding tonsillar pillars and soft palate. It has subsequently gone on to become the most common surgical procedure for the surgical treatment of OSA. The use of UPPP alone in the management of OSA has met with mixed results. Initially, the success rate of UPPP was reported to be less than 40%, with success defined as a reduction of respiratory disturbance index by 50% and an apnea-hypopnea index less than 10 or a respiratory disturbance index less than 20.[2] This low success rate may be due to poor patient selection and misdiagnosis of the level of nocturnal obstruction that UPPP is designed to alleviate.

Alternative methods of the procedure began to come into development. Modifications to the UPPP were designed to reduce the incidence of some of the negative aspects of the procedure. Laser-assisted uvulopalatoplasty (LAUP) was developed using carbon dioxide (CO_2) surgical laser cutting technology to minimize collateral tissue damage that results in less morbidity and postoperative pain compared with UPPP.[3] LAUP utilizes CO_2 surgical laser technology to trim and shorten the uvula while simultaneously tightening and contracting the adjacent soft palatal tissue.

Indications for Use of the Procedures

The retropalatal upper airway has been established as one of the most common areas of obstruction in OSA.[4] The original UPPP procedure was designed to enlarge the retropalatal airway through excision of the tonsils with relocation of the tonsillar pillars in conjunction with a uvulectomy and mucosal closure of the soft palate.

The Friedman staging system has been used to aid in proper patient selection for OSA surgical palatal procedures.[5] This system is based on palate position, tonsil size, and body mass index and may be used to improve the probability of success with these procedures.[6] Stage I patients have palate size of 1 or 2 based on a modified Mallampati scale and tonsil size of 3 or 4 based on the Brodsky scoring system. Stage II patients have a palate position and tonsil size of 3 or 4. Patients with a body mass index greater than 40 kg/m^2 are classified as stage III. The Mallampati classification and Friedman tongue position assessment techniques are significantly correlated with predicting OSA severity.[7] Stage I patients are the best candidates for palatal surgery with a reported success rate of 80.6%, followed by Stage II with a 37.9% success rate of only 8.1%.[6]

Drug-induced sleep endoscopy (DISE) is a technique employed to visualize locations of upper airway obstruction during a drug-induced level of sedation designed to mimic sleep and may be used as a guide in treatment decisions for palatal procedures for OSA. DISE has shown that individuals respond best to UPPP and other palatal procedures for OSA who have grade 3 and 4 tonsillar hypertrophy and anterior-posterior mild/partial collapse at the velum.[8] Conversely, subjects with complete circumferential collapse at the velum and complete anterior-posterior collapse at the tongue base had significantly less chance of success with UPPP or other palatal procedures.

Limitations and Contraindications

The main limitation to the UPPP procedure as a sole procedure is the success rate in unselected OSA patients of only 20% to 25%. Even after appropriately selected patients, UPPP has an unpredictable success rate between 50% and 60% in best cases. The greatest limitation of the isolated UPPP procedure in successful OSA management is a result of upper airway obstruction collapse occurs at more than one site. UPPP as a part of multilevel airway surgery performed in conjunction with other airway procedures in multi- or single-stage fashion has had greater success in OSA management.

Contraindications of palatal surgical procedures are surgery in the presence of pharyngitis, exceptionally large lateral adenoid bands, revision surgery, and cicatrizing and keloid diatheses.[9] Additionally, subjects with complete circumferential collapse at the velum and complete anterior-posterior collapse at the tongue base tend to have less successful outcomes with surgical palatal procedures.[8]

TECHNIQUE: Uvulopalatopharyngoplasty

STEP 1: Pre-operative UPPP Evaluation

Preoperative evaluation must be completed for the point where the soft palate comes in contact with posterior pharyngeal wall. Observation of the palate during gag or phonation for "dimple" where approximation of palate occurs. This point is termed the J point and is usually approximately 2 cm posterior to the edge of the hard palate.

STEP 2: Access to Surgical Site

Under general anesthesia and the patient intubated with an oral RAE endotracheal tube, the patient is positioned with shoulder roll in place and neck extended. A self-retaining mouth gag (such as a Dingman or Crowe-Davis mouth retractor) is placed with care to protect the teeth and tongue. This allows for unobstructed access to the tonsillar pillars and soft palate (Fig. 161.1).

STEP 3: Determine Point of Palatal Incision

Determine the point of palatal incision. A useful intraoperative maneuver is to place a Yankauer suction tip into one nostril while closing off the other side causing a suction in the nasopharynx triggering the palate to move back and close against the pharyngeal wall. This will replicate to some degree the point of closure seen in the awake patient. This area can also be palpated to feel for the edge of the palatal muscles.

STEP 4: Local Anesthesia

Once the incision line is determined, administration of local anesthetic with epinephrine (usually 1% to 2% lidocaine with 1:100,000 epinephrine) to aid in hemostasis is injected into the surgical areas of the palate and tonsillar pillars.

STEP 5: If Tonsil are Present

If tonsils are present, a standard tonsillectomy procedure is performed, generally with coblation (Fig. 161.1). Coblation stands for controlled ablation, a procedure that combines low temperature radiofrequency ablation and saline to allow for gentle and precise tonsil dissection allowing for less risk of injury to surrounding tissue and decreased morbidity. Once the tonsillectomy is completed, a mucosal incision is made curving laterally from the palatal incision to meet the tonsillectomy incisions. If a tonsillectomy had been previously performed, portions of the pillar and underlying scar tissue are removed with careful dissection to avoid damage to the underlying musculature and carotid sheath structures (Fig. 161.2).

STEP 6: Palatal Incision Technique

The palatal incision should be beveled to leave the nasal mucosa longer than the oral mucosa (Figs. 161.3 and 161.4). This allows for closure of the mucosa over the raw surface of the palate and further facilitates opening of the nasopharyngeal inlet. Hemostasis is obtained with bipolar electrocautery (Fig. 161.5)

STEP 7: Closure of Wound

Closure begins by suturing the tonsillar fossae with interrupted 3-0 resorbable sutures (Fig. 161.6). The corners should be closed first with mattress sutures passing through the mucosal edges and superficial layers of muscle. This approach reduces tension on the closure and eliminates the dead space where hematomas can form. The closure then progresses toward the tongue leaving a small opening inferiorly to allow for drainage of any blood.

The palatal incision should then be closed by approximating the nasal and oral mucosal edges together. Care should be taken not to overly tighten the sutures to allow for some edema and avoid dehiscence. The nasopharynx should be irrigated to remove accumulated blood. Suction the hypopharynx and esophagus with a soft catheter to remove any blood. The mouth gag is then removed, and the teeth and tongue are examined for any injury. Long-acting local anesthetic with epinephrine is injected into the surgical site for both pain and hemorrhage control.

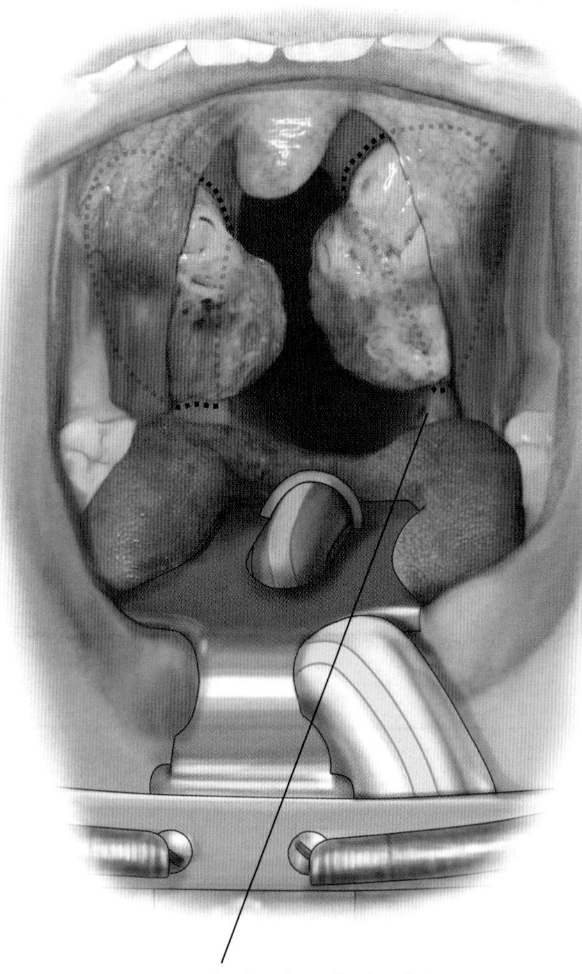

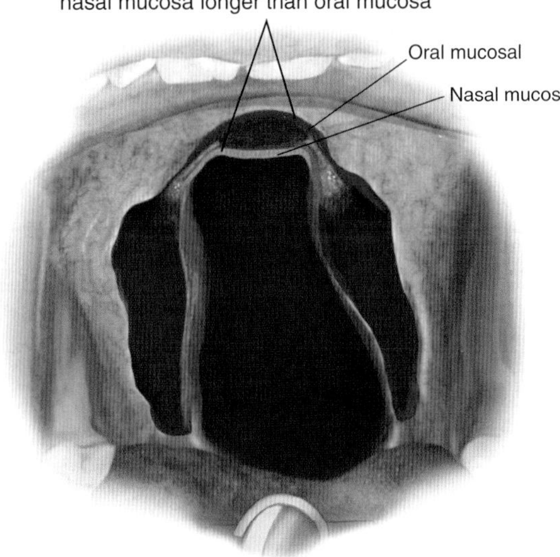

Fig. 161.1 Palatal incisions and dissection for uvulopalatopharyngoplasty (UPPP).

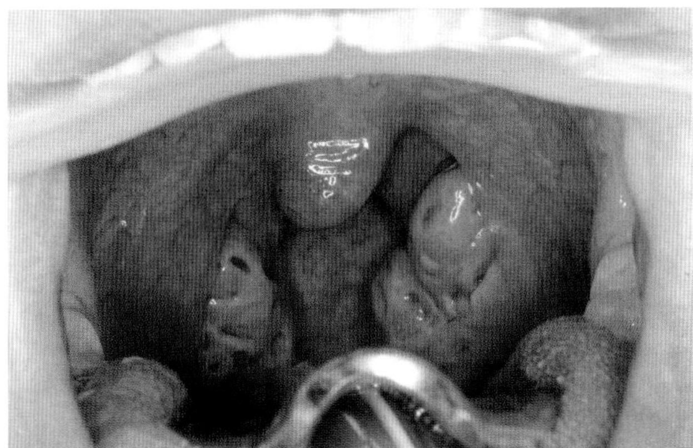

Fig. 161.2 Dingman retractor in place allowing access to tonsillar pillars, soft palate, and uvula.

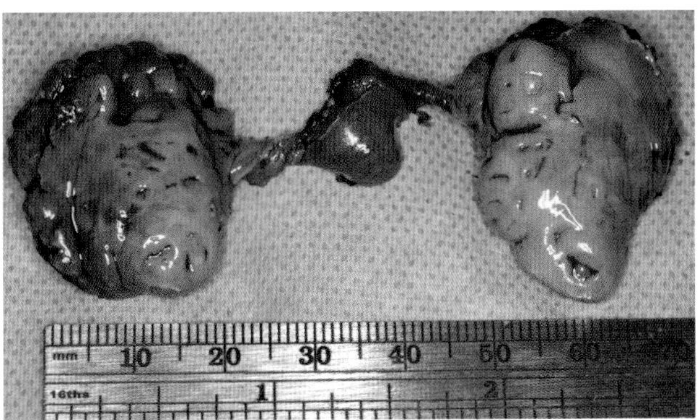

Fig. 161.3 Frontal view of specimen following uvulopalatopharyngoplasty (UPPP) with tonsils and uvula.

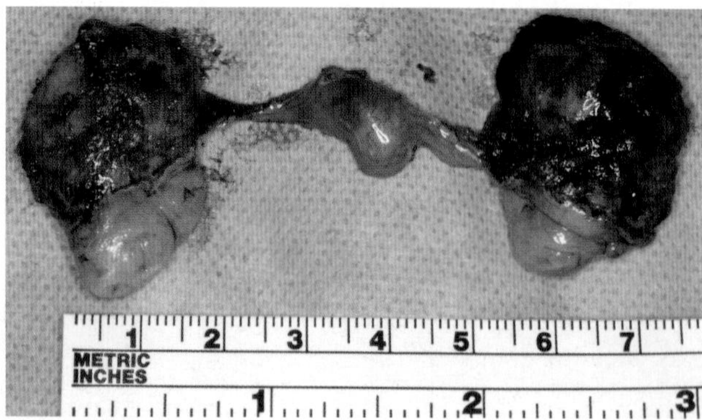

Fig. 161.4 Undersurface of specimen following uvulopalatopharyngoplasty (UPPP) with tonsils and uvula.

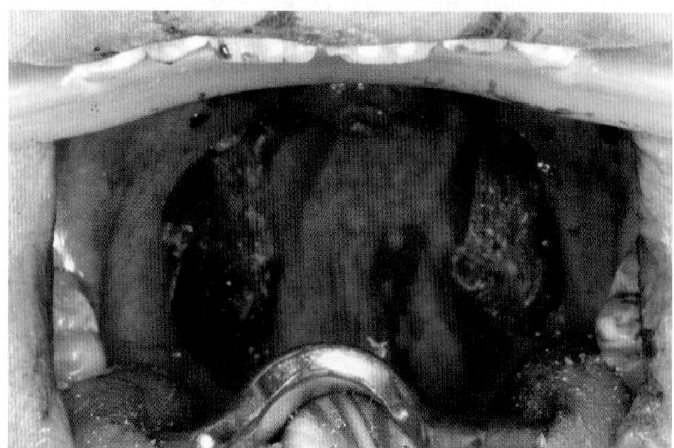
Fig. 161.5 Open wound surface of tonsillar pillars and soft palate following uvulopalatopharyngoplasty (UPPP).

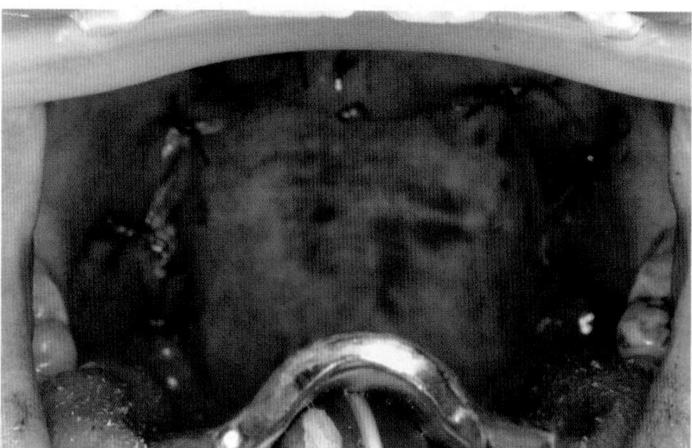
Fig. 161.6 Suture closure after uvulopalatopharyngoplasty (UPPP).

ALTERNATIVE TECHNIQUES

ALTERNATIVE TECHNIQUE 1: Laser-assisted Uvulopalatoplasty

Kamami first published on the use of LAUP for OSA in 1990[10] and showed a high rate of success (40 of 46 patients being classified as responders).[11] LAUP may be performed under outpatient intravenous moderate-to-deep sedation[12,13] or general anesthesia with nasotracheal intubation. A handheld CO_2 laser is used to incise a wedge or crescent trough of soft palate on either side of the uvula, which is then ablated with the laser and removed (Fig. 161.7 and 161.8). The procedure may be performed alone, with or without tonsillectomy or pharyngoplasty, or with concomitant upper airway procedures such as functional rhinoplasty[12] or multilevel pharyngeal surgery consisting of genioglossus advancement and hyoid myotomy.[14]

A meta-analysis of LAUP (with or without tonsillotomy/tonsillectomy/pharyngoplasty) as the sole procedure for OSA showed that the procedure reduced apnea hypopnea index (AHI) by 32% among all patients; while the lowest oxygen saturation only changed minimally with a success rate of 23%, a cure rate of only 8%, and worsening of the AHI of 44%.[15] This leads credence the American Academy of Sleep Medicine's Standards of Practice Committee statement that states that as a sole procedure "LAUP is not recommended for the treatment of sleep-disordered breathing."[16]

ALTERNATIVE TECHNIQUE 2: Radiofrequency-assisted Uvulopalatoplasty

Radiofrequency-assisted uvulopalatoplasty (RAUP) is primarily used for the treatment of snoring (Fig. 161.9). It is surgically similar to LAUP but uses radio frequency instead of a laser. RAUP surgery induces temperatures of 70°C to 85°C with the intention of diminishing the amount of damage to the surrounding tissues. Compared with the LAUP procedure, RAUP has been found to take less time and have less postoperative pain and fewer postoperative complications, such as globus sensation (the feeling of having a lump in the throat) and scar contracture, while maintaining the advantages produced by the LAUP procedure.[17]

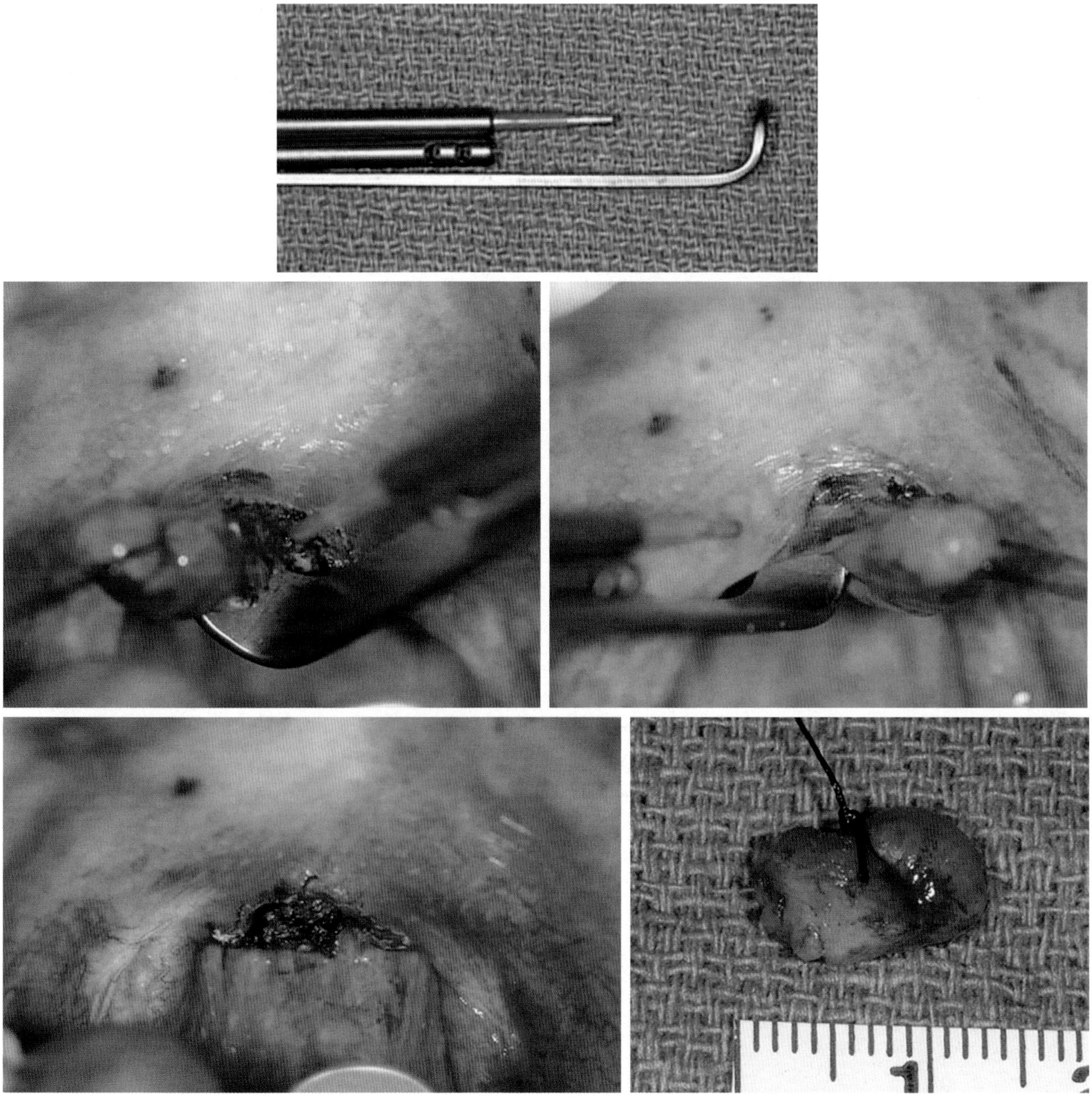

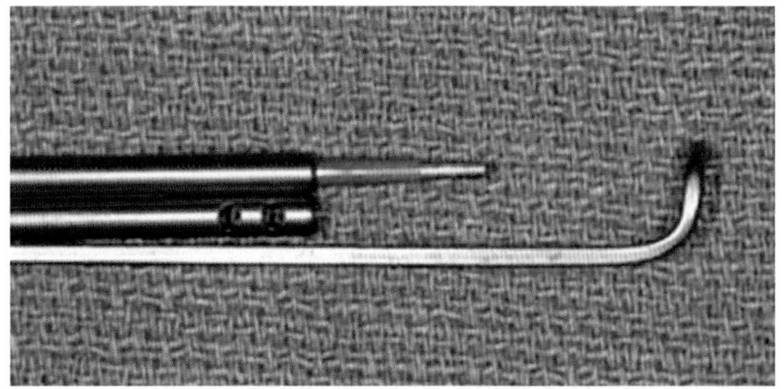

Fig. 161.7 Laser-assisted uvulopalatoplasty (LAUP) procedure sequence for uvulectomy. (Courtesy Dr. Richard Finn)

Avoidance of Intraoperative Complications

Intraoperative bleeding will generally occur from either the tonsillar pillar regions or from the uvula, where the palatal arteries are larger in size.[18] Potential sources of intraoperative bleeding from the tonsillar pillars will include the ascending palatine artery, tonsillar branch of the facial artery, palatine branch of the ascending pharyngeal artery, tonsillar branch of the dorsal lingual artery, and tonsillar branch of the descending palatine artery. The palatal arteries surrounding the uvula include branches of the internal maxillary artery, which are the descending palatine neurovascular bundle that supplies vascularity and sensation to the soft palate.

Applying silver nitrate or local anesthesia infiltration may temporarily stop the bleeding as well. In our experience, all delayed bleeding was secondary to temporary management of bleeding with local anesthesia and silver nitrate application. As a result of these findings, we highly recommend initial chemical cautery or electrocautery followed by suture.

Postoperative Complications

Several postoperative complications may occur from palatal procedures. Medical comorbidity, AHI, and body mass index are risk factors for serious complication after UPPP.[19] A review of 3572 patients treated with UPPP revealed the

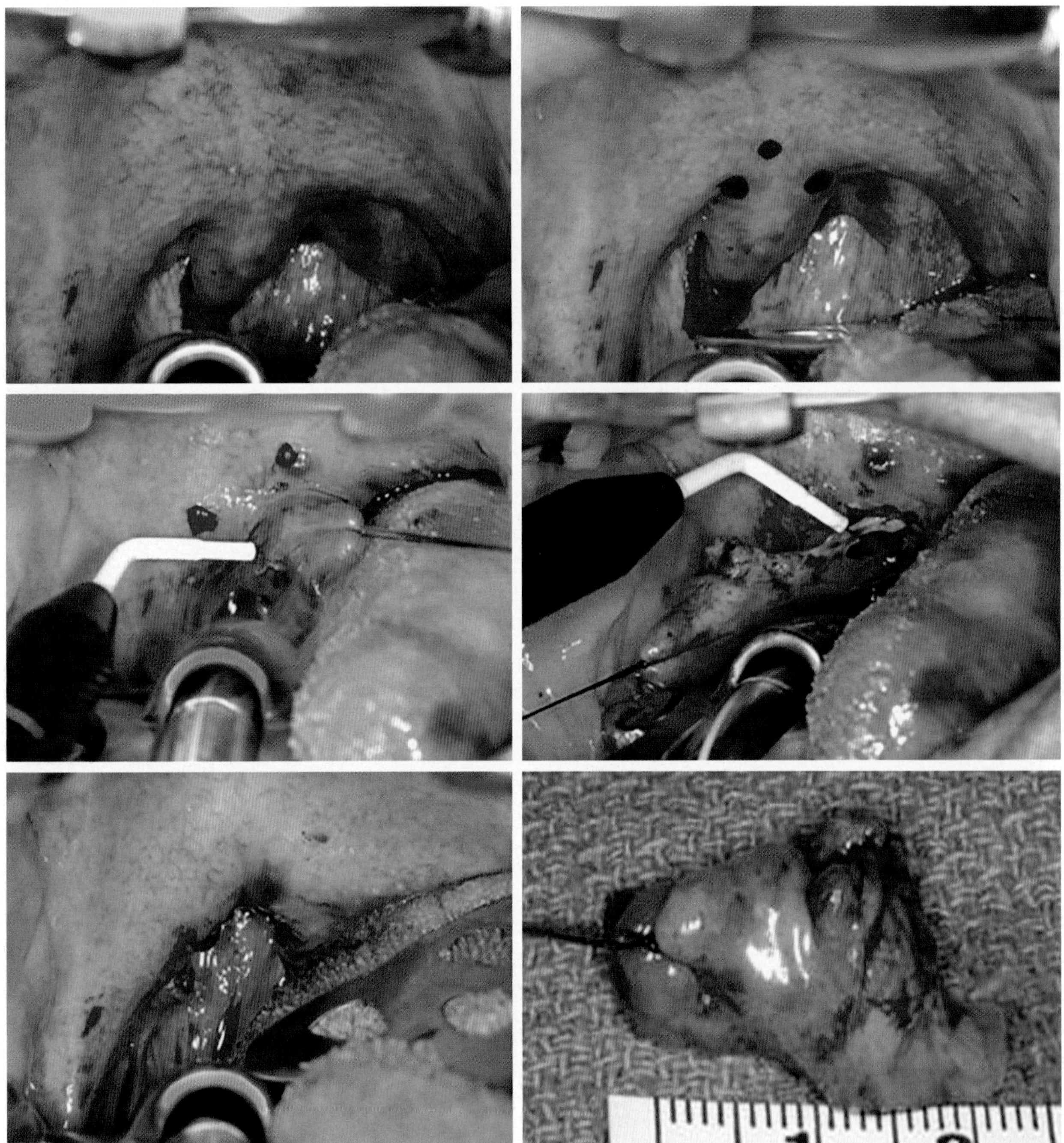

Fig. 161.8 Radiofrequency-assisted uvulopalatoplasty (RAUP) procedure sequence for uvulectomy. (Courtesy Dr. Richard Finn)

incidence of serious complications to be 37.1 per 1000 patients.[20] The most common postoperative complications include bleeding and infection. The incidence of postoperative bleeding is approximately 2% and usually occurs 4 to 8 days after surgery but may occur as late as 12 to 15 days postoperatively. Another relatively common postoperative complication from palatal surgery is velopharyngeal insufficiency (VPI). VPI refers to the inability to temporarily close the communication between the nasal cavity and the mouth that leads to dysfunctional problems with speech, eating, and breathing.[21] The incidence of permanent VPI, severe enough to require surgical intervention, has been shown to be as high as approximately 2% with traditional UPPP methods. If surgical correction of VPI is deemed necessary, the severity of OSA should be considered because OSA will most likely deteriorate following correction.

Nasopharyngeal stenosis is a potentially devasting post-UPPP complication as it may result in significant functional disability and is extremely difficult to correct. Prevention of this complication cannot be overemphasized. Predisposing factors for postsurgical nasopharyngeal stenosis include excessive destruction of palatal mucosa, surgery in the presence of pharyngitis, exceptionally large lateral adenoid bands, revision surgery, and cicatrizing and keloid diatheses.[9] This

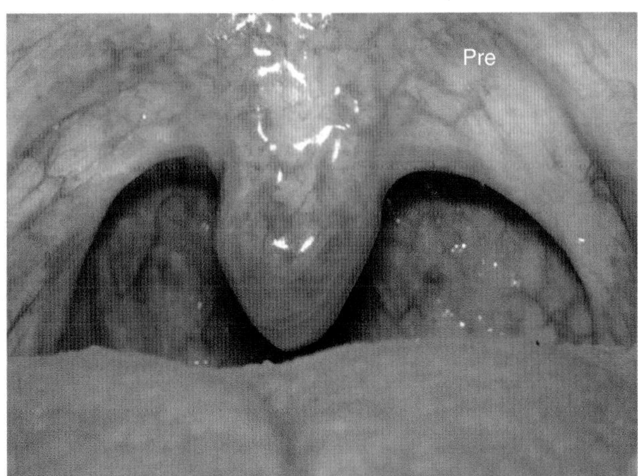

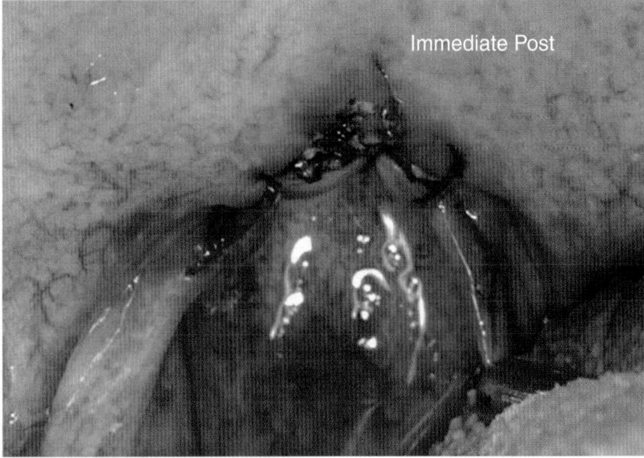

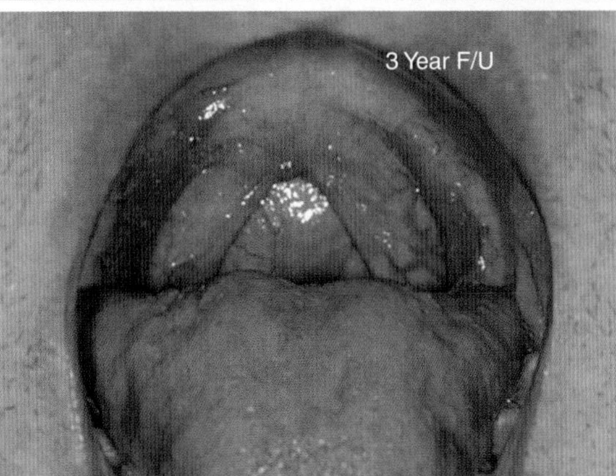

Fig. 161.9 Long-term follow-up of uvulectomy. (Courtesy Dr. Richard Finn)

usually develops 6 to 8 weeks after UPPP with various grades of severity. Mild forms present with adherence of the lateral aspects of the palate to the posterior pharyngeal walls and are usually asymptomatic while more severe forms range from excessive scarring of the velum with a cicatricial band on the posterior pharyngeal wall, with a small opening remaining to complete fusion of the palate to the pharynx. Postoperative mortality from palatal procedures is extremely rare with a 30-day mortality rate in large reviews found to be between 0.02 and 0.2%.[10,22,23]

References

1. Fujita S, Conway W, Zorick F, Roth T. Surgical correction of anatomic azbnormalities in obstructive sleep apnea syndrome: uvulopalatopharyngoplasty. *Otolaryngol Head Neck Surg*. 1981;89(6):923–934.
2. Sher AE, Schechtman KB, Piccirillo JF. The efficacy of surgical modifications of the upper airway in adults with obstructive sleep apnea syndrome. *Sleep*. 1996;19(2):156–177. https://doi.org/10.1093/sleep/19.2.156.
3. DicksonRI,MintzDR.One-stagelaser-assisted uvulopalatoplasty. *J Otolaryngol*. 1996;25(3):155–161.
4. Metes A, Hoffstein V, Mateika S, Cole P, Haight JS. Site of airway obstruction in patients with obstructive sleep apnea before and after uvulopalatopharyngoplasty. *Laryngoscope*. 1991;101(10):1102–1108.
5. Friedman M, Ibrahim H, Bass L. Clinical staging for sleep-disordered breathing. *Otolaryngol Head Neck Surg*. 2002;127(1):13–21. https://doi.org/10.1067/mhn.2002.126477.
6. Friedman M, Ibrahim H, Joseph NJ. Staging of obstructive sleep apnea/hypopnea syndrome: a guide to appropriate treatment. *Laryngoscope*. 2004;114(3):454–459. https://doi.org/10.1097/00005537-200403000-00013.
7. Friedman M, Hamilton C, Samuelson CG, Lundgren ME, Pott T. Diagnostic value of the Friedman tongue position and Mallampati classification for obstructive sleep apnea: a meta-analysis. *Otolaryngol Head Neck Surg*. 2013;148(4):540–547. https://doi.org/10.1177/0194599812473413.
8. Wang Y, Sun C, Cui X, Guo Y, Wang Q, Liang H. The role of drug-induced sleep endoscopy: predicting and guiding upper airway surgery for adult OSA patients. *Sleep Breath*. 2018;22(4):925–931. https://doi.org/10.1007/s11325-018-1730-7.
9. Giannoni C, Sulek M, Friedman EM, Duncan NO III. Acquired nasopharyngeal stenosis: a warning and review. *Arch Otolaryngol Head Neck Surg*. 1998;124(2):163–167. https://doi.org/10.1001/archotol.124.2.163.
10. Kamami YV. Laser CO2 for snoring. Preliminary results. *Acta Otorhinolaryngol Belg*. 1990;44(4):451–456.
11. Kamami YV. Outpatient treatment of sleep apnea syndrome with CO 2 laser, LAUP: laser-assisted UPPP results on 46 patients. *J Clin Laser Med Surg*. 1994;12(4):215–219.
12. Cillo JE Jr, Finn R, Dasheiff RM. Combined open rhinoplasty with spreader grafts and laser-assisted uvuloplasty for sleep-disordered breathing: long-term subjective outcomes. *J Oral Maxillofac Surg*. 2006;64(8):1241–1247. https://doi.org/10.1016/j.joms.2006.04.020.
13. Cillo JE Jr, Finn R. Hemodynamics and oxygen saturation during intravenous sedation for office-based laser-assisted uvuloplasty. *J Oral Maxillofac Surg*. 2005;63(6):752–755. https://doi.org/10.1016/j.joms.2005.02.004.
14. Utley DS, Shin EJ, Clerk AA, Terris DJ. A cost-effective and rational surgical ap-

proach to patients with snoring, upper airway resistance syndrome, or obstructive sleep apnea syndrome. *Laryngoscope*. 1997;107(6): 726–734. https://doi.org/10.1097/00005537-199706000-00005.

15. Camacho M, Nesbitt NB, Lambert E, et al. Laser-Assisted uvulopalatoplasty for obstructive sleep apnea: a systematic review and meta-analysis. *Sleep*. 2017;40(3). https://doi.org/10.1093/sleep/zsx00.
16. Littner M, Kushida CA, Hartse K, et al. Practice parameters for the use of laser-assisted uvulopalatoplasty: an update for 2000. *Sleep*. 2001;24(5):603–619.
17. Lim DJ, Kang SH, Kim BH, Kim HG. Treatment of primary snoring using radiofrequency-assisted uvulopalatoplasty. *Eur Arch Otorhinolaryngol*. 2007;264(7):761–767. https://doi.org/10.1007/s00405-007-0252-x.
18. Madani M. Complications of laser-assisted uvulopalatopharyngoplasty (LA-UPPP) and radiofrequency treatments of snoring and chronic nasal congestion: a 10-year review of 5,600 patients. *J Oral Maxillofac Surg*. 2004;62(11):1351–1362. https://doi.org/10.1016/j.joms.2004.05.213.
19. Kezirian EJ, Weaver EM, Yueh B, Khuri SF, Daley J, Henderson WG. Risk factors for serious complication after uvulopalatopharyngoplasty. *Arch Otolaryngol Head Neck Surg*. 2006;132(10):1091–1098. https://doi.org/10.1001/archotol.132.10.1091.
20. Franklin KA, Haglund B, Axelsson S, Holmlund T, Rehnqvist N, Rosén M. Frequency of serious complications after surgery for snoring and sleep apnea. *Acta Otolaryngol*. 2011;131(3):298–302.
21. Hirschberg J. Results and complications of 1104 surgeries for velopharyngeal insufficiency. *ISRN Otolaryngol*. 2012;2012:181202.
22. Kezirian EJ, Weaver EM, Yueh B, et al. Incidence of serious complications after uvulopalatopharyngoplasty. *Laryngoscope*. 2004;114(3):450–453.
23. Jiang RS, Chang YH. Olfactory loss after uvulopalatopharyngoplasty: a report of two cases with review of the literature. *Case Rep Otolaryngol*. 2014;2014:546317.

CHAPTER 162

Tongue Reduction for Obstructive Sleep Apnea

John M. Nathan, Yuliya Petukhova, and Christopher F. Viozzi

Armamentarium

#15 Scalpel blade and handle
Bite block (or Molt mouth prop)
DeBakey or other tissue forceps
Frasier and Yankauer suction tips
Local anesthetic with vasoconstrictor
Mayo-Hegar needle drivers
Metzenbaum scissors
Monopolar electrocautery with spatula and needle tips (Colorado tip)
Nasal endotracheal tube (PolarPro) tube or armored endotracheal tube (for carbon dioxide laser cases)
Optional—carbon dioxide laser
Shoulder roll or Mayfield adjustable horseshoe headrest
Sutures: 2-0 silk retraction suture, 2-0 and 3-0 Vicryl on taper needle, 2-0 and 3-0 Vicryl on cutting needle

History of the Procedure

The tongue and its impact on orthognathic surgery has been a long-term source of interest for the oral and maxillofacial surgeon performing these procedures. Unfortunately, our understanding of the true impact of the tongue on facial growth and development, its impact on developing skeletal-occlusal relationships, and the degree to which it may interfere short term or long term with orthognathic surgical corrections is a source of ongoing debate.

Tongue reduction for the treatment of obstructive sleep apnea (OSA) has yielded mixed results. Partial glossectomy alone has not proven to be a reliable treatment for OSA; however, tongue reduction in conjunction with multilevel surgery has shown to significantly improve the apnea/hypopnea index, Epworth Sleepiness Scale, snoring visual analog scale, and lowest oxygen saturation.[1] Many different surgical techniques including traditional surgery, and laser-assisted, Coblator-assisted, radiofrequency-assisted, and transoral robotic surgery have been described for the treatment of OSA.[2] In addition, different glossectomy incision designs have also been described to achieve dimensional and volume reduction. The midline glossectomy technique, designed specifically for the treatment of OSA in adults, was first described by Fujita et al. in 1991.[3] Various additional techniques for macroglossia in pediatric patients with Beckwith-Wiedemann syndrome and Down syndrome have also been described.[4] Most incision designs can be performed using the different surgical techniques. Selection of incision design depends on the patient's severity and suspected anatomic location of the obstruction. No technique has been proven to be more effective than the others when treating OSA. This chapter focuses on the keyhole glossectomy that was first described by Morgan et al. in 1993[5]. This technique provides reduction in the transverse and anterior-posterior dimensions.

Indications for Use of the Procedure

In orthognathic/telegnathic surgery, the main indications for reduction of the anterior two-thirds of the tongue are the presence of true macroglossia, defined for the purposes of this chapter as a tongue that is excessive and identified prior to presurgical orthodontic treatment,[6] after presurgical orthodontic treatment is complete, or prior to orthognathic/telegnathic surgery when the postsurgical oral cavity space is still likely to be too diminutive to accommodate the tongue after osseous surgery is completed (whether orthodontics is planned or not).[7]

Limitations and Contraindications

Surgical reduction of the anterior two-thirds of the tongue would not be indicated in cases of tongue habits such as tongue thrusting. This is appropriately managed by speech and language therapists to control the abnormal neuromuscular patterns with therapy. Similarly, excessive oropharyngeal soft tissue such as tonsillar and/or adenoid tissue enlargement should be addressed by excision of those tissues rather than reducing tongue size to accommodate them.

Patient-specific conditions that would contraindicate tongue reduction as described for OSA might include coagulation defects, wound-healing defects (diabetic status, steroid use, previous radiotherapy), previous surgeries with excessive scarring and speech/functional impact, the presence of vascular malformation that has not been interrogated with computed tomography angiography, and neoplastic growths.

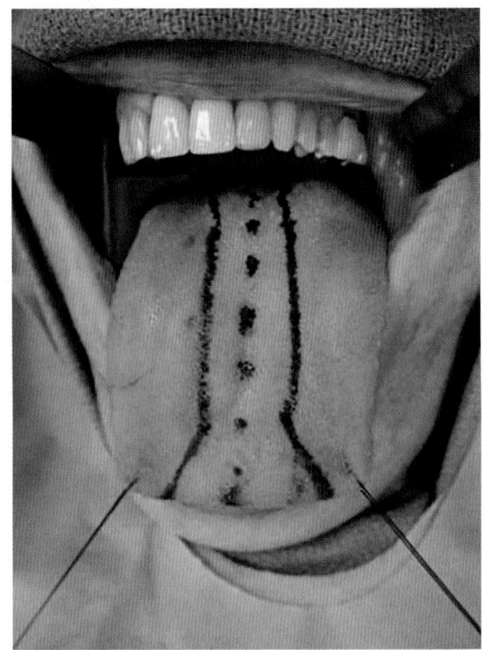

Figure 162.1 Outline of the excision.

TECHNIQUE: Keyhole Glossectomy

STEP 1: Anesthetic Considerations

The patient is prepared in the routine manner for intraoral surgery. General anesthesia with nasotracheal intubation is performed. Our preference is to use a longer, flexible nasal Ring-Adair-Elwyn (RAE) tube to avoid inadvertent intraoperative extubation. In cases where use of a laser is planned, an appropriate protected endotracheal must be used and full laser precautions assured to protect the patient and operating room staff. Intravenous injection of an appropriate edema-reducing dose of dexamethasone as well as intravenous antibiotic is accomplished prior to incision.

STEP 2: Local Anesthesia

A large bite block is inserted on the contralateral side from the surgeon. The tongue is anesthetized with bilateral lingual nerve blocks utilizing 0.5% bupivacaine with 1:200,000 epinephrine. Infiltration anesthesia of the anterior two-thirds of the tongue is deliberately not performed at this point to avoid distorting tongue anatomy.

STEP 3: Outlining Incisions

The excision is outlined with a surgical marker and 2-0 silk sutures placed as traction sutures (Fig. 162.1).

STEP 4: Incision and Removal of Excess Tissue

Initial mucosal incision is made with a #15 scalpel blade, and then needle point electrocautery is used to continue the excision into the muscle (alternatively carbon dioxide laser excision can be utilized). It is critical to be aware of the intended resection dimensions. Anteriorly, full thickness dorsal-to-ventral excision may be desired, transitioning to a partial-thickness dissection as the surgery proceeds posteriorly.

STEP 5: Hemostasis

Hemostasis is ensured at this time using electrocautery. Larger vessels can be isolated and suture tied as necessary but this is uncommon. Injury to the left or right lingual arteries can generally be avoided by adequate knowledge of their position within the tongue. It is important to find and isolate the distal injury in the same manner. Importantly, it is possible to ligate both left and right lingual arteries with causing necrosis as the tongue has an abundant collateral blood supply. It is reasonable at this time to inject epinephrine-containing local anesthesia into the muscle layer (Fig. 162.2).

STEP 6: Closure

Closure is initiated at the tip of the tongue to respect the dorsoventral relationships and to not create any more anatomical distortion than necessary. Deep suturing with 2-0 or 3-0 Vicryl suture on a taper needle or 3-0 chromic can be done but should not be overutilized as these can be a nidus for reaction or infection. Mucosal closure with 2-0 or 3-0 Vicryl suture vertical mattress sutures with wound margin eversion is preferred (Fig. 162.3).

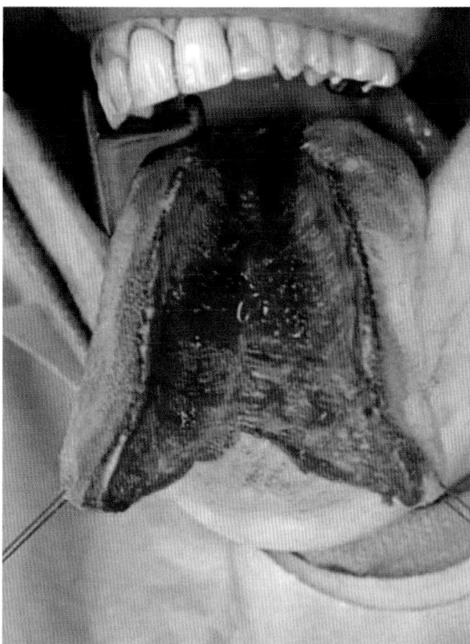

Figure 162.2 Initial mucosal incision with dissection through tongue musculature.

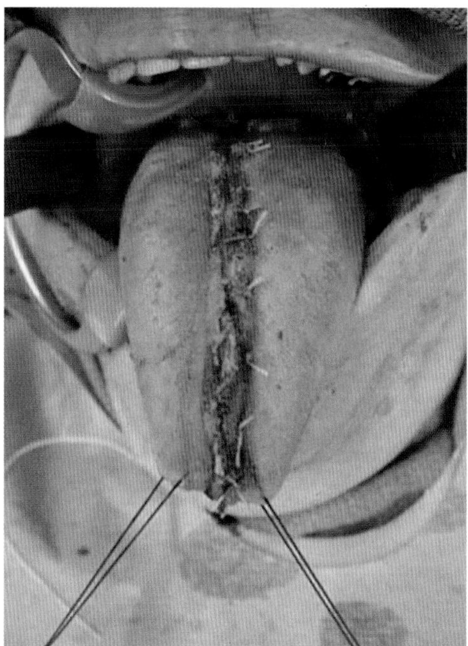

Figure 162.3 Closure is initiated at the tip of the tongue.

TECHNIQUE: Keyhole Glossectomy—*cont'd*

STEP 7: Post Surgical Monitoring

As the surgery concludes, it is important to monitor the surgical site for development of bleeding or hematoma prior to extubation. Normalization of patient's blood pressure is best done prior to initiating closure and is necessary prior to extubation.

STEP 8: Post Surgical Analgesia

Injection of liposomal bupivacaine can be performed at this time if desired for postoperative analgesia. This will provide up to 72 hours of additional analgesia.

ALTERNATIVE TECHNIQUES

There are a large number of alternative and useful techniques to reduce the size of the anterior tongue that have been described in the literature. The fundamental principle used is tissue removal followed by primary closure. Reduction in the transverse, anterior-posterior, or both dimensions can be achieved depending on the incision and excision design. The dimension of reduction needed will dictate the approach and incision design. In most cases, a combination of reduction in the anterior-posterior and transverse dimensions will be needed. We present a review of the multiple techniques below, as each case is unique and may call for a particular technique based on the desired type of reduction.

Wedge-shaped incisions at the tip of the tongue primarily decrease the anterior-posterior dimension and shorten the tongue (Fig. 162.4A).[8] However, the transverse width of the tongue remains unchanged posteriorly. Incision outline is in the shape of an upside-down V or wedge at the anterior tip of the tongue. An outline should be made prior to injection of local anesthetic and distortion of the tongue. A suture passed two to three times through the anterior tip of the tongue can be used in order to distract and control the tongue during excision. The amount of reduction needed should be estimated so that the new anterior tip is housed within the lingual surfaces of the teeth or mandibular alveolus if the patient has no dentition. The incision can be started with a blade, cautery, or laser. The initial incision can have a slight bevel to more easily bring the mucosal margins together for closure. The incision should be carried full thickness from the dorsal surface to the ventral tongue while taking care to control bleeding and to not violate the sublingual or submandibular duct openings. Once appropriate hemostasis is achieved, the tongue should be primarily closed in a layered fashion. The muscles should be closely reapproximated using a long-acting suture such as 2-0 or 3-0 Vicryl. The dorsal and ventral mucosa should be aligned and closed with simple interrupted or interrupted horizontal mattress sutures. Lingual frenectomy can be performed as needed if there is significant tethering of the tongue. Other modified anterior tip reduction

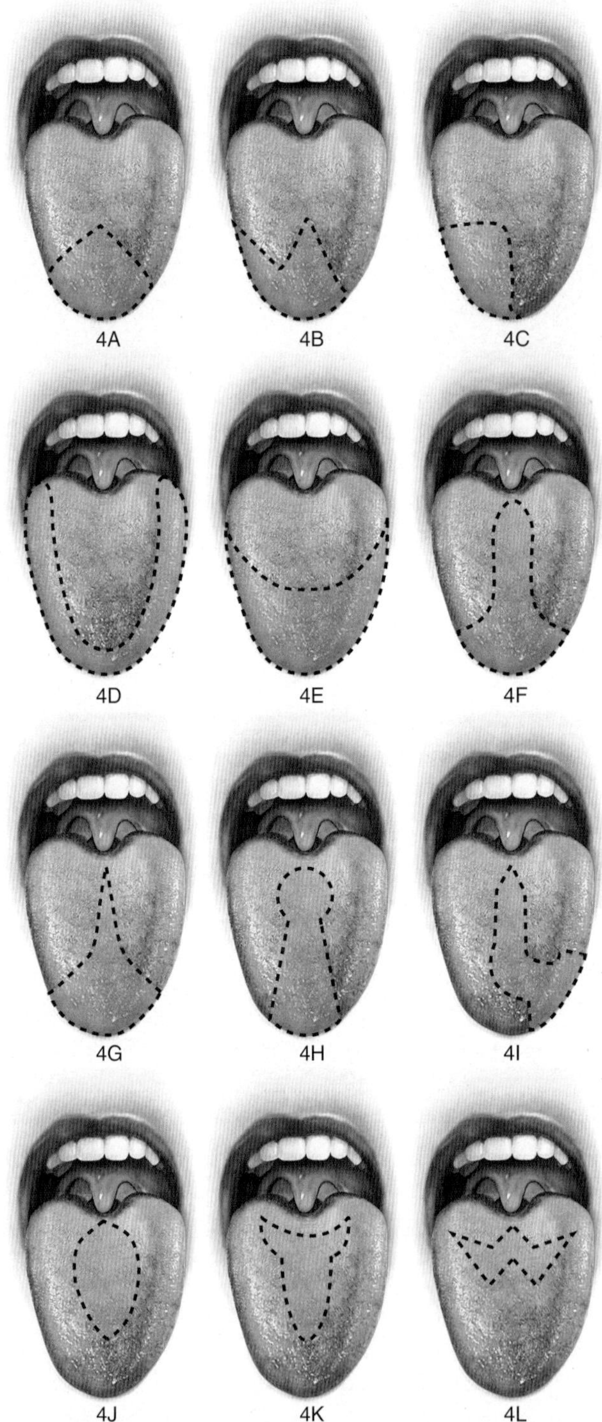

Figure 162.4 Incision shapes. (Redrawn from Wang J, Goodger NM, Pogrel MA. The role of tongue reduction. *Oral Surg Oral Med Oral Pathol Oral Radiol Endod.* 2003;95(3):269–273.)

techniques were described by Austerman and Machtens (Fig. 162.4B and C).[9] These techniques also primarily decrease anterior-posterior length without reducing the width of the tongue. Closure should also be performed in a layered fashion using Vicryl sutures.

Peripheral glossectomy techniques have also been proposed that primarily remove the lateral and anterior margins of the tongue.[10] These techniques will reduce the tongue in the anterior-posterior and transverse dimensions; however, they can potentially leave the tongue immobile and with less functionality. Dingman and Grabb proposed a more extensive peripheral glossectomy that removes more of the anterior tip of the tongue in cases of lymphangioma (Fig. 162.4D and E). Similar considerations should be taken when performing a peripheral glossectomy as compared with anterior wedge resections. Incision is made full thickness with a slight bevel at the mucosa. Care should be taken to avoid duct opening if performing a more extensive anterior tip resection, and closure should be performed in a layered fashion. Closure will bring the dorsal and ventral mucosal surfaces together. The muscular layer and mucosal layer should be closed as separate layers using long-acting resorbable suture as previously described.

Multiple longitudinal resection designs that involve the anterior tip of the tongue have been proposed that reduce both transverse and anterior-posterior dimensions. Egyedi et al., Kole et al., and Davalbhakta et al. all described this technique of performing an anterior tip wedge resection that includes a longitudinal continuation of the resection along the midline of the tongue tapering posteriorly (Fig. 162.4F and G).[11–13] The depth and width of muscle removal from the longitudinal section will depend on the amount of tongue bulk needing removal. Another method named the keyhole design was described by Morgan et al. and Kacker et al. that also narrows and shortens the tongue. As the name describes, the incision design is of a keyhole with the circular portion being located posteriorly on the tongue (Fig. 162.4H).[14,15] This design has consistently shown adequate reduction in both dimensions.[16] These techniques are closed primarily as previously described. An alternative design described by Kruchinksy et al. preserves half of the anterior tip of the tongue with the goal of improved speech and functionality.[17] The strip of preserved tongue is pulled over and sutured to the lateral tongue of the opposite side (Fig. 162.4I). This design helps to maintain integrity of the tip of the tongue.

Other techniques described include longitudinal designs based at the midline of the tongue that do not include the anterior or lateral margins of the tongue. An elliptical design described by Edgerton et al. can be used to narrow the tongue (Fig. 162.4J).[18] The most posterior portion of this design is carried just anterior to the circumvallate papilla. Width will depend on the amount of bulk needing to be removed. This technique primarily reduces the width of the mid-tongue and does not affect the anterior width of the tongue. Harada et al. described a modified elliptical incision with a posteriorly positioned crescent design. This added crescent helps to shorten the tongue (Fig. 162.4K).[19] Mixter et al. described a transverse incision that removes a W-shaped wedge of tissue just anterior to the circumvallate papilla (see Fig. 162.4L). This design primarily shortens the tongue without removing any tip of the tongue. The margins are closed primarily in a layered fashion using Vicryl sutures to reapproximate the muscle and mucosal layers separately.[20]

Avoidance and Management of Intraoperative complications

An in depth understanding of the relevant anatomy of the lingual nerve and artery is critical to the avoidance to the extent possible of injuring these structures during surgery. The reader is directed to the Part I section of the book to gain this information. Should these structures be injured, consideration must be given to ligation of the artery and repair of the nerve respectively. Additionally, the surgeon should ensure not to over or under reduce the tongue during the procedure.

Postoperative Considerations

The major immediate postoperative consideration is focused on airway maintenance. Swelling of the tongue after reduction can be significant despite the use of intraoperative and postoperative steroids. There are some cases that may merit preemptive tracheostomy. Examples include the patient with previous history of difficult intubation or limited jaw range of motion, and patients having additional procedures that will create more sites of oropharyngeal edema (genioglossus surgery, palatal surgery, etc.). Each case will be unique in this regard but consideration prior to surgery is important. However, all patients should be warned of the possibility of perioperative need for a surgical airway.

Pain control can be problematic due to the rich innervation of the oral tongue. The injection of perioperative local anesthetic, including liposomal products can mitigate some of the need for analgesics. Judicious use of opioids is necessary because of the surgical impact on the airway from swelling.

Oral intake of liquids and solids is challenging early on after tongue reduction due to the numbness and changes in anatomy from the procedure. The use of thickened liquids early on with transition to a soft diet as tolerated seems to work well for most patients. It is crucial for patients to understand that altered anatomy will cause these disturbances early on, and that they will improve with time fairly quickly (most patients are doing well within 4 to 6 weeks).

Patients will routinely have an objective articulation disorder after surgery. Due to the adaptability of neuromuscular control, the vast majority will go on to recover good phonetics within 4 to 6 weeks after operation. Despite that, many of these patients will continue to have a subjective (but not objectively verifiable) articulation disorder that is persistent.[21] Reassurance from a speech and language therapist may be necessary to convince patients that they are intelligible and "within the norm" for articulation. Certain patients may be at more risk of these types of subjective issues, including the patient with neurotic behavior, obsessive-compulsive disorder, anxiety and depression, previous abuse, personality disorders, etc. Careful patient selection is key.

References

1. Murphey AW, Kandl JA, Nguyen SA, Weber AC, Gillespie MB. The effect of glossectomy for obstructive sleep apnea: a systematic review and meta-analysis. *Otolaryngol Head Neck Surg*. 2015;153(3):334–342.
2. Calik MW. Treatments for obstructive sleep apnea. *J Clin Outcomes Manag*. 2016;23(4):181–192.
3. Fujita S, Woodson BT, Clark JL, Wittig R. Laser midline glossectomy as a treatment for obstructive sleep apnea. *Laryngoscope*. 1991;101(8):805–809.
4. Cielo CM, Duffy KA, Vyas A, Taylor JA, Kalish JM. Obstructive sleep apnoea and the role of tongue reduction surgery in children with Beckwith-Wiedemann syndrome. *Paediatr Respir Rev*. 2018;25:58–63.
5. Morgan WE, Friedman EM, Duncan NO, Sulek M. Surgical management of macroglossia in children. *Arch Otolaryngol Head Neck Surg*. 1996;122(3):326–329.
6. Hotokezaka H, Matsuo T, Nakagawa M, Mizuno A, Kobayashi K. Severe dental open bite malocclusion with tongue reduction after orthodontic treatment. *Angle Orthod*. 2001;71(3):228–236.
7. Hikita R, Kobayashi Y, Tsuji M, Kawamoto T, Moriyama K. Long-term orthodontic and surgical treatment and stability of a patient with Beckwith-Wiedemann syndrome. *Am J Orthod Dentofacial Orthop*. 2014;145(5):672–684.
8. Hendrick JW. Macroglossia or giant tongue; case report. *Surgery*. 1956;39(4):674–677.
9. Austermann KH, Machtens E. The influence of tongue asymmetries on the development of jaws and the position of teeth. *Int J Oral Surg*. 1974;3(5):261–265.
10. Dingman RO, Grabb WC. Lymphangioma of the tongue. *Plast Reconstr Surg Transplant Bull*. 1961;27:214–223.
11. Kole H. Results, experience, and problems in the operative treatment of anomalies with reverse overbite (mandibular protrusion). *Oral Surg Oral Med Oral Pathol Oral Radiol Endod*. 1965;19:427–450.
12. Egyedi P, Obwegeser H. Zur operativen zungenvereinerung. *Dtsh Zehn Mund Kieferhielk*. 1964;41:16–25.
13. Davalbhakta A, Lamberty BG. Technique for uniform reduction of macroglossia. *Br J Plast Surg*. 2000;53(4):294–297.
14. Kacker A, Honrado C, Martin D, Ward R. Tongue reduction in Beckwith-Weidemann syndrome. *Int J Pediatr Otorhinolaryngol*. 2000;53(1):1–7.
15. Klaiman P, Witzel MA, Margar-Bacal F, Munro IR. Changes in aesthetic appearance and intelligibility of speech after partial glossectomy in patients with Down syndrome. *Plast Reconstr Surg*. 1988;82(3):403–408.
16. Somers E, Samson T. Keyhole tongue reduction. *Operat Tech Otolaryngol Head Neck Surg*. Vol 26. Elsevier; 2015:4.
17. Kruchinsky HV. A new tongue reduction method. *J Oral Maxillofac Surg*. 1990;48(7):756–757.
18. Edgerton M. The management of macroglossia when associated with prognathism. *Br J Plast Surg*. 1950;3(2):117–122.
19. Harada K, Enomoto S. A new method of tongue reduction for macroglossia. *J Oral Maxillofac Surg*. 1995;53(1):91–92.
20. Mixter RC, Ewanowski SJ, Carson LV. Central tongue reduction for macroglossia. *Plast Reconstr Surg*. 1993;91(6):1159–1162.
21. Van Lierde KM, Mortier G, Huysman E, Vermeersch H. Long-term impact of tongue reduction on speech intelligibility, articulation and oromyofunctional behaviour in a child with Beckwith-Wiedemann syndrome. *Int J Pediatr Otorhinolaryngol*. 2010;74(3):309–318.

CHAPTER 163

MMA for Obstructive Sleep Apnea

Yedeh Ying and Peter D. Waite

Armamentarium

#9 Molt periosteal elevator
#15 Scalpel blade
Appropriate sutures
Bone rongeurs
Calipers
Curved Mayo scissors
Double-guarded septal osteotome
Freer elevator
Internal fixation kit (midface and mandible)
"J" strippers
Kirschner wire
Local anesthetic with vasoconstrictor
Mallet
Medium Langenbeck (toe-in)
Monopolar cautery
Needle driver
Pterygoid chisel
Retractors (two)
Round/egg bur
Rowe disimpaction forceps
Safe-edge saw
Sagittal saw
Seldin retractor
Smith spreaders
Spatula osteotome
Straight osteotome
Suture scissors
Woodson elevator

History of the Procedure

Maxillomandibular advancement (MMA) is an effective surgical option for the treatment of obstructive sleep apnea (OSA) in patients who may be noncompliant with continuous positive airway pressure (CPAP) or refractory to other surgical modalities.[1–4] The facial skeleton is advanced as a unit with both upper and lower jaws in occlusive harmony. This increases the pharyngeal and hypopharyngeal airspace to address obstructions in a multilevel manner. Patients who may also have skeletal hypoplasia especially benefit from MMA, although this is not a hard indication. It has been well reported that MMA enlarges the posterior airway space and tightens the upper airway musculature by skeletal advancement strategies.[5–8]

The original Stanford protocol addressed the airway in two phases. Phase 1 surgery involved management of the soft tissues at each distinct level based on the Fujita classification. These procedures include uvulopalatopharyngoplasty, genial tubercle advancement, and hyoid suspension. Patients who then have persistent OSA after phase 1 procedures were then considered for phase 2 surgery, which addressed the facial skeleton.[9,10] MMA is viewed as the most effective and safe treatment of OSA that can predictably lead to improvements in sleepiness, quality of life, sleep-disordered breathing and neurocognitive performance, and a reduction in cardiovascular risk.[11]

Indications for the Use of the Procedure

MMA surgery is indicated under the following conditions:

1. History of clinically significant OSA noncompliance/responsive to conservative therapy (CPAP, splints, etc.)
2. Requires management of the airway at multiple levels (Fujita class II)
3. Medically/psychologically stable and willing to proceed with surgery
4. Positive drug-induced sedation endoscopy (DISE) showing severe lateral pharyngeal wall collapse with circumferential collapse of the velum (Fig. 163.1).[12,13]

Limitations and Contraindications

MMA is contraindicated when there is the absence of hypopharyngeal narrowing (posterior airway space >11 mm), indicating the site of obstruction can be corrected via soft-tissue surgical procedures.[14] Other medical factors such as history of temporomandibular joint derangement, connective tissue disorders, use of antiresorptive/antiangiogenic medications, and coagulopathies may warrant careful consideration of potential risks for complications. Situations that limit the duration of general anesthesia (lung function or cardiac conditions) may also preclude one from undergoing MMA.[15]

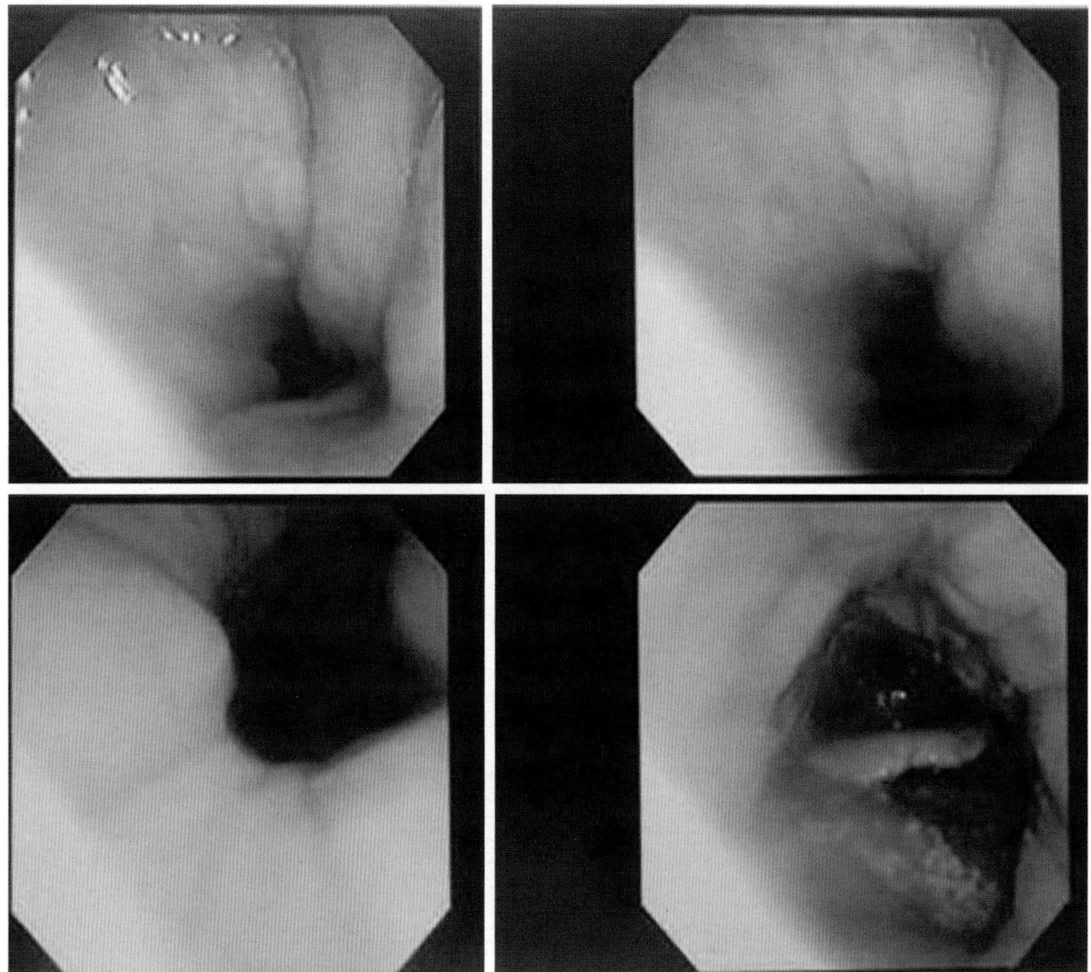

Figure 163.1 Sequential images showing active concentric collapse with narrowing of the lower airway during a preoperative Mueller's maneuver.

TECHNIQUE: Maxillomandibular Advancement Surgery

STEP 1: Presurgical Assessment

Once OSA has been diagnosed and failure of nonsurgical methods attempted, surgical planning should begin. Evaluation of the level of airway collapse can be assessed with awake nasopharyngoscopy, DISE and can highlight advancement movements to focus on. As clinical examination alone is insufficient to assess upper airway changes, standard cephalometric analysis must be included as well. This may include obtaining cone beam computer tomography or traditional two-dimensional imaging. This would include a lateral and anteroposterior radiograph for standardized and objective measurements from known skeletal landmarks for cephalometric analysis.

STEP 2: Determination of Surgical Order

The introduction of virtual surgical planning (VSP) allows for the simulation of the planned movements, which can allow the most stable intermediate splints to be fabricated. Typically, a mandible-first approach leads to a better, more stable advancement splint. Anticipating a counterclockwise rotation can better improve advancement goals while minimizing changes to appearance and cosmetics (Fig. 163.2).

STEP 3: Mandibular Advancement Considerations

The actual technique for bilateral split sagittal split osteotomy is well described elsewhere in the text. These pointers are modifications by these surgeons for our approach to the mandible.

Incision: A mouth prop is placed on the contralateral dentition to aid with exposure. A #15 blade is used starting along the external oblique ridge along the lateral aspect of the anterior border of the ramus. Starting approximately 1 cm above the occlusal plane allows for a full-thickness incision either linearly or with a stepped

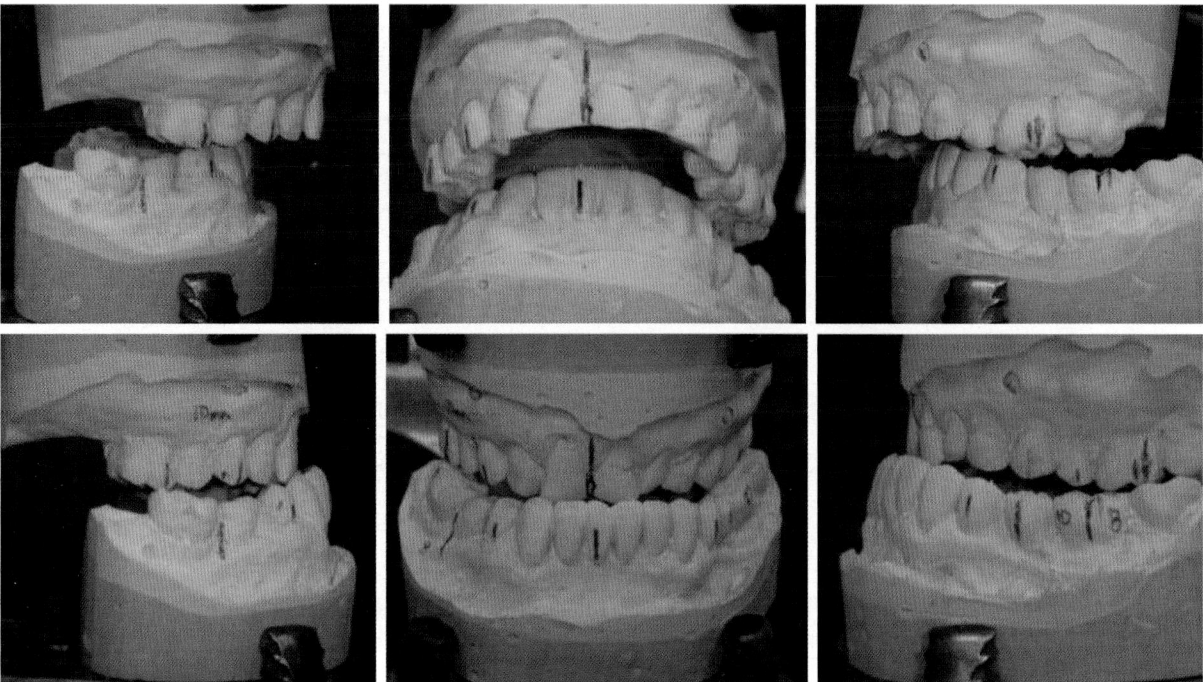

Figure 163.2 Advancing the mandible first allows for a more stable intermediate splint.

TECHNIQUE: Maxillomandibular Advancement Surgery—*cont'd*

incision lateral to the first molar to aid in would closure. Staying lateral will give you a better mucosal cuff for soft-tissue closure and prevent unesthetic scarring at the mucogingival junction.

Dissection: Mucosa and connective tissue dissection is performed subperiosteally laterally up the coronoid, posteriorly to the mandibular border, and inferiorly to the antegonial notch. The wide undermining of the muscular attachments allows for advancement and counterclockwise rotation dependent on the surgical plan. Starting from the medial aspect of coronoid downward along the medial mandible, stay subperiosteal to avoid the lingual nerve. Continue to stay subperiosteal to identify the lingual/mandibular fossa and entry of the inferior alveolar nerve. A nerve hook can be utilized to identify the foramen itself prior to performing osteotomies.

Osteotomies: The authors' preferred technique is to use the standard stepwise chisels to slowly propagate osteotomies along the medial aspect of the mandible from the lingual fossa to the anterior ramus following the external oblique ridge in a "lazy S" fashion to the lateral vertical cut. Care is taken to ensure the bone cut is complete at the inferior border at an angle to prevent unfavorable splits. Surgical planning for large surgical advancements is envisioned for ideal fixation techniques.

Fixation: Large advancement of the mandible with counterclockwise rotation has a greater trend of relapse. Standard fixation can be utilized for fixation of the proximal and distal segments in standard movement. Consideration for combinations of bicortical screws and a monocortical plate or double plating should be made for larger movements (>7 mm) (Fig. 163.3).

STEP 4: Maxillary Osteotomy Considerations

The actual technique is well described for the performance of the Le Fort osteotomies elsewhere in the text. These pointers are modifications by these surgeons for our approach to the maxilla for MMA.

Incision: A #15 blade is used starting 5 to 10 mm above the mucogingival junction in the maxillary vestibule from first molar to first molar. This incision should give access to visualize the maxillary buttresses without violating the buccal fat pad. One should note the location of Stenson's duct to avoid iatrogenic injury. Modification of the incision can be performed with a posterior vertical incision at the zygomatic buttress superiorly to increase the base of the posterior vascular pedicle.

Dissection: Dissection is caried to the infraorbital foramen, medially to the piriform rims, and laterally to the zygomatic buttress. A pocket is then created subperiosteally to the pterygomaxillary fissure and packed with neuropatties to aid with hemostasis and blunt dissection. Care is taken with a Freer elevator to elevate

Continued

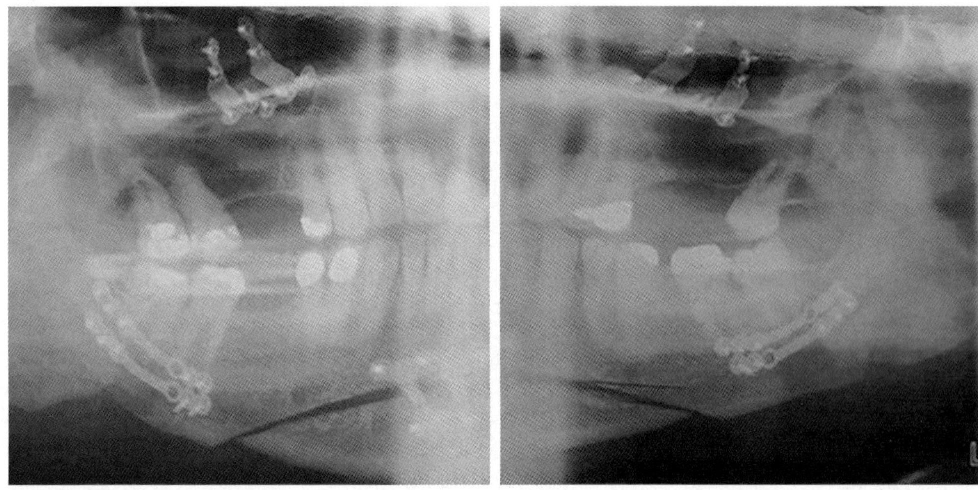

Figure 163.3 Fixation technique of utilizing two mandibular advancement plates for a large advancement.

TECHNIQUE: Maxillomandibular Advancement Surgery—*cont'd*

the mucoperiosteum off the floor of the nose from the septum medially and the inferior turbinate laterally.

Osteotomies: The authors' preferred technique is to use a reciprocating saw starting at the midpoint of zygomaticomaxillary buttress medially to the piriform rim. In order to gain additional counterclockwise rotation, a wedge of bone can be removed starting from the piriform rim and tapered toward the initial osteotomy. This allows for additional impaction to help reduce excess dental show and aid in counterclockwise rotation. Improved bone contact will be found at the piriform buttresses. The standard septal/pterygoid osteotomies are as described before in the chapters on the Le Fort I osteotomies.

Down-fracture/Mobilization: Once osteotomies through the septum, lateral nasal walls, maxilla, and pterygoid junction have been completed, down-fracture with firm steady pressure at the anterior nasal spine and Smith spreaders at the buttresses should easily complete the disjunction. The ideal down-fracture is posterior to the palate and tuberosity. Rowe disimpaction forceps are utilized to ensure adequate release of the posterior soft tissue by rotational movements along all axes. Releasing the soft -tissue attachments can assure adequate advancement if needed. Sacrifice of the descending palatine artery is optional, but many times it may need to be clipped for adequate release. The forceps are not meant to advance the maxilla anteriorly as there is a risk for avulsing the soft-tissue pedicle.

Nasal aperture modifications: Since OSA can be related to turbulent flow through the upper nasal cavity, septoplasty to correct deviation is performed at this time. The cartilage is exposed inferiorly and excised as needed. The maxillary crest can be adjusted if there are interferences that may cause buckling. Interior turbinectomies can be performed at this time in conjunction with enlargement of the piriforms apertures with an egg bur. The nasal septum is then sutured to the anterior nasal spine during closure.

Fixation: The fixation of the maxilla should focus on tightening the pharyngeal dilator musculature while minimizing unesthetic changes of the midface (burying of the teeth with impaction). Typically 1.0-mm L plates that are either prebent or prefabricated are used along the osteotomies at the buttresses. It is of the authors' opinion that prefabricated bent plates fit better and have less stress fractures due to less manipulation. Good bone stock can be found at the piriform and zygoma for fixation screws. Bone grafting along the lateral walls of the sinus is a good place for interpositional grafts, which helps facilitate healing and improve stability (Figs. 163.4 and 163.5).

ALTERNATIVE TECHNIQUE: Digital Workflow With Virtual Surgical Planning

VSP protocols have become the norm with orthognathic surgery. The outcomes following these protocols have been shown to have predictable and accurate results.[16] The planning allows for osteotomies to maximize advancement movements and prediction of counterclockwise rotation and possible interferences. More importantly, the three-dimensional imaging that can be obtained from traditional computed tomography or cone beam computer tomography (CBCT) can identify anatomic sites of obstruction and how to best address advancement and impaction in patients undergoing MMA.

Standard work-up for the sleep apnea patient is performed in the initial setting. A protocol for computer-aided

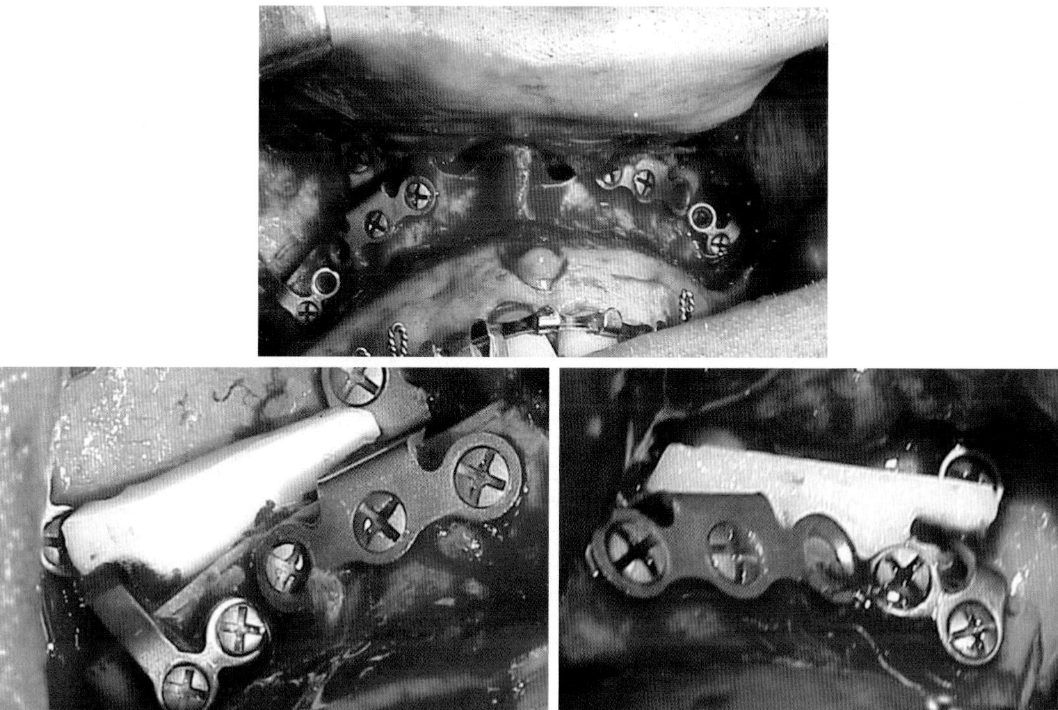

Figure 163.4 Interpositional bone grafting for a large maxillary advancement.

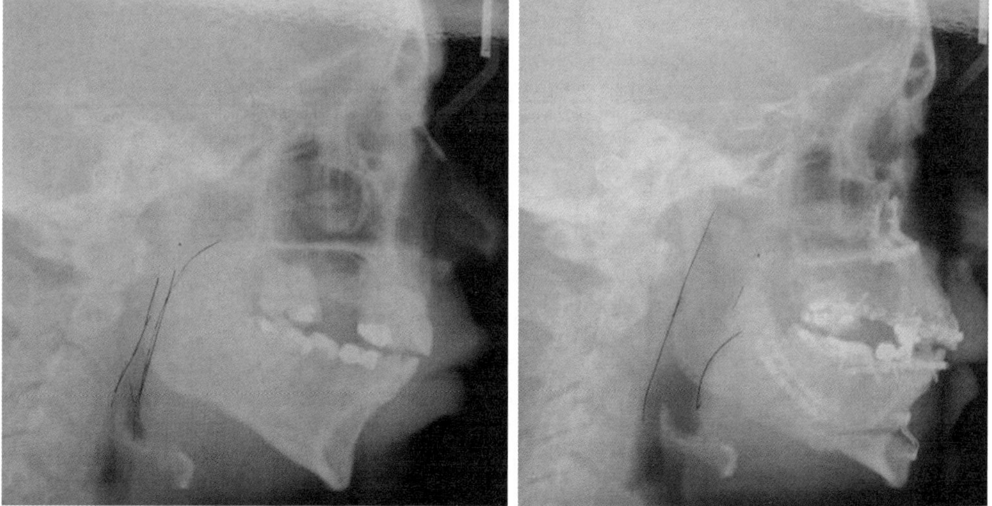

Figure 163.5 With large advancements, significant improvements can be made with impaction of the maxilla anteriorly and gaining further advancement with counterclockwise rotation. Note the change in occlusal plane.

planning has been discussed previously and can be reviewed to incorporate the data into a virtual planning software. It has been shown that in the sagittal plane, posterior airway space (PAS) and airway lengths have been shown to improve after MMA and are associated with improvement of symptoms.[17,18]

With the use of VSP, we have been able to identify the degree of advancement and impaction to measure parameters such PAS, A-point, B-point, etc. and the impacts on the improvement of sleep apnea. The authors would like to achieve specific cephalometric measurements such as a PAS of 6 mm in the occlusal plane and 11 mm at the mandibular plane. More recently, we found optimal surgical change to be 6 mm for A-point, 7.9 mm for upper incisors, 7.6 mm for B-point, 11.2 mm for pogonion, and 10 mm menton for patients treated at our institution. This resulted in maxillary advancements less than 10 mm but was adequate to increase total airway volume by at least 70%.[19] Fig. 163.6 shows that the measurements can be evaluated with VSP, but not all metrics may be possible to achieve in order to maximize PAS. Careful consideration of patient esthetics and function must be balanced with surgeon experience to maximize PAS.

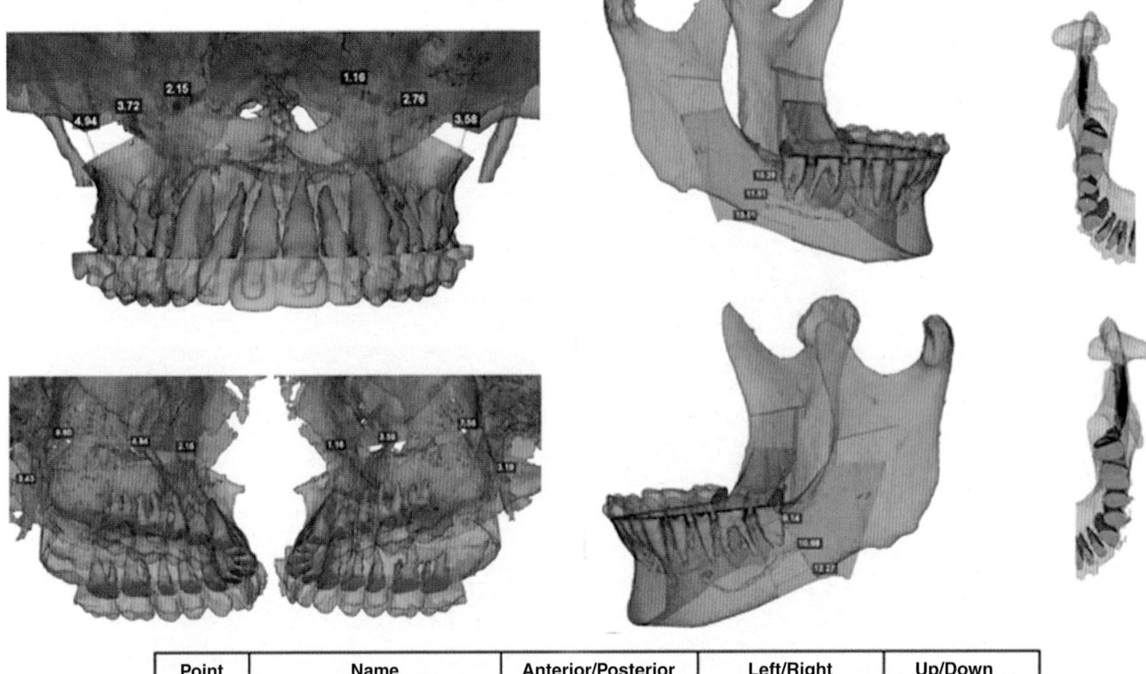

Point	Name	Anterior/Posterior	Left/Right	Up/Down
ANS	Anterior Nasal Spine	0.27mm Anterior	0.85mm Right	1.57mm Up
A	A Point	1.65mm Anterior	0.64mm Right	0.98mm Up
ISU1	Midline of Upper Incisor	6.00mm Anterior	0.00	2.00mm Up
U3L	Upper Left Canine	5.97mm Anterior	0.00	1.06mm Up
U6L	Upper Left Anterior Molar (mesiobuccal cusp)	5.63mm Anterior	0.00	2.65mm Down
U3R	Upper Right Canine	5.75mm Anterior	0.01mm Right	0.07mm Up
U6R	Upper Right Anterior Molar (mesiobuccal cusp)	5.49mm Anterior	0.00	3.80mm Down
ISL1	Midline of Lower Incisor	5.74mm Anterior	0.03mm Right	1.58mm Up
L6L	Lower Left Anterior Molar (mesiobuccal cusp)	5.67mm Anterior	0.01mm Left	2.60mm Down
L6R	Lower Right Anterior Molar (mesiobuccal cusp)	5.34mm Anterior	0.03mm Right	3.64mm Down
B	B Point	9.40mm Anterior	0.53mm Left	0.27mm Up
Pog	Pogonion	12.07mm Anterior	0.93mm Left	0.40mm Up

Figure 163.6 Measurements obtained during virtual surgical planning (VSP) planning. Note the minimal advancement of the maxilla with more focus on counterclockwise rotation to improve airway space in order to minimize impact of patient esthetics.

By virtually planning the degree of impaction of the maxilla, we can anticipate the tooth-to-lip relationship as shown in Fig. 163.7. A secondary benefit will be the visualization of the autorotation of the mandible and achieve predictable advancement of the mandible at the chin point.

Avoidance and Management of Intraoperative Complications

As mentioned in previous chapters, complications with MMA mirror that of single jaw surgery. With the advances of VSP, interferences and nerve positioning can be predicted and osteotomies can be planned to avoid neurosensory injury or malpositioning of the jaws.[20]

Attention to occlusion during the evaluation can aid in stabilization of the intermediate splint. Extraction of third molars allows for a smaller occlusal platform and leveling the occlusion for more stability (Fig. 163.8).

Postoperative Considerations

Although patients are routinely extubated at the end of the procedure, patients must be carefully monitored with continuous pulse oximetry or in the intensive care unit for respiratory complications. Careful administration of long-acting

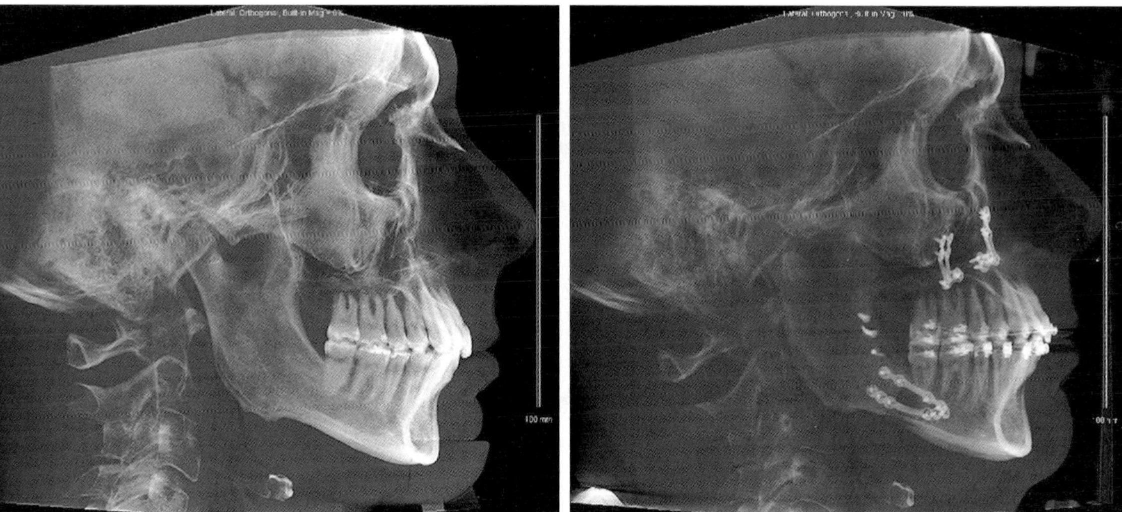

Figure 163.7 Pre- and postoperative imaging of previous case. Note the change in occlusal plane for counterclockwise rotation but a significant increase in posterior airway space (PAS).

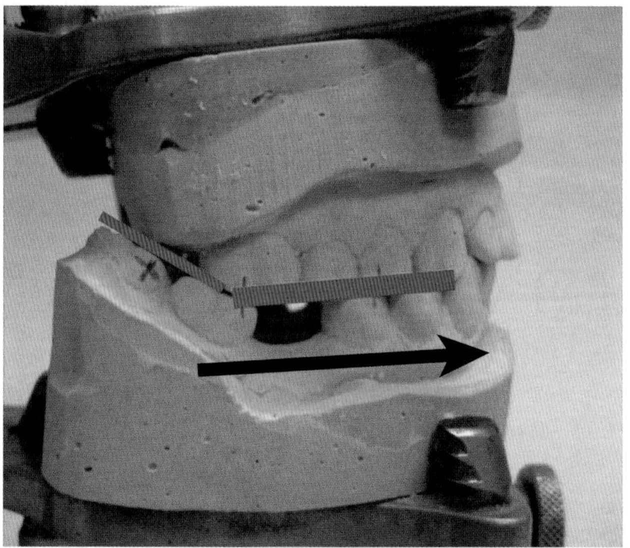

Figure 163.8 Removal of the third molars allows for additional advancement and leveling of the occlusion.

opioids to minimize risk of respiratory depression and strong consideration for nonsteroidal antiinflammatory or nonnarcotic analgesics for pain control is critical in the postoperative setting. Long-acting local anesthetic at the completion of the surgery can also be considered to minimize the need for excess opioid requirements. Facial edema from surgery is managed by intravenous corticosteroids and ensures patency of the airway. Hemostats or wire cutters should be readily available in patients who have temporary maxillomandibular fixation elastics/wires in the setting of significant tongue swelling. Nutritional counselling for a strict non-chewing diet for 6 weeks to allow for initial bony healing is recommended. The long-term stability of MMA has been well described based on predictable movements of the skeleton.[21–23]

MMA is a highly predictable procedure with relatively low risk and morbidity. While radiographically the anatomic airway can be improved by the procedures mentioned previously (see Fig. 163.8), polysomnography is ultimately the metric that defines success (Fig. 163.9).

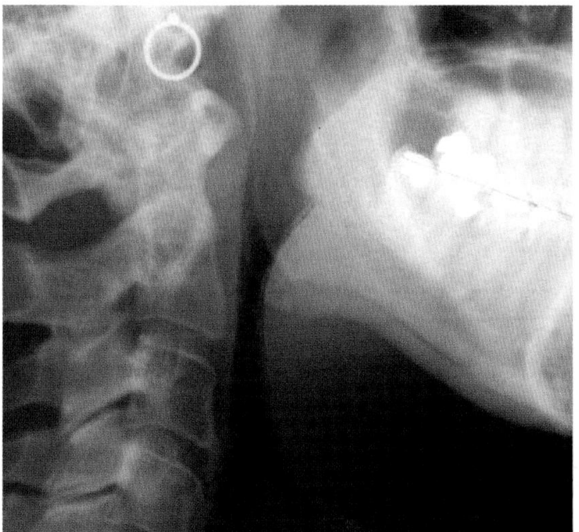

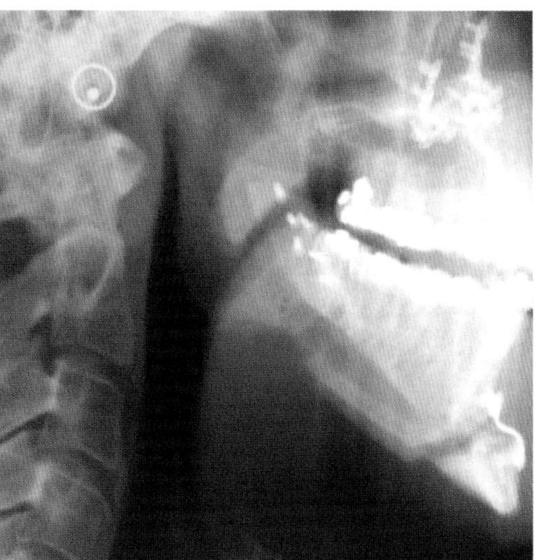

Figure 163.9 Lateral cephalogram of patient demonstrating improvement in posterior airway space but poor improvement in the apnea-hypopnea index/respiratory disturbance index.

References

1. Li KK. Surgical management of obstructive sleep apnea. *Clin Chest Med*. 2003;24(2):365–370.
2. Riley RW, Powell NB. Maxillofacial surgery and obstructive sleep apnea syndrome. *Otolaryngol Clin North Am*. 1990;23(4):809–826.
3. Riley RW, Powell NB, Guilleminault C. Maxillofacial surgery and nasal CPAP. A comparison of treatment for obstructive sleep apnea syndrome. *Chest*. 1990;98(6):1421–1425.
4. Powell NB, Riley RW, Guilleminault C, Murcia GN. Obstructive sleep apnea, continuous positive airway pressure, and surgery. *Otolaryngol Head Neck Surg*. 1988;99(4):362–369.
5. Riley RW, Powell NB, Li KK, Troell RJ, Guilleminault C. Surgery and obstructive sleep apnea: long-term clinical outcomes. *Otolaryngol Head Neck Surg*. 2000;122(3):415–421.
6. Caples SM, Rowley JA, Prinsell JR, et al. Surgical modifications of the upper airway for obstructive sleep apnea in adults: a systematic review and meta-analysis. *Sleep*. 2010;33(10):1396–1407.
7. Won CHJ, Li KK, Guilleminault C. Surgical treatment of obstructive sleep apnea. *Proc Am Thorac Soc*. 2008;5:193.
8. Li KK. Hypopharyngeal airway surgery. *Otolaryngol Clin North Am*. 2007;40(4):845–853.
9. Li KK, Powell NB, Riley RW. Surgical management of obstructive sleep apnea. In: Lee-chiong TL, Sateia MJ, Caraskadon MA, eds. *Sleep Medicine*. Philadelphia, PA: Hanley & Belfus; 2002.
10. Riley RW, Powell NB, Guilleminault C. Obstructive sleep apnea syndrome: a surgical protocol for dynamic upper airway reconstruction. *J Oral Maxillofac Surg*. 1993;51(7):742–747.
11. Boyd SB, Chigurupati R, Cillo Jr JE, et al. Maxillomandibular advancement improves multiple health-related and functional outcomes in patients with obstructive sleep apnea: a multicenter study. *J Oral Maxillofac Surg*. 2019;77(2):352–370.
12. Liu SY, Huon LK, Iwasaki T, et al. Efficacy of maxillomandibular advancement examined with drug-induced sleep endoscopy and computational fluid dynamics airflow modeling. *Otolaryngol Head Neck Surg*. 2016;154(1):189–195.
13. Liu SY, Huon LK, Powell NB, et al. Lateral pharyngeal wall tension after maxillomandibular advancement for obstructive sleep apnea is a marker for surgical success: observations from drug-induced sleep endoscopy. *J Oral Maxillofac Surg*. 2015;73(8):1575–1582.
14. Riley RW, Powell N, Guilleminault C. Current surgical concepts for treating obstructive sleep apnea syndrome. *J Oral Maxillofac Surg*. 1987;45(2):149–157.
15. Li KK, Riley RW, Powell NB, Troell R, Guilleminault C. Overview of phase II surgery for obstructive sleep apnea syndrome. *Ear Nose Throat J*. 1999;78(11):851–857. 854-857.
16. Hsu SS, Gateno J, Bell RB, et al. Accuracy of a computer-aided surgical simulation protocol for orthognathic surgery: a prospective multicenter study. *J Oral Maxillofac Surg*. 2013;71(1):128–142.
17. Fairburn SC, Waite PD, Vilos G, et al. Three-dimensional changes in upper airways of patients with obstructive sleep apnea following maxillomandibular advancement. *J Oral Maxillofac Surg*. 2007;65(1):6–12.
18. Abramson ZR, Susarla S, Tagoni JR, Kaban L. Three-dimensional computed tomographic analysis of airway anatomy. *J Oral Maxillofac Surg*. 2010;68(2):363–371.
19. Kongsong W, Waite PD, Sittitavornwong S, Schibler M, Alshahrani F. The correlation of maxillomandibular advancement and airway volume change in obstructive sleep apnea using cone beam computed tomography. *Int J Oral Maxillofac Implants*. 2021;50(7):940–947.
20. Farrell BB, Franco PB, Tucker MR. Virtual surgical planning in orthognathic surgery. *Oral Maxillofac Surg Clin North Am*. 2014;26(4):459–473.
21. Li KK, Powell NB, Riley RW, Troell RJ, Guilleminault C. Long term results of maxillomandibular advancement surgery. *Sleep Breath*. 2000;4(3):137–140.
22. Reiche-Fischel O, Wolford LM. Posterior airway space changes after double jaw surgery with counter-clockwise rotation. *J Oral Maxillofac Surg*. 1996;54:96.
23. Proffit WR, Turvey TA, Phillips C. The hierarchy of stability and predictability in orthognathic surgery with rigid fixation: an update and extension. *Head Face Med*. 2007;3:21.

CHAPTER 164

Hypoglossal Nerve Stimulation for Obstructive Sleep Apnea

Stanley Yung-Chuan Liu and Allen Huang

Armamentarium

#15 Scalpel blades
2-0 Permanent silk suture on SH (2)
20-gauge angiocath
3-0 Permanent silk suture on RB1 (7)
3M 1012 Drape (critical that this is clear, not frosted)
Collaborative viewing
Fine-tipped instruments: McCabe, Right Angle, Tonsil, Kelly
Gauze

Implants and Accessories

Inspire Generator #3028
Inspire programmer
Inspire Respiratory Sense Lead #4340
Inspire Sleep Remote control #2500
Inspire Stimulation Lead #4063
Karl Storz endoskope VITOM Visualization system for open surgery
Kittner dissection sponges
Local injectable anesthetic
Lone Star elastic stays (4)
Malleable retractor: 5 mm wide
Medtronic Catheter Passer #8591-38
Medtronic NIM Response 3.0 Console
Medtronic Side-by-Side Bipolar Stimulator Probe #8225401
Medtronic Torque Wrench Accessory #3550-80
Medtronic Xomed 18-mm Paired EMG electrodes #8227304
Needle holders

Nonsterile Prep Table

Retractors (Army-Navy, Richardson, Appendiceal, Langenbeck)
Skin marker and ruler
Straight pick-up or curved dissector (DeBakey)

Surgical Instruments

Tongue blade
Ultrasound probe cover
Vessel loops

History of the Procedure

Obstructive sleep apnea (OSA) affects millions of people globally, and nearly 5% to 10% of the US population.[1] The cessation of airflow that leads to hypoxemia during sleep diminishes cognitive function with daytime sleepiness and fatigue. It also increases the risk for stroke, coronary artery disease, hypertension, and congestive heart failure.[2] Our improved understanding of OSA has allowed targeted approaches for surgical treatment.[3] In the updated Stanford sleep surgery algorithm centered around precision in airway phenotyping and continuity of multi-modal interventions, hypoglossal nerve stimulation (HNS) plays a significant role (Fig. 164.1).[3,4]

In early 2001, Schwartz et al. showed a decrease in upper airway collapse through genioglossus stimulation via branch specific selection of the hypoglossal nerve.[5,6] Upper airway therapy through neuromuscular stimulation of the hypoglossal nerve and genioglossus muscle became an option for patients intolerant of first-line therapy, such as positive air pressure (PAP) or oral appliance therapy (OAT).[7,8] By stimulating the medial branches of the hypoglossal nerve, protrusion of the stiffened tongue results in reduced pharyngeal collapse and increased airflow during sleep.[9,10] Several systems of HNS are in various stages of development. Currently, Inspire II (Inspire Medical System, Maple Grove, MN, USA) is the only Food and Drug Administration-approved HNS for OSA. The pivotal Stimulation Therapy for Apnea Reduction (STAR) trial and subsequent studies have continued to establish its safety and efficacy.[11]

Indications for the Use of the Procedure

An attended polysomnogram remains the gold standard diagnostic exam for OSA. Patients typically begin with medical therapy including PAP and OAT. Patients that are intolerant of PAP and OAT may respond to treatment of nasal obstruction.[3] Body mass index (BMI) is another important determinant of treatment efficacy. Patients who elect for surgical treatment may undergo the Riley-Powell phased protocol, starting with interventions for the soft palate and tongue as phase 1.[12] Patients with persistent OSA may be offered maxillomandibular advancement (MMA) for phase 2. Today, OSA patients with concomitant dentofacial deformity or with complete concentric and lateral pharyngeal wall collapse during drug-induced sleep endoscopy (DISE) may be advised to bypass phase 1 and start with MMA.[3,4,13–16]

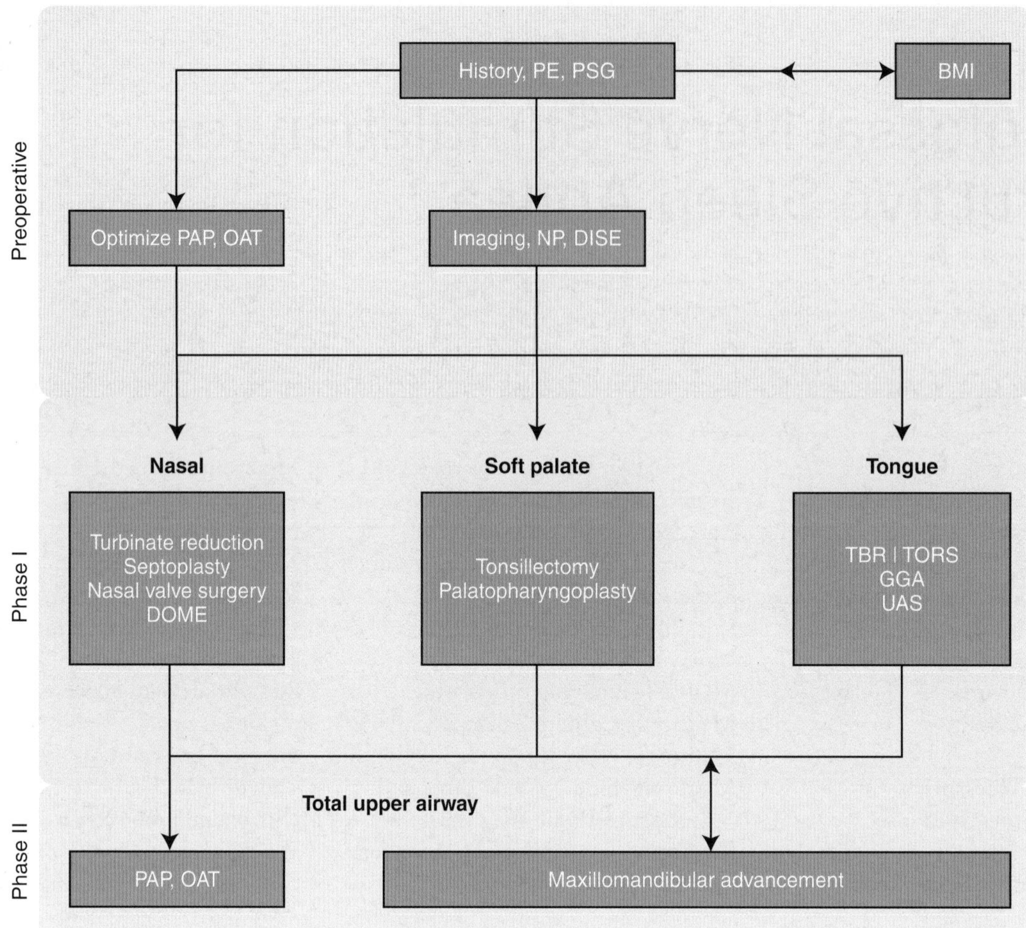

Figure 164.1 Updated Stanford protocol.

Patients who elect to have HNS for OSA management with the Inspire II system need to be adults (1) presenting with an apnea-hypopnea index between 15 and 65 events per hour, with less than 25% being mixed or central apnea, (2) BMI equal to or less than 32 kg/m^2, and (3) absence of complete concentric collapse at the velum during DISE.[9] Pediatric HNS use is undergoing clinical trials for patients with trisomy 21. As OSA is a chronic condition that can relapse, HNS is also attractive for patients previously treated with other forms of sleep surgery.[17] Finally, the ability to titrate neurostimulation for the collapsible airway allows clinicians flexibility in adjusting therapy (Fig. 164.2).[18]

Limitations and Contraindications

Patients with complete concentric palatal collapse (CCC) during DISE, greater than 25% central or mixed apneas, who are pregnant, who require frequent MRI of the torso, or who have preexisting neurologic disorders or anatomic variants are not candidates for the current form of HNS. While CCC of the velum is an exclusion criteria, it can be converted and reversed with palatopharyngoplasty or other procedures, including distraction osteogenesis for maxillary expansion or MMA.[13,19–21] Other limitations of HNS may include cost and availability of ongoing follow-up at certified sleep centers.[15,16] Patients with preexisting insomnia or those who find the therapy to be overstimulating can become frustrated finding a therapeutic setting. Multiple titrations in-office with nasopharyngoscopy, with DISE, or during attended polysomnography may be necessary

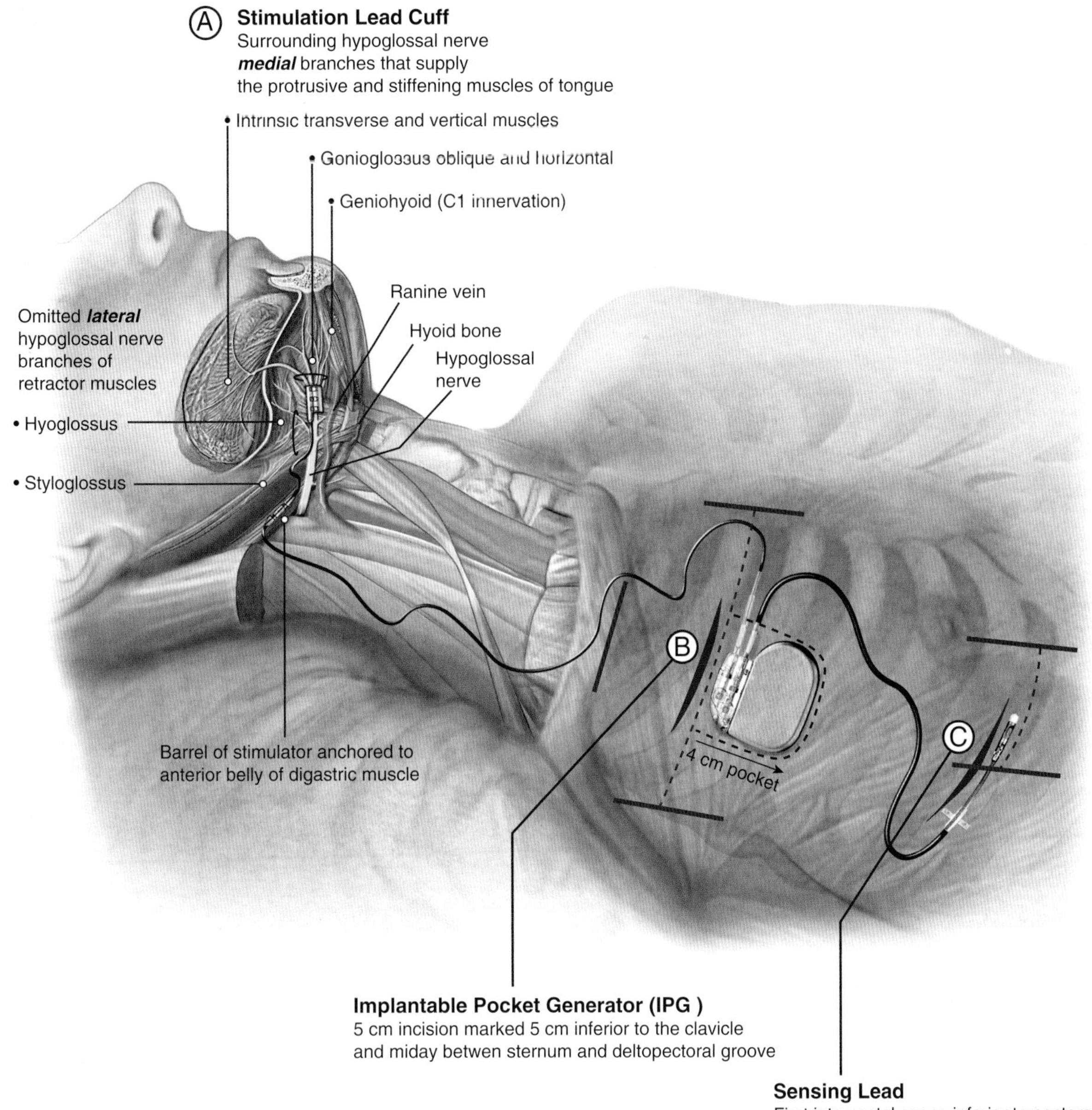

Figure 164.2 Illustration of hypoglossal nerve stimulator.

TECHNIQUE: Hypoglossal Nerve Stimulator Placement

STEP 1: Preparation

The patient is placed in the supine position, with a chest bump beneath the right torso for easier access to the lateral chest wall. Short-acting muscle relaxants, dexamethasone, and preprocedural antibiotics are given. A nerve integrity monitoring (NIM) system (Medtronic, Minneapolis, Minnesota) is set up to monitor tongue movement with sensor leads (Xomed 82273049) and bipolar stimulating probe (Xomed 8225401). The NIM blue electrode is inserted through the floor of the mouth, slightly right of the midline, to include muscles innervated by the medial branches of the hypoglossal nerve. These include protrusive muscles (genioglossus oblique and horizontal) and stiffening muscles (intrinsic transverse and vertical muscles of the tongue). The NIM red electrode is inserted submucosally into the right ventrolateral surface of the tongue to monitor retractor muscles (styloglossus and hyoglossus), which are innervated by the lateral branches of the hypoglossal nerve. A small bite block is then placed on the left side for visualization of tongue movement after implant placement but before closing. Three surgical sites are then marked:

1. For the stimulation lead: A 5-cm incision is marked midway along the length of the right mandible and is midway between the hyoid and mandible, staying 1 cm from the midline.

(Continued)

TECHNIQUE: Hypoglossal Nerve Stimulator Placement—*cont'd*

2. For the implantable pulse generator (IPG) pocket: A 5-cm incision is marked 5 cm inferior to the clavicle and midway between the sternum and deltopectoral groove.
3. For the sensing lead: The first intercostal space inferior to the pectoralis major is usually used for a 5-cm incision approximately 5 cm lateral from a line straight down from the nipple.

The surgical field, including the face, neck, and chest are then prepped in sterile fashion. Sterile towels are secured to isolate the field, and adhesive drapes are used to maintain aseptic technique.

STEP 2: Dissection to the Main Branch of the Hypoglossal Nerve in the Neck

The incision is carried sharply through skin, platysma, and the superficial layer of the deep cervical fascia. Care is taken to protect the marginal mandibular nerve, though the surgical site is anterior to where the nerve courses across the mandible. The submandibular gland is isolated and retracted posterior-superiorly. The posterior border of the mylohyoid muscle is identified, freed, and retracted anteriorly. The anterior belly of the digastric muscle is traced to the digastric tendon and retracted inferiorly. The main trunk of the hypoglossal nerve is usually seen within these boundaries, overlying the hyoglossus muscle. The ranine vein is often encountered and can be ligated if it interferes with isolation of the medial and lateral nerve branch point.

STEP 3: Identification of Medial and Lateral Branches of Hypoglossal Nerve and C1

To identify the C1, medial and lateral branches of the hypoglossal nerve distal to the branch point, NIM stimulation is used. Collaborative viewing for the entire care team is recommended. The author uses a Storz VITOM scope for visualization (Fig. 164.3). A microscope or handheld sinus surgery scope is frequently used by other surgeons for the same purpose. The NIM stimulation begins with the most inferior branches of the main trunk at the branch point. The first branch that may have early or late take-off is usually the C1 nerve that innervates the geniohyoid muscle. As the stimulation is performed in a counterclockwise direction, medial and lateral branches are identified (Fig. 164.4). The lateral branches that retract the tongue are excluded. The medial branches are further freed anteriorly for about 1 cm to clear way for placement of the stimulation lead. Care is taken to minimize overdissection and prevent neuropraxia.

STEP 4: Placing the Stimulation Lead

A vessel loop is placed around the intended inclusion branches and verified with repeat stimulation via NIM probe. The corner of the stimulation lead outer flap is held with a right-angled dissector and placed beneath the medial branches. The shorter outer flap is positioned past the nerve branches such that when the right-angled dissector is released, the medial branches are completely wrapped inside the cuff (Fig. 164.5). Irrigation using a 20-gauge sterile syringe is performed inside the cuff. The barrel of the stimulator cuff is then anchored to the anterior belly of the digastric muscle with two 3-0 silk sutures.

STEP 5: Creating the Implantable Pocket Generator Pocket

The IPG pocket incision is made through skin and subcutaneous tissue superficial to the pectoralis major fascia. Blunt dissection is performed in this plane. The pocket is made roughly 4 cm inferior to the incision.

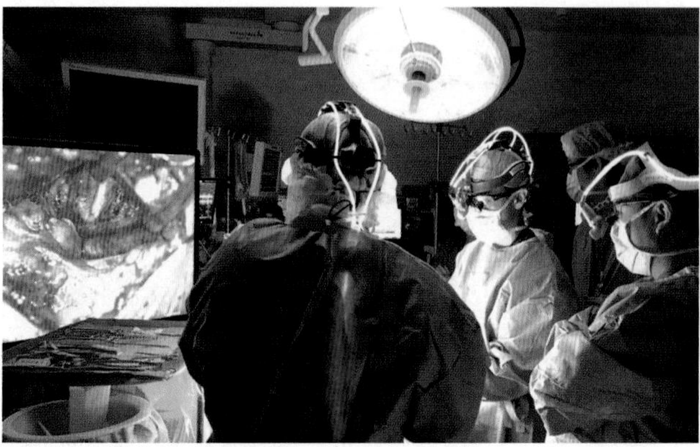

Figure 164.3 Collaborative viewing.

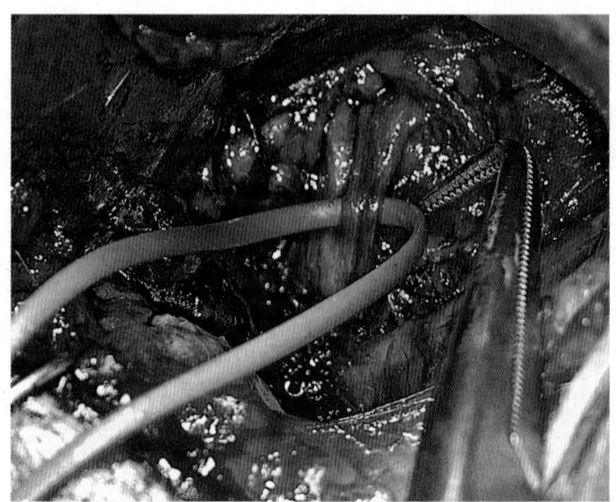

Figure 164.4 Isolation of medial from lateral branches.

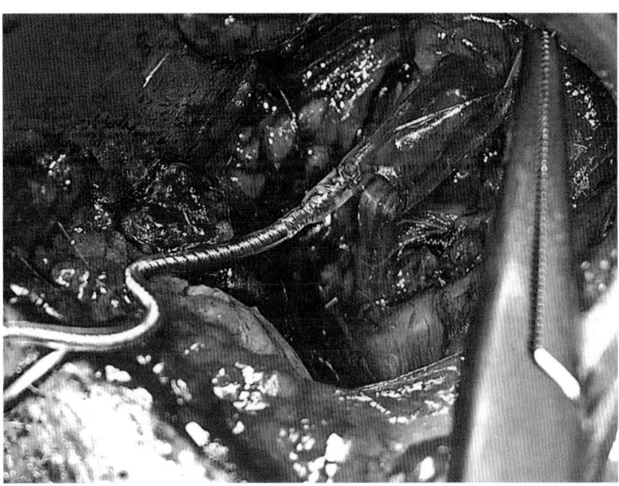

Figure 164.5 Placement of stimulation cuff.

TECHNIQUE: Hypoglossal Nerve Stimulator Placement—*cont'd*

STEP 6: Placement of the Sensing Lead

Incision is made along the right inferolateral chest through skin, subcutaneous tissue, and serratus muscle fibers. A small window is made through the fibers of the external intercostal fibers until the fibers of the internal intercostal muscle are encountered. A narrow malleable retractor is then tunneled approximately 5 cm between the external and internal intercostal muscles for the sensing lead pocket (Fig. 164.6). The sensing lead is grasped on a blue silicone sleeve that protects the hardware. The barrel of the sensing lead is then anchored to the surrounding fascia and serratus muscle using 3-0 silk sutures. The strain relief anchor is left loose until tunneling has been completed.

STEP 7: Tunneling of Sensing and Stimulation Leads to the IPG Pocket

The ideal tunnel device for its length, malleability, and rigidity is the Medtronic Catheter Passer (#8591-38). Prebend the shaft and guide the device within the subcutaneous plane from the inferolateral chest incision to the IPG pocket site, staying superficial to the pectoralis fascia. Special care is needed for patients with breast augmentation. After the passer is fully tunneled through the IPG pocket, the plastic probe is removed and the sensing lead placed into the collet. Then, the tunneling device is withdrawn from the IPG pocket. This allows the sensing lead to be directed into the IPG pocket (Fig. 164.7). The sensing lead is removed from the tunneling device and anchored with strain relief to the fascia at the inferolateral incision site using four 2-0 silk sutures. The length between respiratory lead anchors is calibrated to allow normal range of chest motion. Similarly, the stimulation lead is tunned from the neck incision in a subplatysma plane, over the right clavicle, and through to the IPG pocket. The external jugular vein should be located and avoided during the tunneling process.

(Continued)

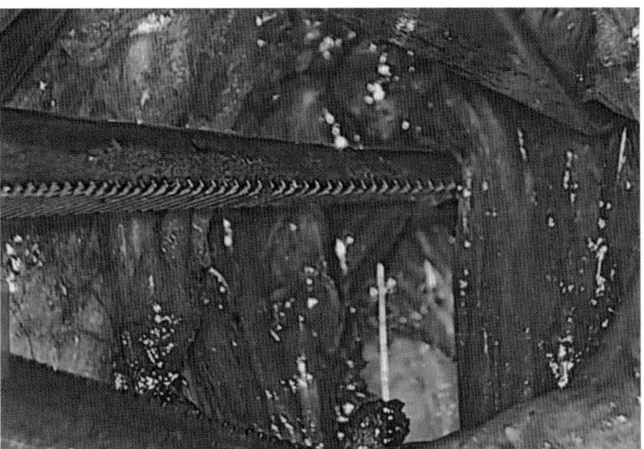

Figure 164.6 Right lateral chest pocket for sensing lead.

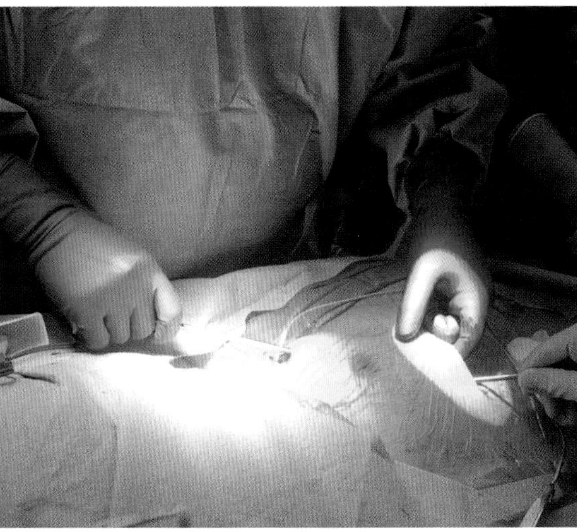

Figure 164.7 Tunnel from sensing lead to IPG pocket.

TECHNIQUE: Hypoglossal Nerve Stimulator Placement—*cont'd*

STEP 8: Connecting Leads to the IPG

After wiping terminal pins of the sensing and stimulation leads with wet and dry gauze, the sensing lead is placed into the inferior IPG port. The lead should protrude beyond the distal connector block. A wrench is used to tighten. This is followed by verifying terminal pin security with a tug back test. This is repeated for the stimulation lead inserted into the superior port. The engraved side of the IPG faces up during insertion into the pocket. Silk sutures (2-0) are threaded through the anchor holes on the IPG and then anchored to the pectoralis major fascia. This forms a V-shaped sling that prevents the IPG from migration and postoperative discomfort.

STEP 9: Confirmation and Closure

Sensing lead function is verified by introducing the telemetry head over the IPG in a sterile fashion. Sensor waveforms should be noted for at least 30 seconds with rise and fall that correspond to inspiration and expiration. Visually confirm tongue protrusion (forward and to the left) starting with 1.0 V, down to 0.5 V, or further below to identify the functional threshold. Program therapy is then turned off to 0.0 V. Surgical sites are closed in layers and a pressure dressing is placed.

Avoidance and Management of Intraoperative Complications

Given the close proximity of the surgical site to the pleural cavity, postoperative radiographs are required to rule out pneumothorax (anteroposterior films for all three implant sites and lateral views for stimulation lead). An arm sling on the side of IPG pocket is recommended for 1 week to restrict upper extremity range of motion. Pain is usually minimal and rarely do patients need narcotic pain medication.

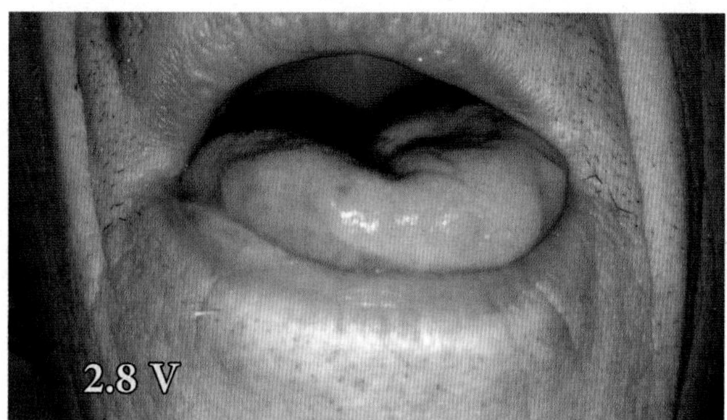

Figure 164.8 Activation and titration in clinic.

Postoperative Considerations

A wound check is performed 7 to 10 days after surgery. The implant is typically activated 1 month after surgery. Patients are then given the remote control to slowly increase the level of stimulation toward the projected therapeutic threshold. A sleep study performed approximately 3 to 6 months after implant placement allows further titration.

Additional adjustments can be performed in-office with the assistance of nasopharyngoscopy (Fig. 164.8). This allows visualization of airway activation. The same thing can be performed during DISE for complex cases. Patient complaints of discomfort with electrical stimulation can be diminished significantly after adjustment.[17] Follow-up includes recommended visits every 6 months to a year to ensure that the therapy addresses patient needs.

Adverse events can be separated into surgical or device-related complications. Surgical adverse events include pneumothorax, infection, prolonged tongue weakness, or inclusion of lateral hypoglossal nerve branches. Device-related adverse events include discomfort from the electrical stimulation, malfunction of the device, or dislodgement of leads. The majority of minor postoperative complications resolve by 1 year, according to the STAR trial.[10]

References

1. Soose RJ, Gillespie MB. Upper airway stimulation therapy: a novel approach to managing obstructive sleep apnea. *Laryngoscope.* 2016;126(suppl 7):S5–S8.
2. Salman LA, Shulman R, Cohen JB. Obstructive sleep apnea, hypertension, and cardiovascular risk: epidemiology, pathophysiology, and management. *Curr Cardiol Rep.* 2020;22(2):6.
3. Liu SY, Wayne Riley R, Pogrel A, Guilleminault C. Sleep surgery in the era of precision medicine. *Atlas Oral Maxillofac Surg Clin North Am.* 2019;27(1):1–5.
4. Liu SY, Awad M, Riley R, Capasso R. The role of the revised Stanford protocol in today's precision medicine. *Sleep Med Clin.* 2019;14(1):99–107.
5. Schwartz AR, et al. Electrical stimulation of the lingual musculature in obstructive sleep apnea. *J Appl Physiol.* 1996;81(2):643–652.
6. Schwartz AR, Bennett ML, Smith PL, et al. Therapeutic electrical stimulation of the hypoglossal nerve in obstructive sleep apnea. *Arch Otolaryngol Head Neck Surg.* 2001;127(10):1216–1223.

7. Caples SM, Rowley JA, Prinsell JR, et al. Surgical modifications of the upper airway for obstructive sleep apnea in adults: a systematic review and meta-analysis. *Sleep*. 2010;33(10):1396–1407.
8. Sawyer AM, Gooneratne NS, Marcus CL, Ofer D, Richards KC, Weaver TE. A systematic review of CPAP adherence across age groups: clinical and empiric insights for developing CPAP adherence interventions. *Sleep Med Rev*. 2011;15(6):343–356.
9. Gupta RJ, Kademani D, Liu SY. Upper airway (hypoglossal nerve) stimulation for treatment of obstructive sleep apnea. *Atlas Oral Maxillofac Surg Clin North Am*. 2019;27(1):53–58.
10. Strollo Jr PJ, Gillespie MB, Soose RJ, et al. Stimulation Therapy for Apnea Reduction (STAR) trial group. Upper airway stimulation for obstructive sleep apnea: durability of the treatment effect at 18 months. *Sleep*. 2015;38(10):1593–1598.
11. Mahmoud AF, Thaler ER. Outcomes of hypoglossal nerve upper airway stimulation among patients with isolated retropalatal collapse. *Otolaryngol Head Neck Surg*. 2019;160(6):1124–1129.
12. Riley RW, Powell N, Guilleminault C. Current surgical concepts for treating obstructive sleep apnea syndrome. *J Oral Maxillofac Surg*. 1987;45(2):149–157.
13. Liu SY, Awad M, Riley RW. Maxillomandibular advancement: contemporary approach at Stanford. *Atlas Oral Maxillofac Surg Clin North Am*. 2019;27(1):29–36.
14. Liu SY, Huon LK, Iwasaki T, et al. Efficacy of maxillomandibular advancement examined with drug-induced sleep endoscopy and computational fluid dynamics airflow modeling. *Otolaryngol Head Neck Surg*. 2016;154(1):189–195.
15. Liu SY, Huon LK, Powell NB, et al. Lateral pharyngeal wall tension after maxillomandibular advancement for obstructive sleep apnea is a marker for surgical success: observations from drug-induced sleep endoscopy. *J Oral Maxillofac Surg*. 2015;73(8):1575–1582.
16. Yu MS, Ibrahim B, Riley RW, Liu SY. Maxillomandibular advancement and upper airway stimulation: extrapharyngeal surgery for obstructive sleep apnea. *Clin Exp Otorhinolaryngol*. 2020;13(3):225–233.
17. Hong SO, Poomkonsarn S, Millesi G, Liu SYC. Upper airway stimulation as an alternative to maxillomandibular advancement for obstructive sleep apnoea in a patient with dentofacial deformity: case report with literature review. *Int J Oral Maxillofac Implants*. 2020;49(7):908–913.
18. Hong SO, Chen YF, Jung J, Kwon YD, Liu SYC. Hypoglossal nerve stimulation for treatment of obstructive sleep apnea (OSA): a primer for oral and maxillofacial surgeons. *Maxillofac Plast Reconstr Surg*. 2017;39(1):27.
19. Oliven A, et al. Effect of coactivation of tongue protrusor and retractor muscles on pharyngeal lumen and airflow in sleep apnea patients. *J Appl Physiol*. 2007;103(5):1662–1668.
20. Liu SY, Riley RW. Continuing the original Stanford sleep surgery protocol from upper airway reconstruction to upper airway stimulation: our first successful case. *J Oral Maxillofac Surg*. 2017;75(7):1514–1518.
21. Liu SY, Hutz MJ, Poomkonsarn S, Chang CP, Awad M, Capasso R. Palatopharyngoplasty resolves concentric collapse in patients ineligible for upper airway stimulation. *Laryngoscope*. 2020;130(12):E958–E962.

CHAPTER 165

Functional Nasal Surgery

Hwi Sean Moon and Neeraj Panchal

Armamentarium

#8 Frazier tip suction
#15 Blade
0-degree or 30-degree endoscope and camera
2-mm osteotome
Adson-Brown tissue forceps
Adson dressing forceps
Afrin-soaked pledgets
Aufricht nasal retractor
Ballenger (right-angle) swivel knife
Blakesley forceps
Boise elevator
Bovie monopolar or bipolar electrocautery
Cartilage grid
Cottle elevator
Cottle mallet
Curved hemostat
Double ball retractor
Freer elevator or suction Freer elevator
Gorney turbinate scissors
Jansen-Middleton forceps
Joseph scissors
Local anesthetic with vasoconstrictor
Microdebrider with small shaver blade
Nasal speculum
Suture materials
Suture scissors

History of the Procedure

The first illustration of nasal surgery dates back to 3500 BC by the Egyptians in a document later known as the *Edwin Smith Surgical Papyrus*. Since its beginning, nasal reconstructive surgery has predominantly involved the manipulation of external bone and the use of external incisions to reshape the nose.[1] It was not until 1887 that John Orlando Roe demonstrated the first closed rhinoplasty using the endonasal approach to correct a nasal tip deformity.[2]

In the early 1900s, Freer and Killian described the submucous resection septoplasty, which became the foundation of modern septoplasty techniques. This endonasal approach involves raising mucoperichondrial flaps and resecting the cartilaginous and bony septum while preserving the L-strut, 1-cm dorsal and caudal margins, to maintain nasal support.[3,4] In 1947, Cottle described the endonasal hemitransfixion incision and advocated for a conservative approach to the nasal septum in order to avoid septal perforations and columellar retraction that are seen with significant cartilage resection.[5] Although Šercer introduced the open transcolumellar rhinoplasty for greater surgical access beyond the nasal septum, the endonasal approach remained to be the mainstay of nasal surgery until the 1970s. It was not until Padovan, Goodman, and Gunter in the 1970s to 90s that the open rhinoplasty regained popularity, especially for cases that require grafting.[6] The spreader graft was described by Sheen in 1984 and remains as the workhorse for augmenting the internal nasal valves.[7] In 1991, Lanza and Stammberger described the first endoscopic nasal surgery.[8]

The history of turbinate surgery deserves a separate mention. Turbinate surgery dates to the last decade of the 19th century. Total turbinectomy, the complete resection of the inferior turbinate, was first described by Hartmann in the 1890s and became one of the most practiced nasal surgery until the early 20th century. However, for decades the procedure was controversial due to its numerous complications including bleeding, atrophic rhinitis, synechiae, and empty nose syndrome. This led to the development of other techniques such as outfracturing the turbinate bone by Killian in 1904, submucosal resection in 1906, and crushing and trimming in the early 1930s, all of which aimed to be less invasive than the total turbinectomy. Turbinate reduction was again recommended beginning in the 1980s owing to newer techniques such as radiofrequency ablation, cryotherapy, and laser reduction.[9,10]

Indications for the Use of the Procedure

The nasal complex serves to warm, humidify, and filter inspired air and is an important structure accounting for 50% of the total upper airway resistance.[11] Nasal obstruction is best described as inadequate airflow between the external nose and nasopharynx due to mechanical impediment within the nasal complex. It is one of the most common outpatient problems and is a common feature in obstructive sleep apnea (OSA).[12] Symptoms of nasal obstruction include difficulty breathing through one or both sides of the nose, mouth breathing, congestion, increased daytime fatigue, snoring, and poor sleep quality, which are independent of OSA.[13] Severity of sleep apnea is assessed by the apnea-hypopnea index (AHI). Nasal obstruction exacerbates symptoms of OSA as evidenced by increased respiratory disturbance index (RDI) and duration of snoring in patients with mild but not moderate to severe OSA.[14]

Nasal obstruction can be broadly categorized into occurring due to anatomic and physiologic causes. Nasal obstruction in most patients with OSA is of anatomic cause that can occur in one or multiple areas of the nasal complex: nasal turbinates, nasal septum, and internal and external nasal valves. One study showed that 85% of OSA patients had turbinate hypertrophy, septal deviation, or nasal valve collapse.[15] In contrast, patients without OSA had a much lower prevalence of anatomic nasal obstruction.[16] Identifying the level of obstruction is best performed using a combination of external examination with a modified Cottle test, anterior rhinoscopy, and nasal endoscopy. External examination provides an assessment of septal deviation and nasal valve compromise. Anterior rhinoscopy or nasal endoscopy can reveal septal deformity and turbinate hypertrophy. Computed tomography scan is not routinely ordered but can serve as a useful adjunct, especially when the etiology of obstruction is not obvious such as in patients with previous nasal surgery or trauma.

There are no standardized means of grading the severity of nasal obstruction. Many surgeons use patient-reported symptoms and clinical findings to achieve diagnosis and determine indications for treatment. Others have advocated the use of the Nasal Obstruction Symptom Evaluation (NOSE) scale. Although not inclusive, the following exam findings have been implicated in anatomic nasal obstruction:

- External nasal dorsum deviation or asymmetric nostrils suggest an underlying septal deviation.
- Patients with prominent nasion to subnasale length but short nasal bones are often predisposed to internal valve collapse.
- During inspiration, deviations at the lateral nasal wall or the nostril suggests dynamic collapse at the internal or external nasal valve, respectively.
- Positive modified Cottle maneuver at the lateral surface of the upper lateral cartilage or the lateral crus of the lower lateral cartilage indicates whether the obstruction is due to internal or external nasal valve competency, respectively.
- The inferior turbinate is generally not in contact with the nasal septum.
- Deviation of the septum can result in compensatory contralateral inferior turbinate hypertrophy.

Functional nasal surgery includes turbinate reduction, septoplasty, and rhinoplasty, which are often combined depending on the areas of obstruction. There are many techniques involving turbinate reduction. While many argue that the submucosal inferior turbinate reduction may be the most effective turbinate surgery, the overarching goal of inferior turbinate surgery is to improve nasal airway while preserving turbinate function.[17] Meanwhile, endonasal septoplasty is typically the preferred approach to treat septal deviations. However, dorsal septal deviations and concomitant correction of internal and/or external nasal valves with grafting usually necessitate the open septorhinoplasty approach for better access and visibility. The overall purpose of functional nasal surgery is to improve nasal breathing by alleviating areas of obstructions while preserving structural integrity.

The first-line treatment of OSA is continuous positive airway pressure (CPAP); however, many patients are nonadherent due to discomfort from the air pressure, nasal congestion, and psychological and social factors.[18] Functional nasal surgery has shown improvement in tolerance of CPAP after nasal surgery, increased duration of CPAP use, and reduced CPAP therapeutic pressure.[19]

Functional nasal surgery can be combined with palate and/or tongue surgery (e.g., uvulopalatopharyngoplasty and genioglossus advancement) as multilevel surgery for OSA patients. One multicenter study showed significant improvement in the Epworth sleepiness scale (ESS) and AHI in patients who underwent nasal surgery as part of the multilevel surgery compared to those without nasal surgery.[20]

Limitations and Contraindications

Limitations

While nasal obstruction plays a role in the pathogenesis of OSA, functional nasal surgery has not been proven significantly effective as a single modality treatment for OSA. A 50% reduction in AHI and a final AHI of 20 per hour or less is defined as a surgical cure. Nasal surgery improves subjective nasal breathing and ESS, but no significant improvement in AHI.[21] Further controlled studies are needed to confirm the direct benefits of functional nasal surgery for patients with OSA.

Physiologic causes of nasal obstruction include inflammatory (e.g., allergic rhinitis), medication-induced (e.g., oxymetazoline), and infectious (e.g., viral), which all manifest as swelling and hypertrophy of the nasal mucosa. There is no test that correlates specifically to the underlying cause of nasal obstruction. Diagnosis of physiologic nasal obstruction can be challenging and requires a thorough consideration of the patient's history, medication or drug use, and other risk factors. Unlike anatomic nasal obstruction that may require surgery, physiologic nasal obstruction requires treatment of the underlying etiology, often including allergy evaluation, saline irrigations, and intranasal or systemic steroid and/or antihistamine. Functional nasal surgery can be offered to patients with allergic rhinitis with persistent obstructive symptoms refractory to medical management.[22]

Contraindications

A contraindication to functional nasal surgery includes poor surgical candidates due to comorbid medical conditions, tobacco or cocaine dependence, body dysmorphic disorder, and those uncertain about surgery. Such patients may benefit from externally applied breathing strips that temporarily splint the nasal valves open.

TECHNIQUE 1: Submucosal Inferior Turbinate Reduction

Submucosal inferior turbinate reduction can be performed under direct visualization or with a nasal endoscopy. When combined with septoplasty or rhinoplasty, turbinate reduction is best performed prior to septorhinoplasty, which otherwise could damage the operated nasal septum during retraction.

STEP 1: General Anesthesia and Preparation of Nose

Submucosal inferior turbinate reduction is typically performed under general anesthesia with the placement of an oral endotracheal tube. The patient is positioned supine in a 15-degree reverse Trendelenburg position to minimize bleeding. The patient is prepped and draped in a normal sterile fashion. 1% lidocaine with 1:100,000 epinephrine is injected along the inferior turbinates and lateral nasal walls for vasoconstriction and hydrodissection in the anteroposterior direction. Oxymetazoline-impregnated cotton pledgets are applied into both nasal passages for added vasoconstriction. Incision is made only after appropriate time has elapsed for adequate vasoconstriction.

STEP 2: Incision and Elevation of Flap

Although the surgery can be performed using a headlight and nasal speculum, endoscopes can offer better visualization. A #15 blade on a long handle is used to make the incision through the periosteum at the anterior head of the inferior turbinate (Fig. 165.1A). Submucoperiosteal planes are identified, and with the aid of a suction Freer elevator for visualization, a flap is raised until the inferior turbinate bone is identified. Once the bony is sounded, the submucosa is circumferentially raised off the bone (Fig. 165.1B).

STEP 3: Removal of Bone and Submucosa

Blakesley forceps are used to remove the inferior turbinate bone partially or completely (Fig. 165.1C). Submucosal soft tissue reduction is performed using a microdebrider shaver blade, initially facing the lateral nasal wall to trim the lateral submucosal tissue. The blade is then rotated 180 degrees to thin the medial submucosal tissue with care not to perforate through the inferior turbinate mucosa (Fig. 165.1D). The anterior aspect of the inferior turbinate must be reduced to alleviate obstruction near the internal nasal valve. The microdebrider is angled parallel to the floor of the nose to avoid inadvertent perforation of the turbinate mucosa.

STEP 4: Lateral Displacement of Inferior Turbinate Bone

If the residual inferior turbinate bone extends medially into the nasal cavity, lateral displacement or outfracturing of the inferior turbinate bone is often performed. This is achieved using a Boise or Freer elevator by applying lateral pressure against the remaining inferior turbinate bone until the bone fractures. Bleeding is controlled with a cotton pledget soaked in topical decongestant. Sutured closure is often not necessary.

ALTERNATIVE TECHNIQUE: Partial Turbinectomy

The anterior head of the inferior turbinate is considered to contribute most to nasal obstruction symptoms. In partial turbinectomy, only the anterior head is resected while preserving the remainder of the turbinate for air humidification. A curved hemostat is used to clamp and create a crush line along the anterior 1 to 2 cm of the inferior turbinate. Then Gorney turbinate scissors are used to remove turbinate tissue just anterior to the hemostat. Once resected, the hemostat is removed, and any bleeding area is carefully cauterized using electrocautery until hemostasis is achieved.

TECHNIQUE 2: Endonasal Septoplasty

Endonasal septoplasty is the preferred approach for conservative resection and preservation of septal cartilage and bone.

STEP 1: General Anesthesia and Preparation of Nose

Endonasal septoplasty is typically performed under general anesthesia with the placement of an oral endotracheal tube. The patient is positioned supine in a 15-degree reverse Trendelenburg position to minimize bleeding and improve visualization of the nasal septum. The patient is prepped and draped in a normal sterile fashion. 1% lidocaine with 1:100,000 epinephrine is injected along the septum bilaterally underneath the mucoperichondrial layer for va-

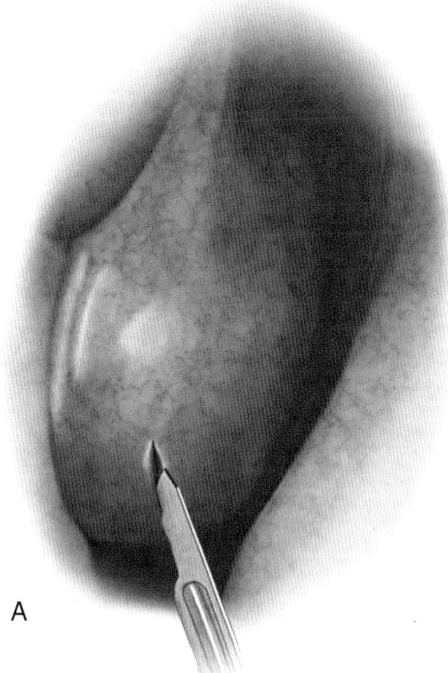
A
Incision through periosteum at anterior head of
the inferior turbinate

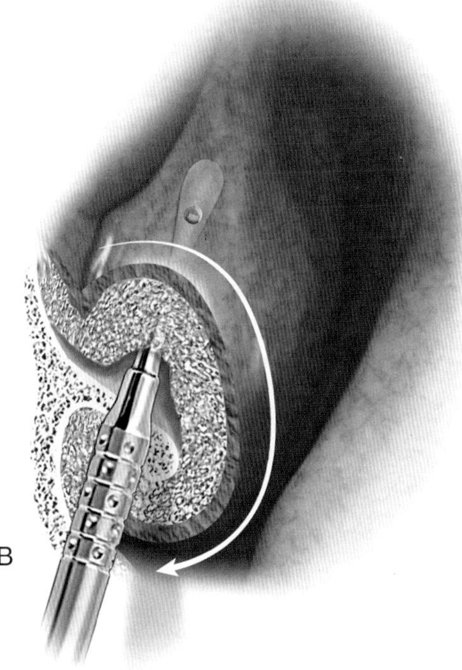
B
Submucosa is circumferentially raised
off the bone

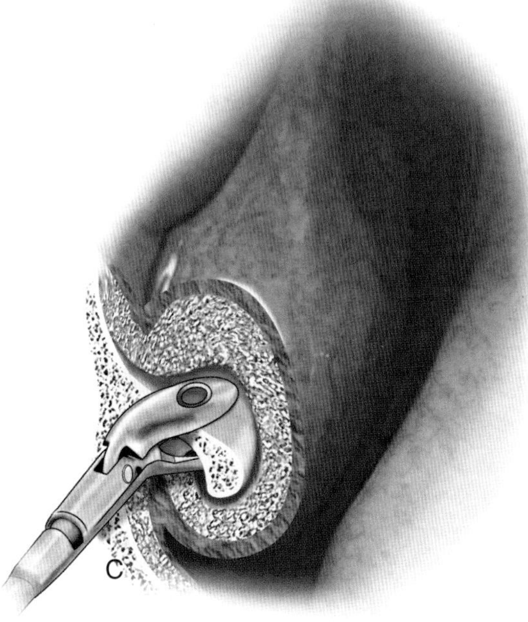
C
Inferior turbinate bone removed partially
or completely with Blakesley forceps

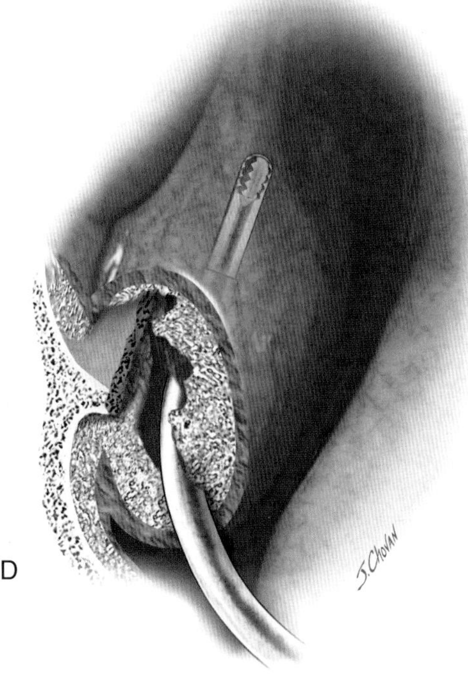
D
Submucosal soft tissue reduction
with microdebrider shaver blade

Figure 165.1 Submucosal Inferior Turbinate Reduction. A. Incision through periosteum at anterior head of the inferior turbinate. B. Submucosa is circumferentially raised off the bone. C. Inferior turbinate bone removed partially or completely with Blakesley forceps. D. Submucosal soft tissue reduction with microdebrider shaver blade.

Continued

TECHNIQUE 2: Endonasal Septoplasty—*cont'd*

soconstriction and hydrodissection in the anteroposterior direction. Oxymetazoline-impregnated cotton pledgets are applied into both nasal passages for added vasoconstriction. Incision is made only after appropriate time has elapsed for adequate vasoconstriction.

STEP 2: Incision

The endonasal approach to the nasal septum includes the hemitransfixion incision over the membranous septum or the Killian incision over the cartilaginous septum (Fig. 165.2). Incision choice depends on the location of the septal deviation and is surgeon dependent. Incision is typically made on the side with the most prominent deflection.

The incision outline is created by retracting the columella with a nasal speculum toward the contralateral nare to expose the caudal septal margin and create tension before making the incision. A #15 blade is used to make a hemitransfixion incision through mucosa and perichondrium to expose the cartilage, which has a white and rough appearance. The incision is often extended to the nasal floor for larger or caudal septal deviations.

A Kilian incision can be used if access to the caudal septum is not necessary or if the septal deviation is within the posterior third of the nasal cavity. Incision is typically made 1 to 2 cm superoposterior to the caudal septum along the cartilaginous septum and anterior to the deviation.

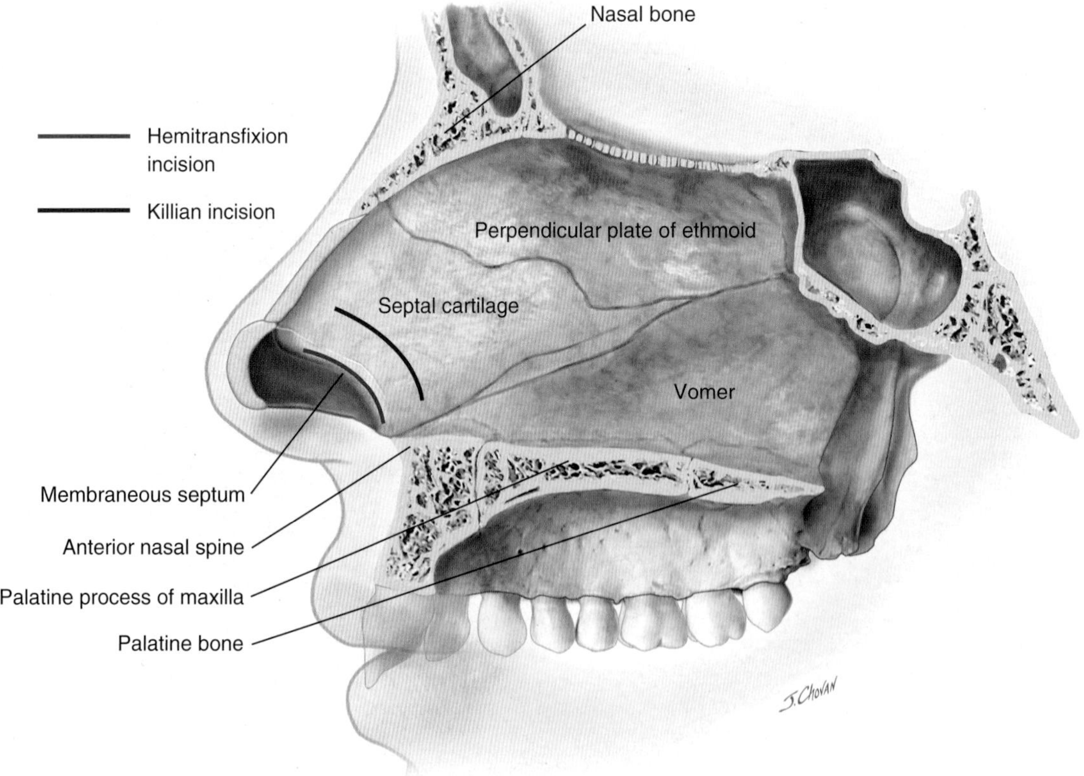

Figure 165.2 Endonasal approaches to the nasal septum.

TECHNIQUE 2: Endonasal Septoplasty—*cont'd*

STEP 3: Elevation of Flap

After incision is made, a full-thickness mucoperichondrial flap is raised, starting with the sharp end of a Cottle elevator. Once in the subperichondrial plane, elevation of the flap is performed with the dull end of a Cottle or Freer elevator. Care must be taken to elevate the flap atraumatically, ensuring that the elevator is always in contact with the septum (Fig. 165.3). Dissection is extended inferiorly toward the floor of the nose, allowing reflection of the periosteum off the nasal crest of the maxilla. Dissection is also extended posteriorly to the vomer-cartilage junction to access any bony deflection.

During elevation, care must be taken when encountering septal deviations or spurs, which can be tightly adherent to the thinned overlying mucosa. To reduce tension and inadvertent tears, flap elevation can be approached superiorly and inferiorly to the septal spur and then connecting the two pockets to release any adhesions.

Next, attention is turned toward the opposite side of the septum. Incision and flap elevation is performed in a similar fashion. If grafting is not planned, a more conservative flap elevation can be performed using a transcartilaginous incision. This incision is typically made 2 mm anterior and inferior to the most caudal aspect of the deviation.

STEP 4: Removal of Obstruction

Once both flaps are raised, the deviated portion of the cartilage is excised using a right-angle swivel knife (Fig. 165.4). Incision starts at the dorsal-most margin of the planned excision and is carried superoposteriorly until bone is sounded. The knife is then carried inferoposteriorly to the maxillary crest and then carried anteriorly paralleling to the superior cut. The deviated cartilage must be removed conservatively with preservation of at least 1 cm at the dorsal and caudal septum (also known as L-strut) to prevent loss of tip support and saddling of the nose (Fig. 165.5). Some surgeons advocate preserving 1.5 cm of L-strut. The cartilage is excised in one piece especially if the cartilage will be used for grafting.

Bilateral subperiosteal dissection is carried superiorly and posterior to identify any bony deviation, which can be removed with Jansen-Middleton forceps. When encroaching onto the perpendicular plate of the ethmoid bone, care must be taken to prevent damage to the cribriform plate, which can result in cerebrospinal fluid (CSF) leak.

Any unused portion of the septum can be placed back within the mucoperichondrial flaps.

STEP 5: Closure and Splints

The surgical site is irrigated and the mucoperichondrial flaps are allowed to redrape and brought to the midline. The hemitransfixion and transcartilaginous incisions are closed using 4-0 plain gut suture with multiple interrupted sutures. A quilting 4-0 mattress suture is passed back and forth from one side of the septum to the other side to approximate the mucoperichondrial flaps together. This is to reduce the dead space between the flaps and prevent septal hematoma formation.

Bacitracin-immersed Doyle splints are placed within the nasal passages to prevent septal hematoma formation.

Continued

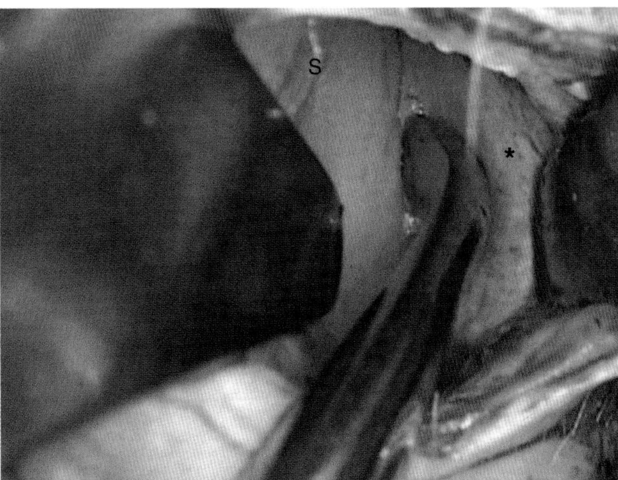

Figure 165.3 Subperichondrial dissection using a Cottle elevator. S: Nasal septum * Full-thickness mucoperichondrial flap. (Reprinted from Myers EN. *Operative Otolaryngology: Head and Neck Surgery*. 3rd ed. Elsevier; 2017:633.)

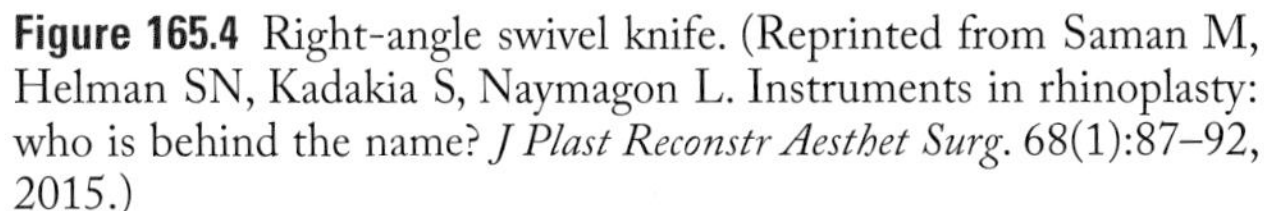

Figure 165.4 Right-angle swivel knife. (Reprinted from Saman M, Helman SN, Kadakia S, Naymagon L. Instruments in rhinoplasty: who is behind the name? *J Plast Reconstr Aesthet Surg*. 68(1):87–92, 2015.)

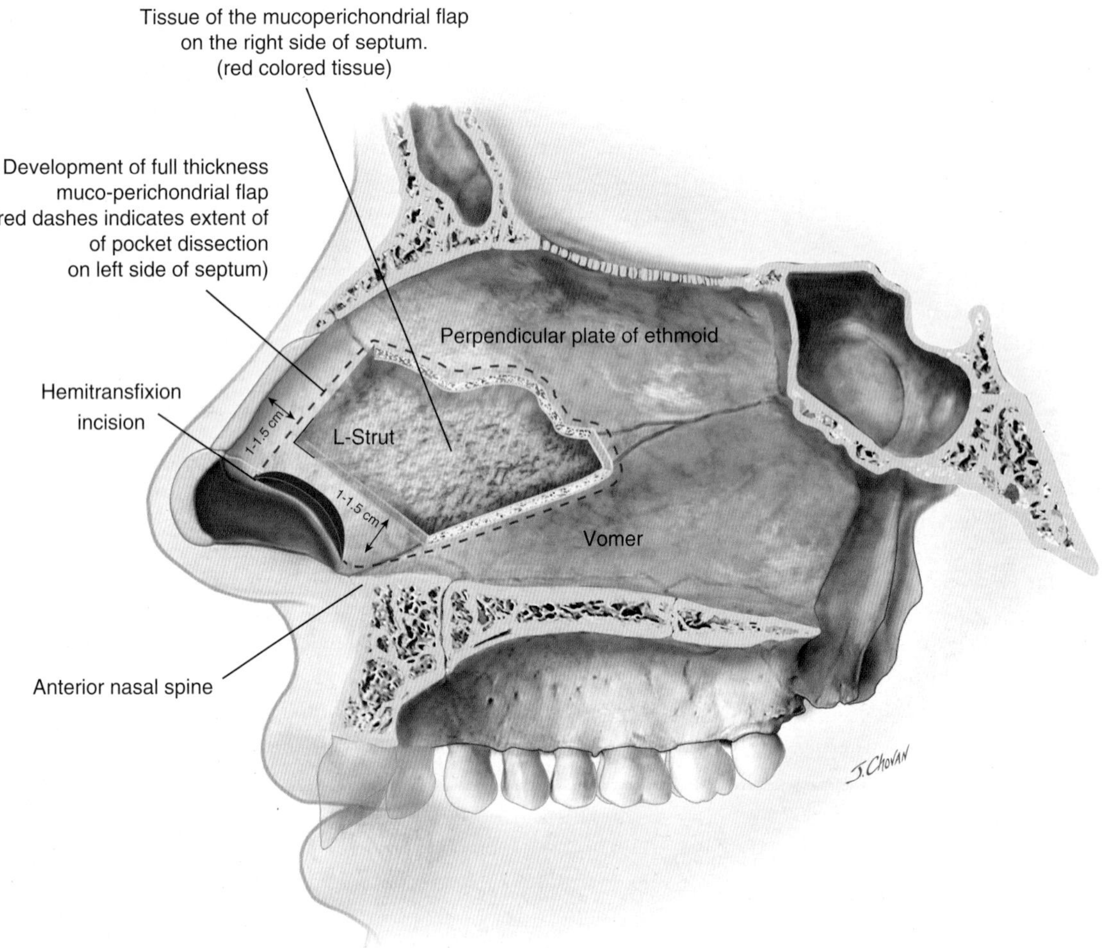

Figure 165.5 Removal of deviated cartilage with preservation of 1-1.5 cm of dorsal and caudal septum (L-strut).

TECHNIQUE 3: Open Septorhinoplasty

The open approach allows superior visibility with a simultaneous approach to the caudal and dorsal septum as well as access to the internal and external valves. The goal of this technique is to relieve nasal obstruction by correcting septal deviation and expanding the nasal valves.

STEP 1: General Anesthesia and Preparation of Nose

Surgery is performed under general anesthesia with the placement of an oral endotracheal tube. The patient is positioned supine in a 15-degree reverse Trendelenburg position to minimize bleeding. The patient is prepped and draped in a normal sterile fashion. A local anesthetic with a vasoconstrictor (usually 1% lidocaine with 1:100,000 epinephrine) is injected depending on the surgical approach and grafting required, in which local anesthetic is injected into the septum, caudal edge of the lateral crus, columellae, dome, and lateral nasal walls. Oxymetazoline-impregnated cotton pledgets are applied into both nasal passages for added vasoconstriction. Incision is made only after appropriate time has elapsed for adequate vasoconstriction.

STEP 2: Incision

The incision outline is created using double ball retractors to create tension before making the incision. A marginal alar incision is made using a #15 blade along the inferior aspect of the lower lateral cartilage (infracartilaginous). The vertical incision along the medial columellar side wall is placed approximately 5 mm

TECHNIQUE 3: Open Septorhinoplasty—*cont'd*

posterior to the cutaneous edge of the columellar skin. A similar marginal incision is made along the opposing nasal passage before the incision is extended toward the columellar, where an inverted-V transcolumellar incision is made halfway between the nasal lobule and subnasale (Fig. 165.6). This area also corresponds to the narrowest portion of the columellae.

STEP 3: Elevation of Skin-Muscle Flap

The nose, in the form of a skin-muscle flap, is degloved superiorly starting at the columellar incision in a subperichondrial plane for direct visualization of the lower and upper lateral cartilages. Elevation of the skin-muscle flap is extended superiorly until the nasal bones are seen where the dissection becomes subperiosteal. An Aufricht nasal retractor can be used for superior retraction of the skin-muscle flap while double-prong skin hooks can be used to retract the cartilage dome inferiorly (Fig. 165.7).

STEP 4: Exposure of Septum

The upper lateral cartilages are freed from their attachments to the dorsal nasal septum and the medial crura of the lower lateral cartilages are separated by severing the transdomal ligaments using a #15 blade. Once the septum is exposed, mucoperichondrial flaps are raised bilaterally starting from the cephalad surface with care to avoid inadvertent tears. A separate transfixion or Killian incision is not necessary with the open approach. The nasal mucoperichondrial flap can be raised as described in the septoplasty section above. Elevation of the mucoperichondrial flap continues superiorly toward the ethmoid, posteriorly toward the vomer bone, and inferiorly toward the maxillary crest, all of which proceed subperiosteally.

Continued

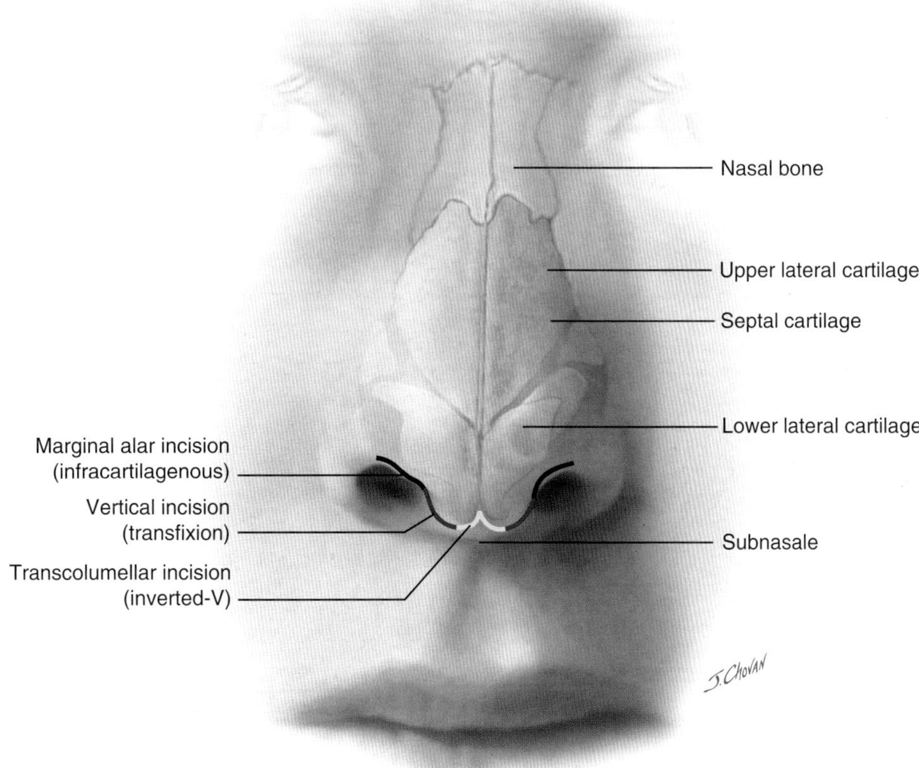

Figure 165.6 Incision design for the open approach.

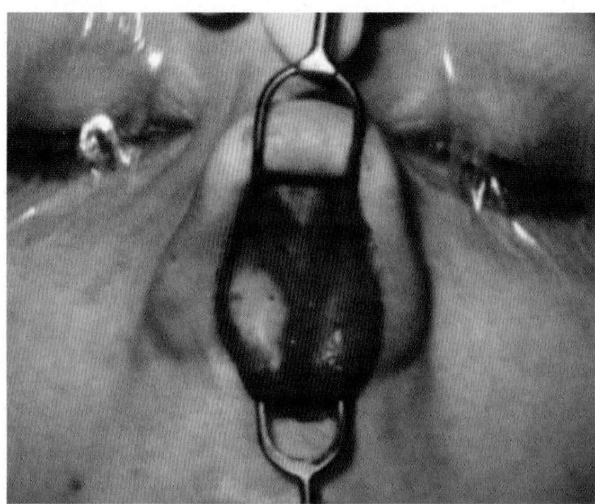

Figure 165.7 Exposure of the lower and upper lateral cartilages. (Reprinted from Myers EN. *Operative Otolaryngology: Head and Neck Surgery*. 3rd ed. Elsevier; 2017.)

TECHNIQUE 3: Open Septorhinoplasty—*cont'd*

STEP 5: Harvest of the Septal Cartilage

Once both flaps are raised, the septal cartilage is harvested with preservation of at least 1 cm at the dorsal and caudal septum to prevent loss of tip support and saddling of the nose. With a right-angle swivel knife, incision starts at the dorsal-most margin of the planned excision and is carried posteriorly until bone is sounded. The knife is then carried inferiorly to the maxillary crest and then carried anteriorly paralleling to the superior cut. The deviated portion of the septal cartilage is removed during the harvest. It is important that enough septal cartilage is available for grafting. The cartilage is excised in one piece and stored in a saline bath for grafting.

If additional grafts are required, auricular cartilage can be harvested.

STEP 6: Removal of Bony Obstruction

If any bony deviation is present, it can be removed conservatively with Jansen-Middleton forceps. A septal osteotomy on the ethmoid can be made with a 2-mm osteotome to prevent the fracturing of the cribriform plate.

Following septoplasty, the surgical site is irrigated and the mucoperichondrial flaps are allowed to redrape and brought to the midline. A quilting 4-0 mattress suture is passed back and forth from one side of the septum to the other side to approximate the mucoperichondrial flaps together. This reduces the dead space between the flaps and thereby the risk of septal hematoma formation.

STEP 7: Spreader Grafts

The harvested septum is typically sectioned for use as spreader grafts, columellar strut graft, and/or alar batten grafts.

Spreader grafts are placed submucosally along the internal nasal valves between the dorsal septum and upper lateral cartilages. This allows lateral displacement of the upper lateral cartilages and opening of the internal nasal valves. The size of each spreader graft typically measures between 20 and 25 mm in length and 5 and 7 mm in height. The width of the graft depends on the width of the harvested septum but is typically 1 to 3 mm. The grafts extend from the bone-cartilage junction to the anterior septal angle. They are often beveled at the ends to maximize the nasal airway and sutured with 4-0 polydioxanone (PDS) suture as horizontal mattresses. The needle must be of adequate size to engage all structures in a single pass. Care must be taken to not cinch down the sutures too tightly and inferiorly, which would buckle the upper lateral cartilages medially. A suspension suture can also be used to correct internal nasal valve narrowing. The upper lateral cartilages are sutured back to the septum using 4-0 or 5-0 PDS (Fig. 165.8).

STEP 8: Columellar Strut Graft

External nasal valve collapse requires reinforcement of the lower lateral cartilages and the alar rim. The columellar strut graft allows concomitant correction of tip projection and external nasal valves. It is typically indicated when the transdomal ligaments are severed during open rhinoplasties. The graft typically measures 20 mm in length and 2.5 mm in width. It is placed between the medial crura and superior to the anterior nasal spine and sutured using 4-0 or 5-0 PDS as a mattress suture (Fig. 165.9).

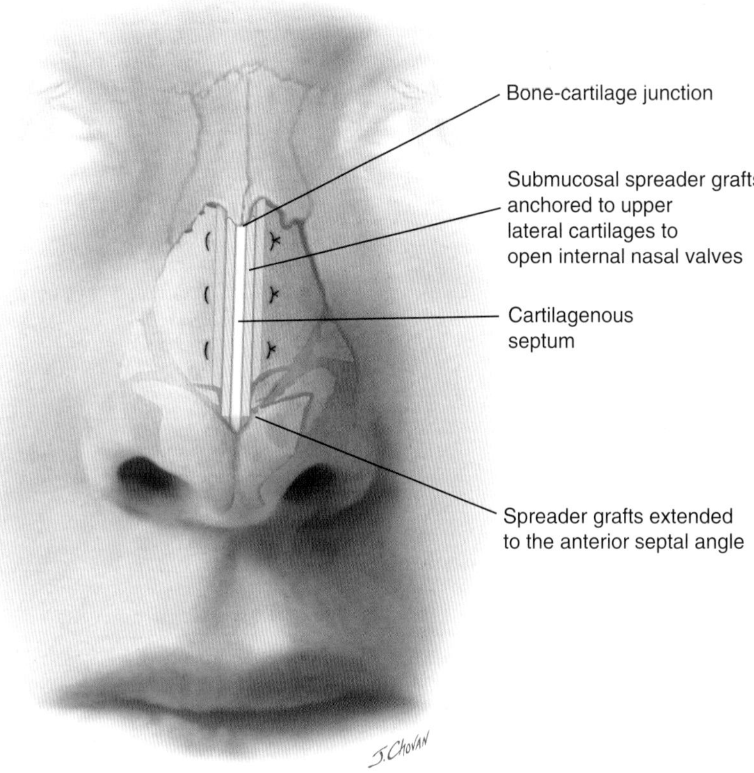

Figure 165.8 Placement of spreader grafts.

TECHNIQUE 3: Open Septorhinoplasty—*cont'd*

STEP 9: Alar Batten Grafts

Alar batten grafts augment the alar rim and provide integrity to the external nasal valves. If adequate lower lateral cartilage structures are observed, repositioning of the lower lateral cartilages to the upper lateral cartilages and septum often opens the external nasal valve. If the lateral crura are weakened, they are reinforced using alar batten grafts. The size of each alar batten graft measures approximately 15 mm in length and the width is typically 4 to 5 mm wider than the existing alar cartilage. These grafts can be placed between nasal mucosa and lower lateral cartilages, anterior to the pyriform aperture and 2 mm superior to the existing alar cartilage, and sutured using 4-0 or 5-0 PDS (Fig. 165.10).

STEP 10: Closure and Splints

The marginal alar incisions are closed using 4-0 or 5-0 plain gut and the columellae with 5-0 or 6-0 prolene with multiple interrupted sutures. Care should be taken not to include the cartilage in the closure to prevent distortion or warping.

Strip tapes are placed over the external nasal skin to reduce postoperative edema. An external nasal splint, usually a Denver or thermoplastic splint, is trimmed, shaped, and then placed over the nose. The internal Doyle splints are placed to prevent septal hematoma and synechia formation.

Continued

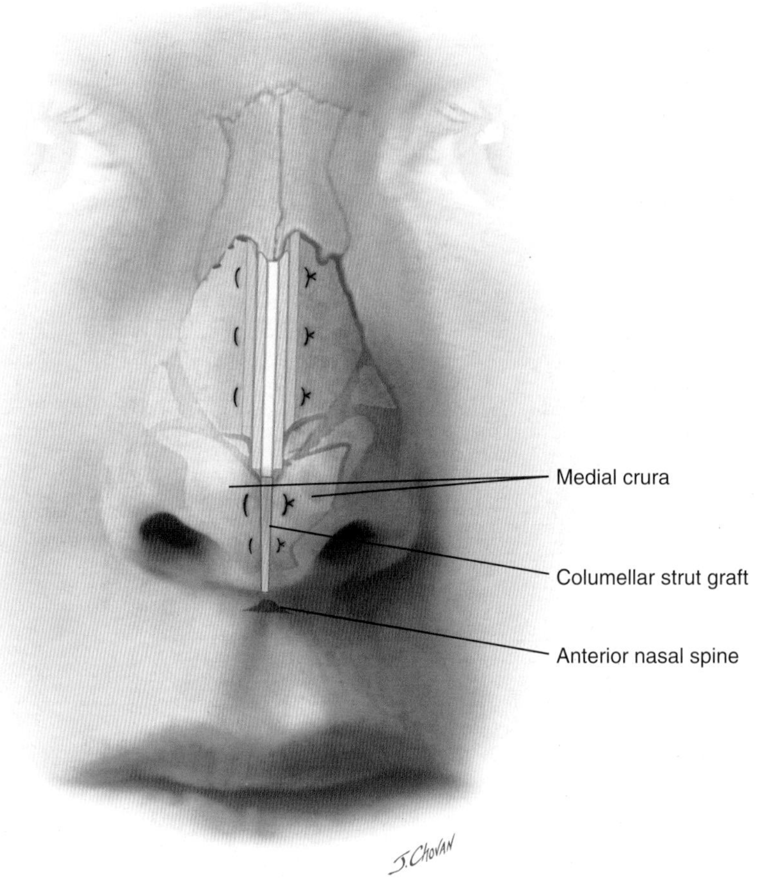

Figure 165.9 Placement of columellar strut graft.

Avoidance and Management of Intraoperative Complications

Bleeding is one of the most common intraoperative complications of nasal surgery and must be promptly recognized and treated. Anterior bleeding from Kiesselbach's plexus is more readily identified and controlled, but posterior bleeding from the posterior ethmoidal and sphenopalatine arteries can be difficult to visualize. Bleeding is often due to inadequate vasoconstriction with local anesthesia or inadvertent mucosal trauma during flap elevation. Adequate use of local anesthesia aids in flap elevation as it hydrodissects the periosteum at the head of the inferior turbinate or mucoperichondrium off the septal cartilage. Injecting topical decongestant with 0.05% oxymetazoline or 4% cocaine prior to making an incision helps reduce bleeding and improves visibility. Nasal packing can aid in hemostasis but requires prompt removal within 48 hours to reduce the risk of toxic shock syndrome. In rare situations, fibrin sealant or arterial embolization may be required.

CSF leakage is an exceedingly rare but serious complication of functional nasal surgery that deserves mention. CSF leak can inadvertently occur during the elevation of the septal mucoperichondrium using a Cottle elevator superiorly beyond the ethmoid roof and subsequently fracturing through the thin cribriform plate. When correcting a high bony septal deviation, a controlled separation of the perpendicular plate using a 2-mm osteotome provides safe separation of the perpendicular plate of the ethmoid bone from the skull base. Early symptoms of CSF leak include positional headaches, rhinorrhea, and metallic postnasal drip. Prompt diagnosis and management is critical to preventing life-threatening complications, including meningitis, brain tissue herniation, or brain abscess. The presence of a halo sign on a pledget is suggestive of a CSF leak and can be confirmed with β-2 transferrin, which takes several days to result. Management of CSF leak includes bed rest, head elevation, sinus precautions, oral diuretics, and meningococcal antibiotic prophylaxis.[23]

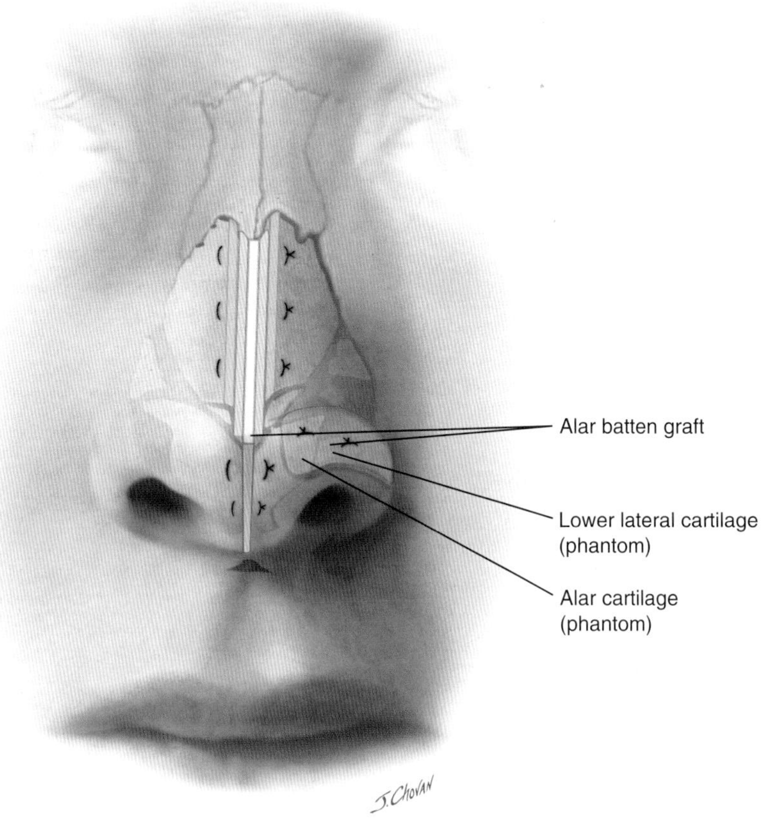

Figure 165.10 Placement of alar batten grafts.

Avoidance and Management of Postoperative Complications

The nasal cavity is colonized with normal bacterial flora, and a breach in the mucous membranes during surgery puts the patient at risk for postoperative infection. Although rare, infection could progress to meningitis, brain abscess, or cavernous sinus thrombosis, all of which are fatal.[24] *Staphylococcus aureus* plays a major role in pathogenesis, and therefore antistaphylococcal antibiotic prophylaxis is recommended postoperatively. The use of nasal packing greater than 48 hours has been implicated in bacteremia and toxic shock syndrome. Patients with fever, hypotension, peripheral rash, and desquamation should be admitted and treated promptly with aggressive resuscitation, empiric antibiotics, and removal and culture of the nasal packing. While it is impossible to prevent every infection, the potential risk of toxic shock syndrome can be mitigated by avoiding nasal packing unless placed to control bleeding.

Septal hematoma is a significant morbidity of septoplasty that occurs due to unrecognized bleeding between the mucoperichondrial flaps following the removal of septal cartilage or bone. Untreated septal hematoma can result in ischemia and necrosis of the remaining septum leading to subsequent loss of nasal support and saddling of the nose. Septal hematoma can also lead to septal abscess, colonized with *S. aureus*, *Haemophilus influenza*, and *Pseudomonas aeruginosa*.[22] Treatment of septal hematoma involves incision and drainage followed by placement of nasal packing. It can be prevented with the intraoperative placement of quilting suture through the mucoperichondrial flaps in a continuous mattress.

Empty nose syndrome is a rare complication of turbinate surgery. It is a form of atrophic rhinitis in which patients who underwent surgery experience sensation of nasal obstruction, dryness, crusting, and pain without objective exam findings. Diagnosis is controversial and challenging. Treatment is similar to that of atrophic rhinitis by keeping the mucosa moist with saline or cool mist humidifier. It is linked to reduced inferior turbinate volume and increased mucosal damage and therefore likely prevented with conservative reduction of the turbinates without using ablative or thermal techniques.[25]

Poor intraoperative techniques can lead to poor functional and aesthetic outcomes. The keystone area is an area of confluence between the septal cartilage, upper lateral cartilages, nasal bones, and perpendicular plate of the ethmoid bone. Violation of the keystone area leads to downward and inward rotation of the anterior septal cartilage with subsequent widening of the nasal base. Saddle nose deformity occurs as a result of aggressive resection of the caudal septum, which can be reduced by maintaining a 1-cm L-strut. It usually takes up to a year of recovery and maturation of soft tissues prior to considering a revision surgery unless significant nasal deformity is noted.

Postoperative Considerations

Functional nasal surgery is generally an outpatient procedure. Pain control is achieved using acetaminophen or low-potency opioid. Nonsteroidal antiinflammatory drugs can be initiated starting on postoperative day 7 once hemostatic. Ice compresses are applied for the first two days, the head is elevated 30 degrees at night, and steroids are prescribed, all to help reduce postoperative swelling. Postoperative antibiotics are prescribed for 7 to 10 days, especially when nasal stents or packings are placed. Saline rinses are recommended to reduce congestion and remove dried blood from the nasal cavity. Afrin can be used to control intermittent nasal bleeds but should not be prescribed for more than 3 days. Vigorous exercise should be avoided for at least 2 weeks. Sinus precautions are recommended for 2 to 3 weeks to prevent barometric pressure changes. Patients are seen within a week after surgery for the removal of splints and sutures.

References

1. Meltzer ES, Sanchez GM. *The Edwin Smith Papyrus: Updated Translation of the Trauma Treatise and Modern Medical Commentaries.* ISD LLC; 2014.
2. Lam SM. John Orlando Roe: father of aesthetic rhinoplasty. *Arch Facial Plast Surg.* 2002;4(2):122–123.
3. Freer OT. The correction of deflection of the nasal septum with minimal traumatism. *JAMA.* 1902;38(10):636–642.
4. Killian G. The submucous window resection of the nasal septum. *Ann Otol Rhinol Laryngol.* 1905;14(2):363–393.
5. Cottle MH, Loring RM. Newer concepts of septum surgery: present status. *Eye Ear Nose Throat Mon.* 1948;27:403.
6. Gunter JP. The merits of the open approach in rhinoplasty. *Plast Reconstr Surg.* 1997;99(3):863–867.
7. Sheen J. Spreader graft: a method of reconstructing the roof of the middle nasal vault following rhinoplasty. *Plast Reconstr Surg.* 1984;73(2):230–239.
8. Stammberger H, Posawetz W. Functional endoscopic sinus surgery. *Eur Arch Oto-Rhino-Laryngol.* 1990;247(2):63–76.
9. Nurse LA, Duncavage JA. Surgery of the inferior and middle turbinates. *Otolaryngol Clin North Am.* 2009;42(2):295–309.
10. Hol MK, Huizing EH. Treatment of inferior turbinate pathology: a review and critical evaluation of the different techniques. *Rhinology.* 2000;38(4):157–166.
11. Ferris BG, Mead J, Opie LH. Partitioning of respiratory flow resistance in man. *J Appl Physiol.* 1964;19:653–658.
12. Krakow B, Foley-Shea M, Ulibarri VA, et al. Prevalence of potential nonallergic rhinitis at a community-based sleep medical center. *Sleep Breath.* 2016;20(3):987–993.
13. Young T, Finn L, Kim H. Nasal obstruction as a risk factor for sleep-disordered breathing. The University of Wisconsin Sleep and Respiratory Research Group. *J Allergy Clin Immunol.* 1997;99(2):S757–S762.
14. Friedman M, Maley A, Kelley K, et al. Impact of nasal obstruction on obstructive sleep apnea. *Otolaryngol Head Neck Surg.* 2011;144(6):1000–1004.
15. Zonato AI, Bittencourt LR, Martinho FL, et al. Association of systematic head and neck physical examination with severity of obstructive sleep apnea-hypopnea syndrome. *Laryngoscope.* 2003;113(6):973–980.
16. Zonato AI, Martinho FL, Bittencourt LR, et al. Head and neck physical examination: comparison between nonapneic and obstructive sleep apnea patients. *Laryngoscope.* 2005;115(6):1030–1034.
17. Larrabee YC, Kacker A. Which inferior turbinate reduction technique best decreases nasal obstruction? *Laryngoscope.* 2014;124:814–815.
18. Sawyer AM, Gooneratne NS, Marcus CL, et al. A systematic review of CPAP adherence across age groups: clinical and empiric insights for developing CPAP adherence interventions. *Sleep Med Rev.* 2011;15:343–356.
19. Camacho M, Riaz M, Capasso R, et al. The effect of nasal surgery on continuous positive airway pressure device use and therapeutic treatment pressures: a systematic review and meta-analysis. *Sleep.* 2015;38(2):279–286.
20. Pang KP, Montevecchi F, Vicini C, et al. Does nasal surgery improve multilevel surgical outcome in obstructive sleep apnea: a multicenter study on 735 patients. *Laryngoscope Investig Otolaryngol.* 2020;5(6):1233–1239.
21. Ishii L, Roxbury C, Godoy A, et al. Does nasal surgery improve OSA in patients with nasal obstruction and OSA? A meta-analysis. *Otolaryngol Head Neck Surg.* 2015;153:326–333.
22. Seidman MD, Gurgel RK, Lin SY, et al. Clinical practice guideline: allergic rhinitis. *Otolaryngol Head Neck Surg.* 2015;152:S1–S43.
23. Onerci TM, Ayhan K, Ogretmenoglu O. Two consecutive cases of cerebrospinal fluid rhinorrhea after septoplasty operation. *Am J Otolaryngol.* 2004;25(5):354–356.
24. Schwab JA, Pirsig W. Complications of septal surgery. *Facial Plast Surg.* 1997;13(1):3–14.
25. Kuan EC, Suh JD, Wang MB. Empty nose syndrome. *Curr Allergy Asthma Rep.* 2015;15(1):493.

CHAPTER 166

Mandibular Distraction in Infancy for Airway Obstruction

Jocelyn M. Shand

Armamentarium

#15 Scalpel blades
Allevyn Ag dressing
Appropriate sutures
Cat paw retractors
Distraction kit and screwdriver
Langenbeck retractors
Local anesthetic with vasoconstrictor
Mallet
Mandibular pediatric distraction appliances
Metzenbaum scissors
Mosquito forceps
Needle electrocautery, bipolar
Osteotomes, fine
Pediatric gel horseshoe headrest and shoulder roll
Periosteal elevators
Steri-Strips
Surgairtome with fine bur (101)
Tegaderm dressing
Tenotomy scissors
Vari-Stim nerve stimulator

History of the Procedure

Distraction osteogenesis has become a useful technique in the armamentarium for the correction of skeletal anomalies. In 1992, McCarthy and colleagues described the use of external distraction appliances for mandibular advancement in the management of hemifacial microsomia.[1] Its application in the management of pediatric obstructive apnea appeared a few years later. In 1994, Moore and associates reported the management of obstructive sleep apnea with mandibular lengthening by distraction osteogenesis in a 6-year-old tracheostomy-dependent patient with Treacher Collins syndrome, with successful decannulation.[2] Since then, many reports have documented the use of mandibular distraction for resolving airway obstruction, achieving early decannulation of tracheotomized children, and improving oral feeding.[3–6]

In 1998, Cohen and colleagues reported on 16 patients who had undergone external mandibular distraction osteogenesis in conjunction with soft tissue procedures to treat medically refractory obstructive sleep apnea. In a group of eight tracheotomy-dependent patients, seven were successfully decannulated and the need for tracheotomy was averted in eight patients.[3]

As experience with the technique increased, the use of distraction osteogenesis evolved from achieving decannulation in tracheotomy-dependent patients to the prevention of long-term airway support with continuous positive airway pressure (CPAP), nasopharyngeal tubes, or tracheotomy placement. Morovic and Monasterio performed mandibular distraction in seven patients, ranging in age from 1 to 18 months, with severe obstructive apnea secondary to mandibular hypoplasia, and two patients had tracheotomies. They reported the avoidance of a tracheotomy in five patients and achieved early decannulation in two tracheotomized patients in a group with congenital craniofacial malformations (five with Pierre Robin sequence and two with Treacher Collins syndrome).[5] Denny and colleagues described their experience with mandibular distraction in neonates; they reported the resolution of upper airway obstruction (UAO) and noted the importance of careful selection of patients.[4,7,8] With time, the appliances were further developed with the introduction of small devices for intraoral pediatric mandibular distraction. In the first decade of the 21st century, a number of pediatric surgeons, such as Denny, Sidman, Smith, Chigurapati, and Monasterio, reported on the outcomes of the use of these appliances in neonates and infants.[4,7–12] Mandibular distraction has since become a recognized approach in carefully selected neonatal and infant patients with severe UAO secondary to micrognathia.[13–15]

Indications for the Use of the Procedure

Infants and children with craniofacial syndromes, such as Pierre Robin sequence, Treacher Collins syndrome or craniofacial microsomia, and syndromic craniosynostosis, often present with varying degrees of UAO. In these anomalies the micrognathic mandible is retropositioned, causing the posterior displacement of the tongue and a concomitant reduction of the oropharyngeal airway that leads to UAO (Fig. 166.1). The degree of respiratory compromise may range from none to significant with potential morbidity and mortality.[16–19] Abramson and colleagues demonstrated by three-dimensional computed tomography (CT) that

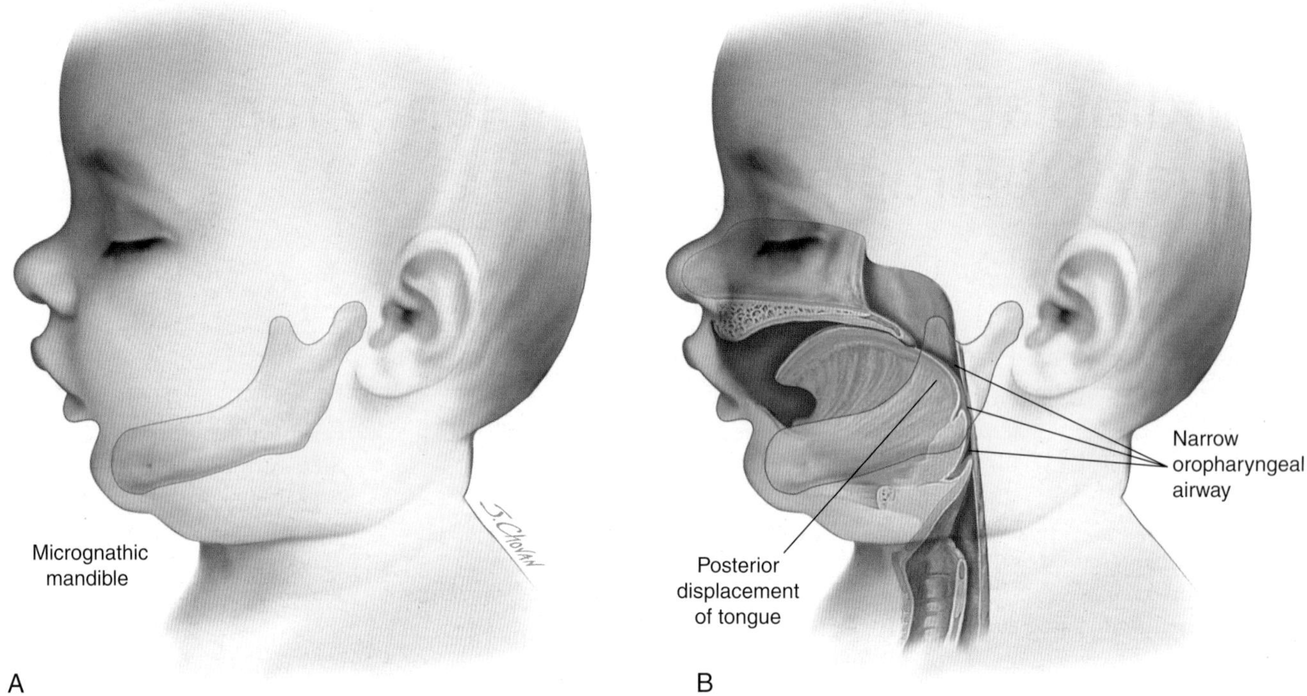

Figure 166.1 Micrognathia (A) and the posteriorly positioned tongue showing narrowing of the oropharyngeal airway (B).

distraction osteogenesis for the management of micrognathia increases airway size, decreases airway length, and alters the airway shape.[20] UAO may result in disturbed sleep, daytime somnolence, and obstructive sleep apnea with the development of cor pulmonale and cardiac failure. An important relationship between airway obstruction and raised intracranial pressure (ICP) is also recognized. Studies have demonstrated that during apnea, elevations in ICP were observed and these elevations in pressure were only observed in relation to the apneic episodes. ICP, central perfusion pressure, and respiratory obstruction appear to interact in a vicious cycle.[21,22] Obstructive sleep apnea (OSA) is also associated with reduced neurocognitive performance in children; however, the etiology is not fully elucidated.[23–27] It has been proposed that neurocognitive deficits may be due to chronicity of OSA that is occurring at the time of rapid neurologic development. It has been reported that infants with obstructive apnea have a higher incidence of abnormal neurologic development in the first year of life than normal infants.[25] In a study on older children (3 to 7 years), a relationship among sleep disordered breathing, increased cerebral blood flow and indices of cognition, and perhaps behavioral function was suggested, but the exact causal relationship has yet to be established.[23]

These infants often have a concomitant failure to thrive, and the relationship among feeding difficulties, failure to thrive, and airway obstruction is now well known.[28,29] Patients with craniofacial syndromes may present with multiple anomalies of the airway involving different parts of the tract. These abnormalities may include glossoptosis, tonsillar or adenoidal hypertrophy, narrowing of the nasopharynx, septal deviation, choanal atresia or stenosis, macroglossia, laryngotracheomalacia, subglottic stenosis, and tracheal anomalies.[30] In addition, the role of central apnea needs to be carefully delineated. The increased sophistication of polysomnography investigations has been important in distinguishing the role of central apnea in the OSA for some patients, and they may not be candidates for distraction as the underlying systemic condition will persist despite surgical intervention.

As the respiratory compromise may have multifactorial causes, a multidisciplinary team approach is essential for the comprehensive evaluation of the airway. This usually involves assessment by specialists in the fields of neonatal and pediatric medicine; respiratory and sleep medicine; ear, nose, and throat medicine; and craniomaxillofacial surgery. Potential investigations may include polysomnography, endoscopy or bronchoscopy, plain films, CT scan, reflux studies, and cardiac investigations as well as electrocardiography and echocardiogram. Depending on the severity of the UAO, a nasopharyngeal tube (NPT), which extends past the level of the tongue base in the oropharynx, may be inserted (Fig. 166.2). There is usually a trial of extubation of the NPT and, if UAO persists, the infant may be a candidate for mandibular distraction (Fig. 166.3).

In a small group of patients with Pierre Robin sequence, UAO may develop following the closure of the cleft palate. It is speculated that these are borderline patients who are only able to maintain airway patency with an unrepaired cleft palate. However, following a palate repair and the resultant change in the airway anatomy, OSA symptoms develop with a plateau or reduction in weight gain, and this requires

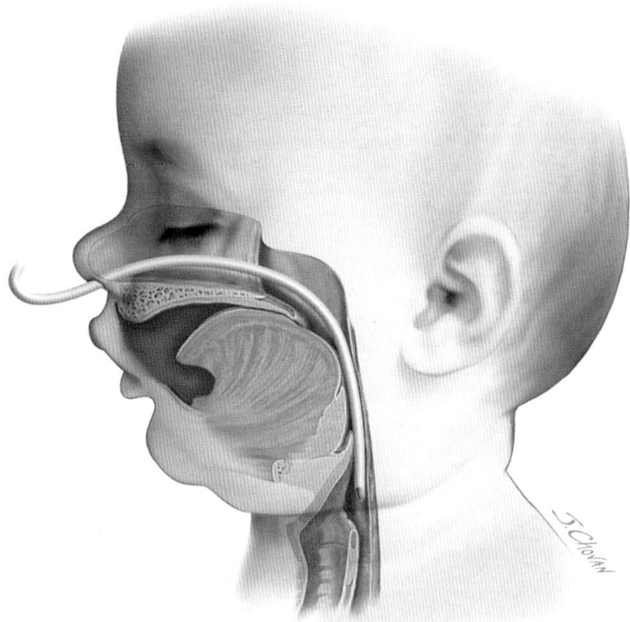

Figure 166.2 A nasopharyngeal tube (NPT) positioned in the pharynx below the level of the obstructing tongue base.

management.[31] Tonsillectomy and adenoidectomy are often first-line interventions, but mandibular distraction may need to be considered to manage UAO in these children.

There are a small number of reports on the anesthetic airway management of patients with UAO and micrognathia following mandibular distraction.[32] In a series of 51 cases, Frawley and associates demonstrated a significant reduction in the incidence of difficult airway management in infants with mandibular hypoplasia (micrognathia) following distraction. The benefit of mandibular distraction was most pronounced in isolated versus syndromic Pierre Robin sequence patients and other syndromes, but it was less marked in those with Treacher Collins syndrome.[32] Brooker and Cooper described the anesthetic management of seven infants, six with Pierre Robin sequence and one with Goldenhar syndrome, who underwent mandibular distraction for UAO. An improvement in laryngoscopic grade was recorded in five Pierre Robin sequence cases but not the patient with Goldenhar syndrome.[33] Hosking and colleagues reported on 240 cases of anesthesia in 35 children with Treacher Collins syndrome. It was noted in this series that the failure to intubate rate was 5% of the planned intubations. It has been suggested that intubation in Treacher Collins syndrome may become more difficult as the patient ages and that airway problems in Treacher Collins syndrome increase with age.[34]

Neonates or infants who are intubated, nasopharyngeal tube dependent, or require airway support with CPAP secondary to severe mandibular hypoplasia/micrognathia are potential candidates for mandibular lengthening with distraction techniques. Similarly, tracheostomy-dependent patients may also be decannulated following advancement of the tongue base. Predictable outcomes have been achieved in patients with Pierre Robin sequence, as the OSA has resolved and feeding has improved with this approach (Fig. 166.4). However, in infants with multiple anomalies or other conditions such as Treacher Collins syndrome or craniofacial microsomia, there is a possibility that obstructive symptoms may redevelop in future years and require additional management.

Limitations and Contraindications

There are limitations to the outcomes that are achievable with distraction osteogenesis for mandibular hypoplasia in certain patient groups. To avoid a tracheotomy or to decannulate a tracheostomy-dependent patient with Treacher Collins syndrome or craniofacial microsomia, mandibular distraction remains a treatment option in selected cases. This option requires appropriate imaging to ensure adequate bone volume to accommodate the appliances. A number of these patients will have significant abnormalities of their mandible with absence or malformation of the ramus/condyle unit, particularly in patients with type IIB and III craniofacial microsomia, Goldenhar syndrome, and Treacher Collins syndrome. These anatomic considerations may preclude distraction, and alternative methods of airway management will need to be considered in these infants.

Patients with concomitant hypotonic or neurologic conditions remain difficult to manage, as despite attempts at surgical correction of mandibular hypoplasia these children will often have persistence of airway obstruction. Similarly, patients with a large component of central apnea resulting in hypoxia and hypoventilation will have limited improvement in their response to mandibular lengthening. Individual patient assessment by a multidisciplinary team to determine the best treatment plan remains imperative. Careful case selection before proceeding with mandibular distraction for UAO results in good outcomes, and there must be recognition that mandibular lengthening may not have a role or benefit in certain cases, even if micrognathia is a feature of the patient's condition.

TECHNIQUE: Posterior Body Osteotomy for Mandibular Distraction

STEP 1: Intubation

Nasoendotracheal intubation with the tube exiting superiorly over the head is the preferred position, as most intensive care units prefer a nasal tube for longer periods of intubation. The infants undergoing mandibular distraction procedures often have a difficult airway (grades III and IV) that may require a video laryngoscope or fiberoptic bronchoscopy-assisted intubation. The tube is taped and secured. The head is placed in the horseshoe headrest and a shoulder roll is positioned (Fig. 166.5A).

Continued

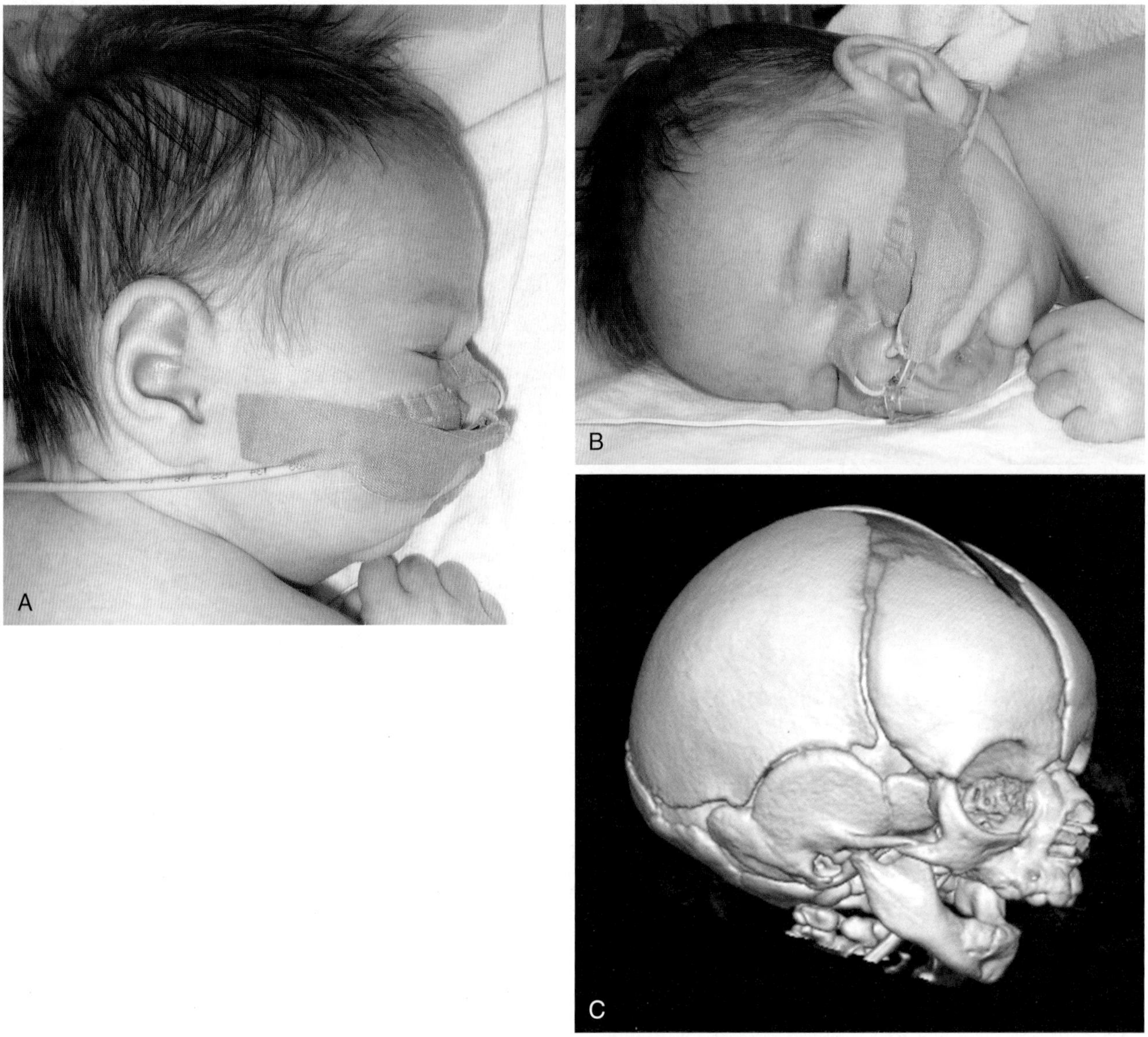

Figure 166.3 **A, B,**Five-week old nasopharyngeal tube-dependent infant with Pierre Robin Sequence and severe micrognathia. **C,** computed tomography (CT) scan demonstatrating mandibular hypoplasia.

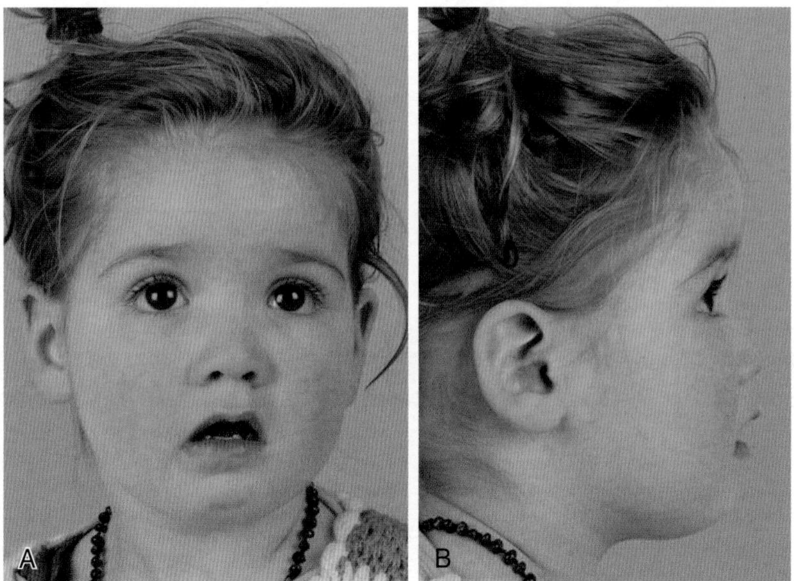

Figure 166.4 **A,** Frontal and **B,** Lateral facial view of a child with Pierre Robin sequence, 2 years after mandibular distraction.

TECHNIQUE: Posterior Body Osteotomy for Mandibular Distraction—*cont'd*

STEP 2: Submandibular Dissection

The skin is prepared with Betadine. Skin marking of the level of the lower border of the mandible is made and an incision line is marked in the submandibular region. Local anesthetic with adrenaline is infiltrated into the submandibular region and on the buccal aspect of the mandible.

A submandibular incision is made with dissection through layers, with the use of a nerve stimulator, and hemostasis of vessels with electrocautery is performed. Dissection down to the periosteum is undertaken, and a horizontal incision made through the periosteum onto the mandible. Using periosteal elevators, the surgeon exposes the buccal aspect of the posterior body, angle, and ramus of the mandible. The lingual periosteal flap is then elevated to expose the antegonal notch and inferior border region.

STEP 3: Insertion of Distraction Appliance

The distraction appliance is positioned on the mandible with the shaft placed below the level of the inferior border. The incision site of the exit point of the activation arm through the skin, in the retromandibular region, is marked. A stab incision is made with a scalpel and mosquito forceps are used to blunt dissect into the surgical site. The activation arm is pulled through the skin incision with the mosquito forceps, and the distraction appliance is positioned onto the surface of the mandible. Temporary self-tapping screws are placed in both foot plates with a screw in each foot plate (Fig. 166.5B).

STEP 4: Corticotomy

The superior margin of the corticotomy is performed with a fine bur curving in a C shape from the junction of the posterior body and ramus. The corticotomy is performed until the level of the appliance is reached. The screws are removed, the appliance is rotated inferiorly out of the way, and the corticotomy is continued inferiorly. The bur cut is made full thickness at the inferior border of the mandible, and it can be continued on the lingual aspect of the mandible that is accessible under direct vision (see Fig. 166.5B).

STEP 5: Mobilization of the Corticotomy

Using osteotomes at the inferior and superior border regions, the corticotomy is mobilized and the mandible separated while preserving the medullary tissue around the inferior alveolar nerve bundle. An osteotome may need to be gently tapped up the lingual cortex to achieve adequate mobilization, and care should be taken not to tear through the lingual periosteum. The distraction appliance is rotated superiorly and repositioned against the bone. The self-tapping screws are replaced into the original screw holes and the remaining screws are placed into the anterior and posterior

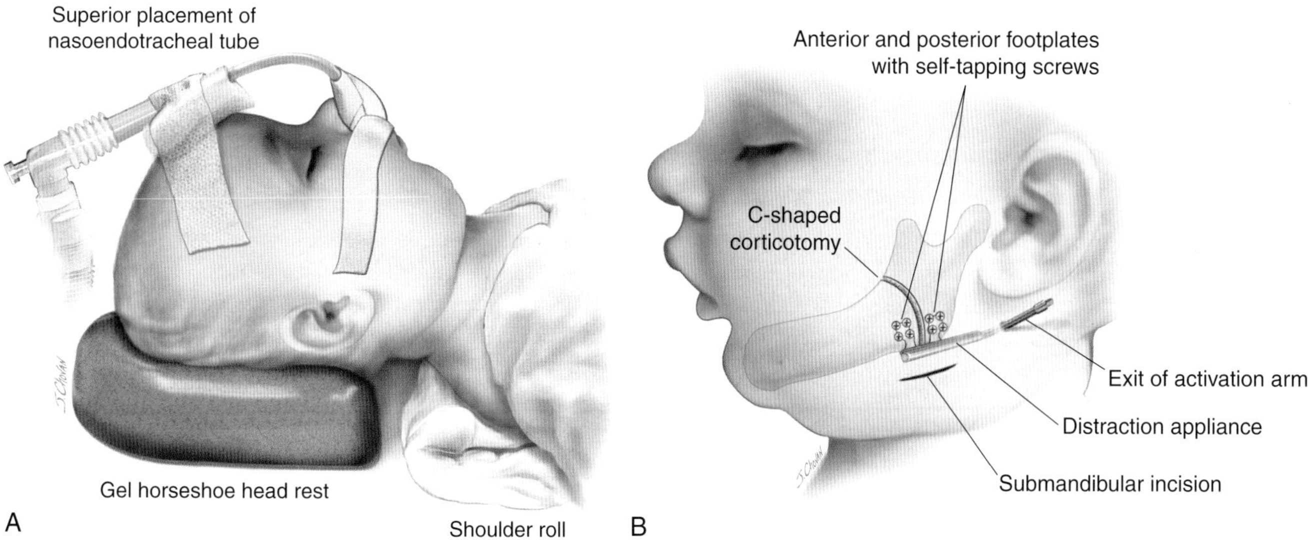

Figure 166.5 **A,** Nasal intubation and positioning of the head in a gel headrest with a shoulder roll. **B,** Placement of the distraction appliance on the posterior body of the mandible, corticotomy, and exit of the activation arm in the retromandibular region.

Continued

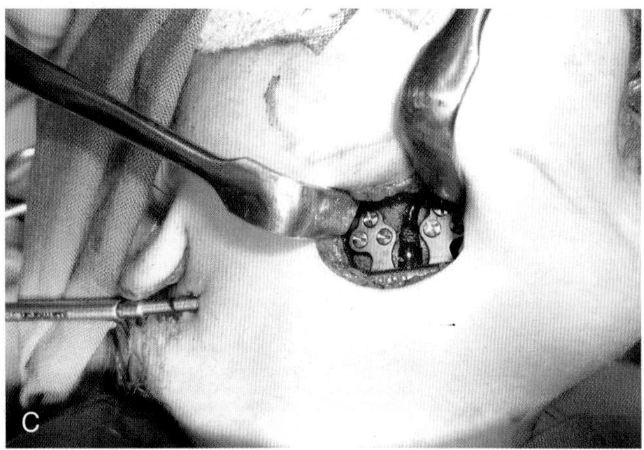

Figure 166.5, cont'd **C,** Intraoperative image showing the opening of the mandibular corticotomy with activation of the distraction appliance, with the interior alveolar nerve bundle preserved.

TECHNIQUE: Posterior Body Osteotomy for Mandibular Distraction—*cont'd*

foot plates. The distraction screwdriver is used to activate the appliance with two to three turns to ensure that the corticotomy site is opening and the appliance is not detaching from the bone. The appliance is then reversed back into the closed position (Fig. 166.5C). Appliances with an anti-relapse rachet will not reverse unless it is deactivated; however, it can be difficult to access the rachet component in the infant as it can be positioned deeper in the retromandibular tissues. Reversal of these appliances back to the closed position may not be achievable and the initial opening can be preserved.

STEP 6: Closure and Dressings

The submandibular wound is closed in layers; 3-0 Vicryl to the periosteum and tissues overlying the appliance, subdermal 4-0 Vicryl, then a continuous 5-0 Monocryl subcuticular suture to the skin. Steri-Strip dressings are applied to the skin, covered by a waterproof plastic dressing (e.g., Tegaderm or Opsite). Around the activation arms, an absorbent, nonadhesive antimicrobial dressing is placed on the skin (e.g., Allevyn Ag). A nasogastric tube should be in situ, and the patient remains nasally intubated and is transferred to the intensive care unit.

STEP 7: Activation of the Distraction Appliance

Each appliance is activated on the first postoperative day. The approach of our unit is to do a two full turn of each appliance (0.3 mm/turn), three times a day (1.8 mm/day), or one 0.5-mm turn three times a day (1.5 mm) depending on the device used. The appliances are activated to the full distance of 15 mm. This process usually takes 7 to 10 days, depending on the device (Fig. 166.5D and E).

ALTERNATIVE TECHNIQUE: Vertical Ramus Osteotomy for Mandibular Distraction

There are some reports of the use of a vertical subsigmoid osteotomy as an alternative to the posterior body corticotomy for mandibular distraction. The advantage of this approach is that there is no risk of damage to the tooth buds. However, this approach appears to have a much higher incidence of trismus that is difficult to manage in the long term, as the advanced segment contains both the coronoid process and mandibular body.

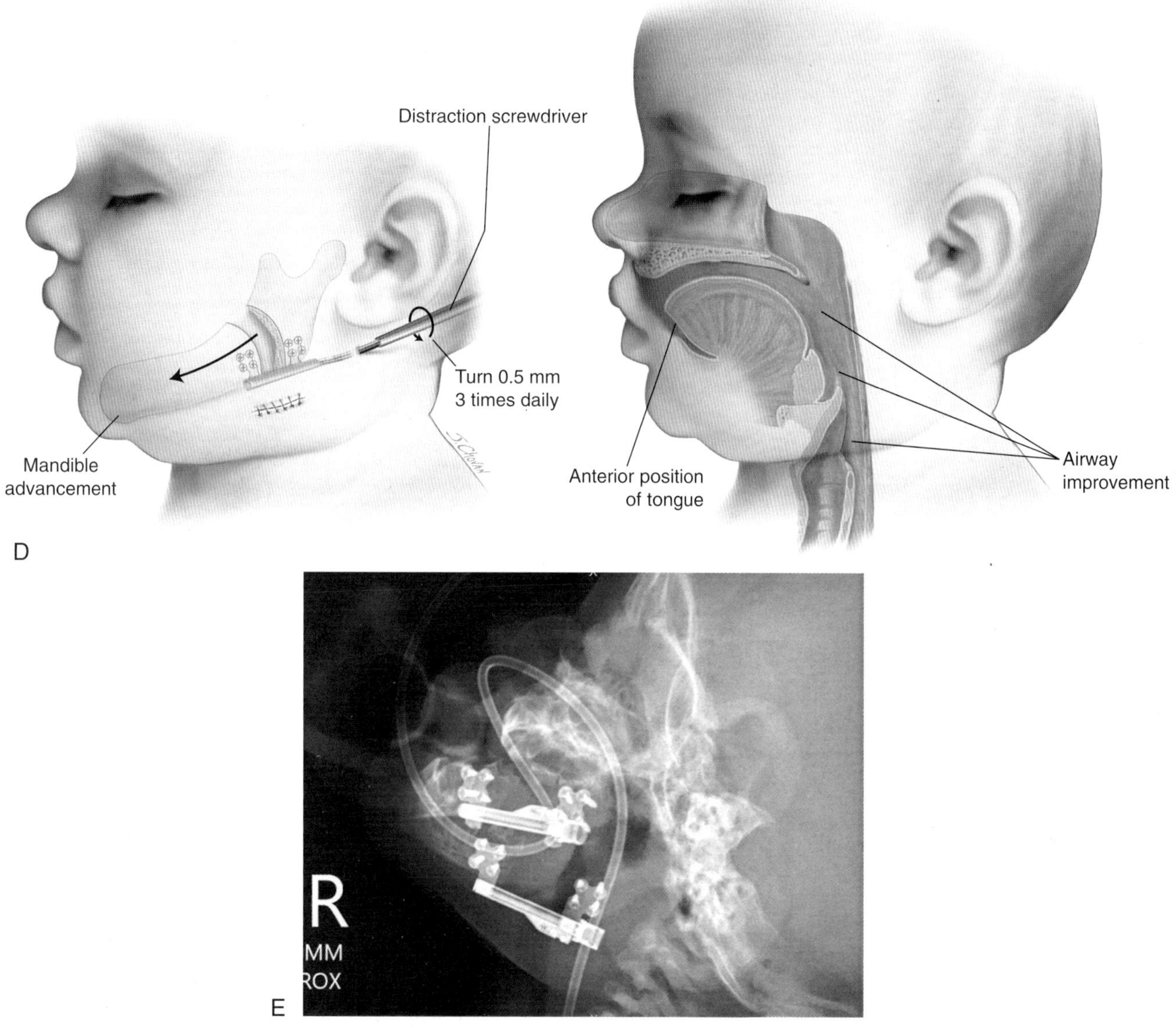

Figure 166.5, cont'd **D,** Lengthening of the mandible following distraction osteogenesis and the resultant anterior position of the tongue and improvement in the airway. **E,** Postdistraction lateral oblique radiographic view of the mandible demonstrating the lengthening of the body of the mandible.

Avoidance and Management of Intraoperative Complications

In neonates and infants, methodical submandibular dissection and control of any bleeding are essential to reduce the need for transfusion. The corticotomy cut should be C-shaped and curved posteriorly away from the tooth buds where possible within the alveolar process. The bony cuts should be monocortical on the buccal and lingual aspects of the mandible to preserve the inferior alveolar nerve bundle within the mandible. Excessive manipulation of instruments at the superior border of the mandible for mobilization of the segments should be avoided to minimize trauma to the developing tooth buds.

In the neonate, in particular, the mandible is relatively "plastic" in nature and rather than a clear mobilization of the segments, the edges of the corticotomy may bend or distort without full separation of the segments. The mandibular segments should be checked for complete separation before application of the device to ensure that the distraction is not impeded by persistent bony attachment, particularly on the lingual aspect.

Postoperative Considerations

The infant remains nasally intubated and is transferred to the intensive care unit for postoperative management. The patients are extubated between day 4 and day 6 postoperatively. Intravenous antibiotics, usually a cephalosporin, are administered at induction and continued for the first 24 to 48 hours.

The distraction appliances are activated on the first postoperative day, with turns performed three times a day until each distraction device is activated its full distance, usually 15 mm. There are longer (20 and 25 mm) pediatric distraction appliances to select if required for individual cases. The activation arm sites are managed with saline washes around the skin margins, and an Allevyn Ag dressing (or a dressing of a similar nature) is fitted around the activation arm against the skin. For appliances with detachable arms, these are removed following the elongation of the mandible and at the completion of distraction. The Steri-Strip and waterproof plastic dressing in the submandibular regions are removed 7 to 10 days postoperatively.

When extubated, the speech pathology unit may review the infant and commence attempts at oral feeding. A phase of oral feeding with supplemental nasogastric feeds will be required, and the duration of this phase varies between patients but may range from weeks to months. In patients with other craniofacial conditions, such as Treacher Collins syndrome and craniofacial microsomia, other factors may influence the ability to feed orally, and some of these patients will require long-term nasogastric feeding or the insertion of a percutaneous endoscopic gastrostomy tube.

The distraction appliances are removed 6 to 8 weeks postoperatively via the previous submandibular incisions.

References

1. McCarthy JG, Schreiber J, Karp N, Thorne CH, Grayson BH. Lengthening the human mandible by gradual distraction. *Plast Reconstr Surg*. 1992;89(1):1–8.
2. Moore MH, Guzman-Stein G, Proudman TW, Abbott AH, Netherway DJ, David DJ. Mandibular lengthening by distraction for airway obstruction in Treacher-Collins syndrome. *J Craniofac Surg*. 1994;5(1):22–25.
3. Cohen SR, Simms C, Burstein FD. Mandibular distraction osteogenesis in the treatment of upper airway obstruction in children with craniofacial deformities. *Plast Reconstr Surg*. 1998;101(2):312–318.
4. Denny A, Kalantarian B. Mandibular distraction in neonates: a strategy to avoid tracheostomy. *Plast Reconstr Surg*. 2002;109(3):896–904.
5. Morovic CG, Monasterio L. Distraction osteogenesis for obstructive apneas in patients with congenital craniofacial malformations. *Plast Reconstr Surg*. 2000;105(7):2324–2330.
6. Williams JK, Maull D, Grayson BH, Longaker MT, McCarthy JG. Early decannulation with bilateral mandibular distraction for tracheostomy-dependent patients. *Plast Reconstr Surg*. 1999;103(1):48–57.
7. Denny AD, Talisman R, Hanson PR, Recinos RF. Mandibular distraction osteogenesis in very young patients to correct airway obstruction. *Plast Reconstr Surg*. 2001;108(2):302–311.
8. Denny A, Amm C. New technique for airway correction in neonates with severe Pierre Robin sequence. *J Pediatr*. 2005;147(1):97–101.
9. Sidman JD, Sampson D, Templeton B. Distraction osteogenesis of the mandible for airway obstruction in children. *Laryngoscope*. 2001;111(7):1137–1146.
10. Smith K, Harnish M. Pediatric sleep apnoea treated with distraction osteogenesis. In: Samchukov ML, Cope JB, Cherkashin AM, eds. *Craniofacial Distraction Osteogenesis*. St Louis, MO: Mosby; 2001.
11. Chigurupati R, Massie J, Dargaville P, Heggie A. Internal mandibular distraction to relieve airway obstruction in infants and young children with micrognathia. *Pediatr Pulmonol*. 2004;37(3):230–235.
12. Monasterio FO, Drucker M, Molina F, Ysunza A. Distraction osteogenesis in Pierre Robin sequence and related respiratory problems in children. *J Craniofac Surg*. 2002;13(1):79–83.
13. Shand JM, Smith KS, Heggie AA. The role of distraction osteogenesis in the management of craniofacial syndromes. *Oral Maxillofac Surg Clin North Am*. 2004;16(4):525–540.
14. Tibesar RJ, Scott AR, McNamara C, Sampson D, Lander TA, Sidman JD. Distraction osteogenesis of the mandible for airway obstruction in children: long-term results. *Otolaryngol Head Neck Surg*. 2010;143(1):90–96.
15. Hicks KE, Billings KR, Purnell CA, et al. Algorithm for airway management in patients with Pierre Robin sequence. *J Craniofac Surg*. 2018;29(5):1187–1192.
16. da Costa AL, Manica D, Schweiger C, et al. The effect of mandibular distraction osteogenesis on airway obstruction and polysomnographic parameters in children with Robin sequence. *J Craniomaxillofac Surg*. 2018;46(8):1343–1347.
17. Adhikari AN, Heggie AA, Shand JM, Bordbar P, Pellicano A, Kilpatrick N. Infant mandibular distraction for upper airway obstruction: a clinical audit. *Plast Reconstr Surg Glob Open*. 2016;4(7):e812.
18. Goldstein JA, Chung C, Paliga JT, et al. Mandibular distraction osteogenesis for the treatment of neonatal tongue-based airway obstruction. *J Craniofac Surg*. 2015;26(3):634–641.
19. Marcus CL, Loughlin GM. Obstructive sleep apnea in children. *Semin Pediatr Neurol*. 1996;3(1):23–28.
20. Abramson ZR, Susarla SM, Lawler ME, Peacock ZS, Troulis MJ, Kaban LB. Effects of mandibular distraction osteogenesis on three-dimensional airway anatomy in children with congenital micrognathia. *J Oral Maxillofac Surg*. 2013;71(1):90–97.
21. Gonsalez S, Hayward R, Jones B, Lane R. Upper airway obstruction and raised intracranial pressure in children with craniosynostosis. *Eur Respir J*. 1997;10(2):367–375.
22. Hayward R, Gonsalez S. How low can you go? Intracranial pressure, cerebral perfusion pressure, and respiratory obstruction in children with complex craniosynostosis. *J Neurosurg*. 2005;102(suppl 1):16–22.
23. Walter LM, Shepherd KL, Yee A, Horne RSC. Insights into the effects of sleep disordered breathing on the brain in infants and children: imaging and cerebral oxygenation measurements. *Sleep Med Rev*. 2020;50:101251.
24. Tabone L, Khirani S, Amaddeo A, Emeriaud G, Fauroux B. Cerebral oxygenation in children with sleep-disordered breathing. *Paediatr Respir Rev*. 2020;34:18–23.
25. Butcher-Puech MC, Henderson-Smart DJ, Holley D, Lacey JL, Edwards DA. Relation between apnoea duration and type and neurological status of preterm infants. *Arch Dis Child*. 1985;60(10):953–958.
26. Piteo AM, Kennedy JD, Roberts RM, et al. Snoring and cognitive development in infancy. *Sleep Med*. 2011;12(10):981–987.
27. Spicuzza L, Leonardi S, La Rosa M. Pediatric sleep apnea: early onset of the 'syndrome'. *Sleep Med Rev*. 2009;13(2):111–122.
28. Smith MC, Senders CW. Prognosis of airway obstruction and feeding difficulty in the Robin sequence. *Int J Pediatr Otorhinolaryngol*. 2006;70(2):319–324.
29. Breugem CC, Evans KN, Poets CF, et al. Best practices for the diagnosis and evaluation of infants with Robin Sequence. A clinical consensus report. *JAMA Pediatr*. 2016;170(9):894–902.
30. Burstein FD, Cohen SR, Scott PH, Teague GR, Montgomery GL, Kattos AV. Surgical therapy for severe refractory sleep apnea in infants and children: application of the airway zone concept. *Plast Reconstr Surg*. 1995;96(1):34–41.
31. Smith D, Abdullah SE, Moores A, Wynne DM. Post-operative respiratory distress following primary cleft palate repair. *J Laryngol Otol*. 2013;127(1):65–66.
32. Frawley G, Espenell A, Howe P, Shand J, Heggie A. Anesthetic implications of infants with mandibular hypoplasia treated with mandibular distraction osteogenesis. *Paediatr Anaesth*. 2013;23(4):342–348.
33. Brooker GE, Cooper MG. Airway management for infants with severe micrognathia having mandibular distraction osteogenesis. *Anaesth Intensive Care*. 2010;38(1):43–49.
34. Hosking J, Zoanetti D, Carlyle A, Anderson P, Costi D. Anesthesia for Treacher Collins syndrome: a review of airway management in 240 pediatric cases. *Paediatr Anaesth*. 2012;22(8):752–758.

Index

Note: Page numbers followed by "f" indicate figures, "t" indicate tables, and "b" indicate boxes.

B

C

E

G

H

J

N

Q

R

W

X

Y

Z